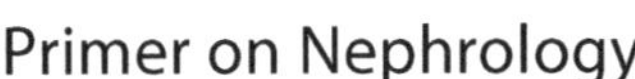

Primer on Nephrology

Mark Harber
Editor

Primer on Nephrology

Second Edition

Volume I

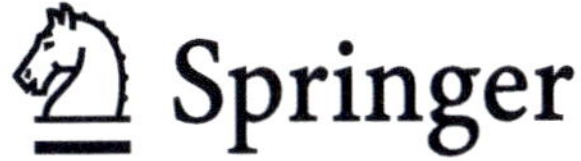

Editor
Mark Harber
Department of Renal Medicine
UCL
London, UK

ISBN 978-3-030-76421-0 ISBN 978-3-030-76419-7 (eBook)
https://doi.org/10.1007/978-3-030-76419-7

This Springer imprint is published by the registered company Springer Nature Switzerland AG
The registered company address is: Gewerbestrasse 11, 6330 Cham, Switzerland

Preface

The forerunner to *Primer in Nephrology*, *Practical Nephrology*, was published in 2014 and aimed to provide a clear, modern account of nephrology with a practical spin. The motivation for the book came from teaching and the acknowledgment that practical experience, examples of real-world nephrology (good and bad), and case discussions are an essential aspect of training. This edition of *Primer in Nephrology* is an update with the same ethos, but hopefully yet more experience imparted. In addition, much has happened both within and outside nephrology since 2014 that has transformed the practice, and this edition addresses major ongoing challenges for our patients and staff as well as key questions for us as nephrologists.

Our knowledge and understanding of acute kidney injury (AKI) have grown substantially, particularly the appreciation of the long-term impacts of moderate to severe AKI on renal function and frailty, with significant implications for patients who survive episodes of AKI. AKI is not only emerging as an important cause of chronic kidney disease (CKD) but CKD is also an important risk factor for AKI. In the context of a massive increase in the global prevalence of CKD, secondary to an aging population with multiple comorbidities, this represents a major test for nephrologists specifically and healthcare providers in general. By way of a medical counterattack, there have been many exciting new treatments in nephrology over the last few years. In particular, the development of GLA-1 receptor agonists and SGLT-2 inhibitors that significantly slow the progression of diabetic nephropathy and markedly mitigate the risk of cardiovascular comorbidities is particularly welcome. The observation that SGLT-2 inhibitors are equally effective in protecting non-diabetic patients with heavy proteinuria from renal progression and cardiovascular disease offers huge potential in combating progressive renal disease. The real challenge for us, however, is implementation of all the measures we know to prevent the development and severe consequences of CKD and cardiovascular co-morbidity. How do we as a specialty tackle major healthcare inequalities and ensure that patients from all backgrounds and in all communities are identified early, supported, and treated to deliver the best outcome?

The COVID-19 pandemic has shaken the world and pummeled health services. It has demonstrated the susceptibility of patients with end-stage renal disease, particularly those with no choice but to attend hospital dialysis as well as those who are immunosuppressed. It has highlighted the critical importance for our patients of prevention of infectious disease in the form of good infection control and vaccination. The early pandemic revealed nephropathies associations with this virus but most strikingly it has reminded us of the importance of appropriate fluid replacement in sepsis; when anxiety about wet lungs, and relative fluid restriction, contributed to a huge surge in hospital AKI. This unintended consequence, in turn, demonstrated the vulnerability of supply chains for acute renal replacement therapy and engendered an unprecedented cooperation between nephrologists and intensivists, working in a less rigid and more dynamic way across regions supporting colleagues outside usual arrangements. We have rapidly learned to assess patients in virtual clinics, been forced to become more fluent with setting ceilings of treatment and guiding patients and families through end-of-life care in profoundly stressful circumstances, as well as adapting to deliver background renal medicine including transplantation, and treatment of autoimmune diseases with the minimum possible risk. It has also reminded us of the selfless dedication, value, and, at times, vulnerability of frontline workers in the healthcare sector. We have learned a great deal over the last 2 years and adapted rapidly in our patient's interests. A key question is how many of the positive aspects of practice will we preserve post pandemic, and will we retain our capacity to innovate imaginatively when things normalize?

The above questions are germane to another, greater global crisis, that of the climate emergency. It is still very difficult to discuss the scientifically backed implications of global warming without seeming to resort to hyperbole. But the bottom line from the 6th International Panel on Climate Change was that "climate change is real, man made, rapid and unprecedented. That temperatures will continue to rise in all scenarios. Species extinction, widespread disease, unlivable heat, ecosystem collapse and cities menaced by rising seas will become painfully obvious before a child born today turns 30." Or put it another way, approximately 1 billion, nearly half the world's population of children, currently live in regions at extreme risk of environmental stresses from flooding to drought, extreme heat, ecosystem collapse, and famine. Low-income countries will bear the brunt initially, but high-income countries are already seeing extreme weather events and a dawning of the disorder this will cause. The multitude of ways climate change will affect patients with kidney conditions are not difficult to imagine, but supply-chain disruption including energy, food, and water will occur. In 2019, there were estimated to be approximately 80 million refugees or internally displace individuals. Extremes of heat, flooding, and famine will inevitably contribute to a huge increase in this number. Optimizing the care of patients with lifelong CKD or those receiving renal replacement therapy as the consequences of climate change or war, will become increasingly demanding, especially for those who are displaced or in high-risk regions. We face the most serious practical, ethical, and financial issues, many of which are not difficult to predict, and yet our collective response has thus far been grossly inadequate.

The healthcare sector is responsible for roughly 5% of CO_2 emissions, and nephrology has a disproportionately large carbon footprint, so we have a particular obligation to address this and start thinking sustainably. The good news is that, as recently demonstrated, we are at our best when free to innovate and invent. In this context, there are huge changes afoot in healthcare with rapidly developing alliances of like-minded people and green nephrology networks aimed at sustainable change and using the financial clout of the healthcare sector to catalyze change in providers. And then there is us, healthcare professionals who have had a crash course in supporting each other and remodeling, who like science, evidence, and facts, the wealth of which mean it is not difficult to predict the challenges ahead. As a profession, we are well regarded and have a responsibility to influence change and change the ethos of the institutions we work in with vigor and urgency.

I hope that this edition not only serves as a useful and engaging text on nephrology but also invites us all to ambitiously reassess practice with the aim of achieving the best possible experience and outcomes for our patients.

Mark Harber
Hampstead
London, UK

Acknowledgments

As with the previous edition, *Practical Nephrology*, I would like to thank again the generosity of the numerous authors who have contributed to this book. For most, clinical practice over the last 2 years has been particularly punishing and all consuming, so I remain especially indebted to all those authors have over the years taught me much of the nephrology I know and who contributed so generously and with such tolerance.

I am also particularly grateful to those who have very generously contributed to the additional material used in the book, especially Sue Car and Peter Topham, Steve Holt and Michael Ci, Mr. Peter Veitch, Arundi Mahendran, Justin Harris, Dominic Yu, Shella Sandoval, Ramesh Batra, Hannah Deltrey-King, Amanda Rea, and David Bishop who have produced videos that demonstrate procedures with much greater clarity than I could have achieved in prose and that I hope will assist doctors in carrying out these procedures with safety and confidence. I would particularly like to thank Paul Sweny for his mentorship and for the gift of his collection of clinical images accumulated over the years of frontline service. Histological images were generously provided by Lauren Heptinstall, Paul Bass, Alec Howie, Catherine Horsfield, and Mared Casey-Owen.

Once again, my heartfelt thanks to our patients who have contributed to this book in so many ways and who remain the key motivation behind this book.

Contents

Volume I

IV Hypertension and Renovascular Diseases

V Glomerular Diseases

Contributors

Ali Abdall-Razak, BSc Imperial College School of Medicine, London, UK
ali.abdall-razak14@imperial.ac.uk

Shahid Abdullah, MBBS, MRCP Salford Royal NHS Foundation Trust, Salford, UK
Manchester Royal Infirmary, Manchester, UK

Asmat Abro, MBBS, MRCP UCL Centre for Nephrology, Royal Free Hospital, London, UK
Department of Renal Medicine and Transplantation, Royal Free Hospital, London, UK
a.abro@nhs.net

Sarah Afuwape Department of Nephrology and Transplantation, Royal Free London NHS Foundation Trust, London, UK
sarah.afuwape@nhs.net

John Agar University Hospital Geelong and Deakin University School of Medicine, Barwon Health, Geelong, VIC, Australia
geerenal@ncable.net.au

Yogita Aggarwal University Hospitals of Coventry and Warwickshire NHS Trust, London, UK
Yogita.Aggarwal@uhb.nhs.uk

Nikita Agrawal North Middlesex University Hospital NHS Trust, London, UK
nikita.agrawal@nhs.net

Ammar Al Midani Department of Nephrology & Transplantation, Royal Free London NHS Foundation Trust, London, UK
ammar.almidani@nhs.net

Inji Alshaer North Middlesex University Hospital NHS Trust, London, UK
Inji.alshaer@nhs.net

Rakesh Anand, BSc, MSc, MBBS, MRCP Royal Free London NHS Foundation Trust, London, UK
rakesh.anand1@nhs.net

Marilina Antonelou Department of Renal Medicine, University College London and Royal Free London NHS Foundation Trust, London, UK
Department of Renal Medicine, University College London, London, UK
Marilina.antonelou@nhs.net

Ravi Armstron Johannesburg, South Africa

Caroline Ashley, BPharm (Hons), FFRPS, FRPharmS Department of Pharmacy, Royal Free London NHS Foundation Trust, London, UK
carolineashley@nhs.net

Domenico Bagordo, MD Nephrology Unit, Sapienza University of Rome, Rome, Italy
d.bagordo@ucl.ac.uk

Richard J. Baker, MBBChir, MA, FRCP, PhD Renal Medicine, St James's University Hospital, Leeds, UK
Richard-j.baker@nhs.net

Simon Ball Queen Elizabeth Hospital, Birmingham, UK
Simon.Ball@uhb.nhs.uk

Ravi Barod Royal Free London, London, UK
r.barod@nhs.net

Jonathan Barratt The John Walls Renal Unit, Leicester General Hospital, University Hospitals of Leicester, Leicester, UK
jb81@le.ac.uk

Chathurika Beligaswatta Department of Renal Medicine, UCL, London, UK
chathurika.beligswatta@nhs.net

Christopher O. C. Bellamy Department of Renal Medicine, Royal Infirmary of Edinburgh, Edinburgh, UK

Sanjay Bhagani Royal Free London Hospital, London, UK
Department of Infectious Diseases/HIV Medicine, Royal Free Hospital, London, UK
s.bhagani@nhs.net

Hannah Blakey Renal Department, Queen Elizabeth Hospital NHS Trust, Birmingham, UK
hannah.blakey2@uhb.nhs.uk

Sarah Blakey Hammersmith Hospital, Imperial College Healthcare NHS Trust, London, UK
sarahblakey@nhs.net

Detlef Bockenhauer University College London, Great Ormond Street Hospital, London, UK
d.bockenhauer@ucl.ac.uk

Ekaterini Boleti Kidney Cancer Centre, Royal Free Hospital, London, UK
ekaterini.boleti@nhs.net

John Booth Royal London Hospital, Department of Nephrology, London, UK
John.booth@bartshealth.nhs.uk

James Brown Department of Respiratory Medicine, Royal Free London NHS Foundation Trust, London, UK
james.brown13@nhs.net

Sinéad Burke Royal Free London NHS Foundation Trust, London, UK
sinead.burke@nhs.net

Áine Burns Royal Free Hospital, London, UK
Aine.burns@nhs.net

Michael X. Cai The Royal Melbourne Hospital, Melbourne, VIC, Australia
Michael.Cai@mh.org.au

Chris J. Callaghan, PhD, FRCS University Department of Surgery, Addenbrooke's Hospital, Cambridge, UK
chris.callaghan@gstt.nhs.uk

Stephanie Camilleri Mater Dei Hospital, Valletta, Malta
Stephanie.b.camillia@gov.mt

Ben Caplin, BSc (Hons), MBChB, PhD UCL Medical School, Royal Free Campus, London, UK
Department of Renal Medicine, UCL Medical School, Royal Free Campus, London, UK
Department of Renal Medicine, University College London, London, UK
b.caplin@ucl.ac.uk

Paul J. Champion de Crespigny The Royal Melbourne Hospital, Melbourne, VIC, Australia
Paul.ChampiondeCrespigny@mh.org.au

Melanie M. Y. Chan, MRCP UCL Department of Renal Medicine, Royal Free Hospital, London, UK
melanie.chan@nhs.net

Rawya Charif, MRCP, MD (Res) Imperial College Kidney and Transplant Centre, Imperial College Healthcare NHS Trust, Hammersmith Hospital, London, UK
Rawya.Charif@nhs.net

Lindsay Chesterton, FRCP, DM Department of Renal Medicine, Royal Derby Hospital, Derby, UK
lindsay.chesterton@nhs.net

Chee Kay Cheung University of Leicester, Leicester, UK
ckc15@le.ac.uk

Roohi Chhabra Royal Free Hospital, London, UK
roohi.chhabra@nhs.net

Stephanie M. Y. Chong Department of Nephrology, Royal Free Hospital, London, UK
Stephanie.chong1@nhs.net

Pratima Chowdary, MBBS, MRCP, FRCPath Katharine Dormandy Haemophilia and Thrombosis Centre, Royal Free London NHS Foundation Trust, London, UK
Department of Haematology, University College London, London, UK
P.chowdary@ucl.ac.uk

Paul Cockwell Department of Renal Medicine, Queen Elizabeth Hospital Birmingham, Birmingham, UK
Paul.Cockwell@uhb.nhs.uk

John O. Connolly, PhD, FRCP UCL Department of Renal Medicine, Royal Free Hospital, London, UK
johnconnolly@nhs.net

Thomas M. F. Connor Oxford Kidney Unit, Churchill Hospital, Oxford, UK
thomas.connor@ouh.nhs.uk

Bryan Conway Department of Renal Medicine, Royal Infirmary of Edinburgh, Edinburgh, UK
Bryan.Conway@nhslothian.scot.nhs.uk

Richard W. Corbett Hammersmith Hospital, Imperial College Healthcare NHS Trust, London, UK
rwcorbett@nhs.net

A. E. Courtney Regional Nephrology & Transplant Unit, Belfast City Hospital, Belfast, UK
aisling.courtney@belfasttrust.hscni.net

Jeff Cove Renal Psychology Service, Royal Free London NHS Foundation Trust, London, UK
j.cove@nhs.net

Alison Craik Freeman Hospital, Newcastle Upon Tyne, UK
alison.craik2@nhs.net

Jennifer Cross Royal Free London NHS Foundation Trust, London, UK
Royal Free Hospital, London, UK
jennifer.cross@nhs.net

John Cunningham UCL Centre for Nephrology, The Royal Free Hospital, London, UK

Sunil K. Daga, MBBS, MRCP (Nephrology), PhD Renal Medicine, St James's University Hospital, Leeds, UK
Sunildaga@nhs.net

Andrew Davenport UCL Centre for Nephrology, Royal Free Hospital, University College London Medical School, London, UK
University College London, London, UK
Andrewdavenport@nhs.net

Sara N. Davison University of Alberta, Edmonton, AB, Canada
Sara.davison@ualberta.ca

Clara Day Renal Department, Queen Elizabeth Hospital Birmingham, Birmingham, UK
clara.day@uhb.nhs.uk

Neeraj Dhaun, MD Centre for Cardiovascular Science, University of Edinburgh, The Queen's Medical Research Institute, Edinburgh, UK
bean.dhaun@ed.ac.uk

Geraint Dingley Wessex Kidney Centre, Portsmouth, UK

Philippa Dodd Whittington Hospital, London, UK
Phillipa.dodd@nhs.net

Gavin Dreyer Barts Health NHS Trust, London, UK

Peter J. Dupont, PhD, FRCPI Department of Renal Medicine, University College London, Royal Free Hospital, London, UK
pdupont@nhs.net

Cathy Egan Moorfields Eye Hospital, London, UK
cathy.egan@nhs.net

Nasirul Jabir Ekbal Royal Free London NHS Foundation Trust, London, UK
Nasirul.Ekbal@nhs.net

Timothy John Ellam Renal Services, The Newcastle upon Tyne Hospitals NHS Foundation Trust, Newcastle upon Tyne, UK
timothy.ellam@nuth.nhs.uk

Rhys Evans University College London, London, UK
rhys.evans@ucl.ac.uk

Stanley Fan Consultant Nephrologists, The Royal London Hospital, Barts Health NHS Trust, London, UK
fan.stanley@bartshealth.nhs.uk

John Feehally University of Leicester, Rutland, UK
jf27@leicester.ac.uk

Raymond Fernando, BSc, PhD Department of Renal Medicine, University College London & The Anthony Nolan Laboratory, Royal Free Hospital, London, UK
raymond.fernando@nhs.net

Richard S. Fish University Hospitals of North Midlands, Stoke-on-Trent, UK
rsfish@doctors.org.uk

Richard J. Fluck, FRCP, MA (Cantab), MBBS Department of Renal Medicine, Royal Derby Hospital, Derby, UK
richard.fluck@nhs.net

Suzanne H. Forbes, MBBS, MRCP, MD Department of Nephrology, The Royal London Hospital, Barts Health NHS Trust, London, UK
Suzanne.Forbes@bartshealth.nhs.uk

Antje Fürstenberg-Schaette Nephrology, Nierenzentrum Stendal-Gardelegen MVZ, Stendal, Germany

Alice Gage Royal Free London NHS Foundation Trust, London, UK
alice.gage1@nhs.net

Daniel Gale, MA, MB, BChir, PhD, FRCP Department of Renal Medicine, University College London, Royal Free Hospital, London, UK
d.gale@ucl.ac.uk

Jack Galliford, MBBS, FRCP Richard Bright Renal Unit, Southmead Hospital, Bristol, UK
Jack.Galliford@nbt.nhs.uk

David Game, MA, PhD, FRCP Department of Nephrology and Transplantation, Guy's Hospital, London, UK
David.Game@gstt.nhs.uk

Conall Mac Gearailt Galway University Hospital, Galway, Ireland
conall.macgearailt@hse.ie

Julian D. Gillmore UK National Amyloidosis Centre, University College London and Royal Free Hospital London NHS Foundation Trust, London, UK
j.gillmore@ucl.ac.uk

Jane Goddard Department of Renal Medicine, Royal Infirmary of Edinburgh, Edinburgh, UK
Unkn2134@meteor.com

Gabrielle Goldet Royal Free Hospital, London, UK
gabrielle.goldet@nhs.net

Antony Goode Department of Radiology, Royal Free Hospital, London, UK
Antony.goode1@nhs.net

Darren Green Vascular Research Group, Manchester Academic Health Sciences Center, University of Manchester, Salford Royal NHS Foundation Trust, Stott Lane, Salford, UK
Unkn524@meteor.com

George H. B. Greenhall, MRCP(Neph.), MBChB, MSc Department of Statistics and Clinical Research, NHS Blood and Transplant, Bristol, UK
georgegreenhall@nhs.net

Pooja Mehta Gudka Renal Services, Department of Pharmacy, Royal Free London NHS Foundation Trust, London, UK
Poojamehta.gudka@nhs.net

Angela D. Gupta, MD Texas Childrens Pediatric Urology Clinic, Houston, TX, USA
agupta45@jhmi.edu

Asheeta Gupta, BSc, BMedSci, BMBS, MRCPCH Department of Nephrology, Birmingham Women's and Children's NHS Foundation Trust, Steelhouse Lane, Birmingham, UK
asheeta.gupta@nhs.net

Sanjana Gupta, MBBS, MSc, MRCP, DPMSA Royal Free and Royal London Hospital, London, UK

University College London, London, UK
sanjana.gupta@ucl.ac.uk

Zoya Hameed, BSc, MBBS, MSc, FRCOphth Royal Free London NHS Foundation Trust, London, UK
Zoya.hameed@nhs.net

Sally Hamour Department of Renal Medicine, University College London and Royal Free London NHS Foundation Trust, London, UK
sallyhamour@nhs.net

Tanzina Haque Royal Free Hospital, London, UK
thaque@nhs.net

Mark Harber, MBBS, PhD, FRCP Department of Renal Medicine UCL, London, UK
mark.harber@nhs.net

Justin Harris Royal Free London NHS Foundation Trust, London, UK
justinharris@nhs.net

Gerlineke Hawkins-van der Cingel Royal Free London NHS Foundation Trust, London, UK
gerlineke.hawkins-vandercingel@nhs.net

Scott R. Henderson UCL Centre for Nephrology, Royal Free Hospital, London, UK
scotthenderson@nhs.net

Heidy Hendra Department of Nephrology & Transplantation, Royal Free London NHS Foundation Trust, London, UK

Royal Free London NHS Foundation Trust, London, UK
heidy.hendra1@nhs.net

Joanne Henry Department of Nephrology and Transplantation, Royal Free London NHS Foundation Trust, London, UK
joannehenry@nhs.net

Lauren Heptinstall Royal Free London NHS Foundation Trust, London, UK
lauren.heptinstall@nhs.net

Sarah Hildebrand Royal Free London NHS Foundation Trust, London, UK
sarah.hildebrand2@nhs.net

Peter Hill West London Renal and Transplant Centre, Hammersmith Hospital, Imperial College Health Trust, London, UK
peter.hill4@nhs.net

Aroon Hingorani UCL Division of Biosciences, London, UK
a.hingorani@ucl.ac.uk

Stephen G. Holt, BSc, MBBS, PhD, FRCP, FRACP The University of Melbourne, School of Medicine, Melbourne, VIC, Australia
steve.holt@mh.org.au

Sally-Anne Hulton, MBBCh, FCP(Paeds)SA, FRCPCH, MD Birmingham Women's Childrens and Children's NHS Foundation Trust, Birmingham, UK
sally.hulton@nhs.net

Rachel K. Y. Hung Department of Nephrology, Royal Free Hospital, London, UK
Royal Free Hospital, Department of Nephrology, London, UK
R.hung@nhs.net

Buddhika Illeperuma Royal Free London NHS Foundation Trust, London, UK
Buddhika.Illeperuma@nhs.net

Ferina Ismail, BSc, MBBS, MRCP, PhD Department of Dermatology, Royal Free London NHS Foundation Trust, London, UK
ferina.ismail@nhs.net

Alan Jaap Department of Diabetes, Royal Infirmary of Edinburgh, Edinburgh, UK
Unkn3134@meteor.com

Aneesa Jaffer Department of Nephrology & Transplantation, Royal Free London NHS Foundation Trust, London, UK
aneesa.jaffer@nhs.net

Paramjit Jeetley Department of Cardiology, Royal Free London NHS Foundation Trust, London, UK
paramjit.jeetley@nhs.net

Sarah Jenkins, FRCP Sheffield Kidney Institute, Sheffield, UK
sarah.jenkins@sth.nhs.uk

Jennie Jewitt-Harris Transplant Links, Camberley, UK
info@transplantlinks.org

Gareth Jones North Middlesex University Hospital NHS Trust, London, UK
gareth.jones14@nhs.net

Philip A. Kalra, MA, MB, BChir, FRCP, MD Vascular Research Group, Manchester Academic Health Sciences Center, University of Manchester, Salford Royal NHS Foundation Trust, Stott Lane, Salford, UK

Department of Renal Medicine, Salford Royal NHS Foundation Trust, Stott Lane, Salford, UK
philip.kalra@srft.nhs.uk

Nigel Suren Kanagasundaram The Newcastle upon Tyne Hospitals NHS Foundation Trust, Newcastle upon Tyne, UK
suren.kanagasundaram@newcastle.ac.uk

Zuze Kawale The Queen Elizabeth Central Hospital, Blantyre, Malawi

Maryam Khosravi Royal Free Hospital, London, UK
m.khosravi@ucl.ac.uk

Ed Kingdon Brighton and Sussex University Hospital Trust, Brighton, UK
Sussex Kidney Unit, Brighton and Sussex University Hospitals NHS Trust, Brighton, UK
ekingdon@nhs.net

David C. Kluth, MD Department of Renal Medicine, Royal Infirmary of Edinburgh, Edinburgh, UK
Centre for Cardiovascular Science, University of Edinburgh, The Queen's Medical Research Institute, Edinburgh, UK
David.Kluth@ed.ac.uk

Ellen Knox Obstetrics Department, Birmingham Women's Hospital, Birmingham, UK
ellen.knox1@nhs.net

Jeevan Kumaradevan Department of Radiology, Whittington Hospital, London, UK
jeevan.kumaradevan@nhs.net

Helen J. Lachmann UK National Amyloidosis Centre, University College London and Royal Free Hospital London NHS Foundation Trust, London, UK
h.lachmann@ucl.ac.uk

Chris Laing Department of Nephrology, University College London, London, UK
UCL Centre for Nephrology, Royal Free Hospital, London, UK
chris.laing@nhs.net

Katie Lane Guy's and St Thomas' NHS Foundation Trust, London, UK
Katie.Lane@nhs.net

Steven Law UCL Department of Renal Medicine, Royal Free Hospital, London, UK
stevenlaw@nhs.net

Ben Lindsey, FRCS Department of Vascular Surgery and Department of Renal Surgery, The Royal Free London NHS Foundation Trust, Hampstead, UK
ben.lindsey@nhs.net

Graham Lipkin Renal Department, Queen Elizabeth Hospital Birmingham, Birmingham, UK
graham.lipkin@uhb.nhs.uk

Mark A. Little Tallaght University Hospital, Dublin, Ireland
MLITTLE@tcd.ie

Rebecca Liu Royal Free Hospital, London, UK
rebecca.liu@nhs.net

Olivia Lucas Barts Cancer Centre, St Bartholomew's Hospital, London, UK
olivia.lucas@nhs.net

Valerie Luyckx University of Cape Town, Cape Town, South Africa
Harvard Medical School, Boston, MA, USA
valerie.luyckx@uzh.ch

Bernadette Lynch Galway University Hospital, Galway, Ireland
bernadette.lynch4@hse.ie

Douglas Macdonald Royal Free Hospital, Department of Gastroenterology, London, UK
douglasmacdonald@nhs.net

Iain C. Macdougall, BSc, MD, FRCP London, UK
iain.macdougall@nhs.net

Iain A. M. MacPhee St George's, University of London, London, UK
imacphee@sgul.ac.uk

Ciara N. Magee UCL Centre for Nephrology, Royal Free Hospital, London, UK
Ciara.magee@nhs.net

Hannah Maple, FRCS, PhD Department of Nephrology and Transplantation, Guy's Hospital, London, UK
Hannah.Maple@gstt.nhs.uk

Stephen D. Marks, MD, MSc, MRCP, DCH, FRCPCH Professor of Paediatric Nephrology and Transplantation, University College London Great Ormond Street Institute of Child Health and Great Ormond Street Hospital for Children NHS Foundation Trust, London, UK
stephen.marks@gosh.nhs.uk

Philip David Mason, BSc, PhD, MBBS, FRCP Oxford Kidney Unit, The Churchill Hospital, Headington, Oxford, UK
Phil.Mason@ouh.nhs.uk

Phil Masson Royal Free Hospital, London, UK
philip.masson@nhs.net

David Mathew Department of Nephrology & Transplantation, Royal Free London NHS Foundation Trust, London, UK
david.mathew2@nhs.net

Alexander P. Maxwell, MD, PhD, FRCP Regional Nephrology Unit, Belfast City Hospital, Belfast, Antrim, UK
Centre for Public Health, Queens University Belfast, Institute of Clinical Sciences, Block B, Royal Victoria Hospital, Belfast, Antrim, Ireland
a.p.maxwell@qub.ac.uk

Patrick H. Maxwell University of Cambridge, Cambridge, UK
Regius@medschl.cam.ac.uk

Stephen P. McAdoo Centre for Inflammatory Disease, Department of Medicine, Imperial College London, London, UK
s.mcadoo@imperial.ac.uk

Fiona McCaig Royal Free London NHS Foundation Trust, London, UK
fionamccaig@nhs.net

Adam McLean, MA, MBBS, FRCP, DPhil Imperial College Kidney and Transplant Centre, Hammersmith Hospital, Imperial College Healthcare NHS Trust, London, UK
AdamMclean@nhs.net

Breeda McManus Barts Health NHS Trust, London, UK
breeda.mcmanus@bartshealth.nhs.uk

Clare Melikian Department of Anaesthesia, Royal Free London NHS Foundation Trust, London, UK
c.melikian@nhs.net

Stephen Mepham Royal Free London NHS Foundation Trust, London, UK
stephen.mepham@nhs.net

Shona Methven, BSc, MBChB, MD, MRCP, FRCP(Edin) Aberdeen Royal Infirmary, Aberdeen, UK
shona.methven@nhs.net

Eve Miller-Hodges, MD Department of Renal Medicine, Royal Infirmary of Edinburgh, Edinburgh, UK

Centre for Cardiovascular Science, University of Edinburgh, The Queen's Medical Research Institute, Edinburgh, UK
Eve.miller-hodges@ed.ac.uk

Shabbir H. Moochhala UCL Department of Renal Medicine, Royal Free Hospital, Royal Free Hospital, London, UK

Royal Free Hospital, London, UK
smoochhala@nhs.net

Frances Mortimer Centre for Sustainable Healthcare, Oxford, UK
frances.mortimer@sustainablehealthcare.org.uk

Fliss E. M. Murtagh Hull York Medical School, University of Hull, Hull, UK
fliss.murtagh@hyms.ac.uk

Vasantha Muthu Muthuppalaniappan Royal Free Hospital, London, UK

Queen Elizabeth Hospital, Birmingham, UK
vasantha.muthuppalaniappan@nhs.net

Anna Nagy Royal Free Hospital, London, UK
anna.nagy@ucl.ac.uk

David Nicol Department of Urology, Royal Marsden Hospital & Institute of Cancer Research, London, UK
davidnicol@nhs.net

Dorothea Nitsch, MD, MSc Department of Non-Communicable Disease Epidemiology, Faculty of Epidemiology and Population Health, London School of Hygiene and Tropical Medicine, London, UK
dorothea.nitsch@lshtm.ac.uk

Aisling O'Riordan Department of Nephrology, St. Vincent's University Hospital, Dublin, Ireland
aisling.oriordan@svhg.ie

Thomas Oates Royal London Hospital, London, UK

Amin Oomatia, MRCP, MBBChir, MA (Cantab) Department of Nephrology, Royal Free London NHS Foundation Trust, London, UK
amin.oomatia@nhs.net

Mared Owen-Casey, MBBCh, FRCPath Histopathology Department, Betsi Cadwaladar University Health Board, Wrexham, UK
mared.owencasey@wales.nhs.uk

Padmasayee Papineni Northwick Park Hospital, London, UK
p.papineni1@nhs.net

Arum Parthipun Department of Radiology, Royal Free Hospital, London, UK
Arum.parthipun@nhs.net

Katharine Pates, MBBS, MBiochem Department of Renal Medicine, UCL Medical School, Royal Free Campus, London, UK
Unknown_54098@Meteor.com

Alan Patrick Department of Diabetes, Royal Infirmary of Edinburgh, Edinburgh, UK
Unkn5134@meteor.com

Ruth J. Pepper Royal Free Hospital, London, UK
UCL Centre for Nephrology, Royal Free Hospital, London, UK
r.pepper@ucl.ac.uk

Alfredo Petrosino Department of Nephrology, Royal Free Hospital, London, UK
alfredo.petrosino@nhs.net

Benedict L. Phillips, BSc (Hons), MSc, MRCS Renal and Transplant Surgery, Guy's Hospital, London, UK
benedict.phillips@nhs.uk

Jennifer Pinney Department of Renal Medicine, Queen Elizabeth Hospital Birmingham, Birmingham, UK
Jennifer.Pinney@uhb.nhs.uk

Liam Plant Department of Renal Medicine, Cork University Hospital & University College Cork, Cork, Ireland
william.plant@ucc.ie

Madhu Potluri, MBCHB, MRCP UK, MRCP Gloucestershire Hospitals NHS Foundation Trust, Cheltenham, UK
madhupotluri@nhs.net

Nithya Prasannan, MBBS, MRCP, FRCPath Katharine Dormandy Haemophilia and Thrombosis Centre, Royal Free London NHS Foundation Trust, London, UK
Department of Haematology, University College London, London, UK

Maria Prendecki Centre for Inflammatory Disease, Department of Immunology and Inflammation, Imperial College London, London, UK
m.prendecki@imperial.ac.uk

Zudin Puthucheary William Harvey Research Institute, Barts and The London School of Medicine and Dentistry, Queen Mary University of London, Royal London Hospital, Barts Health NHS Trust, London, UK
z.puthucheary@nhs.net

Ravindra Rajakariar Barts Health NHS Trust, London, UK
ravindra.rajakariar@bartshealth.nhs.uk

Gayathri Rajakaruna University College London, London, UK
g.rajakaruna@ucl.ac.uk

Ritika Rana Department of Renal Medicine, Queen Elizabeth Hospital Birmingham, Birmingham, UK
Ritika.Rana@uhb.nhs.uk

Andrew Ready University Hospital Birmingham, Birmingham, UK

Transplant Links, Camberley, UK
andrew.ready@uhb.nhs.com

James Ritchie Vascular Research Group, Manchester Academic Health Sciences Center, University of Manchester, Salford Royal NHS Foundation Trust, Stott Lane, Salford, UK
james.ritchie@nca.nhs.uk

Candice Roufosse Imperial College, London, UK
Candice.roufosse@nhs.net

Adam Rumjon, MBBS, PhD, MRCP North Middlesex University Hospital, Sterling Way, London, UK
adamrumjon@nhs.net

Gill Rumsby, PhD, FRCPath UCL Hospitals, London, UK
gill.rumsby@nhs.net

Omid Sadeghi-Alavijeh Royal Free Hospital, London, UK
omid.sadeghi-alavijeh@nhs.net

Alan D. Salama, MBBS, MA, PhD, FRCP University College London, London, UK

Royal Free Hospital, London, UK

UCL Department of Renal Medicine Royal Free Hospital, London, UK
a.salama@ucl.ac.uk

Nasreen Samad Consultant Nephrologists, The Royal London Hospital, Barts Health NHS Trust, London, UK
nareen.samad@bartshealth.nhs.uk

Jennifer Scott Trinity Health Kidney Centre, Dublin, Ireland

Haresh Selvaskandan The John Walls Renal Unit, Leicester General Hospital, University Hospitals of Leicester, Leicester, UK
haresh.selvaskandan@nhs.net

Claire C. Sharpe Department of Inflammation Biology, Faculty of Life Sciences and Medicine, King's College London, London, UK
Claire.sharpe@kcl.ac.uk

Neil S. Sheerin National Renal Complement Therapeutic Centre, Translational and Clinical Research Institute, Newcastle University, Newcastle upon Tyne, UK
neil.sheerin@ncl.ac.uk

Ali M. Shendi, MD Faculty of Medicine, Zagazig University, Zagazig, Egypt

Nephrology Unit, Internal Medicine Department, Faculty of Medicine, Zagazig University, Zagazig, Egypt
ali.shendi@zu.edu.eg

Kin Yee Shiu, MBBS, PhD, FRCP Department of Renal Medicine, University College London, Royal Free Hospital, London, UK
kinyee.shiu@nhs.net

Badri Shrestha, MD, FRCS Sheffield Kidney Institute, Sheffield, UK
badri.shrestha@sth.nhs.uk

Ruth Silverton University College London Medical School, Department of Postgraduate Medical Education, London, UK

Cambridge University Hospitals NHS Foundation Trust, Department of Renal Medicine, Cambridge, UK
ruth.silverton@doctors.org.uk

James Smith, BSc, MBChB, PhD, MRCP Abderdeen Royal Infirmary, Foresterhill, Aberdeen, UK
jsmith82@nhs.net

Reecha Sofat UCL Institute of Health Informatics, London, UK
r.sofat@ucl.ac.uk

Henry Stephens, BSc, PhD Department of Renal Medicine, University College London & The Anthony Nolan Laboratory, Royal Free Hospital, London, UK
h.stephens@ucl.ac.uk

Dinesha Himali Sudusinghe Faculty of Medical Sciences, University of Sri Jayewardenepura, Sri Lanka, Colombo, Sri Lanka

James Tomlinson Royal Free London NHS Foundation Trust, London, UK
James.tomlinson3@nhs.net

Charles R. V. Tomson, MA, BMBCh, FRCP, DM (Oxon) Newcastle upon Tyne Hospitals NHS Foundation Trust, Newcastle upon Tyne, UK

Freeman Hospital, Newcastle upon Tyne, UK
charles.tomson1@nhs.net

Caroline Tulley Royal Free London NHS Foundation Trust, London, UK
caroline.tulley@nhs.net

A. Neil Turner, PhD, FRCP Centre for Inflammation, University of Edinburgh, QMRI, Edinburgh, UK
neil.turner@ed.ac.uk

M. Umaid Rauf Royal Free Hospital, London, UK
m.rauf@nhs.net

Robert Unwin UCL Department of Renal Medicine, Royal Free Hospital, Royal Free Hospital, London, UK
robert.unwin@ucl.ac.uk

Diana Vassallo Vascular Research Group, Manchester Academic Health Sciences Center, University of Manchester, Salford Royal NHS Foundation Trust, Stott Lane, Salford, UK
Unk534@meteor.com

Stephen B. Walsh University College London, London, UK
stephen.walsh@ucl.ac.uk

Elizabeth R. Wan University College London, London, UK
e.mumford@nhs.net

Thuvaraka Ware Department of Nephrology, Royal Free Hospital, London, UK
Royal Free Hospital, London, UK
thuvaraka.ware@nhs.net

Christopher J. E. Watson, MA, MD, FRCS University Department of Surgery, Addenbrooke's Hospital, Cambridge, UK
cjew2@cam.ac.uk

Lakshman Weerasekara Royal Free London NHS Foundation Trust, London, UK
Lakshman.weerasjara@nhs.net

David C. Wheeler, MD, FRCP Department of Renal Medicine, UCL Medical School, Royal Free Campus, London, UK
d.wheeler@ucl.ac.uk

William White Departments of Acute Medicine & Nephrology, Royal London Hospital, London, UK
william.white9@nhs.net

Dilushi Wijayaratne Department of Renal Medicine, UCL, London, UK
Dilushi.Wijajaratne@nhs.net

Martin Wilkie, MD, FRCP Sheffield Kidney Institute, Sheffield, UK
Sheffield Teaching Hospitals NHS, Sheffield, UK
martin.wilkie@nhs.net

Eleri Williams, MB, BChir, MRCP Centre for Inflammation, University of Edinburgh, QMRI, Edinburgh, UK
eleri.williams@doctors.org.uk

Elizabeth Williams Homerton University Hospital, London, UK
eawilliams@doctors.org.uk

Jo Wilson Royal Free Hospitals London NHS Foundation Trust and University of Bath, London, UK
jo.wilson8@nhs.net

Dan Wood, PhD, FRCS (Urol) Adolescent Urology, University College London Hospitals NHS Foundation Trust, London, UK
dan.wood1@nhs.net

Nick Woodward, MBBS, MRCP, FRCR Department of Radiology, Royal Free London NHS Foundation Trust, London, UK
nick.woodward@nhs.net

Dominic Yu Royal Free London NHS Foundation Trust, London, UK
dominic.yu@nhs.net

Assessment of the Renal Patient

Contents

Assessment of the Renal Patient

Maryam Khosravi, Omid Sadeghi-Alavijeh, Phil Masson, and Ben Caplin

Contents

M. Harber (ed.), *Primer on Nephrology*, https://doi.org/10.1007/978-3-030-76419-7_1

1

Learning Objectives

1. To safely assess the unwell patient with renal disease and develop suitable assessments of patients for varying stages of their illness, in order to inform diagnosis and treatment.

Key Points

1. The first question before performing an assessment must be: Is the patient safe? Are they in the appropriate environment? Is there an indication for emergency medical therapy? Do they require urgent renal replacement therapy?
2. Assessment of fluid balance requires integration of multiple sources of clinical, biochemical and radiological information.
3. Taking different approaches to patients who are presenting for the first time versus those well-known to renal services facilitates more organised clinical thinking and better management of time and resource.
4. When assessing the first presentation of a case of renal dysfunction, determining the chronicity is a key factor for deciding on the next steps of management.
5. Attention to the extra-renal sequela of systemic disease can often hint at the diagnosis prior to renal deterioration.

1.1 Introduction

Patients may present to nephrology services with a spectrum of renal disease, from asymptomatic incidental findings to severe renal impairment or electrolyte disturbance in a critically ill patient. Others will have significant comorbidity perhaps alongside previously diagnosed and complex chronic renal disease. These factors mean the assessment of the 'renal patient' can be a challenging proposition to the less (and on occasion the more) experienced physician. There are numerous approaches to the assessment of patients with kidney disease, and practitioners will develop their own style with time. However, a common pitfall for the new nephrologist is the failure to recognise that although attention to detail is essential, the potential to lose the critical aspects of history and examination in a mass of less relevant information is high. One strategy to avoid this is to frame the assessment as a series of questions by asking oneself 'what is the next thing I need to know to guide my management?' The 'practical' approach we outline here is only one of many but one that we find successful in day-to-day practice. We approach the assessment of the renal patient with a series of questions, as illustrated in the flow-diagram (◻ Fig. 1.1) below.

The first priority is to ask if the patient is safe. This question provides the starting point of this chapter. Since an assessment of fluid balance is integral to the patient's clinical safety, as well as many aspects of subsequent diagnosis or management, this is the next focus. Subsequently, it is usually important to clarify whether the patient is already being managed for an underlying kidney condition. The approach to the patient with established kidney disease, for example, a patient receiving dialysis or with inflammatory glomerulonephritis, will be completely different from the approach to the patient who presents with a renal disorder for the first time. In first presentations, the priority will be to establish the underlying cause of the renal disorder. This is the clinical scenario where there is often significant diagnostic uncertainty, representing some of the most interesting and challenging areas of nephrology practice. Patients with established disease often require equally challenging, focused and specific assessment to optimise their management, and this is addressed in the last section of this chapter.

1.2 Urgent Assessment for Renal Emergencies

As with all acutely unwell patients, the priority is assessing and correcting potentially life-threatening physiological dysfunction. For the maintenance of an adequate airway, ventilation and circulation (ABC), urgent renal-specific contributors are likely to relate to intravascular volume depletion or fluid overload (see next section) alongside metabolic disturbance, most usually hyperkalaemia or acidaemia. These latter scenarios may be an indication for urgent renal replacement therapy (RRT) if not responsive to medical treatment. When there is an indication for urgent RRT, attention must be given to the most appropriate mode of delivery and the correct clinical environment in which to deliver it. Requirements will depend on the need for other organ support, and local policies will vary, but the use of any extracorporeal circuit (even with the low blood flows used in continuous therapies such as haemofiltration) risks haemodynamic instability. Adequate (usually invasive) monitoring and access to vasopressors or inotropes are mandatory in those receiving RRT who are cardiovascularly unstable (see ▶ Chap. 12). Critically, the immediate management may depend on whether the acidaemic or hyperkalaemic patient has an immediately remediable medical condition; a patient with urinary retention and potassium of 7.2 mmol/L may be easy to manage medically (following relief of obstruction), whereas a septic oliguric hypotensive patient with a potassium of 5.8 mmol/L is much more likely to need renal replacement imminently.

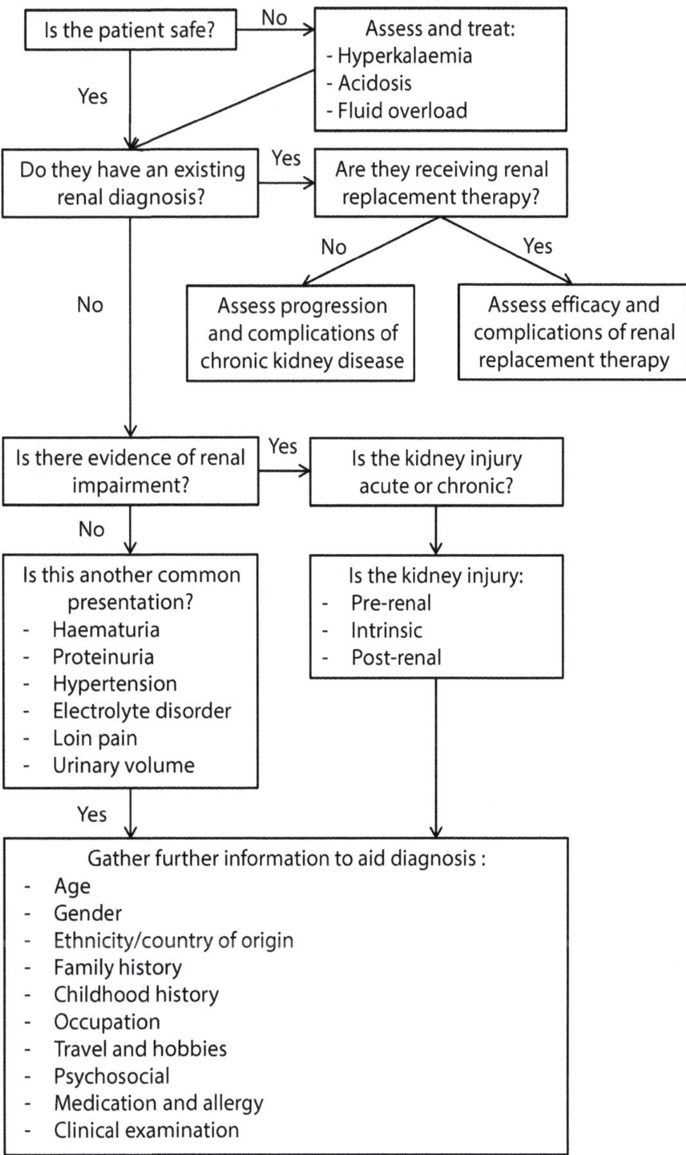

Fig. 1.1 Practical approach to the assessment of a renal patient

1.3 Fluid Assessment

Evaluation of intravascular volume status is critical for the assessment and management of all renal patients. It is especially important as a cause of pre-renal kidney injury and for critically ill patients with hypovolemic shock, as well as being challenging to manage in other forms of shock. Volume assessment is also key in the evaluation of patients with hypertension, nephrotic syndrome or allograft dysfunction, as well as integral in the management of all patients receiving RRT. Abnormalities of intravascular volume are challenging to detect, especially when there is co-existent hypo- or hypertension relating to vascular pressure (e.g. sepsis or pre-eclampsia). Assessment of intravascular volume can be neglected on the general ward and may receive little emphasis during training in some specialities and so should be an essential skill for all nephrologists.

1.3.1 Clinical Assessment

Table 1.1 shows some of the symptoms and signs that have merit in assessing fluid balance. Some such as serial measurement of weight and orthostatic blood pressure should be incorporated into ward observations and encouraged on non-renal wards. Again, where appropriate, some patients such as those discharged home with recovering AKI or nephrotic syndrome may benefit and be empowered by monitoring their own weight and postural blood pressure. Some clinical signs such as peripheral temperature and observation of central veins are

1

Table 1.1 Clinical assessment of fluid status

History	Paroxysmal nocturnal dyspnoea, orthopnoea, increased weight and worsening oedema are relatively sensitive and fairly specific symptoms of fluid overload
	Thirst is a relatively sensitive marker of dehydration or salt overload. A history of significant fluid loss or reduced fluid intake contributes to assessment of fluid balance
Examination	
Pulse	Tachycardia is a non-specific marker of intravascular volume depletion and may be associated with excessive intravascular volume in the context of heart failure
Blood pressure	Relative hypotension (comparison with historical blood pressure) and episodes of documented hypotension (intraoperative, hospital or community based) are always a significant finding in patients with renal dysfunction. Although trends may inform assessment, hypotension is a non-specific marker of intravascular volume depletion
Orthostatic changes	Reflex tachycardia (increase in 30 beats per minute or more) is sensitive for acute large blood loss but insensitive for smaller bleeds or other causes of hypovolaemia and non-specific
	Changes in blood pressure with changes in posture are a useful finding that can be delegated to ward staff. Changes of 20 mmHg in systolic and 10 mmHg in diastolic blood pressure upon change in posture are widely used as significant thresholds
Peripheral temperature	Cool nose, hands or feet at room temperature imply either decreased intravascular volume (low JVP) or cardiac failure (raised JVP). These are not sensitive but easy and reproducible. Unhelpful in patients with peripheral vascular disease or vasodilated patients (sepsis, cirrhosis, thyrotoxicosis)
Jugular venous pressure (JVP)	Operator dependent and highly dependent on body habitus. Raised JVP may represent either increased intravascular volume or high right ventricular filling pressure (cardiac failure, pulmonary hypertension, tricuspid regurgitation or stenosis, restrictive defects, tamponade). Common for ESRD patients with previous access to have internal jugular stenosis or occlusion (including secondary to current line) or SVC obstruction
Oedema	Diurnal variation (feet swollen in the evening, face in the morning) usually rules out any anatomical cause. A bed-bound patient may have normal ankles but several litres in sacral or flank oedema. Oedema will also be influenced by drugs and plasma oncotic pressure
Third heart sound (S3 gallop rhythm)	Indicative of ventricular failure/overload, insensitive
Ascites and pleural effusions	Non-specific and poorly sensitive
Bedside measurements:	
Weight	Extremely useful serial measurement for general nephrology patients as well as those on dialysis with a 'dry weight'. Serial measurements for inpatients extremely valuable measure of total body water (but not intravascular volume)
Urine output	Non-specific but important part of AKI classification and relatively sensitive marker of intravascular volume. Unhelpful as a marker of intravascular volume if AKI from whatever cause or concentrating defect, e.g. post-obstructive diuresis
Documentation of inputs and outputs	Anaesthetic charts, ward charts including drain losses and stool charts can be invaluable if accurate but do not equate to current fluid status
Bedside ultrasound	Inferior vena cava compressibility
Laboratory measurements:	
Urine specific gravity (SG)	High or low SG suggests intravascular depletion or a positive fluid balance; however, acute or chronically injured kidneys lose the ability to concentrate and therefore has limited value
Urinary sodium	A low spot urinary sodium or fractional excretion of sodium is indicative of reduced renal perfusion and can be helpful in differentiating pre-renal (including hepatorenal) from replete intravascular volume but invalid in the face of acute tubular injury, diuretics or dopamine
N-terminal probrain-type natriuretic peptide	Some evidence of correlation with fluid status, particularly in the dialysis population

useful, whereas skin turgor and dryness of mucous membranes are insensitive and non-specific signs.

1.3.2 Bedside Tests

At the bedside, it is important to recognise that dynamic markers of intravascular volume are usually the most informative. In particular, the critical care field has provided some reliable indices for assessment of volume status, since dynamic changes of arterial waveform-derived variables in mechanically ventilated patients have good evidence for accurately predicting volume responsiveness [1]. Furthermore, there is some evidence of a relationship between the amplitude of the arterial pressure wave correlates with pulse oximetry waveform (again in ventilated patients [2]), suggesting this approach might be useful in the assessment of a renal patient managed outside of critical care environment. However, evidence to assess the utility of this approach is lacking.

An alternative method in the spontaneously breathing patient is to use the passive leg raise. By raising the patient's legs from the recumbent position, and back again, the passive leg raise delivers a venous return of approximately 300 ml from the lower body to the right heart of the patient. This test relies on precise execution of the technique and requires direct measurement of cardiac output in real time [3].

Bedside ultrasound is increasingly available and necessary in the acute assessment of unwell patients in the hospital setting. With the necessary training, ultrasound can be a useful tool in fluid assessment since there is good evidence for correlation of inferior vena cava diameter and collapsibility in assessing fluid responsiveness [4–6].

1.3.2.1 Investigations

Chest X-ray can be invaluable in diagnosing or confirming gross fluid overload, but it is not particularly sensitive for mild/moderate overload, and acute lung injury/leaky lungs can occur with no increase in right-sided filling pressure (see ◘ Fig. 1.2a and b).

Bioimpedance is an inexpensive and non-invasive technique to estimate body water. Given the difficulties with clinical assessment of fluid status, the possibility of an easily usable objective measure is attractive. However, as with many of the clinical parameters guiding assessment of fluid balance, a single measurement in an individual patient does not appear to add significant value to clinical assessment. Serial measures may be more valuable, so this technique may be most useful in patients attending chronic dialysis or the outpatient department rather than in the acute situation [7].

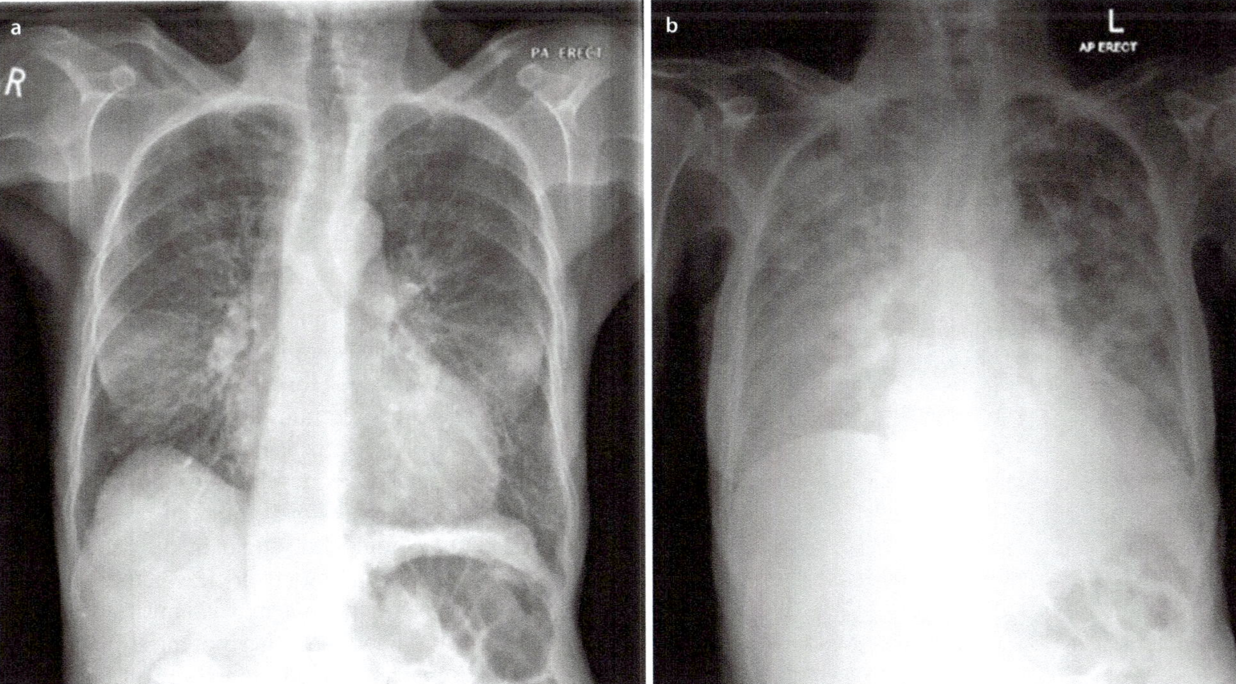

◘ **Fig. 1.2** **a** CXR of a patient with raised left ventricular end-diastolic pressure (LVEDP) showing upper lobe blood diversion, fluid in the fissure and Kerley B lines. This approximately equates to an LVEDP of 18 mmHg or above. **b** Frank pulmonary oedema in the same patient within 24 h in the absence of any filling or cardiac event but in the presence of sepsis. This demonstrates that pulmonary oedema on a CXR is not necessarily indicative of excessive filling pressures per se

Biochemical measures that have been advocated as indices of fluid status such as a 'disproportionately' high urea, raised serum urate or elevated serum lactate also lack sensitivity or specificity. Natriuretic peptides have been shown to be a useful biomarker of volume status in dialysis patients, but in the general adult population, studies are inconclusive and clouded by confounding data [8].

1.4 Assessment of the Patient When the Renal Disorder Has Yet to Be Identified and/or Characterised

1.4.1 Presentation with Renal Impairment

Impaired kidney function is the commonest reason for referral to a nephrologist. Patients may present with symptoms directly related to renal dysfunction (◘ Table 1.2), but these symptoms usually herald advanced renal impairment. More often, referrals follow the incidental finding of renal impairment in blood tests performed following a clinical presentation unrelated to the kidney.

1.4.1.1 Does the Patient Have Acute or Chronic Renal Impairment?

The urgency of further investigation in a patient with impaired kidney function is critically dependent on whether the onset is acute (occurring over days to weeks) or chronic (occurring over months to years). Differentiation of these clinical scenarios is straightforward if previous blood tests are available. The distinction can be more difficult in cases of acute on chronic renal dysfunction where a baseline creatinine that would uncover the time course of the disease is not available. The duration of symptoms can be a useful indicator of chronicity; however, advanced renal impairment can be present for some time before the patient reports the onset of illness. Furthermore, the presence of risk factors or a systemic disorder known to put the patient at risk of kidney disease does not provide definite evidence for the time of onset of any pre-existing renal dysfunction.

The best markers of long-standing (and consequently irreversible) renal impairment are radiological appearances. Bipolar renal diameter <10 cm in combination with increased cortical echogenicity (defined as a higher pixel density in the renal cortex than the liver) is a strong indicator of advanced chronic kidney disease [9]. Exceptions to this rule occur, where the size of chronically diseased kidneys is preserved, most typically in diabetes, but also cystic diseases (such as ADPKD), protein deposition diseases (amyloid), chronic obstruction, xanthogranulomatous pyelonephritis and HIV nephropathy.

Biochemical markers such as potassium, calcium, phosphate, parathyroid hormone and haemoglobin are often described as indicators of chronic renal dysfunction. However, these parameters have limited utility in practice since all can also change rapidly in the context of AKI.

◘ Table 1.2 Symptoms attributable to renal impairment

Uraemia	Anorexia, nausea, pruritis, malaise and sleep disturbance are all common symptoms in ESRD. Patients may also complain of headaches, reduced mental agility, chest pain (pericarditis), prolonged bleeding or bruising
Anaemia	Lethargy, palpitations, shortness of breath (particularly exertional)
Electrolyte disturbance	Palpitations, musculoskeletal pain, cramps, restless limbs, seizures, confusion
Fluid maldistribution or excess	Facial or peripheral swelling, shortness of breath or reduced exercise tolerance, orthopnoea, paroxysmal nocturnal dyspnoea
Urinary symptoms	Oliguria, dysuria, nocturia (a common symptom in CKD), alterations in appearance (colour/froth)

1.4.1.2 Diagnostic Breakdown of Acute or Chronic Renal Dysfunction

Assessment of a patient with AKI is described in detail in ► Chap. 5. However, the classical subdivision into pre-, post- and intrinsic causes of renal impairment is a useful approach in any patient presenting with either acute or chronic renal impairment.

Pre-renal Causes

A 'pre-renal' aetiology implies hypoperfusion of the kidney. This is a critical component of the assessment of patients with AKI as this form of insult is usually associated with an acute presentation. However, renal artery stenosis and chronic hypovolaemia (e.g. in patients with high output stomas) may develop more insidiously and present with CKD. Therefore, potential precipitants of pre-renal injury should be sought in all patients with renal dysfunction. Circulatory shock, whether vasodilatory, cardiogenic or hypovolaemic will invariably lead to an acute injury. These and other potential precipitants of pre-renal impairment are outlined in ◘ Table 1.3.

Post-renal Causes

Post-renal causes of renal impairment are often straightforward to treat which in turn can lead to the full or partial recovery of the associated renal injury.

Furthermore, obstruction is a common and often asymptomatic cause for unexpected deterioration in patients with established medical renal disease.

Although the clinical history or examination (◘ Table 1.4) may suggest an obstructive cause of kidney injury, exclusion of a post-renal cause of renal impairment cannot be made without radiological investigation. A renal ultrasound is the first line of investigation, but there are limitations which should be considered when interpreting the results:

- 'False positives' can occur in cases of chronic dilation of the pelvicalyceal system. Functional imaging (renograms) can be helpful for establishing the significance of anatomical abnormality (but kidney function must be adequate for these to be useful). Renograms with the addition of diuretics using nuclear medicine tracers can be helpful in this context (see ► Chap. 5)
- 'False negatives' can occur in anuric patients, who may not have pelvicalyceal dilatation. If the history is suggestive, more detailed anatomical imaging such as MRI or CT may be helpful. However, a trial of relief of the potential obstruction can be the only way to definitively make a diagnosis in some cases.

Symptomatic changes in urine volume are not usually diagnostically helpful other than abrupt anuria which may point to a bilateral obstruction but can also reflect medical renal disease (see below). Clinical history that might suggest a post-renal causes of kidney dysfunction is shown in ◘ Table 1.4.

Intrinsic Renal Causes

Intrinsic renal causes of AKI and CKD are numerous but can be grouped into broad categories for the purpose of initial assessment (◘ Table 1.5).

Examination of the urine is absolutely critical in establishing the diagnosis of intrinsic renal injury, and this is discussed in detail in ► Chap. 2. In the context of AKI, it is important to recognise that although haematuria and proteinuria may represent a rapidly progressive glomerulonephritis, these same findings can also reflect a chronic underlying glomerular lesion with a concomitant acute deterioration in renal function due to an unrelated cause.

1.4.2 Presentations Other Than with Biochemical Evidence of Change in Renal Function

Although the majority of patients referred for the first time to nephrologists will have a biochemical evidence of renal dysfunction, patients with isolated urinary abnormalities are also often sent for expert review. The assessment of isolated haematuria and proteinuria is discussed in the following chapter. In addition to urinary abnormalities, nephrologists will find themselves faced with diverse clinical syndromes. These syndromes and the logical diagnostic approaches are discussed further in the chapters devoted to these subjects, but some of the more common presentations are discussed briefly below.

1.4.2.1 Haematuria

Haematuria can originate from anywhere along the urinary tract, so it is important to identify coexistent lower urinary tract symptoms in any patient with visible blood in the urine. Intermittent visible haematuria can be temporally associated with an upper respiratory tract infection which is suggestive of IgA nephropathy or related to exercise. Haematuria associated with menses can be seen in patients with endometriosis. Finally, myoglobinuria and haemoglobinuria (both important nonglomerular precipitants of AKI) will often lead to a false-positive dipstick urinalysis for haematuria.

1.4.2.2 Proteinuria

Proteinuria is usually identified on dipstick testing during routine medical examinations or surveillance (e.g. for diabetes) or in the investigation of associated oedema, but patients with nephrotic range proteinuria can on occasion present symptomatically with frothy urine. History of past episodes of dipstick positive proteinuria is helpful but is rarely recalled by patients.

1.4.2.3 Nephrotic Syndrome

The presentation of nephrotic syndrome is usually unambiguous. Diagnostic difficulties can occur in the presence of anuria or advanced renal failure or in the context of other causes for hypoalbuminaemia. For patients with nephrotic syndrome, swelling of the face or 'puffy eyes' in the morning is a common early symptom (and does not occur when an oedematous state is secondary to heart failure), pedal oedema and frothy urine may be noted and fatigue or tiredness are also common complaints. For some individuals, nephrotic syndrome may be precipitated by vaccinations, insect bites or nonspecific infections. The definition, investigation and initial management of nephrotic syndrome are covered in ► Chap. 12.

1.4.2.4 Hypertension

Uncontrolled or unexpected hypertension is a fairly common referral to the nephrologist and is discussed in detail in ► Chap. 27. Beyond emergency care and determining duration, severity and compliance, the main consideration is whether an underlying cause can be

1

Table 1.3 Assessment of potential precipitants of pre-renal kidney injury

Relative hypotension	A drop in BP, for whatever reason, in a normally hypertensive patient
Cardiogenic shock	Risk factors for cardiovascular disease, suggestive of cardiological investigations
Intravascular volume depletion	
Blood loss	
Poor oral intake	In the confused or immobile patient
Fever, sweating, burns	
Vomiting, diarrhoea	Patients with short bowel or high output stomas are at particular risk of volume depletion
Polyuria	Prescribed or non-prescribed diuretics, mannitol
	Central polyuria (intracranial causes) – cerebral salt wasting, diabetes insipidus (DI)
	Tubular dysfunction – Addison's, nephrogenic DI (lithium toxicity), salt-losing nephropathies, hyperglycaemia, diuresis associated with recovery of kidney function
Fluid redistribution with reduced arterial perfusion	
Ascites	Liver disease
Fluid accumulation in the GI tract	Bowel obstruction, post-operative ileus
Oedema secondary to nephrotic syndrome	
Septic/anaphylactic shock	
Drugs Adrenal	Calcium channel blockers, minoxidil, thiazolidinediones, docetaxel, pramipexole Hypoadrenalism – primary or secondary
Local hypoperfusion	
Arterial occlusion	Emboli, most commonly following endovascular intervention; arterial dissection; malignant infiltration
Renal artery stenosis	'Crash' pulmonary oedema caused by sudden reduction of GFR post renin-angiotensin blockade
Venous obstruction	Renal vein thrombosis (consider in association with pro-coagulant states, e.g. nephrotic syndrome), page kidney (subscapular haematoma causing compression) following kidney biopsy

NB patient notes (including anaesthetic records) are invaluable for identifying episodes of relative hypotension, poor IV or oral intake, excessive losses or weight changes

identified and treated (Table 1.6). Such an underlying cause is more likely if hypertension occurs before the age of 40 years (the younger the patient, the greater the likelihood of a secondary cause) or if there is severe end organ damage, accelerated hypertension, sudden worsening or a family history of early hypertension/stroke. However, it is important to recognise that the majority of secondary hypertension relates to underlying renal disease.

1.4.2.5 Loin Pain

Although kidney stones are a common and potentially serious cause of loin pain, pain arising from the kidneys can occur in numerous conditions. The differential diagnosis of causes of loin pain is listed in Table 1.7.

Nephrolithiasis is usually accompanied by severe symptoms although it may only be on direct questioning that patients mention passing 'gravel' (small sand-like material). Working or living in hot, dehydrating environments, with limited access or possibility for adequate hydration, multiple long flights and high salt intake, as well as any dietary precipitants such as betel nut, are associated with stones in epidemiological studies. Any history of obstruction, lithotripsy or stone removal is also clearly important. Identifying if and where any stones have been analysed is very helpful and can expedite appropriate preventative therapy.

Table 1.4 Clinical history suggestive of urinary tract obstruction

Anuria	Suggests bilateral ureteric or bladder outlet obstruction. Beware of non-obstructive causes
Symptoms of bladder outlet obstruction	Urinary frequency, dysuria, poor flow, nocturia, urgency, double micturition, hesitancy, post micturition dribbling, incontinence (overflow obstruction), sensation of incomplete emptying
N.B. Acute urinary retention can be painless with a neuropathic bladder	
Spraying on micturition	Urethral stricture, phimosis or paraphimosis
Loin pain	Any cause of obstruction:
	On micturition (suggestive of vesicoureteral reflux)
	On excessive drinking (suggestive of PUJ obstruction)
Visible haematuria	Nephrolithiasis, malignancy, papillary necrosis
Medications	Anticholinergics, withdrawal of alpha blockers
Disseminated or pelvic malignancy	Systemic symptoms, fevers, weight loss
Iatrogenic obstruction	Pelvic surgery or radiotherapy
Nephrolithiasis	
Pregnancy	Collecting systems can be dilated without functional obstruction
Childhood UTI or enuresis	May suggest congenital abnormalities of the urinary tract
Travel and swimming in at risk waters	Schistosomiasis infection

1.4.2.6 Electrolyte Disorders

The renal physician is often asked to aid in the diagnosis and management of patients with electrolyte abnormalities. Renal tubular syndromes are discussed in detail later in this book although differentiation of renal tubular abnormalities from endocrine, metabolic or gastroenterological aetiologies can be difficult.

Where an abnormal finding is unexpected or sudden, the possibility of an aberrant value should be considered. Recognition of the abnormal lab finding as being the result of blood sampling from a drip arm or patient misidentification can save significant anxiety.

Symptomatology can be non-specific, such as muscle weakness with hyperkalaemia, or classic such as perioral paraesthesia and muscle spasm (latent tetany) in hypocalcaemia. The urgency of investigation and treatment will typically depend on both the severity and the chronicity of any abnormality.

Table 1.5 Approach to intrinsic renal causes of renal dysfunction

Endogenous toxins	Precipitants of rhabdomyolysis, intravascular haemolysis, tumour-lysis syndrome, immunoglobulin light chain precipitation, hyperoxaluria, cholesterol emboli, hypercalcaemia, hyperbilirubinemia
Exogenous toxins	Prescribed medication, illicit drugs, herbal remedies, poisons (e.g. snake bite), sepsis, IV radiocontrast
Glomerular injury	Features to suggest nephritic (or nephrotic) syndrome; haematuria or cola-coloured, recent or current infections; constitutional symptoms consistent with systemic inflammatory or autoimmune disease or malignancy, e.g. fevers, weight loss, ENT symptoms, red eyes, alopecia, rashes, haemoptysis, pleurisy, arthralgia, oedema. Bruising or bleeding in TMA such as HUS
Tubulointerstitial inflammatory	Autoimmune, infiltrative, e.g. lymphoma, or inflammatory, e.g. TB or sarcoid
Any cause of unresolved pre-renal injury	

1.4.2.7 Changes in Urinary Volume

In the absence of disease, urinary volume can vary at least tenfold, so aside from anuria, patients may find it difficult to recognise changes in urinary volume. Oliguria is a manifestation of advanced renal impairment, but acute, absolute anuria is rare; the causes of which are listed in Table 1.8.

Conversely, polyuria can be difficult to distinguish from urinary frequency, but it is important to try and differentiate the two, since the differential diagnosis of polyuria is wide. One approach to assessment is shown in Table 1.9.

1.4.2.8 Renal Manifestation of Multisystem Disorders

Abnormalities of the kidney occur in a large number and diverse range of systemic disorders with vascular, inflammatory, malignant or infective aetiologies. Indeed, where the kidney represents the first clinical manifestation of these disorders, the renal physician may best placed to establish diagnosis with predominantly extra-

Table 1.6 Evaluation of the patient with hypertension

Age of onset	Early onset <40 more suggestive of secondary cause
Compliance	Agents tried, evidence of concordance
Severity/end organ damage	Number of agents, retinopathy, left ventricular hypertrophy/failure, cerebral vascular disease
Any history of renal disease	
Family history	e.g. Liddle's, Gordon's but more usually a family history without diagnosis
Coarctation (cold feet, leg cramps, exercise intolerance)	Congenital heart disease, murmurs or abnormal pulses
Renal artery stenosis	Flash pulmonary oedema, history of macrovascular disease, deterioration in renal function with angiotensin-converting-enzyme inhibitors (ACE-I) or angiotensin receptor blockers (ARB), absent peripheral pulses
Pheochromocytoma	*Episodic*: headache, palpitations (64%) sweating (70%), pallor, hypotension, tremor, flushing, dyspnoea and epigastric pain
Obstructive sleep apnoea	Usually typical history and body habitus
Other endocrine causes	Cushingoid features, signs of acromegaly, etc.

Table 1.7 Pain associated with renal disease

Pyelonephritis	Acute and chronic such as xanthogranulomatous pyelonephritis
Nephrolithiasis	Typically, severe, sudden onset and radiating (loin to groin)
Acute obstruction	Stone, sloughed papillae, blood clot, intermittent PUJ obstruction (particularly after fluid challenge)
Reflux	Occasionally patients describe loin pain on micturition
Wunderlich syndrome	Spontaneous renal haemorrhage from renal carcinoma, angiomyolipoma (renal AML) or arteriovenous malformation
Abdominal pain	Polyarteritis nodosa, infiltration with tumour
Infarction	Arterial or venous occlusion
Loin pain haematuria	Nutcracker syndrome – compression of the left renal vein between the aorta and proximal superior mesenteric artery

renal involvement. In these cases, it is often attention to a comprehensive clinical history and examination that will reveal an underlying disorder (Table 1.10).

1.4.3 Clinical History Relevant to Establishing a Renal Diagnosis

In patients presenting for the first time with a renal syndrome (e.g. a presentation with new renal impairment or an electrolyte disorder), a further clinical history and examination can be pursued. A clear understanding of what brought the patient to seek medical attention alongside a full past-medical and surgical history is essential. Further aspects of the personal, family, social and drug history that might be helpful in establishing a diagnosis are discussed in this section.

1.4.3.1 Age

A patient presenting with ESKD in their 20s is more likely to have an inherited or congenital cause, and it is important to determine if symptoms started in childhood or adolescence. Age may make some diagnoses much less likely. For example, it is very unusual for lupus nephritis to present late in life, whereas primary vasculitis may well present in a patient's eighth or ninth decade. Furthermore, there is an increased prevalence of CKD in the older population, with a greater risk of AKI in the elderly.

1.4.3.2 Gender

Some renal diseases show significant gender bias, and patterns of inheritance may give a significant clue to the diagnosis when a clear family history is available. For example, X-linked conditions like Alport's syndrome and X-linked Anderson-Fabry's disease have a male bias, whereas conditions such as Takayasu's aortitis, fibromuscular dysplasia and systemic lupus erythematosus have a very strong female preponderance.

1.4.3.3 Ethnicity and Country of Origin

Ethnicity and country of origin may be pointers to increased exposure to risk factors for some renal diseases and comorbid conditions that may affect the kidneys; some examples are given in Table 1.11.

1.4.3.4 Family History

With expanding possibilities for genetic testing, a detailed family history can provide the key to unlocking a diagnosis. This is important because it can affect the patient's treatment and their family planning. It also allows the patient's extended family to have a chance of diagnosis, with the possibility of earlier screening for renal impairment in other family

Table 1.8 Causes of acute anuria

Vascular 1. Arterial catastrophe	Aortic dissection or thrombo-embolic event to single functioning kidney
Vascular 2. Venous thrombosis	Bilateral venous thrombosis (e.g. nephrotic syndrome or IVC occlusion)
Urinary obstruction	Bladder outflow, or acute obstruction to single functioning kidney. Rarely bilaterally obstructing ureteric lesions – stones or extra-ureteric masses bilaterally
Urinary leak	Usually traumatic rupture, occasionally after instrumentation or surgery
Intrinsic anti-GBM disease	The most likely intrinsic renal disease causing abrupt anuria
Profound shock	In patients with underlying CKD
Obstruction	Bilateral obstruction or obstruction of single functioning kidney, surgical obstruction
Page kidney	Single functioning kidney
Urinary leak	e.g. Bladder rupture leaking transplant ureter

members. Genetic diagnoses also affect prospects for transplantation and live organ donation from family members. Therefore an accurate family history is a critical component of the renal history and can be swiftly recorded using standardised symbols (Fig. 1.3).

Table 1.12 summarises some of the most common diagnoses that could be associated with genetic renal disease, such that asking about the presence of these can form the basis of a screen for familial disease. Additionally, a family history of unexplained deaths, early death or infant death should be sought, as an indicator of undiagnosed genetic disease.

A pedigree (Fig. 1.2) is essential for accurately recording this information and helping to delineate possible inheritance patterns. If there is known renal disease in the family, then information from the renal unit of affected family members (with consent) can expedite the diagnosis and avoid unnecessary renal biopsy.

The majority of genetic renal diseases are likely to present to paediatric nephrologists with disease onset in childhood. However, patients with less severe disease may transition to adult clinics. Table 1.13a outlines genetic disease that present in infancy, while Table 1.13b highlights diseases that may present later, in adolescence or adulthood.

Table 1.9 Assessment of polyuria

Polyuria associated with thirst	
Increased urinary loss:	
Renal tubular disorders congenital	
Nephrogenic diabetes insipidus	Patients may give a history of extreme water craving [10]
Bartter's syndrome	
Medullary cystic kidney disease	Nephronophthisis, childhood thirst and polyuria
Renal tubular disorders acquired	
Recovery from AKI	
Medication	Lithium, diuretics, etc.
Acquired medullary pathology	Pyelonephritis, obstructive uropathy, sickle cell disease, analgesic nephropathy, light chains
Hypercalcaemia, hypokalaemia	
Osmotic diuresis	Glucose, mannitol, contrast
Endocrine causes	Cranial diabetes insipidus (history of trauma, pituitary or hypopituitary disease), Addison's disease, hyporeninaemic hypoaldosteronism
Without increased urinary loss:	Xerostoma (sicca syndrome) anticholinergic medication
Polyuria without thirst	
Psychogenic polydipsia	
Following fluid loading	Excessive drinking, IV fluids

Table 1.13c reveals the features found in mitochondrial cytopathies with renal involvement. Though rare, 5% of patients with primary mitochondrial disease have renal involvement. This can present as tubular disease, most commonly as Fanconi syndrome; glomerular disease, most often in the form of steroid-resistant nephrotic syndrome and focal segmental glomerulosclerosis; and, finally, interstitial disease, presenting as chronic kidney disease without proximal tubular dysfunction. Most cytopathies present in childhood mainly with myopathy; however, adults with cytopathy and renal disease do present with most having MELAS syndrome (mitochondrial encephalopathy with lactic acidosis and stroke-like episodes syndrome).

1

Table 1.10 Common multisystem disorders with renal involvement

Diabetes	**Diabetic nephropathy**
Atherosclerosis	Large vessel or small vessel renal involvement
Connective tissue disorders	Scleroderma renal crisis Interstitial disease: Sarcoidosis, treatment related (calcineurin inhibitors) Glomerulonephritis: systemic lupus erythematosus; systemic vasculitis, treatment related (gold penicillamine) AA amyloidosis: rheumatoid arthritis
Malignancy (primary or metastatic disease)	Obstruction, hypercalcaemia, tumour lysis syndrome, AL amyloid (paraproteinaemia) Direct infiltration Thrombotic microangiopathy Glomerulonephritis: membranous, breast, lung, GI; minimal change, lymphoma Treatment related
Infections	
Tuberculosis	Sterile pyuria, haematuria, cystitis, nephrolithiasis Interstitial disease Glomerular – MCGN type 2, focal proliferative, amyloid Treatment-associated nephropathy
Enterohaemorrhagic bacteria	Thrombotic microangiopathy
Other bacterial infections	Post-infectious glomerulonephritis
Schistosomiasis	Chronic cystitis, bladder fibrosis, malignancy, ureteric obstruction and vesicoureteric reflux Interstitial fibrosis Glomerulopathy
Blood-borne viruses e.g. Hepatitis B and C; HIV	Disease associated. Glomerular, thrombotic microangiopathy, cryoglobulin Treatment-related nephropathy
Chronic suppurative infection	AA amyloidosis
Gout	Urate nephropathy, uromodulin disorder
Chronic pain	Analgesia use – nephropathy/TIN
Chronic neurological disorder	Bladder dysfunction
Inflammatory bowel disease	Short bowel/ileostomy losses; treatment associated, oxalate nephropathy, AA amyloidosis
Hepatic failure	Hepato-renal syndrome
Ear, nose and throat disorders	Deafness – Alport's, Anderson-Fabry's Epistaxis – cocaine or systemic vasculitis
Pulmonary renal syndromes	Haemoptysis: systemic vasculitis, lupus, anti-GBM syndrome Asthmatic: eosinophilic granulomatosis with polyangiitis

Further information on renal involvement in mitochondrial cytopathies is available elsewhere [11].

1.4.3.5 Childhood History

Any evidence of childhood kidney or urological issues (congenital anomalies of the kidney and urinary tract, pyelonephritis, glomerular disease) even if renal function is normal is associated with a significant increased risk of developing ESRF in later life [12].

An antenatal history may also be important with evidence now highlighting the importance of the intra-uterine environment on consequent renal development and future risk of CKD. A baby born from a mother with medical, behavioural (e.g. smoking), social or environmental comorbidity is more likely to be have a low birth weight and consequently a smaller number of nephrons and be at higher risk for developmental programming of hypertension and renal disease [13].

1.4.3.6 Obstetric History

An abnormal obstetric history can suggest chronic underlying renal disease. Moreover, dipstick urinalysis and blood pressure measurement at booking (usually

■ **Table 1.11** Populations at increased risk of ESRD compared with native population and geography-prevalent nephropathy

UK	South Asian/Black populations have higher rates of diabetic nephropathy and hypertension Possibly chronic TIN in Asian population
USA	African Americans and Hispanics have high rates of diabetic nephropathy and hypertension Pima tribe has high rates of diabetic nephropathy Zuni Pueblo tribe has a broader susceptibility to CKD as well as diabetic nephropathy and glomerulonephritis
Australasia	Aborigines, Maoris and Pacific Islanders have increased rates of diabetic nephropathy and hypertension
Geographically prevalent nephropathy	
Danube river	Balkan nephropathy is chronic tubulointerstitial nephropathy affecting inhabitants in the region of the Danube river. A familial predisposition also exists. There is also a higher prevalence of renal tract tumours in this population
Tunisia and France	Ochratoxin associated with chronic interstitial nephritis
China and Indian subcontinent	Aristolochic acid causing 'Chinese herb nephropathy' Takayasu's arteritis, heavy metal intoxication
Black African and Africans in the Caribbean	Sickle cell nephropathy more prevalent in the geographic distribution of sickle cell disease. Systemic lupus erythematosus (SLE), focal segmental glomerulosclerosis
Africa and Indian subcontinent	Genitourinary tuberculosis in distribution of TB prevalence
Africa	*Schistosoma haematobium* – lower urinary tract disease and glomerulopathy
Africa and South/Central Asia	*Schistosomiasis mansoni* – glomerulopathy
Africa, particularly sub-Saharan Africa	HIV-associated nephropathy
Africa, Australasia and Indian Subcontinent	Post-streptococcal glomerulonephritis
Far East	IgA Nephropathy, SLE, hepatitis B-associated glomerulonephritis
Middle East	Nephrolithiasis
Sri Lanka	Tubulointerstitial disease
Central America	Tubulointerstitial disease
Italy	Hepatitis C-associated kidney disease
Cyprus	CFHR5 nephropathy, thin basement membrane nephropathy, familial Mediterranean fever

12 weeks) and throughout pregnancy may unveil both pregnancy-associated and pre-existing renal conditions. If the patient is not clear about the details, it is worthwhile pursuing via her family practitioner or obstetric unit.

The number of pregnancies, including miscarriages, stage of pregnancy reached and any reason for early delivery can be highly relevant as outlined in ■ Table 1.14.

1.4.3.7 Occupation

Occupation may be a factor in risk of developing some renal conditions (■ Table 1.15). Sometimes, the exposure is not immediately apparent, and a detailed history of both occupation and hobbies is important to avoid continued risk of deterioration.

1.4.3.8 Travel and Hobbies

In addition to considering the patient's geographical origins, a travel history should be completed. This is particularly important history in the context of AKI, and important questions are shown in ▶ Box 1.1. Relevant hobbies include water sports (leptospirosis), pets (hantavirus) and endurance sports (haematuria, rhabdomyolysis).

1

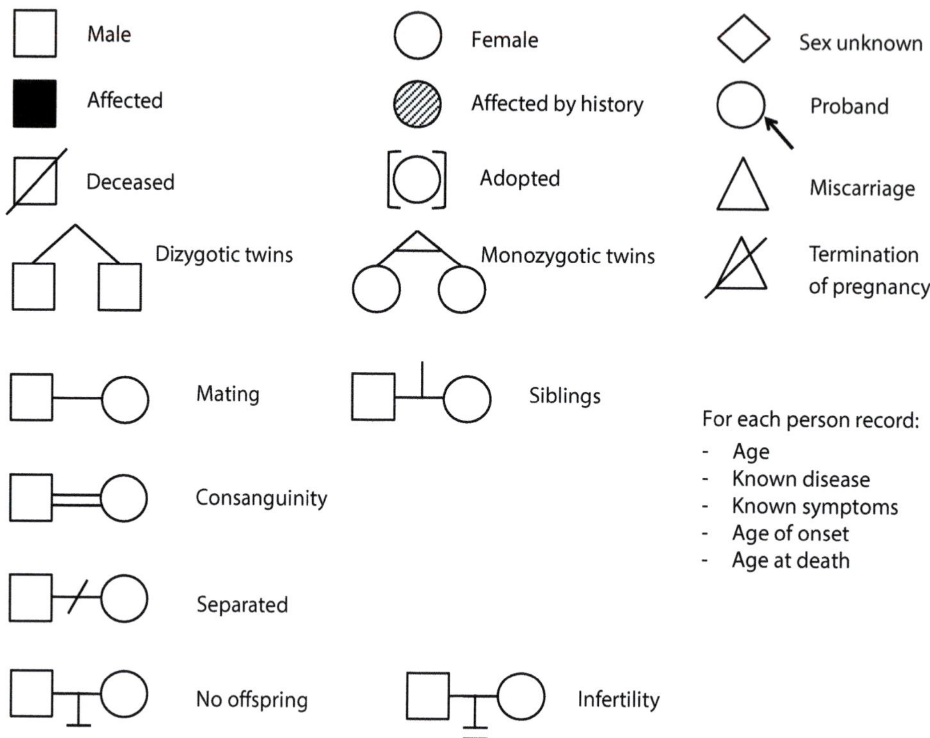

Fig. 1.3 Symbols used for documenting family history. This should be in the family history bit of the chapter see below

Table 1.12 Family history in renal disease

CKD or ESRD (dialysis or transplantation	Cause as identified by renal unit, age of onset or pattern of inheritance
Hypertension and diabetes	Polygenic influence, renal cysts and diabetes (RCAD) syndrome
Stones	Calcium nephrolithiasis
Reflux nephropathy	Dysplastic kidneys, posterior urethral valves (PUV) or any other congenital abnormality of the urogenital tract
Renal tumours	Age of onset, numbers, other malignancies, non-renal malignancies (including pheochromocytoma), epilepsy, learning disabilities, pneumothorax, fibroids, skin lesions – may indicate Von Hippel-Lindau disease (VHL), Birt-Hogg-Dube (BHD), Hereditary leiomyomatosis and renal cell cancer (HLRCC) or tuberous sclerosis complex (TSC)
Sub-arachnoid haemorrhage	May indicate PKD or need for screening if known PKD
Deafness	Female family members may have history of isolated haematuria suggesting X-linked Alport's, Fabry's, autosomal dominant history suggestive of branchio-oto-renal syndromes, MYH9 mutations, mitochondrial disorders, ciliopathies
Microscopic haematuria	X-linked or autosomal recessive Alport's syndrome; thin basement membrane nephropathy; CFHR5 nephropathy; HANAC syndrome; MYH9-associated nephropathies (Epstein/Fechtners syndromes)
Retinitis pigmentosa	Bardet-Biedl syndrome and other ciliopathies; m-mitochondrial disorders
Liver fibrosis and cysts	Autosomal recessive polycystic kidney disease
Heart disease	Fabry's disease; hereditary amyloidosis
Gout	Uromodulin-associated disease (MCKD2)

Table 1.13 Syndromes with renal involvement

Syndrome	Age of presentation/genetics	Renal involvement	Extra-renal manifestations
Syndromes usually lethal in childhood (13A)			
Beckwith-Wiedemann	Infancy Deregulation of imprinting gene expression (epigenetic)	Nephromegaly Structural abnormalities including duplications Cystic changes Nephrocalcinosis Medullary sponge kidney	Exomphalos Macroglossia Macrosomia Hemihyperplasia Anterior linear ear lobe creases Wilms tumour and hepatoblastoma
Branchio-oto-renal	Infancy AD	Renal aplasia and hypoplasia VUR Duplications	Cervical fistulas Ear pits Deafness
Cenani-Lenz syndrome	Infancy AR	Agenesis Hypodysplasia	Syndactyly Oligodactyly Facial dysmorphism
CHARGE syndrome	Infancy AD but many genes not discovered	Genesis Hypoplasia Duplex kidneys UPJO VUR	Coloboma of the eye Heart defects Atresia of the choanae retardation of growth and development Ear abnormalities and deafness
Denys-Drash	Infancy AD	Diffuse mesangial sclerosis Progressive nephrotic syndrome and ESRF	Male pseudohermaphroditism Wilms tumour
Fraser	Infancy AR	Agenesis Renal cystic dysplasia	Cryptophalmos Cutaneous syndactyly Genital malformation Craniofacial anomalies
HDR syndrome (Barakat)	Infancy to adulthood AD	Renal dysplasia	Hypoparathyroidism Sensorineural deafness
Jeune's syndrome	Infancy AR	Cystic kidneys	Skeletal dysplasia Polydactyly Small thorax Liver, pancreatic and retinal involvement
Kallman	Diagnosed after delay in puberty Multiple genes identified	Renal agenesis	Hypogonadotropic hypogonadism Anosmia Obesity
Noonan	Infancy AD	Pelviectasis in utero Ectopia and structural anomalies	Wide spaced eyes Short stature Pulmonary stenosis
MURCS	Females in infancy Unknown cause	Agenesis	Müllerian duct aplasia Cervicothoracic somite
Pallister-Hall	Infancy AD	Dysplasia	Hypothalamic hamartoma Polydactyly Bifid epiglottis Imperforate anus
Renal cysts and diabetes syndrome	Infancy AD	Enlarged kidneys Cysts Dysplasia Agenesis ESRF in childhood	Diabetes in adolescence Autism and schizophrenia Raised GGT

(continued)

1

Table 1.13 (continued)

Syndrome	Age of presentation/genetics	Renal involvement	Extra-renal manifestations
Simpson-Golabi-Behmel syndrome	Infancy X-linked	Duplicated collecting system VUR Large ureter UPJO	Overgrowth Craniofacial abnormalities Organomegaly
Schimke immuno-osseous dystrophy	Infancy AR	Progressive FSGS with nephrotic syndrome leading to ESRF	Shot stature Spondyloepiphyseal dysplasia T-cell deficiency
Townes-Brock	Infancy AD	Renal hypoplasia Renal agenesis Cystic changes VUR ESRF	Imperforate anus Polydactyly Ear abnormalities
Turner	Infancy – female Partial/complete loss of X chromosome	Collecting system malformations Horseshoe kidney	Short stature Ovarian insufficiency Neck webbing Widely spaced nipples Bicuspid aortic valve
Williams	Infancy Hemizygous microdeletion	Bladder diverticula Horseshoe kidney Renal aplasia Hypertension	Elfin facies Systemic arterial stenosis – supravalvular aortic stenosis Cocktail party personality Short stature Hypertension
WAGR	Infancy AD	Late-onset proteinuric nephropathy – link to FSGS	Wilms tumour Aniridia Genitourinary anomalies Mental retardation
Syndromes seen in adult nephrology (13B)			
Alagille syndrome	Majority prior to 6 months of age Autosomal dominant	Renal dysplasia	Chronic cholestasis Cardiac anomalies – pulmonary artery stenosis Butterfly vertebrae Posterior embryotoxon Dysmorphic facies
Alport's	Dependent on mutation, family history and sex X-linked, autosomal recessive (AR), autosomal dominant (AD) and digenic	Microscopic/macroscopic haematuria progressing to proteinuric end-stage renal failure (ESRF)	Sensorineural hearing loss Anterior lenticonus
Bardet-Biedl	Infancy AR	Tubular dysfunction – diabetes Insipidus/acidosis – polyuria Cysts formation and urogenital malformation Interstitial nephritis Glomerular scarring ESRF	Retinal dystrophy Hypogonadism Polydactyly Short statue Obesity
Down	Infancy Trisomy 21	Renal malformations Glomerulopathy	Up slanting palpebral fissures Epicanthic folds Brachycephaly Cognitive impairment Heart abnormalities

Table 1.13 (continued)

Syndrome	Age of presentation/genetics	Renal involvement	Extra-renal manifestations
Nail-Patella syndrome	Infancy AD	GBM dysmorphia – progressive proteinuria and microscopic haematuria – Chronic Kidney Disease (CKD)	Nail hypoplasia or dystrophy Absent patella Elbow abnormalities
Neurofibromatosis type 1	Variable AD	Renal artery stenosis and hypertension	Café-au-lait macules Axillary/inguinal freckling Lish nodules Neurofibromas
Prune belly	Infancy Unknown cause	Urinary tract abnormalities leading to vesicoureteral reflux (VUR), scarring and ESRF	Abdominal muscle deficiency Bilateral cryptorchidism
Renal coloboma	Variable age of onset from infancy to adulthood AD	Renal hypoplasia VUR Cystic dysplasia Focal segmental glomerulosclerosis (FSGS) ESRF	Optic nerve coloboma Optic nerve dysplasia Sensorineural hearing loss
VATER/VACTERL	Infancy Unknown cause	Agenesis Ureteropelvic Junction Obstruction (UPJO) VUR ESRF in early adulthood/late childhood	Vertebral anomalies Anorectal anomalies Ventricular septal defects and congenital heart disease Tracheoesophageal fistula Oesophageal atresia Limb defects
Von Hippel-Lindau	Variable presentation AD	Bilateral renal clear cell carcinomas potentially requiring bilateral nephrectomy	Benign and malignant tumours of the cerebellum, retina, adrenal gland, middle ear, pancreas and broad ligaments
Mitochondrial cytopathies with multisystem involvement (13C)			
Barth syndrome	X-linked	Renal hypoplasia Tubular dysfunction	Cardiomyopathy, mitochondrial myopathy and cyclic neutropenia
Coenzyme Q10 deficiency	AR	Glomerulopathy including FSGS/crescentic GN Proteinuria	Cerebellar ataxia Myopathy Encephalomyopathy
GRACILE	AR	Fanconi syndrome	Growth retardation, amino aciduria, cholestasis, iron overload, lactic acidosis and early death
Leber hereditary optic neuropathy	Maternal	Renal artery aneurysm CKD	Bilateral subacute optic neuropathy Extrapyramidal syndrome Intellectual disability Peripheral neuropathy
Leigh syndrome	X-linked, AR, maternal	Fanconi syndrome CKD	Subacute necrotising encephalomyelopathy
Maternally inherited deafness and diabetes	Maternal	FSGS	Sensorineural deafness Diabetes
			Retinal dystrophy Cardiomyopathy Gastric pathology Short stature

(continued)

1

Table 1.13 (continued)

Syndrome	Age of presentation/genetics	Renal involvement	Extra-renal manifestations
MELAS	Maternal	Proteinuria Nephrotic syndrome ESRF FSGS TIN	Lactic acidosis Stroke-like episodes Hearing loss Seizures Myopathy
NARP	Maternal	Proteinuria CKD to ESRF	Neuropathy, ataxia and retinitis pigmentosa Hearing loss Cardiac conduction defects
Pearson's syndrome	Maternal	Fanconi syndrome Renal cysts	Sideroblastic anaemia Neutropenia Thrombocytopenia Exocrine pancreatic dysfunction

Table 1.14 Obstetric history and renal disease

Multiple miscarriages	Suggestive of anti-cardiolipin antibody syndrome
Hypertension	Stage of pregnancy, severity and number of agents required to treat. Hypertension early in pregnancy, e.g. at booking is highly suggestive of a non-pregnancy-related cause
Proteinuria	Proteinuria (or haematuria) at booking or heavy proteinuria early in pregnancy or prolonged postpartum is very suggestive of underlying renal disease
Pre-eclampsia	Early (<20/40) pre-eclampsia is suggestive of underlying renal disease (20% have underlying CKD). An underlying renal cause is more likely if hypertension worsens in second pregnancy (with the same partner). A history of maternal jaundice suggests haemolysis, elevated liver enzymes and low platelet count (HELLP) or haemolytic uremic syndrome (HUS)
UTIs (lower or pyelonephritis)	Pyelonephritis is more common in pregnancy and may result in renal scarring
Obstetric sepsis/ severe haemorrhage	AKI following either may rarely result in cortical necrosis

Table 1.15 Occupations associated with renal diagnoses

Solvents	Glomerular and tubular pathology
Aniline dye	Urothelial tumours
Sewage workers	Leptospirosis
Outdoor workers in endemic areas	Hantavirus, leptospirosis
Old paint work/plumbing	Lead nephropathy
Occupations with restricted water access	Nephrolithiasis [14]
Metal workers	Heavy metal nephropathy [15]

Box 1.1 Key Travel Questions

- Details of travel, particularly in the previous 12 months
- Particular attention should be paid to the following:
  - Pre-travel vaccinations and malaria prophylaxis
  - Rural vs. urban destinations
  - Unwell contacts
  - Time period between return and onset of symptoms
  - Accommodation and food/drink exposures
  - Fresh water swimming
  - Animal contacts or bites: tick, animal, bird or bat bites and scratches
  - Occupation and hobbies – e.g. water sports or agricultural employment
  - Recent dental work, surgical procedures
  - Sexual history

1.4.3.9 Psychosocial History

There are several aspects of the psychosocial history relevant to the care of the renal patient. There remains a significant excess of CKD in those from socioeconomically disadvantaged groups as well as those with a his-

Table 1.16 Substance misuse

Smoking	Hastens the progression of renal disease associated with both diabetes and hypertension Increased microalbuminuria Increased likelihood of pulmonary haemorrhage in anti-GBM disease
Alcohol	IgA nephropathy in alcoholic liver cirrhosis, rhabdomyolysis Cirrhosis and hepatorenal syndrome
Solvent	Toluene in 'glue sniffing' has been associated with numerous tubular and glomerular lesions
Cocaine	Renal ischaemia, vasculitis or rhabdomyolysis
Heroin	FSGS
Intravenous drug injection	Blood borne viruses Infective endocarditis AA Amyloid
Ketamine	Inflammatory cystitis and obstructive uropathy
Ecstasy/MDMA	Increased risk of rhabdomyolysis
Anabolic steroids	FSGS
Synthetic cannabinoids ("spice")	AKI secondary to acute tubular necrosis and tubulointerstitial nephritis
3-fluorophenmetrazine	Renal ischaemia

tory of mental illness or substance misuse. Educational level, mental health issues, non-prescribed drug use and home circumstances can pose barriers to engagement with medical professionals and delay recognition of ill health, delay initial diagnosis, limit adherence and influence suitability for home therapies. Getting a clear understanding of a patient's psychosocial history is therefore fundamental to the delivery of full and effective care. In addition, there are certain abused substances that have associations with renal disease shown in Table 1.16.

1.4.3.10 Medication and Allergy

The kidneys are susceptible to a wide range of adverse effects from medications and their active metabolites. Different medications may cause toxicity in a variety of sites within the kidney. It is essential to obtain a history of (1) prescription and (2) non-prescription drugs, (3) recreational or illicit drugs and (4) herbal remedies. Ward prescription charts and in-patient procedural records such as anaesthetic charts, as well as redundant completed drug charts, should be reviewed to identify potential toxins in use at the onset of renal dysfunction. Accurately identifying a complete drug history may be time-consuming, but confirming prior use of aminoglycosides, exposure to a common cause of tubulointerstitial nephritis or that a patient is taking a product containing aristolochic acid may be critically important. Key elements of the drug history are shown in ▶ Box 1.2.

Box 1.2 Key Elements of Medication History

- Prescribed medication
  - Start and stop dates
  - Route of administration including preparations such as PR
  - Previous exposures on timeline
- Non-prescribed, over the counter or commercially purchased medication
  - Particularly analgesic and NSAID use which may not be volunteered
  - Include use of creams and gels with consideration to systemic absorption
- Drug interactions
  - Anticipated/dose adjustment/drug level monitoring
- Drug reactions
  - Fever, rash, arthralgia in suspected AIN
  - Defining accuracy of interaction with precipitating drug
  - Reversibility of effect
  - Concomitant administration of prophylaxis for side effects
  - Including IV contrast reaction
- Dietary supplements
  - Creatine-based sports supplements
  - Dieting supplements
  - Nutritional additives
  - Laxatives and diuretics
- Herbal preparations
  - Whenever possible, ascertain the origin, and obtain a sample for analysis since it may contain heavy metals or NSAIDS
  - Consider interactions with prescription medication, for example, via cytochrome P450
- Illicit drug abuse
  - Modality – frequency of needle use and sharing between individuals or participation in needle exchange
  - Route – intravenous or subcutaneous (increased risk of amyloid) associated with thrombophlebitis or cellulitis
  - Risk factors for infective endocarditis
  - Ketamine, cocaine, glue sniffing

1

Table 1.17 Examination tips and renal disease

Habitus	Obesity (OSA), Bardet-Biedl (renal cysts), short stature: Noonan syndrome (short and webbed neck, renal dysplasia), Turner's syndrome (short stature webbed neck, horse-shoe kidney), Down's syndrome (renal dysplasia), lipodystrophy (MPGN), limb abnormalities-VACTERL association. *Any form of CKD in childhood can result in short stature*
Hair	Scaring alopecia (SLE), diffuse alopecia heavy metal poisoning (tacrolimus, steroids), hirsutism (cyclosporine)
Ears	Otitis, inflammation of the pinna with GPA, pre-auricular pit, sensorineural deafness BOR syndrome, Alport's, Anderson-Fabry's, CHARGE syndrome (ear abnormalities)
Nose	Crusting, nasal bridge collapse (GPA) cocaine
Mouth	Dentition (infective endocarditis (IE)), mouth ulcers (vasculitis, SLE, herpes viral infections and fungal infections), macroglossia (useful sign of amyloid)
Polydactyly	Bardet-Biedl
Nails	Periungal fibromas (TSC), dysplastic nails (nail patella syndrome), splinter haemorrhages (IE), Muehrcke's bands (episodes of nephrotic syndrome)
Skin	*Signs of renal disease:* vasculitic rashes, palpable purpura (HSP), palpable subcutaneous nodules/ulcers (PAN), malar flush (SLE), cutaneous lupus erythematosus, alopecia (SLE, tacrolimus), neurofibroma, viral exanthem, erythema nodosum, tracheostomy scar (previous ICU admission), xanthelasma, nicotine stains (atherosclerotic disease); Janeway lesions (endocarditis); bruising (amyloid), livedo reticularis (cholesterol emboli, SLE, anti-cardiolipin syndrome), angiokeratoma (AFD), Raynaud's (SLE, scleroderma, anti-cardiolipin syndrome), facial angiofibromas, ash-leaf macule and shagreen patch (TSC) *Signs of immunosuppression:* purpura, thin skin, gum hypertrophy (cyclosporine), sebaceous gland hyperplasia, actinic keratosis, Kaposi's sarcoma, squamous cell carcinoma, basal cell carcinoma, hypertrichosis (cyclosporine), Cushingoid features and striae (steroids) *Signs of advanced CKD:* Xerosis, acquired perforating dermatosis, porphyria cutanea tarda, calciphylaxis
Eyes	Retinopathy (hypertensive, diabetic); Retinitis pigmentosa/dysplasia (Bardet-Biedl, senior Loken syndrome-nephronophthisis, Jeune's syndrome, Kearns-Sayres mitochondrial cytopathy); uveitis (tubulointerstitial nephritis with uveitis); uveitis, band keratopathy, sicca (Sjogren's syndrome); corneal clouding (cystinosis); lenticonus (Anderson-Fabry's disease, Alport's); proptosis (GPA, IgG-4-related disease); angiomatosis retinae (VHL); coloboma (renal coloboma syndrome CHARGE and COACH syndromes), periorbital bruising (amyloid), iritis, scleritis, retinal vasculitis (vasculitis), drusen (dense deposit disease)
Lymphoproliferative	Lymphadenopathy (tuberculosis, lymphoma); splenomegaly (IE, sarcoid, lymphoproliferative disorder)
CVS	Atrial fibrillation (Emboli), pericardial rub (SLE, infections, uraemic pericarditis), murmur/pacing wire (endocarditis), radiofemoral delay/missing pulses (aortic coarctation/mid-aortic syndrome Takayasu's arteritis); bruits (renovascular disease, fibromuscular dysplasia), ventricular failure (right or left sided)
Chest	Pneumothorax (tuberosclerosis); pleural rub (SLE, vasculitis, infection); asthma (eosinophilic granulomatosis with polyangiitis); pulmonary fibrosis (systemic vasculitis, scleroderma, SLE, Sjogren's, drugs); signs of bronchiectasis (amyloid)
Abdominal	Signs of chronic liver disease (hepato-renal syndrome, viral hepatitis); stoma (high output), absent abdominal musculature (prune belly syndrome)
Neurological	Asterixis/tremor (uremic encephalopathy, calcineurin inhibitor toxicity); hemiparesis (bladder dysfunction, infection-associated amyloid), spina bifida (occulta)
Musculoskeletal	Polyarthropathy (rheumatoid arthritis, SLE, ankylosing spondylitis), monoarthritis (hyperuricaemia), infection including IE, Charcot joint, absent patellae (nail patella syndrome)

1.4.4 Aspects of the Clinical Examination to Help Establish the Cause of a Renal Disorder

A thorough clinical examination is an essential part of the approach to any patient presenting either acutely or to the outpatient department. Accurate fluid assessment will be critical to most presentations to the renal physician and is discussed in detail above. Alongside intravascular volume assessment, other findings on clinical examination can provide an important clue to the aetiology of a renal presentation. These examination findings are summarised in Table 1.17.

1.5 Assessment of the Patient with Known Renal Disease

Many renal conditions are chronic, and it is common to encounter patients who have previously been investigated or treated either locally or in another centre. When a patient is known to suffer from a renal disorder, the aim of the assessment will be usually focused on the management of the underlying condition or associated complications. Those in contact with renal services frequently have complex histories, and the importance of handling the transfers of care, particularly, but not exclusively when transitioning from child to adult services cannot be over-stated (see ▶ Chap. 69). Fortunately, patients are increasingly involved in their own care and have a good understanding of their disease and access to their clinical records. When they do not, it is important to make the effort to trace historical imaging and blood and urine results. In all patients known to have renal disease, the nature and duration of the condition, as well as histological details if available, are an essential starting point of any assessment. Patients with known renal disease will broadly fall into the following groups allowing the clinician to focus their clinical assessment.

1.5.1 Patients with ESKD Treated with Dialysis

Patients with ESKD may have been receiving renal replacement therapy for many years and have been treated with several treatment modalities. Renal physicians will often be integral to the holistic care of patients on dialysis programmes. Therefore, alongside dialysis-related issues, the renal specialist increasingly needs at least a basic understanding of a broad range of medical, surgical and psychiatric problems so that appropriate further expertise can be sought when necessary. When thinking about dialysis-related problems, presentations will commonly be related to dialysis access (including infection) and intradialytic issues (instability, adequacy or complications). Important considerations for the assessment of the patient on dialysis are outlined in ◘ Table 1.18.

◘ **Table 1.18** Clinical assessment specific to the dialysis patient

Underlying cause of ESRF	
Duration of ESRF and different treatment modalities	
Most recent dialysis session and intradialytic problems	Date/duration of last session, problems with treatment, loss of circuit
Dialysis access	Date of formation/insertion, signs of infection, adequate function, position (temporary HD catheters or PD catheters)
PD catheter	
Temporary vascular access for HD	
AVF or AV grafts	
Fluid status	
Dialysis adequacy	URR or KT/V, serum potassium, residual native kidney function, ultrafiltration volumes, intradialytic weight gains (HD), constipation (PD)
Blood pressure control	Anti-hypertensive medication, sodium intake, intradialytic hypotension
Traditional cardiovascular risk factors	Smoking, dyslipidaemia and treatment
Complications of CKD and treatment	Anaemia, bone-mineral disorder
Transplant listing status	May impact on decisions regarding transfusion
Nutritional status	Changes in 'dry weight', may indicate chronic infection or malignancy

1.5.2 Patients with ESKD with Functioning Kidney Transplants

Patients with kidney transplants will often present to their 'home' transplant unit with a transplant related issues and problems not immediately associated with function of the transplant. The management of graft dysfunction will represent a substantial workload for any transplant unit, and again assessment of intravascular volume status is a critical element in the assessment. In addition, the management of immunosuppression-related complications such as infection and malignancy will need attention in transplant patients. ◘ Table 1.19 outlines aspects of clinical assessment important in the patient with a functioning renal allograft.

1.5.3 Patients with ESKD on Conservative Care Programmes

Increasingly, renal units run large and successful conservative care programs. One of the reasons patients may have decided that they do not wish to receive active care for ESKD is to reduce time spent in a medical environment. Although these patients may have decided not to

Table 1.19 Clinical assessment specific to the transplant patient

Underlying cause of ESKD	
Duration of ESKD and different treatment modalities	
Previous transplantation	Date, duration, reason for graft loss
Current transplant	
Donor details	Age, donor type, donor comorbidity/COD
Immunological details	Overall sensitisation (%CRF, donor-specific and non-specific antibodies), mismatch, cross-match details, post-transplant donor-specific antibodies
Surgical details	Cold and warm ischaemic times, arterial and venous anatomy, ureteric anastomosis
Post-operative course	Delayed graft function, infection, rejection, thrombosis, obstruction (stent removal)
Allograft biopsies	Tubular injury, rejection, recurrence if primary disease, degree of fibrosis
Immunosuppressive treatment	Induction, maintenance, treatment for rejection, steroid withdrawal, drug levels
Infection risk and prophylaxis	Donor and recipient viral immunity, prophylaxis, infection history, BK virus
Recent allograft imaging	Ultrasound, MRA/angiography, nuclear medicine
Baseline function	Look out for slow declines over many months
Fluid status	
Evidence of infection	Urine, chest, GI, neurological, atypical organisms
Evidence of malignancy	Weight loss, breast/cervical screening
Blood pressure control	Anti-hypertensive medication, sodium intake
CV risk	Smoking, dyslipidaemia (post-transplant), diabetes
Osteoporosis	Fractures, prophylaxis
Complications of CKD and treatment	Anaemia, bone-mineral disorder

undergo dialysis or transplantation, assessment and prompt management of fluid status, anaemia, bone-mineral disorders, nausea and pain can have a significant impact on quality of life and should be pursued as a priority.

When patients are clearly close to death, the renal physician may need to play an active part in ensuring that the appropriate end-of-life care can be most effective and in the appropriate environment.

1.5.4 Patients with CKD and Significantly Reduced GFRs

Some form of chronic kidney disease is thought to affect between 5% and 10% of the population in Western countries. Nephrologists will often be asked to help manage this group of patients who often have multiple comorbidities. The increasing recognition of the increased risk of AKI in those with CKD as well as the contribution of AKI to the future progression of CKD means that a key focus of the assessment of this group of patients surrounds the management, and prevention, of a further decline in kidney function. The approach to this clinical situation should be similar to that set out in the section on establishing the cause of previously undiagnosed renal impairment.

Patients with CKD also commonly present with fluid overload, and the nephrologist will often be asked for advice. In this group of patients, particular attention should also be paid to appropriate dosing regimens of medications for the patients' GFR. Failure to dose-reduce certain drugs can lead to significant adverse renal and non-renal effects (see ▶ Chap. 56). The management of patients with stable CKD also needs to address the complications of decreased renal function, specifically anaemia, bone mineral disorder and cardiovascular risk, and, at lower GFRs, decision-making around ESKD.

1.5.5 Patients with Inflammatory Renal Diseases or Requiring Immunosuppression

Patients suffering from systemic vasculitis, SLE, nephrotic syndrome or other inflammatory renal conditions will often be taking immunosuppressive drugs. In addition to the issues related to CKD or dialysis, the possibility of disease relapse and the consequences of immunosuppression need to be considered when these patients present to renal services. An approach to this group of patients is outlined in Table 1.20.

1.6 Summary and Conclusion

Patients attending renal specialists present enormous clinical heterogeneity. An approach to the review of patients using a system similar to the one outlined above allows for comprehensive and readily presentable summary of the background and current problems. However, it is only by focusing the assessment on answering the relevant questions at hand that clinical problems will be appropriately prioritised and timely and safe treatment instigated. The critical importance of accurate assessment of intravascular volume status cannot be overemphasised, and this is a skill that can only be learned with repeated practice. Although as experience is gained each clinician will develop their own unique approach to clinical assessment, it is only with a systematic approach that renal physicians will be confident of providing safe, efficient and high-quality care to their patients.

Cases (2–4) Illustrating important points

Table 1.20 Clinical assessment specific to the patient with inflammatory renal disease

Underlying diagnosis	
Duration of disease, relapses, multi-system involvement	
Baseline kidney function	
Renal biopsies	Active disease, chronic fibrosis
Immunosuppressive treatment	Induction, maintenance, steroid withdrawal, drug levels
Evidence of relapse	Extra-renal symptoms and signs
Fluid status	
Infection risk and prophylaxis	Infection history, viral immunity, prophylaxis
Evidence of infection	Urine, chest, GI, neurological, atypical organisms
Evidence of malignancy	Weight loss, breast/cervical screening
Blood pressure control	Anti-hypertensive medication, sodium intake
CV risk	Smoking, statins, diabetes
Osteoporosis	Fractures, prophylaxis
Complications of CKD and treatment	Anaemia, bone-mineral disorder

Case Study

Case 1

A 52-year-old man was referred by the intensive care team on the point of haemofiltration. He was admitted 1 week before with sepsis secondary to biliary obstruction from a common bile duct stone for which he underwent ERCP with stone removal and stenting. Piperacillin-tazobactam was prescribed for *Enterobacter* bacteraemia. His creatinine 6 months earlier was 82 micromole/L but on admission was 300 micromole/L, rising further to 450 micromole/L. The rest of his blood tests are as listed: sodium 160 mmol/L, urea 39 mmol/L, potassium 5.0 mmol/L, haemoglobin 10.0 g/dL, white cell count 15,000 per mcL and C-reactive protein 80 mg/L.

On clinical examination, his blood pressure was 110/80 supported with a low dose of noradrenaline; heart rate was 80 and regular. Respiratory rate was 18, with SaO_2 99% on room air and afebrile. The patient was drowsy but easily rousable and orientated to time, place and person. His peripheries were cool. There was no oedema, and cardiac, respiratory and abdominal examinations were normal. Urine output 20–40 mls/hour and dark.

Upon straight leg raising, there was a 20/10 mmHg increase in his BP as measured by his invasive arterial measurement.

His AKI was felt to have a significant pre-renal component still, and he was given closely monitored fluid challenges followed by IV maintenance fluids and NG water. Within 1 day, the patient's AKI and hypernatremia significantly improved.

This case illustrates the importance of an accurate fluid balance – whenever a patient is being given inotropes and being haemofiltered, the first question you should ask yourself is if the patient is in fact hypovolaemic.

1

Case 2

A 42-year-old man is referred by the stroke unit with a left-sided middle cerebral artery (MCA) infarct leaving him with a right-sided hemiparesis. His renal function on admission was noted to be abnormal with a creatinine of 140 micromole/L (eGFR of 40 mL/min). There was +2 protein and +1 blood. Of note his admission venous blood gas revealed a lactate of 3.8.

On direct questioning, he gave a history of muscle weakness and pain as a child but never sought medical help. His clinical exam was notable for a generalised myopathy, a right-sided hemiparesis and hypertension 178/101. The rest of his blood tests were unremarkable.

A provisional diagnosis of MELAS syndrome was made and subsequently a renal biopsy showing focal segmental glomerulosclerosis. His genetics revealed a MT-TL1 transfer RNA mutation. He subsequently had a live donor transplant 5 years later due to progressive chronic kidney disease. His siblings also undergo genetic screening with appropriate follow-up and counselling.

This case illustrates the importance of a good clinical history, wherever possible, starting with an antenatal history. In this case a CVA in a relatively young person, unexplained renal impairment and lactate make the history of long-standing muscle weakness critical to directing further assessment towards a mitochondrial cytopathy.

Tips and Tricks

(clinical pearls, anything about diagnosis or management that you feel is important to pass on and the sorts of gem you would pass on to your registrars to improve patient are):

1. The passive leg raise is an effective tool for assessing fluid responsiveness.
2. A patient still may have functional obstructive nephropathy even in the presence of normal imaging on ultrasound – when the index of suspicion is high, request functional imaging or cross-sectional imaging of the urinary system followed by formal endoscopic investigation of the urinary tract.
3. Beware of opiates as being a cause of fluid unresponsive hypotension in patients with AKI, or AKI on CKD taking opiate-based pain killers at home.

? Chapter Review Questions

1. The following are causes for chronic kidney disease with preserved renal size except:
   (a) HIV nephropathy
   (b) Diabetic nephropathy
   (c) Polycystic kidney disease
   (d) Chronic glomerulonephritis
   (e) Renal amyloidosis

2. Which of the following is a known intrinsic renal cause of acute anuria?
   (a) Anti-glomerular basement membrane disease
   (b) Membranoproliferative glomerulonephritis
   (c) Cryoglobulinemia
   (d) AL amyloidosis
   (e) Fabry's disease

3. Hearing loss is associated with the following renal disease except:
   (a) Renal coloboma syndrome
   (b) Bartter syndrome
   (c) Bardet-Biedl syndrome
   (d) Fabry disease
   (e) Prune belly syndrome

4. Retinal abnormalities are found in the following renal disease expect:
   (a) CHARGE syndrome
   (b) Turner syndrome
   (c) Alport syndrome
   (d) Membranoproliferative glomerulonephritis type II
   (e) Cystinosis

5. Please mark true or false for the following statements:
   (a) Cocaine users with renal disease are often found to AA amyloid deposition on kidney biopsy.
   (b) Smoking is one of the few protective risk factors for relapse of anti-glomerular basement membrane disease.
   (c) Tachycardia is a non-specific marker of intravascular volume depletion and may be associated with excessive intravascular volume in the context of heart failure.
   (d) Aniline dye exposure puts one at an increased risk of focal segmental glomerulosclerosis.
   (e) Balkan nephropathy is characterised by the formation of multiple renal cysts.

Answers

1. (d) Chronic glomerulonephritis is a cause of bilaterally small kidneys
2. (a) Whilest most causes of intrinsic nephropathy can present sub-acutely, anti-GBM disease can render a patient anuric with alarming rapidity and requires a high index of suspicion to make a timely diagnosis.
3. (e) Prune belly syndrome is triad of partial or complete absence of the abdominal muscles, failure of both testes to descend into the scrotum (bilateral cryptorchidism), and/or urinary tract malformations
4. (b) Turners syndrome does not classically affect the eye. CHARGE syndrome is characterised by coloboma. Alport and MPGN type II patients often have retinal drusen. Cystinosis is characterised by refractile cysteine crystals deposited in the retina.
5. (a) False: – cocaine users can suffer from renal ischaemia, vasculitis or rhabdomyolysis., (b) False: – smoking increases the chances of relapse from anti-GBM disease., (c) True., (d) False: – aniline dye exposure increases the chance of developing urothelial malignancy., (e) False: – Balkan nephropathy is associated with a chronic tubulointerstitial nephritis.

References

1. Marik PE, Cavallazzi R, Vasu T, Hirani A. Dynamic changes in arterial waveform derived variables and fluid responsiveness in mechanically ventilated patients: a systematic review of the literature*. Crit Care Med. 2009;37:2642–7.
2. Cannesson M, Besnard C, Durand PG, Bohé J, Jacques D. Relation between respiratory variations in pulse oximetry plethysmographic waveform amplitude and arterial pulse pressure in ventilated patients. Crit Care. 2005;9:R562–8.
3. Monnet X, Teboul J-L. Passive leg raising: five rules, not a drop of fluid! Crit Care. 2015;19:18.
4. Dipti A, Soucy Z, Surana A, Chandra S. Role of inferior vena cava diameter in assessment of volume status: a meta-analysis. Am J Emerg Med. 2012;30:1414–1419.e1.
5. Feissel M, Michard F, Faller J-P, Teboul J-L. The respiratory variation in inferior vena cava diameter as a guide to fluid therapy. Intensive Care Med. 2004;30:1834–7.
6. Muller L, et al. Respiratory variations of inferior vena cava diameter to predict fluid responsiveness in spontaneously breathing patients with acute circulatory failure: need for a cautious use. Crit Care. 2012;16:R188.
7. Olde Rikkert MG, Deurenberg P, Jansen RW, van't Hof MA, Hoefnagels WH. Validation of multi-frequency bioelectrical impedance analysis in detecting changes in fluid balance of geriatric patients. J Am Geriatr Soc. 1997;45:1345–51.
8. Kumar S, Khosravi M, Massart A, Davenport A. Is there a role for N-terminal probrain-type natriuretic peptide in determining volume status in haemodialysis patients? Nephron Clin Pract. 2012;122:33–7.
9. Moghazi S, et al. Correlation of renal histopathology with sonographic findings. Kidney Int. 2005;67:1515–20.
10. van Lieburg AF, et al. Clinical phenotype of nephrogenic diabetes insipidus in females heterozygous for a vasopressin type 2 receptor mutation. Hum Genet. 1995;96:70–8.
11. Emma F, Salviati L. Mitochondrial cytopathies and the kidney. Nephrol Ther. 2017;13:S23–8.
12. Calderon-Margalit R, et al. History of childhood kidney disease and risk of adult end-stage renal disease. N Engl J Med. 2018;378:428–38.
13. Luyckx V, Nephrology, B. B.-N. R. & 2015, undefined. Birth weight, malnutrition and kidney-associated outcomes—a global concern. nature.com.
14. Goldfarb DS. The exposome for kidney stones. Urolithiasis. 2016;44:3–7.
15. Johri N, Jacquillet G, Unwin R. Heavy metal poisoning: the effects of cadmium on the kidney. Biometals. 2010;23:783–92.

Urine Analysis

Scott R. Henderson and Mark Harber

Contents

M. Harber (ed.), *Primer on Nephrology*, https://doi.org/10.1007/978-3-030-76419-7_2

2

Learning Objectives

1. Urine analysis is cheap, allows early detection of renal disease and is great for teaching.
2. Microscopic examination of urine can be diagnostic sometimes make a rapid diagnosis or exclude others. It may also be used as a biopsy surrogate and guide treatment in patients with ongoing disease.
3. Investigation of haematuria needs a joint approach with urologists.

2.1 Introduction

Formation of urine allows a cheap, non-invasive and novel insight into the pathological processes affecting the kidneys and urinary tract and has been shown to be an essential tool to the practising nephrologist [1–4] and very nicely covered by Fogazzi and colleagues [5]. Urinalysis has evolved from *the art of uroscopy*, practised in medieval times [6], to detailed chemical analysis and microscopy, allowing early detection and differentiation of renal disease. There is significant global variation in practice regarding the emphasis placed on urine analysis, and occasionally missed opportunities for non-invasive diagnosis or as an aid to management. Thus, for trainees, a sound knowledge of and finger-tip access to simple analysis of urine is an important part of the clinical and diagnostic skill set.

2.2 Sample Collection

At the outset, it is important to optimise sample collection: poorly procured samples have little value and may result in inappropriate management (see ► Box 2.1 for guidance on sample collection). It is also important to ensure that samples are delivered without delay for processing; microscopy or cytology samples dispatched at the end of the day and left overnight are likely to be useless and waste lab resources. As a guideline, samples for cytology should ideally reach the laboratory within 2 hours, whereas samples for culture may be refrigerated, if required, for 24 hours at 4 °C. It is therefore worth ensuring that a system is in place for prompt sample delivery and that nursing staff routinely educate patients on how to reliably provide 'clean-catch' midstream urine (MSU) samples.

A variety of clean catch systems are commercially available to reduce contamination although to date, there is very limited evidence of benefit. For those patients unable to co-operate, and in whom urine analysis is important, then alternatives include 'in-out' catheterisation or suprapubic aspiration (common in paediatrics), both of which may be contaminated by erythrocytes, but worth considering when urine analysis is critical.

Indwelling catheter specimens are invariably contaminated by blood and low-level proteinuria. Ileal conduits, urostomies and indwelling catheters are also very frequently (*universally*) colonised with bacteria, and there is little point routinely obtaining samples in the asymptomatic patient except to exclude gross proteinuria or for analysis of electrolytes.

Box 2.1 Health Protection Agency Standard Method of MSU Sample Collection in Men and Women

- Midstream sample of urine is always preferential
- Quality of urine sample determines accuracy of analysis
- Clear instructions should be provided prior to voiding to avoid contamination
- *Males: retract foreskin and clean glans*
- *Females: clean labia and urethral meatus*
- Place container midstream in the flow of urine
- Analysis should be performed as soon as possible to avoid decomposition of cellular elements
- As a general rule, samples should be exposed to minimal light and not be stored at room temperature for longer than 2 hours
- First morning urine provides a concentrated urine sample most likely to contain clinically important elements

Quick link

► http://www.hpa-standardmethods.org.uk/documents/bsop/pdf/bsop41.pdf

2.3 Urine Dipstick

Prior to any testing of a urine sample, physical appearance should be assessed, particularly colour, odour and turbidity as certain circumstances result in specific appearances, as outlined in ◘ Table 2.1. This is a golden, or other colour, opportunity to make a clever diagnosis and impress colleagues. An example is 'purple urine bag syndrome' as shown in ◘ Fig. 2.1 where the production of indoxyl sulphate by certain bacteria (*E. coli, Klebsiella pneumonia* and *Proteus mirabilis*) results in a purple discolouration. There are many other examples where the diagnosis can be made rapidly on the basis of colour such as acute porphyria (darkens to black on standing), dark urine of pigment nephropathies, chyluria (white) (◘ Fig. 2.2), phenol poisoning and alkaptonuria (black/dark). Normal urine is clear when analysed in a transparent container against a white background, and colour ranges from light yellow to dark amber depend-

Table 2.1 Physical characteristics of urine [4, 5]

Colour	Yellow/brown – hyperbilirubinaemia, chloroquine, nitrofurantoin Orange – rifampacin, senna Red/brown – blood, myoglobin, phenytoin, beetroot (anthocyanins), blackberries, rhubarb, chronic lead or mercury poisoning Pink – propofol (especially in alcoholics) Blue – methylene blue, *Pseudomonas* infection, indicanuria Green – propofol, amitriptyline, indomethacin, Phenergan White/milky – chyluria Purple – reaction of bacterial indoxyl sulphate with urine bag Black – ochronosis, porphyria (on standing, pink under UV light), melanomatosis, copper poisoning, chloroquine, primaquine, metronidazole, phenol poisoning, alkaptonuria, tyrosinosis Causes of urine darkening on standing – alkaptonuria, typically when left exposed to open air caused by oxidation and polymerisation of excess homogentisic acid, enhanced with alkaline pH
Odour	Offensive – consider bacterial infection 'Maple syrup' – Maple syrup urine disease Acetone – Diabetic ketoacidosis 'Sweaty feet' – Isovaleric acidaemia
Turbidity	'Cloudy' – high concentration of either leucocytes, erythrocytes, epithelial cells, bacteria or crystals. Consider genital tract contamination (females); white cloudy can occur with phosphaturia (disappears with acetic acid) 'Milky' – lipid-rich material (chyluria); consider abnormal connection between lymphatic and urinary systems (Fig. 2.2) 'Gas' – termed pneumaturia, an important symptom that occurs in the presence of colovesical fistula or emphysematous pyelonephritis 'Frothy' indicative of nephrotic range proteinuria

ing on the amount of urochromes present and solute concentration.

Urine dipstick abnormalities are widely prevalent in both community and hospital practice and is most often the first clue to the presence of renal disease. Careful interpretation of dipstick abnormalities is therefore important and should guide further appropriate investigations and specialist referral. Sample collection is an undervalued yet essential component of urinary examination and should be performed by standard methods as outlined in ► Box 2.1.

A variety of dipstick testing kits are available, but standard combination strips routinely include five or seven of the following tests: *protein*, *blood*, *glucose*, *ketones*, *pH*, *bilirubin* and *urobilinogen*. Other characteristics detected on urine dipstick are *specific gravity* and

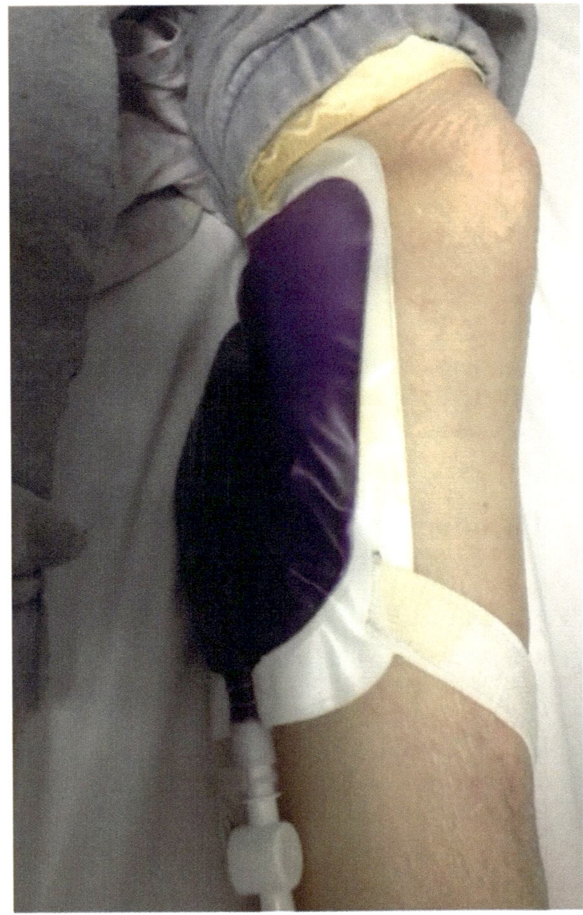

Fig. 2.1 Purple urinary bag syndrome. (Courtesy of Stephen B Walsh)

the presence of *leucocytes* and *nitrites*. Table 2.2 outlines common abnormalities, possible causes and important false-positive situations to consider. Specific urine dipstick tests are also available in specialist practice with the most widely available tests including Micral-Test II® or Microbumintest® (microalbuminuria), Ictotest® (bilirubin), Acetest® (ketones) and Clinistix® (glycosuria only).

An important angle here is the potential for patient involvement; it is very helpful for patients with recurrent nephrotic syndrome or recurrent UTI or those with the need to produce dilute urine (e.g. stone formers) to have access to the appropriate dipstick. This can facilitate early diagnosis or permit virtual review and is an underutilised aspect of urine dipstick.

2

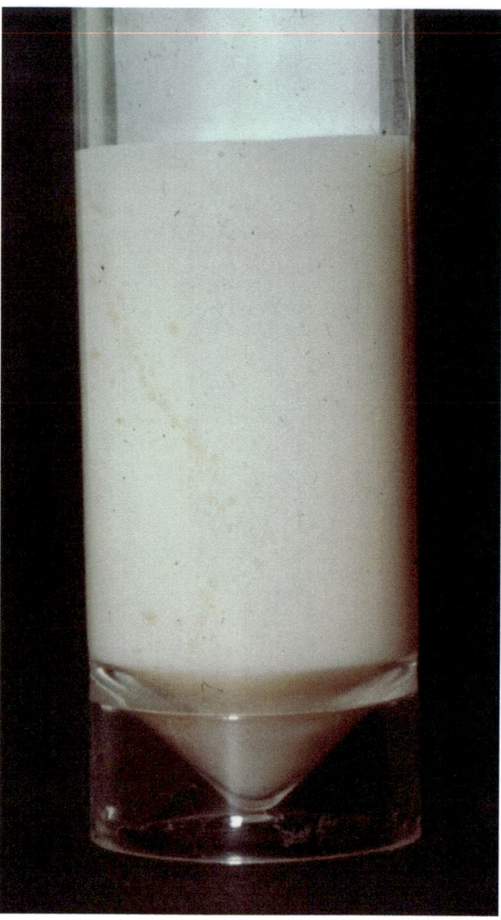

Fig. 2.2 Milky white urine pathognomonic of chyluria

2.4 Urine Microscopy

> Urine...... can provide us day by day, month by month and year by year with a serial story of the major events going on within the kidney.
> Thomas Addis (1948) [3]

Urine microscopy performed by a nephrologist is a cheap, non-invasive and educational test that, in the right setting, can substantially aid the diagnosis of kidney disease [7]. Interestingly, there is a huge variation in practice among nephrologists around the world, some countries retaining an obsessional devotion to urine microscopy, whilst many nephrology practices have long abandoned it as a diagnostic or teaching tool. We aim to persuade nephrologists that in selected patients, it can be extremely helpful. If setting up urine microscopy, before investing in resources, it is worth approaching local laboratories for used centrifuges and microscopes. The requirements are:

1. A centrifuge capable of taking 10 ml samples at 1500 rpm
2. Centrifuge tubes
3. Disposable pipettes
4. Microscope slides
5. Cover slips
6. Microscope (with phase contrast)
7. Appropriate bench space (usually dirty utility room)
8. Individual with responsibility for maintaining equipment

(Draconian penalties for leaving the microscope on or in a mess – optional)

Suitably preparing urine for microscopy is essential to obtaining informative results. A midstream sample should be obtained by the method outlined (▶ Box 2.1) and at least 10 ml urine collected and analysed *within 2 hours*. ▶ Box 2.2 shows how to prepare a urine sample for light microscopy and Table 2.3, technical information on analysing the urine sediment.

The urine sediment may contain a vast number of cellular elements. This section is not an exhaustive atlas, but rather a summary of the important components which should be recognised on examination in association with the relevant clinical syndromes, helping guide the practising nephrologist in the pursuit of diagnosis.

Box 2.2 Preparation of Urine for Microscopy

- Collect 10 ml midstream urine sample in sterile universal container
- Centrifuge 10 ml at 1500 rpm
- Discard supernatant (9.5 ml)
- Re-suspend 500 μl sediment using *Pasteur* pipette
- Transfer 50 μl of urinary sediment to slide
- Apply coverslip (24 × 32 mm)

2.4.1 Isolated Haematuria

Haematuria on dipstick should *always* be confirmed by microscopy to exclude false-positive (pigment nephropathy, hypochlorite solutions, oxidising agents, bacterial peroxidase) and false-negative results (vitamin C, gentisic acid).

New patients over 40 years of age (or younger for those with risk factors for urinary tract malignancy, e.g. previous cyclosphosphamide or aristolic acid exposure) with proven micro- or macroscopic haematuria should be screened for urinary tract malignancy or another cause of lower urinary tract bleeding. There is a strong argument for an integrated uro-nephrology approach to haematuria in this group of patients (Fig. 2.3). Perhaps the most patient-orientated approach is a *haematuria one-stop-shop* where patients are seen and assessed by urologists with urine microscopy, renal blood tests, same day ultrasound of kidneys and bladder and cystoscopy when appropriate. Those deemed not to

Table 2.2 Urinary dipstick abnormalities (*for haematuria and proteinuria see below*)

Specific gravity Normal range 1.002–1.035 NB. Varies according to urine concentration	Polyuria associated with low SG <1.010 Low with polydipsia (psychogenic, beer drinking) and diabetes insipidus Tends to be fixed (c.1.010) in acute tubular injury or CKD High levels (≥1.035) seen in shock and dehydration (appropriately concentrated) Artificially high with glycosuria, proteinuria and following IV contrast *Useful cheap measure of fluid intake for patients with recurrent UTI or stone disease if renal function normal*
pH Normal range 5–8, Western diet pH = ~6	Low pH in acidosis and high protein diet and promotes uric acid and cysteine stone formation High pH in (1) renal tubular acidosis (inappropriately alkaline urine (>5.5) in the face of acidosis) (pH <5.4 excludes distal RTA), (2) low protein/vegetarian diet and (3) urinary tract infection, particularly from urease-producing organisms such as *Proteus mirabilis.* High pH promotes calcium-phosphate deposition
Glucose In normal homeostasis, glucose is not present in urine	Freely filtered at glomerulus, but almost completely reabsorbed at the proximal tubule Causes of glycosuria Pregnancy (normal physiological response) Hyperglycaemia (diabetes mellitus) Impaired proximal tubular reabsorption in isolation (SGLT2 defect)
Ketones In normal homeostasis, ketones are not present in the urine	Ketones are produced following increased metabolism of fat. Ketone bodies (acetoacetic acid, acetone and 3-hydroxybutyrate *not detected*) are freely filtered in the glomerulus Causes of ketonuria Type 1 diabetes mellitus (diabetic ketoacidosis) Starvation states (prolonged fasting, anorexia nervosa)
Bilirubin Urobilinogen gives urine its 'normal' physical appearance	Bilirubin is normally conjugated and excreted into the gastrointestinal tract as a water-soluble molecule. Small bowel bacterial metabolism converts bilirubin to urobilinogen which is then re-absorbed at the distal small bowel lumen and partially excreted in the urine *Positive bilirubin dipstick test* – suggests failure of hepatic conjugation of bilirubin preventing excretion and conversion of urobilinogen *Negative urobilinogen dipstick test* – indicates failure of hepatic excretion of conjugated bilirubin (biliary obstruction)
Nitrites In health, nitrites are excreted in variable amounts, although are undetectable in the majority	Most bacteria convert nitrates to nitrites during growth and replication. Positive nitrite test is suggestive of infection, but a negative test is not exclusive. A minimum time period is required for bacterial transformation Bacteria that do not reduce nitrate compounds include: *Enterococcus* *Pseudomonas* species *Streptococcus faecalis* *Staphylococcus albus* *Neisseria gonorrhoea*
Leucocytes The presence of leucocytes in the urine suggests inflammation or infection *NB may be absent in neutropenia*	Urine dipstick detects the enzymatic reduction of a synthetic ester substrate by urinary neutrophil esterase to a blue derivative in the presence of air Leucocyte esterase reaction has a reported better sensitivity than nitrite testing for the diagnosis of urinary tract infection, but false negatives can occur in the presence of tetracyclines, cephalosporins, glucose, albumin and ketones

have a urological cause for haematuria can then be assessed by a nephrologist in reserved slots on the same day. This takes a bit of organising, but the dividends for the patient and the clinician are obvious in terms of providing an efficient and joined-up approach.

Lower urinary tract bleeding is indicated by erythrocytes (RBC) with essentially normal and homogeneous morphology. In haematuria due to glomerular disease, RBC presumably become distorted as they pass through the glomerular basement membrane and down the tubule resulting in heterogeneous and dysmorphic shapes including acanthocytes, best seen with phase contrast microscopy (Fig. 2.4). A large quantity of dysmorphic red blood cells is suggestive of an aggressive glomerular lesion, whereas scanty dysmorphic RBC are more indicative of a sub-acute GN. The presence of a red blood cell cast (Fig. 2.5) is highly suggestive of an aggressive glomerulonephritis, and to paraphrase the old adage, *one RBC cast makes a Summer*. As this is one of the most important and specific findings in urine microscopy, it is extremely helpful to train the nephrolo-

2

Table 2.3 Technical aspects of urine microscopy

Microscope	Indications
Phase contrast	*Allows best identification of cellular elements, less need for special stains*
Light	*Poor visualisation of contents with low refractive index*
Polarised light	*Positive birefringence allows detection of crystalluria*
Stains	
Wright's	*Lymphocytes*
Papanicolaou's	*'Decoy cells' pathognomic of Bk viruria*
May-Grünwald-Giemsa Hansel's	*Eosinophils*
Prussian blue	*Haemosiderin*

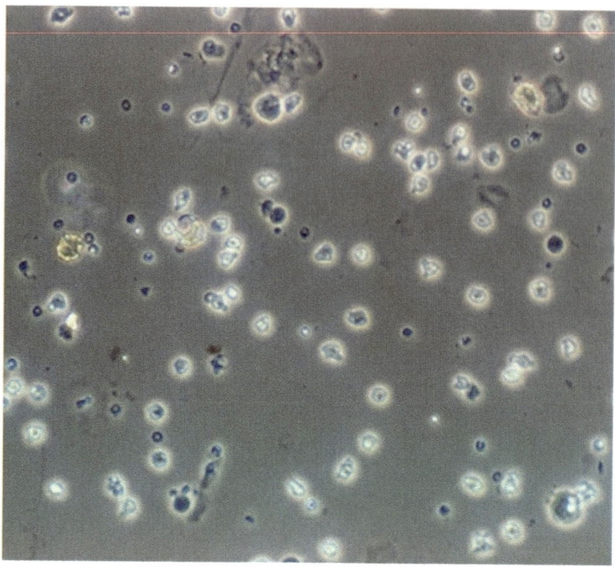

Fig. 2.4 Dysmorphic erythrocytes under polarised light at low power. Red cells showing multiple blebs and extrusions

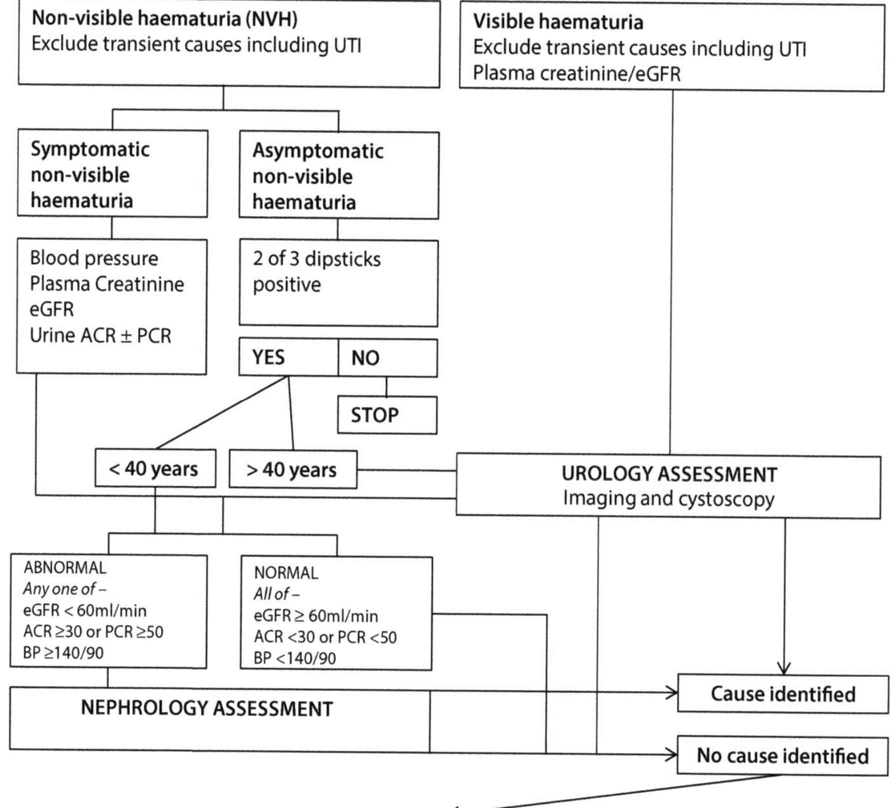

Fig. 2.3 Decision algorithm for the investigation and referral of haematuria. (Adapted from the UK Renal Association Clinical Guidelines [8])

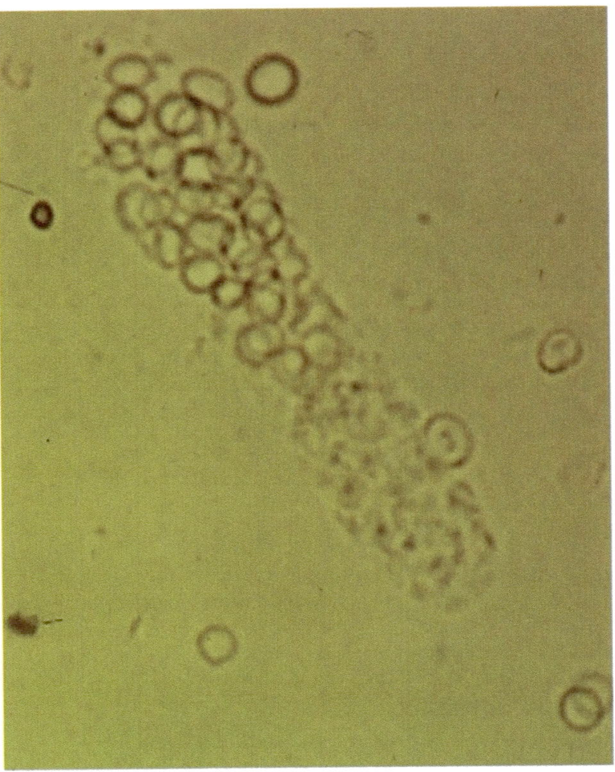

Fig. 2.5 Red cell cast highly suggestive of an active glomerulonephritis

Table 2.4 Semi-quantitative correlation of dipstick proteinuria

	Protein concentration (mg/dL)	Estimated daily protein excretion (g/day)
Trace	5–20	
1+	30	<0.5
2+	100	0.5–1
3+	300	1–2

gist's eye with the urine of patients known to have acute renal vasculitis/lupus.

2.4.2 Isolated Proteinuria

The detection of protein on urine dipstick is affected by (i) concentration (consider specific gravity), (ii) macroscopic haematuria and (iii) urine pH >8.0. Urine dipstick testing does however provide a semi-quantitative measurement of proteinuria as outlined in Table 2.4, but whilst dipstick reagent testing is sensitive to albumin, it has low sensitivity to other proteins, such as tubular proteins and light chain immunoglobulins. Proteinuria should therefore be confirmed by additional testing, and for the vast majority of patients, a random urine protein/creatinine ratio (uPCR) or urine albumin/creatinine ratio (uACR) (monitoring of choice in early diabetic nephropathy) is sufficient for diagnosis and monitoring. Urine ACR and PCR have a non-linear relationship, but it can be helpful to multiple uPCR by 10 to roughly estimate 24-hour protein excretion. Table 2.5 shows correlation between uACR and uPCR as well as estimate of 24-hour protein excretion. Table 2.6 outlines different types of proteinuria with important clinical considerations.

Table 2.5 uACR and uPCR values and relationship with 24-hour protein excretion

uACR	uPCR	g/24 hours	Description
3–30		<0.3	Microalbuminuria
30	50	0.5	Overt proteinuria
70	100	1	
300	350	3.5	Nephrotic range

Although largely superseded by simpler tests, occasionally, 24-hour collections may be helpful for the assessment of proteinuria particularly if combined with other diagnostic tests such as 24-hour sodium, urine volume, creatinine clearance and Bence-Jones proteinuria. It is noteworthy that the value of such tests is diminished if incomplete collection is performed. For 24-hour collections, patients should be given clear guidance and a pre-labelled large volume container and instructed to empty their bladder first thing in the morning (ideally, a non-working day with no heavy exercise) and then collect all urine until the following morning including finishing with an empty bladder on rising.

2.5 Clinical Significance of Urine Diagnostic Tests

2.5.1 Acute Kidney Injury

Urine analysis is absolutely critical in guiding the diagnosis and initial management of patients with AKI, and although the clinical picture is often complex, there are several scenarios when urine analysis can substantially guide or cleverly make the diagnosis [1–5]. It is important that your referring wards and emergency departments try, where possible, to obtain a fresh urine prior to

2

Table 2.6 Types of proteinuria with important clinical considerations

Glomerular proteinuria Predominantly albumin and an early, important indicator of glomerular injury. Standard dipsticks sensitive	*Physiological* – ACR <30 mg/24 hours (but raised acutely if febrile; see below) *Microalbuminuria* – ACR >30–300 mg/24 hours (not detectable with standard dipstick) *Overt proteinuria* – ACR >PCR *Nephrotic range proteinuria* – ACR> PCR>
Tubular proteinuria Suspect with low-level proteinuria especially if uPCR out of proportion to dipstick/uACR, or accompanied by other features of tubular injury/inflammation such as sterile pyuria, or features of Fanconi syndrome	Rarely greater than 100 mg/mmol or 1 g/L Indicated by normal ACR but raised PCR Specific tests for tubular proteins include retinol-binding protein (RBP), α-1 Microglobulin and N-acetyl β glucosamine (NAG) Causes include drug toxicity (e.g. cisplatinum, tenofovir, etc.), causes of acquired tubulointerstitial nephritis, heavy metal poisoning and Dent's disease
Overflow proteinuria	Overproduction of proteins, most commonly light chains Not detected by standard urine dipsticks Negative or low-level dipstick with disproportionate urine PCR may suggest overflow or tubular proteinuria
Benign proteinuria	'Physiological': febrile proteinuria, post-exercise proteinuria Orthostatic proteinuria: Isolated low-level proteinuria, often in young males, possibly associated with 'nutcracker kidney' (arterial compression of renal veins occasionally with loin pain). Proteinuria is absent on rising sample, present after being ambulant so easily diagnosed with paired rising and ambulant uPCRs

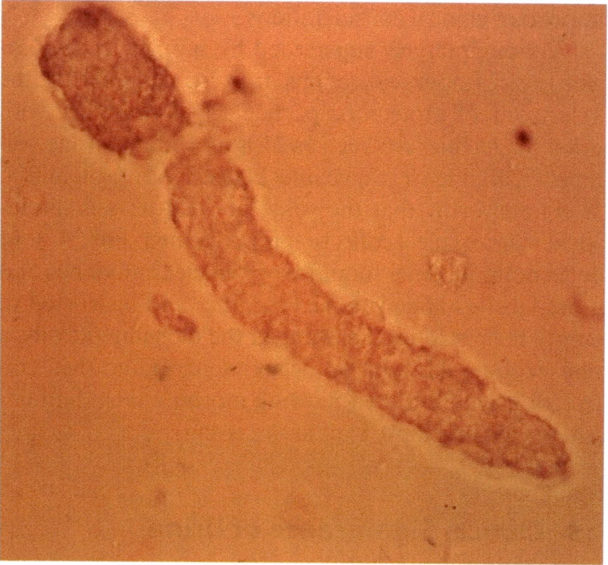

Fig. 2.6 Granular cast

catheterisation (and reliably record residual urine volume on catheterisation).

1. *Acute Tubular Injury*: The majority of AKI is secondary to hypoperfusion-induced acute tubular injury, and in the absence of an intrinsic renal disease, the urine is likely to have minimal haematuria or proteinuria, and urine microscopy therefore reveals large numbers of renal epithelial cells, granular casts (not specific) (Fig. 2.6) and limited numbers of erythrocytes with no red cell casts. Urine festooned with tubular cells is highly suggestive of acute tubular injury, but more often it is the exclusion of an active glomerular lesion that is critical.
2. *Pigment Nephropathy*: This is a great opportunity to make a rapid diagnosis in that myoglobinuria and haemoglobinuria both result in a dark urine and positive Hemastix test, but microscopy will show an absence of RBC. Thus +++ haematuria but no RBC on microscopy is highly suggestive of a pigment nephropathy. If sent rapidly enough, rhabdomyolysis may be confirmed by the presence of myoglobin in the urine, but this is evanescent. Although not strictly urine analysis, intravascular haemolysis can then be cunningly distinguished from rhabdomyolysis by spinning the patient's blood and demonstrating pink serum. Myoglobin and haemoglobin can stain granular and epithelial casts orange/brown, and this can be a late useful clue.
3. *Rapidly Progressive Glomerulonephritis (RPGN)*: The presence of a classical *active urine*, i.e. significant blood and protein on urine dipstick and dysmorphic RBC in large numbers (and ideally a RBC cast), is an extremely helpful contributory evidence for RPGN. Similarly, the absence of any dysmorphic RBC may be very reassuring in a complex patient with AKI.
4. *Acute Interstitial Nephritis (AIN)*: There are no truly discriminatory findings in the urine of patients with AIN, but patients often have low-to-moderate levels of haematuria/proteinuria but can occur with nei-

ther, emphasising the importance of urine microscopy for white blood cells, large amounts of either blood or protein tending to make the diagnosis less likely (e.g. urine PCR >200). Classically AIN is associated with a sterile pyuria, but this finding is neither particularly specific nor sensitive (**visible on Giemsa staining*). Of note, simultaneous measurement of urinary albumin and protein to creatinine ratio allows determination of urinary albumin to total protein ratio, and it has been shown that a measurement of <0.40 is highly sensitive and specific for the diagnosis of AIN [9].

5. *Crystal Nephropathy*: The rhomboid shapes of uric acid crystals in otherwise 'quiet' urine may be indicative of tumour lysis syndrome. Bipyramidal crystals of calcium oxalate may be extensive in acute oxalosis secondary to ethylene glycol ingestion or hyperoxaluria of any cause, although can occur in normal urine. Occasionally, it may be possible to heroically make the diagnosis of drug-induced crystal nephropathy relating to aciclovir, anti-retroviral therapy or antibiotics, such as ciprofloxacin and amoxicillin.

There is a delay in serum creatinine elevation and diagnosis of AKI highlighting the need for better biomarkers of AKI, and there are several under investigation. Neutrophil gelatinase-associated lipocalin (NGAL) is produced by epithelial tissues and undergoes glomerular filtration and tubular reabsorption whilst being produced by distal tubular cells in the setting of ischaemia. Early detection of urinary NGAL is therefore a sensitive and specific marker of ATN, but there is a need to consider increased expression by other epithelial tissues offering confounding factors in some clinical settings. Cystatin C is a cellular protease inhibitor released at a constant rate into the plasma and is freely filtered and reabsorbed by proximal tubular cells. Acute kidney injury therefore causes a rise in urinary cystatin C 12–24 hours after insult. Retinal-binding protein (RBP) follows the same processing and is detectable approximately 12 hours after onset of AKI. In contrast, kidney injury molecule-1 (KIM-1) is produced by proximal tubular cells in response to injury and can be measured in the urine, again detectable 12–24 hours after injury. It should be noted that despite much hope and huge investment, few new urinary biomarkers have yet to demonstrate a clinical benefit and to make it into clinical practice.

In summary, whilst many cases of AKI result from multiple insults, sometimes, careful assessment of the urine can cheaply and non-invasively hone the differential diagnosis significantly or reassuringly exclude some important disease groups.

2.5.2 Chronic Kidney Disease (CKD)

The kidney loses the ability to substantially regulate urine concentration (beyond 1.010) or control pH in CKD. The concentration of creatinine in the urine tends to remain stable with worsening renal function as GFR falls but plasma creatinine rises. Low levels of proteinuria are very common in CKD but substantial proteinuria (3+), especially if combined with haematuria, suggests a primary glomerular lesion. Microscopy of urine in CKD is usually dominated by signs of progressive tubular damage including tubular cell casts, waxy casts, coarse granular casts and leucocytes.

2.5.3 Is There Any Value in Urine Analysis in Suspected CKD?

The role of urine analysis in chronically damaged kidneys is rather more limited than in AKI. However, when faced with a new patient who has marked renal impairment, it is critical to distinguish between AKI and CKD. This is often resolved by detailed clinical history, historical creatinine results or renal ultrasound; however, urine microscopy demonstrating granular and tubular cell casts with an *absence* of acute cellular casts, dysmorphic red cells or features of an 'active urine deposit' may be helpful confirmatory evidence of CKD and exclusion of a rapidly progressive glomerulonephritis or urinary tract infection.

A significant proportion of patients with ESRF have no definite renal diagnosis, and occasionally thoughtful urine analysis in CKD can narrow down the differential diagnosis and sometimes achieve a diagnostic coup and is worth considering in new patients, for example:

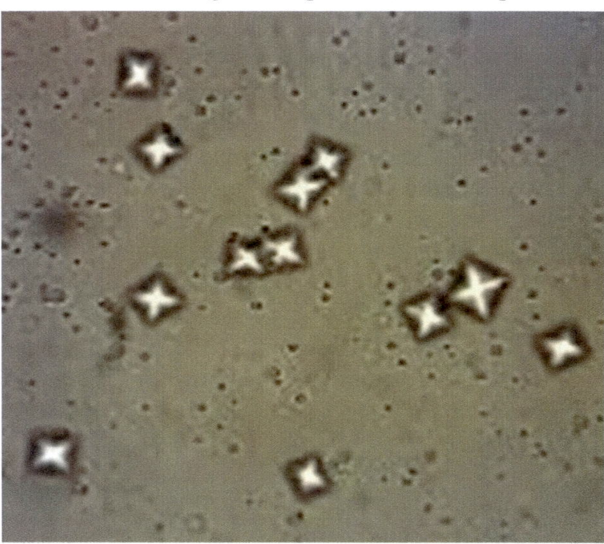

Fig. 2.7 'Maltese cross' crystals on polarised light

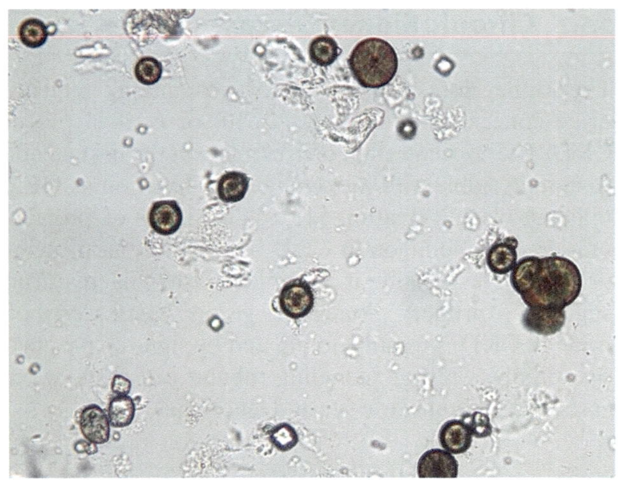

Fig. 2.8 2, 8-Dihydroxyadenine crystals

- The identification of 'Maltese cross' on polarised light microscopy (Fig. 2.7) in a patient with CKD and low-level proteinuria is highly suggestive of Anderson-Fabry's disease but can occur in any heavily nephrotic state. In Anderson-Fabry's disease, these represent myelin bodies free within the urine or within hyaline casts and can be definitively distinguished by electron microscopy.
- Extremely broad *hyaline casts* are said to be indicative of medullary cystic disease or reflux nephropathy and may be helpful in early CKD but can occur in any advanced CKD.
- The oval or bipyramidal crystals of *calcium oxalate* may indicate either acute or chronic hyperoxalaemia although oxalate crystals are a fairly non-specific finding.
- Hexagonal crystals of *cysteine* are always pathological and thus indicate cystinosis if not already identified or isolated cystinuria as a cause of stones.
- *2,8-Dihydroxyadenine crystals* (Fig. 2.8) are indicative of the rare adenine phosphoribosyl-transferase deficiency – an important diagnosis to make in terms of treatment and risk of recurrence [10].
- Urine microscopy (of early morning sample) is a cheap and widely used method for diagnosis of *schistosoma haematobium* in endemic areas and may give the diagnosis in CKD secondary to obstructive uropathy.
- In the setting of CKD, significant blood and glomerular range proteinuria is suggestive of a *sub-acute glomerular disorder* (such as IgA or Alport's syndrome).

2.5.4 Tubular Disorders

The causes of tubular and interstitial disease are numerous, but there are less pathognomic signs on urine microscopy than that found in the context of glomerular injury. Nevertheless, the presence of isolated mild proteinuria should always raise the possibility of a tubular disorder and may be supported by the detection of granular or 'waxy' casts on urine microscopy. In addition, the diagnosis of tubular clinical syndromes is often heralded by urinary abnormalities. Tubular syndromes result from abnormal handling of waste products, electrolytes and hydrogen ions and bicarbonate compounds without a necessary change in GFR.

1. *Renal tubular acidosis* either may be associated with a consistently elevated urine pH (distal RTA, type 4) or may be variable (proximal RTA, type 1) according to changes in bicarbonate reabsorption.
2. *Fanconi syndrome* is associated with reduced urine pH, but rather than an isolated bicarbonate reabsorption defect being present, additional proximal tubular function is impaired. Characteristic urinary abnormalities are phosphaturia, glycosuria (normoglycaemia), uricosuria and aminoaciduria. These abnormalities may be found in association with 'tubular' proteinuria.
3. *Tubular proteinuria* is a term used interchangeably with low-molecular-weight proteinuria and usually implies chronic proximal tubular dysfunction with the abnormal presence of β2-microglobuin, α-microglobulin, retinol-binding protein and Clara cell protein within the urine. Tubular proteinuria is rarely more than 1 g/L and may be indicated by minimal protein on dipstick (detecting albumin) or normal ACR with a raised PCR.
4. *Acute and chronic tubulointerstitial nephritis* as mentioned above tend to be associated with low levels (<1.5 g/L) of proteinuria (PCR ≫ ACR), pyuria (more common in AIN than chronic TIN), occasional eosinophiluria (nice to see but very low sensitivity and uncertain specificity) and sometimes microscopic haematuria.

2.6 Urine Cytology

The utility of urine cytology is variable according to the cellularity and cell content of urine specimens. Samples can be contaminated by degenerative changes, microbes, haematuria or other artefacts. There remains an absence of evidence-based practice and so a lack of consensus clinical guidelines. Nevertheless, the presence of some abnormalities can quickly guide diagnosis and help in the management of certain clinical conditions.

2.6.1 Viruses

Decoy cells in kidney transplant recipients with Bk polyoma viral infection can be detected by urine

Table 2.7 Considerations in the diagnosis of a significant/clinically relevant UTI

	Features suggestive of UTI	Features against clinically relevant UTI
Appearance	Cloudy/turbid/offensive	Clear urine in asymptomatic patient
Urine dipstick	*Leucocyte esterase* positive (sensitive and very specific for pyuria) *Nitrites* (helpful if present but low sensitivity) *Low-level proteinuria/haematuria* (sometimes macroscopic), particularly if not previously present	Negative *leucocyte esterase* and *nitrite* dipstick has a strong negative predictive value (caveats above)
Microscopy	*White cell casts* (rare but important finding as very strong evidence of pyelonephritis) *Pyuria* (for other causes of sterile pyuria, see ► Box 2.3) *Bacteriuria* (if present on high-power field in clean catch, unspun urine, correlates with 10^5 or more bacteria/ml). Two clean catch specimens in asymptomatic woman with 10^5 or more bacteria/ml represents a 95% probability of true bacteriuria	Absence of pyuria (NB pyuria may be absent in neutropenic patients)
Culture	Pure growth of single organism with $>10^5$ cfu/ml	Bacteriuria in the absence of pyuria and/or multiple squamous cells contaminating sample Mixed growth of organisms (bona fide in 5% of UTIs)

microscopy and further confirmed by Simian vacuolating virus 40 immunostaining. Other viral infections show typical cytological features. CMV infection is associated with large basophilic intra-nuclear inclusions surrounded by a halo and margination of chromatin, whilst multinucleated cells with occasional eosinophilic intra-nuclear inclusions can be seen in *herpes virus infection.*

2.6.2 Malignancy

Anaplastic cells in the urine have a high degree of sensitivity and specific for high-grade urothelial cell carcinomas, but increased cellularity and urothelial clusters may be the only finding in low-grade disease. Urine cytology is important in identifying urothelial carcinoma in situ that can sometimes be missed on cystoscopic examination. High nuclear to cytoplasmic ratio with prominent nucleoli points the pathologist in this direction. Clusters of atypical cells are the main finding in transitional cell carcinoma, and cytology helps in tumour grading. Squamous cell carcinoma is rare, but malignant cells have a dense cytoplasm and are orangeophilic. Sheets of uniform glandular cells can be seen in patients with prostate adenocarcinoma. Renal carcinoma cells are rarely shed into the urine.

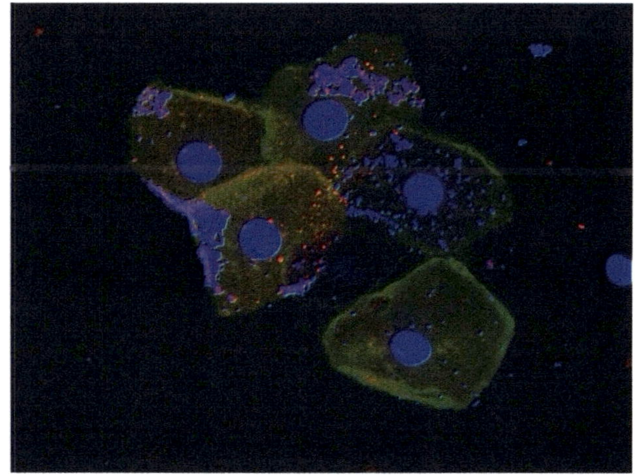

Fig. 2.9 'Clue cells' uroepithelial cells, stained with uroplakin (green) and demonstrating multiple intracellular bacteria. (Courtesy of Jennifer Rohn and Sanchutha Sathiananthamoorthy)

2.7 Urinary Tract Infection (UTI)

The initial appearance of cloudy, offensive urine (especially in a symptomatic patient) may convincingly make a rapid diagnosis of UTI. It is often helpful to see urine at presentation, and it is important to get fresh samples to the laboratory swiftly for culture in order to confirm the diagnosis and guide antimicrobial chemotherapy. Urine analysis findings both in favour and against of a significant/clinically relevant UTI in a MSU specimen are shown in ◘ Table 2.7. Sterile pyuria has to be considered in the differential diagnosis prior to confirmation of bacterial culture as hallmark 'non-specific' features on initial urine analysis may also be explained by the causes of sterile pyuria as outlined in ▶ Box 2.3. Pyelonephritis might be detectable by the presence of white cell casts. More common than this is the presence of 'clue cells' (see ◘ Fig. 2.9), uroepithelial cells infected with uropathogenic bacteria. These can be seen with phase contrast microscopy and are indicative of lower tract infection (often sub-acute).

Considerable thought also needs to be applied to the interpretation of urine from patients with indwelling catheters, ileal conduits and urostomies in that these frequently demonstrate all the features of a urinary tract infection, a result of chronic colonisation, and these samples frequently do not represent clinically relevant UTI.

Box 2.3 Causes of Sterile Pyuria

- Urinary tract infection during or immediately post antibiotics
- Children with pyrexia of non-urinary tract origin
- Urinary tract infection with fastidious organism
- Symptomatic patient but no bacteria:
  - *Neisseria gonorrhoeae, Chlamydia trachomatis*
  - *Mycoplasma genitalium*
- Asymptomatic tuberculosis, fungal infections
- Interstitial nephritis
- Chronic prostatitis
- Papillary necrosis
- Radiation or chemical cystitis
- Renal stones
- Solvent abuse

2.8 Urinary Electrolytes

Measurement of urinary electrolytes and osmolality is often performed in clinical practice in an attempt to guide diagnosis. However, interpretation is complex, compounded by the intricate mechanisms regulating solute excretion and osmolality. It is useful to remember

◘ **Table 2.8** Guide to interpretation of urine electrolytes

	Urinary abnormalities	**Considerations**
Acute kidney injury		
'Pre-renal' volume-deplete AKI Acute tubular necrosis (ATN) Contrast nephropathy Pigment nephropathy Interstitial nephritis	UNa^+ <20 mmol/l, UOsm ↑, FE_{Na}^+ < 1%, FE_{urea} <35% UNa^+ >20 mmol/l, UOsm ↔, FE_{Na}^+ > 3%, FE_{urea} <35% *(Hepatorenal syndrome = UNa^+ < 20 mmolll, FE_{urea} ↓)* FE_{Na}^+ typically <1% *(Also seen in cardiac failure)* Usually 'salt-wasting' state - UNa^+ >20 mmol/l, FE_{Na}^+ > 3%	Abnormalities in urinary electrolytes in AKI reflect disease/damage to renal tubules with concentrating ability usually preserved in 'pre-renal' volume deplete AKI UNa^+ in post-obstructive uropathy is *not* reliable despite volume depletion In any post-operative patient, vasopressin release alters urine concentration ability
Chronic kidney disease		
Crystal nephropathy Renal stone disease Nephrocalcinosis Fanconi syndrome	24-hour urine collection most useful. Need to measure – Volume, calcium (acid preservative), phosphate, oxalate (acid preservative), uric acid (alkaline preservative), sodium, citrate, creatinine (ensure adequate collection), pH In addition, random urine sample to measure Amino acids, β2-microglobulin, glucose Phosphaturia, glycosuria (normoglycaemia), uricosuria and aminoaciduria	Risk factors for calcium stone formation Hypercalciuria, hypocitraturia, hyperoxaluria, hyperuricosuria, RTA *(see also ▶ Chap. 55)*

UNa^+ urine sodium, *UOsm* urine osmolality, *FE_{Na}^+* fractional excretion of sodium, *FE_{Urea}* fractional excretion of urea

$$FE_{Na}{}^+ = \frac{\text{Urine Na}^+ \times \text{Plasma Creatinine}}{\text{Plasma Na}^+ \times \text{Urine Creatinine}} \times 100$$

$$FE_{Na}{}^+ = \frac{\text{Urine Urea} \times \text{Plasma Creatinine}}{\text{Plasma Urea} \times \text{Urine Creatinine}} \times 100$$

that urinary electrolytes and osmolalities do not have fixed 'normal' values but rather parameters, based on the clinical setting.

From a practical perspective, testing is now routinely performed on a 'random' 10 ml clean-catch MSU sample, although certain circumstances require a 24-hour collection. Common indications and clinical scenarios when testing of urinary electrolytes and osmolality is appropriate are outlined in ◘ Table 2.8. However, the physiological principles underpinning water and solute

Case Study

Case 1

A 34-year-old woman under the care of rheumatology with SLE and mixed connective tissue disorder presented with acute kidney injury (stage 2) and hypertension. Urine dipstick testing confirmed the presence of 2+ blood and 2+ protein on a Friday evening. The rheumatology team felt that her presentation represented a flare of SLE with renal involvement and recommended high-dose IV steroids. Urine microscopy, however, demonstrated no evidence of an active glomerulonephritis (no casts and minimal RBCs that were not dysmorphic). On the basis of this, steroids were withheld, and a subsequent renal biopsy demonstrated histology consistent with scleroderma renal crisis. High-dose steroids are not without risk and in this case may well have exacerbated the patient's scleroderma renal crisis. Urine microscopy can sometimes be very effective at ruling in or out an active glomerulonephritis in the context of AKI.

Case 2

A 44-year-old man presented to A&E after collapsing during a half marathon. He had developed bilateral leg pain. He had no significant past medical history and was not taking any regular medications. He was tachycardic but normotensive. There was no neurovascular deficit in either legs, but both calves were very tender on examination. Serum creatinine measured 363 umol/l on arrival with a lactic acidosis. The patient was oliguric. Creatine kinase measured 72,800 U/L. Renal ultrasound scan was normal. Urine analysis showed 3+ blood and 1+ protein. After aggressive fluid resuscitation, renal function improved, and creatine kinase level fell. The use of urine dipstick testing in the case highlights that the detection of blood in urine testing may be a result of myoglobinuria. Myoglobin is freely filtered at the glomerulus and produces a characteristic red-brown urine discolouration. Dipstick is positive for blood, and orthotolidine test is also positive. However, myoglobin has a short half-life, and so pigmenturia may be missed.

Case 3

A 36-year-old man presented to A&E following a deliberate suicide attempt. Regular medications included an antidepressant. He was hypertensive on presentation and displayed signs of poor co-ordination with a GCS of 14/15. He was normoglycaemic but acidotic with a raised anion gap. Serum creatinine measured 120 umol/l. Urine analysis confirmed 1+ protein. Microscopy showed extensive deposition of calcium oxalate bipyramidal crystals of calcium (below ◘ Fig. 2.10).

He later admitted drinking 400 ml of ethylene glycol. Urine microscopy can be particularly useful in identifying some of the causes of AKI, particularly in cases of crystal nephropathy.

Case 4

A 68-year-old woman with type 2 diabetes and hypertension was admitted from clinic with rapidly progressive renal impairment (a rise from a baseline of 180 to 540 in

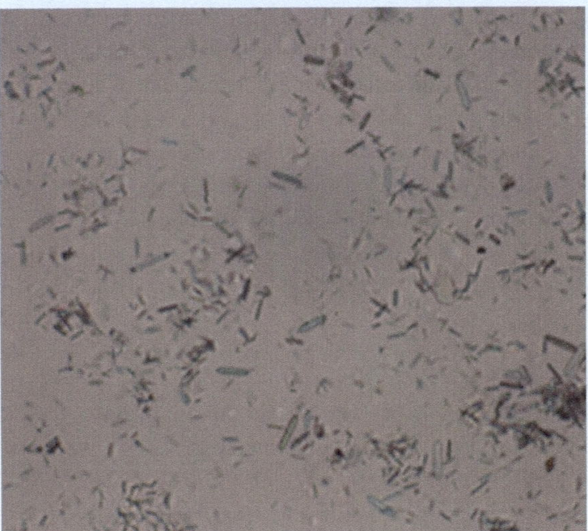

◘ **Fig. 2.10** Numerous calcium oxalate crystals in urine of case 3

2

3 months). She was well, asymptomatic and afebrile, with no obvious pre-renal elements nor obstruction on USS (she had normal-sized kidneys). Urine dipstick was positive for protein 1+, leucocytes 3+ nitrites negative. Urine microscopy demonstrated white cell casts consistent with pyelonephritis, and bilateral pyelonephritis was subsequently confirmed with culture and imaging. Her decline in renal function was originally attributed, in part, to progression of diabetic nephropathy, but her renal function responded well to intravenous antibiotics. Urine microscopy was able to narrow the differential diagnosis and suggest a diagnosis here without the need for a biopsy or missing a potentially reversible cause for progression.

Tips and Tricks

1. Urine analysis remains an important tool available to all clinicians and offers particularly useful information to the practising nephrologist.
2. Persistent micro- or macroscopic haematuria in patients over 40 years of age (or younger for those with risk factors for urinary tract malignancy, e.g. previous cyclosphosphamide or aristolic acid exposure) should be screened for urinary tract malignancy or another cause of lower urinary tract bleeding.
3. Urine dipstick testing is sensitive to albumin but has low sensitivity to other proteins, such as tubular proteins and light-chain immunoglobulins.
4. The presence of haematuria and proteinuria alongside dysmorphic RBCs supports the diagnosis of RPGN.
5. Urine osmolality assesses the action of ADH in the collecting ducts, and urinary sodium is a measure of tubular function.
6. Consider empowering patients with recurrent conditions such as nephrotic syndrome or UTIs to dipstick their urine to speed assessment if relapsing or avoid unnecessary appointments if clear.
7. Consider obtaining and storing urine for drug or poison analysis in patients with intractable hypertension, unexplained electrolyte abnormalities or sick without explanation.

Chapter Review Questions

1. What is the definition of microalbuminuria?
2. Urine dipstick testing has a high sensitivity to detect tubular proteins?
3. The presence of Maltese cross in the urine is suggestive of post-streptococcal glomerulonephritis?
4. Acanthocytes and dysmorphic RBCs are predominantly found in patients with lower urinary tract bleeding.

Answers

1. Microalbuminuria is a term used to describe an increase in the permeability of albumin in the glomerulus. It is an important prognostic marker for kidney disease, particularly diabetes mellitus and hypertension. It is defined as the excretion of more than 30–300 mg albumin in 24 hours.
2. Urine dipstick testing has a high sensitivity for the presence of albumin in urine but not tubular proteins or light-chain immunoglobulins. Specific quantification of retinal binding protein is more sensitive.
3. Anderson-Fabry's disease is associated with the presence of Maltese cross on polarised light microscopy representing myelin bodies.
4. Glomerular disease is characteristically associated with dysmorphic RBCs and acanthocytes.

excretion need to be continually considered; for example, urine osmolality assesses the action of ADH in the collecting ducts and hence water excretion, whilst urinary sodium is a measure of tubular function with the majority of freely filtered sodium being reabsorbed by the renal tubules. ◘ Table 2.8 is intended to be a helpful guide to interpreting urinary electrolytes, rather than an exhaustive atlas.

2.9 Drug and Poison Screening

It is worth remembering urine as an easily accessible material for assaying compliance with medication, drug abuse such as opiates or diuretics and poisons. Obtaining a sample early in patients with intractable hypertension, electrolyte abnormalities consistent with diuretic abuse or anyone presenting acutely unwell but without clear explanation may significantly assist in patient care.

2.10 Summary

Urine analysis remains an important tool available to all clinicians and offers particularly useful information to the practising nephrologist. From initially inspecting the urine to performing routine urine dipstick and microscopy, clinical information is available at each stage and should therefore always be considered as an extension of the physical examination. Cavanaugh and Perazella have produced a definitive review of urine microscopy in kidney disease as part of the core curriculum and recommended reading for enthusiasts (10).

References

1. Bagshaw SM, Haase M, Haase-Fielitz A, Bennett M, Devarajan P, Bellomo R. A prospective evaluation of urine microscopy in septic and non-septic acute kidney injury. Nephrol Dial Transplant. 2012;27(2):582–8.
2. Kanbay M, Kasapoglu B, Perazella MA. Acute tubular necrosis and pre-renal acute kidney injury: utility of urine microscopy in their evaluation- a systematic review. Int Urol Nephrol. 2010;42(2):425–33.
3. Addis T. Glomerular nephritis. Diagnosis and treatment. New York: Macmillan; 1948. p. 2.
4. Berman LB. Urine in technicolor. J Am Med Assoc. 1974;228(6):753.
5. Fogazzi GB, Verdesca S, Garigali G. Urinalysis: core curriculum 2008. Am J Kidney Dis. 2008;51(6):1052–67.
6. Connor H. Medieval uroscopy and its representation on misericords – part 1: Uroscopy. Clin Med. 2001;1(6):507–9.
7. HPA. Investigation of urine. Health Protection Agency. National Standard Method BSOP 41. 2009. http://www.hpa-standardmethods.org.uk/documents/bsop/pdf/bsop41.pdf.
8. BAUS/RA Guidelines. Joint Consensus Statement on the Initial Assessment of Haematuria. Renal Association 2015. http://www.renal.org/Libraries/Other_Guidlines/Haematuria_-_RA-BAUS_consensus_guideline_2015.sflb.ashx.
9. Smith ER, Cai MMX, McMahon LP, Wright DA, Holt SG. The value of simultaneous measurements of urinary albumin and total protein in proteinuric patients. Nephrol Dial Transplant. 2012;27(4):1534–41.
10. Bouzidi H, Lacour B, Daudon M. 2,8-dihydroxyadenine nephrolithiasis: from diagnosis to therapy. Ann Biol Clin (Paris). 2007;65(6):585–92.

Laboratory Tests in Nephrology

Ali M. Shendi

Contents

M. Harber (ed.), *Primer on Nephrology*, https://doi.org/10.1007/978-3-030-76419-7_3

3

Learning Objectives

1. Identifying the different methods of kidney function assessment, pros and cons of each, and how to interpret the results.
2. Multiple filtration markers are in clinical use, each has its own characteristics and clinical applications.
3. Investigating a patient with renal disorder can involve hematologic, immunologic, virologic, and microbiologic investigations.
4. Understanding the clinical applications and limitations of the different tests employed in investigating patients with renal disorders.

3.1 Introduction

Nephrology is a very numerate speciality; not only is much of diagnosis based on tests, but monitoring of disease and response of laboratory tests to treatment is critical to patient management. The introduction of algorithms for the diagnosis of AKI is a prime example of the importance trends in renal tests but also the tip of the iceberg in terms of potential for defining recovery, decline, or diagnoses.

For the nephrologist, the role is to select appropriate tests based on a careful clinical history and examination and to understand the limitations of laboratory tests. Practicing "appropriateness" is complex because it interplays with "patient's safety," "healthcare costs," "clinical decision-making," and "effectiveness." The aim should be to avoid the waste of resources and potential medical errors. Venesection is on the whole safe, but not without hazards, discomfort, and contribution to anemia. There is a considerable price tag associated with blood tests, for example, between 2014 and 2015 in the UK, the Department of Health estimated that 230 million biochemistry and 47 million hematology tests were performed in secondary care at a cost of £415 million pounds with an estimated total cost of blood tests reaching £3 billion pounds per annum. There are very few healthcare systems with more money than they know what to do with, and nephrologists have some responsibility to request tests wisely.

This chapter will give insight into the assessment of kidney function and then provide an overview of the different tests resorted to in order to diagnose kidney disorders and their complications.

3.2 Kidney Function Assessment

Glomerular filtration rate (GFR) is considered the parameter that best reflects overall kidney health and function [1]. GFR can be assessed through direct measurement (measured GFR: mGFR) or GFR estimation (estimated GFR: eGFR); yet both are associated with systematic and random error (bias and imprecision, respectively) and may differ from "true GFR" [2].

3.2.1 Measurement of GFR

GFR is the amount of fluid filtered from glomerular capillaries to the Bowman's space per unit time (≈ 180 L/day; 130 ml/min/1.73 m^2 for men and 120 ml/min/1.73 m^2 for women).

GFR measurement is feasible through recording the clearance of endogenous or exogenous biomarkers. Renal clearance of a biomarker would equal true GFR when it is characterized by appearing in the plasma at a constant rate, and being eliminated only through free glomerular filtration with no protein binding, tubular secretion, or reabsorption. The only ideal biomarker is inulin which is not practical to be used in clinical and research settings [3].

3.2.1.1 Endogenous Markers of GFR

Characteristics of different endogenous markers are illustrated in ◘ Table 3.1.

3.2.1.2 Exogenous Markers of GFR

Exogenous filtration markers whether isotopic (chromium-51-labelled ethylenediaminetetraacetic acid (^{51}Cr-EDTA), technetium-99m-labelled diethylenetriaminepentaacetic acid (^{99}Tc-DTPA), or ^{125}I-iothalamate) or non-isotopic (iohexol or iothalamate) are considered the "gold standard" for GFR measurement in clinical practice. The choice depends on availability and tradition. GFR can be measured by urinary (both urine and plasma concentration) or plasma (only plasma concentration) clearance of these markers. Characteristics are illustrated in ◘ Table 3.3.

3.2.2 Estimation of GFR

GFR-estimating equations are based on serum levels of endogenous filtration markers in combination with other variables (◘ Table 3.3). Guidelines recommend using the CKD-EPI creatinine equation to estimate GFR using standardized creatinine assays. Cystatin C-based equations can be used to validate the diagnosis of CKD when solely based on creatinine-based eGFR: 45–59 ml/min/1.73 m^2 without markers of kidney damage. If eGFRcys/eGFRcreat-cys is also <60 ml/min/1.73 m^2, the diagnosis of CKD is confirmed [4, 8].

Table 3.1 Endogenous filtration markers

Test	Properties	Clinical application	Advantages	Disadvantages
1. Creatinine	MW: ≈113 Da Generated from muscle creatine and phosphocreatine and from dietary meat Proportional to lean body mass No plasma protein binding Free glomerular filtration Proximal tubular secretion (7–10% of urine creatinine) *Methods of measurement:* 1. Alkaline picrate methods: most routine creatinine assays; have interference problems 2. Enzymatic assays: more specific, more expensive, less interference 3. High-pressure liquid chromatography	Most commonly used biomarker for kidney function assessment	Available international standardization using reference material traceable to isotope-dilution mass spectrometry. This led to lower creatinine values by 10–30% Low cost	Not perfect biomarker of GFR: 1. Determined by non-GFR determinants (Table 3.2) 2. Increases when kidney function is reduced by >50%. Below this level, creatinine is not a good representative of kidney function "creatinine-blind range" 3. Lag in change in serum creatinine behind actual GFR in non-steady states (AKI) [4]
2. Urea	MW: ≈60 Da Free glomerular filtration Extensive tubular back diffusion (40–60%)	1. Differential diagnosis of pre-renal AKI and ATN. In pre-renal AKI: Fractional excretion of urea nitrogen decreases ($FE_{UN} \leq 35\%$: "sensitivity 85% and specificity 92%") [5], and BUN/creatinine ratio increases (Reference BUN/Cr, 10:1 to 20:1) 2. Assessment of dialysis adequacy	One of the first indicators used to measure GFR Low cost	Not a reliable marker of GFR: 1. Extensive tubular back diffusion 2. Influenced by non-renal factors: High serum urea in: 1. Volume depletion 2. High protein intake 3. Major GI hemorrhage 4. Catabolic states, muscle breakdown
3. Cystatin C	MW: ≈13.3 kDa Cysteine proteinase inhibitor Produced by all nucleated cells Free glomerular filtration Catabolized by proximal tubular cells	GFR estimation (second filtration marker of clinical relevance)	Weaker association with age, sex, race, and muscle mass than creatinine Available international standardization	Non-GFR determinants: 1. Associated with body mass index, inflammation, diabetes, and surrogates of muscle mass (age, sex, race) [6] 2. Sensitive to changes in thyroid function
4. B_2-microgloblin (β_2M)	MW: ≈11,8 kDa Removed by glomerular filtration >99.9% reabsorbed and catabolized in proximal convoluted tubule	1. Marker for middle molecular weight uremic toxins 2. Incorporated into GFR prediction equations: Under development Less accurate than CKD-EPI equations Do not require demographic variables 3. Indicator of residual renal function in patients with ESRF 4. Risk prediction of all-cause and CV mortality 5. Urinary β_2M can be used to detect tubular injury	Less affected by age, sex, and muscle mass than creatinine and not affected by ethnicity [7]	1. Elevated in inflammatory, infectious, and lymphoproliferative disorders 2. Lack of standardization 3. Poor stability in acidic urine

3

Table 3.2 Non-GFR determinants of creatinine

Factors	Effect on kidney function	
	Decreased creatinine Overestimated eGFR	**Increased creatinine Underestimated eGFR**
1. Creatinine generation	Low muscle mass: elderly, females, malnourished, sarcopenic obesity	Increased muscle mass: athletes, Africans
2. Dietary intake	Vegetarian diet	High meat diet, creatine supplements
3. Drugs interfering with tubular secretion		Trimethoprim, cimetidine, pyrimethamine, salicyclic acid, cobicistat, dolutegravir, fibric acid derivatives
4. Interference with creatinine assay	Bilirubin	Keto acids, glucose, some cephalosporins

Table 3.3 GFR assessment methods

Method	Principle	Advantage	Limitations	References
A. Measured GFR Indicated when eGFR is unreliable including: 1-Patients with abnormal muscle mass or body composition, anorectic, and obese patients. 2-When an exact value of GFR is required: before potential living kidney donation and the use of toxic drugs with narrow therapeutic range. 3-Non-kidney solid organ transplant recipients [4, 8].				
1. Creatinine clearance (CrCl)	CrCl = urine creatinine (mg/dl) X urine volume (ml/24 h)/plasma creatinine (mg/dl) X time interval for collection (1440 min "24-hour collections")	Used when eGFR is not reliable and mGFR is not practical or feasible	1. Overestimates GFR (tubular secretion of creatinine) 2. Errors of 24-hour urine collections	[9, 10]
2. Inulin clearance	IV infusion Timed-urine collections	Gold standard (equals true GFR)	Laborious and expensive; inapplicable	[3, 11]
3. Isotopic GFR	Plasma or urinary clearance			
1. ^{51}Cr-EDTA	Bolus IV	Available in Europe	1. GFR underestimation by 5–15% (tubular reabsorption) 2. Long-term radiation exposure	[12]
2. ^{99m}Tc-DTPA	Bolus IV	Available in US Short $t_{1/2}$ (6 hours), minimizing radiation exposure Minimal tubular reabsorption High counting efficiency of ^{99m}Tc GFR can be measured by dynamic renal imaging, and split kidney function can be determined	1. Potential unpredictable dissociation of ^{99m}Tc and binding to plasma proteins, leading to underestimation of GFR 2. GFR overestimation by plasma clearance, not renal clearance (extrarenal elimination) 3. Chelating kits and Tc generators are not standardized 4. Poor correlation of GFR measured by ^{99m}Tc-DTPA dynamic renal imaging with simultaneous urinary or plasma clearance	[11, 12]
3. ^{125}I-iothalamate	Ionic contrast medium Subcutaneous or bolus IV	Inexpensive	1. Long $t_{1/2}$; long-term radiation exposure 2. GFR overestimation (Tubular secretion) 3. Problems with thyroidal iodine uptake	[11, 12]
4. Non-isotopic GFR	Plasma or urinary clearance			

Table 3.3 (continued)

Method	Principle	Advantage	Limitations	References
Iohexol	Non-ionic contrast medium	1. Inexpensive marker, available, low inter-laboratory variation 2. Low dose of iohexol: safe, no severe adverse events 3. Avoids radiation 4. Low extrarenal clearance	1. Potential allergic reactions and nephrotoxicity 2. Small underestimation of GFR (tubular reabsorption or protein binding (1.5%)) 3. Complex and expensive assay (HPLC)	[13, 14]
Estimated GFR Reliable for clinical decision-making and epidemiological studies in cases of poor renal function. eGFR within 30% of mGFR is satisfactory for clinical interpretation [2] Guidelines recommend to rely on eGFR rather than serum creatinine alone [4, 8] Common limitations include: 1. Limitations of creatinine as endogenous filtration marker 2. Unavoidable differences between eGFR and mGFR 3. Variable performance among different ethnic groups 4. Inaccuracies at high or low kidney functions 5. More accurate in the steady state than in the non-steady state				
1. Cockcroft-Gault equation	The first widely used equation Parameters used: 1. Creatinine 2. Age 3. Weight 4. Gender Clcr (ml/min) = (140 − age) × (wt kg)/72 × scr(mg/100 ml) (× 0.85 if female)	Estimates creatinine clearance without urine collection	1. Imprecise: Does not estimate GFR Current creatinine assay differs from the assays performed to derive the equation 2. Requires measurement of weight (and height for BSA) 3. Influenced by weight: not for very obese persons and pronounced edema	[15]
2. MDRD study equation	The four-variable MDRD equation developed then re-expressed using standardized creatinine to improve GFR prediction Parameters used: 1. Creatinine 2. Age 3. Ethnicity 4. Gender GFR = 175 × standardized $Scr^{-1.154}$ × $age^{-0.203}$ × 1.212 [if black] × 0.742 [if female]	Simple estimates of GFR More accurate than Cockroft-Gault equation	Imprecision: Underestimation of GFR at higher GFR values leading to overestimation of CKD stage 3 prevalence	[16]
3. CKD-EPI creatinine equation	Developed to reduce bias in MDRD-estimated GFR Parameters used: 1. Creatinine 2. Age 3. Ethnicity 4. Gender GFR = 141 × $\min(Scr/\kappa, 1)^{\alpha}$× $\max(Scr/\kappa, 1)^{-1.209}$ × 0.993^{Age} × 1.018 [if female] × 1.159 [if black] *Where:* κ is 0.7 for females and 0.9 for males α is −0.329 for females and −0.411 for males min indicates the minimum of Scr/ κ or 1 max indicates the maximum of Scr/ κ or 1	More accurate than MDRD equation particularly at GFR >60 ml/min/1.73 m^2	Imprecision: underestimates GFR and overestimates CKD prevalence	[17]

(continued)

3

Table 3.3 (continued)

Method	Principle	Advantage	Limitations	References
4. The CKD-EPI cystatin C equation	Parameters used: 1. Cystatin C 2. Age 3. Gender GFR = 133 × min(Scys/0.8, 1) – 0.499 × max (Scys/0.8, 1) – 1.328 × 0.996Age [×0.932 if female] *Where:* min indicates the minimum of Scr/κ or 1, and max indicates the maximum of Scys/κ or 1	Cystatin C is less affected by non-GFR determinants Usually agree with $eGFR_{creatinine}$	1. Not more accurate than creatinine-based estimates 2. Increased laboratory costs	[18]
5. The CKD-EPI creatinine-cystatin C equation	Parameters used: 1. Creatinine 2. Cystatin C 3. Age 4. Ethnicity 5. Gender GFR = 135 × min(Scr/κ, 1)α × max(Scr/κ, 1) – 0.601 × min(Scys/0.8, 1) – 0.375 × max(Scys/0.8, 1) – 0.711 × 0.995Age [×0.969 if female][×1.08 if black] *Where:* κ is 0.7 for females and 0.9 for males α is −0.248 for females and – 0.207 for males min indicates the minimum of Scr/κ or 1 max indicates the maximum of Scr/κ or 1	More accurate eGFR than creatinine or cystatin C alone Confirmatory test for CKD	Increased laboratory costs	[18]

CKD chronic kidney disease, *CrCl* creatinine clearance, *GFR* glomerular filtration rate, *Scr* serum creatinine, *Scys* serum cystatin C, *BSA* body surface area, *BMI* body mass index

3.2.3 Kidney Function Assessment During Pregnancy

Kidney function can be assessed through serial creatinine measurement and less frequently creatinine clearance. No formula has been validated [19].

3.2.4 Kidney Function Assessment During Non-steady State: AKI

Mainly through serial creatinine measurement as measuring GFR is unsuitable for patients in intensive care, and both eGFR and CrCl equations are invalid. Short-timed urine CrCl can be used [20].

3.3 Other Laboratory Investigations for Assessing Patients with Kidney Diseases

Highlights of the main laboratory investigations used to evaluate patients with renal disorders are discussed in Table 3.4.

Table 3.4 Laboratory investigations used to assess patients with kidney diseases

Test	Principles/method of assessment	Clinical application	Sensitivity	Specificity	Advantages	Disadvantages	References
A. Urine analysis Urine analysis including testing for proteinuria has been discussed in ▶ Chap. 2 "Urine Analysis".							
B. Markers of inflammation Inflammatory markers can be used to monitor disease activity in various inflammatory kidney disorders							
Erythrocyte sedimentation rate (ESR)	Measures the distance erythrocytes fall after 1 hour in vertical column of anticoagulated blood under gravity	Surrogate marker of acute phase reaction in inflammatory renal disorders: 1. Monitoring disease activity and response to therapy 2. Prognostic marker Extremely elevated ESR (>100 mm/hr) has very low false-positive rate for serious underlying disease: (1) Infections. (2) Collagen vascular disease. (3) Malignant tumors In proteinuric states: Mild ESR elevations are expected due to hypoalbuminemia; albumin in plasma inhibits erythrocyte sedimentation In patients with CKD: Mild to moderate ESR elevations; ESR gets more elevated in patients with ESRD on dialysis			1. Inexpensive, quick, simple 2. Better inflammatory marker than CRP in autoimmune diseases particularly SLE and some low-grade bone and joint infections	Increases with age, in females, and with pregnancy Affected by other factors, e.g., plasma albumin, size, shape, and number of RBCs and non-acute-phase reaction proteins, e.g., immunoglobulins increase ESR	[21, 22]

(continued)

Table 3.4 (continued)

Test	Principles/method of assessment	Clinical application	Sensitivity	Specificity	Advantages	Disadvantages	References
C-reactive protein (CRP)	Acute-phase protein synthesized by hepatocytes in response to pro-inflammatory cytokines during inflammatory/infectious processes	Non-specific marker of acute-phase reaction in acute inflammatory response and to gauge chronic inflammation and tissue damage			1. More specific and sensitive than ESR 2. Rapid response to inflammation: concentrations exceed 5 mg/l by ≈6 hours and peak ≈48 hours 3. Plasma $t_{1/2}$ is short (≈19 hours)	1. Non-specific 2. Not recommended in SLE activity follow-up SLE is associated with ESR/CRP discordance: CRP is higher at baseline than in general population and during activity than in remission (proposed cutoff: 10 mg/l for active SLE) Synchronous elevation of ESR and CRP during concomitant infections and during flares in patients with serositis and/or arthritis	[22, 23]
C. Immunologic investigations Laboratory assays which evaluate the immune response are valuable in establishing a diagnosis and/or monitoring disease activity of various immune-mediated kidney disorders							
Complements Routinely, serum C3, C4, and possibly CH50 Other analyses performed at specialized laboratories	Play role in pathogenesis of antibody-mediated glomerulonephritis, C3 glomerulopathy, atypical hemolytic uremic syndrome, ischemic-reperfusion injury of transplanted kidney, and antibody-mediated renal allograft rejection	Assessment of complement activity helps the evaluation and follow-up of certain renal disorders: Low C3 and C4 indicate immune complexes-mediated-classic pathway activation, e.g. SLE Low C3 and normal C4 suggest alternative complement pathway (AP) activation, e.g., C3G Normal/low C3, often undetectable C4 in essential and type II mixed cryoglobulinemia Low C3 can be present with AAV; indicates severe disease			Patterns of complement activity characteristic for certain renal disorders	Non-specific Complement is an acute-phase reactant and so may be in the normal range when consumed in the setting of sepsis Complement may be low in the setting of liver failure	[24]

Auto-antibodies							
ANA	Autoantibodies that react with constituents of cell nuclei *Methods of detection:* Indirect immune-fluorescence (IIF): The most widely used initial test using human epidermoid carcinoma cell line (HEp-2) The gold standard for ANA screening If positive ANA (IIF): testing with solid-phase assays (ELISA and RIA) to detect specific auto-antibodies If negative ANA (<1/160): extremely unlikely SLE. Additional antibody testing can be considered	Screening for SLE and other autoimmune diseases *Prevalence:* ANA titer >1:160 in 94–100% and ≥1:80 in ≈99.5% In LN: 100% *Types of ANA:* based on the nuclear antigen: 1. Autoantibodies to DNA (single and double-stranded) and histones 2. Autoantibodies to extractable nuclear antigens (ENA): Smith antigen (Sm), ribonucleoproteins (RNP), SSA/Ro, or SSB/La, Scl-70, Jo-1, and PM1	*SLE:* 93–95.2% (97.8% for ANA titer ≥1:80) *SSc:* 85–93.6% *Sjögren's syndrome:* 48–88.4% *MCTD:* 100% *Drug-induced LE:* 80–95%	*SLE:* 57–83.3% *SSc:* 54–84.2% *Sjögren's syndrome:* 52–86.8%	High sensitivity and negative predictive value	1. Low specificity: high prevalence of low-titer ANAs in healthy individuals (30% at 1:40, 10–15% at 1:80, 5% at 1:160) 2. Not useful for monitoring disease activity or response to therapy	[25–27]
Specific ANAs							
1. Anti-dsDNA		1. Diagnostic for SLE * *Prevalence:* 70–98% of SLE. In LN: 70% 2. Monitoring SLE activity: Associated with more severe disease with renal involvement Correlates with disease activity Titer increase may predict disease relapse	57.3% Sensitivity for active LN: 100%	97.4% Specificity for active LN: 50%	High specificity for SLE; very rare in other pathological conditions and healthy subjects (<0.5%)	Possible false-positive anti-dsDNA using *Crithidia luciliae* assay	[28, 29]
2. Anti-histone		Drug-induced SLE *Prevalence:* 70%; In LN: 37%	55%	69%	Sensitive in drug-induced SLE	Non-specific Little clinical usefulness	[30]
3. Antinucleosome (anti-chromatin) Ab		Diagnosis of SLE: equal specificity, higher sensitivity, and prognostic value than anti-dsDNA *Prevalence:* 61–85%; In LN: 60–90% Associated with SLE disease activity Predicts flares in quiescent lupus	61%	94%	High specificity and sensitivity for SLE; especially if anti-ds-DNA negative		[31]

(continued)

Table 3.4 (continued)

Test	Principles/method of assessment	Clinical application	Sensitivity	Specificity	Advantages	Disadvantages	References
4. Anti-Sm		Diagnosis of SLE * *Prevalence:* 20–40%; In LN: 14%	10–55%	98–100%	High specificity	1. Low sensitivity 2. Static over SLE disease course, difficult to link with clinical manifestations	[28]
5. Anti-SSA/Ro		1. SLE: Associated with photosensitive rash, serositis, hematological manifestations, neonatal lupus erythematosus (complete heart block: more with Anti-SSA/Ro) *Prevalence* Anti-SSA/Ro: 30%; anti-SSB/La: 10% In LN: Anti-SSA/Ro: 31%; anti-SSB/La: 14% 2. Sjögren's syndrome	40%	96%		Low sensitivity	[28, 32]
Anti-SSB/La			25%	97%			
6. Anti-U1-RNP		1. In SLE: associated with arthritis and Raynaud's phenomenon. *Prevalence:* 10–30% 2. Mixed connective tissue disease **Prevalence*: 100%	8–69%	25–82%		Low sensitivity and specificity for SLE	[32]
7. Anti-P ribosomal protein		SLE: Associated with neuropsychiatric manifestations *Prevalence:* SLE: 13–40%; In LN: 6%	36%	97–100%			[32]
8. Anti-Scl-70 (anti-topoisomerase I)		Systemic sclerosis (diffuse) Increased risk of scleroderma renal crisis (SRC)	43% (for diffuse SSc: 37%)	100% (for diffuse SSc: 82%)			[33]
9. Anti-centromere		Systemic sclerosis (limited)	33% (for CREST: 61%)	99.9% (for CREST: 84%)			[33]

10. Anti-RNA polymerase III antibodies		Systemic sclerosis (diffuse with severe cutaneous thickening) * *Prevalence:* 3.8–19.4% Associated with SRC * *Prevalence:* ≈30%	38%	94%	Immunological marker for SRC Diagnosis of SRC sine scleroderma		[32]
Antiphospholipid antibodies (aPL)	Heterogeneous autoantibodies directed to plasma proteins bound to anionic surfaces (phospholipid). The term antiphospholipid is thus misnomer	Diagnosis of antiphospholipid syndrome (APS): at least one positive laboratory test confirmed on two or more occasions at least 12 weeks apart aPL should be tested in autoimmune disorders (SLE) or when there is suspicion of APS *Prevalence* in LN: 20–80%	63% using triple tests IgG aCL and IgG anti-β_2GPI have the highest sensitivity for APS			Poorly standardized; non-specific	[34, 35]
1. Lupus anticoagulant (LA)	Heterogeneous IgG or IgM auto-antibodies: In vitro, interfere with phospholipid-dependent coagulation tests, while in vivo, associated with thromboembolic events and pregnancy complications Detected by functional clotting assays involving screening tests, testing after mixing with normal plasma, and, if abnormal, confirmatory testing after increasing phospholipid concentration	The most widely used tests for aPL * *Prevalence:* 53.6%	44.8%	77.3%	Stronger risk factor for thrombosis than aCL antibodies	1. Lack of gold standards for ideal diagnostic strategy and cutoff values 2. The term lupus anticoagulant is a misnomer	[36]
2. Anti-cardiolipin (aCL)	Detected by ELISA; IgG and IgM isotypes	aCL positivity can be elicited by antibodies to phospholipid-binding proteins in serum samples, sample diluent, and blocking, or directly binding cardiolipin IgG and/or IgM aCL titers must be medium/high: >40 GPL or MPL units or >the 99th percentile calculated in normal subjects * *Prevalence:* 87.9%	IgG: 25.7% IgM: 5.7%	IgG: 94.8% IgM: 98.7%	May detect potentially important antibodies not yet defined	Positivity can be elicited by clinically relevant and/or irrelevant antibodies	[34]

(continued)

Table 3.4 (continued)

Test	Principles/method of assessment	Clinical application	Sensitivity	Specificity	Advantages	Disadvantages	References
3. Anti-beta-2 glycoprotein I (anti-β2GPI)	Detected by ELISA; IgG and IgM, and if negative and APS is still suspected IgA isotypes	Plasma glycoprotein that binds to anionic phospholipids on cell membranes *Prevalence:* IgM: 65%; IgA: 47%	57.1%	79.2%	The only aPL antibodies against specific protein	May identify antibodies different from those relevant to the syndrome	[34, 37]
Anti-C1q antibodies	Autoantibodies against C1q; can result in decreased C1q in SLE	Diagnosis of SLE: *Prevalence:* 30–40% Titers correlate with SLE disease activity Good predicative marker for active LN (40–100%)	28% (In active LN: 87%)	92% (In active LN: 92%)	Associated with hypocomplementemia, disease activity, and renal involvement	Not specific: observed in hypo-complementemic urticarial vasculitis, anti-GBM nephritis, HIV infection	[38]
Antineutrophil cytoplasmic antibodies (ANCA)	Auto-antibodies against antigenic targets in the cytoplasmic granules of neutrophils: myeloperoxidase (MPO) and leukocyte proteinase 3 (PR3) *Methods of detection:* 1. IIF using human neutrophils detects two staining patterns: perinuclear (pANCA) and cytoplasmic (cANCA). Rare Atypical pattern (A-ANCA) combines cytoplasmic and perinuclear or nuclear staining mostly in absence of vasculitis 2. Antigen-specific solid-phase assays (ELISA) for MPO and PR3, the antigenic targets of pANCAs and cANCAs, respectively Antigen-specific assays should be the primary screening method	1. Diagnosis of ANCA-associated vasculitis (AAV): PR3-ANCAs in: 1. ≈2/3 of GPA 2. 25% of MPA MPO-ANCAs in: 1. Majority of MPA 2. ≈25% of GPA 2. Titers are related to disease activity 3. Rising ANCA during remission can predict relapse	*IIF:* *cANCA:* GPA:65–77% MPA: 5–6% *pANCA:* GPA:11–15% MPA:85–89% *Immunoassay* *PR3-ANCA:* GPA:77–81% MPA: 5–9% *MPO-ANCA:* GPA: 9–12% MPA:71–88% *Combining IIF with ELISA* decreased the sensitivities to 67–82%	*IIF:* cANCA: 97–98% pANCA: 81–96% *Immunoassay* PR3-ANCA: 98–99% MPO-ANCA: 96–99 *combining IIF with ELISA:* 98%	1. Available assay standardization. 2. ANCA specificity defines homogeneous groups of AAV patients	1. Large variability between IIF methods 2. ANCAs found in other conditions (e.g., anti-GBM, primary sclerosing cholangitis) 3. Patients diagnosed as having GPA or MPA can be negative for PR3 and MPO-ANCA (11–17% by IIF and 9–16% by immunoassay) 4. Difficult to differentiate P-ANCA (or A-ANCA) patterns from ANA staining on IIF	[39, 40]
Anti-GBM antibodies	Auto-antibodies against the non-collagenous (NC1) domain of $\alpha3$ chain of type IV collagen ($\alpha3$[IV]NC1; "Goodpasture autoantigen") Detected using enzyme immunoassays or bead-based fluorescence assays	Diagnosis of anti-GBM disease (renal limited anti-GBM and the complete Goodpasture syndrome) in patients with RPGN * *Prevalence*: 90%	41.2%	85.4%		Lack of sensitivity. Patients with atypical anti-GBM (≈10%) do not have identifiable circulating antibodies	[41]

Anti-podocytic antibodies							
1. Anti-phospholipase A2 receptor (PLA2R) antibodies	IgG antibodies (predominantly IgG4) that react with PLA_2R, a glycoprotein expressed on normal glomerular podocytes and present in the glomerular immune deposits in patients with IMN	1. Differentiation of IMN from secondary forms and other glomerulopathies * *Prevalence*: 70% of IMN 2. Serum PLA2R-Abs correlate with proteinuria, disease activity, and prognosis: Higher spontaneous remission in negative and low-titer PLA2R-Abs Serial evaluation to monitor response to therapy Pre-transplant PLA2R-Ab could predict recurrence of MN post-transplant	81%. (combined with PLA2R tissue localization: 95.2%)	100% (both serum anti-PLA2R and glomerular PLA2R)	High specificity		[42, 43]
2. Anti-thrombospondin type 1 domain containing 7A (THSD7A)	IgG4 antibody specific for THSD7A, podocyte membrane antigen similar to PLA2R	1. Diagnosis of IMN * *Prevalence:* 3–5% 2. Anti-PLA2R/THSD7A levels correlate with proteinuria, clinical course, and outcomes 3. THSD7A-associated MN characterized by (1) female predominance and (2) association with malignancy					[44]

(continued)

Table 3.4 (continued)

Test	Principles/method of assessment	Clinical application	Sensitivity	Specificity	Advantages	Disadvantages	References
C3 nephritic factor	IgG autoantibody that stabilizes C3 convertase increasing its half-life and inducing uncontrolled activation of AP C5 nephritic factor (C5NeF): IgG autoantibody that prolongs C5 convertase half-life *Methods of detection:* 1. Traditionally, hemolytic assay using sensitized sheep red cells 2. More recent approach: screening for C3NeF using multiple ELISA steps. Where appropriate, further screening for fH resistance or C5 convertase stabilizing antibodies	Identification of autoimmune forms of MPGN * *Prevalence:* 40–50% of IC-MPGN 45–80% of C3G (40–50% in C3GN and 70–80% of DDD) Patients with C3G could have negative C3 and C5 convertase stabilization assays (22%), positive C3bBb convertase stabilization (28.8%), or C5 convertase stabilization assays (10.2%), or both (39%) 71% of patients with isolated C3NeF have DDD, while 72% of patients with C5NeF show C3GN			Strong disease association	1. Uncertain pathogenic significance: Poor correlation with C3 consumption and disease activity Reported in other diseases and healthy individuals 2. Assays: technically complex, lack of standardization. 3. C3NeF are heterogeneous, and assays may detect only subsets	[45]
Cryoglobulins	Immunoglobulins which precipitate below 37 °C and re-dissolve when rewarmed in vitro. Blood samples are transported and processed at 37 °C to avoid premature precipitation. Serum-containing tubes are kept at 4 °C and analyzed at 72 hours Type I cryoprecipitate may appear as early as 24 hours, but mixed cryoglobulins may precipitate after several days. Some laboratories wait 7 days if no precipitate formed initially	Diagnosis of cryoglobulinemia				1. False-negative results: (1) improper handling of sample (not transported at 37 °C). (2) Lipemia interfering with cryoglobulin identification 2. Healthy individuals can have detectable cryoglobulins with unknown significance	[46]
D. Hematologic investigations							

1. Complete blood picture	Assessment of number and morphology of RBCs, hemoglobin levels, platelets, WBCs, and reticulocytes	Essential in the assessment of different kidney disorders. Helps in identifying their etiology and/or complications, for example: Anemia diagnosis and follow-up as a complication of CKD Leukocytosis with elevated inflammatory markers in sepsis-induced AKI Hemolytic anemia with fragmented RBCs and thrombocytopenia in cases of AKI caused by micro-angiopathic hemolytic anemia					
2. Fibrinogen:	Soluble 340-kD protein mainly synthesized by the liver with the central function in hemostasis	*1. Plasma fibrinogen:* 1. Detection of hypo-fibrinogenemia complicating plasma-pheresis 2. Elevated levels predict adverse cardiovascular, stroke, and mortality outcomes in patients with CKD stages 3 and 4 *2. Urinary fibrinogen:* * Elevated in proteinuric kidney diseases *Significantly higher in FSGS than MCD and may be used as biomarker for differentiation * Noninvasive method to monitor kidney fibrosis and prediction of CKD progression			Not present in urine under normal conditions		[47, 48]

(continued)

Table 3.4 (continued)

Test	Principles/method of assessment	Clinical application	Sensitivity	Specificity	Advantages	Disadvantages	References
3. Investigations for amyloidosis and related disorders (▶ Chap. 50, Amyloid and the Kidney): 1. Plasma protein electrophoresis 2. Bence Jones proteinuria 3. Free light chain assays 4. Serum amyloid A protein (SAA)							
E. Investigations for infection-related kidney diseases (microbiology and virology):							
1. Antibodies against streptococcal antigens: 1. ASO titer 2. Anti-hyaluronidase 3. Anti-DNAse		Identify streptococcal infection as the trigger of acute post-streptococcal glomerulonephritis (PSGN) * *Prevalence of high ASO:* 60–72% ASO titers are higher in pharyngitis-associated than pyoderma-associated PSGN Cases following pyoderma are more likely to have raised anti-DNAse than elevated ASO titers	ASO: 97%	ASO: 80%	High sensitivity	Low specificity	[49, 50]
2. Urine culture and antibiotic susceptibility testing for suspected urinary tract infection *(▶ Chap. 54; Urinary Tract Infection)*							
3. Blood culture and antibiotic susceptibility testing for suspected bloodstream infection							
4. Viral screening for hepatitis C, hepatitis B, and human immunodeficiency virus (HIV) infections Surveillance for HCV, HBV, and HIV infection using serologic and\or nucleic acid testing is recommended at the time of initial evaluation of glomerulopathies and CKD and during evaluation for kidney transplantation. Guidelines for viral screening during hemodialysis are discussed in ▶ Chap. 76							

AAV ANCA-associated vasculitis, *ANA* antinuclear antibodies, *aCL* anti-cardiolipin, anti-*β2GPI* anti-beta-2 glycoprotein I, *anti-THSD7A* Anti-thrombospondin type 1 domain containing 7A, *anti-PLA2R* anti-phospholipase A2 receptors, *ANCA* antineutrophil cytoplasmic antibodies, *Anti-GBM* anti-glomerular basement membrane, *ASO* anti-streptolysin O, *C3NeF* C3 nephritic factor, *C5NeF* C5 nephritic factor, *CKD* chronic kidney disease, *CRP* C-reactive protein, *ELISA* enzyme-linked immunosorbent assay, *ESR* erythrocyte sedimentation rate, *GPA* granulomatosis with polyangiitis, *GPL units* IgG phospholipid units, *IIF* indirect immunofluorescence, *IMN* idiopathic membranous nephropathy, *LN* lupus nephritis, *MPA* microscopic polyangiitis, *MPL* units *IgM* phospholipid units, *PSGN* post-streptococcal glomerulonephritis, *RBCs* red blood cells, *RIA* Farr radioimmunoassay, *RNP* ribonucleoprotein, *SSc* systemic sclerosis, *WBCs* white blood cells

Tips, Tricks, and Pitfalls

1. Despite the inevitable difference from true GFR, eGFR is practical and reliable for clinical decision-making in cases of poor renal function. It is not accurate in patients with GFR >60 ml/min/1.73 m^2.
2. It is not possible to routinely refer to mGFR in daily clinical practice. However, it should be requested when eGFR is unreliable including patients with abnormal muscle mass or body composition and when an exact value of GFR is required like before potential living kidney donation and the use of toxic drugs with narrow therapeutic range.
3. Each method of GFR measurement has its own limitations. There is no clear recommendation for one method over the other, and choice would thus depend mainly on availability and tradition.
4. The most accurate creatinine-based GFR estimation equation is CKD EPI, which should be used as the primary equation. Cystatin C-based equations can then to be used as confirmatory.
5. GFR estimation equations cannot be used in patients with AKI or in pregnant ladies. Serial creatinine is the method of choice to monitor kidney function with less frequent reference to creatinine clearance based on short-timed urine collection in AKI and 24-hours collection in pregnancy.
6. CRP is generally used to monitor an inflammatory response. In SLE, though it is higher at baseline than the general population, during flares, it increases but not to the level we would expect. It can be used to detect concurrent infections or in patients with arthritis and/or serositis.
7. Mild-to-moderate elevations of ESR without any other signs or abnormalities are not specific and should not trigger extensive investigations to search for etiology. It should be repeated at some time weeks later.
8. ANA is the most sensitive test to screen for SLE and related autoimmune diseases. It should be performed primarily by IIF, and if positive, ELISA testing to identify disease-specific antibodies is performed.
9. Negative ANA can occasionally be encountered with positive anti-dsDNA. First, ELISA testing for anti-dsDNA can be more sensitive than the IIF used for ANA. Second, *Crithidia luciliae* assay, an IF test, can yield false-positive anti-dsDNA.
10. Antigen-specific solid-phase assays should be used as the primary screening method for ANCA, and if negative but clinical suspicion of vasculitis is high, then IIF can be resorted to.
11. False-negative cryoglobulin is not infrequent mostly due to sample handling/processing error. Thus the test should be repeated in cases with high clinical suspicion.
12. Antiphospholipid antibody testing involves LA, aCL IgM and IgG, and anti-β2GPI IgM and IgG. The three tests should be performed as no one can replace the others. Positivity of one test is sufficient to diagnose antiphospholipid syndrome provided that it is accompanied by clinical criteria and remains positive after 12 weeks.

Case Studies

Case 1

Creatinine of a patient with a stable renal transplant and baseline creatinine of 140 μmol/l (eGFR 43 ml/min/1.73 m^2) who developed a severe inflammatory arthropathy. The fall in creatinine from 140 to 60 μmol/l (and eGFR >90 ml/min/1.73 m^2) was entirely due to muscle loss in this period with subsequent rise in creatinine not a consequence of falling GFR but recovering muscle mass (◘ Fig. 3.1).

Interpretation of creatinine levels and eGFR should thus be judicious in patients with abnormal muscle mass.

Case 2

A 58-year-old man presented with progressively rising serum creatinine up to 406.6 μmol/l (from a baseline of 159.1 μmol/l) after having an AKI following a bout of severe diarrhea (◘ Fig. 3.2). The patient had diabetes, hypertension, and CKD diagnosed as diabetic kidney disease. Investigations showed subnephrotic proteinuria with no hematuria, persistently elevated inflammatory markers (CRP 54 mg/l; ESR 95 mm/first hour), and negative virology and immunology screen and angiotensin-converting enzyme. Serum amyloid A and LDH were significantly elevated. Kidney biopsy was

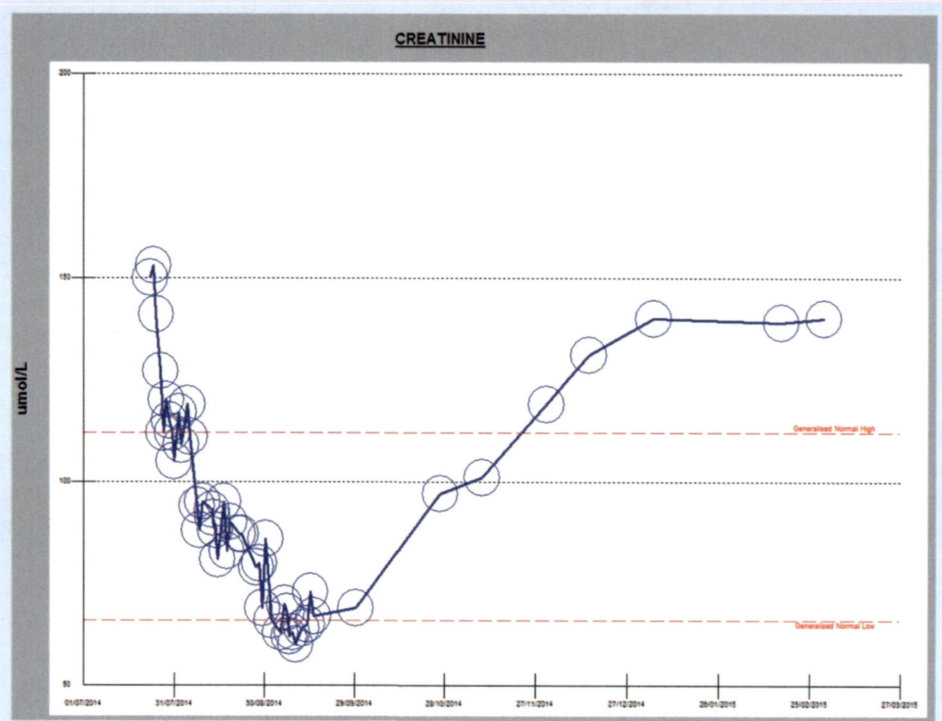

■ **Fig. 3.1** Serum creatinine decline in a patient with stable kidney transplant due to muscle loss during the course of severe inflammatory arthropathy

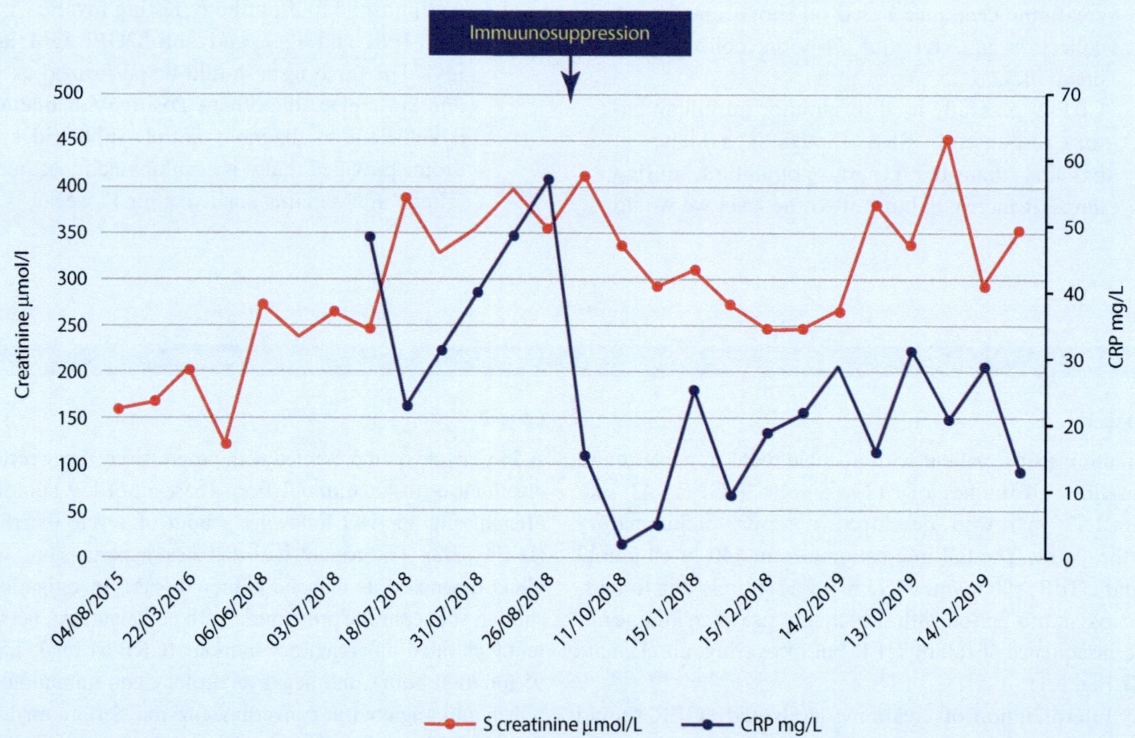

■ **Fig. 3.2** Time course of creatinine and CRP in a diabetic patient with sarcoidosis

denied. PET/CT showed bilateral hypermetabolic pulmonary sub-pleural nodules with hypermetabolic bilateral hilar and mediastinal lymph nodes (◻ Fig. 3.3). True cut biopsy was characteristic for sarcoidosis.

The patient received immunosuppression (prednisolone and MMF) with improvement of the general condition, initial stabilization of kidney functions (3-month creatinine, 247.5 µmol/l; after 15 months, 353 µmol/l), and decline of the inflammatory markers.

An unexplained inflammatory milieu together with progressive deterioration of kidney functions required thorough investigations to identify the underlying etiology.

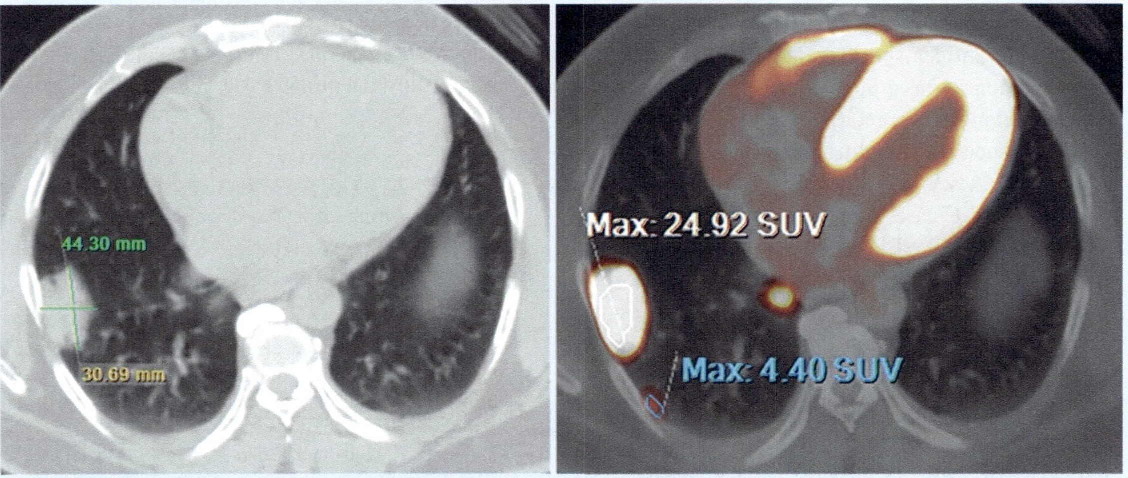

◻ **Fig. 3.3** Sarcoidosis as a cause of progressive CKD diagnosed by PET CT and elevated inflammatory markers. Right lower lung lobe (lateral segment) irregular hypermetabolic sub-pleural soft tissue mass

Nephrologists rely very heavily on blood tests (as well as histology and imaging), and trends in results are critical to both diagnosis and management. It is beholden upon us as a speciality to obtain results of tests done elsewhere that may give a clearer picture of diagnosis and progression as well as rationalizing investigations in our patients to avoid inappropriate testing/phlebotomy. Achieving this balance is not entirely straightforward, but excessive testing is not cost-free for our patients or healthcare systems. Artificial intelligence or IT-based models have huge potential to enhance and rationalize diagnostic testing.

Chapter Review Questions

1. Is it possible to rely on eGFR for kidney function assessment in a potential kidney transplant donor?
2. Which GFR estimation equation is currently recommended to monitor kidney function?
3. Why is ANCA not recommended to be performed using IIF?
4. Can ANA positivity be considered a sin qua non for the diagnosis of SLE?
5. What is the diagnostic utility of anti-PLA2R antibody in idiopathic membranous nephropathy?

Answers

1. No, a potential kidney transplant donor has normal serum creatinine, and all eGFR equations are unreliable in patients with normal serum creatinine where actual GFR is more than 60 ml/min/m^2. This is a typical situation where mGFR should be requested.
2. CKD-EPI creatinine equation is recommended by KDIGO and NICE clinical practice guidelines to estimate GFR. The MDRD study equation has been proven to be more accurate than Cockroft-Gault equation in predicting GFR, and the CKD-EPI equation gives more accurate estimates than the MDRD, particularly in populations with higher mGFR. Clinical practice guidelines have also suggested the use of cystatin C-based equations to validate the diagnosis of CKD in patients who are considered to have CKD solely on the

basis of a creatinine-based eGFR of 45–59 ml/min/1.73 m^2, without albuminuria or other markers of kidney damage. If eGFRcys/eGFRcreat-cys is also <60 ml/min/1.73 m^2, the diagnosis of CKD is confirmed.

3. First, solid-phase assays are generally more sensitive and specific. P-ANCA staining pattern is indistinguishable from ANA nuclear staining pattern, and thus not specific. Also, IIF staining does not provide antigenic specificity, while solid-phase assays are antigen-specific and thus can help define homogeneous groups of AAV patients with different clinical characteristics: MPO and PR3 ANCA-associated vasculitis.
4. No, despite ANA at a titer ≥1:80 is prevalent in ≈99.5% of SLE cases and holding sensitivity of 97.8% to diagnose SLE, some cases can be negative for ANA. The 2019 American College of Rheumatology and European League against Rheumatism classification criteria for SLE positioned ANA positivity (≥1/80) as an entry criterion to diagnose SLE, yet this is still a matter of uncertainty since there remains a subgroup of patients who are persistently ANA negative. Positive anti-dsDNA with negative ANA may occur as the solid-phase assay used for anti-dsDNA and can have higher sensitivity than IIF. Moreover, LN can present without positive SLE serologies (seronegative LN) which may or may not convert to positive ones during follow-up.
5. Anti-phospholipase A2 receptor (PLA2R) antibody is 100% specific for idiopathic membranous nephropathy (IMN); thus, it can reliably diagnose IMN even without a kidney biopsy. The presence and level of serum PLA2R-Abs correlate with proteinuria, disease activity, and prognosis.

References

1. Seegmiller JC, Eckfeldt JH, Lieske JC. Challenges in measuring glomerular filtration rate: a clinical laboratory perspective. Adv Chronic Kidney Dis. 2018;25(1):84–92.
2. Levey AS, Inker LA. Assessment of glomerular filtration rate in health and disease: a state of the art review. Clin Pharmacol Ther. 2017;102(3):405–19.
3. Shannon BJA, Smith HW. The excretion of inulin, xylose and urea by normal and phlorizinized man. J Clin Invest. 1935;14:393–401.
4. Kidney Disease: Improving Global Outcomes (KDIGO) CKD Work group. KDIGO 2012 clinical practice guideline for the evaluation and management of chronic kidney disease. Kidney Int Suppl. 2013;3:1–150.
5. York N. Significance of the fractional excretion of urea in the differential diagnosis of acute renal failure. Kidney Int. 2002;62:2223–9.
6. Stevens LA, Schmid CH, Greene T, Li L, Beck GJ, Joffe MM, et al. Factors other than glomerular filtration rate affect serum cystatin C levels. Kidney Int. 2009;75(6):652–60.
7. Foster MC, Levey AS, Inker LA, Shafi T, Fan L, Gudnason V, et al. Non-GFR determinants of low-molecular-weight serum protein filtration markers in the elderly: AGES-kidney and MESA-kidney. Am J Kidney Dis. 2017;70(3):406–14.
8. NICE guidance: Chronic kidney disease in adults: assessment and management Clinical guideline [CG182] [Internet]. 2015 [cited Jan 6, 2020]. Available from: https://www.nice.org.uk/guidance/cg182/chapter/1-Recommendations#investigations-for-chronic-kidney-disease-2
9. Lam YWF, Banerji S, Hatfield C, Talbert RL. Principles of drug administration in renal insufficiency. Clin Pharmacokinet. 1997;32(1):30–57.
10. Shannon JA. The renal excretion of creatinine in man. J Clin Invest. 1935;14(4):403–10.
11. Soveri I, Berg UB, Bjork J, Elinder CG, Grubb A, Mejare I, et al. Measuring GFR: a systematic review. Am J Kidney Dis. 2014;64(3):411–24.
12. Stevens LA, Levey AS. Measured GFR as a confirmatory test for estimated GFR. J Am Soc Nephrol. 2009; 20(11):2305–13.
13. Delanaye P, Ebert N, Melsom T, Gaspari F, Mariat C, Cavalier E, et al. Iohexol plasma clearance for measuring glomerular filtration rate in clinical practice and research: a review. Part 1: how to measure glomerular filtration rate with iohexol? Clin Kidney J. 2016;9(5):682–99.
14. Delanaye P, Melsom T, Ebert N, Bäck S, Mariat C, Cavalier E, et al. Iohexol plasma clearance for measuring glomerular filtration rate in clinical practice and research: a review. Part 2: why to measure glomerular filtration rate with iohexol? Clin Kidney J. 2016;9(5):700–4.
15. Cockcroft D, Gault H. Prediction of creatinine clearance from serum creatinine. Nephron. 1976;41:31–41.
16. Levey A, Coresh J, Greene T, Stevens L, Zhang Y (Lucy), Hendriksen S, et al. Using standardized serum creatinine values in the modification of diet in renal disease study equation for estimating glomerular. Ann Intern Med. 2006;145(4):247–54.
17. Levey AS, Stevens LA, Schmid CH, Zhang YL, Iii AFC, Feldman HI, et al. A new equation to estimate glomerular filtration rate. Ann Intern Med. 2009;150:604–12.
18. Inker LA, Schmid CH, Tighiouart H, Eckfeldt JH, Feldman HI, Greene T, et al. Estimating glomerular filtration rate from serum creatinine and cystatin C. N Engl J Med. 2012;367(1):20–9.
19. Piccoli GB, Cabiddu G, Attini R, Vigotti F, Fassio F, Rolfo A, et al. Pregnancy in CKD: questions and answers in a changing panorama. Best Pract Res Clin Obstet Gynaecol. 2015;29(5):625–42.
20. Chawla LS, Bellomo R, Bihorac A, Goldstein SL, Siew ED, Bagshaw SM, et al. Acute kidney disease and renal recovery: consensus report of the Acute Disease Quality Initiative (ADQI) 16 Workgroup. Nat Rev Nephrol. 2017;13(4):241–57.
21. Brigden ML. Clinical utility of the erythrocyte sedimentation rate. Am Fam Physician. 1999;60(5):1443–50.
22. Harrison M. Erythrocyte sedimentation rate and C-reactive protein. Aust Prescr. 2015;38(3):93–4.
23. Pepys MB, Hirschfield GM. C-reactive protein: a critical update. J Clin Invest. 2003;111(12):1805–12.
24. Berger SP, Roos A, Daha MR. Complement and the kidney: what the nephrologist needs to know in 2006? Nephrol Dial Transpl. 2005;20(12):2613–9.
25. Solomon DH, Kavanaugh AJ, Schur PH. Evidence-based guidelines for the use of immunologic tests: antinuclear antibody testing. Arthritis Care Res (Hoboken). 2002;47(4): 434–44.

26. Jeong S, Yang D, Lee W, Kim G, Kim H, Ahn HS, et al. Diagnostic value of screening enzyme immunoassays compared to indirect immunofluorescence for anti-nuclear antibodies in patients with systemic rheumatic diseases: a systematic review and meta-analysis. Semin Arthritis Rheum. 2018;48(2):1–9.
27. Meroni PL, Schur PH. ANA screening: an old test with new recommendations. Ann Rheum Dis. 2010;69:1420–2.
28. Cozzani E, Drosera M, Gasparini G, Parodi A. Serology of lupus erythematosus: correlation between immunopathological features and clinical aspects. Autoimmune Dis. 2014;2014:321359.
29. Isenberg DA, Manson JJ, Ehrenstein MR, Rahman A. Fifty years of anti-ds DNA antibodies: are we approaching journey's end? Rheumatology. 2007;46(7):1052–6.
30. Gonza'lez C, Garcia B, Herra O, Gonza M. Anti-nucleosome, anti-chromatin, anti-dsDNA and anti- histone antibody reactivity in systemic lupus erythematosus. Clin Chem Lab Med. 2004;42(3):266–72.
31. Bizzaro N, Villalta D, Giavarina D, Tozzoli R. Are anti-nucleosome antibodies a better diagnostic marker than anti-dsDNA antibodies for systemic lupus erythematosus? A systematic review and a study of meta-analysis. Autoimmun Rev. 2012;12(2):97–106.
32. Didier K, Bolko L, Giusti D, Toquet S, Robbins A, Antonicelli F, et al. Autoantibodies associated with connective tissue diseases: what meaning for clinicians? Front Immunol. 2018;9:541.
33. Reveille JD, Solomon DH. Evidence-based guidelines for the use of immunologic tests: Anticentromere, Scl-70, and nucleolar antibodies. Arthritis Care Res (Hoboken). 2003;49(3):399–412.
34. Pengo V, Banzato A, Bison E, Denas G, Padayattil Jose S, Ruffatti A. Antiphospholipid syndrome: critical analysis of the diagnostic path. Lupus. 2010;19(4):428–31.
35. Miyakis S, Lockshin MD, Atsumi T, Branch DW, Brey RL, Cervera R, et al. International consensus statement on an update of the classification criteria for definite antiphospholipid syndrome (APS). J Thromb Haemost. 2006;4(2):295–306.
36. Moore GW. Recent guidelines and recommendations for laboratory detection of lupus anticoagulants. Semin Thromb Hemost. 2014;40(2):163–71.
37. Parkpian V, Verasertniyom O, Vanichapuntu M, Totemchokchyakarn K, Nantiruj K, Pisitkul P, et al. Specificity and sensitivity of anti-beta2-glycoprotein I as compared with anticardiolipin antibody and lupus anticoagulant in Thai systemic lupus erythematosus patients with clinical features of antiphospholipid syndrome. Clin Rheumatol. 2007;26(10):1663–70.
38. Seelen MA, Trouw LA, Daha MR. Diagnostic and prognostic significance of anti-C1q antibodies in systemic lupus erythematosus. Curr Opin Nephrol Hypertens. 2003;12(6):619–24.
39. Csernok E, Moosig F. Current and emerging techniques for ANCA detection in vasculitis. Nat Rev Rheumatol. 2014;10(8):494–501.
40. Damoiseaux J, Csernok E, Rasmussen N, Moosig F, van Paassen P, Baslund B, et al. Detection of antineutrophil cytoplasmic antibodies (ANCAs): a multicentre European Vasculitis Study Group (EUVAS) evaluation of the value of indirect immunofluorescence (IIF) versus antigen-specific immunoassays. Ann Rheum Dis. 2017;76(4):647–53.
41. Mcadoo SP, Pusey CD. Anti-glomerular basement membrane disease. Clin J Am Soc Nephrol. 2017;12:1162.
42. Radice A, Trezzi B, Maggiore U, Pregnolato F, Stellato T, Napodano P, et al. Clinical usefulness of autoantibodies to M-type phospholipase A2 receptor (PLA2R) for monitoring disease activity in idiopathic membranous nephropathy (IMN). Autoimmun Rev. 2016;15(2):146–54.
43. Beck LHJ, Bonegio RGB, Lambeau G, Beck DM, Powell DW, Cummins TD, et al. M-type phospholipase A2 receptor as target antigen in idiopathic membranous nephropathy. N Engl J Med. 2009;361(1):11–21.
44. Tomas NM, Beck LHJ, Meyer-Schwesinger C, Seitz-Polski B, Ma H, Zahner G, et al. Thrombospondin type-1 domain-containing 7A in idiopathic membranous nephropathy. N Engl J Med. 2014;371(24):2277–87.
45. Paixao-Cavalcante D, Lopez-Trascasa M, Skattum L, Giclas PC, Goodship TH, de Cordoba SR, et al. Sensitive and specific assays for C3 nephritic factors clarify mechanisms underlying complement dysregulation. Kidney Int. 2012;82(10):1084–92.
46. Motyckova G, Murali M. Laboratory testing for cryoglobulins. Am J Hematol. 2011;86(6):500–2.
47. Wang H, Zheng C, Lu Y, Jiang Q, Yin R, Zhu P, et al. Urinary fibrinogen as a predictor of progression of CKD. Clin J Am Soc Nephrol. 2017;12(12):1922–9.
48. Wang Y, Zheng C, Xu F, Liu Z. Urinary fibrinogen and renal tubulointerstitial fibrinogen deposition: discriminating between primary FSGS and minimal change disease. Biochem Biophys Res Commun. 2016;478(3):1147–52.
49. Roy S, Pitcock JA, Etteldorf JN. Prognosis of acute poststreptococcal glomerulonephritis in childhood: prospective study and review of the literature. Adv Pediatr Infect Dis. 1976;23:35–69.
50. Balasubramanian R, Marks SD. Paediatrics and international child health post-infectious glomerulonephritis. Paediatr Int Child Health. 2017;37(4):1–8.

Further Reading and Guidelines

KDIGO guidelines for CKD evaluation and management: https://kdigo.org/guidelines/ckd-evaluation-and-management/.

NICE guidance: Chronic kidney disease in adults: assessment and management Clinical guideline [CG182]: https://www.nice.org.uk/guidance/cg182/chapter/1-Recommendations#investigations-for-chronic-kidney-disease-2.

2019 European League Against Rheumatism/American College of Rheumatology Classification Criteria for Systemic Lupus Erythematosus: https://onlinelibrary.wiley.com/doi/full/10.1002/art.40930.

Kidney Biopsy

Lakshman Weerasekara, Nick Woodward, and Mark Harber

Contents

Supplementary Information The online version of this chapter (https://doi.org/10.1007/978-3-030-76419-7_4) contains supplementary material, which is available to authorized users.

M. Harber (ed.), *Primer on Nephrology*, https://doi.org/10.1007/978-3-030-76419-7_4

Learning Objectives

- To appreciate the indications, contraindications and risks of renal biopsy.
- To illustrate the techniques and alternative approaches of renal biopsy and to consider the entire patient pathway in terms of information and after care.

4

4.1 Introduction

The percutaneous renal biopsy (PRB) was first practiced and described in Denmark by Poul Iverson and Claus Brun in 1951, and despite the advances in other diagnostic tests, it remains critical to the diagnosis, management and prognosis of the renal transplant and many nephrological conditions [1].

In experienced hands using real-time ultrasound and spring-loaded biopsy guns, the procedure has become routine, often performed as a day case, and should have a diagnostic yield of 95% with a significant complication rate of <5% [2]. This chapter will discuss the indications and practical aspects of non-directed renal biopsy.

4.2 Indications and Contraindications for Renal Biopsy

However prosaic biopsies have become, obtaining a suitable diagnostic core safely is a skilled procedure; thus, for those providing a renal biopsy service and those requesting a biopsy, the risk-benefit ratio for the patient remains an important consideration. If the operators are relatively inexperienced and doing infrequent biopsies, then the risk for the patient is likely to be significantly higher, and a renal service needs to mitigate this risk.

As with all invasive procedures, it is of value to define patients as standard or increased risk; while standard risk patients are perfectly capable of having complications, the threshold for requesting a biopsy in an increased risk patient should be higher.

The indications for renal biopsy are shown in ◻ Fig. 4.1, but it is worth noting that there is variation in practice globally; a survey of 166 nephrologist worldwide, while showing strong alignment of practice for biopsing adults with nephrotic syndrome or a rapidly progressive glomerulonephritis, revealed a significant variation in practice for softer abnormalities such as low-level proteinuria and isolated haematuria [3].

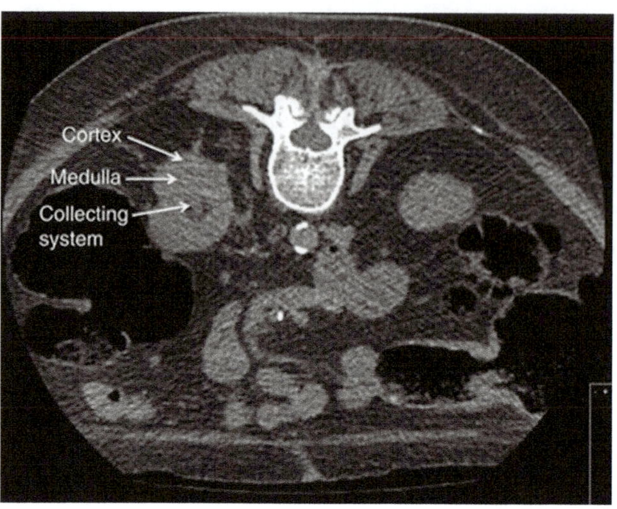

◻ **Fig. 4.1** Prone unenhanced CT at the level of the lower pole of the left kidney

4.3 Indications (See ◻ Table 4.1)

The decision to advocate a renal biopsy will very much be determined by individual circumstances: whether the likely diagnosis can be established without a biopsy, how high risk the treatment for the presumed diagnosis is, and how safely a biopsy could be done. In essence, what is the question being asked in terms of diagnosis, prognosis and response to treatment, and can it be reliably answered without a biopsy? A unit with a fairly inexperienced biopsy service should have a higher threshold for PRB and may benefit from developing skilled urine microscopy.

In the broadest sense, the indications for a biopsy are divided into two: firstly, investigation of specific renal abnormalities (unexplained abnormal urinary sediment or impaired renal function), by far the commonest group, and secondly, to assist in the diagnosis of a suspected multisystem disease with evidence of renal involvement, such as vasculitis or persistent infection.

Acute Kidney Injury: In the majority of cases of AKI, the diagnosis is not in doubt and the acute kidney injury is explained by preceding hypotension, sepsis, or medication especially in the setting of pre-existing CKD; in these circumstances a biopsy is likely to contribute little but hazard. However, there are times when a biopsy can add substantially to the management of AKI (see ◻ Table 4.1):

1. Rapidly progressive glomerular nephritis. In the setting of an active urine deposit, a biopsy may be critical to exclude a rapidly progressive glomerular

Table 4.1 Indications for nondirected renal biopsy

AKI	1. Rapidly progressive AKI
	2. AKI without obvious explanation
	3. AKI in the setting of undiagnosed systemic illness
	4. Failure to recover from AKI
Proteinuria	Nephrotic syndrome in adults
	Steroid-resistant nephrotic syndrome in children
	Moderate unexplained proteinuria with renal impairment or haematuria
Microscopic haematuria	Non-lower urinary tract haematuria with renal impairment and hypertension or in potential live donor or to aid counselling in the setting of a family history
Pyuria	Unexplained pyuria in the context of renal impairment
Tubular dysfunction	Unexplained tubular abnormalities without an obvious aetiology
CKD	Unexplained CKD in the setting of relatively preserved renal size/cortex
Diagnosis and monitoring of systemic disease	Response to treatment and prognosis in, e.g. vasculitis, SLE, myeloma, sarcoid, Sjogren's
Transplantation	Graft dysfunction (exclusion of rejection, recurrent disease, BKV and other infections, quantification of IFTA)
	Protocol biopsy

nephritis for which getting the *correct* treatment urgently has very significant consequences (e.g. anti-GBM disease or infective endocarditis).

2. A proportion of patients will present with AKI in the absence of any obvious hypotension or sufficient comorbidity to fit with the degree of renal impairment, and in these individuals a biopsy may diagnose either a chronic underlying renal disease or an active unanticipated renal disease such as acute interstitial nephritis.
3. Occasionally AKI occurs in the setting of unexplained constitutional illness, and assuming there is convincing evidence of direct renal involvement (haematuria, proteinuria or pyuria), then a renal biopsy may be the most direct approach to a diagnosis (e.g. sarcoid, tuberculosis, systemic vasculitis, cryoglobulinaemia, endocarditis).
4. Finally, in a patient who would be expected to recover renal function within days or a few weeks of a limited renal insult. When this is not the case and the persistence of oliguria is unexpected, then a biopsy may be helpful in determining prognosis of recovery or establishing renal disease such as acute TIN or renal infection. As a rule of thumb, if the patient is still oliguric 6 weeks post-AKI, then a biopsy may be helpful; however, the timing for this would be sooner if the primary insult was mild or the threshold would be higher if there have been multiple significant insults.

Nephrotic syndrome is a common indication for renal biopsy; however, in paediatric practice, it is unusual to biopsy a patient at first presentation as the real issue is whether the nephrotic syndrome is steroid responsive. Thus, patients are only offered a biopsy if they fail to respond to a course of steroids. In adults the equation is very different, for example, a significant proportion of nephrotic adults will have membranous glomerulonephritis, amyloid, or mesangiocapillary glomerulonephritis for which there is no evidence that steroid monotherapy has any benefit. Committing all nephrotic adults to a prolonged course of steroids on speculation would inflict serious side effects with no benefit for a significant proportion, and thus most units have a low threshold for biopsy in adults with nephrotic syndrome. However, in certain nephrotic adults, a renal biopsy can be avoided. For example, in diabetic patients with evidence of long-standing, low-grade proteinuria and/or diabetic eye disease, the nephrotic syndrome would be very much secondary to diabetic nephropathy, and the diagnosis can be made on clinical grounds. Also, in nephrotic adults with suspected systemic amyloidosis the histological diagnosis can often be made by non-invasive techniques such as abdominal wall fat aspiration or SAP scan.

In patients with isolated sub-nephrotic range proteinuria, the indications are more controversial; significant proteinuria in any renal disease is an adverse prognostic factor, and reduction of proteinuria by any means such as control of blood pressure and blockade of the renin angiotensin system improves the prognosis. Therefore, the majority of patients will go on to receive this treatment whatever the underlying condition; however, it is common to biopsy non-diabetic patients with isolated proteinuria >1 g/day or a consistent PCR >100 to exclude other potentially treatable conditions particularly if there is evidence of declining renal function.

Isolated Microscopic Haematuria

It is usual, in patients over 40 with isolated microscopic haematuria, to exclude lower urinary tract disease/malignancy before assuming a renal lesion. The underlying renal pathology is usually either IgA glomerulonephritis, hereditary abnormalities of the GBM (e.g. Alport syndrome) or thin basement membrane disease. In this setting there is very little in the way of specific treatments, and thus benefits of a biopsy predominantly relate to prognosis for the patient (particularly for insurance purposes), especially in the context of potential live donation, and family if excluding a heritable glomerular basement membrane abnormality (GBM) abnormality. In practical terms and in the absence of the indications above, most units will merely recommend observation unless hypertension or renal impairment intervenes; however with newer therapies for IgA and other conditions on the horizon, the benefits of a PRB in this group may increase.

▪ **Pyuria**

It is conventional wisdom to avoid a renal biopsy in the context of a UTI for fear of generating an abscess; however, it is not uncommon of to make a diagnosis of pyelonephritis on a biopsy with a culture-negative MSU, and there is little or no data indicating the degree of risk for abscess formation following a biopsy. Similarly, the diagnosis of renal TB or sarcoid may only be made following a biopsy in a patient with sterile pyuria and renal impairment.

▪ **Tubular Disorders**

It is rare that a biopsy is necessary for the diagnosis of tubular disorders, but very occasionally electron microscopy can reveal the underlying cause, for example, in Fanconi syndrome an underlying mitochondrial cytopathy, dysproteinuria and heavy metal poisoning are worth considering if the primary diagnosis is not obvious.

▪ **CKD**

Patients with CKD 4–5 with small kidneys are at very high risk from a biopsy, and it is much less common that the risk-benefit ratio justifies the investigation. There is a stronger imperative if the primary disease cannot be diagnosed by less-invasive tests, and there is a high likelihood of clinically relevant recurrence post-transplant. In practice this is rare; diseases with significant impact if not identified such as Goodpasture's syndrome, atypical HUS, systemic vasculitis, primary hyperoxalosis and SLE can usually be diagnosed without recourse to a biopsy, and conditions such as IgA which require a biopsy for diagnosis have limited impact post-transplant and would not alter the decision to transplant. However, very rarely conditions with significant impact on a future transplant such as membranoproliferative GN may only be diagnosed via renal biopsy.

▪ **Diagnosis of a Systemic Disease**

Finally, renal biopsy can be critical in establishing a diagnosis in systemic disease, and occasionally repeat biopsy can act as a barometer of disease control in the absence of other less-invasive markers. Most commonly this is in the context of connective tissue diseases such as vasculitis and SLE with an active urine deposit. However, a biopsy may demonstrate deposition of light chains in myeloma and evidence of endocarditis or of HIV-related nephropathy which might provoke a change in management. Similarly, biopsy of enlarged kidneys with dysfunction can diagnose infiltration and escalation of treatment in lymphoproliferative disorders.

4.4 Contraindications

In the majority of patients with significant contraindications to renal biopsy, it is possible to make a diagnosis and management plan based on urine microscopy and other clinical features. However, it is important to note that most of the contraindications to renal biopsy (◘ Table 4.2) are relative, in that if a biopsy is *really* critical to patient management, it is often possible to reduce the risk of a PRB or to use alternative approaches. The coagulopathy of renal failure is covered in ▶ Chap. 75, but a uremic patient is likely to have significant platelet dysfunction, and in practical terms there is no routinely available test (including bleeding time) that can predict this accurately. In uremic patients there is a correlation with the risk of bleeding at haemoglobins below 10 g/dl; thus, in high-risk patients it is common to optimise the risk by dialysis (if dialysis dependent) and transfusion the day before a biopsy. Amyloidosis was said to increase the risk of PRB, but a recent retrospective study has demonstrated no apparent excess in complications.

It is important for the unit to have a robust system in place to ensure that low molecular weight heparins (which will not be detectable with PT and PTT assays) are suspended 24 h prior to biopsy.

Finally, an increasing proportion of renal patients is on anti-platelet agents. Conventionally aspirin is stopped a week before an elective biopsy; however, when given for secondary prevention, there seems to be an increased risk of acute coronary events [4] and cerebrovascular events [5] on stopping aspirin. A recent review suggests stopping clopidogrel 3–5 days prior to surgical procedures and continuing aspirin in general patients [6]. Clearly the risk-benefit ratio needs to be decided on an individual basis with the caveat that a patient with significant cardiovascular morbidity is unlikely to tolerate a substantial bleed very well.

Desmopressin (DDAVP) V2 antagonist results in a release of stored ultra-large von Willebrand factor multimers and factor VIII. The effect lasts from 1 to 24 h and can be used in uremic high-risk patients to promote

Table 4.2 Contra-indications to nontargeted native renal biopsy

contra-indications	
Uncooperative patient	Absolute contraindication if unable or unwilling to cooperate with breath holding. If lacking capacity and biopsy essential, consider biopsy under a general anaesthetic
Uncontrolled bleeding diathesis	Absolute contraindication if uncontrolled, relative if correctable (see coagulation in renal disease ► Chap. 75)
Severe hypertension	Kidney vasculature poorly able to autoregulate even if blood pressure is acutely controlled
Relative contraindications	
Renal mass	Potential risk of neoplastic spread
Polycystic kidneys	High risk and low diagnostic yield
Small end-stage kidneys	Very high risk and low diagnostic yield
Acute bacterial pyelonephritis	Risk of perinephric abscess formation; lower UTI is a relative contraindication
Solitary kidney, horseshoe kidney	Increased risk of dialysis dependence but relatively safe in experienced hands, open or laparoscopic biopsy alternatives
Obstructed kidneys	Increased risk of urinary leak
Uraemia	Relative contraindication, due to platelet dysfunction; where possible correct prior to biopsy and consider DDAVP
Severe obesity	Biopsy becomes technically more difficult and dangerous with increasing obesity. Transjugular, laparoscopic, and open biopsy may offer significant advantage. Consider lateral approach for PRB
Third trimester pregnancy	Relatively contraindicated, dilated system, risk of foetal loss, but rarely necessary after second trimester and before delivery. Consider erect sitting position if essential
Vascular abnormalities	Aneurysms (e.g. PAN), arteriovenous malformations

platelet aggregation. One randomised trial demonstrated a reduction in bleeding and hematoma size with prophylactic DDAVP in PRB [7]. However, it can induce coronary vasospasm in patients with ischemic heart disease, and our practice is to ensure that it is given slowly (>1 h) and only to those with a low risk of coronary disease.

4.5 Procedure PRB

Renal biopsies are now generally obtained using spring-loaded biopsy guns using 14–18 gauge needles (typically 16G for native and 18G for transplants); increasingly, biopsy guns are also disposable, but if using a non-disposable gun, a robust process for post-procedure sterilisation is mandatory. Biopsies should be performed under real-time ultrasound (curvilinear ultrasound probes are preferred as lower-frequency range gives a larger field of view and greater depth than linear probes). The probe should be covered by a sterile, disposable probe cover procedure performed with full aseptic technique.

There is a strong argument for the use of a pre-biopsy checklist (similar to that used in many theatres globally) ensuring correct patient, correct indication, safe clotting and identification of any other anticoagulant issues, family or personal history of bleed disorders, imaging to identify two functioning kidneys, controlled blood pressure, etc.

The technique for native biopsies is beautifully illustrated on the video produced by Dr. Peter Topham and Dr. Sue Carr at Leicester Royal Infirmary (see Video 4.1). The technique for transplant biopsies is slightly different and again nicely illustrated on the video produced by Mr. Peter Veitch and Arundhati M. at UCL Centre for Nephrology (see Video 4.2).

Skewing things in your favour by ensuring a good- and high-resolution US scanner, properly darkened room and good positioning of a relaxed patient is fundamental to success and safety. Figs. 4.1 and 4.2 show CT and ultrasound images of the lower pole of a native kidney in a prone patient.

It is important to note that patients are often, understandably, nervous about the biopsy, and it is also imperative to ensure that the patient is thoughtfully talked through the procedure and reassured.

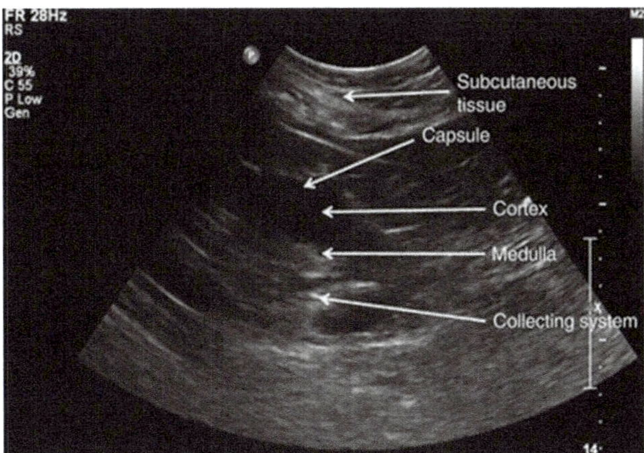

Fig. 4.2 Prone ultrasound, same patient

It is rarely necessary to biopsy a patient in the third trimester, but sometimes a biopsy is required in the second trimester, and if not possible to do this prone, the patient can be sat upright on the bed with arms and head resting on a table. Obese patients can sometimes be biopsied lying laterally with pillows supporting their middle or biopsied from a lateral approach (▶ Case 4.14.1).

4.6 Anatomy and Complications and Consent

Complication rates in the literature vary significantly depending on definition, how studiously they were looked for and how high risk the biopsy is. There is almost certainly a significant publication bias in favour of low rates. What follows is a rough and hopefully reasonable summation of the risks; ultimately complications will depend on local practice and experience, but individuals and units should be audited against these outcomes on a regular basis and quote their complication risks to patients when consenting [8–10].

Temporary local pain and discomfort on administration of local anaesthetic is universal but should subside rapidly, and patients should be prewarned of this. Native renal biopsies tend to be more uncomfortable than biopsy of a superficial denervated renal transplant kidney.

1. Bleeding is the commonest and the major complication of renal biopsy (see ◘ Figs. 4.3, 4.4 and 4.5). In a meta-analysis of 34 studies involving more than 9000 patients who underwent real-time native kidney

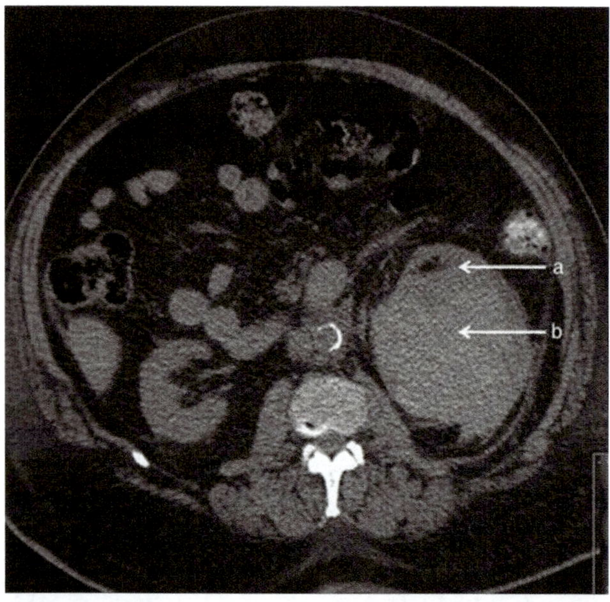

◘ **Fig. 4.3** CT scan of subcapsular haematoma following biopsy of the left kidney. The left kidney (*a*) is displaced anteriorly, secondary to a high-density collection (*b*)

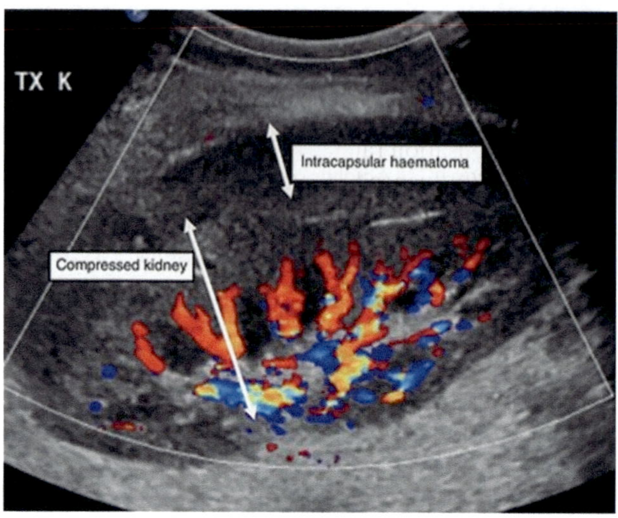

◘ **Fig. 4.4** Intracapsular haematoma causing gross compression of the kidney (Page kidney) and anuria in a transplant recipient. Urine flow was restored instantly with surgical decompression

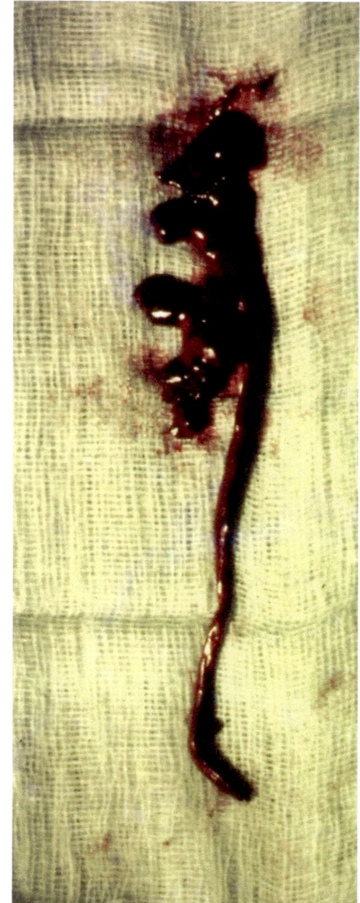

◘ **Fig. 4.5** After a routine biopsy, a patient had difficulty passing urine and macroscopic haematuria was observed. He subsequently passed a clot-cast of his pelvi-calyceal system and ureter, which, understandably elicited anxiety and subsequent awe in near equal measure. He had no further bleeding after this and remained stable

biopsy, the rate of bleeding complications are as follows [11]:

(a) Macroscopic haematuria: 3.5%.
(b) Bleeding requiring transfusion: 0.9%.
(c) Embolisation rate to control bleeding post-PRB: 0.6% (influenced by availability).
(d) Loss of kidney or nephrectomy rate: 0.01% (it is important to discuss this as a potential complication for transplant and solitary kidney biopsy).
(e) Mortality rate associated with PRB: 0.02% (and mostly secondary to bleeding complications but occasionally perforation).

Perirenal haematoma appears to be a very common complication with rates of 57–85%, but for the majority of patients, haematoma in itself appears to have had little consequence. However, rarely a subcapsular haematoma may cause kidney' (see ◘ Figs. 4.3 and 4.4) and, in a single kidney, acute oliguria requiring urgent surgical decompression. The rates of bleeding complications varied according to the risk factors, and high-risk patients had, perhaps not surprisingly, a higher risk of bleeding manifestations than the standard-risk patients.

Statistically significant risk factors for bleeding included use of a 14 gauge needle compared with smaller needles (2.1 vs 0.5%), creatinine over 176, age over 40 and BP >130 mm Hg [11]. In a review of 750 PRBs (with a high complication rate of 13%), a lower haemoglobin (110 vs 120) and higher creatinine (a common observation) were significant risk factors [8].

2. Failure of technique or diagnostic inadequacy of 5% (important to mention this during the consent process).
3. Percutaneous infection with aseptic technique experience suggests that this seems rare and the risk of a renal/perirenal abscess following a biopsy in the presence of urosepsis is difficult to define and rarely consented for.
4. Biopsy of non-renal tissue should be rare; however, it is not unheard of to obtain small bowel with native PRB; anecdotal evidence seems to suggest this is of little consequence. Biopsy of the large bowel, gallbladder or pancreas is rarer but potentially much more serious. The first indication of this may be from the histopathologist, and histology of non-renal offal needs to be reliably and rapidly conveyed to the physicians looking after the patient in which case patients should be carefully reassessed closely monitored and discussed with surgeons and radiology colleagues.
5. Arteriovenous fistulae (AVF) on the other hand appear to be common if specifically screened for. As 95% of AVF appear to resolve spontaneously, this complication tends not to be quoted for when obtaining consent. However, AVF that do not resolve pose a potential hazard for future biopsies, the kidney and potentially the patient in terms of high output (◘ Fig. 4.6) (a bruit over the kidney, persistent haematuria or an otherwise unexplained fall in GFR

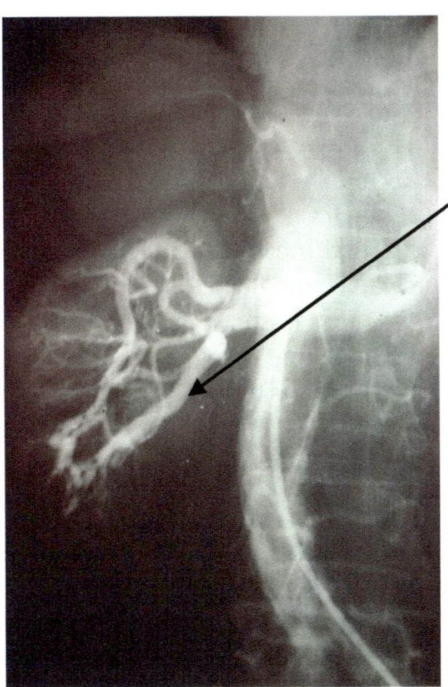

◘ **Fig. 4.6** Angiogram demonstrating a large AV fistula following a native renal biopsy. The only hint of this initially was a post-biopsy deterioration in renal function (creatinine increasing from 104 to 145). The lower half of the kidney had very little perfusion as blood rapidly short-cut to the renal vein. The differential for decline in function was a Page kidney (see below) or an AVM; the latter was suspected by auscultating a loud bruit Embolisation risks permanent loss of perfusion to a significant portion of the kidney, but if not spontaneously resolving, a high output shunt may grow and render the rest of the kidney increasingly ischaemic

secondary to a significant steal from the kidney should raise suspicion).

Acute oligoanuria post-transplant is likely due to the following:

(a) Shock: this is usually pretty obvious.
(b) Clot retention: easily diagnosed by US or catheterisation.
(c) Page kidney: subcapsular haematoma may tamponade the kidney and cause complete anuria in a transplant recipient or patients with a solitary native kidney, but often missed in native biopsies once identified urgent surgical decompression can instantly restore perfusion to a transplant kidney but risks further bleeding by removing any tamponade; the optimum option is to surgically decompress the kidney and perform selective radiological embolisation immediately if haemostasis cannot be achieved. Missed Paged kidney following a native kidney biopsy might cause chronic hypertension, or a step decline in GFR immediately after the biopsy which may persist or improve over time.
(d) Urinary leak: this seems to be a very rare complication but important not to miss. Likely to be associated with raised inflammatory markers and pain, it may be identifiable on delayed film MAG-3. Persistent urinary leak can cause urinoma formation and associated complications.

4.7 Post-Biopsy Monitoring

Typical post-biopsy monitoring would be pulse and blood pressure monitoring as follows: every 15 min for an hour; then if stable, every 30 min for 2 h; then if stable, every hour for 4 h; and then if stable and the patient has passed urine (without haematuria), mobilise and discharge; if an inpatient (high-risk patient), then continue 4-hourly monitoring for 24 hours.

The most critical aspect of post-biopsy monitoring is that nursing and medical staff are familiar with the procedure and are comfortable escalating monitoring and requesting medical review at the first sign of a complication. Performing renal biopsies on wards not familiar with post-biopsy observations and appropriate escalation is to be avoided.

The timing of complications is important and somewhat controversial; one large study detected 38% of complications within 4 h, 67% by 8 h, 89% by 12 h and 91% by 24 h [12]. This data would imply that day-case biopsies would not be safe, yet a third of complications occurring after 8 h does not seem to be general experience, and day-case biopsies in standard-risk patients seem to have a high safety record.

On discharge patients should be educated to avoid heavy exercise and contact sports for at least 10 to 14 days to minimise post-biopsy bleeding risk. We recommend that patients do not drive a vehicle for at least 24 hours post-biopsy.

4.8 Day-Case Vs Inpatient Procedure

In the last two decades, standard-risk PRBs have been increasingly performed as day-case procedures. The published audits seem to have a good safety record, benefits to patients and significant cost savings [9, 12, 13].

There are no standard guidelines for who is suitable for day-case biopsy, but the criteria below seem to have been arrived at independently by several units and represent a reasonable starting place.

Suggested criteria for day-case renal biopsy:

1. Two kidneys ≥10 cm.
2. Blood pressure ≤ 150/90.
3. eGFR ≥30,
4. Hb ≥10 g/dl.
5. Platelets ≥100.
6. INR ≤1.2 PTT ≤1.2.
7. Off aspirin or clopidogrel for 7 days.
8. Lack of significant cardiovascular comorbidity.
9. BMI ≤30 (not significant centripetal obesity).
10. A responsible adult to transport home and at home to provide care and support for 24 h post-transplant.
11. Experienced operator and day ward staff.

The good outcome data presumably, in part, reflects that patients suitable for a day-case biopsy are carefully selected; thus, if the above criteria are breached, then the decision to proceed as a day-case biopsy must be discussed with the patient and should be made at a senior level.

Example of day-case and inpatient renal biopsy pro forma are attached and can be modified for local practice.

For inpatient biopsies it is less easy to be absolutist because there may be compelling reasons to perform a biopsy despite the increased risk, and depending on local expertise, options such as open, laparoscopic or transjugular biopsy might be employed.

4.9 Alternatives to PRB in High-Risk Patients (Table 4.3)

As levels of obesity and comorbidity increase, we will be increasingly faced with high-risk patients. There are a variety of alternatives to stand PRB nicely summarised in a review by Stiles et al. [14].

Table 4.3 Alternatives to PRB in high-risk patients

Technique	Advantages	Disadvantages	Possible indications
Open biopsy	Direct vision, very high diagnostic yield, direct haemostasis, suitable for ventilated patient	General anaesthetic, long recovery and hospitalisation, cost	Single kidney, kidney with multiple cysts, obese patient, patient unable to cooperate with breath holding
Laparo-scopic biopsy	Direct vision, very high diagnostic yield, direct haemostasis, less invasive than open biopsy, suitable for ventilated patient	General anaesthetic, long recovery and hospitalisation, cost	Single kidney, kidney with multiple cysts, obese patient, patient unable to cooperate with breath holding
Transvenous biopsy	Suitable for grossly obese, contractures preventing PRB, abnormal clotting, diagnostic yield 78–97% Suitable for ventilated patient	Contrast load, smaller sample size predominance of medulla	Simultaneous liver kidney biopsy, concomitant with dialysis line placement, obese patient, bleeding diathesis, patient unable to cooperate with breath holding

4.10 Open Renal Biopsy (ORB)

The definitive series of ORB was of 934 patients and reported 100% tissue adequacy with apparently no significant complications [15]. Open (and laparoscopic) approaches offer the distinct advantage of direct vision and direct haemostasis and thus can be helpful in patients with cysts or other focal abnormalities as well as other high-risk patients and those already ventilated. The need for general anaesthetic and significant recovery time however are not justified in standard-risk patients.

4.11 Laparoscopic Renal Biopsy (LRB)

There are several case series of LRB usually in the setting of high-risk patients. As with ORB direct vision means the diagnostic yield approaches 100% and immediate haemostasis can be performed. This offers a significant advantage in patients with a body habitus preventing PRB, mild bleeding disorders or focal abnormalities of the kidney. As with ORB this technique obligates a general anaesthetic but is less invasive, and the recovery time is likely to be less than for an ORB and again can be considered in patients already ventilated on ITU.

4.12 Transvenous Renal Biopsy (TVRB)

Transvenous renal biopsy (TVRB) (usually transjugular) has been reported in the setting of bleeding diathesis [16–19] or obesity [20] (mean BMI 44). The theoretical advantages are that (a) the capsule is less likely to be punctured, (b) any bleeding should be back into the vein, (c) any acute extracapsular bleeds demonstrated at the time can be embolised if significant, (d) tissue can be obtained in patients in whom the percutaneous approach is not feasible, e.g. grossly obese and (e) occasionally it may be combined with TJ liver biopsy in patients with workup for liver disease. Diagnostic yields of 78–97% have been reported and, in the largest study to date, major complications of only 1% [16], but other smaller studies have had significantly higher complication rates, and it is easy to inadvertently perforate the capsule. Since the technique requires a small amount of contrast, the contrast-induced nephropathy is also a potential complication of TVRB. In short TVRB is a useful albeit rarely used technique for high-risk patients if there is sufficient local expertise; however, it is not without risk and remains extremely important to correct coagulopathies as much as possible prior to biopsy.

4.13 Standards for Renal Biopsy

In 2010, the British Association for Paediatric Nephrology published suggested standards for renal biopsy [2] which are also a useful benchmark for adult patients with some amendments to consider (added in italics):

1. All patients should receive an appropriate patient information leaflet (PIL) about the biopsy procedure[1] *(in advance and, ideally, in their first language)* *(the patient or guardian should have a clear understanding of the indication for the biopsy)*.

1 The renal association has produced a PIL available on the website (▶ www.renal.org), and there is a similar PIL available on MedlinePlus and includes Spanish translation.

2. *Complication rates for macroscopic haematuria, transfusion, embolisation and loss of kidney (if single or transplant) should be quoted as part of consent.*
3. For both native and transplant biopsies, ≤3 passes should be achieved in 80% of occasions.
4. There should be adequate tissue for diagnosis on 95% of occasions.[2]
5. Major complications (defined as delay in discharge as a result of post-biopsy complications or requirements for further investigations or monitoring) should be <5% of biopsies.
6. *There should be on-site access to interventional radiology and surgeons experienced in dealing with a major renal bleed.*
7. *Operators should maintain a prospective audit of adequacy and complications.*

Informative, detailed request forms greatly assist the pathologist, while uninformative ones do not; it is thus good practice to ensure that the indication and clinical details are of a high standard.

The workup of a renal biopsy is reviewed in more detail elsewhere [21]; however, assessment requires light microscopy always, immunohistochemistry frequently and electron microscopy occasionally. Although there are many different approaches to technical aspects of these, the most important factor is the competence of the pathologist who is giving a report on the specimen. Different pathologists have their own preferences for the number of sections, whether serial sections are cut, which stains are used, whether immunofluorescence usually on frozen sections or an enzyme method such as immunoperoxidase on paraffin sections is used for immunohistological studies and whether electron microscopy, if available, is necessary on a particular specimen. Importantly if your laboratory processes biopsies for immunoperoxidase, then it is often possible to retrospectively obtain tissue for electron microscopy (see Howie [22]). Renal pathology is a highly specialised field, and it is important to have close liaison between clinicians and pathologists as well as consider presenting difficult cases between renal teams and pathologists.

Finally, pathology MDT meetings are an invaluable liaison between clinicians and pathologists, and it is important to document, in real time (ideally electronically), conclusions of these discussions and consequent treatment plans.

---

2 Adequacy: the general consensus is that for native renal biopsies, 10–15 glomeruli are an optimal number to exclude a focal glomerulonephritis (>20 ideal), but this definition of adequacy may be a little rigid as sometimes it is possible to make the diagnosis on a single glomerulus. Conversely, a sample of less than 10–15 may miss focal disease and therefore be unable to rule out other disease (such as interstitial nephritis or rejection in transplantation). For transplant biopsies, the Banff classification requires >10 glomeruli and two arteries with a minimum of seven glomeruli and one artery. A more pragmatic definition of adequacy is that if the cause of the renal dysfunction is identified, then the sample was adequate, if not, then adequate only if containing ≥10–15 glomeruli.

In the transplant setting, one large study reported a sensitivity for the diagnosis of acute rejection of 91% with a single core and 99% for two cores suggesting that if the index of suspicion for rejection is high then a second core should be taken if possible [23] (Colvin R B 1997 JASN (8) 1930–41).

Case Study

Case 1

A 60-year-old man with a BMI of 51, type 2 diabetes and COPD in the context of heavy smoking was seen with nephrotic syndrome (NS). The abrupt increase in his proteinuria from low-level microalbuminuria made diabetic nephropathy and secondary FSGS seem less likely alternative diagnoses important to exclude. All other blood screenings (including anti-phospholipase A2R antibody) were negative. Given the severity of his NS, it was felt that a biopsy would be in his interests. The combination of his obesity and COPD meant that a prone PRB was not possible and laparoscopic or open biopsy is also unappealing. The two options were felt to be transvenous or left lateral PRB, and the latter was performed with relative ease reducing the distance from >13 cm to approximately 6 cm by adopting a left lateral approach, without complications and demonstrated membranous glomerulonephritis. Imaging (◘ Fig. 4.7) demonstrates how a different angle made the kidney much more superficial and accessible. This patient was clearly at increased risk, not least because of the technical difficulties of a biopsy but also because he was anticoagulated before and after the biopsy due to his NS, and illustrates the importance of weighing up the risk-benefit as well as considering alternatives to conventional PRB.

Case 2

A 50-year-old man underwent a day-case PRB for isolated proteinuria. The biopsy was difficult, and during the biopsy the patient experienced sudden pain in the flank.

The procedure was abandoned, the patient admitted for observation, and a CT with contrast is performed which demonstrated no haematoma and was essentially normal. The following morning the patient appeared well and haemodynamically stable with no change in haemoglobin and on initial inspection well enough to go home, but his CRP was markedly elevated 245. On further assessment he had a pleural effusion on the side of biopsy and mild tenderness in the RUQ and flank. A repeat CT confirms the pleural effusion and demonstrated free fluid in the paracolic gutter. The differential diagnosis included haemothorax, perforated colon, perforated gallbladder, small bowel/duodenal puncture or pancreatic puncture.

The use of contrast CT is critical when assessing post-biopsy complications, in this case ruling out blood and a haemothorax. The absence of blood on the scan and the rapidly rising CRP were highly suggestive of a perforated viscus. The patient was given broad-spectrum antibiotics and taken to theatre where a perforated gallbladder was removed.

A unit that performs enough biopsies will at some point have a serious complication; having a high index of suspicion, close monitoring and a rapid MDT (radiological and surgical) review are critical to reducing the risk posed by such complications.

Case 3

A 38-year-old woman with systemic lupus erythematosus and a creatinine of 123 and two equal-sized kidneys (10.5 cm) underwent an uncomplicated PRB. She was reviewed with the result 10 days later and noted to be hypertensive and with a creatinine of 195. A MAG-3 scan revealed a non-functioning right kidney, and an urgent Doppler ultrasound demonstrated a subcapsular haematoma and minimal diastolic flow although a patent artery. The diagnosis was of a Page kidney: high intra-renal pres-

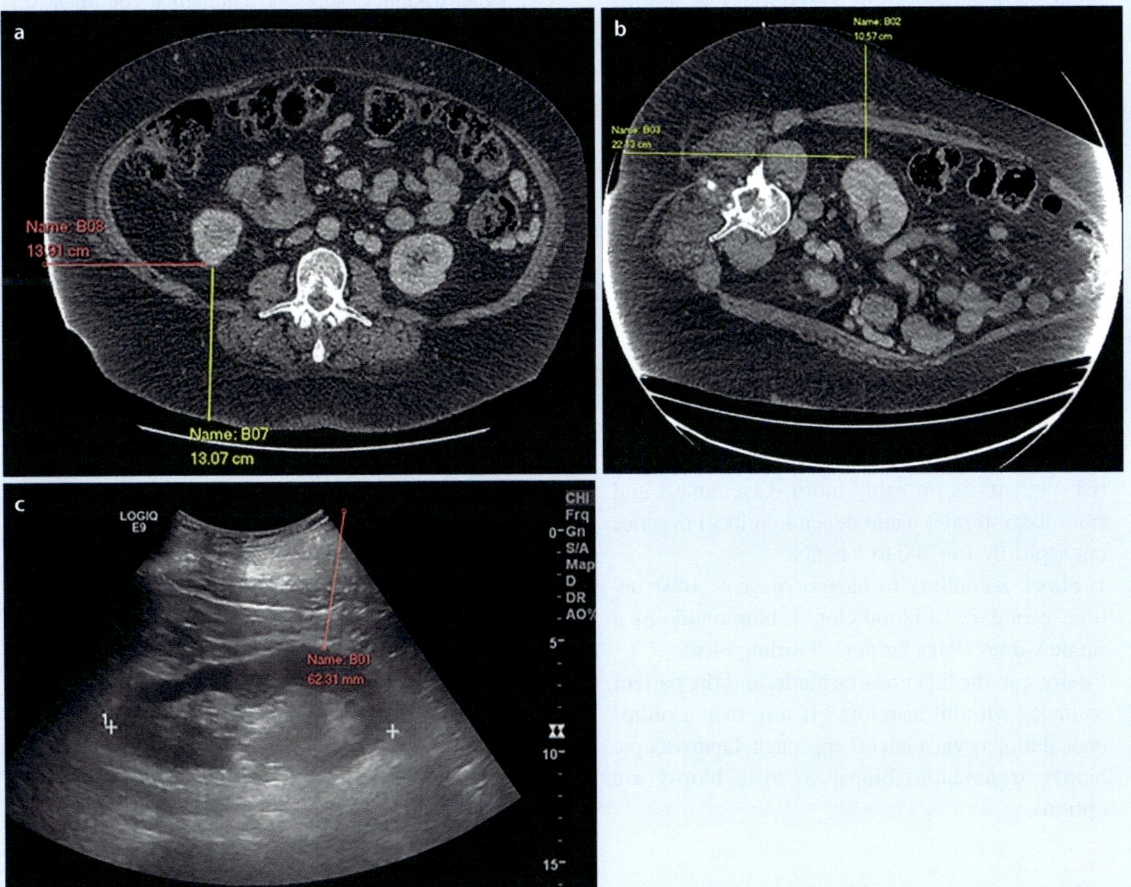

Fig. 4.7 **a** Showing distance from the skin to the lower pole of the kidney. **b** Change in position of the kidney with the patient in lateral position. **c** Shortened distance to the kidney at time of biopsy in left lateral position

sures reducing arterial perfusion. Over the next 4 weeks, her blood pressure settled and renal function improved to a baseline of 140. Subsequent MAG-3 scans showed the right kidney producing 30% of total renal function with no improvement over time.

A Page kidney can easily be missed in a patient with two kidneys and good function. Hypertension and a step increase in creatinine post-biopsy may indicate this complication. In a patient with a single kidney (transplant or otherwise) anuria and a rapid rise in creatinine, it is more obvious and serious. Surgical decompression of the kidney (if identified rapidly) resolves the problem, but decompressing the tamponade may release extensive bleeding, and this needs to be anticipated.

Questions

1. How many glomeruli are felt to be sufficient to exclude a focal process in native kidney and represent an adequate transplant biopsy to exclude rejection?
2. What rates of insufficient tissue for diagnosis, macroscopic haematuria, transfusion and embolisation following biopsy should be quoted?
3. What are the causes of oliguria post-biopsy?
4. What are the options for obtaining renal histology in a morbidly obese patient?

Answers

1. > 20 glomeruli is felt to be required to confidently exclude a focal process and > 10 to exclude rejection in a transplant patient. The diagnostic certainty in diagnosing or excluding rejection increases from 91% with one to 99% with two cores.
2. The answer to this question depends on audit of local practice but in general (a) failure of technique (to obtain sufficient material for diagnosis), 5%; macroscopic haematuria, 3–5%; need for blood transfusion, 1% (quoting 2% in increased risk patients is probably more reasonable); and embolisation rates again depend on local practice but typically 1 in 200 to 1 in 500.
3. 1. Shock secondary to haemorrhage, 2. obstruction secondary to blood clot, 3. tamponade of a single kidney (Page kidney), 4. urinary leak
4. Firstly, can the diagnosis be made, and the patient managed without histology? If not, then a radiological biopsy via a lateral approach, laparoscopic biopsy, transvenous biopsy or open biopsy are options.

References

1. Richards NT, Darby S, Howie AJ, Adu D, Michael J. Knowledge of renal histology alters patient management in over 40% of cases. Nephrol Dial Transplant. 1994;9(9):1255–9.
2. Hussain F, Mallik M, Marks SD, Watson AR. Nephrology on behalf of the BA of P. renal biopsies in children: current practice and audit of outcomes. Nephrol Dial Transplant. 2010;25(2):485–9.
3. Fuiano G. AJKD. 2000;35(3):448–57.
4. Ferrari E, Benhamou M, Cerboni P, Marcel B. Coronary syndromes following aspirin withdrawal: a special risk for late stent thrombosis. J Am Coll Cardiol. 2005;45(3):456–9.
5. Sibon I, Orgogozo JM. Antiplatelet drug discontinuation is a risk factor for ischemic stroke. Neurology. 2004;62(7):1187.
6. O'Connor SD, Taylor AJ, Williams EC, Winter TC. Coagulation concepts update. Am J Roentgenol. 2009;193(6):1656–64.
7. Manno C. Desmopressin acetate in percutaneous ultrasound-guided kidney biopsy: a randomized controlled trial. Am J Kidney Dis. 2010;57(6):850–5.
8. Whittier WL, Korbet SM. Timing of complications in percutaneous renal biopsy. J Am Soc Nephrol. 2004;15(1):142–7.
9. Preda A, Van Dijk L, Van Oostaijen J, Pattynama P. Complication rate and diagnostic yield of 515 consecutive ultrasound-guided biopsies of renal allografts and native kidneys using a 14-gauge Biopty gun. Eur Radiol. 2003;13(3):527–30.
10. Hergesell O, Felten H, Andrassy K, Kühn K, Ritz E. Safety of ultrasound-guided percutaneous renal biopsy-retrospective analysis of 1090 consecutive cases. Nephrol Dial Transplant. 1998;13(4):975–7.
11. Corapi KM, Chen JL, Balk EM, Gordon CE. Bleeding complications of native renal biopsy: a systematic review and meta-analysis. AJKD. 2012;60(1):62–73.
12. Khajehdehi P, Junaid SMA, Salinas-Madrigal L, Schmitz PG, Bastani B. Percutaneous renal biopsy in the 1990s: safety, value, and implications for early hospital discharge. Am J Kidney Dis. 1999;34(1):92–7.
13. Hussain F, Watson A, Hayes J, Evans J. Standards for renal biopsies: comparison of inpatient and day care procedures. Pediatr Nephrol. 2003;18(1):53–6.
14. Stiles KP, Yuan CM, Chung EM, Lyon RD, Lane JD, Abbott KC. Renal biopsy in high-risk patients with medical diseases of the kidney. Am J Kidney Dis. 2000;36(2):419–33.
15. Nomoto Y, Tomino Y, Endoh M, Suga T, Miura M, Nomoto H, Sakai H. Modified open renal biopsy: results in 934 patients. Nephron. 1987;45(3):224–8.
16. See T, Thompson B, Howie A, Karamshi M, Papadopoulou A, Davies N, Tibballs J. Transjugular renal biopsy: our experience and technical considerations. Cardiovasc Intervent Radiol. 2008;31(5):906–18.
17. Cluzel P, Martinez F, Bellin MF, Michalik Y, Beaufils H, Jouanneau C, Lucidarme O, Deray G, Grenier PA. Transjugular versus percutaneous renal biopsy for the diagnosis of parenchymal disease: comparison of sampling effectiveness and complications. Radiology. 2000;215(3):689–93.
18. Misra S, Gyamlani G, Swaminathan S, Buehrig CK, Bjarnason H, McKusick MA, Andrews JC, Johnson CM, Fervenza FC, Leung N. Safety and diagnostic yield of transjugular renal biopsy. J Vasc Interv Radiol. 2008;19(4):546–51.

19. Sarabu N, Maddukuri G, Munikrishnappa D, Martin KJ, Qazi RA, Alvarez A, Schmitz PG. Safety and efficacy of transjugular renal biopsy performed by interventional nephrologists. Semin Dial. 2011;24(3):343–8.
20. Fine DM, Arepally A, Hofmann LV, Mankowitz SG, Atta MG. Diagnostic utility and safety of transjugular kidney biopsy in the obese patient. Nephrol Dial Transplant. 2004;19(7):1798–802.
21. Amann K, Haas CS. What you should know about the work-up of a renal biopsy. NDT. 2006;21:1157–61.
22. Howie AJ. Handbook of renal biopsy pathology. 2nd ed. New York: Springer; 2008.
23. Colvin RB. 1997. JASN (8) 1930-41).

Imaging in Nephrology

Ciara N. Magee, Arum Parthipun, Antony Goode, and Asmat Abro

Contents

M. Harber (ed.), *Primer on Nephrology*, https://doi.org/10.1007/978-3-030-76419-7_5

Learning Objectives

1. To understand the advantages and disadvantages of each imaging modality in order to choose the most appropriate test, based both on the clinical question and pertinent patient factors.
2. To understand the role interventional radiology and nephrology can play in the management of the renal patient.

5

5.1 Introduction

Radiological imaging and interventions are increasingly utilised in the diagnosis and management of patients with renal disorders and merit careful consideration. Wider access to progressively sophisticated imaging techniques has facilitated the incidental identification of a range of renal disorders, while patients with chronic kidney disease can easily accumulate significant radiation, gadolinium and radio-contrast exposures over their lifetime.

In this chapter, we will discuss common diagnostic and interventional radiological procedures, their indications according to clinical scenarios, and the issues to consider when requesting their use in patients with kidney disease; to properly evaluate the clinical question, it is important to understand the benefits, limitations and diagnostic yields of each modality.

5.2 Diagnostic Imaging Governance and Radiation

The majority of diagnostic imaging techniques utilise ionising radiation, in the form of X-rays for plain radiography, computed tomography (CT) or fluoroscopy and gamma rays in nuclear medicine; it is therefore important to consider the risks and potential harm this poses to both patients and staff. The cumulative dose of radiation needs to be considered (Table 5.1), with careful selection of the appropriate investigation at the outset and avoidance of unnecessary repeat studies. A close, cooperative relationship between radiology, nuclear medicine and clinical staff, supported by a regular, formal clinico-radiological multidisciplinary team meeting (MDTM), is critical to the achievement of this. The organisation of a cancer MDTM is tightly defined and subject to peer review for quality assurance, with published guidelines on the conduct of a cancer MDTM for radiologists [1]. Non-cancer MDTMs, such as the nephrology MDTM, are not subject to such tight regulation; however the standards may still be used to guide its organisation. The nephrology MDTM should be attended by both junior and consultant nephrologists and be led by a radiologist with an appropriate interest. Local practice will vary, but in a unit where vascular access for dialysis or kidney transplants are performed, a surgeon who performs these procedures should attend in addition to the nephrology staff. The Royal College of Radiologists recommend that all imaging to be presented at the MTDM should be reviewed by the radiologist beforehand, and where resources allow, a coordinator may be employed to prepare a list of patients. Decisions taken during an MDTM should be recorded in the patient's notes, and the MDTM coordinator may assist with this – where possible, this should be done electronically with the record made visible to all members of the MDTM; the appointment of a nominated chairperson for the MDTM will allow the meeting to progress efficiently.

Table 5.1 Radiation dose for common imaging protocols

Examination	Effective dose (mSv)
1 day of background radiation	0.006
Chest X-ray	0.02
Abdomen X-ray	0.7
CT chest	7
CT pulmonary angiogram	15
CT KUB (low dose)	5
CT abdomen and pelvis	14
CT IVU	28
Nuclear medicine MAG3	2.6
Nuclear medicine DMSA	3.3
Whole-body PET-CT	25

Adverse outcomes related to radiation risk can be divided into deterministic or stochastic effects. Deterministic effects are those which will not happen below a certain threshold dose; once this dose is achieved, the likelihood of the event occurring becomes inevitable; examples include cataracts and skin erythema. These events occur at relatively high doses and are really only of consideration in certain circumstances, for example, complex interventional procedures where there may be a long period of screening over one part of the body. This effect is not cumulative – if the patient undergoes a further procedure in the future, the same dose of radiation is required to develop the complication. Pregnancy requires special attention and precautions, as it is recognised that there is a threshold dose of radiation above which adverse pregnancy and foetal outcomes occur with greater frequency; while the risk of this is greatest in the first trimester, particularly in the first 8 weeks, it is essential to minimise the radiation exposure of any patient who is pregnant. It is also important, however, to ensure that necessary imaging is not denied on a pregnant female; studies indicate that treating physicians and radiologists often overestimate the radiation risk to the foetus from a given investigation [2, 3].

Stochastic effects of radiation relate to the risk of cancer or genetic abnormalities, which increase linearly with the dose of radiation exposure, and can most usefully be measured by the effective dose of radiation. This is a theoretically calculated value that gives a weighted view of the radiation dose to the entire body and is quantified in sieverts; it cannot be measured directly but is instead calculated from the known radiation output. The average expected effective dose for different examinations is shown in ◘ Table 5.1 but may vary according to the equipment and size of the patient. Doses from certain examinations can be orders of magnitude greater than the yearly average background dose for an individual (2.7 mSv), and with serial examinations or multiphase CT, this can constitute significant risk. The risk of developing a fatal cancer is 5% per Sievert (Sv) effective dose or 1:20,000 per millisievert (mSv) and is cumulative, even if there has been a significant time period between exposures.

5.3 Diagnostic Radiology

5.3.1 Ultrasound

Medical sonography uses high-frequency sound waves (>20 kHz) to interrogate tissue reflectivity, thereby determining the nature of a structure, and is particularly useful in distinguishing between solid and cystic lesions: fluid-filled structures (e.g., bladder or cysts) do not reflect any sound, such that sound waves pass through and appear black; bone or calcification reflects sound waves, such that these structures appear white. Its use of tissue reflectivity rather than ionising radiation renders it versatile and capable of providing a myriad of information concerning pathological lesions (◘ Table 5.2); it is also particularly suited to repeat examinations.

From a renal perspective, ultrasound is the first-line examination in both acute kidney injury and chronic kidney disease, to investigate the size and parenchymal thickness of the kidneys and to determine if any structural abnormality, including hydronephrosis, exists. Kidneys are normally less echogenic than either the liver or spleen, and the appearance of increased echogenicity suggests the presence of renal parenchymal disease; this is however a non-specific finding and one which does not correlate with the degree or severity of kidney injury. Ultrasound is also routinely used to guide kidney biopsy and to characterise renal cysts or masses. Duplex ultrasonography combines traditional ultrasound with Doppler ultrasound which can detect the characteristics of blood flow and is thus a useful, non-invasive method of examination of arterial supply and venous drainage of the kidney; it should be the first-line investigation of acute transplant dysfunction. Ultrasound is not diagnostic for pyelonephritis: the kidneys do show changes under ultrasound; however these rarely manifest early, and a normal appearance does not exclude pyelonephritis; the role of ultrasound is better for detecting obstruction or renal/peri-renal abscess or collection secondary to the infection.

The sensitivity and role of ultrasound for different renal pathologies is discussed in ◘ Table 5.2.

5.3.2 CT Scan

Computed tomography (CT) uses X-rays to generate an image based on the density of the tissues being examined and is responsible for a large proportion (approximately 40%) of the annual dose of ionising radiation due to medical exposures.

While most soft tissues within the body attenuate X-rays by the same amount, and therefore appear as the same density or same shade of grey on an unenhanced CT scan, intravenous (IV) contrast agents concentrate in different organs to different degrees and so improve the distinction between tissues and organs. These contrast agents contain iodine, which, due to its relatively high atomic number, appears denser than the body's soft tissues, thereby improving the visualisation of blood vessels or tissues which have a higher blood flow. The sensitivity of CT for different aspects of the renal system is discussed in ◘ Table 5.2. The clinical scenario and question will determine both the need for IV contrast and, consequently, the timing of the scan following injection of the contrast medium. Depending on the suspected pathology, the scan protocol can be tailored so that IV contrast is within the arterial or venous system or delayed so that it is within the ureters or bladder. Examples of some commonly used protocols are shown in ◘ Table 5.3.

Where a radiological examination requires IV contrast, patients need to be assessed for their risk of an adverse reaction (see ◘ Table 5.4). In addition, there are different types of contrast media with differing toxicities, and the selection of agent will depend upon the clinical scenario and risk factors, as discussed below. Non-ionic, low or iso-osmolar iodinated media are five to ten times safer than the older, high osmolar ionic con-

5

Table 5.2 The sensitivity and role of ultrasound, CT scan and MRI for different renal pathologies

		Ultrasound	CT	MRI
Paren-chyma	Mass lesions	20% sensitivity for lesions <1 cm, 70% sensitivity for lesions sized 1–2 cm Allows Bosniak characterisation of cystic lesions. Superior to CT	76% sensitivity for lesions <1 cm, 95% sensitivity for lesions sized 1–2 cm. Allows assessment of fat, calcium and soft tissue content and enhancement pattern with IV contrast	100% sensitivity and 94% specificity for solid mass detection
	Scarring	37–100% sensitivity when compared to DMSA		
Collect-ing system	Calculi	30–90% sensitive for collecting system calculi. Sensitivity poor for small calculi	>90% sensitivity. Also allows assessment of other causes of flank pain	No role
	Tumour	TCC appears as solid hypoechoic mass. Can be mistaken for hydrone-phrosis	89–100% sensitivity for TCC on CT-IVU	No role
	Obstruc-tion	First-line test for diagnosis and grading of hydronephrosis. Excellent visualisation of the pelvicalyceal system when dilated	Sensitive for obstruction and helps demonstrate cause; however US is a better first-line test	MRU increasingly used for anatomical and functional assessment of obstruction
Ureters	Calculi	Poor visualisation of ureters with USS makes detection of calculi difficult. Will show if there is obstruction, hydronephrosis	98% sensitive for ureteric calculi. Also allows demon-stration of inflammatory change which may indicate recent stone passage	
	Tumour	No role	CT-IVU is 96% sensitive and 99% specific for TCC of the ureter. Also allows staging	
	Obstruc-tion			
Bladder	Wall lesions	63% sensitive for bladder tumours; direct visualisation is therefore needed in macroscopic haematuria to exclude bladder wall pathology. Endoscopic ultrasound is more sensitive but invasive	CT-IVU 79% sensitive for bladder wall tumours	Excellent for assessing invasion of tumour beyond bladder and involvement of local structures
	Emptying	Volumetric measurement of bladder pre- and post-micturition is simple and fast. Can also show bladder wall trabeculation, diverticula to suggest chronic outflow obstruction	No role	No role
Vascula-ture		Good for demonstrating general vascularity of the kidney and patency of main renal artery and vein RAS -0–70% sensitivity in experi-enced operators, increasing to >90% for transplant kidneys. Ultrasound does have a role in looking for asymmetry in renal sizes to suggest RAS	Renal perfusion can be assessed as can the renal vasculature Anatomical delineation for pre-transplant assessment	87% sensitive and 69% specific for RAS. Often overestimates degree of stenosis MR venography useful for venous anomalies but also for assessing central thoracic veins when planning tunnelled dialysis catheter insertion or AV fistula formation. MRA and MRV may also be used to assess pelvic vasculature when planning renal transplantation, in conjunction with unenhanced CT (MR does not show calcification in vessels well)

Table 5.3 The characteristics and applications of relevant CT protocols

Protocol	
CT KUB	Typically used to investigate the presence of renal tract calculi Lower dose of radiation used, no IV contrast required Not an optimal study to examine the renal parenchyma or other solid organs
CT abdomen	'Standard' abdominal/pelvic CT Requires IV contrast Timed so that most of the contrast is within the venous system, which allows lesions to be distinguished from normal soft tissue
CT IVU	Multi-phase protocol Unenhanced phase to detect calculi Venous/nephrogenic phase to study the renal parenchyma Delayed phase that displays the collecting system and ureters Radiation dose is relatively high, so patient selection is important
CT angiogram	Requires significant dose of IV contrast Timed so that IV contrast is within the arterial system Frequently used to assess renal arterial anatomy prior to potential live renal transplant donation

Table 5.4 Patients at risk of adverse reactions from intravenous contrast

1. Previous reaction
2. Asthma – Increases risk of a severe reaction by six to ten times
3. Renal impairment (up to date eGFR or creatinine is essential when making a radiology request)
4. Multiple allergies
5. Diabetes – Risk of development of lactic acidosis in patients with renal impairment when taking metformin. Consider stopping metformin for 48 hours after contrast in patients whose eGFR<60 ml/min/1.73m^2

trasts, with non-ionic contrast media reported to have an incidence of severe reactions of 0.04% and very serious reactions of 0.004% (see Table 5.5) [4, 5]. When an adverse reaction occurs, it is recommended that this is explicitly documented (preferably with the use of electronic record systems such as RIS/picture archiving and communication systems [PACS]) so that patients are better prepared for future imaging investigations [6]. The National Institute for Clinical Excellence (NICE) guidelines recommend that before offering iodine-based contrast media to adults for non-emergency imaging, patients are screened for co-existent CKD by measuring eGFR or by checking an eGFR result obtained within the past 3 months [7].

5.3.2.1 Contrast-Associated and Contrast-Induced Acute Kidney Injury (CA-AKI and CI-AKI)

The development of AKI following IV iodinated contrast administration has long been recognised, and until recently, any episode of AKI occurring within 48 hours of contrast administration, following the exclusion of other nephrotoxic factors, was termed contrast-induced nephropathy. In practice, however, it can be difficult to determine when the contrast media is culpable, as there are often several co-existent potential causes of AKI. Recent studies indicate that this has led to an overestimation of the nephrotoxic risk of iodinated contrast media, and in an effort to characterise these cases more clearly, consensus statements from the American College of Radiology (ACR) and the National Kidney Foundation (NKF) have endorsed the terms contrast-associated AKI (CA-AKI) and contrast-induced AKI (CI-AKI) [8].

> CA-AKI describes any AKI (according to the Kidney Disease: Improving Global Outcomes (KDIGO) definition) occurring within 48 hours after the administration of contrast media and is synonymous with the term post-contrast acute kidney injury (PC- AKI) [9].

Neither term indicates a causal link between the administration of intravenous contrast media but rather acknowledges correlation.

> CI-AKI denotes the subset of CA-AKI cases where a causal relationship between the contrast media and episode of AKI can be established.

CI-AKI is due to a combination of afferent arteriolar vasoconstriction and direct toxicity of the contrast media on renal tubular epithelial cells; peak injury (as reflected in serum creatinine) is usually seen 72 hours post-contrast. NICE guidelines recommend that before offering iodine-based contrast media to adults, their risk of acute kidney injury is assessed but that emergency imaging is not delayed [7]. While the primary risk factor for CA-AKI is reduced eGFR, multiple other patient-related risk factors have been reported [10–12] and are listed in Table 5.6; in studies where a diagnosis of CI-AKI could be established, the only evident risk factor was reduced eGFR.

In cases where an increased risk of CA-AKI exists (see Table 5.6), the first consideration is whether a different modality such as MRI, ultrasound or unenhanced CT will answer the clinical question. If contrast must be administered, the management focusses on prevention, as there is no specific treatment established (see Renal Association guidelines for prevention in Table 5.7). The joint ACR/NKF guidelines recommend prophylaxis for patients not undergoing dialysis who have an eGFR <30 mL/min/1.73 m^2 or AKI [8], KDIGO guidelines recommend a threshold of 45 ml/min/1.73m^2, while joint Renal Association (RA)/Royal College of Radiology (RCR) guidelines recommend prophylaxis in patients with an eGFR <40 ml/min/1.73m^2. A recent review of the evidence completed as part of the updated NICE guidelines indicated that oral fluid replacement was non-inferior to IV fluid replacement for prevention of CI-AKI [7] and that routine admission for pre-contrast volume expansion was not therefore indicated in stable outpatients capable of increasing their oral fluid intake. While there are some differences across guidelines as to the level of eGFR at which prophylaxis with IV fluids is indicated, either 0.9% sodium chloride or isotonic bicarbonate may be used as a replacement fluid [6, 7, 12–15]. There are no convincing data to support the use of n-acetyl cysteine (NAC), or any other pharmacological agents, as prophylaxis [6, 7]. Nephrotoxins should be discontinued, where feasible, while consideration may also be given to temporary cessation of angiotensin-converting enzyme (ACE) inhibitors and angiotensin II receptor blockers (ARBs). It is not advised to either commence dialysis or adjust the schedule thereof, on the basis of contrast administration.

Table 5.5 Adverse reactions to intravenous contrast

1. Anaphylactoid
2. Skin reactions, including delayed reactions up to 1 week after IV contrast
3. Thyrotoxicosis in patients with uncontrolled hyperthyroidism due to high iodine content of IV contrast
4. Contrast-induced acute kidney injury (CI-AKI)

Table 5.6 Risk factors for CA-AKI

Chronic kidney disease (adults with an eGFR <40 ml/min/1.73 m^2 are at particular risk)
Diabetes mellitus
Co-incident use of nephrotoxic agents
Reduced renal perfusion (e.g. heart failure)
Hypovolaemia
Hypoalbuminuria
Increasing volume of contrast agent
Intra-arterial administration of contrast medium with *first-pass renal exposure*

Table 5.7 Renal association guidelines for prevention of contrast nephropathy

1. Volume expansion IV 0.9% sodium chloride at a rate of 1 ml/kg/hour for 12 hours pre- and post-contrast OR IV isotonic sodium bicarbonate *NICE guidelines recommend oral hydration regimens in stable outpatients
2. Nephrotoxic drugs Withhold any potentially nephrotoxic drugs, including non-steroidal anti-inflammatory drugs and aminoglycosides Temporary cessation of ACEi/ARB use may be appropriate where a high risk of AKI exists Consider temporarily withholding metformin in patients with an eGFR <60/ml/min/1.73m^2
3. Minimise the volume of contrast media – By selecting the examination appropriate for the clinical question at the outset, the need for multiple radiological investigations, and, accordingly, the volume of contrast media required, can be minimised.
4. Measure renal function In stable patients, eGFR is the preferred measurement; however in patients with AKI, this should not be used. eGFR should be measured pre-examination in those at risk and 48–72 hours post-IV contrast to ensure it has remained stable

5.3.3 Intravenous Pyelography (IVP)

IVP is rarely performed now, as CT is superior for most applications. The IVP is, however, the investigation of choice in the diagnosis of medullary sponge kidney and papillary necrosis, as the superior spatial resolution of film radiography over CT better demonstrates the typical findings of both these conditions.

5.3.4 Magnetic Resonance Imaging (MRI)

MRI utilises the interaction between hydrogen ions (protons) and radiofrequency waves in the presence of a high magnetic field, producing images that are depen-

Table 5.8 Contraindications for MRI scanning with implants

Absolute contraindication	Pacemaker, otic implant, metal in eye or orbit, implanted cardiac defibrillator
Likely contraindication	Heart valve or aneurysm clip installed before 1996
Possible contraindication	Heart valve or aneurysm clip installed after 1996, any type of prosthesis
Usually allowable 6–8 weeks after implantation	Passive implants, weakly ferromagnetic (e.g. coils, filters and stents; metal sutures or staples)
Usually allowable immediately after implantation	Passive implants, non-ferromagnetic (e.g. bone/joint pins, screws or rods)

dent upon the chemical composition of the tissue rather than density. It provides an excellent contrast between soft tissue structures and is superior to CT for the imaging and assessment of tumours and soft tissue masses; it is also often used to investigate the renal vascular system. Its use is complicated, however, by its contraindication in the presence of certain implanted metallic objects; some orthopaedic and cardiac implants can safely be imaged with MRI (Table 5.8), and it is therefore vital to obtain accurate records of any medical, cosmetic or other implants.

Gadolinium-based contrast agents (GBCAs) are widely used in MRI and allow assessment of the enhancement patterns of lesions and visualisation of vessels to assess for anatomy and stenosis. GBCAs work by harnessing the paramagnetic properties of the gadolinium ion; free gadolinium ions are highly toxic but, when formulated as a chelated compound, are rendered safe for use. The incidence of anaphylactoid reactions with gadolinium is <0.01%, with an increased risk in patients with previous reactions, the second reaction often being more severe. Asthma or atopy also confers a 3.7x adverse reaction rate.

5.3.4.1 Nephrogenic Systemic Fibrosis (NSF)

NSF is a rare but serious multi-system disorder characterised by the deposition of collagen in the skin; systemic involvement is also seen, including involvement of the lungs, liver, muscles and heart. There is a well-documented link between exposure to GBCAs and development of NSF; the diagnosis is made using a combination of clinical and pathological factors known as the Girardi criteria [16]. Patients with CKD Stage 5 (eGFR <15 ml/min/1.73m^2) and end-stage kidney disease (ESKD) have a 1–7% chance of developing NSF; repeated exposure confers increased risk. While the exact cause of NSF has not been definitively proven, the hypothesis is that gadolinium ions are released from chelates in GBCAs due to the prolonged clearance time in patients with advanced kidney disease, as a result of displacement of the gadolinium ion by another metallic ion, such as calcium or zinc, in a process known as transmetallation. The gadolinium ion binds with free anions and precipitates out in various tissues resulting in fibrosis. The European Medicines Agency (EMEA) has classified the various GBCAs as low, medium and high risk: GBCAs with linear chelates appear to have greater risk than those with cyclical chelates.

Clinical features include initial pain, pruritus, swelling and erythema, usually starting in the legs. This progresses to thickening and fibrosis of the skin and subcutaneous tissues, characterised by a "woody" texture with development of plaques and associated contractures. Systemic fibrosis, involving the diaphragm, heart, liver and lungs, is also seen. Cachexia may develop, and death occurs in a proportion of patients [12]. Time of onset ranges from the day of exposure to several months. Patients with acute kidney injury, CKD Stage 4 and 5 and ESKD on dialysis are considered higher risk, alongside patients with reduced renal function who have had or are awaiting liver transplantation; patients with CKD 3 (GFR 30–59 ml/min/1.73 m^2) and children aged less than 1 year are considered low risk [12]. In these patient cohorts, alternative imaging tests or MRI without gadolinium should first be considered. If, following review, use of a low-risk agent is deemed appropriate or if it is necessary to use a medium-risk agent, the single lowest dose possible can be used (not to exceed 0.1 mmol/kilogram body weight) and should not be repeated for at least 7 days; use of a high-risk agent is contraindicated.

No cases of NSF have been reported in patients with an eGFR >60 ml/min/1.73 m^2, and it appears that the few cases reported in patients with an eGFR >30 ml/min/1.73 m^2 were associated with an episode of AKI, in which eGFR is inappropriate and misleading. The influence of various possible co-factors in the pathogenesis of NSF is not proven, but both hyperphosphataemia and erythropoietin use are suspected to play a role. Guidance on the use of gadolinium in patients with kidney disease is available from a variety of sources [12, 17].

5.3.5 Nuclear Medicine

Nuclear medicine examinations also involve the use of radiation; however instead of projecting a beam of X-rays through the patient as in plain radiography or CT, a radioactive isotope is chemically bound to a pharmaceutical with affinity for the relevant target tissue; this is then injected into the patient, and as the radioactive isotope decays, radiation is emitted which can be detected. Radioactive isotopes such as technetium-99 m emit gamma rays, and these are detected by a gamma camera, which traditionally and typically produce planar images. However, most gamma cameras can produce a three-dimensional acquisition by rotating around the patient and combining multiple circular views to give a volume image known as single-photon emission tomography (SPECT).

Other radioactive isotopes commonly used in radionuclide imaging, such as fluorine-18, emit positrons which travel noticeably short distances before colliding with electrons in the body, to release two high-energy photons of gamma radiation. These two gamma photons travel in geometrically opposite directions and are detected by the scanner. Positron emitters are used in positron emission tomography (PET) and are commonly combined with CT in PET-CT scanners. PET has the advantage of producing three-dimensional volume images as the scanner can detect the two simultaneously released gamma photons and triangulate their point of origin in the body.

As the radiopharmaceutical can be selected specifically for the tissue of interest, this allows either static or dynamic imaging (as in the case of MAG3) and places a greater emphasis on function rather than anatomical detail. However, the combination of nuclear medicine imaging with CT allows accurate localisation of the administered radioactivity, providing a combination of function and improved anatomical detail. These are performed in PET-CT scanners or SPECT-CT scanners if the isotope used for imaging is a positron emitter or gamma emitter, respectively.

Table 5.9 describes some of the different applications of nuclear medicine examinations to various aspects of the renal system.

Table 5.9 The role of nuclear medicine in renal imaging

Tissue	Pathology	Nuclear medicine imaging
Parenchyma	Pyelonephritis Scarring Split function	DMSA and FDG PET CT DMSA DMSA
Vasculature	Perfusion Renal artery stenosis	MAG3 Captopril renography
Collecting system	Obstruction Reflux	MAG3 Indirect micturating cystoscintigraphy
Others	Pyrexia of unknown origin Occult malignancy or suspected PTLD Suspected IgG4-related retroperitoneal fibrosis	FDG PET-CT FDG PET-CT FDG PET-CT

5.3.5.1 MAG3

MAG3 (mercaptoacetyltriglycine) is chelated with radioactive technetium-99 m to form the radiopharmaceutical. It is cleared from the body by the kidneys primarily by tubular secretion.

This scan is performed as a dynamic renal study to assess renal perfusion, divided function, drainage and ureteric clearance. The patient is initially asked to empty their bladder, and then the radiopharmaceutical is administered while they are on the gamma camera. The whole examination takes about 20–40 minutes after administration of the radiopharmaceutical, during which time acquisitions are taken to show curves of activity related to time within the kidneys, known as a renogram. This is supplemented with static images of the kidneys, ureter and bladder. A diuretic (furosemide 0.5 mg/kg, with a maximum dose of 40 mg, given either 15–20 minutes prior to scanning or 15 minutes after MAG3 injection) is used if there is clinical suspicion of obstruction and if the collecting system is dilated. The diuretic increases the urinary flow rate and will ensure there is drainage in an unobstructed, but dilated collecting system. If the tracer still does not clear from the collecting system despite diuretic administration, this suggests an obstruction to drainage of the collecting system.

The dynamic nature of the scan allows gross assessment of the parenchymal perfusion and morphology and good dynamic visualisation of the parenchymal clearance and collecting system drainage. The differential function between both kidneys can be calculated from the early parenchymal phase of the MAG3, prior to drainage into the collecting system. The differential function calculated from MAG3 is accurate when kidney function is good, but in the context of chronic kidney disease or at the extremes of function, a DMSA is more accurate.

Transplant Kidney MAG 3

MAG3 studies can be performed in transplant kidneys to assess perfusion, parenchymal function and drainage. While routine use of post-transplant MAG3 has been largely superseded by ultrasound Doppler, there remains a role for MAG3 in assessing transplant kidneys in the immediate post-operative period where there is concern for perfusion of the kidney, particularly where multiple arteries exist, or in assessing poor graft function

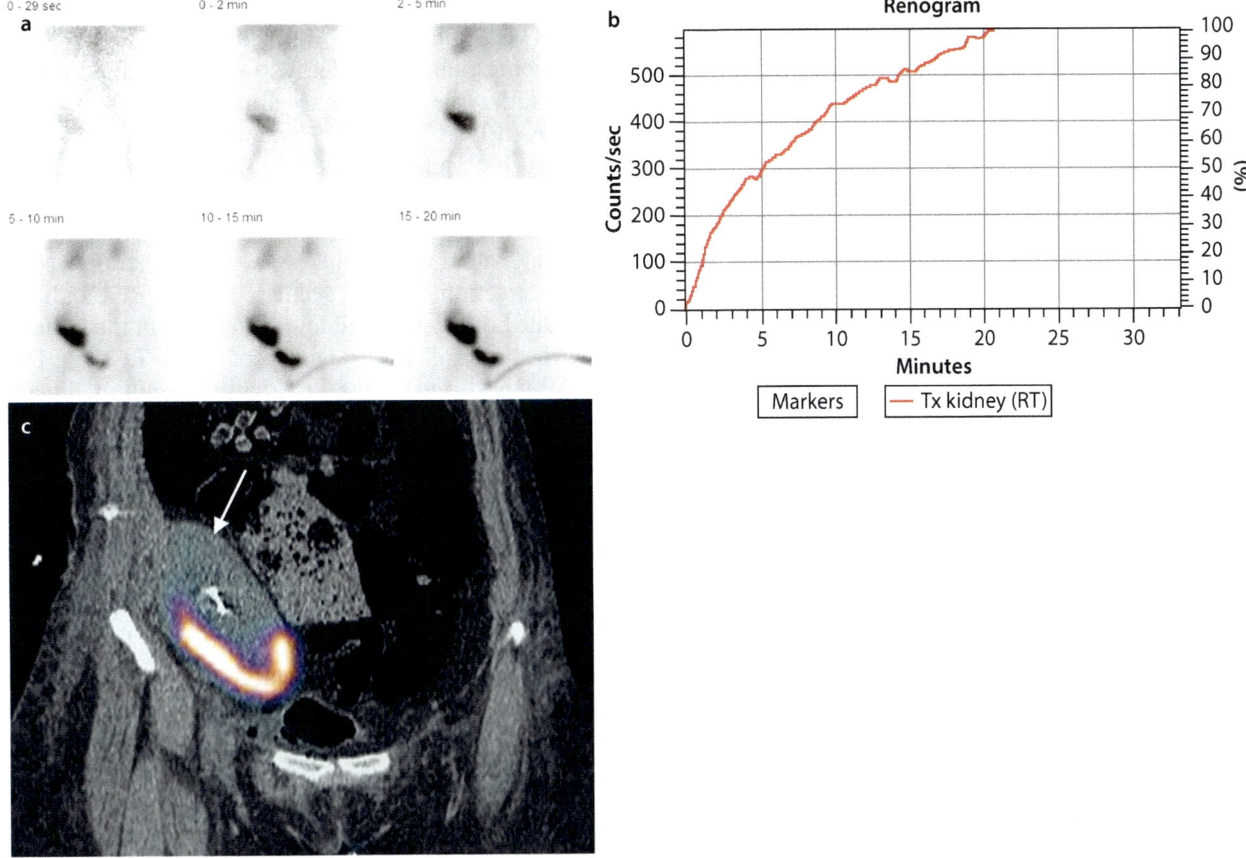

Fig. 5.1 [^{99m}Tc]Tc-MAG 3 renogram in a 3-day post-operative transplant kidney. **a** Serial planar images show normal uptake in the lower pole but absent uptake in the upper pole (arrows). **b** There is a slowly rising time-activity curve over the lower pole indicating poor tubular function. **c** Coronal fused SPECT-CT images of the same kidney show absent uptake in the upper pole due to infarction of an upper pole transplant artery

(Fig. 5.1a–c). Some studies have suggested that MAG3 can differentiate early rejection from acute tubular necrosis in the early post-operative period. The perfusion index, a measure of the blood flow in the transplant kidney relative to the external iliac artery, is usually preserved in acute tubular necrosis. Sequential imaging with MAG3 can be useful in assessing graft function in the post-operative period and is highly sensitive, but non-specific, for evaluating transplant kidney pathology [18]. Finally, because MAG3 is excreted into the collecting system and bladder, it can be used to non-invasively assess for post-operative urine leaks [19].

Indirect Micturating Cystoscintigraphy

As MAG3 is excreted into the collecting system and bladder, a micturating study can be performed to assess for vesicoureteric reflux [20, 21]. This has the advantage over a direct micturating cystogram performed using contrast because catheterisation of the bladder is not required. The study is performed by injecting ^{99}Tc-MAG3 followed by imaging similar to a standard renogram. Once the tracer has drained from the kidneys into the bladder, a second acquisition is performed while the patient micturates into a specially designed commode. Reflux into the kidneys from the bladder is evident by measuring the activity in the kidneys over time and identifying an increase in activity during micturition [22]. Sensitivity for reflux is limited and often only reflux into the kidneys can be identified.

Captopril Renography

Captopril renography involves performing a MAG3 examination before and after administration of an angiotensin-converting enzyme inhibitor, typically captopril. The technique is used to identify renovascular causes of hypertension and renal artery stenosis. Although captopril renography is not as sensitive or specific for renal artery stenosis as MR angiography, it remains a useful examination for renovascular disease in patients with preserved renal function [23], and to a lesser extent patients with chronic kidney disease, in predicting the beneficial effect of revascularisation [24]. Renal artery stenosis is diagnosed if there is a fall in function of one kidney by at least 5% or if there is a delay to peak activity to 10 minutes in one kidney after the administration of captopril [25]. However, if the split function of a single kidney is less than 20% on the baseline study, then captopril renography is unlikely to be accurate, limiting its usefulness in certain patients with chronic kidney disease.

5.3.5.2 DMSA

In this examination, dimercaptosuccinic acid is chelated with technetium-99 m to form the radiopharmaceutical. After injection, this concentrates within the renal cortex and becomes bound to proximal tubular cells; only 10% is excreted into the urine in the first few hours after injection, providing high-resolution images of the renal cortex.

Unlike the dynamic nature of MAG3, DMSA is used to assess the renal parenchyma for anatomy or scarring. As such, it is useful in cases of horseshoe or solitary kidneys or for localisation of an ectopic kidney [26, 27]; it is also used to assess renal scarring and parenchymal damage in acute pyelonephritis in children and adults [28, 29]. The relative function of the two kidneys is also calculated, useful for surgical planning [30]. As DMSA is only minimally excreted in the urine, it can more accurately assess relative function in patients with chronic kidney disease [31] than MAG3.

Once the radiopharmaceutical is injected, the patient waits approximately 3 hours for it to accumulate within the kidneys before images are acquired with a gamma camera. Planar imaging in multiple views is standard practice, but some centres perform SPECT or SPECT-CT to improve anatomical localisation of scarring.

5.3.5.3 PET-CT

The use of PET-CT scans, most often performed using fluorodeoxyglucose (FDG) labelled with fluorine-18, is increasingly widespread. PET-CT has greater spatial resolution compared to SPECT-CT imaging, but the short half-life of ^{18}F (110 minutes) limits its availability. As a glucose analogue, FDG is taken up by cells and phosphorylated but cannot then be further metabolised as it lacks the necessary 2-hydroxyl group present in glucose. FDG uptake is therefore a good indicator of glucose uptake by cells in the body, and organs with high glucose metabolism, such as the brain, myocardium and brown adipocytes, will show increased uptake on PET-CT scans at baseline; tissues with abnormal high metabolic activity, including malignant tumours, will also show increased uptake on FDG PET-CT. Approximately 20% of FDG is eliminated by urinary excretion, with the rest undergoing radioactive decay. As a result, the kidneys and bladder can show intense uptake on PET-CT.

FDG PET-CT is most commonly used in tumour imaging, particularly in the diagnosis, staging and monitoring of Hodgkin's disease, non-Hodgkin's lymphoma, breast cancer, lung cancer, melanoma and gastrointestinal malignancies; it is not generally useful in the detection of renal cell carcinomas (RCCs); however, due both to the high level of uptake in the kidneys and the lack of FDG avidity of most RCCs. FDG PET-CT is also often used to identify occult malignancies in patients with unexpected weight loss or to identify a primary malignancy in patients with metastatic disease.

FDG PET-CT can be used to assess post-transplant lymphoproliferative disease (PTLD) following renal transplant [32, 33] and adds value over other imaging modalities. FDG can identify sites of PTLD in lymph nodes that are not enlarged on anatomical imaging, can aid diagnosis by identifying a target for biopsy and can confirm extranodal sites of disease such as in the liver, lungs and bone that may be occult on other imaging modalities (◘ Fig. 5.2a–c). There is also some evidence that FDG can be used to assess treatment response in PTLD [34].

FDG accumulates in activated leukocytes, and PET-CT can therefore be used to evaluate inflammatory and infectious processes, including the identification of sites of infection in patients with pyrexia of unknown origin [35, 36], and can guide further management such as therapeutic intervention or biopsies. As well as identifying sources of bacterial infection, FDG PET-CT is useful in identifying active TB, sarcoidosis, large vessel vasculitis and Still's disease. It is increasingly used in the diagnosis and management of IgG4-related retroperitoneal fibrosis.

As FDG is excreted by the urinary system, its role in evaluating the kidneys and bladder is somewhat limited by the physiological activity of these organs. However, FDG PET-CT can be used to diagnose transplant pyelonephritis and infected cysts in patients with polycystic kidney disease [37, 38] (◘ Fig. 5.3a–b). Despite a relatively poor sensitivity, the absence of iodinated contrast media in PET-CT makes it a useful examination in patients where the risk of contrast-induced nephropathy is considered excessive (◘ Table 5.10).

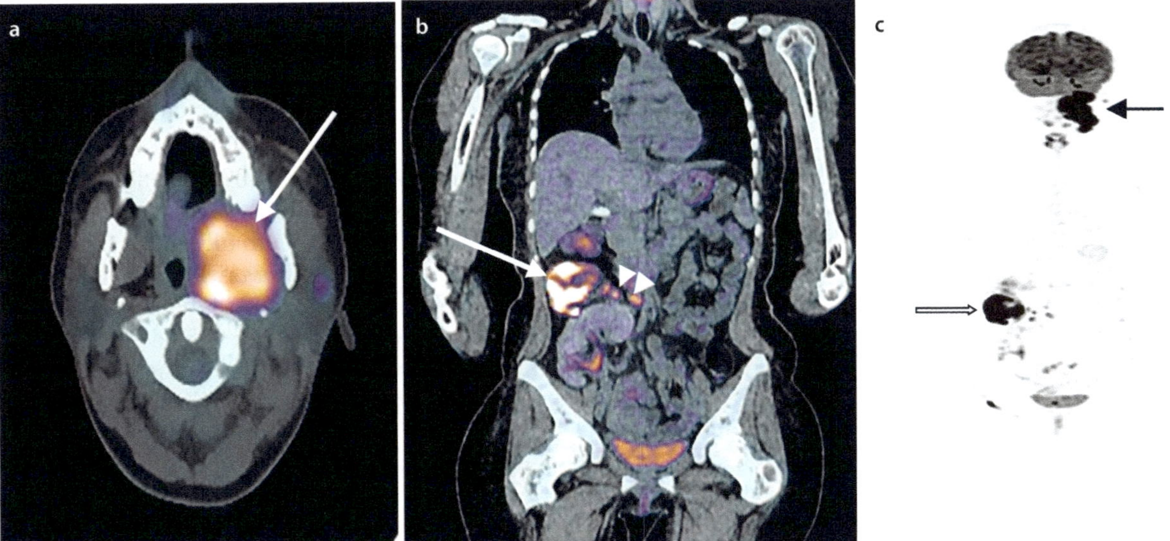

Fig. 5.2 2-[^{18}F]FDG PET-CT images of a 30-year-old transplant recipient with new cervical lymphadenopathy. **a** Axial fused PET-CT image through the level of the oropharynx showing a left tonsillar mass (arrow). **b** Coronal fused PET-CT image showing a caecal mass (arrow) and mesenteric lymphadenopathy (arrow heads). **c** Maximum intensity projection (MIP) imaging in the same patient with a tonsillar mass (arrow) and caecal mass (open arrow). A biopsy confirmed a diagnosis of post-transplant lymphoproliferative disease

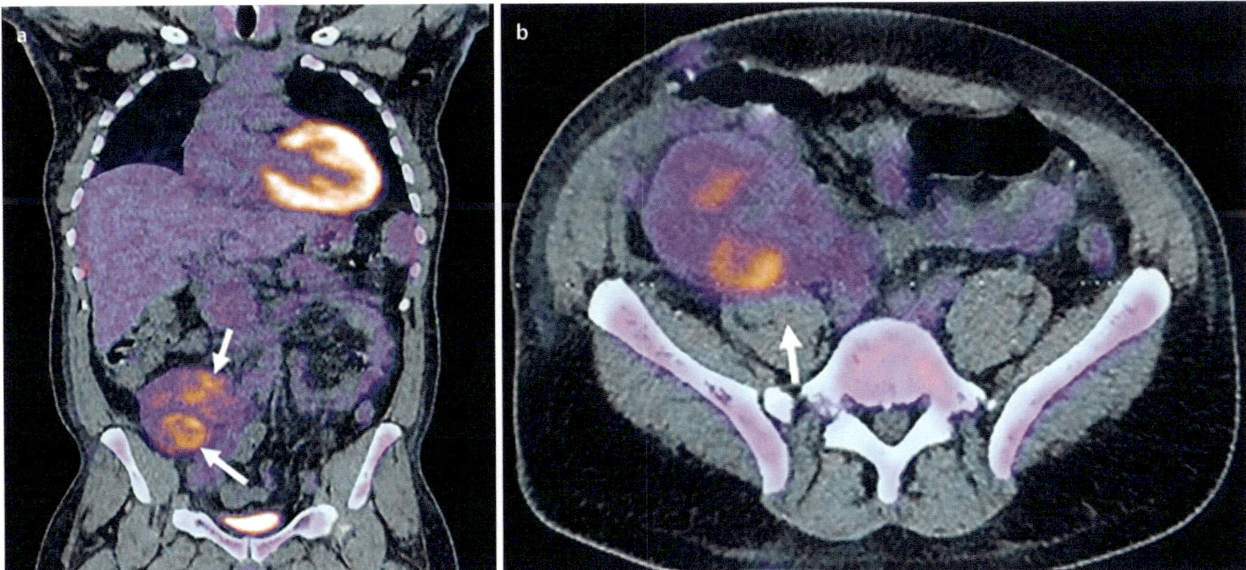

Fig. 5.3 2 [^{18}F]FDG PET-CT scan of a 48-year-old transplant recipient being investigated for pyrexia of unknown origin. **a** Coronal and **b** axial fused PET-CT images show multiple foci of increased uptake in the cortex of the transplant kidney (arrows) which are in keeping with transplant pyelonephritis

5

Table 5.10 General preparation for interventional radiology

Request	
Clinical information	Relevant history and indications, diagnostic question or therapeutic aim. Significant patient history, e.g. confusion, high levels of anxiety, previous procedures, bleeding diathesis, allergies
Need for interpreter	Important and frequently forgotten issue
Infection risk	Hepatitis C and B and HIV, MRSA, VRE ESBL, CPO
Requirements	For example, oxygen, monitoring
Preparation	
IV access	Sufficient size for contrast need
Nil by mouth	If having IV sedation
Coagulation	Haemoglobin, platelets, clotting screen, use of low molecular weight or another prophylactic heparin
Urea and Electrolytes	e.g., degree of hyperkalaemia (particularly important for tunnelled line insertions)
Patient information	Patient information leaflet (ideally in first language), reasons for procedure discussed and explained

5.4 Interventional Radiology

Many renal patients will undergo an interventional radiology (IR) procedure during their treatment course, and it is essential that these are carefully planned to both maximise the benefit and reduce the risk; for pre-dialysis or dialysis patients in particular, consideration should be given to future vascular access needs. The clinical information provided should therefore be comprehensive and relevant so that the radiologist can decide whether the proposed treatment is indicated or indeed feasible. Some general points on clinical information and preparation are listed in (Table 5.11). It is worth noting that many departments will have their own local guidelines which may vary from these.

Common interventional procedures undertaken in patients with kidney disease are described below, including complications that may be encountered.

5.4.1 Fistuloplasty and Venoplasty

This involves accessing a stenotic or occluded segment of a native or prosthetic arteriovenous (AV) fistula and placing a guidewire across the abnormal segment to allow passage of an angioplasty balloon for venous dilatation. Access sheaths may be placed into the fistula vein, into the prosthetic graft or into an internal jugular vein or common femoral vein.

Table 5.11 The advantages and disadvantages of ultrasound, CT, MRI and nuclear medicine are compared in the table 5.10

	Ultrasound	CT	MRI	Nuclear medicine
Advantages	1. Cheap 2. No radiation 3. Can be performed at bedside with portable machine and is therefore useful in unstable patients	1. Multiplanar – CT builds the images using data about the body as a volume; therefore the area of interest can be examined in different planes, and its relationship to other structures can be studied 2. Speed – Modern CT scanners can cover the whole body in a matter of a few seconds, which can be vital for unstable patients 3. Wider and out of hours availability in most centres	1. Good soft tissue contrast 2. No ionising radiation – Preferable for younger patients and for repeat scans to avoid radiation exposure	1. Allows imaging of physiological processes within organs 2. Virtually no contraindications 3. Anaphylactic reactions extremely rare, no risk of contrast-induced nephropathy 4. Safe to use in chronic and end-stage kidney disease

	Ultrasound	CT	MRI	Nuclear medicine
Disadvantages	1. Small field of view (single plane at one time) – The view directly in front of the probe 2. Operator skill and experience dependent 3. Image review – Due to the factors above, an ultrasound can only really be interpreted by the person who has performed it unlike CT or MRI scan where whole sequence of images will be available for later review 4. Patient dependent – Movement, breathing and presence of large amount of subcutaneous fat in obese patients, for example, can affect the image quality	1. Risk of radiation and cancer 2. Artefact – Movement and breathing during the scan can produce blurred images obscuring pathology 3. Poor soft tissue resolution on a plain CT – Although this is improved by the use of IV contrast, this carries its own risks	1. Time – Can take many minutes. Patients are required to lie still 2. Availability – Less readily available due to high cost and time consumption 3. Claustrophobia – The bore of the scanner, inside which the patient is placed for imaging is about 60 cm, smaller than a CT. Wide bore or open MRI scanners are available at specialist institutes, although image quality is usually poorer with these magnets	1. Risk of radiation and additional risk to other patients, carers and staff as body fluids are radioactive with radiopharmaceutical 2. Poor spatial resolution giving low anatomical details; some investigations are therefore combined with CT (e.g. PET-CT and SPECT-CT) to enable spatial localisation of the physiological data shown by the nuclear medicine component 3. Time-consuming to gain necessary data despite recent advancements, as scans aim to look at physiological processes

The procedure is often performed with the use of intravenous sedation and analgesia, as venous dilatation is typically very painful. For a native AV fistula, no antibiotics are given; however for an AV fistula with a prosthetic graft, antibiotic prophylaxis with Gram-positive, Gram-negative and anaerobic cover is commonly given.

▪▪ Complications

- Haemorrhage: this is not usually clinically significant at the puncture site, even when an arterialised segment of fistula vein has been punctured, as manual compression is sufficient to obtain haemostasis.
- Infection: prosthetic grafts at risk; see above for antibiotic prophylaxis.
- Rupture of fistula: risk greatest if there has been very recent surgical revision of the fistula or if there is infection present.
- Central venous perforation: this may occur due to perforation by a guidewire or during angioplasty of a central vein and carries the potential for significant intrathoracic haemorrhage.

5.4.2 Nephrostomy and Antegrade Stent

Antegrade renal drainage may be used to established drainage of an obstructed kidney when retrograde drainage has been unsuccessful or cannot be attempted. There are no data that show either approach to have a superior safety profile, but there are specific situations when retrograde drainage may not be possible. These include extensive distal tumour, ureteric injury and reimplantation of the ureter, e.g. a transplant kidney. Urgent drainage should be considered in an obstructed infected pelvicalyceal (PC) system or obstructed single kidney (including transplant) with acute derangement of renal function.

The procedure requires IV analgesia, sedation and antibiotic prophylaxis.

▪▪ Complications

- Haemorrhage: may be sufficient to threaten kidney or life. Bleeding may occur from the kidney, or from the abdominal wall.
- Infection: puncture of an obstructed infected PC system may result in septic shower and rapid instability of the patient.
- Deterioration in renal function: haemorrhage may lead to loss of the kidney, or renal compression and reduced function, while secondary infection may also cause injury.

5.4.3 Tunnelled Dialysis Catheter

Vascular access for haemodialysis may be performed by radiologists, nephrologists, surgeons or other paramedical staff groups, such as nurses, who have had appropriate training. Patients who have had multiple central venous lines, however, eventually lose access to common sites for line insertion, such as the jugular veins, and there may also be stenoses or occlusions of the brachiocephalic veins, SVC, IVC or iliac veins. These patients may need associated venoplasty to facilitate line insertion, or an unusual access site such as a translumbar or transhepatic inferior vena cava (IVC) line, and some may require insertion of a line surgically, for example, directly into an iliac vein.

Antibiotic prophylaxis is not usually given for line insertion.

5

5.4.4 Percutaneous Peritoneal Dialysis Catheter

While peritoneal dialysis catheters are traditionally inserted surgically under general anaesthetic, they may also be inserted percutaneously, using local anaesthesia. This procedure may be performed by interventional nephrologists or radiologists and is typically confined to patients who have not previously had any abdominal surgery and who may be deemed unfit for general anaesthesia.

5.4.5 Angiography, Angioplasty and Stent Insertion

Renal angiography is used for diagnosis of conditions such as renal vasculitis, fibromuscular dysplasia (FMD) and renal artery stenosis (RAS) and is usually performed via a transfemoral approach. It is safe, with a complication rate of 1% for femoral arterial injury and <1% for renal arterial damage. Mesenteric angiography is often performed at the same time when investigating vasculitis.

Renal angioplasty is indicated for the treatment of fibromuscular dysplasia; however, stent insertion is not performed for this indication due to the potential provocation of neointimal hyperplasia within the stent leading to in-stent re-stenosis.

The finding of the *a*ngioplasty and *st*enting for *r*enal *a*rtery *l*esions (ASTRAL) trial resulted in a large reduction in the number of patients with atherosclerotic renal artery stenosis being treated with angioplasty and stent insertion. The trial showed no benefit of intervention over medical therapy in either preventing deterioration of renal function or treating hypertension. Despite this, there are still situations in which angioplasty with/without stent insertion may be appropriate:

- Transplant renal artery stenosis – intervention may lead to stabilisation of renal function. Stent insertion is not usually performed due to the difficulty in treating in-stent restenosis should this occur.
- Renal artery stenosis with flash pulmonary oedema – stent insertion may reduce episodes of pulmonary oedema.
- New deterioration of renal function in established renovascular disease.
- Severe stenosis and single kidney with significant impairment of renal function.

Many patients with renal disease require peripheral arterial revascularisation. The preparation is the same as for renal angiography, although the complication rate is higher, at 4%, and includes arterial damage or haemorrhage at the puncture site, and distal embolisation following angioplasty, which at worst may be limb-threatening (<1%). Antibiotic prophylaxis is not usually necessary.

5.5 Tips for Requesting Imaging

Requesting imaging can be a daunting process, which can be mitigated by familiarity with local departmental protocols. Most hospitals now have electronic request forms, although handwritten requests remain the norm in some institutions. These request forms are part of the patient's medical record and hence should be clear, accurate and eligible. The request should be made by a registered medical practitioner and discussed with a radiologist if urgent or if there is uncertainty about which investigation is required. It is mandatory that the correct identification and sufficient demographic details, such as name, date of birth and address and hospital number, are provided to ensure the radiology department can correctly identify the patient to avoid unintentional radiation exposure.

The referring person should ensure their full name, contact details and department details are provided so the radiology department can inform them of any urgent results if needed. The request should clearly mention clinical priority such as urgent, routine and planned, which investigation of a specific body part is required and what question is being asked, along with relevant clinical details. To avoid confusion, abbreviations and acronyms should not be used on request forms.

Images are now typically stored electronically and can be retrieved from other institutions, both nationally and internationally; this facilitates longitudinal review of disease or lesions and may avoid the need for repeat imaging, limiting radiation exposure.

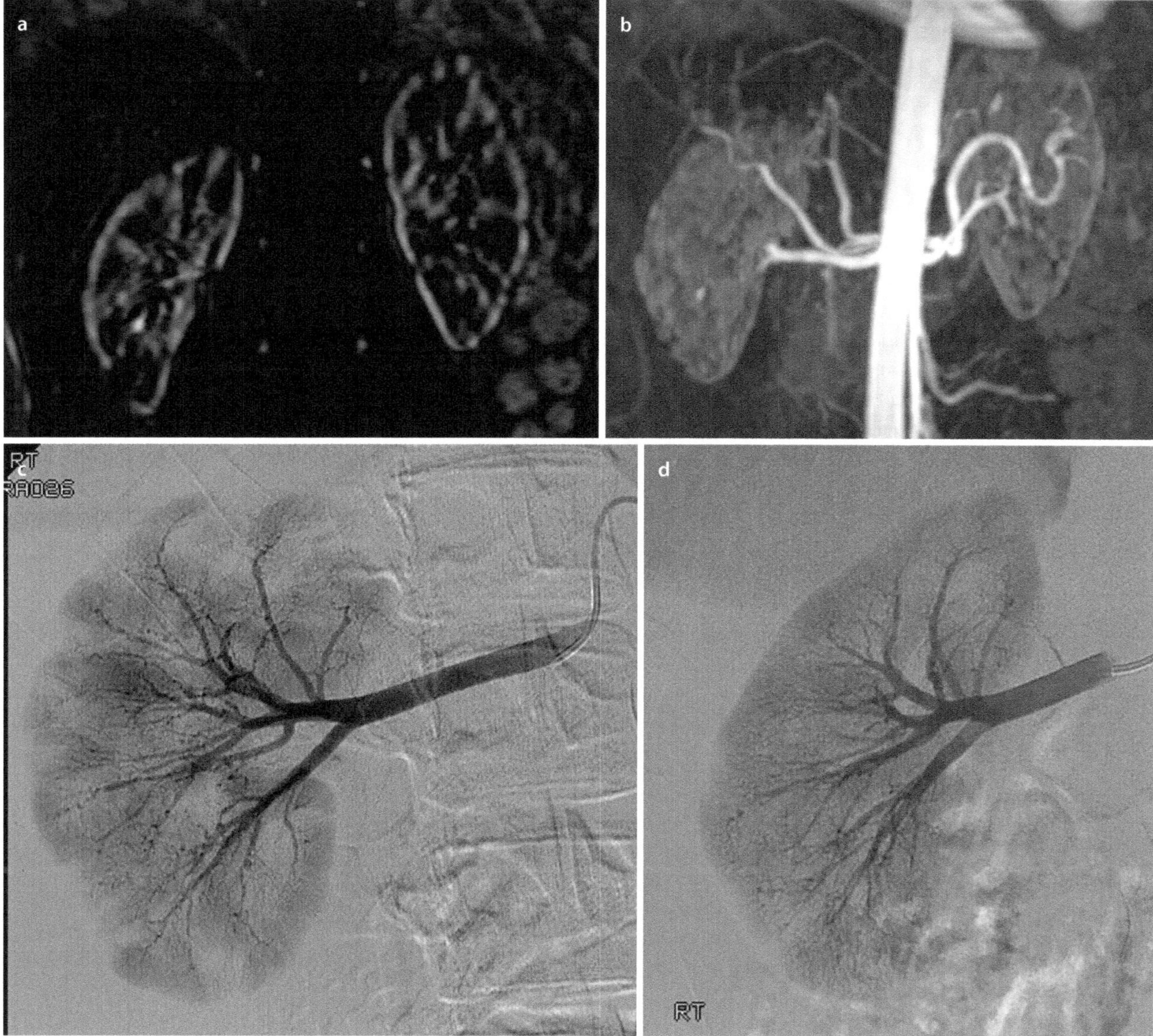

Fig. 5.4 (Case 1) MR angiography shows multiple parenchymal perfusional defects **a.** and normal renal arteries **b.** Renal digital subtraction angiography (DSA) shows multiple small vessel strictures and ectasia typical of polyarteritis nodosa (PAN) **c.** MR angiogram shows improved appearance of renal arterial tree with fewer parenchymal perfusional defects following treatment **d**

5.6 Considerations when Requesting Imaging

When requesting imaging, it is important to inform the patient of the request and discuss any risks involved, including the use of ionising radiation; extra caution should be taken with pregnant patients and children and consideration given to the use of other modalities, including ultrasound or MRI; and informed consent should be taken where its use is unavoidable. Where patients have special needs, including learning difficulties or dementia, particular attention should be paid to their ability to understand the need for an investigation, wherein discussion with their families may be required, and to tolerate a particular investigation or procedure.

5.7 Following up Imaging Reports

It is the legal responsibility of the referring doctor to follow up the results of requested radiological investigations, and failure to read such reports is the most common source of error leading to delay in the diagnosis and management of patients. Urgent or unexpected findings from an imaging report should, however, be explicitly communicated to the referring doctor or team by the reporting radiologist. In most centres, the images can be viewed electronically on a picture archiving and communication system (PACS) where the radiology report is also stored.

Case Study

Case 1

An 18-year-old male presented with accelerated hypertension and microscopic haematuria. There was evidence of kidney injury (creatinine 127 µmol/L) with normal inflammatory markers (CRP 1); cANCA was negative and pANCA was equivocal.

MR angiography was performed to assess for renal artery stenosis or mid-aortic syndrome as a cause of young-onset hypertension; this showed multiple renal parenchymal perfusional defects (◘ Fig. 5.4a) and normal renal arteries (◘ Fig. 5.4b). The patient proceeded to renal digital subtraction angiography (DSA), which showed multiple small vessel strictures and ectasia (◘ Fig. 5.4c) typical of polyarteritis nodosa (PAN). Microaneurysms are often a feature of PAN but were not demonstrated in this case. Following treatment, the renal function returned to normal, and a follow-up angiogram (◘ Fig. 5.4d) showed significant improvement in the appearances of the renal arterial tree with fewer parenchymal perfusional defects. Follow-up DSA is not usually necessary; however as the inflammatory markers were normal, and the antibody profile was equivocal, it was felt to represent the best way of objectively demonstrating a response to treatment in this case.

Case 2

A 73-year-old female presented 3 months following renal transplantation with new-onset graft dysfunction and hypertension. An MR angiogram was performed but did not show renal artery stenosis; on review, however, it was apparent that the MRA didn't include the entire origin of the transplant artery on the scan volume (◘ Fig. 5.5a). A subsequent Doppler US remained suspicious for transplant renal artery stenosis, demonstrating a typical "tardus-parvus" waveform (◘ Fig. 5.5b). A repeat MR angiogram confirmed the presence of renal artery stenosis (◘ Fig. 5.5c). The patient subsequently underwent renal angioplasty resulting in successful treatment of the renal artery stenosis (◘ Fig. 5.5d and e), with improvement in graft function. Transplant renal angioplasty is not routinely followed by stent insertion, although practice varies between centres with little evidence to support either action. Although primary patency rates with stent insertion may be higher, in-stent restenosis is harder to treat effectively than recurrence of a stenosis treated with angioplasty alone.

Case 3

A 38-year-old female was investigated for young-onset hypertension and underwent MR angiography, which showed typical features of fibromuscular dysplasia (FMD) in the left renal artery (◘ Fig. 5.6a). This was confirmed with DSA (◘ Fig. 5.6b) and angioplasty, or the left renal artery was performed, resulting in clinical improvement. The post-angioplasty angiogram usually remains abnormal following angioplasty in FMD (◘ Fig. 5.6c), in contrast to angioplasty of atherosclerotic or post-transplant stenosis. In FMD, however, the disease process involves the generation of extensive intimal synechiae which obstruct the vessel lumen and which are not well demonstrated angiographically; these are broken down during angioplasty resulting in improved flow.

Case 4

A 73-year-old man with a history of right nephrectomy for cancer and known stenosis of the left renal artery presented with uncontrolled hypertension, diuretic-resistant cardiac failure and renal impairment (eGFR 42 ml/min/1.73m^2). MRA (◘ Fig. 5.7a) demonstrated a lesion involving the bifurcation of the main left renal artery with significant stenosis of the origins of both branches. Confirmed on formal angiogram (◘ Fig. 5.7b), the lesion was treated successfully with two "kissing" stents from the main artery into each branch (◘ Fig. 5.7c). Following the procedure, better control of both his hypertension and heart failure was achieved, while his renal function also improved (eGFR 57 ml/min/1.73m^2). Although randomised trials have shown no advantage in renal artery stenting versus medical therapy, the procedure remains indicated in the context of a single kidney with cardiac failure/pulmonary oedema, renal impairment and hypertension, as well as FMD and transplant artery stenosis, as discussed above.

Case 5

A 78-year-old man presented with a short history of left loin pain, sepsis and anuria. CT KUB showed hydronephrosis (◘ Fig. 5.8a) and an obstructing left ureteric calculus (◘ Fig. 5.8b). In view of his comorbidities, the patient was deemed unsuitable to undergo general anaesthesia for retrograde ureteric stent insertion and instead had a nephrostomy inserted with local anaesthesia (◘ Fig. 5.8c). Although a commonly performed procedure, in this case the patient suffered a large haemorrhage complicating the nephrostomy insertion which prolonged the patient's admission and recovery of renal function. The decision to choose retrograde or antegrade drainage should therefore always be made after discussion between the nephrologist, urologist and interventional radiologist to ensure optimal care.

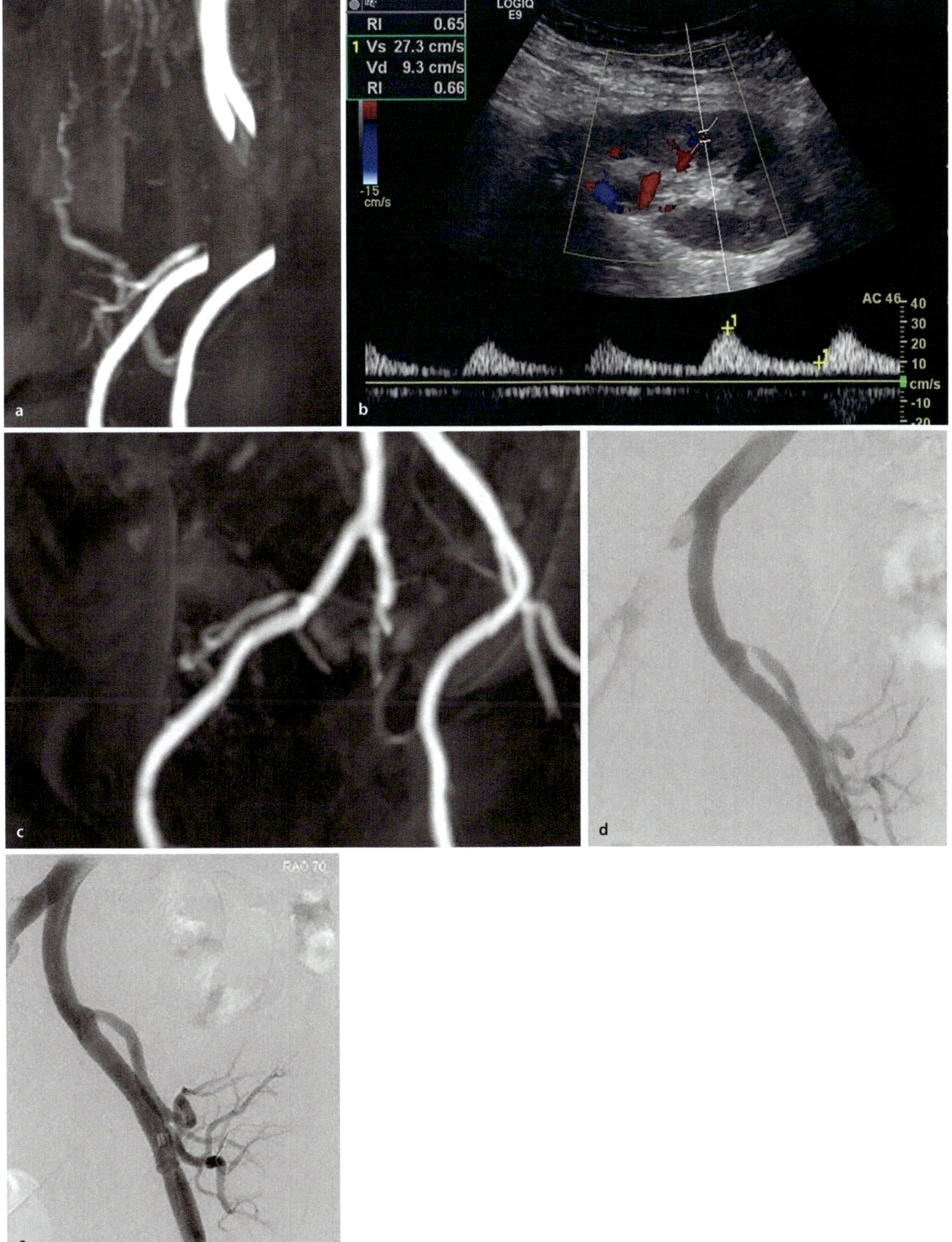

◘ **Fig. 5.5** (Case 2) MR angiogram with no stenosis (but did not include the origin of renal artery **a.** Doppler US showing a typical "tardus-parvus" waveform suspicious for renal artery stenosis **b.** Repeat MR angiogram confirming presence of renal artery stenosis **c.** Renal angioplasty resulting in successful treatment of renal artery stenosis **(d.** and **e.)**

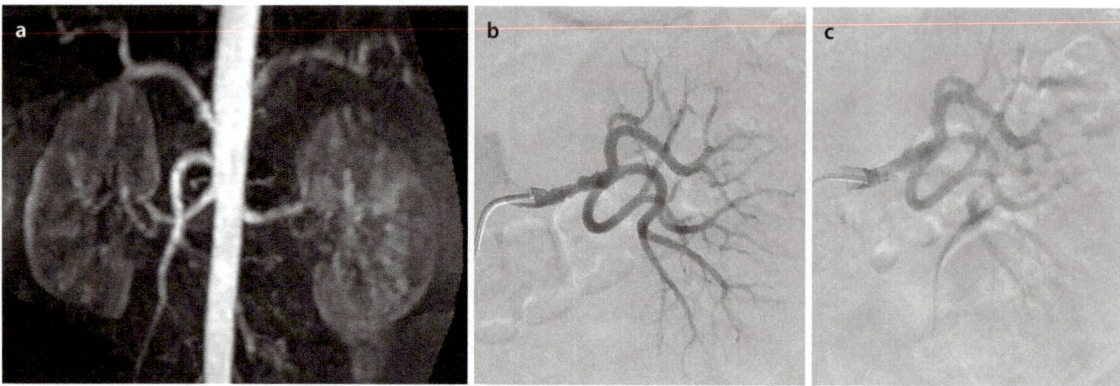

Fig. 5.6 (Case 3) MR angiography showing typical features of fibromuscular dysplasia (FMD) in left renal artery **a.** DSA confirming FMD **b.** Post-angioplasty angiogram which is usually abnormal following successful angioplasty in FMD **c**

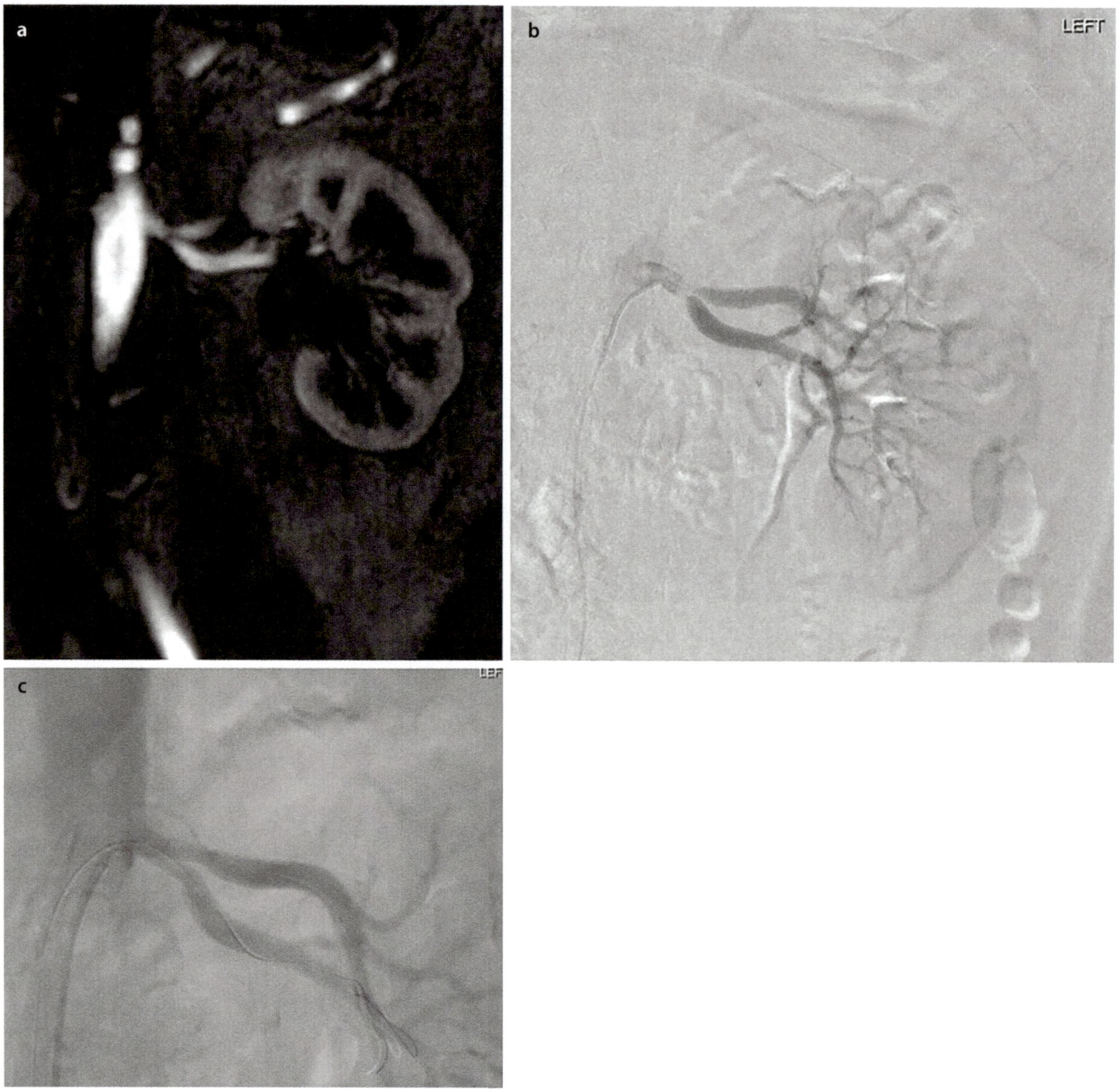

Fig. 5.7 (Case 4) MRA showing a lesion involving the bifurcation of the main left renal artery with significant stenosis of the origins of both branches **a.** confirmation on formal angiogram **b.** successful treatment of the lesion with two "kissing" stents from the main artery into each branch **c**

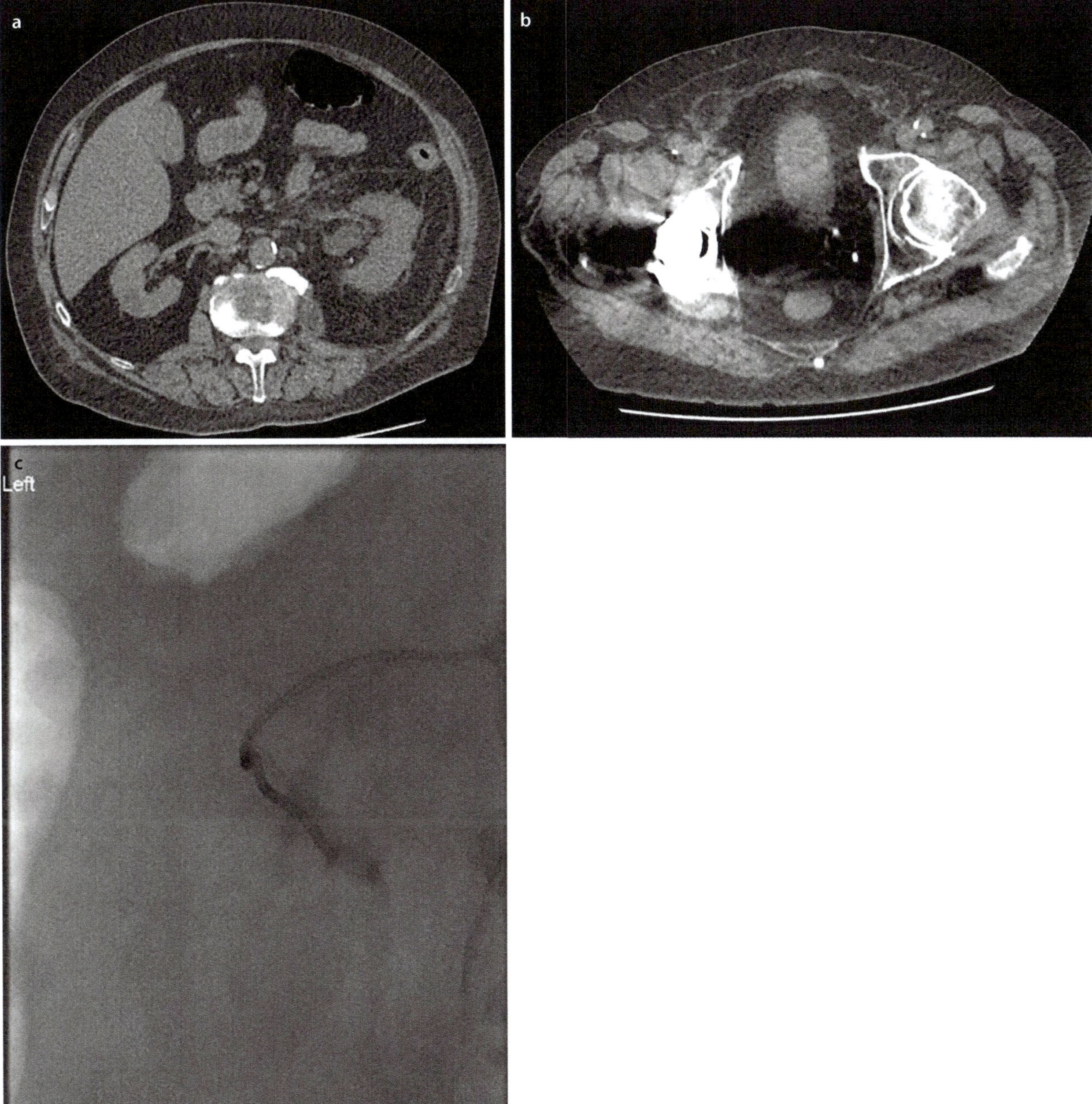

Fig. 5.8 (Case 5) CT KUB showing hydronephrosis **a.** and an obstructing left ureteric calculus **b.** nephrostomy insertion for treatment **c**

Tips and Tricks

1. MR angiography has a high negative predictive value for renal artery stenosis (RAS) in both native and transplant kidneys. Formal catheter angiography is the most sensitive investigation for RAS and allows simultaneous treatment of any lesions through angioplasty, albeit with the small risk of arterial puncture-related complications. Therefore, in cases with a high clinical index of suspicion for RAS with a negative MRA, consider proceeding to catheter angiography.
2. In FMD, the disease process involves the generation of extensive intimal synechiae which obstruct the vessel lumen and which are not well demonstrated angiographically; these are broken down during angioplasty resulting in improved flow and amelioration of symptoms, but the angiographic appearance will remain abnormal.
3. ^{99m}Tc-MAG3 is predominantly cleared by tubular secretion and is used to assess the perfusion, tubu-

lar function and drainage of the kidney. However, the accumulation of the tracer in the collecting system depends on the tubular secretion, so a ^{99m}Tc-MAG3 renogram cannot reliably identify urinary tract obstruction when the function of the kidney is significantly reduced.

4. ^{99m}Tc-DMSA accumulates in the renal cortex and very little is excreted into the collecting system. It cannot be used to assess the drainage of the kidney but is an accurate method of assessing the differential function of two kidneys.
5. ^{18}F-FDG is a commonly used PET tracer that localises in tissues with a high glucose metabolism. Consider a PET-CT scan in patients with suspected post-transplant lymphoproliferative disease or pyrexia of unknown origin.

5.8 Conclusion

There is growing use of radiological diagnostic and interventional procedures in the field of nephrology. With better understanding of the use, indications and complications, these can be safely organised and play enormous role in timely diagnosis and management of renal patients.

Questions

1. Can a normal ultrasound reliably exclude obstructive nephropathy in all the cases?
2. Should renal artery stenting ever be offered to patients with single kidney?

Answers

1. Ultrasound is typically the investigation of choice to rule out obstructive nephropathy, showing hydronephrosis. Occasionally, however, obstructive nephropathy may exist in the absence of hydronephrosis due to encasement of the kidneys by retroperitoneal fibrosis of any aetiology; consider CT KUB where the clinical suspicion for obstruction is high but ultrasound is negative.
2. Although randomised trials have shown no advantage in renal artery stenting versus medical therapy, the procedure remains indicated in the context of a single kidney with cardiac failure/pulmonary oedema, renal impairment and hypertension, as well as FMD and transplant artery stenosis.

References

1. https://www.england.nhs.uk/wp-content/uploads/2020/01/multi-disciplinary-team-streamlining-guidance.pdf
2. Ratnapalan S, Bona N, Chandra K, Koren G. Physicians' perceptions of teratogenic risk associated with radiography and CT during early pregnancy. AJR Am J Roentgenol. 2004;182(5):1107–9.
3. Brent RL. Saving lives and changing family histories: appropriate counseling of pregnant women and men and women of reproductive age, concerning the risk of diagnostic radiation exposures during and before pregnancy.
4. Katayama H, Yamaguchi K, Kozuka T, Takashima T, Seez P, Matsuura K. Adverse reactions to ionic and non-ionic contrast media. A report from the Japanese committee on the safety of contrast media. Radiology. 1990;175:621–8.
5. Hunt CH, Hartman RP, Hesley GK. Frequency and severity of adverse effects of iodinated and gadolinium contrast materials: retrospective review of 456,930 doses. AJR Am J Roentgenol. 2009;193:1124–7.
6. The Renal Association, British Cardiovascular Interventional Society and The Royal College of Radiologists. Prevention of contrast induced acute kidney injury (CI-AKI) in adult patients. London: The Royal College of Radiologists, 2013.
7. Acute kidney injury: prevention, detection and management [A] Evidence review for preventing contrast- induced acute kidney injury. NICE guideline NG148 Evidence reviews December 2019. https://www.nice.org.uk/guidance/ng148/chapter/recommendations.
8. Use of Intravenous Iodinated Contrast Media in Patients with Kidney Disease. Consensus statements from the American College of Radiology and the National Kidney Foundation. Radiology. 2020;294:660–8.
9. American College of Radiology. Manual on contrast media. Version 10.3. Reston, Va: American College of Radiology, 2018. https://www.acr.org/Clinical-Resources/Contrast-Manual. Last Accessed 26 August 2020.
10. Nyman U, Ahlkvist J, Aspelin P, et al. Preventing contrast medium-induced acute kidney injury : side-by-side comparison of Swedish-ESUR guidelines. Eur Radiol. 2018;28(12):5384–95.
11. Palevsky PM, Liu KD, Brophy PD, et al. KDOQI US commentary on the 2012 KDIGO clinical practice guideline for acute kidney injury. Am J Kidney Dis. 2013;61(5):649–72.
12. Faucon AL, Bobrie G, Clément O. Nephrotoxicity of iodinated contrast media: from pathophysiology to prevention strategies. Eur J Radiol. 2019;116:231–41.
13. Royal College of Radiology. Standards for intravascular contrast administration to adult patients. 3rd Ed. 2015. https://www.rcr.ac.uk/sites/default/files/Intravasc_contrast_web.pdf.
14. Hoste EA, De Waele JJ, Gevaert SA, Uchino S, Kellum JA. Sodium bicarbonate for prevention of contrast-induced acute kidney injury: a systematic review and meta-analysis. Nephrol Dial Transplant. 2010;25(3):747–58.
15. Brar SS, Hiremath S, Dangas G, Mehran R, Brar SK, Leon MB. Sodium bicarbonate for the prevention of contrast induced-acute kidney injury: a systematic review and meta-analysis. Clin J Am Soc Nephrol. 2009;4(10):1584–92.
16. Girardi M, Kay J, Elston DM, Leboit PE, Abu-Alfa A, Cowper SE. Nephrogenic systemic fibrosis: clinicopathological definition and workup recommendations. J Am Acad Dermatol. 2011;65:1095–106.

17. http://www.esur.org/fileadmin/content/NSF/NSF-ESUR_Guideline_Final.pdf
18. Carmody E, Greene A, Brennan P, Donohue J, Carmody M, Keeling F. Sequential Tc 99m mercaptoacetyl-triglycine (MAG3) renography as an evaluator of early renal transplant function. Clin Transpl. 1993;7(3):245–9.
19. Goodear M, Barratt L, Wycherley A. Intraperitoneal urine leak in a patient with a renal transplant on Tc-99m MAG3 imaging. Clin Nucl Med. 1998;23(11):789–90.
20. Gordon I, Barratt TM. Detection of vesico-ureteric reflux by indirect radionuclide cystography. Lancet. 1989;2(8671):1108.
21. Gordon I, Peters AM, Morony S. Indirect radionuclide cystography: a sensitive technique for the detection of vesico-ureteral reflux. Pediatr Nephrol. 1990;4(6):604–6.
22. Peters AM, Morony S, Gordon I. Indirect radionuclide cystography demonstrates reflux under physiological conditions. Clin Radiol. 1990;41(1):44–7.
23. Bongers V, Bakker J, Beutler JJ, Beek FJ, De Klerk JM. Assessment of renal artery stenosis: comparison of captopril renography and gadolinium-enhanced breath-hold MR angiography. Clin Radiol. 2000;55(5):346–53.
24. Fernandez P, Morel D, Jeandot R, Potaux L, Basse-Cathalinat B, Ducassou D. Value of captopril renal scintigraphy in hypertensive patients with renal failure. J Nucl Med. 1999;40(3):412–7.
25. Ramsay D, Belton I, Finlay D. A review of captopril renal scintigraphy and its effect on patient management. Nucl Med Commun. 1997;18(7):631–3.
26. Jain TK, Basher RK, Mittal BR, Bhatia A, Rao KL. Follow-up (99m)Tc EC renal dynamic scintigraphy and DMSA-III SPECT/CT in unmasking a masqueraded case of horseshoe kidney. Rev Esp Med Nucl Imagen Mol. 2015;34(6):387–9.
27. Moon EH, Kim MW, Kim YJ, Sun IO. Crossed fused renal Ectopia: presentations on 99mTc-MAG3 scan, 99mTc-DMSA SPECT, and multidetector CT. Clin Nucl Med. 2015;40(10):835–7.
28. Bailey RR, Lynn KL, Robson RA, Smith AH, Maling TM, Turner JG. DMSA renal scans in adults with acute pyelonephritis. Clin Nephrol. 1996;46(2):99–104.
29. Kim SB, Yang WS, Ryu JS, Song JH, Moon DH, Cho KS, et al. Clinical value of DMSA planar and single photon emission computed tomography as an initial diagnostic tool in adult women with recurrent acute pyelonephritis. Nephron. 1994;67(3):274–9.
30. Sattari A, Kampouridis S, Damry N, Hainaux B, Ham HR, Vandewalle JC, et al. CT and 99mTc-DMSA scintigraphy in adult acute pyelonephritis: a comparative study. J Comput Assist Tomogr. 2000;24(4):600–4.
31. Tripathi M, Agarwal KK, Mukherjee A, Thukral P, Damle NA, Shamim SA, et al. 99mTc-DMSA planar imaging versus dual-detector SPECT for the detection of renal cortical scars in patients with CKD-3. Nucl Med Commun. 2016;37(9):911–6.
32. Metser U, Lo G. FDG-PET/CT in abdominal post-transplant lymphoproliferative disease. Br J Radiol. 2016;89(1057):20150844.
33. Takehana CS, Twist CJ, Mosci C, Quon A, Mittra E, Iagaru A. (18)F-FDG PET/CT in the management of patients with post-transplant lymphoproliferative disorder. Nucl Med Commun. 2014;35(3):276–81.
34. Noraini AR, Gay E, Ferrara C, Ravelli E, Mancini V, Morra E, et al. PET-CT as an effective imaging modality in the staging and follow-up of post-transplant lymphoproliferative disorder following solid organ transplantation. Singap Med J. 2009;50(12):1189–95.
35. Kouijzer IJE, Mulders-Manders CM, Bleeker-Rovers CP, Oyen WJG. Fever of unknown origin: the value of FDG-PET/CT. Semin Nucl Med. 2018;48(2):100–7.
36. Solav SV. FDG PET/CT in evaluation of pyrexia of unknown origin. Clin Nucl Med. 2011;36(8):e81–6.
37. McCammack KC, Hawkes NC, Silverman ED, Paz DA. PET/CT appearance of acute pyelonephritis. Clin Nucl Med. 2013;38(7):e299–301.
38. Wan CH, Tseng JR, Lee MH, Yang LY, Yen TC. Clinical utility of FDG PET/CT in acute complicated pyelonephritis-results from an observational study. Eur J Nucl Med Mol Imaging. 2018;45(3):462–70.

IT and Data in Nephrology

Thomas Oates

Contents

M. Harber (ed.), *Primer on Nephrology*, https://doi.org/10.1007/978-3-030-76419-7_6

6

6.1 Introduction

Over the last 10–15 years, healthcare has undergone a significant digital transformation with increasing use of electronic medical records, healthcare information systems, and handheld, wearable, and smart devices. Consequently, many data sources exist digitally – including socio-demographics, medical insurance claims, and procedural billing data in addition to clinical information – yet remain largely underutilized. This diverse wealth of healthcare data offers the potential for optimizing efficient healthcare delivery, directing health policymakers and service commissioners, setting the national research agenda, and improving patient-centred outcomes. This chapter summarizes the current state of play of big data collection, synthesis, and practical applications within nephrology, along with the challenges, risks, and future opportunities it presents.

Learning Objectives

1. To summarize the sources of big data available to nephrologists and the opportunities for analysis and application in terms of research and improving standards and consistency of care.
2. Explore the potential for alerts and AI in nephrology.
3. Discuss the possibility of using social media to improve communication between healthcare professionals and patients.

6.2 Big Data

Definitions of what constitutes big data vary but converge around the five concepts of volume (how much), velocity (how quickly collected), variety (how broad), veracity (how precise), and value (how useful). By 2020, it is estimated that 35 zettabytes of healthcare data, varying in nature from structured to unstructured, will have been collected. Electronic reporting systems increasingly allow dynamic "real-time" continuous data generation and collection. This increasingly large volume and heterogeneous data resource presents major logistical challenges in terms of storage, security, and accuracy (including inconsistencies in coding, missing data, and duplication), as well as difficulties in extraction of useful information using traditional data analytical tools and techniques.

Big data in healthcare collate a wide range of baseline characteristics, exposures, interventions, and outcomes including demographic, physiological, clinical, molecular, and environmental parameters. The main sources of big data are routinely collected administrative databases (including medical insurance and prescription claims), clinical databases (including specialty-specific registries such as the UK Renal Registry (UKRR), the Australia and New Zealand Dialysis and Transplant Registry (ANZDATA), and the US Renal Data System (USRDS)), electronic health record (EHR) data (including the UK Hospital Episode Statistics and the US National Inpatient Sample), and laboratory information system data (including creatinine, estimated glomerular filtration rate [eGFR], and urinary albumin/protein measurements). Other sources include patient-reported data (standardized health surveys, renal patient national surveys, quality of life and patient experience questionnaires collected in clinical studies), biometric data (wearable or sensor generated, device integration), data from social media, medical imaging data, and biomarker data. Accordingly, key stakeholders are as diverse as the data itself and include governmental agencies and large companies; academic groups and technology, biotech, and medical device companies; healthcare providers and payers; not-for-profit foundations; and patient advocacy groups (▫ Table 6.1).

6.3 Big Data in Nephrology

6.3.1 Secondary Care

Specific to nephrology, renal registries, health insurance providers, and clinical investigators (either pharmaceutical companies or academic institutions) constitute the majority of stakeholders collecting large renal patient-focussed datasets. In the United Kingdom (UK), the largest renal-specific registry is the UK Renal Registry (UKRR), a nationwide registry of all patients receiving treatment for end-stage kidney disease in the UK, established in 1995. The UKRR collects demographic, clinical, and treatment data on all people whose native kidney function is not expected to recover and for whom indefinite treatment for end-stage kidney disease (ESKD) is anticipated. UKRR records the aetiology of ESKD and other major comorbidities including cardiovascular events and malignancies, as well as lifestyle risk factors (diabetes and smoking). Renal replacement therapy (RRT) treatments are also recorded, including dates of modality changes and graft function (creatinine measurements) for people with kidney transplants (▫ Table 6.2). Since April 2013, a registry of people experiencing acute kidney injury (AKI) has also been added to the dataset. Similar (and more established) registries exist worldwide including the ANZDATA registry (collecting data since 1977), USRDS (established in 1989, the largest and most comprehensive national end-stage renal disease (ESRD) and chronic kidney disease

Table 6.1 Sources of healthcare big data

Type	Description		Source
Clinical	Electronic medical records	Patient-related information including diagnostic and procedure codes, discharge destinations, medication prescriptions, inpatient complications	Hospitals, clinics, community health services data, social care data
	Diagnostic	Imaging, laboratory results	Laboratories, radiology departments
	Biomarkers	Genomic, proteomic, metabolomic	Universities, diagnostic companies
	Administrative databases	Admission, discharge and transfer data	Healthcare providers, insurance companies
	Renal registries	Demographics, renal-specific diagnoses, treatment/modality history, complications, outcomes	UKRR, ANZDATA, USRDS, ERA-EDTA, OPTN
Claims	Medical insurance claims	Financial medical reimbursement claims	Healthcare providers, insurance companies
	Prescriptions	Prescription reimbursement claims (including drug, dosage, duration, collection)	National pharmacy datasets, insurance companies
Clinical research	Clinical trials	Design parameters (intervention tested, effect size, endpoint)	Universities, pharmaceutical companies, medical journals
Patient-generated	Social media	Web-board discussions	Electronic health portals, social media websites
	Wearable/sensors	Smartphones, fitness monitors, dialysis machine automated feedback systems	Device integration systems, technology firms
	Clinical studies	Quality of life surveys, patient-reported outcome measures	Pharmaceutical companies, universities

UKRR United Kingdom Renal Registry, *ANZDATA* Australia and New Zealand Dialysis and Transplant Registry, *USRDS* United States Renal Data System, *ERA-EDTA* European Renal Association – European Dialysis and Transplant Association

surveillance system worldwide), the European Renal Association – European Dialysis and Transplant Association (ERA-EDTA, established in 1964 though with progressively more European members joining), and the Canadian Organ Replacement Register (CORR).

In addition to compiling routine annual reports on the incidence and prevalence of CKD, ESKD, and RRT patterns, registries are increasingly being used to identify cohorts of people with ESKD with which other datasets of interest are linked, in large-scale cohort studies. These studies harness the power of routinely and prospectively collected, comprehensive data with a long duration of follow-up, helping to make the most efficient use of pre-existing data. Linkage with rare disease registries – such as the National Registry of Rare Kidney Diseases (RaDaR) – allows otherwise prohibitively expensive or time-consuming cohort studies to be conducted.

In the United States (USA), large healthcare companies (including insurers and care providers) also compile large amounts of data on the people they sell services to. Although not a renal-specific dataset, the Kaiser Permanente Research Bank is the second largest biobank in the USA (including between 20 and 50% of each regional area's insured population) with a wealth of de-identified medical record information, health survey results, and bio-specimens available to scientists for genetic, epidemiological, and other research. Multiple cohort studies have been published, both for Kaiser Permanente patients with ESKD and with CKD – an advantage over many of the ESKD registries.

Finally, the pharmaceutical industry (and to a lesser extent, academia) generates ever increasing volumes of data. This data growth is generated from several sources including the research and development (R&D) process itself, retailers, patients, and caregivers. Effectively utilizing these data may help pharmaceutical companies better identify new potential candidate drugs and develop them into effective, approved, and reimbursed medicines more quickly. The European Union (EU) Drug Regulating Authorities Clinical Trials Database

Table 6.2 Nephrology-specific datasets

Source	Description	Additional	Link for further information
Regional or national registry			
UKRR	Demographics, comorbidity, test results, renal replacement therapy treatment details, and medications since 1995	AKI data since August 2013. Data are submitted to the UKRR from 71 adult (and 13 paediatric) renal units on a quarterly basis	► https://www.renalreg.org/
ANZ-DATA	Demographics, cause of renal failure, comorbidity status, date of start of first RRT, history of RRT with dates and changes of modality, treatment Centre, date and cause of death. Bi-national data collection since 1977	Data is collected from all dialysis and transplant units in Australia and New Zealand annually with the census period ending on the 31st of December every year	► http://www.anzdata.org
ANZOD	Data related to organ donation and transplantation including care of donors, quality of transplant organs, and transplant recipient outcomes. Data collected since 1989 in Australia and 1993 in New Zealand	Data collected since 1989 in Australia and 1993 in New Zealand. Data for living kidney donors collected since 2004	► http://www.anzdata.org.au/anzod/v1/indexanzod.html
USRDS	US national data system that collects, analyses, and distributes information about chronic kidney disease and end-stage renal disease established in 1988	Wide measures of incidence, prevalence, outcomes, and financial costs associated with different treatment modalities	► http://www.usrds.org
CORR	Pan-Canadian information system collecting data from hospital dialysis programs, transplant programs, organ procurement organizations, and independent health facilities. Established in 1985		► https://www.cihi.ca/en/canadian-organ-replacement-register-corr
ERA-EDTA	Demographics, cause of renal failure, comorbidity status, date of start of first RRT, history of RRT with dates and changes of modality, treatment Centre, date and cause of death since 1963	Annual data collection from national and regional registries from 36 European countries	► https://era-edta-reg.org
CK-NET	Chinese CKD registry identified from hospital discharge coding recording age, sex, geographic residence, and medical comorbidities	CKD classified according to ten main categories	
Health insurance providers			
Kaiser Permanente	Private US health insurance provider enrolling 20–50% of each regional area's insured population (total membership 11.6 million)	General, pregnancy and cancer cohorts established, with biobanking of saliva, urine, and DNA. Lifestyle and behaviour survey data. Linkage with electronic medical records	► https://researchbank.kaiserpermanente.org/our-research/for-researchers/
ESKD PPS	Part of US Medicare/Medicaid program specifically for funding renal dialysis services	Patient- and facility-level adjusted per treatment payment to ESKD facilities for renal dialysis services provided. Co-interventions (including medications, education) recorded. Clinical outcomes recorded to ensure standard practice and costs across providers	► https://www.cms.gov/Medicare/Medicare-Fee-for-Service-Payment/ESRDpayment/index.html

UKRR United Kingdom Renal Registry; *ANZDATA* Australia and New Zealand Dialysis and Transplant Registry; *USRDS* United States Renal Data System; *ERA-EDTA* European Renal Association – European Dialysis and Transplant Association; *ESKD PPS* End Stage Renal Disease Prospective Payment System

(EudraCT) collates information on interventional clinical trials on medicines conducted in the EU or the European Economic Area (EEA) which started after 2004. Currently, there are 33,690 clinical trials for renal disease registered with a EudraCT protocol. The parallel US-based ▶ ClinicalTrials.gov currently identifies 7701 studies for "kidney diseases" and includes registrations and protocols for interventional and observational studies. In addition to primary analyses, trial data are increasingly used in secondary studies: synthesis of data across multiple RCT of similar interventions in meta-analyses allows more robust estimates of treatment effects (as well as exploration of clinical heterogeneity), and linkage of data from participants in randomized controlled trials (RCT) to either renal-specific registries or other large electronic datasets has allowed nested cohort studies using data linkage to examine long-term outcomes for rare disease and expensive interventions which are beyond the scope of most clinical trials.

Chronic kidney disease (CKD) management often involves primary and secondary care providers working toward the achievement of disparate outcomes dictated by payment systems. As a result, aligning outcomes and facilitating information flow between providers may result in improved quality of care. Basic interventions in earlier stages of CKD may retard progression of CKD and prove to be cost-effective [6].

Medical coding, the process of transforming descriptions of medical diagnoses and procedures into universal numeric codes, has been rapidly enabled by the growth of electronic health records (EHRs). Intelligent use of coded data to examine the efficacy and cost-effectiveness of interventions, track new trends in medical needs, and guide reimbursement of healthcare providers represents one of the key goals of data usage in medicine.

Coding of individuals' disease status, often followed by inclusion in primary care disease registers, may associate with differences in outcomes. Recently, the UK National CKD Audit collected data from over 400,000 patients registered with 1005 primary care practices in the UK [12]. This showed a striking association between lack of a CKD code in patients with CKD and secondary care outcomes. An increasing likelihood of death, unplanned hospital admission, and acute kidney injury was seen in patients with uncoded CKD as eGFR fell. However, given that this was audit data collected only to interrogate CKD, potential confounders cannot be adjusted for, limiting potential conclusions. Additionally, patients with uncoded CKD were less likely to have basic management interventions such as achieving blood pressure targets, quantification of urine protein, and offering of statin treatment [12], suggesting that driving up CKD coding could improve outcomes.

Additionally, there is evidence that the efficacy of technology-enabled interventions subsequent to detection of CKD may differ. A recent randomized trial of 93 primary care practices [15] found that blood pressure control in patients with CKD was significantly improved in practices that were part of an audit-based education intervention scheme compared with those practices using usual care or EHR-based guidelines and prompts about CKD. Audit-based education is a validated quality improvement intervention that depends upon IT systems to extract and make comparisons between practices and against evidence-based guidelines.

Similarly, in the USA – partly as a result of the federal government paying for most dialysis care since 1972 – Medicare's large administrative datasets have had a central role in the evaluation and development of public policy, helping to identify trends in costs, access to dialysis care, and quality of care delivered. Studies using Medicare data – including the Dialysis Outcomes and Practice Patterns Study – have enabled care provider comparisons with the generation of an outcome-focussed national ESKD Quality Incentive Program (QIP) in which key quality metrics (including vascular access, hospitalizations, infections, and use of blood transfusions) determine financial reimbursement in an effort to improve quality of care.

6.4 Using and Analysing Big Data

Big data analytics has the potential to transform clinical pathways for efficient delivery of care, set priorities for patient-centred clinical research, and – by recognizing patterns and detecting disease associations – facilitate autonomous decision-making. In clinical practice, big data analytics can also help in the personalization of predictions of disease trajectory and the estimation of risks and benefits associated with different treatment options and support clinical decision-making aids. Different techniques can be applied to analysing big data depending on the healthcare application (◘ Table 6.3).

Nephrology has been a leader in embracing big data both by design and by necessity. The multiple, recurrent nature of episodic care that nephrologists provide to people with ESKD on RRT – as well as the emerging epidemic of chronic kidney disease – means that nephrologists need to be able to use big data to monitor and ensure equity and quality of service delivery, detect disease, assess benefits and harms of new interventions, and predict likely future healthcare outcomes and needs.

Table 6.3 Big data analytical techniques

Technique	Application
Cluster analysis	Determination of population clusters for targeted screening, detection, and treatment of chronic diseases
Association studies	Detection of risk factor/biomarker/gene-disease or outcome associations
Graph analytics	Comparison of key outcome measures across healthcare providers
Machine learning	Prediction of disease risk
Neural networks	Diagnosis of chronic diseases Prediction of future disease
Data mining	Inductive reasoning and exploratory data analysis

6.4.1 Surveillance of Healthcare Delivery and Service Transformation

6.4.1.1 Improving Service Delivery by Using Data

Evidence suggests that delays in recognition of both acute kidney injury (AKI) [11, 15] and chronic kidney disease (CKD) [22] may be associated with poorer outcomes. Information systems aligned to early detection and alerting of these diagnoses are already available in nephrology.

6.5 AKI Alerts

AKI has been an exemplar field in using IT and data in clinical practice. AKI alerts require a two-step process: first using diagnostic criteria to establish the presence of AKI and then second employing IT solutions to alert clinicians to the diagnosis. The practical application of this process has revealed issues in both steps of this method.

6.5.1 Automated Diagnosis of AKI

The NHS in England has recently produced a national algorithm to automate and standardize the definition of AKI. Different diagnostic criteria for AKI (e.g. the AKIN [16] and the Risk, Injury, Failure, Loss of kidney function, and End-stage kidney disease (RIFLE) [3] criteria) exist, but all require comparison of a serum creatinine result to a baseline value. Numerous approaches to the calculation of a baseline creatinine value have been used (reviewed in [3, 10]) resulting in wide variation in the sensitivity and specificity of detection algorithms. The NHS England algorithm is uncommon in that it is able to compute a baseline value in various ways depending on the availability of recent creatinine measurements. This approach attains better sensitivity than algorithms based upon a single creatinine value [18].

6.5.2 Electronic Alerting

The second part of an alert system is the method by which the detected diagnosis is communicated to relevant clinicians. There is an evolving literature around how best to "alert" clinicians.

A single-centre randomized controlled trial enrolled 2393 patients diagnosed with AKI by an electronic algorithm. The control group received usual care, whilst the intervention group had the AKI diagnosis communicated to a hospital cell phone through a single standardized text message [21]. The trial's primary outcome of death, dialysis, or creatinine rise at 30 days was similar in the two groups. The use of a text message can be labelled as a "passive" type of electronic alerting. Evidence exists that so-called "interruptive" alerts, those in which a specific response, usually in an electronic health record, is required to remove the alert, may be more effective in this context [13].

However, as AKI is a heterogeneous syndrome with many underlying aetiologies, the nature of the definitive action suggested in an interruptive alert requires thought. Currently, there is significant interest in care bundles that mobilize members of a multidisciplinary team to implement a structured set of practices. Care bundles are ultimately designed to improve the processes of care delivery to patients with AKI. There is an evolving evidence base that care bundles in AKI may improve patient outcomes [13, 20], and their use is currently being evaluated in a multi-centre pragmatic clinical trial [19].

6.6 Risk Prediction

Given than 15–20% of the adult population in Westernized countries has CKD stages 3 and greater, identifying those at risk of progression is vital if nephrologists are not to be overwhelmed by this major public health issue. Large population cohort datasets have been used to develop prediction tools for prognosis in CKD including the Grampian Laboratory Outcomes Mortality and Morbidity Study (I and II) and the Kidney Failure Risk Equation (KFRE) which was based on a large Canadian population cohort and validated in more than 30 countries. Whilst renal registries and cohort studies capture a large amount of baseline information, the integration of an ever-increasing availability of patient-level data captured from EHRs has the potential to incorporate dynamically evolving, clinically relevant patient-level data. Newer automated techniques are being developed to extract this longitudinal, unstructured clinical narrative data using natural language processing (NLP), with its incorporation into risk prediction modelling showing improved accuracy of predicting progression of CKD stage 3 to 4, post-operative RRT-requiring AKI, as well as helping define the epidemiology of rare diseases (such as calciphylaxis) without specific international classification of disease (ICD) codes. Within kidney transplantation, models predicting graft loss and mortality have also shown significantly increased efficacy with the inclusion of EHR data including serial laboratory measurements as well as key data extracted using NLP from unstructured text (including Banff scores from biopsy reports, vital signs pre-dating EHR, and social worker assessments). For patients, risk prediction modelling using big data is also being used to create shared clinical decision-making tools. The iChoose Kidney – developed in the USA and recently validated in a Canadian cohort of nearly 30,000 patients with ESKD – aims to help personalize estimates of mortality based on RRT treatment decisions (dialysis versus living or deceased donor kidney transplantation) and help patients make more informed choices.

6.7 What Are the Weaknesses of Big Data?

Medical big data are frequently hard to gain access to, with strict data access and security requirements. Medical big data can be further affected by several sources of uncertainty, such as measurement errors or errors in coding the information buried in textual reports. Analyses are complicated by technical issues, such as missing values, dimensionality, and bias control, and share the inherent limitations of observational studies – namely, the inability to test causality resulting from residual confounding and potential reverse causality. Many challenges, such as the absence of evidence of practical benefits of big data, methodological issues including legal and ethical issues, and clinical integration and utility issues, must be overcome to realize the promise of medical big data as the fuel of a continuous learning healthcare system that will improve patient outcomes and reduce waste in areas including nephrology.

6.8 Networks and Communication

The ongoing revolution in affordability and power of personal computing devices and the scale and accessibility of the Internet has facilitated the formation of novel global networks in many fields. In healthcare, these networks have benefitted both healthcare professionals (HCPs) and patients and their carers. Largely as a result of the growth and acceptance of social media channels, HCPs are now able to exchange ideas, share resources, build relationships, and pursue continued professional development in ways that were previously impossible. Nephrology has been ahead of the curve in this regard, and many formalized education resources are now available (reviewed in [5]).

Meeting the information needs of patients is a core goal for HCPs. Use of online networks and non-traditional communication channels to provide reliable information to patients and to facilitate peer-to-peer support is growing. Whilst social media peer-to-peer support groups exist for many diseases, these groups are augmented by the involvement of medical professionals [8]. In recognition of this, and to balance the concerns HCPs have about taking part in a novel area, common sense guidelines for professional conduct in these groups and communities are now available [7].

There is evidence that patients with the knowledge, skills, and confidence to manage their own health and care may achieve improved health outcomes. This engagement can be formalized through the concept of "patient activation", measured by the Patient Activation Measure (PAM) [9], a licensed product which has been extensively tested and verified across numerous demographic and disease states. The PAM can be a reliable indicator of a number of health outcomes, including medication adherence and disease monitoring. Patient activation may vary over time, and targeted interventions may increase it, raising the possibility that associated outcomes may improve as a result.

In nephrology, PAM data suggests that up to 46% of patients with CKD may report low activation [23] and that less activated patients may not be as able to partake in shared decision-making about their care. Additionally, health literacy (defined as the personal characteristics and social resources needed for individuals and communities to access, understand, appraise, and use information and services to make decisions about health) and PAM are not fully correlated. Indeed, the use of IT tools suggestive of high health literacy, such as patient portals, may not associate with increased PAM [2, 23].

Validated interventions to improve PAM have largely been dependent upon education programmes seeking to help patients adopt healthy behaviour and transform the patient-HCP relationship into a collaborative partnership [4]. Traditionally, these programmes were delivered face to face. Recently, online IT solutions have been used, which have achieved concurrent improvements in PAM and medical endpoints such as HbA1c in patients with diabetes [4, 14] and hospital admissions [1].

Although such programmes may expand access to healthcare, support engagement, and provide durable development in health behaviours, ultimately resulting in improved patient outcomes and cost savings, the relationship between these aspects is complex, and further research is needed to elucidate the relationships between PAM and health literacy, information needs and delivery, and which outcomes to measure before the full potential is reached.

6.9 Conclusions

Systematic community-wide approaches to detection and management of kidney disease have previously shown efficacy [17]. Modern IT presents huge opportunities to enhance collection and analysis of digitized data and information, build networks of relevant professionals and patients, and create new care models in kidney disease, thus expanding and exceeding these previous approaches.

The advances discussed in this chapter suggest an environment that is highly conducive to the development of "learning health systems" in nephrology; systems in which the clinical, scientific, infrastructural, and cultural environment supports improvement and innovation by supporting best practice and capturing new knowledge. If the field of nephrology can harness the potential of IT and data in the near future and coalesce around the idea of learning health systems calibrated to collect key data, focus relentlessly on outcomes, upskill patients in self-care, and engage key HCPs, meaningful improvements in the health of those living with kidney disease are highly likely to result.

References

1. Ahn S, et al. The impact of chronic disease self-management programs: healthcare savings through a community-based intervention. BMC Public Health. 2013;13:1141.
2. Ancker JS, et al. Patient activation and use of an electronic patient portal. Inform Health Soc Care. 2015;40(3):254–66.
3. Bellomo R, et al. Acute renal failure - definition, outcome measures, animal models, fluid therapy and information technology needs: the second international consensus conference of the acute dialysis quality initiative (ADQI) group. Crit Care Soc Crit Care Med. 2004;8(4):R204–12.
4. Bodenheimer T, et al. Patient self-management of chronic disease in primary care. JAMA. 2002;288(19):2469–75.
5. Colbert GB, et al. The social media revolution in nephrology education. Kidney Int Rep. 2018;3(3):519–29.
6. Couser WG, et al. The contribution of chronic kidney disease to the global burden of major noncommunicable diseases. Kidney Int. 2011;80(12):1258–70.
7. Farnan JM, et al. Online medical professionalism: patient and public relationships: policy statement from the American College of Physicians and the Federation of State Medical Boards. Ann Intern Med. 2013;158(8):620–7.
8. Graham-Brown MPM, Oates T. Social media in medicine: a game changer? Nephrology, Dialysis, Transplantation: Official Publication of the European Dialysis and Transplant Association - European Renal Association. 2017;32(11):1806–8.
9. Hibbard JH, et al. Development of the patient activation measure (PAM): conceptualizing and measuring activation in patients and consumers. Health Serv Res. 2004;39(4 Pt 1):1005–26.
10. Horne KL, Selby NM. Recent developments in electronic alerts for acute kidney injury. Curr Opin Crit Care. 2015;21(6):479–84.
11. James MT, et al. Weekend hospital admission, acute kidney injury, and mortality. J Am Soc Nephrol. 2010;21(5):845–51.
12. Kim LG, et al. How do primary care doctors in England and Wales code and manage people with chronic kidney disease? Results from the National Chronic Kidney Disease Audit. Nephrology, Dialysis, Transplantation: Official Publication of the European Dialysis and Transplant Association - European Renal Association. 2018;33(8):1373–9.
13. Kolhe NV, et al. Impact of compliance with a care bundle on acute kidney injury outcomes: a prospective observational study. PLoS One. 2015;10(7):e0132279.
14. Lorig K, et al. Online diabetes self-management program: a randomized study. Diabetes Care. 2010;33(6):1275–81.
15. de Lusignan S, et al. Audit-based education lowers systolic blood pressure in chronic kidney disease: the quality improvement in CKD (QICKD) trial results. Kidney Int. 2013;84(3):609–20.
16. Mehta RL, et al. Acute kidney injury network: report of an initiative to improve outcomes in acute kidney injury. Crit Care Soc Crit Care Med. 2007;11(2):R31.
17. Rayner HC, et al. Does community-wide chronic kidney disease management improve patient outcomes? Nephrology, Dialysis, Transplantation: Official Publication of the European Dialysis and Transplant Association - European Renal Association. 2014;29(3):644–9.
18. Sawhney S, et al. Acute kidney injury-how does automated detection perform? Nephrology, Dialysis, Transplantation: Official Publication of the European Dialysis and Transplant Association - European Renal Association. 2015;30(11):1853–61.
19. Selby NM, et al. Design and rationale of "tackling acute kidney injury", a multicentre quality improvement study. Nephron. 2016;134(3):200–4.
20. Selby NM, Kolhe NV. Care bundles for acute kidney injury: do they work? Nephron. 2016;134(3):195–9.
21. Wilson FP, et al. Automated, electronic alerts for acute kidney injury: a single-blind, parallel-group, randomised controlled trial. Lancet. 2015;385(9981):1966–74.
22. Wouters OJ, et al. Early chronic kidney disease: diagnosis, management and models of care. Nature reviews. Nephrology. 2015;11(8):491–502.
23. Zimbudzi E, et al. Factors associated with patient activation in an Australian population with comorbid diabetes and chronic kidney disease: a cross-sectional study. BMJ Open. 2017;7(10):e017695.

Renal Pathology

Lauren Heptinstall and Paul Bass

Contents

M. Harber (ed.), *Primer on Nephrology*, https://doi.org/10.1007/978-3-030-76419-7_7

Learning Objectives
- To understand the histopathological approach to a renal biopsy.
- To know the differential diagnosis of light microscopic, immunohistological/immunofluorescent and electron microscopic pathological features and patterns of injury.
- To understand the use of some common histological classification systems.

7.1 Introduction

This chapter aims to provide an introduction to medical renal pathology, including native and transplant pathology. Definitions and differentials for the most common pathological features, a description of the various patterns of injury, the immunohistochemical/immunofluorescence and electron microscopic findings of the most commonly seen entities are provided. The most frequently encountered classification systems are described. Some cases are provided at the end of the chapter to provide fully worked examples and to allow the reader to practise their pathological interpretation of renal biopsies.

7.2 The Pathologist's Approach to a Medical Renal Biopsy

Each pathologist will have their own preferences, but the following provides a general outline of how the biopsy will be handled.

7.2.1 Clinical Details

This crucial information will provide the basis for the interpretation of all subsequent findings and often guides the pathologist as to how the tissue should best be utilised. Useful information includes:
- Demographics.
  - Age.
  - Sex.
  - Native/transplant.
- Indication for biopsy.
  - Nephrotic syndrome.
  - Acute kidney injury.
  - Chronic kidney disease.
  - Haematuria.
  - Proteinuria.
  - Transplant dysfunction.
- The result of any previous biopsies.
- Available test results, e.g. autoantibodies.
- If a transplant biopsy:
  - Duration of transplant.
  - Cause of ESKD, if known.
  - Donor information.
    - Living related/altruistic, DCD/DBD.
    - Age.
- The clinical question, e.g. rejection? vasculitis? cause of CKD?

At this stage, the pathologist will decide how the tissue will be treated in the laboratory:
- Urgency.
  - Routine or urgent.
- Whether electron microscopy is required.
  - Samples are ideally taken from the core before the tissue is processed into a wax block to preserve the ultrastructural features (reprocessing tissue from the wax block causes artefacts which can make interpretation difficult).

7.2.2 Initial Sections

Serial 3–5 um sections will be cut from the tissue core. A particular use of serial sections is that many views through a single glomerulus are visible, which allows for better orientation and localisation of lesions. The pathologist will first receive one or two haematoxylin and eosin (H&E) stained slides with between three to six sections on each. At this point further decisions will be made:
- Is there renal tissue?
  - Capsule, cortex, medulla, pelvi-calyceal system, vessels.
  - If not, what is there, and is it pathological? Possibilities include fat, connective tissue, skeletal muscle, liver, adrenal or bowel.
- Is it adequate for diagnosis? (see below).
- If an urgent result is required or the biopsy shows unexpected features (e.g. unexpected vasculitis), a provisional written or verbal report can be issued at this point.

The adequacy of a biopsy will vary depending on the findings; for example, it may be possible to diagnose membranous glomerulopathy with one patent glomerulus, whereas if a lesion is focal, the probability of detection will depend on the number of glomeruli sampled [1].

7.2.3 Further Stains

Further tinctorial stains and immunofluorescence/immunohistochemistry will follow, usually taking 1 to 3 days. A range of complementary stains are used, each of which highlights different aspects of the biopsy. The stains used vary slightly depending on personal preference, but as a guide, these may include the following:

Stain	Staining pattern	Applications
H&E (haema-toxylin and eosin)	Pink cytoplasm Blue nuclei	Overall assessment The most commonly used stain in histopathology
PAS (periodic acid-Schiff)	Pink staining of basement membranes, mesangial matrix, hyaline material	Overall assessment Glomerular cellularity and matrix Hyaline casts, arteriolosclerosis, glomerular deposits
PAMS (periodic acid methenamine silver)	Black staining of collagen (mesangial matrix, basement membranes, fibrosis)	Areas of chronic damage (interstitial fibrosis) Assessment of glomerular capillary walls Mesangial matrix Glomerular sclerosis Tubular basement membranes
HVG/EVG (haema-toxylin/ elastic Van Gieson)	Connective tissue and elastin	Assessment of vessels Areas of chronic damage
Congo red	Positive areas indicating amyloid deposits appear 'salmon pink' with 'apple green' birefringence under polarised light Eosinophil cytoplasm Elastic fibres Calcium phosphate	Identification of amyloid Also useful for: Eosinophils (pink cytoplasm) Interstitial calcium phosphate (pale purple) Vascular elastic lamina (pink)

Other stains that may be used include MSB (Martius scarlet blue) for fibrin, Von Kossa for calcium phosphate and Perl's stain for iron.

7.2.4 Immunohistochemistry and Immunofluorescence

Either immunohistochemistry (IHC) or immunofluorescence (IMF) is used to identify immunoglobulin and complement deposition. Each method has advantages and disadvantages; thus, local preferences and availability will determine which is used. The specific antibodies used will vary slightly, but immunoglobulins (M, A, G), two complement components (C3, C1q or C6–C9) and kappa and lambda light chains are fairly standard in native biopsies. Some centres also routinely use fibrinogen.

The native IHC/MIF panel:

- Immunoglobulin.
  - IgM.
  - IgA.
  - IgG.
- Complement component.
  - C3.
  - C1q.
- Kappa/lambda light chains.

In transplant biopsies, a different panel is used. C4d positivity of the peritubular capillaries is a feature of antibody-mediated rejection. BKV stain highlights tubular epithelial cell nuclei containing viral replication. In some cases, both the native and transplant panels will be used, particularly if there is concern of a recurrent glomerulopathy.

The transplant IHC/IMF panel:

- C4d.
- BKV.

Assessment of positive staining by IHC/IMF includes:

- Glomerular distribution.
  - Focal or diffuse.
  - Segmental or global.
- Glomerular location.
  - Mesangial.
  - Subepithelial capillary wall.
  - Subendothelial capillary wall.
- Extra-glomerular staining.
  - Tubular.
  - Vascular.
- Pattern of staining.
  - Granular (coarse/fine).
  - Linear.
- Intensity of staining.
  - Weak or strong.
  - Dominant or codominant staining (comparing the relative intensity).

7.2.5 Electron Microscopy

Electron microscopic (EM) examination requires separate processing and may take longer than LM and IHC/IMF, and so may be reported at a later date. EM allows for assessment of various features:

- Presence and location of electron dense deposits (usually visible as immunoglobulin/complement positivity on IHC/IMF).

- Presence, morphology and location of organised deposits (e.g. amyloid fibrils).
- Glomerular basement membrane (GBM) thickness and alterations, e.g. duplications.
- Podocyte alterations, e.g. foot process effacement (FPE).
- Identification of other structures, e.g. tubuloreticular inclusions.
- Peritubular capillary alterations, e.g. lamination in transplant biopsies.

The ultrastructural appearances often corroborate the light microscopic and IHC/IMF features and help confirm or provide a more precise diagnosis, but in some cases, EM is essential for a diagnosis to be made:

- Minimal change disease.
- Thin basement membrane disease.
- Fibrillary glomerulopathy (if DNAJB9 IHC is not available).
- Immunotactoid glomerulopathy.
- Alport syndrome.
- Early diabetic glomerulopathy.
- Early membranous glomerulopathy.
- Some cases of Lupus Nephropathy (e.g. lupus podocytopathy).

7.2.6 Reaching a Diagnosis

The combination of the clinical, light microscopic, IHC/IMF and electron microscopic information will allow the pathologist to reach a diagnosis in most cases. Often a summary of findings and discussion explaining the basis for the diagnosis will be useful, and a comparison to any previous biopsies should be included if possible. Many centres will have regular meetings of the nephrologists, transplant surgeons and pathologists, to allow discussion of the findings and to provide in-depth clinicopathological correlation. This is particularly useful in difficult cases, where it may not be possible to reach a definite diagnosis. This situation may arise because the findings are non-specific or complex, the various methodologies have not worked optimally or there is insufficient tissue available to perform all the required tests. In these situations, in discussion with the clinicians, the pathologist will give as definitive a diagnosis as possible.

7.3 What Is Normal?

Within cortical tissue:

Glomeruli (▫ Figs. 7.1 and 7.2)

- Normal size (not noticeably enlarged or shrunken).
- Thin capsule, separate from the glomerular tuft (no adhesions).

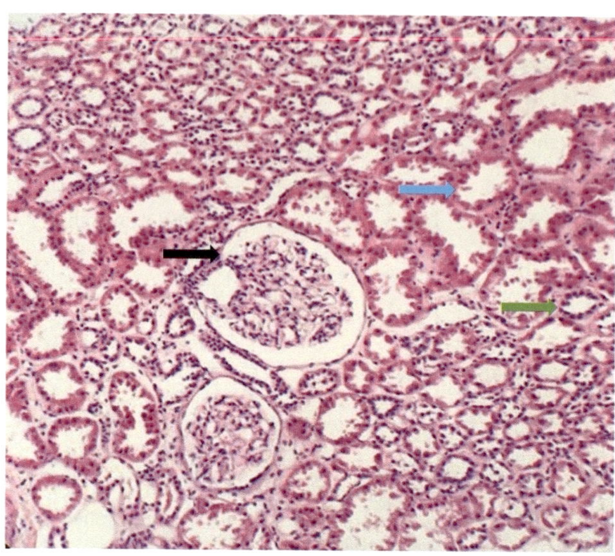

▫ **Fig. 7.1** Normal cortex showing glomeruli (black arrow), proximal tubules (blue arrow), distal tubules (green arrow). Interstitium is inconspicuous. H&E x100

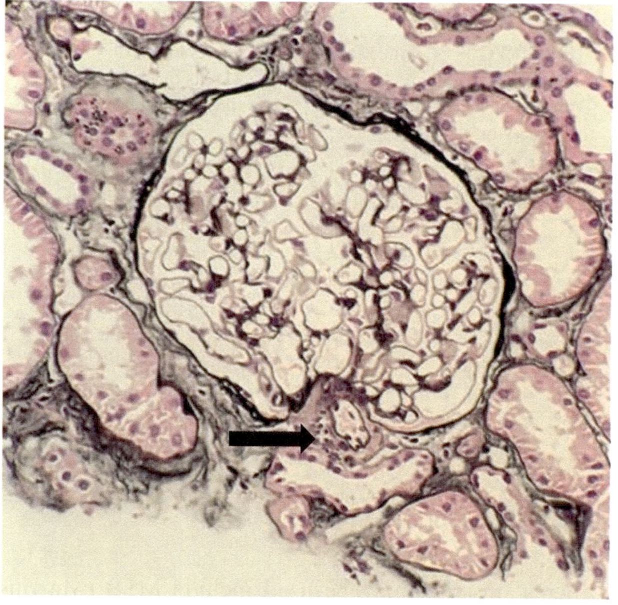

▫ **Fig. 7.2** Normal glomerulus with vascular pole (black arrow). PAMS x400

- A single layer of parietal epithelial cells.
- Glomerular tuft filling the urinary space.
- No cells filling the urinary space.
- Thin, uniform glomerular capillary walls.
- Patent capillary lumens containing occasional red blood cells and endothelial cell nuclei.
- A small amount of mesangial matrix with <4 mesangial cells per peripheral mesangial area (excluding hilar regions).

Tubules

- Back-to-back arrangement of predominantly proximal tubules, with some distal tubules and collecting ducts.
- Proximal tubules; columnar cells with abundant eosinophilic (pink) cytoplasm and an apical brush border.

Interstitium

- Very little or none is visible.

Extra-glomerular Vessels

- Patent arteries, arterioles, veins and capillaries, containing blood.
- No thromboemboli, necrosis, inflammation or degenerative changes (see below).

Within medullary tissue (◘ Fig. 7.3).

Glomeruli

- None are present.

Tubules

- A mixed population of proximal and distal tubules, loops of Henle and collecting ducts.
- Distal tubules; low cuboidal cells with eosinophilic cytoplasm and apical nucleus, lacking a brush border.
- Loops of Henle; very thin epithelial cells, difficult to distinguish from capillaries.
- Collecting ducts; low cuboidal cells with pale cytoplasm, central nucleus and distinct cell borders, lacking a brush border, with a larger lumen.
- Not back-to-back; separated by interstitium.

Interstitium

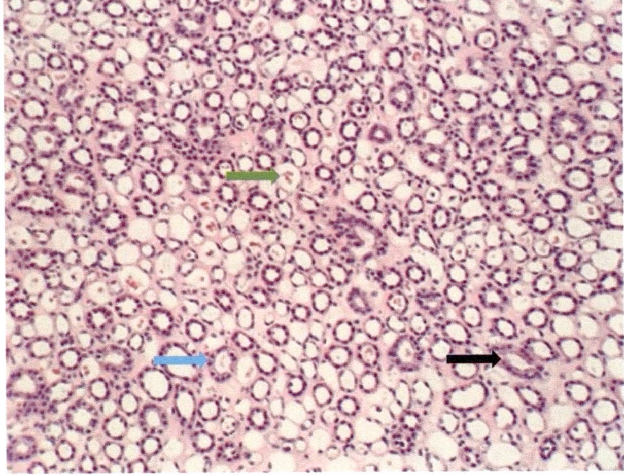

◘ **Fig. 7.3** Normal medulla showing distal tubules (black arrow), collecting ducts (blue arrow) and capillaries (green arrow). H&E x100

- Increased compared to the cortex (particularly within the inner medulla).
- Paucicellular collagenous matrix.
- Contains a few lymphocytes, fibroblasts and vessels.

Normal renal parenchyma will vary in appearance depending on the patient's age. Some age-related chronic damage, known as IFTA (interstitial fibrosis and tubular atrophy), is to be expected in older patients. An estimate of the percentage of chronic damage within the renal cortex can be given using the following equation

Age / 2–10 = % of acceptable sclerosis.

Thus, a biopsy from a 20-year-old patient should have only very minimal chronic damage, whereas one from an 80-year-old patient may have up to 30% IFTA acceptable as a normal feature [2].

7.4 Pathologies of each Compartment

During the assessment of a renal biopsy, each 'compartment' (i.e. glomeruli, tubules, interstitium and extra-glomerular vessels) should be reviewed. As the compartments are interdependent, injury to one will lead to secondary injury in the others, particularly if this injury is long-standing. When there is advanced multicompartmental damage, determining the primary site of injury can be difficult.

7.4.1 Active Versus Chronic

Whether the abnormalities are active/acute or chronic is useful for guiding prognosis and management. Active lesions imply that the injury is current, may benefit from intervention and could recover. Chronic lesions imply that the injury is remote and has healed. These lesions are generally considered irreversible and will not respond to treatment. Chronic lesions are non-specific as the scarring response is similar in any cause of injury, so it can be impossible to determine the original cause if only chronic lesions are present.

Active features	Cellular proliferation within the glomerular tuft (endocapillary and/or mesangial hypercellularity) Cellular proliferation out with the glomerular tuft (parietal epithelial cell proliferation/extracapillary hypercellularity/cellular crescent formation) Necrosis (karyorrhexis, fibrin) Interstitial oedema Inflammation (glomerulitis, tubulitis, interstitial nephritis, vasculitis)
Chronic features	Glomerular sclerosis (segmental or global) Fibrous tissue within the urinary space (fibrous crescents) Interstitial fibrosis and tubular atrophy ('IFTA')

7

7.4.2 Glomerulus

Each glomerulus should be assessed systematically, examining each component (cells and matrix): capsule, the urinary space, capillary walls, capillary lumens, mesangial regions and tubular and vascular poles (where visible) (◻ Figs. 7.4 7.5, 7.6, 7.7, 7.8, 7.9, 7.10, 7.11, 7.12, 7.13, and 7.14).

	Terminology	Definition
Describes all glomeruli	Focal	Involves <50% of all glomeruli
	Diffuse	Involves ≥50% of all glomeruli
Describes one glomerulus	Segmental	Involves <50% of a glomerulus
	Global	Involves ≥50% of a glomerulus

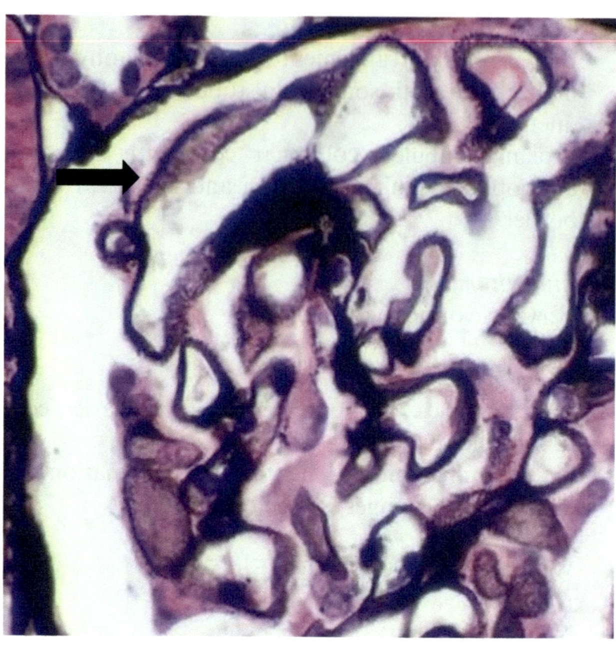

◻ **Fig. 7.4** Subepithelial spikes along capillary walls in a case of membranous glomerulopathy (black arrow). PAMS. x400 original magnification

Glomerulus		
Lesion	***Description***	***Differentials***
Capsule		
Fibrosis	Chronic lesion Thickened, multi-layered membrane best seen on PAMS or PAS	Sclerosed/sclerosing glomeruli Ischaemia
Adhesion	An area of attachment of the glomerular tuft to the capsule	Non-specific, represents a scar implying damage of the tuft has occurred Can be an early feature of FSGS
Rupture	Acute lesion A break in the capsule, usually with associated inflammation and possibly fibrin Best seen on PAMS	Necrotising glomerulonephritis, e.g. ANCA-associated GN, anti-GBM disease, IgA nephropathy
Urinary space, visceral and parietal epithelial cells		
Crescents (a form of extracapillary hypercellularity) (◻ Fig. 7.11)	*Cellularity decreases as fibrosis increases over time, so the proportion of each indicates the age/maturity of the lesion* *Cellular (<25% fibrosis)* Acute lesion Proliferation of parietal epithelial cells extending into the urinary space from the capsule, at least two cells thick. Often includes karyorrhectic debris, inflammatory cells or fibrin from the damaged tuft *Fibrocellular (>25% of cells and fibrosis)* A subacute lesion A mixture of parietal epithelial cells and fibrosis (collagen) *Fibrous (<25% cells)* Chronic lesion Fibrosis in urinary space, containing few/no nuclei. Fibrosis is highlighted on PAMS	*Cellular* Many differentials, particularly vasculitis (ANCA, anti-GBM), immune complex-mediated glomerulopathy, e.g. IgA disease Implies a response of parietal epithelial cells to rupture of a capillary wall *Fibrocellular/fibrous* Non-specific. Healed/healing vasculitis, immune complex-mediated glomerulopathy, ischaemia, sclerosis

Glomerulus		
Lesion	***Description***	***Differentials***
Podocyte/visceral epithelial cell hyperplasia (a form of extracapillary hypercellularity)	Increased number of visceral epithelial cells, which may contain PAS-positive protein resorption droplets	Collapsing FSGS Seen to a lesser extent in many conditions as a non-specific feature (e.g. ischaemia)
Foamy visceral epithelial cells	Podocytes are enlarged with abundant foamy/bubbly cytoplasm	Lysosomal storage disorders, such as Fabry's disease
Capsular drops	Hyaline material attached to the capsule	Diabetic nephropathy
Capillary walls		
Spikes, chains (◘ Fig. 7.4)	Spikes arranged perpendicular to the GBM, extending into the urinary space, or holes (chains) in the capillary wall when viewed obliquely, caused by basement membrane extending between or surrounding subepithelial immune deposits Best seen on PAMS	Membranous glomerulopathy (primary or secondary) Lupus nephropathy (class V) Amyloidosis involving capillary walls causes feathery spike formations/spicules
Double contour ('tram track', splitting, duplication) (◘ Fig. 7.5)	A double-layered appearance of the capillary wall, caused by mesangial interposition and new basement membrane formation inside the original Best seen on PAMS	Subendothelial electron dense deposits: Immune complex-mediated (type I) MPGN, C3 glomerulopathies, SLE, cryoglobulinemia, PIGN Organised deposits, e.g. amyloid, fibrillary, immunotactoid or fibronectin glomerulopathy Chronic endothelial injury: Chronic TMA, pre-eclampsia, transplant glomerulopathy (CAMR)
Wire loop (◘ Fig. 7.7)	Very thick, glassy capillary walls, caused by large subendothelial deposits	An active feature of SLE
Thickening	Thickened capillary walls without definite spikes or double contours	Diabetic nephropathy, an early form of any of the above capillary wall lesions If vacuolated, LCAT deficiency
Hyaline cap	Hyaline material deposited between the glomerular basement membrane and the endothelium, often in sclerotic areas, may occlude the capillary lumen	Diabetic nephropathy Non-specific in sclerosed foci
Endotheliosis	Endothelial cell swelling causing thickened capillary walls and shrinkage of the capillary lumen, which appears bloodless	Pre-eclampsia, eclampsia, other causes of thrombotic microangiopathy (TMA)
Capillary lumen		
Endocapillary hypercellularity (◘ Fig. 7.10)	Lumen narrowed/occluded by cells (can be endothelial and/or inflammatory cells)	Acute PIGN (especially if diffuse and neutrophilic), C3GN, MPGN, SLE, IgA/HSP, vasculitis, infection-associated GN, glomerulitis (ABMR)
Microaneurysm (◘ Fig. 7.13)	Ectasia of capillary loops due to destruction of the mesangial matrix	Diabetic nephropathy Heals to form mesangial nodules
Thrombus (◘ Fig. 7.12)	Occlusion of the lumen by fibrin thrombus	Acute TMA, pre-eclampsia, renal vein thrombosis, sickle cell nephropathy, hyperacute rejection
Hyaline thrombus	A pseudothrombus, composed of cryoglobulins, with the glassy, eosinophilic appearance of hyaline (with IHC/IMF positivity)	Cryoglobulinaemia, an active feature of lupus nephritis
Sickle cells	Dysmorphic, sickle-shaped erythrocytes	Sickle cell disease

Glomerulus		
Lesion	*Description*	*Differentials*
Mesangium		
Proliferation (◘ Fig. 7.9)	More than three cells in a group within a peripheral mesangial area (away from the hilum)	IgA nephropathy, lupus nephritis (class II), secondary membranous glomerulopathy
Increased matrix (◘ Fig. 7.6.)	Diffuse; maintains the normal distribution of the matrix, but more material is present Nodular; rounded areas of matrix with a rim of mesangial cells	Diabetes, amyloid, monoclonal immunoglobulin deposition disease (MIDD), idiopathic nodular glomerulopathy
Mesangiolysis	Injury and destruction of mesangial matrix and cells releasing the anchoring points of adjacent capillary loops, which merge, forming one large, microaneurysmal capillary loop	Diabetes, TMA, malignant hypertension, radiation nephropathy, rarely a non-specific feature of various glomerulonephritides with mesangial deposits
Multicompartmental lesions		
Segmental sclerosis and hyalinosis (◘ Fig. 7.8)	A segment of the glomerular tuft shows increased mesangial matrix with obliteration of capillary loops. Represents a segmental scar May be attached to the capsule forming an adhesion May contain foam cells May be adaptive enlargement of uninvolved glomeruli Begins at the cortico-medullary junction The morphology and location within the tuft determine the variant of FSGS (see 'classification systems') Hyaline is glassy acellular material which often forms part of a sclerosed area. Formed from insudated plasma proteins in response to endothelial injury	FSGS primary or secondary Most commonly a non-specific feature in many types of glomerulonephritis, which should be excluded before giving a diagnosis of FSGS
Global sclerosis	A chronic feature The end point of any glomerular injury Complete replacement of the tuft by fibrosis. Highlighted on PAMS	A non-specific feature Can be accepted as a normal feature depending on patient age and the number of glomeruli involved (see above)
Chronic ischaemic change	Small tuft, urinary space fibrosis (collagen deposition inside the capsule), wrinkled capillary walls (highlighted on PAMS), contracted mesangium, the urinary space may appear enlarged	Chronic hypoperfusion of any cause, e.g. renal artery stenosis, atherosclerosis, thromboemboli Ischaemic glomeruli are often seen as a non-specific feature of many renal diseases
Necrosis (◘ Fig. 7.11)	Cell death (mesangial, epithelial, endocapillary or inflammatory) with associated karyorrhectic debris. Once capillary walls are involved, fibrin deposition, haemorrhage and crescents may be seen	Any highly active glomerulopathy, particularly vasculitic diseases
Hypertrophy	Enlargement of the glomerulus	A compensatory response to nephron loss of any cause Can be a helpful clue to suggest covert FSGS if sclerosing lesions are not evident

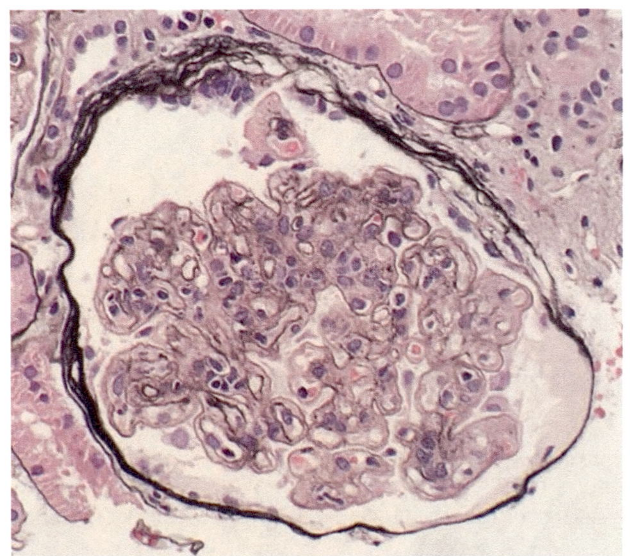

Fig. 7.5 Glomerulus showing diffuse capillary wall double contours in an MPGN. PAMS x400

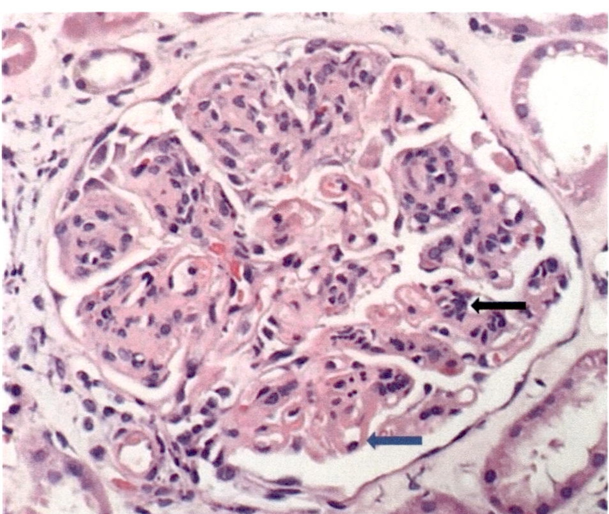

Fig. 7.7 Glomerulus showing an MPGN in a case of lupus nephritis, including mesangial hypercellularity (black arrow) and thickened glomerular capillary loops, including wire loops (blue arrow). H&E. x400

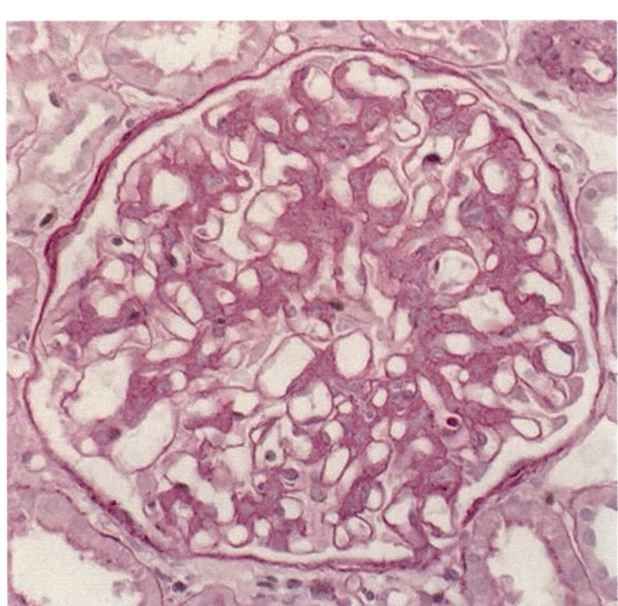

Fig. 7.6 Mesangial matrix expansion in a case of fibrillary glomerulopathy. PAS. X400

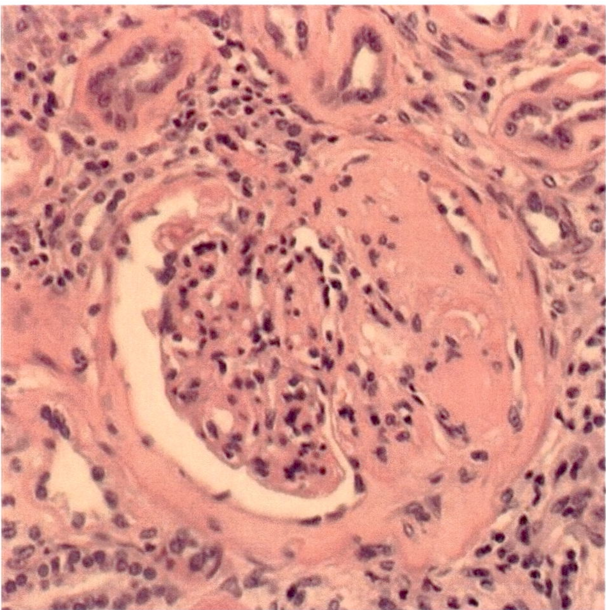

Fig. 7.8 Glomerulus with a segment of sclerosis. Surrounding tubules are atrophic. H&E. x400

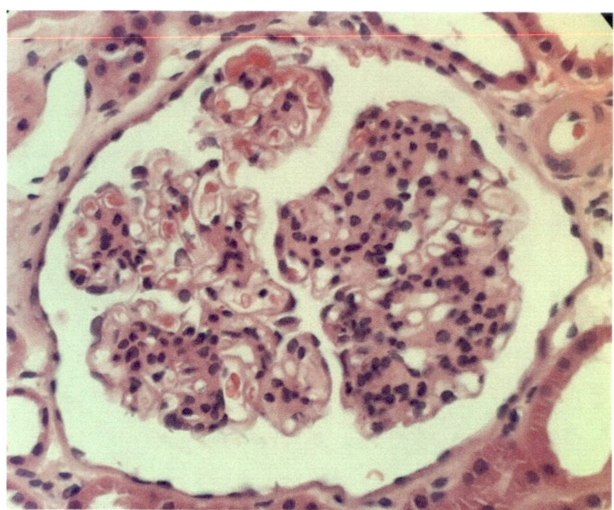

Fig. 7.9 Glomerulus showing mesangial proliferation in a case of IgA nephropathy. H&E. X400

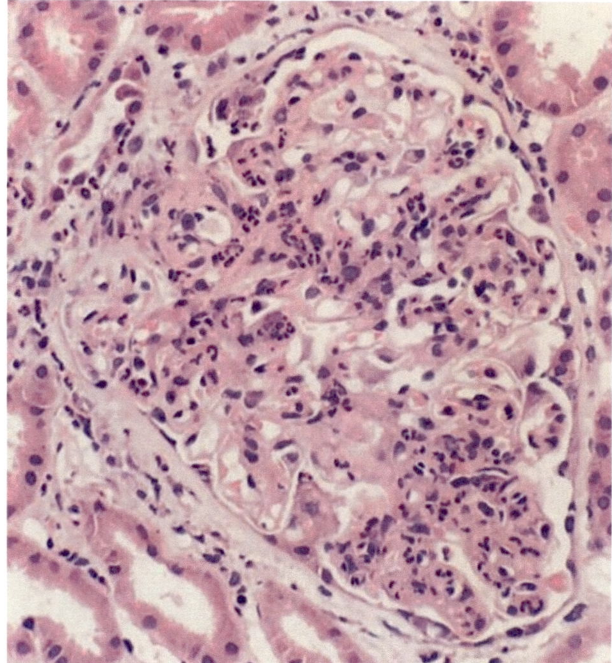

Fig. 7.10 Endocapillary, neutrophilic hypercellularity in a case of post-infectious glomerulonephritis. H&E. x400

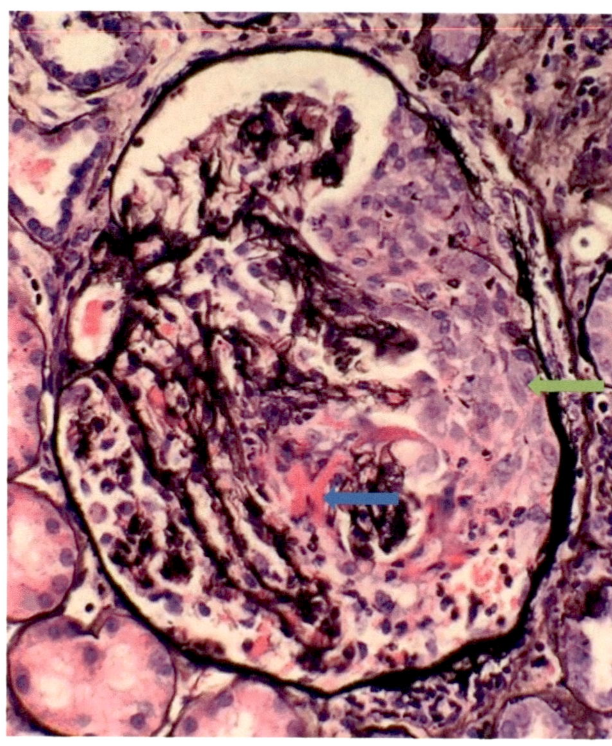

Fig. 7.11 Glomerulus with fibrinoid necrosis (blue arrow) and cellular crescent formation (green arrow). PAMS x400

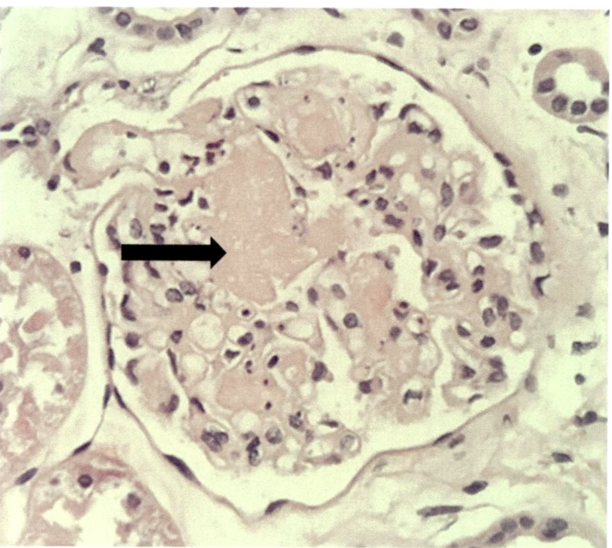

Fig. 7.12 Glomerulus showing fibrin thrombi (black arrow) within capillary loops in a case of acute thrombotic micorangiopathy. H&E. x400

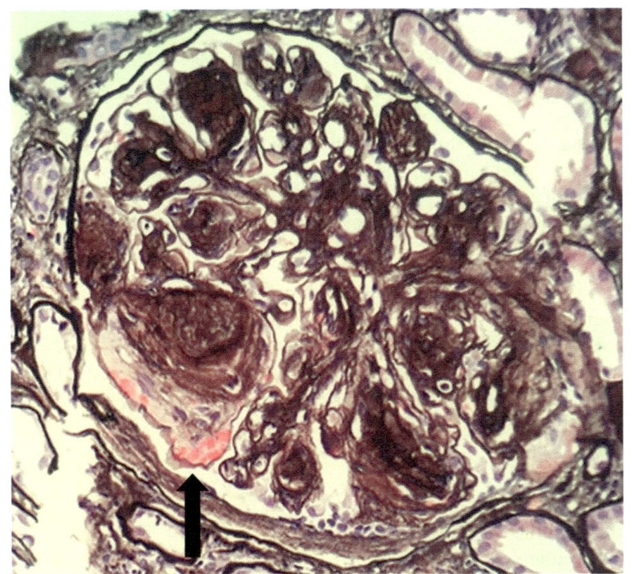

Fig. 7.13 Nodular glomerulopathy with a microaneurysm (arrow) in a case of diabetic nephropathy. PAMS X400

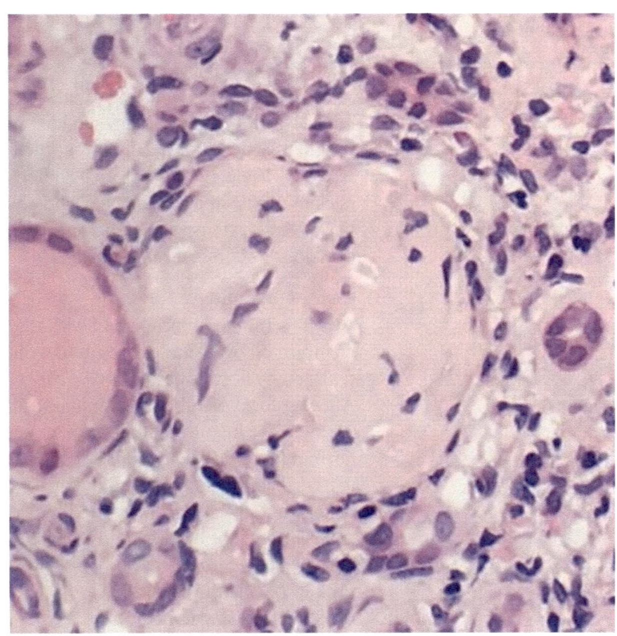

Fig. 7.14 Globally sclerosed glomerulus. H&E x200

7.4.3 Tubules (Figs. 7.15, 7.16, 7.17, 7.18, 7.19, 7.20, and 7.21)

Tubules		
Lesion	***Description***	***Differentials***
Tubular cells		
Acute tubular injury (ATI) (Fig. 7.15) Acute tubular necrosis (ATN) (Fig. 7.18)	ATI – Simplification (loss of the proximal tubular brush border and thinning/flattening of the cytoplasm), luminal ectasia, nuclear enlargement, prominent nucleoli, blebbing/sloughing of cytoplasm into the lumen (forming casts), vacuolisation and variation in cell size and shape ATN – Severe form of ATI involving loss of tubular nuclei and detachment, necrosis and fragmentation of tubular epithelial cells with denudation of the basement membrane Often associated with interstitial oedema	Primary; ATI/ATN due to toxic/ischaemic injury Secondary; acute glomerular injury or vascular injury of any cause Vacuolation may be particularly prominent in ATI due to particular toxins or hyperosmolar injury (hyperkalaemia, mannitol) Histological changes can be mild even in clinically severe AKI ATI can be seen in glomerular and vascular diseases, which should be excluded before giving a diagnosis of ATI
Tubulitis (Fig. 7.16)	Leukocytes (usually lymphocytes) infiltrating tubular epithelial cells (within the tubular basement membrane) with acute tubular injury	TIN (any cause), pyelonephritis, acute T cell-mediated rejection
Crystalline inclusions	Proximal tubular injury (as seen in ATI/ATN), with crystalline or needle-shaped inclusions and cytoplasmic monoclonal light chain deposition. May only be visible on electron microscopy	Light chain proximal tubulopathy
BK viral cytopathic changes	Appearances range from normal to marked cytopathic change (enlarged and hyperchromatic). Causes basophilic intranuclear inclusions Often also see tubulitis and interstitial inflammation	Acute T cell-mediated rejection TIN Other viral infections, e.g. CMV, adenovirus (with different viral cytopathic appearances) ATI/ATN

7

Tubules		
Lesion	***Description***	***Differentials***
Infarction (◘ Fig. 7.18)	Areas of infarction are likely to involve all the compartments within the affected area, which will show coagulative necrosis, meaning that the architecture remains visible, but the cytological details (cytoplasm and nucleus) are lost, leaving a pale, ghostly outline. Often there is also extensive haemorrhage, particularly in infarction due to venous thrombosis	The cause is not usually present in the biopsy, but possibilities include hypoperfusion, vascular thrombosis, thromboembolism or vasculitis, and the included vessels may show evidence of these
Atrophy (◘ Fig. 7.17)	A chronic feature Atrophic tubules appear small with thick basement membranes; over time, these tubules disappear and are replaced by fibrous tissue Another form of tubular atrophy is called 'thyroidisation' (because the histological appearance is similar to that of normal thyroid follicles). These tubules are dilated, with flattened epithelial cells and filled with hyaline cast material Another form of atrophy is endocrine type (because the appearance resembles parathyroid glands); small cuboidal tubular cells with very little/no visible lumen and no thickened basement membrane All types are usually associated with interstitial fibrosis	A non-specific finding, but the pattern of atrophy can help suggest aetiology. Patchy atrophy is classically seen in reflux nephropathy, whereas stripy atrophy suggests chronic CNI toxicity. The endocrine type can suggest renal artery stenosis
Hypertrophy	Large tubules with large tubular epithelial cells and an increased volume of cytoplasm Often also see glomerular hypertrophy	An adaptive change to a reduced number of tubules This may be because the kidney is small relative to body mass (e.g. low birth weight, obesity, some transplants), or due to loss of tubules due to chronic damage
Vacuolation	Fine (small) or coarse (large) vacuoles within the tubular cytoplasm	Can be a non-specific sign of acute tubular injury, specific causes include CNI toxicity, osmotic tubular injury, mannitol, contrast, IVIg, hypo/hyperkalaemia
Resorption droplets	Eosinophilic, PAS-positive, small, round cytoplasmic inclusion, formed from protein	Any cause of glomerular proteinuria
Luminal material		
Casts		
Hyaline casts (◘ Fig. 7.19)	The most common type of cast, composed of Tamm-Horsfall protein. Appear glassy, eosinophilic, PAS-positive and solid	Non-specific, increased in chronically damaged tubules
Myeloma/light chain casts (◘ Fig. 7.20)	Composed of monoclonal immunoglobulins mixed with Tamm-Horsfall protein, appears cracked/fractured/crystalline with a surrounding inflammatory cell reaction (giant cells, macrophages, neutrophils or lymphocytes), usually shows restriction on IHC/IMF for kappa or lambda light chains ATI also seen	Myeloma/plasma cell dyscrasia
Myoglobin casts (◘ Figs. 7.21 and 7.22)	Red/brown granular cast material Myoglobin immunostain positive ATI also seen May see rhabdomyolysis in any skeletal muscle present	Myoglobinuria
Red blood cells or red cell casts (◘ Fig. 7.23)	Red blood cells filling the tubular lumen	A few red blood cells are acceptable as part of biopsy-related trauma Larger numbers may be due to vasculitis or any necrotising glomerulopathy If there is no evidence of this, more levels should be examined

Tubules		
Lesion	***Description***	***Differentials***
Inflammatory cell casts	Inflammatory cells and cellular debris May be an associated interstitial infiltrate and ATI	Pyelonephritis, reflux nephropathy Can be seen occasionally in any cause of interstitial inflammation, e.g. TIN, ACR, GN
Bile casts	Brown cast material, stains with Fouchet, usually with ATI (a rare diagnosis)	Hyperbilirubinaemia of any aetiology
Crystals		
Calcium oxalate crystals (◘ Fig. 7.24)	Fan-shaped colourless crystals within tubules, refractile under polarised light Do not dissolve during processing	A large number are seen in primary hyperoxaluria and ethylene glycol toxicity, whereas less are usually present in secondary hyperoxaluria. A small number can be seen as a non-specific finding in severely damaged/end-stage kidneys
2,8-dihydroxyadenine crystals (2,8-DHA)	Single or clusters of birefringent, brown needle/rod-shaped crystals in tubules, tubular cytoplasm and interstitium, predominantly within the cortex May see an inflammatory cell reaction including giant cells Do not dissolve during processing Appear black on PAMS and blue on trichrome	2,8-Dihydroxyadeninuria
Cystine crystals	Birefringent hexagonal or rhomboid colourless crystals within glomerular and tubular cells and in interstitial macrophages Multinucleated tubular epithelial cells and podocytes and atrophic proximal tubules ('swan neck' deformity) are also seen Crystals dissolve during processing so are best seen in frozen tissue. In processed tissue, empty clefts remain as evidence of crystal deposition	Cystinosis
Monosodium urate crystals (◘ Fig. 7.25)	Clusters of birefringent, needle-shaped crystals in tubules or interstitium, predominantly in the medulla (within collecting ducts) May be surrounded by a granulomatous inflammatory response, forming a tophus Monosodium urate crystals are birefringent and needle-shaped, but dissolve during processing, so are best seen in frozen tissue. In processed tissue, empty clefts remain as evidence of crystal deposition	Uric acid nephropathy/gout
Calcium phosphate deposits	Granular, purple deposits within tubules and interstitium Not birefringent Do not dissolve during processing Stain black on von Kossa	Nephrocalcinosis (hypercalcaemia, hypercalciuria, hyperphosphataemia, hyperphosphaturia of any cause) Occasional incidental calcium phosphate deposits are often seen in areas of chronic damage

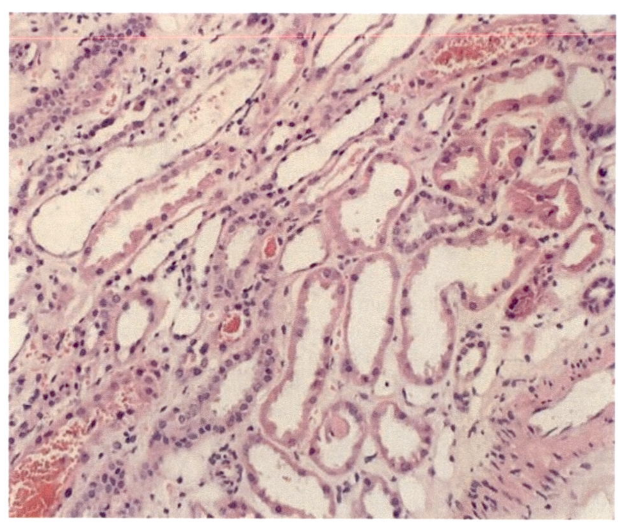

Fig. 7.15 Acute tubular injury and red cell casts in a case of pauci-immune glomerulonephritis. H&E x200

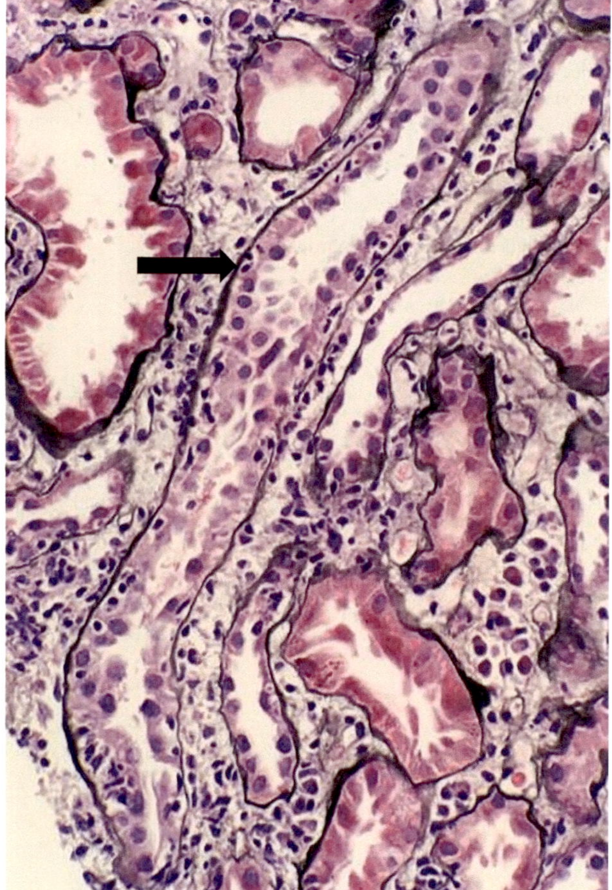

Fig. 7.16 A distal tubule showing infiltration by lymphocytes (tubulitis), in a case of acute cellular rejection. PAMS x200

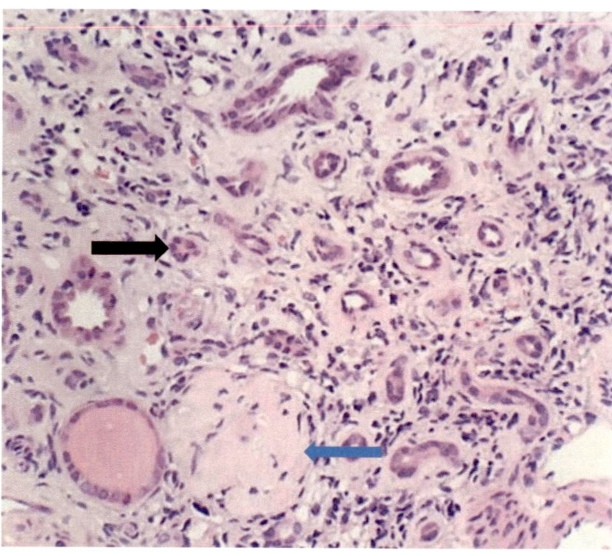

Fig. 7.17 Chronically damaged parenchyma showing atrophic tubules (black arrow), fibrotic interstitium and a globally sclerosed glomerulus (blue arrow). H&E. x100

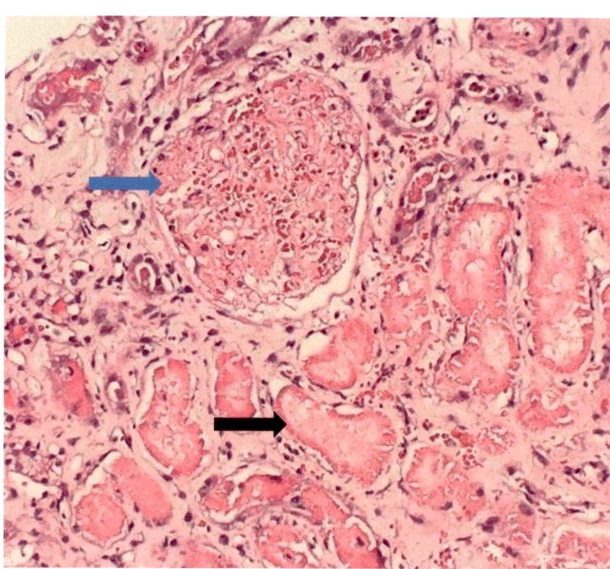

Fig. 7.18 Tubular necrosis (black arrow) and glomerular necrosis (blue arrow) in an area of cortical infarction in a case of active antibody-mediated transplant rejection. H&E. x100

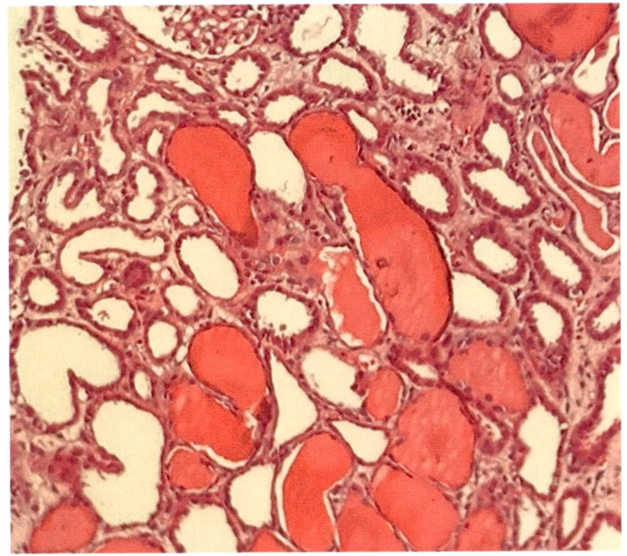

Fig. 7.19 Tubular hyaline casts. H&E X100

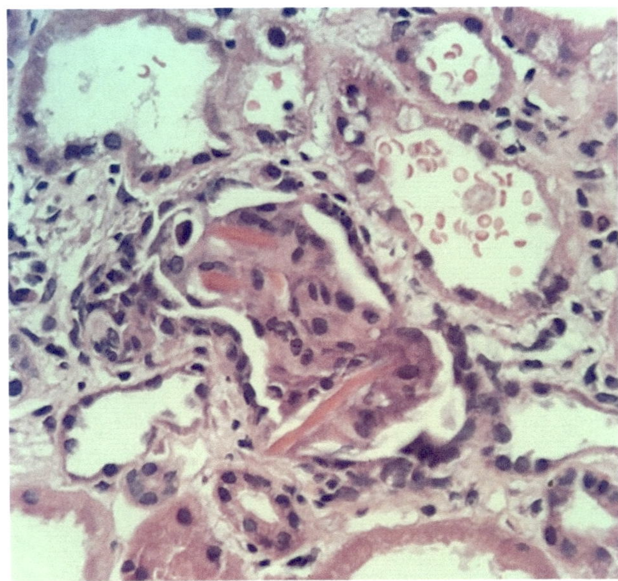

Fig. 7.20 A distal tubule containing angulated cast material with a surrounding multinucleate cell reaction. H&E X400

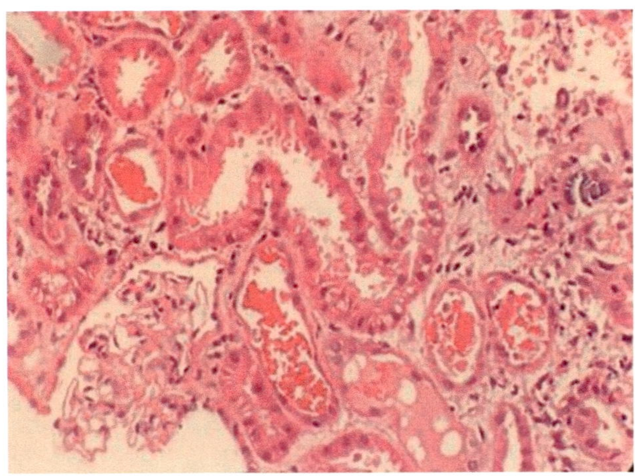

Fig. 7.21 Tubular myoglobin casts in a case of myoglobinuria due to rhabdomyolysis. H&E x200

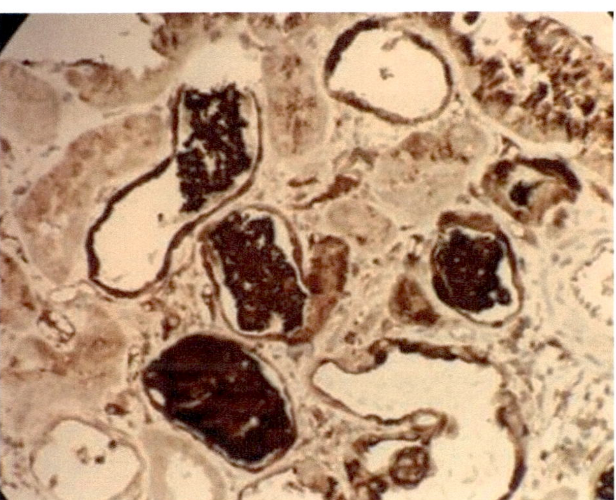

Fig. 7.22 Myoglobin immunohistochemistry showing positive staining of tubular myoglobin casts. x200

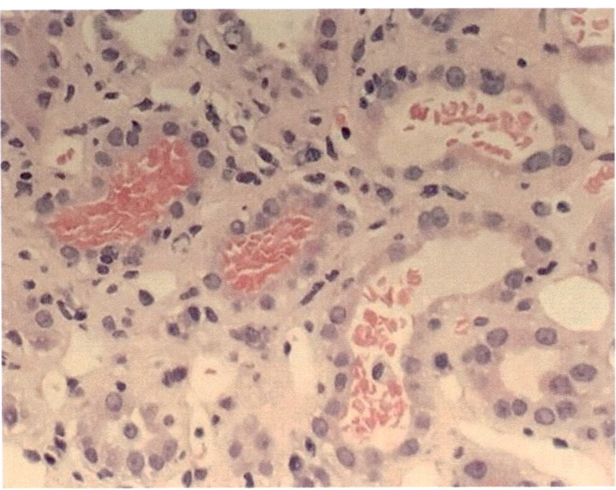

Fig. 7.23 Tubules containing red cell casts in case of crescentic glomerulonephritis. H&E x200

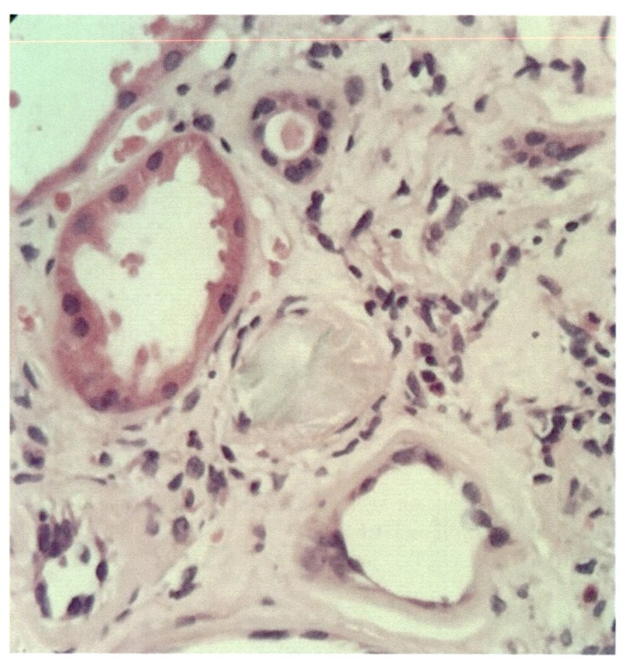

Fig. 7.24 Tubular oxalate crystal. H&E X400

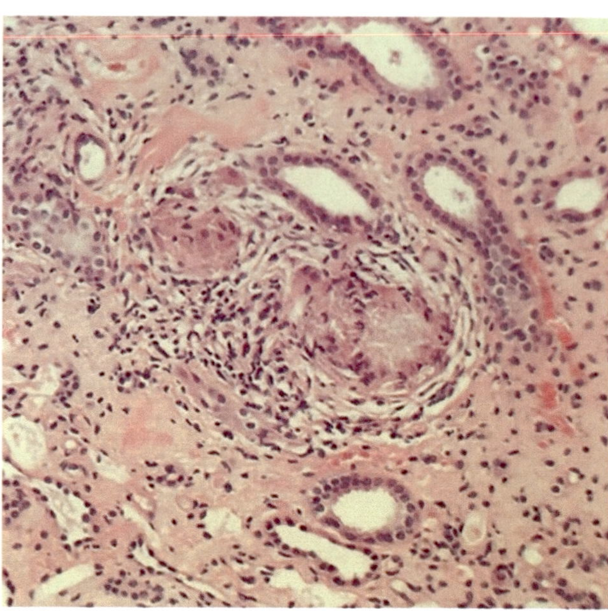

Fig. 7.25 Urate deposition in chronically damaged parenchyma. H&E X100

7.4.4 Interstitium

Interstitium		
Lesion	*Description*	*Differentials*
Inflammation (Fig. 7.26)	Any type of inflammatory cell may be seen. Lymphocytes usually predominate, often with a few plasma cells, but neutrophils, eosinophils, plasma cells or granulomas (aggregates of macrophages) may be conspicuous If inflammatory cells are seen infiltrating tubular epithelial cells, this is tubulointerstitial nephritis Inflammatory cells, particularly lymphocytes, can aggregate in areas of chronic damage (interstitial fibrosis); if it is limited to these areas, it is likely to be non-specific	**Lymphocytes**: Chronic parenchymal damage (e.g. chronic glomerulonephritis) TIN Acute cellular rejection Obstruction Lymphoproliferative disease (neoplastic lymphocytes) **Neutrophils**: Pyelonephritis Light chain cast nephropathy **Eosinophils**: Allergy/drug-related TIN ANCA GN Diabetic nephropathy **Granulomas**: ANCA GN Tuberculosis Fungal infection Sarcoidosis Xanthogranulomatous pyelonephritis Malakoplakia
Oedema	Acute and reversible Pale expansion of the interstitium by fluid, separating adjacent tubules	Any cause of acute parenchymal damage, e.g. ATI, acute TIN, RPGN, acute cellular rejection
Fibrosis (Fig. 7.17)	Chronic and irreversible Eosinophilic expansion of the interstitium, composed of collagen, often contains a few lymphocytes. Entrapped tubules and glomeruli may be atrophic/sclerosed	Any cause of chronic parenchymal damage
Amyloid	Eosinophilic amorphous material may also be seen in the glomerular mesangium and capillary walls, arteriolar walls and surrounding tubules	Amyloidosis
Foam cells	Large cells with central nuclei and abundant multi vacuolated cytoplasm (containing lipid, which is removed during processing) The cells are thought to be of macrophage/monocyte origin	Often seen in any cause of proteinuria, particularly in the nephrotic syndrome (hyperlipidaemia), also in Fabry's disease, Alport syndrome, lipoprotein glomerulopathy
Cellular infiltrate	Rarely, a neoplastic population can be seen infiltrating or replacing the renal parenchyma	Renal neoplasia, myeloma, lymphoma, metastatic carcinoma, adrenal inclusions

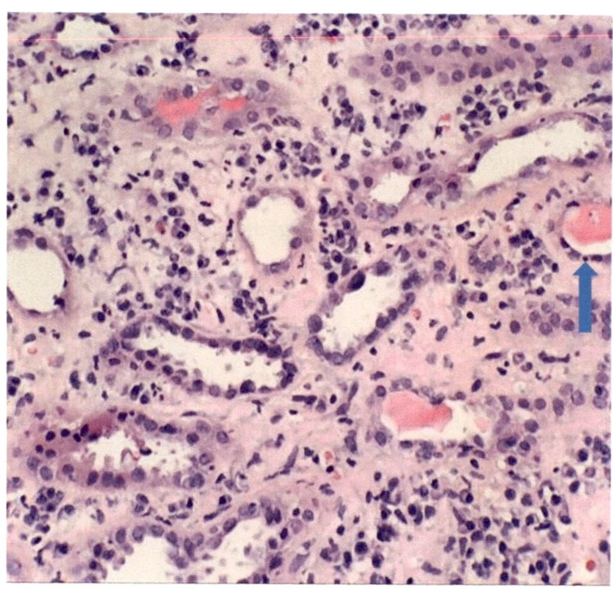

Fig. 7.26 Interstitial inflammation, including lymphocytes, plasma cells and neutrophils, with tubulitis (blue arrow). H&E x400

7

7.4.5 Vascular

Extra-glomerular vessels		
Lesion	*Description*	*Differentials*
Vasculitis (Fig. 7.27)	Inflammation within an arterial/arteriolar wall, with fibrinoid necrosis and schistocytes (fragmented erythrocytes) if severe Inflammation may be lymphocytic, neutrophilic, eosinophilic or granulomatous Can be seen with thrombi, interstitial inflammation, haemorrhage or infarction	Any cause of vasculitis, most commonly seen are ANCA vasculitis, anti-GBM disease, IgA vasculitis
Endothelialitis Endarteritis	Arterial/arteriolar subendothelial lymphocytes, extending through to the media if severe May see reactive (enlarged) endothelial nuclei and subendothelial swelling	Acute vascular rejection
Capillaritis	Increased numbers of leukocytes within peritubular capillaries	Acute antibody-mediated rejection
Thromboemboli	Lumenal material in vessels. Can be fibrin thrombus, atheroma (cholesterol crystals) (rare with others such as fat or tumour cells)	Most commonly embolisation of an atheromatous plaque in atherosclerosis
Hypertensive vasculopathy (Fig. 7.28)	Fibrointimal proliferation with multiplication of the elastic lamina (fibroelastosis), medial thickening of arterioles, hyaline arteriolosclerosis Highlighted on elastin stain	Hypertension (essential or secondary to any cause, including chronic renal disease) Renal artery stenosis Scleroderma
Hyaline arteriolosclerosis (Fig. 7.29)	Eosinophilic, glassy amorphous material within the arteriolar wall	Hypertension Diabetic nephropathy CNI-related, classically 'nodular' in appearance

Extra-glomerular vessels		
Lesion	*Description*	*Differentials*
Accelerated/malignant hypertensive changes (Fig. 7.30)	Fibrinoid necrosis and thrombi, 'onion-skinning' (multilayered intima of arterioles), mucoid intimal thickening (pale bluish acellular matrix material)	Accelerated/malignant hypertension Thrombotic microangiopathy, Scleroderma
Amyloid	Eosinophilic material within the vessel wall, appears red/pink on Congo red stain. When the Congo red stain is viewed under polarised light, amyloid classically shows 'apple green' birefringence Often also present in glomeruli and interstitium	Amyloidosis
Atherosclerosis	Intimal thickening composed of foam cells (lipid-laden macrophages), cholesterol clefts, amorphous material, all present underneath the endothelium	Atherosclerosis
Acute thrombotic microangiopathy (Fig. 7.31)	Endothelial swelling obstructing the lumen, intramural schistocytes (fragmented erythrocytes), fibrin thrombi and fibrinoid necrosis	Many, including HUS, aHUS, TTP, malignant hypertension, pre-eclampsia, scleroderma, antiphospholipid syndrome, acute antibody-mediated rejection

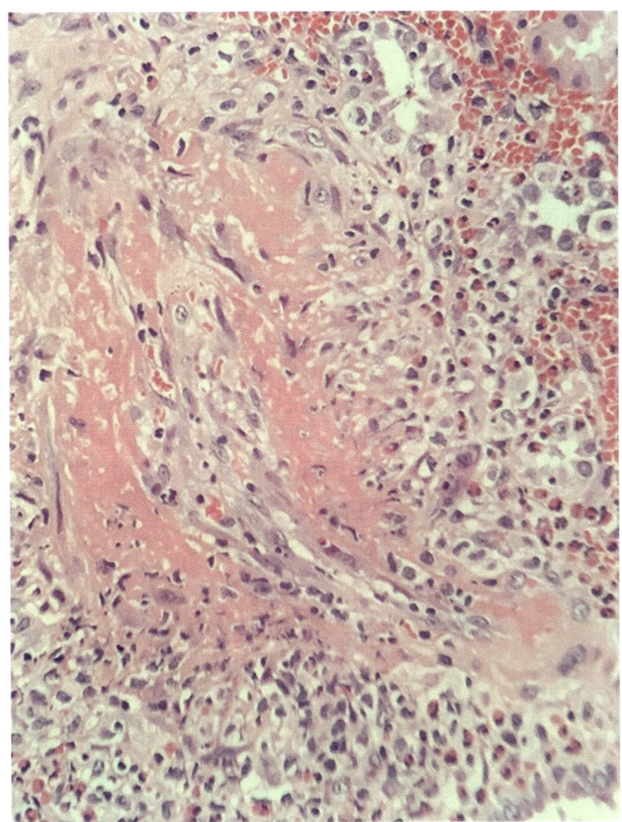

Fig. 7.27 Arterial vasculitis with fibrinoid necrosis in a case of ANCA vasculitis. H&E X100

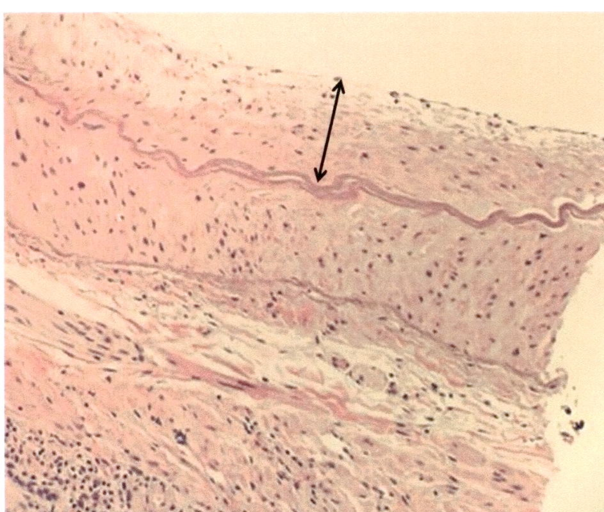

Fig. 7.28 Section of an artery showing fibrointimal proliferation (arrow spans the area of proliferation from the internal elastic lamina to the endothelium) H&E x400

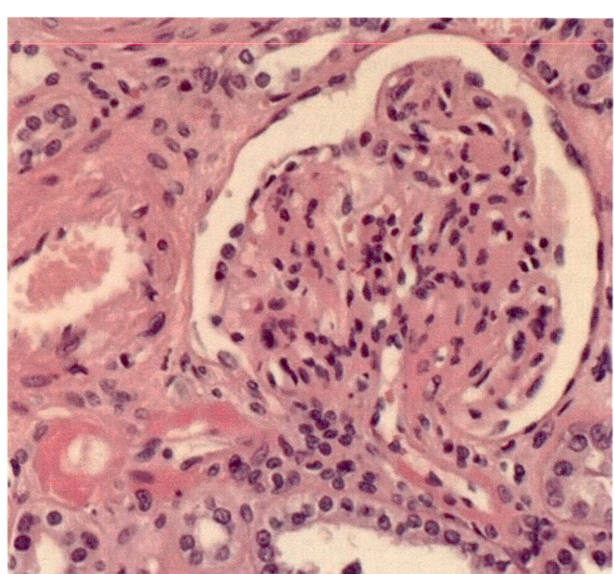

Fig. 7.29 Hyaline arteriolosclerosis of the afferent and efferent arterioles in a case of diabetic glomerulopathy. H&E x400

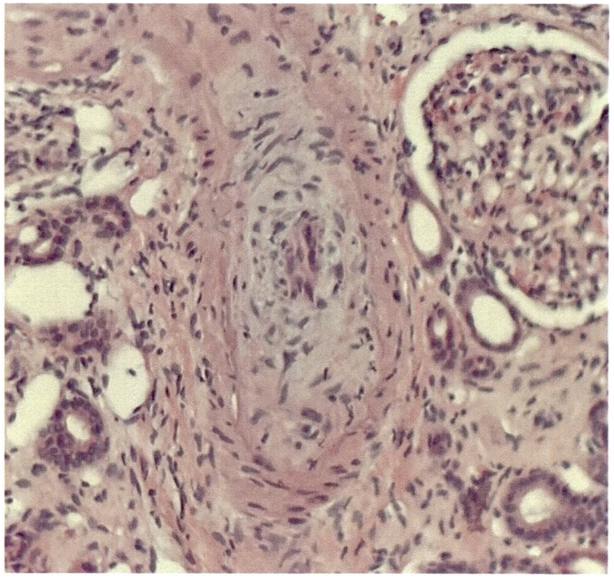

Fig. 7.30 An artery showing mucoid intimal thickening in a case of accelerated hypertension. H&E X100

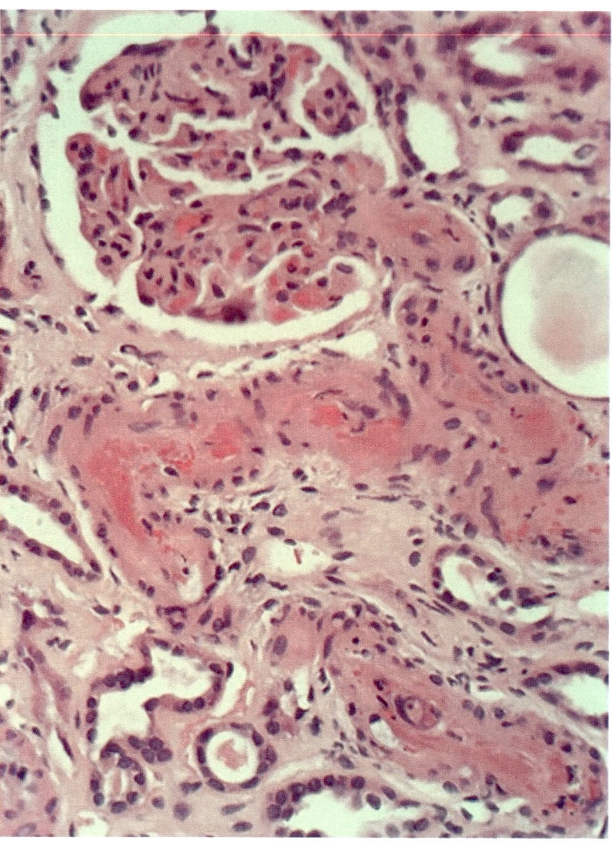

Fig. 7.31 Subendothelial fibrin and fragmented red cells in an arteriole in a case of acute TMA. H&E x200

7.4.6 Patterns of Injury

Once each compartment has been examined for the above features, the glomerular findings can be used to identify a pattern of injury, which provides a differential diagnosis. While this is often helpful, it is important to note that diseases do not always conform to their typical morphology and one disease can have more than one potential pattern (e.g. particularly lupus nephritis). Occasionally, more than one disease process will be present, complicating the interpretation.

Pattern of injury	Differential diagnosis
Normal on light microscopy (◘ Fig. 7.2)	Normal glomerulus No light microscopic change: • Minimal change disease. • Thin basement membrane disease. • Unsampled focal segmental process. • Lupus podocytopathy. • Alport syndrome. Any early/mild glomerulopathy, particularly: • Membranous glomerulopathy. • IgA nephropathy. • Lupus nephritis. • Amyloidosis.
Capillary wall subepithelial 'spikes' (◘ Fig. 7.4)	Membranous glomerulopathy (primary or secondary) Class V lupus nephritis Amyloidosis (spicules)
Endocapillary hypercellularity (◘ Fig. 7.10)	IgA nephropathy/Henoch-Schonlein nephritis Lupus nephritis Acute postinfectious glomerulonephritis (neutrophilic) Cryoglobulinaemic glomerulonephritis C3 glomerulopathy HIV-associated immune complex kidney disease (HIVICK)
Diffuse mesangial matrix expansion (◘ Fig. 7.6)	Monoclonal immunoglobulin deposition disease Amyloidosis Diabetic nephropathy Cryoglobulinaemic GN Immunotactoid GP Fibrillary GN
Nodular mesangial matrix expansion (◘ Fig. 7.13)	Diabetic glomerulosclerosis Monoclonal immunoglobulin deposition disease Amyloidosis Idiopathic nodular sclerosis Advanced MPGN (also shows double contours) Fibronectin glomerulopathy
Mesangial proliferation (◘ Fig. 7.9)	IgA disease/Henoch Schonlein purpura Lupus nephritis class II Late post-infectious glomerulonephritis PGNMID
Membranoproliferative glomerulonephritis (MPGN) (Mesangiocapillary glomerulonephritis) (◘ Fig. 7.7)	Immune complex-related MPGN (of any cause) C3 glomerulopathy (C3 glomerulonephritis or dense deposit disease) Chronic endothelial injury, e.g.TMA Chronic antibody-mediated rejection (transplant glomerulopathy)
Segmental sclerosis (◘ Fig. 7.8)	FSGS (primary or secondary) Sclerosis as part of any glomerular disease
Crescentic glomerulonephritis (◘ Fig. 7.11)	Vasculitic glomerulonephritis: • Pauci-immune/ANCA-related. • Anti-glomerular basement membrane disease. Immune complex-mediated glomerulonephritis: • IgA vasculitis. • Lupus nephritis. • Any MPGN. • PIGN. Can rarely be seen in others, e.g. cryoglobulinaemia, TMA

7.5 Immunohistology and Immunofluorescence

Once a pattern has been identified, immunohistology (IHC) or immunofluorescence (IMF) allows for a more specific diagnosis. The typical glomerular findings are listed in the table below. IHC often show some background staining, which is non-specific, particularly within the mesangial regions and areas of sclerosis.

7

Disease	IHC/IF	Pattern and distribution
Immunoglobulin dominant		
IgA nephropathy (◘ Fig. 7.32)	IgA dominant +/– C3	Granular Mesangial and paramesangial
Membranous glomerulopathy (◘ Fig. 7.33)	IgG +/– C3 (IgA, IgM, C1q + in secondary forms)	Granular Subepithelial capillary wall +/– mesangial (secondary)
Anti-GBM disease (◘ Fig. 7.34)	IgG +/– C3	Linear Capillary wall
Immune complex-related MPGN (◘ Fig. 7.35)	IgG dominant + C3 (IgA, IgM and C1q may also be +)	Coarsely granular Subendothelial capillary wall +/– mesangial
Cryoglobulinaemic glomerulonephritis	Type I – Monoclonal (k > l) with IgG and C3 Type II – Monoclonal IgM (k > l) with polyclonal IgG and C3 Type III – Polyclonal IgG, IgM and C3	Granular Hyaline thrombi, subendothelial capillary walls, mesangial
Fibrillary glomerulonephritis	IgG dominant + C3 DNAJB9+	Coarse granular Mesangial, segmental subendothelial/subepithelial capillary wall
Immunotactoid glomerulonephritis	IgG +/– C3 May be monoclonal	Coarse granular Subendothelial/subepithelial capillary walls, mesangial
Complement dominant		
Post-infectious glomerulonephritis (◘ Fig. 7.36)	C3 +/– IgG (IgA dominant in staphylococcal infections)	Coarse granular Irregular subepithelial 'humps' along capillary walls, mesangial 'Starry sky' pattern
Dense deposit disease	C3 Ig typically negative, can be some focal + but must be C3 dominant	Coarse granular Subendothelial capillary wall and mesangial
C3 glomerulonephritis	C3 Ig typically negative, can be some focal + but must be C3 dominant	Coarse granular Subendothelial/subepithelial capillary wall and mesangial
Immunoglobulin and complement		
Lupus (◘ Fig. 7.35)	IgG IgA IgM C3 C1q (referred to as 'full house')	Granular Mesangial +/–subendothelial/subepithelial capillary wall
Other		
Amyloidosis	AL is monoclonal, usually lambda light chain restriction Subtypes may show SAA+ LECT2+ TTR+	Smudgy Mesangial, capillary wall, interstitial, vascular (same distribution as Congo red positivity)

Disease	IHC/IF	Pattern and distribution
MIDD	Monoclonal, usually kappa	Linear Capillary, mesangial, tubular basement membranes
Collagenofibrotic glomerulopathy	Collagen III +	Mesangium
Negative		
Pauci-immune/ANCA glomerulonephritis (also GPA, EGPA, MPO)	All negative	N/A
Diabetes		
TTP		
FSGS Including HIVAN		
Fabry's disease		
Minimal change disease		
Idiopathic nodular glomerulosclerosis		
Alport syndrome		
Thin basement membrane disease		
Sickle cell glomerulopathy		

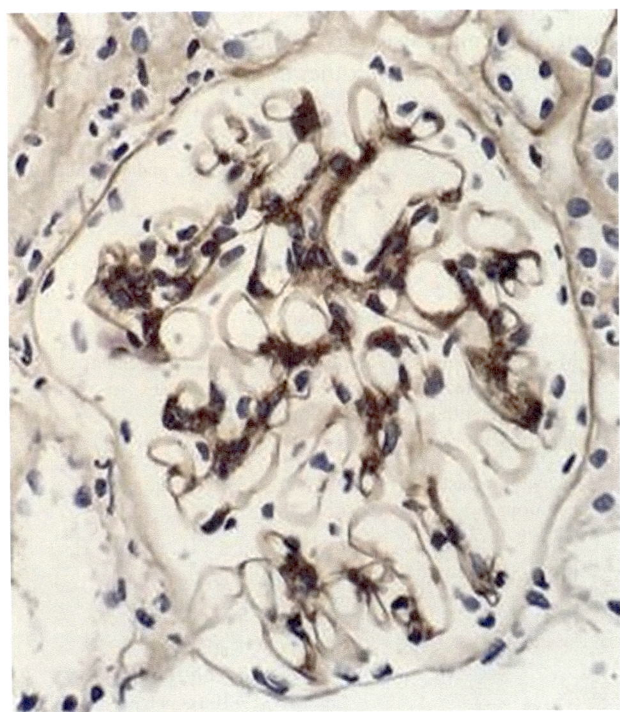

Fig. 7.32 IgA stain showing mesangial staining in a case of IgA nephropathy. X200

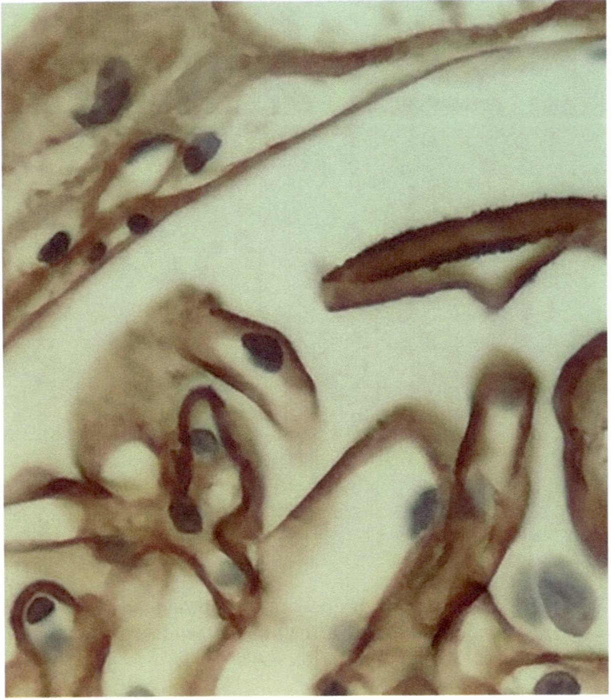

Fig. 7.33 An immunohistochemical stain for IgG shows granular subepithelial capillary wall positivity in a case of membranous glomerulopathy. x400

7

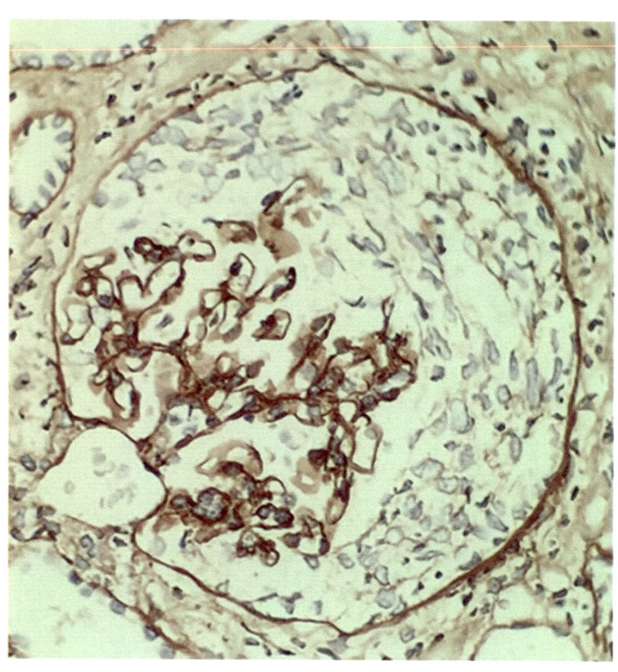

Fig. 7.34 Linear capillary wall positivity for IgG in a glomerulus with a cellular crescent, in a case of anti-GBM disease. X400

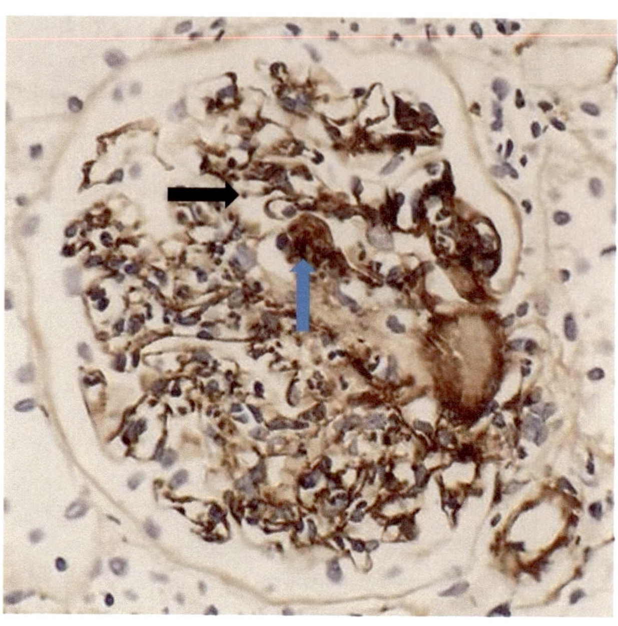

Fig. 7.36 Immunohistochemical stain for C3 shows positive subepithelial humps (black arrow) and granular mesangial positivity (blue arrow) in a case of post-infectious glomerulonephritis. X400

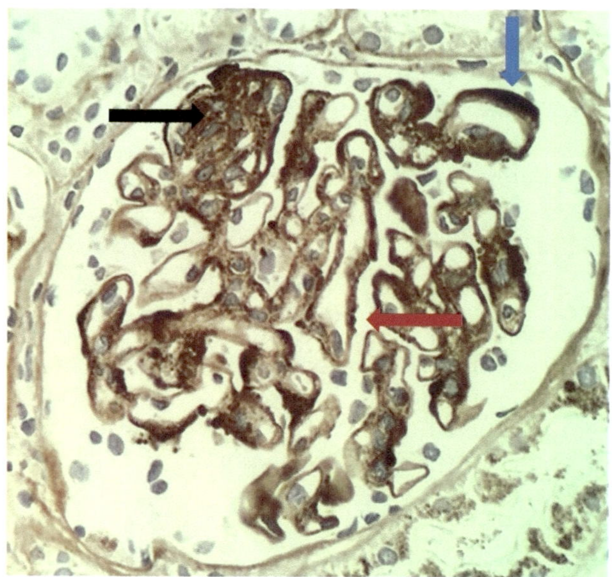

Fig. 7.35 C1q immunohistochemistry showing mesangial (black arrow), subendothelial (blue arrow) and subepithelial (red arrow) positivity in case of lupus nephritis. X400

While the glomerulus is usually the focus for assessment of immunohistology, some pathologies may show significant positivity in other compartments.

Disease	IHC	Pattern and distribution
Tubules		
Light chain cast nephropathy	Kappa or lambda restriction	Pathogenic casts
Monoclonal light chain mediated tubulointerstitial nephritis	Kappa or lambda restriction	Tubular basement membranes
Myoglobin cast nephropathy (Fig. 7.22)	Myoglobin positive	Pathogenic casts
Interstitium		
IgG4 disease	IgG4 positive	Plasma cells Ratio of IgG:IgG4 > 40% or >10 IgG4+ plasma cells per high-power field (x40 objective)

7.6 Electron Microscopic Findings

As stated above, EM is not always crucial for the diagnosis; however, it is helpful to confirm, refine and clarify the light microscopy findings, and in some cases, it is essential. The table below shows a description of the usual findings in the conditions listed. Usually only one or two glomeruli are assessed. As with the other modalities previously discussed, EM findings are not always specific and can be difficult to interpret. Also, focal and segmental lesions may not be represented (◘ Figs. 7.37 and 7.38).

Organised deposits					
	Light microscopy			**Electron microscopy**	
	PAMS	**CR**	**IHC**	**Morphology**	**Distribution of deposits**
Glomerulosclerosis (of any cause, e.g. diabetic glomerulopathy, idiopathic nodular sclerosis)	+	–	Negative (may show non-specific entrapment within sclerosis)	Banded or randomly arranged collagen and precollagen fibrils	Areas of sclerosis
TMA (fibrin deposition)	+	–	Fibrinogen +	Fibrin; 6–8 nm fibrils	Mesangium
Collagenofibrotic/collagen 3 glomerulopathy	+	–	Collagen 3 +	Curved disorganised fibres with periodicity (regular transverse bands at 43–65 nm)	Subendothelium Mesangium
Fibronectin glomerulopathy	–	–	Fibronectin +	12–16 nm fibrils, but often amorphous or granular	Subendothelium Mesangium
Immunotactoid glomerulopathy	–	–	Monoclonal IgG+	10–50 nm microtubules arranged in parallel arrays	Subendothelium Subepithelium Mesangium
Cryoglobulin GN	–	–	IgG, IgM, C3, may be monoclonal (see above)	25–35 nm curved microtubules (not present in every case, can be amorphous)	Subendothelium Mesangium Intraluminal (hyaline thrombi)
Fibrillary GN (◘ Figs. 7.39 and 7.40)	–	–	IgG+ C3+	15–30 nm randomly oriented non-branching fibrils	Subendothelium Subepithelium Mesangium
DM fibrillosis	- (often within + mesangial nodule)	–	–	10–25 nm random fibrils	Mesangium (less argyrophilic areas)
Amyloidosis (◘ Figs. 7.37 and 7.38)	–	+	Subtypes AL, AA, beta-2-microglobulin etc.	8–12 nm randomly oriented non-branching fibrils	Subendothelium Subepithelium Mesangium Tubular basement membranes Arterioles Interstitium

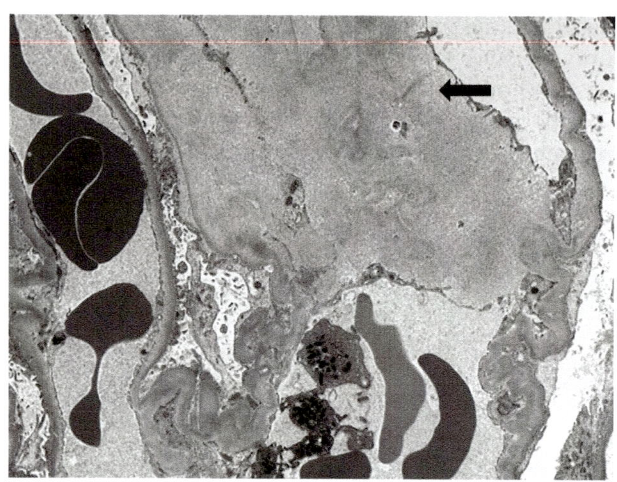

Fig. 7.37 Electron micrograph showing mesangial amyloid deposits (black arrow), in a case of amyloidosis. X1200. (Image courtesy of Leicester Royal Infirmary electron microscopy department)

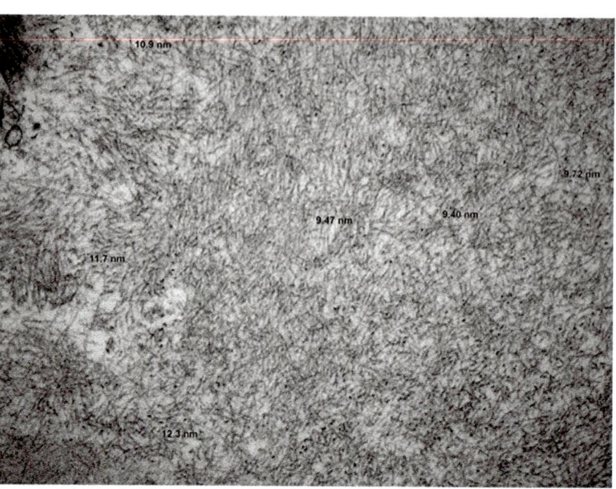

Fig. 7.38 Electron micrograph of amyloid fibrils with measurements, in a case of amyloidosis. X12000. (Image courtesy of Leicester Royal Infirmary electron microscopy department)

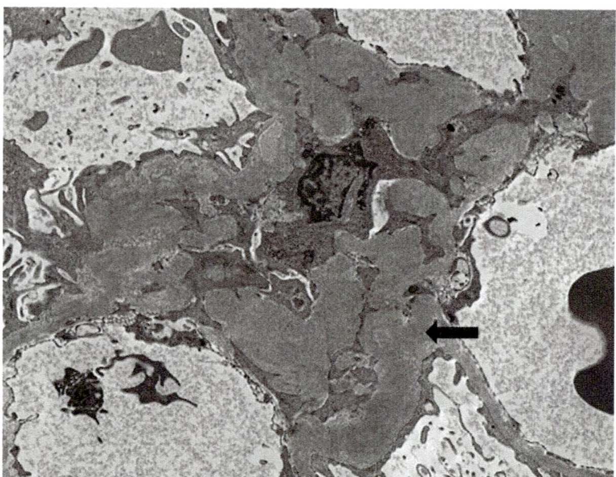

Fig. 7.39 Expanded mesangial region containing organised mesangial deposits (black arrow) in a case of fibrillary glomerulopathy. X1500. (Image courtesy of Leicester Royal Infirmary electron microscopy department)

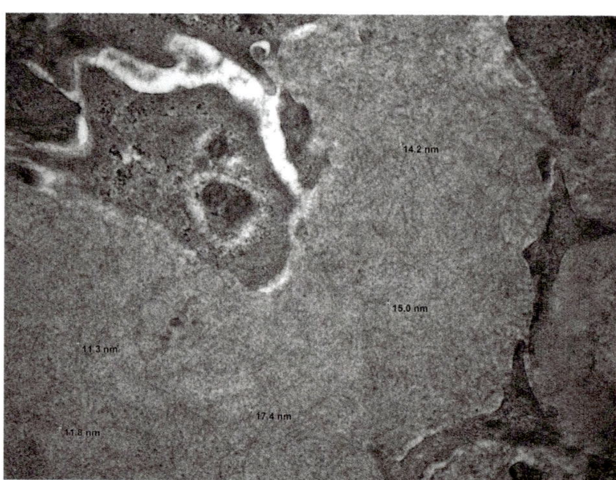

Fig. 7.40 A closer view showing the randomly organised fibrils, with an average diameter of 18 nm, in a case of fibrillary glomerulopathy. X8000. (Image courtesy of Leicester Royal Infirmary electron microscopy department)

Disease	EM Findings
Electron dense deposits (EDD)	
Post-infectious GN (◘ Fig. 7.41)	Subepithelial hump-shaped electron dense deposits (EDD)
Dense deposit disease (◘ Fig. 7.42)	Elongated "ribbon-like" very dense intramembranous and mesangial deposits
C3 glomerulonephritis	Subendothelial, subepithelial (can be hump-like) and mesangial EDD
Lupus nephritis (◘ Fig. 7.43)	Mesangial, subendothelial and subepithelial EDD can all be present. Endothelial cell cytoplasm may contain tubuloreticular inclusions
IgA disease (◘ Fig. 7.44)	Mesangial and paramesangial EDD
Membranous glomerulopathy	Subepithelial EDD Mesangial EDD may be present in secondary forms
PGNMID	Mesangial and subendothelial EDD
Other deposits/materials	
MIDD	Amorphous granular deposits along glomerular basement membrane (GBM), and within mesangium
LCAT deficiency	Lipid inclusions, basement membrane lacunae, striated membranous structures within the mesangium
Lipoprotein glomerulopathy	Capillary loop lipoprotein thrombi; lamellated with lipid vacuoles and granules, FPE
Fabry's disease (◘ Fig. 7.45)	Lamellated lysosomal inclusions (myelin/zebra bodies) particularly within podocytes, but can be seen in all renal cells
BK nephropathy	Intranuclear viral particles 30 to 50 nm diameter (typically seen in tubular epithelial cells)
Tubuloreticular inclusion	Approximately 20 nm organised structures seen in lupus nephritis, viral infection (particularly HIV) and interferon therapy (typically found in the endoplasmic reticulum of endothelial cells)
Structural changes	
Minimal change nephropathy (◘ Fig. 7.46)	Extensive foot process effacement (FPE) of podocytes, typically no other abnormalities
FSGS	Focal FPE overlying areas of sclerosis and in non-sclerotic glomeruli
Thin basement membrane disease (◘ Fig. 7.47)	Diffusely thin GBM (compared with age-matched controls, generally <250 nm in adults [3]).
Alport syndrome	Variably thinned and thickened GBM with a multilaminated, 'basket weave' appearance of the lamina densa
Lupus podocytopathy	Extensive FPE (as in minimal change nephropathy), may see mesangial EDD but no capillary wall EDD
Diabetic nephropathy (◘ Fig. 7.48)	Thickened glomerular basement membrane (often >600 nm), FPE, increased mesangial matrix, hyaline material (can resemble EDD)
Thrombotic microangiopathy	Acute; expansion of the lamina rara interna, endothelial cell swelling; may see fibrin tactoids and thrombi Chronic; duplication of theGBM, mesangial cell interposition
Chronic allograft glomerulopathy (◘ Fig. 7.49)	Duplication of the GBM and lamination of the peritubular capillary basement membranes

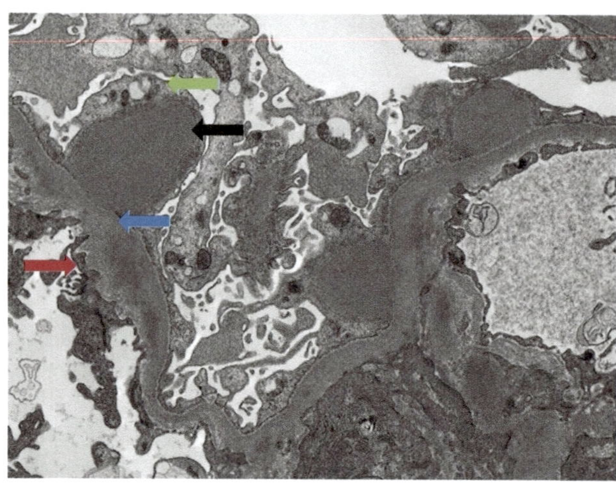

■ **Fig. 7.41** Electron micrograph showing subepithelial hump deposits in a case of post-infectious glomerulonephritis. Black arrow, subepithelial deposit; blue arrow, basement membrane; green arrow, effaced podocyte foot process, X2500. (Image courtesy of Leicester Royal Infirmary electron microscopy department)

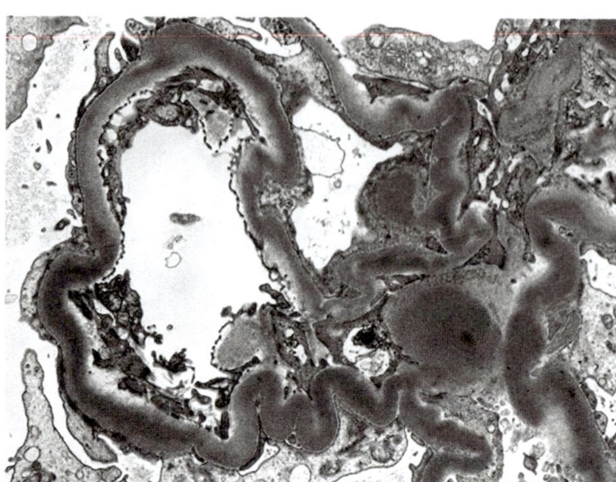

■ **Fig. 7.42** Electron micrograph showing highly dense intramembranous and mesangial deposits. X2500. (Image courtesy of Leicester Royal Infirmary electron microscopy department)

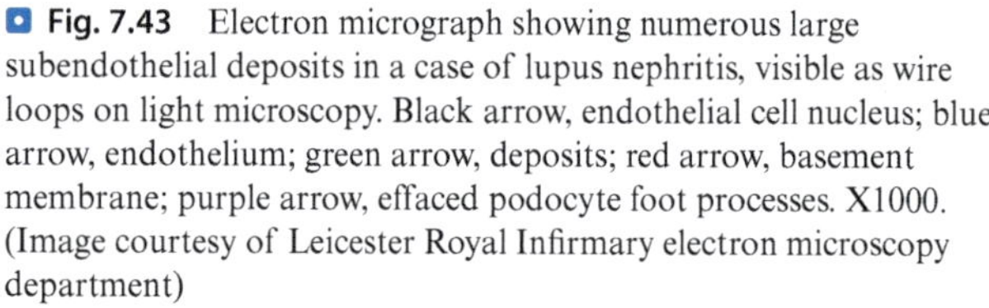

■ **Fig. 7.43** Electron micrograph showing numerous large subendothelial deposits in a case of lupus nephritis, visible as wire loops on light microscopy. Black arrow, endothelial cell nucleus; blue arrow, endothelium; green arrow, deposits; red arrow, basement membrane; purple arrow, effaced podocyte foot processes. X1000. (Image courtesy of Leicester Royal Infirmary electron microscopy department)

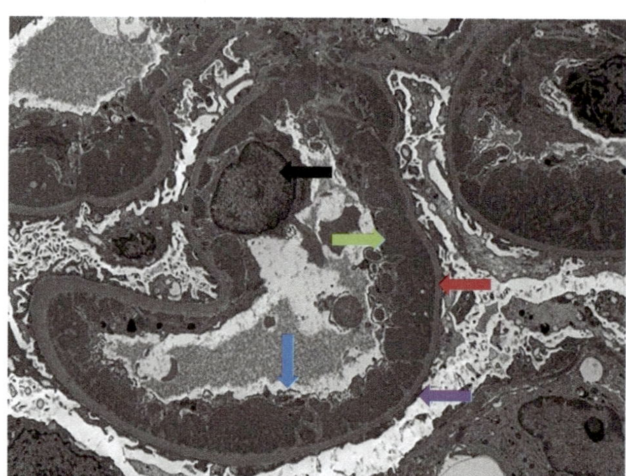

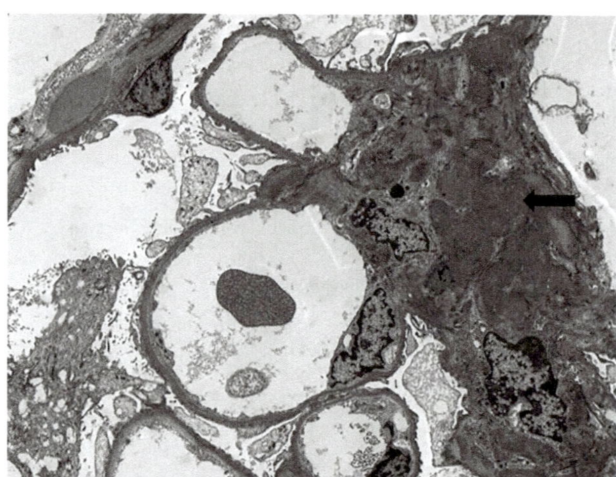

■ **Fig. 7.44** Electron micrograph showing mesangial electron dense deposits (black arrow) in a case of IgA nephropathy. X1000. (Image courtesy of Leicester Royal Infirmary electron microscopy department)

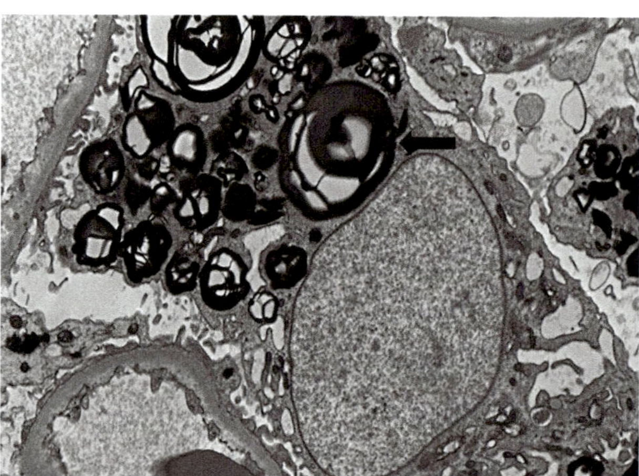

■ **Fig. 7.45** Zebra bodies (black arrow) within podocyte cytoplasm in a case of Fabry's disease. X4400. (Image courtesy of Leicester Royal Infirmary electron microscopy department)

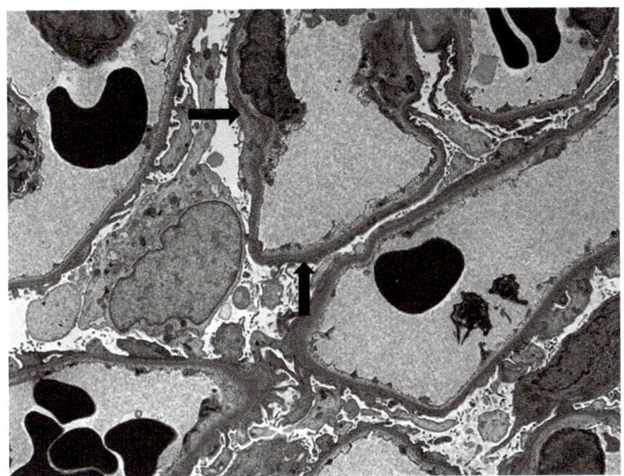

Fig. 7.46 Electron micrograph showing widespread podocyte foot process effacement (black arrows) in a case of minimal change nephropathy. X1000. (Image courtesy of Leicester Royal Infirmary electron microscopy department)

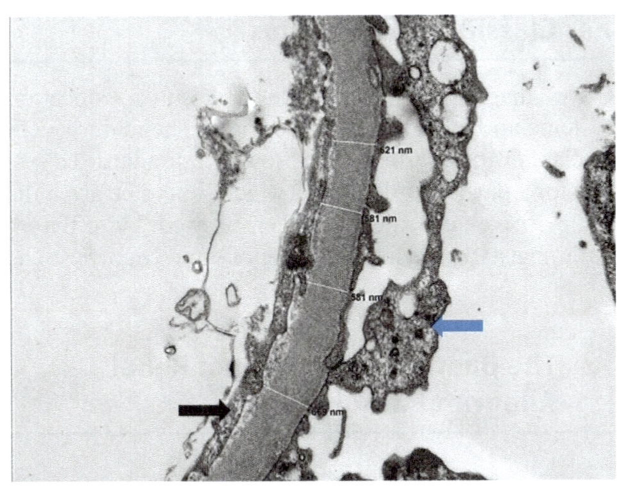

Fig. 7.48 Electron micrograph showing thickened glomerular basement membrane with measurements, in a case of diabetic nephropathy. Blue arrow, effaced podocyte foot process; black arrow, endothelium. X4000. (Image courtesy of Leicester Royal Infirmary electron microscopy department)

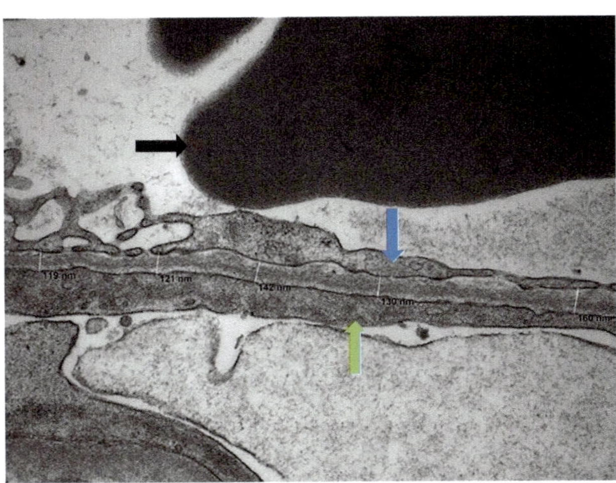

Fig. 7.47 Electron micrograph showing thinning of the glomerular basement membrane. Black arrow, erythrocyte; blue arrow, endothelium; green arrow, effaced podocyte foot process. X8000. (Image courtesy of Leicester Royal Infirmary electron microscopy department)

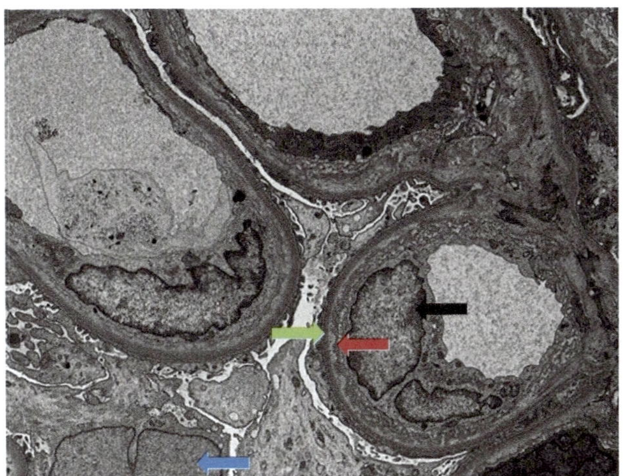

Fig. 7.49 Electron micrograph showing duplication of the glomerular basement membranes, visible as double contours on light microscopy, in a case of transplant glomerulopathy. Black arrow, endothelial cell nucleus; blue arrow, podocyte nucleus; green arrow, original basement membrane; red arrow, reduplicated basement membrane. X1200. (Image courtesy of Leicester Royal Infirmary electron microscopy department)

7.7 Reaching a Diagnosis

Given the variety of features on clinical, light microscopic, IHC/IMF and electron microscopy assessment of renal biopsies, and the fact that very few are specific for a single diagnosis, it is easy to see how each in isolation may not be diagnostic. However, the combination of each of these modalities with the clinical context will usually be sufficient for diagnosis. In some cases, there will be uncertainty, either due to unusual features, a lack of convincing or definitive features, suboptimal functionality of one or more tests or insufficient tissue. While all cases benefit from discussion in a multidisciplinary setting, this is particularly helpful for these ‘difficult’ or less conclusive cases, where the differential and clinical management options can be discussed.

7.8 Classification Systems

Once a diagnosis has been made, a relevant classification system can be applied if appropriate. The main benefit of classification systems is to provide a standardised system for a particular diagnosis, which should be given the same 'score' or category when viewed by different pathologists across hospitals, regions and countries. The standardised approach can be helpful in determining the treatment strategy, e.g. in lupus nephritis, and is useful in research. Potential drawbacks are that not all biopsies will fit neatly into one category; some may show poor concordance and systems change as they are updated. The following are examples of some of the most commonly used. Some are straightforward; others are more complex.

7.9 The Banff Classification of Renal Allograft Pathology [4]

Category 1: Normal biopsy or non-specific changes	
Requires exclusion of any diagnosis from the Banff diagnostic categories 2–4, 6	
Category 2: Antibody-mediated changes (use the diagnostic criteria groups to reach one diagnosis)	
Diagnoses	**Diagnostic criteria groups**
C4d staining without evidence of rejection Banff lesion score C4d > 1 (IF on fresh frozen tissue) OR C4d > 0 (IHC on paraffin-embedded tissue) AND Banff lesion scores t0, v0, no arterial intimal fibrosis with mononuclear cell inflammation in fibrosis and formation of neointima, no criterion from group 1 (AMR activity), no criterion from groups 4 (histologic features of AMR chronicity), no increased expression of thoroughly validated gene transcripts/classifiers in the biopsy tissue strongly associated with AMR	Criteria group 1 AMR activity: Banff lesion score g > 0 in the absence of glomerulonephritis and/or Banff lesion score ptc > 0 in the absence of TCMR or borderline Banff lesion score v > 0 Acute thrombotic microangiopathy in the absence of any other cause Acute tubular injury in the absence of any other apparent cause
Active AMR No criterion of AMR chronicity (criteria group 4) AND At least one criterion from criteria group 1 (AMR activity) AND At least one criterion from criteria group 2 (antibody interaction with tissue) AND At least one criterion from criteria group 3 (DSA or equivalents)	Criteria group 2 antibody interaction with tissue: Banff lesion score C4d > 1 (IF on fresh frozen tissue) OR C4d > 0 (IHC on paraffin-embedded tissue) At least moderate MVI (g + ptc >1) in the absence of recurrent or de novo glomerulonephritis; borderline (diagnostic category 3) or acute T cell-mediated rejection (TCMR; diagnostic category 4). If borderline, acute TCMR or infection is present (Banff lesion scores g + ptc) >1 is not sufficient and Banff lesion score g > 1 is required Increased expression of thoroughly validated gene transcripts/classifiers in the biopsy tissue strongly associated with AMR
Chronic active AMR At least one feature of AMR chronicity (criteria group 4) AND At least one criterion of antibody interaction with tissue (criteria group 2) AND At least one criterion of DSA or equivalents (criteria group 3)	Criteria group 3 DSA or equivalents: DSA (anti-HLA or other specificity) Banff lesion score C4d > 1 (IF on fresh frozen tissue) OR C4d > 0 (IHC on paraffin-embedded tissue) Increased expression of thoroughly validated gene transcripts/classifiers in the biopsy tissue strongly associated with AMR
Chronic AMR Banff 2017 permits the use of this term for biopsy specimens showing TG and/or peritubular capillary basement membrane multilayering in the absence of criterion of current/recent antibody interaction with the endothelium (Criteria Group 2) but with a prior documented diagnosis of Active or Chronic Active or documented prior evidence of DSA	Criteria group 4 histologic features of AMR chronicity Banff lesion score cg > 0 (by LM or EM), excluding biopsies with evidence of chronic thrombotic microangiopathy Seven or more layers in one cortical peritubular capillary and five or more in two additional capillaries, avoiding portions cut tangentially by EM in available Arterial intimal fibrosis of new onset, excluding other causes leukocytes within the sclerotic intima favour chronic AMR if there is not prior history of biopsy-proven TCMR but are not required

Category 3: Suspicious (borderline) for acute TCMR

Foci of Banff lesion score $t > 0$ AND Banff lesions score $i \leq 1$
OR
Foci of Banff lesion score t1 AND Banff lesion score $i \geq 2$

Category 4: TCMR

Acute TCMR IA
Banff lesion score $i \geq 2$
AND
Banff lesion score t2
Acute TCMR IB
Banff lesion score $i \geq 2$
AND
Banff lesion score t3
Acute TCMR IIA
Banff lesion score v1 regardless of Banff lesion scores i or t
Acute TCMR IIB
Banff lesion score v2 regardless of Banff lesion scores i or t
Acute TCMR III
Banff lesion score v3 regardless of Banff lesion scores i or t
Chronic active TCMR grade IA
Banff lesion score $ti \geq 2$
AND
Banff lesion score i-IFTA≥2; other known causes of i-IFTA (e.g. pyelonephritis, BK-virus nephritis, etc.) ruled out
AND
Banff lesion score t2
Chronic active TCMR grade IB
Banff lesion score $ti \geq 2$
AND
Banff lesion score i-IFTA≥2; other known causes of IFTA ruled out
AND
Banff lesion score t3
Chronic active TCMR grade II
Arterial intimal fibrosis with mononuclear cell inflammation on fibrosis and formation of neointima

Category 4: IFTA

Grade I (mild)
Banff lesion score ci1
OR
Banff lesion score ct1
Grade II (moderate)
Banff lesion score ci2
OR
Banff lesion score ct2
Grade III (severe)
Banff lesion score ci3
OR
Banff lesion score ct3

Category 6: Other changes not considered to be caused by acute or chronic rejection

BK virus nephropathy
Post-transplant lymphoproliferative disorder
Calcineurin inhibitor toxicity
Acute tubular injury
Recurrent disease
De novo glomerulopathy (other than TG)
Pyelonephritis
Drug-induced interstitial nephritis

7.9.1 The Oxford Classification of IgA nephropathy [6]

Variable	Score
Mesangial hypercellularity (≥4 cells in a single mesangial area)	≤50% glomeruli M0 >50% glomeruli M1
Endocapillary hypercellularity	Absent E0 Present E1
Segmental glomerulosclerosis	Absent S0 Present S1 (with a comment indicating the presence/absence of podocytopathic features)
Tubular atrophy and interstitial fibrosis	<25% T0 26–50% T1 >50% T2
Cellular/fibrocellular crescents	Absent C0 In at least one glomerulus C1 In >25% of glomeruli C2

7

7.9.2 The Columbia Classification of Focal Segmental Glomerulosclerosis

The diagnosis of FSGS can be problematic, as segmental lesions are non-specific and there are many possible aetiologies (genetic, viral, drug, adaptive, underlying glomerulopathy). This classification can be used in primary or secondary forms and is based on light microscopic features. Given the focal nature of the diagnostic features, it has been suggested that 25 glomeruli and multiple sections are required to reliably detect lesions. The juxtamedullary region is thought to be affected initially; therefore, biopsies ideally will include this area. The NOS variant is the commonest and is thought to develop from the other variants [5].

Variant	Inclusion criteria	Exclusion criteria	Prognosis
FSGS NOS (not otherwise specified)	At least one glomerulus with segmental increase in matrix obliterating the capillary lumina There may be segmental glomerular capillary wall collapse without overlying podocyte hyperplasia	Exclude perihilar, cellular, tip and collapsing variants	Standard
Perihilar variant	At least one glomerulus with perihilar hyalinosis, with or without sclerosis >50% of glomeruli with segmental lesions must have perihilar sclerosis and/or hyalinosis	Exclude cellular, tip and collapsing variants	Good
Cellular variant	At least one glomerulus with segmental endocapillary hypercellularity occulding lumina, with or without foam cells and karyorrhexis	Exclude tip and collapsing variants	Intermediate between collapsing and NOS variants
Tip variant	At least one segmental lesion involving the tip domain (outer 25% of tuft next to the origin of the proximal tubule) The tubular pole must be identified in the defining lesion The lesion must have either an adhesion or confluence of podocytes with parietal or tubular cells at the tubular lumen or neck The tip lesion may be cellular or sclerosing	Exclude collapsing variant Exclude perihilar sclerosis	Excellent Highest rate of complete remission
Collapsing variant	At least one glomerulus with segmental or global collapse and overlying podocyte hypertrophy and hyperplasia	None	Poor Highest rate of ESRD

7.10 ISN/RPS Classification of Lupus Nephritis

The International Society of Nephrology/Renal Pathology Society lupus nephritis classification was originally proposed in 2004 [7], but has recently been updated [8]. Some of the most prominent changes are the elimination of the segmental and global (S/G) subdivisions of class IV, due to poor concordance and uncertain clinical significance, and the introduction of an activity/chronicity index, modified from the NIH activity and chronicity index, to replace the previously used A, C and A/C parameters. Class V can co-exist with class III or IV (i.e. lupus nephritis class III + V).

Classification	Description	Features
Class I	Minimal mesangial lupus nephritis	Normal glomeruli on light microscopy, with immune deposits detectable on IHC/IF
Class II	Mesangial proliferative lupus nephritis	Mesangial hypercellularity (four or more mesangial cells per mesangial region, surrounded by matrix, not including the central or hilar regions)
Class III	Focal lupus nephritis	Active or inactive, focal or global endo-extracapillary glomerulonephritis, involving <50% of glomeruli
Class IV	Diffuse lupus nephritis	Active or inactive, focal or global endo-extracapillary glomerulonephritis, involving ≥50% of glomeruli
Class V	Membranous lupus nephritis	Global or segmental subepithelial immune deposits, with or without mesangial changes
Class VI	Advanced sclerotic lupus nephritis	>90% of glomeruli globally sclerosed, with no residual activity

Modified NIH Activity Index	Definition	Score
Endocapillary hypercellularity	Endocapillary hypercellularity in % of glomeruli: <25% (1+) 25–50% (2+) >50% (3+)	0–3
Neutrophils/karyorrhexis	Neutrophils and/or karyorrhexis in % of glomeruli: <25% (1+) 25–50% (2+) >50% (3+)	0–3
Hyaline deposits	Wire loops or hyaline thrombi in % of glomeruli: <25% (1+) 25–50% (2+) >50% (3+)	0–3
Fibrinoid necrosis	Fibrinoid necrosis in % of glomeruli: <25% (1+) 25–50% (2+) >50% (3+)	(0–3) x2
Cellular/fibrocellular crescents	Cellular/fibrocellular crescents in % of glomeruli: <25% (1+) 25–50% (2+) >50% (3+)	(0–3) x2
Interstitial inflammation	Interstitial leukocytes in % of the cortex: <25% (1+) 25–50% (2+) >50% (3+)	0–3
Total		**0–24**
Modified NIH chronicity index	**Definition**	**Score**
Total glomerulosclerosis	Global and/or segmental glomerulosclerosis in % of glomeruli: <25% (1+) 25–50% (2+) >50% (3+)	0–3
Fibrous crescents	Fibrous crescents in % of glomeruli: <25% (1+) 25–50% (2+) >50% (3+)	0–3
Tubular atrophy	Tubular atrophy in % of the cortical tubules: <25% (1+) 25–50% (2+) >50% (3+)	0–3
Interstitial fibrosis	Interstitial fibrosis in % of the cortex: <25% (1+) 25–50% (2+) >50% (3+)	0–3
Total		**0–12**

7.10.1 The Modified Karpinski Score for Time Zero Renal Transplant Biopsies [9]

This scoring system is one of a number of similar systems used for biopsies taken at implantation of a transplant. The function of these biopsies is to provide a baseline of the condition of the kidney at the time of transplant (donor-related damage), which can be used for comparison on subsequent biopsies. This scoring system should be used in biopsies with more than 20 glomeruli present.

7

Glomerular score
0 – No globally sclerosed glomeruli 1 – <20% 2 – 20–50% 3 – >50%
Tubular score
0 – No atrophic tubules 1 – <20% 2 – 20–50% 3 – >50%
Interstitial score
0 – No interstitial fibrosis 1 – <20% 2 – 20–50% 3 – >50%

Vascular score (use arterial or arteriolar score – Whichever is greater)
0 – No arteriolar narrowing/hyaline arteriolosclerosis 1 – Increased wall thickness less than the diameter of the lumen 2 – Increased wall thickness the same as or slightly more than the diameter of the lumen 3 – Increased wall thickness much greater than the diameter of the lumen or occlusion 0 – No arterial sclerosis/intimal fibroplasia 1 – Increased wall thickness less than the diameter of the lumen 2 – Increased wall thickness the same as or slightly more than the diameter of the lumen 3 – Increased wall thickness much greater than the diameter of the lumen or occlusion

Tips and Tricks

- Look for a second diagnosis, particularly in common conditions such as diabetic or IgA nephropathy.
- Atrophic tubules are generally accepted as the main determining factor of irreversible damage in the kidney and so are a key prognostic indicator [10].
- The percentage of chronic parenchymal damage within a core biopsy is assumed to be representative of the whole kidney, but this is not always the case, particularly in subcapsular samples, which may overestimate the amount of damage [11].

Case Studies

Case 1

Clinical Scenario.

A 73-year-old male with renal impairment, haematuria and proteinuria.

The H&E image (Fig. 7.50) shows a nodular glomerulopathy. Differentials are diabetic glomerulopathy, amyloidosis, monoclonal light chain deposition disease or idiopathic nodular glomerulopathy (a diagnosis of exclusion).

The silver stain (PAMS, Fig. 7.51) shows that the mesangial material is silver negative (excluding diabetic glomerulopathy).

The Congo red stain shows that the mesangial material is Congo red positive and shows ‘apple green’ birefringence under polarised light (Fig. 7.52) diagnostic of amyloidosis.

Light chain immunohistochemistry shows stronger mesangial positivity for lambda than kappa (Fig. 7.53), giving a diagnosis of AL (lambda) amyloidosis.

Diagnosis: AL amyloidosis.

Clinical Correlation: The patient was found to have a plasma cell neoplasm on bone marrow biopsy.

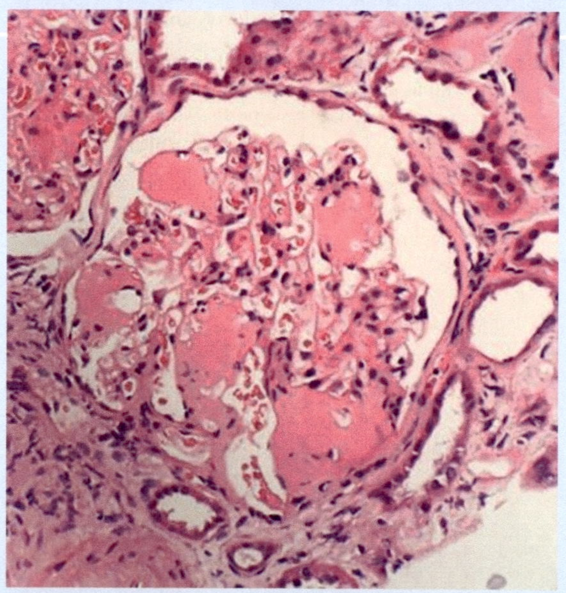

Fig. 7.50 Case 1 H&E. x400

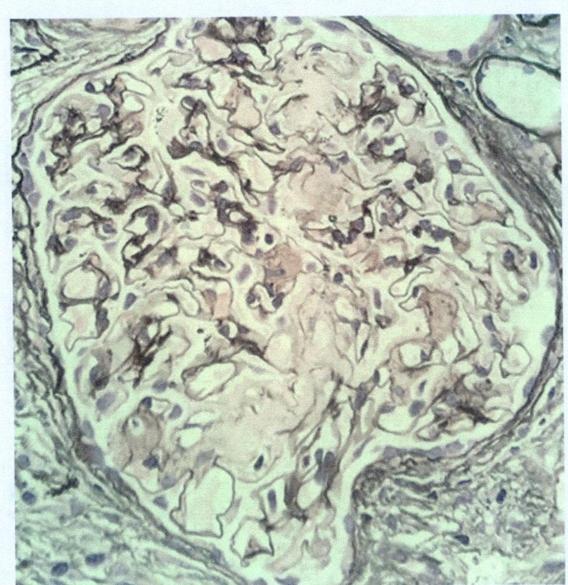

Fig. 7.51 Case 1. PAMS X400

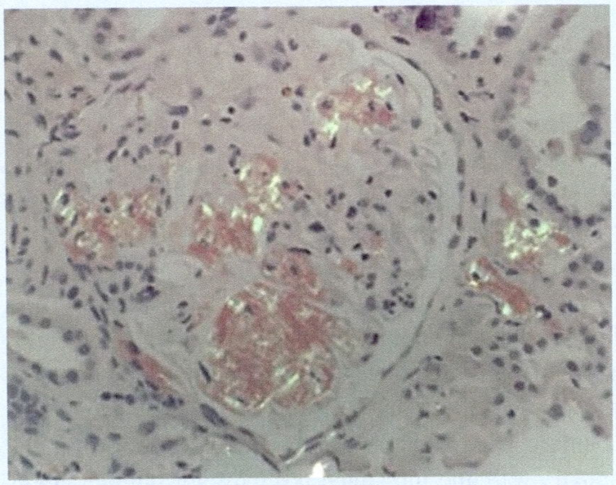

Fig. 7.52 Case 1. Photographed under polarised light. Congo red. X400

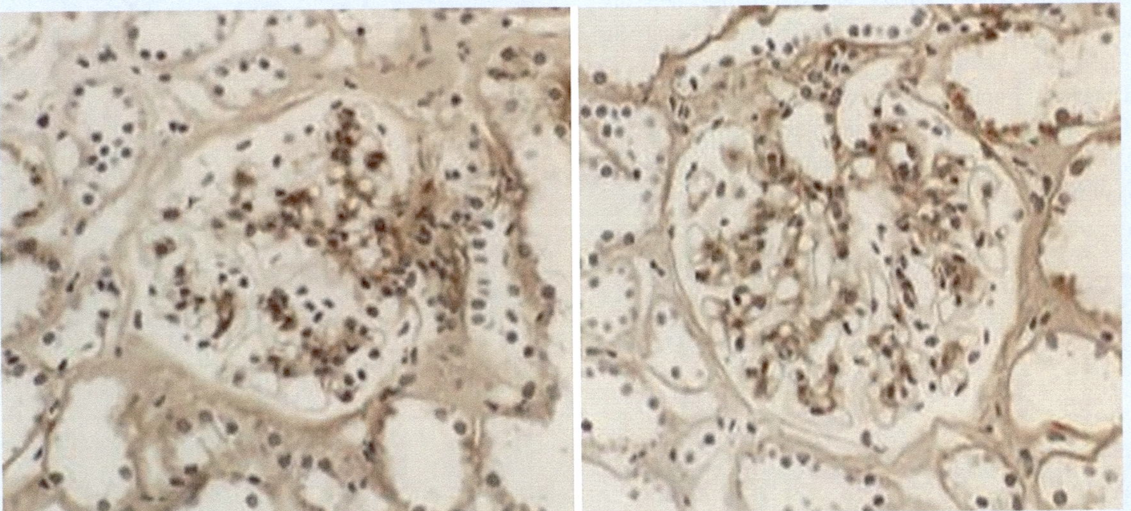

Fig. 7.53 Case 1. Kappa (right) and lambda (left) light chain immunohistochemical stains. X400

7

Case 2

Clinical Scenario.

A 25-year-old lady with increasing proteinuria and low serum complement levels.

The initial H&E (◘ Fig. 7.54) shows a glomerulus with a segment of necrosis and a small cellular crescent. At this point, it is apparent that there is an active glomerular process (necrosis and cellular crescent).

The PAMS stain (◘ Fig. 7.55) demonstrates diffuse, global spike formation along the capillary walls indicating that there are subepithelial deposits producing a membranous pattern.

Immunostains (◘ Figs. 7.56 and 7.57) show granular capillary wall and mesangial positivity for immunoglobulins G, A and M and complement component C3 and C1q. This implies that immune deposits are present both in the capillary walls and the mesangium. The capillary wall deposits are predominantly subepithelial, with occasional subendothelial deposits.

Electron microscopy (◘ Fig. 7.58) shows subepithelial (green arrow), mesangial (black arrow) and occasional subendothelial (blue arrow) electron dense deposits. Tubuloreticular inclusions are seen within endothelial cells (◘ Fig. 7.59).

Diagnosis: Lupus nephritis, class III + V.

Clinical correlation – this lady had positive ANA and dsDNA antibodies and fulfilled clinical criteria for a diagnosis of SLE.

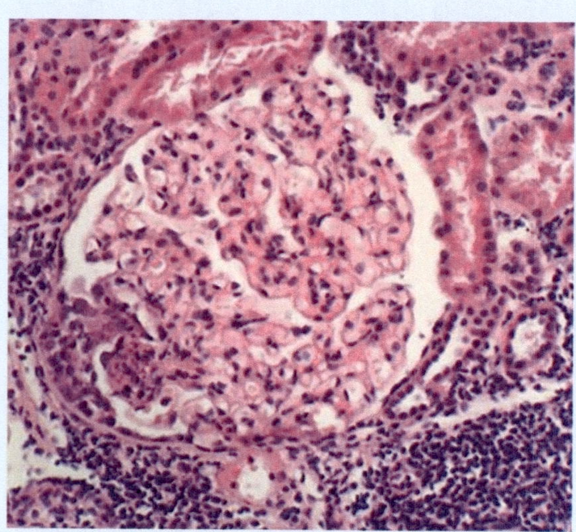

◘ **Fig. 7.54** Case 2. H&E x200

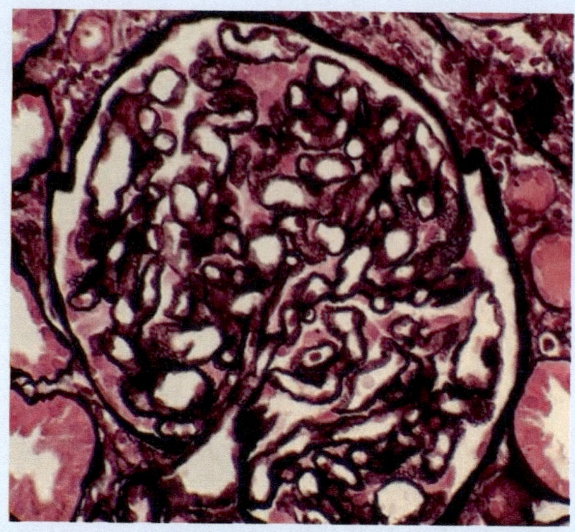

◘ **Fig. 7.55** Case 2. PAMS x400

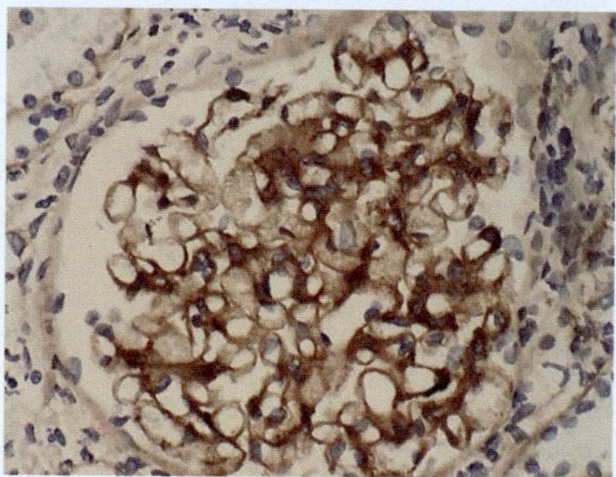

◘ **Fig. 7.56** Case 2. Immunohistochemical stain for IgG. IgA and IgM showed similar patterns of staining. X400

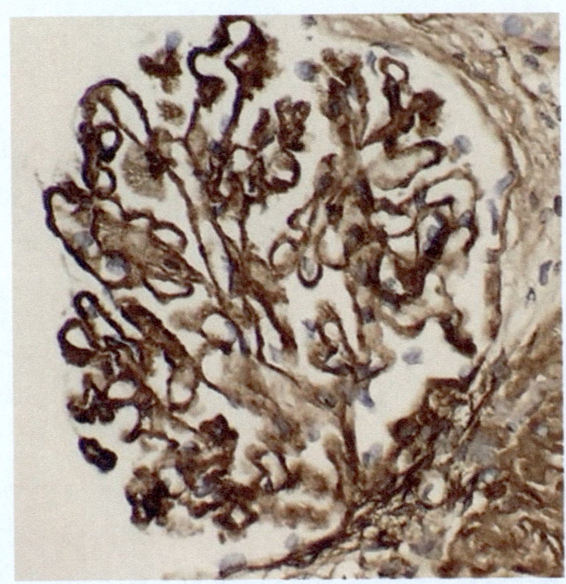

■ **Fig. 7.57** Case 2. Immunohistochemical stain for C3. C1q showed a similar pattern of staining. X400

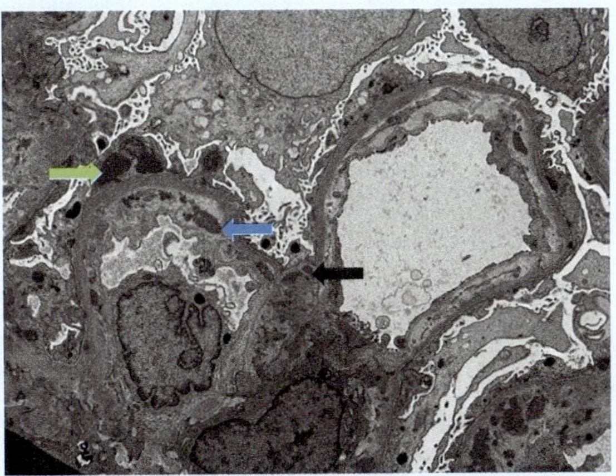

■ **Fig. 7.58** Case 2. Electron micrograph X1200. (Image courtesy of Leicester Royal Infirmary electron microscopy department)

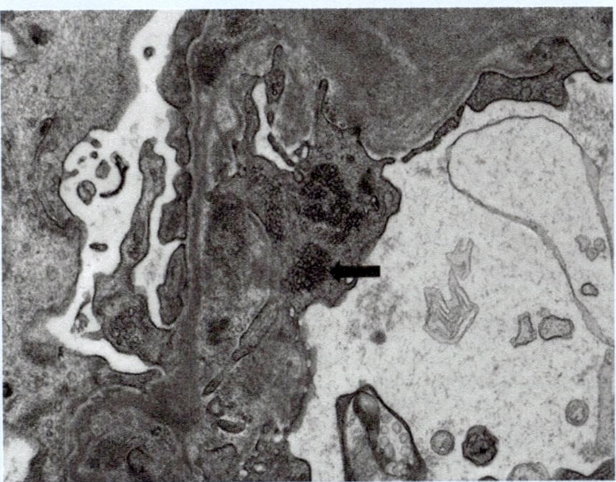

■ **Fig. 7.59** Case 2. Electron micrograph. X5000. (Image courtesy of Leicester Royal Infirmary electron microscopy department)

Case 3

Clinical Scenario.

A 44-year-old man, recipient of a DBD renal transplant 16 months ago. Best creatinine 170, now risen to 236.

Initial H&E sections (Fig. 7.60) show acute tubular injury with some nuclear pleomorphism and focal tubulitis. No acute vascular rejection is seen. There is moderate chronic damage. Some glomeruli (not shown) are poorly perfused but show no other acute changes. At this point, the differential lies between acute cellular rejection and BK nephropathy. Without confirmatory tests, it can be very difficult to reliably distinguish these possibilities. In this case, viral cytopathic changes are present, and further clinical history was sought, making the diagnosis straightforward.

7

Further tests show positive tubular nuclei on BK immunohistology (Fig. 7.61).

Diagnosis: BK nephropathy.

Clinical correlation – this patient was compliant with immunosuppressive therapy, and a serum BK viraemia was identified.

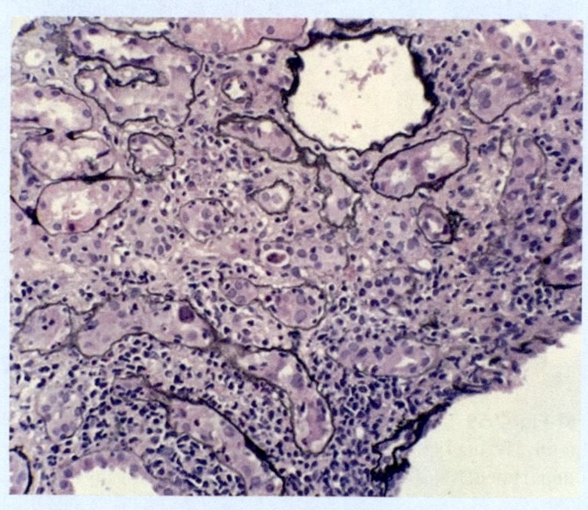

Fig. 7.60 Case 3. PAMS x200

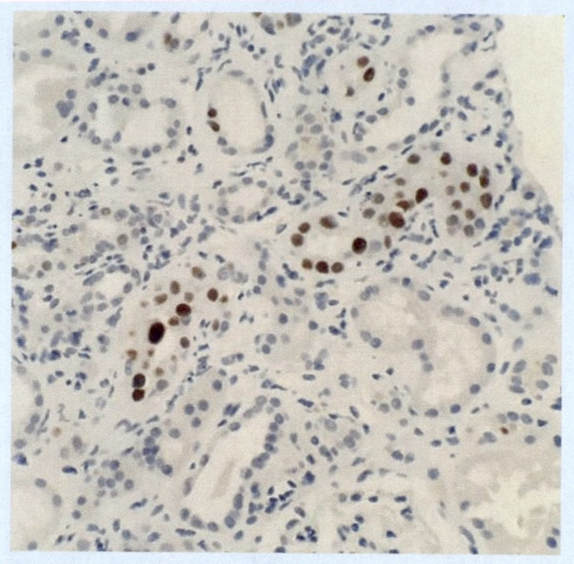

Fig. 7.61 Case 3. Immunohistochemical stain for SV40. X200

Questions

The answers may be found within the text.

1. What is the differential diagnosis for a nodular glomerulopathy?
2. What is the differential diagnosis for glomerular IgA deposition?
3. What is the differential diagnosis for a glomerulopathy with negative IHC/IF?
4. Which feature on a biopsy is generally considered to be the best predictor of long-term outcome?
5. What are the Banff criteria for a diagnosis of acute cellular rejection?

References

1. Corwin HL, Schwartz MM, Lewis EJ. The importance of sample size in the interpretation of the renal biopsy. Am J Nephrol. 1988;8:85–9.
2. Fogo AB, Kashgarian M. Diagnostic atlas of renal pathology. 3rd ed. Philadelphia: Elsevier; 2017. p. 21.
3. Tiebosch ATMG, et al. Thin basement-membrane nephropathy in adults with persistent hematuria. N Engl J Med. 1989;320:14–8.
4. Roufosse C, et al. A 2018 reference guide to the Banff classification of renal allograft pathology. Transplantation. 2018;102:1795–814.
5. Howie AJ, et al. Evolution of nephrotic-associated focal segmental glomerulosclerosis and relation to the glomerular tip lesion. Kidney Int. 2005;67(3):987–1001.
6. Trimarchi H, et al. Oxford classification of IgA nephropathy 2016: an update from the IgA nephropathy classification working group. Kidney Int. 2017;91:1014–21.
7. Weening JJ, et al. The classification of glomerulonephritis in systemic lupus erythematosus revisited. Kidney Int. 2004;65:521–30.
8. Bajema IM, et al. Revision of the International Society of Nephrology/Renal Pathology Society classification for lupus nephritis: clarification of definitions, and modified national institutes of health activity and chronicity indices. Kidney Int. 2018;93:789–96.
9. Karpinski J, et al. Outcome of kidney transplantation from high-risk donors is determined by both structure and function. Transplantation. 1999;67(8):1162–7.
10. D'Amico G. Influence of clinical and histological features on actuarial renal survival in adult patients with idiopathic IgA nephropathy, membranous nephropathy, and membranoproliferative glomerulonephritis: survey of the recent literature.
11. Howie AJ. Handbook of renal biopsy pathology. 2nd ed. New York: Springer; 2008. p. 35.

Acute Kidney Injury

Contents

Acute Kidney Injury Epidemiology and Causes

Dilushi Wijayaratne, Chathurika Beligaswatta, and Mark Harber

Contents

M. Harber (ed.), *Primer on Nephrology*, https://doi.org/10.1007/978-3-030-76419-7_8

Learning Objectives

1. To understand the definition of acute kidney injury.
2. To understand the epidemiology of acute kidney injury in terms of incidence, prevalence and patterns of distribution.
3. To understand the important risk factors for AKI.
4. To understand the pathophysiology and mechanisms of AKI.
5. To identify the common causes and mechanisms of AKI in at-risk patient groups.

8.1 Introduction

Acute kidney injury (AKI) is one of the commonest medical emergencies, and the spectrum of AKI is strongly influenced by environmental, socio-economic and health-care-related factors. AKI carries a high mortality (roughly 20% globally) and is likely to be on the increase, yet as many cases of AKI are preventable protection from death by AKI was recently portrayed as a human right by the International Society of Nephrology initiative for zero preventable deaths from AKI by 2025 (0by25) [1]. Achieving this target will require a new and holistic approach including improvements in health policy and infrastructure, public awareness and education and medical management; nephrologists have a key role to play in promoting these improvements. In this chapter we will define acute kidney injury; describe its epidemiology, pathophysiology and causes; and discuss a few special groups of patients who are particularly at high risk of AKI.

8.2 Definitions and Classifications

The clinical syndrome of acute kidney injury (AKI) is characterised by a sudden decline in glomerular filtration rate (GFR) over a period of hours to days and manifests as retention of fluid and metabolic waste products which are normally excreted by the kidneys. It includes a spectrum of patients ranging from those with minor deviations detected on laboratory testing to those with life-threatening abnormalities of fluid and solute balance. Various groups have attempted to develop a consensus definition for AKI which is sensitive, reliable and convenient and of practical and prognostic value. In 2000 the Acute Dialysis Quality Initiative (ADQI) developed a consensus definition with AKI stratified based on the severity and duration of injury into stages of Risk, Injury, Failure, Loss and End-Stage (RIFLE) disease [2]. The Acute Kidney Injury Network (AKIN) comprising the ADQI group and others later modified this definition [3] based on the recognition that even small changes in serum creatinine are associated with increased mortality. At the same time, the term Acute Kidney Injury (AKI) was introduced to encompass the entire spectrum of renal injury from minor changes in kidney function to dialysis dependency. Most recently the international guideline group Kidney Disease: Improving Global Outcomes (KDIGO) agreed a definition and staging system that harmonises the previous systems proposed by both ADQI and AKIN [4]. It has now been globally adopted and dramatically assisted the identification and quantification of AKI which will permit assessment of the incidence, outcomes and efficacy of therapeutic interventions for AKI.

Under the KDIGO classification scheme, AKI is defined as an abrupt (within 48 hours to 1 week) rise in serum creatinine or as a sustained (more than 6 hours) reduction in urine output. It is further classified into three stages based on the absolute or relative increase in serum creatinine or duration and magnitude of reduction in urine output (Table 8.1). These classifications help define the degree of kidney dysfunction at diagnosis, aid in tracking of the clinical course, are widely validated and have been shown to predict outcomes in diverse patient populations and in large international databases. Under all classification schemes, loss of kidney function requiring dialysis for more than 3 months constitutes end-stage kidney disease.

Table 8.1 KDIGO classification of acute kidney injury (3)

AKI Stage	Serum creatinine criteria	Urine output criteria
1	Increase in serum creatinine of ≥26 μmol/L (0.3 mg/dL) within 48 hours or increase to ≥1.5 to 1.9 x baseline serum creatinine within 1 week	<0.5 mL/kg/hour for >6 consecutive hours
2	Increase in serum creatinine to >2.0 to 2.9 x baseline serum creatinine	<0.5 mL/kg/hour for >12 consecutive hours
3	Increase in serum creatinine greater than threefold from baseline or serum creatinine of ≥354 μmol/L [≥4.0 mg/dL] or commenced on renal replacement therapy irrespective of stage	<0.3 mL/kg/hour for >24 consecutive hours *Or* anuria for 12 hours

8.3 Epidemiology: The Incidence and Burden of AKI

The true worldwide incidence and distribution of AKI is still poorly understood because of under-reporting, regional disparities and differences in definition. More recently, the adoption of KDIGO or KDIGO equivalent definitions of AKI worldwide has brought in some comparable data from regions such as Africa and Southeast Asia, where data was previously scarce. Especially in low-resource settings, much of the data are derived from studies done in tertiary-care hospitals and may not be representative of the total disease burden.

AKI has been reported to affect about 13.3 million people annually, 85% of whom live in developing countries. In high-income countries, it affects 3000–5000 per one million population per year. In a recent meta-analysis of the worldwide epidemiology of AKI, which included 765 studies and over 77 million patients, the pooled incidence of AKI was 21% of hospital admissions with 2% requiring dialysis (11% of all AKI). 80% of AKI was KDIGO stage 1 [1, 5]. The overall pooled mortality was 21%, with those with KDIGO stage 3 AKI, or requiring dialysis having a mortality of 42% and 46%, respectively (◘ Fig. 8.1).

There has been a significant increase in the incidence of reported AKI over the past few decades. Recent data on AKI comes from large databases which use ICD coding or creatinine change criteria to diagnose AKI [7]. This increase, therefore, needs to be interpreted with some caution as it may be partially explained by the changing definitions of AKI, increased awareness and coding of AKI as well as alterations in clinical practice such as increased blood testing or hospital admission. In particular, increased recognition of milder forms of AKI could be the cause of a rising incidence alongside an apparent reduction in mortality. However, beyond a reporting bias, it seems likely that there is a genuine increase in some settings particularly in the setting of an ageing and increasingly comorbid population. If so, this is clearly important for a condition with an average mortality of 20% and no effective treatment other than supportive measures (◘ Fig. 8.2).

The clinical presentation of community-acquired AKI in various parts of the world is influenced by several factors.

1. Geographical location and natural environment.
2. Socio-economic factors.
3. Cultural practices.
4. Health-care services and infrastructure.

8.4 Geographical Location and Natural Environment

In a snapshot of AKI in 72 countries in 2014, 58% of AKI was community-acquired. This was lower in high-income countries (HICs) at approximately 50%,

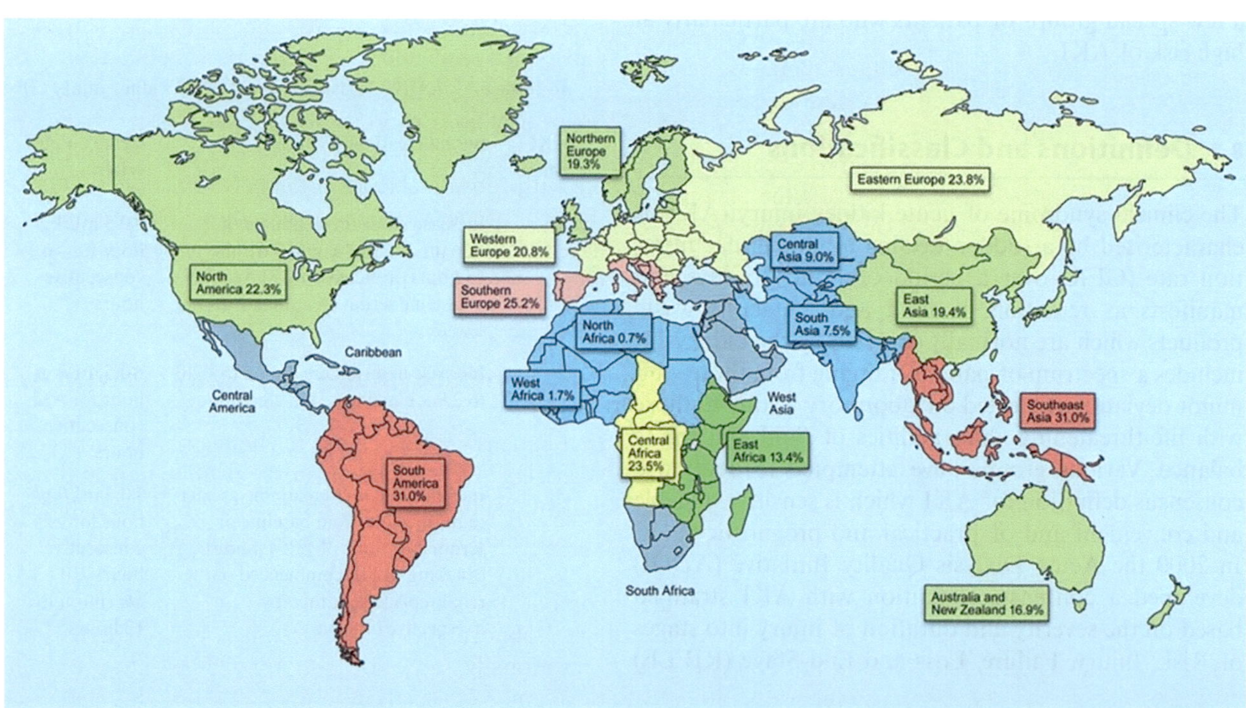

◘ **Fig. 8.1** Global epidemiology of AKI: Published incidence of AKI using KDIGO criteria vary widely across regions. The percentages shown represent the proportion of the hospitalised population with AKI. (Reproduced with permission from *Global epidemiology and outcomes of acute kidney injury*. Nature Review Nephology. 2018; 14:607–625 [6])

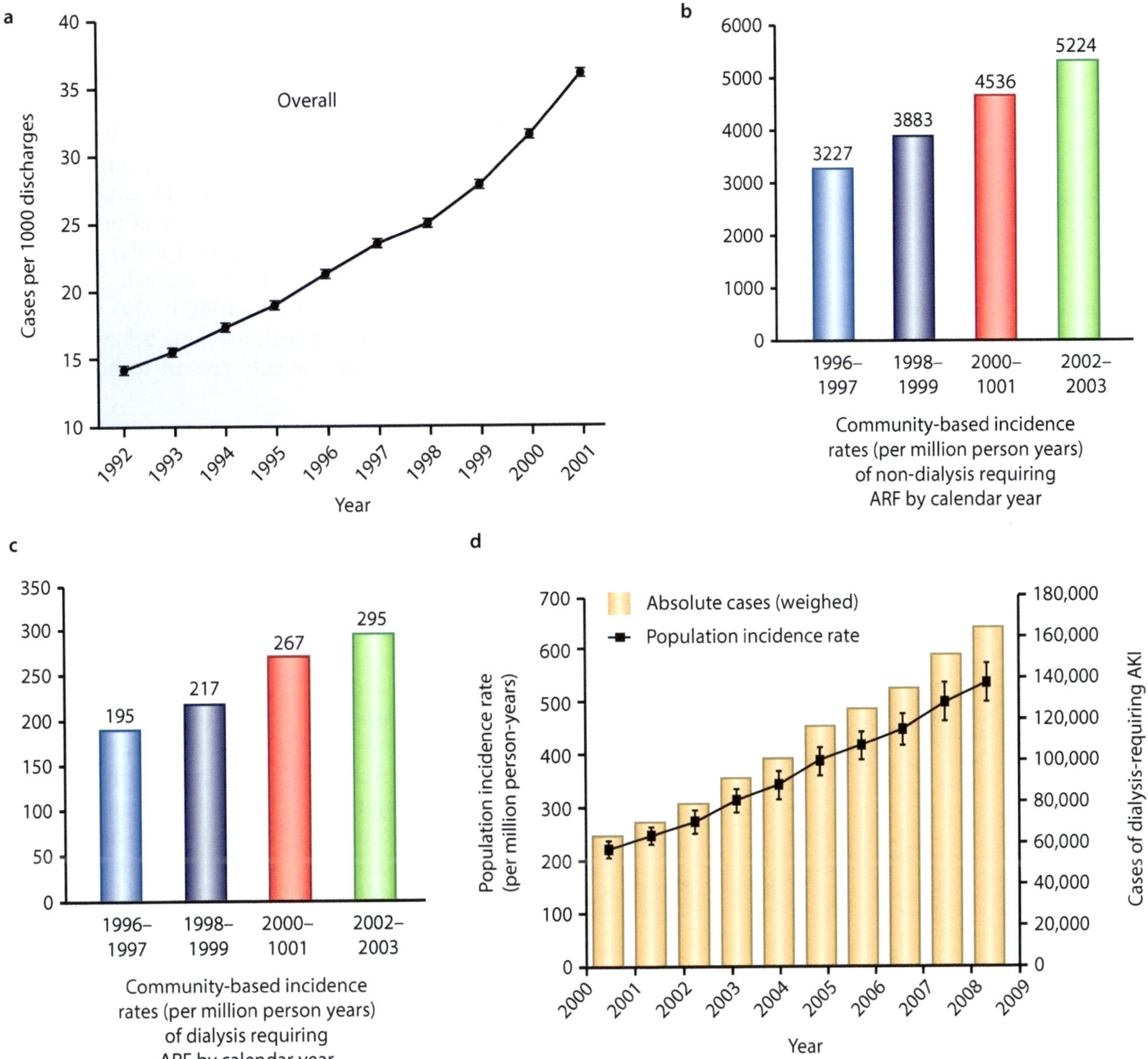

Fig. 8.2 Temporal trends in the hospital-based and population-based incidence of acute kidney injury (AKI). (**a**) Hospital-based incidence in AKI among elderly (aged >65 years) Medicare beneficiaries using administrative codes (USA). (**b, c**) Community-based incidence of non-dialysis- and dialysis-requiring AKI in Northern California (USA) using administrative codes and creatinine-based definitions, respectively. (**d**) Population incidence of dialysis-requiring AKI using the Nationwide Inpatient Sample and US Census data. (Reproduced with permission [7])

compared to 80% in low-income countries (LICs) [8]. Regardless of GDP, hypotension and dehydration were the commonest precipitants of AKI. In LICs, however, this predominantly relates to a single illness such as infectious diseases, obstetric complications or toxins [9]. For LICs in the tropics, severe malaria, diarrhoeal illnesses and nephrotropic infections such as leptospirosis are common and account for a significant burden of AKI. Animal and plant poisons are also, not infrequent, causes of AKI in tropical countries (see below). Intermittently, there are spikes of AKI related to natural disasters such as acute kidney injury due to rapid spread of water-borne infection (e.g. leptospirosis, hantavirus, cholera and other diarrhoeal illnesses following flooding) and traumatic rhabdomyolysis in the setting of earthquakes. In HICs or tertiary centres in LMICs, the pattern is different with much of AKI being related to drugs, trauma, surgery, cardiac illness or other comorbidity in an older population [10]. Importantly, increases in international travel mean that patients may present with AKI secondary to less familiar insults and toxins (Table 8.2).

Table 8.2 A comparison between the characteristics of AKI in high-income countries and low- to middle-income countries [6]

	High-income countries	Low- to middle-income countries
Setting	Secondary care and ITU	Rural health centres and hospital as well as larger urban hospitals and ITUs
Disease spectrum	Associated with comorbidity and multi-organ failure	Often a single disease
Mortality	High	Same or lower than in high-income countries
Population	Elderly	Otherwise healthy young population
Incidence	Increasing	Increasingly apparent
Reporting	Adequate	Under-reported
Expense of treatment	Expensive	Very inexpensive in early stages. Very costly in severe stages
Aetiology	Pre-renal and acute tubular Trauma Sepsis Post-surgical Drug-induced Obstructive nephropathy	Infections: Diarrhoea, malaria, leptospirosis, hantavirus, dengue fever Animal toxins envenomation: Snake bite, multiple hornet or wasp stings Traditional remedies Obstetric emergencies

8.5 Socio-Economic Factors

Regardless of national GDP, the level of education, availability of clean water, sanitation, nutrition, drug and alcohol abuse and access to health care have an impact on the both incidence and aetiology of AKI within a country. For example, acute gastroenteritis complicated by severe dehydration is one of the commonest causes of AKI in low-income countries, influenced by lack of clean water and limited access to health care. While less common in more affluent countries, gastroenteritis remains an important cause of AKI particularly for those with less access to health care, and drug and alcohol dependency remain important risk factors for AKI.

8.6 Cultural Factors

Health beliefs and practices unique to certain populations may alter the spectrum of AKI seen in different parts of the world. Certain natural remedies may be toxic to kidneys in their own right (e.g. starfruit used in treatment of diabetes is known to cause oxalate nephropathy) or may delay the initiation of proven medical interventions such as treatment of malaria or snake bite. The use of agricultural poisons such as organophosphates and paraquat in suicide is also associated with AKI. Differences in health-seeking behaviours may influence if and when patients present to hospital for treatment.

8.7 Health Care-Related

At a national level, adequacy of health budget allocation, health-care human resources and health-care services and hospitals plays a role in the risk related to AKI. Inadequate hospital resources, for instance, in obstetric care, lack of transport facilities, scarcity of educated heath-care workers and physicians and insufficient diagnostic equipment are barriers to successful prevention of AKI in low-income areas. Health-care systems which place importance on screening and early detection of acute kidney injury and protocol-based care may have a higher apparent incidence of AKI due to more detection but hopefully have better outcomes due to more systematic treatment. In HICs, much of AKI is hospital acquired with up to 20% of adults developing AKI when hospitalised for an acute illness in part related to surgery, contrast studies and the use of nephrotoxic drugs. In resource-rich regions, older patients with more medical comorbidities may be considered for more adventurous medical interventions that might not be considered or available in LICs. This group constitutes an inherently "at-risk" population being exposed to often multiple risk factors for AKI in the hospital setting.

8.8 Risk Factors for AKI

For both the community and hospital setting, there are several features that predict a significantly increased risk of AKI. Given the substantial increased mortality associated with AKI, it is clearly important to have systems in place to identify who is at risk. The awareness, for example, among general medical and surgical teams that an elderly patient with cardiac impairment on an angiotensin-converting enzyme inhibitor (ACEI) undergoing surgery is at significant risk of AKI is an important first step in prevention of this serious complication.

As alluded to in the introduction, underlying chronic kidney disease is one of the strongest risk factors for AKI. It is not really surprising that reduced nephron mass and by definition reduced renal reserve have an increased risk of AKI. Even among patients with a relatively well-preserved GFR of 45–49 ml/min per 1.73 m^2, there is on average a twofold increase in AKI compared with subjects with estimated GFR of 60 ml per min per 1.73 m^2 [11]. This risk is further increased by the presence of diabetes or proteinuria [12]. Thereafter, risk factors tend to relate to reduced effective renal arterial perfusion, impaired drainage or direct damage to the remaining nephrons whether that be from intrinsic disease or exposure to external toxins (see below).

The common risk factors for AKI are listed in ▶ Box 8.1. Many of these can occur in the same patient particularly if elderly or frail or with other significant medical conditions.

Box 8.1 Predisposing Risk factors for AKI

1. Pre-existing CKD (especially diabetes, myeloma) and proteinuria.
2. Old age (reduced GFR, reduced renal reserve, comorbidity).
3. Reduced intravascular volume (reduced renal perfusion).
   (a) hypovolaemia (impaired oral intake, haemorrhage, GI losses, renal losses, skin losses),
   (b) reduced effective arterial blood volume (cirrhosis, nephrotic syndrome, third-spacing e.g. pancreatitis, complex fractures, acute lung injury, peritonitis),
4. Impaired cardiac output (reduced renal perfusion).
5. Sepsis (reduced renal perfusion).
6. Prolonged surgery (any, but especially if involving cross clamping of the aorta or renal arteries).
7. Jaundice.
8. Exposure to toxins.
   (a) Endogenous.
   (b) Exogenous.

8.9 Pathophysiology

The kidneys are perhaps uniquely predisposed to injury for four principle reasons. Firstly, in health, kidneys command a huge blood supply in order to achieve filtration requirements. To illustrate this, adult kidneys weigh roughly 0.5% of the total body weight and yet receive 20–25% of the cardiac output (proportionally 3 times greater than that to the heart).

Moreover, the high energy requirements of the tubules (especially the proximal tubule) required for the reabsorption of 98% of the 180 L glomerular filtration per day mean the kidney is second only to the heart in terms of major organ oxygen requirement.

Furthermore, perfusion within the kidney is not evenly distributed with a much larger proportion going to the cortex than the outer medulla. The low medullary perfusion combined with high oxygen consumption in the thick ascending limb results in health of O_2 partial pressures around 10–20 mmHg compared to 50 mmHg in the cortex.

So, although the kidney is remarkably able to maintain renal perfusion and GFR, it is perhaps not surprising that it is vulnerable to injury from ischaemia in the face of reduced perfusion and that renal tubules are specifically more susceptible to perturbations in blood supply or oxygenation.

Finally, the kidneys have unparalleled exposure to endogenous and exogenous toxins in terms of relative perfusion and the secretion, reabsorption and concentration that occurs in the renal tubules. In short, despite important regulatory mechanisms, it is not at all surprising that renal tubular injury is common in the setting of reduced renal perfusion/oxygenation such as in sepsis or cardiac failure and/or when exposed to toxins.

8.10 Morphology

Severe renal hypoperfusion associated with septic abortion, envenomation and severe sepsis or hypotension may result in acute tubular necrosis or cortical necrosis. But it is important to note that most AKI does not result in necrosis (tubular or cortical). In fact, a striking feature of most acute tubular injury (ATI) is how disproportionate the functional impairment maybe compared to the minimal histological changes. Typically, the most common findings are mitochondrial enlargement, loss of PCT brush border with flattening of the distal and

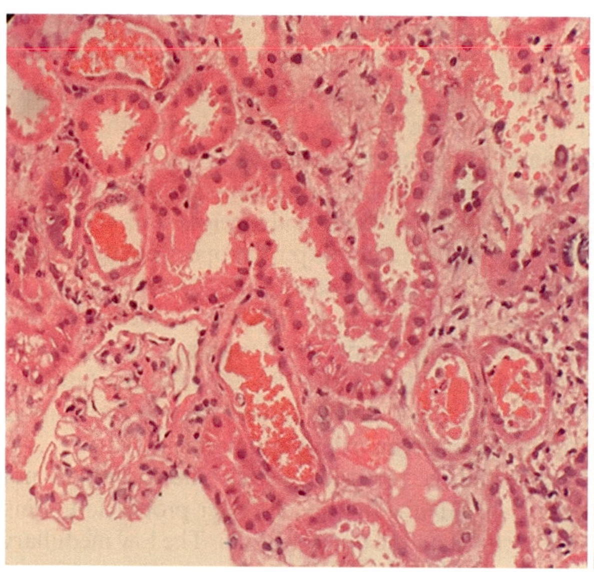

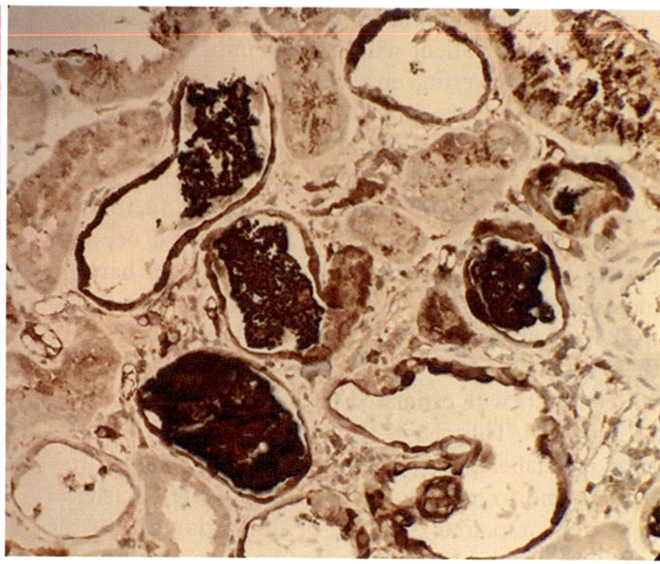

8

Fig. 8.3 (Left) H&E stain of a patient with AKI in the setting of rhabdomyolysis. Biopsy shows marked blebbing of the tubular cells, flattened tubular cells and myoglobin casts, demonstrated clearly in right image stained for myoglobin. Slides courtesy of Lauren Heptinstall

proximal tubular cells with consequent dilatation of the tubules (Swiss cheese appearance) (see Fig. 8.3) and desquamation of epithelial cells. Tubular cells may demonstrate mitosis if recovering or apoptosis with tubular necrosis only in severe injury. There may be cellular casts if the cause is a rapidly progressive glomerulonephritis; granular casts composed of exfoliated tubular cells if the injury is predominantly tubular; pigment casts if myoglobin, haemoglobin or light chain casts present; and crystals if, for example, oxalate is the principle cause. Vacuolisation of the proximal tubular cells if the patient has been exposed to osmotic stress such as mannitol, hyperosmolar contrast, hydroxyethyl starch colloids, sugars and dextrans, for example, with IgG treatment. In addition, there may be interstitial oedema and cellular infiltration with inflammatory cells depending on the aetiology of the AKI. Somewhat surprisingly, there is not yet a morphological score to quantify AKI, and predicting recovery remains very subjective.

8.11 Functional

There are two principal components that contribute to the acute decrease in GFR in AKI, a "vascular" component and a "tubular" component which are intimately connected. Ischaemic injury to the kidney is the most common cause of AKI, but it must be remembered that contributory factors include not only diminished renal blood flow leading to reduced oxygen and substrate delivery but also a relative increase in oxygen demand by the tubular cells. In all forms of AKI, including non-ischaemic, nephrotoxic injury, there is an early and significant reduction in renal blood flow. In health, reduced renal perfusion and GFR result in reduced sodium delivery to the macular densa. This results in afferent renal artery vasodilatation via adenosine and efferent artery vasoconstriction via renin, both of which serve to maintain/increase GFR in a process known as tubular glomerular feedback (Fig. 8.4). However, acute ischaemia is associated with a loss of renal autoregulation, endothelial dysfunction and vasoconstriction rather than the usual autoregulatory renal vasodilatation that occurs in response to decreased renal perfusion. Moreover, outer cortical blood flow is disproportionally reduced, and outer medullary congestion is another prominent feature that may worsen the relative hypoxia in the outer medulla and thus potentiate hypoxic injury (Fig. 8.5).

Pressure in the proximal tubulars increases rapidly partly due to the accumulation of luminal debris or casts. As this pressure increases, the ability of glomeruli to produce filtrate reduces further, and there is trans-tubular back leak of filtrate (see Fig. 8.6) leading to interstitial inflammation. The latter occurs via the production of chemo-attractants by injured epithelial cells that recruit inflammatory cells and potentiate further inflammation [13].

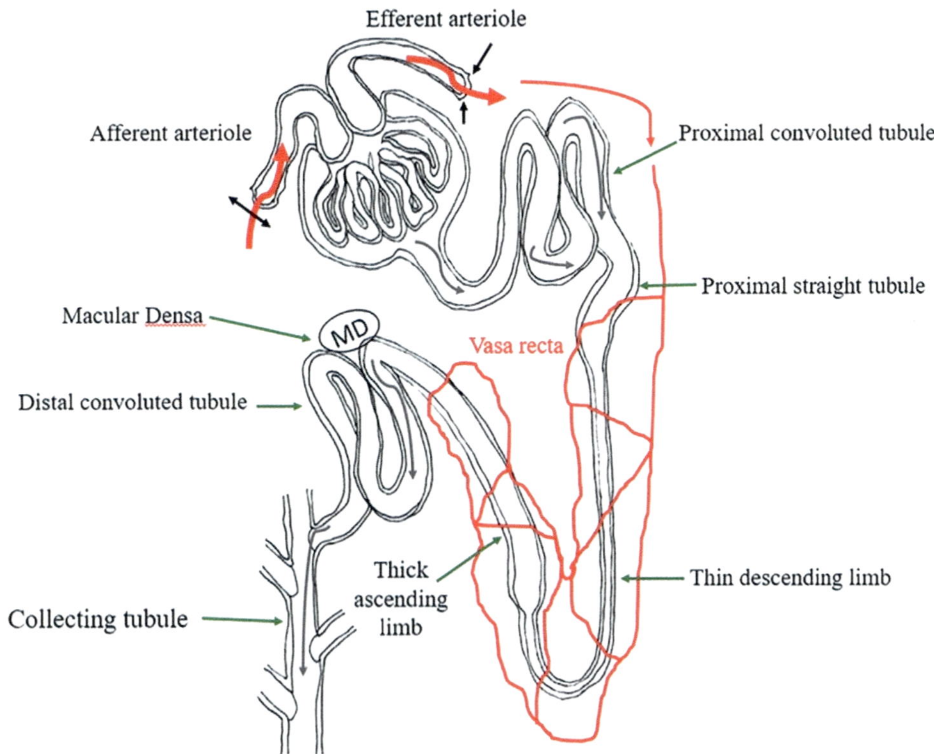

Fig. 8.4 Diagram of the nephron in health. The macular densa (MD) which is situated next to the afferent and efferent arterioles forms part of the juxtaglomerular apparatus (JGA). The JGA also includes the terminal portion of the afferent arteriole with its renin-producing cells and the beginning of the efferent arteriole. In response to reduced sodium concentration in the thick ascending limb of Henle following reduced renal perfusion, the macular densa (MD), which is situated next to the vascular pedicle of the glomerulus and forms part of the causes afferent arteriole dilatation (probably via adenosine and in part mediated through prostaglandins blocked by NSAIDs). Low sodium chloride delivery to the MD also results in release of renin which causes general arteriolar (but especially efferent arteriole) constriction (blocked by RAS inhibition). Vasodilatation of the afferent and vasoconstriction of the efferent arterioles helps maintain glomerular vascular perfusion and GFR

Injury to the PCT cells results in failure to dilute the filtrate by sodium reabsorption. This leads to delivery of higher than normal concentrations of sodium to the DCT, which is sensed by the macular densa and results in a physiological negative feedback loop (tubulo-glomerular feedback (TGF)). The macular densa (situated between the afferent and efferent arterioles of the same nephron) generates adenosine that results in constriction of the afferent arteriole via the A_1 receptor and results in reduction in glomerular filtration. Vasoconstriction and shutting down of the glomeruli in the setting of ischaemia or toxic injury may seem to compound the damage. However, given that the kidney is the funnel for many toxins and that the reabsorption of about 178 L of filtrate a day is dependent on healthy oxygen and energy replete tubules, autoregulated shutdown of glomeruli and temporary oliguria may be an adaptive response to protect the kidney and individual against further deleterious effects of AKI.

8.12 Key Causes of AKI

With an understanding of the pathogenesis of AKI, it is not difficult to appreciate the key reasons a kidney may suffer AKI. The causes of AKI can be grouped into those that lead to decreased renal blood flow (pre-renal acute kidney injury, 40–70% of patients), those that lead to direct renal parenchymal damage (intrinsic acute kidney injury, 10–50% of patients) and those that lead to obstructed flow of urine (post-renal acute kidney injury, 10% of patients). Although not to be missed, AKI secondary to rapidly progressive glomerulonephritis is relatively rare. Very frequently there will be mul-

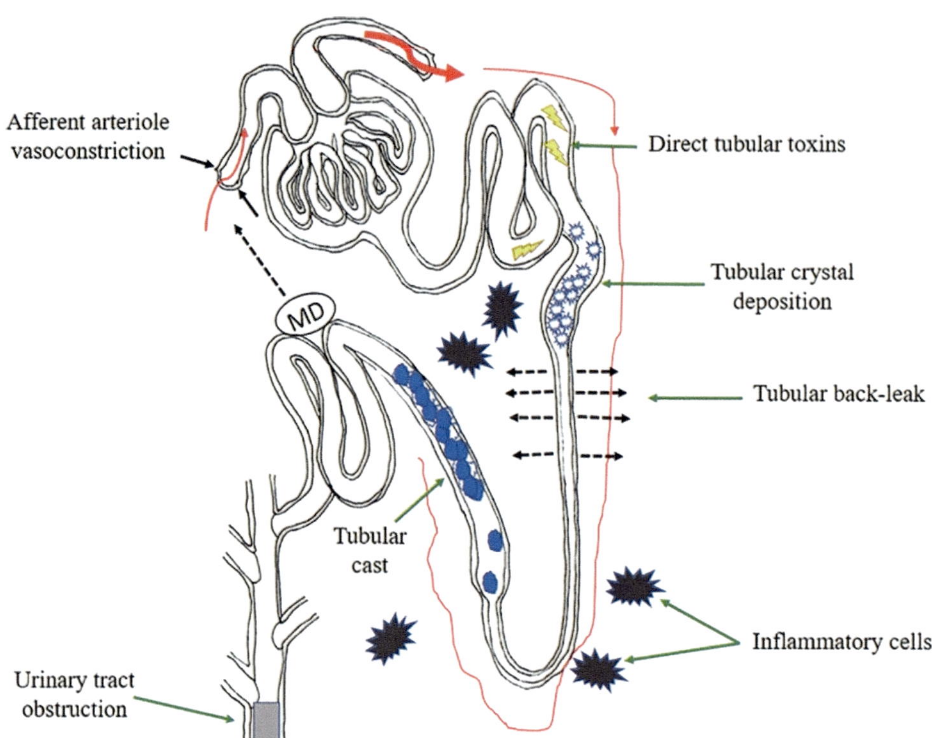

8

Fig. 8.5 Diagram showing pathogenesis of acute tubular injury. In AKI tubular dysfunction from whatever cause may result in increased delivery of sodium chloride to the MD and negative (tubuloglomerular) feedback to the afferent arteriole causing vasoconstriction reducing glomerular perfusion and GFR. Generalised vasoconstriction from sympathetic activity and renin secondary to hypotension further contributes to reduced (especially cortical tubular) blood supply. Filtration of toxins exposes all of the tubule to endogenous or exogenous toxins. Crystals may form in any part of the tubule causing obstruction and inflammation. Similarly tubular casts (most commonly casts from shed tubule-epithelial cells but also red cell casts from glomerulonephritis, pigment casts, myeloma cast, white cell casts) can obstruct the tubules and cause back leak of tubular fluid. Urinary tract obstruction has a similar effect on tubular drainage. Many of these pathways result in activation and recruitment of inflammatory cells which may contribute to further damage

tiple components contributing to renal dysfunction, and rapid identification of the causes is critical (Fig. 8.7).

8.13 Pre-Renal Causes of Acute Kidney Injury

Pre-renal causes are the most common and include any condition that leads to under-perfusion (reduced effective arterial perfusion) of the kidney (see Table 8.3). They can be divided into:

1. Hypovolaemia.
2. Reduced cardiac output.
3. Redistribution of cardiac output (sepsis and hepatorenal syndrome).
4. Impairment of local vascular supply (aortic or renal artery compromise, impairment of renal microcirculation, venous thrombosis or abdominal compartment syndrome).

Renal blood flow and GFR remain roughly constant across a wide range of mean arterial pressures due to changes in pre- and post-glomerular arteriolar resistance. This renal auto-regulation mainly depends on a combination of pre-glomerular arteriolar vasodilatation, mediated by prostaglandins and nitric oxide, and post-glomerular arteriolar vasoconstriction, mediated by angiotensin II. Drugs that interfere with these mediators may provoke pre-renal acute kidney injury. In particular clinical settings, most notably NSAIDs block the normal adaptive response to hypoperfusion mediated by prostaglandins, and RAS inhibition thwarts the second compensatory mechanism to maintain GFR-efferent artery vasoconstriction. This explains why NSAIDs and RAS inhibition can be so problematic in the setting of CKD and acute hypoperfusion such as shock or hepatorenal syndrome.

At-risk populations include older people with atherosclerotic cardiovascular disease, those with pre-existing CKD and those with chronic renal hypoperfusion (e.g. cardiac failure, hepatorenal syndrome, recurrent high fluid losses (usually gastrointestinal or renal)). In critical care units, the most common cause of AKI is sepsis causing systemic vasodilatation and reduced effective renal blood flow despite an increased cardiac output. In tropical and developing countries pre-renal AKI com-

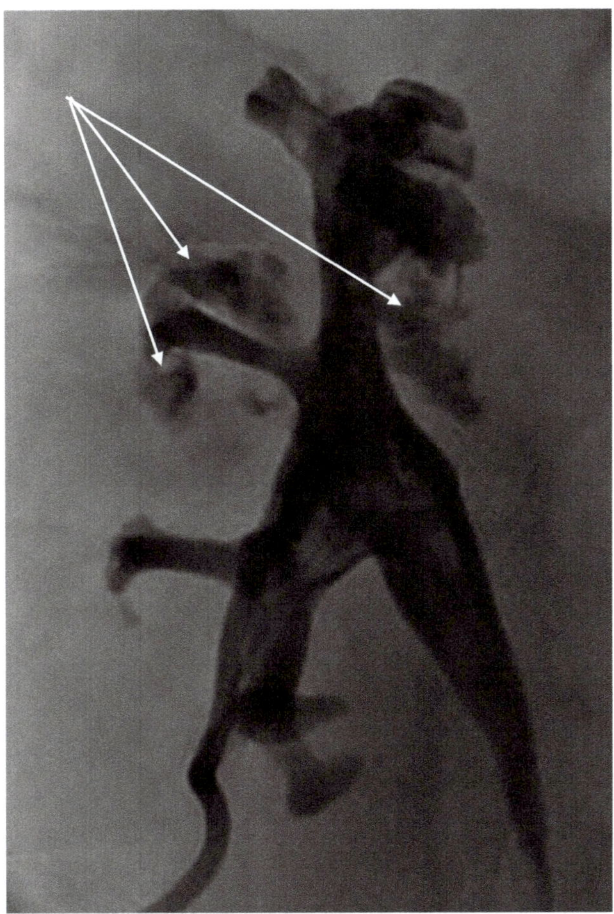

Fig. 8.6 Nephrostogram of a kidney obstructed with clot. Pressure during antegrade study resulting in reverse flow into the collecting tubules and possibly back leak of contrast into the interstitium as a result of back pressure. This gross example illustrates the potential for back leak in the setting of obstruction and increased pressure at a macro level that might be mimicked at a microscopic level with tubular obstruction

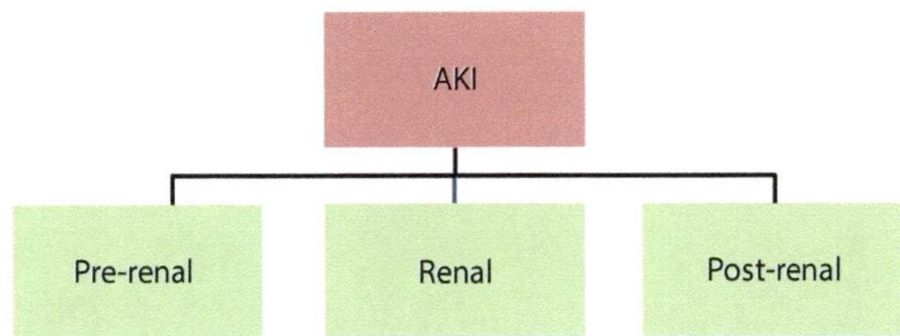

Fig. 8.7 Basic classification of causes of acute kidney injury

monly occurs secondary to dehydration due to diarrhoeal diseases or shock secondary to trauma, affecting a relatively younger population, often children. Much less frequent is local reduction of blood flow in the absence of reduced cardiac output or hypovolaemia, such as embolisation or aortic dissection. Impairment of the microcirculation can occur in the setting of haemolytic uraemic syndrome, vasculitis or other glomerular thrombotic disorders. Finally, although relatively uncommon but under-recognised, abdominal compartment syndrome can have a profound effect on arterial and venous perfusion of the kidney as well as causing functional obstruction (Fig. 8.8).

Table 8.3 Main causes of pre-renal AKI

Causes	Examples
Hypovolaemia	Severe bleeding Volume depletion, for example, gastrointestinal fluid losses, burns, polyuria (post-obstructive, over-diuresis, salt-wasting nephropathy, hyperglycaemia, diabetes insipidus)
Reduced cardiac output	Reduced cardiac output (cardiogenic shock or chronic cardiac failure)
Redistribution of cardiac output	Sepsis Liver cirrhosis Distributive shock ("third spacing"), for example sepsis, anaphylaxis, severe pancreatitis Hypotension secondary to hypotensive medication Nephrotic syndrome
Reduced renal blood flow Increased abdominal pressure	Drugs: Non-steroidal anti-inflammatory drugs (NSAIDs) Selective cyclo-oxygenase 2 inhibitors Angiotensin-converting enzyme (ACE) inhibitors Angiotensin II receptor antagonists Renal artery stenosis, aortic or renal cross clamping, occlusion/dissection (see Fig. 8.8) or embolisation Hepatorenal syndrome Thrombotic microangiopathies, haemolytic uraemic syndrome, acute sickle crisis, vasculitis Abdominal compartment syndrome (reduced perfusion and drainage)

8.14 Intrinsic Acute Kidney Injury

Intrinsic acute kidney injury may be caused by conditions affecting the glomeruli, renal tubules, interstitium or microvasculature. The most important causes are listed in Table 8.4. The majority of "renal" causes of AKI relate to acute tubular injury secondary to ischaemia and toxins. Rapidly progressive glomerulonephritis and interstitial nephritis represent only a small percentage of AKI in HICs. These are covered in detail elsewhere in this book but while relatively uncommon remain an important cause of AKI not to miss.

8

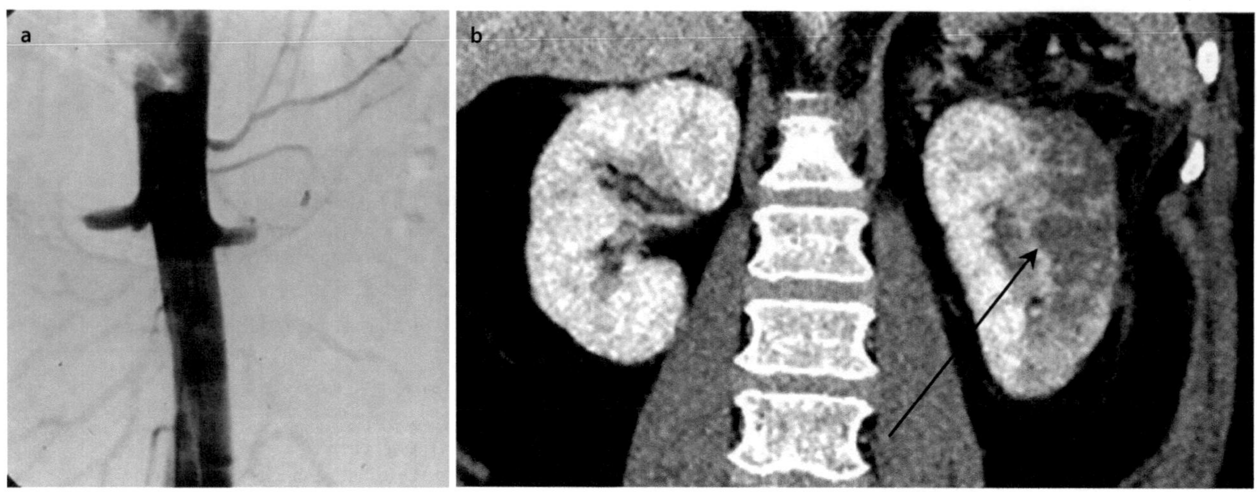

Fig. 8.8 **a** Aortogram of patient who attempted suicide by jumping from a bridge and developed immediate anuric AKI. The study shows abrupt lack of perfusion to both kidneys secondary to dissection of the renal arteries. **b** CT with contrast of kidneys in a patient with atrial fibrillation and sudden onset of loin pain following an embolus to the left kidney and mild AKI. The arrow shows an area or markedly reduced perfusion and localised swelling

Table 8.4 Main causes of intrinsic AKI

Causes	Examples
Glomerular disease	
a. Inflammatory	Post-infectious glomerulonephritis Henoch-Schönlein purpura Systemic lupus erythematosus Antineutrophil cytoplasmic antibody glomerulonephritis Antiglomerular basement membrane disease Cryoglobulinaemic vasculitis
b. Occlusive	Disseminated intravascular coagulopathy Thrombotic microangiopathy, haemolytic uraemic syndrome Malignant hypertension Cholesterol embolism Plasmodium malaria Sickle cell crisis
Tubular injury	Ischaemia secondary to prolonged renal hypoperfusion Toxins: Exogenous Drugs (i) Direct tubulotoxins, e.g. aminoglycosides, amphotericin (ii) crystals (e.g. acyclovir, indinavir, sulphonamides) (iii) vasoconstrictors (e.g. cocaine) Radio contrast Natural toxins (e.g. envenomation, toxic plants, fungi) Heavy metals Crystals, oxalate (e.g. ethylene glycol, star fruit) Endogenous Pigments, myoglobin and haemoglobin Immunoglobulin light chains Hypercalcemia Crystals, urate (e.g. tumour lysis syndrome) and oxalate
Interstitial nephritis	1. Allergic: Drug-induced, e.g. NSAIDs and antibiotics, allopurinol, proton-pump inhibitors 2. Autoimmune: e.g. sarcoidosis, Sjogren's syndrome, tubule-interstitial nephritis with uveitis (TINU), SLE, vasculitis 3. Infectious: Pyelonephritis, leptospirosis, hantavirus, etc. 4. Infiltrative: Lymphoma, etc

8.15 Toxins and AKI

As the organs responsible for elimination of waste products, the kidneys are highly vulnerable to the effects of both endogenous and exogenous toxins.

Endogenous toxins include the haem pigments; myoglobin and haemoglobin, light chains, urate, calcium and oxalate all produced within the body by disease and with direct tubular toxicity. There are undoubtedly other less well-defined exogenous toxins particularly in the setting of systemic illnesses including adverse effects of cytokines in the setting of malignancies such as lymphoma.

8.16 Rhabdomyolysis

Rhabdomyolysis deserves special mention as a cause of AKI induced by an endogenous toxin. It was first described in the victims of crush injury during the 1940–1941 World War II bombing raids in London, and its complications remain significant problems for those injured in disasters such as earthquakes and bombings but also for individuals after excessive activity, muscle compression and following envenomation or drugs.

Rhabdomyolysis is characterised by the leakage of muscle cell contents, including electrolytes, myoglobin, creatine kinase and other proteins, into the circulation. High circulating plasma myoglobin levels (lasting for only 1–6 hours) can cause acute tubular injury and AKI. The cause of rhabdomyolysis is often self-apparent (◘ Fig. 8.10), but if not it may occasionally be due to an inherited muscle enzyme deficit [14]. AKI complicates up to 50% of cases of severe rhabdomyolysis and substantially worsens the prognosis [15]. Rhabdomyolysis is a relatively common cause of AKI, accounting for, or contributing to, 8–15% of cases in the United States [16]. The classic presentation is with myalgia, limb weakness, pigmenturia due to myoglobinuria (very transient) with positive dipstick for blood but without haematuria on microscopy and a markedly raised creatine kinase (CK) (in tens or hundreds of thousands, starting 2–12 hours post insult and peaking between 1 and 3 days). Serum potassium is usually raised (in the presence of renal impairment often dangerously so), and phosphate levels are disproportionately high for the degree of renal impairment and calcium levels low (in part due to sequestration by damaged muscle).

Occasionally patients will present with AKI several days after the event with an unremarkable CK level: (1) subsequent hypercalcaemia, (2) calcification in the affected muscles on x-ray or (3) a bone scan showing uptake in the muscles may make the diagnosis (◘ Fig. 8.9).

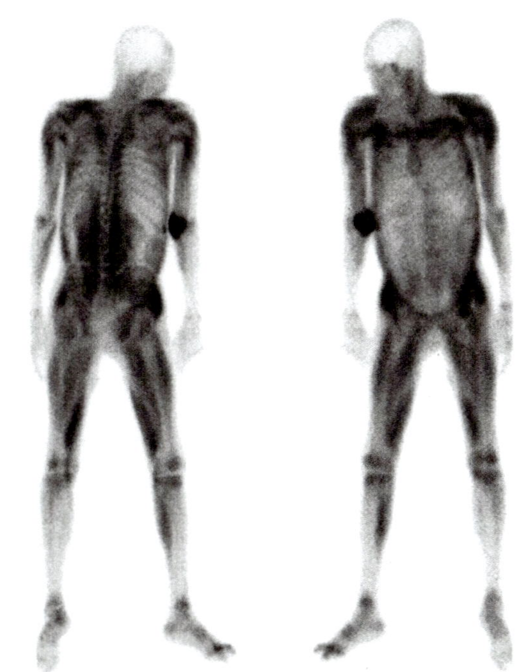

◘ **Fig. 8.9** Rhabdomyolysis visualised with a Tc99-labelled diphosphonate bone scan. Posterior (left) and anterior (right) views. (Reproduced with permission from reference 17)

8.17 Intravascular Haemolysis

In the setting of mild intravascular haemolysis, free haemoglobin is bound to haptoglobin (without consequences to the kidney). In massive intravascular haemolysis, the binding of haptoglobin is exceeded, and free haemoglobin disassociates into αβ dimers which are small enough to be filtered causing cast nephropathy and direct toxicity. Therefore, it only tends to be causes of large sudden intravascular haemolysis that results in AKI (▶ Box 8.2). Intravascular haemolysis can either be from:

(i) An intrinsic cause such as paroxysmal nocturnal haemoglobinuria with spontaneous haemolysis.
(ii) Secondary to an external artificial cause such as mismatched transfusion or drug-induced G6PD deficiency haemolysis.
(iii) Secondary to infections such as malaria.

Transfusion reactions should be very rare, but haemoglobinuria may occur in the face of massive transfusion for other reasons. Haemoglobin in the urine can form obstructive casts in the tubules, with (as in rhabdomyolysis) urine dipsticks strongly positive for blood but in the absence of red cells on microscopy. It may also be a contributing factor in any microangiopathic haemolytic anaemia such as haemolytic uraemic syndrome (HUS) or thrombotic thrombocytopenia purpura (TTP) where

Hyperthermia or hypothermia
Metabolic

Medical causes:
- Hypokalaemia
- Hypophosphataemia
- Hyponatraemia
- Hypothyroidism
- Diabetic ketoacidosis
- Hyperosmolar non-ketotic diabetic coma

Infectious
- Viral (Influenza, adenovirus, echovirus, HIV, EBV, Coxsackie, enterovirus)
- Bacterial (staphylococcus aureus, streptococcus pneumoniae, salmonella) all can cause direct bacterial myositis (typhoid, shigella, e.coli, leptospirosis, legionella, chlostridium perfringes)

Drugs

Direct Injury or hypoxia:

Direct trauma, crush injury, burns, frost-bite, electrocution
Ischaemia secondary to immobility-falls, coma (medical or drug induced), prolonged surgery
Ischaemia secondary to acute vascular insufficiency or compartment syndrome

Excessive muscle activity:

Grand mal fit, status epilepticus, acute psychosis, prolonged myoclonus, dystonia, status asthmaticus

Excessive exercise e.g. marathon running, military training of new recruits

NB Clinically relevant rhabdomyolysis secondary to excessive exercise usually only occurs in the presence of dehydration (or heat stroke) unless underlying medical predisposition

Muscle enzyme defects

Deficiency of glycol(geno)lytic enzymes
- Myophosphorylase deficiency (McArdle's)
- Phosphorylase kinase deficiency
- Phosphorylase mutase deficiency
- Lactate dehydrogenase deficiency

Abnormal lipid
- Carnitine palmitoyltransferase deficiency
- Carnitine deficiency

Miscellaneous
- Neuroleptic malignant syndrome
- Malignant hyperthermia
- Myoadenylate deamine deficiency
- Idiopathic rhabdomyolysis

Rare causes, usually presenting before the age 20. Look out for history of:
- exercise intolerance
- cramps
- intermittent dark urine
- family history (most autosomal recessive)

More than one episode of rhabdomyolysis with minor exercise or no obvious precipitant

If suspicious refer for muscle biopsy

Hypokalaemia, hypophosphataemia and hyponatraemia important predisposing risk factors

Check autoimmune screen including Anti-JO-1

Risk of lipid lowering myositis increased with dual fibrate/statin therapy, dose, concomitant renal or liver disease, hypothyroidism.
Also inhibitors of cytochrome p450 macrolide antibiotics, warfarin, cyclosporine, azoles, digoxin. (Fluvastatin, pravastatin and atorvastatin are metabolised independently of cytochrome p450 and therefore lower risk)

Fig. 8.10 Causes of rhabdomyolysis

the greatest injury relates to microvascular injury, but filtered haemoglobin, exceeding the capacity of circulating haptoglobin, may contribute to the AKI.

Box 8.2 Causes of Intravascular Haemolysis Causing AKI

- Autoimmune haemolytic anaemia – cold type.
- G6PD deficiency.
- Paroxysmal nocturnal haemoglobinuria.
- Reticuloendothelial hyper-reactivity (massive splenomegaly or haemophagocytic syndrome).
- Malaria.
- Transfusion reaction.
- March haemoglobinuria.
- Envenomation (snake bite).
- Burns.
- Drugs: quinine, quinidine, penicillins, methyldopa, clopidogrel, dapsone, ticlopidine.
- Toxins: copper and lead.
- Microangiopathic haemolytic anaemias: HUS, TTP.

8.18 Hyperuricaemia

Hyperuricaemia appears to be a risk factor for AKI in its own right but may in part be as a surrogate for hypovolaemia or CKD. However, it is clearly implicated in tumour lysis syndrome (TLS) which deserves special mention as an oncological emergency. It is most often seen in patients with bulky, rapidly proliferating and treatment-responsive lymphoproliferative malignancies (e.g. acute leukaemias and high-grade non-Hodgkin lymphomas such as Burkitt lymphoma) after chemotherapy, radiation or corticosteroids. TLS may occur spontaneously in the absence of any treatment but is rare in patients with solid tumours. It is particularly important to identify those at risk, especially so in those with pre-existing renal impairment, and monitor their potassium and renal function closely. Risk factors for and clinical markers of TLS are shown in ▶ Box 8.3 and reviewed in reference [18].

Box 8.3 Risk Factors and Clinical Features of Tumour Lysis Syndrome

Risk factors for tumour lysis syndrome

1. High tumour burden (bulky tumour or extensive metastases).
2. High cell lysis potential (rapidly proliferating tumour – LDH is a surrogate marker for this; high cancer cell sensitivity to therapy; intensity of therapy).
3. Pre-existing patient factors (older age; renal impairment; dehydration; acidic urine; hypotension; nephrotoxic drugs).
4. Inadequate supportive care (inadequate hydration; lack of allopurinol or rasburicase prophylaxis).

Clinical markers of tumour lysis syndrome

1. Hyperuricaemia (uric acid >0.4 mmol/L).
2. Hyperphosphataemia (serum phosphate >1.5 mmol/L in adults; >2.1 mmol/L in children).
3. Rapid (sometimes life-threatening) rise in potassium (serum potassium >6.0 mmol/L).
4. Hypocalcaemia (corrected calcium <1.75 mmol/L; ionised calcium <0.3 mmol/L).
5. Raised lactate dehydrogenase.
6. Acute kidney injury.

8.19 Light Chain and Immunoglobulin-Related Disease

Monoclonal gammopathies are an important cause of AKI and can cause intrinsic renal dysfunction in a variety of ways (see ▶ Chaps. 49 and 50) as well as pre-renal secondary to hypercalcaemia, sepsis, immunoglobulin hyperviscosity and hyperuricaemia and post-renal from obstruction. Direct renal involvement may occur with crystal nephropathy, direct PCT toxicity, glomerular disease (amyloid, light chain deposition disease and cast nephropathy (see ◘ Fig. 8.11). Renal impairment at presentation is common, frequently being a combination of CKD and AKI, the latter being a medical emergency.

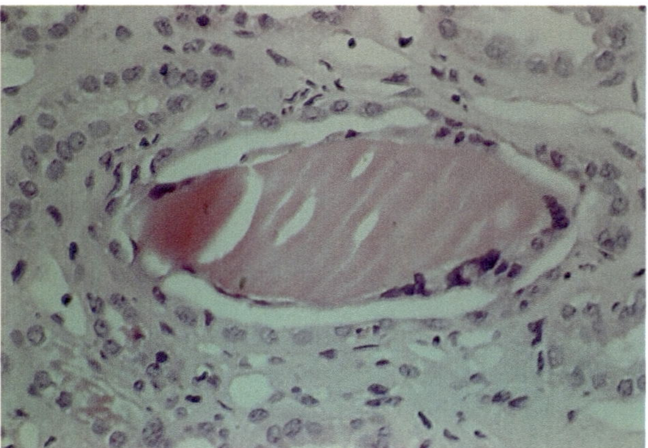

◘ **Fig. 8.11** Pathognomonic myeloma cast demonstrating fracture lines, causing tubular obstruction and an early cellular response

8.20 Hypercalcaemia

Hypercalcaemia from any cause can result in direct tubular injury in part due to vasoconstriction and tubular injury particularly in the medulla with exfoliation of tubular cells and deposition of calcium crystals (nephrocalcinosis). Calcium-induced polyuria may compound the pre-renal element. Hypercalcaemia causing AKI is most frequent in the setting of malignancy and hyperparathyroidism, sarcoidosis and supplementation.

8.21 Oxalosis

Finally, while oxalate nephropathy can occur chronically in the setting of primary hyperoxalosis and from exogenous consumption of toxins (see below), it can also occur secondary to enteric hyperoxalosis particularly in the setting of pancreatic insufficiency or chronic short bowel malabsorption but only in the setting of an intact colon.

8.22 Exogenous Toxins

Exogenous toxins are an important but often under-recognised cause of AKI. These included both natural and artificial toxins. The toxic renal effects may be mediated by a variety of mechanisms including proximal tubular cell damage due to extensive uptake or due to tubular crystal formation as a result of supersaturation of urine.

8.23 Contrast-Associated AKI

Contrast-induced AKI is increasingly referred to as contrast-associated AKI (CAAKI) to reflect there may be a variety of processes contributing to AKI in this setting. It has been considered to be an important complication of the use of iodinated contrast media and is the third commonest cause of hospital-acquired AKI [19], with a reported incidence of 1–2%, typically within 72 hours of receiving contrast media, usually recovering over the following 5 days [20]. However, the threat posed by modern low osmolality and iso-osmolar agents has been significantly challenged in recent years. One meta-analysis including nearly 26,000 patients found no difference in AKI rates (c.6%) for those who had scans with or without contrast and a rate of AKI severe enough to require renal replacement of only 0.3% [21]. Nonetheless, it does appear that large quantities of contrast (>350mls or > 4mls/kg or doses repeated within 73 hours) have the potential to cause or compound AKI and, rarely, individual patients seem to be hypersensitive to contrast, developing AKI with contrast when not apparently at high risk.

Patients at risk include those with:

1. Pre-existing renal impairment (this is the single biggest risk factor).
2. Older age > 75 years.
3. Diabetes mellitus.
4. Volume depletion.
5. Haemodynamic instability.
6. Sepsis.
7. Cardiac failure.
8. Concurrent nephrotoxic medications.
9. Multiple doses of contrast.
10. Large volumes of contrast.
11. Hyperosmolar contrast.

These risk factors have an additive effect and justify the term contrast-*associated* AKI [22]. The pathogenesis is not entirely clear but relates in part to renal microvascular vasoconstriction and direct toxicity to the tubules, particularly in the setting of hyperosmolar agents. Unsurprisingly, pre-existing CKD with a low GFR results in a much higher, per-nephron exposure to the contrast and explains why these patients may be more vulnerable beyond simply having a low GFR.

8.24 Nephrotoxic Drugs

Administration of nephrotoxic drugs has a much stronger association with AKI and has been implicated as a causative factor in up to 25% of all cases of severe AKI in critically ill patients [23]. Retrospective cohort studies of AKI have documented the frequency of drug-induced nephrotoxicity to be approximately 14–26% in adult populations [24, 25]. Nephrotoxicity is a significant concern in paediatrics with 16% of hospitalised AKI events being attributable primarily to a drug.

Although most cases of drug-induced AKI are secondary to tubular toxicity, dugs can damage the kidney in a multitude of ways including microvascular dysfunction, causing acute tubular injury, intrarenal obstruction, interstitial nephritis, nephrotic syndrome and acid-base and fluid electrolytes disorders and occasionally provoke acute glomerulonephritis, the latter increasing with the use of novel chemo- and immunotherapeutics. Given that prescribed medication is ubiquitous among the sick, drug toxicity often compounds other forms of AKI. Some toxicities are predictable and others, particularly allergic responses such as tubule-interstitial nephritis, much less so. The drugs below are worth special mention because of the frequency and predictability of renal injury (◘ Table 8.5).

Table 8.5 Common nephrotoxins

Drug	Comments
Aminoglycosides	Incidence 10–20% Toxic to PCT ATN. Risk factors: High peak serum levels Cumulative dose Frequency and duration of administration Concomitant nephrotoxins 5% of filtered aminoglycoside is actively reabsorbed by the proximal tubule where it is concentrated and causes cellular injury and ATN. As proximal tubular cell uptake of aminoglycosides is saturable, single large doses permit more of the drug to be excreted without undergoing tubular resorption, so reducing cell injury Numerous meta-analyses have shown similar clinical efficacy with once-daily aminoglycoside dosing, though none has shown a significant reduction in nephrotoxicity [26] Patients at increased risk of AKI may be vulnerable to even single doses, with significant consequences [27]
Amphotericin B	Occurs in up to 80% Causes distal tubular injury resulting in hypokalaemia, hypomagnesemia, metabolic acidosis and often polyuric AKI Risk factors: Cumulative dose Dehydration Concomitant nephrotoxins Randomised trials have shown that lipid-based formulations of amphotericin B are significantly less nephrotoxic [28, 29]
Foscarnet	Direct tubular toxicity. Can cause nephrogenic diabetes insipidus
Cidofovir	Predominantly proximal tubular injury
Tenofovir	Mitochondrial injury and proximal tubulopathy with phosphate wasting
Acyclovir	Crystal formation, resulting in tubular obstruction and local inflammation
Indinavir	Crystal formation, resulting in tubular obstruction and local inflammation
Methotrexate	Crystal cause crystal formation, resulting in tubular obstruction and local inflammation
Ciprofloxacin	Crystal formation, resulting in tubular obstruction and local inflammation
Triamterene	Crystal formation, resulting in tubular obstruction and local inflammation
Atazanavir	Crystal formation, resulting in tubular obstruction and local inflammation
Sulphonamides	Crystal formation, resulting in tubular obstruction and local inflammation
Ifosfamide	Cause mitochondrial injury in the PCT resulting in a Fanconi-like pattern with acidosis
Cisplatin	Proximal tubular injury, Fanconi-like syndrome, salt wasting, hypomagnesaemia
Polymyxins	Cause increased tubular permeability swelling and lysis
Calcineurin inhibitors	Afferent artery vasoconstriction through the inhibition of prostaglandin induced dilatation
IVIG	Sucrose carriers associated with intravenous immunoglobulins accumulate in the PCT and cause vacuolisation, cell swelling and injury. A similar pattern is seen with other osmotic agents such as mannitol
HES	Filtered and taken up by the PCT and accumulates within the lysosome causing cellular injury or death

8.25 Recreational Drugs

The rapid growth of illicit drug use is clearly a major public health problem. The kidneys can be injured in diverse ways primarily due to their high degree of filtration and metabolism by the kidneys to potentially toxic by-products and to whatever adulterants the dealer choses to add. Commonly used recreational drugs that cause nephrotoxicity include opiates, anabolic androgenic steroids, synthetic cannabinoids, methamphetamines (ecstasy), cocaine and its levamisole-adulterated counterpart. Other notable nephrotoxic drugs of abuse include toluene-induced renal tubular acidosis, and a more recently described syndrome of AKI seen with bath salts.

8.25.1 Opiates

Heroin (diacetylmorphine, diamorphine) is the most commonly abused drug in this group. There are several renal complications from its abuse. Coma from overdose or underestimated drug potency leads to pressure-induced muscle damage and rhabdomyolysis. There is a high rate of viral, bacterial and fungal contamination associated with intravenous drug misuse, including heroin, and consequently users are at risk of a variety of infections. Glomerulonephritis (GN) may be associated with these chronic infections. Secondary (AA) amyloidosis is seen in chronic parenteral drug users, particularly among those who inject drugs subcutaneously ("skin poppers"). In the 1970s and 1980s, heroin-associated nephropathy (HAN) was described, presenting as nephrotic syndrome and progressing rapidly to end-stage renal failure.

8.25.2 Cocaine and its Levamisole-Adulterated Counterparts

The nephrotoxic effects of cocaine are numerous and are thought to be related to changes in renal haemodynamics, glomerular matrix synthesis, degradation and oxidative stress and induction of renal atherogenesis. Cocaine can cause rhabdomyolysis, and this is probably the most common reason for AKI associated with cocaine use. Cocaine causes vascular smooth muscle constriction and inhibits reuptake of serotonin, norepinephrine and dopamine to promote hypertension and tachycardia. Severe and acute hyponatremia associated with cocaine exposure has been reported, possibly due to stimulation of AVP and subsequent development of a syndrome of inappropriate antidiuretic hormone secretion. Although rare, there are also case reports of cocaine-associated kidney infarction, presumably due to thrombotic or embolic disease, vasospasm, cardiogenic shock or other forms of occlusive large vessel disease, such as dissection, aneurysmal rupture, trauma or vasculitis.

Levamisole-adulterated cocaine use is known to be associated with ANCA-associated vasculitis. Serologically, almost all patients have anti-myeloperoxidase (MPO)-ANCA, and at least half of all patients also have anti-proteinase 3 (PR3)-ANCA. In fact, positivity for both MPO- and PR3-ANCA is now becoming pathognomonic for levamisole-adulterated cocaine exposure. In addition, antinuclear autoantibodies, lupus anticoagulant and low complement levels are detected in most patients.

8.25.3 Ecstasy and Other Amphetamines

Ecstasy is known to cause rhabdomyolysis and/or hyperpyrexia syndrome which can result in acute kidney injury. Drug abusers often drink large quantities of water after taking ecstasy to try to prevent dehydration, and dilutional hyponatraemia results as a consequence.

8.25.4 Anabolic Androgenic Steroids

Renal effects of AAS abuse in humans are primarily described in case reports and small case series. It is known to cause elevations in serum creatinine and substantial proteinuria. The mechanism of renal injury in the setting of AAS abuse is not well established and is likely multifactorial. Hyperfiltration injury is an important factor in the causation of renal damage.

8.25.5 Solvents

The nephrotoxic insult of volatile glues appears to be due principally to toluene. Various renal lesions have been associated with its abuse which include microhaematuria, pyuria and proteinuria, distal renal tubular acidosis and Fanconi's syndrome, urinary calculi, glomerulonephritis, Goodpasture's syndrome, acute tubular injury, hepatorenal syndrome and acute and chronic interstitial nephritis.

8.26 Ethylene Glycol Poisoning

Ethylene glycol (EG) is a sweet-tasting, odourless organic solvent found in many agents, such as anti-freeze, brake fluids and industrial solvents. EG is composed of four organic acids: glycoaldehyde, glycolic acid, glyoxylic acid and oxalic acid in vivo. EG poisoning can result in acute kidney injury (AKI), requiring haemodialysis to restore kidney function. The kidney toxicity of ethylene glycol occurs 24 to 72 hours post ingestion and is caused by a direct cytotoxic effect of glycolic acid. The glycolic acid is then metabolised to glyoxylic acid and finally to oxalic acid. Oxalic acid binds with calcium to form calcium oxalate crystals which may accumulate in the kidneys leading to oliguric or anuric renal failure.

8.27 Heavy Metal Toxicity

Heavy metals are extensively used in agriculture and industrial applications such as production of batteries, pesticides, alloys and textile dyes. Because of its ability to filter, reabsorb and concentrate divalent metals, the kidney is the first target organ of heavy metal toxicity. The most common metals implicated in kidney toxicity are arsenic, barium, cadmium, cobalt, copper, lead, lithium, mercury and platinum. The extent of kidney impairment depends on the nature, the dose and the time of exposure. Both acute and chronic intoxication have been linked to various renal manifestations which include severe renal failure leading occasionally to death, tubular dysfunctions like acquired Fanconi syndrome, tubule interstitial nephritis and chronic kidney disease.

8.28 Natural Toxins

There are a variety of natural toxins that are associated with AKI. These include animal venoms and poisons, mushroom and plant poisons and microbial toxins and tend to have strong geographical associations, being important causes of AKI in some countries.

8.29 Envenomation

Snake bites are a common and important cause of AKI in the tropics of Asia, Africa and Central and Latin America. The common snakes associated with AKI are the Viperidae, which includes the deathly Russell's viper (***Daboia russelii***, ***Daboia siamensis***), seen predominantly in southern and south-eastern Asia, and the ***Bothrops*** and ***Crotalus*** species (▫ Fig. 8.12) commonly seen in central and Southern America, and the sea snakes. In studies done in Asia, snakebites have accounted for 1.2% of total AKI in Thailand, 3% in India and as much as 70% in Myanmar [30]. The victims are predominantly men and agricultural workers.

Snake venom may cause AKI by diverse mechanisms such as acute tubular necrosis secondary to direct nephrotoxicity, profound ischaemia as a result of haemorrhagic shock and intravascular haemolysis or rhabdomyolysis, or thrombotic microangiopathy. In severe cases renal cortical necrosis may result in irrecoverable kidney damage and dialysis dependency.

Envenomation as a cause of AKI from other organisms is much less common but well recognised in defined geographical regions (see ▫ Fig. 8.13).

8.29.1 Plant and Fungal Toxins

Aristolochic acid nephropathy (AAN) was first described in a group of Belgian women who presented with rapidly progressive tubulointerstitial nephritis and

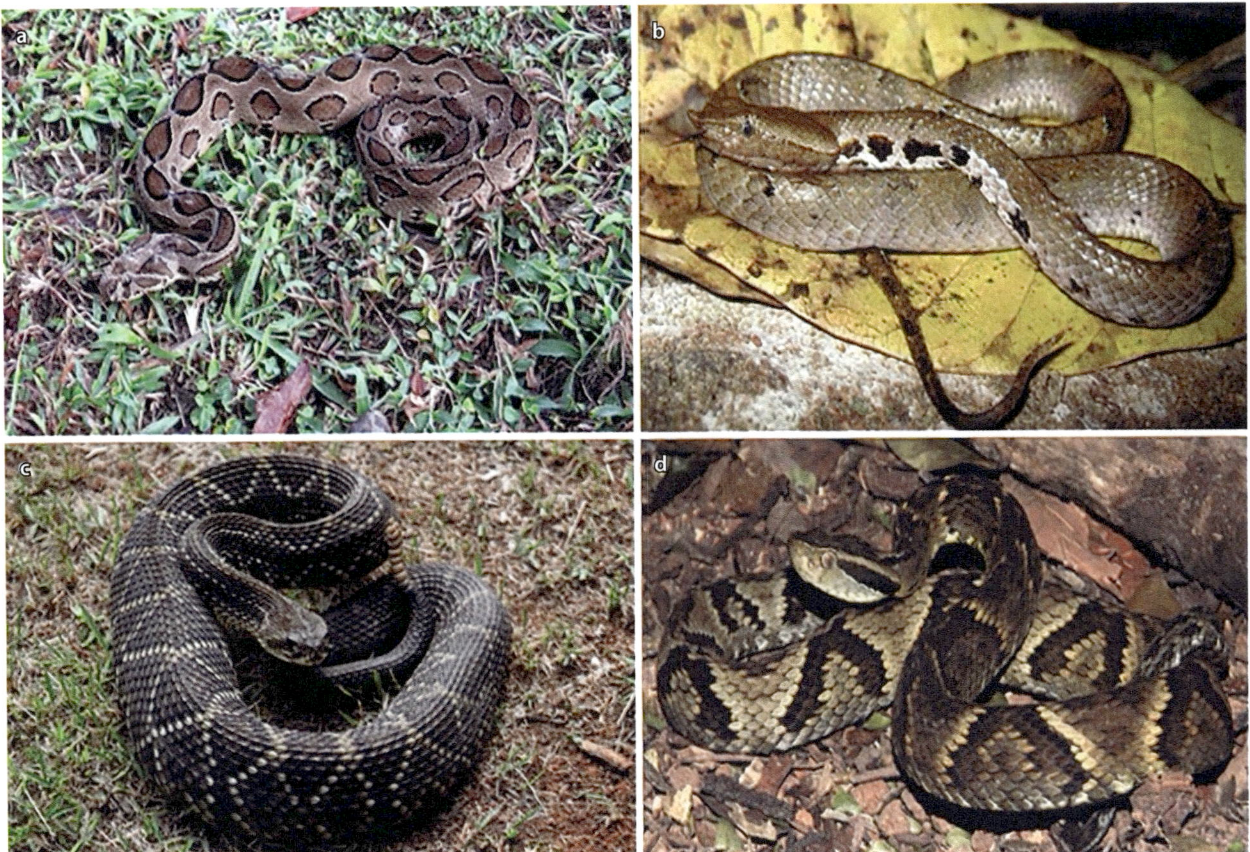

▫ **Fig. 8.12** Common snakes causing acute kidney injury across the world: **a** Russell's viper, **b** hump-nosed viper, **c** *Crotalus*, **d** *Bothrops*. (Source: (**a**,**b**) Anslem de Silva, Herpetologist, Sri Lanka (**c**,**d**) Marcelo Ribeiro Duarte, Assistant Research Biologist, Brazil)

8

Loxosceles spp. Spider
Causes dermonecrosis. Intravascular haemolysis or hypotension leads to AKI. Direct nephrotoxicity may contribute. Found in the Americas, West Indies, Africa 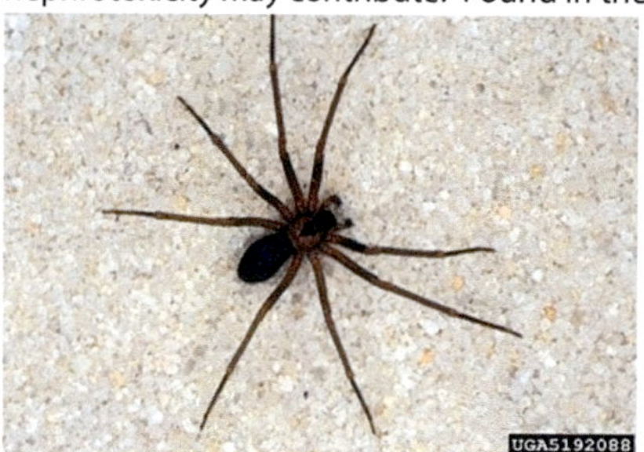 Permission from Florida Division of Plant Industr , Florida Department of Agriculture and Consumer Services, Bugwood.org
Scorpion (eg *Hemiscorpius, Tityus*)
AKI seen secondary to thrombotic microangiopathy, intravascular haemolysis and hypovolaemia. Also associated with acute pancreatitis. Found in the middle east 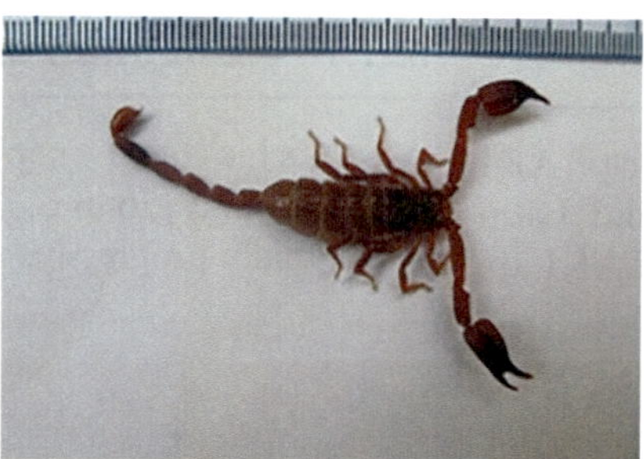 Permission from Mehran Shah, Assistant Professor, Department of Medical Entomology & Vector Control, School of Public Health, Infectious and Tropical Diseases Research Center, Hormozgan Health Institute, Hormozgan University of Medical Sciences, Bandar Abbas, Iran
Carp Gall bladder/ bile
AKI and acute hepatitis following consumption of raw carpgall baldder. Used as a traditional medicine in South East Asia. Toxicity may be due to nephrotoxicity of bile or pre-renal factors
Tussock moth *Lonomia*(caterpillar phase)
Causes severe haemorrhage due to consumptive coagulopathy or fibrinolysis. AKI may be due to haemorrhagic shock and / or ? direct nephrotoxicity.
Multiple Hymenoptera stings (bees, wasps, hornets)-usually mass attacks
Direct nephrotoxicty, hypotension, heme-pigment toxicity (intravascular haemolysis and rhabdomyolysis) 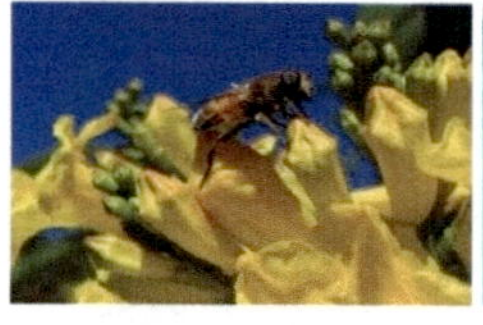 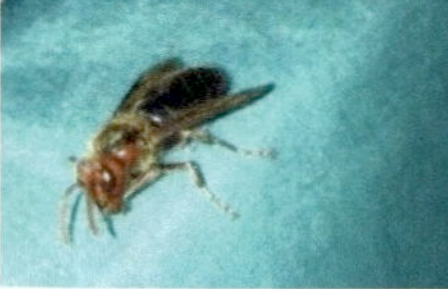 Permission from Sanjay Vikrant, Indhira Gandhi Medical College

Fig. 8.13 Animal toxins associated with acute kidney injury

fibrosis following the consumption of slimming pills containing Chinese herbs. The striking similarity to a form of chronic tubulointerstitial nephritis of unknown cause in the Balkans was noted. Both conditions were linked to the nephrotoxin aristolochic acid giving rise to the name aristolochic acid nephropathy. In the Balkans, the contamination of wheat grain with the seeds of the *Aristolochia clematitis* was identified as the cause. End-stage kidney disease can arise in as little as 1 month, especially after continuous high dose of ingestion, particularly seen in the case of Chinese herbal nephropathy.

Atractyloside is a toxin present in *Callilepis laureola* (Impila), a tuber used as a traditional medicine in South Africa, which causes acute severe hepatic and renal failure with high mortality, especially in children. It is also found in the Mediterranean thistle and the cocklebur. Poisoning is characterised by coma, severe refractory hypoglycemia and metabolic acidosis. Cape aloe is another commonly used traditional medicine that is associated with AKI in South Africa.

Djenkolism is another uncommon cause of AKI caused by ingestion of the Djenkol beans which are native to South-east Asia. Patients present with a rapid onset of abdominal or flank pain, haematuria and AKI. The mechanism of AKI is thought to be a combination of hypersensitivity (toxicity is not dose dependent), direct toxicity and crystal deposition leading to obstruction.

Poisonous mushrooms are a rare but potentially catastrophic cause of AKI (see ◘ Fig. 8.14). The amatoxins of *Amanita* species (*Amanita phalloides*) of mushrooms account for the majority of toxicity related to mushroom poisoning. Presentation is characterised by a latency to the onset of symptoms, GI disturbance, jaundice, coma and death. Direct toxicity results in both hepatic and renal failure. *Gyromitra esculenta* is a form of mushroom found in Eastern Europe and North America. Poisoning is associated with GI symptoms and seizures due to inactivation of GABA-ergic pathways by active metabolites of the toxin gyromitrin. Direct toxicity leads to hepatocellular injury. AKI is often secondary to volume depletion, oxidative damage by reactive metabolites or haem pigment injury caused by intravascular haemolysis. *Cortinarius orellanus* mushrooms contain the toxin orellanine which is concentrated in the kidney and causes interstitial nephritis. It was first described in 1952 in Poland when over 100 local residents suffered poisoning. Toxicity is dose dependent and unforgiving; 20–40% develop irreversible AKI.

8.30 Post-Renal Acute Kidney Injury

Acquired urinary tract obstruction is covered in the chapter by McCaig. It is important to recognise obstructive nephropathy results not only in acute glomerular shutdown but recruitment of inflammatory cells and interstitial inflammation. It is not a benign state: rapid diagnosis and prompt intervention can result in improvement or even complete recovery of

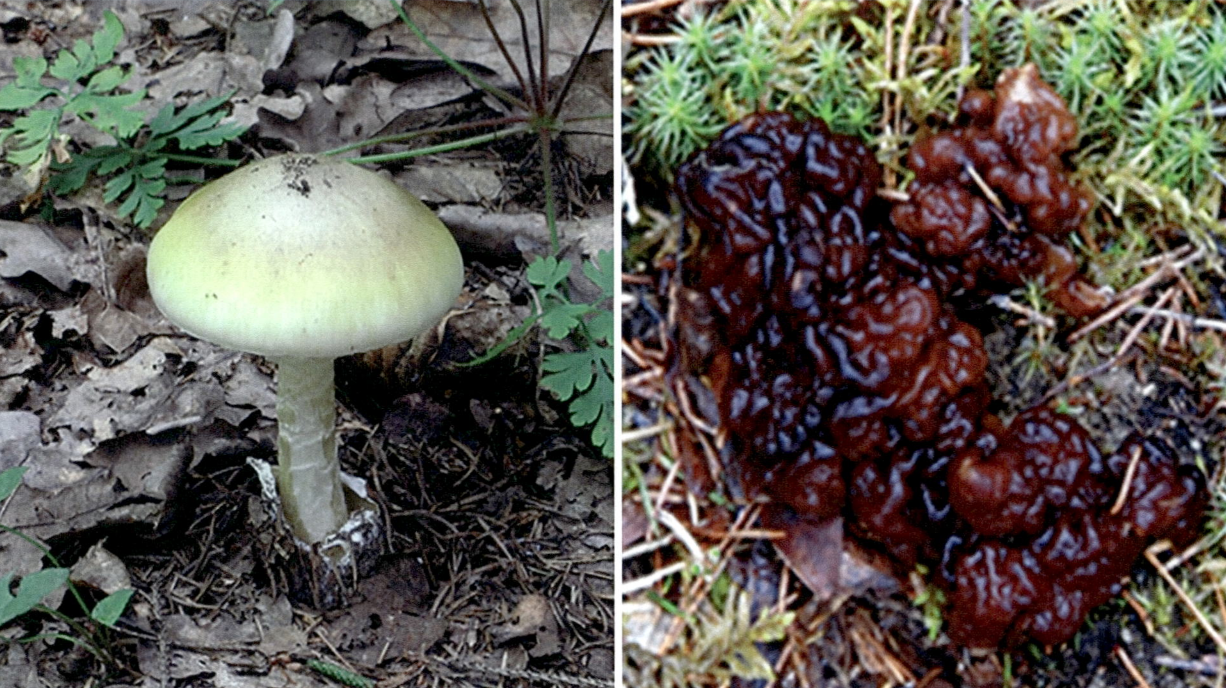

◘ **Fig. 8.14** Poisonous mushrooms associated with acute kidney injury: Left *Amanita phalloides*. Right *Gyromitra esculenta*

Table 8.6 Main causes of post-renal AKI (see ▶ Chap. 57)

Obstructive causes	
Causes	
Intrinsic	Intraluminal Stone, blood clot and papillary necrosis Intramural Urethral stricture (benign or malignant) and bladder tumour
Extrinsic	Prostatic hypertrophy or malignancy Pelvic malignancy Retroperitoneal fibrosis Radiation fibrosis Abdominal compartment syndrome[a]
Non-obstructive causes	
Neuropathic bladder Drugs (e.g. anticholinergics) Abdominal compartment syndrome Immobility Pain Constipation	

[a]Abdominal compartment syndrome is an under-recognised contributor to AKI when the peritoneal cavity pressure is high. The mechanism for causing a fall in GFR is not known but is likely to be due to a combination of renal hypoperfusion, renal vein congestion and impaired urinary drainage [31]

8

kidney function, whereas delay will result in long-term loss of nephrons (Table 8.6).

8.31 Specific Conditions Associated with AKI

There are many diseases associated with a high risk of AKI (see Table 8.7) and groups of patients with a particular spectrum of AKI risk.

8.32 Special Areas

8.32.1 Children

In low-income countries, AKI is predominantly a disease of the young and children, in whom volume-responsive "pre-renal" mechanisms are common [32], and AKI-related mortality is very high despite commonly being due to reversible conditions such as post-streptococcal glomerulonephritis, malaria and diarrhoeal illnesses [33]. In high-income countries, AKI is approximately 20-fold less common in children than in adults. Special considerations in children include a higher likelihood of acute obstructive uropathy due to congenital abnormalities of the kidney and urinary tract. Other causes of AKI that are relatively more common in children include microangiopathies due to underlying damage to kidney endothelial cells, particularly diarrhoea-associated haemolytic uraemic syndrome (HUS) arising from endothelial damage by bacterial endotoxin such as the toxin expressed by *Escherichia coli* 0157 [34]. It is important to remember that childhood AKI may manifest decades later as otherwise unexplained CKD.

8.32.2 Pregnancy (See Chapter on Pregnancy and Renal Disease)

AKI in pregnancy may be due to any disorder that can cause AKI in the general population, but there are additional complications characteristic of each trimester of pregnancy that can result in AKI. During the first trimester, the most common causes are hypovolaemia due to hyperemesis gravidarum or acute tubular injury or cortical necrosis following a septic abortion. Later in pregnancy, a variety of less common disorders can cause AKI. These include acute pyelonephritis, which occurs in 1–2% of pregnancies and can be associated with hypovolaemia and septic shock. The gravid uterus may cause ureteric obstruction, particularly if the pregnancy is multiple or if there is polyhydramnios. Endothelial changes in pregnancy may contribute to a number of conditions including a predisposition to thrombotic microangiopathies (TMA) such as haemolytic uraemic syndrome and thrombotic thrombocytopenic purpura [35]. During the third trimester, catastrophic hypotensive events such as placental abruption or severe postpartum haemorrhage may result in acute cortical necrosis from severe ischaemic injury, and globally this remains an important cause of AKI. Acute fatty liver of pregnancy may be associated with AKI or multi-organ failure. In developing countries, AKI remains a common and potentially preventable cause of maternal mortality, which varies between 6% and 30% in reported series [36].

8.32.3 The Elderly and CKD

The incidence rate of AKI is highest in elderly patients [5], who make up an ever-growing proportion of the general population. Pre-existing CKD is a powerful risk factor although few studies have focused on this

Table 8.7 Some specific conditions associated with AKI

Diabetes:	Hypovolaemia: renal losses HONK and DKA
Urosepsis: Acute sepsis and pyelonephritis	
Obstruction:Secondary to sloughed papilla (papillary necrosis), obstruction: Secondary to autonomic bladder	
Underlying (often subclinical) diabetic nephropathy is a significant contributing risk factor for AKI. NB pyelonephritis may be sub-acute and asymptomatic	
Gastrointestinal:	Acute diarrhoeal illnesses (hypovolaemia +/−sepsis)
	Diarrhoea-associated HUS
	Hypovolaemia secondary to high output ileostomy
	Obstruction secondary to stones in short bowel
	Acute oxalate nephropathy -pancreatic insufficiency or short bowel (check plasma oxalate levels or oxalate on phase contrast microscopy of biopsy)
	Interstitial nephritis secondary to sulphasalazines in inflammatory bowel disease (IBD)
	Chronic diarrhoea often associated with malnutrition, and a low creatinine belies a poor GFR secondary to multiple AKI events
	IBD may have underlying amyloid (proteinuria)
Liver disease:	Reduced effective arterial blood volume
	Hepatorenal syndrome
	Variceal haemorrhage
	Hypovolaemia post paracentesis
	Over diuresis
	Hypoalbuminaemia
	Fulminant hepatitic failure any cause
	Abdominal compartment syndrome
	Infections
	Sepsis, e.g. spontaneous bacterial peritonitis
	Leptospirosis, Legionnaire's disease, hantavirus, hepatitis B and C, etc.
	Reduced effective arterial blood volume
Drugs	Paracetamol, rifampicin, isoniazid, azathioprine, tetracycline, etc.
Toxins	*Amanita phalloides* (mushroom poisoning), Hydrotetracarbon inhalation, etc.
	Jaundice and reduced effective arterial blood volume make patients with chronic liver disease exquisitely sensitive to AKI from other insults such as hypovolaemia, sepsis or nephrotoxic drugs. Abdominal compartment syndrome is an under-recognised contribution to AKI and should be suspected in anyone with a tense abdomen

(continued)

Table 8.7 (continued)

Cardiovascular:	Mmyocardial stunning/decreased cardiac output
	Contrast nephropathy
	Acute cholesterol emboli syndrome
	Renal arterial embolism
	Chronic heart failure
	Atherosclerotic renal artery stenosis
	Takayasu's aortitis and middle aorta syndrome
	Surgery involving cross-clamping suprarenal aorta or renal arteries
	Infective endocarditis
	IVC thrombosis extending to renal vein
	Renal vein thrombosis and pulmonary emboli
Cancer:	Hypercalcaemia
	Tumour lysis syndrome (hyeruricaemia)
	Light chain nephropathy (myeloma)
	Exogenous toxins
	Radiation (fibrosis and TMA)
	Reduced renal perfusion eg hypovolaemia nausea/vomiting/anorexia
	Direct infiltration
	Lymphoma (and PTLD), chronic lymphocytic leukaemia, acute lymphoblastic leukaemia
	Obstruction
	Glomerular lesions
	Minimal change GN (lymphoma)
	Membranous GN (solid organ malignancy)
	TMA

area [37]. AKI in this group is often multifactorial and is pre-disposed to by age-related deterioration in fluid and salt homeostasis, such as reduced thirst response, urine concentrating ability and salt reabsorption. Many of the elderly are on drugs such as NSAIDs, RAAS blockade and diuretics which contribute to pre-renal AKI in the setting of a minor added insult. In older people the commonly used signs to gauge volume depletion can be misleading. Severely ill patients may have gross oedema while at the same time being intravascularly depleted. Malignancy is a commoner cause of AKI in this age group and may be intrinsic, as in the setting of myeloma or obstructive as in the setting of prostatic or other pelvic malignancies. The limitations of serum creatinine to estimate GFR are much more pronounced in the elderly, including its dependence on muscle mass and the presence of multiple drug use and comorbidities [38]. Older age is also associated with a greater risk of non-recovery of renal function back to baseline, which, given the increasing incidence of AKI,

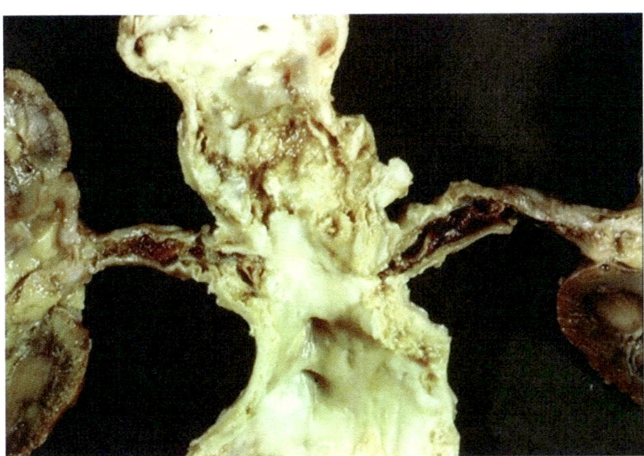

Fig. 8.15 Post-mortem findings in the aorta and renal arteries of an elderly man with CKD 4 who developed irreversible AKI following an acute episode of hypotension. Such cases illustrate the high risk of AKI in patients with poor renal function and significant comorbidity

raises significant public health concerns about the absolute number of elderly people developing incident CKD (Fig. 8.15).

Table 8.8 Types of acute kidney injury in patients with cancer

Cancer-related kidney injury	Obstructive nephropathy – Due to retroperitoneal lymphadenopathy Infiltration of the kidney by the tumour – Common with leukaemia and lymphoma Hypercalcaemia – With hemodynamic acute kidney injury and acute nephrocalcinosis Glomerular diseases – Amyloidosis, minimal change, FSGS, membranous, immunotactoid and fibrillary GN Lysozymuria with direct tubular toxicity in AML or CMML Hemophagocytic lymphohistiocytosis with interstitial nephritis
Treatment-related AKI	Tumour lysis syndrome with acute urate nephropathy Drug-related nephrotoxicity – Acute tubular injury, interstitial nephritis, glomerular disease or thrombotic microangiopathy Intra-tubular obstructions from medication
Other types of injuries	Volume depletion Contrast-induced nephrotoxicity Sepsis and septic shock

8.33 Cancer

As mentioned above, AKI is a common complication in patients with cancer. The incidence and severity depend on the type of cancer and its stage, treatment regimen and other co-existing clinical conditions. The development of AKI is associated with poor prognosis although early recognition and treatment are associated with better outcomes [39]. It is difficult to assess the overall prevalence, but studies carried out in specific diseases such as multiple myeloma have shown that 15–30% of patients have evidence of renal impairment [40]. In a 7-year Danish study of 37,267 incident cases of cancer, the 1-year risk of acute kidney injury, as defined by the Risk, Injury, Failure, Loss of kidney function and End-Stage kidney (RIFLE) disease classification was 17.5%. The 5-year risk for the individual risk, injury and failure categories was 27.0%, 14.6% and 7.6%, respectively. Furthermore, 5.1% of patients in whom acute kidney injury developed required long-term dialysis within 1 year [41]. Important risk factors are volume depletion, older age, use of nephrotoxic drugs, pre-existing renal impairment, renal hypoperfusion (due to cardiomyopathy, nephrotic syndrome or cirrhosis) and large tumour burden. Common causes of malignancy-associated AKI include those resulting from the malignancy itself (e.g. obstruction or infiltration, cast nephropathy in multiple myeloma, paraneoplastic syndromes such as hypercalcaemia), those resulting from treatment (e.g. nephrotoxic drugs, tumour lysis syndrome, interstitial nephritis) and general causes (e.g. volume depletion, sepsis, radiocontrast) (see Table 8.8).

8.34 Summary

It is clear that AKI has a very significant mortality and a high and increasing global incidence. The aetiology of AKI is very dependent on geography and socio-economic factors with young people in LICs, being disproportionally affected by infection and pre-renal AKI, whereas CKD, multimorbidity and medication are much more significant factors in HICs.

8

Case Study

1. A 16-year-old boy presented to hospital with nausea, vomiting and general malaise. He had been camping and drinking moderate amounts of beer in the 3 days before. He denied taking any drugs. He was felt to be euvolaemic but had a creatinine of 1300 and urea of 36. Urine dipstick was bland, and ultrasound showed normal-sized kidneys. 12 hours later, a second boy also presented with similar symptoms and similar findings (a creatinine of 900). It was not immediately clear what had caused the AKIs, but while a drug screen was pending, a further boy appeared with a similar but milder presentation. It became clear that this must have been secondary to an environmental toxin, and on further questioning, it became apparent that the boys had mistaken *Cortinarius orellanus* mushrooms for magic mushrooms. AKI in adolescence in HICs is likely to have very different causes than for older patients. The fact that more than one individual developed AKI makes an environmental toxin very likely, and in this demographic, recreational drugs would be an important cause.
2. An 81-year-old woman was admitted with a fractured neck of femur. She had been found on the floor by her carer having been unable to get up for some hours. She had a past medical history of hypertension ischaemic heart disease with moderate heart failure (treated with an ACEI and diuretic). She also had osteoarthritis for which she took occasional NSAIDs and a previous stroke. On examination she was felt to be septic possibly secondary to cholecystitis and had saturations of 92% and a blood pressure of 92 mmHg systolic on arrival. She was treated with broad-spectrum antibiotics including gentamicin and cautious fluid resuscitation and had a CT with contrast to define the source of sepsis. Her blood pressure remained low for 24 hours, she became oligoanuric, and her creatinine rose from a baseline of 110 to 420 in 3 days. This not unusual case represents multiple comorbidity in the elderly and associated risks of further insults such as reduction in renal perfusion, sepsis and exposure exogenous toxins.
3. A young woman was admitted acutely unwell with abdominal pain and vomiting. She was acidotic with a rising lactate, progressive coagulopathy and oliguria in the context of acute pancreatitis secondary to hypertriglyeridaemia. Her mean arterial pressures were maintained, and an ultrasound demonstrated normal-sized kidneys with no evidence of obstruction. There were no other obvious nephrotoxins or evidence of intrinsic renal disease in this abrupt illness. Her abdomen was very tense on examination (◘ Fig. 8.16) with signs of retroperitoneal haemorrhage. Measurement of intra-abdominal pressure recorded values of 34–48 mmHg (normal 5 mmHg), and a diagnosis of abdominal compartment syndrome (ACS) was made, and she underwent decompressive laparotomy. Compression of the renal veins and obstruction of the collecting system contribute to renal failure.

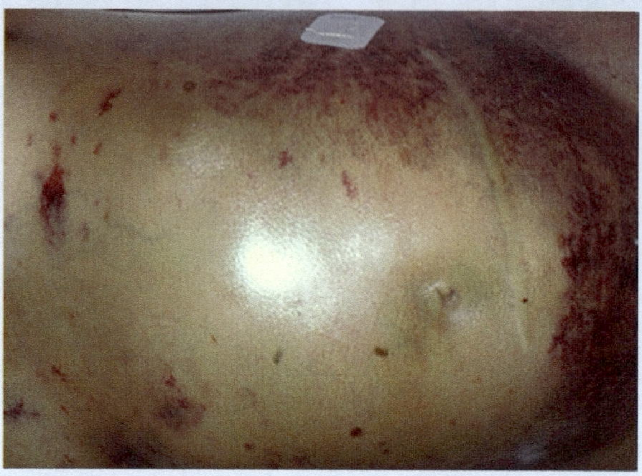

◘ **Fig. 8.16** Tense abdomen with Grey Turner's sign of retroperitoneal (in this case pancreatic) haemorrhage and general coagulopathy. Intra-abdominal pressure was grossly elevated, severely impairing perfusion of intra-abdominal organs including the kidneys as well as causing functional obstruction

ACS is fortunately relatively rare but well recognised following trauma and potentially fatal. This case illustrates the potential causes of pre-, intrinsic and post-renal impairment, in this case the impact of acute venous and urinary obstruction, as potential causes of AKI.

Questions

1. What is the definition of AKI 2 based on urine output?
2. In health approximately what percentage of body weight are the kidneys? What percentage of cardiac output goes to the kidneys, how many litres do the kidneys filter a day, and what percentage of this is reabsorbed?
3. Roughly what percentage of AKI have medication as a contributory element?
4. How does intravascular haemolysis cause AKI?
5. What are the causes of rhabdomyolysis?

Answers

1. A urine output of less than 0.5 ml/kg/hour for more than 12 hours. Ideally this should be based on ideal body weight.
2. In health the kidneys account for approximately 0.5% of body weight and 20–25% of cardiac output and filter approximately 180 L a day of which

98% is reabsorbed. It is, therefore, easy to see how insults to renal perfusion or acute tubular injury can have a profound impact.

3. Medication is contributory to severe AKI in approximately 25% of cases with medication being a significant factor in 14–26% of all AKI in high-income countries.
4. Haemoglobin is toxic to the tubules and causes cast nephropathy; however, free haemoglobin is normally bound by haptoglobin and not filtered. In massive intravascular haemolysis, haptoglobin is overwhelmed, and free haemoglobin splits into alpha-beta dimers that are freely filtered.
5. There are multiple causes of rhabdomyolysis from direct crush/compression of muscle compartments to toxin-related diffuse rhabdomyolysis and intrinsic muscle disorders (see ◘ Fig. 8.10).

References

1. Mehta RL, Cerda J, Burdmann EA, et al. International Society of Nephrology's 0by25 initiative for acute kidney injury (zero preventable death by 2025): a human rights case for nephrology. Lancet. 2015;385:2616–43.
2. Bellomo R, Ronco C, Kellum JA, Mehta RL, Palevsky P. Acute dialysis quality initiative workgroup. Acute renal failure - definition, outcome measures, animal models, fluid therapy and information technology needs: the second international consensus conference of the acute dialysis quality initiative (ADQI) group. Crit Care. 2004;8(4):R204–12.
3. Mehta RL, Kellum JA, Shah SV, Molitoris BA, Ronco C, Warnock DG, Levin A, Acute Kidney Injury Network. Acute kidney injury network: report of an initiative to improve outcomes in acute kidney injury. Crit Care. 2007;11(2):R31.
4. Kidney Disease: Improving Global Outcomes. Clinical practice guideline on acute kidney injury. 2011. www.kdigo.org.
5. Susantitaphong P, Cruz DN, Cerda J, Abulfaraj M, Alqahtani F, Koulouridis I, Jaber BL. World incidence of AKI: a meta-analysis. CJASN. 2013;8(9):1482–93. https://doi.org/10.2215/CJN.00710113.
6. Hoste E, Kellum JA, Selby NM, Zarbock A, Palevsky PM, Bagshaw SM, Goldtein SL, et al. Global epidemiology and outcomes of acute kidney injury. Nature Rev Nephrol. 2018;14:607–25.
7. Siew ED, Davenport A. The growth of acute kidney injury: a rising tide or just closer attention to detail. Kidney Int. 2015;87:46–61. https://doi.org/10.1038/ki.2014.293.
8. Mehta RL, Burdmann EA, Cerdá J, Feehally J, Finkelstein F, et al. Recognition and management of acute kidney injury in the International Society of Nephrology 0by25 global snapshot: a multinational cross-sectional study. Lancet. 2016;387(10032):2017–25. https://doi.org/10.1016/S0140-6736(16)30240-9. Epub 2016 Apr 13.
9. Eswarappa M, Gireesh MS, Ravi V, Kumar D, Dev G. Spectrum of acute kidney injury in critically ill patients: a single center study from South India. Indian J Nephrol. 2014;24(5):280–5. https://doi.org/10.4103/0971-4065.132991.
10. Cerdá J, Lameire N, Eggers P, Pannu N, Uchino S, Wang H, Bagga A, Levin A. Epidemiology of acute kidney injury. CJASN. 2008;3(3):881–6.
11. Hsu CY, Ordoñez JD, Chertow GM, Fan D, McCulloch CE, Go AS. The risk of acute renal failure in patients with chronic kidney disease. Kidney Int. 2008;74(1):101–7. https://doi.org/10.1038/ki.2008.107.
12. Huang TM, Wu VC, Young GH, Lin YF, Shiao CC, Wu PC, et al. Preoperative proteinuria predicts adverse renal outcomes after coronary artery bypass grafting. JASN. 2011;22(1):156–63. https://doi.org/10.1681/ASN.2010050553.
13. Pereira BJ, Narang A, Pereira S, Gupta A, Sakhuja V, Chugh KS. Acute renal failure in infants in the tropics. Nephrol Dial Transplant. 1989;4(6):535–8.
14. Bosch X, Poch E, Grau JM. Rhabdomyolysis and acute kidney injury. N Engl J Med. 2009;361:62–72.
15. Melli G, Chaudhry V, Cornblath DR. Rhabdomyolysis: an evaluation of 475 hospitalized patients. Medicine (Baltimore). 2005;84(6):377–85.
16. Bagley WH, Yang H, Shah KH. Rhabdomyolysis. Intern Emerg Med. 2007;2(3):210–8.
17. Walsh S, Fan SL. Visualising rhabdomyolysis. Lancet. 2009;373(9658):154.
18. Moffett BS, Goldstein SL. Acute kidney injury and increasing nephrotoxic-medication exposure in noncritically-ill children. Clin J American Soc Nephrol. 2011;6(4):856–63.
19. Nash K, Hafeez A. Hou S hospital-acquired renal insufficiency. Am J Kidney Dis. 2002;39(5):930–6.
20. Berns AS. Nephrotoxicity of contrast media. Kidney Int. 1989;36:730–40.
21. McDonald JS, McDonald RJ, Comin J, Williamson EE, Katzberg RW, Murad MH, Kallmes DF. Frequency of acute kidney injury following intravenous contrast medium administration: a systematic review and meta-analysis. Radiology. 2013;267(1):119–28. https://doi.org/10.1148/radiol.12121460. Epub 2013 Jan 14.
22. McCullough PA. Contrast-induced acute kidney injury. J Am Coll Cardiol. 2008;51(15):1419–28.
23. Pannu N, Nadim MK. An overview of drug-induced acute kidney injury. Crit Care Med. 2008;36(4 Suppl):S216–23.
24. Mehta RL, Pascual MT, Soroko S, Savage BR, Himmelfarb J, Ikizler TA, et al. Spectrum of acute renal failure in the intensive care unit: the PICARD experience. Kidney Int. 2004;66(4):1613–21.
25. Hoste EA, Bagshaw SM, Bellomo R, Cely CM, Colman R, Cruz DN, et al. Epidemiology of acute kidney injury in critically ill patients: the multinational AKI-EPI study. Intensive Care Med. 2015;41(8):1411–23.
26. Pannu N, Nadim MK. AN overview of drug-induced acute kidney injury. Crit Care Med. 2008;36(4 suppl):S216–23.
27. Bell S, Davey P, Nathwani D, Marwick C, Vadiveloo T, Sneddon J, Patton A, Bennie M, Fleming S, Donnan PT. Risk of AKI with gentamicin as surgical prophylaxis JASN. 2014;25(11):2625–32. https://doi.org/10.1681/ASN.2014010035.
28. Costa S, Nucci M. Can we decrease amphotericin nephrotoxicity? Curr Opin Crit Care. 2001;7(6):379–83.
29. Eremina V, Jefferson JA, Kowalewska J, Hochster H, Haas M, Weisstuch J, et al. VEGF inhibition and renal thrombotic microangiopathy. N Engl J Med. 2008;358(11):1129–36.
30. Sitprija V. Snakebite nephropathy. Nephrology (Carlton). 2006;11(5):442–8.
31. Askenazi D. Evaluation and management of critically ill children with acute kidney injury. Curr Opin Pediatr. 2011;23(2):201–7.
32. Hsu CY, Mc Culloch CE, Fan D, Ordenez JD, Chertow GM, Go AS. Community-based incidence of acute renal failure. Kidney Int. 2007;72:208–12.

33. Coca SG, Cho KC, Hsu CY. Acute kidney injury in the elderly: predisposition to chronic kidney disease and vice versa. Nephron Clin Pract. 2011;119(Suppl 1):c19–24; Epub 2011 Aug 10.
34. Haase M, Story DA, Haase-Fielitz A. Renal injury in the elderly: diagnosis, biomarkers and prevention. Best Pract Res Clin Anaesthesiol. 2011;25(3):401–12.
35. Ganesan C, Maynard SE. Acute kidney injury in pregnancy: the thrombotic microangiopathies. J Nephrol. 2011;24(5):554–63. https://doi.org/10.5301/JN.2011.6250.
36. Bentata Y, Housni B, Mimouni A, Azzouzi A, Abouqal R. Acute kidney injury related to pregnancy in developing countries: etiology and risk factors in an intensive care unit. J Nephrol. 2011;5(0) https://doi.org/10.5301/jn.5000058.
37. Christiansen CF, Johansen MB, Langeberg WJ, Fryzek JP, Sørensen HT. Incidence of acute kidney injury in cancer patients: a Danish population-based cohort study. Eur J Intern Med. 2011;22:399–406.
38. Howard SC, Jones DP, Pui C-H. The tumor lysis syndrome. N Engl J Med. 2011;364:1844–54.
39. Denker B, Robles-Osorio ML, Sabath E. Recent advances in diagnosis and treatment of acute kidney injury in patients with cancer. Eur J Intern Med. 2011;22(4):348–54.
40. Humphreys BD, Soiffer RJ, Magee CC. Renal failure associated with cancer and its treatment: an update. J Am Soc Nephrol. 2005;16:151–6.
41. Christiansen CF, Johansen MB, Langeberg WJ, Fryzek JP, Sørensen HT. Incidence of acute kidney injury in cancer patients: a Danish population-based cohort study. Eur J Intern Med. 2011;22(4):399–406. https://doi.org/10.1016/j.ejim.2011.05.005; Epub 2011 Jun 8.

Assessment and Investigation of Acute Kidney Injury (AKI)

Maria Prendecki and Ed Kingdon

Contents

M. Harber (ed.), *Primer on Nephrology*, https://doi.org/10.1007/978-3-030-76419-7_9

Learning Objectives

This chapter should enable the reader to:

1. Identify cases of AKI using current diagnostic criteria.
2. Differentiate between pre-renal, post-renal and intrinsic renal disease as causes for AKI using a thorough history and examination.
3. Identify patients in whom further investigations such as immunology testing, renal ultrasound or biopsy is indicated.

9.1 Introduction

The assessment and investigation of a patient with acute kidney injury (AKI) require a careful history, scrutiny of the medical notes, drug charts, observations charts and anaesthetic records, thorough physical examination and interpretation of appropriate investigations including laboratory tests and imaging. It is vital not to miss an underlying, reversible cause of AKI, and often a presumptive diagnosis can be made from clinical history and investigations. The questions that should be evaluated when assessing a patient with AKI are:

1. Are there life-threatening complications of AKI which require immediate intervention?
2. Is this AKI or progressive chronic kidney disease (CKD)?
3. What is the cause of the AKI?
    a. Has the patient been exposed to extrinsic or intrinsic toxins?
    b. What does the urinalysis show?
    c. Is there or has there been a pre-renal insult?
    d. Is there urinary tract obstruction and if present at what site/level?
    e. Are there signs or symptoms or systemic inflammatory disease?

9.2 Standardising Classification of Acute Kidney Injury

Historical definitions of acute renal failure lacked precision. Individual trials and studies of natural history used different biochemical parameters and the criteria for how much these had to change and how quickly were not standardised. However, in 2004, the Risk, Injury, Failure, Loss and End-Stage disease (RIFLE) classification was developed by the Acute Dialysis Quality Initiative (ADQI) [1]. This was modified further in 2007 by the AKI Network report, which proposed standard definitions for AKI stages 1–3 following recognition that even small changes in serum creatinine are associated with poor outcomes [2]. At the same time, the term acute kidney injury (AKI) was introduced to encompass the entire spectrum of renal injury from minor changes in kidney function to dialysis dependence [3]. These scoring systems have been combined to result in the Kidney Disease: Improving Global Outcomes (KDIGO) definition and staging system currently in use [4] (Table 9.1).

Table 9.1 KDIGO, AKIN and RIFLE classifications of AKI

AKI stage	KDIGO	AKI Network	RIFLE	Common urine output criteria
1	Increase in serum creatinine of ≥26 µmol/L (0.3 mg/dL) within 48 hours or increase to ≥1.5 to 1.9 x baseline serum creatinine within 1 week	Increase in serum creatinine 1.5–2x baseline or ≥ 26 µmol/L (0.3 mg/dL) within 48 hours	**Risk:** Increase in serum creatinine ≥1.5x baseline within 7 days, persists for ≥24 hours	<0.5 mL/kg/hour for >6 consecutive hours
2	Increase in serum creatinine to >2.0 to 2.9 x baseline serum creatinine	Increase in serum creatinine 2–3x baseline	**Injury:** Increase in serum creatinine to ≥2x baseline	<0.5 mL/kg/hour for >12 consecutive hours
3	Increase in serum creatinine to greater than threefold from baseline or serum creatinine of ≥354 µmol/L [≥4.0 mg/dL] or commenced on renal replacement therapy irrespective of stage	Increase in serum creatinine>3x baseline or ≥ 354 µmol/L [≥4.0 mg/dL] or commenced on renal replacement therapy	**Failure:** Increase in serum creatinine greater than threefold from baseline or serum creatinine of ≥354 µmol/L [≥4.0 mg/dL] or commenced on renal replacement therapy **Loss:** Loss of kidney function sustained for >4 weeks **ESRD:** ESRD for >3 months	<0.3 mL/kg/hour for >24 consecutive hours OR anuria for 12 hours

9.3 Recognition of Biochemical Changes Suggesting Acute Kidney Injury

Agreement on AKI diagnostic criteria based on the magnitude and timing of changes in serum creatinine has allowed the introduction of algorithms for the automated detection of patients who may have AKI. When biochemical changes are compared with clinical coding of AKI, the specificity of biochemical changes is approximately 90% [5]. However, it is important to remember that imperfections in the techniques available to measure creatinine, biological causes for change in creatinine other than AKI and circumstances under which this approach is not validated may lead to biochemical changes in the absence of a true AKI. Notwithstanding these caveats, automated ascertainment of biochemical changes suggestive of AKI is likely to enhance early recognition of AKI. It is possible that timely identification of a precise AKI phenotype facilitates therapeutic gains using existing and new treatments. There are several limitations to the use of creatinine and urine output for the diagnosis of AKI, and other biomarkers may offer the opportunity to more accurately describe the phenotype of the kidney injury and identify this earlier in the course of the patient's illness. Novel biomarkers in AKI are discussed further below.

9.4 Novel Biomarkers in AKI

There are several limitations to the use of creatinine and urine output for the diagnosis of AKI. For example, the use of drugs which interfere with tubular secretion of creatinine (e.g. trimethoprim) may lead to misdiagnosis of AKI. The use of creatinine in those with very high or low BMI is inaccurate. Additionally, due to renal reserve, creatinine may not rise until a 50% fall in GFR has occurred [6]. As such, there are a number of novel biomarkers which are under investigation to improve early identification and monitoring of AKI for use either in addition to or in replacement of creatinine. These include neutrophil gelatinase-associated lipocalin (NGAL), insulin-like growth factor-binding protein 7 (IGFBP-7), tissue inhibitor of metalloproteinases 2 (TIMP-2), interleukin (IL)-18 and kidney injury molecule-1 (KIM-1). These markers may be elevated prior to serum creatinine, and some are available currently as diagnostic tests, including urinary TIMP-2 and IGFBP-7 in combination as the Nephrocheck test, NGAL and Cystatin C. TIMP2 and IGFBP7 are cell cycle arrest markers and are thought to be present in urine due to increased filtration and proximal tubular leakage in AKI rather than changes at the transcriptional level [7]. NGAL is a component of the innate immune system, and, in AKI, NGAL mRNA is upregulated in the kidney, liver and lungs. Increased transcription and reduced clearance secondary to a fall in in GFR contribute to the observed increases in plasma NGAL in AKI [8]. Cystatin C is an inhibitor of cysteine proteases and is produced by all nucleated cells. It is freely filtered and then reabsorbed and catabolised by the proximal tubule and is less dependent on age, muscle mass and liver function than serum creatinine [8]. The utility of these tests was evaluated using a systematic review and meta-analysis in an NIHR health technology assessment in 2018 [9]. The clinical studies that were reviewed included small studies, and the design of the studies was heterogeneous. The authors concluded that the combined urinary TIMP-2 and IGFBP-7 test appeared to be the most promising of the three with high sensitivity and moderate specificity for AKI in a critical care setting. Plasma NGAL had moderate sensitivity and high specificity for detecting AKI, but there was greater heterogeneity between studies than for the combined urinary TIMP-2 and IGFBP-7 test. There was weaker evidence for urinary NGAL and cystatin C testing with considerable variation between studies. Despite the heterogeneity of reported studies, novel biomarkers have the potential to improve care of patients who are at risk of AKI, and this area warrants further research.

9.5 Clinical Evaluation in Patients with AKI

In a patient with biochemical changes or oliguria characterising AKI, clinical history, examination and near patient testing should be reviewed to generate a diagnosis at the highest hierarchical level possible. This evaluation may also identify signs and symptoms of complications of AKI, such as fluid overload, electrolyte abnormalities, acidaemia or hypertension. Traditionally, causes of AKI are divided into pre-renal, renal and post-renal causes (◘ Fig. 9.1). This classification is helpful in delivering a comprehensive and logical assessment of patients with AKI.

Post-renal causes may be identified by morphological changes on imaging. Mechanical obstruction from within the lumen, within the wall of the urinary tract or obstruction from external compression is a frequent cause of AKI. Rarely obstruction may occur due to a functional cause. Finally, although difficult to diagnose without a biopsy, a proportion of AKI relates to tubular obstruction by non-specific tubular debris accumulation secondary to acute tubular injury or cast nephropathies seen in cases of myeloma cast nephropathy, pigment nephropathies or crystal nephropathies.

A pre-renal cause is suggested when findings in the history, examination or investigations indicate current

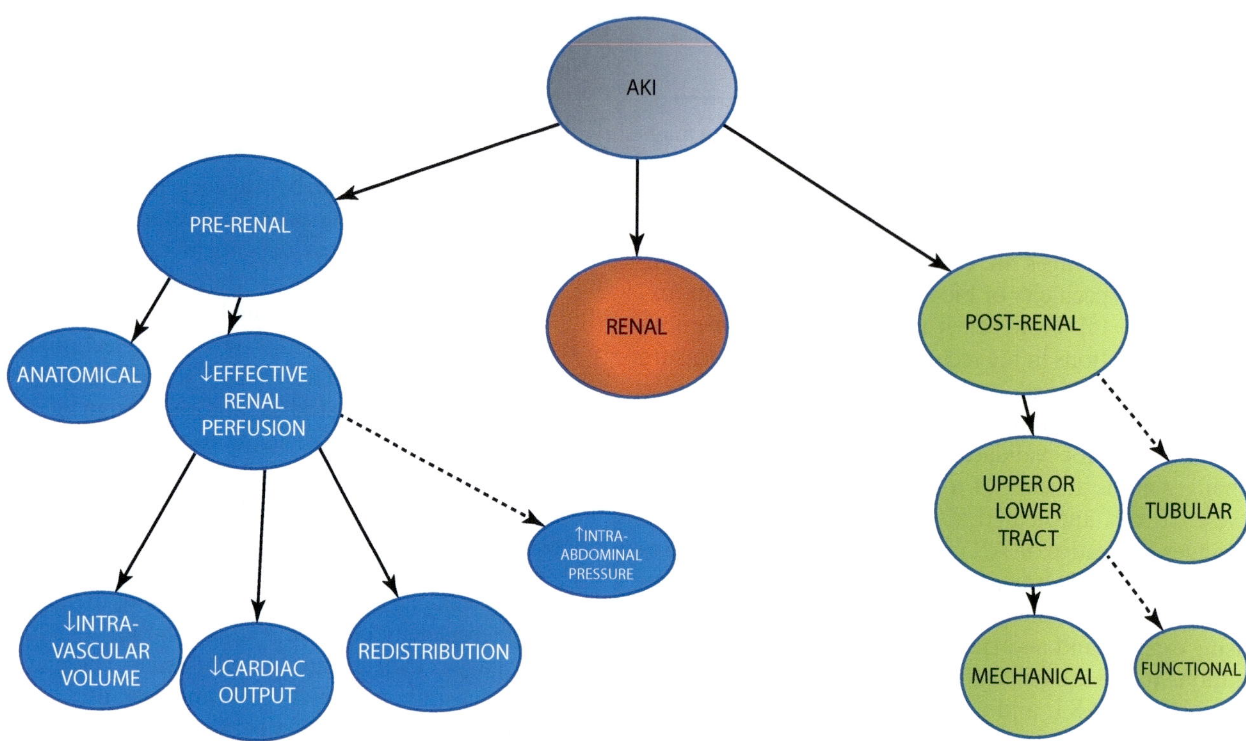

Fig. 9.1 Diagnostic classification for AKI

or recent hypoperfusion of the kidneys. This is usually caused by the presence of one or more of four factors: (a) hypovolaemia, (b) reduced cardiac output (c) regional hypoperfusion associated with splanchnic vasoconstriction and reduced renal perfusion most typically in sepsis or hepatorenal syndrome and (d) less commonly reduced perfusion because of increased abdominal pressure reducing renal venous drainage. Finally, renal hypoperfusion may complicate vascular events including aortic clamping or stenting, renal arterial dissection and occlusion by thrombosis or emboli.

"Renal" or intrinsic causes of AKI can be subdivided into glomerular, vascular, interstitial and tubular (Fig. 9.2). Tubular causes can be further subdivided into extrinsic (exogenous) or intrinsic (endogenous) causes (Fig. 9.3). Urinalysis is often extremely helpful in narrowing the differential diagnosis for AKI. The finding of significant blood and/protein in the urine is much more suggestive of a glomerular/vascular cause, than a tubular or interstitial cause. This is discussed more fully below in the section on near patient testing.

9.5.1 AKI Assessment May be Complicated

It is important to arrive at an accurate and precise diagnosis to ensure timely initiation of treatment for the cause of AKI given the high mortality and morbidity associated with admissions complicated by AKI. It may be that the mechanism of injury is obvious, but for those patients where this is not the case or where patients' recovery does not proceed as anticipated, comprehensive review of live and historical information held in the case notes and other records is very important. This often reveals factors predisposing to AKI and repeated minor insults, the significance of which are much more easily interpreted when a clear sequence of events is described.

Although monitoring of renal function in groups at high risk of CKD has been incentivised in many settings, AKI may occur in patients without prior measurement of renal function. Patients without previous serum creatinine measurements may not trigger the algorithms for automated ascertainment of AKI. In the absence of previous measurements, it is more difficult to categorically distinguish between AKI and progressive CKD.

The clinical setting in which patients from high-income settings with AKI are identified has only limited influence on variation in the aetiology of acute kidney injury. However, obstruction is a more common cause of AKI in community-acquired AKI in high-income countries [10]. For the remainder of the chapter, community- and hospital-acquired AKI are considered together.

Two cases are presented to illustrate the value of comprehensive assessment. The cases highlight the dispersal of helpful information to more than one record that is often seen in a real-world setting. Additionally, it is common for patients to need to be assessed more than once. The nature and precision of the renal diagnosis may change as additional information becomes available.

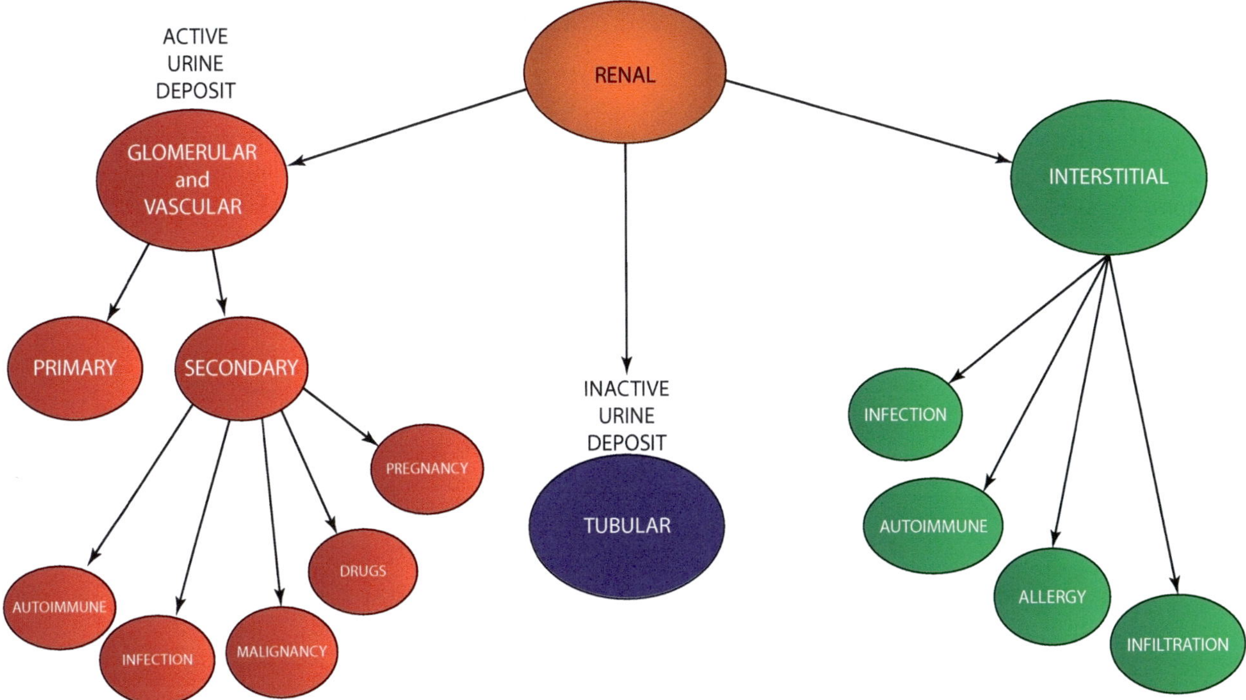

Fig. 9.2 Diagnostic classification for 'renal' AKI

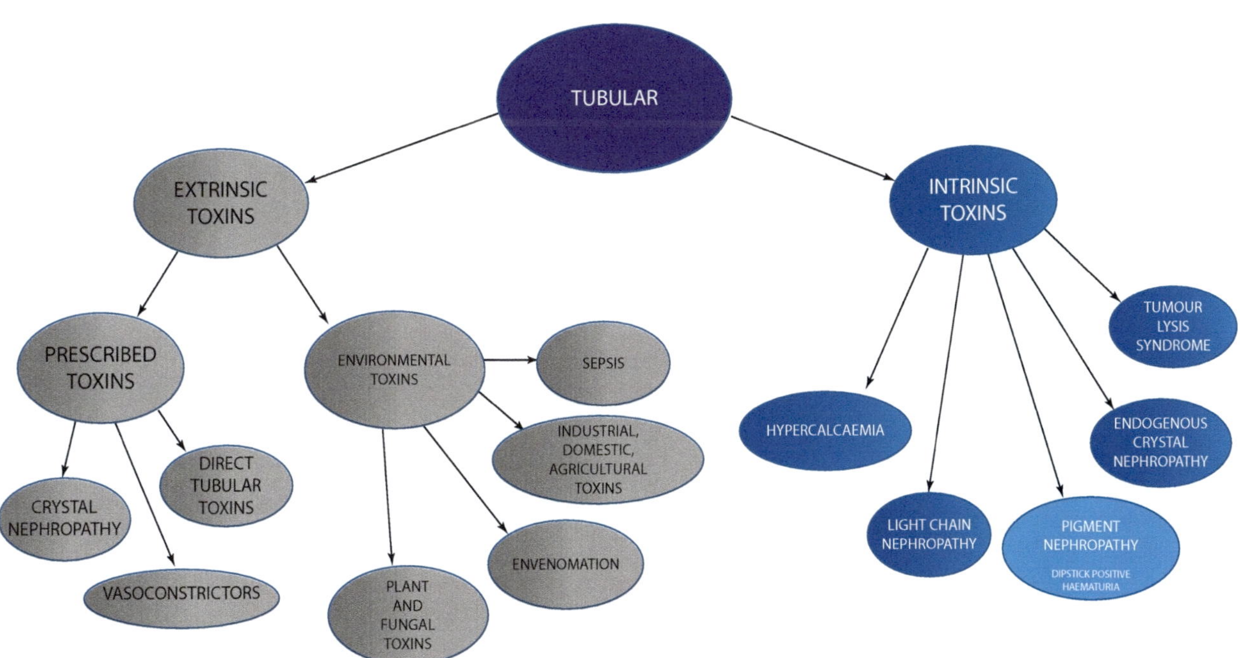

Fig. 9.3 Diagnostic classification for 'renal' AKI where the injury is predominantly tubular in origin. In searching for extrinsic environmental causes, some events such as snake bites may be readily recalled, but a careful history may be required to reveal ingestion of a natural or artificial toxin. In the medical setting, it is important to establish what has been prescribed such as vasoconstrictors and intravenous contrast (in what quantity), which potentially tubule-toxic drugs have been prescribed and in what quantity or what drugs that might precipitate as crystals

Case Study

Case 1

A 68-year-old woman was referred with oliguric AKI. She had a history of hypertension usually treated with two medications but was in good health until being admitted with cholecystitis. At the time of referral to the renal team, the clinicians looking after her team felt that she was euvolaemic. During the 18 hours prior to the referral, she had an average blood pressure averaging 160/78 mmHg, and the severity of her AKI seemed unexplained. However, review of observations from earlier in the admission revealed a prolonged period of relative hypotension for 48 hours in the context of severe infection. Whilst hypotensive, she had received intravenous contrast for a CT scan and one of two doses of amikacin. The chronology of these events in shown in ◘ Fig. 9.4 with contrast administration marked by the blue arrow and amikacin dosing by black arrows.

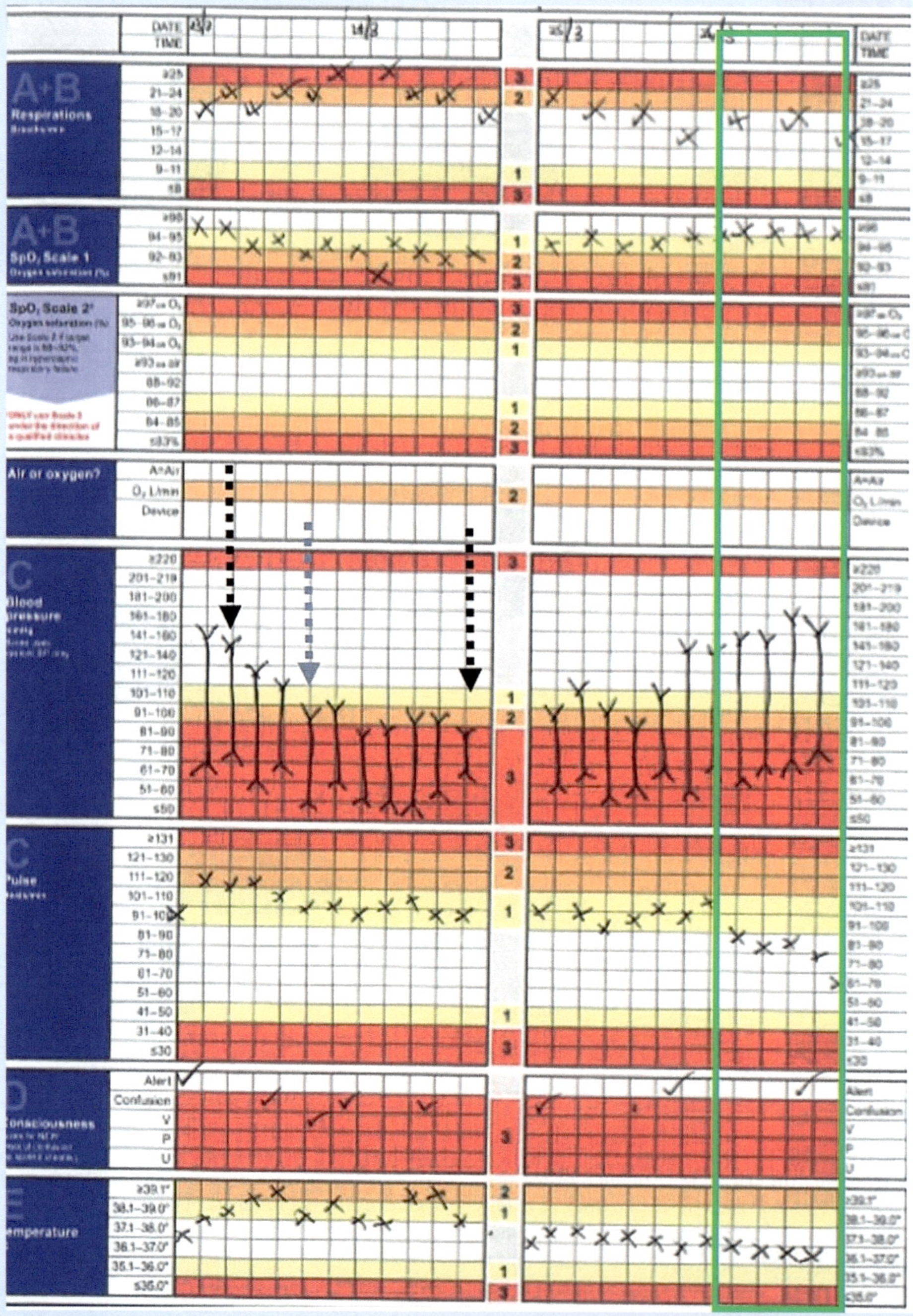

◘ **Fig. 9.4** Observation chart for the patient in case 1. Contrast administration is marked by the blue arrow and amikacin dosing by black arrows

Identifying these insults rendered her AKI much more readily explicable. The patient and the family were reassured without the need for extensive further investigations.

Case 2

The importance of reassessing patients with AKI as additional information becomes available is illustrated in case 2. A 79-year-old woman presented with breathlessness and was found to have AKI on a background of chronic kidney disease (baseline creatinine of 120 mmol/L). Comorbidities included ischaemic heart disease, coronary artery bypass grafting, type 2 diabetes and cardiac failure (echocardiography identified an ejection fraction of 25–30%). At presentation, her serum creatinine was 360 mmol/L. On examination, she had peripheral oedema; admission chest X-Ray is shown in ◘ Fig. 9.5. She was treated for heart failure with diuretics. Post-renal causes of AKI were excluded, and renal size and cortical thickness were seen to be preserved at CT scanning. History and examination did not reveal additional insults. Urinalysis showed isolated proteinuria, and this was quantified in the laboratory (urine protein/creatinine ratio (UPCR) of 270). There were no recent uPCRs for comparison, but the patient was known to have diabetic retinopathy, and the urine albumin/creatinine ratio was known to have been significantly elevated in the past. Renal immunological investigations were unremarkable, and AKI was attributed to cardiorenal syndrome. She was treated with diuretics, and the serum creatinine continued to rise. Ceilings of treatment were discussed by the parent medical team. A consensus was arrived at that renal replacement therapy in the context of cardiorenal syndrome would not extend her life outside the hospital. However, despite the diagnosis of cardiorenal syndrome, the blood pressure was persistently around 160/80, and a repeat echocardiogram showed no deterioration in LVEF. Review of the results of laboratory tests identified disproportionate anaemia. Immunoglobulins and serum protein electrophoresis had been undertaken and were unremarkable. Further tests were undertaken as the AKI remained unexplained. These revealed Bence Jones proteinuria and an excess of serum free light chains (kappa/lambda ratio of 188), and a diagnosis of multiple myeloma with light chain nephropathy was made. Challenging the clinical diagnosis when findings are discordant may prompt additional tests that identify potentially treatable causes of AKI.

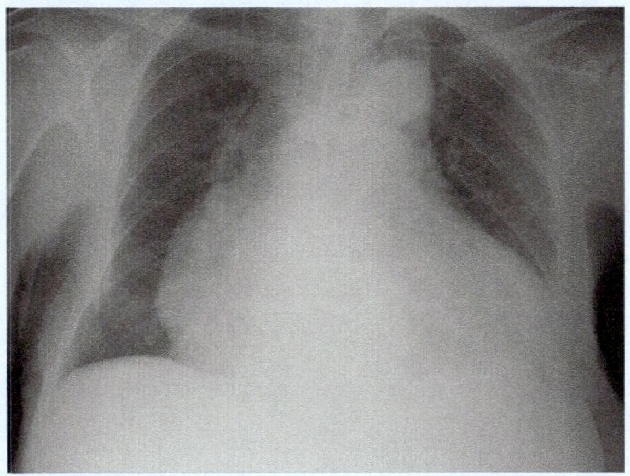

◘ **Fig. 9.5** Chest X-ray at the time of presentation

9.6 History

A detailed history should provide clues to the underlying cause of AKI and will guide further investigations. The history given by patients or carers is usually enhanced by referral documentation and by entries and documentation completed by other clinicians who have cared for the patient. The chronology of the past medical history and temporal relationship between potentially harmful exposures and changes in function are important in evaluation of the aetiology of AKI. In hospital-acquired AKI, assessing the timing of AKI can often be crucial in determining the underlying cause. If blood tests and urine output are being monitored frequently, then the day of an initial creatinine rise or decline in urine output may be preceded a day or two earlier by the underlying insult.

AKI often occurs in patients with substantial comorbidity. The commonest cause of AKI in hospital inpatients is pre-renal failure or acute tubular injury (ATN), and in one large case series, these accounted for nearly 70% of cases, rising to 85% if acute on chronic renal failure was included [11]. It is very common for "pre-renal" AKI to be multifactorial. In the AKI-EPI study of critically ill patients sepsis, hypovolaemia and nephrotoxic drugs were identified as causes of AKI in 90% of cases [12].

A history of fluid loss (either from the patient or the fluid balance chart) from diarrhoea, vomiting, insensible losses or haemorrhage may indicate volume depletion as a likely contributory cause. Consideration of fluid losses is important in patients who are nil by mouth and those where reduced conscious level, difficulty swallowing or initiating drinking increase vulnerability. During the COVID-19 pandemic, an under-appreciation of insensible losses related to fever and tachypnoea may have contributed to a high rate of AKI. There may be a history of interventional procedures or administration

Table 9.2 Differential diagnosis of AKI and key history points

Broad category	Aetiological factor	Risk/vulnerability	Specific questions	Additional sources of information
"Pre-renal" Renal hypoperfusion	Infection	Therapeutic immunosuppression Conditions associated with immunodeficiency Foreign bodies/prostheses IVDU	Fevers Symptoms localizing a focus of acute or chronic infection previous and current immunosuppression	Bedside charts Microbiology results
	Low cardiac output	Cardiogenic (cardio renal syndromes) and obstructive shock		Baseline BP Habitual weight
	Hypovolaemia	Conditions associated with Fluid maldistribution +/– abnormal effective arterial volume Cardiac disease Liver disease Nephrotic syndrome	Diarrhoea and vomiting Overt haemorrhage Periods of fasting or anorexia Diuretic use	Bedside charts: Fluid balance including extra-anatomical fluid losses (drains/fistulae)
Intrinsic renal disease	Systemic or renal limited inflammatory disease		Fever, weight loss, night sweats Mouth ulcers, myalgia, arthralgia, malaise, rashes, epistaxis, red eyes, haemoptysis, sicca symptoms	
	Tubular toxicity		Prescribed and "over-the-counter" medications Rhabdomyolysis Prolonged immobility Compartment syndromes Extreme exercise Myeloma Back pain Cholesterol embolisation Recent angiography, vascular surgery or onset of anticoagulation	
Post-renal	Urinary tract obstruction	Stone disease Prostatic enlargement Malignancy (uterine, cervical, ovarian, prostatic, bladder and ureteric) Solitary kidney	Pain Visible haematuria Post-menopausal bleeding Passage of gravel/grit PU Treated urinary tract infection LUTS – Lower urinary tract symptoms	

9

of intravenous contrast media. Volume of urine output may be helpful in narrowing the differential diagnosis; the presence of complete anuria is usually due to rapidly progressive glomerulonephritis (RPGN), acute cortical necrosis, complete obstruction of the urinary tract or renal infarction. Further suggestions for specific points in the history are summarised in Table 9.2.

A review of medication charts is essential as medications may have been started prior to the recognition of AKI and contributed to its development. This includes (a) medication prescribed in primary care, (b) over-the-counter medication, (c) herbal medications and (d) recreational drugs. Common drug causes of tubulointerstitial disease include antibiotics and proton pump inhibitors (AIN); chemotherapeutic agents (tumour lysis syndrome); and acyclovir (crystal nephropathy). Aminoglycoside antibiotics can cause acute tubular injury via direct toxicity to proximal tubular cells particularly with substantial cumulative exposure. Additionally medications such as ACE inhibitors and angiotensin receptor antagonists may be associated with haemodynamic changes within the kidney and changes in creatinine.

9.7 Examination

Bedside observations in in-patient settings routinely incorporate patient's level of consciousness (AVPU – alert, voice, pain, unresponsive), temperature, blood pressure, pulse rate, respiratory rate and oxygen saturation. Abnormalities in early warning scores which aggregate weighted scores for abnormalities in these physiological parameters segregate with poor outcomes and are used in many healthcare organisations to support decision-making, recognition of deteriorating patients and treatment escalation. A careful assessment of the patients' volume status including pulse rate and volume, blood pressure, postural blood pressure, JVP and peripheral perfusion is essential.

Assessment of peripheral circulation is important but is influenced by cardiac output, arterial tone and intravascular volume. Serial assessments of skin turgor and mucous membranes are more useful than isolated observations.

Signs Assessing Peripheral Perfusion

- Cap refill.
- Peripheral temperature.
- Skin turgor.
- Mucous membrane.

Blood pressure needs to be reviewed in the context of the patient's usual BP and whether they are usually and currently taking antihypertensive drugs. Patients may have significant hypotension relative to their habitual levels and yet have readings that remain within the expected and accepted range.

Response to a fluid bolus with a sustained or transient rise in blood pressure or JVP can be helpful in determining if a patient is volume replete. In a critical care setting with access to appropriate monitoring, variation in stroke volume and pulse pressure and the response to passive leg raising (PLR) can be used to estimate fluid responsiveness.

Postural BP may be more easily replicated than assessment of the JVP and provide useful information.

Postural Blood Pressure

- The initial BP should be measured after lying for at *least five minutes.*
- The second BP should be measured after standing for 1 minute.
- A third BP should be measured after standing for 3 minutes.
- Symptoms of dizziness, light-headedness, vagueness, pallor, visual disturbance, feelings of weakness and palpitations should be documented.
- Postural or orthostatic hypotension is identified by:
  - A drop in systolic BP of 20 mmHg or more (with or without symptoms).
  - A drop to below 90 mmHg on standing even if the drop is less than 20 mmHg (with or without symptoms).
  - A drop in diastolic BP of 10 mmHg with symptoms.

It is important to recognise assessment of intravascular volume status may be an area in which clinicians lack confidence and that frequently repeated assessment following intravenous fluids may be difficult to deliver in hard-pressed clinical settings. It is important to emphasise the difference between signs that reliably indicate increases or decreases in intravascular volume and those that identify fluid maldistribution and elevated total body salt and water. In this context, the internal jugular venous pressure and the presence of a third heart sound are discriminant signs, but clinicians may find these difficult to detect with certainty.

Inspection of the JVP is an important element of the assessment of whether a pericardial effusion is present. A pericardial effusion causing cardiac tamponade would be expected to cause tachycardia, hypotension and a raised JVP [13].

Signs of Tamponade

Tachycardia, Hypotension, Raised JVP.

Pulsus paradoxus – This can be determined using a manual sphygmomanometer. The observer identifies the difference between the peak systolic BP during expiration and the BP at which Korotkoff sounds are audible during inspiration and expiration. When the difference between the two is greater than 10 mmHg, a paradoxical pulse is present.

Kussmaul's sign – A paradoxical rise in jugular venous pressure (JVP) on inspiration, or a failure to observe the expected and appropriate fall in the JVP during inspiration.

^Signs of systemic inflammatory disease are important clues to AKI aetiology in a minority of AKI cases. However, early irreversible loss of function may occur early in the course of these conditions so there is much to be lost by delayed diagnosis and initiation of treatment. Such signs may be found in all systems and comprehensive examination of the skin, eyes and nervous system should be part of AKI assessment.

Signs of Systemic Inflammatory Disease

- Skin, hair and nails: rash, livedo reticularis, splinter hemorrhages, alopecia.
- ENT: mouth ulcers, nasal bridge collapse.
- Eyes: iritis, conjunctivitis, scleritis and episcleritis.
- Nervous system: isolated mononeuropathy, mononeuritis multiplex, cranial nerve lesions.

Other more specific clinical signs may point to the aetiology of AKI such as a drug rash in patients with acute interstitial nephritis (AIN), livedo reticularis (and a history of angiography or cardiac bypass) in cholesterol emboli and anticardiolipin antibody syndromes, clinical evidence of heart failure suggesting cardiorenal syndrome, signs of liver failure or jaundice suggesting consideration of the hepatorenal syndrome, tense ascites causing abdominal compartment syndrome or a palpable bladder from bladder outflow obstruction.

9

9.8 Investigation of AKI

Healthcare providers often recommend an extensive and costly panel of investigations in patients with AKI. The utility of these recommendations and the diagnostic yield are uncertain. It is likely that both will be influenced by consideration of pre-test probabilities [14].

The rationale for testing in AKI is described in ◘ Table 9.3.

9.8.1 Near Patient Testing

9.8.1.1 Urine Dipstick Testing

Urinalysis is a simple, noninvasive and cheap test and should be performed in all patients with AKI. It will inform further investigations. Normal urine dipstick provided the test has been performed correctly makes a glomerular aetiology for AKI much less likely. Unfortunately, prompt performance and recording of urine dipstick abnormalities is not universally achieved. Dipstick haematuria and proteinuria in combination suggest glomerular inflammation. Leucocytes and nitrites are observed in pyelonephritis. Isolated pyuria may be seen in interstitial nephritis.

On occasions, dipstick testing may be misleading. In pigment nephropathies myoglobin or haemoglobin in the urine of patients with rhabdomyolysis or intravascular haemolysis may cause acute tubular injury. In such cases, a dipstick test will be strongly positive for blood but in the absence of a glomerular lesion.

9.8.1.2 Urine Microscopy

Fully automated bright field microscopy is used in microbiology departments with digital imaging software employed to identify cellular and other elements found in un-centrifuged urine. This is an effective means by which to quantify white and red cells in midstream urine samples [15].

It is important to remember that red cells lyse in dilute urine and that this technique may underestimate the incidence of red cells in dilute, alkaline urine and in samples with prolonged transportation to the laboratory. However, haematuria on dipstick urinalysis in the absence of red blood cells at microscopy may be seen in pigment nephropathies such as from rhabdomyolysis or intravascular haemolysis.

Phase contrast microscopy of the re-suspended pellet of a freshly and gently centrifuged urine may, in the hands of an experienced observer, yield information unavailable using automated urine microscopy techniques described above.

Renal presentation	Phase contrast microscopy findings
Acute tubular injury	Renal tubular epithelial cells (RTEC), RTEC casts, coarse granular casts, "muddy brown" casts
Acute interstitial nephritis	White blood cells, WBC casts, RTECs RTEC casts, RBC, occasional RBC casts
Glomerular inflammation	Dysmorphic and isomorphic RBC, RBC casts and WBC casts
Nephrotic syndrome	Lipid droplets, oval fat bodies, lipid laden casts

Isomorphic red cells imply bleeding from the urinary tract sites other than the glomerulus [16]. Eosinophiluria is described as a feature of drug-induced interstitial nephritis. However, it has limited sensitivity and specificity for detecting AIN in the context of biopsy-proven AIN [17].

Table 9.3 Haemoatological, biochemical and microbiology tests to be considered in the investigation of patients with AKI

Laboratory	Test	Notes
Haematology	FBC, blood film	Thrombocytosis and leucocytosis in systemic disease such as ANCA-associated small vessel vasculitis Thrombocytopenia, high reticulocytes and red cell fragments in thrombotic microangiopathy (TMA) MAHA in sepsis-associated disseminated intravascular coagulation (DIC) Eosinophillia in AIN, cholesterol embolisation or eosinophilic granulomatosis with polyangiitis Leucopaenia and thrombocytopaenia in SLE
	Coagulation	Changes in APPT and PT in association with SLE, anti-phospholipid syndrome or DIC Clotting normal in context of thrombocytopaenia in HUS and TTP
Biochemistry	Electrolytes Bone profile	Marked hyperkalaemia in tumour lysis syndrome or rhabdomyolysis Hyperkalaemia, hyperphosphataemia and hypocalcaemia with high CK in rhabdomyolysis Hypercalcaemia in multiple myeloma and metastatic malignancy
	Serum protein electrophoresis (SPE) immunoglobulins Serum free light chains (SFLC)[a] Urine BJP	Diagnostic in plasma cell dyscrasias
	CRP	Elevated in sepsis or infection and systemic inflammatory conditions
	LFTs	Abnormal in underlying liver disease Raised bilirubin in TMA/haemolysis
Virology	Hepatitis B and C, HIV	May be found in patients with AKI and proteinuria Essential screening to mitigate risk of nosocomial infection in all patients who may need RRT/dialysis
Point of care/ near patient testing	ABG	Marked acidosis in rhabdomyolysis or sepsis Mild-moderate acidosis common in all causes of AKI
Microbiology	Blood and urine cultures	If infection suspected

[a]Serum free light chains and protein electrophoresis have high sensitivity for detection of plasma cell dyscrasias and urine immunofixation may not be required unless AL amyloidosis is suspected[b]

[b]Dispenzieri A, Kyle R, Merlini G, Miguel JS, Ludwig H, Hajek R, et al. International Myeloma Working Group guidelines for serum-free light chain analysis in multiple myeloma and related disorders. Leukemia. 2009;23(2):215–24

9.8.2 Further Investigation

9.8.2.1 Urine Biochemistry

Traditionally, differential rises between urea and creatinine and fractional urinary sodium and urea excretion have been used to distinguish pre-renal from intrinsic renal failure due to acute tubular necrosis. These investigations are not often helpful with very limited utility in patients receiving diuretics, those with pre-existing renal or cardiac disease and those with sepsis [18]. More recently, several studies have identified the presence of tubular damage in patients with transient "pre-renal" AKI, and diffuse tubular necrosis may not always be present in intrinsic AKI [19]. Crucially, distinguishing between the two syndromes may be of little impact clinically as even transient "pre-renal" failure is associated with high mortality [20].

9.9 Other Blood Tests

Blood tests are complimentary to a thorough clinical assessment of patients with AKI, and it is frustrating that on occasions, an extremely expensive array of blood tests is undertaken before evaluation of fluid balance, review of the drug chart, dipstick urinalysis and consideration of the patient's escalation plan have been completed. However, in addition to narrowing the differential

Table 9.4 Immunological tests as part of a "renal screen" in patients in whom a glomerular cause of AKI is suspected such as those with blood and protein on urine dipstick

Anti-nuclear antibodies (ANA)	SLE, scleroderma, Sjogrens
Antibodies to extractable nuclear antigens (ENA)	SLE, scleroderma, Sjogrens
dsDNA	SLE
Anti-glomerular basement membrane (GBM) antibodies	Anti-GBM disease
Anti-neutrophil cytoplasmic antibodies (IIF) (ANCA)	ANCA-associated small vessel vasculitis
Antibodies against specific ANCA antigens (proteinase-3 PR3 and myeloperoxidase MPO)	ANCA-associated small vessel vasculitis
Complement components C3 and C4	Immune-complex diseases SLE, endocarditis, chronic deep-seated infection, post-infectious glomerulonephritis, cryoglobulinaemia
ASOT, anti-DNAse B	Post-infectious GN
Rheumatoid factor	Cryoglobulinaemia

9

diagnosis, blood tests may help a number of questions in patients with AKI.

- *Is the patient critically ill and in need of critical care?*
- *Is immediate renal replacement therapy required?*
- *Are additional medications required?*
- *Can invasive tests be performed?*
- *Is there evidence of improvement in renal function?*
- *Are modifications of existing prescriptions required?*

Serial measurements of urea, creatinine and electrolytes should be carried out. The presence of anaemia, hyperphosphataemia and hypocalcaemia may suggest chronic rather than acute kidney injury. However, all of these findings may also be seen in AKI. An assessment of the metabolic consequences of AKI should be made, looking for hyperkalaemia and metabolic acidosis. Other more specific tests directed at investigating the underlying cause of AKI should be guided by the patient's history and clinical situation. These tests are summarised in Tables 9.3 and 9.4.

9.10 Radiology

It is extremely likely that patients admitted to hospital acutely with AKI will have undergone a chest radiograph. Chest imaging may reveal air space shadowing, cardiomegaly, a cardiac silhouette suggestive of a pericardial effusion or mass lesions, all of which are likely to influence management decisions. Air space shadowing may be caused by fluid, infection or blood and may need to be resolved by radiological review with or without additional tests including cross-sectional imaging, echocardiography and measurement of the carbon monoxide transfer coefficient. Chest radiograph findings may change rapidly in patients with pulmonary haemorrhage in pulmonary-renal syndromes, and the authors recommend all patients with AKI and dipstick haematuria have a chest radiograph at presentation.

Renal ultrasound is cheap and noninvasive but can be difficult in some patient habitus and is subject to substantial inter-observer variation. It seems reasonable, albeit poorly evidence-based, to consider the pre-test probability of abnormal findings (features likely to alter the patient's management plan) before making a request. Patients at high risk of obstruction and those with a single functioning kidney are likely to have an ultrasound as part of AKI assessment. In the UK, NICE suggest that ultrasound is unnecessary if another cause of AKI is identified but that it should be performed in all patients with an unexplained AKI within 24 hours and urgently (within 6 hours) when pyonephrosis is suspected [21].

Although the terms are used synonymously, hydronephrosis (dilatation of the pelvicalyceal system) and obstruction are morphological and functional descriptions, respectively, and are not necessarily interchangeable.

Ultrasound may be very useful when distinguishing between acute and chronic renal impairment. Although CKD secondary to HIV, amyloid or diabetes may be associated with enlarged kidneys, patients with CKD often have small kidneys with thinning of the renal cortex. Additionally renal USS in CKD may show increased echogenicity and loss of corticomedullary differentiation.

9.11 Renal Biopsy

Renal biopsy should be considered when the cause of AKI is unclear or if pre- and post-renal causes have been excluded. If a putative diagnosis requiring specific treatments such as glomerulonephritis or interstitial nephritis is suspected, then biopsy should be carried out to guide management. In patients who fail to recover from AKI, renal biopsy is also warranted.

9.12 AKI in Patients with CKD

CKD is a significant independent risk factor for developing AKI, risk increases with increasing severity of CKD, and patients with proteinuria and CKD are at the greatest risk of AKI [22]. When patients with CKD have an episode of AKI, studies have shown that risk of progression to ESRD is increased even if their renal function returns to their usual baseline [23, 24]. The usual approach to clinical assessment of the cause of AKI should be followed in patients with CKD, but both the cause of their underlying renal impairment or treatment and medications they may have received for this should be considered as potential causes.

Tips and Tricks

1. Valuable information may be dispersed amongst the medical record, investigation results and drug and observation charts.
2. Thorough evaluation of a patient with AKI will allow a narrower differential diagnosis and target the most appropriate use of investigations.
3. Assessment of patients with AKI with a pre-renal cause may have had more than one renal insult.
4. Referring clinicians may not always recognise the severity of pre-renal insults.
5. Fluid resuscitation of patients with AKI is likely to need repeated assessment of the patient.
6. It is important to exclude post-renal causes of AKI in patients in whom no other cause of AKI is apparent.
7. Constellations of findings may suggest the need for urgent investigation. Patients with AKI with a prodromal history suggesting systemic inflammatory disease should have a chest X-ray and dipstick urinalysis. Where these yield abnormalities, the need for an acute renal screen is urgent.
8. Early diagnosis of causes of AKI associated with early irreversible loss of function can mean the difference between renal recovery and long-term dialysis.

Questions

- Question 1

A 58-year-old man presented with a 3-month history of weight loss, general malaise and fatigue. On direct questioning, he reported some nasal stuffiness and crusting. He had no significant past medical history. He worked in an office and was a non-smoker.

On examination, his blood pressure was 156/86, RR 18 and HR 82. He had pale conjunctivae and bilateral ankle oedema. His BMI was 17.4. Urinalysis showed blood 3+ and protein 2 + .
Investigations.

Haemoglobin	92 g/L
White cell count	$14.6x10^9/L$
Serum creatinine	200 μmol/L
Serum C-reactive protein	293 mg/L
Chest X-ray	Bilateral patchy air space shadowing

The results of a panel of blood tests to identify the cause of AKI were awaited.
Which investigation is most likely to lead to the underlying diagnosis?
A. Anti-neutrophil antibody.
B. Anti-neutrophil cytoplasm antibody.
C. High resolution CT chest.
D. Complement proteins C3 and C4.
E. Rheumatoid factor antibody.

- Question 2

1. A 78-year-old woman presents with a history of type 2 diabetes presented with an area of cellulitis surrounding a foot ulcer. She was admitted for treatment with intravenous flucloxacillin.

On examination, her blood pressure was 155/90, and she had a purulent ulcer with surrounding erythema. Urinalysis shows blood 2+ and protein 2 + .
Investigations after 2 days of IV antibiotics showed.

Haemoglobin	102 g/L
White cell count	$24.6x10^9/L$
Serum creatinine	350 μmol/L (200 μmol/L on admission, 60 μmol/L 2 weeks prior to admission)
Serum C-reactive protein	312 mg/L

What is the most likely cause of the change in creatinine observed in this case?
A. Diabetic nephropathy.
B. Pre-renal AKI.
C. Infection-related glomerulonephritis.
D. Tubulointerstitial nephritis.

E. Obstruction secondary to papillary necrosis.

- Question 3
  2. A 69-year-old lady presented with an AKI diagnosed by her GP on routine testing due to her history of hypertension. She was asymptomatic, and her only past medical history was hypertension treated with amlodipine. She had a painful right knee on walking for which she had recently been taking ibuprofen. She had no fevers or other systemic symptoms.

On examination, her blood pressure is 128/60 and HR 60.

Investigations

Haemoglobin	132 g/L
White cell count	10.6×10^9/L
Serum creatinine	550 μmol/L
Serum C-reactive protein	1.2 mg/L

9

Phase contrast microscopy was performed.

What urine microscopy finding is most likely?

A. Dysmorphic red cells and red cell casts.
B. Lipid droplets and oval fat bodies.
C. Isomorphic red cells.
D. White cells and white cell casts.
E. Granular casts.

Answers

- Question 1
  Answer: B
  This patient most likely has ANCA-associated small vessel vasculitis, and chest radiograph suggests he may have evidence of pulmonary haemorrhage. Complement proteins will also be useful as consumed C3 and C4 suggest an alternative diagnosis such as endocarditis which it would be important to exclude particularly if he had evidence of a murmur or prior to starting immunosuppression. CT chest should also be performed to investigate chest X-ray findings but will not lead to a definitive diagnosis. Rheumatoid factor and ANA are less helpful in this scenario.
- Question 2
  Answer: C
  The positive urine dipstick for blood and protein would not be expected in diabetic nephropathy, prerenal AKI or TIN. There may be haematuria in papillary necrosis, and she may have baseline diabetic nephropathy to account for the proteinuria, but the patient does not display any of the clinical features of obstruction due to papillary necrosis.
- Question 3
  Answer: D
  There is nothing in the history to suggest an acute glomerulonephritis (A), nephrotic syndrome (B), bleeding from elsewhere in the urinary tract (C) or ATN (E). It is most likely she has acute interstitial nephritis due to NSAID use which would result in white cells and white cell casts in the urine.

References

1. Bellomo R, Ronco C, Kellum JA, Mehta RL, Palevsky P. Acute renal failure - definition, outcome measures, animal models, fluid therapy and information technology needs: the second international consensus conference of the acute dialysis quality initiative (ADQI) group. Crit Care. 2004;8(4):R204–12.
2. Chertow GM, Burdick E, Honour M, Bonventre JV, Bates DW. Acute kidney injury, mortality, length of stay, and costs in hospitalized patients. J Am Soc Nephrol. 2005;16(11):3365–70.
3. Mehta RL, Kellum JA, Shah SV, Molitoris BA, Ronco C, Warnock DG, et al. Acute kidney injury network: report of an initiative to improve outcomes in acute kidney injury. Crit Care. 2007;11(2):R31.
4. 2011. Kidney Disease: Improving Global Outcomes clinical practice guideline on acute kidney injury 2011.
5. Sawhney S, Fluck N, Marks A, Prescott G, Simpson W, Tomlinson L, et al. Acute kidney injury-how does automated detection perform? Nephrol Dial Transplant. 2015;30(11):1853–61.
6. Swan SK. The search continues--an ideal marker of GFR. Clin Chem. 1997;43(6 Pt 1):913–4.
7. Johnson ACM, Zager RA. Mechanisms underlying increased TIMP2 and IGFBP7 urinary excretion in experimental AKI. J Am Soc Nephrol: JASN. 2018;29(8):2157–67.
8. Tsigou E, Psallida V, Demponeras C, Boutzouka E, Baltopoulos G. Role of new biomarkers: functional and structural damage. Crit Care Res Prac. 2013;2013:361078.
9. Hall PS, Mitchell ED, Smith AF, Cairns DA, Messenger M, Hutchinson M, et al. The future for diagnostic tests of acute kidney injury in critical care: evidence synthesis, care pathway analysis and research prioritisation. Health Technol Assess (Winchester, England). 2018;22(32):1–274.
10. Stevens PE, Tamimi NA, Al-Hasani MK, Mikhail AI, Kearney E, Lapworth R, et al. Non-specialist management of acute renal failure. QJM. 2001;94(10):533–40.
11. Liano F, Pascual J. Epidemiology of acute renal failure: a prospective, multicenter, community-based study. Madrid acute renal failure study group. Kidney Int. 1996;50(3):811–8.
12. Go AS, Parikh CR, Ikizler TA, Coca S, Siew ED, Chinchilli VM, et al. The assessment, serial evaluation, and subsequent sequelae of acute kidney injury (ASSESS-AKI) study: design and methods. BMC Nephrol. 2010;11:22.
13. Mansoor AM, Karlapudi SP. Images in clinical medicine. Kussmaul's Sign N Engl J Med. 2015;372(2):e3.
14. Leaf DE, Srivastava A, Zeng X, McMahon GM, Croy HE, Mendu ML, et al. Excessive diagnostic testing in acute kidney injury. BMC Nephrol. 2016;17:9.
15. Cavanaugh C, Perazella MA. Urine sediment examination in the diagnosis and Management of Kidney Disease: Core curriculum 2019. Am J Kidney Dis. 2019;73(2):258–72.
16. Perazella MA, Coca SG, Kanbay M, Brewster UC, Parikh CR. Diagnostic value of urine microscopy for differential diag-

nosis of acute kidney injury in hospitalized patients. Clin J Am Soc Nephrol: CJASN. 2008;3(6):1615–9.
17. Perazella MA, Bomback AS. Urinary eosinophils in AIN: farewell to an old biomarker? Clin J Am Soc Nephrol. 2013;8(11):1841–3.
18. Bagshaw SM, Langenberg C, Bellomo R. Urinary biochemistry and microscopy in septic acute renal failure: a systematic review. Am J Kidney Dis: Off J National Kidney Foundat. 2006;48(5):695–705.
19. Nejat M, Pickering JW, Devarajan P, Bonventre JV, Edelstein CL, Walker RJ, et al. Some biomarkers of acute kidney injury are increased in pre-renal acute injury. Kidney Int. 2012;81(12):1254–62.
20. Uchino S, Bellomo R, Bagshaw SM, Goldsmith D. Transient azotaemia is associated with a high risk of death in hospitalized patients. Nephrology, Dialysis, Transplantation: Official Publication of the European Dialysis and Transplant Association - European Renal Association. 2010;25(6):1833–9.
21. https://www.nice.org.uk/guidance/cg169/chapter/1-Recommendations 2013.
22. Hsu CY, Ordonez JD, Chertow GM, Fan D, McCulloch CE, Go AS. The risk of acute renal failure in patients with chronic kidney disease. Kidney Int. 2008;74(1):101–7.
23. Wu VC, Huang TM, Lai CF, Shiao CC, Lin YF, Chu TS, et al. Acute-on-chronic kidney injury at hospital discharge is associated with long-term dialysis and mortality. Kidney Int. 2011;80(11):1222–30.
24. Bucaloiu ID, Kirchner HL, Norfolk ER, Hartle JE 2nd, Perkins RM. Increased risk of death and de novo chronic kidney disease following reversible acute kidney injury. Kidney Int. 2012;81(5):477–85.

Prevention and Treatment of Acute Kidney Injury

Dinesha Himali Sudusinghe, Yogita Aggarwal, Chris Laing, and Mark Harber

Contents

M. Harber (ed.), *Primer on Nephrology*, https://doi.org/10.1007/978-3-030-76419-7_10

Learning Objectives

In this chapter, we aim to cover:

1. Generic preventative measures that can be employed to reduce the risk of AKI.
2. Treatment options and management of established AKI describing the evidence for those treatments with merit.
3. Specific management of AKI in conditions that benefit from unique treatments:
   - Contrast-induced acute kidney injury.
   - Tumour lysis syndrome.
   - Pigment-induced AKI.
   - Crystal-induced AKI.
   - Envenomation.

10.1 Introduction

Acute kidney injury (AKI) is common and associated with increased morbidity, mortality and extended length of hospital stay. It is recognized not only among hospitalized patients but also in the community. The incidence of AKI varys in different settings; approximately 7 to 18 percent of hospitalized patients, 30 to 70 percent of patients admitted to the intensive care unit (ICU) and 20 to 200 per million population in the community can have AKI [1, 2]. Among patients with AKI, the data suggests that even a modest rise in creatinine of 27 mmol/l can result in a seven-fold increase in mortality adding to poor patient outcome [3].

Recently, AKI and chronic kidney disease (CKD) have been recognized as interconnected entities and may represent a continuum of the same disease process. Thus, AKI survivors can progress to CKD and later end-stage kidney disease (ESRD) requiring dialysis [4]. The exact pathophysiological process linking AKI and CKD remains unclear. However, acute kidney disease (AKD) is recognized as a disease entity which links AKI and CKD (Fig. 10.1) with underlying maladaptive repair leading to chronic inflammation, fibrosis, nephron loss and CKD. Intervention taken during this stage to correct reversible factors of AKI may be important in preventing the disease progression [5]. The presence of pre-existing kidney disease, increased severity and duration

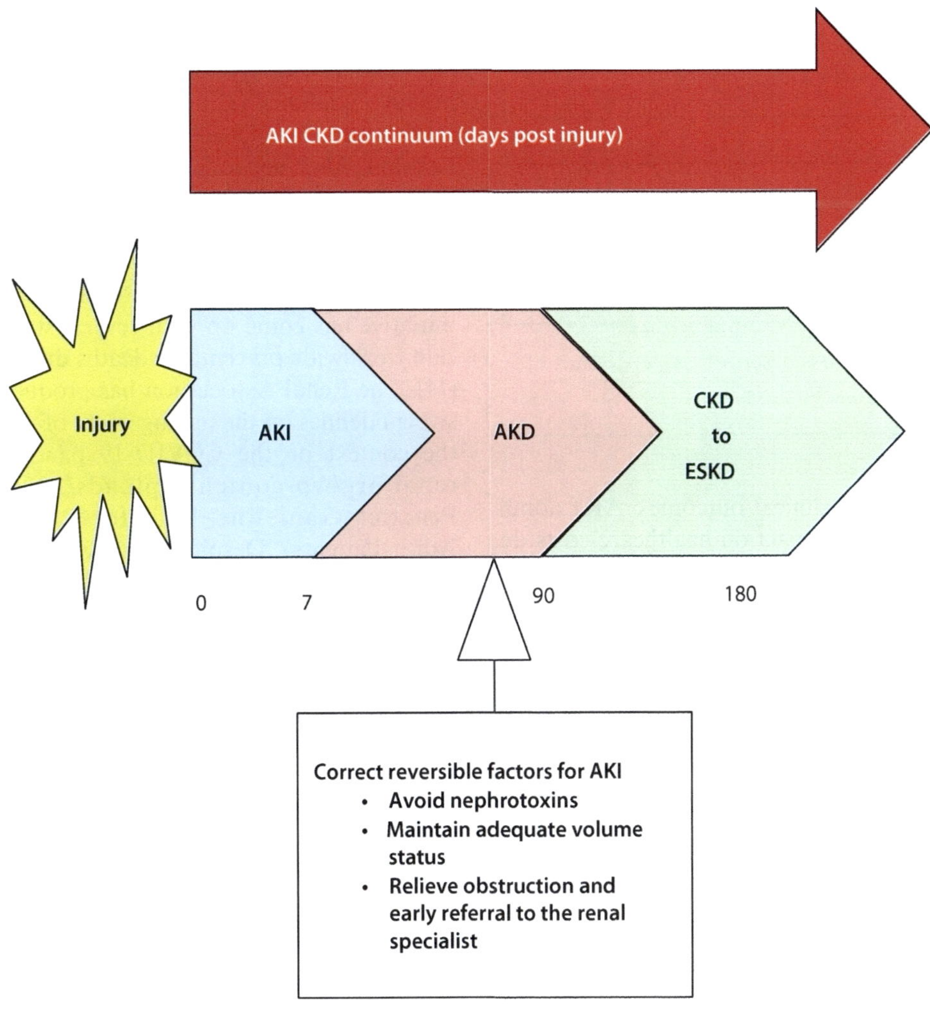

Fig. 10.1 The continuum of acute kidney injury (AKI), acute kidney disease (AKD) and chronic kidney disease (CKD)* [5]

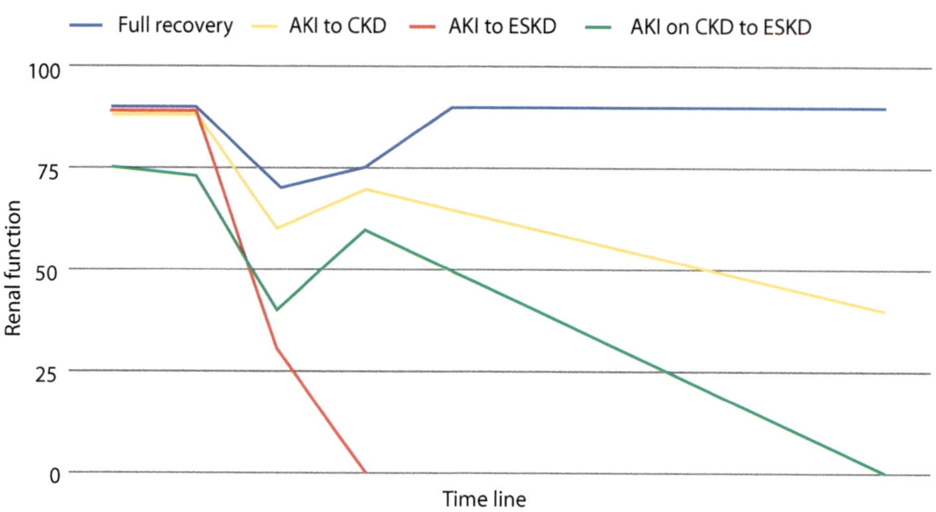

Fig. 10.2 Diagrammatic representation of the natural history of AKI

of AKI are associated with rapid decline in kidney functions following an episode of AKI (Fig. 10.2).

10

> Acute kidney disease is acute or subacute damage or loss of kidney function between 7 and 90 days after initial exposure to acute kidney injury.

> Acute kidney injury is an abrupt decrease in kidney function over 7 days or less.

> Chronic kidney disease is described as persistence of kidney damage beyond 90 days.

In addition to adverse clinical outcomes, AKI admissions have a significant impact on healthcare costs due to prolonged hospital stays. The estimated cost of AKI-related inpatient care to NHS England over a 1-year period is around £1 billion, accounting for about 1% of the NHS budget [6]. This has been brought into sharp relief for all of us given the huge impact of COVID-19 on renal services and ICUs not to mention our patients. UK data shows that one in four patients admitted to ICU in the UK due to COVID-19 requires renal replacement therapy (RRT). These patients had a mortality of up to 80% compared to 44% for those who did not require RRT. Moreover, these patients spent roughly three times as long in ICU compared to those without AKI. The vast spike in AKI and critically ill patients revealed weaknesses in supply chains and resilience in the system, emphasizing the critical importance of prevention in AKI as well as the importance of advanced care planning.

Over the last 10 years, multiple clinical guidelines to prevent AKI have emerged including 2012 KDIGO [7], 'Think Kidneys' in the acute kidney injury best practice guidance [8] and 2019 National Institute for Health and Care Excellence (NICE) guidance [9]. The London AKI network has produced pragmatic and practical guidelines to improve care bundles for the management of patients with AKI which can be modified to suit local practice and London AKI app [10]. The International Society of Nephrology (ISN) '0by25' initiative has come up with several strategies to eradicate worldwide preventable deaths due to AKI by 2025 [11]. The Renal Association has produced comprehensive guidelines on the management of AKI and RRT in the context of the COVID-19 pandemic (▶ https://renal.org/wp-content/uploads/2020/10/Clinical-Practice-Guideline_RRT-for-Critically-Unwell-Adult-Patients). Despite growing wealth of novel and accessible AKI tools and strategies, their implementation into clinical care and application into routine clinical practice have been suboptimal, and much more needs to be done. The National Confidential Enquiry into Patient Outcome and Death (NCEPOD) report, which analysed the deaths of patients in the UK with AKI, found that 30% of AKI-related deaths were avoidable and were a result of significant failures in the delivery of basic care [12]. Thus, AKI remains a significant and preventable endemic challenge, and there is a clear need to improve the awareness of this common condition among healthcare workers and the general public to improve the standards of care.

10.2 Prevention of AKI

Given that there is a notable dearth of effective 'cures' for established AKI, prevention is profoundly important. The NCEPOD report has provided useful recommendations on the prevention and management of AKI after reviewing deaths of patients with AKI in the UK (◘ Fig. 10.3), and it has set a challenging but not an unreasonable target to prevent all avoidable AKIs (and to better manage the unavoidable). The 0by25 initiative focuses on optimum management of AKI considering five domains, namely, risk assessment, early recognition, response, renal support and rehabilitation (◘ Fig. 10.4). Nephrologists can and should have an important impact on implementing these recommendations through training, audit and support as well as contributing to systems that assess risk and identify AKI [12].

Considering current evidence and recommendations, there are four main aspects of prevention: (1) improve awareness, (2) identifying patients at increased risk of AKI, (3) avoidance of renal insult and (4) prophylactic treatment. These themes have underpinned the development of AKI care bundles which have proved useful in reducing the progression of AKI, length of hospital stay and associated mortality [13].

10.2.1 Improve Awareness

This is an often overlooked but a key component in primary prevention. Individuals responsible for healthcare planning must recognize the burden of mortality, disability and cost associated with AKI. To address this issue, a multifaceted approach will be necessary, encompassing education, training and ongoing research coupled with a systematic process to disseminate information. Awareness of AKI needs to improve in all levels of the healthcare system, where educational programs should reach all non-specialist medical practitioners, nurses and allied personnel working in health care.

10.2.2 Identifying Patients at Increased Risk of AKI

The identification of risk factors of AKI is a crucial aspect of care (◘ Table 10.1). Some patients are at greater risk of developing AKI than others. Therefore, there needs to be a systematic and robust mechanism for ensuring that all such patients at risk are identified.

Over the last few years, working alongside the increasing electronic evolution of healthcare systems, there has been a drive to implement AKI e-alerts to assist in the early identification and initiation of treat-

Edited Recommendations from NCEPOD

- All emergency admissions should be assessed for risk of AKI
- All acute admissions should receive adequate senior review (consultant review within 12 hours)
- There should be sufficient critical care and renal beds to allow rapid escalation of care when required
- Undergraduate and post-graduate medical training should include the diagnosis, prevention, and management of AKI

◘ **Fig. 10.4** Focus areas for the 5R (risk assessment, early recognition, appropriate response, renal support and rehabilitation) approach for prevention and management of AKI. (*RIFLE* Risk, Injury, Failure, Loss, End-stage renal disease, *AKIN* Acute Kidney Injury Network, *KDIGO* Kidney Disease: Improving Global Outcomes, *RRT* renal replacement therapy [11])

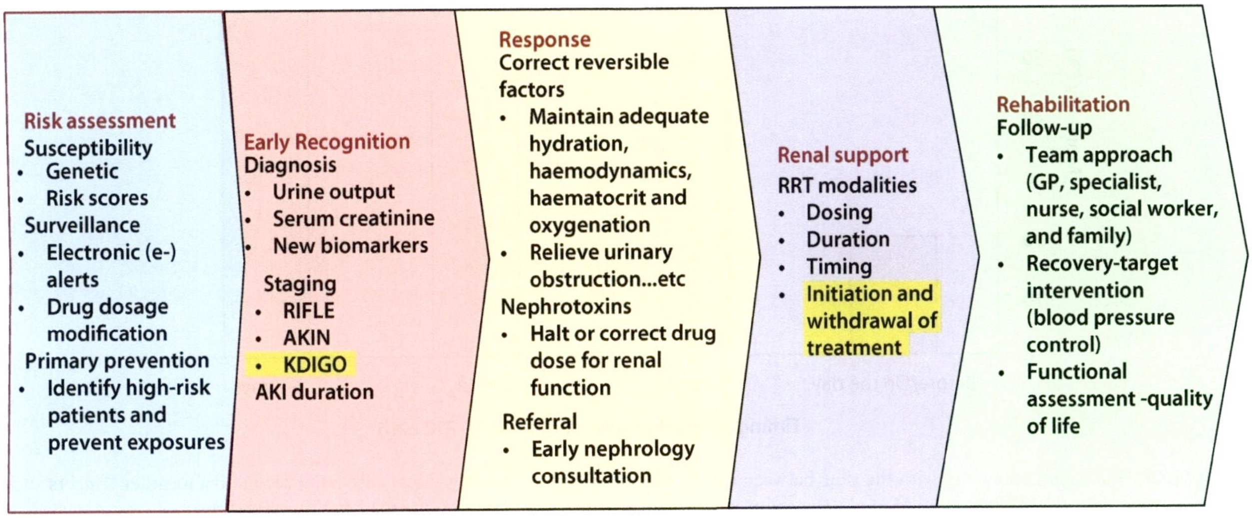

Risk assessment
Susceptibility
- Genetic
- Risk scores

Surveillance
- Electronic (e-) alerts
- Drug dosage modification

Primary prevention
- Identify high-risk patients and prevent exposures

Early Recognition
Diagnosis
- Urine output
- Serum creatinine
- New biomarkers

Staging
- RIFLE
- AKIN
- KDIGO

AKI duration

Response
Correct reversible factors
- Maintain adequate hydration, haemodynamics, haematocrit and oxygenation
- Relieve urinary obstruction...etc

Nephrotoxins
- Halt or correct drug dose for renal function

Referral
- Early nephrology consultation

Renal support
RRT modalities
- Dosing
- Duration
- Timing
- Initiation and withdrawal of treatment

Rehabilitation
Follow-up
- Team approach (GP, specialist, nurse, social worker, and family)
- Recovery-target intervention (blood pressure control)
- Functional assessment -quality of life

◘ **Fig. 10.3** Recommendations from the UK National Confidential Enquiry into Patient Outcome and Death (NCEPOD, 2009) report to prevent AKI [12]

Table 10.1 Common risk factors for development of AKI

Environmental and infrastructure
Insufficient clean water Inadequate health budget Insufficient healthcare human resources
Patient-related
Non-modifiable
Comorbid medical disorders Chronic kidney disease Diabetes Cancer Cardiac impairment Chronic gastrointestinal disease (e.g. decompensated liver disease)
Demographic factors Sex – Female gender Age – Older age Race – Black race
Modifiable
Dehydration Hypotension Malnutrition Sepsis Trauma Burn injury Surgical procedures, e.g. cardiac surgery Nephrotoxins

10

ment to prevent AKI and halt its progression. This system can instantly link into locally adopted AKI clinical guidelines and facilitate earlier and appropriate referral to the nephrology team and has been effective in improving AKI patient outcomes [14, 15]. In one retrospective analysis of patients seen by the critical care outreach team on the basis of other indications, those patients who were seen on the same day as their AKI alert had a much better outcome in terms of mortality or need for renal replacement than those seen on days after the AKI alert (Figs. 10.5 and 10.6). This does not prove that seeing patients with AKI early improves outcomes but does indicate that AKI is a biomarker for sickness, not reviewing patients at the time of their initial AKI alert is associated with a much worse outcome and using AKI alerts to identify patients early is eminently sensible.

10.2.3 Avoidance of Renal Insult

Strategies to avoid exposure to renal insults start with informing patients, their carers and primary care physicians the importance of maintaining adequate hydration, encouraging to check that any medication that is prescribed (or bought over the counter) is kidney-compatible and the importance of seeking assessment early if unwell. Patients can be educated on seeking advice on stopping angiotensin-converting enzyme inhibitors (ACEI), angiotensin receptor blockers

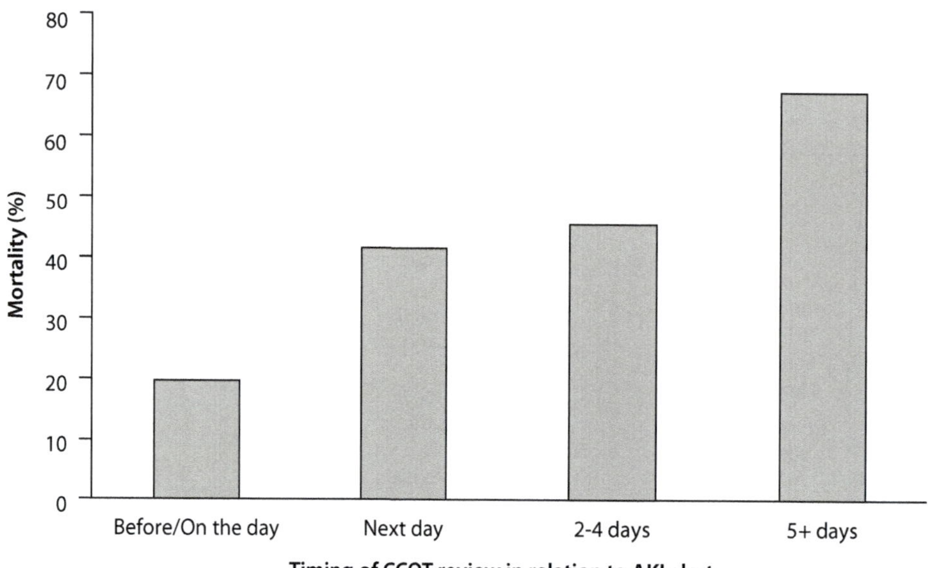

Fig. 10.5 Increasing mortality with the time between initial AKI alert and review by critical care team secondary to other triggers such as hypotension ($p = 0.018$) Prendecki M et al. (Reproduced with permission from postgraduate medical journal [15])

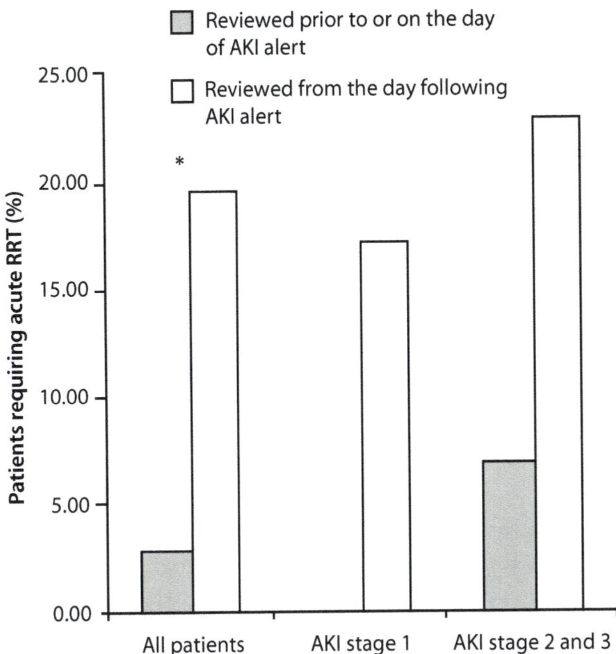

Fig. 10.6 Need for renal replacement therapy in patients reviewed by the critical care outreach team prior to or on the day of the initial AKI alert (grey) vs those seen by critical care the day following the AKI alert ($p = 0.05$) Prendecki M et al. (Reproduced with permission from postgraduate medical journal [15])

(ARBs), sodium-glucose cotransporter-2(SGLT-2) inhibitors and diuretics and avoiding NSAIDs if they develop a condition that makes them prone to acute episodes of hypotension such as vomiting and/or diarrhoea. These points need to be well documented in correspondence and reiterated at the time of administering the prescription. Empowering patients to know about the 'sick day rules' is advocated by the NICE AKI guidelines [9] and healthcare professionals, though the evidence base for such advice reducing AKI and harm is very weak.

In the hospital set-up, it is reasonable to ensure that minimal blood pressure limits are set for routine prescription of anti-hypertensives. Consideration also needs to be given to pharmacokinetics of medications that require dose adjustments. These are typically antimicrobials such as penicillin, aminoglycosides and antivirals, but the list is exhaustive, and thought should be given to every prescribed medication as to their ongoing requirement in the acute setting, duration of treatment and renal dose. There are several specifically renal-adapted resources that can be found either in the BNF or in the Renal Drug Handbook [16], and the increasing adoption of electronic prescribing linked to eGFR should reduce this risk. Where possible, iodinated contrast should be avoided or minimized (detail discussion of contrast-related AKI is discussed under CI-AKI) for patients with risk factors.

Table 10.2 Nephrotoxic medications and endogenous toxins (* TLC tumour lysis syndrome)

Endogenous
Light chains
Hypercalcaemia
Pigment nephropathy – TLS* and oxalate
Exogenous
Antibiotics – Aminoglycosides
Iodinated contrast agents
Non-steroidal anti-inflammatory drugs
Anticancer drugs
Antiretroviral drugs
Calcineurin inhibitors

Early cessation or avoidance of nephrotoxic agents (Table 10.2) is of paramount importance among patients at risk of developing AKI. ACEI, ARB and SGLT-2 inhibitors are not nephrotoxic (and are best not labelled as such) but, like NSAID, can have a profound effect on the kidneys' ability to autoregulate blood flow that it makes sense to consider withholding them in established AKI and/or before a major surgical procedure. There is a caveat here too as ACEI and ARBs have very substantial benefits in reducing cardiovascular mortality (and reducing proteinuria/renal progression); while it is very sensible to stop these, there need to be a strategy for reassessing patients with cardiac failure to decide on timely reintroduction, if appropriate. Having an electronic alert system to flag patients at risk of potentially hazardous medication is helpful. In the absence of intelligent IT solutions, clinical vigilance, training and education of healthcare workers are critical and particularly important in identifying patients at risk.

10.2.4 Prophylactic Treatment

The most generic and fundamental prophylactic treatment of AKI is to maintain good renal perfusion by ensuring optimum blood pressure targets. Hypotension with systolic blood pressure (SBP) <110 mmHg or mean arterial pressure (MAP) <65 mmHg needs to be assessed for consideration for volume expansion with the fluid challenges or early initiation of vasopressors if indicated.

10.3 Resuscitate Intravascular Volume and Restore Renal Perfusion

High-risk patients can be pre-hydrated either orally (with specific instructions, e.g. 'drink 1L before coming to hospital') or parenterally to expand intravascular volume. This is worth considering for anyone at risk of AKI following a surgical procedure, planning use of potentially nephrotoxic agents such as contrast, receiving chemotherapy (ifosfamide, cisplatin, mitomycin) or taking drugs causing crystal nephropathy (acyclovir, indinavir, triamterene, sulphonamides, methotrexate). The type of fluid used for hydration can vary depending on the clinical circumstance.

Early resuscitation with intravenous fluids is fundamental to ameliorate AKI in patients with hypovolemia, and the COVID-19 pandemic has demonstrated the importance of adequate fluid maintenance in those who are sick but not overtly hypovolaemic. Therefore, clinical assessment of fluid status is a crucial step in managing patients at risk of AKI. Timely reversal of volume depletion in patients with pre-renal AKI can improve renal perfusion and prevent progression to acute tubular necrosis (ATN). For instance, the increased rate of AKI in the early stages of COVID-19 has been the impact of 'running patients dry' to avoid provoking adult respiratory distress syndrome. Inadequate resuscitation and maintenance fluids almost certainly contributed to a huge excess of AKI and a global shortage of renal replacement equipment. This huge natural experiment has been an important reminder of the critical importance of maintaining appropriate hydration and intravascular volume. Therefore, the importance of fluid resuscitation should not be underestimated.

Intravenous fluids should be given only when indicated, and it should be prescribed like any other drug that is being prescribed to a patient. For example, it is recommended to consider 'four Ds' of fluid therapy in patients with septic shock, drug, dosing, duration and de-escalation, to avoid volume overload in non-volume-responsive patients [17]. Background history, examination, monitoring charts and investigations are key factors to determine appropriate fluid therapy (▣ Fig. 10.7).

Aggressive fluid therapy can have adverse consequences, and one should be cautious, specifically in patients at risk of fluid overload and progression to pulmonary oedema. A large multicentre study focusing on critically ill patients with AKI has shown that those with fluid overload (10% weight gain) at the time of initiation of dialysis had an odds ratio for death of 2.07 (95% confidence interval of 1.27–3.37). Thus, excessive fluid is dangerous not just by precipitating pulmonary oedema but in terms of mortality [18, 19]. To obtain the best clinical outcomes, serial fluid status assessment in line with the cardiovascular and renal functions are important. Central hemodynamic measurements can be used to assess volume responsiveness in intensive care settings.

History		Examination	Charts	Investigations
PMH -Heart disease -Kidney disease -Liver disease -Diabetes (can affect the type fluid you give)	**Drug history** -Diuretics -Antihypertensives -Nephrotoxic drugs ex:-NSAIDS	**General** -Temperature, -Capillary refill -JVP -Skin turgor -Oedema **Respiratory** -RR -SpO2 **Cardiovascular** -PR and BP (postural drop) - 3rd heart sound **Abdomen** -Ascites -Tender hepatomegaly	**Drug** **Fluid balance** -Input oral/NG/PEG tube/IV fluids/TPN -Output urine, stoma, diarrhoea..etc **Weight** **BP (postural drop)**	-Electrolytes -Blood urea and Scr -Full blood count -Lactate -Albumin -Glucose

▣ **Fig. 10.7** Factors that need to be assessed to determine the type and amount of fluid therapy. PMH (past medical history); NSAID (non-steroidal anti-inflammatory drugs); JVP (jugular venous pressure); RR (respiratory rate); PR (pulse rate); BP (blood pressure); NG (nasogastric); PEG (percutaneous endoscopic gastrostomy); IV (intravenous); TPN (total parenteral nutrition)

10.3.1 How to Determine the Type of Resuscitation Fluid?

There are two major classes of fluids, crystalloid solutions and colloids (◘ Table 10.3). 5% dextrose is not used as a resuscitation fluid due to the risk of severe hyponatremia. Initial choice of replacement fluid therapy depends on the cause of hypovolemia. For instance, blood products are used to treat haemorrhagic shock and crystalloids and colloids containing solutions for the non-haemorrhagic shock.

10.3.1.1 Crystalloids

Normal saline (0.9% saline) is inexpensive, and it is the most used crystalloid solution. It is hyperchloraemic relative to the plasma, and the use of large volumes can lead to hyperchloraemic metabolic acidosis. Hyperchloraemia theoretically can exacerbate AKI due to increased renovascular resistance. Among a group of healthy volunteers, administration of 0.9% saline has been associated with increased extravascular volume and reduced renal perfusion compared to buffered solutions [20]. To explore this association, a study conducted by Yunos et al. comparing normal saline and buffered solutions has shown reduced AKI rates in the buffered solution group (8.4% vs 10%) [21]. In contrast, the SALT trial found no significant difference between both types of fluids [22]. Similar findings were observed in SPLIT study with no difference in AKI in ICU patients receiving buffered solutions and normal saline although this study was criticized for including postoperative patients that received relatively smaller resuscitation volumes (median, 2 L) [23]. The follow-up of the SALT trial, the SMART study, demonstrated similar figures (◘ Table 10.4); however, use of balanced crystalloids resulted in a lower rate of composite outcome of death from any cause, new renal replacement therapy or persistent renal dysfunction [24]. Therefore, buffered crystalloids are a reasonable alternative to normal saline when large volumes of resuscitation fluids are required or if hyperchloraemic acidosis is a concern. It is important to remember that buffered crystalloids are modestly hypotonic and associated with the development of hyponatremia. Thus, the choice between buffered solutions and normal saline is individualized and depends on the patient's biochemical parameters and estimated volume of resuscitation fluid.

◘ **Table 10.3** Types of resuscitation fluids

Types of fluids	
Crystalloids	*Normal saline (0.9% saline)* *Buffered solutions* Lactated Ringer's Plasmalyte Bicarbonate
Colloids	*Synthetic* Hyperoncotic starch, dextran, gelatin *Human albumin* *Blood products* Packed red cells Blood substitutes (FFP, cryoprecipitate)

◘ **Table 10.4** Comparison of AKI rates in SPLIT (Effect of a Buffered Crystalloid Solution vs Saline on Acute Kidney Injury Among Patients in the Intensive Care Unit), SALT (Balanced Crystalloids versus Saline in Noncritically Ill Adults) and SMART (the Isotonic Solutions and Major Adverse Renal Events Trial) trials according to the type of fluids administered (buffered crystalloid group and saline group) [22, 23, 24]

Study	Results	
SPLIT	***N* = 2092**	
AKI in buffered crystalloid group (%)	102 of 1067 (9.6)	*P* = 0.77
AKI in saline group (%)	94 of 1025 (9.2)	
SALT	***N* = 13,347**	
AKI in balanced crystalloid group (%)	315 of 6708 (4.7)	*P* = 0.01
AKI in saline group (%)	370 of 6639 (5.6)	
SMART	***N* = 15,802**	
AKI in balanced crystalloid group (%)	1139 of 7942 (14.3)	*P* = 0.04
AKI in saline group (%)	1211 of 7860 (15.4)	

10.3.1.2 Colloids

Albumin

Albumin appears to be relatively safe in critically ill patients except in patients with a history of traumatic brain injury. A large RCT meta-analysis showed the use of albumin when compared to other fluid solutions in severe sepsis/septic shock was associated with decreased mortality (OR 0.82) [25]. The Saline versus Albumin Fluid Evaluation [SAFE] trial has demonstrated that use of 4% human albumin solution and 0.9% saline has shown similar renal outcome and mortality results and can be used as an alternative or adjunct in fluid resuscitation especially in patients who are at risk of pulmonary oedema with larger volume of replacements fluids

[26]. Furthermore, albumin infusion is also indicated in patients with liver cirrhosis with AKI due to hepatorenal syndrome.

Hydroxyethyl Starch (HES)

The use of starch solutions such as hydroxyethyl starch (HES) remains controversial because hypertonic HES may cause AKI due to osmotic nephrosis. The multicentre 6S Trial (798 patients) [27] and VISEP Trial (537 patients) [28] showed increased mortality rates and AKI with hypertonic HES compared to Ringer's acetate/lactate [29]. However, the CHEST study, enrolling 7000 patients who had been admitted to an intensive care unit, compared HES to isotonic saline and showed a lower overall rate of AKI with 6% HES (iso-oncotic) but more severe AKI with a greater need for renal replacement therapy (RR 1.21) [30]. Therefore, use of HES is not straightforward and should not routinely be used in fluid resuscitation of patients with AKI.

Blood

10

Administration of blood is indicated in patients with pre-renal AKI due to acute blood loss. However, it is important to remember that although the volume of blood being administered may be relatively small compared to traditional fluid resuscitation regimes with crystalloids, higher potassium content and oncotic effects may be sufficient to precipitate the need for premature extracorporeal renal replacement therapy in an oligoanuric patient. The supernatant potassium concentration [K+] of red blood cell (RBC) units is frequently much higher than normal human plasma potassium levels, especially in units nearing the end of their storage life. Consideration for sequential fluid balance assessment following each unit of blood and the use of contemporaneous diuretics reduces the likelihood of complications with transient hyperkalaemia and fluid overload.

10.3.1.3 Comparing Colloids and Crystalloids

There is a lack of evidence to support routine use of colloids to treat pre-renal AKI, and several trials have demonstrated renal toxicity with HES. The Colloid Versus Crystalloid (CRISTAL) study, including 2857 ICU patients [31], showed no difference in RRT requirement or 28-day mortality with colloids and crystalloids. However, it has shown low rates of vasopressor requirement and ventilation in patients treated with colloids. Further, a meta-analysis of 56 randomized control trials has shown no overall difference in mortality between crystalloids and artificial colloids (modified gelatins, HES, dextran) when used for initial fluid resuscitation [32]. Therefore, crystalloids are the preferred intravenous fluid over colloids for treating patients with pre-renal AKI due to non-haemorrhagic causes, and it is cost-effective over colloids.

10.3.2 Maintenance Fluids

Following initial resuscitation, maintenance fluids should be continued to replace the patient's daily requirements of water, electrolytes and glucose. The basic daily needs are water in an amount of 25–30 mL/kg of body weight, 1 mmol/kg potassium, 1–1.5 mmol/kg sodium and glucose or dextrose 5 or 10% (1.4–1.6 g/kg) to avoid starvation ketosis.

10.4 Special Consideration Should be Given to Prophylactic Treatments in the Following Situations

10.4.1 Contrast-Induced Acute Kidney Injury

Contrast-induced acute kidney injury (CI-AKI) is a potentially avoidable cause of AKI in hospitalized patients. It typically occurs within 48–72 hours of contrast administration but can extend up to 7 days. Although the pathogenesis of CI-AKI is not clear, contrast can induce significant vasospasm and direct proximal tubular cell toxicity causing functional impairment or cellular necrosis of tubular cells leading to AKI.

CI-AKI is known to occur at a rate of 25% in patients with risk factors for the development of AKI. Therefore, patients undergoing non-urgent contrast procedures should undergo careful risk assessment (◘ Fig. 10.8), iodinated contrast should be avoided in high-risk patients whenever possible, and alternative imaging options should be considered. However, emergency procedures should not be delayed for risk assessment and can be proceeded with meticulous post-procedure care guided by the renal specialists [33]. In such circumstances where contrast imaging is unavoidable, limiting the dose of contrast to a minimum, using iso-osmolar or low osmolar contrast agents and avoiding repeated doses in quick succession are recommended to avoid CI-AKI. ACE inhibitors, ARBs and metformin should be stopped temporarily and can consider reinstitution after 48 hours if renal functions are back to baseline and remain stable (◘ Fig. 10.9).

According to current evidence, ensuring adequate hydration with intravenous sodium chloride (NaCl) is the cornerstone of prevention of CI-AKI. Intravascular

Risk factors for CI-AKI	
Patient related factors	**Procedure related factors**
• Known/pre-existing renal impairment (CKD of any cause and eGFR less than 40 ml/min/1.73 m2) • Reduced renal perfusion (cardiac or liver impairment, sepsis, hypovolaemia) • Age 75 years or more • Renal transplant • Concomitant nephrotoxins • Multiple myeloma	• Dose of contrast (total volume > 350ml or > 4ml/kg) • Re-institution of contrast within 72 hours of initial administration • Angiography >computer tomography (CT) • High osmolality contrast agents > low or iso-osmolar contrast media

Fig. 10.8 Risk factors for CI-AKI (contrast-induced acute kidney injury) [34]

volume expansion improves renal perfusion and contrast elimination. A recent non-inferiority clinical trial (AMACING) challenges the protective effects of intravenous fluids and results to show that there was no statistical difference between hydration and no hydration groups regarding incidence of AKI. However, the validity of results was not convincing due to under-enrolment, low rate of intra-arterial and interventional procedures and having a higher number of patients with less severe renal impairment [35].

In addition to normal saline, isotonic bicarbonate can be used to hydrate patients to prevent CI-AKI. Theoretically, urinary alkalinization can reduce oxidative free radical generation during contrast procedures. However, the Prevention of Serious Adverse Events Following Angiography (PRESERVE) study demonstrated no additional benefit of bicarbonate compared to isotonic saline. Similar rates of AKI (9.5% versus 8.3%), need for dialysis at 90 days (1.3% versus 1.2%) or persistent kidney impairment by 90 days (1.1 versus 1.0) and death (2.4 versus 2.7) were seen in the bicarbonate and saline treatment groups, respectively [36]. Similarly, oral N-acetylcysteine delivers no clinical benefits [7].

A variety of studies have looked at dialysis or filtration pre- or post-contrast to reduce AKI. A meta-analysis by Cruz et al. showed that haemodialysis, hemofiltration or hemodiafiltration has no benefit in prevention of CI-AKI, preservation of residual renal function, volume overload or osmotically induced electrolyte shift with iodinated contrast. Therefore, dialysis patients can proceed with the next scheduled dialysis session following contrast administration [37].

In summary, condensing vast numbers of papers on CI-AKI, the bottom line is that reducing exposure to contrast in high-risk patients where possible and ensuring adequate hydration pre- and post-contrast, avoiding other concomitant nephrotoxins to prevent CI-AKI and anything else are distractions.

10.4.2 Tumour Lysis Syndrome

Tumour lysis syndrome (TLS) is an oncological emergency and a relatively predictable cause of AKI requiring coordinated management between the oncologist and the nephrologist. AKI is mainly due to metabolic derangement in TLS, and aggressive lymphomas and leukaemias are known to associate with TLS (Fig. 10.10) [38, 39]. Monitoring serum uric acid, potassium, calcium and phosphate within 3 days before and 7 days after is important for early detection and initiation of treatment. Prevention of renal toxicity is important because renal impairment is not only dangerous but can limit the continuation of further chemotherapy.

The main prophylactic therapy in TLS is hydration with isotonic saline or balanced crystalloids. The aim of hydration is to improve renal perfusion and increase urine output (achieve 2 ml/kg/hour) to minimize precipitation of uric acid and calcium phosphate within renal tubules. Diuretics (furosemide) are not routinely recommended and can be only considered to maintain urine output in euvolemic or overloaded patients without obstructive uropathy to achieve desired urine output. Hydration should be continued until there is no evidence of TLS or patients can continue oral fluids to maintain urine output. Urinary alkalinization as a mode of preventive strategy is not recommended as it increases the risk of calcium phosphate deposition in patients with marked hyperphosphataemia.

Pharmacotherapy with hypouricaemic agents (allopurinol or febuxostat) can be used to control uric acid burden. Treatment can be started with allopurinol in

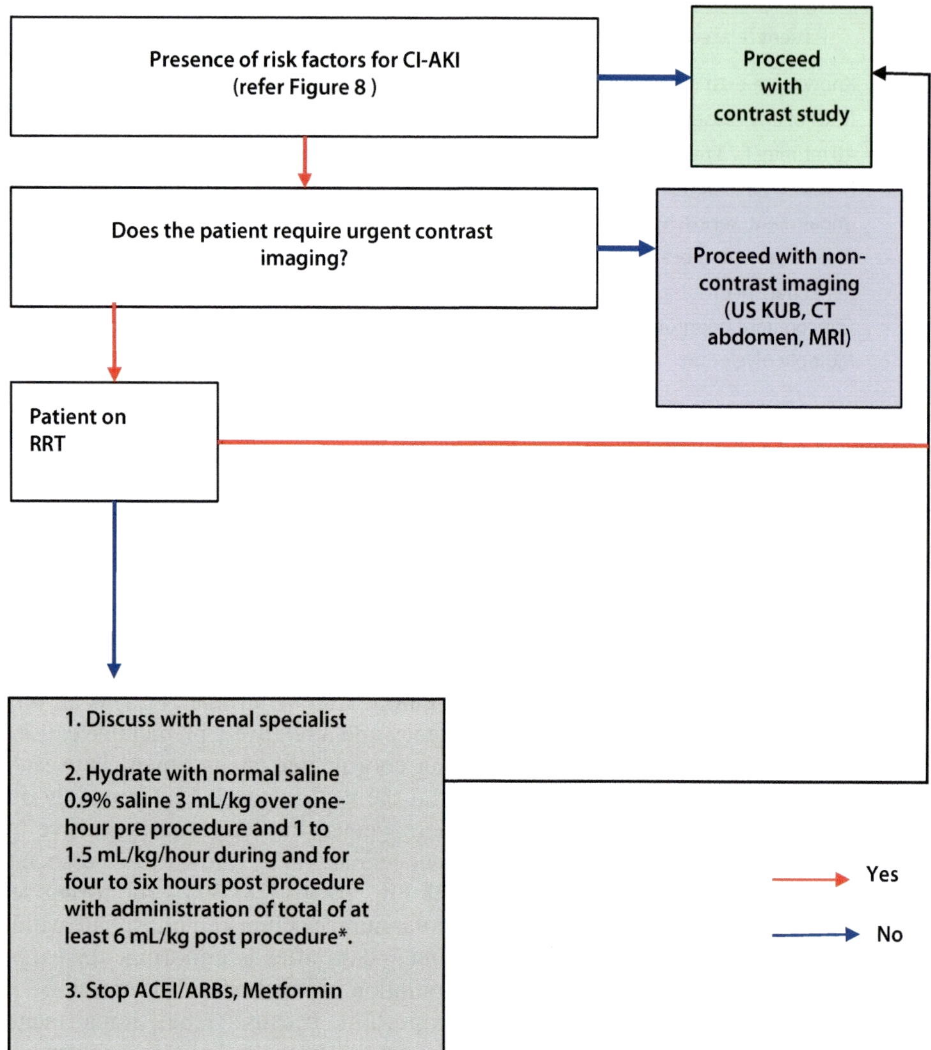

Fig. 10.9 Stepwise approach to prevent CI-AKI (contrast-induced acute kidney injury)

patients with an intermediate risk of TLS and pretreatment uric acid levels <8 mg/dl. Allopurinol dose should be adjusted according to renal functions. However, in high-risk patients (uric acid level >8 mg/dl) with deranged renal functions rasburicase (recombinant urate oxidase) is preferable over allopurinol. It breaks down poorly soluble uric acid to an inactive and more soluble metabolite of uric acid, allantoin, and rapidly reduces uric acid concentration (preferably within 4 hours of initiation of therapy). It is commonly given as a single dose (0.2 mg/kg), and the average duration of therapy is 2 days; however, treatment can be extended up to 7 days depending on biochemical derangements. Febuxostat (xanthine oxidase inhibitor) can be used in patients who cannot tolerate allopurinol and who have renal dysfunction or if rasburicase is unavailable or contraindicated (glucose-6-phosphate dehydrogenase deficiency) [40].

RRT is indicated in patients with established AKI despite optimum supportive therapy. Indications to initiate renal replacement therapy are like those with other causes of AKI. However, a low threshold to initiate dialysis can be considered due to rapid biochemical derangement. HD can remove uric acids as well as phosphates,

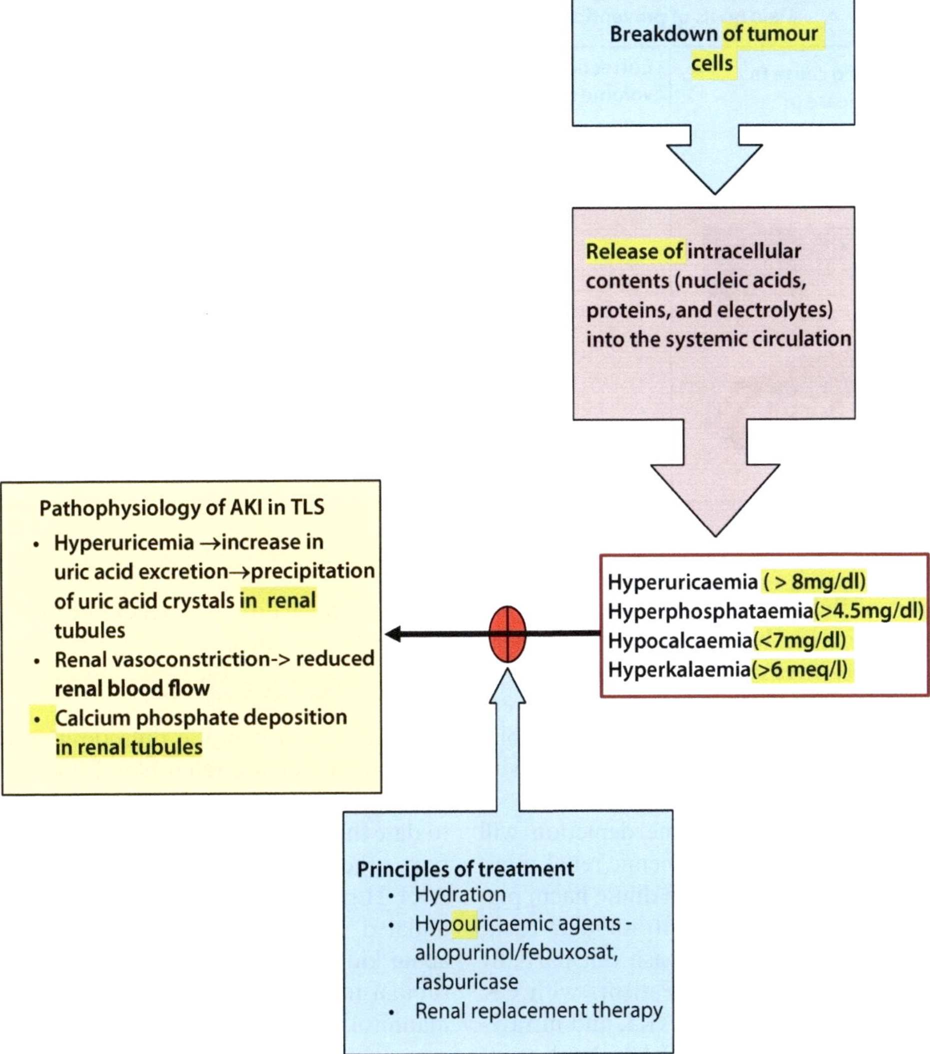

Fig. 10.10 Pathophysiology and principles of treatment in TLS (tumour lysis syndrome)

but CVVHD is better tolerated and effective than intermittent HD to prevent rebound hyperphosphatemia [41].

10.4.3 Pigment-Induced AKI

Pigment-induced AKI is a known complication of rhabdomyolysis and intravascular haemolysis (IVH). Renal injury is thought to be due to intravascular volume depletion and tubular damage from haem pigments. Identifying patients at risk of AKI is important to prevent renal damage. Advanced age, severity of muscle damage or haemolysis, baseline serum creatinine, initial serum phosphate and cause of pigment formation are the main risk factors. Treating the underlying cause of pigment nephropathy is critical in reducing the severity of the AKI as well as reducing long-term damage.

Early initiation of goal-directed therapy is paramount to prevent progression to AKI (Fig. 10.11). Accurate fluid status assessment, monitoring UOP and electrolytes are important to prevent adverse consequences.

10.4.3.1 Volume Resuscitation

Volume depletion is more common in patients with rhabdomyolysis than IVH due to sequestration of fluids within the affected muscles. Therefore, vigorous fluid therapy is the key to prevent AKI and should be started preferably within the first 6 hours of muscle injury at a rate to maintain a urine output of 200 to 300 mL/h. This will require an infusion of around 1.5 L/h of intravenous fluids. Volume status of the patient should be frequently assessed to prevent iatrogenic fluid overload, especially in patients who are not established to have adequate diuresis.

Main goals of prevention of pigment induced renal injury		
Correction of underlying cause to prevent continuous release of haeme pigments Ex. decompression fasciotomy in rhabdomyolysis 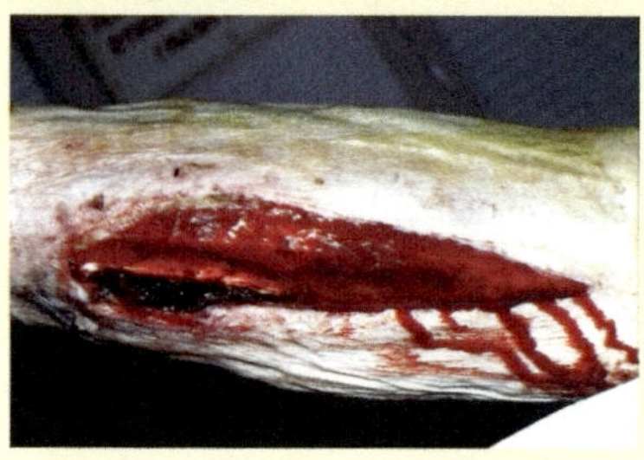	**Correction of intravascular volume depletion with,** • Isotonic saline/balance crystalloids • Isotonic bicarbonate	**Prevention of intratubular cast formation** • Hydration • Urinary alkalinization

Fig. 10.11 Approach to goal-directed therapy to prevent pigment-induced AKI

Specific choice of fluid with a greatest benefit is not clear and isotonic saline can be used as the initial resuscitation fluid. Multiple litres of 0.9% saline can lead to hyperchloraemic metabolic acidosis, which can theoretically decrease urinary clearance of myoglobin. Therefore, balanced crystalloids can be combined with isotonic saline after initial volume resuscitation [42].

Correction of intravascular volume depletion will improve renal perfusion and avoid ischemic renal tubular injury. Increase in urine volume can dilute haem pigments and minimize formation of intratubular casts, and increase in urine flow rate can wash out partially occluded casts within renal tubules. Patients with CK >5000 unit/L are at increased risk of AKI, and intravenous fluids should be continued until CK level starts falling and <5000 units/L. In patients with IVH, hydration should continue until haemolysis is controlled unless the patient develops signs of volume overload.

10.4.3.2 Urinary Alkalinization

Urine alkalinization prevents haem protein precipitation and intratubular cast formation. Therefore, bicarbonate infusions can be considered to hydrate patients in addition to isotonic saline/balanced crystalloids in patients with severe rhabdomyolysis, such as those with serum CK above 5000 unit/l.

Isotonic bicarbonate (1.26% sodium bicarbonate or 150 mL of 8.4 percent sodium bicarbonate mixed with 850 ml of 5 percent dextrose) can be given at a rate of 200 mL/hour to achieve a urine pH of >6.5, and if diuresis is established, the infusion can be continued until CK <5000 unit/l. Close monitoring of serum and urine biochemistry is required to ensure there is no hypocalcaemia, arterial pH is <7.5 and serum bicarbonate is <30 mmol/l. Bicarbonate can precipitate calcium phosphate deposition and worsen the degree of hypocalcaemia, and caution is recommended if patients are already hypocalcaemic [43].

10.4.3.3 Mannitol

Mannitol is an osmotic diuretic which was originally thought to increase renal blood flow, reduce renal cast formation and act as a free-radical scavenger. However, to date there are no randomized controlled trials to support the use of mannitol in pigment-induced AKI. Higher doses of mannitol (>200 g per day or accumulated doses of >800 g) have been associated with acute kidney injury due to renal vasoconstriction and tubular toxicity (osmotic nephrosis), and routine use of mannitol is not recommended. If it is used, plasma osmolality and the osmolar gap should be monitored frequently, and treatment should be discontinued if adequate diuresis is not achieved or the osmolar gap rises above 55 mOsm per kilogram [44].

10.4.3.4 Loop Diuretics

Loop diuretics had been previously used to achieve forced diuresis; however, it is not recommended in rhabdomyolysis except for the medical management of fluid overload. Use of diuretics can worsen urine acidosis, and there is no benefit in mortality, need for dialysis or length of stay in patients with rhabdomyolysis and renal injury.

10.5 Renal Replacement Therapy

RRT, specifically continuous RRT (CRRT), should be considered in patients who are anuric with elevated creatinine or having evidence of life-threatening hyperkalaemia, fluid overload or uraemia. Only 4% to 20% of patients with AKI caused by rhabdomyolysis typically require RRT. CRRT is associated with more stable haemodynamics compared to intermittent RRT and removes myoglobin and other inflammatory molecules. Despite clearance of myoglobin, RRT does not provided additional mortality benefits compared to medical therapy, and it should be considered when life-threatening complications of AKI emerge.

10.5.1 Crystal-Induced AKI

Crystal-induced AKI occurs due to precipitation of intratubular crystals which result in obstruction and occasionally an inflammatory response. In addition to uric acids, drugs and their metabolites and toxins that are poorly soluble in urine can cause crystal-induced nephropathy. Identification of risk factors such as volume depletion, renal insufficiency, liver disease and changes in urinary pH is important, and AKI can be prevented by premedication, hydration, appropriate medication dose adjustment and urinary alkalinization [45].

10.6 Acyclovir

Intravenous acyclovir is rapidly excreted in urine and has a poor solubility. Therefore, acyclovir crystals can be deposited in volume-depleted patients and can result in tubular obstruction and inflammation. Pre- and post-hydration with intravenous fluid aiming for a high urine output (above 75 mL/hour) can reduce rapid development of high tubular lumen acyclovir concentrations and reduce the risk of development of AKI. Oral therapy is usually well tolerated, presumably due to slow acyclovir excretion. Addition of a loop diuretics may facilitate high urine flow rates, but diuretic-induced fluid loss must be replaced. Haemodialysis can remove a substantial amount of acyclovir, but use is limited to correct metabolic consequences of AKI and neurotoxicity. RRT does not prove to reverse or limit the duration of AKI.

10.7 Methotrexate

Methotrexate (MTX) can typically cause non-oliguric AKI when administered in high doses, especially when the patient is volume depleted and the urine is acidic. The plasma creatinine concentration usually peaks within the first week and returns toward baseline level within 1–3 weeks. This is a medical emergency because 80–90 percent of the drug is excreted unchanged in the kidney and delay in excretion of MTX can cause life-threatening adverse effects.

The standard treatment of MTX toxicity is intravenous fluid therapy, urinary alkalinization and leucovorin rescue. Aim of expansion of the intravascular space is to increase urine flow rates to wash out crystals within the tubular lumen to minimize or avoid nephrotoxicity. Current recommendation is to administer intravenous fluid 2.5 to 3.5 litres/m^2 over 2 hours, preferably 12 hours before starting MTX infusion and to continue 24–48 hours afterwards. Early initiation of hydration is paramount to avoid progression to acute tubular necrosis at which point renal recovery will be delayed despite hydration and other measures.

MTX and its metabolites, 7(OH)MTX and DAMPA, are poorly soluble at acidic pH, and urinary alkalinization (pH >7) will help to prevent precipitation of crystals. Therefore, apart from hydration, 40–50 mEq of sodium bicarbonate can be added to each litre of intravenous fluid. This approach can be considered in a non-oliguric patient without evidence of hypocalcaemia and metabolic alkalosis [46].

In addition to above therapeutic strategies, leucovorin rescue is recommended to prevent adverse effects due to MTX toxicity such as myelosuppression and hepatotoxicity. Leucovorin is an active metabolite of folic acid which is an essential coenzyme for nucleic acid synthesis. MTX inhibits nucleic acid synthesis by blocking the activation of folic acid. Thus, leucovorin antagonizes MTX action by providing activated metabolite of folic acid and also by competing with MTX to enter into cells via the same transport process.

A recombinant bacterial enzyme, glucarpidase, is approved by the Food and Drug Administration (FDA) to use in patients with delayed MTX excretion. It is a rescue agent that cleaves MTX into inactive metabolites (DAMPA and glutamate), providing an alternative route of elimination for the drug in patients with nephrotoxicity. A single dose of glucarpidase (50 U/kg i.v. over 5 minutes) reduces plasma methotrexate concentration by 97% or more within 15 minutes. However, it does not have an effect on intracellular MTX; therefore, co-administration with leucovorin is recommended to protect cells until renal recovery. Leucovorin should not be administered within 2 hours before or after a dose of glucarpidase because, like methotrexate, leucovorin is a substrate for glucarpidase and leucovorin efficacy can be reduced if it is given at the same time. In addition to increased extrarenal metabolism of MTX, observational studies have shown that glucarpidase has some effect on early renal recovery. However, further research in this area is needed to assess the optimum timing and likelihood of renal recovery [47].

Therapeutic use of haemodialysis, charcoal haemoperfusion or plasma exchange for drug removal is of limited value due to large volume of distribution, and

MTX is being a protein bound medication. However, high flux haemodialysis and CRRT found to be effective in removal of MTX.

10.8 Indinavir

Indinavir is a protease inhibitor that is used to treat human deficiency virus infection. It can cause kidney damage by crystal deposition and nephrolithiasis.

Indinavir has a low solubility at urinary pH of 6 but is much more soluble at lower pH values. However, acidification of urine is difficult to achieve and potentially harmful; thus, urine acidification is not recommended. Increased fluid intake (around 2–3 L/day) prior to each oral dose may decrease the risk of crystal formation and allows to continue indinavir in approximately 75% of patients [45].

10.8.1 Aminoglycoside-Induced Nephropathy

10

Aminoglycosides deserve special mention as cheap and highly effective bactericidal antibiotics which are particularly useful for initial treatment of sepsis. However, drugs such as gentamicin, tobramycin and amikacin are associated with significant proximal tubular toxicity (and ototoxicity) potentially exacerbating AKI.

The bactericidal effect of aminoglycosides is dependent on the peak dose, whereas toxicity is time-dependent and correlates with trough levels. Aminoglycosides are taken up by the megalin receptor of the proximal convoluted tubule which is saturated at high doses. This means that divided doses have the highest toxicity, while once-daily dosing and a single initial dose have a low risk of nephrotoxicity. Nomograms have been developed for patients with renal impairment including 36- and 48-hour dosing [48]. While we need these antibiotics, inappropriate usage and dosing and poor monitoring are very common [49]. ◘ Table 10.5 suggests some ways in which nephrologists might collaborate with colleagues to reduce the risk of nephrotoxicity from these important drugs. Dialysis removes aminoglycosides and might be considered in patients with toxic levels and poor renal function.

◘ **Table 10.5** Prevention of aminoglycoside-induced nephropathy

Identify patients at risk and avoid if possible	Elderly, hypotensive, known renal impairment, diabetic, already on other nephrotoxins, who had a recent course of aminoglycosides
Review cultures after initial dose	Consider alternative in high-risk patients
Once daily dosing	Clear evidence of enhanced effect and reduced toxicity
Antibiotic control team	Review choice, dose, monitoring and length of treatment
Appropriate monitoring of levels	This is not done well generally – Protocols linking pharmacists, microbiologists and the lab are worth developing
Dose adjustment for renal impairment	The renal drug handbook or e-prescribing tools
Avoid concomitant nephrotoxins	Loop diuretics in high dose, CNIs and any other tubular toxins

10.8.2 Envenomation

10.8.2.1 Snakebite Envenomation

Snakebites are common in tropical countries, especially in the south, southeast Asia and sub-Saharan Africa, and most of the affected individuals are young and engaged in agricultural activities.

AKI is recognized as an independent predictor of mortality, and bite to hospital time or bite to needle time more than 2 hours, hypotension, regional lymphadenopathy, cellulitis, low serum albumin, prolonged bleeding time, prolonged prothrombin time, low haemoglobin and high total bilirubin are found be risk factors for the development of AKI [51]. Therefore, both pre-hospital and in-hospital management are important to prevent progression to AKI (◘ Fig. 10.12).

Bleeding from the bite site (fang mark), swelling or blistering (typical of hump-nosed viper bite) can be seen following snakebites (◘ Fig. 10.13). Community awareness is important to discourage applying tourniquets, local incisions, suction of venom or application of cow dung on the bite site because these measures are associated with adverse complications; especially, use of tight tourniquets is known to increase the risk of renal injury due to rhabdomyolysis [50].

In-hospital management depends on the presence or absence of envenomation, and it is important to identify whether the victim has evidence of systemic envenomation. AKI is known to occur 48–72 hours after snakebite and sometimes can extend up to 3–5 days. Therefore, victims should be closely monitored in the hospital or in the community for development of AKI even if the renal involvement is not evident at presentation. Delay in diagnosis and treatment can lead to irreversible cortical necrosis needing RRT.

AV is the definitive treatment of snakebite and early administration is helpful to prevent complications

Management of snake bite	
Pre-hospital management • Reassurance and attempts to identify the snake • Immobilization of the bitten extremity • Quickly transfer the victim to the nearest hospital	**Avoid** ⊗ • Excessive activity of the affected area • Applying constricting bands over the bitten extremity • Applying suction

In hospital management
• Detail clinical assessment and species identification • Observe up to 24 to 48 hours to look for signs of envenomation • Commence supportive therapy as early as possible • Careful fluid resuscitation in hypotensive patients • Tetanus toxoid • Support systemic involvement - ventilation, renal replacement therapy • Bite site management - wound care, look for evidence of compartment syndrome • Antivenom(AVS) therapy, observe response and determine need for repeat doses

Indications for antivenom		
Local envenomation		**Systemic envenomation**
• Swelling involving more than half of the bitten limb (in the absence of a tourniquet) within 48 hr of the bite • Rapid extension of swelling (Ex: beyond the wrist or ankle within a few hours of bites on the hands or feet) • Enlarged tender lymph nodes draining the bitten limb	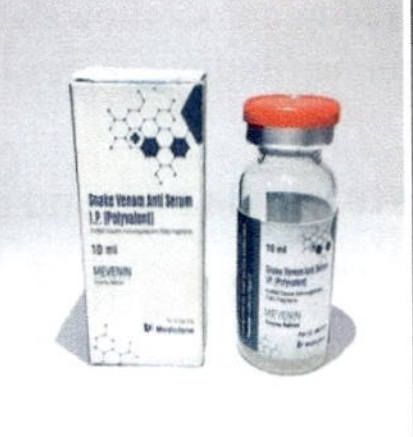	• **Haematological**- spontaneous systemic bleeding • **Neurological**-paresthesia, abnormalities of taste and smell, ptosis, external ophthalmoplegia • **Renal** - haematuria, haemoglobinuria, myoglobinuria, oliguria/anuria • **Cardiovascular** - hypotension, cardiac arrhythmias • **Endocrine** - hyponatraemia, evidence of pituitary insufficiency

Fig. 10.12 Suggested management of snakebite envenomation

(Fig. 10.14). AV is an immunoglobulin purified from plasma of horses or sheep that is hyperimmunized with venoms. It can cause allergic reactions resulting in anaphylactic shock and death. Therefore, AV should be used when there is evidence of systemic envenomation, and prophylactic antivenom in the absence of envenomation is not encouraged. Monovalent antivenom neutralizes the venom of one species of snake, and polyvalent antivenom can neutralize venoms of several different species of snakes [52]. Further, type and dose of AV can vary according to the region. Therefore, administration of AV developed for snakes from a specific geographical location is more effective than giving AV produced for another region. Thus, identification of the snake is important to guide therapy [53].

To date, administration of AV greatly depends on clinical evidence of envenomation, and identification of species is difficult based on symptoms alone. Therefore, most of the patients end up receiving polyvalent AV, which is not the most effective therapy. The development of reliable diagnostic tools to identify species could, therefore, initiate a paradigm shift in the treatment of snakebites [54].

Delay in diagnosis and treatment may lead to oliguric AKI needing RRT. During recovery, they can progress to non-oliguric AKI with polyuria, and measures should be taken to prevent volume depletion and electrolyte imbalances. Patients with delayed renal recovery beyond 4 weeks need a renal biopsy to identify the extent of renal injury and should be referred to the nephrolo-

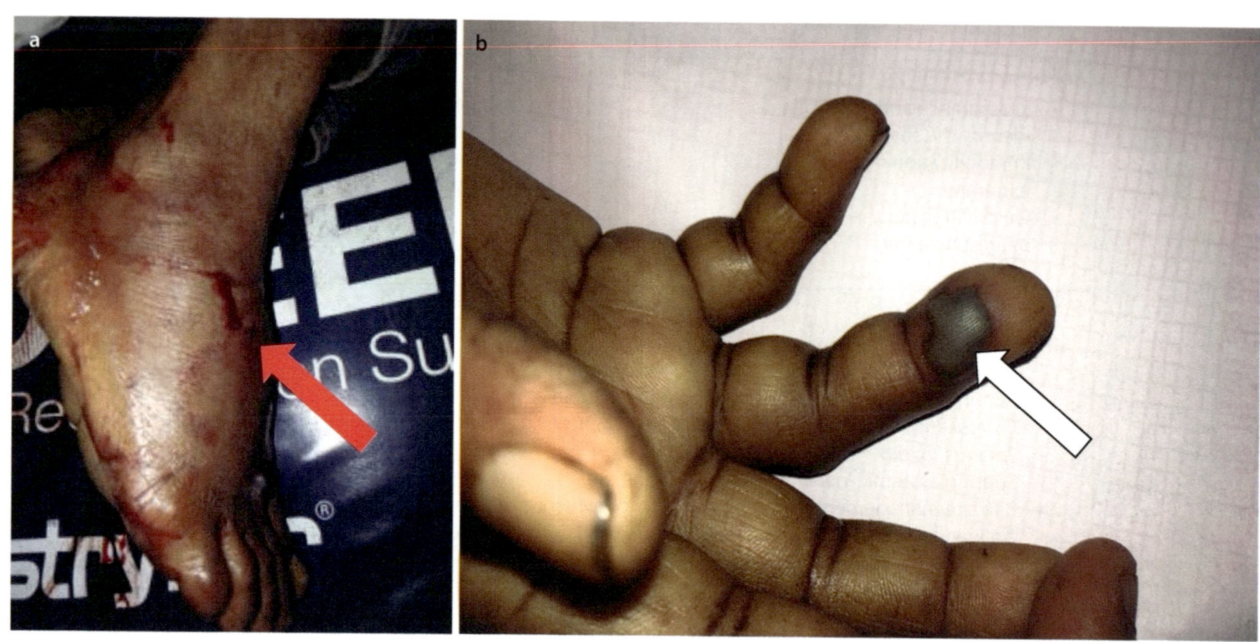

Fig. 10.13 **a** Red arrow points towards bleeding from fang mark following a snakebite, **b** white arrow points blistering following hump-nosed viper bite. (Image courtesy to Anjana Silva and Kalana Maduwage, Sri Lanka)

10

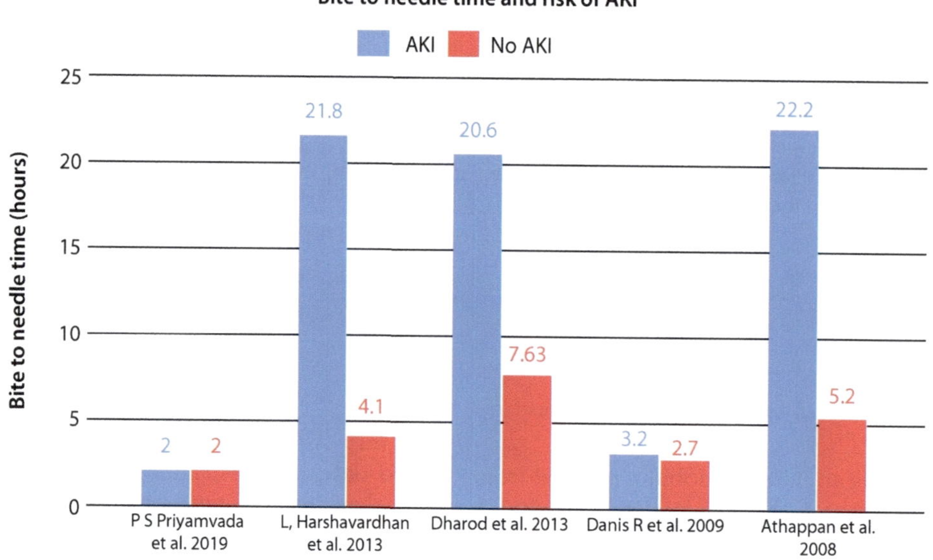

Fig. 10.14 Bite to needle time and risk of development of AKI

gist. Common histological findings are cortical necrosis and acute interstitial nephritis, and glomerulopathy can be seen rarely.

10.9 Hymenoptera Envenomation

Although mass attacks from bees, wasps and hornets are rare, cases remain a serious problem in China, South Asia, Southeast Asia as well as Latin America. Mass attacks can result in AKI, and arterial hypotension following anaphylactic shock is the main cause of AKI following bee stings. Intravascular haemolysis, rhabdomyolysis and direct toxicity of the venom components to the renal tubules are other aetiologies for AKI. The severity of AKI seems to be associated with the number of stings; creatinine levels were reported to be higher in most cases when there were more than 1000 stings [55].

There is no specific treatment for AKI beyond rapid hospitalization, fluid resuscitation and dialysis [56]. Removal of the inoculated stings from the victim's body should be carried out as soon as possible to avoid longer sting-to-skin contact time to prevent higher venom inoculation. The type of removal (by scraping or pinching) is considered irrelevant and should be as fast as possible to shorten exposure time. However, it is important to remove the stinger without squeezing it. Nonetheless, this approach should not delay the medical treatment.

AKI caused by *Hymenoptera* envenomation is associated with high mortality, and avoidance of envenomation is paramount to prevent complications. All patients with a history of severe reactions to insect bites should avoid *Hymenoptera* insects to the best of their ability and should always carry an epinephrine auto-injection pen.

10.9.1 AKI in Pregnancy

Pregnancy can be complicated with AKI from a variety of causes and is a major concern in low-income economies. Aetiology can be related to obstetric complications, pregnancy-specific disorders and miscellaneous causes that are unrelated to pregnancy.

Treatment of obstetric AKI starts with early diagnosis of obstetric emergencies and specific treatment of the emergency. For instance, urgent delivery should be considered in patients with severe pre-eclampsia. Rapid and aggressive intervention may reduce the risk of cortical necrosis, but there is a critical caveat: fluid resuscitation in the setting of pre-eclampsia/eclampsia may run a high risk of invoking pulmonary oedema. Indications for dialysis are similar to the general population.

Detailed discussion of this topic can be found in ▶ Chap. 50. In terms of prevention and treatment of AKI, it is important to establish clear protocols with obstetric departments and facilitate early referral and senior review.

10.10 Treatment of Established or Incipient AKI

Therapeutic approach to treatment of AKI depends on the aetiology of AKI, whether the underlying cause is pre-renal, renal or a post-renal.

10.11 Pre-Renal AKI

The management of pre-renal AKI is mainly restoration of intravascular volume status, and this is discussed under prophylactic therapy.

10.12 Intrinsic Renal Disease

In most cases of intrinsic renal disease, management depends on the underlying cause and is covered in subsequent chapters. As with endogenous toxins, the key is early diagnosis (haematuria, proteinuria or pyuria being important clues) and prompt investigation (several days' wait for an anti-GBM antibody level is not appropriate if Goodpasture's syndrome is the real diagnosis), and urgent nephrological assessment of all patients suspected to have intrinsic renal disease needs to be built into local care pathways. Service level agreements with immunology departments and alerting the nephrologist on call to any positive anti-GBM result will enable early initiation of treatment. Similarly, myeloma kidney is a medical emergency requiring rapid diagnosis and prompt initiation of treatment.

10.13 Post-Renal AKI

The treatment of post-renal causes of AKI is covered in ▶ Chap. 55 and requires rapid identification and timely resolution of the obstruction.

It is worth emphasizing that an infected obstructed urinary tract is a medical emergency and UK guidelines recommend that an ultrasound of the renal tract is performed within 6 hours in a septic patient if pyonephrosis is a possibility. Another circumstance to consider is the contribution of abdominal compartment syndrome (ACS), defined as a sustained pressure >20 mmHg and evidence of organ dysfunction. This is often missed as a contributing factor to AKI in a patient with tense ascites and with tension sutures following a laparotomy or particularly in young patients with acute third spacing in the abdomen secondary to conditions such as pancreatitis in which abdominal pressures can be so high as to not only cause impaired arterial perfusion and venous drainage but visceral infarction. A hand on the abdomen may indicate high pressure, urinary catheter pressures may give some quantification, and rapid consideration of decompression may be required.

Once the AKI is established, the treatment options are limited and mainly supportive. The general management principles are common to all patients: (1) maintaining optimum blood pressure to improve perfusion pressure, (2) treatment of sepsis, (3) careful use of/avoidance of drugs that are not routinely used to prevent or treat AKI, (4) intensive glycaemic control, (5) nutritional support and rehabilitation, (6) management of complications and (7) timely initiation of renal replacement therapy and early referral to a nephrologist [7].

10.13.1 Maintaining Optimum Blood Pressure

It is vital to maintain an optimum mean arterial pressure (MAP) in hypotensive patients to prevent further renal damage. Vasopressors and inotropes should be considered in patients with persistent hypotension despite initial fluid resuscitation. The sepsis and mean arterial pressure (SEPSISPAM) trial targeting a MAP of 80 to 85 mm Hg as compared with 65 to 70 mm Hg in patients with septic shock did not show significant difference in mortality at either 28 or 90 days. However, in patients with a history of chronic arterial hypertension, targeting a mean arterial pressure of 80 to 85 mm Hg was noted to have reduced incidence of AKI and need of renal-replacement therapy compared to low MAP groups. There was no significant difference between groups with regard to overall rate of serious adverse events, but patients in the high MAP target group had significantly more episodes of atrial fibrillation. Thus, blood pressure target should be individualized depending on the premorbid blood pressure, weighing the beneficial effects of greater renal perfusion and potential deleterious effects of vasoconstriction resulting in hypoperfusion of other organs [57].

10

Norephedrine is the first vasopressor of choice in the context of sepsis and hypotension [58]. Dopamine may be particularly useful in patients with compromised systolic function. However, routine use of dopamine over norephedrine as first-line vasopressor support is not recommended as it is less potent and associated with a greater incidence of arrhythmic events and short-term mortality. Despite its persistence in the 'we must do something' armamentarium, there is no evidence for the use of low-dose dopamine to encourage renal function. A large randomized trial and meta-analysis compared low-dose dopamine to placebo and found no difference in the peak serum creatinine, need for renal replacement, urine output, time to recovery of normal renal function and survival [59].

Often patients with intrinsic causes of AKI can present with hypertension. For example, glomerulonephritis is classically present with high blood pressure or accelerated hypertension, and its management is discussed in ▶ Chap. 12. Care with capping the blood pressure is required to avoid cerebral hypoperfusion-related strokes and seizures. Initial BP control in these patients should be with short-acting IV therapies, and later oral medications such as calcium channel blockers and alpha blockers can be used. However, ACEI and ARBS should be avoided until the creatinine has stabilized post-AKI recovery.

10.13.2 Treat Sepsis

Sepsis is a contributing factor for around 50% of AKI and associated with a significantly worse outcome. Prevention of sepsis-associated AKI (S-AKI) is usually impossible due to the presence of AKI at the time of presentation. Therefore, early recognition of AKI in the setting of sepsis is vital to provide optimal treatment and avoid further kidney injury.

The 'surviving sepsis campaign' (SSC guidelines) and proponents of early goal-directed therapy advocate rapid assessment and implementation of treatment care bundles in the setting of sepsis [60]. The SSC guidelines are extensive and have multiple recommendations, but a more digestible bundle, derived from the original guidelines, known as the Sepsis 6 (◘ Fig. 10.15), is straightforward and easy to implement and audit (downloadable as a free app 'sepsis 6').

While these publications were not specifically focused on AKI, implementation of 'sepsis 6' within an hour is associated with decreased mortality and length of hospital and ICU stay [61]. Goal-directed therapy to control the infection by diagnosing the pathogen, early appropriate antibiotic therapy (within 1 hour) and source control with the aid of appropriate investigations remains the backbone of sepsis treatment. Minimizing nephrotoxic agents (special consideration for using aminoglycosides, vancomycin and antifungals), drug dose adjustments according to renal functions and cautious use of contrast in diagnostic evaluation are important in preventing progression of AKI. Supportive care should be initiated immediately (◘ Fig. 10.16), patients who failed to respond to initial therapy will require renal replacement therapy, and this will be discussed under RRT and in detail in ▶ Chap. 10.

10.13.3 Drugs that Are Not Routinely Used to Prevent or Treat AKI

10.13.3.1 Loop Diuretics

Loop diuretics were considered to have a role in protecting the kidney from AKI by decreasing oxygen consumption in the loop of Henle and potentially lessening ischaemic injury. It was believed that furosemide might also hasten recovery of AKI by washing out necrotic debris blocking tubules and by inhibiting prostaglandin dehydrogenase, which reduces renovascular resistance and increases renal blood flow. While theoretically reasonable, clinical evidence would suggest that loop diuretics may precipitate an AKI by precipitating volume depletion. A systematic review by Krzych et al. includ-

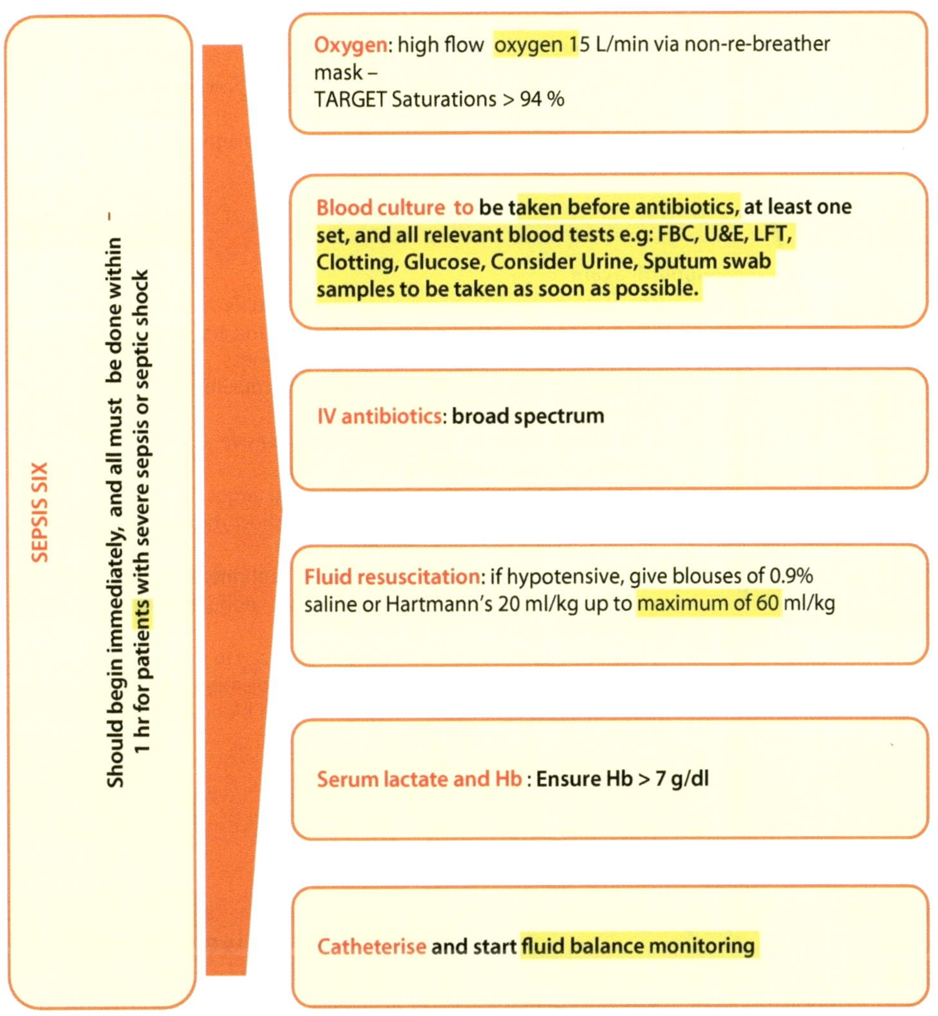

Fig. 10.15 Diagrammatic representation of sepsis 6 care bundle [60]

ing 20 RCTs with over 2600 patients with AKI or at risk of AKI found that furosemide did not have an impact on mortality or need for RRT [62].

It is important to avoid furosemide in acutely hemodynamically unstable patient due to its venodilatory effects. A potential indication for furosemide in patients with AKI is fluid overload with stable blood pressure. While loop diuretics have no role in preventing AKI, they may (typically as an infusion) have a useful role in managing potassium and volume in volume replete patients with established AKI (Table 10.6).

10.14 Dopamine

Dopamine causes renal vasodilation, natriuresis and increased GFR in healthy kidneys. For this reason, it was initially considered to be beneficial in the prevention or treatment of AKI; but this has not been supported by clinical data and use of dopamine to treat AKI is not recommended.

A prospective, double-blind randomized controlled study by Lauschke et al. including 30 intensive care patients with AKI, to investigate the effect of 'low-dose' dopamine on renal resistance indices (determined by Doppler ultrasound), found that 'low-dose' dopamine can worsen renal perfusion in patients with AKI. These findings add to the rationale for abandoning the routine use of 'low-dose' dopamine in critically ill patients [64].

10.15 Fenoldopam, Natriuretic Peptide, Theophylline and Growth Factor Intervention

While all championed in the past, they have no clinically beneficial role in the prevention or treatment of AKI [7].

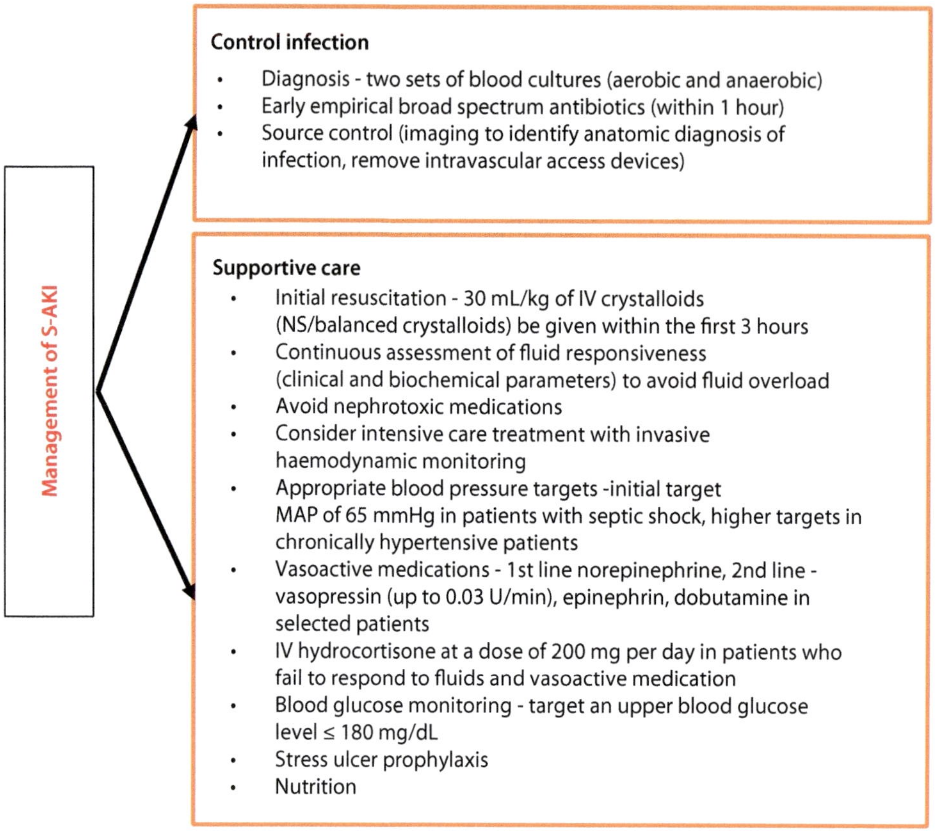

Management of S-AKI

Control infection
- Diagnosis - two sets of blood cultures (aerobic and anaerobic)
- Early empirical broad spectrum antibiotics (within 1 hour)
- Source control (imaging to identify anatomic diagnosis of infection, remove intravascular access devices)

Supportive care
- Initial resuscitation - 30 mL/kg of IV crystalloids (NS/balanced crystalloids) be given within the first 3 hours
- Continuous assessment of fluid responsiveness (clinical and biochemical parameters) to avoid fluid overload
- Avoid nephrotoxic medications
- Consider intensive care treatment with invasive haemodynamic monitoring
- Appropriate blood pressure targets -initial target MAP of 65 mmHg in patients with septic shock, higher targets in chronically hypertensive patients
- Vasoactive medications - 1st line norepinephrine, 2nd line - vasopressin (up to 0.03 U/min), epinephrin, dobutamine in selected patients
- IV hydrocortisone at a dose of 200 mg per day in patients who fail to respond to fluids and vasoactive medication
- Blood glucose monitoring - target an upper blood glucose level ≤ 180 mg/dL
- Stress ulcer prophylaxis
- Nutrition

10

Fig. 10.16 Parallel and sequential steps in the management of sepsis-associated AKI

Table 10.6 Possible roles and pitfalls or harmful effects of using furosemide in patients at risk of or with established AKI [63]

Potential roles of furosemide in AKI	Pitfalls or harmful effects of using furosemide in AKI
To avoid fluid retention in patients with co-existing acute lung injury	An improvement in urine output can be misinterpreted as an improvement in renal function
As part of the therapy for hypercalcaemia and AKI	Limits the use of urinary sodium concentrations to differentiate between hypovolaemia and normo-volaemia
Using urinary response to furosemide as a prognostic test to predict the risk of requiring RRT	Induces ototoxicity at high doses in patients with reduced renal clearance of furosemide
To manage hyperkalaemia	Delay in initiation of RRT

10.15.1 Intensive Glycaemic Control

Hyperglycaemia is associated with worse outcomes in critically ill patients, and initial studies demonstrated significantly reduced rates of AKI and renal replacement therapy in patients treated with intensive insulin therapy. However, subsequent studies have failed to confirm improved outcomes, and intensive insulin arms are associated with increased mortality and episodes of significant hypoglycaemia [65].

Patients with AKI are at risk of severe hypoglycaemia given the kidneys' role in insulin and glucose metabolism. The current evidence is summarized in the KDIGO AKI guidelines, but in essence, the cumulative evidence does not support intensive glycaemic control [7].

10.15.2 Nutrition and Rehabilitation

AKI is a catabolic state, and patients with severe AKI may be in the hospital for weeks, losing substantial amounts of flesh weight, incurring critical illness and neuropathy and becoming depressed. A holistic approach is often an underappreciated yet vital aspect of AKI recovery. Nutrition needs to be considered on a daily basis and nutritional support starts early (ideally within 48 hours), preferably via enteral feeding and aiming for 20–30 kcal/kg/day and protein of 0.8–1 g/kg/day (increasing if on RRT or catabolic) [7].

Mobilization with physiotherapy support (if required) should be instigated as soon as possible. Stable patients on CRRT may benefit from early conversion to intermittent haemodialysis in ICU to permit mobilization. Getting patients into clothes, if possible, out of the ward for breaks, providing talking books, games and clear explanations of projected recovery and future are often somewhat neglected aspects of care in patients recovering from a serious illness.

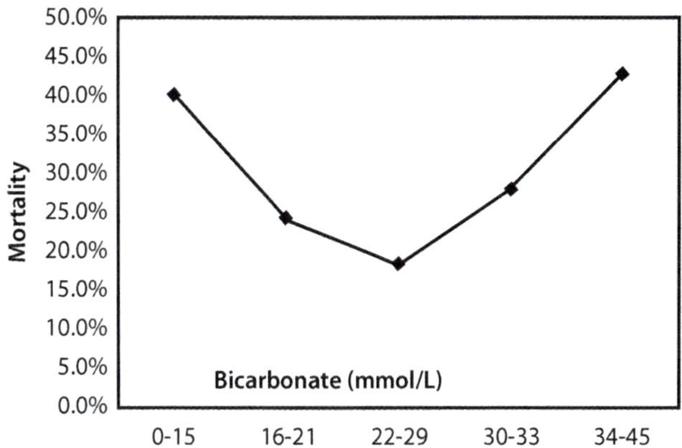

Fig. 10.17 A retrospective study of over 500 patients with AKI, presenting bicarbonate as a predictor of mortality. In those with a bicarbonate <22 mmol/L, mortality was 25.7% compared with 16.9% when bicarbonate was 22–29 mmol/L and 27.5% when >29 mmol/L ($p = 0.047$). This was most pronounced in patients with AKI stage 1; mortality is 24.3% when bicarbonate <22 mmol/L, 12.0% when 22–29 mmol/L and 25.6% when >29 mmol/L ($p = 0.015$). Significantly more patients with an abnormal bicarbonate required ITU admission; 25.7% when <22 mmol/L, 14.7% when 22–29 mmol/L and 24.1% when >29 mmol/L ($p = 0.015$). The need for acute RRT was greatest in those with low bicarbonate compared with the two other groups, 7.3% vs 2.2% vs 1.7% ($p = 0.019$). Prendecki M et al. (Reproduced with permission from postgraduate medical journal [15])

10.15.3 Management and Avoidance of AKI Complications

The NCEPOD enquiry into AKI deaths demonstrated that fluid overload, acidosis and hyperkalaemia were quite common complications of AKI, and despite being predictable hazards these complications were not infrequently missed.

Management of fluid overload has been touched on above, and it is important to actively resuscitate a patient who is intravascularly depleted. Once AKI is established, there is no evidence in favour of pushing fluids beyond maintenance requirements. Ensuring that oliguric patients are not iatrogenically overloaded is important. For those who are fluid overloaded, venodilators such as GTN (as an infusion) may be helpful, and for those who are not anuric but who have pulmonary oedema, they may respond to diuretics (e.g. loop diuretic infusion). Ultimately, RRT may be the only option, but pulmonary oedema is a situation best avoided in the first instance.

Acidosis is a common complication and a predictor of outcome. Fig. 10.17 is from a retrospective study of inpatients with AKI. On the day of the AKI presentation, a single serum bicarbonate measurement predicted patient mortality and renal replacement therapy. This may simply indicate that abnormal bicarbonate levels are a biomarker of sickness, but awareness that the patient with an abnormal bicarbonate is at greater risk is an important alert [14]. Correction of bicarbonate is not straightforward, and rapid corrections are potentially dangerous. However, oral or cautious intravenous bicarbonate solution can be particularly helpful in managing hyperkalaemia and potentially avoiding the need for renal replacement in a patient with the potential for rapid recovery from AKI.

Hyperkalaemia is extremely common in AKI, a common indication for renal replacement therapy, hence, the importance of identifying the problem and causes of hyperkalaemia. Ceasing drugs that might be contributing, treating acidosis and provoking a diuresis in auric patients who are intravascularly replete and insulin and dextrose are often lifesaving, etc.

Newer potassium binders, sodium zirconium and patiromer, appear to be much more effective and rapidly acting than polystyrene sulfonates (e.g. calcium resonium) and may have a role in avoiding dialysis or permitting safe transfer to a dialysis unit if employed early enough but are not a substitute for renal replacement in the setting of pulmonary oedema or uraemic encephalopathy [66].

10.16 Indications for Renal Replacement Therapy

Despite treatment, some patients may progress to severe AKI requiring renal replacement therapy (RRT). Detailed discussion of RRT is discussed in ▶ Chap. 10 and this section gives an overview of RRT in AKI.

Table 10.7 Indications for haemodialysis

Conventional indication for haemodialysis in AKI	
Hyperkalaemia	If resistant to medical treatment
Fluid overload	If resistant to medical treatment
Severe metabolic acidosis	If resistant to medical treatment
Uraemia	Impaired consciousness, pericardial rub
Drug intoxications	Methotrexate, salicylate, lithium, hyperoxalosis

When AKI is complicated with some of the metabolic and volume status-related complications (Table 10.7), the patient needs RRT. However, when severe AKI is not complicated with conventional indications, it is unclear whether the patient may benefit by early initiation of RRT. Commencing RRT may improve the patient's outcome, and there may be a need to anticipate the requirement for RRT in severe AKI. Therefore, is it important to ensure early referral to the ICU or local renal unit to ensure time is factored in for the patient transfer especially if the dialysis unit is at a different hospital.

The current practice is to offer dialysis as clinically indicated due to lack of evidence regarding the most effective timing for initiation of such therapy. Thus, nephrologists identify patients who are not going to recover safely with medical therapy and make a robust plan to provide RRT in a safe and timely manner. A recent multinational randomized controlled trial involving 2927 critically ill patients with AKI compared standard versus accelerated initiation of renal replacement therapy in acute kidney injury (STARRT-AKI). As per the study results, accelerated renal replacement strategy was not associated with a lower risk of death at 90 days compared to standard strategy (relative risk, 1.00; 95% confidence interval [CI], 0.93 to 1.09; $P = 0.92$). Adverse events (mainly hypotension and hypophosphataemia) occurred in 346 of 1503 patients (23.0%) in the accelerated-strategy group and 245 of 1489 patients (16.5%) in the standard-strategy group ($P < 0.001$). Among survivors at 90 days, a higher percentage of patients were continued dependence on renal replacement therapy in the accelerated-strategy group (10.4% vs 6.0%). Thus, this suggests that greater exposure to renal replacement therapy, possibly modified according to baseline risk (e.g. the presence of chronic kidney disease), may compromise kidney repair and the return of baseline kidney function [67].

Table 10.8 Suggested inter-hospital transfer criteria (London AKI network)

Suggested inter-hospital transfer criteria (London AKI network)	
Hyperkalaemia	No ECG changes of hyperkalaemia, potassium ≤6 mmol/L (not transient, i.e. the result of recent insulin and dextrose administration)
Acidosis	pH ≥7.2, venous bicarbonate 12 mmol/L, lactate ≤4 mmol/L
Cardiovascular	Heart rate ≥ 50 and ≤ 120 bpm, systolic blood pressure ≥ 100 mm hg (sustained), mean arterial pressure ≥ 65 mm hg, lactate ≤4 mmol/L
Respiratory	Respiratory rate ≥ 11 bpm and ≤ 26 bpm, saturations ≥94% on not more than 35% oxygen. If required CPAP then independent of this for ≥24 hours
Neurological	Glasgow coma scale ≥12

10.17 Transfer Criteria

Many but not all patients with AKI can be managed locally. For those that cannot and need inter-hospital transfer to a renal unit, then the transfer should be speedy, but clear criteria need to be established regarding patient stability and suitability as death on transfer is not unheard of. The London AKI network generated the following guidelines which are a very useful starting position for negotiation, are common sense and can be modified locally depending on resources (Table 10.8).

10.18 Treatment Escalation Plans and Ceilings of Care

Finally, the COVID-19 pandemic has starkly highlighted the need for an early holistic assessment of patients with serious illness. Nephrologists are increasingly referred to frail patients with significant comorbidity who have developed AKI due to an intercurrent illness. Frequently, the question is 'does this patient need acute renal replacement therapy?' and 'if the renal function did not recover would they be suitable for long-term dialysis?'. These are often exceedingly difficult decisions made at a time when the patient is at their most vulnerable stage, and the decision is often made with limited information. These are challenging decisions and should not be made casually. However, early thoughtful assessment of ceilings of care is important when appropriate and needs to be carefully discussed with the patient and the next of kin. This is an extremely important part of nephrology care with a significant responsibility.

10.19 Outcome of AKI

As stated in the introduction, for a long time the seriousness of AKI was under-estimated, but it is now clear that AKI is associated with extremely high mortality. Roughly 50% of patients with AKI require renal replacement on ICU die, and this rises to nearly 70% if combined with sepsis. In one multicentre multinational study using the RIFLE categorization, renal failure was associated with ten times the relative risk (RR) of death, and 'risk' and 'injury' had a RR of 2.5 and 5.4, respectively [68]. But even outside the setting of critically ill patients, AKI makes its mark. A review of Medicare data from the 1990s showed an average inpatient hospital mortality of roughly 5% in patients who did not develop AKI, but inpatient mortality was three to six times higher in those with AKI, and 90-day mortality was nearly 50% [69]. Increasingly recognized are the long-term renal consequences of AKI. A meta-analysis of studies following children with HUS, previously thought to have no long-term consequences, revealed that at 5–10 years 25% of children had either hypertension, proteinuria or CKD [70]. A meta-analysis in adults dividing AKI into mild, moderate and severe showed a relative risk of subsequent CKD of 2, 3 and 28, respectively [71]. The severity of AKI is thus a key factor, and in one study the need for renal replacement therapy conferred a 500-fold increased risk of developing CKD compared to no AKI [72]. AKI in the setting of CKD is not only very common but confers a fourfold increased risk of ESRD compared to patients with CKD who do not have an episode of AKI.

10.20 Follow-Up of AKI

Given the evidence that even apparently reversible AKI has a significant risk of CKD, it seems sensible to ensure a follow-up. The intensity of follow-up and whether it is done by nephrologists or in primary care depends to a large extent on the recovery from AKI and the likelihood of recurrence. There are not yet clear guidelines on this but there are formulas to predict the risk of CKD. A practical approach would be to ensure that patients with significant AKI but good recovery have blood pressure, urine dipstick and creatinine checked annually. Those without complete recovery may need to be seen and assessed as a one-off in an AKI renal clinic, which permits accurate recording of diagnosis, proteinuria, recovery and risk of CKD. Prospective data sets of AKI will be extremely valuable, and recording episodes of AKI in patients' diagnostic lists is important.

10.21 Summary

AKI is not a benign condition and can have profound short- and long-term consequences for patient morbidity and mortality. There is a huge potential for improving standards of care and patient experience starting with an ongoing audit of AKI management. Nephrologists, through training and teaching, need to raise the profile of AKI, promote systems to develop local protocols and AKI networks, implement straightforward guidance and be responsive to early referrals and transfer of appropriate patients. Remember, AKI-associated deaths are predictable and often preventable.

Tips and Tricks

1. Establishing early warning of AKI is an important first step in prevention. Educating and engaging with other departments to ensure rapid detection and intervention is a key responsibility of nephrologists. It is especially important for nephrologists to be accessible to provide rapid treatment for AKI emergencies such as anti-GBM disease, myeloma kidney or life-threatening complications of AKI.
2. Developing and embedding clear protocols for fluid resuscitation and maintenance with safeguards to avoid overloading volume replete patients is another role that nephrologists should engender.
3. Similarly establishing clear guidelines for the safe management of hyperkalaemia and judicious use of the newer potassium binders may avoid the need for renal replacement, facilitate safe transfer and hopefully reduce the use of insulin/dextrose.
4. Given the high mortality associated with AKI, there is a particular need to establish a patient's wishes and make an early careful, well-informed assessment of ceilings of care. This is particularly key for frail and multiple comorbid patients likely to need renal replacement therapy. Frequent explanation and updates for patients and relatives where appropriate are important components of care.

Questions

1. What is the prophylaxis for tumour lysis syndrome?
2. What are the key components of treating envenomation by snakebite?
3. What is the definition of abdominal compartment syndrome and treatment?
4. Which medications have been shown to improve renal or patient outcomes in acute tubular injury AKI? (a) dopamine (b) mannitol (c) loop diuretic (d) theophylline (e) fenoldopam (f) intensive glycaemic control.
5. What are the approximate mortality figures for hospital-based AKI, 90-day mortality following AKI, AKI requiring renal replacement in ICU and AKI associated with sepsis requiring renal replacement in ICU?

Answers

1. Identification of risk (renal dysfunction, large volume treatment sensitive haematological malignancy), prophylaxis with hydration and prophylactic use of hypouricaemic agents.
2. Management of snakebite out of hospital involves identification of the snake if possible, immobilization of the limb (no tourniquet or suction) and rapid transfer to the hospital. Inpatient care with detailed clinical assessment, bite site care (look for evidence of compartment syndrome and wound management), tetanus toxoid and supportive therapy as early as possible including careful fluid resuscitation in hypotensive patients, most importantly, shortest possible door to needle time for antivenom (if indicated) (specific if species identified or polyclonal AV if not) and ventilation or RRT if required.
3. A sustained intra-abdominal pressure of >20 mmHg and evidence of organ dysfunction. Treatment is supportive, identifying the underlying cause, reversing this if possible either by surgical decompression or paracentesis of ascites.
4. None of the above; *there is no specific treatment* for established AKI apart from supportive therapy for which there is evidence of clinical benefit.
5. Typical figures for mortality associated with AKI are 20%, with higher 90-day mortality of up to 50%; mortality of 50% is a remarkably consistent figure for patients with AKI requiring renal replacement on ICU, and this figure rises if associated with sepsis (70% in one study). Assessment of risk and early prevention are therefore absolutely critical.

10

Case Study

Case 1

A 65-year-old man was admitted collapsed having been found by his carers. He had a history of diabetes, obesity, hypertension, obstructive sleep apnoea and CKD with an estimated baseline eGFR of 35mls/min. He was poorly mobile and required thrice daily support for activities of daily living and was felt to be very frail. On presentation his systolic blood pressure was 75 mmHg, with warm peripheries and abdominal ascites; he was oliguric with an average urine output of 20mls per hour and a creatinine that had risen from a baseline of 170 to 500 μmol/L with a CRP of 300 mg/L. He underwent rapid assessment and triggered the sepsis 6 pathway including urine and ascitic culture. His anti-hypertensive RAAS inhibition stopped and he had initial IV resuscitation and urinary catheterization. He was diagnosed as having spontaneous bacterial peritonitis in the context of cirrhosis and AKI on CKD. His prognosis was assessed, and it was felt that he would be a poor candidate for chronic renal replacement therapy and that he would unlikely return to good quality of life if he needed ventilation, and indeed his medium-term prognosis was felt to be very poor. Consequently, ceilings of treatment were discussed regarding CPR, ventilatory support and renal replacement therapy. However, his daughter disagreed with this assessment and was vigorous in her desire for everything to be done. He was moved to high dependency, fluid challenged with albumin, prescribed terlipressin treated with broad-spectrum antibiotics but avoiding aminoglycosides. Sodium zirconium potassium binder was added early. His ascites was felt to be tense and probably contributed to abdominal compartment syndrome and therefore his AKI. He underwent a therapeutic drainage with albumin intravascular support. Having achieved a systolic blood pressure of 130/65 mmHg within 4 hours, he started passing more urine and over 3 days recovered his renal function.

He had underlying pulmonary hypertension and was therefore dependent on right-sided filling; getting the optimum intravascular volume in a patient who is oliguric and obese and with cirrhosis and pulmonary hypertension is difficult and easier to get right in high dependency.

This case presentation is not uncommon and demonstrates the challenges of managing multiple comorbid patients who are at very high risk of AKI, particularly if they are not previously known to a nephrologist or had advanced care planning. Rapid resuscitation, treatment of sepsis and restoration of renal perfusion avoided profound tubular injury, while controlling potassium bought time for spontaneous recovery without the need for renal replacement therapy. Once recovered there was the opportunity to discuss his wishes and advanced care planning for any future episode. Early rapid holistic assessment of significant AKI is critical.

Case 2

A 79-year-old man presented to his family doctor complaining of blood in his urine. He had symptoms of bladder outflow tract obstruction but little else. Blood tests revealed an increase in baseline creatinine to 160 μmol/L, and he was referred to urology but presented shortly after in urinary retention with a creatinine of 590 μmol/L and potassium of 7.6 mmol/L. A urinary catheter relieved 1.5 L residual, and a non-contrast CT-KUB confirmed a very thick-walled bladder, bilateral upper tract obstruction and blood in the renal pelvis and ureter (◻ Fig. 10.18, a and b). He was assessed as being mildly hypovolaemic, and

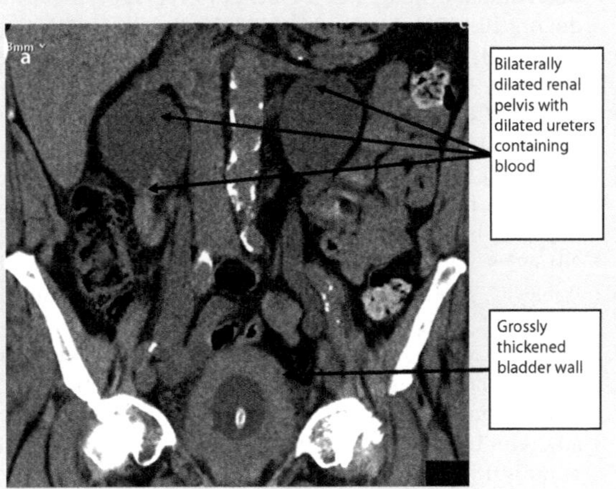

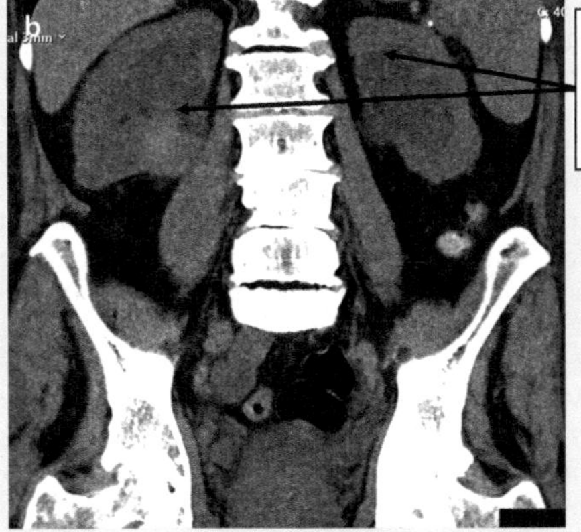

◻ **Fig. 10.18** (**a** and **b**) Images shows bilateral dilatation hydronephrosis and blood in renal pelvis and grossly thickened bladder wall

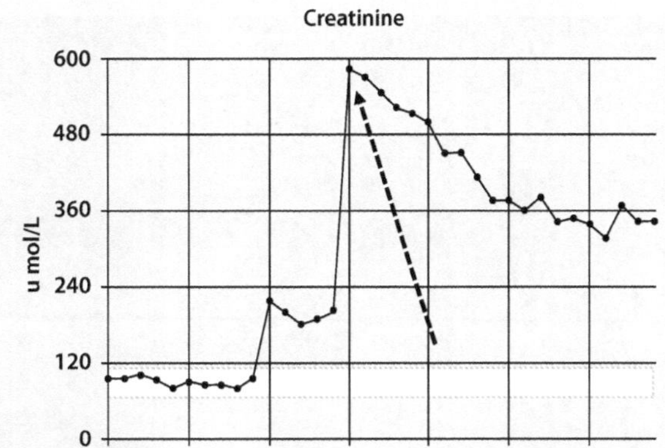

◻ **Fig. 10.19** Fall in creatinine following insertion of the urinary catheter

given a 500 ml fluid challenge, his potassium was medically treated, and once euvolaemic his previous hours' urine output was replaced with crystalloid overnight. This is a relatively safe way of treating post-obstructive diuresis in a patient who is adequately filled for *short periods* initially, providing electrolytes are closely monitored and any drop in urine output provokes a careful reassessment. Over the next few days, his creatinine fell as shown in ◻ Fig. 10.19 (arrow shows catheterization), and he was discharged by the urologists with an indwelling catheter and a diagnosis of bladder outflow tract obstruction secondary to a large prostate but requiring a CT IVU as an outpatient to investigate the pre-catheterization haematuria.

The nephrologists were asked to review his high urine PCR of 4000 mg/dl which raised possibilities of malignancy-associated glomerulonephritis, but uPCR is not possible to interpret in the context of gross haematuria, and transient proteinuria is common in acute obstruction. However, the concern was raised that his creatinine had not fallen as swiftly as one might have expected with decompression of the system and his creatinine had levelled off at a higher than expected level (300 μmol/L). There might be many reasons for failure to recover, but a significant risk is that there was persistent vesico-ureteric obstruction and possibly not just related to a hypertrophied bladder wall (which had been anticipated to resolve spontaneously).

An urgent ultrasound (◻ Fig. 10.20) 2 weeks after the initial catheterization demonstrated persistent bilateral upper tract dilatation. He underwent bilateral nephrostomies with subsequent improvement in creatinine to 125 μmol/L, and the proteinuria disappeared. Widespread bladder tumour was found to be obstructing both ureters. This case illustrates the importance of reassessing a patient if the diagnosis or progress does not fit and ensuring that loose ends are followed up and resolved rapidly.

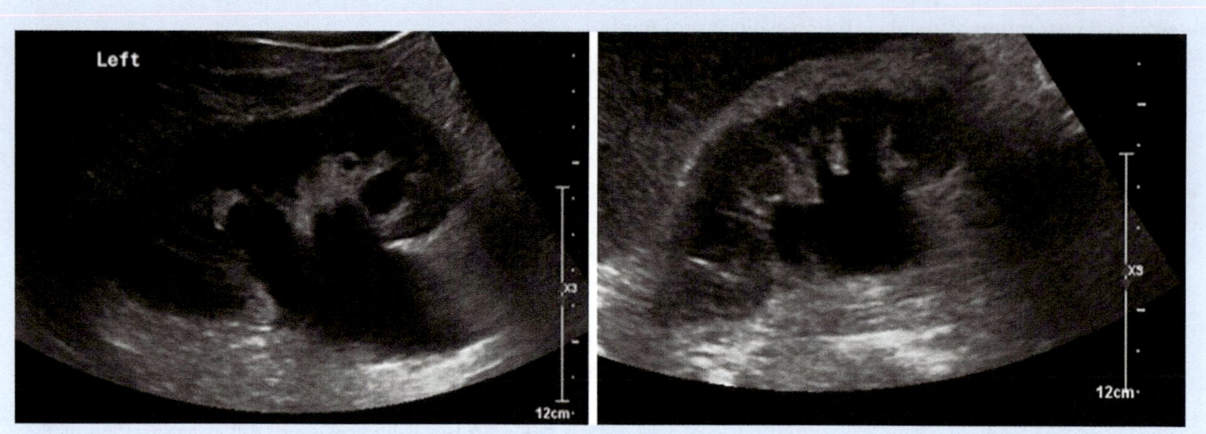

Fig. 10.20 Ultrasound image of the kidneys demonstrating persistent hydronephrosis following initial catheterization

10

References

1. Hoste EA, Bagshaw SM, Bellomo R, et al. Epidemiology of acute kidney injury in critically ill patients: the multinational AKI-EPI study. Intensive Care Med. 2015;41(8):1411–23. https://doi.org/10.1007/s00134-015-3934-7.
2. Finlay S, Bray B, Lewington AJ, et al. Identification of risk factors associated with acute kidney injury in patients admitted to acute medical units. Clin Med (Lond). 2013;13(3):233–8. https://doi.org/10.7861/clinmedicine.13-3-233.
3. Chertow GM, Burdick E, Honour M, Bonventre JV, Bates DW. Acute kidney injury, mortality, length of stay, and costs in hospitalized patients. J Am Soc Nephrol. 2005;16(11):3365–70. https://doi.org/10.1681/ASN.2004090740.
4. Bell M, Chawla LS, Wald R. Understanding renal recovery. Intensive Care Med. 2017;43:924–6. https://doi.org/10.1007/s00134-017-4773-5.
5. Chawla L, Bellomo R, Bihorac A, et al. Acute kidney disease and renal recovery: consensus report of the acute disease quality initiative (ADQI) 16 workgroup. Nat Rev Nephrol. 2017;13:241–57. https://doi.org/10.1038/nrneph.2017.2.
6. Kerr M, Bedford M, Matthews B, O'Donoghue D. The economic impact of acute kidney injury in England. Nephrol Dial Transplant. 2014;29(7):1362–8. https://doi.org/10.1093/ndt/gfu016.
7. Levin A, Stevens PE. Summary of KDIGO 2012 CKD guideline: behind the scenes, need for guidance, and a framework for moving forward. Kidney Int. 2014;85(1):49–61. https://doi.org/10.1038/ki.2013.444.
8. Think Kidneys National AKI programme, review and evaluation report. 2017. https://www.thinkkidneys.nhs.uk. Accessed 04/09/2020.
9. Acute kidney injury: prevention, detection and management NICE guideline [NG148] Published date: 18 December 2019.
10. Connell A, Montgomery H, Martin P, et al. Evaluation of a digitally-enabled care pathway for acute kidney injury management in hospital emergency admissions. NPJ Digit Med. 2019;2(67) https://doi.org/10.1038/s41746-019-0100-6.
11. Mehta RL, Cerdá J, Burdmann EA, et al. International Society of Nephrology's 0by25 initiative for acute kidney injury (zero preventable deaths by 2025): a human rights case for nephrology. Lancet. 2015;385(9987):2616–43. https://doi.org/10.1016/S0140-6736(15)60126-X.
12. NCEPOD 2009.
13. Kolhe NV, Staples D, Reilly T, et al. Impact of compliance with a care bundle on acute kidney injury outcomes: a prospective observational Study. PLoS One. 2015;10(7):e0132279. https://doi.org/10.1371/journal.pone.0132279. Published 2015 Jul 10.
14. Selby NM, Crowley L, Fluck RJ, et al. Use of electronic results reporting to diagnose and monitor AKI in hospitalized patients. Clin J Am Soc Nephrol. 2012;7(4):533–40. https://doi.org/10.2215/CJN.08970911.
15. Prendecki M, Blacker E, Sadeghi-Alavijeh O, et al. Improving outcomes in patients with acute kidney injury: the impact of hospital based automated AKI alerts. Postgrad Med J. 2016;92:9–13.
16. Ashley C. The renal drug handbook: Written by Caroline Ashley. 4th ed. Radcliffe Publishing Ltd; 2014.
17. Malbrain MLNG, Van Regenmortel N, Saugel B, et al. Principles of fluid management and stewardship in septic shock: it is time to consider the four D's and the four phases of fluid therapy. Ann Intensive Care. 2018;8(1):66. https://doi.org/10.1186/s13613-018-0402-x. Published 2018 May 22.
18. Bouchard J, Soroko SB, Chertow GM, et al. Fluid accumulation, survival and recovery of kidney function in critically ill patients with acute kidney injury. Kidney Int. 2009;76(4):422–7. https://doi.org/10.1038/ki.2009.159.
19. Prowle JR, Kirwan CJ, Bellomo R. Fluid management for the prevention and attenuation of acute kidney injury. Nat Rev Nephrol. 2014;10(1):37–47. https://doi.org/10.1038/nrneph.2013.232.
20. Chowdhury AH, Cox EF, Francis ST, Lobo DN. A randomized, controlled, double-blind crossover study on the effects of 2-L infusions of 0.9% saline and plasma-lyte® 148 on renal blood flow velocity and renal cortical tissue perfusion in healthy volunteers. Ann Surg. 2013.
21. Yunos NM, Bellomo R, Taylor DM, et al. Renal effects of an emergency department chloride-restrictive intravenous fluid strategy in patients admitted to hospital for more than 48 hours. Emerg Med Australas. 2017;29(6):643–9. https://doi.org/10.1111/1742-6723.12821.
22. Semler MW, Wanderer JP, Ehrenfeld JM, et al. Balanced crystalloids versus saline in the intensive care unit. The SALT randomized trial. Am J Respir Crit Care Med. 2017;195(10):1362–72. https://doi.org/10.1164/rccm.201607-1345OC.

23. Young P, Bailey M, Beasley R, et al. Effect of a buffered crystalloid solution vs saline on acute kidney injury among patients in the intensive care unit: the SPLIT randomized clinical trial. JAMA. 2015;314(16):1701–10. https://doi.org/10.1001/jama.2015.12334.
24. Semler MW, Self WH, Wanderer JP, et al. Balanced crystalloids versus saline in critically ill adults. N Engl J Med. 2018;378(9):829–39. https://doi.org/10.1056/NEJMoa1711584.
25. Delaney AP, Dan A, McCaffrey J, Finfer S. The role of albumin as a resuscitation fluid for patients with sepsis: a systematic review and meta-analysis. Crit Care Med. 2011;39(2):386–91. https://doi.org/10.1097/CCM.0b013e3181ffe217.
26. Vincent JL, Russell JA, Jacob M, et al. Albumin administration in the acutely ill: what is new and where next? [published correction appears in Crit Care. 2014;18(6):630; Roca, Ricard Ferrer [corrected to Ferrer, Ricard]]. Crit Care. 2014;18(4):231. Published 2014 Jul 16. https://doi.org/10.1186/cc13991.
27. Perner A, Haase N, Guttormsen AB, et al. Hydroxyethyl starch 130/0.42 versus Ringer's acetate in severe sepsis [published correction appears in N Engl J med. 2012;367(5):481]. N Engl J Med. 2012;367(2):124–34. https://doi.org/10.1056/NEJMoa1204242.
28. Brunkhorst FM, Engel C, Bloos F, et al. Intensive insulin therapy and pentastarch resuscitation in severe sepsis. N Engl J Med. 2008;358(2):125–39. https://doi.org/10.1056/NEJMoa070716.
29. Sakr Y, Payen D, Reinhart K, et al. Effects of hydroxyethyl starch administration on renal function in critically ill patients. Br J Anaesth. 2007;98(2):216–24. https://doi.org/10.1093/bja/ael333.
30. Myburgh JA, Finfer S, Bellomo R, et al. Hydroxyethyl starch or saline for fluid resuscitation in intensive care [published correction appears in N Engl J med. 2016 mar 31;374(13):1298]. N Engl J Med. 2012;367(20):1901–11. https://doi.org/10.1056/NEJMoa1209759.
31. Annane D, Siami S, Jaber S, et al. Effects of fluid resuscitation with colloids vs crystalloids on mortality in critically ill patients presenting with hypovolemic shock: the CRISTAL randomized trial [published correction appears in JAMA. 2013;311(10):1071; Régnier, Jean [corrected to Reignier, Jean]; Cle'h, Christophe [corrected to Clec'h, Christophe]]. JAMA. 2013;310(17):1809–17. https://doi.org/10.1001/jama.2013.280502.
32. Perel P, Roberts I. Colloids versus crystalloids for fluid resuscitation in critically ill patients. Cochrane Database Syst Rev. 2007;4:CD000567. https://doi.org/10.1002/14651858.CD000567.pub3. Published 2007 Oct 17.
33. (NICE CIN) (Nice guideline, 2019).
34. American College of Radiology Committee on Drugs and Contrast Media, 2016.
35. Nijssen EC, Rennenberg RJ, Nelemans PJ, et al. Prophylactic hydration to protect renal function from intravascular iodinated contrast material in patients at high risk of contrast-induced nephropathy (AMACING): a prospective, randomised, phase 3, controlled, open-label, non-inferiority trial. Lancet. 2017;389(10076):1312–22. https://doi.org/10.1016/S0140-6736(17)30057-0.
36. Garcia S, Bhatt DL, Gallagher M, et al. Strategies to reduce acute kidney injury and improve clinical outcomes following percutaneous coronary intervention: a subgroup analysis of the PRESERVE trial. JACC Cardiovasc Interv. 2018;11(22):2254–61. https://doi.org/10.1016/j.jcin.2018.07.044. (Weisbord SD, 2018).
37. Cruz DN, Goh CY, Marenzi G, Corradi V, Ronco C, Perazella MA. Renal replacement therapies for prevention of radiocontrast-induced nephropathy: a systematic review. Am J Med. 2012;125(1):66–78.e3. https://doi.org/10.1016/j.amjmed.2011.06.029.
38. Cairo MS, Bishop M. Tumour lysis syndrome: new therapeutic strategies and classification. Br J Haematol. 2004;127(1):3–11. https://doi.org/10.1111/j.1365-2141.2004.05094.x.
39. Howard SC, Jones DP, Pui CH. The tumor lysis syndrome [published correction appears in N Engl J med. 2018 Sep 13;379(11):1094]. N Engl J Med. 2011;364(19):1844–54. https://doi.org/10.1056/NEJMra0904569.
40. Tan HK, Bellomo R, M'Pis DA, Ronco C. Phosphatemic control during acute renal failure: intermittent hemodialysis versus continuous hemodiafiltration. Int J Artif Organs. 2001;24(4):186–91.
41. Edeani A, Shirali A. Tumor lysis syndrome. Am Soc Nephrol, pp. 2016:1–2.
42. Chavez LO, Leon M, Einav S, Varon J. Beyond muscle destruction: a systematic review of rhabdomyolysis for clinical practice. Crit Care. 2016;20(1):135. https://doi.org/10.1186/s13054-016-1314-5. Published 2016 Jun 15.
43. Bosch X, Poch E, Grau JM. Rhabdomyolysis and acute kidney injury. N Engl J Med. 2009;361(1):62–72. https://doi.org/10.1056/nejmra0801327.
44. Long B, Koyfman A, Gottlieb M. An evidence-based narrative review of the emergency department evaluation and management of rhabdomyolysis. Am J Emerg Med. 2019; https://doi.org/10.1016/j.ajem.2018.12.061.
45. Perazella MA. Crystal-induced acute renal failure. Am J Med. 1999;106(4):459–65. https://doi.org/10.1016/s0002-9343(99)00041-8.
46. Feinsilber D, Leoni RJ, Siripala D, et al. Evaluation, identification, and Management of Acute Methotrexate Toxicity in high-dose methotrexate Administration in Hematologic Malignancies. Cureus. 2018;10(1):e2040. https://doi.org/10.7759/cureus.2040.
47. Howard SC, McCormick J, Ching-Hon P, Buddington RK, Harvey RD. Preventing and managing toxicities of high-dose methotrexate. Oncologist. 2016;21:1471–82. https://doi.org/10.1634/theoncologist.2015-0164.
48. Nicolau DP. Antimicrobial agents and chemotherapy, 1995, p. 650–655 Vol. 39, No. 3 1995, American Society for Microbiology Experience with a Once-Daily Aminoglycoside Program Administered to 2,184 Adult Patients.
49. Zahar JR. Inappropriate prescribing of aminoglycosides: risk factors and impact of an antibiotic control team. J Antimicrob Chemother. 2006;58:651–6.
50. BMJ case reports. https://doi.org/10.1136/bcr-2013-202891.
51. Dharod MV, Patil TB, Deshpande AS, Gulhane RV, Patil MB, Bansod YV. Clinical predictors of acute kidney injury following snake bite envenomation. N Am J Med Sci. 2013;5(10):594–9. https://doi.org/10.4103/1947-2714.120795.
52. WHO Guidelines for the Production, Control and Regulation of Snake Antivenom Immunoglobulins EXPERT COMMITTEE ON BIOLOGICAL STANDARDIZATION Geneva, 17 to 21 October 2016.
53. Keyler DE, Gawarammana I, Gutiérrez JM, Sellahewa KH, McWhorter K, Malleappah R. Antivenom for snakebite envenoming in Sri Lanka: the need for geographically specific antivenom and improved efficacy. Toxicon. 2013;69:90–7. https://doi.org/10.1016/j.toxicon.2013.01.022.
54. Williams HF, Layfield HJ, Vallance T, Patel K, Bicknell AB, Trim SA, Vaiyapuri S. The urgent need to develop novel strategies for the diagnosis and treatment of snakebites. Toxins. 2019;11:363.
55. Rhodes A, Evans LE, Alhazzani W, et al. Surviving sepsis campaign: international guidelines for Management of Sepsis and

Septic Shock: 2016. Intensive Care Med. 2017;43:304–77. https://doi.org/10.1007/s00134-017-4683-6.
56. Daniels R, Nutbeam T, McNamara G, Galvin C. The sepsis six and the severe sepsis resuscitation bundle: a prospective observational cohort study. Emerg Med J. 2011;28(6):507–12. https://doi.org/10.1136/emj.2010.095067.
57. Asfar P, Meziani F, Hamel JF, et al. High versus low blood-pressure target in patients with septic shock. N Engl J Med. 2014;370(17):1583–93. https://doi.org/10.1056/NEJMoa1312173.
58. Pollard S, Edwin SB, Alaniz C, Inotropes H, SSC 2012. Vasopressor and inotropic management of patients with septic shock. P & T: A Peer-Reviewed Journal for Formulary Management. 2015;40(7):438–50.
59. Bellomo R, Cass A, Cole L, et al. Intensity of continuous renal-replacement therapy in critically ill patients. N Engl J Med. 2009;361:1627–38.
60. Petros S, John S. Die Sepsisleitlinie der surviving sepsis campaign 2016 [the 2016 surviving sepsis campaign sepsis guideline]. Med Klin Intensivmed Notfmed. 2017;112(5):454–8. https://doi.org/10.1007/s00063-017-0298-5.
61. Daniels R, Nutbeam T, Mcnamara G, et al. The sepsis six and the severe sepsis resuscitation bundle: a prospective observational cohort study. Emerg Med J. 2011;28:507–12.
62. Krzych ŁJ, Czempik PF. Impact of furosemide on mortality and the requirement for renal replacement therapy in acute kidney injury: a systematic review and meta-analysis of randomised trials. Ann Intensive Care. 2019;9(1):85. https://doi.org/10.1186/s13613-019-0557-0. Published 2019 Jul 24.
63. Ho KM, Power BM. Benefits and risks of furosemide in acute kidney injury. Anaesthesia. 2010;65(3):283–93. https://doi.org/10.1111/j.1365-2044.2009.06228.
64. Lauschke A, Teichgräber UK, Frei U, Eckardt KU. 'Low-dose' dopamine worsens renal perfusion in patients with acute renal failure. Kidney Int. 2006;69(9):1669–74. https://doi.org/10.1038/sj.ki.5000310.
65. Study Investigators NICE-SUGAR, Finfer S, Chittock DR, et al. Intensive versus conventional glucose control in critically ill patients. N Engl J Med. 2009;360(13):1283–97. https://doi.org/10.1056/NEJMoa0810625.
66. Dépret F, Peacock WF, Liu KD, et al. Management of hyperkalemia in the acutely ill patient. Ann Intensive Care. 2019;9:32. https://doi.org/10.1186/s13613-019-0509-8.
67. Investigators STARRT-AKI, et al. Timing of initiation of renal-replacement therapy in acute kidney injury. The New England journal of medicine vol. 2020;383(3):240–51. https://doi.org/10.1056/NEJMoa2000741.
68. Uchino S, Kellum JA, Bellomo R, et al. Acute renal failure in critically ill patients: a multinational, multicenter study. JAMA. 2005;294(7):813–8. https://doi.org/10.1001/jama.294.7.813.
69. Xue JL, Daniels F, Star RA, et al. Incidence and mortality of acute renal failure in Medicare beneficiaries, 1992 to 2001.
70. Garg AX, Suri RS, Barrowman N, et al. Long-term renal prognosis of diarrhea-associated hemolytic uremic syndrome: a systematic review, meta-analysis, and meta-regression. JAMA. 2003;290(10):1360–70. https://doi.org/10.1001/jama.290.10.1360.
71. Coca SG, Singanamala S, Parikh CR. Chronic kidney disease after acute kidney injury: a systematic review and meta-analysis. Kidney Int. 2012;81(5):442–8. https://doi.org/10.1038/ki.2011.379.
72. Chawla LS, Amdur RL, Amodeo S, Kimmel PL, Palant CE. The severity of acute kidney injury predicts progression to chronic kidney disease. Kidney Int. 2011;79(12):1361–9. https://doi.org/10.1038/ki.2011.42.

Establishing an AKI Service

Sarah Hildebrand, Rhys Evans, and Ed Kingdon

Contents

M. Harber (ed.), *Primer on Nephrology*, https://doi.org/10.1007/978-3-030-76419-7_11

Learning Objectives

1. Understand variation in AKI outcomes and different models of service provision.
2. Understand that early recognition of AKI is key to facilitating further intervention.
3. Understand the potential role of care bundles in standardising and enhancing care.
4. Appreciate the difficulties in establishing AKI in different healthcare settings.

11.1 Introduction

Admissions including episodes of acute kidney injury (AKI) are associated with significantly increased mortality and prolonged length of stay [1], and AKI is costly for healthcare purchasers and providers. It is estimated that AKI costs between £ 434 and 620 million each year in the NHS in England and Wales [2] and exceeds 200 million Canadian dollars per year in Canada [3]. In addition, patients who survive hospital admissions complicated by AKI are at increased risk of long-term sequelae [4]. A meta-analysis of 82 published studies identified an increased risk of new or progressive chronic kidney disease (CKD) (Hazard ratio (HR) 2.67), end-stage renal disease (ESRD) (HR 4.81) and death (HR 1.80) when outcomes were compared with those for patients without AKI [5].

Acute kidney injury is seen in patients cared for in primary care and under the care of most hospital specialities. Nephrologists will be the primary physicians for a minority of all patients whose in-patient episode includes evidence of AKI [6]. In many settings specialised renal services are delivered using a hub-and-spoke model with concentration of resources in the hub and movement of patients between hub and spoke depending on illness severity and complexity. The influence of configuration of renal services in the UK on outcomes has been examined in a study of emergency admissions with AKI using hospital episode statistics [7]. In this study, access to renal specialist care was associated with variation in outcomes for patients with AKI. The mortality rates for cases coded for AKI were higher in hospital trusts without on-site renal services. Socioeconomic status is also associated with variation in AKI. Analysis of 22 months of adult AKI alerts in Wales demonstrated that deprivation was associated with a higher incidence of AKI, more AKI episodes per patient and greater AKI severity at onset of AKI episode [8]

Given the clinical outcomes of admissions associated with AKI, observed variations in outcome and the very substantial costs of care, it is important to think how services for patients with AKI can be delivered. When planning how to configure services, it is important to review evidence for interventions that may yield benefits and to consider service design and other factors that influence whether such interventions are reliably delivered.

11.2 Service Specifications and Targets for Improvement

Expert consensus panels have published guidance on how to deliver and organise care for patients with AKI [9, 10]. In 2009, the UK National Confidential Enquiry into Patient Outcome and Death (NCEPOD) published the report "Adding Insult to Injury" on AKI management within the UK National Health Service (NHS) (see Table 11.1). The NCEPOD inquiry made recommendations about how services for patients with severe AKI are configured and about access to expert clinicians and renal replacement therapy (RRT) (see Table 11.2).

Consideration of the quality of care for patients with AKI might include elements of clinical practice that need to be incorporated or, if already present, how reliable delivery is monitored and assured. These are service elements for which there is widespread expert support in the context of AKI:

- Identification of patients at risk of AKI.
- Automated ascertainment of patient with AKI.
- Reliable delivery of proven clinical interventions in patients who have dialysis-independent AKI.
- Renal replacement therapy for dialysis-dependent AKI (further discussed in ▶ Chap. 12 Acute Renal Replacement).

AKI is heterogeneous, and although effective, specific treatments exist for a minority of cases, there is no proven pharmaceutical treatment for acute tubular injury associated with one or more of the following; sepsis, hypovolaemia, hypotension and treatment toxicity. It is possible that reliable identification of the patient's AKI phenotype may allow for the design of RCTs to test existing or novel pharmaceutical interventions for a specific AKI phenotype. In the event that some but not all AKI phenotypes are proven to respond to specific rather than supportive measures, establishing a service for AKI patients will require infrastructure and staffing necessary to deliver elaboration of the AKI phenotype in a timely fashion.

When establishing a service, it is worth remembering that the majority of patients with increases in creatinine sufficient to support a diagnosis of AKI have mild changes and that most of these improve without complex interventions. It is possible that the prompt

Table 11.1 NCEPOD recommendations on AKI service provision 2009

Admission and assessment of acute kidney injury	Initial clerking of all emergency patients should include a risk assessment for AKI
	All patients admitted as an emergency (**all** specialties) should have their electrolytes checked routinely on admission and appropriately thereafter
Investigation and Management of acute Kidney injury	Reagent strip urinalysis should be performed on **all** emergency admissions
	Guidance for recognising the acutely ill patient (NICE CG 50) should be disseminated and implemented. In particular **all** acute patients should have admission physiological observations performed
Referral and support	When referral is made for specialist advice from nephrologists prompt senior advice and a review where appropriate is required
	Every hospital should have a written guideline detailing how the clinical areas where patients with AKI are treated (critical care unit, the renal unit and the non-specialist ward) interact to ensure delivery of high-quality, clinically appropriate care for patients with AKI
Recognition of severity of illness	**All** acute admissions should receive adequate senior reviews (with a consultant review within 12 hours of admission)
	There should be sufficient critical care and renal beds to allow escalation of care if appropriate
Organisation of renal services	**All** acute admitting hospitals should have access to either onsite nephrologists or a dedicated nephrology service within reasonable distance of the admitting hospital
	All acute admitting hospitals should have access to a renal ultrasound scanning service 24 hours a day including the weekends and the ability to provide emergency relief of renal obstruction
	All level 3 critical care units should have the ability to deliver renal replacement therapy; and where appropriate these patients should receive clinical input from a nephrologist

and reliable delivery of simple proven interventions has an impact on many domains of the quality of care. In AKI these might include effectiveness, efficiency, avoidable harm, equity, accessibility and patient experience (see Table 11.3). In addition to interventions that can be evaluated as they are introduced, that other healthcare provider attributes including skill mix, staffing density and quality assurance of patient pathways influence outcomes for patients with AKI.

Table 11.2 National Institute for Health and Care Excellence (NICE) AKI Quality Standards 2014

Quality statement 1: *Raising awareness in people at risk*	People who are risk of AKI are made aware of the potential causes
Quality statement 2: Identifying acute kidney injury in people with no obvious acute illness	People who present with an illness with no clear acute and one or more indications or risk factors for AKI are assessed for this condition
Quality statement 3: Monitoring in hospital for people at risk	People in hospital who are at risk of AKI have their serum creatinine and urine output measured
Quality statement 4: Identifying the cause – Urine dipstick test	People have a urine dipstick test performed as soon as AKI is suspected or detected
Quality statement 5: Discussion with a nephrologist	People with AKI have the management of their condition discussed with a nephrologist as soon as possible and with 24 hours of detection if they are at risk of intrinsic renal disease or if they have stage 3 AKI
Quality statement 6	People with AKI who meet the criteria for RRT are referred immediately to a nephrologist or critical care specialist

Table 11.3 Quality domains and measures employed in studies of AKI care

Quality domain	Measure examples
Effectiveness	In-patient mortality, critical care admission, residual chronic kidney disease, residual requirement for RRT
Efficiency	Length of stay, cost of care episode
Patient centred	Patient experience measures (PEM) Delivery of care that is respectful of and responsive to individual patient preferences, needs and values Care close to home
Equity	Unwarranted variation segregating with personal characteristics (gender, ethnicity, geographic location, or socioeconomic status)
Safety	Avoidable harm
Timely	Reducing waits and harmful delays Review within aspirational time window Transfer to tertiary care Centre within specified time frame Critical care RRT for patients with single organ failure

Table 11.4 Heterogeneity of studies designed to evaluate interventions to improve care in patients with AKI

Setting	Design	Interventions	Service reconfiguration
Single acute care organisation	Controlled trial	Identification of patients at risk of AKI	In-reach review by visiting specialist nephrologists at acute sites without on-site renal service
Multiple acute care organisations	QI project	Automated ascertainment of patients with AKI	Post-discharge AKI clinics
Whole system	Observa-tional study	Identification of AKI phenotype	AKI review by specialist AKI nurses (CCOT or AKI-dedicated)
NB *high–/ middle–/ low-income settings*		Reliable delivery of proven clinical interventions in patients with AKI (isolated interventions or as part of a care bundle)	On-site provision of pharmacy and dietetic review at acute sites without on-site renal service
		Educational Initiatives	Remote consultation with nephrologists for acute sites without on-site renal service

The published literature is heterogeneous, and Table 11.4 lists examples of the settings, study design, intervention and service reconfiguration in studies in this area which the authors will refer to in the remainder of this chapter.

11

11.3 Improving Outcomes in AKI: Domains of Care

11.3.1 Identification of Those at Risk of AKI

Models incorporating comorbidity, physiological parameters and variables related to treatment and illness severity factors have been used to estimate risk of developing AKI in a variety of clinical contexts. Precise estimates of risk might inform targeting of particular elements of care in those at highest risk of AKI. Risk scores are available in cardiac and non-cardiac surgery, but there are few examples of clinical implementation [11]

The largest study addressing this question in patients attending for acute medical care found that risk factor modelling offered limited discrimination in identification of patients who would go on to develop hospital-acquired AKI [12]. This is consistent with the earlier finding from a service evaluation study in 4 Welsh medical assessment units that prediction models based on risk factors added little to risk stratification based on age [13]. More recently a controlled before-and-after study has demonstrated reductions in the incidence of hospital-acquired AKI following the deployment of a clinical prediction rule identifying those at risk of AKI alongside electronic alerts for those with AKI [14].

Identifying Patients with AKI and Messaging Clinicians Delivering Their Care.

Physicians may not always recognise the clinical significance of changes in creatinine, and a number of algorithms are available that allow the magnitude and timing of changes in serum creatinine and comparison with baseline levels to be used to identify patients who may have AKI. The specificity of the UK National AKI algorithm is >90% when AKI warning test alerts are compared with clinical coding of AKI in hospital episode statistics [15]. A randomised controlled study comparing electronic AKI alerting (text messaging of the AKI warning test result) to the covering doctor and pharmacist with standard care did not identify improvement in the composite outcome of maximum increase in creatinine, renal replacement therapy or death [16]. Alerting was one of three interventions in the step-wedge Tackling AKI RCT study [17]. This study did not achieve its primary endpoint of a reduction in mortality. In contrast a single centre propensity score matched cohort study found an advantage when alerting was combined with targeted education and use of a care bundle [18]. Prendecki and colleagues explored whether the impact of delayed review of sick patients might be ameliorated by use of an AKI alert system in a retrospective study [19]. They found that an AKI alert would predate recruitment of specialist review by physiological parameters by up to 2 days.

11.3.2 Care Bundles

The Institute for Healthcare Improvement defined a bundle as:

> "a structured way of improving the processes of care and patient outcomes: a small, straightforward set of evidence-based practices that, when performed collectively and reliably, have been proven to improve patient outcomes."

In the context of AKI, there is some variation in which practices or interventions are included in such a bundle and the outcomes against which they are assessed. There is also heterogeneity in the methods used to evaluate these interventions and to deliver evidence of effectiveness: controlled trials, QI and the observational studies [20, 21, 22].

The ambitious RCT study, Tackling AKI [17], tested three interventions in a stepped-wedge design. The study was powered to identify a 20% reduction in in-patient mortality but did not meet its primary endpoint. The study had three interventions: (a) STOP-AKI care bundle (b) e-Alerting of AKI warning test results and (c) an educational package.

Three large well-conducted quality improvement QI projects in the NHS in the Northwest of England also tested the effectiveness of a care bundle in patients with AKI [23–25]. These studies have demonstrated improvements using statistical process control methodology. The interventions tested in the QI studies are summarised in ◘ Table 11.5 alongside the outcome measures described in the studies.

Medication review and assessment and optimisation of fluid balance are frequent components of AKI care bundles. Targeted fluid therapy with frequent reassessment of the patient, provided by the specialist and generalist members of the clinical team, is an important intervention in this context [26]. Patients with severe AKI in whom goal-directed fluid therapy is unsuccessful may require renal replacement therapy

Medication review is an intervention that often follows an AKI warning test result and which is frequently one of the elements in an AKI care bundle. The advent of electronic prescribing, with an integrated AKI alerting system, can highlight medications that require dose adjustment or discontinuation to prevent toxicity [27]. E-alerting systems to tackle AKI can anticipate those at

◘ **Table 11.5** AKI QI projects

	Chandrasekar 2017	Ebah 2017	Sykes 2018
Process measures			
AKI detection		✓	
Fluid assessment		✓	✓
Repeat creatinine following first alert	✓		✓
Expert medication review	✓	✓	
Witholding medicines	✓*		✓**
Patient information leaflet	✓		✓
Written self-management plan prior to discharge	✓		
Dipstick urinalysis	✓		✓
Renal imaging	✓		✓
Discussion with/referral to specialist nephrology service or critical care	✓		✓
Outreach nurse review	✓		
Care bundle documentation	✓		
Care bundle completion		✓	
Design	QIP	QIP	QIP
Outcomes	AKI in-hospital death rate ↓ AKI 30-day mortality↓ LOS↓	AKI LOS↓ HA-AKI incidence↓ AKI days (time to recovery)↓	HA-AKI incidence↓ Proportion of AKI episodes increasing in severity↓

high risk and reduce the risk of AKI. The NINJA system electronically identified children at risk of a drug-related AKI due to nephrotoxin exposure. In the paediatric setting in which routine phlebotomy is judiciously used, identification of high-risk individuals enables either discontinuation of medication or adequate monitoring to ensure any subsequent AKI is promptly identified and managed [28]

11.4 Service Reconfiguration

11.4.1 Which Clinicians Should Review Patients with AKI?

Stage 3 AKI warning test results are a minority of all AKI WTRs, and parenchymal inflammatory renal disease and systemic disease account for a small proportion of cases of AKI. The National Institute for Health and Care Excellence (NICE) has described criteria for renal referral (see ◘ Table 11.6). Questions remain about how best to bring the remaining cases of AKI to the attention of clinicians responsible for care of affected patients, which professional group should review the patients and whether this requires face-to-face review. Telephone-based advice for clinicians managing AKI has been described [29]. Many acute trusts have critical care outreach teams who may be recruited to review patients based on the presence of deteriorating physiological parameters or subjective impressions of patient deterioration. The impact of an AKI outreach team is being investigated in unselected AKI in the Acute Kidney Outreach to Reduce Deterioration and Death (AKORDD) trial: the protocol for a large pilot study [30].

11

◘ Table 11.6 NICE AKI Guidelines 2014 suggests the following indications for renal referral

Indications for renal referral
Stage 3 AKI
Stage 2 AKI with failure to respond to medical treatment
Complications of AKI failing to respond to medical treatment
Indication for dialysis present
A possible systemic inflammatory cause for AKI
Blood or protein on urine dipstick indicating possible intrinsic renal disease

11.4.2 Follow-Up of AKI Patients

Patients who have had an episode of AKI have a greater risk of developing chronic kidney disease (CKD) and progression up to ESRD in the future [31]. Repeated episodes of AKI are associated with progression of CKD and incomplete recovery from an episode of AKI is also associated with a poor prognosis [32]. With these observations in mind, follow-up in specific AKI survivor clinics is well established in some centres [33]. These offer the opportunity to deliver patient education and identify and mange CKD, reconciliation of prescribed medication and rational re-introduction of treatments associated with prognostic gain that are temporarily interrupted at the time of AKI. Nephrologists and nephrology guidelines often advocate specialist follow-up after an episode of AKI. However, there is limited evidence that such follow-up is delivered [34] and uncertainty if such follow-up improves patient outcomes. An uncontrolled study of patients who received transient RRT study for AKI identified a lower mortality in those who were followed up by nephrologists than was observed in those who were not followed [35]. This area merits further investigation.

11.5 Patient and Carer Engagement, Education and Sick Day Rules

Delivery of patient-appropriate educational materials is used as a process measure in some AKI QI projects [36]. Despite this approach being widespread, many AKI survivors' knowledge of their illness and future risks remains limited [37]. AKI survivor clinics may increase AKI literacy amongst survivors [38]. The introduction of "sick day rules", temporary interruption of medications at the time of acute illness, for those at risk of AKI has been the subject of much interest. Qualitative assessments suggest significant challenges when AKI sick day rules are considered in a primary care setting [39], and description of the effect of AKI sick day rules on patient outcomes, unintended consequences and the use of healthcare resources are awaited . The authors are unaware of studies of patient experience of care in AKI or of formal experience-based co-design in this context.

11.6 AKI in a Primary Care Setting

Acute kidney injury may accompany patient episodes that begin outside the hospital (community-acquired AKI) and may complicate hospital admissions. Episodes of AKI beginning more than 48 hours after admission are often termed hospital-acquired AKI (HA-AKI). This is a somewhat arbitrary distinction as almost half of the cases satisfying the CA-AKI criterion had had earlier measurements of creatinine as part of in-patient or emergency department care in the 30 days before CA-AKI diagnosis [40]

A minority of episodes of community-acquired AKI are managed exclusively outside the hospital [41]. Changes in creatinine sufficient to meet the criteria for AKI ascertainment algorithms may be encountered when blood tests are performed in primary care settings, both in response to acute illness and as part of chronic disease surveillance or to guide safe prescribing.

Several elements need to be considered when considering AKI in primary care:

(a) Messaging of AKI warning test result from the biochemistry laboratory to the community-based practitioner.
(b) Timely responses upon receipt of an AKI warning test result in primary care [42].
(c) Management of a patient discharged from the hospital after community-acquired or HA-AKI.

There is evidence that the use of an e-alert has improved response times in the context of community-acquired AKI [43] and of higher rates of creatinine monitoring [44]. However, e-alerts are also associated with higher rates of hospitalisation [44]. National guidance on the nature and timeliness of responses to AKI warning test results in primary care has been informed by a RAND/UCLA Appropriateness Method study [42]. Guidance in this area has been reviewed by the UK Royal College of General Practitioners (RCGP), and a toolkit is available online (▶ https://www.rcgp.org.uk/clinical-and-research/resources/toolkits/acute-kidney-injury-toolkit.aspx). The second phase of an RCGP-sponsored AKI quality improvement project that will focus on post-discharge AKI care and guidelines to support clinical decision-making about follow-up of patients who have sustained AKI is awaited.

11.7 Commissioning AKI Services in a High-Income Setting

The earlier sections of this chapter discuss how configuration of existing services might be influenced by recent published trials, observational studies and QI projects. The UK Think Kidneys website includes useful case studies describing how to establish an AKI service in secondary care. Although these are specific to the English health economy, they do address more widespread challenges associated with management of AKI.

- Lancashire Teaching Hospitals NHS FT.

▶ https://www.thinkkidneys.nhs.uk/aki/wp-content/uploads/sites/2/2016/01/Lancashire-Teaching-Hospitals-NHS-FT-Establishing-an-AKI-Service-in-a-Tertiary-Renal-Centre-.pdf

- Wrightington, Wigan and Leigh NHS FT.

▶ https://www.thinkkidneys.nhs.uk/kquip/wp-content/uploads/sites/5/2016/11/Wrightington-Wigan-Leigh-Case-Study-Improving-Patient-Safety-and-Reducing-Harm1-1.pdf

When commissioning renal services, commissioners may need to consider incidence of AKI, the nature of the local case mix and the need for specialised services to be concentrated in a limited number of tertiary sites or co-terminus with other specialised services. Tertiary-level renal services are able to provide standard ward-based care in addition to renal replacement therapy and in some locations may also be sufficiently well staffed and skilled to deliver critical care functions. However, whatever the complexity of supportive care available, renal units that are servicing a referral practice for a large population are likely to need to offer specialist diagnostic and treatment services, including immunological testing, immunosuppression prescribing and delivery, percutaneous renal biopsy and plasma exchange [45].

The speed with which patients are transferred from critical care facilities offering continuous RRT to specialist renal units is likely to influence time taken to make a definitive diagnosis, critical care bed availability and the cost of an AKI episode.

A tertiary care centre is likely to sit at the hub of a network of secondary care hospitals from which referrals are received. The nephrologist may provide an advice service, often visiting the secondary care centre, and a pathway for patient transfer to the tertiary care centre. These services need to be carefully evaluated in light of the catchment population served to justify capital investment and revenue costs necessary to sustain them.

Many networks publish criteria that determine whether the patient is sufficiently stable to transfer between settings and physical sites. The London AKI network has parameters of these in an openly accessible app (▶ www.healthcreatives.co.uk/work/london-aki-network.html) generated by consensus.

11.8 AKI Services in Low- and Middle-Income Settings

The availability of resources influences healthcare priorities and delivery. This is of particular relevance in kidney disease, as long-term provision of renal replacement therapy for chronic kidney disease is prohibitively expensive in most low- and middle-income countries. AKI, on the other hand, is largely a preventable and treatable condition with relatively limited resource. Establishing an AKI service may support the development of a nephrology service with gains unrelated to AKI, and small improvements in the provision of AKI care can save lives no matter where you are in the world (case history 1).

Managing AKI in low- and middle-income settings provides substantial challenges. These include a lack of education and training of healthcare professionals involved in the management of AKI; a lack of availability of even basic laboratory tests (e.g. serum creatinine) required for the diagnosis of AKI; a patient population at extremely high risk of kidney injury from acute infectious illness on a background of an ongoing epidemic of HIV and emergent cardiovascular disease; and limited resources for AKI monitoring and management, ranging from a lack of basic equipment such as catheter bags to monitor urine output to the provision of renal replacement therapy and critical care.

The International Society of Nephrology (ISN) has made significant efforts to improve AKI service provision in low-income settings worldwide through a number of its programmes focused on education, training, advocacy and research (▶ https://www.theisn.org/programs). These are encompassed within the ISN 0by25 initiative (▶ https://www.theisn.org/all-articles/616-0by25#0by25-initiative), which aims to eliminate preventable deaths from AKI worldwide by 2025 [46]. It has identified a number of potential targets for improvement in AKI care:

- *Risk:* Public health measures may influence the prevalence of infectious disease associated with AKI [47], and socioeconomic and cultural factors may influence health-seeking behaviours putting individuals at a higher risk of more severe AKI.
- *Recognition:* Correctly identifying those at risk of AKI and appropriate use of point-of-care testing are likely to enhance recognition of AKI. Telemedicine may support access to specialist advice and onward referral to more specialist services if required. Repeated measurement of serum creatinine during the course of hospital admission is far less common in developing countries [48], but ongoing assessment is vital in those at high risk of development of AKI during a hospital admission [49].
- *Response:* Smaller renal units, outside large tertiary care centres, support delivery of specialist input in cases of moderately severe AKI that are not referred onwards to tertiary care centres. These function optimally with close liaison with the tertiary care centre, either for knowledge or practical support [50].
- *Renal support:* In low-income settings, on-stie renal replacement therapy is not widely available. However, protocols developed in other settings can be adopted and adapted to enable the initiation of emegency management of AKI (for example acute peritoneal dialysis) and delivery of care underpinned by telemedicine support from dedicated geographically distant renal physicians [51]. Peritoneal dialysis is the most commonly employed modality of renal replacement reflecting resource availability and ease of training for local renal and non-renal physicians [52].
- *Rehabilitation:* Most of the reports are of the outcomes following tertiary-level care for the AKI. A significant proportion of affected individuals do not have a fully recovered renal function [53]. Thus ongoing support and chronic kidney disease management are required to provide optimal kidney care [54].

Case Study

Case 1: Establishing an AKI Service in Blantyre, Southern Malawi

The ISN supported a sister renal centre partnership between Queen Elizabeth Central Hospital (QECH), Blantyre, Malawi, and Barts Health NHS Trust, London, UK, from 2013 to 2019. Prior to this partnership, there was no renal expertise in the region. Establishing an AKI service has been the focus of developing nephrology services more generally in Southern Malawi. Key components of the development of this AKI service have included the following.

1. Establishing the Epidemiology of AKI.

A number of observational studies were undertaken at QECH in medical, paediatric and obstetric cohorts to determine the incidence, aetiologies and outcomes of AKI (Evans et al. BMC nephrol 2017; Cooke et al. BMC nephrol 2018; Evans et al. PDI 2018; Mwanza et al. BMC nephrol 2018). AKI was found to be common (17% of adult medical admissions), predominantly due to preventable and treatable causes (acute infective illness and pre-eclampsia), with poor outcomes despite tertiary care (44% in-hospital mortality with any AKI in adults).

2. Establishing the Need for and Providing Education and Training to Healthcare Professionals.

A survey amongst district and tertiary healthcare workers in Malawi highlighted that 98% of respondents wanted more help in managing patients with AKI (Evans et al. MMJ 2015). Need was greatest in rural areas. An outreach education programme was established, and training sessions have now been undertaken in 14 sites in the southern region (Craik et al., BJRM 2016).

3. Improving Tertiary Renal Services.

An acute haemodialysis service for adult AKI and an acute peritoneal dialysis service for paediatric AKI have been established at QECH, with the help of the ISN Saving Young Lives Program (▶ https://www.theisn.org/programs/saving-young-lives-project). These services are provided free at the point of care, supported by the Malawi Ministry of Health. Both forms of dialysis are feasible and effective; 54 patients underwent haemodialysis from 2014 to 2017 with 37 (68%) recovering to dialysis independence and discharged. Alongside dialysis services, a dedicated in-patient renal ward was opened in 2016, where AKI patients now received specialised in-patient renal care.

4. Researching Novel Diagnostic Tools for the Diagnosis of AKI.

A lack of reliably available serum creatinine tests outside tertiary care centres is a major obstacle to the management of AKI in low-income settings worldwide. Research undertaken at QECH and in community health centres in Malawi demonstrated that a saliva urea nitrogen dipstick performs well in diagnosing and tracking renal function during the management of AKI (Evans et al. KIR 2017 and 2018).

5. Providing Sustainability Through Training of Renal Nurses and Nephrologists.

Sustainability of any new AKI service is paramount, but particularly in low-income settings. The AKI service at QECH is now locally led by Malawian nurses and clinicians who have been trained in the provision of AKI care during exchange visits as part of the sister renal partnership. Malawi's first fully trained nephrologist will return to lead the service later this year having undertaken an ISN fellowship in Cape Town.

Case 2: Implementation of an AKI e-Alert Service in London, UK

The identification of the morbidity, mortality and costs of potentially preventable AKI has directed investment of resources into preventative strategies. The implementation of a national acute kidney injury (AKI) algorithm by NHS England and incorporation of the algorithm into laboratory information management systems (LIMS) have facilitated timely identification of biochemical changes suggesting AKI. The delivery of AKI warning test results to the clinicians has been the subject of an innovative project at the Royal Free Hospital, an 800-bedded teaching hospital in London, UK, with a tertiary renal care centre serving a catchment referral population of 1.5 M. The Royal Free commissioned DeepMind Health™ to develop the "Streams-AKI App", which continually applies the NHS AKI algorithm to a live stream of real-time creatinine data from prevalent hospital in-patients. Alerts for those identified as having an AKI are delivered to hospital-issued mobile devices held by the renal and critical care outreach teams. Alongside the alert, demographic and other clinical information are available. Those thought to have a clinically relevant AKI are discussed with their parent team and have prompt bedside review.

At present, the effectiveness of this service is under evaluation through a multifaceted approach. This includes the quantitative analysis of the clinical outcomes, the financial impact of such an impact and, qualitatively, the acceptability of such a service on the nephrology and critical care staff who are delivering it and the wider hospital team whose patients are being reviewed [55]. The impact of this service transformation on AKI outcomes is yet to be established [56].

Tips and Tricks

- Most AKI is managed without specialist input from nephrology or critical care.
- AKI service configuration may influence patient outcomes.
- Care bundles can provide a framework in which non-specialists are empowered to optimise AKI management.
- Education and training are fundamental. These should focus both on identification and subsequent management of the AKI and awareness of when to refer to specialist services.

Conclusion

The establishment of an AKI service is complex, with no universal consensus as to the optimal way in which this can be done. Providing an infrastructure with rapid identification of AKI and education of individuals involved in their clinical management is key. The manner in which this is done needs to be adapted to the local healthcare setting. The effectiveness of strategies implemented to optimise AKI management needs ongoing evaluation as to their effectiveness.

Questions

1. What additional challenges in AKI service delivery are present in the community setting?
2. What 5Rs are the ISN targets for improvement in AKI management?
3. What role do care bundles have in AKI management?

Answers

1. AKI management requires results to be promptly relayed from laboratory to community clinicians and the ability to undertake a rapid response thereafter. Individuals who have recently returned to community with an AKI from secondary care need additional focus.
2. The targets are risk reduction, recognition, response, renal support and rehabilitation.
3. These provide a framework by which non-specialist clinicians can standardise care and can include, for example, assessment of fluid status, medication review and monitoring.

References

1. Chertow GM, Burdick E, Honour M, Bonventre JV, Bates DW. Acute kidney injury, mortality, length of stay, and costs in hospitalized patients. J Am Soc Nephrol. 2005;16(11):3365–70.
2. Kerr M, Bedford M, Matthews B, O'Donoghue D. The economic impact of acute kidney injury in England. Nephrol Dial Transplant. 2014;29(7):1362–8.
3. Collister D, Pannu N, Ye F, James M, Hemmelgarn B, Chui B, et al. Health Care Costs Associated with AKI. Clin J Am Soc Nephrol. 2017;12(11):1733–43.
4. Coca SG, Singanamala S, Parikh CR. Chronic kidney disease after acute kidney injury: a systematic review and meta-analysis. Kidney Int. 2012;81(5):442–8.
5. See EJ, Jayasinghe K, Glassford N, Bailey M, Johnson DW, Polkinghorne KR, et al. Long-term risk of adverse outcomes after acute kidney injury: a systematic review and meta-analysis of cohort studies using consensus definitions of exposure. Kidney Int. 2019;95(1):160–72.
6. Porter CJ, Juurlink I, Bisset LH, Bavakunji R, Mehta RL, Devonald MA. A real-time electronic alert to improve detection of acute kidney injury in a large teaching hospital. Nephrol Dial Transplant. 2014;29(10):1888–93.
7. Abraham KA, Thompson EB, Bodger K, Pearson M. Inequalities in outcomes of acute kidney injury in England. QJM. 2012;105(8):729–40.
8. Phillips D, Holmes J, Davies R, Geen J, Williams JD, Phillips AO. The influence of socioeconomic status on presentation and outcome of acute kidney injury. QJM. 2018;111(12):849–57.
9. National Clinical Guideline C. National Institute for Health and Clinical Excellence: Guidance. Acute Kidney Injury: Prevention, Detection and Management Up to the Point of Renal Replacement Therapy. London: Royal College of Physicians (UK). National Clinical Guideline Centre; 2013.
10. KDIGO A. Work Group. KDIGO clinical practice guideline for acute kidney injury. Kidney Int Suppl. 2012;2:1–138.
11. Wilson T, Quan S, Cheema K, Zarnke K, Quinn R, de Koning L, et al. Risk prediction models for acute kidney injury following major noncardiac surgery: systematic review. Nephrol Dial Transplant. 2016;31(2):231–40.
12. LobotRi F. Risk prediction for acute kidney injury in acute medical admissions in the UK. QJM. 2019;112(3):197–205.
13. Roberts G, Phillips D, McCarthy R, Bolusani H, Mizen P, Hassan M, et al. Acute kidney injury risk assessment at the hospital front door: what is the best measure of risk? Clin Kidney J. 2015;8(6):673–80.
14. Hodgson LE, Roderick PJ, Venn RM, Yao GL, Dimitrov BD, Forni LG. The ICE-AKI study: Impact analysis of a Clinical prediction rule and Electronic AKI alert in general medical patients. PLoS One. 2018;13(8):e0200584.
15. Sawhney S, Fraser SD. Epidemiology of AKI: Utilizing Large Databases to Determine the Burden of AKI. Adv Chronic Kidney Dis. 2017;24(4):194–204.
16. Wilson FP, Shashaty M, Testani J, Aqeel I, Borovskiy Y, Ellenberg SS, et al. Automated, electronic alerts for acute kidney injury: a single-blind, parallel-group, randomised controlled trial. Lancet. 2015;385(9981):1966–74.
17. Selby NM, Casula A, Lamming L, Stoves J, Samarasinghe Y, Lewington AJ, et al. An Organizational-Level Program of Intervention for AKI: A Pragmatic Stepped Wedge Cluster Randomized Trial. J Am Soc Nephrol. 2019;30(3):505–15.
18. Kolhe NV, Reilly T, Leung J, Fluck RJ, Swinscoe KE, Selby NM, et al. A simple care bundle for use in acute kidney injury: a propensity score-matched cohort study. Nephrol Dial Transplant. 2016;31(11):1846–54.
19. Prendecki M, Blacker E, Sadeghi-Alavijeh O, Edwards R, Montgomery H, Gillis S, et al. Improving outcomes in patients with Acute Kidney Injury: the impact of hospital based automated AKI alerts. Postgrad Med J. 2016;92(1083):9–13.
20. Logan R, Davey P, Davie A, Grant S, Tully V, Valluri A, et al. Care bundles for acute kidney injury: a balanced accounting of

the impact of implementation in an acute medical unit. BMJ Open Qual. 2018;7(4):e000392.
21. Bhagwanani A, Carpenter R, Yusuf A. Improving the management of Acute Kidney Injury in a District General Hospital: Introduction of the DONUT bundle. BMJ Qual Improv Rep. 2014;2(2).
22. Joslin J, Wilson H, Zubli D, Gauge N, Kinirons M, Hopper A, et al. Recognition and management of acute kidney injury in hospitalised patients can be partially improved with the use of a care bundle. Clin Med (Lond). 2015;15(5):431–6.
23. Chandrasekar T, Sharma A, Tennent L, Wong C, Chamberlain P, Abraham KA. A whole system approach to improving mortality associated with acute kidney injury. QJM. 2017;110(10): 657–66.
24. Sykes L, Sinha S, Hegarty J, Flanagan E, Doyle L, Hoolickin C, et al. Reducing acute kidney injury incidence and progression in a large teaching hospital. BMJ Open Qual. 2018;7(4):e000308.
25. Ebah L, Hanumapura P, Waring D, Challiner R, Hayden K, Alexander J, et al. A Multifaceted Quality Improvement Programme to Improve Acute Kidney Injury Care and Outcomes in a Large Teaching Hospital. BMJ Qual Improv Rep. 2017;6(1).
26. Prowle JR, Kirwan CJ, Bellomo R. Fluid management for the prevention and attenuation of acute kidney injury. Nat Rev Nephrol. 2014;10(1):37–47.
27. McCoy AB, Waitman LR, Gadd CS, Danciu I, Smith JP, Lewis JB, et al. A computerized provider order entry intervention for medication safety during acute kidney injury: a quality improvement report. Am J Kidney Dis. 2010;56(5):832–41.
28. Goldstein SL, Mottes T, Simpson K, Barclay C, Muething S, Haslam DB, et al. A sustained quality improvement program reduces nephrotoxic medication-associated acute kidney injury. Kidney Int. 2016;90(1):212–21.
29. Thomas ME, Sitch A, Baharani J, Dowswell G. Earlier intervention for acute kidney injury: evaluation of an outreach service and a long-term follow-up. Nephrol Dial Transplant. 2015;30(2):239–44.
30. Abdelaziz TS, Lindenmeyer A, Baharani J, Mistry H, Sitch A, Temple RM, et al. Acute Kidney Outreach to Reduce Deterioration and Death (AKORDD) trial: the protocol for a large pilot study. BMJ Open. 2016;6(8):e012253.
31. Leung KC, Tonelli M, James MT. Chronic kidney disease following acute kidney injury-risk and outcomes. Nat Rev Nephrol. 2013;9(2):77–85.
32. Sawhney S, Marks A, Fluck N, Levin A, McLernon D, Prescott G, et al. Post-discharge kidney function is associated with subsequent ten-year renal progression risk among survivors of acute kidney injury. Kidney Int. 2017;92(2):440–52.
33. Silver SA, Goldstein SL, Harel Z, Harvey A, Rompies EJ, Adhikari NK, et al. Ambulatory care after acute kidney injury: an opportunity to improve patient outcomes. Can J Kidney Health Dis. 2015;2:36.
34. Karsanji DJ, Pannu N, Manns BJ, Hemmelgarn BR, Tan Z, Jindal K, et al. Disparity between Nephrologists' Opinions and Contemporary Practices for Community Follow-Up after AKI Hospitalization. Clin J Am Soc Nephrol. 2017;12(11):1753–61.
35. Harel Z, Wald R, Bargman JM, Mamdani M, Etchells E, Garg AX, et al. Nephrologist follow-up improves all-cause mortality of severe acute kidney injury survivors. Kidney Int. 2013;83(5):901–8.
36. Kashani K, Rosner MH, Haase M, Lewington AJP, O'Donoghue DJ, Wilson FP, et al. Quality Improvement Goals for Acute Kidney Injury. Clin J Am Soc Nephrol. 2019;14(6):941–53.
37. Siew ED, Parr SK, Wild MG, Levea SL, Mehta KG, Umeukeje EM, et al. Kidney Disease Awareness and Knowledge among Survivors ofAcute Kidney Injury. Am J Nephrol. 2019;49(6): 449–59.
38. Ortiz-Soriano V, Alcorn JL 3rd, Li X, Elias M, Ayach T, Sawaya BP, et al. A Survey Study of Self-Rated Patients' Knowledge About AKI in a Post-Discharge AKI Clinic. Can J Kidney Health Dis. 2019;6:2054358119830700.
39. Martindale AM, Elvey R, Howard SJ, McCorkindale S, Sinha S, Blakeman T. Understanding the implementation of 'sick day guidance' to prevent acute kidney injury across a primary care setting in England: a qualitative evaluation. BMJ Open. 2017;7(11):e017241.
40. Holmes J, Allen N, Roberts G, Geen J, Williams JD, Phillips AO. Acute kidney injury electronic alerts in primary care - findings from a large population cohort. QJM. 2017;110(9): 577–82.
41. Talabani B, Zouwail S, Pyart RD, Meran S, Riley SG, Phillips AO. Epidemiology and outcome of community-acquired acute kidney injury. Nephrology (Carlton). 2014;19(5):282–7.
42. Blakeman T, Griffith K, Lasserson D, Lopez B, Tsang JY, Campbell S, et al. Development of guidance on the timeliness in response to acute kidney injury warning stage test results for adults in primary care: an appropriateness ratings evaluation. BMJ Open. 2016;6(10):e012865.
43. Tollitt J, Flanagan E, McCorkindale S, Glynn-Atkins S, Emmett L. Darby D, et al. Fam Pract: Improved management of acute kidney injury in primary care using e-alerts and an educational outreach programme; 2018.
44. Aiyegbusi O, Witham MD, Lim M, Gauld G, Bell S. Impact of introducing electronic acute kidney injury alerts in primary care. Clin Kidney J. 2019;12(2):253–7.
45. Medcalf JF, Davies C, Hollinshead J, Matthews B, O'Donoghue D. Incidence, care quality and outcomes of patients with acute kidney injury in admitted hospital care. QJM. 2016;109(12): 777–83.
46. Mehta RL, Cerda J, Burdmann EA, Tonelli M, Garcia-Garcia G, Jha V, et al. International Society of Nephrology's 0by25 initiative for acute kidney injury (zero preventable deaths by 2025): a human rights case for nephrology. Lancet. 2015;385(9987): 2616–43.
47. Kashani K, Macedo E, Burdmann EA, Hooi LS, Khullar D, Bagga A, et al. Acute Kidney Injury Risk Assessment: Differences and Similarities Between Resource-Limited and Resource-Rich Countries. Kidney international reports. 2017;2(4):519–29.
48. Zhao Y, Yang L. Perspectives on acute kidney injury strategy in China. Nephrology (Carlton, Vic). 2018;23(4):100–3.
49. Daher EF, Silva Junior GB, Santos SQ, CC RB, Diniz EJ, Lima RS, et al. Differences in community, hospital and intensive care unit-acquired acute kidney injury: observational study in a nephrology service of a developing country. Clin Nephrol. 2012;78(6):449–55.
50. Jha V, Arici M, Collins AJ, Garcia-Garcia G, Hemmelgarn BR, Jafar TH, et al. Understanding kidney care needs and implementation strategies in low- and middle-income countries: conclusions from a "Kidney Disease: Improving Global Outcomes" (KDIGO) Controversies Conference. Kidney Int. 2016;90(6):1164–74.
51. Gordon EJ, Fink JC, Fischer MJ. Telenephrology: a novel approach to improve coordinated and collaborative care for chronic kidney disease. Nephrol Dial Transplant. 2013;28(4): 972–81.
52. Abdou N, Antwi S, Koffi LA, Lalya F, Adabayeri VM, Nyah N, et al. Peritoneal Dialysis to Treat Patients with Acute Kidney Injury-The Saving Young Lives Experience in West Africa: Proceedings of the Saving Young Lives Session at the First International Conference of Dialysis in West Africa, Dakar, Senegal, December 2015. Perit Dial Int. 2017;37(2):155–8.
53. Ponce D, Dias DB, Nascimento GR, Silveira LV, Balbi AL. Long-term outcome of severe acute kidney injury survivors

followed by nephrologists in a developing country. Nephrology (Carlton, Vic). 2016;21(4):327–34.
54. Sobrinho A, da Silva LD, Perkusich A, Pinheiro ME, Cunha P. Design and evaluation of a mobile application to assist the self-monitoring of the chronic kidney disease in developing countries. BMC Med Inform Decis Mak. 2018;18(1):7.
55. Connell A, Montgomery H, Morris S, Nightingale C, Stanley S, Emerson M, et al. Service evaluation of the implementation of a digitally-enabled care pathway for the recognition and management of acute kidney injury. F1000Res. 2017;6:1033.
56. Connell A, Montgomery H, Martin P, Nightingale C, Sadeghi-Alavijeh O, King D, et al. Evaluation of a digitally-enabled care pathway for acute kidney injury management in hospital emergency admissions. NPJ Digit Med. 2019;2:67.

Acute Renal Replacement

Andrew Davenport

Contents

M. Harber (ed.), *Primer on Nephrology*, https://doi.org/10.1007/978-3-030-76419-7_12

Learning Objective

1. To appreciate the indication and timing of dialysis in the setting of AKI.
2. To understand the issues relating to dialysis of patients with acute co-morbidity (such as brain or cardiac injury or significant electrolyte abnormalities).
3. To compare different modalities of renal replacement in the setting of AKI, including elements such as dose and anticoagulation.

12.1 Initiation of Dialysis

The decision when to initiate replacement therapy (RRT) in patients with acute kidney injury (AKI) is extremely variable and tends to be based on empiricism, depending upon the immediate and projected trajectory of the clinical situation, clinician experience and local institutional practices and resources. For example, RRT is typically initiated for oliguria, acidosis and correction of volume overload in the intensive care unit (ICU), whereas in the renal ward, azotaemia and hyperkalaemia are more common triggers to initiate RRT.

The indications for RRT depend on both or either the clinical scenario or biochemical abnormalities and also on whether the situation is expected to improve following appropriate resuscitation or supportive or interventional management, and as such indications may be relative or absolute (Table 12.1). Current clinical practice is to consider initiating RRT in patients with AKI, defined by an abrupt fall of glomerular filtration rate, who are at risk of clinically significant solute imbalance, toxicity or volume overload.

Table 12.1 Clinical and biochemical indications to consider initiation of renal replacement therapy. Rifle criteria relate to changes in baseline serum creatinine [1], discussed in Chap. 8

Indication	Characteristics	Absolute/relative	Trigger to initiate RRT
Azotaemia	Blood urea nitrogen (serum urea)	Relative Absolute	>76 mg/dl (27 mmol/l) >100 mg/dl (35.7 mmol/l) Uraemic pericarditis Uraemic encephalopathy
Metabolic acidosis	pH pH Lactic acidosis	Relative Absolute Absolute	<7.25 and >7.15 <7.15 Secondary to metformin
Anuria/oliguria	RIFLE Class R RIFLE Class I RIFLE Class F	Relative Relative Relative	
Volume overload	Diuretic sensitive Diuretic resistant	Relative Absolute	Need to create space for blood, plasma products, nutrition Refractory pulmonary oedema
Severe hyperkalaemia	<6.5 >6.5	Relative Absolute	ECG – tenting of T waves ECG – additional to T wave changes
Electrolyte abnormalities	Hypo/hypernatraemia Hypo/hyper calcaemia	Relative Absolute	Correction of hyponatraemia prior to liver transplantation Coma, refractory to medical management
Tumour lysis syndrome	Hyperuricaemia Hyperphosphataemia	Relative Absolute	Urate >1.0 mmol/l, phosphate >4.0 mmol/l Failure to respond to medical therapy
Metabolic coma	Urea cycle defects Organic acidaemia, hyperammonaemia	Relative Absolute	Acidaemia Coma, failure to respond to conservative management
Poisoning, drug over dosage	Water-soluble drugs/poisons relative small volume of distribution	Relative Absolute	e.g. Alcohols, lithium depending upon serum concentrations Coma, failure to respond to supportive management
Thermal regulation	Hyperpyrexia Hypothermia	Relative Relative	Temperature >40° <32 °C coma, unresponsive to other therapies

12.2 Does the Timing of RRT Influence Outcome in AKI?

Historic data suggests that "early" initiation of RRT in AKI was associated with improved survival when RRT was started with BUN levels of 100 mg/dl (35.7 mmol/l) or less.

More recently, several retrospective studies reported improved clinical outcomes with earlier institution of dialysis at urea levels <21.5 mmol/l or initiation of CRRT in post-cardiac surgery patients with a urine output of <100 mL/8 hr, and an observational study reported a twofold increased mortality starting RRT at higher urea concentrations. However, a prospective randomized study did not show any survival advantage with early initiation, although this study was somewhat underpowered.

Early introduction of RRT as soon as a patient enters RIFLE-F or AKI stage 3 [2] may be of potential benefit, so that the patient is not exposed to the potential deleterious effects of metabolic abnormalities or volume overload. However, early initiation of RRT could equally cause some patients to suffer complications of RRT, including hypotension, access catheter-associated bacteraemia and anticoagulant induced haemorrhage. In addition, some patients with AKI, especially those with single organ failure, may recover renal function without ever requiring RRT. Indeed, one study from Pittsburgh which followed over 5000 patients admitted to ICU reported that <1% of 2273 who developed RIFLE-I required RRT and only 14% of 1511 who developed RIFLE-F [3].

There have been three prospective studies of early vs later initiation of RRT in the modern era [4–6]. A single-centre study reported a benefit from starting at RIFLE grade 2 vs grade 3 [5], whereas the two multicentre trials showed no benefit from an early start approach, and almost 50% of patients in the delayed start group did not require RRT, suggesting that an early start strategy would lead to treating many patients who would otherwise not require RRT [6]. On the other hand, the early start patients did not appear to suffer any adverse consequences from being treated by RRT [4–6]. In view of the ongoing uncertainty, larger trials have been proposed [7].

Although retrospective and observational studies suggest that "early" initiation of RRT in AKI is associated with improved patient survival, this remains to be confirmed by appropriately powered, prospective multicentre randomized trials. In every day clinical practice, clinicians typically start RRT earlier in critically ill patients with multiple organ failure, than in those with single organ AKI alone "It is important to ensure that the sick oliguric patient who is unlikely to recover function with intravenous fluids alone, is identified early and RRT anticipated rather than precipitated as an emergency".

12.3 When Should RRT Be Withdrawn in AKI?

There have been no formal studies performed as to when to switch patients from CRRT to intermittent dialytic therapies or withdraw RRT. Typically withdrawal of RRT is an empiric decision made by clinicians based on a falling pre-dialysis urea or creatinine concentrations, increasing urine output and general improvement in the clinical condition of the patient. As such, some clinicians favour abrupt cessation, whereas others reduce the dose of CRRT or intermittent dialytic therapies and then if no deterioration in chemistries stop RRT. It is now realized that just as with conventional intermittent haemodialysis, the blood supply to the kidney is reduced when patients are treated by CRRT. This is why patients apparently oligo-anuric whilst on CRRT may suddenly appear to start passing urine when CRRT is stopped. For those undergoing continuous RRT, there may be an advantage transitioning the recovering patient to IHD to permit greater mobility and physiotherapy. Either way, it is important to establish close liaison between ITU and the renal unit who may inherit patients with multiple medical problems.

12.4 Treatment Options for RRT

Whereas in the early 1980s the options for RRT therapy were limited to intermittent haemodialysis (IHD) and peritoneal dialysis (PD), the currently available therapies in the developed world now include various forms of continuous renal replacement therapy (CRRT). ◘ Figure 12.1 shows the difference between convective (haemofiltration) and diffusive (haemodialysis) blood purification techniques. Newer "hybrid" therapies variously termed extended duration dialysis (EDD), sustained low-efficiency dialysis (SLED) and prolonged intermittent renal replacement therapy (PIRRT) and the single batch dialysate Genius® system (Fresenius, Bad Homberg, Germany) [8] (◘ Table 12.2) offer a variety of alternative approaches. In the intensive care setting, a variety of additional therapies are currently being trialled as add-on therapies for treating septic patients including dialyzers designed to enhance endotoxin clearance, additional endotoxin filters and plasma separators with adsorption cartridges.

The significant difference in urea clearance between modalities is emphasized in ◘ Fig. 12.2.

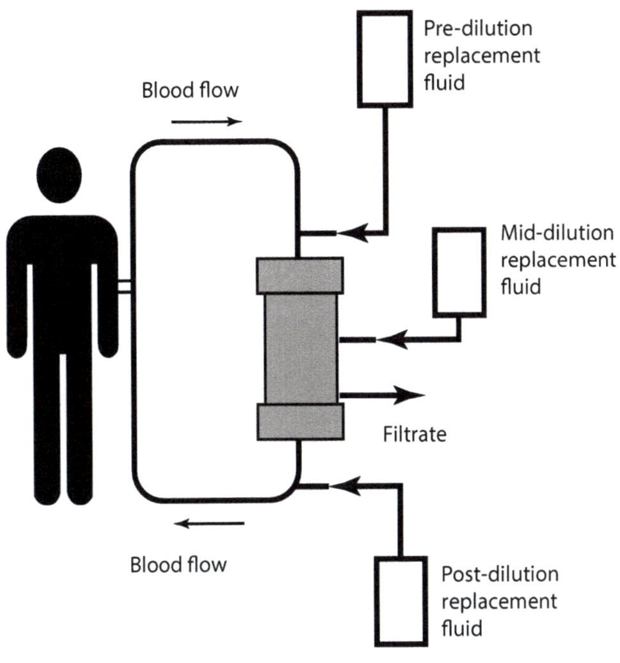

Convective blood purification haemofiltration

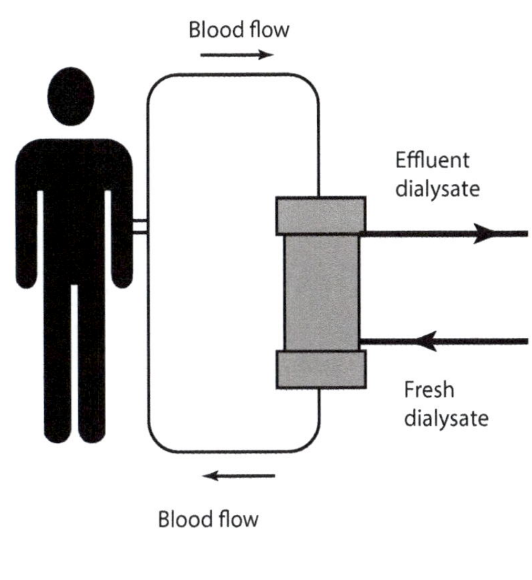

Diffusive blood purification haemodialysis

Fig. 12.1 Comparison of haemodialysis and haemofiltration modalities for acute renal replacement

Table 12.2 Different modalities of renal replacement therapy

Modality	CVVH	CVVHD	CVHDF	PD	PIRRT	IHD
Qb ml/min	100–250	100–250	100–250	None	100–300	200–350
Qd ml/min	None	25–50	25–50	32–50	200–300	300–800
Therapy time h	24	24	24	24	6–12	4–6
Primary solute transport	Convection	Diffusion	Diffusion Convection	Diffusion	Diffusion	Diffusion
Ultrafiltrate l/h	1.5–3.0	Variable	1.5–3.0	Variable	Variable	Variable
Effluent volume l/day	36–72	36–72	36–72	20–25	Variable	Variable
Replacement fluid l/h	1.5–3.0	None	1.5–3.0	None	None	None
Urea clearance ml/min	20–40	25–45	25–45	15–35	90–140	150–180

CVVH continuous veno-venous haemofiltration, *CVVHD* haemodialysis, *CVVHDF* haemodiafiltration, *PD* peritoneal dialysis, *PIRRT* prolonged intermittent renal replacement therapy, *IHD* intermittent haemodialysis

12.5 Does Modality of Renal Replacement Therapy Affect Outcomes?

12.5.1 Mortality

Although it is widely perceived that CRRT is superior to IHD in haemodynamically unstable critically ill adult patients, prospective randomized clinical trials have failed to confirm this supposition. In many of the earlier trials, the more critically ill patients received CRRT rather than IHD, and as such, mortality was greater for patients treated with CVVH [9]. Correcting for illness severity mortality was similar for both modalities.

Seven randomized prospective controlled trials have compared CRRT and IHD. These trials excluded very seriously ill patients with limited life expectancy, and

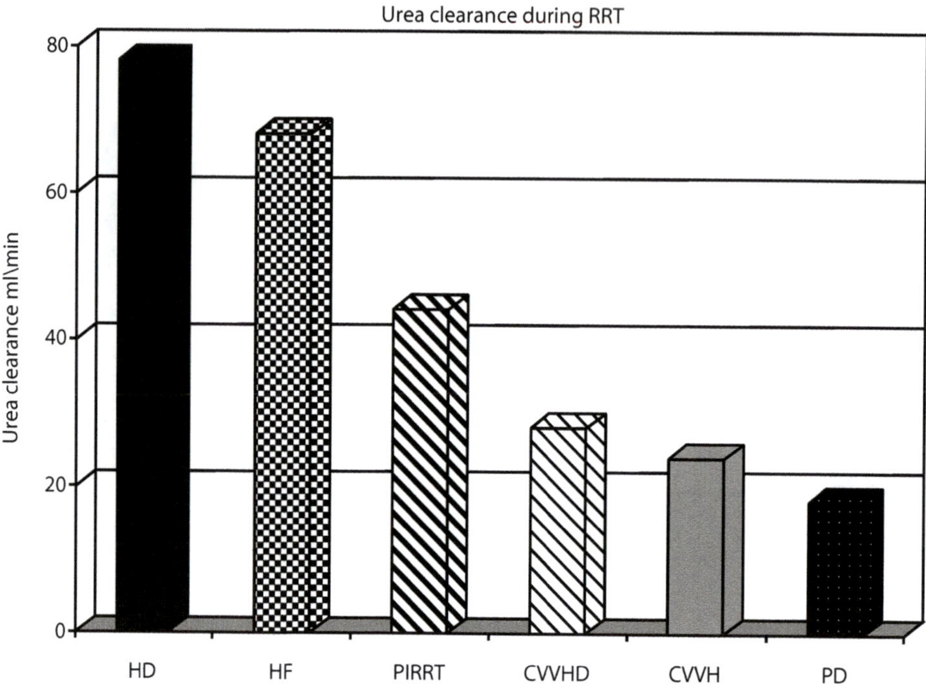

Fig. 12.2 Comparison of clearance between acute renal replacement dialysis modalities

12

also some of the trials had a high crossover of patients, typically CRRT switching to IHD due to recurrent problems with circuit clotting and IHD to CRRT due to hypotension. No trial showed that modality impacted on overall survival. Several trials observed greater cardiovascular stability with CRRT. However, the largest of the these studies, the Hemodiafe study, a multicentre randomized controlled trial of 359 patients, successfully delivered IHD to patients despite marked haemodynamic instability with very little crossover between treatment groups [10]. In this trial, IHD used cooled dialysate combined with a higher dialysate sodium concentration compared to the serum sodium and extended session time to minimize cardiovascular instability during IHD and compared to other studies delivered the highest Kt/V dose in the IHD group.

Although there have been few comparisons of PIRRT and CRRT, those which have been reported have not shown any effect of modality on patient survival [8].

12.5.2 Recovery of Residual Renal Function

Although there was no obvious difference in overall survival, two large prospective observational studies reported greater recovery of residual renal function and dialysis independence in survivors treated by CRRT compared to IHD. One study from the Cleveland Clinic reported that intradialytic hypotension during the first IHD session predicted dialysis dependence in survivors [11], and as many ICU patients have haemodynamic instability and intra-dialytic hypotension during IHD is more likely in hypotensive patients requiring vasopressors, this has led to the suggestion that CRRT may be associated with an increased likelihood for recovery of renal function. Interestingly, in the Hemodiafe study, there were a similar number of hypotensive episodes during both IHD and CRRT and no difference in dialysis dependence in the survivors [10]. As such, the risk of remaining dialysis dependent would appear to be related to episodes of hypotension rather than treatment modality per se.

Studies comparing other forms of RRT have been limited. No studies have directly compared "hybrid" treatments to either IHD or CRRT, although "hybrid" therapies have been shown to provide similar haemodynamic stability and solute control when compared to CRRT. Although peritoneal dialysis is widely used in paediatric practice, more and more units are using various forms of CRRT and hybrid technologies, but as of yet there is no comparative data.

As such, analysis of the currently published studies does not allow evidence-based guidelines for the selection of RRT modality for the treatment of AKI. The modality chosen should therefore be guided by the individual patient's clinical status, local medical and nursing expertise and availability of equipment.

12.6 Tailoring Intermittent Therapies for Patients with Acute Kidney Injury

12.6.1 Haemodialysis

In the 1980s, IHD in the ICU was typically delivered thrice weekly, using bio-incompatible low-flux cellulosic dialyzers, low-sodium, acetate-based dialysate warmed to body temperature and with dialysis machines that did not have accurate volume regulation. However, just as CRRT has developed, so has IHD with the introduction of volumetric dialysis machines, fitted with relative blood volume monitoring, temperature control modules and biofeedback control, along with synthetic high-flux bio-compatible membranes and bicarbonate dialysate. In addition, the importance of daily or at least alternate day extended treatments designed to reduce ultrafiltration requirements coupled with higher sodium and lower dialysate temperatures to reduce the frequency of intradialytic hypotension is now recognized, such that the introduction of this so-called "bundle" effect has been shown to have had a marked impact on reducing IHD-associated hypotension reducing the frequency of intradialytic hypotension to that of CRRT [10].

However, the limitation of these technological advances has to be appreciated. For intermittent haemodialysis/haemodiafiltration, relative blood volume measurements (BVM) which are the cornerstone of biofeedback systems, designed to regulate ultrafiltration rates, coupled with changing dialysate sodium or temperature, depend upon the concept that if the rate of ultrafiltration exceeds plasma volume refill, then haematocrit and whole blood viscosity increase. There are a number of errors that need to be considered. The main error with BVM is determining the starting point, and then as ultrafiltration proceeds, the normal physiological response is to close down small capillaries, but as the haematocrit in these smaller vessels is less than that in the inferior vena cava, blood returning to the central veins is relatively dilute, so minimizing changes recorded by the blood volume monitoring modules. In addition, there is a marked intra-patient variation in response to ultrafiltration, which is more marked in the ICU patient, particularly those with sepsis and liver failure by affecting endothelial function and integrity. As such the changes recorded by these modules lag behind in real time as to what is actually occurring in the body, and although these devices can reduce the frequency and severity of intradialytic hypotension, they cannot prevent hypotension [12].

12.6.2 Haemofiltration

Intermittent haemofiltration (IHF) which was introduced in the late 1970s has mainly been superseded by intermittent haemodiafiltration (IHDF). IHF was reported to reduce the frequency of hypotensive episodes compared to IHD. Initially this was thought to be due to the convective loss of cardio-depressant factors but was more likely to be due to the cooling effect of IHF, as subsequent studies showed that the frequency of intra-treatment hypotension was similar between different dialysis modalities provided the same degree of cooling was achieved. Typically cooling is greater with pre-dilution rather than post-dilution fluid replacement (◘ Fig. 12.1).

IHF as with CRRT requires a sterile replacement solution. IHDF in the outpatient dialysis clinic uses online ultrapure water to reduce costs. Many ICUs only have access to a domestic water supply, rather than the specialized water treatment plant in the chronic haemodialysis unit. However, with the addition of simple particle filters, in combination with carbon filters and portable reverse osmosis machines, some units can provide water of ultrapure quality, when using dialysis machines fitted with ultrafilters.

12.6.3 Continuous Renal Replacement Therapies (CRRT)

CRRT initially started with continuous arterio-venous haemofiltration (CAVH), but as the clearances achieved were often low, then many patients required supplemental haemodialysis sessions to control biochemistries. To improve efficiency, countercurrent dialysate was added, continuous arterio-venous haemodialysis (CAVHD) and then a blood pump to allow veno-venous systems. Initially, there were no specialized replacement solutions or dialysates, so peritoneal dialysates were often used. Over time commercial sterile replacement fluids and dialysates based on extracellular fluid composition became available.

Although CRRT machines are volumetrically controlled, as the fluid management systems are often based on 24-hour periods, then volume errors can occur with reprogramming following repeatedly over riding error messages and replacing circuits due to clotting.

12.6.4 Hybrid Therapies

Hybrid therapies encompass a group of treatments which are essentially based on extending the duration and slowing down the rate of diffusion of IHD. Most regimens use standard IHD machines with slower blood and dialysate flow rates (◘ Table 12.1). There is in addition there are batch IHD machines (NxStage system 1, and Genius®, Fresenius Bad Homberg, Germany) in which the blood and dialysate flows are linked by a single pump, so that the flow rates are of similar magnitude, and this treatment can be extended for more than 12 hours by slowing the flow rates down to 100 ml/min, although 150–200 ml/min is more common in clinical practice. In the USA, there has been increasing use of the NxStage haemodialysis machine in providing dialysis treatments in the ICU. This haemodialysis machine, originally developed for home haemodialysis, can use sterile bagged dialysate or batch dialysate and as with the Genius® benefits from lower dialysate and blood flows [13].

Depending on the design, hybrid therapies can provide diffusive clearances of small solutes such as urea of around 36 ml/kg.h and greater solute clearances of vitamin B12 or beta 2-microglobulin, some 50–66% of that with CRRT. In addition hybrid therapies can also be set up to provide haemodiafiltration, then achieving comparable larger solute clearances to CRRT.

Whereas circuit thrombus formation has been reported in 20–25% of hybrid therapies using standard haemodialysis machines, clotting is much less frequent with the batch dialysate therapies, such as the Genius®. This may be due to the difference in blood pump technology between the systems, with much greater leukocyte and platelet activation with standard occlusive roller pump. Genius® is also reported to reduce the risk of hypotension due to cooling of blood. The NxStage machine does not operate with a venous air detector chamber, a source for thrombus formation in the extracorporeal circuit.

12

12.7 Peritoneal Dialysis

Although the role of peritoneal dialysis for adult AKI is declining in Europe and North America, it is still used in developing countries, for paediatric AKI, particularly post-cardiac surgery, and in patients with single organ failure. Peritoneal dialysis machines are useful but not obligatory. Clearances achieved in paediatric AKI are certainly comparable to those targeted for chronic kidney disease.

However, there have been debates as to whether peritoneal dialysis can provide adequate clearances for treating adult AKI. Traditionally acute peritoneal dialysis was practised by using rapid small volume cycling designed to minimize peritoneal leaks [14], typically 0.5 l cycles with short inflow times of 5 minutes, dwell 20–25 minutes and 5–10 minutes of drainage. However, this type of prescription provided much lower clearances than that achieved by low-volume CRRT. More recently this low-volume rapid cycle prescription has been challenged, with studies from Brazil, using 2 litre fill volumes, with longer dwell times of 65–80 minutes, so allowing greater diffusion of solutes reporting average urea clearances of 17.3 ± 5 ml/min. Peritoneal dialysis can be an effective treatment particularly for patients with single organ failure, such as post-cardiac surgery [15]. However, not all patients may be suitable for peritoneal dialysis due to recent or previous major intra-abdominal surgery and high catabolic demands. Double cuffed catheters can be inserted under local anaesthesia using an open Seldinger technique or closed with direct visualization using peritoneoscopy. Infections can be minimized by covering catheter insertion with prophylactic antibiotics and applying topical antibiotic creams to the exit site. To minimize the risk of early leaks, most centres limit the initial exchange volumes to 750–1000 ml, with a 85% tidal prescription and dwell time of 70–90 minutes and, then providing there are no leaks, increasing the fill volume to 2.0 l for the average 70 kg patient and increasing the dwell time to 90–120 minutes and reducing the tidal component. Initially peritoneal dialysis is continuous 24 hours a day, but a longer dwell using 7.5% icodextrin can be substituted to reduce nursing time and costs. Despite these larger fill volumes, no increase in the frequency of peritoneal leaks has been reported, and similarly the larger intra-peritoneal fill volumes have not been shown to impair alveolar gas exchange or delay weaning from ventilators. In addition, these larger fill volumes have not been reported to increase the risk of ventilator-associated pneumonia, despite increasing intraperitoneal hydrostatic pressure and increasing the risk of reflux. However, as most patients have sepsis, and are fast peritoneal transporters, the majority require dialysate glucose concentrations in excess of 2.0% to achieve adequate ultrafiltration, and as such, this may lead to increase insulin requirements to maintain euglycaemia, particularly for diabetic patients.

Earlier studies using smaller shorter dwells volumes reported an advantage for CRRT over peritoneal dialysis, although the dose of dialysis delivered by peritoneal dialysis was somewhat low. Even so, higher volumes and longer dwell times only achieved clearances similar to those of spontaneous arterio-venous haemofiltration and/or dialysis. Some authors have therefore suggested that peritoneal dialysis may not be able to control chemistries in patients with hypercatabolic AKI, and this has led to the development of novel techniques, such as continuous flow through peritoneal dialysis, with recycling of the peritoneal dialysate effluent.

However, the number of patients suitable for peritoneal dialysis may be limited by surgical procedures, and complications include mechanical leaks and peritonitis (Table 12.3).

12.8 Choosing Dialysis Modality for Patients

In an ideal world, all patients with AKI would have their dialysis tailored to their specific circumstances. However, in practice, no one centre can provide every possible treatment modality, and as such depending upon local

Table 12.3 Comparison of renal replacement modalities: equipment and costs

Modality	Machine technology	Machine costs	Special requirements	Nurse time training	Therapy cost
Peritoneal dialysis	Yes/no	None/++	PD fluid	++	+/++
Intermittent haemodialysis	Yes	+++	Water supply	++++	+
Intermittent haemofiltration	Yes	+++	HF fluids/OL-F Ultrapure water	++++	++++
Intermittent HDF	Yes	+++	Water supply Ultrapure water	++++	+
Hybrid techniques PIRRT	Yes	+++	Water supply	+++++	++
CVVH	Yes	++++	HF fluids	++++++	++++
CVVHD	Yes	++++	HF fluids	++++++	++++
CVVHDF	Yes	++++	HF fluids/OL-F Ultrapure water	++++++	++++++

HF haemofiltration, *OL-F* online fluid production. Costs – assuming no online fluids for CRRT and intermittent haemofiltration

Table 12.4 Theoretical advantages and disadvantages of different renal replacement modalities

Modality	Potential role	Advantages	Disadvantages
PD	Paediatrics Single organ failure Haemodynamically unstable Difficult vascular access	Technically simple No anticoagulation Gradual removal of azotaemic toxins Usually haemodynamically stable Lower financial costs	Low clearances in patients with reduced mesenteric blood flow Unpredictable fluid removal Intact peritoneum required Risk of peritonitis hyperglycaemia and hypostatic pneumonia
CRRT	Haemodynamically unstable patients Patients at risk of raised intracranial pressure	Continuous removal of azotaemic toxins Haemodynamic and intracranial stability Reliable volume control	Slower clearance of toxins and poisons Prolonged anticoagulation Immobilization Hypothermia Financial costs
PIRRT	Haemodynamically unstable patient General ICU patient with AKI	Faster removal of azotaemic toxins than CRRT but slower than IHD more haemodynamically stable than IHD Reduced exposure to anti-coagulation allows time for diagnostic/therapeutic procedures and reduces immobility	Slower clearance of toxins and poisons than IHD Requires dialysate and anticoagulation
IHD	Haemodynamically stable	Rapid removal of azotaemic toxins and poisons Allows time for diagnostic/therapeutic procedures Reduces immobility Reduced anticoagulation requirements Lower financial costs	Requires dialysate Increased risk of hypotension and dialysis disequilibrium with intracranial hypertension

facilities, equipment, staffing and nursing skills, centres should aim to provide high-quality treatment limited to a few modes of RRT.

For example, the risk of intradialytic hypotension is greatest for hypotensive patients requiring vasopressor support, and therefore an alternative treatment to intermittent haemodialysis should be considered. Although CRRT and peritoneal dialysis could be suitable options, mesenteric blood flow is reduced by noradrenalin, so potentially compromising clearances and fluid removal by peritoneal dialysis. CRRT limits patient mobility, so would be not be an ideal option for patients with single organ failure, and peritoneal dialysis may be the preferred option in a patient with extensive burns involving the neck and groins (■ Table 12.4).

12.9 Convection or Diffusion?

When haemofiltration was introduced, haemofilter design differed from that for diffusive clearance for haemodialysis, to maximize hydrostatic pressure-driven convective losses. As such haemofiltration membranes were typically shorter in length, with wider diameter fibres and high flux made from synthetic polymers, whereas dialysis used low-flux cellulosic membranes. This led to increased losses of middle-sized molecular weight solutes with haemofiltration compared to dialysis, with diffusional losses. On the other hand, haemodialysis was a more effective treatment in clearing small solutes, including potassium.

In the intensive care setting, it was hypothesized that convective modes could increase the clearance of larger solutes such as inflammatory cytokines and other inflammatory mediators. However, in clinical practice, much of the observed increased clearance was due to membrane adsorption rather than convective clearance into the ultrafiltrate.

As convection depends upon the bulk movement of water across the haemofilter membrane, convective losses can be increased by increasing hydrostatic pressure and reducing osmolality and haematocrit by adding pre-dilutional fluid (■ Fig. 12.1). However, pre-dilutional fluid reduces concentration gradients which reduces diffusional losses, and as such smaller solute clearances tend to be lower with pre-dilutional fluid replacement compared to post-dilutional fluid replacement. In addition, as some of the fresh pre-dilutional fluid is removed during its first passage through the haemofilter, more fluid is required to achieve solute clearances, so increasing costs.

The development of dialyzers for haemodialysis has produced a newer generation of high-flux modified cellulosic and synthetic membranes, which allow a degree of internal convection even during standard haemodialysis. As such in clinical practice, modern-day dialysis is a diffusional technique with a varying amount of convection, whereas filtration modes are based on convective losses with a varying amount of diffusional clearance.

12.10 Choice of Dialyzer/Haemofilter Membrane

Until relatively recently there was a marked cost difference between unmodified cellulosic (cuprophane), modified cellulosic and synthetic membranes. Laboratory experiments showed that synthetic membranes cause less activation of complement, and mononuclear cells, and the initial industry sponsored studies reported improved patient survival and recovery from AKI with synthetic dialyzer membranes, although later larger randomized trials failed to show a difference. Meta-analyses subsequently showed that although there was a possible patient survival and renal recovery advantage when synthetic membranes were compared to unmodified cuprophane membranes, there was no difference between synthetic and the newer modified cellulosic membranes.

As blood initially flows across the dialyzer, anaphylatoxins, such as C3a and C5a, can be generated along with bradykinin and nitric oxide, resulting in hypotension, which can potentially be profound. This reaction depends upon a number of factors including membrane surface charge, structure, polymer composition and dialyzer design, but also the negative charge from the priming fluid (typically saline), and anticoagulant (heparins). However, in the critically ill patient, this reaction is more dependent upon patient factors, being greatest for those with severe sepsis and acute liver failure, than the choice of dialyzer. However, the prescription of angiotensin-converting enzyme inhibitors and to a lesser extent angiotensin receptor antagonists can increase the risk of hypotensive reactions when commencing dialysis.

As studies of high-flux dialyzers in patients with AKI did not show any advantage, dialyzer manufacturers have further modified membranes for patients with AKI. These newer developments have produced a range of high permeability membranes, termed high cutoff, designed to increase cytokine and inflammatory mediator clearances and also to alter surface composition to increase endotoxin adsorption, as prospective observational studies have reported increased mortality in patients with high plasma cytokines, irrespective of whether they be pro-inflammatory (IL-6) or anti-inflammatory (IL-10). Preliminary trials have failed to demonstrate any advantages for these newer technological developments on patient outcomes. Membrane adsorptive properties can also be used to adsorb heparin, potentially allowing intermittent haemodialysis/haemodiafiltration treatments without the need or a reduction in anticoagulant requirement. Trials of endotoxin absorbing membranes have also failed to demonstrate any improvement in patient survival.

12.11 Dose of Renal Replacement Therapy for AKI

In patients with chronic kidney disease stage 5, treated by regular dialysis, the term "dose" describes urea clearance achieved during RRT. The evidence from chronic kidney disease suggests that although urea per se is not a major azotaemic toxin, failure to achieve a minimum urea clearance target results in increased patient morbidity and mortality. However, the question arises as to whether patients with AKI, who often have increased catabolism, require a greater dose of dialysis, and due to the lack of prospective studies addressing the minimum "dose" of RRT required in AKI, the multi-national Acute Dialysis Quality Initiative (ADQI) consensus panel recommended that patients with AKI receive at least the minimum dose considered appropriate for patients with end-stage renal disease. However, due to the difficulty in assessing the true volume of distribution of urea in patients with AKI, several studies have shown that the delivered dose of IHD can be markedly lower than that prescribed.

There are very few haemodialysis studies, but one prospective study reported improved survival and more rapid recovery of AKI with daily haemodialysis rather than alternate day treatments. However, the increased dose associated with more frequent dialysis was also accompanied by lower ultrafiltration rates and less intradialytic hypotension. Whereas there have been a number of studies investigating the effect of dose in CRRT. Some of which suggested a benefit, particularly for septic AKI patients with greater delivered dose of RRT. For example, Ronco and colleagues randomized 425 patients to one of three CVVH doses, defined by achieved daily ultrafiltration rates of 20 ml/kg.hr, 35 ml/kg.hr and 45 ml/kg.hr [16]. Mortality was markedly lower in the intermediate- and high-dose arms (43% and 42%, respectively) compared to the low-dose arm (59%, $p < 0.001$). Although these findings were supported by some smaller studies, not all studies showed any effect of dose on outcomes.

Two major trials each with more than 1000 patients were devised to try and answer whether the dose of RRT was important in determining outcomes in AKI. The NIH/VA ATN trial stratified patients according to illness severity and randomized the less critically ill patient to standard thrice-weekly haemodialysis to achieve a sessional Kt/V of 1.2 or to six times weekly dialysis [17]. This study showed no differences in outcomes, and paradoxically intradialytic hypotension was greater in the more frequent dialysis group, but this transpired to be due to increased fluid administration and higher ultrafiltration requirements in the more frequent dialysis group. The more critically ill patients were randomized to CRRT prescribed to achieve ultrafiltration rates of 0.35 vs 20 ml/kgh, respectively, and again there were no differences in outcomes between the groups. The RENAL trial compared two doses of haemofiltration, 25 vs 40 ml/kg/h, and again showed no differences in outcomes [18]. Whereas the Ronco study compared delivered CRRT dosages, these latter trials compared prescribed and not delivered doses. Both of these trials reported increased CRRT clotting with the more intensive regimes, and as such the delivered dose of RRT was most likely somewhat lower than that prescribed. Even so taken together, it is unlikely that above a critical threshold of a sessional Kt/Vurea for intermittent treatments and 20 ml/kg/h for CRRT additional treatments do not appear to offer benefit. As it takes time for azotaemic toxins to accumulate, then in AKI, probably correction of volume overload and electrolyte and acid-base disturbances are more important than removing azotaemic solutes above a critical threshold.

In terms of other treatment modalities, there are no studies looking at the optimum dose of peritoneal dialysis required for patients with single organ and/or multiple organ failure; there is a similar paucity of data on the recently introduced PIRRT (Genius®., EDD, and SLED). Preliminary studies suggest that EDD systems have comparable small solute clearances to conventional CRRT, but may be less effective in terms of middle molecule clearances.

12.12 Pulsed High-Volume CRRT or Haemodiafiltration

Although there appears to be no benefit from an increased dosage of RRT, several single-centre reports suggested a benefit of an initial high pulse of RRT, in keeping with ICU policies of initial active fluid resuscitation, as part of early goal-directed therapy, and early administration of antibiotics for sepsis.

It has been suggested that high-volume treatments can help reduce the inflammatory milieu, but equally the improved cardiovascular stability reported could be attributable to increased sympathetic drive secondly to additional cooling, accompanied by positive sodium and calcium balance. The positive outcomes reported with this treatment came from single centres, and the one randomized prospective dual-centre trial of high-dose CRRT was abandoned as there was no observed patient benefit for high-dose therapy.

12.13 Choice of Dialysate and Substitution Replacement Fluid

Studies from both chronic haemodialysis patients and patients with AKI have shown an increased incidence of supraventricular arrhythmias, typically precipitated by a relative reduction in effective plasma volume. These arrhythmias and intra-dialytic hypotension can be ameliorated by using higher sodium dialysate, of around 5 mmol/l above the serum concentration, up to 145 mmol/l, with some reports using even higher gradients, coupled with higher potassium dialysates, so minimizing the serum to dialysate potassium gradient to

2 mmol/l or less, and higher dialysate calcium concentrations between 1.35 and 1.5 mmol/l, although there is a suggestion that a further increase in dialysate calcium concentrations may actually cause cardiovascular instability. In addition, bicarbonate-based dialysates provide greater cardiovascular stability than acetate. Cooling of the dialysate also reduces the risk of intradialytic hypotension. Dialysis machines may have dialysate temperature modules, which can reduce the dialysate temperature to prevent patient warming or an increase in heat energy, as during dialysis, blood skin flow falls, so reducing thermal energy dissipation and increasing core temperature, which if it reaches a critical threshold can cause reflex vasodilatation. Recent studies have shown that greater cardiovascular stability can be achieved by simply cooling the dialysate to 35 °C. One of the differences between haemodiafiltration compared to haemodialysis is the additional cooling achieved with haemodiafiltration, which is greatest with pre-dilution mode.

Lactate and acetate have been used as the primary buffers for both replacement fluids and dialysates for CRRT, due to ease of sterility and prolonged storage life. Lactate and acetate are indirectly metabolized, in the liver and skeletal muscle, through to bicarbonate. The blood lactate level can increase during lactate-based CRRT, if the rate of administration exceeds the rate of metabolism, particularly in patients with pre-existent lactic acidosis and/or impaired hepatic function, potentially contributing to increased protein catabolism and impaired myocardial contractility. Relatively recently, commercially available bicarbonate-buffered fluids have been introduced for CRRT, and although there has been no study showing a significant effect on patient survival, some studies have reported improved cardiovascular stability and control of metabolic acidosis with bicarbonate-based fluids.

12

There are a wide range of commercially available dialysates and replacement fluids for CRRT. As the amount of lactate and chloride is balanced to sodium and other cations, if a fluid has a high chloride concentration, then the lactate concentration will be lower and vice versa. As such the spectrum of fluids available varies from 95 mmol/l of chloride and 46 mmol/l of lactate to 115 mmol/l chloride and 30 mmol/l lactate. As such, after a few days, and more noticeably with higher volume exchanges, patients may potentially develop a hypochloraemic alkalosis with the first electrolyte combination, and conversely a hyperchloraemic acidosis with the second electrolyte composition.

In addition, during purely convective therapies, as the dialyzer membrane is charged, the ratio of a small cation in the ultrafiltrate will be less than that of plasma water, and conversely anions greater. This effect also depends upon whether fluids are replaced in pre-dilution or post-dilution mode. As such sodium and calcium balances are most positive with post-dilutional fluid replacement, whereas chloride gains are greatest with pre-dilutional fluid replacement. Again, as sodium and calcium content of fluids also vary, the actual electrolyte balances will vary with different fluid compositions and ultrafiltration.

12.14 Choice of Anticoagulation During IHD/Hybrid and CRRT

AKI is often associated with systemic inflammation, and as such these patients are more likely to have clotting problems with extracorporeal circuits than chronic kidney disease patients attending for routine haemodialysis. Other systemic anticoagulants may be contraindicated as patients with AKI may have recently undergone surgery or be at increased risk of haemorrhage.

Clotting in the extracorporeal circuit typically occurs in the dialyzer, venous air detector chamber and catheter access. The risk of clotting can be reduced by careful priming to remove air from the circuit, so reducing air-blood interfaces, and using tubing within minimum changes in lumen diameter and joints to minimize areas of turbulence.

12.14.1 Anticoagulation Free Options

Although prefilter normal saline flushes can be used to avoid anticoagulation during intermittent haemodialysis, particularly for short sessions by reducing haemoconcentration during passage through the dialyzer, other options include heparin adsorption to the dialyzer and citrate dialysate. Unfractionated heparin (UFH) is very negatively charged and as such can adsorb to dialyzer membranes. This has led to a number of centres devising their own protocols, recirculating 10–20,000 IU UFH for 30–60 minutes and then rinsing out the circuit to avoid systemic anticoagulation. Taking this one step further, the polyacrylonitrile membrane has been specially modified to increase UFH adsorption and is now commercially available (AN 69ST®) [19], although trials have not shown an advantage over standard no-anticoagulant practices. Citrate is an effective anticoagulant by binding calcium. Formal citrate anticoagulation adds a degree of cost and complexity to CRRT circuits (see ◘ Fig. 12.3), and an alternative is to replace acetate in the dialysate with citrate. As such the patient is exposed to a low concentration of citrate (Citrasate®), which may permit short session systemic anticoagulant free dialysis, or reduced anticoagulant requirements [20].

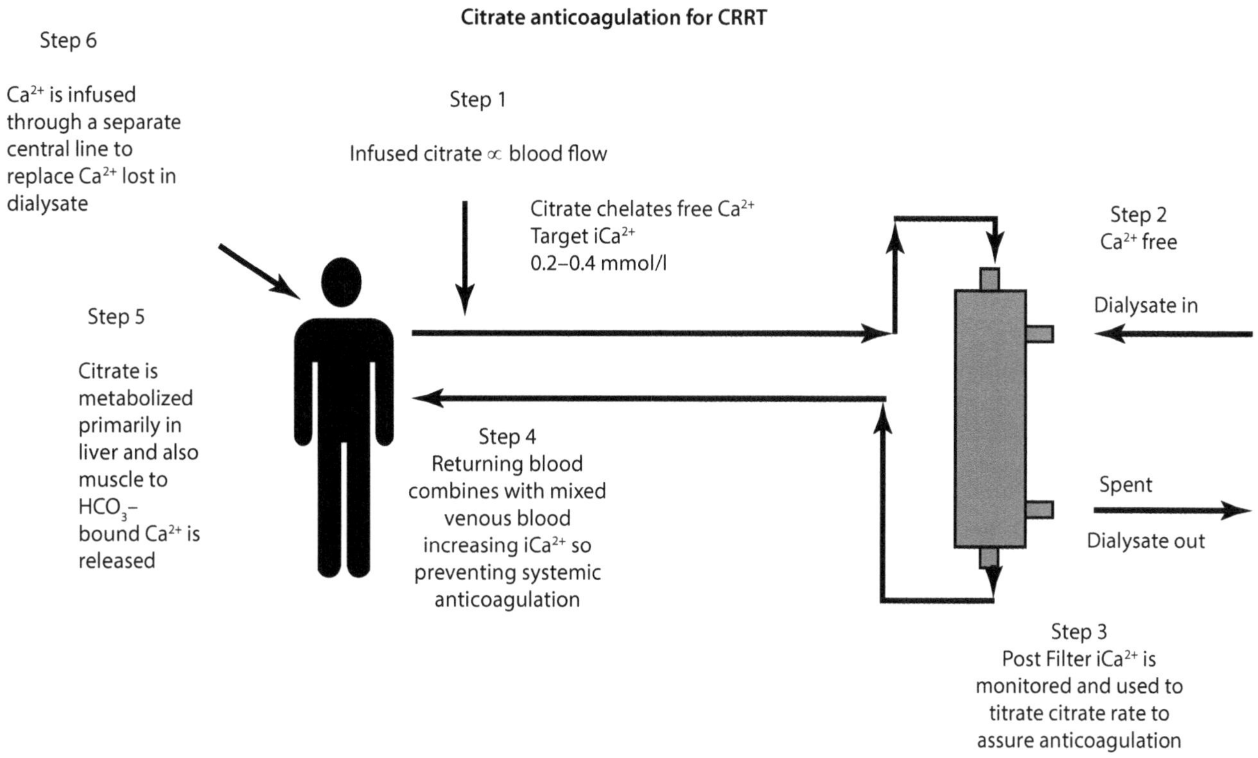

Citrate anticoagulation for CRRT

Step 6

Ca^{2+} is infused through a separate central line to replace Ca^{2+} lost in dialysate

Step 1

Infused citrate ∝ blood flow

Citrate chelates free Ca^{2+}
Target iCa^{2+}
0.2–0.4 mmol/l

Step 2
Ca^{2+} free

Dialysate in

Step 5

Citrate is metabolized primarily in liver and also muscle to HCO_3^- bound Ca^{2+} is released

Step 4
Returning blood combines with mixed venous blood increasing iCa^{2+} so preventing systemic anticoagulation

Spent

Dialysate out

Step 3
Post Filter iCa^{2+} is monitored and used to titrate citrate rate to assure anticoagulation

Fig. 12.3 Shows circuit for continuous citrate anticoagulation with calcium replacement

Anticoagulant free CRRT is possible particularly with careful priming to exclude all air, minimizing circuitry, with pre-dilutional fluid replacement, so minimizing haemoconcentration and also for patients with thrombocytopenia.

12.14.2 Systemic Anticoagulants

UFH is typically administered as a bolus (500–1000 Iu depending on the risk of haemorrhage), and as it has a relatively short half-life then continuously infused (500–1000 IU/h) until 30–60 minutes prior to the end of the session. Low-molecular-weight heparins (LMWHs) have a more prolonged half-life and as such typically are administered as a single bolus (tinzaparin 1500–2500 IU, enoxparin 0.4–0.8 mg/kg depending upon duration of session and risk of haemorrhage). UFH is a series of large molecules, but LMWHs are smaller molecules, and as such there can be loss if administered as a single bolus immediately prior to a high flux or high permeability dialyzer, before it has become protein coated. As such administration into the venous limb of the circuit or delaying the administration into the arterial limb of the circuit by a few minutes reduces LMWH requirements.

UFH remains the most widely used anticoagulant for CRRT. Although an effective anticoagulant for IHD in patients with chronic kidney disease, UFH may be less effective in AKI, as many critically ill patients have reduced levels of anti-thrombin, especially with CRRT. In addition, heparin is associated with a risk of bleeding and with the development of heparin-induced thrombocytopenia (HIT). LMWHs can equally be used for CRRT, with either an initial bolus followed by an infusion or simply starting with a greater infusion rate and then titrated according to anti-Xa activity, aiming for a target of around 0.4 antiXa IU/ml. Regional heparinization protocols, with reversal of heparin by infusion of protamine into the return line, have been developed to prevent systemic anticoagulation and minimize bleeding risk. Unfortunately, these protocols are cumbersome, may be associated with paradoxical increased risk of bleeding if excess protamine is infused and do not alter the risk of HIT. Protamine may cause anaphylaxis, particularly in patients allergic to salmon.

If patients with HIT develop thrombosis, or other major complications, then systemic anticoagulation with either heparinoids, danaparoid, fondiparinux, or direct thrombin inhibitor argatroban is required. If however, patients have HIT antibodies, but no symptoms or signs of thrombosis, then other anticoagulants, including prostacyclin (prostaglandin I_2), nafamostat and citrate, are safe in patients with a history of HIT, provided all exposure to heparin has ceased. In the laboratory there may be cross reaction between the heparinoids and HIT antibodies, although only occasionally has this led to clinical cross reactivity. Heparinoids, such as danaparoid, have an increased half-life in AKI and require anti-factor Xa monitoring. For CRRT, following an initial bolus dose of 1500 anti-Xa U and an infusion rate of 150 U/h which has to be then adjusted to maintain anti-Xa levels between 0.2 and 0.4 IU/ml. Argatroban, derived from l-arginine, requires a continuous infusion, starting at 0.5 ug/kg/min followed by dose adjustment to maintain an aPTTr of 1.8–2.0, and additional dose reduction in liver disease (starting at 0.02 ug/kg/min). The major metabolite of argatroban has biological activity and accumulates with time. In addition, argatroban also prolongs the prothrombin time, and this may complicate the transfer from argatroban to oral warfarin.

12.14.3 Regional Anticoagulants

Over the last decade, citrate has emerged as a very effective regional anticoagulant for CRRT. Citrate is infused into the pre-filter line and works by chelating calcium, aiming for a pre-filter ionized calcium of 0.2–0.4 mmol/l. As such the amount of citrate to be infused depends upon blood flow (▫ Table 12.5). Calcium is then re-infused separately, or into the return line, to maintain a normal systemic ionized calcium [21]. Citrate comes as a sodium salt, either trisodium citrate or acid citrate dextrose, and each citrate molecule is indirectly converted to three bicarbonates, so there can potentially be changes in sodium balance and acid-base status depending upon the citrate load and the ability of the patient to adequately metabolize citrate. Thus, most centres that used citrate developed their own in-house calcium free dialysates and re-infusion fluids. It is only more recently that pharmaceutical and dialysis companies have marketed specialized dialysates and re-infusion fluids designed for citrate systems. The advent of these commercially available fluids for citrate-based anticoagulation has increased the usage in both adult and particularly paediatric practice, where circuit clotting has been a greater clinical problem. There have been few prospective comparative studies of UFH and citrate anticoagulation; in two such CRRT studies, the median circuit survival time was significantly prolonged with citrate (70 hours vs 40 hours and 124 vs 38 hours) with reduced blood transfusion requirement and/or haemorrhage in the citrate groups.

▫ Table 12.5 Citrate dose for varying blood flows (Qb)

Qb ml/min	4% TCA ml/h	ACD-A ml/h
100	175	210
150	262	315
200	350	420
250	438	525
300	525	630

TCA trisodium citrate, *ACD-A* acid citrate dextrose

In AKI, citrate is primarily metabolized in the liver and muscle, so patients with acute liver failure and cardiogenic shock may not be able to adequately metabolize citrate, leading to an increase in total serum calcium, with a lowered ionized calcium, due to an increasing calcium-citrate complexes, termed the calcium gap, and a metabolic acidosis. Citrate accumulation, or toxicity, is likely when the ratio of total serum calcium to ionized calcium exceeds 2.5 [22]. Treatment includes increasing dialysate flow to increase circuit citrate losses, stopping or reducing the rate of citrate infusion and increasing blood flow. On the other hand, excess citrate delivery, which is metabolized through to bicarbonate, can lead to a metabolic alkalosis.

Other regional anticoagulants include prostacyclin (5–10 ng/kg/min), which is a potent vasodilator. As such patients should be made volume replete prior to administration and infusions started at 0.5 ng/kg/min and titrated upwards prior to starting CRRT. In Japan, nafamostat maleate is used as a regional anticoagulant and appears to have similar efficacy and safety profile to citrate.

12.15 Acute Brain Injury

During a standard intermittent outpatient haemodialysis session, the brain swells. This is due to a combination of a relatively faster fall in serum urea compared to that in brain extracellular fluid and astrocytes, which regulate the blood-brain barrier. As water moves some 20 times faster through aquaporin channels than urea through urea transporters, water passes back into the brain along a concentration gradient. In addition, as the effective plasma volume decreases, then middle cerebral artery blood flow falls. In patients with acute traumatic brain injury or acute cerebral oedema, then autoregulation may not be intact, and as such intradialytic hypotension may lead to a fall in cerebral perfusion pressure with increased local cerebral oedema in areas of ischaemia.

As such the two key objectives for RRT in patients with acute brain injury are to maintain cardiovascular stability and avoid a rapid reduction in serum urea.

Patients with intracranial monitoring devices, particularly intraventricular drains and subdural catheters, are at increased risk of local bleeding around these devices if given systemic anticoagulants.

In clinical practice, acute brain injury requiring RRT is encountered in two main scenarios, firstly chronic dialysis patients who have sustained an intracranial haemorrhage or ischaemic stroke and secondly acute traumatic brain injury or cerebral oedema and AKI. As the brain typically takes 10–14 days to adapt to injury, RRT should be modified during this period. In patients with compromised cerebral perfusion pressure (<60 mmHg) or major midline shift on brain scanning, then standard intermittent haemodialysis should be avoided. Peritoneal dialysis is an option, as changes in serum urea are slower than those during intermittent haemodialysis, but dialysates are hyponatraemic, and patients may require additional hypertonic saline. Large-volume cycles, particularly using hypertonic glucose dialysates, can alter cardiac filling by sudden changes in intraperitoneal pressure and compression of the inferior vena cava, and so may lead to sudden falls in cerebral perfusion pressure. As such, tidal exchanges or smaller fill cycle fill volumes are to be preferred. CRRT provides the greatest cardiovascular stability, and haemofiltration is less effective at clearing urea than dialysis and so causes slower reduction. By performing pre-dilution CVVH, patients achieve greater cooling and so are less likely to suffer hypotension, and pre-dilution reduces urea clearance compared to post-dilution. In cases of raised intracranial hypertension, with lower or borderline cerebral perfusion, hypertonic saline infusions can be given during CRRT, to raise serum sodium, or 20% mannitol.

Typically, in cases of AKI following acute traumatic brain injury, or acute cerebral oedema with liver failure, urea and creatinine concentrations are not high, and RRT is initiated for oliguria and metabolic acidosis, so disequilibrium due to too rapid urea shifts is less likely, but maintaining cerebral perfusion pressure and cardiac output are key to patient management, and so dialysis machines equipped with relative blood volume monitoring are preferred. Whereas in cases of acute intracranial haemorrhage in established dialysis patients, then urea levels are often raised, and the major management decision is to balance the risks of early RRT to deferring treatment but then starting with a higher urea and risking greater disequilibrium. Although there have been no randomized trials, most centres aim to maintain the serum urea <15 mmol/l. If haemodialysis is the only modality available, then the rate of change in plasma osmolality can be reduced by using a smaller surface area dialyzer (0.6–0.8 m^2), slowing blood flow to 200 ml/min with a slower dialysate flow of 200–300 ml/min, switching the dialysate flow from counter current to concurrent, and using a dialysate sodium of +5 mmol/l above the serum concentration up to 145 mmol/l. To maintain cardiovascular stability, then the ultrafiltration rate needs to be slowed by extending dialysis session time in combination with higher dialysate sodium, potassium and calcium concentrations, with the dialysate cooled to 35 °C. So, in essence, haemodialysis becomes PIRRT. Pre-dilutional haemodiafiltration would provide additional cooling. Daily treatments would lower ultrafiltration requirements and also help prevent rises in serum urea, leading to a lower time-averaged urea concentration. If there are contraindications to systemic anticoagulation, then pre-dilutional fluid replacement, with either citrate in the dialysate or citrate anticoagulation, would be preferable. Both hypertonic saline and mannitol can be administered during haemodialysis as short infusions.

To minimize the risk of hypotension when first connecting the patient to the extracorporeal circuit, then priming with isotonic bicarbonate, by reducing negative charge, reduces the risk of anaphylatoxin and bradykinin-induced vasodilatation. Similarly, if a bolus of UFH or LMWH is administered into the venous limb of the circuit, this reduces the charge effect from anticoagulants. Some centres prime the circuit with albumin to precoat the dialyzer with proteins prior to directly connecting the patient to the RRT circuit.

12.16 Cardiorenal Syndrome

Increasingly nephrologists are encountering patients with cardiac failure who have developed AKI following an additional insult.

Although cardiorenal syndromes can occur with both acute cardiac and renal dysfunction following drugs or toxins, and acute myocardial infarction, most patients developing a cardiorenal syndrome do so, on a background of both chronic heart and kidney disease [23]. Patients with acute multi-organ dysfunction should preferably be managed in the ICU setting by CRRT. As although peritoneal dialysis is technically possible, low blood pressure in cases of cardiogenic shock will limit mesenteric blood flows, so reducing solute clearances and water removal.

Most patients with heart failure have a normal or increased cardiac output, and only a minority, around 10% with cardiogenic shock and reduced cardiac output [24] (taken from the European Heart Society guidelines on heart failure). As such peritoneal dialysis may be an effective therapy. Increased right-sided cardiac filling pressures contribute to renal dysfunction, and as such fluid removal by peritoneal dialysis using smaller fill volumes may help restore renal function. Typically, these patients behave as fast peritoneal transporters, and 7.5% icodextrin exchanges may be required to achieve ultrafiltration without exposing the patient to hypertonic glucose dialysates. After stabilization some patients can be discharged home on a single overnight icodextrin exchange. However, for some patients, peritoneal dialysis is not initially effective in correcting volume overload, due to increased peritoneal permeability and loss of glucose gradients, and for these patients, CRRT or daily intermittent dialysis or PIRRT is required. Later, when stabilized, these patients may well return to peritoneal dialysis. As outlined above for dialysing patients with brain injury, dialysis needs to be tailored to improve cardiovascular stability and minimize ultrafiltration rates, utilizing machines capable of relative blood volume monitoring. For patients with acute cardiorenal syndromes treated by haemodialysis, there is an increased risk of intra-dialytic hypotension, which may then convert a potentially reversible acute episode into one of established dialysis-dependent kidney failure. The main risk of hypotension is due to an ultrafiltration rate which removes plasma water at a rate faster than tissue fluid can refill the plasma water. Even for a healthy dialysis outpatient, once the ultrafiltration rate exceeds 10 ml/kg/h, the risk of intradialytic hypotension rises exponentially. Thus, to minimize ultrafiltration rates, patients should be dialysed more frequently, ideally daily if possible. The risk of arrhythmias on dialysis depends upon both relative intravascular hypovolaemia and also electrolyte shifts. To minimize electrolyte shifts, patients should be dialysed against a dialysate potassium of at least 2 or 3 mmol/l, to reduce the gradient between serum and dialysate potassium concentration. Dialysate calcium concentrations also affect cardiovascular stability, and although higher dialysate calcium concentrations confer cardiovascular stability over lower concentrations (1.5 vs 1.0 mmol/l), too high a calcium (>1.5 mmol/l) also increases the risk on cardiac instability. Dialysate bicarbonate also affects the flux of ions between the plasma water and cells, and although bicarbonate-based dialysate confers cardiovascular stability compared to acetate-based dialysate, then higher bicarbonate concentrations (>32 mmol/l) and acetate (≥3 mmol/l) increase the risk of electrolyte fluxes. Cooling the dialysate also reduces the risk of intradialytic hypotension. Some dialysis machines can be programmed to provide isothermic dialysis, so as the patient starts to warm up during dialysis due to the relative increase in core blood flow and reduced skin blood flows, the dialysis machine automatically cools the dialysate to prevent any increased body temperature. If this technology is available, then simply setting the dialysate temperature to 35 °C will be equally, if not more, effective. During dialysis, the plasma urea concentration falls exponentially and so reduces plasma osmolality, and this may reduce plasma water refilling rate and so risk intradialytic hypotension. Thus using a higher dialysate sodium can reduce this fall in osmolality and so better maintain blood pressure. Most studies have advocated a dialysate sodium set at 5 mmol/l above serum sodium up to a maximum dialysate sodium of 147 mmol/l. Advances in haemodialysis machine technology have brought a new generation of dialysis machines that can monitor relative blood volume, based on changes in haematocrit or blood viscosity, and can therefore sense if the ultrafiltration rate exceeds plasma refilling. This can be visually displayed allowing the supervising dialysis nurse or technician to respond to sudden changes. The more sophisticated machines have feedback loops which automatically adjust ultrafiltration rate and/or dialysate sodium to these changes, so reducing the risk of intra-dialytic hypotension. When dialysis first starts, the passage of blood across the dialyzer leads to activation of platelets and leukocytes, with pulmonary sequestration and fall in arterial oxygen tension, typically during the first 20 minutes, and this then tends to resolve after 1 hour. In cases of patients who have recently suffered myocardial ischaemia, then supplemental oxygen should be considered to prevent any reduction in arterial oxygen tension. Several reports have advocated haemodiafiltration over haemodialysis due to the additional cooling effect in maintaining cardiovascular stability whilst achieving required ultrafiltration. As fluid volume control is achieved, then cardiac biomarkers such as NTproBNP fall.

12.17 Chronic Cardiorenal Syndromes

Patients who have recovered from a major myocardial infarction or patients with other cardiac pathology, such as cardiac amyloid infiltration, may be left with chronic hypotension and symptomatic dyspnoea. As such, quality of life may be poor, and the decision whether to offer such patients dialysis to help control fluid volume should not be taken lightly. However, if patients can tolerate chronic hypotension and wish to have palliative dialysis, then peritoneal dialysis using a single overnight 2 l exchange of 7.5% icodextrin may help contain volume overload without significantly reducing systemic blood pressure. As patients are often incapacitated, then exchanges may have to be performed by a family member or assistant. Over time, the underlying cardiac pathology will typically progress, and patients may lose residual renal function, so requiring standard peritoneal dialysis. At this stage, the role of palliative peritoneal dialysis should be reassessed, as ultrafiltration volumes are often unpredictable with peritoneal dialysis, leading to periods of volume overload interspersed with hypotensive episodes, as typically patients require higher glucose exchanges to sustain adequate ultrafiltration.

Table 12.6 Dialysis prescription for patients with acute cardiorenal syndrome secondary to myocardial infarction

Modality	Haemodiafiltration preferred to haemodialysis
Frequency	Preferably daily
Duration	3–4 hours
Dialyzer	Small surface area bio-compatible dialyzer
Dialysate	Sodium +5 mmol/l above serum sodium
	Potassium 3 mmol/l
	Calcium 1.35–1.5 mmol/l
	Bicarbonate 32 mmol/l
	Isothermic or cooled dialysate to 35 °C
	Dialysate flow 500 ml/min
Blood pump speed	250–300 ml/min
Ultrafiltration rate	<5 ml/kg/h
Anticoagulation	Depends on whether patient systemically anticoagulated with bivalirudin, low-molecular-weight heparin or antiplatelet agents

Some patients may opt for haemodialysis, but this needs to be viewed as a palliative therapy. As haemodialysis risks exacerbation of hypotension, then patients typically require more frequent dialysis sessions (4–6 × week) to allow adequate volume control. Patients should be dialysed with cooled dialysate and higher potassium and calcium dialysates (Table 12.6), but continuous exposure to high dialysate sodium will lead to increased thirst and weight gains, and as such dialysate sodium should be set to around 140 mmol/l. For patients with excessively low systemic blood pressures (<80 mmHg), then vasoconstrictive agents such as midodrine or terlipressin may prevent intradialytic hypotension, but risk ischaemia to the gastrointestinal tract, and other organs, and these risks have to considered on an individual basis.

12.18 Severe Electrolyte Imbalances

12.18.1 Hyponatraemia in AKI

When asked to provide RRT in a patient with severe hyponatraemia, firstly establish volume status, as if the patient has hypovolaemic hyponatraemia; this should be corrected before initiating RRT, to avoid hypotension during RRT. Peritoneal dialysis uses fixed hyponatraemic dialysates (Na 132/133 mmol/l), and haemodialysis machines are typically designed to deliver dialysates of 136–145 mmol/l, and outside this range, machines would have to recalibrated to provide more hyponatraemic dialysates. Even so this would be prone to errors, and accurate concentrations could not be guaranteed.

Depending upon the clinical situation, dialysis would be designed to increase the serum sodium to 125 mmol/l over the first 12–24 hours. As such only CRRT would allow a slow rise in serum sodium from 110 mmol/l or so compared to peritoneal or intermittent therapies, especially as the risk to pontine demyelination also depends on cerebral oxygen delivery and perfusion [25]. Although the replacement fluids and dialysates for CRRT come with a fixed sodium (typically 138–144 mmol/l), it is possible to tailor the composition of the dialysate/replacement fluid by using a combination of commercial fluids and Hartmann's, dextrose and either 0.9% saline or dextrose saline, to achieve an initial dialysate 5 mmol/l above the serum dialysate (e.g. 5 l of commercial fluid Na 143 mmol/l, 4.0 l Hartmann's with a sodium of 132 mmol/l and 1.0 l of 5% dextrose provide a sodium of 124 mmol/l). Reducing exchange volumes to 1.0 l/hour, and using post-dilution CVVH, also slows the rate of rise in serum sodium. Regular monitoring of the serum sodium allows a controlled rise in serum sodium and determines changes in replacement fluid/dialysate sodium composition, so that a serum sodium of 125 mmol/l is achieved over 24 hours. Thereafter, serum sodium can be steadily increased.

12.18.2 Hypernatraemia

As with hyponatraemia, volume status needs to be assessed, as if the patient has hypovolaemic hypernatraemia, and this should be corrected before initiating RRT due to the risks of hypotension with RRT. Similarly serum sodium concentration should be reduced slowly. Whereas peritoneal dialysis and haemodialysis machines have relatively fixed dialysate sodium concentrations, CRRT allows the possibility of tailoring the dialysate/replacement solution sodium concentration, by adding hypertonic saline to achieve the desired composition.

12.18.3 Hypercalcaemia

In cases of severe hypercalcaemia (>4.0 mmol/l) in moribund patients not responding to standard medical practices, the RRT can be used to reduce the serum calcium and prevent soft tissue calcification. Standard peritoneal dialysates have a fixed calcium concentration of 1.25–1.75 mmol/l, and as this is equivalent to ionized calcium concentrations, these fluids are not hypocalcaemic. Similarly, standard dialysates for haemodialysis start at 1.0 mmol/l and thus will allow calcium clearance with haemodialysis, down to an ionized calcium of 1.0 mmol/l. To increase calcium losses, a large surface area dialyser should be coupled with a prolonged session time, so moving from intermittent haemodialysis to PIRRT. The standard dialysates and fluid replacement fluids designed for CRRT are typically hypercalcaemic, as they were designed for critically ill patients who are often hypocalcaemic. However, following the introduction of citrate as an anticoagulant for CRRT, there are now commercially available fluids designed for citrate which contain no calcium. As such these fluids will correct hypercalcaemia, and a greater calcium loss is achieved with pre-dilution rather than post-dilution mode, with 3 l hourly cycles. If these fluids are not available, then CRRT could be performed using 0.9% saline with potassium and phosphate supplements as appropriate.

12.18.4 Poisoning

RRT should be considered in severe cases of poisoning or drug intoxication that have not responded to standard supportive medical treatment, and patients have serum levels of drugs and/or poisons which are known to result in significant risk of patient mortality and/or organ failure, and also if the rate of extracorporeal clearance exceeds that of endogenous hepatic and/or renal clearance (Table 12.7).

12

Table 12.7 Serum drug/poison concentrations at which extracorporeal removal may be beneficial

Drug	Serum mg/l	Concentration mmol/l
Phenobarbital	100	0.43
Glutethimide	40	0.18
Methaqualone	40	0.16
Salicylates	800	4.4
Theophylline	40	0.22
Paraquat	0.1	0.5
Methanol	500	16
Ethylene glycol	500	8.1
Meprobamate	100	0.46
Lithium acute	4.0	4.0
Lithium chronic	>2.5	>2.5
Phenytoin	30	120
Valproate	1000	7.0

12.18.5 Volume of Distribution

Although RRT is most effective when treating drugs/toxins with a small volume of distribution, they may be a role in treating tissue/protein bound compounds, if a temporary reduction in plasma concentration results in reversal of life-threatening toxic effects.

12.18.6 Haemodialysis and Haemodiafiltration

HD provides rapid clearance for water-soluble drugs/toxins, particularly those of a low-molecular-weight with a small volume of distribution, including alcohols, organic acids (which accumulate in urea cycle defects of metabolism), aminoglycosides, atenolol and lithium (Table 12.8). Larger drugs such as amphotericin (9241 D) can be cleared using high-flux dialyzers and by adding in pre-dilutional HDF. As such HDF is the preferred option for clearing valproate, vancomycin and hirudin. In cases of cardiovascular instability, then CRRT with high-volume exchanges should be considered, but clearances will not be as effective as intermittent HD or HDF.

In cases of drugs which have substantial tissue binding and haemoperfusion is not available, then HD and HDF may still be effective in reducing drug toxicity, provided that session times are prolonged to PIRRT For example, methotrexate can be effectively cleared by extending haemodialysis times to 6 hours and performing two dialysis sessions with only a short break between.

Table 12.8 Drugs and toxins preferentially removed by HD and HP [26]

HD effective	HP effective
Lithium	Lipid soluble
Bromide	Barbiturates
Ethanol	Sedatives
Methanol	Tranquillizers
Ethylene glycol	Theophylline
Salicylates	Paraquat
Antimicrobials	Mushroom
Antivirals	Phenytoin
Valproate	Trichloroethanol
Carbamazepine	Disopyramide
Metformin	

12.18.7 Haemoperfusion

Haemoperfusion (HP) uses a sorbent cartridge, typically carbon or an exchange resin to bind protein-bound drugs or poisons, including arsenic, calcium-channel blockers, benzodiazepines, phenytoin and tricyclic antidepressants (▣ Table 12.7). HP will also remove lipophilic drugs/toxins more effectively than HD [20]. Depending upon the column, there may be an increased risk of hypotension due to bradykinin and nitric oxide generation and increased risk of clotting due to the combination of platelet activation and also the adsorption of the natural anticoagulant protein C, particularly to anionic exchange resins. As such anticoagulants with a predominately anti-platelet effect (prostacyclin, prostanoids and citrate) are more potent anticoagulants than heparins for haemoperfusion.

The key difference between haemoperfusion and HD is that the haemoperfusion cartridge will become saturated depending upon the plasma concentration of the substance to be adsorbed, with a typical cartridge becoming saturated in 4–6 hours. Thus, in cases of severe poisoning, then two HP treatments should be performed in series, with a short break in between, rather than waiting to perform the second haemoperfusion on the following day. Is there a website on how to do haemoperfusion, i.e. it would be helpful to have a how to do it guide – of course not.

Case Study

Case 1

A 65-year-old man with a past history of diabetes and chronic kidney disease who had been receiving thrice-weekly haemodialysis for 24 months was admitted at night with a non-Q wave myocardial infarction. He underwent emergency coronary artery angiography and cardiac angioplasty and stenting and was given fondaparinux and started on aspirin, prasugrel and ramipril. The next morning, the cardiology team contacted the renal team and asked for dialysis treatment, as it was his normal dialysis day. The renal team reviewed the patient; he had a peripheral oxygen saturation of 95% on room air and minimal peripheral oedema, with a blood pressure of 110/70; a jugular venous pulse was not elevated, and there were no pulmonary crackles. His serum creatinine was 800 umol/L with a urea of 30 mmol/l and serum potassium 4.5 mmol/l.

Would you dialyse this man as requested by the cardiology team?

Observational studies from the USA report an increased mortality for patients dialysed post-myocardial infarction. The blood supply to the heart depends upon the diastolic blood pressure. As such, the key to dialysing patients post-myocardial infarction depends upon maintaining oxygen delivery and perfusion pressure to the heart. As such, the key question is whether dialysis is required or could be delayed. In this case, dialysis should be delayed until there is a clinical indication for dialysis. Angiotensin-converting enzyme inhibitors (ACEIs) are cleared by dialysis but increase the risk of increased hypotensive episodes at the start of dialysis as bradykinin is produced when diluted blood crosses the dialyzer membrane. As such, sartans are preferred to ACEIs.

Case 2

A chronic dialysis patient was admitted with bacteraemia due to *E. coli* septicaemia due to urosepsis. She had a blood pressure of 110/60 mmHg compared to her normal pre-dialysis pressure of 160/90 mmHg. She had no clinical signs of extracellular water excess. Her serum creatinine was 800 umol/L with a urea of 30 mmol/l, serum potassium 6.5 mmol/l and sodium of 136 mmol/l. Her outpatient dialysis prescription was a 4-hour dialysis using a dialysate of 136 mmol/l sodium, potassium 2.0 mmol/l and calcium 1.0 mmol/l and dialysate temperature 37.0 °C.

Would you use her standard outpatient dialysis prescription?

This lady is septic with a relatively low blood pressure and is at increased risk of hypotension during dialysis reduced. The risks of hypotension can be reduced by reducing the dialysate temperature to 35.0 °C and increasing the dialysate sodium to 10 mmol/l above the serum sodium concentration, up to a maximum of 145 mmol/l. The risk of arrhythmias is increased by a greater serum to dialysate potassium gradient, and as such a potassium of 2.0 or 3.0 mmol/l would be appropriate. Similarly dialysate calcium concentrations of 1.35–1.5 mmol/l provide greater cardiovascular stability compared to lower or higher calcium dialysate concentrations. Cooler dialysate temperatures cause vasoconstriction and reduce the risk of hypotension, and as such the dialysate temperature should be reduced to 35 °C.

Case 3

A patient unknown to the renal service was admitted by the emergency department confused. He had Kussmaul respiration but was not hypervolaemic, with a blood pressure of 140/80 with a serum urea of 50 mmol/l and serum creatinine of 1800 umol/L; the serum calcium was 1.9 mmol/l and bicarbonate of 16 mmol/l and potassium of 4 mmol/l.

You are asked to dialyse this patient. What dialysis prescription would you prescribe?

This man has long-standing chronic kidney disease and is not volume overloaded. Choosing a high bicarbonate dialysate will increase the risk of hypocalcaemia and hypokalaemia. As such, a lower dialysate bicarbonate of 28 mmol/l with an acetate of 3.0 mmol/l would be appropriate, in combination with a higher dialysate calcium of 1.5 mmol/l and potassium of 3.0 mmol/l. As there is a risk of dialysis disequilibrium, then a shorter dialysis session time of 2 hours, with reduced blood and dialysate flows, should be chosen in combination with a small surface area dialyser and dialysis planned for the following day.

Case 4

A 75-year-old lady who had chronic kidney disease and attended for thrice-weekly haemodialysis was admitted with an acute stroke. She was thrombolysed, and the acute stroke team contacted the dialysis centre as her serum chemistries were as follows, serum urea 25 mmol/l, serum creatinine 650 umol/L and potassium 6.3 mmol/l, and sodium 138 mmol/l, and requested dialysis.

Would you dialyse this patient, and if so what dialysis prescription would you prescribe?

Standard outpatient haemodialysis treatments cause an increase in brain swelling and water content. As such standard dialysis increases the risk of further brain injury. A serum urea >15 mmol/l increases the risk of brain oedema; as such, dialysis is required to reduce further brain swelling and ischaemic injury. There are two key issues: first is minimizing cerebral oedema. This requires a change of dialysis prescription to shorter daily dialysis sessions of 2 hours, coupled with reducing blood and dialysate flows of 250 ml/min and 300 ml/min and a small area dialyzer of 1.5 m^2. The second is to reduce the risk of cerebral ischaemia by reducing the risk of hypotension, as cerebral autoregulation is impaired. This can be done by cooling the dialysate to 35 °C and increasing the dialysate sodium to 10 mmol/l above the serum sodium, up to a maximum of 145 mmol/l.

12

Chapter Review Questions

1. Is there an advantage in starting RRT early in patients with AKI?
2. Is there a benefit from an increased dose of renal replacement therapy in AKI?
3. What are the three main problems with RRT in patients with acute brain injury and how can they be mitigated?
4. Which medications are best removed by haemodialysis and which by haemoperfusion?

Answers

1. Currently, the evidence does not suggest that early RRT improves outcome, and there is evidence that many patients who might not have required RRT would be treated unnecessarily. However, on an individual basis, it is important to ensure that the sick oliguric patient, who is thought unlikely to recover function with intravenous fluids alone, is identified early and RRT anticipated rather than precipitated as an emergency.
2. Although there is conflicting data on balance, there is probably no advantage in high-dose RRT for the management of most patients with AKI. The greater the delivery of the dose of dialysis, there will be greater losses of the electrolytes including phosphate and magnesium, and increased clearance of medicines, such as penicillins, cephalosporins, aminoglycoside and glycopeptin antibiotics and antiepileptics.
3. Rapid reduction in urea can result in an influx of water and brain swelling, middle cerebral artery flows may reduce with volume removal and brain vascular autoregulation is often impaired in the setting of acute injury.

   Avoiding a sharp reduction in urea (e.g. low pump speeds and the use of small dialyzers reduced dialysate flow or concurrent dialysate flow in conjunction with dialysate sodium greater than serum sodium (gentle daily dialysis) and avoiding cardiovascular instability (e.g. gentle daily dialysis, small UF rates and cool higher sodium dialysate).
4. Drugs and poisons with small volume of distribution (e.g. lithium, atenolol, aminoglycosides, alcohols, organic acids and valproate) have potential for significant removal by conventional IHD or CRRT, toxins that are significantly protein bound (such as tricyclic anti-depressants, phenytoin, barbiturates and benzodiazepines, calcium channel blockers and arsenic) will need haemoperfusion therapies to remove significant quantities. However, in the absence of access to haemoperfusion, there may be some benefit in prolonged dialysis to remove any unbound toxins and thus reduce the potential damage.

References

1. Bellomo R, Ronco C, Kellum JA, Mehta RL, Palevsky P, Acute Dialysis Quality Initiative workgroup. Acute renal failure - definition, outcome measures, animal models, fluid therapy and information technology needs: the Second International Consensus Conference of the Acute Dialysis Quality Initiative (ADQI) Group. Crit Care. 2004;8:R204–12.
2. Molitoris BA, Levin A, Warnock DG, Joannidis M, Mehta RL, Kellum JA, Ronco C, Shah S, Acute Kidney Injury Network. Improving outcomes from acute kidney injury. J Am Soc Nephrol. 2007;18:1992–4.
3. Hoste EA, Hoste EA, Clermont G, Kersten A, Venkataraman R, Angus DC, De Bacquer D, Kellum JA. RIFLE criteria for

acute kidney injury are associated with hospital mortality in critically ill patients: a cohort analysis. Crit Care. 2006;10:R73.

4. Wald R, Adhikari NK, Smith OM, Weir MA, Pope K, Cohen A, Thorpe K, McIntyre L, Lamontagne F, Soth M, Herridge M, Lapinsky S, Clark E, Garg AX, Hiremath S, Klein D, Mazer CD, Richardson RM, Wilcox ME, Friedrich JO, Burns KE, Bagshaw SM, Canadian Critical Care Trials Group. Comparison of standard and accelerated initiation of renal replacement therapy in acute kidney injury. Kidney Int. 2015;88(4):897–904.
5. Zarbock A, Kellum JA, Schmidt C, Van Aken H, Wempe C, Pavenstädt H, Boanta A, Gerß J, Meersch M. Effect of early vs delayed initiation of renal replacement therapy on mortality in critically ill patients with acute kidney injury: the ELAIN randomized clinical trial. AMA. 2016;315(20):2190–9.
6. Gaudry S, Hajage D, Schortgen F, Martin-Lefevre L, Pons B, Boulet E, Boyer A, Chevrel G, Lerolle N, Carpentier D, de Prost N, Lautrette A, Bretagnol A, Mayaux J, Nseir S, Megarbane B, Thirion M, Forel JM, Maizel J, Yonis H, Markowicz P, Thiery G, Tubach F, Ricard JD, Dreyfuss D, AKIKI Study Group. Initiation strategies for renal-replacement therapy in the intensive care unit. N Engl J Med. 2016;375(2):122–33.
7. Barbar SD, Binquet C, Monchi M, Bruyere R, Quenot JP. Impact on mortality of the timing of renal replacement therapy in patients with severe acute kidney injury in septic shock: the IDEAL-ICU study (initiation of dialysis early versus delayed in the intensive care unit): study protocol for a randomized controlled trial. Trials. 2014;15:270. https://doi.org/10.1186/1745-6215-15-270.
8. Kielstein J, Kretschmer U, Ernst T, Hafer C, Bahr M, Haller H, Fliser D. Efficacy and cardiovascular tolerability of extended daily dialysis in critically ill patients: a randomized controlled study. Am J Kidney Dis. 2004;43:342–9.
9. Swartz RD, Messana JM, Orzol S, Port FK. Comparing continuous hemofiltration with hemodialysis in patients with severe acute renal failure. Am J Kidney Dis. 1999 Sep;34(3):424–32.
10. Vinsonneau DCC, Combes A, Costa de Beauregard MA, Klouche K, Boulain T, Pallot JL, Chiche JD, Taupin P, Landais P, Dhainaut JF. A prospective, multicentre, randomized clinical trial comparing continuous venovenous hemodiafiltration to intermittent hemodialysis for the treatment of Acute Renal Failure in Intensive Care Unit patients with Multiple Organ Dysfunction Syndrome. Lancet. 2006;368:379–85.
11. Augustine JJ, Sandy D, Seifert TH, Paganini EP. A randomized controlled trial comparing intermittent with continuous dialysis in patients with ARF. Am J Kidney Dis. 2004;44:1000–7.
12. Davenport A. Can advances in hemodialysis machine technology prevent intradialytic hypotension? Semin Dial. 2009;22:231–9.
13. Kohn OF, Coe FL, Ing TS. Solute kinetics with short-daily home hemodialysis using slow dialysate flow rate. Hemodial Int. 2010;14(1):39–46.
14. Phu NH, Hien TT, Mai NT, Chau TT, Chuong LV, Loc PP, Winearls C, Farrar J, White N, Day N. Haemofiltration and peritoneal dialysis in infection-associated acute renal failure in Vietnam. N Engl J Med. 2002;347:895–902.
15. Gabriel DP, Nascimento GV, Caramori JT, Martim LC, Barretti P, Balbi AL. High volume peritoneal dialysis for acute renal failure. Perit Dial Int. 2007;27:277–82.
16. Ronco C, Bellomo R, Homel P, Brendolan A, Dan M, Piccinni P, La Greca G. Effects of different doses in continuous venovenous haemofiltration on outcomes of acute renal failure: a prospective randomised trial. Lancet. 2000;356:26–30.
17. VA/NIH Acute Renal Failure Trial Network, Palevsky PM, Zhang JH, O'Connor TZ, Chertow GM, Crowley ST, Choudhury D, Finkel K, Kellum JA, Paganini E, Schein RM, Smith MW, Swanson KM, Thompson BT, Vijayan A, Watnick S, Star RA, Peduzzi P. Intensity of renal support in critically ill patients with acute kidney injury. N Engl J Med. 2008; 359:7–20.
18. RENAL Replacement Therapy Study Investigators, Bellomo R, Cass A, Cole L, Finfer S, Gallagher M, Lo S, McArthur C, McGuinness S, Myburgh J, Norton R, Scheinkestel C, Su S. Intensity of continuous renal-replacement therapy in critically ill patients. N Engl J Med. 2009;361:1627–38.
19. Brunet P, Frances J, Vacher-Coponat H, Jaubert D, Lebrun G, Gondouin B, Duval A, Berland Y. Hemodialysis without heparin: a randomized, controlled, crossover study of two dialysis membranes (AN69ST and polysulfone F60). Int J Artif Organs. 2011;34:1165–71.
20. Hanevold C, Lu S, Yonekawa K. Utility of citrate dialysate in management of acute kidney injury in children. Hemodial Int. 2010;14(Suppl 1):S2–6.
21. Davenport A, Tolwani A. Citrate anticoagulation for continuous renal replacement therapy (CRRT) in patients with acute kidney injury admitted to the intensive care unit. NDT Plus. 2009;2:439–47.
22. Meier-Kriesche HU, Gitomer J, Kinkel K, DuBose T. Increased total to ionised calcium ratio during continuous venovenous haemodialysis with regional citrate anticoagulation. Crit Care Med. 2001;29:748–52.
23. House AA, Anand I, Bellomo R, Cruz D, Bobek I, Anker SD, Aspromonte N, Bagshaw S, Berl T, Daliento L, Davenport A, Haapio M, Hillege H, McCullough P, Katz N, Maisel A, Mankad S, Zanco P, Mebazaa A, Palazzuoli A, Ronco F, Shaw A, Sheinfeld G, Soni S, Vescovo G, Zamperetti N, Ponikowski P, Ronco C, Acute Dialysis Quality Initiative Consensus Group. Definition and classification of Cardio-Renal Syndromes: workgroup statements from the 7th ADQI Consensus Conference. Nephrol Dial Transplant. 2010;25:1416–20.
24. Bagshaw SM, Cruz DN, Aspromonte N, Daliento L, Ronco F, Sheinfeld G, Anker SD, Anand I, Bellomo R, Berl T, Bobek I, Davenport A, Haapio M, Hillege H, House A, Katz N, Maisel A, Mankad S, McCullough P, Mebazaa A, Palazzuoli A, Ponikowski P, Shaw A, Soni S, Vescovo G, Zamperetti N, Zanco P, Ronco C, Acute Dialysis Quality Initiative Consensus Group. Epidemiology of cardio-renal syndromes: workgroup statements from the 7th ADQI Consensus Conference. Nephrol Dial Transplant. 2010;25:1406–16.
25. Wszolek ZK, McComb RD, Pfeiffer RF, Steg RE, Wood RP, Shaw BW Jr, Markin RS. Pontine and extrapontine myelinolysis following liver transplantation. Relationship to serum sodium. Transplantation. 1989;48:1006–12.
26. Winchester JF, Harbord NB, Rosen H. Management of poisonings: core curriculum 2010. Am J Kidney Dis. 2010;56:788–800.

Useful Web Sites

Acute Dialysis Quality Initiative www.adqi.net.

Acute Kidney Injury Network www.akinet.org.

Continuous Renal Replacement Therapies www.crrtonline.com.

International Society for Peritoneal Dialysis www.ispd.org/lang-en/treatmentguidelines/guidelines.

Kidney Disease Improving Global Outcomes www.kdoqi.org.

National Institute for Clinical Excellence acute kidney injury www.nice.org.uk/nicemedia/live/12959/54435/54435.pdf.

National Confidential Enquiry into Patient Outcomes and Deaths - AKI: Adding Insult to *Injury* Report (2009) www.ncepod.org.uk

Schiffl H, Lang SM, Fischer R. Daily hemodialysis and the outcome of acute renal failure. N Engl J Med. 2002;346:305–10.

Acid Base and Electrolyte Disorders

Contents

Common Electrolyte Abnormalities

Alfredo Petrosino, Domenico Bagordo, Antje Fürstenberg-Schaette, and Chris Laing

Contents

M. Harber (ed.), *Primer on Nephrology*, https://doi.org/10.1007/978-3-030-76419-7_13

Learning Objectives

1. Electrolytes homeostasis is tightly regulated as essential to vital functions: its disturbances are associated with increased morbidity, hospitalisation and mortality.
2. Age, poly-drug therapies and comorbidities are strongly associated with the risk of developing electrolytes disturbances, which are predicted to increase in the future.
3. Understanding the physiology of electrolyte balance and analysis of trends is key to the diagnosis of electrolyte disturbances.
4. The first step in the management of electrolytes disorders should be the identification of life-threatening risks arising from the disorder itself or its correction.

13.1 Introduction

Electrolyte disturbances are common and associated with increased hospitalisation and mortality risk, which increase with both the severity and the number of associated disturbances.

Epidemiology

The epidemiology varies considerably in different settings, and reports are heterogeneous. More than 50% of the 320,000 inpatients in a Chinese tertiary centre were diagnosed with one or more electrolyte disorders, with hyponatraemia being the most common (16.6%), followed by hypokalaemia (13.7%) and hypochloraemia (13.6%). In the Emergency Department, the prevalence of electrolyte abnormalities on admission is reported around 14%, with the great majority developing in the context of other systemic disease. [1, 2] In the community, electrolyte abnormalities may be as common as 15%, hyponatraemia remaining the commonest [3].

Risk Factors

Gastroenteritis is the main cause in paediatric cases. In the adult population, recognised risk factors for electrolytes disorders are age, type 2 diabetes mellitus, respiratory diseases and drugs (mainly diuretics and benzodiazepines). Elderly people are particularly at risk due to increased chances of having multiple risk factors and renal senescence (leading to a decline in the renal handling of solutes and water).

Mortality

All the electrolytes disorders are associated with a substantial two- to fivefold increase in mortality. The risks increases with the severity of the disorder and remains relevant at least up to 1 year after discharge. Hypernatraemia carries the highest mortality (11%–75%) which remains substantial even after the correction of the disorder. Hyperkalaemia follows with a 10% mortality. Acid-base disorders are commonly an associated finding and confer additional mortality risk [4].

Hyponatraemia, hypernatraemia, hypokalaemia and hypercalcaemia are associated with increased length of stay (3 to 6 days on average).

The causality link between electrolytes disturbances and adverse outcomes remains debated. Hyponatraemia offers a paradigmatic example: on one extreme, several critically ill patients develop hyponatraemia without this being the cause of death. At the opposite, rapid changes in plasmatic sodium can be rapidly lethal in otherwise fit people (e.g. hyponatraemia in endurance athletes). In between, some diseases can facilitate the development of hyponatraemia which can increase the risk of death (e.g. increasing the risk of confusion and falls), despite not being the only factor [5, 6].

13.1.1 Approach to Electrolyte Abnormalities

Electrolytes homeostasis depends on a fine regulation of:

1. The body input (enteral or parenteral, excess or deficit?). This is usually difficult to measure, and most of the estimates come from the analysis of urinary excretion.
2. The body output (urine, stool, sweat). Is the output physiologically appropriate in the current state? Kidneys play a pivotal role in tuning excretions.
3. Internal redistribution across body compartments and the ionised and molecule-bound forms (biological actions defined by cellular membranes, proteins and other molecular receptors). The bone represents the biggest storage for many of the electrolytes.

Further steps in the diagnostic workup are:

1. Fluid balance and hydration assessment. Electrolyte concentration is a ratio between the solute (electrolyte) and the solvent (water). A primary alteration in fluid status is often the cause in sodium disturbances.
2. Acid-base status as electrolytes carry an electric charge.
3. Renal function as kidneys are responsible for electrolyte excretion and water and acid-base homeostasis.
4. Additional hormonal tests (renin, aldosterone, cortisol, thyroid function, etc.).

Electrolytes abnormalities can be divided into increased (hyper-) or decreased (hypo-) concentration of an electrolyte (with reference to plasmatic concentrations and not absolute total body quantities).

13.1.2 Sodium and Water Disorders

Sodium is the dominant extracellular cation. Its ability to move across membranes is tightly regulated, and as membranes are almost freely permeable to water, sodium defines and defends the extracellular volume. Changes in extracellular fluid volume elicit compensatory changes in renal sodium handling, while variations in extracelllar osmolarity affect the renal free water clearance. Plasmatic sodium is a ratio (sodium/water), and it is not indicative per se of the total body sodium and water content. Sodium disorders are the result of both sodium and water balance dysregulation (with the latter being most commonly the problem).

13.1.3 Hyponatraemia

Hyponatraemia is defined as a serum sodium of less than 135 mmol/L (severe hyponatraemia loosely being below 125 mmol/L).

Hyponatraemia is one of the commonest electrolyte abnormalities both in the community and in hospital, carries significant morbidity, cost and yet it is often avoidable. One study on 120,000 patients attending a large hospital showed 42.6% of patients had sodium levels below 136 mmol/l either at presentation (28%) or at some point during their stay (14%), with 6.2% below 126 mmol/L and 1.2% below 116 mmol/L. [7] Hyponatraemia is more common in certain settings such as post-operatively and in heart failure, cirrhosis, old age and dementia (Table 13.1). Low body mass, malnourishment, drugs (diuretics, antidepressants, etc.) and comorbidities such as diabetes are other significant risk factors. The disorder is also increasingly recognised among endurance athletes [8].

13.1.4 Clinical Features of Hyponatraemia

The main clinical features are related to hyponatraemic encephalopathy (Fig. 13.1), resulting from osmotic swelling of brain cells due to hypo-osmolar serum. The symptoms are in most cases non-specific, and it is unusual to make the diagnosis before the blood results, but the progression can be very dramatic and quick depending on how rapidly hyponatraemia develops. Lethargy, anorexia, nausea and vomiting, dysgeusia (sweet unpleasant taste in the mouth), impaired concentration, restlessness, irritability, cramps and muscle weakness, increased risk of falls and headaches are just some of the symptoms. Progressively worsening hyponatraemia will result in confusion, disorientation, seizures, coma and ultimately tentorial herniation and

13

Table 13.1 Epidemiology of hyponatraemia: some associations with high incidence (A. Upadhyay 2009)

Cirrhosis	35–50% depending on severity of disease
Heart failure	20% depending on severity of disease
Elderly	Significantly increased risk with age, especially in institutionalised with feeding or fluids (up to 30%)
Thiazides	15% in the elderly and low body weight significant risk factors (apparent within 2 weeks)
Serotonin uptake inhibitors	10–20% (apparent within 2 weeks)
Hospital admissions	Variable depending on environment 5–40% common when associated with diarrhoeal illnesses
Emergency department	3% (hypovolaemia common)
Hospital acquired	15%
Post-operative	(<130 mmol/L) 4–5%
ICU	10–15%
Endurance athletes	Marathon runners 10–20%, severe hyponatraemia ~0.5%
Pneumonia	10%
HIV	Untreated HIV high incidence but also pseudohyponatraemia
Anorexia nervosa	20%
3,4 Metylenedioxymethylamphet-amine	Ecstasy'

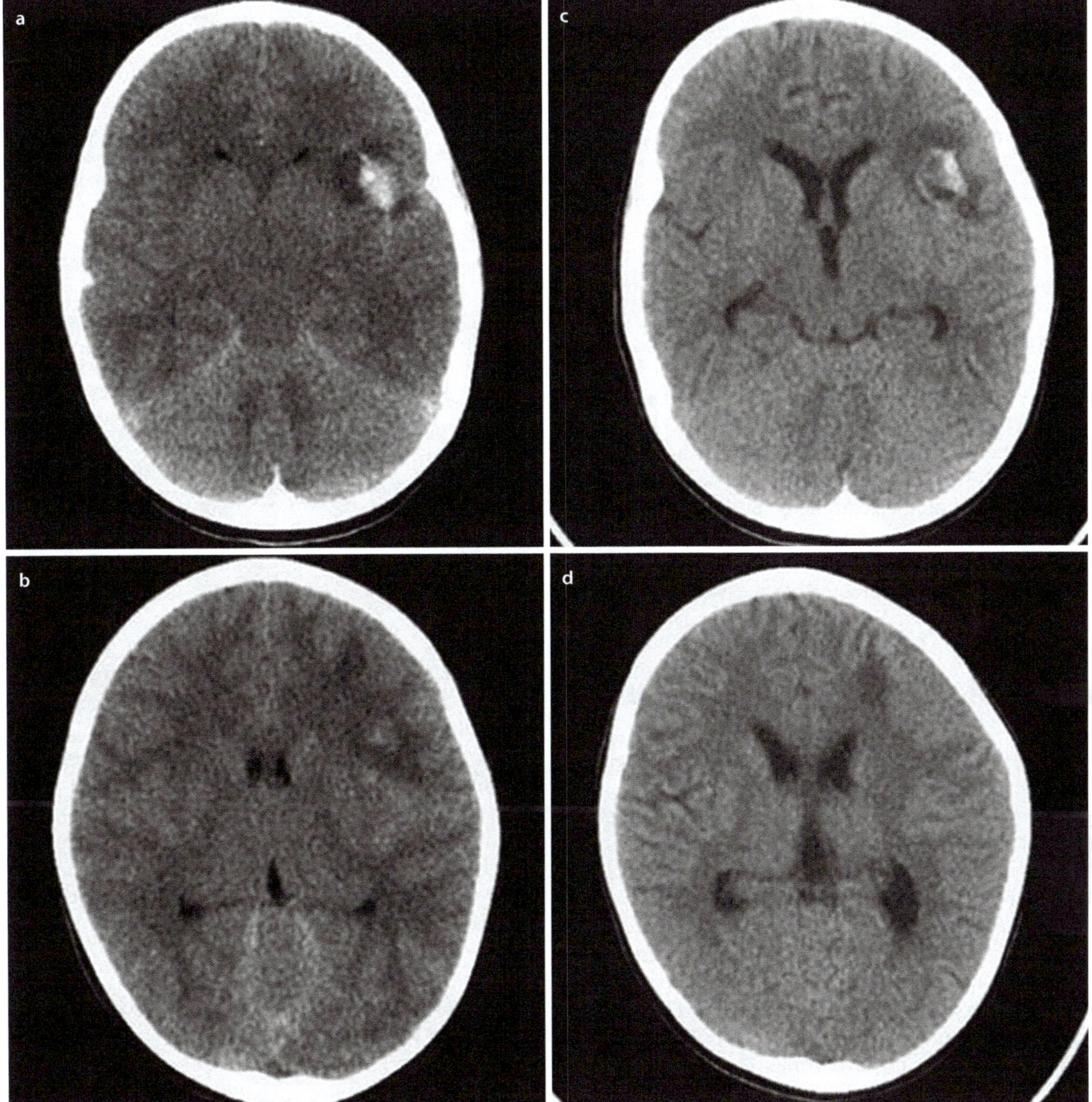

Fig. 13.1 **a** and **b**: Brain CT scan showing diffuse cerebral oedema, effacement of quadrigeminal cistern and loss of sulci in the context of hyponatraemia. **c** and **d**: Resolution after administration of hypertonic saline. (From Carpenter, J. et al. Inadvertent hyponatremia leading to acute cerebral edema and early evidence of herniation. *Neurocrit Care* 6, 195–199 (2007). ► https://doi.org/10.1007/s12028-007-0032-x)

death. Young (pre-menopausal) women, prepubescent children (large brain/skull ratio) and those with associated hypoxia appear to be at greatest risk.

The brain is normally protected from osmotic injury by the regulation of intracellular electrolytes and small organic molecules contributing to osmoregulations (*polyols* such as myoinositol and sorbitol; *amino acids* as taurine, glutamate, aspartate and glycine; and *methylamines* as glycerophosphorylcholine). In hyponatraemia, electrolytes can be transferred out of the neurons rapidly to reduce intracellular osmolality. The reduction in organic intraneural osmolytes, however, takes longer, explaining why sudden drops in sodium (<48 hours) are more dangerous than worse hyponatraemia that develops slowly. Even mild "asymptomatic" hyponatraemia, despite often felt to be harmless, has been shown to have adverse effects not only on the neurological state (with significant delay in response to audiovisual stimuli, increase in errors and a risk of falls) but also on the development of osteoporosis (two- to threefold increase) and fractures [9, 10].

13.1.5 Causes and Differential Diagnosis of Hyponatraemia

Hyponatraemia is an imbalance in the sodium and water ratio. Three common pathophysiology mechanisms are (a) pure increase in total body water (euvolaemia), (b) increase in total body sodium and water (hypervolaemia) and (c) genuine reduction in total body sodium (hypovolaemia). In the majority of cases, however, altered water balance is the driving element rather than sodium losses. Antidiuretic hormone (ADH) modulates free water clearance, defining plasma osmolarity and volume. It often has a key role in hyponatraemia development and should be considered in the diagnostic process distinguishing hyponatraemia that develops in the context of increased (A) or reduced (B) ADH secretion. Of note, ADH is not practical to measure, so its action is deduced by urinary osmolality (high under the antidiuretic effect of ADH).

13.1.5.1 Hyponatraemia with Increased ADH (High Urine Osmolarity)

13

Hyponatraemia can develop in circumstances leading to a "physiologically appropriate" ADH secretion. Low effective arterial blood volume, from an absolute blood volume losses (hypovolaemia, shock, diuretic therapy) or despite an increase in total body fluids in advanced congestive heart failure and cirrhosis, strongly elicits ADH release independently of plasma osmolarity. More rarely ADH is released in the absence of such physiologically appropriate triggers, leading to "syndromes of inappropriate ADH secretion" (or SIADH). In this cases, patients present with feature of ADH excess (high urine osmolarity) and euvolaemia (◘ Table 13.2).

◘ **Table 13.2** Causes of SIADH

Cranial pathology	Stroke, subarachnoid haemorrhage, nasopharynx carcinoma, neuroblastoma, intracranial infiltrative disorders
Chest pathology	Pneumothorax, small cell carcinoma, pneumonia (*legionella*), asthma, cystic fibrosis, respiratory failure with positive-pressure ventilation
Endocrine disorders	Thyroid and parathyroid disorders
Medications	SSRIs, thiazide diuretics, chlorpropamide, tricyclic antidepressants, NSAIDs, carbamazepine, opiates, nicotine, DDAVP, oxytocin, vincristine, cyclophosphamide, ifosfamide, ecstasy
Post-surgical	
Genetic	V2 receptor mutation (nephrogenic syndrome of inappropriate anti-diuresis)
Miscellaneous	Stress, pain, nausea, endurance sports

13.1.5.2 Hyponatraemia with Normal or Decreased ADH (Low Urinary Osmolarity)

In case of low urinary osmolarity, the first step should be to rule out pseudohyponatraemia and osmotic hyponatraemia. Pseudohyponatraemia (falsely low laboratory plasma sodium) occurs with severe hyperlipidaemia (especially triglycerides) and high protein levels (e.g. myeloma or polyclonal gammopathy in HIV). With pseudohyponatraemia, plasma osmolality will be normal as measured by ion-specific electrode (blood gas analyser). "Osmotic" hyponatraemia develops when osmotically active substances (e.g. mannitol, glucose and alcohol) induce an osmotic shift of water from the intracellular to the extracellular compartment. As plasma osmolality is normal (or mildly raised), there is no brain oedema. In hyperglycaemia, the plasmatic sodium concentration can be "corrected" by an increase of 1.6 mEq/l for every 100 mg/dl (5.6 mmol/l) of blood glucose increase above 100 mg/dl.

True hyponatraemia in this context of suppressed ADH can develop in the case of an excessive intake of water that overcomes the maximum free water clearance (see below) (◘ Fig. 13.2).

13.1.6 Assessment and Investigations of Hyponatraemia

Assuming that pseudohyponatraemia and hyperosmolar states have been excluded, then assessment of hyponatraemia requires a careful history of fluid balance, losses and gains, significant comorbidity cranial lesions and cardiac, hepatic, adrenal, thyroid or renal disease. For hospitalised patients, careful review of fluid balance and weights can be diagnostic. The physical assessment needs also to ascertain whether the patient has a raised, normal or low effective arterial blood volume (and this is the main information that we can get from the urinary fractional excretion of sodium).

A physiological response to hyponatraemia requires (a) "central" cessation of thirst and suppression of antidiuretic hormone release and (b) maximal preservation of body sodium (with minimal urinary excretion), aiming

Condition		Sodium/Water imbalance	Disease
Hypo-osmolar hyponatraemia			
Increase EABV (hypervolaemia)		Increased total body sodium < water	
		Increased renin:angiotensin activity	
			Cirrhosis (low urinary sodium)
			Congestive cardiac failure (low urinary sodium)
			Nephrotic syndrome (low urinary sodium)
			Renal failure (high urinary sodium)
Normal EABV (euvolaemia)		Increased total body water	
			Water intoxication, psychogenic polydipsia, excessive beer drinking, ecstasy
			Syndrome of inappropriate ADH (high urinary sodium)
			Medication (thiazides, SSRIs, opiates)
			Hypothyroidism (thyroxine required for maximal free water clearance: high urinary sodium)
			Hypoadrenalism (cortisol required for maximal free water clearance; high urinary sodium)
			Pregnancy
Reduced EABV (hypovolaemia)		Reduced total body sodium > water	
	(d)	**Renal losses** (high urinary sodium)	Diuretics
			Hypoadrenalism
			Salt-losing nephropathies
			Cerebral salt-wasting(excessive BNP)
	(e)	**Extra-renal loses**(low urinary sodium)	Sweating (and water intake) endurance exercise, vomiting, diarrhoea
	(f)	**Low solute intake**	
Hyper-Osmolar and Iso-osmolar hyponatraemia			
		Hyper-osmolar states	Hyperglycaemia, Mannitol
		Iso-osmolar state	Absorption of irrigation fluid
Pseudohyponatraemia			Hyperlipidaemia, high protein (immunoglobulin levels)
Factitious hyponatraemia			Diluted sample eg from drip arm or Munchausen syndrome

Fig. 13.2 Causes of hyponatraemia

Investigation	Comment
Serum electrolytes, glucose and plasma osmolality	to exclude osmotic hyponatraemia
Triglycerides, albumin and total protein	to exclude pseudohyponatraemia
Renal and liver function, urate, brain naturetic peptide	
Urinary sodium	Low (<20mmol/L): associated with cirrhosis, heart failure, nephrotic syndrome, hypovolaemia of any cause and water intoxication High (>20mmol/L): associated with renal loss, SIADH and renal impairment, diuretics
Urine osmolality	
Urinary potassium	
Thyroid function, Adrenal function	Both hormones required for maximal free water clearance

Fig. 13.3 Investigations of hyponatraemia

to maximise electrolyte-free water excretion. Although it may appear easy to identify what is preventing a physiological response to hyponatraemia in hyponatraemic patients, in complex cases with multiple comorbidities, it can be challenging (Figs. 13.3 and 13.4).

Investigations in Fig. 13.3 are a useful but not comprehensive guide.

13

13.1.7 Some Specific Causes of Hyponatraemia

Psychogenic Polydipsia and Beer Potomania

A person with normal diet and kidney function can excrete up to 12–14 L of free water per day (assuming the availability of average solute load to excrete). This amount is rarely achieved, and hyponatraemia secondary to psychogenic polydipsia is rare. Conditions in which the kidney function and (mainly) the osmotic solute load are decreased (poor generation of urea in malnourishment) cause a significant decrease in the maximal free water clearance. Hyponatraemia can then start to develop with a "moderate" fluid intake of just more than 4 L per day (so-called beer potomania and "Tea and toast" syndrome). Moreover with dedicated polydipsia, the counter-current multiplier will get washed out, and the ability to generate free water clearance is further reduced.

Endurance sports are becoming increasingly popular, and "exercise-associated hyponatraemia" (EAH) is common. This is probably the combination of excessive fluid intake and fluid retention secondary to exercise-associated (non-osmotic) ADH release. The latter may be sustained by physical stress and pain, nausea, heath, drugs (NSAIDs) and inflammatory cytokines (interleukin-6). Many athletes with symptomatic EAH present with an unexpectedly increased body weight as sign of fluid overload. Risk factors seem to relate to body size, duration of exercise, fluid intake (most sports drinks are hypotonic) and the use of NSAIDs. Menstruating females would be at increased risk as estrogens may impair the cerebral adaptation to rapid osmolar changes. Clinical manifestations are mainly neurological with cerebral oedema up to brainstem herniation, but non-cardiogenic pulmonary oedema can also present in severe cases. Rapid identification and treatment can save lives: acute hyponatraemia should always be considered in case of collapse in an endurance athlete. IV hypertonic saline is the treatment of choice in severe cases. Drink according to thirst remains the main prevention strategy.

Drugs

Some medication has a particular association; thiazide diuretics and selective serotonin uptake inhibitors both have a high incidence. Again, it is the elderly and low body weight that have the highest risk for this. For thiazides, those gaining weight within 48 hours of starting have increased risk. Fortunately, for both classes of medication, hyponatraemia usually becomes apparent within 2 weeks, and testing at this time in high-risk patients is likely to identify most.

Post-operative hyponatraemia is common and related to SIADH (stress, opiates, pain and nausea result in the non-osmotic release of ADH) combined with fluid intake and can have very severe consequences.

Ecstasy-induced hyponatraemia can cause deaths in otherwise healthy young adults and appears to be a combination of polydipsia and inappropriate ADH secretion. The advice to drink copious quantities of

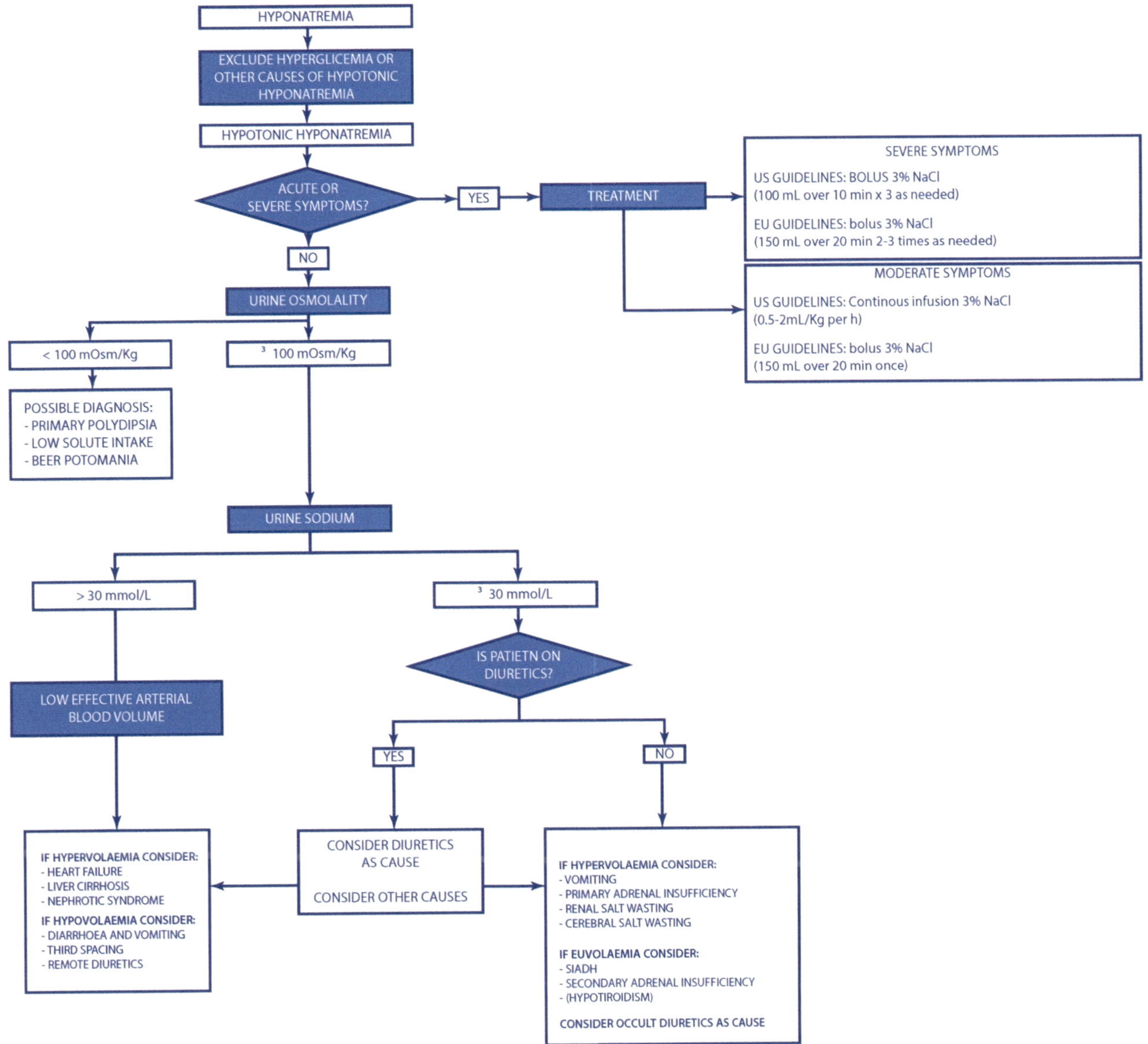

Fig. 13.4 Diagnostic flow chart for hyponatraemia and treatment for acute or life-threatening symptoms. (*SIADH* syndrome of inappropriate secretion of antidiuretic hormone)

water to avoid heat-related illness and rhabdomyolysis is probably inappropriate.

Hyponatraemia in institutionalised elderly is very common, and the cause is multifactorial including polypharmacy, low body weight and low solute intake. It can have a profound effect decompensating patients with comorbidity. Patients receiving IV fluids or medical feeding are particularly at risk. Dissecting the principle cause of hyponatraemia may be very difficult, and identifying the patient at risk is critical.

Syndromes of inappropriate ADH secretion is a relatively common cause of hyponatraemia (Table 13.2). The diagnosis is suggested by hypo-osmolar serum (<275 mmol/L), a relatively high urine osmolality (>100 mmol/L) in a euvolaemic patient as supported by a urinary sodium >20 mmol/L. Other causes of hyponatraemia such as hypothyroidism, hypoadrenalism or renal impairment should however be excluded. The precipitating cause may be obvious such as pneumonia or surgery, but, if not, further steps to consider are suspending any potentially culpable medication and a search for malignancy.

Cerebral salt wasting syndrome (CSWS) is a rare cause of hyponatraemia that may onset after brain injury. An association has been described with aneurysmal subarachnoid haemorrhage but has been described also with head trauma, stroke, intracranial tumours/metastases, viral and bacterial infections and after neurosurgery. The main features are elevated urinary sodium excretion and hypovolaemia. The pathophysiology may be related to natriuresis induced by inappropriate brain-natriuretic-peptide release. The differential diagnosis with SIADH is important as the treatment is substantially the opposite: rehydration and sodium supplements.

13.1.8 Treatment of Hyponatraemia

The main concern with treating hyponatraemia is that rapid correction of serum osmolality causes osmotic dehydration of neural cells (osmotic demyelination syndrome, ODS). Classically at risk is the central pons (*central pontine myelinolysis, CPM*), but extrapontine areas as basal ganglia and cerebellum can be involved as well. Clinical manifestations of CPM usually develop few days after the insult with seizure, altered state of consciousness, changes in gait and respiration up to emotional lability, spastic quadriparesis and pseudobulbar palsy. Having shed organic osmolytes and electrolytes, neurons are particularly vulnerable to an increase in plasma osmolality as reaccumulation of osmolytes (such as the major osmolyte myoinositol) is slower than their loss (uraemia representing an interesting exception where myoinositol reuptake is faster, causing somewhat protection from CPM).

Treatment relies on identifying and addressing the specific causes (sodium deficit, SIADH or sodium and water excess; ◘ Fig. 13.4). The fundamental rules to maintain patient safety and avoid CPM are however very frequent monitoring and slow correction. In a seminal study looking at patients with severe hyponatraemia (<105 mmol/L), no patients who had increments of ≤12 mmol/L in 24 hours or 18 mmol/L in 48 hours suffered neurological injury [11]. The two common limits used in practice are [1] <8–10 (up to 12 according to some Authors) mEq/L in the first 24 hours and <18 mEq/L in the first 48 hours if hyponatraemia is likely to have been present for ≥48 hours. In those with hyponatraemic encephalopathy (seizures, neurological signs, neurogenic pulmonary oedema), the initial correction should be no greater than 8–10 mmol/L/24 hours to be achieved with 100mls of 3% (hypertonic) saline plus or minus an infusion of the same at 1–2 ml/kg/hour. This can be given in conjunction with loop diuretics, but again the concern is that correction may be too rapid if not monitored extremely closely. Oxygenation is important in anyone at risk of hyponatraemic encephalopathy. Non-peptide vasopressin receptor antagonists (vaptans), such as conivaptan (IV) and tolvaptan (oral), offer an elegant way of promoting free water clearance acting on V1a and V2 receptors (tolvaptan more selectively on the latter). They are effective at increasing sodium in euvolaemic and hypervolaemic states and appear safe but contraindicated in hypovolaemia and not the treatment of choice in hyponatraemic emergencies. Patients can become polyuric and over-correct, so close monitoring on initiation is important, and fluid restriction may need to be limited or reversed (caution with patients who do not have free access to fluids and do not use simultaneously with hypertonic saline and diuretics). There is a danger that vaptans will be used willy-nilly, but concerns over liver toxicity, extortionate cost and lack of long-term outcome benefits mean the role of these drugs for long-term conditions is not yet established: it seems likely that in the right setting and if carefully handled, they could be a welcome addition to the therapeutic armamentarium [12].

In summary:

1. Hypovolaemic and sodium-depleted patients: the treatment is usually with saline replacement and treating the underlying cause such as gastrointestinal losses, correcting adrenal or thyroid insufficiency or sodium supplementation in patients with salt-losing nephropathies. Potassium deficits if present should be corrected. Vaptans are contraindicated.
2. Euvolaemic patients: require treatment of the underlying condition and fluid restriction. Demeclocycline (300–600 mg bid, which inhibits cAMP in the collecting duct, inducing nephrogenic diabetes insipidus and AVP resistance) can be used in SIADH, but it is slow acting and potentially nephrotoxic. Urea is another option but is not well tolerated. Vaptans achieve free water clearance without natriuresis or kaliuresis and are well suited to treatment of euvolaemic hyponatraemia if progress is not made with simpler measures. In hyponatraemic emergencies, hypertonic saline and/or loop diuretics are the treatment of choice and should be used as a temporary measure to make a gentle increment in serum sodium while correcting the underlying cause.
3. Salt- and water-overloaded patients: fluid restriction, usually diuretics, and treatment of the underlying condition, in combination with chronic salt restriction. Vaptans have been used to promote free water clearance in these conditions of elevated ADH.

In case of excessively rapid correction of hyponatraemia, sodium re-lowering is supported by the fact that while the neuronal response to hyponatraemia is achieved rapidly (48 hours), the re-accumulation of intracellular osmoles can take 5–7 days. As a result hyponatraemia secondary to excessive sodium re-lowering would have a significantly lower risk of causing cerebral oedema. Furthermore, the process of osmotic demyelination would be reversible to some extent, even after symptom onset. Therefore, it is experts' opinion that sodium re-lowering should be considered [1] after a too rapid correction in high-risk patients (alcohol abuse, cirrhosis, malnutrition, hypokalaemia, initial severe hyponatraemia), aiming for the therapeutic correction targets reported above, and [2] in patients with initial signs of CPM/ODS. Relowering of plasma sodium should be achieved with a combination of desmopressin (2–4 mcg IV or SC every 6 hours) and glucose 5% (3 ml/Kg/h for a 1 mmol/l/h correction of plasmatic sodium), and desmopressin only should be continued after the achievement of target plasma sodium.

Prevention of hyponatraemia is probably underpractised. Important measures would be to vigilate against the routine use of hypotonic solutions post-operatively, identify and closely monitor patients at risk (particularly the elderly and institutionalised), check plasma sodium within 2 weeks of starting thiazides or SSRI and advise endurance athletes to avoid NSAIDs and drink according to thirst.

13.1.9 Outcomes of Hyponatraemia

Hospital-associated hyponatraemia is a universal and independent risk factor for worse outcome, be it worsening ascites in liver disease, readmission with heart failure, admission to ICU and ventilation, length of stay or death. In many cases, this may simply be a reflection of illness, but even so low sodium becomes an important biomarker for risk [13].

13.1.10 Hypernatraemia

Hypernatraemia is defined as a plasma sodium of >145 mmol/L.

This is also relatively common in the hospital setting affecting between 1 and 5% of hospitalised patients and associated with very high mortality (40–75%) when severe. It is caused by either loss of body water or, less commonly, a gain in total body sodium and water. Powerful protective mechanisms usually prevent hypernatraemia, and in the former scenario it is usually related to impaired thirst, reduced access to water, impaired AVP release or impaired AVP responsiveness. Consequently the elderly, confused, debilitated and ventilated and infants are at greatest risk. A list of causes is shown in ◘ Table 13.3 and can be categorised in the same way as hyponatraemia based on EABV. Of note, more than one cause may be in play.

13.1.11 Clinical Features

As with hyponatraemia, symptoms depend on the extent of the abnormality and the rate of change. The brain compensates for hypernatraemia by manipulating intracellular osmolality (increasing intracellular osmolytes in this case). The symptoms and signs are relatively nonspecific including lethargy, muscle weakness, impaired mental ability, confusion, coma and death. Acute hypernatraemia results in osmotic shrinkage of the brain and can result in subarachnoid haemorrhage.

13.1.12 Assessment and Investigation of Hypernatraemia

As with hyponatraemia, hypernatraemia is usually detected either incidentally or in the investigation of a patient who has impaired mental state. A careful his-

◘ **Table 13.3** Causes of hypernatraemia

Increased EABV (hypervolaemia)	Excessive mineralocorticoid activity	e.g. Cushing's syndrome, Conn's usually associated hypokalaemia and hypertension and low urinary sodium
	Excessive salt intake	Hypertonic feed, hypertonic saline, normal saline and colloid have a sodium of 155 mmol/L, high salt load medication (e.g. some antibiotics, sodium bicarbonate, glucocorticoids and mineralocorticoids), associated with high urinary sodium
Normal EABV (euvolaemia)	Renal water loss	Nephrogenic diabetes insipidus
		Central diabetes insipidus
	Extra renal water loss	(with inadequate water intake) insensible losses hyperventilation
Reduced EABV (hypovolaemia)	Renal water losses	Diuretics, osmotic diuresis, vaptans
	Extra renal water loss	Vomiting, diarrhoea, sweating, NG suction

tory (including changes in weights and fluid balance with emphasis on water intake, gastrointestinal losses and polyuria) in conjunction with the assessment of the patient's effective arterial blood volume is key.

A physiologically appropriate renal response to hypernatraemia (that is always associated with increased serum osmolality) would be to produce urine with higher solute concentration than plasma ($U_{osm} > P_{osm}$). When this is confirmed, a non-renal cause of hypernatraemia should be sought. The electrolyte free water clearance (EFWC) gives a similar information: it represents the amount of water without electrolytes that would remain after the hypothetical removal of urinary solutes and of the water volume required for their dilution to plasmatic concentration. In other words, the EFWC is the amount of fluid (positive or negative) necessary to define the observed urinary concentration if we started with the same solute load but at iso-osmolar concentration.

Equation 13.1 Electrolyte free water clearance (EFWC; Posm, plasma osmolality; Uosm, urine osmolality; Uvol, urine volume)

$$EFWC = \frac{Posm - Uosm}{Posm} * Uvol \tag{13.1}$$

Positive EFWC means excretion of electrolyte free water in addition to iso-osmotic urine (so diluted urine), while a negative EFWC means retention of part of the water necessary to iso-osmolarity (with excretion of concentrated urine). Clearly this does not hold true in case of osmotic diuresis (Table 13.4).

Table 13.4 Initial investigation of hypernatraemia

Careful history and examination	GI losses, skin losses or polyuria, history of poor water intake, excessive thirst. Is the patient hypovolaemic?
Plasma urea and electrolytes including calcium	
Plasma osmolality	
Glucose	To exclude non-ketotic hyperosmolar diabetic coma
Urine osmolality	>600 mosmol/kg suggests unreplaced gastrointestinal, renal or insensible losses, sodium overload or a primary defect in thirst
	If 300–600 mosmol/kg, consider the presence of an osmotic diuretic
	<300 mosmol/kg suggests diabetes insipidus
Urine Na⁺	Low urinary sodium (<20 mmol/L) suggestive of extra renal losses or excessive mineralocorticoid activity; raised urinary sodium (>20 mmol/L) suggestive of renal losses (diuretics, salt wasting) or high sodium intake
Water restriction test	If suspicious of diabetes insipidus (DI)
ADH levels	If suspicious of DI (low in cranial DI, normal or high in renal DI)

13.1.13 Water Restriction Test

The water restriction test helps distinguish diabetes insipidus from primary (psychogenic) polydipsia, and furthermore central diabetes insipidus (CDI) from nephrogenic diabetes insipidus (NDI). Water deprivation would normally cause a rise in P_{osm}, which stimulates ADH secretion. ADH then leads to increased renal water reabsorption (via aquaporin-2 water channel insertion in the distal tubule and the collecting duct). Subsequently the U_{osm} will rise to a maximum value of 800–1400mosm/kg, and U_{Volume} will fall to <0.5 ml/min reflecting the maximum ADH effect on the kidney. This is reached when P_{osm} is 285–295mosm/kg.

In individuals with defects in either ADH release (CDI) or ADH effect (NDI), their U_{osm} remains inappropriately low despite a rise in P_{osm} to levels ≥295 mosm/kg.

Test instructions:

- Patient should stop drinking 2 to 3 hours before starting the test. Avoid overnight fluid depletion as severe hypernatraemia and dehydration may occur. Keep nil by mouth during the test.
- Measure baseline U_{osm}, P_{osm}, P_{Sodium} and body weight.
- Measure U_{osm}, U_{Volume} and body weight every hour.
- Measure P_{Sodium} and P_{osm} every 2 hours.

Stop the test once any of the following endpoints are reached:

1. Appropriate response: U_{osm} >600 mosmol/kg.
2. Inappropriate response:
   - U_{osm} is stable on two to three successive hourly measurements despite a rising P_{osm}.
   - P_{osm} exceeds 295 to 300 mosmol/kg.
   - P_{Sodium} is 145 meq/L or higher.
   - Body weight falls below 97% from baseline.

Desmopressin (dDAVP) can then be administered for further differentiation (10 mcg by nasal insufflation or 1–2 mcg intravenously), and U_{osm} and U_{Volume} are monitored every 30 min over the following 2 hours. Desmopressin administration should lead to an increase in U_{osm} of at least 50% or a significant fall in urine output in CDI, but will have no or only little effect in NDI (Table 13.5).

Table 13.5 Water restriction test interpretation [14–16]

Condition	Urine osmolality in mOsm/kg, after water deprivation	U_{osm} rise in response to dDAVP administration
Normal response	>800	No response
Primary polydipsia	>600[a]	No response
CDI	<300	>100% (complete CDI) 15–50% (partial CDI)
NDI	<300	≤45% (partial NDI) No response (complete NDI)

[a]primary polydipsia will be associated with a rise in urine osmolality, usually above 500–600 mosmol/kg, but maximum concentrating ability is frequently impaired in this disorder. This defect may be due to downregulation of the release of AVP in response to hypertonicity in those patients [17]

Test Limitations. The water restriction test establishes the correct diagnosis in 80%; however, the main limitation seems to be the differentiation between partial CDI and primary polydipsia, as some patients with partial CDI have an upregulation of ADH receptors. Those patients are polyuric at normal P_{osm}, but will be able to concentrate their urine normally when P_{osm} rises to 295. They will not respond to dDAVP administration. Hence, they may be mistakenly diagnosed with primary polydipsia. In equivocal cases, a trial of desmopressin may be helpful as patients with partial CDI will get quick relief of the polyuria, whereas patients with primary polydipsia may have some fall in urine output, but if they continue to have excessive water intake, they may develop severe hyponatraemia.

13.1.14 Treatment of Hypernatraemia

In the majority of cases, management consist in treating the underlying cause and supplying adequate free water and/or diuretics (excretion of sodium). The estimated absolute water deficit, below, will give an idea of the amount of water replacement to achieve normal hydration.

$$\text{Absolute water deficit} = \frac{(P-Na+)-(Desired\ P-Na+)}{Desired\ P-Na+} * (\text{Total Body Water})$$

$$\text{Total Body Water} = 0.6 * (\text{Body Weight})$$

(assuming 60% of body weight is water, in the elderly, 50% may be used)

The estimated water deficit is not a prescription for replacement, as it does not account for ongoing renal or other losses. For most patients, correction merely involves providing ready access to water; for the infirm, it may be via NG water or 5% dextrose. Titration with regular measurement and clinical assessment is critical. There are no evidence-based guidelines available for sodium correction in hypernatraemia. Hypovolaemia should be corrected with balanced crystalloid. Experts usually suggest that rapid correction of acute (≤48 hour) hypernatraemia is relatively safe due to neuronal adaption (by increasing osmolytes or retaining electrolytes) and up to a maximum rate of 1 mmol/l/hr. is recommended for very acute cases. In chronic hypernatraemia, however, rapid correction can cause cerebral oedema, and experts support a 0.4 mmol/L/hr. for anything remotely chronic, with a total maximum decrease in sodium of 10 mmol/l in 24 hours. Interestingly, some study found no differences between rapid (>0.5 mmol/L/hr) and slow (0.5 mmol/L/hr) sodium correction in terms of 30 days mortality, seizure nor cerebral oedema [18]. Finally, in hypervolaemic hypernatraemia, diuretics are used in combination with free water to induce negative sodium balance.

13.1.15 Diabetes Insipidus (DI)

DI is relatively rare but can result in severe and recurrent hypernatraemia. On etiological basis, it is classified as central and nephrogenic (Table 13.6). Congenital causes of cranial or pure nephrogenic DI usually present in infancy with dehydration, failure to thrive and hyponatraemia. Children may give a history of drinking water from any source including puddles, and polyuria manifests as urinary frequency, nocturia and enuresis. Urine outputs of up to 20 L can occur (although more commonly less than this), and bladder dysfunction can result from chronic bladder distension. Other genetically acquired renal diseases can also result in predominantly collecting tubule damage and usually a milder version of NDI as the disease progresses. Urine osmolality is low in the face of high plasma osmolality, whereas urinary sodium is variable.

Table 13.6 Causes of diabetes insipidus

Cranial diabetes insipidus (CDI)	
Inherited/congenital	Inherited AD is very rare and resulting from mutations of AVP-NPII, carrier protein neurophysin II and its co-peptide, Wolfram syndrome (DI, DM, optic atrophy and deafness), birth trauma
Acquired	Trauma and vascular head injury (basal skull fracture, subarachnoid haemorrhage, aneurysm), surgery especially hypophysectomy, pituitary apoplexy (Sheehan's syndrome: Postpartum pituitary necrosis, snake bite, profound shock)
	Idiopathic
	Tumour-related: Craniopharyngioma, hypothalamic lesions, metastases, lymphoma, pineal gland tumours, optic gliomas
	Granulomatous and autoimmune conditions: Sarcoidosis, histiocytosis-X
	Infection related: Meningitis, encephalitis, cerebral abscess or systemic shock from sepsis
Inherited	X-linked defect of vasopressin receptor (AVPR2 gene) (90%), rarer still (10%) AR mutation of aquaporin 2 gene (AQP2)
	Medullary cystic disease, juvenile nephronophthisis, ADPKD, Bartter's syndrome, renal dysplasia
Acquired	Drug-induced: Lithium is a very common drug which can cause acute or chronic NDI, amphotericin-B, cidofovir, ifosfomide, demeclocycline and by definition vaptans
	Chronic hypercalcaemia, chronic hypokalaemia
	Amyloidosis, light chain disease, sickle cell disease, recurrent pyelonephritis, any cause of papillary necrosis, post-obstruction, Sjogren's syndrome
"Mixed central and nephrogenic" diabetes insipidus	Placental secretion of enzyme vasopressinase metabolising ADH resulting in a very rare (and spontaneously resolving) complication of third trimester with polyuria

13.1.16 Treatment of DI

CDI is treatable with nasal or oral desmopressin (DDAVP). NDI is more tricky to treat, and addressing any secondary cause is important (treating hypercalcaemia and avoiding culpable medication). Lithium should be stopped or the dose decreased when possible. Alternatively, amiloride may be employed to compete for lithium uptake, potentially reducing its toxicity. A high water intake (with planning for this and toilets) and low-salt and modest protein diet are first line. If symptoms cannot be controlled with these, then thiazide or amiloride diuretics may help induce a mild contraction of the effective arterial blood volume. Non-steroidal anti-inflammatory drugs can be useful for NDI and lithium-induced DI.

Patients need to have a clear understanding of the condition (► www.patient.co.uk/health/diabetes-insipidus), avoid excessive fluid intake while on DDAVP, and keep a close eye on daily weights, especially if unwell. A MedicAlert bracelet of equivalent is very sensible.

Patients with chronic profound polyuria should have surveillance ultrasound to check for functional "high-pressure" obstruction.

13.1.17 Potassium Disorders

Potassium is the main intracellular cation ~*100 mmol/L* (and around 98% of total body potassium is intracellular), which is why necrosis can be associated with fulminant hyperkalaemia. The large gradient between intra- and extracellular compartments is actively maintained by the Na + -K + -ATPase. It is via the Na^+-K^+-ATPase that β_2-adrenoreceptor agonists and insulin act to shift potassium into cells, acidosis and α_1-adrenoreceptor stimulation (increased in CKD) having the opposite effect. The concentration of extracellular potassium is critical as it influences the voltage difference across cell membranes [19]. The proximal tubule is the site of reabsorption of the majority (55%) of filtered potassium via paracellular diffusion and some reabsorption via the Na^+-K^+-$2Cl^-$ co-transporter in the thick ascending limb of the loop of Henle. Potassium is also actively secreted via the ROM-K transporter. Only 10% of filtered potassium reaches the distal convoluted tubule and cortical collecting duct where critical control of potassium secretion occurs.

13.1.18 Hypokalaemia

Oral intake is approximately 100 mmol/day. 95% of potassium excretion is via the kidney and 5% from the colon. Hypokalaemia is relatively uncommon in healthy individuals as in health the kidney is able to avidly retain potassium (less than 15 mmol/day).

> Thus hypokalaemia, defined as serum potassium less than 3.5 mmol/l (moderate 2.5–3.0 mmol/L, severe <2.5 mmol/L).

Is normally the consequence of significant underlying pathology or drug use and is extremely common in hospitals (up to 20% of patients). Mostly this relates to medication, fluid losses, fevers, malnutrition, eating disorders and potassium-lite fluid replacement [19]. Gastrointestinal losses are a common cause of hypokalaemia (and hypomagnesaemia) globally and can be fatal in severe diarrhoea particularly in countries with limited health care. Causes of hypokalaemia are shown in ▫ Table 13.7, and in patients who develop hypokalaemia, multiple associated causes are often detected (such as diarrhoea and diuretic treatment or malnourishment).

The clinical manifestations of hypokalaemia are mainly related to cardiac dysrhythmias (usually below 3.0 mmol/L or higher in those predisposed to dysrhythmias), including atrial or ventricular dysrhythmias, due to increased myocardial excitability, but muscle weakness may also occur (see Appendix 1). Hypokalaemia increases renal ammonia production predisposing to decompensation of hepatic encephalopathy. Acute and chronic hypokalaemia may cause polyuria. Finally chronic hypokalaemia was thought to cause tubulointerstitial damage, but this is somewhat controversial and may merely be an association with the primary causes of hypokalaemia.

Investigation of hypokalaemia (▫ Table 13.8) aims to determine if it is a problem of intra-extracellular redistribution (intracellular uptake), of poor intake or of excessive losses (and in this case if renal or extra-renal losses) of potassium.

Urinary potassium (as total urinary potassium or the quicker "potassium fractional excretion", FE_{K+}, and "transtubular potassium gradient", TTKG) is a useful test to discriminate between renal and non-renal losses. Non-renal losses from any cause (usually the GI tract) will be associated with an appropriately reduced

▫ **Table 13.7** Causes of hypokalaemia

Reduced total body potassium	
Deficient intake	Rare on Western diet but seen in alcoholics, elderly and those with wasting disease such as cancer, may predispose to re-feeding hypokalaemia
Extra-renal losses (low urine potassium (<15 mmol/day)	Chronic or severe acute diarrhoea, laxatives, gastrointestinal and biliary drains, sweating, vomiting[a] (secondary hyperaldosteronism and alkalosis)
Renal losses (high urine potassium)	**Drugs:** Diuretics (loop and thiazide (hypokalaemia more common in women on thiazide) (potent synergistic effect of loop and thiazide in combination), mineralocorticoid and glucocorticoids, medication causing proximal tubular injury, e.g. aminoglycosides, amphotericin-B, cisplantin. Excess licorice
	Primary hyper-reninaemia (high renin and aldosterone) malignant hypertension, renal artery stenosis, coarctation, renin secreting tumour, page kidney **primary hyperaldosteronism** (low renin, high aldosterone), conn syndrome, adrenal hyperplasia, glucocorticoid remediable aldosteronism (GRA) **excess mineralocorticoid activity** Cushing's syndrome, congenital adrenal hyperplasia, apparent mineralocorticoid excess, exogenous mineralocorticoid, licorice **increased delivery of sodium or non-reabsorbable ions to distal nephron** diuretics proximal to connecting tubule and cortical collecting duct (see above), magnesium deficiency, Bartter and Gitelman syndrome, Liddle syndrome, chronic metabolic acidosis including proximal and distal RTA, Fanconi syndrome, ketoacidosis, starvation
Redistributive hypokalaemia	Hyperinsulinaemia, alkalosis, increased beta-adrenergic receptor, alkalosis activation (stress response or beta-agonists for chronic airways disease)
Miscellaneous	Rapid uptake with correction of B12 deficiency, hypokalaemic periodic paralysis, hypothermia, thyrotoxicosis. Overdose of chloroquine, risperidone, quetiapine, barium and caesium
Pseudohypokalaemia	Massive leucocytosis (usually chronic leukaemias) (can be avoided by rapid separation of cells from plasma), artifactual hypokalaemia from drip-arm or poorly flushed central line

[a]vomiting can be associated with high urinary potassium because of secondary hyperaldosteronism

Table 13.8 Investigation of hypokalaemia

History	GI losses, laxatives, diuretics, medication
Examination	EABV, blood pressure, evidence of Cushing's syndrome or macrovascular disease suggestive of RAS, nutritional state
Urea, electrolytes, bicarbonate, osmolality, magnesium	
Urine potassium	**Extra-renal** <15 mmol/day or urine K^+:Urine creatinine <1.5
	Renal >15 mmol/day or urine K^+:Urine creatinine >1.5
	Fractional excretion of potassium: FE_{K+} = (urine K^+ × plasma creatinine/plasma K^+ × urine creatinine) × 100
	Transtubular potassium gradient (TTKG) = (urine K^+ × plasma osmol)/(plasma K^+ × urine osmol)
Urinary chloride	**Low** gastric losses, non-resorbable anions,
	High diuretics, Gitelman, Bartter syndrome, magnesium deficiency
Urinary pH	Alkaline urine with acidosis; RTA
Renin/aldosterone	See Table 13.7
Specialist endocrine tests	
Urine laxative and diuretic screen	If suspicion of illicit use

13

urinary potassium excretion (<15 mmol/24 hours, FE_{K+} <2–6.5% or TTKG <3), whereas a inappropriately high urinary potassium excretion (>15 mmol/24 hrs or FE_{K+} >6.5% or TTKG >3) suggests renal losses and is most commonly the result of kaliuretic medication or proximal convoluted tubule toxicity.

In the context of a renal cause of hypokalaemia, the presence of hypertension suggests either hyperaldosteronism or mineralocorticoid excess (such as accelerated phase hypertension, renal artery stenosis, Conn's, GRA or causes of mineralocorticoid excess such as Cushing's syndrome). Renin/aldosterone levels and specialist endocrine tests may be required. Another useful diagnostic element is urinary chloride: low with gastric losses and non-reabsorbable anions, high with diuretics, magnesium deficiency and Bartter and Gitelman syndromes. Urine diuretic screen and laxative screen can also be useful particularly if hypokalaemia is intermittent.

Non-specific tubular interstitial damage may cause hypokalaemia usually in association with hypovolaemia and secondary (appropriate) hyperaldosteronism. Distal renal tubular acidosis is covered in ▶ Chap. 9, but hypokalaemia is associated with hyperchloraemic acidosis (serum bicarbonate and urine pH). Some rare renal conditions causing hypokalaemia are discussed below.

13.1.19 Some Specific Conditions Causing Hypokalaemia

Bartter and Gitelman syndromes (BS and GS) are rare, inherited tubulopathies characterised by hypokalaemic metabolic alkalosis and hyper-reninaemic hyperaldosteronism. *Bartter syndrome* results from mutations of one of a number of transporters necessary for the proper functioning of the sodium potassium chloride co-transporter (NKCC2) in the thick ascending limb of the loop of Henle. This results in disruption of the normal water-reabsorbing function of the loop and severe salt and water loss. Due to volume depletion, they have aggressive activation of their renin-angotensin-aldosterone system (RAAS) and thus hyperaldosteronism. This results in a metabolic alkalosis and hypokalaemia, which may be severe and commonly has a worse phenotype with lower potassium levels than GS. NKCC2 is the pharmacologic target of loop diuretics, and the biochemical features of Bartter are the same as those found with loop diuretic administration.

Given the variety of different genes that can be involved, the phenotype is quite variable, but patients usually present in infancy with failure to thrive and dehydration, but unlike GS polyhydramnios may be present on antenatal screening. Muscle cramps, polydipsia, polyuria, enuresis, salt craving and nephrocalcinosis may be present depending on the mutation.

There is no curative treatment, and treatment is oral replacement of electrolyte loses with oral potassium and magnesium supplementation as required. Angiotensin converting enzyme inhibition, angiotensin receptor blockade, aldosterone antagonists and potassium sparing diuretics can be helpful in maintaining safe potassium levels. In some patients there is hypersecretion of prostaglandin E_2, and thus, non-steroidal anti-inflammatories are worth trying and maybe helpful. In practical terms management of BS (and GS) can be challenging, as it involves titrating large quantities of tablets in children and adolescents for an indefinite period. Periods of non-compliance and intercurrent illness are not uncommon.

Gitelman syndrome is an autosomal recessive condition with a prevalence of 25 per million population making it one of the commonest inherited tubular disorders. Gitelman syndrome results from inactivating mutations (of which there are many reported) of the SLC12A3 gene encoding for the thiazide-sensitive sodium chloride cotransporter (NCC) in the distal convoluted tubule. As this is distal to the loop, it leaves the free water absorbing mechanism of the loop functional, and the salt and water loss in Gitelman is much less pronounced than in Bartter, and hypokalaemia is typically milder. Again, there is activation of the RAAS and subsequent hyperaldosteronism, causing a metabolic alkalosis and hypokalaemia. Hypomagnesaemia is frequently present and may also be severe.

Patients usually present in late childhood or early adulthood with a coincident illness during which routine blood tests reveal hypokalaemia, but the clinical manifestations are highly variable between families. Clinical features relate to the metabolic upset and include muscle weakness, cramps (often exercise intolerance), tetany, paraesthesia, nocturia, thirst, salt craving, abdominal pain and chondrocalcinosis, and growth retardation may also occur. Blood pressure is often normal or low.

The diagnosis is often delayed, and nephrologists usually see these patients with documented marked hypokalaemia and in keeping with a thiazide-like effect characteristic hypomagnesaemia and hypocalciuria (which distinguishes Gitelman from Bartter). Thiazide diuretics mimic exactly the effect of the mutation, and therefore thiazide abuse (as well as laxative abuse) mimics the condition (easily excluded by toxicology screens if done at the right time). Joint X-rays may show chondrocalcinosis.

There is no specific treatment, and therapy relies on oral salt replacement, with oral potassium and magnesium supplementation (see Bartter); this is often a considerable burden of tablets, and bouts of vomiting can rapidly cause hypokalaemia, so patients need to be counselled on this; there is also the importance of seeking medical aid early and considering wearing a MedicAlert bracelet or equivalent.

Liddle syndrome is an extremely rare autosomal dominant condition caused by mutations of the epithelial sodium channel (EnaC) causing it to be overactive. EnaC is normally activated by aldosterone, so Liddle mimics hyperaldosteronism, causing hypertension (which may be severe), metabolic alkalosis, low renin, hypokalaemia and unlike Conn syndrome characteristically normal or low aldosterone levels. Presentation is usually in childhood. Treatment is with a low-salt diet and amiloride or triamterene, which specifically blocks ENaC improving both hypertension and hypokalaemia. Spironolactone is ineffective because the ENaC activity does not depend on aldosterone, which is suppressed.

Fanconi syndrome (FS) is an inherited or acquired syndrome of generalised proximal tubular dysfunction, causing low-molecular-weight proteinuria, amino aciduria, phosphaturia, uricosuria, glycosuria and bicarbonaturia. Bicarbonate is usually reabsorbed by the proximal tubular cells, but can be less efficiently absorbed in the loop. This means that, as bicarbonate is freely filtered, when bicarbonate falls below approximately 14 mmol/L, it will all be absorbed from the filtrate and disappear from the urine. Bicarbonate is not reabsorbed in the collecting duct and remains in the lumen. As it is an anion, this makes the lumen more electronegative, favouring the secretion of positive potassium ions into the lumen. Thus, Fanconi will cause hypokalaemia only when there is bicarbonate in the urine, e.g. when it first develops or when the Fanconi is treated with enough bicarbonate supplements to increase the serum bicarbonate enough to cause bicarbonaturia.

Clinical features relate to the metabolic impact and include polyuria, polydipsia, muscle weakness, hypophospataemic rickets (in children) or osteomalacia (in adults). Severely affected children fail to thrive, but lesser involvement may be clinically silent.

The causes of inherited and acquired FS are shown in Table 13.9. The diagnosis of FS is usually made by demonstrating a combination of hyperchloraemic metabolic acidosis, hypokalaemia, hypophosphataemia and hypouricaemia with evidence of inappropriate urine losses of phosphate, potassium, bicarbonate and aminoaciduria. Glycosuria in the face of normal serum glucose is suggestive, and a cheap screening test may be negative. Depending on the cause, there is often low-molecular-weight tubular proteinuria (retinol-binding protein, β_2 microglobulin, α_1 macroglobulin). The cause of FS needs to be established and treatable secondary causes excluded.

The treatment of FS is to treat the underlying condition where possible (remove potential drug causes, e.g. immunosuppression for Sjogren's syndrome, treatment of plasma cell dyscrasia). Otherwise treatment is to replace bicarbonate, phosphate, vitamin D and if necessary potassium aiming for a bicarbonate above 20 mmol/L and a potassium >3 mmol/L.

Table 13.9 Causes of Fanconi syndrome

Genetic	Cystinosis, Wilson's disease, Lowe's (X-linked) (oculocerebral syndrome), Dent's disease (X-linked), Tyrosinaemia (type 1), Galactosaemia, glycogen storage diseases, hereditary fructose intolerance, mitochondrial disorders
Acquired	**Heavy metals:** Arsenic, lead, mercury and cadmium poisoning/toxicity
	Drugs: Tenofovir, adefovir, aminoglycosides, ifosfamide
	Light chain diseases: Amyloid, multiple myeloma, light chain deposition disease
	Interstitial nephritis: Sjogren's syndrome, other causes of interstitial nephritis

Dent's disease comprises a heterogeneous group of rare X-linked proximal tubulopathies associated with nephrolithiasis, nephrocalcinosis (75%), hypercalciuria (95%) and hypophosphataemia low-molecular-weight proteinuria. It results from mutations in CLCNS (encoding for the chloride/hydrogen exchanger) in Dent's disease-1 or mutations in OCRL-1 encoding for phosphatidylinositol bisphosphate 5-phosphatase in Dent's disease-2. As yet there is no clear genotype/phenotype correlation and there is considerable variation between families, some patients presenting with incomplete FS and low-molecular-weight proteinuria may be the only clue.

Clinical features are of proximal tubular dysfunction, Fanconi syndrome, hypercalciuria, nephrocalcinosis and low-molecular-weight proteinuria (beta-2 microglobulin, retinol-binding protein). Detection of low-molecular-weight proteinuria can be a useful screening test in female carriers. Dent's disease is one of the few causes of nephrocalcinosis associated with end-stage renal disease, and 30–80% of affected males require renal replacement therapy between the third and fifth decade of life which is thus an important (albeit rare) cause of unexplained renal failure. Renal transplantation is curative.

Lowe's syndrome is a very rare (estimated at roughly 1 in a million) X-linked oculocerebrorenal syndrome with a similar renal phenotype to Dent's disease also resulting from mutations of the OCRL gene encoding the PIP phosphatase involved in endosomal trafficking. Aside from a relatively mild FS and metabolic acidosis, male patients develop severe cataracts antenatally, glaucoma is common and visual deficit is almost universal. Hypotonia results in severe motor developmental delay, and scoliosis is common often resulting in chest infections. Severe hypophosphataemia may result in rickets. Although rare, this condition is relevant to adult nephrologists as patients may live to middle age, often have complex needs, and patients have been successfully transplanted [20].

Glucocorticoid remedial hyperaldosteronism (or type 1 familial hyperaldosteronism) is a rare autosomal dominant disease caused by a mutation resulting in a chimeric CYP11B1/CYP11B2 gene. This causes aldosterone synthetase in the zona glomerulosa of the adrenal cortex to become sensitive to ACTH and inappropriately upregulated. A happy consequence of this is that it also becomes suppressible by physiological doses of glucocorticoid. As this is a condition of hyperaldosteronism, there is hypertension, metabolic acidosis and hypokalaemia. Clinical features include fatigue, headaches, muscle cramps, polyuria and consequent polydipsia. The condition is usually diagnosed in childhood or adolescence as part of the investigation of secondary hypertension.

Apparent mineralocorticoid excess is a rare autosomal recessive syndrome of juvenile hypertension associated with a metabolic alkalosis and hypokalaemia but with a low serum aldosterone. It is caused by mutations in the HSD11B2 gene encoding for 11β-hydroxysteroid dehydrogenase type 2. This enzyme normally converts cortisol to cortisone (temporary inhibition of 11β-hydroxysteroid dehydrogenase type 2 is how excessive liquorice is thought to cause hypertension). This conversion is important as cortisol activates the mineralocorticoid receptor as powerfully as aldosterone, and the plasma cortisol concentration is orders of magnitude higher than aldosterone. AME is also glucocorticoid responsive and may be treated with dexamethasone, which suppresses endogenous cortisol production without stimulating the mineralocorticoid receptor, or by inhibiting ENaC using amiloride, or the receptor itself with eplenerone or spironolactone. AME secondary to excess liquorice ingestion just requires a little more restraint in the confectionary department.

13.1.20 Treatment of Hypokalaemia

As most potassium is intracellular, low serum potassium often represents a profound deficit in total body potassium, potassium of <3.0 and <2.0 representing deficits of ~200 and 300 mmol of potassium, respectively, and thus it may take several days to become replete [19].

Administration of IV potassium is helpful especially when depletion is severe, when oral intake is insufficient or unreliable and in hypokalaemic emergencies such as arrhythmias. Intravenous potassium chloride may be given peripherally in normal saline or 5% dextrose at a rate of up to 10 mmol/h. The risk of phlebitis limits faster infusion via a peripheral route, whereas rates of up to 40 mmol/h are felt to be safe via a central line with cardiac monitoring.

Potassium may be given orally as potassium chloride and potassium citrate, titrated against response with the caveat that effervescent potassium is poorly tolerated in large amounts (dose should be split) and slow release potassium has the nasty habit of accumulating before absorption and causing oesophageal ulcers if taken before bedtime. Treating the underlying causes, be they extra-renal or renal in origin, is obviously important as is correcting any concomitant hypomagnesaemia. In chronic potassium-wasting conditions (such as Gitelman, Barrter and renal Fanconi syndrome, syndromes of mineralocorticoid excess or diuretic dependence), other strategies including the use of ACE inhibitors and potassium-sparing diuretics amiloride and spironolactone may need to be considered.

13.1.21 Hyperkalaemia

Hyperkalaemia (>5 mmol/L)

Is relatively uncommon in the general population but relatively common in patients with renal disease or who are taking drugs which limit renal excretion. The efficacy of renin-angiotensin blockade in proteinuric renal disease and cardiac failure has resulted in "clinic hyperkalaemia" being a frequent occurrence. Values of more than 6.0 mmol/l are viewed as medical emergencies, while values greater than 6.5 mmol/l are genuinely life-threatening although patients with CKD and chronically high total potassium seem to tolerate higher levels.

Pseudohyperkalaemia is usually the result of a red cell or platelets leak of potassium in extracted blood as a result of direct haemolysis, platelet activation in blood tube (Fig. 13.5) or cell leakage (haematological disease, infectious mononucleosis or inherited red cell membrane abnormalities; see Table 13.10).

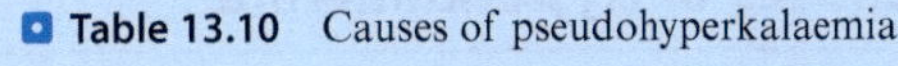

Table 13.10 Causes of pseudohyperkalaemia

Sample taking and processing:	Traumatic venesection with red blood cell lysis or sample squirted through needle into bottle
	Contamination with anticoagulant from another sample (potassium EDTA)
	Increased release from muscles during venesection (excessive hand clenching, prolonged tourniquet time)
	Cell death during long delay/storage prior to analysis (more common with out of hospital samples)
Predisposing medical conditions:	**Marked leucocytosis such as chronic leukaemias**
	Thrombocytosis
	Hereditary and acquired red cell disorders predisposing to cell lysis including familial pseudohyperkalaemia

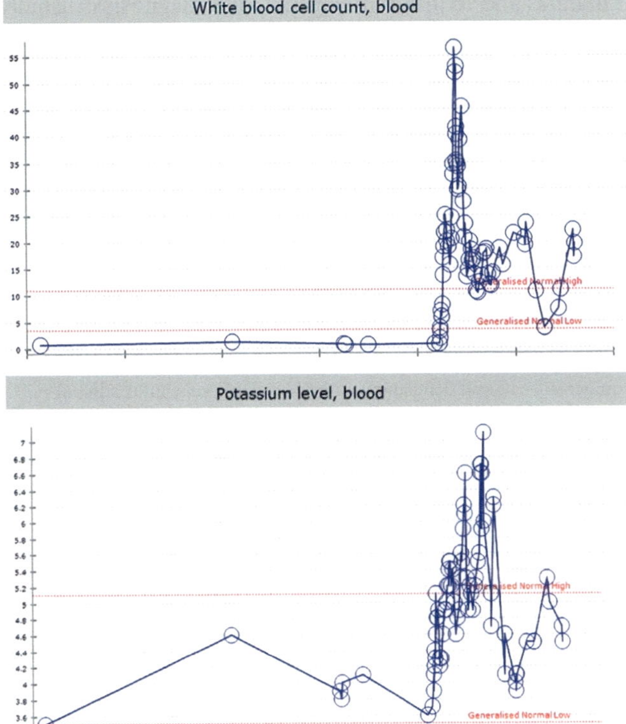

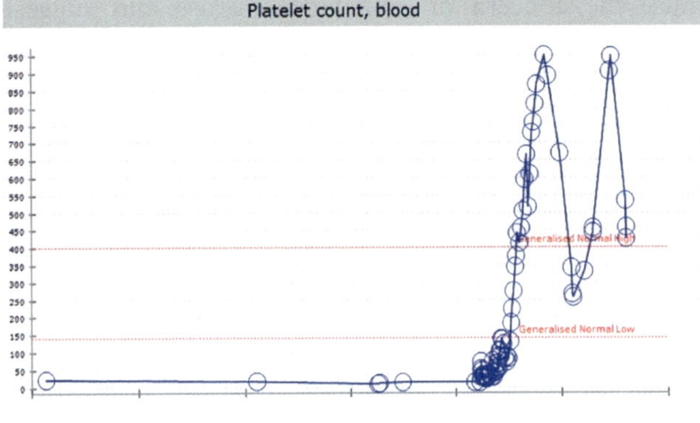

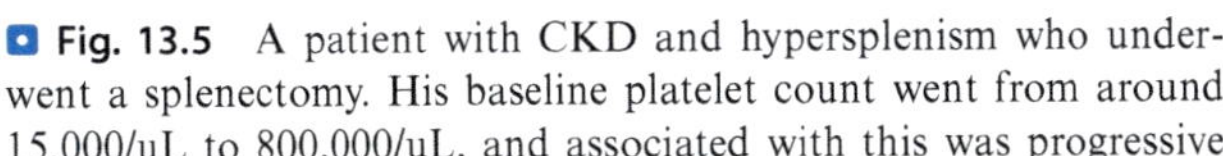

Fig. 13.5 A patient with CKD and hypersplenism who underwent a splenectomy. His baseline platelet count went from around 15,000/uL to 800,000/uL, and associated with this was progressive hyperkalaemia (up to 7 mmol/L) despite a significant improvement in GFR. Blood analysed from a lithium heparin tube gave a value almost 2 mmol/L less than the EDTA sample

13.1.22 Causes of Hyperkalaemia

Causes of hyperkalaemia are reported in ◘ Table 13.11. Of note a reduced GFR is a key risk factor as are drugs that reduce renal potassium excretion. Dietary excess only really comes into play if a patient is predisposed by reduced renal excretion. Less common are endocrine causes of reduced urinary potassium loss such as mineralocorticoid deficiency (Addison's disease, resulting in aldosterone deficiency) or pseudohypoaldosteronism (aldosterone resistance), and, as with hypokalaemia, redistributive shifts between ECF and ICF can result in significant changes in serum levels.

13.1.23 Assessment and Investigation of Hyperkalaemia

A thorough clinical assessment, including drug and dietetic history as well as volume status, is essential, but an ECG takes precedence in the setting of severe hyperkalaemia as this will establish whether the patient is at imminent risk of life-threatening bradycardia, asystole and death (see Appendix 1). "Regular Really Wide Complex Tachycardia" (◘ Fig. 13.6) with QRS >200 ms and an only moderate elevation in heart rate should raise the concern of a metabolic cause and suggest the use of IV calcium and sodium bicarbonate rather than antiarrhythmic drugs [21]. Pseudohyperkalaemia should be excluded in unexpectedly hyperkalaemic patients, particularly in the absence of ECG changes (see ◘ Table 13.10). Here a fresh sample should be rapidly spun and separated (avoiding haemolysis or ongoing red cell potassium leakage).

24-hour urinary potassium excretion is the gold standard and will differentiate renal from non-renal hyperkalaemia; <20 mmol/24 hrs, in the face of hyperkalaemia, suggests a problem with renal excretion. Alternatively, and more conveniently, potassium excretion can be assessed using the transtubular potassium gradient (◘ Table 13.8) from a spot urinary potassium. A value of less than 5 in the face of hyperkalaemia is abnormal, while a value of >7 is considered appropriate (unreliable with a very dilute urine or urinary sodium >25 meq/L. [22] If renal potassium excretion is reduced, in the face of a normal GFR, the patient must then be investigated for hypoaldosteronism or aldosterone resistance.

Gordon's syndrome pseudohypoaldosteronism (type II) is a rare inherited mutation of WNK1 or WNK4 genes resulting in gain of function and increased inhibition or the thiazide-sensitive sodium chloride co-transporter. This results in excess sodium and chloride retention, hyperkalaemia, hyperchloraemic metabolic acidosis and low renin hypertension which can become severe by the third decade. Aldosterone levels are high not low due to impaired feedback. It may be associated with short stature, dental abnormalities and reduced intelligence. The diagnosis is usually made by paediatricians but renin/aldosterone levels and fractional excretion of sodium or TTKG (low). Treatment is with a low-salt diet and thiazide diuretics.

13

◘ **Table 13.11** Causes of hyperkalaemia

Reduced renal loss (low urinary potassium)	**Drugs:** Angiotensin converting enzyme inhibitors (ACEi), angiotensin receptor antagonists (ARBs), beta-blockers, aldosterone receptor antagonists (spironolactone, eplerenone? Sp), potassium-sparing diuretics (amiloride, triamterene), calcineurin inhibitors (CNIs), trimethoprim, non-steroidal anti-inflammatories (NSAIDs), heparin
	Endocrine: Addison's disease (aldosterone/mineralocorticoid deficiency), some forms of congenital adrenal hyperplasia
	Renal: Most causes of reduced GFR, type I renal tubular acidosis and type IV renal tubular acidosis, Gordon's syndrome (pseudohypoaldosteronism)
Excessive production	Rhabdomyolysis, intravascular haemolysis, massive transfusion (especially incompatible transfusion), tumour lysis syndrome, significant tissue infarction (especially if impaired renal function), severe exercise
Redistributive	Acidosis, beta-blockade, insulin deficiency, digoxin toxicity, suxamethonium muscle relaxant, hyperkalaemic periodic paralysis
Reduced non-renal losses	Rarely clinically relevant, but constipation can worsen hyperkalaemia in patients with reduced GFR
Excessive intake	Only usually relevant in context of reduced renal excretion (but becomes a common, and avoidable, cause in patients with ESRD or supplemented patients with AKI), the notable exception being lethal injection. Lo-salt condiment has high levels of potassium and not suitable for patients with reduced GFR
Pseudohyperkalaemia	See ◘ Table 13.10

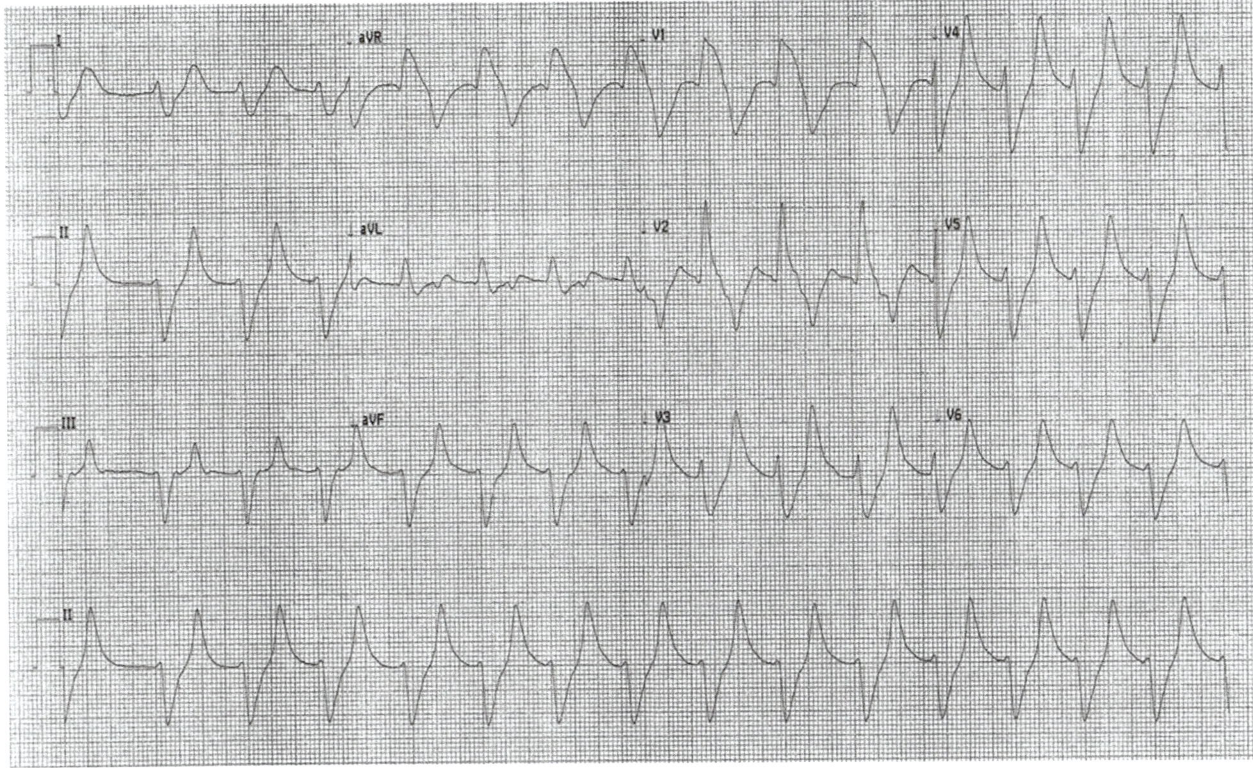

Fig. 13.6 ECG changes in patient with severe hyperkalaemia (8.2 mmol/L). Standard 12-lead ECG (25 mm/s, 10 mm:1 mV). Ventricular rate 100 bpm, QRS 208 ms

13.1.24 Management of Hyperkalaemia

The management of hyperkalaemia (Table 13.12, Fig. 13.7) depends on the severity of the disorder and the presence of ECG changes. Acutely reducing plasma potassium by redistribution is just a temporary measure, and initiating treatment that will reduce total body potassium is crucial. It is not unusual for patients to be given repeated doses of insulin and dextrose without appropriate measures to resolve the underlying problem. Moreover, it needs to be made clear that in an oliguric, hyperkalaemic patient with AKI or ESRD, early plans need to be made for renal replacement therapy unless there is a rapidly reversible element.

Sodium polystyrene sulfonate (SPS) is an oral resin which binds potassium in the large intestine approved by FDA in 1958 for chronic hyperkalaemia. One gram of SPS exchanges 0.5–1 mEq of potassium. Although his role in acute settings is less clear, its use is widespread after cardiac membrane stabilisation and administration of drugs to increase intracellular shift of potassium. Its main side effects are electrolyte disturbances (e.g. hypokalaemia, hypomagnesaemia, hypocalcaemia) and gastrointestinal symptoms (nausea, vomiting, constipation and diarrhoea up to gastrointestinal bleeding, ulceration, perforation and ischemic colitis). The association with sorbitol is reported at increased risk of complications. A recent retrospective cohort study by Noel et al. showed a twofold higher 30-day risk of gastrointestinal events for SPS users with an absolute risk of 1 in 1000. The commonest gastrointestinal events was intestinal ischemia and thrombosis, followed by ulceration and perforation. Nevertheless, due to limitations of this study (no dose-dependent information, no investigations on chronic SPS administration, no SDS-sorbitol association evaluation), the safety characteristics of SPS remain unclear [24].

New potassium binders have been recently approved, such as patiromer and sodium zirconium cyclosilicate (Table 13.13). They showed promising results in studies on their long-term efficacy and safety in chronic hyperkalaemia with less adverse events compared to SPS. Furthermore, these drugs may prevent the discontinuation of renin-angiotensin-aldosterone system blockers, often limited by hyperkalaemia in people with advanced CKD [25].

13.1.25 Calcium Disorders

Calcium is the most abundant mineral in the body. The majority of total body calcium is stored in the skeleton with the remainder overwhelmingly intracellular, where its effects are regulated by calmodulin. Extracellular cal-

Table 13.12 Treatment of hyperkalaemia

Cardiac stabilisation	If ECG changes, then IV **calcium gluconate** 10 ml of 10% instant effect can be repeated
Redistribution (combination treatment more effective)	**Insulin and dextrose**: 50 ml of 50% dextrose with 10 units of insulin IV effect with 15 minutes effect lasting for about 4 hours
	Beta$_2$-agonists: Nebulised but high dose required, e.g. salbutamol 10–20 mg (drop in K^+ 0.6 and 0.85 mmol/L)
	Correction of acidosis: With bicarbonate both redistributes potassium and can lead to sustained reduction in the setting of CKD with chronic acidosis
Reduce/stop intake	Stop supplements and dietary excess (consider dietary review)
Stop/suspend/reduce potassium-sparing medication	ACEI, ARB, aldosterone antagonists, NSAID, trimethoprim, heparin, CNIs
Lowering total body potassium:	
1. Renal losses	**Diuresis:** Loop diuretics (plus or minus thiazides if poor renal function) thiazides for CNI-induced hyperkalaemia
	Mineralocorticoid: Fludrocortisone, for patients with adrenal insufficiency supplementing hydrocortisone and fludrocortisone
Gastrointestinal losses	**Binders:** e.g. calcium resonium very limited evidence (should be given with laxatives which may be more effective than resins)
	Laxatives: An important and under-used method of reducing total body potassium in a tight corner (NB ensure laxative does not contain potassium)
2. Renal replacement therapy	**Haemofiltration, haemodialysis or acute peritoneal dialysis** highly effective at reducing total body potassium

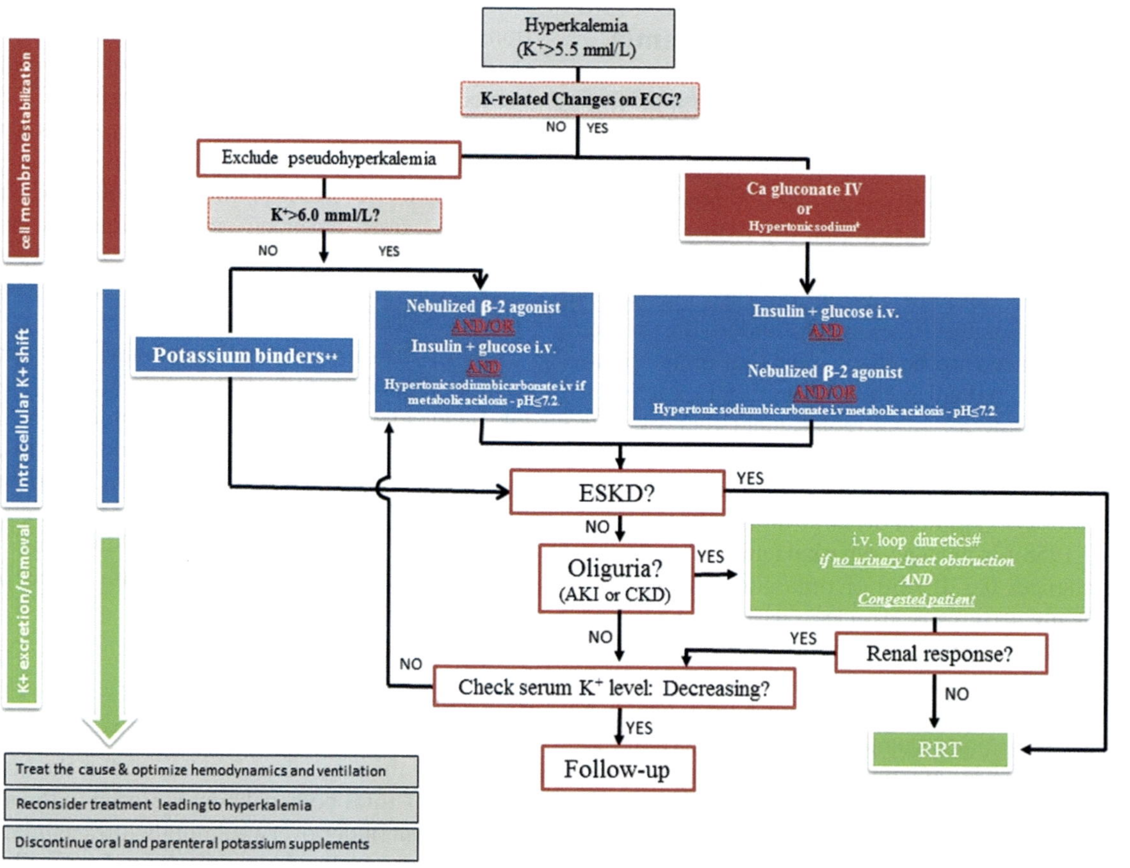

Fig. 13.7 Suggested algorithm for hyperkalaemia. *In case of *Digitalis* intoxication or hypercalcemia. (**Sodium zirconium cyclosilicate and patiromer when available, kayexalate if not available. ESKD end-stage kidney disease, AKI acute kidney injury, CKD chronic kidney disease, RRT renal replacement therapy [23])

Table 13.13 Characteristics of potassium-binding agents for their treatment of hyperkalaemia (Adapted from Bianchi S and Regolisti G, 2019) [26]

Drung	Sodium polystyrene sulphonate	Patiromer	Sodium zirconium cyclosilicate
Molecule	Non-specific cation-binding, sodium-containing organic resin	Selective, calcium-containing sodium-free, organic polymer	Highly selective, sodium- and zirconium-containing, inorganic crystalline silicate
Mechanism of action	Non-specific binding of K in exchange for sodium	Non-specific binding of K in exchange for calcium	Selective K binding in exchange for sodium
Formulation/route	Oral/rectal suspension	Oral suspension	Oral suspension
Site of action	Colon	Distal colon	Entire intestinal tract
Onset of effect	1–6 h	7 h	1 h
Dose	15–60 g/day	8.4–25.2 g/day	5–15 g/day
Common adverse events	GI intolerance Hypokalaemia Hypocalcaemia Hypernatraemia	GI intolerance Hypokalaemia Hypomagnesaemia	GI intolerance Hypokalaemia Oedema
Possible severe adverse events	Colonic necrosis	None	None

cium is either protein bound, ionised (the active form) or complexed with phosphate, citrate, bicarbonate or sulphate. The total body calcium is closely regulated and determined by the balance of gut uptake and renal excretion with bones being a large reservoir. Regulation is via the parathyroid glands (via the calcium-sensing receptor (CaSR; see ▶ Chap. 50). [27] Most calcium assays measure total (bound and unbound) calcium correcting for albumin levels using the following formula:

Adjusted Calcium (mmol/L) = measured serum calcium (mmol/L) + 0.02 × [40-serum albumin (g/L)]

This becomes inaccurate if the patient is very acidotic, with paraproteinaemia and at extremes of albumin. Changes in ionised calcium are significant clinically and can be obtained via blood gas analysers although in practical terms most diagnosis and decisions are made on the corrected calcium.

13.1.26 Hypercalcaemia

Hypercalcaemia (corrected calcium >2.6 mmol/L)

Is a relatively common disorder, affecting around 1% of the population. Often patients have chronically, mildly elevated levels, but occasionally they present with severe hypercalcaemia (≥3.5 mmol/L) and life-threateningly high levels, sometimes precipitating AKI.

13.1.27 Causes of Hypercalcaemia

The causes of hypercalcaemia are shown in Table 13.14 with malignancy and primary hyperparathyroidism accounting for more than 90% of cases. Malignancy can cause hypercalcaemia in a variety of ways in part through the production of PTH-related protein (PTHrP), typically through solid malignancies with metastases, classically breast and squamous cell carcinoma. Alternative mechanisms include malignancy-associated cytokine release (IL-6, IL-1, TGF-β, RANK), direct bones involvement, prolonged immobility and increased macrophage production of 1,25 $(OH)_2$ vitamin D with some haematological malignancies. More than 40% of all hypercalcemia cases presenting to the Emergency Department may be secondary to cancer, and these patients have a 50% 30-day mortality.

13.1.28 Clinical Features of Hypercalcaemia

Non-specific symptoms such as malaise, anorexia, nausea and vomiting, depression and lethargy often predominate and may be subtle if the hypercalcaemia is not severe and particularly if chronic as with primary

Table 13.14 Causes of hypercalcaemia

Malignancy	PTHrP (squamous cell carcinoma, breast malignancy), pro-inflammatory cytokine release, immobilisation, direct bone involvement (multiple myeloma), increased synthesis of 1,25 $(OH)_2$ vitamin D (lymphoma)
Hyperparathyroidism	
Primary	85% single adenoma> primary hyperplasia, multiple endocrine neoplasia (MEN), parathyroid carcinoma
Tertiary	Exacerbated by high doses of vitamin D, aluminium intoxication and adynamic bone disease
Granulomatous diseases	Classically TB and sarcoidosis but potentially any chronic inflammatory process involving accumulation of macrophages (sometimes unmasked by vitamin D supplementation)
Vitamin D intoxication	Hypervitaminosis D, food faddists but not uncommon iatrogenic cause in patients with CKD on large doses of supplements
Vitamin A intoxication	
Aluminium intoxication	
Medication	Thiazides, lithium, excess antacid ingestions (milk-alkali syndrome)
Endocrine causes	Addison's disease, acromegaly, hyperthyroidism, phaechromocytoma
Familial hypocalciuric hypercalcaemia	Secondary to calcium-sensing receptor mutations
Prolonged immobilisation	Unusual as a sole cause; Paget's disease only causes hypercalcaemia in the immobile patient
Recovery phase of rhabdomyolysis	Hypercalcaemia 1–2 weeks post AKI may be the only clue as to the aetiology of missed rhabdomyolysis

hyperparathyroidism. Renal effects include polyuria, thirst, renal failure, nephrocalcinosis and kidney stones (most commonly associated with primary hyperparathyroidism as chronic). Bone pain is common but often non-specific; however, worsening bone pain in known malignancy should provoke a calcium check. Pruritus and conjunctivitis may also occur. Neurological complications include depression, inability to concentrate, confusion, reduced neural excitability resulting in neurological depression, ataxia, upper motor neurone signs and (in severe cases) coma as well as reduced smooth and striated muscle movement. Constipation is a common feature in part due to reduced smooth muscle activity. Hypercalcaemia induces increased gastrin secretion, and peptic ulcers can occur as can pancreatitis. Cardiotoxicity may also occur in severe hypercalcaemia with ECG changes including short QT interval and ST changes mimicking acute coronary syndrome (see Appendix 1).

13.1.29 Assessment and Investigation of Hypercalcaemia

A history of long-standing symptoms especially stones is suggestive of primary hyperparathyroidism, whereas constitutional symptoms of malignancy may suggest this as a primary cause (although symptoms of hypercalcaemia may mimic neoplasia). Rarely there may be a family history of MEN or familial hypocalciuric hypercalcaemia. Examination may reveal signs of malignancy, granulomatous conditions, an underlying endocrine cause or very rarely (but very satisfyingly) corneal calcification. As with all electrolyte disorders, volume status needs to be assessed. Blood tests should include PTH level, alkaline phosphatase, phosphate, albumin, total proteins and renal function (magnesium and potassium will be important for subsequent management). In general hyperparathyroid patients have inappropriately high PTH and a low phosphate. In such cases parathyroid ultrasound and radioisotope scanning may be performed. If the PTH is not suppressed in the face of hypercalcaemia, then the patient has primary or tertiary hyperparathyroidism (the caveat being that some patients have this and a secondary cause such as malignancy). If the PTH is suppressed, then a more detailed assessment of secondary causes is warranted, e.g. serum ACE (unhelpful if on ACEI), 25(OH) vitamin D, paraproteins, Bence Jones proteinuria, protein electrophoresis and immunofixation, chest X-ray and where appropriate further imaging with mammogram, CT scanning or gallium. An ECG is necessary to exclude any electrophysiological changes.

Of note, in some occasions, total calcium level may be very high in the context of a normal ionised calcium and usually no manifestations of hypercalcaemia. This is defined as pseudohypercalcaemia and usually arises in the presence of a circulating factor that can bind calcium (such as additional albumin, paraproteins or additional immunoglobulins like in Waldenstrom macroglobulinaemia, or citrate in case of citrate overload during CRRT regional citrate anticoagulation).

13.1.30 Treatment of Hypercalcaemia

The treatment of hypercalcaemia is directed at restoring intravascular volume and treating the underlying cause. Severe and symptomatic hypercalcaemia requires urgent corrective therapy with most agreeing that a calcium above 3.4 mmol/L requires admission and urgent correction. Cessation of contributing medication (antacids, thiazides, lithium, vitamin D supplements) is appropriate. Volume expansion with normal saline promotes a diuresis and is calciuric; in fact anything promoting a natriuresis promotes calciuresis. Once euvolaemia has been achieved, saline may be given in tandem with intravenous or oral loop diuretics, promoting renal losses further. In hypercalcaemia due to sarcoidosis, other granulomatous disease, vitamin D intoxication and some malignancies, prednisolone therapy is effective and of course is part of the treatment of adrenal insufficiency. Bisphosphonates (pamidronate and etidronate) can be given to inhibit bone resorption although are relatively contraindicated in patients with GFR <30 mL/min, and a judgment call needs to be made on the risk/benefit in patients with severe hypercalcaemia and low GFR. Subcutaneous calcitonin also blocks bone resorption and increases urinary calcium excretion by inhibiting calcium reabsorption and can be useful in severe acute hypercalcaemia.

The calcimimetic agent cinacalcet has been shown to lower calcium in hyperparathyroidism related to reduced GFR, although surgical parathyroidectomy remains the standard UK approach in the absence of contraindications to surgery and occasionally should be considered as an urgent procedure. Finally, severe hypercalcaemia around 4 mmol/L or above (lower if ECG changes) may be better treated by acute renal replacement therapy, especially if the patient has significant AKI or CKD, which is highly effective at temporarily reducing calcium levels.

13.1.31 Hypocalcaemia

Hypocalcaemia (corrected calcium <2.1 mmol/L)

Is less common than hypercalcaemia but familiar to nephrologists in the setting of CKD and nutritional deficiency and very common among hospital inpatients. Severe hypocalcaemia (<1.75 mmol/L) can have life-threatening consequences in terms of seizures and cardiac arrhythmias.

13.1.32 Causes of Hypocalcaemia

The commonest cause of hypocalcaemia is artifactual and relates to a low serum albumin, and the corrected calcium and ionised calcium should be normal if no deficiencies. Parathyroid hormone level (PTH) can be useful in dividing possible aetiologies especially if chronic but may be less discriminatory in acute illnesses such as burns or pancreatitis. Beyond renal disease as a cause of hypocalcaemia, vitamin D deficiency is epidemic and may be a contributing factor with other causes of hypocalcaemia (◘ Table 13.14). "Hungry bone syndrome" is worth special mention as it occurs in renal practice following parathyroidectomy in patients with tertiary hyperparathyroidism and can result in life-threatening hypocalcaemia. It results from reduced bone resorption, a marked influx of calcium into calcium-depleted bones and reduced calcium absorption from the gut secondary to a fall in PTH. Advanced age, hypomagnesaemia, vitamin D deficiency and size of gland removed are risk factors, but it is largely dependent on how severe the parathyroid bone disease is and occurs in 25–90% of those patients with radiological evidence of hyperparathyroidism compared to only 0–6% of those without radiological change [28] (◘ Table 13.15).

13.1.33 Clinical Features of Hypocalcaemia

Perioral paraesthesia and numbness, dystonia, bronchospasm, laryngospasm, seizures, tetany and respiratory arrest are well-known neuromuscular features of severe hypocalcaemia. Prolonged QTc, heart block and flat T waves, reduced PR interval and U waves, heart block, Torsades de Pointes and ventricular fibrillation are cardiovascular sequelae (see Appendix 1). Chronic hypocalcaemia may be associated with rickets and/or osteodystrophy, basal ganglia calcification, poor dentition and cataracts. More moderate hypocalcaemia may also be associated with more subtle symptoms chronically such as depression, irritability, muscle cramps and dementia. Chvostek's sign (ipsilateral facial muscle contraction on tapping of the facial nerve) and Trousseau's sign (hand and wrist flexion on inflating a blood pressure cuff above systolic blood pressure) may confirm a clinical suspicion of significant hypocalcaemia.

Table 13.15 Causes of hypocalcaemia

High PTH	**Renal failure** (falling 1α (OH) vitamin D and rising phosphate)
	25 (OH) vitamin D deficiency (UV exposure, short-bowel syndromes, malabsorption, liver disease)
	Pseudohypoparathyroidism resistance to PTH (Albright hereditary osteodystrophy (type 1a) short fourth and fifth metacarpals and round facies)
Low/normal PTH	**Magnesium deficiency (severe)** (lowers PTH secretion and end-organ resistance)
	Hypoparathyroidism: Post-operative parathyroidectomy (acute "Hungrey bones") (chronic PTH deficiency with removal of all four glands), post-operative thyroidectomy/neck trauma, infiltrative malignancy, autoimmune (including part of polyglandular syndrome-1, haemochromatosis, DiGeorge syndrome (thymic aplasia and absent parathyroid glands), Barakat (HDR) syndrome (hypoparathyroidism, sensorineural deafness and renal disease (dysplasia, reflux, cystic)), idiopathic hypoparathyroidism
Hyperphosphataemia	Rhabdomyolysis (acutely), tumour lysis syndrome, phosphate supplements (IV, oral, rarely phosphate enema's in patients with CKD)
Medication	Cinacalcet, bisphosphonates, loop diuretics, proton pump inhibitors, cisplatin, phenobarbital, phenytoin
Miscellaneous	Acute pancreatitis, burns, sepsis, massive transfusion
Artifactual	Low albumin (correction for serum albumin or ionised calcium give true status)
Redistributive	Alkalosis (e.g. hyperventilation)

13.1.34 Investigation of Hypocalcaemia

Albumin, total protein and bicarbonate help confirm genuine hypocalcaemia. PTH, vitamin D, phosphate, renal function and magnesium are useful first-line tests. Amylase, creatine kinase and exclusion of malabsorption and liver disease may be helpful if no obvious cause. Osteomalacia may be apparent on X-rays. The presence of a low PTH in the absence of surgical removal requires further investigation (see Table 13.14).

13

13.1.35 Treatment of Hypocalcaemia

Depends largely on the underlying cause, but acute, symptomatic hypocalcaemia should be treated with intravenous calcium (e.g. 10% calcium gluconate) which may need repeat doses or an infusion, for example, in the setting of "hungry bone syndrome". This syndrome tends to cause a nadir of calcium at 2–4 days post-operatively but may continue for significantly longer. IV calcium supplements are usually necessary initially transferring to oral calcium (often calcium carbonate but taken *after* meals to avoid reducing phosphate) 6–12 g/day. Correction of magnesium is important, and large doses of 1,25 (OH) vitamin D are necessary. Pre-treatment with high doses of vitamin D pre-surgery for several days and bisphosphonate pre-op, if high PTH is present, appears to significantly reduce the severity of post-operative hypocalcaemia although the evidence base for the use of bisphosphonates is limited.

Stopping causative drugs, correcting magnesium deficiency and treatment with calcium and vitamin D are helpful with any cause of hypocalcaemia. Thereafter maintenance is with calcium and vitamin D: calcitriol if significant CKD and colecalciferol if 25(OH) vitamin D deficient. Deficiencies in diet, sun exposure and malabsorption should be addressed where possible. Severe hyperphosphataemia and hypocalcaemia may be corrected with dialysis in, for example, rhabdomyolysis or tumour lysis syndrome. Getting the dose of IV and/or oral calcium supplements right can be tricky, as the requirements alter and close monitoring is essential in severe hypocalcaemia.

13.1.36 Phosphate Disorders

Over 99% of total body phosphate is intracellular (muscles and visceral) as well as bone (where it forms a key structural component). It is the most abundant intracellular anion and essential for normal cell structure and membrane integrity, nucleic acid synthesis and metabolism, buffering and energy metabolism via ATP synthesis and is crucially involved in activation of intracellular molecules involved in signalling and metabolism. Phosphate is abundant in most diets and absorbed predominantly in the duodenum and upper jejunum via passive transcellular uptake as well as active sodium-phosphate coupled transport. Gut absorption is increased by hypophosphataemia and 1,25 (OH) vitamin D via upregulation of the sodium-phosphate cotransporter.

Total body phosphate balance is in part regulated by gut uptake and exchange with bone and largely maintained by the kidney. Phosphate being freely filtered but the vast majority (>75%) is actively reabsorbed in the proximal convoluted tubule via a sodium-phosphate cotransporter. Some additional phosphate reabsorption occurs in the distal convoluted tubule. Renal excretion of phosphate is influenced by several factors including GFR (with impaired excretion once the kidney reaches CKD3b and progressively so with further decline), dietary intake, 1,25 (OH) vitamin D, PTH and phosphatonins such as fibroblast growth factors 23 (FGF-23, a bone-derived phosphatonin) and 7 (FGF-7), secreted frizzled-related protein-4 (sFRP-4) and klotho (anti-ageing protein produced mainly by the kidney) [29].

The skeleton is a critical storage of phosphate but also highly dependent on adequate supplies for healthy mineralisation and remodelling of the bone, which is now considered as a sophisticated inner sensor connecting several functions and pathological pathways, such as osteoporosis, CKD-mineral bone disorders (CKD-MBD), inflammation response and aging ("inflammaging"). Indeed, the so-called bone marrow niche has been recently described as a bone marrow functional which a complex interplay between bone cells and hematopoietic cells takes place, leading to the deep cross-talk of immune system with bone under the influence of several chemokines (IL-17, IL-1b, TGF-β, TNF-α, etc.) [30, 31].

Finally, like potassium, phosphate can translocate between the intracellular and extracellular compartments under the influence of insulin with a potential role in acute disease as described in the refeeding syndrome.

13.1.37 Hypophosphataemia

Hypophosphataemia (0.65–0.81 mmol/L mild, 0.32–0.64 mmol/L moderate and <0.32 mmol/L severe)

Is common in hospitalised patients (up to 5%) particularly so in malnourished patients (especially once being fed), alcoholism, malabsorption, acute sepsis, ITU admission (most with continuous filtration) and patients with diabetic ketoacidosis.

13.1.38 Causes of Hypophosphataemia

Causes of hypophosphataemia are shown in ◘ Table 13.12 and can broadly be separated into renal causes (increased excretion), gastrointestinal causes (decreased absorption) and redistributive. Renal causes can be further subdivided into those secondary to FGF-23 and those not; this is not a very practical division as clinical assays for FGF-23 are not readily available in most health settings but do add a certain something. Medication is thought to be a contributing factor in a significant proportion of cases, and malnourished patients are substantially predisposed.

The majority of inherited renal causes causing phosphate wasting are diagnosed in childhood, but autosomal dominant hypophosphataemic rickets can present in adulthood with bone pain and osteomalacia. Presentation of acquired renal wasting depends on the cause or insult, resulting in either a selective or, more commonly, diffuse proximal convoluted tubular dysfunction. Not infrequently a combination of factors is present in patients with malabsorption, malnutrition or alcoholism, and such patients with depleted total body phosphate levels are at very high and predictable risk of refeeding syndrome (◘ Table 13.16).

▪ Refeeding Syndrome (RFS)

This is the result of restoration of nutrition after prolonged/severe starvation. This usually develops in the first 72 hours after nutrition is restarted and can have rapidly life-threatening consequences. Main features are hyperglycaemia and dropping of serum potassium, magnesium and phosphate levels and of micronutrients (especially thiamine or vitamin B1). This is often associated with hypernatraemia and fluid overload that may become clinically relevant up to pulmonary oedema. After a few days, lipolysis increases, subsequently leading to raised levels of free fatty acids in the circulation.

The re-introduction of glucose in a catabolic state causes the suppression of ketogenesis and a new increase in insulin. The resulting activation of anabolic processes drive intracellular shifts of glucose, water and electrolytes with potential sharp drop of plasmatic levels.

Severe acute electrolyte disorders can cause cardiac arrhythmias, neuromuscular disorders including rhabdomyolysis, haemolysis and severe respiratory failure. Vitamin B1 deficiency can cause neurological and cardiovascular disorders (Wernicke encephalopathy and Beriberi). Prevention may be sought with lower energy rate feeding start and prophylactic electrolyte and high-dose vitamin B1 supplementation in association with intensive monitoring of electrolytes and fluid balance to prevent fluid overload.

13.1.39 Clinical Features of Hypophosphataemia

The majority of hypophosphataemia is asymptomatic with perhaps non-specific weakness, paraesthesia and fatigue. Severe hypophosphataemia can result in proximal myopathy, rhabdomyolysis and respiratory failure

Table 13.16 Causes of hypophosphataemia

Renal	
Inherited phosphate-wasting disorders	Autosomal dominant hypophosphataemic rickets (via impaired metabolism of FGF-23) (variable age of presentation may appear in early adulthood), autosomal recessive hypophosphataemic rickets (dentin matrix protein-1 (DMP1) via impaired inhibition of FGF-23), X-linked hypophosphataemic rickets (phosphate regulating endopeptidase (PHEX) mutation via FGF-23), childhood rickets and inappropriately low or normal vitamin D, X-linked *dominant*.
	Hereditary hypophosphataemic rickets with hypercalciuria (defect of NaPi2 co-transporter, increased vitamin D levels and risk of stones)
Proximal tubular disorders	Fanconi syndrome (see Table 13.6), Dent's disease, cystinosis
Medication/drugs	Diuretics (acetazolamide, loop and thiazide diuretics), cisplatin, ifosfamide, tetracyclines, aminoglycosides, tenofovir, adefovir, imatinib, streptozocin, toluene, mannitol (pseudohypophosphataemia), IV iron maltose
Post-transplant	FGF-23 mediated usually short term
Tumour-induced osteomalacia (TIO)	Mostly benign mesenchymal tumours via FGF-23
Fibrodysplasia	May be associated with endocrine abnormalities and café au lait spots in McCune-Albright syndrome (facial or long bone asymmetry)
Hyperparathyroidism/vitamin D deficiency	Reduced sodium/phosphate co-transporter expression
Gastrointestinal	Malnutrition from any cause, chronic alcoholism (common), eating disorders, short-bowel syndrome, chronic phosphate binders (especially in context of improving renal function)
Redistributive	Refeeding syndrome, insulin and or glucose infusion, respiratory alkalosis, salicylate poisoning, catecholamines, diabetic ketoacidosis, post partial hepatic resection
Miscellaneous	Post-dialysis (especially in malnourished patients) with continuous renal replacement therapy (HDU/ITU), bisphosphonates

13

as well as acute cardiomyopathy. Intravascular haemolysis, depressed white cell function and neurotoxicity in the form of neuropathy, metabolic encephalopathy and seizures can also occur in very advnaced deficiency. More chronic cases in adults and those often occurring with milder levels of hypophosphataemia result in osteomalacia with diffuse bone pain and fracture risk. On the other hand, in children with inherited forms of hypophosphataemia, rickets and growth retardation are common.

13.1.40 Assessment and Investigation of Hypophosphataemia

Hypophosphataemia is often a surrogate marker for malnutrition, or renal proximal tubular disease, and investigations should include an overall assessment of the patient's nutritional status and clinical features of tubular disorders as well as signs of osteomalacia, rickets and proximal myopathy (Table 13.17).

Unless the cause of hypophosphataemia is obvious, then renal excretion of phosphate is helpful in distinguishing between renal and extra-renal. If renal, then further tests for diffuse proximal tubular disease such as Fanconi syndrome are warranted. Family history is essential in children and young adults with isolated phosphate wasting who should be offered genetic screening.

13.1.41 Treatment of Hypophosphataemia

The underlying cause of hypophosphataemia should be established and, where possible this, treated (e.g. vitamin D supplementation, cessation of tubular toxins

■ **Table 13.17** Investigation of hypophosphataemia

Urea, creatinine and electrolytes	Phosphate, magnesium, calcium, potassium, glucose
Acid-base	Venous bicarbonate or arterial blood gases (may reflect proximal tubular acidosis, respiratory alkalosis)
Liver function	Evidence of liver disease, GGT for alcoholism, ALP for osteomalacia
PTH and vitamin D	Hyperparathyroidism, vitamin D deficiency
Urine phosphate	**Extra-renal** <10 mmol/day
	Renal >20 mmol/day
	Fractional excretion of phosphate: $FE_{phosphate}$ = (urine phosphate × plasma creatinine/plasma phosphate × urine creatinine) × 100
$FE_{Phosphate}$ >20% renal wasting	$FE_{Phosphate}$ <20% deficiency, gastrointestinal wasting or redistribution
Nutritional status/ gastrointestinal disease	Overall nutritional state and evidence of malabsorption (low BMI or recent poor intake increases risk of refeeding syndrome), vitamin and trace elements
Imaging of the skeletal system	Focused X-rays or bone densitometry as appropriate in chronic hypophosphatemia
Imaging for tumours	In otherwise unexplained renal phosphate wasting to exclude TIO

such as tenofovir if feasible, resolution of malabsorption). Acute mild-to-moderate hypophosphataemia can usually be managed with high-phosphate foods with or without oral phosphate supplements (although diarrhoea is a common and frequently limiting side effect of phosphate supplements). The evidence base for dosing in acute moderate-to-severe hypophosphataemia is somewhat limited [32]; anticipation, close monitoring and common sense are probably the best guides. IV phosphate should be considered in patients with severe (<0.32 mmol/L) acute hypophosphataemia particularly if they already have cardiorespiratory compromise (e.g. ventilated patients), those with a predisposition to seizures or those unable to take enteral feed. As always, with electrolyte abnormalities, the response depends on the stability of the deficit and the direction of travel: for example, those with hypophosphataemia with ongoing losses such as continuous renal replacement therapy or anticipated re-feeding syndrome in a sick patient are likely to need IV supplements (or phosphate addition to the dialysate/reinfusate for patients on CRRT), whereas a healthy post-transplant patient with a level of 0.30 mmol/L, who is able to take a high-phosphate diet, vitamin D and oral supplements, may not need to be given IV phosphate, particularly if it is clear that level has reached a nadir and is no longer falling. An important caveat with supplementation, especially intravenous, is that it can worsen hypocalcaemia and hypomagnesaemia, both of which must be corrected and monitored, and over-aggressive poorly monitor supplementation may result in phosphate-induced AKI (which does not look good for a nephrologist).

If there is associated vitamin D deficiency, then supplementation is essential (patients with malabsorption, starvation or alcoholism, sufficient to cause hypophosphataemia, are likely to have multiple vitamin and other nutritional deficiencies as well). Resection of the causative tumour is curative in tumour-induced osteomalacia (TIO) and induced hypophosphataemia [33].

13.1.42 Hyperphosphataemia

Hyperphosphataemia, serum phosphate >1.5 mmol/l

Is uncommon in the general population but omnipresent in advanced CKD (in the absence of phosphate lowering measures) (see ▶ Chap. 50). Acute hyperphosphataemia can occur, usually in the setting of significant cell death or inappropriate supplementation. In both scenarios, this is much more likely to occur with impaired renal function (■ Table 13.18).

13.1.43 Clinical Features of Hyperphosphataemia

The major clinical consequence of hyperphosphataemia is related to the presence of calcium-phosphate deposits in target organs which may manifest as conjunctivitis or tenosynovitis. It is usually asymptomatic but if chronic

Table 13.18 Causes of hyperphosphataemia

Reduced renal excretion[a]	AKI and CKD, hypoparathyroidism, pseudohypoparathyroidism (PTH promotes phosphate excretion), acromegaly (increased tubular reabsorption)
Cell lysis	Tumour lysis syndrome (TLS), rhabdomyolysis, significant infarction, intravascular haemolysis and extravascular haemolysis (e.g. extensive haematoma). High LDH, lactate, urate, potassium and creatine kinase may be raised depending on cause
Excess intake	Inappropriate supplementation (especially IV phosphate) and phosphate enemas can cause an acute rise in phosphate and thus can be hazardous in patients with significant renal impairment especially those with pre-existing vascular calcification. Intake of phosphate-rich foods (see ▶ chap. 54) is rarely an issue in patients with normal renal function but commonplace in patients with advanced CKD
Vitamin D intoxication	Rare cause of hyperphosphataemia in the general population but contributory in patients with CKD (vitamin D (25 (OH) and 1, 25 (OH) levels may be helpful
Redistributive	Acidosis promotes shift from extracellular to intracellular location

[a]Reduced GFR significant predisposition to all other causes

will lead to calcium-phosphate deposition in multiple tissues, the most significant being vascular and with important cardiovascular consequences including calciphylaxis (see ▶ Chap. 51). Occasionally and particularly in dialysis patients, a large hard mass may develop in the soft tissue (Teutschlander's disease) sometimes secondary to calcification of a haematoma. This is often painful and may ulcerate, but X-ray imaging usually makes the diagnosis fairly evident and rules out more sinister causes. Sudden acute hyperphosphataemia may lead to acute tissue calcification, hypocalcaemia and acute kidney injury.

13

13.1.44 Treatment of Hyperphosphataemia

Treatment needs to be directed at the underlying cause and in the case of CKD covered in ▶ Chaps. 50 and 54. Management of acute and severe hyperphosphataemia involves prevention in the setting of TLS (see ▶ Chap. 30) and volume expansion to promote renal excretion (if good renal function), with the possible addition of loop diuretic to promote renal excretion (with monitoring of calcium). Although the evidence base is weak, there is at least a good theoretical argument for acute haemodialysis or haemofiltration in the setting of tumour lysis syndrome or rhabdomyolysis associated with hyperphosphataemia in the context of AKI and is worth considering, especially if potassium is becoming bothersome.

In patients with CKD, management relies on patient engagement with the issue, excellent and clear education on how to have a good and culturally relevant low-phosphate diet and the purpose and importance of phosphate binders (see ▶ Chaps. 50 and 54).

13.1.45 Magnesium Disorders

Magnesium is the second intracellular cation after potassium and is a co-factor of several enzymatic reactions, and it is involved in the regulation of ion membrane transport (e.g. for K and Ca), having a critical role in a series of biological processes including mitochondrial function, inflammation, neuromuscular and cardiac electrical activity and blood pressure regulation.

Of the total body content of magnesium (around 26 g), nearly 99% are located in the bones (60%), 20% skeletal muscle and 19% soft tissues, leaving only 1% in the extracellular fluid. Serum magnesium (0.3% of total) is ionised for nearly two thirds, and only in a smaller proportion is bound to proteins and other anions. Magnesium balance is maintained by dietary intake and absorption (small intestine via TRPM6 channel, influenced by calcium steroids and PTH) and renal excretion with limited shift between the intra- and extracellular pools and the bone.

Good sources of Mg are green leafy vegetables, such as spinach, nuts, brown rice, wholegrain bread and cocoa. Proton pump inhibitors can decrease Mg absorption. Magnesium is passively reabsorbed mainly in the thick ascending limb of the loop of Henle but also in the distal convoluted tubule via an active mechanism. Renal excretion has a primary role in finely tuning the balance, and it is influenced by extracellular fluid volume, GFR, magnesium, calcium and phosphate levels, acid-base status, PTH and glucagon.

13.1.46 Hypomagnesaemia

The current reference range for plasmatic magnesium is 0.70–1.05 mmol/L.

> Hypomagnesaemia (Mg <0.7 mmol/l)

Appears to be quite common in hospitalised patient with an incidence of up to 10%.

These reference values have been put in question lately for two main reasons. First, they were assumed from a healthy population of the NHANES I cohort (1974) rather than based on clinical outcomes (and with all the limits of a "historical" control). Second, significant evidence now supports the idea of subclinical magnesium deficiency and of advantages of higher magnesium levels beyond those target values. Available evidence suggests 0.85 mmol/l as new cutoff for hypomagnesaemia [34].

13.1.47 Causes of Hypomagnesaemia

Hypomagnesaemia is most commonly related to gut losses followed by renal losses or a combination of the two, and dietary deficiency is relatively rare except in alcoholics, the malnourished and the hospital setting (Table 13.19).

Table 13.19 Causes of hypomagnesaemia

Gastrointestinal losses	Acute or chronic diarrhoea, prolonged vomiting, nasogastric drainage, short bowel syndrome of any cause, malabsorption of any cause acute or chronic pancreatitis, non-magnesium containing laxative abuse
Renal losses	
Acquired renal causes	**Drugs:** Loop or thiazide diuretics especially in combination, drugs causing tubular injury, especially aminoglycosides, cisplatin, foscarnet, amphotericin B
	Others proton pump inhibitors, calcineurin inhibitors
	Endocrine: Hyperthyroidism, hyperaldosteronism, hypoparathyroidism (particular risk post-parathyroidism with "hungry bone syndrome")
	High urine output: Osmotic diuresis, post-obstructive diuresis any polyuric state
Genetic renal causes	Gitelman syndrome, Barrter syndrome, congenital magnesium wasting (TRPM6-Mg^{2+} channel), familial hypomagnesaemia with hypercalciuria and nephrocalcinosis, isolated dominant hypomagnesaemia with hypocalciuria.
Redistributive	Movement from ECF to ICF occurs in refeeding and insulin treatment of diabetic ketoacidosis
Inadequate intake	Chronic malnutrition (especially if associated with diarrhoea), alcoholism, parentral fluids/feed without magnesium

13.1.48 Clinical Features of Hypomagnesaemia

These are principally related to neuromuscular and cardiac toxicity, being magnesium necessary to generate a transmembrane potential, generate ATP for ionic transporters and regulate K outward via the inwardly rectifying potassium channels. The latter role is lost in the case of intracellular Mg depletion which causes increased intracellular K losses and risk for cardiotoxicity. Neurological involvement may occur with only mildly reduced levels 0.5–0.7 mmol/L with weakness, apathy, depression, confusion and paraesthesia, and as with hypocalcemia, Chvostek's and Trousseau's signs may be apparent. It is important to note that even mildly low levels may result sufficient to precipitate seizures or dysrhythmias in patients with a predisposition or who have concomitantly low calcium levels (or potassium levels). More severe deficiency, usually <0.5 mmol/L, may manifest as prolonged QT, U-waves and T wave changes (ST depression, see Appendix 1). Supraventricular tachyarrhythmias may occur, and classically Torsade de Pointes is the ventricular tachycardia, but fibrillation is also a significant complication. Tetany, seizures, respiratory muscle weakness, confusion, altered mental state and coma become increasingly likely with falling levels.

Further long-term effects of magnesium in mortality are related to potential role for heart remodelling and congestive heart failure, hypertension, endothelial dysfunction and vascular calcifications. These may be explained in part by the fact that magnesium may have phosphate-binding activity in the gut and may interact with calcium-sensing receptor leading to improved endothelial dysfunction as shown in patients with CKD [35].

13.1.49 Assessment and Investigation of Hypomagnesaemia

History targeted at potential causes, principally GI or renal losses including drugs likely to promote magnesium wasting (Table 13.19). Bloods including urea, creatinine and electrolytes, calcium, phosphate, liver function, pancreatic enzymes, alcohol, glucose, albumin and total proteins should be performed. Protein levels will influence the measurement of total plasma magnesium, so as with calcium a low serum albumin requires correction of magnesium upwards. If hypomagnesaemia is confirmed, it is useful to assess the fractional excretion of magnesium in a spot urine with simultaneous plasma level using the following equation:

$$FEMg = (UMg \times PCr) / (PMg \times UCr \times 0.7) \times 100$$

In hypomagnesaemia, daily excretion of more than 1 mmol (on 24-hour collection) or a fractional excretion >2% represents renal wasting [23, 36].

Treatment of acute severe hypomagnesaemia is via intravenous magnesium sulphate bolus and/or infusion but also correction of any associated hypocalcaemia and hypokalaemia, both of which are very commonly associated electrolyte abnormalities. More chronic therapy involves treating the underlying cause, where possible, and supplementing with oral magnesium salts such as magnesium glycerophosphate, magnesium oxide and magnesium carbonate although diarrhoea is a common side effect. Lesser maintenance doses are required for patients with CKD, and levels need to be monitored.

13.1.50 Hypermagnesaemia

Hypermagnesaemia is defined as a serum magnesium of greater than 0.9 mmol/l.

It is rare, and signs and symptoms are unusual below a serum level of 1.5–2 mmol/L. As the kidney has huge reserve for excreting magnesium, it is somewhat uncommon outside the setting of CKD.

Noticeably, no symptom is observed for magnesium levels below 2.0 mmol/L, and an increasing number of reports suggest better outcomes in populations (including CKD) with higher magnesium levels, with a benefit for all-cause mortality (and in particular for cardiovascular mortality and sudden death) directly related to Mg levels, as discussed, even above the current upper reference value.

Causes of hypermagnesaemia are shown in Table 13.16 and divided into reduced excretion, excessive intake and release from cell death.

13.1.51 Clinical Features of Hypermagnesaemia

These relate principally to neuro- and cardiotoxicity (bradycardia, prolonged QT, widening of QRS complex) (see Appendix 1). Paraesthesia and hyporeflexia occur as an early feature, as well as flushing nausea and vomiting. In very severe cases, hypotension, hypocalcaemia, paralysis, ileus, urine retention, coma, heart block and ventricular fibrillation may occur.

Perhaps the most important aspect of investigation is the index of suspicion, i.e. checking the magnesium level particularly in patients with CKD and those likely to be chronically consuming high levels of magnesium-containing products. Fractional excretion of magnesium in the face of hypermagnesaemia may indicate whether there is failure of excretion or excessive intake/production. However, in renal impairment, it is likely to be a combination of factors, and it is necessary to get a careful history of prescribed and non-prescribed medication, illicit use of laxatives and exclusion of other secondary causes (see Table 13.20).

13.2 Treatment of Hypermagnesaemia

Treatment consists of removing any oral or IV intake and treating secondary causes, which is usually sufficient if no neurological signs or ECG changes. IV calcium will counteract acute cardiac and neurotoxicity thereafter IV fluids with or without loop diuretics (supplemented calcium and potassium as necessary). Dialysis is highly effective at acutely reducing magnesium and rarely necessary outside significant renal impairment but worth considering for patients with treacherously high levels or CKD.

Table 13.20 Causes of hypermangesaemia

Reduced renal excretion	Renal impairment (acute or chronic)
	Hypothyroidism
	Lithium therapy
	Addison's disease
	Hyperparathyroidism
	Familial hypocalciuric hypercalcaemia
Excessive intake	Antacids, laxatives (including Epsom salts), IV magnesium (e.g. pre-eclampsia, milk-alkali syndrome, magnesium enemas)
Excessive production	Tumour lysis, crush injury, rhabdomyolysis

Conclusions

Good confidence in the management of basic electrolyte disturbances is an essential skill for any physician as these problems are common, associated with considerable morbidity and mortality and predicted to increase in the future. Medical emergencies directly related to the electrolyte disorders or potentially arising from their treatment should be promptly spotted when defining the treatment plan. Identification of precipitating causes (often multiple) and careful monitoring of treatment effects with the right timing allow for a safe clinical management in most cases of electrolyte disorders.

Case Studies

Case 1

A 50-year-old patient underwent cardiac surgery for mitral valve replacement due to severe mitral regurgitation secondary to myocardial infarction. Lab tests showed a substantially normal biochemistry. After an uneventful valve replacement, he was admitted to the post-surgical ITU, where he received IV hydration, opioids and paracetamol for pain. Three days after, the patient was referred to the renal team due to a significantly decreased urinary output (from 2500 to 700 ml/24 h) with dark-orange urine in absence of haematuria or proteinuria on the urine dip. On examination, the patient was neurologically appropriate and showing no features of haemodynamic instability. He looked to be in an overall good clinical condition apart from moderate peripheral oedema but with preserved capillary refill time; the repeated laboratory tests were as follows:

- **FBC:** Hb 13,4 g/dL, WBC 4700/mcL, RBC 5 mln/mcL, HCT 43%, PLT 300000/mcL.
- **Biochemistry**: P-osmolality 275 mOsm/Kg, BUN 10 mg/dL, Na + 124 mEq/L, K+ 3.5 mEq/L, glucose 109 mg/dL, bicarbonates 24 mEq/L.
- **Urine**: U-osmolality 250 mOsm/Kg, Na + 35 mEq/L, SG 1025.

In this case, the patient developed hyponatraemia in the contest of a reduction in the urinary output and with a urine osmolality lower then plasma osmolality (inadequate response to a hypo-osmolar state). The first step in the clinical assessment of hyponatraemia should be the identification of clinical emergencies: is there any new neurological symptom requiring urgent treatment? Second, we should aim to identify the causes of the disorder: in this case hyponatraemia could be a combination of post-operative fluid intake and a clear over-production of ADH, possibly due to chest surgery and pain.

Case 2

A 68-year-old woman presented to A&E complaining of chest tightness and severe fatigue. She was brought in by the ambulance crew on a wheelchair as unable to stand due to leg weakness over the previous few days. The daughter reported also a history of significant weight loss and persistent sickness for which the patient had been unable to eat hardly anything. ECG showed a moderate and wide complex tachycardia. Laboratory tests were still pending; when on a blood gas, the following results were noted: Na + 130 mEq/L, K+ 8.2 mEq/L, creatinine 4 mg/dL, bicarbonate 18 mmol/L and ionised calcium 1.0 mmol/L.

Despite concomitant hyponatraemia, the key element to address is severe hyperkalaemia which would require urgent treatment especially in the context of ECG changes suspected for metabolic toxicity. When seen by the emergency physician, the patient was prescribed with 10 ml of calcium gluconate IV in rapid infusion and with 500 ml of sodium bicarbonate over 4 hours.

ECG changes recovered few seconds after IV calcium administration.

Which is the other relevant question to ask in order to plan any further management of hyperkalaemia? A key element would be to know if the patient is passing urine as this would be the only reliable way to decrease the total body content of potassium apart from renal replacement therapies.

Case 3

A 65-year-old man was admitted to the Emergency Department for fatigue and widespread body pain worsening over the last 4 months. No other symptoms where reported apart from some constipation. There was no significant past medical history. Observations were in the normal range. Lab tests showed as follows: Hb 8.0 g/dL, WCC 2000/ul, Plts 99,000/ul, ESR 47 mm/h, creatinine 2 mg/dL, Na and K in normal range, Ca 16.5 mg/dL, albumin 3.8 g/dL, phosphate 2.2 mg/dL, iPTH 3 pg/mL and 25 (OH)Vit D3 4 nmol/L.

The emergency physician after noticing severe derangement in calcium levels requested for ECG which showed no significant changes. After further discussion with his senior colleague, a blood gas was requested, and this showed a normal ionised calcium. As a result, the senior physician requested for a haematological opinion.

Why was the total calcium so high? The likely explanation is the presence of calcium-binding substances in the bloodstream. In this case it is mandatory to look for paraproteins, and myeloma becomes the main working diagnosis.

Tips and Tricks of Electrolyte Disorders

- Relative urinary electrolyte concentrations are often very helpful in swiftly distinguishing between renal and extra-renal loss of electrolytes.
- Acute electrolyte abnormalities tend to be more dangerous than those that develop over time, and establishing the rate and direction of travel is of critical clinical relevance in determining speed and vigour of correction.
- Establishing close and frequent monitoring of serious electrolyte abnormalities is vital to avoid failure to correct or over-rapid correction; hence patients with significant electrolyte abnormalities need to be in a place of safety.
- Artificial intelligence or just slick IT reporting of results with early intervention by wise and experienced experts is likely to improve patient care, and nephrologists should have a role in developing a safe service.
- Patients with long-term predisposition to electrolyte abnormalities may need MedicAlert bracelets or equivalent as well as clear instructions and streamlined access to medical review if they become unwell.

13

Questions

1. Which are the complications of chronic hyperphosphataemia?
2. What is the therapeutic approach for a patient presenting with severe hypokalaemia and arrhythmias?
3. Which are the main characteristics of the so-called hungry bone syndrome?
4. Which is a major issue with the treatment of hyponatraemia?
5. What is Bartter syndrome?

Answers

1. Chronic hyperphosphataemia can stimulate vascular media calcification, with severe cardiovascular consequences. Moreover, these calcium-phosphate deposits can manifest as conjunctivitis and tenosynovitis.
2. Therapy is based on intravenous potassium chloride, in normal saline or 5% dextrose. Using a peripheral route, rate is up to 10 mmol/h. If a central line is available, rate can be faster, up to 40 mmol/h. Cardiac monitoring and frequent potassium assessments are essential.
3. Hungry bone syndrome includes a series of conditions, such as the rapid, deep and prolonged hypocalcaemia associated with hypophosphataemia and hypomagnesaemia, after parathyroidectomy in patients with severe hyperparathyroidism. It is a relatively uncommon but serious adverse effect of parathyroidectomy. Treatment relies on intravenous calcium supplementation (with following shift to oral calcium), correction of hypomagnesaemia. Vitamin D is also essential after parathyroidectomy, but it can also be administered pre-operatively, together with bisphosphonates.
4. Rapid correction of hyponatraemia can cause a rapid rise in serum osmolality and subsequent osmotic dehydration of neural cells with central pontine myelinolysis. This is a serious condition which manifests with seizure and altered state of consciousness, up to spastic quadriparesis and reduction of respiratory function.

   Suggested correction rates are <8–10 mEq/L in the first 24 hours and <18 mEq/L in the first 48 hours.
5. Bartter syndrome is caused by mutations of a number of transporters necessary for the proper functioning of the sodium potassium chloride co-transporter in the thick ascending limb of the loop of Henle. Disruption of the normal water-reabsorbing function of the loop causes severe salt and water loss with the activation of renin-angiotensin-aldosterone system and thus hyperaldosteronism, resulting in metabolic alkalosis and hypokalaemia.

References

1. Giordano M, Ciarambino T, Castellino P, Malatino L, Di Somma S, Biolo G, Paolisso G, Adinolfi LE. Diseases associated with electrolyte imbalance in the ED: age-related differences. Am J Emerg Med. 2016;34:1923–6.
2. Schlanger LE, Bailey JL, Sands JM. Electrolytes in the aging. Adv Chronic Kidney Dis. 2010;17:308–19.
3. Liamis G, Rodenburg EM, Hofman A, Zietse R, Stricker BH, Hoorn EJ. Electrolyte disorders in community subjects: prevalence and risk factors. Am J Med. 2013;126:256–63.
4. Wang Y, Hu J, Geng X, Zhang X, Xu X, Lin J, Teng J, Ding X. A novel scoring system for assessing the severity of electrolyte and acid-base disorders and predicting outcomes in hospitalized patients. J Investig Med. 2019;67:750–60.
5. Hoorn EJ, Zietse R. Hyponatremia and mortality: how innocent is the bystander?: figure 1. CJASN. 2011;6:951–3.
6. Chawla A, Sterns RH, Nigwekar SU, Cappuccio JD. Mortality and serum sodium: do patients die from or with hyponatremia? Clin J Am Soc Nephrol. 2011;6:960–5.
7. Hawkins RC. Age and gender as risk factors for hyponatremia and hypernatremia. Clin Chim Acta. 2003;337:169–72.
8. Upadhyay A, Jaber BL, Madias NE. Epidemiology of hyponatremia. Semin Nephrol. 2009;29:227–38.
9. Decaux G. Is asymptomatic hyponatremia really asymptomatic? Am J Med. 2006;119:S79–82.
10. Schrier RW. Does "asymptomatic hyponatremia" exist? Nat Rev Nephrol. 2010;6:185.
11. Sterns RH, Cappuccio JD, Silver SM, Cohen EP. Neurologic sequelae after treatment of severe hyponatremia: a multicenter perspective. J Am Soc Nephrol. 1994;4:1522–30.

12. Lehrich RW, Ortiz-Melo DI, Patel MB, Greenberg A. Role of Vaptans in the Management of Hyponatremia. Am J Kidney Dis. 2013;62:364–76.
13. Waikar SS, Mount DB, Curhan GC. Mortality after hospitalization with mild, moderate, and severe hyponatremia. Am J Med. 2009;122:857–65.
14. Miller M. Recognition of partial defects in antidiuretic hormone secretion. Ann Intern Med. 1970;73:721.
15. Zerbe RL, Robertson GL. A comparison of plasma vasopressin measurements with a standard indirect test in the differential diagnosis of polyuria. N Engl J Med. 1981;305:1539–46.
16. Rose BD, Post TW (2001) Clinical physiology of acid-base and electrolyte disorders, 5th ed. McGraw-hill, medical pub. Division, New York.
17. Moses AM, Clayton B. Impairment of osmotically stimulated AVP release in patients with primary polydipsia. Am J Phys Regul Integr Comp Phys. 1993;265:R1247–52.
18. Chauhan K, Pattharanitima P, Patel N, et al. Rate of correction of hypernatremia and health outcomes in critically ill patients. Clin J Am Soc Nephrol. 2019;14:656–63.
19. Unwin RJ, Luft FC, Shirley DG. Pathophysiology and management of hypokalemia: a clinical perspective. Nat Rev Nephrol. 2011;7:75–84.
20. Schurman SJ, Scheinman SJ. Inherited cerebrorenal syndromes. Nat Rev Nephrol. 2009;5:529–38.
21. Mattu A. How do you avoid a clean kill with wide complex tachycardias? Essentials of Emergency Medicine. 2017;2017. https://youtu.be/UXh8PS9dtmoo
22. West ML, Marsden PA, Richardson RM, Zettle RM, Halperin ML. New clinical approach to evaluate disorders of potassium excretion. Miner Electrolyte Metab. 1986;12:234–8.
23. Dépret F, Peacock WF, Liu KD, Rafique Z, Rossignol P, Legrand M. Management of hyperkalemia in the acutely ill patient. Ann Intensive Care. 2019;9:32.
24. Noel JA, Bota SE, Petrcich W, Garg AX, Carrero JJ, Harel Z, Tangri N, Clark EG, Komenda P, Sood MM. Risk of hospitalization for serious adverse gastrointestinal events associated with sodium polystyrene sulfonate use in patients of advanced age. JAMA Intern Med. 2019;179:1025.
25. Meaney CJ, Beccari MV, Yang Y, Zhao J. Systematic review and meta-analysis of Patiromer and sodium zirconium Cyclosilicate: a new armamentarium for the treatment of Hyperkalemia. Pharmacotherapy. 2017;37:401–11.
26. Bianchi S, Aucella F, De Nicola L, Genovesi S, Paoletti E, Regolisti G. Management of hyperkalemia in patients with kidney disease: a position paper endorsed by the Italian Society of Nephrology. J Nephrol. 2019;32:499–516.
27. Carmeliet G, Cromphaut SV, Daci E, Maes C, Bouillon R. Disorders of calcium homeostasis. Best Pract Res Clin Endocrinol Metab. 2003;17:529–46.
28. Witteveen JE, van Thiel S, Romijn JA, Hamdy NAT. THERAPY OF ENDOCRINE DISEASE: hungry bone syndrome: still a challenge in the post-operative management of primary hyperparathyroidism: a systematic review of the literature. Eur J Endocrinol. 2013;168:R45–53.
29. Covic A, Vervloet M, Massy ZA, et al. Bone and mineral disorders in chronic kidney disease: implications for cardiovascular health and ageing in the general population. Lancet Diab Endocrinol. 2018;6:319–31.
30. Mazzaferro S, Cianciolo G, De Pascalis A, Guglielmo C, Urena Torres PA, Bover J, Tartaglione L, Pasquali M, La Manna G. Bone, inflammation and the bone marrow niche in chronic kidney disease: what do we know? Nephrol Dial Transplant. 2018;33:2092–100.
31. Mazzaferro S, Bagordo D, De Martini N, Pasquali M, Rotondi S, Tartaglione L, Stenvinkel P; ERA-EDTA CKDMBD working group. Inflammation, oxidative stress, and bone in chronic kidney disease in the osteoimmunology era. Calcif Tissue Int. 2021;108(4):452–60.
32. Imel EA, Econs MJ. Approach to the Hypophosphatemic patient. J Clin Endocrinol Metabol. 2012;97:696–706.
33. Felsenfeld AJ, Levine BS. Approach to treatment of hypophosphatemia. Am J Kidney Dis. 2012;60:655–61.
34. Leenders NHJ, Vervloet MG. Magnesium: a magic bullet for cardiovascular disease in chronic kidney disease? Nutrients. 2019; https://doi.org/10.3390/nu11020455.
35. Costello RB, Elin RJ, Rosanoff A, et al. Perspective: the case for an evidence-based reference interval for serum magnesium: the time has come. Adv Nutr. 2016;7:977–93.
36. Agus ZS. Hypomagnesemia. J Am Soc Nephrol. 1999;10:1616–22.

Acid-Base Disorders

Elizabeth R. Wan and Stephen B. Walsh

Contents

M. Harber (ed.), *Primer on Nephrology*, https://doi.org/10.1007/978-3-030-76419-7_14

Learning Objectives

This chapter aims to teach:

1. An understanding of the physiological principles of acid-base homeostasis
2. An approach that is clinically useful to approaching a patient with a disorder of acid-base balance
3. An understanding of the principles of treating patients with disturbances of acid-base physiology

14.1 Introduction

Disorders of acid base homeostasis and their treatment are often a source of confusion in clinical practice; this is not helped by the varied nomenclature, the different ways of measuring and classifying acid base disorders and the rationale for treating them.

This chapter outlines the methods of classifying and diagnosing different acid base disorders and their treatment. Included at the end is a section detailing the management of some individual disorders that merit special consideration.

14.2 Determination of Respiratory/ Metabolic Acidosis/Alkalosis

The Henderson-Hasselbalch equation (Fig. 14.1) dictates that the blood pH is determined by the ratio of the serum bicarbonate and the $_{P}CO_2$. If either of these values are lowered or raised, then the blood pH will be altered; if the pH is altered by the serum bicarbonate concentration, the process is a *metabolic* acidosis or alkalosis; if the $_{P}CO_2$ change alters the pH, then it is a *respiratory* acidosis or alkalosis (see Side Bar).

14.3 Compensation (Respiratory/ Metabolic)

As the pH is affected by both bicarbonate and $_{P}CO_2$, a simple alteration in one of these variables is usually *compensated* by a change in the other in order to mitigate the effect on the blood pH.

When a metabolic disorder causes the bicarbonate to fall (metabolic acidosis) or rise (metabolic alkalosis), there is a compensatory respiratory response to change the $_{P}CO_2$ in the same direction as the bicarbonate (i.e. to maintain the bicarbonate/ $_{P}CO_2$ ratio) and thus to minimise the effect on the blood pH. This is achieved by increasing or decreasing the respiratory rate and is therefore a rapid compensation, starting as soon as 30 minutes after the serum bicarbonate falls.

$$pH = 6.1 + \log([HCO_3^-]/(0.03 \times pCO_2))$$

Fig. 14.1 The modified Henderson-Hasselbalch equation

On the other hand, when a respiratory disorder causes the $_{P}CO_2$ to rise (respiratory acidosis) or fall (respiratory alkalosis), there is a similar compensatory rise or fall in the serum bicarbonate. This is achieved by either an increase or decrease in the rate of acid secretion by the renal tubule (which generates bicarbonate for the circulation). This is a much slower response than respiratory compensation, taking 3–5 days to complete; this means that the degree of compensation can be taken as a guide to the chronicity of the respiratory disorder; acute disorders will have little or no metabolic compensation; chronic ones will have full metabolic compensation.

It is important to note that in simple acid base disorders, compensatory respiratory or metabolic responses do not return the blood pH to normal, with the possible exception of mild chronic respiratory acidosis or alkalosis, which may be fully compensated, to give a low normal or high normal blood pH, respectively. Thus, a normal blood pH in the presence of significantly altered serum bicarbonate and $_{P}CO_2$ may well indicate a *mixed* acid-base disorder.

14.4 Respiratory Acid-Base Disorders

These are caused by ventilatory disturbances, which alter the $_{P}CO_2$ and thus the blood pH.

14.5 Respiratory Acidosis

As stated before, respiratory acidosis can be divided into acute and chronic by the degree of metabolic compensation that accompanies them.

Acute respiratory acidosis will have little or no metabolic compensation and will occur when an abrupt interruption in ventilation occurs; this can be either due to decreased central nervous stimulation (e.g. sedative drugs), neuromuscular failure of ventilatory effort (e.g. myasthenia crisis, Guillain-Barré, flail chest) or acute airway obstruction (e.g. acute asthma, inhaled foreign object) (see ► Box 14.1).

Chronic respiratory acidosis will have a much more pronounced metabolic compensation, in some cases, enough to normalise the blood pH. Conditions which cause it are more likely to be long-standing and ongoing, in the same categories as above: central nervous (e.g.

14

cerebral disease), neuromuscular (e.g. amyotrophic lateral sclerosis, muscular dystrophy), structural/mechanical (e.g. severe obesity, thoracic deformities) and chronic airway obstruction (e.g. chronic obstructive pulmonary disease) (see ▶ Box 14.1).

Box 14.1 Causes of Respiratory Acid-Base Disturbances

- Acute respiratory acidosis
  - Decreased CNS stimulation
    - Sedative drugs
  - Neuromuscular ventilatory failure
    - Guillain-Barre
    - Myasthenic crisis
  - Structural/mechanical ventilatory failure
    - Flail chest
    - Tension pneumothorax
  - Airway obstruction
    - Acute asthma
    - Inhaled foreign object
- Chronic respiratory acidosis
  - Decreased CNS stimulation
    - Cerebral disease
  - Neuromuscular ventilatory failure
    - Amyotrophic lateral sclerosis
    - Muscular dystrophy
  - Structural/mechanical ventilatory failure
    - Severe obesity
    - Thoracic deformities
  - Chronic airway obstruction
    - Tracheal stenosis
    - Chronic obstructive pulmonary disease
- Acute respiratory alkalosis
  - Increased CNS stimulation
    - Anxiety/psychiatric causes
    - Drugs (e.g. aspirin)
    - Subarachnoid haemorrhage
  - Increased ventilation
    - Mechanical overventilation of an intubated patient
- Chronic respiratory alkalosis
  - Increased CNS stimulation
    - Stroke
    - Increased hypoxic drive (e.g. high altitude)

14.6 Respiratory Alkalosis

This will be caused by hyperventilation and the resultant excessive fall in the $_{P}CO_2$.

Acute respiratory alkalosis will have little or no metabolic compensation and can be due to central nervous stimulation of ventilation (e.g. psychiatric/anxiety, drugs, subarachnoid haemorrhage) or mechanical over-ventilation (e.g. over-ventilating an intubated patient).

Chronic respiratory alkalosis will be more fully compensated metabolically and may be due to central nervous system disease (e.g. stroke) or increased hypoxic drive (e.g. high altitude, conditions with decreased alveolar gas exchange) (see ▶ Box 14.1).

14.7 Metabolic Acidosis

Metabolic acidosis can be caused by one of three main mechanisms: increased acid production, increased bicarbonate loss and decreased renal excretion of acid (see ▶ Box 14.2).

Increased acid production/ingestion:

1. Lactic acidosis (e.g. hypoperfusion, metformin, alcohol, malignancy)
2. Ketoacidosis (e.g. diabetic ketoacidosis, alcohol, fasting)
3. Ingested acid (e.g. Salicylate poisoning, ethylene glycol ingestion, toluene)

Increased Bicarbonate Losses

1. Bicarbonate loss through diarrhoea or ureteric diversion, or any other cause of loss of pancreatic, biliary or intestinal secretions
2. Renal bicarbonate loss in the proximal tubule in proximal renal tubular acidosis

Decreased Renal Acid Excretion

1. A specific failure of acid secretion in the distal renal tubule (distal renal tubular acidosis)
2. Reduced acid excretion in generalised renal failure

Box 14.2 Causes of Metabolic Acidosis

- Increased acid production/ingestion
  - Lactic acidosis
    - Hypoperfusion (secondary to any cause, e.g. hypovolaemia, cardiac failure, sepsis)
    - Alcohol
    - Malignancy
    - Metformin
    - Nucleoside reverse transcriptase inhibitors (e.g. stavudine, didanosine)
  - Ketoacidosis
    - Diabetic ketoacidosis
    - Alcohol
    - Fasting
  - Ingested acid
    - Methanol

- Ethylene glycol
- Salicylate
- Toluene
- Increased bicarbonate losses
  - GI loss
    - Diarrhoea
    - Ureteric diversion
  - Renal loss
    - Proximal renal tubular acidosis
- Decreased renal acid excretion
  - Acute or chronic renal failure
  - Distal renal tubular acidosis

14.8 Anion Gap (with Albumin Correction)

The cause of a metabolic acidosis can be difficult to determine, so it may be helpful to see if there are any unusual and therefore unmeasured ions that might be contributing to the acidosis. This is the reason for calculating the *anion gap.*

The anion gap is the difference between the amount of measured cations and measured anions.

The main measured cations are sodium and potassium; the main measured anions are chloride and bicarbonate.

The standard anion gap is usually (Na + K) – (Cl + HCO_3).

As the potassium concentration is small, it is often omitted from the equation.

The normal anion gap depends to a certain extent on the reference ranges in the local laboratory but is usually in the range of 7–13 mmol/L, or on average 4 mmol/L lower (3–9 mmol/L) if potassium is not used in the calculation.

The anion gap is helpful because it will be increased if there is a fall in unmeasured cations (such as calcium or magnesium), or, much more importantly and more markedly, an increase in unmeasured anions, such as ketones (beta-hydroxybutyrate in diabetic ketoacidosis), lactate (in lactic acidosis) and ingestion of exogenous acids (e.g. ethylene glycol, methanol or salicylate).

The largest part of the normal anion gap is due to albumin, which is an unmeasured anion. Therefore, hypoalbuminaemia will decrease the anion gap (by approximately 1 mmol/L for every 4 mmol/L drop in albumin); this is a potential cause for confusion, especially in critically ill patients who tend to have low albumin concentrations.

There is a correction factor that should therefore be used in hypoalbuminaemic patients:

$$\text{Anion gap} = (\text{Na} + \text{K}) - (\text{Cl} + \text{HCO}_3) + (0.25 \times (\text{normal albumin} - \text{observed albumin}))$$

14

The causes of a high anion gap metabolic acidosis are summarised in ▶ Box 14.3. An anion gap of 25 mmol/L or over is strongly suggestive of one of these disorders.

The main causes are:

1. Lactic acidosis with increased lactate in shock, sepsis or malignancy.
2. Diabetic ketoacidosis with increased beta-hydroxybuyrate.
3. Ingestion of acids:
   1. Methanol with formate as the principal unmeasured anion
   2. Ethylene glycol with glycolate and oxalate comprising the unmeasured anions
   3. Aspirin with ketones and lactate as the unmeasured anions

And less commonly:

4. Renal failure, which may cause a normal or increased anion gap acidosis, the latter through the retention of sulphate, phosphate and urate.
5. Much more rarely, some inherited and acquired metabolic conditions may cause a high anion gap acidosis (see ▶ Box 14.3).

Box 14.3 Causes of a High Anion Gap Acidosis

- Lactic acidosis
- Ketoacidosis
  - Diabetic ketoacidosis
  - Alcoholic ketoacidosis
  - Starvation ketoacidosis
- Ingestion of acid
  - Ethylene glycol (also propylene glycol and diethylene glycol)
  - Salicylate
  - Methanol
- Renal failure
- Toxins
  - Iron
  - Isoniazid

- Toluene
- Inherited causes
  - Glutathione synthetase deficiency
- Other acquired causes
  - Pyroglutamic acid accumulation (rarely with glutathione depletion following paracetamol ingestion)

14.9 Base Excess

Base excess is probably familiar to most from blood gas measurements and is a different way of classifying acid-base disorders. The concept of base excess was to introduce a measure of the metabolic component of an acid-base disturbance that is independent of the respiratory component, replacing [HCO_3^-]. BE actually represents the amount of acid or alkali that must be added to 1 l of blood (at a pCO_2 of 40 mmHg) to achieve a pH of 7.4. If the blood is alkalotic, acid is required, and the BE is positive (there is a 'base excess'); if the blood is acidotic, then alkali is required, and the BE is negative (there is a base deficit). Most blood gas analysers compute standardised BE using pH, pCO_2 and haemoglobin.

Thus, metabolic disorders are defined by changes in the BE and respiratory disorders by changes in pCO_2. The base excess approach is therefore complemented by calculation of the anion gap.

Pros BE measures the contribution of all extracellular buffers to a metabolic acidosis or alkalosis; it is simple, and a blood gas analyser is able to measure all three relevant variables.

Cons the unreliability of the standardisation equation in oedematous patients [1] and the fact that it is only independent from acute changes in the pCO_2; chronic changes in pCO_2 provoke compensatory changes in renal acidification, altering the BE [2].

14.10 Stewart Hypothesis/Physiochemical Approach

In 1983, a chemist called Peter Stewart formulated a different model of acid-base disorders known as the 'physiochemical approach' or more recently as the 'Stewart hypothesis'.

He proposed that the [H^+] (and thus the pH) of living organisms is governed by the changes in the dissociation of water induced by the presence of 'strong ions' (ions that are fully dissociated at physiologic pH), as well as the pCO_2 and the presence of non-volatile weak acids.

This approach uses three primary variables, the strong ion difference (*SID*), the total concentration of weak acids (**A_{tot}** which includes proteins and phosphate) and the **pCO_2**.

The SID is the sum of the strong cations (Na^+, K^+, Ca^{2+} and Mg^{2+}) minus the sum of the strong anions (Cl^-, SO_4^- and anions of organic acids). Because they are present in the largest amount, this means that Na^+ and Cl^- are the main determinants of SID.

To be used clinically, one must measure the blood pH and pCO_2 and determine the A_{tot} and two formulations of the SID. The subtraction of strong anions from strong cations yields the apparent SID (**SID_a**); the second formulation of SID, the effective SID (**SID_e**), represents the fact that the SID must be balanced electrically by the sum of the concentrations of the other measured anions (HCO_3^-, PO_4^- and albumin). Thus, under normal conditions, the sum of these anions should equal the SID_a. Thus, the SID_e = [HCO_3^-] + [PO_4^-] + [albumin] and is usually estimated from the blood pH, pCO_2 and the plasma concentrations of albumin and phosphate using a nomogram.

If there is a discrepancy between the SID_a and SID_e, then there must be an excess of an unmeasured ion. The SID_a minus the SID_e is called the strong ion gap (**SIG**) and is used as an estimate of unmeasured anions in the same way as the anion gap.

The Stewart approach therefore defines six acid-base disorders based on disturbances on its three main variables. Abnormal SIDe or A_{tot} indicate the presence of metabolic acid-base disorders; a low SIDe indicates a metabolic acidosis, and a high SIDe indicates a metabolic alkalosis. A high A_{tot} indicates metabolic acidosis (hyperalbuminaemic acidosis) and a low A_{tot} a metabolic alkalosis (hypoalbuminaemic alkalosis). Increases and decreases in pCO_2 indicate a respiratory acidosis and alkalosis, respectively, as expected.

Pros Some data suggest that SIG predicts the risk of death in critically ill patients better than the anion gap, base excess or serum lactate [3, 4]; however, most studies have not identified any diagnostic or prognostic advantage of the Stewart approach over other approaches in these patients [5, 6].

Cons The Stewart approach needs additional measurements of multiple ions and the use of specialised software, increasing the potential for error. Also, the interpretation of SID is tricky as SIDa and SIDe have different connotations; and despite the central contention in the Stewart approach that HCO_3^- is irrelevant, it is one of the main components of SIDe.

Also, the classification of metabolic acid-base disorders is overly complex (e.g. metabolic acidosis can be associated with normal SIDa, low SIDa, normal SIG, high SIG or high A_{tot}).

Whilst the classical and base excess methodologies keep a clear distinction between diagnosis and cause, the Stewart approach tries to do both at once which can be misleading; the concept of A_{tot} acidosis and alkalosis is largely groundless [7]; in vivo, there is no evidence that changes in serum albumin correlate with changes in pCO_2 or pH [8]. The assertion that SID and A_{tot} mechanistically determine $[HCO_3^-]$ is based on mathematics, not biology and as such does not satisfactorily establish cause and effect, and experimental evidence for just such cause and effect is lacking [8].

14.11 Treatment of Metabolic Acidosis

The general principles of treating metabolic acidosis is the treatment of the underlying disorder and the restoration of the normal extracellular pH.

In the acute setting, the extracellular pH can be normalised with alkali therapy, usually sodium bicarbonate; with an aim to increase the serum pH to greater than 7.2, the point at which the serious and acute consequences of acidosis should not occur.

However, this guideline does not apply in all cases, especially where the anion will be metabolised to bicarbonate during recovery (see special cases, lactic acidosis and ketoacidosis, below).

14

In adequately ventilated patients with acute severe acidaemia, an appropriate replacement regime would be 1–2 mmol/kg sodium bicarbonate as an intravenous bolus with a repeat dose after 30–60 minutes if the pH is still less than 7.1.

In chronic acidosis, oral alkali treatment, usually with sodium bicarbonate, is given with the aim of raising the serum bicarbonate to 22–24 mmol/L with the aim of bone protection and often volume expansion.

In the setting of metabolic acidosis, a major site for the buffering of the excess hydrogen ions is in the intracellular compartment. This will tend to cause an efflux of potassium in order to maintain electroneutrality. The plasma potassium concentration will rise by an average of 0.6 mmol/L for every reduction in pH of 0.1. However, this average is of a wide range (0.2–1.7 mmol/L) [9], so the response of the plasma potassium cannot be reliably predicted, and therefore calculation is no substitute for vigilant monitoring.

As calcium binds with albumin in competition with hydrogen ions, pH changes can alter the amount of ionised calcium ions. The amount of ionised calcium present will increase in a variable manner as the serum pH falls; in metabolic acid base disturbances, the increment may be as great as 0.83 mmol/L ionised calcium per 0.03 pH [10].

14.12 Metabolic Alkalosis

Metabolic alkalosis can be caused by loss of bicarbonate, either from the GI tract or renally, by inappropriate secretion of renal acid or by ingestion of exogenous base.

14.12.1 GI Acid Loss

The stomach secretes HCl and to a lesser extent, KCl. Production of HCl in the stomach does not cause alkalosis as it is matched by bicarbonate secretion by the pancreas, which is stimulated by acid reaching the duodenum [11]. This stimulus is missing in the case of vomiting or NG tube drainage, and so alkalosis can occur. Urinary chloride conservation will occur in this setting, and so the urinary chloride concentration will be very low (<25 mmol/L); this can be an important clue if the vomiting is surreptitious.

14.12.2 Renal Acid Loss

Inappropriate renal acid secretion sufficient to cause a metabolic acidosis requires aldosterone excess and/or increased sodium and chloride delivery to the cortical collecting duct. Aldosterone increases the amount of ENaC present in the collecting duct increasing the absorption of sodium as well as the activity of the acid secreting $vH^+ATPase$. Rapid absorption of sodium and the slow absorption of chloride generate lumen electronegativity, increasing the amount of H^+ (and K^+) secreted.

14.12.3 Mineralocorticoid Excess

Therefore, any primary cause of mineralocorticoid excess will tend to lead to a metabolic alkalosis, usually with hypertension.

14.12.4 Increased Sodium Delivery

Diuretic use, surreptitious or otherwise will lead to metabolic alkalosis. These patients will tend to be volume contracted and thus also have a high aldosterone concentration. Urinary chloride concentration will be high during the duration of action of the drug and thereafter will be very low as the kidney appropriately retains chloride.

A similar picture will occur with either Bartter or Gitelman syndromes, which are caused by genetic inactivation of the loop of Henle sodium potassium and chloride cotransporter (**NKCC2**) and the distal convoluted tubule sodium and chloride cotransporter (**NCC**), respectively. NKCC2 is the target of loop diuretics, and NCC is the target of thiazide diuretics, which is the reason that loop diuretics cause the same biochemical picture as Bartter and thiazides mimic Gitelman.

14.12.5 Exogenous Base

Metabolic alkalosis may occur with the ingestion of large amounts of bicarbonate (or any anion that is metabolised to HCO_3^-, e.g. acetate or citrate).

Thus, alkalosis can occur after ingestion of large amounts of bicarbonate or citrate and large blood transfusions (when anticoagulated with acid citrate dextran), after FFP administration after plasmapheresis or with crack cocaine (which is mainly comprised of alkaline 'free base').

14.12.6 Contraction Alkalosis

The term contraction alkalosis is still used occasionally and therefore deserves some explanation; it theoretically occurs after the loss of relatively large volumes of bicarbonate free fluid, which raises the plasma bicarbonate concentration as there is contraction of the extracellular fluid whilst the quantity of extracellular bicarbonate in solution remains constant.

Examples include rapid fluid removal with diuretics in oedematous patients, sweat losses in patients with cystic fibrosis and congenital chloride diarrhoea.

The difficulty with this concept is that other mechanisms to account for the alkalosis can be invoked in all of these cases, increased sodium delivery to the CCD with diuretics, increased aldosterone concentrations in volume contraction with cystic fibrosis and chloride depletion in congenital chloride diarrhoea (bicarbonate excretion depends on chloride reabsorbtion in the CCD).

14.13 Treatment of Metabolic Alkalosis

Metabolic alkalosis is surprisingly common and well tolerated, however as a persistent alkalosis will promote hypokalaemia, which may be problematic in the acutely unwell, and will also depress the respiratory drive, which is challenging for those with pulmonary disease.

The treatment of a metabolic alkalosis will aim for three goals:

- *Correction of chloride loss*. Chloride is exchanged for bicarbonate in the distal tubule and is required for bicarbonate secretion. Increasing chloride delivery to the distal tubule will therefore facilitate the renal elimination of bicarbonate.
- *Correction of hypovolaemia*. This will remove the stimulus for sodium conservation that causes more bicarbonate to be resorbed in the proximal tubule. Therefore, volume replacement with *intravenous sodium chloride* is very effective.
- *Correction of hypokalaemia*. Potassium will displace intracellular hydrogen ions which move into the extracellular space in order to maintain electroneutrality. These hydrogen ions will then buffer excess bicarbonate, ameliorating the alkalaemia.

In oedematous patients, it may not be safe to give IV sodium chloride, in which case, *potassium chloride* may be helpful if the patient is hypokalaemic. Alternatively, renal bicarbonate wasting can be facilitated by giving *acetazolamide*, which will also act as a weak diuretic. Finally, in critically ill patients who prove resistant to acetazolamide, *intravenous hydrochloric acid* can be used via a central vein. This requires very careful monitoring, and should not be attempted without senior and experienced supervision.

14.14 Special Cases

- ***Renal Tubular Acidosis***

  Chronic Metabolic Acidosis AG/N

  Distal renal tubular acidosis (*dRTA* or type 1 RTA) is caused by failure of the acid secreting alpha intercalated cell of the CCD to secrete acid. This failure is most often caused by autoimmune disease (typically *Sjögren syndrome*, but also SLE, RA or hypergammaglobulinaemia from any cause) or genetic disease (mutations of the basolateral anion exchanger 1 (*AE1*), carbonic anhydrase 2 (*CA2*) or the apical proton pump (inactivating mutation of the *A4 or B1 subunit of vH⁺ATPase*, the forkhead trranscription factor FOXI1 and the WD repeat-containing protein WDR72). Genetic dRTA is rare, with the possible exception of dRTA causing AE1 mutations in Southeast Asia, where they are somewhat more common [12]. Acquired causes are a little more common, the commonest being Sjögren syndrome: dRTA is reported in up to 25% of Sjögren series [13].

This failure to secrete acid into the urine results in an *alkaline urine* despite a possible *metabolic acidosis*, *osteomalacia/low bone mineral density* from chronic acidosis, (which may cause growth retardation and rickets in children), *hypercalciuria*, *nephrocalcinosis* and *kidney stone* formation (calcium phosphate stones, as $CaPO_4$ precipitates at an alkaline pH) and renal potassium losses leading to *hypokalaemia*. The severity of the clinical features varies greatly, even in the same families with hereditary disease. Patients can be asymptomatic and have problems with recurrent kidney stones, through to life-threatening hypokalaemia or end-stage renal disease from nephrocalcinosis. (*See* ◘ Fig. 14.2)

An alkaline urine pH (>5.3) in the presence of a metabolic acidosis is diagnostic of dRTA; however, the acidification defect may not be enough to provoke a systemic acidosis (termed *incomplete dRTA*); in this case, a urinary acidification test can be used to make the diagnosis, either by testing urinary acidification in response to a furosemide and fludrocortisone challenge [14] or to ammonium chloride [15], which directly provokes systemic acidaemia.

Correction of the acidaemia will correct the growth retardation seen in children and protect bone from osteopenia; it will diminish the stone formation/nephrocalcinosis risk and also reduce urinary potassium wasting. This may be achieved with oral sodium bicarbonate (typically 1–3 g/day in divided doses). If hypokalaemia is a problem, oral potassium citrate (9 g/day as solution in divided doses) may be used.

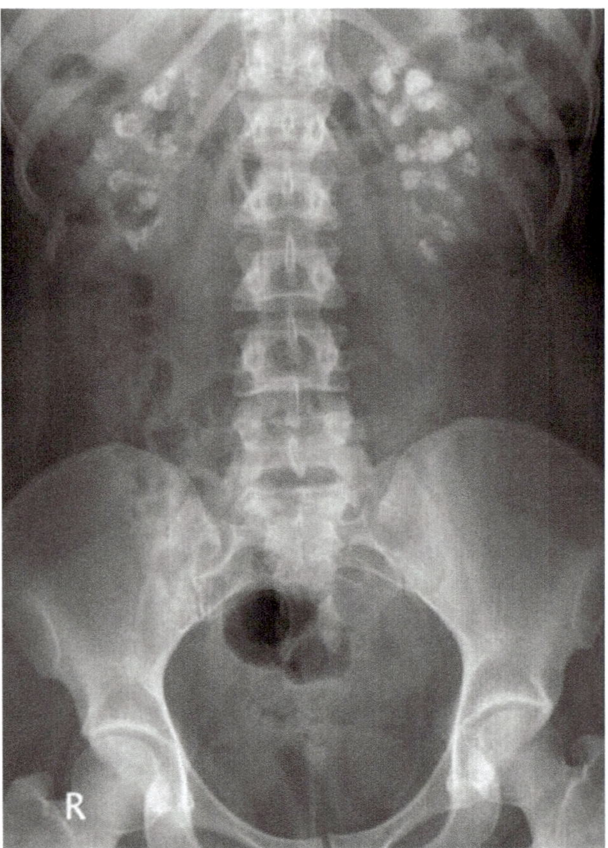

◘ **Fig. 14.2** Nephrocalcinosis on plain abdominal radiograph

Proximal renal tubular acidosis (*pRTA* or type 2 RTA) is caused by a failure of bicarbonate reabsorption in the proximal tubular cell. It is usually accompanied by generalised transport failure of that cell; the resulting *glycosuria, phosphaturia, uricosuria, aminoaciduria and tubular proteinuria* are known as the *renal Fanconi syndrome*. It is usually caused by proximal tubular *toxicity* (e.g. tenofovir, lead), myeloma or Wilson disease (see ► Box 14.4). Two hereditary forms have been described. Although the acidosis is usually milder than in dRTA due to the acidaemia being self-limiting (due to bicarbonate being absorbed in the loop of Henle and collecting duct when the serum concentration falls below approximately 14 mmol/L), administration of oral bicarbonate provokes an immediate bicarbonate diuresis, so that the amount of oral bicarbonate required to stay ahead of the increased urinary losses is typically much higher than that needed in dRTA and may be as high as 10–15 g bicarbonate a day. This also enhances urinary potassium losses, so increased potassium supplementation may be needed when commencing bicarbonate replacement, replacing up to half of the alkali as potassium citrate is a good strategy. Serum bicarbonate and potassium concentrations must be monitored and doses titrated to achieve target levels.

Box 14.4 Causes of pRTA with Fanconi Syndrome

- Hereditary causes:
  - Wilson disease
  - Lowe syndrome
  - Cystinosis
  - Tyrosinaemia
  - Galactosaemia
  - Von Gierke disease (glycogen storage type 1)
  - Hereditary fructose intolerance
  - Carbonic anhydrase 2 mutations
- Acquired causes:
  - Myeloma
  - Drugs (tenofovir, ifosfamide and carbonic anhydrase inhibitors, e.g. acetazolamide and topiramate)
  - Heavy metals (lead, cadmium, mercury, copper)
  - Paroxysmal nocturnal haemoglobinuria

- ***Ureteric Diversion***

  Chronic/acute metabolic acidosis AG/N

  Ureters may be implanted into the sigmoid colon (ureteric diversion) or a short section of ileum that opens onto the anterior abdominal wall (uretoileostomy), or a section of colonic tissue may be used to augment a dysplastic bladder (clam cystoplasty).

  A normal anion gap acidosis is frequent in these situations [16] and is due to two factors. Firstly and most importantly, the chloride bicarbonate cotransporter anion exchanger 2 (AE2) is present on colonic and ileal epithelium. Urinary chloride in contact with this epithelium will be absorbed via AE2, and bicarbonate will therefore be excreted into the urine, causing bicarbonaturia in proportion to the amount of chloride presented in the urine. Therefore, intravenous sodium chloride will make this acidosis worse by increasing the concentration of urinary chloride. Secondly, the gut epithelium can absorb ammonium, both that already present in the urine and that formed by urea splitting microorganisms resident in the epithelium. Ammonium is converted to ammonia by the liver, and this may cause hyperammonaemic encephalopathy if there is liver disease or urosepsis with a urea splitting bacteria. This is an important differential diagnosis in a patient with a ureteric diversion or augmented bladder presenting with an acute confusional state. Such a presentation should prompt a measurement of the serum ammonia concentration. Metabolic acidosis is much less likely with uretoileostomy, due to the short exposure the urine has to gut epithelium. The development of metabolic acidosis in these patients usually occurs when there is an anastomotic stenosis, causing increased exposure of the gut epithelium to the urine [17]. This should prompt a loopogram and surgical opinion, if appropriate.
- ***Ketoacidosis***

  Acute Metabolic Acidosis AG: High

  Diagnosis of ketoacidosis depends on detection of ketonuria (usually via urine dipsticks) or ketonaemia (via a serum beta-hydroxybutryate assay, if available), in the presence of a high anion gap metabolic acidosis.

  In ketoacidosis of any cause, bicarbonate is replaced by an inorganic anion, mainly beta-hydroxybutyric acid. This is a physiologically important anion and will be mainly metabolised to bicarbonate eventually. Therefore, there is no imperative to remove the anion, and the underlying disorder should be treated, and the ketoacidosis will resolve as normal physiology reasserts itself.

  In diabetic ketoacidosis, this means that fluid replacement, insulin therapy and correction of electrolyte abnormalities (importantly hypokalaemia) take precedence over correction of the acidosis.

  Evidence for benefit for bicarbonate replacement in DKA is lacking [18, 19]; however, no randomised trials have been performed on DKA patients with severe acidosis (pH < 6.9). There are concerns about using bicarbonate therapy in DKA:

  – There is some evidence that giving bicarbonate may delay the recovery from the ketosis; this was suggested by one very small study of seven patients in which bicarbonate administration delayed recovery from ketosis by 6 hours [20], although this was not the case in a randomised study of bicarbonate treatment in DKA with less severe acidosis [19].

  Insulin treatment will cause the ketoacids to eventually be metabolised to bicarbonate, and thus bicarbonate administration during treatment may lead to eventual metabolic alkalosis.

  However, there are potential benefits for bicarbonate therapy in DKA:

  Patients have impaired cardiac contractility and vasodilatation with a serum pH of less than 7.0; therefore, alkali therapy in this cohort may improve tissue perfusion; this effect is unlikely to be significant above a pH of 7, as insulin therapy will rapidly improve pH in any case.

  If the serum potassium is dangerously high, then intravenous bicarbonate will act to shunt some of the extracellular potassium intracellularly, lowering the serum potassium concentration.

  The ketoacidosis seen in alcoholic patients can be severe, whilst that seen in fasting patients rarely is (bicarbonate levels rarely fall below 14 mmol/L).

  This reflects the additional burden of pathophysiology present in the alcoholic ketoacidotic patient; a lack of carbohydrates reduces insulin secretion and raises glucagon, whilst alcohol inhibits liver gluconeogenesis and stimulates lipolysis contributing to increased ketoacid formation. Ethanol metabolism to acetaldehyde and then acetic acid will also contribute to the acidosis.

  It may be difficult in the alcoholic patient with a high anion gap metabolic acidosis to distinguish between alcoholic ketoacidosis, diabetic ketoacidosis and methanol or ethylene glycol poisoning. It is therefore essential to take a careful history, demonstrate ketoacidosis, perform urinalysis (for oxalate crystals) and measure serum levels of possible toxins, if the assays are available.

  In fasting and alcoholic ketoacidosis, as in DKA, correction of the underlying metabolic defect will lead to metabolism of the ketoacids and resolution of the acidosis. In both cases, this is achieved by infusion of dextrose to increase insulin and decrease glucagon secretion and saline to volume expand the patient. In alcoholics, it is important to give intravenous (or intramuscular) thiamine before IV dextrose to prevent precipitating Wernicke encephalopathy or Korsakoff psychosis.

- ***Lactic Acidosis***

  Acute Metabolic Acidosis AG: High

  Like ketoacidosis, in lactic acidosis, the lactate replaces bicarbonate. Once the stimulus for lactic acid production is removed, lactate is metabolised to bicarbonate, ending the acidaemia.

  This means that the role of alkali therapy in lactic acidosis is limited to control of acute acidosis. There is some evidence [21, 22] that acidosis impairs cardiac contractility, and in severe acidosis, acute therapy with intravenous bicarbonate may improve tissue perfusion.

  However, there a number of reasons to be cautious with bicarbonate replacement in lactic acidosis:
  - Fluid overload and post-treatment metabolic alkalosis when the excess lactate is converted to bicarbonate, as with ketoacidosis.
  - CO_2 retention may be a problem in patients with compromised cardiac and pulmonary function, as bicarbonate buffers excess hydrogen ions, CO_2 is formed, and normally this would be eliminated via the lungs; if the pulmonary circulation is inadequate to vent the CO_2, it will be retained [23], adding an additional acid burden.
  - It has been proposed that intravenous bicarbonate could cause a paradoxical drop in intracellular pH [24], worsening hepatic lactate metabolism and cardiac contractility [22]. This was based on isolated cell experiments, and several lines of evidence show that this is probably not the case in vivo [25].
  - Bicarbonate therapy may cause a fall in serum ionised calcium by increasing calcium binding to albumin [26]; this could potentially worsen cardiac contractility.

  Thus, much like in ketoacidosis, the role for bicarbonate therapy is probably only for the acute control of severe acidaemia (~pH 7.1).

- ***Ingestion of Methanol or Ethylene Glycol***

  Acute Metabolic Acidosis AG: High

  Both methanol and ethylene glycol poisoning tend to occur in the setting of ethanol substitution, either deliberate (i.e. drinking methylated spirits or deliberate self-harm) or accidental (i.e. methanol contamination of domestically distilled alcohol or occult ethylene glycol substitution in illegally produced spirits).

  Unlike ketoacidosis and lactic acidosis, the inorganic anions generated in methanol or ethylene glycol poisoning are not metabolised to bicarbonate; they are toxic and must be removed. Therefore, treatment is much more active in these cases.

  Both methanol and ethylene glycol are both relatively harmless alcohols (both can cause sedation), but they both form very toxic metabolites when oxidised by alcohol dehydrogenase and (to a lesser extent) aldehyde dehydrogenase.

  Methanol is metabolised to *formate*. Formate toxicity causes visual impairment from optic disc oedema and direct retinal damage, leading eventually to permanent *blindness*, as well as *injury to the basal ganglia*, probably via mitochondrial toxicity [27].

  Ethylene glycol is metabolised to *glycolate*, glyoxalate and *oxalate*. These metabolites cause *acute kidney injury*, mainly from tubular injury caused by glycolate, but also via oxalate precipitation in the kidney. The kidney injury will further delay the elimination of the ethylene glycol. Hypocalcaemia may occur due to calcium oxalate precipitation.

  Inhibition of alcohol dehydrogenase is an important strategy, to prevent metabolism of the parent alcohols to their toxic metabolites. *Fomepizole* is an alcohol dehydrogenase inhibitor, which is superior to ethanol therapy, is safe and easy to administer. Alternatively, alcohol dehydrogenase can be competitively inhibited by *ethanol* which has a higher affinity for alcohol dehydrogenase than either methanol or ethylene glycol. However, it is vastly inferior to fomepizole, as it is difficult to administer, monitor and adjust; it is irritant to veins and most importantly causes central sedation, possibly leading to obtundation and airway compromise. Although this is only effective if done early, co-ingestion with ethanol is very common and will delay the appearance of the toxic metabolites, so it is worth attempting inhibition even hours after ingestion.

  Alkalinisation: both formate and glycolate and/or oxalate are more likely to penetrate their target cell membranes when they are protonated (and therefore uncharged), and this is more likely to occur when the patient is acidaemic. There is thus a clear rationale for alkalinisation with bicarbonate in these patients, especially as the metabolic acidosis in these cases is often severe (bicarbonate often as low as 8 mmol/L). Intravenous bicarbonate should be given with an aim for an arterial pH of 7.35.

  Haemodialysis is the best way to rapidly clear both the parent alcohols and their toxic metabolites.

It should be started rapidly in a case of suspected methanol or ethylene glycol poisoning, and the patient has evidence of acidaemia, and end organ damage (renal failure or visual impairment) confirmatory levels of methanol or ethylene glycol should not delay treatment. Repeated courses of haemodialysis may be necessary in massive overdoses or in those whom renal failure results from ethylene glycol poisoning. Haemodialysis may also shorten the course of alcohol dehydrogenase inhibitor therapy. Haemodialysis may not be necessary in ethylene glycol ingestion if fomepizole has been given, there is no acidaemia (i.e. there is little or no glycolate circulating), and renal function remains normal.

- ***Aspirin Overdose***

  Acute (Rarely Chronic) Respiratory Alkalosis/Metabolic Acidosis AG: High

  Aspirin (and other salicylates, such as salicylic acid and methyl salicylate) is common and can cause multiple toxic effects (tinnitus, nausea and vomiting, altered mental state and seizures, tachyarrhythmias, acute lung and liver injury), including a complex acid-base disturbance.

  Salicylates directly stimulate the respiratory centre causing hyperventilation and *respiratory alkalosis*. This is followed by a high anion gap *metabolic acidosis*, caused by accumulation of organic anions, including lactate and ketoacids. Approximately a third of salicylate overdoses are a part of mixed overdoses, often with respiratory depressants, so the respiratory alkalosis may be ameliorated, or a respiratory acidosis may be present in these cases.

  Salicylate is also uncharged when protonated and able to cross cell membranes; thus, acidaemia will increase its delivery to target tissues.

  Alkalinisation of serum and urine is therefore desirable, not just to reduce tissue penetration but also to enhance the renal elimination of the salicylate. Intravenous bicarbonate should be given, even if there is a mild respiratory alkalosis.

  Haemodialysis removes salicylate and should be considered in patients with cerebral or pulmonary oedema, renal failure, depressed level of consciousness, a very high salicylate level (>700 mg/dL) and clinical deterioration despite good supportive treatment.

- ***Chronic Renal Failure***

  Chronic Metabolic Acidosis AG: N

  Excess acid consumed in the diet is excreted renally, mainly as ammonium. In chronic kidney disease, as the GFR falls, the ammonium production per nephron increases to maintain normal acid excretion; however, this compensation starts to fail at about a GFR of 40–50 mls/min. After this, there will be a net retention of acid, which may progress to a significant metabolic acidaemia.

  Even in salt- and water-retaining patients with advanced chronic renal failure, oral sodium bicarbonate is well tolerated [28], and treatment of the acidosis has three main aims:

  Retardation of the progression of renal impairment. Oral bicarbonate supplementation has been shown to retard the progression of CKD in acidotic CKD patients compared to patients receiving no bicarbonate supplementation [29]. The mechanism for this effect is not clear.

  Bone protection. As a chronic acidosis, the acidosis of CKD causes calcium and phosphate leeching from the bone in order to buffer the extra hydrogen ions. Preventing this by bicarbonate supplementation may delay the onset of osteopenia, in dialysis patients at least [30].

  Improved nutritional status. Acidosis in CKD can cause muscle wasting and weakness, probably by a direct effect of the acidaemia in stimulating genes that promote muscle proteolysis, an effect ameliorated by bicarbonate [31]. Bicarbonate is also beneficial in preventing the growth retardation caused by chronic acidosis in children with CKD.

- ***Surreptitious Vomiting***

  Chronic Metabolic Alkalosis AG: N

  The urinary sodium concentration is often used as an indicator of volume status. However, it should be borne in mind that in acute metabolic alkalosis, the urine concentration of both sodium and potassium is high, even if there is volume depletion. In fact, the urinary losses of potassium are the main cause of hypokalaemia in vomiting, and the potassium loss in vomitus itself is minimal.

  In this setting a much better indicator of volume depletion is the urinary chloride concentration, which will be low as the kidney appropriately retains chloride, both for volume expansion and due to the hypochloraemia due to chloride loss in the vomitus.

  In protracted vomiting, the reabsorbative capacity of the nephron is increased in order to deal with the increased filtered load of bicarbonate; at this point, the urinary concentrations of sodium and potassium will become very low, and the urine pH will fall.

- ***Surreptitious Diuretic Abuse***

  Chronic Metabolic Alkalosis AG: N/high

  As mentioned above, the biochemical profile of a patient taking a loop diuretic is identical to that of Bartter syndrome, and the profile of someone taking a thiazide is the same as that of Gitelman syndrome. If a patient is taking either of these drugs surreptitiously, they may present as either of these conditions.

The only biochemical clue may come from the urine; patients with either Bartter or Gitelman have constant inappropriate urinary losses of chloride. Patients on loop or thiazide diuretics will also have inappropriately high urinary chloride losses, but only during the duration of action of the diuretic, during which time, the diuretic should be detectable in the urine. After this time, the urinary chloride will fall precipitously, as the kidney tries to conserve chloride, and the diuretic will be undetectable.

- ***Sudden Relief of Hypercapnoea***

  Acute Metabolic Alkalosis AG: N

  Chronic hypercapnoea will cause an appropriate compensatory metabolic increase in renal hydrogen ion secretion. Sudden correction of the hypercapnoea (e.g. by mechanical ventilation) can cause metabolic alkalosis due to the sustained high serum concentration of HCO_3^-. This may be enough to increase cerebral pH and cause a neurological deficit or even death [32]. As chloride is exchanged for bicarbonate in the cortical collecting duct, and hypercapnoeic patients may have a chloride deficit [33], it is often necessary to administer IV sodium chloride to allow the excess bicarbonate to be excreted.

14.15 Worked Case Example

A 60-year-old woman was visiting family in the UK. She had been unwell with vomiting and fever for 2 weeks and saw a GP who gave her antibiotics for a urinary tract infection.

She had a background of previous renal stones, high blood pressure, recurrent urine infections and a bladder operation 20 years before. She would normally intermittently self-catheterise, but had not done so since arriving in the UK. She took sodium docusate, omeprazole and lisinopril.

On assessment, she was unwell with a temperature of 37.2 °C. She was obese with BMI 41, drowsy and confused. Her vital signs showed pulse 85, BP 150/80, JVP -1 cm, oxygen saturations 99% on room air and respiratory rate 32. Her heart sounds were normal, chest was clear and abdomen was soft, with a lower abdominal scar. She had been catheterised with a residual volume of 1300 ml and was now passing 100 ml/hr urine.

Her blood results are shown in Table 14.1.

What is the acid-base disturbance?

She has a primary metabolic acidosis with incomplete respiratory compensation.

What are the likely causes?

We can narrow down the potential causes of a metabolic acidosis by calculating the anion gap. Note that the albumin is normal, and does not therefore need to be corrected for. In practice, the potassium is often excluded from the equation because it is too small to be significant.

Table 14.1 Blood results for worked case

U&Es		Full blood count		ABG on air	
Urea	31.1	Haemoglobin	10.2		
Creatinine	344	White cell count	16	pH	7.037
Sodium	148	Platelets	163	pCO_2	1.52
Potassium	4.3	Clotting	Normal	pO_2	15.9
Chloride	126			Bicarbonate	4
Glucose	7.2				
Corrected calcium	2.05				
Phosphate	2.00				
Albumin	41				
C-reactive protein	50				

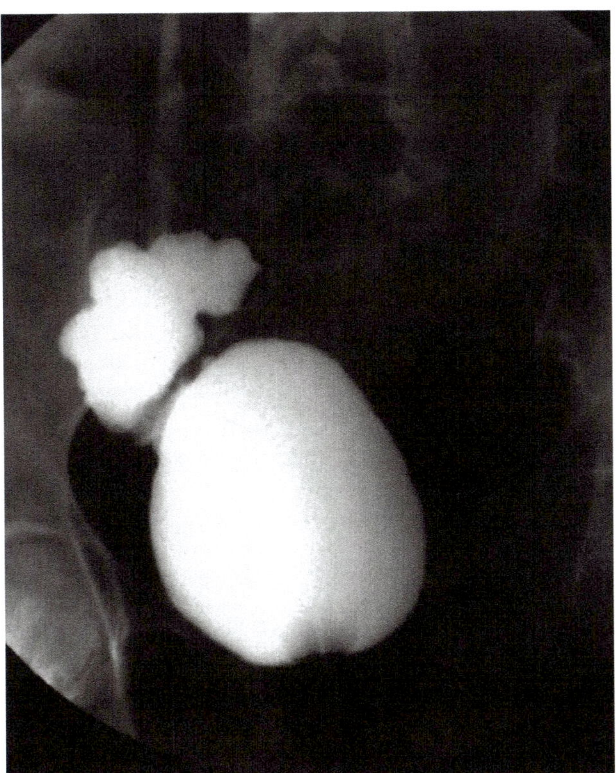

Fig. 14.3 Cystogram demonstrating colo-vesical fistula

$$\text{Anion Gap}\quad (148)-(126+4)=18$$

This is normal, suggesting that there is NOT a large increase in unmeasured anions. Causes of a normal anion gap metabolic acidosis include gastrointestinal bicarbonate losses, renal tubular acidosis (1, 2 and 4), *ureteric diversion, post-treatment of ketoacidosis and carbonic anhydrase inhibition.*

Review the cystogram (Fig. 14.3). Why has she deteriorated?

This image shows a colovesical fistula, with abnormal flow of urine from the bladder into the bowel. This would explain her symptoms of recurrent UTIs and loose stool. This could be a long-term complication from her previous bladder surgery.

In this scenario, the acidosis is equivalent to that caused by ureteric diversion (e.g. with an ileal conduit). The degree of acidosis is determined by the length of contact between the bowel and the urine, in this case prolonged due to failure to self-catheterise, and the segment of bowel involved. In health, the bowel secretes sodium in exchange for hydrogen and bicarbonate in exchange for chloride. When exposed to urine, the bowel reabsorbs ammonia, ammonium, hydrogen and chloride. This leads to a hyperchloraemic metabolic acidosis. Any component of acute kidney injury (in this case both pre- and post-renal) will further reduce the body's ability to excrete acid. The blood ammonia levels would be high if checked.

Chapter Review Questions

1. What is the problem with a patient having a well-tolerated metabolic acidosis?
2. Metabolic alkalosis: how common is it, and how serious?
3. Why does the renal Fanconi syndrome only cause a mild-moderate metabolic acidosis? What is the problem with correcting this mild acidosis with bicarbonate supplementation?
4. What are the principles of treating poisoning with ethylene glycol or methanol?
5. You have an acidotic patient admitted on the intensive care unit, and the intensivist wants to discuss the patient's physiology in terms of the strong ion gap. How will you explain to them the weaknesses of the Stewart hypothesis?

Answers

1. Although there have been a number of potential problems posited to be associated with a chronic and well-tolerated metabolic acidosis (negative inotropic effects, decreased protein synthesis), these are mainly based on animal data. Patients with chronic, well-tolerated metabolic acidosis (e.g. with dRTA) get bone demineralisation (osteomalacia in adults, rickets in children) as the only obvious negative effect.
2. This is the most common acid-base disturbance in hospitalised patients, due to problems such as prolonged vomiting, diuretic use and hypokalaemia. Extremely severe cases can cause agitation, delirium, seizures and coma, but this is uncommon; it is almost never serious enough to cause clinical consequences outside of those with pre-existing respiratory depression.
3. Absorption of bicarbonate occurs mainly in the proximal convoluted tubule; this is therefore disrupted in the renal Fanconi syndrome. However, the disturbance can be compensated by reabsorption of bicarbonate later on in the tubule, including in the loop of Henle and collecting duct (beta-intercalated cells), which together can reab-

sorb ~15 mmol/L of bicarbonate from the filtrate. This ensures the serum concentration will not fall lower than that in Fanconi syndrome. Supplementing patients with oral bicarbonate delivers more bicarbonate to the filtrate and urine. However, large doses are needed (e.g. more than 16 g/24 hours). Also, once the reabsorption mechanism is saturated, the additional bicarbonate anions in the tubules create a lumen electronegative potential which can only be equalised by secreting a cation, in this case potassium. Thus, bicarbonate supplementation can cause hypokalaemia.

4. Methanol and ethylene glycol are both alcohols whose metabolites are poisonous. They are both metabolised by alcohol dehydrogenase. The first goal of therapy is to inhibit alcohol dehydrogenase and cause a lower rate of generation of those metabolites. This should be done with non-competitive inhibitors like fomepizole rather than with competitive inhibitors like ethanol, as dosing is safer, and patients will already have alcohol intoxication from their poisoning. Second, the toxic metabolites (formate and oxalate, respectively) cross cell membranes best when they are chargeless (i.e. they are proton bound), so increasing the systemic pH of the patients will help reduce the cell toxicity of the metabolites. Lastly, the parent alcohols and their toxic metabolites are all small molecules that will cross a dialyser membrane and can therefore be dialysed out. Poisoning with ethylene glycol or methanol is therefore an indication for emergency haemodialysis.
5. Classical acid base theory has been well validated and accepted in clinical correlation, whereas the Stewart hypothesis is less well validated, and may correlate less well with clinical findings. Also, in classical acid base theory, different classifications relate to different biological pathologies (respiratory alkalosis, raised anion gap metabolic acidosis, etc.). The six main classifications that Stewart dictates are overly complex and do not break up into distinct pathologies in the same way. Finally, Stewart's strong ion difference is calculated from multiple measurements, usually with software, leading to accumulation of measurement error.

14

Definitions (Side Bar)

Acidemia	An arterial pH below the normal range (<7.36)
Alkalaemia	An arterial pH above the normal range (>7.44)
Acidosis	A process that tends to lower the extracellular fluid pH. This can be caused by a fall in the serum bicarbonate (HCO_3) concentration or a rise in ${}_{P}CO_2$
Metabolic acidosis	A disorder that causes a reduction in the serum HCO_3 concentration and pH
Respiratory acidosis	A disorder that causes an elevation in arterial ${}_{P}CO_2$ and a reduction in pH
Alkalosis	A process that tends to raise the extracellular fluid pH. This can be caused by an elevation in the serum HCO_3 concentration and/or a fall in ${}_{P}CO_2$
Metabolic alkalosis	A disorder that causes an elevation in the serum HCO_3 concentration and pH
Respiratory alkalosis	A disorder that causes a reduction in arterial ${}_{P}CO_2$ and an increase in pH
Simple acid-base disorders	One of the four acid-base disorders with or without the appropriate compensatory response
Mixed acid-base disorder	Having two (or more) of the above disorders at the same time

References

1. Schwartz WB, Relman AS. A critique of the parameters used in the evaluation of acid-base disorders. "Whole-blood buffer base" and "standard bicarbonate" compared with blood pH and plasma bicarbonate concentration. N Engl J Med. 1963;268:1382–8.
2. Madias NE, Adrogue HJ, Horowitz GL, Cohen JJ, Schwartz WB. A redefinition of normal acid-base equilibrium in man: carbon dioxide tension as a key determinant of normal plasma bicarbonate concentration. Kidney Int. 1979;16(5):612–8.
3. Balasubramanyan N, Havens PL, Hoffman GM. Unmeasured anions identified by the Fencl-Stewart method predict mortality better than base excess, anion gap, and lactate in patients in

the pediatric intensive care unit. Crit Care Med. 1999;27(8):1577–81.
4. Kaplan LJ, Kellum JA. Initial pH, base deficit, lactate, anion gap, strong ion difference, and strong ion gap predict outcome from major vascular injury. Crit Care Med. 2004;32(5):1120–4.
5. Cusack RJ, Rhodes A, Lochhead P, Jordan B, Perry S, Ball JA, et al. The strong ion gap does not have prognostic value in critically ill patients in a mixed medical/surgical adult ICU. Intensive Care Med. 2002;28(7):864–9.
6. Dubin A, Menises MM, Masevicius FD, Moseinco MC, Kutscherauer DO, Ventrice E, et al. Comparison of three different methods of evaluation of metabolic acid-base disorders. Crit Care Med. 2007;35(5):1264–70.
7. Siggaard-Andersen O, Fogh-Andersen N. Base excess or buffer base (strong ion difference) as measure of a non-respiratory acid-base disturbance. Acta Anaesthesiol Scand Suppl. 1995;107:123–8.
8. Kurtz I, Kraut J, Ornekian V, Nguyen MK. Acid-base analysis: a critique of the Stewart and bicarbonate-centered approaches. Am J Physiol Renal Physiol. 2008;294(5):F1009–31.
9. Adrogue HJ, Madias NE. Changes in plasma potassium concentration during acute acid-base disturbances. Am J Med. 1981;71(3):456–67.
10. Oberleithner H, Greger R, Lang F. The effect of respiratory and metabolic acid-base changes on ionized calcium concentration: in vivo and in vitro experiments in man and rat. Eur J Clin Investig. 1982;12(6):451–5.
11. Perez GO, Oster JR, Rogers A. Acid-base disturbances in gastrointestinal disease. Dig Dis Sci. 1987;32(9):1033–43.
12. Khositseth S, Bruce LJ, Walsh SB, Bawazir WM, Ogle GD, Unwin RJ, et al. Tropical distal renal tubular acidosis: clinical and epidemiological studies in 78 patients. QJM. 2012;105(9):861–77.
13. Poux JM, Peyronnet P, Le Meur Y, Favereau JP, Charmes JP, Leroux-Robert C. Hypokalemic quadriplegia and respiratory arrest revealing primary Sjogren's syndrome. Clin Nephrol. 1992;37(4):189–91.
14. Walsh SB, Shirley DG, Wrong OM, Unwin RJ. Urinary acidification assessed by simultaneous furosemide and fludrocortisone treatment: an alternative to ammonium chloride. Kidney Int. 2007;71(12):1310–6.
15. Wrong O, Davies HE. The excretion of acid in renal disease. Q J Med. 1959;28(110):259–313.
16. Mundy AR. Metabolic complications of urinary diversion. Lancet. 1999;353(9167):1813–4.
17. McDougal WS. Metabolic complications of urinary intestinal diversion. J Urol. 1992;147(5):1199–208.
18. Lever E, Jaspan JB. Sodium bicarbonate therapy in severe diabetic ketoacidosis. Am J Med. 1983;75(2):263–8.
19. Morris LR, Murphy MB, Kitabchi AE. Bicarbonate therapy in severe diabetic ketoacidosis. Ann Intern Med. 1986;105(6):836–40.
20. Okuda Y, Adrogue HJ, Field JB, Nohara H, Yamashita K. Counterproductive effects of sodium bicarbonate in diabetic ketoacidosis. J Clin Endocrinol Metab. 1996;81(1):314–20.
21. Narins RG, Cohen JJ. Bicarbonate therapy for organic acidosis: the case for its continued use. Ann Intern Med. 1987;106(4):615–8.
22. Orchard CH, Kentish JC. Effects of changes of pH on the contractile function of cardiac muscle. Am J Phys. 1990;258(6 Pt 1):C967–81.
23. Adrogue HJ, Rashad MN, Gorin AB, Yacoub J, Madias NE. Assessing acid-base status in circulatory failure. Differences between arterial and central venous blood. N Engl J Med. 1989;320(20):1312–6.
24. Adrogue HJ, Madias NE. Management of life-threatening acid-base disorders. First of two parts. N Engl J Med. 1998;338(1):26–34.
25. Goldsmith DJ, Forni LG, Hilton PJ. Bicarbonate therapy and intracellular acidosis. Clin Sci (Lond). 1997;93(6):593–8.
26. Cooper DJ, Walley KR, Wiggs BR, Russell JA. Bicarbonate does not improve hemodynamics in critically ill patients who have lactic acidosis. A prospective, controlled clinical study. Ann Intern Med. 1990;112(7):492–8.
27. Wallace KB, Eells JT, Madeira VM, Cortopassi G, Jones DP. Mitochondria-mediated cell injury. Symposium overview. Fundam Appl Toxicol. 1997;38(1):23–37.
28. Husted FC, Nolph KD, Maher JF. NaHCO3 and NaC1 tolerance in chronic renal failure. J Clin Invest. 1975;56(2):414–9.
29. de Brito-Ashurst I, Varagunam M, Raftery MJ, Yaqoob MM. Bicarbonate supplementation slows progression of CKD and improves nutritional status. J Am Soc Nephrol. 2009;20(9):2075–84.
30. Lefebvre A, de Vernejoul MC, Gueris J, Goldfarb B, Graulet AM, Morieux C. Optimal correction of acidosis changes progression of dialysis osteodystrophy. Kidney Int. 1989;36(6):1112–8.
31. Bailey JL, Wang X, England BK, Price SR, Ding X, Mitch WE. The acidosis of chronic renal failure activates muscle proteolysis in rats by augmenting transcription of genes encoding proteins of the ATP-dependent ubiquitin-proteasome pathway. J Clin Invest. 1996;97(6):1447–53.
32. Rotheram EB Jr, Safar P, Robin E. Cns disorder during mechanical ventilation in chronic pulmonary disease. JAMA. 1964;189:993–6.
33. Schwartz WB, Hays RM, Polak A, Haynie GD. Effects of chronic hypercapnia on electrolyte and acid-base equilibrium. II. Recovery, with special reference to the influence of chloride intake. J Clin Invest. 1961;40:1238–49.

Hypertension and Renovascular Diseases

Contents

Approach to Hypertension: Diagnosis and Investigation

Roohi Chhabra, Reecha Sofat, Aroon Hingorani, and Jennifer Cross

Contents

M. Harber (ed.), *Primer on Nephrology*, https://doi.org/10.1007/978-3-030-76419-7_15

Hypertension is one of the most common chronic medical conditions and the single most important preventable cause of premature death in developed countries. It presents a significant burden of disease to society as persistent uncontrolled hypertension is associated with coronary artery disease, cerebrovascular disease and renal impairment. The prevalence of hypertension rises with age, affecting 60% of the population over the age of 60. Among young adults (18–39 years), approximately 20% of men and 15% of women have been diagnosed with hypertension in the USA. Forty-five percent of the adult population worldwide has hypertension, and recent estimates suggest that this number may increase by as much as 15–20% by 2025 [1].

Most cases of hypertension are idiopathic or essential with no identifiable underlying cause. In 5–10% of cases, hypertension is related to an underlying disorder or secondary; this is termed secondary hypertension which is most commonly related to diseases of the kidney such as diabetic nephropathy but also vascular and endocrine disorders. Given the magnitude and importance of hypertension as a risk factor for cardiovascular and renal disease, this chapter will discuss the approach to defining and diagnosing hypertension before discussing the approach to investigation of patients with suspected resistant and secondary hypertension.

Definition

Hypertension is arbitrarily defined as a persistently elevated arterial blood pressure with a current threshold exceeding 140/90 mmHg in adults.

Accelerated hypertension (also known as malignant hypertension) is a severe increase in blood pressure ≥180/120 mmHg associated with new or progressive end-organ damage such as retinopathy.

Learning Objectives

The aims of this chapter are to explore the causes of complex or difficult to manage hypertension and to understand the diagnostic approach to patients with complex or multi-agent hypertension.

15.1 Introduction

Hypertension is the most prevalent, modifiable risk factor for cardiovascular disease (CVD), stroke, chronic kidney disease (CKD), heart failure and peripheral arterial disease.

The risk of death, myocardial infarction (MI) and stroke has a continuous relationship on a log scale with both systolic and diastolic blood pressure (BP), though the relationship is steeper for stroke than MI. As an indication of the strength of the relationship, for those between 40 and 69 years for every 20/10 mmHg rise in BP above 115/70 mmHg, cardiovascular risks roughly double [2] (◘ Fig. 15.1). The converse is also true; reduction of blood pressure by 20/10 mmHg approximately halves the risk of cardiovascular events. BP also shows a continuous, independent relationship with CKD, heart failure and peripheral artery disease. According to the Global Burden of Disease 2000 study, approximately 50% of strokes and MIs can be attributed to hypertension and an estimated 7.6 million deaths per year (13.5% of all deaths worldwide) [3].

The relationship between CKD and hypertension is complex, given the kidney's role in regulation of body fluid volumes and BP homeostasis. More than 80% of CKD patients are hypertensive and teasing out whether the hypertension is primary, and the cause of the CKD can be a challenge. However, data from cohort studies in patients with hypertension and no baseline renal disease demonstrate a graded relationship between increasing BP and the development of CKD [4] suggesting that it relates to BP control.

15.2 Defining Hypertension and Setting Treatment Thresholds

BP has a well-recognised skewed normal distribution in the population, and given the continuous log linear relationship with cardiovascular and renal disease, down to at least a level of 115/70 mmHg [2], the BP cut-off that defines 'hypertension' is arbitrary.

Definitions of hypertension and treatment thresholds and targets have been issued by more than 100 organisations worldwide including the National Institute of Clinical Excellence (NICE) in the UK [5], the American Heart Association (AHA) [6], European Societies of Hypertension (ESH) and Cardiology (ESC) [7, 8], Japanese Society of Hypertension (JSH) [9] and the World Health Association (WHO) [10].

◘ Table 15.1 summarises the definitions of hypertension used in these particular guidelines. All of these sample guidelines agree that the term hypertension be applied to a patient with a clinic BP of ≥140/90 mmHg. However, BP is further subdivided using a variety of terms such as optimal, normal, high-normal, prehypertension and grades (or stages) 1–3.

Treatment thresholds and targets differ between guidelines, but there is clear consensus in all guidelines delineating between low- and higher-risk groups. High-risk groups are those with additional cardiovascular risk factors, including diabetes mellitus (DM), established CKD, pre-existing cardiovascular disease (including cerebrovascular, heart disease and peripheral arterial disease), subclinical end-organ damage (◘ Table 15.2) or a '10 year

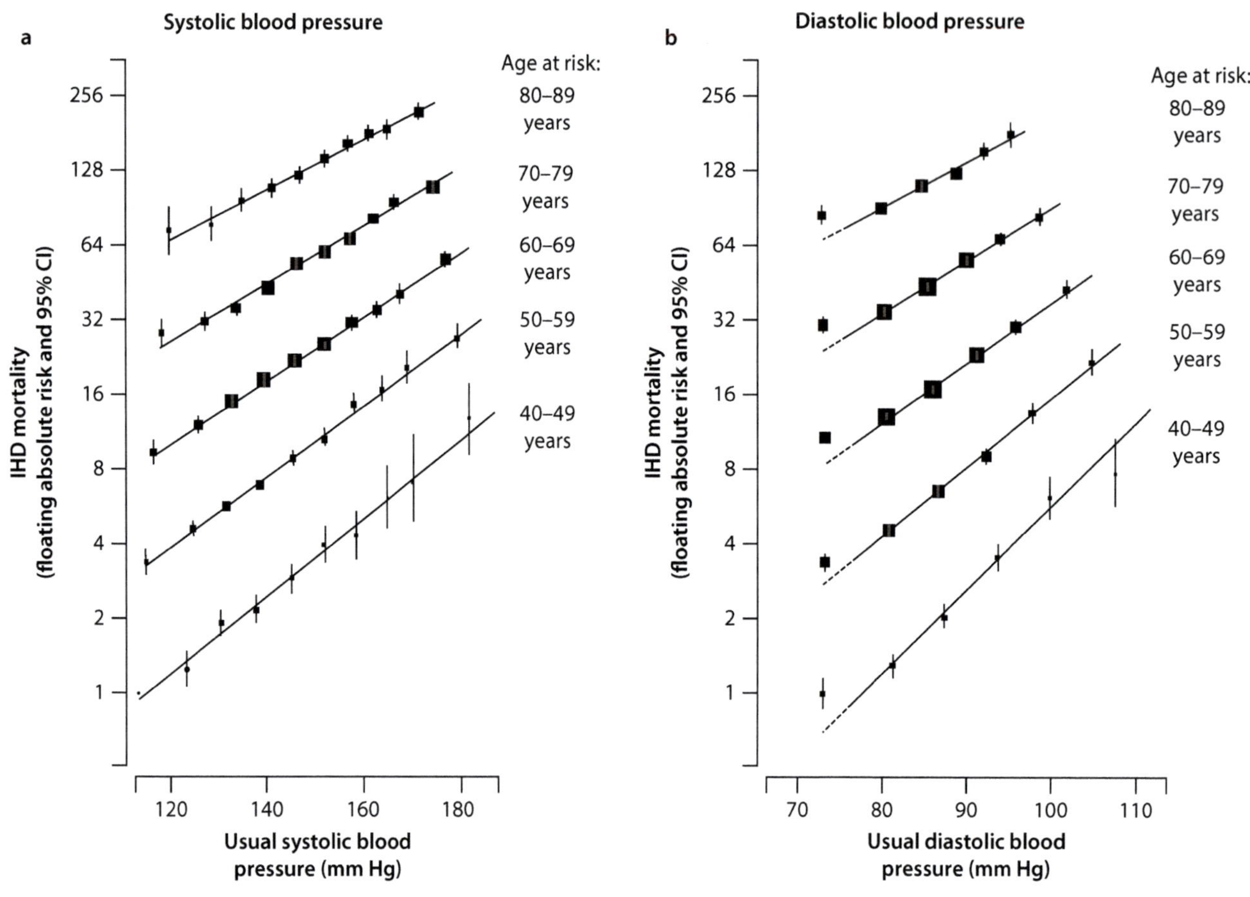

Fig. 15.1 Association between blood pressure and ischaemic heart disease

15

Table 15.1 Definitions of hypertension in international guidelines

Term	Clinic sBP	Clinic dBP
NICE 2011 [10]		
Stage 1 hypertension	140–159	90–99
Stage 2 hypertension	160–179	100–109
Severe hypertension	≥180	≥110
JSH 2009 [13], *ESH 2007* [12], *WHO 2007* [14]		
Optimal BP	<120	<80
Normal BP	120–129	80–84
High-normal BP	130–139	85–89
Grade 1 hypertension	140–159	90–99
Grade 2 hypertension	160–179	100–109
Grade 3 hypertension	≥180	≥110
AHA 2007 [11]		
Pre-hypertension	130–139	80–89
Hypertension	≥140	≥90

cardiovascular risk' of a predefined level (Table 15.3). The summary of the baseline investigations required to make a reasonable assessment of cardiovascular risk for a patient with hypertension is listed in ► Box 15.1.

Box 15.1 Initial Investigations in a Patient with Hypertension

- Blood electrolytes, creatinine and eGFR
- Fundoscopy
- Random blood glucose
- Serum total and HDL cholesterol
- Urine strip for protein (and blood)
- Weight and height for BMI
- 12 lead ECG

15.3 Defining Thresholds in Low-Risk Patients

As described, a low-risk patient is one with no history of DM or vascular disease in any territory, with no evidence of subclinical end-organ damage and a low cal-

Table 15.2 Investigation of subclinical end-organ damage

Abnormality	Investigations[a]	Suggested threshold[b]	Evidence[c]
Heart			
Left ventricular hypertrophy	*ECG*	Sokolow-Lyon >38 mm	Havranek EP et al. (15)
	Echocardiogram	LVMI $M \geq 125$ g/m^2, $W \geq 110$ g/m^2	Milani RV et al. (16)
Arteries			
Carotid intima-media thickening (IMT)	Ultrasound Doppler carotid	IMT >0.9 mm	Zanchetti A et al. (17)
Renal			
Low estimated glomerular filtration rate (eGFR) (MDRD formula)	*Serum eGFR*	<60 ml/min/1.73 m^2	Tsioufis C et al. (18)
Microalbuminuria	*Urine dip*	1+ protein (proceed to measure of quantity)	
	Random urine: albumin/creatinine ratio	$M > 22$ $W > 31$ mg/g creatinine	Cirillo M et al. (19)
	24-hour urine collection	30–300 mg/24 h	
Cerebrovascular			
Small vessel ischaemia	MRI	Presence of cerebrovascular lesions	Kearney-Schwartz A et al. (20)
Retinal			
Hypertensive retinopathy	*Fundoscopy*	≥Grade 2 changes	Kim GH et al. (21)

[a]Investigations in bold are first-line and should be performed in all patients; others may have a role in selected patients
[b]Thresholds (other than fundoscopy) taken from 2007 ESH guidelines [12]
[c]Reference provided is an example of a study demonstrating an association between the end-organ damage in question and cardiovascular end-points

culated 10-year cardiovascular risk. In general, such patients are underrepresented in clinical trials, as the selection of high-risk patients maximises event rate and thus the power of trials. Furthermore, most trials are of a short duration (4–5 years), whereas the additional life expectancy for middle-aged hypertensives is 20–30 years. Consequently, there is a lack of high-quality evidence and therefore consensus regarding treatment thresholds in this cohort.

In the largest overview of blood pressure treatment trials conducted by Law et al. [11], all patients who achieved a sustained BP reduction over 5 years of 5–6 mmHg in systolic BP recorded a reduction in coronary events by approximately 20% and strokes by 40% [11]. The percentage reductions in CVD events and stroke were similar in people with or without cardiovascular disease regardless of blood pressure before treatment (to a nadir of 110 mmHg systolic). This is in keeping with evidence from prospective observational studies that predict lowering BP by this degree confers a similar magnitude of protection [2]. The authors of this review suggested that their results indicated the importance of lowering blood pressure in everyone over a certain age (55 years old), rather than in just those with higher-risk profile.

Despite this data, guidelines differ in their recommendations for low-risk individuals.

All guidelines agree that treatment should be commenced when the clinic BP is >160/100 mmHg. However, there is variance. The guidelines produced by NICE, WHO and JSH do not recommend treatment in this group when BP is between 140 and 160 mmHg [5, 9, 10]. However, the ESH and the AHA [6, 7] do recommend treatment if BP is uncontrolled by lifestyle measures.

Table 15.3 10-year cardiovascular risk calculators

Calculator	Notes	Data fields	URL
Framingham	Based on the long-standing prospective Framingham cohort studies Included in AHA guidelines Risk calculated after cumulative points total (based on series of charts)	BP Age Sex Diabetes Smoking LDL cholesterol Total cholesterol HDL cholesterol	► http://www.framinghamheartstudy.org/risk/coronary.html
QRISK	Based on data collected by general practitioners in NHS Online risk calculator	BP Age Sex Ethnicity Smoking Diabetes Family history Renal function AF On BP Rx Rheumatoid arthritis Cholesterol/HDL ratio BMI	► http://www.qrisk.org/
WHO	Included in WHO/ISH guidelines A series of region-specific prediction charts Lest number of fields required	BP Sex Age Diabetes Smoking Total cholesterol Region	► http://www.who.int/cardiovascular_diseases/guidelines/PocketGL.ENGLISH.AFR-D-E.rev1.pdf

15.4 Measuring Blood Pressure and Diagnosing Hypertension

The extremely large evidence base on which the treatment for hypertension is based, including cohort studies with approximately one million participants and randomised studies in over 500,000 individuals [11], is based on using clinic BP measurements. Such measurements are cheap and readily available and require no specialised training or equipment over and above what is usually available in a clinic setting, and treatment based on these measurements is cost-effective, worldwide.

However, BP can be highly variable and is influenced by multiple factors including the time of day, posture, stress, pain, room temperature, etc. Indeed, even with serial back-to-back measurement, BP reproducibly falls. Thus, one-off clinic readings, even performed under ideal conditions, may give limited information about a patient's BP and thus cardiovascular risk. In order to overcome this limitation, multiple measurements over time are required to make a diagnosis, and this is advocated in multiple guidelines. However, increasing emphasis is being put on the value of ambulatory blood pressure measurement (ABPM) in diagnosing hypertension.

15.5 Ambulatory Blood Pressure Measurement (ABPM) in the Diagnosis of Hypertension

ABPM requires a patient wearing a cuff and bladder connected to electronic sensors which measures BP by the oscillometric technique. Serial BP measurements are performed (usually every 30–60 minutes), while going about their daily routine, over a period of time (usually 24 hours). This allows their diastolic and systolic blood pressures to be plotted over time and allows calculation of various measures, including mean ambulatory BP over 24 hours, diurnal variation (by comparing mean BP at night with the daytime mean) and the overall range and variability of BP.

Of nine cohort studies identified by the NICE 2011 clinical guideline, eight (including over 25,000 patients) found that mean 24-hour blood pressure values derived from ABPM were more strongly associated with and therefore more accurately predict cardiovascular events than standard clinic measurements [5].

The authors of the NICE guideline were persuaded to recommend (somewhat contentiously) that ABPM be used in all patients with a clinic BP greater than 140/90 mmHg to confirm the diagnosis of hypertension [5], but not to use ABPM in monitoring the response to treatment. At present, of the major hypertension guidelines, only NICE have recommended using ABPM to make the diagnosis of hypertension in all patients. Other international guidelines recommend its use in a more targeted fashion. Other indications for its use include investigating patients with suspected resistant, white coat or masked hypertension and monitoring response to treatment, particularly when there is a concern regarding iatrogenic hypotension.

Although the predictive value of ABPM is well established, there is no randomised evidence to guide the selection of an average BP threshold at which treatment would be indicated. In an effort to address this, Head et al. [13] compared mean 24-hour BP and mean daytime BP (n = 8575) with clinic BP in a different cohort (n = 1693), and using least product regression analysis established that clinic BP was 6/3 mmHg higher than daytime mean ambulatory BP and 10/5 mmHg higher than 24-hour mean ambulatory BP. The differences were more marked at higher BPs. On the basis of this data, the ABPM daytime equivalent to 140/90 mmHg in guidelines is 135/85 [10].

The overall impact of utilising ABPM more frequently in clinical practice is yet to be fully appreciated.

15.6 Home Blood Pressure Monitors

An alternative to ABPM is home monitoring where patients have their own home BP monitoring device which allows for similar benefits to ABPM as well as other potential benefits, such as allowing patients to assess their response to antihypertensive medications and providing frequent measurements over longer periods of time. It has been shown that the use of self-monitoring to titrate antihypertensive medication leads to significantly lower BP than titration guided by clinic readings.

Home BP monitors have been immensely useful during the difficult times of the SARS-CoV-2 pandemic as they allowed for virtual patient assessment and limited unnecessary patient visits to hospital, helped reduce the risk of infection compared to clinic machines and are likely to form an increasing part of remote management. However, concerns have been raised that such monitors may cause anxiety and obsessive behaviours and that the readings may be subject to observer prejudice and may produce unreliable readings. An approach that may be taken is regular testing three times weekly, ignoring the first reading and repeating at 2-minute intervals while the BP is above target and once achieving target to reduce the frequency of monitoring to weekly or even monthly. Recording BP at home may be regarded as a healthy lifestyle choice to confirm control and monitor treatment efficacy and provides patients with control recording results in smart phone apps and is an effective way of communicating results over time to primary and secondary care. Various apps exist that will in future allow us to download this data set to healthcare systems.

15.7 Resistant Hypertension

Resistant hypertension is defined as hypertension (clinic BP >140/90 mmHg) despite treatment with a rational combination of at least three antihypertensive agents, or controlled hypertension on four agents including a diuretic. It excludes non-adherence. Cohort studies suggest a prevalence of 10–15% among those diagnosed with hypertension [14]. Apparent resistant hypertension may be due to white coat hypertension (WCH) and poor adherence with prescribed medication, which may be as common as 50% of cases or due to a secondary cause. Careful clinical evaluation of patients with suspected resistant or secondary hypertension is critical as the diagnosis may significantly alter treatment. A list of suggested first-line investigations in patients with resistant hypertension is presented in ▪ Table 15.4.

▪ **Table 15.4** Suggested first-line investigations in resistant hypertension

Cause	First-line investigation(s)
White coat hypertension	24-hour ABPM
Poor adherence	Directly observed therapy OR Measurement of serum/urinary levels of antihypertensives
Renal parenchyma disease	Blood electrolytes, creatinine and eGFR Urine strip for protein and blood
Renal artery stenosis	CT or MR renal angiogram
Primary aldosteronism	Plasma renin (+/– aldosterone) Cross-sectional imaging of adrenal gland (can be done concurrently with CT/MR renal angiogram)
Cushing's syndrome	24-hour urinary cortisol, single-dose dexamethasone suppression test
Pheochromocytoma	Plasma-free metanephrines/catecholamines OR Urine-free metanephrines/catecholamines

15.8 White Coat Hypertension

WCH or 'isolated clinic hypertension' is a condition in which BP measured in clinic is hypertensive, but that measured out of the clinic is normal where the introduction of routine ABPM or home monitors allows its identification. This phenomenon is observed in approximately 30% of patients with a clinic BP >140/90 mmHg [15], and the prognosis of these patients is good compared with those with sustained hypertension. However, whether or not the patients with WCH should be treated with antihypertensives is controversial.

Several studies have linked WCH with subclinical end-organ damage including left ventricular hypertrophy and proteinuria; however, these findings have not been reproduced across all studies. Multiple longitudinal studies suggest that WCH increases the long-term risk of stroke, cardiovascular events and all-cause mortality but to a significantly lesser degree than sustained hypertension. The relative risk of WCH versus sustained hypertension is nicely demonstrated in the Kaplan-Meier curves derived from the PAMELA study (◘ Fig. 15.2) [16].

Thus, patients with WCH appear to have an intermediate risk of cardiovascular events, compared with normotensives and hypertensives. Several reasons for this increased risk have been proposed, most notably that BP variation (inherently higher in those with white coat hypertension) is itself an independent risk factor for cardiovascular events and that over time, a significant proportion of patients with WCH develop sustained hypertension.

ABPM is the investigation of choice to investigate whether a patient has WCH.

15

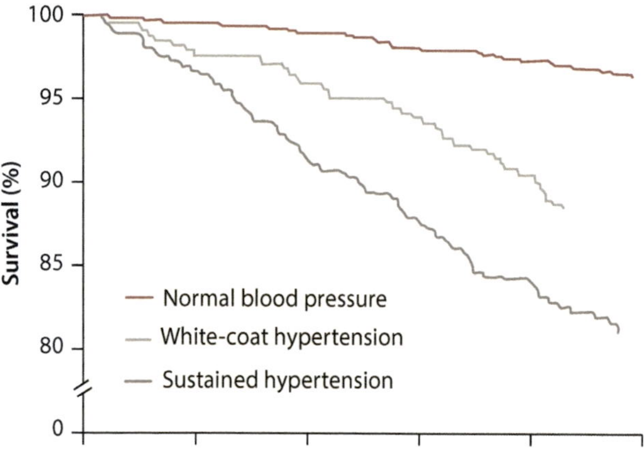

◘ **Fig. 15.2** Kaplan-Meier curves depicting the survival of patients with normal BP (red), WCH (light grey) and sustained hypertension (dark grey)

15.9 Masked Hypertension

Masked hypertension or isolated ambulatory hypertension is the inverse of WCH, in which clinic BP measurements are <140/90 mmHg, whereas the mean BP on ABPM is elevated (>135/85 mmHg). This occurs in approximately 15% of the population [17], and since the associated cardiovascular risk is similar to that of sustained hypertension, it represents a significant diagnostic challenge. A high index of suspicion is warranted in patients with a normal clinic BP who have multiple cardiovascular risk factors and evidence of organ damage.

15.10 Adherence

Poor adherence is a major cause of lack of blood pressure control and, along with WCH, accounts for the majority of patients who appear to have resistant hypertension. Retrospective analyses indicate that up to 40% of patients with newly diagnosed hypertension will discontinue their medication the first year of treatment [18] and over 5–10 years this figure may rise to over 60 [19]. Adherence or compliance with medication is complex and is commonly not deliberate. Assessing adherence is difficult. Patients rarely report it and often wish to comply but cannot comply. Several strategies have been developed to overcome this, including directly observed therapy and measurement of urinary or serum antihypertensive levels. Directly observed therapy may necessitate an admission to a day ward or overnight inpatient stay and should be conducted with caution – giving multiple prescribed antihypertensives to a patient who has not been taking them in the community may cause profound and life-threatening hypotension; thus giving only 1–2 agents initially is advised.

Once this diagnosis is established, management can be a challenge, but focusing on patient's motivations and considering side-effect profiles of available antihypertensives should both form part of the strategy. Educating the patient about the condition as well as using patient-centred techniques such as motivational interviewing is likely to increase adherence [20].

It is important to explore and determine possible non-intentional (e.g. forgetfulness) and intentional (e.g. unhelpful beliefs about medication-taking) lapses in medication-taking behaviours. In one study conducted at the Royal Free Hospital, renal unit, the Medication Adherence Report Scale (MARS) [21] demonstrated discrepancies between patients' reported antihypertensive treatment adherence and their corresponding urine analysis with approximately one-fifth of the patients under-reporting their non-adherence. Furthermore, conflict between patients' concerns and worries about taking medication and their beliefs about its necessity in managing their blood pressures was shown in the beliefs about medicines questionnaire (BMQ) with this 'conflict' being greater than that found in similar studies of medication-taking in other long-term conditions [22].

15.11 Secondary Hypertension

Secondary hypertension is hypertension in which there is an identifiable cause. It is thought to account for up to 10% of patients with hypertension although this figure is likely to increase with the increasing prevalence of chronic kidney disease and obesity. In addition to patients with apparently resistant hypertension, secondary causes should be considered in those who present:

1. Young (<40 years)
2. With accelerated hypertension/hypertensive emergencies
3. Have suddenly worsening hypertension
4. Severe end-organ damage
5. Family history of early onset hypertension/stroke

Secondary causes of hypertension may be split into four broad groups: (i) renal, (ii) endocrine, (iii) drugs (see ► Box 15.2) and (iv) 'other causes'. A comprehensive summary of these is presented in ◘ Table 15.5. The most important of these will now be discussed.

Box 15.2 Drugs Which Increase BP

- Oestrogens (e.g. in contraceptives)
- Non-steroidal anti-inflammatory drugs
- COX-2 inhibitors
- Weight-loss agents (amphetamine-related)
- Stimulants (e.g. cocaine)
- Mineral and glucocorticoids
- Antiparkinsonian agents (serotoninergic)
- Monoamine oxidase inhibitors (serotoninergic)
- Anabolic steroids
- Sympathomimetics including decongestants
- Migraine treatments (triptans – serotoninergic)
- Calcineurin inhibitors

15.12 Renal Causes of Secondary Hypertension

These can be broadly divided into (a) diseases of renal parenchyma, (b) renovascular hypertension and (c) distal tubular disorders.

◘ **Table 15.5** Causes of secondary hypertension

Condition	Symptom/sign
Renal	
Renal parenchymal disease	Mostly asymptomatic
Renal artery stenosis	Renal bruit, rise in serum creatinine >30% after initiation of angiotensin-converting enzyme inhibitor
Distal tubular disorders	Mostly asymptomatic
Endocrine	
Primary aldosteronism	Mostly asymptomatic
Pheochromocytoma	Episodic headaches, sweating, palpitations, flushing
Cushing's syndrome	Moon faces, central obesity, easy bruising
Hypothyroidism/hyperthyroidism	Symptoms of hypothyroidism or hyperthyroidism, e.g. gain/loss of weight, cold/heat intolerance
Hyperparathyroidism	Bone pain, stones, abdominal pain, constipation
Acromegaly	Headache, visual field defects, macroglossia
Carcinoid syndrome	Cutaneous flushing, venous telangiectasia, diarrhoea, bronchospasm
Other	
Coarctation of aorta	Radio-femoral delay
Obstructive sleep apnoea	Daytime somnolence, fatigue, obesity
Obesity	Mostly asymptomatic
Pregnancy (pre-eclampsia)	Headache. Blurring of vision, fluid retention
Medication	See ► Box 15.2
Familial dysautonomia	Sensorimotor neuropathy, sympathetic storm

15.12.1 Renal Parenchymal Disease

Renal parenchymal disease is the most common cause (50–75%) of secondary hypertension. Hypertension may occur in the course of glomerulonephritis, vasculitis and almost any cause of reduced GFR. The mechanisms leading to hypertension in kidney disease includes impaired urinary sodium and water excretion resulting in volume overload, excessive release of vasoconstrictors (renin, angiotensin II) and sympathetic activation.

CKD itself is associated with a marked escalation of cardiovascular risk increase; thus, all patients with newly diagnosed hypertension should have serum urea, creatinine and electrolytes measured and an estimation of glomerular filtration rate (eGFR) as well as a urine dip for protein, erythrocytes and leucocytes. There should be a robust referral pathway for patients with renal impairment or an abnormal urine sediment.

15.12.2 Renovascular Hypertension (See Chap. 17 on Renal Vasculature)

Renal artery stenosis (RAS) is a common cause of secondary hypertension. The vast majority is atheromatous in origin and risk factors include long-standing hypertension, diabetes, smoking and dyslipidaemia.

Its prevalence in the general hypertension population is approximately 2–5% and is more than 30% in patients undergoing cardiac catheterisation and may account for up to 14% of patients with end-stage renal failure. The culprit stenoses are of the conduit renal arteries and are most commonly caused by atherosclerotic plaques but may also be the result of vasculitis, neurofibromatosis, congenital bands and extrinsic compression.

In a young patient with RAS, it is important to consider fibromuscular dysplasia (FMD) as a potential cause. FMD is a noninflammatory, non-atherosclerotic disorder that leads to arterial stenosis, and most frequently involved are the renal and carotid arteries. It is more common in young women in the third and fourth decade, and its aetiology remains unknown, although various hormonal, mechanical and genetic factors have been suggested. The angiographic appearance of FMD is classified as multifocal FMD, where the classic 'string-of-beads' appearance is seen typically in the middle and distal two-thirds of the main renal artery (unlike atheromatous RAS which is usually ostial), and focal FMD, where a concentric, smooth, band-like focal stenosis is seen. FMD is highly responsive to revascularisation with angioplasty and should be attempted in those with evidence of symptomatic disease (renovascular hypertension and renal atrophy).

Classically, RAS is suggested by the presence of hypertension, fluid overload, an abdominal bruit though this is very poor at discerning, progressive deterioration of renal function, acutely worsening renal function after the introduction of an angiotensin-converting enzyme (ACE) inhibitor (poor sensitivity and specificity) and episodes of unexplained flash pulmonary oedema or angina.

The gold-standard diagnostic test is intravenous contrast-enhanced digital subtraction angiography. However, non-invasive tests are often sufficient in confirming the diagnosis. Due to its wide availability and low cost, ultrasonography and colour Doppler studies are often the first imaging study used to investigate RAS; however, results are operator-dependent, and stenotic lesions are often missed. Preferable imaging modalities are computed tomography (CT) and magnetic resonance (MR) angiography. Both have sensitivities over 90%, and the choice of modality may be guided by factors such as renal function and the presence of implanted devices. MRI tends to overestimate RAS particularly if there is generalised vascular calcification.

Rarer causes of renovascular hypertension include middle-aortic syndrome, Takayasu's arteritis, which primarily affects women in 80–90% of cases and may be expected in case of absent or diminished peripheral pulses, most commonly at the level of radial arteries.

Other rare causes include page kidney (acute hypertension secondary to intra capsular haematoma) and suprarenal coarctation of the aorta.

15.12.3 Coarctation of the Aorta

Coarctation is a rare but important cause, representing about 6–8% of all congenital heart disease and 1 in 2500 births [30]. It is seven times more common in white than Asian children. Patients may present as children or adolescents with symptoms of dyspnea, leg cramps on exercise, chest pain, fainting and shortness of breath but are increasingly identified earlier because of other congenital heart disease or as investigation of mid-systolic murmur (radiating to the back). Making the diagnosis is critical as untreated there is 80% mortality by 50 years. Cool feet and poor lower limb pulses are a strong clue; radio-femoral delay and unequal blood pressure in limbs are non-invasive and useful simple clinical examinations (◘ Figs. 15.3 and 15.4).

15.12.4 Distal Tubular Disorders

Rare, inherited dysfunctions of the distal renal tubule can cause increase sodium absorption and hypertension. The most important of these is Liddle's syndrome.

Liddle's syndrome is the result of mutations in the genes which encode the amiloride-sensitive epithelial sodium channel (ENaC) in the distal nephron which increases both the numbers and activity of the channels. This results in increased sodium and water retention and therefore hypertension. It is inherited in an autosomal dominant fashion and is probably the most common type of monogenic hypertension. It usually presents in

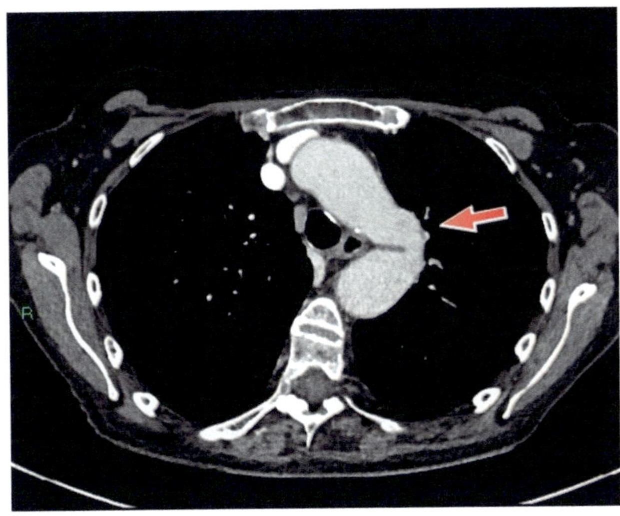

Fig. 15.3 Aortic coarctation, contrast CT thorax. (Image courtesy of Dr. Mohammad Khosh Zaban, Radiologist at Royal Free Hospital)
A 54-year-old Caucasian gentleman presented with exertional dyspnea. His past medical history was significant for dyslipidaemia, diabetes and hypertension. His hypertension was poorly controlled despite a combination of antihypertensive agents. On examination, his blood pressure was 160/90 mmHg in both arms, heart rate 70 beats per minute. Femoral pulses were weak and delayed compared to radial pulse

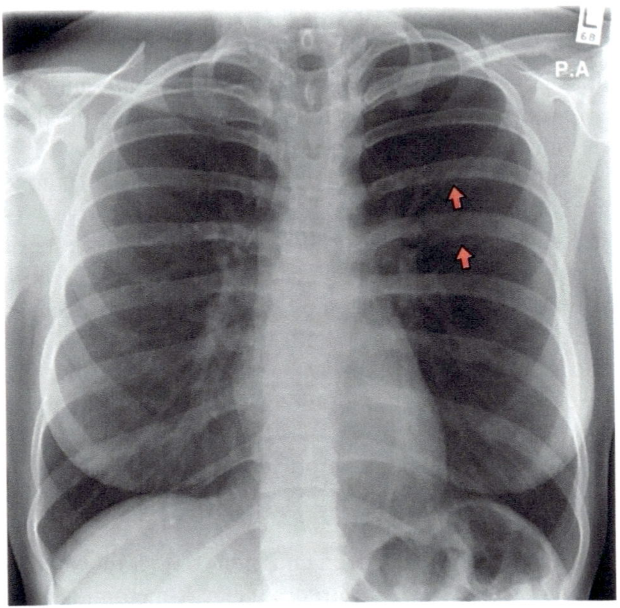

Fig. 15.4 Rib notching, chest X-ray. (Image courtesy of Dr. Mohammad Khosh Zaban, Radiologist at Royal Free Hospital)

childhood or early adulthood with hypertension and hypokalaemia. A key diagnostic feature is that plasma renin and aldosterone levels are markedly suppressed. Treatment includes dietary salt restriction and inhibitors of the ENaC such as amiloride.

Another, familial autosomal disease of the distal nephron is Gordon's syndrome (pseudohypoaldosteronism type II). Gain-of-function mutations in the thiazide-sensitive sodium chloride co-transporter result in excessive sodium and chloride reabsorption, hypertension and hyperkalaemia.

15.13 Endocrine Causes of Secondary Hypertension

There a multiple endocrine causes of secondary hypertension which should be considered in any secondary work-up. In addition to mineralocorticoid excess, Cushing's syndrome and pheochromocytoma which are all detailed below, hypertension may also be a feature of the following endocrine disorders:

1. Hyper- and hypothyroidism: In hyperthyroidism, free T3 dilates peripheral arterioles leading to fall in systemic vascular resistance and fall in effective arterial volume. This causes stimulation of renin angiotensin system. In hypothyroidism, there is increased salt sensitivity and renal sodium reabsorption leading to expansion of blood volume [23].
2. Hyperparathyroidism: It has been proposed that abnormal calcium metabolism may lead to alteration of vascular tone and result in increased total peripheral vascular resistance [24].
3. Acromegaly: There is increased peripheral vascular resistance due to chronic IGF-1 excess [25].
4. Carcinoid syndrome: Predominantly due to serotonin release by tumour cells.

15.13.1 Mineralocorticoid Excess

Mineralocorticoid excess results in increased renal sodium reabsorption and hypertension. It is most often the result of primary aldosteronism.

Primary aldosteronism is characterised by overproduction of the mineralocorticoid aldosterone. Approximately 30% are due to adrenal adenomas, with the majority being due to bilateral adrenal hyperplasia. Rarely it may be due to unilateral adrenal hyperplasia.

The incidence of primary aldosteronism may be as high as 20% in patients with resistant hypertension, and primary aldosteronism is the commonest curable cause of secondary hypertension. Hypokalaemia is not a reliable indicator as less than 15% may present with this finding [26], and thus previous studies which were reliant on this finding to make the diagnosis grossly underestimated its prevalence. Although not ubiquitous, it is an important signal to trigger investigation.

Table 15.6 Effect of antihypertensives on serum renin and aldosterone levels

Drug Group	Examples	Effect on renin	Effect on aldosterone	Comments
Beta blockers	Atenolol, bisoprolol, metoprolol	↓	↓	Generally consistent effect
Potassium-sparing diuretics	Amiloride, spironolactone	↑	↑	Very large increases in renin
ACE inhibitors	Enalapril, perindopril, Ramipril	↑	↓	Large increases in renin. Effect on aldosterone less consistent
Thiazide (and thiazide-like) diuretics	Bendroflumethiazide, chlorthalidone, metolazone	↑	↑	Consistent effect with renin, more variable with aldosterone
Loop diuretics	Bumetanide, frusemide	↑	⟷/↓	Only small changes seen
Calcium channel antagonists	Amlodipine, felodipine, nifedipine	⟷/↓/↑	⟷/↓/↑	Variable, unpredictable effects
Alpha channel antagonists	Doxazosin, indoramin, tamsulosin	Non-significant	Non-significant	Best when measuring renin and aldosterone

A good initial screening test is measurement of plasma renin levels, with or without the addition of plasma aldosterone levels and calculation of a renin/aldosterone (R/A) ratio.

A suppressed renin and elevated aldosterone – resulting in an elevated ratio (>800) is suggestive of primary aldosteronism; however, a ratio >2000 with aldosterone >250 pmol/L makes the diagnosis almost certain in the absence of polluting drugs which must be omitted prior to testing as the results may be uninterpretable.

However, this test must be interpreted with caution in the elderly or black patients who tend to have lower renin levels and those on drugs which interfere with the renin-angiotensin-aldosterone pathway (Table 15.6). This is clearly a common problem in patients with resistant hypertension that may be on several of these agents. Ideally, the antihypertensives are stopped between 2 and 6 weeks prior to the measurement of serum renin and aldosterone levels. Beta blockers have the biggest impact and make the ratio uninterpretable as they prevent renin release. Alpha-blockers, diltiazem, or hydralazine can be used to treat the hypertension during this period. Calcium channel blockers have unpredictable effects on renin and aldosterone but are nonetheless commonly used to control blood pressure in such patients. Spironolactone has a long-acting effect and should be omitted for 6 weeks prior to testing. Time of day, posture and serum potassium levels are other important factors which may affect renin. Ideally potassium should be corrected into the normal range, and R/A ratio following normal saline infusion is said to be more specific. Test is positive if aldosterone (pmol/L)/Renin (mcg/L/hr) (ARR) >550 and aldosterone >416 pmol/L.

15

Confirmatory functional tests involve aldosterone suppression utilising oral or intravenous salt loading, fludrocortisone or captopril, although these are seldom used in practice. The ARR criterion is highly suggestive of primary aldosteronism, but in equivocal cases, a saline suppression or captopril challenge test is more discerning. CT or MR imaging is required to identify the presence of an adenoma. The absence of adenoma does not exclude the diagnosis, and in a small minority of cases, visible adenomas are not the source of aldosterone.

Subsequently, adrenal vein sampling (AVS) allows for confirmation and localisation of the primary aldosteronism to one or both adrenals. The success rate of this procedure depends on accurate cannulation of both adrenal veins. The adequacy of AVS is determined by the ratio of cortisol concentration in the adrenal vein and in the inferior vena cava. AVS is a technically challenging procedure that should be carried out by an experienced practitioner.

AVS is particularly important as identified adenomas may be non-functioning or may in fact be the result of nodular hyperplasia.

More recently, positron emission tomography (PET) CT, utilising the radiotracer (11) C-metomidate, a potent inhibitor of adrenal steroidogenic enzymes, has been developed as a non-invasive alternative to adrenal vein sampling [27].

Rarer causes of mineralocorticoid excess include the following:

1. Congenital adrenal hyperplasia – Defects in 11-hydroxylase and 17-hydroxylase (key enzymes in the production of adrenal steroids) result in excessive

accumulation of intermediate products with mineralocorticoid activity. In addition to hypertension, patients have genital ambiguity.

2. Glucocorticoid-remediable aldosteronism – A rare autosomal dominant disorder in which a fusion of two genes results in aldosterone production being stimulated by adrenocorticotropic hormone (ACTH).
3. Apparent mineralocorticoid excess – A rare autosomal recessive disorder in which an inactivating mutation of the 11 B-hydroxysteroid dehydrogenase type II enzyme allows cortisol to activate the mineralocorticoid receptor.
4. Exogenous mineralocorticoid excess – May be the result of fludrocortisone administration or excess licorice ingestion.

15.13.2 Cushing's Syndrome

Cushing's syndrome is caused by excess glucocorticoids, which is most commonly iatrogenic. It may also be due to over production of ACTH by the pituitary gland (Cushing's disease) or by production of cortisol by a tumour of the adrenal gland or rarely by ectopic release from another organ or gland. The syndrome affects <0.1% of the total population but causes hypertension in approximately 80% of those affected [28].

Screening tests include 24-hour urinary cortisol excretion (sensitivity 76–100%, specificity 95–98%) and the single-dose (1 mg) dexamethasone suppression test (sensitivity 95%, specificity 86%) where a normal response is suppression of serum cortisol to less than 50 nmol/L. Positive results should be confirmed by performing at least one other tests or midnight cortisol. Prednisolone should be stopped at least 24 hours prior to the test as it cross reacts with assays and has a half-life of 3.5 hours and so takes 16–18 hours to be adequately cleared from the circulation.

Subsequent localising tests include plasma ACTH, long dexamethasone suppression tests and the corticotrophin-releasing hormone stimulation test.

15.13.3 Pheochromocytoma

Pheochromocytoma is a rare cause of secondary hypertension accounting for <0.5% of patients with hypertension (*M*/*F* 2:1), but some case series have reported an incidence of 4% in patients with resistant hypertension [29]. Approximately 85% arise from the adrenal glands, with the remainder, termed 'paragangliomas' arising from extra-adrenal chromaffin tissue, typically in the abdomen, urinary bladder or mediastinum. They can be inherited, often as part of a multiple endocrine neoplasia syndrome or acquired.

The diagnosis should be suspected in patients who report episodic headaches, palpitations (64%) and sweating (70%) in addition to hypertension. Episodic pallor, tremor, flushing, epigastric pain, dyspnea, syncope and hypotension are also important though less common findings. It can also present with hypokalaemia. Of note, previous cohort studies have suggested that up to 70% of such patients are hypertensive, but since many are now picked up incidentally, hypertension is only a feature in approximately half. Screening tests (in order of sensitivity) include plasma-free metanephrines (99%), urinary fractionated metanephrines (97%), urinary and plasma catecholamines (85%), urinary total metanephrines (77%) and vanillylmandelic acid (VMA) (64%) (◘ Fig. 15.6).

Confirmatory tests include glucagon stimulation and clonidine suppression tests, and cross-sectional imaging is required to localise the tumour. In the case of extra-adrenal tumours, isotopic scanning with meta-iodobenzylguanidine (MIBG) can be of use.

15.14 Other Causes of Secondary Hypertension

There are several other secondary causes of hypertension which are listed in ◘ Table 15.5. Obstructive sleep apnoea and obesity are particularly important causes which will now be discussed further.

15.14.1 Obstructive Sleep Apnoea

There is a strong association between obstructive sleep apnoea (OSA) and hypertension (present in 50–90% of patients with OSA and with increasing severity, the associated hypertension is more difficult to control). The proposed mechanism to explain this association is that intermittent hypoxaemia induces a sustained increase in sympathetic nervous system activity, which intern raises blood pressure by well-described mechanisms. The cardiovascular risk of OSA is a significant and an important cause of hypertension not to miss. Loss or reversal of nocturnal dipping (the usual 10% drop in BP at night) may be prominent, and a clue but history or body habitus of OSA should prompt exclusion of OSA as a contributor to hypertension as correction can sometimes have a marked effect on hypertension and cardiovascular risk.

15.14.2 Obesity

Although not strictly considered a secondary cause of hypertension, obesity is a strong independent risk factor for hypertension. Furthermore, observations that there are an increasing number of children and adolescents with hypertension are likely attributed to the rising prevalence of obesity. In 2010, 16.9% of children and adolescents in the USA were obese, which was significantly higher than a decade before [31] and has been driven by diet and lifestyle changes. If this trend continues there will be an epidemic of hypertension and other obesity-related comorbidities in western countries.

15.14.3 Familial Dysautonomia

Familial dysautonomia (FD) is a rare hereditary sensory and autonomic neuropathy (type III) and is also known as Riley-Day syndrome. It is caused by a point mutation in the IKBKAP gene. It is characterised by dramatic blood pressure instability due to baroreflex failure. Other signs and symptoms include impaired swallowing leading to aspiration pneumonia, diminished pain and temperature perception, impaired proprioception, optic neuropathy and corneal opacities, leading to visual loss.

The excessive BP variability over time leads to target organ damage and decline in eGFR. A cardinal feature of FD is hypertensive vomiting attack which occurs when stimuli increase sympathetic outflow and catecholamine release continues unopposed. Common triggers include infection, illness, emotions or surgery.

Orthostatic hypotension is also a feature of FD as the normal reflex increase of sympathetic outflow on standing is absent. However, syncope is infrequent and usually suggests volume depletion or an alternate cause.

15.15 Conclusion

As hypertension is the most important modifiable risk factor for cardiovascular and renal disease, an understanding of its diagnosis and thresholds for treatment is crucial to impact on cardiovascular and renal disease. National and international published guidelines provide a useful framework for the diagnosis of hypertension, but differences in approach exist. When measuring blood pressure and making decisions to treat, considerations include not only the measured clinic blood pressure but an overall assessment of cardiovascular risk, end-organ damage (clinical or subclinical) and the need for 24-hour ABPM. Further considerations and investigations of secondary causes are required in those that present young, with accelerated hypertension or apparent resistant hypertension.

15

Case Study

Case 1

A 45-year-old male with no past medical history presented with a 4-month history of headaches and generalised weakness. On examination, physical examination was unremarkable apart from a BP of 190/105 mmHg, which was initially treated with a calcium channel blocker. Initial investigation revealed Na 132 mmol/L, K 3.3 mmol/L, urea 4 mmol/L, Cr 100 µmol/L and bicarbonate 36 mmol/L. In view of hypertension and hypokalaemic alkalosis, an aldosterone to renin ratio was checked and was found to be consistent with the suspected diagnosis of primary hyperaldosteronism. An abdominal CT showed slight enlargement of the left adrenal gland (◘ Fig. 15.5). This was followed by adrenal vein sampling which confirmed left-sided lateralisation of plasma aldosterone concentration. A left adrenalectomy was performed which had a good clinical and biochemical response. Treatment includes medical therapy with mineralocorticoid receptor antagonist for bilateral disease and adrenalectomy for unilateral aldosterone producing adenoma.

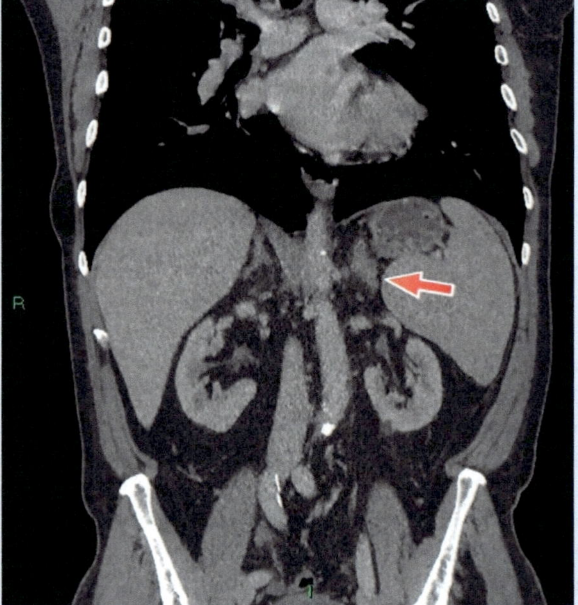

◘ **Fig. 15.5** Primary aldosteronism (Conn's syndrome), left adrenal adenoma, CT adrenals. (Image courtesy of Dr. Mohammad Khosh Zaban, Radiologist at Royal Free Hospital)

Case 2

A 46-year-old male with no past medical history presents with episodic headaches, sweating, palpitations and

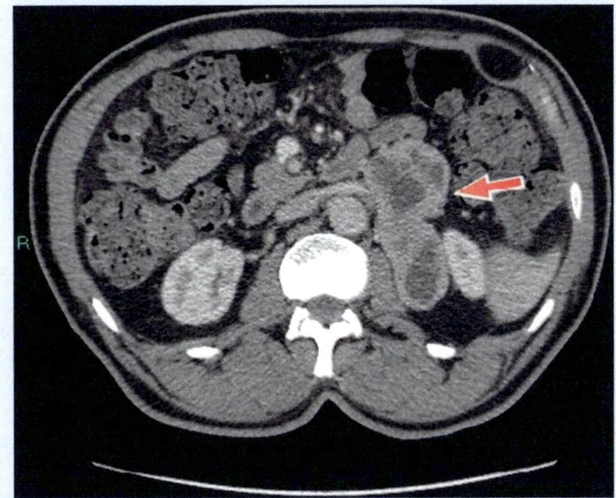

■ **Fig. 15.6** Pheochromocytoma, CT adrenals. (Image courtesy of Dr. Mohammad Khosh Zaban, Radiologist at Royal Free Hospital)

tremor. On examination, his blood pressure was elevated at 170/92 mmHg, heart rate 117 beats per minute and respiratory rate of 20 breaths per minute. He was diaphoretic. His 24-hour urine metanephrine excretion was elevated at 39.69 umol/24 hours and urine normetanephrines elevated at 13.67 umol/24 hours.

Case 3

A 35-year-old woman was diagnosed with hypertension, refractory to treatment with three antihypertensive agents. All routine serum and urine tests performed as part of work-up for secondary hypertension were normal. A magnetic resonance angiography (MRA) of renal arteries was performed which demonstrated beaded aneurysms in the mid-portion of the right main renal artery representing the classic 'string-of-beads' appearance of fibromuscular dysplasia (■ Fig. 15.7). She underwent percutaneous transluminal balloon angioplasty of the right renal artery. Three months post-procedure, the patient was normotensive and off all antihypertensive agents.

FMD is rare but should be considered in a young patient with resistant hypertension.

Treatment for patients with FMD may include medical therapy and surveillance or endovascular therapy for

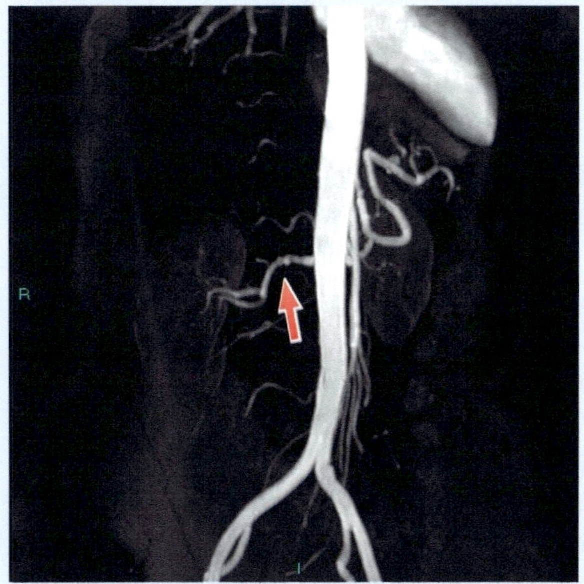

■ **Fig. 15.7** Renal artery stenosis due to fibromuscular dysplasia, MRA renal. (Image courtesy of Dr. Mohammad Khosh Zaban, Radiologist at Royal Free Hospital)

stenosis, depending on the nature and location of vascular lesions.

Case 4

A 42-year-old obese Asian gentleman presented with a 1 day history of acute severe headache. He was previously healthy and well and had no past medical history but complained of morning headache for 1 month, fatigue and excessive daytime somnolence. Physical examination revealed a blood pressure of 220/110 mmHg. He had a neck circumference of 40 cm. Investigations for secondary work-up for hypertension including bloods and imaging were unremarkable. Renal ultrasound, chest X-ray and CT brain were normal. Fundoscopy was normal. He was treated as hypertensive urgency.

He was sent for polysomnography due to his history of daytime somnolence which confirmed sleep apnoea. He was successfully treated with continuous positive airway pressure (CPAP), and his blood pressure also improved with strict adherence to CPAP treatment.

OSA may be an important, treatable cause of secondary hypertension and must be considered.

Chapter Review Questions

1. In which patients should secondary hypertension be considered?
2. Outline the causes of secondary hypertension.
3. Name two rare distal tubular disorders associated with hypertension.
4. Which class of drugs prevents renin release and must be stopped prior to measuring renin-aldosterone ratio while investigating for primary aldosteronism?
5. Which drugs do not interfere with renin/aldosterone production and can be used to treat hypertension while investigating for primary aldosteronism?

Answers

1. In younger patients (<40 years) who present with hypertensive emergencies or have accelerated hypertension with end-organ damage or those who have a strong family history of early onset hypertension.
2. *Renal*: Renal artery stenosis, renal parenchymal disease

   Endocrine: Primary hyperaldosteronism (Conn's syndrome), Cushing's syndrome, acromegaly, hyper-/hypothyroidism and hyperparathyroidism, pheochromocytoma,

   Arterial: Coarctation of the aorta

   Other: Obstructive sleep apnoea
3. Liddle's syndrome, Gordon's syndrome
4. Beta blockers
5. Alpha-blockers, calcium channel blockers and hydralazine

Tips and Tricks

1. When non-adherence is identified, giving ownership of blood pressure control as part of a healthy lifestyle to patients increases adherence and thus, outcome
2. Listen to patient's objections to specific drug types, and work with them to find a regime that they can tolerate to support adherence
3. Home BP monitoring can support healthy behaviours and adherence
4. Hypokalaemia in the absence of a diuretic or onset of hypertension under the age of 40 should precipitate a thorough search for secondary causes of hypertension

References

1. Kearney PM, Whelton M, Reynolds K, Muntner P, Whelton PK, He J. Global burden of hypertension: analysis of worldwide data. Lancet. 2005;365(9455):217–23.
2. Lewington S, Clarke R, Qizilbash N, et al. Age-specific relevance of usual blood pressure to vascular mortality: a meta-analysis of individual data for one million adults in 61 prospective studies. Lancet. 2002;360:1903–13.
3. Lawes CMM, Vander Hoorn S, Rodgers A. Global burden of blood-pressure-related disease, 2001. Lancet. 2008;371:1513–8.
4. Hsu C, McCulloch CE, Darbinian J, et al. Elevated blood pressure and risk of end-stage renal disease in subjects without baseline kidney disease. Arch Intern Med. 2005;165:923–8.
5. NICE. CG127 hypertension: NICE guideline. http://publications.nice.org.uk/hypertension-cg127. Accessed 24 Aug 2012.
6. Rosendorff C, Black HR, Cannon CP, et al. Treatment of hypertension in the prevention and management of ischemic heart disease a scientific statement from the American Heart Association Council for high blood pressure research and the councils on clinical cardiology and epidemiology and prevention. Circulation. 2007;115:2761–88.
7. Mancia G, De Backer G, Dominiczak A, et al. 2007 Guidelines for the management of arterial hypertension: the task force for the management of arterial hypertension of the European Society of Hypertension (ESH) and of the European Society of Cardiology (ESC). Eur Heart J. 2007;28:1462–536.
8. Mancia G, Laurent S, Agabiti-Rosei E, et al. Reappraisal of European guidelines on hypertension management: a European Society of Hypertension Task Force document. J Hypertens. 2009;27:2121–58.
9. Chapter 2. Measurement and clinical evaluation of blood pressure. Hypertens Res. 2009;32:11–23.
10. World Health Organization. Prevention of cardiovascular disease : guidelines for assessment and management of total cardiovascular risk. World Health Organization. 2007.
11. Law MR, Morris JK, Wald NJ. Use of blood pressure lowering drugs in the prevention of cardiovascular disease: meta-analysis of 147 randomised trials in the context of expectations from prospective epidemiological studies. BMJ. 2009;338 https://doi.org/10.1136/bmj.b1665.
12. De Galan BE, Perkovic V, Ninomiya T, et al. Lowering blood pressure reduces renal events in type 2 diabetes. J Am Soc Nephrol. 2009;20:883–92.
13. Head GA, Mihailidou AS, Duggan KA, et al. Definition of ambulatory blood pressure targets for diagnosis and treatment of hypertension in relation to clinic blood pressure: prospective cohort study. BMJ. 2010;340:c1104.
14. De la Sierra A, Segura J, Banegas JR, et al. Clinical features of 8295 patients with resistant hypertension classified on the basis of ambulatory blood pressure monitoring. Hypertension. 2011;57:898–902.
15. Mancia G, Facchetti R, Bombelli M, et al. Long-term risk of mortality associated with selective and combined elevation in office, home, and ambulatory blood pressure. Hypertension. 2006;47:846–53.

16. Sega R, Trocino G, Lanzarotti A, et al. Alterations of cardiac structure in patients with isolated office, ambulatory, or home hypertension: data from the general population (Pressione Arteriose Monitorate E Loro Associazioni [PAMELA] study). Circulation. 2001;104:1385–92.
17. Hansen TW, Jeppesen J, Rasmussen S, et al. Ambulatory blood pressure monitoring and risk of cardiovascular disease: a population based study. Am J Hypertens. 2006;19:243–50.
18. Caro JJ, Speckman JL, Salas M, et al. Effect of initial drug choice on persistence with antihypertensive therapy: the importance of actual practice data. CMAJ. 1999;160:41–6.
19. Van Wijk BL, Klungel OH, Heerdink ER, et al. Rate and determinants of 10-year persistence with antihypertensive drugs. J Hypertens. 2005;23:2101–7.
20. Palacio A, Garay D, Langer B, et al. Motivational interviewing improves medication adherence: a systematic review and meta-analysis. J Gen Intern Med. 2016;31:929–40.
21. Chan AHY, Horne R, Hankins M, Chisari C. The Medication Adherence Report Scale (MARS-5): a measurement tool for eliciting patients' reports of non-adherence. Br J Clin Pharmacol. 2020;86(7):1281–8.
22. Horne R, Weinman J, Hankins M. The beliefs about medicines questionnaire: the development and evaluation of a new method for assessing the cognitive representation of medication. Psychol Health. 1999;14(1):1–24.
23. Berta E, Lengyel I, Halmi S, et al. Hypertension in thyroid disorders. Front Endocrinol (Lausanne). 2019;10:482. Published 2019 Jul 17. https://doi.org/10.3389/fendo.2019.00482.
24. Schiffl H, Lang SM. Hypertension secondary to PHPT: cause or coincidence? Int J Endocrinol. 2011;2011:974647. https://doi.org/10.1155/2011/974647.
25. Ramos-Leví AM, Marazuela M. Bringing cardiovascular comorbidities in acromegaly to an update. How should we diagnose and manage them? Front Endocrinol (Lausanne). 2019;10:120. Published 2019 Mar 7. https://doi.org/10.3389/fendo.2019.00120.
26. Stowasser M, Gordon RD, Gunasekera TG, et al. High rate of detection of primary aldosteronism, including surgically treatable forms, after 'non-selective' screening of hypertensive patients. J Hypertens. 2003;21:2149–57.
27. Burton TJ, Mackenzie IS, Balan K, et al. Evaluation of the sensitivity and specificity of (11) C-metomidate positron emission tomography (PET)-CT for lateralizing aldosterone secretion by Conn's adenomas. J Clin Endocrinol Metab. 2012;97:100–9.
28. Newell-Price J, Bertagna X, Grossman AB, et al. Cushing's syndrome. Lancet. 2006;367:1605–17.
29. Martell N, Rodriguez-Cerrillo M, Grobbee DE, et al. High prevalence of secondary hypertension and insulin resistance in patients with refractory hypertension. Blood Press. 2003;12:149–54.
30. Kenny D, Hijazi ZM. Coarctation of the aorta: from fetal life to adulthood. Cardiol J. 2011;18:487–95.
31. Ogden CL, Carroll MD, Kit BK, et al. Prevalence of obesity and trends in body mass index among US children and adolescents, 1999-2010. JAMA. 2012;307:483–90.

Further Reading

https://www.nice.org.uk/guidance/ng136/chapter/Recommendations#diagnosing-hypertension.

Management of High Blood Pressure

M. Umaid Rauf and Jennifer Cross

Contents

M. Harber (ed.), *Primer on Nephrology*, https://doi.org/10.1007/978-3-030-76419-7_16

Learning Objectives

1. To explore the treatment of high blood pressure with lifestyle modifications and various drug classes to prevent end-organ damage and identification of the indications and contraindications of specific drug groups when making decisions about treatment initiation and escalation.
2. To describe the management of hypertensive crises and its aim to reduce end-organ damage.
3. To appreciate that achieving BP targets in a substantial proportion of patients is difficult because it is usually asymptomatic, no gain is immediately discernible to patients for decades and commencing treatment usually commits the patient to lifelong daily medication in the majority often in youth when there is likely to be the greatest gain. Its management is akin to convincing patients to invest in a health pension. Pay now to protect yourself from the unknown later with no guarantee that it will be effective.

16.1 Introduction

Treatment of blood pressure in the context of renal disease is important for several reasons. If unchecked it is a common cause of end-stage kidney disease (EKD); high BP is a consequence of renal disease and impacts upon many other organ systems; and finally hypertension is a major modifiable risk factor for CVD which in turn is the main cause of mortality and morbidity in individuals with EKD. The approach to treatment of BP should be similar in those with and without established renal disease. For the most part, antihypertensives that are efficacious and reduce risk in groups without renal failure, often excluded from major cardiovascular trials, broadly seem to benefit at least as much and possibly more in groups with renal failure as the event rate in these individuals is considerably higher.

Randomised controlled trials (RCTs) demonstrate BP reduction, whether achieved by diet, lifestyle or drug therapy, and reduce the risk of CHD, stroke and EKD. Review of RCTs of drugs that demonstrate effective BP lowering demonstrates that a 5-year sustained reduction of 5–6 mm Hg reduces coronary events by 20% and stroke by 40% [1]. This is in keeping with evidence from prospective observational studies that predict lowering BP confers the same magnitude of protection [2]. There has been much discussion about specific drugs and their efficacy in reducing cardiovascular risk, but the overall signal from the evidence appears to be that it is more important to achieve blood pressure lowering than to focus on which drug is used to achieve it.

16.2 Non-pharmacological Management of Hypertension

Many patients, particularly those age group under 40 and some patients from BAME groups, find the concept of committing to lifelong antihypertensive agents daunting and would prefer a more natural solution. In general this is adequate in only the minority, but supporting this avenue of treatment initially goes a long way to creating a cooperative therapeutic relationship between clinician and patient to support engagement in self-testing and ownership of this long-term condition which in turn increases compliance when and if pharmacological interventions are required. A number of non-pharmacological interventions have been shown to be effective in randomised controlled trials, producing sustained reductions in blood pressure. These measures can therefore be a useful first strategy for lowering BP in individuals, particularly where no end-organ damage has been identified. *Lifestyle modifications offer the potential to lower BP in a simple, inexpensive, effective manner and also improve a range of other health-related outcomes (e.g. alteration in lipid profile resulting from diet and exercise and liver function through moderation of alcohol intake).*

Such measures include:

1. Salt (reducing sodium intake from 10 g/d to 5 g/d leads to a ~5/3 mm Hg reduction in BP) [3, 4]: Recommendation is for lowering salt intake to <90 mmol (<2 g) per day of sodium (corresponding to 5 g of sodium chloride), unless contraindicated. Salt retention is associated with high BP in patients with CKD. The vast majority of salt is not added to food but instead found in everyday food. In a typical western diet, a lunch of a ham and cheese sandwich and a packet of crisps constitutes the majority of your daily salt intake.
2. Alcohol (reduction is dependent upon initial consumption) [5]: Recommended alcohol intake to no more than two standard drinks, units, per day for men and no more than one unit for women.
3. Weight: Recommend healthy weight corresponds to BMI 20–25. On average you can expect a 1–2 mm Hg BP for every kg above an ideal BMI [6]. In CKD patients, weight reduction also confers other health benefits including reduction in urine albumin or protein levels, an independent negative prognosticator, improved lipid profile and increased insulin sensitivity and reduction in hepatic steatosis which is a common incidental finding in hypertension. The impact of weight control in the management of hypertension is demonstrated in a meta-analysis of 57 studies that showed improvement and resolution of hypertension after bariatric surgery in morbidly obese

patients, defined as BMI >40 kg/m^2 or BMI >35 kg/m^2 with significant comorbidities [7].

4. Exercise: Thrice weekly aerobic exercise results in an average reduction of ~3/4 mm Hg [8]. The KDIGO 2012 guidelines recommend undertaking exercise for at least 30 minutes five times per week to optimise cardiovascular health and reduce blood pressure.
5. Diet: A diet rich in fresh fruit and vegetables, whole grains and low-fat dairy products, with reduced content of total and saturated fat, is effective in blood pressure lowering by approximately 11 mm Hg. Dietary potassium supplementation (~ 3500–5000 mg/d) through consumption of high-potassium foods reduces BP by 4/5 mm Hg. This is limited in advanced renal impairment because of the risks of potassium supplementation resulting in accumulation in renal impairment below a GFR of 25 ms/ min [9]. The Dietary Approaches to Stop Hypertension (DASH) eating pattern is well established to reduce BP, by 6.7/3.5 mm Hg [10].
6. [11–13] Fish oil supplementation is similarly effective although the mechanism is unclear.
7. A variety of psychosocial stressors (e.g. occupational stress, poor social support); negative personality traits like anxiety, anger and depression; and reduced sleep duration/quality, in association with sleep apnoea, have also been associated with high BP.
8. A number of environmental exposures, including loud noises (e.g. traffic), colder temperatures (e.g. winter), higher altitudes and air pollutants, exacerbate high BP.
9. Although nicotine in cigarette smoke is a vasodilator initially, in the medium term it is associated with rebound vasoconstriction, and although precise mechanisms are unclear, the same applies to many recreational substances such as marijuana and cocaine, in particular, that both result in vasoconstriction, especially cocaine which can be associated with hypertensive crises and severe acute renal failure. Cigarette and recreational substance use effect on overall cardiovascular risk is multiplicative and is eminently modifiable as a risk factor making advice on cessation a routine part of care.

16

16.2.1 Role of Evidenced Natural Therapies as Antihypertensive Agents

The increasing role of Complementary and Alternative Medicine (CAM) in treatment of various health conditions including hypertension relates to a number of factors including de-medicalising long-term conditions, health belief systems held by patients who need to integrate management into their lifestyle. Natural remedies are perceived as safe, holistic and inexpensive and provide a sense of authority and control over health, independent of conventional medicine and the sickness role. Several clinical trials have demonstrated efficacy of natural herbs in BP lowering. The mechanisms of action are attributed primarily to their effect on vascular smooth muscle generating a variety of intermediaries including nitric oxide (NO). They also combat pathological damage to vessels by reversing endothelial dysfunction resulting from imbalance between vasodilators (NO, PGI2) and vasoconstrictors (Enthothelin-1, thromboxane, PDGF) and also by modifying ROS (reactive oxygen species) generated by various pathological states [14].

Some widely used herbs in the treatment of hypertension and CVD, validated by randomised control trials, include:

1. Garlic
2. Beetroot
3. Tea (black and green)
4. Berberine
5. Hawthorns
6. Saffron
7. Roselle
8. Black cumin
9. Ginseng

Some of the most scientifically persuasive evidence exists for beetroot and other food stuffs high in nitrates such as celery, cabbage and other leafy green vegetables including spinach and some lettuce. Dietary inorganic nitrates eaten enter the circulation rapidly; some of them are absorbed and then resecreted in a concentrated form in saliva, a process known as the enterosalivary nitrate circulation. Bacteria in the mouth convert inorganic nitrate to nitrite [15] which is swallowed and then absorbed into the circulation where it acts as a substrate for conversion to NO resulting in vasodilation and cardiovascular protection [16]. Professor Ahluwalia's group demonstrated that supplementation of dietary nitrate (6.4 mmol nitrate daily equivalent to a glass of beetroot juice daily) for 4 weeks was associated with robust, sustained and clinically meaningful reductions in BP (measured by clinic, ambulatory and home methods) of ~8/4 mm Hg, an effect magnitude broadly in line with a single antihypertensive agent at full dose [17].

16.3 Drugs Used to Lower Blood Pressure

There are seven broad classes of antihypertensive drugs although the British National Formulary lists ~50 BP agents. Four drug classes dominate prescribing in the UK: angiotensin-converting enzyme (ACEi) inhibitors and angiotensin receptor blockers (ARBs) (A-class drugs), β-blockers (B-class drugs), calcium channel blockers (CCBs) (C-class drugs) and diuretics (D-class drugs). Each class has a differing mechanism of action [18], but all classes have been shown in RCTs to be effective in reducing the risk of cardiovascular and renal pathological outcomes.

Evidence from review of short-term trials (with blood pressure as the outcome) indicate that all classes of blood pressure-lowering drugs at either standard, half or quarter standard doses result in broadly comparable reductions in BP [19]. Combinations of drugs from different classes at low dose may provide a way of achieving additive or in some combinations multiplicative reductions in blood pressure with the possible advantage of a reduction in dose-related mechanism-based adverse effects, which are important causes of discontinuation of therapy [19].

Generic drugs are available for all the major drug classes. Reduced acquisition costs of drugs translate into cost savings to health providers, provided branded medications are avoided (from within these major classes). Newer agents available currently (e.g. aliskiren) or in the future can only be rationally prescribed if there are persuasive reasons to think that they are superior to existing generic drugs for which there is little evidence currently.

The evidence base for the efficacy of BP-lowering drugs from all the major classes reducing not just blood pressure itself but cardiovascular and renal outcomes is large, numbering ~150 RCTs over four decades. Broadly there are three types of trials conducted. Those that test active treatments versus placebo were the first trial to be performed in the 1940s to 1960s (long-term trials are no longer ethical because of the established benefits of BP-lowering), then those that test a more versus a less intensive BP-lowering regime and, lastly, trials of one active drug versus another so-called head-to-head trials. The first two categories of trial answer questions about the efficacy of BP lowering on outcome. However, differences between classes might be inferred by exploring evidence for heterogeneity in effect sizes across trials of different agents. The third category of trial investigates class- or drug-specific differences in efficacy. To ensure a fair test in a head-to-head trial of this type, the achieved BP in the two arms of such a trial *must* be similar, to allow that differences in outcome/event rates are not simply due to BP differences between the two arms. Two recent overviews [1, 20] have both interpreted the evidence in the context of achieved BP reductions and emphasised the similarity in effectiveness of different BP-lowering drugs in the prevention of cardiovascular outcomes with two possible exceptions: beta-blockers may have a class-specific advantage in reducing recurrent CHD events in patients who have suffered an MI, and dihydropyridine calcium channel blockers may have an advantage over other classes in the prevention of stroke. The number of patients with kidney disease in these trials is small, but it seems reasonable to extrapolate the findings to patients with kidney disease.

16.4 Controversies in Blood Pressure Management

Despite this evidence there continue to be controversies in the pharmacological management of BP. Until 2006, international guidance on BP management was largely uniform. The message was clear, and the recommendation was that the overarching benefit of antihypertensive medication is in lowering BP rather than the specific features of the drug used to achieve it. Subsequent to the publication of influential trials and meta-analysis [21, 22], guidance in England and Wales has evolved. As a consequence pharmacological updates of joint guidance issued by the National Institute for Health and Care Excellence (NICE) and the British Hypertension Society (BHS) have led to recommendation of A-class drugs as initial treatment in those <55 years and C-class drugs in those >55 years of age, while B-class drugs have been relegated to being a third- or fourth-line option. In the most recent NICE/BHS guidelines (▶ http://www.nice.org.uk/CG127), D-class drugs were relegated to a third-line option because they were considered to be less effective in reducing BP variability than C-class drugs. The rationale for the emphasis of updated guidelines on drug choice rather than BP reduction can be summarised as follows:

1. BP-lowering drugs differ in their BP-lowering efficacy in younger and older patients: drugs that target the renin-angiotensin system (A-/B-class drugs) are considered to be more effective in lowering BP in younger patients (aged under 55 years) than in older patients where renin concentration tends to be lower and C-/D-class drugs are considered more effective.
2. Differences exist in the efficacy and safety of different BP-lowering drug classes in different age and disease groups. Specifically:

- B-class (β-blockers) and D-class (thiazide diuretics) increase the risk of type 2 diabetes.
- B-class (β-blockers) in general and atenolol in particular confer less protection from stroke than other drug classes but greater protection post-myocardial infarction.
- A-class drugs confer a specific advantage, over and above BP-lowering, in protection from renal disease thought to relate to the reduction in transglomerular

pressure and the concomitant proteinuria which is an independent negative prognosticator.

3. Apparent differences in cardiovascular outcomes between the different drug classes may arise as a result of differences in their effect on diabetes risk, their effect on central (aortic) compared to peripheral (brachial artery) BP and their effect on BP variability.

However, the extent to which these proposals are supported by the evidence is debatable. The European and US guidelines on the treatment of hypertension remain largely similar to the pre-2006 UK guidance unswayed by the preceding arguments.

a. **Age as a Determinant of BP-Lowering Response to Different Drug Classes**

Recommendations that BP is best lowered with A-class drugs in patients aged under 55 years (in whom an activated renin-angiotensin system may be an important mechanism) and D-class diuretics or C-class calcium channel blockers in older patients (because sodium retention, with suppression of the renin-angiotensin system, may be more important) were based primarily on the findings of a mechanistic study ($n = 36$) that rotated young patients through monthly treatment with each of four main classes of BP-lowering drugs and assessed the effect on BP [23]. Since renin declines with age [24], and the major drug classes differ in their effect on the renin-angiotensin system [25], age has been proposed as a proxy for stratifying the response of BP medications on cardiovascular outcomes. However, on the few occasions when potential effect modification by age of the effect of BP treatment on cardiovascular outcomes has been evaluated, no major differences have been observed [20]. Similar analyses using renin concentrations (now possible with a rapid, cheap assay [26]) have yet to be conducted, and this therefore remains a hypothesis.

16

b. **β-Blockers and Stroke Prevention**

Two sources of evidence were influential in the relegation of B-class β-blockers from first-line treatment of the NICE guidance: the 2005 Anglo-Scandinavian Cardiovascular Outcomes Trial (ASCOT) [21] and three meta-analyses examining the efficacy of β-blockers in prevention of cardiovascular events, published in 2005–2006 [22, 27, 28]. ASCOT was a randomised trial comparing a C-class drug (amlodipine)-based treatment regimen (with addition of perindopril and then doxazosin if required) with a B-class drug (atenolol)-based treatment regimen (with the addition of bendroflumethiazide and then doxazosin if required) to achieve a BP <140/90 mm Hg. The trial was terminated early on the advice of the data safety monitoring committee because of a significant treatment difference in favour of patients randomised to the C-class-based regimen for two secondary endpoints (stroke and total cardiovascular events). There was no evidence of a difference in the primary endpoint of non-fatal myocardial infarction or fatal coronary heart disease. BP after intervention was lower in the group randomised to amlodipine compared to atenolol by on average 2/3 mm Hg throughout the trial. The trialists' analysis suggested the BP difference was insufficient to explain the disparity in event rates, but others have reached the opposite conclusion [29].

A subsequent meta-analysis examined trials comparing B-class drugs with other BP-lowering drugs [22]. Stroke risk was 16% higher (95% CI 4–30%) among patients randomised to B-class drugs than in those taking other drug classes. A number of other meta-analyses reached similar conclusions [27, 28]. However, they are all sensitive to the requirement to include only including RCT and did not take full account of differences in achieved BP between treatment arms. These limitations are borne out by a re-analysis [30] suggesting that achieved BP favoured the comparator drug over B-class drugs in all instances, which may explain the apparent benefit of other BP drugs over β-blockers. The BP disparity is unlikely to be because β-blockers are inherently less effective at lowering BP than other drugs but rather because achieving a precisely equivalent BP reduction in two arms of a comparator trial is extremely difficult.

The pairwise meta-analyses conducted by Law et al. [1] and that by the Blood Pressure Lowering Treatment Trialists' Collaboration [17] now supersede these studies. They examined the efficacy of all major BP drug classes (not just B-class drugs) in the context of the achieved reductions in BP. The Blood Pressure Lowering Treatment Trialists' Collaboration incorporated information from 190,606 participants across 31 treatment trials and concluded that all classes of drug were broadly equivalent with respect to protection from major cardiovascular events if achieved BP was taken into account. The investigators found a log-linear association between BP reduction and the relative risk of cardiovascular events, in keeping with predictions from observational studies. A second analysis by Law and colleagues, which included information from 147 published trials among 464,000 participants, concluded that the protective effect of lowering BP on coronary heart disease was the same for all drug classes in primary prevention, with the possible exception of the effect of C-class drugs on stroke [1]. The authors considered that this probably accounted for most of the apparent disadvantage of B-class drugs in stroke protection, because C-class calcium channel blockers had been the most common comparator drug in trials of B-class drugs.

c. **BP-Lowering Drugs and the Risk of Type 2 Diabetes**

Patients receiving B- or D-class drugs rather than A-class drugs are at higher risk of diabetes. But what is the magnitude of the blood glucose increase; by how much is the absolute risk of diabetes increased; and, importantly, how does this affect the risk of cardiovascular events?

In the ASCOT trial, diabetes risk was increased among people randomised to the B-class arm (atenolol-bendroflumethiazide) (the hazard ratio comparing C-class (amlodipine) with B-class (atenolol) was 0.70, 95% CI 0.63–0.78, equating to a risk difference of 11 per 1000 people over 5 years). However the average absolute difference in blood glucose concentration was only 0.2 mmol/L (SD 2.08 mmol/L, $P < 0.0001$). The substantial increase in the risk of diabetes arises because an average increase in glucose of as little as 0.2 mmol/L leads to an increase in the proportion of people marginally exceeding the diagnostic fasting blood glucose threshold of 7 mmol/L and therefore being classified as diabetic.

The evidence is less than compelling that this small average increase in glucose translates to a net reduction in protection from stroke or coronary heart disease. Recent overviews of prospective observational studies [31, 32] indicate that although the risk of coronary heart disease is linearly and modestly increased above a fasting glucose value of 5 mmol/L, the risk of stroke is substantially raised only at fasting glucose values well above 7 mmol/L [32].

In the ALLHAT trial (in which 33,357 patients were randomised to A-class (lisinopril), C-class (amlodipine), or D-class (chlorthalidone)), there was a difference in blood glucose of 0.16 mmol/L in the amlodipine group compared with the chlorthalidone group with an odds ratio for diabetes of 0.73 (0.58–0.91) [33]. Yet the hazard ratio for stroke after 4.9 years of follow-up was 0.93 (0.82–1.06). There was a very small BP disparity between the chlorthalidone and amlodipine arms (mean difference for amlodipine versus chlorthalidone 0.8 mm Hg systolic ($P = 0.03$)). This suggests that the observed differences in the risk of stroke in these trials are more likely to be explained by between-arm differences in BP rather than glucose level. The relevance of the small average increase in glucose is further brought into doubt by results of recent trials which indicate that, after 5 years follow-up, tight glucose control does not necessarily lead to a reduction in cardiovascular event rates [34].

d. **A-Class Drugs and Protection from Renal Disease**

UK guidance [35, 36] has encouraged the use of drugs that specifically block the renin-angiotensin system (including ACEi and ARBs) as first-line treatment to reduce proteinuria and slow the progression of renal disease. The recommendation, initially for those with diabetes and evidence of renal impairment, is now more generally applied even to those without diabetes. These recommendations evolved following randomised trials of A-class ACEi and subsequently ARBs that demonstrated a reno-protective effect. Implicit in the interpretation of the guidance is that inhibition of the renin-angiotensin system with ACEi/ARBs has specific reno-protective effects beyond lowering BP alone. However the RCTs on which this guidance was based compared ACEi and ARBs against placebo rather than another BP-lowering agent. Given that systemic BP is a major determinant of the progression of renal disease [37] and that BP differences are inevitable when comparing placebo with BP-lowering drugs, the between-treatment-arm BP differences may confound the observed effects on renal outcomes in placebo-controlled trials of ACEi/ARBs.

A previous systematic review and meta-analysis of RCTs investigated the effect of different classes of antihypertensive drugs on the progression of renal disease [38]. ACEi/AR0Bs, when compared to other BP-lowering drugs, stratified by degree of BP lowering, yielded a relative risk of 0.74 (95% CI 0.59–0.92), in the group with greatest degree of BP lowering (−6.9 mm Hg), and a RR of 0.9 (95% CI 0.72–1.12) in the group with the smallest degree of BP lowering (1.5 mm Hg), reinforcing the major role of BP differences as the mechanism to explain the observed benefits of A-class drugs over other antihypertensive drug classes on renal outcomes. Smaller studies demonstrated a smaller overall benefit in renal endpoints. There was little evidence of an advantage in the diabetic subgroup, in which the relative risk for end-stage renal failure was 0.89 (95% CI 0.74–1.07). Despite these findings, and the lack of large trials, the UK (and in this instance other international guidelines) recommends the use of A-class drugs first line to treat hypertension and retard progression of renal disease [35, 39]. This may be an example of a widely applied drug policy that over-reached its evidence base; it is an academic point given that most patients with kidney disease will require combination antihypertensive treatment.

16.5 Antihypertensive Treatment and Proteinuric Kidney Disease

Proteinuria is an independent predictor of poor outcome in renal disease, the development of renal disease in hypertension and cardiovascular events independent of blood pressure control. Protein, once it leaked through the basement membrane, is a direct tubular toxin. Various classes of antihypertensives have consistently been shown to slow progression of renal disease in proteinuric CKD, and by extension it seems logical that drugs which preferentially reduce proteinuria may retard progression of renal disease and reduce cardiovascular risk.

ACE inhibitors are established first-line therapy in proteinuric CKD as studied in AASK and REIN trials conducted in non-diabetic CKD populations which demonstrated a reduction in proteinuria in the treatment arm. ARBs have similar reno-protective effect, as evaluated in RENAAL and IDNT trials [40].

Combination therapy is sometimes used to decrease proteinuria, if not controlled by a single agent. Besides ACEi/ARBs combination, non-dihydropyridine CCBs and aldosterone antagonists have been studied and established as second-line drugs; however, the side effect profile requires close monitoring as hyperkalaemia in CKD population is common. KDIGO 2020 hypertension guidelines recommend against the use of dual RAAS blockade because of the significant risk of increased incidence of AKI with the combination in the context of unpredictable intercurrent illness.

Given the grave prognostic implications for cardiovascular and renal outcomes of heavy proteinuria, selecting antihypertensive agents that reduce proteinuria should be a major consideration.

16

16.5.1 Antihypertensive Effects of SGLT-2 Inhibitors

A quantum change in the management of proteinuric diabetic and recently non-diabetic [41] proteinuric renal disease has been the introduction of SGLT-2 inhibitors which have a modest antihypertensive effect.

The sodium glucose linked transporter-2 (SGLT-2) inhibitors like empagliflozin and canagliflozin, designed to reduce blood glucose with renal wasting, also consistently reduce blood pressure in a type 2 diabetic patient. The mechanism may include persistent negative caloric balance resulting in weight loss, osmotic diuresis, synergistic natriuretic activity with diuretics, improvement of endothelial function, reduction of vascular stiffness and inhibition of the sympathetic nervous system [42]. Because of the harmful cardiovascular effects of predecessor novel diabetes drugs, when SGLT-2 inhibitors were introduced, cardiovascular outcomes were carefully monitored, and somewhat unexpectedly the class demonstrated a reduction in cardiovascular events. It is unclear whether this is an effect of its blood pressure-lowering effect. Although this is an exciting potential opportunity for a novel agent to reduce cardiovascular risk in high-risk groups, use in hypertensives and those with renal impairment in the absence of diabetes remains unproven, and their use is not currently justified.

e. **Effectiveness of Thiazides in Prevention of Cardiovascular Events**

   The 2011 NICE guidance relegated diuretics (D-class drugs) from first to third choice. Diuretics as a class are among the most widely studied of all BP-lowering drugs and remain the preferred first-line agent for high BP treatment in the USA [43]. The prominence given to C-class calcium channel blockers over D-class diuretics was based on recent analysis of observational studies that BP variability might be more predictive of adverse cardiovascular outcomes than usual BP and that C-class drugs reduce BP variability to a greater extent than D-class drugs [44]. However, the evidence base for the relationship between usual BP and cardiovascular outcomes far exceeds that for BP variability, and no randomised trial has tested the influence of a reduction in BP variability on cardiovascular outcomes. The recommendation to use D-class thiazide-like diuretics rather than D-class thiazide diuretics was based on the interaction of these agents with carbonic anhydrase, which is no longer the major therapeutic target of these drugs.

f. **Aldosterone Antagonists and Resistant Hypertension**

   The efficacy of moderate dose of spironolactone as monotherapy has been studied in trials, and it has proved to improve BP in stage 2 essential hypertension [45]. However its side effect profile including metabolic profile disturbance, gynaecomastia (dose related), renal impairment and hyperkalaemia has limited its utilisation in low doses in resistant (~3 agents) hypertension. Its role as a fourth agent in treatment of uncontrolled hypertension was evaluated among participants of ASCOT trial [46].

   PATHWAY 2 RCT established spironolactone as the most effective add-on drug in treating resistant hypertension, partly due to its diuretic effect [47]. There is much less data with the alternative aldosterone antagonist eplerenone in this setting, but it is said to produce significantly less gynaecomastia (0.5%) than spironolactone (10%), and this makes it worth considering in male patients who might benefit from this class of drug.

16.6 Other Classes of Antihypertensives

Beyond the four main classes of antihypertensives, nephrologists often reach for alternatives either in the face of intractable hypertension or difficult side effects. Of these the most commonly used are alpha-blockers which have a good side effect profile as long as not short acting (in which case symptomatic postural hypotension is extremely common). The direct vasodilator hydralazine has a particular niche in the treatment of heart failure and is felt to be relatively safe in pregnancy but not particularly potent. Minoxidil, the other direct vasodilator, seems more potent but dosing is frequently limited by peripheral oedema, with hirsutism.

Centrally acting alpha adrenergic agents such as clonidine, methyldopa and guanfacine induce peripheral sympatho-inhibition and have their place (clonidine in ICU, methyldopa in pregnancy), but side effects including sedation, impotence and dry mouth limit their use. Newer drugs in this class such as moxonidine and rilmenidine seem to have a better side effect profile. It is important to remember that sudden discontinuation of clonidine can cause severe rebound hypertension.

16.7 Antihypertensives in Dialysis Population

The first line in management of hypertension in a dialysis patient is volume control. This starts with salt restriction, diuretics and reducing dry weight on dialysis.

Beta-blockers, mainly due to their positive impact on cardiovascular disease burden in this patient population, are generally preferred as first-line pharmacological intervention to treat hypertension. The Hypertension in Hemodialysis Patients Treated with Atenolol or Lisinopril (HDPAL) trial showed sustainable reduction in blood pressure in patients on maintenance haemodialysis with left ventricular hypertrophy over a period of 1 year, in atenolol treatment arm [48].

16.8 Management of Hypertensive Crises

A hypertensive crisis or emergency is defined as an acute elevation of blood pressure in the presence of acute, ongoing or rapidly deteriorating end-organ damage (shown in ◘ Table 16.1).

◘ **Table 16.1** Summary of hypertensive crises, signs and symptoms associated with their presentation and pharmacological approach for each

Hypertensive emergency	Important signs/symptoms	Key investigations	Preferred agent
Hypertensive encephalopathy	Headache, altered conscious level, seizures, focal neurological signs, haemorrhage/exudates and papilloedema on fundoscopy	MRI of the brain	Labetalol
Dissecting aortic aneurysm	Chest and back pain, BP in both arms, palpation of all peripheral pulses	CT or MRI of the aorta	Labetalol, GTN (only after labetalol to counter reflex tachycardia)
Acute ventricular failure with pulmonary oedema	Breathlessness, gallop rhythm, raised JVP, third heart sound, inspiratory crackles on auscultation	CXR, echo may be useful	GTN
Acute myocardial ischaemia/infarction	Chest pain, diaphoresis, breathlessness	ECG, cardiac enzymes	GTN, labetalol, esmolol
Eclampsia	Visual fields, headaches, altered mental state, acute stroke, abdominal pain, heart failure, oliguria		Labetalol (and delivery)
Acute kidney injury	Oliguria, uraemia, electrolyte-associated arrhythmias	Urea, creatinine, electrolytes, urinalysis	Labetalol, nicardipine
Sympathetic crisis (cocaine induced)	Labile blood pressure	Toxicology screen	Verapamil/diltiazem/nicardipine
Catecholamine associated crisis	Labile blood pressure with associated flushing	Urine catecholamines	Phentolamine

Hypertensive crisis most commonly presents as a complication of intrinsic or essential hypertension and can result from non-adherence with prescribed antihypertensive medication, but a larger proportion of this group have a secondary underlying cause which should be sought. It is important to distinguish hypertensive emergencies from severe hypertension without *acute* end-organ damage. While the latter does involve intensive treatment, it does not require immediate parenteral therapy and may be the difference between inpatient and outpatient management. Most hypertensive emergencies are associated with a systolic blood pressure (SBP) of greater than 180 mm Hg or a diastolic blood pressure (DBP) of greater than 110 mm Hg. Rarely it presents with more normal blood pressure readings in the context of specific patient groups who have experienced a rapid acceleration of BP such as the preeclamptic or those with thrombotic microangiopathy or conditions resulting in renal ischaemia such as dissection or HCV-related cryoglobulinaemia. Hypertensive crises require rapid introduction of controlled, modest blood pressure reduction over time, ideally with relatively non-potent, short-acting, parenteral therapy that can be titrated minute to minute. A high dependency setting is ideal with a high nursing ratio with arterial blood pressure and cardiac monitoring available. Rapid normalisation of blood pressure can result in end-organ hypoperfusion ischaemia or infarction. In the first 2 hours of management, a reduction in BP of 20% is appropriate; thereafter a reduction of 10% magnitude each day until 160/90 is reached, and in general conversion to an oral regime can be commenced and further escalation can be achieved in the outpatient area with weekly appointments. In the setting of arterial dissection, more rapid control is justified for organ salvage as hypertension is usually the driver for further dissection.

16

In contrast to the management of chronic hypertension, where there is a mature evidence base, there are no large randomised trials in the setting of hypertensive emergencies. This is likely to be due to the small numbers of individuals presenting in this way (1% of all those with hypertension) and the heterogeneity of the presentation (◘ Table 16.1). Management is therefore based on consensus rather than evidence.

16.9 Pathophysiology

Pathophysiology of hypertensive crises is not well understood. A crisis can develop de novo or can complicate an underlying primary or secondary cause of hypertension. The vast majority of hypertensive crises appear to occur in patients with background hypertension, the exceptions being eclampsia and de novo nephritic syndrome. A key first step is thought to be a rapid increase in systemic vascular resistance (SVR) precipitated by vasoconstrictor substances (e.g. noradrenalin, angiotensin II) or relative hypovolaemia. Like many other biological systems, the endothelium attempts to compensate by release of vasodilators to counter increases in SVR. However sustained hypertension overwhelms compensatory mechanisms, leading to further endothelial dysfunction, increase in vascular permeability, fibrinoid necrosis of the vessel wall, activation of platelet aggregation and the coagulation cascade. Activation of these systems can promote further inflammation of the endothelium, thrombosis and vasoconstriction.

16.10 Determination of Precipitant for Hypertensive Crises Is Crucial to Prevent Recurrence

Non-adherence to prescribed antihypertensive medications is the most common precipitating factor, but others to look for include use of prescribed, over-the-counter or illicit drugs (e.g. cocaine, amphetamines, sympathomimetic agents, nonsteroidal anti-inflammatory drugs and high-dose steroids). Patients with acute glomerulonephritis such as lupus, preeclampsia, phaeochromocytoma or scleroderma renal crisis may present with hypertensive urgency/emergency. Acute stroke or heart failure can be both cause and consequence of severe hypertension.

Further testing should be considered for secondary causes of hypertension if no precipitant is identified, such as renovascular disease, primary aldosteronism, glucocorticoid excess, phaeochromocytoma and, in younger patients, coarctation of the aorta [49].

Assessment and Clinical Evaluation A targeted history and examination supported by key laboratory and imaging investigations are essential. Salient features in any evaluation should establish pre-existing hypertension, its treatment, control and adherence to medication, concurrent clinical conditions that could precipitate a hypertensive crises and drugs including prescribed, over-the-counter or illicit such as cocaine. Examination should focus on identifying syndromes where rapid intervention can be life-saving (aortic dissection, eclampsia, hypertensive encephalopathy, acute renal failure, pulmonary oedema) as a priority but should not preclude a full examination as other complications may also be present. Assessment should be made of BP in both arms, in the supine, seated and standing position if possible, to determine volume status. Cardiac compromise in particular left ventricular failure can be assessed by examination of the jugular venous pressure, the presence of a gallop rhythm and/or fourth heart sound and presence of inspiratory crackles on auscultation of the lungs. Hypertensive encephalopathy can be detected by assessment of the conscious level, assessment of focal neurology and grades III or IV hypertensive retinopathy. Assessment and symmetry of all pulses should also be made and is particularly important where aortic dissection is suspected.

Investigations Bedside tests should include urine analysis to identify glomerulonephritis and electrocardiogram to assess ischaemic changes and in particular ST segment elevation which can be present in both acute myocardial infarction and aortic dissection. A chest radiograph in the presence of clinical signs and symptoms of left ventricular failure or aortic dissection can indicate a widened mediastinum (computed tomography (CT) aortogram or a magnetic resonance imaging (MRI) being the investigation of choice). In individuals presenting with hypertensive encephalopathy, CT brain imaging may be helpful to rule out intracranial haemorrhage or large infarcts although magnetic resonance imaging (MRI) is more sensitive to changes associated with hypertensive encephalopathy with typical findings of cerebral oedema and white matter changes. These can be extensive or more localised to the posterior part of the brain (occipital and parietal lobes), when it is known as posterior reversible encephalopathy syndrome (PRES) (see Fig. 16.1). PRES can however be also due to other causes such as calcineurin inhibitors, thrombotic microangiopathies and HIV. Changes associated with PRES as well as hypertensive encephalopathy are potentially reversible with treatment of the underlying cause. Blood tests should include renal function, electrolytes, LDH and a full blood count/platelet count with a peripheral blood film to exclude a thrombotic microangiopathic anaemia.

16.11 Therapeutic Approach to Hypertensive Crisis

In the absence of randomised evidence, consensus guidance recommends lowering mean arterial pressure by no more than 20–25% within a period of minutes up to 2 hours or a decrease in DPB to 100–110 mm Hg. This is best achieved by parenteral administration of blood pressure-lowering agents that are short acting and titratable. The one instance when more rapid BP reduction is indicated is aortic dissection, where BP lowering should be achieved within 10 minutes, whereas in all other crises an arbitrary time to achieve BP control of 1 hour is often used. Once endpoints are reached and maintained, patients can be commenced on oral maintenance therapy while parenteral agents are weaned off. End-organ vessels are often grossly abnormal with narrowed lumens but also unable to autoregulate and cannot vasodilate or compensate normally for precipitous hypoperfusion;

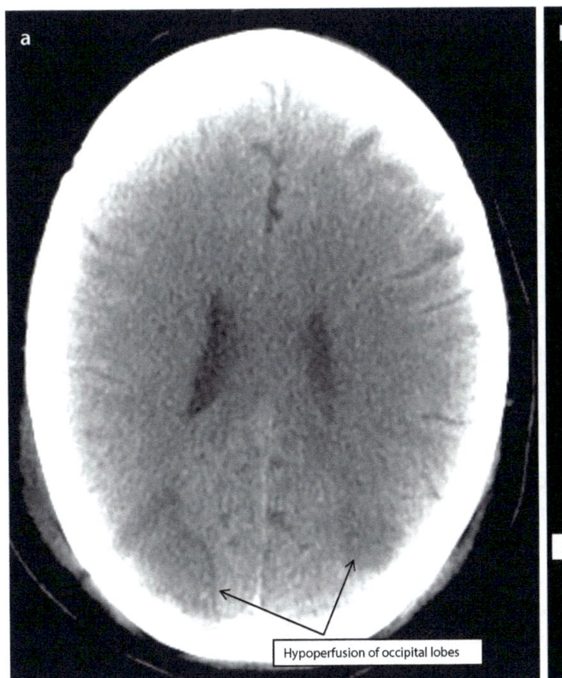

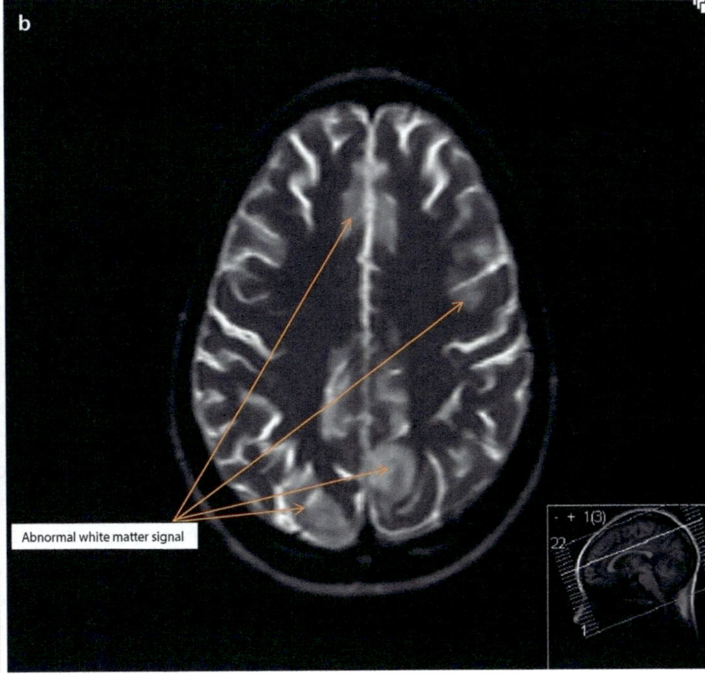

Fig. 16.1 **a** CT scan of a patient with CKD who developed bilateral cortical blindness with a blood pressure of 165/105 mm Hg. The scan shows bilateral hypoperfusion consistent with posterior reversible encephalopathy syndrome (PRES) and patient went on to recover her vision. **b** MRI scan showing extensive white matter changes in a 21-year-old with systemic lupus erythematosus and a blood pressure of 230/140 mm Hg

therefore over-zealous or poorly monitored blood pressure reduction carries a significant risk [49]. In acute ischaemic stroke, BP reduction to <185/110 mm Hg is warranted if thrombolytic therapy is indicated. If thrombolytic therapy is not indicated and there is no acute end-organ damage other than stroke, no intervention is indicated for the first 48–72 hours.

In cases of acute intra-cerebral haemorrhage in known hypertensives and those with underlying vascular abnormalities, decrease SBP to 140–150 mm Hg within 1 hour if systolic BP is in the range of 150–220 mm Hg.

Cases of increased intracranial pressure due to massive intracranial bleed warrant more liberal approach (keep SBP <180 mm Hg).

16.12 Pharmacological Agents

Agents for the management of hypertensive crises need to be fast acting, rapidly reversible and titratable with minimal adverse effects. In the absence of one ideal agent, knowledge of the pharmacological properties of agents that are available can be used to tailor treatments for a given clinical situation. Parenteral preparations of most drug classes are available with preferred options in UK-based practice being beta-blockers (labetalol and esmolol) and nitric oxide donors (glyceryl trinitrate).

Beta-blockers (esmolol and labetalol) are often the preferred drug, as they are short acting (esmolol within 60 seconds and labetalol within 5 minutes) and are the drug of choice where cardiac output, heart rate and blood pressure are all increased. They achieve control of systemic vascular resistance, lowering this without reduction in total peripheral blood flow. They are the agents of choice in aortic dissection, eclampsia (labetalol does not cross the placenta) and myocardial ischaemia (in the absence of left ventricular failure).

16

Glyceryl trinitrate (GTN) is the nitric oxide donor commonly used in the UK. It acts by venodilation with effects on arterial tone only at higher doses. It therefore achieves its therapeutic effect by reducing preload and cardiac output but can cause a reflex tachycardia and significant hypotension, which may be disadvantageous in certain hypertensive crises (myocardial ischemia, aortic dissection). However, given the short duration of action and plasma half-life, the advantage of GTN is that unwanted effects are rapidly reversible. GTN can be particularly useful in individuals presenting with hypertensive crises associated with left ventricular failure. Sodium nitroprusside, another nitric oxide donor, also acts by reducing venous tone, with more of an effect on arterial tone, reducing both pre- and post-load. Like GTN it has a rapid onset of action, with a short duration of action and plasma half-life, but like GTN it also can be associated with reflex tachycardia and precipitous BP falls. The other disadvantage of nitroprusside is the association with cyanate or thiocyanate toxicity and the need to protect from light, if used over days, particularly in individuals with hepatic or renal dysfunction. This should be offset by use of the drug over a short period of time and a dose not exceeding 2 microgram/kg/min. If needed at higher doses, concurrent thiosulphate infusions can be considered.

Other useful agents include hydralazine, calcium channel blockers and dopamine-1 receptor agonists. Hydralazine acts by vasodilation but can cause precipitous BP falls and has a 12-hour half-life. Because of this prolonged and somewhat unpredictable effect on blood pressure and inability to titrate dose to BP, it is no longer used first line but can be reserved for more complex refractory cases with careful administration and monitoring. Parenteral preparations of calcium channel blockers are available (nicardipine), which act by vasodilation. These are more water soluble than nifedipine, whose use in the setting of hypertensive emergencies or urgencies can cause sharp falls in BP when chewed and swallowed, an effect which can last up to 8 hours, and is therefore not recommended. In contrast nicardipine given as an intravenous infusion has a rapid onset of action (5–15 minutes) with a duration of 4–6 hours. It can therefore be titrated to BP, although the shorter-acting beta-blockers and nitric oxide donors are of greater use for rapid titration.

The dopamine receptor agonist fenoldopam has been approved by the Food and Drug Administration (FDA) for hypertensive emergencies. Although similar to dopamine in mechanism, fenoldopam is a much more specific agonist at peripheral dopamine-1 receptors. Like dopamine it increases renal blood flow and promotes natriuresis. It can be given by the intravenous route and has a rapid onset of action (5 minutes), with a duration of action of 30–60 minutes. It may therefore be useful in hypertensive crises with a renal cause, in order to maintain renal blood flow.

Prostacyclin has a very short half-life and often used in the treatment of scleroderma renal crisis.

Hypertensive emergencies require rapid diagnosis and immediate treatment in a place of safety. Recognition of the underlying clinical syndrome is essential to guide both clinical and pharmacological management. BP lowering in hypertensive emergencies should be carried out in a high dependency setting where close nursing, cardiac and arterial monitoring are available. Drugs that are short acting with a short half-life are preferable so that doses can be titrated to BP.

It is important to differentiate between hypertensive emergency and hypertensive urgency (acute severe hypertension without target-organ damage) since these patients can be cared for as outpatients. Treatment with guideline-concordant long-acting medications should be started, resumed or adjusted, and follow-up should be scheduled within 1–7 days. Intravenous medications are not advised in this context.

16.13 Resistant Hypertension and Non-adherence to Antihypertensives

Resistant hypertension is defined as failure to achieve a guideline-driven blood pressure of less than 140/90 mm Hg in patients who are adherent to maximally tolerated doses of at least three antihypertensive drugs, including a diuretic appropriate for kidney function [50].

16.14 Delivery of Hypertension Treatment

It is worth spending time considering how to deliver not just treatment but monitoring and responsive adjustments for a patient with hypertension. This is particularly key in the management of 'resistant hypertension' that is usually due to one of two causes (a) poor compliance or (b) undiagnosed secondary cause of hypertension.

In order to diagnose a secondary cause of resistant hypertension, non-adherence to antihypertensive medications as well as white coat hypertensive effect should be excluded. Medication non-compliance is highly prevalent among patients with apparent resistant hypertension, so much that an estimated 50–80% of hypertensive patients who are prescribed antihypertensive medications demonstrate suboptimal adherence [51].

Few factors contributing to non-adherence are large pill burden, dosing complexity, expense, high frequency of adverse reactions with multidrug antihypertensive regimens, poor patient-clinician relationship and clinician inertia with reduced insistence on adherence when patients are consistently non-adherent.

Exclusion of non-adherence should include frank and non-judgemental clinician-patient discussion, monitoring of prescription refills and pill counts and, if available, biochemical assay of drugs or their metabolites in urine or plasma.

A patient-centred approach in decision-making helps in improving adherence to antihypertensive medications. Effective strategies include preference for once daily dosing and using fixed-dose combination agents when available, using low-cost and generic antihypertensives and consolidating refills.

Educating patients, their families and caregivers about hypertension, the consequences of hypertension and the possible adverse effects of medications is of vital importance. Robust systems to maintain contact with patients for ongoing follow-up and monitoring including tele- and e-communication may be helpful. Patients should be encouraged to integrate pill taking into their routine activities of daily living with the use of adherence support tools such as reminders, pillboxes, etc.

16.15 Role of RDN (Renal Denervation) in Management of Resistant Hypertension

The role of sympathetic nervous system is pivotal in the pathogenesis of primary hypertension and had been an area of interest for potential treatment of drug-resistant hypertension with emergence of renal sympathetic denervation therapy.

However, after encouraging results from initial clinical trials, a large randomised control trial (SYMPLICITY HTN-3) could not meet its primary efficacy endpoint, that is, office BP reduction; hence the use of renal denervation for treatment of resistant hypertension is not recommended in routine clinical practice [52].

16.15.1 Overview of Treatments of Major Causes of Secondary Hypertension

1. Primary Hyperaldosteronism: 20% prevalence in confirmed cases of resistant hypertension. There should be low index of suspicion to investigate for it in any patient with unexplained high BP and low serum potassium levels. Medical management by aldosterone antagonists (selective preferably, e.g. eplerenone) is preferred and laparoscopic adrenalectomy for unilateral adenomas with ~50% complete cure [51].
2. Phaeochromocytoma: Up to 4% prevalence in resistant hypertension and should be high index of suspicion to investigate. Ninety percent are adrenal catecholamine-secreting tumours. Laparoscopic removal of tumour is the only option after diagnosis. Peri-operative management such as combined α- and β-blockade, a high-sodium diet and fluid hydration is recommended for at least a week before surgery to prevent intraoperative BP instability and to reverse volume contraction. β-Blockade alone can result in paradoxical pressor responses. Postoperatively, close follow-up is needed for the possibility of recurrence or metastasis, especially with the inherited forms.
3. Cushing's Syndrome: RAS blockade with ACEi/ARBs/potassium-sparing diuretics treats 50% of

medically managed Cushing's syndrome-related hypertension. Adrenergic blockade and calcium channel blockers in combination can be effective. Definitive treatment is surgical excision of underlying cause of hypercortisolism.

4. Renovascular Disease: Almost 20% of hypertensive patients undergoing coronary catheterisations are found to have renovascular disease, having unilateral or bilateral stenosis [50]. ASTRAL and CORAL trials didn't show any benefit of endovascular renal artery stenting/balloon angioplasty over optimal medial therapy in management of atherosclerotic renovascular disease. On the contrary, treatment of choice for renovascular disease due to fibro-muscular dysplasia is percutaneous renal angioplasty (PTRA) with or without stenting.
5. Obstructive Sleep Apnoea (OSA): 55–85% prevalence of OSA in resistant hypertension has been reported in different studies. Sympathetic stimulation along with enhanced upper airway resistance plays crucial role; elevated aldosterone levels have also been consistently observed. Continuous positive airway pressure (CPAP) is the treatment of choice. Beta-blockers and spironolactone are reasonable options to manage hypertension in OSA [53].

16.16 Riley-Day Syndrome: A Complex Scenario

[54] Riley-Day syndrome, also referred to as familial dysautonomia (FD), is a genetic disease with extremely labile blood pressure due to baroreflex deafferenation. High incidence of CKD in these patients had previously been attributed to recurrent arterial hypotension and renal hypoperfusion.

However, hypertension precedes kidney disease in these patients as evident by histopathological findings of kidney biopsies. Moreover, increased blood pressure variability and mineralocorticoid treatment accelerate the progression of renal disease.

These findings warrant new treatment guidelines to delay the progression of renal disease in these patients. Aggressive management of hypertension along with non-pharmacological measures like head-up sleeping and physical counter manoeuvers to treat orthostatic hypotension should be implemented.

Delay in progression of CKD in these patients with tight control of BP in a recent trial presents even more challenging scenario, because antihypertensive drugs may worsen symptoms of orthostatic hypotension. It will be an intriguing idea to evaluate if renal denervation can have any benefit in management of this one particular condition.

16

Chapter Review Questions

1. Which class of antihypertensives has more evidence in prevention of stroke in hypertension?
2. What is the arbitrary recommendation for BP lowering in most hypertensive emergencies?
3. Which condition warrants rapid BP lowering, within 10–20 minutes, in hypertensive crisis?
4. What is the potential disadvantage of nitroprusside administration in treatment of hypertensive emergency?
5. What should be ruled out before the diagnosis of resistant hypertension?

Answers

1. Calcium channel blockers
2. Reduction by 20% in the first 2 hours
3. Acute aortic dissection
4. Cyanide toxicity
5. Non-adherence to antihypertensive drugs

Tips and Tricks

- Poor compliance is a common cause of treatment failure; therefore also consider this and consider assaying urine medication levels and/or observed dosing of medication in patients on multiple agents who fail to achieve a good blood pressure (with the caveat that a completely non-compliant patient given several prescribed antihypertensives simultaneously may have a profound drop in blood pressure).
- It is critical for medical teams to distinguish between a hypertensive crisis (requiring urgent parenteral treatment and high dependency monitoring) and severe hypertension without acute end-organ damage (which requires immediate attention but not parenteral antihypertensives).
- Over-zealous correction of blood pressure in patients with a thrombotic microangiopathy may result in worse renal function and prolonged dialysis dependence.
- Generally we are poor at achieving blood pressure targets in the CKD and transplant populations; electronic alerts, setting a target blood pressure with the patient and regular audits are all helpful strategies for focusing effort.
- The commonest cause of 'secondary' hypertension is renal disease (which should be apparent to a nephrologist) but after that primary hyperaldosteronism which should be considered in the setting of hypokalaemia and may offer simple definitive treatment.

Conclusion

A simple approach to BP management is therefore summarised below. The evidence for the approaches described in this table have been discussed throughout this chapter. The key concepts are to encourage non-pharmacological lifestyle strategies for lowering BP and overall cardiovascular risk in all, identification of a target blood pressure and introduction of pharmacological intervention if targets are not met with lifestyle measures. The overarching goal of BP management should be reduction of BP regardless of the agent used to achieve this.

An evidence-based guide to treating high blood pressure

Who to treat	Anyone older than 55 will benefit from BP lowering[a] Anyone with a prior cardiovascular event Anyone with evidence of end-organ damage, irrespective of BP level Anyone with severe elevation of BP[b]
What to treat with	Diet and lifestyle for all BP-lowering medication, consider contraindications and potential dual beneficial effects (losartan is uricosuric so useful if gout is also present), use any drug and titrate up. Add combination agents considering synergies and dose tolerability
What treatment target	The lower the BP achieved without producing symptoms of hypotension, the better. In general <130/80 > 75% of the time Address other cardiovascular risk factors

[a]Lifestyle advice: first, reduce salt and alcohol intake, lose weight, increase aerobic exercise and fruit/vegetable and oily fish consumption

[b]Investigate for secondary causes of raised BP, particularly in the young; if all are negative, proceed to directly observed therapy to ensure non-adherence as a cause of persistently elevated BP despite presumed adequate therapy

Case Study

Case 1

A 56-year-old man, with past medical history of hypertension and active smoker, presented to A&E with dizziness and moderate central chest pain radiating through the back for the last 6 hours. He reported recent bouts of self-resolving chest pains over the last week. ECG with paramedics showed ST depressions in lateral leads. His BP was 230/125 mm Hg and pulse 80 beats/min. Physical exam revealed a fourth heart sound, a diastolic murmur and inter-arm BP difference of >20 mm Hg. IV access was obtained and initial blood sent. He was started with IV labetalol with aggressive management target of BP. Troponins were elevated to 60 ng/L (normal: <14). Other laboratory tests were normal. CXR showed slight widening of mediastinum, and patient was moved to ITU for invasive monitoring. An urgent CT chest confirmed ascending aortic dissection. Vascular and cardiothoracic teams were involved, and surgical correction of dissection was undertaken. It shows the importance of physical exam and high index of suspicion for aortic dissection because it can mimic acute coronary event, management of which may be highly detrimental for underlying aortic dissection.

Case 2

A 63-year-old woman, with known hypertension, on amlodipine and atenolol, presented to A&E with two episodes of witnessed generalised tonic conic seizures. She was post-ictal, though her son reported a 3-day history of her having occipital headaches and blurred vision. Also reported is her spotty adherence with antihypertensives. She had her airway secured with Guedel's airway. Her BP was 232/135 and heart rate 85 bpm. Her GCS was 10/15. Auscultation of heart revealed fourth heart sound. Fundoscopy revealed arteriolar narrowing, cotton wool spots and papilloedema. Rest of physical examination was unremarkable. Initial bloods including electrolytes were normal. ECG showed LV strain pattern and CXR was normal. Her emergency CT head showed heterogeneous areas of low attenuation in posterior parieto-occipital regions bilaterally with no acute haemorrhage or infarction. These findings were consistent with PRES (posterior reversible encephalopathy syndrome), precipitated by non-adherence to antihypertensive medications. She was started on IV labetalol infusion with target reduction of BP by 20–25% during first hour and was transferred to high dependency unit for close monitoring.

Case 3

A 40-year-old lady, being diagnosed with diffuse systemic sclerosis a year ago, was being referred from rheumatology clinic to A&E on account of high BP. She was recently being started on steroids. She was monitoring her BP at home over the last week that showed a persistent rise despite being started on antihypertensive. She also reported 3-day history of fatigue, decreased urine output and ankle swelling. Her BP upon presentation was 185/105 mm Hg. Her physical exam revealed tight perioral skin and chronic skin ulceration and induration of digits. Auscultation of the lungs revealed bibasal fine crackles. Her initial blood results showed serum creatinine

220 umol/L and urea 18 mg/dL. Full blood count revealed Hb of 10 g/dL and platelets of 125 × 10*9/L. LDH was slightly raised and there are no fragments observed on peripheral film. Urine showed active sediment. Acute renal screen was sent. She was immediately started on ACEI and moved to high dependency unit. Her presentation was likely due to scleroderma renal crisis (SCR) causing malignant hypertension and AKI. Thrombotic microangiopathic picture was secondary to high BP itself; however, index of suspicion for other causes of AKI with active urine should be high. Prognosis of SRC depends upon methodical BP control prior to onset of irreversible kidney damage; hence prompt recognition and treatment are critical.

Acknowledgement Special Acknowledgements to Authors of First Edition:

Hingorani, A., Sofat, R., Cross, J.

References

1. Law MR, Morris JK, Wald NJ. Use of blood pressure lowering drugs in the prevention of cardiovascular disease: meta-analysis of 147 randomised trials in the context of expectations from prospective epidemiological studies. BMJ. 2009;338:b1665.
2. Lewington S, Clarke R, Qizilbash N, Peto R, Collins R. Age-specific relevance of usual blood pressure to vascular mortality: a meta-analysis of individual data for one million adults in 61 prospective studies. Lancet. 2002;360(9349):1903–13.
3. He FJ, MacGregor GA. Effect of longer-term modest salt reduction on blood pressure. Cochrane Database Syst Rev. 2004;(3):CD004937.
4. Hooper L, Bartlett C, Davey SG, Ebrahim S. Advice to reduce dietary salt for prevention of cardiovascular disease. Cochrane Database Syst Rev. 2004;(1):CD003656.
5. Xin X, He J, Frontini MG, Ogden LG, Motsamai OI, Whelton PK. Effects of alcohol reduction on blood pressure: a meta-analysis of randomized controlled trials. Hypertension. 2001;38(5):1112–7.
6. Horvath K, Jeitler K, Siering U, Stich AK, Skipka G, Gratzer TW, Siebenhofer A. Long-term effects of weight-reducing interventions in hypertensive patients: systematic review and meta-analysis. Arch Intern Med. 2008;168(6):571–80.
7. Wilhelm SM, Young J, Kale-Pradhan PB. Effect of bariatric surgery on hypertension. Ann Pharmacother. 2014;48(6):674–82.
8. Fagard RH, Cornelissen VA. Effect of exercise on blood pressure control in hypertensive patients. Eur J Cardiovasc Prev Rehabil. 2007;14(1):12–7.
9. Whelton PK, Carey RM, Aronow WS, Casey DE Jr, Collins KJ, Dennison Himmelfarb C, DePalma SM, Gidding S, Jamerson KA, Jones DW, MacLaughlin EJ, Muntner P, Ovbiagele B, Smith SC Jr, Spencer CC, Stafford RS, Taler SJ, Thomas RJ, Williams KA Sr, Williamson JD, Wright JT Jr. 2017 ACC/AHA/AAPA/ABC/ACPM/AGS/APhA/ASH/ASPC/NMA/PCNA guideline for the prevention, detection, evaluation, and management of high blood pressure in adults: executive summary: a report of the American College of Cardiology/American Heart Association Task Force on Clinical Practice Guidelines. Hypertension. 2018;71:1269–324.
10. Carey RM, Calhoun DA, Bakris GL. Resistant hypertension: detection, evaluation, and management: a scientific statement from the American Heart Association. Hypertension. 2018;72:e53–90.
11. Appel LJ, Miller ER 3rd, Seidler AJ, Whelton PK. Does supplementation of diet with 'fish oil' reduce blood pressure? A meta-analysis of controlled clinical trials. Arch Intern Med. 1993;153(12):1429–38.
12. Geleijnse JM, Giltay EJ, Grobbee DE, Donders AR, Kok FJ. Blood pressure response to fish oil supplementation: metaregression analysis of randomized trials. Journal of hypertension. 2002;20(8):1493–9.
13. Morris MC, Sacks F, Rosner B. Does fish oil lower blood pressure? A meta-analysis of controlled trials. Circulation. 1993;88(2):523–33.
14. Chrysant SG, Chrysant GS. Herbs used for the treatment of hypertension and their mechanism of action. Springer Science+Business Media, LLC; 2017. Published online: 18 September 2017 #.
15. Webb AJ, Patel N, Loukogeorgakis S, et al. Acute blood pressure lowering, vasoprotective, and antiplatelet properties of dietary nitrate via bioconversion to nitrite. Hypertension. 2008;51:784–90. https://doi.org/10.1161/HYPERTENSIONAHA.107.103523.
16. Kapil V, Milsom AB, Okorie M, et al. Inorganic nitrate supplementation lowers blood pressure in humans. Hypertension. 2010;56:274–81. https://doi.org/10.1161/HYPERTENSIONAHA.110.153536.
17. 2008 amrita Ahluwalia prof of clin Pharm Wm Harvey institute Barts health with Adrian Hobbs and Magdi Yacoob. Ghosh SM, Kapil V, Fuentes-Calvo I, et al. Enhanced vasodilator activity of nitrite in hypertension novelty and significance. Hypertension. 2013;61.
18. Rang HP, Dale MM. Rang and Dale's pharmacology. 7th ed. Edinburgh: Elsevier Churchill Livingstone; 2012.
19. Law MR, Wald NJ, Morris JK, Jordan RE. Value of low dose combination treatment with blood pressure lowering drugs: analysis of 354 randomised trials. BMJ. 2003; 326(7404):1427.
20. Turnbull F, Neal B, Ninomiya T, Algert C, Arima H, Barzi F, Bulpitt C, Chalmers J, Fagard R, Gleason A, Heritier S, Li N, Perkovic V, Woodward M, MacMahon S. Effects of different regimens to lower blood pressure on major cardiovascular events in older and younger adults: meta-analysis of randomised trials. BMJ. 2008;336(7653):1121–3.
21. Dahlof B, Sever PS, Poulter NR, Wedel H, Beevers DG, Caulfield M, Collins R, Kjeldsen SE, Kristinsson A, McInnes GT, Mehlsen J, Nieminen M, O'Brien E, Ostergren J. Prevention of cardiovascular events with an antihypertensive regimen of amlodipine adding perindopril as required versus atenolol adding bendroflumethiazide as required, in the Anglo-Scandinavian Cardiac Outcomes Trial-Blood Pressure Lowering Arm (ASCOT-BPLA): a multicentre randomised controlled trial. Lancet. 2005;366(9489):895–906.
22. Lindholm LH, Carlberg B, Samuelsson O. Should beta blockers remain first choice in the treatment of primary hypertension? A meta-analysis. Lancet. 2005;366(9496):1545–53.
23. Dickerson JE, Hingorani AD, Ashby MJ, Palmer CR, Brown MJ. Optimisation of antihypertensive treatment by crossover

rotation of four major classes. Lancet. 1999;353(9169):2008–13.
24. Belmin J, Levy BI, Michel JB. Changes in the renin-angiotensin-aldosterone axis in later life. Drugs Aging. 1994;5(5):391–400.
25. Seifarth C, Trenkel S, Schobel H, Hahn EG, Hensen J. Influence of antihypertensive medication on aldosterone and renin concentration in the differential diagnosis of essential hypertension and primary aldosteronism. Clin Endocrinol. 2002;57(4):457–65.
26. de Bruin RA, Bouhuizen A, Diederich S, Perschel FH, Boomsma F, Deinum J. Validation of a new automated renin assay. Clin Chem. 2004;50(11):2111–6.
27. Bradley HA, Wiysonge CS, Volmink JA, Mayosi BM, Opie LH. How strong is the evidence for use of beta-blockers as first-line therapy for hypertension? Systematic review and meta-analysis. J Hypertens. 2006;24(11):2131–41.
28. Khan N, McAlister FA. Re-examining the efficacy of beta-blockers for the treatment of hypertension: a meta-analysis. CMAJ. 2006;174(12):1737–42.
29. Staessen JA, Birkenhager WH. Evidence that new antihypertensives are superior to older drugs. Lancet. 2005;366(9489):869–71.
30. Sofat R, Casas JP, Grosso AM, Prichard BN, Smeeth L, MacAllister R, Hingorani AD. Could NICE guidance on the choice of blood pressure lowering drugs be simplified? BMJ. 2012;344:d8078.
31. Lawlor DA, Fraser A, Ebrahim S, Smith GD. Independent associations of fasting insulin, glucose, and glycated haemoglobin with stroke and coronary heart disease in older women. PLoS Med. 2007;4(8):e263.
32. Sarwar N, Gao P, Seshasai SR, Gobin R, Kaptoge S, Di Angelantonio E, Ingelsson E, Lawlor DA, Selvin E, Stampfer M, Stehouwer CD, Lewington S, Pennells L, Thompson A, Sattar N, White IR, Ray KK, Danesh J. Diabetes mellitus, fasting blood glucose concentration, and risk of vascular disease: a collaborative meta-analysis of 102 prospective studies. Lancet. 2010;375(9733):2215–22.
33. Barzilay JI, Davis BR, Cutler JA, Pressel SL, Whelton PK, Basile J, Margolis KL, Ong ST, Sadler LS, Summerson J. Fasting glucose levels and incident diabetes mellitus in older nondiabetic adults randomized to receive 3 different classes of antihypertensive treatment: a report from the antihypertensive and Lipid-Lowering Treatment to Prevent Heart Attack Trial (ALLHAT). Arch Intern Med. 2006;166(20):2191–201.
34. Patel A, MacMahon S, Chalmers J, Neal B, Woodward M, Billot L, Harrap S, Poulter N, Marre M, Cooper M, Glasziou P, Grobbee DE, Hamet P, Heller S, Liu LS, Mancia G, Mogensen CE, Pan CY, Rodgers A, Williams B. Effects of a fixed combination of perindopril and indapamide on macrovascular and microvascular outcomes in patients with type 2 diabetes mellitus (the ADVANCE trial): a randomised controlled trial. Lancet. 2007;370(9590):829–40.
35. Type 2 diabetes: national clinical guideline for management in primary and secondary care (update). National Collaborating Centre for Chronic Conditions London: Royal College of Physicians 2008.
36. NICE. CG73 Chronic Kidney Disease. National Institute for Clinical Excellence.
37. Hsu CY, McCulloch CE, Darbinian J, Go AS, Iribarren C. Elevated blood pressure and risk of end-stage renal disease in subjects without baseline kidney disease. Arch Intern Med. 2005;165(8):923–8.
38. Casas JP, Chua W, Loukogeorgakis S, Vallance P, Smeeth L, Hingorani AD, MacAllister RJ. Effect of inhibitors of the renin-angiotensin system and other antihypertensive drugs on renal outcomes: systematic review and meta-analysis. Lancet. 2005;366(9502):2026–33.
39. Consensus statement on management of early CKD. Royal college of Physicians of Edinburgh and Renal Association. 2007.
40. Sarafidis PA, Khosla N, Bakris GL. Antihypertensive therapy in the presence of proteinuria. Am J Kidney Dis. 2007;49(1):12–26.
41. Heerspink HJL and Others. https://doi.org/10.1056/NEJMoa2024816 | September 24, 2020 study of over 4000 non diabetic patients with CKD and moderate to heavy proteinuria.
42. Wilcox CS. Antihypertensive and renal mechanisms of SGLT2 (sodium-glucose linked transporter 2) inhibitors. Hypertension. 2020;75(4):894–901. https://doi.org/10.1161/HYPERTENSIONAHA.119.11684. Epub 2020 Mar 2.
43. Chobanian AV, Bakris GL, Black HR, Cushman WC, Green LA, Izzo JL Jr, Jones DW, Materson BJ, Oparil S, Wright JT Jr, Roccella EJ. Seventh report of the Joint National Committee on prevention, detection, evaluation, and treatment of high blood pressure. Hypertension. 2003;42(6):1206–52.
44. Rothwell PM, Howard SC, Dolan E, O'Brien E, Dobson JE, Dahlof B, Sever PS, Poulter NR. Prognostic significance of visit-to-visit variability, maximum systolic blood pressure, and episodic hypertension. Lancet. 2010;375(9718):895–905.
45. Junemaitre X, Chatellier G, Kreft-Jais C, Charru A, Devries C, Plouin P-F, et al. Efficacy and tolerance of spironolactone in essential hypertension. Am J Cardiol. 1987;60(10):820–5. https://doi.org/10.1016/0002-9149(87)91030-7.
46. Chapman N, Dobson J, Wilson S, Dahlof B, Sever PS, et al. Effect of spironolactone on blood pressure in subjects with resistant hypertension. Hypertension. 2007;49(4):839–45.
47. Williams B, MacDonald TM, Morant S, Webb DJ, Sever P, McInnes G, et al. Spironolactone versus placebo, bisoprolol, and doxazosin to determine the optimal treatment for drug-resistant hypertension (PATHWAY-2): a randomised, double-blind, crossover trial. Lancet. 2015;386(10008):2059–68.
48. Agarwal R, Sinha AD, Pappas MK, Abraham TN, Tegegne GG. Hypertension in hemodialysis patients treated with atenolol or lisinopril: a randomized controlled trial. Nephrol Dial Transplant. 2014;29(3):672–81. https://doi.org/10.1093/ndt/gft515.
49. Caren G Solomon, M.D., M.P.H., Editor. Peixoto AJ. Acute severe hypertension. N Engl J Med. 2019;381:1843–52.
50. Calhoun DA, Jones D, Textor S, Goff DC, Murphy TP, Toto RD, White A, Cushman WC, White W, Sica D, Ferdinand K, Giles TD, Falkner B, Carey RM. Resistant hypertension: diagnosis, evaluation, treatment: a scientific statement from the American Heart Association Professional Education Committee of the Council for High Blood Pressure Research. Hypertension. 2008;51:1403–19.
51. Carey RM, Calhoun DA, Bakris GL, Brook RD, Daugherty SL, et al. Resistant hypertension: detection, evaluation, and management: a scientific statement from the American Heart Association. Hypertension. 2018;72(5):e53–90.
52. Lobo MD, de Belder MA, Cleveland T, et al. Joint UK societies' 2014 consensus statement on renal denervation for resistant hypertension. Heart. 2015;101:10–6.
53. Faselis C, Doumas M, Papademetriou V. Common secondary causes of resistant hypertension and rational for treatment. Int J Hypertens. 2011;2011:1–17.
54. Norcliffe-Kaufmann L, Axelrod FB, Kaufmann H. Developmental abnormalities, blood pressure variability and renal disease in Riley Day syndrome. J Hum Hypertens. 2013;27(1):51–5.

Disease of the Renal Vessels

Diana Vassallo, James Ritchie, Darren Green, and Philip A. Kalra

Contents

M. Harber (ed.), *Primer on Nephrology*, https://doi.org/10.1007/978-3-030-76419-7_17

Learning Objectives

1. To learn about non-atheromatous and atheromatous renal artery disease, focusing in more detail on fibromuscular dysplasia (FMD) and atherosclerotic renovascular disease (ARVD)
2. The role of renal revascularization in management of ARVD in light of recent RCT data

17.1 Renal Artery Disease

17.1.1 Introduction

In the Western world, 90% of renal artery stenosis (RAS) is due to atheromatous disease, with fibromuscular disease accounting for the majority of the remainder. Elsewhere, vasculitic stenosis is more prevalent. Clinical presentation, patient management and prognosis for renal function depend on the aetiology of the underlying renovascular disease.

17.1.2 Non-atheromatous Renal Artery Stenosis

17.1.2.1 Vasculitis

In Indian and South Asian populations, almost 60% of RAS cases are vasculitic, whereas in Caucasian populations, this is extremely rare. Takayasu's arteritis is the most common form of vasculitis in Asia and affects females more than males with ratios of up to 9:1 reported. Presentation is typically before the fifth decade of life. The disease follows two clinically distinct phases. The first phase is inflammatory with mononuclear leukocytes and scattered multinucleated giant cells observed within the vessels on histological examination. The second is described as 'pulseless disease' in which progressive fibrosis results in stenoses. The diagnosis is often delayed as symptoms are often non-specific but should be considered in young Asian women with constitutional symptoms such as fevers, arthralgia, hypertension and an acute phase response (raised ESR/CRP). In the chronic phase, features of end-organ ischaemia predominate such as claudication and difficult hypertension. If suspected it is important to check blood pressures in all limbs and examine across the vascular tree for bruits, and whole-body MRA is helpful in assessing the extent of involvement (Fig. 17.1). The territory of blood vessel affected further describes the disease. Within the Indian population, Takayasu's disease of the descending thoracic and abdominal aorta is the most common pattern. This explains the high incidence of associated RAS.

17

In the acute or inflammatory phase of the disease, Takayasu's is treated using corticosteroids +/– cyclophosphamide or methotrexate or increasingly with biologicals such as anti-TNF-α monoclonal antibodies. However, due to limitations in local health care in developing countries, the majority of patients present with secondary hypertension in the chronic pulseless phase of disease. In this context, revascularization is an appropriate intervention, with combined clinical and angiographic success rates of over 90% following balloon angioplasty reported [1].

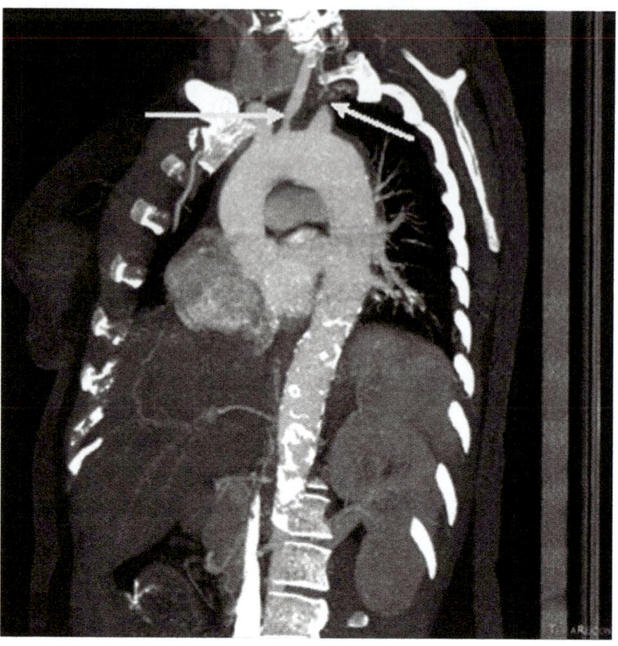

Fig. 17.1 Takayasu's arteritis in a young Asian woman with difficult hypertension and undetectable pulses in the left arm. The images show occlusion of the left subclavian artery (1) near its origin and stenosis of the left common carotid (surrounded by inflammatory tissue) (2)

17.1.2.2 Fibromuscular Disease

Fibromuscular disease (FMD) accounts for approximately 10% of diagnosed cases of RAS in Western populations. Fibromuscular dysplasia (FMD) describes several idiopathic, segmental, non-atherosclerotic, non-inflammatory diseases of arterial wall musculature, causing stenosis of small- and medium-sized arteries.

Clinical Features

The commonest presenting symptoms of FMD are hypertension and headache. Clinical presentation of FMD is diverse depending on the arterial bed involved, and the US FMD registry has also highlighted sex-related differences in presentation. Women present with symptoms and signs of carotid or vertebral artery involvement (e.g. pulsatile tinnitus, neck pain, cervical bruit) more frequently than men, whereas men are more likely to display symptoms and signs consistent with renal artery involvement (e.g. flank or abdominal pain, renal impairment or renal infarction) [2]. Given that FMD commonly co-exists in more than one vascular bed (74% in ≥2 vascular beds), it is recommended that diagnosis of FMD should prompt screening in other vascular beds [3, 4]. The US FMD registry highlighted delayed diagnosis with a mean time between clinical presentation and diagnosis of 3.6 ± 7.4 years. Clinical scenarios that should raise the suspicion of FMD are shown in ◘ Table 17.3.

Epidemiology

The true general population prevalence of clinically significant fibromuscular dysplasia (FMD) is not known, but estimates are in the order of 0.4%. Asymptomatic FMD is more common. A recent review of 4 angiographic studies of 3181 asymptomatic potential kidney donors found FMD in 139 subjects (4.4%) [5].

FMD can present across a wide age range (5–83 years) with peak age of diagnosis at 52 years. Men present at a similar age to women. The overall prevalence of arterial dissections and aneurysms in patients with FMD is 20%.

Extrarenal FMD is more common than previously thought. Renal arteries are most commonly involved in 75–80% of cases. Cranio-cervical arteries (e.g. carotid and vertebral arteries) are involved in 75% of cases. Two-thirds of renal artery FMD have co-existent cranio-cervical involvement and vice versa. FMD can be seen in any small- or medium-sized arteries including lower extremities (60%), mesentery (26%) and upper extremities (16%) and rarely in coronary arteries [3]. Based on these data, guidelines now recommend that FMD found in any arterial bed should prompt screening for FMD elsewhere.

Aetiopathology

FMD is neither inflammatory nor atherosclerotic, with the cause(s) poorly elucidated. Although the vast majority of affected patients are female (at a ratio of 9:1), the reason is unclear, with no evidence of a link between increased oestrogen exposure (including from use of oral contraceptives) and development of disease.

Genetic factors almost certainly play a part in the development of FMD, most likely a dominant trait with variable penetrance. However, limited patient numbers make it hard to reach firm conclusions about genetic linkage. Reports of a familial link in 11% of FMD patients are not consistently duplicated, and other data have rebutted a potential link with alpha-1-antitrypsin deficiency. Work into other potential genetic factors is ongoing as is investigation of a 'two-hit' hypothesis, with some data describing higher rates of disease and more severe disease in smokers (although again conflicting reports exist) [6].

FMD can lead to a variety of abnormal artery morphologies including stenosis, a beaded appearance, aneurysms and dissections. FMD is usually found in the middle and distal parts of the renal artery distinct from atherosclerosis which is most often proximal (◘ Fig. 17.1). A histological classification is based on the predominantly involved arterial layer, but biopsies are rarely warranted, and the American Heart Association recommends an angiographic classification based broadly on multifocal or focal involvement (◘ Table 17.1) [4].

◘ Table 17.1 Histological and angiographic classification of fibromuscular dysplasia (FMD) (adapted from)

Type	Frequency (%)	Histology	Angiographic appearance	Angiographic classification
Medial fibroplasia (common)	85–100	Heterogenous collagen deposition with fragmented internal elastic lamina resulting in multiple small aneurysms. Interspersed with localized regions of fibrotic narrowing	'String of beads' with bead diameter larger than normal vessel lumen (Fig.17.2)	Multifocal
Perimedial fibroplasia (rare)		Collagen deposition in outer half of media but does not extend beyond external elastic lamina	'String of beads' with bead diameter more narrower than the normal vessel lumen	
Medial hyperplasia (rarest)		True smooth muscle hyperplasia with no fibrosis	Stenosis without beading appearance	Focal
Intimal	<10 (more common in children)	Intimal concentric collagen deposition	Concentric or long smooth stenosis	
Adventitial	<1	Dense collagen replaces the fibrous adventitia and may extend into surrounding tissues	Smooth stenosis or diffuse attenuation of lumen	

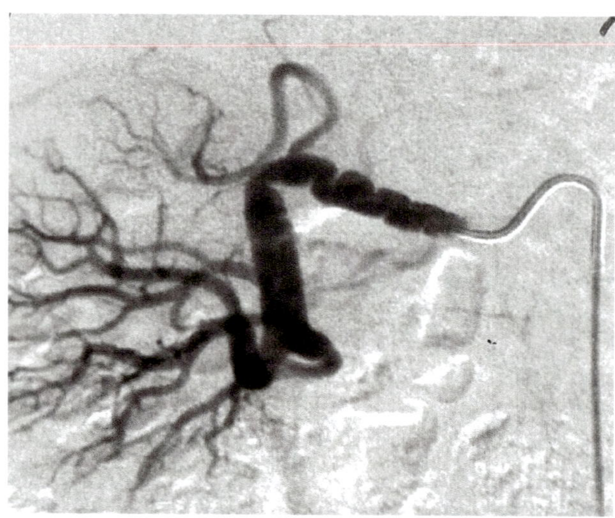

Fig. 17.2 Direct angiography in fibromuscular disease *Medial fibroplasia causing multiple stenoses giving rise to the classical 'string of beads' appearance*

Diagnosis

Direct angiography is the gold standard investigation for identifying FMD (Fig. 17.2), although the invasive nature of this test means that as described below, indirect methods such as computed tomography angiography (CTA) and magnetic resonance angiography (MRA) are generally accepted to be first-line investigations. The major limitation of indirect angiography is poor specificity in identifying branch vessel disease.

Differential Diagnosis

The angiographic appearance of FMD easily distinguishes it from atheromatous disease, and the non-inflammatory nature of the condition facilitates the use of simple blood markers of inflammation (e.g. CRP/ESR) in distinguishing it from a vasculitic aetiology. A more challenging differential diagnosis is segmental arterial mediolysis. This is a poorly understood condition that may actually be a sub-type of FMD. Here, spontaneous arterial occlusion, aneurysm formation and dissection can all occur – typically associated with severe pain from infarction of visceral organs. The acute onset pain and presentation in a more elderly population (50–80 years old) help distinguish segmental arterial mediolysis from FMD.

17

Treatment

Historically, percutaneous transluminal coronary angioplasty (PCTA) without stenting has been considered as first-line therapy for hypertension secondary to FMD. However, no form of revascularization (surgical or percutaneous) has ever been compared to medical therapy in a randomized controlled trial (RCT). With the primary aim of therapy being to control blood pressure, patient age (perhaps a surrogate marker of disease duration) appears to be an important factor. In patients aged younger than 30 years, PCTA for FMD has a cure rate (defined as blood pressure <140/90 mmHg off anti-hypertensive medications) in excess of 60%. This progressively falls to under 15% in patients aged older than 60 years [7]. It is unclear whether the reduced cure rate represents an evolution of the natural history of the disease process or an increased incidence of co-existent primary hypertension with older age. Current opinion favours managing older patients with medical therapy and reserving PCTA for cases in which blood pressures cannot be controlled or renal function begins to deteriorate [2]. For young patients with both newly diagnosed hypertension and FMD, PCTA may be more appropriate as first-line therapy. With regard to medical therapy, all patients, including asymptomatic FMD, should have empirical treatment with anti-platelet therapy [4]. The role of statins in patients with FMD is not clear, but general atherosclerosis risk prevention advice and smoking cessation should be advocated in these patients [8]. Adequate blood pressure control can usually be achieved with antihypertensive agents such as renin-angiotensin-aldosterone system (RAS) antagonists (angiotensin-converting enzyme inhibitors [ACEi] or angiotensin receptor blockers [ARBs]). Registry data will describe long-term outcomes and better inform treatment decisions in the future. Figure 17.3 suggests a basic treatment algorithm.

17.1.3 Atheromatous Renal Artery Disease

The umbrella term renal artery stenosis is useful to describe physical loss of luminal diameter but fails to distinguish between atheromatous and non-atheromatous causes. A more specific term is atheromatous renovascular disease (ARVD).

Most clinical studies of ARVD have considered the respective roles of revascularization and medical therapy. The open surgical techniques pioneered in the 1950s and 1960s have been almost entirely replaced by percutaneous approaches. Percutaneous interventions were introduced in the 1980s and have evolved with improvements in technology from angioplasty alone to angioplasty and stenting, or primary stenting, which offer higher rates of long-term vessel patency. Despite these continued improvements, *no RCT has ever demonstrated superiority of an interventional approach over standard medical therapy for clinical outcomes such as progressive renal dysfunction, cardiovascular or renal events or mortality*. However, many questions remain, as the ARVD population *cannot* be considered a single homogenous group.

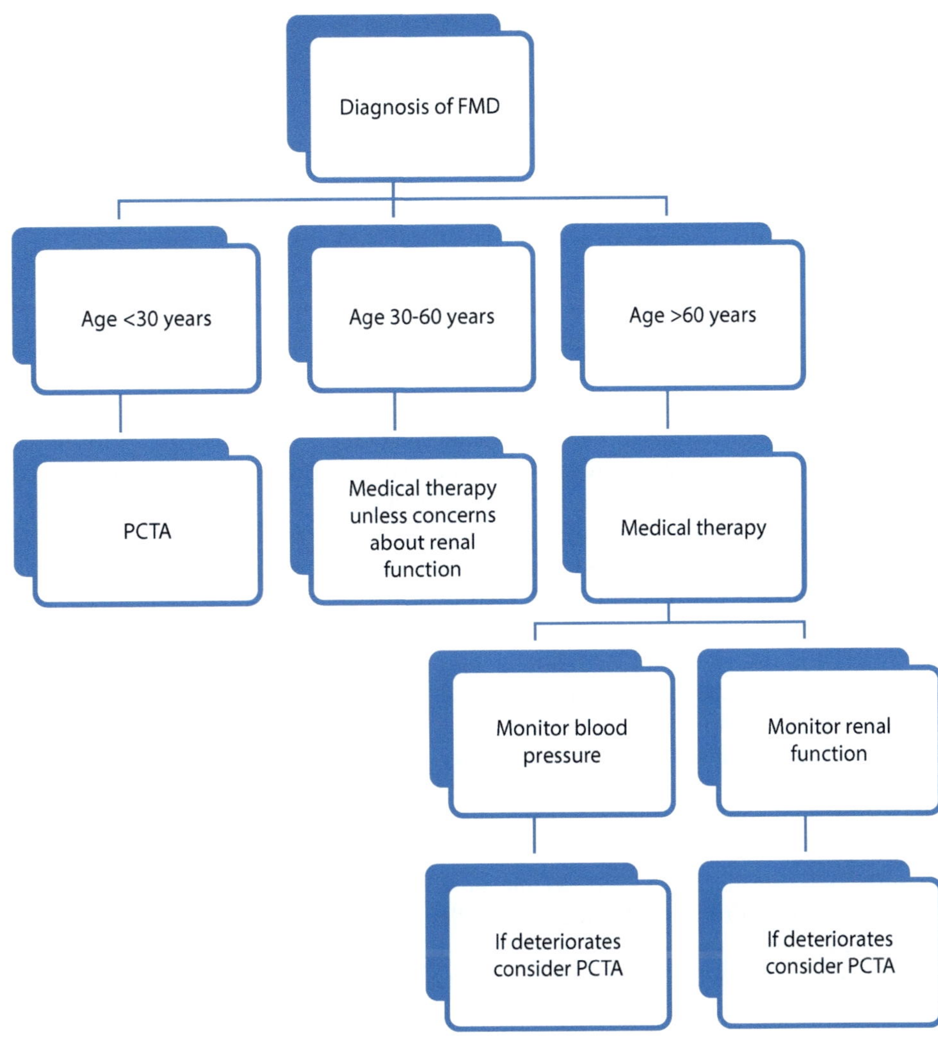

Fig. 17.3 Potential management algorithm for fibromuscular disease

17.1.3.1 Clinical Features

Subclinical

ARVD is often diagnosed incidentally during coronary or peripheral angiography. In these patient groups, cardiovascular event rates are worse in those with incidental ARVD compared to those without [9].

Renovascular and Refractory Hypertension

Atherosclerotic RAS accounts for only 2% of all cases of hypertension, but it is a more common cause of refractory hypertension (8–14%). Conversely, hypertension is almost universal with 95% prevalence in those diagnosed with ARVD. Epidemiology studies can only show associations and cannot determine causality or natural history. In individual patients, hypertension might be one of several atherosclerotic factors causing the development of the ARVD. On the other hand, renovascular hypertension refers to hypertension as a consequence of RAS-induced activation of the renin-angiotensin-aldosterone system that may resolve upon restoring patency with a procedure. In this sense, renovascular hypertension is a retrospective diagnosis.

Ischaemic Nephropathy/Progressive Chronic Kidney Disease

The most common presentation of ARVD is stable chronic kidney disease (CKD) with hypertension. With modern anti-atherosclerosis therapy, the average annual decline of eGFR in ARVD is around 1–2 ml/min/1.73m^2/year, similar to most other causes of CKD [10]. However this disguises the 12–22% with rapid renal functional loss in contemporary clinical trials [11]. Risk prediction for this important minority remains challenging.

Acute Kidney Injury

As with all forms of CKD, those with ARVD have increased risks of developing AKI from all causes. This is more likely with a greater severity stenosis to a single functional kidney or bilateral disease. A few specific causes worth noting are:

- Cholesterol embolization of atheroma after angiography or revascularization procedures or commencing anticoagulation
- Contrast-induced nephropathy
- Treatment with RAS antagonists in patients with physiologically significant RAS, due to dilatation of the efferent glomerular arteriole with a greater than expected decline in GFR

Use of RAS antagonists such as ACEi and ARBs is complex and depends on context. A highly activated RAS can be both a consequence and cause of RAS that is associated with a more rapid long-term decline in GFR. While major randomized controlled trials have established that RAS antagonists help preserve renal function in patients with diabetic and non-diabetic proteinuric kidney disease [12, 13], the evidence that these agents provide the same benefit in patients with ARVD is less robust [14]. Use of RAS antagonists in patients with ARVD has been associated with concerns related to increased risk of AKI [15]. However, it is also clear that RAS antagonists can optimize cardiac status and prevent cardiovascular events in this patient population with cardiovascular disease and cardiac structural abnormalities [16] and can improve overall survival [17, 18]. On starting RAS antagonists, a short-term and stable decline in GFR is hemodynamically and physiologically expected. Diagnosis of AKI requires a larger than expected decline in GFR. The UK National Institute of Healthcare Excellence guidance advice on starting RAS antagonists in CKD recommends to stop or reduce the drug if creatinine rises >30% or eGFR falls >25% from baseline and to exclude hemodynamically stressful risk factors such as volume depletion and NSAID use [19]. If ARVD is not already identified, it should be suspected and diagnostic imaging considered. Use of RAS antagonists should be temporarily withheld during an intercurrent illness or prior to administering iodinated contrast agent.

Cardiorenal Syndromes Including Flash Pulmonary Oedema

Flash pulmonary oedema (FPO) refers to a dramatic form of acute decompensated heart failure. The seminal description by Pickering showed a strong association with RAS particularly if bilateral or to a single functioning kidney [20]. Patients with ARVD have chronically elevated left ventricular and atrial pressures due to chronic hypertension, diastolic dysfunction, left ventricular hypertrophy and fluid retention associated with highly activated RAAS. This leads to increased ventricular wall stress (afterload) and back reflection of the ventricular pressure into the left atrial and pulmonary capillaries [21]. Flash pulmonary oedema remains a strong indication for renal revascularization, and such patients have not typically been included in clinical trials as discussed further below. Chronic heart failure and coronary atherosclerosis are also frequent associations with ARVD.

17.1.3.2 Epidemiology

Many cases of ARVD are clinically silent, making it difficult to accurately estimate disease prevalence. Interpretation of available data is complicated both by temporal changes in availability of diagnostic tools and also by changes in attitudes towards use of these resources following publication of 'negative' RCTs such as the Angioplasty and Stenting for Renal Artery Lesions (ASTRAL) trial and the Cardiovascular Outcomes in Renal Atherosclerotic Lesions (CORAL) study [22, 23]. With these caveats considered, the most definite statement that can be made is that ARVD is not rare in the general population aged older than 65 years (annual incidence 0.5%; prevalence 7%) and is recognized as a primary cause of ESKD in a proportion of these patients (annual incidence of ESKD due to ARVD, 1.3–1.7%; prevalence, 0.7–1%) [24]. Ethnicity is not a significant factor in the development of ARVD.

Populations enriched with other vascular disease have higher rates of ARVD. Given the anatomical proximity of the abdominal aorta and the iliac vessels to the renal arteries, it is unsurprising that 20% and 40% of patients with atheromatous disease in these respective areas have ARVD. However, the association extends to more distant vascular beds, with high rates of ARVD found in patients with carotid (10%) and coronary (40%) disease [25].

17.1.3.3 Aetiopathology

Despite the significant associations with other vascular pathologies, the effects of classical risk factors for development of atherosclerosis are less clear in ARVD than, e.g. coronary artery disease. Although the associations of CKD with smoking and diabetes may skew the data, single-centre comparison of patients investigated for ARVD did not describe a difference in smoking rates or prevalence of diabetes mellitus between patients with normal or abnormal renal angiograms. This is despite higher rates of other vascular disease in the patients found to have ARVD [26]. The surprising lack of effect of smoking is confirmed in other data, but systematic reviews appear to suggest that increased rates of ARVD are observed in diabetic patients [25].

Given that patients with a single kidney can have an eGFR in the normal range, it is not immediately clear why unilateral RAS should lead to loss of renal function. Indeed, the renal vasculature is highly adapted for filtration, and renal blood flow is in excess of the metabolic needs of that kidney. Compensatory arteriovenous shunting, tubulo-glomerular feedback and neuro-hormonal inputs form part of a complex autoregulation that maintains renal oxygenation across a wide range of blood flows [27]. Studies using latex casts and hemodynamic measurements indicate measurable hypoxia only occurs when a renal artery stenosis (RAS) is 70–80% by angiographic assessment [28]. Loss of renal function in ARVD is probably twofold: direct hemodynamic consequences of significant reduction in renal perfusion and a consequence of an ischemic cascade of neuro-humoral activation, inflammation, oxidative stress, capillary rarefaction and fibrosis that might persist despite perfusion being restored [29]. Thus there is likely a threshold at which restoring blood flow cannot reverse this vicious cycle of hypoxic consequences, and this may explain the negative results of ASTRAL and CORAL.

Thus it is most likely that renal parenchymal damage, secondary to 'flow-independent' effects of the stenosis (e.g. hypertension/micro-emboli), is the main arbiter of functional loss. In support of this, there is no correlation between degree of stenosis and level of proteinuria in ARVD, but an inverse relationship between eGFR and proteinuria, where proteinuria acts as a surrogate marker of the degree of irreversible renal parenchymal damage. Indeed observational studies have shown that the level of proteinuria is a possible marker of likelihood of improvement in eGFR following revascularization. Even minor elevations (>0.6 g/24 hours) correspond to large reductions in the chance of renal functional benefit from intervention [30, 31].

Table 17.2 Diagnostic imaging techniques for renovascular disease

Technique	Advantages	Disadvantages
Duplex ultrasound	Entirely non-invasive No contrast or radiation Able to monitor disease progression	Time-consuming Operator dependent Technical failure rate >10% (bowel gas, obesity, etc.)
Computed tomography angiography	Widely available tool Reproducible results Most sensitive technique	Contrast and radiation exposure. Risk of contrast nephropathy Calcified vessels can limit interpretability of images Can over-estimate stenosis
Magnetic resonance angiography	No risk of contrast nephropathy No radiation Reproducible images	Can over-estimate stenosis Risk of nephrogenic systemic fibrosis

17.1.3.4 Diagnosis

As for any patient with CKD, measurement of baseline blood pressure, renal function and proteinuria should be performed. However, the key decision in the investigation for ARVD is which imaging modality is most appropriate.

Renal Artery Imaging

Advances in imaging technology have allowed a shift in focus from anatomical to functional imaging of RAS to assess hemodynamic significance and the functional viability of the renal parenchyma. ARVD can be diagnosed by several techniques. None are perfect, with a trade-off between risk and the ability to determine functional significance and a response to treatment (Table 17.2).

- X-ray angiography is the reference standard technique, but this is invasive and reserved for planned intervention (Fig. 17.4). It is now well recognized that visual estimates from these 2D images have poor inter-observer variability and poor correlation to quantification of the images offline. Furthermore, this quantitative stenosis grading still correlates poorly with functional severity as measured by pressure or flow changes. Reasons for such discrepancies are largely due to the inaccuracy in assessing complex 3D fluid dynamics from static 2D images that ignore effects of plaque length, geometry, radiolucency and post-stenotic microvascular resistance. There are some small studies showing promising data using trans-lesional pressure gradients, but they require validation against clinically important outcomes.
- Computed tomographic angiography (CTA) (Fig. 17.5) and gadolinium-enhanced magnetic resonance angiography (MRA) are the current mainstay of diagnostic techniques with near equivalent accuracy. Their use is restricted in patients with estimated GFR <30 ml/min due to respective risks of contrast-induced nephropathy and nephrogenic systemic fibrosis. These risks are acceptably low if preventive protocols are followed.
- Duplex ultrasound is inexpensive, not associated with any risks to patients with estimated GFR <30 ml/min and non-invasive with potential to determine hemodynamic significance. However, it is the least accurate and most operator dependent. Advances in contrast-enhanced ultrasound may improve accuracy, but to date only preliminary data are available.
- Captopril renography is rarely used, but radioisotope studies to determine single-kidney GFR (SK-GFR) remain the reference standard technique for measured GFR.
- In research centres, novel CT methods allow the estimation of single-kidney GFR and perfusion with the caveat of greater ionizing radiation exposure.

Renal functional magnetic resonance imaging (MRI) shows great promise given its inherent value in tissue characterization using relaxation times. Techniques such as relaxometry, velocity-encoding, blood oxygen level-

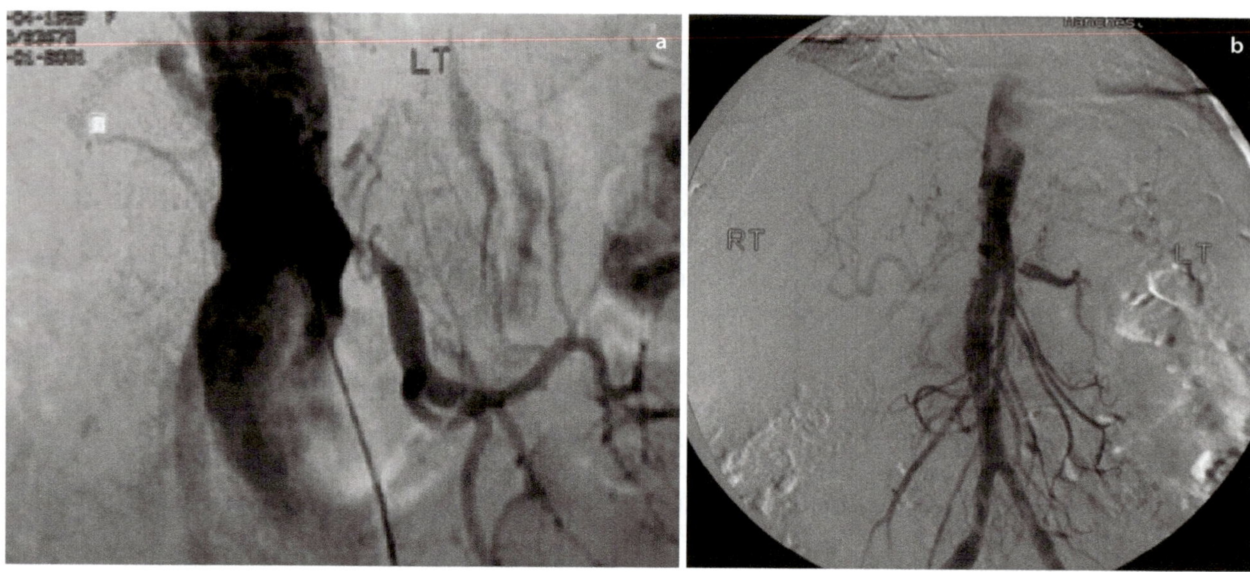

Fig. 17.4 Direct angiography in atherosclerotic renal vascular disease. **a** – *70% left renal artery stenosis.* **b** – *Right renal artery occlusion and 98% left renal artery stenosis*

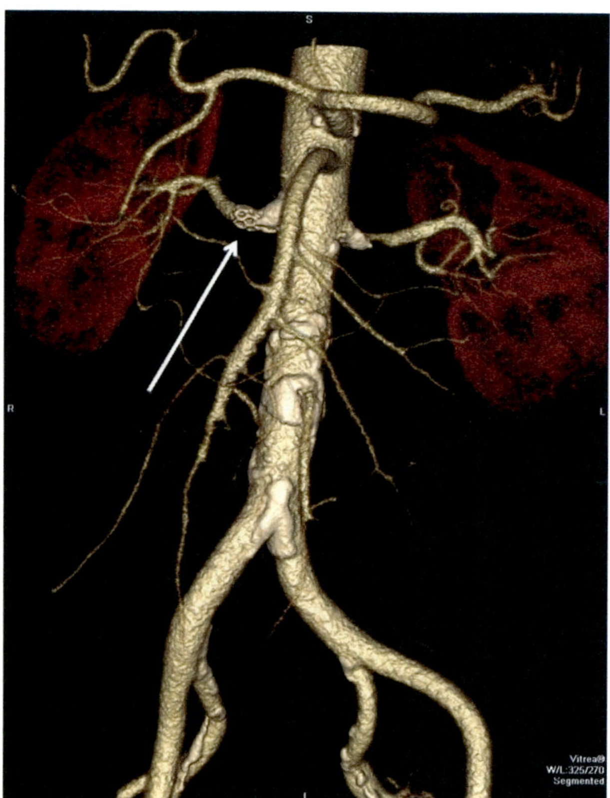

Fig. 17.5 Computed tomography angiography in atherosclerotic renal vascular disease. *Reconstructed CT angiogram demonstrating patent left renal artery and patent right renal artery stent (arrow)*

dependent (BOLD) imaging, volumetry, arterial-spin labelling and single-kidney GFR by dynamic contrast enhancement allow a comprehensive evaluation of renal artery haemodynamics and tissue characterization. However much of this is confined to research studies or expert centres, and standardized protocols in multi-centre studies are required to enable the evidence base to mature and test the clinical utility of such protocols [32].

Cardiac Imaging

In over 95% of patients with ARVD, an abnormality of either left ventricular function or structure can be demonstrated on transthoracic echocardiography, with risk of deterioration in all these parameters over time [33]. Baseline cardiac imaging is therefore an appropriate request. Currently this is of more prognostic than therapeutic benefit. Randomized data comparing cardiac structural and functional outcomes between medical and interventional therapy in patients with ARVD have interestingly not shown any significant differences between the two treatment arms [34, 35]. This is again similar to the lack of differences in primary outcome measures noted in the two main RCTs ASTRAL and CORAL. As explained below, potential explanations include the clinical heterogeneity of the ARVD patient population and the underrepresentation of 'high-risk' ARVD patients in these studies.

17.1.3.5 Differential Diagnosis

It is important to recognize that RAS is not the sole cause of asymmetrical kidney sizes, with primary renal dysplasia and reflux nephropathies typically resulting in asymmetric organs. Unlike FMD, ARVD tends to affect the proximal or ostial part of the renal artery.

17.1.3.6 Treatment

Revascularization

As of 2021, there have been nine RCTs published looking at different revascularization modalities and comparing medical therapy with or without percutaneous revascularization in ARVD. These studies are summarized in Table 17.3. A range of clinical outcome measures, rate of change in renal function and blood pressure and hard

Table 17.3 Controlled studies comparing different revascularization modalities and medical therapy for the management of atherosclerotic renovascular disease

Author	Year	Patients (*n*)	Inclusion criteria	Follow-up in months	Treatment modality	Primary end-point	Key clinical outcomes	Comments
Weibull et al. [62]	1993	58	Non-diabetic ≤70 years Untreated BP ≥160/100 mmHg Significant unilateral RAS Serum creatinine <300 umol/L	24	29 – PTRA 29 – surgery	Technical success, primary and secondary patency and changes in BP and renal function from baseline	Diastolic BP <90 mmHg – secondary results [b]: PTRA 5/29 (17%), Surgery 5/29 (17%) Secondary improved/stable renal function [b]: PTRA 83%, surgery 72% $p = 0.53$ Complications: PTRA 5/29 (17%), surgery 9/29 (31%) $p = 0.17$ Primary patency rate at 24 months: PTRA – 75%, surgery – 96%	Given the tight inclusion criteria and the highly selected population, it was unclear whether the clinical benefit observed following both interventions could be extrapolated to the general population of patients with ARVD
Plouin et al. [63]	1998	49	<75 years of age Diastolic BP >95 mmHg CrCl ≥50 ml/min Significant unilateral RAS	6	23 – PTRA 26 – medical treatment	Blood pressure at 6 months and change from baseline	No statistical difference between mean ambulatory BP at 6 months and average reduction in BP between the two groups Complications: PTRA 6/23 (26%), medical 2/25 (8%)	PTRA resulted in a reduced antihypertensive medication use at 6 months; however it was associated with a higher risk of complications
Webster et al. [64]	1998	55	<75 years Diastolic BP ≤95 mmHg ≥50% Unilateral/bilateral stenosis sCr <500 umol/L	3–54	25 – PTRA 30 – medical treatment	Blood pressure at 6 months and change from baseline	A statistically significant drop in BP ($p < 0.05$) was detected only in patients with bilateral disease randomized to PTRA There were no significant differences in renal function or survival between groups	BP fell significantly following the 4-week run-in period with standardized antihypertensives in both groups

(continued)

Table 17.3 (continued)

Author	Year	Patients (*n*)	Inclusion criteria	Follow-up in months	Treatment modality	Primary end-point	Key clinical outcomes	Comments
Van de Ven et al. [65]	1999	85	≥50% ostial ARVD BP >160/96 mmHg Positive captopril renography or increase in sCr of ≥20% with ACEi	6	42 – PTRA 43 – PTRAS	Primary success rate and patency rate at 6 months	Primary success rate [c]: PTRA 24/42 (57%), PTRAS 37/42 (88%) Restenosis at 6 months: PTRA 11/23 (48%), PTRAS 5/35 (14%) Complications: PTRA 18/42 (43%), PTRAS 21/42 (50%) Diastolic BP <90mmHg[a]: PTRA 2/41 (5%), PTRAS 6/40 (15%) Improved renal function[d] PTRA 4/41 (10%), PTRAS 5/40 (13%)	PTRAS was technically more successful than PTRA, whereas 12 patients who underwent PTRA required secondary PTRAS due to failed primary PTRA. This argued for primary PTRAS for ostial atherosclerotic RAS
Van Jaarsveld et al. [44]	2000	106	< 75 years sCr ≤200umol/L Diastolic BP ≥95 mmHg Unilateral or bilateral >50% RAS	12	56 – PTRA 50 – medical treatment	Blood pressure at 3 and 12 months after randomization	No significant differences between the two groups at 12 months, in terms of both renal function and BP control	PTRAS may only be of benefit in controlling blood pressure in patients with bilateral renal artery disease
Bax et al. [36] (STAR)	2009	140	Unilateral or bilateral ostial ARAS ≥50% CrCl <80 ml/min Controlled BP <140/90 mmHg for 1 month	24	76 – medical Rx 64 – medical Rx + PTRAS (intervention group)	20% or greater decrease in estimated creatinine clearance compared with baseline	>20% decrease in CrCl from baseline: 16/76 (22%) medical Rx, 10/62 (16%) intervention group Deaths: 6/74 (8%) medical Rx, 5/62 (8%) intervention group	Significant number of PTRAS-related complications: 2/62 (3%) – periprocedure mortality 1 death secondary to infected haematoma ESKD needing dialysis in one patient

Wheatley et al. (ASTRAL) [22]	2009	806	Unilateral or bilateral 'substantial' ARAS Uncertainty regarding benefit from revascularization	33.6 (median)	403 – medical Rx 403 – medical Rx + PTRAS (95%) or PTRA (intervention group)	Change in renal function (measured by the mean slope of the reciprocal of serum creatinine) from baseline	BP control: No statistically significant difference in systolic BP; diastolic BP was lower in the medically treated group ($p = 0.06$) ESKD: 30/403 (8%) intervention group; 31/403 (8%) medical Rx CVE: 141/403 (35%) intervention group, 145/403 (36%) medical Rx Deaths: 103/403 (26%) intervention group; 106/403 (26%) medical Rx	Revascularization was associated with serious adverse events in 23/403 (6.7%) patients, including two deaths and three amputations; revascularization conferred no advantage over optimal medical therapy
Marcantoni et al. [34] (RAS-CAD)	2012	84	Unilateral/bilateral RAS >50%–≤80% IHD and elective coronary angiography	12	41 – Medical therapy 43 – Medical therapy + PTRAS (intervention group)	Change in echocardiographic LVMI from baseline	Controlled[a] or improved BP control: 75% - Intervention group; 81% - medical Rx Deaths: 2/43 (4.6%) Intervention group; 2/41 (4.9%) medical Rx CVE: 11/43 (25.6%) Intervention group; 11/41 (26.8%) medical Rx	LVMI, a surrogate cardiovascular end-point, decreased by equivalent amounts in both groups

(continued)

17

Table 17.3 (continued)

Author	Year	Patients (n)	Inclusion criteria	Follow-up in months	Treatment modality	Primary end-point	Key clinical outcomes	Comments
Cooper et al. [23] (CORAL)	2014	947	Unilateral or bilateral ARAS ≥60%	43 (median)	480 – medical Rx 467 – medical Rx + PTRAS (95%) or PTRA (intervention group)	Composite end-point of death from cardiovascular or renal causes, myocardial infarction, stroke, hospitalization from congestive heart failure, progressive renal impairment or need for renal replacement therapy	Composite primary end-point 169/472 (35.8%)-medical Rx; 161/459 (35.1%)-intervention group ($p = 0.58$) Deaths: 63/459 (13.7%) – intervention group 76/472 (16.1%) – medical Rx ($p = 0.2$) ESKD: 16/459 (3.5%) – intervention group 8/472 (1.7%) – medical Rx ($p = 0.11$)	Revascularization conferred no benefit over optimal medical treatment in terms of clinical outcomes

[a]Without antihypertensive medication

[b]The results achieved following intervention in the event of restenosis

[c]Patency after the first intervention

[d]sCr decreased by >20% from baseline

ACEi angiotensin-converting enzyme inhibitor, *ARAS* atherosclerotic renal artery stenosis, *ARVD* atherosclerotic renovascular disease, *BP* blood pressure, *ESKD* end-stage kidney disease, *IHD* ischaemic heart disease, *PTRA* percutaneous transluminal renal angioplasty, *PTRAS* percutaneous transluminal renal angioplasty and stenting, *RAS* renal artery stenosis, *RF* renal function, *sCr* serum creatinine

end-points such as death, cardiovascular events and progression to renal replacement therapy have been assessed. No trial has shown a conclusive benefit of revascularization over medical therapy for any outcome measure.

The first three trials published between 1998 and 2000 used angioplasty alone. Subsequently, it was established that better long-term angiographic outcomes occurred when angioplasty was coupled with bare metal stenting (PTRAS). This technique was therefore adopted for more recent trials [22, 23, 36]. This difference in interventional technique limits direct comparison between RCTs. Small patient numbers, short follow-up periods and low rates of statin/renin-angiotensin blockade use in early trials further limit their applicability to current practice. The largest two landmark studies, ASTRAL and CORAL, provide the most robust data about the role of revascularization and, despite the limitations of both studies, had an important impact on the current management of ARVD:

- The Angioplasty and Stenting for Renal Artery Lesions (ASTRAL) trial was based in the UK and Australasia and randomized 806 patients with ARAS to either medical therapy alone or medical therapy with revascularization. Patients were included into the study if they had significant stenosis in at least one renal artery and their clinician was uncertain that revascularization would be of benefit. This inclusion criterion received significant criticism as criteria for revascularization were not established and the functional significance of stenosis was not assessed; indeed, out of the entire study population, 40% were found to have low-grade stenosis (50–70%) at angiography, while 17% of patients randomized to stenting were not revascularized either due to non-significant degrees of stenosis at angiography (8%) or patient refusal [11]. After a median of 34 months follow-up, there was no between-group difference in the primary outcome of renal function nor for secondary outcomes of blood pressure control, cardiovascular event rates or mortality (secondary end-points) [22]. Safety analysis noted a 6.8% rate of significant complications in the revascularized arm.
- The US-based Cardiovascular Outcomes in Renal Atherosclerotic Lesions (CORAL) study randomized 947 patients to stenting and best medical therapy or best medical therapy alone. The original design of CORAL aimed to overcome the shortcomings of ASTRAL; only patients with haemodynamically confirmed severe renal artery stenosis and a systolic BP of 155 mmHg or higher despite use of at least two antihypertensive agents were intended to be recruited. The degree of stenosis was standardized by means of an angiographic 'core lab' evaluation and translesional gradient measurement, and severe stenosis was defined as either at least 80% but less than 100%

Example clinical scenarios

Scenario	Actions	
Patient aged <30 years presenting with hypertension	Examine for bruits Indirect angiography to investigate for FMD	Good candidate for angioplasty if angiogram shows FMD
Patient with eGFR 20 ml/min and asymmetric kidneys on ultrasound	Do not expose to gadolinium. Image renal vessels with either DUS or CTA	Consider admission for hydration for CTA
Elderly patient with chronic CKD stage 3 and renal artery stenosis	Address lifestyle factors – e.g. smoking, diabetic control	Prescribe angiotensin blockade as first-line blood pressure control. Commence statin and consider anti-platelet agent
Patient presenting with recurrent acute onset pulmonary oedema	Assess left ventricular function. If systolic function is preserved, perform indirect renal angiography	If significant bilateral renal artery stenosis, consider referral for revascularization
Patient with suspected renal artery stenosis and previously preserved renal function presenting acutely dialysis dependent	Doppler imaging of renal vessels	Refer for renal artery angioplasty and stenting
Greater than 25% reduction in eGFR following initiation of angiotensin blockade to treat chronic heart failure	Consider volume state and concurrent nephrotoxic drugs Indirect renal angiography	If significant stenosis and no other culprit medications, consider revascularization
Patient with uncontrolled symptoms of CHF and renal artery stenosis	Review echocardiograms regarding LVMI	If uncontrolled symptoms, increased LVMI and significant stenosis, consider revascularization

FMD fibromuscular disease, *DUS* duplex ultrasound, *CTA* computed tomography angiography, *CHF* chronic heart failure, *LVMI* left ventricular mass index

angiographic stenosis or 60–80% stenosis with a trans-lesional systolic pressure gradient of at least 20 mmHg. However, patient recruitment proved to be very slow, and hence these inclusion criteria were relaxed such that by the end of the study average angiographic stenosis was 66% (very similar to ASTRAL), and only 20% of patients had >80% stenosis [11, 37]. The primary end-point was a composite of major cardiovascular events, progressive deterioration in renal function and death from cardiovascular or renal causes. Again, after a median follow-up of 43 months, revascularization did not confer any clinical benefit over medical therapy on its own [23].

Both the ASTRAL and CORAL trials received criticism due to selection bias: patients had well-preserved renal function at recruitment in CORAL (eGFR 58 ml/min/1.73m^2), and high-risk patients with uncontrolled hypertension, rapidly deteriorating renal function or recurrent flash pulmonary oedema, more likely representing clinically significant stenosis, were under-represented in both studies. We have undertaken a single-centre observational retrospective study of 237 patients with at least 50% RAS and one or more of the above 'high-risk features', 24% of whom were treated with revascularization. Clinical outcomes for this subset of patients were compared to those of patients who were treated exclusively medically. Results showed that revascularization was associated with improved outcomes in patients with either flash pulmonary oedema or with a combination of rapidly declining kidney function and uncontrolled hypertension [38].

We have published another recent observational study that confirms that revascularization appears to be of benefit in a sub-group of high-risk patients with rapidly deteriorating renal function either in the context of critical stenosis (≥70% bilaterally) or <1 g/day baseline proteinuria, a surrogate marker of well-preserved parenchyma [39] (◘ Fig. 17.6a). Previous work from our research group forged the concept of 'hibernating parenchyma', that is, viable renal parenchyma that has not yet undergone the irreversible changes associated with ARVD and hence retains the possibility to recover function post-revascularization (◘ Fig. 17.6b, c). Studies which have related the isotopic GFR of the kidney with RAS to its parenchymal volume (measured by MRI) suggest that selecting organs with the highest volume-GFR ratio can potentially select patients most likely to improve renal function following PTRAS [40]. Although increased mortality is observed in patients with higher degrees of stenosis, a direct causal link cannot be made, due

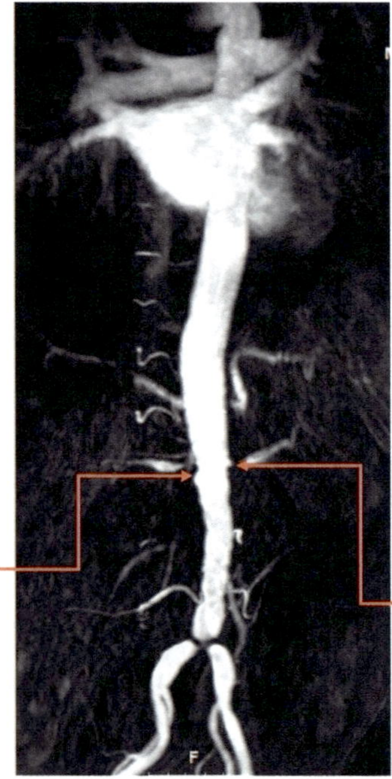

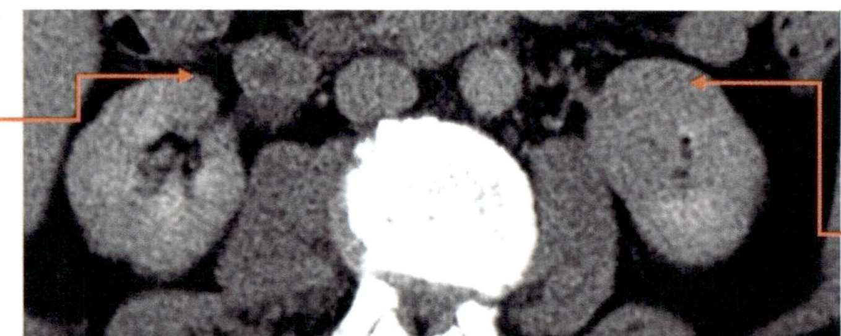

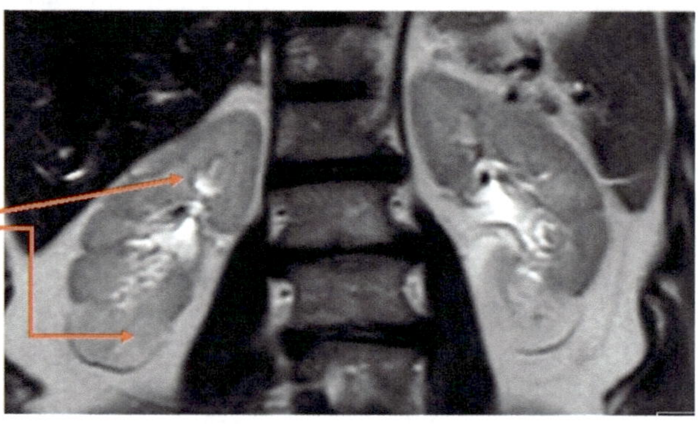

17

◘ **Fig. 17.6** **a** Angiogram of a 41-year-old male smoker who presented with severe hypertension, a creatinine of 90 and pulmonary oedema. The angiogram demonstrates bilateral tight proximal renal artery stenosis with post-stenotic dilatation (arrows). Despite evidence of good adherence, he had multiple admissions with hypertension (c.220/120 mmHg) and pulmonary oedema on five antihypertensives including maximum dose ACEi. **b** The CT with contrast demonstrated marked differential perfusion with significant areas of hypoperfusion consistent with 'hibernating renal parenchyma'. **c** MRA also demonstrates differential perfusion of 'hibernating' renal parenchyma. Crucially both the CT and MRA show good sized kidneys with preserved renal cortex. Following bilateral renal angioplasty and stenting, his blood pressure returned to 140/90 on ACEi alone

to increased co-existent coronary disease in these patients. Sub-analyses of patients with >70% RAS in RCT data have not shown any difference in outcome following PTRAS than in patients with a lower percentage stenosis. Again, selection bias affects interpretations of the RCT data, but RAS severity especially when considered in isolation is not considered a reliable guide to intervention.

It is hoped that recent advances in imaging technology will enable accurate characterization of functional renal tissue in ARVD with the aim of identifying patients who may benefit from revascularization in a timely manner.

In Which of the Following Scenarios Is Revascularization to Be Considered?

Stable CKD or Incidentally Diagnosed ARVD

Available evidence does not support revascularization for patients with stable CKD. Real-world experience has duplicated trial findings, emphasizing the need to focus on appropriate medical therapy for these patients. Acceptance of this finding is important to minimize risk of complications from intervention (discussed below). While incidentally diagnosed ARVD could be considered to be the same as ARVD with stable CKD, specific outcome data exist for patients found to have RAS during another angiographic procedure. In line with trial data, when incidental cases of ARVD were compared between those that were revascularized and those who were not, no difference was seen in terms of blood pressure or renal function at 12 months.

The overall lack of benefit from revascularization when examining renal dysfunction as a primary outcome measure is almost certainly due to the slow rate of loss of renal function seen in ARVD. The annual eGFR loss associated with ageing is around 0.7 ml/min/1.73 m^2/year, with the average rate of loss in ARVD only slightly higher than this. As such, any longitudinal difference in renal function between medical and interventional groups would be subtle and require an RCT to be powered to very high patient numbers to identify a statistical difference.

Acute and Chronic Heart Failure

Approximately 5% of patients with ARVD present with flash pulmonary oedema. Although this patient group has yet to be investigated in an RCT or case control series, this presentation is accepted as an indication for PTRAS [17]. Despite the lack of high-grade evidence, this approach is appropriate based on what data are available – an unmatched series of 39 patients with FPO showed a significant reduction in hospitalization rates following revascularization from 2.4/year to 0.3/year [41].

As discussed above, significant cardiac structural changes are observed in ARVD, and over 30% of elderly patients with chronic heart failure (CHF) have co-existent ARVD [42]. With examples of cardiac structural benefit described following revascularization, and a case series describing improved NYHA status and reduced hospitalization rates following intervention [42], there is interest in the potential role of PTRAS in the treatment of chronic heart failure [43]. In spite of this, both the cardiac imaging substudies of ASTRAL and the Stenting of Renal Artery Stenosis in Coronary Artery Disease (RAS-CAD) study have not shown any significant cardiac structural or functional improvement between revascularized and non-revascularized patients [34, 35]. As explained above, selection of relatively 'low-risk' patients is an important limitation for both studies, but to date revascularization is not considered to play a role in the management of chronic heart failure.

Renin-angiotensin blockade is recognized as an important therapy in treatment of both CHF and ARVD with morbidity and mortality benefits. Though angiotensin-converting enzyme inhibitors and angiotensin II receptor blockers are well tolerated in ARVD, there remains a small group of patients for whom these treatments are associated with a significant decline in renal function. Revascularization can allow safe use of renin-angiotensin blockade in previously intolerant patients [20]. As such intervention can be considered a tool to facilitate optimal medical therapy.

Rapid Loss of Renal Function and Refractory Hypertension

Refractory hypertension (defined as a blood pressure >160/90 mmHg despite three or more different antihypertensive agents) is considered by some as a potential indication to revascularize a patient with RAS. In part, this position is supported by an early RCT published by the Dutch Renal Artery Stenosis Intervention Cooperative Study Group (DRASTIC) [44]. Although the study was not powered to examine this end-point, patients saw reductions in their blood pressure from an average of 190/111 mmHg at 3 months to 169/102 mmHg at 12 months suggesting that further studies with this group are warranted. Within ASTRAL, a limited prespecified analysis of patients with rapidly declining renal function (greater than a 20% or 100 μmol/L increase in serum creatinine in the 12 months before enrolment into the study) was performed. For the 96 patients fitting these criteria, there was a non-significant reduction in serum creatinine at 12 months in the revascularization group compared to the medical group. As described above, two small retrospective observational analyses suggest that patients with rapidly deteriorating renal function and uncontrolled hypertension can gain benefit from revascularization especially if there is evidence of well-preserved renal parenchyma with low levels of proteinuria. Larger studies or data from an international ARVD registry would add clarity.

17.1.3.7 Complications of Revascularization

Although there is a possibility that minor complications (e.g. discomfort) may be over-reported in RCT data, it is clear that PTRAS has potentially serious side effects and should not be undertaken lightly. Some of the more common complications associated with PTRAS in contemporary medical practice include groin haematoma, renal artery dissection, cholesterol embolization, renal artery rupture, contrast-induced nephropathy and aortic dissection.

Meta-analysis of 687 patients represented in data published between 1991 and 1998 found that 9% of renal angioplasty procedures resulted in a serious complication (e.g. significant blood loss, renal infarction, loss of renal function), with an overall 1% mortality rate. The more recent RCT quoted a lower rate of serious adverse events (6.8% in ASTRAL and 5.2% in CORAL), although two deaths were reported in the ASTRAL trial. The reported rate of the more common complications mentioned above is between 0.5% and 10%.

17.1.3.8 Medical Therapy

Given the overall 'negative' findings in trials of revascularization versus medical therapy in ARVD, an understanding of appropriate use of pharmacotherapy is vital. Despite this, a lack of concordance between trials makes it difficult to define optimal medical therapy. We would suggest that renin-angiotensin blockade in conjunction with statin therapy should be considered first-line treatment for all patients with ARVD, with anti-platelet agents strongly considered on a case by case basis. These interventions have benefits in excess of blood pressure and proteinuria reduction and should be complimented by general measures to manage risk in CKD such as smoking cessation advice, good diabetic control and taking exercise.

17

Renin-Angiotensin Blockade

The importance of tight blood pressure control is well recognized in all-cause CKD, with a widespread appreciation that blockade of the RAAS provides renal benefits in excess of those delivered solely by the associated blood pressure reduction. As explained above, in ARVD these agents reduce both blood pressure and risk of mortality to a greater extent than other antihypertensive agents.

Second-Line Treatment of Hypertension

For ARVD patients with blood pressure not controlled by RAAS inhibition, data on second- and third-line agents is scarce. CORAL has defined thiazide diuretics as a second-line agent (replaced by loop diuretics where there is advanced renal dysfunction), with beta-blockers and calcium channel blockers as third-line agents. Although no outcome data support use of diuretics in ARVD, the understanding that resistant hypertension in CKD is often due to underuse of diuretics, and especially that salt-water retention is increased by RAAS overstimulation, makes these agents a logical choice.

Support for use of beta-blockade comes from recognition of increased local sympathetic and adrenergic activity in ARVD. This local increase is associated with elevated serum noradrenaline concentrations which have been linked to both reduced eGFR and the increased cardiovascular mortality. There are some data which suggest that beta-blockade following revascularization leads to improved renal functional outcomes and lower rates of restenosis. Renal artery denervation, which has been shown (in a non-ARVD population) to reduce peripheral blood pressure, may be helpful, but as yet there are no data in the ARVD population to support its use.

Statins

The evidence supporting statin therapy in ARVD has a clear narrative. Though early case reports describing regression of stenosis with statin therapy have not been duplicated, it is certain that rate of progression of stenosis is slowed. In addition, statin-treated patients (even with a normal lipid profile) have been shown to have lower rates of death and progression to dialysis [45].

Revascularized patients also benefit from treatment with statins, with a reduction in risk of death of over 80%. Although the mechanism of benefit is not clear, it is most likely achieved through a composite effect of reduced renal fibrosis, reduced left ventricular hypertrophy and the wider cardiovascular advantages of these agents.

Anti-platelet Therapy

The historical perspective of anti-platelet therapy in all forms of atheromatous disease makes an objective assessment of the role of these agents in ARVD challenging. With the co-existent burden of vascular disease in ARVD, the use of anti-platelets is easy to justify. Although the DOPPS study did not identify a benefit of aspirin therapy in dialysis-dependent patients, sub-analysis of patients with mild to moderate CKD in primary prevention studies have shown significant reduction in the rate of vascular events, albeit with a significant increase in bleeding risk [46]. Less information is available regarding alternative agents such as clopidogrel (which may have reduced pharmacological activity in CKD).

The time point for which there is definitive evidence for anti-platelet agents in ARVD is at time of intervention. The amount of micro-emboli released during stenting is significantly reduced by clopidogrel loading in combination with aspirin therapy (although the long-term functional benefits are not yet established).

17.1.3.9 Future Treatment Options

The negative findings of RCTs were not predicted due to a range of case reports and series describing benefit from intervention. As explained above, it is likely that selection bias accounts for the bulk of this discrepancy. Hence more focused selection of patients and risk stratification likely to benefit from revascularization (discussed below) may be an important approach. A simple risk calculator has been designed by our centre and is freely available. Although this requires further validation in larger ARVD populations, this risk calculator shows that a small number of easily obtained variables can help predict clinical outcomes and encourage a patient-specific therapeutic approach [47].

In addition to an increased recognition of the need for accurate clinical phenotyping, there is the potential that serum biomarkers could aid selection of patients most likely to benefit. Of a range of markers under investigation, the most promising thus far is brain natriuretic peptide (BNP). Studies assessing BNP level in relation to blood pressure response from revascularization have shown that patients with a BNP level >50 pg/ml (average baseline eGFR 66 ml/min/1.37m^2) have a higher likelihood of a blood pressure reduction following PTRAS. This finding is more marked in patients with a >70% stenosis or refractory hypertension [48]. A small retrospective observational study performed at our centre showed that only patients with NT-proBNP levels above a standard cut-off (300 pg/ml) gained benefit from revascularization with regard to all adverse end-points compared to medically managed patients.

Novel revascularization techniques have also been explored as a way of improving patient outcomes. The Sirolimus-Eluting vs. Bare Metal Low Profile Stent for Renal Artery Treatment trial failed to demonstrated significant benefit of drug-eluting stents at 2 years. More promising is the use of embolic protection devices (EPD). Crossing a renal artery lesion with an undeployed stent risks causing disruption of the stenosis and release of downstream emboli. These emboli may contribute to the rapid eGFR losses noted when patients with CKD stage 1 or 2 undergo revascularization. Dual anti-platelet therapy at the time of PRTA can reduce the proportion of patients with distal embolization from 50% to 36% [49], but use of downstream EPD to capture larger particles is an attractive proposition. In a small pilot RCT where these devices have been deployed in conjunction with glycoprotein IIa/IIIb inhibition, significant improvements in eGFR have been seen at 1 month (compared with eGFR reductions in other treatment groups); however further studies are required before these devices form part of routine clinical practice [50].

As mentioned above, novel functional magnetic resonance imaging (MRI) techniques such as blood oxygen level-dependent magnetic resonance imaging (BOLD-MRI) may play a role in risk stratification by estimating the degree of intrarenal hypoxia to identify critically ischaemic kidneys with potentially viable or 'hibernating' parenchyma.

Increased understanding of the complex pathogenesis of renal parenchymal injury in ARVD raises the possibility of novel therapeutic strategies. Cell-based therapies have been proposed to counteract the inflammatory milieu and oxidative stress typically found in the post-stenotic kidney, in order to prevent irreversible loss of renal microvascular architecture and help improve clinical outcomes. Some strategies that are still at an experimental stage include targeting mitochondrial injury, which appears to play a major role in mediating both renal and cardiac remodelling in ARVD and infusion of vascular growth factors, endothelial progenitor cells or mesenchymal stem cells to stimulate angiogenesis and modulate the inflammatory milieu [51–54].

17.2 Renal Artery Embolic Disease

17.2.1 Cholesterol Emboli

Cholesterol embolization occurs when cholesterol crystals are released following the rupture of an atheromatous plaque. These crystals can occlude any small vessel, precipitating a multisystem disorder. Although the true incidence and prevalence are unknown, cholesterol embolization is typically described as a disease of the over-60s (with a male preponderance) and may account for between 5% and 10% of cases of acute kidney injury within this demographic.

17.2.1.1 Clinical Features

As with vasculitis, disease presentation depends entirely on the vessels involved. Severe acute kidney injury is relatively rare, with only the minority of patients having a significant abrupt rise in serum creatinine within a few days of an interventional procedure. Mostly there is slow, progressive loss of renal function spread over a period in excess of 4 weeks. This is suggestive of two distinct pathologies – the first where a large crystal burden causes acute vascular occlusion within the kidney and a second where there is either slow sustained emboli release or a regional inflammatory response to emboli dispersed to the kidney.

In patients with renal involvement, the two other most commonly affected organ systems are the skin (presenting with livedo reticularis, blue toes, purpura, ulceration and gangrene) and the gastrointestinal tract (presenting with non-specific abdominal pain, bleeding, ischemic bowel, pancreatitis). Neurological manifestations are less common and harder to define, but where retinal embolization occurs, this should dramatically raise the index of suspicion for the diagnosis.

17.2.1.2 Aetiopathology and Epidemiology

Given the link between cholesterol embolization and pre-existing atheromatous disease, it is unsurprising that risk factors are common between these conditions (age over 60 years, hypertension, diabetes, smoking history, Caucasian). More clinically relevant are the precipitants for embolization, which *have* changed over time. While 20–30 years ago spontaneous plaque rupture was almost the sole cause, the greatly increased use of interventional endovascular techniques has resulted in over 75% of contemporary cases being iatrogenic. Coronary angiography appears to carry the highest risk, with approximately 20 cases per 1000 procedures. Additionally, anticoagulation can precipitate cholesterol emboli, although this is a rare complication [55].

17.2.1.3 Diagnosis

It is highly likely that many minor or clinically asymptomatic cases of cholesterol embolization go undetected, especially following endovascular revascularization therapy. However, the presence of acute/subacute renal dysfunction in the context of a clear precipitant and other signs of peripheral embolization is sufficient to confirm the diagnosis of cholesterol embolization. Where this triad does not exist (and if retinal emboli cannot be demonstrated on fundoscopy), tissue is required to make a definitive diagnosis and exclude conditions such as small vessel vasculitis. Renal biopsy is the gold standard test (providing a positive diagnosis in over 75% of cases – . Fig. 17.7), but samples from other areas, e.g. skin, can be valuable if this is contraindicated.

Prior to biopsy, there are few serum markers of diagnostic use, but new-onset proteinuria (assuming no co-existing renal disease cause) may be suggestive. A relationship between cholesterol embolization and hypocomplementaemia is not consistently reported, and the presence of this should perhaps direct more attention to the possibility of other diagnoses such as subacute bacterial endocarditis. Of more clinical use is the presence of systemic eosinophilia, which, although transient, is commonly seen at high levels where there is cholesterol embolization. This finding, although sensitive, is not specific and should also prompt consideration of acute interstitial nephritis if there has been a newly introduced medication.

17

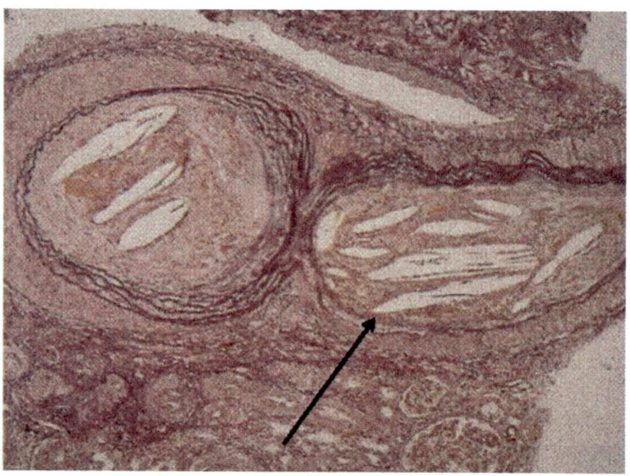

Fig. 17.7 Renal biopsy showing cholesterol emboli. *Renal biopsy demonstrating small vessel cholesterol athero-emboli (arrow)*

17.2.1.4 Treatment

There is no definitive treatment for cholesterol embolization, and between 40 and 60% of patients suspected to have the diagnosis require acute dialysis with a significant proportion remaining dialysis dependent. Withdrawal of any clear precipitant is a vital first step. Thereafter, the mainstay of treatment is statin therapy. Although there is a lack of randomized data or a mechanistic explanation, there is good, prospective, evidence that these agents reduce risk for ESKD [56]. There is no large-scale evidence of benefit for corticosteroids, and use is often limited to patients with severe multisystem disease.

17.2.2 Renal Artery Thromboembolism

Renal artery thromboembolism, if not immediately treated, leads to irreversible renal parenchymal damage and loss of renal function. Unfortunately, due to the non-specific nature of the symptomatology and the rarity of the condition, this is often a delayed diagnosis.

17.2.2.1 Clinical Features and Diagnosis

Most patients are aged over 60 years and present with severe acute onset flank/abdominal pain, which can be associated with a fever and nausea and vomiting. There is no gender or racial preponderance.

While the presence of new-onset dipstick haematuria/proteinuria is supportive of renal thromboembolism, the key to making the diagnosis is a high index of clinical suspicion and expedient angiographic imaging (either direct angiography or CTA, as USS has very low sensitivity). When reviewing imaging it should be understood that up to 10% of cases present with bilateral thrombi.

17.2.2.2 Aetiopathology

The primary source of emboli causing renal infarction is cardiac (typically left atrial clots secondary to atrial fibrillation), although cases linked to sickle cell disease and septic emboli are reported.

17.2.2.3 Treatment

The rarity of the condition makes treatment recommendations difficult. Prompt initiation of anticoagulation with i.v. heparin (followed by warfarin when stable) is the accepted first step, followed by percutaneous thrombolysis or thrombectomy as soon as possible. Renal functional prognosis is highly dependent on speed of diagnosis and treatment [57].

17.3 Renal Vein Disease

Diseases of the renal veins are rare and mainly limited to three disease presentations.

17.3.1 Renal Vein Thrombosis

17.3.1.1 Clinical Features

Where RVT is acute, occlusive and bilateral, AKI will develop. However, most patients slowly develop a progressive thrombus, allowing the development of a collateral venous system. These two distinct pathologies account for the disparity in reported incidence of venous thrombo-embolic events in patients with membranous nephropathy when considering overt clinical presentations (less than 10%) versus those identified by screening (50–80%) [58].

The key symptom of an acute thrombus is loin or flank pain, typically associated with a fever, nausea and vomiting or occasionally presenting as pulmonary emboli. Leucocytosis and dipstick haematuria are common, making pyelonephritis a key differential diagnosis. Cross-sectional imaging may show a significantly swollen kidney (explaining the loin pain) with perinephric stranding (see ◘ Fig. 17.8). The diagnosis can be easily missed on ultrasound unless the renal vein is specifically studied with Doppler.

Chronic thrombi are usually non-occlusive and asymptomatic and characterized by increased proteinuria and subtle alterations in renal function.

17.3.1.2 Aetiopathology

In adults, renal vein thrombosis (RVT) most commonly occurs in the context of nephrotic level protein loss, typically in association with membranous nephropathy. However, associations with other glomerular diseases (e.g. lupus), malignancy (e.g. renal cell carcinoma) and hypercoagulable states (e.g. protein C and S deficiency, postpartum) are also described. While the risk of all types of thrombo-embolic events is elevated in nephrotic states, RVT is one of if not the most common. Why this should be the case is uncertain, but reduced renal vein pressures and increased local thrombin production secondary to glomerular injury are two proposed factors.

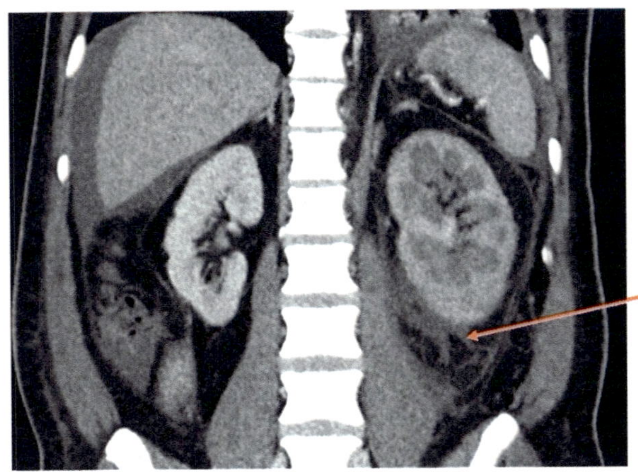

◘ **Fig. 17.8** Acute left renal vein thrombosis demonstrating a modest increase in length but grossly enlarged kidney, reduced perfusion and marked perinephric stranding (arrow). Many of these features in particular the general enlargement can be missed by an inexperienced ultra-sonographer, and it is important to consider a diagnosis of RVT even in the context of an apparently normal ultrasound scan

17.3.1.3 Treatment

There is no defined *gold standard* treatment strategy for renal vein thrombosis. The decision will depend mainly on local expertise and experience but also in part on which kidney is affected (with the left kidney less likely to rupture in the setting of acute venous occlusion due to a pre-existing collateral drainage system). Thrombolysis can be considered where there are bilateral renal vein thrombi or pulmonary embolus, with medical anticoagulation (using warfarin or low molecular weight heparin) then used as chronic therapy. These agents can be utilized as first-line therapy in less severe cases. Interventional approaches including percutaneous thrombectomy, surgical venous bypass and nephrectomy are available. However, these approaches tend to be reserved for cases of extensive clot or where there is risk of capsular rupture.

17.3.2 Renal Vein Stenosis

Very rarely the renal vein can suffer a non-occlusive stenosis resulting in proteinuria and/or reduced function. The diagnosis is easily missed and may only be picked up incidentally in the venous phase of contrast studies (see ◘ Fig. 17.9).

17.3.3 Left Renal Vein Entrapment Syndrome

Left renal vein entrapment (also referred to as the 'nutcracker syndrome') results from entrapment of the

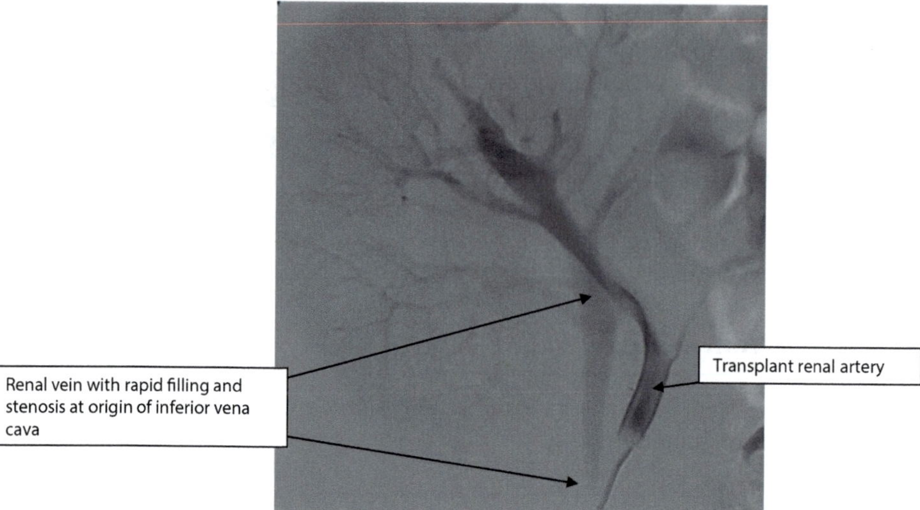

Fig. 17.9 Renal vein stenosis in a renal transplant with an arteriovenous fistula. Angiogram shows very rapid (almost simultaneous) venous return and a venous stenosis at the point of the inferior vena cava

renal vein between the abdominal aorta and the superior mesenteric artery. The presentation can be at any age and is classically with left flank pain (which can extend to the left testicle) with non-visible or visible haematuria or orthostatic proteinuria. Diagnosis can be made either by ultrasound or computed tomography imaging.

Treatment of the 'nutcracker syndrome' is dependent on the severity of symptoms. In the most extreme cases, renal vein stenting, surgical venous bypass and autotransplantation have all been used [59].

17.4 Lymphatic Disease

Cystic dilatation of renal lymphatic channels, renal lymphangiomatosis (also called cystic lymphangioma or renal lymphangiectasia), is an exceptionally rare condition in which the renal lymphatics fail to adequately drain, resulting in structural malformations. The kidneys can enlarge to such a size that they may mimic polycystic disease or cause an obstructive uropathy. As there is minimal effect on renal function, management is normally conservative. The exception is during pregnancy in which the condition may be exacerbated to the point of requiring percutaneous drainage [60].

17

17.5 Questions and Answers

A 65-year-old male is referred for investigation of lower limb claudication pains. His past medical history includes diabetes, longstanding hypertension, angina and a previous transient ischaemic attack. He is also a lifelong smoker. His symptomatic claudication arises after walking for approximately 200 m on the level. He is receiving an angiotensin-converting enzyme inhibitor (ACEi), which was commenced about 2 months before referral, and he also receives a diuretic and a calcium antagonist at full dosage to optimize his blood pressure. On examination he is noted to have bilateral ilio-femoral bruits but palpable pedal pulses. His blood pressure remains sub-optimally controlled at 170/90 mmHg. He is commenced on an alpha-blocker (Doxazosin).

Following the clinic visit, you review his blood results and notice that there has been a deterioration in his renal function with the serum creatinine increasing from 120 to 180 μmol/L and estimated glomerular filtration rate (eGFR) decreasing from 58 to 36 mL/min since the time of referral.

Chapter Review Questions

1. Which statement(s) support(s) your suspicion that the patient has underlying renovascular disease?
   A. Longstanding hypertension.
   B. There is difficulty in controlling the blood pressure with three different antihypertensive drugs.
   C. There was a relatively rapid deterioration of renal function between the time of referral and the first clinic visit.
   D. He is an arteriopath with symptoms of lower limb claudication pains.

2. What would be the most appropriate investigation(s) to decide whether the hypertension has a renovascular origin?
   A. Direct intra-arterial angiography
   B. Renography with captopril provocation
   C. Magnetic resonance angiography (MRA)

D. Computerized tomography angiogram (CTA)
E. Duplex ultrasound of the renal arteries

3. What is the most appropriate revascularization approach for the renal artery stenosis?
   A. Aortorenal bypass
   B. Thromboendarterectomy
   C. Percutaneous transluminal angioplasty (PTA) with stent
   D. PTA alone
   E. Nephrectomy

4. Which are the most frequent serious complications seen after renal artery PTA?
   A. Arterial rupture
   B. Occlusion
   C. Cholesterol microembolization
   D. Contrast-related acute kidney injury
   E. Groin haematoma
   F. All of the above

5. Which of the following would be most appropriate for his future management?

   A. Regular clinic review with attention to medical control of blood pressure and vasculoprotective therapy
   B. Repeat renal artery imaging with possible repeat left renal artery stenting
   C. Right renal artery PTA and stenting
   D. Surgical revascularization of the left kidney

Answers

1. B and D. Haemodynamically -significant renovascular disease leads to neurohumoral activation and upregulation of the renin- angiotensin system leading to hypertension that can prove resistant to medical management. This gentleman has numerous atherosclerotic risk factors, and up to a quarter of patients with peripheral vascular disease have been found to have incidental ARVD.
2. C and D. Both MRA and CTA are non-invasive and have been shown to have an almost equivalent performance to direct intra-arterial angiography, with sensitivities and specificities >90%. Given that his eGFR is >30 ml/min, he is not at high risk of Ccontrast-induced nephropathy or Nnephrogenic systemic fibrosis. Currently there is insufficient evidence to support the routine discontinuation of angiotensin-converting enzyme inhibitors (ACE-Ii) or angiotensin receptor blockers (ARBs) in stable outpatients. However in acutely ill patients at an increased risk of developing AKI, it is suggested that withholding ACEi-I and ARBs should be considered on an individual patient basis [61]. In this situation, the ACEi-I was withheld given the acute on chronic kidney injury.

   In this patient, magnetic resonance imaging showed diffuse aorto-iliac disease. There was a 90% stenosis with post- stenotic dilatation at the ostium of the left renal artery, and the kidney was 10 cm in length. On the right hand side, there were two renal arteries,; the smaller of these exhibited a 50% renal artery stenosis (RAS). The kidney measured 11 cm in length. Given the rapidly deteriorating renal function, uncontrolled hypertension and anatomically severe stenosis in the left renal artery, this patient fell into the 'high-risk' category, and it was decided to proceed with intervention.
3. C. The most appropriate revascularization technique is percutaneous transluminal angioplasty (PTA) with stent.
4. F. Renal Aartery PTA is a potentially hazardous intervention associated with significant complications. The prevalence of these complications in contemporary clinical practice is around 0.5 – 10%.

   The patient underwent percutaneous angioplasty with bare- metal stent placement in the left renal artery. The right renal artery was not amenable to endovascular intervention. The procedure progressed without complications, and the patient was sent home the day after treatment in good condition.

   He was reviewed again after 2 weeks at which stage his creatinine had improved to 140 μmol/L (eGFR 49 mL/min). His blood pressure (165/90) control had improved to some extent.
5. A. The most appropriate long-term management plan for this gentleman would be aggressive control of his atherosclerotic risk factors with appropriate vasculoprotective therapy that includes a statin, aspirin, and, once kidney function is stable, re-introduction of renin- angiotensin blockade. Clinic reviews should focus on optimization of blood pressure and glycaemic control together with smoking cessation advice. Further intervention on the left renal artery is not warranted; however he is at risk of developing in-stent restenosis in the future especially if his atherosclerotic risk factors are not adequately controlled. Open surgical revascularization techniques are very rarely performed nowadays. Intervention on the right renal artery is not needed given that the degree of stenosis (50%) is not of any haemodynamic or functional significance.

Tips, Tricks and Pitfalls

- FMD affects multiple vascular beds with diverse presentations. Diagnosis of FMD in one vascular bed should prompt vascular imaging for FMD involvement in others.
- Although FMD is 91% female predominant, males present more frequently with arterial dissections and aneurysms.
- Angioplasty in FMD is more successful in controlling blood pressure than in atherosclerotic RAS especially in younger patients with recent-onset hypertension.
- The latest and largest RCTs performed in ARVD show that revascularization does not confer added benefit to optimal medical treatment in unselected populations. There are well-described caveats of underrepresentation of high-risk patients that were the most likely to benefit from revascularization.
- Renin-angiotensin blockade has been shown to improve cardiovascular outcomes and survival in patients with ARVD; NICE guidance recommends stopping or reducing the drug if creatinine rises >30% or eGFR falls >25% from baseline and to exclude hemodynamically stressful risk factors.

17.6 Conclusion

FMD may be more common than previously thought, and the diagnosis of the condition in one vascular bed should prompt vascular imaging for FMD involvement in others. Prognosis is favourable with good therapeutic response to PCTA especially in patients <60 years. ARVD is a heterogenous condition with variable clinical outcomes in different patients. While optimized medical vascular therapy remains the mainstay of management of this condition, new information about the complex pathophysiology of this condition highlights the importance of a more individualized and patient-centred approach. It is hoped that novel diagnostic and risk stratification techniques will help identify patients who may potentially benefit from revascularization while avoiding this potentially hazardous intervention in others.

17

References

1. Sharma S, Gupta H, Saxena A, et al. Results of renal angioplasty in nonspecific aortoarteritis (Takayasu disease). J Vasc Interv Radiol. 1998;9(3):429–35.
2. Kim ESH, Olin JW, Froehlich JB, et al. Clinical manifestations of fibromuscular dysplasia vary by patient sex: a report of the United States registry for fibromuscular dysplasia. J Am Coll Cardiol. 2013;62(21):2026–8. https://doi.org/10.1016/j.jacc.2013.07.038.
3. Olin JW, Froehlich J, Gu X, et al. The United States registry for fibromuscular dysplasia: results in the first 447 patients. Circulation. 2012;125(25):3182–90. https://doi.org/10.1161/CIRCULATIONAHA.112.091223.
4. Sharma AM, Kline B. The United States registry for fibromuscular dysplasia: new findings and breaking myths. Tech Vasc Interv Radiol. 2014;17(4):258–63. https://doi.org/10.1053/j.tvir.2014.11.007.
5. Plouin P-F, Perdu J, La Batide-Alanore A, Boutouyrie P, Gimenez-Roqueplo A-P, Jeunemaitre X. Fibromuscular dysplasia. Orphanet J Rare Dis. 2007;2:28. https://doi.org/10.1186/1750-1172-2-28.
6. Olin JW, Sealove BA. Diagnosis, management, and future developments of fibromuscular dysplasia. J Vasc Surg. 2011;53(3):826–36. https://doi.org/10.1016/j.jvs.2010.10.066.
7. Trinquart L, Mounier-Vehier C, Sapoval M, Gagnon N, Plouin PF. Efficacy of revascularization for renal artery stenosis caused by fibromuscular dysplasia: a systematic review and meta-analysis. Hypertension. 2010;56(3):525–32. https://doi.org/10.1161/HYPERTENSIONAHA.110.152918.
8. Olin JW, Gornik HL, Bacharach JM, et al. Fibromuscular dysplasia: state of the science and critical unanswered questions: a scientific statement from the American Heart Association. 2014;129 https://doi.org/10.1161/01.cir.0000442577.96802.8c.
9. Amighi J, Schlager O, Haumer M, et al. Renal artery stenosis predicts adverse cardiovascular and renal outcome in patients with peripheral artery disease. Eur J Clin Investig. 2009;39:784–92. https://doi.org/10.1111/j.1365-2362.2009.02180.x.
10. Ritchie J, Green D, Alderson HV, Chiu D, Sinha S, Kalra PA. Risks for mortality and renal replacement therapy in atherosclerotic renovascular disease compared to other causes of chronic kidney disease. Nephrology (Carlton). 2015;20:688–96. https://doi.org/10.1111/nep.12501.
11. Herrmann SMS, Saad A, Textor SC. Management of atherosclerotic renovascular disease after Cardiovascular Outcomes in Renal Atherosclerotic Lesions (CORAL). Nephrol Dial Transplant. 2014;30(3):366–75.
12. Lewis E, Clarke W, Berl T, et al. Renoprotective effect of the angiotensin-receptor antagonist irebesartan in patients with nephropathy due to type 2 diabetes. N Engl J Med. 2001;345(12):851–60.
13. Wright JTJ, Bakris G, Greene T, et al. Effect of blood pressure lowering and antihypertensive drug class on progression of hypertensive kidney disease. JAMA - J Am Med Assoc. 2002;288(19):2421–31. https://doi.org/10.1001/jama.288.19.2421.
14. Rahman M, Pressel S, Davis BR, et al. Renal outcomes in high-risk hypertensive patients treated with an angiotensin-converting enzyme inhibitor or a calcium channel blocker vs a diuretic: a report from the antihypertensive and lipid-lowering treatment to prevent heart attack trial (AL). Arch Intern Med. 2005;165(8):936. https://doi.org/10.1001/archinte.165.8.936.
15. Onuigbo MAC, Onuigbo NTC. Worsening renal failure in older chronic kidney disease patients with renal artery stenosis concurrently on renin angiotensin aldosterone system blockade: a prospective 50-month Mayo-Health-System clinic analysis. QJM. 2008;101(7):519–27. https://doi.org/10.1093/qjmed/hcn039.
16. Brugts JJ, Boersma E, Chonchol M, et al. The cardioprotective effects of the angiotensin-converting enzyme inhibitor perindopril in patients with stable coronary artery disease are not modified by mild to moderate renal insufficiency. Insights from the EUROPA trial. J Am Coll Cardiol. 2007;50(22):2148–55. https://doi.org/10.1016/j.jacc.2007.08.029.

17. Losito A, Errico R, Santirosi P, Lupattelli T, Scalera GB, Lupattelli L. Long-term follow-up of atherosclerotic renovascular disease. Beneficial effect of ACE inhibition. Nephrol Dial Transplant. 2005;20(8):1604–9.
18. Chrysochou C, Foley RN, Young JF, Khavandi K, Cheung CM, Kalra PA. Dispelling the myth: the use of renin-angiotensin blockade in atheromatous renovascular disease. Nephrol Dial Transplant. 2012;27(4):1403–9. https://doi.org/10.1093/ndt/gfr496.
19. National Institute for Health and Care Excellence. Acute Kidney Injury.
20. Pickering TG, Herman L, Devereux RB, et al. Recurrent pulmonary oedema in hypertension due to bilateral renal artery stenosis: treatment by angioplasty or surgical revascularisation. Lancet. 1988;2(8610):551–2. https://doi.org/10.1016/S0140-6736(88)92668-2.
21. Messerli FH, Bangalore S, Makani H, et al. Flash pulmonary oedema and bilateral renal artery stenosis: the Pickering syndrome. Eur Heart J. 2011;32(18):2231–5. https://doi.org/10.1093/eurheartj/ehr056.
22. Wheatley K, Ives N, Gray R, et al. Revascularization versus medical therapy for renal-artery stenosis. N Engl J Med. 2009;361(20):1953–62.
23. Cooper CJ, Murphy TP, Cutlip DE, et al. Stenting and medical therapy for atherosclerotic renal-artery stenosis. N Engl J Med. 2014;370(1):13–22.
24. Kalra PA, Guo H, Kausz AT, et al. Atherosclerotic renovascular disease in United States patients aged 67 years or older: risk factors, revascularization, and prognosis. Kidney Int. 2005;68(1):293–301. https://doi.org/10.1111/j.1523-1755.2005.00406.x.
25. de Mast Q, Beutler J. The prevalence of atherosclerotic renal artery stenosis in risk groups: a systematic literature review. J Hypertens. 2009;27(7):1333–40.
26. Shurrab A, Mamtora H, O'Donoghue D, Waldrek S, Kalra P. Increasing the diagnostic yield of renal angiography for the diagnosis of atheromatous renovascular disease. Br J Radiol. 2001;74(879):213–8.
27. Carlstrom M, Wilcox CS, Arendshorst WJ. Renal autoregulation in health and disease. Physiol Rev. 2015;95(2):405–511. https://doi.org/10.1152/physrev.00042.2012.
28. Textor SC, McKusick MM, Misra S, Glockner J. Timing and selection for renal revascularization in an era of negative trials: what to do? Prog Cardiovasc Dis. 2009;52(3):220–8. https://doi.org/10.1016/j.pcad.2009.10.001.
29. Saad A, Herrmann SMS, Crane J, et al. Stent revascularization restores cortical blood flow and reverses tissue hypoxia in atherosclerotic renal artery stenosis but fails to reverse inflammatory pathways or glomerular filtration rate. Circ Cardiovasc Interv. 2013;6(4):428–35. https://doi.org/10.1161/CIRCINTERVENTIONS.113.000219.
30. Chrysochou C, Cheung C, Durow M, et al. Proteinuria as a predictor of renal functional outcome after revascularization in atherosclerotic renovascular disease (ARVD). QJM. 2009;102(4):283–8.
31. Vassallo D, Ritchie J, Green D, Chrysochou C, Blunt J, Kalra PA. The importance of proteinuria and prior cardiovascular disease in all major clinical outcomes of atherosclerotic renovascular disease - a single-center observational study. BMC Nephrol. 2016;17(1) https://doi.org/10.1186/s12882-016-0409-1.
32. Odudu A, Vassallo D, Kalra PA. From anatomy to function: diagnosis of atherosclerotic renal artery stenosis. Expert Rev Cardiovasc Ther. 2015;13(12) https://doi.org/10.1586/14779072.2015.1100077.
33. Wright J, Shurrab A, Cooper A, Kalra P, Foley R, Kalra P. Left ventricular morphology and function in patients with atherosclerotic renovascular disease. J Am Soc Nephrol. 2005;16(9):2746–53.
34. Marcantoni C, Zanoli L, Rastelli S. Effect of renal artery stenting on left ventricular mass: a randomised clinical trial. Am J Kidney Dis. 2012;60(1):39–46.
35. Ritchie J, Green D, Chrysochou T, et al. Effect of renal artery revascularization upon cardiac structure and function in atherosclerotic renal artery stenosis: cardiac magnetic resonance sub-study of the ASTRAL trial. Nephrol Dial Transplant. 2017;32(6):1006–13.
36. Bax L, Woittiez A, Kouwenberg H, et al. Stent placement in patients with atherosclerotic renal artery stenosis and impaired renal function. Ann Intern Med. 2010;150(12):840–8.
37. Textor SC, McKusick MM. Renal artery stenosis: if and when to intervene. Curr Opin Nephrol Hypertens. 2016;25(2):144–51.
38. Ritchie J, Green D, Chrysochou C, Chalmers N, Foley RN, Kalra PA. High-risk clinical presentations in atherosclerotic renovascular disease: prognosis and response to renal artery revascularization. Am J Kidney Dis. 2014;63(2):186–97.
39. Vassallo D, Ritchie J, Green D, Chrysochou C, Kalra PA. The effect of revascularization in patients with anatomically significant atherosclerotic renovascular disease presenting with high-risk clinical features. Nephrol Dial Transplant. 2018;33(3) https://doi.org/10.1093/ndt/gfx025.
40. Chrysochou C, Green D, Ritchie J, Buckley DL, Kalra A. Kidney volume to GFR ratio predicts functional improvement after revascularization in atheromatous renal artery stenosis. PLoS One. 2017;12(6):e0177178.
41. Kane G, Xu N, Mistrik E, Roubicek T, Stanson A, Garovic V. Renal artery revascularization improves heart failure control in patients with atherosclerotic renal artery stenosis. Nephrol Dial Transplant. 2010;25(3):813–20.
42. MacDowall P, Kalra P, O'Donoghue D, Waldek S, Mamtora H, Brown K. Risk of morbidity from renovascular disease in elderly patients with congestive cardiac failure. Lancet. 1998;352(9121):13–6.
43. Green D, Ritchie J, Chrysochou C, Kalra P. Revascularization of atherosclerotic renal artery stenosis for chronic heart failure versus acute pulmonary oedema. Nephrology. 2018;23(5):411–7.
44. Van Jaarsveld BC, Krijnen P, Pieterman H, et al. The effect of balloon angioplasty on hypertension in atherosclerotic renal artery stenosis. Dutch Renal Artery Stenosis Intervention Cooperative Study Group. N Engl J Med. 2000;342(14):1007–14.
45. Silva V, Martin L, Franco R, et al. Pleiotropic effects of statins may improve outcomes in atherosclerotic renovascular disease. Am J Hypertens. 2008;21(10):1163–8.
46. Jardine MJ, Ninomiya T, Perkovic V, et al. Aspirin is beneficial in hypertensive patients with chronic kidney disease: a post-hoc subgroup analysis of a randomized controlled trial. J Am Coll Cardiol. 2010;56(12):956–65. https://doi.org/10.1016/j.jacc.2010.02.068.
47. Vassallo D, Foley R, Kalra P. Design of a clinical risk calculator for major clinical outcomes in patients with atherosclerotic renovascular disease. Nephrol Dial Transplant. 2019;34(8):1377–84.
48. Staub D, Zeller T, Trenk D, et al. Use of B-type natriuretic peptide to predict blood pressure improvement after percutaneous

revascularisation for renal artery stenosis. Eur J Vasc Endovasc Surg. 2010;40(5):599–607.
49. Kanjwal K, Cooper C, Virmani R, et al. Predictors of embolization during protected renal artery angioplasty and stenting: role of antiplatelet therapy. Catheter Cardiovasc Interv. 2010;76(1):16–23.
50. Cooper CJ, Haller ST, Colyer W, et al. Embolic protection and platelet inhibition during renal artery stenting. Circulation. 2008;117(21):2752–60. https://doi.org/10.1161/CIRCULATIONAHA.107.730259.
51. Eirin A, Ebrahimi B, Kwon SH, et al. Restoration of mitochondrial cardiolipin attenuates cardiac damage in swine renovascular hypertension. J Am Heart Assoc. 2016;5(6):pii: e003118. https://doi.org/10.1161/JAHA.115.003118.
52. Iliescu R, Fernandez SR, Kelsen S, Maric C, Chade AR. Role of renal microcirculation in experimental renovascular disease. Nephrol Dial Transplant. 2010;25(4):1079–87.
53. Chade AR, Zhu X-Y, Krier JD, et al. Endothelial progenitor cells homing and renal repair in experimental renovascular disease. Stem Cells. 2010;28(6):1039–47. https://doi.org/10.1002/stem.426.
54. Eirin A, Zhu X-Y, Krier JD, et al. Adipose tissue-derived mesenchymal stem cells improve revascularization outcomes to restore renal function in swine atherosclerotic renal artery stenosis. Stem Cells. 2012;30(5):1030–41.
55. Scolari R, Ravani P. Atheroembolic renal disease. Lancet. 2010;375(9726):1650–60.
56. Scolari F, Ravani P, Gaggi R, et al. The challenge of diagnosing atheroembolic renal disease: clinical features and prognostic factors. Circulation. 2007;116(3):298–304. https://doi.org/10.1161/CIRCULATIONAHA.106.680991.
57. Lopez V, Glauser J. A case of renal artery thrombosis with renal infarction. J Emerg Trauma Shock. 2010;3(3):302.
58. Lionaki S, Derebail VK, Hogan SL, et al. Venous thromboembolism in patients with membranous nephropathy. Clin J Am Soc Nephrol. 2012;7(1):43–51. https://doi.org/10.2215/CJN.04250511.
59. Kurklinsky AK, Rooke TW. Nutcracker phenomenon and nutcracker syndrome. Mayo Clin Proc. 2010;85(6):552–9. https://doi.org/10.4065/mcp.2009.0586.
60. Ozmen M, Deren O, Akata D, Akhan O, Ozen H, Durukan T. Renal lymphangiomatosis during pregnancy: management with percutaneous drainage. Eur Radiol. 2001;11(1):37–40.
61. Lewington A, MacTier R, Hoefield R, Sutton A, Smith D. Prevention of contrast induced acute kidney injury (CI-AKI) in adult patients. The Renal Association. https://doi.org/10.1017/CBO9781107415324.004.
62. Weibull H, Bergqvist D, Bergentz SE, Jonsson K, Hulthén L, Manhem P. Percutaneous transluminal renal angioplasty versus surgical reconstruction of atherosclerotic renal artery stenosis: a prospective randomized study. J Vasc Surg. 1993;18(5):841–50; discussion 850–852.
63. Plouin P-F, Chatellier G, Darné B, Raynaud A, Study G for the EMM vs A (EMMA). Blood pressure outcome of angioplasty in atherosclerotic renal artery stenosis: a randomized trial. Hypertension. 1998;31(3):823–9.
64. Webster J, Marshall F, Abdalla M, et al. Randomised comparison of percutaneous angioplasty vs continued medical therapy for hypertensive patients with atheromatous renal artery stenosis. J Hum Hypertens. 1998;12(5):329–35.
65. Van De Ven PJG, Kaatee R, Beutler JJ, et al. Arterial stenting and balloon angioplasty in ostial atherosclerotic renovascular disease: a randomised trial. Lancet. 1999;353(9149):282–6.

Internet Resources

Contrast nephropathy risk calculator: http://www.qxmd.com/calculate-online/nephrology/contrast-nephropathy-post-pci.

The Fibromuscular Dysplasia Registry: http://www.fmdsa.org.

Glomerular Diseases

Contents

Management of the Nephrotic Patient: The Overall Approach to the Patient with Nephrotic Syndrome

Gabrielle Goldet and Ruth J. Pepper

Contents

M. Harber (ed.), *Primer on Nephrology*, https://doi.org/10.1007/978-3-030-76419-7_18

Learning Objectives

1. To appreciate that NS has potentially life-threatening complications such as infection, AKI and thromboembolism and that strategies minimising the risk of these complications are a critical aspect of NS management.
2. To note that in children initial treatment may be empirical as most NS is steroid-sensitive, but in adults the potential causes of nephrotic syndrome is much wider and much less likely to be steroid-responsive. Consequently, in adults a renal biopsy is much more critical for management.
3. NS can result from genetic or acquired causes, and the glomerular lesion may be a primary glomerular disorder, or secondary to systemic diseases. Differentiating the causes is key to management; most secondary NS will improve with treatment of the underlying disease.
4. Careful fluid balance is essential in the management of these patients whether in hospital or in the community, and patients should be empowered and supported to be involved.

Definition

The definition of nephrotic syndrome is oedema, with protein excretion quantified at a urine protein creatinine ratio of ≥300 mg/mmol [1] (>3.5 g/day in adults) or >3+ protein on urine dipstick with a serum albumin of less than 25 g/l. [2].

18.1 Introduction

Any patient presenting with oedema and/or a low albumin should have prompt urine analysis performed, and the presence of proteinuria in the dipstick should then be quantified with a urine protein creatinine ratio (PCR). It is an important diagnosis for non-nephrologists to make as it can carry a significant morbidity and requires specialist management. In children, minimal change disease is the most common cause of nephrotic syndrome followed by FSGS, with membranous nephropathy accounting for less than 5% of cases [2]. The majority of children will respond to steroids (steroid-sensitive nephrotic syndrome). However, a significant proportion will relapse or become steroid-dependent. Frequently relapsing NS syndrome is defined as two or more relapses within 6 months or four or more within 12 months.

Steroid-dependent NS is defined as two consecutive relapses occurring while attempting to wean steroids to a low dose, or within 2 weeks of cessation of steroids. Steroid resistance is defined as persistent proteinuria despite 8 weeks of high-dose steroids [3]. In adults, causes of nephrotic syndrome are more diverse with patterns such as membranous nephropathy and other secondary causes increasing in incidence [4], highlighting the importance of the kidney biopsy for diagnosis in adults with NS.

18.2 The Podocyte

Minimal change disease and FSGS are now known to be podocytopathies, with podocyte injury the key pathological feature of disease. Podocytes are the cells located on the outer (urinary) aspect of the glomerular capillary wall and are also known as visceral glomerular epithelial cells. Podocytopathies are diseases where the cell that is primarily injured/dysfunctional is the podocyte. In health, the glomerular capillary wall is relatively impermeable to protein, and its selective sieving action is maintained via a complex tripartite structure involving podocytes on the outside, glomerular endothelial cells on the inside and the glomerular basement membrane in between the two cellular layers. Podocytes have a specialised structure comprising a cell body, primary and secondary processes (◘ Fig. 18.1a). The secondary processes interdigitate together, and the slits they form, analogous to the teeth of a zipper, are the filtration slits through which glomerular filtration occurs. Each is bridged by a slit diaphragm. The complex architecture of the podocyte is maintained by actin fibres arranged throughout the cytoplasm of the cell, and when there is foot process effacement, the distribution of actin fibres is markedly deranged (◘ Fig. 18.1b). The selective filtration function of the glomerular capillary wall is then disrupted, and proteinuria results. Podocytes have a very limited capacity for repair or regeneration [5], so that when podocytes are irreversibly damaged or lost, they are not adequately replaced, proteinuria continues and progressive loss of kidney function can supervene. A proportion of patients with steroid-resistant disease will have a single-gene mutation, resulting in an abnormality of the podocyte [6] (◘ Fig. 18.2).

18.3 Causes of Nephrotic Syndrome

NS may be due to an underlying primary renal disease such as minimal change disease, membranous nephropathy or primary focal segmental glomerulosclerosis or secondary to a more systemic illness and are covered in detail in their respective chapters. It is important to note here that the spectrum of diseases causing NS changes significantly with demographics in particular age (◘ Fig. 18.3).

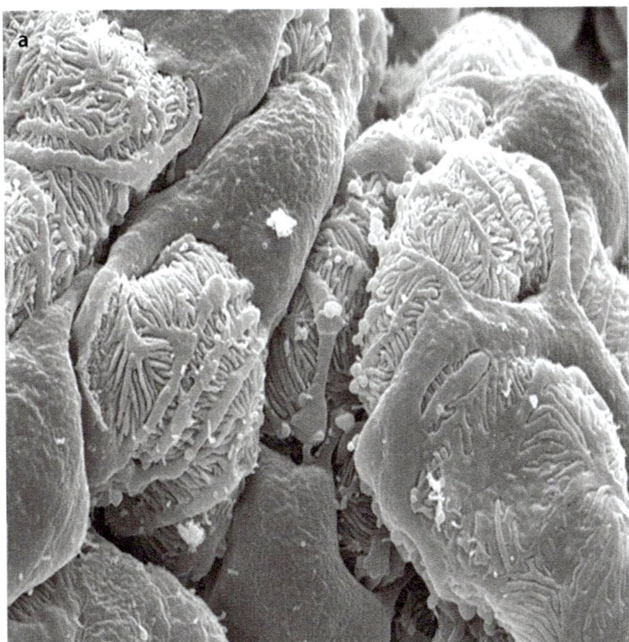

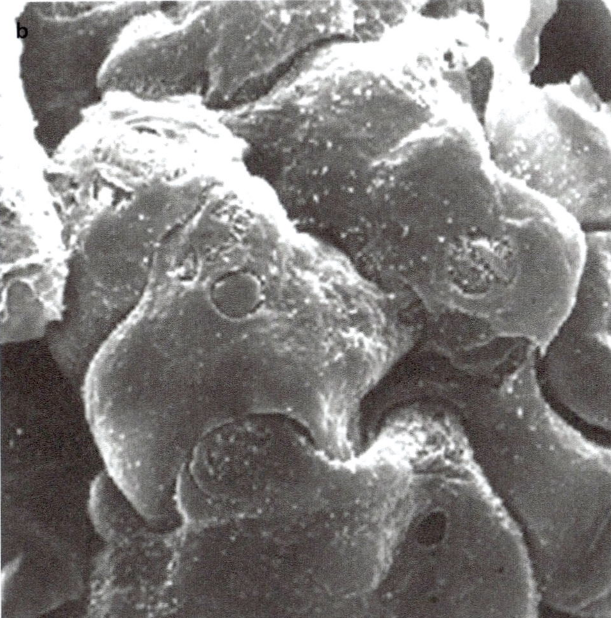

Fig. 18.1 Scanning electron micrograph of external (urinary) aspect of normal human glomerular capillary showing podocyte cell bodies (*), primary (1°) and secondary (2°) processes. (**a**) demonstrates a normal podocyte. (**b**) demonstrates a podocyte in nephrotic syndrome and the loss of normal architecture with foot process effacement

In adults, primary membranous nephropathy (PMN) is the most common cause of nephrotic syndrome, with some series describing 20–37% of cases of nondiabetic adults presenting with nephrotic syndrome, with an increasing incidence in patients aged over 60 years old [12] the majority of which have autoantibodies to M-type phospholipase A-2 receptor [13]. A proportion of patients with membranous nephropathy will have a secondary process, for example, driven by infection, autoimmune disease such as lupus, as well as drugs and malignancy.

Minimal change disease in adults is responsible for about 10–15% of cases of nephrotic syndrome. This is in contrast to children greater than 1 year old up to puberty, in which minimal change disease will account for 70–90% of cases of nephrotic syndrome [7]. In older children the incidence does start to decrease and accounts for about 50% of cases of nephrotic syndrome.

The incidence of FSGS has increased in the 1990s compared to 1970s (15% increasing to 35% in one study). There is also an ethnic variation with FSGS, with an increased incidence in African-American patients compared to Caucasian ethnicity [10]. This is supported in other renal biopsy studies of patients presenting with nephrotic-range proteinuria, with African-American patients having a FSGS incidence of 57% compared to 23% in a Caucasian population [14]. African-American patients with FSGS may have mutations in the apolipoprotein L1 (*APOL1*) gene, but this is not routinely analysed.

Although IgA nephropathy is a common glomerulonephritis, it does not often cause nephrotic syndrome. Membranoproliferative (mesangiocapillary) glomerulonephritis is a recognised cause of the nephrotic syndrome but is relatively rare and is usually is a secondary process being driven by a primary cause. It is crucial to make the correct diagnosis of the cause of nephrotic syndrome, as there are differences in treatment as well as rates of CKD and progression to ESRF.

Alternatively, NS may be due to a secondary process such as diabetes mellitus, autoimmune diseases (lupus), amyloid and the paraproteinaemias; a virally driven process (hepatitis B, hepatitis C or HIV), medication, or a paraneoplastic process with treatment of these secondary causes focused on the underlying cause. This demonstrates the importance of a detailed and thoughtful assessment.

18.4 Inherited Causes

The unifying factor in most genetically mediated podocyte disorders seems to be disruption of the actin cytoskeleton: in 85% of cases of steroid-resistant nephrotic syndrome (SRNS) presenting by the age of 3 months and 66% of cases presenting by the 1st year of life, a recessive mutation in just four genes has been demonstrated (*NPHS1*, *NPHS2*, *LAMB2*, *WT1*) [15]. Nephrin (*NPHS1*) is a signalling molecule located at the slit diaphragm that forms an integral part of the glomerular

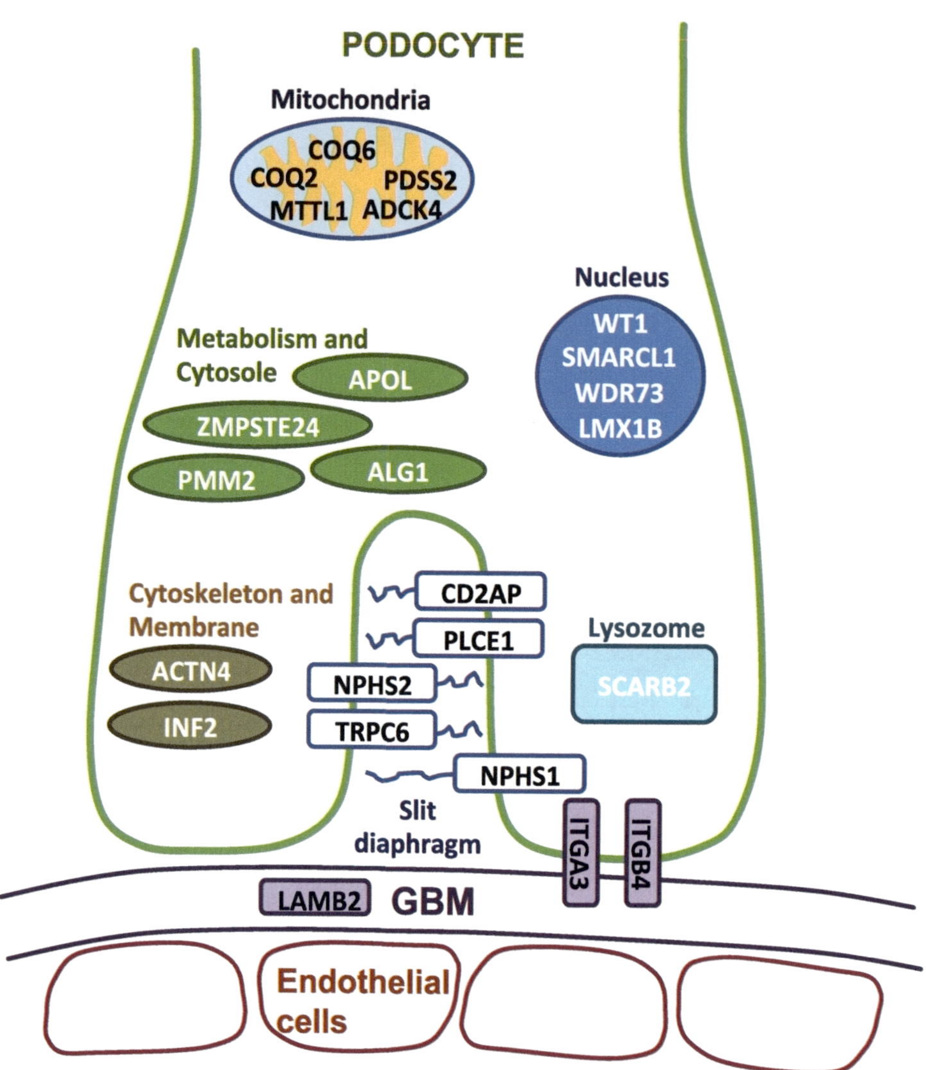

Fig. 18.2 Diagram representing the podocyte, glomerular basement membrane (GBM), endothelial cells and common gene mutations causing nephrotic syndrome

The defective gene-resulting mutated protein pairs are as follows: (mitochondria) ADCK4 AarF domain containing kinase 4, COQ2 coenzyme Q2, COQ6 Coenzyme Q6, MTTL1 mitochondrial tRNA 1, PDSS2 prenyl diphosphate synthase subunit 2, (nucleus) WTI Wilms' tumour protein 1, SMARCL1 SMARCA-like protein, WDR73 WD repeat-containing protein 73, LMX1B LIM homeobox transcription factor 1β, (metabolism and cytosol) ALG1 asparagine-linked glycosylation 1, APOL1 apolipoprotein L1, PMM2 phosphomannomutase 2, ZMPSTE24 zinc metalloproteinase STE24, (cytoskeleton and membrane) ACTN4 α-actinin 4, INF2 inverted formin 2, (lysosome) SCARB2 lysosomal integral membrane protein type 2, (slit diaphragm) NPHSE1 nephrin, NPHSE2 podocin, CD2AP CD2-associated protein, PLCE1 phospholipase C epsilon 1, TRPC6 transient receptor potential channel C6, (GBM) LAMB2 laminin β2, ITGA3 integrin α3, ITGB4 integrin β4

filtration barrier. Mutations in podocin are associated with steroid-resistant nephrotic syndrome and mutations in the cation channel TRPC6, leading to constitutive activity of the channel and unregulated calcium entry into the cell, seem to exert some or all of their effects via alterations in the actin cytoskeleton and therefore in the cell shape [16, 17].

A single-gene cause of SRNS presenting before the age of 25 years has been demonstrated in 29.5% of patients [18]. A genetic diagnosis is significant as this may result in a specific intervention, for example, SRNS caused by mutations in the Q_{10} pathway, which may respond to coenzyme Q_{10} treatment. Additionally, a high risk of progression to ESRF has been demonstrated in genetic SRNS with a lower risk of disease recurrence in transplantation [8]. Therefore genetic testing (and appropriate counselling) is crucial for young patients and their families. Genetic screening is being introduced nationally and should be considered for steroid-resistant nephrotic syndrome presenting at any age. Additionally, in those patients with FSGS, screening should be considered if immunosuppression or transplantation is being considered especially in the context of a family history of syndromic features.

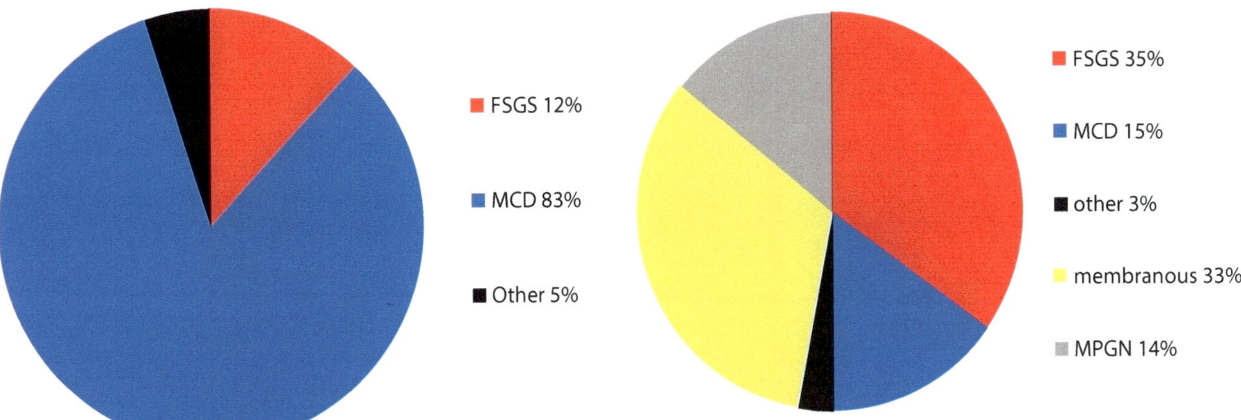

Fig. 18.3 Pie charts demonstrating relative causes of nephrotic syndrome due to primary glomerulonephritides in both children (i) and adults (ii). (i) In children MCD, 83%; FSGS, 12%; other 5%. Other in children includes diffuse mesangial sclerosis (DMS), progressive mesangial sclerosis (PMS), collapsing glomerulopathy (CG) and membranous nephropathy [7, 8]. (ii) FSGS, 35%; membranous nephropathy, 33%; MCD, 15%; MPGN, 14%; other, 3%. Other in adults includes amyloid nephropathy, IgA, chronic glomerulonephritis, nephrosclerosis, C1q nephropathy and fibrillary glomerulonephritis [9–11]

18.5 Investigations

The initial investigations for patients with nephrotic syndrome (see Table 18.1) are aimed to (1) confirm the presence of nephrotic syndrome, (2) elucidate primary or secondary cause and (3) prepare the patients for a kidney biopsy to allow a definitive diagnosis. Urine dipstick with quantification of proteinuria with a urine protein creatinine ratio (uPCR) along with renal function and albumin will confirm the nephrotic state with a uPCR of 300–350 mg/mmol defining nephrotic-range proteinuria.

Table 18.1 Table to demonstrate investigations in nephrotic syndrome

Confirming diagnosis	Urine dipstick, urine protein creatinine ratio, renal function, liver function tests
Investigation secondary causes	Full blood count, bone profile, autoantibodies (ANA, dsDNA, complement C3 and C4), ENA, immunoglobulins, serum-free light chains, serum and urine electrophoresis, glucose, C-reactive protein, virology (HIV, hepatitis B and C)
Investigating complications	Vitamin D, thyroid function tests, lipids Consider CT-PA or V/Q scan if PE suspected, CXR may show pleural effusions, Doppler renal vessels if renal vein thrombosis suspected, Doppler lower legs exclude DVT
Additional tests	Anti-phospholipase A-2 receptor antibody If malignancy suspected: targeted investigations (imaging, endoscopy)
Preparing for renal biopsy	MSU, coagulation screen, renal tract US scan
Genetic testing in SRNS	Podocyte panel of genes

18.6 Treatment and General Management

KDIGO (kidney disease improving global outcomes) clinical practice guidelines for glomerulonephritis provides guidance in the treatment of glomerular disease and is used as an aid in decision-making, with clinicians taking account individual patient preference and patient factors [19]. The treatment of specific causes of NS are covered in their respective chapters, but clear and consistent advice on salt restriction (high-salt diets impair the impact of RAS blockade, increase oedema and result in more rapid progression to ESRD in proteinuric patients), regular monitoring of weight, postural blood pressure, urine dipstick and urine PCR for inpatient and outpatient care is critical. A guide dry weight is often helpful to discuss a mechanism with the patient by which diuretics and antihypertensives can be adjusted depending on response.

Nephrotic syndrome may or may not be associated with hypertension. Blood pressure control is important, but the benefit is disproportionately so the greater the amount of proteinuria.

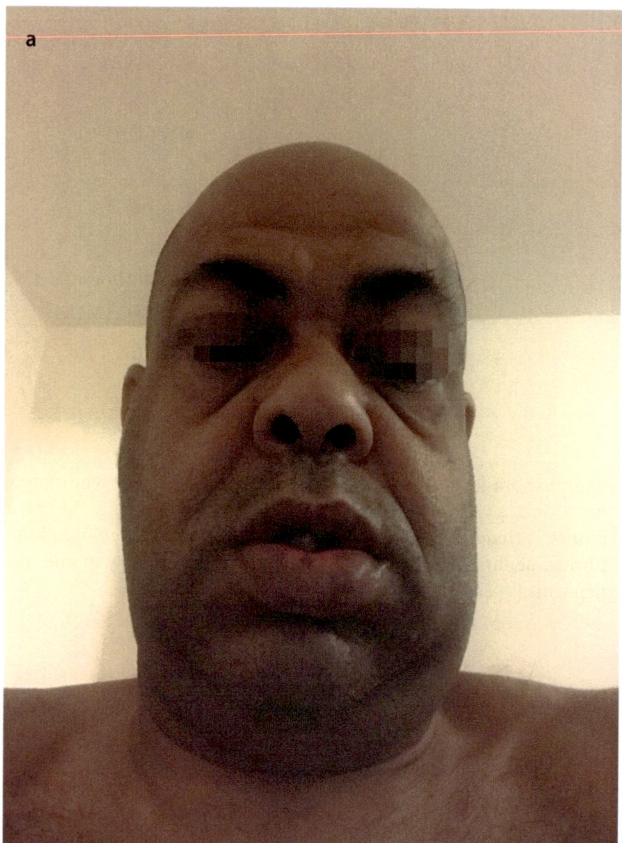

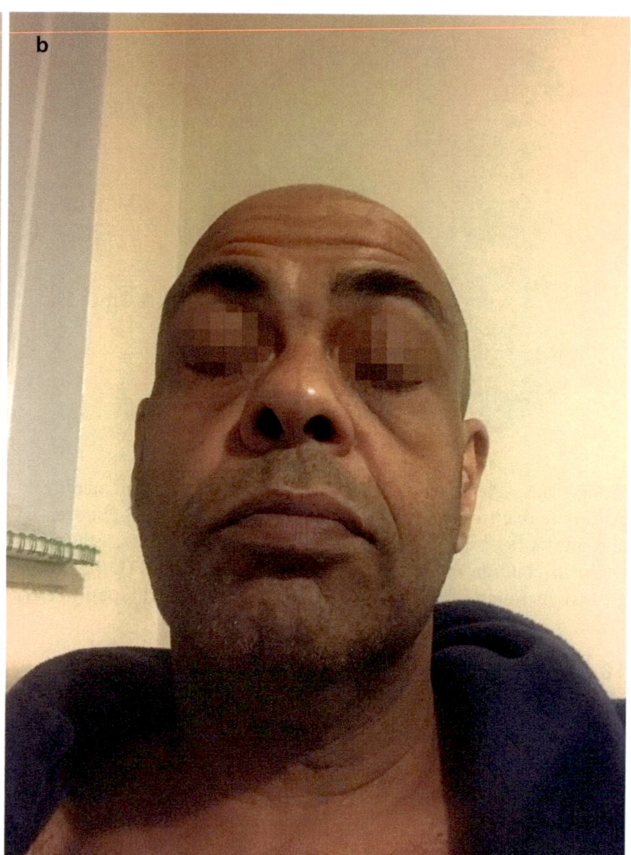

Fig. 18.4 (**a**) Significant oedema at relapse. (**b**) Remission

General measures in the nephrotic patient with significant oedema include salt and fluid intake restriction along with diuretic therapy (management of oedema in NS is covered in the following chapter). Figure 18.4 demonstrates the significant oedema patients with nephrotic syndrome can suddenly develop, with (i) taking at time of relapse and (ii) at time of remission.

Renin and angiotensin inhibition, with either ACE-I or ARB, is important in reducing proteinuria (and hypertension) in patients who are not volume deplete and who are unlikely to go into rapid remission. In the setting of CKD, the greater the proteinuria, the more a patient is likely to benefit from RAS blockade. Due to the potential adverse effect of reducing GFR especially in the patient with significant hypoalbuminaemia, care must be taken to monitor the renal function following initiation. Non-dihydropyridine calcium channel blockers also reduce proteinuria (by up to 30%), and mineralocorticoid receptor antagonists may have an additive effect.

Calcineurin inhibitors also have an antiproteinuric effect beyond any immunomodulatory role, in part through afferent artery vasoconstriction. They can be very useful in the setting of intractable proteinuria but run the risk of contributing to AKI and progressive CKD if not handled with careful monitoring and modest target trough levels. The KDIGO guidelines recommend initially tacrolimus doses of 0.05–0.1 mg/kg/day in two divided doses, with the doses tapering to maintain remission in minimal change disease with a dose of 0.1–0.2 mg/kg/day in FSGS with an initial target of 5–10 ng/ml (6–12 nmol/l) with slow tapering once remission achieved. For membranous nephropathy, the dose of tacrolimus recommended is 0.05–0.075 mg/kg/day in two divided doses.

18.7 Steroid Side Effect Prophylaxis

For patients with significant doses of glucocorticoids, as one-off or especially repeated courses, bone prophylaxis should be considered and ultimately bone density assessed. Prophylaxis against candida and gastritis also need to be covered. Patients should be forewarned about increased appetite and weight gain including strategies to reduce this including careful eating and regular exercise.

This is important for several reasons not least because patients may be understandably distressed by the weight gain induced by steroids and reluctant to be compliant a second time around.

18.8 Personal Treatment Plan (PTP)

For patients with recurrent relapses, it is vital to support patients and their families and encourage their engagement through education and explanation. Providing patients with urine protein sticks (along with daily weight measurement) allowing early identification of a relapse and to contact their nephrologist early to prevent a full-blown relapse and avoid hospital admission.

For those in whom a relapse can be managed with early institution of treatment, a personal treatment plan may avoid an unnecessary admission via the emergency department and treatment by non-specialists. Agreeing a PTP with the patient or their family goes some way towards self-determination.

An example of a PTP might be:

3+ or 4+ protein on dipstick for 3 consecutive days in a patient known to have frequently relapsing steroid sensitive nephrotic syndrome

Arrange urgent blood and urine tests
Prompt initiation of prednisolone 60mg (with gastric and bone protection)
Albumin <20, arrange prophylactic anti-coagulation

Early clinic review if uncomplicated
If unwell/AKI/NS complicated by sepsis: urgent admission

Clear plan to reduce prednisolone and frusemide once remission achieved.

18.9 Causes of Relapse or Treatment Resistance

A significant proportion of patients with nephrotic syndrome, especially minimal change, will continue to have frequently relapsing disease. Additionally some patients with nephrotic syndrome may become steroid-resistant. At times of relapses, or of treatment non-response, a detailed history and further investigations may be appropriate.

18.10 Complications of Nephrotic Syndrome

18.10.1 Thrombosis and Nephrotic Syndrome

Thrombosis is a well-known complication of nephrotic syndrome. There are several important factors contributing to this hypercoagulable environment. These include urinary loss of antithrombin III, protein C, protein S and tissue factor pathway inhibitor as well as alterations in procoagulants such as fibrinogen, factor V and VIII, von Willebrand factor with increased platelet reactivity and changes in fibrinolysis [20]. Albumin has been demonstrated to play a critical role in platelet aggregation, with platelet activation inversely correlating with the level of albumin in the serum [21].

Very low serum levels of antithrombin III have been demonstrated in children with complications such as DVT and PE. These thrombotic complications have been demonstrated when the levels are 75% below normal with an albumin of less than 20 g/L [22]. Membranous nephropathy is well-recognised to result in a higher thrombotic risk compared to the other causes of nephrotic syndrome. One study has demonstrated the risk of thrombotic events (DVT, renal vein thrombosis (RVT) and PE) in membranous was significantly higher (7.9%) compared to FSGS (3%) and IgA nephropathy (0.4%) [23]. The risk of thrombosis events is highest in the 1st 6 months of presentation. The highest risk of RVT is observed in membranous nephropathy (accounting for 37% of cases of a RVT), with a clinically significant risk in MPGN (occurring in 26% of cases of RVT) and minimal change (in 24% cases of RVT) [24]. This increased risk of DVT and or RVT has been demonstrated when the albumin level is <20–25 g/l. However, thromboembolism can still occur with a more mildly reduced level of albumin [25]. There is no clear consensus or randomised trial data of when to initiate prophylactic anticoagulation. Generally, low-molecular-weight heparin or warfarin is used in patients with membranous nephropathy with an albumin less than 20–25 g/l. Prophylaxis in other causes of nephrotic syndrome due to the high thrombotic risk is also initiated [26]. In those patients with a thrombotic event, it seems sensible to continue with anticoagulation for the duration of nephrotic syndrome. In those patients with minimal change nephropathy in which a response to treatment may occur in a few weeks, prophylaxis with heparin is more appropriate than warfarin. The dose of warfarin may change depending on albumin levels, and higher doses of heparin are likely due to the loss of antithrombin III in the urine. For patients with relapsing NS who have had previous thromboembolism, then a personal treatment plan that involves early anticoagulation is worth considering.

18.10.2 Infection

Infection is a well-recognised cause of morbidity and mortality in patients with nephrotic syndrome. Low levels of IgG from urinary loss and changes in complement are recognised as well as alterations in neutrophil phagocytosis and T-cell function [27]. Spontaneous bacterial peritonitis, for example, caused by *Streptococcus pneumoniae*, is a recognised and serious complication of nephrotic syndrome, and in children, administration of pneumococcal vaccination is recommended [28].

Immunodeficiency is compounded if immunotherapy is used in an attempt to treat the NS, and patients should be investigated aggressively for infection if unwell including blood cultures, ascitic tap (spontaneous bacterial peritonitis) and commenced rapidly on antibiotics if febrile.

Patients should be tested for varicella-zoster immunity as infection in the immunocompromised can be life-threatening. Vaccination can be considered in patients in remission. Data from children has demonstrated although this is a live vaccine, it is safe and effective in children in remission or on alternate low-dose steroids [29]. Following exposure to non-immune patients, prophylactic varicella-zoster immune globulin can be given. However, a Cochrane review concluded there is no strong evidence on the effectiveness of other prophylactic interventions to prevent infection in patients with nephrotic syndrome [30].

18

18.10.3 Acute Kidney Injury

Risk factors for AKI in patients with nephrotic syndrome include older age (e.g. AKI is less common in children with minimal change disease compared to adults), male gender, hypertension and heavy proteinuria with a low albumin [31]. An episode of AKI is not uncommon during either the presentation or relapse of nephrotic syndrome, and there are several potential causes (see Table 18.2). The commonest cause relates to glomerular hypoperfusion, which is usually secondary to hypotension, reduced intravascular volume and blockade of the RAS. Other causes may include the use of nephrotoxic drugs (such as calcineurin inhibitors) or contrast which is usually apparent, but renal vein thrombosis and abdominal compartment syndrome secondary to tense ascites need to be excluded. Additionally, patients treated with ciclosporin or tacrolimus should have drug levels carefully monitored due to the known nephrotoxic effects of these drugs.

Proteinuria also has a deleterious effect on the proximal tubular epithelial cells, with the persistence of proteinuria known to be a poor prognostic factor in progression of chronic kidney disease. Proteinuria, with the filtration of macromolecules such as albumin and immunoglobulins, can have a direct toxic effect via the dysregulation of signalling pathways of proximal tubular epithelial cells with the resultant inflammatory milieu and stimulation of pro-apoptotic pathways [32].

For the reason above as well as the risk of thromboembolic disease, it is critical to keep patients with severe NS under close observation by checking for signs of intravascular depletion such as hypotension, cool peripheries, significant weight loss, cramps and serial chemistry results. Critically, patients or their carers need to be involved in their management by weighing themselves and reporting significant changes in weight as well as being instructed to suspend ACE-I and/or ARB if, for example, they get gastroenteritis.

Table 18.2 Causes of relapse/non-response

Steroid-resistant	Consider genetic causes especially in younger patients, or a positive family history
Relapse of a secondary cause of NS	Has the underlying disease reoccurred, e.g. malignancy and membranous, lymphoma and minimal change
Treatment resistance	Non-adherence
Low drug levels of ciclosporin or tacrolimus	Drug interactions
Oedema	Poor absorption of diuretics
Vaccinations	Well-recognised to be a relapse trigger
Viral infections	Typically upper respiratory tract infections known to trigger relapses

18.11 Progressive Renal Impairment

The risk of progressive renal impairment depends on the underlying cause of nephrotic syndrome as well as the burden of drugs such as ciclosporin and tacrolimus. Minimal change disease is not a cause of CKD or ESRF, and if this occurs, a diagnosis of FSGS must be considered. Additionally, the long-term use of ciclosporin or tacrolimus, which may have been required to stop recurrent relapses, is a well-recognised cause of CKD in patients with minimal change disease.

With steroid-resistant nephrotic syndrome and heavy proteinuria, a significant proportion of patients will require renal replacement therapy within 5 years of their diagnosis with about 30–50% of the patients with less severe proteinuria at 10 years surviving without renal replacement therapy. Repeated episodes of AKI during times of relapse are also a recognised factor for increasing the risk of CKD in the future.

In those patients with CKD, addressing the reversible, modifying factors of CKD known to cause progression is key to their management with the aggressive control of blood pressure vital. In those proteinuric patients, the benefit of treatment with ACE-I or ARB (independent of the blood pressure lowering effects) has been demonstrated, with clear beneficial effects with respect to preserving GFR and a lower rate of decline in GFR [33]. There is a correlation between the reduction in proteinuria with therapy and the decreased progression of renal disease [34]. Along with these medications, adherence to a low-salt diet is also vital, as a high salt intake will additionally impair the anti-proteinuria action of ACE-I and ARBs (◘ Table 18.3).

◘ **Table 18.3** Causes of AKI in nephrotic syndrome

Prerenal intravascular depletion	Can occur acutely. Also, when a patient is entering remission and remains on high-dose diuretics. Patients on ACE-I or ARB may be susceptible
Acute tubular injury	Following on from a prerenal insult. Also may occur secondary to hypotension
Renal vein thrombosis	Often clinically silent. More common in membranous and with albumin less than 20 g/l. May present with loin pain, haematuria or just a decrease in GFR
Interstitial nephritis	May be related to medication: PPI, NSAIDs, antibiotics, diuretics
Renal vascular compression	Tense ascites increasing intra-abdominal pressure and reduced renal perfusion
Progression of renal disease	Rapid progression of the underlying cause
Calcineurin inhibitor toxicity	

18.12 Dyslipidaemia

Abnormalities of lipids in nephrotic syndrome increase the risk of atherosclerosis and are a significant risk factor for vascular disease. This abnormality in lipids correlates with the degree of proteinuria. Cholesterol, triglycerides and apolipoprotein B (ApoB)-containing lipoproteins have been demonstrated to be increased in patients with nephrotic syndrome, with changes in the composition as well as the function of these lipoproteins. The total cholesterol to HDL cholesterol ratio is increased in patients with nephrotic syndrome [35]. There are several different mechanisms in the pathogenesis of the dyslipidaemia of nephrotic syndrome. These include defective lipoprotein lipase activity as well as decreased hepatic lipase activity and increases in fatty acid biosynthesis due to increased expression of enzymes involved in this process. There is an increase in production of LDL, with resulting increase in LDL and cholesterol levels [36]. Loss of lecithin-cholesterol acyltransferase (LCAT) from urinary loss as well as low albumin and a reduction in hepatic HDL docking receptor and increased plasma cholesterol ester transfer protein levels lead to increased triglyceride content of HDL and contribute to the abnormalities in HDL seen in nephrotic syndrome [37].

Additionally, the treatments used in nephrotic syndrome may also have a deleterious effect on a patient's lipid profile. Corticosteroids are used in the treatment of nephrotic syndrome and have also been demonstrated to cause hyperlipidaemia through different mechanisms. Calcineurin inhibition with drugs such as tacrolimus and ciclosporin, with a higher risk in ciclosporin, treated patients in which there is an increase in LDL cholesterol [38].

The significance of dyslipidaemia is acceleration of atherosclerosis as well as dyslipidaemia being a risk factor for thrombosis complications [39].

No clear guidelines exist for the treatment of the lipid abnormalities in nephrotic syndrome, but given accelerated atherosclerosis in patients with very high cholesterol, it is common practice to treat with HMG CoA reductase inhibitors unless the patient is likely to go into rapid remission.

18.13 Nutrition and Endocrine

Along with loss of albumin, patients with nephrotic syndrome lose other proteins in the urine. This has several implications. There is decreased level of bioavailable vitamin D in patients with nephrotic syndrome [40]. Abnormalities in thyroid function are also well-recognised due to urinary loss of thyroid hormones and thyroxine binding globulin [41].

Anaemia in the context of nephrotic syndrome with preserved renal function is additionally recognised even in the context of iron and erythropoietin administration. There are several mechanisms to explain this effect. There is loss of iron and transferrin in the urine of nephrotic patients as well as loss of erythropoietin. It is also recognised that loss of the copper carrier ceruloplasmin may also be contributing to anaemia [42]. Levels of vitamin B6 have also been demonstrated to be low in nephrotic syndrome [43]. Thiamine deficiency has been demonstrated in patients with heart failure due to frusemide and increased urinary loss [44].

There should be emphasis on the important of salt and fluid restriction in those overloaded patients, with a low threshold for measuring haematinics, thyroid function and vitamins with adequate replacement.

Tips and Tricks

For many patients NS is a chronic and sometimes debilitating and for others a relapsing condition interfering with education, work and family life. A review of thrombotic risk is crucial. An often underdeveloped but crucial part of management is patient involvement and streamlined pathways for complications or relapses. There may be many patients in the young adult/transition clinics with relapsing nephrotic syndrome, and a youth worker is a valuable contribution to the management of these patients.

All suitable patients should be encouraged to (a) get scales and weigh themselves on a regular basis monitoring trends and reporting significant changes, (b) monitor home blood pressure and postural blood pressure (guiding the success of hypertensive control and identifying over diuresis) and (c) monitoring urine dipstick for those patients with steroid-responsive NS both for remission and early identification of relapse. Generally a relapse is defined as 3+ or 4+ of protein present on the urine dipstick, and monitoring at home allows the very early detection of a relapse. Our practice has been to define remission as 3 consecutive days with no protein present on the urine dipstick.

A well-informed patient with recurrent steroid-responsive NS is likely to find self-monitoring and liaison with the nephrologist more efficient than multiple routine appointments. Similarly, it should be possible to establish an individualised patient plan for most patients with relapsing NS that avoids or reduces the need for emergency admission and permits rapid nephrology review.

Case Study

Case 1

A 67-year-old male presented with a 2-month history of increasing oedema. He underwent a kidney biopsy for nephrotic-range proteinuria, which was reported as MCD. Steroids were commenced. Over the following 2 years, he had recurrent relapses and became steroid-dependent. This leads to complications including diabetes mellitus and significant weight gain. As a result, treatment with tacrolimus was started with partial response. This was followed by a decline in his renal function. At this point, he underwent a second renal biopsy to investigate a possible alternative diagnosis and assess the extent of CNI-induced damage. This demonstrated FSGS. A diagnosis of FSGS had been missed on the 1st biopsy when it was rereviewed. This diagnosis was strongly suspected due to the partial response to immunosuppression. It is critical to make this diagnosis as this puts the patient at significant risk of CKD and end-stage renal failure. It is also helps to prognosticate poor treatment response.

Case 2

An 18-year-old female is referred to the transition clinic with a diagnosis of FSGS. As a child she had undergone treatment with steroids, tacrolimus, cyclophosphamide and rituximab. None of these medications had resulted in a response. She was of short stature, which indicated her significant steroid exposure during childhood and also had low bone density. She had abnormal renal function as a result of her underlying disease, which had been resistant to treatment. She had received oral cyclophosphamide in childhood, which would have hopefully impacted a minimal amount on her fertility compared older, adult females receiving this treatment. Upon transfer she underwent genetic tests to identify a possible underlying genetic mutation as this would have been important with respect to a lower risk of disease recurrence postrenal transplantation. She found it very difficult to come to terms with her illness and imminent preparation for renal replacement therapy. A youth worker was involved in her transition, and she also received input from the renal psychology team.

Case 3

A 20-year-old man with steroid-sensitive, frequently relapsing minimal change had been on tacrolimus therapy for many years with unsuccessful cessation of therapy due to recurrent relapses requiring high-dose steroids. He was subsequently treated with rituximab. This enabled tacrolimus therapy to be weaned and stopped and allowed a prolonged period relapse-free without tacrolimus therapy. 1 year after rituximab, he was treated again with rituximab to ensure a prolonged period of B-cell depletion and disease remission.

Case 4

A 30-year-old patient with MCD was known to relapse when her prednisolone was tapered down to less than 5 mg. She would then develop venous thromboembolisms. A PTP, through which she would be provided with instant DVT prophylaxis and an early increase in her glucocorticoid dose, was instituted. This demonstrated the merit of this approach in terms of avoiding admissions and missing work and possibly also reducing the total dose of steroids administered to her.

Case 5

A 60-year-old woman with diabetes mellitus, diabetic retinopathy and albuminuria was shown to have a sudden increase in her proteinuria. Blood tests including virology, PLA2R-antibody testing and an autoimmune screen were negative. A biopsy demonstrated membranous nephropathy. A cause for this glomerulopathy was sought, and a lung malignancy was thus found, thus demonstrating how an increase in proteinuria in a diabetic patient should not simply be attributed to diabetes mellitus, especially if the increase is sudden.

Chapter Review Questions

1. What are the genetic mutations associated with NS, and by what mechanism do they cause protein leak?
2. For whom is genetic testing indicated?
3. Name the reasons why might patients with nephrotic syndrome develop AKI? And how would you exclude them?
4. What are the risk factors for progression to ESRD?

Answers

1. The glomerular filtration barrier consists of the endothelial cells, the glomerular basement membrane and the podocyte. The podocyte is key to the maintenance of the glomerular filtration barrier with secondary processes of the podocyte interdigitating together. These processes are connected together by a slit diaphragm. Actin fibres within the cytoplasm of the podocyte are integral to maintaining the structure of the cell. *NPHS1*-encoding nephrin was the first mutation detected in patients with congenital nephrotic syndrome. Nephrin is a signalling protein located in the slit diaphragm illustrating the important of the slit diaphragm in maintaining the filtration barrier. *NPHS2*-encoding podocin also has a role in the slit diaphragm. Subsequently over 50 proteins have been identified including WT1 (a transcription factor important in kidney development). Generally, the mutations can be divided into those proteins involved in the podocyte cytoskeleton (actin binding and regulatory proteins, with mutations causing changes in the cell shape of the podocyte), proteins involved in the interaction between the podocyte and glomerular basement membrane (integrin and laminin), podocyte mitochondrial proteins (coenzyme Q10 pathway) and nuclear and transcription factors. In some cases, an isolated renal phenotype is present, or in others extra-renal features may be present.
2. Genetic screening should be offered to any patient with steroid-resistant nephrotic syndrome. The younger the age of presentation with steroid-resistant nephrotic syndrome, the more likely a genetic mutation may be detected. Even in young adults (patients presenting before the age of <25 years), a genetic cause is identified in 29.5%. This has implications for response to treatment as well as the risk of recurrence post-transplantation.

Other indications for genetic testing include a positive family in any age group, a history of consanguinity or the presence of extra-renal features suggestive of a syndrome. Patients with FSGS in which transplantation is being considered should also be offered genetic testing.

3. There are many reasons for AKI in patients with nephrotic syndrome. This may be due to overuse of diuretics; hence careful monitoring is required with attention to the weight of the patient (in relation to their dry weight) as well as the presence of oedema. The patients with a low albumin are at risk of a renal vein thrombosis. There may also be a concomitant crescentic glomerulonephritis that has been recognised along with a membranous GN; hence those patients with an unexplained rapid increase in creatinine will need a repeat renal biopsy. Additionally, those older, male patients with a background of atherosclerotic disease tolerate the disturbances in fluid balance and nephrotic syndrome poorly and may present with an AKI and acute tubular injury alongside nephrotic syndrome. Patients on tacrolimus (or ciclosporin) should have regular monitoring of drug levels with advice about foods to avoid and education about the numerous drug interactions.
4. Those patients who are resistant to immunosuppression (SRNS) are at risk of disease progression. The risk of ESRF is greater in those with heavy proteinuria, with a shorter time to reach ESRF compared to those with less heavy proteinuria in SRNS. Those patients with poorly controlled blood pressure are also at increased risk for progression. Prolonged treatment with CNIs also risks accruing chronic damage and CKD.

References

1. Chapter 3: Steroid-sensitive nephrotic syndrome in children. Kidney Int Suppl (2011). 2012;2(2):163–71.
2. Eddy AA, Symons JM. Nephrotic syndrome in childhood. Lancet. 2003;362(9384):629–39.
3. Noone DG, Iijima K, Parekh R. Idiopathic nephrotic syndrome in children. Lancet. 2018;392(10141):61–74.
4. Floege J, Amann K. Primary glomerulonephritides. Lancet. 2016;387(10032):2036–48.
5. Mathieson PW. Update on the podocyte. Curr Opin Nephrol Hypertens. 2009;18(3):206–11.
6. Bierzynska A, Saleem M. Recent advances in understanding and treating nephrotic syndrome. F1000Res. 2017;6:121.
7. Vivarelli M, et al. Minimal change disease. Clin J Am Soc Nephrol. 2017;12(2):332–45.
8. Preston R, Stuart HM, Lennon R. Genetic testing in steroid-resistant nephrotic syndrome: why, who, when and how? Pediatr Nephrol. 2017.
9. Hull RP, Goldsmith DJ. Nephrotic syndrome in adults. BMJ. 2008;336(7654):1185–9.
10. Haas M, et al. Changing etiologies of unexplained adult nephrotic syndrome: a comparison of renal biopsy findings from 1976–1979 and 1995–1997. Am J Kidney Dis. 1997;30(5):621–31.
11. Orth SR, Ritz E. The nephrotic syndrome. N Engl J Med. 1998;338(17):1202–11.
12. Couser WG. Primary membranous nephropathy. Clin J Am Soc Nephrol. 2017;12(6):983–97.
13. Beck LH Jr, et al. M-type phospholipase A2 receptor as target antigen in idiopathic membranous nephropathy. N Engl J Med. 2009;361(1):11–21.
14. Korbet SM, et al. The racial prevalence of glomerular lesions in nephrotic adults. Am J Kidney Dis. 1996;27(5):647–51.
15. Hinkes BG, et al. Nephrotic syndrome in the first year of life: two thirds of cases are caused by mutations in 4 genes (NPHS1, NPHS2, WT1, and LAMB2). Pediatrics. 2007;119(4):e907–19.
16. McCarthy HJ, Saleem MA. Genetics in clinical practice: nephrotic and proteinuric syndromes. Nephron Exp Nephrol. 2011;118(1):e1–8.
17. Tian D, et al. Antagonistic regulation of actin dynamics and cell motility by TRPC5 and TRPC6 channels. Sci Signal. 2010;3(145):ra77.
18. Sadowski CE, et al. A single-gene cause in 29.5% of cases of steroid-resistant nephrotic syndrome. J Am Soc Nephrol. 2015;26(6):1279–89.
19. Summary of recommendation statements. Kidney Int Suppl (2011). 2012;2(2):143–53.
20. Barbano B, et al. Thrombosis in nephrotic syndrome. Semin Thromb Hemost. 2013;39(5):469–76.
21. Remuzzi G, et al. Platelet hyperaggregability and the nephrotic syndrome. Thromb Res. 1979;16(3–4):345–54.
22. Citak A, et al. Hemostatic problems and thromboembolic complications in nephrotic children. Pediatr Nephrol. 2000;14(2):138–42.
23. Barbour SJ, et al. Disease-specific risk of venous thromboembolic events is increased in idiopathic glomerulonephritis. Kidney Int. 2012;81(2):190–5.
24. Singhal R, Brimble KS. Thromboembolic complications in the nephrotic syndrome: pathophysiology and clinical management. Thromb Res. 2006;118(3):397–407.
25. Glassock RJ. Prophylactic anticoagulation in nephrotic syndrome: a clinical conundrum. J Am Soc Nephrol. 2007;18(8):2221–5.
26. Pincus KJ, Hynicka LM. Prophylaxis of thromboembolic events in patients with nephrotic syndrome. Ann Pharmacother. 2013;47(5):725–34.
27. Charlesworth JA, Gracey DM, Pussell BA. Adult nephrotic syndrome: non-specific strategies for treatment. Nephrology (Carlton). 2008;13(1):45–50.
28. Gipson DS, et al. Management of childhood onset nephrotic syndrome. Pediatrics. 2009;124(2):747–57.
29. Furth SL, et al. Varicella vaccination in children with nephrotic syndrome: a report of the Southwest Pediatric Nephrology Study Group. J Pediatr. 2003;142(2):145–8.
30. Wu HM, et al. Interventions for preventing infection in nephrotic syndrome. Cochrane Database Syst Rev. 2012;(4):CD003964.
31. Smith JD, Hayslett JP. Reversible renal failure in the nephrotic syndrome. Am J Kidney Dis. 1992;19(3):201–13.
32. Baines RJ, Brunskill NJ. Tubular toxicity of proteinuria. Nat Rev Nephrol. 2011;7(3):177–80.
33. Maione A, et al. Angiotensin-converting enzyme inhibitors, angiotensin receptor blockers and combined therapy in patients

with micro- and macroalbuminuria and other cardiovascular risk factors: a systematic review of randomized controlled trials. Nephrol Dial Transplant. 2011;26(9):2827–47.

34. Jafar TH, et al. Angiotensin-converting enzyme inhibitors and progression of nondiabetic renal disease. A meta-analysis of patient-level data. Ann Intern Med. 2001;135(2):73–87.
35. Joven J, et al. Abnormalities of lipoprotein metabolism in patients with the nephrotic syndrome. N Engl J Med. 1990;323(9):579–84.
36. Agrawal S, et al. Dyslipidaemia in nephrotic syndrome: mechanisms and treatment. Nat Rev Nephrol. 2018;14(1):57–70.
37. Vaziri ND. HDL abnormalities in nephrotic syndrome and chronic kidney disease. Nat Rev Nephrol. 2016;12(1):37–47.
38. Chakkera HA, Sharif A, Kaplan B. Negative cardiovascular consequences of small molecule immunosuppressants. Clin Pharmacol Ther. 2017;102(2):269–76.
39. Jackson SP, Calkin AC. The clot thickens--oxidized lipids and thrombosis. Nat Med. 2007;13(9):1015–6.
40. Aggarwal A, et al. Bioavailable vitamin D levels are reduced and correlate with bone mineral density and markers of mineral metabolism in adults with nephrotic syndrome. Nephrology (Carlton). 2016;21(6):483–9.
41. Mario FD, et al. Hypothyroidism and nephrotic syndrome: why, when and how to treat. Curr Vasc Pharmacol. 2017;15(5):398–403.
42. Iorember F, Aviles D. Anemia in nephrotic syndrome: approach to evaluation and treatment. Pediatr Nephrol. 2017;32(8):1323–30.
43. Mydlik M, Derzsiova K. Erythrocyte vitamin B1, B2 and B6 in nephrotic syndrome. Miner Electrolyte Metab. 1992;18(2–5):293–4.
44. Katta N, Balla S, Alpert MA. Does long-term furosemide therapy cause thiamine deficiency in patients with heart failure? A focused review. Am J Med. 2016;129(7):753 e7–753 e11.

Management of Extracellular Fluid Volume in the Nephrotic Patient

Liam Plant

Contents

M. Harber (ed.), *Primer on Nephrology*, https://doi.org/10.1007/978-3-030-76419-7_19

Learning Objectives

1. To understand the mechanisms underlying the salt retention and expansion of ECF volume that occurs in NS.
2. To understand the nuanced differences between these mechanisms and those underlying other salt-retaining states such as CHF and CKD.
3. To understand the interactions between intake, excretion and regulatory factors in salt balance in man.
4. To understand the sites of actions of commonly used classes of diuretic (saliuretic) agents and the factors that alter pharmacokinetics and pharmacodynamics.
5. To formulate rational and dynamic strategies of dietary salt restriction, sequential nephron blockade and (where appropriate) specific disease-modifying treatments to rapidly, sufficiently and sustainably control ECF volume expansion in NS.

19.1 Introduction

Nephrotic syndrome (NS) is a relatively less common manifestation of kidney disease [1]. In childhood it is most commonly due to minimal change disease. Most cases in adults are due to primary glomerular diseases, but some are due to secondary glomerular diseases such as diabetes, systemic lupus erythematosus or amyloidosis [1]. Cardinal clinical features are proteinuria, hypoalbuminaemia and oedema.

In all cases, expansion of extracellular fluid (ECF) volume is a troublesome symptom. This can be very disabling, with peripheral oedema, pulmonary oedema, gut oedema and ascites. If disease-specific therapies do not rapidly induce a remission, it is often difficult to bring these symptoms under control with generic therapies. Patients with NS may then seem to be 'diuretic-resistant', in much the same way as some patients with chronic heart failure (CHF) or chronic kidney disease (CKD) are considered to so be [2].

However, it may be a mistake to view all oedematous patients who are 'slow' to respond to initial therapies as being 'the same' just because the general principles of therapy are similar [2, 3]. It is important to recognise that the pathophysiological basis of oedema differs between different underlying conditions and this may have implications for choices in therapy. Furthermore, differences in drug pharmacokinetics and pharmacodynamics influence response to treatment [2–6].

An example of the increasing interest in more precise characterisation and treatment of oedematous states has been that focused on acute decompensated heart failure (ADHF) and associated cardio-renal syndromes (CRS) [7]. This acknowledges pathophysiological interactions between the heart and the kidney as well as the effects of neurohumoral activation [8]. Salt restriction, use of diuretics and use of other agents are demonstrated to exhibit a complex interplay in such cases. Some of these factors will overlap with the pathophysiology/treatment of ECF volume expansion in NS; some will not. Important trials on how to use diuretics in ADHF have been published [9]. The findings of these studies may not translate directly to strategies for treating oedematous NS patients.

19.1.1 What Are the Clinical Goals of Disease-Specific Management of NS?

These are dealt with elsewhere in this book and relate to inducing a remission of proteinuria and preserving glomerular filtration rate. There are extensive reviews and guidelines on potential therapies to induce remission/reduce proteinuria [10]. All make reference to the necessity for salt restriction and use of diuretics, but there is heterogeneity in clinical practice strategies, with a need to individualise such treatments. Consensus on how to achieve this is not prominent in the literature; in one very extensive guideline [10], the word 'diuretic' appears only 13 times in a 15-page document!

How we describe 'diuretics' may influence how we understand and use them. The commonly used diuretic agents are (in almost all cases) highly selective inhibitors of a variety of ion transporters expressed on the luminal surface of renal tubular cells. Successful use leads to a reduction in sodium (and usually also chloride) absorption with a consequent loss of sodium in the urine (*natriuresis*), within a broader loss of salt in the urine (*saliuresis*) and an associated loss of water in the urine (*diuresis*).

19.2 Clinical Features

Nephrotic syndrome is marked by the triad of:an expanded ECF volume, manifest as oedema (This may be peripheral only or extend to pleural effusions, pulmonary oedema or ascites. It may occur with normal renal function or with CKD - especially if it is a feature of a worsening diabetic nephropathy); urinary protein excretion typically exceeding 3 g/day, and low serum albumin concentration which may fall below 20 g/dl in severe cases.

19

19.3 Epidemiology

New cases of NS occur with an estimated annual incidence of 3 new cases per 100,000 in adults and 2 new cases per 100,000 in children [1].

19.4 Aetiopathology

19.4.1 Why Do Nephrotic Patients Become Oedematous?

The traditional explanation has been that proteinuria leads to hypoalbuminaemia, causing a decrease in plasma oncotic pressure. The consequent imbalance in Starling forces across the capillary wall causes fluid to 'leak' into the interstitium. Effective hypovolaemia follows, and this triggers activation of the renin-angiotensin-aldosterone, sympathetic nervous and arginine vasopressin systems, with inhibition of the release of atrial natriuretic peptide. All of this leads to secondary renal salt and water retention [3, 11].

However, observations in clinical cases and in experimental models call this 'underfill' hypothesis into question, and whilst it may play some role, particularly at the onset of NS, opinion now favours a greater role for a specific renal salt retention process coupled with an alteration in capillary permeability independent of changes in oncotic gradients [11, 12].

No compelling and consistent explanation for the dysregulation in sodium balance in NS has yet been universally accepted, but it is notable that many studies indicate an upregulation of epithelial sodium channel (ENaC) expression in the distal nephron, independent of aldosterone and other systemic hormones [12]. Recent studies postulate a role for plasminogen and plasmin, both of which appear in proteinuric urine. It is postulated that, in NS, plasminogen enters the urine through more permeable glomerular capillaries; that it is then activated to plasmin by urokinase; and that plasmin activates distal nephron epithelial sodium (ENaC) channels [13]. Thus, a prominent aspect of NS is a particular salt avidity in the distal nephron, mediated through ENaC and occurring in concert with other mechanisms (possibly reflecting the 'underfill' hypothesis) enhancing salt retention at other sites.

19.5 Diagnosis

The diagnosis is made based on the clinical triad of oedema, hypoalbuminaemia and proteinuria. Other conditions (e.g. SLE or diabetes mellitus) may co-exist.

19.6 Treatment

19.6.1 What Are the Clinical Goals of Generic Management of NS?

The primary objective of generic therapy is to initiate and sustain an increased natriuresis/saliuresis/diuresis until the patient has returned to clinical euvolaemia. It should then be easier to maintain homeostasis at the new desired steady state, particularly if dietary salt restriction is appropriately introduced.

Whilst the NS persists, total body salt and water will not decrease unless excretion exceeds intake. Dietary sodium intake frequently exceeds 100 mmol/day (~6 g salt/day). Thus, for example, a patient will need to excrete 300 mmol of sodium over and above that needed to balance this daily intake if s/he is to lose 2 kg of excess ECF volume.

Whilst salt avidity persists, this requires the use of (various) natriuretic agents – usually referred to as 'diuretics', with specific pharmacokinetic and pharmacodynamic properties, in different doses and combinations.

Dietary sodium intake also needs to be restricted, ideally to <80 mmol/day, but this may be difficult to achieve. Most salt intake is not 'elective' but occurs because of addition in food processing. Furthermore, many patients find diets containing less than 80 mmol/day of sodium to be bland and unpalatable.

Unexpected failure to lose weight/ECF volume in a patient on a seemingly appropriate diuretic dose should prompt enquiry into salt intake. Measurement of 24-h sodium excretion may help. A patient passing 150 mmol/day or more but not losing weight is likely to have salt intake in excess of the reduced target.

19.6.2 What Are the Different Classes of Diuretics and How Do They Work?

Diuretics are different classes of drugs that inhibit sodium reabsorption at different sites along the nephron. By increasing natriuresis they achieve clinical benefit [2–6]. However, clinical goals may not always be easily achieved.

Site of action classifies the commonly used agents (▫ Table 19.1). Although most (60–70%) filtered sodium is reabsorbed in the proximal tubule, agents acting at this site (e.g. acetazolamide) are of relatively little clinical use in oedematous states because the increased sodium loss here is offset by increased reabsorption further down the nephron, especially in the thick ascending loop of Henle. The same principle applies to the proximal tubular effect of some thiazide diuretics.

Table 19.1 Classes of diuretic agents

Class	Examples	Site of action
Loop diuretics	Furosemide Bumetanide	Thick ascending loop of Henle (TALH)
Thiazide-type diuretics Thiazide-like diuretics	Hydrochlorothiazide Bendroflumethiazide Chlorthalidone Metolazone Indapamide	Distal convoluted tubule (DCT)
Potassium-sparing diuretics	Amiloride Triamterene	Cortical collecting duct (CCD)
Selective aldosterone receptor antagonists (SARA)	Spironolactone Eplerenone	Cortical collecting duct (CCD) – Principal cells

Table 19.2 Ion transporters/channels

Transporter	Role	Location
Organic anion transporter (OAT1)	Secretion of loop diuretics and thiazide-type/like diuretics into tubular lumen	Proximal convoluted tubule
Organic cation transporter	Secretion of potassium-sparing diuretics into tubular lumen	Proximal convoluted tubule
Sodium-potassium-2 chloride transporter (NKCC2) *Solute carrier family 12 A1 (SCL12A1)*	Site of action of loop diuretics	Thick ascending loop of Henle
Sodium-chloride cotransporter (NCC) *Solute carrier family 12 A3 (SCL12A3)*	Site of action of thiazide/thiazide-like diuretics	Distal convoluted tubule
Epithelial sodium channel (ENaC)	Site of action of amiloride and triamterene	Cortical collecting duct (Principal cells) *Expression influenced by activation of aldosterone receptor*

Loop diuretics (e.g. furosemide, bumetanide) are organic anions, secreted into the tubular lumen by the organic anion transporter (OAT1) in the proximal tubule (Table 19.2). They act on the luminal aspect of the thick ascending loop of Henle where they exhibit high affinity for the chloride-binding site of the sodium-potassium-2 chloride (NKCC2) transporter – a member (SCL12A1) of the solute carrier family 12 group of proteins [2, 4–6] (Table 19.2). This directly inhibits sodium and chloride reabsorption and indirectly leads to decreased reabsorption of calcium and magnesium. Up to 20% of filtered sodium can be excreted using these agents.

Thiazides and related compounds (e.g. bendroflumethiazide, hydrochlorothiazide, chlorthalidone, metolazone, indapamide) are organic anions also secreted by OAT1 in the proximal tubule. They act on the distal tubule and connecting segment where they bind to a number of transporters, principally the chloride-binding site of the sodium-chloride cotransporter (NCC) – another member (SCL12A3) of the solute carrier family 12 protein group – directly inhibiting sodium reabsorption [2, 4–6] (Table 19.2). This indirectly increases calcium reabsorption. The maximum natriuresis achievable is less than that achieved with loop diuretics, but a combination of these classes can be especially potent [14].

19

The potassium-sparing diuretics include amiloride, triamterene and spironolactone. These have slightly different modes of action. Amiloride and triamterene are organic cations secreted into the lumen of the proximal tubule and acting on the luminal aspect of the epithelial sodium channel (ENaC) in the cortical collecting duct [2, 4–6] (Table 19.2). Spironolactone and eplerenone, by contrast, enter the principal cells of the cortical collecting duct from the plasma and interfere with the activation of the intracellular aldosterone receptor. This leads to a reduction in the activity of the baso-lateral sodium-potassium ATPase and a reduction in luminal expression of ENaC (Table 19.2).

19.6.3 What Are the Pharmacokinetic Barriers to Achieving Therapeutic Objectives?

The primary driver of pharmacological natriuresis (other than with SARA drugs) is the rate of excretion of diuretic into the tubular fluid. This relationship exhibits a threshold phenomenon, following which the rate of

Table 19.3 Pharmacokinetic barriers to achieving therapeutic goals

Problem	Response
Decreased oral bioavailability *More likely with gut oedema*	Increase drug dose Uses drug with higher oral bioavailability Administer drug intravenously
Hypoproteinaemia (which increases the volume of distribution of agents within the circulation) *More likely with nephrotic syndrome*	As above
Interference with proximal tubule excretion by organic anions/other medications *More likely with cirrhosis/CKD*	As above
Decreased GFR/cardiac output *More likely with CKD/CHF*	As above

sodium excretion reflects diuretic excretion in a linear dose-dependent pattern [4–6]. Failure to deliver a sufficient dose of diuretic to exceed the natriuretic threshold may be described as 'diuretic resistance' but more usually reflects a failure to appreciate pharmacokinetic principles (Table 19.3).

Most prescribing choices to address pharmacokinetic issues involve administering larger doses of diuretic or enhancing bioavailability.

The first step is to ensure that an adequate dose of diuretic enters the bloodstream and is delivered to the kidney for excretion into the tubular lumen. Diuretics differ in their oral bioavailability. The oral bioavailability of furosemide ranges from 20% to 70%, decreasing with increased gut oedema. On the other hand, bumetanide has an oral bioavailability approaching 80%. When faced with a very oedematous patient, administering a higher dose of oral furosemide, switching to oral bumetanide or administering furosemide intravenously are all rational therapeutic choices.

Loop and thiazide diuretics are transported bound to albumin and other plasma proteins. In NS, levels of albumin and other plasma proteins are often extremely low, and the consequent increased volume of distribution decreases the amount delivered to the kidney [15]. Increasing the dose administered is the appropriate response to this; coadministration of albumin with diuretic has not been consistently demonstrated as being of additional benefit [16–18].

Diuretics compete with other anions for excretion by OAT1 into the proximal tubule [3–6]. Such anions accumulate particularly in the presence of renal failure and hepatic failure. In such circumstances the expected dose-response to loop and thiazide diuretics may be less than anticipated. Certain drugs (such as cimetidine) also compete for excretion. This problem does not occur with spironolactone, which does not require to be excreted into the tubular lumen, and its diuretic effect is thus less affected by liver failure.

A fall in GFR, particularly when combined with a low cardiac output, will decrease diuretic delivery and also reduce the initial filtered sodium load making a substantial natriuresis even more difficult to achieve.

It was previously postulated that urinary protein bound to diuretic in the tubular lumen decreased its effectiveness. This view has not been substantiated by experimental studies [19].

Therefore, there are many factors active in NS that act as additional pharmacokinetic 'hurdles' to achieving a degree of diuretic excretion sufficient to initiate a natriuresis. In most circumstances, increasing the prescribed dose or otherwise enhancing the bioavailability of that dose is the appropriate strategy. An illogical, but common, error is to repeat the same ineffective dose more frequently. If there is doubt as to whether or not a natriuresis has been initiated, measurement of 24-h sodium excretion (or even 6-h excretion following diuretic administration) is a rational choice.

19.6.4 What Are the Pharmacodynamic Barriers to Achieving Therapeutic Objectives?

Once a natriuresis is initiated, it needs to be sustained until the patient has been restored to the desired steady state. Once diuretics are administered and natriuresis achieved, there is a rapid functional and structural response in the nephron that acts to reduce the degree of enhanced natriuresis [2–6]. This can be viewed as 'diuretic blunting' and reflects pharmacodynamic principles.

Most of the adaptation occurs downstream from the site of action of the initially deployed diuretic. Changes in the expression and activity of transporters in the distal tubule and the cortical collecting duct occur within days [3–6]. It is now apparent that allelic variations, particularly in the genes encoding for the SLC12A3 protein (NCC) and the β-subunit of the SCNN1 protein (ENaC) (Table 19.2), may explain variance in response between patients [20].

In addition, there is evidence that chronic exposure to both loop and thiazide/thiazide-like diuretics increases the expression of their respective target transporters as well as of OAT1 [21].

The clinician needs to anticipate these changes. In the first instance, once a natriuresis has been initiated, one can prescribe the effective dose more frequently. Although the response to consecutive doses will progressively decline, more net natriuresis will be achieved with twice daily, thrice daily or a continuous infusion of diuretic. It is unclear if a continuous infusion achieves a greater daily natriuresis than the same total dose given as boluses [5, 22].

However, the most effective strategy to adopt is the early initiation of sequential nephron blockade, using a combination of diuretic agents to target multiple sites down the nephron [2–6]. This blocks the adaptation in the distal tubule and cortical collecting duct to the increased luminal sodium delivery following inhibition of the NKCC2. Combination of loop diuretics with thiazide/thiazide-like diuretics is effective, even in the presence of advanced renal dysfunction and in advanced heart failure [14, 23]. In addition, the early prescription of potassium-sparing diuretics will minimise the kaliuresis/hypokalaemia that will occur with successful blockade of the NKCC2/NCC systems [2–6]. Given the key role of ENaC activation in the aetiopathology of NS, early prescription of amiloride is also a plausible strategy.

There is now also some interest in supplementing the use of standard natriuretic agents with human atrial natriuretic peptide analogues such as carperitide [24]. These are not yet part of the mainstay of therapy.

Tips, Tricks and Pitfalls

1. On clinical examination, first determine the probable extent of ECF volume expansion; express this in kg; set a target weight to be achieved at which one can anticipate that the patient will be restored to euvolaemia.
2. Initiate dietary sodium restriction to a target of 80 mmol/day or less (a trained dietician is very helpful for this).
3. Administer a loop diuretic, selecting agent/dose/mode of administration based on degree of oedema, level of hypoproteinaemia, level of renal and cardiac function and presence of liver disease.
4. Progressively increase the dose until a natriuresis is initiated (either on clinical evidence or with a measurement of urinary sodium excretion).
5. Once natriuresis is established, administer the same dose more frequently, or as a continuous infusion.
6. Rapidly (within 2–3 days, or immediately if the patient has already been on loop diuretics for some time) initiate sequential nephron blockade with thiazide/thiazide-like agents and potassium-sparing diuretics.
7. When choosing between thiazide/thiazide-like diuretics, consider duration of action when used in combination with loop diuretics (indapamide/metolazone are longer acting than bendroflumethiazide/hydrochlorothiazide).

Case Study

A 39-year-old female patient with Type 1 diabetes and diabetic nephropathy was transferred from the Diabetes service. She was massively oedematous, with a serum albumin of 14 g/dl and a 24-h protein excretion of 16 g/day. Serum creatinine concentration was 200umol/l. Her weight had continued to rise on a dose of 120 mg p.o. furosemide, which had been increased to twice daily without benefit.

The renal dietician assisted her with reducing her dietary sodium intake to <100 mmol/day. She was converted to 100 mg twice daily of iv furosemide administered 2 and 6 h after administration of 5 mg of bendroflumethiazide. A natriuresis was initiated. Two days later she was also prescribed amiloride 5 mg daily.

With this regimen, her weight dropped by 8 kg over 10 days; she was converted to 3 mg of bumetanide twice daily whilst remaining on her other medications. She became clinically euvolaemic despite there being no change in her serum albumin concentration or urinary protein excretion.

This illustrates the 'classical' strategy employed to control ECF volume in NS.

Conclusion

Failure to control ECF volume in NS usually stems from insufficient dietary sodium restriction, an insufficient initial dose of loop diuretic to initiate natriuresis and insufficiently rapid introduction of sequential nephron blockade to maintain natriuresis. In some cases, patience is needed with frequent adjustments of medication doses and timings; fastidiousness usually achieves the desired objective.

Chapter Review Questions

1. What is the time to onset of effect and duration of effect with iv furosemide?
2. Are there any strategies other than salt restriction and sequential nephron blockade that can increase natriuresis in NS?
3. Which diuretic agents limit magnesiuria and hypomagnesaemia?

Answers

1. Onset 5 mins; duration 2 h. This compares with an onset of effect after 30–60 mins and a duration of onset of 6–8 h with p.o. furosemide. If a patient takes p.o. bendroflumethiazide (onset 1–2 h; duration 6–12 h) at the same time that iv furosemide is given, the combined effect will not occur in synchrony.
2. Previous studies suggested that an equivalent dose of diuretic given by intravenous infusion as opposed to bolus doses was associated with greater natriuresis – it is now felt that it was the need to lie recumbent whilst having the infusion that led to greater natriuresis. Consideration can be given to the beneficial effects of recumbency on natriuresis.
3. Successful inhibition of the NKCC2 transporter will lead to increased magnesiuria; however, increased sodium delivery to the distal nephron consequent to inhibition of the NCC transporter typically leads to more hypomagnesaemia. This effect is mitigated by amiloride, but not by spironolactone.

References

1. Hull RP, Goldsmith DJA. Nephrotic syndrome in adults. BMJ. 2008;336:1185–9.
2. Plant L. Clinical use of diuretics. In: Barratt J, Harris K, Topham P, editors. Oxford desk reference nephrology, Chap 18.3. Oxford: Oxford University Press; 2009. p. 708–12.
3. Qavi AH, Kamal R, Schrier RW. Clinical use of diuretics in heart failure, cirrhosis and nephrotic syndrome. Int J Nephrol. 2015:1–9.
4. Brater DC. Pharmacology of diuretics. Am J Med Sci. 2000;319:38–50.
5. Brater DC. Update in diuretic therapy: clinical pharmacology. Semin Nephrol. 2011;31:483–94.
6. Sica DA. Diuretic use in renal disease. Nat Rev Nephrol. 2012;8:100–9.
7. Acute Dialysis Quality Initiative (ADQI) consensus group. Cardio-renal syndromes: an executive summary from the consensus conference of the Acute Dialysis Quality Initiative (ADQI) Consensus Conference. Contrib Nephrol. 2010;165:54–7.
8. Ronco C, Cicoira M, McCullough PA. Cardiorenal syndrome type 1: pathophysiological crosstalk leading to combined heart and kidney dysfunction in the setting of acutely decompensated heart failure. J Am Coll Cardiol. 2012;60:1031–42.
9. Felker GM, Lee KL, Bull DA, Redfield MM, Stevenson LW, Goldsmith SR, LeWinter MM, Deswal A, Rouleau JL, Ofili EO, Anstrom KA, Hernandez AF, McNulty SE, Velazquez EJ, Kfoury AG, Chen HH, Givertz MM, Semigran MJ, Bart BA, Mascette AM, Braunwald E, O'Connor CM, for the NHLBI Heart Failure Clinical Research Network. Diuretic strategies in patients with acute decompensated heart failure. N Engl J Med. 2011;364:797–805.
10. Kidney Disease: Improving Global Outcomes (KDIGO) Glomerulonephritis Work Group. KDIGO clinical practice guideline for glomerulonephritis. Kidney Int. 2012;2(Suppl):139–74.
11. Rondon-Berrios H. New insights into the pathophysiology of oedema in nephrotic syndrome. Nefrologia. 2011;31:148–514.
12. Doucet A, Favre G, Deschenes G. Molecular mechanism of edema formation in nephrotic syndrome: therapeutic implications. Pediatr Nephrol. 2007;22:1983–90.
13. Svenningsen P, Bistrup C, Friis UG, Bertog M, Harteis S, Krueger N, Stubbe J, Nørregrad Jensen O, Thiesson HC, Uhrenholt TR, Jespersen B, Jensen BL, Korbmacher C, Skøtt O. Plasmin in nephrotic urine activates the epithelial sodium channel. J Am Soc Nephrol. 2009;20:299–310.
14. Fliser D, Schröter M, Neubeck M, Ritz E. Coadministration of thiazides increases the efficacy of loop diuretics even in patients with advanced renal failure. Kidney Int. 1994;46:482–8.
15. Pichette V, Geadah D, du Souich P. Role of plasma protein binding on renal metabolism and dynamics of furosemide in the rabbit. Drug Metab Dispos. 1999;27:81–5.
16. Akcicek F, Yalniz T, Basci A, Ok E, Mees EJ. Diuretic effect of furosemide in patients with nephrotic syndrome: is it potentiated by intravenous albumin? BMJ. 1995;310:162–3.
17. Fliser D, Zurbrüggen I, Mutschler E, Bischoff I, Nussburger J, Franek E, Ritz E. Coadministration of albumin and furosemide in the nephrotic syndrome. Kidney Int. 1999;55:629–34.
18. Chalasani N, Gorski JC, Horlander JC, Craven R, Hoen H, Maya J, Brater DC. Effects of albumin/furosemide mixtures on responses to furosemide in hypoalbuminemic patients. J Am Soc Nephrol. 2001;12:1010–6.
19. Agarwal R, Gorski JC, Sundblad K, Brater DC. Urinary protein binding does not affect response to furosemide in patients with nephrotic syndrome. J Am Soc Nephrol. 2000;11:1100–5.
20. Vormfelde SV, Sehrt D, Toliat MR, Schirmer M, Meineke I, Tzvetlov M, Nürnberg P, Brockmöller J. Genetic variation in

the renal sodium transporters NKCC2, NCC, and ENaC in relation to the effects of loop diuretic drugs. Clin Pharmacol Ther. 2007;82:300–9.
21. Jim JH. Long-term adaptation of renal ion transporters to chronic diuretic treatment. Am J Nephrol. 2004;24:595–605.
22. Salvador DR, Rey NR, Ramos GC, Punzalan FE. Continuous infusion versus bolus injection of loop diuretics in congestive heart failure. Cochrane Database Syst Rev. 2005;(3):CD003178.
23. Channer KS, McLean KA, Lawson-Matthew P, Richardson M. Combination diuretic treatment in severe heart failure: a randomized controlled trial. Br Heart J. 1994;71:146–50.
24. Kanzaki M, Wada J, Kikumoto Y, Akagi S, Nakao K, Sugiyama H, Makino H. The therapeutic potential of synthetic human atrial natriuretic peptide in nephrotic syndrome: a randomized controlled trial. Int J Nephrol Renovasc Dis. 2012;5:91–6.

Minimal Change Disease

Philip David Mason

Contents

M. Harber (ed.), *Primer on Nephrology*, https://doi.org/10.1007/978-3-030-76419-7_20

Learning Objectives

1. Minimal change disease is a common cause of nephrotic syndrome in children and adults.
2. Biopsy of patients with nephrotic syndrome is indicated for adults but only for children who do not respond to steroids.
3. Understand the initial treatment and management of relapsing disease.

20.1 Introduction

Minimal change disease (MCD) and focal segmental glomerulosclerosis (FSGS) have traditionally been considered to have different aetiologies although it has been suggested that they are different manifestations of the same disease but reflecting the intensity of podocyte injury [1].

MCD is the cause of the nephrotic syndrome in ~90% of children aged under 10 years (most common age 2–7 years), about 50–70% of older children and 20–35% of adults. The incidence in boys is twice that in girls although there is no gender difference in adolescents or adults. The reported incidence varies geographically. In the UK it has been reported to be as low as 1 per million but up to 27 per million in the USA. It is commoner in Indo-Asians and Native Americans but is rarer in Black Africans (who are much more likely to have FSGS with steroid-resistant nephrotic syndrome). Since children with nephrotic syndrome are very likely to have MCN, they are not usually biopsied, and the term steroid-responsive nephrotic syndrome is used if they respond to steroids.

20.2 Aetiology and Pathogenesis

In a minority of patients, nephrotic syndrome with MCD is associated with a secondary factor, and some of the most frequent are listed in Table 20.1 (a more comprehensive list can be found in Reference [2]).

Table 20.1 Factors associated with the onset of nephrotic syndrome in minimal change disease

Drugs
Nonsteroidal anti-inflammatory drugs
Lithium: rare (usually causes chronic interstitial nephritis)
Interferon-α
Gold: rare (usually associated with membranous nephropathy)
Allergies
Pollens
House dust
Insect stings
Immunisations
Malignancies
Hodgkin's disease
Mycosis fungoides
Chronic lymphocytic leukaemia: uncommon (usually associated with MPGN)
Following haematopoietic stem cell transplants

MCN, in common with FSGS, profoundly affect podocyte structure and function and are often referred to as podocytopathies. In normal glomeruli, the filtration barrier to protein is provided by a combination of size barriers and charge selectivity so that neutral molecules larger than 4–4.5 nm are excluded. Albumin molecules are smaller but are excluded because as anionic molecules they are repelled by the normal negative charge on the epithelial cells and glomerular basement membrane (GBM) (predominantly heparan sulphate). In MCD and FSGS, the clearance of small neutral molecules is actually less than normal, suggesting that the large albumin filtration is primarily the result of loss of GBM surface charge. The cause of this is uncertain, and the presence of circulating cationic factors (which may result in a generalised increased capillary permeability) remains controversial. The characteristic podocyte foot process fusion is seen in other patients with heavy proteinuria suggesting that these changes may be secondary. Finding foot process fusion in children dying of kwashiorkor with severe hypoalbuminaemia, but no proteinuria, and the absence of foot process fusion in patients with heavy proteinuria with early recurrent FSGS following transplantation would support this.

MCD is thought to have an immune aetiology and is likely to be a systemic condition rather than an intrinsic disease of the kidney. Before corticosteroids were found to be effective, the nephrotic syndrome often remitted in children who contracted measles, which is known to be a potent inhibitor of cell-mediated immunity. MCD is associated with lymphomas (especially Hodgkin's disease) and atopy (in some series in up to 30% of children) and responds to immunosuppressive drugs. There are also many reports of abnormal humoral and cellular immunity in patients with MCD during relapse and sometimes in remission as well, but not in those with other causes of nephrotic syndrome. Finally, there is an association (in some ethnic groups) with HLA-DR7 in steroid-responsive individuals. There are many anecdotal reports of MCD relapse following exposure to an allergen in sensitive individuals. As a result, patients with identified food allergies have been managed with exclusion diets with reported complete or partial remissions and relapse following reintroduction of the offending food. However, even if the relationship is real, it is possible that the allergic events merely trigger relapse, as may infections.

A primary podocyte abnormality may be involved. Podocyte expression of CD80 (B7.1) has been reported in patients with MCD and the soluble molecule found in their urine [3], and experimentally, CD80 expression by podocytes results in shape change and the development of proteinuria.

There is circumstantial evidence that a circulating factor is involved in the pathogenesis. Lymphocyte-derived cytokines have been proposed but remain elusive, and T regulatory cells have been reported to be abnormal in MCD and that there is generalised activation of T cells during active disease. In one small study, plasma haemopexin (an acute phase reactant found in human plasma) was increased in MCD patients in relapse with some evidence of an altered isoform [4]. It is unclear how this relates to clinical disease although the authors suggest that protease inhibitors might normally mask its activity. Reduced levels of dystroglycans (adhesion molecules believed to anchor podocytes to the GBM) have also been reported in MCD, with normalisation following corticosteroid treatment. Evidence of a circulating factor in humans is also supported by the observation that proteinuria resolved within days following transplantation from a cadaveric donor with MCD [5].

Experimental studies have implicated T lymphocyte-derived IL-13 in causing the proteinuria by a mechanism involving induction of CD80 in the podocyte, and this cytokine is associated with allergic states, and MCD may be triggered by vaccination or exposure to an allergen in sensitive individuals [6].

20.3 Natural History

- A relapsing–remitting course is common and more frequent in children.
- Those presenting at an earlier age are more likely to have a longer disease course before long-term remission occurs (see Fig. 20.1).

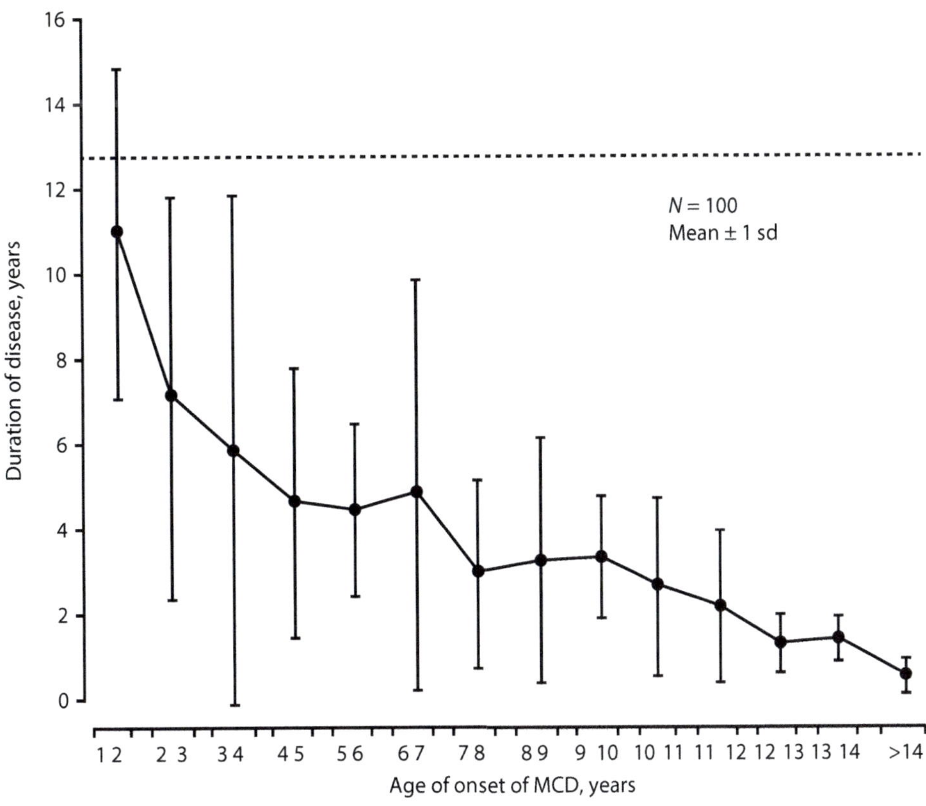

Fig. 20.1 Long-term outcome in childhood-onset minimal change disease. The duration of disease is inversely related to the age of presentation. (Reproduced with permission from Trompeter et al. [8])

- Relapse occurs in >2/3 of children and about half relapse more than four times, usually following steroid cessation or reduction. If relapse occurs during steroid reduction, the patient is described as steroid-dependent.
- <5% of children with MCD enter adulthood still relapsing, although the younger the onset of the first attack, the longer the child is likely to continue having relapses [7].
- In general, increasing time since last relapse reduces the risk of further relapse, but occasionally adults relapse after an interval of >10 years.
- MCD does not progress to renal failure, although a number of patients with this diagnosis are found to have FSGS on subsequent biopsies. It is unclear whether the focal nature of the disease resulted in the correct diagnosis being missed on the initial biopsy or whether evolution from MCD to FSGS occurs.

20.4 Clinical Features and Complications

The symptoms and clinical signs are the same as those for the nephrotic syndrome from any cause, but it is worth noting:

- A fairly rapid onset of oedema is common with increased risks of hypovolaemia (especially in children).
- Severe fluid retention exceeding 3% of the body weight and often much more.
- 60% of presentations and relapses follow an infection (most often upper respiratory tract); however, minor infections are common in children, and following remission most infections do not trigger a relapse, so it is uncertain whether or not these are of causative significance.
- Children commonly present with pleural effusions, ascites and hepatomegaly and may present with abdominal pain.
- Pericardial effusions may occur, but pulmonary oedema is uncommon except following treatment with albumin or with coexisting cardiac disease.
- Oedema is gravitational, but a puffy face is common and genital swelling may be very uncomfortable, especially in men. Gross oedema may result in ulceration, and infection of dependent skin and lacerations and needlestick punctures may weep fluid profusely.
- Striae commonly appear even without steroids.
- Bowel oedema may cause diarrhoea, and increased capillary leak has been suggested as a mechanism for losing protein via the gut.
- Other clinical features include white nails, sometimes in bands (Muehrcke's bands) correlating with periods of clinical relapse. Rarely xanthomata are associated with gross hyperlipidaemia.
- Microscopic haematuria is rare.
- Hypertension is present in 30–43% of adults [8] and in 14–21% of children, when compared with age- and sex-matched blood pressure reference ranges [9]. This usually resolves during remission, especially in children. Hypertension is sometimes associated with expansion of the intravascular volume but may paradoxically be secondary to hypovolaemia and activation of the renin–angiotensin axis.
- AKI is present or develops in ~18% of patients.
- Other complications, as for any cause of nephrotic syndrome, include thromboembolism, infection and hyperlipidaemia.

20.5 Diagnosis and Differential Diagnosis

The clinical diagnosis of nephrotic syndrome is usually obvious, with oedema and heavy proteinuria, usually without microscopic haematuria on urine dipstick testing. The differential diagnosis is that of nephrotic syndrome and requires a renal biopsy to make a definitive diagnosis. In patients with conditions that may be associated with the nephrotic syndrome (e.g. diabetes or amyloidosis), the decision to biopsy needs to be carefully considered.

20.6 Investigations

20.6.1 Routine Investigations

Hyaline and sometimes lipid casts may be seen on urine microscopy. There is nephrotic-range proteinuria (>3.5 g/24 h in adults or >40 mg/h per m^2 in children or a protein/creatinine ratio >350 mg/mmol).

Routine blood biochemistry confirms hypoalbuminaemia and hyperlipidaemia. Hyponatraemia may be present even before treatment, and elevated urea and creatinine are more common in adults.

Usually the IgG level is low, IgM is normal or raised and serum complement levels are normal. In children, steroid-responsive MCD is usually associated with 'selective' proteinuria of smaller molecules including albumin and transferrin but not of larger molecules such as immunoglobulins and ferritin. A selectivity index can be derived from the ratio of IgG to albumin clearance:

$$\text{Selectivity index (SI)} = \frac{[\text{IgG}]_U\,[\text{Albumin}]_S}{[\text{IgG}]_S\,[\text{Albumin}]_U}$$

where U and S are the concentrations in urine and serum. A SI of <0.1% indicates 'highly selective' proteinuria, and an SI of >0.2% is 'non-selective'. This is of limited clinical value since highly selective proteinuria is less common in adult MCD and does not influence a decision to treat with steroids. However, highly selective proteinuria, when present, does indicate that MCD is more likely to be the diagnosis, and some argue that such patients should be given a trial of steroids without a renal biopsy.

Children presenting under 1 yr or with syndromic features and steroid non-responders should have genetic testing.

20.7 Renal Biopsy

In children (especially <12 years), renal biopsy is unnecessary unless the patient does not respond to corticosteroid treatment. In adults, since steroid-responsive disease is less likely (<30%) and a wide differential diagnosis for nephrotic syndrome exists, a renal biopsy is recommended to establish the diagnosis. In the absence of a specific contraindication to steroid therapy, some argue that a therapeutic trial of steroids should be given, reserving renal biopsy for nonresponders. However, adults with steroid-responsive nephrotic syndrome may take up to 12 weeks before induction of remission and so the morbidity from steroids does become significant outweighing the small risks of a renal biopsy. Even when there is a typical biopsy appearance, it is always important to consider whether the patient may have a secondary cause of MCD.

20.8 Histopathology

- Classically completely normal glomeruli on light microscopy and immunohistology with podocyte foot process effacement on electron microscopy (◘ Fig. 20.2) as the only (but nonspecific finding) abnormality.
- Mild mesangial hypercellularity is now accepted as an infrequent finding, as are small amounts of mesangial IgG, complement C3 and occasionally IgA (partly based on patients whose clinical course is indistinguishable from classical MCD). Mesangial hypercellularity may be a predictor of steroid resistance and a poorer prognosis.
- The presence of mesangial IgM is considered by some to define a separate entity (see below).

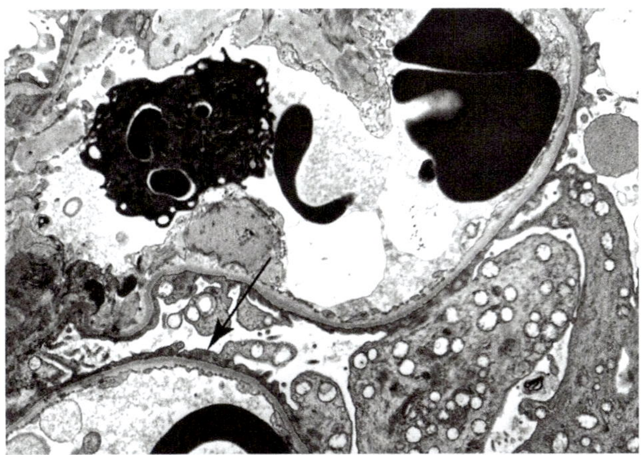

◘ **Fig. 20.2** Podocyte foot process fusion in minimal change disease. The epithelial cells (*arrows*) are completely effaced along the glomerular basement membranes (electron micrograph ×6000). (Courtesy of Prof Ian Roberts, Oxford University Hospitals NHS Trust)

- Hyaline casts obstructing tubules, foam cells and appearances consistent with acute tubular injury may be seen, especially if AKI is present at the time of biopsy.

20.9 Management

As described in the chapter on the general management of nephrotic syndrome, all patients should receive general management of the nephrotic syndrome to control oedema with fluid and salt restriction and diuretics (used less often in children because of the greater risk of hypovolaemia). Consideration should be given to prophylaxis against thrombosis (especially when the serum albumin level is <20g/L) and infection and, in nonresponders, control of hyperlipidaemia [10].

More than 90% of patients with MCD respond to steroids, although there is considerable variation in the recommended doses and duration and when to introduce second-line treatments, reflecting the dearth of adequate controlled trials. Therefore, the recommendations here are pragmatic and justified, where possible, by evidence from clinical trials.

20.10 Childhood Minimal Change Disease

The ISKDC recommends that the first episode should be treated with oral prednisolone 60 mg/m^2/day or 2 mg/kg to a maximum of 60 mg/day (calculated on estimated 'dry' weight). Response rates are 75% within 2 weeks, 80–85% within 4 weeks and over 90% within 8 weeks (◘ Fig. 20.4). Assuming urinary remission, steroids should be continued at the initial dose for 6 weeks followed by a switch to alternate-day dosing at 1.5 mg/kg (maximum 40 mg per day) for 6 weeks, but subsequent tapering is no longer recommended [11, 12]. Children should remain on steroids for 3–4 months, which is associated with a lower 1-year relapse rate compared with those receiving steroids ≤2 months (19% v. 64%, respectively) based on several studies and a meta-analysis [13, 14]. The 2-year sustained remission rate is 49% with a 29% frequent relapse rate although this is higher in younger children. The KDIGO recommendations published in 2021 now recommend a shorter course of high dose steroids (8–12 weeks), which are noninferior to longer courses [15, 16].

For children still proteinuric after 4 weeks on steroids, there is anecdotal evidence that either increasing the steroid dose or giving an intravenous pulse of methylprednisolone (1 g/1.73 m^2) improves the probability of inducing a remission. However, it is important to consider reasons for treatment failure including noncompliance and poor absorption from an oedematous bowel, especially in the presence of diarrhoea, both of which would make intravenous steroids logical. Even in the absence of diarrhoea, prescription of non-enteric-coated steroid formulations is recommended, since occasionally enteric-coated tablets are poorly or not absorbed.

20.11 Diagnosis and Treatment of Initial and Infrequent Relapses

Daily urine testing should continue after remission in order to detect and treat relapses early. Relapse should be diagnosed on the basis of dipstick 3+ proteinuria for 3 consecutive days. The first relapse is treated with a 2nd induction course of steroids but of shorter duration, for instance, halving the dose after 3 consecutive days of a dipstick-negative/1+ urine for 4 weeks and then stopping is probably as effective as a more prolonged course.

Subsequent relapses may be treated similarly or by tapering the prednisolone to 15 mg/m^2 on alternate days and continuing for 12–18 months (assuming this is above the 'steroid threshold' at which relapse occurs in that individual). Clearly the acceptability of this approach depends on the 'steroid threshold'.

20

20.12 Frequent Relapsers and Steroid-Dependent MCD

There is wide variation in the management of frequent relapsers and children who become steroid-dependent, relapsing as the steroid dose is reduced. There is a paucity of controlled data, but generally 'second-line' drugs are used to avoid steroid toxicity, most commonly alkylating agents (cyclophosphamide and chlorambucil), levamisole, ciclosporin or tacrolimus and, more recently, rituximab.

Alkylating agents were originally first-line, although increasingly other agents are now being tried first, mainly because of the potential side effects of alkylating agents (immediately infection and alopecia, and subsequently sterility [17], haemorrhagic cystitis and longer-term risks of hematologic malignancy). Although these are small for a 3-month course, they need to be balanced against the fact that MCD is usually self-limiting and the permanent remission rate is not very high. On the basis of one but not all studies, cyclophosphamide (2–2.5 mg/kg daily) for 12 weeks is more effective than an 8-week course, giving a 2-year remission rate of 60% versus 30% [18]. Younger children are less likely to have a sustained response to cyclophosphamide (Fig. 20.3). Chlorambucil (0.2 mg/kg daily) for 2 months appears to have a similar effect to cyclophosphamide and, apart from not provoking haemorrhagic cystitis, has similar adverse effects. Frequent relapsers are more likely to have a long-term remission following an 8-week course of cyclophosphamide or chlorambucil than steroid-dependent children (75% versus 35%). Second courses are not recommended as they are less effective, and the cumulative dose of 150–250 mg/kg [17] is likely to be exceeded.

During treatment with cyclophosphamide or chlorambucil, blood counts should be checked weekly and dose reductions made to avoid cytopenias. Herpes zoster infection is potentially catastrophic, serostatus must be

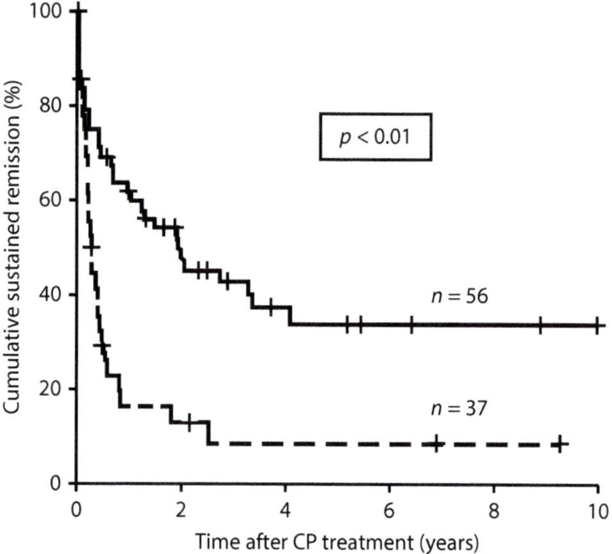

Fig. 20.3 Older children are more likely to respond to cyclophosphamide than younger children. Sustained remission in older (*solid line*) and younger (<5.5 years, *dotted line*) children following cyclophosphamide treatment. (Reproduced with permission from Vester et al. [19])

checked on starting treatment and in case of unavoidable contact with active zoster, children should be given hyperimmune immunoglobulin and antivirals.

Azathioprine has no proven role in the management of children with MCD and was ineffective in a randomised trial. Mycophenolate has also studied in RCTs and may be effective, but inferior to ciclosporin with a higher relapse rate [20].

Ciclosporin (up to 150 mg/m^2 or 4 mg/kg per day with initial target trough levels of 50–150 ng/ml) is generally effective in children with both steroid-dependent and frequently relapsing nephrotic syndrome [21]. Unfortunately relapse within 3 months of stopping treatment is very common, and there is a risk of nephrotoxicity, even with careful monitoring of blood levels, renal function and blood pressure control. The aim of therapy is that ciclosporin will maintain steroid-free remission until the underlying disease remits. The optimum duration of therapy is not established, but treatment for 1–2 years followed by its slow withdrawal is recommended. Limited reports suggest that tacrolimus is as effective as ciclosporin and is used especially when side effects are a problem (especially hypertrichosis or gingival hypertrophy), but diabetes may be more common. Tacrolimus use is only supported by observational studies with no randomised controlled trials in MCD and so should be second-line.

The choice between a calcineurin inhibitor and cyclophosphamide needs to be individualised and may be influenced by the frequency of relapses and how quickly the child responds to steroids, and often the relative side effects are discussed with the parents. Also relevant is that younger children are less likely to have a sustained remission after cyclophosphamide (◘ Fig. 20.3).

The antihelminthic drug levamisole (2.5 mg/kg on alternate days for 3 months) has been shown to be effective [22]. However, relapse within 3 months of stopping the drug is very common although, as with ciclosporin, it may provide a relatively nontoxic alternative to steroids until spontaneous remission of the condition occurs.

Rituximab appears to be effective and seems to be associated with a more prolonged remission and a lower incidence of side effects than cyclophosphamide in children frequently relapsing and steroid-dependent MCD. This has been demonstrated in two randomised controlled trials although the follow-up was only 1 year [23, 24] and similar results in an observational study with longer follow-up [25]. Other studies have failed to demonstrate efficacy, and an adequately powered randomised controlled trial with longer follow-up is needed. In the UK NICE has approved rituximab use for children with MCD but not for adults.

Although there continue to be many unresolved issues, the clinical setting may suggest an obvious approach to frequent relapsers. For instance, a child who presents at a very young age (and is, therefore, statistically likely to continue to relapse for many years) and who is a frequent relapser but not steroid-dependent may stand to benefit more from an alkylating agent than an older, steroid-dependent patient.

20.13 Adult Minimal Change Disease

With few adequate controlled studies in adults, treatment recommendations are extrapolated from the paediatric experience, but lower doses of oral prednisolone (1 mg/kg daily up to 80 mg/day) are traditionally prescribed. The response rate is lower than in children, and up to 25% do not respond despite 3–4 months of treatment [26] (◘ Fig. 20.4). The reasons for this are likely to include lower relative doses of steroids and higher chance of underlying FSGS, missed on the original biopsy, which is more often steroid-resistant.

After 1 week of urinary remission, the prednisolone dose is halved for 4–6 weeks, followed by further tapering to stop after a further 4–6 weeks aiming, as in children, for a total steroid course of 3–4 months (extrapolation from paediatric data and not evidence-based in adults). Steroid treatment should be combined with gastric protection (an H2 blocker or proton pump inhibitor) and bone protection with a bisphosphonate.

A recent (small) RCT suggested similar response to standard prednisolone and tacrolimus [32], but only 50% of the latter achieved remission by 8 weeks and maximum response only after 26 weeks. A Chinese RCT compared standard steroids to tacrolimus and half-dose (0.5 mg/kg) prednisolone response rate was still a little less than standard treatment but with a lower relapse rate to the end of the study (only 24 weeks and patients were still on tacrolimus) [33]. However, a recent RCT has demonstrated that tacrolimus can now be recommended first line for patients with a contraindication to corticosteroids [33].

20.14 Relapse

The relapse rate is slightly lower than in children (30–50%), and older adults have fewer relapses and are less likely to require second-line agents [27]. It is important to remember that transient non-nephrotic relapses may occur, so treatment should await confirmation of relapse with 3–5 consecutive days of proteinuria >2+ on urine dipstick and weight gain, the development of oedema or a fall in plasma albumin. Initial relapses are treated with prednisolone (1 mg/kg up to 80 mg/day) but with a much

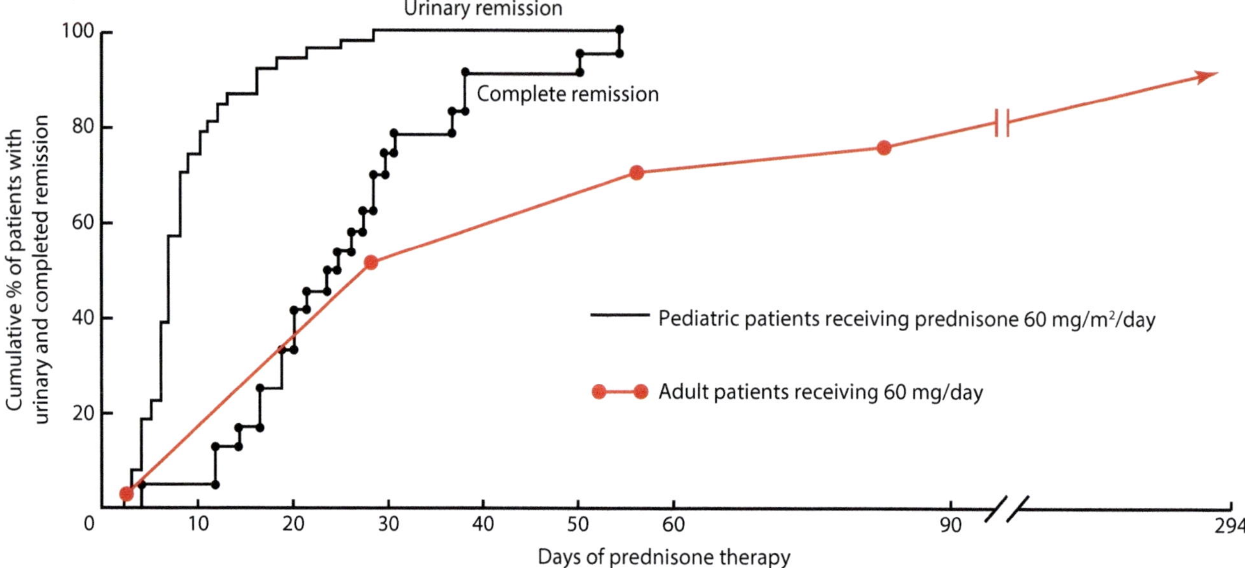

Fig. 20.4 Corticosteroid responses in children and adults. (Adapted from [13, 26])

more rapid tapering after urinary remission is achieved (e.g. halving dose every 5 days until 10–15 mg/day and then reduce by 5 mg/day every 5 days until stopped).

Second-line treatments are given to frequently relapsing patients and those who are steroid-dependent (who relapse as the steroid dose is reduced but remain in remission as long as a 'threshold' dose is maintained). As in children, cyclophosphamide or calcineurin inhibitors are used. A permanent remission is achieved with cyclophosphamide more often than in children (75 and 66% at 2 and 5 years, respectively) [26], and based on the paediatric data, a 12-week course (2 mg/kg of ideal body weight up to 175 mg/day) may be more effective than 8 weeks. Adults may be less susceptible to gonadal damage, and men can be given the opportunity to bank sperm prior to treatment. IV cyclophosphamide has not been adequately evaluated in MCN (one study in children concluded 6 monthly pulses was less effective the historical 3-month oral cyclophosphamide).

Ciclosporin (4–6 mg/kg/day, aiming for 50–150 ng/ml) and tacrolimus (target levels 4–6 ng/ml) are alternatives (and may be preferred in younger adults) or can be used if cyclophosphamide fails. Relapse usually follows dose reduction or withdrawal, but since immunosuppression-free remission eventually occurs in up to 75% of patients, it is an effective strategy to maintain patients non-nephrotic. There are no controlled studies to inform the best length of time on ciclosporin. My practice is to treat for 1 year and then taper the dose gradually to stop over 4–6 months. Relapse would indicate a longer course of treatment. Since nephrotoxicity is more common after >1-year treatment [28], careful monitoring of renal function and ciclosporin levels is essential, and if the GFR falls, a biopsy is indicated to distinguish between calcineurin inhibitor toxicity or the development of FSGS. Tacrolimus is similarly effective and useful for patients with side effects from ciclosporin.

Reports of the use of mycophenolate and rituximab are, as for children, anecdotal and need to await further studies. The largest published study of rituximab in adult steroid-dependent or frequently relapsing MCN suggests that a significant proportion of patients (65%) maintained a remission for >2 years, and it appeared to be more effective when given in remission [29]. However, the study was retrospective, and although patients were adults, 12/17 had developed NS as children. Evidence remains anecdotal [30, 31] and controlled prospective trials are needed.

A small proportion of patients with repeated relapses, even if they remain steroid-dependent, but more often if they become steroid-dependent or resistant are shown to have FSGS of repeat biopsy. These patients then develop progressive chronic kidney disease and, eventually, renal failure.

20

20.15 'Minimal Change' Appearance with Non-nephrotic Proteinuria and Normal Albumin

Steroid treatment is not indicated, but hypertension should be treated with an ACE inhibitor or angiotensin II receptor antagonist. Proteinuria and renal function should be monitored with re-biopsy in case of increased proteinuria of reduced renal function.

Case Study

Case 1

A 34-year-old Afro-Caribbean woman presented with acute onset of nephrotic syndrome. She had no significant past medical history but was obese with a BMI of 42. Her blood pressure was higher than expected for her age at 145/90. She had renal impairment with a creatinine of 298 μmol/L (eGFR 23 ml/min, corrected for ethnicity), albumin of 11 g/L and a urinary PCR of 1150 mg/mmol. A renal biopsy confirmed minimal change disease with some acute tubular injury, and she was treated with prednisolone at 80 mg/day. She went into remission after 6 weeks with a creatinine falling to 59 μmol/L (eGFR >100 ml/min), and her blood pressure normalised (115/70). Unfortunately she stopped her steroids precipitously 2 weeks after her remission as she was feeling well and relapsed within 2 weeks. She responded promptly to reinduction with steroids, but over the next year had 2 more relapses and was treated with a 3-month course of cyclophosphamide, and she remains in remission 5 years later.

This case represents a fairly typical clinical course with mild hypertension that resolved when the patient went into remission. Acute kidney injury is present or develops in about one in five patients although rarely requires dialysis but usually recovers quickly on treatment. Reducing or stopping steroids rapidly after remission often results in relapse. Frequent relapses were cured following a 3-month course of cyclophosphamide.

Case 2

A 3-year-old male child presented with nephrotic syndrome aged 2 years 9 months. He was treated with steroids and rapidly went into remission. He had recurrent relapses over the next 9 years all of which were steroid-sensitive. A kidney biopsy at this stage confirmed minimal change disease. After discussion with his parents (now aged 12 years), he started ciclosporin, which kept him in remission but with occasional relapses, and a biopsy 2 years later again confirmed minimal change disease but with some interstitial fibrosis, and the ciclosporin was stopped. He transferred to the adult service age 17. Frequent nephrotic relapses continued, and although these remained generally steroid-sensitive, he never went into complete remission with PCRs of around 50 mg/mmol. He and his parents were not keen to try cyclophosphamide. His kidney function deteriorated, and a further biopsy showed FSGS, and over the next 2 years, his chronic kidney disease progressed until he required dialysis.

Children who present at a very young age with nephrotic syndrome due to minimal change nephropathy are most likely to have frequent relapses for the longest period of time, not infrequently extending into adulthood as in this patient. The later biopsy did show evidence of FSGS. This case is slightly unusual in that such patients usually become steroid-resistant.

Case 3

A 34-year-old female presented with acute nephrotic syndrome with a creatinine of 48 μmol/L, serum albumin of 9 g/L and a urinary PCR of 800 mg/mmol. The renal biopsy confirmed minimal change disease, and she was treated with prednisolone and responded within 4 weeks and continued a tapering dose of prednisolone for a further 10 weeks. She relapsed 6 months later and then had two further relapses within 6 weeks of completing each course of steroids although responded promptly. She was anxious about taking cyclophosphamide in view of the possible effect on her fertility especially in view of her age and opted for treatment with ciclosporin. She was monitored for 3 months and maintained normal renal function, normal blood pressures and ciclosporin levels of 75–100 ng/ml. After 18 months of treatment, the ciclosporin dose was gradually tapered and stopped over 6 months. She remains in remission after 6 years of follow-up.

Cyclophosphamide is more likely to cause reduced fertility in older women. Some patient relapse after tapering of stopping the ciclosporin and this can be restarted and a further attempt to stop made at a later time (usually more than a year).

Tips and Tricks

1. If patients relapse during steroid tapering, check compliance, as some patients are eager to get off steroids. It is worth emphasising the importance of following the steroid wean, especially after the initial treatment.
2. Patients who have had MCD often get a non-nephrotic increase in proteinuria, especially associated with minor infections, which settle spontaneously, so only treat proper nephrotic relapses with weight gain with oedema with nephrotic-range proteinuria and hypoalbuminuria. [Some patients religiously check urine with dipsticks and get anxious about positives and request steroids despite no other symptoms].
3. If a patient becomes steroid-dependent or steroid-resistant, consider another biopsy as it is possible that the condition has developed into FSGS.

4. Monitor ciclosporin/tacrolimus levels and aim for the lowest effective dose. If the creatinine rises without high CNI levels, a biopsy is necessary to determine if the cause is CNI toxicity, presence of FSGS or other (e.g. tubulointerstitial nephritis).

Chapter Review Questions

1. When is a biopsy necessary in a patient presenting with nephrotic syndrome?
2. Are there any clinical tests that can be used to predict that MCD is the cause of a patient's nephrotic syndrome without a biopsy?
3. Since cyclophosphamide often results in a long-term remission of MCD, why shouldn't this be offered to all patients with relapsing disease?

Answers

1. Generally a biopsy is recommended for all adults with nephrotic syndrome since, as compared to children, MCD is less likely to be the diagnosis. Arguably in young adults, some clinicians have suggested a trial of steroids first, but this would expose a significant number of patients with another cause of nephrotic syndrome to unnecessary high steroid exposure. Diabetics may become nephrotic, and if this follows relatively low-level proteinuria before, a biopsy is worth doing as this may demonstrate MCD (or other cause of nephrotic syndrome).
2. Yes, by measuring the selectivity index of the proteinuria. Highly selective proteinuria does indicate that MCD is more likely to be the diagnosis (and therefore steroid-responsive). However, this is of limited clinical value since highly selective proteinuria is uncommon in adult MCD and children are treated with steroids without a biopsy anyway.
3. Management of relapsing MCD needs to be discussed with the patient (and parents of children) as they may have views about the consequences of repeated steroid courses, cyclophosphamide side effects – especially infertility even though the risks are low, or relatively long-term treatment with ciclosporin and its side effects.

References

1. Maas RJ, Deegens JK, Smeets B, Moeller MJ, Wetzels JF. Minimal change disease and idiopathic FSGS: manifestations of the same disease. Nat Rev Nephrol. 2016;12(12):768–76.
2. Glassock RJ. Secondary minimal change disease. Nephrol Dial Transplant. 2003;18 Suppl 6:vi52–8.
3. Garin EH, Diaz LN, Mu W, Wasserfall C, Araya C, Segal M, et al. Urinary CD80 excretion increases in idiopathic minimal-change disease. J Am Soc Nephrol. 2009;20(2):260–6.
4. Bakker WW, van Dael CM, Pierik LJ, van Wijk JA, Nauta J, Borghuis T, et al. Altered activity of plasma hemopexin in patients with minimal change disease in relapse. Pediatr Nephrol. 2005;20(10):1410–5.
5. Ali AA, Wilson E, Moorhead JF, Amlot P, Abdulla A, Fernando ON, et al. Minimal-change glomerular nephritis. Normal kidneys in an abnormal environment? Transplantation. 1994;58(7):849–52.
6. Abdel-Hafez M, Shimada M, Lee PY, Johnson RJ, Garin EH. Idiopathic nephrotic syndrome and atopy: is there a common link? Am J Kidney Dis. 2009;54(5):945–53.
7. Clement LC, Avila-Casado C, Mace C, Soria E, Bakker WW, Kersten S, et al. Podocyte-secreted angiopoietin-like-4 mediates proteinuria in glucocorticoid-sensitive nephrotic syndrome. Nat Med. 2011;17(1):117–22.
8. Trompeter RS, Lloyd BW, Hicks J, White RH, Cameron JS. Long-term outcome for children with minimal-change nephrotic syndrome. Lancet. 1985;1(8425):368–70.
9. Waldman M, Crew RJ, Valeri A, Busch J, Stokes B, Markowitz G, et al. Adult minimal-change disease: clinical characteristics, treatment, and outcomes. Clin J Am Soc Nephrol. 2007;2(3):445–53.
10. Lin R, McDonald G, Jolly T, Batten A, Chacko. A systematic review of prophylactic anticoagulation in nephrotic syndrome. Kidney Int Rep. 2020;5(4):435–47.
11. Ehrich JH, Brodehl J. Long versus standard prednisone therapy for initial treatment of idiopathic nephrotic syndrome in children. Arbeitsgemeinschaft fur Padiatrische Nephrologie. Eur J Pediatr. 1993;152(4):357–61.
12. Gipson DS, Massengill SF, Yao L, Nagaraj S, Smoyer WE, Mahan JD, et al. Management of childhood onset nephrotic syndrome. Pediatrics. 2009;124(2):747–57.
13. Short versus standard prednisone therapy for initial treatment of idiopathic nephrotic syndrome in children. Arbeitsgemeinschaft fur Padiatrische Nephrologie. Lancet. 1988;1(8582):380–3.
14. Hodson EM, Willis NS, Craig JC. Corticosteroid therapy for nephrotic syndrome in children. Cochrane Database Syst Rev. 2007;(4):CD001533.
15. Lombel RM, Gipson DS, Hodson EM, O. Kidney Disease: Improving Global. Treatment of steroid-sensitive nephrotic syndrome: new guidelines from KDIGO. Pediatr Nephrol. 2013;28(3):415–26.
16. Rovin BH, et al. Executive summary of the KDIGO 2021 guideline for the management of glomerular diseases. Kidney Int. 2021;100(4):753–79.
17. Trompeter RS, Evans PR, Barratt TM. Gonadal function in boys with steroid-responsive nephrotic syndrome treated with cyclophosphamide for short periods. Lancet. 1981;1(8231):1177–9.
18. Cyclophosphamide treatment of steroid dependent nephrotic syndrome: comparison of eight week with 12 week course. Report of Arbeitsgemeinschaft fur Padiatrische Nephrologie. Arch Dis Child. 1987;62(11):1102–6.
19. Vester U, Kranz B, Zimmermann S, Hoyer PF. Cyclophosphamide in steroid-sensitive nephrotic syndrome: outcome and outlook. Pediatr Nephrol. 2003;18(7):661–4.
20. Querfeld U, Weber LT. Mycophenolate mofetil for sustained remission in nephrotic syndrome. Pediatr Nephrol. 2018;33(12):2253–65.

21. Niaudet P, Broyer M, Habib R. Treatment of idiopathic nephrotic syndrome with cyclosporin A in children. Clin Nephrol. 1991;35 Suppl 1:S31–6.
22. Levamisole for corticosteroid-dependent nephrotic syndrome in childhood. British Association for Paediatric Nephrology. Lancet. 1991;337(8757):1555–7.
23. Iijima K, Sako M, Nozu K, Mori R, Tuchida N, Kamei K, et al. Rituximab for childhood-onset, complicated, frequently relapsing nephrotic syndrome or steroid-dependent nephrotic syndrome: a multicentre, double-blind, randomised, placebo-controlled trial. Lancet. 2014;384(9950):1273–81.
24. Ravani P, Magnasco A, Edefonti A, Murer L, Rossi R, Ghio L, et al. Short-term effects of rituximab in children with steroid- and calcineurin-dependent nephrotic syndrome: a randomized controlled trial. Clin J Am Soc Nephrol. 2011;6(6):1308–15.
25. Webb H, Jaureguiberry G, Dufek S, Tullus K, Bockenhauer D. Cyclophosphamide and rituximab in frequently relapsing/steroid-dependent nephrotic syndrome. Pediatr Nephrol. 2016;31(4):589–94.
26. Nolasco F, Cameron JS, Heywood EF, Hicks J, Ogg C, Williams DG. Adult-onset minimal change nephrotic syndrome: a long-term follow-up. Kidney Int. 1986;29(6):1215–23.
27. Tse KC, Lam MF, Yip PS, Li FK, Choy BY, Lai KN, et al. Idiopathic minimal change nephrotic syndrome in older adults: steroid responsiveness and pattern of relapses. Nephrol Dial Transplant. 2003;18(7):1316–20.
28. Melocoton TL, Kamil ES, Cohen AH, Fine RN. Long-term cyclosporine A treatment of steroid-resistant and steroid-dependent nephrotic syndrome. Am J Kidney Dis. 1991;18(5):583–8.
29. Munyentwali H, Bouachi K, Audard V, Remy P, Lang P, Mojaat R, et al. Rituximab is an efficient and safe treatment in adults with steroid-dependent minimal change disease. Kidney Int. 2013;83(3):511–6.
30. Miyabe Y, Takei T, Iwabuchi Y, Moriyama T, Nitta K. Amelioration of the adverse effects of prednisolone by rituximab treatment in adults with steroid-dependent minimal-change nephrotic syndrome. Clin Exp Nephrol. 2016;20(1):103–10.
31. Mallat SG, Itani HS, Abou-Mrad RM, Abou Arkoub R, Tanios BY. Rituximab use in adult primary glomerulopathy: where is the evidence? Ther Clin Risk Manag. 2016;12:1317–27.
32. Chin HJ, Chae DW, Kim YC, An WS, Ihm C, Jin DC, Kim SG, Kim YL, Kim YS, Kim YG, Koo HS, Lee JE, Lee KW, Oh J, Park JH, Jiang H, Lee H, Lee SK. Comparison of the efficacy and safety of tacrolimus and low-dose corticosteroid with high-dose corticosteroid for minimal change nephrotic syndrome in adults. J Am Soc Nephrol. 2020 (in press).
33. Medjeral-Thomas NR, et al. Randomized, controlled trial of tacrolimus and prednisolone monotherapy for adults with de novo minimal change disease: a multicenter, randomized, controlled trial. Clin J Am Soc Nephrol. 2020;15(2):209–218.

Focal Segmental Glomerulosclerosis

Philip David Mason

Contents

M. Harber (ed.), *Primer on Nephrology*, https://doi.org/10.1007/978-3-030-76419-7_21

Learning Objectives

1. FSGS a more common cause of nephrotic syndrome adolescents and young adults. It is important to understand this disease is different from FSGS on biopsy without heavy proteinuria or nephrotic syndrome
2. A trial of treatment with high-dose steroids is necessary since complete or partial response significantly improves the prognosis
3. FSGS commonly recurs following transplantation, and this needs to be tested for and treated with plasma exchange

21.1 Introduction and Epidemiology

Primary FSGS is the cause of nephrotic syndrome in <10% of children under 10 years, the middle aged and the elderly but is the diagnosis in up to 20% of nephrotic adolescents and young adults. It has an incidence of about two per million in a white European population [1] but is commonest cause in adult African Americans, and the incidence appears to be rising [2]. Overall, it is the cause of renal failure in about 2.5% of patients on renal replacement therapy in the USA, but this is more than 10% in younger patients [3].

It is important to remember that FSGS is defined by histopathology and the clinical presentation with nephrotic syndrome. Similar histopathologic appearances are seen in patients with non-nephrotic proteinuria who have other conditions with different prognoses and are, therefore, managed differently.

21.2 Aetiology and Pathogenesis

FSGS, in common with minimal change disease (MCD), is a podocytopathy affecting podocyte structure and function as described in Chapter [MCD]. The close clinical relationship between MCD and FSGS has led some to suggest a shared pathogenesis and may be different manifestations of the same disease but reflecting the intensity of podocyte injury [4]. The non-sclerotic regions of glomeruli in FSGS are indistinguishable from MCD, and patients with FSGS sometimes have a diagnosis of MCD in initial biopsy. This may merely be a reflection of early disease and sampling error, but there are well-documented cases of patients with steroid-sensitive MCD developing into FSGS after many years of relapses.

Nephrotic FSGS is sometimes found in association with a wide range of other conditions and genetic mutations (Table 21.1). These include a variety of infections, non-renal conditions and pre-existing renal diseases. These secondary forms of FSGS are more likely if the proteinuria is not in the nephrotic range, are often associated with podocyte injury or result from

Table 21.1 Secondary FSGS

Genetic
Autosomal recessive (usually present in childhood):
NPHS1 (nephrin)[a], NPHS2 (podocin)[b], NPHS3 (phospholipase Cε1), CD2-associated protein, MYO1E (non-muscle myosin)
Autosomal dominant (usually present in older children, adolescents and adults):
TRPC6 (Ca channel), ACTN4 (a-actinin-4), INF2 (formin)[c]
Uncertain:
APOL1[d]
Viral infections
HIV (collapsing FSGS, HIV-associated nephropathy [HIVAN])
Rarely CMV and parvovirus
Drugs
Heroin (sometimes also with HIV)
Lithium
Pamidronate
γ-Interferon
Sulphasalazine
Anabolic steroids (possibly by hyperfiltration)
'Adaptive' in response to hyperfiltration
Obesity
Reduced nephron mass (e.g. subtotal nephrectomy)
Renal dysplasia
Reflux nephropathy
Congenital heart disease (cyanotic)
Sickle cell anaemia
Chronic allograft (transplant) nephropathy

[a]Most common cause of Finnish congenital nephrotic syndrome
[b]Most common genetic cause of SRNS in children
[c]Most common cause of adult familial FSGS—usually non-nephrotic
[d]Mutations confer resistance to *Trypanosoma brucei* but predispose (uncertain aetiology) to FSGS

adaptive changes in response to glomerular loss from scarring resulting in hyperfiltration [5].

Nephrotic FSGS may also be a consequence of genetic mutations, which usually present in childhood and mostly encode podocyte proteins involved with the actin cytoskeleton and integrity of the slit diaphragm [6]. At least 38 genes have now been identified [7]. Sadowski et al. reported nearly 30% children had an identified gene mutation and was more common in the younger patients (69% of those presenting younger than 3 months and 50% presenting at 4–12 months of age) [8]. Mutations are also increasingly being discovered in adults onset FSGS [9].

Evidence for a circulating factor in FSGS is more substantial than in MCD, mainly based on the high incidence of recurrence following transplantation, with heavy proteinuria developing sometimes within hours (with resolution reported in one case report of an affected transplant after retransplantation into a second recipient [10]). In another case report, transmission of heavy proteinuria to the foetus of a mother with FSGS resolved rapidly after delivery [11]. Following transplantation the histologic picture is initially MCD later developing into FSGS. Plasma exchange and elution with protein A or anti-IgG columns can lead to temporary remission in transplant recurrence of FSGS, and eluates from the columns may induce proteinuria [12]. A soluble factor that causes increased protein permeability in cultured human glomeruli has also been described [13]. Although not definitively characterised, cardiotrophin-like cytokine-1 (structurally similar to interleukin-16) is a potential candidate, and upregulated receptors have been demonstrated on the podocytes of patients with recurrent disease [14]. Upregulated expression of transforming growth factor-β (TGF-β), a pro-fibrotic cytokine, has been described in patients with FSGS, but it is unclear whether this is a primary or secondary phenomenon. Yu et al. reported CD80 may be upregulated in some patients and abatacept (CTLA4-Ig which binds CD80 and blocks T-cell activation) induced remission [15], but further studies have resulted in contradictory findings [16].

In 2013 it was reported that soluble urokinase-type plasminogen activator receptors (suPAR) were present in two-thirds of patients with FSGS and high levels seem to be predictive of recurrence following transplantation [17]. It is believed that the suPAR activates β3 integrin, which plays a major role in anchoring the podocyte to the GBM, resulting in dysregulation. However, further studies have cast doubt on suPAR as the underlying causative factor and may be merely a biomarker [18].

21.3 Natural History and Complications

- The incidence of progressive renal failure in primary FSGS is often quoted as around 50%, although there may be variation in the exact diagnostic criteria.
- The prognosis is clearly related to the level of proteinuria and the response to treatment [19] (◘ Figs. 21.1 and 21.4).
- Non-nephrotic patients with normal plasma albumin and proteinuria of <3 g/day have a 10-year incidence of renal failure of just 10–15%, but many of these will have secondary FSGS.

The complications of FSGS are generally the same as for any cause of nephrotic syndrome and include infection (especially with encapsulated bacteria and including spontaneous bacterial peritonitis particularly in children), life-threatening venous or arterial thrombosis, AKI (especially adults).

21.4 Clinical Features

The symptoms and clinical signs are the same as those for the nephrotic syndrome from any cause, but it is worth noting:

- Severe fluid retention exceeding 3% of the body weight and often much more.
- As in MCD, oedema is gravitational, but a puffy face is common, and genital swelling may be very uncomfortable, especially in men. Gross oedema may result in ulceration and infection of dependent skin and lacerations, and needlestick punctures may weep fluid profusely.
- Striae commonly appear even without steroids.
- Bowel oedema may cause diarrhoea, and increased capillary leak has been suggested as a mechanism for losing protein via the gut.
- Other clinical features include white nails, sometimes in bands (Muehrcke's bands) correlating with periods of clinical relapse. Rarely xanthomata are associated with gross hyperlipidaemia.
- Microscopic haematuria is more common in FSGS than MCD.
- Hypertension is more common, especially with impaired function [20].
- AKI is present or develops in ~18% of patients with MCD.
- Other complications, as for any cause of nephrotic syndrome, include thromboembolism, infection and hyperlipidaemia.

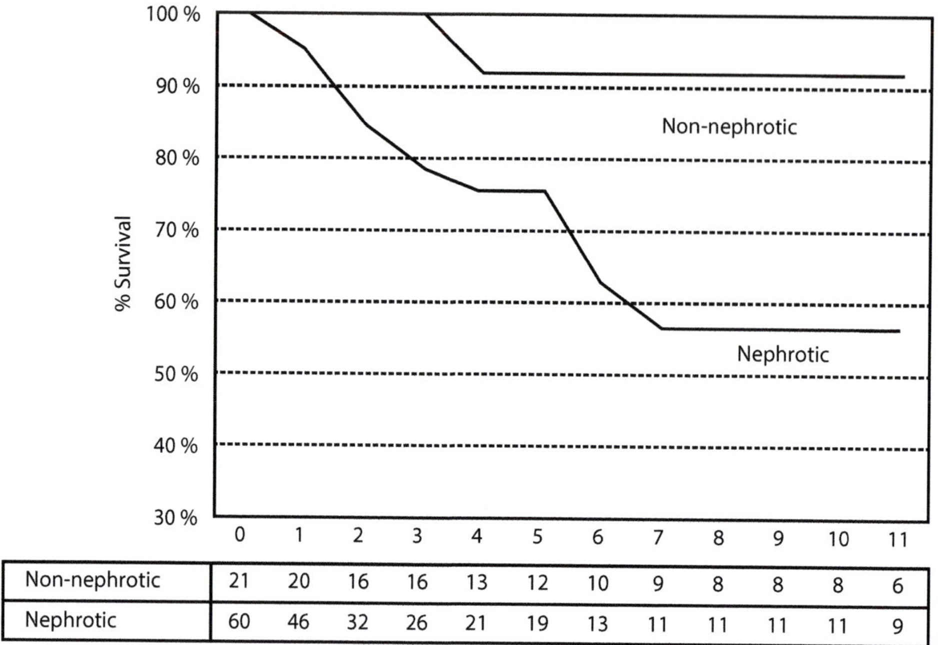

	0	1	2	3	4	5	6	7	8	9	10	11
Non-nephrotic	21	20	16	16	13	12	10	9	8	8	8	6
Nephrotic	60	46	32	26	21	19	13	11	11	11	11	9

Fig. 21.1 Prognosis in primary focal segmental glomerulosclerosis. The risk of developing renal failure is related to the extent of proteinuria. Those with nephrotic-range proteinuria are much more likely to develop renal failure than those with low-grade proteinuria. The figures indicate the number of at-risk patients at different time points. (Reproduced with permission from Rydel et al. [19])

21.5 Diagnosis and Differential Diagnosis

The clinical diagnosis of nephrotic syndrome is usually obvious, with oedema and heavy proteinuria microscopic haematuria may be present. The differential diagnosis is that of nephrotic syndrome and requires a renal biopsy to make a definitive diagnosis.

21.6 Investigations

21.6.1 Routine Investigations

Hyaline and sometimes lipid casts may be seen on urine microscopy. There is nephrotic-range proteinuria (>3.5 g/24 h in adults or >40 mg/h per m^2 in children or a protein/creatinine ratio >350 mg/mmol).

Routine blood biochemistry confirms hypoalbuminaemia and hyperlipidaemia. Hyponatraemia may be present even before treatment, and elevated urea and creatinine are more common in adults.

Usually IgG levels are low and IgM is normal or raised. Serum complement levels are normal.

21.7 Histopathology

21.7.1 Light Microscopy

- As the name implies, there is focal segmental glomerular scarring (Fig. 21.2). Typically juxta-medullary glomeruli are affected first, and so it is possible to miss the diagnosis if there are only a few glomeruli in the biopsy sample, and a glomerulus containing a sclerotic segment may be missed on a single section (examination of serial sections increase the incidence of lesions [21]).
- Glomerular capillaries in affected segments are obliterated by acellular matrix and hyaline deposits, sometimes with adhesions to Bowman's capsule.
- As more glomeruli are affected as the disease progresses, there is more global sclerosis with tubular atrophy with the development of interstitial fibrosis. A diagnosis of FSGS in a nephrotic patient might be suggested by focal tubular atrophy and interstitial fibrosis with normal looking glomeruli (especially with a small biopsy specimen), in which case serial sections may reveal the typical glomerular changes.

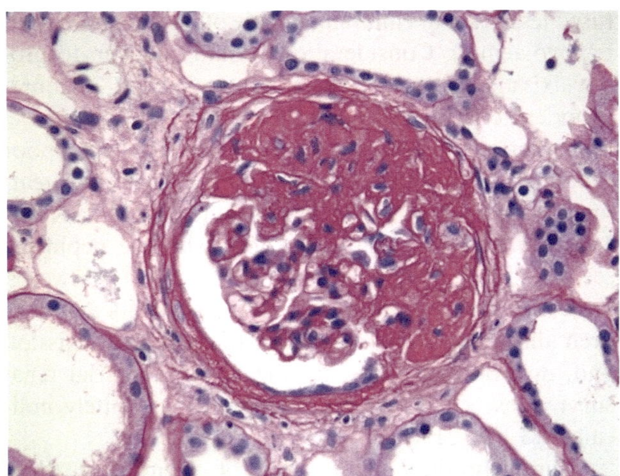

Fig. 21.2 Light microscopic appearances in focal segmental glomerulosclerosis. Segmental scars with capsular adhesions in otherwise normal glomeruli [periodic acid—Schiff, ×300]. (Courtesy of Prof Ian Roberts, Oxford University Hospitals NHS Trust)

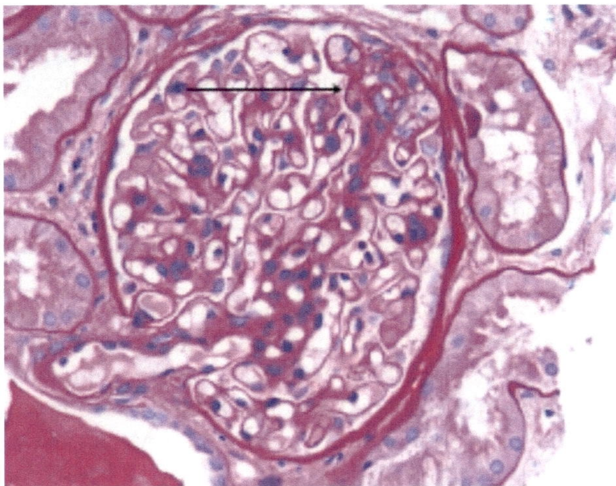

Fig. 21.3 The glomerular 'tip' lesion. A glomerulus in a renal biopsy from an adult with steroid-responsive nephrotic syndrome. The glomerular tuft is normal away from the tubular origin, but at the tubular origin, there is adhesion to Bowman's capsule with protrusion into the tubular lumen (methenamine silver stain ×300). (Courtesy of Prof Ian Roberts, Oxford University Hospitals NHS Trust)

21.8 Immunofluorescence

- Sclerotic segments are often positive for IgM and C3 complement (thought to be a nonspecific consequence of the injury, possibly caused by passive trapping of large molecules in damaged capillary loops).

21.9 Electron Microscopy

- Foot process fusion of non-sclerotic segments and unaffected glomeruli may be indistinguishable from that seen in MCD, but diffuse foot process fusion predominates in the sclerotic segments, with partial effacement in surrounding apparently normal lobules.

21.10 Histologic Variants of Primary FSGS

There is considerable overlap in the descriptions of histologic variants of FSGS and uncertainty as to whether they should be regarded as distinct entities.

- *Collapsing variant* (best defined histologically variant): segmental sclerotic lesions are associated with glomerular tuft collapse and clinically associated with nephrotic syndrome and rapidly progressive AKI similar to HIV and bisphosphonate-associated FSGS. The prognosis is significantly worse with resistance to treatment and usually rapid decline in renal function.
- *Glomerular 'tip' lesion*: segmental scars are described as 'hilar' when related to the vascular pole, 'peripheral' when opposite the tubular pole or 'intermediate'. The 'tip' lesion refers to peripheral segmental sclerosis adjacent to the tubular pole of Bowman's capsule, often with adhesions or synechiae to Bowman's capsule and may prolapse into the proximal tubular lumen (Fig. 21.3). The glomerular capillary loops adjacent to the proximal tubule may be dilated, with accumulation of foamy cells. 'Tip' lesions are seen in other proteinuric conditions including normal glomeruli consistent with MCD (more often in adults than children), which may explain why they have been reported to be more likely to be steroid-responsive with a better long-term prognosis. However, most series do not support an association with a better prognosis, possibly reflecting a more widespread use of the term 'tip' lesion when glomerular changes at the tubular origin occur in other glomerular disorders with proteinuria, including membranoproliferative glomerulonephritis and IgA nephropathy (and renal transplants).

The most important reason to recognise the lesion is to prevent a misdiagnosis of a proliferative glomerulonephritis.

- *The cellular variant*: characterised by podocyte hyperplasia and proliferation, often overlying segmental scars or areas of collapsed capillary loops, sometimes with endocapillary hypercellularity, foam cells, leukocytes and nuclear debris, mimicking proliferative glomerulonephritis. Clinicopathologic correlates of this variant are variable.

- *Mesangial hypercellular variant*: there are contradictory data regarding the significance of this, but many consider mesangial hypercellularity to be an intermediate step in the evolution (progression) of MCD to FSGS.
- *IgM nephropathy*: Patients with mesangial deposits of IgM, usually with minor mesangial hypercellularity, are more likely to be associated with haematuria (usually microscopic) and less likely to respond to steroids (50% compared with 90% for MCD). However, since IgM deposits are seen in MCD, FSGS and mesangial proliferative glomerulonephritis in a similar proportion of patients, it may not be a specific entity in its own right. Similar arguments apply to the rarer finding of mesangial complement C1q deposition, sometimes labelled as C1q nephropathy.

21.11 Management

As described in the chapter on the general management of nephrotic syndrome, all patients should receive general management of the nephrotic syndrome to control oedema with fluid and salt restriction and diuretics (used less often in children because of the greater risk of hypovolaemia). Consideration should be given to prophylaxis against thrombosis and infection and, in nonresponders, control of hyperlipidaemia.

Traditionally, FSGS has been thought to have a poor prognosis, with a low rate of response to steroid treatment and about 50% of patients progressing to ESRD in 10 years [22] although only those who are nephrotic seem to be at particular risk (◘ Fig. 21.1). However, since up to 40% of nephrotic patients (adults and children alike) respond to steroids with complete remission and, in those who respond, the 5-year actuarial renal survival exceeds 95% [19], treatment is definitely indicated (◘ Fig. 21.4).

Currently there is no way of identifying those patients who will respond. The only (retrospective) factor identified in published studies seems to be the duration of steroid treatment, but recommended protocols vary widely. For example, one study showed that 87% of responders received 60 mg prednisolone for 1 month and 67% for 2 months and that the median response time was 3.7 ± 2 months [23].

A pragmatic approach is to treat nephrotic adults with FSGS with prednisolone, 1 mg/kg daily for at least 3 months (2 months in children) after considering patient comorbidities and possible contraindications and after discussion with the patient. Responders, in whom the proteinuria reduces or remits, are treated with

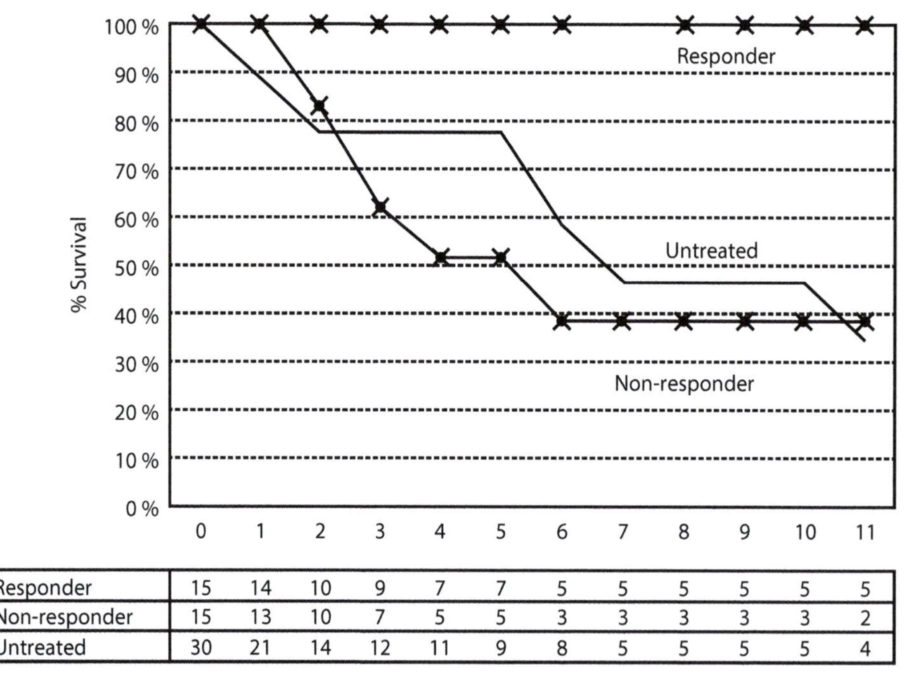

	0	1	2	3	4	5	6	7	8	9	10	11
Responder	15	14	10	9	7	7	5	5	5	5	5	5
Non-responder	15	13	10	7	5	5	3	3	3	3	3	2
Untreated	30	21	14	12	11	9	8	5	5	5	5	4

◘ **Fig. 21.4** Renal survival is good in patients with FSGS who respond to steroids. (Reproduced with permission from Rydel et al. [19])

reducing doses for about 6 months, whilst the steroids are tapered and stopped within 4 weeks in nonresponders. Steroid treatment should be combined with gastric protection (an H2 blocker or proton pump inhibitor) and bone protection with a bisphosphonate. Patients should be monitored for steroid side effects and decisions to abandon treatment need to be made on an individual basis.

Frequent relapsers and those who become steroid-dependent may benefit from a 3-month course of cyclophosphamide [24], but steroid-unresponsive patients rarely, if ever, obtain a sustained remission [24, 25], and so the risks outweigh the benefits.

Ciclosporin is sometimes effective, especially in the steroid-dependent patients, and although, as in the MCD patients, relapse usually follows withdrawal of the drug [22], it may have a role in those patients with refractory nephrotic syndrome. There are several randomised controlled trials of ciclosporin, including patients with steroid-resistant FSGS [22]. Treated patients received ciclosporin for 6 months, followed by gradual withdrawal. Only 20% of patients achieved complete remission, but a further 60% had a partial remission, although there were many relapses following dose reduction. There have been anecdotal reports that patients kept in remission for 12 months can then have ciclosporin successfully withdrawn without relapse [26].

Currently the largest randomised trial of ciclosporin includes only 49 adults: all patients were steroid-resistant (and 40% had also received cyclophosphamide) and received prednisolone (0.15 mg/kg/day) and 6 months of either ciclosporin (3.5 mg/kg/day adjusted to trough levels 125–225 ng/ml) or placebo. Complete (12%) or partial (58%) remission followed in the ciclosporin arm compared with 4% (combined) in the placebo group. Although 60% of responders relapsed within a year following the end of the trial medication, the remainder was still in remission at last follow-up (up to 4 years), and the treated cohort had a significantly lower rate of progression of renal failure [27].

Based on these limited data, I treat steroid nonresponders with ciclosporin (aiming for trough levels of 150–200 ng/ml) for 6 months if remission is not achieved but continue for 1 year with tapering over 3–6 months if remission does occur. This takes advantage of the proven long-term beneficial effects of 6 months of ciclosporin with control of nephrotic syndrome. Ciclosporin is restarted in patients who subsequently relapse again but with careful monitoring of renal function.

Other approaches that have been tried include tacrolimus and very aggressive regimens such as prolonged courses of daily cyclophosphamide (up to 2 years), extended therapy with pulse steroids and intravenous cyclophosphamide or cyclical treatments with corticosteroids and chlorambucil, similar to that introduced by Ponticelli for the treatment of membranous nephropathy. More recently mycophenolate and rituximab have been reported by several groups to be effective, but no controlled trials are available, and the risks of potentially toxic treatments need to be carefully weighed against likelihood of success and alternatives, even if these include progression to ESRD with medical or surgical nephrectomy for intractable and debilitating nephrotic syndrome. All patients, whilst proteinuric, especially those who are steroid-resistant should receive angiotensin-converting enzyme (ACE) inhibitors or ARBs to reduce proteinuria and treatment for hyperlipidaemia.

21.12 Focal Segmental Glomerulosclerosis with Non-nephrotic Proteinuria

Careful evaluation is required to exclude secondary FSGS in those with non-nephrotic proteinuria. There is no convincing evidence that these patients are steroid-responsive and the risks of treatment outweigh the benefits.

21.13 Transplant Recurrence

Recurrence is common after transplantation, but because the label FSGS may often include non-nephrotic native renal disease, an accurate proportion is difficult to assess. It is often reported to be 20% but is probably higher (~40%) for patients with true nephrotic FSGS. Recurrence is more likely with rapid progression in native kidneys, previous recurrence following transplantation (up to 80%) and paediatric recipients [28].

Recurrence may be evident early, even within hours, although the median time to appearance is 14 days and acute renal failure and acute rejection are common. Because of the evidence that a circulating agent is pathogenic in FSGS, patients with recurrent disease following transplantation have been managed with plasma exchange. There is no doubt that plasma exchange can reduce proteinuria, although the response is not absolutely reliable but has been reported in many case reports and small series [29] and a systematic review and meta-analysis [30]. The best chance of a lasting response occurs when plasma exchange is initiated as soon as possible after the appearance of proteinuria and in those whose recurrence is in the first few weeks after transplantation [30]. The effect can be dramatic and long-lasting, but unfortunately the nephrotic syndrome frequently recurs within a few months of discontinuing plasma exchange, and there is much less evidence that a further course of plasma exchange is useful. Some have suggested that pre-emptive plasma exchange is logical, especially for those with a rapid course in native kidneys, but others have found no benefit [31]. High-dose ciclosporin and rituximab (and more recently ofatumumab) have been tried anecdotally with mixed results.

I generally treat with daily plasma exchange for 7 days; if improvement occurs continue with reducing frequency depending on response, but sometimes treatments are continued for weeks with plasma exchange associated with reduction in proteinuria and improvement or preservation of renal function.

Case Study

Case 1

A 37-year-old male presented with nephrotic syndrome with a creatinine of 102 μmol/L (eGFR 66 ml/min), serum albumin 14 g/L and a urinary PCR of 780 mg/mmol. His blood pressure was 138/78. A renal biopsy demonstrated FSGS. He was treated with high-dose steroids and made a partial response with a serum albumin increasing to 28 g/L with a urinary PCR of 115 mg/mmol. He was maintained on a tapering dose of steroids for 4 months. After withdrawal of steroids, his proteinuria continued at a similar level for about 2 years, after which it increased with worsening of his nephrotic syndrome symptoms. He was tried on ciclosporin, but this only resulted in a small reduction in proteinuria, but his creatinine increased to 154 μmol/L (eGFR 43 ml/min) and so was discontinued. Over the next 6 years, kidney function gradually deteriorated until he started dialysis and then received a living donor kidney transplant from his wife. He developed heavy proteinuria on day 6 post-transplant, and the creatinine increased from 116 μmol/L to 145 μmol/L over the next 2 days. At the onset of heavy proteinuria, plasma exchange was started, and he had seven treatments over the next 10 days. Proteinuria initially reduced but increased again and after a second course of plasma exchange proteinuria settled but remained significant with a urinary PCR of 200 mg/mmol, but his renal function improved with a creatinine falling to 119 μmol/L. He is now 2 years post-transplant and continues to have the same level of proteinuria but with stable renal function and he has minimal oedema.

About 50% of patients who get recurrent FSGS in a transplant do respond to plasma exchange. A minority end up with little or no proteinuria. Those that do not respond at all to not always lose their transplant from recurrent disease in a short space of time in the transplant may last several years. Patients who have had graft loss from recurrent FSGS are more than 80% likely to have recurrence in the second transplant but do not always lose the transplant in a short space of time, and so transplantation is usually offered with appropriate counselling.

Case 2

A 58-year-old female presented with sudden onset of nephrotic syndrome with normal renal function with a creatinine of 88 μmol/L and serum albumin 17 g/L with heavy proteinuria (urinary PCR at 950 mg/mmol). She was hypertensive with a blood pressure of 159/94. Renal biopsy demonstrated FSGS, and she was given a trial of high-dose steroids (60 mg/day of prednisolone). After 8 weeks of treatment, there was little change in her condition with an albumin of 20 g/L urinary PCR 480 mg/mmol. Since a nephrotic syndrome was difficult to control despite maximal ACE inhibition and high-dose diuretics, she was tried on ciclosporin which she did not tolerate because of side effects and was changed to tacrolimus, but these treatments had little or no effect on the proteinuria, but her renal function was declining with a creatinine of 239 μmol/L (eGFR 19 ml/min). She was re-biopsied, and this showed extensive FSGS with more than 30% interstitial fibrosis and tubular atrophy. There were some changes consistent with calcineurin inhibitor toxicity, but there was no improvement in function when the tacrolimus was withdrawn. She had a progressive further decline in renal function and started dialysis 3 months later.

This picture is seen in up to one-half of patients with this diagnosis although this rapid progression is seen less often. However, since there is some circumstantial evidence that patients with very rapid decline (less than 1 year from diagnosis to dialysis) are more likely to have rapid recurrence following transplantation, she has been advised to delay transplantation (she has willing potential living donors) for at least a year.

Tips and Tricks

1. Make sure the diagnosis of FSGS is associated with the nephrotic syndrome rather than a secondary FSGS. Childhood FSGS, especially <2 year is likely to have a genetic cause and should not be treated with steroids.
2. The progression of chronic kidney disease in FSGS (as in most kidney diseases) is related to the level of proteinuria, and so it is important to reduce this if possible. Even a partial response to steroids or a calcineurin inhibitor will reduce the rate of decline of kidney function. Always remember to also maximise ACEI/ARB treatment to reduce proteinuria.
3. Calcineurin inhibitors are effective in some patients, but careful monitoring of renal function is important, and a decline should lead to consideration of a further biopsy to determine if disease progression or CNI toxicity is to blame.
4. Patients who progress rapidly to kidney failure (especially in <1 year) should be counselled about the risk of recurrence in a transplant, and most clinicians would recommend waiting at least a year before transplanting, although the evidence is anecdotal.

Chapter Review Questions

1. Why are there some reports of patients with FSGS having low-level proteinuria with better long-term outcomes?
2. If a patient with severe nephrotic FSGS hasn't responded to steroids, is it worth trying cyclophosphamide?
3. The histopathologist reports a patient's biopsy as showing a collapsing FSGS pattern. What clinical implications does this have?
4. A patient initially has a good response to steroids but frequently relapses but continues to respond. What would you recommend as second-line treatment?

Answers

1. A FSGS pattern on a renal biopsy may represent scarring as a result of another pathology such as a burnt out focal segmental glomerulonephritis or even reflux or diabetic nephropathy or following hyperfiltration as a result, e.g. of obesity (see ▫ Table 21.1). Such patients rarely have nephrotic-range proteinuria, and their clinical course is different from 'primary' nephrotic FSGS described in this chapter.
2. No, the limited evidence (only case reports and small series) suggests this isn't effective, and so the risks probably out way the potential benefits. In this situation it is worth a trial of ciclosporin, especially if the nephrotic syndrome is difficult to control with ACEI/ARB and diuretics.
3. This pattern is usually associated with a secondary cause, most commonly HIVAN and pamidronate treatment (see ▫ Table 21.1). It is also seen more often without an identified secondary cause in patients of African origin. It is usually resistant to treatment and progresses rapidly to renal failure, but a trial of steroids is recommended, and there are case reports of complete remission. It is also seen occasionally after parvovirus infection when the prognosis is better.
4. Yes, although the evidence is not very strong so needs to be discussed with the patient regarding potential side effects. The alternative would be a trial of ciclosporin or tacrolimus. Obviously it is also important to always maximise ACEI/ARB treatment and manage hypercholesterolaemia.

References

1. Schena FP. Survey of the Italian Registry of Renal Biopsies. Frequency of the renal diseases for 7 consecutive years. The Italian Group of Renal Immunopathology. Nephrol Dial Transplant. 1997;12(3):418–26.
2. Haas M, Meehan SM, Karrison TG, Spargo BH. Changing etiologies of unexplained adult nephrotic syndrome: a comparison of renal biopsy findings from 1976–1979 and 1995–1997. Am J Kidney Dis. 1997;30(5):621–31.
3. Kitiyakara C, Eggers P, Kopp JB. Twenty-one-year trend in ESRD due to focal segmental glomerulosclerosis in the United States. Am J Kidney Dis. 2004;44(5):815–25.
4. Maas RJ, Deegens JK, Smeets B, Moeller MJ, Wetzels JF. Minimal change disease and idiopathic FSGS: manifestations of the same disease. Nat Rev Nephrol. 2016;12(12):768–76.
5. D'Agati VD. Pathobiology of focal segmental glomerulosclerosis: new developments. Curr Opin Nephrol Hypertens. 2012;21(3):243–50.
6. Rood IM, Deegens JK, Wetzels JF. Genetic causes of focal segmental glomerulosclerosis: implications for clinical practice. Nephrol Dial Transplant. 2012;27(3):882–90.
7. Rosenberg AZ, Kopp JB. Focal segmental glomerulosclerosis. Clin J Am Soc Nephrol. 2017;12(3):502–17.
8. Sadowski CE, Lovric S, Ashraf S, Pabst WL, Gee HY, Kohl S, et al. A single-gene cause in 29.5% of cases of steroid-resistant nephrotic syndrome. J Am Soc Nephrol. 2015;26(6):1279–89.
9. Liu J, Wang W. Genetic basis of adult-onset nephrotic syndrome and focal segmental glomerulosclerosis. Front Med. 2017;11(3):333–9.
10. Gallon L, Leventhal J, Skaro A, Kanwar Y, Alvarado A. Resolution of recurrent focal segmental glomerulosclerosis after retransplantation. N Engl J Med. 2012;366(17):1648–9.

11. Kemper MJ, Wolf G, Muller-Wiefel DE. Transmission of glomerular permeability factor from a mother to her child. N Engl J Med. 2001;344(5):386–7.
12. Dantal J, Godfrin Y, Koll R, Perretto S, Naulet J, Bouhours JF, et al. Antihuman immunoglobulin affinity immunoadsorption strongly decreases proteinuria in patients with relapsing nephrotic syndrome. J Am Soc Nephrol. 1998;9(9):1709–15.
13. Savin VJ, Sharma R, Sharma M, McCarthy ET, Swan SK, Ellis E, et al. Circulating factor associated with increased glomerular permeability to albumin in recurrent focal segmental glomerulosclerosis. N Engl J Med. 1996;334(14):878–83.
14. McCarthy ET, Sharma M, Savin VJ. Circulating permeability factors in idiopathic nephrotic syndrome and focal segmental glomerulosclerosis. Clin J Am Soc Nephrol. 2010;5(11):2115–21.
15. Yu CC, Fornoni A, Weins A, Hakroush S, Maiguel D, Sageshima J, et al. Abatacept in B7-1-positive proteinuric kidney disease. N Engl J Med. 2013;369(25):2416–23.
16. Novelli R, Benigni A, Remuzzi G. The role of B7-1 in proteinuria of glomerular origin. Nat Rev Nephrol. 2018;14(9):589–96.
17. Wei C, El Hindi S, Li J, Fornoni A, Goes N, Sageshima J, et al. Circulating urokinase receptor as a cause of focal segmental glomerulosclerosis. Nat Med. 2011;17(8):952–60.
18. Saleem MA. What is the role of soluble urokinase-type plasminogen activator in renal disease? Nephron. 2018;139(4):334–41.
19. Rydel JJ, Korbet SM, Borok RZ, Schwartz MM. Focal segmental glomerular sclerosis in adults: presentation, course, and response to treatment. Am J Kidney Dis. 1995;25(4):534–42.
20. Nephrotic syndrome in children: prediction of histopathology from clinical and laboratory characteristics at time of diagnosis. A report of the International Study of Kidney Disease in Children. Kidney Int. 1978;13(2):159–65.
21. Fuiano G, Comi N, Magri P, Sepe V, Balletta MM, Esposito C, et al. Serial morphometric analysis of sclerotic lesions in primary "focal" segmental glomerulosclerosis. J Am Soc Nephrol. 1996;7(1):49–55.
22. Korbet SM. Primary focal segmental glomerulosclerosis. J Am Soc Nephrol. 1998;9(7):1333–40.
23. Banfi G, Moriggi M, Sabadini E, Fellin G, D'Amico G, Ponticelli C. The impact of prolonged immunosuppression on the outcome of idiopathic focal-segmental glomerulosclerosis with nephrotic syndrome in adults. A collaborative retrospective study. Clin Nephrol. 1991;36(2):53–9.
24. Siegel NJ, Gaudio KM, Krassner LS, McDonald BM, Anderson FP, Kashgarian M. Steroid-dependent nephrotic syndrome in children: histopathology and relapses after cyclophosphamide treatment. Kidney Int. 1981;19(3):454–9.
25. Tarshish P, Tobin JN, Bernstein J, Edelmann CM Jr. Cyclophosphamide does not benefit patients with focal segmental glomerulosclerosis. A report of the International Study of Kidney Disease in Children. Pediatr Nephrol. 1996;10(5):590–3.
26. Meyrier A, Noel LH, Auriche P, Callard P. Long-term renal tolerance of cyclosporin A treatment in adult idiopathic nephrotic syndrome. Collaborative Group of the Societe de Nephrologie. Kidney Int. 1994;45(5):1446–56.
27. Cattran DC, Appel GB, Hebert LA, Hunsicker LG, Pohl MA, Hoy WE, et al. A randomized trial of cyclosporine in patients with steroid-resistant focal segmental glomerulosclerosis. North America Nephrotic Syndrome Study Group. Kidney Int. 1999;56(6):2220–6.
28. Keith DS. Therapeutic apheresis rescue mission: recurrent focal segmental glomerulosclerosis in renal allografts. Semin Dial. 2012;25(2):190–2.
29. Artero ML, Sharma R, Savin VJ, Vincenti F. Plasmapheresis reduces proteinuria and serum capacity to injure glomeruli in patients with recurrent focal glomerulosclerosis. Am J Kidney Dis. 1994;23(4):574–81.
30. Kashgary A, Sontrop JM, Li L, Al-Jaishi AA, Habibullah ZN, Alsolaimani R, Clark WF. The role of plasma exchange in treating post-transplant focal segmental glomerulosclerosis: a systematic review and meta-analysis of 77 case-reports and case-series. BMC Nephrol. 2016;17(1):104.
31. Gonzalez E, Ettenger R, Rianthavorn P, Tsai E, Malekzadeh M. Preemptive plasmapheresis and recurrence of focal segmental glomerulosclerosis in pediatric renal transplantation. Pediatr Transplant. 2011;15(5):495–501.

Membranous Nephropathy

Sanjana Gupta and Alan D. Salama

Contents

M. Harber (ed.), *Primer on Nephrology*, https://doi.org/10.1007/978-3-030-76419-7_22

Key Points

1. Membranous nephropathy can be either primary or secondary. These can be difficult to differentiate between at presentation.
2. The cause of most primary membranous nephropathy is now known to be autoimmune with two identified autoantigens, phospholipase A2 receptor and thrombospondin type-1 domain-containing 7A.
3. Antibodies to these antigens correlate with clinical outcomes and may help in stratifying management decisions.
4. Treatment options should include supportive therapy initially, in case of spontaneous remissions followed by immunosuppressive therapy after 6 months if no remission has occurred, although optimal regimens remain to be defined.
5. Routine use of PLA2R antibody measurements may alter our understanding of likelihood of spontaneous relapses and responses to therapies.

22.1 Introduction

Membranous nephropathy (MN) is the most common cause of nephrotic syndrome in adults, with an incidence of approximately ten cases per million population per year [1]. Identical clinical presentations and histological appearances can occur whether the condition is autoimmune (historically termed primary or idiopathic) or secondary to other aetiological factors, such as drugs, infections or tumours (see ◘ Table 22.1). Careful assessment to exclude a secondary cause is needed for each new patient. If a secondary cause can be identified, the prognosis is frequently dependent on that of the underlying condition, and management should be directed towards that condition: causative drugs should be stopped, infections eradicated and tumours treated if possible. Successful treatment of the underlying cause may lead to resolution of the secondary MN.

22.2 Epidemiology

MN has a male preponderance (2.2:1), is increasingly common after the 4th decade and is rare in children (incidence <5%). There is very little global variation in incidence of autoimmune membranous nephropathy (AMN) which represents roughly 70–80% of all membranous glomerulonephritis. The incidence of secondary MN relates to the prevalence of the underlying condition. Consequently, and in contrast to AMN, secondary causes of MN are a significant cause of nephrotic syndrome in developing countries, where individuals are more commonly prone to developing infections [2]. Although familial cases have been reported, these are rare. A large number of secondary diagnoses have been associated with MN; however, few have clear proof of causality, which may come in the form of identifying antigens within the kidney or resolution of the MN following treatment of the underlying condition.

Several forms of glomerulonephritis are associated with malignancy; however, MN has the strongest association. Approximately 10% of patients with MN have an underlying malignancy, and 70% of patients with carcinoma and nephrotic syndrome have MN. Lung and gastrointestinal carcinomas predominate with risk factors being over the age of 65 and greater than 20 pack year smoking history [3], although various other tumours have also been identified (◘ Table 22.1).

22.3 Pathogenesis

The pathogenesis of AMN is like many other autoimmune conditions, with genetically predisposed individuals developing antibodies to self-proteins, which in this case are expressed by the renal podocytes.

Although animal models of MN, termed Heymann nephritis, have been established for a long time, it was clear that the inciting antigen in the rodent model was not the cause of human AMN [4]. The first major advance in discovering the aetiology of AMN was the description of neonatal MN due to alloimmunisation against neutral endopeptidase (NEP) [5]. NEP-expressing babies, born to NEP-deficient mothers who had developed anti-NEP antibodies induced by an immune response to paternal NEP from a previous pregnancy, developed transient neonatal MN due to transplacental transfer of the anti-NEP IgG. However, NEP was not the autoantigen in sporadic AMN. Subsequently, the seminal paper by Beck et al. reported that 70% of patients with idiopathic MN had autoantibodies directed against phospholipase A2 receptor-1 (PLA2R) [6]. This has been confirmed by many other groups and in different ethnic populations. Next a second antigenic target was identified, thrombospondin type-1 domain-containing 7A (THSD7A) [7]. This is a less common antigenic target with antibodies against THSD7A found in approximately 5% of all AMN cases. Further additional antigens with correlating antibodies have been identified; neutral endopeptidase (NEP) [8], neural epidermal growth factor-like1 protein (NELL-1) [9], serine protease high-temperature requirement A serine peptidase 1 (HTRA1) [10], protocadherin 7 (PCDH7) [11] and semaphorin 3B (Sema3B) [12]. It is likely that further antigens may be found accounting for the remaining cases of AMN.

Table 22.1 Causes of membranous nephropathy

Autoimmune (idiopathic or primary) MN 70–80%	Serum Anti-PLA2R Antibody Histological immunostaining of renal tissue Exclusion of secondary causes
Secondary MN	
Malignancy Associated:	Thorough clinical assessment in all patients for symptoms or signs of neoplasia. Consider clinically appropriate investigations to exclude malignancy.
1. Carcinomas Lung Gastric Oesophageal Renal Prostate Breast Colon Ovary Oropharyngeal 2. Others Lymphoproliferative: Lymphomas and CLL Melanoma Mesothelioma Wilm's Tumour Schwannoma Neuroblastoma Hepatic adenoma	
Infection Associated:	Hepatitis B by far the commonest cause world-wide Hepatitis B sAg, eAg, delta, HIV, Hepatitis C, Syphilis serology, Blood film, Schistosomiasis, Hydatid and Microfilaria serology
Hepatitis B Hepatitis C HIV Syphilis Malaria Schistosomiasis Filariasis Leprosy Hydatid	
Autoimmune Associated:	Autoimmune disease usually clinically apparent but following tests appropriate on all patients with MN, Anti-nuclear antibody, complement (C_3/C_4), ENA screen, dsDNA, Rheumatoid factor, Thyroid function tests and anti-thyroid antibodies
Systemic Lupus Erythematosus Rheumatoid Arthritis Grave's Disease Hashimoto's Thyroiditis Sjogren's Syndrome Mixed Connective Tissue Disorder Ankylosing Spondylitis Scleroderma Myasthenia Gravis Bullous Pemphigoid Dermatomyositis Primary Biliary cirrhosis Guillain-Barre Syndrome	
Alloimmune Associated:	
Transplant glomerulopathy/*de novo* MN	Donor specific antibodies
Graft vs Host Disease	

Anti-PLA2R antibody levels correlate with disease activity and with response to treatment [13]. Testing for anti-PLA2R antibody has now become routine in many hospitals and can be measured serially. Utilised in this way, it can be used to guide treatment duration. PLA2R1 is expressed by podocytes, but it is not yet clear how the immune response develops against podocyte PLA2R1. Renal tissue anti-PLA2R immunostaining can predate serological detection of the anti-PLA2R antibody, suggesting that renal binding occurs first, with subsequent overspill of anti-PLA2R antibody into the circulation. This may also explain some cases of anti-PLA2R antibody negativity in patients with AMN. Podocytes are targeted by the anti-PLA2R antibodies and injured through complement activation, via the classical and lectin pathways.

The genetic basis of AMN was demonstrated by a genome-wide association study using three European populations [14]. The genetic regions associated with disease encoded *PLA2R1* on chromosome 2 and genes in the human leucocyte antigen locus on chromosome 6, specifically, *HLA-DQA1*. These regions and nearby genes have been replicated as susceptibility markers in other ethnicities. The strength of the association was greatest with *HLA-DQA1* with an odds ratio of 20.2; however, if both variants (*HLA-DQA1* and *PLA2R1*) were present, the odds ratio increased to 78.5. To date there is no research to demonstrate the direct causation with these variants.

22.4 Clinical Features

The most common presenting feature of MN is nephrotic range proteinuria, found in 80% of patients, while the remainder has non-nephrotic range proteinuria [15]. Renal impairment is unusual at presentation, and if present other causes of acute kidney injury should be excluded. Microscopic haematuria can be present in 45% of cases, but red cell casts are rare unless associated with other renal pathology such as lupus nephritis or anti-GBM disease. Hypertension can be present due to severe salt and fluid retention. Patients may have features suggestive of a secondary cause such as symptoms and signs of underlying malignancy, SLE, rheumatoid arthritis or an infective disease (see ◘ Table 22.1). For MN associated with malignancy, the two conditions are usually identified within 12 months of each other with 80% of malignancies being present before or at time of the diagnosis of nephrotic syndrome.

22

The risk of thromboembolic disease is highest in MN compared to all other causes of nephrotic syndrome [16] and greatest for AMN. Both arterial and venous thromboembolism are more common, with the risk greatest in the first 6 months of diagnosis and correlation with serum albumin levels, being greatest in those with albumin levels below 28 g/L [17]. The published rates vary, but approximately 20% of patients will have a deep vein thrombosis, 11% pulmonary embolism and 35% renal vein thrombosis [18].

22.5 Histopathology

MN is a discrete pathological entity (◘ Fig. 22.1) which can only be identified by renal biopsy and histological analysis including electron microscopy. The glomerular capillary wall is expanded, but the cellularity of the glomerulus is not typically increased (◘ Fig. 22.1a). Immune deposits including IgG and complement are found in a granular distribution along the glomerular capillary wall (◘ Fig. 22.1b). Anti-PLA2R antibody immunostaining has the same pattern as the immune deposits and is present in up to 70% of all AMN patients. Anti-PLA2R immunostaining is more sensitive than antibody titres and can be utilised to assist differentiation between primary and secondary MN [19]. THSD7A immunohistochemistry has also very recently proven to be of clinically significant use in identifying a subset of AMN [20] (◘ Fig. 22.1c). Electron microscopy shows electron dense deposits in the sup-epithelial space adjacent to the foot processes of the podocytes (◘ Fig. 22.1d), (see also separate chapter on podocytopathies).

22.6 Remission

AMN has a variable natural history, with around a third of patients undergoing spontaneous remission and having an excellent long-term prognosis, a third remaining stable with ongoing proteinuria but the final third experiencing progressive deterioration of excretory renal function and developing advanced chronic kidney disease with all its associated morbidity and mortality. Spontaneous remission can occur even in those heavily nephrotic (>12 g per day of proteinuria) and can take over 2 years to occur [21]. Greater use of anti-PLA2R antibody testing may influence our understanding of likelihood of spontaneous remissions in different groups and allow better patient stratification. There is a clear prognostic advantage of inducing either a partial or complete remission with improved long-term renal outcome. Complete remission has the added advantage of reducing the risk of relapse and improved patient survival.

The difficulty with the critical assessment and comparison of studies in MN has been that different studies utilise different criteria for remission. Remission criteria that are now considered standard practice are as follows [22]:

- Complete remission: proteinuria <0.3 g per day with a stable glomerular filtration rate (GFR)
- Partial remission: >50% reduction in proteinuria and total proteinuria <3.5 g per day with stable GFR

22.7 Management

22.7.1 Non-immunosuppressive Treatment

General supportive treatment, as for all other causes of nephrotic syndrome, should be given. This includes dietary salt restriction, renin-angiotensin system blockade (even in the absence of hypertension), blood pressure management if hypertensive, cholesterol lowering therapy, diuretics for oedema control and smoking avoidance. Prophylactic anticoagulation is administered in most UK renal units in patients with severe hypoalbuminaemia (at or below 2.5 g/dL or 25 g/L). Secondary causes of MN should be screened for, and the underlying condition should be treated. It is also important to consider vaccination against encapsulated bacteria and consideration of antibiotic prophylaxis in those with persistent hypogammaglobulinaemia and documented infectious episodes. This treatment should be used in both AMN and secondary MN.

22.7.2 Risk Stratification

The most useful way to tailor treatment is based on the patients' risk category for renal progression or complications. The classification of risk still used is the historical model from 1997 [23]. Interestingly, recent research has

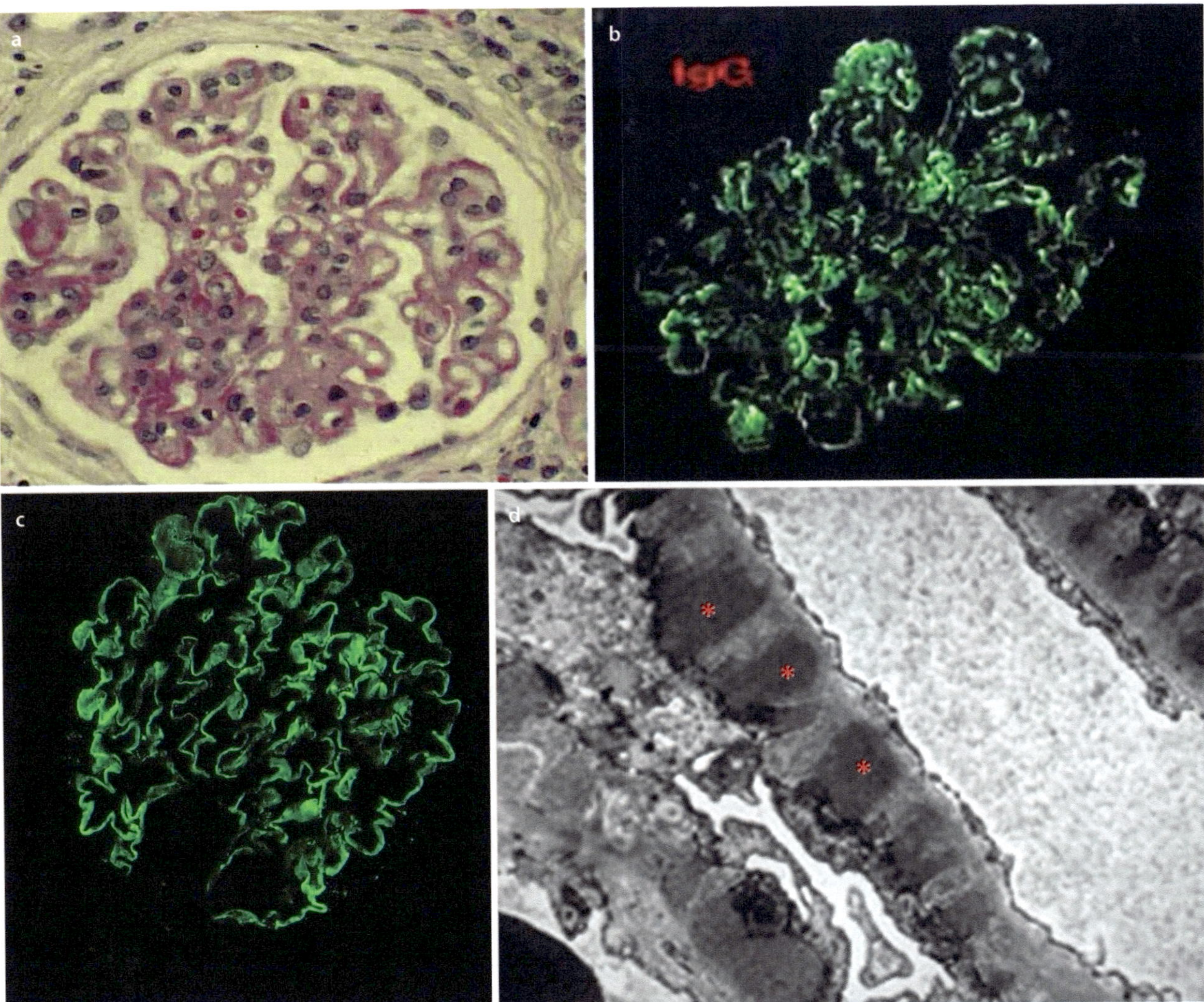

Fig. 22.1 Renal biopsy appearances of membranous nephropathy. (**a**) Light microscopy (haematoxylin and eosin stain). (**b**) Immunofluorescence, in this case for IgG but similar appearances typically seen for C3 and anti-PLA2R. (**c**) Global granular capillary wall staining for THSD7A by immunofluorescence. (Courtesy of Dr Shree Sharma, Arkana Laboratories, USA). (**d**) Electron microscopy: electron dense deposits are shown by asterisks *

demonstrated that risk criteria have not changed significantly [22]. The most recent addition to risk stratification has been anti-PLA2R antibody status.

22.7.2.1 Low Risk

Low-risk patients are aged less than 50 years, with normal renal function, without fibrosis on histology, with lower levels of proteinuria (less than 4 g per day) and have low serum anti-PLA2R antibody levels. For these patients, non-immunosuppressive anti-proteinuric treatment (NIAT) is recommended, in addition to the treatment measures discussed above.

22.7.2.2 Medium to High Risk

Patients with a medium to higher risk are older and have abnormal renal function with fibrosis on their histology, declining renal function, proteinuria (greater than 8 g per day) or persistent proteinuria greater than 4 g per day after 6 months of treatment and/or severe symptoms or complications. These patients should be treated with NIAT, and in most instances clinicians would wait for 6 months for signs of remission, prior to initiating immunosuppressive treatment.

22.7.3 Immunosuppressive Treatment

The goal of immunosuppression is to induce remission, but immunosuppressive treatment is not without risk, and patients should be counselled about the risks and benefits so they can make an informed decision. The gold-standard regimen for treatment of AMN remains the KDIGO guidelines due to a lack of an alternative proven superior regime [24]; see links for clinical trials below.

The KDIGO guidelines advocate use of the 'Ponticelli regimen' for high-risk patients. This comprises a 6-month course of treatment alternating 30-day cycles starting with intravenous methylprednisolone (1 g) daily for 3 days followed by oral prednisolone (0.5 mg/kg/day) for the remainder of the month. In the second month, patients receive an alkylating agent (either cyclophosphamide 0.5 mg/kg/day or chlorambucil 0.15–0.2 mg/kg/day) orally and then repeat the cycle by returning to the steroid regimen.

Alternative regimes exist, such as the 'modified restrictive Ponticelli' regimen that is more practical and continuous with an option of excluding the intravenous methylprednisolone thereby making it easier to administer orally and exclusively at home. Prednisolone is administered (1 mg/kg/day, maximum 60 mg, tapering per clinical response) with cyclophosphamide (1.5–2 mg/kg/day) for a maximum of 6 months. The risk with alkylating agents remains infections, increased risk of malignancy and infertility. Male patients should be sperm banked if possible prior to therapy and ovarian protection strategies offered to women of child bearing age.

Calcineurin inhibitors (ciclosporin 3.5–5 mg/kg/day or tacrolimus 0.05–0.075 mg/kg/day) with low-dose steroids (prednisolone 0.15 mg/kg/day) reduce proteinuria and induce remission. They should be reserved for patients who are not suitable for or fail alkylating agents. A minimum treatment duration of 6 months is advocated, and often longer treatment durations are required. It is important to the monitor therapeutic drug levels in the initial phase when starting treatment. As there is a very high risk of relapse when calcineurin inhibitors are stopped, it is recommended that they are continued for a minimum of 1 year after remission. A small decline in renal function should be expected, but more severe impairment should prompt treatment cessation.

There is no evidence that steroids alone, or mycophenolate mofetil has any role in the treatment of AMN, yet they are still used in instances when neither an alkylating agent or a calcineurin inhibitor is suitable. Adrenocorticotrophic hormone therapy is hypothesised to have an additional beneficial direct action on podocytes, but clinical studies using this agent have been on small cohorts with unconvincing results [25].

Rituximab is currently of interest in AMN as a result of studies that have demonstrated efficacy; however, no studies have yet shown superiority over other treatments. Rituximab depletes B-cell lymphocytes, which are involved in disease pathogenesis through autoantibody production, antigen presentation to T cells and production of pro-inflammatory cytokines. There are different dosage regimens in use in studies – either 1 g given twice, 2 weeks apart, or 375 mg/m^2 weekly for four doses. Follow-up doses are sometimes required at 6 months, as niches of B cells can persist following rituximab therapy [26]. There is increasing evidence for the safety profile of rituximab, especially compared to alkylating agents. The recent MENTOR trial compared calcineurin inhibitors versus rituximab and demonstrated non-inferiority with a safer side effect profile [27]. However, there has not been a randomised controlled trial of cyclophosphamide versus rituximab. A recent study comparing the use of rituximab against a historical cohort of patients treated with cyclophosphamide demonstrated no difference in remission rates but a better side effect profile with rituximab. Patients in both groups were not matched as the cyclophosphamide group had higher risk disease [28]. Another comparative study of cohorts treated with rituximab compared with a separate cohort treated with cyclophosphamide demonstrated that complete immunological remission was more common in the cyclophosphamide group and that RTX was less able to induce disappearance of anti-PLA2R antibodies in those patients with higher (than 152 RU/ml) anti-PLA2R starting levels [29]. Further direct evidence is required to prove rituximab superiority to current cheaper and effective treatments. A trial directly comparing rituximab to cyclophosphamide should be informative [30].

Novel agents such as anti-CD38 monoclonal antibodies (daratumumab) or proteasome inhibitors (bortezomib) are possible alternatives as they deplete plasma cells, the producers of autoantibodies [26]. Another treatment currently being investigated in phase II trials is immunoadsorption. The extracorporeal removal of immunoglobulins including the pathogenic anti-PLA2R antibodies is proposed to prevent patients' exposure to toxic non-specific immunosuppressive treatment [31].

22.8 Recurrent and De Novo MN Following Transplantation

Recurrent AMN is found in the renal allografts with recurrence rates of 10% at 5 years and 16% at 10 years [32]. After disease recurrence, the 5-year allograft survival rate is significantly reduced to 59% [32]. Anti-PLA2R antibodies were not routinely measured until recently, and so the current paradigm is that antibody titres should be undetectable at the time of transplantation, to avoid the risk of disease recurrence. De novo AMN in a transplanted kidney is apparent in up to 2% of all transplants. The reason for this is not clear but may be associated with donor-specific antibodies (HLA or non-HLA).

22.9 AMN and Other Autoimmune Diseases

AMN may be found in association with other autoimmune conditions such as anti-GBM disease, ANCA-associated vasculitis, thyroid disease and of course SLE.

22.10 Summary

MN is a common cause of nephrotic syndrome in adults and associated with significant morbidity. Distinguishing AMN from secondary MN is critical, and anti-PLA2R antibodies and PLA2R histology immunostaining help identify AMN. Meaningful clinical studies are required to determine best and safest treatment strategies to prevent side effects from toxic treatment as well as improving outcomes to reduce rates of end stage kidney disease.

Case Study

Case 1

A 53-year-old man was diagnosed with AMN and treated successfully with tacrolimus for 1.5 years which induced a complete remission. Twelve months later he presented with increasing oedema and was found to have declining renal function, microscopic haematuria and proteinuria. Repeat renal biopsy showed a crescentic glomerulonephritis, with linear IgG staining on immunohistochemistry. Serology subsequently revealed positive anti-GBM antibodies, with a titre of 150 IU/ml (NR < 15).

Case 2

A 60-year-old man presented with nephrotic syndrome, but normal renal function and renal biopsy confirmed AMN. His anti-PLA2R antibodies were strongly positive with a titre of 120 IU/ml. He was treated with losartan and simvastatin, and after six months without any signs of remission, he was started on tacrolimus, which induced a partial remission. However, following withdrawal of therapy 1 year later, he relapsed and was treated with rituximab. This induced a remission and reduction in anti-PLA2R antibody titre, to 60 IU/ml. Following a second course of rituximab, his anti-PLA2R antibodies became negative, and he entered a complete remission.

Case 3

A 52-year-old man presented to the accident and emergency department short of breath and tachycardic. He was found to have bilateral pulmonary emboli on CT chest. He was treated with low-molecular-weight heparin. Investigations revealed low serum albumin at 21 g/L, proteinuria with a urinary protein creatinine ratio of 890 mg/mmol and preserved renal function with a creatinine of 90 mcmol/l. As he was anticoagulated for his pulmonary emboli, a PLA2R antibody was sent (which was subsequently found to be negative) and was started on tacrolimus. He was screened for possible malignancies with a CT scan of chest, abdomen and pelvis, PSA and faecal occult blood screen. He entered disease remission, and following 2 years of treatment had his tacrolimus tapered successfully.

22.11 Seminal Papers

1. Beck LH, et al. M-type phospholipase A2 receptor as target antigen in idiopathic membranous nephropathy. *N Engl J Med.* 2009;361:11–21.
2. Tomas NM, et al. Thrombospondin type-1 domain-containing 7A in idiopathic membranous nephropathy. *N Engl J Med.* 2014;371:2277–87.
3. Stanescu HC, et al. Risk HLA-DQA1 and PLA2R1 alleles in idiopathic membranous nephropathy. *N Engl J Med.* 2011;364:616–26.
4. van de Logt A-E, et al. Immunological remission in PLA2R-antibody–associated membranous nephropathy: cyclophosphamide versus rituximab. *Kidney Int.* 2018;93:1016–1017.

Tips and Tricks

- Biopsy is important in differentiating causes of nephrotic syndrome, for which treatment may vary considerably.
- Negative anti-PLA2R antibodies do not exclude the diagnosis of membranous GN.
- Remember to consider other diagnoses alongside membranous GN in those with renal impairment, such as anti-GBM disease or ANCA-associated vasculitis.

Chapter Review Questions

1. Can SLE patients with a class V lupus nephritis have positive anti-PLA2R antibodies? (Yes, in 5% there appear to be positive antibodies.)
2. Should anticoagulation be used in all heavily nephrotic patients? (Risk is greatest with MN and should be guided by serum albumin, which if <25 g/L should be initiated.)
3. If renal function deteriorates in an AMN patient, is this always due to progression of CKD? (No, secondary crescentic changes may occur and may require additional therapies.)

References

1. McGrogan A, Franssen CFM, de Vries CS. The incidence of primary glomerulonephritis worldwide: a systematic review of the literature. Nephrol Dial Transplant. 2011;26(2):414–30.
2. Menon S, Valentini RP. Membranous nephropathy in children: clinical presentation and therapeutic approach. Pediatr Nephrol Berl Ger. 2010;25(8):1419–28.
3. Leeaphorn N, Kue-A-Pai P, Thamcharoen N, Ungprasert P, Stokes MB, Knight EL. Prevalence of cancer in membranous nephropathy: a systematic review and meta-analysis of observational studies. Am J Nephrol. 2014;40(1):29–35.
4. Farquhar MG, Saito A, Kerjaschki D, Orlando RA. The Heymann nephritis antigenic complex: megalin (gp330) and RAP. J Am Soc Nephrol. 1995;6(1):35–47.
5. Debiec H, Nauta J, Coulet F, van der Burg M, Guigonisy V, Schurmans T, et al. Role of truncating mutations in MME gene in fetomaternal alloimmunisation and antenatal glomerulopathies. Lancet. 2004;364(9441):1252–9.
6. Beck LH, Bonegio RGB, Lambeau G, Beck DM, Powell DW, Cummins TD, et al. M-type phospholipase A2 receptor as target antigen in idiopathic membranous nephropathy. N Engl J Med. 2009;361(1):11–21.
7. Tomas NM, Beck LH, Meyer-Schwesinger C, Seitz-Polski B, Ma H, Zahner G, et al. Thrombospondin Type-1 domain-containing 7A in idiopathic membranous nephropathy. N Engl J Med. 2014;371(24):2277–87.
8. Debiec H, Guigonis V, Mougenot B, et al. Antenatal Membranous Glomerulonephritis Due to Anti–Neutral Endopeptidase Antibodies. N Engl J Med. 2002;346(26):2053–60. https://doi.org/10.1056/NEJMoa012895.
9. Sethi S, Debiec H, Madden B, et al. Neural epidermal growth factor-like1 protein (NELL-1) associated membranous nephropathy. Kidney Int. Published online October 7, 2019. https://doi.org/10.1016/j.kint.2019.09.014.
10. Al-Rabadi LF, Caza T, Trivin-Avillach C, et al. Serine Protease HTRA1 as a Novel Target Antigen in Primary Membranous Nephropathy. J Am Soc Nephrol. 2021;32(7):1666–81. https://doi.org/10.1681/ASN.2020101395.
11. Sethi S, Madden B, Debiec H, et al. Protocadherin 7–Associated Membranous Nephropathy. J Am Soc Nephrol. 2021;32(5):1249–61. https://doi.org/10.1681/ASN.2020081165.
12. Sethi S, Debiec H, Madden B, et al. Semaphorin 3B–associated membranous nephropathy is a distinct type of disease predominantly present in pediatric patients. Kidney Int. 2020;98(5):1253–64. https://doi.org/10.1016/j.kint.2020.05.030.
13. Hoxha E, Thiele I, Zahner G, Panzer U, Harendza S, Stahl RAK. Phospholipase A2 receptor autoantibodies and clinical outcome in patients with primary membranous nephropathy. J Am Soc Nephrol. 2014;ASN.2013040430.
14. Stanescu HC, Arcos-Burgos M, Medlar A, Bockenhauer D, Kottgen A, Dragomirescu L, et al. Risk HLA-DQA1 and PLA2R1 alleles in idiopathic membranous nephropathy. N Engl J Med. 2011;364(7):616–26.
15. Glassock RJ. Diagnosis and natural course of membranous nephropathy. Semin Nephrol. 2003;23(4):324–32.
16. Kerlin BA, Ayoob R, Smoyer WE. Epidemiology and pathophysiology of nephrotic syndrome–associated thromboembolic disease. Clin J Am Soc Nephrol. 2012;7(3):513–20.
17. Lionaki S, Derebail VK, Hogan SL, Barbour S, Lee T, Hladunewich M, et al. Venous thromboembolism in patients with membranous nephropathy. Clin J Am Soc Nephrol. 2012;7(1):43–51.
18. Nickolas TL, Radhakrishnan J, Appel GB. Hyperlipidemia and thrombotic complications in patients with membranous nephropathy. Semin Nephrol. 2003;23(4):406–11.
19. Svobodova B, Honsova E, Ronco P, Tesar V, Debiec H. Kidney biopsy is a sensitive tool for retrospective diagnosis of PLA2R-related membranous nephropathy. Nephrol Dial Transplant. 2013;28(7):1839–44.
20. Sharma SG, Larsen CP. Tissue staining for THSD7A in glomeruli correlates with serum antibodies in primary membranous nephropathy: a clinicopathological study. Mod Pathol. 2018;31(4):616–22.

21. Polanco N, Gutiérrez E, Covarsí A, Ariza F, Carreño A, Vigil A, et al. Spontaneous remission of nephrotic syndrome in idiopathic membranous nephropathy. J Am Soc Nephrol. 2010;21(4):697–704.
22. Thompson A, Cattran DC, Blank M, Nachman PH. Complete and partial remission as surrogate end points in membranous nephropathy. J Am Soc Nephrol. 2015;ASN.2015010091.
23. Cattran DC, Pei Y, Greenwood CM, Ponticelli C, Passerini P, Honkanen E. Validation of a predictive model of idiopathic membranous nephropathy: its clinical and research implications. Kidney Int. 1997;51(3):901–7.
24. KDIGO Work Group. KDIGO clinical practice guideline for glomerulonephritis. Kidney Int Suppl. 2012;2(2):140–274.
25. Hladunewich MA, Cattran D, Beck LH, Odutayo A, Sethi S, Ayalon R, et al. A pilot study to determine the dose and effectiveness of adrenocorticotrophic hormone (H.P. Acthar® Gel) in nephrotic syndrome due to idiopathic membranous nephropathy. Nephrol Dial Transplant Off Publ Eur Dial Transpl Assoc Eur Ren Assoc. 2014;29(8):1570–7.
26. Barbari A. Continuing the paradigm shift in the treatment of idiopathic membranous nephropathy. Nat Rev Nephrol. 2017;13(11):720.
27. Fervenza FC, Gipson DS, Kretzler M, Radhakrishnan J, Hebert LA, Gipson PE, et al. A multi-center randomized controlled trial of rituximab versus cyclosporine in the treatment of idiopathic membranous nephropathy (MENTOR). In: High-Impact Clinical Trials [Internet]. 2017 [cited 2018 Aug 29]. Available from: https://www.asn-online.org/education/kidneyweek/2017/program-abstract.aspx?controlId=2831149.
28. van den Brand JAJG, Ruggenenti P, Chianca A, Hofstra JM, Perna A, Ruggiero B, et al. Safety of rituximab compared with steroids and cyclophosphamide for idiopathic membranous nephropathy. J Am Soc Nephrol. 2017;28(9):2729–37.
29. van de Logt A-E, Dahan K, Rousseau A, van der Molen R, Debiec H, Ronco P, et al. Immunological remission in PLA2R-antibody–associated membranous nephropathy: cyclophosphamide versus rituximab. Kidney Int. 2018;93(4):1016–7.
30. Scolari F, Ravani P. Rituximab versus steroids and cyclophosphamide in the treatment of idiopathic membranous nephropathy - full text view - ClinicalTrials.gov [Internet]. [cited 2018 Sep 11]. Available from: https://clinicaltrials.gov/ct2/show/NCT03018535.
31. Hamilton P, Kanigicherla D, Hanumapura P, Walz L, Kramer D, Fischer M, et al. Peptide GAM immunoadsorption therapy in primary membranous nephropathy (PRISM): phase II trial investigating the safety and feasibility of peptide GAM immunoadsorption in anti-PLA2R positive primary membranous nephropathy. J Clin Apheresis [Internet]. [cited 2018 Jun 1];0(0). Available from: https://onlinelibrary.wiley.com/doi/abs/10.1002/jca.21599.
32. Allen PJ, Chadban SJ, Craig JC, Lim WH, Allen RDM, Clayton PA, et al. Recurrent glomerulonephritis after kidney transplantation: risk factors and allograft outcomes. Kidney Int. 2017;92(2):461–9.

Links

KDIGO guidelines, https://kdigo.org/guidelines/gn/.

Rare Renal provides patient information for membranous nephropathy patients. http://rarerenal.org/patient-information/membranous-nephropathy-patient-information.

MENTOR trial results prepublication from the American Society of Nephrology Kidney Week. https://www.asn-online.org/education/kidneyweek/2017/program-abstract.aspx?controlId=2831149.

Membranoproliferative Glomerulonephritis and C3 Glomerulopathy

Daniel Gale and Mared Owen-Casey

Contents

M. Harber (ed.), *Primer on Nephrology*, https://doi.org/10.1007/978-3-030-76419-7_23

Key Points

1. MPGN and C3 glomerulopathy are rare diseases that usually result from systemic disorders that lead to excess antibody production (such as chronic infectious or autoimmune disease in MPGN) or complement dysregulation (such as a C3 nephritic factor or complement gene mutation in C3 glomerulopathy).
2. MPGN and C3 glomerulopathy present with proteinuria, frequently with one or more of nephrotic syndrome, haematuria and progressive renal dysfunction.
3. On immunostaining, MPGN is characterised by antibody and complement deposition in the glomerulus, whereas in C3 glomerulopathy complement C3 is deposited without significant immunoglobulins.
4. There are no therapies of proven efficacy in these disorders, although it is likely that in some cases immunosuppression is of benefit.
5. Since they usually result from systemic disorders, renal transplantation in MPGN and C3 glomerulopathy is often complicated by recurrent disease.

Learning Objectives

1. Understand how MPGN and C3G are diagnosed and classified.
2. Understand current knowledge about their aetiology and pathogenesis.
3. Understand which investigations to perform in patients diagnosed with these disorders.
4. Understand approaches to their treatment.

23.1 Introduction

The terms membranoproliferative glomerulonephritis (MPGN) and mesangiocapillary glomerulonephritis (MCGN) are interchangeable and refer to the light microscopic appearances of cellular proliferation in the mesangial regions of the glomeruli, with expansion of both cells and mesangial matrix, accompanied by thickening of the glomerular capillary walls. Rather than being a specific disease, MPGN is a morphological pattern which is associated with a wide range of distinct (and usually systemic) diseases. Recent developments in the understanding of these conditions emphasise the importance of establishing underlying disorder.

23.2 Definition and Classification: MPGN and C3 Glomerulopathy

The first description of MPGN) as a distinct histomorphological entity was in 1961 [1]. MPGN was at first subdivided purely on the basis of light microscopic morphology, but the introduction of electron microscopy and immunostaining in the 1960s led to the classical subdivision into 'type 1', 'type 2' and 'type 3' MPGN (see Table 23.1). Using this system, a diagnosis of type 2 MPGN prompted the search for complement alternative pathway dysregulation, and a diagnosis of type 1 or type 3 MPGN suggested excessive or aberrant immunoglobulin production. Although this categorisation proved clinically useful, in recent years improved understanding of the pathophysiology of MPGN has led to the move towards classifying proliferative GN according to the underlying clinicopathological process, rather than relying entirely on the morphological features seen in the kidney biopsy. This has been driven by three crucial observations: firstly, while the degree of inflammatory change (e.g. mesangial hypercellularity and crescent formation) seen on kidney biopsy is correlated with renal prognosis, histomorphological type per se is not [2]. Secondly, the morphological changes defining 'type 1' MPGN sometimes occur *without* the deposition of immunoglobulins, and in these cases, evidence of dysregulation of the complement alternative

Table 23.1 Traditional classification of membranoproliferative glomerulonephritis (MPGN) by location of electron dense deposits

MPGN type	Electron microscopic appearances	Typical immunostaining	Serum complement	Other
1	Discrete electron dense material in mesangium and *subendothelial* GBM	IgG ± IgA ± IgM + C3 + C1q	Normal ± reduced C4 and C3	Infections, autoimmune disease, cryoglobulinaemia
2	Dense transformation of GBM lamina densa	C3 only	Reduced C3, normal C4	C3NeF
3	*Subendothelial* and *subepithelial* GBM electron dense deposits	IgG ± IgA ± IgM + C3 + C1q	Normal ± reduced C4 and C3	Infections, autoimmune disease, cryoglobulinaemia

pathway is frequently present [3]. The third observation was that dense transformation of the GBM (regarded as pathognomonic of 'type 2 MPGN') is more often seen without the accompanying light microscopic changes of MPGN, leading to the unsatisfactory diagnosis of 'type 2 MPGN without MPGN' in a number of cases [4].

These considerations have led to the introduction of the term 'C3 glomerulopathy' which encompasses the disorders in which complement C3 accumulates in the kidney in the absence of significant immunoglobulin deposition there. This is the hallmark of complement alternative pathway dysregulation and represents pathophysiology, prognosis and underlying aetiology which are distinct from those cases of proliferative GN in which strong immunostaining for immunoglobulin is seen in the glomerulus, whatever the morphology may be by light or electron microscopy. Differential diagnoses suggested by biopsy appearances are summarised in ◘ Fig. 23.1, and the patterns associated with specific diseases are shown in ◘ Table 23.2.

In addition to immune-mediated proliferative glomerulonephritis and C3 glomerulopathies, light microscopic appearances resembling MPGN are sometimes seen in patients with chronic thrombotic microangiopathies (TMAs). In this situation there is no deposition of immunoglobulin or complement in the glomeruli – rather there is accumulation of electron-lucent, flocculent material (thought to be composed of fibrin and its breakdown products) beneath the endothelial cells). This can result in capillary wall thickening and other light microscopic features resembling MPGN. Electron microscopy easily distinguishes this from the dense, osmiophilic basement membrane deposits seen in immune complex GN or C3 glomerulopathies. Causes

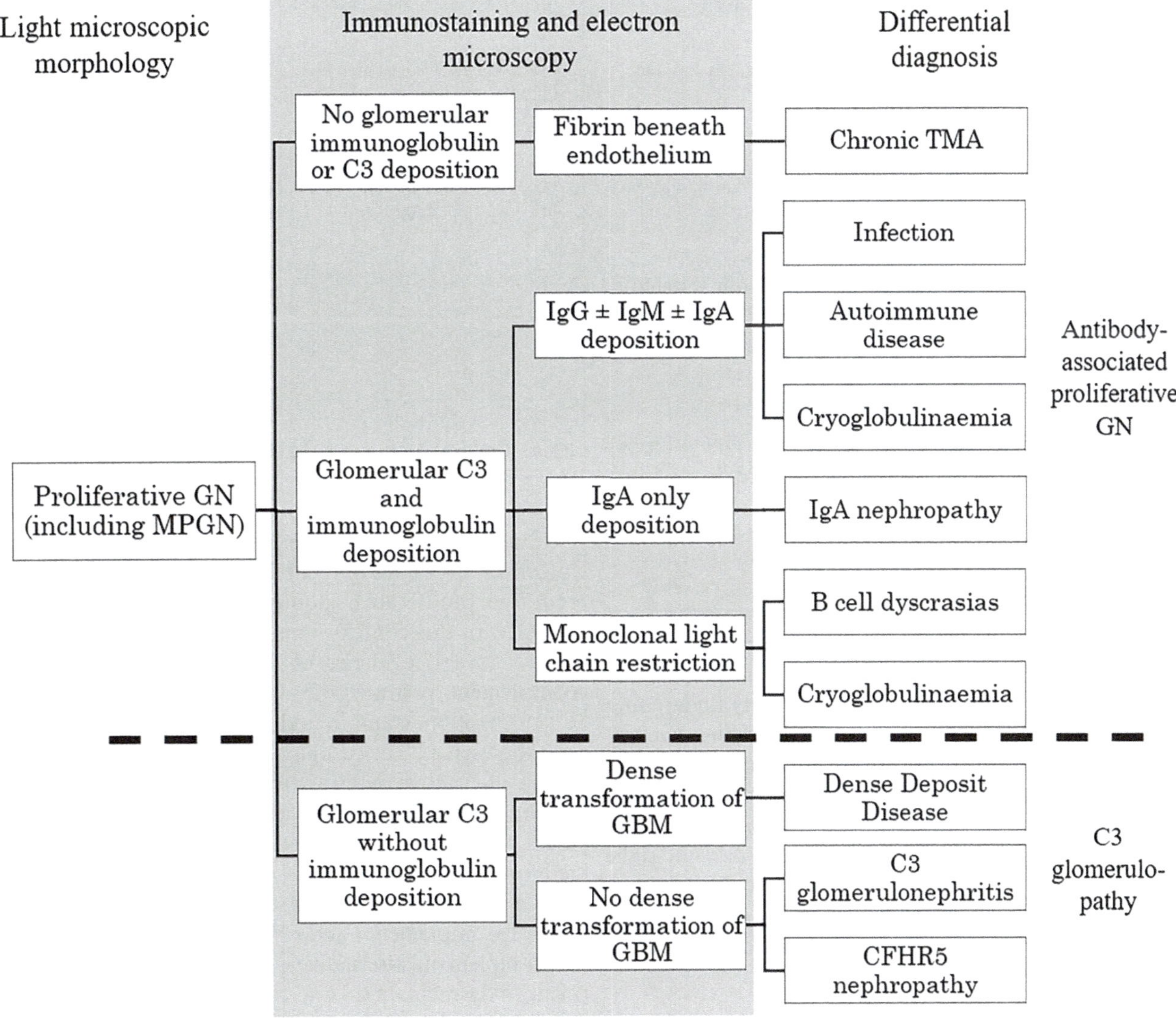

◘ **Fig. 23.1** Histological categorisation and commoner causes of proliferative glomerulonephritis (GN); GBM glomerular basement membrane, CFHR5 Complement Factor H-related 5, TMA thrombotic microangiopathy

Table 23.2 Histological characteristics of different diseases causing MPGN pattern. Diagnosis, light microscopy, immunofluorescence and electron microscopy. The term 'C3 glomerulopathy' encompasses both DDD and C3 glomerulonephritis

Immune complex membranoproliferative glomerulonephritis (IC-MPGN)	Global and diffuse mesangial proliferation and glomerular hypercellularity, doubled GBMs with mesangial interposition. The glomerulus may have a distinct lobular/nodular appearance	IgG and C3 +/– IgM on the inside of glomerular capillary walls with occasional mesangial deposits	Subendothelial deposits and occasional mesangial deposits
Acute postinfectious glomerulonephritis	Global and diffuse increase in mesangial matrix and cellularity with an infiltrate of neutrophils within capillary loops	Coarse C3 and IgG on the outside of glomerular capillary loops	Irregular and variably sized electron dense subepithelial deposits that appear as humps
Dense deposit disease (DDD)	Normal, mild or variable mesangial proliferation with thickened GBMs without spikes. Often the GBM does not stain strongly with silver and has a more characteristically brown colour with no doubling of the GBM. The main differential diagnosis to consider on H&E is membranous nephropathy	Coarse, granular C3 deposition in glomerular capillary walls, with scant or no immunoglobulins. Sometimes complement can also be seen within mesangium, Bowman's capsule and within tubular basement membranes	Intramembranous electron dense deposits often with ring-like mesangial deposits and corresponding deposits within Bowman's capsule and tubular basement membranes
C3 glomerulonephritis (C3GN)	Variable increase in mesangial matrix and cellularity	Complement C3 deposited in GBMs and mesangium with minimal immunoglobulins	Discrete subendothelial, subepithelial and/or mesangial electron dense deposits
Cryoglobulinaemic glomerulonephritis	Global and diffuse mesangial proliferation, mesangial hypercellularity, doubled basement membranes with acellular eosinophilic material in capillary loops, possibly representing cryoprecipitate, occasionally vasculitic changes are seen in glomeruli	Intraluminal glomerular capillary IgM +/– IgG, kappa/lambda	Organised subendothelial deposits often with a recognisable substructure

of TMAs which may result in these kidney biopsy appearances are summarised in Table 23.3.

23.3 Epidemiology

The incidence of MPGN varies significantly across the world with higher rates in developing countries. MPGN is diagnosed in approximately 2% patients undergoing renal biopsy in the UK and is the underlying primary glomerulopathy in 5–10% patients with nephrotic syndrome. However, up to 29% of biopsies in countries such as Romania or Nigeria show MPGN [5, 6]. While comparisons between different countries are difficult since reporting of, indications for and access to renal biopsy can vary markedly, longitudinal data suggest that rates are falling over time [6–8] probably related to reduction in chronic infection-related MPGN.

23.4 Aetiology and Pathophysiology

Excessive or prolonged immunological stimulation and antibody production (whether as a consequence of infection, autoimmunity or blood cell dyscrasias) can result in proliferative glomerulonephritides, including MPGN. In this context, immunostaining of the kidney biopsy reveals evidence of activation of the classical complement pathway (i.e. C1q deposition) alongside C3 in the kidney and in addition to the immunoglobulins themselves. The recognition that isolated activation of the alternative pathway (see Fig. 23.2) is sufficient to cause proliferative GN with deposition of complement C3 (in the absence of immunoglobulin or C1q) reinforces the view that renal complement activation per se is sufficient to cause disease. Furthermore, abnormalities of Complement Factor H (CFH, a central regulator of complement alternative pathway activity) are sufficient to dysregulate C3 and can result in MPGN.

Table 23.3 Causes of thrombotic microangiopathy

Disease	Investigations
Thrombotic thrombocytopaenic purpura	ADAMTS13 activity <5% of normal
Haemolytic uraemic syndrome	STEC PCR; mutation screening: *CFH*, *CFI*, *C3*, *MCP (CD46)*, *CFB*
Pre-eclampsia/eclampsia	Evidence of current or very recent pregnancy
Antiphospholipid syndrome	Anti-cardiolipin antibodies, lupus anticoagulant
Accelerated hypertension	
Systemic sclerosis	ANAs: Anti-Scl-70/RNP
Systemic lupus erythematosus	ANAs: Anti-dsDNA; C3/C4
Allograft rejection	Donor-specific antibodies
Drugs (e.g. cyclosporin A, tacrolimus, gemcitabine)	
Radiation exposure	

STEC Shiga toxin-producing *E. coli*, *ANA* antinuclear antibodies, *CFH* Complement Factor H, *MCP* membrane cofactor protein, *FB* Factor B

In this paradigm, the histomorphological changes that define MPGN can be viewed as the downstream consequence of renal complement activation, which may be caused either by increased antibody production (leading to the generation of antibody-antigen complexes) or by defects in the regulation of the complement system itself. In clinical practice, determining which of these processes is driving the renal disease is crucial in determining the appropriate therapy.

23.5 Antibody-Associated Proliferative GN

Proliferative and membranoproliferative GN associated with glomerular antibody deposition can occur in a very wide range of diseases, with examples given in Table 23.4. In approximately 1/3 of patients, immune complexes are detectable in the circulation, but it is important to recognise that most people with such circulating complexes do not develop a GN. The extent to which characteristics of the antigen, immune complexes, local glomerular characteristics, variation in complement regulators or other factors determine which patients develop renal inflammation in this context is unknown (Figs. 23.3 and 23.4).

23.5.1 Clinical Features

The clinical manifestations of MPGN are varied and in part dependent on the underlying disease. However, very approximately one third of patients with MPGN present with the nephrotic syndrome. Another third present with haematuria and sub-nephrotic range proteinuria which is often detected because of symptoms related to primary pathology (such as infection or cryoglobulinaemia; see below). Of the remaining third, patients may present with chronic progressive renal impairment or less commonly with acute kidney injury. Microscopic haematuria is present in the majority of patients, some of whom also report episodes of macroscopic haematuria. High blood pressure in adults with MPGN is common and can be complicated by severe or accelerated phase hypertension. A respiratory tract infection often precedes an acute presentation.

23.5.2 Proliferative GN in Infectious Diseases

Chronic infections are known to be associated with proliferative glomerulonephritis, and, in general, the mechanism is thought to depend on generation of large amounts of antibody-antigen complexes. Although the overall risk of GN is low, some infections, such as endocarditis and viral hepatitis (with or without associated cryoglobulinaemia; see below), seem particularly prone to result in this type of renal injury: infection with *Schistosoma mansoni* is one of the commoner causes of MPGN worldwide, possibly because hepatosplenic disease diverts blood away from the Kupffer cells, allowing increased exposure of the systemic circulation (including the kidney) to the immune complexes that are generated in response to the infection.

Occasionally, glomerular inflammation is seen several days after an acute bacterial (typically streptococcal) infection. In this postinfectious glomerulonephritis, presentation is typically with haematuria, proteinuria (sometimes in the nephrotic range) and renal impairment, with or without oliguria, some 7–14 days following a bacterial infection. The disease is usually self-limiting, although supportive renal replacement therapy may be needed in some cases. Serological tests for antibodies against bacterial antigens such as streptolysin O and DNase B may be positive, and hypocomplementaemia

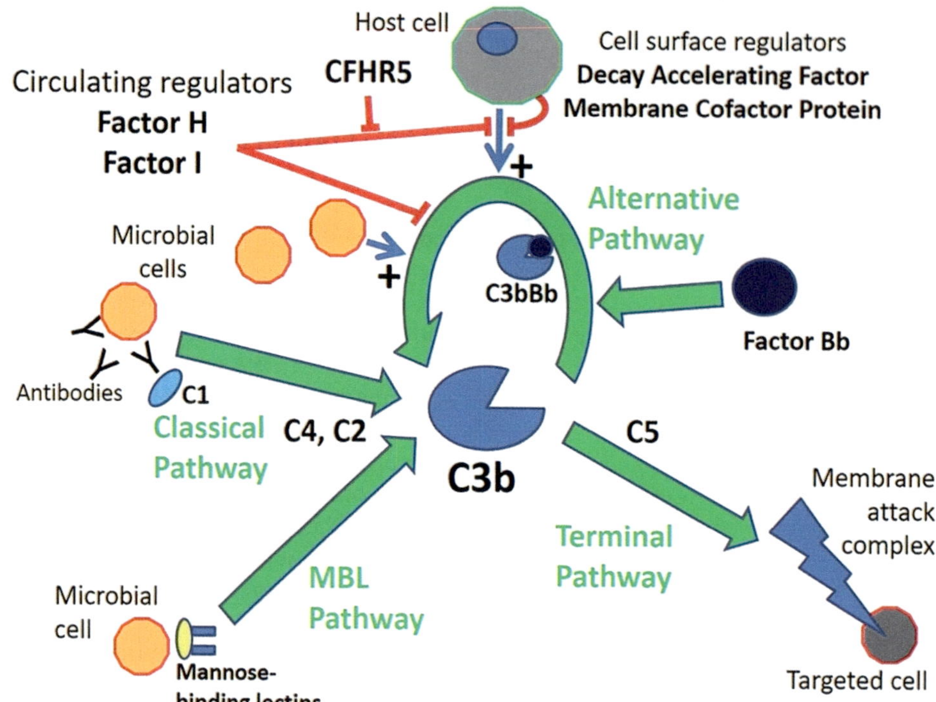

Fig. 23.2 The complement system
The complement system is a cascade of circulating proteases which plays a pivotal role in defence against infection. In humans, complement has a number of functions, including innate recognition and destruction of invading micro-organisms; opsonisation (labelling of foreign material for phagocytosis); activation of cellular immunity; and as an effector system for the destruction of antibody-coated micro-organisms. Complement therefore bridges innate and adaptive mechanisms of immune defence. Activation of complement occurs via three pathways, termed the classical, mannose-binding lectin (MBL) and alternative (AP) pathways. All result in the cleavage of the abundant circulating protein C3 to form the active C3b.
The Classical Pathway
Antibody-antigen complexes are recognised by the circulating proteins C1q, r and s to form the C1qrs complex which recruits and cleaves the circulating complement proteins C4 and C2 (releasing the small C4a anaphylatoxin fragment that causes enhanced vascular permeability, histamine release and recruitment of immune cells) to result in the C4b2a complex bound to the cell surface. C4b2a is a C3 convertase which is able to cleave C3 to form C3a (an anaphylatoxin) and the active C3b.
The Mannose-Binding Lectin (MBL) Pathway
Mannose groups on bacterial cell surfaces are recognised by circulating mannose-binding lectin (MBL) proteins which bind to form a complex which, similar to the C1qrs complex, is able to recruit and cleave C4 and C2, producing the C4b2a C3 convertase.
The Alternative Pathway (AP)
C3b is continuously generated by low-grade cleavage of the abundant plasma protein C3 by water hydrolysis – a process known as AP tickover. In the alternative pathway, C3b binds Factor B which is cleaved by factor D to result in the non-covalently bound C3bBb complex – a C3 convertase that is able to catalyse the cleavage of C3 to form more C3b. This completes a positive feedback loop which amplifies generation of C3b and which is further amplified by the presence of an appropriate biological surface (such as a cell membrane). In addition to catalysing C3 cleavage, the C3b also acts as an opsonin (labelling the cell to which it is bound for phagocytosis) and forms part of the complex which cleaves circulating C5 to activate the terminal complement pathway.
The Terminal Pathway
The binding of C3b to either of the C3 convertases (C4b2a or C3bBb) produces a C5 convertase which catalyses the cleavage of the circulating protein C5 to release C5a (an anaphylatoxin) and C5b which initiates the terminal pathway, leading to the recruitment of the tubular membrane attack complex (MAC) which lyses the cell by forming a pore (composed of C6–9) in its surface.
Alternative Pathway Regulation
In order to prevent runaway activation of its positive feedback loop, the AP requires tight regulation. This is achieved in by a number of mechanisms, including cleavage of C3b and acceleration of decay of the C3bBb complex, and effected by a range of regulators, including Factor I and Factor H, which prevent over-activation of the pathway both in the circulation and at host surfaces. The *Complement Factor H (CFH)* gene is situated immediately upstream from its 5 homologues, the *CFH-related* genes 1–5. The proteins encoded by these genes (FHR1–5) are also present in the circulation (although are much less abundant than Factor H), and some have complement deregulating activity.

is common. However, because some bacterial antigens (or antibodies directed against them) may stabilise the alternative pathway C3 convertase, low serum C3 is not always accompanied by low serum C4 in this condition.

Kidney biopsy typically shows diffuse proliferation of mesangial cells with prominent neutrophil infiltration and large, hump-like deposits on the subepithelial side of the GBM on electron microscopy. Glomerular immunostaining is usually positive for IgG, IgM, C1q and C3 although occasionally immunostain positivity for C3 alone is seen. The pathophysiology of postinfectious glomerulonephritis is not completely understood,

Table 23.4 Causes of immune complex proliferative glomerulonephritis

Disease category	Examples	Additional investigation(s)
Chronic infections	Viral – Hepatitis B, hepatitis C, HIV ± cryoglobulinaemia type 2	Viral serology; RF; cryoglobulins; C3/C4
	Bacterial – Endocarditis, infected shunt or prosthesis, abscess	Blood cultures; imaging; transoesophageal echo
	Protozoal – Malaria, schistosomiasis	Blood film; serology
	Other – Mycoplasma, mycobacterial	Cultures; imaging
Autoimmune diseases	Systemic lupus erythematosus (SLE)	ANAs: Anti-dsDNA; C3/C4
	Sjögren's syndrome ± cryoglobulinaemia	ANAs: Anti-Ro/La
	Rheumatoid arthritis	Rheumatoid factor (RF)
	Scleroderma	ANAs: Anti-Scl-70/RNP
	Coeliac disease	Endoscopy; anti-endomysial abs
Paraprotein deposition diseases	Cryoglobulinaemia type 1	Serum protein electrophoresis; serum free light chain assay/immunofixation; bone marrow biopsy; imaging
	Waldenström's macroglobulinaemia	
	Immunotactoid glomerulopathy	
	Lymphoproliferative disease	
	Leukaemia	
	Malignant neoplasms	
Inherited complement deficiency	C2 deficiency leading to bacterial infections and SLE	CH_{50}, C3/C4
Chronic liver disease	Cirrhosis and alpha1-antitrypsin deficiency	Liver biopsy, A1AT levels
Renal allograft rejection		Donor-specific antibodies
Unknown (formerly 'idiopathic')	Fibrillary glomerulonephritis	

ANA Antinuclear antibodies, *RF* rheumatoid factor, CH_{50} complement haemolytic activity

but it has been postulated that some bacterial antigens become deposited in the GBM, perhaps as a consequence of their physico-chemical properties, and it is the aggressive immunological response to these antigens, including local complement activation, which causes the renal inflammation.

23.5.3 Cryoglobulinaemic GN

Cryoglobulins are immunoglobulins which reversibly precipitate at a temperature of 4 °C. Cryoglobulinaemia is subdivided into three types, based on clonality (see Table 23.5): type 1 arises as a result of an aberrant, usually IgM-producing, plasma cell clone (e.g. in multiple myeloma or Waldenstrom's macroglobulinaemia). Type 2 comprises monoclonal (usually IgM) bound to polyclonal (usually IgG) immunoglobulins and is most commonly found in people with serological evidence of hepatitis C virus infection and/or lymphoproliferative disorders. In type 3 cryoglobulinaemia, there is a complex of polyclonal immunoglobulins and can also be seen in the context of hepatitis C infection, other infections, autoimmune disorders and paraneoplastic syndromes. In type 2 and type 3 cryoglobulinaemia (collectively referred to as mixed cryoglobulinaemias), tests for rheumatoid factor are positive, since the IgM antibody (whether monoclonal or polyclonal) binds to the Fc region of IgG.

The association of cryoglobulins with viral infections is well-recognised, with detectable mixed cryoglobulinaemia reported in 15–20% of people infected with HIV and as many as 50% of those infected with hepatitis C (HCV) [9, 10]. In addition to lymphoprolif-

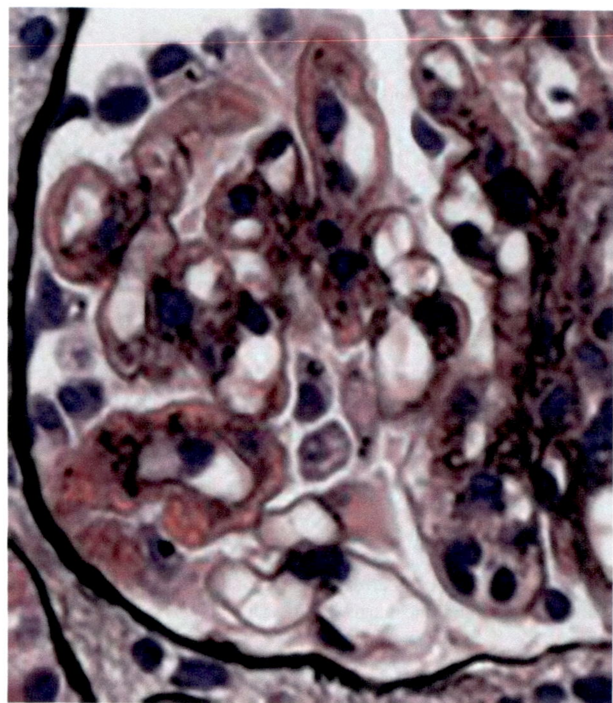

Fig. 23.3 Subendothelial membranoproliferative glomerulonephritis – silver
Part of a glomerulus at high magnification showing doubled basement membranes on silver staining with mesangial interposition, subendothelial immune deposits and increase in mesangial matrix

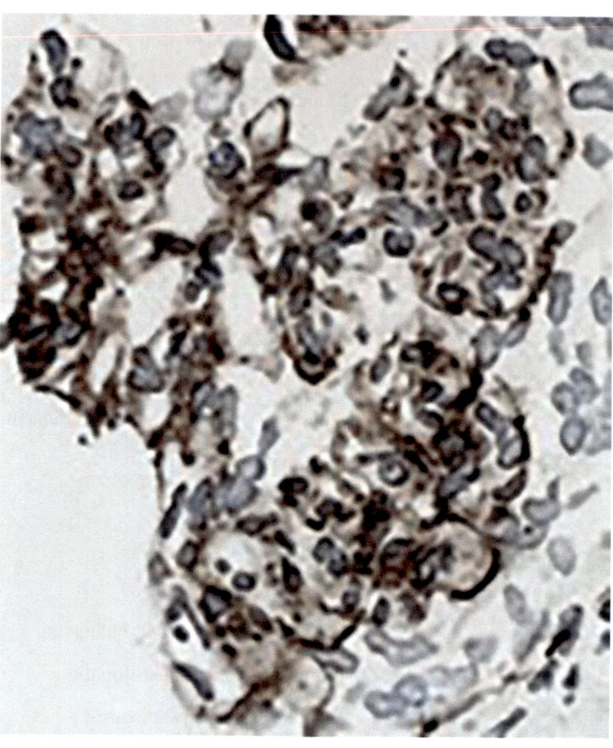

Fig. 23.4 Subendothelial membranoproliferative glomerulonephritis – C9
Immunoperoxidase method to detect C9 (complement component C9 is in the same distribution as C3 but is technically easier to detect than C3 in immunoperoxidase method) shows heavy, granular deposition along the inside of glomerular capillary loops. Similar deposits would be seen with IgG

Table 23.5 Types of cryoglobulinaemia. Rheumatoid factor, RF

	Clonality	Associations
Type 1	Monoclonal (usually IgM)	Multiple myeloma, Waldenstrom's macroglobulinaemia
Type 2	Monoclonal IgM bound to polyclonal IgG	Hepatitis C, lymphoproliferative disordershepatitis C, HIV, other infections, autoimmune diseases, cancers
Type 3	Polyclonal IgM bound to polyclonal IgG	

erative and infectious diseases, cryoglobulinaemia may sometimes occur in the context of autoimmune diseases, with approximately 45% HCV negative cases of mixed cryoglobulinaemia in one series occurring in patients with Sjögren's syndrome [11]. Clinically significant cryoglobulinaemic disease, however, is only apparent in a proportion of patients in whom a cryoglobulin is detectable serologically.

Cryoglobulins may precipitate anywhere in the body, leading to local complement activation and thrombus formation. Clinically this may manifest as Meltzer's classic triad of palpable purpura, joint pain and muscle weakness, but other manifestations, including neuropathy, may be present. Renal involvement in cryoglobulinaemia usually presents with proteinuria, microscopic haematuria and renal impairment. Nephrotic syndrome is seen in approximately 20% patients, and around one third of patients have concurrent extra-renal disease at time of presentation. Importantly, over half the patients with HCV-related cryoglobulinaemic MPGN have normal or near normal liver function tests at presentation. Consumption of complement components resulting in reduced plasma levels of C4 and sometimes C3 is frequently seen in active cryoglobulinaemic disease making levels of C3 and C4 excellent screening tests for cryoglobulinaemia. In addition, CH_{50}[1] and C1q levels may also be reduced, again reflecting classical complement pathway activation.

Kidney biopsy in cryoglobulinaemic GN can show typical features of MPGN, but there may also be prominent glomerular hypercellularity with massive infiltra-

1 Complement haemolytic activity: patient serum across a range of dilutions is used to lyse antibody-coated sheep erythrocytes. Lack of haemolysis at a given dilution suggests deficiency of complement component(s).

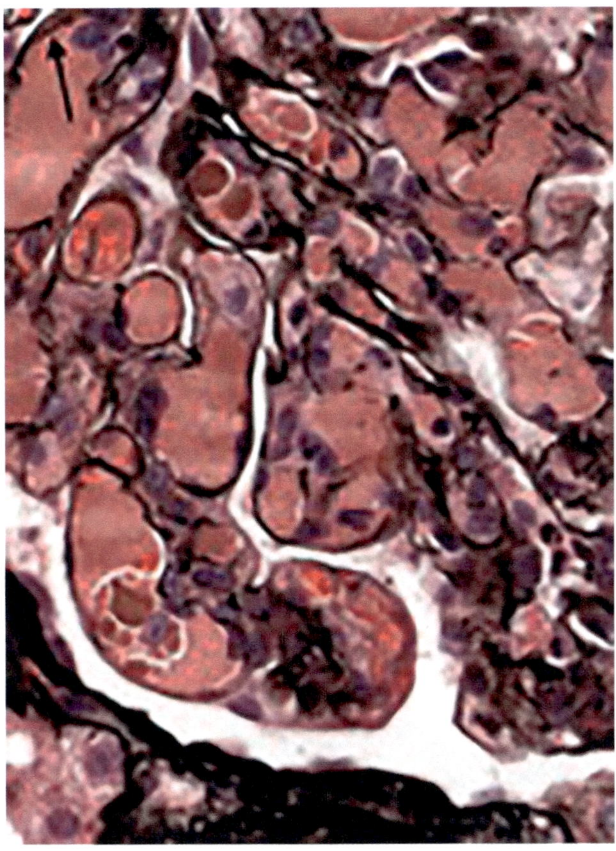

Fig. 23.5 Cryoglobulinaemic glomerulonephritis – silver Glomerulus from the renal biopsy specimen of a patient with cryoglobulinaemic glomerulonephritis showing eosinophilic, acellular deposits within the majority of capillary loops and occasional doubled basement membranes, arrowed

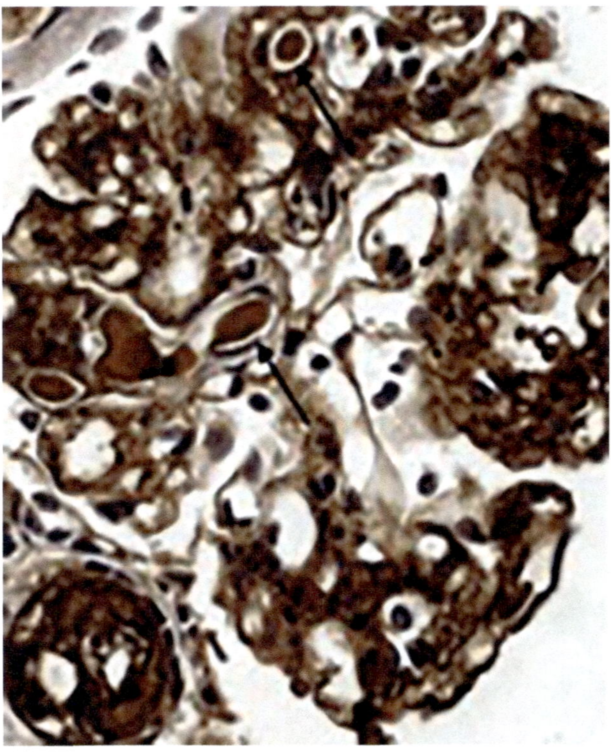

Fig. 23.6 Cryoglobulinaemic glomerulonephritis – IgM Immunoperoxidase method to detect IgM shows aggregates of IgM in several capillary loops

tion of macrophages or accumulation of eosinophilic material in intraluminal thrombi which probably represent cryoprecipitate within the glomerular capillaries (Figs. 23.5 and 23.6). In approximately one third of patients, there is also associated small- and medium-sized vessel vasculitis [12]. Cryoglobulinaemic MPGN is usually rather indolent, and progression to end-stage renal disease is seen in around 10% of patients, usually over 10 years or more although often accompanied by severe hypertension. Therapy is usually aimed at treating the underlying cause, for example, by clearing hepatitis C virus infection or suppressing any clonal haematological disorder.

23.5.4 Autoimmune Disease and Proliferative GN

Renal involvement is seen in a variety of systemic autoimmune diseases in which there are circulating antibody-autoantigen complexes. While glomerular changes of MPGN may be present, more commonly proliferation is confined to the either the mesangial regions or the capillaries of the glomerular tuft. In this context, positive immunostaining for IgA (but not other immunoglobulins) is diagnostic of IgA nephropathy, and immunostaining for IgA, IgG and IgM is compatible with lupus nephritis (Figs. 23.7 and 23.8). Occasionally, proliferative glomerulonephritis with staining for IgM but not IgA or IgG is seen, and this is sometimes termed IgM nephropathy, although clinical data in this condition are lacking, presumably due to its rarity. In all of these proliferative glomerulonephritides, immunostaining for C1q and C3 is typically positive, reflecting complement activation via the classical pathway.

23.5.5 Treatment of Immune Complex-Associated Glomerulonephritis

Renal prognosis in proliferative GN is ultimately dependent on the course of the underlying disease process responsible. While blood pressure control and angiotensin blockade may delay progressive renal scarring in the presence of hypertension and/or proteinuria from a variety of causes, identification and treatment of any underlying lymphoproliferative, infective or autoimmune

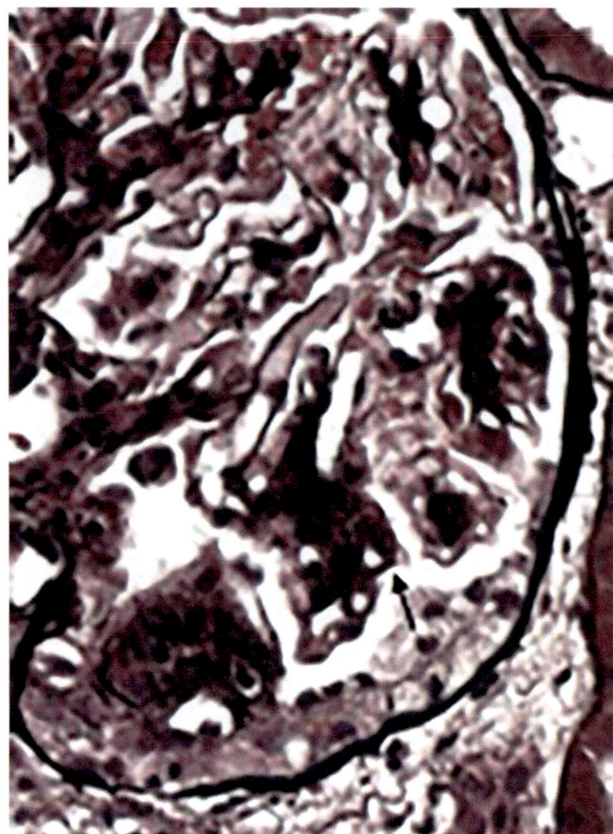

Fig. 23.7 Lupus nephritis – silver
Glomerulus showing features of lupus nephritis seen as a subendothelial membranoproliferative pattern with mesangial increase and occasional doubled basement membranes, arrowed

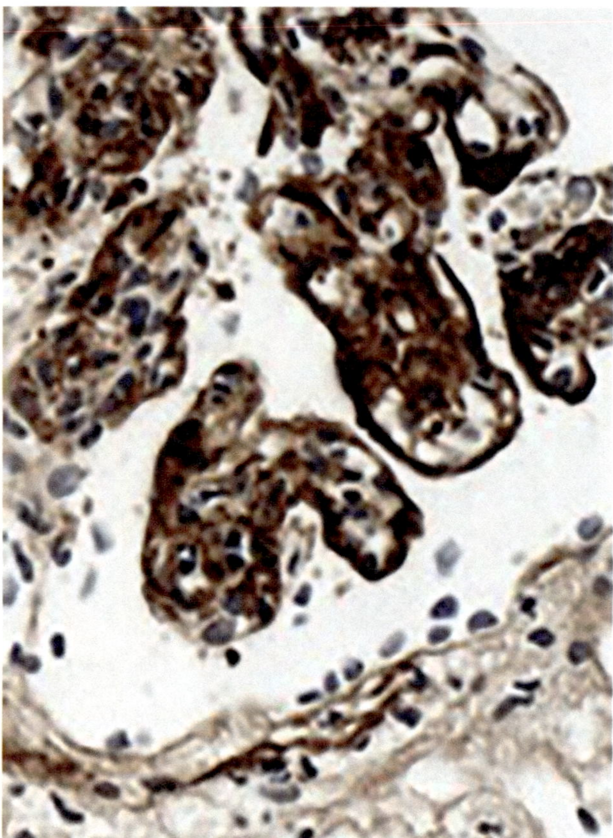

Fig. 23.8 Lupus nephritis – C9
Immunoperoxidase method to detect C9 shows heavy deposition within mesangium and glomerular basement membranes. Similar deposition of IgG, IgM and IgA would also be seen

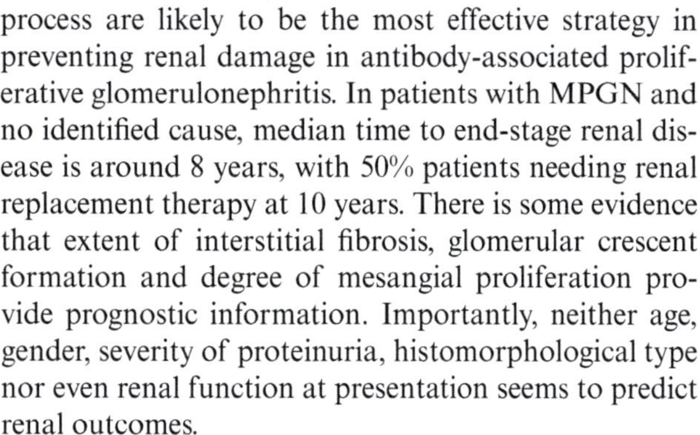

process are likely to be the most effective strategy in preventing renal damage in antibody-associated proliferative glomerulonephritis. In patients with MPGN and no identified cause, median time to end-stage renal disease is around 8 years, with 50% patients needing renal replacement therapy at 10 years. There is some evidence that extent of interstitial fibrosis, glomerular crescent formation and degree of mesangial proliferation provide prognostic information. Importantly, neither age, gender, severity of proteinuria, histomorphological type nor even renal function at presentation seems to predict renal outcomes.

The evidence base for any treatment in MPGN where a cause is not identified is extremely limited in part because of its rarity and partly because most studies failed to differentiate between the underlying diseases causing the MPGN [13]. Alternate day corticosteroids have been advocated on the basis of small observational studies. One of the few randomised controlled trials (RCTs) investigated the use of steroids in children with MPGN type 1 and showed some evidence of a beneficial effect of alternate day prednisolone (40 mg/m^2) in those with heavy proteinuria and good function (61% had stable function vs 12% of controls) leading to the recommendation that steroids should be tried in this group [14]. However, there have been no subsequent RCTs. In the 1980s antiplatelet agents in the form of aspirin and dipyridamole were thought to be beneficial, but this has not been supported by clinical trials and has not gained widespread acceptance. Antiproliferative agents have been reported to have some success in small observational studies with limited follow-up but have never been tested in RCTs. In the face of this paucity of data, the KDIGO guidelines suggest that in idiopathic MPGN in the context of frank nephrotic syndrome and declining function, it is reasonable to give a trial of corticosteroids and either cyclophosphamide or mycophenolate mofetil for no more than 6 months initially. It may be that immunosuppressive therapy ameliorates some of the glomerular damage caused by macrophage and neutrophil infiltration in severe disease and a closely monitored trial of immunosuppressive therapy in unexplained MPGN where the kidney biopsy shows substantial glomerular infiltration by immune cells and interstitial fibrosis is not too advanced can often be justified.

23.5.6 Recurrence Post-Transplantation

In view of the systemic nature of these diseases, it is not surprising that they can recur following renal transplantation. Reduction of antibody production is likely to reduce the risk to the allograft, and ability to achieve this will depend on the underlying disease process in each patient. In patients with MPGN and no identified cause, the risk of post-transplantation disease recurrence is greater in younger patients and is correlated with the degree of mesangial proliferation and crescent formation at presentation [2].

23.5.7 C3 Glomerulopathies

It is known that proliferative GN can occur without significant deposition of immunoglobulins or C1q in the glomerulus. While this pattern of immunostaining is characteristic of DDD (formerly known as type 2 MPGN), it is now recognised that it can occur without dense transformation of the GBM (producing appearances which would have formerly been categorised as type 1 or type 3 MPGN). In addition, the degree of inflammatory change and endocapillary proliferation can be subtle (perhaps depending on the timing of the biopsy), so the term C3 glomerulopathy also applies to those cases in which there is not enough proliferative change in the biopsy to be categorised as membranoproliferative GN (◘ Figs. 23.9 and 23.10). This umbrella term is useful because it provides the specific implication that the disease results from complement alternative pathway dysregulation. C3 glomerulopathy can be subdivided into dense deposit disease (DDD), C3 glomerulonephritis (C3GN) and CFHR5 nephropathy and although is usually sporadic can occasionally be seen as a familial disorder, in which case a monogenic cause should be considered.

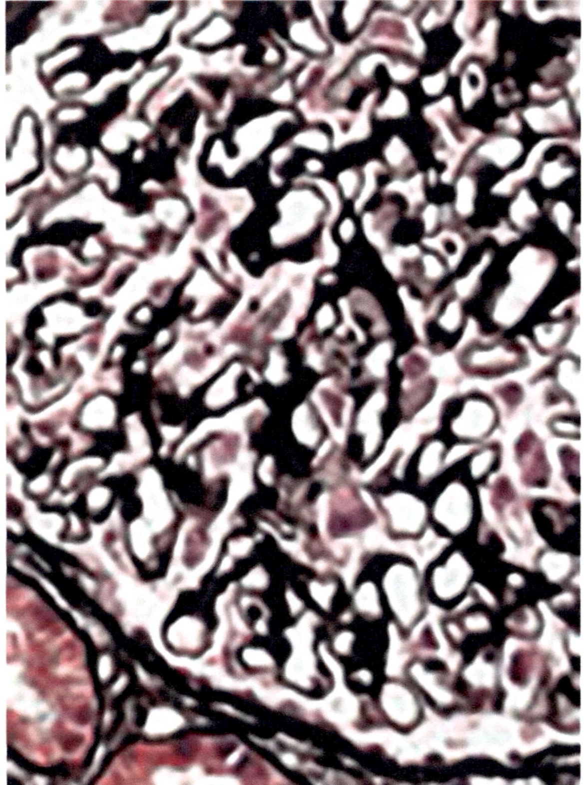

◘ **Fig. 23.9** C3 glomerulopathy – silver
Glomerulus at high magnification showing mild increase in mesangial matrix on silver staining and no thickening or doubling of the glomerular basement membrane

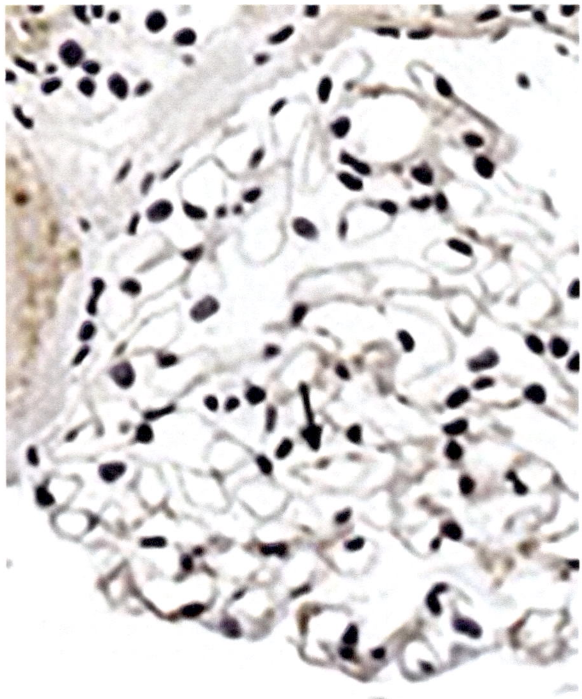

◘ **Fig. 23.10** C3 glomerulopathy – C9 immunoperoxidase
Glomerulus at high magnification. An immunoperoxidase method to detect C9 shows irregular, granular deposits within glomerular basement membranes consistent with the diagnosis of C3 glomerulopathy

23.5.8 Dense Deposit Disease

Dense deposit disease (DDD, formerly known as type 2 MPGN) is diagnosed by observing the characteristic dense transformation of the lamina densa of the GBM (◘ Figs. 23.11, 23.12 and 23.13). This may be accompanied by the morphological appearances of MPGN, but more often there is more subtle evidence of glomerular inflammation. DDD is a rare disease, affecting around 2–3 per million population. It can occur at any age although is more common in children, accounting for around 15–20% MPGN in those under 18 years. Clinical presentation is most often with proteinuria, which may be accompanied by the nephrotic syndrome and microscopic haematuria. There is slowly progressive renal impairment with approximately 50% patients needing renal replacement therapy within 10 years of

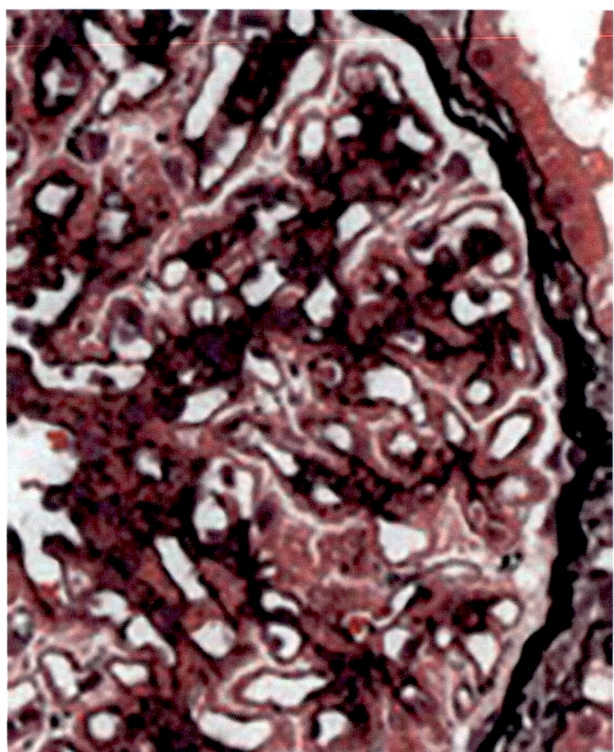

Fig. 23.11 Dense deposit disease – silver
Glomerulus at high magnification showing marked thickening of the majority of glomerular basement membranes. However, unlike membranous nephropathy, the thickening is irregular and no spikes are seen. Also, the thickened glomerular basement membranes (GMB) fail to take the silver stain well, whereas in membranous nephropathy the GBMs appear black

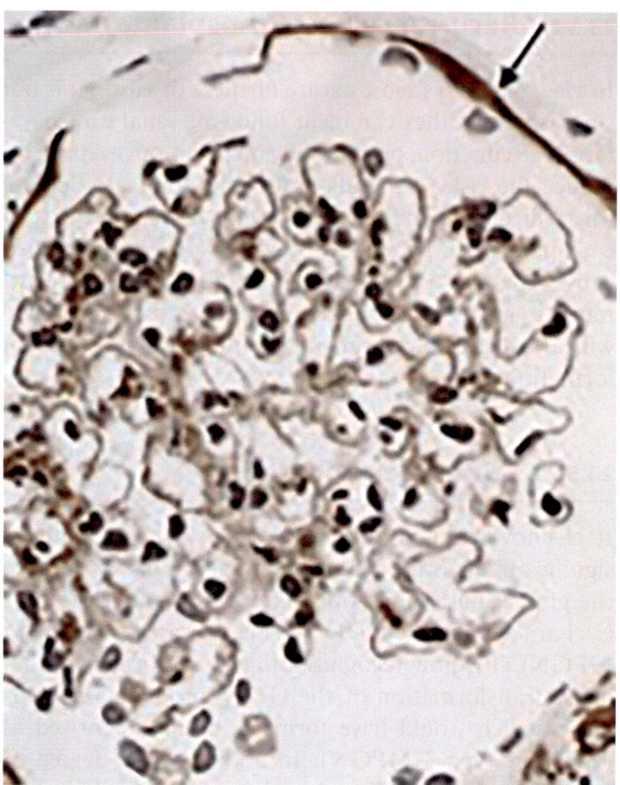

Fig. 23.12 Dense deposit disease – C9 immunoperoxidase
Immunoperoxidase method to detect C9 shows an irregular deposition of granular deposits in glomerular basement membranes. Also, heavy deposition is seen in Bowman's capsule, arrowed

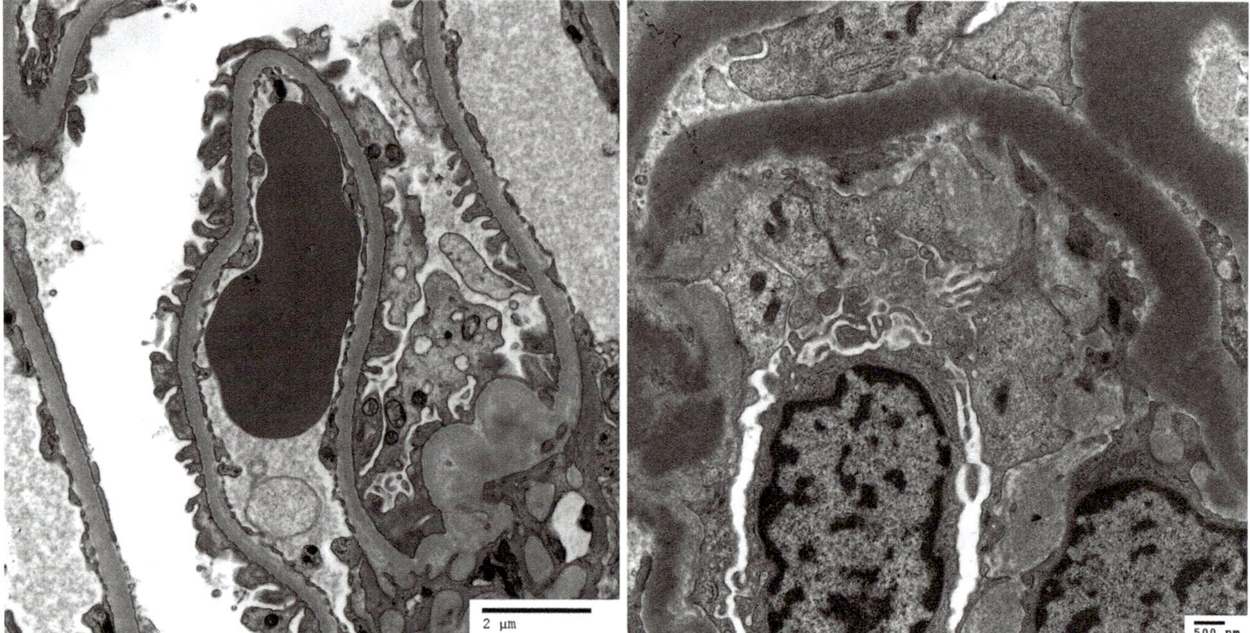

Fig. 23.13 Dense deposit disease – electron microscopy
Electron micrographs showing a normal glomerular capillary loop (right) and dense deposit disease (left) associated with electron dense transformation of the glomerular basement membrane

diagnosis: poor prognostic features are greater age and greater degree of renal impairment at diagnosis. The disease often recurs following kidney transplantation with over 50% graft loss at 5 years reported. This reflects the systemic nature of the disease. Interestingly, although the disease (with very few exceptions, outlined below) is almost never familial, a notable increase in the frequency of type 1 diabetes mellitus (DM1) among relatives of patients with DDD has been reported, consistent with the existence of shared genetic risk factors for the two diseases.

23.5.9 Aetiology and Pathophysiology of DDD

DDD is associated with systemic over-activation of the complement alternative pathway, and its causes are summarised in ▶ Box 23.1. In up to 80% of patients with DDD, an autoantibody which recognises the C3bBb alternative pathway convertase (called a C3 nephritic factor or C3NeF) is detectable in the circulation. This antibody prevents the normal dissociation and degradation of the C3 convertase, causing runaway activation of the alternative pathway in the circulation and depletion of C3. The presence of a C3NeF is detected by functional assays using, for example, sheep erythrocyte lysis or C3a generation in vitro as an indicator for enhanced complement activating ability of patient serum. Circulating C4 levels are typically normal since the classical pathway is not activated. In patients with DDD in whom a C3NeF is not detectable, antibodies which bind to both C3b and Factor B have occasionally been identified. In a handful of other C3NeF-negative cases, autoantibodies against Complement Factor H have been detected. Whether these autoantibodies are causal is not completely clear at present, and their utility as a diagnostic tool (in DDD) is not known. Of note, C3NeFs are identified in up to 25% of cases of IC-MPGN and 20–40% of C3GN, suggesting either that different C3NeFs activate complement in different ways or that there is overlap between these different conditions [15, 16]. In addition, antibodies termed C4NeFs or C5NeFs that stabilise the C4 or C5 convertases, respectively (usually in addition to the C3 convertase), have been documented in some patients, although it is not yet clear whether assays for these factors represent a clinically useful biomarker. DDD sometimes occurs in association with a monoclonal gammopathy, raising the possibility that circulating monoclonal immunoglobulins, in some circumstances, can lead to complement alternative pathway dysregulation.

Rarely, individuals with DDD have been identified who are homozygous (or compound heterozygous) for mutations in the *CFH* gene and in whom plasma CFH levels are undetectable. This leads to unregulated complement alternative pathway activity in the circulation and depletion of plasma C3 in the absence of a C3NeF. Of note, this contrasts with individuals heterozygous for mutations (usually in the C-terminal two domains) of Factor H which impair its ability to bind to host surfaces. In these patients, fluid phase complement regulation is relatively preserved (and plasma C3 levels may be normal). but complement dysregulation at endothelial surfaces results in thrombotic microangiopathy, and the clinical presentation is with atypical haemolytic uraemic syndrome (aHUS). A crucial further insight into the pathophysiology of the disease has come from the description of a single family in which a particular heterozygous mutation of *C3* co-segregates with DDD. The mutant C3 allele in this family (termed $C3_{923\Delta DG}$) is able to cleave the wild-type C3 and is resistant to degradation by Factor H in the circulation but not by membrane cofactor protein at host surfaces, leading to complement dysregulation particularly in the fluid phase, and resulting in DDD [17]. This illustrates that resistance of C3 to Factor H-mediated degradation is sufficient to cause DDD.

Box 23.1 Causes of dense deposit disease (DDD)

Causes of DDD
C3NeF (80%)
Homozygous CFH mutations (very rare)
Activating C3 mutation (case reports)

Other associations with DDD
Factor B autoantibodies
Complement factor H autoantibodies
Monoclonal gammopathy

23.5.10 Systemic Manifestations of DDD

DDD is associated with the accumulation of retinal deposits (also containing C3) in Bruch's membrane (which separates the retinal pigment epithelium from the choroid) which manifest clinically as drusen. Visual loss may occur (typically over two to three decades) usually as a consequence of retinal atrophy and sometimes associated with subretinal neovascular membrane formation. Consequently, ophthalmological assessment and review are recommended for patients diagnosed with DDD.

DDD in the presence of a C3NeF can also be associated with acquired partial lipodystrophy, which is selective destruction of the adipocytes in the top half of the body. Importantly, acquired partial lipodystrophy has not been reported in humans (or animals) with DDD resulting from genetic deficiency of CFH, implying a direct effect of the C3NeF itself in causing the adipocyte damage, rather than this being a manifestation of systemic complement alternative pathway dysregulation per se. Partial lipodystrophy can precede renal disease by some years and is sometimes noticed acutely following an otherwise minor infection, suggesting that cytokine release or other manifestations of immunological activation can trigger adipocyte damage in the disease.

23.5.11 C3 Glomerulonephritis

C3 glomerulonephritis (C3GN) is defined by the presence of glomerular complement C3 deposition and inflammation in the absence of significant immunoglobulin deposition or dense transformation of the GBM. MPGN is present in some, but not all, biopsies and is not required to make the diagnosis. C3GN is rare, accounting for less than 10% of proliferative GN but is significantly more common than DDD in adult practice. Clinical presentation is highly variable and may be with microscopic or intermittent macroscopic haematuria and/or proteinuria which may be in the nephrotic range. Renal dysfunction tends to be mild, at least in the early stages, and, until recently, this was regarded as a benign disease. A small proportion of patients exhibit hypocomplementaemia (low C3 with normal C4), and a C3NeF is detectable in 20–40% of patients with C3GN.

23.5.12 CFHR5 Nephropathy

By far the commonest monogenic cause of C3 glomerulopathy is CFHR5 nephropathy, a highly penetrant autosomal dominant disease which is particularly common in Cypriots (affecting approximately 1:6000 of the population of the country). CFHR5 nephropathy is caused by mutation of *CFHR5* (*Complement Factor H-related 5,* a homologue of *CFH*) leading to duplication of the N-terminal two domains and the production of an elongated version of the FHR5 protein encoded by the gene [18]. Although the histological and ultrastructural features overlap with C3GN (◘ Fig. 23.14), the characteristic clinical and molecular findings have led to its categorization as a separate disease. CFHR5 nephropathy is characterised clinically by microscopic haematuria with episodes of macroscopic haematuria and acute renal dysfunction occurring at times of upper respiratory tract (synpharyngitic) or other infections. Mild to moderate proteinuria is seen late in the disease, and the nephrotic syndrome is not a feature. Circulating complement C3 and C4 levels are normal and progressive renal impairment occurs in late adulthood, with >80% men (but <20% women) developing kidney failure (see ◘ Table 23.6). The reason for this sexual dimorphism is not understood. Kidney biopsies in patients with CFHR5 nephropathy invariably shows discrete electron dense deposits in the subendothelial GBM, as well as deposits in mesangial regions, with occasional subepithelial deposits seen in some patients. Light microscopic appearances are characterised by mesangial expansion and proliferation, with usually rather mild capillary wall changes.

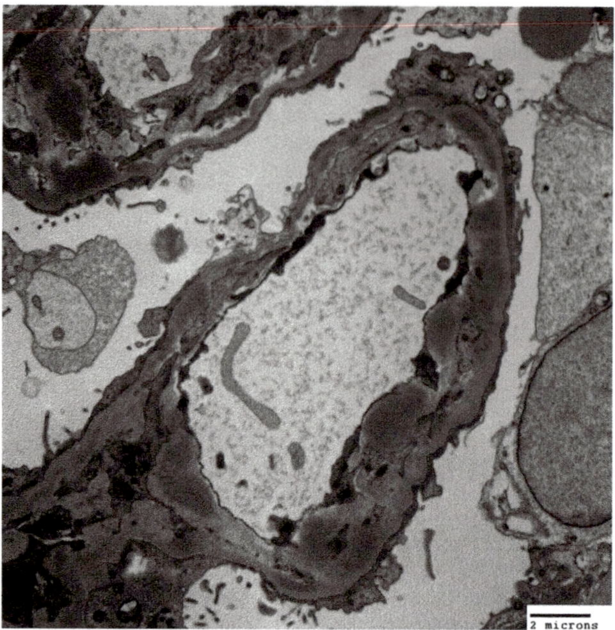

◘ **Fig. 23.14** CFHR5 nephropathy – electron microscopy Electron micrograph showing discrete electron dense deposits in the subendothelial glomerular basement membrane and mesangium in a patient with CFHR5 nephropathy

Although renal allograft survival in patients with CFHR5 nephropathy is generally very good, the disease recurs following transplantation. While this observation proves that CFHR5 nephropathy results from a systemic factor, extra-renal manifestations of the disease have not been reported, again suggesting that the FHR5 protein may have a particular role in the kidney. Mechanistic studies suggest that FHR5, in common with some of the other FHRs, competitively antagonises Factor H at surfaces (i.e. in the glomerulus) and thus deregulates complement there. Mutations that elongate FHR5 can enhance this complement deregulating activity, leading to glomerular inflammation. Genetic rearrangements that elongate other FHR proteins have also been

Table 23.6 C3 glomerulopathies: clinical and laboratory features. Nephrotic syndrome, NS; C3 nephritic factor, C3NeF

	Dense deposit disease	C3GN	CFHR5 nephropathy
Typical features	Proteinuria and renal impairment	Variable proteinuria ± haematuria	Haematuria and renal impairment
Other features	Haematuria and NS	Occasional NS or renal impairment	Synpharyngitic macroscopic haematuria
Inheritance	Usually sporadic. Rare familial cases reported	Sporadic	Autosomal dominant
Gender distribution	More common in females	–	More severe disease in males
Serum C3	Low	Low or normal	Normal
Serum C4	Normal or transiently low	Normal or transiently low	Normal
Autoantibody	C3NeF (80%)	C3NeF (20–40%)	Antibodies absent
Extra-renal manifestations	Ocular drusen Partial lipodystrophy	None reported	None reported
Diagnostic finding	Dense transformation of GBM	–	CFHR5 mutation
Post-transplant recurrence	Typical, with 50% graft loss at 5 years	Variable	Universal – But rarely causes graft loss

reported in other rare families with C3 glomerulopathy, implying that these proteins can play an important role in complement regulation in the kidney.

An important clinical observation which is shared by many disorders of complement alternative pathway regulation (including DDD, C3GN and aHUS) is that otherwise trivial stimulation of the immune system (for instance, by a minor infection) can trigger overt flares of disease and significant kidney damage.

23.5.13 Genetics of MPGN and C3 Glomerulopathy

Although rare variants in the range of complement genes implicated in aHUS have been reported in small, uncontrolled cohorts of patients with nonfamilial C3GN, DDD and immune complex MPGN, convincing evidence that the frequency of such variants is increased compared with the general population is lacking. In addition, a monogenic cause would be inconsistent with the usually nonfamilial nature of the disease, the increased prevalence of DM1 among relatives of those with DDD and of course the presence of a C3NeF in many patients with these disorders. A recent genome-wide association study identified association of all of DDD, C3GN and antibody-associated MPGN (including those with and without a documented C3NeF) with a particular HLA haplotype (incorporating alleles DQA1*05:01, DQB1*02:01 and DRB1*03:01) that is also associated with DM1 and coeliac disease, likely explaining the co-occurrence of the conditions in the same families and suggesting that, in nonfamilial cases at least, autoimmunity (i.e. the generation of a C3NeF) plays the key role in the aetiologies of all these disorders [16]. This contrasts with the monogenic complement regulation defects (such as CFHR5 nephropathy) in familial cases, in which a primary defect of the complement system is responsible.

23.5.14 Investigation of C3 Glomerulopathies

Diagnosis of a C3 glomerulopathy (i.e. DDD or C3GN) in a patient should prompt investigation of alternative pathway regulation. Tests for paraproteinaemia, complement C3, complement C4 and C3 nephritic factor are widely available and should be performed in all such patients. In patients with a C3 glomerulopathy who may have Cypriot ancestry, a genetic test for the Cypriot mutation should be performed since CFHR5 nephropathy is common in this population (available at the Institute of Child Health in London, ▶ http://www.labs.gosh.nhs.uk/laboratory-services/genetics/tests/cfhr5-nephropathy). Additional tests such as serum Complement Factor H and Factor I levels and tests for autoantibodies against Factor B and Factor H should be considered if a C3NeF is not identified. Given the high frequency of rare complement gene variants in healthy populations (estimated at around 6%), the clinical significance of rare missense variants in these genes in patients with C3G is not understood, so genetic testing (including analyses to detect copy number variation) of *CFH*, *CFHR1-5* and *C3* should usually be performed only where there is a family history of the disease.

23.5.15 Treatment of C3 Glomerulopathies

Although it is generally presumed that blood pressure control and angiotensin system blockade should be introduced to delay progression of renal damage, there is currently no proven therapy for DDD, C3GN or CFHR5 nephropathy. Since the diseases are rare and rather slowly progressive, robust clinical trial data in humans are lacking. Strategies aimed at supressing the immune system (e.g. using steroids or antiproliferative agents such as mycophenolate mofetil) may have some beneficial effects on renal inflammation. Where a C3NeF is detected, plasma exchange, immunosuppression, cytotoxic therapy or B-cell depletion (for instance, using the chimeric anti-CD20 monoclonal antibody rituximab) may reduce its levels, but trials have not been published showing a clinical benefit of these approaches. It is important to recognise that the C3NeF is playing a different role from that played by circulating antibodies in most autoimmune diseases – only tiny quantities of C3NeF are needed to stabilise the C3 convertase and activate the positive feedback loop of the alternative pathway: thus strategies to deplete C3NeF must be very efficacious indeed if they are to normalise complement regulation in the circulation.

In patients with a genetic cause for C3G (e.g. in individuals with deficiency of *CFH* or a *CFHR5* lengthening mutation), plasma infusion or exchange is sometimes thought to be beneficial, presumably by removal of the mutant FHR protein or supplementation of missing Factor H. Interventions which minimise the frequency of intercurrent infections (such as tonsillectomy in children) have also been reported to provide benefit in CFHR5 nephropathy, which is consistent with the role that infection plays in precipitating acute deterioration of renal function in the disease.

Eculizumab, a humanised monoclonal antibody directed against C5, blocks the terminal complement pathway. The drug is effective and licenced for use in aHUS, but reports of its use in C3G (in very small numbers of patients) have shown a mixed response, and this treatment is not widely used for this indication.

Recurrence of C3G following transplantation is a well-recognised complication with estimates of the risk of graft loss to recurrent disease ranging between 30% and 80%, with the risk likely higher in younger people. Loss of an allograft to recurrent disease does not guarantee that future transplants will have the same fate, but such patients should be regarded as being at higher risk of subsequent allograft loss and counselled accordingly. Unlike aHUS, no cases of de novo MPGN or C3G following living-related kidney donation have been described, so there is no clear rationale for genetic testing prior to living donor transplantation in nonfamilial cases.

23.6 Summary

Activation of complement can lead to kidney damage with histological appearances ranging from mild proliferative changes to membranoproliferative glomerulonephritis. Complement may be activated via the classical pathway (as a consequence of antibody-antigen complex formation) or by defects in the regulation of the alternative pathway. Excessive complement dysregulation in the circulation is associated with dense deposit disease, whereas complement dysregulation at endothelial surfaces typically leads to atypical haemolytic uraemic syndrome. For reasons which are not yet completely understood, some defects which result in complement dysregulation at surfaces can result in C3 glomerulonephritis instead.

Treatment of these kidney diseases relies on identification and correction of the aetiological factor(s). It is hoped that development of novel drugs that allow the modulation of complement activity directly may provide completely new ways to treat these disorders.

Case Study

A 24-year-old woman was found to have abruptly increased proteinuria (>1.5 g/day) and renal impairment (creatinine 160) during routine monitoring for her type 1 diabetes mellitus, which had been diagnosed aged 5. Blood pressure was low-normal on an angiotensin 2 receptor blocker, and blood sugar control using insulin had been excellent for many years, without previous evidence of diabetic nephropathy, retinopathy or other complications. There was no other past medical history. Her mother had been treated for rheumatoid arthritis, but there was no additional family history of renal or autoimmune disease that she was aware of.

Investigations showed reduced complement C3 at 0.57 g/L (normal range 0.8–1.6) but normal C4, autoimmune and virology screens. A kidney biopsy showed multisegmental glomerular capillary wall thickening and wrinkling with marked multisegmental mesangial expansion associated with moderate hypercellularity. Immunostains were negative for immunoglobulins but showed discrete, variably sized C3-positive granules (including 'hump-like' structures) on capillary walls and granules within mesangial regions, and electron microscopy revealed diabetic-type glomerular basement thickening as well as numerous intramembranous (Fig. 23.15), as well as subendothelial and mesangial, electron dense deposits and a diagnosis of C3G (likely dense deposit disease), was made. Assays for C3 nephritic factor were initially negative, but subsequent immunological testing over a 6-year period showed the presence of a C3NeF on 3 out of the 12 occasions it was tested and C3 levels that varied from just below to just within the normal range. Proteinuria and serum creatinine fluctuated over this time period without any trend or correlation with C3/C3NeFs being appreciable.

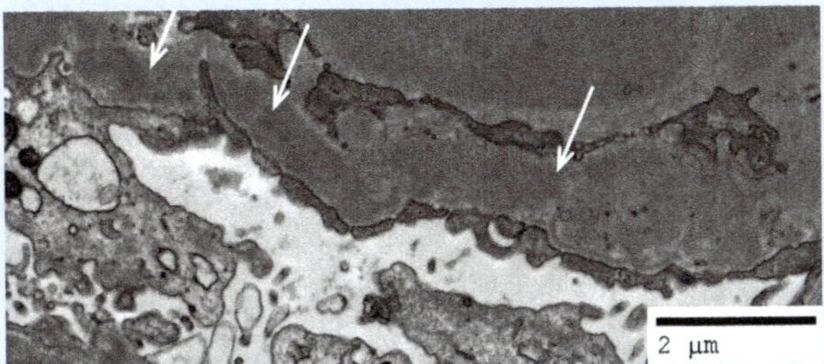

Fig. 23.15 C3 glomerulopathy case – electron microscopy Electron micrograph showing smudgy electron dense patches (arrows) within the glomerular basement membrane

This case illustrates (1) the coincidence of C3G with autoimmune (type 1) diabetes mellitus in the same patient (2) that it is not always possible to distinguish C3GN and DDD with complete certainty; (3) the C3NeF assay may be negative initially, but subsequent assays may reveal its presence, and (4) disease progression may be too slow to be detectable, even over prolonged follow-up, in the absence of immunomodulatory therapy.

Tips, Tricks and Pitfalls

1. In patients with C3 glomerulopathy, assays for C3 nephritic factor should be performed multiple times during follow-up because, since only tiny amounts of the antibody can be sufficient to cause disease, not all assays are sensitive enough to detect low but clinically important levels of C3 nephritic factor.
2. Because rare, missense variants in complement genes are present in 6–10% of the general population, identification of such a variant in a patient with MPGN or C3G is seldom helpful: genetic testing should therefore be reserved for familial cases.
3. Even where a patient has lost one or more allograft to recurrent disease, successful (i.e. recurrence free) transplantation is still possible subsequently.

Chapter Review Questions

1. What are the three different types of cryoglobulinaemia and what underlying diseases are they associated with?
2. What are the causes of thrombotic microangiopathy?
3. What are the clinical characteristics of dense deposit disease (DDD)?
4. What disease entities are encompassed by the term C3 glomerulopathy?

Answers

1. Type 1 monoclonal IgM associated with Waldenstrom's macroglobulinaemia, type 2 monoclonal IgM bound to polyclonal IgG associated with hepatitis and lymphoproliferative disorders and type 3 polyclonal IgM bound to polyclonal IgG associated with hepatitis C, HIV, other infections, autoimmune diseases, cancers.
2. Haemolytic uraemic syndrome, thrombocytopenia purpura, pre-eclampsia, systemic lupus erythematosus, antiphospholipid syndrome, scleroderma renal crisis, accelerated hypertension, radiotherapy, antibody-mediated allograft rejection and some drugs such as tacrolimus and cyclosporin.
3. DDD is very rare and can occur at any age, but it is more common to present in children with proteinuria, progressive renal impairment and often nephrotic syndrome. 80% are associated with C3NeF antibody, drusen and lipodystrophy.
4. DDD and C3 glomerulonephritis and CFHR5.

References

1. Habib R, Michielsen P, et al. In: Wolstenholme GEW, Cameron MP, editors. Clinical, microscopic and electron microscopic data in the nephrotic syndrome of unknown origin. Ciba Foundation Symposium - renal biopsy: clinical and pathological significance. Chichester: John Wiley & Sons Ltd; 1961. p. 70–102.
2. Little MA, Dupont P, et al. Severity of primary MPGN, rather than MPGN type, determines renal survival and post-transplantation recurrence risk. Kidney Int. 2006;69(3):504–11.

3. Servais A, Fremeaux-Bacchi V, et al. Primary glomerulonephritis with isolated C3 deposits: a new entity which shares common genetic risk factors with haemolytic uraemic syndrome. J Med Genet. 2007;44(3):193–9.
4. Walker PD, Ferrario F, et al. Dense deposit disease is not a membranoproliferative glomerulonephritis. Mod Pathol. 2007;20(6):605–16.
5. Abdurrahman MB, Aikhionbare HA, et al. Clinicopathological features of childhood nephrotic syndrome in northern Nigeria. Q J Med. 1990;75(278):563–76.
6. Covic A, Schiller A, et al. Epidemiology of renal disease in Romania: a 10 year review of two regional renal biopsy databases. Nephrol Dial Transplant. 2006;21(2):419–24.
7. Hanko JB, Mullan RN, et al. The changing pattern of adult primary glomerular disease. Nephrol Dial Transplant. 2009;24(10):3050–4.
8. Woo KT, Chan CM, et al. The changing pattern of primary glomerulonephritis in Singapore and other countries over the past 3 decades. Clin Nephrol. 2010;74(5):372–83.
9. Cicardi M, Cesana B, et al. Prevalence and risk factors for the presence of serum cryoglobulins in patients with chronic hepatitis C. J Viral Hepat. 2000;7(2):138–43.
10. Bonnet F, Pineau JJ, et al. Prevalence of cryoglobulinemia and serological markers of autoimmunity in human immunodeficiency virus infected individuals: a cross-sectional study of 97 patients. J Rheumatol. 2003;30(9):2005–10.
11. Matignon M, Cacoub P, et al. Clinical and morphologic spectrum of renal involvement in patients with mixed cryoglobulinemia without evidence of hepatitis C virus infection. Medicine. 2009;88(6):341–8.
12. D'Amico G. Renal involvement in hepatitis C infection: cryoglobulinemic glomerulonephritis. Kidney Int. 1998;54(2):650–71.
13. Levin A. Management of membranoproliferative glomerulonephritis: evidence-based recommendations. Kidney Int Suppl. 1999;70:S41–6.
14. Tarshish P, Bernstein J, et al. Treatment of mesangiocapillary glomerulonephritis with alternate-day prednisone--a report of the International Study of Kidney Disease in Children. Pediatr Nephrol. 1992;6(2):123–30.
15. Servais A, Noël LH, et al. Acquired and genetic complement abnormalities play a critical role in dense deposit disease and other C3 glomerulopathies. Kidney Int. 2012;82(4):454–64.
16. Levine AP, Chan MMY, et al. Large-scale whole-genome sequencing reveals the genetic architecture of primary membranoproliferative GN and C3 glomerulopathy. J Am Soc Nephrol. 2020;31(2):365–73.
17. Martínez-Barricarte R, Heurich M, et al. Human C3 mutation reveals a mechanism of dense deposit disease pathogenesis and provides insights into complement activation and regulation. J Clin Invest. 2010;120(10):3702–12.
18. Gale DP, et al. Identification of a mutation in complement factor H-related protein 5 in patients of Cypriot origin with glomerulonephritis. Lancet. 2010;376(9743):794–801.

Further Reading

Goodship THJ, et al. Atypical hemolytic uremic syndrome and C3 glomerulopathy: conclusions from a "Kidney Disease: Improving Global Outcomes" (KDIGO) Controversies Conference. Kidney Int. 2017;91(3):539–51.

Sethi S, Fervenza FC. Membranoproliferative glomerulonephritis: pathogenetic heterogeneity and proposal for a new classification. Semin Nephrol. 2011;31(4):341–8.

IgA Nephropathy and IgA Vasculitis

Haresh Selvaskandan, Chee Kay Cheung, and Jonathan Barratt

Contents

M. Harber (ed.), *Primer on Nephrology*, https://doi.org/10.1007/978-3-030-76419-7_24

Learning Objectives

1. IgA nephropathy is the commonest reported cause of primary glomerulonephritis worldwide; incidence varies with geography and race.
2. IgA nephropathy most commonly presents in young adults and is associated with slowly progressive renal impairment in the majority of cases with 30% of affected individuals developing end-stage renal disease within 20 years of diagnosis.
3. Treatment focusses on optimisation of supportive measures, most importantly blood pressure control and renin-angiotensin blockade. There is little evidence for efficacy of immunosuppressants in IgA nephropathy.
4. IgA vasculitis (Henöch-Schonlein purpura) is a rare vasculitis, most commonly seen in children, that presents as a multisystem disorder.
5. IgA vasculitis is commonly self-limiting, and immunosuppression is reserved only for those patients with rapid deterioration in renal function.

24.1 Introduction

Immunoglobulin A nephropathy (IgAN) is the commonest reported primary glomerulonephritis worldwide. It was first described by the Parisian pathologist Jean Berger in 1968, at a time in which immunofluorescence was starting to become readily available. IgAN is defined by predominant mesangial IgA deposition and can have a spectrum of clinical presentations. Despite running a benign course in most patients, it remains a leading cause of progressive kidney disease globally. Its incidence also peaks among young adults, and 30% of patients progress to end-stage renal disease within 20 years of diagnosis.

Closely related to IgAN is IgA vasculitis (Henoch-Schönlein purpura). This less commonly seen disease is more frequently found in children. It is a systemic small-vessel vasculitis, characterised by IgA deposition in the skin, joints, gut and kidney, leading to a characteristic set of symptoms of rash, arthralgia, abdominal pain and nephritis. The renal biopsy in a patient with IgA vasculitis is indistinguishable from IgAN.

> The defining feature of IgA nephropathy and IgA vasculitis-associated nephritis is the predominant deposition of immunoglobulin A in the glomerular mesangium.

24.2 IgA Nephropathy

24.2.1 Clinical Features

IgA nephropathy can present on a clinical spectrum. Most patients present with either:

- Visible haematuria, typically 12–72 hours after a mucosal infection. Such infections are thought to trigger nephritogenic IgA immune complex production (commonly upper respiratory tract infections and less commonly gastrointestinal or urinary tract infections).
- Incidental finding of non-visible haematuria +/– proteinuria (e.g. on testing for insurance purposes or occupational screening).

More rarely, patients may present with:

- Acute kidney injury (either due to red cell cast tubular obstruction secondary to massive haematuria or a crescentic glomerulonephritis)
- Overt nephrotic syndrome
- Chronic kidney disease
- End-stage renal disease
- Malignant hypertension

Although IgA nephropathy can follow a benign course, a proportion of patients do develop progressive renal disease culminating in end-stage renal disease. The perceived risk of progressive disease is heavily influenced by biopsy practice. For example, in centres where there is a low threshold for renal biopsy (e.g. isolated non-visible haematuria), the cohort of patients diagnosed with IgAN will be biased towards those with a lower risk of progressive renal disease.

However, it is generally accepted that:

- Less than 10% of patients will have complete resolution of urinary abnormalities.
- Episodes of visible haematuria become less frequent with time.
- 30% of patients will progress to end-stage renal disease within 20 years of diagnosis.

24.2.2 Epidemiology

The reported incidence of IgAN is highly variable across the globe. It is most commonly reported in Asian populations, is regarded as a rare disease in Caucasians and is extremely uncommon in people of African origin. The cause of this variation is likely to be multifactorial but may in part simply be due to differences in screening policies for asymptomatic urinary abnormalities and variations in biopsy practice [1]. Japan, for instance, has an annual school screening program, which may contribute to higher incidences resulting from a detection of cases that may have otherwise been subclinical. Subclinical IgAN is estimated to occur in 2–3% of Caucasians but up to 16% of the general Asian population [2].

Patients can present at any age, although incidence peaks in the second and third decades. There is a 2:1 male to female predominance in North American and Western European populations, which is not observed in Asian populations.

24.2.3 Aetiopathology

The defining feature of IgAN is mesangial deposition of IgA. Human IgA exists in two isoforms, IgA1 and IgA2, which can each exist as monomers (single molecules) or polymers (most commonly dimers; two IgA molecules linked by a peptide 'J-chain'). It is predominantly polymeric IgA1 that is found in the mesangium of IgAN patients. IgA1 contains a hinge region, which is rich in serine, proline and threonine residues. These amino acids can be variably glycosylated giving rise to a range of IgA1 *O*-glycoforms in the serum (◘ Fig. 24.1). Unusual for a serum protein, the IgA1 hinge region carries *O*-linked oligosaccharides in addition to the more commonly seen *N*-linked sugars which are present on virtually all serum proteins.

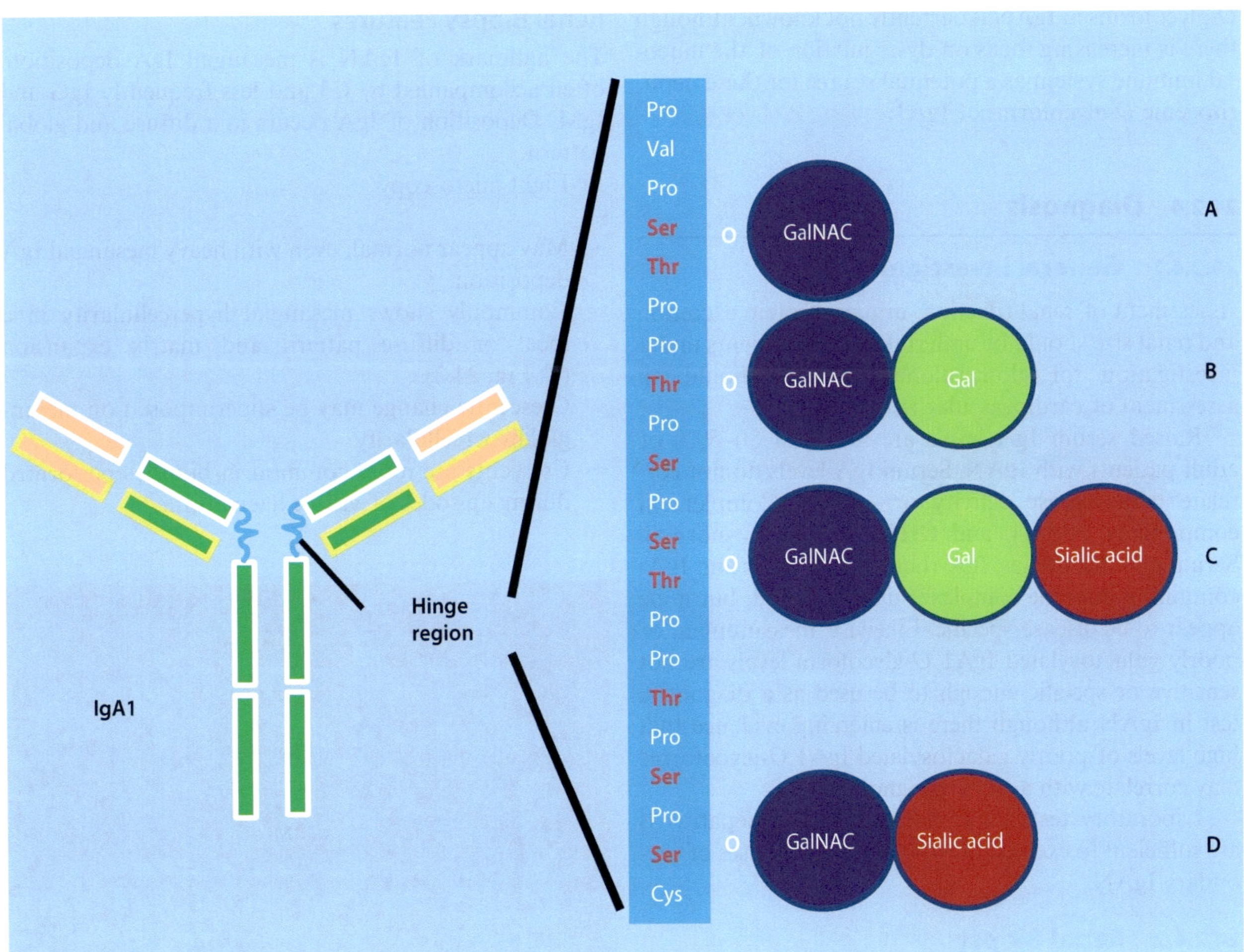

◘ **Fig. 24.1** The IgA1 molecule showing the position of the hinge region *O*-glycans. Serine (Ser) and threonine (Thr) residues in the hinge region provide nine potential *O*-linked glycosylation sites; although to date only six are known to be occupied by *O*-glycans. It is still not known which amino acids are occupied by *O*-glycans and whether it is the same amino acids for all *O*-glycoforms of IgA1. The IgA1 *O*-glycans are all based on *N*-acetylgalactosamine (GalNAC) units in *O*-linkage with serine or threonine (**a**). GalNAC which may be extended either with galactose (Gal) alone (**b**) or with Gal and sialic acid (**c**). Alternatively, the GalNAC may simply carry a sialic acid (**d**)

Changes in the composition of the *O*-linked sugars at the IgA1 hinge region are the most consistent finding in patients with IgAN across the world, with changes having been seen in patient cohorts from North America, Europe and Asia [3]. The key change is an increase in the serum of IgA1 *O*-glycoforms that contain less galactose. This increase in poorly galactosylated IgA1 *O*-glycoforms is believed to play a central role in the pathogenesis of IgAN. It is believed poorly galactosylated IgA1 *O*-glycoforms form high-molecular-weight circulating immune complexes, either through self-aggregation or through generation of IgG and IgA hinge region specific autoantibodies. These high-molecular-weight immune complexes are prone to mesangial deposition resulting ultimately in mesangial cell proliferation, release of pro-inflammatory mediators and glomerular injury [4]. Why there should be an increase in the levels of poorly galactosylated IgA1 *O*-glycoforms in IgAN is currently not known, although there is increasing focus on dysregulation of the mucosal immune system as a potential source for these nephritogenic *O*-glycoforms of IgA1.

24.2.4 Diagnosis

24.2.4.1 General Investigations

Assessment of renal function, urinary protein excretion and renal size should be undertaken in all patients under investigation for glomerulonephritis, as should an assessment of cardiovascular risk.

Raised serum IgA levels are found in 30–50% of adult patients with IgAN. Serum IgA levels do not correlate with disease activity or severity. Complement components C3, C4, and CH50 are usually normal. Serum autoantibodies, IgA-rheumatoid factor and IgA-containing immune complexes may be found, but none appear to be disease-specific. Likewise, measurement of poorly galactosylated IgA1 *O*-glycoform levels are not sensitive or specific enough to be used as a diagnostic test in IgAN although there is emerging evidence that high levels of poorly galactosylated IgA1 *O*-glycoforms may correlate with a worse prognosis.

Laboratory tests for liver function and hepatitis B are sufficient to exclude the most common causes of secondary IgAN.

24.2.4.2 Renal Biopsy

IgAN can only be diagnosed with a renal biopsy; however, in some cases where IgAN is one of the most likely diagnoses, e.g. in isolated non-visible haematuria [5], many nephrologists would not now routinely perform a renal biopsy, although these patients will require careful follow-up (see below).

When to Consider Doing a Renal Biopsy in Suspected IgAN?

Most clinicians would consider performing a renal biopsy in the context of normal renal imaging and the following:

- Proteinuria >1 g/24 h ± haematuria without impaired renal function
- Impaired renal function with or without haematuria ± proteinuria (any level)
- Acute kidney injury

Occasionally, patients with IgAN develop acute on chronic renal failure, and a renal biopsy may be necessary to distinguish acute tubular necrosis (due to red cell cast tubular obstruction secondary to massive haematuria) from a crescentic transformation of IgAN.

Renal Biopsy Features

The hallmark of IgAN is mesangial IgA deposition, often accompanied by C3 and less frequently IgG and IgM. Deposition of IgA occurs in a diffuse and global pattern.

Light microscopy:

- May appear normal, even with heavy mesangial IgA deposition.
- Commonly shows mesangial hypercellularity in a focal or diffuse pattern and matrix expansion (Fig. 24.2).
- Crescentic change may be superimposed on mesangial hypercellularity.
- Crescents are more common in biopsies performed during episodes of visible haematuria.

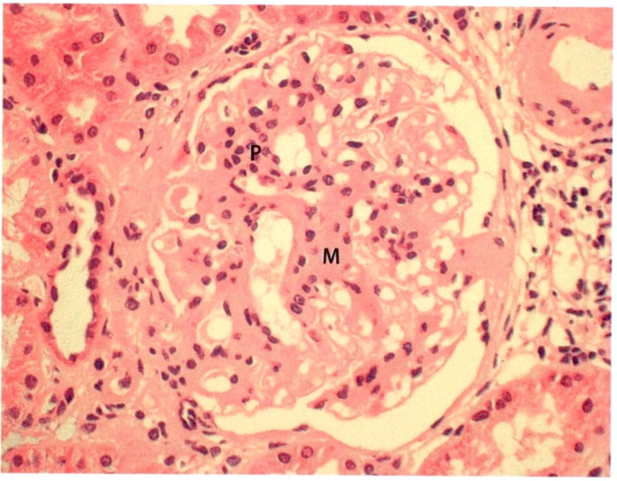

Fig. 24.2 A renal biopsy showing mesangial proliferation (P) and expansion of the mesangial extracellular matrix (M) in a patient with IgA nephropathy

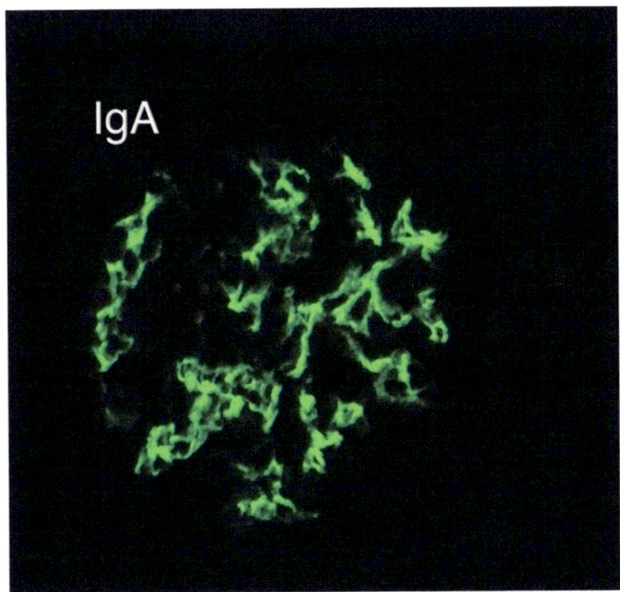

Fig. 24.3 A renal biopsy showing immunofluorescent staining for IgA in a patient with IgA nephropathy

- Tubulointerstitial changes are similar to other forms of progressive glomerulonephritis with tubular atrophy and interstitial fibrosis.

Immunohistology:

- Mesangial staining for IgA is the defining feature of IgAN (Fig. 24.3).
- IgA deposits may extend beyond the mesangium to the glomerular capillaries. This finding is associated with a worse prognosis.
- IgA is the sole deposited immunoglobulin in 15% of cases.
- Other immunoglobulins may also be deposited: IgG (50–70% of cases) and IgM (31–66% of cases), although staining is usually less intense than IgA. The presence of IgG and IgM has no prognostic significance.
- C3 deposition is usually also present.

Electron microscopy:

- Mesangial and para-mesangial electron-dense deposits are often seen and correspond to IgA immune complex deposition (Fig. 24.4).
- Capillary loop deposits may be seen and are usually subendothelial but may be intramembranous or subepithelial. These are associated with a worse prognosis.
- The size, shape, quantity and density of the deposits vary between glomeruli.

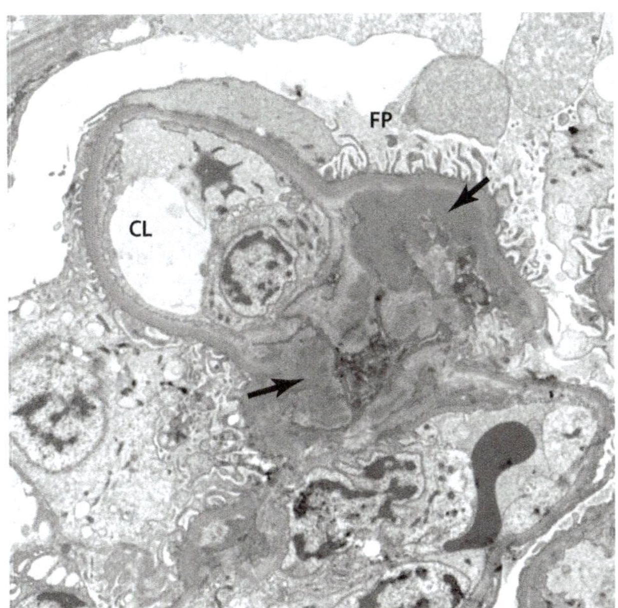

Fig. 24.4 An electron micrograph of a portion of a glomerulus (CL capillary lumen, FP foot processes) showing electron-dense immune complex deposits (arrowed) within the mesangium

- Glomerular basement membrane (GBM) abnormalities are seen in 15–40%, and are associated with heavy proteinuria, more severe glomerular changes and crescent formation.
- A group of patients have thinning of the GBM indistinguishable from thin membrane disease. It remains unclear whether the clinical course of these patients is altered.

The Oxford Classification of IgA Nephropathy

In 2009, a consensus on the pathologic classification of IgAN was published by the International IgA Nephropathy Network and the Renal Pathology Society (the Oxford Classification). Clinical data and renal biopsies were obtained from 265 patients followed for a median of 5 years. The first part of this work identified histological variables which could be interpreted with a high degree of reproducibility between different pathologists [6]. The second part was a retrospective analysis identifying renal biopsy features that correlated most strongly with clinical outcome, independent of known clinical risk factors including the presence of hypertension, impaired renal function at diagnosis and degree of proteinuria [7]. Following a number of validation studies and new studies evaluating additional lesions, the Oxford Classification was reviewed and updated in 2017 such that it now comprises the MEST-C score (Table 24.1):

Table 24.1 The Oxford Classification of IgA nephropathy. Scoring should be assessed on periodic acid-Schiff-stained sections. For a precise definition of each parameter, see [7, 9]

Histological variable	Definition	Score
Mesangial hypercellularity	Mesangial hypercellularity score	*M*0 ≤ 0.5 *M*1 > 0.5
Endocapillary hypercellularity	Hypercellularity due to increased number of cells within glomerular capillary lumina causing narrowing of the lumina	*E*0 absent *E*1 present
Segmental glomerulosclerosis	Any amount of the tuft involved in sclerosis, but not involving the whole tuft or the presence of an adhesion	*S*0 absent *S*1 present
Tubular atrophy/interstitial fibrosis	Percentage of cortical area involved by the tubular atrophy or interstitial fibrosis, whichever is greater	*T*0 0–25% *T*1 26–50% *T*2 > 50%
Crescent	Percentage of glomeruli with crescenteric changes	*C0* No crescents *C1* ≥ 1 Glomerular Crescent *C2* ≥ 25% Crescents

- *M*esangial hypercellularity
- *E*ndocapillary hypercellularity
- *S*egmental glomerulosclerosis
- *T*ubular atrophy/interstitial fibrosis
- *C*rescents

The predictive value of these biopsy features is similar in both adults and children [8]. This classification system now forms an integral part of the evaluation of a renal biopsy in IgAN [9].

24.2.5 Differential Diagnosis

24.2.5.1 Differentiating Between Causes of Isolated Non-visible Haematuria

Urine microscopy in non-visible haematuria due to glomerular disease will typically show dysmorphic red cells, and there may also be red cell casts. Non-visible haematuria in glomerulonephritis is often also accompanied by proteinuria, and there may also be pre-existing evidence of renal disease with a reduced GFR and development of hypertension.

The three main differential diagnoses of persistent isolated non-visible haematuria due to glomerular disease are:

1. IgA nephropathy
2. Alport syndrome
3. Thin basement nephropathy

Features that may help distinguish between these disorders include:

- Episodes of visible haematuria – this may occur in IgAN or Alport syndrome but is uncommon in thin basement membrane disease.
- Family history
  - Alport syndrome is associated with a family history of end-stage renal disease and deafness. It is most commonly X-linked (80%) but may be autosomal recessive (15%) and rarely autosomal dominant (5%).
  - Thin basement nephropathy is commonly inherited in an autosomal dominant manner.
  - A family history of IgAN is uncommon.

Differentiation between these three disorders does however ultimately require a renal biopsy. As the likelihood of the biopsy altering the clinical management of a patient with isolated non-visible haematuria is low, many nephrologists would elect not to biopsy this patient group. The prognosis for most patients with isolated non-visible haematuria is good, although patients with IgAN and Alport syndrome may later develop progressive kidney disease, heralded by the development of proteinuria and renal impairment. Therefore, these patients require long-term follow-up. Thin basement membrane disease typically has a more benign course; however, patients with a COL4A3 or COL4A4 mutation will have a disease course similar to patients with hereditary nephritis.

24.2.5.2 Other Causes of Recurrent Visible Haematuria

Recurrent visible haematuria in the over 40s should always raise the suspicion of a urinary tract malignancy, and it is essential initial investigations exclude this as a cause of the haematuria. In terms of IgA nephropathy, visible haematuria classically occurs around *1–3 days* after an upper respiratory tract infection, whereas in post-streptococcal glomerulonephritis it classically occurs around *2 weeks* after streptococcal infection.

24.2.5.3 Differential Diagnosis of Mesangial IgA Deposition on Renal Biopsy

The four principle differential diagnoses of mesangial IgA deposition are:

1. IgA nephropathy (renal-limited disease).
2. IgA vasculitis (Henoch-Schönlein purpura nephritis – there will be manifestations of an extra-renal vasculitis affecting skin, joints, gut).
3. Lupus nephritis (mesangial deposition of IgA, along with other immunoglobulin classes and complement, is a feature of lupus nephritis, but the distinctive clinical and serologic features usually make this diagnosis obvious).
4. IgA-dominant postinfectious glomerulonephritis (often associated with methicillin-sensitive and methicillin-resistant *Staphylococcus aureus* infection. This disease is marked by severe glomerular changes on renal biopsy, nephrotic range proteinuria and rapid decline in renal function with many patients developing irreversible ESRD).

24.2.5.4 Secondary IgAN

Mesangial IgA deposition may occur secondary to a number of other diseases, and the renal biopsy appearances are often indistinguishable from primary IgAN [10]. The course of the renal disease is however typically very different with most patients rarely progressing to end-stage renal disease.

Diseases associated with mesangial IgA deposition include:

- Chronic liver disease, particularly alcoholic liver disease (possibly due to impaired clearance of IgA immune complexes by the liver).
- HIV/AIDS (associated with a high serum IgA concentration).
- Coeliac disease (no clear explanation but a gluten-free diet may lead to a short-term reduction in proteinuria and improvement in renal function).
- IgA vasculitis (Henoch-Schönlein purpura).
- IgA-dominant postinfectious glomerulonephritis

Treatment of secondary forms of IgAN should be based on treating the primary disease.

24.2.6 Treatment

Despite advances in the understanding of the pathogenesis of IgAN, there is still no intervention available to prevent production of nephritogenic IgA, its glomerular deposition or progression of the disease. Current treatment strategies therefore centre on modulating downstream immune and inflammatory events and can be thought of as generic strategies applicable to all chronic glomerulonephritides. These generic strategies include:

- Weight optimisation
- Smoking cessation
- Blood pressure control
- Renin-angiotensin blockade
- Dietary sodium restriction

Weight optimisation, smoking cessation and blood pressure control can aid IgAN patients independent of their cardiovascular benefits. Extremes of body mass index and smoking both correlate with poorer outcomes in IgAN, with smoking exerting its negative effects in a dose-dependent manner [11]. As with all other causes of CKD, cardiovascular risk factors should also be addressed.

Several randomised controlled trials have shown that renin-angiotensin blockade, with an angiotensin converting enzyme inhibitor (ACEi) or angiotensin II receptor blocker (ARB) to control hypertension and reduce proteinuria to less than 0.5 g/day, is beneficial in slowing progression of proteinuric IgAN [12–14]. Although the combination of using both ACEi and ARB reduces proteinuria in IgAN, long-term beneficial effects on renal survival have not been demonstrated, and the safety of this approach has been questioned by the ONTARGET study [15]. Dietary salt restriction may augment the antiproteinuric effects of renin-angiotensin blockade [16].

24.2.6.1 The Patient with Non-visible Haematuria and <0.5 g/Day Proteinuria

No specific therapy is advised, although long-term follow-up in primary care is recommended to identify development of increasing proteinuria, renal impairment and hypertension.

24.2.6.2 The Patient with Recurrent Visible Haematuria

No specific treatment is required for patients with recurrent visible haematuria, and there is no role for prophylactic antibiotics. Tonsillectomy reduces the frequency of acute episodes of visible haematuria where tonsillitis is the provoking factor and has its advocates, especially in Japan, as a treatment to reduce progression to

ESRD. However, data from clinical trials is conflicting, and larger studies are needed before any conclusion can be drawn regarding the role of tonsillectomy in preserving long-term renal function in IgAN [17–19].

24.2.6.3 The Patient with >0.5 g/Day Proteinuria and Slowly Progressive IgAN

The risk of progressive IgAN correlates with the degree of proteinuria. Patients with less proteinuria have improved renal survival, and reducing proteinuria improves prognosis, according to registry data [20].

There are a number of patients who will continue to have proteinuria in excess of 0.5 g/day and declining renal function despite maximal tolerated doses of ACEi and/or ARB. In these patients, current evidence regarding additional therapy is controversial. The 2012 KDIGO guidelines for management of IgAN state that the following should not be offered to treat IgAN:

- Tonsillectomy
- Mycophenolate mofetil
- Cyclophosphamide
- Azathioprine
- Anticoagulation or antiplatelet agents

Mycophenolate mofetil (MMF) has been studied in a number of small RCTs, but results have been inconsistent, and a recent meta-analysis of these trials concluded that there is no significant benefit of MMF in reducing proteinuria in IgAN [21]. There does appear to be a disparity between the effect of MMF in Caucasian (no effect) and Asian (some renoprotection reported) IgAN, and further studies are needed to evaluate this further. In Asia MMF is often used as a steroid-sparing agent in situations where corticosteroids are planned to be used.

Based on low-quality evidence, the 2012 KDIGO guidelines suggest the following may be considered:

- Corticosteroids
- Fish oil

The KDIGO guidelines for the management of glomerulonephritis are currently being reviewed, and new guidelines are expected in 2020–2021.

Corticosteroids

A 6-month course of corticosteroids in patients with persistent proteinuria >1 g/day despite renin-angiotensin blockade and preserved renal function (eGFR > 50 ml/min) may slow progression of renal decline.

Pozzi et al. showed that treatment of patients with IgAN with a course of corticosteroids reduced proteinuria and prevented progression to ESRD over a 10-year period [22]. However, the high-dose corticosteroid regimen used 'pulsed' methylprednisolone (1 g daily for 3 days at induction and at the beginning of months 2 and 4), and alternate day prednisolone (0.5 mg/kg) for 6 months is felt by many clinicians to carry unacceptable toxicity, although only minor side effects were reported in this study. Additionally, renin-angiotensin blockade was only used in a minority of patients, although usage was evenly distributed between both treatment groups.

Studies by Manno et al. and Lv et al. evaluated the effect of corticosteroids plus renin-angiotensin blockade versus renin-angiotensin blockade alone in patients with preserved renal function (mean eGFR around 100 ml/min/1.73m^2) and proteinuria (>1 g/day) [23, 24]. In the study by Manno et al., a combination of an ACEi and 6 months oral prednisolone led to fewer patients reaching the combined end point of doubling of serum creatinine or ESRD compared to those treated with ACEi alone. Lv et al. demonstrated a reduction of patients reaching the primary endpoint of a 50% increase in serum creatinine in the combination ACEi and corticosteroid arm compared to ACEi alone (3% versus 24%).

These studies have, however, been criticised as they required ACEi and ARBs to be stopped prior to commencement in the trial, and therefore there was a lack of a suitable run-in period to allow for optimisation of supportive treatment prior to administration of corticosteroids. Patients entering into the corticosteroid treatment arm may therefore have benefited from optimised supportive care alone. The STOP-IgAN trial was designed to address this [14]. Patients with persistent proteinuria >0.75 g/d despite optimised supportive management for 6 months were randomised to either continue supportive therapy or receive additional immunosuppressive therapy (corticosteroids if eGFR ≥60 mL/min, corticosteroids plus cyclophosphamide/azathioprine if eGFR <60 ml/min). The STOP-IgAN study demonstrated:

- A third of patients in the run-in phase with 'persistent proteinuria' responded to rigorous application of supportive management alone, demonstrating the value of this strategy.
- While corticosteroids induced remission of urine abnormalities in more patients than those receiving supportive therapy alone (17% vs 5%), this did not translate into renoprotection as there was no difference in eGFR at the end of the study between the groups.
- Immunosuppressive therapies were associated with more adverse effects, including weight gain and infections.

In parallel, results from the TESTING study that compared methylprednisolone against placebo highlighted the significant side effects associated with immunosuppression in IgAN [25]. In this study recruitment was halted because of the high levels of opportunistic infections in the treatment arm. Intriguingly, there did appear to be a renoprotective effect of methylprednisolone, albeit at a dose that was shown to be toxic. A low-dose TESTING study is currently recruiting.

The STOP-IgAN and TESTING studies highlight the importance of having a full and frank discussion with the patient before embarking on immunomodulatory therapy, particularly corticosteroids.

Fish Oil

Conflicting data exists regarding the use of prescription strength fish oil. Fish oil is widely prescribed for IgAN in certain centres and appears to be safe, although tolerability is a major issue due to a fishy odour to the breath and perspiration and increased flatulence. In one RCT patients randomised to receive fish oil (compared to placebo) had better preservation of renal function over a median of 6-year follow-up [26]. However, this finding has not been reproduced in other RCTs, and a meta-analysis concluded that the available evidence is inconclusive [27]. Further studies in this area are required before a definitive recommendation can be made.

Experimental and Future Therapies

There has been a welcome rise in the number of clinical trials being undertaken to evaluate the safety and efficacy of novel and repurposed therapeutic agents in IgAN [28]. Agents currently being evaluated include:

- Mucosal targeted corticosteroid: targeted release formulation (TRF)-budesonide
- B cell-directed therapies: blisibimod, atacicept, belimumab
- Spleen tyrosine kinase inhibition: fostamatinib
- Complement inhibitors: Lectin pathway (OMS721), alternative pathway (LNP023), final common pathway (avacopan)

Perhaps the most well advanced of these in 2018 is TRF-budesonide which was evaluated in the phase 2 NEFIGAN trial which investigated the efficacy and safety of TRF-budesonide in 150 patients with IgAN. Treatment with TRF-budesonide significantly reduced proteinuria above that achieved with supportive management and reported no statistically significant differences in adverse effects between the treatment and placebo group. However, the stringency with which supportive measures were optimised in this study was unclear, as the decline in eGFR observed in the placebo group was greater than what would otherwise be expected [29].

The Patient with Acute Kidney Injury

IgAN patients who develop AKI and fail to respond to simple supportive measures should have a renal biopsy to differentiate between the two most common causes of AKI in IgAN:

Acute Tubular Necrosis with Intratubular Erythrocyte Casts

This requires supportive care only. Recovery to baseline GFR is usual; however, some patients may be left with irreversible tubulointerstitial scarring.

Crescentic IgAN

Patients with rapidly progressive loss of renal function, active glomerular inflammation and crescents on renal biopsy and no significant chronic damage may be treated in a similar way to other forms of crescentic GN, i.e. high-dose corticosteroids, cyclophosphamide and plasma exchange. Evidence for treatment of crescentic IgAN is derived from small case series and retrospective data [30]. Response to treatment is worse in crescentic IgAN than in other forms of crescentic glomerulonephritis, and renal survival is estimated to be only 50% at 1 year and 20% at 5 years. This may be the consequence of significant pre-existing chronic damage at the time of a crescentic transformation, thereby reducing the chances of a response to immunosuppression.

24.2.6.4 The Patient with Nephrotic Syndrome

Nephrotic syndrome in association with mesangial IgA deposition may be due to advanced glomerular scarring as a consequence of longstanding IgAN and therefore reflect established CKD or an acute podocyte injury indistinguishable from minimal change disease, occurring in a patient with coincidental IgAN. A renal biopsy is clearly the key to distinguishing between these two extremes, and in particular electron microscopy should be performed. Patients with IgAN, nephrotic syndrome, minimal glomerular scarring and podocyte effacement typical of minimal change disease should be treated as minimal change disease [31].

24.2.7 Follow- up

Patients with IgAN and CKD1-3 may be followed up in primary care. On discharge from nephrology services, clear guidance should be provided to the primary care physician regarding frequency of renal function, urine dipstick and blood pressure monitoring. This will be dictated by local guidelines; however, we would suggest this should be performed at least annually.

Patients with CKD 4–5 require follow-up in a nephrology clinic.

24.2.8 Special Circumstances in IgAN

24.2.8.1 Transplantation

Recurrence of IgA deposition following renal transplantation is common, affecting up to 50% of grafts within 5 years [32]. Graft failure due to recurrence of IgAN is however relatively rare and most often occurs in patients who have had a rapidly progressive course in their native kidneys, e.g. crescentic IgAN. There is little evidence that the choice of post-transplant immunosuppression protocol modifies the risk of recurrence although analysis of the Australia and New Zealand Dialysis and Transplant Registry (ANZDATA) suggests recurrent disease is more common in patients who undergo steroid withdrawal [33]. There is also no evidence to support any specific therapy regimen once recurrent IgAN has been diagnosed following renal transplantation although a single-centre retrospective analysis has suggested that ACEi/ARB treatment may reduce the rate of decline of allograft function in recurrent IgAN [34].

24.2.8.2 Pregnancy

As with other forms of glomerulonephritis, renal prognosis is worse in pregnancy (see Pregnancy and Renal Disease Chapter) when there is:

- Renal impairment (serum creatinine>150 μmol/L)
- Proteinuria (>1 g/day)
- Hypertension (on treatment or BP >140/90)

Patients should receive appropriate pre-conception counselling. ACEi and ARBs along with teratogenic immunosuppressive agents (e.g. cyclophosphamide, MMF) should be stopped prior to planned conception or at the earliest indication of pregnancy. Once pregnant, patients should receive careful monitoring in a combined renal-obstetric clinic.

24.3 IgA Vasculitis (Henoch-Schönlein Purpura)

24.3.1 Introduction

IgA vasculitis (IgAV) is the commonest form of systemic vasculitis in children and is characterised by IgA deposition in affected blood vessels. The renal lesion is a mesangioproliferative glomerulonephritis with mesangial IgA deposition, indistinguishable from IgAN.

24.3.2 Clinical Features

IgAV is a multisystem disease. The classical tetrad of symptoms in IgAV are:

1. Palpable purpuric rash
2. Arthritis/arthralgia
3. Abdominal pain
4. Renal disease

Symptoms appear in any order and can evolve over a few days to weeks [35].

The *rash* is classically distributed on extensor surfaces, with sparing of the trunk and face. It typically appears in crops and is symmetrically distributed (◘ Fig. 24.5).

Polyarthralgia is common and is usually transient and migratory. There is often swelling and tenderness but without chronic destructive damage.

Gastrointestinal symptoms often appear after the rash. Abdominal pain is usually mild and transient but may be severe and lead to gastrointestinal haemorrhage, bowel ischaemia, intussusception and perforation (◘ Fig. 24.6).

Renal involvement typically manifests as transient asymptomatic invisible haematuria and/or proteinuria. More severe complications, such as nephrotic syndrome or rapidly progressive deterioration of renal function, occur less frequently and tend to occur in adults more often than in children.

Rarely, IgAV can be associated with other features more commonly seen with the ANCA-associated small-vessel vasculitides including pulmonary haemorrhage (◘ Fig. 24.7).

The renal disease that accompanies IgAV is often transient and self-limiting in nature, with haematuria or

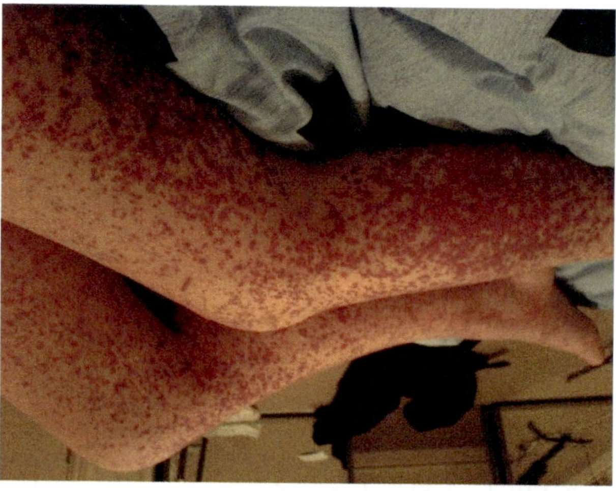

◘ **Fig. 24.5** Typical appearance of the leukocytoclastic vasculitis of IgA vasculitis

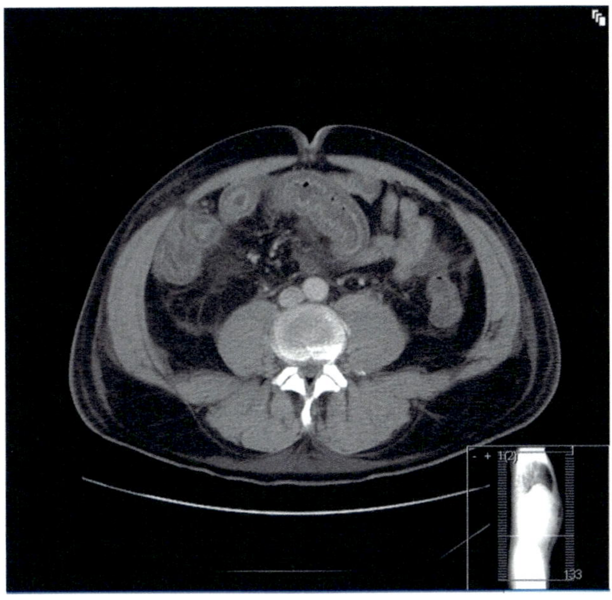

Fig. 24.6 CT scan showing marked oedema of the small bowel in a patient with IgA vasculitis and abdominal pain

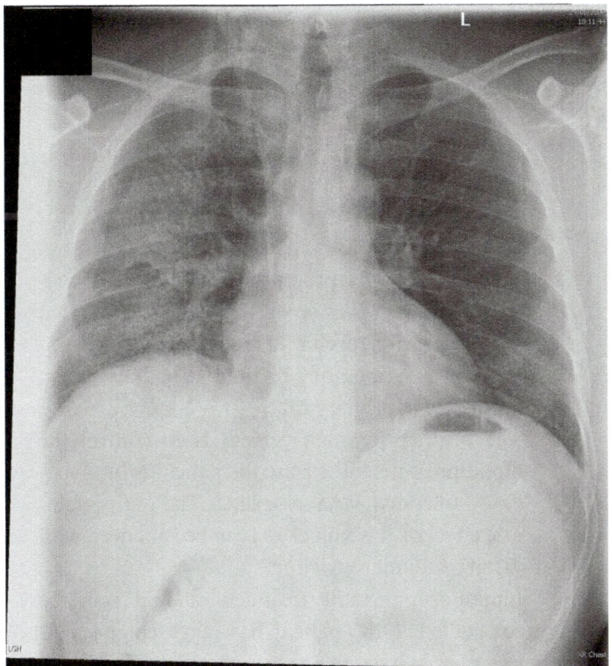

Fig. 24.7 Extensive right-sided alveolar shadowing due to pulmonary haemorrhage in a patient with IgA vasculitis and crescentic glomerulonephritis (note the vascular catheter in place for dialysis and plasma exchange)

proteinuria typically resolving within weeks of presentation. AKI due to crescentic IgAV is more common than crescentic IgAN (although still uncommon) and tends to occur early in the course of the disease. The long-term outlook of patients who have transient IgAV is generally very good. However, up to 10% of patients with IgAV will develop ESRD [36].

24.3.3 Epidemiology

Although IgAV may occur at any age, it is most common during childhood, between the ages of 3 and 15. There is a slight male predominance. Most cases occur in the winter, spring and autumn months, which may be due to its association with preceding upper respiratory tract infections.

24.3.4 Aetiopathology

The exact cause of IgAV remains unknown. There are, however, many factors which suggest there are common pathogenic pathways operating in IgAV and IgAN [37]:

- Identical twins have been reported, where one presents with IgAN and the other with IgAV.
- IgAV developing on a background of IgAN is described in both adults and children.
- Both diseases share similar findings on renal biopsy and also changes in the complement of serum IgA1 *O*-glycoforms.
- There is a similar association between mucosal infection and presentation of disease.

24.3.5 Diagnosis

In children, a clinical diagnosis is often made without the need to proceed to a renal biopsy.

In adults, the differential diagnoses are wide and include other forms of small-vessel vasculitides such as ANCA-associated vasculitis, cryoglobulinaemia and systemic lupus erythematosus. These should be distinguished on the basis of clinical, serological and histological findings.

24.3.5.1 Investigations

General Investigations

Assessment of renal function, urinary protein excretion and renal size should be undertaken in all patients under investigation for glomerulonephritis, as should an assessment of cardiovascular risk.

As in IgAN raised serum IgA levels are found in 30–50% of adult patients with IgAV. Serum IgA levels do not correlate with disease activity or severity. Similarly, changes in the levels of poorly galactosylated IgA1 *O*-glycoform levels are not sensitive or specific enough to be used as a diagnostic test in IgAV.

Confirmation of the clinical diagnosis requires histological evidence of IgA deposition in affected tissue, often the skin or kidney.

Skin Biopsy

Biopsy of the skin rash typically shows a leukocytoclastic vasculitis. IgA immune complex deposition can be seen by immunofluorescent staining; however, detection of IgA is unreliable, and if a tissue diagnosis is required, then a renal biopsy should be performed if there is clear evidence of nephritis.

Renal Biopsy

Renal biopsy is usually reserved for adult cases of diagnostic uncertainty, or when a child presents with more severe renal involvement. Histological features are the same as those for IgAN; however, in IgAV there will also be extra-renal manifestations of disease [38].

24.3.6 Treatment

There is little evidence to guide the treatment of IgAV, and what is available is derived from small retrospective case series [36].

Patients with haematuria, proteinuria and mild renal impairment do not require any specific treatment, and the nephritis usually resolves spontaneously.

In patients with crescentic IgAV, typified by a rapidly progressive loss of renal function, and systemic manifestations of small-vessel vasculitis, there is limited evidence that high-dose corticosteroids may be beneficial. Regimes include pulsed methylprednisolone followed by a 3-month course of oral prednisolone [39, 40]. Although there is some evidence that mycophenolate mofetil may act as a possible steroid-sparing agent [41], there is currently no conclusive evidence that other immunosuppressive agents, including cyclophosphamide or azathioprine, or other interventions such as plasmapheresis have any beneficial effect on outcome.

24.3.7 Follow- up

Patients should be monitored as for IgAN. As with other forms of glomerular disease, those patients with persistent proteinuria are at highest risk of developing progressive CKD [42].

24.3.8 Special Circumstances in IgAV

24.3.8.1 Transplantation

Renal transplantation is the treatment of choice in patients with ESRD due to IgAV. As with IgAN recurrence of mesangial IgA deposition may occur, while loss of the graft due to recurrence is less common and tends to occur in patients who had an aggressive original disease [43, 44]. Renal transplantation should be delayed for 12 months from date of presentation.

24.3.8.2 Pregnancy

Evidence from cohort studies of children with IgAV suggest that all women with a history of IgAV should be carefully monitored during pregnancy, even if they had no evidence of renal disease at the time of diagnosis as they are increased risk of developing hypertension and proteinuria [45].

Tips, Tricks and Pitfalls

1. IgAN incidence varies geographically and among races, being most common in those from East Asia.
2. Patients over the age of 40 with persistent haematuria should be investigated for urinary tract malignancy.
3. Familial IgAN is very rare, and therefore a family history of haematuria should trigger investigation for a type IV collagen disorder (Alport or thin membrane disease).
4. IgAN is a slowly progressive disease, and long-term follow-up is essential to detect development of hypertension, decline in renal function or development/worsening of proteinuria. Follow-up can take place in primary care.
5. The priority for management is to control the blood pressure and ensure the patient is on maximally tolerated RAS blockade. The antiproteinuric effect of RAS blockade can be enhanced with dietary sodium restriction.
6. Immunosuppressant treatment should only be considered if the patient has persistent proteinuria>1 g/24 h despite measures outlined in [5] and has preserved renal function (eGFR>20 ml/min/1.73m^2)
7. There is no evidence for the use of azathioprine, mycophenolate mofetil or cyclophosphamide in IgAN patients.
8. The evidence for efficacy of corticosteroids is very weak, while the frequency of adverse events is predictable and high. Any decision to start corticosteroids in IgAN MUST involve a full and frank

discussion with the patient describing the risks and benefits of such a treatment strategy, accepting that adverse events are much higher when the eGFR is 20–50 ml/min/1,73m^2.

9. Although serum immunoglobulin A levels are increased in up to 50% of patients with IgAN and IgAV, it is not a marker of disease activity or severity.
10. Most cases of IgAV are self-limiting, and immunosuppression should be reserved for patients with rapidly deteriorating renal function.

Case Study

Case 1

A 27-year-old female originally from China was found to have isolated non-visible haematuria on routine screening for employment insurance. She was otherwise well. The eGFR was 78 ml/min/1.73m^2. There was no family history of renal disease or deafness. Over the proceeding 6 months, the haematuria persisted, blood pressure and eGFR remained normal and there was no proteinuria on urine dipstick testing. She was discharged back to primary care, with the advice to have her blood pressure, urinalysis and renal function checked annually. Indications to refer back to nephrology were development of overt proteinuria or hypertension and decline in eGFR<60 ml/min/1.73m^2.

This case illustrates a typical presentation of likely IgA nephropathy in which observation alone is appropriate. In the majority of cases, the condition follows a benign course, and re-evaluation is only needed if signs of progressive disease manifest. A biopsy was unlikely to alter management.

Case 2

A 19-year-old male presented with visible haematuria 2 days following an episode of tonsillitis. The visible haematuria resolved spontaneously, but there was persistent non-visible haematuria and proteinuria. Quantification of the proteinuria revealed 1.34 g/24 h. The eGFR was 69 ml/min/1.73m^2. Blood pressure was 118/65 mmHg. A renal biopsy confirmed a diagnosis of IgA nephropathy. An ACE inhibitor was commenced (ramipril 2.5 mg/d) with step-wise dose escalation to the maximally tolerated dose (ramipril 7.5 mg/d). He could not tolerate ramipril 10 g/d due to symptomatic hypotension. 4 months following presentation, he was reassessed: 0.41 g/24 h proteinuria, eGFR 60 ml/min/1.73m^2, BP 107/63 mmHg. Non-visible haematuria persisted.

This case highlights the value of conservative measures and ACE inhibition in patients with IgA nephropathy to reduce proteinuria and the risk of disease progression. There was no indication in this case for immunosuppression. This patient requires long-term annual follow-up either in nephrology or primary care.

Case 3

A 12-year-old female presented with generalised arthralgia and a florid purpuric rash affecting her lower limbs. There was no fever, neck stiffness or photophobia. Platelet count was normal. Urinalysis demonstrated non-visible haematuria and proteinuria. eGFR was 58 ml/min/1.73m^2. IgA vasculitis was suspected. She was given analgesia for the arthralgia. It was not felt necessary to perform either a skin or renal biopsy as the rash was typical for IgA vasculitis. With conservative management the rash and arthralgia resolved over 2 weeks, and the haemoproteinuria over the proceeding 4 weeks.

This case is typical for presentation of IgA vasculitis in the paediatric population, where a clinical diagnosis is normally made and a biopsy only performed if symptoms/urine abnormalities persist. In most cases of IgA vasculitis no specific treatment is required.

Conclusion

IgAN and IgAV with nephritis are characterised by mesangial IgA deposition. Globally, IgAN is the most commonly reported glomerulonephritis. IgAN can follow a benign course; however, 30% of patients progress to end-stage renal disease within 20 years of diagnosis. Management centres on controlling the blood pressure and minimising proteinuria with maximally tolerated blockade of the renin-angiotensin system. The evidence for immunosuppression in IgAN is extremely weak. A number of clinical trials of novel therapeutic agents are underway and may provide new options for managing IgAN over the next 5 years. IgA vasculitis (Henoch-Schönlein purpura) is a rare form of vasculitis related to IgA nephropathy. It is a multisystem disease that can affect the skin, joint, gut and kidney. IgA vasculitis can be self-limiting, and management with immunosuppression is usually instigated only in cases of rapid renal function decline.

Chapter Review Questions

1. Do all patients with persistent non-visible haematuria require a renal biopsy?
2. Should renin-angiotensin system antagonists be initiated in all patients with IgAN?
3. Does recurrent visible haematuria require specific treatment?
4. Is there a role for corticosteroids in IgAN?
5. Should you treat all cases of IgA vasculitis with immunosuppression?

Answers

1. No. In the absence of hypertension, proteinuria or a deteriorating renal function, the prognosis of non-visible haematuria is good, and thus a biopsy will not alter management. Urological investigations must be considered in the context of persistent haematuria in patients above the age of 40.
2. No. Renin-angiotensin blockade should be employed when the patient has hypertension and/or overt proteinuria (>0.3 g/24 h). There is no indication to start these drugs in a patient with isolated non-visible haematuria and normal blood pressure.
3. No. Visible haematuria will settle spontaneously. There is no evidence for benefit of prophylactic antibiotics. In Japan where tonsillectomy is routinely performed for IgAN, it is reported that the frequency of episodes of visible haematuria reduced post-tonsillectomy; however, there is no evidence this is related to improved renal survival, and therefore tonsillectomy is not recommended outside Japan.
4. Corticosteroids should only be considered in patients with persistent proteinuria >1 g/24 h despite 3 months of both maximally tolerated RAS blockade and blood pressure control (BP < 130/80 mmHg) and an eGFR>20 ml/min/1.73m^2. If corticosteroids are being considered, there must be a full and frank discussion with the patient about the potential risks (multiple) and variable evidence of benefit of using corticosteroids in IgAN.
5. No. IgA vasculitis tends to remit spontaneously in most cases in children and adults. Indications for immunosuppression include a rapidly progressive glomerulonephritis (RPGN), pulmonary haemorrhage and gastrointestinal haemorrhage secondary to gut involvement. The immunosuppressive regimen used is usually the same as that used to treat ANCA-associated vasculitis.

References

1. D'Amico G. Natural history of idiopathic IgA nephropathy: role of clinical and histological prognostic factors. Am J Kidney Dis. 2000;36(2):227–37.
2. Suzuki K, Honda K, Tanabe K, Toma H, Nihei H, Yamaguchi Y. Incidence of latent mesangial IgA deposition in renal allograft donors in Japan. Kidney Int. 2003;63(6):2286–94.
3. Barratt J, Smith AC, Feehally J. The pathogenic role of IgA1 O-linked glycosylation in the pathogenesis of IgA nephropathy. Nephrology (Carlton). 2007;12(3):275–84.
4. Barratt J, Feehally J. Primary IgA nephropathy: new insights into pathogenesis. Semin Nephrol. 2011;31(4):349–60.
5. Topham PS, Harper SJ, Furness PN, Harris KP, Walls J, Feehally J. Glomerular disease as a cause of isolated microscopic haematuria. Q J Med. 1994;87(6):329–35.
6. Roberts ISD, Cook HT, Troyanov S, Alpers CE, Amore A, Barratt J, et al. The Oxford classification of IgA nephropathy: pathology definitions, correlations, and reproducibility. Kidney Int. 2009;76(5):546–56.
7. Cattran DC, Coppo R, Cook HT, Feehally J, Roberts ISD, Troyanov S, et al. The Oxford classification of IgA nephropathy: rationale, clinicopathological correlations, and classification. Kidney Int. 2009;76(5):534–45.
8. Coppo R, Troyanov S, Camilla R, Hogg RJ, Cattran DC, Cook HT, et al. The Oxford IgA nephropathy clinicopathological classification is valid for children as well as adults. Kidney Int. 2010;77(10):921–7.
9. Trimarchi H, Barratt J, Cattran DC, Cook HT, Coppo R, Haas M, et al. Oxford Classification of IgA nephropathy 2016: an update from the IgA Nephropathy Classification Working Group. Kidney Int. 2017;91(5):1014–21.
10. Pouria S, Barratt J. Secondary IgA nephropathy. Semin Nephrol. 2008;28(1):27–37.
11. Orth SR, Stöckmann A, Conradt C, Ritz E, Ferro M, Kreusser W, et al. Smoking as a risk factor for end-stage renal failure in men with primary renal disease. Kidney Int. 1998;54(3):926–31.
12. Coppo R, Peruzzi L, Amore A, Piccoli A, Cochat P, Stone R, et al. IgACE: a placebo-controlled, randomized trial of angiotensin-converting enzyme inhibitors in children and young people with IgA nephropathy and moderate proteinuria. J Am Soc Nephrol. 2007;18(6):1880–8.
13. Praga M, Gutiérrez E, González E, Morales E, Hernández E. Treatment of IgA nephropathy with ACE inhibitors: a randomized and controlled trial. J Am Soc Nephrol. 2003;14(6):1578–83.
14. Rauen T, Eitner F, Fitzner C, Sommerer C, Zeier M, Otte B, et al. Intensive supportive care plus immunosuppression in IgA nephropathy. N Engl J Med. 2015;373(23):2225–36.
15. Mann JFE, Schmieder RE, McQueen M, Dyal L, Schumacher H, Pogue J, et al. Renal outcomes with telmisartan, ramipril, or both, in people at high vascular risk (the ONTARGET study): a multicentre, randomised, double-blind, controlled trial. Lancet. 2008;372(9638):547–53.
16. Suzuki T, Miyazaki Y, Shimizu A, Ito Y, Okonogi H, Ogura M, et al. Sodium-sensitive variability of the antiproteinuric efficacy of RAS inhibitors in outpatients with IgA nephropathy. Clin Nephrol. 2009;72(4):274–85.
17. Piccoli A, Codognotto M, Tabbi M, Favaro E, Rossi B. Influence of tonsillectomy on the progression of mesangioproliferative glomerulonephritis. Nephrol Dial Transplant. 2010;25(8):2583–9.

18. Wang Y, Chen J, Wang Y, Chen Y, Wang L, Lv Y. A meta-analysis of the clinical remission rate and long-term efficacy of tonsillectomy in patients with IgA nephropathy. Nephrol Dial Transplant. 2011;26(6):1923–31.
19. Feehally J, Coppo R, Troyanov S, Bellur SS, Cattran D, Cook T, et al. Tonsillectomy in a European cohort of 1,147 patients with IgA nephropathy. Nephron. 2016;132(1):15–24.
20. Reich HN, Troyanov S, Scholey JW, Cattran DC. Remission of proteinuria improves prognosis in IgA nephropathy. J Am Soc Nephrol. 2007;18(12):3177–83.
21. Xu G, Tu W, Jiang D, Xu C. Mycophenolate mofetil treatment for IgA nephropathy: a meta-analysis. Am J Nephrol. 2008;29(5):362–7.
22. Pozzi C, Andrulli S, Del Vecchio L, Melis P, Fogazzi GB, Altieri P, et al. Corticosteroid effectiveness in IgA nephropathy: long-term results of a randomized, controlled trial. J Am Soc Nephrol. 2004;15(1):157–63.
23. Manno C, Torres DD, Rossini M, Pesce F, Schena FP. Randomized controlled clinical trial of corticosteroids plus ACE-inhibitors with long-term follow-up in proteinuric IgA nephropathy. Nephrol Dial Transplant. 2009;24(12):3694–701.
24. Lv J, Zhang H, Chen Y, Li G, Jiang L, Singh AK, et al. Combination therapy of prednisone and ACE inhibitor versus ACE-inhibitor therapy alone in patients with IgA nephropathy: a randomized controlled trial. Am J Kidney Dis. 2009;53(1):26–32.
25. Lv J, Zhang H, Wong MG, Jardine MJ, Hladunewich M, Jha V, et al. Effect of oral methylprednisolone on clinical outcomes in patients with IgA nephropathy: the TESTING randomized clinical trial. JAMA. 2017;318(5):432–42.
26. Donadio JV, Grande JP, Bergstralh EJ, Dart RA, Larson TS, Spencer DC. The long-term outcome of patients with IgA nephropathy treated with fish oil in a controlled trial. Mayo Nephrology Collaborative Group. J Am Soc Nephrol. 1999;10(8):1772–7.
27. Strippoli GFM, Manno C, Schena FP. An "evidence-based" survey of therapeutic options for IgA nephropathy: assessment and criticism. Am J Kidney Dis. 2003;41(6):1129–39.
28. Yeo SC, Liew A, Barratt J. Emerging therapies in immunoglobulin a nephropathy. Nephrology (Carlton). 2015;20(11):788–800.
29. Fellström BC, Barratt J, Cook H, Coppo R, Feehally J, de Fijter JW, et al. Targeted-release budesonide versus placebo in patients with IgA nephropathy (NEFIGAN): a double-blind, randomised, placebo-controlled phase 2b trial. Lancet. 2017;389(10084):2117–27.
30. Tumlin JA, Hennigar RA. Clinical presentation, natural history, and treatment of crescentic proliferative IgA nephropathy. Semin Nephrol. 2004;24(3):256–68.
31. Lai KN, Lai FM, Ho CP, Chan KW. Corticosteroid therapy in IgA nephropathy with nephrotic syndrome: a long-term controlled trial. Clin Nephrol. 1986;26(4):174–80.
32. Floege J. Recurrent IgA nephropathy after renal transplantation. Semin Nephrol. 2004;24(3):287–91.
33. Clayton P, McDonald S, Chadban S. Steroids and recurrent IgA nephropathy after kidney transplantation. Am J Transplant. 2011;11(8):1645–9.
34. Courtney AE, McNamee PT, Nelson WE, Maxwell AP. Does angiotensin blockade influence graft outcome in renal transplant recipients with IgA nephropathy? Nephrol Dial Transplant. 2006;21(12):3550–4.
35. Saulsbury FT. Henoch-Schönlein purpura in children. Report of 100 patients and review of the literature. Medicine (Baltimore). 1999;78(6):395–409.
36. Sanders JT, Wyatt RJ. IgA nephropathy and Henoch-Schönlein purpura nephritis. Curr Opin Pediatr. 2008;20(2):163–70.
37. Davin JC, Ten Berge IJ, Weening JJ. What is the difference between IgA nephropathy and Henoch-Schönlein purpura nephritis? Kidney Int. 2001;59(3):823–34.
38. Gedalia A. Henoch-Schönlein purpura. Curr Rheumatol Rep. 2004;6(3):195–202.
39. Niaudet P, Habib R. Methylprednisolone pulse therapy in the treatment of severe forms of Schönlein-Henoch purpura nephritis. Pediatr Nephrol. 1998;12(3):238–43.
40. Balow JE. Renal vasculitis. Curr Opin Nephrol Hypertens. 1993;2(2):231–7.
41. Ren P, Han F, Chen L, Xu Y, Wang Y, Chen J. The combination of mycophenolate mofetil with corticosteroids induces remission of Henoch-Schönlein purpura nephritis. Am J Nephrol. 2012;36(3):271–7.
42. Sano H, Izumida M, Shimizu H, Ogawa Y. Risk factors of renal involvement and significant proteinuria in Henoch-Schönlein purpura. Eur J Pediatr. 2002;161(4):196–201.
43. Ponticelli C, Glassock RJ. Posttransplant recurrence of primary glomerulonephritis. Clin J Am Soc Nephrol. 2010;5(12):2363–72.
44. Meulders Q, Pirson Y, Cosyns JP, Squifflet JP, van Ypersele de Strihou C. Course of Henoch-Schönlein nephritis after renal transplantation. Report on ten patients and review of the literature. Transplantation. 1994;58(11):1179–86.
45. Ronkainen J, Nuutinen M, Koskimies O. The adult kidney 24 years after childhood Henoch-Schönlein purpura: a retrospective cohort study. Lancet. 2002;360(9334):666–70.

Resources and Patient Information

The International IgA nephropathy network. https://www.iigann.com/.

Vasculitis UK. http://www.vasculitis.org.uk/about-vasculitis/henoch-schonlein-purpura.

ANCA-Associated Systemic Small-Vessel Vasculitis

Jennifer Scott and Mark A. Little

Contents

M. Harber (ed.), *Primer on Nephrology*, https://doi.org/10.1007/978-3-030-76419-7_25

Learning Objectives

1. ANCA-associated vasculitis (AAV) is a rare autoimmune disease, which results in rapidly progressive kidney impairment and immune-mediated destruction of other organs. It is an important differential diagnosis of the 'pulmonary-renal syndrome'.
2. It is associated with the development of characteristic autoantibodies directed against epitopes on the myeloperoxidase or proteinase-3 molecules, which are abundant proteins in neutrophils and monocytes.
3. It is characterised by a necrotising pauci-immune small-vessel vasculitis, with a relapsing and remitting course.
4. Treatment involves immunosuppression to induce and maintain remission.
5. AAV is associated with increased morbidity and mortality, both as a consequence of the disease itself, and the toxic immunosuppression therapy required.

25.1 Introduction

The vasculitides are inflammatory disorders of blood vessels that can be classified as primary or secondary and as localised or systemic. Vasculitis may be localised (single-organ vasculitis) or affect several organ systems (systemic vasculitis).

The secondary vasculitides generally involve small blood vessels and hence can involve the glomerulus resulting in glomerulonephritis. Importantly, they are often associated with immune complex deposition in the vessel walls, which can be demonstrated on immunofluorescence (Table 25.1).

The primary systemic vasculitides are rare inflammatory disorders affecting blood vessels of varying sizes in multiple organs without an identifiable cause. The American College of Rheumatology (ACR) criteria or Chapel Hill Consensus Conference definitions are widely used to describe the systemic vasculitis; the latter characterises these according to the predilection for the size of the smallest blood vessel affected, i.e. small, medium or large vessel [1]. Small-vessel vasculitides primarily affect blood vessels smaller than arteries, i.e. arterioles, venules and capillaries, and are of particular interest to nephrologists given their propensity to cause glomerular inflammation and acute kidney injury. Of note, medium or large vessels may also be affected in microscopic polyangiitis (MPA) or granulomatosis with polyangiitis (GPA, formerly known as Wegener's granulomatosis); the syndrome is defined by the size of the smallest vessel affected.

Henoch-Schönlein purpura (IgA vasculitis), cryoglobulinaemic vasculitis, anti-glomerular basement membrane (anti-GBM) disease and hypocomplementemic urticarial vasculitis (anti-C1q vasculitis) are primary small-vessel vasculitides that are associated with immune complex deposition. MPA, GPA and eosinophilic granulomatosis with polyangiitis (EGPA, formerly known as Churg-Strauss syndrome) are primary small-vessel vasculitides that are termed 'pauci-immune' as they are not associated with immune complex deposition. They share similar pathological features and a clinical association with anti-neutrophil cytoplasmic antibodies (ANCA) and are therefore termed ANCA-associated vasculitides (AAV). Although rare, they are the most frequent cause of rapidly progressive glomerulonephritis (RPGN) and are important as they are commonly fatal or result in severe organ damage when left untreated. Despite the improvement in outcomes with the use of immunosuppression, AAV still carries a 2.7-fold increased risk of death [2] and, untreated, has an 80% 1-year mortality [3]. AAV is associated with increased morbidity, specifically due to infection, cardiovascular disease and malignancy, both in association with the disease itself and its toxic treatments.

This chapter focuses on the clinical presentation, pathogenesis, diagnosis and management of ANCA-associated vasculitis (AAV).

Table 25.1 Causes of secondary vasculitis

Disease category	Examples
Connective tissue disease	Rheumatoid arthritis, systemic lupus erythematosus (SLE), Behcet's disease
Infection	Bacterial endocarditis, Neisseria meningitides, hepatitis B and C (often secondary to cryoglobulins), HIV
Drugs	Drug-induced immune complex vasculitis, serum sickness vasculitis
Malignancy	Carcinoma, lymphoproliferative and myeloproliferative disorders

25.2 Clinical Presentation

AAV is a rare systemic autoimmune disease, which can affect multiple organ systems. It is characterised by necrotising small-vessel vasculitis with a relapsing and remitting course.

The clinical presentation of a patient with AAV therefore varies depending on the pattern of organ involvement (◘ Table 25.2). There are four distinct clinicopathological syndromes associated with AAV [4]:

1. Granulomatosis with polyangiitis (GPA)
2. Microscopic polyangiitis (MPA)
3. Eosinophilic granulomatosis with polyangiitis (EGPA)
4. Single-organ AAV (e.g. renal-limited AAV)

Classification of systemic vasculitis has traditionally been confusing with little consensus between centres. Criteria for diagnosis were developed by the American College of Rheumatology (ACR) in 1990, but these do not recognise a small-vessel subtype of polyarteritis nodosa [5]. The Chapel Hill Consensus Conference (CHCC) proposes definitions for AAV (GPA, MPA and EGPA) that were primarily based on histology (not always practical to obtain), and not intended for use as diagnostic criteria in the clinical setting [1, 4]. The CHCC were revised in 2012 and now recognise the contribution of the ANCA test to the classification [4].

◘ Table 25.2 Clinical manifestations of ANCA-associated systemic vasculitis

Organ system	Clinical manifestations
Kidney	Microscopic haematuria, proteinuria, progressive renal impairment, oligoanuric renal failure
Respiratory tract	Cough, haemoptysis, pulmonary infiltrates, cavitating lung granulomata, alveolar capillaritis with pulmonary haemorrhage
ENT	Nasal crusting, sinusitis, hearing loss (conductive and sensorineural), laryngotracheal granulomatous inflammation causing subglottic stenosis, chondritis of the auricle or nasal cartilage
Skin	Purpuric rash, painful erythematous nodules, focal skin necrosis/ulceration
Musculoskeletal	Myalgia and migratory arthritis
Ocular	Episcleritis, scleritis, orbital granuloma, proptosis
Gastrointestinal	Gastrointestinal bleeding, abdominal pain
Nervous system	Mononeuritis multiplex, peripheral neuropathy, stroke
Constitutional symptoms	Fever, general malaise, weight loss and anorexia

Although the ACR and CCHC criteria are widely used, there was no consensus on how they should be applied clinically, when diagnosing a patient with suspected AAV. A consensus methodology has since been published with a proposed diagnostic algorithm, which incorporates the ACR and CHCC definitions [6] (◘ Fig. 25.1).

A non-specific prodrome is common in AAV, which can precede other organ manifestations of the disease by several months. The constellation of signs and symptoms are often misidentified, resulting in delayed and incorrect diagnoses. Constitutional symptoms include fever, anorexia, weight loss and general malaise, reflecting the underlying inflammatory nature of this disease. A purpuric vasculitic rash and arthralgia are also very common and often associated with symmetrical, migratory small joint polyarthritis (◘ Fig. 25.2).

The kidneys and lungs are the two organ systems most commonly and extensively injured in AAV. Hence, AAV is an important cause of the 'pulmonary-renal syndrome'. Vasculitis in the kidney may progress to a necrotising crescentic glomerulonephritis with haematuria (often with urinary red cell casts) and rapidly progressive renal failure. Lung involvement is varied depending on the particular clinicopathological syndrome (see below) but in its most severe form leads to development of pulmonary capillaritis with consequent alveolar haemorrhage, an important cause of early mortality in this condition (◘ Fig. 25.3).

The different clinicopathological syndromes of AAV may present with typical clinical features and different patterns of organ involvement at the time of diagnosis (◘ Table 25.3):

- *GPA* is classically associated with granulomatous inflammation of the upper respiratory tract, which produces a variety of ENT symptoms including nasal crusting, hearing loss (conductive and sensorineural), sinusitis and occasionally a saddle-shaped nasal deformity as a result of necrotising inflammation in the cartilaginous nasal septum. Seventy-seven percent of patients with GPA have upper respiratory tract symptoms at the time of diagnosis compared to 29% of patients with MPA [7]. Ultimately, 86% of patients with GPA will develop renal disease at some point in their disease although this is less common at presentation than in MPA (see below).
- If there is no clinical evidence of granulomatous inflammation or eosinophilic vasculitis, the AAV syndrome is termed *MPA*. It is important to note that granulomatous inflammation may emerge at a later time point, at which stage the diagnosis will

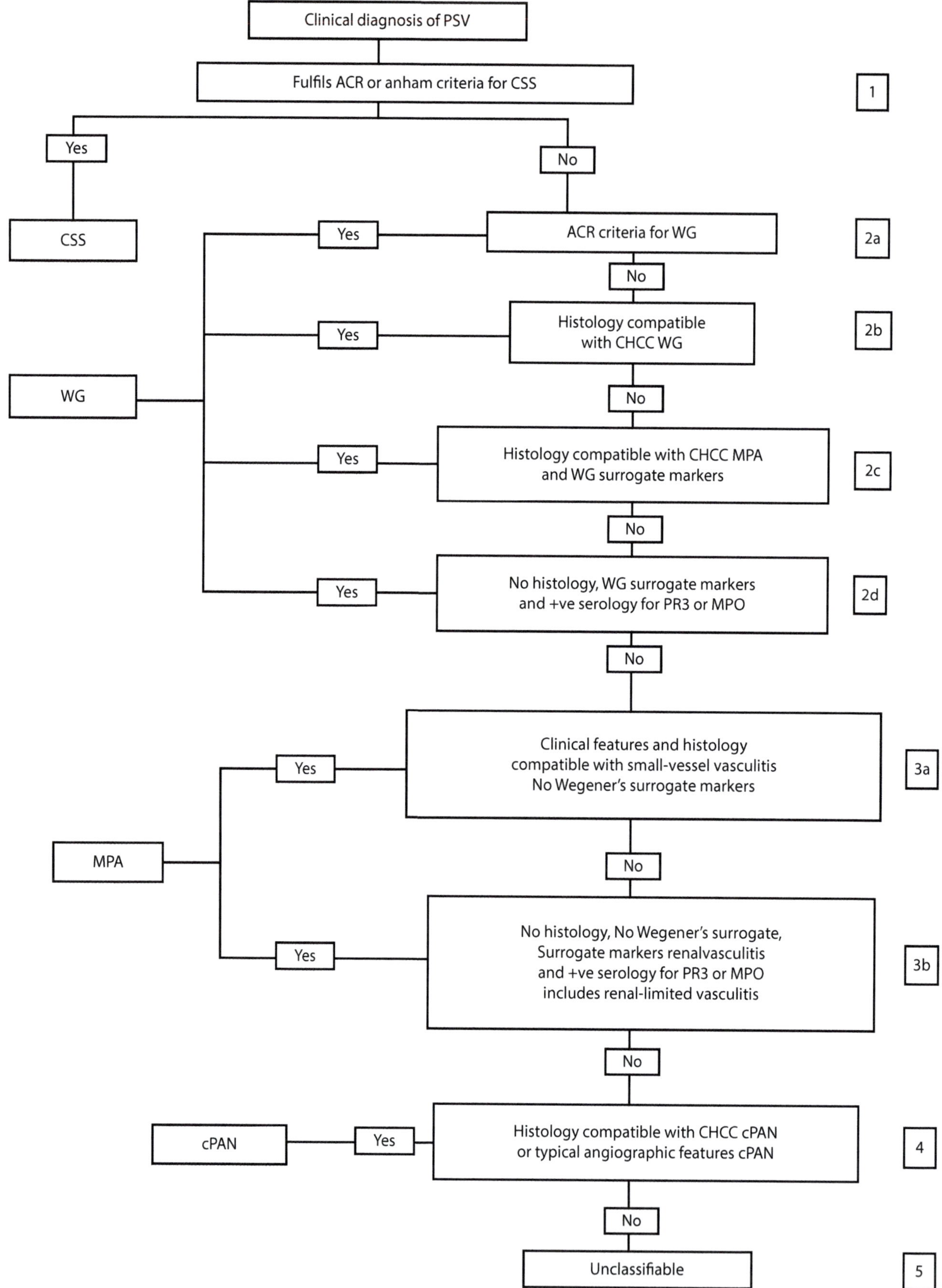

Fig. 25.1 EMEA algorithm for pragmatic classification of systemic small-vessel vasculitis. (Adapted from Watts et al. [6])

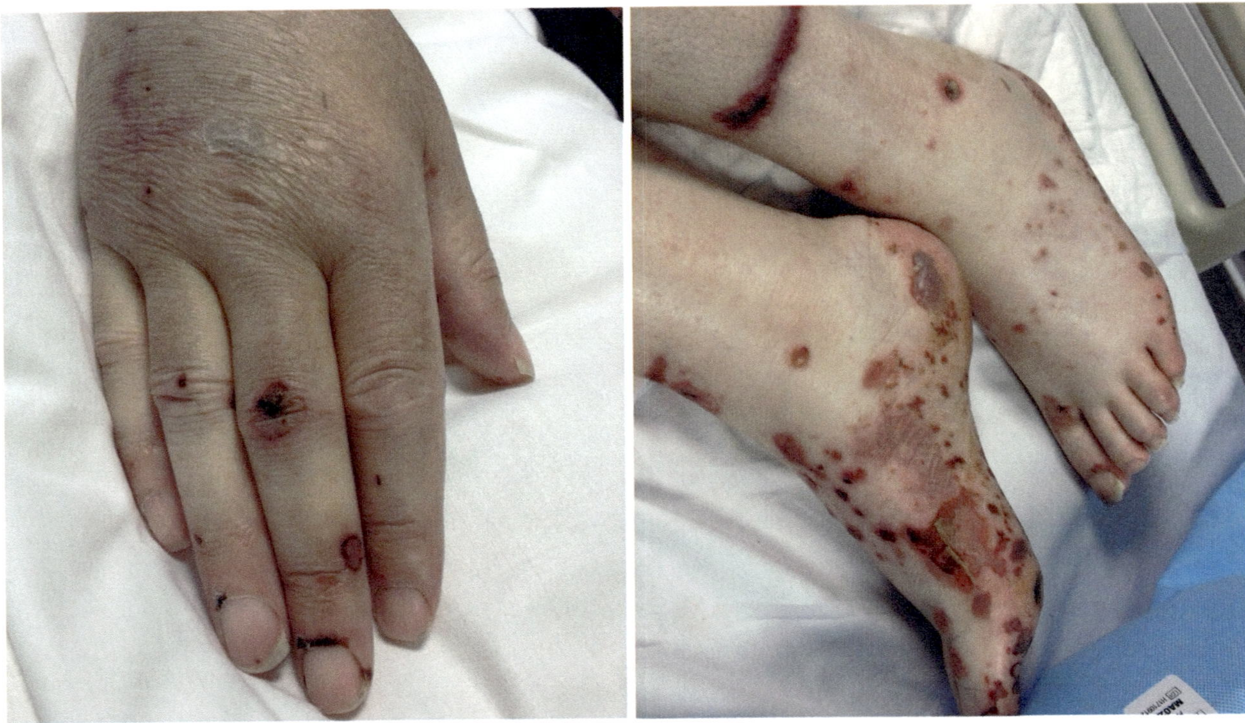

Fig. 25.2 Leukocytoclastic skin vasculitis typical of small-vessel vasculitis; in the context of AAV, this would be pauci-immune, differentiating it from Henoch-Schönlein purpura

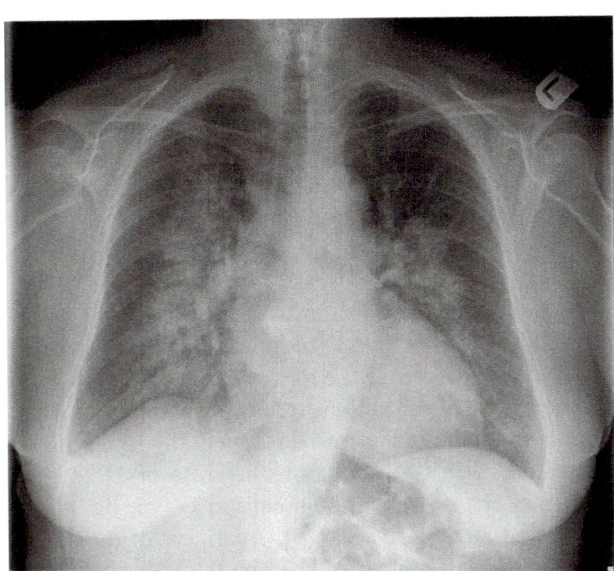

Fig. 25.3 Chest X-ray showing alveolar haemorrhage in a patient with MPO-ANCA vasculitis

change to GPA. Extra-renal organ involvement in MPA is generally less common than in GPA. Patients tend to present with renal disease, which is more common at the time of diagnosis in MPA than in GPA (92% vs 77%), possibly as they present later in the disease because the renal disease is largely asymptomatic until advanced.

- Some patients may present with disease limited to the kidney (causing a pauci-immune crescentic glomerulonephritis). This renal-limited disease is considered MPA, unless evidence of granulomatous inflammation develops subsequently.
- *EGPA* displays clinical features of (1) late onset asthma and wheeze (>95%) with (2) variable peripheral blood eosinophilia accounting for >10% of leukocytes (100%, although disappears rapidly with treatment of asthma with glucocorticoids so may be missed) and evidence of (3) end-organ damage secondary to vasculitis. Rhinitis, with nasal polyposis and hearing loss is often present. End-organ disease is manifested as skin granulomas or palpable purpura (60%), mononeuritis multiplex (75%), pauci-immune crescentic glomerulonephritis (25%) and cardiac disease (pericarditis/myocarditis/valvular lesions/coronary arteritis, 40%). It is not uncommon for patients to have chest symptoms with eosinophilia for months or years before developing overt vasculitis. Renal involvement is less common compared to GPA and MPA, and the association with ANCA is much weaker, although those with renal disease tend to have positive ANCA serology.

25

Table 25.3 Characteristics of AAV clinicopathological syndromes

Characteristic	GPA	MPA	EGPA
Granulomatosis	+	–	+
Eosinophilia	–	–	+
Asthma	–	–	+
Upper respiratory tract (URT)/ ENT symptoms	+ (77%)	+ (29%)	+ (nasal polyps common)
Lower respiratory tract (LRT) symptoms (e.g. pulmonary haemorrhage)	+ (85%)	+	+
Renal Involvement	77%	92%	Less common (25%, bad prognostic sign)
Other common features			Skin (60%), mononeuritis multiplex (75%), cardiac involvement (40%), GI
Limited subtypes	URT/LRT/eye	Renal-limited	URT/LRT
ANCA subtype	PR3 (–ve in 40% of limited GPA)	MPO (70%), PR3 can occur	MPO (30–38%) [8], increased ANCA positivity with presence of renal disease
Incidence	Increased in the UK vs China/Japan (14.3 vs 2.1/ million adults)	Increased in China/Japan vs the UK (18.2 vs 6.5/million adults)	2.4 million/year (least common)

25.3 Epidemiology

The estimated overall annual incidence of AAV is 13–20 cases/million with a prevalence of 46–184 cases per million [9]. Most studies indicate a Caucasian preponderance [9]. Incidence increases with age with a peak age of onset between 65 and 74 years [10]. Studies suggest that, in contrast to other autoimmune diseases, AAV does not display a female predominance [10], and in fact, most studies report a slight male majority [9].

Some epidemiological studies indicate an increasing incidence of GPA and MPA [9]. The reasons for this are not clear but are almost certainly partly due to increased awareness of the disease, better case definition and enhanced availability of ANCA testing. Clinician experience suggests that there appears to be a seasonal peak in incidence in Spring, but this is not uniformly supported by formal epidemiological studies [11].

The incidence of clinicopathological syndromes of AAV differs according to geographical location. GPA is more common in Northern Europe, whereas MPA is more common in the south [12], suggesting an impact of latitude on pathogenesis. There is also variability in the distribution of AAV subtypes by location. GPA predominates in the UK, while MPA is more common in Japan [13]. EGPA is significantly less common than GPA and MPA, with an annual incidence of 0.5–2.0/ million [14]. The environmental triggers of AAV are not completely understood but are thought to include infections, weather, radiation, silica, drugs and pollutants [9].

Although AAV is a rare disease, it is the most common cause of RPGN and accounts for 4% of all cases of end-stage renal disease (ESRD). It carries a significantly greater mortality rate than other autoimmune diseases and many malignancies. It is generally fatal if left untreated, with a 1-year mortality rate of 80%. Even with modern treatment regimens, 15% of die within 1 year and 36% by 5 years [15]. Treatment of the disease with immunosuppressive therapy is a double-edged sword as it is associated with a high rate of adverse events. One study demonstrated that death within 1 year of presentation was three times more likely to be attributable to an adverse event related to treatment than to active vasculitis [16].

The costs of managing this group of patients are disproportionate to the frequency of the condition. The average first year costs to the NHS of treating AAV is £8000 and £4000/annum thereafter (D Jayne, unpublished data).

25.4 Diagnosis of ANCA-Associated Vasculitis

The diagnosis of AAV requires a combination of clinical, radiological, serological and pathological features. The histological hallmark is necrotising small-vessel vasculitis, and this is still considered necessary for definitive diagnosis.

Renal involvement with rapidly progressive glomerulonephritis (RPGN) carries a high risk of progression to irreversible end-stage renal failure and is associated with a high risk of patient death if not treated promptly. It is therefore essential to make an early and accurate diagnosis of AAV so that appropriate treatment can be administered without delay. Rapid loss of renal function in association with clinical features of glomerulonephritis should be considered a medical emergency.

All patients with suspected RPGN should therefore have appropriate urgent serological investigation and be considered for renal biopsy to obtain histological confirmation of the diagnosis. If the kidneys are not involved, every effort should be made to obtain a sample of affected tissue for histological analysis, although this is seldom rewarding in cases of isolated sino-nasal disease, in whom the often observed absence of a positive ANCA test may lead to significant diagnostic uncertainty.

25.4.1 Use of ANCA Testing in Diagnosis

25.4.1.1 Indirect Immunofluorescence

ANCA were originally described by the staining pattern produced by autoantibodies to neutrophil cytoplasmic proteins, as detected by indirect immunofluorescence (IIF) using ethanol-fixed neutrophils. Two distinct patterns of staining were identified: cytoplasmic staining (c-ANCA) and perinuclear (p-ANCA) staining. Additional ANCA-staining patterns are now recognised including 'atypical c-ANCA' (with homogenous flat cytoplasmic fluorescence) and combination p- and c-ANCA staining.

c-ANCA positivity correlates with antibodies to proteinase-3 (PR3), a serine protease enzyme, and is primarily associated with GPA. p-ANCA positivity correlates with antibodies to myeloperoxidase (MPO), a lysosomal peroxidase enzyme, and is associated with MPA and Churg-Strauss syndrome, in general. Overlap between ANCA specificity and clinicopathological syndromes exists. Both the PR3 and MPO antigens are expressed in neutrophil and monocyte cytoplasmic granules.

Staining of the perinuclear region by p-ANCA in patients with AAV and anti-MPO antibodies is an artefact of ethanol fixation. This makes the neutrophil granule membranes permeable and results in a redistribution of positively charged cytoplasmic granular proteins, i.e. MPO, onto the surface of the negatively charged nucleus, resulting in a perinuclear-staining pattern, which outlines the neutrophil multilobed nucleus. By comparison, patients with PR3 antibodies have a c-ANCA-staining pattern where the nucleus appears as a 'ghost', and the cytoplasm between the lobes of the neutrophil nucleus is accentuated (◘ Fig. 25.4 and ◘ Table 25.4).

This artefactual perinuclear staining caused by antibodies to MPO in ethanol-fixed neutrophils may closely resemble the staining pattern produced by anti-nuclear (ANA) antibodies, resulting in a 'false-positive' p-ANCA result. Equally, p-ANCA-positive patients who are also strongly positive for ANA antibodies may have the subtle perinuclear staining masked by strong homogenous nuclear staining produced by the ANA antibody.

25.4.1.2 Enzyme-Linked Immunosorbent Assay (ELISA)

Historically, any suspected new AAV diagnosis was initially screening using IIF and then confirmed with ELISA for PR3 and MPO, to confirm the identity of the autoantigen. However, in recent years, immunosorbent assays with improved sensitivity and specificity are commercially available and can be run on automated platforms. Therefore, an International Consensus Statement in 2017 recommended performing a high-quality ELISA for PR3- and MPO-ANCAs as the preferred screening tool for suspected cases of AAV (GPA or MPA), without the routine use of IIF [17]. This approach has not yet fully entered clinical practice. Immunosorbent assays have an additional quantitative benefit over prior binary results from IIF. The likelihood ratio for AAV increases with increasing levels of PR3- and MPO-ANCAs [18]. High pretest probability is also important to avoid false positives – clinical indications for ANCA testing are listed in ◘ Table 25.5 [17]. As no test is absolute, in patients with a high clinical suspicion and a negative ANCA result, a diagnosis of AAV cannot be excluded. A significant number of patients with small-vessel vasculitis, particularly those with disease limited to the nose and sinuses (and about 10% of those with renal disease), are negative for ANCA. Testing by another method (e.g. another immunoassay or IIF) can increase sensitivity in this situation [17]. It is also recommended to perform biopsies of the affected organs in these seronegative patients, to improve the diagnostic yield. The recommended pathway is documented in ◘ Fig. 25.5.

Although the International Consensus Statement only refers to ANCA testing in suspected GPA or MPA, positive ANCA tests are also found in 30–38% of

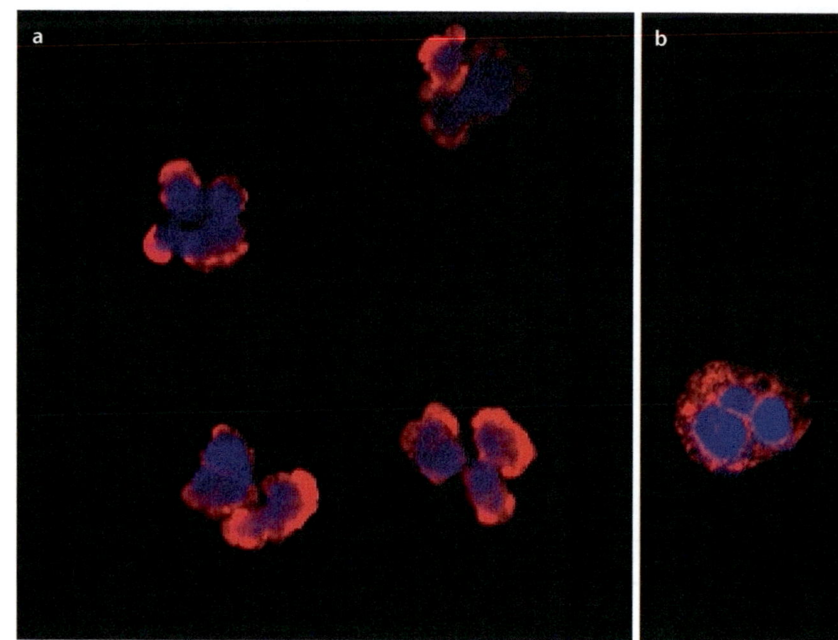

Fig. 25.4 Indirect immunofluorescence staining of neutrophils by antibodies contained within the serum of patients with (**a**) anti-myeloperoxidase antibody-positive MPA displaying a p-ANCA-staining pattern and (**b**) anti-proteinase-3 antibody positive GPA, displaying a c-ANCA-staining pattern

Table 25.4 Potential pitfalls with use of indirect immunofluorescence ANCA testing in clinical practice

Test finding	Potential pitfalls
Positive p-ANCA	In addition to anti-MPO antibodies, p-ANCA may be observed in the presence of antibodies to lactoferrin, elastase, cathepsin G, catalase, bactericidal permeability inhibitor, lysozyme and beta-glucuronidase
Positive p-ANCA	May be confused with a positive ANA
Positive p-ANCA	Associated with non-vasculitic conditions, e.g. inflammatory bowel disease, cystic fibrosis, autoimmune hepatitis
Negative ANCA with clinical vasculitis	Relatively common with ENT-limited disease; 10% of multisystem disease is also ANCA-negative
Positive c-ANCA	Usually indicative of systemic vasculitis but may be seen in chronic cocaine use with nasal septum destruction

Table 25.5 Clinical indications for ANCA testing [17]

Clinical indications
Glomerulonephritis
Pulmonary haemorrhage, especially pulmonary-renal syndrome
Cutaneous vasculitis with systemic features
Multiple lung nodules
Chronic destructive upper airway disease
Chronic sinusitis/otitis
Subglottic tracheal stenosis
Mononeuritis multiplex or other peripheral neuropathy
Retro-orbital mass
Scleritis

patients with EGPA [8], and in 20–35% of patients with anti-GBM disease [19], the majority of which are specific for MPO.

False-positive ANCA results can occur in patients with (1) chronic infection (e.g. tuberculosis, hepatitis C and infective endocarditis), (2) malignancies (e.g. non-Hodgkin lymphoma), (3) gastrointestinal disease (e.g. inflammatory bowel disease, primary sclerosing cholangitis and inflammatory liver diseases) and, most notably, (4) exposure to certain drugs (e.g. cocaine, hydralazine, propylthiouracil and minocycline). Therefore, decisions about treatment should be based on clinical, pathological and radiological features, in addition to serological testing, rather than relying on the ANCA results alone. Of particular concern is the exclusion of infections noted above prior to commencement of treatment, due to the harmful consequences of immunosuppression in this cohort.

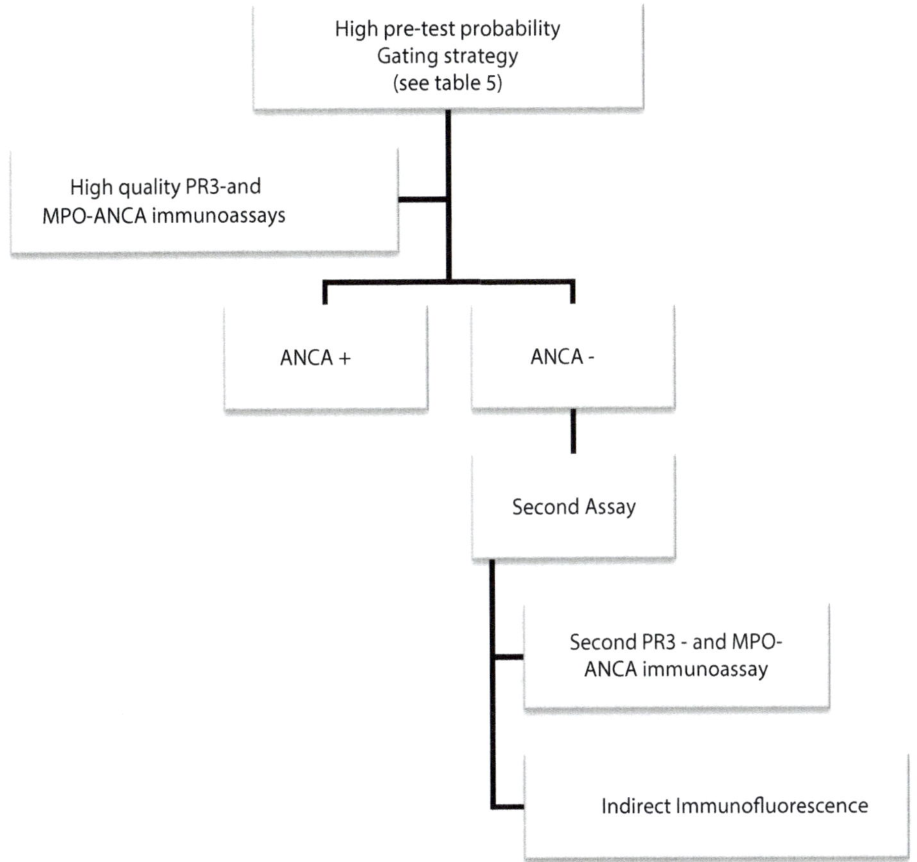

Fig. 25.5 Recommended diagnostic algorithm. (Adapted from Bossuyt et al. [17])

25.4.1.3 Renal Biopsy

A positive MPO- or PR3-ANCA result, in the context of clinical evidence of RPGN with active urinary sediment, provides sufficient evidence to diagnose probable AAV and initiate treatment in a timely fashion. However, renal biopsy is the gold standard for diagnosis and is useful to:

1. Confirm the diagnosis of pauci-immune focal necrotising glomerulonephritis (i.e. associated with the paucity of immune deposits on immunofluorescence and/or electron microscopy).
2. Establish the activity and extent of glomerulonephritis.
3. Assess the degree of chronic irreversible glomerular, interstitial and tubular damage, all of which will influence management with respect to the choice and intensity of induction immunosuppressive therapy.

25.5 Classification of Disease Severity

At presentation, patients should have a clear assessment of disease severity in order to guide appropriate induction therapy. The EULAR recommendations [20] on the management of AAV suggest that disease severity should be assessed at diagnosis. This has recently been simplified into three categories 'non-organ-threatening disease', 'organ or life-threatening disease' and 'rapidly progressive renal failure or pulmonary haemorrhage'. Immunosuppression regimens for induction and maintenance of remission, in patients with AAV, are dependent on the degree of disease severity. Refractory disease is defined as progressive disease, unresponsive to initial therapy – there are particular management recommendations with regard to this disease subgroup (see management section).

During follow-up it is important that patients' symptoms are attributed correctly to either current disease activity or organ damage in order to guide appropriate treatment. Given the rarity of AAV, patients should ideally receive expert assessment from specialists in dedicated vasculitis centres using standardised assessment tools to assess disease activity and damage, i.e. The Birmingham Vasculitis Activity Score (BVAS) and the Vasculitis Damage Index (VDI), respectively. (► http://golem.ndorms.ox.ac.uk/calculators/bvas.html)

25.6 Pathology

AAV is characterised histologically by necrotising small-vessel vasculitis. Renal involvement by the vasculitic process results in fibrinoid necrosis of glomerular capillaries and arterioles supplying the glomerular tuft with consequent inflammatory glomerular necrosis and crescent formation (◘ Fig. 25.6). Early lesions demonstrate segmental glomerular necrosis with or without adjacent small crescents. This may progress to global glomerular necrosis with large circumferential crescents in acute, severe disease. Glomerular capillaries rupture at sites of fibrinoid necrosis resulting in haemorrhage into Bowman's space, microscopic haematuria and the clinical appearance of urinary red cell casts. Patients with MPA tend to display more chronic, scarred lesions than those with GPA, perhaps reflecting the more frequent delay in diagnosis in the absence of granulomatous lesions.

Renal involvement in AAV is differentiated histologically from other causes of acute glomerulonephritis by the relative paucity or absence of glomerular deposits of immunoglobulin or complement demonstrated by immunofluorescent staining or electron microscopy (hence the term "pauci-immune" vasculitis). It is also often possible to distinguish severe glomerulonephritis due to AAV from that due to anti-glomerular basement membrane disease by the focal nature of the glomerular lesion: it is not uncommon to find an entirely normal appearing glomerulus adjacent to one that has been destroyed, whereas other causes of RPGN tend to affect all glomeruli equally. In addition, the glomerular lesions in AAV may vary significantly in age, with acute lesions interspersed with globally sclerosed glomeruli.

Fibrinoid necrosis of small vessels also occurs in other organs, resulting in tissue ischaemia, which causes a range of other clinical manifestations. For example, alveolar capillaritis in the lung may result in pulmonary

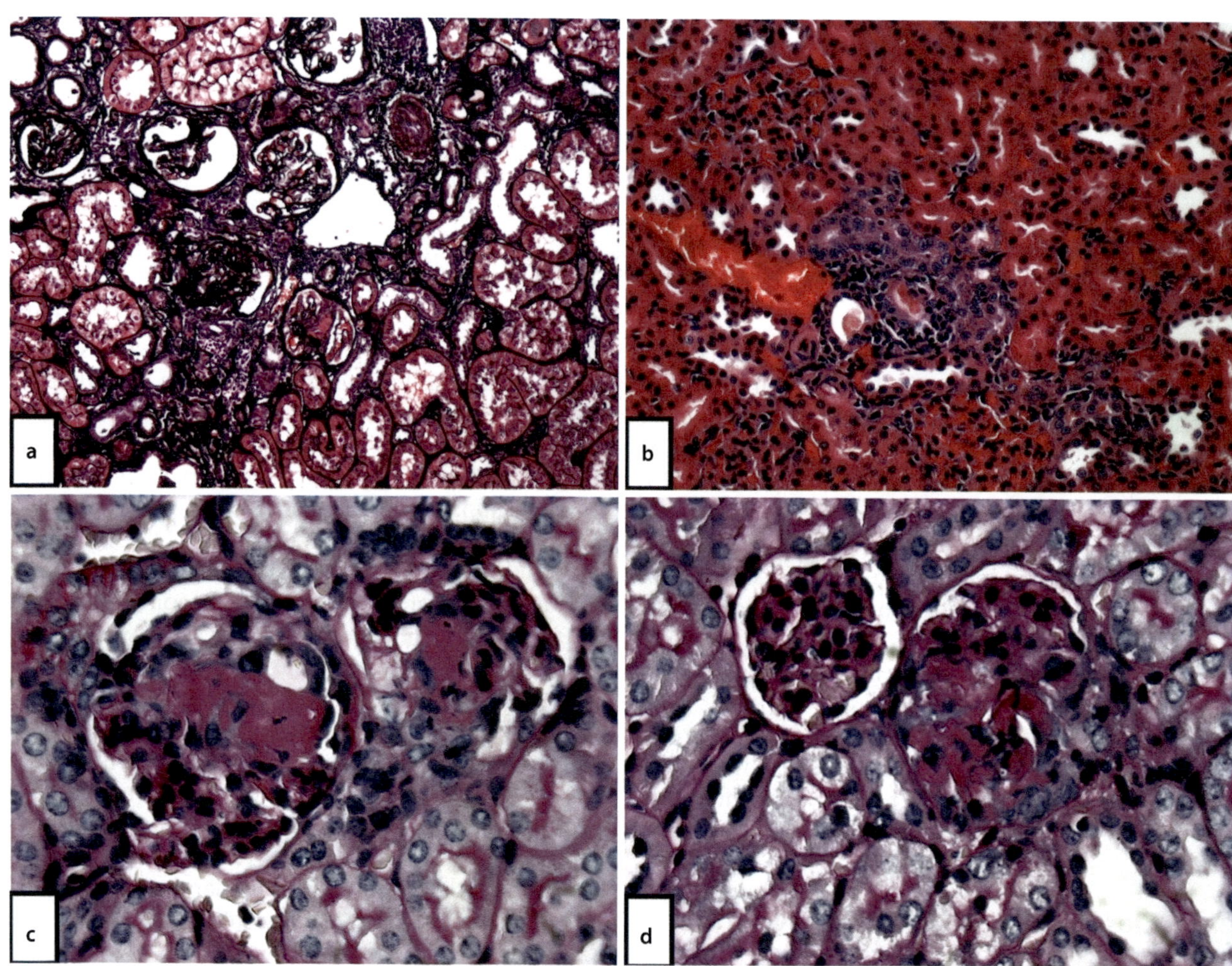

◘ **Fig. 25.6** (**a**) Focal necrotising glomerulonephritis with bridging interstitial scarring (×200, PAS-silver stain); (**b**) typical red cell tubular cast with associated inflammatory infiltrate (×200, H&E); (**c**) focal necrotising glomerulonephritis (×600, PAS); (**d**) crescentic glomerulonephritis (×600, PAS)

haemorrhage, inflammation of dermal venules in the skin causes palpable purpura and involvement of epineural arteries causes mononeuritis multiplex. The perivascular inflammatory infiltrate comprises neutrophils, macrophages and T cells; an infiltrate composed primarily of eosinophils ('eosinophilic vasculitis') is diagnostic of EGPA.

Patients with GPA and EGPA also display necrotising granulomatous inflammation. This is characterised by zones of tissue necrosis surrounded by a mixed inflammatory infiltrate consisting of neutrophils, lymphocytes, monocytes, macrophages and multinucleated giant cells. This inflammatory process causes tissue destruction in the upper respiratory tract in patients with GPA, resulting in sinusitis, conductive hearing loss and nasal deformity due to destruction of the cartilaginous nasal septum. Eosinophils may also be seen in the inflammatory infiltrate in these granulomatous lesions in both GPA and EGPA but are usually more prominent in the latter.

In 2010, the Berden histopathological classification system [21] was introduced to categorise glomerular lesions, in an effort to predict renal prognosis in a standardised fashion. Three categories of glomerular lesions – focal, crescentic and sclerotic – are determined by the percentage of normal glomeruli, cellular crescents and globally sclerotic glomeruli, respectively. The fourth category, mixed, comprises biopsies without a predominant glomerular phenotype. Tissue should be assessed under light microscopy and scored for glomerular lesions in the following order: ≥50% globally sclerotic, ≥50% normal, ≥50% cellular crescents (◘ Fig. 25.7). Consensus exists with the best and worst prognosis associated with the focal and sclerotic class, respectively [22]. Prognosis of the crescentic and mixed forms varies across studies.

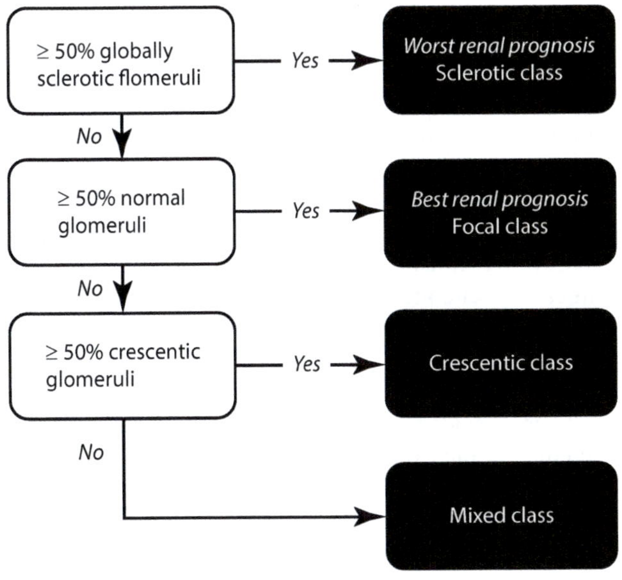

◘ **Fig. 25.7** Histopathological classification. (Adapted from [21])

25.7 Pathogenesis

The aetiology of AAV is not fully understood. Evidence suggests a complex interaction of polygenic susceptibility, epigenetic influences and environmental triggers. It is considered an autoimmune disease given the specific association with ANCA: autoantibodies directed against enzymes (PR3 and MPO) stored in the granules and lysosomes of neutrophils and monocytes.

25.7.1 Genetic Factors

A genome-wide association study (GWAS) demonstrated a strong genetic association with ANCA subtype (PR3/MPO), rather than the clinical syndrome [23] suggesting that they could potentially be distinct autoimmune syndromes. There is a tight association between polymorphisms in the HLA-DPB01 allele, as well as associations with the serpina1, prtn3 and ptpn22 genes, all of which are only seen within the PR3-ANCA-positive cohort [24].

25.7.2 Environmental Factors

Epidemiological data supports a strong environmental impact, although the exact nature of these triggers is unknown. Variables include seasonality, latitude (as discussed in epidemiology), infections and environmental dusts (e.g. silica).

25.7.2.1 Silica Exposure

Exposure to silica dust has been associated with several autoimmune disorders, including AAV. Case-control studies suggest that 22–46% of patients with AAV have previously been exposed to silica and there is an association between AAV with jobs such as farming, sandblasting, textile work and drilling, which are associated with high exposure to crystalline silica dust [25, 26]. Interestingly, there was a significant rise in the incidence of AAV in the aftermath of the Kobe earthquake in 1996, and this has been attributed to the release of large quantities of silica and other industrial dusts.

The mechanism by which silica triggers AAV is not known. It induces apoptosis of neutrophils in a dose-dependent manner [27], and silica may trigger an inflammatory reaction through accelerated apoptosis of neutrophils and alveolar macrophages. MPO released by neutrophils can be taken up by activated alveolar macrophages and may be presented to T- and B-lymphocytes resulting in the development of anti-MPO antibodies and, hence AAV [28].

25.7.2.2 Bacterial Infections

Bacterial infections, particularly with *Staphylococcus aureus*, have been associated with disease relapse in GPA. Patients with chronic nasal carriage of *S. aureus* are more likely to have disease relapses [29], and there is evidence that maintenance treatment with co-trimoxazole can reduce the frequency of disease relapse by 60% in patients with GPA and granulomatous inflammation of the upper respiratory tract [30].

There is some evidence that patients with PR3-ANCA vasculitis have antibodies to complementary PR3 (cPR3, the peptide translated from the antisense DNA strand of the PR3 gene), as well as to the autoantigen PR3, found in the granules of neutrophils [31], although these findings have not been reproduced in other studies [32]. Peptides from cPR3 share homology with peptides from *S. aureus* and other infectious pathogens. It has therefore been proposed that infection with *S. aureus* may induce cPR3 antibodies and, subsequently, PR3-ANCAs by means of an antibody-idiotypic network [28, 33].

Additional evidence for the role for infection and molecular mimicry with microbial peptides in the pathogenesis of AAV comes from the observation that 90% of patients with active focal necrotising glomerulonephritis (FNGN) have intermittent autoantibodies to lysosomal membrane protein-2 (LAMP-2). These antibodies cross-react with FimH, a bacterial adhesin which shares 100% homology with an epitope of human LAMP-2. Infections with fimbriated pathogens (e.g. *E. coli* and *K. pneumoniae*) may therefore induce production of autoantibodies to LAMP-2 through molecular mimicry. There are numerous other case reports describing a multitude of potential infectious triggers, such as *Enterococcus* and Epstein-Barr virus [9]; however, further evidence is required to assess causation.

25.7.2.3 Drugs

Several drugs have been associated with the development of ANCA and subsequent AAV, most notably propylthiouracil. Others include hydralazine, D-penicillamine, minocycline and cocaine. Most of these have potent epigenetic effects, which is likely to be the mechanism by which they increase risk of autoimmunity.

25.7.3 Role of ANCA in the Pathogenesis of AAV

There is increasing evidence from clinical, in vitro and in vivo studies that ANCA have a pathogenic role in the development of AAV. Numerous studies have demonstrated that ANCA activate neutrophils inappropriately and animal model work has proven that anti-MPO antibodies can cause systemic vasculitis in mice and rats.

Perhaps the most convincing evidence comes from a case report describing the development of pulmonary haemorrhage and glomerulonephritis associated with elevated MPO-ANCA titres in a neonate, thought to be caused by transplacental transfer of IgG MPO-ANCA from a mother with active MPA [34].

Disease activity correlates well with ANCA titres in some patients with AAV [35] with some longitudinal observational studies suggesting that clinical remission is associated with falling ANCA titres, and increasing ANCA titres predict clinical relapse with a sensitivity of 79% and a specificity of 68% [28]. This may provide supportive evidence of the pathogenic role of these antibodies, although much controversy exists in this area [28, 36–38]. At present, there is insufficient evidence to support the use of ANCA titre alone as a guide to therapy but rather as an adjunct to the clinical picture. Indeed, some patients can attain full clinical remission in the face of persistently elevated ANCA levels. Conversely, some patients may have significantly raised ANCA titres, with no clinical disease – this should trigger close observation for the onset of symptoms. ANCA titres are also useful in assessing possible relapse. Multiple studies demonstrate that disease relapse, in patients who are ANCA-positive at diagnosis, is associated with a persistent or renewed positive ANCA, in 80–100% of cases [39]. This is particularly the case in those with capillaritis (i.e. glomerulonephritis or alveolar haemorrhage); the RAVE trial demonstrated a rise in PR3-ANCA is associated with an increased risk of relapse in this patient group [40]. In addition, it is widely agreed that PR3-AAV is associated with a higher rate of relapse [39, 41]. However, ANCA titres must be interpreted in the context of other clinical, biochemical and histological parameters and therefore can be viewed as an 'alert signal'. Therefore, at present, the use of rising ANCA titres to guide treatment remains experimental [41].

There is evidence from randomised trials that plasma exchange (which removes circulating IgG ANCA) and rituximab (monoclonal anti-CD20 antibody which depletes peripheral B cells) are effective in treating severe AAV. Treatment with rituximab is associated with a decline in ANCA titres, and observational studies suggest that reconstitution of peripheral B cells may precede clinical relapse. The efficacy of these treatments, which are targeted at antibody removal, provides indirect evidence of the pathogenic role of ANCA in AAV.

25.8 Management

Morbidity and mortality is a result of both the destructive, inflammatory disease process itself and of the high-intensity immunosuppression required to induce and maintain remission of this disease. AAV, particularly GPA, is characteristically a relapsing disease with each relapse causing cumulative destructive inflammation and organ damage. Hence most patients with AAV require long-term immunosuppression to maintain remission, although the optimal duration of treatment is unknown.

Treatment of AAV is divided into two phases:

- *Induction* with high-intensity immunosuppression to induce remission as quickly as possible and avoid irreversible organ damage
- *Maintenance* of remission with lower-intensity immunosuppression to prevent disease flares while minimising adverse effects of the treatment itself

Evidence-based management of AAV is summarised in an algorithm in Fig. 25.8 [20] and general approaches described in the following sections. Details of immunosuppressive regimens, which are similar to those used for anti-GBM disease and SLE, are provided in Chaps. 27, 28 and summarised in Chap. 29.

25.8.1 Induction Therapy

Conventional treatment of active AAV with renal involvement, aiming to induce disease remission, is comprised of high-dose corticosteroids and cyclophosphamide (CYC). This regimen induces remission in up to 80% of patients but is associated with significant toxicity and infectious complications. Therefore several clinical trials have been performed to establish effective treatment regimens using other immunosuppressive agents, with the aim of reducing treatment-related toxicity.

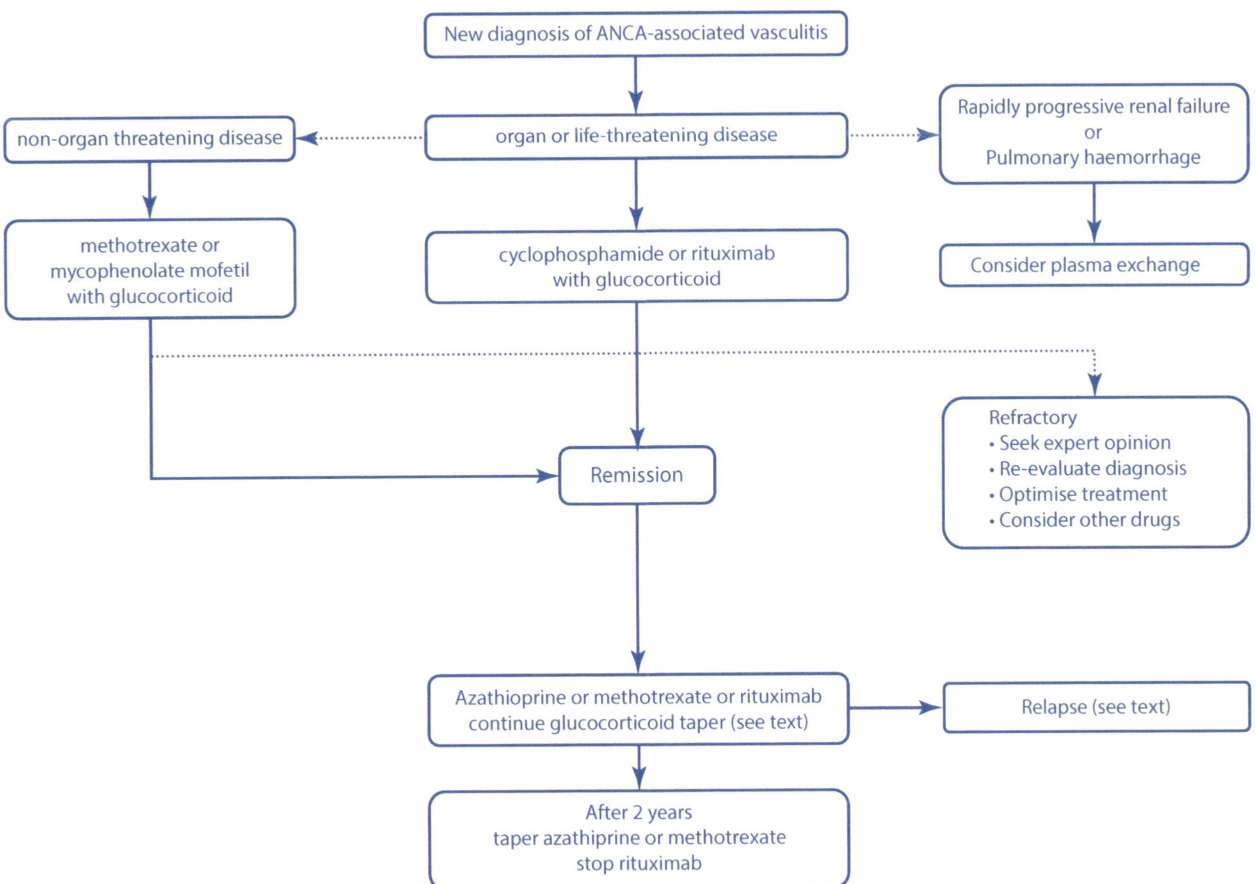

Fig. 25.8 EULAR algorithm for disease management. (Adapted from [20])

25.8.1.1 Organ- or Life-Threatening Disease

Glucocorticoid AND

(a) *Cyclophosphamide (CYC) OR*
(b) *Rituximab (RTX)*

Patients with AAV presenting with organ- or life-threatening disease should receive induction therapy with corticosteroids combined with CYC or RTX [42]. The intensity and duration of induction therapy are important factors in determining the risk of subsequent relapse. For example, pulsed intravenous (IV) cyclophosphamide regimens employ approximately half the dose of oral regimens (CYCLOPS) [43]; this is associated with equivalent rates of remission and survival but higher long-term relapse rates [44]. The lower cumulative dose in the CYCLOPS protocol is associated with reduced rates of infertility, leucopenia and bladder-related complications. It is probable that most patients will do well with lower cumulative dose pulsed CYC, although those at high risk of frequent relapses (anti-PR3-positive and/or large granulomatous disease burden) may benefit from a daily oral induction CYC regimen. The standard dosing for oral CYC is 2 mg/kg/day (maximum 200 mg/day), and IV CYC is 15 mg/kg (maximum 1.2 g/pulse), given three times 2 weeks apart, and then once every 3 weeks for 3–6 months (CYCLOPS). CYCAZAREM demonstrated that the majority (77%) of patients develop remission within 3 months, while almost all (93%) are in remission within 6 months – again supporting the reduced cumulative CYC dose [45]. Dosing adjustments should also incorporate age and renal function. Anti-emetic therapy should be a routine adjuvant to CYC, as well as oral or IV fluids on the day of infusion to dilute CYC metabolites in the urine, and hence limit injury to the urothelium [20]. The use of MESNA, to reduce bladder complications, is controversial but should be considered.

RTX has entered guidelines as an alternative first-line treatment to CYC, since the recent publication of two randomised controlled trials. RITUXVAS compared CYCLOPS regimen to RTX plus low-dose IV CYC and GCC, in severe renal disease [42, 46]. RAVE, on the other hand, compared RTX with PO CYC and GCC [42], in patients with more preserved renal function. Remission rates, degree of renal impairment and adverse events were equivalent between RTX and CYC, except in relapsing disease, where RTX was superior. Dosing in these trials was 375 mg/m^2 weekly for 4 weeks. An alternative regimen is two infusions of 1 g a fortnight apart. The most common side effect of RTX is hypogammaglobulinaemia, which may require IV immunoglobulin therapy.

The choice between RTX and CYC is guided by the desire to protect fertility, the presence of contraindications to CYC, perceived patient frailty or injured bone marrow. Those at high risk of adverse events may do better not receiving cyclophosphamide, although clinical trials of rituximab have disappointingly failed to provide robust evidence in favour of this presumed safety benefit. The main limitation to RTX use is cost and therefore access, as well as the unknown long-term efficacy and safety outcomes. It is also important to remember that experience with RTX alone (i.e. without combined CYC) in severe disease is limited.

Various glucocorticoid dosing schedules exist. EULAR recommends 1 mg/kg/day, with maximum of 80 mg/day [20]. The PEXIVAS trial (Plasma Exchange and Glucocorticoids for Treatment of Anti-neutrophil Cytoplasm Antibody-Associated Vasculitis) [47] recently revealed preliminary data demonstrating that a reduced glucocorticoid dose (target of 5–7.5 mg by week 16) is non-inferior to a 'standard' regime (target of 10–15 mg by week 16), with fewer serious infections.

25.8.1.2 Rapidly Progressive Renal Failure or Pulmonary Haemorrhage

Patients presenting with dialysis-dependent renal failure, Cr > 500 μmol/L or pulmonary haemorrhage may benefit from adjunctive therapy in addition to standard treatment with CYC or rituximab and oral corticosteroids, including:

- High-dose IV methylprednisolone (three daily doses at 10–15 mg/kg)
- Plasma exchange (60 ml/kg × 7 exchanges)

The rationale for plasma exchange and rituximab is partially based on their antibody-depleting properties, which makes theoretical sense given the evidence for the pathogenic role of circulating ANCA. Very few patients with such severe disease were included in trials examining the efficacy of rituximab, so most clinicians would default to use of cyclophosphamide in these settings. In the RITUXVAS trial (the only such trial to include patients with severe disease), each dose of rituximab was accompanied by a dose of intravenous cyclophosphamide. The full benefit, however, is clearly due to additional, more complex mechanisms. The MEPEX trial supported a benefit of plasma exchange *over* high-dose methylprednisolone [48], although this clear benefit disappears on long-term follow-up [49]. Of note, the global PEXIVAS trial (Plasma Exchange and Glucocorticoids for Treatment of Anti-neutrophil Cytoplasm Antibody-Associated Vasculitis) [47], has just released preliminary data. It demonstrated, in severe AAV, that plasma exchange does not improve composite end point of death or end-stage renal disease. There is still potential benefit of plasma exchange in patients with combined positive ANCA and anti-glomerular basement membrane (GBM) antibodies and therefore should still be used in this circumstance.

Unlike those with anti-GBM disease, patients presenting with dialysis-dependent renal failure often achieve renal recovery and independence from dialysis with appropriate high-intensity immunosuppression. However, there is a clear need to balance the risk of treatment-related toxicity with the potential benefit of organ recovery; histology on renal biopsy is useful in assessing this risk/benefit ratio [50]. Severe tubular atrophy and a low percentage of normal glomeruli on renal biopsy should prompt caution in administering high-intensity immunosuppression as treatment for renal vasculitis as the risk of treatment-related mortality likely exceeds the potential benefit in these patients.

25.8.1.3 Non-organ-Threatening Disease

Methotrexate (MTX) or mycophenolate mofetil (MMF), in combination with glucocorticoids, is recommended for remission-induction of non-organ-threatening AAV. MTX may be used with similar efficacy to CYC in this circumstance. The NORAM trial [51] demonstrated reduced treatment-related toxicity with MTX but higher relapse rates and increased time to remission, compared to CYC. Patients should receive concomitant therapy with folic acid to minimise MTX toxicity. MTX 20–25 mg/week, oral or parenteral, is recommended [20]. Dose adjustments for renal impairment should be made, which often limits its use.

Mycophenolate mofetil (MMF) is another alternative to CYC, in non-organ-threatening disease [52], although there is no published trial data to guide its use.

25.8.1.4 Standard Prophylaxis

All patients receiving induction immunosuppression for AAV should receive standard prophylaxis to minimise infections complications, gastric ulceration and bone resorption including:

- Trimethoprim/sulphamethoxazole (Septrin): 800/1600 mg alternate days or 400/80 mg daily.
- Systemic antifungal prophylaxis therapy should be considered in patients receiving intense immunosuppression. Patients should perform daily self-inspection of the mouth to detect mucosal candidiasis early.
- Hepatitis B, annual influenza and 5-yearly pneumococcal vaccination (twice in lifetime) vaccination are recommended.
- Gastric protection agent, e.g. proton-pump inhibitor (PPI).
- Calcium/vitamin D supplementation.

These medications should be administered as part of the induction therapy regimen in all patients. For female patients receiving CYC, who wish to maximise subsequent fertility, ovarian protection with a GnRH agonist such as goserelin is employed by some centres, although without strong evidence to support the practice. Similarly, sperm banking can be used in younger men, if this can be arranged without delaying the induction therapy.

Guidelines addressing infection prophylaxis varies, and therefore each clinician should seek out local guidance. Some guidelines recommend measuring HIV, HBV and syphilis serology (Brazilian Society of Rheumatology), as well as tuberculosis screening, before immunosuppression (British Society for Rheumatology, BSR). Varicella zoster vaccine, or indeed any live vaccine, should not be given while a patient is immunosuppressed, but titres should be measured and immunoglobulin given if exposure risk is significant (BSR). Female patients should be considered for cervical intraepithelial neoplasia (CIN) screening and HPV vaccination according to age-specific local guidance.

25.8.2 Maintenance Therapy

Up to 50% of patients with AAV will relapse despite appropriate high-intensity induction therapy [53]. Maintenance therapy aims to reduce the risk of disease relapse while minimising the adverse events associated with long-term immunosuppression. Therapy generally consists of low-dose glucocorticoids with a second steroid-sparing agent:

- Azathioprine (2 mg/kg/day)
- Methotrexate (0.3 mg/kg/wk increasing to 25 mg weekly), if tolerated
- Mycophenolate mofetil (2 g/day)
- Rituximab (500 mg every 6 months)

The optimum duration of maintenance immunosuppression remains unclear. In general, given the relapsing nature of AAV, it should be continued for at least 2 years, although some centres stop after 6 months, and it may be required indefinitely in patients with frequent relapses. Consideration should be given to extending maintenance to 5 years in patients with high-risk of relapse (◘ Table 25.5) [54]. The REMAIN trial investigating the rate of relapse associated with 2- or 4-year maintenance therapy provided a clear signal of increased relapse with the shorter maintenance therapy duration [55].

Azathioprine (AZA) is now widely used for maintenance therapy. It is as effective as CYC at maintaining remission and is a less toxic drug (CYCAZAREM) [45].

Methotrexate is as effective as azathioprine at maintaining disease remission and associated with a similar rate of adverse events (WEGENT) [56]. It is contraindicated in patients with significant renal impairment and is therefore more frequently used as maintenance therapy in non-organ-threatening disease.

Mycophenolate mofetil (MMF) has been used in AAV as maintenance therapy, but data from the IMPROVE trial [57] suggests it is less effective (as well as being much more expensive) than AZA in maintaining disease remission. It is recommended as second-line maintenance therapy in relapsing disease or patients intolerant of AZA.

Rituximab is emerging as an important remission maintenance agent, particularly for those with anti-PR3-positive disease. The MAINRITSAN trial compared low-dose RTX in GPA/MPA to AZA for remission maintenance after induction with pulsed CYC and found more sustained remission in the RTX arm, with no difference in adverse events [58]. MAINRITSAN2 is underway in an effort to establish dosing frequency and indication for treatment guided by ANCA titre or B-cell reconstitution. The RITAZAREM trial is also underway to compare RTX 1 g maintenance with AZA in patients who received RTX induction; a preliminary report confirms the effectiveness of rituximab at inducing remission in relapsing AAV [59]. The maintenance component of this trial has not yet reported. There are concerns regarding repeated use of rituximab, notably progressive hypogammaglobulinaemia and a possible increased risk of progressive multifocal leukoencephalopathy.

Patients with GPA with localised upper respiratory tract disease should receive trimethoprim/sulphamethoxazole (Septrin) in addition to other maintenance therapy as there is evidence this decreases the frequency of disease relapse [30]. Treatment guidelines and links to current active trials are maintained on the EUVAS website (▶ http://www.vasculitis.org).

25.8.3 Refractory Disease

Refractory disease should be managed in a vasculitis centre. It is defined as increased or unchanged disease activity after 4 weeks of standard therapy, lack of response (i.e. <50% reduction in BVAS) after 6 weeks of therapy or chronic persistent disease (one major or three minor BVAS items) after 12 weeks of treatment [60]. It is crucial to ensure the correct diagnosis has been made, that treatment has been optimised and that infection, comorbidities, malignancy and chronic damage have been ruled out as potential causes of 'refractory disease'. Once confirmed, the alternative to the initial induction regime should be trialled (i.e. if CYC used at initial induction, now use RTX) [20]. In cases where RTX is not an option and IV pulsed CYC was used initially, daily oral CYC can be used [61]. In patients with persistent low-level disease activity, who fail to achieve remission, IV immunoglobulin may be of benefit [20].

25.8.4 Relapsed Disease

Due to meticulous follow-up, disease relapse is often diagnosed earlier in the course than the initial disease presentation. Major relapses can be treated the same as standard induction treatment. It is worth noting that RTX was more effecting than CYC in treating relapsed disease in the RAVE trial [42]. One should also be cognisant of the CYC cumulative dose, especially if used as part of the initial induction regime – it should not exceed 25 g (and ideally <15 g) [62]. Minor relapses can be treated by increasing the dose of maintenance immunosuppression (i.e. GCC and/or AZA/MTX).

25.8.5 Future Therapy

Significant research into optimisation of treatment strategy in AAV continues. Specifically, the current focus is on the personalisation of immunosuppression therapy to the individual, in an attempt to maximise disease control and minimise toxic complications associated with treatment. Various strategies are being explored, including steroid minimisation and the use of avacopan (CLEAR trial [63]: investigating the use of oral C5a receptor inhibitor to replace high-dose glucocorticoids in induction therapy) and the use of belimumab as add-on treatment to AZA/MTX and GCC in maintenance therapy (BREVAS trial).

25.8.6 Monitoring and Follow-up

All patients should be followed up closely in, or in collaboration with an expert vasculitis (see below). Typically, three monthly follow-up is standard for patients in remission; however, this is variable, and individual patient factors must be considered. Clinicians should be aware of patients with increased risk of relapse, listed in ◘ Table 25.6.

Follow-up should include a focused clinical history and examination, looking for signs and symptoms of

Table 25.6 Factors associated with higher rates of disease relapse [41]

Predictors of relapse
PR3-ANCA positivity
Newly positive or rising ANCA titre (especially in patients with history of capillaritis)
GPA
Lung/upper respiratory tract involvement
Lower serum creatinine at presentation
Cardiovascular involvement
Nasal carriage of *Staphylococcus aureus*
HLA-DPB1*04:01 (homozygous >heterozygous, independent of ANCA specificity, although seen more frequently in those with PR3-AAV) [64]

disease relapse, as well as side effects of treatment. In particular, one should assess for any incident diabetes mellitus, as a consequence of glucocorticoid therapy, as well as routine assessment of traditional cardiovascular risk factors, given the association of increased risk among those with AAV. Clinicians should also be astute to the increased risk of thromboembolic disease, particularly during periods of disease activity. Blood pressure measurement and urinalysis (looking for blood or protein) are routine. Laboratory investigations should include (at a minimum) white blood cell count (WCC, as leucopenia is a common side effect of treatment), renal function, liver function tests (LFTs) and C-reactive protein (CRP), while serial ANCA titres may be useful in selected cases (as discussed above). Serum immunoglobulin measurements, prior to each course of RTX, are also recommended. For those at increased risk of osteoporosis, screening with bone densitometry should be considered, and fracture risk should be estimated (e.g. ▸ https://www.sheffield.ac.uk/FRAX/). Haematuria, in patients previously treated with CYC, should prompt urology review, for consideration of cystoscopy, to rule out bladder cancer [20].

AAV is a treatable but chronic, relapsing-remitting disease, which can significantly affect a patient's quality of life. A holistic approach to treatment is recommended, in which the patient is at the centre of the process. A clear non-jargon explanation of the condition, treatment, side effects and prognosis should be given. Patients should be encouraged to take ownership of their disease, as this enables them to recognise potential relapse episodes early, resulting in timely treatment and therefore limitation of further morbidity. Patient support groups and smartphone apps, to assist disease monitoring, are useful complimentary aids.

25.9 Special Considerations

25.9.1 The Elderly or Frail Patient

Not surprisingly, the elderly have significantly higher early mortality rates in AAV compared to younger patients. In fact, age and serum creatinine at diagnosis are by far the strongest independent predictors of death, and elderly patients are at particular risk of treatment-related toxicity. Therefore the risk/benefit ratio of high-intensity treatment vs the potential benefit of organ and patient survival should be considered prior to administration of induction therapy. Treatment regimens in most of the EUVAS trials used dose reduction of up to 50% in those >70 years. It is worth noting that the risk/benefit equation almost always weighs on the side of administering some immunosuppression (rather than none) and that elderly patients also have a high risk of morbidity and death if they require long-term dialysis therapy.

25.9.2 The Young Woman Wishing to Have a Family

Women of child-bearing age may wish to avoid cyclophosphamide as prolonged exposure is associated with infertility. In these patients, rituximab may be used in preference to cyclophosphamide as part of induction therapy. However, the risk of infertility is smaller with modern low cumulative dose CYC regimens, compared to when the drug was administered for several years, and it is important to emphasise strongly the profound effect that severe chronic renal failure has on fertility. Most women who recover renal function after receiving CYC as treatment for vasculitis will subsequently be able to bear children. It is important not to compromise on treatment intensity when managing a young woman with severe systemic vasculitis. Pregnancy can be considered after 6 months of remission, in consultation with an obstetrician specialising in high-risk pregnancy. AZA is the preferred maintenance agent, if required, as MTX, MMF and RTX are potentially teratogenic.

25.9.3 The Septic Patient

The patient who presents with active AAV and coincident infection is extremely challenging to manage. Firstly, it is critical to ensure that the AAV is not occurring secondary to the infection. This is particularly true of patients with infectious endocarditis. In practice, this means treating both conditions and keeping an open mind as the condition evolves, with frequent reassessment of the vasculitis activity and spread of infection. If a suspicion lingers that the episode of vasculitis was secondary to infection, it may be possible to carefully withdraw immunosuppression early after the infection has been cured, with very close monitoring of vasculitis activity. In those who are overtly septic, intense immunosuppression is likely to lead to patient death from overwhelming sepsis. In these cases intravenous immunoglobulin therapy (1–2 g/kg) may suppress vasculitis activity without compromising the immune response to the infection. RTX has been shown to be safe in the context of severe infection [65].

25.10 The Vasculitis Unit

AAV is a complex multisystem rare disease and consequently falls prey to many of the factors that hamper care in other rare diseases:

- Lack of awareness among clinicians leading to a delay in diagnosis
- Lack of access to the most recently developed therapies and diagnostic tools
- Poorly coordinated care with inadequate communication and integration between the specialties that a patient with vasculitis will encounter
- Requirement for the patient to travel to numerous clinics at different times
- Lack of ancillary support, such as clinical psychology and social work

Therefore, there is a strong rationale for development of regional centres of excellence linked to local units ('hub and spoke' model) at which a patient can attend for a 'one-stop shop' assessment with access to a multidisciplinary team. This includes:

- Ready access to ENT assessment with nasendoscopy
- An infusional therapy unit for administering CYC (with appropriate governance to ensure this is delivered safely)
- Respiratory team input with ability to provide rapid access to bronchoscopy
- Dermatology team input with facilities for diagnostic skin biopsy
- Ready access to neurology and facilities for sural nerve biopsy
- Excellent immunology services, with rapid turnaround of serological tests

The key person in coordinating such a clinical service efficiently and acting as a first port of call for patients is the clinical nurse specialist, who, with the assistance of carefully designed algorithmic protocols, would be able to manage immunotherapy, provide initial clinical assessments and coordinate multispecialist input. Procedures should be in place for recording the amount and type of immunosuppression delivered to an individual patient. This provides the capability to calculate cumulative CYC dose received and to audit the use of expensive biologic agents. The principal factor in determining treatment of relapsing vasculitis is the cumulative dose of CYC received previously.

Case Study

Case 1

A 58-year-old male had presented to multiple medical professionals over the preceding 5 months. This included diagnosis and treatment of sinusitis, hearing loss due to 'waxy ears', multiple lower respiratory tract infections, weight loss and generalised fatigue. On routine blood testing, a creatinine level of 430 μmol/l was noted, with urine dipstick positive for blood and protein. He was hypertensive and euvolaemic. Renal ultrasound was normal. Acute screen was sent urgently. Results included ANCA-positive, anti-PR3 titre 65 (NR <3) and anti-GBM titre 46 (NR <5). Kidney biopsy demonstrated pan-necrotising crescentic glomerulonephritis with linear staining of the basement membrane for IgG. He remained non-oliguric and avoided haemodialysis. He was commenced on glucocorticoids and IV cyclophosphamide and received seven plasma exchanges. Creatinine level has stabilised at 330 μmol/l. One month later he presented with right lower limb pain and swelling. A right deep venous thrombosis was diagnosed.

This case highlights the multisystem presentation that is often misdiagnosed, leading to delayed diagnosis and treatment. One should always be alert to the possibility of small-vessel vasculitis when a variety of systems are involved. It is also important to arrange timely processing of both ANCA and anti-GBM titres where small-vessel vasculitis is suspected, as dual positivity exists and urgent treatment with immunosuppression and plasma exchange is imperative. This case also highlights the increased risk of venous thromboembolism in this cohort, which anecdotally appears to be the highest in those with dual positive disease (i.e. ANCA and anti-GBM positivity).

Case 2

A 64-year-old lady presented feeling generally unwell, 3 kg weight loss and epistaxis. She had a history of PR3-AAV, diagnosed 3 years ago, with pulmonary and renal involvement at initial presentation. Her anti-PR3 titre had become negative after induction therapy with glucocorticoids and IV cyclophosphamide. Given her anti-PR3 status and pulmonary involvement conveying increased risk of relapse, she was maintained on azathioprine for 3 years. This presentation occurred 4 months after azathioprine was tapered off. Urine dipstick was positive for blood and protein, and anti-PR3 titre was elevated at 43, with a small creatinine level rise to 180 µmol/l (baseline 120 µmol/l). She was commenced on induction therapy, including glucocorticoids and IV cyclophosphamide. Renal function recovered to 140 µmol/l, and she felt systemically improved after two doses on cyclophosphamide. She developed persistent leucopenia that delayed administration of further doses. Four weeks later she complained of significant mid-back pain that began acutely 1 week previously. X-ray revealed thoracic vertebral compression fractures, a presumed complication of steroid therapy. She was rapidly tapered off corticosteroids and remains on azathioprine. This case highlights the relapsing nature of the disease and the need for close follow-up of these patients. Although guidelines exist to guide therapy, one must always individualise this to the patient in front of you. Elderly patients are at increased risk of adverse effects, as seen in this case. It is important to reduce immunosuppression therapy when these complications occur.

Case 3

A 46-year-old previously fit and well university lecturer presented with shortness of breath and haemoptysis, with a recent history of upper respiratory and sinus symptoms. He had a cough productive of heavily blood-stained purulent sputum. Blood pressure was 230/150, urine dipstick was positive for +3 protein, +2 blood and creatinine level was rising past 250 µmol/l. Chest X-ray revealed widespread alveolar infiltrates, and pO2 level on room air was 5.2 kPa, necessitating the use of non-invasive ventilation. He was ANCA-, ANA -and anti-GBM-negative. Echocardiogram revealed a dilated left ventricle with ejection fraction of 37%. Urgent kidney biopsy showed severe microangiopathy with 'onion skin' appearance of intra-renal vessels and approximately 45% interstitial fibrosis. There was no evidence of glomerulonephritis. He was treated with antibiotics, diuretics and antihypertensive agents, with a diagnosis of pneumonia complicating acute pulmonary oedema in the context of hypertensive cardiac failure and hypertensive nephrosclerosis. This case highlights the importance of keeping an open mind in the face of seemingly clear vasculitic pulmonary-renal syndrome; although primary systemic small-vessel vasculitis can be ANCA and anti-GBM antibody negative, this was a flag that other pathologies may be at play and focused attention on cardiac function.

Tips and Tricks (Table 25.7)

Table 25.7 'Tips of the trade' in managing systemic vasculitis

Scenario	Salutary tips
A patient presenting with fever, systemic illness and positive anti-MPO serology	Look very carefully for endocarditis and tuberculosis: multiple blood cultures and echocardiography
Intensive induction therapy of a patient with dialysis requiring renal failure	Once the GFR drops below 15 ml/min, the risk of adverse event risk rises rapidly. If adverse events start accumulating, *pull back on therapy rapidly*
Young woman with dialysis requiring renal vasculitis who wants to maintain fertility	Consider using rituximab in place of CYC, but do not compromise on therapy intensity; the priority is to recover renal function
Very scarred kidney in a patient requiring dialysis	Early withdrawal of immunosuppression, but *beware extra-renal disease*
Rapidly progressive renal vasculitis with lung disease	Measure anti-GBM antibodies as well as ANCA, up to 30% of anti-MPO patients are also anti-GBM positive. Treat as 'rapidly progressive renal failure'
ENT clinic	Introduce routine urine dipstick testing for patients with sino-nasal disease to pick up glomerulonephritis in a timely fashion

(continued)

Table 25.7 (continued)

Scenario	Salutary tips
Multidisciplinary clinics	AAV affects many organs and patients probably have improved outcomes if cared for in a clinic setting that attempts to join up various services, such as rheumatology, nephrology, ENT, clinical psychology and immunology. This may involve running a joint clinic
Pulsed intravenous CYC	This is logistically more difficult to deliver than daily oral CYC but has several advantages: lower cumulative dose with equivalent remission-induction efficacy and improved compliance (you know the patient has received it). It is worth setting up the infrastructure required
Want to use pulsed therapy but logistically difficult in a given unit	Oral pulses (given over 3 days) are probably as effective as intravenous pulses
Dialysis-dependent, when to transplant?	Consider after 12 months of clinical remission. Persistent ANCA positivity is not a contraindication
Rising ANCA in an asymptomatic patient	Increase vigilance to look for any evidence of new organ dysfunction; treat the clinical features, not the blood test

Chapter Review Questions

1. A 63-year-old gentleman presents with acute kidney injury (creatinine 347 μmol/L) and an active urine sediment (i.e. blood and protein on urinalysis). Other than some fatigue, he is asymptomatic. ANCA, including PR3 and MPO, and anti-GBM serology are all negative. Could this still be AAV?
2. What is the first-line treatment for AAV when initially presenting with rapidly progressive renal failure and pulmonary haemorrhage?
3. A 72-year-old female is being treated for relapse of PR3-GPA with pulsed IV CYC and glucocorticoids. She presents 3 months later with persistent leucopenia and significant back pain. Renal function has returned to baseline, despite some persistent proteinuria, and PR3 is now negative. MRI spine reveals an osteoporotic fracture of T12. What is the best course of management now?

Answers

1. Renal biopsy demonstrated a pauci-immune crescentic necrotising small-vessel vasculitis, suggesting a diagnosis of AAV. The lack of extra-renal symptoms implies it is renal-limited disease, which can occur as a subtype of MPA. ANCA-negative AAV is also a recognised phenomenon, accounting for about 10% of cases. The use of highly sensitive and specific immunosorbent assays to screen for PR3 and MPO has become increasingly the first line screening tool for suspected AAV cases. As no test is absolute, in patients with a high clinical suspicion and a negative ANCA result, a diagnosis of AAV cannot be excluded, and renal biopsy is warranted, as in this case.
2. Induction treatment should include IV CYC (dose adjusted for age and renal function) or RTX, with IV methylprednisolone (followed by high-dose oral glucocorticoid) and/or plasma exchange. In practice, both are administered in tandem. Studies show RTX is superior for relapsing disease.
3. This lady presents with complications of treatment, namely, leucopenia secondary to CYC, and an osteoporotic fracture as a result of significant glucocorticoid use. Her increased age predisposes her to increased adverse effects from toxic immunosuppression. Her return of renal function to baseline and the conversion of anti-PR3 to negative are reassuring. Persistent proteinuria likely reflects a degree of chronic damage. At this point, a rapid reduction in glucocorticoids is warranted, with no further CYC therapy. When leucopenia resolves and providing thiopurine methyltransferase (TPMT) levels are normal, azathioprine would be a reasonable choice of maintenance immunosuppression.

References

1. Jennette JC, Falk RJ, Andrassy K, Bacon PA, Churg J, Gross WL, et al. Nomenclature of systemic vasculitides. Proposal of an international consensus conference. Arthritis Rheum. 1994;37(2):187–92.
2. Tan JA, Dehghan N, Chen W, Xie H, Esdaile JM, Avina-Zubieta JA. Mortality in ANCA-associated vasculitis: ameta-analysis of observational studies. Ann Rheum Dis. 2017;76(9):1566–74.
3. Walton EW. Giant-cell granuloma of the respiratory tract (wegener's granulomatosis). Br Med J. 1958;2(5091):265–70.

4. Jennette JC, Falk RJ, Bacon PA, Basu N, Cid MC, Ferrario F, et al. 2012 Revised International Chapel Hill consensus conference nomenclature of vasculitides. Arthritis Rheum. 2013;65(1):1–11.
5. Fries JF, Hunder GG, Bloch DA, Michel BA, Arend WP, Calabrese LH, et al. The American College of Rheumatology 1990 criteria for the classification of vasculitis. Summary. Arthritis Rheum. 1990;33(8):1135–6.
6. Watts R, Lane S, Hanslik T, Hauser T, Hellmich B, Koldingsnes W, et al. Development and validation of a consensus methodology for the classification of the ANCA-associated vasculitides and polyarteritis nodosa for epidemiological studies. Ann Rheum Dis. 2007;66(2):222–7. https://doi.org/10.1136/ard.2006.054593.
7. Lane SE, Watts RA, Shepstone L, Scott DG. Primary systemic vasculitis: clinical features and mortality. QJM. 2005;98(2):97–111.
8. Mouthon L, Dunogue B, Guillevin L. Diagnosis and classification of eosinophilic granulomatosis with polyangiitis (formerly named Churg-Strauss syndrome). J Autoimmun. 2014;48–49:99–103.
9. Watts RA, Mahr A, Mohammad AJ, Gatenby P, Basu N, Flores-Suárez LF. Classification, epidemiology and clinical subgrouping of antineutrophil cytoplasmic antibody (ANCA)-associated vasculitis. Nephrol Dial Transplant. 2015;30:i14–22.
10. Watts RA, Lane SE, Bentham G, Scott DG. Epidemiology of systemic vasculitis: a ten-year study in the United Kingdom. Arthritis Rheum. 2000;43(2):414–9.
11. Aries PM, Herlyn K, Reinhold-Keller E, Latza U. No seasonal variation in the onset of symptoms of 445 patients with Wegener's granulomatosis. Arthritis Rheum. 2008;59(6):904.
12. Mohammad AJ, Jacobsson LT, Westman KW, Sturfelt G, Segelmark M. Incidence and survival rates in Wegener's granulomatosis, microscopic polyangiitis, Churg-Strauss syndrome and polyarteritis nodosa. Rheumatology (Oxford). 2009;48(12):1560–5.
13. Fujimoto S, Watts RA, Kobayashi S, Suzuki K, Jayne DRW, Scott DGI, et al. Comparison of the epidemiology of anti-neutrophil cytoplasmic antibody-associated vasculitis between Japan and the UK. Rheumatology. 2011;50(10):1916–20.
14. Watts RA, Scott DG. L32. ANCA vasculitis over the world. What do we learn from country differences? Presse Med. 2013;42(4 PART2):591–3.
15. Little MA, Nazar L, Farrington K. Outcome in glomerulonephritis due to systemic small vessel vasculitis: effect of functional status and non-vasculitic co-morbidity. Nephrol Dial Transplant. 2004;19(2):356–64.
16. Little MA, Nightingale P, Verburgh CA, Hauser T, De Groot K, Savage C, et al. Early mortality in systemic vasculitis: relative contribution of adverse events and active vasculitis. Ann Rheum Dis. 2010;69(6):1036–43.
17. Bossuyt X, Cohen Tervaert JW, Arimura Y, Blockmans D, Flores-Suárez LF, Guillevin L, et al. Position paper: revised 2017 international consensus on testing of ANCAs in granulomatosis with polyangiitis and microscopic polyangiitis. Nat Rev Rheumatol. 2017;13(11):683–92. https://doi.org/10.1038/nrrheum.2017.140.
18. Bossuyt X, Rasmussen N, van Paassen P, Hellmich B, Baslund B, Vermeersch P, et al. A multicentre study to improve clinical interpretation of proteinase-3 and myeloperoxidase anti-neutrophil cytoplasmic antibodies. Rheumatology (United Kingdom). 2017;56(9):1533–41.
19. Hellmark T, Segelmark M. Diagnosis and classification of Goodpasture's disease (anti-GBM). J Autoimmun. 2014;48–49:108–12.
20. Yates M, Watts RA, Bajema IM, Cid MC, Crestani B, Hauser T, et al. EULAR/ERA-EDTA recommendations for the management of ANCA-associated vasculitis. Ann Rheum Dis. 2016;75(9):1583–94.
21. Berden AE, Ferrario F, Hagen EC, Jayne DR, Jennette JC, Joh K, et al. Histopathologic classification of ANCA-associated glomerulonephritis. J Am Soc Nephrol. 2010;21(10):1628–36.
22. Binda V, Moroni G, Messa P. ANCA-associated vasculitis with renal involvement. J Nephrol. 2018;31(2):197–208.
23. Lyons PA, Rayner TF, Trivedi S, Holle JU, Watts RA, Jayne DRW, et al. Genetically distinct subsets within ANCA-associated vasculitis. N Engl J Med. 2012;367(3):214–23.
24. Merkel PA, Xie G, Monach PA, Ji X, Ciavatta DJ, Byun J, et al. Identification of functional and expression polymorphisms associated with risk for antineutrophil cytoplasmic autoantibody-associated vasculitis. Arthritis Rheumatol. 2017;69(5):1054–66.
25. Beaudreuil S, Lasfargues G, Laueriere L, El Ghoul Z, Fourquet F, Longuet C, et al. Occupational exposure in ANCA-positive patients: a case-control study. Kidney Int. 2005;67(5):1961–6.
26. Hogan SL, Satterly KK, Dooley MA, Nachman PH, Jennette JC, Falk RJ. Silica exposure in anti-neutrophil cytoplasmic autoantibody-associated glomerulonephritis and lupus nephritis. J Am Soc Nephrol. 2001;12(1):134–42.
27. Leigh J, Wang H, Bonin A, Peters M, Ruan X. Silica-induced apoptosis in alveolar and granulomatous cells in vivo. Environ Health Perspect. 1997;105 Suppl 5:1241–5.
28. Chen M, Kallenberg CG. ANCA-associated vasculitides--advances in pathogenesis and treatment. Nat Rev Rheumatol. 2010;6(11):653–64.
29. Stegeman CA, Tervaert JW, Sluiter WJ, Manson WL, de Jong PE, Kallenberg CG. Association of chronic nasal carriage of Staphylococcus aureus and higher relapse rates in Wegener granulomatosis. Ann Intern Med. 1994;120(1):12–7.
30. Stegeman CA, Tervaert JW, de Jong PE, Kallenberg CG. Trimethoprim-sulfamethoxazole (co-trimoxazole) for the prevention of relapses of Wegener's granulomatosis. Dutch Co-Trimoxazole Wegener Study Group. N Engl J Med. 1996;335(1):16–20.
31. Pendergraft WF 3rd, Preston GA, Shah RR, Tropsha A, Carter CW Jr, Jennette JC, et al. Autoimmunity is triggered by cPR-3(105-201), a protein complementary to human autoantigen proteinase-3. Nat Med. 2004;10(1):72–9.
32. Tadema H, Kallenberg CG, Stegeman CA, Heeringa P. Reactivity against complementary proteinase-3 is not increased in patients with PR3-ANCA-associated vasculitis. PLoS One. 2011;6(3):e17972.
33. Kallenberg CG, Tadema H. Vasculitis and infections: contribution to the issue of autoimmunity reviews devoted to "autoimmunity and infection". Autoimmun Rev. 2008;8(1):29–32.
34. Bansal PJ, Tobin MC. Neonatal microscopic polyangiitis secondary to transfer of maternal myeloperoxidase-antineutrophil cytoplasmic antibody resulting in neonatal pulmonary hemorrhage and renal involvement. Ann Allergy Asthma Immunol. 2004;93(4):398–401.
35. Boomsma MM, Stegeman CA, van der Leij MJ, Oost W, Hermans J, Kallenberg CG, et al. Prediction of relapses in Wegener's granulomatosis by measurement of antineutrophil cytoplasmic antibody levels: a prospective study. Arthritis Rheum. 2000;43(9):2025–33.
36. Birck R, Schmitt WH, Kaelsch IA, van der Woude FJ. Serial ANCA determinations for monitoring disease activity in patients with ANCA-associated vasculitis: systematic review. Am J Kidney Dis. 2006;47(1):15–23.

37. Kerr GS, Fleisher TA, Hallahan CW, Leavitt RY, Fauci AS, Hoffman GS. Limited prognostic value of changes in antineutrophil cytoplasmic antibody titer in patients with Wegener's granulomatosis. Arthritis Rheum. 1993;36(3):365–71.
38. Stegeman CA. Anti-neutrophil cytoplasmic antibody (ANCA) levels directed against proteinase-3 and myeloperoxidase are helpful in predicting disease relapse in ANCA-associated small-vessel vasculitis. Nephrol Dial Transplant. 2002;17(12):2077–80.
39. Staegeman CA. Anti-neutrophil cytoplasmic antibody (ANCA) levels directed against proteinase-3 and myeloperoxidase are helpful in predicting disease relapse in ANCA-associated small-vessel vasculitis. Nephrol Dial Transplant. 2002;17(12):2077–80.
40. Fussner LA, Hummel AM, Schroeder DR, Silva F, Cartin-Ceba R, Snyder MR, et al. Factors determining the clinical utility of serial measurements of antineutrophil cytoplasmic antibodies targeting proteinase 3. Arthritis Rheumatol. 2016;68(7):1700–10.
41. Kemna MJ, van Paassen P, Damoiseaux JGMC, Cohen Tervaert JW. Maintaining remission in patients with granulomatosis with polyangiitis or microscopic polyangiitis: the role of ANCA. Expert Opin Orphan Drugs. 2017;5(3):207–18.
42. Stone JH, Merkel PA, Spiera R, Seo P, Langford CA, Hoffman GS, et al. Rituximab versus cyclophosphamide for ANCA-associated vasculitis. N Engl J Med. 2010;363(3):221–32.
43. de Groot K, Harper L, Jayne DR, Flores Suarez LF, Gregorini G, Gross WL, et al. Pulse versus daily oral cyclophosphamide for induction of remission in antineutrophil cytoplasmic antibody-associated vasculitis: a randomized trial. Ann Intern Med. 2009;150(10):670–80.
44. Harper L, Morgan MD, Walsh M, Hoglund P, Westman K, Flossmann O, et al. Pulse versus daily oral cyclophosphamide for induction of remission in ANCA-associated vasculitis: long-term follow-up. Ann Rheum Dis. 2012;71:955–60.
45. Jayne D, Rasmussen N, Andrassy K, Bacon P, Tervaert JW, Dadoniene J, et al. A randomized trial of maintenance therapy for vasculitis associated with antineutrophil cytoplasmic autoantibodies. N Engl J Med. 2003;349(1):36–44.
46. Jones RB, Furuta S, Tervaert JWC, Hauser T, Luqmani R, Morgan MD, et al. Rituximab versus cyclophosphamide in ANCA-associated renal vasculitis: 2-year results of a randomised trial. Ann Rheum Dis. 2015;74(6):1178–82.
47. Walsh M, Merkel PA, Peh CA, Szpirt W, Guillevin L, Pusey CD, et al. Plasma exchange and glucocorticoid dosing in the treatment of anti-neutrophil cytoplasm antibody associated vasculitis (PEXIVAS): protocol for a randomized controlled trial. Trials. 2013;14:73.
48. Jayne DR, Gaskin G, Rasmussen N, Abramowicz D, Ferrario F, Guillevin L, et al. Randomized trial of plasma exchange or high-dosage methylprednisolone as adjunctive therapy for severe renal vasculitis. J Am Soc Nephrol. 2007;18(7):2180–8.
49. Walsh M, Casian A, Flossmann O, Westman K, Hoglund P, Pusey C, et al. Long-term follow-up of patients with severe ANCA-associated vasculitis comparing plasma exchange to intravenous methylprednisolone treatment is unclear. Kidney Int. 2013;84(2):397–402.
50. de Lind van Wijngaarden RA, Hauer HA, Wolterbeek R, Jayne DR, Gaskin G, Rasmussen N, et al. Chances of renal recovery for dialysis-dependent ANCA-associated glomerulonephritis. J Am Soc Nephrol. 2007;18(7):2189–97.
51. De Groot K, Rasmussen N, Bacon PA, Tervaert JW, Feighery C, Gregorini G, et al. Randomized trial of cyclophosphamide versus methotrexate for induction of remission in early systemic antineutrophil cytoplasmic antibody-associated vasculitis. Arthritis Rheum. 2005;52(8):2461–9.
52. Jones R, Harper L, Ballarin J, Blockmans D, Brogan P, Bruchfeld A. A randomized trial of mycophenolate mofetil versus cyclophosphamide for remission induction of ANCA-associated vasculitis. Presse Med. 2013;42(4):678–9.
53. de Joode AAE, Sanders JSF, Rutgers A, Stegeman CA. Maintenance therapy in antineutrophil cytoplasmic antibody-associated vasculitis: who needs what and for how long? Nephrol Dial Transplant. 2015;30(suppl_1):i150–i8.
54. Ntatsaki E, Carruthers D, Chakravarty K, D'Cruz D, Harper L, Jayne D, et al. BSR and BHPR guideline for the management of adults with ANCA-associated vasculitis. Rheumatology (Oxford). 2014;53(12):2306–9.
55. Karras A, Pagnoux C, Haubitz M, Groot K, Puechal X, Tervaert JWC, et al. Randomised controlled trial of prolonged treatment in the remission phase of ANCA-associated vasculitis. Ann Rheum Dis. 2017;76(10):1662–8.
56. Pagnoux C, Mahr A, Hamidou MA, Boffa JJ, Ruivard M, Ducroix JP, et al. Azathioprine or methotrexate maintenance for ANCA-associated vasculitis. N Engl J Med. 2008;359(26):2790–803.
57. Hiemstra TF, Walsh M, Mahr A, Savage CO, de Groot K, Harper L, et al. Mycophenolate mofetil vs azathioprine for remission maintenance in antineutrophil cytoplasmic antibody-associated vasculitis: a randomized controlled trial. JAMA. 2010;304(21):2381–8.
58. Guillevin L, Pagnoux C, Karras A, Khouatra C, Aumaitre O, Cohen P, et al. Rituximab versus azathioprine for maintenance in ANCA-associated vasculitis. N Engl J Med. 2014;371(19):1771–80.
59. Smith RM, Jones RB, Specks U RITAZAREM coinvestigators, et al. "Rituximab as therapy to induce remission after relapse in ANCA-associated vasculitis". Ann Rheum Dis. 2020;79:1243–49. https://doi.org/10.1136/annrheumdis-2019-216863.
60. Hellmich B, Flossmann O, Gross WL, Bacon P, Cohen-Tervaert JW, Guillevin L, et al. EULAR recommendations for conducting clinical studies and/or clinical trials in systemic vasculitis: focus on anti-neutrophil cytoplasm antibody-associated vasculitis. Ann Rheum Dis. 2007;66(5):605–17.
61. Seror R, Pagnoux C, Ruivard M, Landru I, Wahl D, Riviere S, et al. Treatment strategies and outcome of induction-refractory Wegener's granulomatosis or microscopic polyangiitis: analysis of 32 patients with first-line induction-refractory disease in the WEGENT trial. Ann Rheum Dis. 2010;69(12):2125–30.
62. Tesar V, Hruskova Z. Limitations of standard immunosuppressive treatment in ANCA-associated vasculitis and lupus nephritis. Nephron Clin Pract. 2014;128(3–4):205–15.
63. Jayne DRW, Bruchfeld AN, Harper L, Schaier M, Venning MC, Hamilton P, et al. Randomized trial of C5a receptor inhibitor avacopan in ANCA-associated vasculitis. J Am Soc Nephrol. 2017;28(9):2756–67.
64. Hilhorst M, Arndt F, Joseph Kemna M, Wieczorek S, Donner Y, Wilde B, et al. HLA-DPB1 as a risk factor for relapse in antineutrophil cytoplasmic antibody-associated vasculitis: a cohort study. Arthritis Rheumatol. 2016;68(7):1721–30.
65. Gregersen JW, Chaudhry A, Jayne DR. Rituximab for ANCA-associated vasculitis in the setting of severe infection. Scand J Rheumatol. 2013;42(3):207–10.

Patient Information and Guidelines

Vasculitis UK: http://www.vasculitis.org.uk/.

Vasculitis Foundation: www.vasculitisfoundation.org.

UKIVAS: http://rarerenal.org/rare-disease-groups/vasculitis-rdg/.

EUVAS: http://www.vasculitis.org.

Birmingham Vasculitis Activity Score calculator: http://golem.ndorms.ox.ac.uk/calculators/bvas.html.

Renal Involvement in Large- and Medium-Vessel Vasculitis

Stephen P. McAdoo

Contents

M. Harber (ed.), *Primer on Nephrology*, https://doi.org/10.1007/978-3-030-76419-7_26

26

Learning Objectives

1. Medium and large-vessel vasculitis typically present with constitutional symptoms, systemic inflammatory responses and features of vascular insufficiency in the territory of affected vessels. There are no validated diagnostic criteria, and diagnosis is usually made on a combination of clinical, laboratory, histopathological and, increasingly, non-invasive imaging findings.
2. Hypertension and renal insufficiency may arise as a complication of aortic and renal artery involvement, particularly in Takayasu arteritis and polyarteritis nodosa.
3. Aneurysm formation and rupture may present with haematuria, loin pain and life-threatening bleeding in polyarteritis nodosa.
4. In addition to medical therapy, endovascular or surgical intervention may be required for significant steno-occlusive or aneurysmal lesions, including those of the renal artery.
5. Significant glomerular disease is uncommon in large- and medium-vessel vasculitis and should alert physicians to the possibility of alternative diagnoses.

Table 26.1 Chapel Hill Consensus Conference Nomenclature of Vasculitides. (Modified from [1])

Large vessel		Giant cell arteritis
		Takayasu arteritis
Medium vessel		Polyarteritis nodosa
		Kawasaki disease
Small vessel	ANCA-associated	Microscopic polyangiitis
		Granulomatosis with polyangiitis
		Eosinophilic granulomatosis with polyangiitis
	Immune-complex SVV	Anti-GBM disease
		Cryoglobulinaemic vasculitis
		IgA vasculitis
		Hypocomplementaemic urticarial vasculitis

Abbreviations: *ANCA* anti-neutrophil cytoplasm antibody, *SVV* small-vessel vasculitis, *GBM* glomerular basement membrane

26.1 Introduction

The systemic vasculitides are a group of heterogeneous disorders characterised by inflammation of blood vessel walls. They may manifest clinical features as a result of lost vessel wall integrity, aneurysmal change and bleeding, or more commonly through compromise of lumen patency, as a result of wall swelling or scarring, thrombosis or dissection, giving rise to tissue ischaemia and infarction. The exact manifestations will depend upon the size, type and location of the affected vessels, the severity of inflammation and patterns of tissue injury unrelated to vasculitis.

A number of approaches for classifying and defining the systemic vasculitides have been proposed, the most well-known being the Chapel Hill Consensus Conference (CHCC) Nomenclature of Vasculitides, first published in 1994 and revised in 2012 (Table 26.1) [1]. The major categorisation in this system is based on size of blood vessel involved. Large-vessel vasculitis (LVV), therefore, is characterised by the involvement of the aorta and its major branches; medium-vessel vasculitides affect the main visceral arteries; and in small-vessel vasculitis, inflammation of the intraparenchymal arteries, arterioles, capillaries and their analogous veins predominates. It is important to recognise, however, that any vessel size can be affected in all three major categories of vasculitis. Indeed, in an individual patient with LVV, a greater number of medium-sized vessels may be affected (owing to their greater number) than are large vessels.

Small-vessel vasculitides with capillaritis are frequently complicated by glomerulonephritis, though this is uncommon in LVV. More frequently, large- and medium-vessel vasculitis may cause renal impairment through involvement of the aorta, the main renal artery and the interlobar arteries, resulting in ischaemia, impaired glomerular filtration and hypertension and possible cortical necrosis.

26.2 General Approach to Patients with Large- and Medium-Vessel Vasculitis

26.2.1 Clinical Assessment

In all forms of vasculitis, constitutional symptoms are frequently reported, such as lethargy, anorexia, weight loss, low-grade fever and arthralgia. Specific symptoms of tissue or organ ischaemia will be determined by the site of affected vessels and may include claudication, visual disturbance, angina, dyspnoê and neurological deficits. Rarely, patients may present with life-threatening vascular events such as dissection or vessel rupture.

Examination of patients with suspected LVV should include comprehensive assessment of blood pressure and arterial pulsation in all extremities and auscultation for vascular bruits. Carotidynia may indicate the presence of carotid artery inflammation. Cardiac examination may reveal aortic valve insufficiency as a complication aortitis in several forms of LVV.

26.2.2 Laboratory Findings

An acute phase response is common in all forms of vasculitis, including elevations in serum C-reactive protein (CRP) and erythrocyte sedimentation rate (ESR). Leucocytosis, thrombocytosis, normochromic normocytic anaemia and polyclonal hypergammaglobulinaemia may also be present. Other markers of inflammation, including serum amyloid A, may be raised, though these are not currently in routine clinical use. It should be noted, however, that the absence of an inflammatory response does not exclude a diagnosis of LVV and that these markers are frequently normal in the presence of active arterial inflammation.

At present, there are no specific circulating biomarkers for the large- or medium-vessel vasculitides, though the work-up of suspected patients will often include testing for anti-nuclear antibodies (ANA), anti-neutrophil cytoplasm antibody (ANCA), rheumatoid factor, complement, cryoglobulins and protein electrophoresis, to exclude other conditions that may mimic LVV.

26.2.3 Imaging

A variety of non-invasive imaging techniques are now used in the diagnosis and assessment of patients with suspected LVV (◘ Table 26.2), though the optimum modality, as well as the use of imaging for monitoring disease activity and response to treatment, remains somewhat controversial. The European League Against Rheumatism (EULAR) recently proposed a set of recommendations relating to the use of imaging in LVV in clinical practice [2].

26.2.4 Classification and Diagnostic Criteria

It should be noted that the CHCC nomenclature provides names and definitions for the various forms of vasculitis, rather than diagnostic criteria for use in clinical practice. In 1990, the American College of Rheumatology (ACR) published a series of classification criteria that aimed to differentiate patients with a given form of vasculitis from patients with other vasculitides, largely for the purpose of classifying patients for research studies [3]. Like the CHCC nomenclature, they are not intended to be used as diagnostic criteria to direct clinical management, though they may highlight important features (◘ Table 26.3). In addition, these classification criteria predate the discovery of ANCA, and the recent expansion of non-invasive imaging in vasculitis, such that they have striking limitations in current practice. To date, there are no validated diagnostic criteria for the most common forms of large- and medium-vessel vasculitis, including giant cell arteritis, Takayasu arteritis and polyarteritis nodosa. Important diseases to consider in the differential diagnosis of these conditions are listed in ◘ Table 26.4.

26.3 Giant Cell Arteritis

Definition

Giant cell arteritis (GCA), also sometimes known to as temporal arteritis, is defined in the CHCC 2012 nomenclature as arteritis, often granulomatous, usually affecting the aorta and/or its major branches, with a predilection for the branches of the carotid and vertebral arteries, often involving the temporal artery, and with onset usually in patients older than 50 years.

In practice, GCA is a heterogeneous condition, and there have been attempts to define sub-phenotypes of disease, including 'classical' cranial GCA (where the external carotid artery and its branches, including the posterior ciliary arteries which supply the optic nerve, are predominantly involved) and 'extra-cranial' or large-vessel GCA (LV-GCA, where the aorta and first-order large supra-aortic vessels are affected, with or without classical cranial involvement) [4]. There is also a well-recognised association with polymyalgia rheumatica (PMR), an inflammatory condition characterised by pain and stiffness in the shoulder and hip girdles. PMR occurs in approximately 50% of patients with GCA, and conversely GCA is found in approximately 15% of patients with PMR, either at the time of diagnosis or a subsequent event, though the precise nature of this relationship is not fully understood [5].

26.3.1 Epidemiology and Aetiology

GCA is the most common primary vasculitis worldwide, with highest incidence amongst populations of Northern European descent, in whom the incidence

Table 26.2 Imaging modalities employed in large- and medium-vessel vasculitis

Modality	Uses and findings	Advantages	Disadvantages
CDU	Assessment of vessel wall and lumen patency, in particular for temporal, carotid, axillary and femoral arteries Stenoses and occlusions Loss of pulsation Hypoechoic, circumferential wall thickening ('halo' sign) Aneurysms	Inexpensive No radiation exposure Better resolution for smaller vessels than MRA or CTA Repeatable	Operator-dependent Not suitable for assessing non-superficial vessels (e.g. thoracic aorta)
MRI/MRA	Assessment of vessel wall and lumen patency, in particular for the aorta and its major branches Circumferential wall thickening Contrast enhancement Wall oedema	No radiation exposure Acquired images Repeatable	Poor resolution for small vessels May overestimate vascular occlusions Expense Contraindicated with metallic devices or implants Relative contraindication for gadolinium contrast in renal impairment Claustrophobia
CTA	Assessment of vessel wall and lumen patency, in particular for the aorta and its major branches Circumferential wall thickening and oedema Contrast enhancement May detect calcifications	May differentiate vascular and perivascular structures Acquired images	Radiation exposure Iodinated contrast exposure Poorer resolution than CDU
FDG-PET	Combines functional information from PET and anatomical information from CT Increased FDG uptake indicates metabolic activity May alter following treatment	Whole body assessment Most sensitive imaging method for detecting early vessel inflammation	Vascular uptake of FDG not specific for vasculitis (e.g. may not discriminate atherosclerotic lesions) No information on vessel wall structure or lumen patency Evaluation of cranial and renal vessels not feasible Expense High radiation exposure
Conventional angiography	Lumen patency assessment Stenosis and occlusion Microaneurysms	Excellent resolution Central blood pressure recording Potential for therapeutic intervention	No assessment of vessel wall Iodinated contrast exposure Complications of arterial access

Abbreviations: *CDU* colour Doppler ultrasonography, *MRI* magnetic resonance imaging, *MRA* magnetic resonance angiography, *CTA* computerised tomography angiography, *FDG* 18F-fluorodeoxyglucose, *PET* positron emission tomography

ranges from 18 to 29 per 100,000 people over the age of 50, with peak incidence in the 8th decade [5]. Females are more commonly affected than males, at a ratio of approximately 3:1. There is particular predilection amongst those of Scandinavian ancestry, suggesting a genetic predisposition to disease. There has been consistent association with the inheritance of class II MHC molecules, in particular with *HLA-DRB1*04* alleles [6]. Associations with genes encoding cytokines and their receptors (e.g. *TNF*, *IFNG*, *IL6*), molecules associated with endothelial function (e.g. *ICAM1*, *VEGF*) and regulators of innate immunity (e.g. *TLR4*, *MPO*) have also been described. Reports of seasonal variation in disease onset and epidemiological associations with some infections, such as *Mycoplasma pneumonia* and parvovirus B19, suggest that infectious or environmental factors may act to incite disease in genetically susceptible individuals, though there is no consistent evidence of any particular micro-organism as a direct trigger [7].

Table 26.3 1990 American College of Rheumatology Classification Criteria for Systemic Vasculitides

Disease	Criteria	Criteria threshold	Sensitivity[a] (%)	Specificity[a] (%)
Giant cell arteritis [48]	Age at disease onset >50 years New headache Temporal artery abnormality Elevated ESR Abnormal artery biopsy	3 of 5	93.5	91.2
Takayasu arteritis [49]	Age at disease onset <40 years Claudication of the extremities Decreased brachial artery pulse BP difference < 10 mmHg Bruit over subclavian arteries or aorta Arteriogram abnormality	3 of 6	90.5	97.8
Polyarteritis nodosa [50]	Weight loss >4 kg Livedo reticularis Testicular pain or tenderness Myalgias, weakness or leg tenderness Mononeuropathy or polyneuropathy Diastolic BP >90 mmHg Elevated BUN or creatinine Hepatitis B virus Arteriographic abnormality Biopsy of small or medium-sized artery containing PMN	3 of 10	82.2%	86.6%

Abbreviations: *ESR* erythrocyte sedimentation rate, *BP* blood pressure, *BUN* blood urea nitrogen, *PMN* polymorphonuclear neutrophils

[a]Sensitivity and specificity refer to ability to discriminate a given form of vasculitis from patients with other forms of vasculitis, rather than unselected populations. These criteria are used for classification rather than diagnostic purposes

Table 26.4 Possible large- and medium-vessel vasculitis mimics

Atherosclerosis including chronic peri-aortitis	
IgG4-related disease	
Fibromuscular dysplasia	
Post-radiation therapy	
Congenital conditions	Aortic coarctation
	Mid-aortic syndrome
Infectious diseases	Mycotic aneurysms
	Cardiovascular syphilis
	Tuberculosis
	Leprosy
	HIV
Inherited connective tissue diseases	Marfan syndrome
	Ehlers Danlos syndrome
	Pseudoxanthoma elasticum
	Loeys Dietz syndrome

26.3.2 Clinical and Laboratory Features

Symptoms of classical cranial GCA include headache, jaw and tongue claudication, scalp tenderness and visual disturbances including amaurosis fugax and diplopia. Clinical examination may reveal enlarged, thickened or tender temporal arteries, with absence of pulsation. An acute phase response is often present.

These features may be less prominent or absent in LV-GCA, where patients may present with constitutional symptoms in addition to symptoms of peripheral arterial insufficiency, usually in the upper extremities. Vascular bruits and pulse discrepancies may be evident on clinical examination. The finding of a regurgitant aortic murmur may indicate the development of ascending aortic aneurysm and dilatation of the aortic valve. Specific clinical features of large-vessel compromise in LV-GCA, however, may not be evident, and patients may present only with constitutional or PMR symptoms. In these cases, a heightened index of clinical suspicion with low threshold for dedicated vascular imaging is required in order to identify subclinical large-vessel disease.

26

26.3.3 Pathology

Prior to the uptake of advanced non-invasive imaging techniques, temporal artery biopsy was regarded as an essential gold standard for diagnosis of GCA, particularly in those with symptoms of cranial arteritis. In acute disease, focal granulomatous panarteritis, typically with multinucleate giant cells, intimal hyperplasia and rarely luminal thrombosis, may be observed. These lesions may be scattered irregularly ('skip lesions') in affected vessels, and thus adequate sampling (segments >1 cm) is required to avoid false-negative results. In the chronic phase of disease, inflammatory lesions may evolve to fibrosis with resultant vessel narrowing.

In patients with LV-GCA without symptoms of cranial arteritis, temporal artery biopsy is reported to have lower sensitivity than in patients with cranial manifestations, though a systematic, prospective study of temporal artery biopsy in LV-GCA has not been conducted. Given the arterial distribution of vessel involvement in LV-GCA, targeted tissue sampling is often not possible, and diagnosis relies on the use of appropriate imaging methods.

26.3.4 Imaging

Recent EULAR guidelines suggest use of colour Doppler ultrasound (CDU) of the temporal artery as the first-line imaging modality in patients with suspected cranial GCA, assuming adequate expertise and prompt availability of testing [2]. The typical finding is of homogenous, hypoechoic, circumferential wall thickening (the 'halo' sign), and vessel stenosis or occlusion may also be seen. High-resolution MRI of the cranial vessels may identify mural inflammation and is an alternative imaging modality where CDU is not readily available or inconclusive. In patients where there is high clinical suspicion of cranial GCA and compatible imaging findings, diagnostic temporal artery biopsy may not be necessary.

In patients with suspected LV-GCA, a variety of imaging modalities may be used to identify mural inflammation or luminal changes in extra-cranial arteries, which may support the diagnosis. These include MRI, CT and FDG-PET (◘ Table 26.2). CDU may be less useful, given its limited access to the thoracic aorta.

Some guidelines recommend baseline CTA or MRA imaging in all patients with newly diagnosed GCA [8], given the frequency of aortic involvement, though the use of this screening approach has not been evaluated prospectively.

26.3.5 Treatment

Prompt initiation of therapy in confirmed or suspected GCA is essential, given that the majority of adverse ischaemic complications, such as visual loss, occur prior to receiving treatment. Corticosteroids have been the mainstay of treatment for several decades, usually initiated at high dose (0.75–1 mg/kg.day) for a period of 4 weeks, followed by gradual taper over 1–2 years. The majority of patients demonstrate prompt resolution of clinical symptoms and inflammatory response following corticosteroid treatment, though it should be noted that steroid-related adverse events are very common (occurring in almost 90% of cases [9]) and appear to be related to both cumulative exposure and patient age. In addition, relapses or steroid dependency is frequently observed, occurring in 40–60% of patients. In these cases, there is limited evidence to support the use of conventional alternative immunosuppressives such as methotrexate (or azathioprine where methotrexate is contraindicated or not tolerated) [10].

A number of biologic therapies have been studied in the treatment of GCA [11]. Tocilizumab, an IL6 receptor alpha antagonist, has shown clinical efficacy and a corticosteroid-sparing effect in a large randomised control trial [12] and is now licensed for treatment of GCA in the USA and Europe. Other biologic therapies undergoing investigation in GCA include ustekinumab (an IL12/IL23 blocking monoclonal antibody) and abatacept (a selective T-cell co-stimulation blocker). Clinical studies have failed to show benefit of anti-TNFα therapy in GCA.

26.3.6 Renal Involvement in GCA

Significant renal involvement is thought to be uncommon in GCA. A pooled analysis of historical post-mortem series found that arteritis of the main renal artery was present in 32% of cases [13], though reports of clinically apparent renovascular involvement are uncommon [14]. Renal artery involvement has not been specifically addressed in the more recent imaging studies [15]. These patients usually receive conventional treatment as for LV-GCA, and percutaneous revascularisation may be considered in cases where main renal artery disease is associated with resistant hypertension or progressive renal impairment [16].

Asymptomatic microscopic haematuria is not uncommon in GCA, being reported in 33–48% of patients in retrospective series [17, 18]. The largest of these series reported low rates of concomitant proteinuria, preserved renal function and resolution of haematuria in 71% of cases after corticosteroid treatment. In the small number of cases in whom urinary red cell morphology was assessed (n = 7), dysmorphic cells were seen in all. However, it is unclear whether the microscopic haematuria in these cases was related to indolent intra-renal vasculitis, glomerulonephritis or other pathology, as renal biopsy was not performed.

In this regard, there are rare case reports and small series of severe glomerulonephritis in patients with GCA [19–22]. Histopathological lesions include fibrinoid glomerular necrosis, crescent formation and vasculitis of the renal arterioles and small arteries, lesions more typical of ANCA-associated small-vessel vasculitis. Conversely, temporal artery involvement had been documented in patients diagnosed with granulomatosis with polyangiitis [23, 24]. Many of these reports, however, predate the routine use of ANCA testing, and the pathological lesion of granulomatous vessel wall inflammation may be indistinguishable in the two diseases, so whether these cases of glomerulonephritis represent true manifestations of GCA, possible 'overlap' syndromes, or a casual association of disease entities, remains unclear. Renal biopsy is recommended in patients with GCA demonstrating persistent urinary abnormalities, and when severe pauci-immune glomerulonephritis is confirmed, induction treatment with cytotoxic therapy in addition to corticosteroids should be considered, in order to prevent long-term renal morbidity.

Finally, there are rare reports of AA-type amyloidosis in GCA, with both renal and systemic involvement. A systematic review identified 11 cases in the literature and suggests that the development of amyloidosis confers adverse renal outcomes and poor overall survival [25].

26.4 Takayasu Arteritis

Definition

Takaysu arteritis is defined as arteritis, often granulomatous, predominantly affecting the aorta and/or its major branches, usually with onset in patients younger than 50 years.

The disease shares some epidemiological, clinical and histopathological features with GCA, which has led some authors to suggest that the two conditions represent spectrums of the same disease [26]. There are, however, important differences, emphasised below, such that most regard these diseases as distinct entities.

26.4.1 Epidemiology and Aetiology

Takayasu arteritis was first described in Japanese populations, where it currently has an estimated incidence of one to two per million per year, though it is now recognised to occur worldwide. The annual incidence of Takayasu arteritis in the UK, for example, is estimated to be 0.8 per million [27]. It is more common in women (80–90% of cases), and age of onset is usually between 10 and 40 years, the major epidemiological feature that distinguishes it from GCA. Disease susceptibility and severity are consistently associated with inheritance of the *HLA-B*52:01* allele in populations of multiple ethnicities (in contrast to the class II association observed in GCA). Additional associations with polymorphisms in other class I HLA genes and genes encoding pro-inflammatory (e.g. *IL6*, *IL12B*) and regulatory immune responses (e.g. *LILRB*, *IL38*) have been reported [28]. Of note, polymorphisms in *KDM4C* (a gene encoding a histone demethylase involved in the epigenetic control of gene expression) were recently associated with susceptibility to a number of large and small-vessel vasculitides, including Takayasu arteritis [29]. A number of putative bacterial and viral infectious triggers have been suggested for Takayasu arteritis, though no micro-organism has been robustly implicated in disease onset.

26.4.2 Clinical and Laboratory Features

Takayasu arteritis tends to have indolent presentation, and its detection is often delayed, such that stenotic vascular abnormalities may be well established at first diagnosis. Constitutional symptoms are common in the initial phase. Symptoms of arterial insufficiency will depend on the territories affected; common manifestations include limb claudication (30–80%); hypertension, and where the cranial arteries are affected, headache (50–70%); syncope (4–19%); visual disturbance (15–35%); and potentially stroke (3–22%). Angina and gastro-intestinal and respiratory symptoms may be present when the coronary, mesenteric and pulmonary vasculatures are involved, respectively. Carotidynia (tenderness of the carotid artery) is present in up to 30% of cases. Absent or weak peripheral pulses, discrepant blood pressure measurements and vascular bruits may also be evident on clinical examination. The presence of an acute phase response may support a clinical diagnosis of Takayasu arteritis; however, these tests do not reliably reflect disease activity and are frequently normal in the presence of active arterial inflammation.

26.4.3 Pathology

Takayasu arteritis is characterised by transmural infiltration of arterial walls by inflammatory cells including lymphocytes, monocytes and neutrophils. Multinucleate giant cells and granulomata are typically found in the tunica media. This inflammation may progress to sclerosis, developing from the adventitial layer, which can occlude the vessel lumen. This may be compounded by intimal fibroplasia. Less commonly, destruction of the elastic lamina and tunica media may result in aneurysm formation with the affected vessel wall. The disease may be confluent or patchy, with areas of normal vasculature separated by disease affected segments.

Tissue biopsy, however, is rarely used in the diagnosis of Takayasu arteritis, given the pattern of vascular involvement and technical difficulty of performing large-vessel biopsy. Tissue samples, however, may be obtained during revascularisation or surgical procedures and may inform subsequent treatment decisions based on the observed activity of disease.

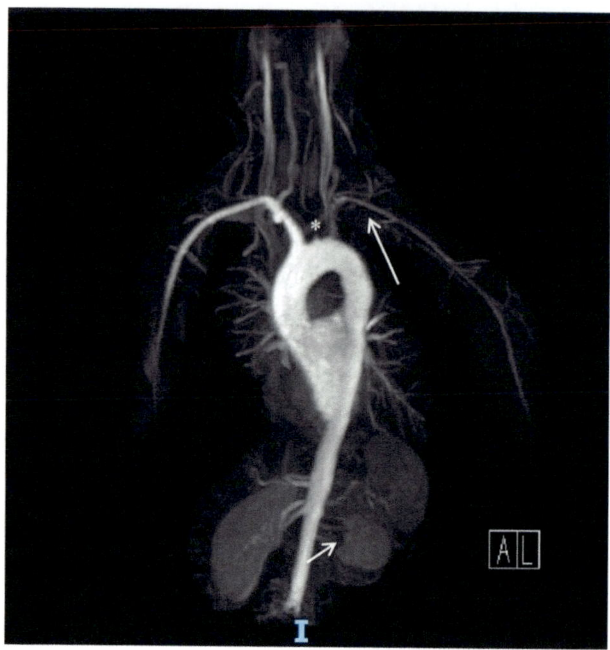

Fig. 26.1 *Magnetic resonance angiogram in Takayasu arteritis*, showing occlusion of the left common carotid artery (star) and narrowing of the left subclavian artery (long arrow). There is proximal stenosis affecting the left renal artery resulting in a small ischaemic left kidney (short arrow). (Image provided by Prof Justin Mason, Imperial College London)

26.4.4 Imaging

Arterial imaging studies are essential for corroborating a diagnosis of Takayasu arteritis and for determining the extent and pattern of vascular involvement. Current guidelines recommend contrast-enhanced MR imaging as first-line modality [2] (Fig. 26.1). This had the advantage of delineating both luminal and inflammatory vessel wall changes, while avoiding radiation exposure in young patients. CT, FDG-PET and CDU may also be used, though the latter has limited utility for imaging non-superficial vessels. These non-invasive imaging techniques have largely superseded conventional intraarterial angiography for the diagnosis of Takayasu arteritis, though their role in monitoring disease activity and for long-term follow-up of vessel changes remains undefined.

26.4.5 Treatment

As in GCA, corticosteroids are the mainstay of therapy, with a suggested initial prednisolone dosage of 0.5–1 mg/kg daily. Relapses and corticosteroid dependence are, however, common, and between 46% and 84% of patients will require a second immunosuppressive agent in order to achieve sustained remission with acceptable corticosteroid doses. There are no randomised trial data regarding the use of conventional steroid-sparing agents in Takayasu arteritis, though uncontrolled studies suggest that methotrexate, azathioprine and mycophenolate mofetil could be considered. Promising results have been observed with biologic therapies including anti-TNFα agents (in contrast to GCA) and tocilizumab, and these agents may have a role in relapsing or resistant disease [11].

In addition to medical therapy, patients may require revascularisation procedures for symptomatic steno-occlusive disease, or aneurysmal lesions with risk of rupture [30]. Percutaneous angioplasty may be preferred to surgical intervention, though complex, lengthy or heavily scarred lesions may not be amenable to catheter-based approaches, and restenosis rates are high. Ideally, interventions should be performed after a period of immunosuppressive treatment when vessel wall inflammation is quiescent.

26.4.6 Renal Involvement in Takayasu Arteritis

Hypertension is common in Takayasu arteritis (occurring in >50% of cases), and it may be the initial clinical manifestation in a significant proportion. The aetiology of hypertension is multifactorial, arising as a complication of aortic or renal artery disease driving hyperreninism, carotid baroreceptor hyposensitivity, loss of vessel wall elasticity, vascular endothelial dysfunction and/or of corticosteroid treatment. Somewhat paradoxically, the diagnosis of hypertension in Takaysu's arteritis may be overlooked in the presence of bilateral subclavian artery involvement. Indeed, a recent Chinese study found that previously unrecognised hypertension was detected at intraarterial angiography in 16% of such cases [31]. The same study found that renal artery lesions were present in 70% of hypertensive Takayasu patients, thoracic aortic lesions in 26%, abdominal aortic lesions in 21% and mixed pathology in 26%.

In unselected Takayasu arteritis cohorts, renal artery involvement remains common, with reported incidences between 10% and 60%, and it appears to be more frequent in Asian populations compared to those of European descent [32]. Disease is often ostial and proximal, frequently with co-existent involvement of the perirenal aorta. Bilateral renal artery involvement may occur in approximately 50% of cases. The severity of renal artery stenosis correlates with the frequency of hypertension, and inversely with estimated glomerular filtration rate, somewhat in contrast to atherosclerotic renovascular disease (ARVD).

The optimum treatment for hypertension resistant to medical therapy secondary to renal artery involvement in Takayasu arteritis is unclear, owing to the rarity of the disease and a lack of controlled, prospective studies; data derived from studies in ARVD are likely not applicable, given differences in patient demographics and disease pathogenesis. A recent meta-analysis of studies that compared conventional balloon angioplasty to endovascular stenting suggested that these approaches were equally efficacious for improving renovascular hypertension but that the risk of restenosis was significantly higher following stenting compared to balloon angioplasty [33]. The main limitation of percutaneous approaches includes suboptimal correction of long, irregular, potentially fibrotic lesions and recoiling of ostial lesions. A further meta-analysis of retrospective observational studies (giving low-moderate quality evidence) suggested that restenosis is less common with surgical rather than percutaneous interventions, though the former carry a higher risk of complications [34]. A number of surgical approaches have been described, including aorto-renal bypass, aortic reimplantation, arterioplasty and autotransplantation to the iliac vessels [35]. In practice, the choice of intervention requires careful consideration of lesion anatomy and risk of complications in individual patients.

Few studies have investigated urinary abnormalities or renal histopathology in Takayasu arteritis. In a large Chinese cohort, the prevalence of proteinuria was estimated to be approximately 9%, which has been attributed to hypertensive or ischaemic glomerulopathy. In keeping with this suggestion, an autopsy-based study of 25 cases found histopathological features of long-standing arterial hypertension or renal ischaemia in all [36]. In addition, however, specific features of glomerulonephritis were found in 14. The most common pattern was mild diffuse mesangial proliferative GN, occurring in ten patients, and this associated with a larger extent of vascular inflammatory cell infiltrate, suggesting a possible relationship between these phenomena. The frequency of specific glomerular lesions in this report is perhaps higher than expected, though it is possible that findings in these post-mortem cases are not representative of a general Takayasu arteritis population.

There are case reports of a variety of other primary glomerular disorders, such as IgA nephropathy, crescentic glomerulonephritis and membranous glomerulonephropathy, occurring in patients with Takayasu arteritis, though these likely reflect coincidental rather than causal relationships. As reported in GCA, cases of secondary AA amyloidosis have been described in patients with Takayasu arteritis.

26.5 Polyarteritis Nodosa

Definition

Polyarteritis nodosa (PAN) is a systemic necrotising vasculitis of medium or small arteries without glomerulonephritis or vasculitis in arterioles, capillaries or venules. It is not associated with ANCA.

It should be noted that historical descriptions of PAN, prior to the introduction of ANCA testing in the 1990s and the widespread recognition of microscopic polyangiitis (MPA) as a distinct clinical entity, may have included a significant proportion of patients with other vasculitides, and they should be interpreted accordingly.

26.5.1 Epidemiology and Aetiology

The annual incidence of PAN is estimated to be 0–1.6 cases per million in European populations [37]. It most commonly presents in middle age, with a peak incidence in the sixth decade. There is a slight male preponderance. Pan has a well-recognised association with hepatitis B, with disease onset typically occurring 4 months after infection [38], and the incidence of PAN is increased in regions of endemic HBV infection. Loss of function mutations in *ADA2*, the gene encoding the enzyme adenosine deaminase 2, has been associated with the development of a PAN-like illness, with onset in childhood or adolescence [39].

26.5.2 Clinical and Laboratory Features

Patients often present with constitutional inflammatory symptoms, in association with multisystem vascular involvement. Cutaneous manifestations such as purpura, erythematous nodules and livedo reticularis are common (>50%; ◘ Fig. 26.2), along with neuropathy (mononeuritis multiplex or asymmetrical motor and sensory polyneuropathy; 75%) and gastro-intestinal disease (abdominal pain, rectal bleeding; 40%) [40]. Less commonly, the central nervous system (20%), heart (10%) or testes (20%) are involved.

Laboratory tests may reveal an acute phase response, and testing for hepatitis infection and serologies associated with other forms of vasculitis (ANCA, ANA) should be undertaken.

26.5.3 Pathology

PAN predominantly affects medium-sized muscular arteries, occasionally smaller arteries, and in contrast to many other forms of vasculitis, veins are not affected. Focal and segmental fibrinoid necrosis is seen, characteristically at vessel branching points, with a mural and perivascular infiltrate of neutrophils and monocytes (◘ Fig. 26.3). Leucocytoclasia may be observed, while granulomata are not a feature. Intra-luminal thrombosis formation may contribute to vessel occlusion. Disruption of the external elastic lamina may result in aneurysmal dilatation (◘ Fig. 26.3b). In more advanced lesions, vascular remodelling results in intimal hyperplasia and fibrotic changes within the vessel wall.

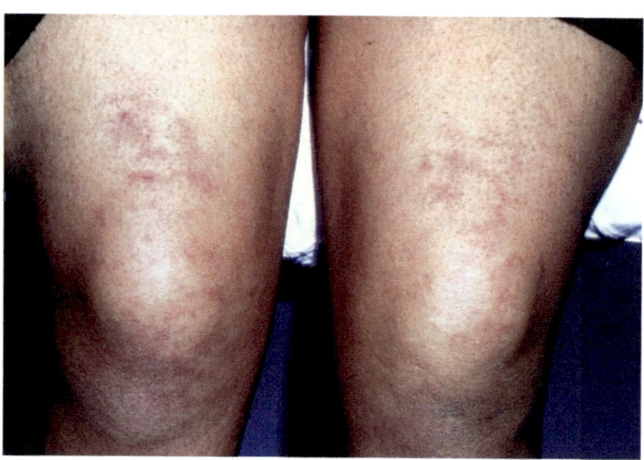

◘ **Fig. 26.2** Classic livedo reticularis rash in a patient with polyarteritis nodosa. (Image provided by Dr Mark Harber, University College London)

Frequently biopsied sites in clinical practise include the skin (including subcutaneous fat containing medium-sized arteries), nerves and muscles, though the latter may lack diagnostic sensitivity. Renal biopsy may be considered, though there slightly increased risk of bleeding due to vessel rupture.

26.5.4 Imaging

Selective arteriography is the imaging modality of choice for evaluating PAN (◘ Fig. 26.4). Arterial saccular or fusiform microaneurysms (1–5 mm in diameter) are typically seen, often in association with vascular ectasia, luminal irregularity, stenosis or occlusion. Non-invasive angiographic techniques (CTA, MRA) may also be used, particularly with continued improvements in imaging resolution, and they may have a role in monitoring disease progression or response to treatment while avoiding repeated invasive angiography.

26.5.5 Treatment

Patients presenting with mild disease, such as constitutional symptoms or with isolated cutaneous involvement, may be treated initially with oral corticosteroids alone. Approximately 50%, however, will require addition of a second immunosuppressive agent for refractory or relapsing disease, and one small prospective trial suggested that azathioprine and pulsed intravenous cyclophosphamide were equally efficacious in this setting, though the latter may be associated with a higher rate of adverse events [41].

There are no randomised controlled studies of therapeutic approaches for patients with severe disease manifestations, including significant visceral, renal or neurological involvement, specifically in patients with PAN alone. EULAR guidelines recommend cyclophosphamide and corticosteroids in combination for remission-induction [42], an approach supported by historical observational studies that suggest improved outcome and survival with cytotoxic treatment, and follow-up of randomised trials that included patients with PAN (in addition to other vasculitides including EGPA and MPA). There are limited data on the ideal dose, route and duration of cyclophosphamide treatment, and regimens analogous to those used in other forms of necrotising vasculitis are often used [43, 44].

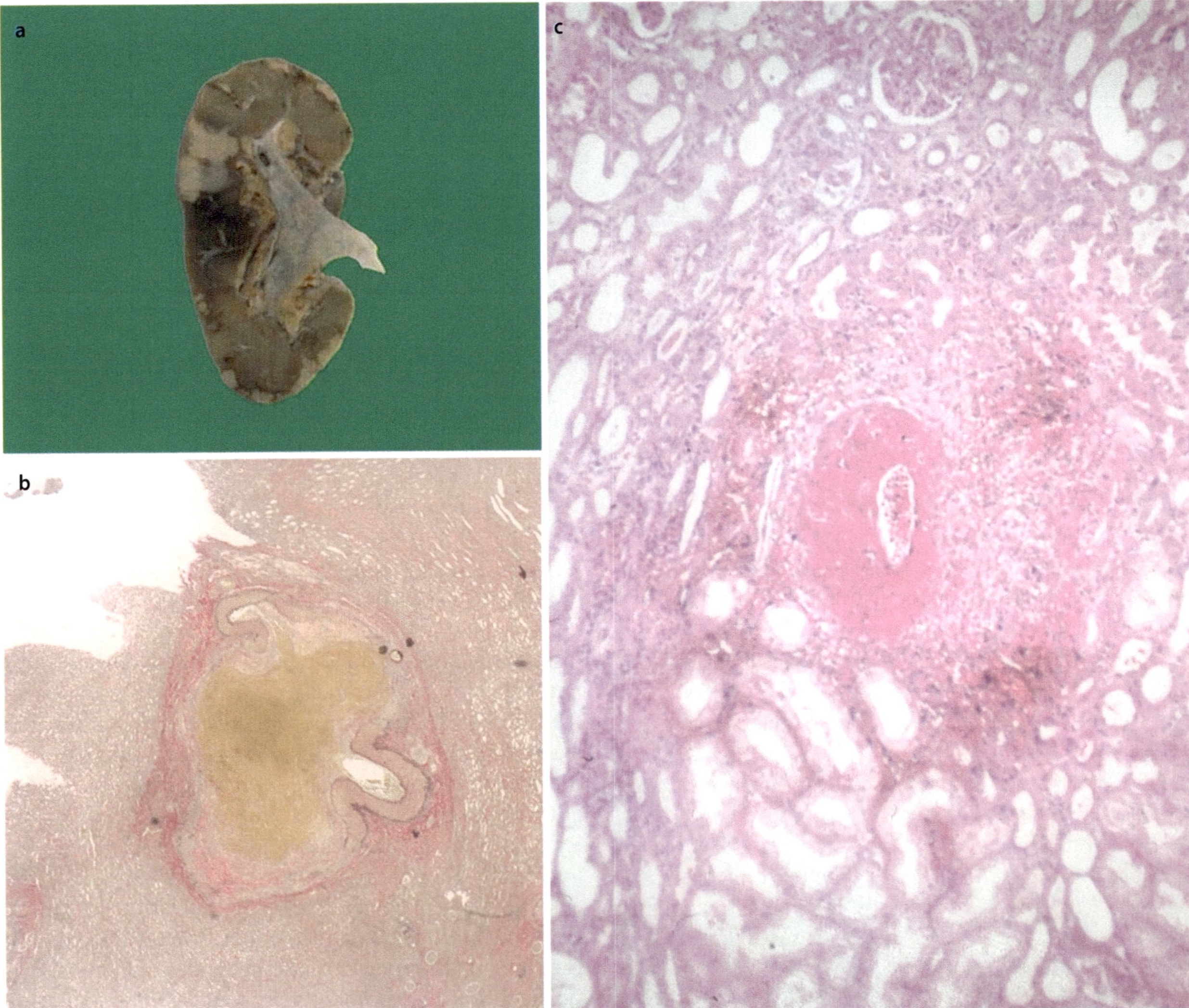

Fig. 26.3 Renal pathology in polyarteritis nodosa. (**a**) Multiple wedge-shaped cortical infarcts in a post-mortem kidney specimen. (**b**) Necrotising arteritis in a large muscular interlobar artery, with disruption of external elastic lamina and early aneurysm formation. (**c**) Circumferential necrotising arteritis and perivascular inflammation in an arcuate artery. (Images provided by Professor Terry Cook, Imperial College London)

One small randomised trial found that relapse rates were higher in patients who received 6 versus 12 monthly doses of intravenous cyclophosphamide; however this study included a high proportion of patients with microscopic polyangiitis [45]. Remission-maintenance treatment is usually offered for 18–24 months, though the risk of relapse in PAN appears to be lower than in other forms of vasculitis; a large retrospective study, for example, found that 21.8% of patients relapsed during average follow-up of 5.7 years [40]. There are limited data on the use of biologic therapies such a rituximab or tocilizumab in the treatment of PAN.

The treatment of HBV-associated PAN requires both antiviral therapy and immunosuppression directed to the severity of disease manifestations. Plasmapheresis may be considered as an adjunct in acute disease to reduce immunosuppressive burden in patients with active viraemia [38].

26.5.6 Renal Involvement in PAN

The kidney is the most commonly affected visceral organ in PAN. Historical and autopsy series report renal involvement in up to 75% of cases, though contemporaneous studies report lower frequencies of approximately 50% [40], perhaps due to recent changes in classification criteria for systemic vasculitides.

The renal, interlobar and arcuate arteries may be affected, resulting in cortical ischaemia and infarction

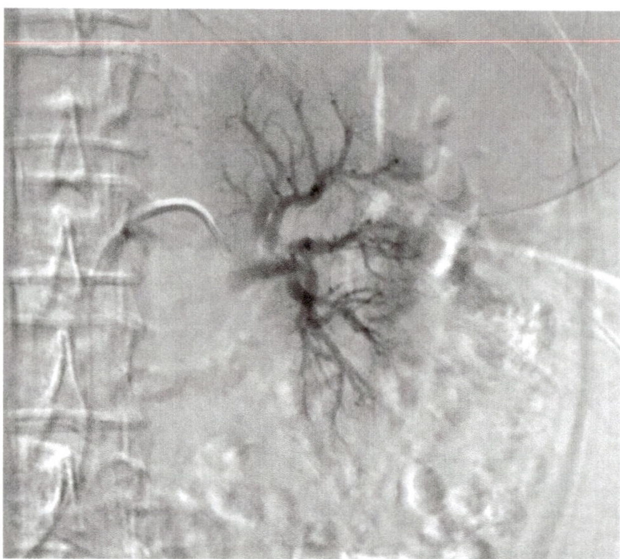

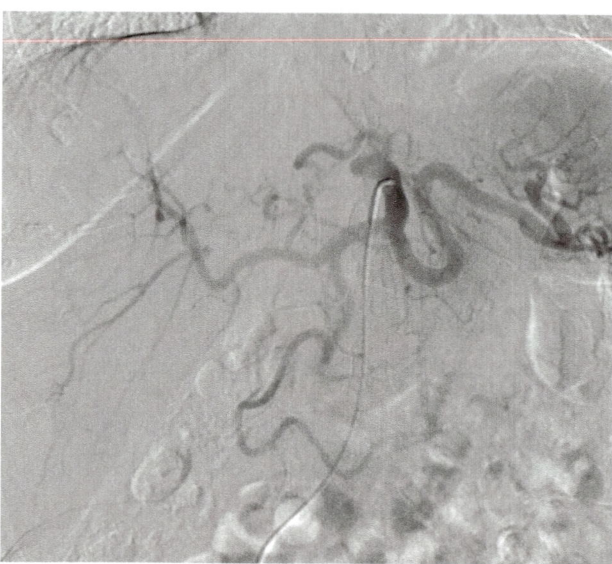

◘ **Fig. 26.4** *Renal and mesenteric angiography in polyarteritis nodosa*, demonstrating multiple arterial microaneurysms, with a predilection for vessel branching points. (Images provided by Professor Alan Salama, University College London)

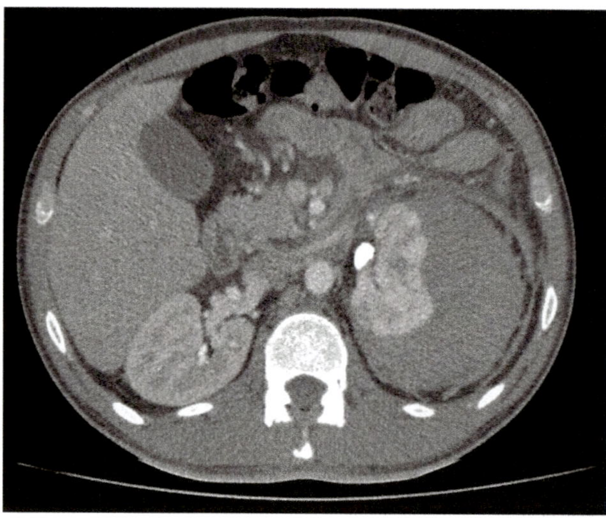

◘ **Fig. 26.5** Large perinephric haemorrhage following aneurysm rupture in a patient with polyarteritis nodosa

(◘ Fig. 26.3). Chronic glomerular ischaemia may result in hyper-reninaemic hypertension and progressive loss of GFR, though oliguric acute kidney injury is uncommon. Rupture of arterial aneurysms may present with visible haematuria and loin pain. Rarely, life-threatening parenchymal or retroperitoneal bleeding may occur (◘ Fig. 26.5). By definition, the glomerular capillaries are spared in PAN, and thus significant proteinuria, dysmorphic erythrocyturia and glomerulonephritis are not a feature, and their presence should alert to the possibility of an alternative or second diagnosis.

PAN is an uncommon cause of end-stage renal disease. The European Renal Association-European Dialysis and Transplant Association (ERA-EDTA) registry identified 112 patients with a diagnosis of polyarteritis who underwent renal transplantation between 1982 and 1990 [46]. Three-year patient (77% versus 91%) and allograft (60 versus 69%) survivals were poorer than in those receiving transplantation for other primary renal diseases, and 13% of graft failures were attributed to recurrent disease. This study, however, predates refined definitions of PAN and MPA, and it likely includes a high proportion of patients who would now be recognised as having MPA. While it does not comment on the timing of renal transplantation relative to disease diagnosis or remission status, surgery is usually delayed until 1 year after disease control in AAV [47].

Case Study

Case 1

A 78-year-old female presented with lethargy, weight loss, myalgias, temporal headache and a moderate inflammatory response, CRP 31.5 mg/L, ESR 74 mm/hr. A temporal artery biopsy revealed focal inflammation of the intima and media, with occasional giant cells, compatible with a diagnosis of GCA. Following treatment with high-dose oral corticosteroids, she had prompt resolution of her symptoms and inflammatory response, and steroids were weaned after 1 year. Three years later she re-presented with recurrence of constitutional symptoms, without headache. She was found to have an acute phase response and a nephritic urine sediment. Renal biopsy revealed a focal and segmental pauci-immune necrotising glomerulonephritis. Concurrent testing for ANCA demonstrated high-titre anti-PR3 antibodies. She was treated with rituximab and corticosteroids, resulting sustained clinical remission after 1 year. In retrospect, her initial presentation could be compatible with a diagnosis of granulomatosis with poylangiitis (GPA) without initial renal involvement (noting that ANCA were not determined at first presentation); alternatively, this patient may have sequential diagnoses of GCA and GPA. This case illustrates the diagnostic challenge in vasculitis, and the utility of kidney biopsy in the presence of urinary abnormalities.

Case 2

A 24-year-old male presented to the emergency department with acute severe flank pain, followed by an episode of syncope. Blood tests revealed a haemoglobin of 59 g/L, CRP 157 mg/L, creatinine 92 umol/L. Urgent cross-sectional imaging demonstrated a large perinephric haemorrhage (◘ Fig. 26.5). Subsequent CT angiography demonstrated multiple small aneurysms in both kidneys, the spleen and the pancreas. Further history revealed a diagnosis of early-onset hypertension, and multiple attendances to hospital with abdominal pain in the preceding year, for which no clear cause had been found. Testing for hepatitis viruses was negative. He received treatment with pulsed intravenous cyclophosphamide and oral corticosteroids for a diagnosis of PAN. This case illustrates the initial non-specific features of PAN and the rare occurrence of life-threatening bleeding following aneurysm rupture.

Case 3

A woman in her early 20s initially presented with headache, visual disturbance and a raised acute phase response without constitutional symptoms. After initial recovery her condition flared and was complicated by myocarditis with significant hypertension. Following supportive treatment, she recovered, only to represent a year later with carotidynia and symptoms suggestive of cerebral ischemia including transient loss of consciousness and intermittent visual disturbance. Blood tests revealed a moderate rise in ESR and CRP. She was referred to rheumatology where subsequent imaging revealed Takayasu arteritis with thoracic aortitis, proximal stenoses affecting the great vessels and stenosis affecting the proximal coeliac trunk and the left renal artery resulting in a small ischaemic left kidney (◘ Fig. 26.1).

Conclusion

The large and medium vasculitides are a heterogenous and challenging group of diseases. In the absence of validated diagnostic criteria, a combination of clinical, laboratory and non-invasive imaging findings, with or without tissue biopsy, are used to make a diagnosis. Glomerular disease is uncommon, though renovascular involvement is frequent, particularly in patients with Takayasu arteritis and PAN. In addition to immunosuppressive and medical therapy, these cases require expert multidisciplinary management from rheumatologists, nephrologists and vascular surgeons for the management of symptomatic steno-occlusive or aneurysmal lesions. In the future, it is hoped that increased awareness of disease, coupled to improvements in imaging and the use of novel biologic treatments, will lead to earlier diagnosis and improved outcomes for patients with these rare diseases.

? Chapter Review Questions

1. A 32-year-old woman presents with a 6-month history of lethargy, weight loss and headache. In the past month, she reports a dull ache in her left arm. Examination reveals tenderness of the carotid artery and absent pulsation in the left radial and brachial artery. Which is the preferred vascular imaging modality?
   - Contrast-enhanced CT angiography
   - Intraarterial angiography
   - Contrast-enhanced MR angiography
   - Colour Doppler ultrasound
   - 18F-fluorodeoxyglucose PET CT

2. A 53-year-old Caucasian man presents with rash, abdominal pain and diarrhoea. He reports weight loss, generalised arthralgia and a low-grade fever for the preceding 4 weeks. Examination reveals blood pressure of 192/112 and weakness of right wrist extension with numbness on the dorsum of the right hand. Urinalysis is positive for blood 3+, negative for protein, leucocytes and nitrites. Blood test show an elevated erythrocyte sedimentation rate of 69 mm/hr, C-reactive protein 45 mg/L and serum creatinine of 145 μmol/L. Anti-nuclear antibodies (ANA), anti-neutrophil cytoplasm antibodies (ANCA) and rheumatoid factor are negative. Which test will provide most diagnostic information?

- Renal biopsy
- Skin biopsy
- Nerve conduction studies
- Mesenteric angiography
- Colonoscopy

3. A 35-year-old non-smoking woman presents following a transient loss of motor function in the right upper limb lasting for 15 minutes. She describes 3-month history of headache and neck pain. Examination reveals blood pressure 185/105, with renal and carotid bruits, but is otherwise unremarkable. Urinalysis is negative, and bloods tests show a normal full blood count, serum creatinine 72 μmol/L, ESR <10 mm/hr, CRP <1 mg/L. CT angiography demonstrates irregular "string of beads" appearances of the left renal and left carotid artery. Which is the most likely underlying diagnosis?
   - Fibromuscular dysplasia
   - Takayasu arteritis
   - Atherosclerotic disease
   - Polyarteritis nodosa
   - Ehlers Danlos syndrome

4. A 72-year-old woman presents with myalgia and temporal headache. She has a pronounced inflammatory response, and temporal artery biopsy confirms a granulomatous panarteritis. She is treated with oral prednisolone 60 mg daily for 1 month, with prompt response to treatment, followed by a gradual corticosteroid taper. On reducing her prednisolone dose to 20 mg daily, she develops recurrence of her symptoms and elevated inflammatory markers, requiring repeat high-steroid therapy. On further attempts to wean corticosteroids, she is unable to achieve a dose lower than 20 mg daily while controlling her symptoms. Proven next line therapy is:
   - Methotrexate
   - Tocilizumab
   - Cyclophosphamide
   - Infliximab
   - Azathioprine

Answers

1. This patient presents with typical features of Takayasu arteritis. Current guidelines recommend contrast-enhanced MR angiography as first-line imaging in suspected cases [2]. This has the advantage of providing comprehensive, high-resolution assessment of both lumen patency and of vessel walls (unlike intraarterial angiography), while avoiding radiation exposure associated with CT scanning in young patients. Colour Doppler ultrasound may demonstrate diagnostic features in the upper limb vessels, but cannot provide a comprehensive assessment of the thoracic aorta and its branches.
2. This patient's presentation is suggestive of a diagnosis of polyarteritis nodosa. All of the above investigations may be considered, though the highest diagnostic yield will be provided by intraarterial angiography, which typically demonstrates saccular or fusiform microaneurysms (1–5 mm in diameter) in medium-sized arterial vessels. Renal biopsy is relatively contraindicated due to hypertension and associated bleeding risk. Nerve conduction studies and colonoscopy may provide supporting evidence of neuropathy or colitis, respectively, though features may be non-diagnostic. Skin biopsy may show histologic features of PAN, though it will not confirm the presence of visceral involvement.
3. The radiographic findings are typical of multifocal fibromuscular dysplasia, an idiopathic noninflammatory, non-atherosclerotic arteriopathy that can affect both the renal and carotid arteries. It shares demographic and clinical features with Takayasu arteritis (both having a predilection for young females), for which it is an important differential diagnosis, though the absence of preceding constitutional symptoms and an inflammatory response in this patient makes the latter diagnosis (as well as polyarteritis nodosa) less likely in the context of these typical imaging findings. Atherosclerotic disease is unlikely given the patient's young age and her lack of cardiovascular risk factors.
4. This patient has refractory giant cell arteritis. Tocilizumab has been shown to have a steroid-sparing effect in a large randomised controlled trial in GCA [12]. Alternative immunosuppressants such as methotrexate and azathioprine are often used in steroid-dependent disease, though controlled data are lacking. There is no evidence for the use of anti-TNFα therapy in the treatment of GCA.

Acknowledgements Professors Justin Mason (Imperial College London), Terry Cook (Imperial College London) and Alan Salama (University College London) for pathology and radiographic images.

References

1. Jennette JC, Falk RJ, Bacon PA, et al. 2012 revised international Chapel Hill consensus conference nomenclature of vasculitides. Arthritis Rheum. 2013;65(1):1–11.
2. Dejaco C, Ramiro S, Duftner C, et al. EULAR recommendations for the use of imaging in large vessel vasculitis in clinical practice. Ann Rheum Dis. 2018;77(5):636–43.
3. Fries JF, Hunder GG, Bloch DA, et al. The American College of Rheumatology 1990 criteria for the classification of vasculitis. Summary. Arthritis Rheum. 1990;33(8):1135–6.
4. Koster MJ, Matteson EL, Warrington KJ. Large-vessel giant cell arteritis: diagnosis, monitoring and management. Rheumatology. 2018;57(suppl_2):ii32–42.
5. Dejaco C, Brouwer E, Mason JC, Buttgereit F, Matteson EL, Dasgupta B. Giant cell arteritis and polymyalgia rheumatica: current challenges and opportunities. Nat Rev Rheumatol. 2017;13(10):578–92.
6. Carmona FD, Gonzalez-Gay MA, Martin J. Genetic component of giant cell arteritis. Rheumatology. 2014;53(1):6–18.
7. Nordborg E, Nordborg C. Giant cell arteritis: epidemiological clues to its pathogenesis and an update on its treatment. Rheumatology. 2003;42(3):413–21.
8. Hiratzka LF, Bakris GL, Beckman JA, et al. 2010 ACCF/AHA/AATS/ACR/ASA/SCA/SCAI/SIR/STS/SVM Guidelines for the diagnosis and management of patients with thoracic aortic disease: Executive summary: a report of the American College of Cardiology Foundation/American Heart Association Task Force on Practice Guidelines, American Association for Thoracic Surgery, American College of Radiology, American Stroke Association, Society of Cardiovascular Anesthesiologists, Society for Cardiovascular Angiography and Interventions, Society of Interventional Radiology, Society of Thoracic Surgeons, and Society for Vascular Medicine. Anesth Analg. 2010;111(2):279–315.
9. Proven A, Gabriel SE, Orces C, O'Fallon WM, Hunder GG. Glucocorticoid therapy in giant cell arteritis: duration and adverse outcomes. Arthritis Rheum. 2003;49(5):703–8.
10. Dasgupta B, Borg FA, Hassan N, et al. BSR and BHPR guidelines for the management of giant cell arteritis. Rheumatology. 2010;49(8):1594–7.
11. Muratore F, Pipitone N, Salvarani C. Standard and biological treatment in large vessel vasculitis: guidelines and current approaches. Expert Rev Clin Immunol. 2017;13(4):345–60.
12. Stone JH, Tuckwell K, Dimonaco S, et al. Trial of tocilizumab in giant-cell arteritis. N Engl J Med. 2017;377(4):317–28.
13. Greene GM, Lain D, Sherwin RM, Wilson JE, McManus BM. Giant cell arteritis of the legs. Clinical isolation of severe disease with gangrene and amputations. Am J Med. 1986;81(4):727–33.
14. Lambert M, Weber A, Boland B, De Plaen JF, Donckier J. Large vessel vasculitis without temporal artery involvement: isolated form of giant cell arteritis? Clin Rheumatol. 1996;15(2):174–80.
15. Cid MC, Prieto-Gonzalez S, Arguis P, et al. The spectrum of vascular involvement in giant-cell arteritis: clinical consequences of detrimental vascular remodelling at different sites. APMIS Suppl. 2009;127:10–20.
16. Both M, Jahnke T, Reinhold-Keller E, et al. Percutaneous management of occlusive arterial disease associated with vasculitis: a single center experience. Cardiovasc Intervent Radiol. 2003;26(1):19–26.
17. Manna R, Cristiano G, Todaro L, Latteri M, Gasbarrini G. Microscopic haematuria: a diagnostic aid in giant-cell arteritis? Lancet. 1997;350(9086):1226.
18. Vanderschueren S, Depoot I, Knockaert DC, Verbeken EK, Zaman Z, Bobbaers H. Microscopic haematuria in giant cell arteritis. Clin Rheumatol. 2002;21(5):373–7.
19. Truong L, Kopelman RG, Williams GS, Pirani CL. Temporal arteritis and renal disease. Case report and review of the literature. Am J Med. 1985;78(1):171–5.
20. Canton CG, Bernis C, Paraiso V, et al. Renal failure in temporal arteritis. Am J Nephrol. 1992;12(5):380–3.
21. Lenz T, Schmidt R, Scherberich JE, Grone HJ. Renal failure in giant cell vasculitis. Am J Kidney Dis. 1998;31(6):1044–7.
22. Medvedev G, Al-Shamari AE, Copland MA, Magil AB. Isolated renal giant cell arteritis. Am J Kidney Dis. 2002;40(3):658–61.
23. Small P, Brisson ML. Wegener's granulomatosis presenting as temporal arteritis. Arthritis Rheum. 1991;34(2):220–3.
24. Nishino H, DeRemee RA, Rubino FA, Parisi JE. Wegener's granulomatosis associated with vasculitis of the temporal artery: report of five cases. Mayo Clin Proc. 1993;68(2):115–21.
25. Legault K, Shroff A, Crowther M, Khalidi N. Amyloidosis and giant cell arteritis/polymyalgia rheumatica. J Rheumatol. 2012;39(4):878–80.
26. Maksimowicz-McKinnon K, Clark TM, Hoffman GS. Takayasu arteritis and giant cell arteritis: a spectrum within the same disease? Medicine (Baltimore). 2009;88(4):221–6.
27. Watts R, Al-Taiar A, Mooney J, Scott D, Macgregor A. The epidemiology of Takayasu arteritis in the UK. Rheumatology. 2009;48(8):1008–11.
28. Renauer P, Sawalha AH. The genetics of Takayasu arteritis. Presse Med. 2017;46(7–8 Pt 2):e179–87.
29. Carmona FD, Coit P, Saruhan-Direskeneli G, et al. Analysis of the common genetic component of large-vessel vasculitides through a meta-Immunochip strategy. Sci Rep. 2017;7:43953.
30. Mason JC. Surgical intervention and its role in Takayasu arteritis. Best Pract Res Clin Rheumatol. 2018;32(1):112–24.
31. Qi Y, Yang L, Zhang H, et al. The presentation and management of hypertension in a large cohort of Takayasu arteritis. Clin Rheumatol. 2018;37(10):2781–8.
32. Chen Z, Li J, Yang Y, et al. The renal artery is involved in Chinese Takayasu's arteritis patients. Kidney Int. 2018;93(1):245–51.
33. Jeong HS, Jung JH, Song GG, Choi SJ, Hong SJ. Endovascular balloon angioplasty versus stenting in patients with Takayasu arteritis: a meta-analysis. Medicine (Baltimore). 2017;96(29):e7558.
34. Jung JH, Lee YH, Song GG, Jeong HS, Kim JH, Choi SJ. Endovascular versus open surgical intervention in patients with Takayasu's arteritis: a meta-analysis. Eur J Vasc Endovasc Surg. 2018;55(6):888–99.
35. Vijayvergiya R, Sharma A, Kanabar KP, Sihag BK. Renal autotransplantation for the management of renal artery in-stent restenosis in an adult patient with Takayasu arteritis. BMJ Case Rep. 2018;2018:bcr2018226236.
36. de Pablo P, Garcia-Torres R, Uribe N, et al. Kidney involvement in Takayasu arteritis. Clin Exp Rheumatol. 2007;25(1 Suppl 44):S10–4.
37. Watts RA, Robson J. Introduction, epidemiology and classification of vasculitis. Best Pract Res Clin Rheumatol. 2018;32(1):3–20.
38. Guillevin L, Lhote F, Cohen P, et al. Polyarteritis nodosa related to hepatitis B virus. A prospective study with long-term

observation of 41 patients. Medicine (Baltimore). 1995;74(5):238–53.
39. Navon Elkan P, Pierce SB, Segel R, et al. Mutant adenosine deaminase 2 in a polyarteritis nodosa vasculopathy. N Engl J Med. 2014;370(10):921–31.
40. Pagnoux C, Seror R, Henegar C, et al. Clinical features and outcomes in 348 patients with polyarteritis nodosa: a systematic retrospective study of patients diagnosed between 1963 and 2005 and entered into the French Vasculitis Study Group Database. Arthritis Rheum. 2010;62(2):616–26.
41. Ribi C, Cohen P, Pagnoux C, et al. Treatment of polyarteritis nodosa and microscopic polyangiitis without poor-prognosis factors: a prospective randomized study of one hundred twenty-four patients. Arthritis Rheum. 2010;62(4):1186–97.
42. Mukhtyar C, Guillevin L, Cid MC, et al. EULAR recommendations for the management of primary small and medium vessel vasculitis. Ann Rheum Dis. 2009;68(3):310–7.
43. de Groot K, Harper L, Jayne DR, et al. Pulse versus daily oral cyclophosphamide for induction of remission in antineutrophil cytoplasmic antibody-associated vasculitis: a randomized trial. Ann Intern Med. 2009;150(10):670–80.
44. Jayne D, Rasmussen N, Andrassy K, et al. A randomized trial of maintenance therapy for vasculitis associated with antineutrophil cytoplasmic autoantibodies. N Engl J Med. 2003;349(1):36–44.
45. Guillevin L, Cohen P, Mahr A, et al. Treatment of polyarteritis nodosa and microscopic polyangiitis with poor prognosis factors: a prospective trial comparing glucocorticoids and six or twelve cyclophosphamide pulses in sixty-five patients. Arthritis Rheum. 2003;49(1):93–100.
46. Briggs JD, Jones E. Renal transplantation for uncommon diseases. Scientific Advisory Board of the ERA-EDTA Registry. European Renal Association-European Dialysis and Transplant Association. Nephrol Dial Transplant. 1999;14(3):570–5.
47. Little MA, Hassan B, Jacques S, et al. Renal transplantation in systemic vasculitis: when is it safe? Nephrol Dial Transplant. 2009;24(10):3219–25.
48. Hunder GG, Bloch DA, Michel BA, et al. The American College of Rheumatology 1990 criteria for the classification of giant cell arteritis. Arthritis Rheum. 1990;33(8):1122–8.
49. Arend WP, Michel BA, Bloch DA, et al. The American College of Rheumatology 1990 criteria for the classification of Takayasu arteritis. Arthritis Rheum. 1990;33(8):1129–34.
50. Lightfoot RW Jr, Michel BA, Bloch DA, et al. The American College of Rheumatology 1990 criteria for the classification of polyarteritis nodosa. Arthritis Rheum. 1990;33(8):1088–93.

Resources and Patient Information

Vasculitis UK: http://www.vasculitis.org.uk/.

United Kingdom and Ireland Vasculitis Registry: https://research.ndorms.ox.ac.uk/ukivas/.

Vasculitis Foundation: https://www.vasculitisfoundation.org/.

Vasculitis Clinical Research Consortium: https://www.rarediseasesnetwork.org/cms/vcrc.

Goodpasture's or Anti-glomerular Basement Membrane (GBM) Disease

Alan D. Salama

Contents

M. Harber (ed.), *Primer on Nephrology*, https://doi.org/10.1007/978-3-030-76419-7_27

27

Learning Objectives

To understand the basis of anti-GBM disease, its presentation, associations and management.

Key Points

1. Anti-GBM disease is a rare cause of acute kidney injury but requires prompt diagnosis to prevent end-stage renal disease.
2. It often presents with a pulmonary-renal syndrome but may be renal limited.
3. It is often is found in association with ANCA positivity.

27.1 Introduction

Goodpasture's disease is the term for a pulmonary-renal syndrome associated with rapidly progressive glomerulonephritis[1] and anti-glomerular basement (GBM) membrane antibodies and is used alongside the term anti-GBM disease. The eponym was coined by Stanton and Tange in 1958 after their report of patients with the condition and their recognition that they were similar to the cases published 37 years earlier by Ernest Goodpasture, an American pathologist who described the clinical constellation of pulmonary haemorrhage and renal failure, during the 1918–1919 influenza pandemic. In the USA, Goodpasture's syndrome is often used to refer to any cause of pulmonary-renal syndrome, while Goodpasture's disease is limited to those patients with anti-GBM antibodies.

Goodpasture's disease is a rare, rapidly progressive autoimmune condition leading to acute kidney injury and lung haemorrhage. It is vitally important to make a rapid diagnosis as early recognition and treatment can lead to significantly better clinical outcomes. Delayed therapy may make renal recovery unlikely and can be associated with significantly greater morbidity and higher mortality. There are many examples of delay in treatment resulting in irreversible renal failure, and it is thus critical to have robust processes for rapid diagnosis, transfer and treatment.

27.2 Clinical Features

Goodpasture's disease has a bimodal distribution with peaks of incidence in the third and sixth decades and has a slight male predominance [1]. It generally presents with a rapidly progressive decline in renal function in association with pulmonary haemorrhage in over half the patients, most frequently smokers (see ◘ Fig. 27.1) [2]. While isolated glomerulonephritis is well recognised, it can also rarely present as isolated pulmonary haemorrhage, although urinary abnormalities may be detected if looked for carefully. Patients have limited systemic features, which mostly relate to anaemia and renal impairment and manifest as generalised fatigue and malaise, but in some cases weight loss may also be found. This is in contrast to the main differential diagnosis of systemic anti-neutrophil cytoplasm antibody (ANCA)-associated vasculitis, in which systemic features are much more common (see ◘ Table 27.1).

Goodpasture's disease may present with complete anuria, in up to a fifth of cases [3], and this symptom should raise suspicion of the diagnosis (along with consideration of outflow obstruction and renal venous or arterial thrombosis). Rarely patients may present with macroscopic haematuria or loin pain related to renal oedema. Despite the target autoantigen being found in the lung, kidney, ear, eye and brain, symptoms are generally limited to the pulmonary-renal systems.

Goodpasture's disease rarely relapses, unlike ANCA-associated vasculitis, and in those few cases that do, there is more frequently a relapse of pulmonary haemorrhage in those with provoking factors such as infection or fluid overload, or recurrent exposure to factors such as smoking or solvent/hydrocarbon exposure [4, 5].

27.3 Epidemiology

Goodpasture's disease is 10–20 times less common than systemic ANCA-associated vasculitis, with an incidence of 0.5–1.5 cases /million population. However, it accounts for almost a fifth of the cases of rapidly progressive glomerulonephritis. It is common in white populations but is clearly found in other ethnic groups including Japanese and Chinese, in whom it appears to have similar genetic susceptibility traits. There are recognised genetic and environmental risk factors, with one of the strongest human leukocyte antigen (HLA) associations with disease, as over 90% of patients carry the HLA DRB1*1501 or *0401 alleles [6]. There are also negative associations with HLA DRB1*01 and DRB1*07, with these alleles being under represented in the Goodpasture's patients. The reason for the relative susceptibility and protective effects of these alleles is somewhat clearer as it appears that while both DRB1*1501 and DRB1*0701 bind the Goodpasture antigen, the immunodominant disease-causing epitopes are only effectively presented by the DRB1*1501 allele [7]. In addition, recent reports demonstrated

1 Rapidly progressive glomerulonephritis denotes a precipitous decline in renal function (doubling of creatinine) in less than 3 months due to crescentic glomerulonephritis.

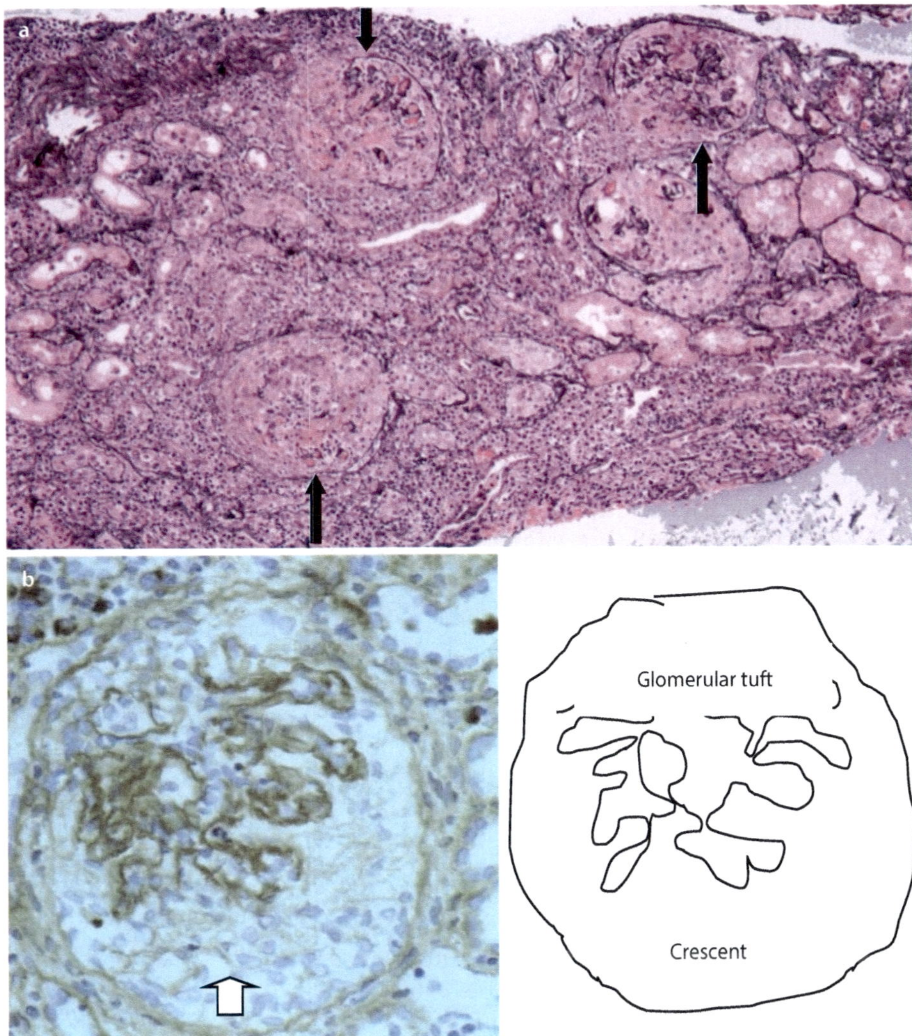

Fig. 27.1 **a** Low-power silver stain of a kidney biopsy from a patient with anti-GBM disease demonstrating widespread crescentic glomerulonephritis(arrows) with lesions all appearing of similar vintage (×100 magnification). **b** Immunoperoxidase staining for IgG on a renal biopsy from a patient with anti-GBM disease demonstrating fine smooth linear deposition along the basement membrane and a surrounding crescent(arrowhead) which is clearly compressing the glomerular tuft

Table 27.1 Comparison of clinical and pathological features of Goodpasture's disease and ANCA associated vasculitis

Goodpasture's disease	ANCA-associated vasculitis
May present with rapidly progressive renal failure and anuria	May present with rapidly progressive renal failure
Systemic prodromal symptoms uncommon	Systemic prodromal symptoms common, except in cases of renal limited vasculitis
Dialysis dependency at presentation rarely associated with renal recovery	Dialysis dependency at presentation associated with renal recovery in 50–60% cases
Pulmonary haemorrhages in 50–70% cases	Pulmonary haemorrhage in 25%
Anti-GBM Ab-positive Concurrent ANCA positivity in 30–47% cases	Anti-GBM negative, ANCA-positive in 95% cases
Glomerular crescents of similar age	Glomerular lesions of various ages
Linear immunoglobulin deposition along GBM	Pauci-immune

polymorphisms in the inhibitory Fc (immunoglobulin) receptor FCγRIIB and copy number variation in activatory FcγRIIIA receptors in Chinese patients with anti-GBM disease, suggesting that these conferred increased risk of disease through augmented Fc receptor signalling. Despite these immunological susceptibility factors, Goodpasture's disease does not form part of a generalised autoimmune phenotype. However, in over 30% of cases, there may be a concurrent ANCA detected, mostly a perinuclear (P)-ANCA with anti-myeloperoxidase reactivity [8]. Less often, Goodpasture's disease may follow on from membranous nephropathy [9] or systemic lupus erythematosus [10], while rare cases have also been reported following lithotripsy treatment for renal calculi [11]. It is assumed that in these cases, the primary damage to the glomerular basement membrane, which may have been mechanical or inflammatory, allows exposure of collagen chain neo-epitopes which then induces an immune response directed against the GBM.

27.4 Diagnosis

Diagnosis relies on renal biopsy demonstrating crescentic glomerulonephritis with linear immunoglobulin deposition along the basement membrane (see ◘ Fig. 27.2). This is predominantly IgG, but rare cases of other immunoglobulin classes predominating have been reported, some of which may bind alternative GBM antigens. Less intense linear basement membrane staining with IgG may occasionally be seen in patients with diabetes, systemic lupus erythematosus, myeloma or transplanted kidney, but these are not associated with crescent formation. Unlike ANCA-associated glomerulonephritis, crescents in anti-GBM disease appear of the same age – without evidence of old and new lesions as it does not follow the same stuttering course as ANCA-associated disease.

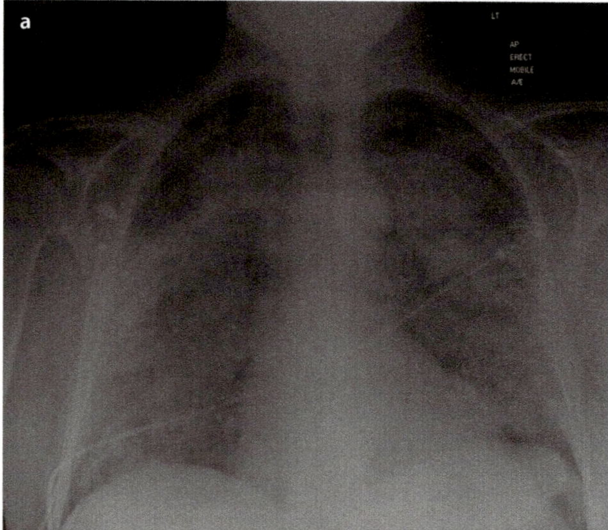

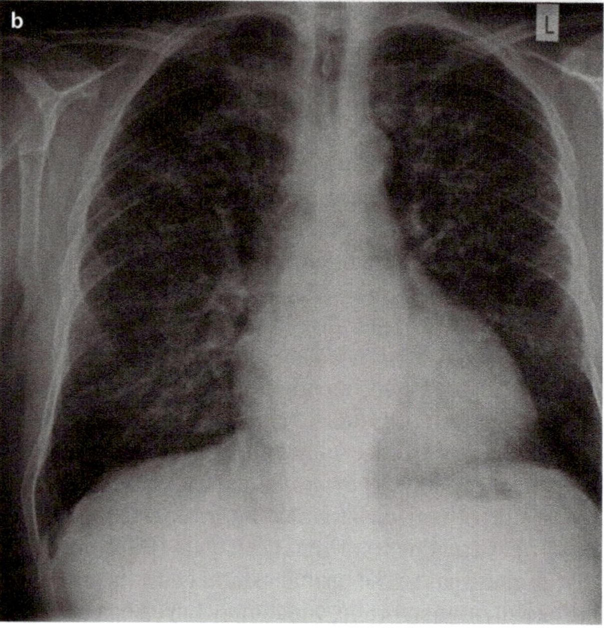

◘ **Fig. 27.2** **a** Chest radiograph of a patient with Goodpasture's disease demonstrating pulmonary haemorrhage with relative sparing of costophrenic angles and **b** 3 days later following immunosuppression with steroids and cyclophosphamide and plasmapheresis

Pulmonary haemorrhage in the absence of significant haemoptysis may be diagnosed on the basis of chest radiography with an elevated gas transfer coefficient (KCO) or by bronchoscopy. Suspicion should arise if there is an iron deficiency anaemia with no other obvious source of blood loss and a consistent chest radiograph. Serial KCO measurements may be useful in the monitoring of resolution of pulmonary haemorrhage. Serology to assay anti-GBM antibodies is helpful, as the assay is sensitive and specific. However, there are two common pitfalls. False positivity may occur in cases of polyclonal gammopathy – such as in acute viral infections(often HCV or HIV) [12] and may require confirmation with Western blotting (not routinely performed in clinical laboratories); false negativity may rarely occur, for reasons that are not clear, but a small number of patients have been described in whom typical biopsy features are found, but circulating anti-GBM antibodies are not detected by standard methodology such as ELISA [13] . Finally, rare cases of IgA anti-GBM antibody-mediated disease have been reported, and these would not be detected on standard anti-GBM ELISA. In all these cases, renal biopsy is critical to refute or confirm the diagnosis.

It is also critical to test all ANCA-positive patients presenting with rapidly progressive glomerulonephritis for anti-GBM antibodies, as some will be double positive. This group of patients behave like anti-GBM disease as regards renal recovery (i.e. less likely to recover if presenting with dialysis dependency, unlike ANCA-associated vasculitis in which 50–60% will recover independent renal function) but have extra-renal relapses like ANCA-associated vasculitis patients, which may necessitate maintenance immunosuppression. Curiously, there may be a dichotomy between the ANCA and anti-GBM autoantibodies, with the ANCA fluctuating during disease remission, but with the anti-GBM generally remaining negative.

Some laboratories batch sera for testing in immunological assays. This is clearly of no use if a timely diagnosis is to be made; therefore it is important to discuss the urgency of the assay with the clinical immunology laboratory as many can perform rapid assays when requested if they appreciate the urgency of a particular clinical situation. All patients with a rapidly progressive decline in renal function, with active urinary sediment should have an urgent anti-GBM assay performed, and the result obtained from the immunology lab within 24–48 hours. Furthermore it is worth establishing a standard operating procedure whereby the immunology laboratories within the renal unit's catchment urgently communicate any positive anti-GBM to the nephrologist on call, who can urgently discuss the case with the relevant clinical team.

Finally, since many patients may present at times when the routine laboratory is not open, there may be some utility in having rapid assay kits (such as the QuickCard – which are also available for PR3 – and MPO-ANCA), which require the addition of serum to a supplied buffer, which can be done on the wards, if there is an available centrifuge. These should not replace standard testing (formal confirmation with a standard laboratory assay is still required) but may represent a good interim measure to dictate whether emergency plasmapheresis should be instituted.

27.5 Immunology

The adult GBM is formed from a network of specialised type IV collagen molecules, consisting of α3, α4 and α5 chains. The Goodpasture antigen is present in the non-collagenous 1 (NC1) domain of the α3 chain of type IV collagen (α3(IV)NC1). Two main antibody epitopes are closely co-localised in the intact molecule, and these are sequestered under normal conditions, suggesting that tolerance is broken after exposure of the cryptic epitopes to the immune system. The anti-GBM antibodies are mostly IgG1 although some IgG4 antibodies are also found. Less commonly, other immunoglobulins may predominate such as IgA. The anti-GBM antibodies are almost never detected in normal individuals using conventional assays, making the test a highly sensitive and specific assay. Anti-GBM antibodies are closely associated with disease activity and were shown to transfer disease to experimental animals in classic experiments some 40 years ago. However, there is evidence for both humoral and cellular autoimmunity in patients, with both antibodies and T cells reactive to the α3(IV)NC1 [14]. In part the lack of disease relapse, unlike the high incidence in ANCA-associated vasculitis, is due to the early and persistent development of regulatory antigen specific T-cell populations [15].

27.6 Treatment

Treatment consists of general measures such as avoiding fluid overload and stopping smoking – which may precipitate pulmonary haemorrhage. The rare cases of relapse, with pulmonary haemorrhage, were in patients who returned to smoking after their initial illness. The mainstay of treatment is with specific immunosuppression using oral corticosteroids and cyclophosphamide with additional plasmapheresis performed daily for 14 days or until antibody levels are undetectable, whichever comes first (Table 27.2). Steroids should be started at 1 mg/Kg, maximum 60 mg, although there are no trial data to support this specific dosage regimen, and withdrawn by 6 months. Cyclophosphamide should be given for 2–3 months at a starting dose of 2–3 mg/Kg/day, rounded down and dose-adjusted in the elderly (over 60 years) to use 1–1.5 mg/Kg. Prophylactic treatment to prevent infectious, metabolic and gastric complications is also required (see Table 27.2). Plasmapheresis was first introduced by the Hammersmith Hospital group in the 1970s, following their report of seven patients treated

Table 27.2 Treatment of anti-GBM disease

Plasma exchange	Daily 50 mls/Kg, maximum 4-L exchange, for 4.5% human albumin solution. Replace 300–600 mL albumin with fresh plasma within 3 days after invasive procedure (e.g. biopsy) or in patients with pulmonary haemorrhage Continue for 14 days or until antibody levels are fully suppressed Withhold if platelet count is <70 × 10^9/mL, fibrinogen <1 g/L or haemoglobin is <9 g/dL. Watch for coagulopathy, hypocalcaemia and hypokalaemia.
Cyclophosphamide	Daily oral dosing at 2–3 mg/kg/day (round down to nearest 50 mg; use 1–1.5 mg/kg/day in patients >60 years) Stop if white cell count is less than 4 × 10^9/mL, and restart at lower dose when count increases to >4 × 10^9/mL Treat for 2–3 months; 2 months in elderly Pulsed IV cyclophosphamide has not been tested formally but is equivalent in ANCA-associated vasculitis
Prednisolone	Daily oral dosing at 1 mg/kg/day (maximum, 60 mg) Reduce dose weekly to 20 mg by week 6 and then more slowly. Should be off steroids by 6 months There is no evidence of benefit of IV methylprednisolone, but consider if plasma exchange not immediately available
Prophylactic treatments	Use oral nystatin 1 ml qds or fluconazole 50 mg od to prevent oral thrush Use ranitidine or proton-pump inhibitor for steroid-promoted gastric ulceration Use cotrimoxazole 480 mg daily or 960 mg three times a week for *Pneumocystis jiroveci* pneumonia Use calcium-D3, two tablets a day as bone protection
Dialysis regimen	Avoid fluid overload by ensuring dry weigh is carefully assessed and maintained. Albumin solutions contain significant sodium loads which should be factored in, when considering ultrafiltration volumes

27

with steroids, cyclophosphamide and plasmapheresis [16], in which they demonstrated a rapid decline in anti-GBM antibodies, and improvement in renal function in those patients who were not dialysis-dependent at presentation. Surprisingly, there has only been one randomised trial investigating whether there is any additional benefit of plasmapheresis to conventional immunosuppressive therapy. This consisted of 17 patients, all treated with steroids and cyclophosphamide with 8 receiving additional plasmapheresis, every 3 days. In these eight patients, antibody removal was more rapid, and renal function showed greater improvement. However, the two groups of patients were not well matched at onset, as serum creatinine and percentage crescent involvement on biopsy were lower in the plasmapheresis group [17]. The currently accepted protocol has evolved from these data based on the outcomes reported from institutions with significant experience in the management of such patients. Clearly, novel treatments may be of equal benefit, but there have been no formal trials comparing intravenous pulsed cyclophosphamide, rituximab ciclosporin A or mycophenolate mofetil. However, there are anecdotal reports of all of these agents being used with variable outcomes [18–22], but these have tended to be used in patients in whom cyclophosphamide has failed or has led to complications, and so they cannot be recommended as first-line therapies. Ongoing trials with IgG-cleaving enzymes (IdeS) that attenuate IgG effector functions are ongoing and could provide alternative or adjunctive therapeutic approaches in the future.

27.7 Outcomes

Retrospective cohort studies have confirmed that renal outcome is dependent on the severity of the renal damage at presentation, with those patients with greater severity of glomerular disease (based on the crescent score) and worse renal function having the highest degree of end-stage renal failure at 1 year despite immunosuppressive therapy [2] (see Table 27.3). All series demonstrate that patients with serum creatinine levels greater than 600 mcmol/l had the worst outcome with regard to renal survival at 1 year. In the largest series reported by Levy [2], those with presenting creatinine >500 mcmol/l and requiring dialysis at presentation fared the worst with few regaining independent renal function (see Table 27.3), despite treatment. Those with creatinine >500 mcmol/l but not requiring immediate (within 72 hours of presentation) dialysis had better renal outcomes than those who required immediate dialysis upon presentation. Finally, those patients with less severe glomerular damage and better preserved renal function(creatinine <500 mcmol/l) have excellent

Table 27.3 Renal outcomes in Goodpasture's disease patients according to presenting creatinine levels

Study	Patients	Percentage with independent renal function at 1 year according to presenting serum creatinine (μmol/l)		Reference
		<600	>600	
Levy	71	95[a]	8[b]	[2]
Daly	40	20	0	[32]
Bouget	14	50	0	[33]
Walker	22	82	18	[3]
Johnson	17	69	0	[17]

[a]In this study less than 500 μmol/l and [b]dialysis-dependent with creatinine >500 μmol/l

short (1-year)- and long (20-year)-term renal outcome following immunosuppressive therapy [2] and should be treated with standard therapy or modified regimens if contraindications to standard therapy are found. Recent outcomes from a national analysis in Ireland demonstrate overall higher rates of ANCA co-positivity and poorer recovery of renal function with over 70% of patients reaching ESRD [23]. Similar poor outcomes were reported in retrospective cohort analysis in the UK [24, 25], with up to 84% dialysis dependency at 1 year and less than 5% of those dialysis-dependent at presentation achieving independent renal function at long-term follow up, while the best clinical predictor of poor outcome was found to be oligoanuria (<500mls/day) on the day of diagnosis [24], again emphasising the need for early diagnosis.

27.8 When Not to Treat?

Since data demonstrate that patients presenting with dialysis dependency and 100% crescents, i.e. crescents in all glomeruli on the section, do not tend to recover independent renal function, if diagnosis is delayed and patients are already dialysis-dependent with extensive crescentic change on biopsy, many practitioners would not treat with immunosuppression unless there was coexistent pulmonary haemorrhage. However, there are patients who do not present requiring dialysis but develop dialysis dependency in the early hospitalisation period. These may well benefit from immunosuppression, and the decision should be made based on a balanced assessment of the individual risk of immunosuppression.

In some circumstances, such as those patients with a living kidney donor, even with dialysis dependency and 100% crescents, treatment may be warranted to allow more rapid elimination of anti-GBM antibodies and early transplantation. In the absence of immunosuppressive therapy, anti-GBM antibodies may persist for up to 3 years [26].

27.9 Transplantation

Early experience of transplantation in the face of positive anti-GBM antibodies resulted in rapid disease recurrence [27]. It is therefore essential that transplantation is deferred until there has been a prolonged period of anti-GBM antibody negativity, and using this approach recurrence is rare [8]. Although there are no trial data to guide this period of time, we and others wait 6 months from the time of first antibody negativity, before proceeding. Persistent low-level anti-GBM antibody has been removed prior to transplantation by immunoadsorption, with those patients who could not have antibody successfully removed not undergoing transplantation [26]. Cases of late anti-GBM disease recurrence following cessation of transplant maintenance immunosuppressive therapy or following viral infection have been reported, but are uncommon [28, 29]. If recurrence does occur, augmented immunosuppressive treatment may be used but is successful in only a minority of cases [29].

27.10 Anti-GBM Disease in Alport's Disease Following Transplantation

Alport's disease arises from mutations in the type IV collagen chains found in the glomerular basement membrane, which is the α5 (IV) chain in the X-linked form of disease. Following transplantation of a kidney containing a normal α5(IV) chain, an alloimmune response to the collagen IV chain can arise and lead to development of anti-GBM antibodies. While this can be found in up to 20% of patients, only 5–6% go on to develop a crescentic glomerulonephritis which tends to be extremely difficult to treat, even with augmented immunosuppression [30]. Once this anti-collagen response has developed, subsequent transplantation is increasingly likely to result in disease recurrence.

While monitoring Alport's patients who have undergone renal transplantation, it is important to realise that many anti-GBM assays are now using recombinant α3 (IV) and not whole GBM as a substrate. They will therefore not detect anti-α5 (IV) antibodies, to which the transplanted X-linked Alport's patient will react to [31].

Case Studies

Case 1

57-year-old with a 2-month history of feeling generally unwell. Found to have a creatinine of 436 at general practitioners; urine dipstick positive for blood and protein. Normal renal tract ultrasound. Acute screen sent. Anti-GBM titre of 650 (NR < 10). Required haemodialysis for fluid overload and started on cyclophosphamide and high-dose prednisolone. Maintained his urine output. Required 21 plasma exchanges to bring anti-GBM antibody down to normal range. There was then a later mild rebound with anti-GBM titre increasing which took further 2 months to return to normality, with ongoing oral cyclophosphamide (◘ Fig. 27.3).

Case 2

A 71-year-old woman with heart failure was admitted with breathlessness and raised CRP. She was treated with diuretics but found to have no other signs of decompensated heart failure. Urine grew a fully sensitive *E. coli*, for which she was treated. Baseline creatinine 90 mcmol/l. She was discharged with declining renal function and rising CRP (creatinine 131mcmol/l, CRP 42). Readmitted unwell with creatinine of 425mcmol/l, CRP 92. Treated with further antibiotics. When creatinine reached 530, and anuric, referred to renal team. Acute screen sent, but results not returned urgently. Biopsy confirmed anti-GBM disease and subsequently found to have anti-GBM titre of >900 AU. Had two doses of cyclophosphamide and then decided to stop immunotherapy. Did not recover independent renal function.

Case 3

A 38-year-old man with pleural and pericardial effusions thought to be due to mycobacterial tuberculosis, treated empirically with quadruple anti-TB therapy, who subsequently developed acute kidney injury, with 3 + blood and 3 + protein on urinalysis. Required dialysis on transfer to renal unit. Initially thought to be due to anti-TB medication, with negative acute renal screen (including anti-GBM antibody) but subsequent biopsy revealing crescentic change in all glomeruli, and linear staining of IgA along GBM, without IgG. Remained dialysis-dependent despite a trial of immunotherapy and plasmapheresis.

27

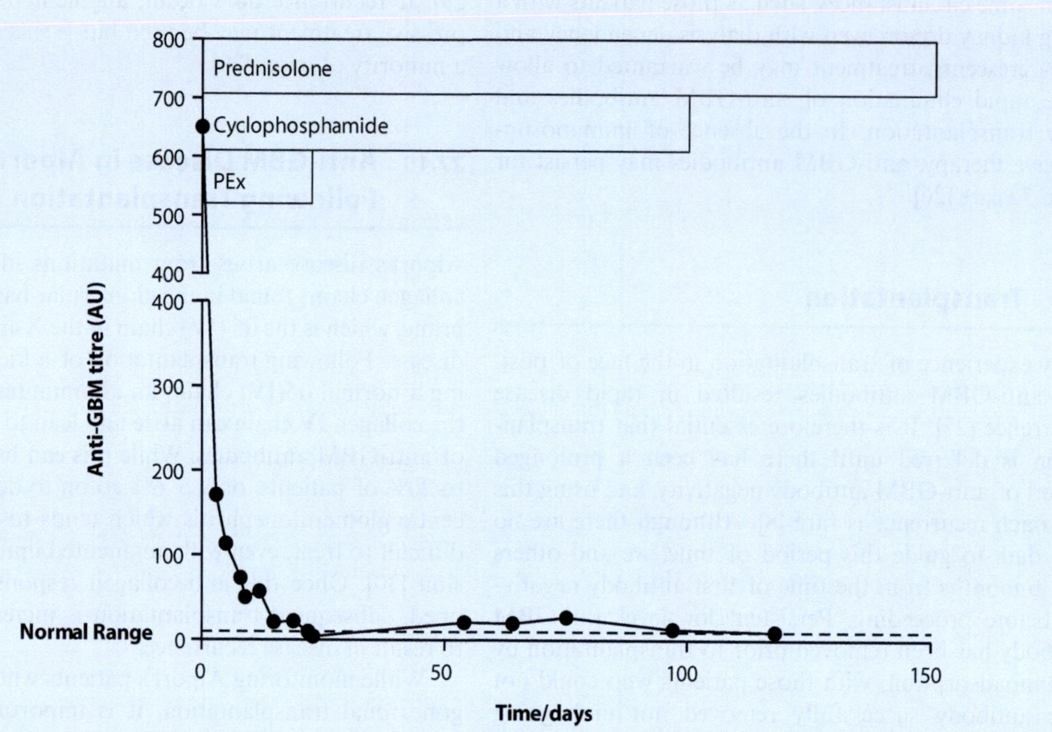

Fig. 27.3 Changes in anti-GBM titre with treatment of patient 1, demonstrating rapid decline in autoantibody titre with plasma exchange and ongoing immunosuppression

Tips and Tricks

1. Early diagnosis can potentially make a difference between renal recovery and dialysis dependency. Classical features of pulmonary-renal syndrome may be absent; rapidly declining renal function in a patient without a clear explanation and with blood and protein in urine should prompt urgent anti-GBM assay. Aim to get result back same day.
2. Complete anuria is rare outside of obstruction or severe nephritis. Consider anti-GBM disease in anyone with complete anuria. Send test urgently.
3. Consider pulmonary haemorrhage in any patient with unexplained anaemia and pulmonary air-space shadowing.
4. If history compatible, in a patient with rapidly declining renal function and inability to obtain anti-GBM titre, consider starting blind immunosuppression with high-dose steroids.
5. Always check for ANCA in patient with anti-GBM disease.

Questions

1. Is a biopsy ever required in patients with positive anti-GBM antibodies?
2. Can a negative anti-GBM antibody exclude anti-GBM disease?
3. Why do Alport's disease patients not develop pulmonary haemorrhage post-transplantation if they generate an anti-GBM antibody?
4. Should immunotherapy ever be offered to an anti-GBM patient who is established on dialysis and has no evidence of pulmonary haemorrhage?

Answers

1. Yes, a biopsy may be needed despite positive anti-GBM antibodies being detected. There are cases where anti-GBM antibodies may represent false positives, or may not bind the GBM in the kidney or the renal biopsy may show mild glomerular disease but severe tubular injury explaining the renal impairment and prospects for recovery are good.
2. It's a good screening test, but rare cases of serum negativity but biopsy evidence of anti-GBM are

reported. In addition, non-IgG or non-alpha 3(IV)-directed antibodies may not be picked up by modern immunoassays. In cases of unexplained RPGN, consider early biopsy.

3. Alpha 5 (IV) is not expressed in the lungs, so there is no target for the anti-a5 (IV) antibodies.
4. Yes, in cases of potential living donors, it will allow resolution of the anti-GBM antibody quicker and could allow early transplantation (6 months following persistent antibody negativity).

References

1. Salama AD, Levy JB, Lightstone L, Pusey CD. Goodpasture's disease. Lancet. 2001;358(9285):917–20.
2. Levy JB, Turner AN, Rees AJ, Pusey CD. Long-term outcome of anti-glomerular basement membrane antibody disease treated with plasma exchange and immunosuppression. Ann Intern Med. 2001;134(11):1033–42.
3. Walker RG, Scheinkestel C, Becker GJ, Owen JE, Dowling JP, Kincaid-Smith P. Clinical and morphological aspects of the management of crescentic anti-glomerular basement membrane antibody (anti-GBM) nephritis/Goodpasture's syndrome. Q J Med. 1985;54(213):75–89.
4. Levy JB, Lachmann RH, Pusey CD. Recurrent Goodpasture's disease. Am J Kidney Dis. 1996;27(4):573–8.
5. Bowley NB, Steiner RE, Chin WS. The chest X-ray in antiglomerular basement membrane antibody disease (Goodpasture's syndrome). Clin Radiol. 1979;30(4):419–29.
6. Fisher M, Pusey CD, Vaughan RW, Rees AJ. Susceptibility to anti-glomerular basement membrane disease is strongly associated with HLA-DRB1 genes. Kidney Int. 1997;51(1):222–9.
7. Ooi JD, Chang J, O'Sullivan KM, et al. The HLA-DRB1*15:01-restricted Goodpasture's T cell epitope induces GN. J Am Soc Nephrol. 2013;24(3):419–31.
8. Levy JB, Hammad T, Coulthart A, Dougan T, Pusey CD. Clinical features and outcome of patients with both ANCA and anti-GBM antibodies. Kidney Int. 2004;66(4):1535–40.
9. Sano T, Kamata K, Shigematsu H, Kobayashi Y. A case of anti-glomerular basement membrane glomerulonephritis superimposed on membranous nephropathy. Nephrol Dial Transplant. 2000;15(8):1238–41.
10. Savige JA, Dowling J, Kincaid-Smith P. Superimposed glomerular immune complexes in anti-glomerular basement membrane disease. Am J Kidney Dis. 1989;14(2):145–53.
11. Xenocostas A, Jothy S, Collins B, Loertscher R, Levy M. Anti-glomerular basement membrane glomerulonephritis after extracorporeal shock wave lithotripsy. Am J Kidney Dis. 1999;33(1):128–32.
12. Szczech LA, Anderson A, Ramers C, et al. The uncertain significance of anti-glomerular basement membrane antibody among HIV-infected persons with kidney disease. Am J Kidney Dis. 2006;48(4):e55–9.
13. Salama AD, Dougan T, Levy JB, et al. Goodpasture's disease in the absence of circulating anti-glomerular basement membrane antibodies as detected by standard techniques. Am J Kidney Dis. 2002;39(6):1162–7.
14. Salama AD, Chaudhry AN, Ryan JJ, et al. In Goodpasture's disease, CD4(+) T cells escape thymic deletion and are reactive with the autoantigen alpha3(IV)NC1. J Am Soc Nephrol. 2001;12(9):1908–15.
15. Salama AD, Chaudhry AN, Holthaus KA, et al. Regulation by CD25+ lymphocytes of autoantigen-specific T-cell responses in Goodpasture's (anti-GBM) disease. Kidney Int. 2003;64(5):1685–94.
16. Lockwood CM, Rees AJ, Pearson TA, Evans DJ, Peters DK, Wilson CB. Immunosuppression and plasma-exchange in the treatment of Goodpasture's syndrome. Lancet. 1976;1(7962):711–5.
17. Johnson JP, Moore J Jr, Austin HA 3rd, Balow JE, Antonovych TT, Wilson CB. Therapy of anti-glomerular basement membrane antibody disease: analysis of prognostic significance of clinical, pathologic and treatment factors. Medicine (Baltimore). 1985;64(4):219–27.
18. Uezu Y, Kiyatake I, Tokuyama K. A case of Goodpasture's syndrome with massive pulmonary hemorrhage ameliorated by cyclophosphamide pulse therapy. Nihon Jinzo Gakkai Shi. 1999;41(5):499–504.
19. Arzoo K, Sadeghi S, Liebman HA. Treatment of refractory antibody mediated autoimmune disorders with an anti-CD20 monoclonal antibody (rituximab). Ann Rheum Dis. 2002;61(10):922–4.
20. Kiykim AA, Horoz M, Gok E. Successful treatment of resistant antiglomerular basement membrane antibody positivity with mycophenolic acid. Intern Med. 2010;49(6):577–80.
21. Merkel F, Weber M. Successful use of cyclosporin A in progressive anti-glomerular basement membrane nephritis. Nephrol Dial Transplant. 2000;15(10):1714–5.
22. Wechsler E, Yang T, Jordan SC, Vo A, Nast CC. Anti-glomerular basement membrane disease in an HIV-infected patient. Nat Clin Pract Nephrol. 2008;4(3):167–71.
23. Canney M, O'Hara PV, McEvoy CM, et al. Spatial and temporal clustering of anti-glomerular basement membrane disease. Clin J Am Soc Nephrol. 2016;11(8):1392–9.
24. Alchi B, Griffiths M, Sivalingam M, Jayne D, Farrington K. Predictors of renal and patient outcomes in anti-GBM disease: clinicopathologic analysis of a two-centre cohort. Nephrol Dial Transplant. 2015;30(5):814–21.
25. Antonelou M, Oliveira B, Baumann A, Blunden M, Harber M. A two-centre cohort experience of anti-GBM disease. JASN. 2017;28:745A.
26. Flores JC, Taube D, Savage CO, et al. Clinical and immunological evolution of oligoanuric anti-GBM nephritis treated by haemodialysis. Lancet. 1986;1(8471):5–8.
27. Wilson CB, Dixon FJ. Anti-glomerular basement membrane antibody-induced glomerulonephritis. Kidney Int. 1973;3(2):74–89.
28. Fonck C, Loute G, Cosyns JP, Pirson Y. Recurrent fulminant anti-glomerular basement membrane nephritis at a 7-year interval. Am J Kidney Dis. 1998;32(2):323–7.
29. Sauter M, Schmid H, Anders HJ, Heller F, Weiss M, Sitter T. Loss of a renal graft due to recurrence of anti-GBM disease despite rituximab therapy. Clin Transpl. 2009;23(1):132–6.
30. Browne G, Brown PA, Tomson CR, et al. Retransplantation in Alport post-transplant anti-GBM disease. Kidney Int. 2004;65(2):675–81.
31. Dehan P, Van den Heuvel LP, Smeets HJ, Tryggvason K, Foidart JM. Identification of post-transplant anti-alpha 5 (IV)

collagen alloantibodies in X-linked Alport syndrome. Nephrol Dial Transplant. 1996;11(10):1983–8.
32. Daly C, Conlon PJ, Medwar W, Walshe JJ. Characteristics and outcome of anti-glomerular basement membrane disease: a single-center experience. Ren Fail. 1996;18(1):105–12.
33. Bouget J, Le Pogamp P, Perrier G, et al. [Anti-basement-membrane antibody mediated, rapidly progressive, glomerulonephritis. Diagnostic and therapeutic strategy based on a retrospective study of 14 cases]. Ann Med Interne (Paris) 1990; 141(5): 409–15.

27

Patient Information and Guidelines

Rare Renal UK; see http://rarerenal.org/clinician-information/vasculitis-clinician-information/

UKIVAS: http://www.vasculitis.org.uk/about-vasculitis/anti-gbm-goodpastures-disease

Systemic Lupus Erythematosus, Antiphospholipid Syndrome and the Kidney

Eve Miller-Hodges, Christopher O. C. Bellamy, David C. Kluth, and Neeraj Dhaun

Contents

M. Harber (ed.), *Primer on Nephrology*, https://doi.org/10.1007/978-3-030-76419-7_28

28.1 Systemic Lupus Erythematosus

Learning Aims

1. SLE is a chronic multi-system disease that frequently affects the kidney.
2. Immunosuppressive treatment is required to prevent the progression of end-stage renal disease (ESRD).
3. SLE is a major cardiovascular risk factor.
4. Fertility, pregnancy and contraception require specific management in women with SLE.

28

28.1.1 Introduction

Systemic lupus erythematosus (SLE) is a chronic multi-system autoimmune disorder. Kidney involvement is common and is a major contributor to disease morbidity and mortality. At presentation, up to 50% of patients with SLE will have clinical evidence of renal involvement with haematuria, with or without proteinuria. Renal excretory function is often normal. During follow-up, renal involvement will be evident in >60%, with an even greater representation amongst children and young adults.

Definition

Lupus nephritis is an inflammation of the kidneys caused by SLE. It most commonly affects the glomeruli, but can also affect the tubulointerstitium and vasculature.

28.1.2 Clinical Features

In general, the identification of lupus nephritis follows on from the diagnosis of SLE. Symptoms of SLE include alopecia, arthralgia, epilepsy, haematological abnormalities (anaemia, lymphopenia, thrombocytopenia), mouth ulcers, skin rash (discoid, malar or photosensitive rashes), serositis and Raynaud's phenomenon. Hypertension is also often present. However, lupus nephritis should be considered in any multi-system disease (particularly in young females) with unexplained haematuria and proteinuria.

All patients with known SLE should undergo regular urinalysis for haematuria and proteinuria to allow early detection of lupus nephritis, which is usually clinically silent. Proteinuria can be quantified using a spot protein-to-creatinine ratio or an albumin-to-creatinine ratio. Serum creatinine is frequently within the normal range at presentation, even in the presence of significant inflammatory disease, but may be elevated compared to baseline (see ▶ Cases 28.1 and 28.2). About 50% of patients will present with a reduction in glomerular filtration rate (GFR) and occasionally with acute kidney injury (AKI).

28.1.3 Epidemiology

The majority of individuals affected by SLE are women of child-bearing age, although diagnosis is often after the age of 40 in Europeans [1]. The prevalence ranges from 20 to 150 cases per 100,000 population, with the highest prevalence reported in Brazil. In the United Kingdom, the prevalence is almost 1 in 1000, with a female predominance of 9:1 [1]. Numbers appear to be increasing, as the disease is recognised more readily and as survival increases. SLE is more common in people of African, Hispanic or Asian ancestry, who also experience greater organ involvement. The 10-year survival is ~70%, with the major causes of death being infection, cardiovascular disease and cancer. In the United Kingdom, approximately one-third of patients develop lupus nephritis, which tends to occur early (within the first 3 years following diagnosis) [2, 3]. Current treatments have improved the 5-year renal survival to 50–95%.

28.1.4 Aetiopathology

SLE is characterised by polyclonal B-cell activation and the presence of autoantibodies, particularly directed against nuclear components, leading to inflammation in multiple body systems. The aetiology of SLE is unclear, but it is likely multifactorial, incorporating several environmental, genetic, hormonal and immunoregulatory factors. Generation of autoantibodies and subsequent tissue deposition of immune complexes – some passively trapped in the glomeruli and others attached to glomerular structures – lead to glomerulonephritis. Subsequent complement fixation initiates an inflammatory and cytotoxic reaction. The autoantibodies may themselves be cytotoxic.

Renal lupus can manifest in several different ways, which may exist concurrently. These include *glomerulonephritis*, *vasculopathy* and *tubulointerstitial disease* (see ◘ Table 28.1).

28.1.4.1 Glomerular Disease

The pattern of injury in lupus glomerulonephritis reflects the glomerular compartments in which immune deposits accumulate. Immunofluorescence labelling of renal biopsies reveals that the deposited immunoglobulins are of multiple classes and that they activate the classical pathway of complement activation, with C1q

Table 28.1 ISN/RPS histological classification of lupus nephritis

Class I	Normal glomeruli by light microscopy but mesangial immune deposits on immunofluorescence
Class II	Purely mesangial hypercellularity of any degree or mesangial expansion by light microscopy, with mesangial immune deposits
Class III	Focal proliferative lupus glomerulonephritis <50% glomeruli affected
Class IV	Diffuse proliferative lupus glomerulonephritis >50% glomeruli affected Disease may be segmental (IV-S or global IV-G)
Class V	Membranous lupus glomerulonephritis
Class VI	Advanced sclerotic lupus glomerulonephritis >90% glomeruli globally sclerosed with no disease activity

deposition. The deposition of complexes in multiple glomerular compartments (mesangial, sub-endothelial and sub-epithelial) is characteristic of lupus glomerulonephritis.

- *Mesangial* immune complex deposition alone is typical of milder disease. This leads to a histological pattern similar to IgA nephropathy, with mesangial hypercellularity and mesangial matrix accumulation. Clinically, this pattern of disease typically gives microscopic haematuria, sub-nephrotic range proteinuria and preserved renal function [4].
- *Sub-endothelial* immune deposits result in leucocyte accumulation, endothelial cell injury and proliferation. Over time, with repeated injury, remodelling of the glomerular capillary wall produces chronic changes of reduplication of the glomerular basement membrane and mesangial cell interposition into the capillary wall (mesangiocapillary pattern).
- *Sub-epithelial* disease immune deposits produce a membranous reaction in the capillary wall analogous to membranous nephropathy. Clinically, this is associated with heavy proteinuria. Although kidney function is usually preserved initially, there often follows a gradual decline in glomerular filtration rate (GFR) [5].

28.1.4.2 Vasculopathy

Renal vascular complications are frequent in lupus nephritis, and their presence may profoundly alter the clinical course and treatment of the disease. They include:

- *Vascular immune complex deposits in the intima and media of small arteries and arterioles*: common and without prognostic significance [6].
- *Non-inflammatory necrotising vasculopathy (lupus vasculopathy)*: intimal and luminal mixed immune deposits, fibrin and other plasma proteins; uncommon but associated with class IV nephritis and a poor prognosis [7].
- *Thrombotic microangiopathy*: may be seen independently of lupus glomerular disease, especially in those with the antiphospholipid syndrome; variable prognosis [8].
- *Renal vasculitis*: inflammatory destructive vasculitis often with fibrin deposits; this is rare and not well characterised [9].
- *Renal vein thrombosis*: more common in the presence of the nephrotic and antiphospholipid syndromes.

28.1.4.3 Tubulointerstitial Disease

In ~50% of individuals with lupus nephritis, immune complexes may be found in the tubular basement membrane [10]. This tubulitis is common in active disease. In more chronic disease, the interstitium is expanded with collagen fibrosis. Rarely, acute tubulointerstitial nephritis may be the first presentation of lupus renal disease, presenting as AKI.

28.1.5 Diagnosis

The cardinal features of lupus nephritis are haematuria, proteinuria and impaired renal function. The diagnosis is supported by the presence of autoantibodies. The vast majority of patients with SLE are positive for the antinuclear antibody (ANA), often with a titre of >1:160. However, ANA may also be positive in Sjögren's syndrome, scleroderma and rheumatoid arthritis, all of which may also have renal involvement. Depending upon the titre, the false-positive rate in healthy volunteers varies from ~30% with ANA titres of 1:40 (high sensitivity, low specificity) to as little as 3% with ANA titres of 1:320 (low sensitivity, high specificity). More specific serological tests are anti-double-stranded DNA antibody (anti-dsDNA) and anti-Smith antibody (anti-Sm). Compared to ANA, the sensitivity of these is much lower at about 75% and 25%, respectively. The presence of a high titre of anti-dsDNA increases the likelihood of lupus nephritis. Other autoantibodies (anti-Ro, anti-La and anti-RNP antibodies) are less specific for SLE. However, as anti-Ro and anti-La antibodies can cause neonatal lupus syndrome and congenital heart block, they should be measured, especially prior to pregnancy.

Hypocomplementaemia is often found at presentation with lupus nephritis (see ▶ Cases 28.1 and 28.2). Normal complement levels carry a high negative predictive value (>90%) to exclude active renal disease [11]. Hypocomplementaemia may also occur in other glomerulonephritides, including post-infectious glomerulonephritis and cryoglobulinaemic vasculitis. All patients with SLE should also be tested for antiphospholipid syndrome (see below).

A renal biopsy is required to confirm the diagnosis. Histopathological examination using light, immunofluorescent and electron microscopy is required to determine the class of disease and to guide treatment.

28.1.5.1 Prognosis of Lupus Nephritis

The factors that predict poorer prognosis at disease presentation include:

Non-renal Factors

- Male sex
- Haematological features (thrombocytopenia and leucopenia)
- Younger age
- Persistent hypocomplementaemia
- Persistently raised dsDNA antibodies after treatment
- Antiphospholipid antibodies

Renal Factors

- Abnormal renal function at presentation
- Failure of renal response to treatment
- Renal flares of disease

28.1.6 Treatment of Lupus Nephritis

Although SLE may involve any compartment of the kidney, glomerular involvement is the best studied and correlates well with presentation, course and treatment of the disease [12]. In 2004, the International Society of Nephrology (ISN) and the Renal Pathology Society (RPS) revised the World Health Organization (WHO) classification of lupus glomerulonephritis [13]. Current treatment for lupus glomerulonephritis – and studies of newer therapies – is guided by ISN/RPS histological disease class, with appropriate consideration given to clinical parameters and degree of renal impairment. Updates to these classifications have been recommended, to better define terminology, and provide activity and chronicity indices to apply to all classes, but these remain under evaluation [14].

28.1.6.1 Conservative, Non-immunosuppressive Therapy Is Appropriate for ISN/RPS Class I and II Lupus Glomerulonephritis

Class I disease means that glomeruli look normal by light microscopy but have mesangial immune deposits on immunofluorescence and/or electron microscopy. Class II is similar but with mesangial proliferation also apparent on light microscopy [13]. In general, patients with class I and II disease do not require renal-specific treatment. Most will have an excellent prognosis. The only exception to this is the small group of lupus patients who develop minimal change disease or a lupus podocytopathy [15–17]. These patients respond well to a short course of high-dose corticosteroids (1 mg/kg/day to a maximum dose of 80 mg/day) similar to conventional minimal change disease.

28.1.6.2 Mycophenolate Mofetil and Corticosteroids for Proliferative Lupus Glomerulonephritis (ISN/RPS Classes III and IV)

Class III and IV disease means that glomerular capillaries show endocapillary or extracapillary proliferation or have sufficiently severe sub-endothelial immune deposits as to be appreciable by light microscopy alone. Mesangial disease is not a consideration. The differences between the classes are arbitrarily whether fewer (class III) or more than (class IV) half the glomeruli in an adequate biopsy sample show any of these changes. These abnormalities may affect some or most of each individual diseased glomerulus. And each class is subclassified according to whether more of the diseased glomeruli have segmental (IV-S) or global (IV-G) disease.

Corticosteroids and cyclophosphamide (CYC) have been the cornerstone of immunosuppressive treatment for severe lupus nephritis for several decades. However, mycophenolate mofetil (MMF) is now considered the first-line treatment for class III and IV lupus nephritis.

CYC, although not licensed for SLE, is effective at treating lupus nephritis. It is unclear whether oral or intravenous CYC is more effective, but intravenous therapy is associated with a lower cumulative dose and less frequent cytopenias, enables enhanced bladder protection and avoids problems of non-adherence. Although earlier studies suggested that a greater cumulative CYC dose – usually alongside steroid treatment – may prevent more disease relapses and lead to a better long-term GFR [18], it was clear that this was associated with clinically unacceptable side effects such as infection, ischaemic and valvular heart disease, avascular necrosis, osteoporosis and premature menopause. Thus, more recent clinical studies have focused on achieving a high disease induction rate with fewer side effects.

The Euro-Lupus attempted to minimise CYC toxicity but maintain efficacy in their study of 90 patients with diffuse or focal proliferative lupus nephritis or membranous plus proliferative disease [19]. Patients were randomised to either six monthly pulses of intravenous CYC (0.5–1 g/m^2), followed by a pulse every third month, or to a shorter treatment course of 500 mg of intravenous CYC every 2 weeks for six doses (cumulative dose 3 g), followed by azathioprine maintenance therapy thereafter. Both arms of the study were as effective in achieving the various renal and extra-renal endpoints, but the shorter treatment was associated with a lower rate of infections. It is noteworthy that this trial was mostly performed in white subjects, and so the results should only be extrapolated to other populations with caution. However, the 10-year follow-up data continue to suggest no differences between the two groups [20].

MMF is the new standard of care for proliferative lupus nephritis [21–26]. The first good evidence of its efficacy was from a Chinese study in 42 patients randomised to receive either 12 months of MMF (2 g/day for 6 months, followed by 1 g/day for 6 months) or 6 months of oral CYC (2.5 mg/kg/day), followed by 6 months of azathioprine (1.5 mg/kg/day) [21]. Both groups received a tapering course of steroids. At 12 months, there were no differences between the MMF and CYC groups in terms of complete remission (81% vs. 76%), partial remission (14% vs. 14%) and relapses (15% vs. 11%). However, infections were less common with MMF, and mortality was associated with CYC alone (0% vs. 10%). Longer-term follow-up has shown similar rates of chronic kidney disease (CKD – defined as doubling of serum creatinine) as well as similar rates of relapse and relapse-free survival. Importantly, MMF is associated with lower infection rates than CYC (13% vs. 40%), and mortality remained a feature of only the CYC group [22].

A second study supporting the use of MMF was reported in 2005 [23]. The study was in 140 patients (of whom >50% were African American) with proliferative (classes III and IV) and membranous (class V) lupus nephritis. There were two groups randomised to either monthly intravenous pulses of CYC or MMF up to 3 g/day, each with a tapering dose of corticosteroids over 6 months. Although this study was powered to be a non-inferiority study, complete and partial disease remissions were significantly more common with MMF at 6 months than with CYC (52% vs. 30%). MMF had a better side effect profile, and there were no differences between the two treatments in terms of incidence of renal failure, ESRD or mortality at 3 years.

The most recent study supporting the use of MMF in lupus nephritis was published in 2009 [25]. This was a large (by lupus nephritis standards) international, multicentre study in 370 patients. It again compared monthly pulses of CYC against MMF up to 3 g/day. At 6 months, complete and partial remission rates were similar between the CYC and MMF arms (53% vs. 56%), with similar improvements in renal (GFR, serum creatinine, proteinuria and urine sediment) and non-renal parameters (reduction in dsDNA titres, normalisation of complement and increase in serum albumin). There was also no difference in mortality between the two groups. A recent Cochrane review supports the use of MMF (2–3 g/day) above cyclophosphamide for induction treatment and above azathioprine for maintenance therapy, although the level of certainty remains low. [27]

Therefore, our current practice is to treat patients with class III or IV lupus nephritis with MMF (2–3 g/day) and corticosteroids (0.5–1 mg/kg daily, tapering over months) (see ▶ Case 28.1). However, intravenous CYC may still have a role for those with more severe disease, marked by crescentic changes on biopsy and more rapidly declining renal function (see ▶ Case 28.2).

28.1.6.3 Hydroxychloroquine for Lupus Nephritis

Hydroxychloroquine is often used to treat the skin and joint manifestations of SLE. There is also evidence that it protects against progression and relapse of all classes of lupus nephritis. It is our standard practice to put all patients with lupus nephritis on this adjunctive therapy (200–400 mg/day). Hydroxychloroquine is well tolerated but can cause retinopathy. Patients should have ophthalmology review before initiation of treatment and advised about changes in visual acuity. Ophthalmology follow-up should be every 3–5 years whilst on treatment.

28.1.6.4 Rituximab for Lupus Nephritis

Rituximab, the anti-CD20 monoclonal antibody that depletes B cells, shows promise in the management of lupus nephritis, particularly as rescue induction therapy for those patients who have failed with either CYC or MMF [28, 29]. Two recent randomised controlled trials investigated a role for rituximab as add-on therapy to standard of care with rather disappointing results. The first of these compared rituximab and placebo, in addition to standard care, in 257 patients with moderate to severe active SLE but without clinically overt nephritis [30]. No differences were seen between placebo and rituximab in any of the endpoints studied. The LUNAR study randomised 140 patients with severe lupus nephritis to either rituximab or placebo on a background of MMF and tapering corticosteroids. Although more patients achieved complete or partial remission in the rituximab arm than in the placebo, there were no differences in the primary clinical endpoint at 1 year [31]. Although the data currently available do not support the routine use of rituximab in lupus nephritis, this may be down to trial design – with rituximab added to standard therapy in reasonably small numbers of patients with a short follow-up period. Anecdotally, the early use of rituximab has also allowed a reduction in corticosteroid use [32]. However, a randomised clinical trial (RITUXILUP) comparing induction with rituximab 2 × 1 g, a single dose of 500 mg methylprednisolone and MMF 2 g/daily with a standard induction regimen of MMF 3 g/daily plus tapering oral corticosteroids 0.5 mg/kg/day was terminated early due to difficulties recruiting patients not already on maintenance steroids. Thus, rituximab may well have a role in treating resistant patients, in preventing flares or in reducing the number of doses of other immunosuppressive medications, but further studies are required.

Overall, there remains significant uncertainty about the most effective treatments for lupus nephritis, particularly due to heterogeneity in treatment regimens, and the small number of clinical trials.

28.1.6.5 Maintenance Therapy for Proliferative Lupus Nephritis

Once remission has been achieved, the longer-term goals of maintenance therapy are:

- To prevent disease flares
- To avoid smouldering disease activity that may result in irreversible renal damage
- To prevent long-term side effects of treatment

Although the long-term use of immunosuppressive therapy is well established in lupus nephritis [26, 33, 34], the choice of agent, its dose, duration and potential for infertility and teratogenicity should be considered on an individual patient basis.

Corticosteroids remain the major component of maintenance therapy for lupus nephritis. However, given their potential side effects, the dose should be minimised and appropriate bone and gastric prevention given. Although there are no studies of maintenance therapy in lupus nephritis that do not include corticosteroids, there are no data that tell us at which point these agents should be stopped. Current KDIGO guidelines suggest tapering steroids over 6–12 months and continuing low-dose steroids for at least a further year once in the maintenance phase [35].

The long-term use of CYC is to be avoided given its risks of haemorrhagic cystitis, bladder cancer, infertility and early menopause. Both azathioprine and MMF are effective maintenance agents in lupus nephritis [36, 37]. Their equivalent efficacy has been shown in the MAINTAIN trial, which looked at 105 patients with class III (31%), class IV (58%) and class V (10%) lupus nephritis and followed them up for 3 years [38]. Here, induction was with intravenous CYC with patients randomised to azathioprine (mean maximum daily dose 124 mg) or MMF (mean maximum daily dose 2 g). The rates of all primary and secondary endpoints, including remission, steroid withdrawal and disease flares, were equal amongst the two groups. In contrast to this, the ALMS study published in 2011 showed MMF to be superior to azathioprine in terms of renal benefits [39]. This may be due to differences in racial contribution (MAINTAIN involved only Europeans, whereas ALMS a mixture of patients, some of whom were non-Caucasians, who may be more likely to respond to MMF) and the larger size of the ALMS study. Nevertheless, azathioprine in doses of 1–2.5 mg/kg/day is safe over a long period of time [40]. Macrocytosis, leucopenia and interactions with allopurinol are all potential side effects, alongside the obvious risk of infection with all immunosuppressive agents. Furthermore, azathioprine has only a small oncogenic potential, and pregnancy during maintenance azathioprine is relatively safe. Although MMF has a similar long-term toxicity profile, it should not be used during pregnancy, which is a major consideration given that many patients with lupus nephritis are women of child-bearing age. MMF should also be avoided during breastfeeding. Our practice is to routinely use MMF as maintenance therapy unless pregnancy is planned in the short term. We would then electively switch to azathioprine as part of preconception planning.

28.1.6.6 Treatment of Membranous (ISN/RPS Class V) Lupus Glomerulonephritis

Class V, or membranous, lupus nephritis is histologically characterised by widespread sub-epithelial immune deposits. A few such deposits are often present in class III or IV disease without particular clinical significance, but if they affect >50% of the glomerular capillaries in >50% of glomeruli, then class V disease is diagnosed alongside class III/IV. The optimal management of pure class V membranous lupus nephritis remains unclear. Patients who have sub-nephrotic range proteinuria, or nephrotic range proteinuria but without the nephrotic syndrome, and pure class V disease usually do very well and may require no more than standard renin-angiotensin system blockade. For those with the nephrotic syndrome, treatment is often as for idiopathic membranous nephropathy, although there are no evidence-based guidelines regarding treatment.

In a study of 42 patients with membranous lupus nephritis, patients were randomised to cyclosporine and steroids for 11 months, monthly intravenous CYC for

6 months and steroids, or steroids alone [41]. At 1 year, the achieved remission rates were 27% with steroids alone, 60% with CYC and 83% with cyclosporine. Remission occurred quicker with cyclosporine, but there were fewer relapses with CYC [42]. Subgroup analyses of the MMF vs. CYC trials for induction therapy in lupus nephritis show that for those patients with pure membranous nephritis, MMF is as effective as CYC in achieving disease control [23, 25]. Thus, there are several options for class V lupus nephritis associated clinically with the nephrotic syndrome, but further trials are needed. Given the recent data supporting the use of rituximab in idiopathic membranous nephropathy [43], this may be another attractive option in class V lupus nephritis and has been shown to be effective in small, observational studies [44].

28.1.6.7 Newer Agents for the Treatment of Lupus Nephritis

A number of immunomodulatory biological agents have been studied for the treatment of SLE. These are largely for proliferative (classes III and IV) nephritis and as add-on therapy to current standard of care – either MMF or CYC. However, the only agent that has met its primary endpoint in phase III clinical trials, but in non-renal lupus, has been belimumab [45].

Ocrelizumab is a fully humanised anti-CD20 monoclonal antibody and was therefore anticipated to have a better outcome and safety profile than rituximab. However, the trial investigating the potential benefits of ocrelizumab in lupus nephritis was stopped early due to an unexpected number of infections in the active treatment arm.

Abatacept is a selective T-cell co-stimulation modulator, currently licensed for use in adult rheumatoid arthritis and juvenile idiopathic arthritis. It binds to a protein on antigen-presenting cells preventing them from activating T cells, a crucial step in the development of glomerulonephritis. However, the ACCESS trial comparing the addition of abatacept or placebo to low-dose CYC did not show any benefit at either 24 weeks or 1 year [46]. A similar lack of benefit was found when combining abatacept with MMF [47].

In 2011, belimumab was the first drug to be licensed for the treatment of active lupus in over 50 years. It is a fully humanised, monoclonal antibody that binds to soluble B lymphocyte stimulator, which contributes to B-cell proliferation and differentiation. Two large, phase III clinical trials have demonstrated increased response rates in those who received belimumab in addition to standard care, in moderate-severe non-renal SLE. Belimumab is now recommended by NICE for patients with persistent disease activity despite standard treatment.

However, these studies did not include patients with overt lupus nephritis. Its efficacy in lupus nephritis has been shown in a small number of case reports [48], but the true clinical value remains to be demonstrated in ongoing clinical trials (BLISS-LN) [49].

Targeting the innate immune system using interferon-targeted therapies offers an alternative strategy to anti-T- and B-cell therapies. A number of biological agents that target type 1 interferons have been tested in phase II clinical trials, including sifalimumab and anifrolumab, with encouraging results in a subset of patients. However, they do appear to confer an increased risk of herpes zoster infections [50].

28.1.6.8 Clinical Follow-Up After Initiation of Treatment

The frequency of clinical follow-up will vary depending on diagnosis and therapy. A response to treatment will be shown by a reduction in proteinuria, fall in, or stabilisation of, serum creatinine and resolution of microscopic haematuria. Although it is encouraging to see a fall in anti-dsDNA antibodies, these have a relatively poor correlation with clinical response. As lupus nephritis has an indolent onset, it can take some months for maximum response to occur (unlike ANCA-associated vasculitis). Whilst proliferative (classes III and IV) lupus nephritis may resolve completely, membranous nephropathy (class V) may show an even slower response to treatment and residual proteinuria is common. Therefore, at least 1 year is required to determine the effectiveness of treatment, and some patients may continue to improve after this (see ▶ Case 28.2). If the response to therapy is considered inadequate, a repeat renal biopsy should be performed to establish the nature of any ongoing disease and to determine the extent of chronic renal damage. Clinical follow-up may be in renal, rheumatology or dermatology clinics. In non-renal clinics, all patients should have their urinalysis and renal function checked. A change in either should trigger a referral to a specialist renal service. Serial anti-dsDNA and complement levels are useful, as changing levels may herald a future flare of lupus nephritis [51].

There is no consensus on the length of immunosuppressive therapy. In part, this will depend on the degree of response to treatment. Most patients will receive immunosuppression for 3–5 years, but with earlier discontinuation of steroids (after 18 months to 2 years). A further renal biopsy before stopping immunosuppression should be considered, so that the extent of background injury and the presence of ongoing disease can be determined. This will help inform subsequent treatment decisions. Half of patients will experience disease relapses, and so long-term follow-up is advised.

28.1.7 Cardiovascular Risk

SLE is one of the strongest known risk factors for cardiovascular disease (CVD), which is one of the leading causes of death in patients with lupus [52]. The risk of a woman under the age of 45 with SLE developing atherosclerosis, even in the absence of renal involvement, is 50-fold greater than that of an age-matched control. A number of traditional and non-traditional risk factors contribute. Hypertension, impaired glucose tolerance and altered lipid profiles are common and exacerbated by chronic corticosteroid use. CVD burden is also significantly increased in patients with chronic inflammatory conditions. The development and progression of CKD further increase CVD risk. Thus, alongside immunosuppressive treatment of the nephritis, CVD risk should be assessed and treated aggressively in all patients with SLE, with or without nephritis.

We recommend all patients with SLE (both with and without nephritis) be treated with an angiotensin-converting enzyme (ACE) inhibitor or an angiotensin receptor blocker. These agents are first line for achieving optimum blood pressure (BP) control in proteinuric CKD. They reduce intra-glomerular pressure, lower systemic BP, reduce proteinuria and delay CKD progression. Emerging data suggest that ACE inhibitors may also delay the development of renal involvement in SLE [53]. In this study, the use of ACE inhibitors was also associated with a decreased risk of disease activity. The use of hydroxychloroquine is also recommended as it improves lipid profiles and inhibits platelet aggregation [54].

28.1.8 Pregnancy and Reproductive Health

Fertility may be affected by SLE. The major cause of infertility is CYC-associated premature ovarian failure, and so pre-treatment fertility preservation should be considered in all pre-menopausal women prior to CYC use. Ovarian stimulation to preserve oocytes is controversial due to the risk of thrombosis and/or disease flare [55]. Some evidence exists, mainly in cancer patients receiving CYC, for the use of LH-releasing hormone analogues that work by inhibiting ovarian function during CYC treatment [56]. In vitro fertilisation can be used in patients with SLE, and a recent study has demonstrated similar pregnancy outcomes to the general population, albeit few of the women included had significant renal involvement [57].

There are a number of factors to consider when a patient with SLE wants to have a baby. Pregnancy in women with lupus nephritis is associated with an increased risk of foetal loss and with worsening of the renal and extra-renal manifestations of SLE. Pre-eclampsia is also a frequent complication of pregnancy in SLE, and differentiating between pre-eclampsia and active disease can be extremely difficult. Maternal SLE is also associated with an increased risk of premature delivery and intrauterine growth restriction. There may be an increased risk of learning disabilities in the offspring, especially in males.

The prognosis for both mother and child is best when the disease, including renal disease, has been quiescent for at least 6 months prior to the pregnancy. We would recommend a pre-pregnancy renal biopsy to confirm histological disease activity. If the patient is prescribed maintenance therapy, this should be converted to azathioprine with or without corticosteroids. Hydroxychloroquine should be continued during pregnancy to reduce the risk of flares, potentially improve placental function and reduce the risk of complete heart block in babies born to mothers with anti-Ro antibodies [58]. Accordingly, all women with anti-Ro and anti-La antibodies should be offered foetal echocardiography from approximately 16 weeks' gestation [59]. Thrombotic risk should be assessed, and thrombotic prophylaxis with low-molecular-weight heparin offered to those with antiphospholipid syndrome and/or significant proteinuria [55]. All women should be offered low-dose aspirin from 12 weeks to reduce the risk of pre-eclampsia and may benefit from this being started pre-conception [59]. Breastfeeding is feasible for most women with SLE, and steroids, azathioprine, enalapril, amlodipine and aspirin may all be used safely during lactation [55].

Effective contraception and appropriate contraceptive counselling should be offered to all pre-menopausal women with SLE. Oestrogen-containing hormonal contraceptives are usually avoided, due to the risk of hypertension, thrombosis and disease flares. However, a number of progesterone-based methods are suitable, including the progesterone-only pill, Mirena IUD and subdermal implant.

28.1.9 Case Studies

Tips and Tricks

1. Consider lupus nephritis in any patient, particularly young women, with multi-system disease and haematuria and/or proteinuria.
2. Ensure all patients with SLE have regular urinalysis and checks of renal function and blood pressure.
3. Lupus nephritis is unlikely in the absence of hypocomplementaemia.
4. Immune complex deposition in multiple compartments within the kidney is characteristic of lupus nephritis.
5. Pregnancy outcomes in lupus are best with careful pre-conception planning.
6. Ensure all women of reproductive age are using appropriate contraception.

28.2 Antiphospholipid Syndrome (APLS)

28.2.1 Introduction

Antiphospholipid syndrome is a unique form of autoantibody-induced thrombophilia, characterised by recurrent (arterial and venous) thrombosis and pregnancy complications. The syndrome arises due to endothelial cell, monocyte and platelet activation by antiphospholipid antibodies with anti-β2-glycoprotein 1 activity. Endothelial cells then express a number of adhesion molecules and together with monocytes upregulate the production of tissue factor. Activation of platelets results in an increase in their expression of glycoprotein 2b-3a and synthesis of thromboxane A2. Endothelial cell, monocyte and platelet activation results in a prothrombotic state and, alongside complement activation, provokes thrombosis. This usually occurs in the presence of a second hit such as infection or surgery. Traditional cardiovascular risk factors such as smoking, inflammation or oestrogen therapy may play an important role at this point – such factors are present in >50% of patients with the APLS.

28.2.2 Clinical Manifestations

Thromboses, in particular venous thromboembolism, are the most frequent manifestation of the APLS. Importantly, by comparison to other thrombophilias, thrombosis may occur in any vascular bed. Arterial thrombosis occurs most frequently in the central nervous system, usually in the form of a stroke or transient ischaemic attack. Less common presentations include venous sinus thrombosis, myelopathy, chorea, migraine and epilepsy.

Anticardiolipin antibodies are also associated with cognitive impairment in SLE. Considerable interest, and controversy, has focused on the relationship between APLS and cognitive impairment. Cognitive deficits range from subtle findings to transient global amnesia to permanent and profound cognitive impairment. The cognitive deficits reported in APLS are sometimes but not always associated with white matter lesions.

Other clinical manifestations of the APLS include cardiac valvular disease – the mitral valve is more commonly affected than the aortic; regurgitation more common than stenosis. Renal involvement in the APLS has only been described relatively recently [60]. Thrombotic microangiopathy is the commonest feature of APLS nephropathy, but other histological findings include fibrous intimal hyperplasia and focal cortical atrophy. A typical presentation of APLS nephropathy is hypertension with (often sub-nephrotic range) proteinuria and renal insufficiency. Other clinical features of the APLS include haemolytic anaemia, thrombocytopenia, skin involvement with livedo reticularis – present in ~25% of patients with APLS and a marker of patients at risk of arterial thrombosis – avascular bone necrosis and adrenal insufficiency. Obstetric complications of the APLS include recurrent miscarriage, foetal death, severe pre-eclampsia and placental insufficiency.

Clinically, the most severe, but fortunately the most infrequent, form of the syndrome is catastrophic APLS characterised by widespread small vessel thrombosis with multi-organ failure. Catastrophic APLS is associated with a >50% mortality.

28.2.3 Epidemiology

About 40% of patients with SLE have antiphospholipid antibodies, but <40% of those will eventually have thrombosis. However, thrombotic APLS is regarded as a major adverse prognostic factor in SLE. In women with recurrent miscarriage (~1% of the general population), APLS is eventually diagnosed in 10–15%.

28.2.4 Diagnosis

The diagnosis of APLS relies on specific clinical manifestations alongside laboratory evidence of a circulating antiphospholipid antibody [61].

28

28.2.4.1 Clinical Criteria

- Vascular thrombosis – arterial, venous or small vessel
- Pregnancy morbidity – one or more of:
- One or more deaths of a healthy foetus at 10 or more weeks' gestation
- One or more premature births of a healthy baby before 34 weeks' gestation because of eclampsia or pre-eclampsia
- Three or more unexplained consecutive spontaneous abortions before 10 weeks' gestation

28.2.4.2 Laboratory Criteria

Demonstration on two more occasions at least 12 weeks apart of:

- Lupus anticoagulant
- Anticardiolipin antibody (IgM or IgG)
- Anti-β2-glycoprotein 1 antibody (IgM or IgG)

Antibodies directed against phosphatidylserine-prothrombin complex, those of IgA subtype and anti-prothrombin antibodies currently remain excluded from these criteria. The IgG subclass of antibody confers a greater risk of thrombosis than do those of IgM or IgA subtype.

28.2.5 Treatment

The goal of therapy is to prevent thrombosis either in those individuals with antiphospholipid antibodies who have already had a thrombotic event (secondary prevention) or in those who without previous thrombosis (primary prevention).

Current treatment for secondary prevention in those individuals presenting with a first venous thrombosis is with lifelong anticoagulation, usually with warfarin, with a target INR of 2.0–3.0. For those who have had recurrent venous thrombosis or arterial thrombosis, a higher INR may be desirable.

Current recommendations for primary prevention of APLS are not clear. However, the annual thrombotic risk of patients with SLE and antiphospholipid antibodies is about 3–4%, and so we would recommend the use of low-dose daily aspirin in these patients. Importantly, other vascular risk factors should be treated aggressively in all patients with antiphospholipid antibodies.

Tips and Tricks

1. Check all patients with SLE for the presence of antiphospholipid antibodies (lupus anticoagulant, anticardiolipin antibody and/or anti-β2-glycoprotein 1 antibody).
2. Catastrophic APLS can be precipitated by a 'trigger' such as disruption to usual anticoagulation, surgery, infection or, importantly, renal biopsy (and the sub-therapeutic anticoagulation this entails).

28.3 Resources and Patient Information

28.3.1 For Professionals

► http://www.rheumatology.org/practice/clinical/classification/

► http://www.eular.org/index.cfm?framePage=/recommendations_management.cfm

28.3.2 For Patients

► http://www.lupusuk.org.uk

► http://www.arthritiscare.org.uk

Questions

1. Does ANA positivity confirm a diagnosis of SLE?
2. How would you treat a young woman with creatinine 63 μmol/L, urine protein/creatinine ratio 63 mg/mmol and evidence of endocapillary proliferation in less than half her glomeruli on renal biopsy?
3. What specific treatments should be avoided in women with SLE planning a pregnancy?
4. What specific treatments are recommended for women with SLE planning a pregnancy?

Answers

1. No – although the vast majority of patients with SLE are positive for the anti-nuclear antibody (ANA), it can also be found in Sjögren's syndrome, scleroderma and rheumatoid arthritis. Importantly, a low titre of ANA (1:40) can be found in up to 30% of healthy volunteers.
2. Despite the seemingly preserved renal function (and it would be important to calculate the estimated GFR in this case, as young women should have very low creatinine levels) and moderate pro-

teinuria, this patient has class III lupus nephritis. We would recommend induction immunosuppression with corticosteroids (prednisolone 40 mg daily) and MMF 1 g twice daily to achieve remission.

3. MMF is teratogenic and so contraindicated in pregnancy. Ideally, patients should be swapped to azathioprine 3–6 months prior to conception, to ensure their disease remains in remission, despite the change in therapy. ACE inhibitors are contraindicated in the second and third trimesters of pregnancy and, however, appear not to cause birth defects in early pregnancy. Therefore, for women with significant proteinuria, it may be appropriate to keep ACE inhibition going until the woman has a positive pregnancy test. Cyclophosphamide and rituximab cannot be used in pregnancy.
4. Hydroxychloroquine should be continued during pregnancy, as it reduces the risk of disease flares and the risk of neonatal lupus syndrome and/or congenital heart block. All women with lupus should take 75 mg aspirin from 12 weeks, and in some women, this should be started preconception. Folic acid (400 mcg daily) and vitamin D supplementation should also be prescribed prior to and during pregnancy.

Case 28.1

A 19-year-old Caucasian woman presented with swelling of her ankles and a purpuric rash over both legs. She had recently returned from a holiday in Spain and noticed feeling lethargic with aching joints. She had recently started taking oral tetracycline for acne. Initial investigations showed:

Haematology	Biochemistry	Urinalysis	Immunology
Hb 109 g/L	Urea 6.2 mmol/l	Blood +++	ANA 1/640 (speckled pattern)
WCC 5.6 × 10^9/l	Creatinine 102 µmol/l (no previous measure)	Protein +++	dsDNA 22 U/ml
Platelets 109 × 10^9/l	ALT 225 U/l	Protein/creatinine ratio 924 mg/mmol	ENA negative
	Albumin 22 g/l	MSU negative	Positive lupus anticoagulant
	CRP 87 mg/L		C3 0.61 g/L C4 0.14 g/L

A renal biopsy was performed (◘ Fig. 28.1a, b) which showed a diffuse, segmental and global, necrotising and proliferative glomerulonephritis, with one crescent. There was no evidence of chronic renal damage. These changes were consistent with WHO class IV lupus nephritis. The patient was treated with a tapering course of oral corticosteroids and MMF 2 g/day. She was also started on prophylactic low-dose aspirin. Clinical improvement was rapid alongside an improvement in renal function, liver enzymes and proteinuria (◘ Fig. 28.1c). MMF was tapered to 1 g/day after 2 years and all immunosuppression stopped after a total of 3 years' treatment. The patient had a disease relapse 3 months following this and was re-commenced on oral corticosteroids – which were gradually tapered to zero – and MMF on which she remains at last clinic review.

28

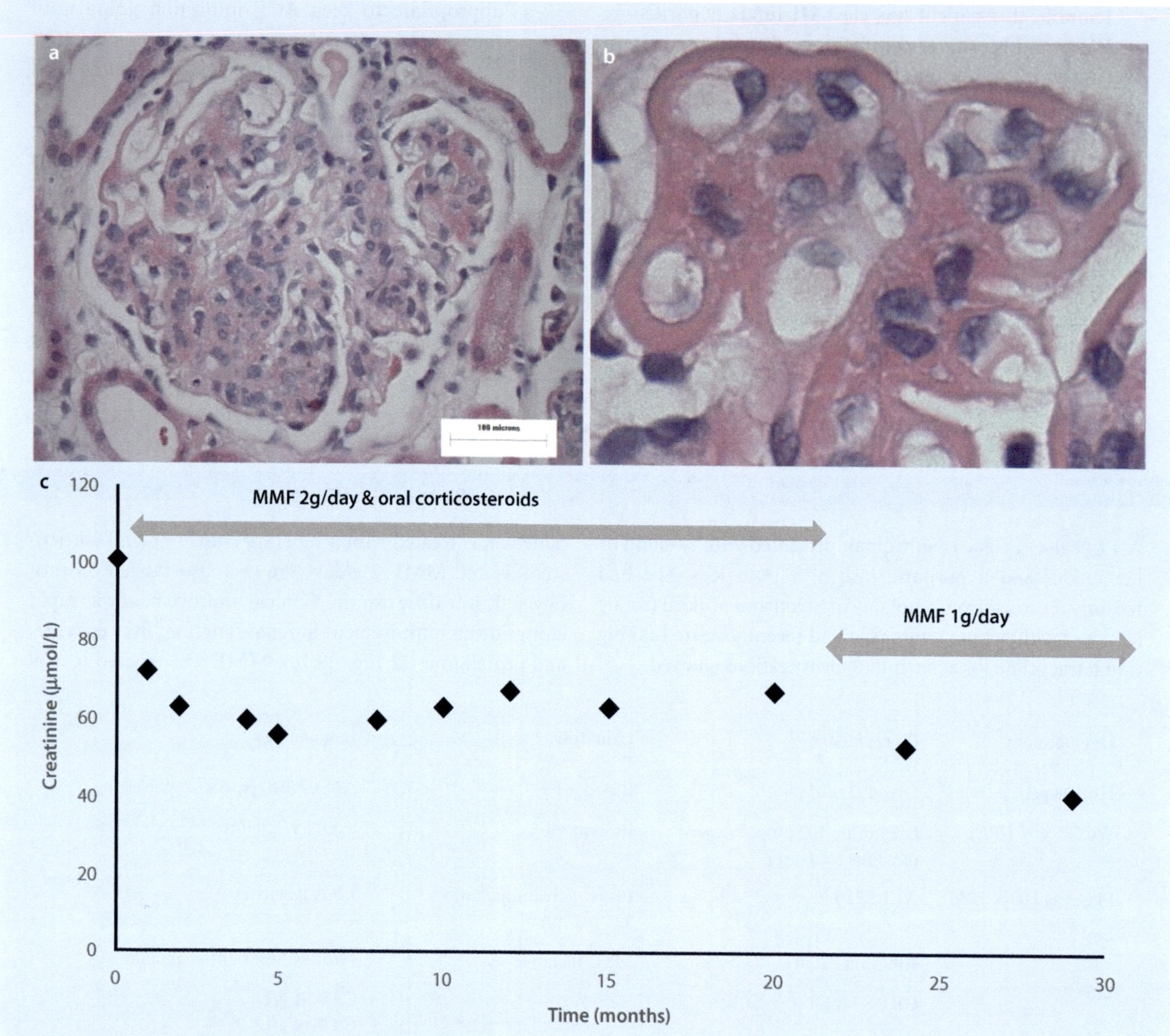

Fig. 28.1 **a** Glomerulus with global proliferation (>50% of the tuft area) (H&E stain). **b** Glomerular tuft (H&E stain) showing "wire loop" capillary walls thickened due to immune deposits. **c** Change in serum creatinine following diagnosis. There is a rapid fall, even with what seems only a minor elevation in serum creatinine at presentation

Case 28.2

A 37-year-old female presented with arthralgia, lethargy and alopecia. She was of Chinese origin and had one child. She had been diagnosed 10 years earlier with idiopathic thrombocytopenic purpura and treated with oral corticosteroids alone. Five years later, she had presented with lethargy, night sweats, fevers, cough and mouth ulcers, with a high titre of dsDNA antibodies. She was given a diagnosis of SLE and treated with oral corticosteroids and hydroxychloroquine. She had been well for the last 2 years. Initial investigations showed:

Haematology	Biochemistry	Urinalysis	Immunology
Hb 102 g/L	Urea 7.2 mmol/l	Blood +++	dsDNA >200 U/ml
WCC 3.1 × 10^9/l	Creatinine 90 µmol/l (previously 54)	Protein +++	C3 0.21 g/L C4 0.02 g/L
Platelets 87 × 10^9/l	CRP 34 mg/L	Protein/creatinine ratio 575 mg/mmol	
		MSU negative	

A renal biopsy was performed (Fig. 28.2a, b) which showed a diffuse, segmental and global, necrotising and proliferative glomerulonephritis, with crescents. There was no evidence of chronic damage. These changes were in keeping with WHO class IV lupus nephritis. Given the prominent crescents, the patient was treated with a tapering dose of oral corticosteroids alongside six doses of intravenous CYC. The patient was then switched to MMF 2 g/day as maintenance therapy. There was a rapid and sustained improvement in the patient's symptoms and biochemical parameters (Fig. 28.2c, d). After 12 months of MMF, the dose was reduced from 2 g to 1 g/day and the patient was continued on this long term. Note that serum creatinine and proteinuria continued to improve even after 12 months of treatment.

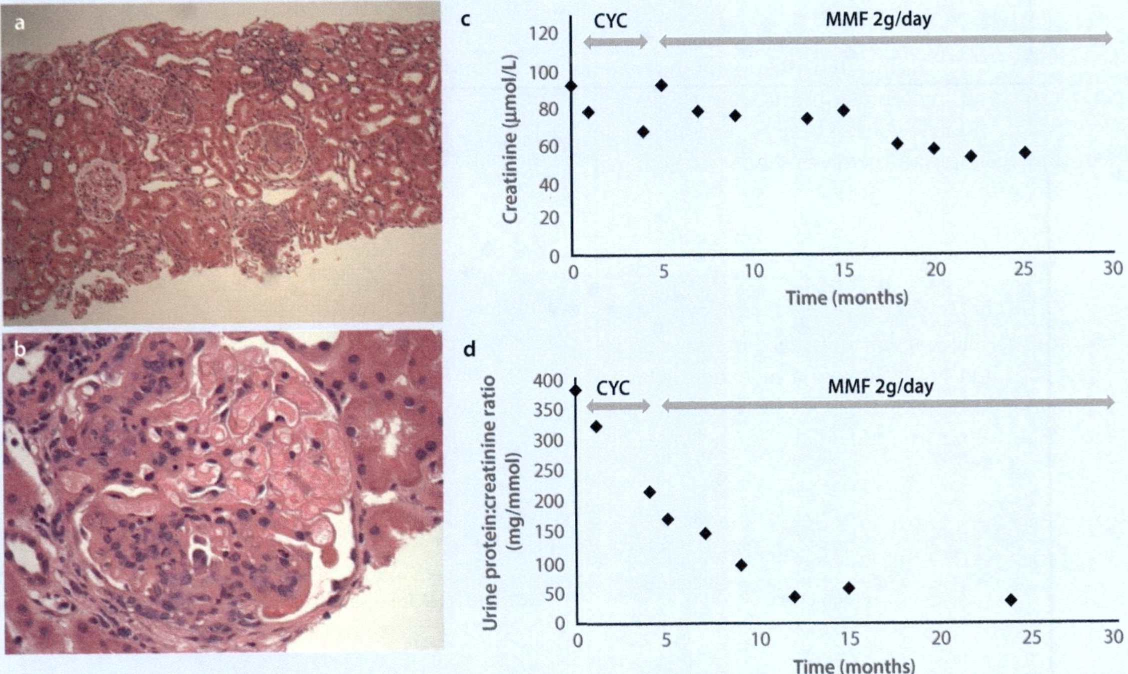

Fig. 28.2 **a** Kidney cortex (H&E stain) at low magnification, showing segmental abnormalities in 4 of 5 glomeruli but minimal chronic tubulointerstitial damage. **b** Glomerulus at high magnification (H&E stain), showing marked proliferation affecting just over 50% of the tuft area (i.e. global). **c** Improvement in serum creatinine following treatment with intravenous cyclophosphamide at induction, followed by MMF for maintenance treatment. Renal function continues to improve for almost 2 years after starting treatment. **d** Reduction in proteinuria following treatment

28

Case 28.3

A 31-year-old woman with a long history of SLE presented to the renal clinic prior to planning a pregnancy. She had received multiple treatments for relapsing lupus nephritis over the preceding 10 years but was not currently taking any immunosuppression. She had blood and protein on urine dipstick. Whilst undergoing investigations, including renal biopsy, to ascertain the level of disease activity, she became pregnant. The renal biopsy was consistent with class IV lupus nephritis, so she was treated with azathioprine, prednisolone and hydroxychloroquine. Early pregnancy was uneventful, but by 30 weeks, she had become increasingly proteinuric with worsening hypertension and eventually became profoundly nephrotic (◘ Fig. 28.3a, b). She delivered a small but healthy baby by emergency Caesarian section at 36 weeks. She continued to have nephrotic range proteinuria following delivery and was treated with corticosteroids, azathioprine and enalapril. Proteinuria improved but remained elevated, with a protein/creatinine ratio of 100–150 mg/mmol. Following cessation of breastfeeding, she was switched from azathioprine to MMF and proteinuria completely resolved. Steroids were successfully weaned, and she has been maintained on MMF until a recent switch to azathioprine prior to planning her next pregnancy.

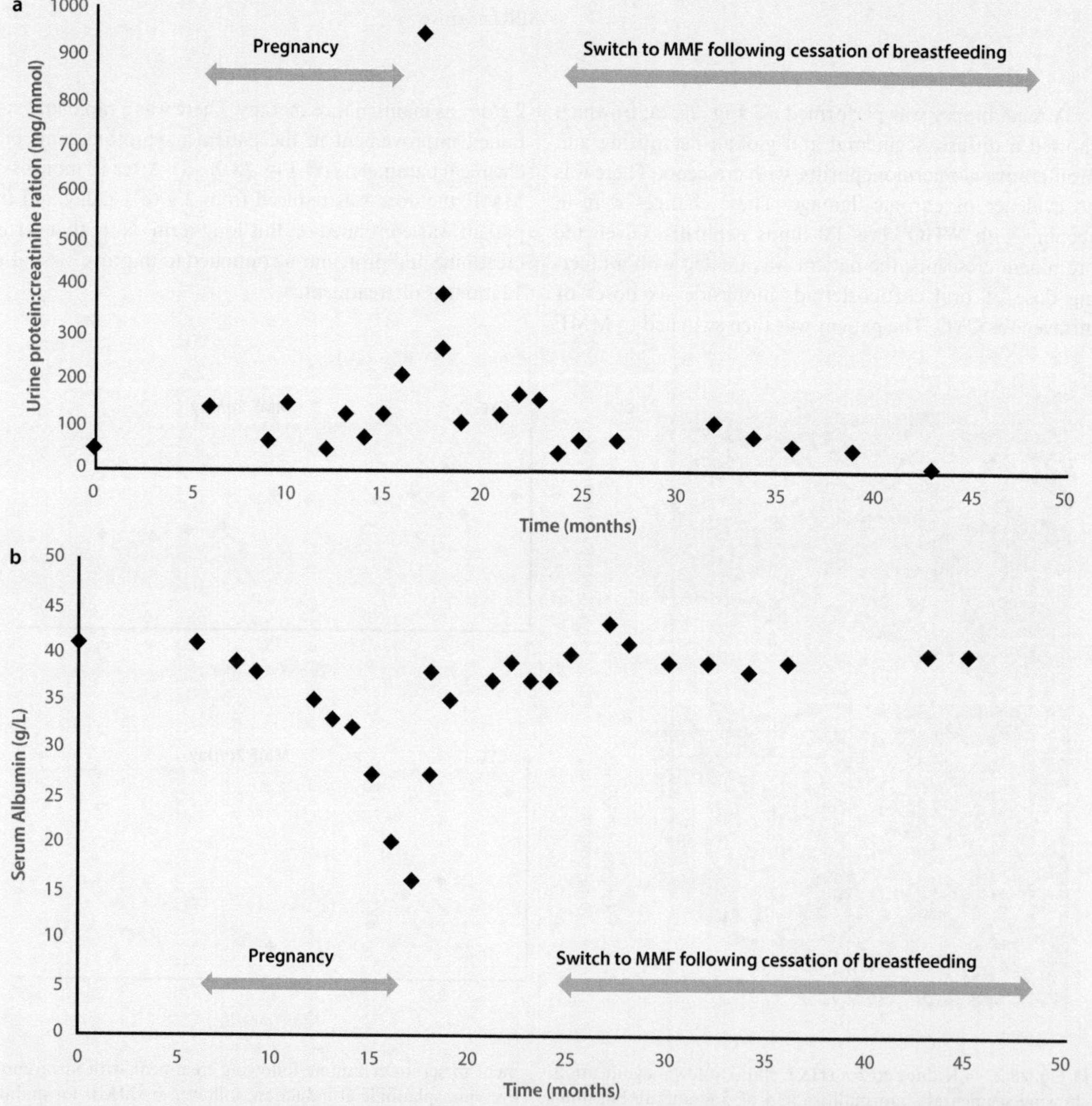

◘ **Fig. 28.3** **a** Proteinuria increasing during pregnancy, and persisting, at a lower level, until the switch to MMF at 8 months post-partum. **b** Serum albumin falls significantly during late pregnancy with the development of frank nephrotic syndrome

References

1. Rees F, Doherty M, Grainge M, Davenport G, Lanyon P, Zhang W. The incidence and prevalence of systemic lupus erythematosus in the UK, 1999–2012. Ann Rheum Dis. 2016;75:136–41.
2. Yee CS, Su L, Toescu V, et al. Birmingham SLE cohort: outcomes of a large inception cohort followed for up to 21 years. Rheumatology. 2015;54:836–43.
3. Croca SC, Rodrigues T, Isenberg DA. Assessment of a lupus nephritis cohort over a 30-year period. Rheumatology. 2011;50:1424–30.
4. Berden JH. Lupus nephritis. Kidney Int. 1997;52:538–58.
5. Austin HA, Illei GG. Membranous lupus nephritis. Lupus. 2005;14:65–71.
6. Pirani CL, Olesnicky L. Role of electronmicroscopy in the classification of lupus nephritis. Am J Kidney Dis. 1982;2:150–63.
7. Tsumagari T, Fukumoto S, Kinjo M, Tanaka K. Incidence and significance of intrarenal vasculopathies in patients with systemic lupus erythematosus. Human Pathol. 1985;16:43–9.
8. Banfi G, Bertani T, Boeri V, et al. Renal vascular lesions as a marker of poor prognosis in patients with lupus nephritis. Gruppo Italiano per lo Studio della Nefrite Lupica (GISNEL). Am J Kidney Dis. 1991;18:240–8.
9. Grishman E, Venkataseshan VS. Vascular lesions in lupus nephritis. Modern Pathol. 1988;1:235–41.
10. Cameron JS. Lupus nephritis. J Am Soc Nephrol. 1999;10:413–24.
11. Bertsias GK, Tektonidou M, Amoura Z, et al. Joint European League Against Rheumatism and European Renal Association-European Dialysis and Transplant Association (EULAR/ERA-EDTA) recommendations for the management of adult and paediatric lupus nephritis. Ann Rheum Dis. 2012;71:1771–82.
12. Markowitz GS, D'Agati VD. Classification of lupus nephritis. Curr Opin Nephrol Hypertens. 2009;18:220–5.
13. Weening JJ, D'Agati VD, Schwartz MM, et al. The classification of glomerulonephritis in systemic lupus erythematosus revisited. J Am Soc Nephrol. 2004;15:241–50.
14. Bajema IM, Wilhelmus S, Alpers CE, et al. Revision of the International Society of Nephrology/Renal Pathology Society classification for lupus nephritis: clarification of definitions, and modified National Institutes of Health activity and chronicity indices. Kidney Int. 2018;93:789–96.
15. Dube GK, Markowitz GS, Radhakrishnan J, Appel GB, D'Agati VD. Minimal change disease in systemic lupus erythematosus. Clin Nephrol. 2002;57:120–6.
16. Kraft SW, Schwartz MM, Korbet SM, Lewis EJ. Glomerular podocytopathy in patients with systemic lupus erythematosus. J Am Soc Nephrol. 2005;16:175–9.
17. Han TS, Schwartz MM, Lewis EJ. Association of glomerular podocytopathy and nephrotic proteinuria in mesangial lupus nephritis. Lupus. 2006;15:71–5.
18. Illei GG, Austin HA, Crane M, et al. Combination therapy with pulse cyclophosphamide plus pulse methylprednisolone improves long-term renal outcome without adding toxicity in patients with lupus nephritis. Ann Intern Med. 2001;135:248–57.
19. Houssiau FA, Vasconcelos C, D'Cruz D, et al. Immunosuppressive therapy in lupus nephritis: the Euro-Lupus Nephritis Trial, a randomized trial of low-dose versus high-dose intravenous cyclophosphamide. Arthritis Rheumatol. 2002;46:2121–31.
20. Houssiau FA, Vasconcelos C, D'Cruz D, et al. The 10-year follow-up data of the Euro-Lupus Nephritis Trial comparing low-dose and high-dose intravenous cyclophosphamide. Ann Rheum Dis. 2010;69:61–4.
21. Chan TM, Li FK, Tang CS, et al. Efficacy of mycophenolate mofetil in patients with diffuse proliferative lupus nephritis. Hong Kong-Guangzhou Nephrology Study Group. New Engl J Med. 2000;343:1156–62.
22. Chan TM, Tse KC, Tang CS, Mok MY, Li FK. Long-term study of mycophenolate mofetil as continuous induction and maintenance treatment for diffuse proliferative lupus nephritis. J Am Soc Nephrol. 2005;16:1076–84.
23. Ginzler EM, Dooley MA, Aranow C, et al. Mycophenolate mofetil or intravenous cyclophosphamide for lupus nephritis. New Engl J Med. 2005;353:2219–28.
24. Walsh M, James M, Jayne D, Tonelli M, Manns BJ, Hemmelgarn BR. Mycophenolate mofetil for induction therapy of lupus nephritis: a systematic review and meta-analysis. Clin J Am Soc Nephrol. 2007;2:968–75.
25. Appel GB, Contreras G, Dooley MA, et al. Mycophenolate mofetil versus cyclophosphamide for induction treatment of lupus nephritis. J Am Soc Nephrol. 2009;20:1103–12.
26. Lee YH, Woo JH, Choi SJ, Ji JD, Song GG. Induction and maintenance therapy for lupus nephritis: a systematic review and meta-analysis. Lupus. 2010;19:703–10.
27. Tunnicliffe DJ, Palmer SC, Henderson L, et al. Immunosuppressive treatment for proliferative lupus nephritis. Cochrane Database Syst Rev. 2018;6:CD002922.
28. Lu TY, Ng KP, Cambridge G, et al. A retrospective seven-year analysis of the use of B cell depletion therapy in systemic lupus erythematosus at University College London Hospital: the first fifty patients. Arthritis Rheumatol. 2009;61:482–7.
29. Melander C, Sallee M, Trolliet P, et al. Rituximab in severe lupus nephritis: early B-cell depletion affects long-term renal outcome. Clin J Am Soc Nephrol. 2009;4:579–87.
30. Merrill JT, Neuwelt CM, Wallace DJ, et al. Efficacy and safety of rituximab in moderately-to-severely active systemic lupus erythematosus: the randomized, double-blind, phase II/III systemic lupus erythematosus evaluation of rituximab trial. Arthritis Rheumatol. 2010;62:222–33.
31. Rovin BH, Furie R, Latinis K, et al. Efficacy and safety of rituximab in patients with active proliferative lupus nephritis: the Lupus Nephritis Assessment with Rituximab study. Arthritis Rheumatol. 2012;64:1215–26.
32. Lightstone L. Minimising steroids in lupus nephritis–will B cell depletion pave the way? Lupus. 2013;22:390–9.
33. Flanc RS, Roberts MA, Strippoli GF, Chadban SJ, Kerr PG, Atkins RC. Treatment of diffuse proliferative lupus nephritis: a meta-analysis of randomized controlled trials. Am J Kidney Dis. 2004;43:197–208.
34. Zhu B, Chen N, Lin Y, et al. Mycophenolate mofetil in induction and maintenance therapy of severe lupus nephritis: a meta-analysis of randomized controlled trials. Nephrol Dial Transplant. 2007;22:1933–42.
35. Chapter 12: Lupus nephritis. Kidney Int Suppl (2011) 2012;2:221–32.
36. Contreras G, Pardo V, Leclercq B, et al. Sequential therapies for proliferative lupus nephritis. New Engl J Med. 2004;350:971–80.
37. Contreras G, Tozman E, Nahar N, Metz D. Maintenance therapies for proliferative lupus nephritis: mycophenolate mofetil, azathioprine and intravenous cyclophosphamide. Lupus. 2005;14 Suppl 1:s33–8.
38. Houssiau FA, D'Cruz D, Sangle S, et al. Azathioprine versus mycophenolate mofetil for long-term immunosuppression in lupus nephritis: results from the MAINTAIN Nephritis Trial. Ann Rheum Dis. 2010;69:2083–9.
39. Dooley MA, Jayne D, Ginzler EM, et al. Mycophenolate versus azathioprine as maintenance therapy for lupus nephritis. New Engl J Med. 2011;365:1886–95.

28

40. Ginzler E, Sharon E, Diamond H, Kaplan D. Long-term maintenance therapy with azathioprine in systemic lupus erythematosus. Arthritis Rheumatol. 1975;18:27–34.
41. Austin HA 3rd, Illei GG, Braun MJ, Balow JE. Randomized, controlled trial of prednisone, cyclophosphamide, and cyclosporine in lupus membranous nephropathy. J Am Soc Nephrol. 2009;20:901–11.
42. Cattran DC, Alexopoulos E, Heering P, et al. Cyclosporin in idiopathic glomerular disease associated with the nephrotic syndrome: workshop recommendations. Kidney Int. 2007;72:1429–47.
43. Waldman M, Austin HA 3rd. Treatment of idiopathic membranous nephropathy. J Am Soc Nephrol. 2012;
44. Chavarot N, Verhelst D, Pardon A, et al. Rituximab alone as induction therapy for membranous lupus nephritis: a multicenter retrospective study. Medicine. 2017;96:e7429.
45. Oon S, Huq M, Godfrey T, Nikpour M. Systematic review, and meta-analysis of steroid-sparing effect, of biologic agents in randomized, placebo-controlled phase 3 trials for systemic lupus erythematosus. Semin Arthritis Rheum. 2018;
46. Group AT. Treatment of lupus nephritis with abatacept: the abatacept and cyclophosphamide combination efficacy and safety study. Arthritis Rheumatol. 2014;66:3096–104.
47. Furie R, Nicholls K, Cheng TT, et al. Efficacy and safety of abatacept in lupus nephritis: a twelve-month, randomized, double-blind study. Arthritis Rheumatol. 2014;66:379–89.
48. Margiotta DPE, Basta F, Batani V, Afeltra A. Belimumab and low-doses of mycophenolate mofetil as induction therapy of class IV lupus nephritis: case series and literature review. BMC Nephrol. 2018;19:54.
49. Dhaun N, Kluth DC. Belimumab for systemic lupus erythematosus. Lancet. 2011;377:2079–80; author reply 80–1.
50. Kalunian KC. Interferon-targeted therapy in systemic lupus erythematosus: is this an alternative to targeting B and T cells? Lupus. 2016;25:1097–101.
51. Petri M, Singh S, Tesfasyone H, Malik A. Prevalence of flare and influence of demographic and serologic factors on flare risk in systemic lupus erythematosus: a prospective study. J Rheumatol. 2009;36:2476–80.
52. Bernatsky S, Boivin JF, Joseph L, et al. Mortality in systemic lupus erythematosus. Arthritis Rheumatol. 2006;54:2550–7.
53. Duran-Barragan S, McGwin G Jr, Vila LM, Reveille JD, Alarcon GS, cohort LamU. Angiotensin-converting enzyme inhibitors delay the occurrence of renal involvement and are associated with a decreased risk of disease activity in patients with systemic lupus erythematosus–results from LUMINA (LIX): a multiethnic US cohort. Rheumatology. 2008;47:1093–6.
54. Croca S, Rahman A. Atherosclerosis in systemic lupus erythematosus. Best Pract Res Clin Rheumatol. 2017;31:364–72.
55. Wiles K, Lightstone L. Glomerular disease in women. Kidney Int Rep. 2018;3:258–70.
56. Lambertini M, Ceppi M, Poggio F, et al. Ovarian suppression using luteinizing hormone-releasing hormone agonists during chemotherapy to preserve ovarian function and fertility of breast cancer patients: a meta-analysis of randomized studies. Ann Oncol. 2015;26:2408–19.
57. Orquevaux P, Masseau A, Le Guern V, et al. In vitro fertilization in 37 women with systemic lupus erythematosus or antiphospholipid syndrome: a series of 97 procedures. J Rheumatol. 2017;44:613–8.
58. Gordon C, Amissah-Arthur MB, Gayed M, et al. The British Society for Rheumatology guideline for the management of systemic lupus erythematosus in adults. Rheumatology. 2018;57:e1–e45.
59. Andreoli L, Bertsias GK, Agmon-Levin N, et al. EULAR recommendations for women's health and the management of family planning, assisted reproduction, pregnancy and menopause in patients with systemic lupus erythematosus and/or antiphospholipid syndrome. Ann Rheum Dis. 2017;76:476–85.
60. Amigo MC, Garcia-Torres R, Robles M, Bochicchio T, Reyes PA. Renal involvement in primary antiphospholipid syndrome. J Rheumatol. 1992;19:1181–5.
61. Miyakis S, Lockshin MD, Atsumi T, et al. International consensus statement on an update of the classification criteria for definite antiphospholipid syndrome (APS). J Thromb Haemostasis. 2006;4:295–306.

Practical Immunosuppression Guidelines for Patients with Glomerulonephritis

Ruth J. Pepper and Alan D. Salama

Contents

M. Harber (ed.), *Primer on Nephrology*, https://doi.org/10.1007/978-3-030-76419-7_29

Learning Objectives

1. Immune-mediated renal disease often requires immunosuppression, so appropriate pathways and protocols need to be in place to ensure immunosuppression is delivered safely.
2. Increasing age and renal failure are associated with greatest risk of treatment-related complications such as leucopenia and opportunistic infections.
3. Newer treatment regimens increasingly focus on steroid sparing/minimisation and alternatives to the traditional use of drugs such as cyclophosphamide.
4. Plasmapheresis may have a more limited role in induction therapy in the context of high-dose glucocorticoids.

29

29.1 Introduction

Many forms of glomerular disease are immune mediated and are therefore treated with immunosuppression. The particular regimen that is used may vary depending on the underlying condition, but many protocols are based on combination therapy using glucocorticoids and a second agent, which has historically often been cyclophosphamide. With the introduction of newer immunosuppressive agents, including biologics, these protocols have been modified for different conditions and, in only some cases, tested in randomised controlled trials. Certain protocols are based on oral therapies and can easily be delivered safely as outpatients; others require infusions which necessitate careful co-ordination of day case admissions and outpatient monitoring to allow early recognition of potential adverse events. Particular agents appear to have heightened risks for particular adverse effects and require specific screening and/or prophylaxis consideration. Regardless of the actual regimen used, there are some general principles that apply to delivering a safe immunosuppressive service. In this chapter, we discuss practical issues surrounding immunosuppression in glomerular disease.

29.2 Protocol Constituents

29.2.1 Cyclophosphamide

The risks of cyclophosphamide are believed to be outweighed in severe life- or organ-threatening conditions; however, it is important to make patients aware of potential toxicities (see ▶ Appendix for example of a cyclophosphamide consent sheet). Limiting the patient's total exposure is desirable, as adverse events are related to cumulative dose and there are significant increases in haematological and bladder malignancies once total exposure exceeds 36 g [1].

Cyclophosphamide may be used orally (at doses of 2–3 mg/kg), for example, in anti-GBM disease or intravenously as pulses every 2–3 weeks depending on the protocol, for example, in the EUROLUPUS regimen, which is based on low-dose short-duration cyclophosphamide, or the CYCLOPS vasculitis regimen, which uses higher doses for a longer duration.

There is ample evidence that pulsed intravenous treatment induces remission as rapidly in as many patients as daily oral therapy but exposes the patients to lower drug levels and thus is associated with fewer leucopenic episodes [2]. Long-term lower doses of cyclophosphamide are associated with higher relapse rates in certain conditions [3, 4]. While the data are available to confirm benefit in SLE and ANCA-associated vasculitis(AAV), no direct comparisons have, or will likely to be, performed in anti-GBM disease. Therefore, many practitioners still utilise oral cyclophosphamide in anti-GBM disease based on established protocols.

Mesna is a compound administered to reduce the risk of haemorrhagic cystitis by binding and inactivating the urotoxic metabolite of cyclophosphamide such as acrolein in the bladder. However, with modern dosage regimens of intravenous cyclophosphamide, the incidence of haemorrhagic cystitis is low, and the use of mesna as a bladder protectant may be unnecessary [5]. In addition, there may be reactions to the mesna itself, and thus some units have abandoned the routine use of mesna. Encouraging oral input (assuming the patient is not oligo-anuric) to maintain a good urine output and reduce the concentration of bladder accumulating metabolites is useful.

Dose adjustments should be made based on age and renal function. A schema for dose reduction of pulsed intravenous cyclophosphamide as used in ANCA-associated vasculitis is shown in ◘ Table 29.1, while if daily oral treatment is used, the dose should be reduced by 25% if >60 years and 50% if >70 years.

Cyclophosphamide should be withheld if the total WCC is less than 4×10^9, and oral doses should be reduced by 50 mg if the white count is trending downwards, to avoid the development of episodes of leucopenia. Weekly WCC checks are mandatory while on oral cyclophosphamide for the first month, twice-weekly for the second month and monthly thereafter for the first year.

Pulsed therapy dosage should be adjusted depending on nadir WCC and checked 7–10 days after treatment. We ensure that a recent (within 1 week) blood test is available prior to delivering the next dose.

Table 29.1 Intravenous cyclophosphamide regimen used in systemic vasculitis demonstrating dose adjustment for both age and renal function

Age (years)	Creatinine μmol/L	
	<300	>300
<60	15 mg/kg/pulse	12.5 mg/kg/pulse
60–70	12.5 mg/kg/pulse	10 mg/kg/pulse
>70	10 mg/kg/pulse	7.5 mg/kg/pulse

Taken from Ref. [2]
Patients with a nadir leucocyte count of 2–3 × 10^9/L had a dose reduction of 20%. Dose reduced by 40% in those who had a nadir leucocyte count of 1–2 × 10^9/L.
Omit pulse if WBC nadir <1 × 10^9/L and consider g-CSF administration and antibiotic prophylaxis

Table 29.2 Steroid reducing protocol

Prednisolone **(non-enteric coated) protocol**	**Starting dose: 1 mg/kg daily orally**
Week 1	50 mg (<50 kg), 60 mg (50–75 kg), 75 mg (>75 kg)
Week 2	25 mg, 30 mg, 40 mg
Weeks 3–4	20 mg, 25 mg, 30 mg
Weeks 5–6	15 mg, 20 mg, 25 mg
Weeks 7–8	12.5 mg, 15 mg, 20 mg
Thereafter steroid reductions depending on patient's response	2.5 mg dose reduction every 2 weeks
Weeks 15–19	5 mg in all weight groups

If pulsed methylprednisolone is given, starting dose of steroid could be reduced (reduced dose PEXIVAS protocol)

Prophylaxis for *Pneumocystis jirovecii* with low-dose co-trimoxazole is required in CYP-treated patients. This can be delivered as 480 mg daily or 960 mg three times a week. In cases of co-trimoxazole allergy, monthly nebulised pentamidine may be used instead. Anti-emetics such as ondansetron 8 mg or granisetron 1–2 mg should be given 30 minutes pre- and 12 hours post-infusion.

29.2.2 Glucocorticoids

Steroids (glucocorticoids) have been the mainstay of treatment for nearly all immune-based diseases, and this is true of most glomerular diseases. The dose regimens used in glomerular diseases have been highly variable and mostly decided on empirically without any comparative trial data. There are two main ways of delivering steroids by intravenous bolus (using methylprednisolone or dexamethasone) or by daily or alternate-day oral medication (using prednisolone or methylprednisolone). These are clearly not mutually exclusive. Conventionally, in adult practice, steroids are taken daily and doses of 1 mg/kg, with a maximum starting dose of 60 mg, of prednisolone are commonly used to induce remission. The speed of taper and decision to wean completely or not are highly variable in clinical practice. One strategy commonly used for weaning is shown in Table 29.2. Recent data from the PEXIVAS study demonstrates a benefit with regard to infection and severe adverse reactions in using a more rapid taper, with no reduction in efficacy [6]. If pulses of methylprednisolone are used, and there is an anxiety regarding steroid toxicity, then it may be possible to reduce the initial dose of oral prednisolone, to start at 30 mg/day, although there are no available trial data to support this approach at present. Pulsed methylprednisolone has been delivered at doses of 250–1000 mg/day over three consecutive days, again without ever comparing the efficacy of differing doses. It is probably reasonable to limit pulses to a total of 1.5 g of methylprednisolone, as it is generally believed that much of the early morbidity following immunosuppression induction may relate to steroid usage. Pulsed steroid use appears to negate any benefit of additional plasmapheresis (at least in the management of ANCA-associated vasculitis), although early studies suggested that plasmapheresis was associated with better early renal recovery compared with pulsed methylprednisolone, but this effect was not sustained [7]. Combining the two in severe disease appears to lead to greater complications without providing additional benefit [8].

29.2.3 Glucocorticoid Avoidance

Many groups have refined treatment protocols to minimise the dose and duration of corticosteroids. One such strategy has been the combination of low-dose intravenous cyclophosphamide, rituximab and a very short duration of corticosteroids in AAV [9] or the combination of rituximab and MMF without any oral steroids in lupus nephritis [10]. Recently, the PEXIVAS trial in AAV demonstrated a reduced total dose and more rapid taper of corticosteroids was not inferior to the 'standard' dose regimen and resulted in fewer serious infections. In addition, the development of non-glucocorticoid agents for disease induction has been piloted in AAV (see complement inhibitors below).

29

29.2.4 Infection, Bone and Gastric Prophylaxis

Prevention of steroid side effects warrants prophylactic treatment with regard to gastric, bone and fungal complications. All patients on high-dose steroids should receive gastric protection with proton pump inhibitors or H2 antagonists. Bone protection with calcium D3 combination (1 g of calcium/day) and consideration for bisphosphonate use if renal function allows and if there is any pre-existing bone mineral density loss. Fungal prophylaxis may be in the form of nystatin suspension or low-dose fluconazole (but confirm no possible drug interaction with other immunosuppressants such as calcineurin inhibitors). Pneumocystis prophylaxis, with co-trimoxazole, dapsone or nebulised pentamidine, is warranted in patients treated with cyclophosphamide or rituximab. Recent appreciation of an increased risk of reactivation of certain viruses, especially hepatitis B, has prompted recommendations for prophylaxis depending on the type and dose of immunosuppressives and appears to be most important in those patients at risk (e.g. HBV core antibody positive) treated with rituximab [11].

29.2.5 Plasmapheresis

Plasmapheresis removes a number of plasma proteins that may contribute to disease pathogenesis, including autoantibodies, immune complexes, complement components, clotting factors and microparticles derived from inflammatory or endothelial cells. There are two main ways of performing plasmapheresis, using a plasmafilter or a centrifugal bowl. The advantage of the former is that it is easily performed by most dialysis nurses, but the filter may limit removal of larger molecules such as IgM; by contrast, bowl centrifugation has the advantage of removing all plasma components, but may be limited in availability in certain units. Further modifications of these techniques exist including the double filtration plasmapheresis (DFPP) method, which returns some of the smaller plasma molecules (such as albumin) to the patient, necessitating less replacement fluid; cryofiltration which is when the plasmapheresis is performed at lower temperatures in an attempt to increase removal of immune complexes; and plasma absorption when specific affinity columns are used to allow greater removal of certain molecules such as immunoglobulin (using protein A columns).

Replacement fluid should be in the form of 4.5% albumin, unless there is a bleeding tendency, a recent invasive procedure or the procedure is aimed at replacing a missing factor, such as in atypical HUS where an abnormal complement factor may be contributing to disease. In those oligo-anuric or anuric patients, the salt load from the 4.5% albumin solution can be considerable, and increased fluid removal with subsequent dialysis may be necessary to prevent fluid overload.

The dose of plasmapheresis should be calculated based on plasma volume or body weight, and typically 1–1.5 plasma volumes are exchanged per session (generally 50–60 ml/kg). It is important to review the delivered dose that is achieved, as failure to respond may be due to inadequate plasma exchange.

Plasmapheresis has been shown to be of benefit in anti-GBM disease, when it is delivered for 14 exchanges or until the anti-GBM antibody is negative. Early trial data also suggested a benefit in patients with ANCA-associated vasculitis (AAV) and severe renal involvement (creatinine >500 μmol/L) [12, 13], although there was no long-term benefit with regard to renal failure or death [7]. However, a recently concluded trial (PEXIVAS) compared plasma exchange in patients with severe AAV and concluded the plasma exchange, in addition to pulsed methylprednisolone, did not reduce the composite endpoint of mortality or ESRD. Subgroup analysis may yet suggest benefit in patients with pulmonary haemorrhage [6].

There is no evidence for a benefit of plasmapheresis in SLE [14] or in other forms of rapidly progressive glomerulonephritis, but it is often used in such patients with renal deterioration in the hope that there may be some benefit (see RPGN below).

29.2.6 Fertility Sparing Measures and Pregnancies

Fertility impairment is related to the use of cyclophosphamide and is in part related to the age of the patient and the pre-treatment sperm viability or ovarian function. It is therefore always best to sperm bank men of child-bearing age, prior to cyclophosphamide treatment, and discuss ovarian protection or egg harvesting in women. Practically, the induction therapy for egg harvesting is not suited to acutely ill patients who may need to start cyclophosphamide therapy urgently, and so a more favoured approach is the use of gonadotropin-releasing hormone (GnRH) analogues prior to the use of cyclophosphamide treatment, which may be appropriate in female patients up to the age of 40 years [15]. The use of goserelin monthly (3.6 mg) or three monthly is generally adequate for induction of chemical menopause. There are no data, however, confirming that this approach results in a better proportion of patients with preserved fertility, but many practitioners use such an approach nonetheless. The EUROLUPUS

Table 29.3 Drug modifications in those planning pregnancy

Can be continued in pregnancy	Needs to be discontinued	Uncertain
Azathioprine Steroids Tacrolimus or ciclosporin A Hydroxychloroquine IVIG	Mycophenolate mofetil/MPA Cyclophosphamide ACE inhibitors/ARB Statins	Rituximab

low-dose intravenous cyclophosphamide regimen has been demonstrated not to impact the ovarian reserve in patients as assessed by serum levels of anti-Mullerian hormone [16].

In those planning a pregnancy, this should be ideally delayed for a period such as 6 months following the last dose of cyclophosphamide. The patient should also have had a period of disease remission for several months before planning a pregnancy. Certain maintenance immunosuppressives can be continued, while others need to be stopped or switched to more appropriate equivalents. Examples of drugs that can be or cannot be continued in pregnancy are shown in Table 29.3.

29.2.7 Rituximab and Other B Cell-Targeted Therapies

This anti-CD20 monoclonal antibody, first introduced for the treatment of lymphoma, is now extensively used in autoimmunity and in many forms of glomerular disease. It is administered as a slow intravenous infusion with steroid and antihistamine premedication (methylprednisolone 125 mg and chlorpheniramine). Infusion reactions are the most common adverse event. B cell depletion is generally achieved after one dose but may be less efficacious if significant monoclonal is lost in the urine, in nephrotic states. B cell numbers can be checked following administration. It may be administered as two infusions 2 weeks apart (each of 1 g) or as a four-dose weekly regimen of 375 mg/m^2. Both appear to be equally efficacious in glomerular disease.

Secondary hypogammaglobulinaemia may result, and the more severe this is, the more likely the patient will develop an infectious complication. IgG levels should be monitored in case levels are low and replacement immunoglobulin may be required. Rituximab has also been demonstrated to be effective as maintenance treatment in AAV with higher rates of remission compared to azathioprine [17]. The fully humanised anti-CD20 monoclonal antibody ofatumumab and obinutuzmab have been used successfully in patients with lupus nephritis and AAV in patients unresponsive or intolerant due to infusion reactions to rituximab.

Belimumab, a monoclonal antibody directed against the B cell-activating factor (BAFF or BLyS), has recently obtained both FDA and NICE approval as an add-on treatment in patients with SLE; however, it is not indicated in patients with severe lupus nephritis. Current trials are either ongoing to investigate the use of a combination of belimumab with rituximab in both lupus nephritis and AAV, as BAFF levels increase following rituximab therapy and may predispose to disease relapse when B cell repopulation occurs.

29.2.8 MMF and Azathioprine

MMF is extensively used as induction therapy in SLE and has been shown to be of equal efficacy in inducing remission in lupus nephritis as cyclophosphamide – with better tolerability in certain ethnic groups (such as African-Americans and Hispanics). Some centres advocate therapeutic drug monitoring, although many trials treated to a particular dose. Starting at a lower dose and increasing rapidly may allow for fewer gastrointestinal side effects.

Azathioprine requires no such dose adjustments, but thiopurine methyltransferase (TPMT) levels may be checked prior to commencing therapy as this can allow dose adjustment in patients likely to suffer bone marrow toxicity, with low TPMT activity. Care should be taken if patients are on allopurinol as this increases azathioprine toxicity. Monitoring of liver function tests and a full blood count regularly will help prevent hepatitis and leucopenia. Azathioprine is infrequently used for induction therapy, but rather as a common maintenance agent. It is more effective than MMF in vasculitis maintenance, with significantly longer time of relapse-free remission in patients treated with azathioprine compared to MMF.

29.2.9 Complement Antagonism

Animal models and clinical data have implicated complement in various glomerular diseases, including pauci-immune small vessel vasculitis. Avacopan is an oral selective C5a receptor inhibitor and has recently been trialled in the treatment of AAV demonstrating non-inferiority to corticosteroids when used with a cyclophosphamide- or rituximab-based induction regimen [18, 19].

29.3 Protocols for Particular Glomerular Diseases

29.3.1 Rapidly Progressive Glomerulonephritis

Rapidly progressive glomerulonephritis (RPGN) is defined as sudden loss of renal function, with halving of GFR within 3 months. Prompt diagnosis and treatment is crucial to prevent irreversible loss of renal function. Histologically, RPGN is caused by a crescentic glomerulonephritis, which is due to severe glomerular injury, as a result of rupture of the glomerular capillary loop basement membrane. Crescentic glomerulonephritis is generally defined as having more than 50% of glomeruli involved with crescents, which are identified by the presence of at least two layers of cells in Bowman's space.

RPGN can be commonly categorised into being caused by:

- Anti-glomerular basement membrane (GBM) disease
- Immune complex glomerulonephritis
- Pauci-immune glomerulonephritis, associated with ANCA in most cases

The standard of care has long been steroids and cyclophosphamide, with trials in pauci-immune GN demonstrating that newer regimens using lower doses of cyclophosphamide delivered as intravenous pulses provide equal efficacy and fewer adverse events such as leucopenia. New trials in AAV have demonstrated that induction therapy with rituximab is as effective as cyclophosphamide [20, 21], while studies in SLE have failed to demonstrate benefit of additional RTX therapy above standard treatment [22, 23]. Since there have been few randomised studies of the treatment of other causes of RPGN, we are left to extrapolate protocols from these studies.

29.3.1.1 Anti-GBM Disease

Treatment should be initiated immediately in those in whom it is appropriate. Recommendations are to initiate daily plasma exchange for a total of 14 sessions or until the anti-GBM antibody has disappeared. Plasma exchange should be against human albumin solution, unless there has been a recent renal biopsy or active bleeding, and then it should be replaced in part (300–600 ml) with fresh frozen plasma (FFP) [24]. Long-term immunosuppression is not required due to the monophasic nature of the disease, with cyclophosphamide treatment recommended for 2–3 months and steroid for no more than 6–9 months (see ◘ Table 29.4).

29.3.1.2 Immune Complex Glomerulonephritis

This describes the formation of immune deposits, which contain immunoglobulins, complement and other proteins within the glomerulus resulting in glomerular injury. There are several underlying causes of a RPGN with immune complex deposition histologically.

IgA Nephropathy (IgAN) and IgA Vasculitis (IgAV or Henoch-Schönlein Purpura)

While there are data demonstrating the efficacy of immunosuppression with steroids in patients with IgAN with moderate proteinuria (1–3.5 g/day) and mild renal

◘ **Table 29.4** Treatment regimen for anti-GBM disease [24]

Drug/treatment	Dose	Duration
Corticosteroids	1 mg/kg/day (max 60 mg/day)	6–9 months
Cyclophosphamide	Oral: 2–3 mg/kg Dose reduction in >55 years	2–3 months
Plasma exchange	Human albumin solution; 50 ml/kg max 4 L	At least 14 days or till anti-GBM antibody normalised
Prophylaxis	Nystatin or fluconazole Calcium D3 PPI or H2 antagonist Septrin 480 mg daily or 960 mg three times a week	For duration of high-dose steroids For duration of cyclophosphamide

impairment (serum creatinine ≤1.5 mg/dl) [25], evidence is lacking for the treatment of a crescentic IgAN. A rapidly progressive course with crescents has been treated with a regimen based on that for systemic vasculitis using combination steroids and cyclophosphamide. A small study of 12 patients with a crescentic, progressive disease treated with pulsed steroids and monthly cyclophosphamide resulted in a reduction in proliferative lesions and proteinuria and stabilisation in renal function [26]. In some young patients with crescentic IgA or IgAV and a rapid renal decline, plasmapheresis has also been used with variable results. Recent data has suggested no benefit of rituximab in IgA disease [27] but a steroid sparing capacity in patients with IgAV [28].

Lupus Nephritis

Renal involvement frequently occurs in SLE, with proliferative lesions (classes III and IV) having a poorer outcome than mesangial lesions (class II). The treatment regimen can be considered in two parts: induction therapy and maintenance. However, there are limited published data on treating crescentic lupus nephritis or SLE causing a RPGN.

The old NIH high-dose pulsed cyclophosphamide (CYP) regimen [29] has for the most part been abandoned, and there are now two significant protocols to consider. The first is the EUROLUPUS protocol [30]. The EUROLUPUS trial consisted of predominantly Caucasian patients with proliferative lupus nephritis, including those patients with glomerular crescents, and compared low-dose CYP with standard high-dose (NIH) CYP. This trial provided evidence for a short, low-dose course of intravenous cyclophosphamide (500 mg every 2 weeks for 3 months) followed by azathioprine (2–2.5 mg/kg/day) which was initiated 2 weeks after the last dose of CYP, as well as corticosteroids [30]. The dose of steroids was initially started at 1 mg/kg/day, with a gradual taper down to 5–7.5 mg after approximately 6 months of therapy.

The second is based on the use of mycophenolate mofetil (MMF) at a target dose of 3 g/day [31], in conjunction with prednisolone starting at 60 mg/day. Although a recent multi-centre trial failed to demonstrate MMF *superiority* over intravenous cyclophosphamide (0.5–1 g/m^2 6 monthly pulses), the two drugs induced similar rates of remission and MMF treatment was associated with significantly fewer serious adverse events. In addition, differences in response to these immunosuppressants were found in different ethnic groups, with MMF proving more effective than cyclophosphamide in Black and Hispanic patients [31].

After the completion of induction therapy, patients are prescribed maintenance treatment to aim to reduce the risk of flares. This treatment should be continued for some time although exactly how long is debated. Similar to the induction treatment trials, there seems to be an ethnic variation in the response to treatment. In a predominantly Caucasian cohort, MMF (2 g/day) was not superior to azathioprine (2 mg/kg per day) with respect to renal flares, doubling of creatinine or infectious complications [32]. However, in the ALMS study, which included more of the high-risk Black patients, MMF was superior to azathioprine at maintaining disease remission [33].

Various uncontrolled studies have demonstrated promising results with rituximab for patients with lupus nephritis [34] including those with refractory/relapsing disease [35]. However, a large multi-centre, randomised trial (LUNAR) investigating the use of rituximab alongside steroids and MMF in proliferative lupus nephritis failed to demonstrate additional impact of rituximab [23]. Currently, rituximab may be considered an option for those with refractory, relapsing disease or intolerant of first-line therapies. However, an anti-BLyS (B-lymphocyte stimulator) monoclonal antibody, belimumab, has been shown to be effective in a recent SLE trial demonstrating improvements in a number of disease domains and has recently been licensed for the treatment of SLE [36]. The treatment options are summarised in ◘ Table 29.5.

Post-Infectious Glomerulonephritis (PIGN)

Infections can result in glomerulonephritis, with a variety of different histological manifestations. Bacteria such as *Staphylococcus aureus* and Streptococci as well as infective endocarditis are well recognised as underlying causes of an infection-related glomerulonephritis, which may manifest as a RPGN with crescentic or vasculitic lesions seen on renal biopsy. The association between staphylococcal infections and IgA nephropathy is now well established. Antibiotic therapy is clearly crucial in these infectious diseases, while there may be a role for corticosteroids under certain circumstances. However, overall, no correlation between steroid use and renal outcome has been demonstrated [37], so this issue remains controversial.

29.3.1.3 Pauci-Immune Glomerulonephritis

This describes the appearance on renal biopsy in which there is little or no glomerular staining of immunoglobulins, which most commonly is associated with anti-neutrophil cytoplasm antibody (ANCA), and represents the most likely cause of a RPGN in adults [38]. Like the treatment of SLE, the treatment of AAV consists of induction and maintenance. Renal function and age are important predictors of outcome. Cyclophosphamide

Table 29.5 Treatment in lupus nephritis (class III, IV)

Drug	Dose	Investigations	Caution
MMF	Titrate aiming to 3 g/day (induction) 2 g/day (maintenance)	WCC: stop if neutropenic	Teratogenic
Cyclophosphamide EUROLUPUS: outpatient infusions	500 mg IV every 2 weeks for 3 months	WCC: 10–14 days after last dose; hold dose if WCC <4	Mesna optional, dose 20% of CYP dose Ovarian protection with GnRHa may be beneficial
Corticosteroids	60 mg/day: taper decreasing to ≤10 mg by 24 weeks		Gastric protection Bone protection
Azathioprine	2 mg/kg	TPMT activity: low levels will require decreasing the dose FBC, LFTs: monitor after initiation of therapy	Can replace MMF as maintenance therapy if pregnancy being considered
Consider:			
Rituximab	1 g days 1 and 15	Peripheral B count (CD19) to assess depletion	Prevention of infusion reaction give methylprednisolone 125 mg
Belimumab	Days 0, 14, 28, then every 28 days		

has been part of the gold standard induction agent for many years, although its use at high doses for prolonged periods resulted in significant adverse effects. Treatment regimens have been refined over the years to reduce the total cumulative dose of cyclophosphamide. Numerous EUVAS (European Vasculitis Study Group) trials have investigated optimal regimens for different disease states. The CYCLOPS trial included patients with a serum creatinine <500 μmol/L and demonstrated that the combination of pulsed intravenous cyclophosphamide and oral steroids was as effective at inducing disease remission as an oral cyclophosphamide regimen but induced fewer episodes of leucopenia [2], although long-term follow-up has shown that this intravenous regimen is associated with increased relapses [3]. Table 29.1 demonstrates the intravenous dosing regimen used in this study.

The MEPEX study investigated patients with more advanced renal failure (serum creatinine >500 μmol/L) and demonstrated the benefits of plasma exchange, alongside oral cyclophosphamide and corticosteroids in renal recovery at 3 months and 1 year [12]. However, long-term follow-up of this study cohort suggested no benefit at 5 years with regard to a combined endpoint of ESRD or death. This was confirmed in the randomised PEXIVAS trial, demonstrating that in patients treated with pulsed corticosteroids and cyclophosphamide or rituximab, plasmapheresis provided no benefit using the same endpoint. However, subgroup- and meta-analysis have suggested a possible benefit in those patients with pulmonary haemorrhage or advanced renal failure [39].

There is now an increasing use of intravenous cyclophosphamide in this group of patients with severe renal failure to reduce the incidence of leucopenia, with patients receiving 6–10 pulses of cyclophosphamide. The dose of steroids is usually started at 1 mg/kg, with tapering to a dose of 10–15 mg/day by 3 months and 5 mg by 1 year. Maintenance therapy consists of long-term immunosuppression following the period of induction therapy. The CYCAZAREM trial demonstrated that cyclophosphamide at 3–6 months could be safely substituted for azathioprine (2 mg/kg/day) [40], while a study demonstrated that MMF is not as effective as azathioprine in maintenance therapy [41], and so should be reserved for patients who cannot tolerate azathioprine.

There is an increasing use of rituximab in patients with AAV, with two randomised trials providing evidence that its use as induction therapy is equivalent to that of cyclophosphamide [20, 21]. The RAVE trial compared oral cyclophosphamide with rituximab, excluding those with severe renal failure (creatinine >4 mg/dl), although patients with less severe renal disease were included [20] and demonstrated equivalence of RTX and CYP but superiority of RTX for those with relapsing disease. RITUXVAS

Table 29.6 Induction and maintenance doses of immunosuppressive agents in ANCA-associated vasculitis

Therapy	Dose	Specific investigations that modify dose/therapy
Cyclophosphamide	MEPEX oral: 2–3 mg/kg Age >60 years 2 mg/kg	WCC: <4 withhold drug WCC: 4–5 reduce dose Prophylaxis as for anti-GBM disease
Rituximab	Either 375 mg/m^2 × 1/week for 4 weeks Or 1 g at day 1 and day 15	May monitor CD19 count: adequate peripheral blood depletion <0.005 × 10^9 WCC: neutropenia reported following chronic use Monitor immunoglobulins; hypogammaglobulinaemia common
Azathioprine	1–2 mg/kg	TPMT activity: Low levels require decreasing the dose to 1 mg/kg FBC, LFTs: monitor after initiation of therapy
Mycophenolate Mofetil	2 g/day	WCC: stop if neutropenic Reduce dose WCC <4
Methotrexate	0.03 mg/kg/week Starting at 10–15 mg/week	Check LFT, WCC alt weeks to begin with Annual CXR Procollagen III may be helpful in monitoring for liver damage Add folic acid 5 mg weekly taken 2 days after MTX

included those with severe (dialysis-dependent) renal involvement and demonstrated the rituximab regimen not to be inferior [21]. Both the 375 mg/m^2 × 1/week for 4 weeks (regimen in RAVE and RITUXIVAS) and 1 g repeated after 2 weeks appeared equally effective. With regard to maintenance therapy, the MAINRITSAN trial included patients with AAV who entered remission following induction therapy with cyclophosphamide and compared rituximab (500 mg days 0 and 14, followed by months 6, 12 and 18) with azathioprine for maintenance. This trial demonstrated higher rates of sustained remission with rituximab [17]. The RITAZAREM trial compared repeated doses of rituximab to azathioprine in relapsing disease in patients who have undergone induction therapy with rituximab, and showed reduced relapse rates in rituximab treated patients [42].

Case Study

Case 1

A 72-year-old man presented with haemoptysis and is found to have a significant AKI (creatinine 350 μmol/L with blood and protein on urine dipstick). An acute screen demonstrated a high titre of PR3-ANCA, and treatment was started with steroids and cyclophosphamide. Following discharge, the patient completed 6 cycles of intravenous cyclophosphamide as an outpatient. He was then readmitted with shortness of breath, cough and fever. Antibiotics were commenced without much of an improvement, and a CT scan demonstrated bilateral lung infiltrates with ground glass changes. Antibiotic treatment was broadened to include cover for *Pneumocystis jiroveci* (PJP). A bronchoscopy was performed which confirmed the diagnosis.

Case 2

A 47-year-old woman presented with dialysis-dependent AKI, positive MPO-ANCA and a renal biopsy consistent with AAV. Treatment with plasma exchange, haemodialysis, steroids and cyclophosphamide was initiated, and she remained dialysis dependent. Due to missing outpatient appointments, her steroids were not tapered according to schedule. Shortly after presentation, she developed a fever, raised inflammatory response and diarrhoea. Further investigations demonstrated very high levels of CMV DNA by PCR. Treatment was initiated with valganciclovir with regular monitoring of CMV during close follow-up. As there had been no renal recovery, immunosuppression was decreased with the cessation of cyclophosphamide therapy.

Case 3

A 32-year-old female patient with known SLE and class IV lupus nephritis had received several courses of rituximab therapy to treat her renal disease. Her blood tests demonstrated persistent low levels of IgG (<3) with a history of persistent chest infections. In view of the persistent low IgG and recurrent infections, regular treatment with IVIG was initiated. This then allowed further treatment of rituximab during lupus flares.

29

Table 29.6 shows the treatment options in AAV.

Tips and Tricks

1. Consider rituximab induction therapy as an alternative to cyclophosphamide therapy, especially in those patients with relapsing PR3-ANCA vasculitis.
2. In AAV patients treated with rituximab induction, those who remain B cell depleted and ANCA negative are at low risk of relapse.
3. Check hepatitis serology prior to starting immunosuppression and consider lamivudine prophylaxis in those patients who are hepatitis B core antibody positive with regular monitoring of hepatitis B surface antigen. Additionally, a patient's Varicella Zoster virus (VZV) status is important, as if naïve and exposed, to VZV the immunocompromised state may result in life-threatening infection. VZV immunoglobulin can be administered in VZV-naïve patients on immunosuppression.
4. PJP prophylaxis should be used for 3–6 months following rituximab and for the duration of cyclophosphamide therapy.
5. In patients requiring cyclophosphamide, the low-dose EUROLUPUS regimen is effective and exposes patients to low overall doses of the drug, and therefore, this can be extended or repeated if needed. Generally, we try and minimise total cyclophosphamide dosage, and it is good to keep a running total of overall dose exposure so as to prevent excessive doses. Doses of 10–20 g may be necessary for severe relapsing patients.

Chapter Review Questions

1. Can tacrolimus be added to steroids and MMF in the treatment of lupus nephritis?
2. A patient with newly diagnosed SLE, blood and protein in the urine is pregnant. Should you perform a kidney biopsy, and what treatments could she have?
3. A newly diagnosed young female AAV patient has an IgG level of 6.5 g/l (NR 7–16). Can you treat her with rituximab induction, or should she have cyclophosphamide?

Answers

1. Yes, in cases of class V or III/IV + V lupus nephritis, tacrolimus can be added to patients with a significant nephrotic syndrome. Generally, tacrolimus therapy is then subsequently weaned and stopped after 12–24 months of treatment to avoid long-term exposure to calcineurin inhibition therapy.
2. Kidney biopsies can be performed safely in pregnant women early in the pregnancy if clinically indicated and are associated with change in management in up to 45% of patients. In the case of a newly diagnosed lupus patient with possible nephritis, the severity of the kidney disease would be helpful to counsel her with regard to renal outcomes, need for medication and pregnancy progress and outcomes. She could be treated with azathioprine, tacrolimus (especially if significantly proteinuric), corticosteroids and hydroxychloroquine.
3. Yes, she can have rituximab. Approximately 20% of patients with AAV have some degree of hypogammaglobulinaemia at presentation. This does increase with regular rituximab therapy, but if she has not suffered infections, she can be induced with rituximab and only considered for prophylactic antibiotics or IVIG replacement if she develops recurrent infectious illnesses with worsening hypogammaglobulinaemia. Some clinical immunology services will test response to vaccines to decide if IVIG replacement is necessary.

Appendix: Information for Renal Patients Receiving Cyclophosphamide Therapy

This information sheet describes cyclophosphamide, how it is administered and some of the side effects it may cause. Please ask a member of staff if you want information about other alternatives to treatment with cyclophosphamide or if you have any other questions.

How Is It Given?

Cyclophosphamide can be given by injection into a vein (intravenously) or as a tablet. Your doctor will agree with you as to which the best route is for you to receive the drug.

Tablets may have to be taken for a number of months; the intravenous infusion is generally given every 2–4 weeks. The length of the treatment will depend on your condition and response to treatment, but it generally lasts 3–4 months.

If you are receiving the intravenous infusion, you will attend the renal day ward. You will need to stay for up to 2 hours, although generally it takes less time.

How Does Cyclophosphamide Work?

Cyclophosphamide works by depressing ('damping down') your immune system. The aim of the treatment is to reduce the inflammation that is causing the problem with your affected organs such as kidneys, lungs or nose.

What Are the Possible Side Effects?

Nausea and vomiting may occur if you take cyclophosphamide. This can be controlled by giving you anti-sickness (anti-emetic) tablets as needed.

Increased risk of infection is a result of the suppression of white blood cell production in your bone marrow. White blood cells help to fight infection. Your levels of white blood cells will be monitored. If you develop a temperature, fever or any signs of infection, please contact either the ward or your GP. You should also report any bruising/bleeding or excessive tiredness. You will be given an antibiotic tablet (or nebuliser if you cannot tolerate the tablets) to stop certain infections, but this will not prevent *all* infections.

Bladder irritation is a possible side effect if you are receiving intravenous cyclophosphamide. Symptoms include blood in the urine and symptoms of cystitis. You may be given a drug called mesna during the intravenous infusion that will help to prevent this occurring. If you notice any blood in your urine after discharge home, please contact the ward.

Hair thinning may occur. This is not permanent and will grow back after treatment.

Mouth sores may develop if you are taking the tablets and you will be given a supply of mouth lozenges to help prevent this. Good oral and dental hygiene is important.

Contraception and fertility should be discussed with your doctor or nurse as cyclophosphamide may affect your ability to conceive or father a child. With a standard treatment course, the risk of this happening is relatively small. Women may find their periods altered and men may wish to discuss sperm banking.

Cyclophosphamide and Pregnancy

Cyclophosphamide may cause several different birth defects if it is taken either at the time of conception or during pregnancy. Be sure that you practice effective birth control with a barrier method of contraception while you are being treated with cyclophosphamide. Tell your doctor right away if you think you have become pregnant while taking cyclophosphamide.

If you become unwell while being treated with cyclophosphamide

If you become unwell or develop a temperature above 37.5 °C, you must let your doctors know. Please contact your clinic consultant (through switchboard), or the renal day ward during working hours, or the on-call renal registrar out of hours, who can be reached through switchboard.

If you require any further information or advice, please ask either your doctor or nurse.

Contact Details

Call main switchboard........................

Renal pharmacy...............................

Vasculitis/lupus clinic ....

If you would like a large print or audio version of this information, please ask a member of staff.

References

1. Faurschou M, Sorensen IJ, Mellemkjaer L, et al. Malignancies in Wegener's granulomatosis: incidence and relation to cyclophosphamide therapy in a cohort of 293 patients. J Rheumatol. 2008;35(1):100–5.
2. de Groot K, Harper L, Jayne DR, et al. Pulse versus daily oral cyclophosphamide for induction of remission in antineutrophil cytoplasmic antibody-associated vasculitis: a randomized trial. Ann Intern Med. 2009;150(10):670–80.
3. Harper L, Morgan MD, Walsh M, et al. Pulse versus daily oral cyclophosphamide for induction of remission in ANCA-associated vasculitis: long-term follow-up. Ann Rheum Dis. 2012;71(6):955–60.
4. Pepper R, Chanouzas D, Tarzi R, et al. Intravenous cyclophosphamide and plasmapheresis in dialysis dependent ANCA associated vasculitis. J Am Soc Nephrol. 2011;22:560A.
5. Monach PA, Arnold LM, Merkel PA. Incidence and prevention of bladder toxicity from cyclophosphamide in the treatment of rheumatic diseases: a data-driven review. Arthritis Rheum. 2010;62(1):9–21.
6. Walsh M, Merkel PA, Peh CA, et al. Plasma exchange and glucocorticoids in severe ANCA-associated vasculitis. N Engl J Med. 2020;382(7):622–31.
7. Walsh M, Casian A, Flossmann O, et al. Long-term follow-up of patients with severe ANCA-associated vasculitis comparing plasma exchange to intravenous methylprednisolone treatment is unclear. Kidney Int. 2013;84(2):397–402.
8. Chanouzas D, McGregor JAG, Nightingale P, et al. Intravenous pulse methylprednisolone for induction of remission in severe ANCA associated Vasculitis: a multi-center retrospective cohort study. BMC Nephrol. 2019;20(1):58.
9. Pepper RJ, McAdoo SP, Moran SM, et al. A novel glucocorticoid-free maintenance regimen for anti-neutrophil cytoplasm antibody-associated vasculitis. Rheumatology (Oxford). 2019;58:260–8.
10. Oon S, Huq M, Godfrey T, Nikpour M. Systematic review, and meta-analysis of steroid-sparing effect, of biologic agents in randomized, placebo-controlled phase 3 trials for systemic lupus erythematosus. Semin Arthritis Rheum. 2018;48:221–39.
11. Reddy KR, Beavers KL, Hammond SP, Lim JK, Falck-Ytter YT, American Gastroenterological Association I. American Gastroenterological Association Institute guideline on the prevention and treatment of hepatitis B virus reactivation during

29

immunosuppressive drug therapy. Gastroenterology. 2015;148(1):215–9; quiz e16–7.
12. Jayne DR, Gaskin G, Rasmussen N, et al. Randomized trial of plasma exchange or high-dosage methylprednisolone as adjunctive therapy for severe renal vasculitis. J Am Soc Nephrol. 2007;18(7):2180–8.
13. Johnson JP, Moore J Jr., Austin HA 3rd, Balow JE, Antonovych TT, Wilson CB. Therapy of anti-glomerular basement membrane antibody disease: analysis of prognostic significance of clinical, pathologic and treatment factors. Medicine (Baltimore). 1985;64(4):219–27.
14. Lewis EJ, Hunsicker LG, Lan SP, Rohde RD, Lachin JM. A controlled trial of plasmapheresis therapy in severe lupus nephritis. The Lupus Nephritis Collaborative Study Group. N Engl J Med. 1992;326(21):1373–9.
15. Henes M, Henes JC, Neunhoeffer E, et al. Fertility preservation methods in young women with systemic lupus erythematosus prior to cytotoxic therapy – experiences from the FertiProtekt network. Lupus 2012;21(9):953–8.
16. Tamirou F, Husson SN, Gruson D, Debieve F, Lauwerys BR, Houssiau FA. Brief report: the euro-lupus low-dose intravenous cyclophosphamide regimen does not impact the ovarian reserve, as measured by serum levels of anti-Mullerian hormone. Arthritis Rheumatol. 2017;69(6):1267–71.
17. Guillevin L, Pagnoux C, Karras A, et al. Rituximab versus azathioprine for maintenance in ANCA-associated vasculitis. N Engl J Med. 2014;371(19):1771–80.
18. Jayne DRW, Bruchfeld AN, Harper L, et al. Randomized trial of C5a receptor inhibitor avacopan in ANCA-associated vasculitis. J Am Soc Nephrol. 2017;28(9):2756–67.
19. Jayne DRW, Merkel PA, Schall TJ, Bekker P. For the ADVOCATE Study Group* Avacopan for the Treatment of ANCA-Associated Vasculitis. N Engl J Med. 2021;384:599–609.
20. Stone JH, Merkel PA, Spiera R, et al. Rituximab versus cyclophosphamide for ANCA-associated vasculitis. N Engl J Med. 2010;363(3):221–32.
21. Jones RB, Tervaert JW, Hauser T, et al. Rituximab versus cyclophosphamide in ANCA-associated renal vasculitis. N Engl J Med. 2010;363(3):211–20.
22. Merrill JT, Neuwelt CM, Wallace DJ, et al. Efficacy and safety of rituximab in moderately-to-severely active systemic lupus erythematosus: the randomized, double-blind, phase II/III systemic lupus erythematosus evaluation of rituximab trial. Arthritis Rheum. 2010;62(1):222–33.
23. Rovin BH, Furie R, Latinis K, et al. Efficacy and safety of rituximab in patients with active proliferative lupus nephritis: the lupus nephritis assessment with rituximab study. Arthritis Rheum. 2012;64(4):1215–26.
24. Levy JB, Turner AN, Rees AJ, Pusey CD. Long-term outcome of anti-glomerular basement membrane antibody disease treated with plasma exchange and immunosuppression. Ann Intern Med. 2001;134(11):1033–42.
25. Pozzi C, Andrulli S, Del Vecchio L, et al. Corticosteroid effectiveness in IgA nephropathy: long-term results of a randomized, controlled trial. J Am Soc Nephrol. 2004;15(1):157–63.
26. Tumlin JA, Lohavichan V, Hennigar R. Crescentic, proliferative IgA nephropathy: clinical and histological response to methylprednisolone and intravenous cyclophosphamide. Nephrol Dial Transplant. 2003;18(7):1321–9.
27. Lafayette RA, Canetta PA, Rovin BH, et al. A randomized, controlled trial of rituximab in IgA nephropathy with proteinuria and renal dysfunction. J Am Soc Nephrol. 2017;28(4):1306–13.
28. Lundberg S, Westergren E, Smolander J, Bruchfeld A. B cell-depleting therapy with rituximab or ofatumumab in immunoglobulin A nephropathy or vasculitis with nephritis. Clin Kidney J. 2017;10(1):20–6.
29. Austin HA 3rd, Klippel JH, Balow JE, et al. Therapy of lupus nephritis. Controlled trial of prednisone and cytotoxic drugs. N Engl J Med. 1986;314(10):614–9.
30. Houssiau FA, Vasconcelos C, D'Cruz D, et al. Immunosuppressive therapy in lupus nephritis: the Euro-Lupus Nephritis Trial, a randomized trial of low-dose versus high-dose intravenous cyclophosphamide. Arthritis Rheum. 2002;46(8):2121–31.
31. Appel GB, Contreras G, Dooley MA, et al. Mycophenolate mofetil versus cyclophosphamide for induction treatment of lupus nephritis. J Am Soc Nephrol. 2009;20(5):1103–12.
32. Houssiau FA, D'Cruz D, Sangle S, et al. Azathioprine versus mycophenolate mofetil for long-term immunosuppression in lupus nephritis: results from the MAINTAIN Nephritis Trial. Ann Rheum Dis. 2010;69(12):2083–9.
33. Dooley MA, Jayne D, Ginzler EM, et al. Mycophenolate versus azathioprine as maintenance therapy for lupus nephritis. N Engl J Med. 2011;365(20):1886–95.
34. Pepper R, Griffith M, Kirwan C, et al. Rituximab is an effective treatment for lupus nephritis and allows a reduction in maintenance steroids. Nephrol Dial Transplant. 2009;24(12):3717–23.
35. Melander C, Sallee M, Trolliet P, et al. Rituximab in severe lupus nephritis: early B-cell depletion affects long-term renal outcome. Clin J Am Soc Nephrol. 2009;4(3):579–87.
36. Manzi S, Sanchez-Guerrero J, Merrill JT, et al. Effects of belimumab, a B lymphocyte stimulator-specific inhibitor, on disease activity across multiple organ domains in patients with systemic lupus erythematosus: combined results from two phase III trials. Ann Rheum Dis. 2012;71(11):1833–8.
37. Nasr SH, Markowitz GS, Stokes MB, Said SM, Valeri AM, D'Agati VD. Acute postinfectious glomerulonephritis in the modern era: experience with 86 adults and review of the literature. Medicine (Baltimore). 2008;87(1):21–32.
38. Jennette JC. Rapidly progressive crescentic glomerulonephritis. Kidney Int. 2003;63(3):1164–77.
39. Walsh personal communication, Prendecki M, McAdoo SP, Pusey CD. Is there a role for plasma exchange in anca-associated vasculitis? Current treatment options in rheumatology. 2020;6:313–24.
40. Jayne D, Rasmussen N, Andrassy K, et al. A randomized trial of maintenance therapy for vasculitis associated with antineutrophil cytoplasmic autoantibodies. N Engl J Med. 2003;349(1):36–44.
41. Hiemstra TF, Walsh M, Mahr A, et al. Mycophenolate mofetil vs azathioprine for remission maintenance in antineutrophil cytoplasmic antibody-associated vasculitis: a randomized controlled trial. JAMA. 2010;304(21):2381–8.
42. Smith R, Jayne D, Merkel PA. OP0026 A randomized, controlled trial of rituximab versus azathioprine after induction of remission with rituximab for patients with anca-associated vasculitis and relapsing disease. Oral PresentationsVasculitis. 79(1): http://doi.org/10.1136/annrheumdis-2020-eular.2717.

Infections and the Kidney

Elizabeth Williams, Padmasayee Papineni, Sanjay Bhagani, and Mark Harber

Contents

M. Harber (ed.), *Primer on Nephrology*, https://doi.org/10.1007/978-3-030-76419-7_30

30

Learning Objectives

1. Infectious causes of renal disease are common, and the growing global population with CKD is more at risk of AKI in the setting of sepsis; prevention and rapid diagnosis of sepsis in renal patients are vital.
2. A good travel history including activities, occupation and what area (urban or rural) is very important for differential diagnosis in undiagnosed renal disease.
3. Infections can cause renal disease via a variety of mechanisms including pre-renal, post-renal, direct renal involvement, as a consequence of persistent infection or a post-infectious phenomenon. Periodically, kidney dysfunction will be the diagnostic clue leading to the diagnosis of persistent infection elsewhere in the body.
4. Some persistent infections may mimic autoimmune disease and neoplastic disease and are an important consideration in the differential diagnosis.

30.1 Introduction

Infections are an important cause of renal dysfunction and can cause this through a variety of mechanisms (see ◘ Table 30.1). Most commonly, this is in the form of acute kidney injury (AKI) as collateral damage in (1) acute severe sepsis but also may occur due to (2a) direct infection of the renal parenchyma (see also ▶ Chap. 54) or (2b) obstruction secondary to involvement of the urinary tract. Renal impairment may result as a secondary phenomenon which can either be (3a) post-infectious (classically post-streptococcal glomerulonephritis (GN)) or as a result of (3b) persistent infection such as endocarditis or chronic viral infections (hepatitis B, hepatitis C and HIV are discussed separately in the following chapter). There is often a significant degree of overlap in these processes; for instance, while the vast majority of AKI secondary to Covid-19 infection is secondary to indirect injury resulting in acute tubular injury, the virus does demonstrate renal tropism, and renal invasion seems to be associated with proximal tubular injury, and possibly other glomerular lesions can co-exist.

By identifying the infective agent and its persistence is important for treatment and prognosis. The secondary effects of infection – resulting in glomerulonephritis, interstitial nephritis or obstruction – are responsible for a large burden of renal disease worldwide.

With increasing globalisation and travel, the epidemiology of infection-related renal disease is changing; in this chapter, we focus on those significant diseases found globally that may present to renal physicians. However, it should not be forgotten that renal patients will be more prone to some infections (particularly nosocomial) and more vulnerable to complications of non-specific sepsis, such as AKI.

◘ Table 30.1 Mechanisms of renal impairment secondary to infection

1. AKI secondary to indirect consequence of acute sepsis	Usually bacterial but can occur as a consequence of severe viral infection, e.g. SARS-CoV-2 (Covid-19) infection, viral haemorrhagic fevers, fungaemia or protozoal infection, e.g. falciparum malaria. Associated with exotoxins and endotoxins (such as myoglobin or haemoglobinuria)
2a. Direct infection of the kidney	Usually acute or chronic bacterial pyelonephritis but particularly in the immunocompromised can be viral, fungal or mycobacterial, typically causing interstitial nephritis
2b. Direct infection of the urinary tract	Obstruction secondary to schistosomiasis or tuberculosis
3a. Indirect effects of infection – post-infectious	Usually immune complex mediated following successful immune response, classically post-streptococcal glomerulonephritis but may also cause interstitial nephritis and haemolytic uraemic syndrome (HUS) (*E. coli* O157:H7). Typically with spontaneous resolution but may provoke autoimmune disease (e.g. vasculitis) secondary to molecular mimicry
3b. Indirect effects of infection – persistent infection	Usually immune complex mediated from persistent chronic antigen exposure and resulting in glomerulonephritis classically secondary to sub-acute bacterial (or fungal) infection such as endocarditis, shunt nephritis, osteomyelitis but also secondary to chronic viral infections such as hepatitis B, hepatitis C and HIV. Spontaneous resolution does not occur until underlying pathogen is eradicated. Long-term infection may also result in AA amyloid, immunotactoid, cryoglobulinaemia and fibrillary involvement

A detailed assessment is important in cases of AKI related to infection (see ▶ Box 30.1). Key points in the assessment include travel history, recent unwell contacts, specific activities (e.g. water sports, hiking/camping, caving, visits to farms), sexual history and drug history including, if any, prophylactic medication taken, e.g. antimalarials or antibiotics. Significant examination findings include bite marks, rashes, hepatosplenomegaly and lymphadenopathy. As discussed below, it is important to have a high index of suspicion and where possible distinguish between post-infectious and ongoing infection as the management is different.

Box 30.1 Key Features in History and Examination in a Patient Suspected of Infection-Related Renal Disease

History

- *Details of travel*: particularly in the previous 12 months, but also country of origin/birth (e.g. schistosomiasis may be asymptomatic). Particular attention should be paid to the following:
  - Pre-travel vaccinations and malaria prophylaxis
  - Rural vs. urban
  - Unwell contacts
  - Time period between return and onset of symptoms
  - Accommodation and food/drink exposures
  - Freshwater swimming and other activities
  - Animal contacts or tick bites
- *Details of domestic activities*:
- Unwell contacts
- Occupation and hobbies – e.g. water sports or agricultural employment
- Recent dental work, surgical procedures
- Tick, animal, bird or bat bites and scratches
- Domestic pets
- Sexual history

Symptoms

- Fevers and rigors (pattern of fever not particularly helpful)
- Night sweats
- Skin rashes
- Arthralgia, myalgia or arthritis
- Mouth ulcers, pharyngitis, cough
- Headaches, especially if associated with fevers and/or accompanied by focal neurological symptoms, meningeal irritation symptoms
- Diarrhoea
- Urinary symptoms suggestive of infection – dysuria, frequency, haematuria, abdominal or flank pain
- Urethral discharge and/or perineal ulcers
- Acute respiratory infection

Signs and examination findings

- Systemic inflammatory response syndrome (SIRS)
- Peripheral stigmata of infective endocarditis
- Skin rash or changes (e.g. purpuric rash or mottled skin changes of severe sepsis)
- Choroidoretinitis
- Oropharyngeal ulcers or candidiasis
- Palpable lymphadenopathy
- New cardiac murmurs
- Hepatosplenomegaly
- Acute arthritis, especially mono-arthritis involving large joints
- Meningism, focal neurological deficits, abrupt change in mental status
- Severe respiratory infection

30.2 Non-specific Acute Kidney Injury

AKI secondary to the effects of sepsis is common and broadly correlates with the severity of the insult or volume loss if associated with diarrhoea. For example, a fulminant streptococcus A infection in previously healthy young adults may result in marked AKI accompanied by thrombocytopenia and shock. Similarly, profound shock secondary to *Neisseria meningitidis* (C > B) can result in severe AKI or cortical necrosis (◘ Fig. 30.1).

Much less commonly bacterial infection with enteropathogenic *E. coli* and *Shigella* can also cause AKI (and occult CKD) via the production of Shiga toxin. Diarrhoea-associated HUS (dHUS) is covered in more detail in Chap. 51, but the high levels of Gb3 glycolipid expression in the renal vascular endothelium make the kidney particularly vulnerable to perturbation of the renal microvasculature as well as secondary to the effects of intravascular haemolysis. Although rare compared to AKI secondary to other forms of sepsis, dHUS is the commonest cause of AKI in children in higher-income countries and perhaps because of the disproportionate impact on the kidney may be associated with a greater risk of long-term CKD.

With the exception of hantavirus, AKI is not the predominant feature of viral haemorrhagic fevers (VHFs) but can be seen in severe cases, and, in common with most sepsis, AKI is associated with marked acute tubular injury (and mild self-limiting mesangial proliferation). However, the high incidence of other VHFs will inevitably result in a significant incidence AKI by way of collateral damage; for instance, the World Health Organization (WHO) estimates that there are 500,000 dengue haemorrhagic fevers resulting in 20,000 deaths per annum, and many of these patients will incur some degree of AKI particularly if they have underlying CKD.

The WHO estimates that between 2000 and 2015, the incidence of clinical falciparum malaria has fallen by over a third and deaths by 60%. Nonetheless, malaria (almost exclusively falciparum although very rarely reported with vivax) remains an important, potentially avoidable cause of AKI (1) [1]. Non-immune adults are particularly at risk [2], with AKI rates of 30–40% in

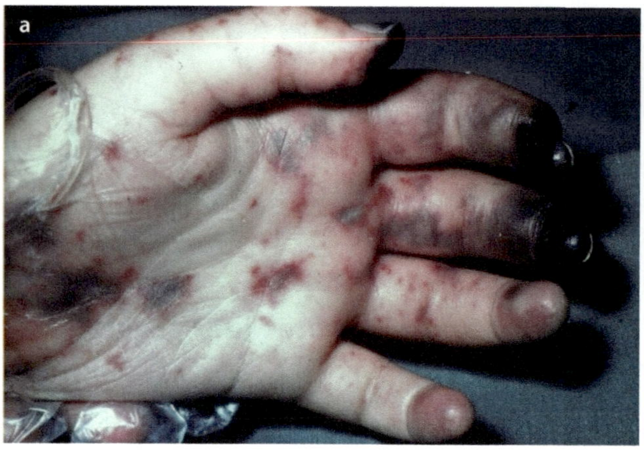

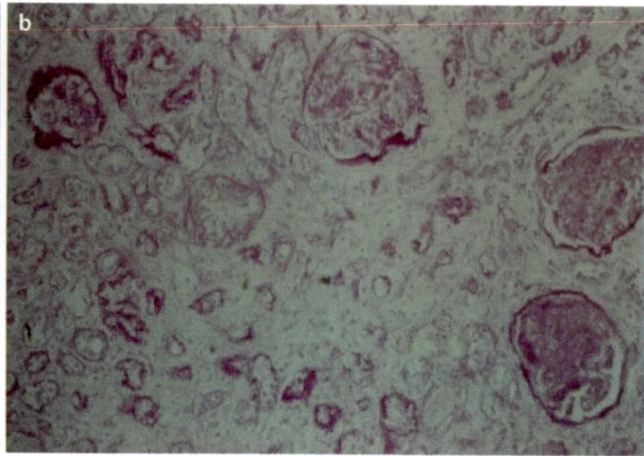

Fig. 30.1 (**a**) Necrotic fingers in a patient with meningococcal sepsis and AKI. The severity of the ischaemic injury to the kidneys was sufficient to cause cortical necrosis. (**b**) Renal biopsy of the same patient on failure to recover from his AKI. Showing the ghostly outline and/or complete loss of normal renal architecture. He required long-term dialysis dependence and illustrated the profound effect of a short episode of severe sepsis on the renal microcirculation

Europeans with a parasitaemia of >5%, the level of parasitaemia being an important risk factor [3]. The rates of AKI secondary to falciparum malaria in endemic areas are less well defined but appear to be much lower at around 3–5% in adults; however, because of the prevalence of malaria, this still represents a significant cause of AKI and if present still augurs a poor prognosis. Hypotension, hyperbilirubinaemia, intravascular haemolysis and hypoxia (although unlike in the cerebral vessels, schizonts do not adhere to and block renal vasculature) all contribute to the acute tubular injury which is the predominant finding; however, mild mesangial proliferation with transitory glomerular proteinuria and tubulointerstitial nephritis do occur. Finally, massive intravascular haemolysis (resulting in blackwater fever) secondary to the use of quinine (also reported with the use of artesunate) for the treatment of falciparum malaria is an important cause of AKI. The pigment nephropathy associated with intravascular haemolysis results in a greater incidence/risk of AKI than would otherwise be attributed to sepsis alone (Fig. 30.2a) [4]. Early diagnosis and effective antimalarial treatment with artesunate are critical, as is avoiding excessive fluid replacement; these patients are at high risk of cerebral and pulmonary oedema (both associated with a high mortality rate). Renal replacement therapy reduces mortality in malaria-associated AKI, and planning provision for this is important given the good prospects for rapid renal recovery. In addition, ready access to acute dialysis is likely to promote the restrained use of IV fluids. Patients treated with intravenous artesunate should be followed up to detect late haemolytic events. Black urine secondary to intravascular haemolysis is a pretty strong diagnostic clue as to the cause of AKI but may clear very rapidly (within 24 hours) and if missed urine microscopy might reveal haemoglobin casts (Fig. 30.2b) or as acute tubular injury and haemosiderin deposition on biopsy (Fig. 30.2c).

30.2.1 Covid-19 (SARS-CoV-2) and Other Severe Respiratory Viruses

Middle East respiratory syndrome (MERS) and SARS-CoV were both associated with a higher mortality than SARS-CoV-2 of approximately 10–37%. In this setting of severely ill patients, AKI rates of up to 27% were reported with the impression that this degree of AKI was commensurate with collateral renal damage in very sick patients. However, it was recognised that the ACE2 receptor and dipeptidyl peptidase-4, both highly expressed in the kidney, acted as ligands for MERS, SARS-CoV and, subsequently, SARS-CoV-2 viruses permitting direct entry to the kidney.

Following initially low rates of reported AKI associated with Covid-19 in Wuhan, China, much higher rates of AKI have been noted elsewhere in patients presenting to hospital, with rates between 25% and 37% in secondary care and up to 90% of those in ICU requiring ventilation. Proteinuria and microscopic haematuria are common in patients but heavy proteinuria relatively rare or transient. Understandably very few patients had renal biopsies, and the majority that have been reported were from autopsy samples. These have predominantly revealed severe, non-specific acute tubular injury. Lymphocytic infiltration and oedema were also common findings with thrombotic occlusion of capillary loops secondary to microthrombi also reported in these

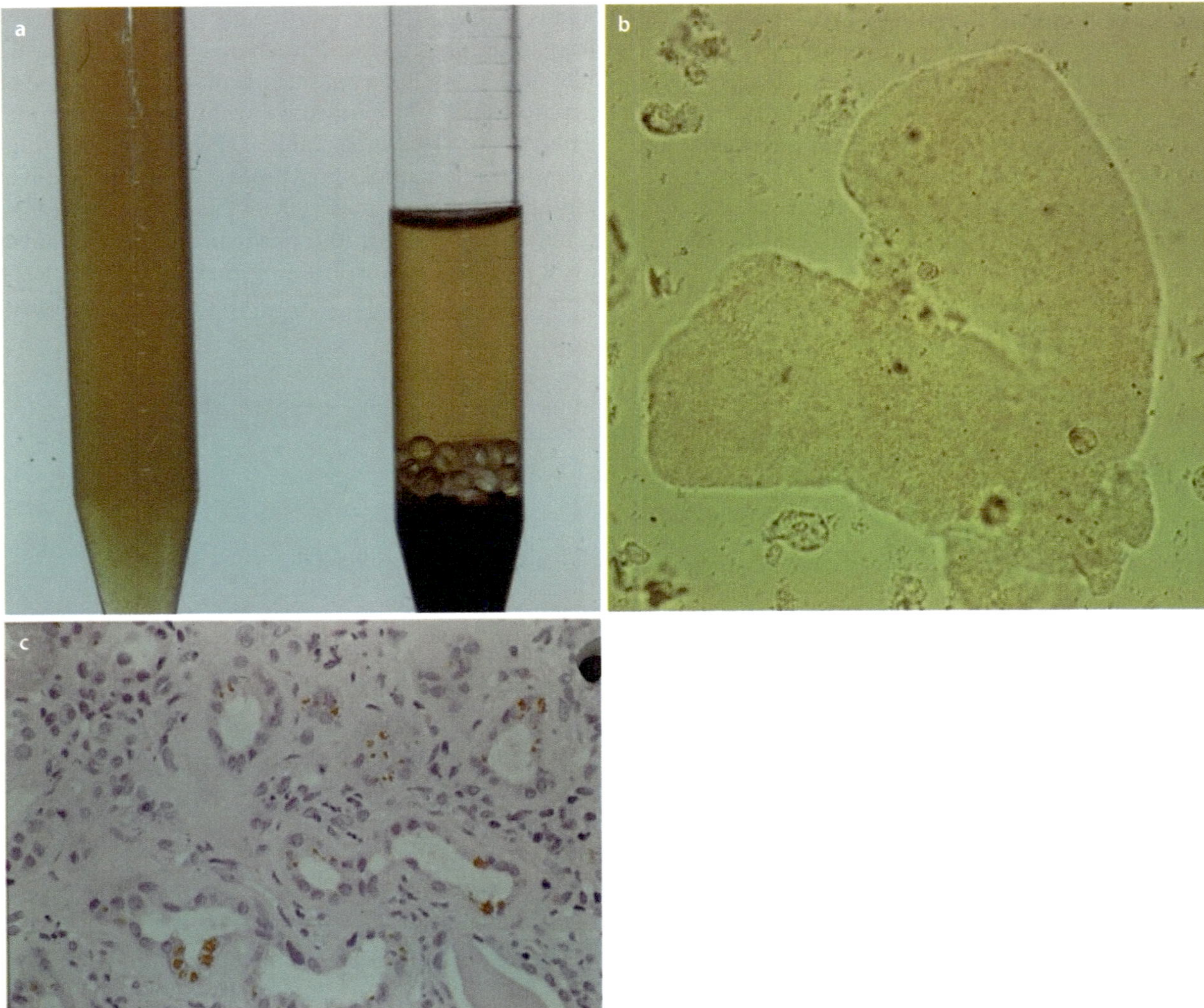

Fig. 30.2 (**a**) Haemoglobinuria in acute falciparum malaria. Urine on right, spun urine from patient with blackwater fever compared with normal urine (right). (**b**) Haemoglobin cast (large homogeneous and acellular) in a patient with high-level parasitaemia and 'blackwater fever'. The patient's urine was clear at presentation with AKI, 3 days after acute malaria and 'dark urine'. (**c**) Renal biopsy of a patient with blackwater fever and AKI. Renal biopsy performed 10 days after AKI shows acute tubular injury and haemosiderin (brown) deposited in the tubules secondary to exposure to large quantities of haemoglobinuria

cohorts. Viral RNA and presumed virus have also been identified from infected kidneys. In the few cases where biopsies have been performed in less critically ill patients (presumably selected because of a presentation less consistent with secondary acute kidney injury), collapsing focal segmental glomerulosclerosis (cFSGS) does seem to be a genuine association, albeit relatively rarely. This would fit with the known associations between cFSGS and some viral infections such as parvovirus and HIV and may have more to do with a systemic cytokine response.

In addition, it is clear small numbers of patients have clearly presented with a Fanconi-like picture with leak of low molecular weight proteins, amino acids, uric acid and phosphate associated with acidosis, presumably secondary to the disproportional direct viral invasion of the proximal tubular epithelial cells.

Approximately 5% of patients with Covid-19 infection need hospitalisation, often in the setting of poor fluid intake, increased fluid losses, generalised sepsis, hypoxia, right heart failure and 'cytokine storm'. Anecdotally, an initial, and understandable, approach of 'running patients dry' to avoid adult respiratory distress syndrome in the UK almost certainly contributed to a huge incidence of AKI in Covid-19-infected patients.

While direct involvement of Covid-19 remains controversial, it seems highly likely that the vast majority of AKI in this setting relates to non-specific, 'indirect' acute tubular injury.

30.3 Direct Renal Involvement

The commonest direct infection of the kidneys is ascending infection by uropathogenic bacteria in the form of pyelonephritis (see ▶ Chap. 54). Less commonly, the kidney can be directly infected by haematogenous spread organisms resulting in an acute or sub-acute interstitial nephritis (TIN). In systemic sepsis with bacteria such as *Staphylococcus aureus*, the kidney may develop multiple micro-abscesses along with all other organs, although disproportionate renal blood flow is likely to result in a great burden of infection. There are other infections, however, that are more renal specific or 'nephrotropic'. The infective causes of interstitial nephritis are listed in ◘ Table 30.2 and include examples where the pathological process is driven by direct infiltration but also others where the interstitial nephritis may be a post-infectious phenomenon without direct involvement. It is worth noting that while the role of some infectious agents causing TIN is well established,

◘ Table 30.2 Infective causes of interstitial nephritis

Viruses:	Investigations and associations
1. HIV	HIV RNA
2. Hepatitis A, B and C	Hepatitis A serology, BsAg or hepatitis B DNA, hepatitis C RNA
3. Cytomegalovirus[a]	CMV PCR
4. Hantavirus	Serology in reference lab, interstitial haemorrhage on biopsy
5. Epstein-Barr virus[a]	EBV PCR, *may* involve granulomata
6. Adenovirus[a]	Adenovirus DNA
7. Herpes simplex[a]	HSV DNA
8. Measles[a]	Clinical features usually obvious
9. Polyomavirus[a]	Typically in significantly immunocompromised, *may* involve granulomata, BKV PCR and SV40 large T cell stain
10. SARS-CoV-2	Lymphocytic interstitial nephritis in the setting of acute tubular injury
Bacteria:	
1. *Mycobacterium tuberculosis*	Classically associated with caseating granulomata (AFB rarely seen but diagnostic)
2. Brucellosis	Serology, *may* involve granulomata
3. Leptospirosis	Usually apparent from clinical picture, may be associated with tubular defect, polyuria
4. *Campylobacter jejuni*	Usually history of significant diarrhoea, stool culture positive
5. *Legionella*	Usually associated with pneumonia
6. Salmonellosis	Usually history of significant diarrhoea, may involve granulomata
7. *Yersinia pseudotuberculosis*	Stool culture
8. *Escherichia coli*	Blood, urine or stool culture depending on source
9. *Streptococcus* species	Blood cultures
10. *Staphylococcus* species	Blood cultures
11. *Chlamydia* species	Serology
12. *Mycoplasma* species	Paired serology may be helpful
Parasites:	
1. *Toxoplasma*	May involve granulomata
2. *Leishmania donovani*	Associated with concentrating defect and polyuria

[a]Typically clinically significant disease only in immunocompromised patients

other reported associations are often based on little more than case reports and circumstantial evidence, so remains fairly speculative.

It is often difficult to differentiate an interstitial nephritis secondary to a primary infection from an antibiotic-induced interstitial nephritis. Identification of granulomata may help guide the diagnosis, but this is not a great discriminator as it can occur with some antibiotic reactions. Ultimately, thorough dissection of drug history and sequential blood results may be the only way to prevent repeating renal injury or avoiding antibiotics inappropriately.

Viral infection of the kidney in the immunocompromised is covered in the chapter on post-transplant infection, and with the exception of hantavirus and hepatitis viruses, it is very unusual in immunocompetent individuals for viral infections to cause a clinically significant interstitial nephritis. It is difficult to know how clinically significant the findings of interstitial nephritis in post-mortem samples in patients with SARS-CoV-2 but likely that interstitial nephritis is damaging. The finding of normally opportunistic organisms causing renal infection in patients on immunosuppression Infections: direct renal involvement warrants exclusion of HIV, lymphopenia and hypogammaglobulinaemia from other causes and congenital immunodeficiency syndromes as a first line. Very rarely primary EBV and CMV infections can lead to AKI as part of the acute sepsis syndrome seen in a minority of immunocompetent patients.

30.3.1 Hantavirus

AKI is common in patients with viral haemorrhagic fevers although usually as collateral damage of severe sepsis in dengue, Lassa fever and Crimean-Congo haemorrhagic fever, whereas *Hantavirus* spp. (zoonotic RNA viruses of the Bunyaviridae family) cause a clinical syndrome in which renal failure predominates.

There are various subtypes of hantavirus, with prevalence differing depending on geographical area with specific rodent reservoirs and disease spectrums and severity. Two main severe syndromes predominate: haemorrhagic fever with renal syndrome (HFRS, also called nephropathia epidemica (NE)) (Asia and Europe), which will be discussed here, and hantavirus cardiopulmonary syndrome (HCPS or HPS) (Americas), which is much less common than HFRS but has a higher mortality [5].

Hantavirus is transmitted by inhalation of the virus in aerosols from urine or faeces of infected rodents, particularly in the dry summer season; human-to-human transmission is extremely rare. Commonly, the subtypes Puumala (Scandinavia and Western Europe) and Dobrava (Balkans) are carried by the bank mole and yellow-necked field mouse, respectively, whereas Hantaan and Seoul are found in China and South Korea (striped field mouse and rats, respectively) [6]. The WHO estimates that 150,000–200,000 people worldwide are hospitalised due to HFRS each year (men more commonly than women), and surveillance suggests that HFRS incidence is increasing. Occupational and leisure history [7] is important as sewage workers, sweepers, forest workers and farmers have a high rate of seropositivity as do water sports enthusiasts, suggesting that sub-clinical infections are much more common than overt HFRS [8].

Clinically, there are various clinical presentations varying from mild influenza-like symptoms to life-threatening illness, with an incubation period of usually 2–4 weeks but ranging from 4 to 42 days. There may be signs of bleeding, mainly petechiae or bleeding from the GI tract, and patients can have disseminated intravascular coagulopathy and thrombocytopenia. HFRS typically has five phases:

1. Febrile phase: non-specific symptoms such as headache, myalgia, back pain, abdominal pain, fevers, nausea and vomiting, lethargy and blurred vision – usually lasting 3–7 days.
2. Hypotensive/septic phase: patients often will have a degree of renal impairment at this stage – usually lasts a few hours up to 2 days.
3. Oliguric phase: oliguric acute renal failure; there may also be evidence of haemorrhage (e.g. conjunctival) – usually lasts 3–7 days.
4. Diuretic phase: the patient becomes polyuric – can last from a few days to several weeks.
5. Convalescent phase: blood results and urine output normalise; this last phase can last a few months [9, 10].

While a useful description, not all patients neatly fit this pattern; cases vary in severity, and patients presenting late may offer few clues other than a history of presumed viral illness. In addition to renal dysfunction, a raised WBC, moderate elevation in transaminases, microscopic haematuria and proteinuria are common, and complement levels may be low. A major clue is the presence of marked thrombocytopenia with normal clotting and without evidence of thrombotic microangiopathy (although leptospirosis can present in a similar way). However, if the patient presents later, the platelet count may have recovered, and some degree of abnormal clotting is not uncommon. There is a marked increase in vascular permeability, endothelial dysfunction, acute tubular injury, interstitial oedema and classi-

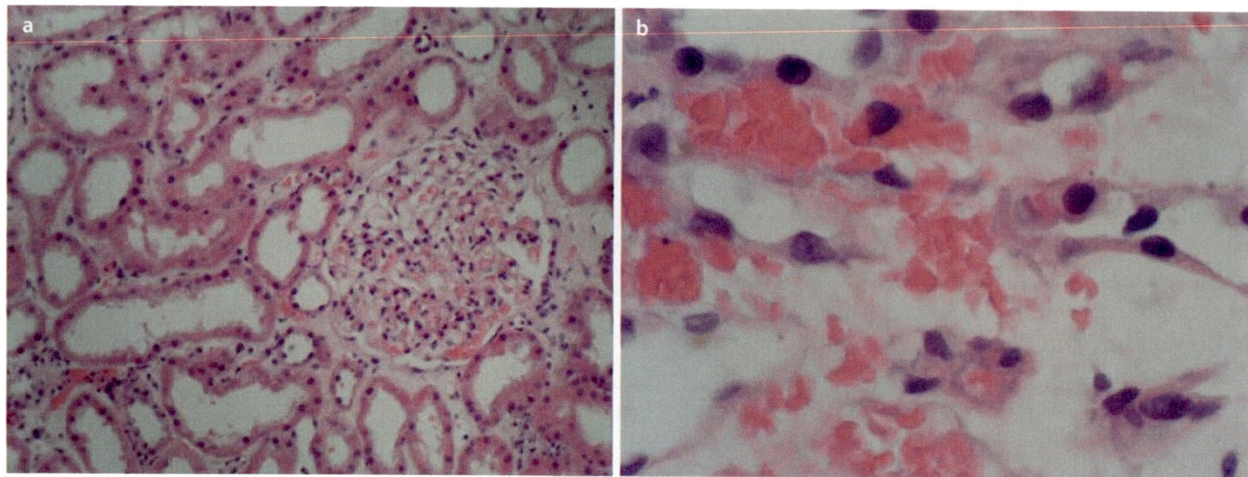

Fig. 30.3 (**a**, **b**) Renal biopsy of a patient with hantavirus infection: (**a**) low power showing marked acute tubular injury and some erythrocytes in the interstitium and (**b**) high power of interstitial haemorrhage

cally interstitial haemorrhage in the outer medulla, which is highly suggestive of the diagnosis (see Fig. 30.3) [11]. Serological tests for IgM and IgG against hantavirus are confirmatory, and in the early phase, peripheral blood RT-PCR may detect virus. Microscopic haematuria, raised AST level and raised leucocyte count at the time of admission are useful predictors of patients who are at risk of developing oliguric renal failure [12].

Management consists of excluding other causes of viral haemorrhagic fevers, bacterial sepsis and MAHA, and treatment is supportive with renal replacement therapy required in ~10%, and ribavirin may be helpful [13]. Most patients' renal function and blood pressure return to baseline, but some remain with a degree of renal impairment and hypertension. Mortality from HFRS is between 1% and 15%, Dobrava virus having a worse prognosis than Puumala virus infection [6].

30.3.2 Leptospirosis

Leptospirosis is a zoonosis caused by the spirochete (gram-negative bacteria) *Leptospira interrogans*. Leptospirosis should be suspected in a patient with non-specific prodrome who then develops AKI and disproportionate hyperbilirubinaemia, particularly with an 'at risk' history. Infections in humans are usually transmitted from rats and domesticated livestock through contact with animal urine usually in contaminated water through breaches in the skin or mucous membranes. *Leptospira interrogans* is almost ubiquitous, but leptospirosis is more common in the tropics due to farming practices, flooding and infection and is more common during rainy seasons or after hurricanes when it can be a common cause of AKI [14]. There is a significant male preponderance (4:1), and this likely relates to sex bias in at-risk employment such as farmers, fish workers, miners, slaughterhouse workers and the military [15]. The incidence in Western countries is falling but does still occur. In the UK, there are approximately 50–60 cases in England and Wales (50% acquired abroad) each year. Worldwide, it is one of the leading zoonotic causes of morbidity particularly in resource-poor countries with approximately a million cases and approximately 60,000 deaths per annum. In Western countries, the proportion of cases that are travel acquired is increasing significantly [16], with a shift from work-related to leisure-acquired infection particularly in those partaking in adventure sports; for example, outbreaks have been reported after triathlons and isolated cases related to pets [17].

Incubation period can range from 2 to 26 days (average 10 days) with the length of illness averaging 14 days. Symptoms are often non-specific in the first week with fevers, malaise, headache, meningism, anorexia, nausea, vomiting, diarrhoea and abdominal, chest and back pain. Physical signs such as hepatomegaly, splenomegaly, rash, jaundice and conjunctival suffusion typically occur in the second week [18]. Weil's disease is the presence of jaundice and AKI in a patient with serologically confirmed leptospirosis infection and occurs in around 5–10% of those infected, less commonly in children. The second phase of the disease is immunologically mediated and may be associated with a myositis, AKI, myocarditis and gastrointestinal and pulmonary (a poor prognostic sign) haemorrhage. Thrombocytopenia occurs in 50% often associated with a neutrophilia, but leucocytopenia can also occur. Liver transaminases are often minimally to moderately raised (<200 U/l), but hyperbilirubinaemia is disproportionate and a vital clue. Low-level proteinuria and haematuria are common, and AKI is non-oliguric in about 50%, often with hypokalaemia. Creatine kinase is elevated in roughly 50%. Diagnosis is made on culture from the blood early in the disease or by serology. Urine cultures may become positive from the second week of illness and may remain so for up to 30 days after resolution of symptoms. Newer PCR-based assays are increasingly being used to diagnose infection [19].

Secondary factors for the development of AKI in leptospirosis include hypotension, hypovolaemia, jaundice and rhabdomyolysis. The main finding on biopsy is interstitial nephritis, oedema and acute tubular injury; mild mesangial proliferation in common with many infectious diseases may be present early on. The predominant site of direct injury by leptospira in the kidney is the proximal convoluted tubule with decreased activity of the sodium-hydrogen co-transporter proximally and NKCC co-transporter in the thick ascending limb. Therefore, sodium and water transport across the tubule wall is impaired causing polyuria and hypokalaemia secondary to more potassium (and magnesium) being excreted distally [20].

Treatment is largely supportive as the condition is usually self-limiting. The role of antibiotics is controversial, and a systematic review concluded that there was insufficient evidence to indicate the benefit of antibiotics in established disease [21]. Antibiotics are only beneficial in the early phase of the disease. If the patient is able to take oral medications, then doxycycline 100 mg twice a day is a good choice as it also covers rickettsial diseases which are an important differential diagnosis. Cefotaxime and ceftriaxone are good intravenous alternatives. Benzylpenicillin is no longer recommended as first-line therapy since it will not cover rickettsiosis. Antibiotic therapy is usually given for 5–7 days.

Mortality figures for Weil's disease vary significantly depending on the series and case mix but amounts to roughly 5–15%. Advanced age, alcohol abuse, oliguria, presence of arrhythmias and jaundice have been shown to be predictors of severe leptospirosis infection [22]. For those who survive, good renal recovery is the norm.

30.3.3 Brucellosis

Brucellosis is a zoonosis caused by *Brucella* spp., most commonly *Brucella melitensis*. Human infection is normally acquired after contact with fluids from infected domestic animals and livestock or derived food products such as unpasteurised milk and cheese particularly in the Mediterranean region. There is little literature on brucellosis causing renal involvement, and it appears to be relatively uncommon but may manifest as cystitis, interstitial nephritis, glomerulonephritis and renal abscess [23, 24]. The diagnosis is often missed as the multitude of symptoms associated with brucellosis such as fevers, malaise, sweating, headaches and bone and joint pain may mimic autoimmune conditions or malignancy. Renal parenchymal involvement is predominantly a granulomatous tubulointerstitial nephritis but can also be associated with indirect involvement secondary to persistent infection in the form of a glomerulopathy associated with *Brucella* endocarditis or membranoproliferative glomerulonephritis (MPGN) sometimes appearing many months after initial symptoms [25].

Diagnosis can normally be confirmed by culture or serology. *Brucella* can be cultured from blood, bone marrow or other appropriate fluids with bone marrow aspirate having the highest yield for positive cultures. There is a significant risk of aerosol transmission in microbiology laboratories; therefore, staff must be informed of the possibility of brucellosis so that the cultures can be incubated in appropriate isolation facilities and appropriately prolonged. A diagnosis can also be made on the basis of an appropriate clinical syndrome together with rising antibody titres on serological tests. *Brucella* antibodies may persist long after recovery of infection, so caution is needed in interpreting serological tests in the context of chronic infection and relapsing infection and in patients from endemic areas.

Treatment is generally with a combination of antibiotics that include doxycycline, rifampicin and aminoglycoside.

30.3.4 Syphilis

The incidence of syphilis caused by *Treponema pallidum* is on the increase in Western Europe and the USA particularly in men who have sex with men [26]. There are well-documented cases of renal involvement associated with secondary syphilis, although this does not result in a high incidence of renal disease. Presentation may be with the classical maculopapular rash involving palms and soles, and proteinuria which may be nephrotic range. The commonest histological pattern is membranous GN [27], but MPGN, PRGN and interstitial nephritis have been described as having solid renal lesions due to syphilitic gumma. Although rare, it is important to exclude treponemal infection as part of the screening for unexplained renal involvement as the treatment is simple and effective. Diagnosis is established by the presence of IgM/IgG by ELISA tests. IgG antibodies persist for life. Positive ELISA IgM needs to be interpreted with care; although a positive IgM reflects active infection, IgM antibodies can persist for 12–18 months post-treatment. Most laboratories will therefore perform a quantitative non-treponemal test (VDRL or RPR). In cases of active infection, RPR titres will be elevated. RPR levels decrease appropriately following successful treatment and can be used to diagnose re-infections or inadequately treated infections.

The choice, route and length of therapy will depend on the stage of disease. Treatment is most commonly with intramuscular benzathine penicillin or PO doxycycline, but inpatients can be treated with IV benzylpenicillin. Treatment should be managed by clinicians experienced in treating syphilis [28].

30.3.5 Visceral Leishmaniasis

This is a zoonosis caused by *Leishmania donovani* and *Leishmania infantum*. It is endemic in tropical and subtropical and Mediterranean countries and transmitted by sandflies. It is known as 'kala-azar', meaning 'black fever' in Hindi. Visceral leishmaniasis is associated with a variety of renal lesions including MPGN, membranous glomerulonephritis or amyloid, but the most characterist finding is a tubulointerstitial nephritis [29]. The interstitial nephritis may be associated with a concentrating deficit (possibly secondary to decreased aquaporin 2 expression), and RTA secondary to PCT injury may occur as a consequence of pentavalent antimonials or amphotericin therapy. Definitive diagnosis is by demonstrating intracellular parasites in histological tissue, usually bone marrow or liver biopsy specimens or splenic aspirates (now rarely performed because of the risk of significant splenic injury). Serological tests using the rK39 antigen have a high specificity, although sensitivities may be variable. Treatment with intravenous amphotericin is often first-line therapy, although the recent availability of miltefosine may offer a reasonable oral alternative [30].

30.4 Direct Involvement: Obstruction

A few infectious agents can impact on the kidney by mechanical obstruction; for instance, *Wuchereria bancrofti* can cause chyluria due to obstruction of renal lymphatics (Fig. 30.4). Chyluria is reported to occur in 2–10% of those infected, but for most, chyluria is intermittent and clinically unimportant; for a few, however, it can result in heavy protein loses and wasting [31]. Most notably, however, obstruction secondary to infection is ureteric or secondary to bladder involvement, tuberculosis and schistosomiasis being the major global causes.

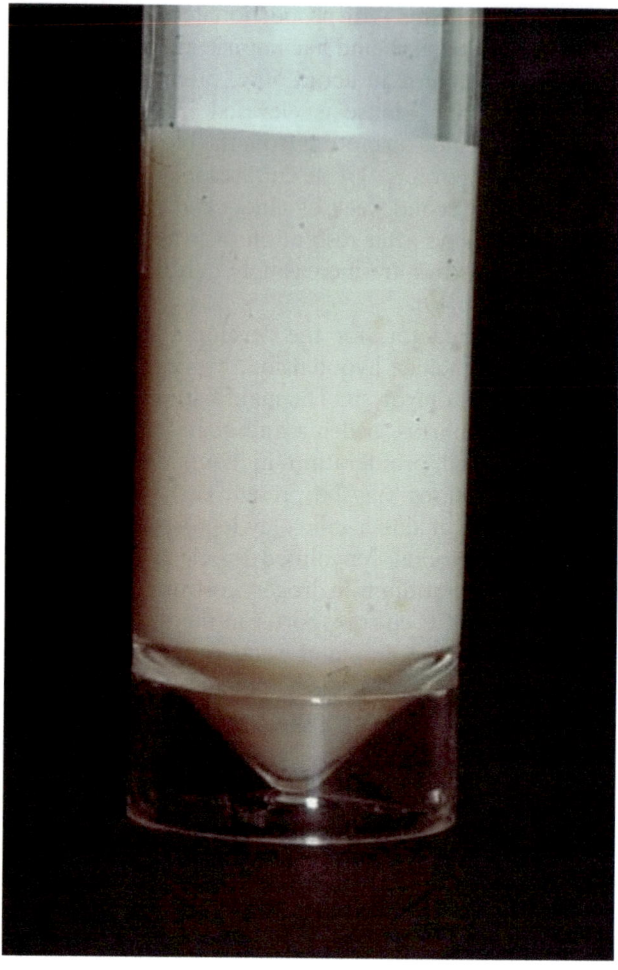

Fig. 30.4 Pathognomonic milky-white urine of chyluria secondary to obstructed renal lymphatics

30.4.1 Schistosomiasis (Bilharziasis)

Schistosomiasis is caused by *S. japonicum* (Southwest Asia), *S. mansoni* (South America and sub-Saharan Africa) and *S. haematobium* (Middle East and sub-Saharan Africa). An estimated 200 million people are infected, 85% of whom live in Africa, resulting in an annual attributed death rate of 20,000 worldwide. *S. mansoni* and *S. japonicum* have both been associated with glomerular lesions especially in the setting of hepatosplenomegaly secondary to portal hypertension. These include MPGN with C3, IgM, IgG and IgA as well as FSGS, cryoglobulinaemia and amyloid deposition. The histological patterns of schistosomal glomerulopathies have been classified into clinicopathological groups that principally assist in determining prognosis. Polyclonal gammopathy, eosinophilia and hypocomplementaemia are suggestive, and *Salmonella* co-infection has been associated with exacerbation of glomerulonephritis. The isolation of *Salmonella* spp. from urine should prompt investigations for schistosomiasis. For most patients, subtle glomerular lesions seem to be much more common than clinical overt nephropathy.

The greatest burden of renal disease, however, results from the urological involvement of *S. haematobium*. The majority of patients clear infection, but 10% develop a chronic type IV delayed hypersensitivity reaction to schistosomal eggs and develop bladder ulcers, granulomatous interstitial cystitis, fibrosis and, in some patients, squamous cell (or less commonly transitional cell) carcinoma. Clinically, patients initially present with macroscopic haematuria often accompanied by dysuria and symptoms suggestive of cystitis. Following this, patients may be relatively asymptomatic while there is progressive fibrosis and calcification of the bladder but can go on to chronic bladder ulcers and cystitis. The bladder can become contracted due to fibrosis or obstructed, and hence recurrent urinary tract infections are a common complication (◘ Fig. 30.5). Renal dysfunction is predominantly secondary to the diseased bladder with fibrosis of the vesicoureteric junction and either upper tract obstruction or development of megaureters with reflux. Chronic and recurrent urinary tract infection may result in chronic pyelonephritis with the development of chronic interstitial nephritis with time [32].

The diagnosis of schistosomiasis relies on a combination of appropriate geographical exposure together with radiological/clinical signs and symptoms and specific tests. A peripheral blood eosinophilia often triggers testing in asymptomatic patients with appropriate epidemiological exposure. Microscopy of end-stream urine specimens and rectal biopsies or stool specimens may be helpful in identifying eggs but is dependent on egg burden and expertise of the microscopist. *Schistosoma* serological tests do not differentiate between previous exposure and current infection and may be difficult to interpret in patients from endemic areas.

Treatment is aimed at eradicating the adult worms and has no effect on already deposited eggs. It is, however, worthwhile doing since adult larvae can live for many years and may continue to produce eggs throughout their life. Praziquantel is the treatment of choice and is safe and well tolerated. It is important to treat any concomitant *Salmonella* infection especially in the setting of a glomerular lesion. There is no effective treatment to reverse the egg-induced interstitial cystitis and fibrosis, so management of established disease should include monitoring of patients with significant bladder involvement for renal dysfunction (UTI and obstruction) as well as surveillance for bladder carcinoma. Fibrotic high pressure, contracted bladders or obstructed upper tracts may need surgical drainage or diversion. Limited evidence suggests that transplantation is safe (assuming low pressure drainage of the bladder) but these patients experience higher levels of UTI post-transplant [33].

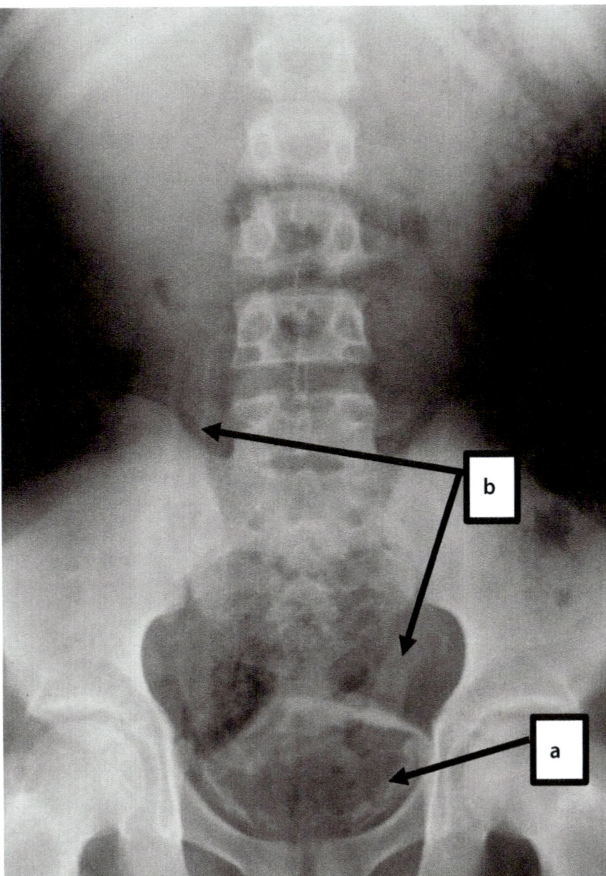

◘ **Fig. 30.5** A plain radiograph showing a calcified and fibrosed bladder (**a**) with grossly dilated and calcified ureters (**b**) in a patient with long-standing schistosomiasis who presented with CKD and recurrent UTIs

30.5 Indirect (Secondary) Renal Effects of Infection

As stated, there are numerous examples of renal dysfunction as a secondary effect of the immune response to infection, and broadly these can be divided into post-infectious and persisting (or ongoing infection). Although interstitial nephritis can be a feature, glomerular pathology is more common, and pathogens associated with glomerular nephritis are shown in ◘ Table 30.3.

Table 30.3 Infective causes of glomerulonephritis

Viral:	
1. Hepatitis B	Membranous GN, MPGN, polyarteritis nodosa
2. Hepatitis C	MPGN, MPGN with cryoglobulinaemia, membranous GN, fibrillary GN
3. HIV	HIVAN collapsing FSGS, immune complex GN (MPGN, lupus-like) FSGS, thrombotic microangiopathy, IgA
4. Coxsackie B	Mesangial proliferative (rare)
5. Influenza A/B/H1N1	Reported but more commonly causes AKI secondary to rhabdomyolysis and systemic sepsis
6. Epstein-Barr virus	Crescentic and leucocytoclastic reported but rare, TIN more common
7. Measles	MPGN, mesangial proliferation more common in patients with sub-acute sclerosing pan-encephalitis
8. Mumps	Mesangial proliferative (rare)
9. Parvovirus	Collapsing FSGS or post-infectious pattern, HSP, MPGN, thrombotic microangiopathy, cryoglobulinaemia
10. Cytomegalovirus	Rare: membranous, FSGS, MPGN, HUS, link with IgA now controversial; all less common than TIN
11. Varicella zoster	Mesangial proliferative, renal vasculitis, HUS reported clinically significant disease seems very rare
12. Rubella	Mesangial proliferative (rare)
13. ECHO	Mesangial proliferative (rare)
14. SARS-CoV-2	Collapsing FSGS associated with infection, glomerular capillary microthrombi
Bacterial:	
1. *Staphylococcus* species	Especially *S. aureus* and usually in the setting of active, ongoing infection
2. *Streptococcus* species	Especially group A, *S. pyogenes*, *S. pneumoniae* and viridans; both post-infectious GN and secondary to active infection
3. *Salmonella* species	Typhi, paratyphi and enteritides; predominantly induces a TIN but glomerulonephritis is well described
4. *Coxiella burnetii*	MPGN with or without cryoglobulinaemia especially in the setting of endocarditis
5. *Leptospira* species	Case reports of GN but predominantly ATI and TIN
6. *Yersinia enterocolitica*	Post-infectious pattern
7. *Mycoplasma pneumoniae*	Post-infectious pattern, rapidly progressive GN
8. *Legionella*	Case reports of proliferative GN but predominantly TIN and ATI
9. *E. coli* 0157:H7	HUS
10. *Campylobacter jejuni*	HUS
11. *Neisseria*	Case reports of GN associated with gonorrhoea and meningitides but vast majority associated with AKI
12. *Treponema pallidum*	Congenital and secondary syphilis associated with membranous GN
13. *Brucella abortus*	MPGN (rare)
14. *Mycobacterium leprae* and TB	Amyloid

■ Table 30.3 (continued)

Fungal:	
1. *Candida*	
2. *Histoplasma capsulatum*	
3. *Coccidioides immitis*	
Protozoal:	
1. *Plasmodium malariae*	Evidence of nephrotic syndrome secondary to *P. malariae* circumstantial and no longer convincing
2. *Toxoplasma gondii*	Rapidly progressive GN, congenital nephrotic syndrome (pyrimethamine inhibits tubular secretion of creatinine)
3. *Trypanosoma cruzi, brucei*	
4. *Leishmania donovani*	MPGN, amyloid, ATI (urinary concentrating defect) and TIN
5. *Strongyloides stercoralis*	MPGN
Heleminthic:	
1. Schistosoma species	MPGN, amyloid, FSGS
2. Wucheria bancrofti	Amyloid, MPGN (rare)
3. Onchocera volvulus	MPGN
4. Loa loa	Membranous GN, MPGN, FSGS

30.5.1 Post-Infectious Renal Disease

Renal dysfunction as an indirect effect of the immune response to infection is classically exemplified by acute post-streptococcal glomerulonephritis but also occurs as the phenomenon of haematuria following upper respiratory tract infections (as with IgA nephropathy) and more rarely following pneumonia or gastroenteritis secondary to other infectious agents such as *Streptococcus pneumoniae*, *Salmonella* spp. and *Mycoplasma pneumoniae*. It is worth reiterating that synpharyngitic haematuria (and proteinuria) occurs rapidly (within 1–3 days) of upper respiratory tract infections with IgA, whereas post-infectious glomerulonephritis from other causes typically occurs 1–2 weeks after the primary infection and post-infectious glomerulonephritis is likely to be accompanied by hypocomplementaemia and a raised anti-streptolysin O (ASO titre) if due to a streptococcal infection.

There are other post-infectious associations in nephrology thought to be driven by molecular mimicry; the infectious antigen provoking a cross-reactivity autoimmune response to a similar autoantigen. For example, there is an association between antibodies to human lysosomal membrane protein (LAMP-2) and the development of ANCA-positive vasculitis following infection with *E. coli* expressing FimH adhesion molecules which have a homologous epitope.

Relapses of vasculitis are more common in patients with nasal carriage of *S. aureus*, although whether this is as a result of molecular mimicry or a non-specific superantigen effect is not clear.

30.5.2 Acute Post-Streptococcal Glomerulonephritis (APSGN)

APSGN remains the most common cause of nephritis worldwide, but the epidemiology over the past 40 years has changed significantly, and it is now relatively rare as a childhood infection in resource-rich countries. It is estimated that there are nearly half a million cases of APSGN globally with an incidence of 10–30 per 100,000/year (0.3 per 100,000/year in Europe), although severe cases of rapidly progressive glomerulonephritis represent <1%. The vast majority occur in children at a mean age of 7 and in the developing world making it still the commonest cause of acute nephritis in children although it is rare in children below the age of 2. There is a second peak in incidence in those over 60 years with a predisposition to those with co-morbidity, alcohol or parenteral drug abuse and is strongly associated with social deprivation. Rates are falling significantly in China and South America with persistently high rates in sub-Saharan Africa and the Indian sub-continent [34].

APSGN occurs secondary to nephritogenic strains of group A streptococcal infection such as pharyngitis/tonsilitis/upper respiratory tract or skin infection, but there have been reported outbreaks due to group C streptococcal infection (*S. zooepidemicus*) from unpasteurised milk [35]. Typically, APSGN is a disease of the socioeconomically disadvantaged and frequently occurs in clusters and epidemics especially following skin infection and commonly associated with scabies and skin sores [36].

30.5.3 Aetiopathogenesis

Only some strains of *S. pyogenes* have nephritogenic potential, and this is attributable to two nephritogenic antigens: nephritis-associated plasmin receptor (NAPlr) and streptococcal pyrogenic exotoxin B (SPEB). Both of these are capable of activating complement via the alternative pathway, inducing the production of IL-6 and MCP-1 by mesangial cells (promoting immune recruitment) and both capable of inducing an antibody response in the host. It has been assumed that the pathogenesis of APSGN is akin to serum sickness with circulating immune complexes to the nephritogenic antigens depositing in the kidney; however, there is still debate about the precise mechanism of the damage to the kidney as C3 (alternative pathway activation) is deposited before IgG complexes [37]. Other possibilities include IgG binding to the GBM secondary to molecular mimicry or in situ deposition of IgG to streptococcal antigens trapped in the kidney.

30.5.4 Clinical Features

Typically, there is a latency of 1–2 weeks after pharyngitis before features of APSGN develop, but it is usually later after skin infections at around 3–6 weeks. History of an infection is an important diagnostic clue; however, approximately 20% of serologically positive household contacts in APSGN epidemics do not show signs of the original streptococcal infection. Patients usually present with oedema, haematuria which may be macroscopic (classically cola coloured) and hypertension (80–90%). Hypertensive crises including encephalopathy are relatively common in childhood presentations. Autoimmune haemolytic anaemia is also reported but a relatively rare complication of APSGN. Proteinuria is usually subnephrotic with nephrotic syndrome in <4%, although said to be more common in adults. Less than 1% develop rapidly progressive glomerulonephritis with crescent formation; however, renal impairment is common especially in the elderly, and patients may present with congestive cardiac failure. For most patients, symptoms resolve spontaneously within 2 weeks, although the microscopic haematuria and proteinuria often persist a little longer.

Blood cultures and swabs may be positive for *S. pyogenes*, but ASOT, anti-hyaluronidase and anti-DNase antibodies are more sensitive. Glomerular haematuria is universal and red blood cell casts are common. One of the most useful diagnostic pointers is a depressed C3 level (typically C4 is normal) which frequently falls before the onset of any clinical features of APSGN and is one of the last tests to return to normal and so may suggest the diagnosis in a late presentation and help differentiate from IgA or pauci-immune vasculitis.

A renal biopsy is rarely necessary, but if performed typically demonstrates a diffuse hypercellularity (proliferative) of the endothelium (resulting in reduced perfusion) and mesangium with infiltration of the tuft with neutrophils (see ◘ Fig. 30.2). Immunohistochemistry reveals deposits of IgG, C3 (but not C4 or C1q) in the mesangium and glomerular capillary wall with pathognomonic sub-epithelial humps on electron microscopy, although sub-endothelial deposits can also occur in the disease. A small proportion of patients can have a more fulminant course with >50% crescents and a RPGN (◘ Fig. 30.6).

Management is largely supportive with sodium and water restriction and diuretics. Haemodialysis is rarely required but may be needed in severe acute renal failure. Appropriate antibiotic therapy such as penicillin is sometimes given to those with APSGN as often it is difficult to know if the streptococcal infection is ongoing, although there is currently no convincing evidence of benefit. Prophylactic antibiotics, however, are indicated in epidemic areas and in close contacts of those affected as early antibiotic therapy in group A streptococcal infections appears to reduce the risk of developing APSGN.

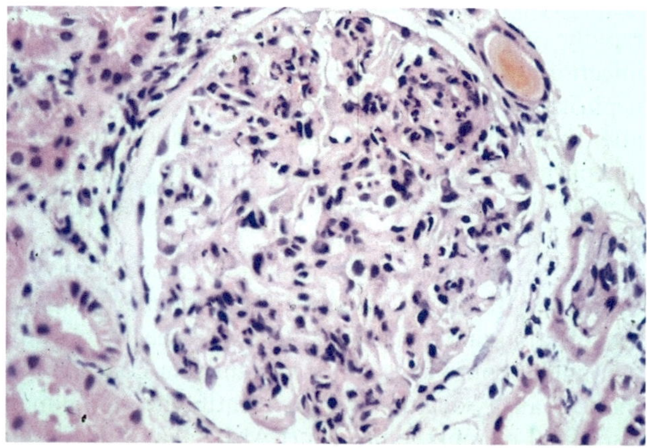

◘ **Fig. 30.6** Light microscopy of post-streptococcal glomerulonephritis with proliferative, hypercellular glomerulus rich in neutrophils

Overall mortality is less than 1% globally representing about 5000 (potentially preventable) deaths per year, 97% of which are in resource-poor countries. The short-term prognosis for the majority is usually very good in children but worse in the elderly with other co-morbidities. In these patients, mortality can be up to 25% and a significant proportion seem to progress to CKD. Of the elderly patients that do survive but have persistent nephrotic range proteinuria, around 75% will go on to develop chronic renal failure [38]. Progression to end-stage renal failure (ESRF) occurs in less than 2% of all patients with PSGN, with less than 1% of children progressing to ESRF after PSGN. Consequently, APSGN has been largely considered benign; however, it has been speculated that childhood APSGN might permanently reduce nephron mass and contribute to the huge burden of CKD in Aboriginal communities that also have a high burden of diabetes and hypertensive renal disease [39]. Recurrence of PSGN is uncommon but has been reported.

30.5.5 Parvovirus

Although the incidence of parvovirus B19 infection in industrialised countries is falling, it is increasingly recognised as a cause (albeit rare) of post-infection (and possibly persistent infection)-related glomerulonephritis, perhaps related to the virus' predilection for vascular endothelium. Nephrotic and nephritic presentations have been described a week or so after initial influenza-like symptoms, often associated with arthralgia, but in adults less commonly associated with the classical rash. A wide range of histological patterns that have been described include collapsing FSGS, MPGN, endocapillary proliferative glomerular lesions, HSP, thrombotic microangiopathy vasculitis and mixed essential cryoglobulinaemia. Deposition of IgM, IgG, C3 and C1q has all been reported. The spectrum of histological patterns associated with parvovirus B19 infection makes it worth considering screening for this infection. Post-infectious GN secondary to parvovirus is largely self-limiting with excellent clinical outcome, although mixed essential cryoglobulinaemia may require further treatment [40].

30.6 Persistent Infection

In contradiction to self-limiting post-infectious renal disease, which is a consequence of the successful immunological response to a pathogen, renal disease secondary to persistent infection is a result of ongoing immunological defence and unlikely to resolve until the infection is treated. Common causes include hepatitis B, hepatitis C and HIV and are shown in ◘ Table 30.4. Globally, some tropical diseases such as filariasis are also implicated.

30.6.1 Malaria

In the 1970s, it was felt that a significant proportion of childhood nephrotic syndrome in sub-Saharan Africa was related to chronic malarial infection principally with *Plasmodium malariae* (quartan malarial nephropathy (QMN)). The evidence for this was largely circumstantial, and even if QMN was a significant clinical entity, it seems a rare beast these days [41]. In practical terms, any patient with nephrotic syndrome in the tropics ought to have a malaria screen and positive results treated, but it should no longer be assumed that malaria is the principal cause of nephrotic syndrome.

◘ Table 30.4 Renal disease as indirect consequence of persistent infection

Viruses:	
1. HIV	HIVAN collapsing FSGS, immune complex GN (MPGN, lupus-like) FSGS, thrombotic microangiopathy, IgA
2. Hepatitis B	Membranous GN, MPGN (with or without cryoglobulinaemia, polyarteritis nodosa
3. Hepatitis C	MPGN (with or without cryoglobulin), membranous GN, cryoglobulinaemic vasculitis, fibrillary GN
4. Cytomegalovirus	Rarely associated with cryoglobulinaemia
Bacterial:	
1. *Staphylococcus* species	Especially *S. aureus*: cellulitis; endocarditis; osteomyelitis; line, wire and shunt infections; pneumonia
2. *Streptococcus*	Cellulitis, endocarditis, pneumonia
3. Other bacteria	Visceral abscess; endocarditis; osteomyelitis; line, wire and shunt infections
4. *Mycobacterium tuberculosis, leprae*	Amyloid
Fungal	
Spirochetes	
Parasites	Filarial infection

30.6.2 Filariasis

A variety of filarial infections can result in a variety of renal diseases mostly via indirect effects, although as mentioned above, *Wuchereria bancrofti* can result in renal lymphatic obstruction with chyluria and significant proteinuria. *Onchocerca volvulus*, *Loa loa*, *Wuchereria bancrofti* and *Brugia malayi* have all been associated with glomerular lesions, although the incidence of significant renal involvement is probably very low. MPGN, diffuse proliferative, minimal change and membranous and collapsing FSGS have all been documented, with occasional microfilariae seen in all parts of the kidney [42].

The other common scenario in which glomerulonephritis results from ongoing infection relates to chronic bacterial infection such as endocarditis, osteomyelitis, visceral abscess as well as infections of foreign bodies. This was classically described in the context of 'shunt nephritis' but increasingly likely to result from infected pacing wires, defibrillators, tunnelled central venous catheters or other foreign bodies. Glomerulonephritis secondary to chronic bacterial infection has a changing demographic and is increasingly likely to occur in older patients with co-morbidity including diabetes, those hospitalised for prolonged periods and with medium-term medical implants such as central venous lines. It is also increasingly common secondary to intravenous and subcutaneous drug abuse.

Renal involvement may take weeks to develop and may be underdiagnosed as these patients, particularly hospitalised ones, often have multiple renal insults including potentially nephrotoxic medication and sepsis. Declining renal function especially associated with de novo haematuria and proteinuria should raise suspicion even in patients with low-grade infections such as diabetic osteomyelitis. The differential diagnosis of AKI in patients with chronic bacterial infection is complicated by raised inflammatory markers, anaemia and false-positive and secondary ANCA but includes (1) acute tubular injury from whatever cause (the commonest), (2) TIN (especially drug induced), (3) vasculitis (GPA/MPA), (4) IgA/HSP, (5) cryoglobulinaemia, (6) post-infectious GN and (7) GN secondary to persistent infection (including *Staphylococcus aureus*-associated glomerulonephritis (SAAGN)).

Features in favour of GN secondary to persistent bacterial infection such as endocarditis include polyclonal increase in Igs especially IgG, hypocomplementaemia, splenomegaly and circulating immune complexes, and if an ANCA is positive, then anti-PR3 tends to be at a relatively low titre (see Table 30.5).

Table 30.5 Discriminating findings in setting of AKI

	Splenomegaly	Polyclonal IgG	C3	C4	Circulating immune complexes	Serology
Endocarditis	Yes	Yes	Low	Low	Yes	Secondary ANCA (low titre), RhF and cryoglobulins very common
SAAGN	No	Yes	Normal	Normal	Yes	Polyclonal Ig increase
GPA/MPA	No	+/–	Normal	Normal	No	Primary ANCA
IgA/HSP	No	No	Normal	Normal	No	Negative, IgA may be raised
Post-infectious	Occasionally	No	Low	Low or normal	Yes	ASO if *streptococcus* IgM response to other infections
Cryoglobulinaemia	Occasionally	Yes	Normal	Low	Yes	RhF
SLE	Yes	Yes	Low	Low	Yes	ANA, dsDNA, ENA, polyclonal
Drug-induced TIN	No	No	Normal	Normal	No	Nil
Acute tubular injury	No	No	Normal	Normal	No	Nil
Cholesterol emboli	No	No	Low		No	Nil

A renal biopsy is often a challenge in septic patients and thereforeurine microscopy is sometimes very helpful in differentiating ATI or TIN from an active proliferative glomerular lesion.

Infective endocarditis is an important cause of secondary glomerulonephritis with approximately a quarter of patients developing an acute glomerulonephritis, although a much higher incidence has been reported particularly in the setting of *Staphylococcus aureus* infections. The demographic of IE is changing in industrialised countries, and *S. aureus* infection is now commoner than *viridans* group streptococcal infections in part due to intravenous drug abuse and medical use of central venous access, vascular grafts and cardiac devices. Haemodialysis patients, in particular, have very high risk of IE. A multitude of other organisms causing IE with glomerulonephritis have been documented including *Coxiella burnetii* (Q fever), *Streptococcus bovis* (associated with bowel pathology), *S. pyogenes*, *S. mitis*, *S. mutans*, *Staphylococcus epidermidis*, *Pseudomonas* spp., *Chlamydia psittaci*, *Brucella* spp., *Bartonella* spp., *Enterococcus faecalis*, *Candida* and even mycobacteria species. Renal involvement is manifest with microscopic haematuria, sub-nephrotic range proteinuria and usually renal impairment, although this may be subtle if previously normal function. Patients may have episodes of macroscopic haematuria and flank pain suggesting emboli which are common. A third of necropsy specimens demonstrate embolic damage which may result in cortical necrosis and scarring or renal abscesses. Microscopically, lesions range from focal segmental proliferative glomerulonephritis to a diffuse exudative proliferative GN with crescents, although MPGN and membranous GN have been described. IgM, IgG and C3 are ubiquitous with sub-endothelial and sub-epithelial deposits.

The renal prognosis is very variable (mortality of IE is about 30%) and largely dependent on early identification and effective treatment of the IE. There is no specific treatment of the secondary glomerulonephritis apart from avoiding nephrotoxins and maintaining vigilance for drug-induced interstitial nephritis. There are case reports and small series advocating the use of steroids or plasma exchange in diffuse proliferative GN, but there is no substantial evidence to support either. In practical terms, some nephrologists do treat aggressive endocarditis with either or both, and it boils down to individual risk versus benefit.

As alluded to above, acute glomerulonephritis with IgA deposition is increasingly recognised as a unique complication of staphylococcal infections [43]. Known as *Staphylococcus aureus*-associated glomerulonephritis (SAAGN), this recently identified clinical entity is almost certainly increasing and significantly underdiagnosed [44]. The emerging prevalence is associated with an ageing population with co-morbidity and in the setting of chronic or sub-acute infections such as cellulitis, line infection, osteomyelitis or visceral abscesses. Renal involvement may occur weeks after the start of the infection and is usually manifest as haematuria, proteinuria (sometimes nephrotic range) and renal dysfunction, often acute renal failure. It may also be associated with palpable purpura which can be confused with vasculitis, HSP or drug-induced cause of renal injury. Although SAAGN is associated with a polyclonal increase in IgM, IgG and IgA (possibly related to the superantigen stimulation of *S. aureus* on T cells), complement levels are normal in 70% of cases, and this may be an important discriminator. While IgG, C3 and IgM may also be present, IgA is predominant, and the histological appearances can be almost indistinguishable from IgA nephropathy with mesangial hypercellularity with or without crescents. Sub-endothelial humps indicate SAAGN rather than IgA; thus, electron microscopy may be helpful in differentiating the two conditions. The management consists of considering and making the diagnosis in the first place and excluding other potential causes of AKI. This is important for a variety of reasons not least as it may alert the clinician to the possibility of sub-clinical low-grade infection such as osteomyelitis and the importance of eradicating an ongoing infection, which is the treatment of this condition.

Shunt nephritis is immune complex-mediated GN secondary to chronic infection of ventriculoatrial or ventriculojugular shunts. It occurs in about 1% of those with ventriculovascular shunts (much less so with ventriculoperitoneal shunts) and thus is rare but important to consider in any patient with ventriculovascular access [45]. *S. aureus* or *S. epidermidis* and also other less virulent skin commensals are the main culprits.

Clinically, renal involvement is with microscopic haematuria, proteinuria, hypertension and AKI usually in the setting of low-grade fevers and hypocomplementaemia (cryoglobulins and rheumatoid factor may also be present). Glomerulonephritis may occur weeks or years after the insertion of the shunt, and as fairly indolent organisms may be involved, the diagnosis may be delayed, and significant damage accrued. Typically, the renal pattern is that of MPGN with IgM, IgG and C3; mesangial proliferation; and sub-endothelial deposits. Management relies on making the diagnosis and treating the primary infection, often entailing removal and replacement of the shunt. There is no specific treatment for the renal lesion, and thus it makes sense for patients with VA/VJ shunts to have their urine dipped, especially if they become unwell.

Glomerulonephritis associated with persistent infection also occurs secondary to bacteria other than *S. aureus* in the setting of visceral abscesses, osteomyelitis and line infections. The clinical history is similar to that of SAAGN, and renal involvement is usually weeks after the onset of the infection and may be mild or severe. Almost all histological patterns have been associated with this, but diffuse or focal proliferative lesion and MPGN seem the commonest.

While antibiotics have no role in the treatment of post-infectious renal disease, they are critical in the resolution of renal disease secondary to persistent infection – thus, identification of an ongoing infective cause is essential, and aggressive pursuit of culture-negative endocarditis or other deep-seated infection with repeated sampling, biopsies for culture and 16 s ribosomal RNA analyses are all important.

30.7 Summary

The causes of acute kidney injury described in this chapter are relatively uncommon in industrialised nations, but the epidemiology of some of these conditions is changing with evolving demographics and travel, and a high index of suspicion is required in unexplained renal disease. A thorough history when the patient is first seen, particularly noting any travel history and activities that may have exposed the patient to these infections, will help list the differential diagnosis and therefore aid appropriate investigations. On an international scale, infections are responsible for a huge burden of potentially avoidable or recoverable kidney disease and represent an important challenge for the renal community.

Case Study

Case 1

A 27-year-old lawyer attended A + E with maculopapaular rash.

On palms and soles (▪ Fig. 30.7), inguinal lymphadenopathy and pedal oedema. His urine dip showed 3+ protein and no blood. Serum albumin was 24 g/L, creatinine 124 μmol/L, and urea 9 mmol/L. He underwent renal biopsy which showed membranous nephropathy. After direct questioning, he stated that he had unprotected sex with three casual male partners in the last 3 months. HIV, hepatitis B and hepatitis C serology negative. Treponemal antibody positive with an RPR of 1:512. He was diagnosed with secondary syphilis and treated with a stat dose of intramuscular benzathine penicillin 2.4 MU.

His rash resolved, and renal function and urine dipstick returned to normal. Secondary syphilis is rare but increasing particularly in men who have sex with men and is an important diagnosis to make as eminently treatable.

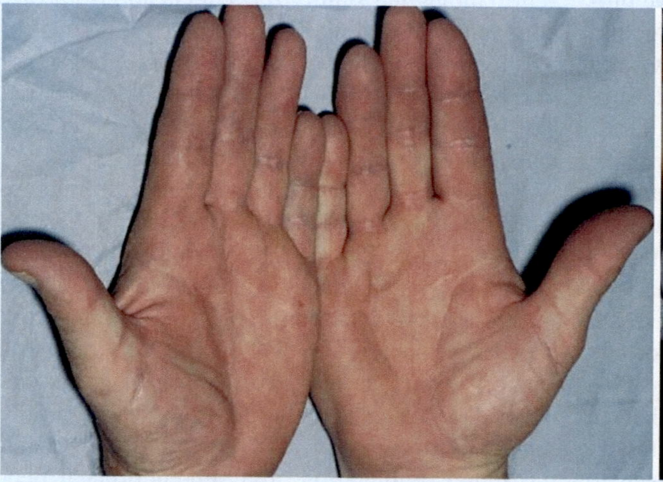

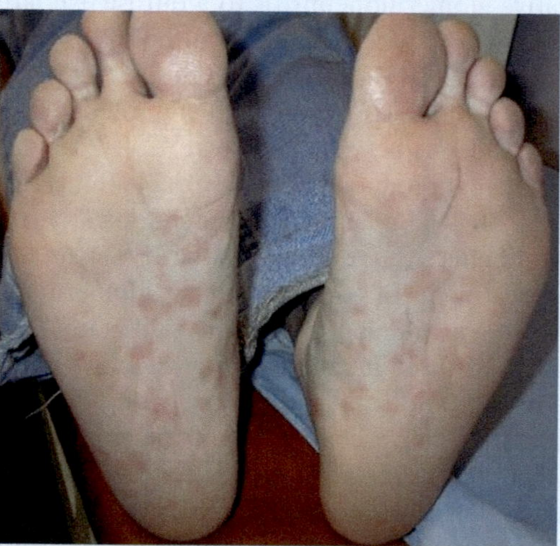

▪ **Fig. 30.7** Classic maculopapaular rash on palms of hands and soles of feet found in secondary syphilis. Photographs courtesy of Dr. Parameswaran Sashidharan

Case 2

A 32-year-old man presented to his GP with headache, myalgia, anorexia and fevers for the preceding 10 days; he was jaundiced and had conjunctival suffusion. He was referred to the medical assessment unit, where on further questioning he stated that he had completed a triathlon 3 weeks before. Blood tests revealed acute kidney injury with a urea of 21 mmol/L, a creatinine of 320 micromol/L and a potassium of 3.1 mmol/L. His bilirubin was 180 micromol/L and ALT was 110 IU/L. Viral hepatitis serology was negative. Urine dipstick showed 1+ protein and 1+ blood. He was managed with IV fluids, electrolyte replacement and fluid balance monitoring. He was started on doxycycline 100 mg twice a day while awaiting results. His blood cultures grew *Leptospira interrogans*. Although the differential is wide, the combination of AKI with hyperbilirubinaemia, conjunctival suffusion and a low potassium is highly suggestive of leptospirosis. Possible exposure because of occupation or leisure activities, in this case freshwater swimming, is contributory evidence in favour of the diagnosis.

Case 3

A 72-year-old ex-smoker was referred to nephrology with new onset nephrotic syndrome, an albumin of 19 and a urine PCR of 2000. She was being followed up for monoclonal gammopathy of unknown significance and had undergone an aortic valve repair and graft repair for a thoracic aorta aneurysm 12 months before and spent several months in hospital recovering from this. Hepatitis C, hepatitis B and HIV negative, normal complement levels, immunology screen including anti-phospholipase A2R antibody negative. She had an ESR of 80 and a CRP of 47.

Her renal biopsy demonstrated amyloid changes initially attributed to her paraprotein, but further staining demonstrated AA amyloid. Multiple blood cultures were negative. A transoesophageal ECHO failed to demonstrate any evidence of endocarditis, but a CT-PET scan showed the aortic graft to be very FDG avid indicating infection (◘ Fig. 30.8a). An amyloid SAP scan also showed uptake in the graft (◘ Fig. 30.8b). In the absence of any positive cultures and a recognition that she would not tolerate replacement of the graft, she was commenced on lifelong doxycycline with a fall in inflammatory markers and proteinuria.

Case 4

A 73-year-old man with diabetes, ischaemic heart disease and peripheral vascular disease who had been in hospital for 5 weeks with a community-acquired chest infection and foot ulcers with cellulitis was referred to the renal team with a creatinine rising progressively from 127 to 352. He had a pacemaker and had bilateral lower limb angiograms 5 days before the referral plus several courses of antibiotics. On examination, he appeared rather frail but not hypovolaemic and with a good blood pressure. There were no peripheral signs of endocarditis or rashes. Urine dipstick had 3+ blood, 2+ protein and 1+ leucocytes.

He was anaemic and had a CRP of 49 and an ESR of 70. The MSU had no growth and serum complements were normal as was a screen for ANCA, ANA, rheumatoid factor, ASO titre was negative. There were no paraproteins but a polyclonal gammopathy. Virology for blood-borne viruses was also negative. Blood cultures and ECHO were negative. A renal biopsy demonstrated florid IgA nephropathy consistent with SAAGN. The differential in cases like this is very wide even if all pre- and post-renal causes are ruled out. Apart from contrast nephropathy and cholesterol emboli (both of which may have occurred after the renal function started to deteriorate), the differential includes persistent infection (endocarditis, pacing wire infection, osteomyelitis) post-infectious (e.g. following cellulitis), potentially an interstitial nephritis secondary to antibiotics and autoimmune conditions such as vasculitis and cryoglobulinaemia. Normal complement levels effectively ruled out the cryoglobulinaemia and make endocarditis and post-infectious GN less likely. Polyclonal gammopathy does suggest either an ongoing infection or an autoimmune disease (made less likely with negative serology). Ultimately, a biopsy was required to definitively define the cause of renal impairment and in this case led to a diagnosis of *S. aureus* osteomyelitis.

30

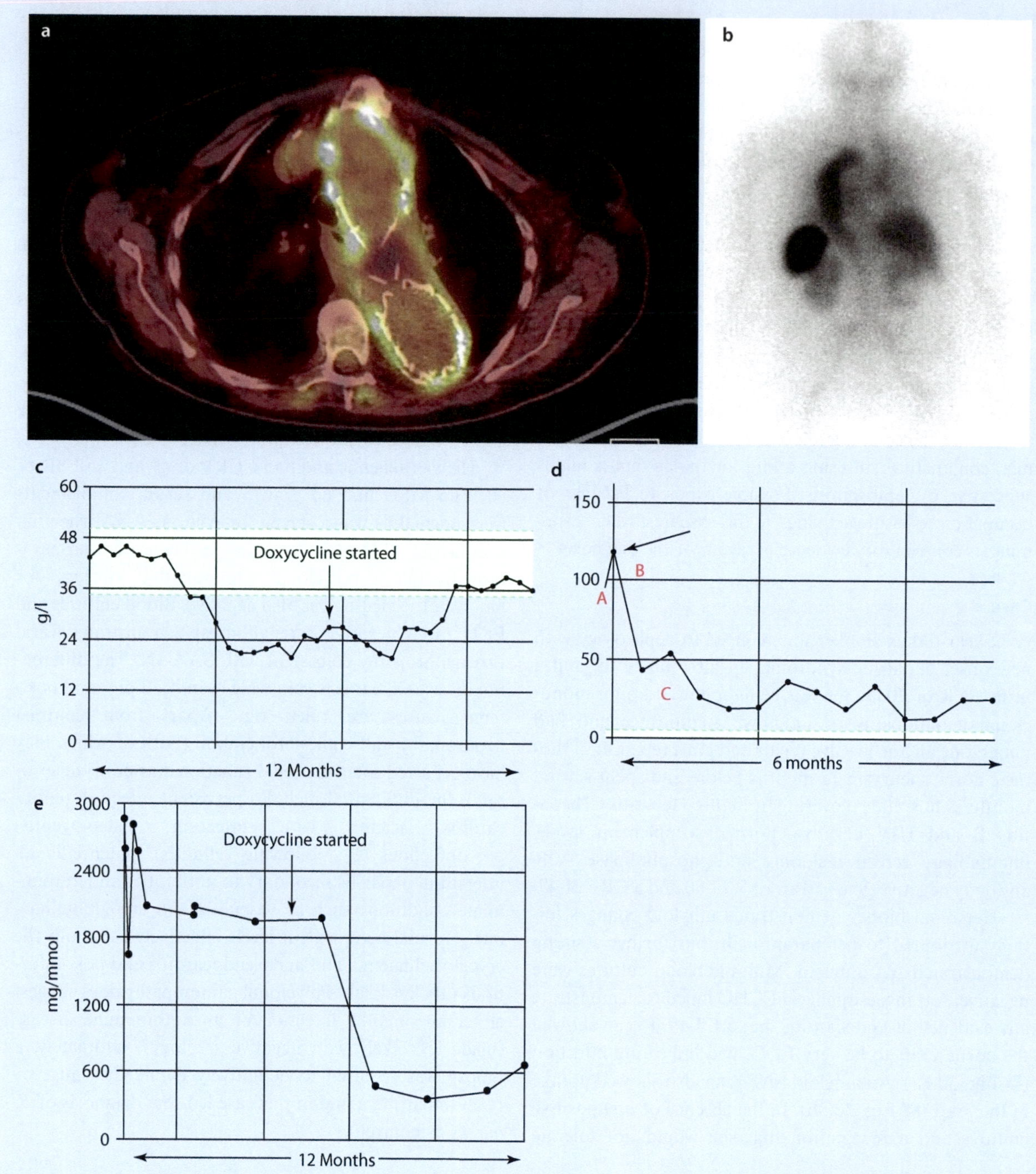

Fig. 30.8 (**a**) CT-PET scan demonstrating intense FDP uptake in the aortic graft. (**b**) Serum amyloid P scan demonstrating uptake in the liver, spleen, kidneys and aortic graft. (**c**) Serum Albumin pre- and post-antibiotics. (**d**) C-reactive protein and serum amyloid protein following initiation of antibiotics. (**e**) Urinary protein following initiation of antibiotics

Tips and Tricks

1. Direct questioning on sexual and travel history is very useful as patients may not deem it relevant.
2. Testing for and managing infections must always be done in conjunction with the local infectious diseases/microbiology and/or virology teams. Public Health England's Rare and Imported Pathogens Laboratory (RIPL) are happy to discuss appropriate tests in accordance with travel history, exposure(s) and clinical syndromes. Details can be found at ▶ https://assets.publishing.service.gov.uk/government/uploads/system/uploads/attachment_data/file/714550/SPATH039RIPL_User_Manual_May_2018.pdf.
3. Three negative malarial blood films are needed to exclude malaria in a patient with a history suggestive of malaria.
4. A patient readmitted following an apparently successful course of antibiotics, with a recurrence of CRP within a short period, may well have an underlying nidus of bacterial infection that has been inadequately treated. Identification of the source and either removing it or prescribing an appropriate course of antibiotics to eradicate the infection is critical to avoid recurrent partial treatment and increasing antibiotic resistance.

Chapter Review Questions

1. What is the most common causative agent for infective endocarditis?
2. What is the most appropriate drug treatment for schistosomiasis? And what two long-term complications might patients with schistosomiasis haematobilium develop?
3. How soon after streptococcal pharyngitis does APSGN (acute post-streptococcal glomerulonephritis) typically occur, and how does this compare to the haematuria of IgA following an URT infection?
4. Which viral haemorrhagic fever pathogen causes acute kidney injury as the predominant feature of the presentation? And what are the key features?
5. What is the treatment of visceral leishmaniasis? And what renal lesion is most common with leishmaniasis?

Answers

1. *Staphylococcus aureus*
2. Praziquantel. Obstructive uropathy and ureteric reflux secondary to a non-compliant fibrous bladder and an increased risk of squamous cell carcinoma of the uroepithelial tract
3. 1–2 weeks after streptococcal infection compared with 1–3 days for IgA
4. Hantavirus, AKI following a viral prodrome and marked thrombocytopenia with preserved clotting, interstitial haemorrhage on biopsy
5. Amphotericin and tubulointerstitial nephritis

References

1. Plewes K, Turner GDH, Dondorp AM. Pathophysiology, clinical presentation, and treatment of coma and acute kidney injury complicating falciparum malaria. Curr Opin Infect Dis. 2018;31(1):69–77.
2. Kurth F, Develoux M, Mechain M, et al. Severe malaria in Europe: an 8-year multi-centre observational study. Malar J. 2017;16:57.
3. Plewes K, Royakkers AA, Hanson J, Hasan MM, Alam S, Ghose A, et al. Correlation of biomarkers for parasite burden and immune activation with acute kidney injury in severe falciparum malaria. Malar J. 2014;13:91.
4. Rodriguez-Valero N, Castro P, Martinez G, Marco Hernandez J, Fernandez S, Gascon J, Nicolas JM. Blackwater fever in a non-immune patient with *Plasmodium falciparum* malaria after intravenous artesunate. J Travel Med. 2018;25(1):tax094.
5. Clement J, Maes P, Van Ranst M. Hemorrhagic fever with renal syndrome in the new, and hantavirus pulmonary syndrome in the old world: Paradi(se)gm lost or regained? Virus Res. 2014;187:55–8.
6. Jonsson CB, Figueiredo LTM, Vapalahti O. A global perspective on hantavirus ecology, epidemiology, and disease. Clin Microbiol Rev. 2010;23(2):412–41.
7. Lovrić Z, Kolarić B, Kosanović Ličina M, Tomljenović M, et al. An outbreak of haemorrhagic fever with renal syndrome linked with mountain recreational activities in Zagreb, Croatia, 2017. Epidemiol Infect. 2018;146(10):1236–9.
8. Muñoz-Zanzi C, Saavedra F, Otth C, Domancich L, Hott M, Padula P. Serological evidence of hantavirus infection in apparently healthy people from rural and slum communities in Southern Chile. Freed EO, ed. Viruses. 2015;7(4):2006–13.
9. Faulde M, Sobe D, Kimmig P, Scharninghausen J. Renal failure and hantavirus infection in Europe. Nephrol Dial Transplant. 2000;15(6):751–3.
10. Jiang H, Du H, Wang LM, Wang PZ, Bai XF. Hemorrhagic fever with renal syndrome: pathogenesis and clinical picture. Front Cell Infect Microbiol. 2016;6:1.
11. Ferluga D, Vizjak A. Hantavirus nephropathy. J Am Soc Nephrol. 2008;19(9):1653–8.
12. Kim YK, Lee SC, Kim C, Heo ST, Choi C, Kim JM. Clinical and laboratory predictors of oliguric renal failure in haemorrhagic fever with renal syndrome caused by Hantaan virus. J Infect. 2007;54(4):381–6.
13. Huggins JW, et al. Prospective, double-blind, concurrent, placebo-controlled clinical trial of intravenous ribavirin therapy of hemorrhagic fever with renal syndrome. J Infect Dis. 1991;164(6):1119–27.
14. Mehta K, Pajai A, Bhurke S, Shirkande A, Bhadade R, D'Souza R. Acute kidney injury of infectious etiology in monsoon season: a prospective study using acute kidney injury network criteria. Indian J Nephrol. 2018;28(2):143–52.
15. World Health Organization. Human leptospirosis: guidance for diagnosis, surveillance and control. Geneva: World Health Organization; 2003.

16. de Vries SG, Visser BJ, Stoney RJ, et al. Leptospirosis among returned travelers: a GeoSentinel site survey and multicenter analysis—1997–2016. Am J Trop Med Hyg. 2018;99(1):127–35.
17. Monahan A, Miller I, Nally J. Leptospirosis: risks during recreational activities. J Appl Microbiol. 2009;107:707–16.
18. Haake DA, Levett PN. Leptospirosis in humans. Curr Top Microbiol Immunol. 2015;387:65–97.
19. Riediger IN, Stoddard RA, Ribeiro GS, et al. Rapid, actionable diagnosis of urban epidemic leptospirosis using a pathogenic *Leptospira lipL32*-based real-time PCR assay. PLoS Negl Trop Dis. 2017;11(9):e0005940.
20. Araujo ER, Seguro AC, Spichler A, Magaldi AJ, Volpini RA, De Brito T. Acute kidney injury in human leptospirosis: an immunohistochemical study with pathophysiological correlation. Virchows Arch. 2010;456:367–75.
21. Brett-Major DM, Coldren R. Antibiotics for leptospirosis. Cochrane Database Sys Rev. 2012;(2):CD008264.
22. Dassanayake DL, Wimalaratna H, Nandadewa D, Nugaliyadda A, Ratnatunga CN, Agampodi SB. Predictors of the development of myocarditis or acute renal failure in patients with leptospirosis: an observational study. BMC Infect Dis. 2012;12:4.
23. Bakri FG, Wahbeh A, Mahafzah A, Tarawneh M. Brucella glomerulonephritis resulting in end-stage renal disease: a case report and a brief review of the literature. Int Urol Nephrol. 2008;40(2):529–33.
24. Li J, Li Y, Wang Y, Huo N, et al. Renal abscess caused by Brucella. Int J Infect Dis. 2014;28:26–8.
25. Provatopoulou S, Papasotiriou M, Papachristou E, Gakiopoulou H, Marangos M, Goumenos DS. Membranoproliferative glomerulonephritis in a patient with chronic brucellosis. Kidney Res Clin Pract. 2018;37(3):298–303.
26. Solomon MM, Mayer KH. Evolution of the syphilis epidemic among men who have sex with men. Sex Health. 2015;12(2):96–102.
27. Gamble CN, Reardan JB. Immunopathogenesis of syphilitic glomerulonephritis: elution of antitreponemal antibody from glomerular immune-complex deposits. NEJM. 1975;292(9):449–54.
28. Kingston M, French P, Higgins S, McQuillan O, Sukthankar A, Stott C, McBrien B, Tipple C, Turner A, Sullivan AK. Syphilis guidelines revision group 2015. UK national guidelines on the management of syphilis 2015. Int J STD AIDS. 2016;27(6):421–46.
29. Clementi A, Battaglia G, Floris M, Castellino P, Ronco C, Cruz DN. Renal involvement in leishmaniasis: a review of the literature. NDT Plus. 2011;4(3):147–52.
30. Olliaro PL, Guerin PJ, Gerstl S, Haaskjold AA, Rottingen JA, Sundar S. Treatment options for visceral leishmaniasis: a systematic review of clinical studies done in India, 1980–2004. Lancet Infect Dis. 2005;5(12):763–74.
31. Abeygunasekera AM, Sutharshan K, Balagobi B. New developments in chyluria after global programs to eliminate lymphatic filariasis. Int J Urol. 2017;24:582–8.
32. Barsoum RS, Esmat G, El-Baz T. Human schistosomiasis: clinical perspective: review. J Adv Res. 2013;4(5):433–44.
33. Mahmoud KM, Sobh MA, El-Agroudy AE, Mostafa FE, Baz ME, Shokeir AA, Ghoneim MA. Impact of schistosomiasis on patient and graft outcome after renal transplantation: 10 years' follow-up. Nephrol Dial Transplant. 2001;16(11):2214–21.
34. Jackson SJ, Steer AC, Campbell H. Systematic review: estimation of global burden of non-suppurative sequelae of upper respiratory tract infection: rheumatic fever and post-streptococcal glomerulonephritis. Tropical Med Int Health. 2011;16(1):2–11.
35. Sesso R, Pinto SW. Epidemic glomerulonephritis due to Streptococcus zooepidemicus in Nova Serrana, Brazil. Kidney Int. 2005;68:S132–6.
36. Svartman M, Finklea J, Potter E, Poon-King T, Earle D. Epidemic scabies and acute glomerulonephritis in Trinidad. Lancet. 1972;299(7744):249–51.
37. Rodriguez-Iturbe B, Batsford S. Pathogenesis of poststreptococcal glomerulonephritis a century after Clemens von Pirquet. Kidney Int. 2007;71(11):1094–104.
38. Hoy WE, White AV, Dowling A, Sharma SK, Bloomfield H, Tipiloura BT, Swanson CE, Mathews JD, McCredie DA. Post-streptococcal glomerulonephritis is a strong risk factor for chronic kidney disease in later life. Kidney Int. 2012;81(10):1026–32.
39. White AV, Hoy WE, McCredie DA. Childhood post-streptococcal glomerulonephritis as a risk factor for chronic renal disease in later life. Med J Aust. 2001;174(10):492–6.
40. Waldman M, Kopp JB. Parvovirus B19 and the kidney. Clin J Am Soc Nephrol. 2007; 2(Supplement 1):S47–56.
41. Olowu WA, Adelusola KA, Adefehinti O, Oyetunji TG. Quartan malaria-associated childhood nephrotic syndrome: now a rare clinical entity in malaria endemic Nigeria. Nephrol Dial Transplant. 2009;25(3):794–801.
42. Van Velthuysen ML, Florquin S. Glomerulopathy associated with parasitic infections. Clin Microbiol Rev. 2000;13(1):55–66.
43. Wehbe E, Salem C, Simon JF, Navaneethan SD, Pohl M. IgA-dominant Staphylococcus infection-associated glomerulonephritis: case reports and review of the literature. NDT Plus. 2011;4(3):181–5.
44. Wang SY, Bu R, Zhang Q, Liang S, Wu J, Liu XG, Cai GY, Chen XM. Clinical, pathological, and prognostic characteristics of glomerulonephritis related to staphylococcal infection. Medicine. 2016;95(15):e3386.
45. Harland TA, Winston KR, Jovanovich AJ, Johnson RJ. Shunt nephritis: an increasingly unfamiliar diagnosis. World Neurosurg. 2018;111:346–8.

Links

UK Malaria Treatment Guidelines 2016. https://www.journalofinfection.com/article/S0163-4453(16)00047-5/pdf.

UK National Guidelines on the Management of Syphilis 2015. https://www.bashhguidelines.org/media/1148/uk-syphilis-guidelines-2015.pdf.

World Health Organization. http://www.who.int/.

Centers for Disease Control and Prevention. https://www.cdc.gov.

Blood-Borne Viruses and the Kidney

Rachel K. Y. Hung, Douglas Macdonald, Sanjay Bhagani, Mark Harber, and John Booth

Contents

M. Harber (ed.), *Primer on Nephrology*, https://doi.org/10.1007/978-3-030-76419-7_31

Learning Objectives

1. Renal disease in HIV can be due to direct HIV-mediated injury of renal tissue, consequences of immunodeficiency or toxicity of medication including combined antiretroviral therapy. As HIV treatment improves, ageing HIV patients are at an increased risk of kidney disease from common comorbid conditions, namely diabetes and hypertension.
2. Renal disease in hepatitis C tends to occur in chronic infection and is commonly associated with cryoglobulinaemia. Hepatitis B is strongly associated with membranous glomerulonephritis or membranoproliferative glomerulonephritis and can present as polyarteritis nodosa.

31

31.1 Introduction

The main blood-borne viruses HIV, hepatitis B (HBV) and hepatitis C (HCV) are responsible for a huge burden of renal disease worldwide. These chronic infections produce a complex and fascinating spectrum of kidney diseases which have the potential to cause end-stage kidney disease (ESKD). New advances in antiviral treatment are altering the epidemiology of these diseases and in many cases permitting near-normal life expectancy. With this has come both new renal disorders secondary to antiviral toxicity and also an increasing population of 'well' patients with ESKD and chronically suppressed virus raising new challenges for transplantation.

31.2 Human Immunodeficiency Virus and the Kidney

The widespread use of combination antiretroviral therapy (cART) in HIV has dramatically enhanced patient survival and reduced the incidence of AIDS, but also altered the spectrum of renal disease encountered in Western populations (Table 31.1) [1]. Rates of HIV-associated acute kidney injury (AKI) have more than halved in the cART era, parallel to a decline in severe infection episodes [2, 3]. The incidence of HIV's archetypal renal lesion, HIV-associated nephropathy (HIVAN), has also diminished. In turn, rates of multifactorial CKD have risen, driven by increasing average patient age and prevalence of common comorbidities such as hypertension and diabetes. Specific nephrotoxicities of cART have also emerged.

HIV-positive patients should be screened for renal disease by means of eGFR measurement, urinalysis and protein/creatinine ratio (uPCR) at diagnosis, prior to starting cART and at periodic intervals no greater than 1 year [4]. Patients with risk factors for CKD (black race, hypertension or cardiovascular disease, diabetes, viral hepatitis, family history or potentially nephrotoxic mediations) need enhanced surveillance.

Table 31.1 The spectrum of renal disease encountered in patients infected with HIV

HIV associated	Examples
HIVAN Immune complex kidney disease Thrombotic microangiopathy Diffuse infiltrative lymphocytic syndrome	See Table 31.3
HIV treatment associated	
ART nephropathy	Proximal tubulopathy with TDF Crystallopathy with indinavir Granulomatous TIN with atazanavir
Immune reconstitution inflammatory syndrome (IRIS)	
Immunodeficiency associated	See Table 31.4
Anti-microbial toxicity	Tubulointerstitial nephritis or ATI with antibiotics
Renal parenchymal infection	Tuberculous granulomatous interstitial nephritis Viral nephropathies, e.g. CMV
Neoplasia	Infiltration, e.g. by lymphoma
Other commonly encountered conditions	
Immune complex kidney disease	HBV-associated membranous nephropathy HCV-associated mesangiocapillary GN
Non-collapsing FSGS (NOS or hilar variants)	
Acute tubular injury	Hypovolaemia, sepsis, nephrotoxic drugs
Diabetic or hypertensive kidney disease	
AA amyloid	Associated with injection drug use

TDF tenofovir disoproxil fumarate, *TIN* tubulointerstitial nephritis, *CMV* cytomegalovirus, *ATI* acute tubular injury, *HBV* hepatitis B virus, *HCV* hepatitis C virus, *FSGS* focal segmental glomerulosclerosis, *NOS* not otherwise specified

■ **Table 31.2** Common nephrotoxic medications encountered in the management of HIV

Drug	Renal adverse effect
Antibiotics	
Co-trimoxazole (Septrin)	Acute TIN, ATI, hyperkalaemia
Aminoglycosides, e.g. gentamicin	ATI
Sulphadiazine	Crystalluria, nephrolithiasis
Rifampicin	Acute TIN
Antivirals	
Acyclovir	Crystallisation with tubular obstruction
Foscarnet	ATI, crystalline glomerulonephritis, RTA
Anti-fungals	
Amphotericin	ATI, proximal tubular dysfunction
Antiretrovirals	
Indinavir	Nephrolithiasis, chronic TIN
Atazanavir	Nephrolithiasis, granulomatous TIN
TDF (NtRTI)	Proximal tubular dysfunction, ATI
NRTIs, e.g. didanosine	Lactic acidosis

TIN tubulointerstitial nephritis, *ATI* acute tubular injury, *RTA* renal tubular acidosis, *TDF* tenofovir disoproxil fumarate

31.2.1 Acute Kidney Injury (AKI)

Common precipitants for AKI in HIV include sepsis, hypovolaemia or exposure to potentially nephrotoxic medication, often during treatment for opportunistic infection (■ Table 31.2). Risk factors include prior chronic kidney disease (CKD) and a greater degree of immunodeficiency [5]. Less common causes include acute presentations of HIVAN or HIV immune complex glomerulonephritis, HIV-associated thrombotic microangiopathy and non-drug-induced tubulointerstitial nephritis or parenchymal infection (■ Table 31.2). Tenofovir disoproxil fumarate (TDF) may exacerbate kidney injury, and alternative antiretroviral drugs (ARVs) should be used in AKI stage 2 or 3 [6]. Doses of renally excreted ARVs must be actively adjusted during AKI or renal recovery. Diagnostic kidney biopsy may be required when injury is severe or sustained and a clear cause is not identifiable. Indications for renal replacement therapy in AKI are the same as those for non-infected individuals.

31.2.2 HIV-Associated Thrombotic Microangiopathy

Thrombotic microangiopathy (TMA) is an uncommon but well-recognised complication of HIV, typified by the presence of microangiopathic haemolytic anaemia, thrombocytopaenia, elevated lactate dehydrogenase and renal impairment and/or neurological symptoms. TMA may present at any stage of HIV infection but is more common in advanced disease. HIV p24 antigen has been detected within endothelial cells during TMA, suggesting that HIV may directly incite endothelial injury [7]. ADAMTS13 activity may be depressed, typically in conjunction with detectable anti-ADAMTS13 antibodies. Other potential secondary causes of TMA may co-exist, including CMV viraemia or drug exposures (e.g. rifampicin).

Where possible, a kidney biopsy should be performed to confirm thrombotic microangiopathy as the cause of renal failure, although thrombocytopaenia may preclude this. Management is based on treatment strategies for TMA in non-infected individuals as no prospective trials have been performed in HIV. Plasma exchange (with plasma replacement) is widely used as first-line therapy albeit with inconsistent outcomes among published studies. Antiretroviral therapy should be initiated early to counteract any ongoing endothelial injury attributable to the virus and should be administered post-plasma exchange. Excellent outcomes have been reported for a regimen of plasma exchange, corticosteroids and early antiretroviral therapy in a cohort of patients with TMA and low ADAMTS13 activity [8].

31.2.3 HIV-Associated Nephropathy (HIVAN)

First described among the AIDS populations of New York and Miami in 1984, the 'collapsing glomerulopathy' of HIVAN is almost exclusively seen in HIV-infected patients of black African or Caribbean ancestry. Although HIVAN has declined in the era of widespread cART use, the prevalence among black HIV-infected patients in the UK remains 1%, with estimates among sub-Saharan African populations significantly higher [9, 10].

31.2.3.1 Aetiology and Pathogenesis

Viral nucleic acids can be identified in human renal epithelial cells in biopsies from patients with HIVAN, and these cells appear to be able to support local replication, although the virus can also be detected in the absence of clinical disease.

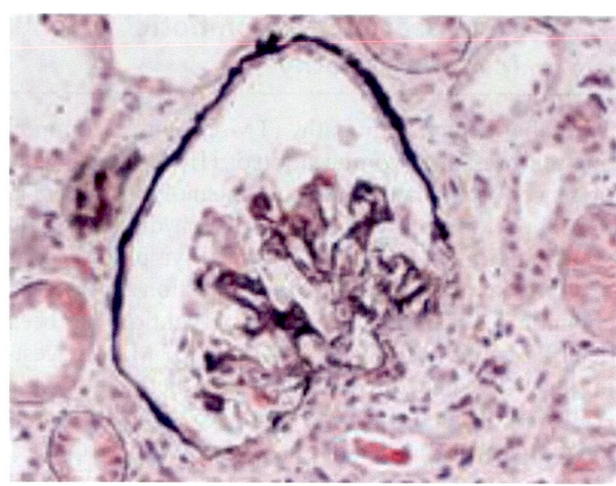

Fig. 31.1 Collapsing glomerulopathy of HIVAN

31

Virtual confinement of disease to those of African ancestry suggests a marked genetic predisposition and a strong association has been found with polymorphisms in *APOL1*, the gene encoding *Apolipoprotein L1* (*APOL1poll*), with disease risk following a recessive pattern of inheritance. Only kidney disease-associated *APOL1* variants lyse the parasite *Trypanosoma brucei rhodesiense* (responsible for the disease African sleeping sickness) in vitro, suggesting that these variants may have proliferated under pressure of positive selection [11].

31.2.3.2 Clinicopathologic Characteristics

Classical disease comprises heavy proteinuria (often nephrotic range) with renal impairment, minimal oedema and relative normotension. CD4 count is typically <200 cells/μl at presentation, although cases have been described early in disease, including at seroconversion. Recent studies have shown that typical histological lesions of HIVAN may be found on biopsy in patients exhibiting only microalbuminuria, although the natural history of disease in such cases is unknown. Ultrasound classically shows bilaterally enlarged echogenic kidneys. No non-invasive test has sufficient specificity for HIVAN, and definitive diagnosis requires renal biopsy.

The hallmark histological lesion of HIVAN is 'collapse' of the glomerular tuft, defined by severe retraction of glomerular capillary walls resulting in loss of patency of capillary lumens, and often best appreciated on silver stain (Fig. 31.1). This is accompanied by podocyte swelling and hyperplasia, often sufficiently florid to obliterate Bowman's space as 'pseudocrescents'. Lesions may evolve into a more typical pattern of focal segmental glomerulosclerosis (FSGS) not otherwise specified (NOS) over time. Tubulointerstitial disease is a prominent feature, with 'microcyst' formation – cylindrically dilated tubules containing large proteinaceous casts – and a lymphocyte-rich interstitial infiltrate. Positive immunostaining is confined to variable IgM and complement deposition in collapsed segments and, to a lesser extent, the mesangium, without significant electron-dense deposits on electron microscopy. Endothelial tubulo-reticular inclusion bodies are frequently seen.

31.2.3.3 Treatment and Prognosis

Treatment recommendations for HIVAN are largely derived from retrospective cohort studies or case series. General measures include careful control of blood pressure, aiming for levels <130/80 ideally with an angiotensin receptor blocker (ARB). Despite current best therapy, rates of progression to ESKD remain high.

31.2.3.4 Antiretroviral Therapy

HIVAN incidence has fallen markedly since widespread introduction of cART and new cases among patients in stable care in the UK are rare [9]. Numerous published cases have reported stabilisation or improvement of disease, including histological changes, with the commencement of cART. Cohort studies examining the effect of cART on renal outcomes in HIVAN have yielded conflicting results, however. The benefits of treatment are likely to be greatest in those with less established interstitial fibrosis and atrophy, and failure to stratify for this may explain some of the heterogeneity in study outcomes. Current guidance is for initiation of cART in all patients where HIVAN is confirmed, regardless of CD4 count [4].

31.2.3.5 Corticosteroids

The majority of published studies examining the effect of steroids on disease progression in HIVAN have reported benefit, but most were conducted before the routine administration of cART or considerably small patient numbers in retrospective analyses. Cases where serial biopsies have been performed before and after steroid therapy suggest a particular amelioration of tubulointerstitial inflammation. A recent small randomised controlled trial from South Africa suggested that the addition of corticosteroids to cART in the initial treatment of cART-naïve patients presenting with HIVAN may lead to a greater increase in GFR (but without additional benefit on proteinuria) but at the expense of an increased risk of severe infection and death [12]. Current guidelines suggest reserving therapy for those in whom concomitant opportunistic infection has been excluded and with a progressive decline in renal function despite cART [13].

Table 31.3 Immune complex kidney disease in HIV

Histological pattern	Important secondary causes/associations in HIV
HIV immune complex kidney disease (HIVICK)	
Membranous GN	Syphilis, HBV, neoplasia
IgA nephropathy	Chronic liver disease
Post-infectious GN	Streptococcal infection, staphylococcal infection (may be IgA predominant), other bacterial, fungal, viral or parasitic disease
Mesangiocapillary GN	HCV, HBV, chronic infection (e.g. SBE), SLE, drugs (e.g. interferon-alpha)
Immunotactoid or fibrillary GN	HCV, neoplasia
Lupus-like nephritis	SLE

HBV hepatitis B virus, *HCV* hepatitis C virus, *SBE* subacute bacterial endocarditis, *SLE* systemic lupus erythematosus

31.2.4 Immune Complex Kidney Disease

Immune complex kidney disease (ICKD) is characterised by the presence of immune deposits on immunostaining, typically accompanied by electron-dense deposits on electron microscopy. A variety of glomerular histological patterns have been described in association with HIV infection (Table 31.3). Patients are more likely to be non-black or co-infected with viral hepatitis, although ICKD does occur in black populations and can co-exist with HIVAN. Clinical presentations mirror the spectrum seen in glomerulonephritis in the non-HIV population: from asymptomatic dipstick haemo-proteinuria in early IgA or mesangial proliferative lesions, to nephrotic syndrome in membranous nephropathy, to hypertension and rapidly progressive renal failure in crescentic proliferative disease.

Patients with HIV are frequently hypergammaglobulinaemic, and circulating immune complexes can be detected in the majority of patients. Immune complexes eluted from biopsy material of patients with ICKD have confirmed the presence of HIV antigens such as p24 within the kidney, and it is likely that HIV represents the primary pathogenic factor in some cases [14]. However, ICKD may precede acquisition of HIV (e.g. IgA disease, lupus nephritis) or may be precipitated by factors other than the HIV (e.g. hepatitis B and C, other opportunistic infections or drugs), meaning a careful evaluation is required to formulate the most appropriate management plan.

31.2.4.1 HIV Immune Complex Kidney Disease (HIVICK)

The term HIVICK has been used to describe a unique histological pattern observed in HIV, characterised predominantly by mesangial hyperplasia with mesangial and sub-epithelial immune deposits, with features intermediate between post-infectious and incompletely expressed membranous glomerulopathies [15]. Sub-epithelial deposits may be large and produce a characteristic 'ball in cup' appearance on light and electron microscopy, while immunohistochemistry shows variable staining of deposits for IgA, IgM, IgG and C3. Lack of consensus when classifying HIV ICKD in studies has limited understanding of the clinical characteristics and natural history of this lesion and, indeed, of whether it represents a discrete disease entity.

31.2.4.2 Lupus-Like Nephritis

Several small studies have described cases of ICKD in HIV resembling lupus nephritis with 'full house' immunoglobulin and complement deposits (including C1q), but in the absence of serological evidence of SLE. Histological features overlap those of HIVICK but frequently include prominent sub-endothelial deposits (sometimes forming 'wire loops') and diffuse or focal endocapillary proliferation. Patients are typically nephritic with microscopic haematuria and marked renal impairment at presentation. Lupus-like nephritis is associated with a high incidence of ESKD by 1 year of diagnosis.

31.2.4.3 Treatment

Management should begin with careful consideration of alternative causes for an immune complex lesion beyond HIV per se which may direct specific treatment (Table 31.3).

No controlled trials have examined specific treatment strategies in HIV ICKD. While initiation of cART has been reported to retard or reverse ICKD in published case reports, cohort studies do not robustly demonstrate a benefit. Such studies have featured small numbers or considered ICKD grouped with other miscellaneous non-HIVAN disease, preventing identification of ICKD sub-groups which may potentially benefit from control of replication. In light of data supporting a pathogenic role for HIV in some cases of ICKD, and the prevailing immune dysregulation attributable to disease, most physicians would currently start cART on diagnosis regardless of CD4 count or viral load (VL).

Other immunomodulatory drugs, including corticosteroids, have not been systematically tested in this area.

31.2.5 Tubulointerstitial Pathology

Tubulointerstitial disease encountered in HIV includes acute tubular injury, frequently attributable to drugs or ischaemic injury consequent on infection, tubulointerstitial nephritis (TIN), drug crystallopathy or functional tubular abnormalities such as that seen with TDF (▫ Table 31.4).

A broad range of conditions may incite acute or chronic tubulointerstitial inflammation in HIV including drug exposures, opportunistic infection, neoplasia and certain specific immune dyscrasias (▫ Table 31.4). Clinical assignment of disease to the tubulointerstitial compartment is often difficult as patients frequently exhibit heavy proteinuria (>1 g/day) and microscopic haematuria, even in the absence of a discernible glomerular lesion [16]. The classic triad of fever, rash and pyuria seen with drug-induced acute TIN is rare in the context of HIV, although peripheral eosinophilia is frequent [16]. Diagnosis of TIN in HIV requires careful consideration of the prevailing degree of immunodeficiency, temporal relationship to drug exposures and work-up for systemic disease present in other organ systems to ensure the correct treatment is instigated.

31.2.6 Diffuse Infiltrative Lymphocytosis Syndrome (DILS)

DILS is a Sjögren-like multi-system disorder of HIV characterised by oligoclonal CD8+ T cell expansion and consequent organ infiltration [17]. Affected individuals may be of any ethnicity or gender, often present some years after HIV diagnosis and, although viraemic, typically have preserved CD4 cell counts and a low incidence of opportunistic infection. DILS incidence has fallen markedly in the post-cART era suggesting a protective effect of viral suppression. Parotid enlargement, often accompanied by sicca symptoms, is almost universal, while extra-glandular disease may include lymphadenopathy, lymphocytic interstitial pneumonitis, cranial or peripheral neuropathies, hepatitis and renal involvement. Renal disease manifests as florid tubulointerstitial infiltration of CD8+ T cells with progressive renal impairment and subsequent fibrosis if untreated. Treatment should include instigation or optimisation of cART to attain viral suppression, theoretically diminishing the stimulus for CD8+ T cell proliferation. Most clinicians will also use adjunctive corticosteroids in the presence of significant renal disease.

▫ **Table 31.4** Differential diagnosis of tubulointerstitial inflammation in HIV

Cause	Clinical or histological pointers to diagnosis
Drugs	
Anti-microbials (e.g. Septrin, rifampicin, β-lactams) Antiretrovirals (abacavir, indinavir) General, e.g. NSAIDs, PPIs	Temporal relationship to drug introduction Clinical response to drug withdrawal Fever and rash unusual, eosinophilia common Often eosinophil infiltrate on biopsy Chronic scarring inflammation and leucocyturia with indinavir
Bacterial infection	
Mycobacterial disease	May be signs of extra-renal disease (e.g. pulmonary infiltrates, lymphadenopathy); granulomatous inflammation on biopsy; specific mycobacterial stains and PCR may be negative despite active disease
Ascending urinary tract infection	Positive urine cultures; neutrophil-rich infiltrate in acute infection with tubular casts
Viral infection	
CMV Adenovirus EBV BK virus (rare in HIV)	CD4 often <100; extra-renal disease may be evident (e.g. retinitis, pneumonitis with CMV); viral inclusion bodies often seen on biopsy and specific immunohistochemistry or in situ hybridisation for viral nucleic acids are diagnostic
Fungal and parasitic infections	
Cryptococcus *Candida* Microsporidia	Occur in conjunction with disseminated disease in the context of severe immunodeficiency (CD4 <100)
Lymphoma	Often extra-renal disease (e.g. lymphadenopathy); infiltrating lymphocytes atypical in morphology
HIVAN	Associated microcystic tubular dilatation, typical collapsing glomerular lesion usually evident
Immune disorders of HIV	
DILS	Parotid enlargement; CD4 often >200; CD8-dominant lymphocytic infiltrate
IRIS	Recent introduction of cART; usually underlying mycobacterial infection; often granulomatous inflammation with CD4+ lymphocytic infiltrate

NSAID non-steroidal anti-inflammatory drugs, *PPI* proton pump inhibitors, *PCR* polymerase chain reaction, *EBV* Epstein-Barr virus, *DILS* diffuse infiltrative lymphocytosis syndrome, *IRIS* immune reconstitution inflammatory syndrome

31.2.7 Immune Reconstitution Inflammatory Syndrome (IRIS)

IRIS describes a syndrome of 'paradoxical' organ inflammation seen while adaptive immunity recovers during antiretroviral treatment, targeted most frequently against residual or occult infectious antigens [18]. Clinical presentation largely corresponds to target organs involved by the inciting infection (e.g. ocular disease with CMV, pneumonitis with pneumocystis) where disease appears to worsen after initial improvement with anti-microbials. Affected patients typically have low (<50 cells/μl) CD4 counts when cART is initiated with rapid viral suppression and immune reconstitution; median time of presentation in the largest retrospective cohort was 46 days [19]. While as many as 30% of patients experience some form of IRIS, renal involvement is rare and largely reported in the context of mycobacterial infection. Histology shows a tubulointerstitial mononuclear cell infiltrate, which may be granulomatous, with CD4+ T cells predominating. cART can usually be continued in such circumstances with addition of oral corticosteroids, which may be tapered after robust clinical improvement. Anti-microbial therapy should be continued if active infection persists.

31.3 Renal Complications of Antiretroviral Therapy

The widespread use of cART has revolutionised outcomes in HIV, but with it has come a broad range of adverse effects including renal toxicities. Certain ARVs such as rilpivirine, cobicistat, ritonavir and dolutegravir inhibit tubular secretion of creatinine, leading to a predictable and benign rise in serum creatinine and fall in eGFR, which may result in misdiagnosis of CKD if not taken into account. This phenomenon is characterised by a 'step change' in serum creatinine within 1 month of starting therapy, without other evidence of renal disease (e.g. proteinuria) or further progressive rise in creatinine over time. Drug interactions between ARVs and other medications are common, and it is essential to make careful checks when prescribing. The Liverpool HIV Drug Interactions checker is a comprehensive and useful tool for this purpose (▶ https://www.hiv-druginteractions.org/). Renally excreted ARVs like zidovudine and lamivudine need careful dose monitoring and adjustment in a patient with CKD.

Three drugs have received most attention as potential nephrotoxins: TDF, indinavir and atazanavir. All three have been associated with an increased risk of developing CKD in a recent large European cohort study, and periodic monitoring for emergence of kidney disease should be performed in all patients on cART [20].

31.3.1 Indinavir

Nephrolithiasis is a common and well-recognised side effect of the now scarcely used protease inhibitor (PI) indinavir, with crystalluria present in up to 65% of patients. Manifestations include classical renal colic with radiolucent stones, a syndrome of flank pain and dysuria in the absence of discrete calculi and a more sinister insidious scarring tubulointerstitial nephritis associated with persistent pyuria and driven by intra-parenchymal crystallisation. Nephrolithiasis can in part be combated by maintenance of good oral water intake (>1.5 L/day), while persistent leucocyturia or new renal impairment should prompt discontinuation.

31.3.2 Atazanavir

Atazanavir is a well-tolerated and commonly used once daily PI. Like indinavir, it has the potential to crystallise and form calculi albeit much less frequently (around 1%). Granulomatous tubulo-interstitial nephritis with atazanavir is correspondingly rare but well-recognised, and a low threshold for discontinuation should be applied in the event that eGFR declines. In contrast, the second-generation PI darunavir has not been linked to renal dysfunction.

31.3.3 TDF

TDF is an acyclic nucleotide reverse transcriptase inhibitor (NtRTI) with activity against both HIV and hepatitis B virus, frequently used in first-line cART regimens. Biochemical features of toxicity are those of a partial or complete Fanconi syndrome, variably comprising glycosuria, phosphaturia, hypouricaemia, aminoaciduria, renal tubular acidosis and low molecular weight proteinuria. Reduced eGFR is a variable finding and may reflect reversible impairment of tubular creatinine secretion, AKI or established CKD with persistent severe toxicity. Risk factors for tenofovir toxicity include older age, lower BMI, prior CKD and use of other nephrotoxic medications. Concomitant use of the NRTI didanosine may enhance tenofovir toxicity and is not recommended, while ritonavir-boosted protease inhibitor regimens have also been associated with increased tenofovir plasma levels and toxicity, requiring vigilance when used [21].

Mild toxicity is frequently asymptomatic, but manifestations of severe injury include osteomalacia with bone pain (consequence of phosphate wasting) or AKI. Renal biopsy in AKI reveals acute proximal tubular damage with giant and misshapen mitochondria on electron microscopy, suggesting this organelle as the primary target for toxicity.

31

Table 31.5 Schema for monitoring of proximal tubular function during TDF therapy (adapted from Hall et al. and European Aids Clinical Society Guidelines)

Screening tests	Frequency
1. eGFR 2. Urine protein/creatinine ratio 3. Urine glucose 4. Urinary fractional excretion of phosphate[a] 5. Tubular proteinuria (e.g. retinol-binding protein)[b]	Baseline 3 monthly for 1 year Twice-yearly thereafter
Additional survey for proximal renal tubulopathy if any of 1–5 abnormal: Serum bicarbonate and urinary pH (bicarbonate <21 and urinary pH >5.5 suggest RTA[c]) Urinary fractional excretion of uric acid (abnormal >0.1 on a fasted morning spot urine sample) Serum potassium and urinary potassium excretion Consider DEXA scan if evidence of renal phosphate wasting	
Consider stopping if: Significant and sustained changes in 1–4 Syndrome of proximal renal tubulopathy with no other cause Progressive deterioration in tubular proteinuria	

[a]Abnormal >0.2 (>0.1 if serum phosphate <0.8 mmol/L). Monitoring fractional excretion of phosphate is preferable to serum phosphate, as hypophosphataemia may be a late event and accompanied by established bone demineralisation. It is important to exclude vitamin D deficiency which may provoke phosphaturia through secondary hyperparathyroidism

[b]Retinol-binding protein (RBP) is a low molecular weight protein, freely filtered by the glomerulus and reabsorbed in the proximal tubule. Elevated levels reflect proximal tubular dysfunction and may be grossly deranged in tenofovir toxicity

[c]Urinary pH may still fall below 5.5 in proximal RTA as distal urinary acidification mechanisms remain intact. An elevated urinary pH in the context of systemic acidaemia would however suggest a renal acidosis

Tenofovir-induced proximal tubular dysfunction is typically reversible if detected promptly and the drug withdrawn. Monitoring eGFR and urinalysis alone are insufficient and must be combined with more specific tests of proximal tubular function (see Table 31.5).

In 2017, tenofovir alafenamide (TAF) was approved for the treatment of HIV. A prodrug of tenofovir, TAF's conversion to its active form occurs largely intracellularly resulting in much lower blood levels and improved renal and bone safety parameters compared to TDF. TAF's safety remains to be proven in patients with previous or current TDF-induced tubulopathy. NHS England has commissioned TAF for use in patients with chronic kidney disease (defined as CKD stage G3, or stage G2 with A3 proteinuria) where abacavir is not a suitable alternative.

31.4 Hepatitis C

31.4.1 Epidemiology

The global prevalence of hepatitis C (HCV) is vast with an estimated 71.1 million infected individuals (1%) in 2015 and a particularly high prevalence in Asia, the Middle East and North Africa (Fig. 31.2). Since the discovery of the virus in 1988, reports rapidly emerged of associated renal disease as well as cryoglobulinaemia, Sjögren's syndrome and lymphoproliferative disorders. The association with cryoglobulinaemia is particularly striking with evidence of type II (monoclonal IgM to polyclonal IgG) or type III (polyclonal IgM to polyclonal IgG) cryoglobulinaemia observed in 20–56% of those with hepatitis C, while 90% of all type II cryoglobulinaemia is attributable to HCV. Cryoglobulinaemia tends to be a late presentation of HCV, however, and curiously only a minority (≤25%) of those patients who develop cryoglobulinaemia develop overt renal disease. HCV can also affect the kidney in the absence of cryoglobulinaemia with immune deposits often detectable within the kidney even in the absence of overt disease [22].

The natural history of HCV is variable. It is estimated that 5–40% of adults infected with HCV clear the virus spontaneously. Spontaneous clearance is almost always within the first 6 months after infection and rarely occurs after the first year. Of those with chronic infection, 20–30% will progress to end-stage liver disease in 20–30 years' time.

31.4.2 Clinical Presentation

HCV-associated renal disease tends to present in the fifth and sixth decades and in the setting of chronic infection. There are a variety of renal pathologies associated with hepatitis C (see ▶ Box 31.1) with clinical manifestations determined by the renal lesion. Typical presentations are with microscopic haematuria and proteinuria with renal impairment, but rapidly progressive glomerulonephritis (RPGN), AKI and nephrotic syndrome can also occur. Patients with cryoglobulinaemia-related renal disease may present with signs or symptoms of extra-renal vasculitis such as arthralgia, abdominal pain (mesenteric vasculitis), purpura or neuropathy.

Polyclonal hypergammaglobulinaemia is common, with low complement C4, C1q and CH50 and variably depressed C3. Detectable cryoglobulinaemia is present in 60–70%, with the presence of rheumatoid factor and low complement C4 being a strong surrogate marker.

It is important to note that hepatitis C antibody (Ab) assays can produce false negatives particularly in patients with renal failure, cryoglobulinaemia or immu-

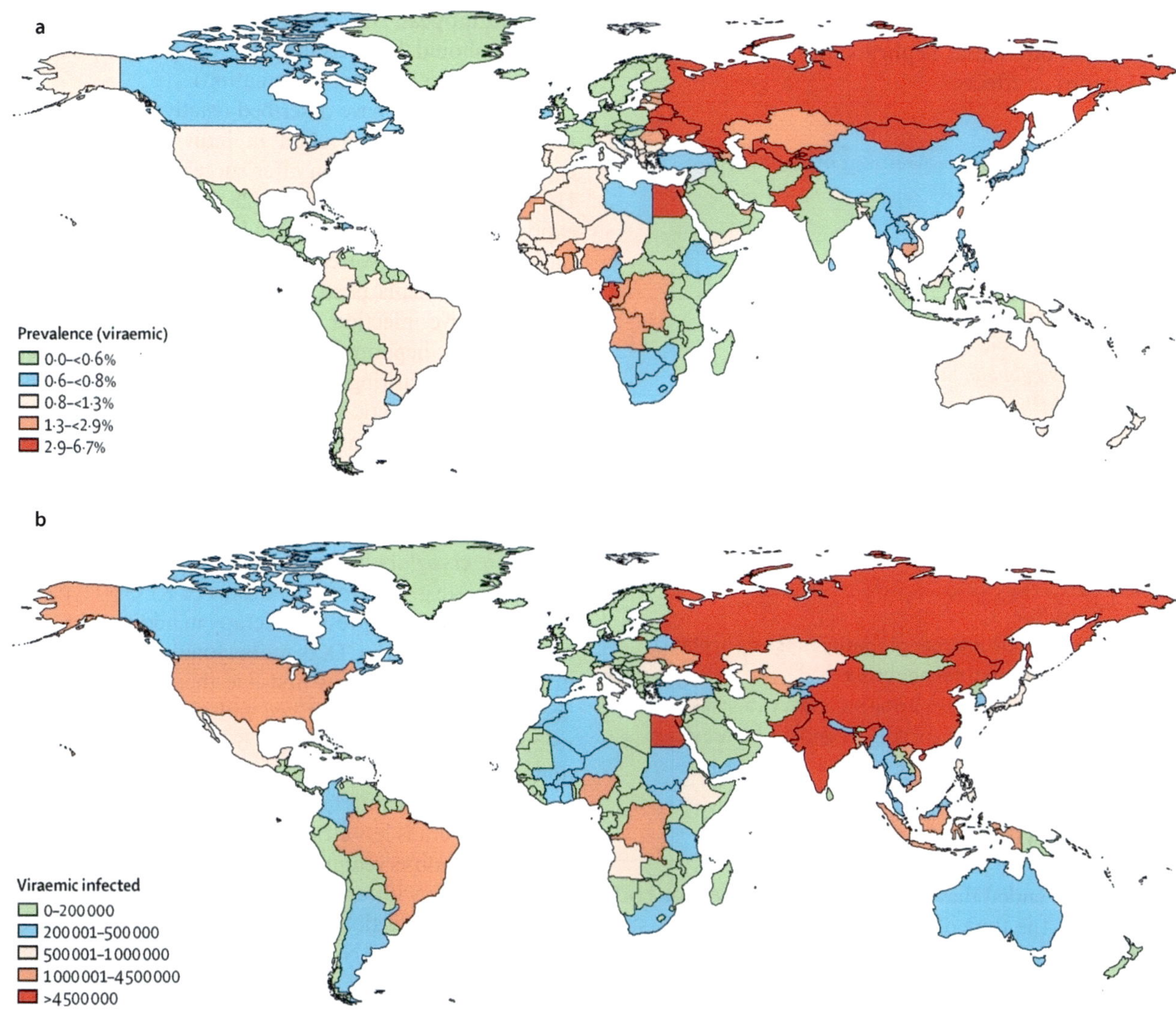

Fig. 31.2 Prevalence of hepatitis C worldwide in 2015. Prevalence of viraemic people by country **a** and absolute number of viraemic individuals **b**. (Reproduced with permission from Blach et al. [23])

nosuppression [24]. Where there is a high index of suspicion for HCV infection and the HCV-Ab test is negative, an HCV RNA test should be carried out.

31.4.3 Pathology

The predominant renal lesion in HCV is membranoproliferative glomerulonephritis (MPGN) which can also occur independently of detectable cryoglobulinaemia. Other glomerular lesions such as interstitial nephritis and necrotising small vessel vasculitis (especially in association with cryoglobulinaemia) have all been reported [25, 26] (see ▶ Box 31.1). The finding of membranous glomerulonephritis should prompt consideration of hepatocellular carcinoma (sought by checking α-fetoprotein and liver imaging). Lymphoma may develop in up to 10% of patients with cryoglobulinaemia and rarely may present as minimal change nephropathy.

It has been difficult to detect HCV antigens histologically in renal lesions, and a direct role of HCV antigens in renal disease is unproven. MPGN is usually associated with deposition of IgM, IgG and C3 in the mesangium and capillary walls. Electron microscopy is important in establishing the diagnosis by demonstrating sub-endothelial deposits and may also reveal cryoglobulin deposition. Fibrillary and immunotactoid glomerulonephritis, although rare, have both been documented with HCV and again emphasise the importance of electron microscopy in the assessment. Crescentic nephritis can occur in the setting of underlying MPGN or in the context of a necrotising vasculitis (usually cryoglobulin associated) or fibrillary GN. Thrombotic microangiopathy has been reported (predominantly post-transplant), and hepatitis C is an infrequent cause of isolated interstitial nephritis, possibly due to direct viral cytotoxic effects. .

Box 31.1 Renal Involvement in Hepatitis C

Glomerular

Cryoglobulin positive
- MPGN
- Fibrillary
- Immunotactoid
- Amyloid

Cryoglobulin negative
- MPGN
- Membranous GN (exclude hepatocellular carcinoma)
- FSGS
- Mesangial deposits
- Amyloid (if associated with IV or SC drug abuse)

Vasculitic

Thrombotic microangiopathy (post-transplant)

Tubulointerstitial nephritis
- Interstitial nephritis secondary to virus
- Interstitial nephritis secondary to interferon

31

31.4.4 Treatment and Outcome

It is recommended that all patients are screened for HCV infection at the time of initial evaluation of CKD, start of dialysis or evaluation of kidney transplantation using a hepatitis C antibody immunoassay, followed by ribonucleic acid testing (HCV RNA) if the immunoassay is positive. All patients with HCV-associated renal disease or any CKD patient found to be infected with HCV on screening should be evaluated for antiviral therapy.

Treatment of HCV previously consisted of pegylated interferon and ribavirin with poor efficacy and high adverse event rates in CKD. This was contraindicated after renal transplantation due to the increased risk of rejection or direct nephrotoxicity.

The advent of direct-acting antivirals (DAAs) has heralded a major breakthrough in HCV treatment, with close to 100% cure rates and mild and infrequent side effects. The latest KDIGO guidelines [27] recommend using an interferon-free regimen chosen in consultation with a hepatologist and tailored to HCV genotype, viral load, previous treatment history, drug interactions, GFR, stage of hepatic fibrosis, kidney or liver transplant candidacy and overall comorbidities. With the emergence of third-generation pan-genotypic DAAs, guidelines are simplifying. Both the American Association for the Study of Liver Diseases (AASLD) and the European Association for the Study of the Liver (EASL) should be consulted for the most up-to-date information (see patient information).

Several reports have described reactivation of hepatitis B virus (HBV) infection in individuals previously exposed to HBV infection after successful treatment for HCV with DAA-based therapy [28, 29]. Markers of HBV exposure or active infection should be assessed before initiation of HCV DAA treatment, particularly in immunosuppressed patients post-renal transplantation. Patients without active infection of HBV but evidence of prior exposure (e.g. hepatitis B core antibody positive) should be actively monitoring for HBV reactivation using HBV DNA and liver function tests every 12 weeks during DAA therapy and for 6 months thereafter. Patients with active HBV infection not on treatment should also be monitored for rising viral loads or abnormal liver function tests which may indicate HBV treatment initiation.

Severe cryoglobulinaemia or HCV-associated glomerular disease (e.g. nephrotic syndrome or RPGN) typically requires immunosuppressive therapy in addition to DAA treatment. The anti-CD20 monoclonal antibody rituximab is recommended as first-line therapy by KDIGO, and is commonly co-prescribed with corticosteroids. This recommendation is supported by data from two randomised controlled trials of rituximab combination therapy with pegylated interferon-alpha. The role of rituximab in the DAA era is less clear, with rapid reductions in vasculitis scores observed in prospective observational studies of patients with cryoglobulinaemic vasculitis treated with DAA therapy alone [30]. While paradoxical flares of cryoglobulinaemic GN were often reported in the interferon era, this appears rare with DAAs, and the current consensus is that antiviral treatment should not be delayed. Antiproteinuric agents such as ACEi/ARBs should be used along with other antihypertensive drugs and diuretics where appropriate to achieve the recommended blood pressure targets for patients with CKD.

Survival in HCV-infected patients with ESKD on dialysis is reduced compared to kidney transplant recipients. DAAs allow for successful clearance of HCV in nearly all patients before and after transplantation; therefore, all eligible HCV-infected ESKD patients should be considered for transplantation. The use of DAAs in kidney transplant recipients requires careful consideration and monitoring due to potential drug interactions with immunosuppressive agents used in transplantation. As most of these agents are metabolised via the cytochrome P450 pathway in the liver, substrate competition can occur with DAAs which undergo the same metabolic pathway. The 'HEP Drug Interactions' website is a useful resource for the latest guidance on potential drug interactions with DAAs (▸ https://www.hep-druginteractions.org).

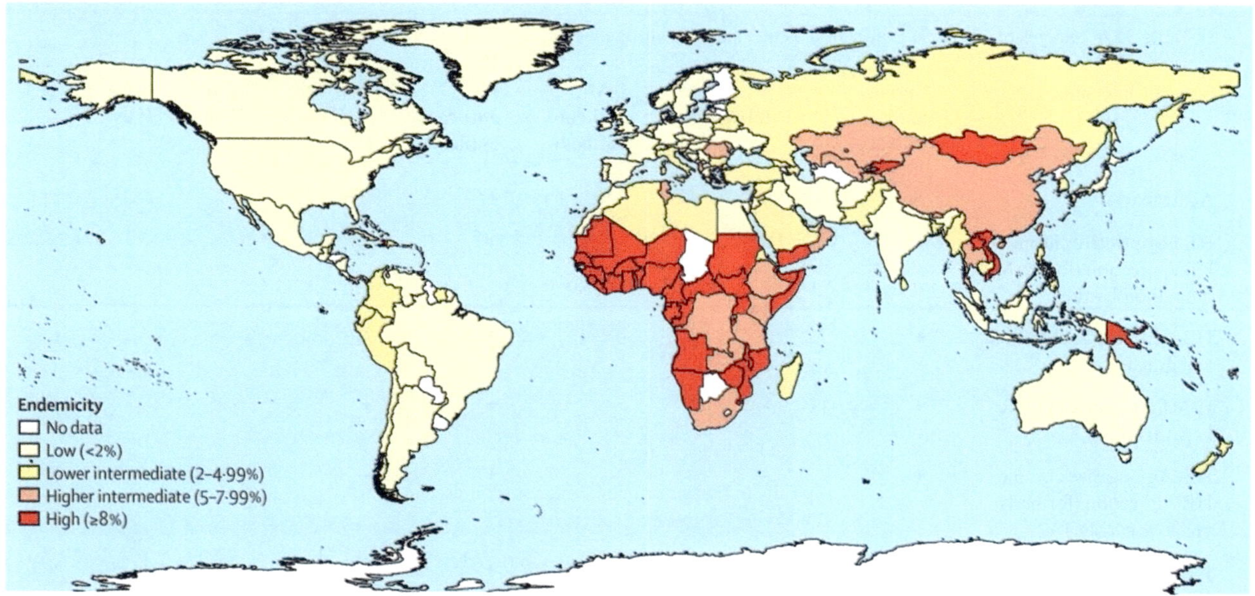

Fig. 31.3 Global endemicity of HBV from 1957 to 2013. (Reproduced with permission from Schweitzer et al. [31])

31.5 Hepatitis B

31.5.1 Epidemiology

Approximately 257 million people are chronically infected with hepatitis B virus (HBV) worldwide exceeding the prevalence even of HCV (see Fig. 31.3). In Africa, exposure to HBV is approaching 100%, and (depending on age of exposure) roughly 10% go on to develop chronic disease, and of these, 3% develop nephropathy.

Table 31.6 shows the relationship between the different phases of disease and the serological tests, HBV DNA levels and serum ALT.

31.5.2 Clinical Manifestations

Renal involvement secondary to HBV can manifest in a variety of ways (see ▶ Box 31.2), most commonly as a membranous glomerulonephritis and less frequently MPGN [32]. Membranous GN is much more common in children and has a marked male predominance which is unexplained. Presentation may be with nephrotic range proteinuria, oedema and less commonly hypertension with renal impairment. A history of clinically overt hepatitis is rare in children. In children, the prognosis is good with most cases resolving spontaneously, but this appears less likely to happen in adults unless viraemia is suppressed. Remission of membranous GN seems to correlate well with the disappearance of HBV e antigenaemia [33].

Complement levels may be low in both MPGN and membranous GN. Cryoglobulinaemia is much less common than with hepatitis C but does rarely occur and can be associated with MPGN.

In addition to these well-recognised presentations of chronic HBV infection, serum sickness (arthralgia, fever, rash (maculopapular), malaise, acute hepatitis) can develop at the time of seroconversion and may come to the attention of the nephrologist if accompanied by microscopic haematuria and proteinuria.

The other unusual presentation of HBV infection is polyarteritis nodosa (PAN) which occurs in a tiny proportion of patients recently infected, possibly as a result of self-antigen mimicry (there have been case reports of PAN following HBV vaccination). The French Vasculitis Study Group reviewed the clinical findings of 384 patients with PAN presenting over a 30-year period of which 123 patients had HBV-associated PAN [34]. They noted 66% of patients had renal involvement which was universally an ANCA-negative medium vessel vasculitis and no patients in this cohort had glomerulonephritis. HBV-associated PAN was frequently accompanied by neuropathy, orchitis and hypertension. It is worth noting that even with the use of antivirals, this group had a mortality of 34% (which was worse than non-HBV-associated PAN), with age >65, hypertension and abdominal pain being adverse prognostic indicators.

Table 31.6 Stages of hepatitis B infection as measured by antigenaemia, antibodies, viral DNA and ALT

Stage of infection	Surface antigen (HBsAg)	'e' antigen (HBeAg)	IgM anti-core antibody	IgG anti-core antibody	Hepatitis B virus DNA	Anti-HBe	Anti-HBs	ALT
Acute (early)	+	+	+[a]	+/–	++	–	–	↑↑↑
HBeAg-positive chronic HBV infection (formerly 'immunotolerant')	+	+	–	+	++	–	–	N[b]
HBeAg-positive chronic hepatitis B	+	+	–	+	+	–	–	↑
HBeAg-negative chronic hepatitis B	+	–	–	+	+	+	–	↑
HBeAg-negative chronic HBV infection (formerly 'inactive carrier')	+	–	–	+	–	+	–	N
HBsAg-negative phase (formerly 'resolved' or 'immune')	–	–	–	+	–	+/–	+/–	N
HBsAg vaccination	–	–	–	–	–	–	+	N

[a]In very early infection, the IgM anti-core can be negative and by definition so can the IgG
[b]*N* = normal

31

Box 31.2 Renal Involvement in Hepatitis B

Glomerular

Cryoglobulin negative

Membranous GN

MPGN

Mesangial proliferation (with serum sickness)

IgA

Cryoglobulin positive

MPGN

Vasculitic

Polyarteritis nodosa

Treatment related

Proximal tubular dysfunction/Fanconi syndrome secondary to tenofovir

31.5.3 Pathology

There seems to be a strong association between HBV e antigenaemia and membranous GN, whereas both HBV e and s antigens are thought to contribute to the aetiopathology of MPGN. The appearance of hepatitis B-associated membranous GN is similar to idiopathic disease, but atypical features such as mesangial expansion may be present. With HBV-associated membranous nephropathy, MPGN or IgA, it may be possible to detect hepatitis B antigens by immunostaining or PCR, and this may help to distinguish between primary and secondary GN.

31.5.4 Treatment and Outcome

Antiviral treatment represents the cornerstone of therapy in HBV-associated renal disease. The KDIGO guidelines recommend that patients with HBV-associated renal disease should be treated according to standard treatment guidelines. Interferon (IFN) and nucleoside analogues (NA) (lamivudine, emtricitabine, telbivudine and entecavir (ETC)) and nucleotide analogues (adefovir and tenofovir) all have activity against HBV. Finite (48 weeks) treatment with IFN-alpha is associated with consistently higher anti-HBe seroconversion than with NAs at 1 year, but similar rates of eAg seroconversion at 5 years. However, IFN is contraindicated in patients with decompensated cirrhosis, autoimmune disease and uncontrolled severe depression or psychosis. It has greater efficacy in certain HBV genotypes (A/B) and in younger patients with high degrees of liver necro-inflammation and lower viral loads. It is also poorly tolerated and carries a risk of rejection in renal

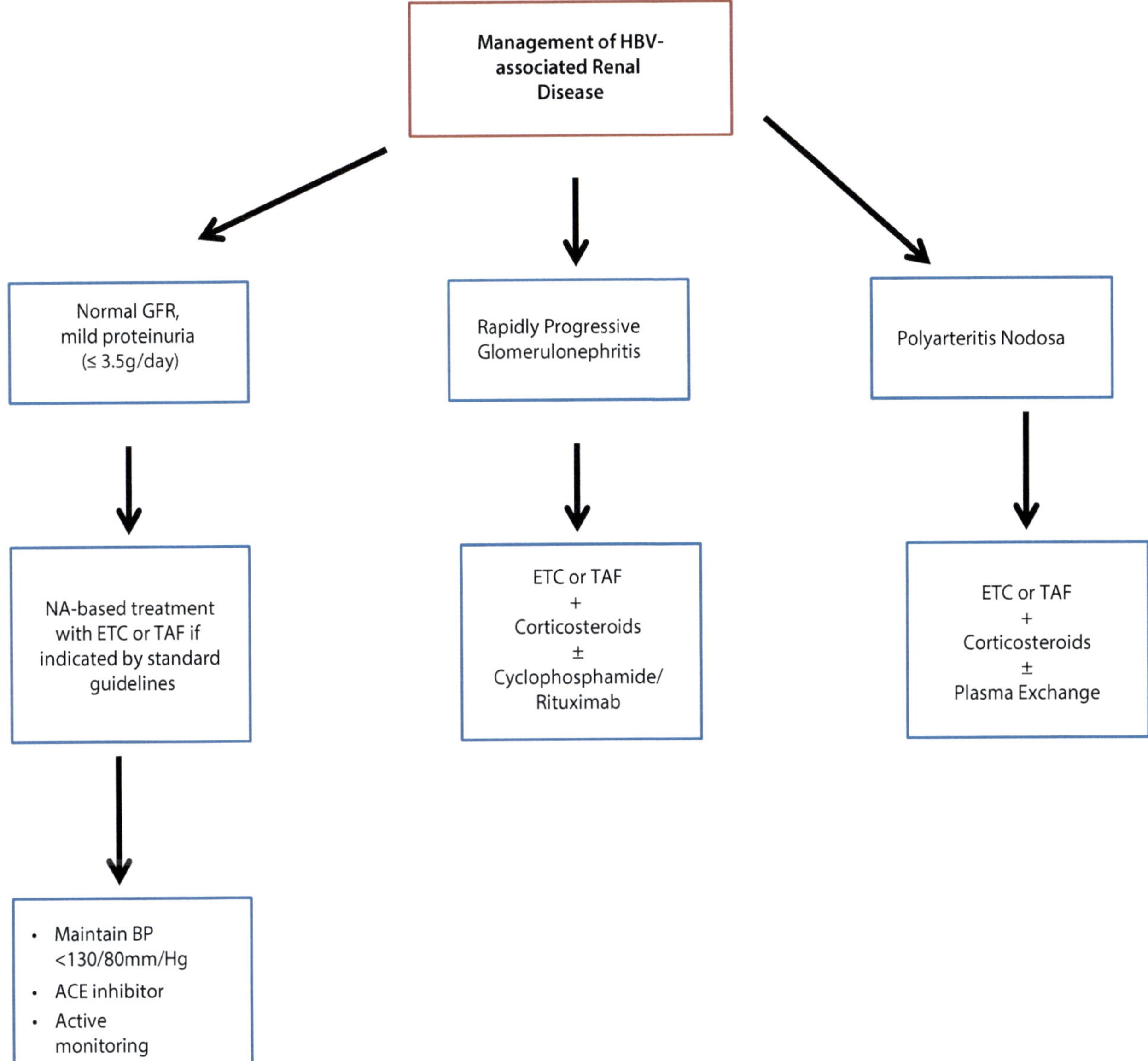

Fig. 31.4 Treatment of HBV-associated renal disease. ETC entecavir, NA nucleoside analogue, TAF tenofovir alafenamide. (Adapted from Pipili et al. [37])

transplant recipients. The nucleoside analogues lamivudine, emtricitabine and telbivudine all have a low genetic barrier to resistance and therefore should be avoided as monotherapy. Adefovir and tenofovir disoproxil fumarate (TDF) have both been associated with Fanconi syndrome and cumulative renal toxicity. Minimising consequences of HBV infection is of paramount importance, and NAs with a high genetic barrier to HBV resistance are typically the best options for HBV-positive patients with CKD. Tenofovir alafenamide (TAF) is a novel prodrug of tenofovir with superior absorption to tenofovir disoproxil fumarate (TDF) and can be administered at approximately tenfold lower doses with similar bioavailability for tenofovir in hepatocytes. TAF-based treatment has been approved in HIV patients with renal impairment. Prospective randomised studies of TAF versus TDF in hepatitis B monoinfection have reported lower rises in creatinine in the TAF group at 2 years [35].

The indication for treatment in HBsAg-positive patients is determined by viral load, the presence or absence of liver inflammation (as determined by aminotransferases and/or biopsy), the stage of liver disease (determined by liver biopsy or non-invasive fibrosis assessment) and risk factors for hepatocellular carcinoma (HCC). Thresholds for initiation of treatment according to these criteria change frequently, and the latest American Association for the Study of Liver Diseases (AASLD), the European Association for the Study of the Liver (EASL) or the Asian Pacific Association for the Study of the Liver (APASL) should be consulted.

The goal of treatment is to lower the risk of liver fibrosis progression and/or HCC through sustained suppression of viral replication. HBsAg seroconversion and HBV DNA clearance is the ideal result but rarely achieved, and suppression of virus replication (with or without eAg seroconversion) is often sufficient to induce proteinuria remission with preservation of renal function. Nucelos(t)ide therapy may need to be lifelong for many patients regardless of the presence of renal disease, although finite therapy may be possible for patients who achieve HBsAg or HBeAg loss and anti-HBe seroconversion [36]. EASL guidelines (2017) recommend the use of entecavir (if lamivudine naïve) or TAF in HBsAg-positive dialysis patients or transplant recipients. Entecavir requires dose adjustment in patients with an eGFR <50 mL/min. TAF does not require a dose adjustment if eGFR >15 mL/min.

While antiviral monotherapy may be sufficient to treat HBV-associated nephropathy in patients who do not have severe or life-threatening disease, additional treatment strategies are required for those with RPGN and PAN (◘ Fig. 31.4). Corticosteroids with or without cyclophosphamide or rituximab (for suppression of vasculitis) and plasma exchange (for removal of circulating immune complexes) may be useful for improving kidney function and disease manifestations. If immunosuppressive therapy is administered, all HBsAg-positive patients should receive pre-emptive NA therapy, ideally 2 weeks before, during and for at least 6–12 months after completing immunosuppressive therapy.

There is hugely encouraging data showing almost complete eradication of childhood MN secondary to hepatitis B following universal vaccination programmes, and a similar approach to control other infective agents may well have comparable benefits.

31.6 HTLV1 and 2

There are a smattering of case reports of glomerular lesions in patients with HTLV1 and 2 infection including lupus-like nephropathy, TINU and MPGN. It is difficult to be clear if these are genuine associations, and although one might expect glomerular disorders in patients with chronic viraemia, the rarity of these reports given the global prevalence of HTLV infection (3.8% of Japanese dialysis patients) suggests HTLV-associated renal disease is rare.

Case Study

Case 1

A 49-year-old Zimbabwean black African male with no past medical history is diagnosed with HIV-1 infection on first contact with medical services in the UK. He is asymptomatic aside from mild ankle swelling and oral candida noted on examination. His blood pressure is 147/82. Blood tests disclose a creatinine of 170 μmol/L, an albumin of 29 g/L and a urine protein/creatinine ratio of 450 mg/mmol. His CD4 count is 136 cells/μl and HIV viral load 54,000 copies/mL. Urinalysis showed protein 4+, blood 2+ and nil else, while an ultrasound showed bilateral echogenic and enlarged kidneys. A kidney biopsy was performed and revealed collapsing glomerulopathy, accompanied by tubular dilatation with microcysts, characteristic of HIVAN (◘ Fig. 31.5).

In this patient with untreated HIV and advanced immunodeficiency, likely causes for renal disease are direct HIV-mediated renal injury or consequences of immunodeficiency (e.g. renal parenchymal infection). Heavy proteinuria, microscopic haematuria and hypoalbuminaemia all point towards a glomerular locus of disease. While the diagnosis in this instance was HIVAN, HIV immune complex kidney disease (ICKD) may present almost identically, and the two entities can only be separated on renal biopsy. Both HIVAN and ICKD are indications to start cART, although if significant tubular atrophy and fibrosis are present on biopsy at the time of diagnosis, many patients will continue to progress towards ESKD regardless of viral control.

Case 2

A 72-year-old Ugandan man presents with a 3-month history of lethargy and weight loss. A new diagnosis of HIV is made with a CD4 count of 25 cells/μl and a viral load of 1.1 million copies/mL. At this attendance, serum creatinine was 113 μmol/L and urine protein/creatinine ratio 54 mg/mmol. He was started on cART: tenofovir disoproxil fumarate (TDF), ritonavir-boosted darunavir and lamivudine, with co-trimoxazole for PCP prophylaxis. Six weeks later, he represents with widespread lymphadenopathy, hepatosplenomegaly, fevers and night sweats. CRP was 150 mg/L, creatinine 230 μmol/L with 1+ protein and 1+ blood on urinalysis, corrected calcium level 2.85 mmol/L and repeat CD4 count 150 cells/μl. Bacterial cultures of urine and blood were sterile, while renal ultrasound confirmed normal sized,

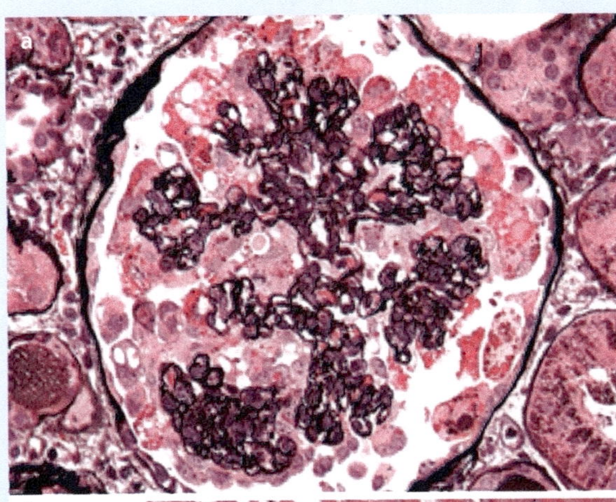

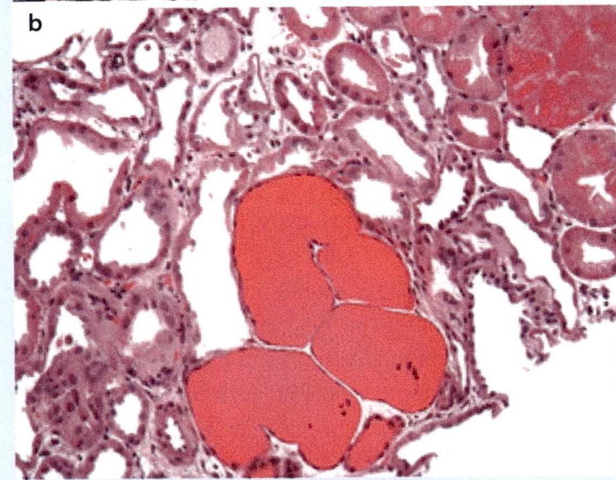

Fig. 31.5 **a** Silver stain of renal biopsy showing a global collapse of capillary loops accompanied by 'pseudocrescent formation' and **b** dilated tubules with microcyst formation

unobstructed kidneys. Serum creatinine failed to fall despite appropriate IV fluid therapy and discontinuation of co-trimoxazole and TDF. A core lymph node biopsy was undertaken and tissue stained positive for acid-fast bacilli with mycobacterium tuberculosis subsequently grown on culture. A kidney biopsy was performed: this showed non-caseating granulomata with acute tubular injury and a CD4 cell-rich interstitial infiltrate (Fig. 31.6).

The patient has developed a renal immune reconstitution inflammatory syndrome (IRIS) in the context of disseminated tuberculosis. IRIS is most commonly seen in individuals presenting with advanced immunodeficiency in whom commencement of cART triggers a rapid increase in CD4 T cell numbers; organ injury corresponds to the location of 'planted' microbial antigen, most commonly mycobacteria in the context of renal disease. This patient should be started on anti-tuberculous chemotherapy together with oral corticosteroids. In most cases, cART can be continued without interruption.

Case 3

A 41-year-old white male presents with rib pain. He was diagnosed with HIV-1 8 years ago and is currently taking TDF, emtricitabine and efavirenz with good viral control. He is also hypertensive taking amlodipine. Blood tests disclose a creatinine 125 μmol/L, urea 6 mmol/L, albumin 45 g/L, phosphate 0.59, CD4 750 cells/μL and viral load <40 copies/mL. His urine protein/creatinine ratio was 95 mg/mmol and an albumin/creatinine ratio was 12 mg/mmol. A urine dip showed protein 1+, glucose + and nil else. An X-ray revealed a pseudo-fracture (Looser's zone) in his scapula, suggestive of osteomalacia (Fig. 31.7).

This patient has developed hypophosphataemia, glycosuria and presumed low molecular weight proteinuria (evidenced by the elevated uPCR and near-normal uACR) consistent with Fanconi syndrome. The most likely culprit in this scenario is TDF. Inhibition of mitochondrial DNA replication in proximal tubular cells may be involved in the pathogenesis of TDF-induced nephropathy. Hypophosphataemia results from renal phosphate wasting and leads to osteomalacia with bone pain and pseudo-fractures in the most severe cases. TDF-induced tubulopathy has been reported in both patients with normal and impaired baseline renal function. A decline in renal function frequently precedes overt toxicity (perhaps due to the consequent increase in blood tenofovir levels), and other risk factors include white ethnicity, older age and co-administration with a ritonavir-boosted protease inhibitor. Patients on TDF require regular checks both of renal function (to pre-empt toxicity in patients with a declining eGFR) and markers of tubular toxicity (particularly uPCR, serum phosphate and urinalysis for glycosuria). Patients on TDF should be switched to TAF-based cART if they develop evidence of renal impairment, hypophosphataemia or accelerated bone-density loss.

Case 4

A 65-year-old man was referred to the renal unit with an acute onset of severe peripheral oedema. He has a past medical history of diabetes mellitus, hypertension and HCV genotype 1 infection 10 years ago and had received

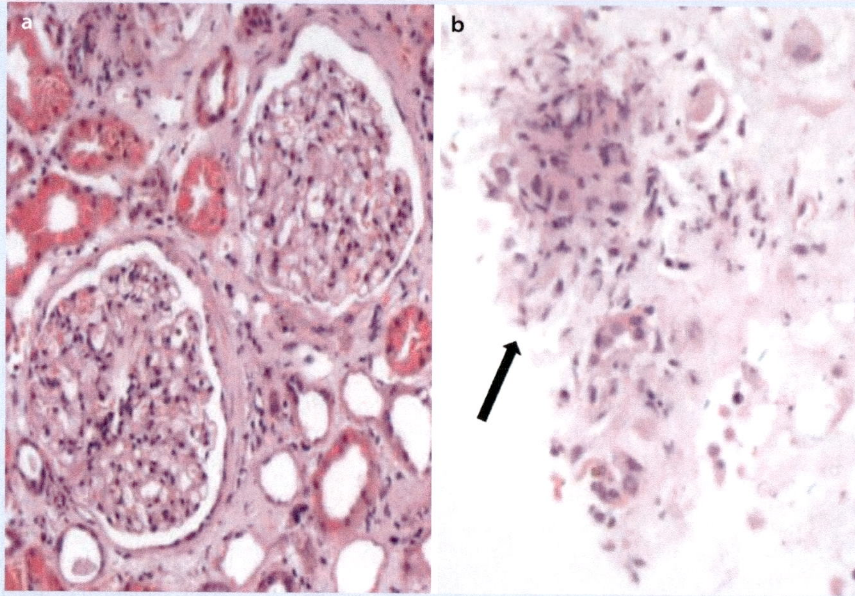

Fig. 31.6 Renal biopsy tissue (haematoxylin and eosin stain). **a** Two representative glomeruli. The upper glomerulus is slightly shrunken, but otherwise morphologically normal. Infiltrating lymphocytes can be seen in the surrounding interstitium. **b** Non-caseating granuloma (shown by arrow)

31

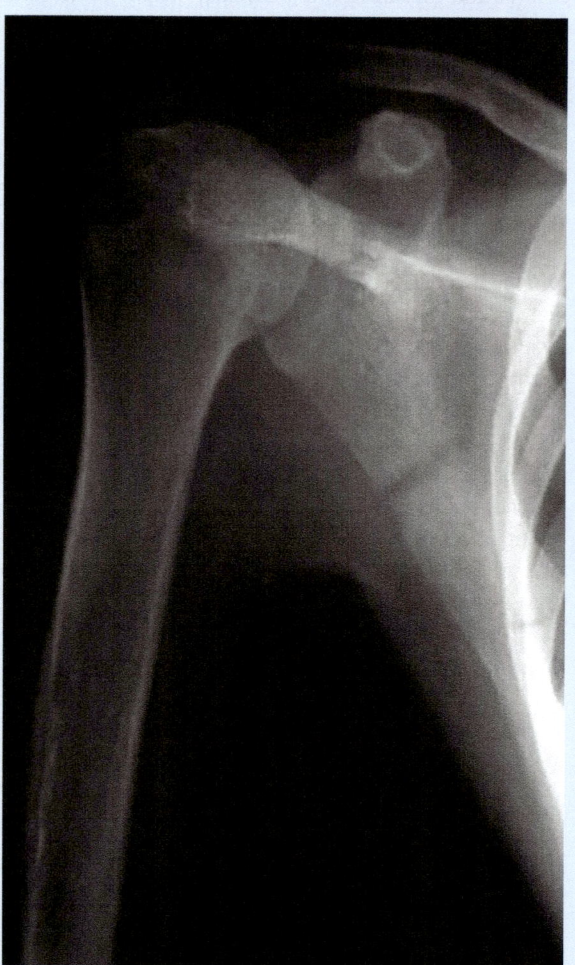

Fig. 31.7 Fracture of the scapula, also known as Looser's zone

pegylated interferon and ribavirin treatment. Treatment was discontinued 1 year later as he developed interferon-induced depression. On examination, he had severe oedema in his extremities but no purpura, arthritis or neuropathy. A urine dip showed blood 3+ and protein 3+; a urine protein/creatinine ratio done was 950 mg/mmol. Blood tests revealed HCV RNA levels of one million IU/L, a creatinine of 370 μmol/L with an eGFR of 15 mL/min/1.73 m^3, hypocomplementaemia with a C3 level of 45 mg/dL and a C4 level of 8 mg/dL, a raised rheumatoid factor, IgM-κ paraproteinemia and cryoglobulinaemia. Subsequent immunoelectrophoresis revealed a type II cryoglobulinaemia with a monoclonal IgM-κ, polyclonal IgG and polyclonal IgA. A kidney biopsy done showed features characteristic of MPGN. Immunofluorescence revealed segmental deposits of IgG, C3, IgM and κ along the glomerular capillary wall. This patient had developed HCV-associated MPGN with a new onset of nephrotic syndrome and rapidly progressive glomerulonephritis. He should be started on a ribavirin-free DAA regimen due to his impaired GFR. As he is heavily nephrotic and developed an acute deterioration in kidney function, the KDIGO guidelines recommend addition of an immunosuppressive therapy, rituximab being first line with or without plasma exchange. The evidence of using plasma exchange is poor, but rapid removal of circulating cryoglobulins could theoretically help prevent further kidney injury. Corticosteroids should also be given in conjunction with rituximab. Renal recovery is possible with clearing of the virus, but he is at high risk of relapse should he have a rare viral relapse (~2%) and should be closely monitored post-DAA treatment so that re-treatment with second-line DAA agents can be initiated if needed.

Tips and Tricks

1. HIVAN only occurs in people of black African or Caribbean ancestry, while HIV immune complex kidney disease may be seen in patients of any ethnicity.
2. The urine dipstick is a poor predictor of the renal 'compartment of injury' (i.e. glomerular or tubulointerstitial) in patients with HIV, meaning a kidney biopsy is often required for concrete diagnosis.
3. Undiagnosed TDF tubular toxicity may present as bone pain and fractures; a new formulation of tenofovir (TAF) is now available which appears to reduce these adverse effects.
4. Direct-acting antivirals (DAAs) have replaced interferon and ribavirin for the first-line treatment of hepatitis C.
5. Consider a diagnosis of hepatocellular carcinoma (liver imaging, serum AFP) in a patient with hepatitis C who develops membranous nephropathy.
6. Nucleoside analogues (NA) with a high genetic barrier to resistance are considered the treatment of choice for HBV in patients with advanced CKD.

31.7 Conclusion

Hepatitis B, hepatitis C and HIV are all major contributors to global renal disease and unrecognised infection should be considered in the diagnostic work of all patients with glomerulonephritis or unexplained AKI or CKD. The mainstay of the treatment of these secondary glomerulonephritides is control or eradication of virus, now eminently achievable with all three viruses, and should be undertaken in collaboration with specialists.

Chapter Review Questions

1. By what mechanism does hepatitis B induce membranous nephropathy?
2. What risk factors predispose to atazanavir-induced renal impairment?
3. Should cART be started on all patients with HIV and an impaired eGFR?

Answers

1. Membranous nephropathy is an immune complex renal disease characterised by the presence of subepithelial deposits seen on immunostaining or electron microscopy examination of the biopsy. In idiopathic disease, the commonest cause is an antibody-antigen reaction between circulating anti-phospholipase A2 receptor (PLA2R) antibody and PLA2R expressed on podocytes in the kidney. In hepatitis B-associated membranous nephropathy, hepatitis B antigens (in particular sAg and eAg) which lodge in the sub-epithelial space of the glomerulus leading to in situ formation of immune complexes are thought to provoke the epithelial cell injury and basement membrane remodelling typical of the disease. Hepatitis B antigens may be detected either by immunostaining or PCR and can help to discriminate between primary and secondary diseases.
2. Atazanavir can cause crystalluria which may induce urolithiasis. Predisposing factors include pre-existing hepatic or renal impairment, alkaline urine, hyperbilirubinaemia (thought to indicate a slower metabolisation of atazanavir) and chronic active hepatitis. The combined use of TDF and atazanavir contributes to a greater decline in eGFR. Atazanavir has also been associated with both acute tubulointerstitial nephritis, where AKI develops rapidly (weeks), and chronic tubulointerstitial nephritis (months to years); the latter may lead to progressive CKD with granulomatous inflammation and intrarenal precipitation of atazanavir crystals seen on biopsy.
3. Yes. While additional investigations (e.g. a kidney biopsy) may be required to determine the precise cause of renal impairment and may direct additional treatments (e.g. corticosteroids in the context of DILS or IRIS), there is no circumstance under which the initiation of cART would be precluded. Since the publication of the START study, showing benefits for initiation of cART even when CD4 cell counts are relatively preserved, there is a broad mandate for starting all newly diagnosed patients on treatment at diagnosis, including those with CKD. Doses of renally excreted ARVs need careful adjustment for eGFR, and those which can potentially cause super-added renal toxicity (e.g. TDF, atazanavir) should be avoided.

References

1. Palella FJ Jr, Delaney KM, Moorman AC, et al. Declining morbidity and mortality among patients with advanced human immunodeficiency virus infection. HIV Outpatient Study Investigators. N Engl J Med. 1998;338:853–60.
2. Li Y, Shlipak MG, Grunfeld C, Choi AI. Incidence and risk factors for acute kidney injury in HIV infection. Am J Nephrol. 2012;35:327–34.
3. Buchacz K, Baker RK, Palella FJ Jr, et al. AIDS-defining opportunistic illnesses in US patients, 1994-2007: a cohort study. AIDS. 2010;24:1549–59.
4. EACS (European AIDS Clinical Society) Guidelines for treatment of HIV infected adults in Europe. 2011. Available at http://www.europeanaidsclinicalsociety.org/images/stories/EACS-Pdf/EACSguidelines-v6.0-English.pdf.

5. Ibrahim F, Naftalin C, Cheserem E, et al. Immunodeficiency and renal impairment are risk factors for HIV-associated acute renal failure. AIDS. 2010;24:2239–44.
6. Tourret J, Deray G, Isnard-Bagnis C. Tenofovir effect on the kidneys of HIV-infected patients: a double-edged sword? J Am Soc Nephrol. 2013;24:1519–27.
7. del Arco A, Martinez MA, Pena JM, et al. Thrombotic thrombocytopenic purpura associated with human immunodeficiency virus infection: demonstration of p24 antigen in endothelial cells. Clin Infect Dis. 1993;17:360–3.
8. Hart D, Sayer R, Miller R, et al. Human immunodeficiency virus associated thrombotic thrombocytopenic purpura--favourable outcome with plasma exchange and prompt initiation of highly active antiretroviral therapy. Br J Haematol. 2011;153:515–9.
9. Post FA, Campbell LJ, Hamzah L, et al. Predictors of renal outcome in HIV-associated nephropathy. Clin Infect Dis. 2008;46:1282–9.
10. Wyatt CM, Meliambro K, Klotman PE. Recent progress in HIV-associated nephropathy. Annu Rev Med. 2012;63:147–59.
11. Genovese G, Friedman DJ, Ross MD, et al. Association of trypanolytic ApoL1 variants with kidney disease in African Americans. Science. 2010;329:841–5.
12. Wearne N, Swanepoel CR, Duffield MS, et al. The effects of add-on corticosteroids on renal outcomes in patients with biopsy proven HIV associated nephropathy: a single centre study from South Africa. BMC Nephrol. 2019;20:44.
13. Gupta SK, Eustace JA, Winston JA, et al. Guidelines for the management of chronic kidney disease in HIV-infected patients: recommendations of the HIV Medicine Association of the Infectious Diseases Society of America. Clin Infect Dis. 2005;40:1559–85.
14. Kimmel PL, Phillips TM, Ferreira-Centeno A, Farkas-Szallasi T, Abraham AA, Garrett CT. Brief report: idiotypic IgA nephropathy in patients with human immunodeficiency virus infection. N Engl J Med. 1992;327:702–6.
15. Gerntholtz TE, Goetsch SJ, Katz I. HIV-related nephropathy: a South African perspective. Kidney Int. 2006;69:1885–91.
16. Parkhie SM, Fine DM, Lucas GM, Atta MG. Characteristics of patients with HIV and biopsy-proven acute interstitial nephritis. Clin J Am Soc Nephrol. 2010;5:798–804.
17. Kazi S, Cohen PR, Williams F, Schempp R, Reveille JD. The diffuse infiltrative lymphocytosis syndrome. Clinical and immunogenetic features in 35 patients. AIDS. 1996;10:385–91.
18. Hirsch HH, Kaufmann G, Sendi P, Battegay M. Immune reconstitution in HIV-infected patients. Clin Infect Dis. 2004;38:1159–66.
19. Shelburne SA, Visnegarwala F, Darcourt J, et al. Incidence and risk factors for immune reconstitution inflammatory syndrome during highly active antiretroviral therapy. AIDS. 2005;19:399–406.
20. Mocroft A, Kirk O, Reiss P, et al. Estimated glomerular filtration rate, chronic kidney disease and antiretroviral drug use in HIV-positive patients. AIDS. 2010;24:1667–78.
21. Hall AM, Hendry BM, Nitsch D, Connolly JO. Tenofovir-associated kidney toxicity in HIV-infected patients: a review of the evidence. Am J Kidney Dis. 2011;57:773–80.
22. McGuire BM, Julian BA, Bynon JS Jr, et al. Brief communication: glomerulonephritis in patients with hepatitis C cirrhosis undergoing liver transplantation. Ann Intern Med. 2006;144:735–41.
23. Blach S, Zeuzem S, Manns M, et al. Global prevalence and genotype distribution of hepatitis C virus infection in 2015: a modelling study. Lancet Gastroenterol Hepatol. 2017;2:161–76.
24. Barsoum RS. Hepatitis C virus: from entry to renal injury--facts and potentials. Nephrol Dial Transplant. 2007;22:1840–8.
25. Kamar N, Izopet J, Alric L, Guilbeaud-Frugier C, Rostaing L. Hepatitis C virus-related kidney disease: an overview. Clin Nephrol. 2008;69:149–60.
26. Fabrizi F, Plaisier E, Saadoun D, Martin P, Messa P, Cacoub P. Hepatitis C virus infection, mixed cryoglobulinemia, and kidney disease. Am J Kidney Dis. 2013;61:623–37.
27. KDIGO. 2018 clinical practice guideline for the prevention, diagnosis, evaluation, and treatment of hepatitis C in chronic kidney disease. Kidney Int Suppl. 2018;8:91–165.
28. Chen G, Wang C, Chen J, et al. Hepatitis B reactivation in hepatitis B and C coinfected patients treated with antiviral agents: a systematic review and meta-analysis. Hepatology. 2017;66:13–26.
29. Mucke MM, Backus LI, Mucke VT, et al. Hepatitis B virus reactivation during direct-acting antiviral therapy for hepatitis C: a systematic review and meta-analysis. Lancet Gastroenterol Hepatol. 2018;3:172–80.
30. Gragnani L, Visentini M, Fognani E, et al. Prospective study of guideline-tailored therapy with direct-acting antivirals for hepatitis C virus-associated mixed cryoglobulinemia. Hepatology. 2016;64:1473–82.
31. Schweitzer A, Horn J, Mikolajczyk RT, Krause G, Ott JJ. Estimations of worldwide prevalence of chronic hepatitis B virus infection: a systematic review of data published between 1965 and 2013. Lancet. 2015;386(10003):1546–55.
32. Bhimma R, Coovadia HM. Hepatitis B virus-associated nephropathy. Am J Nephrol. 2004;24:198–211.
33. Gilbert RD, Wiggelinkhuizen J. The clinical course of hepatitis B virus-associated nephropathy. Pediatr Nephrol. 1994;8:11–4.
34. Pagnoux C, Seror R, Henegar C, et al. Clinical features and outcomes in 348 patients with polyarteritis nodosa: a systematic retrospective study of patients diagnosed between 1963 and 2005 and entered into the French Vasculitis Study Group Database. Arthritis Rheum. 2010;62:616–26.
35. Agarwal K, Brunetto M, Seto WK, et al. 96 weeks treatment of tenofovir alafenamide vs. tenofovir disoproxil fumarate for hepatitis B virus infection. J Hepatol. 2018;68:672–81.
36. EASL clinical practice guidelines: Management of chronic hepatitis B virus infection. J Hepatol 2012;57:167–85.
37. Pipili CL, Papatheodoridis GV, Cholongitas EC. Treatment of hepatitis B in patients with chronic kidney disease. Kidney Int. 2013;84:880–5.

Patient Information and Guidelines

American Association for the Study of Liver Diseases (AASLD): https://www.aasld.org/

European Association for the Study of the Liver (EASL): https://easl.eu/

Liverpool Hepatitis Drug Interactions: https://www.hep--druginteractions.org

Liverpool HIV Interactions: https://www.hiv-druginteractions.org/checker

Terrence Higgins Trust: tht.org.uk

31

Tubulointerstitial Disease

Contents

Acute Tubulointerstitial Nephritis

Vasantha Muthu Muthuppalaniappan and Simon Ball

Contents

M. Harber (ed.), *Primer on Nephrology*, https://doi.org/10.1007/978-3-030-76419-7_32

Learning Objectives

- To emphasise the importance of recognising AIN as a common cause of AKI
- Understanding the wide clinical presentation and causes of AIN
- Diagnostic conundrum in establishing a diagnosis
- Current evidence on available treatment options
- Tips and tricks when approaching a case of suspected AIN
- Helpful factors to establish prognosis and long-term outlook

32.1 Introduction

32

Acute tubulointerstitial nephritis was first described in 1898 by William Thomas Councilman in the setting of diphtheria and scarlet fever whereby he had observed lymphoid and plasma cell infiltrates in the renal interstitium.

The term tubulointerstitial nephritis encompasses a wide range of disorders in which the focus of renal inflammation is extra-glomerular. The diagnosis is made by renal biopsy, almost invariably undertaken to investigate deranged renal function. The histological appearances may be divided into acute interstitial nephritis (AIN) and chronic interstitial nephritis (CIN) (covered in the next chapter) on the basis of the degree of tubulointerstitial atrophy and fibrosis and the extent and distribution of the inflammatory infiltrate. These two entities are therefore contiguous, and diagnostic categorisation in the 'histological middle ground' will often be influenced by the history and recognition of a plausible underlying aetiology.

Chronic kidney disease is also accompanied by tubulointerstitial atrophy and fibrosis regardless of the underlying cause, the severity of which is the histological feature that correlates best with progression to end-stage renal failure (ESRF). In this setting, inflammatory cells can also be detected in areas of interstitial atrophy and fibrosis. The challenge sometimes is to distinguish between infiltrates in areas of secondary damage and those where the tubulointerstitial infiltrate is the primary pathology causing CIN.

These observations with respect to the precision of histological definition are in practice more of a problem for the execution of studies and the authoring of reports than for everyday clinical practice. This is illustrated by the difficulties in consistent description of interstitial nephritis in a well-defined setting such as renal transplant rejection, despite the considerable efforts of Banff consensus meetings. This does not however preclude the generation of consistent results from transplant centres.

32.2 Acute Interstitial Nephritis

32.2.1 Aetiology and Pathogenesis

Tubulointerstitial inflammation may be a manifestation of non-specific local tissue damage or immune recognition of a neo-antigen, whether exogenous or endogenous in origin. In AIN, the cellular immune response seems to predominate, although there are rare cases in which anti-tubular basement membrane antibodies can be detected. Causative factors linked to AIN include idiosyncratic responses to drugs, infection, multisystem inflammatory diseases and tubulointerstitial nephritis with uveitis (TINU). Their representation in different biopsy series is highly variable, perhaps reflecting differences in practice and in demographics; however, the most commonly identified aetiological factor is usually an idiosyncratic adverse drug reaction. The exact mechanism of drug-induced AIN is not truly understood, but there appears to be an allergic hypersensitivity mechanism. It is unclear which components of the immune system contribute to this hypersensitivity reaction, but both cell-mediated and immune humoral mechanisms have been implicated.

32.2.2 Epidemiology

The incidence of AIN is thought to be 1–6% of all renal biopsies [1]. However, the percentage rises to 10–27% when analysis is restricted to renal biopsies performed in the setting of acute kidney injury (AKI) [2, 3]. This rise can be accounted for by the increasing use of renal biopsy in modern practice as well as more renal biopsies being performed in older patients with AKI. The distribution of the underlying cause of AIN (see Fig. 32.1) may differ according to age. A multicentre study from Spain published in 2012 reports an increase in the incidence of AIN in recent years particularly so in those aged over 65 years (12.3%) [1, 4]. Patients greater than 65 years of age are more likely to have drug-induced interstitial nephritis and less likely to have AIN related to autoimmune or systemic disease. It may be that there is a real increase in AIN, possibly as a consequence of an increased widespread use of medications such as proton pump inhibitors (PPIs) and non-steroidal anti-inflammatory drugs (NSAIDs). Although AIN is a rare complication of these medications, they are used by millions and are therefore amongst the most common agents implicated in the causation of AIN. PPI use is approximately three times more common and NSAID use twice as common in patients with AIN than in controls [5].

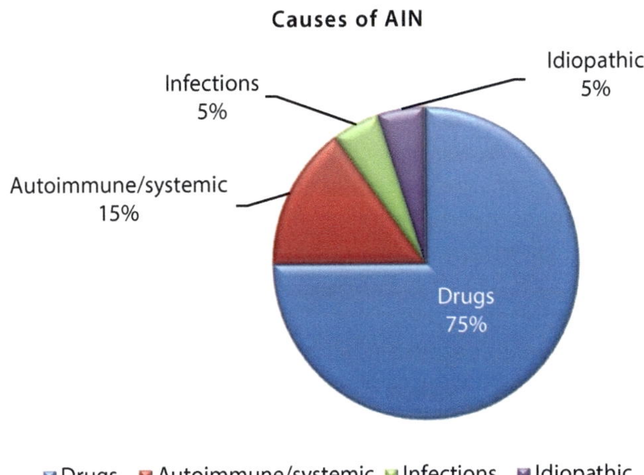

Fig. 32.1 Causes of AIN in Western countries according to frequencies from renal biopsy series [1]

The true incidence of AIN may still be underestimated as many cases are diagnosed based on clinical judgement whereby the offending agent is stopped and improvement in renal function is observed. In some cases, especially in the elderly where there is polypharmacy, the offending agent is often not clear and multiple agents are being stopped at the same time to observe any recovery in renal function. Often elderly and frail patients are treated empirically without being subjected to a renal biopsy. Therefore, how many of these patients truly have AIN on biopsy is not known. Approximately 23–58% of patients with AIN will need renal replacement therapy (RRT) and up to 44% will require ongoing RRT. It is important to have a high index of suspicion in drug-induced AIN as any attempt to rechallenge without renal function monitoring may result in severe AKI and worst-case irreversible renal damage and scarring as often the clinical signs are subtle in these cases.

The likelihood of AIN underlying an episode of AKI is of course significantly increased by prior exposure to relevant drugs or evidence of multisystem inflammatory diseases. Specific causes of AIN also exhibit ethnic variability: mycobacterial AIN is most commonly seen in the South Asian community in the United Kingdom as is interstitial nephritis with no determined cause. AIN in sarcoidosis is also reportedly associated with black ethnicity; however, this may not be any greater than the underlying disease itself. There are few data to suggest ethnic disparities in the occurrence of drug-induced interstitial nephritis, but it seems increasingly likely that there are HLA associations.

32.2.3 Clinical Manifestations

The precise mode of presentation differs between AIN of different causes. In multisystem disease and acute infectious illnesses, biochemical derangement is often detected during routine monitoring. In other situations such as idiosyncratic responses to commonly used medications, there may be a presentation with uraemia, fluid overload and hypertension. There *may* be extra-renal manifestations such as a (i) pyrexia, (ii) rash, (iii) arthralgia and (iv) eosinophilia accompanying these idiosyncratic responses, reflecting a hypersensitivity reaction. The classical triad which includes fever, rash and eosinophilia/eosinophiluria which was observed with methicillin-induced AIN is only seen in one-third of patients with AIN. Each component of the triad is present in 70–100%, 30–50% and 15–20% of AIN cases, respectively [6].

Table 32.1 Clinical and laboratory features in drug-induced AIN

Aetiological agent	Frequency in renal biopsy series
Acute KI	100%
Acute KI requiring dialysis	40%
Arthralgia	45%
Skin rash	22%
Pyrexia	36%
Non-visible haematuria	67%
Visible haematuria	5%
Proteinuria	93%
Nephrotic range proteinuria	2.5%
Nephrotic syndrome	0.8%
Eosinophilia	35%
Eosinophiluria	66%

This is reproduced from Reference [18] and will therefore need permissions

Pyrexia is a common finding in cases with AIN. The rash often observed is a maculopapular rash. The mode of presentation in two large series from Ireland and Spain in which drugs were the causative agent in 116/121 is shown in Table 32.1. In the United Kingdom, at least in the 1980s [2] and 1990s [7, 8], reports from centres serving populations of diverse ethnicity suggest only a third of cases of AIN were associated with idiosyncratic drug reactions and in these series extra-renal manifestations were significantly less common.

Drug-induced AIN typically presents as non-oliguric AKI which usually develops after 7–10 days after drug exposure but shorter in drug rechallenge and maybe longer in certain drug exposure, up to 4 months, e.g.

NSAIDs and proton pump inhibitor [9, 10]. An early presentation within days of drug initiation seems likely to represent a secondary response. There are no hard and fast rules, but since many cases arise in the setting of polypharmacy, deduction of plausible temporal relationships provides some evidence of likely causation. It is, therefore, important to get a clear drug history, if necessary, from the primary practitioner or other third party, ideally with previous exposure and preceding renal tests.

32.2.4 Diagnosis and Investigation

32.2.4.1 Urinary Analysis

32

Eosinophiluria is defined by >1% of WBC in urine which is detected by a Hansel or Wright stain. It is associated with AIN in the absence of other disease processes which include cystitis, prostatitis, pyelonephritis, atheroembolic renal disease, acute tubular necrosis and rapidly progressive glomerulonephritis. Eosinophiluria has a poor predictive value in establishing a diagnosis of AIN due to its poor sensitivity at 31% with a low positive predictive value of 16% and specificity at 68% [11]. The use of Wright's stain is less sensitive than the Hansel stain when looking for eosinophiluria. It is imperative to remember that eosinophiluria is also associated with acute tubular necrosis, post-infectious glomerulonephritis, atheroembolic disease, urinary tract infections, prerenal AKI and prostatitis.

Other urinary sediments that raise the possibility of AIN include renal tubular epithelial cell casts reflecting a tubular cell injury with/without necrosis and white cell casts in the absence of infection.

Proteinuria is usually mild and often less than 1 g/day with a significant fraction of the proteinuria consisting of low molecular weight proteins (e.g. immunoglobulin light chains, beta2 microglobulin, lysozyme, peptide hormones). Low molecular weight proteinuria is common, and the uPCR can be disproportionally higher than the uACR. This is because in normal conditions, proteins of low molecular weight are re-absorbed by the proximal tubules and only a small amount is excreted. However, in AIN (a disease involving tubular structures), this function is impaired and leads to the characteristic tubular proteinuria. Analysis of low molecular weight proteins (such as urinary retinol-binding protein (uRBP), beta2 microglobulin (β_2M) or α_1-microglobulin) may indicate a tubular origin and be strongly suggestive of AIN.

Similarly, *haematuria* is usually non-visible and low level on conventional stick urinalysis. Visible haematuria was reported in early reports of methicillin-induced AIN but is now rare. Importantly, this means that patients sometimes present with a raised creatinine but 'quiet urine' the assumption being that there is not an acute inflammatory process, identification of sterile pyuria may be the only clue to an acute pathology.

There may be defects in tubular handling of water, sodium and hydrogen ions resulting in nephrogenic diabetes insipidus, salt-losing nephropathy, renal tubular acidosis (RTA) and Fanconi syndrome, which can all lead to the initial presentation. In particular, type 1 RTA is a relatively common (~10%) manifestation of Sjögren's syndrome (a lower than expected venous bicarbonate and relatively alkaline urine may hint at this), whilst impaired renal function is less common [12].

32.2.4.2 Blood Analysis

The finding of eosinophilia in patients with AIN, even drug induced, has insufficient predictive value to contribute significantly to the initial diagnostic algorithm. However, if present, it can help define a likely aetiology when there are multiple offending drugs, particularly in patients who have spent significant time in secondary care. Evidence of eosinophilia is only seen in 25–35% of cases, but the absence of eosinophilia does not exclude a diagnosis of AIN [3, 13]. Retrospective analysis of the eosinophil count can be used to define a likely time frame for the immune response often more precisely than renal function in patients who have been critically ill. For example, in patients found to have AIN following prolonged illness and AKI initially attributed to acute tubular injury, a retrospective finding of progressive eosinophilia can help identify candidate drugs and perhaps more importantly help exclude others. This has real value since these patients have often been exposed to multiple agents.

Most patients would have a rise in serum creatinine in AIN prompting further investigation of their AKI with approximately 23–58% requiring renal replacement therapy at presentation [14–16]. Screening for autoimmune and infectious aetiologies may aid diagnosis of AIN. This will generally include a screen for ANCA, ANA, ENA (including SS-A and SS-B (anti-Ro and anti-La), Igs, protein electrophoresis (polyclonal gammopathy being an important clue to autoimmune or infectious causes) and complement levels. Raised IgG or IgG4 levels or hypergammaglobulinaemia with low serum complement level may suggest an IgG4-related disease or hypocomplementaemic interstitial nephritis. Serum ACE may be helpful in the diagnosis of sarcoid. Specific serological testing and screening for mycobacterial infection (EMU and ELISPOT) and other causative organisms outlined in ◘ Table 32.2 may help ascertain a non-drug-induced AIN.

Table 32.2 Infections causing tubulointerstitial nephritis

Virus	Bacteria	Others
Hantaviridae	*Legionella*	*Leishmania*
Epstein-Barr virus	*Leptospira*	*Toxoplasma*
HIV	*Mycobacterium tuberculosis*	
Measles	*Streptococcus*	
Polyomavirus	*Brucella*	
Cytomegalovirus	*Mycoplasma*	
Adenovirus	*Chlamydia*	
Herpes simplex virus	*Salmonella*	
Hepatitis A	*Yersinia*	
Hepatitis B	*Campylobacter*	
Hepatitis C	*Rickettsia*	
	Strep species	
	Staph species	

32.2.4.3 Imaging

A CXR or HRCT may be helpful in diagnosing AIN thought to be caused by TB or sarcoid. The renal ultrasound in cases of AIN may show increased cortical echogenicity or enlarged kidneys but is otherwise noncontributory. Enlarged kidneys noted on ultrasound may be an inviting clue to the presence of an acute inflammatory interstitial nephritis which can be assessed further with a CT. ^{67}Ga scanning has been reported to distinguish between AIN and acute tubular injury (ATI), which may be of some use in special cases in which renal biopsy is contraindicated and the likely differential diagnosis is ATI.

32.2.4.4 Renal Biopsy and Histology Findings

None of the clinical manifestations or investigations are diagnostic of AIN. In patients presenting de novo with renal impairment, this is not a significant challenge because in practice, presentation with unexplained renal failure and normal-sized kidneys would indicate a renal biopsy, providing the diagnosis which is also the current gold standard for establishing AIN.

On biopsy, inflammatory cells can be seen invading the interstitium, breaching the tubular basement membrane and evoking a tubulitis (Fig. 32.1). The pathological process of AIN is often patchy except in severe cases and does not involve the glomeruli or vessels. These distinct features are important when discriminating for SLE or vasculitis-induced AIN. Cells are predominantly T cells and macrophages, but classically eosinophils may be present (although are not specific); B cells and neutrophils are also often present. Granulomas and giant cells may occur and suggest particular underlying aetiologies (see Tables 32.2 and 32.3) (Figs. 32.2 and 32.3). Predominant neutrophilia on the biopsy may suggest an infectious cause of AIN. A lymphocytic dominance is seen in NSAID-induced AIN.

In most cases, renal histology does not identify an underlying aetiology. Even *Mycobacterium tuberculosis*-associated AIN rarely demonstrates caseating granulomata with positive Ziehl-Neelsen staining. Consideration of the clinical context, the precise histology and corroborating information including screening for autoimmune and infectious aetiologies is required. It is prudent to assess the renal biopsy for interstitial fibrosis and tubular atrophy as the extent of these findings on the biopsy sample is associated with renal recovery and variable degree of CKD.

Immunofluorescence (IF) and electron microscopy may not aid or provide any additional information or diagnostic value in drug-induced AIN. However, IF in anti-TBM disease would reveal linear deposits of IgG along the TBM.

Diagnostic Challenges

The most frequent diagnostic challenge is to consider AIN in patients who have other causes of CKD or AKI and to thereby expedite investigation by renal biopsy.

In the case of CKD, the presence of proteinuria gives useful information. The presence of proteinuria with renal dysfunction would usually indicate renal biopsy; conversely, in diabetes mellitus, it may be the absence of proteinuria that suggests an alternative diagnosis such as AIN. There may be little proteinuria in hypertensive ischaemic nephropathy, and the indications for renal biopsy will be informed by the history, rate of change of renal function, renal size and the presence of a candidate cause of AIN.

In the case of AKI with a putative diagnosis of acute tubular necrosis (ATN), alternative diagnoses should be considered if renal failure is out of keeping with degree of physiological disturbance or unexpectedly prolonged. This would indicate further investigation by renal biopsy. An unexpected rash or eosinophilia might also lower the threshold for early biopsy in patients otherwise thought to have ATN.

As mentioned previously, on rare occasions where renal biopsy is precluded (generally by an absolute need for anti-coagulation), then a gallium scan may give some valuable information; however, this is rare.

32

Table 32.3 Medications and AIN

NSAIDs	Antimicrobials	Anticonvulsants	Chemotoxic drugs	Others
Ibuprofen	Penicillins	Phenytoin	Checkpoint inhibitors (ipilimumab, pembrolizumab, nivolumab, atezolizumab)	Allopurinol[1]
Indomethacin	Sulphonamides	Valproate	Cisplatin	H_2 receptor antagonists, e.g. cimetidine[1]
Diclofenac	Rifampicin	Lamotrigine	Tyrosine kinase inhibitors	Phenindione[1]
Piroxicam	Quinolones	Carbamazepine	Pemetrexed	Furosemide and other loop diuretics
COX-2 inhibitors	Vancomycin	Phenobarbitone	BCG	Proton pump inhibitors
Salicylates (Aspirin)	Teicoplanin		Ifosfamide	TNF inhibitors
Mefenamic acid	Tetracyclines			Azathioprine
Naproxen	Cephalosporins			Quinine
Celecoxib and rofecoxib	Isoniazid			Thiazides
Mesalazine	Ethambutol			Phenindione and warfarin
	Nitrofurantoin[1]			Calcium channel blockers
	Tetracyclines			

A wide range of medications have been implicated in AIN; therefore, any medication should be considered as a potential cause. Those shown have consistently been reported in case series and/or case-control studies.
[1]Reported association with granulomatous AIN

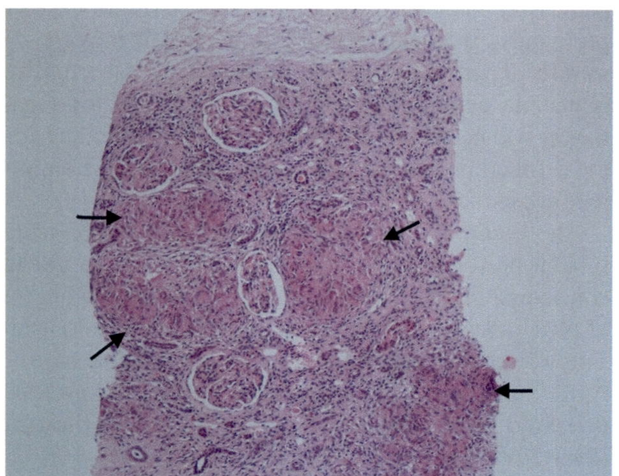

Fig. 32.2 Medium power renal biopsy showing intense acute TIN with diffuse inflammatory cells and gross granulomata in a patient with AKI and a calcium of 3.9 mmol/L detected after starting vitamin D supplements

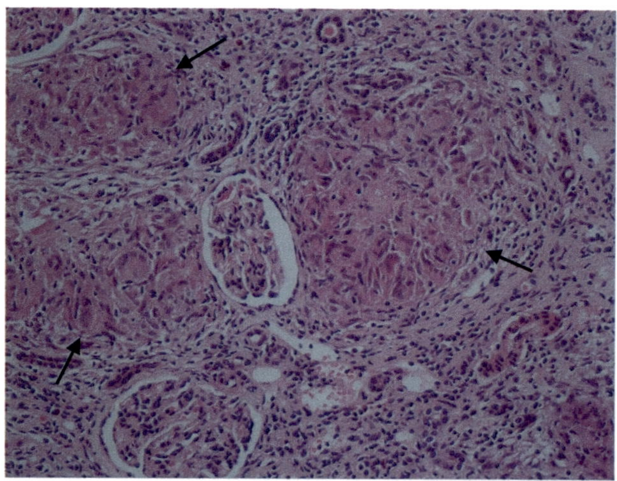

Fig. 32.3 High power image of a giant cell in a patient with acute TIN

32.2.4.5 Biomarkers Still in Research Phase

Monitoring of sensitive urinary markers of tubulointerstitial damage, such as neutrophil gelatinase-associated lipocalin, liver-type fatty acid-binding protein and kidney injury molecule-1, has been suggested as a non-invasive test to evaluate early damage and evolution of interstitial nephritis [17].

32.2.5 Causes of AIN

Drugs by far are the commonest cause of AIN also known as an allergic reaction account for 70–75% of all AIN from biopsy series [13, 18]. Antibiotics (30–50%) are the main culprit, followed by NSAIDs and proton pump inhibitors. Any drug can cause AIN, and knowledge of these drug reactions has come from case reports/studies and retrospective series supported by biopsy findings of AIN. Checkpoint inhibitors (anti-CTLA-4 antibody and anti-PD-1 inhibitors) which are used in various forms of cancer have recently been shown to cause AIN. However, these drugs are more commonly associated with other immune-related adverse events such as dermatitis, colitis, pneumonitis and hepatitis. In fact, nephrotoxicity tends to develop more frequently as a consequence of the above side effects. Drug-related AIN is idiosyncratic and not dose dependent, and recurrence of exacerbation can occur with a second exposure of the same or related drug which occurs more rapidly when rechallenged (refer to Case History 1). Drugs that can cause AIN are also often associated with other side effects which are worth noting as this may help with identifying the offending drug. AIN caused by drugs can occur up to an average of 2 weeks or even longer after starting the medication. See ◘ Table 32.3 for an extensive list of drugs that can cause AIN.

Multisystem diseases associated with AIN account for 10–20% of cases [13, 18]. AIN is often part of a multisystem disease, and renal manifestations may be the quickest route to the diagnosis. Many of these conditions are covered elsewhere in more detail, but it is worth noting that renal limited AIN can occur as an early manifestation of what might normally be classified a multisystem disease.

Sarcoidosis is associated with renal granulomata very commonly; however, clinical manifestation of AIN is relatively uncommon [19]. A more common cause of renal impairment is hypercalcaemia. There are reports that some forms of glomerular disease are more common in those with sarcoidosis; however, this remains to be proved. In recent years, a sarcoid-like illness has been associated with the use of anti-TNF therapy, and this has been documented to cause a granulomatous interstitial nephritis. Although evidently rare, given increasingly widespread use of this class of agents, then this may be increasingly recognised in patients with rheumatoid and inflammatory bowel disease, in both of which there are a number of other potential causes of renal impairment.

Sjögren's syndrome is commonly associated with renal tubular acidosis, but approximately 4% of patients with primary Sjögren's syndrome develop overt renal disease, half of whom have AIN and the others glomerular disease [20]. Thus, it is important to enquire about dry eyes or mouth which is an important clue being the predominant presenting symptom in Sjogren's.

IgG4-related disease (IgG4-RD) is a systemic fibroinflammatory immune-mediated condition. IgG4-RD is characterised by elevated levels of serum IgG4 (seen in two-thirds of patients), lymphoplasmacytic and IgG4 plasma cell-positive infiltrates in a range of organs with variable degree of fibrosis that has a characteristic 'storiform' pattern [21, 22]. There is a typical pattern of progressive expansile interstitial fibrosis in affected tissues and a plasma cell-rich TIN frequently with eosinophils. It is most often associated with 'autoimmune' pancreatitis; however, there can be widespread organ involvement with inflammatory masses, sialadenitis, sclerosing cholangitis, aortitis and retroperitoneal fibrosis. The pathogenesis of this condition is poorly understood but consistent with an autoimmune or an allergic disorder. One-third of cases are associated with an AIN that manifests most often with AKI, however can present as a renal mass. A retrospective study from Australia showed that IgG4-related TIN represented 1% of the total renal biopsies performed over a 10-year period with 13% of all biopsies showing TIN [23]. The majority of data pertaining to IgG4 TIN comes from two series of renal biopsies: a Japanese and an American cohort [24, 25]. Renal involvement of IgG4-RD causes hypocomplementaemia, but the mechanism causing low C3/C4 levels is not entirely clear. Tubular basement membrane immune complexes are also common. Treatment of IgG4-RD is with corticosteroid therapy and B cell depletion in steroid resistant or intolerant cases [26]. Maintenance therapy with low-dose prednisolone and/or azathioprine, MMF, calcineurin inhibitors are necessary in multiorgan disease and relapse with elevated serum IgG4 levels [26].

Since IgG4-RD is a relatively newly identified and defined disease, further improved understanding of the pathogenesis is still needed to help guide diagnosis and treatment.

Systemic lupus erythematosus Tubulointerstitial inflammation is a common and prognostically significant manifestation of the SLE which correlates highly with renal progression but not with other features of disease activity [27]. In a small number of patients, interstitial nephritis is a predominant feature, and this is commonly associated with a renal tubular acidosis.

Granulomatosis with polyangiitis (GPA) (formally known as Wegener's granulomatosis) may also be manifest as an AIN usually in association with, but sometimes without, glomerular inflammation [28].

TIN with uveitis (TINU) syndrome is rare and has a female bias (3:1) and a median age of onset of 15, although cases presenting in middle age are well documented. The condition accounts for 5–10% of all AIN [13, 18]. Presentation is initially with TIN in two-thirds of patients, 20% TIN with uveitis and only 15% initially as uveitis. In some cases, onset seems to be drug induced. Other common features reported include fever, weight loss, rash, arthralgia, myalgia, anorexia and malaise. Renal involvement may manifest as renal impairment, concentrating defects or features of the Fanconi syndrome. The presumed aetiology is immune dysregulation with T cell infiltration, but recently IgG antibodies have been demonstrated against tubular epithelial cells, and predictably HLA associations are emerging. The TIN of TINU is usually treated with steroids but may resolve spontaneously and generally has a good prognosis, although in one group, 15% of patients developed CKD. The prognosis of the uveitis (which is usually anterior) is less good in that it is much more likely to relapse chronically.

32.2.6 Infectious Diseases Associated with AIN

A myriad of infectious diseases have been reported causing renal disease and specifically with AIN (these conditions are covered in more detail in the chapter 'Infection and the Kidney'). Infectious diseases causing AIN are seen in 4–10% of all AIN cases [13, 18]. Whilst with some such as tuberculosis, hantavirus and leptospirosis the aetiology is clear, causality with some other infectious agents is not yet proven.

Acute pyelonephritis is characterised by neutrophil inflammation centred on tubules generally considered to be consequent upon an ascending bacterial infection, although this may not always be proven. Although this could reasonably be considered a form of interstitial nephritis, it is by convention considered separately.

Tubulointerstitial nephritis can complicate various systemic infections (see ◘ Table 32.2). In a large ethnically diverse, urban UK practice, over the course of the last 10 years, we have observed relatively few cases definitely attributable to infection; these have been due to *Mycobacterium tuberculosis* and leptospirosis. The causation of AIN will however inevitably be significantly affected by the location and population served by any centre.

Mycobacterium tuberculosis can affect the urinary tract in various ways; however, one important manifestation is as a granulomatous interstitial nephritis. This may present with unexplained renal impairment usually with a fever, but sometimes remarkably few other symptoms. The microbiological diagnosis may not be immediately established, the granulomas are not necessarily caseating and the Ziehl-Neelsen stain is usually negative. The diagnosis may only become apparent at a later date or be inferred from a beneficial response to antituberculous chemotherapy.

Leptospirosis can result in AIN. The incidence of renal failure varies widely in different series but is common. Other features include presentation with a 'flu-like illness', particularly with disproportionate jaundice, thrombocytopenia in some with a bleeding diathesis and multisystem involvement including pulmonary and central nervous system involvement.

Hantavirus in Europe typically causes nephropathia epidemica, in which a 'flu-like illness' is accompanied by AKI and thrombocytopenia. Travel to endemic areas may identify the risk [29], perhaps most likely from Central and Eastern Europe. AIN can be striking and is often associated with interstitial haemorrhage.

In *HIV infection*, a post-mortem series of HAART experienced patients found that 5/89 patients had interstitial nephritis. The most common cause of interstitial nephritis in this group appears to be drug associated but only rarely is this attributable to components of HAART and more commonly due to NSAIDs and co-trimaxazole.

Epstein-Barr virus is occasionally associated with an AIN, usually as part of a systemic disease [30]. Reports that AIN of undetermined cause may be significantly contributed to by EBV infection [31] seem not to have been supported by subsequent studies [32].

BK virus is a polyomavirus that causes interstitial nephritis sometimes granulomatous in renal transplant patients and occasionally in other immunosuppressed patients (in whom it may also cause a haemorrhagic cystitis). The diagnosis is made by renal biopsy; however, quantification of viral DNA in the plasma by polymerase chain reaction (PCR) or examination of the urine for decoy cells provides non-invasive means of predicting those at risk. It presents with deteriorating renal function, and the diagnosis is made by renal biopsy. The backbone of treatment is reduction of immunosuppression. Various other treatments have been tried, although none have yet been proven to be effective.

Pyelonephritis (covered in detail in Chap. 54) is commonly due to an ascending bacterial infection from the lower urinary tract which is commonly seen in young women who are sexually active or in adults with diabetes, renal stones or if immunocompromised. Patients often present with fevers, flank pain and urinary symptoms. Urinalysis often would reveal a pyuria with white cell casts and positive urine culture. The key features of the renal biopsy in pyelonephritis are the dominant presence of neutrophils rather than lymphocytes which are classically observed in AIN due to hypersensitivity reaction.

32.2.7 Treatment of AIN

The treatment of AIN depends upon a thorough clinical investigation of potential underlying causes, some of which have been discussed above. AIN associated with the aforementioned multisystem inflammatory diseases is invariably treated with corticosteroids, in some instances with additional immunosuppression.

32.2.7.1 Management of Allergic AIN or Drug-Induced AIN

Drug-induced AIN requires early identification and immediate withdrawal of the likely offending agent. Corticosteroid treatment has been used to expedite the rate and extent of renal recovery in drug-induced AIN. However, the role of corticosteroids remains controversial as evidence from retrospective studies that were generally small in size was conflicting. A study of 61 patients with drug-induced AIN undertaken in Spain has suggested that better outcome was associated with earlier corticosteroid treatment [33]; however, the retrospective nature of this analysis means that no recommendation can be conclusive. A similar-sized study from Ireland suggests no benefit [3]; however, the delay in corticosteroid administration was up to 3 weeks in this study. Further studies since have demonstrated long-term favourable outcomes in those treated with corticosteroids [16, 33, 34]. Early treatment with corticosteroids (within the first 5–7 days) after discontinuation of the offending drug can reduce the amount of tubulointerstitial fibrosis that develops and association with better recovery of renal function [33, 35, 36].

There are no prospective studies or established guidelines till date suggesting the use of corticosteroids routinely, but it seems reasonable to recommend that if used, corticosteroids should be introduced early. Several authors have recommended an early pulse of corticosteroids for 3 days, followed by a reducing course of oral prednisone (0.5–1 mg/kg/day) over ~6 weeks [18], whilst others (conventional dosing strategy) have recommended prednisolone at 1 mg/kg (maximum dose of 60 mg orally) with a view to taper over the next 2–3 months [16]. Regardless of the initial dose of steroids, Gonzalez and colleagues suggested continuing prednisolone at 1 mg/kg for the first 4–6 weeks as most recovery in renal function occurs within this time frame.

There has also been emerging evidence and anecdotal reports suggesting benefit from mycophenolate mofetil [37], cyclophosphamide and cyclosporine [38], though the evidence on these treatments remains sparse.

32.2.7.2 Prognosis and Long-Term Outcome of Drug-Induced AIN

The long-term outcome of AIN, especially drug induced, is good. A study from Japan noted that the recovery of AIN occurs in two phases: an initial rapid phase of recovery over 6–8 weeks, followed by a slower phase recovery which can last up to 1 year to ascertain baseline renal function [39]. Longer duration of exposure to the offending drug is associated with worse chance of renal function recovery [14]. Increased age and persistence of AKI for >3 weeks, but not severity of AKI, are associated with worse long-term outcomes [13, 10].

Adverse prognostic factors in AIN recovery include [14, 39]:

- Diffuse (versus patchy) inflammation on biopsy
- Excess number of neutrophils (1–6%); extent
- Severity of interstitial fibrosis and/or tubular atrophy
- Smaller kidneys on ultrasound had poorer response to steroids

These factors were found to correlate most closely with the final glomerular filtration rate. A considerable proportion of affected patients with AIN; up to 36% of patients with AIN develop CKD [13]. Therefore, patients with AIN should have long-term follow-up with a clinician for blood pressure and renal function monitoring.

If a drug is suspected of causing AIN, then it is imperative that the patient is aware they are allergic to this drug, and if there is doubt about an important agent, such as penicillin, then it is critical that the practitioner is aware and monitors renal function within a few days of any rechallenge. Nephrologists have the responsibility of ensuring that this information is clearly imparted.

Tips and Tricks when Approaching a Case of Suspected AIN

- Consider AIN if there is a temporal relationship of drug, infection or systemic process with a progressive rise in serum creatinine. Remember that manifestation of drug-induced AIN differs for different drugs but generally an average latency period of 10–14 days has been suggested.
- Always look for extra-renal manifestations or other haematological or biochemical abnormalities which can help point out towards the offending drug.
- Think AIN is abnormal urinary sediment with evidence of pyuria, non-nephrotic range proteinuria and eosinophiluria.
- Always try to identify the offending agent and withdraw and assess serum creatinine.

- Consider renal biopsy if suitable and no contraindications.
- Consider corticosteroid therapy if no contraindications at a suggested dose of 1 mg/kg/day tapered over 2–3 months if nil improvement in serum creatinine with conservative measures.
- Think of the presence and/or extent of interstitial fibrosis with scarring if poor response with corticosteroid therapy.

Summary and Key Points

- AIN is a hypersensitivity reaction leading to inflammation of the renal interstitium.
- Commonly caused by drugs, infections and autoimmune and systemic conditions.
- Presents with acute kidney injury +/– classic presentation of hypersensitivity (maculopapular rash, eosinophilia/eosinophiluria, fever) +/– proteinuria (less than 1 g/day) +/– haematuria.
- Resolution of symptoms is with withdrawal of the offending drug or treatment of the underlying cause if not due to medications.
- Definitive diagnosis is made via renal biopsy as other investigations (laboratory and imaging) lack specificity and sensitivity.

Management consists of supportive care, careful fluid balance, withdrawal of offending drugs and corticosteroid therapy.

32

32.3 Summary

AIN and CIN represent diverse pathologies with a range of aetiologies. The main diagnostic challenge lies in considering these potential pathologies, particularly in an older population with underlying CKD associated with hypertension and renal ischaemia. Supportive therapy, rapid identification and removal of potential drug causes whilst excluding autoimmune or infectious causes are the mainstay of management. Proper randomised controlled trials of treatments for AIN are surely needed.

Case Study

Case 1

A 75-year-old man presented non-specifically unwell with AKI 3 (creatinine 830 μmol/L) and hyponatraemia (sodium 124 mmol/L). He was otherwise haemodynamically stable and had only 1+ of protein in his urine with no evidence of pre- or post-renal (renal sizes normal) causes or sepsis. He was on no over-the-counter medication but was prescribed a calcium channel blocker, beta blocker, thiazide diuretic and proton pump inhibitor (PPI). He had also finished a course of penicillin for a community-acquired chest infection. A renal biopsy confirmed an acute tubulointerstitial nephritis (TIN) which was presumed to be drug induced. His renal function improved rapidly with conservative measures. A review of previous blood tests demonstrated a previous milder episode of AKI, 3 years before (see ◘ Fig. 32.4). Reviewing the medications with his practitioner, it was clear that this correlated with a course of PPI for indigestion and not related to penicillin or thiazide, although the connection has not been made at the time. It is not always possible to determine which medication is responsible for an AIN, and avoiding key drugs for life on speculation may result in disadvantage to the patient. A thorough review of the drug history and biochemistry may identify a candidate drug or, as in this case, allow a stratification of the risk from multiple candidate drugs.

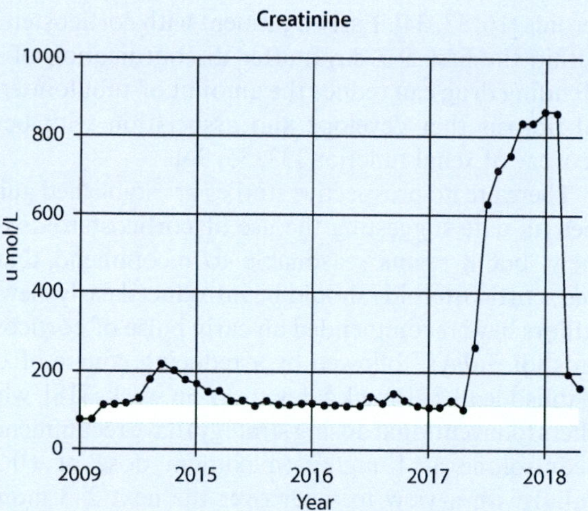

◘ **Fig. 32.4** Serial creatinine results since 2009 with a rise in creatinine correlating to a course of PPI completed for indigestion in 2014 and restarting of PPI in May 2017 leading to a progressive decline in renal function which improved following withdrawal of the offending drug

Case Study

Case 2

A 16-year-old male presented to the emergency department with a 3-week history of loin pain associated with coryzal symptoms. He took several ibuprofen tablets as analgesia. His temperature was 38 degrees with a creatinine of 97 μmol/L at presentation which gradually increased to 203 μmol/L over 7 days. Blood pressure (BP) was 140/65. He complained of visual disturbance with redness of his eyes. Clinically, he had bilateral anterior uveitis following an ophthalmology review. Urine dip was benign. Erythrocyte sedimentation rate (ESR) and C-reactive protein (CRP) were raised, but there were no signs of active infection. An ultrasound of the kidneys revealed bilateral enlarged kidneys. A renal biopsy confirmed the suspicion of tubulointerstitial nephritis and uveitis (TINU). He was treated with high-dose corticosteroids, and his renal function had returned to baseline of normal. Even though ibuprofen can cause AIN, the clinical scenario in this case was in keeping with TINU rather than a drug-induced AIN.

Case 3

A 54-year-old Afro-Caribbean male with a background history of hypertension was referred to the renal clinic with progressive rise in his serum creatinine over the past year from a baseline creatinine of 80 μmol/L to 280 μmol/L. He reported unintentional weight loss of approximately 10 kg over a year with no other symptoms to report. BP was 136/90. Clinical examination revealed several palpable clavicular lymph nodes bilaterally. There were no other abnormalities found otherwise. Urinalysis revealed trace protein and trace of blood. Haematological findings showed a normocytic anaemia with a haemoglobin level of 10.5 g/dL. Blood chemistry revealed a creatinine of 325 μmol/L and a corrected calcium level of 3.2 with a suppressed parathyroid hormone (PTH) level. Liver function tests were normal. He was admitted to the renal department to treat the hypercalcaemia whilst being investigated for an AKI. Myeloma screen was negative. A serum angiotensin-converting enzyme (ACE) and 1,25-dihydroxyvitamin D level was raised. A renal biopsy showed numerous granulomas in the interstitium which were non-caseating with multinucleated giant cells. Immunofluorescence and acid-fast bacilli staining were negative. The patient was treated with 30 mg of prednisolone per day with an improvement in the serum creatinine to 150 μmol/L and normal calcium levels after a year of treatment.

Case 4

A 70-year-old Asian male was referred to the diagnostic clinic with a 1-year history of a progressive rise in creatinine associated with a significant weight loss of 5 kg. His creatinine a year ago was 90 μmol/L but had risen to 150 μmol/L at the time of referral. He suffers from diabetes which has been well controlled over the past 2 years with no known micro- or macrovascular complication. His urine analysis showed protein 1+ and blood 2+ with a urine protein/creatinine ratio of 110 mg/mmol. Other abnormalities noted on his bloods included a raised eosinophil count, elevated IgG, low complement levels with no evidence of cryoglobulinaemia and raised rheumatoid factor levels. The remaining autoimmune and virology screen was unremarkable. Imaging of his renal tract demonstrated normal-sized kidneys. A renal biopsy revealed a plasma cell-rich tubulointerstitial nephritis with fibrosis and infiltrating eosinophils. Immunostaining for IgG4 showed infiltration of IgG4+ plasma cells in the interstitium confirming a diagnosis of IgG4-related disease. The patient was initiated on 30 mg of prednisolone per day which was tapered after 4 weeks with an improvement in his renal function to his baseline creatinine. A PET scan had excluded any other organ involvement of IgG4-related disease. He remains in remission without any steroids for maintenance. The case highlights the importance of recognising the possibility of an alternative diagnosis in this 70-year-old male with diabetes as the clinical presentations, the absence of diabetes-related micro-/macrovascular complications and the urinalysis do not entirely support the probability of diabetes-related renal disease. Subsequent abnormalities detected from the renal screen had steered towards a renal biopsy to investigate other possible causes for this patient's renal dysfunction.

Chapter Review Questions

1. What is the commonest offending drug that can cause an allergic AIN?
   (a) NSAIDs
   (b) Antibiotics
   (c) Proton pump inhibitor (PPI)
   (d) Checkpoint inhibitors (CPI)
2. Which clinical feature below is not commonly associated with AIN?
   (a) Fever
   (b) Visible haematuria
   (c) Arthralgia
   (d) Proteinuria

3. What is the best diagnostic test available to establish a diagnosis of AIN?
   (a) ^{67}Ga scanning
   (b) Renal biopsy
   (c) Eosinophiluria
   (d) Analysis of low molecular weight protein in urine

4. What is the treatment if drug-induced AIN is suspected?
   (a) Stop offending drug
   (b) Corticosteroid therapy
   (c) Mycophenolate mofetil
   (d) Cyclosporine

5. Which of the statements below are incorrect with regard to IgG4-related disease and TIN?
   (a) Complement levels are normal
   (b) Treatment is with corticosteroids
   (c) Serum IgG4 levels are elevated
   (d) Rituximab can be considered in steroid resistant or relapsing cases

Answers

1. All the drugs listed can cause an AIN. However, the commonest culprit is antibiotics, followed by NSAIDs, then PPI and CPI. The common immune-related adverse events from the CPI group of chemotherapy agents are endocrinopathies (thyroiditis), colitis, pneumonitis, hepatitis, cardiotoxicities and neurological. Renal adverse event from CPI is rare but increasingly recognised 3–10 months after treatment initiation. The use of corticosteroids in addition to stopping the immunotherapy agent is the usual mainstay of treatment for patients with severe kidney injury.
2. Visible haematuria is not a common feature associated with AIN. However, microscopic haematuria is often seen in AIN.
3. The definitive diagnosis of AIN is confirmed by a renal biopsy. A diagnostic renal biopsy would predominantly feature interstitial lymphocytic infiltrate with occasional plasma cells and variable eosinophilia, interstitial oedema and tubulitis. In most cases, the underlying cause of AIN may not be identified.
4. Stopping the offending drug is the key measure when AIN is suspected. Corticosteroid treatment has been used to expedite the rate and extent of renal recovery in drug-induced AIN. For AIN due to CPI, corticosteroids are the mainstay of treatment based on observational data.
5. Reduced complement levels are often observed in IgG4-related disease with renal involvement. Serum IgG4 levels are elevated and useful for initial screening but have a poor diagnostic utility as often IgG4 levels can be affected by other disease conditions as well. Corticosteroids are the first-line agent for inducing remission in active IgG4-related disease. Rituximab is the commonest biological agent used in IgG4-related disease.

References

1. Goicoechea M, Rivera F, Lopez-Gomez JM. Increased prevalence of acute tubulointerstitial nephritis. Nephrol Dial Transplant. 2013;28(1):112–5. https://doi.org/10.1093/ndt/gfs143.
2. Farrington K, Levison DA, Greenwood RN, et al. Renal biopsy in patients with unexplained renal impairment and normal kidney size. Q J Med. 1989;70(3):221–33. https://doi.org/10.1093/oxfordjournals.qjmed.a068317.
3. Clarkson MR, Giblin L, O'Connell, et al. Acute interstitial nephritis: clinical features and response to corticosteroid therapy. Nephrol Dial Transplant. 2004;19(11):2778–83. https://doi.org/10.1093/ndt/gfh485.
4. Lopez-Gomez JM, Rivera F. Renal biopsy findings in acute renal failure in the cohort of patients in the Spanish Registry of Glomerulonephritis. Clin J Am Soc Nephrol. 2008;3(3):674–81. https://doi.org/10.2215/CJN.04441007.
5. Leonard CE, Freeman CP, Newcomb CW, et al. Proton pump inhibitors and traditional nonsteroidal anti-inflammatory drugs and the risk of acute interstitial nephritis and acute kidney injury. Pharmacoepidemiol Drug Saf. 2012;21(11):1155–72. https://doi.org/10.1002/pds.3329.
6. Eknoyan G. Acute tubulointerstitial nephritis. In: Schrier RW, Gottschalk CW, editors. Diseases of the kidney. 6th ed. Boston: Little, Brown; 1997. p. 1249–72.
7. Ball S, Cook T, Hulme B, Palmer A, Taube D. The diagnosis and racial origin of 394 patients undergoing renal biopsy: an association between Indian race and interstitial nephritis. Nephrol Dial Transplant. 1997;12(1):71–7. https://doi.org/10.1093/ndt/12.1.71.
8. Ball S, Lloyd J, Cairns T, Cook T, Palmer A, Cattell V, et al. Why is there so much end-stage renal failure of undetermined cause in UK Indo-Asians? QJM. 2001;94(4):187–93. https://doi.org/10.1093/qjmed/94.4.187.
9. Harmark L, van der Wiel HE, de Groot MC, van Grootheest AC. Proton pump inhibitor-induced acute interstitial nephritis. Br J Clin Pharmacol. 2007;64(6):819–23. https://doi.org/10.1111/j.1365-2125.2007.02927.x.
10. Rossert J. Drug-induced acute interstitial nephritis. Kidney Int. 2001;60(2):804–17. https://doi.org/10.1046/j.1523-1755.2001.060002804.x.
11. Ruffing KA, et al. Eosinophils in urine revisited. Clin Nephrol. 1994;41(3):163–6.
12. Maripuri S, Grande JP, Osborn TG, Fervenza FC, Matteson EL, Donadio JV, et al. Renal involvement in primary Sjogren's syndrome: a clinicopathologic study. Clin J Am Soc Nephrol. 2009;4(9):1423–31. https://doi.org/10.2215/CJN.00980209.
13. Baker RJ, Pusey CD. The changing profile of acute tubulointerstitial nephritis. Nephrol Dial Transplant. 2004;19(1):8–11. https://doi.org/10.1093/ndt/gfg464.
14. Muriithi AK, Leung N, Valeri AM, et al. Biopsy proven acute interstitial nephritis, 1993-2011: a case series. Am J Kid Dis. 2014;64:558–66. https://doi.org/10.1053/j.ajkd.2014.04.027.
15. Valluri A, Hetherington L, McQuarrie E, et al. Acute tubulointerstitial nephritis in Scotland. Q J Med. 2015;108(7):527–32. https://doi.org/10.1093/qjmed/hcu236.

16. Prendecki M, Tanna A, Salama AD, et al. Long-term outcome in biopsy-proven acute interstitial nephritis treated with steroids. Clin Kidney J. 2017;10(2):233–9.
17. Tuwabara T, Mori K, Mukoyama M, et al. Urinary neutrophil gelatinase-associated lipocalin levels reflect damage to glomeruli, proximal tubules, and distal nephrons. Kidney Int. 2009;75:285–94. https://doi.org/10.1038/ki.2008.499.
18. Praga M, Gonzalez E. Acute interstitial nephritis. Kidney Int. 2010;3(77):956–61. https://doi.org/10.1038/ki.2010.89.
19. Gobel U, Kettritz R, Schneider W, Luft F. The protean face of renal sarcoidosis. J Am Soc Nephrol. 2001;12(3):616–23.
20. Goules A, Masouridi S, Tzioufas AG, Ioannidis JP, Skopouli FN, Moutsopoulos HM. Clinically significant and biopsy-documented renal involvement in primary Sjogren syndrome. Medicine (Baltimore). 2000;79(4):241–9.
21. Deshpande V, Zen Y, Chan JK, Yi EE, Sato Y, Yoshino T, et al. Consensus statement on the pathology of IgG4-related disease. Mod Pathol. 2012;25(9):1181–92. https://doi.org/10.1038/modpathol.2012.72.
22. Carruthers MN, Khosroshahi A, Augustin T, et al. The diagnostic utility of serum IgG4 concentrations in IgG4 related disease. Ann Rheum Dis. 2015;74:14–8. https://doi.org/10.1136/annrheumdis-2013-204907.
23. Mac K, Wu XJ, Mai J, et al. The incidence of IgG4-positive plasma cells staining TIN in patients with biopsy-proven tubulointerstitial nephritis. J Clin Pathol. 2017;70:483–7. https://doi.org/10.1136/jclinpath-2016-203905.
24. Saeki T, Nishi S, Imai N, et al. Clinicopathological characteristics of patients with IgG4-related tubulointerstitial nephritis. Kidney Int. 2010;78(10):1016–23. https://doi.org/10.1038/ki.2010.271.
25. Raissian Y, Nasr SH, Larsen CP, et al. Diagnosis of IgG4-related tubulointerstitial nephritis. J Am Soc Nephrol. 2011;22(7):1343–52. https://doi.org/10.1681/ASN.2011010062.
26. Khosroshahi A, Wallace ZS, Crowe JL, Akamizu T, Azumi A, Carruthers MN, et al. International consensus guidance statement on the management and treatment of IgG4-related disease. Arthritis Rheumatol. 2015;67:1688–99. https://doi.org/10.1002/art.39132.
27. Hsieh C, Chang A, Brandt D, Guttikonda R, Utset TO, Clark MR. Predicting outcomes of lupus nephritis with tubulointerstitial inflammation and scarring. Arthritis Care Res. 2011;63(6):865–74. https://doi.org/10.1002/acr.20441.
28. Banerjee A, McKane W, Thiru S, Farrington K. Wegener's granulomatosis presenting as acute suppurative interstitial nephritis. J Clin Pathol. 2001;54(10):787–9.
29. Fhogartaigh CN, Newsholme W, Kinirons M, Tong W. An emerging infectious cause of renal impairment in the UK. BMJ Case Rep. 2011;2011:bcr0620114326. https://doi.org/10.1136/bcr.06.2011.4326.
30. Cataudella JA, Young ID, Iliescu EA. Epstein-Barr virus-associated acute interstitial nephritis: infection or immunologic phenomenon? Nephron. 2002;92(2):437–9. https://doi.org/10.1159/000063320.
31. Becker JL, Miller F, Nuovo GJ, Josepovitz C, Schubach WH, Nord EP. Epstein-Barr virus infection of renal proximal tubule cells: possible role in chronic interstitial nephritis. J Clin Invest. 1999;104(12):1673–81. https://doi.org/10.1172/JCI7286.
32. Mansur A, Little MA, Oh WC, Jacques S, Nightingale P, Howie AJ, et al. Immune profile and Epstein-Barr virus infection in acute interstitial nephritis: an immunohistochemical study in 78 patients. Nephron Clin Pract. 2011;119(4):c293–300. https://doi.org/10.1159/000329671.
33. Gonzalez E, Gutierrez E, Galeano C, Chevia C, de Sequera P, Bernis C, et al. Early steroid treatment improves the recovery of renal function in patients with drug-induced acute interstitial nephritis. Kidney Int. 2008;73(8):940–6. https://doi.org/10.1038/sj.ki.5002776.
34. Raza MN, Hadid M, Keen CE, et al. Acute tubulointerstitial nephritis, treatment with steroid and impact on renal outcomes. Nephrology. 2012;17:748–53. https://doi.org/10.1111/j.1440-1797.2012.01648.x.
35. Perazella MA. Diagnosing drug-induced AIN in the hospitalized patient: a challenge for the clinician. Clin Nephrol. 2014;81:381–8. https://doi.org/10.5414/CN108301.
36. Praga M, Sevillano A, Auñón P, González E. Changes in the aetiology, clinical presentation and management of acute interstitial nephritis, an increasingly common cause of acute kidney injury. Nephrol Dial Transplant. 2015;30:1472–9. https://doi.org/10.1093/ndt/gfu326.
37. Preddie DC, Markowitz GS, Radhakrishnan J, et al. Mycophenolate mofetil for the treatment of interstitial nephritis. Clin J Am Soc Nephrol. 2006;1:718–22. https://doi.org/10.2215/CJN.01711105.
38. Zuliani E, Zwahlen H, Gilliet F, et al. Vancomycin-induced hypersensitivity reaction with acute renal failure: resolution following cyclosporine treatment. Clin Nephrol. 2005;64:155–8. https://doi.org/10.5414/CNP64155.
39. Kida H, Abe T, Tomosugi N, Koshino Y, Yokoyama H, Hattori N. Prediction of the long-term outcome in acute interstitial nephritis. Clin Nephrol. 1984;22:55–60.

Acquired Chronic Tubulointerstitial Nephritis

Heidy Hendra, Mark Harber, and Ben Caplin

Contents

M. Harber (ed.), *Primer on Nephrology*, https://doi.org/10.1007/978-3-030-76419-7_33

Learning Objectives

1. Acquired chronic tubulointerstitial disease (or aCIN) is typically caused by medium- to long-term exposure to exogenous nephrotoxins, although infectious, autoimmune and metabolic causes of aCIN are well described.
2. There are epidemic levels of forms of aCIN in a number of low- and middle-income countries affecting working-age adults in agricultural communities though the specific cause(s) remains unclear.
3. Avoidance/withdrawal of precipitating factors remains the most effective strategy for reducing the impact of these diseases.

33.1 Introduction

Chronic interstitial fibrosis represents the final common pathway of almost all progressive kidney disease including chronic glomerular disease and genetic renal disease (e.g. autosomal dominant polycystic kidney disease). Furthermore, both the tubule and interstitium are a common site of acute kidney injury, whether due to ischaemic, toxic tubular injury or inflammatory interstitial disease. However, the tubulointerstitial compartment can also be the primary site of a progressive chronic renal injury, both due to genetic disease and acquired causes. This chapter will outline the heterogeneous group of disorders that can be classified as acquired chronic interstitial nephritis, focusing specifically on the known causes of disease and the clusters of disease currently of unknown cause that represent a major cause of morbidity and mortality in a number of low-income settings.

33

Definitions

Acquired chronic interstitial nephritis (aCIN) refers to the heterogeneous group of conditions that lead to progressive tubulointerstitial scarring and loss of excretory renal function. As all forms of chronic kidney disease (CKD) that cause loss of glomerular filtration rate (GFR) will involve the tubulointerstitial compartment, aCIN (at least for the purposes of this chapter) includes only those conditions where this compartment is the primary site of injury. Differentiation from acute interstitial nephritis is primarily by biochemical trajectory and and abscence of significant inflammation on renal biopsy, although clearly there is substantial clinical and aetiological overlap between these two syndromes. Finally inherited forms of chronic interstitial nephritis, which may be clinically and pathologically indistinguishable from aCIN, have recently been reclassified as autosomal dominant tubulointerstitial kidney disease and are discussed in detail in chapter 34.

33.2 Clinical Features, Diagnosis and Differential Diagnosis

Unless presenting as part of a multisystem disorder, the consequences of aCIN may well go unnoticed by patients for many years. Unlike glomerular disease, chronic interstitial disease typically presents without abnormalities detectable on urine analysis. Similarly, hypertension is not common in aCIN and may only appear as a late sign. Hence, most patients will come to the attention of medical professionals through, often incidental, findings of a low or declining estimate of the GFR. Exposure to potential risk factors for aCIN should then be sort from the clinical history (◘ Table 33.1).

Although low-level albuminuria is described, albumin/creatinine ratios above 30 mg/mmol would provide evidence against an underlying aCIN particularly in those with preserved kidney function (e.g. an estimated glomerular filtration rate (eGFR) >30 mL/min/1.7 m^2). Low-molecular-weight proteinuria (e.g. retinol-binding protein or neutrophil gelatinase-associated lipocalin) has been suggested as a potential marker of these diseases, but robust evidence as to the sensitivity and specificity of these molecules is lacking for most causes of aCIN. Urinary concentrating defects or electrolyte abnormalities can also be early signs of aCIN.

Ultrasound typically demonstrates small but otherwise unremarkable symmetrical kidneys, although several causes of aCIN have characteristic appearances on imaging in advanced disease (see below). Renal biopsy will provide histological confirmation of aCIN (◘ Fig. 33.1), but as any chronic glomerulonephritis will also cause interstitial fibrosis, a diagnosis of aCIN

◘ **Table 33.1** Key points in the clinical history of a patient with aCIN

Country and region of origin
Current and previous occupation
Travel history
Drinking water source
Lifetime use of analgesics and types
Other medication history, specifically lithium and calcineurin inhibitors
Treatment for malignancy, focusing on radiotherapy and cytotoxics
Previous gastroenterological surgery
History of eating disorder
Use of herbal remedies
Potential predisposition to intravascular volume depletion

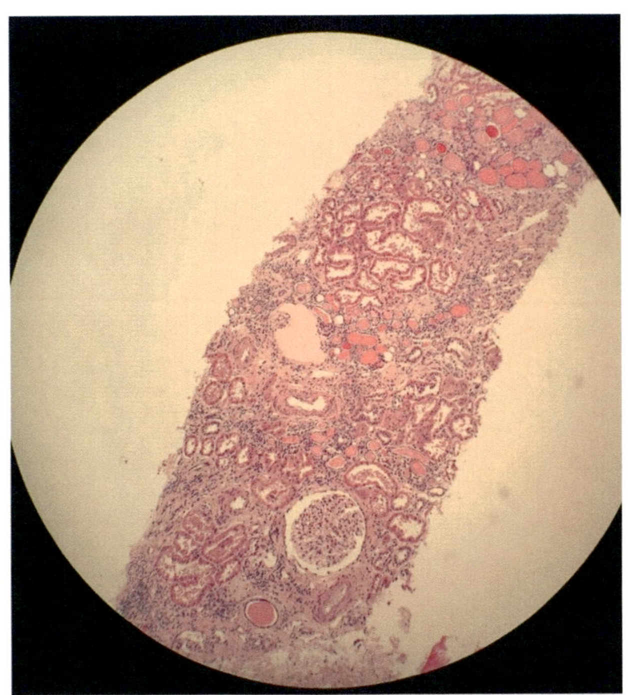

Fig. 33.1 Typical histology in acquired chronic interstitial nephritis. Haematoxylin and eosin ×20. Note severe tubular damage with preservation of glomeruli. The aetiology of disease in this case remains unknown. (Images courtesy of Lauren Heptinstall, Royal Free London)

should only be made in the absence of evidence of primary glomerular disease on biopsy, or at least the absence of glomerular involvement significant enough to cause the degree of interstitial changes. Furthermore, although aCIN can be identified on biopsy, pathognomonic changes that identify the underlying cause are present in only a minority of cases (see below). Differentiation from acute interstitial nephritis is usually on biochemical trajectory, although conditions leading to aCIN will typically not present with an acute inflammatory infiltrate on renal biopsy. The different causes of aCIN are outlined in Table 33.2 and discussed, along with notable features and management, by aetiology below.

To further complicate matters, renal biopsy is often not performed in (or is inaccessible to) patients and populations with aCIN, meaning diagnoses are usually made on clinical grounds alone, usually as a diagnosis of exclusion. This makes systematic descriptions of the epidemiology, and investigations of the causes of aCIN, particularly challenging.

33.3 Epidemiology

Among the most developed regions of the world, aCIN is probably an uncommon cause of CKD and end stage kidney disease (ESKD) outside of specific high-risk pop-

Table 33.2 Causes of acquired chronic interstitial disease[a]

Drugs	Metals	Phyto-/ mycotoxins	Infection	Others	CKD of undetermined cause
Lithium	Cadmium	Aristolochic acid	Tuberculosis	Eating disorder associated	
Phenacetin	Lead	(Ochratoxin)	Chronic bacterial infection in certain populations	Ileostomy associated	
(Other compound or acetaminophen-based analgesics)	(Mercury)		(Other infections)	Radiation nephritis	
Calcineurin inhibitors	(Arsenic)				
Platinum-based chemotherapy					

[a]Evidence for the factors in parentheses as a cause of aCIN are supported by limited data (e.g. the evidence may suggest these factors may be the cause of acute rather than chronic interstitial nephritis or derive from animal models)

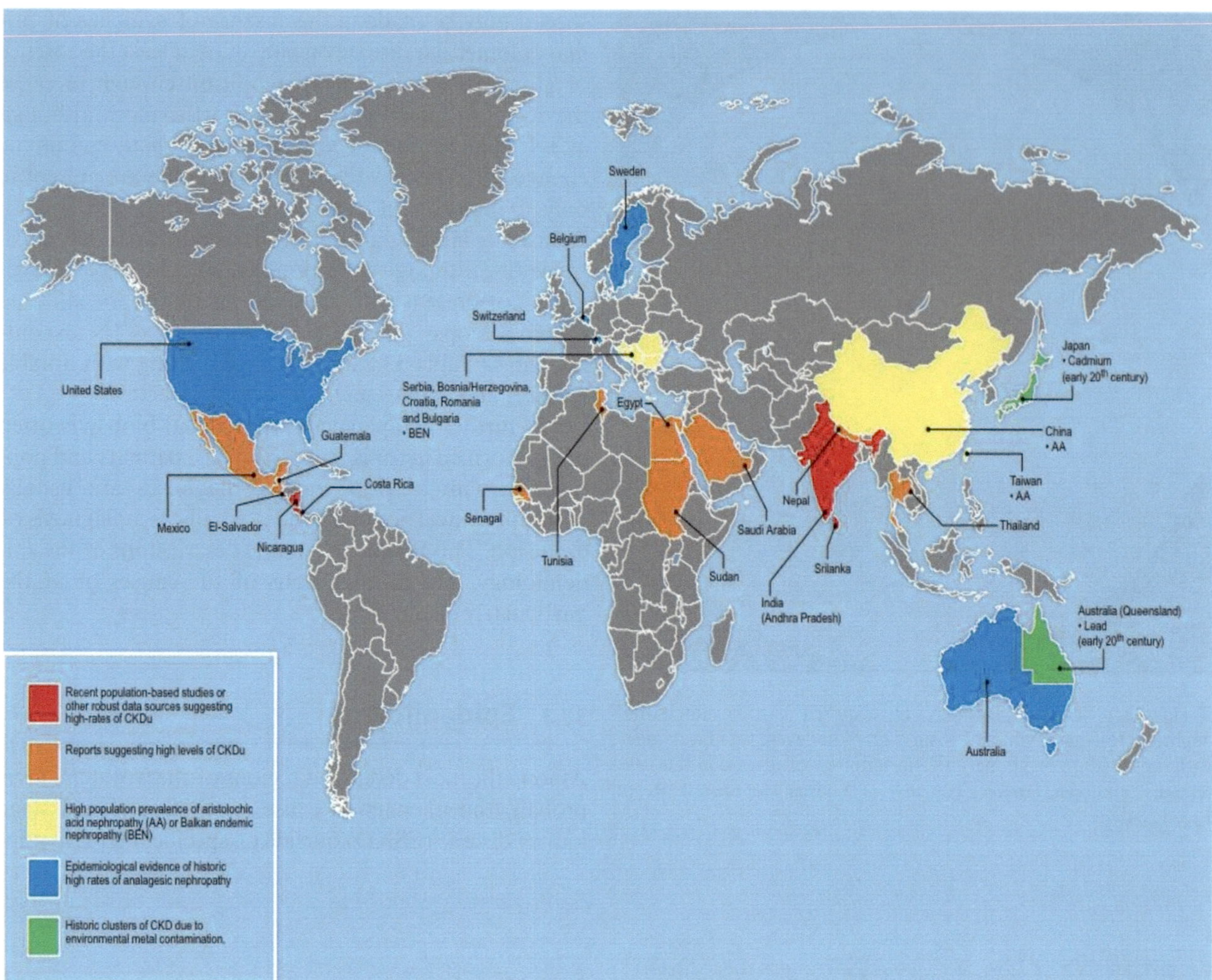

Fig. 33.2 Global distribution of acquired chronic interstitial nephritis. Red: Recent population-based evidence of high rates of CKDu (Mesoamerican nephropathy or chronic interstitial nephritis in agricultural communities); Orange: Reports of possible high rates of CKDu; Yellow: High population prevalence of aristolochic acid nephropathy or Balkan endemic nephropathy; Blue: Historic high rates of analgesic nephropathy; Green: Historic clusters of CKD due to environmental metal contamination

ulations or clusters of disease due to known causes (see below Fig. 33.2). For example, the UK Renal Registry suggests only 18% of incident ESKD patients have a primary renal disease diagnosis of 'other' (the category that would include aCIN but also a number of other unrelated diagnostic entities; Fig. 33.3), although in some regions, patients with aCIN, who have not been biopsied, may fall into an 'unknown' category, making robust estimates of the prevalence difficult to establish.

There are regions where known causes of aCIN contribute, or have contributed, to a substantial burden of ESKD, for example, aCIN secondary to *Aristolochia* in the Balkans [1] or phenacetin in Australia [2]. However, more recently, there is an increasing recognition of aCIN of unknown cause that has reached epidemic levels in areas of South Asia and Central America (and perhaps elsewhere) where the prevalence of impaired kidney function (a single value of eGFR <60 mL/min/1.7 m^2) is close to 20% in some communities [3]. This clinical syndrome is described as CKD of undetermined cause (CKDu). Figure 33.2 illustrates regions where clusters aCIN due to known causes as well as CKDu have been reported.

33.4 Aetiopathology, Features and Management

33.4.1 Drugs

33.4.1.1 Lithium

Lithium therapy is associated with a number of renal disorders including (most commonly) diabetes insipidus, a more generalised tubular dysfunction, CKD and acute kidney injury in overdose. Additional complica-

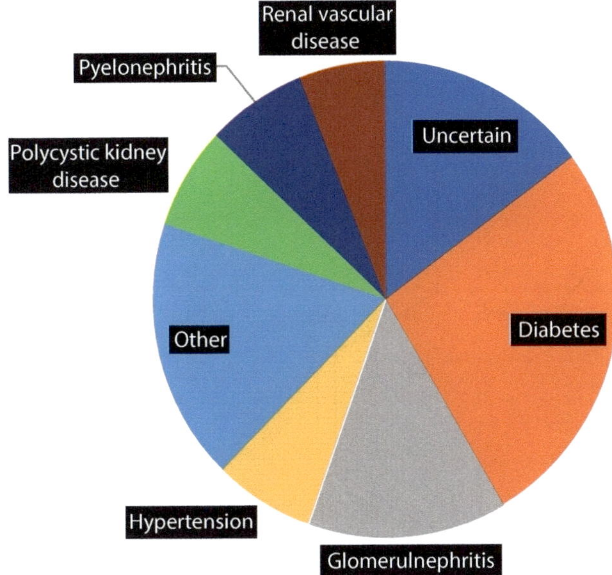

Fig. 33.3 Primary renal disease in those starting ESKD in the UK. (Data from the UK Renal Registry 2017)

tions of long-term lithium exposure include hyperparathyroidism with hypercalcaemia.

Bipolar disorder, in common with other serious mental disorders, is a risk factor for all forms of chronic kidney disease (CKD) [4], but there is clearly an increased risk of renal dysfunction specifically associated with lithium use. European population-based studies have demonstrated risks of CKD are approximately doubled with long-term lithium use after accounting for other risks of renal disease [5, 6]. Histologically, the use of this drug is associated with a chronic interstitial fibrosis which is often histologically apparent even with a creatinine in the normal range. Microcystic lesions associated with tubules are described but are a non-specific sign with similar appearances in a number of other tubulointerstitial disorders. Clinically, the rate of renal decline tends to be slow, however, and overall numbers reaching ESKD low. Estimates from Sweden suggest ~0.5% of the lithium-treated population reach ESKD and those with lithium-induced ESKD make up less than 1% of the renal replacement therapy (RRT) population [7]. Key aspects of management include close monitoring to maintain lithium within the relatively narrow therapeutic window, annual surveillance of eGFR and avoidance of other nephrotoxins. Risks of drug withdrawal in those with declining eGFR but well-controlled mental health symptoms may be significant, and these decisions should usually only be made in partnership with the patient and their other relevant care providers. Early identification may be important, and there is evidence that guidelines on the annual screening of patients on lithium are not always followed. There is no specific treatment for lithium-induced chronic intersitial nephritis (CIN), but avoiding other nephrotoxic agents and early treatment of hypercalcaemia would seem prudent. Although there is good pre-clinical evidence that amiloride blocks lithium uptake into the tubular cell, this agent has not been robustly evaluated in the management of lithium-induced CIN.

33.4.1.2 Analgesic Nephropathy

A number of analgesics have been implicated in forms of aCIN. Importantly, this is a clinical entity distinct from both the predictable vasoconstriction-mediated non-steroidal anti-inflammatory drugs (NSAIDs) induced acute tubular injury and the idiosyncratic acute forms of acute interstitial nephritis or nephrotic syndrome induced by the same class of drugs. Indeed, it is aniline analgesics and compound preparations rather than NSAIDs that are implicated in analgesic nephropathy (AN). Phenacetin, a now-discontinued metabolic precursor of acetaminophen (paracetamol), was associated with a substantially increased risk of developing abnormal kidney function [2]. In Australia, in the 1970s, around 20% of all patients starting dialysis had been diagnosed as analgesic nephropathy. The risk appears dose dependent with disease typically occurring after the ingestion of these drugs over many years (estimated as at least 3000 doses) with presentation typically in the sixth and seventh decades. Although the incidence of disease has declined where phenacetin has been withdrawn, there remains a strong association at the population level between self-reported lifetime acetaminophen use and loss of eGFR, and furthermore, aspirin use has been proposed as an exacerbating factor in this relationship [8, 9].

AN has a clinical presentation and histology typical of aCIN with interstitial fibrosis, particularly in the medulla. However, papillary necrosis/calcification and indented or irregular kidney contours on imaging are particularly characteristic of disease (although similar appearances occur in sickle-cell-associated kidney disease). Management rests entirely on withdrawal of the implicated agents.

33.4.1.3 Other Drugs

Calcinuerin inhibitors such as Cyclosporin A, and perhaps to a lesser extent tacrolimus, are an important cause of aCIN with high blood levels a clear risk factor for decline in GFR. The use of these drugs is ubiquitous in renal transplantation where multiple insults can lead to interstitial fibrosis. However, the well-documented development of aCIN in non-renal solid organ transplantation and other non-kidney-related immune conditions after treatment with these agents confirms the potential for nephrotoxicity with long-term use.

Platinum-based chemotherapy is also associated with aCIN in a dose-dependent manner. Although there is some evidence the thiosulphate amifostine may protect against kidney damage, lower doses and the availability of alternative chemotherapeutic agents may be more effective measures in preventing renal injury.

33.4.2 Metals

Dense or 'heavy' metals, specifically lead, cadmium, mercury and arsenic, have been implicated in kidney disease. The renal tubule has an important role in the reabsorption of these elements from the filtrate either via specific transmembrane transporters or endocytosis of protein bound ions. Evidence for renal toxicity derives from a number of sources. Poisoning with these metals will lead to tubular dysfunction, membranous nephropathy (in the case of mercury) [10] or acute tubular injury [11–13], and animal studies support the nephrotoxic potential of these molecules. However, robust evidence for a clinically important causal role in aCIN derives from episodes of environmental lead and cadmium pollution with a clear temporal link to clusters of renal failure.

High levels of childhood lead exposure in the early twentieth century in Queensland, Australia, led to an excess of CKD and the histopathological lesions consisted of marked tubulointerstitial fibrosis [14]. Similarly, environmental cadmium pollution led to the epidemic of "itai-itai" disease [15] or cadmium-induced aCIN with osteomalacia. These substances are also found in a number of traditional remedies and may be responsible for isolated cases of aCIN. Although the pathophysiology of metal-induced aCIN is poorly understood, diagnosis is usually made through documentation of occupational and/or social history of exposure as well as direct measurement of metals in biosamples. Low-molecular-weight proteinuria has also been described as a useful early marker of nephrotoxic exposure [16].

Finally, higher levels of exposure (though not at the levels observed in the historic episodes described above) to these metals in population studies have been shown to be associated with an incident of CKD [17], and furthermore, ESKD patients have been shown to demonstrate higher levels of some of these metals than matched controls in a number of studies [18, 19]. However, whether the metal is a primary cause of disease, an exacerbating factor in other forms of CKD or merely a surrogate for other exposures remains unclear.

33.4.3 Phytotoxins and Mycotoxins

33.4.3.1 Aristolochic Acid

Aristolochic acids (AAs) originate from flowering plants of the birthwort family (Fig. 33.4). The nephrotoxicity of these substances in rodents was described in the 1980s [20] and proposed as a cause of human disease. However, it was only when there was an outbreak of renal failure among women consuming Chinese herbal products in the 1990s that the clinical relevance of AAs was confirmed in the form of aristolochic acid nephropathy (AAN). Subsequent to this, it has been become clear, both from epidemiological and biopsy-based studies, that herbal preparations containing AAs are an important cause of CKD in China and Taiwan, as well leading to clusters of disease elsewhere, are an important cause of CKD in China and Taiwan [21]. Furthermore, evidence has accumulated that wheat flour contaminated by AAs also underlies Balkan endemic nephropathy, a disease that had been reported to be occurring as early as the 1950s in the farming villages surrounding the tributaries of the Danube River [1].

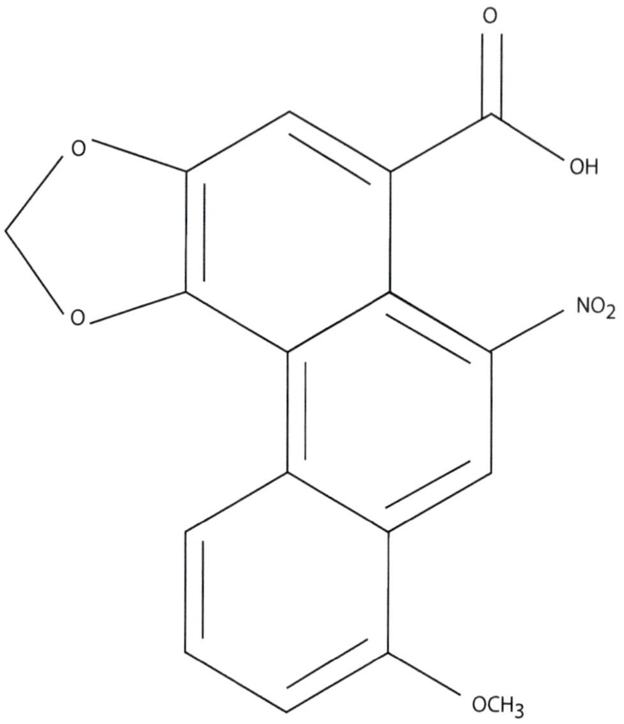

O
OH
O
O
NO_2
OCH_3

Fig. 33.4 Structure of aristolochic acid

AAN presents with progressive chronic renal impairment, but AAs also lead to urothelial malignancy in around 40% of those with confirmed renal disease [22]. Renal biopsy typically demonstrates cortical interstitial fibrosis in the absence of a substantial inflammatory infiltrate. Although there is good evidence to suggest that the formation of covalent DNA adducts which lead to mutations in the TP53 tumour-suppressor gene underlies the development of urinary tract malignancy, the mechanisms underlying progressive renal fibrosis are not clearly understood. The presence of these DNA adducts in tissue specimens, although technically challenging to demonstrate, provides a definitive diagnosis. Both GFR decline and risk of malignancy appear to be associated with dose-dependent exposure to AAs, and management of renal disease mainly consists of general measures alongside withdrawal/avoidance of the causative agent. However, despite the absence of significant inflammation on biopsy, some experts have advocated a therapeutic trial of corticosteroids in those with preserved renal function [23]. Surveillance for urological malignancy (6-monthly urine cytology alongside annual cross-sectional imaging and cystourethroscopy) with nephroureterectomy in those with abnormalities (or prophylactically prior to transplant listing in those receiving dialysis) is also integral to the management of these patients.

33.4.3.2 Ochratoxin

The ochratoxins are a group of pentaketide toxins derived from *Aspergillus* and *Penicillium* species of fungi [24]. Ochratoxin exposure is reported to be high across North Africa; however, although ochratoxin is a well-characterised nephrotoxin in animals, robust evidence for a role in human aCIN remains sparse. For example, serum levels in outpatients with a diagnosis of chronic interstitial nephritis without an attributable cause were higher than those with CKD due to other diagnoses or heathy controls in a study from Tunisia [25].

33.4.4 Infection

33.4.4.1 Tuberculosis

Despite the development of successful antimycobacterial chemotherapy over half a century ago, tuberculosis (TB) remains a global health problem with disease widely prevalent not only in low-income countries but also among at-risk groups in Europe and the USA. Involvement of the genitourinary tract, which almost always occurs through haematological spread from the lungs, occurs in around one-fifth of those with pulmonary disease [26]. Although patients with renal TB can complain of localising symptoms, presentation is more typically with non-specific constitutional upset. Diagnosis can be challenging as traditional microscopy (smear) and culture has poor sensitivity. Immune responses are typically attenuated in those with CKD, meaning tuberculin skin testing is unreliable though interferon gamma release assays may have better sensitivity. Molecular biological diagnosis may soon be routinely available and become the gold standard. Classic changes on imaging occur in advanced disease, but renal biopsy is usually unequivocal with interstitial fibrosis and caseating granuloma with or without acid-fast bacilli. Treatment for renal tuberculosis should follow society guidelines though dose adjustment for some agents is required in those with reduced GFR.

33.4.4.2 Other Infections

Multiple other infections, including hanta and polyoma viruses, leptospirosis and atypical mycobacteria can also lead to acute and subacute forms of interstitial nephritis (see ▶ Chap. 32). Whether any of these pathogens are also responsible for a significant clinical burden of aCIN is less clear, although there is evidence of chronic urinary tract carriage of a number of these organisms. Furthermore, chronic and/or recurrent pyelonephritis due to infection with uropathogens can undoubtedly lead to aCIN, although this does not appear to be a substantial clinical problem outside of renal transplantation, those with anatomically abnormal urinary tract (see ▶ Chap. 56) or an inherited or acquired defect in bacterial killing (see ▶ Chap. 54).

33.4.5 Radiation Nephritis

Radiation-induced kidney injury has been described following treatment of a number of malignancies including gynaecological cancers, lymphomas and sarcomas as well as following total body irradiation prior to bone marrow transplantation. Renal syndromes associated with radiation range from acute kidney injury with thrombotic microangiopathy to a slowly progressive aCIN which may present many years after therapy [27]. Overall incidence has been falling in parallel to improvements in dosing and targeting of radiotherapy and the increasing range of alternative cancer treatments.

33.4.6 Eating Disorders and Gastrointestinal Diversion

Eating disorders are associated with a wide range of renal presentations including acute kidney injury, electrolyte disturbance, recurrent urinary tract infection, nephrolithiasis and aCIN [28]. The pathophysiology underlying aCIN is likely multifactorial with recurrent pre-renal injury, hypokalaemia (with or without the use of laxatives), kidney stones and infection all potentially playing a role. Although evidence from large studies is absent, the risk of end-stage renal disease appears extremely high among these patients [29]; however, prevalent advanced renal impairment can be easily missed in this group as creatinine-based GFR estimating equations will substantially overestimate kidney function [30]. Consistent with the concept that severe chronic/repetitive pre-renal injury and/or electrolyte disturbance is an important risk for eGFR decline in general, and perhaps aCIN in particular, CKD has been reported to occur up to four times more frequently in those with surgical ileostomies (high-output stoma) compared to well-matched (albeit relatively elderly patients with comorbidities) controls [31]. These conditions are discussed further in ▶ Chap. 43.

33.4.7 Other Causes

There are a number of autoimmune, metabolic and systemic inflammatory disorders that present with an acute or chronic tubulointerstitial involvement, either primarily or as part of a mixed picture (e.g. systemic lupus erythematosus or diabetic kidney disease). These are covered in detail either in dedicated sections or in the chapter on acute interstitial nephritis.

33.4.8 Chronic Kidney Disease of Undetermined Cause

33

Notwithstanding the diagnostic uncertainty as to the precise cause of disease even where aCIN is identified on biopsy, this group of conditions is a relatively rare cause of CKD in many populations, particularly in high-income regions. Clusters of high prevalence of aCIN due to *known causes* occur globally and are discussed above, but it is also increasingly clear that forms of aCIN of *unknown cause* are responsible for a huge burden of (often untreated) ESKD in a number of populations in low- and middle-income countries (◻ Fig. 33.2). The umbrella term CKD of undetermined cause (CKDu) is useful to describe the epidemic levels of aCIN of unknown aetiology, specifically in Central America, where it is termed Mesoamerican nephropathy (MeN) [32], and Sri Lanka, where it is labelled as chronic interstitial nephritis in agricultural communities (CINAC) [33]. It should be emphasised that CKDu, a highly prevalent aCIN occurring in low- and middle-income settings, is not synonymous with the ESKD of unknown causes reported in the renal registries of high-income countries which likely represents a heterogeneous group of conditions including chronic undiagnosed glomerulonephritis, congenital abnormalities and vascular disease. However, the relationship between CKDu in low- and middle-income countries and the clusters of aCIN of unknown aetiology occurring in specific populations living in other higher-income parts of the world is unclear, for example, the excess of CKD seen in those of Guajarati origin in the UK [34].

As discussed in the 'Epidemiology' section above, CKDu is currently the leading cause of death among working-age men in Nicaragua [35]. The disease presents as a typical aCIN with little in the way of positive clinical findings until uraemia develops, although symptoms of hyperuricaemia are often particularly prominent in advanced MeN. The natural history of CKDu is poorly described, but evidence from Central America suggests MeN is a highly aggressive disease [36] and anecdotally young men will progress from a serum creatinine in the normal range to ESKD in as little as 5 years.

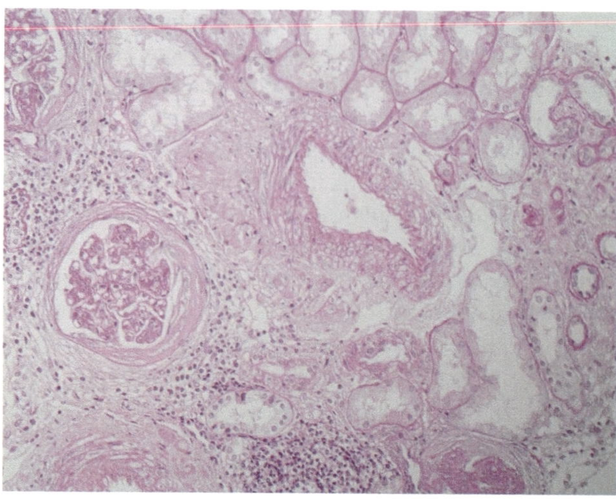

◻ **Fig. 33.5** Renal biopsy from a patient with Mesoamerican nephropathy. PAS stain ×20. The biopsy demonstrates areas of tubular atrophy and interstitial fibrosis along with periglomerular fibrosis but without evidence of glomerular cell proliferation. Some interstitial inflammation is seen in scarred areas. (Image courtesy of Annika Wernesson and Julia Wijkstrom, Karolinska Institute, Sweden)

Although renal biopsy is not routinely available in most communities impacted by CKDu, these have been performed in the research context [37, 38]. Histopathology (◻ Fig. 33.5) is remarkably similar between endemic areas (Central America versus Sri Lanka) and demonstrates tubulointerstitial damage, fibrosis, signs of glomerular ischaemia (but no proliferation or immune complex deposition) and typically low levels of inflammatory infiltrate.

Proposed causes of these diseases are wide ranging and include recurrent pre-renal injury and heat stress (due to extremely poor work conditions), agrichemical toxicity, metal exposure, as yet unidentified infection, myco- or phytotoxins, nephrotoxic drugs or contaminated alcohol, and underlying genetic predisposition, all either individually or in combination. However, despite over a decade of research efforts, conclusive evidence as to the cause of disease (or diseases, as despite the similarities CKDu may represent a number of different conditions) remains absent.

Tips, Tricks and Pitfalls

Patients with aCIN may well be asymptomatic without hypertension or urinary abnormalities on routine screening.

Presentation may be with incidental low eGFR (even within the normal range but low for age).

Renal biopsy may not provide a clear diagnosis, and a thorough social, medical, travel and occupational history is key to establishing the cause of disease.

Chapter Review Questions

1. What can be an early sign of aCIN?
2. What is the commonest renal adverse effect of lithium therapy, and how common is it for patient who is receiving long-term lithium treatment to progress to ESKD?
3. What would one see on CT in patients with analgesic nephropathy?
4. Which heavy metal exposure has been reported to cause membranous nephropathy?
5. Aristolochic acid can lead to urothelial malignancy in some patients with renal disease. Which mutation underlies this development?

Answers

1. Patients with aCIN typically present without clear symptom. Proteinuria, haematuria and hypertension are often absent; however, urinary concentrating defects or electrolyte abnormalities can be an early sign of aCIN.
2. Nephrogenic diabetes insipidus (NDI) is the commonest renal adverse effect of lithium therapy as it occurs in up to 40% of patients. A study from Sweden estimated ~0.5% of the lithium-treated population reach ESKD and those with lithium-induced ESKD make up less than 1% of the RRT population.
3. Characteristics of analgesic nephropathy in CT are papillary necrosis/calcification and indented or irregular kidney contours; however, one should beware in mind that similar appearances can be found in patients with sickle-cell-associated kidney disease.
4. While many metals have been implicated in aCIN, mercury is also associated with membranous nephropathy.
5. Formation of covalent DNA adducts which lead to mutations in the TP53 tumour-suppressor gene underlies the development of urinary tract malignancy in patients taking aristolochic acid.

Case Studies

1. A 29-year-old was referred by his GP when found to be anaemic (haemoglobin of 81) when presenting to donate blood. He was a bit tired and would pass urine once a night, but was otherwise asymptomatic and no history of renal injury, no past medical history and no family history of note. He had no prescribed, over-the-counter, recreational or homeopathic medication. Examination revealed a well-looking individual with a blood pressure of 125/73. Urinalysis reveled 1+ protein, with no white blood cells on urine microscopy, blood tests demostrated creatinine 430micromol/L, urea 21 mmol/L, normal calcium, ESR 6mm/hr, CRP 3mg/L. Virology, immunology and myeloma screen were all clear. An ultrasound revealed smallish (9 cm) kidneys with a normal bladder.

   A biopsy subsequently showed relatively preserved glomeruli with disproportionate chronic tubulointerstitial damage. The original cause was not identified, but minimal findings on the dipstick, nocturia and a good/low blood pressure (in the absence of a pre- or post-renal cause) are strongly suggestive of an aCIN. Active autoimmune, allergic and infectious causes would seem unlikely given the lack of inflammatory response and a presumptive diagnosis of aCIN might have been made without a biopsy.
2. A 41-year-old self-employer IT technician from Bangladesh was referred to clinic for investigation of abnormal renal function (130micromol/L). He had a history of investigations for abdominal pain, malaise and weight loss for which no cause was found and general malaise. He had been taking some traditional medicines. On examination, he had a non-specific macular rash predominantly on the palms and soles of his feet but also on both forearms and neck. Investiagtions demonstrated a urine protein 1+ on urinalysis (urine protein: creatinine ratio 84) with no blood, urea 12.5mmol/L, bicarbonate 17mmol/L, haemoglobin 79g/L. Further screening demonstrated a proximal tubular acidosis as part of Fanconi's syndrome. The kidney lesion was attributed to chronic heavy metal toxicity, which was confirmed on both blood and hair samples and thought to be due to exposure to ground water or the herbal remedy. Heavy metal poisoning typically presents with non-specific symptoms such as malaise, disproportionate anaemia (as in this case), tubular disorders and rashes. In chronic arsenic poisoning, a macular rash on the palms and soles is characteristic.
3. A 62-year-old tennis coach and retired professional tennis player was referred with a low eGFR (27 mls/min and creatinine of 220micromol/L). With the exception of two hip and one knee replacement, he had no significant medical history and remained very fit. The urine was inactive with minimal proteinuria.

Kidneys were 8.5 cm bilaterally on ultrasound. On direct questioning, he had a heavy consumption of analgesics for much of his professional career (exceeding the 3000 doses typically associated with analgesic nephropathy). A non-contrast CT demonstrated characteristic lobulated appearance consistent with AN. As with many aCIN progression of AN appears to be relatively slow once the causative agent is withdrawn, particularly in the absence of high-level proteinuria.

33.5 Conclusion

Acquired chronic tubulointerstitial disease represents a heterogeneous group of disorders which although a generally rare cause of CKD in high-income countries are responsible for clusters of ESKD due to known causes in a number of regions. Furthermore, forms of aCIN without a known cause prevalent in low- and middle-income countries are increasingly recognised as a significant global health problem. Identification of the causative agent can be challenging but is critical as amelioration of renal decline rests on avoidance of the relevant exposures.

References

1. Bamias G, Boletis J. Balkan nephropathy: evolution of our knowledge. Am J Kidney Dis. 2008;52(3):606–16.
2. Dubach UC, Rosner B, Pfister E. Epidemiologic study of abuse of analgesics containing phenacetin. Renal morbidity and mortality (1968–1979). N Engl J Med. 1983;308(7):357–62.
3. Peraza S, et al. Decreased kidney function among agricultural workers in El Salvador. Am J Kidney Dis. 2012;59(4):531–40.
4. Iwagami M, et al. Severe mental illness and chronic kidney disease: a cross-sectional study in the United Kingdom. Clin Epidemiol. 2018;10:421–9.
5. Close H, et al. Renal failure in lithium-treated bipolar disorder: a retrospective cohort study. PLoS One. 2014;9(3):e90169.
6. Kessing LV, et al. Use of lithium and anticonvulsants and the rate of chronic kidney disease: a nationwide population-based study. JAMA Psychiat. 2015;72(12):1182–91.
7. Bendz H, et al. Renal failure occurs in chronic lithium treatment but is uncommon. Kidney Int. 2010;77(3):219–24.
8. Curhan GC, et al. Lifetime nonnarcotic analgesic use and decline in renal function in women. Arch Intern Med. 2004;164(14):1519–24.
9. Fored CM, et al. Acetaminophen, aspirin, and chronic renal failure. N Engl J Med. 2001;345(25):1801–8.
10. Becker CG, et al. Nephrotic syndrome after contact with mercury. A report of five cases, three after the use of ammoniated mercury ointment. Arch Intern Med. 1962;110:178–86.
11. Gerhardt RE, et al. Chronic renal insufficiency from cortical necrosis induced by arsenic poisoning. Arch Intern Med. 1978;138(8):1267–9.
12. Katsuma A, et al. Acute renal failure following exposure to metallic mercury. Clin Nephrol. 2014;82(1):73–6.
13. Sathe K, Ali U, Ohri A. Acute renal failure secondary to ingestion of ayurvedic medicine containing mercury. Indian J Nephrol. 2013;23(4):301–3.
14. Inglis JA, Henderson DA, Emmerson BT. The pathology and pathogenesis of chronic lead nephropathy occurring in Queensland. J Pathol. 1978;124(2):65–76.
15. Emmerson BT. "Ouch-ouch" disease: the osteomalacia of cadmium nephropathy. Ann Intern Med. 1970;73(5):854–5.
16. Nogawa K, Kido T. Biological monitoring of cadmium exposure in itai-itai disease epidemiology. Int Arch Occup Environ Health. 1993;65(1 Suppl):S43–6.
17. Hsu LI, et al. Arsenic exposure from drinking water and the incidence of CKD in low to moderate exposed areas of Taiwan: a 14-year prospective study. Am J Kidney Dis. 2017;70(6):787–97.
18. Hellstrom L, et al. Cadmium exposure and end-stage renal disease. Am J Kidney Dis. 2001;38(5):1001–8.
19. Sommar JN, et al. End-stage renal disease and low level exposure to lead, cadmium and mercury; a population-based, prospective nested case-referent study in Sweden. Environ Health. 2013;12:9.
20. Mengs U. Acute toxicity of aristolochic acid in rodents. Arch Toxicol. 1987;59(5):328–31.
21. Yang CS, et al. Rapidly progressive fibrosing interstitial nephritis associated with Chinese herbal drugs. Am J Kidney Dis. 2000;35(2):313–8.
22. Nortier JL, et al. Urothelial carcinoma associated with the use of a Chinese herb (Aristolochia fangchi). N Engl J Med. 2000;342(23):1686–92.
23. Gokmen MR, et al. The epidemiology, diagnosis, and management of aristolochic acid nephropathy: a narrative review. Ann Intern Med. 2013;158(6):469–77.
24. Malir F, et al. Ochratoxin A: 50 years of research. Toxins (Basel). 2016;8(7):191.
25. Zaied C, et al. Presence of ochratoxin A in Tunisian blood nephropathy patients. Exposure level to OTA. Exp Toxicol Pathol. 2011;63(7–8):613–8.
26. Abbara A, Davidson RN, Medscape. Etiology and management of genitourinary tuberculosis. Nat Rev Urol. 2011;8(12):678–88.
27. Cohen EP, Robbins ME. Radiation nephropathy. Semin Nephrol. 2003;23(5):486–99.
28. Bouquegneau A, et al. Anorexia nervosa and the kidney. Am J Kidney Dis. 2012;60(2):299–307.
29. Zipfel S, et al. Long-term prognosis in anorexia nervosa: lessons from a 21-year follow-up study. Lancet. 2000;355(9205):721–2.
30. Delanaye P, et al. Cystatin C or creatinine for detection of stage 3 chronic kidney disease in anorexia nervosa. Nephron Clin Pract. 2008;110(3):c158–63.
31. Li L, et al. Ileostomy creation in colorectal cancer surgery: risk of acute kidney injury and chronic kidney disease. J Surg Res. 2017;210:204–12.
32. Correa-Rotter R, Wesseling C, Johnson RJ. CKD of unknown origin in Central America: the case for a Mesoamerican nephropathy. Am J Kidney Dis. 2014;63(3):506–20.
33. Jayasumana C, et al. Chronic interstitial nephritis in agricultural communities: a worldwide epidemic with social, occupational and environmental determinants. Nephrol Dial Transplant. 2017;32(2):234–41.
34. Ball S, et al. Why is there so much end-stage renal failure of undetermined cause in UK Indo-Asians? QJM. 2001;94(4):187–93.
35. Cohen J. Mesoamerica's mystery killer. Science. 2014;344(6180):143–7.

36. Gonzalez-Quiroz M, et al. Decline in kidney function among apparently healthy young adults at risk of Mesoamerican nephropathy. J Am Soc Nephrol. 2018.
37. Wijkstrom J, et al. Morphological and clinical findings in Sri Lankan patients with chronic kidney disease of unknown cause (CKDu): similarities and differences with Mesoamerican Nephropathy. PLoS One. 2018;13(3):e0193056.
38. Wijkstrom J, et al. Clinical and pathological characterization of Mesoamerican nephropathy: a new kidney disease in Central America. Am J Kidney Dis. 2013;62(5):908–18.

Further Reading/Guidelines

Bipolar disorder: assessment and management 2014 NICE: https://www.nice.org.uk/guidance/cg185.

British Thoracic Society: guidelines for the prevention and management of Mycobacterium tuberculosis infection and disease in adult patients with chronic kidney disease: https://www.brit--thoracic.org.uk/document-library/clinical-information/tuberculosis/tb-guidelines/guidelines-in-adult-patients-with-tuberculosis-and-chronic-kidney-disease/.

Genetic Tubulointerstitial Disease and Nephronophthisis

Alice Gage, Buddhika Illeperuma, and Mark Harber

Contents

M. Harber (ed.), *Primer on Nephrology*, https://doi.org/10.1007/978-3-030-76419-7_34

Learning Objectives

1. To cover and appreciate the nature, epidemiology and diagnosis of autosomal dominant tubulointerstitial renal diseases
2. To cover the nature, diagnosis and characteristics of autosomal recessive nephronophthisis conditions

Definition

ADTKD is a group of conditions characterised by chronic tubulointerstitial disease and progressive chronic kidney disease (CKD) in the context of a bland urine, with an autosomal dominant pattern of inheritance.

Nephronophthisis (NPHP) is a group of ciliopathies commonly causing end-stage renal disease in childhood and adolescence, characterised by chronic tubulointerstitial disease and progressive CKD in the context of a bland urine with an autosomal recessive pattern of inheritance.

34

34.1 Introduction

In 2015, KDIGO produced a consensus report which proposed the current classification of ADTKDs to replace previous nomenclature which included 'medullary cystic kidney disease' as well as providing guidance on diagnosis and management which has enhanced awareness and understanding of these conditions [1]. The main genes associated with ADTKD are *UMOD*, *MUC1*, *REN* and *HNF1B*, although new mutations and genes allied to this group continue to be discovered. They share an inconspicuous renal presentation, with the not infrequent occurrence of cysts which can be cortical or medullary and do not usually result in renal enlargement. However, there are some clinical clues to indicate the pathological process and differentiate between the individual diseases (◘ Fig. 34.1). The current state of knowledge with ADTKDs is very nicely reviewed by Devuyst et al. [2].

These conditions range from rare to very rare, although it is likely that they are underdiagnosed given the paucity of constitutional symptoms or urinary findings that normally trigger investigation. A recent analysis of patients with end-stage renal failure in Ireland found a prevalence of 0.54% with a mutation consistent with ADTKD; this group comprised 42.6% *MUC1*, 32.5% UMOD and 13% *NHF1-ß* mutations [3]. An increased awareness of these conditions is likely to result in a greater prevalence and earlier diagnosis as well as the discovery of new mutations.

Inherited renal ciliopathies include ADPKD, X-linked disorders such as oral-facial-digital syndrome and a heterogeneous but important group of autosomal recessive conditions such as ARPKD (discussed elsewhere) and nephronophthisis. Nephronophthisis also results in progressive Chronic kidney disease (CKD) characterised by interstitial fibrosis and tubular atrophy (IFTA) and sometimes microcytes as a result of genetic disorders of the cilium. Urine analysis in these patients is also bland and often shows concentration defects. Nephronophthisis is the commonest monogenic cause of ESRD in the first three decades of life. Moreover, in 10–20% of cases, nephronophthisis is associated with significant syndromic findings that result in a much earlier diagnosis as well as long-term disability.

Between nephronophthisis and ADTKD, there is a moderate portion of chronic kidney disease that needs diagnosis and management.

34.2 ADTKD

Autosomal dominant tubulointerstitial kidney diseases (ADTKD).

34.3 ADTKD-UMOD

Uromodulin (also known as Tamm-Horsfall glycoprotein) is a genuinely fascinating molecule produced solely in the kidney and with pleiotropic roles [4]. These include preventative roles in stone formation by reducing aggregation of calcium in super-saturated filtrate and urinary tract infection by binding to uropathogenic *E. coli* inhibiting bacterial adhesion to uroepithelial cells. It is also involved in salt and water regulation via the NKCC2 co-transporter and potassium ROMK channel as well as being implicated in innate immunity and immune regulation within the kidney. In this context, variants of uromodulin have been associated with a propensity to stone formation, CKD and hypertension in the general population.

ADTKD-UMOD is probably the commonest form of ADTKD, with one UK study finding a prevalence of 2% in ESRD patients [5]. It results from mutations in the uromodulin gene that are mostly missense mutations causing disruption of conserved cysteine residues and resulting in misfolding of the mature protein.

34.3.1 Aetiology and Pathogenesis

Misfolded uromodulin is abnormally trafficked with reduced expression on the apical surface of the epithelial cell and progressive accumulation in the endoplasmic reticulum particularly in the thick ascending limb (TAL). This results in ER stress, apoptosis, progressive interstitial fibrosis, tubular atrophy, microcyst formation and a secondary inflammatory infiltrate.

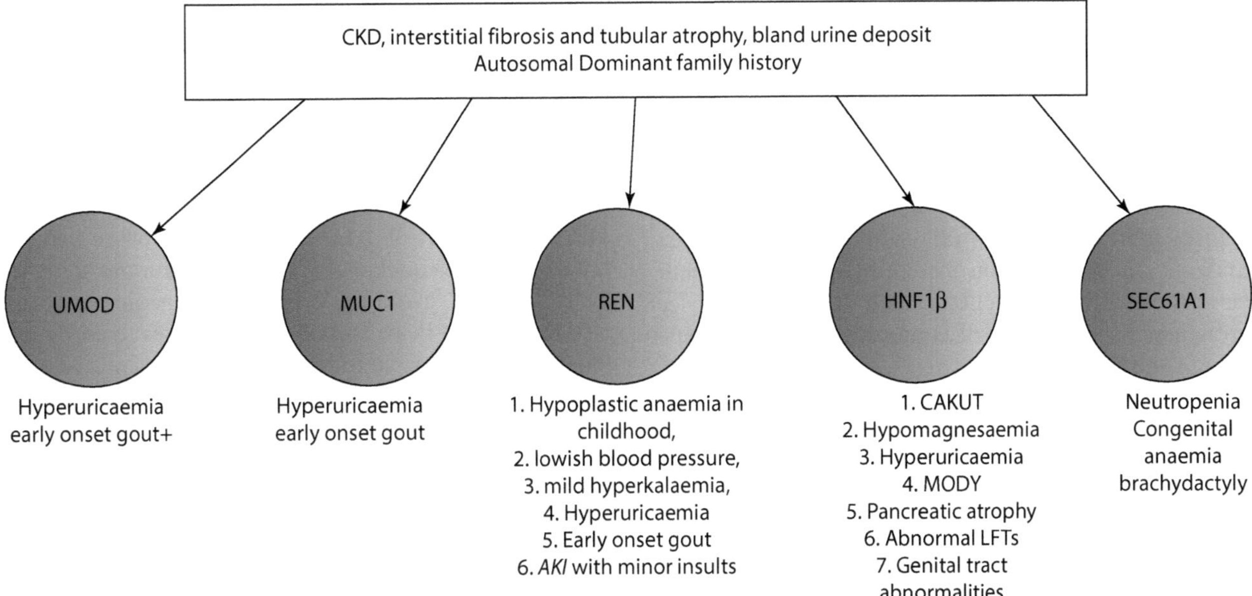

Fig. 34.1 Genes associated with ADTKD and associated clinical features. All are associated with CKD, minimal proteinuria/bland urine and an autosomal dominant family history, although the phenotype may vary significantly in *NHF1-β* so as to appear unrelated kidney conditions. CAKUT congenital abnormalities of the kidney and urinary tract, MODY maturity-onset diabetes of the young

34.3.2 Clinical Features

In common with all ADTKDs, the presentation of ADTKD-UMOD is usually unflamboyant, with progressive CKD, a bland urinary sediment, an absence of hypertension and a mild urinary concentration defect. Hyperuricaemia (70%) and gout (50–75%) are common. Gout tends to be early onset (mean age 21), and men are often worse affected [6]. The clinical course is very variable, but the median age of ESRD is in the mid-50s. Cysts are seen in a proportion of patients, but their absence should not be considered strong evidence against the diagnosis. As mentioned previously, this is one reason why the old name of 'medullary cystic kidney disease type 2' has been retired. In addition, the absence of early onset gout in many people with the disorder has rendered the alternative name of 'familial juvenile hyperuricaemic nephropathy' similarly unhelpful.

34.3.3 Diagnosis

The diagnosis is most likely to be made in the context of a family history of early onset gout and CKD consistent with autosomal dominance by a nephrologist with a high index of suspicion. The kidneys are likely to be normal in size or small and may have some cysts (without renal enlargement). Renal biopsy is not diagnostic but likely to show IFTA as the predominant feature in the context of relatively well-preserved glomeruli. Although not a standard test, it may be possible to demonstrate excess uromodulin by immunofluorescence or to demonstrate low levels of urinary uromodulin. A definitive diagnosis is likely to rely on genetic testing.

34.3.4 Treatment

There is no specific treatment for ADTKD-UMOD apart from normal supportive measures for progressive CKD. As with most tubulointerstitial disease, hypertension is not a major feature and diuretics may exacerbate hyperuricaemia. Management of hyperuricaemia with xanthine oxidase inhibitors makes sense in controlling gout, although there is no data to suggest that it slows progression. Uricosurics such as benzbromarone or losartan (but probably not salicylic acid) might also be helpful. Renal transplantation is curative (with disease recurrence in an allograft not described), but potential familial live donors need genetic screening to exclude the diagnosis.

34.4 ADTKD-MUC1

ADTKD-MUC1 results from a mutation in the *MUC1* gene that encodes the membrane-bound mucoprotein Mucin-1 [10]. The result is progressive chronic kidney disease in the context of bland urinary sediment. It is a rare condition, although recent data suggests a prevalence similar to that of ADTKD-UMOD.

34.4.1 Aetiology and Pathogenesis

Mucin-1 is a membrane-bound mucoprotein found on the apical surface of epithelial cells in many tissues including reproductive organs, glandular tissue and the renal tubules. The protein has an extracellular domain, which includes a variable number of Mucin repeats, a transmembrane domain and a cytoplasmic tail that can undergo phosphorylation mediating several intracellular processes. Its functions include promoting cell growth and survival as well as preventing pathogen invasion of the cell [8].

In ADTKD-MUC1, there is a single cytosine adenine insertion in the variable number tandem repeat which encodes the extracellular Mucin repeat part of the protein. The aberrant protein Mucin-1–frameshifted (MUC1-fs) is unable to serve its intended protective function and accumulates in the cytoplasm leading to premature cell death [9]. This causes progressive nephron loss and therefore chronic kidney disease. Interestingly, in ADTKD-MUC1, this effect is isolated to renal tubular cells and not seen in other tissues.

34

34.4.2 Clinical Features

ADTKD-MUC1 is notable for its lack of distinctive characteristics [10], and this almost certainly contributes to a relatively late age of initial diagnosis (40 years). Individuals present with an elevated serum creatinine and bland urinary sediment in the context of a family history of autosomal dominant kidney disease. Hyperuricaemia and gout do occur but to a lesser degree than in ADTKD-UMOD, and again renal cysts are sometimes observed in affected individuals (hence the older name of medullary cystic kidney disease type 1 that has now fallen out of use). However, they do not have any other biochemical or imaging abnormalities to point towards a specific diagnosis. The kidneys are normal or small in size depending on the degree of chronic kidney disease. Biopsy findings are also non-specific with features of interstitial fibrosis, tubular atrophy and vasculopathy with minimal inflammation. While the mutations demonstrate complete penetrance, the age of progression to end-stage renal failure varies widely from 20 to 60 years (average 51) [7].

34.4.3 Diagnosis

There needs to be a high suspicion of a diagnosis of ADTKD-MUC1 in an individual with progressive CKD and a family history of autosomal dominant kidney disease in the absence of significant cystic disease on imaging [7]. However, genetic testing showing a heterozygous mutation in the *MUC1* sequence is currently the best way to confirm a diagnosis [8].

34.4.4 Treatment

The management of ADTKD-MUC1 is based around preventing the sequelae of CKD. Maintaining adequate hydration and avoiding nephrotoxic medications are also important. If an individual progresses to end-stage renal failure, transplantation is a curative intervention and good outcomes have been reported in this patient group. Given the mode of inheritance and variable age of development of CKD, family members who come forward for live donor transplantation should undergo genetic testing to determine their status.

34.5 ADTKD-REN

ADTKD-REN is a rare but interesting group of diseases resulting from mutations in the renin gene leading to progressive CKD with a bland urinary sediment. There are some clinical features that make it more distinguishable.

34.5.1 Aetiology and Pathogenesis

These conditions result from mutations in either the renin promoter, prosegment or mature renin peptide. Renin is expressed throughout the renal tubule and juxtaglomerular apparatus. In normal circumstances, preprorenin is translocated to the endoplasmic reticulum where it is cleaved to form prorenin and some is translocated to the lysozyme and cleaved to form active renin. Mutations of the promoter and prosegment lead to failure of normal translocation and processing, resulting in reduced functional renin and an accumulation of mutated peptide in the ER. This stresses the ER causing apoptosis, premature cell death and ultimately CKD.

Patients with mutations solely affecting the mature renin peptide probably avoid or incur less cell death from deposition of abnormal peptide but will share the characteristics of a low renin state.

34.5.2 Clinical Features

Reduced renin levels result in clinical features that may give useful diagnostic clues. An early feature is mild to moderate anaemia which is hypoproliferative and associated with low erythropoietin levels. This may present in the second year of life and if apparent in the context of CKD tends to be out of proportion with eGFR. The anaemia may improve or disappear in adolescence secondary to the increase in sex hormones. The hyporeninaemic state results in a lowish blood pressure and a propensity for pre-renal AKI with relatively mild insults or a disproportionate drop in eGFR with NSAIDs. Patients tend to have mildly elevated serum potassium levels. They may also have hyperuricaemia and therefore can present with gout. Patients with mutations involving the renin promoter or prorenin segment tend to have slowly progressive CKD, reaching end-stage renal failure at an average age of 52, w hereas those with abnormalities of the mature renin peptide are more likely to present earlier with gout in their 20s with a greater range of age at the time of development of end-stage renal disease (median age of 64).

34.5.3 Diagnosis

Unexplained childhood anaemia, episodes of unexpected AKI, mild hypotension, mild hyperkalaemia and gout early in life are all suggestive and should be enquired about particularly in the context of reduced eGFR and a family history. These features, although subtle, should give a pretty high index of suspicion, but the definitive diagnosis is through genetic testing as biopsy findings are non-specific but may show IFTA in the context of normal glomeruli.

34.5.4 Treatment

Protecting the patient's intravascular volume by avoiding a low-salt diet makes sense, and fludrocortisone is helpful in maintaining intravascular volume. Theoretically, fludrocortisone will have a negative feedback on renin production and therefore slow injury to tubules from denatured proteins, although to date clinical benefit has not been proven. Patients should also avoid NSAIDs and volume depletion and may benefit from uric acid reduction with xanthine oxidase inhibitors. Transplantation is curative.

34.6 ADTKD-HNF1B

Mutations of the *HNF1B* gene, which encodes Hepatocyte Nuclear Factor-1-β, are associated with renal disease in two main ways: (a) via a variety of congenital abnormalities of the kidney and urinary tract (CAKUT) and tubular development and (b) later in life with ADTKD, fibrosis and tubular atrophy presenting as slowly progressive CKD. *HNF1B* mutations are also associated with extra-renal manifestations including maturity-onset diabetes of the young (MODY), abnormal liver function tests and genital tract abnormalities.

34.6.1 Aetiology and Pathophysiology

How *HNF1B* mutations result in adult renal disease has not been fully elucidated but includes abnormal epithelial-mesenchymal transformation, aberrant TGF-β expression and mitochondrial disease [11].

34.6.2 Clinical Features

Despite the autosomal dominant inheritance of *NHF1-β* mutations, the diagnosis is often difficult as there can be a large variation in clinical presentation. Even within one family, individuals can present with seemingly isolated developmental abnormalities of the kidney and urinary tract. Renal manifestations in adulthood include CKD minimal proteinuria, hypomagnesaemia and renal cystic change that can result in renal enlargement (in which situation patients may be misdiagnosed with the far more common autosomal dominant polycystic kidney disease).

Extra-renal manifestations that are helpful in raising the diagnosis are MODY (initially non-insulin-dependent diabetes before 25 years) with CT findings of pancreatic atrophy. Unexplained raised liver function tests are relatively common, and some patients may have early hyperparathyroidism and autism or develop chromophobe renal cell carcinoma. Ultrasound scans of older children with *NHF1-β* suggest that abnormal corticomedullary differentiation is common (78%) is are hyper-echoic kidneys (50%), with subcortical cysts detectable in 70% and around a third of kidneys small at presentation (REF). However, this represents patients scanned at an early age presumably because of some aspect of presentation or family history. Findings may be less clear in those patients destined to develop ESRD in late adulthood.

34.6.3 Diagnosis

The diagnosis may be suggested by the family history, a low magnesium or high uric acid level, although none of this is pathognomonic. MODY is an important clue, and a review of an abdominal CT specifically for pancreatic atrophy might be indicative as might be persistently abnormal liver function tests with normal synthetic function and no alternative explanation or genital abnormalities. Renal biopsy is likely to show disproportionate IFTA but relatively preserved glomeruli which should raise ADTKD as a diagnosis but is not diagnostic. The definitive diagnosis is based on genetic testing.

34.6.4 Treatment

There is no specific treatment for ADTKD-*NHF1-β* mutations, but it makes sense to educate and support the patient in avoiding obesity and avoiding drugs that are diabetogenic. Transplantation is curative for renal manifestations but with a presumably high risk of NODAT in patients with pancreatic atrophy treated with CNIs and steroids.

34.7 Rarer Forms of ADTKD

There are a small number of rare pedigrees described with other mutations resulting in tubulointerstitial kidney disease. Mutations of the alpha-subunit of *SEC61* have been shown to be associated with abnormal translocation through the ER and accumulation of abnormal SEC61 in the tubular epithelial cells. These mutations are associated with a rare phenotype of small kidneys, simple cysts and neutropenia.

34

34.7.1 Mitochondrial Cytopathy-Related Interstitial Renal Disease

Until now, the most common presentation of mitochondrial DNA diseases involving the kidney has been Fanconi syndrome with case reports of FSGS and steroid-resistant nephrotic syndrome. However, a study of a large pedigree of maternal inherited tubulointerstitial disease recently identified a mutation causing functional impairment of mitochondrial tRNA. The phenotype was not associated with Fanconi syndrome or any systemic neurological deficit. Given the huge metabolic workload of the kidney and the relatively subtle presentation of this form of mitochondrial disorder, it would not be surprising if further mitochondrial mutations are found to result in tubulointerstitial disease. The biggest diagnostic clue here was maternal transmission [12].

34.7.2 Nephronophthisis

Nephronophthisis is a heterogeneous (and expanding) group of ciliopathies with autosomal recessive inheritance that are important because they are the commonest cause of ESRD in the first three decades of life (◘ Fig. 34.2). They are, not infrequently, associated with extra-renal manifestations that result in significant disability. The proteins encoded by NPHP 1-13 are all expressed either in the primary cilia, the centrosome or basal bodies at the base of cilia in renal epithelial cells. This may result predominantly in renal disease or in a proportion of patients serious extra-renal consequences and responsible for a growing variety of clinical manifestations such as Joubert, Jeune, Meckel-Gruber and Bardet-Biedl syndromes with tapetoretinal degeneration (retinitis pigmentosa) and progressive blindness a common feature (20%). The understanding of the mutations causing these diseases is improving rapidly and is comprehensively reviewed by Devlin and Sayer [13].

The commonest (comprising 20%) of the nephronophthisis is NPHP-1 and ranges from 1:10,000 live births in Finland to 1:50,000 in Canada but seemingly less common elsewhere. As a group, they are responsible for between 2% and 15% of ESRD in children and usually diagnosed early in life.

34.7.3 Aetiology and Pathophysiology

As with ADTKD, a variety of genetic mutations result in a common pathway of renal epithelial cell disease. In nephronophthisis, the common pathway is via ciliary dysfunction. NPHP mutations impair intracellular signalling resulting in dysregulated tissue growth and development of cysts. Histology demonstrates interstitial fibrosis and atrophy, tubular cysts, thickened/multilayered basement membranes, relatively well-preserved glomeruli (although secondary atrophy occurs with progression) and with limited inflammation [14].

34.7.4 Clinical Features

The clinical features are somewhat heterogeneous depending on the mutations involved and severity of renal dysfunction. Urinary concentration disorder may be an early symptom with polyuria and polydipsia. Renal dysfunction is usually associated with normotension (perhaps not with NPHP-2) and a bland urine and normal or small kidneys on ultrasound. Cysts may be apparent but they are usually small. Retinitis pigmentosa typically presents with loss of night vision and then progressive visual loss. Those with other extra-renal manifestations may present very early with learning difficulties and cerebellar, hepatic, ocular or psychomotor signs. The key features of some eponymous syndromes linked with NPHP are shown in ◘ Table 34.1.

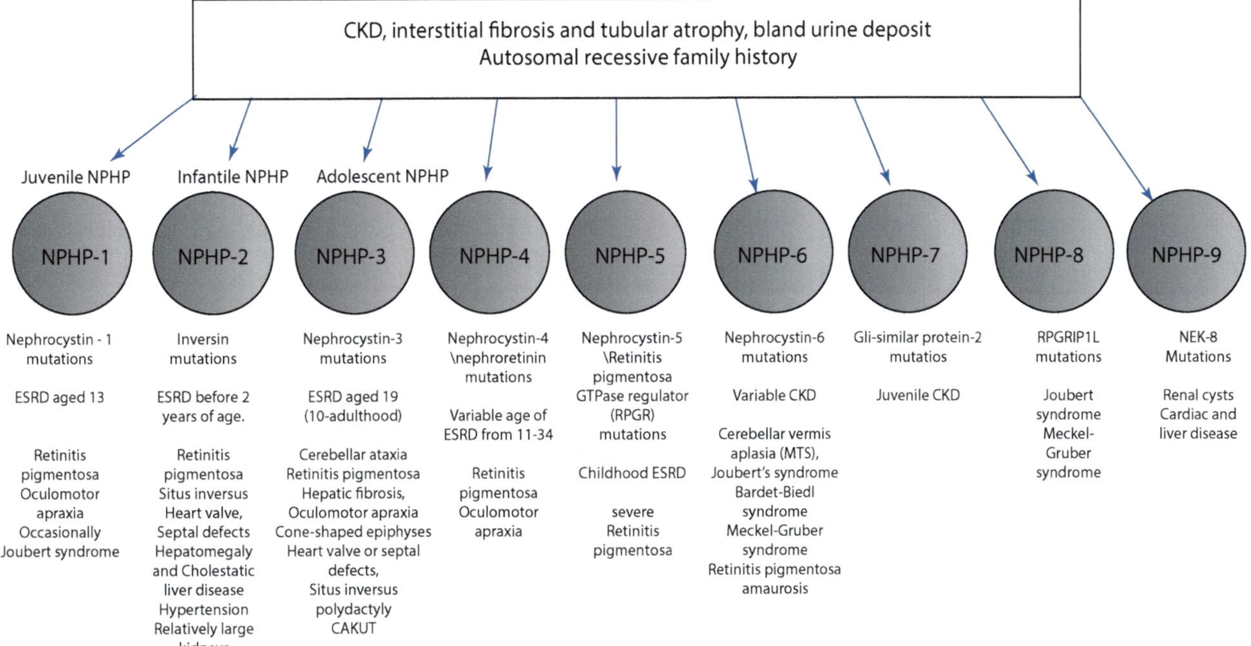

Fig. 34.2 Characteristics of the first nine NPHPs demonstrating common themes in terms of CKD and extra-renal manifestations including Senior-Loken syndrome (combination of NPHP and retinitis pigmentosa (20%)). MTS molar tooth sign, CAKUT congenital abnormalities of the kidney and urinary tract, ESRD end-stage renal disease

Table 34.1 Eponymous Nephronophthisis and their extra-renal manifestations

Senior-Loken syndrome	Retinitis pigmentosa
Leber's congenital amaurosis	Retinal dystrophy
Joubert syndrome	Hypotonia, developmental delay, ataxia, hyperpnoea and sleep apnoea, polydactyly, low-set ears, hypertelorism, cleft lip/palate, ptosis; c haracteristic 'molar tooth sign' on MRI of the midbrain; early non-renal presentation
Bardet-Biedl syndrome	Obesity, retinitis pigmentosa, polydactyly and hypogonadism
Cogan syndrome	Ocular motor apraxia
Mainzer-Saldino syndrome	Cerebellar ataxia, skeletal dysplasia, retinal dystrophy
Jeune syndrome	Small thoracic cavity secondary to short ribs and small chest, abnormal pelvis, polydactyly; e arly non-renal presentation and short life expectancy
Meckel-Gruber syndrome	Pulmonary hypoplasia, occipital encephalocoele, hepatic developmental defects; l ethal in infancy

34.7.5 Diagnosis

The diagnosis of NPHP is usually made by paediatricians either because of extra-renal presentation or in the context of renal impairment. The combination of retinitis pigmentosa and CKD would be highly suggestive or more extreme neurological manifestations may raise suspicion of the diagnosis alongside other clues such as situs inversus suggestive of a ciliopathy or the 'molar tooth sign' on MRI of elongated cerebellar peduncles pathognomonic of Joubert syndrome. Ultimately, neither renal imaging nor biopsy is diagnostic, and genetic screening should be undertaken.

34.7.6 Treatment

There is currently no treatment for the nephronophthisis beyond renal replacement therapy and, ideally, transplantation. For those patients with extra-renal manifestations, considerable thought needs to be put into coordinating long-term care and support.

34.7.7 Oral Facial Dactyly Syndrome

Another very rare ciliopathy associated with polycystic renal disease and hypertelorism, facial asymmetry, syndactyly or polydactyly, agenesis of the corpus callosum, cleft palate or bifid tongue, missing incisors.

Mutations of the OFD-1 gene are X-linked lethal in males and usually diagnosed in females via the constellation of clinical features and confirmed by X-rays of the hand which show irregular radiolucent patches and spicules on the metacarpals and phalanges.

Tips and Tricks

1. The main tip is to maintain an enquiring mind when assessing a patient with unexplained CKD and, most importantly, to always take a detailed family history. This should include enquiries into consanguinity (particularly important for AR conditions), and evidence of maternal or X-linked transmission is important.
2. Checking urate levels and enquiring about early onset gout, an absence of hypertension or evidence of urinary concentration deficit, while not specific, are all suggestive of ADTKDs. Enquire about a family history of MODY, low magnesium, genital tract abnormalities for *NHF1-β* or mild hyperkalaemia, or minimally provoked AKI and childhood anaemia for REN if the possibility of ADTKD arises. Transplantation is curative for both ADTKD and nephronophthisis, but live donation needs to be accompanied with careful assessment and genetic testing of potential donors.
3. It is worth liaising with your local geneticist to agree referral criteria and for updates on conditions that can be screened for and their clinical correlates.

34.8 Summary

Together, the collection of diseases encompassed by nephronophthisis and ADTKD represents an important cause of ESRD. For children with nephronophthisis, this not only brings ESRD into their lives at an early stage but for some with extra-renal manifestations, additional significant disabilities. Identifying these conditions and supporting both patients and their families for the long haul, offering genetic counselling and ensuring successful transition are key aspects of care.

It is likely that many cases of ADTKD are underdiagnosed and that new mutations will be discovered for both ADTKD and nephronophthisis. As genetic screening becomes cheaper and more widely available, it should be increasingly adopted as a diagnostic tool.

34

Case Study

Case 1

A 35-year-old man from Somalia was referred by his family doctor following blood tests to investigate fatigue, showing an eGFR of 15 ml/min. He had been separated from his family for a while and was not aware of any family history. He was normotensive and slim and his examination was unremarkable. Urine dipstick was bland and a renal ultrasound reported normal size kidneys with the appearance of CKD with reduced corticomedullary differentiation. Acute and chronic screen for secondary causes of renal failure was negative, but he had moderately raised liver function tests. A MRCP and liver screen was unremarkable. He received a deceased donor renal transplant and developed diabetes post-transplant. A review of an abdominal CT scan a few years prior demonstrated atrophy of the tail of the pancreas, and a retrospective review of pre-transplant bloods showed a low magnesium and high uric acid levels.

A presumptive diagnosis of *NHF1-β* was made and confirmed by genetic testing. Although the diagnosis had little impact for the patient, the autosomal dominant nature of the mutation had important implications for his family as well as an explanation for his abnormal liver function tests.

Chapter Review Questions

1. What are the clinical characteristics of REN?
2. At what age do patients with NPHP 1-3 typically reach end-stage renal disease?
3. What are the functions of uromodulin (Tamm-Horsfall protein)?
4. What is cheaper, a renal biopsy or genetic testing for NPHP/ADTKD?

Answers

1. REN is characterised by a hyporeninaemic state resulting in anaemia in childhood (hypoplastic), mild hyperkalaemia, hyperuricaemia, lowish blood pressure, AKI with minor provocation and progressive CKD with a bland urine.
2. NPHP-1, known as juvenile form, reaches ESRD at roughly 13 years; NPHP-2, known as infantile form, results in renal failure very early, typically 1 year but always before 2. NPHP-3, adolescent form, reaches ESRD at an average of 19 years but ranging from 10 to adulthood.
3. It has roles inhibiting stone formation, urinary tract infection, innate immunity, immune regulation and water regulation by the kidney.
4. A bit depends on the local costs of genetic screening, but genetic screening, if not already cheaper (and less invasive), is likely to become much cheaper than a renal biopsy.

Acknowledgements Acknowledgement to Professor D Gale for advice and comments.

References

1. Eckardt KU, Alper SL, Antignac C, et al. Autosomal dominant tubulointerstitial kidney disease: diagnosis, classification, and management – a KDIGO consensus report. Kidney Int. 2015;88:676–83.
2. Devuyst O, Olinger E, Weber S, et al. Autosomal dominant tubulointerstitial kidney disease. Nat Rev Dis Primers. 2019;5(1):60.
3. Cormican S, Connaughton DM, Kennedy C, et al. Autosomal dominant tubulointerstitial kidney disease (ADTKD) in Ireland. Ren Fail. 2019;41(1):832–41.
4. Devuyst O, Olinger E, Rampoldi L. Uromodulin: from physiology to rare and complex kidney disorders. Nat Rev Nephrol. 2017;13:525–44.
5. Gast C, Marinaki A, Arenas-Hernandez M, et al. Autosomal dominant tubulointerstitial kidney disease UMOD is the most frequent non polycystic genetic kidney disease. BMC Nephrol. 2018;19:301.
6. Bollée G, Dahan K, Flamant M, et al. Phenotype and outcome in hereditary tubulointerstitial nephritis secondary to UMOD mutations. Clin J Am Soc Nephrol. 2011;6:2429–38.
7. Bleyer AJ, Kmoch S. Autosomal dominant tubulointerstitial kidney disease, MUC1-related. 2013 Aug 15 [updated 2016 Jun 30]. In: Adam MP, Ardinger HH, Pagon RA, et al., editors. GeneReviews® [Internet]. Seattle: University of Washington, Seattle; 1993–2020.
8. Gale DP, Kleta R. *MUC1* makes me miserable. J Am Soc Nephrol. 2018;29(9):2257–8.
9. Dvela-Levitt M, Kost-Alimova M, Emani M, et al. Small molecule targets TMED9 and promotes lysosomal degradation to reverse proteinopathy. Cell. 2019;178(3):521–535.e23.
10. Knaup KX, Hackenbeck T, Popp B, et al. Biallelic expression of Mucin-1 in autosomal dominant tubulointerstitial kidney disease: implications for nongenetic disease recognition. J Am Soc Nephrol. 2018;29(9):2298–309.
11. Chan SC, Zhang Y, Shao A, et al. Mechanism of fibrosis in *HNF1B*-related autosomal dominant tubulointerstitial kidney disease. J Am Soc Nephrol. 2018;29(10):2493–509.
12. Connor TM, Hoer S, Mallett A, Gale DP, Gomez-Duran A, et al. Mutations in mitochondrial DNA causing tubulointerstitial kidney disease. PLoS Genet. 2017;13(3):e1006620.
13. Devlin LA, Sayer JA. Renal ciliopathies. Curr Opin Genet Dev. 2019;56:49–60.
14. Hildebrandt F, Attanasio M, Otto E. Nephronophthisis: disease mechanisms of a ciliopathy. J Am Soc Nephrol. 2008;20(1):23–35.

Patient Information Websites

Autosomal dominant tubulointerstitial kidney disease (ADTKD): https://rarerenal.org/patient-information/adtkd-patient-information/

Nephronophthisis (NPHP): https://rarerenal.org/patient-information/nphp-patient-information/

Nephrology Interface

Contents

Rheumatological Conditions and the Kidney

Conall Mac Gearailt, Áine Burns, and Bernadette Lynch

Contents

M. Harber (ed.), *Primer on Nephrology*, https://doi.org/10.1007/978-3-030-76419-7_35

Learning Objectives

1. To educate about renal complications of rheumatological conditions
2. To inform about potential renal adverse events subsequent to treatment of rheumatological conditions
3. To focus on the epidemiology, pathophysiology and clinical presentation of conditions such as scleroderma and rheumatoid arthritis and their renal manifestations
4. To provide a useful reference for nephrologists dealing with patients with rheumatological disease in day-to-day clinical practice
5. To aim to encourage a closer working relationship between rheumatology and nephrology in order to improve patient outcomes

35.1 Introduction

In this chapter, we aim to educate about renal complications of rheumatological conditions. We also discuss complications of therapies which may occur from treatment. We focus on the renal manifestations of scleroderma, rheumatoid arthritis as well as other rheumatological disorders, demonstrating the epidemiology, pathophysiology and clinical manifestations of these conditions. The presentation of renal complications may present acutely, such as in scleroderma renal crisis, or decades later, as in secondary amyloidosis in rheumatoid arthritis. We aim to illuminate the most pertinent information relating to the kidney in the field of rheumatology. This will be a useful aid to any nephrologist given the proximity of the study of nephrology and rheumatology.

35.2 Scleroderma and the Kidney

Systemic sclerosis (SSc) is a debilitating, chronic, systemic, autoimmune disease of unknown cause. It is classified as limited or diffuse dependent on skin involvement. The incidence and prevalence of SSc vary in different populations where it seems to be more prevalent in the United States (286 cases per million adults) than in Europe (31 cases per million adults) with an annual incidence of 1–20 cases per million. SSc is three times more common in females than males and typically presents between the ages of 30 and 60 years [1]. Typical skin features of SSc are well described and include skin thickening, sclerodactyly, finger pulp pitting, fingertip ulceration, digital gangrene and telangiectasia, some of which are illustrated in Figs. 35.1 and 35.2. SSc causes vascular damage, immune activation and inflammation, culminating in fibrosis which is responsible for the clinical manifestations of the disease [2]. Table 35.1 summarizes the prevalence of extra-renal clinical manifestations seen in SSc.

35.3 Definition of SRC

Scleroderma renal crisis (SRC) is characterized by the development of accelerated hypertension and acute kidney injury (AKI). The definition of SRC is summarized in ► Box 35.1. SRC usually occurs relatively early (within the first 4 years) in the course of aggressive skin disease but has also, rarely, been reported to occur in those without obvious or occasionally preceding skin change and is the presenting feature of this disease in 22% of SSc patients. Although modulators of the renin-angiotensin system have improved the outcome in SRC, this complication still carries very significant morbidity with many patients rendered permanently dependent on dialysis, and mortality still approaches 25% even in specialist centres [3].

Box 35.1 Renal Crisis Classification

Definition of SRC

- New onset of blood pressure >150/85 mmHg obtained at least twice over a 24 hour period
- Documented decrease in the renal function as defined by a decrement of >30% in the calculated glomerular filtration rate (eGFR)

Corroborative features

- Microangiopathic haemolytic anaemia
- Hypertensive retinopathy
- New onset of urinary RBCs (other causes having been excluded)
- Flash pulmonary oedema
- Oliguria or anuria
- Typical renal biopsy features (Fig. 35.4)

35.4 Epidemiology of Scleroderma Renal Crisis

The reported incidence of scleroderma renal crisis (SRC) in SSc patients varies depending on whether limited disease is included, but is likely to occur in approximately 10% of patients with diffuse systemic disease. The presence of RNA polymerase antibodies and recent initiation or intensification of steroid therapy (>15 mg per day) together with rapidly progressing skin scores

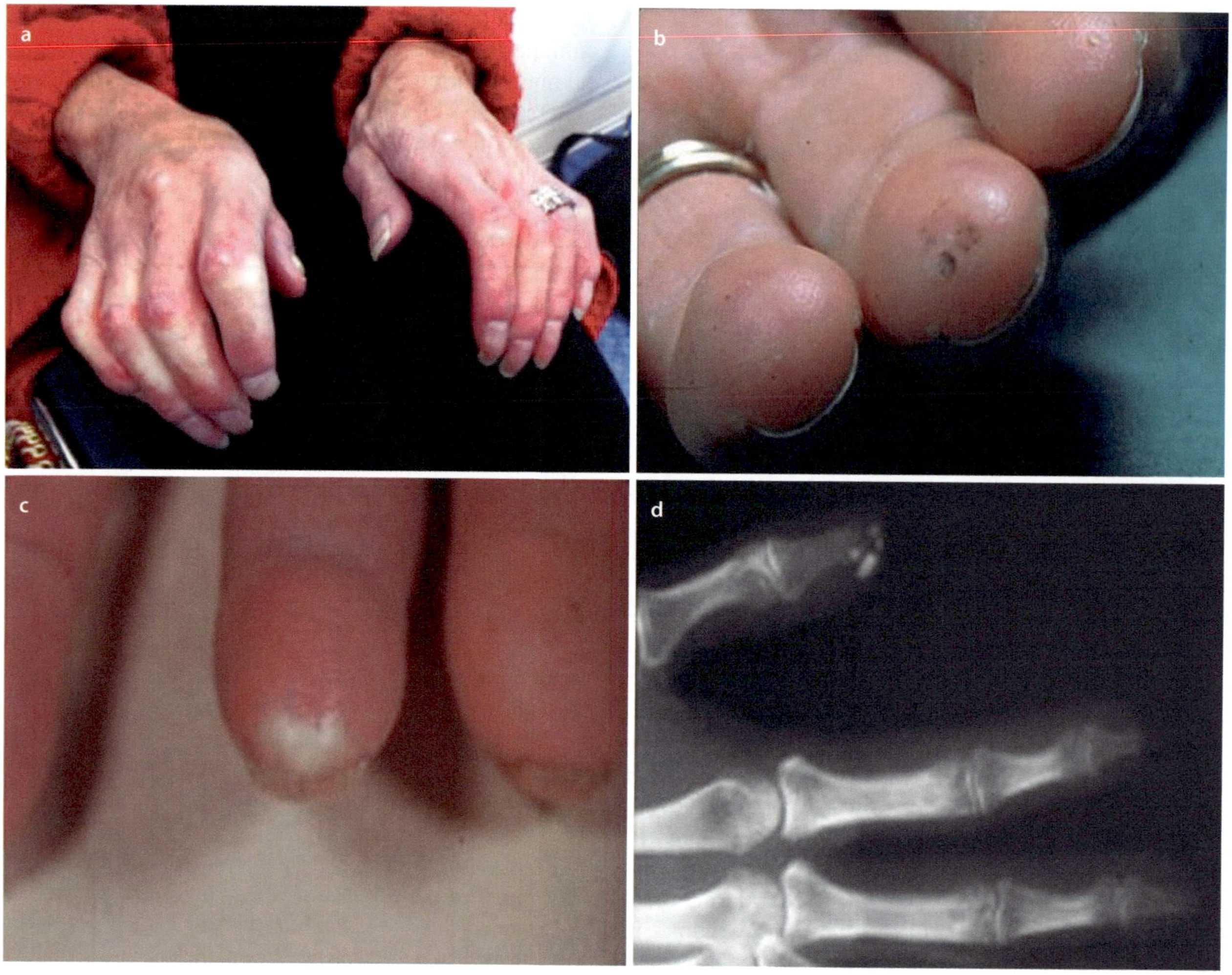

Fig. 35.1 Clinical features of scleroderma showing typical shiny, atrophic skin and Raynaud's of hands **a** with dry ulcers at the tip of middle finger **b** and calcinosis **c** which is illustrated on plain radiograph of the hand at the thumb **d**

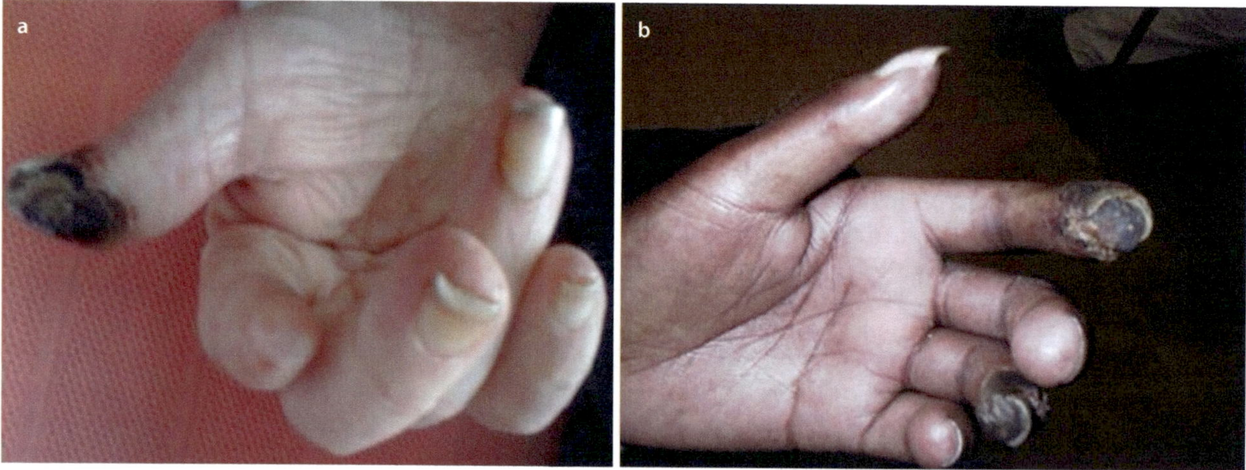

Fig. 35.2 Gangrenous thumb **a** and index and ring finger with telangiectasia of the palm and thumb **b**

Table 35.1 Prevalence of extra-renal manifestations of SSc

Clinical manifestation	Prevalence (%)
Interstitial lung disease	40
Pulmonary arterial hypertension	7–12
Cardiac	20–25
Oesophageal dysmotility	75–90
Stomach involvement	≥50
Small bowel	40–70
Colon	20–50
Anorectal	50–70

are all recognized as risk factors. The prevalence of RNA polymerase antibodies in patients whose disease is progressing to renal crisis is at least five times as high as the prevalence in patients without disease progression.

35.5 Clinical Presentation of SRC

A typical patient undergoing a SRC presents with new or worsening hypertension or its consequences such as headache, blurred vision (with grade 3–4 retinopathy) and hypertensive encephalopathy. If not adequately treated, hypertensive encephalopathy can progress to cerebral haemorrhage, coma and death. However, with timely and appropriate management, hypertensive encephalopathy and its clinical and neuroimaging consequences are potentially fully reversible. During a SRC, a patient can also present with progressive breathlessness (pulmonary oedema or congestive heart failure) and/or palpitations with evidence of biochemical renal impairment. Oligo-anuria, low urinary sodium and high urine specific gravity may be present in early, untreated stages. The hypertensive crisis usually, but not exclusively, occurs in a patient with known SSc during a phase of rapidly worsening skin disease. ► Box 35.2 outlines the presenting features of 110 patients undergoing SRC in a large cohort of British SRC patients. Systemic vascular resistance is up to five times normal, and stroke volume may be reduced by as much as 50%. Consequently (although restrictive cardiomyopathy and myocardial ischaemia may also be important), in an effort to maintain cardiac output, the patient often develops extreme tachycardia. Pulmonary arterial wedge pressures are high, and pulmonary oedema may ensue. Proteinuria may be present on urine analysis. Some patients undergoing a renal crisis have evidence of the underlying profound vasculopathy with digital gangrene developing in tandem with the SRC.

Box 35.2 Presenting Features of 110 Patients Undergoing SRC in a British Cohort

General observations

- Frequency of SRC – 12% dcSSc and 2% lcSS
- Median duration of SSc at the time of SRC was 7.5 months (0–200)
- 66% had SRC within 1 year of diagnosis of SSc
- SRC was the presenting feature in 22%
- 59% treated with steroids within 1 month prior to diagnosis

Presenting statistics

- Mean BP 193/114
- Median creatinine 200 mmol/L
- 50% thrombocytopenia
- 31% ECHO EF <55%

35.6 Aetiology and Pathogenesis of SRC

The sequence of events leading to a SRC is not fully understood. A number of risk factors for the development of SRC have been identified (► Box 35.3). Patients with specific autoantibody profiles are over-represented. Steroids [4] and cyclosporine are well recognized to precipitate crises. This may reflect increased vascular shear stresses consequent on salt and water retention and vascular endothelial injury, respectively. Analgesics (NSAIDs) arguably via their anti-prostaglandin effects together with pain secondary to digital ischaemia (perhaps mediated by adrenaline or other vasoactive substances) as well as increased sensitivity to cold stimuli or temperature changes are all reported as relevant.

Box 35.3 Published Risk Factors for Developing SRC

- Anaemia
- New cardiac events
- Steroid usage >15 mg
- Cyclosporine A treatment
- Diffuse skin disease, high skin score or large joint contractures
- Rapidly progressive skin disease
- RNA polymerase antibodies
- <4 years since scleroderma onset (rare in patients >4 years)
- ACE gene polymorphism
- Cocaine

35.7 Diagnosis

The cardinal feature of SRC is sustained (usually severe) hypertension, and evidence of AKI may be present. Intravascular haemolysis has been found in 50% of SRC patients and is confirmed by the presence of reduced platelet counts, anaemia, reduced haptoglobin levels, red cell fragments and schistocytes on blood film together with very elevated lactate dehydrogenase (LDH) levels (often >2000) and normal clotting.

CXR may reveal evidence of pulmonary oedema or pulmonary fibrosis. An enlarged cardiac silhouette might result from a peri-cardial effusion. Echocardiography is useful to exclude clinically significant effusions, to assess pulmonary pressures and to measure ejection fractions and identify any co-existing valvular abnormalities. Most patients presenting with SRC have non-significant peri-cardial effusions. Troponin and BNP may be useful indicators of myocardial ischaemia and failure, respectively.

Nailfold capillaroscopy and cold pressor testing (◘ Fig. 35.3) can be very helpful in those patients who do not have a known or obvious diagnosis of SSc at presentation or in whom the skin changes are minimal or absent.

35.8 Pathology

The renal pathological findings in SRC are indistinguishable from any other cause of accelerated hypertension [2]. Vessels show profound intimal proliferation that may occlude the vessel lumen completely and fibrinoid necrosis may be present in vessel walls. Glomeruli collapse with wrinkling of the basement membrane (◘ Fig. 35.4). The prognostic value of measurements of renal scarring does not seem to follow the patterns seen in other renal diseases [5–8].

35.9 Pathogenesis

The aetiology of SSc is unknown, but much evidence supports an autoimmune basis for its development. Vascular dysfunction is thought to be one of the initiating steps in SSc and is mediated by cytokines produced by activated lymphocytes and by antibodies against endothelial cells. It is believed that this immunological activity leads to an exaggerated production of fibroblasts and abnormal collagen build-up. Genetic and environmental factors are likely to be relevant, but their exact role has yet to be determined.

The autoantibodies identified in scleroderma patients correlate with distinct subsets of the disease. These autoantibodies often have a relatively high specificity, but their sensitivity is moderate. ◘ Table 35.2 summarizes these autoantibodies and their correlation with disease subsets.

35.10 Management

The outcome of SRC has greatly improved in the last half century. Increased awareness of this complication with regular BP measurements (especially in susceptible groups) allows earlier diagnosis with improved outcomes [12–14]. Renal biopsies are considered to be helpful (to exclude other pathologies and assess prognosis) but should be delayed until the patient's BP is well controlled and platelet counts have recovered.

In the era before treatment with inhibitors of the renin-angiotensin-aldosterone system, 1-year mortality approached 100% although. More recent series report survival rates of 70–80%, although significant numbers still become dialysis dependent following SRC. Renal recovery typically occurs very slowly with median time to dialysis independence of 9 months (1–34 months). Following discontinuation of dialysis, Penn et al. have

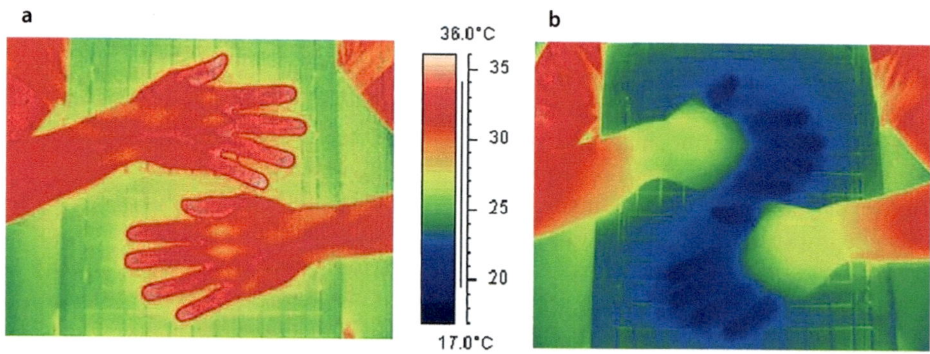

◘ **Fig. 35.3** Cold pressor testing, performed by asking a patient to immerse their hands in cold water for 1 minute, and a thermography study is performed after 10 minutes to assess rewarming. Normal **a** and abnormal **b** response suggestive of Raynaud's. (Courtesy of Kevin Howell, Department of Rheumatology, Royal Free Hampstead)

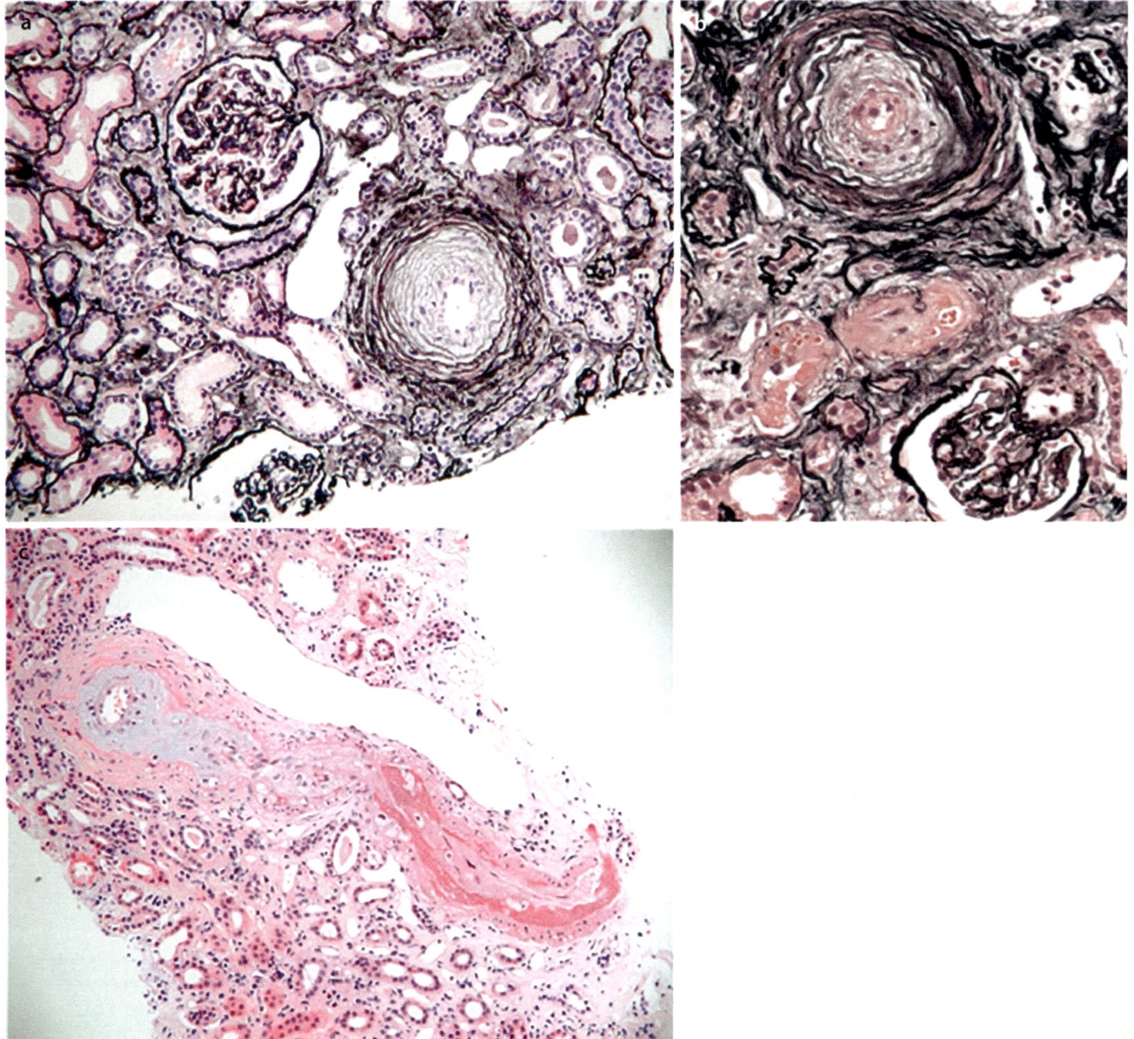

■ **Fig. 35.4** Histological appearances of a typical renal biopsy taken following an SRC. Severe acute small vessel vasculopathy: Panels **a** and **b** (silver stain) show shrunken collapsed glomeruli with wrinkling of basement membranes particularly panel **b**. Interlobular arteries show virtual occlusion by loose concentric intimal thickening (onion skinning). Panel **c** (Haemotoxylin & Eosin stain) is a longitudinal section through a very abnormal, almost completely occluded vessel. (Images courtesy of Professor AJ Howie, Department of Histopathology, Royal Free Hampstead)

■ **Table 35.2** Frequency and clinical associations of hallmark systemic sclerosis (SSc)-associated autoantibodies [9–11]

Autoantibodies	Frequency (%)	Subset associations	Organ complication associations
Anti-centromere	16–40	lcSS	Protective for PF and SRC
Anti-topoisomerase I	9–39	dcSSc > lcSS	PF; SDV
Anti-RNA polymerase	4–25	dcSSc	SRC
Anti-Th/To	0.2–7	lcSS	PF; PH
Anti-U3 RNP	1–6	dcSSc > lcSS; SSc overlap with PM/DM	PH
Anti-U11/U12 RNP	1.6–5	dcSSc = lcSS	PF, GI involvement
Anti-PM-Scl	0–7	SSc overlap with PM/DM or RA	PF

dcSSc diffuse cutaneous systemic sclerosis, *lcSS* limited cutaneous systemic sclerosis, *PH* pulmonary hypertension, *PF* pulmonary fibrosis, *PM/DM* polymyositis/dermatomyositis, *SDV* severe digital vasculopathy, *SRC* scleroderma renal crisis, *RA* rheumatoid arthritis, *GI* gastrointestinal

documented further improvement in renal function (3 mL/min/pa) occurring in their long-term follow-up study of a UK cohort.

Acute management involves general supportive care with thoughtful BP control. Prompt BP control is essential if hypertensive encephalopathy or cardiac decompensation dictates it. Otherwise, moderate steady reduction in BP (10% reduction in systolic BP per day) is likely to optimize chances of renal recovery. The use of an ACEI or ARB in the early stages is now standard, and there is evidence that continuation of these agents even if the patient becomes dialysis dependent improves the chances of recovering sufficient renal function to become dialysis independent. Intravenous vasodilators, especially prostaglandin inhibitors, are effective in the short term, and the latter may have the added advantage of discouraging platelet/vascular endothelial activation. Such agents can be titrated effectively in very sick patients to reduce systemic vascular resistance (SVR) and increase stroke volume (SV) with consequent slowing of heart rate and improvement of cardiac index and cardiac failure. Such careful management can be facilitated using oesophageal Doppler or Swan-Ganz monitoring in an ITU setting. In severely tachycardic patients, beta blockers may be contraindicated as the increased heart rate maintains cardiac output in the setting of such high SVR and reduced SV.

For dialysis dependent patients, renal transplantation is an option, but careful consideration needs to be given to the timing of transplantation as renal recovery can occur up to 2 years following a SRC [15, 16]. Similarly, a suitable immunosuppressive agent needs to be selected bearing in mind that cyclosporine (CYA) can precipitate SRC. Furthermore, co-existing cardiac and pulmonary disease may dictate suitability for listing. ▶ Box 35.4 summarizes the long-term outcomes of a large cohort from one centre with a SRC.

Box 35.4 Long-Term Outcome of SRC [15]

Long-term survival following SRC

- 82% – 1 year
- 74% – 2 years
- 71% – 3 years
- 59% – 5 years
- 47% – 10 years
- Most common in the dialysis recovery group
- The dialysis and recovery group had the best prognosis
- No correlation between age at the time of SRC and death
- Prognosis was worse in males (17% 10-year survival)

Table 35.3 Renal disease in SSc other than SRC

Renal disease	Clinical findings	Renal biopsy
ANCA-associated GN	Progressive renal failure Mild hypertension Proteinuria MPO antigen	Crescentic GN
Penicillamine-associated renal Dx	Rare Progressive renal failure 40% mortality	Membranous GN
Asymptomatic renal injury	10–55% of SSc patients Proteinuria seen in 25% Co-morbidities contributing to renal failure include CCF, GI involvement, medication exposure and dehydration	

ANCA antineutrophil cytoplasmic antibodies, *GN* glomerulonephritis, *MPO* myeloperoxidase, *CCF* congestive cardiac failure, *GI* gastrointestinal

35.11 Renal Disease in SSc Other than SRC

Clinically, SRC should be suspected when AKI develops in SSc patients. Nevertheless, AKI occurring in SSc patients is not always due to SRC. Table 35.3 summarizes other causes of renal disease in SSc.

Tips and Tricks in Managing Scleroderma Renal Crisis SRC

Scenario	Salutary Tip
Any patient with accelerated or malignant hypertension	Consider scleroderma renal crisis. This can happen with little or no skin disease which may develop later. You may see a few telltale telangiectasia. About 22% of patients are diagnosed with scleroderma at the same time as they present with SRC
Who might develop SRC	About 10% of SSC patients develop SRC (2% with lcSS and 12% with dcSSc). Rapidly progressive skin disease and autoantibody profiles (RNA polymerase III) may help predict which patients are more likely to develop SRC
A scleroderma patient who has recently been prescribed steroids for rheumatological overlap symptoms	Steroids are known to trigger SRC. Any scleroderma patient starting steroids or taking an increased dose should have their BP carefully monitored and controlled, preferably with ACEI or ARB

Scenario	Salutary Tip
During a scleroderma crisis, the patient's vasculature is very stiff and cannot tolerate large shifts in intravascular fluid. A patient's systemic vascular resistance may increase very rapidly, dramatically reducing cardiac output	Be very careful when administering fluids as pulmonary oedema can be precipitated very easily. Give very slowly preferably while paying attention to physiology: CVP, pulse rate, stroke volume, cardiac output
New patients with SRC	Aim to reduce BP relatively slowly (10% per day) unless the patient is fitting or in pulmonary oedema when BP needs to be reduced rapidly (lower MAP by 20% or to a diastolic pressure of 100–110 mmHg during the first hour). This will improve the chances of inducing recovery of renal function
A new SRC patient. What agents should I use to bring down BP during the immediate crisis	Systemic vascular resistance is very high. This is usually renin and angiotensin mediated; hence, ACEI and ARBs are the most appropriate treatment, although iloprost works well to reduce BP and inhibit platelet aggregation as well as smooth vascular endothelium. The dose of iloprost can easily be titrated to target BP. Short-acting ACEs, e.g. captopril, can also be useful as doses can be titrated more rigidly, but do not worry any ACEI better than none. GTN and labetalol can be used, but avoid cardio-selective beta blockers for reasons outlined below
Tachycardia during a SCC	Many patients undergoing SRC develop marked sinus tachycardia. This is a physiological response to the very reduced stroke volumes as the ventricle aims to pump against massive SVR. Aim to reduce the SVR and the tachycardia will settle. Do not use beta blockers as CO will be reduced and your patient may collapse
Low platelet counts with evidence of microangiopathic haemolytic anaemia (MAHA)	Do not be tempted to transfuse with platelets. This will resolve when BP settles and transfused platelets can aggravate the MAHA
Nutrition	Gut involvement in scleroderma is very common as is bacterial overgrowth. During a SRC, pay attention to nutrition from an early stage. A PEG may be beneficial. Consider early and sometimes repeated eradication of bacterial overgrowth
In the months after a SRC BP seems to be settling	You may need to reduce the amount of anti-hypertensive medication a patient is taking (as renal blood vessels remodel). Get the patient to monitor their own BP and aim to titrate the BP meds to achieve target BP. Stop Ca channel blockers and alpha blockers retaining the ACEI or ARB if possible as the latter drugs encourage vascular remodelling and the evidence suggests that renal recovery is more likely to occur if these agents are continued
A patient who remains dialysis dependent following a renal crisis	Recovery of renal function occurs in approx. 40% of dialysis-dependent post-SRC patients, but recovery is very slow and can occur up to 18–24 months after starting dialysis. You may want to delay listing on renal transplant waiting list
Which modality of dialysis to use in the event of AKI	Continuous therapies (CVVHD/CVVHF) are very useful during an acute crisis. Peritoneal dialysis provides a gentle therapy which has the advantage of avoiding intravascular volume fluid shifts, but individual patient's hands (contractures) or occasionally the severely thickened abdominal skin may preclude this choice

35.12 Renal Disease in Mixed Connective Tissue Disease

Criteria for the diagnosis of mixed connective tissue disease (MCTD) include the presence of a positive anti-U1-RNP autoantibody, the presence of either swollen fingers or Raynaud syndrome and features of at least two of the following connective tissue diseases: systemic lupus erythematous (SLE), systemic sclerosis (SSc) and polymyositis (PM) [17].

Renal manifestations of MCTD have been reported in 11–40% of patients (most commonly membranous glomerulonephritis), but severe renal disease is rare [17–20]. Anti-U1-RNP antibodies, which are present in all patients with MCTD by definition, may be protective against the development of diffuse proliferative glomerulonephritis. Patients who have renal disease in MCTD have more systemic manifestations than those without. ► Box 35.5 outlines the types of renal disease seen in patients with MCTD. Overlap in scleroderma patients and a few cases of renal crisis, with abrupt onset of severe hypertension and renal dysfunction, have been reported. The histological findings on renal biopsy of these patients are identical to that seen in scleroderma renal crisis; similarly, patients with scleroderma and MCTD may develop membranous nephropathy. There are a few case reports of patients who developed acute renal failure contemporaneously with an exacerbation of MCTD.

Box 35.5 Types of Renal Disease in MCTD

Membranous glomerulonephritis (commonest)
Mesangial proliferative glomerulonephritis (common)
Membranoproliferative glomerulonephritis
Focal and segmental glomerulosclerosis
Scleroderma renal crisis
Renal infarcts (associated with anti-cardiolipin antibody syndrome) (rare)
Renal amyloidosis (rare)
Minimal change disease (rare)
Collapsing glomerulopathy (very rare)

35

35.13 Renal Disease in Polymyositis and Dermatomyositis

The inflammatory myopathies, polymyositis (PM), dermatomyositis (DM) and inclusion body myositis (IBM), are rare diseases with an annual incidence of 2–7 per one million people with a female preponderance (3:1) and a peak incidence at 50–60 years.

Renal involvement is rare in patients with PM/DM and predominantly secondary to rhabdomyolysis causing acute tubular injury secondary to the effect of myoglobinuria [21]. The glomerular lesion most commonly associated with PM is mesangial proliferative glomerulonephritis. However, there are reports of patients with PM who developed rapidly progressive GN. Membranous GN is more commonly associated with DM and highly unlikely in PM. Proteinuria and microscopic haematuria are observed in renal disease associated with PM. ◘ Table 35.4 summarizes the common findings observed in renal disease in myositis. Treatment is aggressive fluid resuscitation and alkalization in order to avoid acidosis, hyperkalaemia and the need for dialysis. The use of renin-aldosterone antagonists have also been shown to prevent proteinuria and progression of chronic kidney disease.

35.14 Renal Disease in Sjögren's Syndrome

Sjögren's syndrome (SS) is characterized by lymphocytic infiltrates of salivary and tear glands leading to ocular and mouth dryness. It is reported to affect 0.1–0.6% of the general adult population with a female preponderance (female-to-male ratio at least 9:1). The peak incidence of the disease occurs after the menopause in the mid-50s.

Renal involvement in SS is frequent, and 16–67% of patients have manifestations such as interstitial nephritis or glomerulonephritis [22–25]. Interstitial nephritis is the commonest renal lesion in primary SS and occurs early in the disease process with lymphocytic infiltration into and subsequent tubular atrophy and fibrosis. Glomerulonephritis (GN) is rare in primary SS and usually occurs late in the disease. It is thought to be due to immune complex deposition in the glomeruli. Three histological types of GN have been reported in SS: membranoproliferative (MP) GN, mesangioproliferative GN and membranous GN. The histology of each of these is summarized in ◘ Table 35.5.

◘ **Table 35.4** Findings observed in renal disease in PM and DM

	Polymyositis	Dermatomyositis
Acute tubular injury Rhabdomyolysis	Yes	Yes
Type of GN	Mesangioproliferative GN	Membranous GN
Immune deposits in kidney	Yes	Yes
Onset of myositis and GN concurrent	Yes	Yes

■ **Table 35.5** Renal histological subtypes in SS

Type	Histology
Interstitial nephritis	Interstitial infiltrate which can develop into interstitial atrophy and fibrosis
Type I MPGN	Predominance of subendothelial deposits
Type II MPGN	Predominance of intramembranous deposits
Type III MPGN Burkholder type	Subepithelial and subendothelial deposits and mesangial dense deposits
Type III MPGN Strife type	Intramembranous and subendothelial deposits with marked basement membrane irregularities
Mesangioprolif-erative GN	
Membranous GN	

■ **Table 35.6** Types of renal disease in SS, associations and outcome

Type	Interstitial nephritis	Glomerulonephritis
Inci-dence	Most frequent	Very rare
Associa-tions	Renal tubular acidosis	Cryoglobulinaemia and vasculitis
Renal failure	Infrequent	Common
Outcome	Good	Associated with increased morbidity and mortality

■ Table 35.6 summarizes the types of renal disease in SS, their clinical presentation and outcome. Interstitial disease typically manifests as hyposthenuria (excretion of urine of low specific gravity due to an inability of the tubules of the kidneys to produce concentrated urine) and type I or type II renal tubular acidosis. Type I renal tubular acidosis is commoner. There is no consensus on the treatment of tubulointerstitial nephritis (TIN) in SS, but our local practice is to use medium-dose steroids and a steroid-sparing agent such as azathioprine, using the acute phase response, IgG level and pyuria as markers of disease activity.

GN is rare in SS. The outcomes in these patients are diverse, but patients tend to have a less favourable outcome. Renal failure is common, and it is often associated with cryoglobulinaemia and vasculitis. There are no controlled studies about treatment of secondary glomerulonephritis in SS.

35.15 Renal Disease in Sarcoidosis

Sarcoidosis is a multisystemic inflammatory disorder of unknown aetiology characterized by the presence of epithelioid non-caseating granulomas in involved organs. It has a worldwide distribution, with the highest geographic prevalence in Northern Europe. Sarcoidosis is slightly more prevalent in women with a peak incidence between 20 and 40 years of age, with a second peak in women over the age of 50.

Kidney involvement in sarcoid is rare (0.7–1%) and is usually diagnosed after lung disease is already evident. It occurs in chronic sarcoidosis and is very rare in acute sarcoidosis. Renal sarcoidosis can result in nephrotic syndrome, tubulointerstitial disease or glomerulonephritis but AKI secondary to hypercalcaemia is more common than direct renal involvement (■ Table 35.7) [26–28].

35.15.1 Hypercalcaemia and Hypercalciuria

Hypercalcaemia and hypercalciuria are the commonest renal abnormalities seen in sarcoidosis. Hypercalcaemia affects 10–20% of patients and can cause AKI or CKD secondary to nephrocalcinosis. Dysregulated calcium and vitamin D metabolism can occur in sarcoidosis as pulmonary macrophages often express 1-α hydroxylase not subject to the normal feedback mechanisms observed in calcium metabolism. Hypercalcaemic episodes can be precipitated by sun exposure because of vitamin D synthesis in skin. Hypercalcaemia causes

■ **Table 35.7** Types of renal dysfunction in sarcoidosis

Renal involvement	Prevalence (%)
Hypercalcaemia	Common
Hypercalciuria (+/– stones)	Very common
Renal tubular dysfunc-tion	Common
Granulomatous interstitial nephritis	Very small percentage of clinically relevant cases
Glomerular disease	Rare
Renovascular disease	Rare
Obstructive uropathy	Rare

afferent arteriolar vasoconstriction, decreasing renal blood flow and GFR. It can cause tubular necrosis leading to urinary sodium wasting and symptomatic polyuria and dehydration. Untreated, hypercalcaemia can lead to nephrocalcinosis and CKD.

Hypercalciuria is the commonest renal abnormality in sarcoidosis. It is due to an increased calcium load at the glomerulus, along with suppression of PTH secretion by calcitriol, thus diminishing tubular reabsorption of calcium. Hypercalciuria predisposes to calcium oxalate nephrolithiasis.

35.15.2 Renal Tubular Dysfunction

Tubular function may be affected with impaired concentrating ability and water reabsorption with abnormal renal acidification. This may cause polyuria or frank nephrogenic diabetes insipidus. Tubular abnormalities and polyuria usually improve with corticosteroid treatment.

35.15.3 Granulomatous Interstitial Nephritis

Granulomatous interstitial nephritis (GIN) represents the classic renal lesion of sarcoid with non-caseating granulomatous inflammation. Although it is found in a large number of kidneys at autopsy in patients with sarcoidosis, it only represents a very small percentage of clinically relevant cases of renal failure. GIN can present as either AKI or CKI. The granulomatous inflammatory infiltrate is confined primarily to the renal cortex. GIN responds well to corticosteroids. There is no standard dosing protocol, but 1 mg/kg/day of oral prednisolone is the most frequent starting regimen. In one case series of 94 patients, only seven patients required dialysis therapy either initially or shortly after presentation, despite treatment with corticosteroids.

35.15.4 Glomerular Disease

Glomerular disease in sarcoidosis is very rare and can present with different associated lesions; the commonest is membranous nephropathy. Sarcoidosis has been reported with many glomerulonephritides, including immunoglobulin A nephropathy, crescentic glomerulonephritis, minimal change disease and focal segmental glomerulosclerosis. Renal amyloid can also occur. There are no particular guidelines for treatment, but corticosteroids are often used.

35.15.5 Renovascular and Obstructive Uropathy

Renovascular disease is rare in sarcoidosis and can be associated with severe hypertension caused by renal artery stenosis from granulomatous angiitis or renal artery encasement by an external inflammatory mass. Urethral, ureteral or bladder obstruction caused by direct sarcoid involvement of these structures is rare.

35.16 Renal Disease in Rheumatoid Arthritis

Rheumatoid arthritis (RA) has a prevalence of approximately 1–2% and is two to three times more prevalent in females than males. The kidney is rarely directly involved in RA but may be compromised by therapies such as non-steroidal anti-inflammatory drugs (NSAIDs) and disease-modifying anti-rheumatic drugs (DMARDs) such as gold and penicillamine. Renal involvement in RA is characterized principally by secondary amyloidosis and side effects of medication, however renal lesions directly due to the disease itself are infrequent [29, 30].

Glomerulonephritis and interstitial renal disease are uncommon in the absence of vasculitis (◘ Table 35.8).

The frequency of amyloidosis in RA has been reported to range from 5% to 13.3% in cases confirmed by biopsy and from 14% to 26% in cases confirmed by autopsy. A clinical diagnosis of amyloidosis is usually suspected with the onset of proteinuria, renal insufficiency and diarrhoea. Renal impairment may progress

◘ **Table 35.8** Types of renal disease in rheumatoid arthritis

Renal disease	
AA amyloidosis	
Type 1 Type 2	Rapid decline in function Insidious decline in function
IgA mesangial GN Membranous GN	Commonest histopathological type Secondary to gold or penicillamine
Interstitial renal disease	Associated with drugs
Type 2 mixed cryoglobulinaemia	Rare
Rheumatoid vasculitis	Very rare; diffuse necrotizing GN

GN glomerulonephritis

to end-stage renal disease which is a major contributor to death in this disease [31, 32].

In patients with RA and AA amyloidosis, two distinct clinical courses in terms of renal function have been identified. In type 1 disease, renal function deteriorates rapidly reaching ESRF within 5 years. Type 2 disease is more insidious, and renal function does not worsen significantly in 5 years. In type 2 disease, amyloid deposits were found around blood vessels and were absent in the glomerulus.

The relationship between IgA, IgA-RF and renal disease in patients with RA is not clear, but the affinity of IgA for mesangium, skin and synovium might explain the clinical presentation of RA with mesangial IgA glomerulonephritis. A striking association of IgM-RF with mesangial glomerulonephritis has been described. It is suggested that a functional deficiency or defect in the renal mesangium to remove IgM-RF-IgG complexes could lead to these mesangial lesions.

Renal involvement due to cryoglobulins is very rare in patients with RA. Type II mixed cryoglobulinaemia is the commonest type. It occurs when cryoglobulins form circulating immune complexes. Rheumatoid vasculitis, a severe necrotizing polyangiitis, may sometimes complicate the course of long-standing RA, but renal involvement (diffuse necrotizing GN) is less common in this form of vasculitis.

35.17 Treatment of Renal Disease in RA

It is important to distinguish between renal dysfunction secondary to active rheumatoid arthritis, a drug reaction or other unrelated causes of AKI or CKD, and often this can only be achieved by renal biopsy. In essence, treatment of the former is by control of disease activity. There are a number of case reports and series that have successfully used etanercept in the treatment of AA amyloidosis with renal involvement. There are no guidelines for the treatment of IgA nephritis, but cyclophosphamide has been used successfully in cases of deteriorating renal function and IgA nephritis.

35.18 Renal Disease in Ankylosing Spondylitis (AS)

Renal disease in AS is relatively common with a reported prevalence of 10–35%. Table 35.9 outlines the different types of glomerular involvement seen in AS. Renal disease can also be caused by treatments such as NSAIDs, sulphasalazine and azathioprine, which can cause tubulointerstitial nephritis.

Amyloidosis is more prevalent in aggressive and active AS and in older patients with long-standing disease. Clinically, amyloid nephropathy causes proteinuria, which can progress to nephrotic syndrome and renal insufficiency. There is very little data available on the treatment of renal amyloidosis; some case reports suggest a potential role of TNF inhibitors in improving AA amyloidosis, but probably the most effective intervention is early detection by ensuring screening for proteinuria in rheumatology clinics and getting control of inflammatory processes.

Table 35.9 Types of renal disease seen in AS

Type of renal disease	Prevalence
Secondary amyloidosis (AA)	Commonest
IgA nephropathy	Second commonest
Mesangioproliferative GN	Rare
Focal segmental GS	Very rare
Focal proliferative GN	Very rare

GN glomerulonephritis, *GS* glomerulosclerosis

35.19 Renal Disease in Behcet's Disease

Behcet's disease is a rare systemic inflammatory condition of unknown aetiology found most prominently in a Middle Eastern and Central Asian population. The condition can affect multiple systems including the eyes, skin, genitalia, musculoskeletal, cardiovascular, neurological and also the kidneys. It has an equal male-to-female preponderance. Autoantibodies are generally negative.

Renal disease is generally rare. The most common renal presentation is with mild nephritis. This is generally of limited clinical significance. However, monitoring is recommended in order to assess for potential disease progression. Secondary amyloidosis may also occur in Behcet's rarely and colchicine may be helpful in these cases.

35.20 Rheumatological drugs and kidney disease

Finally, some of the medication used in rheumatological disease can cause renal disease or need modification of dose to avoid generalised toxicity (Table 35.10). It is important to assess the medication history in patients with chronic musculoskeletal disorders and unexplained renal impairment as well as ensuring that doses are adjusted and renal function monitored in patients with impaired renal function.

Table 35.10 Rheumatological drugs and kidney disease

Drug	Indication	Renal complications	Comments
NSAIDs	OA, RA, ankylosing spondylitis	Acute tubular necrosis	Use for shortest possible duration; complications common; avoid in renal impairment
Methotrexate	RA, PsA, JIA	Renal insufficiency	Uncommon; reduce dose in renal impairment; avoid in severe renal disease
Sulphasalazine	RA, inflammatory arthritis with associated bowel disease	Proteinuria	Ensure adequate fluid intake
Mycophenolate mofetil	Lupus nephritis, vasculitis	Haematuria; raised serum creatinine	No dose adjustment needed
Leflunomide	RA, PsA	Hypertension	Avoid in renal failure due to lack of data
Penicillamine	RA, JIA, Wilson's disease	Proteinuria, haematuria	Used infrequently; dose reduction in renal impairment; avoid use with NSAIDs
Janus kinase inhibitors (tofacitinib, baricitinib)	RA, PsA	No known renal complication	Reduce dose if eGFR <30
Anti-TNF inhibitors (adalimumab, etanercept, infliximab, certolizumab, golimumab)	RA, PsA, AxSpA	Glomerulonephritis in case reports	No renal adjustment
IL-6 inhibitors (tocilizumab)	RA, JIA, GCA	Nephrolithiasis: uncommon	No renal adjustment
CD20 depletion therapy (rituximab)	RA, SLE, vasculitis		No renal adjustment
Allopurinol	Gout prophylaxis	Reduced excretion	Dose adjustment in renal disease
Febuxostat	Gout prophylaxis		No adjustment; avoid in IHD
Colchicine	Acute gout	Reduced excretion	Dose adjustment in renal disease; avoid in severe renal impairment
Bisphosphonates (alendronate, zoledronic acid, ibandronic acid)	Osteoporosis	Reduced excretion	Avoid if eGFR <30 mL/min
Denosumab	Osteoporosis	Increased hypocalcaemia risk	Use with caution if eGFR <30 mL/min
Teriparatide	Osteoporosis	Nephrolithiasis	Avoid in severe renal impairment

NSAIDs non-steroidal anti-inflammatory drugs, *OA* osteoarthritis, *RA* rheumatoid arthritis, *PsA* psoriatic arthritis, *JIA* juvenile idiopathic arthritis, *AxSpA* axial spondyloarthropathy; *GCA* giant cell arteritis, *IHD* ischaemic heart disease

35

Tips and Tricks

Scenario	Salutary Tip
Long-standing rheumatoid arthritis, new peripheral oedema, urine dip positive for protein	Check eGFR and PCR and think secondary amyloidosis
Gout and renal disease	Consider switching to febuxostat if eGFR<30 mL/min and difficulty reducing uric acid below 360 μmol/L. Caution is needed as associated increased risk of ischaemic heart disease with febuxostat
Myositis and renal disease	Rare. Consider rhabdomyolysis and check urinary myoglobins

Case Study

Case 1

A 51-year-old lady, originally from India, presented to the rheumatology review clinic with a 30-year history of rheumatoid arthritis. Her past medical history is significant for hyperlipidaemia. Her medications consist of aspirin 75 mg, atorvastatin 20 mg, prednisolone 5 mg once a day and paracetamol 1 g TDS/PRN. She has no known ischaemic heart disease. She describes significantly worsening SOB with associated swelling of her lower limbs. On examination, she has long-standing RA changes with no active synovitis. Pitting oedema is present to mid thighs. ECG shows normal sinus rhythm with no ischaemic changes. Urine dip shows 3+ protein. Bloods reveal eGFR 31 mL/min/1.73 m^2 and proBNP 132 pg/mL. Urine PCR was 230 mg/mmol. She was seen in clinic by both a nephrologist and rheumatologist and was subsequently diagnosed with secondary amyloidosis secondary to long-standing RA.

Case 2

A 72-year-old lady presented to the emergency department with a 3-day history of headache, a 1-week history of increasing SOB and a 1-month history of a new third digit necrotic ulcer on her right hand. She reports a history of hypothyroidism, asthma and Raynaud's. Her medications include levothyroxine 75 mcg and salbutamol PRN. She recently received a course of tapering steroids for an exacerbation of asthma. On exam, she has a necrotic ulcer on the tip of her third digit of her left hand. She has obvious Raynaud's phenomenon with multiple calcinosis on both hands. Telangiectasia is present on her hands and face. She also has a noticeable chest wall rash. Her respiratory exam reveals fine bibasal creps. Neurological examination is normal. Her blood pressure is 198/100 and heart rate is 134. Sinus tachycardia on ECG. Creatinine 250 μmol/L (90 μmol/L 6 months previously), eGFR 26 mL/min (72 mL/min on most recent bloods). Chest X-ray shows changes consistent with pulmonary oedema. Scleroderma renal crisis is diagnosed, and the patient is treated with aggressive blood pressure management with ACE inhibitors.

Case 3

A 63-year-old man presents to rheumatology clinic for review. He reports ongoing pain in his left MTP 1 joint which is tender to touch. His past medical history is significant for gout, OSA, HTN, type 2 diabetes mellitus and chronic kidney disease. His medications include allopurinol 200 mg, linagliptin 5 mg and lercanidipine 10 mg. He reports good medication compliance. On exam, he has a tender left MTP 1 joint in foot with associated erythema. He also has gouty tophi of his right second and third MCP joints of his right hand. Bloods include a uric acid of 450 μmol/L and an eGFR of 28 mL/min. Upon discussion with his rheumatologist, the decision is taken to switch from allopurinol to febuxostat 80 mg. He is also given a short course of tapering steroids for his acute flare.

35.21 Conclusion

As demonstrated in this chapter, renal disease is common in many rheumatological conditions. Disease severity may vary from minimal in conditions such as Behcet's to life threatening in scleroderma. Simple measures may be undertaken such as ensuring a urine dip is assessed in clinic in order to identify at-risk patients. Other measures include close blood pressure monitoring. ANCA screening is also necessary in patients with fever, fatigue, weight loss or any other features clinically suggestive of small vessel vasculitis. Cooperation ideally in the form of multidisciplinary meetings is needed between rheumatologists and nephrologists. This integrated care model will assist in more informed clinical management and ultimately may lead to improved clinical outcomes.

? Chapter Review Questions

1. Which of the following is the most common extra-renal manifestation of systemic sclerosis?
   A. Interstitial lung disease
   B. Pulmonary arterial hypertension
   C. Oesophageal dysmotility
   D. Cardiac involvement
   E. Small bowel involvement

2. Which of the following statements is correct?
   A. The risk of gout increases with worsening kidney disease
   B. Uric acid levels above 500 should be treated
   C. Febuxostat is the first-line therapy if eGFR <60
   D. Synovial fluid in gout reveals positively birefringent crystals
   E. Pseudogout is more common in renal disease than gout

3. Which of the following is the most common histopathological finding on biopsy in renal disease with rheumatoid arthritis?
   A. Membranous glomerulonephritis
   B. Focal proliferative glomerulonephritis
   C. Focal segmental glomerulosclerosis
   D. IgA mesangial glomerulonephritis
   E. Interstitial fibrosis

4. Which of the following statements is incorrect?
   A. Anti-U1-RNP antibodies may be protective against the development of diffuse proliferative glomerulonephritis
   B. Renal involvement in polymyositis tends to be caused by rhabdomyolysis
   C. Glomerulonephritis is rare in Sjögren's disease
   D. Renal sarcoidosis may result in nephrotic syndrome
   E. Behcet's disease is more common in males

5. Which of the following drugs used in rheumatology requires a renal dose adjustment?
   A. Golimumab
   B. Febuxostat
   C. Tofacitinib
   D. Rituximab
   E. Tocilizumab

Answers

1. C
2. A
3. D
4. E
5. C

References

1. Barnes J, Mayes MD. Epidemiology of systemic sclerosis: incidence, prevalence, survival, risk factors, malignancy, and environmental triggers. Curr Opin Rheumatol. 2012;24:165–70.
2. Batal I, Domsic RT, Medsger TA, Bastacky S. Scleroderma renal crisis: a pathology perspective. Int J Rheumatol. 2010;2010:543704.
3. Wasner C, Cooke CR, Fries JF. Successful medical treatment of scleroderma renal crisis. N Engl J Med. 1978;299(16):873–5.
4. Trang G, Steele R, Baron M, Hudson M. Corticosteroids and the risk of scleroderma renal crisis: a systematic review. Rheumatol Int. 2012;32:645–53.
5. Batal I, Domsic RT, Shafer A, Medsger TA, Kiss LP, Randhawa P, et al. Renal biopsy findings predicting outcome in scleroderma renal crisis. Hum Pathol. 2009;40(3):332–40.
6. Shanmugam VK, Steen VD. Renal disease in scleroderma: an update on evaluation, risk stratification, pathogenesis and management. Curr Opin Rheumatol. 2012;24:669–76.
7. Steen VD, Medsger J. Long-term outcomes of scleroderma renal crisis. Ann Intern Med [Internet]. 2000;133(8):600–3.
8. Cannon PJ, Hassar M, Case DB, Casarella WJ, Sommers SC, LeRoy EC. The relationship of hypertension and renal failure in scleroderma (progressive systemic sclerosis) to structural and functional abnormalities of the renal cortical circulation. Med (United States). 1974;53(1):1–46.
9. Codullo V, Cavazzana I, Bonino C, Alpini C, Cavagna L, Cozzi F, et al. Serologic profile and mortality rates of scleroderma renal crisis in Italy. J Rheumatol. 2009;36(7):1464–9.
10. Moinzadeh P, Nihtyanova SI, Howell K, Ong VH, Denton CP. Impact of hallmark autoantibody reactivity on early diagnosis in scleroderma. Clin Rev Allergy Immunol. 2012;43(3):249–55.
11. Nihtyanova SI, Parker JC, Black CM, Bunn CC, Denton CP. A longitudinal study of anti-RNA polymerase III antibody levels in systemic sclerosis. Rheumatology (Oxford). 2009;48(10):1218–21.
12. D'Angelo WA, Fries JF, Masi AT, Shulman LE. Pathologic observations in systemic sclerosis (scleroderma). A study of fifty-eight autopsy cases and fifty-eight matched controls. Am J Med. 1969;46:428–40.
13. Denton CP, Lapadula G, Mouthon L, Müller-Ladner U. Renal complications and scleroderma renal crisis. Rheumatology (Oxford). 2009;48(Suppl 3):iii32–5.
14. Hudson M, Baron M, Lo E, Weinfeld J, Furst DE, Khanna D. An international, web-based, prospective cohort study to determine whether the use of ACE inhibitors prior to the onset of scleroderma renal crisis is associated with worse outcomes – methodology and preliminary results. Int J Rheumatol. 2010;2010:347402.
15. Penn H, Howie AJ, Kingdon EJ, Bunn CC, Stratton RJ, Black CM, et al. Scleroderma renal crisis: patient characteristics and long-term outcomes. QJM. 2007;100:485–94.
16. Pham PTT, Pham PCT, Danovitch GM, Gritsch HA, Singer J, Wallace WD, et al. Predictors and risk factors for recurrent scleroderma renal crisis in the kidney allograft: Case report and review of the literature. Am J Transplant. 2005;5:2565–9.
17. Radstake TR, Gorlova O, Rueda B, Martin JE, Alizadeh BZ, Palomino-Pakozdi A, Nihtyanova S, Moinzadeh P, Ong VH, Black CM, Denton CP. Clinical and serological hallmarks of systemic sclerosis overlap syndromes. J Rheumatol. 2011;38(11):2406–9.
18. Pakozdi A, Nihtyanova S, Moinzadeh P, Ong VH, Black CM, Denton CP. Clinical and serological hallmarks of systemic sclerosis overlap syndromes. J Rheumatol. 2011;38(11):2406–9.
19. Ortega-Hernandez OD, Shoenfeld Y. Mixed connective tissue disease: an overview of clinical manifestations, diagnosis and treatment. Best Pract Res Clin Rheumatol. 2012;26:61–72.
20. Pope JE. Other manifestations of mixed connective tissue disease. Rheum Dis Clin N Am. 2005;31:519–33.
21. Cucchiari D, Angelini C. Renal involvement in idiopathic inflammatory myopathies. Clin Rev Allergy Immunol. Humana Press Inc. 2017;52:99–107.
22. Adam FU, Torun D, Bolat F, Zumrutdal A, Sezer S, Ozdemir FN. Acute renal failure due to mesangial proliferative glomerulonephritis in a pregnant woman with primary Sjögren's syndrome. Clin Rheumatol. 2006;25(1):75–9.
23. Cortez MS, Sturgill BC, Bolton WK. Membranoproliferative glomerulonephritis with primary Sjögren's syndrome. Am J Kidney Dis. 1995;25(4):632–6.
24. Sun IO, Hong YA, Park HS, Choi SR, Kang SH, Chung BH, et al. Type III membranoproliferative glomerulonephritis in a patient with primary Sjögren's syndrome. Clin Nephrol. 2013;79(2):171–4.
25. Vitali C, Bombardieri S, Jonsson R, Moutsopoulos HM, Alexander EL, Carsons SE, et al. Classification criteria for Sjögren's syndrome: a revised version of the European criteria proposed by the American-European Consensus Group. Ann Rheum Dis. 2002;61:554–8.
26. Berliner AR, Haas M, Choi MJ. Sarcoidosis: the nephrologist's perspective. Am J Kidney Dis. 2006 Nov;48(5):856–70.

27. Holmes J, Lazarus A. Sarcoidosis: extrathoracic manifestations. Dis Mon. 2009;55:675–92.
28. Pastor E, Arriero JM, Gutiérrez AI, Barroso ME, Noguera RJ, Muñoz C, et al. Renal failure as first manifestation of familial sarcoidosis. Eur Respir J. 2010;36:1485–7.
29. Boers M, Croonen AM, Dijkmans BAC, Breedveld FC, Eulderink F, Cats A, et al. Renal findings in rheumatoid arthritis: clinical aspects of 132 necropsies. Ann Rheum Dis. 1987;46(9):658–63.
30. Kuroda T, Tanabe N, Kobayashi D, Sato H, Wada Y, Murakami S, et al. Programmed initiation of hemodialysis for systemic amyloidosis patients associated with rheumatoid arthritis. Rheumatol Int. 2011;31(9):1177–82.
31. Uda H, Yokota A, Kobayashi K, Miyake T, Fushimi H, Maeda A, et al. Two distinct clinical courses of renal involvement in rheumatoid patients with AA amyloidosis. J Rheumatol. 2006;33(8):1482–7.
32. El Maghraoui A. Extra-articular manifestations of ankylosing spondylitis: prevalence, characteristics and therapeutic implications. Eur J Int Med. Elsevier B.V. 2011;22:554–60.

Hepatology and the Kidney

Aisling O'Riordan and Thuvaraka Ware

Contents

M. Harber (ed.), *Primer on Nephrology*, https://doi.org/10.1007/978-3-030-76419-7_36

Learning Objectives

1. To understand the causes and risk factors for hepatorenal syndrome and the interaction of AKI, CKD and chronic liver disease (CLD)
2. To appreciate the differential diagnosis of hepatorenal diseases and the management of HRS

36.1 Definition and Classification of Renal Dysfunction in Cirrhosis

Traditionally when discussing renal impairment in the context of liver disease, a lot of focus has been put on HRS definition and diagnosis [3, 4]. However, there are other causes of renal dysfunction in this patient population, and HRS is often a diagnosis of exclusion. Definitions and classifications for AKI and CKD have also evolved over the years [5, 6] to include both rising creatinine and falling urine output. These were applied to cirrhotic patients in a 2015 update on the diagnosis and management of AKI by the International Club of Ascites (ICA) (Table 36.1). Although the ICA adopts an AKI staging system based on changes in serum creatinine levels over 1 week, urine output was excluded as it was not felt to be relevant in patients with cirrhosis, many of whom are oliguric. The ICA classification has been validated in patients with cirrhosis where development of AKI is associated with increased mortality.

Table 36.1 Diagnostic criteria and staging for acute kidney injury (AKI) in patients with cirrhosis

Definition of AKI	Increase in serum creatinine by >26.5 μmol/L within 48 hours or an increase in creatinine by ≥50% from baseline that has, or is presumed to have, occurred within the preceding 7 days	
Baseline creatinine	The most recent serum creatinine value prior to the episode of AKI, taken in the preceding 3 months. If this is not available, then the admitting creatinine can be used	
Stages of AKI	1	Increase in creatinine by ≥26.6 μmol/L or an increase by 1.5–2-fold from baseline
	2	Increase in creatinine by two- to threefold from baseline
	3	Increase in creatinine >3-fold from baseline or an acute rise over a threshold of 353.6 μmol/L or the need for renal replacement therapy

Adapted from Angeli et al. [7]

An estimated glomerular filtration rate (eGFR) <60 ml/min for >3 months is deemed to be the threshold for CKD in those with cirrhosis [7].

36.2 Definition and Classification of Hepatorenal Syndrome

Hepatorenal syndrome is a critically important cause of AKI in patients with cirrhosis. Previously, threshold values of at least a twofold increase in creatinine to a level >221 μmol/L were needed, but now HRS-AKI can be diagnosed when the patient has >/= stage 2 AKI and also meets the criteria detailed in ▶ Box 36.1. This change has not yet been updated in some guidelines [8, 9]. Hepatorenal syndrome was classically divided into types 1 and 2 depending on the severity and acuity of renal dysfunction (Table 36.2a). Type 1 is now referred to as HRS type of AKI (HRS-AKI) and is an acute, rapidly progressive illness with a very poor prognosis without a liver transplant (LT). HRS type 2 is a less severe condition, traditionally defined using the same criteria as HRS type 1, but was more gradual in onset and had a creatinine threshold for diagnosis of >133 μmol/L. It is often characterised by diuretic-resistant ascites that is less amenable to pharmacological interventions. Hepatorenal syndrome type 2 is a specific form of CKD, and a new term, HRS type of chronic kidney disease (HRS-CKD), has been proposed [2, 4, 7, 10–13].

Box 36.1 Diagnostic Criteria of Hepatorenal Syndrome (HRS)

- Diagnosis of liver disease with cirrhosis, portal hypertension and ascites
- No response to 2 days of diuretic withdrawal and administration of intravenous albumin 1 g/kg of body weight to a maximum of 100 g/day
- The absence of other potential causes of renal dysfunction, e.g. shock or nephrotoxic drug use (e.g. non-steroidal anti-inflammatories, aminoglycosides, iodinated contrast)
- No evidence of parenchymal renal damage* based on the following:
- Proteinuria (>500 mg/day)
- Microscopic haematuria (>50 red blood cells per high-powered field)
- Normal renal ultrasound scan

*Caution as patients may still have some structural damage such as tubular injury. Adapted from Angeli et al. [7]

Table 36.2 Classification and Clinical Feature of HRS

a. Classification of hepatorenal syndrome		
	HRS-AKI (formerly type 1)	**HRS-CKD (formerly type 2)**
Rate of onset	Rapid	Slow and progressive
Precipitating factors	Peritonitis, haemorrhage, acute hepatitis, non-steroidal use, over-diuresis	Precipitating events (as per HRS-AKI) but it can occur spontaneously
Approximate median survival	1 month	6.7 months
b. Clinical features of hepatorenal syndrome (more severe in HRS-AKI)		
Stigmata of liver disease	**Renal**	**Systemic**
Jaundice Palmer erythema Clubbing Spider naevi Bruising Hepatosplenomegaly Hepatic encephalopathy Gynaecomastia Ascites (refractory)	Oedema Oliguria Bland urinary sediment Does not improve with withdrawal of diuretics/ volume expansion	Hypotension Tachycardia Fever in peritonitis Features of malnourishment

Adapted from Salerno et al. [4]

36.3 Incidence

The incidence of renal impairment depends on the aetiology. For example, post paracetamol overdose, the incidence of AKI is as high as 75%. Using the definitions outlined above, the incidence of AKI in hospitalised patients with cirrhosis is 19–54%. There is a broad differential, but HRS is the principal aetiology in 12–18% of cases. In 1993, a study showed that HRS occurred in 18% of patients with cirrhosis and ascites at 1 year and 39% at 5 years [14–17]. Chronic kidney disease occurs in about 1% of those with cirrhosis, and HRS-CKD occurs in between 16% and 61% of those with HRS [2, 12].

36.4 Differential Diagnosis for Renal Dysfunction in Those with Liver Disease

This is broad and is summarised in Table 36.3. Getting the diagnosis correct has critical implications for patient management and prognosis. There is often a shared underlying aetiology causing both the renal and liver disease. Essentially, pre-renal and intrinsic renal causes predominate, and pre-existing renal conditions should always be considered, with HRS often a diagnosis of exclusion [1, 4, 15, 17–19].

36.5 Pathophysiology of HRS

Hepatorenal syndrome is a functional renal impairment characterised by a number of haemodynamic abnormalities. The pathogenic mechanisms outlined below probably integrate, and these are broadly illustrated in Fig. 36.1.

36.5.1 Peripheral Arterial Vasodilation

The peripheral arterial vasodilation seen with portal hypertension plays a key role in the pathogenesis of HRS. As the liver progressively fibroses, intrahepatic portal pressure increases, leading to splanchnic pooling. Nitric oxide release from the splanchnic vasculature endothelium also increases, due to portal hypertension-induced shear stress or bacterial translocation and cytokine-induced increased nitric oxide synthase activity, resulting in local vasodilation. These circulatory changes have been confirmed in studies where increased blood flow in the superior mesenteric artery was demonstrated compared with the femoral, correlating with the degree of liver dysfunction. The consequence of this splanchnic pooling is a reduction in effective arterial blood volume and vascular resistance [1, 4, 19].

Table 36.3 Differential diagnosis for renal impairment in a patient with liver disease

Pre-renal	Volume depletion or inadequate fluid resuscitation from, for example, excessive diuresis and large volume paracentesis Gastrointestinal haemorrhage Diarrhoea from excessive laxative use Septic shock Drugs, e.g. non-steroidal anti-inflammatory agents Hepatorenal syndrome
Renal	Acute tubular injury from persistent hypoperfusion, nephrotoxins (e.g. contrast, aminoglycosides, calcineurin inhibitors, paracetamol or salicylate overdose), very high levels of bilirubin or microorganisms Drug- or toxin-induced interstitial nephritis from, for example, antibiotics, proton pump inhibitors and poisonous mushrooms Glomerular disease related to the cause of the underlying liver disease (e.g. alcohol, viral hepatitis) De novo glomerulonephritis: IgA, membranous or membranoproliferative glomerulonephritis Other causes with proteinuria/haematuria including diabetes, myeloma, amyloid, vasculitis Conditions that can affect the liver and kidney: Drug or poison toxicity (e.g. paracetamol overdose) Hypersensitivity reaction to, for example, antibiotics Infectious diseases (e.g. hantavirus, leptospirosis, hepatitis B or C virus) Sickle cell disease Metabolic syndrome linked with non-alcoholic steatohepatitis, hypertension and diabetes-induced renal disease HELLP syndrome Polycystic kidney and liver disease
Post-renal	Obstruction (rare)

Abbreviations: HELLP, haemolysis, elevated liver enzymes, low platelets

36

36.5.2 Haemostatic Compensatory Mechanisms

To maintain homeostasis in response to the above, there is baroreceptor-mediated activation of the renin-angiotensin-aldosterone and sympathetic nervous systems with subsequent release of anti-diuretic hormone resulting in sodium and water retention. Baroreceptors are principally located in the aortic arch and carotid sinus; however, they are also present in other organs including the liver. Here, there is evidence for a hepatorenal baroreflex whereby afferent hepatic pressure sensors can influence renal blood flow, GFR and salt and water excretion via neurohormonal mechanisms that increase renal sympathetic activity. Renal blood flow may be preserved in the early stages of cirrhosis when local vasodilators such as prostaglandins and nitric oxide can overcome the vasoconstrictor effects, but as liver disease progresses, this equilibrium cannot be maintained, and renal hypoperfusion and HRS can ensue. Vasoconstriction is not isolated to the kidney but has been shown in other vascular beds too. However, the splanchnic vascular bed escapes the effects of the potent vasoconstrictors due to the local concentration of vasodilators. In addition to the factors already mentioned, an inadequate adrenal response to stress such as sepsis is also thought to play a role in the pathophysiology of HRS [1, 3, 19, 20].

36.5.3 Cirrhotic Cardiomyopathy

The increased sympathetic nervous system leads to a hyperdynamic circulation with tachycardia and increased cardiac output to overcome the decreased systemic vascular resistance and blood pressure. However, as liver disease progresses and when additional demands are placed on cardiac function, e.g. with infection, cardiac response may be inadequate despite the absence of known cardiac disease. This has been described as cirrhotic cardiomyopathy where there is reduced cardiac contractility, diastolic dysfunction and electrophysiological abnormalities. The pathophysiology of this blunted cardiac response may be due to some underlying cardiac hypertrophy and fibrosis, increased production of negatively inotropic mediators or functional changes in the cardiomyocyte plasma membrane properties. These changes are potentially reversible post-LT [19, 21].

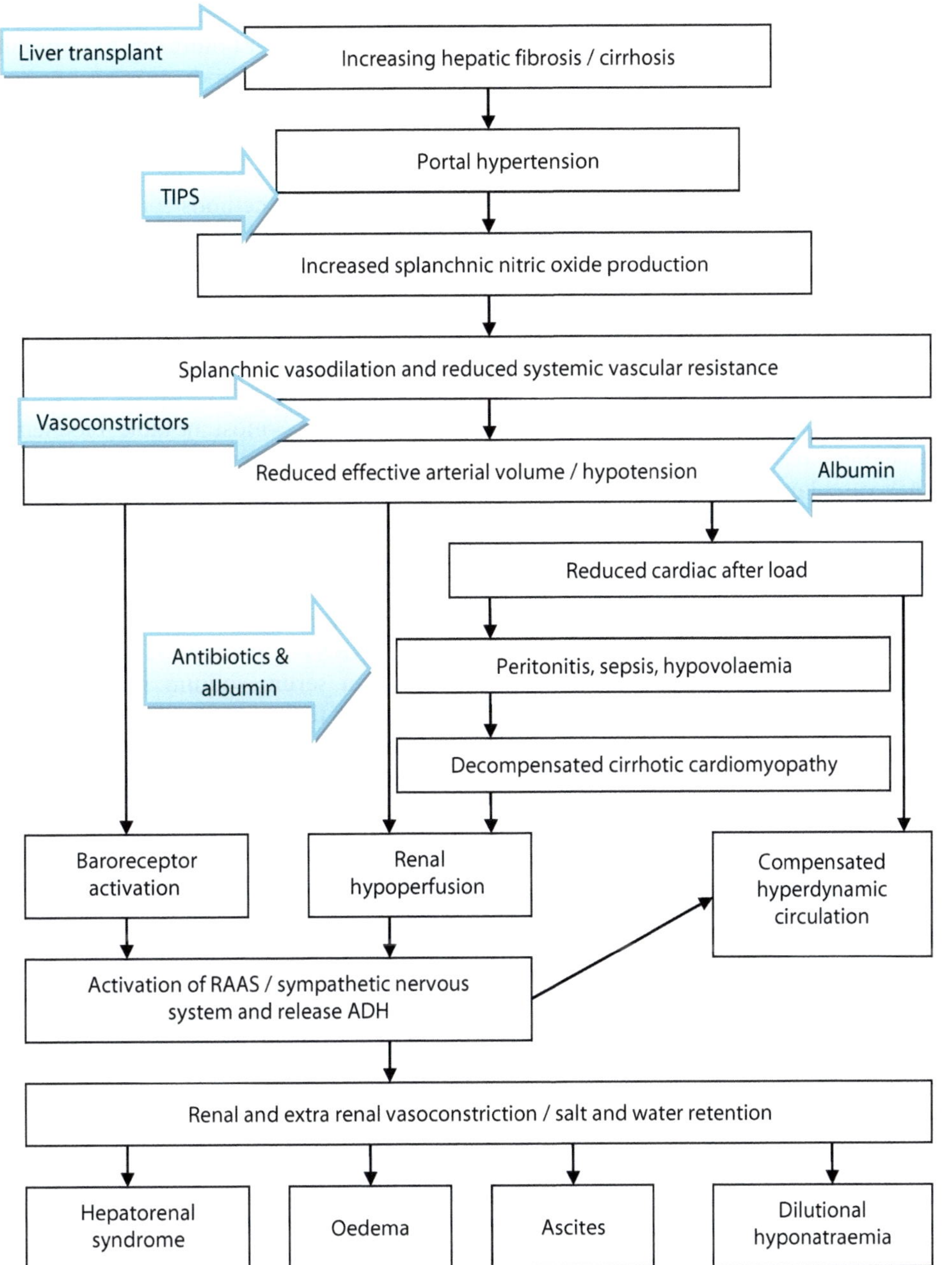

Fig. 36.1 Pathophysiology of hepatorenal syndrome and treatment options. *Abbreviations*: TIPS transjugular intrahepatic portosystemic shunt, RAAS renin-angiotensin-aldosterone system, ADH anti-diuretic hormone

36.6 Clinical Evaluation of Liver Patients with Renal Dysfunction

The key things to determine when assessing a patient include a history of any known renal and liver disease, the aetiology and chronicity of these illnesses including the presence of cirrhosis or signs of portal hypertension. Precipitating events such as a change in medications, haemorrhage, infection, recent diarrhoea or vomiting, or large volume paracentesis, should be ascertained.

Hepatorenal syndrome is an important cause to exclude and is characterised by a constellation of clinical features, outlined in Table 36.2. Most patients will give a long history of chronic liver disease, with ascites being a prominent feature. Depending on the speed of onset and severity of the renal dysfunction, HRS can be classified into HRS-AKI and HRS-CKD, as outlined above. The latter can suddenly progress to HRS-AKI after a precipitating event [2, 7].

On examination, volume assessment is key to the evaluation of patients with renal dysfunction. Hypotension and tachycardia are features of volume depletion and sepsis. A low mean arterial blood pressure <80 mmHg is also seen in HRS-AKI due to splanchnic pooling. This can also be precipitated by factors such as diuretics, paracentesis, sepsis or blood loss. The hypotension is typically accompanied by tachycardia, a manifestation of the hyperdynamic circulation. The haemodynamic changes are not always confined to the kidney, and other vascular beds may also be involved with a reduced cardiac output and encephalopathy in more severe cases. Stigmata of chronic liver disease will usually be evident in those with HRS. Clinical signs of an underlying infection such as peritonitis should be elucidated to enable prompt treatment. Impaired natriuresis is a feature of HRS, and an inability to excrete free water results in peripheral oedema and ascites, and this is typically diuretic resistant. Patients may develop oligo-anuria with a urine output <500 ml/day. Pulmonary oedema can occur in this setting but is not a typical feature of HRS. A bland urinary sediment is characteristic given the functional nature of the renal impairment in HRS, although patients with liver disease may have a number of possible causes for underlying CKD including glomerulonephritis, so haematuria, proteinuria and urinary casts should be excluded. Finally, the skin should be evaluated for signs of a vasculitis rash that can be seen in those with viral hepatitis-related cryoglobulinaemia [3, 4, 22].

36.7 Investigations

Renal function needs to be monitored carefully in those with liver disease, particularly when there is diuretic-resistant ascites, hyponatraemia, peritonitis or gastrointestinal haemorrhage. However, creatinine is a notoriously poor indicator of renal function in patients with cirrhotic liver failure due to poor nutrition, reduced hepatic creatinine production and muscle mass, leading to a delay in diagnosing and treatment based on the traditional creatinine threshold [1]. Commonly used eGFR equations overvalue true GFR, when compared to radio-isotopic methods potentially. This makes the application of the usual CKD stages based on eGFR alone problematic. However, despite these reservations, creatinine and eGFR are currently the easiest and most widely available tools for the assessment of renal function. Cystatin C is also problematic and influenced by clinical factors [13, 23, 24].

One of the most notable biochemical features of HRS is hyponatraemia. Water retention can exceed that of sodium, and so a dilutional hyponatraemia develops in about two-thirds of patients. This parameter can be useful in differentiating HRS from other aetiologies of renal impairment such as acute tubular necrosis. Natriuresis is impaired so one of the other classical findings in HRS is a urinary sodium <10 mmol/L in the context of a serum sodium <135 mmol/L and a urine osmolality that is greater than that of serum [8, 20, 22].

To help distinguish HRS from other parenchymal causes of renal impairment in cirrhotics, a number of tests can be useful (Table 36.4a). A urinary protein-creatinine ratio should be performed if the dipstick is positive along with examination of urinary sediment for casts. If the proteinuria is found to be >500 mg/dL and there is microscopic haematuria (>50 urinary red cells per high-powered field) or any other clinical features to suggest parenchymal renal disease, then consider an alternative diagnosis. However, HRS can develop in the context of a pre-existing renal condition, so this must be taken into account. If no contraindications exist, a renal biopsy may be useful in this scenario to help determine the underling aetiology. This is particularly so if a combined liver and kidney transplant is being considered, as the degree of renal fibrosis will help predict renal prognosis post-LT and avoid unnecessary renal transplantation in those with HRS. The latter is characterised by a lack of significant parenchymal histological changes and typically recovers with LT alone.

Table 36.4a Renal investigations in hepatorenal syndrome – typical results

Laboratory (serum)	Laboratory (urine)	Radiology	Procedures
Creatinine at least × 2 above baseline Sodium <130 mmol/L	Proteinuria <500 mg/day Sodium <10 mEq/L Red blood cells <50 per high-powered field	Normal renal ultrasound	Normal renal histopathology

Table 36.4b Caption

Conditions that cause both renal and liver disease	Some useful investigations
Hepatorenal syndrome	See Table 36.4a
Toxin or drug toxicity or hypersensitivity	Toxicology screen Eosinophilia Urine microscopy may show muddy brown casts Kidney biopsy
Hepatitis B or C virus-related glomerulonephritis	Hepatitis B surface antigen Hepatitis C antibody, PCR or antigen Urine protein-creatinine ratio Urine microscopy for red cell casts Cryoglobulins, rheumatoid factor and complement levels Kidney biopsy
Leptospirosis	Culture Microscopic agglutinin test Polymerase chain reaction
Hantavirus	Anti-hantaviral IgM
Sickle cell disease	Haemoglobin electrophoresis
HELLP syndrome (haemolysis, elevated liver enzymes, low platelets)	Full blood count Blood film looking for red cell fragments or schistocytes Haptoglobins Reticulocytes Lactate dehydrogenase Liver function tests
Polycystic kidney and liver disease	Abdominal ultrasound

As with all other causes of renal impairment, performing a renal ultrasound scan should be a priority to evaluate for evidence of parenchymal disease and to exclude obstruction.

A summary of some useful investigations for conditions that cause both renal and liver dysfunction is outlined in Table 36.4b [1–4, 13, 25].

36.8 Precipitating Factors, Prevention and Initial Therapy

Acute kidney injury is frequently triggered by complications such as peritonitis, acute alcoholic hepatitis and gastrointestinal haemorrhage. Hence, prompt diagnosis and effective treatment is imperative to prevent progression [7].

As previously alluded to, NSAIDs inhibit renal perfusion and so should not be used in those with cirrhosis. Other drugs such as aminoglycosides and angiotensin-converting enzyme inhibitors should also be avoided, where possible. Radiological contrast should be administered with caution in those at risk of developing AKI. Typically, ascites is initially treated with fluid and sodium restriction, but diuretics especially aldosterone antagonists are frequently required. However, overzealous diuresis can have a negative impact on renal perfusion and hence precipitate AKI. Aldosterone antagonists can precipitate dangerous hyperkalaemia and so should be used with caution in those with poor renal function. Preventative strategies include regular monitoring of renal function for all those on diuretics [1, 19].

If renal function does deteriorate, then the first step is to correct intravascular volume depletion, preferably with 1 g/kg albumin per day. This acts as a circulatory expander and may also have antioxidant properties, so is the fluid of choice for resuscitation in all patients with AKI-HRS. Diuretic doses should be reduced or even stopped. In this scenario, the optimum treatment for ascites is paracentesis, with appropriate albumin support for those who require removal of large volumes of over 5 L (8 g/L of ascites drained). Without albumin, approximately 20% will develop HRS. Paracentesis may also relieve raised intra-abdominal pressure impeding renal venous return. There needs to be a low threshold for hospital admission in patients with deteriorating renal function aiming to restore renal perfusion. Some may require high dependency or intensive care unit support to facilitate close monitoring of vital signs and urine output. Adrenal insufficiency may be an exacerbating factor in some, and hydrocortisone administration may also have a role [1, 8, 9, 15].

In a third of cases, HRS is triggered by bacterial peritonitis and is associated with increased cytokine release. Therefore, rapid diagnosis and treatment of any sepsis, including peritonitis, is imperative. Along with antibiotic therapy, albumin administration has also been shown to decrease the risk of HRS from 30.6% to 8.3% compared with controls. This is felt to be due to an improvement in haemodynamics and renal perfusion along with antioxidant effects. For high-risk patients, the use of antibiotic prophylaxis with norfloxacin or ceftriaxone helps to reduce the risk of spontaneous bacterial peritonitis and HRS and improves survival [1, 8, 9, 19, 26, 27].

For those with CKD and liver disease, the key factors in patient management and prevention of progression include those mentioned above, but also attention needs to be given to the management of the underlying cause of the CKD (e.g. diabetes, hepatitis-related glomerulonephritis). Blood pressure should be controlled, and proteinuria minimised, where possible.

36.9 Treatment of AKI and AKI-HRS

If the preventative and initial management strategies outlined above fail and AKI develops secondary to HRS, then several therapies are available. The elimination of creatinine thresholds from the diagnostic criteria should allow for earlier intervention. The key treatment options in the management of HRS depend on the stage of AKI present (▶ Box 36.2) [7, 15].

Box 36.2 Treatment of HRS-CKD

- Diuretics for ascites initially but withdraw if diuretic resistant
- Water and sodium restrict (80–120 mmol/day) for ascites
- Evaluate for sepsis or other precipitants and treat appropriately
- Large volume paracentesis (>5 L) with albumin (8 g/L) support if diuretic-resistant ascites
- Antibiotic prophylaxis if at high risk of bacterial peritonitis with, for example, norfloxacin 400 mg/day
- Consider transjugular intrahepatic portosystemic shunt in appropriate patients
- Little data to support the use of vasoconstrictors and albumin unless renal function is deteriorating and HRS-AKI develops
- Evaluate for liver transplantation

36

36.9.1 Vasoconstrictors and Albumin

As splanchnic vasodilation rather than renal vasoconstriction is the initial circulatory derangement, vasoconstrictors are the pharmacological treatment of choice for HRS-AKI, improving renal function and patient survival. They have also been evaluated in HRS-CKD, but information there is limited. A number of agents have been shown to be effective, either alone or in combination with albumin, but terlipressin, an analogue of the vasopressin V1 receptor, is the most commonly used. A meta-analysis of 18 randomised controlled trials demonstrated that terlipressin resulted in reversal of HRS in 42% versus 15.4% in the placebo group. The relative risk of death was 0.63. It is important to evaluate cardiac risk prior to the initiation of these agents. Relapse after cessation of terlipressin is rare and usually responds to re-treatment. Alpha-1 adrenergic receptor agonists such as midodrine and noradrenaline can also be effective in reversing HRS. Noradrenaline has been compared to terlipressin, and both are equally effective in terms of renal recovery and patient mortality, although the former is less expensive and has fewer side effects. Octreotide is a glucagon inhibitor with vasoconstrictive effects on the splanchnic circulation. When given with midodrine, it has had a positive effect on renal haemodynamics, although benefits were inferior to terlipressin in a randomised controlled trial [1, 8, 13, 28, 29].

36.9.2 Transjugular Intrahepatic Portosystemic Shunt (TIPS)

Here, a metal stent is inserted to bridge the portal and central venous systems aimed at reducing portal hypertension. It is principally used in the treatment for refractory variceal bleeding and diuretic-resistant ascites. One study demonstrated an improvement in renal function in 75% of patients and a mean patient survival of 92 versus 12 weeks in those who underwent TIPS compared with a control group. Patients need to be carefully selected, as a TIPS can result in deterioration in those with severe liver failure, development of congestive cardiac failure or hepatic encephalopathy. In certain scenarios, TIPS does have a role, as in those with HRS and refractory ascites or as an adjunct to vasoconstrictors and albumin while awaiting LT. It may also be an option to prolong survival in those for whom transplantation is contraindicated [8, 13, 19, 30].

36.9.3 Renal Replacement Therapy (RRT) and Artificial Liver Support

End-stage renal failure can develop in both those with AKI and CKD complicating cirrhosis or fulminant hepatic failure. In this case, initiation of RRT and the modality of treatment need to be considered on a case-by-case basis.

Renal replacement therapy may be necessary as a bridge to LT where other treatments have failed. However, a recent study has shown 85% mortality at 6 months post-initiation of RRT in non-listed patients, so careful consideration should be given to initiation of this treatment in this patient group. There may be a role for a time-limited trial of RRT in these individuals if they are not critically ill. Post-transplant, complete renal recovery is usual in patients with HRS-AKI, even in those who have required RRT pre-operatively [31].

Indications for RRT are similar to those for other AKI populations including intractable hyperkalaemia, metabolic acidosis, uraemia and fluid overload. The RRT modality needs to be selected on an individual patient basis. Delivery of RRT can be difficult in those with liver failure for a number of reasons. Coagulopathy and thrombocytopaenia can make gaining vascular access a challenge. Another barrier to the use of intermittent haemodialysis is haemodynamic instability and hypotension. For this reason, continuous RRT is often favoured in patients with HRS-AKI as it allows for more gentle fluid removal, correction or hyponatraemia and other electrolyte disturbances and reduces the likelihood of raised intracranial pressure. Furthermore, the removal by continuous RRT of pro-inflammatory cytokines such as tumour necrosis factor and interleukins 1 and 6 may also be of potential benefit. However, there is no conclusive evidence to support continuous over intermittent therapies for all patients, and the modality should be decided on a case-by-case basis [1, 13, 19, 32].

Another technique that is available is extracorporeal albumin dialysis. This was developed to treat liver failure as a bridge to recovery or LT. The most widely used method is the molecular adsorbent re-circulating system, or MARS. Meta-analysis suggests a survival advantage in those with acute liver failure. Currently, these devices are not in widespread use [8, 13, 19, 33].

36.9.4 Transplantation

The prognosis for patients with HRS is dreadful, and a LT is the best treatment for a meaningful recovery. There is a clear benefit with LT compared with other therapies as it alleviates the underlying liver disease with a progressive improvement in the circulatory derangements post-transplantation, thereby usually restoring renal function. The negative impact of HRS on patient survival is highlighted by the fact that serum creatinine is a key variable in the Model for End-Stage Liver Disease (MELD) score, used to prioritise patients awaiting LT. The number of patients receiving combined liver and kidney transplants rose by 300% in the United States following the introduction of this score in 2002. However, a renal transplant is an inappropriate treatment for HRS unless they also meet the following suggested criteria. Although there are no standard criteria, some indications for combined liver and kidney transplantation are detailed in ◻ Table 36.5. Ideally, patients being considered for a combined transplant should undergo a renal biopsy, provided that it is safe to do so. The presence of >30% renal fibrosis prior to transplantation is likely to lead to a further decline in renal function with the introduction of calcineurin inhibitors post-LT and the development of post-operative AKI. Typically, between 12% and 80% of patients experience AKI in the post-LT period, depending on severity and the definition that is used. It is crucial that any decisions regarding single or dual transplantation are made jointly by the renal and liver teams and on a case-by-case basis [8, 13, 25, 34, 35].

◻ **Table 36.5** Suggested criteria for combined liver and kidney transplant

Patients eligible for liver transplantation with one of the following renal indications:	AKI with GFR <25 ml/min or dialysis dependant for over 6 weeks
	CKD with GFR <35 ml/min or dialysis dependant at the time of listing
	Inherited metabolic disorders

Abbreviations: AKI, acute kidney injury; CKD, chronic kidney disease; GFR, glomerular filtration rate measured by modified diet in renal disease equation or creatinine or radiopharmaceutical clearance

36.9.5 Treatment of Hepatitis B and C in Renal Patients

In patients with glomerular disease, AKI or CKD due to underlying viral hepatitis, it is important to treat the underlying cause. Huge advances have been made in this area in recent times, particularly in relation to hepatitis C virus treatment. Previously, treatment of patients on dialysis or post-transplant with this infection was problematic or impossible because of intolerable side effects or increased risk of rejection. The timing of treatment and drug selection is complex and beyond the scope of this chapter, but guidelines have been published by the European Association for the Study of the Liver (EASL) diseases with details on how to treat those with CKD, on dialysis and pre- and post-renal transplantation [36, 37]. It is important to emphasise that some commonly used drugs need to be avoided or the dose reduced when treating patients with CKD or on dialysis.

36.10 Patient and Renal Outcomes

Without a LT, patient survival with HRS is very poor. Median patient survival for those with HRS-AKI (formerly type 1) is usually as short as 2–4 weeks, while it is 6.7 months in those with HRS-CKD (formerly type 2). HRS-AKI remains an independent predictor of mortality irrespective of the MELD score, further highlighting the negative impact that HRS has on patient outcome [31, 38]. As previously mentioned, vasoconstrictor therapy and liver transplantation do have a positive influence on survival [1, 28]. However, even post-LT, patient survival at 1, 3 and 5 years is inferior in those with HRS compared with those without and survival is particularly poor in patients who remain on dialysis post-LT [39, 40].

The aetiology of renal failure is also important, as HRS is linked to increased mortality compared to other causes of renal failure. Three-month patient survival was 15% with HRS, significantly less than that seen with other causes of renal dysfunction [41]. However, if patients are RRT dependant, survival in those with HRS was not shown to be significantly different to those with a diagnosis of acute tubular necrosis [31].

36

Recovery of renal function following a LT alone is usual after 3–6 weeks, but it may take longer and is not guaranteed in all patients. Between 6% and 10% of patients remain dialysis dependant, and this figure has been reported to be as high as 25% compared with <1% in patients without HRS. Up to 42% of HRS patients continue to have some degree of CKD, but renal function declines in the non-HRS population too with 18% having an eGFR <15 ml/min at 5 years post-LT. This depends on a number of underlying risk factors including age, co-morbidities or pre-existing CKD. The use of calcineurin inhibitors may have further deleterious effects [39, 42, 43].

36.11 Conclusion

Renal dysfunction, including HRS, is a common and very serious complication of cirrhotic liver disease. Therapeutic advances have led to significant improvements in patient outcomes, and as such it is no longer always a terminal complication. However, without the option of LT, the prognosis remains grim for those with HRS-AKI, and the challenge for the nephrologist is the careful and rapid assessment of patients for reversible components and other causes for renal disease. New diagnostic criteria will help to facilitate this. It is critical to establish whether each patient with both renal and liver failure is suitable for a LT or whether a combined liver kidney transplant may be more appropriate in a small number of patients. Getting this right is likely to have a huge impact on the patient's outcome.

Key Points of the Chapter

1. There is a new approach to the diagnosis of hepatorenal syndrome (HRS).
2. A new treatment algorithm has been introduced for the management of HRS type of acute kidney injury.
3. HRS is a functional type of renal failure that is usually reversible post-liver transplant.
4. Albumin and vasoconstrictors are key pharmacological treatment options, and without liver transplantation, prognosis remains very poor.

Tips and Tricks

1. Be aware of the patients who are at risk of developing hepatorenal syndrome (HRS) and take steps to prevent it where possible.
2. The creatinine threshold of 122 μmol/L for the diagnosis of HRS-AKI has been abandoned so treatment can commence earlier.
3. Use albumin for fluid resuscitation.
4. Consider other causes of AKI and CKD in patients with cirrhosis before diagnosing HRS, which is a diagnosis of exclusion.

Abbreviations: *AKI* acute kidney injury, *CKD* chronic kidney disease.

Chapter Review Questions

1. What conditions cause both kidney and liver disease?
2. How is hepatorenal syndrome now defined?
3. Describe the types of hepatorenal syndrome.
4. What is the approach to the treatment of acute kidney injury in patients with liver disease?
5. What are some of the indications for combined liver and kidney transplantation?

Case Study

Case 1

A 53-year-old female was admitted with decompensated cirrhosis due to alcoholic liver disease. She was on the waiting list for liver transplantation but had deteriorating renal function and oliguria. She was disorientated and very oedematous with significant ascites despite high-dose loop diuretics and so was undergoing intermittent large volume paracentesis supported by albumin infusions. Her blood pressure was 100/70 mmHg, pulse rate 98 beats per minute and temperature 37.5°C. A dipstick urinalysis revealed trace proteinuria and blood and no casts were seen on microscopy. Significant lab results were as follows:

Selected laboratory parameters	At the time of initial renal review	On discharge from hospital
Sodium (mmol/L)	130	139
Potassium (mmol/L)	4.8	4.5
Urea (mmol/L)	35	8.1
Creatinine (μmol/L)	204	79
Bilirubin (μmol/L)	201	21
International normalised ratio	1.7	1.1
Platelet count (×10^9/L)	84	178
Urine protein-creatinine ratio (mg/mmol)	47	Not available
Urinary sodium (mmol/L)	19	Not available

She had a negative immunology and myeloma screen. A renal ultrasound was unremarkable. A diagnosis of HRS-AKI was made. The diuretics were stopped, and she was started on albumin and terlipressin intravenously. Despite this, there was little improvement clinically or biochemically, and she decompensated following an episode of sepsis, becoming more confused with haemodynamic instability. She was transferred to the intensive care unit where she was started on intravenous antibiotics for suspected bacterial peritonitis and continuous RRT. She improved significantly, and the antibiotics were stopped a week later. The encephalopathy also resolved, but she remained oliguric and so remained on continuous RRT. She underwent a liver transplant a week later which was without complications and made a full renal recovery. This case demonstrates the fulminant deterioration that can befall a patient with chronic liver disease and the urgency of treatment as well as the potential for good renal recovery when HRS is cured.

Case 2

A 27-year-old female presented to an accident and emergency department with a reduced level of consciousness, malaise and nausea. She had no significant past medical or surgical history of relevance and was not on any regular medications. The history revealed that she had taken a staggered, inadvertent paracetamol overdose over the preceding week for flu-like symptoms and musculoskeletal pain. Socially she drank 5 units of alcohol per week for the preceding 6 months but previously drank more heavily, up to 40 units a week. Her initial blood results are illustrated in the table below, and she also had a paracetamol level of 125 mg/L. She was commenced on acetylcysteine and intravenous fluids, transferred to the intensive care unit and intubated for a falling Glasgow Coma Scale. She was commenced on inotropes for haemodynamic instability and continuous renal replacement therapy for oliguric renal failure and metabolic acidosis. Her condition progressively deteriorated, and after discussion with the hepatology service, she was listed for a super urgent liver transplant. The liver transplant went ahead 2 days later, and the surgery was uncomplicated. She remained in the intensive care unit and on continuous RRT for another week before being commenced on intermittent haemodialysis. She was eventually discharged to the ward and continued to require dialysis for another week before this could be stopped. Her discharge bloods are indicated below. Renal recovery often lags behind hepatic recovery in paracetamol overdose not needing a liver transplant, but either way, in a young patient, the renal prognosis is likely to be good.

Selected laboratory parameters	Prior to liver transplant	On hospital discharge
Sodium (mmol/L)	131	135
Potassium (mmol/L)	5.3	4.1
Urea (mmol/L)	14.1	2.7
Creatinine (μmol/L)	347	85
Albumin (g/l)	25	28
Bilirubin (μmol/L)	68	22
Aspartate aminotransferase (IU/L)	11,487	35
Alanine transaminase (IU/L)	8044	110
Lactate	14	
pH	7.01	7.35
International normalised ratio	4.7	0.99
Haemoglobin	9.1	9.7
Platelet count (×10^9/L)	57	187
Urine protein-creatinine ratio (mg/mmol)	58	Urine dip negative

References

1. Gines P, Schrier RW. Renal failure in cirrhosis. N Engl J Med. 2009;361(13):1279–90.
2. Wong F, Nadim MK, Kellum JA, Salerno F, Bellomo R, Gerbes A, et al. Working party proposal for a revised classification system of renal dysfunction in patients with cirrhosis. Gut. 2011;60(5):702–9.
3. Arroyo V, Gines P, Gerbes AL, Dudley FJ, Gentilini P, Laffi G, et al. Definition and diagnostic criteria of refractory ascites and hepatorenal syndrome in cirrhosis. International Ascites Club. Hepatology. 1996;23(1):164–76.
4. Salerno F, Gerbes A, Gines P, Wong F, Arroyo V. Diagnosis, prevention and treatment of hepatorenal syndrome in cirrhosis. Gut. 2007;56(9):1310–8.
5. KDIGO clinical practice guideline for acute kidney injury. Kidney International Supplements. 2012;2(1).
6. Levey AS, Eckardt KU, Tsukamoto Y, Levin A, Coresh J, Rossert J, et al. Definition and classification of chronic kidney disease: a position statement from Kidney Disease: Improving Global Outcomes (KDIGO). Kidney Int. 2005;67(6):2089–100.
7. Angeli P, Ginès P, Wong F, Bernardi M, Boyer TD, Gerbes A, et al. Diagnosis and management of acute kidney injury in patients with cirrhosis: revised consensus recommendations of the International Club of Ascites. J Hepatol. 2015;62(4):968–74.
8. EASL clinical practice guidelines on the management of ascites, spontaneous bacterial peritonitis, and hepatorenal syndrome in cirrhosis. J Hepatol. 2010;53(3):397–417.
9. Runyon BA. Introduction to the revised American Association for the Study of Liver Diseases Practice Guideline on management of adult patients with ascites due to cirrhosis 2012. Hepatology. 2013;57(4):1651–3.
10. Solé C, Pose E, Solà E, Ginès P. Hepatorenal syndrome in the era of acute kidney injury. Liver Int. 2018;38(11):1891–901.
11. National Kidney Foundation. K/DOQI clinical practice guidelines for chronic kidney disease: evaluation, classification, and stratification. Am J Kidney Dis. 2002;39(2 Suppl 1):S1–266.
12. Bucsics T, Krones E. Renal dysfunction in cirrhosis: acute kidney injury and the hepatorenal syndrome. Gastroenterol Rep (Oxf). 2017;5(2):127–37.
13. Nadim MK, Kellum JA, Davenport A, Wong F, Davis C, Pannu N, et al. Hepatorenal syndrome: the 8th international consensus conference of the Acute Dialysis Quality Initiative (ADQI) Group. Crit Care. 2012;16(1):R23.
14. Fagundes C, Barreto R, Guevara M, Garcia E, Solà E, Rodríguez E, et al. A modified acute kidney injury classification for diagnosis and risk stratification of impairment of kidney function in cirrhosis. J Hepatol. 2013;59(3):474–81.
15. Angeli P, Rodríguez E, Piano S, Ariza X, Morando F, Solà E, et al. Acute kidney injury and acute-on-chronic liver failure classifications in prognosis assessment of patients with acute decompensation of cirrhosis. Gut. 2015;64(10):1616–22.
16. Gines A, Escorsell A, Gines P, Salo J, Jimenez W, Inglada L, et al. Incidence, predictive factors, and prognosis of the hepatorenal syndrome in cirrhosis with ascites. Gastroenterology. 1993;105(1):229–36.
17. Betrosian AP, Agarwal B, Douzinas EE. Acute renal dysfunction in liver diseases. World J Gastroenterol. 2007;13(42):5552–9.
18. Gines P, Guevara M, Arroyo V, Rodes J. Hepatorenal syndrome. Lancet. 2003;362(9398):1819–27.
19. Wadei HM, Mai ML, Ahsan N, Gonwa TA. Hepatorenal syndrome: pathophysiology and management. Clin J Am Soc Nephrol. 2006;1(5):1066–79.
20. Oliver JA, Verna EC. Afferent mechanisms of sodium retention in cirrhosis and hepatorenal syndrome. Kidney Int. 2010;77(8):669–80.
21. Moller S, Henriksen JH. Cardiovascular complications of cirrhosis. Gut. 2008;57(2):268–78.
22. Cardenas A. Hepatorenal syndrome: a dreaded complication of end-stage liver disease. Am J Gastroenterol. 2005;100(2):460–7.
23. Gonwa TA, Jennings L, Mai ML, Stark PC, Levey AS, Klintmalm GB. Estimation of glomerular filtration rates before and after orthotopic liver transplantation: evaluation of current equations. Liver Transpl. 2004;10(2):301–9.
24. Puthumana J, Ariza X, Belcher JM, Graupera I, Ginès P, Parikh CR. Urine interleukin 18 and lipocalin 2 are biomarkers of acute tubular necrosis in patients with cirrhosis: a systematic review and meta-analysis. Clin Gastroenterol Hepatol. 2017;15(7):1003–13.e3.
25. Eason JD, Gonwa TA, Davis CL, Sung RS, Gerber D, Bloom RD. Proceedings of consensus conference on simultaneous liver kidney transplantation (SLK). Am J Transplant. 2008;8(11):2243–51.
26. Cardenas A, Gines P, Uriz J, Bessa X, Salmeron JM, Mas A, et al. Renal failure after upper gastrointestinal bleeding in cirrhosis: incidence, clinical course, predictive factors, and short-term prognosis. Hepatology. 2001;34(4 Pt 1):671–6.
27. Salerno F, Navickis RJ, Wilkes MM. Albumin infusion improves outcomes of patients with spontaneous bacterial peritonitis: a meta-analysis of randomized trials. Clin Gastroenterol Hepatol. 2013;11(2):123–30.e1.
28. Gluud LL, Christensen K, Christensen E, Krag A. Systematic review of randomized trials on vasoconstrictor drugs for hepatorenal syndrome. Hepatology. 2010;51(2):576–84.
29. Wang H, Liu A, Bo W, Feng X, Hu Y. Terlipressin in the treatment of hepatorenal syndrome: a systematic review and meta-analysis. Medicine (Baltimore). 2018;97(16):e0431.
30. Brensing KA, Textor J, Perz J, Schiedermaier P, Raab P, Strunk H, et al. Long term outcome after transjugular intrahepatic portosystemic stent-shunt in non-transplant cirrhotics with hepatorenal syndrome: a phase II study. Gut. 2000;47(2):288–95.
31. Allegretti AS, Parada XV, Eneanya ND, Gilligan H, Xu D, Zhao S, et al. Prognosis of patients with cirrhosis and AKI who initiate RRT. Clin J Am Soc Nephrol. 2018;13(1):16–25.
32. Davenport A. Continuous renal replacement therapies in patients with liver disease. Semin Dial. 2009;22(2):169–72.
33. He GL, Feng L, Duan CY, Hu X, Zhou CJ, Cheng Y, et al. Meta-analysis of survival with the molecular adsorbent recirculating system for liver failure. Int J Clin Exp Med. 2015;8(10):17046–54.
34. Kamath PS, Wiesner RH, Malinchoc M, Kremers W, Therneau TM, Kosberg CL, et al. A model to predict survival in patients with end-stage liver disease. Hepatology. 2001;33(2):464–70.
35. Formica RN, Aeder M, Boyle G, Kucheryavaya A, Stewart D, Hirose R, et al. Simultaneous liver-kidney allocation policy: a proposal to optimize appropriate utilization of scarce resources. Am J Transplant. 2016;16(3):758–66.
36. European Association for the Study of the Liver. Electronic address: easloffice@easloffice.eu; European Association for the Study of the Liver. EASL recommendations on treatment of hepatitis C 2018. J Hepatol. 2018;69(2):461–511.
37. European Association for the Study of the Liver. Electronic address: easloffice@easloffice.eu; European Association for the Study of the Liver. EASL 2017 clinical practice guidelines on the management of hepatitis B virus infection. J Hepatol. 2017;67(2):370–98.

38. Alessandria C, Ozdogan O, Guevara M, Restuccia T, Jimenez W, Arroyo V, et al. MELD score and clinical type predict prognosis in hepatorenal syndrome: relevance to liver transplantation. Hepatology. 2005;41(6):1282–9.
39. Ruiz R, Barri YM, Jennings LW, Chinnakotla S, Goldstein RM, Levy MF, et al. Hepatorenal syndrome: a proposal for kidney after liver transplantation (KALT). Liver Transpl. 2007;13(6):838–43.
40. Davis CL, Feng S, Sung R, Wong F, Goodrich NP, Melton LB, et al. Simultaneous liver-kidney transplantation: evaluation to decision making. Am J Transplant. 2007;7(7):1702–9.
41. Martin-Llahi M, Guevara M, Torre A, Fagundes C, Restuccia T, Gilabert R, et al. Prognostic importance of the cause of renal failure in patients with cirrhosis. Gastroenterology. 2011;140(2):488–96. e4
42. Marik PE, Wood K, Starzl TE. The course of type 1 hepatorenal syndrome post liver transplantation. Nephrol Dial Transplant. 2006;21(2):478–82.
43. Ojo AO, Held PJ, Port FK, Wolfe RA, Leichtman AB, Young EW, et al. Chronic renal failure after transplantation of a nonrenal organ. N Engl J Med. 2003;349(10):931–40.

Chronic Kidney Disease: Cardiovascular Complications

Katharine Pates, Ben Caplin, and David C. Wheeler

Contents

M. Harber (ed.), *Primer on Nephrology*, https://doi.org/10.1007/978-3-030-76419-7_37

Learning Objectives

1. This chapter explores the prevalence of CVD in patients with renal disease and aims to illustrate the complex and intimate relationship between renal and cardiovascular disease.
2. We aim to illustrate the differences between atherosclerotic vascular disease and vascular disease related to CKD and cover the management of classical and renal cardiovascular risk factor including the profound impact of CKD and proteinuria on cardiovascular risk as well as the importance of cardiac disease on renal outcome.

37.1 Epidemiology of CVD in CKD

Both reduced kidney function and albuminuria are associated with increased cardiovascular mortality. In a comprehensive population-based study, the risk of a cardiovascular event was 1.4 and 3.4 times greater in patients with CKD stage 3a and stage 5, respectively [1]. Furthermore, outcomes for CKD patients suffering cardiovascular events are worse than for those with normal kidney function [2]. Thus, cardiovascular events represent the most important avoidable cause of morbidity and mortality in patients with impaired kidney function.

37

37.2 The Association Between CKD and CVD

The interrelationship between CVD and CKD is complex and involves both atherosclerotic and non-atherosclerotic changes (◘ Fig. 37.1). Risk factors including hypertension, smoking and diabetes have been linked to the progression of both CKD and cardiovascular disease, suggesting that there may be common pathogenic mechanisms [3]. However, CKD itself, or its complications such as hyperphosphataemia, may also play an important causal role in the development of cardiovascular diseases. Impaired kidney function and albuminuria/proteinuria have been implicated in the pathogenesis of a wide range of cardiovascular syndromes including heart failure, sudden cardiac death and stroke [4]. Furthermore, a causal role for the kidney in cardiovascular disease is supported by the stepwise increase in the risk of adverse cardiac events at lower levels of kidney function and the reduction in risk following successful kidney transplantation.

The term 'cardiorenal syndrome' has been used to describe the broad spectrum of diseases in which heart and kidney dysfunction overlap. In a classification proposed in the Consensus Conference by the Acute Dialysis Quality Group 2008 [5], cardiorenal syndrome is divided into cardiorenal and reno-cardiac depending on the principal driver of the disease. Each is then further subdivided into acute and chronic. A final type encompasses cardiorenal disease caused by systemic disease.

Therefore, cardiovascular disease and CKD often coexist and may be causally linked. As in individuals with normal kidney function, optimal management of cardiovascular disease in CKD patients requires risk stratification and attention to the management of risk factors. At the present time, it is unclear whether alternative strategies that target 'non-traditional' risk factors associated with CKD, such as hyperphosphataemia or hyperparathyroidism, are worthwhile.

37.3 Atherosclerotic and Non-atherosclerotic Disease in the CKD Population

37.3.1 Atherosclerosis

The high co-prevalence of shared risk factors such as diabetes mellitus means that atherosclerosis is an important cause of cardiovascular disease in patients with kidney disease [6]. The process of plaque formation, rupture and vessel occlusion is likely to be similar in those with and without CKD. Furthermore, atherosclerosis is a systemic disease, meaning that plaque formation in the arterial supply to one organ (e.g. in the coronary arteries) (◘ Fig. 37.2d) is likely to reflect coexistent disease in the arterial supply to other organs (e.g. in the renal, carotid or femoral arteries).

37.3.2 Left Ventricular Disease

Echocardiographic studies suggest that a large proportion of patients with CKD have structural heart disease, rising from 30% of patients with CKD stage 2 to 75% in those with stage 4 [7]. This usually manifests as left ventricular hypertrophy (◘ Fig. 37.2c). Although coronary artery occlusion will cause segmental infarction as in those with normal kidney function, there may also be ultrastructural abnormalities of the heart, such as myocardial fibrosis in those with abnormal kidney function. Whether these changes reflect the consequences of ischaemia secondary to coronary microvascular disease or a specific effect of metabolites that accumulate in CKD remains unclear. In addition, there is now evidence that hypotension during haemodialysis may contribute to recurrent cardiac ischaemia providing another mechanism to drive structural damage to the heart [8].

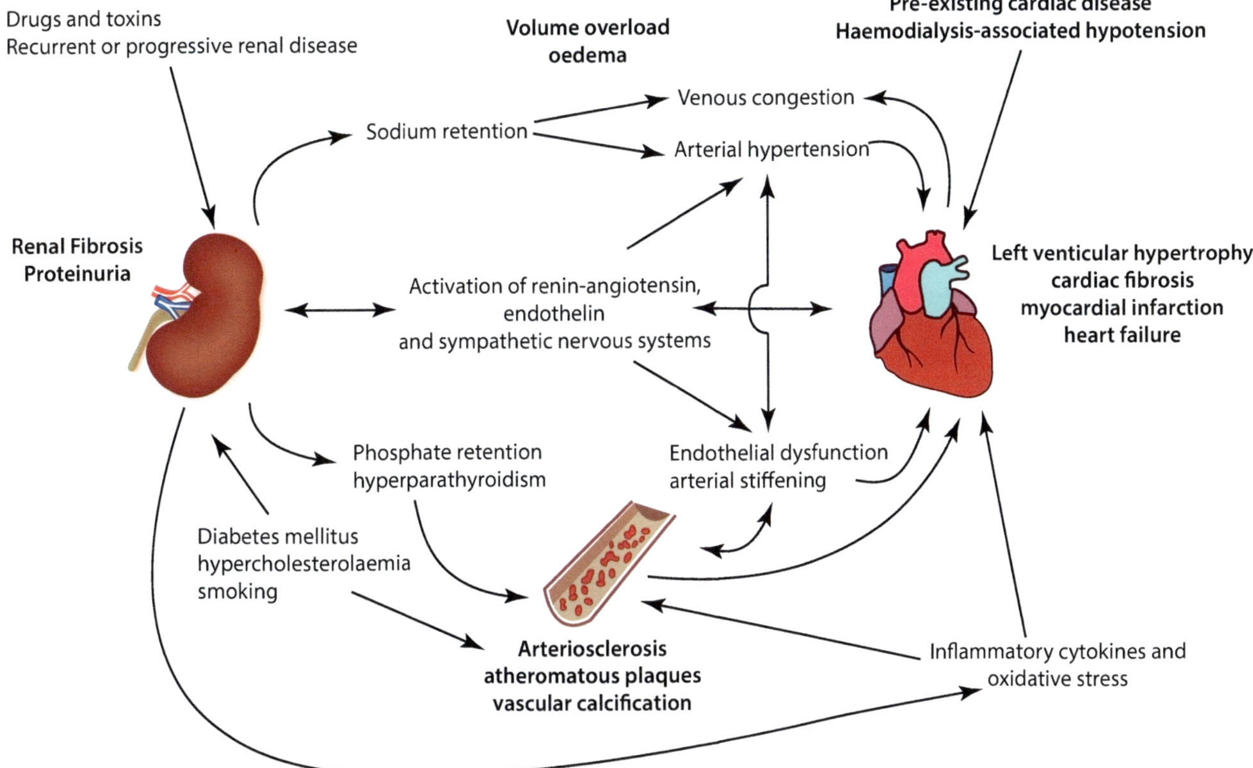

Fig. 37.1 Mechanisms of CV disease in CKD

37.3.3 Arterial Stiffening

The compliance of the arterial tree lessens with normal ageing, but this process is accelerated in patients with CKD. Complaint arteries improve perfusion throughout the cardiac cycle by accommodating the maximal pressure during systole and maintaining blood flow during diastole. Arterial stiffening may manifest as a widened pulse pressure, meaning that although the systolic pressure may be high, the diastolic pressure is low (e.g. a blood pressure of 160/60 mmHg). Both structural and functional changes are thought to lead to arterial stiffening. For example, thickening of the arterial wall (Fig. 37.2e), with or without calcification, will reduce vessel elasticity.

37.3.4 Arterial Calcification

Arterial calcification is a recognised feature of atherosclerosis but is particularly common in CKD. Calcium can be deposited both in atherosclerotic plaques (which are found in the intima of the artery) and within the medial layer of the vessel wall (Fig. 37.2a, b, e). Medial calcification in particular is likely to be associated with arterial stiffening. It is generally accepted that deposition of calcium in soft tissues is a feature of the CKD-bone mineral disorder and may be exacerbated by treatment strategies aimed at preventing secondary hyperparathyroidism such as administration of calcium-based phosphate binders.

37.4 Approach to Cardiovascular Syndromes in Patients with Kidney Disease

37.4.1 Cardiac Ischaemia

37.4.1.1 Aetiology and Clinical Presentation

The presentation of ischaemic heart disease may be atypical in CKD. For example, syncope, arrhythmia, sudden onset of symptoms of left ventricular failure or even isolated hypotension should prompt further investigation to look for underlying coronary ischaemia.

Patients on haemodialysis may also be exposed to asymptomatic chronic myocardial ischaemia. As discussed above, there are well-documented reductions in cardiac perfusion during dialysis in response to removal of circulating volume. This may be particularly damaging in patients with non-compliant arteries and limited left ventricular functional reserve and may cause myocardial stunning and hibernation, leading to progression of chronic myocardial injury.

37

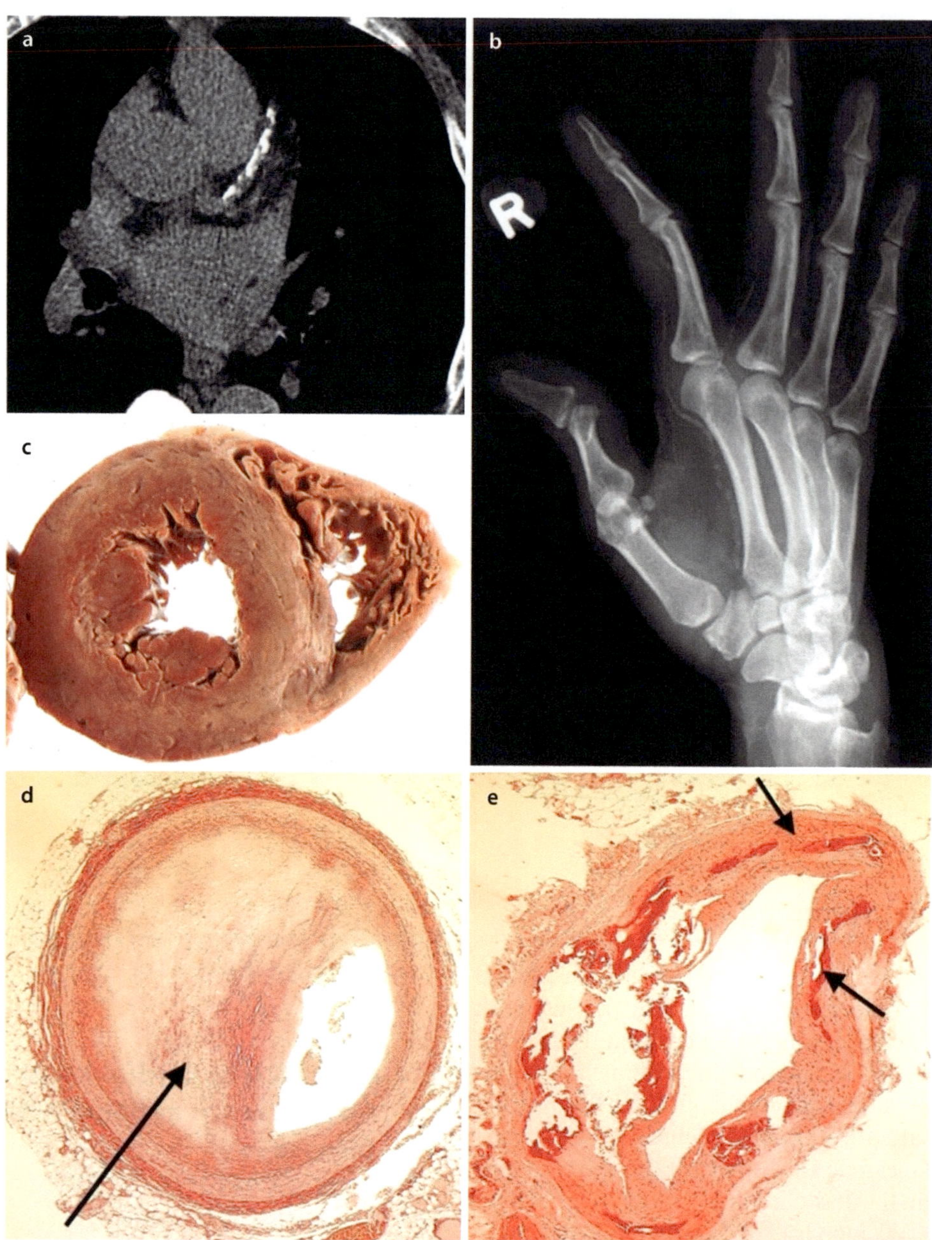

Fig. 37.2 Cardiovascular changes in CKD patients. **a** An electron beam CT scan of the heart in a patient with CKD demonstrating calcium in the left anterior descending coronary artery. **b** Plain x-ray of the hand in a patient on haemodialysis showing calcification of the deep branches of the radial artery as well as osteopaenia of the small bones of the hand. **c** Post-mortem specimen of the heart from a patient with CKD demonstrating left ventricular wall thickening (Courtesy Dr. Paul Bass, Consultant Pathologist, Royal Free London). **d** Histological section of a diseased atherosclerotic artery showing obstructive lipid-filled subintimal plaque (*arrow*; ×300 H&E). **e** Histological section of arteriosclerotic artery demonstrating arterial wall thickening and medial calcification (*arrows*; ×300 H&E). (**d**, **e**: Courtesy Professor Mary Sheppard, Department of Cardiovascular Pathology, St George's University of London)

Patients with CKD who sustain a myocardial infarction may present with ST elevation on ECG, however atypical ECG changes are common. Patients with multiple previous episodes of cardiac ischaemia may have signs of previous infarction on ECG and the manifestations of any new ischaemia on the tracing may not be obvious.

Raised levels of troponin T (cTnT) and troponin I (cTnI) are thought to reflect myocardial injury and are now routinely used to select patients for invasive investigations such as coronary angiography. However, patients with impaired kidney function may have raised blood levels of cardiac troponins, even in the absence of an acute coronary syndrome (Fig. 37.3).

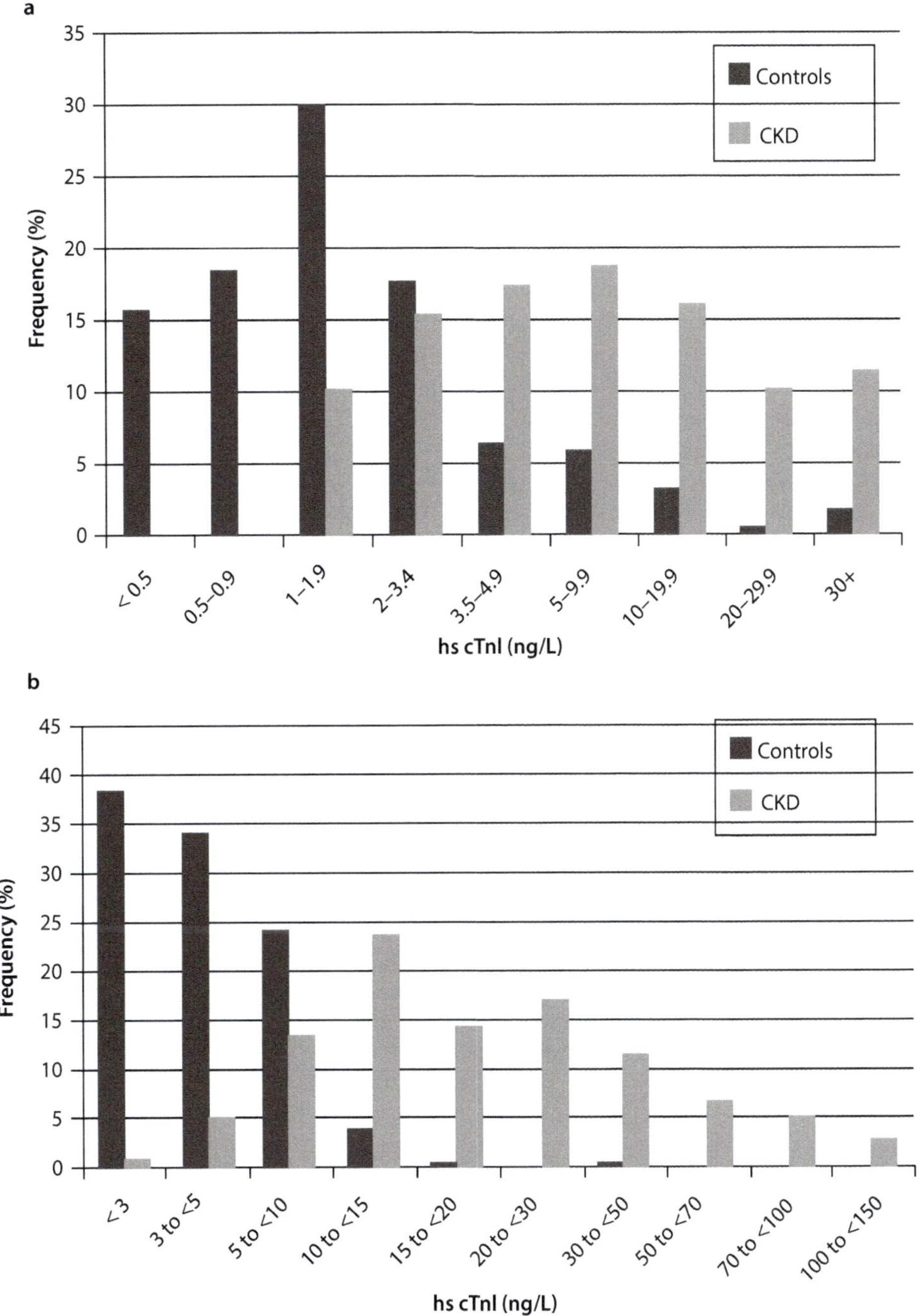

Fig. 37.3 Troponin levels in patients with CKD but without acute coronary syndrome. Distribution of highly sensitive troponin I (**a**) and highly sensitive troponin T (**b**) in 148 subjects with CKD and 288 healthy controls. (Reprinted with permission from DeFilippi et al. [8])

As kidney function declines, circulating cardiac troponin levels increase, with the majority of patients having raised cTnT and a minority having a cTnI above the normal range [9]. These high levels of cardiac troponins have been attributed to (a) failure of clearance of troponin breakdown products via the kidney, (b) subclinical myocardial injury and (c) noncardiac production of the proteins. This presents difficulties when interpreting raised troponin levels in patients with chronic kidney disease, but the following generalisations can be made:

- Elevated troponin T and troponin I concentrations should be interpreted with caution in CKD patients.
- A single measurement cannot be used to stratify a patient's risk in the same way as in those with normal kidney function.

- Troponin concentrations predict poor outcomes including cardiovascular death in patients with CKD. The higher the troponin, the greater the risk of death.
- An acute rise in cardiac troponin (>20% above baseline) is likely to reflect an acute myocardial injury.

In patients receiving haemodialysis, the dialysis process itself may influence troponin levels, but the magnitude of this effect may be dependent on the type of dialysis membrane used [10].

37.4.1.2 Diagnostic Imaging

Angiography remains the investigation of choice for detecting athero-occlusive disease of the coronary and peripheral vessels. Other imaging modalities such as CT angiography may soon become the standard approach for visualisation of arterial plaque. Coronary CT also allows assessment of the vessel wall, so the overall degree of coronary calcification can also be quantified. CT angiography requires contrast administration with the associated risks. Iodinated radiocontrast used in digital subtraction and CT angiography can lead to acute kidney injury. This is generally mild and reversible if adequate precautions are taken before the procedure (hydration, temporary omission of ARBs, ACEi and diuretics), although the potential to damage residual kidney function in patients approaching dialysis must be taken into account when planning these investigations.

37

Given that myocardial disease may occur in the absence of occlusive plaque, cardiac functional studies can be useful in patients with advanced CKD. Possible approaches include myocardial perfusion scanning or stress echocardiography, and there is evidence that the latter of these two approaches can provide useful prognostic information [11].

37.4.1.3 Treatment

Emergency Reperfusion

In patients without impaired kidney function, primary percutaneous transluminal coronary angioplasty (PTCA) improves outcomes following ST-segment elevation myocardial infarction (or acute coronary syndromes with evidence of myocardial injury) compared to conservative treatment. Although the magnitude of this benefit may be reduced as kidney function declines [12], reperfusion is considered first-line treatment in most dialysis centres and the benefits of reperfusion are likely to outweigh any risk to the kidney from radiocontrast in almost all clinical scenarios.

Where PTCA is not available, thrombolysis using t-PA or streptokinase is an alternative approach to reperfusion. There is no reason to assume that patients with renal impairment should not benefit from thrombolysis. However, it should be remembered that patients receiving dialysis are generally at higher risk of bleeding than those with normal kidney function.

As discussed above, the haemodialysis procedure itself can lead to reductions in myocardial perfusion. Haemodialysis should be avoided during and immediately following acute coronary ischaemia unless there are absolute indications such as hyperkalaemia or fluid overload. Some nephrologists also suggest that the haemodialysis prescription should be modified in the period immediately following an acute coronary event in order to maximise cardiovascular stability with short daily treatment times, low blood flow, minimal ultrafiltration and a high sodium concentration in the dialysis fluid (see ▶ Chap. 59).

Delayed/Elective Intervention

Although PTCA appears relatively safe in patients with moderate CKD, as in patients with normal kidney function, there have been no studies showing a positive impact on clinical outcomes when compared to maximising medical therapy in this group [13].

In subgroup analyses of CKD patients entered into trials comparing PTCA to coronary artery bypass grafting, there are no differences in the rate of death, stroke and myocardial infarction between these two approaches, although revascularisation rates are substantially lower following surgery [14]. However, the risks of major surgery are high in patients with additional comorbidities, and postoperative death is more frequent in dialysis patients. Therefore, the choice as to whether to proceed to PTCA or to refer for CABG should be determined by clinical judgement in the absence of good quality evidence.

Medical Therapy

Anticoagulant treatment is routinely administered to patients presenting with acute coronary syndromes. There is no reason to assume that these agents will be less effective in patients with CKD. There is an increased risk of bleeding among patients with CKD stages 4–5 and in addition, the low-molecular-weight heparins accumulate in advanced kidney disease. Newer direct-acting anticoagulants may have a more favourable risk-to-benefit ratio than warfarin according to the limited data available, but there are no data from prospective randomised trials.

Antiplatelet agents such as clopidogrel and glycoprotein IIa/IIIb inhibitors have not been shown to benefit patients with CKD when added to aspirin in the context of acute coronary syndromes. Data from post hoc analyses of large trials suggest that the addition of these agents does not reduce the incidence of further cardiovascular events or death, but increases the risk of serious bleeding [15]. Therefore, optimal medical therapy in the secondary prevention of ischaemic heart disease consists of aspirin in addition to renin-angiotensin system inhibition, beta-blockade and statin therapy. There is no evidence indicating that beta-blockade or drugs targeting of the renin-angiotensin system are any less effective in patients with CKD, therefore given the increased prevalence of IHD, the number of patients needed to treat to gain benefit is likely to be smaller. However, observational studies suggest that despite this likely benefit, patients with CKD are less likely to receive evidence-based medical management following acute coronary syndromes as compared to patients with normal kidney function [16].

37.4.2 Cardiovascular Causes of Shortness of Breath

37.4.2.1 Aetiology and Clinical Presentation

Symptoms and signs of pulmonary oedema may present diagnostic difficulty in CKD patients who can develop sodium and water overload due to a failure of natriuresis, independently of left ventricular dysfunction. Additionally, CKD patients with left ventricular failure secondary to structural abnormalities, such as LV hypertrophy, or ischaemic damage (due to coronary artery occlusion or microvascular disease) will also develop secondary salt and water retention. More rarely, a disruption of cardiac rhythm can precipitate pulmonary oedema. Many patients with CKD, particularly in the advanced stages (stages 4–5), present with a combination of left ventricular dysfunction and fluid overload and may need hospitalisation to optimise management.

Chest x-ray may show evidence of engorged pulmonary vessels (and the ECG may reveal a left ventricular strain pattern). The polypeptide N-terminal pro-brain natriuretic peptide (nt-proBNP) is a highly sensitive marker of cardiac stretch and left ventricular failure in patients with a normal GFR. nt-proBNP is cleared by the kidney, and levels are higher in CKD, with a stepwise increase as GFR falls, but whether additional mechanisms (reflecting the burden of cardiac pathology) are also responsible for the higher levels observed in patients with CKD is controversial. Therefore, although nt-proBNP levels correlate with LV dysfunction in patients with mild and moderate CKD, the upper limit of normal for the assay should be increased in this group of patients. Levels of nt-proBNP are highest in dialysis patients and do not necessarily show an independent association with LV dysfunction in this group [16], although serial measurements may provide useful additional information as to changes in total body salt and water overload. As in the case of troponin, the dialysis procedure may influence circulating concentrations of this marker, and whatever the mechanisms of elevation in patients with CKD, higher levels of nt-proBNP predict adverse outcomes.

Echocardiography is a useful non-invasive investigation in CKD patients with pulmonary oedema. Evidence of reduced left ventricular ejection fraction suggests underlying cardiac dysfunction. However, abnormal left ventricular geometry is common in CKD patients as a result of chronic pressure and volume overload, cardiac ischaemia and fibrosis, but many patients will be found to have diastolic dysfunction on echocardiography. Assessment of left ventricular function is further complicated in patients receiving haemodialysis by the effects of changes in volume status and the potential for myocardial stunning. Thus, the timing of the investigation with reference to the dialysis session may be an important factor in interpreting the result. Based on these considerations, assessment of cardiac function by echocardiography in a dialysis-dependent patient can only be reliable once intravascular volume status has been optimised.

37.4.2.2 Acute Treatment

As in the patient with normal kidney function, the treatment of acute pulmonary oedema in CKD includes maintaining gas exchange and venodilation, followed by salt and water removal. Nitrates remain the mainstay of venodilatory therapy and intravenous therapy allows minute-by-minute titration according to arterial blood pressure.

Loop diuretics, which have both natriuretic and vasodilatory effects when given intravenously, are also useful in CKD patients, except in those who are anuric. Higher doses of loop diuretics are often required when GFR is reduced as compared to when kidney function is normal. These large doses (e.g. 500 mg of frusemide/furosemide) are best given by continuous infusion over a 24 h period as rapid injection of large doses of these drugs can cause deafness. Additional blockade of sodium reabsorption in the distal nephron with thiazide or potassium-sparing diuretics will lead to enhanced natriuresis. Careful monitoring is required when using this combined approach, which can lead to rapid intravascular volume depletion with associated organ dysfunction. In addition, acidosis and hyperkalaemia often complicate the use of potassium-sparing diuretics in those with CKD.

In patients who are dialysis dependent or acutely oliguric, ultrafiltration may be required and should be initiated in a timely fashion. In the acute setting and in situations where the metabolic disturbance is limited, isolated ultrafiltration without dialysis will improve cardiovascular stability and may be the treatment of choice. Furthermore, where diagnostic doubt exists as to the aetiology of the shortness of breath in a dialysis patient, a therapeutic trial of ultrafiltration may be useful. Removal of as little as 500 mL of ultrafiltrate can acutely improve symptoms if due to pulmonary oedema.

Prevention of recurrent pulmonary oedema usually requires attention to both cardiac and renal factors. Management of fluid overload in non-dialysis-dependent CKD patients includes salt restriction and diuretic therapy, sometimes requiring combinations of loop and thiazide or potassium-sparing agents. Care must be taken to avoid over-diuresis, progressive prerenal dysfunction and biochemical deterioration. Regular review of volume status and blood biochemistry along with patient education and daily home monitoring of weight are important strategies. Ultimately, failure of volume control in a CKD patient may be the primary indication for initiating long-term RRT.

Both ACE inhibitors and beta-blockers are likely to have a valuable role in the management of left ventricular failure in CKD, with beneficial effects on cardiac remodelling and clinical outcomes. The roles of spironolactone and newer aldosterone antagonists have not been adequately defined in patients with impaired kidney function. Sodium-glucose cotransporter inhibitors may also improve heart failure outcomes in patients with type 2 diabetes and CKD and are currently undergoing assessment in clinical trials.

37.4.3 Arrhythmia and Sudden Death

37.4.3.1 Aetiology and Clinical Presentation

37

Atrial fibrillation (AF) is the commonest cardiac rhythm disturbance in CKD patients, complicating an estimated 16–21% of patients with CKD not on dialysis and 15–40% of those on dialysis (reference from Turakhaj et al.). AF increases mortality risk in CKD and may also increase the risk of progression to end-stage kidney disease. The effect on stroke and other outcomes related to AF are more difficult to determine due to the numerous shared risk factors between CKD and AF. For example, both CKD and AF are risk factors for stroke; however, whether the relationship is independent or interdependent is currently unknown. Other cardiac rhythm disturbances are less common and less extensively studied, but may also present with syncope or other consequences of hypotension.

The risk of sudden cardiac death in patients with CKD is high, accounting for 25–29% of all-cause mortality in haemodialysis patients, with the annual rate higher than that seen in heart failure and post-infarction patients [17]. The risk in non-haemodialysis CKD patients is also much higher than the general population and is comparable to that of post-infarction patients. The underlying mechanism, however, as to whether the fatal rhythm disturbances are bradyarrhythmias or tachyarrhythmias is poorly understood. Risk factors for sudden cardiac death include the long-standing pathophysiological abnormalities to which CKD patients are exposed and provide targets for intervention, for example, hypertension due to hypervolaemia and sympathetic overactivity, or electrolyte disturbances with rapid ion shifts associated with dialysis.

The role of biomarkers such as troponins and brain natriuretic peptides in risk stratification requires further study, as does the role of prolonged cardiac monitoring such as the Holter system or implantable recording devices.

37.4.3.2 Treatment

Indications for rate vs. rhythm control in AF are the same in CKD patients as for those in the general population. However, the burden of comorbidities in CKD patients and a higher prevalence of potential contraindications for anti-arrhythmic drugs (such as structural heart disease or electrolyte imbalances) increases the importance of individualised decision making [18]. There are no randomised controlled trials specifically comparing rate vs. rhythm control in patients with CKD or ESKD.

A large trial assessing safety and clinical outcomes of catheter ablation of AF in patients with CKD showed that catheter ablation is more effective than anti-arrhythmic drugs alone for maintenance of sinus rhythm, with similar short- and long-term complication rates [19]. Anticoagulation in the primary prevention of AF-associated stroke is discussed in detail below.

As with other arrhythmias, electrolyte disturbance should be corrected where possible and exacerbating drugs withdrawn. Investigations to exclude occult coronary ischaemia should be considered. Primary and secondary prevention using implantable defibrillators in CKD indicates some benefit, although the long-term risk vs. benefit balance requires further study.

37.4.4 Noncardiac Athero-occlusive Disorders

37.4.4.1 Aetiology and Clinical Presentation

Both stroke and peripheral arterial disease are more common in CKD patients than in age- and gender-matched controls, and as discussed above, the arteries of these patients may be structurally and functionally abnormal. As well as an increased prevalence of atherosclerotic disease, increased vascular stiffness leads to reduced peripheral perfusion, and calcification of arteries may impact on the success of revascularisation strategies (both angioplasty and bypass).

The standard investigation for occlusive carotid stenosis and peripheral vascular disease is digital subtraction angiography. In obtaining consent for these procedures, the patient must be aware of the risk of radiocontrast-induced nephropathy, and pre-procedure precautions should be taken.

37.4.4.2 Treatment

Secondary prevention strategies for noncardiac atherosclerotic events include risk factor optimisation, for example, blood pressure and cholesterol lowering. This is discussed in detail below, but certain invasive interventions require specific attention.

Thrombolysis for Stroke

Thrombolysis for acute stroke in patients with normal kidney function presenting within 4.5h is currently a routine part of clinical practice. No evidence for an increased risk of bleeding has been observed in patients with moderate CKD, although the benefits of thrombolytic therapy in this group have not been specifically addressed. As discussed in the section on coronary reperfusion above, the increased risk of bleeding complications must be considered when offering thrombolytic therapy to patients receiving dialysis. No randomised controlled trials of thrombolysis for acute stroke in patients receiving haemodialysis have been published, and opinion on the appropriateness of this treatment remains divided.

Carotid Endarterectomy for Prevention of Stroke

The benefits of endarterectomy in those with symptomatic high-grade carotid stenosis may extend to patients with impaired kidney function, but the ratio of risk to benefit has not been properly defined in patients with ESRD.

37.4.4.3 Dialysis Around Acute Stroke

Haemodialysis leads to brain swelling, with documented changes in brain volume of around 3% attributable to the procedure [20]. Therefore, most physicians would attempt to avoid haemodialysis immediately after acute brain injury unless there was an absolute life-threatening indication such as hyperkalaemia or pulmonary oedema. Dialysis prescriptions can be designed to maximise stability as described in ▶ Chaps. 80 and 81, and systemic anticoagulation should be avoided, particularly in those with intracerebral haemorrhage or when the nature of the stroke has not been determined.

37.4.4.4 Outcomes of Interventions for Critical Limb Ischaemia

As with all other atherosclerotic diseases, outcomes for patients with limb ischaemia caused by peripheral vascular disease worsen with declining kidney function. Patients on dialysis have some of the highest rates of amputation and other complications from peripheral vascular disease with over 13% of incident haemodialysis patients going on to experience lower-limb amputation in one American cohort study [21]. As with other forms of vascular disease, risk factors should be managed, but there are currently no evidence-based medical therapies for critical limb ischaemia. Furthermore, there are no randomised controlled trials investigating different interventional management strategies and decisions regarding angioplasty, bypass and amputation must be made on an individual patient basis. Involvement of the multidisciplinary team is critical in such decision making, which should involve close liaison between vascular, infectious diseases and nephrology teams.

37.5 Prevention of Cardiovascular Complications in Patients with Kidney Disease

37.5.1 Traditional Vascular Risk Factors and Treatment

37.5.1.1 Blood Pressure

Control of blood pressure has been shown to both reduce the risk of cardiovascular events and retard progression of kidney dysfunction in patients with CKD. Current guidelines recommend a systolic pressure of ≤140 mmHg and a diastolic pressure of ≤90 mmHg, except in patients with urinary albumin-to-creatinine ratio greater than 30 mg/mmol (i.e. microalbuminuria and macroalbuminuria) when this target should be reduced to ≤130/80 mmHg, regardless of the presence or absence of diabetes. In a large randomised controlled trial (Systolic Blood Pressure Intervention Trial (SPRINT)), intensive blood pressure lowering in patients with mild-to-moderate CKD and hypertension (but without diabetes) to systolic <120 mmHg compared to <140 mmHg reduced the rates of cardiovascular events and all-cause mortality without evidence of a deleterious effect on CKD progression [22]. This again suggests the need for individualised decision making, particularly in elderly patients in whom overtreatment of blood pressure may exacerbate postural hypotension and lead to falls.

37.5.1.2 Salt Restriction

Blood pressure control can be more difficult in patients with moderate-to-severe CKD and is complicated by a degree of salt and water overload. Salt restriction, which can improve blood pressure in those with normal kidney function, may have an even more important role in those with renal dysfunction. Reducing salt intake in patients with CKD is therefore critical for control of blood pressure, proteinuria and oedema. There is evidence that patients with CKD have a reduced taste sensation for

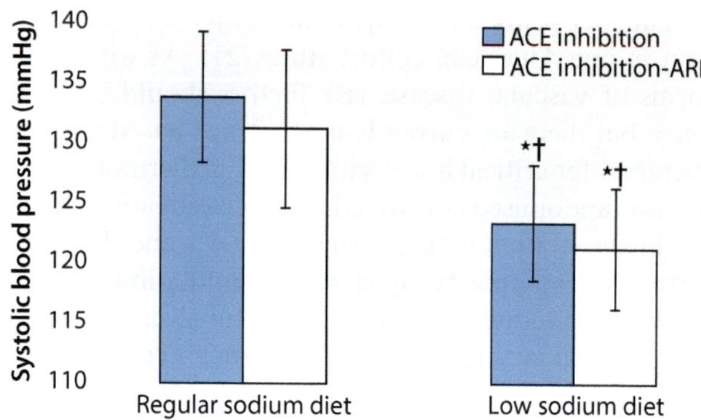

Fig. 37.4 Impact of sodium intake on blood pressure. Fifty-two patients with nondiabetic nephropathy taking an ACE inhibitor received four phases of treatment: ARB or placebo in addition to either regular or a low-sodium diet, each for 6 weeks. Sodium restriction led to a greater reduction in SBP than addition of an ARB. (Reproduced from Slagman et al. [24] with permission)

salt. Importantly, salt restriction, even of relatively short duration (1 week), leads to an increased sensitivity to salt [23]. This means that patients can be reassured that although their food may taste bland during the initial period following salt restriction, gustatory sensation will normalise with time. In controlled trials in subjects with CKD, randomisation to salt restriction targeting 50 mMol Na^{2+}/day (~3 g salt), results in a similar or greater reduction in BP than the addition of another class of antihypertensive medication, even though in reality patients generally only manage to reduce their intake to around 100 mMol Na^{2+}/day [24, 25] (Fig. 37.4).

37

37.5.1.3 Renin-Angiotensin Blockade

Inhibitors of the renin-angiotensin system are effective antihypertensive agents. These agents have additional cardiovascular benefits as well as the potential to reduce albuminuria and retard the rate of decline of kidney function, possibly independent of blood pressure lowering. Although there is currently no clear evidence to support the use of one class of these agents over another, nor evidence supporting combination treatment with ACEis and ARBs, patients with CKD or proteinuria should receive one of these agents unless there are strong contraindications (such as a history of angioneurotic oedema associated with ACE inhibitors).

The nature of action of ACE inhibitors and angiotensin receptor blockers means that the initiation of treatment is often associated with a reduction in GFR. Biochemical tests should be repeated 1–2 weeks following initiation or a dose increase, and although there will often be a small rise in serum creatinine, this reflects the underlying beneficial mechanism of action of these agents and should not lead to discontinuation of treatment. A serum creatinine rise reflecting a drop in GFR of up to 25% is generally accepted assuming that there is a subsequent stabilisation. Hyperkalaemia can also complicate the use of these agents, and dietary potassium restriction will often be needed in those with a low eGFR. Severe hyperkalaemia may necessitate withdrawal of these agents.

A further challenge in blood pressure control is the increase in arterial stiffness seen in many CKD patients. The correct therapeutic approach to a high systolic BP in association with a low diastolic BP is unclear. The risk of reducing cardiac perfusion, which occurs largely in diastole, must be balanced by attempts to reach target systolic blood pressures with serial escalation of antihypertensive therapy.

Thus, management of high BP in patients with CKD is a difficult clinical problem. Dietetic input along with a regimen of multiple antihypertensive agents, including a diuretic, may be required in an individual patient (Table 37.1). Patient education, along with home monitoring, may be particularly beneficial in some patients, improving adherence and preventing overtreatment.

37.5.1.4 Cholesterol

Typical patterns of dyslipidaemia vary with different causes and stages of CKD (Table 37.2), however, treatment with cholesterol-lowering agents leads to a substantial reduction in cardiovascular events in patients with stage 3–5 CKD. In the Study of Heart and Renal Protection (SHARP), a randomised controlled study in subjects with CKD (including dialysis patients), patients receiving simvastatin 20 mg with ezetimibe 10 mg (rather than placebo) suffered almost one-fifth fewer atherosclerotic cardiovascular events over a 5-year follow-up period with no safety concerns (Fig. 37.5) [26].

Evidence as to whether cholesterol reduction reduces the risk of cardiovascular disease specifically in patients with CKD stage 5 is less clear. In two randomised trials recruiting only dialysis patients, statin therapy did not result in a clear reduction in cardiovascular events [27, 28]. However, based on data from an extended follow-up of patients in a trial comparing fluvastatin to placebo, which demonstrated a 20% reduction in cardiac events over approximately 6.5 years [29], most clinicians use statins in kidney transplant recipients, particularly when LDL cholesterol levels are elevated. More recent trials of PCSK9 inhibitors have demonstrated that larger reductions in cholesterol are achievable in patients with stage 2–3 CKD, who seem to gain similar benefits in terms of cardiovascular risk reduction when compared to those with normal kidney function [30].

Table 37.1 Cardiovascular medication in CKD

	Evidence for benefits/harms in CKD	Practical use in CKD
Aspirin	Likely benefit in the prevention of both primary and secondary CV events in CKD	No dose adjustment necessary
Other antiplatelet agents	Clopidogrel appears to be of limited in benefit/efficacy in those with reduced GFR and may be associated with an increased risk of bleeding. Evidence base is poor for other ADP receptor blockers and glycoprotein IIa/IIIb inhibitors	Several glycoprotein IIa/IIIb inhibitors require dose adjustment in patients with reduced GFR
Warfarin	Possibly useful for primary prevention of stroke in patients with atrial fibrillation and moderate CKD. Significant increased risk of bleeding observed and doubt as to overall benefit when used as primary prevention of stroke in patients receiving haemodialysis	No specific dose alteration required but care with drug interactions required
Heparins	Reduce early ischaemic events in acute coronary syndromes. LMWH accumulates in renal impairment. Increased bleeding seen with use of enoxaparin in CKD	Dose reduction of LMWH in CKD. Factor Xa monitoring or unfractionated heparin may be preferred in severe renal impairment
Oral factor Xa inhibitors	May be a useful alternative to heparins and warfarin. Efficacy in stroke and systemic embolism prevention non-inferior to warfarin with GFR 30–50 mL/min; however, significant reduction in major bleeding events seen with apixaban and edoxaban. Unknown effects with GFR <30 mL/min	May require dose reduction in CKD
Renin-angiotensin blockade (ACEi/A2 blockers/ renin inhibitors)	Possible cardiovascular benefits, both in primary and secondary prevention and probable benefit in slowing of decline in kidney function. No clear evidence for combined use of ACE, ARB or renin inhibitors	Monitoring of biochemistry required following commencement or dose increases. Hyperkalaemia can occur and may require dose adjustment or withdrawal. Stable increases in serum creatinine of 20–30% are generally thought to be acceptable
Beta-blockers	Possible benefit in patients with heart failure and CKD and in secondary prevention post-MI. Can be used for rate control in atrial fibrillation	Most agents dosed as in normal renal function but may need to commence at low doses
Diuretics	Thiazide diuretics are useful antihypertensive agents in mild and moderate CKD. Addition of loop diuretics to other antihypertensive therapy is a useful therapeutic strategy in moderate-to-severe CKD. High doses of loop diuretics for the treatment of oedema may be required in advanced CKD	Thiazides may become less effective as GFR falls. Combination therapy with loop and thiazide diuretics recommended in CKD stages 4 and 5. Hyperkalaemia and acidosis may complicate the use of potassium-sparing diuretics in CKD
Calcium channel blockers	Similar benefit in terms of primary prevention of cardiovascular events as compared to ACE inhibitors and diuretics in hypertensive patients with CKD. Dihydropyridines may exacerbate proteinuria	No specific dose adjustments
Digoxin	Can be used for rate control in atrial fibrillation	Standard loading dose, but low maintenance doses required in CKD. Risk of accumulation and toxicity so monitoring levels is essential. Not removed in haemodialysis patients
Cholesterol-lowering agents	Proven benefits of statin plus ezetimibe combination in primary prevention of atherosclerotic CV disease in stage 3–5 CKD. Probable benefit in patients receiving haemodialysis and following kidney transplantation	No evidence for increased statin toxicity in CKD when used in low doses, even when used in combination with ezetimibe. Fibrates should be avoided in patients with stage 4–5 CKD. High doses of statins best avoided because of the potential for muscle injury

(continued)

Table 37.1 (continued)

	Evidence for benefits/harms in CKD	Practical use in CKD
Sodium-glucose cotrans-porter-2 inhibitor (SGLT-2i)	Proven benefit in reducing cardiovascular risk, slowing progression of albuminuria and reducing blood pressure in patients with diabetes and eGFR >30 m;/min/1.73^2. Benefits in more advanced CKD need to be proven. Effect on kidney function may be independent of glycaemic effects (which are lost as GFR declines)	

Table 37.2 Patterns and management of dyslipidaemia in patients with kidney disease

Syndrome	Typical pattern of dyslipidaemia	Management
Nephrotic syndrome	Hypercholesterolaemia due to elevated LDL	Treat underlying glomerular disease if possible
		Reduce proteinuria with ACEi and/or ARB
		Prescribe statin
Chronic kidney disease stages 1–2	Lipid profile usually normal in the absence of albuminuria	Regardless of starting cholesterol, consider statin to reduce risk of CV disease
Chronic kidney disease stages 3–5	Hypertriglyceridaemia with low HDL due to reduced clearance of triglyceride-rich VLDL and chylomicrons. Cholesterol usually normal	Benefits of reducing triglycerides with fibrates unproven
		Focus on reducing CV risk by lowering cholesterol with statins
		Avoid maximum doses of statin by adding ezetimibe

LDL low-density lipoprotein, *VLDL* very-low-density lipoprotein, *HDL* high-density lipoprotein, *CV* cardiovascular

37.5.1.5 Cigarette Smoking

Smoking is associated with an approximate 50% increased risk of new cardiovascular events in dialysis patients [29]. Therefore, reductions in cardiovascular events, as well as fewer cases of respiratory and malignant disease, would be predicted with smoking cessation. CKD patients who smoke should be encouraged to give up and offered appropriate support to do so as required. Care should be taken with pharmacological adjuncts that assist smoking cessation, and dose reductions may be required in advanced CKD.

37.5.1.6 Diabetes

Tight glycaemic control has been shown to reduce cardiovascular complications in the context of diabetes, with the effects lasting many years beyond the intervention. Furthermore, it has been shown to protect against the development of progressive nephropathy (ADVANCE trial) [31]. The benefit appears greatest in those with preserved renal function and good blood pressure control, with intermediate effects in CKD stages 1 and 2, and lesser effects in CKD stage 3 or lower. Therefore, early intensive control of blood glucose must be integral to strategies aimed at preventing cardiovascular events and disease progression in patients at the early stages of CKD. In patients receiving renal replacement therapy, the optimal level of blood glucose control still needs to be defined, with observational studies suggesting that both high and very low HbA1c levels are associated with adverse outcomes.

A reduction in cardiovascular risk that may be independent of glycosuria has been shown with SGLT-2 inhibitors [32]. Data from cardiovascular outcome trials of these agents also shows an effect on reducing blood pressure and body weight and slowing the progression of renal disease. This suggests a role for SGLT-2 inhibitors in addition to that of effective glucose control.

37.5.1.7 Antiplatelet Agents

Aspirin reduces the risk of future cardiovascular events and there is some evidence that this benefit extends to patients with impaired kidney function. In a subgroup analysis of the Hypertension Optimal Treatment, randomisation to aspirin was associated with an estimated reduction of 20 major cardiovascular events but 7.5 more major bleeding episodes per 1000 patient years [33]. Therefore, although the exact groups who will benefit have not been well defined and although the risk of bleeding in CKD may be increased, aspirin may be

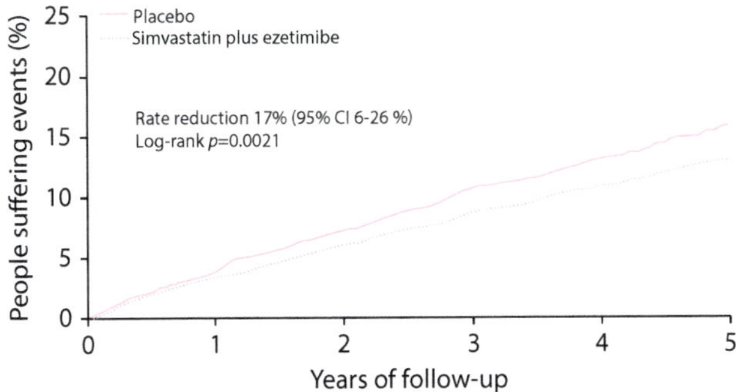

Fig. 37.5 Risk of cardiovascular events in CKD subjects randomised to simvastatin/ezetimibe combination or placebo. (Reproduced from Baigent et al. [26] with permission)

appropriate for secondary prevention of cardiovascular events in CKD. Evidence for the use of alternative antiplatelet agents such as clopidogrel for primary prevention of cardiovascular events in patients with CKD is lacking.

37.6 Prevention of Stroke in Chronic Atrial Fibrillation

In patients with normal kidney function, when anticoagulation is indicated for the prevention of stroke or embolism in atrial fibrillation, warfarin has previously been the therapy of choice. However, a number of randomised trials that have compared the direct oral anticoagulants (DOACs) to warfarin have shown that they are non-inferior to warfarin in the prevention of stroke and embolism in atrial fibrillation, with a reduction in fatal bleeding events and probable reduction in haemorrhagic stroke. As such, DOACs are increasingly being used as the anticoagulant of choice. In patients with CKD, the benefits of warfarin on stroke risk reduction have also been observed [34], with warfarin prescription associated with a 24% relative risk reduction. However, in patients receiving haemodialysis, warfarin treatment has been associated with a doubling in risk of intracerebral haemorrhage [35], so the risks of treatment may well outweigh the benefits in this group. Although aspirin therapy may be indicated for the prevention of cardiac events in this group, it does not appear to be associated with a reduced risk of stroke. With a GFR of 30–50 mL/min, as for those with normal kidney function, the efficacy of the DOACs apixaban and edoxaban in stroke and systemic embolism prevention is non-inferior to warfarin, with a significant reduction in major bleeding events. The effects in patients with a GFR <30 mL/min have not been systematically studied.

37.7 Interventions for Kidney-Related Risk Factors

37.7.1 Albuminuria

Albuminuria is an important independent risk factor for cardiovascular events, even in patients with preserved kidney function. Approaches aimed to reduce blood pressure, such as salt restriction and renin-angiotensin blockade, will also reduce albuminuria.

37.7.2 Nephrotic Syndrome

As well as being prone to venous thromboembolism (discussed in ▶ Chap. 1), patients with nephrotic syndrome are also at greater risk of cardiovascular events such as stroke or coronary heart disease, with an estimated fivefold increased risk of myocardial infarction compared to the general population [36]. Reduction in cardiovascular risk in the context of albuminuria relies on achieving remission or even partial remission where possible. Although no good evidence is available, control of other risk factors such as hypercholesterolaemia and hypertension may also help reduce the risk of vascular events. The routine use of aspirin would seem appropriate, although there is no evidence base for this. Formal anticoagulation is also used in severely hypoalbuminaemic patients as prophylaxis against venous thromboembolism, and whether this has a role in preventing arterial disease is unclear.

37.7.3 Bone Mineral Disorder/ Hyperphosphataemia

Derangements in mineral metabolism occur even in patients with stage 3–5 CKD as part of the bone mineral disorder (see ▶ Chap. 3). Although increases in calcium and phosphate are associated with an increased risk of cardiovascular events, whether this relationship is directly causal and the degree to which different treatment strategies alter this risk is not known. A large randomised trial that measured the effect of the calcimimetic agent cinacalcet in patients with moderate-to-severe secondary hyperparathyroidism who were undergoing haemodialysis showed no significant reduction in either the risk of death or the risk of non-fatal cardiovascular events [37].

37.7.4 Medications

Several medications used in the treatment of kidney disease have adverse cardiovascular profiles. Most commonly used in kidney transplant recipients, calcineurin inhibitors are known to impact on cardiovascular risk factors. Ciclosporin use is associated with an increase in blood pressure and tacrolimus with an increased risk of diabetes. Similarly, corticosteroids can lead to insulin resistance, weight gain and hypertension. Other drugs that modify cardiovascular risk factors include sirolimus (lipid abnormalities) and antiretrovirals used in HIV treatment (lipid abnormalities).

37.7.5 Evidence for Other Proposed Kidney-Associated Risk Factors

A number of circulating markers that potentially contribute to vascular disease in the context of CKD have been identified. These include homocysteine, uric acid, reactive oxygen species and endogenous inhibitors of nitric oxide synthesis. Although increased levels of all of these substances are associated with both reduced kidney function and cardiovascular events, evidence for a causal role remains inconclusive to date.

37

There have been a number of small, unblinded studies showing benefits associated with targeting these non-traditional risk factors however, the results from larger high-quality controlled trials have been negative. For example, in the case of homocysteine, there are a number of studies reporting that increases are independently associated with future cardiovascular events in CKD [38], and there is also a simple therapeutic intervention, folic acid, which has been shown to reduce levels. However, evidence from several good quality randomised trials demonstrate that treatment with folic acid does not reduce the risk of cardiovascular events in CKD patients [39]. Therefore, although there are several proposed novel mediators of cardiovascular risk in CKD, the gap between exploratory studies and evidence-based intervention remains.

37.8 Conclusions

Cardiovascular events are increased in CKD patients when compared to patients with normal kidney function reflecting a wide range of underlying vascular and myocardial diseases. Management of cardiovascular risk in an effort to prevent these events should be initiated in early CKD and includes blood pressure reduction, statin therapy and optimisation of diabetes. Management of clinical cardiovascular events in CKD patients should be based on strategies of proven benefit in the general population, taking into account additional risks that result from a reduced eGFR. Ongoing trials in patients with CKD and analysis of CKD subsets recruited into cardiovascular trials are likely to inform future practice in this area.

Case Study
Case 1

A man in his mid-60s with a long-standing stable renal transplant and past history of ischaemic heart disease became unwell following a community-acquired chest infection. He was treated for the chest infection but developed symptoms and signs of heart failure. He had several admissions and increases in diuretics but remained dyspnoeic and had a relentless rise in creatinine from a baseline of 200 μmol/l with a trajectory strongly predicting the need for dialysis within 6–12 months (see red line figure). His renal dysfunction was felt to be secondary to cardiorenal syndrome, and he underwent cardiac resynchronisation with dual pacing, a further increase in diuretics and endovascular mitral valve repair for marked MR. His symptoms improved markedly, and his renal function stabilised (albeit with the typical pre-renal saw-toothed pattern) with a creatinine averaging 300 μmol/l for 6 years. While one would always strive to optimise the treatment of cardiac failure, this illustrates the profound impact on renal function of achieving the best possible control of heart failure in patients with cardiorenal syndrome.

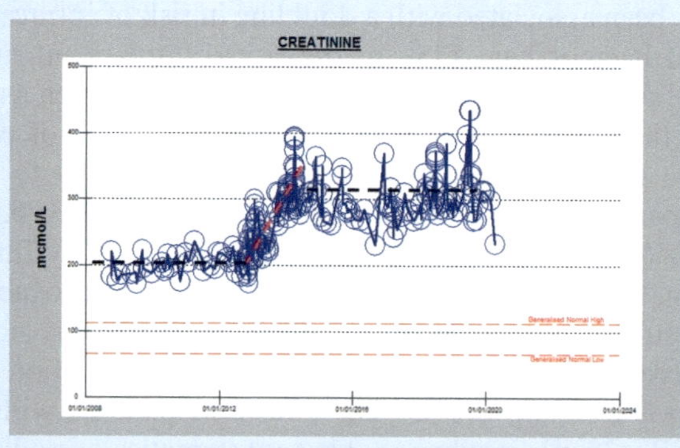

Case 2

A 67-year-old man with type 2 diabetes for 10 years and myocardial infarction 2 years ago was referred to the renal clinic with an eGFR that had fallen from 90 to 58 in 6 months and an ACR of 405 mg/ml (CKD G2A3). Current medication was a thiazide diuretic and a sulphonylurea. He was hypertensive at 145/95 and obese with a BMI of 38 (118 kg) and had a cardiac ejection fraction of 35%. These features put at extremely high risk of rapid progression of CKD and cardiovascular risk. He had tried losing weight many times before without success and had given up trying. His cardiac failure was managed by switching thiazide to loop diuretic and ACE inhibitor which was titrated to maximum tolerated; he was prescribed aspirin and a beta-blocker. He was given thorough advice on a low-salt diet and support on weight loss dieting. His sulphonylurea was switch to a biguanide (metformin) and an SGLT-2 inhibitor with the plan for bariatric surgery if no significant and sustained weight loss within a year. In 1 month, he lost 6 kg (felt mostly to be salt and water) but a further 12 kg over the following year with metformin, SGLT-2 inhibitor and lifestyle changes. His blood pressure stabilised at 135/75, proteinuria reduced to an ACR of <100 and his ejection fraction improved to 50%. The improvement in his cardiovascular risk factors will have very significantly improved is predicted time to dialysis and cardiovascular survival. Intense input to address these issues and choosing diabetic medication that assisted weight loss had a significant and positive impact on his drive to continue to lose weight and improve his lifestyle. The other key issue here is the importance of addressing these issues early when the benefit is likely to be much greater.

Tips and Tricks

1. Nephrologists have an important role in returning patients to RAAS inhibition if and where possible for the management of proteinuria or cardiac failure, following cessation due to AKI or hyperkalaemia. Consider ways of building a review of such patients and supervised reintroduction of these important drugs where appropriate.
2. Many renal patients will have cardiovascular comorbidity and vice versa. It is important to have good communication with your cardiologists and consider joint multidisciplinary team meeting with agreed targets, for example, on blood pressure, smoking cessation, lipid management, reduction in proteinuria and weight as well as disease modifying drugs from RAAS inhibition to SGLT-2 inhibitors.
3. Early transplant with a good kidney is one of the most effective strategies for reducing cardiovascular death if done early, so identifying patients with CKD who are suitable for transplantation and listing early (pre-emptively) and encouraging live donors is very much in the patient's interest.

Chapter Review Questions

1. Which stroke prophylaxis is more likely to be associated with intracerebral bleeding DOACs or warfarin in patients on dialysis?
2. Roughly what percentage of patients will die a sudden cardiac death?
3. What is the approximate risk benefit of aspirin as secondary prevention in CKD?
4. How common is sudden cardiac death (SCD), dysrhythmia, in dialysis patients?
5. Clinically what is the most available indicator of arterial stiffness?

Answers

1. DOACs are associated with a lower rate of intracerebral bleeding than warfarin.
2. Sudden death is 25–30% of all-cause mortality in dialysis patients, thus a common cause of death.
3. In CKD secondary prevention with aspirin was associated with an estimated reduction of 20 major cardiovascular events but 7.5 more major bleeding episodes per 1000 patient years.
4. SCD is the cause of death in roughly 25–30% of dialysis patients, which is higher than that in post-infarct or cardiac failure patients.
5. A persistently wide pulse pressure (high systolic but low normal diastolic).

References

1. Go AS, Chertow GM, Fan D, et al. Chronic kidney disease and the risks of death, cardiovascular events, and hospitalization. N Engl J Med. 2004;351:1296–305.
2. Herzog CA, Ma JZ, Collins AJ. Poor long-term survival after acute myocardial infarction among patients on long-term dialysis. N Engl J Med. 1998;339:799–805.
3. Whaley-Connell AT, Sowers JR, Stevens LA, et al. CKD in the United States: Kidney Early Evaluation Program (KEEP) and National Health and Nutrition Examination Survey (NHANES) 1999–2004. Am J Kidney Dis. 2008;51:S13–20.
4. Sarnak MJ, Levey AS. Cardiovascular disease and chronic renal disease: a new paradigm. Am J Kidney Dis. 2000;35:S117–31.
5. Ronco C, McCullough PA, Anker SD, et al. Cardio-renal syndromes: report from the consensus conference of the acute dialysis quality initiative. Eur Herart J. 2010;31:703–11.
6. Wanner C, Amann K, Shoji T. The heart and vascular system in dialysis. Lancet. 2016;388:276–84.

7. Park M, Hsu CY, Li Y, et al. Associations between kidney function and subclinical cardiac abnormalities in CKD. J Am Soc Nephrol. 2012;23:1725–34.
8. McIntyre CW, Burton JO, Selby NM, et al. Hemodialysis-induced cardiac dysfunction is associated with an acute reduction in global and segmental myocardial blood flow. Clin J Am Soc Nephrol. 2008;3:19–26.
9. Defilippi C, Seliger SL, Kelley W, et al. Interpreting cardiac troponin results from high-sensitivity assays in chronic kidney disease without acute coronary syndrome. Clin Chem. 2012;58:1342–51.
10. Lippi G, Tessitore N, Montagnana M, et al. Influence of sampling time and ultrafiltration coefficient of the dialysis membrane on cardiac troponin I and T. Arch Pathol Lab Med. 2008;132:72–6.
11. Bergeron S, Hillis GS, Haugen EN, et al. Prognostic value of dobutamine stress echocardiography in patients with chronic kidney disease. Am Heart J. 2007;153:385–91.
12. Szummer K, Lundman P, Jacobson SH, et al. Influence of renal function on the effects of early revascularization in non-ST-elevation myocardial infarction: data from the Swedish Web-System for Enhancement and Development of Evidence-Based Care in Heart Disease Evaluated According to Recommended Therapies (SWEDEHEART). Circulation. 2009;120:851–8.
13. Sedlis SP, Jurkovitz CT, Hartigan PM, et al. Optimal medical therapy with or without percutaneous coronary intervention for patients with stable coronary artery disease and chronic kidney disease. Am J Cardiol. 2009;104:1647–53.
14. Ix JH, Mercado N, Shlipak MG, et al. Association of chronic kidney disease with clinical outcomes after coronary revascularization: the Arterial Revascularization Therapies Study (ARTS). Am Heart J. 2005;149:512–9.
15. Palmer SC, Di Micco L, Razavian M, et al. Effects of antiplatelet therapy on mortality and cardiovascular and bleeding outcomes in persons with chronic kidney disease: a systematic review and meta-analysis. Ann Intern Med. 2012;156: 445–59.

37

16. Fox CS, Muntner P, Chen AY, et al. Use of evidence-based therapies in short-term outcomes of ST-segment elevation myocardial infarction and non-ST-segment elevation myocardial infarction in patients with chronic kidney disease: a report from the National Cardiovascular Data Acute Coronary Treatment and Intervention Outcomes Network registry. Circulation. 2010;121:357–65.
17. Turakhia MP, Blankestijn PJ, Carrero JJ, et al. Chronic kidney disease and arrhythmias: conclusions from a kidney disease: improving global outcomes (KDIGO) controversies conference. Eur Heart J. 2018;39(24):2314–25.
18. Garlo KG, Steele DJR, Nigwekar SU, Chan KE. Demystifying the benefits and harms of anticoagulation for atrial fibrillation in chronic kidney disease. Clin J Am Soc Nephrol. 2019;14: 125–36.
19. Ullal AJ, Kaiser DW, Fan J, et al. Safety and clinical outcomes of catheter ablation of atrial fibrillation in patients with chronic kidney disease. J Cardiovasc Electrophysiol. 2017;28(1):39–48.
20. Walters RJ, Fox NC, Crum WR, et al. Haemodialysis and cerebral oedema. Nephron. 2001;87:143–7.
21. Plantinga LC, Fink NE, Coresh J, et al. Peripheral vascular disease-related procedures in dialysis patients: predictors and prognosis. Clin J Am Soc Nephrol. 2009;4:1637–45.
22. Cheung AK, Rahman M, Reboussin DM, et al. Effects of intensive blood pressure control in CKD. J Am Soc Nephrol. 2019;30(8):1523–33.
23. Kusaba T, Mori Y, Masami O, et al. Sodium restriction improves the gustatory threshold for salty taste in patients with chronic kidney disease. Kidney Int. 2009;76:638–43.
24. Slagman MC, Waanders F, Hemmelder MH, et al. Moderate dietary sodium restriction added to angiotensin converting enzyme inhibition compared with dual blockade in lowering proteinuria and blood pressure: randomised controlled trial. BMJ. 2011;343:d4366.
25. Vogt L, Waanders F, Boomsma F, et al. Effects of dietary sodium and hydrochlorothiazide on the antiproteinuric efficacy of losartan. J Am Soc Nephrol. 2008;19:999–1007.
26. Baigent C, Landray MJ, Reith C, et al. The effects of lowering LDL cholesterol with simvastatin plus ezetimibe in patients with chronic kidney disease (Study of Heart and Renal Protection): a randomised placebo-controlled trial. Lancet. 2011;377:2181–92.
27. Fellstrom BC, Jardine AG, Schmieder RE, et al. Rosuvastatin and cardiovascular events in patients undergoing hemodialysis. N Engl J Med. 2009;360:1395–407.
28. Wanner C, Krane V, Marz W, et al. Atorvastatin in patients with type 2 diabetes mellitus undergoing hemodialysis. N Engl J Med. 2005;353:238–48.
29. Holdaas H, Fellstrom B, Cole E, et al. Long-term cardiac outcomes in renal transplant recipients receiving fluvastatin: the ALERT extension study. Am J Transplant. 2005;5:2929–36.
30. Charytan DM, Sabatine MS, Pedersen TR, et al. Efficacy and safety of evolocumab in chronic kidney disease in the FOURIER trial. J Am Coll Cardiol. 2019;73(23):2961–70.
31. ADVANCE Collaborative Group. Intensive blood glucose control and vascular outcomes in patients with type 2 diabetes. N Engl J Med. 2008;358(24):2560–72.
32. Mahaffey KW, Jardine MJ, Bompoint S, et al. Canagliflozin and cardiovascular and renal outcomes in type 2 diabetes and chronic kidney disease in primary and secondary cardiovascular prevention groups: results from the randomized CREDENCE trial. Circulation. 2019; https://doi.org/10.1161/CIRCULATIONAHA.119.042007. [Epub ahead of print].
33. Jardine MJ, Ninomiya T, Perkovic V, et al. Aspirin is beneficial in hypertensive patients with chronic kidney disease: a post-hoc subgroup analysis of a randomized controlled trial. J Am Coll Cardiol. 2010;56:956–65.
34. Olesen JB, Lip GY, Kamper AL, et al. Stroke and bleeding in atrial fibrillation with chronic kidney disease. N Engl J Med. 2012;367:625–35.
35. Winkelmayer WC, Liu J, Setoguchi S, et al. Effectiveness and safety of warfarin initiation in older hemodialysis patients with incident atrial fibrillation. Clin J Am Soc Nephrol. 2011;6: 2662–8.
36. Mahmoodi BK, ten Kate MK, Waanders F, et al. High absolute risks and predictors of venous and arterial thromboembolic events in patients with nephrotic syndrome: results from a large retrospective cohort study. Circulation. 2008;117: 224–30.
37. EVOLVE trail investigators. Effect of cinacalcet on cardiovascular disease in patients undergoing dialysis. N Engl J Med. 2012;367:2482–94.
38. Moustapha A, Naso A, Nahlawi M, et al. Prospective study of hyperhomocysteinemia as an adverse cardiovascular risk factor in end-stage renal disease. Circulation. 1998;97:138–41.
39. Jardine MJ, Kang A, Zoungas S, et al. The effect of folic acid based homocysteine lowering on cardiovascular events in people with kidney disease: systematic review and meta-analysis. BMJ. 2012;344:e3533.

Management of Diabetic Nephropathy

Bryan Conway, Jane Goddard, Alan Jaap, and Alan Patrick

Contents

M. Harber (ed.), *Primer on Nephrology*, https://doi.org/10.1007/978-3-030-76419-7_38

Learning Objectives

1. DN is the most common cause of end-stage renal disease (ESRD), but more patients will die of cardiovascular disease than reach dialysis; therefore, management of cardiovascular risk factors is essential.
2. Modestly elevated albuminuria (microalbuminuria) is the earliest clinical indicator of nephropathy and is associated with increased cardiovascular risk.
3. Less stringent glycaemic control is recommended for those with more advanced kidney disease as the increased risk of hypoglycaemia usually outweighs potential benefits.
4. Glucagon-like peptide-1 (GLP-1) receptor agonists and sodium-glucose co-transporter 2 (SGLT-2) inhibitors convincingly reduce renal and cardiovascular events including delaying progression of CKD and development of ESRD.
5. Inhibition of the renin-angiotensin-aldosterone axis is first-line therapy for patients with evidence of albuminuria, but blockade with two or more agents is not recommended due to the risk of hyperkalaemia and acute kidney injury.

38.1 Introduction

Diabetic nephropathy (DN) remains the single most common cause of end-stage renal disease (ESRD) in developed nations and is of increasing importance in developing countries. The deleterious effect of diabetes on kidney function is reflected in the 12-fold increase in the incidence of ESRD in men with diabetes compared with their non-diabetic counterparts [1]. Nephrologists will see increasingly large numbers of patients with diabetes who have CKD, are on dialysis or have had a renal transplant; therefore, the development of integrated systems to best manage their care to a high standard is a key priority. New developments in the treatment of diabetes with significant cardiovascular and renal benefits are transforming the management of diabetic patients and have emphasised the need for early, focused and coordinated care.

> Diabetic nephropathy can be defined as a triad of albuminuria, evolving hypertension and progressive decline in renal function in patients with diabetes, often in association with other microvascular complications and in the absence of evidence of alternative renal diagnoses.

38.2 Epidemiology

Towards the end of the last millennium, there was a dramatic rise in the incidence of ESRD due to DN in developed countries, chiefly as a consequence of the increased prevalence of type 2 diabetes [2, 3]. However, since 2000, the incidence of ESRD due to DN has broadly stabilised, in large part due to improvements in the treatment of diabetes. Indeed, over the last few decades, the prevalence of overt nephropathy in patients who have had type 1 diabetes for 30 years has fallen from 30% historically to 15% in recent cohort studies and to as little as 9% in clinical trials [4].

There is a marked international variation in the incidence of ESRD due to diabetic nephropathy. For example, in the USA, the incidence of ESRD due to diabetic kidney disease is almost 162 per million population (45% of total ESRD) [2], while in the UK, the incidence is much lower, at 29 per million population (28% of total ESRD) [3]. This may be partly attributed to a lower proportion of the UK population being of high-risk ethnicities; however, additional factors may also be important as Caucasian patients with diabetes and stage 3 or 4 chronic kidney disease (CKD) in the USA have a threefold greater risk of progressing to ESRD compared to Caucasians in Norway [5]. Measures of quality of pre-dialysis care, including timely referral to nephrologists, were superior in Norway, illustrating the importance of developing systems that integrate primary care, diabetologists and renal physicians in the management of persons with diabetes and kidney disease.

Of particular concern is the increasing prevalence of obesity, diabetes and DN in developing countries [6]. Accurate assessment of the true prevalence of DN in developing countries is difficult. For example, CKD due to DN is more prevalent in the Indian subcontinent than in developed countries; however, a much smaller proportion of patients with DN receive renal replacement therapy, as relatively few patients are accepted onto government-funded ESRD programmes. As few people in developing countries can afford health insurance or dialysis, it is likely that the majority of patients with ESRD due to DN will unfortunately die of renal failure [7]. Hence, the challenge is to develop education, screening and management programmes for diabetes and hypertension and to ensure access to subsidised medications. Guidelines tailored to a resource-poor setting should be developed, and these may need to include less stringent glycaemic targets and initially focus on those with moderate-to-severe hypertension. In countries with limited resources, focus is typically directed towards acute, symptomatic conditions; however, successful chronic disease management programmes have been reported, notably in Cuba, where the well-developed primary care system has produced some of the highest levels of attainment of target blood pressure control in the world [8].

38.3 Aetiology and Pathogenesis

38.3.1 Genetic Factors

While poor glycaemic and blood pressure control are risk factors for nephropathy, it is well recognised that some patients with diabetes develop nephropathy despite good glycaemic and blood pressure control, while conversely others who have poorly controlled risk factors remain free of renal disease. This suggests that subsets of people with diabetes may be genetically predisposed to, or protected from, developing nephropathy. A role for genetic susceptibility is supported by differences in prevalence in various ethnic groups, with the proportion of patients with diabetes who develop nephropathy being much higher in Blacks, Hispanics and indigenous populations such as the Pima Indians [9]. In addition, diabetic nephropathy tends to cluster within families, with the risk of DN being greater if there is a parental history of hypertension or cardiovascular disease [10]. Unfortunately, the specific genes that confer susceptibility to, or protection from, diabetic nephropathy have yet to be conclusively established.

38.3.2 Glycaemic Control

The Diabetes Control and Complications Trial (DCCT) confirmed a causal link between poor glycaemic control and overt nephropathy [11] and the development of CKD [12] in patients with type 1 diabetes. Similar data for patients with type 2 diabetes were generated from the UK Prospective Diabetes Study (UKPDS) [13].

38.3.3 Hypertension

In the UKPDS, tight blood pressure control was at least as effective as glycaemic control in preventing nephropathy [14]. Indeed, the pre-eminent role of hypertension in promoting progression to advanced diabetic kidney disease is perhaps best illustrated by an experiment of nature. In patients with diabetes and co-existing unilateral renal artery stenosis, there was no pathological evidence of DN in the kidney downstream of the stenosis, despite severe nephropathy in the contralateral kidney, suggesting that transmission of systemic hypertension to the diabetic glomerulus is a prerequisite for the development of advanced nephropathy [15].

38.3.4 Renin-Angiotensin System Activation

The intra-renal renin-angiotensin-aldosterone system (RAAS) is activated in patients with diabetes, resulting in an increase in systemic and intraglomerular pressure, which in turn may exacerbate proteinuria [16]. In addition, angiotensin II may directly promote inflammation and increase matrix deposition by activating cytokines such as transforming growth factor-β [17]. Hence, there are theoretical advantages for inhibiting RAAS activity, above and beyond lowering of blood pressure. This theory has been supported by the results of clinical trials in which the reduction in the rate of decline in renal function observed with RAAS inhibition remains significant even after correcting for changes in blood pressure [18].

38.4 Natural History and Pathogenesis

Diabetic nephropathy is a slowly progressive disease, typically taking at least 15–20 years from the diagnosis of diabetes to reach end-stage kidney disease. The natural history of DN may be divided into five phases as described by Mogensen (Table 38.1) [19]. The cardinal features are a triad of:

1. Progressive albuminuria: ranging from upper limit of normal, through microalbuminuria to nephrotic-range proteinuria.
2. Evolving hypertension: subtle abnormalities such as loss of nocturnal dipping precede and predict the onset of albuminuria [20]; blood pressure progressively increases, and by the time stage 4 CKD is reached, three or more agents are often required to achieve the target blood pressure [14].
3. Declining renal function: in type 1 diabetes, an initial hyperfiltration phase is often observed, which may predict the onset of microalbuminuria; this is followed by an insidious decline in renal function towards end-stage kidney disease.

38.4.1 Pathological Features

The glomerular pathology in DN has been classified by the Renal Pathology Society into four stages: (1) increase in basement membrane thickness, (2) increased mesangial matrix deposition, (3) nodular glomerulosclerosis and (4) global glomerulosclerosis. An example of the

Table 38.1 Stages of diabetic kidney disease

Stage	Duration of diabetes (years)	Blood pressure (mmHg)	Proteinuria (albumin/creatinine ratio mg/mmol)	Renal function (ml/min/1.73 m^2)	Pathology
1. Hyperfiltration	<3	Normal	<3	>100	Glomerulomegaly
2. Silent	3–5	Loss of nocturnal dipping	<3	100	Increased basement membrane thickness
3. Minimally elevated albuminuria (also known as microalbuminuria)	5–10	Borderline increase	3–30[a]	100	Increased mesangial deposition
4. Overt nephropathy	10–20	Overt hypertension	>30 to overtly nephrotic	15–100	Mild (nodular) glomerulosclerosis and tubulointerstitial fibrosis
5. End-stage kidney disease	>20	Overt hypertension	>30 to overtly nephrotic	<15	Marked glomerulosclerosis and tubulointerstitial fibrosis

Modified from Mogensen [19]
[a]2.5–30 in males or 3.5–30 mg/mmol in females

classical Kimmelstiel-Wilson nodule is shown in Fig. 38.1a. The close relationship between diabetic nephropathy and cardiovascular disease is evident from the observation that features of small vessel injury are common, including intimal arteriolar hyalinosis (Fig. 38.1b) and glomerular fibrin caps, which are due to the insinuation of plasma proteins into the vessel wall. These findings are highly suggestive, but not pathognomonic, of DN as they may also be observed in non-diabetic patients with severe obesity. Tubular atrophy, tubulointerstitial fibrosis and inflammation are also observed, and the severity of tubulointerstitial disease is the best predictor of clinical outcome [21].

38.5 Diagnosis

The first clinical evidence of diabetic nephropathy is the onset of modestly elevated albuminuria (also known as microalbuminuria) defined as an albumin/creatinine ratio in the range of 2.5–30 mg/mmol for males and 3.5–30 mg/mmol for females in at least two out of three successive measurements. Annual screening for microalbuminuria should be performed within 5 years of the diagnosis of type 1 diabetes and from the time of diagnosis in patients with type 2 diabetes, as latent diabetes may have been present for some time prior to diagnosis in the latter. DN is usually diagnosed on clinical grounds, with relatively few patients undergoing renal biopsy, which is reserved for those patients with features of atypical disease (Table 38.2). The predominant rationale for performing renal biopsy is atypically fast progression of disease, such as a sudden increase in proteinuria or a rapid decline in renal function, as such features suggest the presence of another renal pathology (see ▶ Case 1). Retinopathy is present in up to 80% of patients at the time of diagnosis of nephropathy; therefore, the absence of retinopathy highlights the need to consider an alternative diagnosis, but on its own, it is rarely an indication for biopsy. Similarly, non-visible haematuria may be observed in up to 20% of patients with diabetic kidney disease, with a minority of these patients demonstrating an alternative pathology on renal biopsy [22, 23]. Importantly, people over 50 years old who have unexplained non-visible haematuria should be referred for further urological investigation.

While microalbuminuria is classically recognised as the earliest clinical marker of diabetic nephropathy, a reduction in renal function may occasionally be observed in normoalbuminuric patients with type 1 diabetes, often in association with typical structural changes of DN and no evidence of alternative pathology [24]. In type 2 diabetes, almost 75% of patients who have an eGFR <60 ml/min/1.73 m^2 remain normoalbuminuric [25]. Here, the absence of microalbuminuria may reflect the more heterogeneous nature of renal injury in type 2 diabetes, with a higher prevalence of non-diabetic renal disease such as hypertensive and ischaemic nephrosclerosis. These findings highlight that, in addition to screening for albuminuria, an assessment of renal function should be performed on an annual basis in patients with both type 1 and type 2 diabetes.

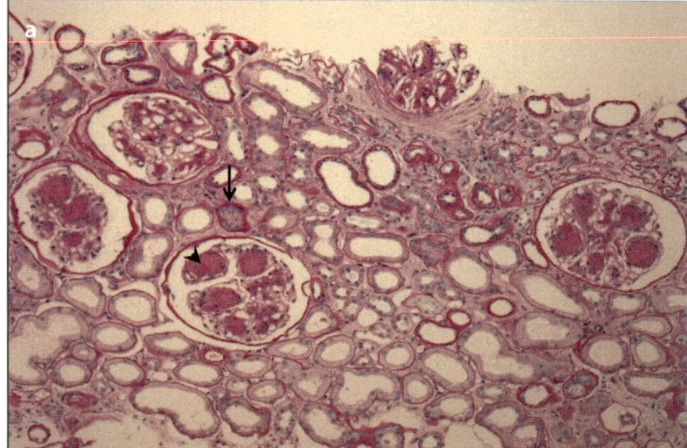

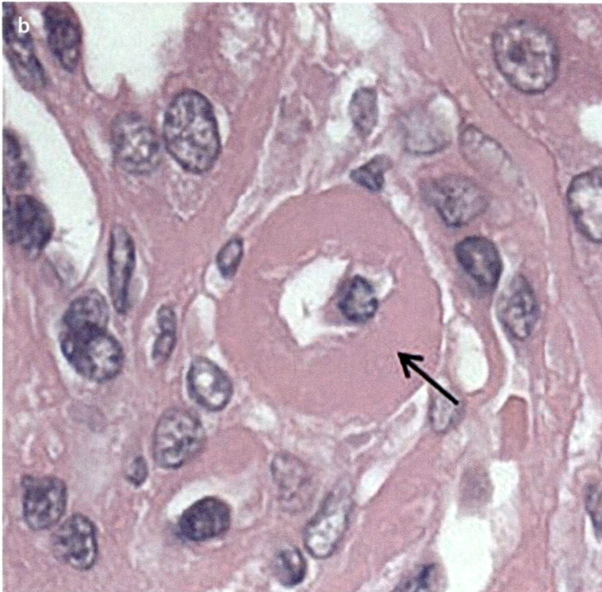

Fig. 38.1 Renal biopsy from a patient with diabetic nephropathy demonstrating **a** classical nodular glomerulosclerosis (Kimmelstiel-Wilson lesion, arrowhead), tubular atrophy and tubulointerstitial fibrosis including thickening of the tubular basement membrane (arrow); **b** arteriolar hyalinosis (arrow). (Images courtesy of Dr. Chris Bellamy, Consultant Pathologist, Royal Infirmary of Edinburgh)

Table 38.2 Clinical features that may indicate the need for renal biopsy

Rapid increase in proteinuria
Rapid decline in renal function
Presence of haematuria
Absence of retinopathy
Presence of systemic symptoms

38

38.6 Management

Recent KDIGO guidelines offer a comprehensive overview of the management of patients with diabetic nephropathy [26]. The ultimate aim is to reduce the rate of progression of nephropathy and the incidence of cardiovascular disease. Studies have suggested that regression of diabetic nephropathy may occur following intensive blood sugar and blood pressure control. In a study of almost 400 patients with type 1 diabetes and microalbuminuria, only 15% progressed to overt proteinuria after 6 years of follow-up, with 40% regressing to normoalbuminuria and the remaining 45% exhibiting persistent microalbuminuria [27]. Factors that predicted regression included tight blood glucose and blood pressure control and low levels of lipidaemia. Even structural changes previously considered irreversible, such as moderate glomerulosclerosis and tubulointerstitial fibrosis, may regress with prolonged normalisation of blood glucose levels following successful pancreatic transplantation [28].

38.7 Lifestyle Factors

All patients should be encouraged to stop smoking, lose weight and take regular exercise. Smoking exacerbates the already high risk of cardiovascular disease in patients with diabetes and kidney disease and may also synergise with poor glycaemic control to increase the rate of decline in renal function [29]. Weight loss and exercise may assist attempts to control glycaemia, but may also have independent beneficial effects on the kidney. For example, in patients with type 1 diabetes, each 10 cm increase in waist circumference is associated with a one-third greater risk of developing microalbuminuria, independent of the effects on glycaemic control [30]. While bariatric surgery has been shown to markedly improve glycaemic control [31], no randomised controlled studies have assessed its role in preventing progression of diabetic kidney disease. Reducing dietary salt can be very effective, though it is challenging to achieve. In a randomised trial, a low-salt diet (6 g/day) resulted in an 11 mmHg reduction in systolic BP and potentiated the anti-proteinuric effects of ACE inhibition compared with a normal salt diet (11 g/day) [32].

38.8 Glycaemic Control

Tight glycaemic control is beneficial in reducing the risk of developing DN and other microvascular complications. In people with type 1 diabetes, the DCCT demonstrated that a reduction in mean HbA1c, from 75 mmol/mol (9.0%) to 53 mmol/mol (7.0%) for a 6-year period, resulted in a 39% reduction in the development of microalbuminuria and a 54% reduction in the development of frank proteinuria [11]. Long-term follow-up of patients from the DCCT has shown that this early reduction in albuminuria translates into a subsequent reduction in the risk of CKD (eGFR <60 ml/min/1.73 m^2) [12]. The UKPDS in type 2 diabetes demonstrated similar findings, with a reduction in mean HbA1c from 63 mmol/mol (7.9%) to 53 mmol/mol (7.0%) being associated with an absolute risk reduction of developing microalbuminuria (11%), proteinuria (3.5%) and a doubling in serum creatinine over 12 years (2.5%) [13].

Long-term follow-up of patients from both the DCCT and UKPDS trials has suggested that the beneficial effect of a period of tight control, in terms of the development of complications, persists for many years. In the DCCT cohort, only 9% of intensively treated patients had developed frank nephropathy after 30 years of type 1 diabetes, compared with 25% who were conventionally treated [4]. In the UKPDS, after a median period of 17 years of follow-up, patients from the intensively treated cohort demonstrated a 24% reduction in the risk of developing microvascular disease [4]. These findings were noted in spite of the fact that the glycaemic control in the 'intensively treated' and 'conventionally treated' cohorts from both studies converged quite quickly after the cessation of the active treatment phase. This suggests a considerable 'legacy effect' from a period of tight glycaemic control in both type 1 and type 2 diabetes, and that efforts to optimise control in the first few years after developing diabetes may well pay considerable dividends in reducing the incidence of future complications, even if control slips at a later stage.

Although there is good evidence that tight glycaemic control in both type 1 and type 2 diabetes is associated with a significantly reduced risk of developing diabetic nephropathy, the benefit of this is less clear cut in patients with established nephropathy. Some studies, including the DCCT [11], indicate that maintaining tight glycaemic control will reduce the risk of developing or rate of progression of nephropathy in patients who already have microalbuminuria. No randomised controlled studies have clearly indicated that intensive glycaemic control slows progression once there is overt proteinuria and a falling glomerular filtration rate. There are, however, observational data suggesting that, even in well-established CKD, the decline in renal function may occur at a more rapid rate in those with poor glycaemic control [17]. In addition, maintaining good metabolic control may reduce the risk of development or progression of other microvascular complications of diabetes. However, in patients with established CKD, aiming for an HbA1c level below 53 mmol/mol (7.0%) does not seem to be associated with any additional benefits in terms of reducing all-cause and cardiovascular mortality. Furthermore, there is some evidence, notably from the ACCORD study, that intensive glycaemic control in patients with CKD can be associated with increased cardiovascular mortality, with no evident beneficial effect on the progression of the renal disease [33]. Recent guidelines therefore suggest that a target HbA1c range of 58–62 mmol/mol (7.5–7.8%) is appropriate for patients with type 1 diabetes and CKD stage 3 or 4, with a realistic target for patients with type 2 diabetes with a similar degree of CKD being 52–58 mmol/mol (6.9–7.5%) for those not requiring insulin and 58–68 mmol/mol (7.5–8.5%) for those on insulin therapy, reflecting the increased risks of hypoglycaemia in insulin-treated patients with CKD [34]. A target range of 58–68 mmol/mol (7.5–8.5%) is probably appropriate for all patients with CKD stage 5, or those on dialysis, irrespective of type of diabetes or blood glucose-lowering therapy. Optimal glycaemic targets therefore need to be considered on an individual patient basis.

In terms of prevention of DN, it appears that it is the level of glycaemia achieved, rather than the drugs used to achieve this, which is paramount. The UKPDS included cohorts treated with insulin, two different sulphonylureas and metformin. All achieved similar levels of glycaemia throughout the duration of the study, and there were no significant differences between the groups in terms of microvascular outcomes [13]. Managing glycaemia in the context of chronic kidney disease does, however, present several other challenges, especially in relation to the choice of glucose-lowering drugs and dose modification. Recently, however, this field has been truly transformed following several large-scale trials with sodium-glucose co-transporter inhibitors and glucagon-like peptide-1 receptor agonists which have marked renal and cardiovascular protective effects over and above their glycaemic effects.

38.9 Choice of Blood Glucose-Lowering Drugs in Chronic Kidney Disease

A plethora of large RCTs have resulted in new guidelines promoting the early use of drugs that impact on the complications of diabetes, principally cardiovascular and renal disease [26, 35].

38.9.1 Metformin

Since the publication of the UKPDS, metformin has become the most widely prescribed oral hypoglycaemic agent in patients with type 2 diabetes. This is predominantly because, in a subgroup of 342 overweight and obese patients randomised to intensive therapy with metformin, there was less weight gain and a reduction in all-cause mortality and in a number of major cardiovascular outcomes, including stroke, in comparison to conventional therapy [36]. Although similar trends were seen in patients who were randomised to intensive therapy with sulphonylureas or insulin, the results in these arms of the study did not attain statistical significance. Given the fact that cardiovascular disease is the major cause of excess morbidity and mortality in people with type 2 diabetes, these findings led to a dramatic increase in the prescription of metformin, and for some time it has been the oral hypoglycaemic of choice in overweight and obese patients.

A concern has been that metformin and its metabolites are predominantly renally excreted and thus will accumulate in renal impairment. Furthermore, there is a well-established link between metformin and lactic acidosis, although to what extent metformin is directly causative remains a matter of some speculation. What is clear, however, is that the risk of lactic acidosis increases in the context of acute kidney injury which, in turn, is much more common in those with pre-existing CKD.

Previously, metformin was widely used by diabetologists in patients whose serum creatinine was 150–200 μmol/l, with few problems. Routine reporting of eGFR, however, initially led to recommendations that metformin be discontinued in stage 3 CKD. In many cases, this demonstrated just what an effective glucose-lowering agent metformin is in obese patients with type 2 diabetes. Frequently, patients who had had excellent glycaemic control on metformin alone became hyperglycaemic when this drug was stopped. Other oral agents proved less effective and often led to significant weight gain. Insulin was frequently required, but despite the use of large doses due to insulin resistance, resultant glycaemic control remained inferior to that achieved on metformin.

38

Such issues have led to a reassessment of the use of metformin in the context of CKD. There is currently general agreement that metformin should usually be avoided when the eGFR drops below 30 ml/min/1.73 m^2 but it is safe in most patients with an eGFR >45 ml/min/1.73 m^2. Between 30 and 45 ml/min/1.73 m^2, regular monitoring of renal biochemistry is recommended, and if renal function is steadily declining, it is appropriate to stop metformin before the eGFR falls to <30 ml/min/1.73 m^2 [37]. Furthermore, as is recommended with ACE inhibitors and angiotensin receptor blockers, patients taking metformin should temporarily discontinue the drug when a situation arises which might lead to a short-lived deterioration in renal function, e.g. if the patient is suffering from vomiting or diarrhoea or is undergoing a radiological study involving the administration of contrast agents. What is currently less clear is whether it can be safe in some circumstances, specifically when the rate of decline in renal function is very slow, to continue with metformin therapy even when the eGFR drops below 30 ml/min/1.73 m^2, with appropriate monitoring.

38.9.2 Sulphonylureas and Meglitinides

These drugs bind to specific, but different, receptors on the pancreatic beta cell and directly stimulate insulin secretion. As such, they are inevitably associated with a risk of hypoglycaemia, and this risk increases in the context of CKD. This is partly due to the accumulation of these drugs and their metabolites, as the sulphonylureas are predominantly renally excreted with the exception of gliquidone. Longer-acting sulphonylureas, such as glibenclamide, are probably best avoided completely, and the dose of other shorter-acting agents may need to be reduced. All patients with CKD on sulphonylurea therapy should be provided with the equipment to perform regular home capillary blood glucose monitoring, given the increased risk of hypoglycaemia.

Meglitinides, with their shorter duration of action than sulphonylureas, have been promoted largely in relation to targeting post-prandial hyperglycaemia, but have not been widely embraced, at least in the UK, due to the need for multiple daily dosing. These drugs may, however, be considered as a useful alternative to sulphonylureas in the context of CKD, especially repaglinide, which is predominantly hepatically metabolised.

38.9.3 Pioglitazone

Pioglitazone is now the only thiazolidinedione available in the UK. It is a peroxisome proliferator-activated receptor-gamma (PPARγ) agonist, with multiple metabolic effects, including increasing insulin sensitivity. It is metabolised by the liver and is hence potentially a useful drug in patients with CKD. However, pioglitazone is associated with fluid retention and contraindicated in the presence of congestive cardiac failure. More recently identified concerns with pioglitazone relate to an increased fracture risk, especially in post-menopausal women [38] and a possible increase in bladder cancer.

38.9.4 Insulin

In addition to patients with type 1 diabetes, many patients with type 2 diabetes who develop CKD will have had diabetes for a long period of time and will already be on insulin therapy due to declining beta-cell function, with or without additional oral hypoglycaemic drugs. As the liver and kidneys are the major sites of insulin clearance/degradation, the half-life of insulin is prolonged in patients with CKD, and therefore there is a greater risk of hypoglycaemia with insulin therapy. The healthy kidney is responsible for approximately one-quarter of the body's gluconeogenesis; therefore, a reduction in gluconeogenesis in patients with CKD adds to the hypoglycaemia risk. Additionally, in patients with both type 1 and type 2 diabetes of long duration, there is an increased prevalence of reduced or absent awareness of hypoglycaemic symptoms, with a corresponding increase in the frequency of severe hypoglycaemic episodes. Hence, many patients on insulin will need to have their doses dramatically reduced as their renal function declines and some, even those with type 1 diabetes, will have very low insulin requirements.

38.10 Newer Glucose-Lowering Drugs

38.10.1 Glucagon-Like Peptide-1 (GLP-1) Agonists

These drugs mimic native GLP-1 and have multiple actions, including stimulation of glucose-dependent insulin secretion and inhibition of glucagon secretion. They also delay gastric emptying and increase satiety. Despite the fact that they need to be administered by subcutaneous injection, GLP-1 agonists have an established role in the treatment of type 2 diabetes because, in addition to improving glycaemic control, they are one of the few classes of hypoglycaemic drugs available which promote weight loss.

There is emerging evidence that treatment with GLP-1 agonists is associated with improved cardiovascular outcomes [39, 40]. In a recent study, patients with type 2 diabetes treated with the GLP-1 agonist liraglutide, which has predominantly extra-renal clearance, had reduced cardiovascular mortality, with subgroup analysis confirming greater benefits in those with eGFR <60 ml/min/1.73 m^2. Further large studies were reviewed in a meta-analysis of over 56,000 patients, which demonstrated that GLP-1 agonists reduced all-cause mortality by 12%, non-fatal MI by 9%, hospitalisation for heart failure by 9% and stroke by 16% [41]. There was also a significant reduction in a composite renal endpoint (falling GFR, rising albuminuria, death by renal cause or ESRD) with a HR of 0.83 [41]. Recently, oral semaglutide has become available, but this appears to be less potent than most injected GLP-1 agonists.

38.10.2 Dipeptidyl Peptidase-4 (DPP-4) Inhibitors

DPP-4 is the enzyme which inactivates GLP-1; therefore, DPP-4 inhibitors enhance GLP-1 levels by slowing down its degradation, but unlike the currently available GLP-1 agonists, these drugs are active orally. They are generally well tolerated and weight neutral; however, clinical experience is that they are often rather less potent glucose-lowering agents than other available drugs, and our own experience has been that gastrointestinal side effects, such as nausea and vomiting, may be more common with these agents in patients with CKD. Several drugs in this class are potentially useful even in patients with advanced CKD. Linagliptin is safe in all degrees of renal impairment, including ESRD, and no dose reduction is required. Other drugs in the class, including alogliptin, saxagliptin, sitagliptin and vildagliptin, can be used in moderate-to-severe renal impairment, although reductions in dose are required.

38.10.3 Sodium-Glucose Co-transporters

Most filtered glucose is reabsorbed by the SGLT-2 co-transporter in the proximal tubules; therefore, SGLT-2 inhibitors reduce HbA1c by promoting glycosuria, with the calorie loss having an added benefit of promoting weight loss. In addition, by inhibiting sodium reabsorption, they modestly reduce blood pressure. Finally, the increased delivery of sodium to the distal tubule may reduce glomerular pressure through tubulo-glomerular feedback. All of these mechanisms may explain the emerging cardiovascular and renal benefits of this class of drugs. SGLT-2 inhibitors have been shown to reduce heart failure in addition to cardiovascular death and all-cause mortality [42, 43]. Data from the EMPA-REG Renal study has also demonstrated a 61% reduction in the onset or worsening of DN, 44% relative risk reduction in doubling of serum creatinine and 55% reduction in the need for renal replacement therapy in patients with type 2 diabetes with an eGFR >30 ml/min/1.73 m^2 treated with empagliflozin [44]. A post hoc analysis in the CANVAS study suggested that canagliflozin also has renoprotective effects, with reductions in the progression of albuminuria and a composite renal endpoint being reported [43]. The CREDENCE study [45] specifically looked at the renal impact of SGLT-2 inhibitors. This landmark study of 4400 patients analysed the effect of adding canagliflozin to patients with type 2 diabetes and evidence of nephropathy. Addition of canagliflozin resulted in a highly significant 30% reduction in a composite endpoint of ESRD, doubling of creatinine or death (from renal or cardiovascular cause), with the benefit likely to be greatest in those with greater proteinuria. In the DAPA-CKD trial, patients with and without diabetes were initiated on dapagliflozin down to a minimum eGFR of 25ml/min/1.73m^2. In those assigned to dapagliflozin, there was a 44% reduction in the composite renal outcome which included a 50% decline in kidney function, end-stage renal disease or death from renal causes. Interestingly, the effect of dapagliflozin was similar in patients with and without diabetes, confirming that most of the renoprotective properties of SGLT2i are independent of blood glucose control. Indeed the glucose-lowering effect of these drugs is likely to be diminished in patients with more advanced CKD. By promoting an osmotic diuresis, these drugs reduce intravascular fluid volume, although no increase in AKI was observed in the clinical trials above. SGLT-2 inhibitors modestly increase the risk of urogenital candidal infection, and there is also a minimally increased risk of bacterial ascending urinary tract infection, which would clearly be undesirable in the context of CKD. In addition, the CANVAS trial found an unexpected increase in distal lower limb amputations in the canagliflozin treatment group [43], which is important, given the high risk of peripheral vascular disease in patients with CKD due to DN.

38.11 Blood Pressure Control

38

Tight blood pressure control is at least as important as glycaemic control in slowing progression of diabetic kidney disease. In the UKPDS, an improvement in blood pressure from 154/87 to 144/82 resulted in a 37% reduction in the incidence of microvascular events [14]. However, in contrast to the management of hyperglycaemia, where tight glycaemic control results in a reduced incidence of nephropathy that persists long after the end of the DCCT [46] and UKPDS trials [4, 47], the benefit of tight blood pressure control tends to recede with time [48], emphasising the need for strict ongoing blood pressure control in preventing progressive DN.

The target blood pressure for patients with diabetes is controversial and may depend on the type of diabetes and the presence of proteinuria. In general, a reasonable target would be to reduce blood pressure to below 140/80 mmHg in those without albuminuria and 130/80 mmHg in those with albuminuria. However, extrapolating from the evidence obtained in non-diabetic patients from the Modification of Diet in Renal Disease Study [49], those with a protein excretion of >1 g/day may benefit from a lower BP target of 125/75 mmHg. Polypharmacy is often required to achieve the target blood pressure – e.g. 29% of patients in the tight BP control arm of the UKPDS trial required three or more antihypertensive agents [14].

38.11.1 Proteinuria as a Specific Target

In clinical trials, the risk of adverse renal outcomes increases linearly with the level of baseline proteinuria, and a reduction in proteinuria is associated with a reduced risk of renal events such as ESRD [50, 51]. Proteinuria is primarily modified by blood pressure reduction, though RAAS-active drugs may have additional anti-proteinuric effects by selectively reducing intraglomerular pressure. For example, in patients with type 2 diabetes, irbesartan has been shown to have anti-proteinuric and renoprotective effects that are greater than other antihypertensive agents [52] and independent of blood pressure reduction [18]. Specific targeting of proteinuria reduction in a ‘regression’ clinic, with sequential add-on of antihypertensive agents, reduced the rate of decline in renal function in patients with nephrotic-range proteinuria at baseline [53]. The rate of decline in renal function was lowest in those who achieved <1 g/day of proteinuria; however, this was much harder to achieve in patients who had a primary renal diagnosis of diabetic nephropathy. The CREDENCE study demonstrated that SGLT-2 inhibitors are effective in reducing renal decline (and cardiovascular mortality) in patients with marked proteinuria (urine protein/creatinine ratio of 300–5000) [45]. Hence, proteinuria may act as a marker of treatment efficacy, and we advocate monitoring of proteinuria routinely in the clinic, aiming to reduce proteinuria by at least 50% although, in reality, the lower the better.

38.11.2 Choice of Antihypertensive Agent

38.11.2.1 Renin-Angiotensin System Blockade

As noted in the previous section, ACE inhibitors and angiotensin II receptor blockers (ARBs) have the ability to reduce intraglomerular pressure by preferentially dilating the efferent arteriole, and they may also counter angiotensin II-mediated pro-inflammatory changes in the kidney.

▪▪ Normoalbuminuria

A meta-analysis of 16 trials that included over 7000 normoalbuminuric patients with both type 1 and type 2 diabetes suggested that ACE inhibitors prevented microalbuminuria even in patients without hypertension [54]. However, a recent study in normoalbuminuric patients with type 1 diabetes found that while RAAS blockade reduced the incidence of retinopathy, it did not reduce the onset of microalbuminuria and importantly it did not alter the degree of mesangial matrix accumulation observed on serial renal biopsies [55]. Furthermore, a meta-analysis of patients with type 2 diabetes found that there was no benefit of RAAS blockade compared with other antihypertensive agents in the absence of albuminuria [56]. On the basis of current evidence, RAAS blockade cannot be recommended for primary prevention of nephropathy, although it may be indicated for other reasons such as to prevent retinopathy and cardiovascular disease. In particular, in the absence of another indication, we generally do not use ACE/ARB as first-line therapy in elderly patients with normoalbuminuria, as they are more likely to have renovascular disease than diabetic nephropathy as a cause for their renal failure and hence are less likely to benefit, but are at an increased risk of AKI.

▪▪ Microalbuminuria

Renin-angiotensin system blockade is indicated in patients with microalbuminuria even when clinic blood pressure is in the normal range. RAAS inhibition reduces the rate of progression from microalbuminuria to overt nephropathy and increases the rate of regression to normoalbuminuria in patients with type 1 diabetes [7]. These findings were only partially attenuated following correction for blood pressure, indicating an additional, blood pressure-independent effect of renin-angiotensin blockade [57]. Similarly, irbesartan prevents progression from microalbuminuria to macroalbuminuria in patients with hypertension and type 2 diabetes [58].

▪▪ Overt nephropathy

RAAS inhibition should also be the antihypertensive therapy of choice in patients with overt proteinuria, as randomised controlled trials indicate that they reduce the risk of a doubling in creatinine [52]. Again the effect of ACE inhibitors and ARBs in this context is likely to be at least in part independent of their blood pressure-lowering effect. Indeed, in the Irbesartan DN Trial (IDNT), irbesartan therapy resulted in a 23% reduction in doubling of creatinine or the development of ESRD compared with amlodipine, despite blood pressure being comparable between the groups [52]. There is no good evidence as to whether the use of an ACE inhibitor or an ARB is preferable. The bulk of evidence for type 1 nephropathy is for ACE inhibitors, while in type 2 nephropathy, most trials have employed ARBs. A direct comparison of ACE inhibitors and ARBs in type 2 diabetes suggested similar efficacy [59]; therefore, given the substantial experience of the use of ACE inhibitors, we generally advocate ACE inhibitors as first-line agents, with ARBs reserved for those who do not tolerate ACE inhibitors, usually on account of cough.

▪▪ Advanced nephropathy

As the risks of hyperkalaemia and AKI due to RAAS blockade increase at low levels of renal function, a key question is at what level of renal function, if at all, RAAS blockade should be discontinued? One study demonstrated that in patients with a mean GFR of 26 ml/min/1.73 m^2, a moderate dose of benazepril reduced progression to dialysis with no increase in the incidence of hyperkalaemia [60]. However, this study was conducted in a Chinese population, where potassium intake may be much lower than in Western societies. Conversely, a recent study has indicated that, in patients with very advanced CKD, stopping RAAS blockade may facilitate an increase in glomerular filtration and delay the onset of dialysis [61]. The role of RAAS blockade in patients with advanced renal failure may become clearer when the results of the STOP-ACEi trial emerge in the next couple of years.

▪▪ Hyperkalaemia

Patients with DN and CKD frequently develop hyperkalaemia due to concomitant type 4 distal renal tubular acidosis, and this may limit the use of RAAS blockade. While it is reasonable to consider reducing the dose or stopping RAAS blockade when the serum potassium concentration exceeds 6 mmol/L, this may be associated with poor renal outcome, particularly in patients with heavy proteinuria (see ▶ Case 2). Therefore, our practice is to keep patients on RAAS blockade as long as possible if they have overt proteinuria, using a combination of low-potassium diet, kaliuretic diuretics and treatment of acidosis where applicable. The development of new potassium binders, such as patiromer or sodium zirconium, which can reduce serum potassium by approximately 1 mmol/L in patients with hyperkalaemia [62], may enable RAAS blockade to be continued safely; however, the benefit of this strategy on hard endpoints has yet to be established.

▪▪ Initiation of RAAS blockade

In all patients, the risk of an acute deterioration in renal function or hyperkalaemia is greatest soon after starting or increasing the dose of RAAS blockade; therefore, renal function should be checked within 7–10 days of dose adjustments. Some decline in renal function is to be expected, and indeed a meta-analysis of clinical trials suggested that the greater the initial decline in renal function, the better the long-term renal outcome [63]. The risk of a rapid decline in renal function is greatest in those with intravascular volume depletion or where the renal auto-regulation system is inhibited, such as in patients on concomitant diuretic therapy or following prescription of a non-steroidal anti-inflammatory agent. Patients should be warned to stop RAAS blockade prior to major surgery or if they develop fever, vomiting or diarrhoea (sick day rule). Specific issues in the use of RAAS blockade in patients with diabetic nephropathy are considered in 'Tips and Tricks'.

■■ Dual RAAS blockade

Dual RAAS blockade, using an ACE inhibitor and ARB together, may have added benefit in lowering proteinuria compared with monotherapy [64], but cannot be recommended in patients with DN due to the increased risk of hyperkalaemia and AKI. In the ONTARGET trial, the combination of an ACE inhibitor and ARB resulted in an increased incidence of doubling of creatinine, dialysis or death [65]. The VA NEPHRON-D trial randomised patients with type 2 diabetes and proteinuria, who were already taking an ARB, to the addition of an ACE inhibitor or placebo. Dual therapy did not reduce adverse renal or cardiovascular outcomes, but there was an increased risk of hyperkalaemia and AKI [66].

■■ Direct renin inhibitors

Although the direct renin inhibitor aliskiren has been shown to act synergistically with ACE inhibitors/ARBs to reduce proteinuria [67], the ALTITUDE trial, which examined the efficacy of adding aliskiren to standard ACE inhibitor/ARB therapy in patients with type 2 diabetes and CKD, was stopped prematurely due to an increase in stroke, renal failure, hyperkalaemia and hypotension in the aliskiren arm [68]. Therefore, the addition of direct renin inhibitors to patients with DN who are taking ACE/ARB is not recommended.

38

■■ Aldosterone antagonists

The addition of spironolactone, eplerenone [69] or the non-steroidal mineralocorticoid antagonist finerenone [70] to ACE inhibition further reduces proteinuria. The FIDELIO-DKD trial randomised patients with overt proteinuria and eGFR 25–75 who were already on maximum RAAS blockade tolerated to finerenone or placebo. Those in the finerenone arm had an 18% reduction compared with the placebo arm in the composite endpoint of 40% reduction in eGFR or death due to renal disease. Unlike the studies with combination of ACE and ARB, there was no increase in the risk of AKI, however the study medication was stopped due to hyperkalaemia in 2.3% of patients in the finerenone arm, compared with only 0.9% of patients in the placebo arm. Furthermore, the risk of hyperkalaemia may be greater with aldosterone antagonists than with other RAAS inhibitors, for which there is a mitigating safety mechanism in that hyperkalaemia per se promotes release of aldosterone to induce a kaliuresis. This risk was highlighted by the fact that, following publication of the Randomised Aldactone Evaluation Study (RALES), a fourfold increase in the number of prescriptions of spironolactone was associated with an increase in the number of hospital admissions due to severe hyperkalaemia [71]. At present, we tend to reserve spironolactone only for patients who have resistant hypertension, concomitant cardiac failure or heavy proteinuria and preserved renal function.

38.11.2.2 Other Antihypertensive Agents

■■ Diuretics

Loop and thiazide diuretics are a very useful adjunct to RAAS blockade in patients with diabetes. Combination therapy further reduces blood pressure, mitigates against hyperkalaemia and potentiates the anti-proteinuric effect of ACE inhibitors.

■■ Non-dihydropyridine calcium channel blockers

As with RAAS blockade, these agents may have specific anti-proteinuric properties [72] and indeed may synergise with ACE inhibitors to reduce proteinuria [73]. We would reserve this class of agents for patients who continue to have proteinuria despite RAAS blockade and who have no cardiovascular indications for β-blockade.

38.12 Cardiovascular Risk

In patients with diabetes, the presence of renal disease confers an increased risk of cardiovascular disease. For example, in the UKPDS, there was a progressive increase in the risk of cardiovascular death with advancing nephropathy, with annual mortality rates ranging from 0.7% in normoalbuminuric patients to 2.0%, 3.5% and 12.1% in those with modestly elevated albuminuria, proteinuria or elevated creatinine/on renal replacement therapy (RRT), respectively [74]. In general, the use of statins in patients with diabetes results in a reduction in cardiovascular events, irrespective of whether they have a prior history of cardiovascular disease or elevated baseline LDL cholesterol levels [75]. Similar results were observed in the subset of patients with diabetes and CKD. Combination treatment with simvastatin and ezetimibe reduced cardiovascular events by 22% in patients with diabetes and CKD in the SHARP study, with an excess risk of myopathy of only 2 per 10,000 per patient years of treatment, although there was no reduction in the risk of doubling of creatinine or need for RRT [76]. Hence, to prevent cardiovascular events, statins should be routinely prescribed in patients with diabetes and kidney disease, unless they are at very low risk of cardiovascular events (e.g. those <40 years old).

38.13 Multifactorial Interventions

Holistic management of multiple renal and cardiac risk factors represents the ideal model of care. An excellent study from the Steno Diabetes Centre demonstrated that, in patients with type 2 diabetes treated over approximately 8 years, targeting multiple risk factors, e.g. lifestyle modifications (low-fat diet, moderate exercise, smoking cessation), tight control of blood glucose, blood pressure and serum lipids and use of aspirin, resulted in a reduction in mortality and a >50% reduction in the risk of developing overt nephropathy. These beneficial effects were sustained more than 13 years after the initial study visit [77]. A practical example of a successful multifactorial interventional strategy is illustrated in ► Case 3.

38.14 Models of Service

As a consequence of trial evidence, we would advocate target-driven multifactorial intervention for all patients with diabetic kidney disease. A key question is how the clinical service should be designed to achieve this and improve outcomes for patients with diabetes and kidney disease with maximal efficiency. Approximately 25% of patients with type 2 diabetes have an eGFR <60 ml/min/1.73 m^2 [25]; therefore, it is impractical, and indeed unnecessary, for all these patients to be under nephrological care. Nonetheless, retrospective studies have demonstrated that when patients are referred to a specialist service, such as a Joint Renal Diabetes clinic or clinics run exclusively by diabetologists or nephrologists with a special interest in DN, clinical targets are more likely to be achieved, and this is associated with a reduction in the rate of progression of renal disease [78]. A key factor in establishing a successful Joint Renal Diabetes clinic remains effective collaboration between enthusiastic diabetologists and nephrologists.

For maximum efficiency of care, there should be strict criteria for acceptance into such clinics, aiming to recruit those who are at greatest risk and therefore most likely to gain benefit (◘ Fig. 38.2). Electronic information technology (IT) systems may aid identification of patients at high risk of renal complications, who can then be recruited proactively to such clinics. Systematic screening using electronic IT systems may reduce the rate of acceptance onto RRT programmes by up to 30% and increase the number of patients who start dialysis with vascular access in place [79].

In addition, consideration should be given to the flow of patients through the clinic. Non-traditional clinic models such as nurse-specialist or pharmacist-led cardiovascular risk reduction clinics may facilitate more frequent review in order to achieve risk factor targets more rapidly. Once target values for risk factors are achieved, and if renal function stabilises, patients may be discharged to general diabetes clinics with clear parameters for re-referral. Conversely, those with advanced kidney disease may migrate to a specialist low clearance clinic.

Decisions on the optimal mode of care at a local level should be made in conjunction with nephrologists, diabetologists and primary care physicians, and an example of a possible system of management is given in ◘ Fig. 38.2.

38.15 Management of Patients with Diabetes on Renal Replacement Therapy (RRT)

38.15.1 Dialysis

Once a patient with DN reaches end-stage renal failure, mortality is high compared to other patients on dialysis (e.g. in those aged 45–64 years, the 5-year survival is only 32% vs. 67% for glomerulonephritis) [80]. Evidence for multifactorial intervention in patients with diabetes on dialysis is lacking. However, by extrapolation, lifestyle factors and blood pressure control should impact on cardiovascular risk and all-cause mortality and should be maintained when a patient transitions to RRT. The importance of tight blood glucose control is less clear cut, with one recent large observational study suggesting no major association between HbA1c and outcomes after correction for confounding factors [81], whereas another similar study with different methodologies reached the opposite conclusion [82]. As previously discussed, recent guidelines have supported relaxing targets for glycaemic control in patients on dialysis [6]. In any case, trying to maintain stability of glycaemic control in this group of patients can be quite challenging, with erratic swings in blood glucose levels being common, in particular hyperglycaemia post-dialysis due to increased insulin clearance during haemodialysis and/or the glucose load in peritoneal dialysis solutions. These issues may be best managed by separate input from renal and diabetes teams, as renal priorities will not necessarily 'cross over' seamlessly with diabetes targets at this stage of the disease process. However, it is important to stress to patients, particularly those commencing haemodialysis, involving frequent visits to the hospital, the importance of regular attendance at diabetes clinics,

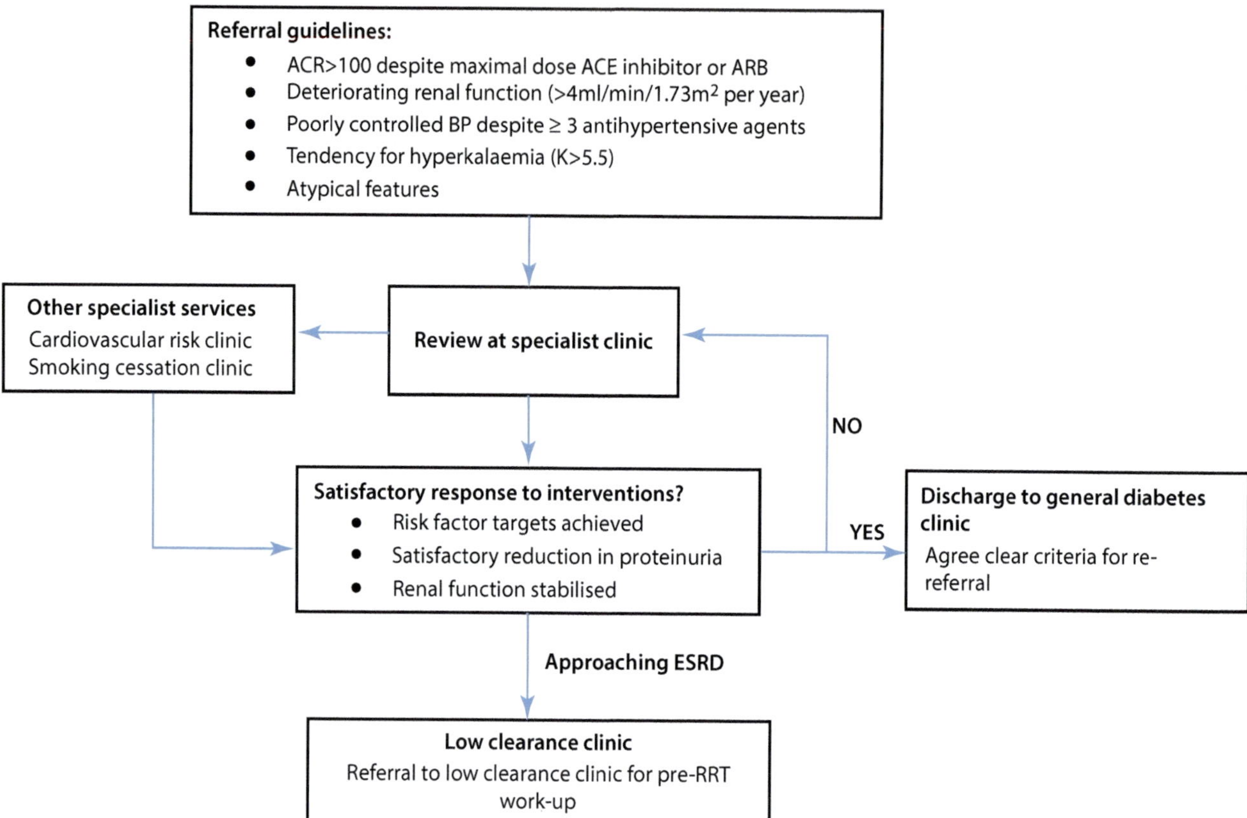

Fig. 38.2 Potential model of care pathways through a specialist diabetic kidney disease clinic

38

including eye and foot screening. Foot screening is particularly important given the high rate of lower limb amputation in diabetes patients receiving RRT, and initiatives where regular foot checks are performed as part of routine care in dialysis units have been shown to reduce amputation rates.

38.15.2 Transplantation

While the survival rate on dialysis of patients with a primary renal diagnosis of DN is poor, it can be dramatically improved by renal transplantation. Patients with ESRD due to DN who receive a transplant will have a projected lifespan of 19 years, compared to 8 years for those who remain on dialysis on the transplant waiting list [2]. Indeed, patients with DN are likely to gain the most benefit from transplantation, with projected survival increasing by 17 years and 14 years for those aged 20–39 years and 40–59 years, respectively, compared to increases of 11 years and 7 years in non-diabetic patients [83]. While transplantation confers an increased risk of early death in patients with DN, largely due to peri-operative mortality, it requires only 181 days for this early increase in risk to be outweighed by the subsequent survival advantages of transplantation, compared with 356 days in non-diabetic patients [83]. Therefore, transplantation should be the mode of choice for RRT, in patients with DN who are deemed medically fit; however, more rigorous cardiac investigations, potentially including angiography, may be necessary to attempt to minimise the increase in peri-operative mortality. Furthermore, as patients with diabetes and overt proteinuria are at high risk of progression to end-stage kidney disease, the prospect of future transplantation should be considered early in the course of the disease, including steps such as minimising blood transfusion.

A key issue when considering transplantation is whether to perform a kidney transplant in isolation or simultaneous pancreas and kidney transplantation. While the latter has much greater peri-operative risks, the improvement in metabolic control conferred by successful pancreas transplantation is associated with improved patient survival beyond the 10th year after transplantation, when compared to patients who have received a live donor renal transplant (HR 0.55, $p = 0.005$), mainly due to a reduction in cardiovascular mortality [84]. The risk/benefit ratio may be particularly attractive for younger patients and those with unstable glycaemic control, who are prone to recurrent, severe episodes of ketoacidosis and/or hypoglycaemia.

38.16 Conclusion

DN remains the commonest cause of ESRD. Biopsy to confirm diagnosis is only required in atypical presentations, most notably when proteinuria is rapidly increasing or renal function rapidly declining. Tight glycaemic and blood pressure control is paramount, with RAAS blockade essential for those with proteinuria. New agents such as GLP-1 receptor agonists and SGLT-2 antagonists [85] also significantly improve renal and cardiovascular outcomes and are particularly important to consider in patients with proteinuria, obesity or heart failure. More patients die of cardiovascular disease than progress to ESRD; therefore, cardiovascular risk factors need to be addressed.

There is now a huge amount that we can offer patients with diabetes, and there is a responsibility to offer an efficient and comprehensive early review of patients with proteinuria as these patients stand the most to lose from neglect and the most to gain from focused intervention and treatment.

Case Study

Case 1

A 23-year-old man, who had type 1 diabetes since the age of 7 years, was referred with leg swelling, new onset proteinuria (protein/creatinine ratio 652 mg/mmol) and low serum albumin (16 g/L). His glycaemic control was generally good (typical HbA1c 60 mmol/mol (7.6%)), and he had no microalbuminuria at his last diabetes clinic attendance 4 months prior to referral. The abrupt onset of nephrotic-range proteinuria was felt to be too rapid for a diagnosis of DN; therefore, he underwent renal biopsy which showed focal and segmental glomerulosclerosis and podocyte foot effacement. His proteinuria abated with high-dose steroids, although he has had a number of relapses of nephrotic syndrome since.

Conclusion: DN presents with slowly progressive albuminuria evolving from modestly elevated albuminuria, through proteinuria to nephrotic syndrome over a period of years, not weeks or months, so the abrupt onset of severe proteinuria warrants a renal biopsy, as this significantly altered management in this case.

Case 2

A 28-year-old lady, who had type 1 diabetes for 13 years, was referred to the Joint Renal Diabetes clinic with poorly controlled blood pressure, overt proteinuria and declining renal function (see ◘ Fig. 38.3). Aggressive control of blood pressure with five antihypertensive agents was instituted, and although glycaemic control remained poor, proteinuria was markedly reduced and renal function declined only slowly over the next 10 years. Unfortunately, serum potassium was measured at 6.1 mmol/L in the community, and her lisinopril was discontinued. This led to a marked increase in proteinuria by the time she attended for her next clinic review. Lisinopril was reintroduced but led to AKI and was again withdrawn in the community. Unfortunately, she rapidly progressed to ESRD. This is a good example of how effective RAAS blockade can be in patients with DN and heavy proteinuria. In our view, it may have been better to recheck potassium and if still high to introduce additional measures to control potassium such as a low-potassium diet, a potassium binder or sodium bicarbonate therapy (she was already on a thiazide diuretic), rather than to stop the ACE inhibitor as a first-line response.

Case 3

A 56-year-old man was referred to the Joint Renal Diabetes clinic with poorly controlled blood pressure, high-grade proteinuria and declining renal function (see ◘ Fig. 38.4). A diagnosis of progressive DN was made on clinical grounds, and he was referred to the cardiovascular risk clinic for rapid intensification of risk factor management over the first year. The lisinopril dose was maximised, and two additional antihypertensive agents were added, leading to a marked reduction in proteinuria. Lifestyle changes were adopted, including smoking cessation and exercise (walking 1.5 miles each day), and he has achieved 8 kg weight loss, all of which will have had beneficial effects on his cardiovascular risk factor profile. While his renal function continued to decline for the first 3 years, potentially due to the haemodynamic effects of blood pressure lowering and RAAS blockade, it has now been stable for the last 3 years. This is an example of successful multifactorial intervention – had the initial trajectory of decline in renal function been maintained, he would have required dialysis within 5 years of his first clinic attendance, whereas aggressive intervention has resulted in him remaining at stage 3 CKD.

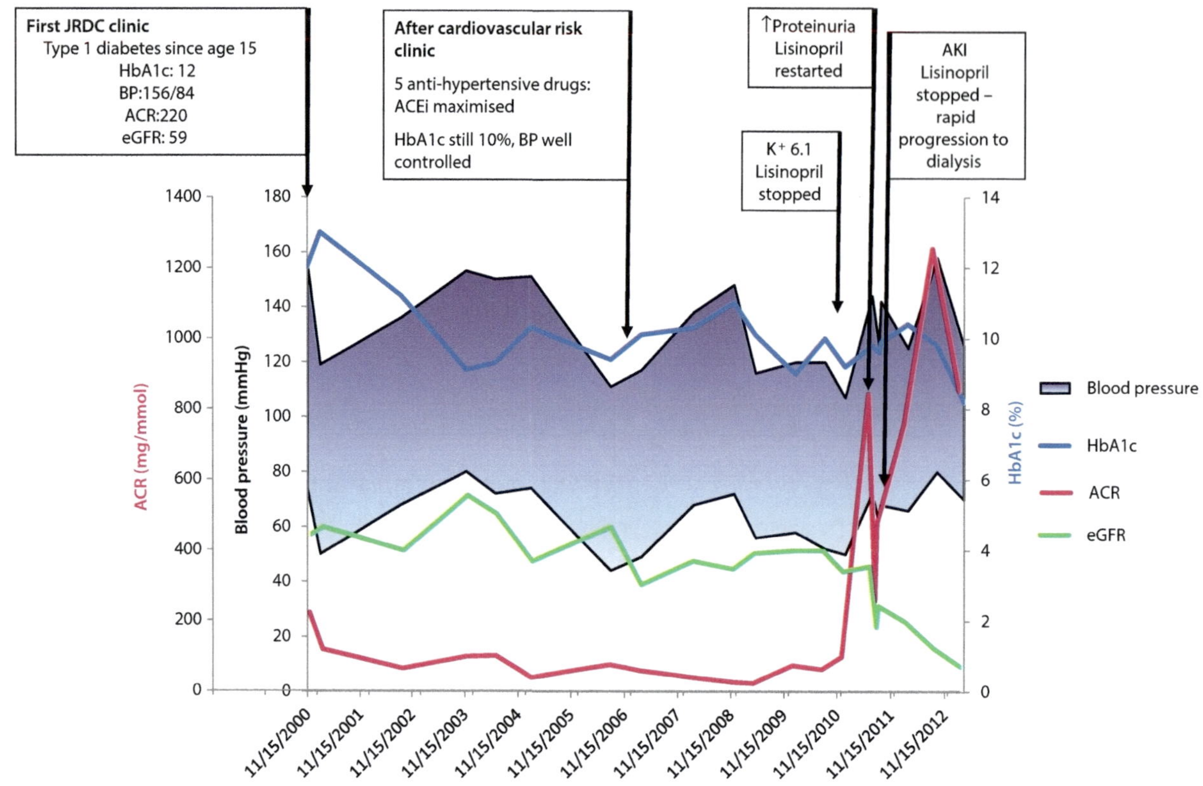

Fig. 38.3 Evolution of blood pressure, proteinuria and renal function in a young woman with type 1 diabetes, demonstrating how withdrawal of ACE inhibitor due to moderate hyperkalaemia resulted in a marked increase in proteinuria and a rapid decline in renal function

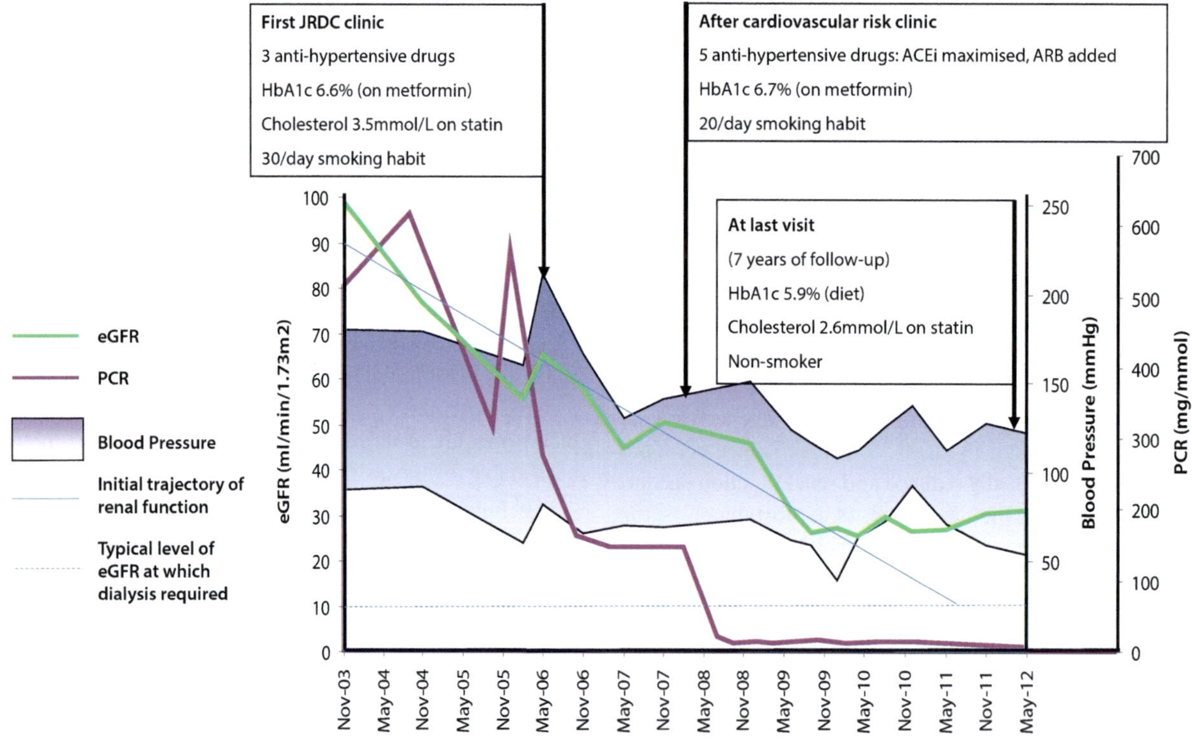

Fig. 38.4 Demonstration of how a multifactorial management strategy reduced proteinuria and led to long-term stability of renal function in a man with type 2 diabetes who had been referred to the Joint Renal Diabetes clinic with nephrotic-range proteinuria and declining renal function

- **Tips and Tricks**

1. RAAS blockade is much more effective when combined with a low-salt diet.
2. Advise a check of renal function within 7–10 days of starting therapy or increasing the dose of an ACE inhibitor/ARB.
3. Warn the patient to stop the drug transiently should they become unwell, e.g. fever, vomiting or diarrhoea.
4. In patients with heavy proteinuria, but who have a tendency for hyperkalaemia, try to maintain RAAS blockade by controlling potassium with a thiazide diuretic, or add sodium bicarbonate if the patient is acidotic. Provide advice on a low-potassium diet and consider the use of potassium binders such as patiromer or sodium zirconium.
5. Warn females of reproductive age to plan to stop ACE inhibitors/ARBs (in consultation with their primary care physician) if they are planning to get pregnant or, in the event of an unplanned pregnancy, to stop as soon as the pregnancy is confirmed.
6. Consider discontinuing therapy in patients with advanced nephropathy and resistant hyperkalaemia, to increase filtration in residual nephrons and delay the need for dialysis.
7. It is important to build a system that asks why is this patient with type 2 diabetes and proteinuria not on optimum treatment, e.g. a low-salt diet, RAAS inhibition, SGLT-2 inhibition and GLP-1 agonists, targeted blood pressure, smoking cessation and exercise programmes, etc.

? Chapter Review Questions

1. Is a biopsy ever required to make the diagnosis?
2. At what level of renal function should metformin be discontinued?
3. What should the target HbA1c be in patients who are on dialysis?

✓ Answers

1. A biopsy is rarely required to make the diagnosis of DN, but it is useful to exclude alternative diagnoses when the clinical course is atypical, in particular when the rate of rise in proteinuria or rate of deterioration in renal function is more rapid than would be expected.
2. This is a tricky balance between the increased risk of rare, but life-threatening, side effects, such as lactic acidosis, at lower levels of renal function and the risk of weight gain, worsening glycaemic control and potentially the need for insulin therapy following withdrawal of metformin. It is our practice not to withdraw metformin if eGFR >30 ml/min/1.73 m^2, unless it was close to that level and falling quickly. When eGFR falls below 30 ml/min/1.73 m^2, we carefully consider the options. However, if the rate of deterioration of renal function is very slow, we would consider reducing the dose and having a discussion with the patient explaining the risks and benefits. Importantly, if the patient is to remain on metformin, we routinely provide a 'sick day rules' card, advising them to stop metformin (and ACE inhibitors/ARBs, NSAIDs and diuretics) transiently if they become unwell.
3. The target HbA1c should be relaxed in patients on dialysis as there is an increased risk of hypoglycaemia due to the accumulation of oral anti-hyperglycaemic agents and endogenous or exogenous insulin, and this risk exceeds any potential long-term benefit of tight glycaemic control. The Association of British Clinical Diabetologists-Renal Association guidelines recommend an HbA1c target of 58–68 mmol/mol (7.5–8.5%).

References

1. Brancati FL, Whelton PK, Randall BL, Neaton JD, Stamler J, Klag MJ. Risk of end-stage renal disease in diabetes mellitus: a prospective cohort study of men screened for MRFIT. Multiple risk factor intervention trial. JAMA. 1997;278(23):2069–74.
2. USRDS 2016 annual data report: atlas of chronic kidney disease and end-stage renal disease in the United States. National Institutes of Health, National Institute of Diabetes and Digestive and Kidney Diseases, Bethesda, 2016.
3. UK Renal Registry annual report 2016. https://www.renalregorg/reports/2016-nineteenth-annual-report/.
4. Nathan DM, Zinman B, Cleary PA, et al. Modern-day clinical course of type 1 diabetes mellitus after 30 years' duration: the diabetes control and complications trial/epidemiology of diabetes interventions and complications and Pittsburgh epidemiology of diabetes complications experience (1983-2005). Arch Int Med. 2009;169(14):1307–16.
5. Hallan SI, Coresh J, Astor BC, et al. International comparison of the relationship of chronic kidney disease prevalence and ESRD risk. J Am Soc Nephrol. 2006;17(8):2275–84.
6. Hossain P, Kawar B, El Nahas M. Obesity and diabetes in the developing worldDOUBLEHYPHENa growing challenge. New Engl J Med. 2007;356(3):213–5.
7. Jafar TH. The growing burden of chronic kidney disease in Pakistan. New Engl J Med. 2006;354(10):995–7.
8. Ordunez-Garcia P, Munoz JL, Pedraza D, Espinosa-Brito A, Silva LC, Cooper RS. Success in control of hypertension in a low-resource setting: the Cuban experience. J Hypertension. 2006;24(5):845–9.
9. Pavkov ME, Knowler WC, Hanson RL, Nelson RG. Diabetic nephropathy in American Indians, with a special emphasis on the Pima Indians. Curr Diab Rep. 2008;8(6):486–93.
10. Freire MB, Ferreira SR, Vivolo MA, Oliveira JM, Zanella MT. Familial hypertension and albuminuria in normotensive type I diabetic patients. Hypertension. 1994;23(1 Suppl):I256–8.
11. The Diabetes Control and Complications Trial Research Group. The effect of intensive treatment of diabetes on the

development and progression of long-term complications in insulin-dependent diabetes mellitus. The Diabetes Control and Complications Trial Research Group. New Engl J Med. 1993;329(14):977–86.
12. de Boer IH, Sun W, Cleary PA, et al. Intensive diabetes therapy and glomerular filtration rate in type 1 diabetes. New Engl J Med. 2011;365(25):2366–76.
13. Intensive blood-glucose control with sulphonylureas or insulin compared with conventional treatment and risk of complications in patients with type 2 diabetes (UKPDS 33). UK Prospective Diabetes Study (UKPDS) Group. Lancet. 1998;352(9131):837–53.
14. UK Prospective Diabetes Study Group. Tight blood pressure control and risk of macrovascular and microvascular complications in type 2 diabetes: UKPDS 38. UK Prospective Diabetes Study Group. Brit Med J. 1998;317(7160):703–13.
15. Beroniade VC, Lefebvre R, Falardeau P. Unilateral nodular diabetic glomerulosclerosis: recurrence of an experiment of nature. Am J Nephrol. 1987;7(1):55–9.
16. Miller JA. Impact of hyperglycemia on the renin angiotensin system in early human type 1 diabetes mellitus. J Am Soc Nephrol. 1999;10(8):1778–85.
17. Ketteler M, Noble NA, Border WA. Transforming growth factor-beta and angiotensin II: the missing link from glomerular hyperfiltration to glomerulosclerosis? Annu Rev Physiol. 1995;57:279–95.
18. Pohl MA, Blumenthal S, Cordonnier DJ, et al. Independent and additive impact of blood pressure control and angiotensin II receptor blockade on renal outcomes in the irbesartan diabetic nephropathy trial: clinical implications and limitations. J Am Soc Nephrol. 2005;16(10):3027–37.
19. Mogensen CE, Christensen CK, Vittinghus E. The stages in diabetic renal disease. With emphasis on the stage of incipient diabetic nephropathy. Diabetes. 1983;32(Suppl 2):64–78.
20. Lurbe E, Redon J, Kesani A, et al. Increase in nocturnal blood pressure and progression to microalbuminuria in type 1 diabetes. New Engl J Med. 2002;347(11):797–805.
21. Gilbert RE, Cooper ME. The tubulointerstitium in progressive diabetic kidney disease: more than an aftermath of glomerular injury? Kidney Int. 1999;56(5):1627–37.
22. Lopes de Faria JB, Moura LA, Lopes de Faria SR, Ramos OL, Pereira AB. Glomerular hematuria in diabetics. Clin Nephrol. 1988;30(3):117–21.
23. Matsumura N, Hanatani M, Nishino T, et al. The clinico-pathological significance of hematuria in diabetics. Nihon Jinzo Gakkai Shi. 1994;36(9):1036–45.
24. Caramori ML, Fioretto P, Mauer M. Low glomerular filtration rate in normoalbuminuric type 1 diabetic patients: an indicator of more advanced glomerular lesions. Diabetes. 2003;52(4):1036–40.
25. Conway BR, Manoharan D, Manoharan D, et al. Measuring urinary tubular biomarkers in type 2 diabetes does not add prognostic value beyond established risk factors. Kidney Int. 2012;82(7):812–8.
26. KDIGO 2020 Clinical Practice Guideline for Diabetes Management in Chronic Kidney DiseaseKidney Disease: Improving Global Outcomes (KDIGO) Diabetes Work Group practice guideline. 98(4 Suppl):S1–S115, 1 Oct 2020. https://www.kidney-international.org/article/S0085-2538(20)30718-3/fulltext.
27. Perkins BA, Ficociello LH, Silva KH, Finkelstein DM, Warram JH, Krolewski AS. Regression of microalbuminuria in type 1 diabetes. New Engl J Med. 2003;348(23): 2285–93.
28. Fioretto P, Steffes MW, Sutherland DER, Goetz FC, Mauer M. Reversal of lesions of diabetic nephropathy after pancreas transplantations. New Engl J Med. 1998;339:69–75.
29. Scott LJ, Warram JH, Hanna LS, Laffel LM, Ryan L, Krolewski AS. A nonlinear effect of hyperglycemia and current cigarette smoking are major determinants of the onset of microalbuminuria in type 1 diabetes. Diabetes. 2001;50(12):2842–9.
30. de Boer IH, Sibley SD, Kestenbaum B, et al. Central obesity, incident microalbuminuria, and change in creatinine clearance in the epidemiology of diabetes interventions and complications study. J Am Soc Nephrol. 2007;18(1):235–43.
31. Schauer PR, Bhatt DL, Kirwan JP, et al. Bariatric surgery versus intensive medical therapy for diabetes – 5-year outcomes. New Engl J Med. 2017;376(7):641–51.
32. Slagman MC, Waanders F, Hemmelder MH, et al. Moderate dietary sodium restriction added to angiotensin converting enzyme inhibition compared with dual blockade in lowering proteinuria and blood pressure: randomised controlled trial. Brit Med J. 2011;343:4366.
33. Action to Control Cardiovascular Risk in Diabetes Study Group, Gerstein HC, Miller ME, Byington RP, et al. Effects of intensive glucose lowering in type 2 diabetes. New Engl J Med. 2008;358(24):2545–59.
34. Association of British Clinical Diabetologists-Renal Association. Managing hyperglycaemia in patients with diabetes and diabetic nephropathy-chronic kidney disease. British Journal of Diabetes. 2018;18(2):78–89.
35. Buse JB, Weler D, Tsapai A, et al. 2019 update to management of hyperglycaemia in type 2 diabetes 2018: a consensus report by the American Diabetes Association (ADA) and the European Association for the Study of diabetes (EASD). Diabetologia. 2020;63:221–8.
36. Effect of intensive blood-glucose control with metformin on complications in overweight patients with type 2 diabetes (UKPDS 34). UK Prospective Diabetes Study (UKPDS) Group. Lancet 1998;352(9131):854–65.
37. Lipska KJ, Bailey CJ, Inzucchi SE. Use of metformin in the setting of mild-to-moderate renal insufficiency. Diabetes Care. 2011;34(6):1431–7.
38. Colhoun HM, Livingstone SJ, Looker HC, et al. Hospitalised hip fracture risk with rosiglitazone and pioglitazone use compared with other glucose-lowering drugs. Diabetologia. 2012;55(11).:2929–.
39. Marso SP, Daniels GH, Brown-Frandsen K, et al. Liraglutide and cardiovascular outcomes in type 2 diabetes. New Engl J Med. 2016;375(4):311–22.
40. Mann JFE, Orsted DD, Brown-Frandsen K, et al. Liraglutide and renal outcomes in type 2 diabetes. New Engl J Med. 2017;377(9):839–48.
41. Kristensen SL, Rorth R, Jhund PS. Cardiovascular mortality and kidney outcomes with GLP-1 receptor agonists in patients with type 2 diabetes: a systematic review and meta-analysis of cardiovascular outcome trials. Lancet Diabetes Endocrinol. 2019;7:776–85.
42. Zinman B, Wanner C, Lachin JM, et al. Empagliflozin, cardiovascular outcomes, and mortality in type 2 diabetes. New Engl J Med. 2015;373(22):2117–28.
43. Neal B, Perkovic V, Mahaffey KW, et al. Canagliflozin and cardiovascular and renal events in type 2 diabetes. New Engl J Med. 2017;377(7):644–57.
44. Wanner C, Inzucchi SE, Lachin JM, et al. Empagliflozin and progression of kidney disease in type 2 diabetes. New Engl J Med. 2016;375(4):323–34.

45. Perkovic V. Canagliflozin and renal outcomes in type 2 diabetes and nephropathy. New Engl J Med. 2019;380(24):2295–306.
46. Group DER, de Boer IH, Sun W, et al. Intensive diabetes therapy and glomerular filtration rate in type 1 diabetes. New Engl J Med. 2011;365(25):2366–76.
47. Holman RR, Paul SK, Bethel MA, Matthews DR, Neil HA. 10-year follow-up of intensive glucose control in type 2 diabetes. New Engl J Med. 2008;359(15):1577–89.
48. Holman RR, Paul SK, Bethel MA, Neil HA, Matthews DR. Long-term follow-up after tight control of blood pressure in type 2 diabetes. New Engl J Med. 2008;359(15):1565–76.
49. Peterson JC, Adler S, Burkart JM, et al. Blood pressure control, proteinuria, and the progression of renal disease. The Modification of Diet in Renal Disease Study. Annals Int Med. 1995;123(10):754–62.
50. de Zeeuw D, Remuzzi G, Parving HH, et al. Proteinuria, a target for renoprotection in patients with type 2 diabetic nephropathy: lessons from RENAAL. Kidney Int. 2004;65(6):2309–20.
51. Atkins RC, Briganti EM, Lewis JB, et al. Proteinuria reduction and progression to renal failure in patients with type 2 diabetes mellitus and overt nephropathy. Am J Kidney Dis. 2005;45(2):281–7.
52. Lewis EJ, Hunsicker LG, Clarke WR, et al. Renoprotective effect of the angiotensin-receptor antagonist irbesartan in patients with nephropathy due to type 2 diabetes. New Engl J Med. 2001;345(12):851–60.
53. Ruggenenti P, Perticucci E, Cravedi P, et al. Role of remission clinics in the longitudinal treatment of CKD. J Am Soc Nephrol. 2008;19(6):1213–24.
54. Strippoli GF, Craig M, Schena FP, Craig JC. Antihypertensive agents for primary prevention of diabetic nephropathy. J Am Soc Nephrol. 2005;16(10):3081–91.
55. Mauer M, Zinman B, Gardiner R, et al. Renal and retinal effects of enalapril and losartan in type 1 diabetes. New Engl J Med. 2009;361(1):40–51.
56. Bangalore S, Fakheri R, Toklu B, Messerli FH. Diabetes mellitus as a compelling indication for use of renin angiotensin system blockers: systematic review and meta-analysis of randomized trials. Brit Med J. 2016;352:438.
57. The ACE inhibitors in Diabetic Nephropathy Trials Group. Should all patients with type 1 diabetes mellitus and microalbuminuria receive angiotensin-converting enzyme inhibitors? A meta-analysis of individual patient data. Annals Int Med. 2001;134(5):370–9.
58. Parving HH, Lehnert H, Brochner-Mortensen J, Gomis R, Andersen S, Arner P. The effect of irbesartan on the development of diabetic nephropathy in patients with type 2 diabetes. New Engl J Med. 2001;345(12):870–8.
59. Barnett AH, Bain SC, Bouter P, et al. Angiotensin-receptor blockade versus converting-enzyme inhibition in type 2 diabetes and nephropathy. New Engl J Med. 2004;351(19):1952–61.
60. Hou FF, Zhang X, Zhang GH, et al. Efficacy and safety of benazepril for advanced chronic renal insufficiency. New Engl J Med. 2006;354(2):131–40.
61. Ahmed AK, Kamath NS, El Kossi M, El Nahas AM. The impact of stopping inhibitors of the renin-angiotensin system in patients with advanced chronic kidney disease. Nephrol Dial Transplant. 2010;25(12):3977–82.
62. Weir MR, Bakris GL, Bushinsky DA, et al. Patiromer in patients with kidney disease and hyperkalemia receiving RAAS inhibitors. New Engl J Med. 2015;372(3):211–21.
63. Bakris GL, Weir MR. Angiotensin-converting enzyme inhibitor-associated elevations in serum creatinine: is this a cause for concern? Arch Int Med. 2000;160(5):685–93.
64. Mogensen CE, Neldam S, Tikkanen I, et al. Randomised controlled trial of dual blockade of renin-angiotensin system in patients with hypertension, microalbuminuria, and non-insulin dependent diabetes: the candesartan and lisinopril microalbuminuria (CALM) study. Brit Med J. 2000;321(7274):1440–4.
65. Mann JF, Schmieder RE, McQueen M, et al. Renal outcomes with telmisartan, ramipril, or both, in people at high vascular risk (the ONTARGET study): a multicentre, randomised, double-blind, controlled trial. Lancet. 2008;372(9638):547–53.
66. Fried LF, Emanuele N, Zhang JH, et al. Combined angiotensin inhibition for the treatment of diabetic nephropathy. New Engl J Med. 2013;369(20):1892–903.
67. Parving HH, Persson F, Lewis JB, Lewis EJ. Hollenberg NK Aliskiren combined with losartan in type 2 diabetes and nephropathy. New Engl J Med. 2008;358(23):2433–46.
68. Parving HH, Brenner BM, McMurray JJ, et al. Cardiorenal end points in a trial of aliskiren for type 2 diabetes. New Engl J Med. 2012;367(23):2204–13.
69. Epstein M, Williams GH, Weinberger M, et al. Selective aldosterone blockade with eplerenone reduces albuminuria in patients with type 2 diabetes. Clin J Am Soc Nephrol. 2006;1(5):940–51.
70. Bakris GL, Agarwal R, Chan JC, et al. Effect of finerenone on albuminuria in patients with diabetic nephropathy: a randomized clinical trial. JAMA. 2015;314(9):884–94.
71. Juurlink DN, Mamdani MM, Lee DS, et al. Rates of hyperkalemia after publication of the Randomized Aldactone Evaluation Study. New Engl J Med. 2004;351(6):543–51.
72. Bakris GL, Copley JB, Vicknair N, Sadler R, Leurgans S. Calcium channel blockers versus other antihypertensive therapies on progression of NIDDM associated nephropathy. Kidney Int. 1996;50(5):1641–50.
73. Bakris GL, Barnhill BW, Sadler R. Treatment of arterial hypertension in diabetic humans: importance of therapeutic selection. Kidney Int. 1992;41(4):912–9.
74. Adler AI, Stevens RJ, Manley SE, Bilous RW, Cull CA, Holman RR. Development and progression of nephropathy in type 2 diabetes: the United Kingdom Prospective Diabetes Study (UKPDS 64). Kidney Int. 2003;63(1):225–32.
75. Colhoun HM, Betteridge DJ, Durrington PN, et al. Primary prevention of cardiovascular disease with atorvastatin in type 2 diabetes in the Collaborative Atorvastatin Diabetes Study (CARDS): multicentre randomised placebo-controlled trial. Lancet. 2004;364(9435):685–96.
76. Baigent C, Landray MJ, Reith C, et al. The effects of lowering LDL cholesterol with simvastatin plus ezetimibe in patients with chronic kidney disease (Study of Heart and Renal Protection): a randomised placebo-controlled trial. Lancet. 2011;377(9784):2181–92.
77. Gaede P, Lund-Andersen H, Parving HH, Pedersen O. Effect of a multifactorial intervention on mortality in type 2 diabetes. New Engl J Med. 2008;358(6):580–91.

78. Joss N, Ferguson C, Brown C, Deighan CJ, Paterson KR, Boulton-Jones JM. Intensified treatment of patients with type 2 diabetes mellitus and overt nephropathy. QJM. 2004;97(4):219–27.
79. Rayner HC, Hollingworth L, Higgins R, Dodds S. Systematic kidney disease management in a population with diabetes mellitus: turning the tide of kidney failure. BMJ Qual Saf. 2012;20:903–10.
80. Scottish Renal Registry Report 2016. http://www.srrscotnhsuk/Publications/docs/scottish-renal-registry-report-2016-web-pdf?34.
81. Williams ME, Lacson E Jr, Teng M, Ofsthun N, Lazarus JM. Hemodialyzed type I and type II diabetic patients in the US: characteristics, glycemic control, and survival. Kidney Int. 2006;70(8):1503–9.
82. Kalantar-Zadeh K, Kopple JD, Regidor DL, et al. A1C and survival in maintenance hemodialysis patients. Diabetes Care. 2007;30(5):1049–55.
83. Wolfe RA, Ashby VB, Milford EL, et al. Comparison of mortality in all patients on dialysis, patients on dialysis awaiting transplantation, and recipients of a first cadaveric transplant. New Engl J Med. 1999;341(23):1725–30.
84. Morath C, Zeier M, Dohler B, Schmidt J, Nawroth PP, Opelz G. Metabolic control improves long-term renal allograft and patient survival in type 1 diabetes. J Am Soc Nephrol. 2008;19(8):1557–63.
85. Heerspink HJL, Stefánsson BV, Correa-Rotter R, Chertow GM, Greene T, Hou F-F, Mann JFE, McMurray JJV, Lindberg M, Rossing P, Sjöström D, Toto RD, Langkilde A-M, Wheeler DC, DAPA-CKD Trial Committees and Investigators. Dapagliflozin in patients with chronic kidney disease. N Engl J Med. 2020;383(15):1436–46. https://doi.org/10.1056/NEJMoa2024816.

38

The Endocrine System and the Kidney

Rachel K. Y. Hung, Stephanie M. Y. Chong, and Mark Harber

Contents

M. Harber (ed.), *Primer on Nephrology*, https://doi.org/10.1007/978-3-030-76419-7_39

Learning Objectives

1. The effects of renal diseases and medications on endocrine hormones require close monitoring especially in patients with CKD.
2. Endocrine disorders and their treatments can impact on the kidneys and vice versa.
3. Strategies and protocols for combined and coordinated care of patients with endocrine and renal disease between both specialties are required for optimisation of patient management and outcome.

39.1 Introduction

The endocrine functions of the kidney are predictably impaired with progressive renal impairment. However, other non-renal-derived hormones are also influenced by changes, which occur in CKD (Table 39.1). The mechanisms of endocrine abnormalities include altered hormone binding and tissue responsiveness, decreased synthesis and reduced metabolic clearance of hormones due to the failing kidney and alterations of homeostatic signalling.

Conversely, disorders and treatment of endocrine disease can impact on the kidney. The most devastating of these is diabetes, which has a profound global impact and is currently the commonest cause of ESRD in many countries. Approximately 40% of affected individuals will develop diabetic nephropathy, which manifests commonly as albuminuria, impaired GFR or both [1, 2]. This is covered extensively in the chapter 'Diabetes and the Kidney'.

Table 39.1 Mechanism of endocrine dysfunction in CKD

Mechanism	Impact
Increased circulatory hormone	**Decreased GFR resulting in impaired renal clearance** • Glucagon • Fasting levels found to be 5× higher in patients on HD than controls • Prolactin • 5–6× higher prolactin levels seen when eGFR<15 • Insulin • 30–80% of endogenous insulin is filtered in the kidney; reduced clearance occurs when eGFR falls below 40 • Growth hormone • 2.5× higher mean GH levels seen in advanced CKD, with a 2× longer endogenous GH mean half-life • Leptin **Increased secretion of hormone** • Parathyroid hormone • Growth hormone **Accumulation of metabolites** • Parathyroid hormone • Calcitonin • Prolactin
Decreased circulatory hormone	**Decreased secretion by the kidney** • 1,25-dihydroxy vitamin D3 • Erythropoietin **Decreased secretion by non-renal endocrine glands** • Testosterone • Oestrogen • Progesterone
Decrease in target organ hormone sensitivity	**Altered target responses** • Growth hormone • Insulin • Parathyroid hormone • Erythropoietin • 1,25-dihydroxy vitamin D3

39

39.2 Pharmacotherapy Interactions in Kidney and Endocrine Diseases

Drugs used in treating endocrine disorders can impact on the kidneys and vice versa. Examples of such interactions are listed below in Tables 39.2 and 39.3.

39.3 Impact of Renal Disease on the Endocrine System

39.3.1 Nephrotic Syndrome

39.3.1.1 Thyroid

The nephrotic syndrome is associated with urinary loss of protein macromolecules including albumin and hormone-binding proteins leading to metabolic derangements including thyroid, vitamin D and calcium metabolism [3]. Approximately 50% of nephrotic patients with a preserved glomerular filtration rate will have low total thyroxine(T4) concentrations due to urinary losses of thyroxine-binding globulin (TBG) and other thyroid hormone-binding proteins (transthyretin and albumin) [4, 5]. Serum triiodothyronine (T3) may also be low due to decreased binding. Despite this, the physiologically important serum free T4, T3 and thyrotropin (TSH) concentrations are usually normal, with a normal T3:T4 ratio; hence nephrotic patients are typically clinically euthyroid. Conversely, patients who are on thyroxine therapy or have limited thyroid reserves may become hypothyroid due to urinary losses of T4. In addition,

Table 39.2 Impact of drugs used in endocrinology on the kidneys

Drug	Use	Mechanism	Kidney disease
Propylthio-uracil	To treat hyperthyroidism	Unclear; likely to trigger immune complex deposition	ANCA-associated vasculitis Acute interstitial nephritis Lupus nephritis
GnRH agonists[a]	Prostate cancer	Unclear but likely causes metabolic changes leading to glomerular injury; loss of protective vasodilation effect of testosterone	AKI CKD
Iodinated contrast	Used in various radiological examinations and interventional procedures	Unclear, but likely due to haemodynamic effects of contrast media, effects of reactive oxygen species and direct tubular cellular toxicity	AKI (contrast-induced nephropathy)

[a]To date only reported when used as androgen deprivation therapy in men with prostate cancer

Table 39.3 Impact of drugs used in renal diseases on the endocrine system

Drug	Use	Mechanism	Endocrine function
Alemtuzumab	Induction agent for kidney transplantation	↑ Risk of autoimmunity; emergence of TSH receptor antibodies	Autoimmune thyroiditis
Thiazides	Diuretic	↓ Urinary calcium excretion	Hypercalcaemia in those with hyperparathyroidism
Glucocorticoids (high dose)	Immunosuppressant for kidney transplantation and various renal diseases	↓ TSH secretion ↓ TBG levels	↓ T4, T3 and TSH by 18–50%
Co-trimoxazole	Prophylaxis against PCP for kidney transplant recipients	↓ Thyroglobulin iodination ↑ Insulin release from pancreatic cells (sulphonamide mimics sulphonylureas)	↓ T4 levels by 5–10% Hypoglycaemia (especially if renal impairment present)
Heparin	Anticoagulant during haemodialysis	Activates lipoprotein lipase ↑ Serum free fatty acids concentration ↑ Displacement of T4 from TBG	Spurious ↑ free T4 by 130–520%
Furosemide (high dose)	Loop diuretic	↓ T4 binding of TBG	Spurious ↓ FT4 and T4 by 10–30%
Iodinated contrast	Used in various radiological examinations and interventional procedures	Exposure to large iodide load; iodine used as substrate for thyroid hormone production	Thyroid storm Acute destructive thyroiditis

nephrotic syndrome has been associated with autoimmune thyroid diseases, such as Graves' disease, where antithyroid antibodies have been demonstrated within glomerular immune deposits. Both Hashimoto's thyroiditis and Graves' disease have also been associated with membranous nephropathy.

Annual thyroid function assessment is recommended in nephrotic individuals when first diagnosed, especially since progressive reduction in renal clearance may exacerbate thyroid dysfunction. Steroids given to nephrotic patients can also lower serum T3 and TSH concentrations, with an increase in rT3 concentrations. Serum T4 is the best marker for thyroid status in these patients and, if low, should be treated as clinically significant hypothyroidism.

39.3.1.2 Vitamin D and Calcium

Urinary losses of vitamin D-binding protein (VDBP) by the nephrotic glomeruli [6] lead to concurrent renal excretion of calcidiol (the precursor of calcitriol that is primarily bound to VDBP). However, the effect of these changes of vitamin D on calcium homeostasis is uncertain. Whilst this leads to reduced total serum calcium levels, physiologically important free calcium concentration remains normal due to concurrent hypoalbuminaemia resulting in a reduction in calcium binding capacity. However, some patients may develop hypocalcaemia secondary to low serum calcitriol concentrations. These patients exhibit a fall in ionised calcium concentrations and an elevation in serum parathyroid concentrations that can subsequently lead to bone disease characterised by mixed osteomalacia and osteitis fibrosa [7, 8].

39.3.1.3 Glucocorticoid Metabolism

Urinary losses of cortisol-binding globulin (CBG) may lead to reduced serum cortisol in nephrotic patients [9]. The ACTH simulation test in these patients may hence be affected due to low cortisol levels associated with urinary losses of CBG. However, symptomatic hypocortisolism does not occur as the percentage of unbound cortisol is increased and serum free cortisol levels are normal.

39.3.2 Chronic Kidney Disease

39.3.2.1 Hypothalamic-Pituitary-Gonadal Axis

CKD causes derangement of the hypothalamic-pituitary-gonadal axis and affects males and females differently. These are summarised in ◘ Table 39.4. The effects of CKD on the hypothalamic-pituitary-gonadal axis in women are illustrated in ◘ Fig. 39.1.

◘ **Table 39.4** The effects of CKD on the hypothalamic-pituitary-gonadal axis

Hormone	Female	Male	Mechanism
FSH	N	↑	Males: impaired spermatogenesis Females: normal in premenopausal females but with a decreased FSH/LH ratio
LH	↑	↑	• Loss of normal pulsatile release • Basal plasma concentrations raised due to decreased renal clearance and catabolism Males: low testosterone levels inhibit GnRH Females: impaired oestradiol feedback causes LH surge leading to anovulation and infertility
Prolactin	↑	↑	Decreased renal clearance Inadequate dopaminergic inhibition Prolactin accumulation inhibits pulsatile secretion of GnRH • Males: reduced testosterone synthesis • Females: amenorrhoea, lowers levels of oestradiol
Oestradiol	↓	N	• Levels normally preserved or low but will be Lower with hyperprolactinaemia
Progesterone	↓	–	• Release during second half of menstrual cycle reduced due to defective follicle luteinisation
Testosterone	–	↓	• Reduced due to defective release of GnRH and LH

39

39.3.3 The Somatotropic Axis

39.3.3.1 Growth Hormone (GH) and Insulin-Like Growth Factor

CKD induces a state of GH resistance and not GH deficiency. Decreased numbers of GH receptors in target organs and uraemia-related alterations in intracellular signal transduction at the post-receptor level lead to GH resistance [10]. Concurrent increase of GH secretion in response to this and reduced clearance due to a falling GFR cause elevated serum GH concentrations in children and adults with CKD. Changes in nutritional intake and metabolic acidosis can also affect GH secretion. Insulin-like growth factor-1 (IGF-1) is stimulated by GH and is mainly secreted by the liver. Its free concentration in serum decreases with progression of CKD mainly due to the elevation of IGF-binding proteins -1, -2, -4 and -6 that binds free IGF-1. The overall contribution of GH to growth retardation in children with CKD is difficult to quantify as growth retardation in CKD is multifactorial including inadequate protein and calorie intake, persistent metabolic acidosis, calcitriol deficiency, renal osteodystrophy, uraemic toxins and drug toxicity.

39.3.3.2 Thyroid Function

Thyroid dysfunction and goitre development are more prevalent in patients with CKD due to uraemia-impaired peripheral metabolism of thyroid hormones [5]. Subclinical hypothyroidism is the most common thyroid disorder in CKD patients with low T3 levels (◘ Table 39.5). This is secondary to impaired conversion of T4 to T3 due to metabolic acidosis and malnutrition. Mineral deficiencies can also reduce T3 levels as GFR declines; selenium modulates the conversion of T4 to T3 (via iodothyronine deiodinase activity)

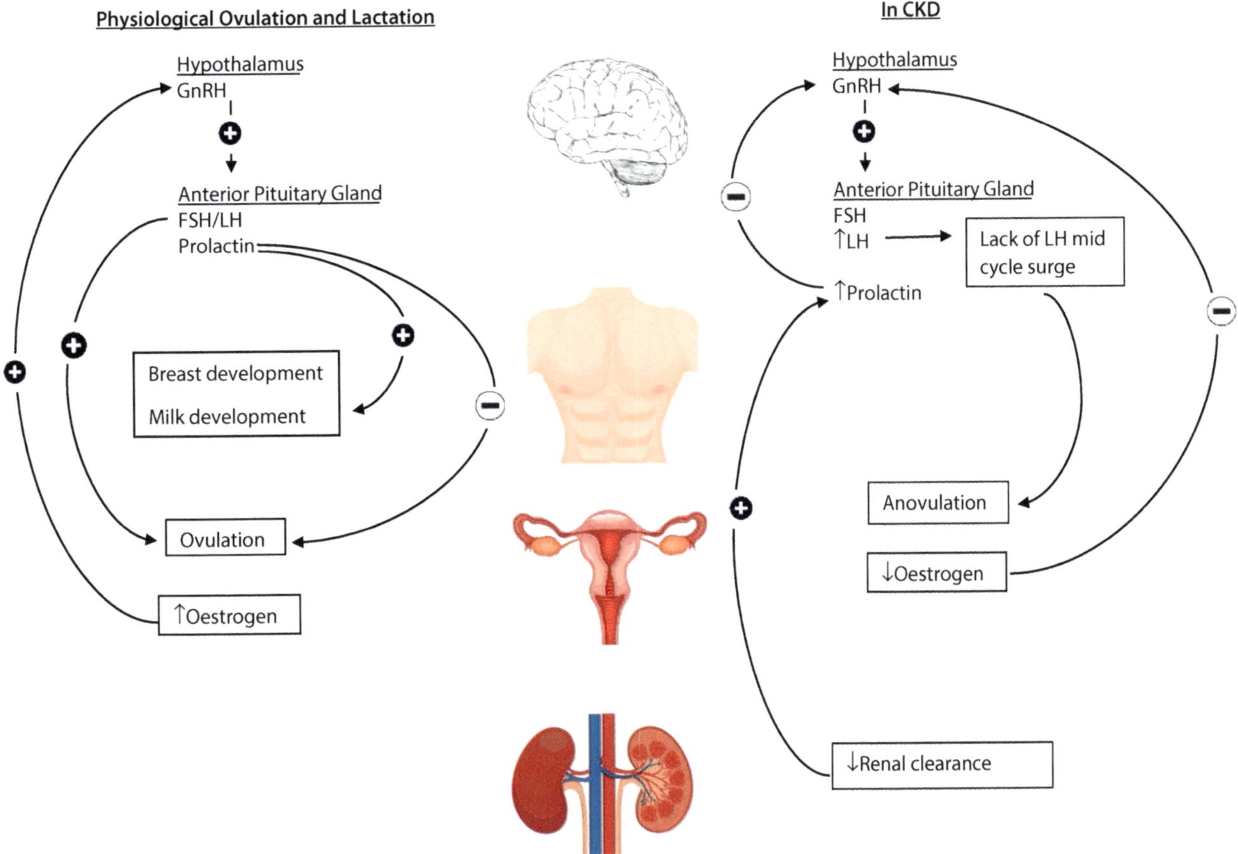

Fig. 39.1 Effects of CKD on hormones of the hypothalamic-pituitary-gonadal axis

Table 39.5 Thyroid function changes in patients with CKD, other chronic diseases and primary hyperthyroidism and hypothyroidism

	TSH	T4	T3	rT3
Chronic kidney disease	N	N, ↓	↓	N
Other chronic disease (non-kidney/thyroid)	N	N, ↓	↓	↑
Primary hypothyroidism	↑	↓	↓	N, ↓
Primary hyperthyroidism	↓	↑	↑	N, ↑

and is a problem particularly in chronic haemodialysis patients. However, the serum concentration of reverse T3 (rT3), an isomer of T3, remains normal despite decreased renal clearance in CKD patients as compared to patients with other non-renal chronic diseases. One possible explanation could be increased cellular uptake and redistribution of rT3 from the vascular to extravascular space [11] in CKD patients. Replacement of selenium in chronic haemodialysis patients likewise does not affect thyroid hormone profile. TSH concentrations tend to be normal in CKD patients despite a tendency of lower T3 and T4 concentrations. This is due to several factors: dysregulation of the hypothalamic-pituitary-thyroid axis where the pituitary receptor response to TRH is blunted resulting in decreased TSH production, impaired renal clearance leading to prolongation of TSH half-life and a disruption of the normal daily rhythm of TSH release (consisting of a peak in late evenings and early mornings) with a concomitant reduction in nocturnal TSH surge [11, 12].

39.3.3.3 Primary Hyperthyroidism and Hypothyroidism

The prevalence of hyperthyroidism in CKD patients is similar to that of the general population. Hyper- and hypothyroidism are associated with several renal abnormalities (Fig. 39.2). When hyperthyroidism is treated, the GFR reverts to normal. However, if left untreated, hyperthyroidism can accelerate CKD via increasing intra-glomerular pressure, proteinuria, free radical generation and RAAS activation predisposing to renal

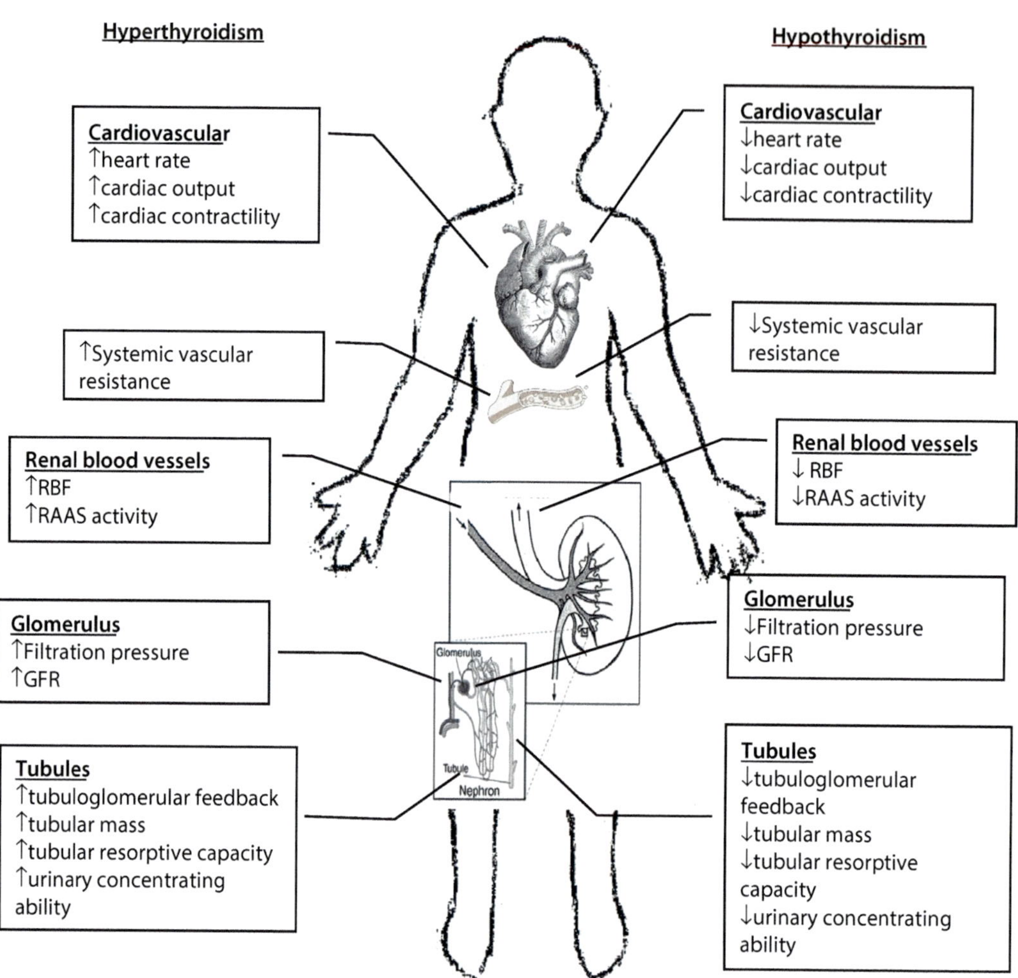

Fig. 39.2 Haemodynamic and renal effects of thyroid underactivity and overactivity

39

fibrosis. Hyperthyroidism also contributes to anaemia and can lead to EPO resistance.

The prevalence of hypothyroidism increases from 5% to 23.1% when GFRs of >90 mls/min/1.73 m^3 fall to <30 mls/min/1.73 m^3. This is likely due to a reduction in iodide excretion, resulting in an increase in serum inorganic iodide level and thyroid gland iodine content leading to gland enlargement, goitre development and hypothyroidism in patients with ESRD. There is an increased frequency of thyroid nodules and thyroid carcinoma, which may be associated with secondary hyperparathyroidism, a common condition in CKD patients [13]. Hypothyroidism is also associated with higher mortality in dialysis patients due to hypothyroid-induced cardiovascular disease.

Chronic haemodialysis patients may have low thyroid hormone levels with maintained euthyroid state due to a compensatory influence of cellular transport of thyroid hormones. A 24-hour transient increase in T4 occurs due to the use of heparin as an anticoagulant, which competes with T4 at the binding site of the hormone-binding protein. Evaluation of thyroid function should be done before heparin administration, prior to commencing the dialysis session. In patients on peritoneal dialysis (PD), TBG, T4 and T3 are lost in the PD effluent. However, losses are relatively minor (10% of T4 and 1% of T3) and easily compensated for.

39.3.3.4 Insulin and Glucagon

The kidney removes about 30–80% of insulin per day. Approximately 60% of insulin is cleared via glomerular filtration and 40% by extraction from the peritubular vessels. When GFR falls below 40 mls/min/1.73 m^3, insulin clearance is reduced thus decreasing the insulin requirement in diabetic patients with CKD [14]. Peripheral insulin resistance also worsens with the fall of GFR and is improved once renal replacement therapy is started. The pathogenesis of insulin resistance is postulated to be due to metabolic acidosis, chronic inflammation, increased RAAS activity and also increased concentration of glucagon and growth hormone in patients with CKD [15].

39.3.4 Renin Angiotensin Axis

Renal artery stenosis is the archetypal endocrine renal disease. Although other organs are essential for production of angiotensinogen (liver) and activation (lung), the entire cascade is precipitated by renin production from the juxtaglomerular apparatus in the kidney in response to a reduction in blood flow, for example, as a result of progressive arterial occlusion from atherosclerotic disease or fibromuscular dysplasia. The consequence is a rise in angiotensin II and aldosterone, which drive salt and water retention and systemic vasoconstriction and hypertension.

39.3.5 Hypothalamic-Pituitary-Adrenal Axis (HPA)

Patients with CKD take glucocorticoids for various reasons including treatment for their primary renal disease, post transplantation or other systemic diseases. Exogenous glucocorticoids exert negative feedback to the HPA axis by suppressing corticotropin-releasing hormone (CRH) secretion that in turn suppresses corticotropin (ACTH) secretion. Chronic usage leads to adrenal atrophy and loss of cortisol secretory capability. Abrupt cessation or too rapid withdrawal of glucocorticoids can cause symptoms of adrenal insufficiency, which may manifest as an Addisonian crisis (see ◘ Fig. 39.3 below).

More commonly, patients can incur functional adrenal insufficiency when steroids are not boosted at the time of an intercurrent illness or stressful events, e.g. undergoing surgery. The symptoms and signs tend to be much subtler particularly in the setting of CKD where the patient is somewhat protected against mineralocorticoid insufficiency and may simply manifest as loose stools, general malaise and slow recovery after an illness. Cortisol stress tests are complicated by ongoing steroid ingestion, and in practical terms it is often simpler to give a short trial of boosted (2–3 times normal dose) steroids.

In a proportion of renal patients with nephrectomies, particularly in those with ADPKD, it is important to document if the adrenal gland was inadvertently removed at the time of surgery. The need for steroid replacement therapy or where it is contraindicated (e.g. von Hippel-Lindau patients with phaeochromocytomas) (◘ Fig. 39.4) has to be clearly documented in medical records to avoid precipitation of crises.

The time taken for recovery of the HPA axis after stopping glucocorticoids following prolonged use is variable and influenced by factors such as dose, time of day and duration of drug use. Drugs that affect the cytochrome P450 enzyme pathway can also lead to changes in serum level of glucocorticoids. Enzyme inhibitors exert incomplete inhibition of cortisol biosynthesis; conversely potent inducers will result in significantly less bioavailable cortisol in patients on long-term glucocorticoids.

39.4 The Effect of CKD on Common Endocrine Medications

39.4.1 Antidiabetics

Diabetes mellitus is a growing epidemic and the leading cause of chronic kidney disease worldwide. Clinicians are faced with treating diabetics with varying degrees of renal insufficiency, and it is important to be aware of how clearance of antidiabetic medications are affected by the GFR (◘ Table 39.6).

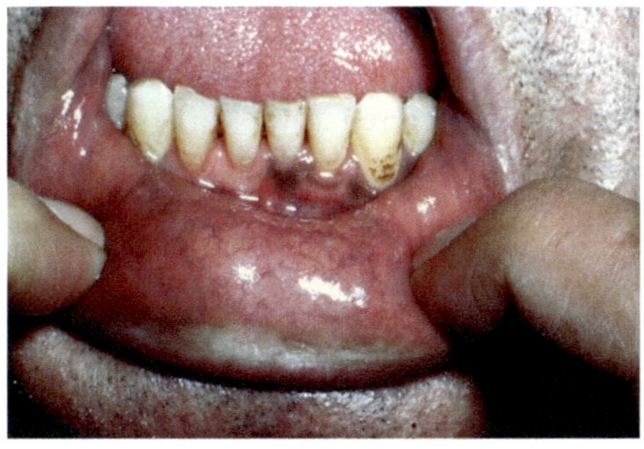
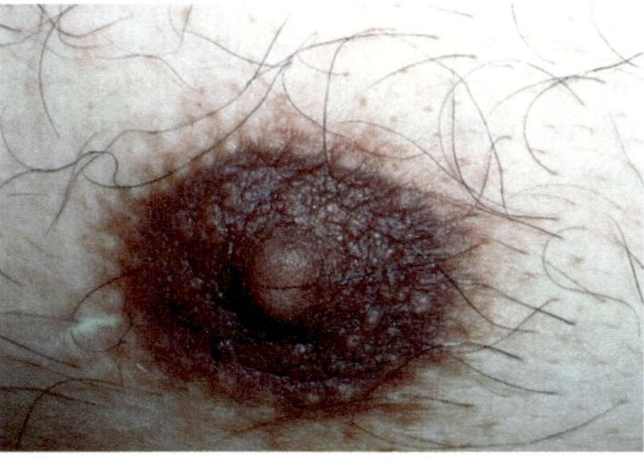

◘ **Fig. 39.3** Hyperpigmentation of the nipple and gums in a long-standing renal transplant recipient who had abruptly stopped steroid maintenance 6–8 weeks before presenting to the clinic and 10 days following a car accident. He complained of malaise, tiredness and loss of appetite. He was hypotensive with a postural drop in blood pressure. Blood tests revealed a rise in creatinine and a potassium of 6.7 mmol/L. The combination of chronic adrenal suppression and a very stressful event was sufficient to cause an Addisonian crisis, which responded rapidly to steroid replacement

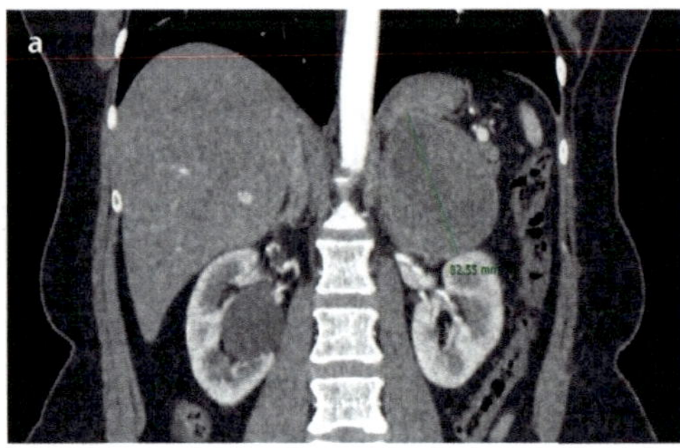
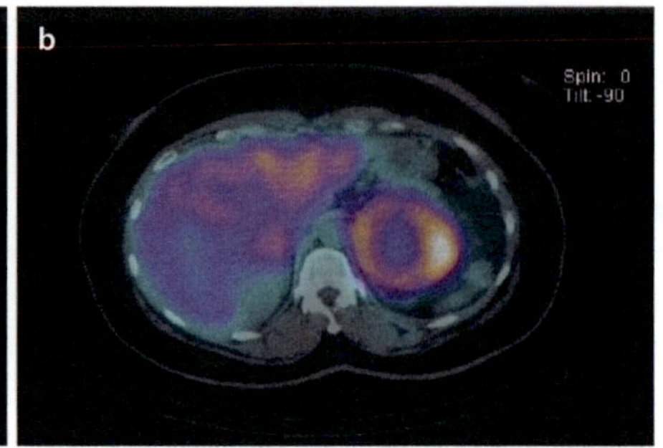

Fig. 39.4 Adrenal mass consistent with a phaeochromocytoma. A 38-year-old female patient presents with headaches and occasional palpitations. She has a history of von Hippel-Lindau disease that manifested as retinal angiomas (bilateral amaurosis at the age of 16) and cerebellar hemangioblastomas (ataxia at the age of 26). She also suffers from hypertension diagnosed 6 years ago that is controlled with antihypertensive medications. On admission, she had evidence of orthostatic hypotension and raised plasma norepinephrines, and a CT scan revealed a 82.5 mm mass above her left kidney **a** that corresponded to an area of increased uptake in a MIBG scintiscan **b**

39.5 Systemic Diseases Affecting the Endocrine System and Kidneys

Many inherited and acquired conditions affect multiple organ systems resulting in a wide spectrum of clinical disease with varying degrees of severity. The common conditions are listed below (Table 39.7). Rarer conditions resulting in inborn errors of metabolism often affect all tissues and can lead to endocrine and renal dysfunction; some of these conditions are listed below (Tables 39.8 and 39.9).

39.6 Impact of Endocrine Diseases on the Kidney

39

Certain endocrine diseases lead to renal complications. They are listed in Table 39.10.

39.7 Endocrine-Mediated Renal Disease

The relationship between endocrine hormones (in particular the RAAS) and the kidney are unique. Imbalance of hormones can lead to undesired systemic manifestations; these are listed in Table 39.11 and further discussed in the chapter 'Genetic Chronic Tubulointerstitial disease'.

39.8 Integrated Care in Endocrine and Renal Diseases

39.8.1 Joint Clinics

Patients with renal complications of endocrine disease often have complex multisystem disease and will benefit from multidisciplinary shared care including clinicians from each specialty as well as dieticians and specialist nurses. However, a large cohort remains managed by individual specialties dependent on the predominant pathology.

The best example of integrated care is the now widespread combined diabetes renal clinics that have been consistently shown to reduce the progression to end-stage kidney disease and improve diabetic control which is further supported by extensive national joint guidelines on management. The use of certain drugs that act primarily in the kidney, e.g. SGLT2 inhibitors which have recently been approved by NICE as an antidiabetic, combined with emerging evidence of its use to treat heart failure, will greatly benefit from a cross-speciality setting. In addition, there are existing multidisciplinary pathways focussing on disorders including MEN and neuroendocrine tumours. Patients should ideally be referred at the earliest opportunity to be co-managed by both specialities to allow for optimal outcome.

Table 39.6 The use of endocrine medications in CKD

Drug	Metabolism	Recommendations in CKD
Antidiabetics		
Insulin	Increased half-life with GFR decline	Dosing altered to individual's response and need
Metformin	Excreted unchanged in urine	GFR < 30: contraindicated by manufacturer guidelines GFR 30–44: maximum 1000 mg
Sulphonylureas	Actively metabolised in the liver and renally cleared	Use in caution with GFRs <60 due to risk of hypoglycaemia
Thiazolidinediones	Fully metabolised by the liver	Can be used in CKD Main side effects include water retention, bone loss and increased fracture rates
Alpha-glucosidase inhibitors	Metabolised in GI tract; ~ 34% excreted by the kidney	Avoid in GFR <25
Dipeptidyl peptidase-4 (DPP4) inhibitors		
Sitagliptin	80% cleared by the kidney	GFR 30–50: reduce dose by ½ GFR <30: reduce dose by ¼
Saxagliptin	Excreted via urine and can be removed via dialysis	GFR <50: reduce dose by ½
Linagliptin	Minimal amounts cleared by the kidney	Safe to use in CKD with no dose adjustment
Sodium-glucose co-transporter 2 (SGLT2) inhibitors		
Canagliflozin	Actively metabolised in the liver and renally cleared	GFR < 30: avoid; if already taking, to continue medication even if new drop in GFR to < 30
Dapagliflozin		Avoid in GFR < 30
Empagliflozin		Avoid in GFR < 30
Glucagon-like peptide (GLP-1) receptor agonists		
Exenatide	Renally cleared followed by proteolytic degradation 84% reduction in clearance in CKD [16]	GFR < 50: use with caution GFR < 30: avoid
Liraglutide	No specific organ identified as major route of elimination	No dose adjustment required
Hormone agonists		
Oestrogen	Mainly metabolised in the liver	No dose adjustment required
Leuprorelin (GnRH agonist)	Degraded by peptidases and excreted in urine	Increased risk of AKI when used in men with prostate cancer as androgen deprivation therapy Increased risk of ovarian hyperstimulation in women on dialysis
Hormone antagonists		
Anti-oestrogens (e.g. tamoxifen) Anti-androgens (e.g. cyproterone) Enzyme inhibitors (e.g. anastrozole)	Metabolised in the liver with varying degrees of elimination by the kidney	No dose adjustment required

Table 39.7 Systemic conditions with endocrine and renal manifestations

Condition	Presentation
Cystic fibrosis	Autosomal recessive disorder resulting in mutation of the cystic fibrosis transmembrane conductance receptor (CFTR)
	Endocrine manifestations
	Progressive pancreatic exocrine failure leading to fat malabsorption due to deficiency in digestive enzymes resulting in steatorrhoea, malnutrition and deficiency in fat-soluble vitamins A, D, E and K Pancreatic endocrine failure leading to diabetes mellitus
	Renal manifestations [17]
	Nephrolithiasis and nephrocalcinosis (enteric hyperoxaluria) Toxicity from recurrent aminoglycoside exposure due to frequent *pseudomonal* infections AA amyloidosis secondary to chronic infection Diabetic nephropathy Recurrent infection-related episodes of acute tubular injury
Multiple endocrine neoplasia type 1	Autosomal-dominant mutations in the tumour suppressor gene MEN1, which encodes a 610-amino acid protein, menin [18], leading to a predisposition to tumour formation in: **P**arathyroid gland **P**ituitary (anterior) **P**ancreas
	Endocrine manifestations
	Primary hyperparathyroidism Anterior pituitary tumours – most commonly prolactinomas (20%), although GH-, ACTH- and TSH-secreting tumours are also seen Neuroendocrine tumours of the gut and pancreas, most commonly gastrin (Zollinger-Ellison syndrome) and less commonly, insulinomas Carcinoid tumours – typically thymic and usually inactive as compared with sporadic forms
	Renal manifestations
	Hypercalcaemia-related volume depletion and nephrocalcinosis
Multiple endocrine Neoplasia type 2	Autosomal-dominant abnormality of the *RET* proto-oncogene on chromosome 10 MEN2A: parathyroid hyperplasia (in classic form or with Hirschsprung disease or cutaneous lichen amyloidosis and familial forms) MEN2B: phaeochromocytoma and medullary thyroid carcinoma but without parathyroid disease
	Endocrine manifestations
	Hyperparathyroidism – typically diffuse hyperplasia Medullary thyroid carcinoma – often younger onset and more aggressive phenotype
	Renal manifestations
	Hypercalcaemia-related volume depletion and nephrocalcinosis

Table 39.7 (continued)

Condition	Presentation
Sjogren's syndrome	Autoimmune rheumatological multisystem disorder characterised by sicca symptoms (dry mouth/eyes) with keratoconjunctivitis or mikulicz syndrome (parotid and lacrimal gland hyperplasia) Endocrine manifestations Autoimmune thyroiditis; anti-thyroid antibodies commonly seen Chronic atrophic gastritis associated with hypopepsinogenaemia and antiparietal cell antibodies Pancreatic insufficiency – rarely clinically significant Renal manifestations Chronic tubulointerstitial nephritis Renal tubular acidosis (RTA) – type 1 distal (Fanconi syndrome); mechanism uncertain but could be from an absence of H+/ATPase in intercalated cells of the collecting ducts seen in one biopsy series [19] or due to autoantibodies against carbonic anhydrase II leading to reduced H + production [20] and may be seen with nephrocalcinosis and/or nephrolithiasis Nephrogenic diabetes insipidus [21] Hypokalaemia without RTA secondary to salt wasting-driven hyperaldosteronism [22] Immune-mediated glomerulonephritis – most commonly membranoproliferative glomerulonephritis and membranous nephropathy, although other glomerular lesions and nephrotic syndrome have also been seen on renal biopsies [23] Cryoglobulinaemia
Sarcoidosis	Multisystem non-caseating granulomatous disorder Endocrine manifestations [24] Cranial diabetes insipidus and hyperprolactinaemia most commonly seen in hypothalamo-hypophyseal infiltration (affecting 5%); may also result in hypothyroidism, hypoadrenalism, diabetes insipidus and SIADH Thyroid infiltration uncommon but increased autoimmune thyroid disease seen Fertility and menstrual abnormalities due to granulomatous infiltration of the testes, ovaries and uterus Renal manifestations Interstitial nephritis Hypercalcaemia-related volume depletion and nephrocalcinosis and nephrolithiasis (calcium oxalate) Tubular dysfunction including type 1 distal RTA Glomerular disease (uncommon) Obstruction secondary to retroperitoneal lymphadenopathy/fibrosis
Amyloidosis	Extracellular deposition of insoluble amyloid fibrils Two types: AA and AL amyloidosis Endocrine manifestations [25] Thyroid goitre Gonadal dysfunction Hypoadrenalism Renal manifestations Proteinuric CKD secondary to glomerular amyloid deposition (more common with AA amyloidosis)
Sickle cell disease	Inherited point mutation of beta-globin gene resulting in abnormally structured haemoglobin (HbSS) Endocrine manifestations Diabetes mellitus (only if iron overload) Renal manifestations Recurrent prerenal episodes of acute kidney injury during sickle crises Medullary infarction and papillary necrosis Nephrogenic diabetes insipidus Glomerular lesions – most commonly FSGS Renal medullary carcinoma Drug toxicity (recurrent courses of antibiotics, analgesics and contrast agents)

(continued)

Table 39.7 (continued)

Condition	Presentation
Human immunodeficiency virus	A lentivirus that causes AIDS (acquired immunodeficiency syndrome)
	Endocrine manifestations
	Hypoadrenalism
	Renal manifestations
	Glomerular pathology (HIV-associated nephropathy, HIV immune complex kidney disease, HIV-associated thrombotic microangiopathy, lupus nephritis) Tubulo-interstitial pathology (diffuse infiltrative lymphocytosis syndrome, immune reconstitution inflammatory syndrome)

Table 39.8 Metabolic conditions with endocrine and renal manifestations

Condition	Presentation
Fabry disease	X-linked lysosomal storage disorder related to deficiency of alpha galactosidase A and resulting accumulation of globotriaosylceramide in multiple organs
	Endocrine manifestations [26]
	Hypothyroidism Infertility Subclinical adrenal insufficiency
	Renal manifestations
	Progressive CKD with proteinuria and/or haematuria (usually progresses to end-stage renal failure in adulthood) due to glycosphingolipid accumulation in podocytes, mesangial cells and vascular endothelium Characteristic lysosomal lamellar cytoplasmic inclusions seen on electron microscopy of renal biopsies (Zebra bodies)
Primary hyperoxaluria (PH)	Autosomal recessive disorder resulting in defects in the enzymes responsible for conversion of glyoxalate to glycine (PH1) or glycolate (PH2) and resultant excess conversion to oxalate
	Endocrine manifestations [26]
	Hypothyroidism
	Renal manifestations
	Excess urinary oxalate excretion leading to nephrolithiasis (calcium oxalate) Nephrocalcinosis
Cystinosis	Autosomal recessive disorder of lysosomal cystine transportation leading to intracellular accumulation
	Endocrine manifestations [26]
	Hypothyroidism Diabetes mellitus
	Renal manifestations
	Type 1 distal RTA (Fanconi syndrome) Progressive CKD from cystine deposition in renal parenchyma

Table 39.8 (continued)

Condition	Presentation
Bardet-Biedl syndrome (and Laurence-Moon syndrome)	Autosomal recessive inherited condition resulting in short stature, weight gain, polydactyly, visual impairment and hypertension Laurence-Moon syndrome has a similar phenotype but occurs with spinocerebellar degeneration Endocrine manifestations Hypogonadism Diabetes mellitus Renal manifestations Vesicoureteric reflux Congenital renal dysplasia and calyceal abnormalities
Alström syndrome	Rare autosomal recessive condition leading to an inborn error of metabolism arising from a defect in the ALMS1 gene Endocrine manifestations [26] Type 2 diabetes Hypogonadism Hypopituitarism and GH deficiency Renal manifestations Progressive CKD
Central diabetes insipidus	A lack of antidiuretic hormone (ADH) due to damage to the pituitary gland or hypothalamus Can occur due to head injury, surgery or tumours Endocrine manifestations ADH low or absent Renal manifestations Polyuria exceeding 10 L/24 hours Hypernatraemia
Nephrogenic diabetes insipidus	Failure of kidney to respond to a normal release of ADH by the pituitary. Can occur due to: *Acquired causes* Drugs: lithium, cidofovir, amphotericin Other diseases: Sickle cell, amyloidosis, ADPKD, Bartter syndrome, Sjogren's syndrome *Hereditary causes* X-linked recessive mutation of AVPR2 gene Autosomal-dominant and recessive mutation of AQP2 gene Endocrine manifestations ADH normal or raised Renal manifestations Polyuria Hypernatraemia

Table 39.9 Other conditions with endocrine and renal manifestations

Condition	Presentation
Sheehan's syndrome	Hypopituitarism caused by ischaemic necrosis postpartum due to hypovolaemia secondary to haemorrhage or hypotension Severe septic shock Envenomation following snake bites
	Endocrine manifestations
	Varying degrees of hypopituitarism depending on area affected, but at least 75% of pituitary have to be infarcted Growth hormone and prolactin secretion most commonly affected (90–100%). Cortisol, ADH gonadotrophin and TSH deficiencies range from 50 to 100%
	Renal manifestations
	AKI in the setting of systemic shock AKI secondary to chronic adrenal insufficiency Cortical necrosis (any systemic shock severe enough to cause cortical necrosis may cause pituitary infarction and vice versa)
Phaeochromocytoma (Fig. 39.4)	Neuroendocrine tumour of the chromaffin cells from the medulla of the adrenals
	Endocrine manifestations
	Part of MEN 2 syndrome Symptoms of sympathetic nervous system hyperactivity secondary to excess secretion of catecholamines
	Renal manifestations
	Part of von Hippel-Lindau syndrome Hypertension Low renin and aldosterone levels AKI in setting of Cardiogenic shock Intravascular depletion Rhabdomyolysis (due to muscle ischaemia from hypertensive crisis) MAHA (rare)

39

Table 39.10 Renal complications of endocrine diseases

Condition	Hormone	Renal manifestation
Hypothyroidism	Thyroxine ↓	Reversible reduction in GFR Hyponatraemia
Cushing's	Cortisol ↑	Hypertension
Addison's	Aldosterone ↓	Hyperkalaemia Hyponatraemia Hypovolaemia Hypotension Acute kidney injury (although GFR commonly preserved) [27]
Hyperaldosteronism	Aldosterone ↑	Hypertension Reversible increase in GFR Hypokalaemia (variable) Hypomagnesaemia

(continued)

Table 39.10 (continued)

Condition	Hormone	Renal manifestation
Acromegaly[47]	Growth hormone/IGF1 ↑	Increased GFR and hyperfiltration Nephromegaly – average longitudinal diameter of 148.3 mm [28] Nephrolithiasis
Congenital adrenal hyperplasia	Cortisol (11-deoxycortisol)↓	Salt losing nephropathy in infancy with failure to thrive, dehydration, hyperkalaemia and hyponatraemia
Renin secreting tumours	Renin ↑	Hypertension Hypokalaemia Metabolic alkalosis
Diabetes mellitus	Insulin ↓ or normal	Diabetic nephropathy
Hyperparathyroidism	Parathyroid hormone ↑	Hypercalcaemia-related volume depletion and nephrocalcinosis
Autosomal-dominant hypocalcaemic hypercalcinuria	Parathyroid hormone ↓	Nephrolithiasis Hypomagnesaemia Hyperphosphataemia
Oncogenic osteomalacia (Fig. 39.5)	Phosphatonin ↑ FGF23 ↑ MEPE↑	Bone pain Hypophosphataemia Normal PTH and serum calcium
X-linked hypophosphataemic rickets	FGF23 ↑ Osteopontin ↓ Calcitriol ↓ MEPE↑	Rickets Hypophosphataemia Nephrocalcinosis
Pseudohypoparathyroidism	PTH ↑ Calcitriol ↓	Hypocalcaemia Hyperphosphataemia

FGF 23 fibroblast growth factor-23, *MEPE* matrix extracellular phosphoglycoprotein

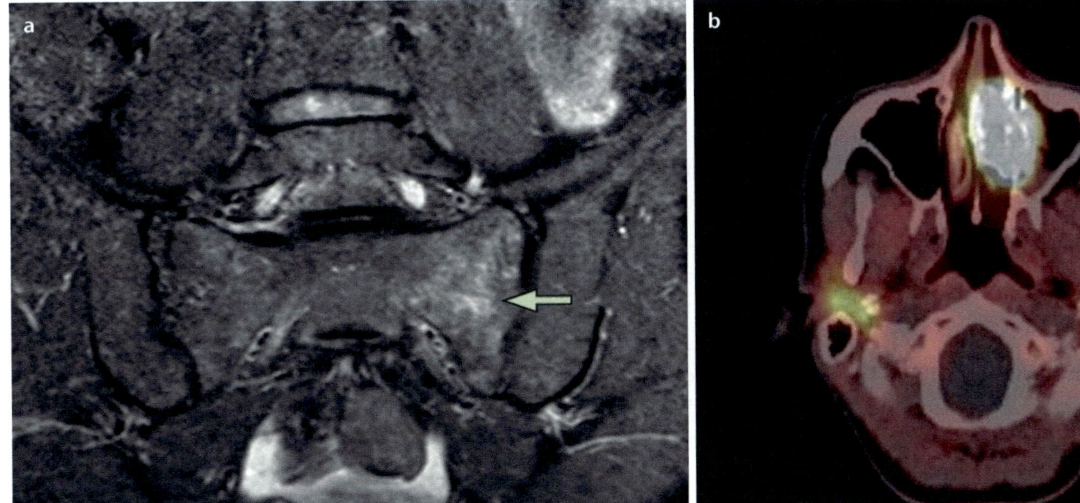

Fig. 39.5 Oncogenic osteomalacia. Radiological findings in a young female patient presenting with isolated hypophosphataemia and pelvic stress fractures (**a**; MRI sacrum with stress fracture indicated by the arrow), which was misdiagnosed as vitamin D deficiency. Subsequent hyperphosphaturia was diagnosed on a calculated fractional excretion of phosphate of 42%. A raised FGF23 level and radiological evidence of an intense uptake in soft tissue lesion in the left nasal cavity and ethmoid sinus detected using PET CT **b** with a radiolabelled octreotide analogue (68Ga-DOTATATE) confirmed the diagnosis of a phosphaturic mesenchymal tumour leading to osteogenic osteomalacia. (Reproduced with permission from Mumford et al. [29])

Table 39.11 Renal manifestations directly caused by RAAS disturbance

Condition	Hormone	Renal manifestation
Bartter syndrome [30]	Renin ↑ Aldosterone ↑	Hypotension Polyuria Hypokalaemia metabolic alkalosis Hypocalcaemia
Gitelman syndrome [30]	Renin ↑ Aldosterone ↑	Hypomagnesaemia Hypokalaemia metabolic alkalosis (mild)
Liddle syndrome	Aldosterone ↓	Hypertension Hypokalaemia metabolic alkalosis (mild)
Renal artery stenosis	Renin ↑ Aldosterone ↑	Hypertension Renal impairment; particularly with RAS blockade Hypokalaemia Salt/water retention

39

Case Study

Case 1

A 32-year-old manager presented to his GP with chronic exhaustion and general malaise making it difficult for him to work. He appeared well and fit with no obvious abnormality. Initial bloods showed a normal full blood count and chemistry apart from an ALT of 101 U/L, creatinine of 141 μmol/L and an estimated eGFR of 53 mL/min/1.73 m^2. His urine was negative on dipstick and further renal screening tests (and renal ultrasound) were unremarkable apart from a CPK of 7020 U/L. Thyroid function tests revealed an unrecordable T4 and TSH of >100. With supplementation, the ALT returned to normal within a month, but his attendance was infrequent and increments in thyroxine irregular as a result. It took over a year to reach a baseline creatinine of 80 μmol/L (eGFR of >90) (Fig. 39.6). This illustrates not only the frustrations of poor attendance but the fact that marked hypothyroidism alone reduced his eGFR by approximately 50%.

Case 2

A 50-year-old woman with hyperthyroidism was treated with carbimazole, with correction of her thyroid profile. This was associated with simultaneous rebound of her serum creatinine to baseline triggering an 'AKI alert' (Figs. 39.7, 39.8). Hyperthyroidism is associated with an increase in renal blood flow and glomerular filtration, causing a lower reading of serum creatinine than normal. It is important to note this and anticipate a rise back to normal levels to avoid unnecessary investigations into an acute kidney injury.

Case 3

A 13-year-old girl was admitted to a hospital in Sri Lanka following a bite from a Russell's viper. There had been a delay of over 24 hours in getting to the hospital as the family had sought help from a traditional healer first. She became oliguric and required dialysis for 6 weeks after where she recovered renal function but had stage 4 CKD. At the age of 15, her parents sought medical advice, reporting that their daughter was becoming increasingly withdrawn and fatigued and they were concerned with her growth and development. On direct questioning, she reveals that she had become isolated at school because she had not developed the secondary sexual characteristics of her peers. Further radiological (Fig. 39.9) and biochemical testing demonstrated pituitary failure, which was subsequently supplemented and she rapidly improved. It is likely that this patient suffered severe shock leading to renal cortical necrosis requiring a period of dialysis when bitten by the snake 2 years ago. Pituitary necrosis (Sheehan's syndrome) would have occurred during the same period leading to hypopituitarism. Sheehan's syndrome is typically associated with obstetric sepsis or haemorrhage, but its development is not an unusual consequence following snakebites.

Tips/Tricks

1. Always measure thyroid function at the start of dialysis, before heparin is given.
2. Have a high index of suspicion for primary hypothyroidism in patients with CKD as they exhibit similar signs and symptoms.
3. Be aware that changes of insulin doses and other glucose lowering medication may be required as CKD advances due to reduced renal clearance of these drugs.
4. Consider the impact of prescribing drugs metabolised by cytochrome p450 on the pituitary axis in patients on long-term corticosteroids.
5. Always consult with a renal pharmacist when prescribing any medication in patients with CKD.
6. Consider an underlying endocrine diagnosis when presented with a patient with electrolyte abnormalities, particularly in the context of renal stones.

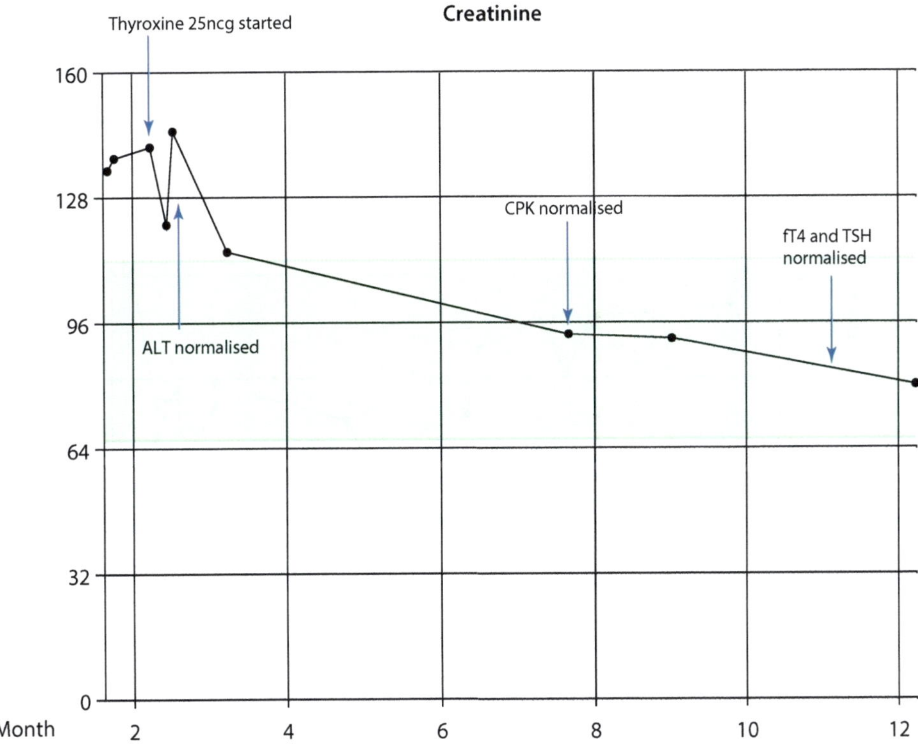

Fig. 39.6 Graph showing reduction of creatinine when thyroxine therapy was started. However, normalisation of creatinine, T4 and TSH levels look over a year due to intermittent attendance

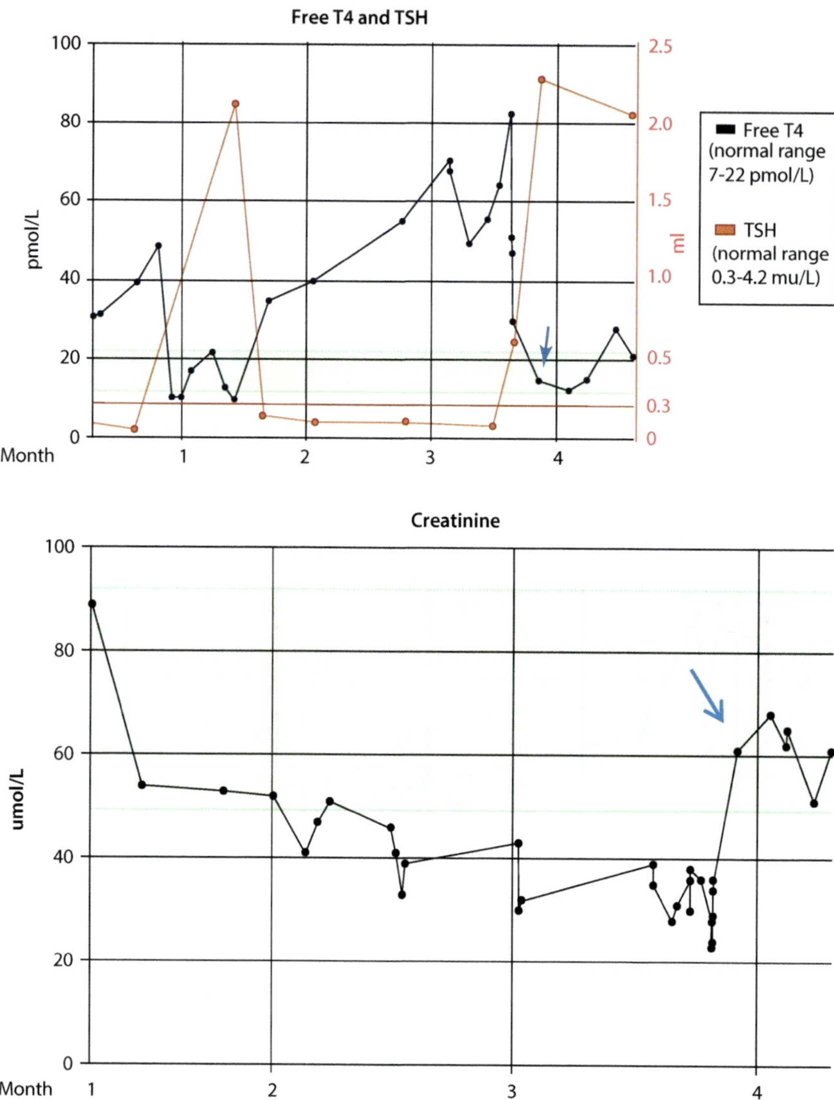

39

Fig. 39.7 and 39.8 These two graphs show the patient's fall in creatinine levels (Fig. 39.7) as free T4 levels rise (Fig. 39.8). The correction of free T4 levels corresponds with an abrupt rise in the patient's creatinine to baseline (blue arrows)

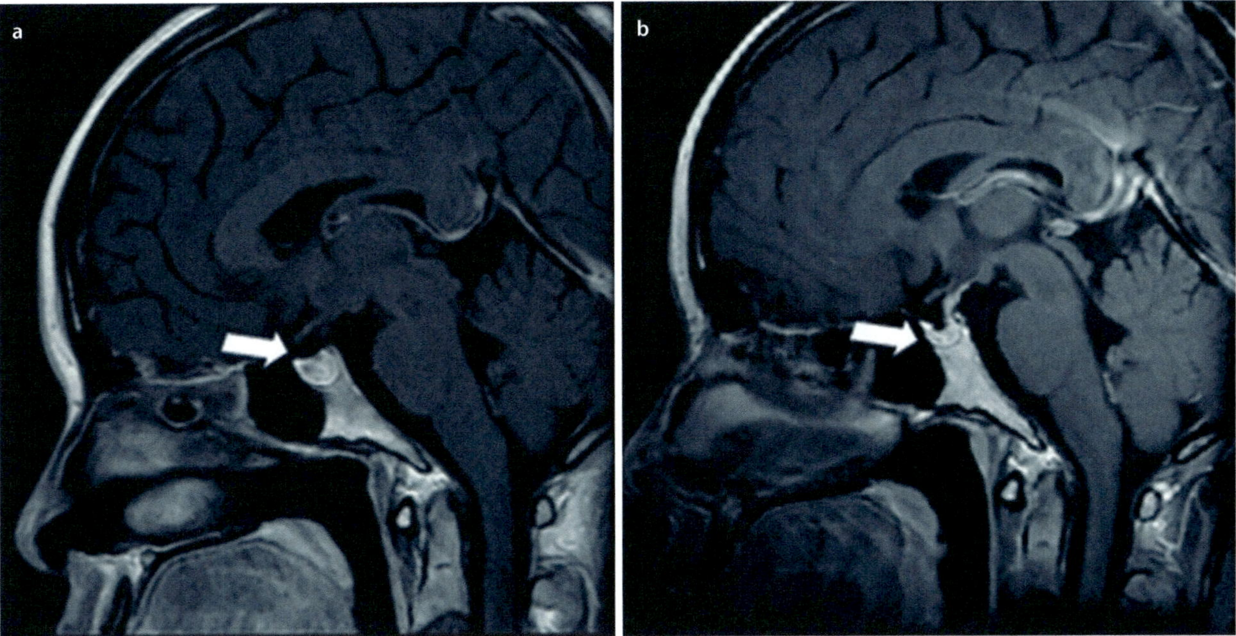

Fig. 39.9 Gadolinium-enhanced T1-weighted magnetic resonance image of the pituitary gland showing a normal gland **a** and a marked diminution in the pituitary gland consistent with necrosis **b**. (Free access from Matsuzaki et al. [31])

39.9 Conclusion

The kidney plays a crucial role in hormonal homeostasis of the body, and diagnosis of endocrine disorders may be obscured in patients with renal disease. The management of endocrine disorders in patients with CKD requires careful consideration and more often than not will benefit from a multidisciplinary approach.

Chapter Review Questions

1. Are treatments for hypogonadism required in patients with CKD?
2. Should vitamin D supplementation be routinely given to patients with nephrotic syndrome?
3. How is insulin degradation in the kidney affected by CKD?
4. How does hyperthyroidism lead to an increase in GFR?
5. Should children with CKD and growth impairment be given recombinant growth hormone treatment?

Answers

1. Yes if they are symptomatic or have osteoporosis. In premenopausal women with CKD, the oral contraceptive pill or oestradiol/progestin replacement therapy is first line. In men, the recommended therapy is testosterone. In postmenopausal women, oestrogen is no longer considered first-line therapy due to an increased risk of breast cancer, coronary heart disease, stroke and venous thromboembolism.
2. No. It may only be beneficial to nephrotic patients with persistently low serum ionised calcium concentrations or in patients who are on steroids for over 3 months.
3. Insulin is freely filtered in the kidney. Approximately 60% is cleared via glomerular filtration and 40% by extraction from the peritubular vessels. Clearance rate of insulin is only affected with a substantial reduction in GFR (to less than 15–20 ml/min) as concomitant increase in peritubular insulin uptake compensates for reduced filtration. However, at GFRs <20 ml/min, insulin clearance falls dramatically, and this is accompanied with a fall in hepatic insulin metabolism.
4. Hyperthyroidism increases renal blood flow and GFR by 18–25%. Intrarenal vasodilatation is mediated by an increase in nitric oxide production directly by the thyroid hormones and indirectly by high arterial pressure-related endothelial shear stress. Activation of the RAAS also contributes to an increased GFR.
5. Yes. Evidence shows that recombinant growth hormone therapy improves growth in children in all clinical situations, in patients with CKD but prerenal replacement therapy, those on dialysis

and those who have received transplantation. However, all other potentially modifiable factors will need to be corrected, e.g. nutritional intake, metabolic acidosis, renal bone osteodystrophy, anaemia, fluid and electrolyte abnormalities. The goal in recombinant growth hormone therapy is to achieve normal final height.

References

1. de Boer IH, Rue TC, Hall YN, Heagerty PJ, Weiss NS, Himmelfarb J. Temporal trends in the prevalence of diabetic kidney disease in the United States. JAMA. 2011;305:2532–9.
2. Tong A, Sainsbury P, Chadban S, et al. Patients' experiences and perspectives of living with CKD. Am J Kidney Dis. 2009;53:689–700.
3. Harris RC, Ismail N. Extrarenal complications of the nephrotic syndrome. Am J Kidney Dis. 1994;23:477–97.
4. Feinstein EI, Kaptein EM, Nicoloff JT, Massry SG. Thyroid function in patients with nephrotic syndrome and normal renal function. Am J Nephrol. 1982;2:70–6.
5. Iglesias P, Diez JJ. Thyroid dysfunction and kidney disease. Eur J Endocrinol. 2009;160:503–15.
6. Alon U, Chan JC. Calcium and vitamin D homeostasis in the nephrotic syndrome: current status. Nephron. 1984;36:1–4.
7. Malluche HH, Goldstein DA, Massry SG. Osteomalacia and hyperparathyroid bone disease in patients with nephrotic syndrome. J Clin Invest. 1979;63:494–500.
8. Goldstein DA, Haldimann B, Sherman D, Norman AW, Massry SG. Vitamin D metabolites and calcium metabolism in patients with nephrotic syndrome and normal renal function. J Clin Endocrinol Metab. 1981;52:116–21.
9. bernard db. Controversies in nephrology, Vol 9, The nephrotic syndrome. New York: Churchill Livingstone; 1982.
10. Wiezel D, Assadi MH, Landau D, et al. Impaired renal growth hormone JAK/STAT5 signaling in chronic kidney disease. Nephrol Dial Transplant. 2014;29:791–9.
11. Mohamedali M, Reddy Maddika S, Vyas A, Iyer V, Cheriyath P. Thyroid disorders and chronic kidney disease. Int J Nephrol. 2014;2014:520281.
12. Abdel-Rahman EM, Mansour W, Holley JL. Thyroid hormone abnormalities and frailty in elderly patients with chronic kidney disease: a hypothesis. Semin Dial. 2010;23:317–23.
13. Klyachkin ML, Sloan DA. Secondary hyperparathyroidism: evidence for an association with papillary thyroid cancer. Am Surg. 2001;67:397–9.
14. Liao MT, Sung CC, Hung KC, Wu CC, Lo L, Lu KC. Insulin resistance in patients with chronic kidney disease. J Biomed Biotechnol. 2012;2012:691369.
15. Siew ED, Ikizler TA. Insulin resistance and protein energy metabolism in patients with advanced chronic kidney disease. Semin Dial. 2010;23:378–82.
16. Linnebjerg H, Kothare PA, Park S, et al. Effect of renal impairment on the pharmacokinetics of exenatide. Br J Clin Pharmacol. 2007;64:317–27.
17. Yahiaoui Y, Jablonski M, Hubert D, et al. Renal involvement in cystic fibrosis: diseases spectrum and clinical relevance. Clin J Am Soc Nephrol. 2009;4:921–8.
18. Thakker RV, Newey PJ, Walls GV, et al. Clinical practice guidelines for multiple endocrine neoplasia type 1 (MEN1). J Clin Endocrinol Metab. 2012;97:2990–3011.
19. Cohen EP, Bastani B, Cohen MR, Kolner S, Hemken P, Gluck SL. Absence of H(+)-ATPase in cortical collecting tubules of a patient with Sjogren's syndrome and distal renal tubular acidosis. J Am Soc Nephrol. 1992;3:264–71.
20. Takemoto F, Hoshino J, Sawa N, et al. Autoantibodies against carbonic anhydrase II are increased in renal tubular acidosis associated with Sjogren syndrome. Am J Med. 2005;118:181–4.
21. Nagayama Y, Shigeno M, Nakagawa Y, et al. Acquired nephrogenic diabetes insipidus secondary to distal renal tubular acidosis and nephrocalcinosis associated with Sjogren's syndrome. J Endocrinol Investig. 1994;17:659–63.
22. Wrong OM, Feest TG, MacIver AG. Immune-related potassium-losing interstitial nephritis: a comparison with distal renal tubular acidosis. Q J Med. 1993;86:513–34.
23. Evans R, Zdebik A, Ciurtin C, Walsh SB. Renal involvement in primary Sjogren's syndrome. Rheumatology (Oxford). 2015;54:1541–8.
24. Porter N, Beynon HL, Randeva HS. Endocrine and reproductive manifestations of sarcoidosis. QJM. 2003;96:553–61.
25. Ozdemir D, Dagdelen S, Erbas T. Endocrine involvement in systemic amyloidosis. Endocr Pract. 2010;16:1056–63.
26. Vantyghem MC, Dobbelaere D, Mention K, Wemeau JL, Saudubray JM, Douillard C. Endocrine manifestations related to inherited metabolic diseases in adults. Orphanet J Rare Dis. 2012;7:11.
27. Talbott JH, Pecora LJ, Melville RS, Consolazio WV. Renal function in patients with Addison's disease and in patients with adrenal insufficiency secondary to pituitary pan-hypofunction. J Clin Invest. 1942;21:107–19.
28. Auriemma RS, Galdiero M, De Martino MC, et al. The kidney in acromegaly: renal structure and function in patients with acromegaly during active disease and 1 year after disease remission. Eur J Endocrinol. 2010;162:1035–42.
29. Mumford E, Marks J, Wagner T, Gallimore A, Gane S, Walsh SB. Oncogenic osteomalacia: diagnosis, localisation, and cure. Lancet Oncol. 2018;19:e365.
30. Shaer AJ. Inherited primary renal tubular hypokalemic alkalosis: a review of Gitelman and Bartter syndromes. Am J Med Sci. 2001;322:316–32.
31. Matsuzaki S, Endo M, Ueda Y, et al. A case of acute Sheehan's syndrome and literature review: a rare but life-threatening complication of postpartum hemorrhage. BMC Pregnancy Childbirth. 2017;17:188.

Dermatology in Kidney Disease

Ferina Ismail and Rakesh Anand

Contents

M. Harber (ed.), *Primer on Nephrology*, https://doi.org/10.1007/978-3-030-76419-7_40

Learning Objectives

1. Clinical presentation and management of the most frequently encountered skin conditions associated with renal disease.
2. Early recognition of skin cancers and their particular importance in the renal transplant population.
3. Strategies for skin cancer prevention in renal transplant recipients.

40.1 Introduction

A wide variety of skin conditions arise in patients with chronic kidney disease (CKD). These are sometimes related to the underlying pathologic process causing the renal disease but are also frequently associated with the uraemic state itself. Cutaneous examination of patients with CKD has shown an almost 100% prevalence of skin disorders in dialysis populations [1], with a marked impact on quality of life [2]. In addition, there is over a 100-fold increase in the incidence of certain types of skin cancer in renal transplant recipients, placing a significant burden on healthcare resources as well as causing significant morbidity and in some cases mortality [3]. Early recognition of these skin problems can therefore avert such complications, making a basic knowledge of the dermatological conditions arising in the setting of renal disease extremely valuable to practising nephrologists.

The cutaneous manifestations of renal disease may be broadly divided into three general categories: (1) skin manifestations of diseases associated with chronic kidney disease (▶ Box 40.1), (2) skin manifestations of diseases associated with renal involvement (◘ Table 40.1) and (3) skin conditions associated with renal transplantation.

Box 40.1 Skin Conditions Associated with Chronic Kidney Disease (Those Highlighted in Bold Discussed Further in Text)

Uraemic pruritus
Calciphylaxis
Nephrogenic systemic fibrosis
Acquired perforating dermatosis
Porphyria cutanea tarda
Hyperpigmentation
Xerosis
Cutaneous infections (bacterial/fungal/viral)
Purpura
Alopecia
Nail changes

◘ **Table 40.1** Skin manifestations of diseases associated with renal involvement

Systemic disorder	Skin manifestations
Diabetes mellitus	Necrobiosis lipoidica, perforating dermatosis, eruptive xanthomas
Systemic lupus erythematosus (SLE)	Photosensitivity, malar erythema, cutaneous LE lesions, diffuse alopecia, vasculitis
Henoch-Schönlein purpura	Palpable purpura
Wegener granulomatosis/polyarteritis nodosa (PAN)	Palpable purpura, subcutaneous nodules, livedo reticularis, ulcers
Systemic sclerosis	Acral or diffuse sclerosis, CREST syndrome, Raynaud's phenomenon
Amyloidosis	Purpura, xanthomatous papules, scleroderma-like changes
Anderson-Fabry disease	Angiokeratomas
HIV	Eosinophilic folliculitis, Kaposi's sarcoma
Cholesterol emboli	Livedo reticularis, petechiae, purpura
Hepatitis C	Purpura, porphyria cutanea tarda, lichen planus, cutaneous PAN
Tuberous sclerosis	Facial angiofibromas, ash-leaf macule, shagreen patch, periungual fibromas

40.2 Skin Conditions Associated with Chronic Kidney Disease

Examination of the skin and nails can reveal abnormalities in patients with end-stage renal disease that precede dialysis or kidney transplantation. Chronic renal failure, regardless of its cause, often produces xerosis, pruritus, hyperpigmentation and nail changes. Although the majority of dermatological conditions in CKD are relatively benign, a few skin diseases have the potential to cause serious morbidity and mortality. It is these conditions which are discussed in more detail in this chapter (▶ Box 40.1).

40.3 Uraemic Pruritus

With improvements in dialysis and the development of biocompatible dialysis membranes, the prevalence of uraemic pruritus (UP) has declined in the past decade. Despite this, a significant proportion of haemodialysis patients still report itching which can have a significant effect on quality of life as it causes considerable discomfort, anxiety, depression and sleeping disorders. In addition, UP is increasingly recognised as an indicator of increased mortality risk in patients with CKD [4].

UP is characterised by daily bouts of itching that tend to worsen at night and may prevent sleep. The itch may be generalised or localised to one area, most often the back, abdomen, head and arms. The skin may appear normal or dry (xerosis), associated with signs of chronic scratching, including excoriations, superimposed infections, nodular prurigo, eczema and lichenification. No single treatment has been shown to be overwhelmingly effective, and whilst the evidence is limited, the first steps in management are to optimise dialysis efficacy, control calcium-phosphate and PTH levels and correct any coexistent anaemia. Dry skin can be managed by applying regular emollients and by using soap substitutes. Phototherapy using UVB may be used for severe uraemic pruritus. Oral antihistamines and systemic steroids are generally not effective, though capsaicin cream, topical calcipotriol and oral gabapentin have all shown some benefit in UP [5].

The pathophysiology of UP is complex with several theories postulated. Increased understanding of the nervous pathways has allowed novel agents to be tested. For example, opioid receptor agonists (e.g. nalfurafine) have been shown to be effective in some patients with CKD, but there have been mixed results. Other agents trialled in UP include thalidomide, mirtazapine and 5-HT3 receptor antagonists such as ondansetron, again with limited evidence for their use. Kidney transplantation usually results in resolution of UP.

40.4 Calciphylaxis

Calciphylaxis or calcific uraemic arteriolopathy is a painful necrotising disorder, which is potentially life-threatening. It is associated with an estimated 1-year survival rate of 45%, with death predominantly due to infectious complications. Its incidence is estimated to be around 4% in patients on dialysis and less than 1% in patients with CKD. Risk factors for the development of calciphylaxis include obesity, diabetes, female sex, white ethnicity, time on renal replacement therapy and the use of warfarin [6]. Other factors reported to be associated with calciphylaxis include the use of vitamin D analogues, calcium-containing phosphate binders and glucocorticosteroids.

Clinical presentation is characterised by progressive cutaneous ulceration on a background of livedo reticularis-like skin changes (◘ Fig. 40.1). There is a predilection for sites with large amounts of subcutaneous fat such as the abdomen, buttocks and thighs, with the evolution of painful subcutaneous purpuric plaques, which subsequently develop in to necrotic ulcers often covered by eschars. Pain may precede the appearance of skin lesions. Prompt recognition and diagnosis enables timely initiation of therapy leading to improved prognosis. A skin biopsy is preferable though the histological features are not pathognomonic. Calciphylaxis should be differentiated from warfarin-induced skin necrosis, vasculitis and pyoderma gangrenosum.

Management involves optimising dialysis, often increasing the frequency of sessions, diligent wound care, as well as normalising biochemical abnormalities including parathyroidectomy in the presence of raised PTH levels. Cinacalcet may be effective for control of patients with secondary hyperparathyroidism. Sodium

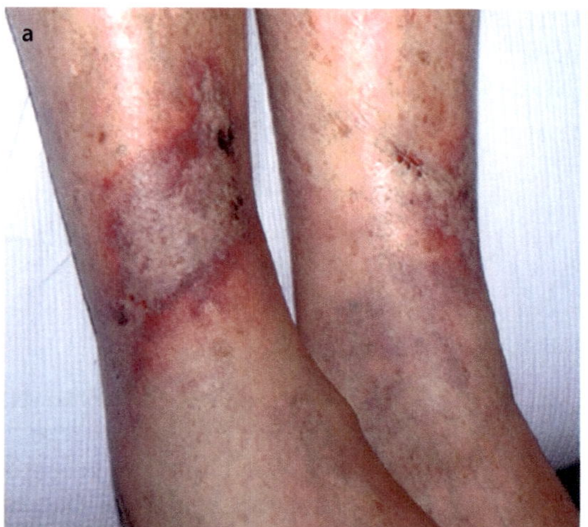

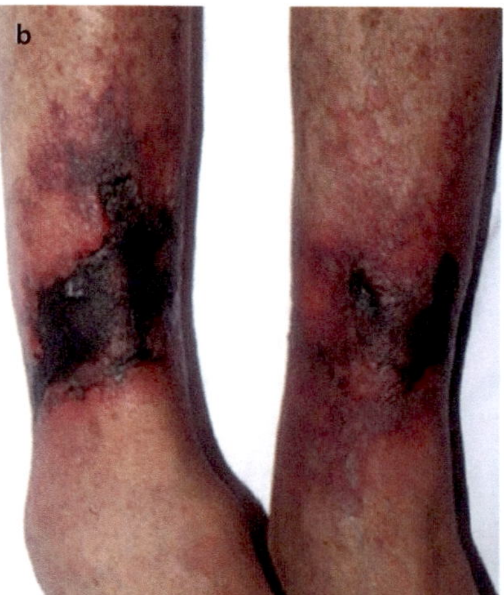

◘ **Fig. 40.1** Calciphylaxis at initial presentation (**a**) and 1 week later (**b**)

thiosulphate during dialysis at a dose of 5–25 g i.v. has also shown to be effective and works by chelating calcium from soft tissue [7]. This may need to be continued for a period of weeks to months, in association with the above measures.

40.5 Nephrogenic Systemic Fibrosis

Nephrogenic systemic fibrosis (NSF) is a scleroderma-like condition that occurs in patients with CKD and is characterised by skin thickening and fibrosis, as well as systemic involvement of major organs such as the heart and lungs. Major clinical criteria include symmetrically distributed indurated plaques and nodules, particularly on the upper and lower limbs, associated with joint contractures and restriction of movement. There is often red/brown discolouration of the skin with orange-peel thickening (peau d'orange). Mean age of onset is 46 years, with equal sex incidence. Exposure to gadolinium-based contrast media is associated with the development of NSF in patients with CKD [8], with a very variable interval of signs of NSF, ranging from 2 days to 18 months post-gadolinium exposure. Diagnosis is confirmed by skin biopsy which demonstrates thickened collagen and proliferation of CD34+ spindle cells.

There is currently no effective treatment for NSF, and prevention by avoidance of, or limited exposure to, gadolinium in patients with CKD (see chapter on imaging) is key [9]. Various therapeutic options have been reported including phototherapy, imatinib, extracorporeal photopheresis and sodium thiosulphate. There is no reported clinical benefit of 'prophylactic' haemodialysis for the prevention of NSF in patients receiving gadolinium-enhanced scans. Measures directed towards preventing contractures and maintaining mobility include physiotherapy and deep tissue massage.

40.6 Acquired Perforating Dermatosis

Acquired perforating dermatosis (APD), or Kyrle disease, occurs in approximately 10% of haemodialysis (HD) patients, with a strong association with diabetes mellitus. APD is also linked with other medical conditions such as hepatitis, thyroid disease, malignancies and HIV. It is characterised by papules with a central hyperkeratotic plug, mainly localised to the trunk, proximal extremities, scalp and face (◘ Fig. 40.2). Lesions are pruritic and difficult to treat. Often the clinical presentation is typical though histological findings include the presence of epidermal invaginations with a central keratotic plug. Treatment options include emollients, potent topical steroids, topical or systemic retinoids and UVB phototherapy.

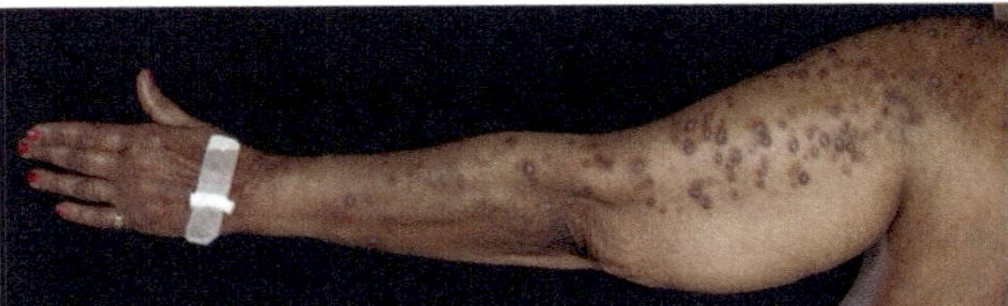

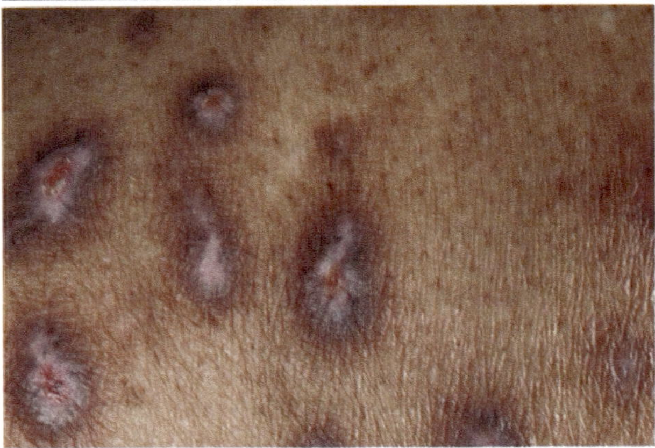

◘ **Fig. 40.2** Perforating dermatosis

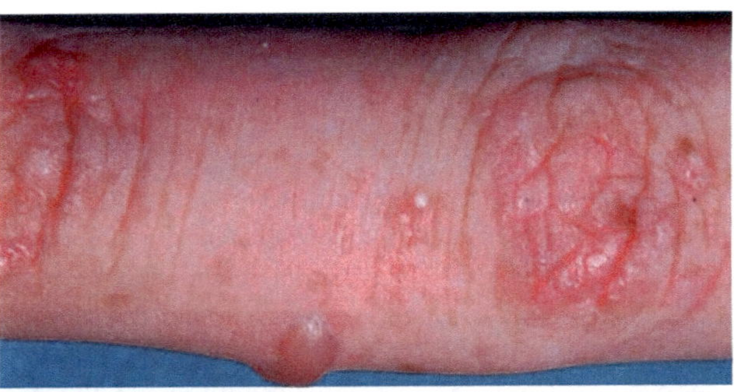

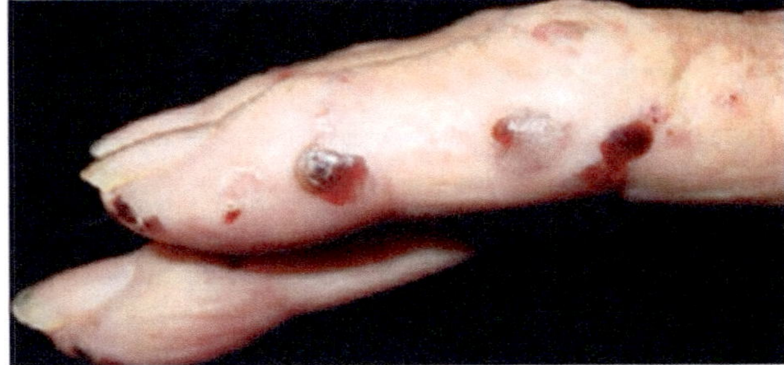

◘ **Fig. 40.3** Porphyria cutanea tarda

40.7 Porphyria

The porphyrias are a group of inherited or acquired disorders of the enzymes involved in the haem biosynthetic pathway. Porphyria cutanea tarda (PCT) is associated with end-stage renal disease and HD and commonly presents as bullae on the dorsal aspects of the hands and sun-exposed sites, which often heal with scarring (◘ Fig. 40.3). This is frequently accompanied by facial hyperpigmentation and hypertrichosis. The sporadic form of PCT occurs in approximately 5% of patients on dialysis and can be precipitated by alcohol, oestrogens, hepatitis B or C infections or HIV. Pseudoporphyria is a condition clinically and histologically identical to PCT but characterised by normal serum and urine porphyrin levels. It is triggered by medications, e.g. amiodarone, tetracyclines and naproxen. Photoprotection is the mainstay of managing such patients via the use of sunscreens and clothing.

40.8 Skin Manifestations of Diseases Associated with Renal Involvement

40.8.1 Lupus Erythematosus

The various clinical types of cutaneous lupus erythematosus (CLE) may be subdivided according to the risk of systemic involvement and clinical outcome. With the advent of immunological testing, groups such as subacute cutaneous lupus have been described [10], and the role of drugs in the development of lupus has also been identified. Broadly speaking, CLE may be classified into three subsets: (1) chronic CLE (CCLE), of which the most common manifestation is that of discoid lupus (DLE); (2) acute CLE (ACLE); and (3) subacute CLE (SCLE). Significant systemic involvement occurs in up to 28% of patients with CCLE with a higher proportion of patients with SCLE (◘ Fig. 40.4) having the diagnostic criteria for systemic lupus but with mild systemic disease. Severe renal disease is uncommon [11, 12]. Mucocutaneous abnormalities occur in around 85% of patients with SLE. Clinically, chronic discoid lesions tend to lead to scarring with more acute and subacute lesions resolving with pigmentary change. Ordinary histology is poor at differentiating between the subtypes of CLE with direct immunofluorescence positive in ~80% of involved skin. Potent topical steroids are usually the mainstay of treatment of skin lesions, along with photoprotection (SPF 50+ with UVA protection) and hydroxychloroquine. Patients with CLE require accurate clinicopathological correlation, not least to attempt to answer the question of the progression of cutaneous disease to systemic disease.

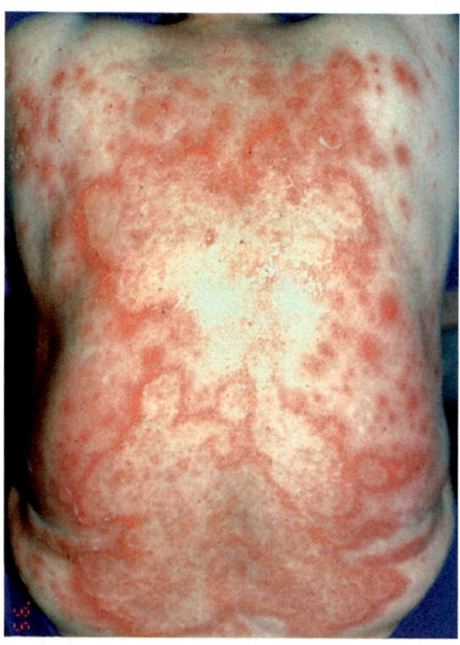

◘ **Fig. 40.4** Subacute cutaneous lupus erythematosus

40.8.2 Cutaneous Vasculitis and Renal Disease

Vasculitides can be classified based on the size of the vessel affected. Small-vessel vasculitides include Henoch-Schönlein purpura (HSP) and ANCA-associated vasculitis. Ninety percent of cases of HSP affect children and renal involvement may not be apparent at the initial diagnosis (◘ Fig. 40.5). Although occurring rarely in adults, the sequelae of disease tend to be more severe with more significant renal impairment. ANCA-associated vasculitis includes Wegener's granulomatosis with skin disease occurring in 14–77% of patients and is associated with a higher frequency of renal involvement [13, 14]. Cutaneous lesions include palpable purpura most commonly on the lower legs, subcutaneous nodules and ulcers. Polyarteritis nodosa (PAN) is a medium- and small-vessel disease, which may be systemic or solely cutaneous. Skin lesions occur in 25–50% of patients with systemic PAN and include livedoid changes (◘ Fig. 40.6) and ulceration attributed to a necrotising vasculitis, with subcutaneous nodules formed by aneurysms of superficial blood vessels. Renal involvement occurs in 25–60% of systemic PAN and is a poor prognostic indicator.

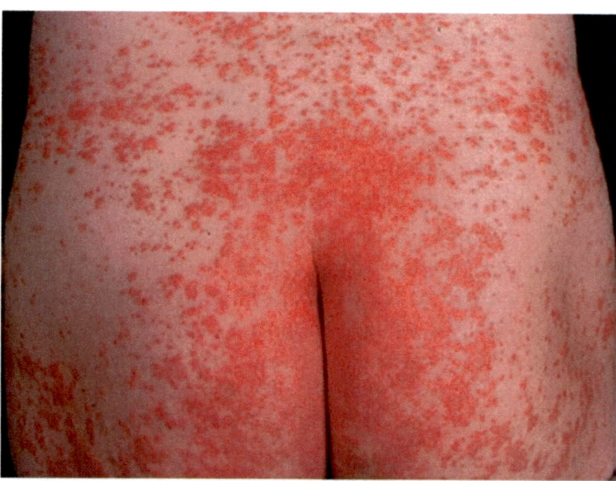

◘ **Fig. 40.5** Henoch-Schönlein purpura

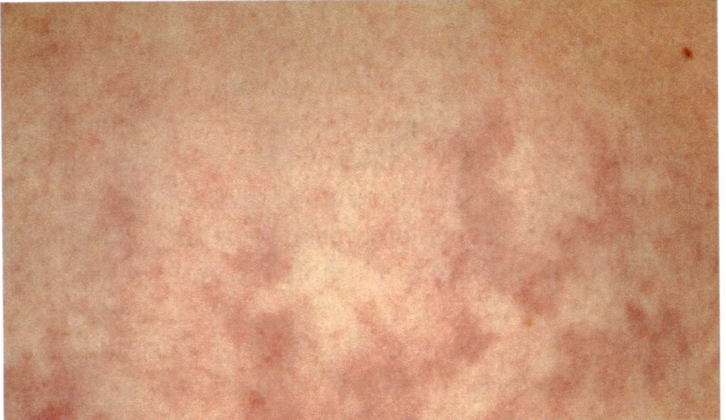

Fig. 40.6 Livedoid changes of PAN

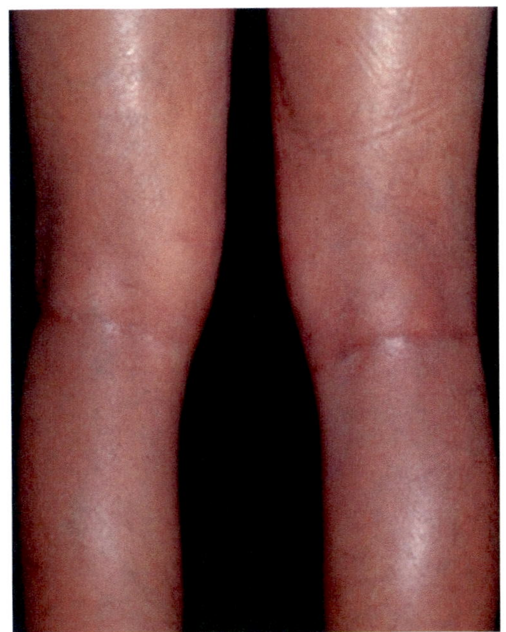

Fig. 40.7 Systemic sclerosis

40.8.3 Systemic Sclerosis

The clinical separation of scleroderma into 'diffuse' and 'limited' is based on whether truncal skin or proximal parts of the extremities are involved (diffuse) or the induration is limited to the face and distal extremities (limited) [15]. In general, diffuse disease carries a worse prognosis but overlap does exist between the two subtypes. Patients with limited disease tend to have features of CREST syndrome (calcinosis, Raynaud's phenomenon, oesophageal involvement, sclerodactyly, telangiectasia). With sclerosis of the skin, there is often symmetric cutaneous induration and thickening caused by progressive accumulation of excess collagen, frequently associated with itching (Fig. 40.7). This is often coupled with diffuse facial hyperpigmentation, as well as localised areas of complete pigment loss with sparing of the perifollicular skin. Telangiectasias are most common in patients with CREST syndrome, particularly on the palms and lips. Capillary abnormalities in the proximal nail fold are present in over 90% of patients, characterised by capillary loss alternating with dilated loops, which can be visualised with a dermatoscope. First-line agents for cutaneous disease include the use of either potent topical steroids or topical tacrolimus ointment, with the addition of either mycophenolate mofetil or methotrexate. These may be helpful particularly for localised and early-stage disease. Phototherapy, particularly UVA, may also be used, as well as exercises and physiotherapy to maintain mobility.

40.8.4 Amyloidosis

In amyloidosis, normally, soluble plasma proteins are deposited in the extracellular space in an abnormal insoluble fibrillar form. Amyloidosis may be a systemic condition or solely localised to the skin. Cutaneous manifestations are common in systemic amyloidosis, particularly the AL type, and are reported in up to 40% of patients [16]. The lesions usually reflect capillary infiltration and fragility with petechiae and purpura (Fig. 40.8). Xanthomatous papules are frequent, and other cutaneous lesions include hyperpigmented keratotic lesions, scleroderma-like changes, alopecia and nail dystrophy. Bullous amyloidosis has also been described. Generalised infiltration of cutaneous tissues frequently causes the appearance of skin thickening with loss of facial wrinkles and can limit mouth opening.

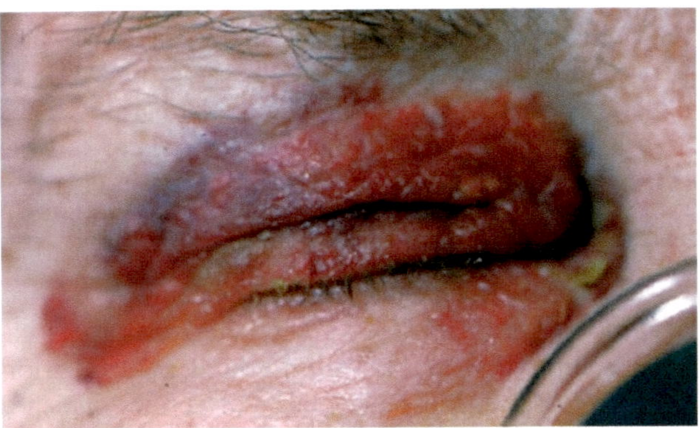

Fig. 40.8 Purpura associated with amyloidosis

40.8.5 Anderson-Fabry Disease

Anderson-Fabry disease is an X-linked lysosomal storage disorder arising from mutations in the GAL A gene. Deficiency of the enzyme galactosidase A results in the accumulation of globotriaosylceramide (Gb3) within

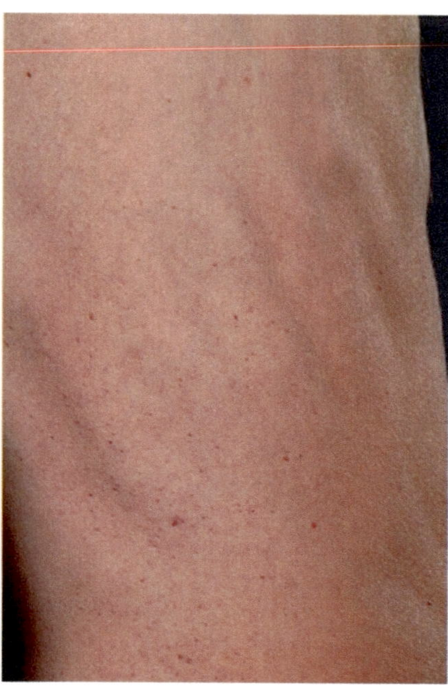

Fig. 40.9 Fabry disease

cellular lysosomes throughout the body. The cutaneous hallmark of Fabry disease is angiokeratoma, which is present in approximately 70% of males and 39% of females. Sites of predilection include the bathing trunk area and genitals in males and the trunk in females (Fig. 40.9). Lips, oral mucosa, umbilicus and extremities may also be affected [17]. Patients with angiokeratoma have higher overall disease severity scores than those without cutaneous vascular lesions. A proportion of Fabry patients also have characteristic facial features including prominent supraorbital ridges, periorbital puffiness, eyelid ptosis, bushy eyebrows, widened nasal bridge, fuller lips and prognathism [18]. Other less well-recognised cutaneous manifestations are sweating abnormalities, lower limb oedema, lymphoedema and Raynaud's phenomenon.

40

40.8.6 HIV

Patients with HIV are prone to a variety of skin manifestations, which can be attributed to an increased susceptibility to various types of infection, e.g. bacterial, viral and fungal, as well as to inflammatory dermatoses and cutaneous malignancies (Kaposi's Sarcoma will be discussed in the renal transplantation and skin disease section below). The predominant cutaneous markers of HIV include eosinophilic/itchy folliculitis, sebopsoriasis, nodular prurigo, acquired ichthyosis and skin photosensitivity. HIV-associated eosinophilic folliculitis is characterised by recurrent episodes of follicular papulopustules, which are often itchy. The lesions predominantly occur on the scalp, face and upper trunk and are observed in HIV-infected patients with a CD4 count of less than 300 cells/mm^3. Histologically, eosinophils are present around the follicular epithelium. Treatment of the underlying HIV infection with a rise in the CD4+ cell count may lead to resolution of the lesions. Other treatment options include topical steroids, UVB phototherapy, oral tetracycline antibiotics and oral isotretinoin.

ESRD in the context of HIV is often multifactorial. With advances in antiretroviral therapy (ART) and improving prognosis of those living with HIV, renal transplantation is no longer an absolute contraindication. Studies have demonstrated comparable patient and graft outcomes comparing HIV-infected patients on ART and uninfected patients [19]. However, there is limited data on the long-term complications of transplant immunosuppression in this population, and whether more opportunistic skin infections, inflammatory dermatoses and skin cancers are observed in this patient population remains to be seen.

40.9 Skin Conditions Associated with Renal Transplantation

Various cutaneous manifestations arise in renal transplant recipients (RTRs), which are mainly attributable to post-transplant immunosuppression. The dermatological complications of immunosuppressive therapy can broadly be divided into drug-specific dermatoses and skin conditions associated with the immunosuppressed state itself, namely, infection and malignancy (Table 40.2). There is also a group of miscellaneous skin conditions, which are not directly related to the immunosuppression or drugs but observed more frequently in the transplant population. Skin conditions are a significant problem in renal transplant patients with their frequency in one study reported to be 95% [20], with a major impact on quality of life [2]. There is an increasing number of older people undergoing renal transplants. Ageing has complex effects on the immune system, and this combination of immunosenescence and immunosuppressive therapy is likely to lead to a rise in the number of skin conditions, in particular skin malignancies.

40.10 Drug-Specific Dermatoses in Transplantation

The well-documented drug-specific skin manifestations are listed in Table 40.2. Acne (Fig. 40.10) in RTRs can often be severe and disfiguring, and as such it is

Table 40.2 Skin conditions associated with renal transplantation

Drug-specific dermatoses	Skin manifestations of immunosuppression			Miscellaneous
Hypertrichosis (cyclosporin)	*Infection*	*Pre-malignant*	*Malignant*	Skin tags
Gingival hypertrophy (cyclosporin)	Viral warts	Actinic keratoses	Squamous cell carcinoma	Melanocytic naevi
Acne (steroids/sirolimus)	Fungal infections (e.g. onychomycosis, pityriasis versicolor)	Bowen's disease	Basal cell carcinoma	Seborrhoeic dermatitis
Sebaceous gland hyperplasia (cyclosporin)	Folliculitis		Melanoma	Seborrhoeic keratoses
Cushingoid features (steroids)	HSV/VZV		Merkel cell carcinoma Kaposi sarcoma	

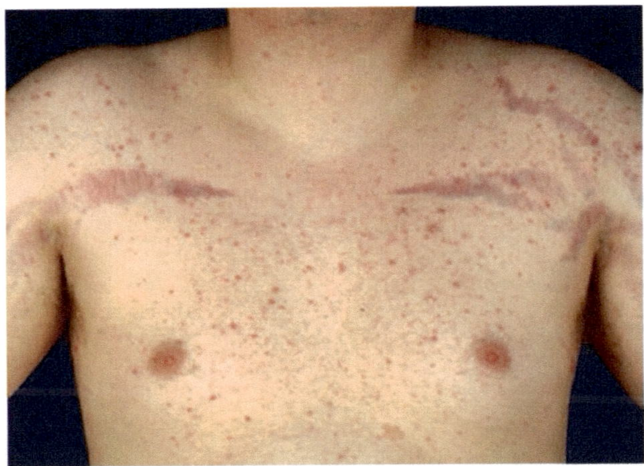

Fig. 40.10 Steroid-induced acne and striae

Table 40.3 Skin infections associated with renal transplantation

Infective skin manifestations of immunosuppression		
Bacterial	***Viral***	***Fungal***
Folliculitis	Viral warts (HPV)	Onychomycosis
Impetigo	HSV/VZV	Pityriasis versicolor
Necrotising fasciitis	Molluscum contagiosum (poxvirus)	Deep fungal infections
Atypical mycobacteria		

important to treat lesions promptly in order to minimise the subsequent risk of scarring. First-line agents for patients with mild to moderate acne include topical agents, such as benzoyl peroxide, and topical antibiotics such as erythromycin or clindamycin. Use of oil-free or water-based moisturisers and cosmetics should also be recommended. More severe cases of acne may warrant treatment with systemic agents, under the supervision of both dermatologists and nephrologists. These include oral tetracyclines for a minimum of 2–3 months, in combination with suitable topical treatment, or if this fails, then the use of the oral retinoid isotretinoin. The latter may only be prescribed by a dermatologist with close monitoring of lipids and liver function, as well as enrolling women of childbearing age into a pregnancy prevention programme due to its teratogenicity. Most courses of isotretinoin last for 5–6 months but may often be longer, depending on the dose used and how well it is tolerated. Any scope for reducing the dose of the offending agents (particularly steroids) should also be considered.

Sebaceous gland hyperplasia can often be disfiguring for patients and are characterised as small yellow papules, often on the forehead and cheeks. They may be treated with gentle cautery, though lesions often recur. Low-dose oral retinoids may be considered if very extensive.

40.11 Skin Infections in Solid Organ Transplantation

Infections of the skin in transplant recipients are common and can be caused by bacteria, mycobacteria, fungi and viruses (Table 40.3). They can be challenging to diagnose and treat as they may have an atypical appearance secondary to the effects of immunosuppression. Human papillomavirus (HPV)-related cutaneous and anogenital viral warts are very common. They are often numerous and recalcitrant to treatment (Fig. 40.11). A number of therapeutic options are available, including chemical or physical destruction, treatments that enhance the local immune response and antiproliferative therapy (Table 40.4). Reduction in immunosuppression where possible may be curative. No treatment is also an option, and indications for treatment will depend on the level of discomfort, cosmetic embarrassment and risk of malignancy. An immune response is essential for clearance, and immunocompromised individuals may never show wart clearance. The HPV vaccine may play a role in both prevention and treatment of warts. However, data on the immunogenicity and efficacy of the vaccines in the transplant population is lacking [21].

Pityriasis versicolor is a common fungal infection in transplant recipients and is characterised by flat, scaly, hyper- or hypopigmented patches which predominantly occur on the trunk (Fig. 40.12). The mainstay

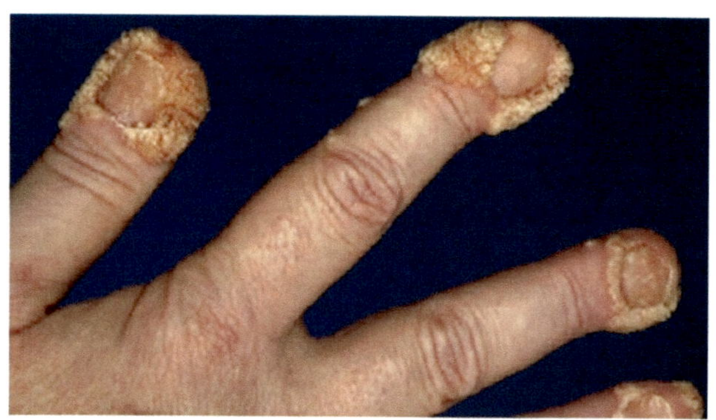

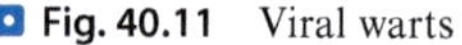

Fig. 40.11 Viral warts

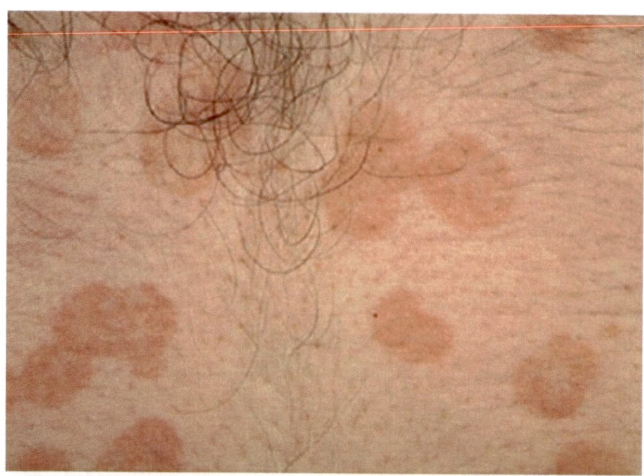

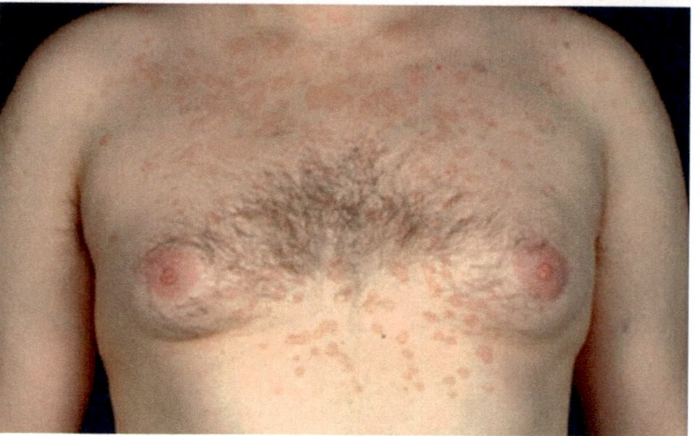

Fig. 40.12 Pityriasis versicolor

Table 40.4 Treatment options for viral warts

Treatments for viral warts	
Destructive	*Antiproliferative*
Topical salicylic acid[a]	Podophyllin/podophyllotoxin
Cryotherapy[a]	Intralesional bleomycin
Thermocautery/curettage and cautery	Retinoids: topical and systemic
Chemical cautery: silver nitrate	Topical 5-fluorouracil[a]
Laser: CO_2/pulsed dye	Occlusotherapy
Photodynamic therapy	Vitamin D analogues, e.g. maxacalcitrol
Topical phenol	Dithranol
Topical cantharidin	Topical cidofovir
Trichloroacetic acid	
Immune stimulation	*Virucidal*
Topical imiquimod[a]	Topical formaldehyde
Contact immunotherapy: diphencyprone	Topical glutaraldehyde
Cimetidine	

[a]Most commonly used first-line therapies

of treatment is with topical antifungal agents such as ketoconazole shampoo, which may be used as a wash. More resistant cases may be treated with oral itraconazole, again in liaison with the nephrologist. Fungal nail infections (onychomycosis) also frequently occur, particularly affecting the large toenails, and are notoriously difficult to treat. Again, if asymptomatic, no treatment is acceptable, since they are rarely more than a cosmetic problem. If treatment is desired, application of a nail lacquer (e.g. amorolfine) may be suggested. Systemic antifungals such as terbinafine are generally avoided since prolonged courses are required which are ultimately often unsuccessful in treating fungal nail infections adequately.

40.12 Premalignant and Malignant Skin Conditions

RTRs are at significant increased risk of cutaneous malignancy compared to the general population. Non-melanoma skin cancers (NMSC), in particular squamous cell carcinoma (SCC) and basal cell carcinoma (BCC), are by far the most common, affecting more than half of organ transplant recipients during their long-term course [3]. NMSCs in RTRs not only place a significant burden on healthcare resources but also cause significant morbidity for individuals as rates are over 100 times that of the general population and tumours are often multiple and more aggressive [3]. Studies have shown that after the first cutaneous SCC, multiple subsequent skin cancers develop in 60–80% of RTRs within 3 years [22]. It is predicted that NMSC incidence will continue to escalate relentlessly as a clinical problem in RTRs as an inevitable consequence of continuing improvements in long-term graft survival. Immunosuppression and HPV have been implicated as possible cofactors in transplant skin carcinogenesis, but cumulative exposure to ultraviolet radiation remains the dominant risk factor [23]. Sunscreen use has been shown to significantly reduce the incidence of cutaneous SCC in immunocompetent individuals with the incidence of SCC lower in the sunscreen group than in the no daily sunscreen group (1115 vs 1832 per 100,000; 0.61 [0.46–0.81]), which is the only robust RCT for cutaneous SCC prevention [24]. Primary and secondary prevention campaigns have accordingly emphasised the importance of photoprotection and self-surveillance. Where possible, a reduction in immunosuppression should be considered as a means of attempting to reduce the incidence and subsequent complications of such tumours.

Many precancerous conditions can be treated by non-surgical means, for example, by spraying liquid nitrogen (cryotherapy), applying a topical agent such as 5-fluorouracil or 5% imiquimod as well as photodynamic therapy (PDT). Daylight PDT is a newer, more convenient and tolerable form of PDT used to treat multiple precancerous actinic keratosis (AKs)/areas of field change on the face and scalp. Results have been comparable with conventional PDT in the general population, though there are currently very limited studies in the transplant cohort.

Most skin cancers themselves can be removed by a minor surgical procedure performed under a local anaesthetic, which is often curative. Aggressive margin control is required, and as such Mohs micrographic surgery is often the treatment of choice for difficult BCCs and SCCs on the face. This is a scar-minimising surgical technique, which enables microscopic examination of all the surgical margins at the time of surgery, thus ensuring complete removal of the tumour whilst sparing as much normal skin as possible. Since most skin cancers arise on sun-exposed sites, e.g. the face, prompt diagnosis potentially minimises the extent of surgery and subsequent scarring. More importantly, rapid treatment reduces the risk of possible tumour spread with certain types of skin cancer.

40.13 Actinic Keratoses (Solar Keratoses)

These are precancerous skin lesions which are characterised by pink/red scaly patches, on sun-exposed sites. The most commonly affected areas are the face and backs of the hands, with confluent areas of involvement known as field change (◘ Fig. 40.13). There has been a lack of evidence in transplant recipients to suggest that treating AK/field change actually prevents progression to SCC, though currently it is standard practice to do so. A RCT by Weinstock et al. demonstrated a 75% risk reduction in SCC development following the use of topical 5% fluorouracil cream to treat AKs on the head and neck of high-risk immunocompetent individuals [25].

40.14 Basal Cell Carcinomas (BCC or Rodent Ulcers)

These are slow-growing, often pearly-pink lesions that typically arise on sun-exposed sites (◘ Fig. 40.14). They seldom, if ever, spread; however, if left untreated, they can erode the skin, eventually leading to ulceration and local invasion. Surgical removal is the mainstay of treat-

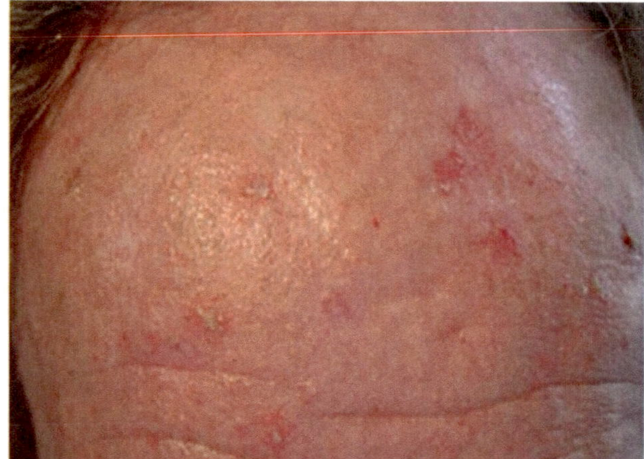

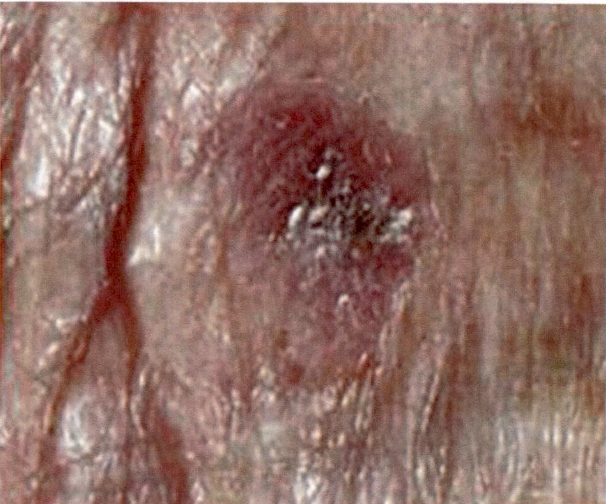

Fig. 40.13 Actinic keratoses

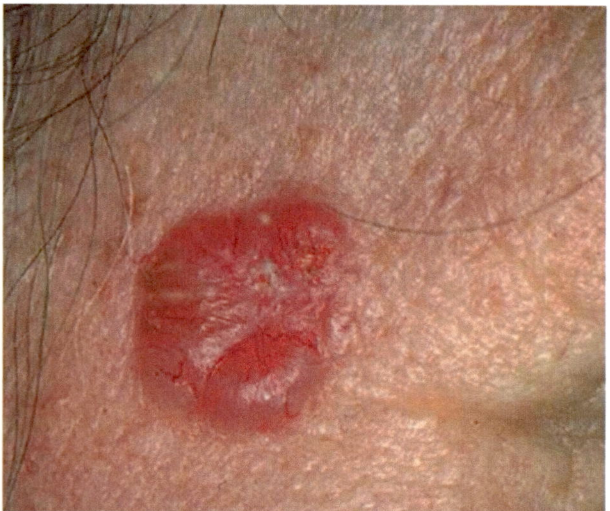

Fig. 40.14 Basal cell carcinoma

40

ment, though other options include local radiotherapy, as well as cryotherapy, topical agents such as imiquimod cream and PDT, for certain superficial subtypes of BCC.

40.15 Squamous Cell Carcinoma (SCC)

SCCs frequently appear as a scaly crusted area of skin, with a red, inflamed base and are often ulcerated (Fig. 40.15). A painful enlarging lump is suspicious for SCC, predominantly occurring on sun-exposed sites, particularly on the ears, lips and backs of the hands. This is the most frequent type of skin cancer in organ transplant patients and, if left untreated, has the potential to metastasise, with a 7% metastatic risk overall. SCCs are best treated by prompt surgical removal. Chemoprevention with the systemic retinoid acitretin has been reported to lead to a significant reduction in SCC development in RTRs and is often used in high-risk individuals with >1 cutaneous SCC. In a retrospective study of 28 RTRs receiving continuous retinoid treatment, a significant mean reduction of 1.46 SCCs occurred in the first year of treatment, 2.24 SCCs by the second year and 2.14 SCCs in year 3. This reduction was sustained, but nonsignificant, at years 4 and later, indicating a loss of efficacy in the chemopreventive properties of acitretin. In addition, a 'rebound' phenomenon is also recognised, whereby interruption of acitretin treatment leads to a relapse in tumour development [26]. A randomised trial of oral nicotinamide 500 mg twice daily for 12 months in immunocompetent patients with a history of $\geq$ 2 NMSCs found a 20% reduction in the number of new BCCs and a 30% reduction in the number of new SCCs in the nicotinamide group, compared with the placebo group [27]. Data on solid organ transplant recipients is limited to small studies but does show promise. Larger randomised trials are needed to determine whether nicotinamide is effective as a chemopreventive agent in renal transplant recipients; however, as it is well tolerated and has a limited side-effect profile, it may be considered.

There is evidence to suggest that switching from calcineurin inhibitors to sirolimus in RTRs with at least one previous cutaneous SCC is associated with a lower risk of subsequent skin cancers [28]. The number of SCCs was lower by a factor of 3.4 in the sirolimus group than in the calcineurin-inhibitor group. Survival free of cutaneous squamous cell carcinoma was significantly longer in the sirolimus group than in the calcineurin-inhibitor group, with a relative risk in the sirolimus group of 0.56. There was however a much higher rate of adverse events in patients converted to sirolimus.

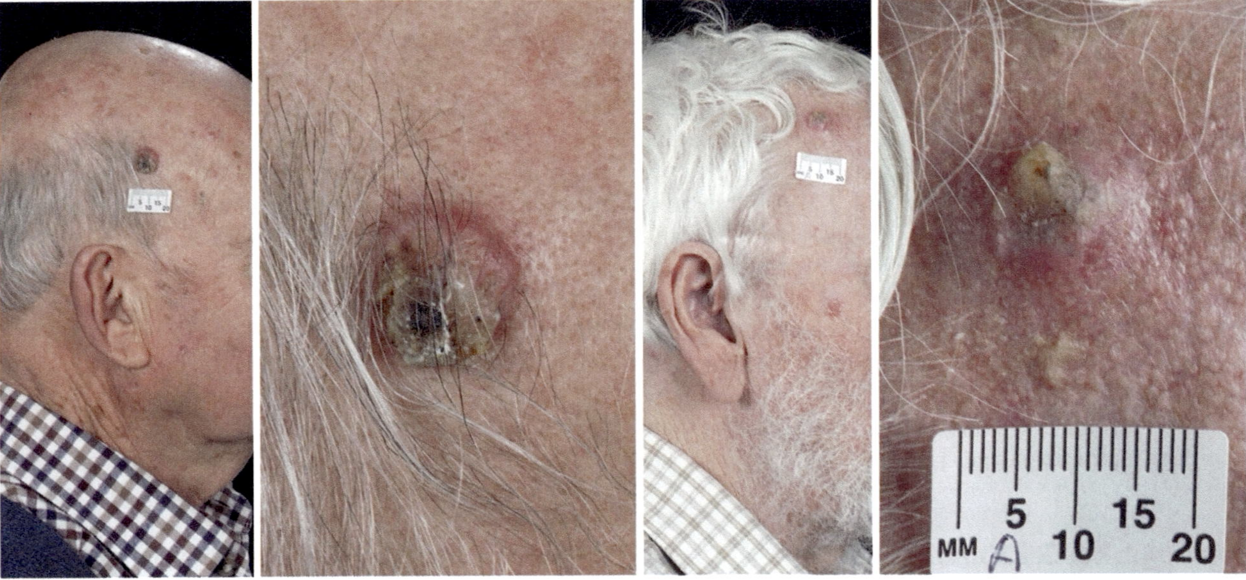

Fig. 40.15 Cutaneous squamous cell carcinoma

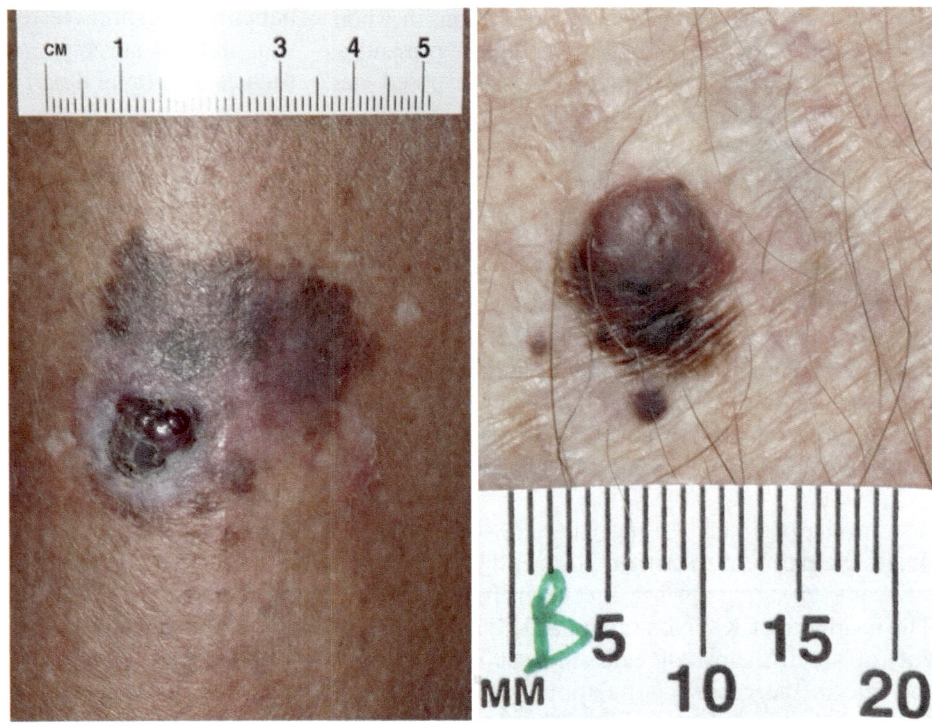

Fig. 40.16 Cutaneous melanoma

40.16 Melanoma

Melanomas occur less commonly than BCCs and SCCs, with an eight- to tenfold increased risk in RTRs, though are potentially more aggressive if not detected early. They are usually characterised as an irregular brown or black lesion, which may start in a pre-existing mole or appear on previously normal skin (Fig. 40.16). Any change in a mole, or any new mole occurring for the first time after the age of 30, should be urgently assessed by a dermatologist with a view to surgical excision. A multicentre European study reported a worse prognosis for stage II disease compared with the general population [29].

The management of melanoma in organ transplant recipients usually parallels that of melanoma in immunocompetent patients. Early-stage melanoma can be managed with surgical excision. Immunosuppression should be reduced to the minimal regimen necessary to maintain organ tolerance in more advanced stage melanomas. With the advent of immunotherapy in the management of metastatic melanoma over recent years, OTRs with advanced malignancies have been largely excluded from clinical trials testing the safety and efficacy of these therapies. Chae et al. reviewed the available data describing immune checkpoint blockade in the OTR population assessing the risk of allograft rejection associated with the various treatment regimens. They found that CTLA-4 inhibitors have been used safely and successfully in selected patients, whilst PD-1 inhibitors were associated with a higher risk of allograft rejection. Further clinical experience and larger clinical trials involving immune checkpoint inhibitors as monotherapies or combinatorial therapies are needed to develop regimens that optimise the antitumour immune response and minimise the risk of graft rejection in organ transplant patients [30].

40.17 Merkel Cell Carcinoma

Merkel cell carcinoma (MCC) is a rare yet aggressive skin tumour occurring around 10 times more commonly in RTRs compared to the general population, in whom it has a significantly worse prognosis. It often presents as an asymptomatic solitary red nodule on sun-exposed sites, most commonly the head and neck, with ~70% rate of metastasis and a 5-year survival of <50% (◘ Fig. 40.17). They are of neuroendocrine origin and 80% are associated with the clonal integration of the Merkel cell polyomavirus (MCPyV) [31]. Management is predominantly surgical, with the use of adjuvant radiotherapy for local disease. Further research on the role of MCPyV may offer hope for more targeted approaches to MCC treatment and prevention. The PD L1 antibody Avelumab, an immune checkpoint inhibitor, has been approved by NICE in 2018 as first-line treatment for advanced or metastatic MCC, though OTRs were excluded from initial studies.

40.18 Kaposi's Sarcoma

The incidence of Kaposi's sarcoma (KS) among recipients of solid organs is greater than 400 to 500 times the rate in the general population, with clinical presentation in transplant patients often confined to the skin. KS is a tumour of endothelial origin and presents as purple papules, plaques and nodular lesions, most often on the lower legs and commonly associated with lymphoedema (◘ Fig. 40.18). Visceral involvement occurs in 25–30% of OTRs. KS is especially prevalent in Mediterranean and African populations and is related to HHV8. Serostatus at the time of transplant is the most important risk factor associated with post-transplant KS, with a mean duration of onset 13 months post-transplantation. The main approach to managing transplant-associated Kaposi's sarcoma is to reduce or even discontinue immunosuppressive therapy, which usually causes skin lesions to regress, although it carries a risk of acute rejection of the graft. KS generally recurs when immunosuppressive therapy is reintroduced or after a second transplantation. In a study of 15 renal transplant recipients, it was found that sirolimus inhibits the progression of dermal KS when given at the usual immunosuppressive dose, with remission induced in all 15 subjects within 3 months [32]. Thus, switching to an mTor inhibitor such as sirolimus is recommended, with a >70% response rate within 3 months. Further treatment options for patients unresponsive to revision of immunosuppression include surgery, radiotherapy or chemotherapy such as liposomal doxorubicin.

40.19 Specialist Transplant Skin Clinics

The need for post-transplant skin cancer surveillance has been recognised in many international expert consensus guidelines. In the UK, the National Institute for Health and Clinical Excellence recommend surveillance in dedicated dermatology clinics [33], and it has been shown that such clinics significantly improve compliance with sun protection and skin cancer awareness [34]. Other guidelines in Europe and the USA also advise specialist full skin examination of RTRs every 6–12 months; however, these recommendations do not take account of individual risk nor the needs of practising clinicians with limited resources. The effectiveness and cost-benefit of skin surveillance in RTRs is unknown, and as such, a surveillance model for skin cancer in RTRs has been proposed by Harwood et al. [35], based on a 22-year prospective study of more than 1000 patients. They define surveillance intervals that enable close follow-up of higher-risk individuals with routine follow-up of those at

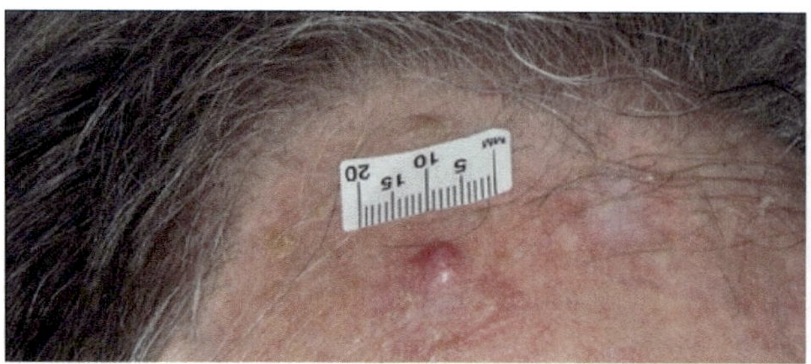

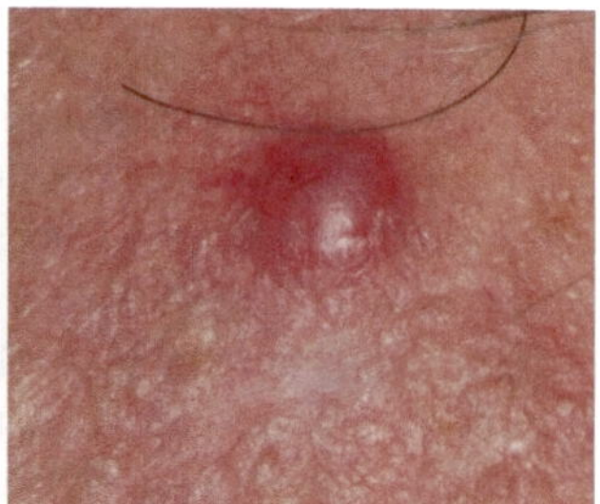

◘ **Fig. 40.17** Merkel cell carcinoma

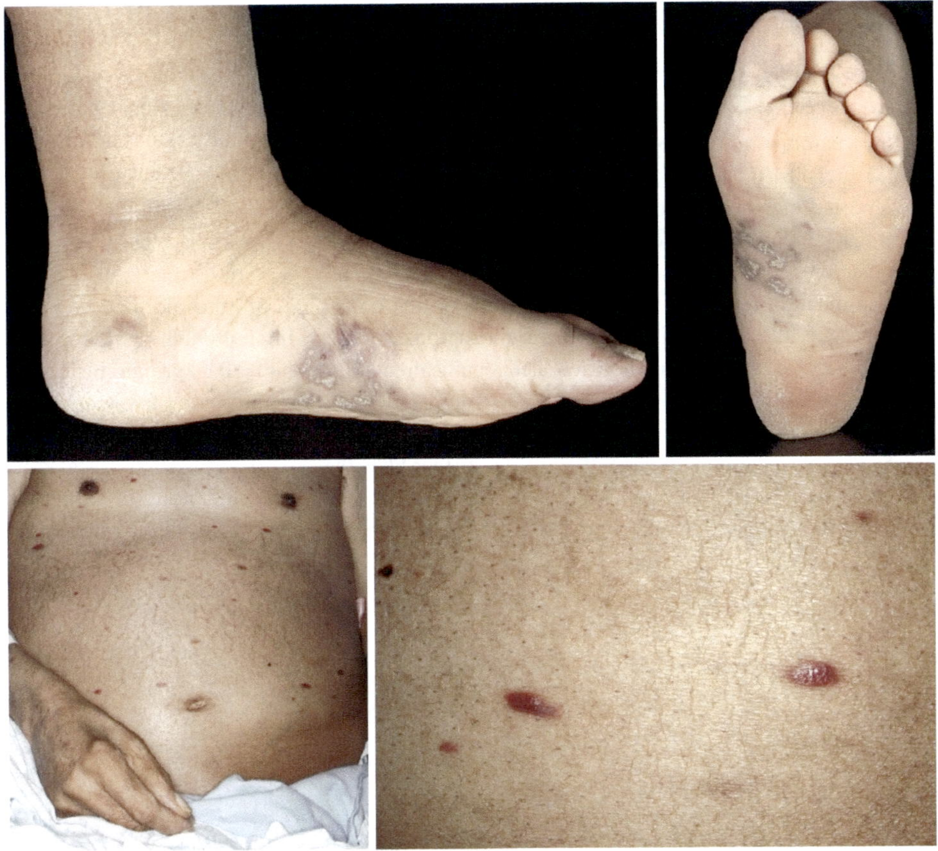

Fig. 40.18 Cutaneous Kaposi's sarcoma

much lower risk. This risk stratification is based upon a number of patient characteristics, including skin phototype, age at transplantation, sunburn history and history of confirmed skin cancer. Garrett et al. evaluated the risk factors for post-transplant skin cancer in a large multicentre study, with elevated risk imparted by increased age, fair skin type and male sex. Understanding the risk factors and trends in post-transplant skin cancer is fundamental to targeted screening and prevention [36]. This is of practical use to those setting up transplant skin clinics, facilitating targeted surveillance and active management to those who need it most.

Any such service should involve a multidisciplinary approach with close interaction between dermatologists, transplant clinicians, plastic surgeons/dermatology surgeons, medical/clinical oncologists, pathologists, clinical nurse specialists and primary care physicians. The relationship between dermatologists and transplant clinicians enables discussion of potential revision of immunosuppression in high-risk individuals as well as the potential need for systemic agents to be introduced. The role of a specialist nurse should also be highlighted, in particular facilitating urgent access for patients as well as undertaking nurse-led surveillance clinics and patient education in relation to photoprotection and skin cancer awareness. Preferably, primary prevention of skin cancers should be emphasised from the outset, i.e. to all patients on transplant waiting lists.

40.20 Conclusions

Dermatological conditions in patients with renal disease are extremely common and varied. Having a basic understanding of these is essential, as early recognition and management can have a huge impact both on the physical and psychological well-being of these patients. Within the transplant population, the clinical presentation of skin conditions can often be difficult to recognise and challenging to treat, and skin cancers in particular are frequently multiple and more aggressive. Published data regarding management of skin diseases in this patient cohort is limited or anecdotal and is predominantly extrapolated from guidelines in immunocompetent individuals. It is therefore essential that further research within this population is undertaken and that there exists a collaborative relationship between renal and dermatology clinicians. Dedicated dermatology clinics are essential for managing this complex group of patients in order to improve both morbidity and mortality from the rising incidence of skin diseases within this population.

Case Study

Case 1

A 59-year-old Caucasian man developed a rapidly enlarging painful nodule on the back of the left hand (◘ Fig. 40.19). He worked for many years as a builder and reported significant occupational sun exposure. He was transplanted 7 years prior and was on maintenance immunosuppression of mycophenolate mofetil and tacrolimus. Examination revealed areas of field change on the dorsal aspect of the hands with a tender erythematous nodule. Further full skin examination revealed significant photodamage on the face and scalp. The lesion from the dorsum of the left hand was excised and confirmed to be a SCC. Twelve months later, he developed a further SCC the on scalp. At that point, the renal team were consulted to consider reducing immunosuppression and to commence acitretin as SCC chemoprevention. In addition, areas of field change were aggressively treated with topical 5-FU as secondary skin cancer prevention, and strict sun protection practices were reinforced. The patient was kept under 3–6 monthly surveillance in a transplant dermatology clinic.

Case 2

A 58-year-old man presented with a 2-year history of an intensely itchy eruption on the trunk, arms and legs. He had a background history of ESRD secondary to diabetic nephropathy for which he was on peritoneal dialysis for over 2 years.

Examination revealed widespread erythematous papules and nodules with a keratotic centre on the upper limbs, lower limbs and trunk (◘ Fig. 40.20). A skin biopsy

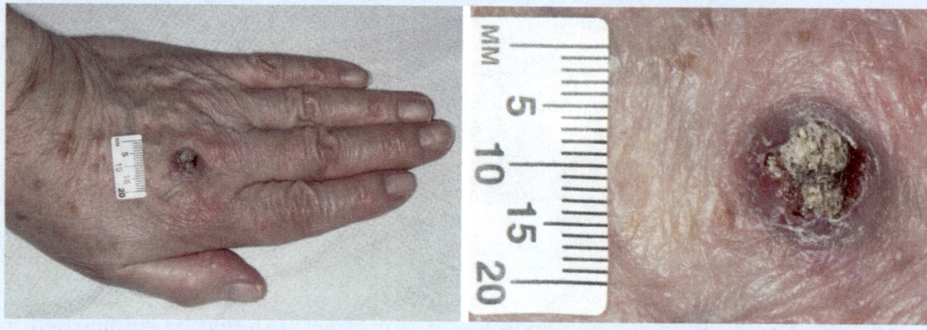

◘ **Fig. 40.19** Cutaneous squamous cell carcinoma

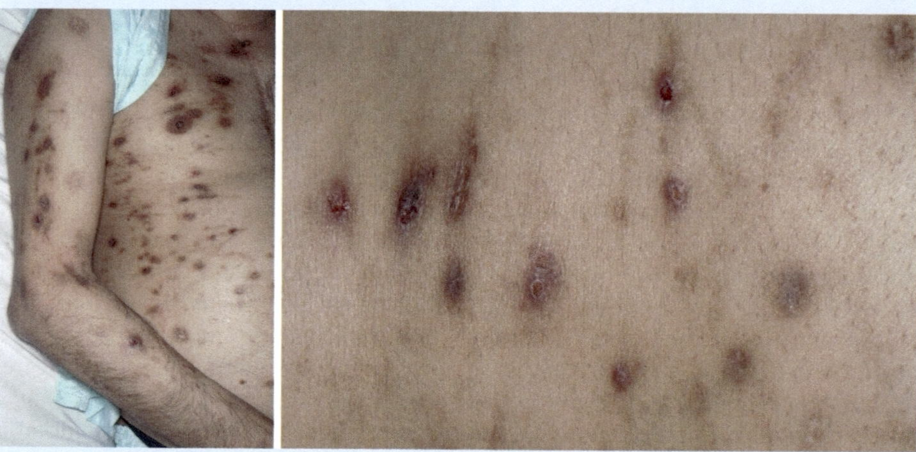

◘ **Fig. 40.20** Perforating collagenosis

revealed a ruptured epidermis with elimination of dermal material, and special stains confirmed the diagnosis of perforating collagenosis.

Management included the regular use of emollients and potent topical steroids for symptomatic relief. Given the extent of the lesions, he was commenced on TL01 (narrow band UVB) phototherapy following which he had further limited improvement.

Case 3

A 52-year-old woman of Kenyan origin presented with a 1-year history of an evolving painful cutaneous eruption around a functioning fistula on her left arm associated with marked oedema, 18 months following a second kidney transplant. She was otherwise clinically well with no systemic symptoms and maintained on tacrolimus and mycophenolate mofetil. Examination revealed multiple palpable purple confluent papules and plaques around the fistula site on her left arm, with oedema and tenderness (◘ Fig. 40.21). Full skin examination was otherwise unremarkable. A diagnostic skin biopsy revealed vascular channels lined with atypical endothelial cells amongst a network of extravasated red cells and hemosiderin deposition, consistent with Kaposi's sarcoma. This was further supported by positive immunostaining for HHV8. She went on to have full body imaging which excluded visceral involvement.

Her immunosuppression was modified with the gradual reduction of tacrolimus and the introduction of sirolimus, with maintenance of her graft function. The cutaneous lesions resolved within 3 months of switching her immunosuppression.

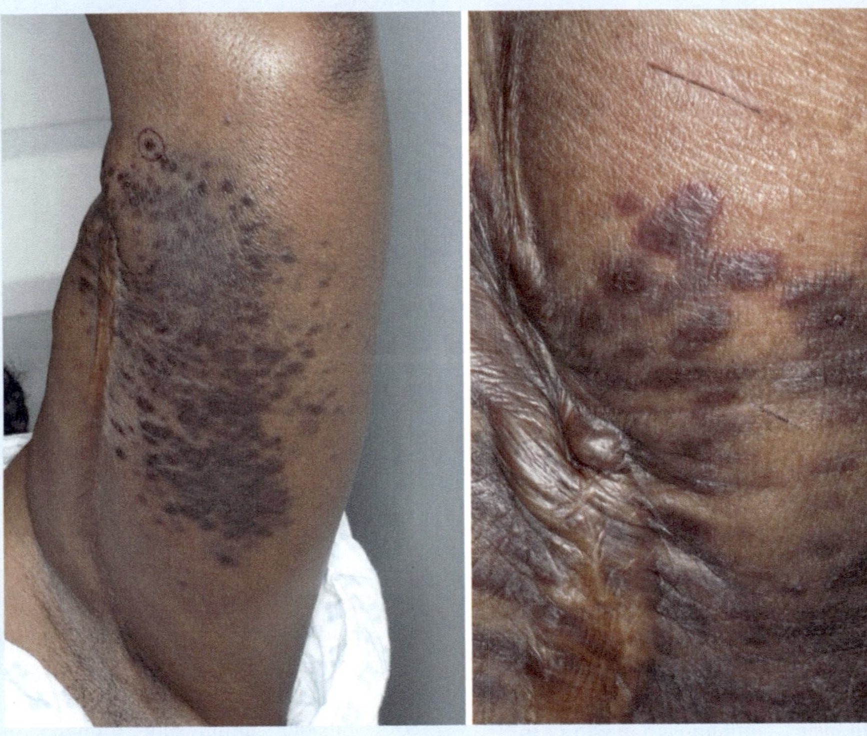

◘ **Fig. 40.21** Cutaneous Kaposi's sarcoma at a fistula site

Case 4

A 68-year-old woman was admitted to hospital with a 3-month history of progressive bilateral breast pain and necrotic ulceration. She noted this first began with darkening of the skin with a 'woody' feeling within the breast. This then began to break down centrally and ulcerate, leaving a thick overlying black crust. She had end-stage renal disease secondary to hypertension and type 2 diabetes and had been on haemodialysis for 10 years.

Examination revealed dusky red mottling over the breasts with a livedoid pattern at the periphery. Centrally there were black eschars on both breasts and across the abdomen. The surrounding skin was indurated and exquisitely tender (◘ Fig. 40.22). A deep incisional skin biopsy was performed on the left breast, which showed ulceration and necrosis with calcification of small- to medium-sized vessels and intravascular thrombi, as well as diffuse calcification of small capillaries in the subcutaneous fat. These changes were consistent with the diagnosis of calciphylaxis.

The frequency of dialysis was increased with immediate effect. Intravenous infusions of sodium thiosulfate were administered during dialysis and meticulous wound care administered, with a gradual improvement in the cutaneous lesions over a 4-month period.

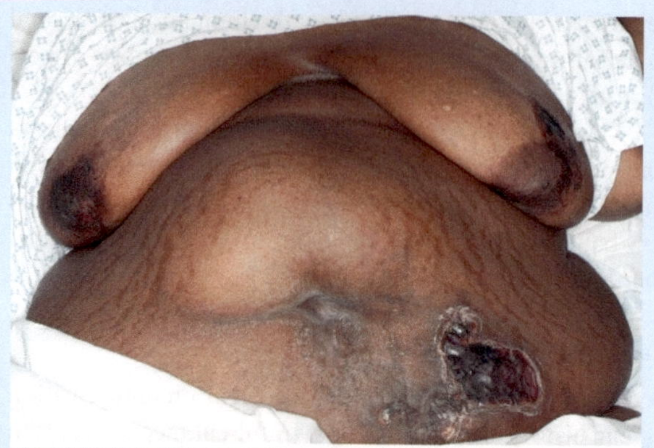

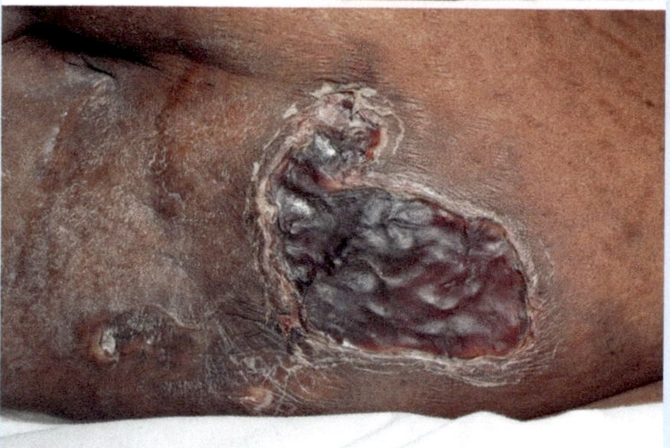

◘ **Fig. 40.22** Calciphylaxis

40

Tips and Tricks

1. Regular use of emollients and soap substitutes in patients with ESRD can minimise symptoms of pruritus.
2. Consider phototherapy for treatment of uraemic pruritus/perforating collagenosis unresponsive to topical treatments.
3. Painful skin ulceration on a background of livedoid change is likely to be calciphylaxis, which requires prompt multidisciplinary treatment.
4. Consider minimising immunosuppression in patients with recalcitrant viral warts +/− low-dose oral retinoids.
5. Sebaceous hyperplasia and acne are common benign skin conditions particularly related to cyclosporine and tacrolimus, which often cause significant patient morbidity, and may be managed by low-dose oral retinoids.
6. Reinforce sun protection measures early, particularly in higher risk RTRs whilst on the transplant waiting list.
7. More regular skin surveillance is required in RTRs at greater risk for skin cancers, i.e. fair skin phototype, older age at transplantation (>50y), duration and intensity of immunosuppression and significant UV exposure.
8. Painful and/or rapidly enlarging nodules require prompt excision. Always be suspicious of cutaneous SCC.
9. Consider minimising immunosuppression in patients with >1 SCC +/− evidence of significant photodamage.
10. KS may present as lymphoedema +/− palpable purplish plaques, predominantly on the lower legs. HHV8 serostatus at time of transplant is the most important risk factor for its development.
11. Consider switching to sirolimus in patients with post-transplant KS.

Chapter Review Questions

1. What is the management strategy for uraemic pruritus?
2. What are the main differentials to consider for a rapidly enlarging nodule on a UV-exposed site in a RTR?
3. What are the most commonly used topical agents for the treatment of cutaneous viral warts?
4. How is troublesome acne managed in renal transplant recipients?
5. What primary, secondary and tertiary prevention methods could be employed to reduce the skin cancer burden in transplant recipients?

Answers

1.
   - Ensure adequate dialysis
   - Normalise calcium-phosphate and PTH levels
   - Correct anaemia
   - Regular emollients
   - Topical capsaicin/calcipotriol
   - Consider UVB phototherapy
2.
   - SCC (usually painful)
   - MCC
   - Amelanotic melanoma

   N.B. Whatever the cause, this should prompt urgent dermatology referral.
3.
   - Destructive, e.g. salicylic acid, cryotherapy
   - Antiproliferative, e.g. 5-FU
   - Immune stimulation, e.g. imiquimod
   - Virucidal, e.g. formaldehyde

   See Table 40.4
4.
   - Avoid over-moisturising skin.
   - Topical benzoyl peroxide or topical antibiotic, e.g. erythromycin/clindamycin.
   - Consider oral tetracycline such as lymecycline for 3 months.
   - In more severe cases, consider oral retinoid (isotretinoin) and even reduction in immunosuppression.
5.
   - Primary prevention:
     - Pre-transplantation screening
     - Patient education concerning sun protection and skin self-examination
   - Secondary prevention:
     - Post-transplantation surveillance
     - Treatment of precancerous lesions
   - Tertiary prevention:
     - Choice and modulation of immunosuppressive therapy, i.e. reduce immunosuppression to the lowest possible safe dose and consider alternative agents, e.g. sirolimus.
     - Consider oral chemoprevention, e.g. acitretin, nicotinamide.

Acknowledgements Professor Catherine Harwood and Dr. Cate Orteu kindly provided many of the clinical photographs and contributed to sections 'Skin Conditions Associated with Renal Transplantation' and 'Skin Manifestations of Diseases Associated with Renal Involvement' of this chapter, respectively.

References

1. Udayakumar P, Balasubramanian S, Ramalingam KS, Lakshmi C, Srinivas CR, Mathew AC. Cutaneous manifestations in patients with chronic renal failure on haemodialysis. Indian J Dermatol Venereol Leprol. 2006;72(2):119–25.
2. Moloney FJ, Keane S, O'Kelly P, Conlon PJ, Murphy GM. The impact of skin disease on renal transplantation on quality of life. Br J Dermatol. 2005;153(3):574–8.
3. Euvrard S, Kanitakis J, Claudy A. Skin cancers after organ transplantation. N Engl J Med. 2003;348(17):1681–91.
4. Narita I, Alchi B, Omori K, Sato F, Ajiro J, Saga D, Kondo D, Skatsume M, Maruyama S, Kazama JJ, Akazawa K, Gejyo F. Aetiology and prognostic significance of severe uraemic pruritus in chronic haemodialysis patients. Kidney Int. 2006;69:1626–32.
5. Millington GWM, Collins A, Lovell CR, Leslie TA, Yong ASW, Morgan JD, Ajithkumar T, Andrews MJ, Rushbook SM, Coelho RR, Catten SJ, Lee KYC, Skellett AM, Affleck AG, Exton LS, Mohd Mustapa MF, Levell NJ. British Association of Dermatologists' guidelines for the investigation and management of generalized pruritus in adults without an underlying dermatosis, 2018. Br J Dermatol. 2018;178(1):34–60.
6. Nigwekar SU, Thadhani R, Brandenburg VM. Calciphylaxis. N Engl J Med. 2018;378(18):1704–14.
7. Peng T, Zhuo L, Wang Y, Jun M, Li G, Wang L, Hong D. A systematic review of sodium thiosulfate in treating calciphylaxis in chronic kidney disease patients. Nephrology (Carlton). 2018;23(7):669–75.
8. Broome DR. Nephrogenic systemic fibrosis associated with gadolinium based contrast agents: a summary of the medical literature reporting. Eur J Radiol. 2008;66(2):230–4.
9. The Royal College of Radiologists – Standards for intravascular contrast administration to adult patients. 2015. https://www.rcr.ac.uk/sites/default/files/Intravasc_contrast_web.pdf.

10. Sontheimer RD. Subacute cutaneous lupus erythematosus: 25-year evolution of a prototypic subset (subphenotype) of lupus erythematosus defined by characteristic cutaneous, pathological, immunological, and genetic findings. Autoimmun Rev. 2005;4(5):253–63.
11. Gronhagen CM, Fored CM, Granath F, Nyberg F. Cutaneous lupus erythematosus and the association with systemic lupus erythematosus: a population-based cohort of 1088 patients in Sweden. Br J Dermatol. 2011;164:1335–41.
12. Chong BF, Song J, Olsen NJ. Determining risk factors for developing systemic lupus erythematosus in patients with discoid lupus erythematosus. Br J Dermatol. 2012;166:29–35.
13. Walsh JS, Gross DJ. Wegener's granulomatosis involving the skin. Cutis. 1999;64(3):183–6.
14. Frances C, Du LT, Piette JC, et al. Wegener's granulomatosis. Dermatological manifestations in 75 cases with clinicopathologic correlation. Arch Dermatol. 1994;130(7):861–7.
15. Moinzadeh P, Denton C, Krieg T, Black C. Fitzpatrick's dermatology in general medicine, vol. 2, sect. 27. 8th ed. 2012. p. 1942–57.
16. Kyle RA, Gertz MA. Primary systemic amyloidosis: clinical and laboratory features in 474 cases. Semin Hematol. 1995;32(1):45–59.
17. Orteu CH, Jansen T, Lidove O, Jaussaud R, Hughes DA, Pintos-Morell G, Ramaswami U, Parini R, Sundur-Plassman G, Beck M, Mehta AB, FOS Investigators. Fabry disease and the skin: data from FOS, the Fabry outcome survey. Br J Dermatol. 2007;157(2):331–7.
18. Hogarth V, Hughes D, Orteu CH. Pseudoacromegalic facial features in Fabry disease. Clin Exp Dermatol. 2013;38(2): 137–9.
19. Stock PG, Barin B, Murphy B, Hanto D, Diego JM, Light J, Davis C, Blumberg E, Simon D, Subramanian A, Millis JM, Lyon GM, Brayman K, Slakey D, Shapiro R, Melancon J, Jacobson JM, Stosor V, Olson JL, Stablein DM, Roland ME. Outcomes of kidney transplantation in HIV-infected recipients. N Engl J Med. 2010;363(21):2004–14.
20. Lugo-Janer G, Sanchez JL, Santiago-Delphin E. Prevalence and clinical spectrum of skin diseases in kidney transplant recipients. J Am Acad Dermatol. 1991;24:410–4.
21. Kwak EJ, Julian K, AST Infectious Diseases Community of Practice. Human papillomavirus infection in solid organ transplant recipients. Am J Transplant. 2009;9(Suppl 4):S151–60.
22. Wisgerhof HC, Edelbroek JR, de Fijter JW, Haasnoot GW, Claas FH, Willemze R, Bavinck JN. Subsequent squamous- and basal-cell carcinomas in kidney transplant recipients after the first skin cancer: cumulative incidence and risk factors. Transplantation. 2010;89(10):1231–8.
23. Hofbauer GF, Bouwes Bavinck JN, Euvrard S. Organ transplantation and skin cancer: basic problems and new perspectives. Exp Dermatol. 2010;19(6):473–82.
24. Green A, Williams G, Neale R, Hart V, Leslie D, Parsons P, Marks GC, Gaffney P, Battistutta D, Frost C, Lang C, Russell A. Daily sunscreen application and betacarotene supplementation in prevention of basal-cell and squamous-cell carcinomas of the skin: a randomised controlled trial. Lancet. 1999;354(9180):723–9.
25. Weinstock MA, Thwin SS, Siegel JA, Marcolivio K, Means AD, Leader NF, Shaw FM, Hogan D, Eilers D, Swetter SM, Chen SC, Jacob SE, Warshaw EM, Stricklin GP, Dellavalle RP, Sidhu-Malik N, Konnikov N, Werth VP, Keri JE, Robinson-Bostom L, Ringer RJ, Lew RA, Ferguson R, JJ DG, Huang GD, Veterans Affairs Keratinocyte Carcinoma Chemoprevention Trial (VAKCC) Group. Chemoprevention of basal and squamous cell carcinoma with a single course of fluorouracil, 5%, cream: a randomized clinical trial. JAMA Dermatol. 2018;154(2):167–74.
26. Harwood CA, Leedham-Green M, Leigh IM, Proby CM. Low-dose retinoids in the prevention of cutaneous squamous cell carcinomas in organ transplant recipients: a 16-year retrospective study. Arch Dermatol. 2005;141(4):456–64.
27. Chen AC, Martin AJ, Choy B, Fernández-Peñas P, Dalziell RA, McKenzie CA, Scolyer RA, Dhillon HM, Vardy JL, Kricker A, St George G, Chinniah N, Halliday GM, Damian DL. A phase 3 randomized trial of nicotinamide for skin-cancer chemoprevention. N Engl J Med. 2015;373(17):1618–26.
28. Euvrard S, Morelon E, Rostaing L, Goffin E, Brocard A, Tromme I, Broeders N, del Marmol V, Chatelet V, Dompmartin A, Kessler M, Serra AL, Hofbauer GF, Pouteil-Noble C, Campistol JM, Kanitakis J, Roux AS, Decullier E, Dantal J, TUMORAPA Study Group. Sirolimus and secondary skin-cancer prevention in kidney transplantation. N Engl J Med. 2012;367(4):329–39.
29. Matin RN, Mesher D, Proby CM, McGregor JM, Bouwes Bavinck JN, del Marmol V, Euvrard S, Ferrandiz C, Geusau A, Hackethal M, Ho WL, Hofbauer GF, Imko-Walczuk B, Kanitakis J, Lally A, Lear JT, Lebbe C, Murphy GM, Piaserico S, Seckin D, Stockfleth E, Ulrich C, Wojnarowska FT, Lin HY, Balch C, Harwood CA. Skin Care in Organ Transplant Patients, Europe (SCOPE) group. Melanoma in organ transplant recipients: clinicopathological features and outcome in 100 cases. Am J Transplant. 2008;8(9):1891–900.
30. Chae YK, Galvez C, Anker JF, Iams WT, Bhave M. Cancer immunotherapy in a neglected population: the current use and future of T-cell-mediated checkpoint inhibitors in organ transplant patients. Cancer Treat Rev. 2018;63:116–21.
31. Feng H, Shuda M, Chang Y, Moore PS. Clonal integration of a polyomavirus in human Merkel cell carcinoma. Science. 2008;319(5866):1096–100.
32. Stallone G, Schena A, Infante B, Di Paolo S, Loverre A, Maggio G, Ranieri E, Gesualdo L, Schena FP, Grandaliano G. Sirolimus for Kaposi's sarcoma in renal-transplant recipients. N Engl J Med. 2005;352:1317–23.
33. National Institute for Health and Clinical Excellence. Improving outcomes for people with skin tumours including melanoma: the manual (2006 guidance). http://www.nice.org.uk/nicemedia/live/10901/28906/28906.pdf.
34. Ismail F, Mitchell L, Casabonne D, Gulati A, Newton R, Proby CM, Harwood CA. Specialist dermatology clinics for organ transplant recipients significantly improve compliance with photoprotection and levels of skin cancer awareness. Br J Dermatol. 2006;155(5):916–25.
35. Harwood CA, Mesher D, McGregor JM, Mitchell L, L-Green M, Raftery M, Cerio R, Leigh IM, Sasieni P, Proby CM. A surveillance model for skin cancer in organ transplant recipients: a 22-year prospective study in an ethnically diverse population. Am J Transplant. 2013;13(1):119–29.
36. Garrett GL, Blanc PD, Boscardin J, Lloyd AA, Ahmed RL, Anthony T, Bibee K, Breithaupt A, Cannon J, Chen A, Cheng JY, Chiesa-Fuxench Z, Colegio OR, Curiel-Lewandrowski

C, Del Guzzo CA, Disse M, Dowd M, Eilers R Jr, Ortiz AE, Morris C, Golden SK, Graves MS, Griffin JR, Hopkins RS, Huang CC, Bae GH, Jambusaria A, Jennings TA, Jiang SI, Karia PS, Khetarpal S, Kim C, Klintmalm G, Konicke K, Koyfman SA, Lam C, Lee P, Leitenberger JJ, Loh T, Lowenstein S, Madankumar R, Moreau JF, Nijhawan RI, Ochoa S, Olasz EB, Otchere E, Otley C, Oulton J, Patel PH, Patel VA, Prabhu AV, Pugliano-Mauro M, Schmults CD, Schram S, Shih AF, Shin T, Soon S, Soriano T, Srivastava D, Stein JA, Sternhell-Blackwell K, Taylor S, Vidimos A, Wu P, Zajdel N, Zelac D, Arron ST. Incidence of and risk factors for skin cancer in organ transplant recipients in the United States. JAMA Dermatol. 2017;153(3):296–303.

Patient Information and Guidelines

Further information for transplant patients, as well as patients awaiting an organ transplant, can be obtained via the British Association of Dermatologists website: http://www.bad.org.uk

Other useful websites include the following:

- After Transplantation – Reduce Incidence of Skin Cancer (AT-RISC Alliance): http://at-risc.org/Home.aspx
- British Society for Skin Care in Immunocompromised Individuals (BSSCII): http://www.bsscii.org.uk
- International Transplant Skin Cancer Collaborative (ITSCC): http://www.itscc.org/
- Skin Care in Organ Transplant Patients Europe (SCOPE): http://www.scopenetwork.org/index.htm

The Nervous System and the Kidney

Anna Nagy, Geraint Dingley, and Rebecca Liu

Contents

M. Harber (ed.), *Primer on Nephrology*, https://doi.org/10.1007/978-3-030-76419-7_41

Learning Objectives

1. To identify multisystem diseases which have both renal and neurological manifestations
2. To develop an awareness of why renal function maybe become impaired in the context of neurological disorders and their treatments.
3. To outline the neurological complications of common renal diseases and their treatments and to develop a strategy for their prevention, investigation and treatment

41.1 Introduction

The kidney and nervous system may be mutually affected by systemic disease processes and also by the side effects of therapeutics directed towards each organ. The risk of stroke and small vessel disease is substantially increased in hypertensive patients with CKD, and there are other specific neurological complications that are strongly or exclusively associated with renal disease, such as PRES, uraemic encephalopathy, dialysis amyloid myelopathy and dialysis dementia. In addition, many patients with CKD will coincidentally have long-term neurological disorders requiring coordinated care, support for disability and advanced care planning for those with progressive neurological impairment. This chapter will explore diseases that may benefit from joint management between nephrologist and neurologist and delineate a practical approach to neurological presentations in renal patients.

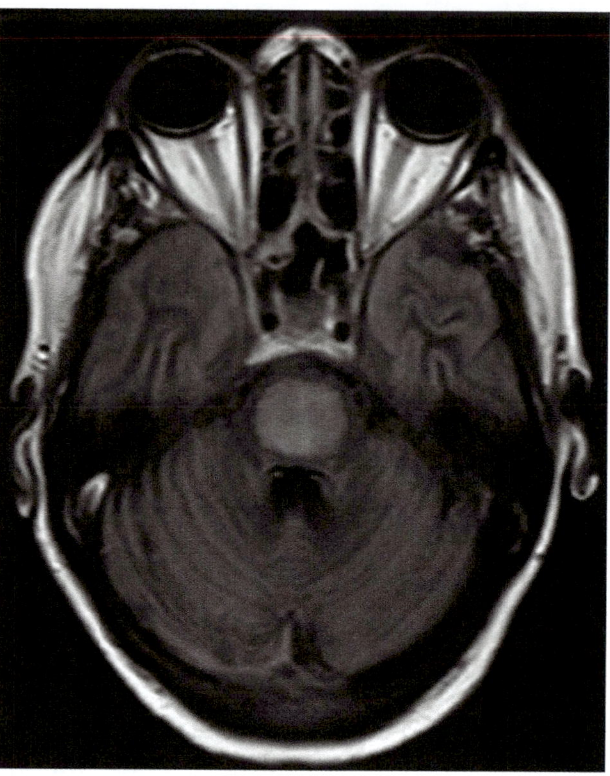

Fig. 41.1 Patient with central pontine myelinolysis. MRI demonstrating central pontine confluent hyperintense lesion on T2 and FLAIR. Changes are symmetrical with no mass effect. (Image courtesy of Dr. Vera Kyriakou)

41.2 Multisystem Diseases Affecting Both the Nervous System and Kidney

41

A variety of genetically determined and acquired systemic diseases exhibit both neurological and renal features. Clinically, the recognition of characteristic neurological features such as mononeuropathy multiplex in Churg-Strauss syndrome may aid swift diagnosis. Similarly, knowledge of the neurological associations of specific renal conditions may alert the nephrologist to possible causes of neurological dysfunction such as central pontine myelinolysis associated with over rapid correction of hyponatraemia (Fig. 41.1), or facilitate pre-emptive screening, such as MRA in high-risk patients for cerebral aneurysm in ADPKD or cerebral tumours in tuberosclerosis complex (Fig. 41.2).

Frequently, the consequences of neurological and renal involvement are chronic and debilitating and necessitate colleagues to provide integrated care, coordinated clinics and MDT working. Table 41.1 lists some of the many conditions that share both renal and neurological disease (Table 41.1).

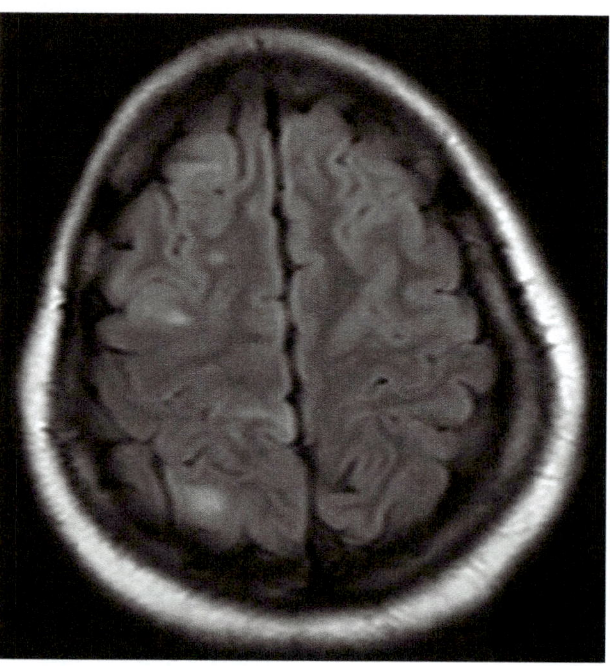

Fig. 41.2 Axial FLAIR MRI brain showing disseminated highly epileptogenic cortical and subcortical hyperintense tubers in patient with tuberous sclerosis

Table 41.1 Genetic, immune-mediated and mitochondrial disorders with nephrological and neurological consequences

Disease	Neurological signs/involvement	Renal involvement	Comment
Genetic diseases			
Polycystic kidney disease	Intracranial aneurysm, particularly berry aneurysms in circle of Willis seen in 5–15% PKD patients. Greater risk of rupture compared to sporadic aneurysms. Increased risk of embolic stroke due to mitral and aortic valve lesions	Multiple kidney cysts, progressive CKD, ESRF requiring RRT	Targeted screening for patients with adult PKD and family history of ICA or SAH with time-of-flight MRA [1]
Alport syndrome	Progressive bilateral sensorineural hearing loss, lenticonus, keratoconus, cataracts	Haematuria progressing to haematoproteinuria, CKD and ESRF often by 40 years old. Severity often consistent within a family	
Fabry's disease	Cerebral vasculopathy, acroparesthesia exacerbated by extremes of temperature and physical exertion, small fibre neuropathy, dysautonomia	Renal failure due to accumulation of glycosphingolipids in small blood vessels	Also characterised by skin angiokeratomas. Death usually in the fifth decade due to uraemia or cerebrovascular disease
Von Hippel-Lindau disease	Retinal angiomatosis and CNS haemangioblastoma in 80% of patients (predominantly in cerebellum and spinal cord)	RCC, seen in 24–45% of VHL patients. Renal cysts	Require regular screening of retina, kidneys and neuroaxis for early detection of tumours. Death usually from metastatic RCC or cerebellar haemangioblastomas
Wilsons	Movement disorders (tremor, chorea, dystonia, extrapyramidal features), dysarthria, cognitive impairment, neuropsychiatric	Haematuria, nephrolithiasis (rare). Fanconi syndrome. Hepato-renal syndrome in CLD	Kayser Fleischer rings seen in 85–100% of patients with neurological involvement
RCC	Spinal cord and cerebral metastases [2] paraneoplastic neuropathy, limbic encephalopathy	Bilateral nephrectomy may lead to dialysis dependence	
Alstrom syndrome	Cone-rod dystrophy, learning disabilities, nystagmus, bilateral sensorineural hearing loss	Slowly progressive kidney failure	
Ciliopathies			
Nephronophthisis	Tapetoretinal degeneration, oculomotor apraxia	Polyuria and polydipsia, progressing to ESRF requiring RRT	Most common genetic cause of childhood kidney failure
Joubert syndrome	Cerebellar and brainstem development abnormalities, hyperpnea, sleep apnoea, hypotonia, seizures and developmental delay	Cystic kidney disease	
Senior Loken syndrome	Retinal dystrophy	Nephronophthisis	
Leber congenital amaurosis	Nystagmus, impaired pupillary responses, early visual loss, keratoconus	Interstitial nephropathy, salt wasting and progressive CKD [3]	
Cogan syndrome	Corneal inflammation, vertigo, tinnitus, hearing loss	Systemic vasculitis in 15% causing renal failure	

(continued)

Table 41.1 (continued)

Disease	Neurological signs/involvement	Renal involvement	Comment
Tuberous sclerosis	Epilepsy, learning disability, hydrocephalus, brain lesions (subependymal nodules, cortical tubers (Figs. 41.2 and 41.3)	Renal involvement in 40–80% of cases. Renal cysts and angiomyolipomas causing pain, renal failure and haemorrhage)	Characteristic skin lesions, pulmonary lymphangioleiomyomatosis, liver, lung and pancreatic cysts, TSC-associated neuropsychiatric disease
Galloway syndrome	Microcephaly, learning disability	Nephrotic syndrome	
Ehlers-Danlos syndrome	Cerebral aneurysms predisposing to SAH. Bilateral carotid artery FMD in 65% of patients with increased risk TIA, stroke and carotid dissection	Renal infarction. FMD affects renal arteries in 85% of patients and leads to hypertension	
Cystinosis	Corneal cystinosis causing blindness, dysphagia, myopathy	Renal Fanconi syndrome, ESRF	
Primary hyperoxaluria	Peripheral neuropathy	Recurrent kidney and bladder nephrolithiasis leading to CKD and ESRF	
Neurofibromatosis	NF1: multiple neurofibromas, lisch nodules NF2: bilateral vestibular schwannoma	Renal artery stenosis, pheochromocytomas, hypertension	
Hereditary sensory and autonomic neuropathies	Progressive cognitive impairment, distal sensory neuropathy, hearing loss.	Renal failure due to amyloidosis or reflux	
Riley-Day syndrome (familial dysautonomia)	Progressive sensorimotor neuropathy with sympathetic autonomic dysfunction	Glomerulosclerosis and CKD	Orthostatic hypotension and bladder dysfunction may cause recurrent AKI and progressive CKD
Immune-mediated diseases			
Diabetes mellitus	Commonest cause of neuropathy in developed countries. Distal symmetrical sensorimotor axonal neuropathy, autonomic neuropathy, carpal tunnel, mononeuritis multiplex, diabetic amyotrophy, cranial neuropathies	Development of characteristic nodular glomerulosclerosis, vascular disease and progressive CKD. Presence of diabetes and CKD significantly increases cardiovascular morbidity and mortality	
Granulomatosis with polyangiitis (previously Wegener's granulomatosis)	28% of patients develop neurological complications due to granuloma leading to basilar meningitis, temporal lobe dysfunction, venous sinus occlusion and cranial neuropathies [4]	Rapidly progressive glomerulonephritis leading to CKD and ESRF	Necrotising granulomatous small vessel vasculitis involving respiratory tract, perforation of nasal septum, saddle nose
Microscopic polyangiitis	Peripheral neuropathy, mononeuropathy multiplex	Rapidly progressive glomerulonephritis leading to CKD and ESRF	
Eosinophilic granulomatosis with polyangiitis (Churg-Strauss)	Highest incidence of peripheral and central nervous systems of all ANCA-associated vasculitides. Peripheral neuropathy is almost ubiquitous and mononeuropathy multiplex affects around 80% [5]	Kidney involvement less common than other ANCA-associated vasculitides	
Sjogren's syndrome	Cranial neuropathies especially trigeminal neuropathy, dorsal root ganglionopathies, autonomic neuropathy	Acute/chronic tubulointerstitial nephritis due to lymphocytic infiltrate	Sicca symptoms. Increased risk of B-cell non-Hodgkins lymphoma

Table 41.1 (continued)

Disease	Neurological signs/involvement	Renal involvement	Comment
SLE	Very common, affecting up to 75% of patients. Headache, seizures, cognitive impairment. If associated anticardiolipin antibodies, increased thrombotic risk. Rarely peripheral lesions	Lupus nephritis (classes I–V)	
TTP	Altered mental status, generalised headache, focal deficits, visual disturbance and seizures secondary to platelet microthrombi	Microangiopathic haemolytic anaemia, microscopic haematuria, acute kidney injury and CKD	
APLS	Recurrent venous and arterial thrombosis	Antiphospholipid associated nephropathy, renal artery stenosis, renal vein thrombosis, CKD, hypertension	May be primary or secondary. Obstetric complications
Systemic sclerosis	Headache, seizures, cognitive impairment, peripheral and autonomic neuropathy	Renal crisis, malignant hypertension, ARF, hypertension	
Scleroderma	Headache and seizures in localised scleroderma en coup de sabre	Scleroderma renal crisis – accelerated hypertension, renal impairment, thrombotic microangiopathy	
Rheumatoid arthritis	Atlanto-axial subluxation, carpal tunnel syndrome, axonal sensorimotor neuropathy, vasculitic neuropathy	AA amyloidosis, membranous and mesangioproliferative GN. Drug-related membranous nephropathy and interstitial disease	
Mitochondrial disorders			
MELAS	Encephalomyopathy, stroke like episodes, seizures, dementia	Renal failure, FSGS [6]	
Kearns-Sayre syndrome	Ophthalmoplegia, ataxia, proximal muscle weakness, deafness	Renal failure, RTA, Bartter-like syndrome, Fanconi syndrome [6]	
Mitochondrial depletion syndrome	Encephalomyopathy, myopathy, seizures	RTA, nephrocalcinosis [6]	

41.3 Neurological Diseases and Medications Which Affect the Kidney

41.3.1 Spinal Cord Disorders

Congenital and acquired spinal cord damage may lead to bladder dysfunction and indirectly to kidney disease. Risk of renal insufficiency increases with the following: indwelling urethral catheter, advanced age, time since spinal cord injury and vesicoureteric reflux from detrusor sphincter dyssynergia and raised bladder pressures. Patients are at risk of developing reflux nephropathy, hydronephrosis and pyelonephritis. Careful history and evaluation, including imaging, are vital for all patients with a neurogenic bladder. Renal failure in patients with spinal cord disease can be avoided by maintaining low post-void residual volumes, avoidance of indwelling catheters, care with nephrotoxic drugs and prompt treatment of sepsis. Most patients are managed with clean technique intermittent catheterization and oral anticholinergic medications. The UK NICE guidance suggests offering video-urodynamic investigations to people known to have high risk of renal complications (e.g. spina bifida and spinal cord injury) but not to those with low risk (e.g. most people with multiple sclerosis) [7]. Patients with spinal cord injury should be assessed and followed up by a urologist.

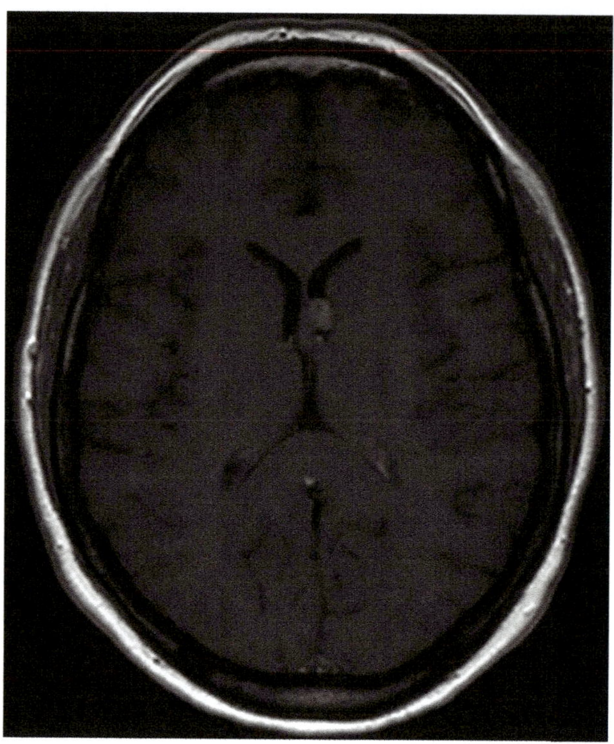

Fig. 41.3 Axial MRI brain with contrast showing enhancing subependymal nodule in the anterior horn of the left lateral ventricle. Subependymal nodules are seen in nearly all tuberous sclerosis patients and calcify with age. They may give rise to supependymal giant cell astrocytomas (SEGAs) during childhood and adolescence

41.3.2 Rhabdomyolysis

Extensive muscle necrosis and release of intracellular muscle constituents resulting in AKI can be seen with a number of neurological conditions. Important neurological causes of rhabdomyolysis include metabolic and mitochondrial myopathies, inflammatory myopathies and excessive muscular activity, as seen in status epilepticus and dystonia. Seizures can also rarely cause rhabdomyolysis through a localised compartment syndrome. An underlying inherited metabolic or mitochondrial myopathy should be suspected if there is a history of recurrent episodes of rhabdomyolysis after exertion, fasting or viral illness; exercise intolerance with cramps, fatigue and pigmenturia; or family history of rhabdomyolysis or exercise intolerance. Helpful pointers include the type of exertional activity, presence or absence of interictal weakness or raised creatine kinase and second wind phenomenon. Patients with an underlying inflammatory myopathy, e.g. polymyositis or dermatomyositis, may present subacutely with features of systemic autoimmunity.

41.3.3 Medications

Medications used to treat neurological disease may adversely affect the kidney, especially in vulnerable patient groups.

The most common interaction in clinical practice is probably nephrotoxicity due to crystal nephropathy and tubulointerstitial nephritis with intravenous aciclovir in patients being treated for encephalitis. Pre-hydration is recommended prior to infusion and renal impairment is generally reversible following discontinuation of therapy. Oral aciclovir and ganciclovir are both associated with lower risk (Table 41.2).

41.4 Neurological Manifestations of Kidney Disease

Patients with CKD may develop central and peripheral neurological complications such as cognitive disorders [8], dementia [9], cerebrovascular diseases [10] and peripheral neuropathy. Conventional risk factors for vascular disease (such as old age, hypertension, diabetes, dyslipidaemia and atrial fibrillation) drive these neurological disorders in CKD through microvascular disease [11].

41.4.1 Encephalopathy

41.4.1.1 Uraemic Encephalopathy

Uraemic encephalopathy is seen in advanced kidney failure and demonstrates a fluctuating course. Early symptoms may be subtle and picked up on specific tests of attention, but these can progress to emotional lability, stupor, visual hallucinations, delirium, seizures and coma, if renal replacement therapy is not implemented in a timely manner. Seizures are usually bilateral tonic-clonic in nature, although focal motor seizures may also occur. In keeping with a metabolic encephalopathy, patients may present with multifocal myoclonus, asterixis, tremor and pyramidal signs. Focal signs, e.g. hemiparesis, may also be seen.

The onset and severity of uraemic encephalopathy broadly parallels the degree of renal impairment, but factors including age, coexisting comorbidity and speed and severity of renal dysfunction may influence the threshold at which symptoms present.

Biochemical changes, including alterations in water transport, brain oedema, disturbances of the blood-brain barrier, impaired synaptic function and changes in cerebral metabolism, have been implicated in the patho-

Table 41.2 Neurological medications associated with renal side effects

Medication	Neurological indication	Renal side effects and considerations
Aciclovir	Viral herpes encephalitis	AKI due to distal intra-tubular crystal nephropathy. Dose reduction needed in renal impairment.
Acetylcholinesterase inhibitors (donepezil, galantamine, rivastigmine, pyridostigmine)	Dementia, neuromuscular junction disorders	May cause urinary retention and worsen bladder outflow obstruction. Rivastigmine may require dose reduction Pyridostigmine is renally excreted and requires reduced dose in renal impairment
Anticholinergics (trihexyphenidyl, procyclidine, oxybutynin, solifenacin, tolterodine)	Movement disorders including Parkinson's disease and dystonia Overactive bladder in MS	Prostatism and urinary retention Excreted in urine and caution is advised in renal impairment
COMT inhibitors (entacapone, tolcapone)	Parkinson's disease	Rhabdomyolysis
Carbamazepine	Epilepsy (generalised and focal)	SIADH-like effect leading to fluid retention and hyponatraemia
Gabapentin	Focal epilepsy, neuropathic pain	Acute renal failure (rare)
Ergot-based dopamine agonists (bromocriptine, cabergoline)	Parkinson's disease, rarely used in current practice	Retroperitoneal fibrosis
Non-steroidal anti-inflammatories	Migraine, other headache disorders	Interstitial nephritis, papillary necrosis, AKI on CKD
Phenytoin	Epilepsy	Interstitial nephritis (rare)
SNRIs (venlafaxine, duloxetine),	Neuropathic pain, mood disorders	Rhabdomyolysis
TCAs (amitriptyline, nortriptyline)	Psychiatric disorders, migraine prophylaxis	Urinary retention and exacerbation of prostatic hypertrophy
Typical antipsychotics (haloperidol, sulpiride)	Tic disorders, behavioural disturbance in neurodegenerative disease	Urinary retention

physiology. Subsequent histopathological changes with extracellular deposition of amyloid protein in senile plaques occur, possibly mediated by aluminium from diet and phosphate binding drugs [12] Imaging studies may show cytotoxic oedema, particularly in subcortical grey and white matter, midbrain and mesial temporal lobes. Chronic renal impairment may be associated with cerebral atrophy. The EEG typically demonstrates prominence of slow waves, intermittent frontal rhythmic theta activity and paroxysmal, bilateral, high-voltage delta waves. Triphasic waves may appear in the frontal regions [13]. CSF analysis may show an aseptic meningitis and raised CSF protein of up to 1 g/l [14].

Uraemic encephalopathy typically improves with the initiation of renal replacement therapy, and improvement in neurological and cognitive function is normally appreciable within 48 hours of starting treatment, although subtle attentional, memory and perceptual deficits may persist. Failure to respond within this time frame should prompt investigations for an alternative diagnosis.

41.4.1.2 Hypertensive Encephalopathy

Hypertensive encephalopathy is characterised by cerebral oedema in the context of severe hypertension and reflects failure of cerebral autoregulation, leading to vascular damage and damage of the vascular endothelium. The clinical picture is often of gradually worsening headache, nausea and vomiting, cortical blindness and other visual symptoms, which, if left untreated, may progress to confusion, seizures and coma.

When imaging reveals oedema to the occipital and parietal lobes, the term PRES (posterior reversible encephalopathy syndrome) maybe applied [15]. Changes are seen both cortical and subcortical and may extend beyond a strictly posterior distribution (Fig. 41.4). When primarily pontine abnormalities are observed, the term hypertensive brainstem encephalopathy is used [16]. Management of hypertensive crisis is covered elsewhere in this book, but gradual (avoiding precipitant falls) control of blood pressure and reduction or withdrawal of immunosuppressive agent are associated with good recovery.

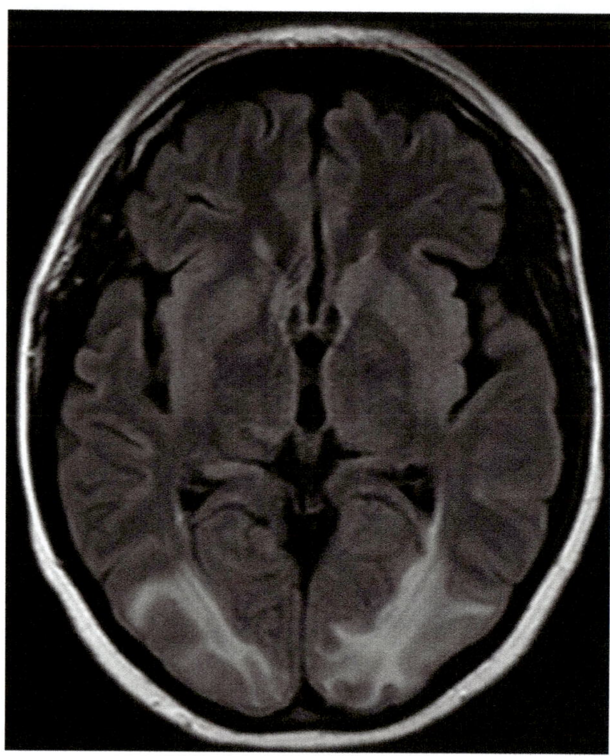

Fig. 41.4 Axial FLAIR image of patient with PRES showing abnormal signal involving subcortical white matter of the posterior occipital lobes and inferior parietal lobes bilaterally. (Image courtesy of Dr. Vera Kyriakou)

41.4.1.3 Neuropathy

Uraemic polyneuropathy is common and seen in up to 70% adults with renal dysfunction [17]. The most common cause is due to the uraemic milieu found in CKD and typically develops below a GFR of 12 mL/min/1.73m^2 [18]. This 'uraemic polyneuropath' is a symmetrical length-dependent axonal sensorimotor polyneuropathy with secondary segmental demyelination [19]. Patients present with loss of proprioception and vibration sense and absent ankle reflexes and progress to limb weakness. Motor nerve involvement with progressive distal atrophy and weakness and small fibre involvement may follow. Commencement of RRT, folic acid, vitamin B supplementation and neuropathic agents may help symptoms. Successful renal transplantation reverses autonomic dysfunction in all but the most severe neuropathies.

Where peripheral neuropathy is clinically out of proportion to the level of renal impairment, other causes including systemic vasculitides and diabetes should be considered.

Mononeuropathies are also common in patients with CKD. Carpal tunnel syndrome (CTS) is particularly prevalent, seen in 6–31 percent of patients with CKD [18] and caused by compression from local amyloid, calcific atherosclerosis, uraemic damage to median nerve, increased extracellular volume leading to nerve ischaemia and increased susceptibility to pressure palsies. CTS typically presents with pain or numbness along the distribution of the median nerve, often worse at night.

Mononeuropathies may also be related to diabetes or iatrogenic, attributable to vascular access surgery [20]; this is considered in ▶ Sect. 41.8.

The most commonly involved cranial nerve in uraemia is the vestibulocochlear nerve. Variable degrees of hearing loss can be seen, which reverse with dialysis or transplantation [21].

41.4.2 Myopathy

Proximal limb weakness and wasting are common in the uraemic state and usually develop when the glomerular filtration rate declines below 25 mL/min. In the absence of peripheral neuropathy, the knee jerks are preserved and may be brisk. Creatine kinase is usually normal and EMG shows a non-inflammatory myopathic picture. Muscle biopsy is non-specific with atrophy of type 2 muscle fibres [22]. The pathogenesis of uraemic myopathy is unclear but is likely multifactorial and related to uraemic toxins, vitamin D metabolic abnormalities, secondary hyperparathyroidism, insulin resistance, malnutrition, changes in mitochondrial metabolism and sedentary lifestyle. There is no specific treatment; it may be prevented with high-quality dialysis and effects ameliorated with aerobic exercise, management of secondary hyperparathyroidism and treatment of anaemia [23].

41.5 Stroke

Patients with CKD are at significantly increased risk of cerebrovascular morbidity and mortality. The risk of stroke is particularly increased in patients with CKD and AF, and the risk of stroke increases with falling GFR and increases with degree of proteinuria [24]. Patients with CKD may exhibit enhanced calcification in carotid plaques, which have greater risk of rupture and increased stroke severity due to impaired cerebral perfusion. It is important to consider specific diseases such as Fabry's or mitochondrial cytopathies in young patients presenting with stroke.

Atrial fibrillation is a risk factor for ischaemic stroke; however, warfarin demonstrates significant lability in the context of haemodialysis, and its use is associated with a significantly elevated risk of intracranial bleeding [25, 26].

In the immediate post-stroke period, the haemodialysis patient will require specialised dialysis regimes to prevent haemorrhagic transformation or stroke extension due to hypoperfusion. Principles of care are to minimise the rate of change of urea and osmolality and to maintain cardiovascular stability. The dialysis prescription should reflect a combination of reduced blood and dialysate flow across a small surface dialyser and a shortened treatment session time [27]. Extra dialysis sessions may be necessary to ensure an adequate solute clearance and may need to continue for up to 2 weeks whilst the ischaemic brain injury stabilises.

Cerebral venous sinus thrombosis is a rare complication of nephrotic syndrome. In line with the more common types of venous thromboses, e.g. DVT and renal thrombosis, thrombosis typically occurs early on in the course of the disease. Risk is increased with severe hypoalbuminaemia and membranous nephropathy. Thrombosis is usually located in the superior sagittal sinus, and MR Venogram is the imaging modality of choice.

41.5.1 Cognitive Impairment and Dementia

CKD is associated with high rates of cognitive impairment, and the severity of CKD is associated with greater risk [8]. Each 10 mL/min/1.73m^2 decrease in eGFR is associated with 11% increased prevalence of impairment [28]. There is increasing evidence that cognitive impairment is related to vascular disease manifest as cerebral microinfarcts, microhaemorrhages and accumulating white matter disease [29]. In addition to chronic hypertension, dyslipidaemia and diabetes, high levels of oxidative stress, high cystatin C levels and endothelial dysfunction contribute to accelerated small vessel disease and cognitive decline in chronic kidney disease.

Dialysis dementia is an important but now rare cause of cognitive deterioration. This is discussed in ▶ Sect. 41.8.

41.6 Common Neurological Presentations in the Renal Patient

41.6.1 Confusion

The differential diagnosis is vast in the CKD patient presenting with confusion and should be guided by the onset of symptoms, associated features and type of kidney disease.

Differential	Associated features
Sepsis	
Systemic	Delirium due to general sepsis: pneumonia, urinary sepsis, endocarditis Dialysis-related sepsis: peritoneal and haemodialysis
CNS	Opportunistic organisms causing meningitis/encephalitis: fungal, viral, TB (◘ Figs. 41.5 and 41.6) Cerebritis, cerebral abscess, septic emboli
Drugs	Opiate accumulation Hyponatraemia due to diuretics Hypoglycaemia due to insulin accumulation. Beta lactam toxicity Aciclovir-induced encephalopathy Erythropoietin causing hypertensive encephalopathy
Metabolic	Uraemic encephalopathy Wernicke's encephalopathy Electrolyte disturbance
Vascular	Subdural haematoma Ischaemic stroke, intracerebral haemorrhage Cerebral venous sinus thrombosis PRES (related to hypertension, immunosuppressive medication)
Inflammatory/ autoimmune	Related to underlying systemic inflammation, e.g. SLE, Sjogren's

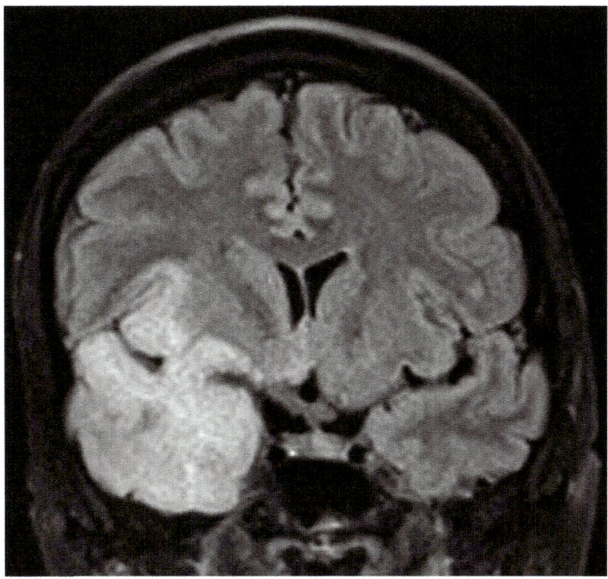

◘ **Fig. 41.5** Patient with herpes simplex encephalitis showing abnormal FLAIR signal throughout the right temporal lobe with oedema and extension into the inferior frontal lobes, limbic system and insular cortex

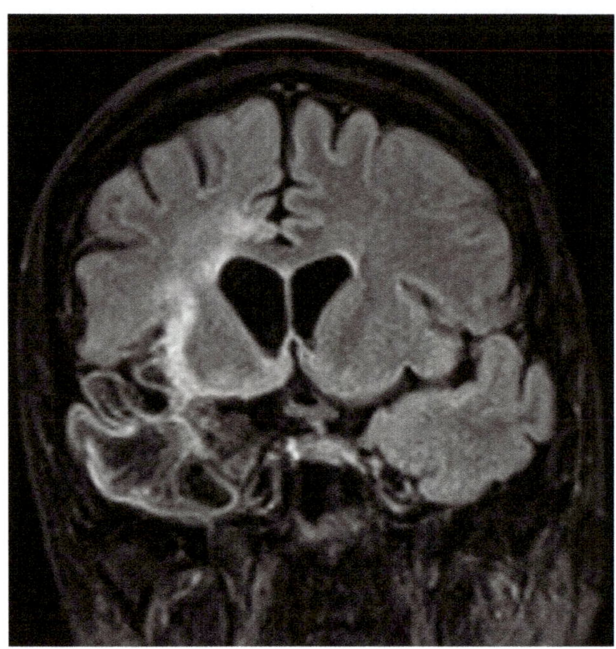

Fig. 41.6 Follow-up scan shows encephalomalacia and gliosis in previously affected areas. (Images courtesy of Dr. Vera Kyriakou)

41.6.2 Seizures

In all patients presenting with seizures, particularly with focal neurology, a primary neurological diagnosis, such as stroke, SDH or intracranial infection, should be considered, given the increased risk of these conditions in renal patients. All causes of an encephalopathy listed above can potentially lead to seizures.

Seizures in the setting of end-stage renal disease may be related to complications of disease or treatment and may occur in earlier stages of disease due to metabolic disturbance or hypertension. Generalised seizures in the context of a uraemic encephalopathy are an indication for dialysis.

In patients with CKD, electrolyte disturbance is a common cause of seizures, particularly hyponatraemia and hypocalcaemia. Seizures generally occur with a sodium concentration below 115 mmol, although risk is increased if sodium falls precipitously. Acute hypocalcaemia as a complication of parathyroidectomy can be associated with bilateral tonic-clonic seizures, focal motor or absence seizures. Patients undergoing parathyroidectomy should be preloaded with 1.25 hydroxyvitamin D. Hypomagnesaemia should be corrected intravenously, alongside calcium replacement, as sulphate anions may bind calcium and aggravate hypocalcaemia.

Hypoglycaemia or hyperglycaemia in the context of suboptimal diabetic control or sepsis may precipitate seizures in patients with renal disease.

In the dialysis patient with epilepsy, timing of AED treatment may lead to subtherapeutic levels; levetiracetam, phenobarbital and primidone are water-soluble and poorly protein bound and therefore readily removed by dialysis. Dosing needs to be appropriately timed and supplemental doses given following dialysis. Marked fluctuations in serum levels may lead to loss of seizure control, and these AEDs are therefore best avoided. Phenytoin, carbamazepine and sodium valproate are poorly dialysed and require no changes. Levetiracetam, gabapentin and, to a lesser extent, topiramate are almost exclusively eliminated by the kidneys and should be avoided in CKD to prevent accumulation and toxicity. CKD and other hypoalbuminaemic states result in increased displacement of highly protein-bound drugs, e.g. phenytoin and valproate, and therefore free serum drug concentrations, if available, should be measured.

Convulsive seizures can also be directly related to complications of dialysis, e.g. dialysis disequilibrium syndrome, prolonged intradialytic hypotension or air embolism.

41.6.3 Movement Disorders

In the context of encephalopathy, patients may present with asterixis: multifocal, action-induced jerks. Uraemia also triggers spontaneous action myoclonus and stimulus-sensitive myoclonus, which can be treated with benzodiazepines. Water-electrolyte imbalance can cause dysfunction of the lower brainstem reticular formation with jerks accompanied by fasciculations, muscle twitches and seizures.

Because opiates depend on renal excretion, opiate toxicity is a common, characteristic and avoidable cause of twitching (often accompanied by confusion) in patients with significant renal impairment. Electronic prescribing linked to eGFR should prevent this, but anticipation of the risk when other teams are prescribing for patients with advanced CKD is important.

Common immunosuppressive drugs used in both renal transplant and renal vasculitis patients can cause movement disorders. Both tacrolimus and cyclosporin are associated with tremor and cerebellar ataxia and peripheral neuropathy.

Movement disorders may additionally result from structural pathology caused by vascular or metabolic complications, e.g. basal ganglia stroke and extrapontine myelinolysis.

Restless leg syndrome (RLS), the irresistible urge to move the lower limbs, particularly at night, is common in CKD patients and associated with significantly reduced quality of life. It is likely multifactorial due to anaemia, iron deficiency, hypercalcaemia and alterations of CNS dopamine and opioid activity. Dopamine-blocking medications such as metoclopramide are associated with increased rates of RLS. The symptoms can be treated through correction of iron [30] and exercise [31]. Clonazepam and gabapentin may improve symptoms [32], and dopamine agonists can be used but may lead to augmentation of symptoms. Short, daily dialysis also reduces prevalence, and renal transplant is associated with symptomatic improvement.

Cramping is a common complication of haemodialysis treatment. The causes are multifactorial but changes in plasma osmolality and extracellular fluid volume are thought to play a significant role. Initial measures should include minimising intradialytic weight gain and reducing ultrafiltration rate of dialysis. Conservative measures such as application of heat and massage to the local area may also be helpful. Pharmacological measures may include a trial of vitamin E [33], use of gabapentin [34] and short-acting benzodiazepines such as clonazepam.

41.6.4 Headache

Haemodialysis headache occurs in around 5% of HD patients and is probably related to intradialytic hypotension and changes in urea and magnesium concentrations. Patients develop bilateral throbbing or non-pulsatile headache lasting less than 4 hours, typically towards the end of haemodialysis sessions. Diagnosis requires at least two episodes of acute headache, which develop during dialysis session, worsen with dialysis and resolve within 72 hours of completing dialysis. The symptoms completely cease following transplantation. Commonly used renal drugs, e.g. alpha-1 blockers, directly acting vasodilators and calcium channel blockers may also contribute to headaches in patients with CKD.

41.7 Renal Treatments and Drugs with Neurological Side Effects

41.7.1 Dialysis

Dialysis complications are common but may present non-specifically [35]. Haemodialysis is more likely to be associated with haemodynamic instability than peritoneal dialysis and more commonly associated with headaches. Dialysis disequilibrium syndrome results from cerebral oedema triggered by more rapid falls in osmolality in serum than CNS. Urea gradient causes more water to move into CNS resulting in raised intracranial pressure. It is a particularly important consideration in patients starting HD with serum urea above 60 who are rapidly dialysed over short periods. Symptoms occur during or immediately after HD, including headache, vomiting, disorientation and progression to seizures, coma and even death. Prevention of these side effects is achieved by targeting a reduction of no more than 30% in serum urea in the first dialysis session. Metabolic derangement can also be seen with the rapid correction of chronic hyponatraemia with haemodialysis, leading to osmotic demyelination of the pons and extrapontine areas. This is usually manifested by altered consciousness and convulsions and can be avoided by lowering dialysate sodium, short duration HD with small surface area dialysers and low flow rate (◘ Fig. 41.1).

Intracerebral haemorrhage is a significant cause of morbidity and mortality in haemodialysis patients; risk factors include chronic uraemia leading to platelet dysfunction, intradialytic anticoagulation and hypertension. In one retrospective study, the prevalence of non-traumatic SDH in HD patients was 0.4% with incidence of 189 per 100,000 patients [36]. The presentation can be atypical with gait ignition failure, confusion and ataxia.

Although uncommon, it is important to consider treatable nutritional causes of confusion in dialysis patients, particularly chronic malnourished patients. Fortunately, thiamine is only lightly plasma protein bound and therefore not readily dialysed. However, classical presentation with ophthalmoplegia may be absent, and a high index of suspicion is required. There is also some evidence to suggest that high-flux HD patients are at increased risk of B12 deficiency through increased losses during dialysis and reduced dietary intake [37].

Dialysis amyloid myelopathy is a rarely observed complication where spinal cord compression develops following chronic haemodialysis. Myelopathy develops secondary to the formation of fibroligamentous rings caused by extradural amyloid derived from beta-2 microglobulin. A progressive myelopathy may require surgical treatment. Amyloid deposition is also seen in dialysis arthropathy, bone cysts and recurrent carpal tunnel syndrome.

Peripheral nerve injury is a risk associated with vascular access surgery required for dialysis. The proximity of median nerve to brachial artery makes it susceptible during the formation of brachiocephalic fistulae. Median nerve compression may result from haematoma and pseudoaneurysm during surgery or following repeating cannulation and require urgent management. Neuropathy of the median nerve occurs chronically in up to 10% of arteriovenous fistula surgery with 'steal' phenomenon and depleted blood supply causing axonal loss, particularly in the setting of diabetes or severe peripheral vascular disease. Management of an ischaemic monomelic neuropathy involves urgent ligation of the fistula.

Dialysis dementia was described in the 1970s and was strongly linked to prolonged exposure to aluminium in municipal water supplies and aluminium-containing phosphate binders. Symptoms start with mixed dysarthria and dysphasia and rapidly progress with more severe language dysfunction, myoclonic jerks, ataxia and seizures. Reduction of aluminium by means of reverse osmosis has markedly reduced the incidence of dialysis dementia. Given the availability of other non-aluminium phosphate binders now available, clinical guidelines advise against long-term use of aluminium-containing phosphate binders [20, 21]. Desferrioxamine is a chelating agent, which is used in the treatment of aluminium toxicity.

41.7.2 Renal Transplantation and the Immunosuppressed Patient

Almost one third of renal transplant recipients will develop neurological complications [38]. Surgical complications at the time of transplantation include neuropraxis of the femoral and lateral cutaneous nerve of the thigh from intraoperative retraction.

Drug-induced suppression of cell-mediated immunity renders patients at increased risk of opportunistic infections, but it is worth reiterating that such patients should be managed with due diligence and with a low threshold for excluding neurological infections due to their blunted inflammatory response to sepsis. In addition, calcineurin inhibitors have a significant burden of minor neurological symptoms. Tremor is said to occur in up to 40% patients on cyclosporine, sleep disturbance is common and less commonly patients may develop a sensory neuropathy and myopathy. Calcineurin inhibitors may be associated with a reversible posterior leukoencephalopathy syndrome. Early recognition, reduction or withdrawal of the immunosuppressive agent and institution of antihypertensive medication is associated with an excellent clinical outcome.

Rejection encephalopathy, usually seen within 3 months of transplantation, is characterised by headache, confusion and seizures in the context of systemic features of graft rejection. Cytokine release during the rejection process is thought to be implicated.

Post-transplant lymphoproliferative disorders may be driven by EBV, and cases with neurological involvement may present with headaches, seizures, altered mental state and focal neurological deficits. There is CNS involvement in 10–15% of cases. Prognosis depends on the extent of disease dissemination.

41.7.3 Medications Commonly Used in Nephrology and Dosing Considerations

Medication	Neurological complication	Considerations in prescribing/dosing
Penicillins and cephalosporin-related antibiotics	Seizures	Only at high doses. Dose reduction in severe renal impairment. Penicillins removed by HD/HDF but not by PD
Gentamicin	Aminoglycoside antibiotic associated with ototoxicity and vestibular failure. Ototoxicity is more prevalent in those patients receiving a prolonged course of treatment	Extending the dose interval to >24 hours. Regular monitoring of serum levels and dose adjustments
Erythropoietin	Hypertensive encephalopathy, seizures	Less common with lower doses of EPO prescribed. Avoid EPO in severe and uncontrolled hypertension
Meperidine	Seizures	Caused by accumulation of toxic metabolite, normeperidine
Metoclopramide	Seizures	Decrease seizure threshold. No change in dosing required. May increase blood ciclosporin levels
Theophylline	Seizures	Seizures in overdose. Dose reduction not required in renal impairment. 50% of dose removed by HD
Ertapenem/meropenem	Seizures	Competitive inhibition of GABA receptors. Dose reduction necessary in renal impairment. Give after dialysis
Aciclovir	Seizures	Dose reduction required in renal impairment. Interactions with tacrolimus, mycophenolate and ciclosporin

41

Medication	Neurological complication	Considerations in prescribing/dosing
Carbamazepine	Seizures	Seizures in overdose. Dose reduction not required in renal failure. May reduce ciclosporin levels and effect of corticosteroids
Lithium	Seizures	Seizures in overdose. Lithium should be preferably avoided in renal impairment. Otherwise, close monitoring is necessary. Loop and thiazide diuretics reduce lithium excretion.
Gabapentin/ pregabalin	Vertigo/sedation/ataxia	Dose reduction required in renal impairment. Dialysed. Give after haemodialysis on dialysis days
Levetiracetam	Vertigo, nausea, diplopia	Dose reduction required in renal impairment. Readily dialysed, therefore 250–500mgs supplemental dose needed post dialysis
Benzodiazepines	Sedation	Active metabolites are renally excreted. Dose reduction advised in renal impairment. Not removed by HD or PD
Opioids	Sedation and twitching	Active metabolites of morphine and diamorphine accumulate in renal impairment. Fentanyl is predominantly metabolised in the liver to the inactive metabolite norfentanyl and maybe preferable to morphine derivatives
Calcineurin inhibitors (cyclosporine/ tacrolimus)	Tremor (fine resting or action), headaches, paraesthesia, mood changes, seizures, ataxia, motor deficits, posterior reversible encephalopathy syndrome	May be present even with therapeutic levels
Corticosteroids	Proximal myopathy, anxiety, psychosis, headache, fever and lethargy on withdrawal	Prednisolone metabolism accelerated by carbamazepine, barbiturates and phenytoin.
OKT3 monoclonal antibody	Aseptic meningitis, encephalopathy	Increases cyclosporine levels
Sunitinib	Posterior reversible encephalopathy syndrome [39]	Case reports only

41.8 Mental Health in Kidney Disease

Psychiatric illness is common among patients with end-stage renal failure, particularly those on haemodialysis compared with those treated conservatively or post transplantation. The psychiatric disorders most frequently observed include affective disorders (particularly depression), anxiety, suicide, organic brain disease such as dementia and delirium, drug-related disorders such as alcoholism, psychoses and personality disorders [40]. Steroids and other immunomodulating drugs can result in insomnia, mood swings, mania, behavioural problems, severe depression and psychosis in 5–18% patients [41].

Depression is under-recognised and undertreated in CKD. Patients with CKD are 1.5–3 times more likely to require inpatient psychiatric treatment than patients with other chronic disorders. Contributing factors may include the following: the feeling of total dependency on a dialysis machine, restrictions on diet and fluid, poor quality of life, reduced employment and limited functional capacity. Untreated depression may impact on treatment compliance, nutritional status, impaired immune function and increased suicide rates. Patients may require psychotropic drugs and psychotherapy and benefit from a MDT approach. Some psychotropic drugs require dose changes in both CKD and dialysis patient, e.g. paroxetine can lead to seizures at higher doses, venlafaxine may cause hypertension at higher doses and mirtazapine can be sedating. Lithium is the treatment of choice for bipolar disease but can be nephrotoxic, associated with nephrogenic diabetes and CKD due to chronic interstitial nephritis and distal renal tubular acidosis. Progression of kidney disease can occur despite discontinuation of lithium.

Case Study

Case 1

A 54-year-old lady who had undergone a simultaneous kidney and pancreas transplantation 5 months previously and who was maintained on tacrolimus and mycophenolate mofetil immunosuppression presented to the emergency department with a 3-day history of progressive worsening headache, confusion and disorientation. Blood pressure was 170/100 and physical examination revealed bilateral pyramidal signs, cortical blindness, dysphasia and clonus. Blood tests were unremarkable. EEG was consistent with a metabolic encephalopathy and MRI was consistent with PRES. Lumber puncture was unremarkable. Antihypertensive treatment was commenced, and tacrolimus was switched to sirolimus. The patient made a slow but complete recovery over 6 weeks. Blood pressure at 6 weeks was 140/60 after the withdrawal of her antihypertensive medication.

Case 2

A 74-year-old lady who had been on maintenance haemodialysis for many years reported a progressively worsening, unpleasant sensation in both her legs over the preceding months. The sensation was worse at night or after any long period of lying down. The sensation was improved by movement but was causing significant sleep deprivation and a marked deterioration in her quality of life. Her partner commented that whilst asleep, she exhibited involuntary, jerking movements of the legs. Neurological examination was unremarkable. Blood tests demonstrated a Hb of 120 g/L in the context of a ferritin of 50. Markers of dialysis adequacy were satisfactory. A diagnosis of restless legs and periodic limb movements was postulated. The patient was advised to restrict her caffeine intake and to take regular exercise. She received treatment with intravenous iron and was started on 25 mg pregabalin, which was doubled 1 month later. Within 2 months, her symptoms had significantly improved and her sleep pattern had returned to normal.

Case 3

An 80-year-old gentleman receiving maintenance haemodialysis complained of increasing somnolence, fatigue and dizziness. Collateral history confirmed unsteadiness and clumsiness at home and also slurring of speech at times. Physical examination revealed depressed reflexes, past pointing bilaterally and evidence of mild dysarthria. The patient was deemed too unsteady to return home and was admitted for investigation and observation. Subsequent review of his repeat prescription demonstrated that gabapentin 300 mg tds had been commenced some 3 weeks previously when the patient had consulted a physician with regard to neuropathic pain along the distribution of his sciatic nerve. The dose and frequency of gabapentin was reduced to 300 mg after every dialysis session. The neurological signs and symptoms gradually improved over the subsequent 10 days, and the patient was discharged home.

Tips and Tricks

EEG: The EEG will show triphasic waves and diffuse slow activity in dialysis dementia, metabolic encephalopathy and seizures (Fig. 41.7). In acute uraemic encephalopathy, EEG changes are usually more severe and may help to distinguish from non-convulsive status epilepticus. There may be focal dysfunction in HSV encephalitis and tacrolimus-related encephalopathy.

LP: Lumbar puncture is essential for the diagnosis of encephalopathy. The CSF in uraemia will show pleocytosis and raised protein concentration in 50% patients, and protein may also be raised in PRES. Lymphocytic pleocytosis would point towards a viral encephalitis.

NCS/EMG: Nerve conduction studies show predominantly axonal neuropathy in uraemic neuropathy although sensory, and motor conduction velocities are often reduced. CKD patients may develop GBS type neuropathy with conduction block, slowing and prolonged F wave latencies. EMG in uraemic myopathy is usually normal.

Neurotoxicity with some drugs such as opiates and aciclovir in severe CKD is very predictable, and local education on dose reduction/avoidance or electronic prescribing should significantly reduce this risk.

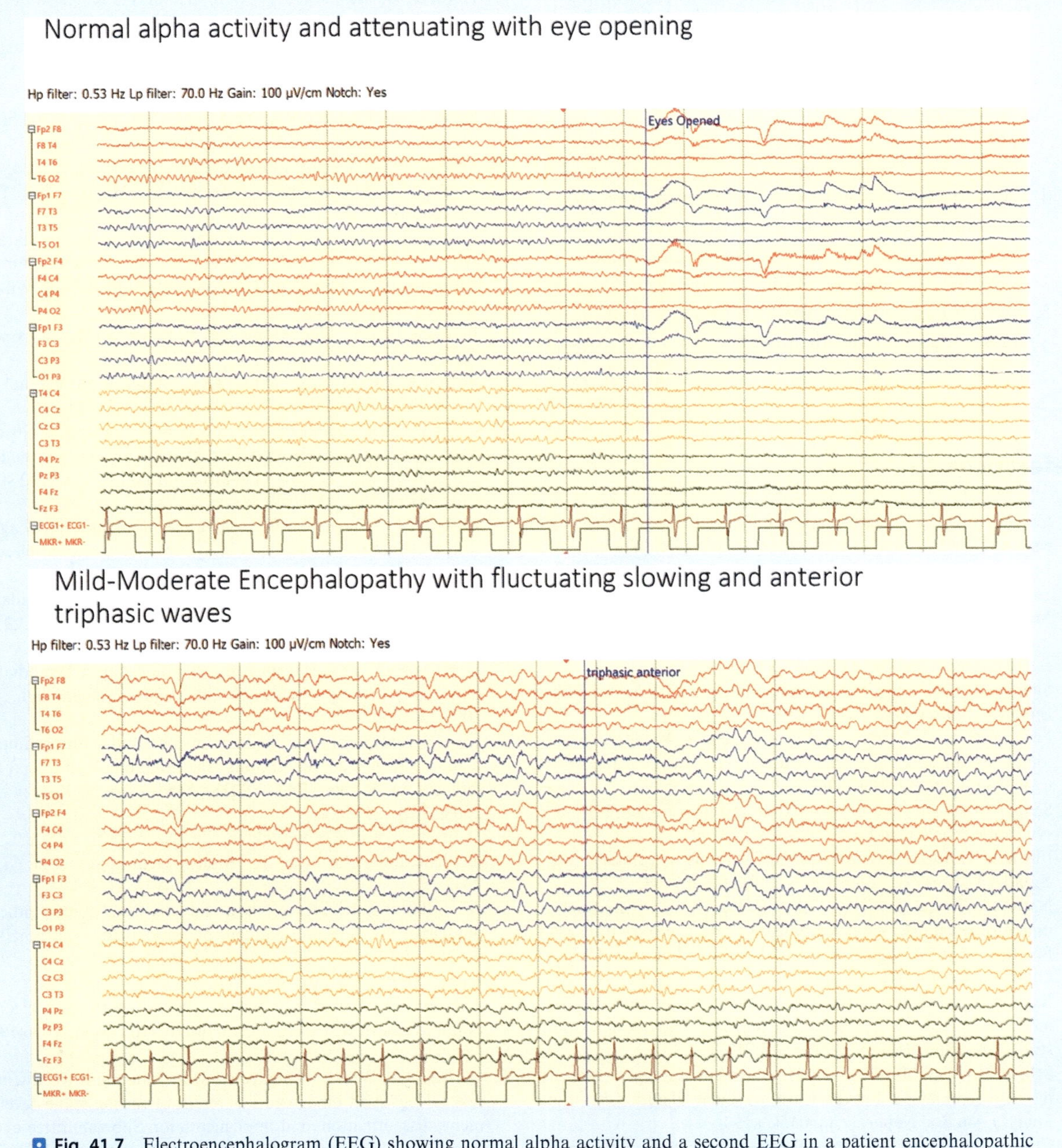

Fig. 41.7 Electroencephalogram (EEG) showing normal alpha activity and a second EEG in a patient encephalopathic with severe uraemia

Chapter Review Questions

1. Should all ADPKD patients be screened to exclude intracerebral aneurysms?
2. Which of the ANCA-associated vasculitides is most commonly associated with neurological complications, and what is the most common neurological complication?
3. Can suprasacral spinal cord injuries cause urological dysfunction? Which patients should be screened?
4. What is the mechanism of aciclovir-induced AKI?
5. What are the cognitive features of uraemic encephalopathy?

Answers

1. No. Low level evidence, based on expert consensus, currently recommends no systematic screening and targeted screening in patients with good life expectancy who have a family history of aneurysm or haemorrhage, with previous rupture, high-risk profession or anxiety.
2. Churg-Strauss syndrome has the highest incidence of neurological involvement. Most commonly, this is a peripheral neuropathy, with 80% of patients showing signs of mononeuropathy multiplex.

3. Yes. Patients with suprasacral spinal cord injury often have detrusor overactivity and high bladder pressures through detrusor sphincter dyssynergia. The UK NICE guidance suggests offering video-urodynamic investigations to people known to have high risk of renal complications, e.g. spinal cord injury or spina bifida.
4. AKI develops due to obstructive nephropathy, with intratubular precipitation of crystals. It may be preventable with appropriate volume expansion prior to administration.
5. Attentional deficits in the early stages with progress to delirium and then decreased level of consciousness.

References

1. Chapman AB, et al. Autosomal-dominant polycystic kidney disease (ADPKD): executive summary from a Kidney Disease: Improving Global Outcomes (KDIGO) Controversies Conference. Kidney Int. 2015;88(1):17–27.
2. Malik MT, Kazmi SJ, Turner S. Teaching NeuroImages: Intradural, intramedullary spinal cord metastasis from primary renal cell carcinoma. Neurology. 2018;90(10):e911–2.
3. Sharma K, et al. Leber's congenital amaurosis with nephropathy. Indian J Ophthalmol. 1994;42(2):83–4.
4. Nishino H, et al. Neurological involvement in Wegener's granulomatosis: an analysis of 324 consecutive patients at the Mayo Clinic. Ann Neurol. 1993;33(1):4–9.
5. Sehgal M, et al. Neurologic manifestations of Churg-Strauss syndrome. Mayo Clin Proc. 1995;70(4):337–41.
6. Finsterer J, Scorza FA. Renal manifestations of primary mitochondrial disorders. Biomed Rep. 2017;6(5):487–94.
7. National Clinical Guideline Centre (UK). Urinary incontinence in neurological disease: management of lower urinary tract dysfunction in neurological disease. London: National Clinical Guideline Centre (UK); 2012.
8. Kurella M, et al. Chronic kidney disease and cognitive impairment in the elderly: the health, aging, and body composition study. J Am Soc Nephrol. 2005;16(7):2127–33.
9. Seliger SL, et al. Moderate renal impairment and risk of dementia among older adults: the Cardiovascular Health Cognition Study. J Am Soc Nephrol. 2004;15(7):1904–11.
10. Chillon JM, Massy ZA, Stengel B. Neurological complications in chronic kidney disease patients. Nephrol Dial Transplant. 2016;31(10):1606–14.
11. Zoccali C, et al. The systemic nature of CKD. Nat Rev Nephrol. 2017;13(6):344–58.
12. Candy JM, et al. Aluminium accumulation in relation to senile plaque and neurofibrillary tangle formation in the brains of patients with renal failure. J Neurol Sci. 1992;107(2):210–8.
13. Brenner RP. The electroencephalogram in altered states of consciousness. Neurol Clin. 1985;3(3):615–31.
14. Raskin NH. Neurological aspects of renal failure. In: Aminoff MJ, editor. Neurology and general medicine. 1st ed. New York: Churchill Livingstone; 1989.
15. Hinchey J, et al. A reversible posterior leukoencephalopathy syndrome. N Engl J Med. 1996;334(8):494–500.
16. Kitaguchi H, et al. A brainstem variant of reversible posterior leukoencephalopathy syndrome. Neuroradiology. 2005;47(9):652–6.
17. Herbert H, Schaumburg ARB, Thomas PK. Disorders of peripheral nerves. Philadelphia: F.A. Davis; 1991.
18. Krishnan AV, Kiernan MC. Uremic neuropathy: clinical features and new pathophysiological insights. Muscle Nerve. 2007;35(3):273–90.
19. Raskin NH, Fishman RA. Neurologic disorders in renal failure (first of two parts). N Engl J Med. 1976;294(3):143–8.
20. Dyck PJ, et al. Segmental demyelination secondary to axonal degeneration in uremic neuropathy. Mayo Clin Proc. 1971;46(6):400–31.
21. Fraser CL. Neurological manifestations of the uremic state. In: Arieff A, Griggs R, editors. Metabolic brain dysfunction in systemic disorders. Philadelphia: Lippincott Williams and Wilkins; 1992. p. 500.
22. Bautista J, et al. Dialysis myopathy. Report of 13 cases. Acta Neuropathol. 1983;61(1):71–5.
23. Brouns R, De Deyn PP. Neurological complications in renal failure: a review. Clin Neurol Neurosurg. 2004;107(1):1–16.
24. Go AS, et al. Impact of proteinuria and glomerular filtration rate on risk of thromboembolism in atrial fibrillation: the anticoagulation and risk factors in atrial fibrillation (ATRIA) study. Circulation. 2009;119(10):1363–9.
25. Elliott MJ, Zimmerman D, Holden RM. Warfarin anticoagulation in hemodialysis patients: a systematic review of bleeding rates. Am J Kidney Dis. 2007;50(3):433–40.
26. Vazquez E, et al. Ought dialysis patients with atrial fibrillation be treated with oral anticoagulants? Int J Cardiol. 2003;87(2–3):135–9; discussion 139–41.
27. Davenport A. Practical guidance for dialyzing a hemodialysis patient following acute brain injury. Hemodial Int. 2008;12(3):307–12.
28. Kurella Tamura M, et al. Kidney function and cognitive impairment in US adults: the Reasons for Geographic and Racial Differences in Stroke (REGARDS) Study. Am J Kidney Dis. 2008;52(2):227–34.
29. Helmer C, et al. Chronic kidney disease, cognitive decline, and incident dementia: the 3C Study. Neurology. 2011;77(23): 2043–51.
30. Allen RP, et al. Evidence-based and consensus clinical practice guidelines for the iron treatment of restless legs syndrome/Willis-Ekbom disease in adults and children: an IRLSSG task force report. Sleep Med. 2018;41:27–44.
31. Aukerman MM, et al. Exercise and restless legs syndrome: a randomized controlled trial. J Am Board Fam Med. 2006;19(5): 487–93.
32. Winkelman JW, et al. Practice guideline summary: treatment of restless legs syndrome in adults: report of the guideline development, dissemination, and implementation Subcommittee of the American Academy of Neurology. Neurology. 2016;87(24): 2585–93.
33. Roca AO, et al. Dialysis leg cramps. Efficacy of quinine versus vitamin E. ASAIO J. 1992;38(3):M481–5.
34. Serrao M, et al. Gabapentin treatment for muscle cramps: an open-label trial. Clin Neuropharmacol. 2000;23(1):45–9.
35. Karunaratne K, et al. Neurological complications of renal dialysis and transplantation. Pract Neurol. 2018;18(2):115–25.
36. Power A, et al. High but stable incidence of subdural haematoma in haemodialysis--a single-centre study. Nephrol Dial Transplant. 2010;25(7):2272–5.
37. Chandna SM, et al. Low serum vitamin B12 levels in chronic high-flux haemodialysis patients. Nephron. 1997;75(3):259–63.
38. Patchell RA. Neurological complications of organ transplantation. Ann Neurol. 1994;36(5):688–703.
39. Duchnowska R, et al. Severe neurological symptoms in a patient with advanced renal cell carcinoma treated with sunitinib. J Oncol Pharm Pract. 2013;19(2):186–9.

40. Kimmel PL, et al. Psychiatric illness in patients with end-stage renal disease. Am J Med. 1998;105(3):214–21.
41. Cerullo M. Corticosteroid-induced mania: Prepare for the unpredictable. Curr Psychiatry 2006 [cited 2016 22/6/16]; Available from: https://www.mdedge.com/psychiatry/article/62206/mental-health/corticosteroid-induced-mania-prepare-unpredictable.

Patient Information and Guidelines

NICE clinical guideline CG148: urinary incontinence in neurological disease: assessment and management. August 2012.

Ophthalmology and the Kidney

Marilina Antonelou, Zoya Hameed, Ali Abdall-Razak, Cathy Egan, and Detlef Bockenhauer

Contents

M. Harber (ed.), *Primer on Nephrology*, https://doi.org/10.1007/978-3-030-76419-7_42

Learning Objectives

1. To provide an overview of important associations between renal and major eye diseases
2. To highlight ocular manifestations of renal insufficiency related to chronic kidney disease itself or its treatment
3. To emphasise the need for close collaboration of the two subspecialties for the diagnosis and prevention of disease

42.1 Introduction

The association between renal disease and blindness was first reported in the middle of the nineteenth century. Although the causes for the link were not known, it is now appreciated that there are several causes for this association. Firstly, disturbances in embryogenesis can lead to anatomic and functional abnormalities in the two organs. There are also multiple proteins that are of importance in both organs, dysfunction of which therefore also leads to oculorenal disease [1]. In addition, there are storage disorders, where accumulation of a metabolite can cause both renal and ocular dysfunction. Critically, given the global burden of CKD, retinal microvascular disease has been shown to be predictive of CKD development and therefore retinal imaging offers nephrologist significant potential for assessing and monitoring risk. Conversely, patients with CKD are at higher risk for age-related macular degeneration (AMD), diabetic retinopathy, glaucoma and cataract. Hypertensive retinopathic changes can be particularly severe in renal failure with accelerated hypertension being a much greater frequency than the general population. The chronic kidney disease in the Chronic Renal Insufficiency Cohort (CRIC) Study group examined retinal photographs of 1936 individuals with varying stages of chronic kidney disease and found 45% had retinal diseases that required ophthalmologic follow-up, while 3% had serious eye lesions that required urgent treatment. This group also reported in patients with CKD 4 and 5 three times greater risk of retinopathy than in patients with a normal eGFR [1]. Given that retinopathy is often asymptomatic in its most treatable stage and delay in diagnosis can result in a significant increase in the risk of visual loss, there is a need for joined up assessment and management of patients with eye and renal disease.

42.2 Acquired Eye Disease

42.2.1 Hypertensive Retinopathy

Hypertensive retinopathy was first described by Marcus Gunn in the nineteenth century in a series of patients with hypertension and renal disease and has long been regarded as a risk indicator for systemic morbidity and mortality. Given the intimate link between kidney disease and hypertension both in terms of pathogenesis, management and outcome, identification and assessment of hypertensive retinopathy have perhaps greater potential than generally appreciated.

42.2.1.1 Pathophysiology

The retinal circulation undergoes a series of pathophysiological changes in response to elevated blood pressure. The initial response to elevated blood pressure is diffuse and localised vasospasm of the retinal arterioles with generalised and focal arteriolar narrowing. Arteriolar narrowing is seen in the early phase and is a defining sign of hypertensive retinopathy and reflects vasoconstriction as an autoregulatory response. If the blood pressure remains persistently elevated, structural changes develop in the arterioles such as intimal thickening, hyperplasia of the media wall and hyaline degeneration. These changes that eventually lead to sclerosis compress adjacent venules resulting in arteriovenous nicking and alterations in the arteriolar light reflex ('copper wiring') [2] .

This is followed by an exudative stage, in which there is disruption of the blood-retina barrier, necrosis of the smooth muscle and endothelial cells, exudation of blood and lipids and retinal ischaemia. These changes manifest in the retina as microaneurysms, haemorrhages, hard exudates and cotton wool spots (◘ Fig. 42.1a and b). Swelling of the optic disc may occur at this time and usually indicates severely elevated blood pressure (i.e. malignant (accelerated phase) hypertension (◘ Fig. 42.1c)) [3].

Acute elevations in blood pressure that overwhelm the compensatory tone actually harm the choroidal circulation more than the retinal circulation due to the sympathetic innervation of choroid. Chronic blood pressure elevation can lead to hypertensive choroidopathy generally seen in younger patients with pliable vessels that are not yet sclerotic from long-standing hypertension [4].

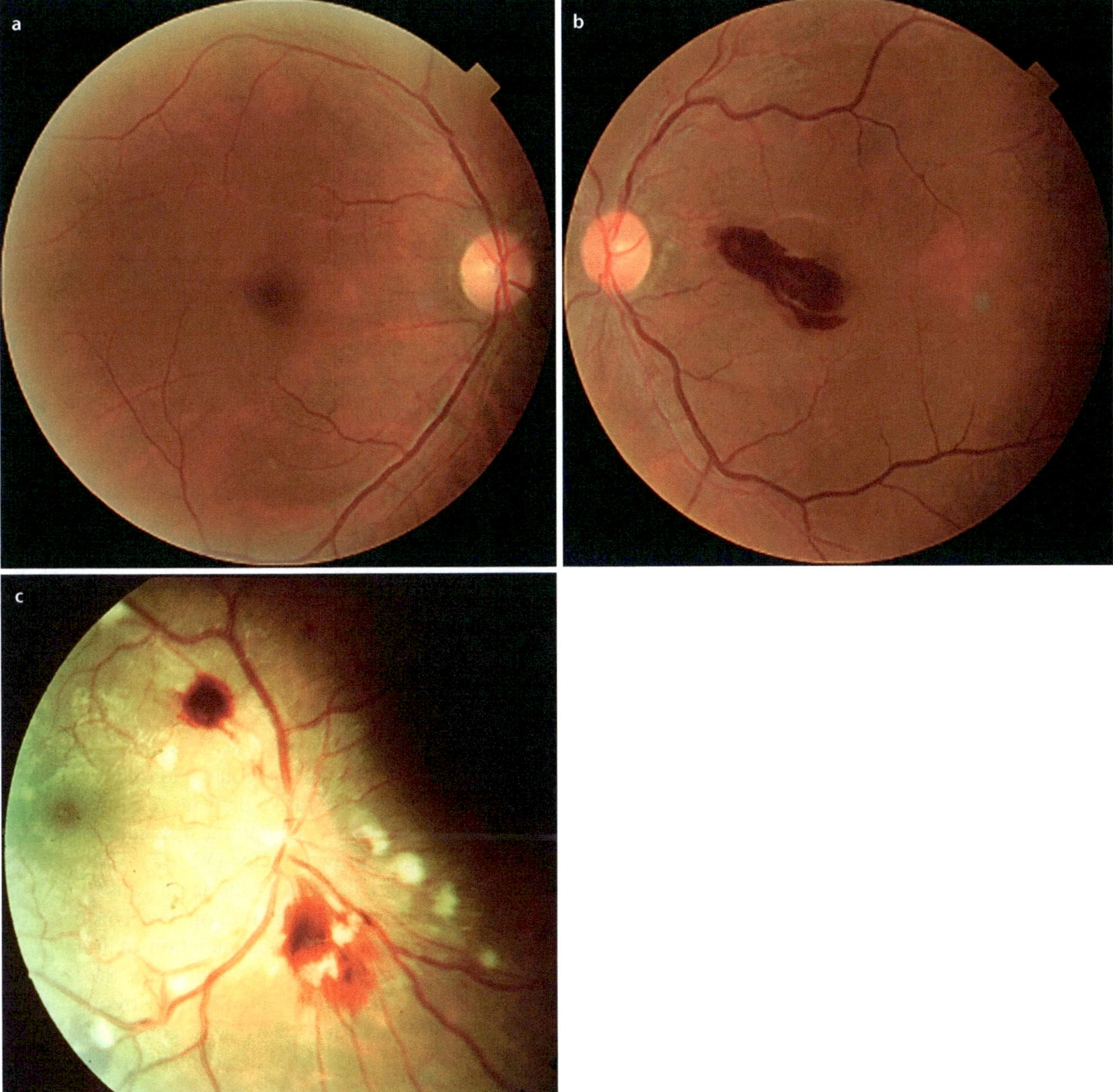

Fig. 42.1 Fundus photograph showing copper wiring' of vessels **a** with haemorrhage **b** in the left eye. **c** Grade IV hypertensive retinopathy with retinal haemorrhages, cotton wool spots and papilloedema

42.2.1.2 Epidemiology

Hypertensive retinopathy is seen in 6–15% of non-diabetic adults aged older than 40 years. Isolated retinal haemorrhages and/or microaneurysms are the most commonly observed signs (5.7–8%) with presence of cotton wool spots being relatively uncommon (0.2%). Some studies suggest that the incidence of generalised arteriolar narrowing is as high as 25% among hypertensive people. The prevalence varies according to the populations being studied with a prevalence of 7.7% in African Americans, which is nearly twice as high than the prevalence in whites (4.1%) [5].

The strongest evidence of the usefulness of an evaluation of hypertensive retinopathy for risk stratification is based on its association with stroke and coronary artery disease. The Atherosclerosis Risk in Communities Study (ARIC), a multicentre study, showed that some signs of retinopathy (retinal haemorrhages, microaneurysms and cotton wool spots) were associated with a risk of newly diagnosed clinical stroke that was 2–4 times as high as that for patients who did not have these signs after adjusting for all other risk factors [6]. Retinal microvascular abnormalities are associated with renal dysfunction, suggesting that common systemic microvascular processes may underlie the development of microvascular damage in the eye and kidneys. In the ARIC study, individuals with retinopathy were twice more likely to develop renal dysfunction than individuals without these abnormalities.

Renal physicians could consider retinal morphology when assessing cardiovascular disease risk in people with CKD based on the work of the CRIC study, which found that worsening of hypertensive retinopathy was associated with an increased risk of incidence of CVD (OR 1.66) [7].

42.2.1.3 Aetiology

Retinal vascular calibre changes reflect cumulative responses to aging, cardiovascular risk factors, inflammation, nitric oxide-dependent endothelial dysfunction and other processes [8]. Data from recent population-based studies suggest that retinal arteriolar and venular calibre changes may reflect different vascular pathophysiological processes that link to a range of demographic factors (e.g. age, race/ethnicity); systemic medical conditions (e.g. blood pressure, diabetes); inflammation, nitric oxide-dependent endothelial dysfunction and lifestyle factors (e.g., smoking); and genetic factors.

42.2.2 Diabetic Retinopathy (DR)

42.2.2.1 Epidemiology

Diabetic retinopathy is the most common ophthalmic complication of diabetes mellitus and was the most common cause of visual impairment in working age adults in the UK until recently [9].

42

In a UK cohort of 7.7 million patients, the prevalence of DR was 48.4% in the population type 1 diabetes mellitus (T1DM) and 28.3% in the population with type 2 diabetes mellitus (T2DM) [10]. Among patients with T2DM, the relative risk of DR varied significantly by region and was increased for older age groups, in men. The risk of severe DR increased in South Asian and more socio-economically deprived groups. Fundoscopic changes may be found at diagnosis due to a potentially long pre-diagnosis period of hyperglycaemia. Within 20 years, 60% of non-insulin-dependent diabetics have some degree of retinopathy.

42.2.2.2 Pathogenesis

Hyperglycaemia and hyperglycaemia-associated pathways such as oxidative stress, the formation of advanced glycation end products, upregulation of protein kinase C, increased polyol pathway flux and focal leucostasis may be important [11].

The initial response to hyperglycaemia is dilatation of the retinal blood vessels. These blood flow changes are considered to be a metabolic autoregulation to increase retinal metabolism in diabetic subjects. Pericyte loss is another hallmark of the early events of DR. Since pericytes are responsible for providing structural support for capillaries, loss of them leads to localised outpouching of capillary walls. This process is associated with microaneurysm formation, which is the earliest clinical sign of DR [12]. In addition to pericyte loss, apoptosis of endothelial cells and thickening of the basement membrane are also detected during advancing disease, which collectively contribute to the impairment of the blood retina barrier, capillary occlusion and ischaemia. Retinal ischaemia/hypoxia leads to upregulation of VEGF through activation of hypoxia-inducible factor 1 (HIF-1). Progressive disease is characterised by diabetic macular oedema or retinal and optic nerve neovascularisation (proliferative diabetic retinopathy) as a result of chronic ischaemia and the upregulation of vascular endothelial growth factor (VEGF) (◘ Fig. 42.2). Diabetic macular oedema is the main cause of visual loss in patients with diabetic retinopathy. This describes the sub- and intra-retinal accumulation of fluid in the macula as a consequence of breakdown of the BRB.

Aberrant vessels may bleed into the vitreous causing sudden vision loss. End-stage disease consists of fibrotic tractional bands and retinal detachment or neovascular glaucoma.

Current treatment strategies for DR aim at managing the microvascular complications. Early-stage disease is reversible or can be stabilised with improved systemic control of hyperglycaemia and blood pressure. Late-stage disease management will include combinations of intravitreal injections of pharmacologic agents, laser photocoagulation and vitreous surgery. Intravitreal administration of anti-VEGF agents is currently the mainstay of therapy for diabetic macular oedema and some neovascular complication.

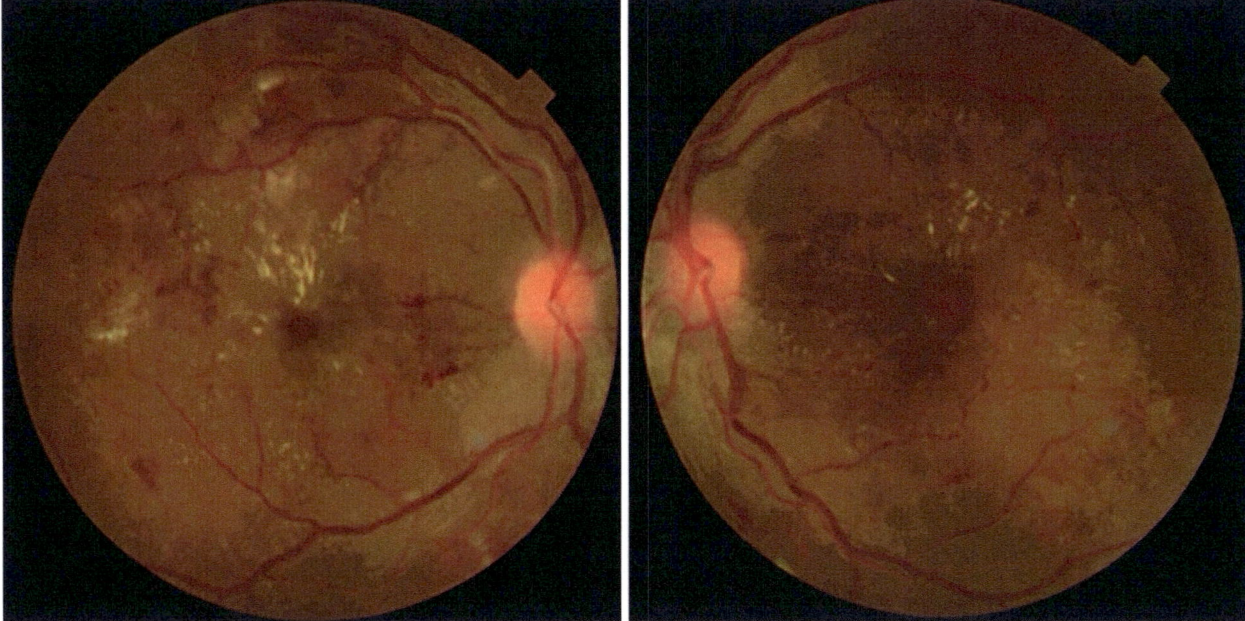

Fig. 42.2 Fundal photograph showing advanced proliferative diabetic retinopathy with visible microaneurysms, haemorrhages, hard exudates and neovascularisation. Macular oedema is likely to be present on a 3D examination of the eyes

42.2.2.3 Risk Factors

In patients with T1DM, higher HbA1c, HbA1c variability, age of onset of T1DM and total cholesterol were independently associated with the risk of DR development, and a protective association was found for HDL cholesterol. Mean HbA1c and presence of albuminuria were associated with progression of DR [13]. In T2DM, age and duration of diabetes are associated with DR development whereas modifiable risk factors include the obesity, hypertension, renal function and total cholesterol.

There are other manifestations of vascular disease manifest in the eye from xanthelasma in the eyelids as a marker of hypercholesterolaemia to retinal arteriolar cholesterol emboli (Fig. 42.3) and macroaneurysms as well as retinal artery occlusions and retinal vein thrombosis.

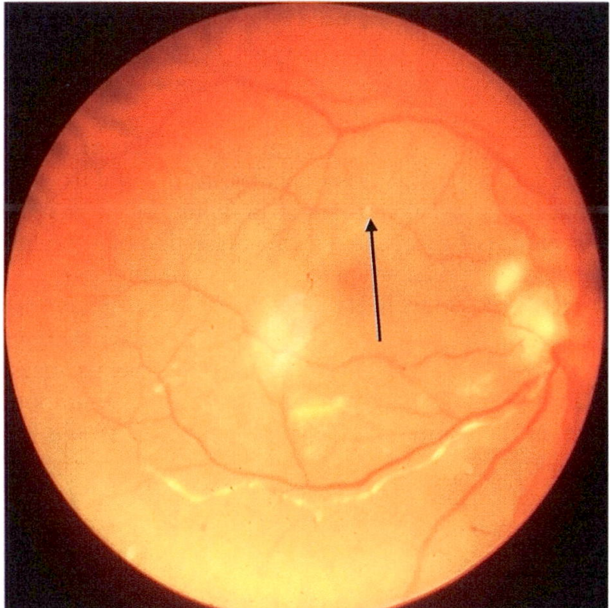

Fig. 42.3 Cholesterol embolus in a patient with extensive vascular disease following a coronary angiogram. There is a reduction in calibre of some of the retinal arteries and a consequent diminution of venous vessels. It is sometimes possible to see cholesterol emboli (arrow) indicative of embolic showering that may have occurred in other organs such as the kidney

42.2.3 Inflammatory Diseases of the Eye in Kidney Disease

There are a variety of acquired inflammatory lesions in the eye that can have associations and, therefore diagnostic importance, with renal diseases. Broadly, these can be divided into eye involvement in systemic autoimmune disease, infection (usually in the context of immunosuppression), syndromes and allergy (usually drug) or toxicity related. These associations are important as they may be useful biomarkers of a flare or renal disease or the harbinger of a systemic disease that can involve the kidney.

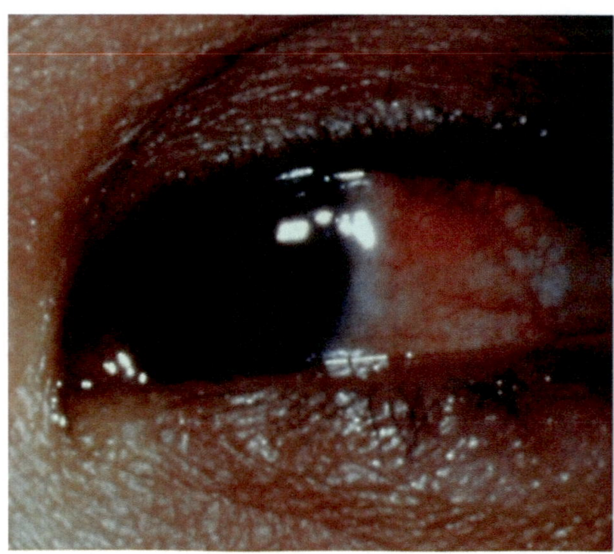

■ Fig. 42.4 Scleritis as the presenting feature in a patient with a flare of micropolyangiitis

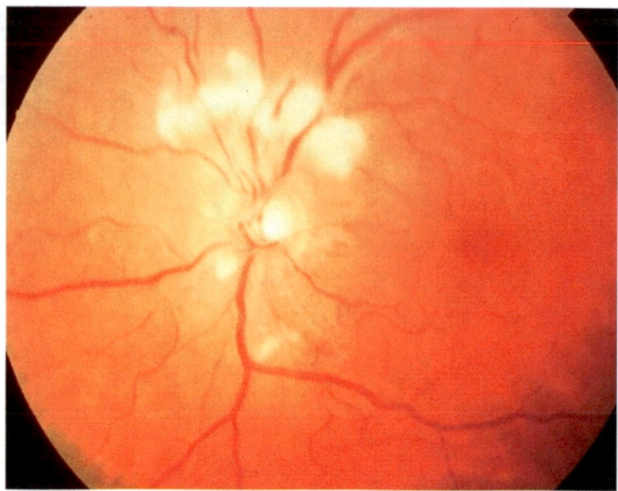

■ Fig. 42.5 Retinal image of retinal vasculitis in a patient with granulomatous polyangiitis who presented with multiple symptoms, including loss of vision

Keratitis (inflammation of the cornea) for nephrologists occurs in the immunocompromised, most commonly related to herpes simplex. The cornea is also involved as part of the sicca syndrome in Sjogren's syndrome ('Do you have dry eyes?' being an important diagnostic question) and sarcoidosis and as corneal dystrophy (verticillata) in Fabry disease.

Episcleritis, typically presents with a red eye (inflammation of superficial vessels and some discomfort. This clinical sign usually occurs in isolation, but in a small percentage of cases can be a manifestation of vasculitis (micropolyangiitis or granulomatous polyangiitis).

Scleritis is more likely to be painful, has a greater risk of progressing to loss of vision and is more strongly associated (c.50%) with an underlying systemic illness (■ Fig. 42.4) – typically, rheumatological conditions and, in the context of renal disease, vasculitis and less commonly SLE.

42

Uveitis can be anterior (involving the iris/ciliary body) which may have symptoms of pain and photosensitivity and is associated with redness at the limbus and cells in the aqueous, intermediate (involving the vitreous/ciliary body) or posterior, involving the choroid/retina. Posterior uveitis is more commonly painless. It is associated with systemic inflammatory conditions in roughly 40% of cases. The retinal vessels may also be involved in systemic vasculitis and be an important diagnostic clue. Most commonly the underlying diagnoses are spondyloarthritidies, such as ankylosing spondylitis and Behcet's syndrome, but from the renal perspective, sarcoidosis, tubulo-interstitial nephritis and uveitis and vasculitis (■ Fig. 42.5) and occasionally Sjogren's syndrome and SLE are underlying diagnoses.

Infectious causes of uveitis are myriad, most notably CMV and herpetic viruses such as HSV and HZV in the immunocompromised and syphilis and tuberculosis.

Granulomatous polyangiitis can also present as proptosis secondary to a retro-orbital mass or vasculitic involvement of optic and orbital nerves.

One anomaly in ocular and renal disease is Goodpasture's syndrome. The target antigen in Goodpasture's syndrome is the alpha 3 chain of type IV collagen, which is present in the basement membranes of the glomerulus, the alveoli and the eye. However, eye involvement in this 'pulmonary renal syndrome' is rarely reported, being limited to non-rheumatogenous retinal detachments subretinal neovascularisation and lesions related to hypertension [14, 15].

Thus, several inflammatory eye conditions with potential for renal involvement may present to the ophthalmologist as the harbinger of renal disease or relapse. Having a system that involves urine analysis for patients with scleritis or uveitis and an established referral pathway is worth considering.

42.3 Inherited Eye Disease

There are a number of inherited disorders that can affect both the eye and the kidney [16]. In general, these can be separated into disorders of organogenesis, disorders of structure and function and metabolic disorders, which lead to accumulation of substances harmful to both organs. Awareness of these multi-organ manifestations is important, so that the diagnosing specialist can counsel and refer appropriately.

42.3.1 Developmental Disorders

These are typically caused by mutations in transcription factors important for normal development of both organs, such as PAX2 and LMX1B (◘ Table 42.1). Manifestations highlight the specific role of these transcription factors. PAX2 plays an important role in early renal development and mutations are therefore commonly associated with renal malformations, especially hypoplasia. The typical eye manifestation is col-

◘ **Table 42.1** Common kidney conditions that affect the eye

	Eye manifestations	Renal manifestation
Systemic disease		
Diabetes	Common: retinopathy (95% and 60% prevalence in patients with type 1 and type 2 diabetics, respectively, with disease duration of over 20 years), cataract (2–5 times more at risk than general population), glaucoma, keratopathy Rare: optic nerve disease	Diabetic nephropathy (see text)
Hypertension	Retinal microvasculature: hypertensive retinopathy, choroidopathy, optic neuropathy Vascular abnormalities: venous occlusive disease, retinal arteriolar macroaneurysm formation and embolic events PRES: reversible vasogenic oedema in the posterior brain, which primarily arises from autoregulation failure and endothelial dysfunction. There are a number of causes that may lead to the development of PRES such as malignant hypertension, pre-eclampsia/eclampsia and malignancy. Studies have indicated that patients with CKD are more likely to develop PRES due to presumed endothelial dysfunction	Hypertensive nephropathy (see text)
Multiple myeloma	Cysts of the ciliary body (33–50%), retinal vascular lesions including retinal arteriole and venous occlusion (up to 66%) [29]	Light chain nephropathy and cast nephropathy, amyloid, heavy chain nephropathy, acute tubular injury secondary to hypercalcaemia
Autoimmune		
ANCA-associated vasculitis	Granulomatosis with polyangiitis (GPA): scleritis (16–38%), conjunctivitis (4–16%), nasolacrimal obstruction, episcleritis, orbital myositis, retinal vasculitis, ulcerative keratitis Microscopic polyangiitis: scleritis, conjunctivitis, episcleritis, retinal vasculitis, ulcerative keratitis Eosinophilic Granulomatosis with polyangiitis (EGPA): episcleritis, conjunctivitis, neuroophthalmic manifestations, myositis, retinal vasculitis, ulcerative keratitis	Renal Vasculitis, crescentic glomerulonephritis
Systemic lupus erythematosus (SLE)	Eye involvement in 20–40% of cases. Keratoconjunctivitis sicca is the most common presentation, while retinopathy and choroidopathy are most associated with visual loss. Also conjunctivitis, episcleritis, scleritis, uveitis, and keratitis	Lupus nephropathy (I–V)
Tubulo-interstitial nephritis and uveitis (TINU)	Uveitis that may proceed or follow TIN	Acute tubulo-interstitial nephritis with mononuclear cell Infiltration of the interstitium
Sarcoid	Dry eyes, optic neuritis, cranial nerve palsies, lid inflammation and uveitis (up to 20% of patients)	Acute tubulo-interstitial nephritis with mononuclear cell Infiltration of the interstitium, acute tubular injury secondary to hypercalcaemia
Polyarteritis nodosa	Retinal artery thrombosis	Renal micro infarction

(continued)

Table 42.1 (continued)

	Eye manifestations	Renal manifestation
Dense deposit disease	Drusen (deposits containing C3 in Bruch's membrane)	Membranoproliferative glomerulonephritis, progressive renal failure
Hereditary		
Alport's *COL4A3, COL4A4, COL4A5*	Dot-and-fleck retinopathy (unimpaired vision). Anterior lenticonus (misshapen lens)	Haematuria, proteinuria, progressive renal impairment
Von Hippel-Lindau syndrome	Retinal angioma 45–60% of cases	Renal cell cancer, phaeochromocytoma
Nail patella *LMX1B*	Glaucoma	Haematuria, proteinuria, CKD
Senior-Loken syndrome	Retinitis pigmentosa, retinal aplasia	Renal dysplasia
Bardet-Biedl syndrome	Retinitis pigmentosa, night blindness proceeding to complete blindness	Cystic and dysplastic changes (nephronophthisis)
Lowe syndrome *OCRL*	Congenital cataracts, infantile glaucoma, corneal keloid	Renal Fanconi syndrome
Joubert syndrome	Retinal dystrophy, dysregulated eye movements, coloboma	Renal dysplasia
Papillorenal (renal-coloboma) syndrome *PAX2*	Wide clinical variation but manifest in retinal coloboma; failure of development closure of choroid fissure leading to optic dysplasia (vessels emerge from edge of a large optic disc (rather than the middle), retinal defects and retinal vessels may be abnormal or absent. Iris coloboma	Renal hypo- or dysplasia, ureteric reflux, renal cysts
Pierson *LAMB2*	Small pupils unresponsive to light, progressive blindness	Congenital nephrotic syndrome and renal impairment
Metabolic		
Fabry disease	Corneal verticillata (asymptomatic opacities seen with a slit lamp)	Proteinuria, polyuria and polydipsia, progressive chronic kidney disease
Primary hyperoxaluria	Diffuse oxalate deposition in the retina 'flecked retinopathy'	Nephrocalcinosis, urolithiasis and progressive chronic kidney disease
Cystinosis	Cystine crystal deposits in all parts of the eye but particularly the anterior chamber. Photophobia, band keratopathy, poor colour vision and glaucoma may develop	Nephrocalcinosis. Hyperchloraemic metabolic acidosis, hypophosphataemia Hypocalcaemia, proteinuria, renal Fanconi syndrome, progressive chronic kidney disease
Infection		
Leptospirosis	Conjunctival suffusion (and often jaundiced sclerae)	Acute kidney injury
Metastatic infection	Roth or Litten spots (white-centred (leucocytes and fibrin) retinal haemorrhages said to be present in 2% of bacterial endocarditis, conjunctival haemorrhage, choroidoretinitis and endo-ophthalmitis (the latter two more associated with fungaemia))	Proliferative glomerulonephritis, micro-infarction
Syphilis	Syphilitic involvement of the eye (e.g. scleritis, posterior uveitis, or optic neuritis) can range from subacute to chronic	Membranous glomerulonephritis in secondary syphilis

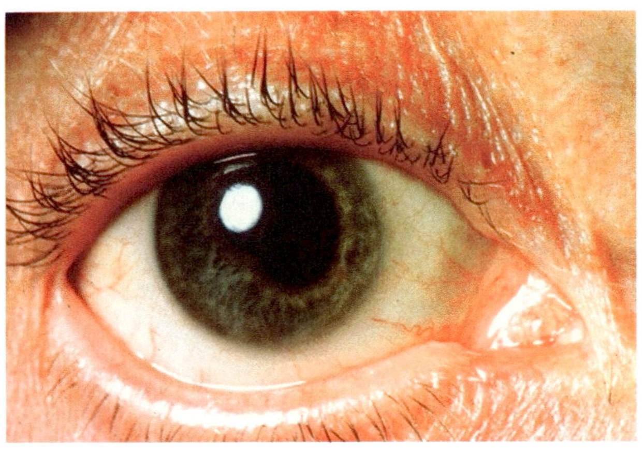

◘ **Fig. 42.6** Coloboma, a maldevelopment of the iris which may be associated with CHARGE syndrome (*CHD7* mutations) or papillorenal syndrome (*PAX2* mutations)

oboma (◘ Fig. 42.6) [17]. In contrast, LMX1B is involved in the organisation of the glomerular basement membrane and mutations (e.g. nail-patella syndrome) manifest with nephrotic range proteinuria, whereas the ocular manifestation is typically open-angle glaucoma [18].

42.3.2 Disorders of Structure and Function

Ciliopathies commonly affect the kidney and eye due to the important role of cilia in both organ systems. The photoreceptors in the eye possess a specialised cilium, involved in photon capture and initiation of the signalling cascade initiating the visual process [19]. Consequently, ciliopathies are commonly associated with retinopathies, such as retinitis pigmentosa in Bardet-Biedl syndrome. In the kidney, epithelial cells in all nephron segments possess cilia, which are involved in a variety of processes. Common renal manifestations of ciliopathies include cystic kidney disease, including nephronophthisis and cystic dysplasia [20].

Lowe syndrome, also known as oculocerebrorenal syndrome is caused by mutations in *OCRL*, encoding a phosphoinositol-5-phosphatase, involved in endocytic recycling [21]. Ocular manifestations include congenital cataracts and glaucoma, whereas the renal phenotype is characterised by a proximal tubulopathy and progressive CKD [22].

Alport syndrome and related type 4 collagenopathies are caused by mutations in genes encoding subunits of type 4 collagen, an important structural component in the basement membranes of the glomerulus, as well as of the lens, cornea and retina [23]. Consequently, clinical manifestations in the eye include lenticonus, but also corneal dystrophy and maculopathy, whereas in the kidney glomerular dysfunction predominates, typically haematuria and proteinuria.

Pierson syndrome is caused by mutations in *LAMB2*, encoding laminin ß2, another important structural component of the glomerular basement membrane. Consequently, renal manifestations are characterised by glomerular dysfunction, especially congenital nephrotic syndrome. LAMB2 is also expressed in neuromuscular junctions and the typical ocular manifestation is microcoria due to dysplastic ciliary muscles [24].

42.3.3 Metabolic

There are several metabolic disorders, where accumulation of a substrate can affect multiple organ systems, including the kidney and eye (◘ Table 42.2). These include the lysosomal storage disorders cystinosis and Fabry disease. Cystinosis, caused by mutations in *CTNS*,

◘ **Table 42.2** Chronic kidney disease and the eye

Haemodialysis	
Conjunctival erythema	Red eyes of uraemia – high plasma phosphate levels induce corneal and conjunctival precipitation of calcium pyrophosphate
Metastatic calcification	Band keratopathy – calcium deposition across the anterior surface of the cornea. Associated with elevations of the serum concentration of calcium or calcium-phosphate product (see ◘ Fig. 42.8)
Uraemic amaurosis/transient cortical blindness	Profound uraemia in association with preserved pupillary contraction on light exposure and normal fundoscopic findings. This abnormality clears within 24–48 hours of initiating dialytic therapy
Raised intraocular pressure	Removal of urea and other solutes reducing serum osmolality more rapidly than ocular osmolality, steep gradient in the presence of ocular-blood barrier
Anterior ischaemic optic neuropathy	Intradialytic hypotension and anaemia
Kidney transplantation	
Opportunistic ocular infections	A variety of infections can involve the eye in patients who are immunosuppressed for renal conditions such as glomerular disorders or transplantation. Most commonly herpes simplex virus and ophthalmic involvement of varicella zoster but potentially CMV, HHV8, listeria, nocardia, mycobacteria, fungi such as *Cryptococcus neoformans*, candida and aspergillus infections, as well as parasites such as toxoplasmosis
Medications used in CKD	
Hydroxychloroquine	Retinopathy with 7.5% prevalence in individuals with more than 5-year exposure

Cyclosporine and interferon	Evanescent cortical blindness
Cidofovir for BKV	Anterior uveitis
Corticosteroids	Posterior subcapsular cataract
Sulphadiazine	Shock of wheat crystals
Steroids	Elevated intra-ocular pressure, 'development of steroid cataract' is dose and duration dependent (15 mg of oral prednisolone for a year)

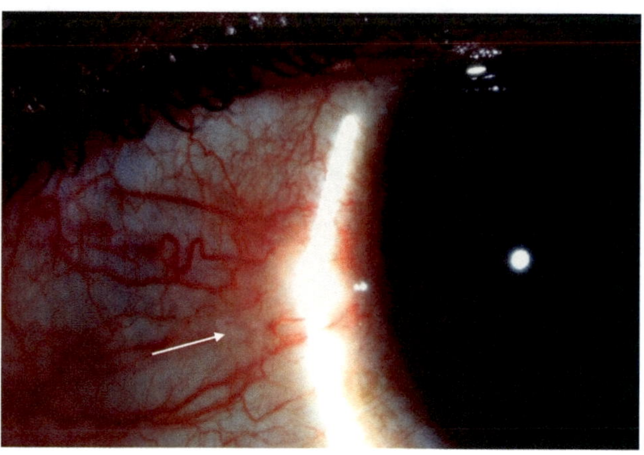

Fig. 42.8 Ectopic calcification (arrow) in a dialysis patient presenting with red eyes. The patient had very poor phosphate control and hypercalcaemia

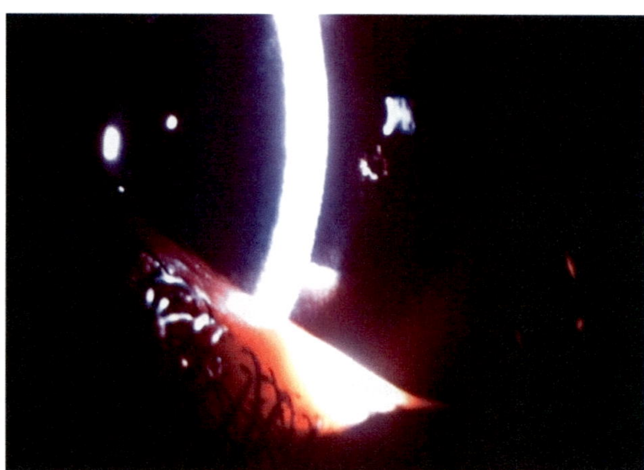

Fig. 42.7 Cystine crystals cannot normally be seen with the naked eye or with an ophthalmoscope, although patients with significant cystine deposits in the eye will often have red irritable eyes. The image here is from a slit lamp examination demonstrating and monitoring cystine deposition in the cornea

encoding a lysosomal cystine transporter is characterised by cystine crystal deposition essentially in every organ system. If not adequately treated, ocular manifestation includes photophobia and keratopathy (Fig. 42.7) but later also retinopathy. Renal manifestation includes Fanconi renotubular syndrome and progressive CKD [25] (Fig. 42.7).

42

Fabry disease is caused by mutations in *GLA*, encoding alpha-galactosidase A. Dysfunction of the enzyme results in accumulation of globotriaosylceramide [26] In the eye, this can lead to corneal dystrophy, whereas renal manifestations are characterised by proteinuria and progressive CKD.

Primary hyperoxalurias (PH) are caused by mutations in genes involved in oxalate metabolism [27]. Eye manifestation is typically only seen in the most severe form, PH1, caused by mutations in *AGXT*, encoding the enzyme alanine glyoxidase aminotransferase. Renal manifestations are primarily in the form of urolithiasis, but in more severe cases end-stage kidney disease can ensue. Without renal excretion of oxalate, there is widespread oxalate deposition in essentially every organ system, which in the eye can lead to crystalline retinopathy and optic neuropathy [28].

42.4 Managing the Patient with CKD and Visual Impairment

Service levels agreements between nephrology and ophthalmology for patients that have been on long-term medications with ocular implications, such as screening for hydroxychloroquine retinopathy, should be straightforward to establish. Some units off joined clinics for patients with vasculitis and other oculo-renal conditions such as VHL syndrome.

A nephrologists should discuss systems for screening urine in patients in ophthalmology clinics with chronic or aggressive uveitis or scleritis to exclude renal involvement and a robust system for rapid renal referral in the face of an abnormal urine deposit.

Some low clearance clinics offer annual diabetic retinopathy screening; given the high prevalence of diabetes (and hypertension) among patients on dialysis, offering ophthalmology review in haemodialysis units would likely improve communication and offer a more patient-focussed service.

For patient on peritoneal dialysis, Baxter has introduced Braille keys and a voice recognition software in certain peritoneal dialysis machines that can allow blind or visually impaired patients to communicate information to the instrument, set-up or modify therapy or even to send a message from instrument through an electronic mail or over the Internet to an on-call clinician.

Case Study

Case 1

A 47-year-old male with insulin-dependent diabetes mellitus and stage 5 CKD attends the low clearance clinic complaining of (visual symptoms). He is hypertensive and fluid overloaded. He has a right AV fistula in place and decision is made to start on haemodialysis. Following three consecutive days of haemodialysis, his visual symptoms improved. ◘ Figure 42.9 shows his optical coherence tomography before and after his third haemodialysis session.

Diabetic macular oedema is the prevailing cause of visual loss in patients with diabetic retinopathy. This describes the sub- and intra-retinal accumulation of fluid in the macula as a consequence of breakdown of the blood retina barrier. High urine albumin-to-creatinine ratio (UACR) and low eGFR diabetic retinopathy in these patients.

Case 2

A 46-year-old patient with SLE attends clinic complaining of blurring of her vision and difficulty reading. She has been on hydroxychloroquine 200 mg bd for 12 years. ◘ Figure 42.10 shows her fundus photograph and autofluorescence.

Hydroxychloroquine retinopathy is characterised by a maculopathy with a 'bullseye' appearance and symptoms include a paracentral or central visual-field scotomata. Patients at increased risk of developing retinopathy include those taking tamoxifen, with renal impairment or concomitant retinal disease and a longer duration of treatment. Cessation of treatment, though unsuccessful in reversing the damage caused, is the basis on which further visual loss is prevented.

Any patients on hydroxychloroquine complaining of blurred vision, decreased central vision or difficulty read-

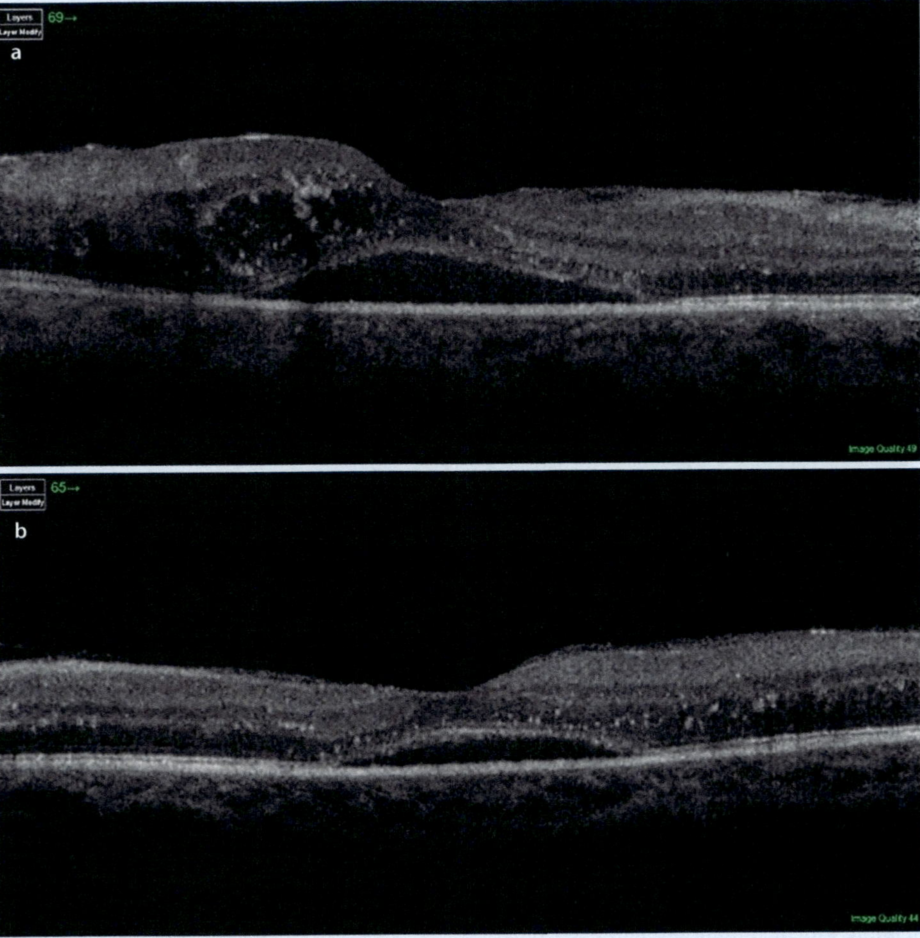

◘ **Fig. 42.9** Optical coherence tomography (OCT) scan of diabetic macular oedema in retina. **a** Pre-dialysis. **b** Post-dialysis

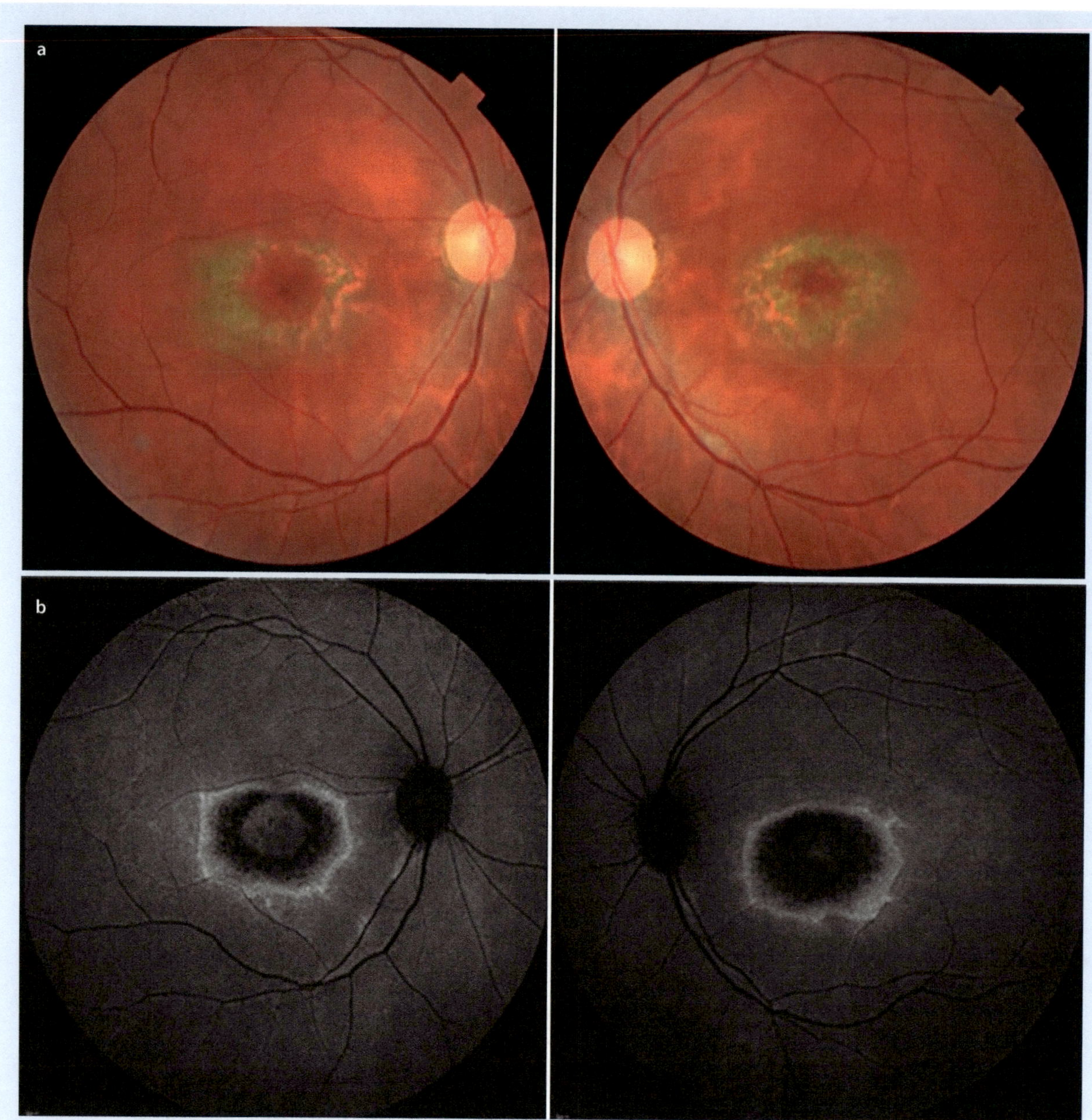

Fig. 42.10 Fundus **a** photograph and **b** autofluorescence of bullseye maculopathy

ing should be referred to an ophthalmologist for assessment. The presence of risk factors warrants annual ophthalmic follow-up.

Case 3

This 29-year-old asymptomatic female had a kidney biopsy for deteriorating renal function and proteinuria that was compatible with membranoproliferative glomerulonephritis (positive immunofluorescence for complement C3 and IgG). Drusen have been described in MPGN as diffuse and often evenly spaced resembling drusen in age-related macular degeneration (AMD) but they are rarely observed in subjects below the age of 50 years. The drusen in MPGN are similar to glomerular deposits in their subepithelial location and their composition from complement components and immunoglobulins. Thickened Bruch's membrane in the young is also seen in MPGN (Fig. 42.11).

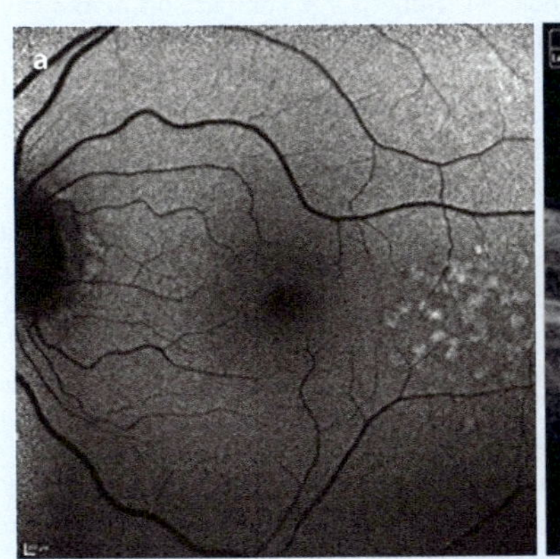

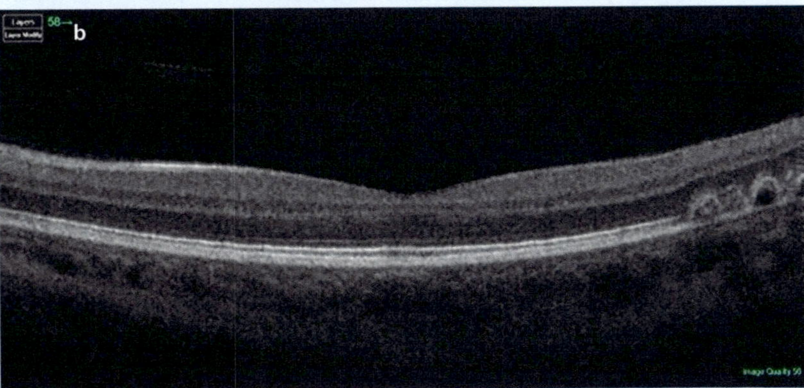

Fig. 42.11 **a** and **b** Autofluorescence showing drusen. Diffuse thickening pf Bruch's membrane with nodular elevations at sites of drusen on optical coherence tomography of the macula

Tips and Tricks

- The ocular manifestations of kidney disease can be a result of the disease itself, or its treatment and ophthalmoscopy are an important but often neglected part of clinical assessment in nephrology. There are several specific renal diseases that can be readily diagnosed by careful ophthalmic examination, expediting the management of the patient and potentially avoiding further unnecessary investigations. Providing ready access to good ophthalmoscopes and expecting that fundoscopy is part of new patient assessment is critically important.
- Systemic immunosuppression can lead to eye-threatening complications including opportunistic ocular infections; awareness of this and the need for rapid ophthalmology assessment are an important parts of patient/staff education.
- Encouraging urinalysis and early renal support/referral for patients under ophthalmologists with recurrent or aggressive scleritis or uveitis are worth considering. Similarly young patients with drusen or renal angiomas which might indicate mesangioproliferative glomerulonephritis or Von Hippel Lindau syndrome, should trigger urine dipstick and further assessment.
- Patients with SLE on hydroxychloroquine need a robust system for retinal screening.
- Patients with diabetic retinopathy (and other chronic eye clinics that require follow-up) are likely to benefit from coordinated follow-up ideally minimising trips and maximising communication. Providing ophthalmology assessment at dialysis units and renal clinics would be a thoughtful way of enhancing the experience for our patients, and providing access to support and resources for our patients on renal replacement therapy should be a standard aspect of care offered to our patients.

Chapter Review Questions

1. Should we heparinise patients with diabetic retinopathy during haemodialysis?
2. What are the differences between scleritis and episcleritis?
3. What are the key ocular features of (a) Fabry disease, (b) von Hippel-Lindau syndrome, (c) Sjogren's syndrome, (d) Bardet-Biedl syndrome, (e) Dense deposit disease
4. How does HD affect glaucoma?

Answers

1. Haemodialysis patients are at risk of ophthalmologic bleeding given their high rate of diabetes and hypertension. A series of 66 haemodialysis patients with proliferative diabetic retinopathy who received heparin with dialysis had no increased bleeding complications with vitrectomy compared with reported rates in similar studies in patients with diabetes not on dialysis therapy [11]. Another study cited a patient with a spontaneous hyphema who had recently received 10,000 IU of heparin with dialysis, but a subsequent 66 haemodialysis patients who received the same dose or more heparin did not have such a complication [12]. Again, the data are limited, but heparin does not appear to increase ophthalmologic bleeding.
2. While both can be associated with systemic disease, this is much more likely with scleritis (and uveitis) than episcleritis. The former is typically more painful rather than mildly irritating.
3. Corneal verticillata, (b) retinal angiomas, (c) sicca syndrome (dry eyes) and keratitis, (d) retinitis pigmentosa, (e) drusen.
4. Oncotic pressure increases due to ultrafiltration because large proteins, such as albumin and globulin, cannot cross the membranes. The colloid gra-

dient between plasma and interstitial fluid moves water from the interstitial and aqueous humour to plasma fluid. These changes in oncotic pressure and ultrafiltration lead to a decline in IOP at the end of dialysis. IOP change is greater with a higher plasma albumin level and degree of ultrafiltration.

In the eyes with glaucoma, narrow angles or impaired aqueous outflow, acute rises in IOP during HD could occur much more frequently than in normal patients. Lower plasma osmolarity, compared to aqueous humour osmolarity, and a relative increase in aqueous humour-urea concentration may contribute to increases in IOP. Observed differences in IOP fluctuations may also result from differences in dialysis technique and duration.

42.5 Summary

The eye offers a unique window onto the body's microcirculation that can aid both diagnosis and monitoring of common conditions but also can be of very significant diagnostic value in the setting of some renal diseases both inherited and acquired.

There is potential to improve the patient pathway between our two specialties and expedite diagnosis and treatment.

42

References

1. Grunwald JE, Alexander J, Ying G-S, Maguire M, Daniel E, Whittock-Martin R, et al. Retinopathy and chronic kidney disease in the chronic renal insufficiency cohort (CRIC) study. Arch Ophthalmol. 2012;130:1136–44.
2. Bhargava M, Ikram MK, Wong TY. How does hypertension affect your eyes? J Hum Hypertens. 2012;26:71–83.
3. Wong TY, Mitchell P. Hypertensive retinopathy. N Engl J Med. 2004;351:2310–7.
4. DellaCroce JT, Vitale AT. Hypertension and the eye. Curr Opin Ophthalmol. 2008;19:493–8.
5. Yin WT, Ronald K, Duncan BB, Javier NF, Klein Barbara EK, Couper DJ, et al. Racial differences in the prevalence of hypertensive retinopathy. Hypertension. 2003;41:1086–91.
6. Wong TY, Klein R, Couper DJ, Cooper LS, Shahar E, Hubbard LD, et al. Retinal microvascular abnormalities and incident stroke: the Atherosclerosis Risk in Communities Study. Lancet. 2001;358:1134–40.
7. Grunwald JE, Pistilli M, Ying GS, Maguire MG, Daniel E, Whittock-Martin R. Progression of retinopathy and incidence of cardiovascular disease: findings from the Chronic Renal Insufficiency Cohort Study. Br J Ophthalmol. 2020; bjophthalmol-2019-315333; https://doi.org/10.1136/bjophthalmol-2019-315333.
8. Sun C, Wang JJ, Mackey DA, Wong TY. Retinal vascular caliber: systemic, environmental, and genetic associations. Surv Ophthalmol. 2009;54:74–95.
9. Liew G, Michaelides M, Bunce C. A comparison of the causes of blindness certifications in England and Wales in working age adults (16–64 years), 1999–2000 with 2009–2010. BMJ Open. 2014;4(2):e004015. https://doi.org/10.1136/bmjopen-2013-004015.
10. Mathur R, Bhaskaran K, Edwards E, Lee H, Chaturvedi N, Smeeth L, et al. Population trends in the 10-year incidence and prevalence of diabetic retinopathy in the UK: a cohort study in the Clinical Practice Research Datalink 2004-2014. BMJ Open. 2017;7(2):e014444. https://doi.org/10.1136/bmjopen-2016-014444.
11. Wang W, Lo ACY. Diabetic retinopathy: pathophysiology and treatments. Int J Mol Sci. 2018;19
12. Ejaz S, Chekarova I, Ejaz A, Sohail A, Lim CW. Importance of pericytes and mechanisms of pericyte loss during diabetes retinopathy. Diabetes Obes Metab. 2008;10:53–63.
13. Schreur V, van Asten F, Ng H, Weeda J, Groenewoud JMM, Tack CJ, et al. Risk factors for development and progression of diabetic retinopathy in Dutch patients with type 1 diabetes mellitus. Acta Ophthalmol. 2018;96:459–64.
14. Jampol LM, Lahov M, Albert DM, Craft J. Ocular clinical findings and basement membrane changes in Goodpasture's syndrome. Am J Ophthalmol. 1975;79(3):452–63. https://doi.org/10.1016/0002-9394(75)90622-4.
15. Rowe PA, Mansfield DC, Dutton GN. Ophthalmic features of fourteen cases of Goodpasture's syndrome. Nephron. 1994;68(1):52–6. https://doi.org/10.1159/000188087.
16. Russell-Eggitt I, Bockenhauer D. The blind kidney: disorders affecting kidneys and eyes. Pediatr Nephrol. 2013;28(12):2255–65.
17. Dziarmaga A, Quinlan J, Goodyer P. Renal hypoplasia: lessons from Pax2. Pediatr Nephrol. 2006;21(1):26–31.
18. Harita Y, et al. Spectrum of LMX1B mutations: from nail-patella syndrome to isolated nephropathy. Pediatr Nephrol. 2017;32(10):1845–50.
19. Chen HY, et al. Retinal disease in ciliopathies: recent advances with a focus on stem cell-based therapies. Transl Sci Rare Dis. 2019;4(1–2):97–115.
20. Devlin LA, Sayer JA. Renal ciliopathies. Curr Opin Genet Dev. 2019;56:49–60.
21. Nussbaum RL, Suchy SF. The oculocerebral syndrome of Lowe (Lowe syndrome). In: Scriver C, et al., editors. The metabolic and molecular basis of inherited disease. New York: McGraw-Hill; 2001. p. 6257–66.
22. Bockenhauer D, et al. Renal phenotype in Lowe Syndrome: a selective proximal tubular dysfunction. Clin J Am Soc Nephrol. 2008;3(5):1430–6.
23. Savige J, et al. Ocular features in Alport syndrome: pathogenesis and clinical significance. Clin J Am Soc Nephrol. 2015;10(4):703–9.
24. Bredrup C, et al. Ophthalmological aspects of Pierson syndrome. Am J Ophthalmol. 2008;146(4):602–11.
25. Nesterova G, Gahl WA. Cystinosis: the evolution of a treatable disease. Pediatr Nephrol. 2012;
26. Chan B, Adam DN. A review of Fabry disease. Skin Therapy Lett. 2018;23(2):4–6.
27. Hoppe B. An update on primary hyperoxaluria. Nature reviews. Nephrology, 2012.
28. Small KW, Letson R, Scheinman J. Ocular findings in primary hyperoxaluria. Arch Ophthalmol. 1990;108(1):89–93.
29. Knapp AJ, Gartner S, Henkind P. Multiple myeloma and its ocular manifestations. Surv Ophthalmol. 1987;31(5):343–51. https://doi.org/10.1016/0039-6257(87)90119-6.

Gastroenterology and the Kidney

Sarah Blakey and Richard W. Corbett

Contents

M. Harber (ed.), *Primer on Nephrology*, https://doi.org/10.1007/978-3-030-76419-7_43

Learning Objectives

This chapter will cover:

1. Systemic diseases where the GI tract and kidneys may be affected
2. Renal conditions which arise directly from primarily GI diseases and their treatment
3. Safe prescription of laxatives including bowel preparation for patients with renal disease

43.1 Introduction

While as compared to, for instance, pulmonary-renal syndromes, disease processes affecting both the gastrointestinal (GI) system and the kidneys are less commonly recognised and may not be so clearly linked by a common pathophysiological mechanism. However, despite this, there are a number of diseases where GI pathology predominates, yet an association with renal disease is recognised; alternatively, there are a number of renal conditions where pathology arises secondary to the GI pathology or its treatment. This chapter also covers the safe use of laxatives in renal disease and lists some of the common side effects of medications used in the treatment of renal disease.

43.2 Systemic Diseases Involving the Kidney and GI System

A number of systemic conditions will affect both the gastrointestinal system and the kidneys as well as potentially other organs. While the list in Table 43.1 is by no means comprehensive, it includes commonly recognised areas where pathology may result in multi-organ involvement (Fig. 43.1). A few conditions warrant further discussion.

43.2.1 Diabetes Mellitus

Diabetes is widely recognised as a major cause of renal impairment; however, gastrointestinal symptoms arising from both type 1 and type 2 diabetes is equally prevalent and higher than in the general population [1]. Broadly, symptoms arise from disruption of the brain-gut axis both peripherally (predominantly autonomic) and centrally (perception and generation of symptoms). The disordered gut motility that arises from diabetes leads to both gastroparesis in the upper GI tract and diarrhoea or conversely constipation in the lower GI tract. Symptoms may be further compounded by medications used to treat the underlying condition, including metformin, lipase inhibitors and GLP-1 receptor agonists (e.g. exenatide, liraglutide).

Table 43.1 Systemic diseases involving the kidney and GI system

Systemic disease	Renal manifestations	GI manifestations
Diabetes mellitus	Diabetic nephropathy: proteinuria, renal impairment	Autonomic neuropathy with gastroparesis, constipation
Coeliac disease	IgA nephropathy; haematuria, proteinuria, renal impairment	Malabsorption, small bowel lymphoma
Atherosclerosis	Renal artery stenosis, ischaemic nephropathy; renal impairment	Abdominal pain, diarrhoea, gastrointestinal bleeding
Systemic lupus erythematosus	Lupus nephritis; haematuria, proteinuria, renal impairment	Pancreatitis, mouth ulcers, abdominal pain
Amyloidosis	Nephrotic syndrome; proteinuria, renal impairment	Diarrhoea, malabsorption, gastrointestinal bleeding and obstruction
Autosomal dominant polycystic kidney disease	Loin pain, macroscopic haematuria, renal impairment	Polycystic liver disease, diverticular disease, herniae
IgA vasculitis (Henoch-Schönlein purpura)	IgA-like nephropathy: haematuria, proteinuria, renal impairment	Abdominal pain, intestinal bleeding, nausea and diarrhoea
Small-vessel vasculitis (ANCA-associated vasculitis)	Pauci-immune glomerulonephritis, renal impairment, microscopic haematuria, proteinuria	Abdominal pain, gastrointestinal bleeding, diarrhoea
Medium-vessel vasculitis (polyarteritis nodosa)	Necrotising arteritis, renal impairment, microscopic haematuria	Intestinal necrosis and perforation, abdominal pain
Scleroderma	Scleroderma renal crisis, proteinuria, microscopic haematuria, renal impairment	Oesophageal and small bowel dysmotility
Fabry's disease	Renal impairment, microscopic haematuria, proteinuria	Abdominal pain, nausea and diarrhoea

43

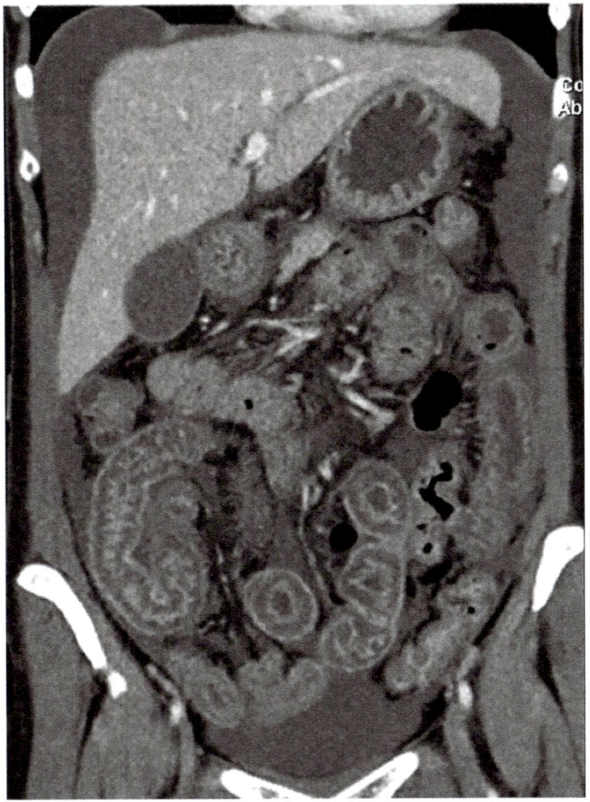

Fig. 43.1 Abdominal CT demonstrating severely oedematous loops of the small bowel. This 50-year-old woman presented with acute gastrointestinal symptoms including diffuse pain and was found to have low complement levels and raised ANA and dsDNA. She had significant proteinuria. After extensive investigation for other causes, including infection, she was diagnosed as having systemic lupus erythematosus and her symptoms and proteinuria rapidly resolved with steroids

43.2.2 Coeliac Disease

Coeliac disease should be considered within the differential for the patient with type 1 diabetes and diarrhoea given the autoimmune association. Equally, IgA nephropathy is frequently seen in patients with coeliac disease, and a greater number still will have glomerular IgA deposition on renal biopsy without manifest renal insufficiency.

43.2.3 Vasculitis

Multisystem involvement is common in vasculitis; however, it is small-vessel (ANCA-associated), medium-vessel and IgA vasculitis (Henoch-Schönlein purpura), which are predominantly responsible for combined GI and renal manifestations. Polyarteritis nodosa (PAN) is associated initially with symptoms of mesenteric angina, resulting from necrotising inflammation, which, in more severe disease, may lead to ischaemic gut and ultimately perforation with a predilection for the small bowel. In ANCA-associated small-vessel vasculitis, there may be bowel involvement, though it is rarely as dramatic as that associated with PAN and can involve both the large and small bowel.

Of all the vasculitides, it is IgA vasculitis that most commonly has GI involvement. Overt purpura is seen in almost all patients, with many having gastrointestinal symptoms alongside renal and joint involvement. In children the condition is often self-limiting, though bowel intussusception may occur; in contrast, in older patients, intussusception is uncommon, but the renal sequelae may be more severe with a more aggressive loss in renal function, including progression to established renal failure [2].

43.3 Renal Pathology Arising from GI Disease

A range of primary GI diseases either directly or as a complication of treatment can result in renal pathology; these are listed in Table 43.2.

43.3.1 Secondary Hyperoxaluria

Oxalate is a ubiquitous small molecule, which appears to have no clear useful role in humans yet is highly

Table 43.2 Renal complications of gastrointestinal disease

Gastrointestinal disease	Renal complication	Mechanism
Inflammatory bowel disease	Proteinuria, renal impairment	AA amyloidosis
	Oxalate nephropathy, nephrolithiasis	Secondary hyperoxaluria
	Nephrolithiasis	Secondary hyperoxaluria, reduced urinary volume
	Tubulointerstitial nephritis	Drug induced (5-ASA compounds, mesalazine)
	Progressive renal impairment, prerenal acute kidney injury	High-output stoma
	IgA nephropathy	Unclear
Small bowel resection	Oxalate nephropathy, nephrolithiasis	Secondary hyperoxaluria
Upper GI	Tubulointerstitial nephritis	Drug induced (proton pump inhibitor)

corrosive with strong chelating properties. It is ingested in abundance in a broad range of foods that include coffee, tea, spinach and rhubarb, while a small quantity is produced endogenously. In healthy individuals, free oxalate appears to bind to calcium in the small bowel before passing through the large bowel to be egested as calcium oxalate [3]. A small quantity is broken down by *Oxalobacter formigenes*, an enteric anaerobe, which may have some controlling oxalate homeostasis in individuals consuming a high burden of oxalate [4]. Any unbound oxalate is absorbed in the large bowel before being excreted in the urine along with any endogenously produced oxalate.

While hyperoxaluria may occur due to inborn errors of metabolism (primary hyperoxaluria), hyperoxaluria may also arise due to increased enteric absorption or excess oxalate intake (secondary hyperoxaluria). Gastrointestinal diseases, which predispose to steatorrhoea and malabsorption, are implicated. In this setting excess free fatty acids competitively bind calcium (saponification) in the small bowel lumen, inhibiting the formation of calcium oxalate. The excess free oxalate is then absorbed in the colon, a process enhanced further by the presence of free fatty acids and bile salts.

Conditions in which malabsorption occurs, including inflammatory bowel disease, small bowel resections for malignancy and Roux-en-Y gastric bypass surgery for obesity [5], have all been associated with hyperoxaluria. However, for this to occur, an intact colon is required; patients with malabsorption and a stoma proximal to the colon will not develop enteric hyperoxaluria [6].

Hyperoxaluria results both in oxalate nephropathy and nephrolithiasis. The former leads to a progressive renal impairment as the consequence of tubular crystalline deposits of calcium oxalate and tubular fibrosis. Crystallisation of calcium oxalate in the collecting ducts and urothelial system manifests as oxalate stones (nephrolithiasis). Furthermore, in patients with a high-output stoma or other causes of diarrhoea, which predispose to volume depletion, the resultant glomerular filtrate may be supersaturated with oxalate hastening the process.

Management once identified can be difficult, and oxalate nephropathy may be irreversible. Key steps in limiting progression of disease are as follows: limiting the dietary intake of oxalate, use of calcium supplementation with meals to increase calcium binding and maintaining a dilute urine through adequate volume intake. While supplementation with *O. formigenes* has been considered a potential route for treatment, it has enjoyed limited success.

43.3.2 High-Output Stoma

The normal gastrointestinal tract may produce in excess of 4 L of intestinal secretions, including saliva, pancreaticobiliary secretions and gastric acid. In patients who undergo the formation of a small bowel stoma, 15% may develop a high-output stoma defined by a stoma output in excess of 2 L/day [7]. The most common reason for which is a short remaining length of the small intestine (<200 cm), though infection, prokinetic drugs, opiate withdrawal and recurrent inflammatory bowel disease may all be implicated.

These patients are particularly susceptible to episodes of recurrent hypovolaemic prerenal acute kidney injury due to the loss of both water and sodium. With a high-output stoma, the ability to concentrate sodium is lost within the jejunum, and sodium will leak precipitously into jejunal fluid, which has a sodium concentration of around 100 mmol/L [8]. Hypomagnesaemia also ensues due to both secondary hyperaldosteronism and impaired gastrointestinal absorption of magnesium, though hypokalaemia only occurs in those patients with very short jejunal remnants.

While, given the high sodium and water losses, thirst may be a major symptom for patients with a high-output stoma, consumption of hypotonic fluids will compound sodium losses, exacerbating the cycles of volume depletion. Seemingly paradoxically, the key to resolving the fluid losses is to reduce the consumption of hypotonic fluids (<500 ml/day) [9] . Equally, hypertonic fluids will result in greater stoma output. Since jejunal sodium absorption is coupled with glucose absorption, individuals benefit from the intake of >1 L/day of a glucose-saline solution, where the sodium concentration is comparable to the jejunal concentration of sodium (90–120 mmol/L), which for some may be at the limits of palatability.

43.3.3 AA Amyloidosis

AA amyloid is an uncommon (<1% incidence) but significant complication of inflammatory bowel disease, which predominantly manifests as proteinuric/nephrotic renal disease [10]. Crohn's disease appears to be more commonly associated than ulcerative colitis, possibly due to the inflammatory nature of Crohn's. Control of inflammation may result in resolution of the nephrotic state in some patients; however, a number of patients will progress to established renal failure.

43.3.4 IgA Nephropathy

IgA nephropathy, while the most common glomerulonephritis, nonetheless appears to have an increased association with inflammatory bowel disease. IgA nephropathy is the most common finding in this group of patients with inflammatory bowel disease who undergo a renal biopsy [11]. This observation is strengthened by the identification of genes in patients with IgA nephropathy, which are implicated in the development of inflammatory bowel disease or in the maintenance of the gut mucosa and its response to pathogens.

43.3.5 Drug-Induced Injury

43.3.5.1 5-ASA Compounds

There is a strong association between nephrotoxicity and the use of 5-aminosalicylic acid (5-ASA) medications (including sulphasalazine and mesalazine) to treat inflammatory bowel disease [12]. While toxicity can occur at any time, it occurs most frequently within the first 12 months after initiation and does not appear to be dose related. The incidence is less than 0.5% of all the patients taking 5-ASA compounds, but the lack of temporal association with commencement of the drug underlines the need for regular monitoring of renal function. When biopsied, the predominant renal lesion is an interstitial nephritis, though, in many patients, withdrawal of 5-ASA medication results in resolution of the renal injury.

While both sulphasalazine and the more recent 5-ASA compounds are dependent on different pharmacological attributes to ensure maximal drug delivery to the large bowel, neither appears to be associated with a greater risk.

43.3.5.2 Proton Pump Inhibitors

Given that proton pump inhibitors are amongst the most commonly prescribed class of drugs, it is unsurprising that, aside from antibiotics, they are most widely implicated in the development of an interstitial nephritis. Given their ubiquity, assessing the incidence of nephrotoxicity is difficult. However, in epidemiological cohort studies, its use as compared to H2-receptor antagonists is, over 5 years, associated with higher rates of decline in renal function and development of end-stage renal failure [13].

43.3.5.3 Calcineurin Inhibitors

Ciclosporin and, to a lesser extent, tacrolimus both have a role in the management of inflammatory bowel disease. Their effect is manifested through both acute and chronic effects on the renal vasculature. While low-dose ciclosporin use (oral dose of $\leq$5 mg/kg/day) has not been associated with significant nephrotoxicity, higher doses and intravenous administration have been. Equally, extended durations of therapy (longer than 6 months) and high trough levels (greater than 100–200 ng/ml) are both adversely associated with nephrotoxicity when used for the treatment of inflammatory bowel disease [14].

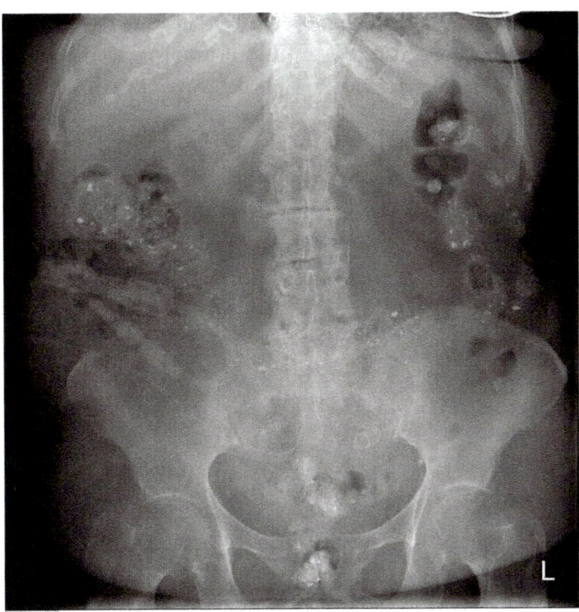

Fig. 43.2 Abdominal plain film with hyper-dense deposits of lanthanum carbonate throughout the large bowel. This plain film was done to check the position of the peritoneal dialysis catheter, which does not lie in the pelvis as expected for optimal catheter function. Within the large bowel, there is evidence of constipation and hyper-dense opacities. Lanthanum is a rare-earth metal with a density similar to barium and is used in the form of lanthanum carbonate as a dietary phosphate binder. Gastrointestinal side effects of most phosphate binders include constipation and abdominal pain, lanthanum is no exception

43.4 Use of Laxatives in Chronic Kidney Disease

Constipation is a common symptom in patients with chronic kidney disease and of particular concern in those patients receiving peritoneal dialysis, where constipation can result in mechanical and infectious complications. The aetiology is multifactorial, with low fibre intake, fluid restriction, reduced mobility and some disease-specific medications all playing a role (Fig. 43.2). While lifestyle modifications, where possible, should be the first-line intervention (increase in fluid intake and physical activity), laxatives are often required. Table 43.3 outlines the safe use of laxatives in chronic kidney disease.

43.4.1 Bowel Preparation for Colonoscopy

The most concerning complication of laxative use is the development of acute phosphate nephropathy. This can occur with the use of oral sodium phosphate solutions as bowel preparation for colonoscopy, with a greater risk in the elderly and those with chronic kidney disease [15]. In those who develop a profound acute kidney injury, this is typically identified a month following colonoscopy, though it may present within a few days of colonoscopy. Renal biopsy findings are of widespread tubular calcium phosphate deposits. While many will recover, a number are left dialysis dependent.

Given this, in patients with underlying renal disease, guidelines advocate the use of solely polyethylene glycol-based bowel preparation. While this can be of a significant volume, use of smaller volumes (2 L rather than 4 L) is associated with poorer bowel preparation and a greater incidence of incomplete colonoscopic studies [16].

Table 43.3 Safe use of laxatives in CKD

Laxative class	Medication	Safety	Notes
Bulk-producing agents	Fibre, ispaghula husk	With caution	Requires a significant volume of fluid to avoid intestinal obstruction. May affect absorption of other medications
Stool softeners	Docusate sodium	Safe	Requires adequate fluid intake
Stimulants	Senna, bisacodyl, sodium picosulphate	Safe	Tolerance may result
Osmotic laxatives	Lactulose, polyethylene glucose	Safe	
	Milk of magnesia, magnesium sulphate	Do not use	Risk of hypermagnesaemia
	Sodium phosphate (oral)	Do not use	Risk of hyperphosphataemia and phosphate nephropathy
Enemas	Glycerin, bisacodyl	Safe	
	Sodium phosphate (enema)	With caution	Risk of significant phosphate absorption with repeated use

Case Study

Proton Pump Inhibitor-Induced Tubulointerstitial Nephritis

A 58-year-old Nepalese woman was commenced on omeprazole by her GP after complaining of vomiting. The vomiting resolved; however, she subsequently lost around 25 kilograms in weight over a 4-month period. There were no other systemic symptoms. A blood test was performed as part of investigations into her weight loss. This demonstrated a severe acute kidney injury, with serum creatinine of 1121 umol/L (from a baseline of 41 umol/L on blood tests taken 6 months earlier) (Fig. 43.3). Urine dipstick was newly positive for blood and 1+ protein (uPCR 46 mg/mmol). Imaging showed 12.5 cm unobstructed kidneys. Standard serological tests were unremarkable.

43

A renal biopsy demonstrated moderate active tubulointerstitial nephritis (TIN) without granuloma. The temporal association would suggest this occurred as a result of omeprazole, which is less likely to be associated with the classic triad of fever, rash and eosinophilia than other causes of TIN. Alongside antibiotics and non-steroidal anti-inflammatories, proton pump inhibitors are the most common cause of a drug-induced interstitial nephritis.

She was switched to ranitidine for gastric protection, and given the severity of her TIN, high-dose oral steroids were commenced. Within 3 months, her serum creatinine had dropped to 105 umol/L. Her weight loss subsequently resolved.

Oxalate Nephropathy

During post-surgical follow-up, a 77-year-old man was identified to have a progressive renal impairment with a rise in serum creatinine from 90 umol/L to a peak of 400 umol/L. A year earlier, he had undergone a Whipple's procedure (pancreatoduodenectomy) for a presumptive carcinoma of the pancreas, which proved ultimately to be histologically benign. He had experienced a number of diarrhoeal illnesses in the post-operative period.

On assessment, his urine sediment was bland and kidneys were 10 cm and 11 cm in size. Renal biopsy was undertaken and revealed widespread acute and chronic tubular injury, with oxalate crystals within several tubules (Fig. 43.4), consistent with oxalate nephropathy. His renal function deteriorated rapidly, and he was established on dialysis before dying 18 months later.

Fat malabsorption in patients with pancreatic insufficiency leads to increased binding of calcium by free fatty acids and leads to higher levels of unbound oxalate available for absorption within the colon. This has also been seen to occur with the use of orlistat, a gastrointestinal

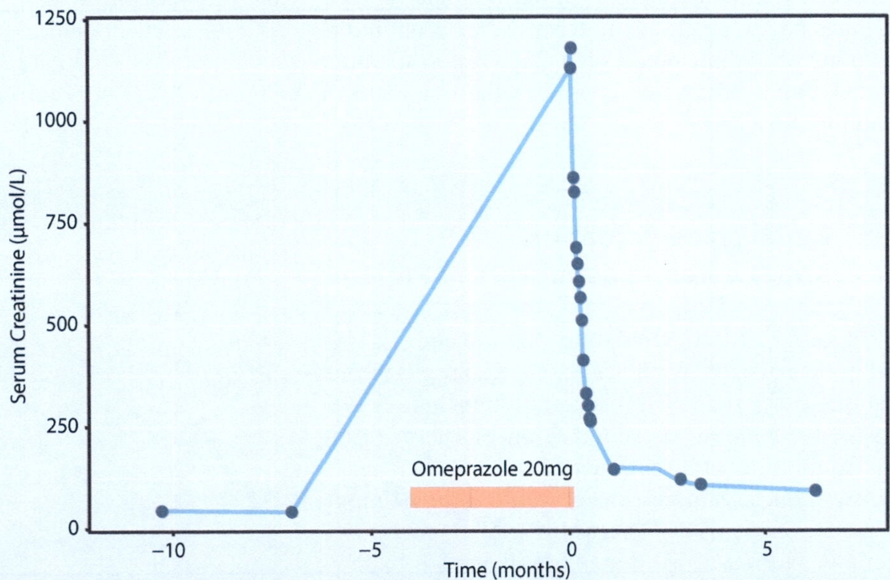

Fig. 43.3 Renal function in a patient with a tubulointerstitial nephritis related to omeprazole exposure and treated with steroids

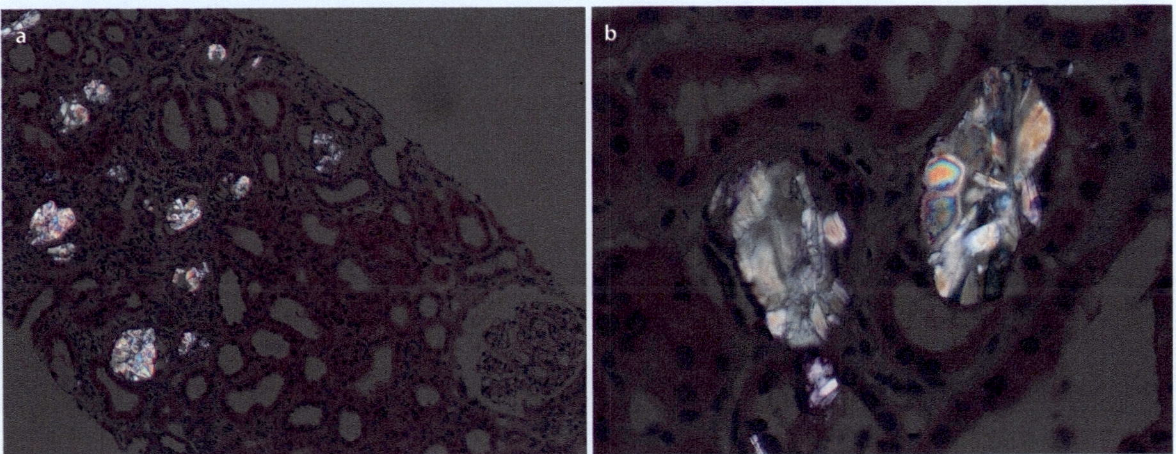

Fig. 43.4 Birefringent crystals of calcium oxalate in tubules on renal biopsy on low-power **a** and high-power **b** view (Images courtesy of Dr. Candice Roufosse)

lipase inhibitor, which prevents the absorption of dietary fats. Renal tubular crystallisation of calcium oxalate may be compounded by associated fluid losses and dehydration secondary to diarrhoea.

Unfortunately, oxalate nephropathy often rapidly progresses in the advanced stages due to the rapid deposition of calcium oxalate crystals within the kidney at a low GFR. Key steps to avoiding progression are adoption of a low-oxalate diet, the use of calcium-based supplements with meals to bind free oxalate and avoiding dehydration.

Short Bowel Syndrome

A 63-year-old woman had developed abnormal renal function and multiple episodes of AKI, following emergency end ileostomy formation for small bowel obstruction. She had a 44-year history of Crohn's disease, managed with steroids and azathioprine. She had undergone associated interventions and complications, including previous total colectomy, small bowel strictures requiring dilatation and enterocutaneous fistulae.

Her kidneys were normal in size and urinary sediment was bland. Stoma output was intermittently very high and unmanageable with St Mark's solution and loperamide. Clinically, she was persistently hypovolaemic and occasionally tetanic, owing to profound hypomagnesaemia and resulting hypocalcaemia. Ad hoc management with intravenous fluid did not achieve adequate correction of volume and electrolytes, with progressive rise in serum creatinine despite loss of muscle mass, causing concern for

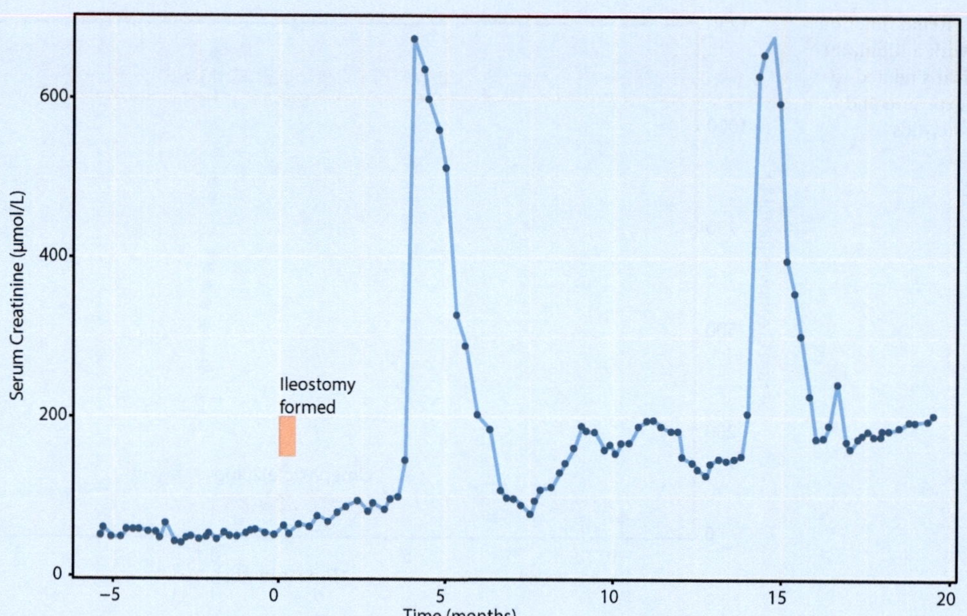

Fig. 43.5 Progressive renal impairment in a patient with a high-output ileostomy, following emergency surgery for Crohn's disease. Chronic hypovolaemia compounded by two severe episodes of acute kidney injury resulted in a rapid, progressive and potentially irreversible decline in underlying renal function

progressive and irreversible tubular fibrosis (Fig. 43.5). Ultimately, a multidisciplinary approach was taken, and the patient was trained to administer parenteral fluids along with oral electrolyte replacement at home. Her nutritional needs were met without the use of total parenteral nutrition.

Given the absence of a colon to reabsorb oxalate, hyperoxaluria was not implicated in this patient but may frequently occur in those with a short gut. Managing patients with progressive renal impairment and high-output stomas requires good communication between the patient's nephrologist and a gastroenterologist – ideally, the latter should have an interest in intestinal failure. While home parenteral fluids via a tunnelled central venous catheter may be a drastic step, in some patients it may be required to avoid long-term dialysis.

43

An approach to the patient with a high-output ileostomy or jejunostomy is suggested in Fig. 43.6. It is a common error for patients to be encouraged to increase their oral intake of either hypotonic solutions (such as water), which causes large stomal sodium losses, or hypertonic fluids (containing artificial sweeteners or glucose), which can also cause stomal losses of water and sodium. Initial treatment begins, paradoxically, with patients restricting their oral intake of fluid. In those with output <1200 ml/day, then, oral sodium replacement may be adequate; in those who have higher outputs, then, patients are advised to sip a 1 L glucose-saline solution with a sodium concentration of at least 90 mmol/l (such as a St Mark's solution) across the day (Fig. 43.7).

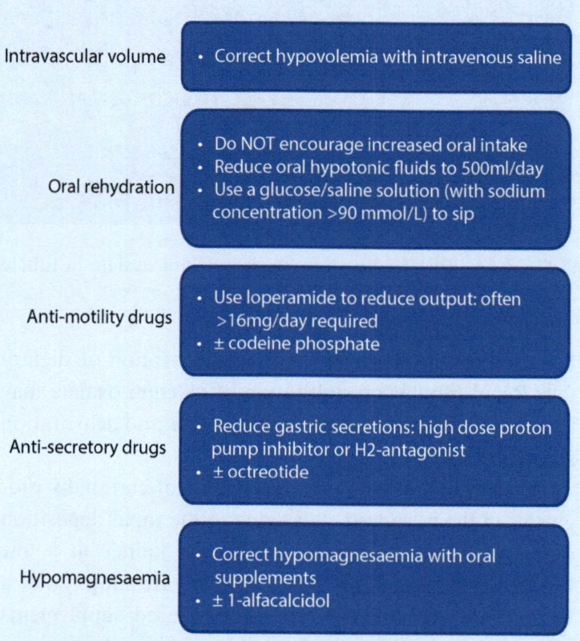

Fig. 43.6 A sequential approach to managing the patient with a high-output ileostomy, particularly in the setting of acute kidney injury. (Derived from [17])

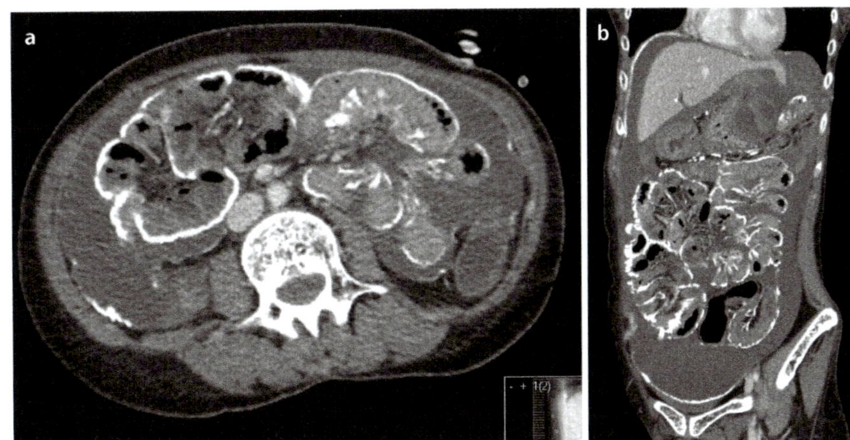

Fig. 43.7 Abdominal CT of a patient with encapsulating peritoneal sclerosis (EPS). Mural and peritoneal calcification, tethering of intestinal loops and ascites, all indicative of EPS, are present. While associated with the use of peritoneal dialysis, the condition may also rarely arise in the context of tuberculosis and other inflammatory conditions. Patients frequently experience recurrent bouts of subacute bowel obstruction and pain. (**a**) axial section (**b**) saggital section

Chapter Review Questions

1. What are the risks for patients who have undergone small bowel resection of consuming high levels of chocolate, spinach or miso in their diets?
2. An elderly woman presents with an acute kidney injury, a skin rash and bloody diarrhoea. What is the most likely diagnosis?
3. What advice would you give to a patient with a high-output stoma and an acute kidney injury in respect of oral intake?
4. What laxatives should not be used in bowel preparation for colonoscopy for patients with advanced renal impairment?
5. Name two classes of medications that are used for the treatment of gastrointestinal disease but which may be implicated in the development of tubulointerstitial nephritis?

Answers

1. These foods are all recognised to have a high level of oxalate. Consumption at high levels in the diet of patients with a short bowel risks the development of renal oxalate stones and oxalate nephropathy.
2. IgA vasculitis (Henoch-Schönlein Purpura).
3. Reduce oral intake and ideally sip a glucose-saline solution with >90 mmol/L saline concentration. Advising patients with a high-output ileostomy to increase their oral intake may exacerbate fluid losses from the stoma.
4. Oral sodium phosphate solutions and the use of laxatives with high phosphate content, risk the development of acute phosphate nephropathy.
5. Proton pump inhibitors (e.g. omeprazole) and 5-aminosalicylic acid compounds (e.g. mesalazine).

References

1. Jones KL, Du YT, Talley NJ, Horowitz M, Rayner CK. Gastrointestinal symptoms in diabetes: prevalence, assessment, pathogenesis, and management. Diabetes Care. 2018;41(3):627–37.
2. Pillebout E, Thervet E, Hill G, Alberti C, Vanhille P, Nochy D. Henoch-Schönlein Purpura in adults: outcome and prognostic factors. J Am Soc Nephrol. 2002;13(5):1271–8.
3. Harper J, Mansell MA. Treatment of enteric hyperoxaluria. Postgrad Med J. 1991;67(785):219–22.
4. Stewart CS, Duncan SH, Cave DR. Oxalobacter formigenes and its role in oxalate metabolism in the human gut. FEMS Microbiol Lett. 2004;230(1):1–7.
5. Kumar R, Lieske JC, Collazo-Clavell ML, Sarr MG, Olson ER, Vrtiska TJ, et al. Fat malabsorption and increased intestinal oxalate absorption are common after Roux-en-Y gastric bypass surgery. Surgery [Internet]. 2011;149(5):654–61. https://doi.org/10.1016/j.surg.2010.11.015.
6. Dobbins JW, Binder HJ. Importance of the colon in enteric hyperoxaluria. N Engl J Med. 1977;296(6):298–301.
7. Baker ML, Williams RN, Nightingale JMD. Causes and management of a high-output stoma. Color Dis. 2011;13(2):191–7.
8. Nightingale JMD, Lennard-Jones JE, Walker ER, Farthing M. Jejunal efflux in short bowel syndrome. Lancet [Internet]. 1990;336(8718):765–8. Available from: https://www.sciencedirect.com/science/article/pii/014067369093238K.
9. Tsao SKK, Baker M, Nightingale JMD. High-output stoma after small-bowel resections for Crohn's disease. Nat Clin Pract Gastroenterol Hepatol. 2005;2(12):604–8.
10. Hawkins PN, Lachmann HJ, Rowczenio D, Gibbs SDJ, Sattianayagam PT, Pinney JH, et al. Inflammatory bowel disease and systemic AA amyloidosis. Dig Dis Sci. 2013;58(6):1689–97.
11. Ambruzs JM, Walker PD, Larsen CP. The histopathologic spectrum of kidney biopsies in patients with inflammatory bowel disease. Clin J Am Soc Nephrol [Internet]. 2014;9(2):265–70. Available from: http://cjasn.asnjournals.org/cgi/doi/10.2215/CJN.04660513.
12. Gisbert JP, González-Lama Y, Maté J. 5-Aminosalicylates and renal function in inflammatory bowel disease. Inflamm Bowel Dis [Internet]. 2007;13(5):629–38. Available from: https://academic.oup.com/ibdjournal/article/13/5/629-638/4644696.
13. Xie Y, Bowe B, Li T, Xian H, Balasubramanian S, Al-Aly Z. Proton pump inhibitors and risk of incident CKD and progression

to ESRD. J Am Soc Nephrol [Internet]. 2016;27(10):3153–63. Available from: http://www.jasn.org/cgi/doi/10.1681/ASN.2015121377.

14. Oikonomou KA, Kapsoritakis AN, Stefanidis I, Potamianos SP. Drug-induced nephrotoxicity in inflammatory bowel disease. Nephron - Clin Pract. 2011;119(2):89–96.
15. Markowitz GS, Stokes MB, Radhakrishnan J, D'Agati VD. Acute phosphate nephropathy following oral sodium phosphate bowel purgative: an underrecognized cause of chronic renal failure. J Am Soc Nephrol. 2005;16(11):3389–96.
16. Hassan C, Bretthauer M, Kaminski MF, Polkowski M, Rembacken B, Saunders B, et al. Bowel preparation for colonoscopy: European Society of Gastrointestinal Endoscopy (ESGE) guideline. Endoscopy. 2013;45(02):142–55.
17. Nightingale J, Woodward JM. Guidelines for management of patients with a short bowel. Gut. 2006;55(SUPPL. 4):1–12.

Respiratory Medicine and the Kidney

Marilina Antonelou, James Brown, and Sally Hamour

Contents

M. Harber (ed.), *Primer on Nephrology*, https://doi.org/10.1007/978-3-030-76419-7_44

Learning Objectives

1. To highlight respiratory complications in patients with renal insufficiency related to chronic kidney disease itself or its treatment
2. To provide an overview of important associations between renal and respiratory diseases
3. To emphasise the need for close collaboration of the two subspecialties for the diagnosis and prevention of disease

44.1 Introduction

From the early stages of embryonic development, foetal urine plays an important role in lung growth through hydrodynamic pressure on airway expansion. During late gestation the kidney is a major source of proline. Urinary proline aids collagen formation in the lung, and insufficient levels of proline secondary to oligohydramnios seen in renal agenesis, urinary tract obstruction, bilateral renal aplasia and cystic kidney disease might explain the associated pulmonary hypoplasia [1].

In later life, lung and kidney functions are closely related in both health and disease. Respiratory changes help to mitigate the systemic effects of renal acid-base disturbances, and the reverse is also true. Chronic renal failure may affect respiratory function and the intrathoracic structures. The lungs and kidneys have similarities in their basement membranes, explaining why both are important target organs in various autoimmune disorders. Additionally, both the lungs and the kidneys rely on the function of cilia, which may explain why certain genetic syndromes affect both organs.

This chapter first reviews the respiratory complications of patients with renal insufficiency. How chronic kidney disease and its treatment may affect respiratory function and the intrathoracic structures is described. It then provides a brief overview of the large group of diseases that affect both the lungs and the kidneys.

44.2 Respiratory Complications of Chronic Renal Failure

44.2.1 Pulmonary Oedema

44

Pulmonary oedema is the most common respiratory complication in patients with renal failure. The aetiology is multifactorial and may result from hypervolaemia, low serum albumin and increased capillary permeability [2]. The characteristic radiographic 'butterfly' or 'batwing' appearance of the oedematous exudates, found in 10% of patients with pulmonary oedema, represents central non-gravitational distribution of alveolar oedema and is explained largely by diversion of blood flow to more central areas of the lung, which are supplied by the shortest arterial pathway (Fig. 44.1). Pulmonary congestion in patients with chronic renal failure is associated with a restrictive pattern on pulmonary function testing, and reduced lung volumes can also be observed on spirometry. These abnormalities have been demonstrated to improve or resolve with haemodialysis [1].

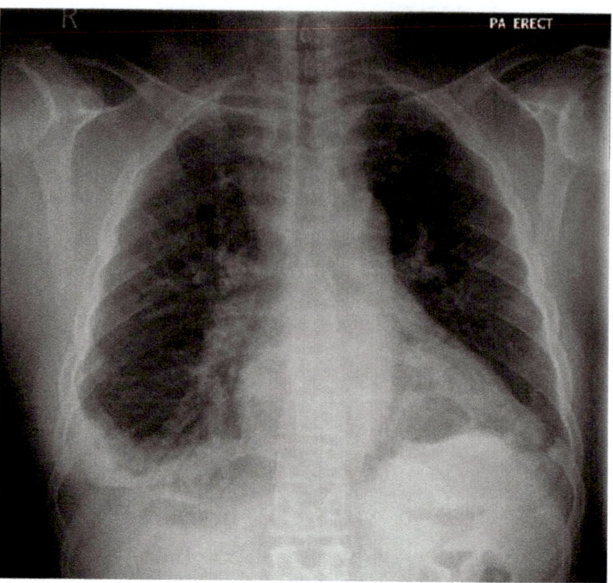

Fig. 44.1 Postero-anterior chest radiograph showing pulmonary oedema in a haemodialysis patient with high intradialytic weight gains. The heart is enlarged, and there are bilateral pleural effusions. There is vascular prominence of both hila with upper zone and venous distribution

44.2.2 Pleural Effusion

Symptomatic pleural effusion is also common in patients with chronic kidney disease (CKD) with a reported prevalence of 6.7% in an Indian cohort of 430 patients. Heart failure, TB and uraemic effusions accounted for 41.9%, 25.5% and 19.4%, respectively [3]. Uraemic patients have increased susceptibility to exudative pleural effusions, as a result of inflammation ('uraemic pleuritis'). Effusions may be large and bilateral and can be haemorrhagic and may often resolve spontaneously within weeks of their appearance. Differentiating TB from uraemic effusion requires a combined clinical and pathological approach, and this differentiation is necessary for proper management, especially if transplantation is being considered. In addition, in patients with CKD on high doses of diuretics, the distinction between transudative and exudative effusion based on the Light's criteria is not always reliable [4].

In transudative effusions, repeated aspiration is not advisable with pleural infection, pneumothorax, patient discomfort and time and expense of repeated procedures being important considerations. Pleurodesis could be recommended for some patients after aspiration if the effusion recurs, medical interventions (fluid restriction, diuretics) have failed and the patient remains symptomatic.

Hydrothorax is an uncommon but well-recognised complication of peritoneal dialysis. It usually presents as an acute right-sided pleural effusion biochemically similar to the dialysate. Structural defects in the tendinous diaphragm are often found in the cases of hydrothorax, and contrast or isotopic peritoneography may be helpful in localising the pleuroperitoneal fistula. Pleural fluid analysis typically detects a high glucose concentration, and contrast imaging reveals tracer uptake transgressing the diaphragm. Treatment requires temporary cessation (6 weeks) of peritoneal dialysis, and transition to haemodialysis until peritoneal dialysis can be retried.

44.2.3 Tuberculosis

Immunodeficiency is associated with CKD and appears to have a multifactorial aetiology (oxidative stress, uraemic inflammation, functional abnormalities in immune cells). Defects in cell-mediated immunity worsen with progression of CKD, leaving dialysis patients susceptible to infectious complications [5].

Active TB is one of these complications and can result from progression of *Mycobacterium tuberculosis* infection after recent exposure or reactivation of latent TB infection. Seven- to fiftyfold increased risk of tuberculosis has been observed in patients with chronic renal failure and on dialysis [6]. This increased risk appears to be related, in part, to demographic characteristics, with country of birth being a particularly important risk factor in dialysis populations. Transplant recipients are also at high risk of active TB, related in part to post-transplantation immunosuppressive medications that specifically target T cell-mediated immunity, which is critical to maintaining latency in patients with *M. tuberculosis* infection.

The clinical presentation of TB in dialysis and kidney transplant patients is often insidious and atypical. Patients frequently present with systemic symptoms, such as fever, anorexia and weight loss, and extrapulmonary disease is observed in as many as 60% to 80% of cases [7].

TB screening in populations with end-stage renal disease (ESRD) can detect asymptomatic or minimally symptomatic active TB early in the disease course, thus limiting potential spread. It may also detect latent TB infection, enabling the initiation of preventive therapy for patients at the highest risk of the development of active disease. Screening for latent TB is via immune assays, including the traditional tuberculin skin test (TST) and the newer interferon gamma release assays (IGRAs). TST and IGRA tests are not useful for the diagnosis or exclusion of active TB [6].

Preventative treatment is effective in reducing the development of TB by 60% to 90% in immunocompetent individuals [8]. This is typically with 6 months of isoniazid or 3 months of isoniazid and rifampicin (if drug-drug interactions do not preclude the use of rifampicin) [9]. Due to the increased risk of drug-induced hepatitis, latent TB treatment is not normally recommended in those over the age of 65. The standard quadruple therapy regimen is recommended in patients with CKD or a kidney transplant with active TB, with ethambutol being avoided in patients with severe renal insufficiency or on dialysis due to the increased risk of ocular toxicity.

44.2.4 Respiratory Viruses

Patients with kidney disease, especially ESRF, are a high-risk population for contracting influenza with resulting increased mortality rates [3]. The benefits of vaccinating patients on dialysis against influenza have been well demonstrated, as evidenced by up to 25% decreased rates of mortality in haemodialysis patients and up to 34% decreased rates of mortality in peritoneal dialysis patients [10]. It has therefore become routine practice to administer the influenza vaccine to patients on dialysis. However, the impaired immunity in these patients can result in an impaired immune response to vaccinations, such that the sero-protection rate in the dialysis population with standard influenza vaccines is 47% compared to 81% in the general population [11].

Severe acute respiratory syndrome coronavirus-2 (SARS-CoV-2) is a novel coronavirus which gave rise to a global pandemic in December 2019, resulting in significant morbidity and mortality within vulnerable populations, including patients with advanced CKD and ESRF. Classic lung appearances are of atypical pneumonia, characterised by bilateral ground-glass opacities on computer tomography (◘ Fig. 44.2). Post-mortem reports of kidney tissue in patients with SARS-CoV-2 that presented with AKI have predominantly revealed acute tubular necrosis with viral inclusions found within tubular cells, lymphocytic infiltration and endotheliitis [12, 13].

Several other opportunistic organisms, including *Cytomegalovirus*, *Pneumocystis jirovecii* and *Aspergillus*, can cause respiratory complications in transplant recipients on immunosuppression, and they are discussed elsewhere in the book.

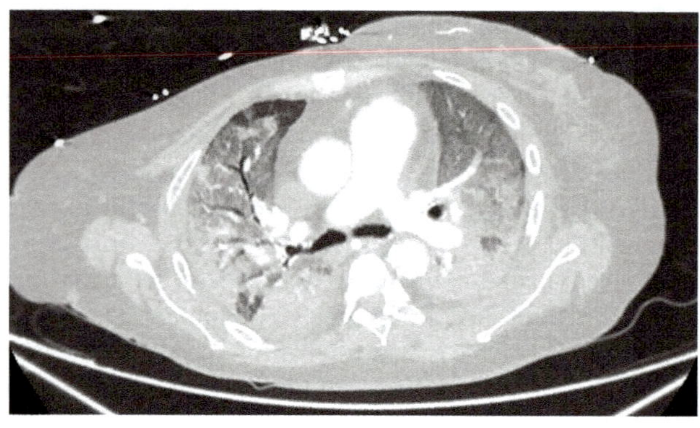

Fig. 44.2 CT chest of a haemodialysis patient who tested positive for SARS-CoV-2. Extensive consolidation throughout both the lungs, which is most dense within the lower lobes and dependent portions of the lungs bilaterally, but with further extensive ground-glass opacification involving the remainder of the lung fields

44.2.5 Pulmonary Embolism

Patients with CKD and especially those on dialysis have complex alterations in their haemostasis and may develop both thrombotic and bleeding complications. Until a decade ago, the prevailing view was that the bleeding propensity may protect dialysis patients from venous thromboembolic events. Since then, large community studies have reported a twofold increased risk for venous thromboembolism (VTE) in patients with CKD, dialysis patients and transplant recipients compared with those with normal renal function [14, 15].

The mechanisms linking CKD with VTE are unknown. VTE is a particularly common complication in patients with nephrotic syndrome. The aetiology is multifactorial and involves increased prothrombotic factors (fibrinogen) and presence of procoagulant factors in patients with SLE and antiphospholipid syndrome, decreased anticoagulant factors (urinary losses of antithrombin III, proteins C and S), haemoconcentration, endothelial cell dysfunction and enhanced platelet activation and aggregation. Larger studies, with data on proteinuria in the absence of nephrotic syndrome, are needed to evaluate the haemostatic mechanisms mediating the association between CKD and VTE.

44.2.6 Dialysis-Associated Hypoxaemia

44

Dialysis-induced hypoxaemia is characterised by decreased alveolar ventilation in response to diffusion of CO_2 into the dialysate. As CO_2 diffuses into the dialysate, the CO_2 content in venous blood falls, leading to a decrease in hypercapnic ventilatory drive and subsequent decrease in minute ventilation and alveolar PO_2 [16]. The magnitude of PO_2 drop varies with chemical composition of the dialysate, with a smaller drop when bicarbonate containing dialysate is used instead of acetate, so, nowadays, with the wider use of bicarbonate buffer, it is not a very common clinical phenomenon. Hypoxaemia affects the heart by direct and reflex effects on the circulation. Although myocardial contractility appears to remain unchanged from hypoxia in healthy individuals, when coronary artery disease is present, chronic hypoxia may precipitate left ventricular dysfunction.

44.2.7 Sleep-Disordered Breathing

The prevalence of severe sleep-disordered breathing has been reported in 20% of patients with advanced CKD and between 50 and 83% in patients on dialysis [17]. There is data to suggest that a lower estimated glomerular filtration rate (eGFR) is associated with more severe sleep apnoea in CKD patients, independent of age, gender and BMI. Sleep-disordered breathing typically results in daytime somnolence, as well as observed apnoea and irregular breathing while asleep. It is important to identify as treatment can result in significant improvements in quality of life and, if untreated, may contribute to cardiovascular morbidity.

The aetiology of sleep-disordered breathing in ESRF is multifactorial relating to risk factors, such as increased body mass index (BMI), fluid overload and a greater disturbance of central breathing control. In particular, ESRF may cause central destabilisation of ventilatory control and upper airway occlusion. Other causes that have been suggested include anaemia, upper airway uraemic myopathy, neuropathy, uraemic toxins and inflammatory cytokines, increased extracellular fluid volume leading to narrowed upper airway, leptin resistance and changes in chemoreceptor sensitivity [18].

There is a strong link between sleep apnoea and nocturnal hypoxaemia and cardiovascular complications such as left ventricular hypertrophy in patients with CKD and ESRF. Uraemia and fluid overload are strong predictors of increased obstructive apnoea-hypopnea index. Nocturnal haemodialysis might reduce episodes of sleep apnoea in the presence of fluid overload [19]. Treatment with continuous positive airway pressure is effective for obstructive sleep apnoea.

44.2.8 Chronic Obstructive Pulmonary Disease (COPD)

COPD is associated with 41% increased risk for all-cause mortality and fourfold increased risk for respiratory-related deaths amongst those with CKD. It is a frequent and underdiagnosed comorbidity in patients with ESRF, with reported prevalence as high as 46% in patients on dialysis [20].

The reason for the coexistence of COPD in ESRF is multifactorial. Smoking is a major risk factor with studies suggesting that chronic low-grade inflammation that follows ESRF may affect the lung epithelium [21]. In addition, patients with COPD may have coexistent diabetes or hypertension, possibly increasing the risk of CKD. Accumulated evidence from animal models and patients with AKI suggests that pro-inflammatory cytokines associated with atherosclerosis and neutrophil proteins, such as neutrophil gelatinase-associated lipocalin (NGAL) released during episodes of AKI, are mediators of lung injury. NGAL may drive COPD epithelial mesenchymal transitions and could reflect the state of systemic inflammation in COPD [9–12]. Interestingly, a study recently revealed that 10.7% of patients who recovered from AKI requiring temporary dialysis were concomitantly diagnosed with COPD, 1 year after index hospitalisation (compared to 2–3% in the general population) [22].

▫ Table 44.1 provides an overview of important associations between autoimmune and genetic renal and respiratory diseases.

▫ Table 44.1 Autoimmune and genetic disorders that affect both the lungs and kidneys

Autoimmune disorders	
Goodpasture syndrome (anti-GBM disease)	40–60% of patients present with diffuse alveolar haemorrhage (DAH); they tend to be younger and smokers. In almost three quarters of the cases, pulmonary haemorrhage precedes or coincides with glomerular disease
Granulomatosis with polyangiitis	Single or multiple pulmonary nodules and masses in 70% of patients tend to be peripheral and contain air bronchograms. Ground-glass halos due to perilesional haemorrhage. Nodules will cavitate in 50% of patients (▫ Fig. 44.3), and infection (tuberculosis, staphylococcal abscess) is an important differential here. DAH in 8–36%
Eosinophilic granulomatosis with polyangiitis	90% of patients present with asthma in the second and third decade of life. Pulmonary lobules, peripheral ground glass and interlobular septal thickening
Systemic lupus erythematosus (SLE)	Pulmonary involvement in 50 to 70% of SLE patients and presenting feature in 4 to 5% of patients. 12% will have accumulated an element of permanent lung damage at 10-year follow-up. Pulmonary complications are broad and include pleural disease (45%), interstitial lung disease (up to 15%), vasculitis with DAH in 1–5%, pulmonary embolism (9%), pulmonary hypertension (up to 17.5%), shrinking lung syndrome (1%) [23]
Systemic sclerosis (SSc)	75% of patients have interstitial lung disease, under 50% pulmonary hypertension. Patients with SSc with diffuse cutaneous involvement can develop fatal isolated pulmonary arterial hypertension. This complication occurs disproportionately more often in patients with serum anti-U3RNP antibody [24]
IgG4-related disease	Pulmonary involvement in over 20% of patients including peribronchial inflammation, discrete nodules, reticulation or septal thickening and consolidation [25]
Sarcoidosis	Pulmonary involvement is seen in over 90% with renal involvement affecting less than 3% of patients with sarcoidosis. Pulmonary manifestations include paratracheal and bilateral hilar lymphadenopathy, pulmonary infiltrates with fissural nodularity that can progress to fibrosis, often with a mid to upper zone predisposition; however, changes can be diverse [26]
Genetic disorders	
Tuberous sclerosis (TSC)	*Lymphangioleiomyomatosis* (LAM): found almost exclusively in women – proliferation of atypical smooth muscles, resulting in vascular and airway obstruction and cystic lung formation. The invading cells contain inactivating mutations in tuberous sclerosis proteins that result in mammalian target of rapamycin complex 1 (mTORC1) pathway-driven cellular proliferation, hence the therapeutic role of sirolimus. LAM is associated with mediastinal lymphangiomas, chylous pleural effusions and spontaneous pneumothorax (▫ Fig. 44.4). LAM may replace nearly the entire lung parenchyma and necessitate lung transplantation; it may also recur after transplantation. *Angiomyolipomas (AMLs)*: benign and soft-tissue-containing lesions found mainly in the kidney (85% of patients with TSC) but are also seen in up to 50% of patients with sporadic LAM. Lesions greater than 4 cm are at risk of spontaneous haemorrhage *Multifocal micronodular pneumocyte hyperplasia:* solid or ground-glass pulmonary nodules between 2 and 14 mm in size (tiny pulmonary hamartomas), in 40–60% of patients with TSC, affects men and women equally [27, 28]

(continued)

Table 44.1 (continued)

Autosomal dominant polycystic kidney disease (ADPKD)	Lung involvement is not a frequent feature of ADPKD, patients do have a higher incidence of bronchiectasis, though typically mild [29]
Birt-Hogg-Dubé syndrome (BHD)	Autosomal dominant monogenic disorder caused by constitutional mutations in the *FLCN* gene that codes for the protein folliculin. Lung cysts are the hallmark of the lung involvement, causing an increased risk of spontaneous pneumothorax. The most severe manifestation of the syndrome is the predisposition to renal cell carcinoma [30]
Sickle cell disease	Acute: acute chest syndrome, characterised by acute chest pain, fever and pulmonary consolidations; likely related to a combination of pulmonary infarcts and pneumonia. Chronic: pulmonary hypertension in one-third of sickle cell patients, with substantial mortality [31]

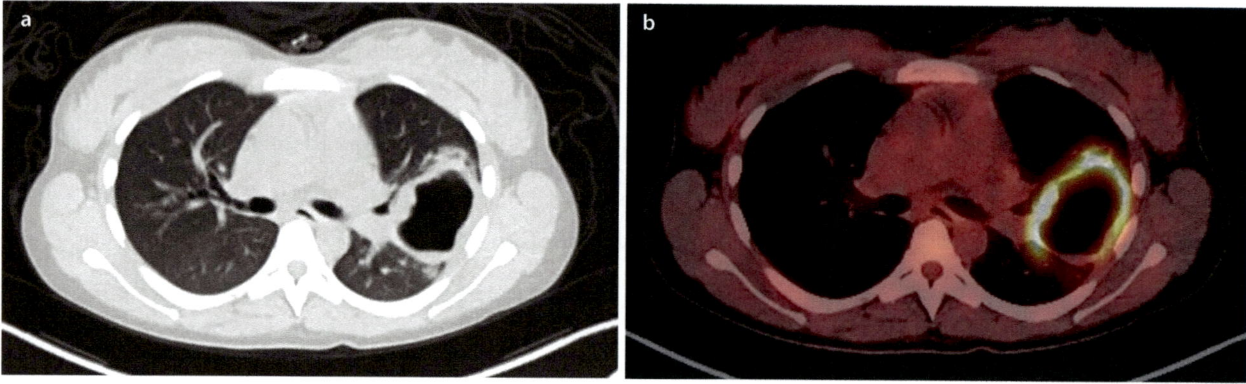

Fig. 44.3 Fluorodeoxyglucose (FDG)-positron emission tomography (PET) **a** in a patient with PR3-ANCA vasculitis with pulmonary involvement showing a large cavitating pulmonary lesion **b** exhibiting intense mural FDG avidity

44.2.9 Pulmonary-Renal Syndrome

The term pulmonary-renal syndrome (PRS), as first described by Ernest Goodpasture in 1919, is used to describe the occurrence of renal failure in association with respiratory failure, characterised by rapidly progressive glomerulonephritis (RPGN) and diffuse alveolar haemorrhage (DAH) secondary to an underlying autoimmune process. DAH is one of the strongest predictors of mortality in patients with RPGN caused by antineutrophil cytoplasmic antibody (ANCA)-associated vasculitis (AAV) and anti-GBM disease, increasing the relative risk by up to 8.6-fold in patients with AAV [32]. Table 44.2 shows radiological and histological features as well as causes of pulmonary-renal syndrome.

Table 44.2 Distinguishing characteristics and causes of pulmonary-renal syndrome

Radiological appearances	Bilateral widespread ground-glass opacification in both the upper and lower lobes on computer tomography (Fig. 44.5)
Histological features	Glomerular crescents on renal biopsy and pulmonary capillaritis on lung biopsy
Autoimmune causes of PRS	ANCA-associated vasculitis (56–77.5%) Anti-glomerular basement disease (12.5–17.5%) [33] Also lupus vasculitis, IgA vasculitis (less than 5% of cases), antiphospholipid syndrome
Non-autoimmune causes of DAH with renal impairment	AKI with pulmonary oedema Infection Leptospirosis *Staphylococcus aureus* *Legionella pneumophila* Hantavirus Malaria Thromboembolic disease

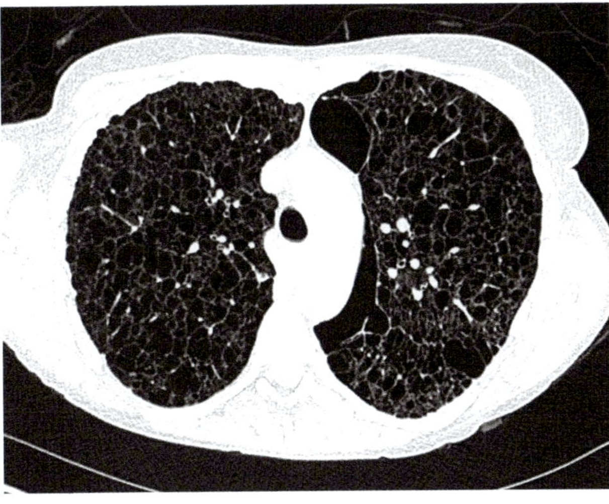

Fig. 44.4 High-resolution CT scan of the chest of a 29-year-old female with tuberous sclerosis reveals multiple well-defined, thin-walled cysts scattered throughout both the lungs, consistent with lymphangioleiomyomatosis

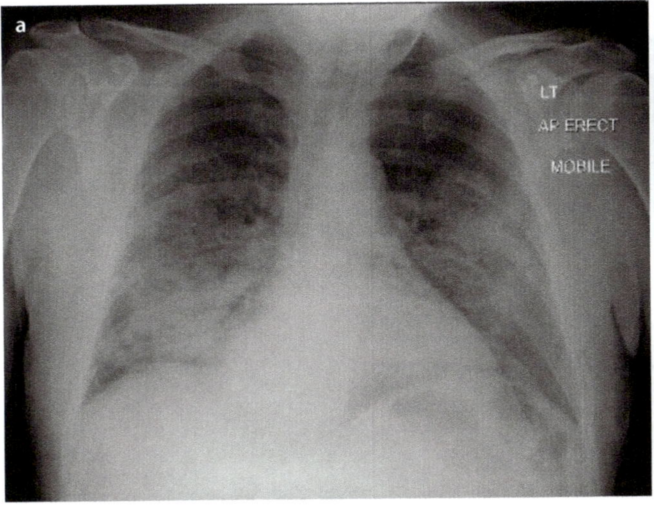

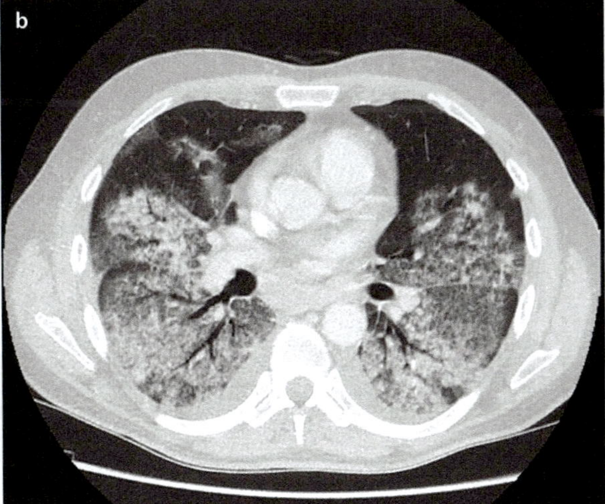

Fig. 44.5 Chest radiograph **a** and chest CT **b** of a patient with PR3-ANCA vasculitis who presented with acute kidney injury and haemoptysis. **a** Bilateral perihilar nodular consolidation is seen, which is most marked in both midzones. **b** The chest CT of the same patient confirms bilateral perihilar consolidation and mediastinal adenopathy. The radiographic differential is wide and includes infection, including atypical infections and pneumocystis pneumonia if there is a history of immunocompromise

Case Study

Case 1

A 33-year-old woman presents with progressively worsening dyspnoea of 2 days. Her medical history was significant for systemic lupus erythematosus. A PD catheter was placed 8 weeks prior, and she began PD. She started on continuous ambulatory PD (CAPD) with 6 hours dwell time and 4–5 exchanges per day. She initially tolerated PD well while on 2.2 L fill volumes; however, over the last 2 days, her drain volume had reduced to 1.8 L. Physical examination was remarkable for right-sided basilar crackles with no other signs of fluid overload.

Her presentation CXR demonstrated the presence of large right-sided pleural effusion (◘ Fig. 44.6a). Right-sided thoracentesis was performed; the pleural fluid analysis is shown in ◘ Table 44.3.

Pleural-fluid glucose concentration that is greater than that of serum is most probably due to pleuroperitoneal leak.

◘ Figure 44.6b shows resolution of the pleural effusion after drainage of the peritoneal fluid. CT peritoneography can confirm the diagnosis as contrast material leaks from the peritoneal into the right pleural space.

PD-related hydrothorax is an important complication of PD with incidence of 1.6–10%.

Case 2

A 67-year-old Bangladeshi man with a background of type 2 diabetes, hypertension and benign prostatic hyperplasia presented to a district general hospital with complaints of feeling unwell and dark urine for 10 days despite a week's course of co-amoxiclav from his GP. His urine dipstick showed +3 protein, +3 blood, his renal US showed normal-sized kidneys and his CXR bilateral alveolar shadowing. His creatinine was 500 μmol/L with no baseline value available out of hours. He was treated with intravenous co-amoxiclav for presumed partially treated UTI and chest consolidation. Over the next 2 days, he became hypoxic, and his urine output reduced. His anti-GBM titre was positive, and he was transferred to a tertiary renal centre for plasma exchange and immunosuppressive treatment.

The peak incidence of anti-GBM disease is in the third and sixth decades, and there is a male preponderance. If untreated, anti-GBM disease is life-threatening, with irreversible kidney damage and respiratory failure. Over 50% of patients present beyond the point at which renal recovery is possible. In particular, renal recovery at 1 year in patients that presented with dialysis-dependent renal failure has been reported to be only 17% [34]. In addition, despite the widespread availability of diagnostic tests,

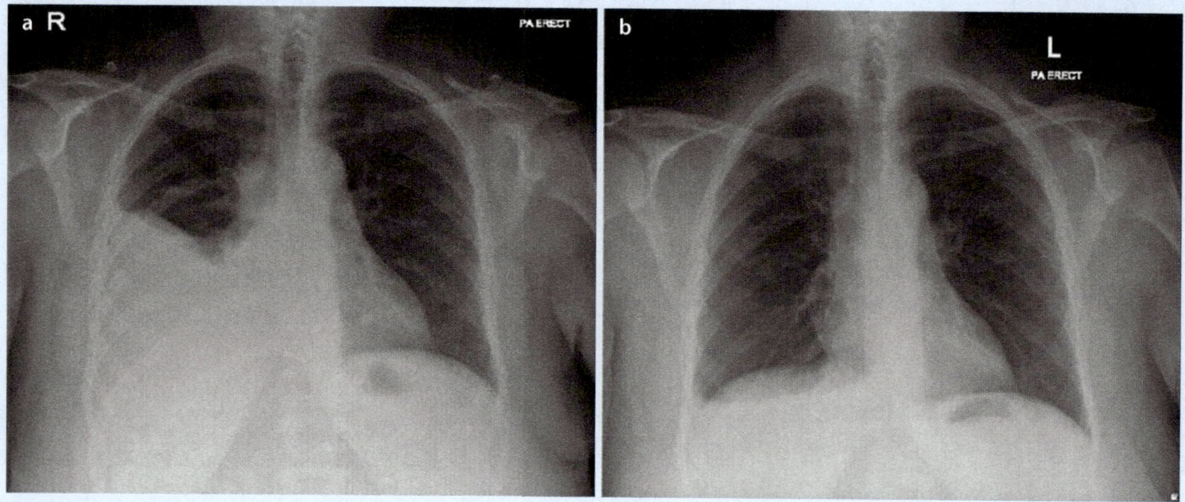

◘ **Fig. 44.6** **a** Moderate right pleural effusion with atelectasis in the right midzone and volume loss in the right lower lobe **b** which resolves after the peritoneal fluid is drained

Table 44.3 Pleural fluid analysis of PD patient in ▶ Case 1 presenting with worsening dyspnoea

Protein	0.2 g/dL
Lactate dehydrogenase	16 U/L
Glucose	16 mmol/L
Serum glucose	6 mmol/L
pH	7.64

delayed establishment of the correct diagnosis and thus transfer to treatment centres results in many patients requiring permanent renal replacement therapy. In part, this is due to the rarity of the disease and confounding clinical factors that can potentially explain the cause of acute kidney injury (AKI).

Case 3

A woman in her early 40s presented with worsening shortness of breath, wheeze and productive cough for 1 week. She had a left nephrectomy as an adolescent for a ruptured AML, with a spontaneous right-sided pneumothorax occurring post-operatively. She was a non-smoker and had no history of seizures or learning difficulties. On examination of the chest, there was equal air entry. Multiple small red-brown papules were noted over the central part of the face, consistent with adenoma sebaceum. General examination was otherwise unremarkable.

High-resolution CT scan of the chest revealed multiple well-defined, thin-walled cysts scattered throughout both the lungs, consistent with lymphangioleiomyomatosis (LAM) (◘ Fig. 44.1). LAM diagnosis is typically delayed by 3–5 years as more common dyspnoea causes, such as asthma or chronic obstructive pulmonary disease, are often diagnosed initially. The two most common presenting symptoms of LAM are dyspnoea on exertion and spontaneous pneumothorax. Pneumothorax has been reported in 40–80% of patients with LAM.

Taking this history into consideration, the differential diagnoses of LAM and TSC should be considered, given the association between AMLs and LAM [35].

Tips and Tricks

- The presence of impaired renal function in patients with pulmonary nodules or consolidation could suggest a vasculitis, IgG4-related disease, or sarcoidosis. Interstitial opacities are most commonly seen in systemic sclerosis, sarcoidosis, and IgG4 disease.
- Around 50% of patients with CKD have reduced skin test responsiveness to the tuberculin skin test. Therefore, a negative tuberculin skin test in a patient with CKD does not exclude latent TB infection.
- In patients with pulmonary-renal syndrome, immunological testing should be carried out early but should not delay treatment, where diagnosis has been made by clinical features and other relevant investigations.
- Consider lymphangioleiomyomatosis (LAM) and tuberous sclerosis in female patients of childbearing age with dyspnoea, particularly with a history of recurrent pneumothorax, epilepsy or angiomyolipomas.

Chapter Review Questions

1. What are the indications for treatment of latent TB?
2. What are the respiratory considerations and contraindications for renal transplantation?
3. How do you screen and test for sleep-disordered breathing in patients with CKD?

Answers

1. Decisions for initiation of treatment or chemoprophylaxis for TB should be made at a multidisciplinary level, involving referral to and assessment by a specialist with an interest in TB, such as a chest and/or infectious disease physician.

   According to the current NICE TB guidelines [9], patients with latent TB that have CKD or receive dialysis are at increased risk to develop active disease. Other groups that have been identified as high risk to progress to active TB are patients with HIV, diabetes, solid organ transplant recipients and patients on immunosuppression.

   There is a high level of anergy to purified protein derivative (PPD) used in tuberculin skin testing (TST) in patients with CKD, giving a high false-negative rate, and for this reason TST is not recommended. Some guidelines recommend the use of interferon gamma release assays, but the evidence for this in patients with CKD is limited [36]. In many units, assessment for latent TB includes history of previous not adequately treated TB or suggestive CXR findings of previous TB, close contact with TB or immigration from a highly endemic country.

For patients undergoing renal transplantation, treatment of latent TB could be considered if transplanted in a highly endemic country or if the organ donor is from a highly endemic country.

2. Guidelines recommend that all patients with CKD at stage 5 or 4 with progressive disease likely to require renal replacement therapy within 6 months should be considered for transplantation [37, 38]. A minority of patients with ESRF are deemed unsuitable for transplantation. Respiratory considerations and contraindications to renal transplantation include:
   - Active infection such as TB
   - Active pulmonary malignancy
   - Patients requiring home oxygen therapy
   - Uncontrolled asthma
   - Severe cor pulmonale

   Severe COPD/pulmonary fibrosis or restrictive disease with any of the following parameters [38]:
   - Best FEV1 <25% predicted value
   - PO2 room air <8 kPa with exercise desaturation SaO2 <90%
   - More than 4 lower respiratory tract infections in the last 12 months
   - Moderate disease with evidence of progression

3. Sleep-disordered breathing, and in particular sleep apnoea, is present in more than 50% of patients with CKD; however, it remains under-recognised. In addition to the high prevalence of sleep-disordered breathing in the CKD population, the importance of prompt recognition is its association with cardiovascular mortality in this population, making early referral to a chest specialist essential.

   Most individual signs and symptoms have limited utility in determining the likelihood of sleep apnoea, and no clinical feature is sufficiently sensitive or specific to confirm or exclude the diagnosis. A variety of clinical prediction scores have been evaluated using common signs and symptoms of SDB relating to snoring, observed apnoea, body mass index, age, neck circumference, gender and sleepiness, which are easily obtained and interpreted. Unfortunately, their sensitivity is generally much higher than their specificity [39]. An example of such questionnaires used in clinical practice is the STOP-Bang score for assessment of obstructive sleep apnoea (OSA) [40].

   The diagnosis of sleep-disordered breathing is based upon the presence or absence of related symptoms, as well as the frequency of respiratory events during sleep as measured by polysomnography.

44.3 Summary

Pulmonary and renal physiology are intimately related in both health and disease. Collaboration between the two specialties is essential to not only aid management and monitoring of common conditions that affect patients with chronic kidney disease but also offer a significant diagnostic value in the setting of inherited and acquired renal diseases.

References

1. Turcios NL. Pulmonary complications of renal disorders. Paediatr Respir Rev. 2012;13:44–9. https://doi.org/10.1016/j.prrv.2011.04.006.
2. Pierson DJ. Respiratory considerations in the patient with renal failure. Respir Care. 2006;51:413–22.
3. Ray S, Mukherjee S, Ganguly J, Abhishek K, Mitras S, Kundu S. A cross-sectional prospective study of pleural effusion among cases of chronic kidney disease. Indian J Chest Dis Allied Sci. 2013;55:209–13.
4. Romero-Candeira S, Fernández C, Martín C, Sánchez-Paya J, Hernández L. Influence of diuretics on the concentration of proteins and other components of pleural transudates in patients with heart failure. Am J Med. 2001;110:681–6. https://doi.org/10.1016/s0002-9343(01)00726-4.
5. Carrero JJ, Stenvinkel P. Inflammation in end-stage renal disease--what have we learned in 10 years? Semin Dial. 2010;23:498–509. https://doi.org/10.1111/j.1525-139X.2010.00784.x.
6. Tuberculosis and chronic renal disease. PubMed – NCBI n.d. https://www.ncbi.nlm.nih.gov/pubmed/12535299. Accessed 20 Jan 2019.
7. Segall L, Covic A. Diagnosis of tuberculosis in dialysis patients: current strategy. Clin J Am Soc Nephrol. 2010;5:1114–22. https://doi.org/10.2215/CJN.09231209.
8. Currie AC, Knight SR, Morris PJ. Tuberculosis in renal transplant recipients: the evidence for prophylaxis. Transplantation. 2010;90:695–704. https://doi.org/10.1097/TP.0b013e3181ecea8d.
9. Overview | Tuberculosis | Guidance | NICE n.d.. https://www.nice.org.uk/guidance/ng33. Accessed 16 July 2020.
10. Wang I-K, Lin C-L, Lin P-C, Liang C-C, Liu Y-L, Chang C-T, et al. Effectiveness of influenza vaccination in patients with end-stage renal disease receiving hemodialysis: a population-based study. PLoS One. 2013;8:e58317. https://doi.org/10.1371/journal.pone.0058317.
11. Chang Y-T, Wang J-R, Lin M-T, Wu C-J, Tsai M-S, Wen-Chi CL, et al. Changes of immunogenic profiles between a single dose and one booster influenza vaccination in hemodialysis patients - an 18-week, open-label trial. Sci Rep. 2016;6:20725. https://doi.org/10.1038/srep20725.

12. Diao B, Wang C, Wang R, Feng Z, Tan Y, Wang H, et al. Human kidney is a target for novel severe acute respiratory syndrome coronavirus 2 (SARS-CoV-2) infection. MedRxiv. 2020.:2020.03.04.20031120; https://doi.org/10.1101/2020.03.04.20031120.
13. Infection TLEC, May 02;3951417-1418 E in C-19 L 2020, Varga Z, Flammer AJ, Steiger P, Haberecker M, et al. Endothelial cell infection and endotheliitis in COVID-19. PracticeUpdate n.d. https://www.practiceupdate.com/content/endothelial-cell-infection-and-endotheliitis-in-covid-19/99774. Accessed 2 June 2020.
14. Wattanakit K, Cushman M, Stehman-Breen C, Heckbert SR, Folsom AR. Chronic kidney disease increases risk for venous thromboembolism. J Am Soc Nephrol. 2008;19:135–40. https://doi.org/10.1681/ASN.2007030308.
15. Zoccali C, Mallamaci F. Pulmonary embolism in chronic kidney disease: a lethal, overlooked and research orphan disease. J Thromb Haemost. 2012;10:2481–3. https://doi.org/10.1111/jth.12046.
16. Munger MA, Ateshkadi A, Cheung AK, Flaharty KK, Stoddard GJ, Marshall EH. Cardiopulmonary events during hemodialysis: effects of dialysis membranes and dialysate buffers. Am J Kidney Dis Off J Natl Kidney Found. 2000;36:130–9. https://doi.org/10.1053/ajkd.2000.8285.
17. Huang H-C, Walters G, Talaulikar G, Figurski D, Carroll A, Hurwitz M, et al. Sleep apnea prevalence in chronic kidney disease - association with total body water and symptoms. BMC Nephrol. 2017;18:125. https://doi.org/10.1186/s12882-017-0544-3.
18. Unruh ML, Sanders MH, Redline S, Piraino BM, Umans JG, Hammond TC, et al. Sleep apnea in patients on conventional thrice-weekly hemodialysis: comparison with matched controls from the sleep heart health study. J Am Soc Nephrol. 2006;17:3503–9. https://doi.org/10.1681/ASN.2006060659.
19. Ogna A, Forni Ogna V, Mihalache A, Pruijm M, Halabi G, Phan O, et al. Obstructive sleep apnea severity and overnight body fluid shift before and after hemodialysis. Clin J Am Soc Nephrol CJASN. 2015;10:1002–10. https://doi.org/10.2215/CJN.08760914.
20. Chronic obstructive pulmonary disease in patients with end-stage kidney disease on hemodialysis - Plesner - 2016 - Hemodialysis International - Wiley Online Library n.d.. https://onlinelibrary.wiley.com/doi/full/10.1111/hdi.12342. Accessed 6 May 2019.
21. Sjöberg B, Qureshi AR, Anderstam B, Alvestrand A, Bárány P. Pentraxin 3, a sensitive early marker of hemodialysis-induced inflammation. Blood Purif. 2012;34:290–7. https://doi.org/10.1159/000342630.
22. Wu C-H, Chang H-M, Wang C-Y, Chen L, Chen L-W, Lai C-H, et al. Long-term outcomes in patients with incident chronic obstructive pulmonary disease after acute kidney injury: a competing-risk analysis of a nationwide cohort. J Clin Med. 2018;7 https://doi.org/10.3390/jcm7090237.
23. Hannah JR, D'Cruz DP. Pulmonary complications of systemic lupus erythematosus. Semin Respir Crit Care Med. 2019;40:227–34. https://doi.org/10.1055/s-0039-1685537.
24. Sacks DG, Okano Y, Steen VD, Curtiss E, Shapiro LS, Medsger TA. Isolated pulmonary hypertension in systemic sclerosis with diffuse cutaneous involvement: association with serum anti-U3RNP antibody. J Rheumatol. 1996;23:639–42.
25. Matsui S. IgG4-related respiratory disease. Mod Rheumatol. 2019;29:251–6. https://doi.org/10.1080/14397595.2018.1548089.
26. Ungprasert P, Ryu JH, Matteson EL. Clinical manifestations, diagnosis, and treatment of sarcoidosis. Mayo Clin Proc Innov Qual Outcomes. 2019;3:358–75. https://doi.org/10.1016/j.mayocpiqo.2019.04.006.
27. Hammer MM, Shetty AS, Sheybani EF, Bhalla S. Diseases and syndromes that affect the lungs and the kidneys: a radiologic review. Curr Probl Diagn Radiol. 2017;46:216–24. https://doi.org/10.1067/j.cpradiol.2016.06.001.
28. Gupta N, Henske EP. Pulmonary manifestations in tuberous sclerosis complex. Am J Med Genet C Semin Med Genet. 2018;178:326–37. https://doi.org/10.1002/ajmg.c.31638.
29. Driscoll JA, Bhalla S, Liapis H, Ibricevic A, Brody SL. Autosomal dominant polycystic kidney disease is associated with an increased prevalence of radiographic bronchiectasis. Chest. 2008;133:1181–8. https://doi.org/10.1378/chest.07-2147.
30. Tomassetti S, Carloni A, Chilosi M, Maffè A, Ungari S, Sverzellati N, et al. Pulmonary features of Birt-Hogg-Dubé syndrome: cystic lesions and pulmonary histiocytoma. Respir Med. 2011;105:768–74. https://doi.org/10.1016/j.rmed.2011.01.002.
31. Dimitrios F, Athanasios A. Pulmonary hypertension associated with hemoglobinopathies. Circulation. 2011;123:1227–32. https://doi.org/10.1161/CIRCULATIONAHA.110.988089.
32. Haworth SJ, Savage CO, Carr D, Hughes JM, Rees AJ. Pulmonary haemorrhage complicating Wegener's granulomatosis and microscopic polyarteritis. Br Med J Clin Res Ed. 1985;290:1775–8.
33. West SC, Arulkumaran N, Ind PW, Pusey CD. Pulmonary-renal syndrome: a life threatening but treatable condition. Postgrad Med J. 2013;89:274–83. https://doi.org/10.1136/postgradmedj-2012-131416.
34. McAdoo SP, Tanna A, Hrušková Z, Holm L, Weiner M, Arulkumaran N, et al. Patients double-seropositive for ANCA and anti-GBM antibodies have varied renal survival, frequency of relapse, and outcomes compared to single-seropositive patients. Kidney Int. 2017;92:693–702. https://doi.org/10.1016/j.kint.2017.03.014.
35. Gosein MA, Ameeral A, Konduru SKP, Dola VNS. Tuberous sclerosis presenting with spontaneous pneumothorax secondary to lymphangioleiomyomatosis; previously mistaken for asthma. BMJ Case Rep. 2013;2013 https://doi.org/10.1136/bcr-2013-009969.
36. Anibarro L, Trigo M, Feijoó D, Ríos M, Palomares L, Pena A, et al. Value of the tuberculin skin testing and of an interferon-gamma release assay in haemodialysis patients after exposure to M. tuberculosis. BMC Infect Dis. 2012;12:195. https://doi.org/10.1186/1471-2334-12-195.
37. Dudley C, Bright R, Harden P. Assessment of the potential kidney transplant recipient. 5th ed. UK Renal Association; 2010. www.renal.org/guidelines
38. British Columbia (BC) Renal Agency guidelines. Absolute contraindications to kidney transplantation. Dec 2017, bcrenalagency.ca.
39. Santos RSS, Motwani SS, Elias RM. Chronic kidney disease and sleeping disordered breathing (SDB). Curr Hypertens Rev. 2016;12:43–7.
40. Chung F, Abdullah HR, Liao P. STOP-Bang questionnaire: a practical approach to screen for obstructive sleep apnea. Chest. 2016;149:631–8. https://doi.org/10.1378/chest.15-0903.

Ageing and the Kidneys

Stephanie M. Y. Chong, Rachel K. Y. Hung, and William White

Contents

M. Harber (ed.), *Primer on Nephrology*, https://doi.org/10.1007/978-3-030-76419-7_45

Learning Objectives

1. To understand the challenges posed by the ageing CKD population
2. To appreciate that physiological and psychosocial differences impact on the management of older patients with kidney disease, necessitating an individualised approach to their management
3. To recognise that frailty is often the greatest predictor of patient outcome in the elderly rather than the modality or adequacy of renal replacement therapy

45.1 Introduction

The World Health Organization (WHO) estimates that by 2050 the proportion of the world's population over the age of 60 will have nearly doubled from that in 2015, from 12% to 22%. In the UK the number of people over 60 is expected to reach 18.5 million by 2025. This will result in an increasingly polymorbid population (75% of 75-year-olds in the UK have more than one long-term condition [1], 30% with CKD; ◘ Fig. 45.1) and exponential rises in healthcare usage.

45.2 Ageing and Chronic Kidney Disease (CKD)

Ageing is associated with senescence of tissues. In the kidneys this results in an approximately 50% reduction in functional nephron mass by the age of 70 when compared to 29–30-year-olds (◘ Fig. 45.2), with a parallel decline in glomerular filtration rate (GFR). The structural changes seen in ageing are evident from studies of tissue from living donor kidneys, which demonstrate typical features such as tubular atrophy, glomerulosclerosis, interstitial fibrosis and athero- and arteriosclerosis (◘ Figs. 45.3 and 45.4). When added to the accrued damage from diseases, such as diabetes and hypertension, these result in an increased risk of CKD. There is also an increased predisposition to acute kidney injury due to toxicity from renally excreted drugs and ischaemic insults.

The relationship between increasing age and prevalence of CKD is based on an estimated GFR (eGFR) cut-off of 60 ml/min/1.73 m^2, as defined by the Kidney Disease Improving Global Outcomes (KDIGO) guidelines. This does not acknowledge the decline in kidney function with physiological ageing. In the original studies of age-related GFR changes in healthy subjects, a sequential reduction in GFR from 122.8 ± 16.4 ml/min/1.73 m^2 to 65.3 ± 20.4 ml/min/1.73 m^2 was found in patients in their 20s and 80s, respectively [5]. In a series of over 1000 healthy American kidney donors, GFR declined by 8 ml/decade after the age of 45 [6]. GFR is typically estimated using the MDRD and CKD-EPI equations, both of which were formulated using a study population under the age of 70. Additionally, they assume unvarying muscle mass, despite body composition changing with age.

It is likely that we have neither a reliable nor validated method of estimating GFR in the older population and that our standard cut-offs for CKD should be age adjusted. That said, the KDIGO eGFR cut-off was determined by a large meta-analysis looking at mortality, cardiovascular risk, risk of end-stage renal disease and progressive CKD, and a subgroup analysis of >65-year-olds included in the study showed similar

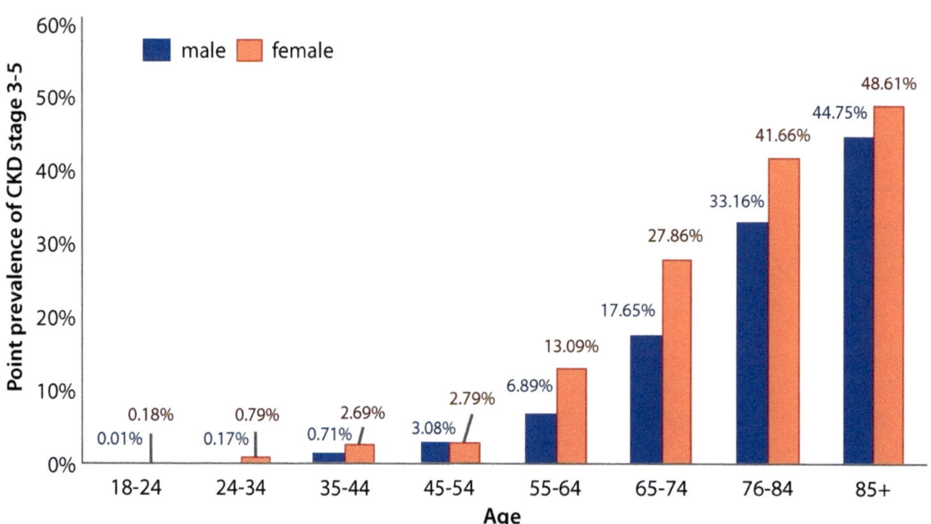

◘ **Fig. 45.1** Estimated CKD stage 3–5 prevalence amongst 38,262 adults in England between 1998 and 2003. (Reproduced using data from Stevens et al. [2])

45

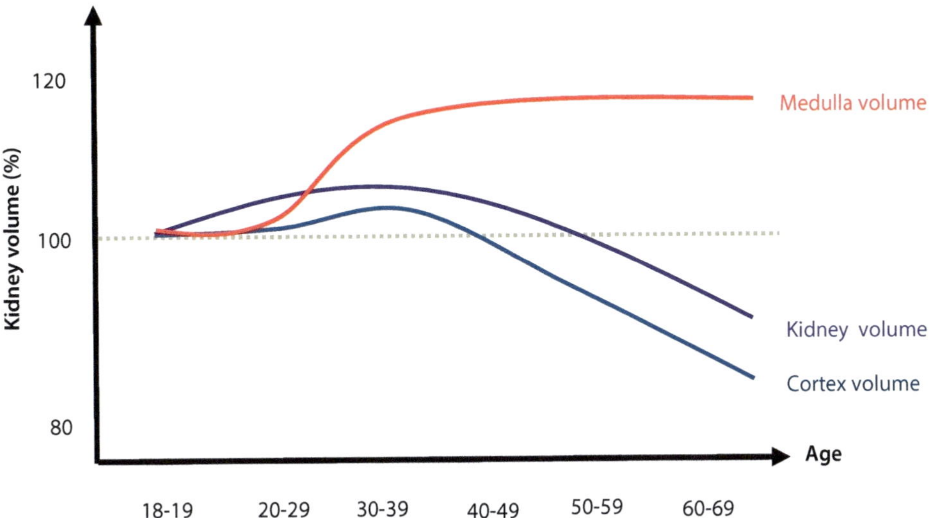

Fig. 45.2 *Effect of age on total kidney, cortical and medullary volumes* based on histology from living kidney donors. Cortical volume declines, whereas medullary volume increases, making total kidney volume relatively stable until about 50 years of age. (Modified from O'Neill et al. [3])

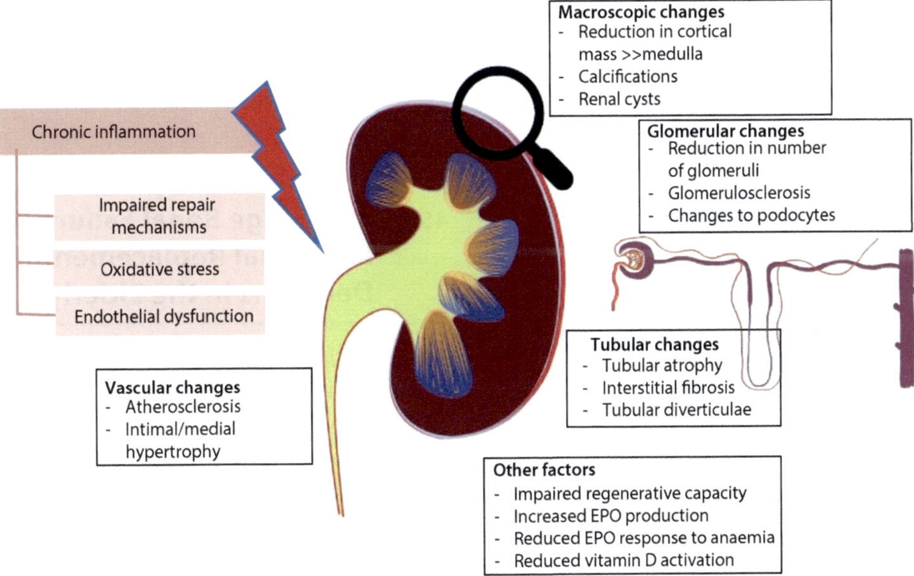

Fig. 45.3 Ageing-related changes in the kidney. (Adapted from Bolignano et al. [4])

increases in risk in all the aforementioned categories at an eGFR less than 60 ml/min/1.73 m^2.

45.3 Ageing and the Management of Chronic Kidney Disease (CKD)

The management of CKD has evolved over the last decade to focus on targets for the management of complications, such as anaemia and mineral bone disease, and with planning and preparing for dialysis or transplantation in its later stages. There is also increasing emphasis on reducing cardiovascular risk by controlling hypertension, diabetes and hyperlipidaemia. These therapeutic targets are generally derived from clinical trials that exclude older patients (and thus lack a solid evidence base to support their implementation in this population) and have end points that are not as relevant (or even detrimental) to their care. For example, major CKD trials, such as AASK [7] and REIN2 [8], included patients only up to the age of 70, with a mean age of 54 years old.

Older patients are often polymorbid and may suffer from one or more of the 'geriatric syndromes', making

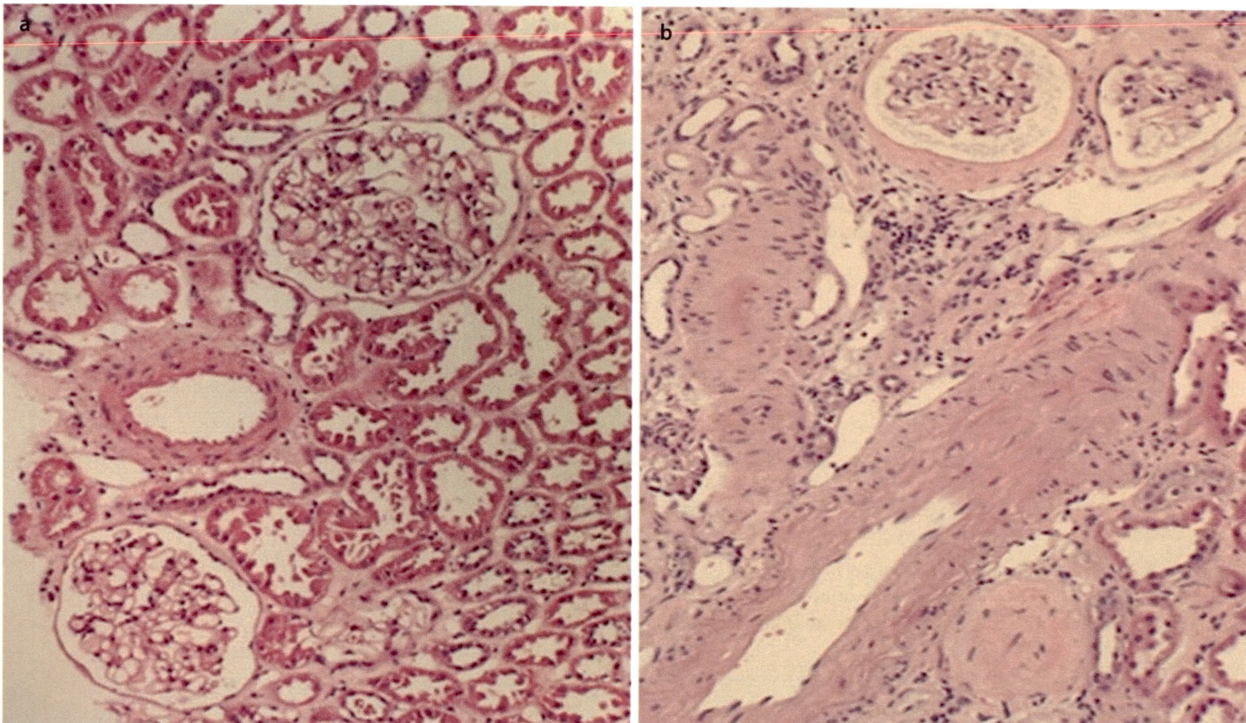

Fig. 45.4 Renal histology showing normal kidney histology in a young **a** and old **b** patient using haematoxylin and eosin staining. Note the thickening of the vessel wall, sclerosed glomerulus and flattening of the tubules in **b**. (Images courtesy of the Royal Free Hospital London, Histopathology Department)

application of standardised care challenging. In addition, many of these syndromes occur more commonly and severely in the context of CKD and frequently coexist. These include cognitive impairment and delirium, falls, polypharmacy, depression, immobility and frailty. Frailty (a phenotype partly defined by weight loss, muscle weakness and fatigue) is especially associated with adverse outcomes in geriatric populations [9].

Several factors should be considered when applying standardised treatment targets to elderly patients, one being the potential harmful impact of interventions: for example, aggressive blood pressure control can lead to postural hypotension and falls. Treatment priorities are often different in the ageing population: these may include maintaining mobility and independence, alleviating symptoms and suffering and maintaining social relationships. Furthermore, whilst hospital admission to expedite investigations and instigate aggressive treatment may improve outcomes for a younger patient, elderly patients will decondition rapidly and have higher risks of delirium and hospital-acquired infections, leading to prolonged hospital stays, pressure sores, low mood and reduced functional status at discharge (Table 45.1).

45.4 End-Stage Renal Failure (ESRF) and Renal Replacement Therapy Decisions in the Elderly

Starting dialysis therapy in later life does not carry the same mortality benefit seen in younger patients (Fig. 45.5). However, within each age cohort, there is a wide degree of variation in life expectancy, with no validated method of predicting good outcomes on dialysis (although high frailty scores and low BMI have been associated with increased mortality in elderly dialysis patients [16]). Choices regarding dialysis become increasingly difficult in the context of mild to moderate cognitive impairment, when judgements about 'quality of life' come into question, and complex family and ethical issues need to be considered.

Whilst there appears to be a modest survival benefit with dialysis (Fig. 45.6), there are many potential drawbacks, including the tolerability of treatments, increased hospital attendance and admissions and an increased likelihood of dying in hospital. Some studies have suggested an increase in symptom burden upon starting dialysis, with a stepwise decline in functional ability with each hospital admission.

Table 45.1 Challenges of managing CKD in an ageing population

Treatment focus	Considerations	Risks
Hypertension, salt and water management	Frequent presentation with isolated systolic hypertension (ISH) with preserved or low diastolic BP due to increased vascular stiffness; it is clear that ISH carries similar CV risks [1]; however, reducing diastolic BP will reduce cardiac perfusion and lead to increased CV events when lowered excessively (i.e. <60 mmHg) Good RCT evidence of benefit in terms of mortality, CV outcomes and CKD progression on patients >80 [10]. However, other studies suggest BP control in this group may in fact cause harm [11] Immobility may affect ability to monitor change in weight and may mask fluid accumulation	Treatment may increase falls due to postural hypotension or increase fatigue and confusion Predisposition ischaemic renal injuries, due to age-related vasculopathy, leading to acute kidney injury (AKI) and hyperkalaemia with Renin-Angiotension system (RAS) blockade
Diabetes control	Visual impairment, loss of dexterity and memory loss may hinder ability to monitor blood sugar levels	Under-recognition or awareness of hypoglycaemia
	Often poor eating habits which may make insulin dose prediction difficult	Increased frequency of hospitalisation
Cardiovascular risk management	*RAS blockade* Pre-existing vascular changes in ageing will predispose to ischaemia from RAS inhibitor-induced reduction in glomerular blood flow	As above
	Beta blockers No study has demonstrated clear benefit of beta blockade in hypertension treatment in the elderly, although does have benefit in heart failure or cardiac ischaemia	Treatment may increase falls due to postural hypotension
	Aspirin therapy Mortality benefit seen in a large trial but was associated with a twofold higher risk of non-fatal major bleeding complications [12]	Increased risk of bleeding, particularly upper gastrointestinal bleeds
	Anticoagulation Large trials of older individuals demonstrate superiority of novel oral anti-coagulant drugs (NOACs) to warfarin [13–15] in reducing cerebrovascular events and also reducing need for hospital attendance for monitoring; however, most studies excluded patients with an eGFR <25 Poor mobility may result in infrequently attendance for international normalised ratio (INR) monitoring Polypharmacy may result in altered efficacy of the anticoagulants Older individuals are prone to falls and head injuries	Increased risk of bleeding, particularly upper gastrointestinal bleeds and catastrophic intracranial bleeds. In this group, this can frequently lead to prolonged hospital stays, significant morbidity and irreversible loss of function
CKD mineral bone disease	May have swallowing difficulties or poor appetite, affecting compliance with phosphate binders May be housebound and therefore likely to have lower levels of vitamin D	May worsen bowel symptoms such as constipation

Whilst it is suggested that most elderly patients would choose quality of life over longevity, it is not clear what strategy is best to achieve this goal. Further trials are needed to ascertain the right treatment options in this group, including better assessment tools to predict outcomes on dialysis, such as frailty scores, which will help guide clinicians, patients and families in decision-making. One such strategy may be to incorporate the

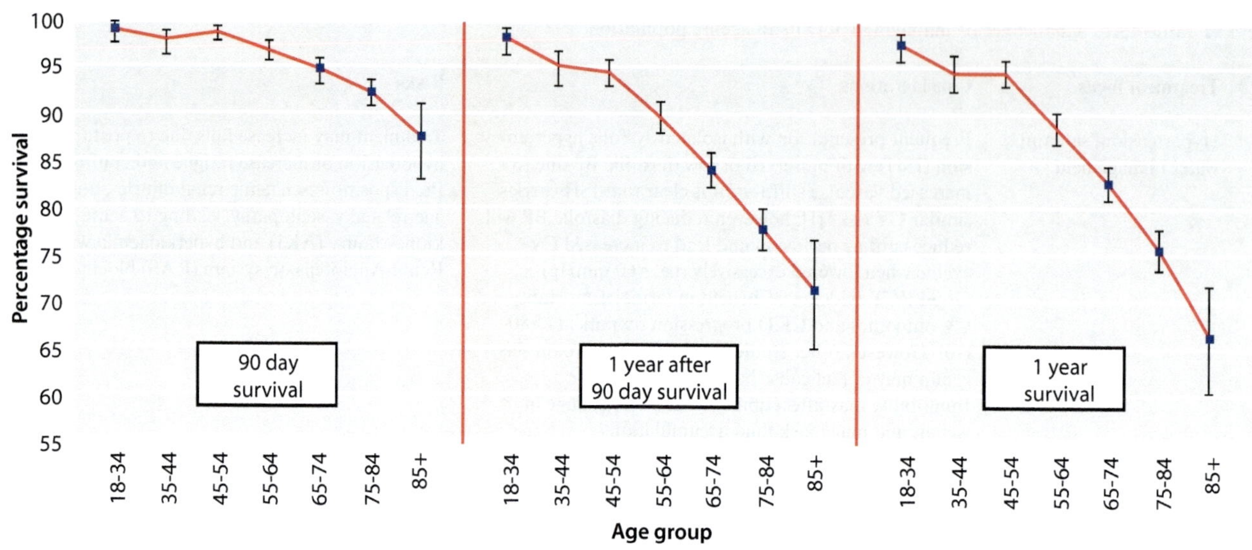

Fig. 45.5 UK renal registry data on unadjusted survival of incident RRT patients by age (2014 cohort). (Open access article by Methven et al. [17])

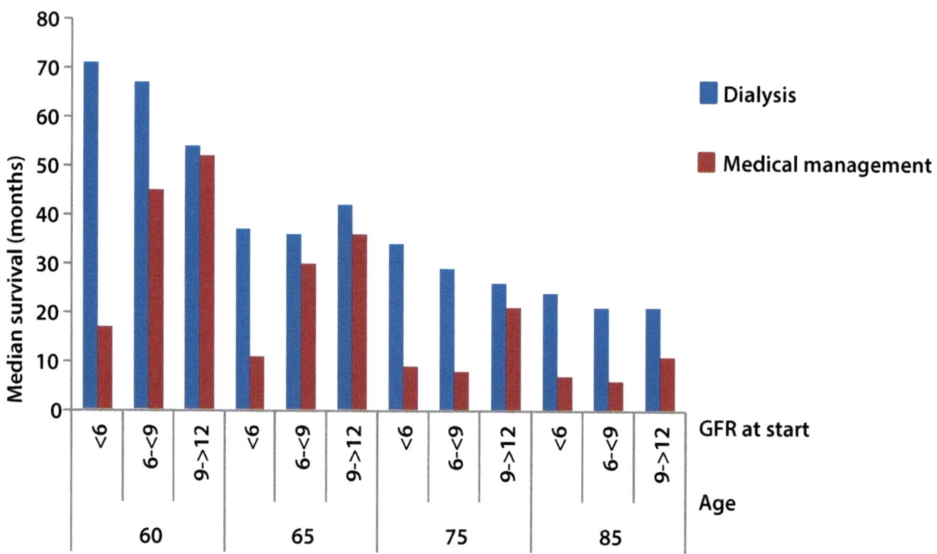

Fig. 45.6 Mortality difference between patients randomised to dialysis therapy compared with medical management in different age groups, subdivided by eGFR at initiation of therapy. This data suggests that initiating dialysis at a higher eGFR results in a diminished mortality benefit compared to medical management, whereas starting dialysis at an eGFR of <6 had a greater mortality benefit, albeit a difference of only 19–26 months. (Reproduced using data from 73 349 US veterans from Tamura et al. [18])

comprehensive geriatric assessment (GCA) into the process. The GCA is a validated tool, which has been beneficial in the assessment of elderly surgical candidates and may be a useful adjunct when making these decisions. There has also been increasing use of augmented dialysis strategies, such as reduced frequency dialysis, which has been shown to improve quality of life for patients rather than regimes with aim to achieve the standard targets of dialysis adequacy (Table 45.2).

45.5 Ageing and Transplantation

45.5.1 Patient and Allograft Outcomes

There is an overall increased survival in older patients after kidney transplantation compared to those who remain on dialysis [19]. However, special considerations should be made when considering transplantation in an older individual (Fig. 45.7). As older recipients are

Table 45.2 Pros and cons of RRT modalities in the elderly

	Haemodialysis	Peritoneal dialysis	Transplant	Conservative care
Pros	Improved solute clearance and ultrafiltration Readily available No training required for patient/carer Short treatment time	Retained independence Assisted service available Minimal haemodynamic compromise More physiological Treatment often tailored to suit lifestyle	Improved quality of life May allow return to social activities, travel and work Reduced dietary and fluid restrictions	Better focus on symptom management Least invasive to lifestyle Few hospital visits Improved recognition of dying and advanced care planning
Cons	Requires frequent hospital attendance Need for vascular access Increased infection risk from indwelling vascular catheters Rapid fluid and electrolyte shifts Requires systemic anticoagulation Dietary and fluid restrictions	Noisy machines/disturbed sleep Risk of peritonitis Long duration of treatment Poor solute clearance and unreliable ultrafiltration Catheter dysfunction Change to physical appearance Requires space for storage of PD fluid Dietary and fluid restrictions	Increased perioperative risks due to comorbidities Increased mortality in initial post-operative period Exposure to immunosuppression and increased infection/malignancy risk Frequent hospital visits Risk of perioperative complications	No life expectancy benefit

more likely to die with a functioning graft, some argued that older donor kidneys or extended criteria donor (ECD) kidneys should be preferentially offered to older recipients. In Europe, the Eurotransplant Senior Program (ESP) initiative is aimed at reducing waiting times for older patients. Kidneys from donors >65 years of age are allocated to recipients >65 years of age within a small geographical area to minimise cold ischaemic time. The 15-year outcome from this showed that despite a higher complication rate (mainly due to atherosclerotic vascular disease of the recipient and donor), the patient and allograft survival are comparable with younger patients. However, both the patient and allograft survival in older kidney transplant recipients (KTRs) who received ECD kidneys are worse when compared to those who received standard criteria donors (SCD) or living donor kidneys, even when adjusted for other donor and recipient factors and pre-transplant dialysis vintage. Renal function at 1 year is similarly worse in older KTRs, who had received an ECD kidney, as compared to a SCD or living donor kidney [20, 21]. Overall, SCD and living donor transplantation is preferred for older patients, but ECD transplantation should be offered to those without a living donor who otherwise will have a very long wait for a SCD kidney.

45.5.2 Rejection

Acute rejection rates are overall lower in older transplant recipients, likely due to decreased immunocompetence. However, preventing acute rejection is critical in older KTRs as rejection can have a greater impact on long-term graft survival in the older compared to younger recipients.

45.5.3 Comorbidities and Frailty in the Older KTR

Frailty increases risks of adverse post-operative outcomes and is a predictor of prolonged hospital stays and early hospital readmission. It has also been identified to be the best predictor of 30-day post-operative complications independent of age and is an independent risk factor for mortality.

45.5.4 Immunosuppressive Therapy

The innate and adaptive immune systems change with age, as do the pharmacokinetics and pharmacodynamics of immunosuppressive drugs. Older KTRs have been found to

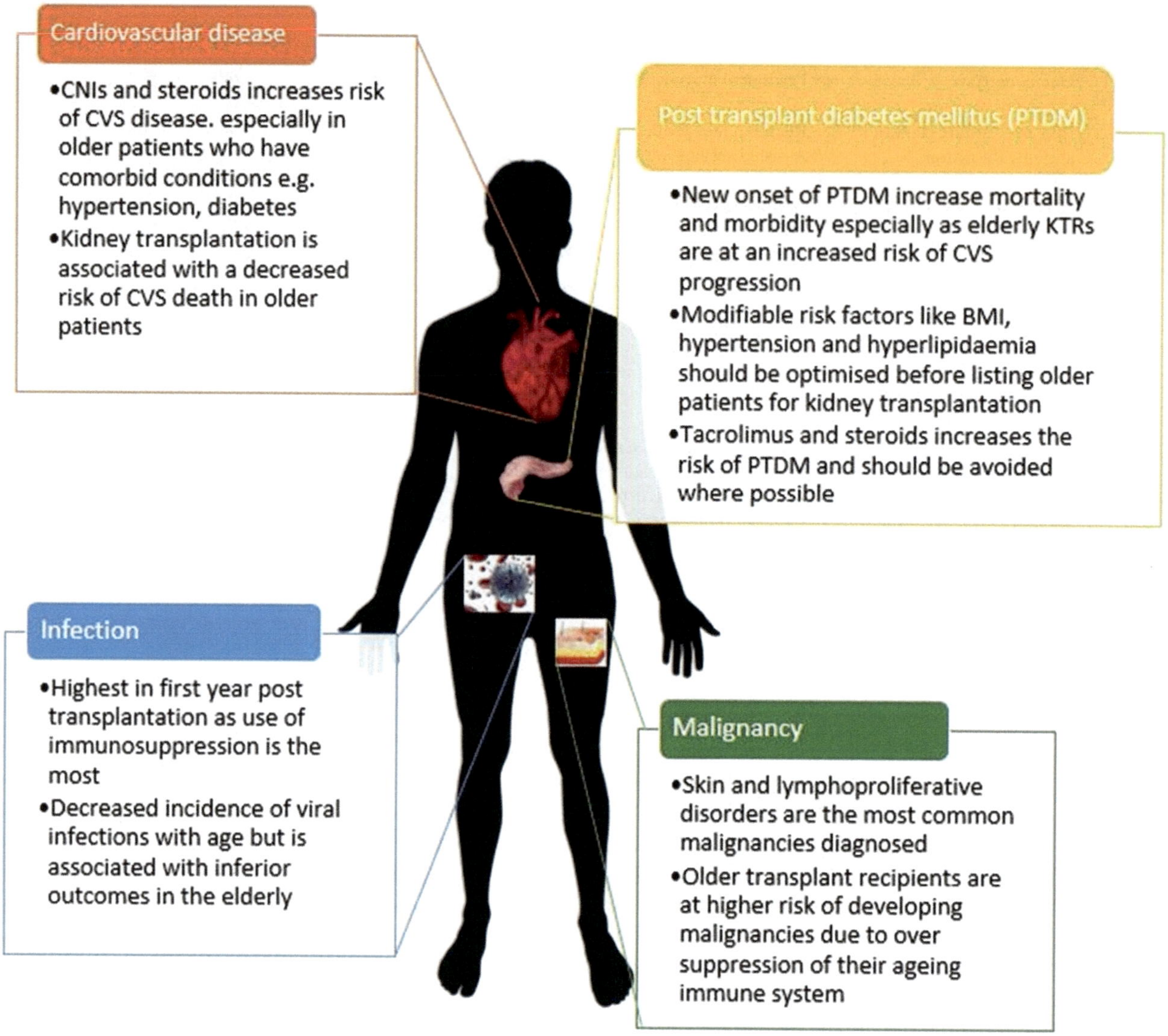

Fig. 45.7 Comorbidities in the older kidney transplant recipient

require significantly lower doses of cyclosporine to achieve similar plasma drug concentrations than young recipients [22]. High calcineurin inhibitor (CNI) peak levels have nephrotoxic potential that can hasten graft failure especially in ECD kidneys. Age-related reduction in hepatic and renal clearance is compounded by factors, such as frailty, comorbidity and polypharmacy, resulting in drug interactions and changes in availability and distribution. For instance, mycophenolate mofetil (MMF) clearance decreases with falling renal function, albumin levels and haemoglobin – all of which are affected in older transplant recipients. MMF usage is also associated with a higher incidence of opportunistic infections (viral, fungal and mycobacterial) [23] in the elderly. The clinical implication of immunosuppressive therapy in older KTRs is clearly significant, but few studies have looked into the impact of these drugs in this age group. Ideally, age-specific immunosuppressive protocols should be developed to optimise both the patient and graft survival and reduce overall morbidity.

45.6 Individualisation of Treatment and Palliative Care

Older patients benefit from an individualised and multidisciplinary approach to care. The treatment priorities of an older patient often centre around social needs and quality of life rather than the standard outcomes of mortality and disease progression that is often used to guide treatment. Some centres in the USA, such as Mount Sinai in New York, have pioneered a multidisciplinary geriatric renal service for patients over the age of 60 with geriatric syndromes, which focuses on both dialysis and non-dialysis therapies and addresses many of the geriatric syndromes and symptom management. Their main focus is on improving quality of life, maintaining independence and avoiding hospital attendances.

The National Service Framework for Renal Services calls for renal patients to have a timely evaluation of their prognosis and information about the choices available to them. High-quality palliative care should be accessible at all stages of patient care, and systems in place to recognise patients who are struggling or declining on dialysis, and for providing opportunities to discuss withdrawal. Anticipatory prescribing for symptom control should be adapted to take renal function into account and an end of life care plan built around an individual's needs and wishes should be made accessible to everyone involved in their care, including family members (see Palliative Care chapter).

Case Study

Case 1

A 76-year-old man is referred to the low clearance clinic with a stable eGFR of 30 ml/min/1.73 m^2. He has a history of type 2 diabetes, symptomatic heart failure, atrial fibrillation and hypertension with a resting BP of 170/80 and his HbA1c is 7.4%. He lives at home with his wife and manages his activities of daily living independently. He is currently taking metformin, ramipril, bisoprolol, atorvastatin and sodium bicarbonate tablets. This man has advancing CKD with isolated systolic hypertension and is at high risk of stroke (as per his CHADS-VASC score of 5). His ramipril dose should be up-titrated to achieve a systolic BP of <140 mmHg but to avoid a DBP of <60, which was associated with increased risk of cardiovascular event in the SHEP study [24]. He should be offered anticoagulation with a novel oral anti-coagulant (NOAC), but other factors, such as fall risk, should be considered. He should then be monitored closely for deterioration in renal function, at which time metformin and NOAC treatment should be reviewed as there is limited data available on anticoagulation in advanced renal failure. He should not be offered aspirin therapy as there is increasing evidence that there is no benefit in primary prevention and excessive bleeding risks have been demonstrated with concurrent anticoagulant use. His diabetes control should not be intensified as this has been associated in increased mortality risk in the ACCORD trial [25]. He should be given advice on lifestyle modification including salt restriction, diet and exercise.

Case 2

A 69-year-old patient who received a kidney transplant 3 years ago presents to clinic feeling generally unwell. His blood tests come back showing a Hb of 98 g/dl, a creatinine of 180mcmol/l from a baseline of 150mcmol/l and a Cytomegalovirus (CMV) titre of 10,000 copies/ml. He has a history of diabetes with diabetic nephropathy leading to ESRF, hypertension and gout and continues to smoke ten cigarettes a day. His maintenance immunosuppression includes tacrolimus (with levels of 6–8) and mycophenolate mofetil 500 mg twice daily, and he never suffered from graft rejection before. This patient has CMV viraemia that warrants urgent treatment with antivirals. The rise in his creatinine is likely secondary to the viraemia, but in the context of a raised CNI level, CNI toxicity should also be considered if that was a true trough level. Given his advancing age and likely immunosenescence, his risk of rejection is low. Therefore, using conventional immunosuppression targets will put him at elevated risk of infections unnecessarily. CMV infection is associated with a significantly increased relative risk of cardiovascular (CVS) disease in older KTRs, and this patient's CVS risk factors, such as diabetes and hypertension, should be well-controlled. He should also be provided support to stop smoking.

Tips and Tricks

1. Consider how therapeutic interventions might confer no benefit to, and even adversely affect, elderly patients.
2. Always assess fall risk, including a postural BP measurement, before up-titrating BP medications, and avoid intensive blood pressure control in very frail patients, especially if non-ambulant and particularly if the pretreatment diastolic BP is low.
3. The use of frailty scores and taking into consideration BMI and comprehensive geriatric assessment can be a useful tool in guiding decisions regarding renal replacement therapy.
4. Changes in the ageing immune system, pharmacokinetics and pharmacodynamics of immunosuppressive drugs used necessitates careful consideration when prescribing immunosuppression for older recipients.
5. A comprehensive evaluation of prospective older transplant recipients should include not only premorbid conditions but also baseline cognition and physical function.
6. Consider additional treatment goals such as independence and quality of life when managing elderly patients.

Chapter Review Questions

1. Should ACE/ARB inhibitors be used as first-line antihypertensive therapy for patients with diabetes-related CKD in the elderly?
2. What is the best anticoagulant to use for stroke prevention in atrial fibrillation (AF) for older patients with CKD?
3. Which type of donor kidney is preferred for older recipients?
4. What is the major cause of graft loss in older KTRs?

Answers

1. Not necessarily: The European Society of Hypertension and the American Heart Association both advise that it is the degree of BP control rather than the agent that had the greatest effect on improving outcomes. In the ALLHAT trial, lisinopril was less effective than chlorthalidone at improving cardiovascular end points. Although trials including IDNT and RENAAL both suggested renoprotective benefits of RAS blockade in type 2 diabetes, it is clear that elderly patients are at higher risk of AKI episodes, electrolyte disturbance and orthostatic hypotension, which should all be considered before commencing RAS blockade. However, all the major heart failure trials included large numbers of older patients and suggested that they would have the same benefit as a younger cohort, which may on balance mean that ACE/ARB therapy would be preferred where possible.
2. Evidence supports the use of NOACs rather than warfarin. Apixaban is the favoured choice due to the lowest proportion of renal clearance (27%)[46] and superiority to warfarin in stroke/VTE prevention seen in the ARISTOTLE trial and, more importantly, reduced risk of major bleeding (HR 0.5).[29]
3. The best patient and graft survival outcomes in older KTRs are in those who receive living donor kidneys. However, older patients who receive ECD kidneys still have better outcomes than those who remain on dialysis.
4. The major cause of graft loss in older KTRs is patient death with a functioning allograft. CVS disease and infection remain the predominant cause of death in older KTRs. A majority of infections occur in the first 6 months post transplantation.

45

References

1. Barnett K, Mercer SW, Norbury M, Watt G, Wyke S, Guthrie B. Epidemiology of multimorbidity and implications for health care, research, and medical education: a cross-sectional study. Lancet (London, England). 2012;380:37–43.
2. Stevens PE, O'Donoghue DJ, de Lusignan S, et al. Chronic kidney disease management in the United Kingdom: NEOERICA project results. Kidney Int. 2007;72:92–9.
3. O'Neill WC. Structure, not just function. Kidney Int. 2014;85:503–5.
4. Bolignano D, Mattace-Raso F, Sijbrands EJ, Zoccali C. The aging kidney revisited: a systematic review. Ageing Res Rev. 2014;14:65–80.
5. Davies DF, Shock NW. Age changes in glomerular filtration rate, effective renal plasma flow, and tubular excretory capacity in adult males. J Clin Invest. 1950;29:496–507.
6. Poggio ED, Rule AD, Tanchanco R, et al. Demographic and clinical characteristics associated with glomerular filtration rates in living kidney donors. Kidney Int. 2009;75:1079–87.
7. Wright JT Jr, Bakris G, Greene T, et al. Effect of blood pressure lowering and antihypertensive drug class on progression of hypertensive kidney disease: results from the AASK trial. JAMA. 2002;288:2421–31.
8. Ruggenenti P, Perna A, Loriga G, et al. Blood-pressure control for renoprotection in patients with non-diabetic chronic renal disease (REIN-2): multicentre, randomised controlled trial. Lancet. 2005;365:939–46.
9. Fried LP, Tangen CM, Walston J, et al. Frailty in older adults: evidence for a phenotype. J Gerontol A Biol Sci Med Sci. 2001;56:M146–56.
10. Beckett NS, Peters R, Fletcher AE, et al. Treatment of hypertension in patients 80 years of age or older. N Engl J Med. 2008;358:1887–98.

11. Poortvliet RK, de Ruijter W, de Craen AJ, et al. Blood pressure trends and mortality: the Leiden 85-plus Study. J Hypertens. 2013;31:63–70.
12. Hansson L, Zanchetti A, Carruthers SG, et al. Effects of intensive blood-pressure lowering and low-dose aspirin in patients with hypertension: principal results of the Hypertension Optimal Treatment (HOT) randomised trial. HOT Study Group. Lancet (London, England). 1998;351:1755–62.
13. Patel MR, Mahaffey KW, Garg J, et al. Rivaroxaban versus warfarin in nonvalvular atrial fibrillation. N Engl J Med. 2011;365:883–91.
14. Agnelli G, Buller HR, Cohen A, et al. Apixaban for extended treatment of venous thromboembolism. N Engl J Med. 2013;368:699–708.
15. Hohnloser SH, Hijazi Z, Thomas L, et al. Efficacy of apixaban when compared with warfarin in relation to renal function in patients with atrial fibrillation: insights from the ARISTOTLE trial. Eur Heart J. 2012;33:2821–30.
16. Alfaadhel TA, Soroka SD, Kiberd BA, Landry D, Moorhouse P, Tennankore KK. Frailty and mortality in dialysis: evaluation of a clinical frailty scale. Clin J Am Soc Nephrol. 2015;10:832–40.
17. Methven S, Steenkamp R, Fraser S. UK renal registry 19th annual report: chapter 5 survival and causes of death in UK adult patients on renal replacement therapy in 2015: national and centre-specific analyses. Nephron. 2017;137(suppl 1):117–50.
18. Kurella Tamura M, Desai M, Kapphahn KI, Thomas IC, Asch SM, Chertow GM. Dialysis versus medical management at different ages and levels of kidney function in veterans with advanced CKD. J Am Soc Nephrol. 2018;29:2169.
19. Oniscu GC, Brown H, Forsythe JL. How great is the survival advantage of transplantation over dialysis in elderly patients? Nephrol Dial Transplant. 2004;19:945–51.
20. Frei U, Noeldeke J, Machold-Fabrizii V, et al. Prospective age-matching in elderly kidney transplant recipients--a 5-year analysis of the Eurotransplant Senior Program. Am J Transplant. 2008;8:50–7.
21. Gill J, Bunnapradist S, Danovitch GM, Gjertson D, Gill JS, Cecka M. Outcomes of kidney transplantation from older living donors to older recipients. Am J Kidney Dis. 2008;52:541–52.
22. Falck P, Asberg A, Byberg KT, et al. Reduced elimination of cyclosporine A in elderly (>65 years) kidney transplant recipients. Transplantation. 2008;86:1379–83.
23. Johnson DW, Nicol DL, Purdie DM, et al. Is mycophenolate mofetil less safe than azathioprine in elderly renal transplant recipients? Transplantation. 2002;73:1158–63.
24. Prevention of stroke by antihypertensive drug treatment in older persons with isolated systolic hypertension. Final results of the Systolic Hypertension in the Elderly Program (SHEP). SHEP Cooperative Research Group. JAMA 1991;265:3255–64.
25. Margolis KL, O'Connor PJ, Morgan TM, et al. Outcomes of combined cardiovascular risk factor management strategies in type 2 diabetes: the ACCORD randomized trial. Diabetes Care. 2014;37:1721–8.

Patient Information and Guidelines

http://www.who.int/news-room/fact-sheets/detail/ageing-and-health

https://www.england.nhs.uk/ourwork/ltc-op-eolc/older-people/improving-care-for-older-people/

The Renal Patient in Critical Care - The ICU: Renal Interface

Katie Lane, Zudin Puthucheary, and Nasirul Jabir Ekbal

Contents

M. Harber (ed.), *Primer on Nephrology*, https://doi.org/10.1007/978-3-030-76419-7_46

Learning Objectives

The learning objectives of this chapter are to understand that

1. Outcome predictors, e.g. APACHE, SOFA scores, used in critical care tend to overestimate mortality in dialysis patients and should be used with caution.
2. Patients with end-stage renal disease (ESRD) have a better ICU and hospital mortality when compared with patients with AKI requiring renal replacement therapy.
3. End-of-life informed decision-making in elderly dialysis patients prior to hospitalisation could prevent unnecessary, aggressive medical interventions and improved use of conservative care pathways.
4. Care of patients with ESRD requires good communication between both the intensive care and nephrology teams from vascular access to medication prescriptions.
5. Renal patients in critical care are at higher risk of muscle wasting and require early intensive rehabilitation.

46.1 Introduction

With the increase in prevalence of chronic kidney disease and the availability of long-term renal replacement therapy, the proportion of patients with pre-existing renal dysfunction developing acute critical illness and necessitating admission to critical care has progressively increased. In the UK, the requirement for an ICU bed is fourfold greater amongst renal patients than the general population. Renal patients also have a higher ICU readmission rate, longer hospital stay and greater overall hospital mortality [1].

The management of the 'critically ill chronic renal patient' has thus become an everyday challenge for both nephrologists and intensive care specialists. The aim of this chapter is to describe the common problems encountered when managing renal patients admitted to critical care and cover aspects of physiology affected by critical illness leading to an acquired functional disability, focussing on the specific interaction related to pre-existing renal failure. This then offers a roadmap to recovery and rehabilitation planning in these patients.

Whilst renal patients are admitted to the ICU for diverse reasons, several predictable frequent causes are found in the literature. Cardiogenic pulmonary oedema, sepsis and management post-cardiac arrest typically account for most admissions to critical care in ESRD, respectively. Predictably, patients with ESRD admitted for elective surgery have a lower mortality when compared with non-surgical admissions and patients undergoing emergency surgery. It is important to distinguish mortality rates in ICU admissions of patients with established end-stage renal failure from those of patients presenting in acute kidney injury (KDIGO 3) requiring renal replacement therapy, in whom in-hospital mortality is nearly fourfold greater [2]. Illness severity scores in critical care (e.g. APACHE II and III and SAPS II) also tend to overestimate illness severity amongst patients on long-term renal replacement therapy (RRT) and should therefore be used with caution for prognostication in patients with ESRD. Thus, patients with ESRD frequently benefit from admission to ICU despite multiple co-morbidities [3].

46.2 Patient-Led Care

As inclusion in long-term renal replacement therapy (RRT) programmes has increased worldwide, so have the age, co-morbidity and frailty of included patients. Advanced care planning for severe illness amongst frailer patients is crucial. Fewer than 10% patients on RRT report having spoken about goals and values and wishes in the context of their illness, despite almost 90% wanting to do so. Likely reasons for this disparity are physician concerns they will upset their patient, uncertainty about predicting outcomes, lack of training and insufficient time to broach the subject. The penalty for missing such end-of-life conversations results in elderly dialysis patients undergoing invasive procedures and aggressive treatments focussed on prolonging life when survival may not be consistent with their personal preferences. Where such discussions do occur, there is an enhanced quality of life for the patient and their family, an enhanced goal-consistent care with greater use of palliative care facilities and an increased likelihood of death out of the hospital setting, mostly without an increase in patient anxiety or distress [4].

46.3 Common Problems in Patients with ESRD on ICU

46.3.1 Access

Arteriovenous fistulae and grafts are inappropriate means of access for continuous renal replacement therapy (CRRT) as prolonged needle placement can damage the access and relatively low flow speeds increases the risk of thrombosis. Instead, a temporary dialysis catheter should be placed for the initiation of RRT. Good communication between the nephrology and critical care team is vital for information regarding previously known central venous stenosis that can maximise success and minimise complications particularly when prompt vascular access is urgently required. If the patient is likely to require prolonged ICU admission, the temporary catheter should be replaced with a cuffed tunnelled dialysis catheter to prevent multiple catheter insertions, as it is imperative to preserve existing venous access in an obtunded patient with few remaining access options. Subclavian vein dialysis catheter placement should be carefully considered, and placement of peripherally inserted central venous catheters (PICC) remains controversial in patients with ESRD, as this site carries the highest risk of subsequent central vein stenosis [5]. In addition, due consideration is necessary prior to placement of temporary venous access on an ipsilateral iliac vein to a functioning renal transplant to reduce risk of graft thrombosis or unintentional arterial injury and thus this site is best avoided.

Pre-existing tunnelled haemodialysis catheters should not be used for routine drug administration to minimise infection and thrombosis risk, although in extremis, they can provide a useful means of immediate wide bore access. Communication between ICU and nephrology staff is important to ensure the line is locked with appropriate antibacterial anticoagulant agent e.g. sodium citrate (DuraLock-C™) after use, as many ICUs may use sodium chloride 0.9% alone to lock lines.

46.3.2 Renal Replacement Therapy for Critically Ill Patients with ESRF

There are no prospective comparative studies of CRRT over intermittent HD (IHD) for the patients in ESRF on ICU. Therefore, the decision regarding the chosen modality is often a pragmatic one based on staff expertise and equipment availability. IHD requires access to an online water supply that meets stringent water purity standards and is provided by a reverse osmosis (RO) system. The necessary piping is usually unavailable in the ICU; however, IHD can be provided using a portable RO connected to a purpose-built water connection at the bedside [6]. Shared protocols detailing patient cohorts suitable for either IHD and continuous veno-venous haemofiltration (CVVH) or CVVH only on the ICU should be discussed and agreed between the intensive care and nephrology teams. The advantage of IHD is that existing vascular access can be used without the need for additional temporary access; however, in situations of haemodynamic instability and multi-organ failure, CRRT is preferable to minimise further alterations in blood pressure and fluid shifts. Similarly, in the context of acute brain injury or elevated intracranial pressure, e.g. in trauma or patients with fulminant hepatic failure, CRRT is recommended for maintaining cerebral perfusion pressure to avoid exacerbating neurological dysfunction [7].

Peritoneal dialysis (PD) may be continued in established patients during critical illness. However, difficulty fine-tuning fluid shifts, a tendency for hypo-osmolar hyponatraemia due to the inability to excrete a free-water load, intra-abdominal pressure considerations, impaired nutrition and thermoregulation have limited its use, and usually temporary extracorporeal renal therapy is established in the acute setting unless in extreme circumstances in patients unable to have CVVH due to a complete lack of vascular access. In addition, technical aspects and a thorough understanding of the PD prescription are factors that play key roles in achieving adequate PD. Notwithstanding, when the recovery phase of critical illness starts, patients who were on maintenance IHD or PD therapies prior to ICU admission can restart, with intermittent therapies facilitating mobilisation and rehabilitation. An exception is breach of the peritoneal cavity due to acute abdominal injury, leading to the inability to perform PD and requirement for conversion to extracorporeal therapy.

46.3.3 Nutrition in ICU

Malnutrition, often a chronic problem in patients with end-stage renal disease, is exacerbated in the setting of acute illness. Calculation of energy and protein requirements is complicated during critical illness, particularly when a patient requires RRT. Some RRT fluids contain energy substrates (citrate, glucose, lactate) that must be accounted for to prevent overfeeding and problems with glycaemic control. Citrate-mediated filtration can provide an additional 300 kcal/day to a patient. The use of concentrated renal feeds (e.g. Nepro®HP – which also contains the highest protein concentration of the supplements – Abbot Laboratories Ltd) in patients unable to self-feed can minimise volume overload. Water-soluble vitamin loss may also be severe during CRRT, particularly in those with suboptimal enteral absorption. In such circumstances, parenteral supplementation may be required. No supplementation of fat-soluble vitamins is usually required.

46.3.4 Electrolyte Abnormalities

46.3.4.1 Hyperkalaemia

The management of a patient with ESRD and severe hyperkalaemia can be challenging. Over ninety percent of potassium excretion occurs via the kidneys, with the remainder occurring via the gut. Priorities of care are to stabilise the myocardium where there is evidence of cardiac conduction abnormality, whilst preparing an urgent means of RRT to reduce total body potassium concentration. Hyperkalaemia leads to suppression of impulse generation by the sino-atrial node and reduced conduction by the AV node and Purkinje system. This results in bradycardia, conduction blocks and ultimately cardiac arrest if left untreated.

The ideal initial treatment for severe hyperkalaemia in ESRD is high-flow haemodialysis or haemodiafiltration to rapidly reduce serum potassium to a safer level, followed by a gentler and gradual removal of potassium, all of which should be done in an environment with close continuous cardiac monitoring and regular reassessment of blood biochemistry, preferably with point-of-care testing. Frequently, there are locally determined practical limitations that preclude optimal care. For example, a physician may need to decide whether rapid haemodialysis of a patient with an established functional fistula or graft on an inpatient haemodialysis unit (albeit with less ability to monitor the patient and fewer nursing staff) would overall be safer than the inherent delay of ICU admission, temporary dialysis catheter insertion and slower potassium removal of CRRT, despite the presence of a higher nurse-to-patient ratio enabling closer monitoring and better access to point-of-care testing. Regardless of location, a patient should receive close cardiac monitoring for several hours after HD. Blood glucose concentration must also be closely observed in patients who have received insulin to temporise hyperkalaemia to ensure hypoglycaemia is treated promptly. If a patient has sustained a hyperkalaemic cardiac arrest, subsequent ICU admission is strongly advised.

Insufficiently expedient institution of RRT to remove potassium can lead to rebound hyperkalaemia in patients with ESRD and minimal renal function: potassium moved intracellularly with insulin therapy leaks back into the extracellular space where it remains due to the lack of renal function. Therefore, it is important to monitor closely for rebound. More recently, sodium zirconium cyclosilicate and Patiromer have been recommended for acute life-threatening hyperkalaemia in adults in emergency care alongside standard care described above [8]. These may have a key role in avoiding the need for RRT in patients with recovering AKI or permitting safe transfer of dialysis patients from institutions that lack dialysis facilities to a dialysis unit thus avoiding the need for ICU admission and acute vascular access.

Some propose that high potassium gradients and consequent rapid potassium shifts put the patient at higher risk of myocardial arrhythmias than hyperkalaemia per se [9]. There are no studies to guide serum potassium reduction targets in hyperkalaemia, but serial monitoring of ECG morphology can be a useful guide. It is important to ensure that post-IHD hypokalaemia (whilst awaiting equilibration of total body potassium that may well remain high) is not overzealously treated by the critical care team (used to supplementing potassium to achieve a target of 4–4.5 mmol/L). Conversely, it may be necessary to replace sustained significant hypokalaemia and hypophosphataemia, induced by CRRT.

46.3.4.2 Hypocalcaemia

Patients with advanced CKD may have hypocalcaemia due to altered calcium-phosphate balance and impaired vitamin D activation. If treated with sodium bicarbonate for the management of acidosis or hyperkalaemia, exacerbated hypocalcaemia can worsen precipitating tetany, seizures and cardiac arrhythmias. In addition, the use of citrate anticoagulation for RRT may exacerbate underlying hypocalcaemia due to the chelation of serum calcium. Treatment of hypocalcaemia is with bolus and/or infusion of calcium gluconate or chloride through a large vein to avoid thrombophlebitis. Coincident hypomagnesaemia may also require treatment.

46.4 Medication in the ICU in Patients with ESRD

46.4.1 Drug Dosing

Drug dosing in a critically ill patient is complex. In the case of antimicrobials, under- and overdosing can have significant adverse consequences for the patient. Alterations in extracellular volume, protein binding and renal and hepatic function can also significantly alter the concentration of drugs and their efficacy. Drug removal frequently varies with modality of renal replacement therapy, blood flow rate, filter surface area and age. There is large individual variability in vancomycin pharmacokinetic and pharmacodynamic target attainment in ICU patients. As a result, it is essential to seek the expert advice of a critical care renal pharmacist. Therapeutic drug monitoring should be used for antimicrobials particularly aminoglycosides and glycopeptides to prevent toxicity in patients with reduced renal function.

46.4.2 Rationalisation of Medication

Multiple medications, though may be indicated and be of benefit, increase the burden of polypharmacy in chronic kidney disease. However, on admission to ICU, these medications often continue to be prescribed by the intensive care team, in-part due to unfamiliarity of their use and/or their mechanism of action. One example are phosphate binders. Phosphate has a molecular weight of only 95 Daltons and is therefore easily cleared by CVVH as the longer treatment time allows greater phosphate transfer leading to hypophosphataemia, even in patients with renal disease. Therefores, medication to reduce phosphate absorption from the gut become redundant. Similarly, erythropoiesis-stimulating agent (ESA) therapy act has a delayed mechanism of action (typically 3–4 days), and many critically ill patients present with ESA resistance due to the presence of inflammatory mediators impairing erythropoietin cell proliferation. ESA use may be appropriate in selected patients in whom blood transfusion is not appropriate for religious reasons (e.g. Jehovah's witnesses). Intravenous (IV) iron does not reduce transfusion requirements in the general critical care population and may even inflict cellular oxidative stress or increase infection risk by invading microorganisms [10]. However, in patients with ESRD, IV iron may be a useful adjunct in the recovery stage of critical illness after the sepsis and systemic inflammatory response have been treated. Thus, the need for medications used to treat anaemia of chronic renal disease should be reviewed in the acute stages of critical illness.

46.5 Patient with Renal Transplant in Critical Care

46.5.1 Acute Phase

Post-transplant care is widely protocolised and in many centres patients return to a monitored area on a specialised ward, rather than routinely requiring critical care admission. When a patient requires ICU admission post-operatively, particular attention to communication with the multidisciplinary team will be needed to ensure the usual focus on timely medication dosing and avoidance of establishing central access close to the renal transplant. A clear plan to inform the renal team of sudden decreases in urine output will be important to ensure vascular problems are investigated and dealt with expediently. Where a patient is unable to take immunosuppressant medication by mouth, the need for nasogastric access or alternative sublingual or intravenous preparations should be anticipated. The timing of therapeutic drug monitoring should be explained to nursing staff that may be less familiar with protocols to ensure accurate drug concentrations are available for dose alteration.

46.5.2 Chronic Phase

Severe sepsis is a common cause of death amongst renal transplant recipients. A frequent dilemma is whether some or all the immunosuppressant medication should at least temporarily be withheld. Although there is general acceptance of the benefit of short-term reduction in immunosuppression in life-threatening infections, there is little consensus of what should be withheld and the duration. There is no definite evidence that immunosuppressant reduction at the time of infection reduces mortality, but there is little evidence that it leads to increased transplant rejection [11]. Nephrologists and ICU consultants need to carefully weigh the risks and benefits of reducing or maintaining immunosuppression; significant loss of renal transplant function is associated with an important reduction in life expectancy, as is a death secondary to sepsis. However, early definitive respiratory tract sampling (ideally obtaining bronchoscopic washings sent for fungal and viral screens) should be encouraged if safe to do so, given the broad range of potential pathogens including opportunistic ones and the advantages of timely targeted therapy.

The remainder of this chapter discusses recovery from critical illness with issues specific to patients with renal failure and the critical outreach: renal interface.

46.6 Critical Illness Recovery

Mortality from critical illness is decreasing worldwide resulting in increasing numbers of critical illness survivors However, this survival is not cost-free: long-term disability is common amongst this cohort with 50% of survivors not returning to work within the first year and 30% of those of a working age needing caregiver assistance to manage their activities of daily living [12]. This disability is primarily physical in nature, because of significant muscle wasting (rates of 2–3% a day) and the inability of interventions during critical illness to ameliorate this. Physical disabilities can persist for up to 5 years post critical illness and are associated with an increased risk of death [13]. Overlaying this are the cognitive deficits seen because of critical illness, loss of short-term memory, difficulty in complex task planning, depression and post-traumatic stress disorders. These are both contributors to the poor quality of life in survivors and confounders in engagement with rehabilitation.

All of this is relevant to patients suffering from chronic renal failure who become critically ill and survive. Prognostication of survival and morbidity in these patients is more complex than the average critically ill patient because of multiple factors:

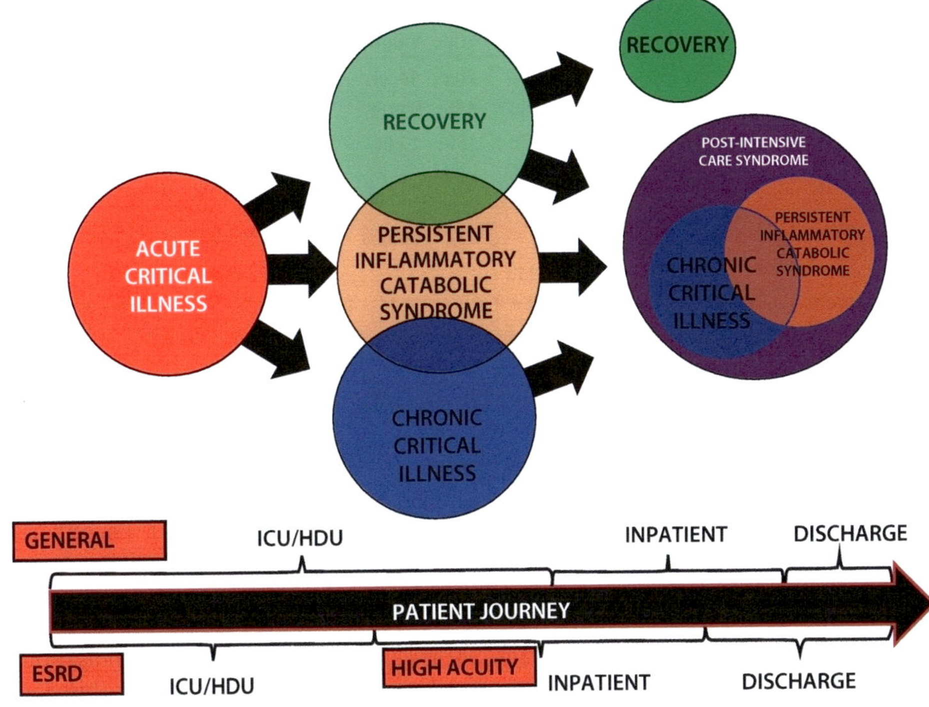

Fig. 46.1 Journey to recovery in general and nephrology critical illness survivors

- As discussed above, acute illness scores often overestimating mortality in ESRD.
- Clinical frailty is associated with both mortality and morbidity in the critically ill [14] and patients with ESRD often fulfil frailty criteria.
- Newly emerging intermediate syndromes such as chronic critical illness and persistent inflammatory catabolic syndrome are likely to exist in patients undergoing ward-based therapy post intensive care discharge (Fig. 46.1).
- The overall prevalence of delirium on the inpatient hospital setting is estimated between 14 and 24% [15].

46.7 Skeletal Muscle Mass

Acute skeletal muscle wasting occurs rapidly in critical illness and is related to severity of illness: Greater organ dysfunction results in greater muscle wasting, with rates of 2–3% loss per day [16]. This is underpinned by altered protein homeostasis. In the acute phase, muscle protein synthesis is depressed and recovery variable over time. In chronic critical illness, rates of muscle protein breakdown are seen to rise. Associated with this quantitative loss is a qualitative loss; myonecrosis is seen in up to 40% of patients, with an associated fasciitis, likely further contributing to loss of function. Patients with renal dysfunction are specifically at risk of muscle wasting and the functional consequences of low muscle mass because of interactions between predisposing factors and the physiology of critical illness.

46.8 Baseline Muscle Mass and Function

Low baseline muscle mass and quality are associated with both critical illness mortality and subsequent decreased independence. This is unsurprising, given that, all things being equal, muscle mass is the major determinant of muscle function. Both loss of muscle mass and function are well described in chronic stable kidney disease, which places these patients at high risk of subsequent functional disability [17].

Increasingly the critical care community is aware that the presence of pre-existing chronic diseases results in a differential trajectory of recovery from those without. Patients with renal disease therefore will require a combination of different rehabilitation strategies and different recovery goals compared to previously healthy individuals. Defining this population is crucial for the development of clinical programmes, and the clinical definitions of frailty are being increasingly demonstrated to be useful in doing so. Figure 46.2 demonstrates the impact of pre-existing clinical frailty on discharge destinations of critical illness survivors [14].

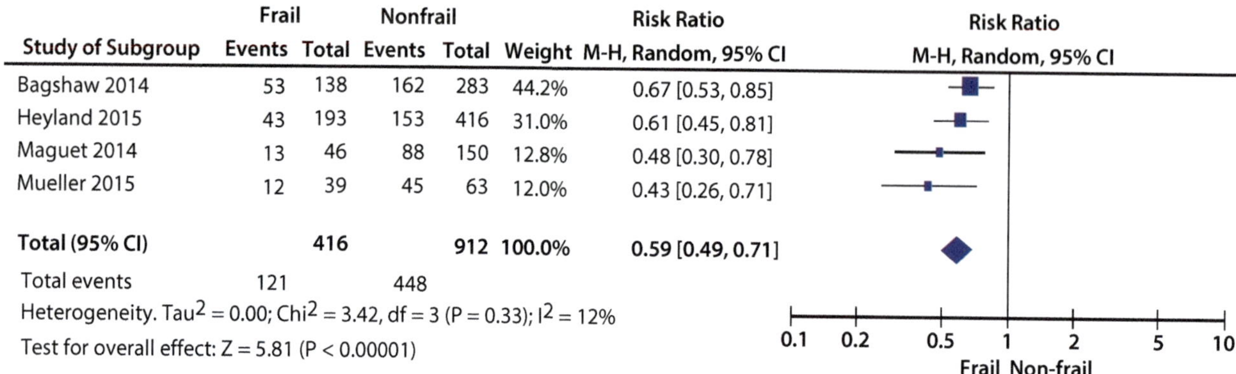

Fig. 46.2 Meta-analysis of discharge destination studies in critically ill patients with and without clinical frailty. From Muscedere Intensive Care Medicine 2017 [14]

46.9 Altered Protein Homeostasis

Muscle mass is maintained by protein homeostasis, a balance between muscle protein synthesis and muscle protein breakdown. In humans, protein synthesis is the process primarily affected by stimuli, both adverse and favourable. In the acute phase of critical illness, muscle protein synthesis is depressed and recovers variably over time. In chronic critical illness, rates of muscle protein breakdown are seen to rise patients with renal disease who are then at further at risk of the consequences and drivers of altered protein homeostasis, with decreased protein synthesis having been described in stable chronic kidney disease [18]. The same factors affect both acute and chronic decreased muscle protein synthesis and need to be addressed for muscle mass to be gained.

46.10 Immobilisation

In bed-rest models, a week of immobilisation results in a decrease in muscle protein synthesis and an appreciable reduction of muscle mass. Importantly this predisposes the patient to further, accelerated muscle mass loss and affects skeletal muscle metabolism. Reversing the effects of immobilisation (acutely) requires resistance exercise, the simple provision of nutrition alone cannot do so. Whilst the exact amount of time required will vary between patients, it is likely to be in the order of minutes per day [19]. This can be seen in the clear differences between patients mobilised early versus those who are not in randomised controlled trials; return to independent functionals status occurred in 59% in the interventional group compared with only 35% in the control group [20]. Incorporating mobilisation into daily care is not straightforward, with multiple barriers existing (Fig. 46.3). These barriers include lack of education regarding the importance of mobilisation, unfounded safety concerns and poor teamworking [21].

A major step forward is the realisation amongst clinicians that mobilisation is a therapeutic intervention and encouraging this, e.g. in sitting patients out of bed for meals, will improve patient outcomes.

46.11 Inflammation

Systemic inflammation suppresses muscle protein synthesis, as does intramuscular inflammation. Whilst both occur during critical illness, persistent low-grade inflammation occurs in survivors and is seen post-hospital discharge [22]. In addition to the immunosuppressive effects, persistent inflammation represents a major physiological barrier to physical recovery, in that it impedes muscle protein synthesis and amino acid uptake by skeletal muscle, rendering exercise and nutritional interventions ineffective. Post-intensive care, patients with chronic kidney disease have multiple causes for persistent inflammation. This may be related to critical illness (persistent unexplained inflammation), secondary to new infections, the result of systemic inflammatory diseases common in this population or lastly as a feature of chronic kidney disease. Regardless of the aetiology, a cause for such inflammation needs to be ascertained and treated to allow recovery of normal protein homeostasis.

46.12 Age

Elderly patients demonstrate anabolic resistance, whilst basal muscle protein synthetic rates are similar to that of younger patients, their synthetic response to resistance

Barriers	Enablers
Diagnosis & illness severity, age & comorbidities **Sedation, delirium & pain** **Pt psychological state (e.g. motivation)**	• Sedation, delirium & pain management • Patient goal setting & family involvement • Sleep
Physiological stability **Concern for line safety & risk of line removal** **concern for risk of HCP or caregiver injury**	• Establish institutional safety guidelines for PA • Removal / secure of lines • Education re: safety with lines in situ and PA
Poor culture, teamwork, & leadership **Lack of expertise & skill training** **Need for physician orders prior to rehap**	• Develop positive culture, MDT team meetings • Interprofessional expertise / skill training • Ward rounds & site visits to est programs • Routine mobility orders • Designated leaders & discipline champions
Motivations & beliefs regarding the benefit / harm of PA interventions	• Education re: importance & benefit of PA • Positive experiences / storytelling of success
Lack of funding & access to PT services **Lack of equipment, resources & staffing** **Lack of time & competing priorities**	• Automatic referral pathways for PA interventions • Illustrate cost saving benefit / business case • Dedicated equipment & staffing • Coordination of schedules within MDT • Mobility protocol, ABCDE bundle & mobility team

Fig. 46.3 Barriers and enablers of mobilisation. From Parry et al. Intensive Care Medicine 2017 [21]

exercise amino acid intake is blunted, in addition is the blunting of muscle protein breakdown to insulin [23]. Elderly patients thus require either more frequent (exercise) or greater concentrations (amino acids) to achieve a similar synthetic response. Whilst age is a non-modifiable risk factor, it remains an important factor in rehabilitation and recovery planning. Separate, tailored interventions are likely to be needed, unlike in younger individuals.

46.13 Acidosis

The effect of metabolic acidosis on muscle mass and protein homeostasis in patients with kidney disease has been well described, as has the reversal of these effects with therapeutic sodium bicarbonate [24]. Metabolic acidosis impairs muscle protein synthesis, and whilst trial data are conflicting as regards the response to acidosis derangement in adults, this is likely to be an over-simplification. No single intervention is likely to correct muscle protein homeostasis in the setting of the complex physiology of chronic renal disease. Rather, a complex or multifaceted intervention is likely to be needed. Correction of acute or chronic metabolic acidosis is most likely to be part of this.

46.14 Interventions to Increase Anabolism and Recovery

Neither trials of increased nutritional delivery in acute critical illness nor early exercise has delivered improvements in functional outcomes or mortality. Once functional deficits are established, they have proven to be difficult to reverse or ameliorate emphasising the need for novel approaches to *primary prevention*. Therefore, patients with chronic kidney disease admitted as in-patients should be treated as being (by definition) at risk of muscle wasting in the same fashion as the elderly and those suffering from chronic obstructive pulmonary disease.

Mobilisation and resistance exercise should be part of the daily in-patient routine, with an 'opt-out' approach taken by the clinical team as opposed to requiring a daily prescription. Amino acid intake and specifically essential amino acids are required for muscle protein synthesis. Exercise without amino acids is a catabolic stimulus and detrimental to patients. In the absence of specific data pertaining to nutrition and muscle gain post critical illness, clinical practise should be in line with the kidney disease outcomes quality initiative, delivering 0.6 g protein/kg/day in non-dialysed patients and 1.2/kg/day for patients undergoing haemodialysis

[25]. Ideally this would be timed to occur post exercise to maximise the synergistic effects on muscle protein synthesis. In the elderly patient, this would be even more efficient if delivered in equitable portions across the day, again maximising synthetic opportunities.

46.15 The Role of Sleep and Delirium in Facilitating and Preventing Rehabilitation

On discharge from ICU, patients frequently suffer from disturbed sleep. This is multi-factorial, because of high levels of noise, poor light management within the ICU, lack of direct sunlight or routine, pharmacological treatment and delirium [26]. The culmination of this is a combination of reversed sleep/wake cycles, poor concentration and engagement with staff and rehabilitation. Whilst hyperactive delirium is commonly recognised, hypoactive delirium is not and often mistaken for sleep, contributing to the issues surrounding sleep deprivation listed above.

Patients with stable kidney disease suffer from both alterations in normal sleep patterns and quality [27] with a high incidence of delirium [28]. The addition of a critical illness therefore represents an acute-on-chronic effect, which, in addition to affecting patients' health-related quality of life, will prevent engagement with rehabilitation and therefore impede recovery. Several measures have been proposed to improve sleep quality. Fundamental to this is the environmental set up, light and noise regulation on the ward needs to be enforced, as does the timings of nursing observations and drug rounds, ensuring that these occur early in the evening [26].

A daily routine and diary are useful aid in orientation and structure provision, as is exposure to direct sunlight. The use of earplugs and sleep masks can aid uninterrupted sleep and transition to deeper stage sleep and rapid-eye movement sleep, both necessary for well-being. Lastly, patients should be screened regularly for delirium. In the setting of a high-acuity patient, the Confusion Assessment Method for the ICU (CAM-ICU) score would seem useful in capturing those with both hyper- and hypoactive delirium. Using the CAM-ICU assessment tool, patients are screened for an acute change or fluctuating course of mental status together with inattention and either altered consciousness or disorganised thinking [29]. If the above criteria are met, the patient is CAM-ICU positive and requires management of delirium, a goal in its own right, in addition to facilitating rehabilitation. A full discussion on the pathophysiology, incidence and management of delirium is beyond the scope of this chapter, though it is of clear relevance.

46.16 Anticipation of Deterioration (the ICU Outreach): Renal Interface

Whilst some risks for readmission and adverse outcomes are fixed and intrinsic to the renal patient, some risks may be modifiable. Therefore, it is good practice to identify and intervene early in patients at risk of deterioration through use of a SBAR or I-PASS multidisciplinary handover on the renal ward (Fig. 46.4). Evidence for effective resident handovers is associated with a reduction in medical error rate of 23% from a pre-intervention period to the post-intervention period [30]. Similarly, it is important to ensure robust processes are in place for post-discharge review of ICU survivors to renal wards who are often frail and at risk of subsequent readmission.

46.17 Conclusion

In summary, rehabilitation strategies for patients who survive critical care remain suboptimal. Many experience significant and persistent physical, cognitive and post-traumatic problems after discharge. For patients with complex co-morbidities such as ESRD, the after-

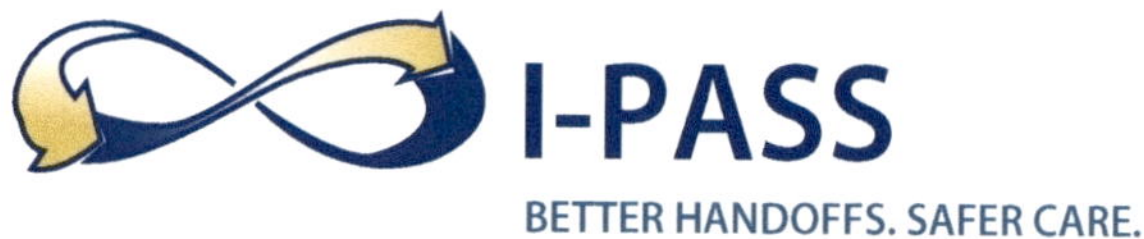

I	Illness Severity	• Stable, "watcher," unstable
P	Patient Summary	• Summary statement • Evens leading up to admission • Hospital course • Ongoing assessment • Plan
A	Action List	• To do list • Time line and ownership
S	Situation Awareness and Contingency Planning	• Know what's going on • Plan for what might happen
S	Synthesis by Receiver	• Receiver summarizes what was heard • Asks questions • Restates key action/to do Items

Fig. 46.4 Elements of the I-PASS mnemonic. From Waltz et al. Curr Pediatr Rep 2019 [30]

care needs are even more fraught with a greater likelihood of long-term difficulties. Therefore, optimisation of recovery as a goal of therapy rather than just survival has gained increasing importance with the role of the multidisciplinary team, with the full spectrum of clinical skills (from medical to occupational therapy) needed to offer a fully holistic approach to patients with such complex rehabilitation needs.

Case Study

Case 1

An 83-year-old male patient had been dialysing for 11 years. He began to report a number of falls to and from his haemodialysis sessions. He also was noted to have difficulty with ultrafiltration during dialysis sessions despite being over his dry weight and a raised BNP. An echocardiogram conducted showed that he had critical aortic stenosis with an AV gradient of 0.6. He declined intervention and over a period of 6 months had admissions with breathlessness and pulmonary oedema. An advanced care planning meeting was conducted with the patient, his dialysis consultant and his son (his next of kin). The patient's priorities of care were discussed. He stated that he understood the difficult situation that he faced – untreatable aortic valve disease with a failing left ventricle causing recurrent pulmonary oedema unable to be treated with ultrafiltration. He opted for ongoing dialysis as he was at that time not ready to withdraw from dialysis but knew that this would soon be inevitable and ceiling of ward-based care placed should he be admitted to hospital. This was documented in his notes and a community do not resuscitate order completed. Three months after this conversation, he was admitted again with pulmonary oedema but was so hypotensive that ultrafiltration was not possible. In view of the discussions documented in the advanced planning meeting, the hospital team were able to have frank discussions with his son who was prepared for his death, and the decision was made to stop dialysis with end-of-life care measures instituted under the guidance of the palliative care team. He died peacefully with his family around him.

This care illustrates that advanced care meetings are invaluable in preventing unnecessary, invasive treatments and interventions in elderly dialysis patients when survival may not be consistent with their personal preferences.

Case 2

A 65-year-old patient with ESRF secondary to diabetes was admitted with line sepsis. Unfortunately, he went on to develop multi-organ failure. Despite his acute respiratory distress syndrome resolving by day 6, he remained ventilator dependent, and on day 10, on awakening he was diagnosed with ICU-AW. He was noted to have a poor cough. A percutaneous tracheostomy was performed at day 12, and respiratory weaning commenced. By day 20 he had been weaned to nocturnal CPAP but suffered from hypoactive delirium. A secondary chest infection necessitated full ventilation again, and he was eventually decannulated by day 40. His cough remained poor, and he was noted to be dysphagic, requiring ongoing nasogastric feeding. He was discharged to the renal ward on day 60. He was too disabled to be discharged home as he struggled to mobilise from bed to chair. He was eventually discharged to a nursing home. His family later communicated to the renal team that the patient would have never wished to have such a poor quality of life and with hindsight had he known the eventual outcome would have never wished to have been admitted to the intensive care unit.

This case illustrates the impact of muscle wasting on critically ill patients, and survival is likely to come with significant physical disability.

Tips and Tricks

Notwithstanding their complexity, patient with end-stage renal failure, despite chronic co-morbidity, often benefits from ICU admission, and therefore long-term dependence on dialysis should not prejudice against prompt referral to critical care in the event of an acute illness. Critical care therapy is not just about ventilation; ensure that all options regarding organ support e.g. vasopressor support and high-flow nasal cannula therapy, are discussed with a senior intensive care physician prior to a decision to decline critical care admission.

However, it is crucial to recognise that due to its chronic nature, patients with pre-existing renal dysfunction know much about their co-morbidities and have insight into their disease and prognosis. It is important to explain escalation therapies, e.g. CPR in the event of a cardio-respiratory arrest or admission to ICU due to an acute illness. This is best discussed in the calm of an outpatient clinic rather than the chaos of an emergency room. Know your patients' attitudes and preferences with a focus on quality of life and goal-consistent care in critical illness and end-of-life situations. Clearly document these in an advanced care plan for others to see when the moment inevitably arises!

Chapter Review Questions

1. What is the most common cause of admission to critical care for dialysis patients?
2. Which is the best central venous access for patients with a functioning renal transplant?
3. What are the common arrythmias associated with hyperkalaemia seen in patient with end-stage renal disease?
4. What is the major physiological process that leads to muscle wasting in critical care or dialysis patients?
5. What is required in addition to adequate nutrition to increase muscle mass and improve function?

Answers

1. Due to the increased risk of cardiovascular disease amongst patients with chronic kidney disease and the increased risk of fluid overload particularly in anuric patients, pulmonary oedema is the most common cause for ICU admission.
2. The latest KDOQI guidelines state the following order of preference for venous access: RIJV, RIFV and LIJV followed by subclavian vein. However, it is important that in renal transplant patients (the renal transplant is usually placed in the right iliac fossa), the right femoral vein is best avoided as cannulation of the ipsilateral iliac vein to a functioning renal transplant may increase the risk of graft thrombosis or unintentional arterial injury.
3. Hyperkalaemia is common in patients with dialysis, particularly if compliance with dialysis and/or dietary potassium restriction is poor. Due to its chronicity, arrythmias may not be seen until the presence of severe hyperkalaemia. A serum potassium over 7.0 mmol/L is associated with conduction abnormalities e.g. bundle branch block. The presence of sinus bradycardia or slow atrial fibrillation heralds imminent depression of electrical activity and in dialysis patients signifies that urgent renal replacement is required.
4. Decreased muscle protein synthesis is the major abnormality, not increased muscle protein breakdown.
5. Resistance exercise and sleep.

References

1. Hutchison CA, Crowe AV, Stevens PE, Harrison DA, Lipkin GW. Case mix, outcome and activity for patients admitted to intensive care units requiring chronic renal dialysis: a secondary analysis of the ICNARC Case Mix Programme Database. Crit Care. 2007;11(2):1–14.
2. Chan O, Ostermann M. Outcomes of chronic hemodialysis patients in the intensive care unit. Crit Care Res Pract. 2013;2013:715807.
3. Arulkumaran N, Annear NMP, Singer M. Patients with end-stage renal disease admitted to the intensive care unit: systematic review. Br J Anaesth. 2013;110(1):13–20.
4. Mandel E, Bernacki REBS. Serious illness conversations in ESRD. Clin J Am Soc Nephrol. 2017;12(5):854–63.
5. Lok C, et al. KDOQI Clinical Practice Guideline for Vascular Access: 2019 Update. Am J Kid Dis. 2020;75(4):S1–S164.
6. Ronco C, Bellomo R, Kellum J, Ricci Z. Critical care nephrology. 3rd ed. Philadelpha, Elsevier.
7. Karkar A, Ronco C. Prescription of CRRT: a pathway to optimize therapy. Ann Intensive Care. 2020;10:32.
8. Rosano G, Spoletini I, Agewall S. Pharmacology of new treatments for hyperkalaemia: patiromer and sodium zirconium cyclosilicate. Eur Heart J Suppl. 2019;21(Suppl A):A28–33.
9. Santoro A, Mancini E, London G, Mercadal L, Fessy H, Perrone B, et al. Patients with complex arrhythmias during and after haemodialysis suffer from different regimens of potassium removal. Nephrol Dial Transplant. 2008;23(4):1415–21.
10. Litton E, Lim J. Iron metabolism: an emerging therapeutic target in critical illness. Crit Care. 2019;23(1):81.
11. Shih C, Tarng D, Yang W, Yang C. Immunosuppressant dose reduction and long-term rejection risk in renal transplant recipients with severe bacterial pneumonia. Singap Med J. 2014;55(201):372–7.
12. Wischmeyer PE, Puthucheary Z, San Millán I, Butz D, Grocott MPW. Muscle mass and physical recovery in ICU: innovations for targeting of nutrition and exercise. Curr Opin Crit Care. 2017;23(4):269–78.
13. Herridge MS, Tansey CM, Matté A, et al. Functional disability 5 years after acute respiratory distress syndrome. New Engl J Med. 2011;364(14):1293–304.
14. Muscedere J, Waters B, Varambally A, et al. The impact of frailty on intensive care unit outcomes: a systematic review and meta-analysis. Intensive Care Med. 2017;43(8):1105–22.
15. Fong TG, Tulebaev SR, Inouye SK. Delirium in elderly adults: diagnosis, prevention and treatment. Nat Rev Neurol. 2009 Apr;5(4):210–20.
16. Puthucheary ZA, Rawal J, McPhail M, et al. Acute skeletal muscle wasting in critical illness. JAMA. 2013;310(15):1591–600.
17. Fried LF, Lee JS, Shlipak M, et al. Chronic kidney disease and functional limitation in older people: health, aging and body composition study. J Am Geriatr Soc. 2006;54(5):750–6.
18. Bohe J, Rennie MJ. Muscle protein metabolism during hemodialysis. J Ren Nutr. 2006;16(1):3–16.
19. Gibson JN, Smith K, Rennie MJ. Prevention of disuse muscle atrophy by means of electrical stimulation: maintenance of protein synthesis. Lancet. 1988;2(8614):767–70.
20. Schweickert WD, Pohlman MC, Pohlman AS, et al. Early physical and occupational therapy in mechanically ventilated, critically ill patients: a randomised controlled trial. Lancet. 2009;373(9678):1874–82.
21. Parry SM, Knight LD, Connolly B, Baldwin C, Puthucheary Z, Morris P, Mortimore J, Hart N, Denehy L, Granger CL. Factors influencing physical activity and rehabilitation in survivors of critical illness: a systematic review of quantitative and qualitative studies. Intensive Care Med. 2017;43(4):531–42.
22. Yende S, D'Angelo G, Kellum JA, et al. Inflammatory markers at hospital discharge predict subsequent mortality after pneumonia and sepsis. Am J Respir Crit Care Med. 2008;177(11):1242–7.
23. Wilkes EA, Selby AL, Atherton PJ, et al. Blunting of insulin inhibition of proteolysis in legs of older subjects may contribute to age-related sarcopenia. Am J Clin Nutr. 2009;90(5):1343–50.
24. Stein A, Moorhouse J, Iles-Smith H, et al. Role of an improvement in acid-base status and nutrition in CAPD patients. Kidney Int. 1997;52(4):1089–95.

25. National KF. K/DOQI clinical practice guidelines for chronic kidney disease: evaluation, classification, and stratification. Am J Kidney Dis. 2002;39(2 Suppl 1):S1–266.
26. Bion V, Lowe A, Puthucheary Z, Montgomery H. Reducing sound and light exposure to improve sleep on the adult intensive care unit: an inclusive narrative review. J Intensive Care Soc. 2017:1–9.
27. Iliescu EA, Coo H, McMurray MH, et al. Quality of sleep and health-related quality of life in haemodialysis patients. Nephrol Dial Transplant. 2003;18(1):126–32.
28. Murray AM, Pederson SL, Tupper DE, et al. Acute variation in cognitive function in hemodialysis patients: a cohort study with repeated measures. Am J Kidney Dis. 2007;50(2):270–8.
29. Gusmao-Flores D, Salluh JI, Chalhub RÁ, Quarantini LC. The confusion assessment method for the intensive care unit (CAM-ICU) and intensive care delirium screening checklist (ICDSC) for the diagnosis of delirium: a systematic review and meta-analysis of clinical studies. Crit Care. 2012;16(4):R115.
30. Walz A, Emrath E, Mack E. Communication in the PICU: handoffs of care. Curr Pediatr Rep. 2019;7:123–9.

Patient Information and Guidelines

Booklet for patients advanced kidney disease planning for end-of-life care; https://heeoe.hee.nhs.uk/sites/default/files/nhs_advanced_kidney_disease_planning_for_end_of_life_care_booklet_dnacpr_info_entry_pg_30.pdf

Oncology and the Kidney

Olivia Lucas, Steven Law, and Mark Harber

Contents

M. Harber (ed.), *Primer on Nephrology*, https://doi.org/10.1007/978-3-030-76419-7_47

Learning Objectives

1. To understand the incidence and prognosis of malignancy in patients with renal disease.
2. To learn the causes of renal dysfunction associated with malignancy.
3. To assess the causes of renal dysfunction associated with cancer treatment.
4. To appreciate the need for a holistic multidisciplinary team approach for patients with cancer and renal disease.

47.1 Introduction

> The relationship between malignancy and renal disease is complex and bidirectional, with both conditions increasing the risk, and worsening the outcome, of the other.

Cancer can affect the kidney in three main ways: (1) direct involvement via infiltration of the kidney or urinary tract causing obstructive nephropathy, (2) treatment-related nephrotoxicity (direct toxicity or due to treatment complications) and (3) glomerular, tubular or other disorders secondary to remote tumour effects. In addition, malignancy can complicate decisions regarding renal replacement therapy.

End-stage renal disease, dialysis and renal transplantation are each associated with a higher incidence of cancer and a worse oncological prognosis. Furthermore, many of the symptoms of malignancy can mimic the non-specific symptoms of advanced renal disease, causing diagnostic delay and more advanced disease at diagnosis. Investigation of suspected malignancy frequently involves contrast media and is often delayed or avoided in the setting of impaired renal function. Treatment choices may be limited by renal function and dosing more cautious. Patients with end-stage renal disease have a poorer survival than the general population even prior to the impact of a cancer diagnosis.

Given these issues, a multidisciplinary approach is essential to optimise outcomes in this complex patient group.

47.2 Epidemiology

Patients with cancer are at high risk of acute kidney injury (AKI) [1]. A Danish study of 37,267 cancer patients demonstrated an 18% 1-year risk of acute kidney injury with 5% of these patients requiring long-term haemodialysis within one year [2]. Causes of AKI include those seen in the non-cancer population, with additional cancer-specific factors (◘ Fig. 47.1). The incidence of AKI is higher in certain cancer types, such as kidney cancer (44%), multiple myeloma (32%) and liver cancer (33%), and AKI is independently associated with mortality, which worsens further with increasing AKI stage [2, 3]. AKI occurs in up to 53% of cancer patients requiring intensive care with 32% of these requiring renal replacement therapy and 6% of survivors requiring chronic dialysis [4, 5]. Despite this, a small cohort study showed that having cancer had no impact on mortality from AKI requiring renal replacement therapy, after adjustment for acute illness severity and patient characteristics [6].

Chronic kidney disease (CKD) is common in patients with cancer and frequently impacts treatment. A multicentre observational study found 57% of patients had abnormal renal function prior to commencing treatment, with 53% of anti-cancer treatments requiring dose adjustment [7]. CKD can also develop following diagnosis and throughout treatment (◘ Fig. 47.1). For example, in haematopoietic stem cell transplantation, one-third develop CKD within 10 years, and CKD can develop following nephrectomy for renal cancer.

47.3 Renal Disease Impact on Cancer Risk

The incidence of cancer is higher compared to the general population in patients with albuminuria, with end-stage renal disease, on pre-renal replacement therapy, on haemodialysis (1.5 fold) and following transplantation (3–5 fold) [8–10]. Pre-dialysis, the incidence of non-Hodgkin lymphoma, Kaposi sarcoma and cancer of the lip, colon and thyroid is significantly increased [9]. On dialysis, stomach, small intestine, liver, breast, renal and lung cancers are added to this list [11]. After transplantation, the incidence of all forms of malignancy increases with 18 sites having a greater than three-fold increase in risk. Thirteen of these have suspected viral aetiologies, including human papillomavirus (HPV), Epstein-Barr virus (EBV), hepatitis viruses and human herpesvirus 8 (HHV8) [9]. The most important risk factor for post-transplant malignancy is the overall immunosuppression burden, including immunosuppressive treatment given pre-transplant; other risk factors include: [12]

- Increasing age.
- Donor transmission (<0.03%).
- Sun exposure.
- Cadaveric donor – especially post-transplant lymphoproliferative disorder (PTLD) and genitourinary cancers.
- Rejection episodes.

47

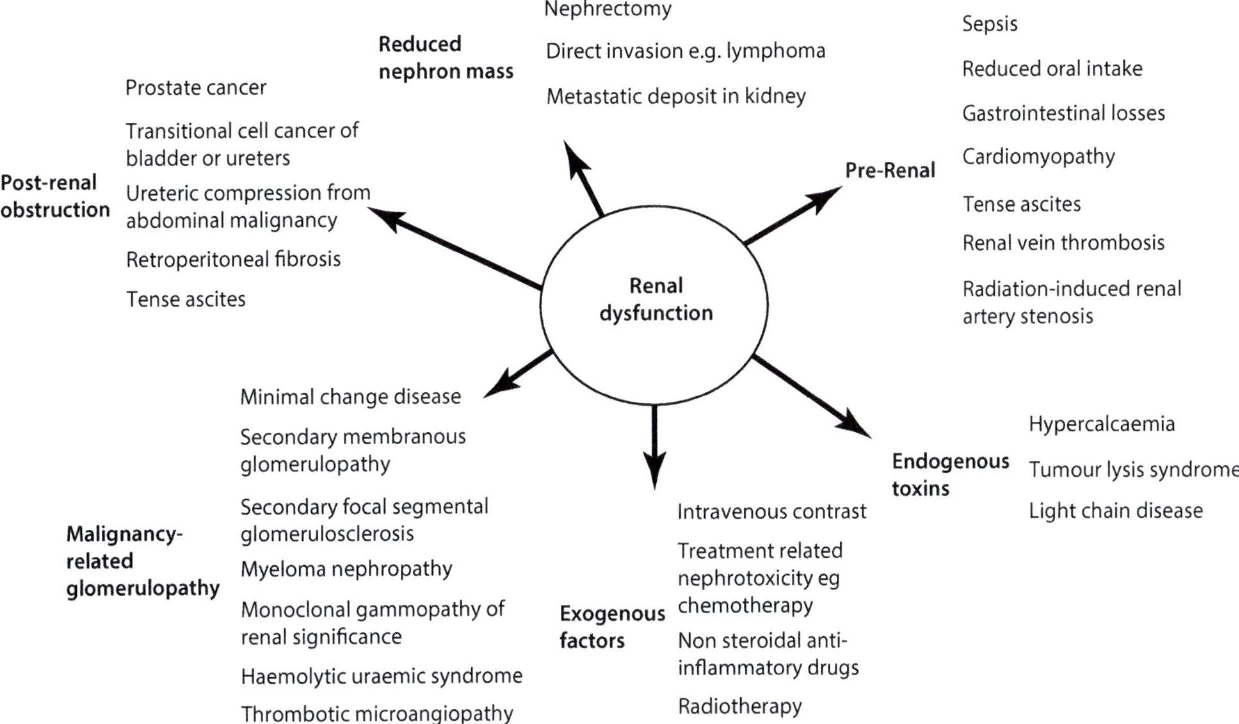

Fig. 47.1 Causes of renal dysfunction in patients with malignancy

- Previous cancer in the recipient (3–4 times more likely to die of cancer post-transplant).
- Viral infections: >50% of PTLD cases are EBV-related (positive donor to negative recipient increases PTLD risk 20-fold [13]); HHV8, HPV, hepatitis viruses and Merkel cell polyomavirus are also carcinogenic.
- Increased dialysis vintage.
- Use of T-cell depleting induction agents.
- Maintenance immunosuppression dose.

47.4 Renal Disease Impact on Cancer Prognosis

Impaired renal function is associated with worse prognosis in cancer patients and impacts cancer treatment. Unfortunately, cancer outcomes are significantly worse for patients with even modest impairment of renal function. An eGFR less than 60 mL/min/1.73m^2 is a significant independent risk factor for death from cancer, with cancer-specific mortality increasing 18% for every 10 mL/min/1.73m^2 of eGFR decline [14]. AKI during treatment is associated with reduced treatment dose intensity, reduced progression-free survival and increased overall mortality [15, 16].

In addition, renal transplantation is associated with poorer cancer outcomes. Post-transplantation, cancer is diagnosed at a later stage compared to the general population and has a worse prognosis, including for common cancer types such as breast, colon, lung and prostate cancer [17]. Outcomes are unsurprisingly tumour specific; for example, following renal transplantation 5-year survival from colorectal cancer is 27% compared to 75% in the general population, and transplant recipients with breast cancer have a 40% excess mortality compared to the general population [18]. In a Dutch study of 12,805 renal transplant recipients, 7% were diagnosed with cancer, of whom 81% died from cancer, with 69% dying with a functional graft. The median survival following a cancer diagnosis was 2.1 years compared to 8.3 years in matched controls without cancer [19].

47.5 Malignancy as a Cause of Renal Disease

There are a multitude of diagnostic possibilities when a patient with malignancy presents with renal dysfunction (Fig. 47.1). Causes can be categorised into three major groups: (i) directly tumour-related, due to direct renal involvement (e.g. due to renal cancer or lymphomatous infiltration) or obstructive nephropathy from retroperitoneal lymph nodes or pelvic malignancy; (ii) treatment-related, due to direct renal toxicity from exogenous agents such as chemotherapy or treatment-related complications such as sepsis or dehydration; and (iii) paraneoplastic, for example due to endogenous agents causing tubular injury or glomerular disease, or due to hypercoagulability-related renal vein thrombosis. It is critical to monitor renal function closely and be responsive in terms of dose adjustment in the face of changing renal function.

47.5.1 Treatment-Related Renal Dysfunction

47.5.1.1 Chemotherapy

Traditional chemotherapy remains the mainstay of treatment for most solid and haematological malignancies. Different chemotherapy agents are associated with different renal toxicities (Table 47.1). Important examples include the following:

Table 47.1 Examples of cancer therapies that cause different renal pathologies

Site of renal injury	Renal pathology	Associated cancer therapy
Renal vasculature	Haemodynamic AKI (capillary leak syndrome)	IL-2
	Thrombotic microangiopathy	Anti-angiogenesis drugs (e.g. bevacizumab, sunitinib), gemcitabine, cisplatin, mitomycin C, vincristine, interferon (IFN), radiotherapy
Glomeruli	Minimal change disease	IFN, pamidronate
	Focal segmental glomerulosclerosis	IFN, pamidronate
	Lupus-like nephritis	Ipilimumab
Tubulointerstitium	Acute tubular injury	Platinum-based chemotherapy (e.g. cisplatin), zoledronate, ifosfamide, pemetrexed, imatinib
	Acute interstitial nephritis	Small molecule TKIs (e.g. sunitinib, sorafenib), pemetrexed, checkpoint inhibitors (PD-1 inhibitors, CTLA-4 inhibitors)
	Crystal nephropathy	Methotrexate
	Fanconi syndrome	Cisplatin, ifosfamide, pemetrexed, imatinib
	Salt-wasting	Cisplatin, azacitidine
	Magnesium-wasting	Cisplatin, cetuximab, panitumumab
	Nephrogenic diabetes insipidus	Cisplatin, ifosfamide, pemetrexed

Agents Causing Predominately Tubular Toxicity

- Platinum-containing compounds (e.g. carboplatin, cisplatin) are used in solid organ malignancies including ovarian, lung, cervical, germ cell and bladder cancers. Cisplatin is dose-limited due to nephrotoxicity with progressive renal dysfunction in 50% of patients [20, 21]. It commonly causes acute tubular injury and longer-term interstitial fibrosis, and is also associated with renal magnesium wasting [20, 22]. Rarely it also causes tubulopathies and thrombotic microangiopathy (TMA) [23]. Nephrotoxicity is generally reversible but can be permanent [22]. Strategies to reduce these risks include pre-hydration, vigilant monitoring for dehydration after administration, avoidance of concomitant nephrotoxics and accurate renal function measurements (EDTA testing and regular renal function tests) with appropriate dose adjustment [21].
- Ifosfamide is an alkylating agent used for various cancers including sarcomas, testicular cancer and lymphoma. Nephrotoxicity is the major toxic effect of this drug, including acute tubular injury, tubulopathy and Fanconi syndrome [20]. The AKI is often reversible but can be permanent [23].
- Pemetrexed is an anti-folate agent used to treat mesothelioma and non-small cell lung cancer. It causes acute tubular injury and tubulopathy, which is usually reversible [24].
- High-dose methotrexate is an anti-folate agent used to treat high-grade lymphoma and some germ cell tumours. It is associated with AKI, which reduces renal clearance and can subsequently lead to severe methotrexate toxicity [20]. AKI is predominately due to crystal nephropathy, with methotrexate and its metabolite 7-OH-methotrextate precipitating in the distal tubules [23]. Prevention includes aggressive hydration, urinary alkalinisation with urinary pH monitoring, methotrexate level monitoring and leucovorin (folinic acid) which reduces the incidence of nephrotoxicity to <2% [23]. Glucarpidase is a carboxypeptidase enzyme which rapidly reduces methotrexate levels by 98% and is indicated when patients have toxic methotrexate levels, deteriorating renal function and no response to supportive measures, and are at risk of life-threatening toxicity [25, 26]. High-flux haemodialysis has been shown to reduce methotrexate levels, but much less effectively, with significant rebound when stopped [27].

Agents Causing Predominately Glomerular Toxicity

- Gemcitabine, used for solid tumours such as lung, pancreas, bladder and breast tumours, is nephrotoxic predominately due to TMA with an incidence of up to 2.2%. Risk factors include previous use of mitomycin C and higher total drug dose [20, 23]. Treatment is supportive and recovery variable [23].
- Mitomycin is an antibiotic with anti-tumour activity used in some gastrointestinal tumours. It can cause dose-dependent renal toxicity due to TMA [20].

47.5.1.2 Radiotherapy

The incidence of direct radiation nephritis has reduced dramatically with effective shielding of the kidneys, but when tumours are located near the kidney, collateral damage is likely. This can result in acute radiation nephritis, an aggressive and progressive nephropathy occurring 6–12 months after radiation exposure which is associated with proteinuria, hypertension and renal impairment. Light microscopy demonstrates endothelial cell swelling and mesangiolysis with capillary wall microaneurysmal change. Over time the areas of mesangiolysis become collagen filled imparting a lobular appearance to the glomeruli, and there is reduplication of the glomerular basement membrane due to subendothelial expansion. Fibrinoid necrosis of small vessel walls is seen. Acute radiation nephritis has a poor prognosis and no known effective treatment.

Chronic radiation nephritis appears to be slightly more indolent and is characterised by tubulointerstitial fibrosis and CKD. Hypertension has been reported as a lone finding, as has accelerated phase hypertension, with some suggestion that this may be related to radiation-induced small vessel renal artery stenosis. Even with effective shielding, total body irradiation (TBI) may cause renal dysfunction by provoking a chronic thrombotic microangiopathy (TMA).

47.5.1.3 Targeted Treatment

Targeted therapies are the cornerstone of precision medicine and have revolutionised cancer treatment; however, nephrotoxicity is common (Table 47.1). Examples include:

- Immune checkpoint inhibitors (CTLA-4 and PD-1 or PD-L1 inhibitors such as ipilimumab, nivolumab and pembrolizumab) are associated with acute interstitial nephritis and less commonly a lupus-like nephritis, minimal change disease or TMA [20, 28]. AKI occurs in 13–29% with onset 2–3 months into treatment for ipilimumab and 3–10 months for anti-PD-1 therapy [28–30]. Treatment is with steroids and cessation of drug where appropriate; most cases are responsive to steroids if identified and treated early [31]. Both CTLA-4 and PD-1 inhibitors are associated with renal transplant rejection, occurring 1 to 8 weeks into treatment, with a high incidence of graft loss [32].
- Bevacizumab, an anti-angiogenic humanised monoclonal antibody against vascular endothelial growth factor, is used in solid organ tumours including colorectal, ovarian and primary brain tumours. It is associated with hypertension and AKI, with the primary renal pathology being TMA [20, 23, 33].
- Cetuximab, an epidermal growth factor receptor monoclonal antibody, is used in epithelial malignancies, including colorectal, lung and head and neck tumours and is associated with renal magnesium wasting, often requiring intravenous replacement [34].
- Small molecule tyrosine kinase inhibitors, such as sunitinib commonly used for renal cell carcinoma, are associated with hypertension, acute interstitial nephritis and TMA [20, 23].

47.5.1.4 Supportive Treatment

During the management of solid organ and haematological malignancies, patients are inevitably exposed to a variety of non-cancer treatments with direct nephrotoxic effects; common examples include contrast media, antibiotics (aminoglycosides), antivirals (foscarnet, aciclovir, ganciclovir, cidofovir), anti-fungals (amphotericin), non-steroidal anti-inflammatory drugs and bisphosphonates (pamidronate, zoledronate).

47.5.1.5 Treatment-Related Complications

Cancer treatments cause a myriad of complications which in turn can cause renal disease. For example, pre-renal AKI can be caused by chemotherapy-induced vomiting and diarrhoea leading to dehydration or chemotherapy-related neutropenic sepsis. Chemotherapy can also increase the risk of thrombosis, including renal vein thrombosis.

47.5.1.6 Treatment Adjustments in Renal Disease

Chemotherapy is predominantly metabolised by the kidneys and/or liver. Renal impairment and uraemia can suppress liver enzymes, reducing the liver metabolism of certain agents [35]. Abnormal renal function increases the risk of systemic and nephrotoxicity from chemotherapy, as well as the risk of sub-therapeutic dosing if dose adjustments are not correctly implemented. Pre-treatment renal function should be measured using glomerular filtration rate rather than creatinine; this can be achieved using standard calculations of creatinine clearance or nuclear medicine tests such as chromium-51 EDTA clearance. Close monitoring throughout the course of treatment is essential with prompt reaction to deteriorating renal function. This should include consideration of other causes of renal dysfunction (e.g. gastrointestinal losses, infection, NSAIDs) and then dose adjustment or treatment delay or cessation as appropriate. CKD stage V, haemodialysis and peritoneal dialysis patients require special consideration with regard to volume status and electrolyte management. For this reason, multidisciplinary team working is crucial. Chemotherapy dosing advice can be found in the renal drug handbook for patients with CKD, haemodialysis and peritoneal dialysis [36].

47.5.2 Endogenous Toxins and Paraneoplastic Renal Dysfunction

47.5.2.1 Hypercalcaemia

Hypercalcaemia is common in cancer, occurring in up to 30% of all cancer patients during the clinical course of their disease. It is most common in later-stage malignancy and is generally associated with poorer prognosis. The estimated yearly prevalence of hypercalcaemia for all cancers is 1.46% to 2.74%, and it is four times more prevalent in stage IV cancer [37]. It is most commonly associated with multiple myeloma, lung cancer and renal cell carcinoma but is also regularly encountered in cancers of the head and neck, breast, ovary and colon [37]. It is frequently caused by excessive tumour secretion of parathyroid hormone-related protein, but is also caused by bone metastasis-related release of osteoclast activating factors and by excessive production of calcitriol [38].

Hypercalcaemia can cause acute and chronic renal disease. Renal manifestations of hypercalcaemia include nephrogenic diabetes insipidus, renal vasoconstriction, distal renal tubular acidosis, nephrolithiasis and tubular dysfunction [39]. It can also cause nephrocalcinosis due to calcium oxalate or calcium phosphate deposition in the tubulointerstitium, causing acute or chronic kidney injury, sometimes with progressive renal dysfunction [40].

Treatment of the underlying cancer is important in correcting hypercalcaemia. Additional therapies are often also required, particularly if severe. The mainstay of acute hypercalcaemia treatment is intravenous fluids and bisphosphonate therapy. Bisphosphonate therapy can be continued regularly for long-term control. Pamidronate and zoledronate are both used and generally take 2–4 days to take effect. Of note, both need to be used with caution in renal impairment due to potentially nephrotoxic effects, and dose reduction may be required. Second-line treatments include calcitonin, steroids (sometimes used in lymphoma to reduce calcitriol production) and denosumab. Denosumab is a human monoclonal antibody which blocks osteoclast formation through the inhibition of RANK-ligand, and is used for refractory hypercalcaemia or if bisphosphonates are contraindicated due to severe renal impairment.

47.5.2.2 Tumour Lysis Syndrome

Tumour lysis syndrome (TLS) is an important and often preventable cause of AKI and constitutes a medical emergency. It occurs when there is mass lysis of tumour cells, either spontaneously or in response to treatment, leading to hyperuricaemia, hyperkalaemia, hyperphosphataemia and hypocalcaemia. It is much more common in haematological than non-haematological malignancies, but can occur in solid tumours (e.g. metastatic germ cell tumours). The incidence varies depending on the definition used, but approximately 10% of patients with acute lymphocytic leukaemia (ALL) develop severe uric acid nephropathy, as do roughly 5% of patients with non-Hodgkin's lymphoma (NHL), with half of these becoming anuric. Both uric acid and phosphate are thought to play a role in the AKI associated with cell lysis, and a spot urinary urate/creatinine ratio of >1 is suggestive of the diagnosis. Risk factors are shown in Table 47.2 and clinical markers in Table 47.3.

Table 47.2 Risk factors for tumour lysis syndrome

1. Patient factors
a. Increasing age, acidic urine, hypotension and renal impairment
b. Concomitant nephrotoxic medications
2. Inadequate supportive care
a. Dehydration
b. No allopurinol or rasburicase prophylaxis
3. High tumour burden
a. Bulky tumour
b. Extensive metastases
4. High cell lysis potential
a. Rapidly proliferating tumour – LDH is a surrogate marker for this
b. High cancer cell sensitivity to therapy
c. Intensity of therapy
d. High white blood cell count

Table 47.3 Clinical markers of tumour lysis syndrome

1. Hyperuricaemia (uric acid >0.4 mmol/L)
2. Hyperphosphataemia (serum phosphate >1.5 mmol/L in adults; >2.1 mmol/L in children)
3. Rapid onset hyperkalaemia (serum potassium >6.0 mmol/L)
4. Hypocalcaemia (corrected calcium <1.75 mmol/L; ionised calcium <0.3 mmol/L)
5. Raised lactate dehydrogenase
6. Acute kidney injury

Table 47.4 Lymphoproliferative causes of glomerular deposition diseases

1. Light chain cast nephropathy
2. AL amyloid
3. Monoclonal immunoglobulin deposition disease (MIDD)
a. Light chain deposition disease
b. Heavy chain deposition disease
4. Cryoglobulinaemia (type 1 and type 2)
5. Macroglobulinaemia-monoclonal IgM Waldenstrom's or multiple myeloma
6. Immunotactoid GN (0.1% of biopsies)
7. Fibrillary GN (1% of biopsies)
8. Monoclonal gammopathy (POEMS[a])

[a]POEMS polyneuropathy, organomegaly, endocrinopathy, monoclonal gammopathy and skin involvement

TLS may occur spontaneously in patients with a heavy burden of disease, but more typically occurs 3–7 days after treatment, though severe hyperkalaemia may be present earlier. Without treatment there is a risk of fulminant hyperkalaemia, arrhythmias, seizures and anuric renal failure, with oligo-anuric patients being particularly at risk of these life-threatening complications. Appropriate treatment includes supportive care and intense monitoring of high-risk patients, in conjunction with rasburicase (see below). There is no evidence that alkalinisation of the urine is helpful (urate is more soluble with higher pH), possibly because xanthine, hypoxanthine and calcium phosphate are less soluble in alkaline urine. There are no trials to support early dialysis but urate and phosphate are rapidly cleared by haemodialysis, and so there is a logical argument for early renal replacement therapy (RRT). In a patient with pre-existing renal failure, it is important to anticipate metabolic mayhem and thus prepare for timely RRT.

The incidence of TLS has been dramatically reduced by prophylaxis with pre-hydration and urate reduction treatments. Allopurinol (a xanthine oxidase inhibitor) inhibits the oxidation of hypoxanthine to xanthine (and then to urate) and is used in prophylaxis. Rasburicase (recombinant urate oxidase) catalyses the oxidation of urate to allantoin (5–10x more soluble) which is excreted harmlessly by the kidney. It reduces urate levels within 4 hours and can be used both as prophylaxis and treatment. As allopurinol prevents the formation of urate (which is the substrate for rasburicase), they should not be prescribed together. Rasburicase is significantly more expensive but appears much more effective; in one randomised controlled trial, rasburicase reduced urate by 86% compared to 12% with allopurinol, and it has been shown to result in better renal function and reduced need for dialysis [41]. Hypersensitivity reactions are not infrequent, anti-oxidase antibodies can be induced with repeated treatments and it is contraindicated in G6PD-deficient patients.

47.5.2.3 Paraneoplastic Phenomenon in Lymphoproliferative Disorders

Acute kidney injury can also occur as a paraneoplastic phenomenon related to lymphoproliferative disorders. This is often in association with multi-organ dysfunction and may be the presenting feature before the underlying diagnosis is made. An example of this is Castleman's disease, which is a non-neoplastic B-cell proliferative disorder associated with renal and systemic effects related to excess IL-6 production. This condition may precede the onset of NHL.

Immunoglobulin-Related Renal Disease

Acute kidney injury and CKD are common accompaniments to endogenous, pathological immunoglobulin production either via glomerular deposition (see ▶ Chap. 50 on Amyloid) or secondary to the toxic effects of excess light and heavy chains (see ▶ Chap. 49 on myeloma). In short, light chains, heavy chains and immunoglobulins can form casts, crystals, fibrils or granular deposits in the kidney; these conditions are termed monoclonal gammopathies of renal significance.

Glomerular disorders secondary to lymphoproliferative disorders (LPD) are relatively common, and whilst there is overlap, they can be divided into (a) glomerular deposition diseases secondary to abnormal production of immunoglobulin components (Table 47.4) and (b) paraneoplastic glomerulonephritides without apparent excess of immunoglobulin production.

Patients with glomerular deposition diseases may present with AKI or other renal syndromes such as nephrotic syndrome (secondary to renal amyloid, membranoproliferative glomerulonephritis (MPGN) or membranous nephropathy), rapidly progressive glomer-

Table 47.5 Characteristics and differential diagnosis of glomerular deposition diseases

	AL amyloid	Immunotactoid glomerulonephritis	Fibrillary glomerulonephritis	Cryoglobulin	MIDD
Congo red	+ve	−ve	−ve	−ve	−ve
Pattern	Fibrillary random	Microtubules, stacks of hollow cylinders	Fibrils, randomly distributed	Fibrillary organised (microtubular) or random Can be curvilinear	Small dense granules
Size	8–15 nm	20–90 nm; mostly 25–35 nm	12–30 nm	25–35 nm	
Immunoglobulin	Monoclonal AL light chain	Monoclonal or oligoclonal, IgG, C3	Usually polyclonal IgG4 > IgG1, C3	Monoclonal	
Associations	LPD	LPD (exclude SLE and cryoglobulin) HIV	Hepatitis C, SLE, cryoglobulin, LPD	LPD, hepatitis C	LPD

ulonephritis (fibrillary GN) or just sub-acute renal impairment. Clinically, nephrotic syndrome occurs in 1–2% of patients with chronic lymphocytic leukaemia (CLL), predominantly associated with an MPGN pattern, but membranous nephropathy, minimal change nephropathy, amyloid deposition, focal segmental glomerulosclerosis (FSGS), crescentic glomerulonephritis and light chain deposition disease can all occur. MPGN is usually associated with cryoglobulinaemia, but may be associated with neither cryoglobulins nor complement activation but instead with IgG deposition in the form of immunotactoid glomerulonephritis.

As well as non-haematological causes, cryoglobulinaemia has been associated with NHL, Hodgkin's lymphoma (HL), CLL, multiple myeloma (MM), chronic myelocytic leukaemia (CML), Waldenstrom's macroglobulinaemia (WM), Castleman's disease, myelodysplasia, thrombotic thrombocytopaenic purpura (TTP) and cold agglutinins. Thus the presence of any monoclonal cryoglobulin requires full haematological assessment. Cryoglobulinaemia secondary to LPD tends to be predominantly type 1, which less frequently presents with vasculitis and purpura compared with types 2–3 but more commonly presents with veno-occlusive disease.

The pattern of deposition on electron microscopy may help to differentiate the underlying pathology: amyloid, cryoglobulin, fibrillary and immunotactoid glomerulonephritis all have a fibrillary pattern, whereas light and heavy chain deposition diseases have a granular pattern. Distinguishing immunoglobulin deposition can be difficult, and it is important to ensure that Congo red staining and electron microscopy are done and fibrils are measured. Differentiating characteristics of immunoglobulin deposition diseases are shown in Table 47.5.

Fibronectin glomerulopathy, collagenofibrotic glomerulopathy, TMA, systemic lupus erythematosus and diabetes mellitus can all be associated with organised deposits, and the distinguishing features are covered in an excellent review by Guillermo and Turbat-Herrera [42].

Glomerulonephritis in Lymphoproliferative Disease

Glomerulonephritides are well documented in association with lymphomas and chronic leukaemias, and rarely occur in association with acute leukaemia. As described above, glomerulonephritis secondary to glomerular deposition of excess immunoglobulin products is common. Paraneoplastic glomerulonephritis without apparent excess of immunoglobulins can also occur in association with haematological malignancies (Table 47.6). Management is focussed on identifying and treating the underlying haematological malignancy. Remission rates for secondary glomerulonephritides are good if the underlying driver is successfully cured.

Minimal change nephropathy (MCN) is the classic glomerulonephritis associated with HL and NHL, occurring in about 1% of cases. FSGS is also associated but at a tenth of the frequency of MCN. As patients with MCN secondary to lymphoma are often steroid resistant, it is important to reassess all steroid-resistant patients with MCN for underlying lymphoma. The diagnosis of lymphoma may not be apparent for months after the appearance of nephrotic syndrome. Approximately 70% of patients presenting with MCN secondary to lymphoma have constitutional symptoms (e.g. fever, night sweats), and 90% have an acute phase response; these signs and symptoms can be used to aid diagnosis [43].

Table 47.6 Glomerulonephritis associated with lymphoproliferative disorders without apparent paraprotein production

Lymphoproliferative disorder	Type of glomerulonephritis
Hodgkin/non-Hodgkin lymphomas	Minimal change, FSGS
CLL/hairy cell leukaemia	MPGN with or without cryoglobulin, membranous
T cell lymphoma (Sezary syndrome, mycosis fungoides)	IgA
Chronic myelomonocytic leukaemia	Various glomerulonephritides
Myelofibrosis/polycythaemia rubra vera/essential thrombocythaemia	FSGS (secondary)

Chronic lymphocytic leukaemia and hairy cell leukaemia (HLL) are predominantly associated with MPGN and monoclonal production of immunoglobulin with or without cryoglobulinaemia (see section Glomerulonephritis in Lymphoproliferative Disease above) but also, to a much lesser extent, membranous glomerulonephritis which may show a fibrillary pattern in the sub-epithelial deposits.

Hyperviscosity

In addition to direct infiltration and cryoglobulin deposition, Waldenstrom's macroglobulinaemia (and IgM multiple myeloma) may result in hyperviscosity syndrome and thus risk of renal arteriovenous thrombosis of any sized vessel, including an acute glomerular capillary thrombosis. As with all the above disorders, the primary aim is to identify any underlying haematological disorder and treat this directly rather than the resultant secondary renal disease.

47.5.2.4 Glomerulonephritides in Solid Cancers

In addition to the range of glomerulonephritides associated with lymphoproliferative disorders, paraneoplastic glomerulonephritis can rarely be associated with solid tumours. Membranous nephropathy is the most frequently reported solid tumour-associated paraneoplastic glomerulonephritis, although minimal change disease, membranoproliferative glomerulonephritis, IgA nephropathy and IgA vasculitis can also occur [44].

Cancer-associated membranous nephropathy is most commonly associated with lung and gastric carcinomas but also with renal carcinoma, prostate cancer and thymoma, amongst others. In a series of patients with membranous nephropathy, cancer was found in approximately 10%, with risk factors for finding cancer including age >65 years and a >20 pack year smoking history [45]. Thromboembolic disease occurred in 25% of cancer-associated membranous nephropathy compared to 7% in primary membranous nephropathy. Findings suggesting a secondary cause of membranous nephropathy include negative immunostaining for M-type phospholipase A2 receptor (PLA2R) and thrombospondin type 1 domain-containing protein 7A (THSD7A) antigens, negative serum PLA2R and THSD7A antibodies and a preference towards a mixed IgG1, IgG2 and IgG3 subclass staining pattern, rather than IgG4 dominant [46].

It is important to screen for malignancy in all patients with glomerulonephritis and clinical or pathological features suggestive of a secondary cause. There are no formal screening guidelines and screening should be driven by a patient's individual risk factors; [43] a small study of patients with membranous nephropathy also highlighted a potential role for 18F-fluorodeoxyglucose positron emission tomography/computed tomography (FDG-PET/CT) in identifying occult malignancy [47]. Treatment is aimed at the underlying malignancy, and the development of proteinuria following successful treatment should prompt investigations for potential recurrence.

47.5.2.5 Renal Vein Thrombosis

Cancer causes a hypercoagulable state, which in turn increases the risk of renal vein thrombosis. This can cause acute kidney injury or chronic kidney disease. Renal cell carcinomas can extend into the renal veins and can be associated with tumour thrombus in 4–25% of cases [48].

47.5.2.6 Cancer-Associated Thrombotic Microangiopathy

Cancer-associated thrombotic microangiopathy (TMA) is characterised by microvascular thrombosis, thrombocytopaenia and resultant end-organ ischaemic damage, commonly affecting the kidneys. It can be caused by malignancy itself (particularly in mucinous adenocarcinomas and widely disseminated malignancy), or it can be a complication of cancer therapy (see Sect. 47.5.1 on chemotherapy and targeted agents) [49].

47.5.3 Renal Impairment Due to Direct Tumour Involvement

Renal impairment can be caused by obstruction anywhere in the urinary tract secondary a pelvic tumour or retroperitoneal malignant lymph nodes. The kidneys can also be directly involved, for example in renal cell carcinoma or in metastatic disease which encases or invades the kidneys. Direct infiltration of the kidneys does occur in some lymphoproliferative diseases. This is often noted as part of the staging workup but may be the presenting feature with impaired renal function and diffuse kidney enlargement (often associated with negative urinalysis) (◘ Fig. 47.2). Arterial or venous tumour thrombosis can also occur due to direct tumour infiltration. Early imaging including ultrasound and Doppler studies to exclude obstruction or arteriovenous thrombosis is crucial in patients with renal dysfunction and an underlying malignancy.

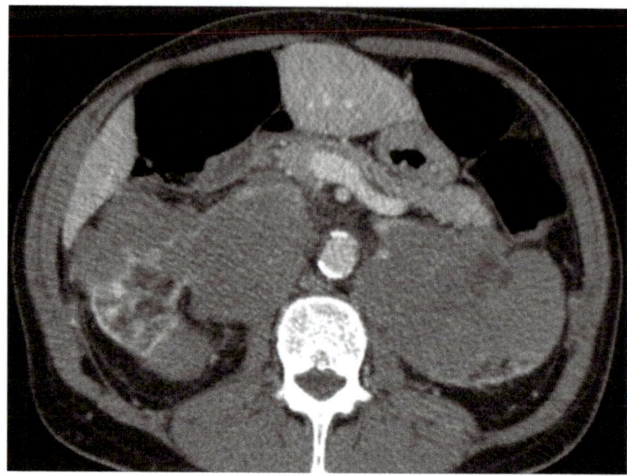

◘ **Fig. 47.2** Computed tomography (CT) scan of the abdomen in a patient with bilateral renal infiltration from LPD

Direct kidney infiltration in lymphoproliferative disease is common post-transplantation, where graft involvement from PTLD is frequent with early presentations, but rarer with late PTLD. A retrospective analysis of 668 patients presenting with lymphoproliferative disorders demonstrated radiologically apparent renal involvement in 3% of cases of NHL, 1.2% of cases of multiple myeloma and 4.9% of cases of other lymphoma, but interestingly with no cases in HL ($n = 41$) [50]. At autopsy, histological evidence of renal involvement by cancer cells seems to be extremely common in leukaemia (60–90%) and NHL (up to a third), but may not be apparent macroscopically, and often does not seem to contribute significantly to renal injury [51].

47.6 Renal Replacement Therapy in Malignancy

Determining escalation of care and the appropriateness of acute or chronic renal replacement therapy in patients with advanced cancer is complex. Key cancer-specific factors include the cancer type, prognosis, impact on quality of life and treatment options. With advances in therapy even patients with incurable metastatic cancer can still have a prognosis of several years. Important renal considerations include the cause and chronicity of renal impairment, the potential for improvement in renal function, the impact on quality of life of long-term renal replacement and whether survival or quality of life are likely to be improved compared with conservative management. Ultimately extensive patient and family discussion, with multidisciplinary renal, oncology and palliative care input is crucial to optimise patient care.

47.7 Renal and Oncology Multidisciplinary Care

As described in this chapter, the links between cancer and renal disease are complex and bidirectional. Renal disease increases the risk of malignancy, impacts cancer treatment options and worsens overall prognosis. Cancer and its treatment can cause both acute and chronic renal impairment through a range of pathologies and can complicate renal replacement therapy decision and delivery. Given this complexity, it is vital to take a patient-centred multidisciplinary approach to optimise patient care. This collaborative approach can vastly improve the patient experience if appointments, scans and blood tests are co-ordinated in order to minimise hospital visits.

Case Study

Case 1

A 62 year-old male presented with nephrotic syndrome following a recent diagnosis of mesenteric and splenic thrombosis which was treated with anticoagulation. His background includes chronic obstructive pulmonary disease, hypertension, monoclonal gammopathy of undetermined significance (MGUS) and obesity. Renal biopsy demonstrated membranous nephropathy, and further investigation demonstrated a limited pulmonary lesion which was confirmed as a lung squamous cell carcinoma on complete resection. His nephrotic syndrome was managed conservatively, and at one year his protein creatinine ratio fell to 100 from 1900. On a further visit, he was found to be nephrotic again and, despite a normal chest X-ray, a CT chest demonstrated the following (◘ Fig. 47.3).

This case demonstrates that malignancy-associated nephrotic syndrome can take months to resolve despite removal of the underlying cause. It also highlights the paraneoplastic nature in this case with proteinuria being a useful biomarker for recurrent disease.

Case 2

A 69-year-old male with metastatic non-small cell lung cancer is referred from oncology with a creatinine of 285 μmol/L from a baseline of 100 μmol/L. He started pembrolizumab immunotherapy two months prior. He has hypertension and takes amlodipine only; his examination is normal. His urinalysis showed 1+ proteinuria only, and his remaining investigations were unremarkable, including a negative renal screen and a normal kidney ultrasound. Renal biopsy showed acute interstitial nephritis. Pembrolizumab was stopped and high-dose corticosteroids were started leading to improvement in renal function. Immune checkpoint inhibitors are being increasingly used in oncology and are associated with acute kidney injury, typically with minimal proteinuria, and occasionally progressing to end-stage renal disease. Acute interstitial nephritis is the most common histology finding and most cases respond well to steroids and withdrawal of the offending agent if appropriate [28].

Case 3

A 54-year-old female with a history of radiotherapy for gynaecological malignancy several years previously presented with hypertensive urgency and acute kidney injury. Magnetic resonance imaging demonstrated bilateral renal artery stenosis, likely related to the previous radiotherapy (◘ Fig. 47.4). Both the acute kidney injury and hypertension improved with bilateral stenting, although recurred requiring further stenting a year later.

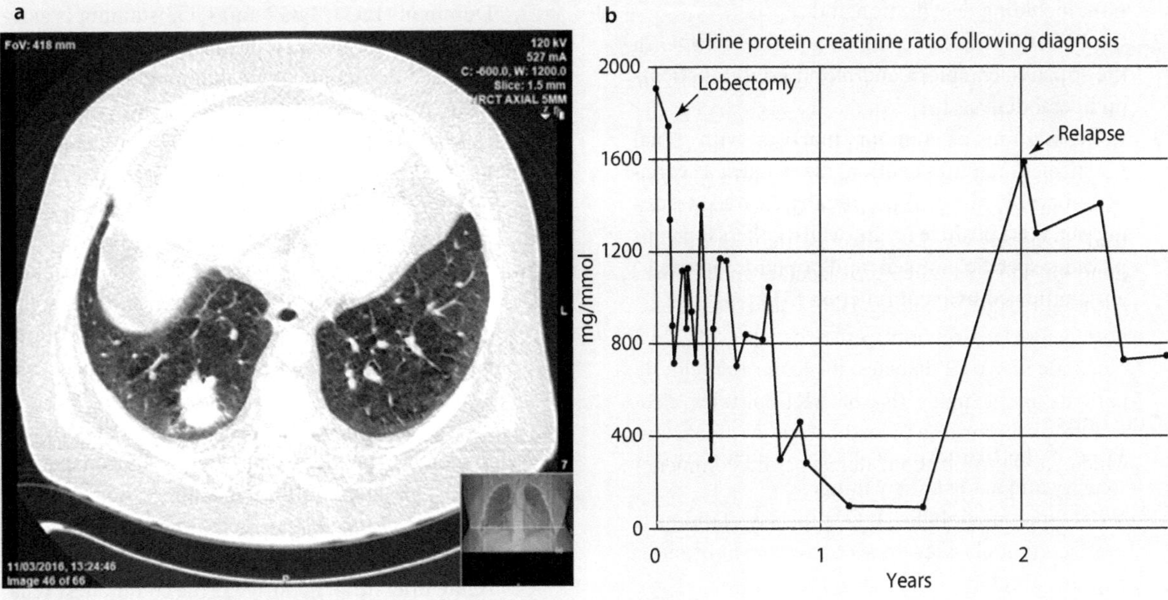

◘ **Fig. 47.3** **a** Spiculated lesion in the right lower lobe suspicious of recurrent lung carcinoma; **b** protein creatinine ratio change from diagnosis, through lobectomy, and cancer recurrence

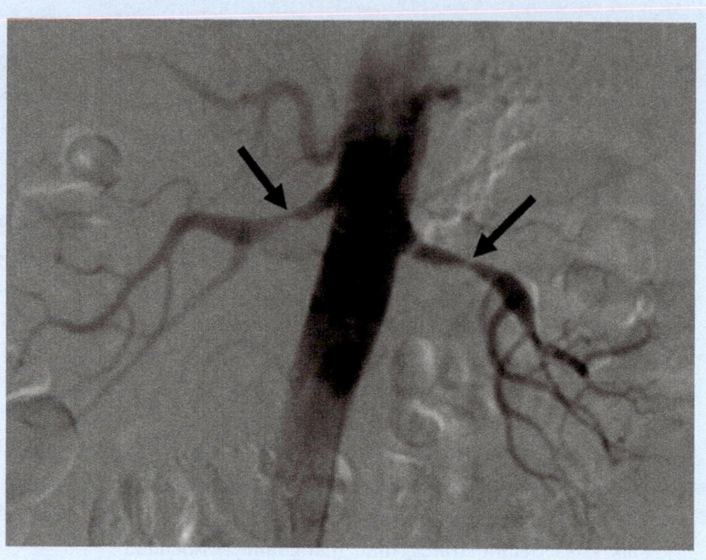

Fig. 47.4 Magnetic resonance angiography demonstratng bilateral renal artery stenosis (arrowheads) in a patient presenting with hypertensive urgency and acute kidney injury with previous pelvis radiotherapy

Tips and Tricks

1. Patients on chemotherapy may have cancer or treatment-specific causes of acute kidney injury but can also commonly develop acute kidney injury for the same reasons as the general population, including dehydration and sepsis.
2. On PET CT, there is a higher uptake of FDG in the soft tissues, spleen and blood pool in patients on haemodialysis [52].
3. Interpretation of tumour markers with renal impairment requires caution; many (such as carcinoembryonic antigen) are renally cleared, resulting in a false positive result, whilst others (such as prostate-specific antigen and alpha-fetoprotein) are unaffected by renal function [53].

Questions

1. What is the treatment of choice in methotrexate toxicity and acute kidney injury?
2. What immunoglobulin IgG subclass staining is most commonly seen in secondary membranous nephropathy?
3. What are risk factors for developing tumour lysis syndrome?
4. What is the most important risk factor for malignancy following transplantation?
5. What is the most common renal histology finding with immune checkpoint inhibitor usage?

Answers

1. Glucarpidase is the treatment of choice in methotrexate toxicity associated with acute kidney injury not responding to supportive measures. It is a carboxypeptidase enzyme which rapidly reduces methotrexate levels by 98%.
2. Dominant IgG1, IgG2 and IgG3 staining is associated with secondary membranous nephropathy whereas dominant IgG4 staining is associated with primary membranous nephropathy. The absence of PLA2R and THSD7A antigens and serum antibodies also suggests a secondary cause of membranous nephropathy, and cancer screening should be considered.
3. Risk factors for tumour lysis syndrome include increasing age, dehydration, absence of allopurinol or rasburicase prophylaxis, bulky tumour, metastatic disease, more intense treatment and more rapidly proliferating tumours.
4. Overall immunosuppressive burden is the primary risk factor for malignancy following transplantation. This includes immunosuppression use pre-transplant and augmented immunosuppression for rejection episodes.
5. Acute interstitial nephritis is the commonest renal histology finding with immune checkpoint inhibitor usage. Lupus-like nephritis, minimal change disease, TMA and acute rejection in kidney transplant recipients can also be found.

Conclusion

This chapter has reviewed the complex and bidirectional relationship between malignancy and the kidney. Cancer can both directly and indirectly cause a range of acute and chronic renal diseases. Renal dysfunction can affect cancer incidence, treatment and outcomes. This complex interaction necessitates multidisciplinary care in patients with both oncological and renal problems.

References

1. Rosner MH, Perazella MA. Acute kidney injury in patients with cancer. N Engl J Med. 2017;376(18):1770–81.
2. CF, Christiansen MB, Langeberg WJ, Fryzek JP, Sørensen HT. Incidence of acute kidney injury in cancer patients: a Danish population-based cohort study. Eur J Intern Med. 2011;22(4):399–406.
3. Kang E, Park M. Park PG, et al. Acute kidney injury predicts all-cause mortality in patients with cancer. 2019;8(6):2740–50.
4. Soares M, Salluh J, Carvalho MS, Darmon M, Rocco JR. Spector NJJCO. Prognosis of critically ill patients with cancer and acute renal dysfunction. 2006;24(24):4003–10.
5. Libório AB, Libório AB, Abreu KLS, et al. Predicting hospital mortality in critically ill cancer patients according to acute kidney injury severity. Oncology. 2011;80(3–4):160–6.
6. Darmon M, Thiery G, Ciroldi M, Porcher R, Schlemmer B, Azoulay É. Should dialysis be offered to cancer patients with acute kidney injury? Intensive Care Med. 2007;33(5):765–72.
7. Launay-Vacher V, Oudard S, Janus N, et al. Prevalence of renal insufficiency in cancer patients and implications for anticancer drug management. Cancer. 2007;110(6):1376–84.
8. Jørgensen L, Heuch I, Jenssen T, Jacobsen BK. Association of albuminuria and cancer incidence. J Am Soc Nephrol. 2008;19(5):992–8.
9. Vajdic CM, McDonald SP, McCredie MRE, et al. Cancer incidence before and after kidney transplantation. JAMA. 2006;296(23):2823–31.
10. M Zeier WH, Wiesel M, Lehnert T, Ritz E. Malignancy after renal transplantation. Am J Kidney Dis. 2002;39(1).
11. Lin MY, Kuo MC, Hung CC, et al. Association of dialysis with the risks of cancers. PLoS One. 2015;10(4):e0122856.
12. Sprangers B, Nair V, Launay-Vacher V, Riella LV, Jhaveri KD. Risk factors associated with post–kidney transplant malignancies: an article from the cancer-kidney international network. Clin Kidney J. 2017;11(3):315–29.
13. Walker RCPC, Marshall WF, Strickler JG, Wiesner RH, Velosa JA, Habermann TM, Daly RC, McGregor CG. Pretransplantation seronegative Epstein-Barr virus status is the primary risk factor for posttransplantation lymphoproliferative disorder in adult heart, lung, and other solid organ transplantations. The Jounral of Heart and Lung Transplantation. 1995;14(2):214–21.
14. Iff S, Craig JC, Turner R, Chapman JR, Wang JJ, Mitchell P, Wong G. Reduced estimated GFR and cancer mortality. Am J Kidney Dis. 2013;63(1):23–30.
15. Péron J, Neven A, Collette L, Launay-Vacher V, Sprangers B, Marreaud S. Impact of acute kidney injury on anticancer treatment dosage and long-term outcomes: a pooled analysis of European Organisation for Research and Treatment of Cancer trials. Nephrol Dial Transplantat. 2020;
16. Salahudeen AK, Doshi SM, Pawar T, Nowshad G, Lahoti A, Shah P. Incidence Rate, Clinical Correlates, and Outcomes of AKI in Patients Admitted to a Comprehensive Cancer Center. 2013;8(3):347–54.
17. Miao Y, Everly JJ, Gross TG, et al. De novo cancers arising in organ transplant recipients are associated with adverse outcomes compared with the general population. Transplantation. 2009;87(9).
18. Chapman JR, Webster AC, Wong G. Cancer in the transplant recipient. Cold Spring Harb Perspect Med. 2013;3(7):a015677.
19. van de Wetering J, Roodnat JI, Hemke AC, Hoitsma AJ, Weimar W. Patient survival after the diagnosis of cancer in renal transplant recipients: a nested case-control study. Transplantation. 2010;90(12).
20. Ilya G. Glezerman aEAJ. Chemotherapy and Kidney Injury. American Society of Nephrology Online Curricula. 2016.
21. Hayati F, Hossainzadeh M, Shayanpour S, Abedi-Gheshlaghi Z, Beladi Mousavi SS. Prevention of cisplatin nephrotoxicity. J Nephropharmacol. 2015;5(1):57–60.
22. Pabla N, Dong Z. Cisplatin nephrotoxicity: mechanisms and renoprotective strategies. Kidney Int. 2008;73(9):994–1007.
23. Perazella MA. Onco-nephrology: renal toxicities of chemotherapeutic agents. Clin J Am Soc Nephrol. 2012;7(10):1713–21.
24. IG Glezerman MCP, Mr V, Seshan SV. Kidney tubular toxicity of maintenance pemetrexed therapy. Am J Kidney Dis. 2011;58(5): 817–20.
25. Ramsey LB, Balis FM, O'Brien MM, et al. Consensus Guideline for Use of Glucarpidase in Patients with High-Dose Methotrexate Induced Acute Kidney Injury and Delayed Methotrexate Clearance. 2018;23(1):52–61.
26. Widemann BC, Schwartz S, Jayaprakash N, et al. Efficacy of Glucarpidase (carboxypeptidase G2) in patients with acute kidney injury after high-dose methotrexate. Therapy. 2014;34(5):427–39.
27. Kitchlu A, Shirali AC. High-flux hemodialysis versus glucarpidase for methotrexate-associated acute kidney injury: What's best? J Onco-Nephrol. 2019;3(1):11–8.
28. Cortazar FB, Marrone KA, Troxell ML, et al. Clinicopathological features of acute kidney injury associated with immune checkpoint inhibitors. Kidney Int. 2016;90(3):638–47.
29. Shirali AC, Perazella MA, Gettinger S. Association of Acute Interstitial Nephritis with Programmed Cell Death 1 inhibitor therapy in lung cancer patients. Am J Kidney Dis. 2016;68(2):287–91.
30. Wanchoo R, Karam S, Uppal NN, et al. Adverse renal effects of immune checkpoint inhibitors: a narrative review. Am J Nephrol. 2017;45(2):160–9.
31. Perazella MA, Sprangers B. AKI in Patients Receiving Immune Checkpoint Inhibitors. 2019;14(7):1077–9.
32. Perazella MA, Shirali AC. Nephrotoxicity of cancer immunotherapies: past. Present and Future. 2018;29(8):2039–52.
33. Mason NT, Khushalani NI, Weber JS, Antonia SJ, McLeod HL. Modeling the cost of immune checkpoint inhibitor-related toxicities. 2016;34(15_suppl): 6627.
34. Tejpar S, Piessevaux H, Claes K, et al. Magnesium wasting associated with epidermal-growth-factor receptor-targeting antibodies in colorectal cancer: a prospective study. Lancet Oncol. 2007;8(5):387–94.
35. Dreisbach AW, Lertora JJL. The effect of chronic renal failure on drug metabolism and transport. Expert Opin Drug Metab Toxicol. 2008;4(8):1065–74.
36. Coroline Ashley AD. The renal drug handbook: the ultimate prescribing guide for renal practitioners. 5th ed; 2018.
37. Goldner W. Cancer-Related Hypercalcemia. 2016;12(5):426–32.
38. Vakiti AMP. Malignancy-related hypercalcemia. StatPearls Publishing; 2019.
39. Mirrakhimov AE. Hypercalcemia of malignancy: an update on pathogenesis and management. N Am J Med Sci. 2015;7(11):483–93.
40. Shavit L, Jaeger P, Unwin RJ. What is nephrocalcinosis? Kidney Int. 2015;88(1):35–43.

41. Goldman SC, Holcenberg JS, Finklestein JZ, et al. A randomized comparison between rasburicase and allopurinol in children with lymphoma or leukemia at high risk for tumor lysis. Blood. 2001;97(10):2998–3003.
42. Herrera GA, Turbat-Herrera EA. Renal Diseases With Organized Deposits: An Algorithmic Approach to Classification and Clinicopathologic Diagnosis. 2010;134(4):512–31.
43. Plaisier E. Ronco P. Screening for Cancer in Patients with Glomerular Diseases. 2020;15(6):886–8.
44. Lien Y-HH, Lai L-W. Pathogenesis, diagnosis and management of paraneoplastic glomerulonephritis. Nat Rev Nephrol. 2011;7(2):85–95.
45. Lefaucheur C, Stengel B, Nochy D, et al. Membranous nephropathy and cancer: epidemiologic evidence and determinants of high-risk cancer association. Kidney Int. 2006;70(8):1510–7.
46. De Vriese AS, Glassock RJ, Nath KA, Sethi S, Fervenza FC. A Proposal for a Serology-Based Approach to Membranous Nephropathy. 2017;28(2):421–30.
47. Feng Z, Wang S, Huang Y, Liang X, Shi W, Zhang B. A follow-up analysis of positron emission tomography/computed tomography in detecting hidden malignancies at the time of diagnosis of membranous nephropathy. Oncotarget. 2016;7(9):9645–51.
48. Aeddula HRMNR. Renal vein thrombosis. StatPearls Publishing; 2019.
49. Govind Babu K, Bhat GR. Cancer-associated thrombotic microangiopathy. Ecancermedicalscience. 2016;10:649.
50. Bach AG, Behrmann C, Holzhausen HJ, et al. Prevalence and patterns of renal involvement in imaging of malignant lymphoproliferative diseases. 2012;53(3):343–8.
51. Schwartz JB, Shamsuddin AM. The effects of leukemic infiltrates in various organs in chronic lymphocytic leukemia. Hum Pathol. 1981;12(5):432–40.
52. Toriihara A, Kitazume Y, Nishida H, Kubota K, Nakadate M, Tateishi U. Comparison of FDG-PET/CT images between chronic renal failure patients on hemodialysis and controls. Am J Nucl Med Mol Imaging. 2015;5(2):204–11.
53. Coppolino G, Bolignano D, Rivoli L, Mazza G, Presta P, Fuiano G. Tumour markers and kidney function: a systematic review. Biomed Res Int. 2014;2014:647541.

Red Cells and the Kidney

Claire C. Sharpe

Contents

M. Harber (ed.), *Primer on Nephrology*, https://doi.org/10.1007/978-3-030-76419-7_48

Learning Objectives

1. Chronic kidney disease is an increasingly prevalent complication of sickle cell disease in developed countries.
2. Patients should be screened for risk factors and early signs of renal damage and managed appropriately.
3. Renal replacement therapy including renal transplantation should be considered early in patients with sickle cell disease approaching end-stage kidney disease.
4. Other red cell disorders associated with acute or chronic intravascular haemolysis are associated with both acute kidney injury and chronic kidney disease.

48.1 Haemoglobinopathies

48.1.1 Introduction

The haemoglobinopathies are inherited single-gene disorders affecting the synthesis (thalassaemias) or structure (e.g. sickle cell disease) of a globin chain of the haemoglobin tetramer. Worldwide, sickle cell disease (SCD) is the most common congenital haematological condition and is increasingly becoming a major cause of renal impairment. The thalassaemias are also a common group of autosomal recessive conditions; however, whilst SCD is a qualitative defect in globin synthesis, thalassaemias reflect a quantitative defect in globin synthesis, which lead to ineffective erythropoiesis. Whilst both conditions result in anaemia, haemolysis per se is not a feature of the thalassaemias, and so the impact on the kidney is much less. Here, we will review the renal complications of red cell disorders with an emphasis on sickle cell disease.

48.1.2 Sickle Cell Disease

48.1.2.1 Epidemiology

Sickle cell disease is endemic in malaria-prevalent (or previously prevalent) regions due to the protective nature of the carrier state, including sub-Saharan Africa, India, Saudi Arabia and the Mediterranean (Turkey, Greece and Italy). Across equatorial Africa, the prevalence of the sickle cell trait (SCT, heterozygous carriers) ranges between 10% and 40% and decreases to between 1% and 2% on the North African coast and <1% in South Africa. However, migration has led to SCD becoming increasingly common in non-endemic regions, for example, there are over 12,000 sufferers of sickle cell disease living in the UK and approximately 72,000 in the USA. Twenty-five percent of babies born with SCD worldwide are born outside of sub-Saharan Africa [1].

Renal involvement in SCD is well recognised, and chronic kidney disease (CKD) secondary to sickle cell nephropathy (SCN) is becoming more prevalent as the life expectancy of patients with SCD improves. Undoubtedly, environmental factors play a role in disease severity as well as co-inherited genes and other risk factors for the development of chronic kidney disease (CKD). The onset is insidious and microalbuminuria, an early manifestation of SCN, reaches a prevalence of approximately 60% in those over 45, although only 4–12% of patients with SCD will develop the serious and life-threatening complication of end-stage renal disease.

> Sickle cell nephropathy can be defined as any renal complication directly related to the presence of sickle cell disease. It is associated with sickling of red blood cells in the vasa recta and is characterised by hyperfiltration in the young, progressive proteinuria and declining renal function in adults (■ Fig. 48.1).

48.1.2.2 Pathogenesis

The sickle haemoglobin mutation (haemoglobin S, or HbS) results in the replacement of the normal glutamine by valine in the sixth position of the β-globin subunit, thereby changing the configuration of the haemoglobin tetramer molecule in the homozygous person from $\alpha 2\beta 2$ to $\alpha 2\beta^S 2$. SCD also occurs in those heterozygotes when HbS coexists with another abnormal or missing β-chain (e.g. HbC ($\alpha 2\beta^S\beta^C$) or HbSβ thalassemia ($\alpha 2\beta^S$). During cellular or tissue hypoxia, dehydration or oxidative stress, the mutated β-globin chains of the HbS molecule tend to polymerise, resulting in changes to the shape of the red blood cell (RBC). This leads to a characteristic crescent or sickle, which increases its rigidity and results in vaso-occlusion and premature destruction (haemolysis).

The pathogenesis of sickle cell nephropathy (SCN) is intimately related to the circulation of the kidney. Although in health the kidneys receive approximately 25% of the cardiac output, the vessels (vasa recta) that supply the medulla of the kidney branch off early from the efferent arteriole, taking only a fraction of the total renal blood flow. The relatively sluggish but intricate cir-

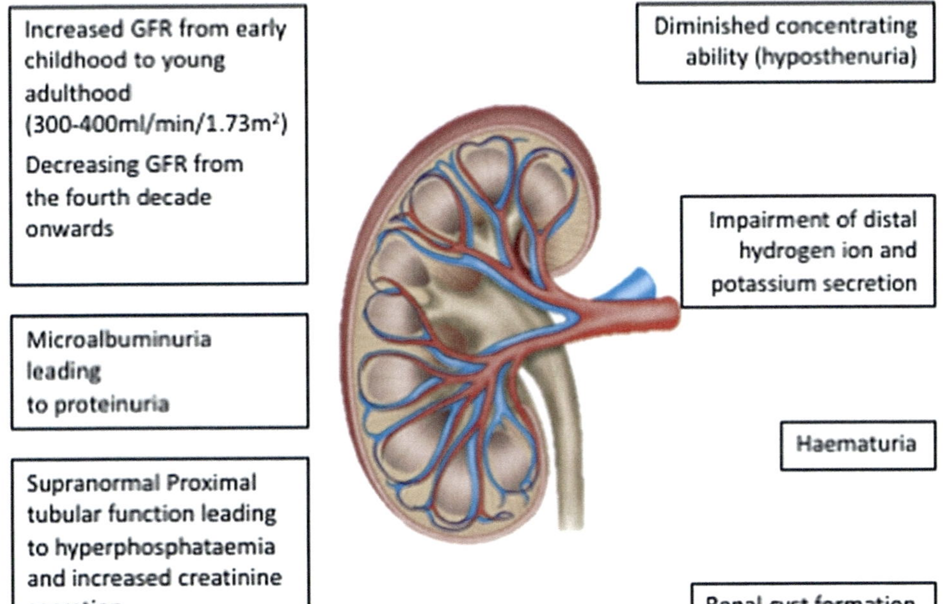

Fig. 48.1 Clinical features of sickle cell nephropathy

culation of the inner medulla is critical to maintaining the counter current multiplier system of the loop of Henle, which drives water and solute reabsorption and allows for effective urinary concentration. The resulting hypoxia, acidosis and hyperosmolarity of the inner medulla makes it an ideal environment for the polymerisation of deoxygenated haemoglobin S. Over time, repeated cycles of sickling and sludging cause micro-infarcts and ischaemic injury, leading to the chronic microvascular disease that is apparent in established SCN. In parallel with this, cortical renal blood flow and glomerular filtration rate (GFR) are increased in response to anaemia and vasodilation leading to hyperfiltration, proteinuria, glomerulosclerosis and tubulointerstitial fibrosis, which herald the onset of progressive CKD. In addition, when red blood cells haemolyse, free haemoglobin, a highly potent nitric oxide scavenger, is released into the circulation. The reduction in free nitric oxide leads to localised vasoconstriction, which is thought to underlie the pathogenesis of pulmonary hypertension, priapism, leg ulceration and stroke and is also likely to be involved in the progression of CKD. Local activation of hypoxia inducible factor 1α (HIF1α) upregulates the expression of endothelin-1 which, in the presence of reduced nitric oxide, leads to an increase in reactive oxygen species and vasoconstriction, thus feeding into a cycle of chronic medullary hypoxia [2].

48.1.2.3 Clinical Features

Hyperfiltration

Glomerular hypertrophy is ubiquitous in SCD and has been reported in children as young as 1–3 years old. Increased renal growth is observed from infancy in children with SCD and accompanies the early rise in glomerular filtration rate (GFR) [3]. GFR continues to rise throughout childhood and early adulthood, often exceeding 200 ml/min/1.73m^2. This may be partially accounted for by an increased cardiac output driven by anaemia, although the elevated GFR is not reversed by repeated red cell transfusion [4]. Localised prostaglandin release and an increase in nitric oxide synthase in response to hypoxia both result in an increase in total renal blood flow, and inhibition of prostaglandin synthesis with indomethacin has a significant negative impact on GFR [5]. Heme oxygenase-1 (HO-1) has also been demonstrated to be upregulated in injured kidneys (and indeed other tissues) in response to ongoing haemolysis in SCD. HO-1 is responsible for the conversion of heme to biliverdin with the subsequent release of carbon monoxide (CO). Both biliverdin and CO at these levels are potent antioxidants, and the carbon monoxide acts locally as a vasorelaxant, thus increasing both total renal blood flow and GFR [2]. However, in contrast to diabetic nephropathy, this hyperfiltration is not associated with an increase in systemic blood pressure, as patients with sickle cell disease tend to have reduced systemic vascular resistance and hence lower mean arterial pressure when compared with age- and ethnicity-matched controls [6].

Although it is not clear whether early or prolonged hyperfiltration is pathogenic in the aetiology of CKD, it is very common; 71% of adults were found to have an estimated GFR (eGFR) ≥140 ml/min/1.73m^2 in a cross-sectional study [7]. Although only a small proportion of these patients develop end-stage renal disease (ESRD), GFR does begin to decline in most people with SCD over the age of 30, and in a study of an elderly cohort of patients in Jamaica those who had died over the age of 60, chronic renal failure was cited as the major cause of death in 43%, making CKD the most frequent fatal complication in this age group [8]. Although this is circumstantial evidence, in CKD due to SCN it is probable that hyperfiltration plays a role in the pathogenesis of progressive renal dysfunction.

Microalbuminuria and Proteinuria

The appearance of albumin in the urine is an early manifestation of SCN. It can be detected from late childhood onwards and is detectable in approximately 28% of patients in the 15–26 age group, 38% in the 26–35 s, 50% in the 36–45 s and >60% in the over 46 s [7]. In some patients, microalbuminuria can develop into heavier proteinuria (protein: creatinine ratio (PCR) >50 mg/mmol) occasionally reaching the nephrotic range. Although full-blown nephrotic syndrome is uncommon (at about 4%), when it does occur it is associated with a very poor renal prognosis. One rare cause of sudden-onset nephrotic syndrome that has been described in patients with SCD is recent infection with human parvovirus B19 (HPV B19). In cases that have been biopsied early, the collapsing variant of focal segmental glomerulosclerosis (FSGS) has been found (with or without evidence of direct HPV B19 infection). Although the nephrotic syndrome per se spontaneously resolves without the need for corticosteroids, it is often followed by persistent proteinuria and slowly progressive renal dysfunction [9].

Tubular Abnormalities

Hyposthenuria (inability to concentrate urine under conditions of water deprivation) is a common phenomenon in people with SCD and often leads to enuresis in children and marked dehydration. It is caused by sickling in the vasa recta leading to microthrombi, infarction and collateral formation of blood vessels. As a consequence, there is a defect in the countercurrent exchange mechanism leading to insufficient trapping of solute in the inner medulla and abnormalities in renal water conservation. Increased endothelin-1 (ET-1) release results in vasoconstriction but also promotes natriuresis via stimulation of ET type b receptors in the renal collecting ducts [10]. Although hyposthenuria is reversible by blood transfusion until the age of 10, after this age it becomes irreversible and is associated with a permanently damaged microvasculature.

SCD is also associated with both proximal and distal tubular abnormalities. The increase in sodium and water loss from the collecting ducts leads to a reactive increase in sodium and water reabsorption by the proximal tubule. This reabsorption of sodium is the driving force for the reabsorption of other solutes, such as phosphate and β2-microglobulin, often causing hyperphosphataemia. Other solutes have a marked increase in proximal tubular secretion, such as creatinine and uric acid. Up to 30% of the total creatinine excretion can arise from tubular secretion, and so creatinine-based formulas for GFR can significantly overestimate renal function. Cystatin C has been demonstrated to be a more accurate surrogate marker of renal function in both adults and children with SCD, and hence its use is more likely to detect early decline in renal function [11].

In contrast, impaired medullary perfusion can cause distal tubule dysfunction, leading to acidosis that arises from diminished availability of ammonium. Hyperkalaemia is a common phenomenon in patients with SCD and has been attributed to hyperchloremic metabolic acidosis linked to a type IV renal tubular acidosis or resistance of the distal tubule to aldosterone [2].

Haematuria

Haematuria is common both in SCD and SCT. It can range from microscopic and painless, through visible and painless to visible and painful. It is usually self-limiting but can occasionally be severe enough to require transfusion. Small microinfarcts are often the cause of minor bleeding, but full renal papillary necrosis (RPN) with sloughing of the ischaemic papilla can lead to severe haemorrhage and obstruction and may be complicated by superadded infection. RPN can sometimes be diagnosed by ultrasonography, but CT urography (or intravenous urography if CT is unavailable) and direct ureteroscopy have a much higher diagnostic rate (◘ Fig. 48.2). The management of haematuria is usually conservative and limited to good hydration, pain relief and antibiotics if necessary. Patients with sickle cell disease also have an increased susceptibility to bacterial infections due to impaired immunity from autosplenectomy and an opsonic antibody deficiency. Bacteriuria was found to be present in 26% of children with SCD presenting with fever in Nigeria and UTI complicated pregnancy in 12% of mothers with SCD in a large UK cohort [12, 13].

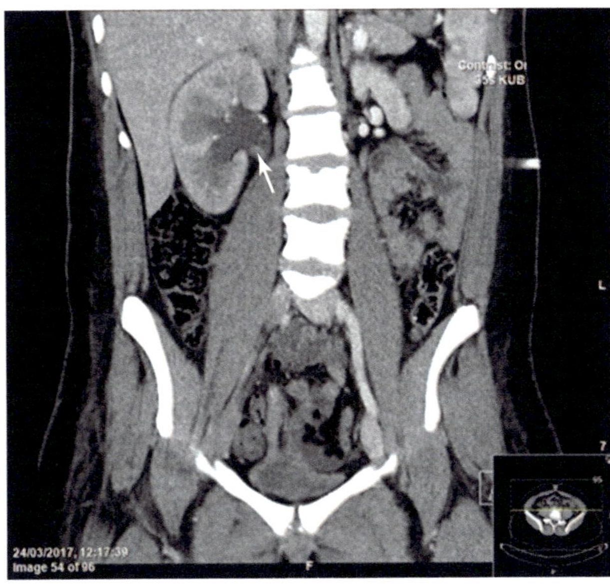

Fig. 48.2 A CT image demonstrating a right-sided hydronephrosis with a soft tissue mass in the renal pelvis caused by sloughing of an infarcted renal papilla. This patient presented with loin pain and visible haematuria

One rare but devastating complication of both SCD and, more commonly, the heterozygous state sickle cell trait (SCT) is renal medullary carcinoma, a cancer specific to patients with sickle haemoglobinopathies. It is a highly aggressive cancer that can occur in children as young as 2. It is most often metastatic at presentation and universally fatal within 2 years of presentation. The tumour is typically located deep in the parenchyma, unlike Wilms' tumour or renal cell carcinoma. Immunohistochemical analysis for epithelial cell markers (e.g. CAM 5.5), epithelial membrane antigen and cytokeratin may assist in diagnosis [14].

48.1.2.4 Clinical Syndromes of Renal Impairment

Acute Kidney Injury

Volume depletion due to inability to concentrate urine makes patients with SCD susceptible to AKI, and repeated episodes of AKI lead to irreversible organ damage and CKD [15]. These patients are more prone to further episodes of AKI, which is reported as a complicating factor in 2–8% of hospital admissions with painful VOC or acute chest syndrome (ACS). The severity of the AKI appears to be directly related to the severity of the acute sickling crisis [16]. Other causes of AKI are rhabdomyolysis, sepsis and drug nephrotoxicity. Less common causes are renal vein thrombosis and hepatorenal syndrome (caused by sickle cell disease related hepatic failure).

Progressive Chronic Kidney Disease

As life expectancy of patients with SCD increases, progressive CKD is becoming an increasingly large problem. Although hypertension is less common in patients with SCD than in an age- and ethnicity-matched cohort, when it is present, it has a marked impact on the rate of progression of CKD [17]. Other predictors of progressive CKD include haematuria; high levels of haemolysis; inheritance of the Bantu, or Central African Republic; β-globin gene cluster haplotype; and younger age at onset of CKD. New insights in to co-inheritance genetic modifiers in both Afro-Caribbean patients and those with SCD can also help us to stratify patients according to risk of progression of CKD [18].

Sickle Cell Trait and CKD

Patients who are heterozygote for the sickle cell gene have approximately 40% of their red cell haemoglobin is HbS with the rest being normal HbA and are said to have sickle cell trait (SCT). In general, these patients have normal haemoglobin levels and do not suffer from symptoms of haemolysis or vaso-occlusion. However, there have been case reports of catastrophic vaso-occlusive crises and sudden death in young people with SCT under extreme adverse conditions, such as excessive exercise or exposure to severe hypoxia. Non-malignant microscopic and macroscopic haematuria are reported more frequently in patients with SCT than in the general population, and older patients exhibit a loss of urinary concentrating ability. Renal medullary carcinoma is more common in patients with SCT than SCD, though the reasons for this are unclear. Patients who co-inherit SCT and adult polycystic kidney disease (APKD) have a more rapid decline to ESRD than family members with APKD who do not carry an HbS gene [19]. Whether having SCT alone is a risk factor for progressive CKD has been debated. One recent study in the USA using data from five large prospective studies of African Americans concluded that patients with SCT had an odds ratio (OR) of developing incident CKD of 1.76, an OR of experiencing a decline in renal function of 1.32 and an OR of having albuminuria of 1.86 compared with non-carriers [20]. In contrast, in a separate study of 3258 African Americans with ESRD secondary to type 2 diabetes, non-diabetic ESRD or controls, no association with SCT and ESRD was detected [21].

48.1.2.5 Investigations

The population at risk of developing SCN is also at risk of other diseases that affect the kidneys, including lupus nephritis, various forms of glomerulonephritis, blood-borne viruses, renal carcinoma, myeloma and renal stones. This differential should be considered when investigating a patient with SCD and new-onset proteinuria or haematuria. Although we don't investigate every patient with SCD and microalbuminuria (ACR >3.5 mg/mmol), patients with a protein to creatinine ratio >50 mg/mmol should be evaluated for other causes of CKD, and if any of these investigations are positive or the patient's signs and symptoms do not conform to those expected within the natural history of SCN as described above, they should be referred for further renal or urological evaluation. In particular, patients with sudden onset of nephrotic syndrome, warrant renal biopsy to look for causes other than SCN [15].

Imaging

Imaging should always be considered in the diagnosis of visible haematuria as described above. Renal iron deposition has been noted on magnetic resonance scans in patients with SCD but appears not to be related to liver iron concentration, a marker of total body iron load. Renal iron does appear to be correlated with markers of haemolysis but has not been shown to be associated with renal dysfunction or degree of albuminuria [22]. Simple renal cysts occur more frequently, are more abundant and develop at a younger age in patients with SCD than ethnically matched controls, though the significance of this is unknown [23].

Renal Histology

There is no pathognomonic lesion that defines SCN. Glomerular hypertrophy with distended capillaries is universally found but is not confined to those who have developed microalbuminuria or proteinuria. Focal and segmental glomerular sclerosis (FSGS) is the most common lesion associated with proteinuria but is not specific to SCN. Other lesions that have been noted on biopsy include thrombotic microangiopathy (TMA) and membranoproliferative glomerulonephritis (MPGN), lesions also not exclusive to SCN [24]. The only frequently demonstrated interstitial lesion is the presence of abundant haemosiderin granules in proximal tubular epithelial cells. As with all causes of progressive CKD, interstitial fibrosis and tubular atrophy predominate in the later stages.

48.1.2.6 Management of Sickle Cell Nephropathy

The management of sickle cell nephropathy can be divided into specific therapies, targeting sickle cell disease and the general management of chronic kidney disease.

Therapies for Treating Sickle Cell Disease

Sickle cell nephropathy is a chronic complication of SCD; therefore, strategies designed to alleviate the severity of SCD are likely to impact upon the development of SCN.

Blood transfusions, either intermittent or regular, are an established treatment for the management of both acute and chronic complications of sickle cell disease and are regularly used for stroke prevention, in the treatment of acute chest crisis and pulmonary in hypertension. However, there is little evidence for the benefits of long-term blood transfusions for the prevention of renal complications. In a recent comparison of children with SCD on chronic transfusion programmes compared to non-transfused cohorts, it was concluded that chronic transfusion is associated with a lower prevalence of albuminuria [25]. Previous studies, however, found no difference in the number of children receiving chronic transfusion when comparing those with microalbuminuria to those without [26].

Hydroxycarbamide (HC, also known as hydroxyurea) is a cytotoxic, antimetabolite approved for use in SCD. Although it has pleotropic effects, it primarily acts to increase levels of foetal haemoglobin which serve to dilute the levels of HbS and reduce risk of polymerisation. Clinical benefits include lower rates of pain, acute chest syndrome and need for blood transfusion. Long-term usage has been associated with improved growth and development in children and reduced overall mortality and morbidity in adults [27, 28]. Although some small studies have suggested that it may also be efficacious both in the treatment of children with established SCN and also in preventing its onset, the BABY HUG study (a phase III randomised, placebo-controlled, double-blind study of 193 patients starting HC in infancy between 9 and 17 months) was unable to prove this [29]. Subsequent prospective observational data collected from the Hydroxyurea Study of Long-Term Effects (HUSTLE) has demonstrated a reduction in hyperfiltration in children treated at the maximum tolerated dose over a 3-year period, but no change in albuminuria was detected. [3]

The only curative treatment currently available for sickle cell disease is allogeneic haematopoietic cell transplantation (HCT). It is usually reserved for children with major complications such as stroke and is not widely available. Although it is probable that HCT recipients who have a good outcome are likely to be protected from developing SCN, most published studies exclude those with established renal disease from receiving this treatment. One small study evaluating the use of

HCT in 10 adults with SCD included three patients with renal dysfunction. After an average of 30 months of follow-up, it was noted that HCT neither exacerbated nor ameliorated the progression of renal disease [30]. There have also been case reports describing HCT as safe in adults with end-stage renal disease (ESRD) and a promising study demonstrating safety of non-myeloablative peripheral blood stem cell transplantation (PBSCT) in patients with chronic organ damage including ESRD [31].

Whilst not a treatment for SCD per se, good management of acute and chronic pain is of paramount importance to patients and clinicians alike. Conflicts over choice and frequency of medications frequently lead to a loss of trust and break down of relations, and so it is vitally important to plan and have mutual agreement of pain management strategies in advance. The added burden of CKD has implications for the use of numerous analgesics including non-steroidal anti-inflammatory drugs (NSAIDs) and opiate-based medications. NSAIDs are effective and generally well-tolerated painkillers. They have the advantage of not causing drowsiness or constipation and are not habit-forming. They should however be avoided in patients with CKD 3–5 (though can be used in patients on dialysis in moderation). Their mechanism of action results in inhibition of prostaglandin synthesis, molecules that are intricately involved in maintaining borderline renal perfusion, and therefore they accelerate decline in GFR and medullary ischaemia. Opiates are often required for pain relief in SCD and should not be withheld if indicated. In advanced CKD, however, accumulation secondary to reduced excretion can occur, and so careful monitoring of dose and side effects is required. Advance pain-management planning involving both haematologists and nephrologists is the ideal situation.

Therapies for Treating Chronic Kidney Disease

In common with other causes of proteinuric CKD, it seems logical to attempt aggressive treatment of hypertension and reduction of proteinuria with blockade of the renin-angiotensin system. Although studies designed to demonstrate the benefit of ACE inhibition in SCN have been small and short term, the results of these have been positive in reducing proteinuria and hyperfiltration [32]. In our own practice, we generally recommend the introduction of an ACEi or angiotensin receptor blockers (ARBs) when a patient has a urinary protein/creatinine ratio persistently above 100 mg/mmol. We have noticed an additional benefit reported by patients that when prescribed these medications they experience a reduction in their frequency of nocturia, presumably due to the reduction in GFR that these drugs impart.

Management of Advanced Chronic Kidney Disease

Despite optimal treatment as outlined above, a proportion of patients with SCN will develop progressive CKD. Chronic anaemia and tissue hypoxia are strong drivers for erythropoietin (epo) synthesis, and SCD patients with normal kidney function often have epo levels well-above the normal range. However, as the GFR falls, their ability to produce sufficient levels of endogenous epo also begins to decline. Erythropoiesis-stimulating agents (ESAs) can be useful, particularly in combination with HC in patients who are intolerant of HC alone due to reticulocytopenia. Patients with CKD stage 3–4 often require very high doses of ESAs to have an impact on haemoglobin (Hb) levels. Although Hb targets should be lower than in the general CKD population (<10 mg/dl) due to the increased risk of triggering vaso-occlusive crises, they are still rarely achieved, and most patients become transfusion dependent by the time they reach end-stage renal disease (ESRD). It is often beneficial to continue ESA therapy after the commencement of dialysis, however, as this can prolong the interval between red cell transfusions and minimise the risk of iron overload [15, 33].

In patients who develop progressive renal dysfunction secondary to SCN, the rate of decline can be quite rapid once the GFR falls below 40 ml/min/1.73m^2, and so timely preparation for renal replacement therapy (RRT) is very important. Multiple admissions to hospital often result in very poor peripheral veins, so access planning needs to be commenced early and with expert input. Outcome data for patients with SCN on dialysis are few, but Powars reported that ESRD is associated with a very poor prognosis as not only was the average age of those reaching ESRD very young (23.1 in those with HbSS disease) but also the mean time to death after reaching ESRD was only 4 years despite being on haemodialysis [34]. More recently, a Saudi Arabian study reported that those with SCD and ESR D suffered more infectious complications, lived on average for only 27 months after commencing RRT and were significantly younger when they died compared to patients with ESRD of other causes [35]. A larger-scale comparison using the US Renal Data System looking at all patients who commenced RRT in the 1990s found that not only was SCN an independent risk factor for death, worse even than diabetes, but also patients with SCD were much less likely to receive a kidney transplant [36]. More recently, a 5-year study of patients with SCD receiving haemodialysis in France reported similar findings [37].

Despite there being may be many obstacles in the path to kidney transplantation, it is probably the modality that offers the best outcome for patients with SCD requiring RRT. Although long-term graft and patient survival are not quite as good as for patients with other causes of renal failure, the prognosis for individuals with SCN is far better after transplantation with a projected 7-year survival of 67% (vs. 83% for other African American) when compared with a 10-year survival of only 14% for those who remain on dialysis [38].

Management of the Transplanted Patient

In our experience, the major complications following transplantation in patients with SCD are sepsis, an increase in painful crises and acute renal sickling. Although we do not specifically tailor induction and maintenance immunosuppression for these patients, their increased susceptibility to infection should be borne in mind when considering the management of acute rejection. Patients with ESRD receiving RRT experience very few painful crises, probably due to severe anaemia and relatively frequent blood transfusions. Following transplantation delayed graft function (DGF) is common, but once renal function improves, there is a significant rise in the haemoglobin, which is often accompanied by an increase in the number of painful crises experienced by the patients [39]. Acute intra-renal sickling has been demonstrated as a cause for a sudden deterioration in renal function post-transplantation in homozygote SCD and, interestingly, also in heterozygotes (Fig. 48.3) [40]. To minimise the risk of DGF, VOC and recurrent SCN, we now recommend patients with SCD receive regular exchange blood transfusion

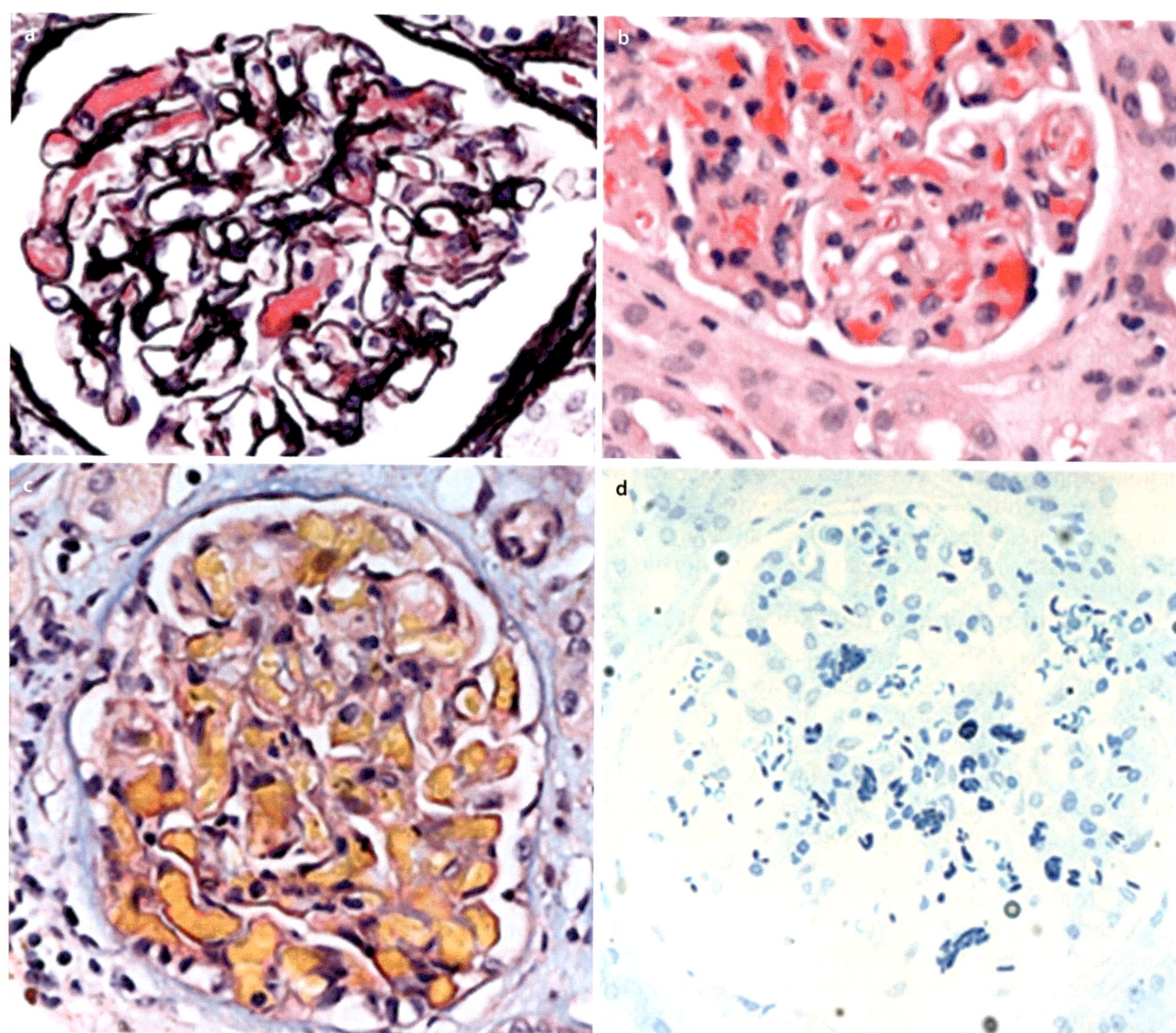

Fig. 48.3 Acute sickle glomerulopathy in a kidney transplant. a biopsy of a kidney transplant demonstrating glomerular capillary tufts congested with sickle shaped red blood cells. **a** silver stain, **b** haematoxylin and & eosin, **c** Picro-Mallory Trichrome, **d** toluidine blue

(EBT) with a view to reducing the HbS to <30% as soon as they are placed on the cadaveric waiting list (or pre-operatively in living donor transplantation), and we continue this for the life of the transplant. Although this exposes patients to more blood than top-up transfusion alone, we have not found it to be associated with an increased level of anti-HLA antibodies or an increased rate of rejection [41].

Case Studies

Case 1

A 22-year-old man with HbSS SCD presented feeling tired and lethargic and was found to have a haemoglobin of 35 g/l which had fallen from a steady-state average of 70–80 g/l. Further investigations revealed a white cell count of 11.7 × 10 [9]/l, a platelet count of 356 × 10 [9]/l, a reticulocyte count of zero, a serum creatinine of 64 μmol/l and positive serology for human parvovirus B19 IgM, suggesting current or recent infection. He was diagnosed with transient red cell aplasia (TRCA) and managed with top-up transfusion for 10 days until his haemoglobin recovered. Fourteen weeks later, he presented to the clinic complaining of leg swelling for a few weeks and periorbital oedema. He had a serum albumin of 19 g/l, creatinine of 72 μmol/l, a urinary protein to creatinine ratio (PCR) of 1128 mg/mmol, a haemoglobin of 71 g/l and positive HPVB19 IgG serology. He was diagnosed with new-onset nephrotic syndrome and was treated cautiously with diuretics and heparin for thromboprophylaxis. He underwent a renal biopsy which showed non-collapsing FSGS and 15–20% interstitial fibrosis and tubular atrophy (IFTA). It did not stain positive for HPVB19. He was commenced on an ACE inhibitor to a maximum tolerated dose (limited by serum hyperkalaemia). Over the next 2–3 months, his serum albumin recovered to 36–38 g/l and his oedema resolved. His serum creatinine rose to 100–110 μmol/l, and he remained significantly proteinuric with a PCR of 200–300 mg/mmol. This illustrates a case of HPVB19-induced nephrotic syndrome. Late biopsy often misses the collapsing FSGS and acute parvovirus infection but shows the sequelae of FSGS and IFTA. Although the nephrotic syndrome recovers spontaneously, patients are left with significant proteinuria and are at risk of progressive CKD. The dose of ACEi is often limited by hyperkalaemia.

Case 2

A 38-year-old man with HbSS SCD suffered from frequent painful VOC requiring admission to hospital 4–6 times a year. He also suffered with AKI during most admissions which resolved with hydration and pain management, but over the previous year, his baseline steady-state serum creatinine had risen from 140 μmol/l to 210 μmol/l. His steady-state haemoglobin was 75–80 g/l, and his urinary PCR was 280 mg/mmol. He was commenced on hydroxycarbamide (HC), which was gradually increased to 1.5 g/day, and an ACEi, which was titrated according to his serum potassium level. Over the next 4 months, his haemoglobin rose to 85 g/l and his % foetal Hb rose from 2% to 20%. His urinary PCR fell to 100 mg/mmol, and he remained well and out of hospital with no painful VOC. His serum creatinine plateaued at 160 μmol/l and remained stable for several years. This case illustrates the link between painful VOC and AKI. Although there is little evidence that HC can directly protect the kidneys from damage caused by sickling, preventing frequent admissions associated with AKI can prevent progression of underlying CKD and enable ACEi to be taken regularly resulting in lowering of proteinuria.

Case 3

A 32-year-old solicitor who had HbSS SCD and had been on peritoneal dialysis for 2 years underwent cadaveric renal transplantation from a non-heart beating donor. His haemoglobin on arrival in hospital was 56 g/l, and he received a top-up transfusion prior to surgery. He was given basiliximab as an induction agent and standard immunosuppression with tacrolimus, mycophenolate mofetil (MMF) and corticosteroids. Post-operatively, he experienced delayed graft function and continued dialysis for 2 weeks. During this period, he was commenced on exchange blood transfusion (EBT). Four weeks post-transplantation, he had a functioning graft with a stable creatinine of 230–240 μmol/l giving him an eGFR of 35 ml/min. He continues regular EBT and his renal function has remained stable for 5 years. He has had no episodes of rejection. This case illustrates the risk of delayed graft function in patients with SCD undergoing renal transplantation. Although the eventual graft function was only moderate, it has been stable for several years following the commencement of EBT.

Tips and Tricks

1. Prescribing ACEi or ARBS in the evening can reduce nocturia resulting in a better night's sleep.
2. Creatinine-based formulas for estimation of GFR (e.g. MDRD) overestimate renal function in patients with SCD due to enhance proximal tubular excretion of creatinine. Relative change rather than absolute values may detect changes in renal function earlier.
3. Patients who choose not to have blood transfusions (e.g. Jehovah's Witnesses) may need parenteral iron to maximise the effect of ESA therapy.
4. When using the MDRD formula to estimate renal function in advanced CKD, the 1.2 multiplication factor applied in Afro-Caribbean patients may overestimate renal function in patients with SCD due to their relatively low muscle mass. If in doubt, measure the true GFR using a gold standard method.
5. When making decisions regarding dialysis modality, consider the benefits of an AV fistula if regular EBT is to be recommended. Patients who choose peritoneal dialysis may still benefit from the formation of an AVF for this reason.

Conclusion

Good communication between the haematologists and nephrologists caring for patients with SCN is imperative. Timely management can minimise the risk of progression of CKD, whilst advanced planning in those approaching ESRD increases the well-being of the patient whilst they are on dialysis and prepares them for transplantation. This not only reduces early complications but also maximises graft function and long-term outcomes. As there is little evidence base for the best way to manage these patients, decisions should be made in discussion with the patient and the multidisciplinary team on a case-by-case basis. Some of the choices available together with their pros and cons are highlighted in ◘ Table 48.1.

48.2 Other Red Cell Disorders

48.2.1 Thalassaemia

There are two genetic loci for α-globin and thus 4 genes in diploid cells. Defects of all four α-genes results in hydrops foetalis and death. Alpha-thalassaemia resulting from defects of 1 or 2 α-globin genes results in very mild or subclinical disease and can in some circumstances be protective against haemolysis when co-inherited with β-globin abnormalities [7]. Defects in 3 α-genes leads to haemoglobin H disease. In general, this disease is relatively mild with affected individuals having stable haemoglobins of around 90 g/l. However, sudden acute haemolysis can occur, often in combination with acute infection, and may lead to acute kidney injury [42].

Beta-thalassaemia syndromes are characterised by genetic abnormalities in beta-globin chain synthesis. In β-thalassaemia major, synthesis of β-globin chains is severely impaired as both genes are affected, whilst α-chain synthesis remains normal. This imbalance in globin chain synthesis results in ineffective erythropoiesis and severe anaemia. Affected individuals require regular transfusion to survive, resulting in chronic iron overload and the necessity for ongoing iron chelation therapy.

Although red cell survival is reduced, intravascular haemolysis is not a feature of this disease, and so the toxic effects of free heme are not manifest. However, shortened red cell lifespan, rapid iron turnover and tissue deposition of excess iron are major factors responsible for chronic organ failure. Cardiopulmonary and reticuloendothelial dysfunction are common, but direct kidney involvement is less apparent. Although renal failure per se is uncommon, tubular abnormalities are detectable in many patients, even in childhood, and are probably related to renal iron deposition. One recent 10-year follow-up has concluded that long-term renal functional decline is uncommon in patients with normal tubular function. However, in those with evidence of tubular damage in childhood (elevated phosphaturia and high levels of uricuria) the rate of decline of GFR in adulthood is greater than in those with normal tubular function and greater than that expected for age

Table 48.1 Treatment options for patients with SCN; their pros and cons

Treatment option	Pros	Cons
Commencing ACEi or ARB for proteinuria in a young person with an eGFR>90 and BP <130/80 mmHg	Reduces proteinuria and may reduce risk of progression to CKD based on evidence in other proteinuric renal diseases Reduces nocturia	New medication for life in a young person Risk of hyperkalaemia so needs monitoring Little research undertaken in this patient group
Commencing hydroxycarbamide for progression of CKD in patients without frequent VOC	May improve foetal Hb levels and reduce intrarenal sickling and hypoxia May improve patient Well-being	No evidence that HC reduces progression of CKD in SCD May have unwanted side effects
Commencing ESAs to improve Hb in patients with eGFR<60 ml/min	May improve Hb and Well-being May allow a higher dose of HC to be tolerated	May not work, needs high doses May need extra iron supplementation if ferritin low (i.e. in patients who have had a low number of blood transfusions) May cause VOC if Hb rises too high (rare)
Commencing EBT on patients on the waiting list for a cadaveric renal transplant	HbS% kept below 30 improves fitness for surgery and reduces intercurrent illness and suspension from the list No need for top-up transfusion or EBT immediately prior to surgery Reduced risk of DGF and early intra-renal sickling May lead to reduced iron overload in patients who require frequent top-up transfusion	Increased exposure to blood risks, increase in anti-HLA antibodies and a positive cross-match High use of a precious resource Good venous access needed for effective EBT (AVFs should be used if needled by experience staff)
Commencing EBT on patients post renal transplant	Removes the risk of frequent painful crises Reduces intrarenal sickling and may improve the longevity of the graft	Increased exposure to blood risks an increase in anti-HLA antibodies and a positive cross match Patients may become highly sensitised and difficult to retransplant in the future May lead to iron overload if continued for years

ACEi angiotensin converting enzyme inhibitor, *ARB* angiotensin receptor blocker. *HC* hydroxycarbamide, *VOC* vaso-occlusive crisis, *EBT* exchange blood transfusion. *AVF* arteriovenous fistula, *DGF* delayed graft function, *HLA* human leucocyte antigen, *CKD* chronic kidney disease, *SCD* sickle cell disease, *ESA* erythropoiesis stimulating agent

alone [43]. Although iron chelation is an important aspect of management for patients with β-thalassaemia, many chelators (deferoxamine (iv or sc) or deferiprone (oral)) require normal renal function for the chelated iron to be excreted. Deferasirox is an orally active and hepatically excreted iron chelator frequently used in patients with iron overload. Unfortunately, it is nephrotoxic and can lead to renal dysfunction or the Fanconi syndrome in patients with clinical or subclinical renal impairment and so is not licenced for use in patients with established kidney disease.

One rare complication of chronic, severe anaemia (due to thalassaemia or other red cell disorders) is over-stimulation of the bone marrow leading to extra-medullary haematopoiesis (EMH). This usually occurs in the reticuloendothelial system but can occasionally occur in other tissues including the kidney. Renal lesions may be asymptomatic but can be complicated by spontaneous haemorrhage requiring treatment. EMH can be avoided by adequate red cell transfusion and iron supplementation where indicated.

Table 48.2 Haemolytic anaemias known to be associated with kidney disease. AKI: acute kidney injury, CKD: chronic kidney disease

Haemolytic anaemia	Associated with AKI	Associated with CKD
Acute transfusion haemolysis	Yes	No
Autoimmune	Yes	No
Paroxysmal cold haemoglobinuria (PCH)	Yes	No
Glucose-6-phospahte dehydrogenase (G6PD) deficiency	Yes	No
Drug reactions	Yes	No
Insect/snake bite	Yes	No
Malaria	Yes	Yes
Paroxysmal nocturnal haemoglobinuria (PNH)	Yes	Yes

48.3 Haemolytic Anaemias

There are many causes of haemolytic anaemia, some of which result in acute and/or chronic kidney disease (Table 48.2). Free heme-containing proteins cause renal injury via a number of mechanisms including oxidative stress, vasoconstriction (through scavenging of nitric oxide), chronic inflammation and haemosiderin deposition. ABO incompatible blood transfusion used to be the most common cause of haemolysis-associated AKI, but this is becoming increasingly rare with the advent of robust blood banking and dispensing practices. However, usually insignificant and untested for antibodies may rarely cause acute haemolysis if a patient is unwittingly transfused with incompatible blood. [44]

Autoimmune haemolytic anaemia, if severe, may also cause AKI, though other concurrent conditions such as dehydration or sepsis are often exacerbating features. Paroxysmal cold haemoglobinuria (PCH) is a self-limiting, postinfectious, cold-agglutinin-mediated form of haemolytic anaemia, which occurs in children, is occasionally associated with AKI and needs to be distinguished from paroxysmal nocturnal haemoglobinuria. Other causes of haemolysis associated with kidney injury include malaria, paroxysmal nocturnal haemoglobinuria, glucose-6-phosphate dehydrogenase deficiency, drug reactions and snake and insect bites.

48.3.1 Paroxysmal Nocturnal Haemoglobinuria

48.3.1.1 Epidemiology and Pathogenesis

Paroxysmal nocturnal haemoglobinuria (PNH) is a rare condition with a prevalence in the region of 16 pmp in the UK and a mean age of onset of approximately 34, though it can occur at any age [45]. It is an acquired haematopoietic disorder that arises from a somatic mutation of the phosphatidylinositol glycan class A (PIG-A) gene in one or more haematopoietic stem cells, followed by non-malignant clonal expansion. This leads to a deficiency of glycosylphosphatidylinositol (GPI)-anchored molecules including CD55 (decay accelerating factor) and CD59 (inhibitor of membrane reaction) in the plasma membrane. These are important regulatory proteins that inhibit the formation of the complement membrane attack complex and thus prevent complement-mediated cell lysis. PNH red bloods cells are consequently more susceptible to both intravascular and extravascular haemolysis and the resultant cell-free haemoglobin leads to the clinical manifestations of the disease as it exceeds the capacity of the body's natural scavenging molecule, haptoglobin to remove it from the circulation.

48.3.1.2 Clinical Manifestations

Paroxysmal nocturnal haemoglobinuria is typically characterised by episodic haemolytic anaemia in association with dark discoloration of the urine in the absence of red cells, most notably in the first urine voided in the morning. It is of varying severity and occurs either in isolation (classic PNH) or in association with aplastic anaemia or myelodysplastic syndrome. Other clinical manifestations include venous thrombosis often affecting the hepatic and mesenteric veins, episodic dysphagia, abdominal pain and kidney disease, both acute and chronic.

48.3.1.3 Renal Disease

When the binding capacity of haptoglobin is exceeded, haemoglobin dimers circulate in the plasma and are filtered by renal glomeruli. The dimers are resorbed in the proximal tubules and degraded, and the iron is stored as ferritin in the epithelium of the proximal tubules. Severe and sudden haemolysis often occurs in conjunction with gastroenteritis and the combination of heavy haemoglobinuria and dehydration can lead to AKI. Management is thus supportive including rehydration, and the kidney injury is usually self-limiting [46].

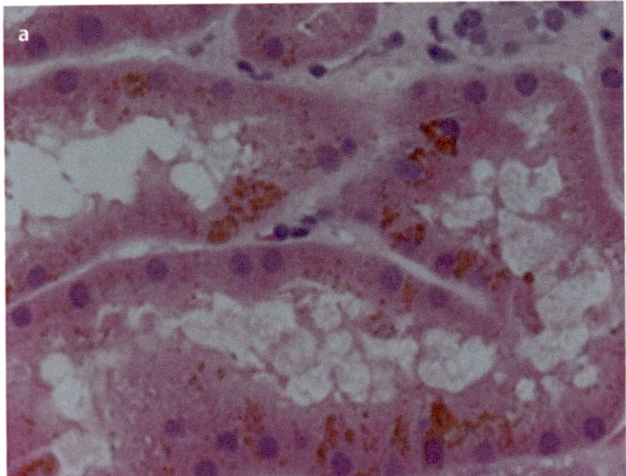

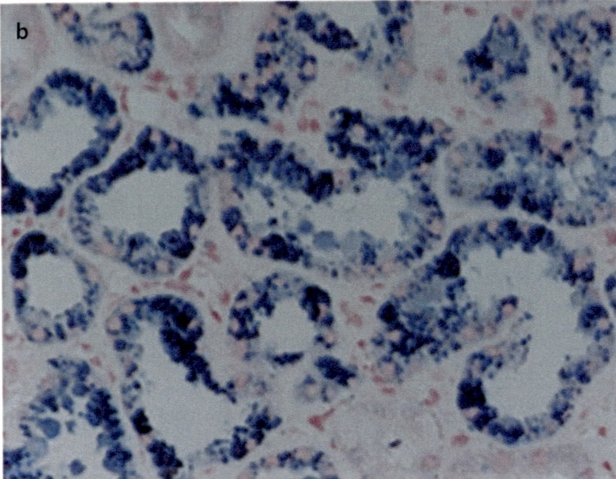

Fig. 48.4 **a** x600 H&E. Golden-coloured haemosiderin in the cytoplasm of the tubular epithelial cells of a patient with intravascular haemolysis. **b** x400 Perls-stained section to demonstrate the iron in the haemosiderin-laden tubular epithelial cell cytoplasm. The iron granules are stained blue in this preparation

Paroxysmal nocturnal haemoglobinuria is, however, a chronic disease with repeated episodes of haemolysis associated with complications such as venous thrombosis. Chronic cortical infarcts leading to urinary concentrating abnormalities is common as is proteinuria in patients with long-standing PNH. CKD stages 3–5 has been shown to be present in 20% of patients, and many of these become dialysis dependent.

48.3.1.4 Investigations

Paroxysmal nocturnal haemoglobinuria should be considered in patients who have an acquired, coombs (direct antiglobulin) negative haemolytic anaemia. This is usually associated with haemoglobinuria, haemosiderinuria, elevated serum lactate dehydrogenase levels and reduce haptoglobin levels. Granulocytes and platelets may also be reduced as they can be derived from the effected haematopoietic clone. Specific tests for PNH include the Ham test in which complement is activated by reducing the pH of fresh serum to 6.4, leading to red blood cell lysis. The gold standard test, however, involves detection a population of cells deficient in the GPI-anchored proteins CD55 and CD59 using monoclonal antibodies followed by flow cytometry [47]. Renal biopsy invariably demonstrates haemosiderosis with iron deposition in the proximal tubular cells (Fig. 48.4). Other features may include interstitial inflammation and fibrosis [48]. The renal iron deposition can also be clearly identified by magnetic resonance imaging (MRI), which typically shows reversed renal cortex-medulla differentiation on T(1)-weighted images and substantial loss of cortical signal intensity on both T(1)- and T(2)-weighted images [49].

48.3.1.5 Treatment

Although a proportion of patients (10–15%) go into spontaneous remission, the only curative treatment for the remaining patients is haematopoietic cell transplantation. However, the treatment of PNH has been transformed over the last 10 years by the development of eculizumab, a humanised monoclonal antibody that binds to the C5 component of complement and inhibits terminal complement activation. This drug not only improves the signs and symptoms associated with the disease but also improves life expectancy, although there is a subgroup of patients whose response to treatment is suboptimal. Eculizumab has specifically been shown to improve or stabilise kidney function in patients with established renal disease secondary to PNH and is also effective at managing other manifestations of the disease in patients on renal replacement therapy [50].

48.3.2 Malaria

The most common pattern of renal disease associated with malaria is acute kidney injury caused by *P. falciparum* (and rarely *P. vivax*) infection in adults and children (malarial acute renal failure, MARF). Although uncommon in native inhabitants in endemic regions, it affects 25–30% of non-immune non-natives who become infected [51]. The pathogenesis of MARF is multifactorial but occurs alongside severe haemolysis in approximately 70% of cases. This may be associated with intense jaundice, which, along with haemoglobinuria, leads to the dark discoloration of urine known as "black water fever". This is a severe complication of malaria, often occurring in a context of multiorgan failure, and has a high mortality rate. With supportive treatment and

Table 48.3 Drugs to be avoided in patients with G6PD deficiency

Drugs unsafe for all patients with G6PD deficiency	Drugs unsafe in some patients with G6PD deficiency
Acetanilide	Aspirin in high doses
Dapsone and other sulfones	Chloroquine (acceptable in acute malaria and malaria prophylaxis)
Furazolidone	Menadione, water-soluble derivatives
Methylthioninium chloride (methylene blue)	Probenecid
Nalidixic acid	Quinidine (acceptable in acute malaria)
Naphthalene (mothballs, henna)	Quinine (acceptable in acute malaria)
Niridazole	
Nitrofurantoin	
Phenazopyridine	
Phenylhydrazine	
Primaquine	
Quinolones	
Sulfonamides	
Toluidine blue	
Trinitrotoluene	
Uricase (rasburicase, pegloticase)	

eradication of the infection, renal recovery is common in patients who survive the acute illness but may die as access to dialysis is limited.

48.3.3 Glucose-6-Phosphate Dehydrogenase Deficiency

Glucose-6-phosphate dehydrogenase (G6PD) deficiency is a common X-linked genetic disorder that, like the haemoglobinopathies, has survived due to its protective nature against malaria infection. G6PD is central in the antioxidant defence of the red blood cell, and hence, affected individuals suffer acute haemolytic anaemia when exposed to drugs with a high redox potential or following ingestion of fava beans [52]. Severe acute haemolysis has, on rare occasions, been associated with episodes of acute kidney injury. [53] Table 48.3 includes a list of drugs to be avoided in patients with G6PD, though this is not exhaustive [54, 55].

Questions

- Is a renal biopsy ever required in the diagnosis of SCN?
- Is hydroxycarbamide effective at increasing the foetal haemoglobin level in every patient?
- Are patients with SCD more likely to be hypertensive than age- and ethnically matched controls?
- Are patients with beta-thalassaemia syndromes at increased risk of CKD?
- What percentage of adults with SCD develop albuminuria and what proportion develop ESRD?

Answers

1. Yes, if the presentation is atypical or a screen for other renal diseases is positive such as lupus nephritis.
2. No, only between 60 and 70% of patients respond to hydroxycarbamide.
3. No, patients with SCD generally have a lower blood pressure than matched controls. However, when hypertension is present, it accelerates CKD and should be treated aggressively.
4. No, there is no significant haemolysis in these conditions and no increased risk of CKD.
5. Albuminuria reaches a prevalence of approximately 60% in those over 45, although only 4–12% of patients with SCD will develop end-stage renal disease.

Patient Information and Guidelines

Standards for the clinical care of adults with sickle cell disease 2018-09-16.

▸ https://www.sicklecellsociety.org/sicklecellstandards/

References

1. Piel FB, Patil AP, Howes RE, Nyangiri OA, Gething PW, Dewi M, Temperley WH, Williams TN, Weatherall DJ, Hay SI. Global epidemiology of sickle haemoglobin in neonates: a contemporary geostatistical model-based map and population estimates. Lancet. 2013;381:142–51.
2. Nath KA, Hebbel RP. Sickle cell disease: renal manifestations and mechanisms. Nat Rev Nephrol. 2015;11:161–71.
3. Aygun B, Mortier NA, Smeltzer MP, Shulkin BL, Hankins JS, Ware RE. Hydroxyurea treatment decreases glomerular hyperfiltration in children with sickle cell anemia. Am J Hematol. 2013;88:116–9.
4. van Eps S. LW, Schouten, H, La Porte-Wijsman, LW, Struyker Boudier, AM: the influence of red blood cell transfusions on the hyposthenuria and renal hemodynamics of sickle cell anemia. Clin Chim Acta. 1967;17:449–61.

5. de Jong PE, de Jong-Van Den Berg TW, Sewrajsingh GS, Schouten H, Donker AJ. Statius van Eps, LW: the influence of indomethacin on renal haemodynamics in sickle cell anaemia. Clin Sci (Lond). 1980;59:245–50.
6. Pegelow CH, Colangelo L, Steinberg M, Wright EC, Smith J, Phillips G, Vichinsky E. Natural history of blood pressure in sickle cell disease: risks for stroke and death associated with relative hypertension in sickle cell anemia. Am J Med. 1997;102:171–7.
7. Day TG, Drasar ER, Fulford T, Sharpe CC, Thein SL. Association between hemolysis and albuminuria in adults with sickle cell anemia. Haematologica. 2012;97:201–5.
8. Serjeant GR, Serjeant BE, Mason KP, Hambleton IR, Fisher C, Higgs DR. The changing face of homozygous sickle cell disease: 102 patients over 60 years. Int J Lab Hematol. 2009;31:585–96.
9. Quek L, Sharpe C, Dutt N, Height S, Allman M, Awogbade M, Rees DC, Zuckerman M, Thein SL. Acute human parvovirus B19 infection and nephrotic syndrome in patients with sickle cell disease. Br J Haematol. 2010;149:289–91.
10. Nakano D, Pollock D. New concepts in endothelin control of sodium balance. Clin Exp Pharmacol Physiol. 2011;
11. Huang SH, Sharma AP, Yasin A, Lindsay RM, Clark WF, Filler G. Hyperfiltration affects accuracy of creatinine eGFR measurement. Clin J Am Soc Nephrol. 2011;6:274–80.
12. Mava Y, Ambe JP, Bello M, Watila I, Nottidge VA. Urinary tract infection in febrile children with sickle cell anaemia. West Afr J Med. 2011;30:268–72.
13. Oteng-Ntim E, Ayensah B, Knight M, Howard J. Pregnancy outcome in patients with sickle cell disease in the UK--a national cohort study comparing sickle cell anaemia (HbSS) with HbSC disease. Br J Haematol. 2015;169:129–37.
14. Alvarez O, Rodriguez MM, Jordan L, Sarnaik S. Renal medullary carcinoma and sickle cell trait: a systematic review. Pediatr Blood Cancer. 2015;62:1694–9.
15. Sharpe CC, Thein SL. How I treat renal complications in sickle cell disease. Blood. 2014;123:3720–6.
16. Lebensburger JD, Palabindela P, Howard TH, Feig DI, Aban I, Askenazi DJ. Prevalence of acute kidney injury during pediatric admissions for acute chest syndrome. Pediatr Nephrol. 2016;31:1363–8.
17. Gordeuk VR, Sachdev V, Taylor JG, Gladwin MT, Kato G, Castro OL. Relative systemic hypertension in patients with sickle cell disease is associated with risk of pulmonary hypertension and renal insufficiency. Am J Hematol. 2008;83:15–8.
18. Saraf SL, Shah BN, Zhang X, Han J, Tayo BO, Abbasi T, Ostrower A, Guzman E, Molokie RE, Gowhari M, Hassan J, Jain S, Cooper RS, Machado RF, Lash JP, Gordeuk VR. APOL1, alpha-thalassemia, and BCL11A variants as a genetic risk profile for progression of chronic kidney disease in sickle cell anemia. Haematologica. 2017;102:e1–6.
19. Shaw C, Sharpe CC. Could sickle cell trait be a predisposing risk factor for CKD? Nephrol Dial Transplant. 2010;25: 2403–5.
20. Naik RP, Derebail VK, Grams ME, Franceschini N, Auer PL, Peloso GM, Young BA, Lettre G, Peralta CA, Katz R, Hyacinth HI, Quarells RC, Grove ML, Bick AG, Fontanillas P, Rich SS, Smith JD, Boerwinkle E, Rosamond WD, Ito K, Lanzkron S, Coresh J, Correa A, Sarto GE, Key NS, Jacobs DR, Kathiresan S, Bibbins-Domingo K, Kshirsagar AV, Wilson JG, Reiner AP. Association of sickle cell trait with chronic kidney disease and albuminuria in African Americans. JAMA. 2014;312:2115–25.
21. Hicks PJ, Langefeld CD, Lu L, Bleyer AJ, Divers J, Nachman PH, Derebail VK, Bowden DW, Freedman BI. Sickle cell trait is not independently associated with susceptibility to end-stage renal disease in African Americans. Kidney Int. 2011;80: 1339–43.
22. Vasavda N, Gutierrez L, House MJ, Drasar E, St Pierre TG, Thein SL. Renal iron load in sickle cell disease is influenced by severity of haemolysis. Br J Haematol. 2012;157:599–605.
23. Meeks D, Navaratnarajah A, Drasar E, Jaffer O, Wilkins CJ, Thein SL, Sharpe CC. Increased prevalence of renal cysts in patients with sickle cell disease. BMC Nephrol. 2017;18:298.
24. Maigne G, Ferlicot S, Galacteros F, Belenfant X, Ulinski T, Niaudet P, Ronco P, Godeau B, Durrbach A, Sahali S, Lang P, Lambotte O, Audard V. Glomerular lesions in patients with sickle cell disease. Medicine (Baltimore). 2010;89:18–27.
25. Alvarez O, Nottage K, Simpson LM, Wood J, Davis BR, Fuh B, Sarnaik S, Aygun B, Helton K, Ware RE. Kidney function of transfused children with sickle cell anemia: baseline data from the TWiTCH study with comparison to non-transfused cohorts. Am J Hematol. 2017;92:E637–9.
26. Becton LJ, Kalpatthi RV, Rackoff E, Disco D, Orak JK, Jackson SM, Shatat IF. Prevalence and clinical correlates of microalbuminuria in children with sickle cell disease. Pediatr Nephrol. 2010;25:1505–11.
27. de Montalembert M, Brousse V, Elie C, Bernaudin F, Shi J, Landais P. Long-term hydroxyurea treatment in children with sickle cell disease: tolerance and clinical outcomes. Haematologica. 2006;91:125–8.
28. Voskaridou E, Christoulas D, Bilalis A, Plata E, Varvagiannis K, Stamatopoulos G, Sinopoulou K, Balassopoulou A, Loukopoulos D, Terpos E. The effect of prolonged administration of hydroxyurea on morbidity and mortality in adult patients with sickle cell syndromes: results of a 17-year, single-center trial (LaSHS). Blood. 2010;115:2354–63.
29. Alvarez O, Miller ST, Wang WC, Luo Z, McCarville MB, Schwartz GJ, Thompson B, Howard T, Iyer RV, Rana SR, Rogers ZR, Sarnaik SA, Thornburg CD, Ware RE. Effect of hydroxyurea treatment on renal function parameters: results from the multi-center placebo-controlled baby hug clinical trial for infants with sickle cell anemia. Pediatr Blood Cancer. 2012;
30. Hsieh MM, Kang EM, Fitzhugh CD, Link MB, Bolan CD, Kurlander R, Childs RW, Rodgers GP, Powell JD, Tisdale JF. Allogeneic hematopoietic stem-cell transplantation for sickle cell disease. N Engl J Med. 2009;361:2309–17.
31. Horwitz ME, Spasojevic I, Morris A, Telen M, Essell J, Gasparetto C, Sullivan K, Long G, Chute J, Chao N, Rizzieri D. Fludarabine-based nonmyeloablative stem cell transplantation for sickle cell disease with and without renal failure: clinical outcome and pharmacokinetics. Biol Blood Marrow Transplant. 2007;13:1422–6.
32. Sasongko TH, Nagalla S, Ballas SK. Angiotensin-converting enzyme (ACE) inhibitors for proteinuria and microalbuminuria in people with sickle cell disease. Cochrane Database Syst Rev. 2013:CD009191.
33. Little JA, McGowan VR, Kato GJ, Partovi KS, Feld JJ, Maric I, Martyr S, Taylor JG, Machado RF, Heller T, Castro O, Gladwin MT. Combination erythropoietin-hydroxyurea therapy in sickle cell disease: experience from the National Institutes of Health and a literature review. Haematologica. 2006;91:1076–83.
34. Powars DR, Elliott-Mills DD, Chan L, Niland J, Hiti AL, Opas LM, Johnson C. Chronic renal failure in sickle cell disease: risk factors, clinical course, and mortality. Ann Intern Med. 1991;115:614–20.
35. Saxena AK, Panhotra BR, Al-Arabi Al-Ghamdi AM. End-stage sickle cell nephropathy: determinants of reduced survival of patients on Long-term Hemodialysis. Saudi J Kidney Dis Transpl. 2004;15:174–5.

36. Abbott KC, Hypolite IO, Agodoa LY. Sickle cell nephropathy at end-stage renal disease in the United States: patient characteristics and survival. Clin Nephrol. 2002;58:9–15.
37. Nielsen L, Canoui-Poitrine F, Jais JP, Dahmane D, Bartolucci P, Bentaarit B, Gellen-Dautremer J, Remy P, Kofman T, Matignon M, Suberbielle C, Jacquelinet C, Wagner-Ballon O, Sahali D, Lang P, Damy T, Galacteros F, Grimbert P, Habibi A, Audard V. Morbidity and mortality of sickle cell disease patients starting intermittent haemodialysis: a comparative cohort study with non- sickle dialysis patients. Br J Haematol. 2016;174:148–52.
38. Scheinman JI. Sickle cell disease and the kidney. Nat Clin Pract Nephrol. 2009;5:78–88.
39. Sharpe CC, Thein SL. Sickle cell nephropathy - a practical approach. Br J Haematol. 2011;155:287–97.
40. Kim L, Garfinkel MR, Chang A, Kadambi PV, Meehan SM. Intragraft vascular occlusive sickle crisis with early renal allograft loss in occult sickle cell trait. Hum Pathol. 2011;
41. Willis J, Awogbade M, Howard J, Breen C, Abbas A, Harber M, Shindi A, Andrews P, Galliford J, Shah S, Sharpe CC. Outcomes following kidney transplantation in patients with sickle cell disease with and without exchange blood transfusion. Kidney Int Suppl.
42. Fucharoen S, Viprakasit V. Hb H disease: clinical course and disease modifiers. Hematology Am Soc Hematol Educ Program. 2009:26–34.
43. Lai ME, Spiga A, Vacquer S, Carta MP, Corrias C, Ponticelli C. Renal function in patients with beta-thalassaemia major: a long-term follow-up study. Nephrol Dial Transplant. 2012;
44. Irani MS, Richards C. Hemolytic transfusion reaction due to anti-IH. Transfusion. 2011;51:2676–8.
45. de Latour RP, Mary JY, Salanoubat C, Terriou L, Etienne G, Mohty M, Roth S, de Guibert S, Maury S, Cahn JY, Socie G. French Society of, H, French association of young, H: Paroxysmal nocturnal hemoglobinuria: natural history of disease subcategories. Blood. 2008;112:3099–106.
46. Qi K, Zhang XG, Liu SW, Yin Z, Chen XM, Wu D. Reversible acute kidney injury caused by paroxysmal nocturnal hemoglobinuria. Am J Med Sci. 2011;341:68–70.
47. Borowitz MJ, Craig FE, Digiuseppe JA, Illingworth AJ, Rosse W, Sutherland DR, Wittwer CT, Richards SJ. Guidelines for the diagnosis and monitoring of paroxysmal nocturnal hemoglobinuria and related disorders by flow cytometry. Cytometry B Clin Cytom. 2010;78:211–30.
48. Rachidi S, Musallam KM, Taher AT. A closer look at paroxysmal nocturnal hemoglobinuria. Eur J Intern Med. 2010;21:260–7.
49. Rimola J, Martin J, Puig J, Darnell A, Massuet A. The kidney in paroxysmal nocturnal haemoglobinuria: MRI findings. Br J Radiol. 2004;77:953–6.
50. de Fontbrune S. F, Peffault de Latour, R: ten years of clinical experience with Eculizumab in patients with paroxysmal nocturnal Hemoglobinuria. Semin Hematol. 2018;55:124–9.
51. Barsoum RS. Malarial acute renal failure. J Am Soc Nephrol: JASN. 2000;11:2147–54.
52. Mason PJ, Bautista JM, Gilsanz F. G6PD deficiency: the genotype-phenotype association. Blood Rev. 2007;21:267–83.
53. Schuurman M, van Waardenburg D, Da Costa J, Niemarkt H, Leroy P. Severe hemolysis and methemoglobinemia following fava beans ingestion in glucose-6-phosphatase dehydrogenase deficiency: case report and literature review. Eur J Pediatr. 2009;168:779–82.
54. Beutler E. G6PD deficiency. Blood. 1994;84:3613–36.
55. Society RP. British national formulary. BMJ Group and Pharmaceutical Press; 2011.

Multiple Myeloma and the Kidney

Ritika Rana, Paul Cockwell, and Jennifer Pinney

Contents

M. Harber (ed.), *Primer on Nephrology*, https://doi.org/10.1007/978-3-030-76419-7_49

Learning Objectives

1. All patients with unexplained AKI should be screened for a monoclonal protein (paraprotein). This screen should include serum protein electrophoresis and a serum or urinary free light chain assay.
2. A monoclonal gammopathy can produce renal disease regardless of the quantity of paraprotein or whether the underlying cause is benign or malignant.
3. Paraprotein-related renal diseases can present as AKI, progressive proteinuric renal disease, and/or as Fanconi syndrome.
4. Prompt commencement of chemotherapy is crucial in MM and AKI, and patients with MGRS usually require chemotherapy.

49.1 Introduction

Multiple myeloma (MM) is a bone marrow cancer caused by clonal expansion of plasma cells. These clonal plasma cells usually produce monoclonal immunoglobulin (MIg), also called a paraprotein. MM is classified by the type of abnormal immunoglobulin (Ig) produced, and diagnostic criteria are based on organ involvement (a myeloma defining event) or a high tumour burden. Patients with MM often have a delayed diagnosis; a recent study showed that patients had an average of three visits to their primary care physician before referral to a hospital specialist [1].

Renal impairment is a common complication of MM. Up to 50% of patients with MM have an eGFR <60 ml/min/1.73m^2 at presentation and around 20% have sufficient severity of renal impairment to classify this involvement as a myeloma defining event (a serum creatinine >2 mg/dl (173 μmol/l)) [2, 3]. Kidney biopsy series report that up to 90% of severe acute kidney injury (AKI) in myeloma is caused by cast nephropathy. Around 3.5% of patients with new presentation MM require dialysis treatment for AKI [4]. Severe renal impairment is an adverse determinant of patient survival, and survival improves if there is an early recovery of renal function [5].

An urgent timeline is crucial in patients who present with AKI and a co-incident paraprotein. Delays in diagnosis and treatment can be the difference between life-long dialysis and recovery of independent renal function, with a profound impact on patient survival.

Definitions of common terms used in monoclonal disorders are summarised below:

Monoclonal cells: A group of cells produced from a single aberrant cell of B-cell lineage (usually a plasma cell) by repeated cellular replication.

Monoclonal protein (M protein) or monoclonal immunoglobulin (MIg) or paraprotein: Abnormal Ig or its components (heavy chain or light chain) present in the serum or urine; produced by an abnormal monoclonal proliferation of a plasma cell or another cell of B-cell lineage.

Dysproteinaemia: An abnormality of the monoclonal Ig content of blood.

Monoclonal disease: A monoclonal protein is present in the blood or urine, and there is tissue damage associated with that protein.

Monoclonal gammopathy: A disturbance in the Ig production as a result of clonal proliferation of cells in the B lymphocyte lineage.

Plasma cell dyscrasia: A monoclonal proliferation of plasma cells.

Monoclonal gammopathy of undetermined significance: Asymptomatic premalignant clonal disorder of a plasma cell or other cells of B-cell lineage, considered to be a precursor of MM or related lymphoplasmacytic malignancies and does not cause end-organ damage.

Monoclonal gammopathy of renal significance (MGRS): Non-malignant proliferation of plasma cells producing a paraprotein causing a distinct renal injury.

Novel chemotherapy agents: Agents introduced into widespread clinical practice for chemotherapy for MM since 2005; they work by targeting novel biological processes. These drugs include bortezomib, thalidomide, and lenalidomide.

49.2 Clinical Features

The signs of MM can be both local and systemic. Infiltration of bone marrow (BM) with clonal plasma cells may result in anaemia, leucopenia, thrombocytopenia, and immune paresis, with a high risk of subsequent infections. Bone involvement leads to hypercalcemia and lytic lesions, and tumour masses arising from the bones may result in spinal cord compression or nerve root compression [6]. If MM involves extramedullary organs, which is rare, the symptoms are similar to those of a solid tumour arising from the involved organ [6]. Systemic clinical features include malaise, weight loss, recurrent infections, consequences of hypercalcemia, and bone pain.

Some patients present with AKI without obvious signs of myeloma, although a disease-related trigger (e.g. hypercalcaemia, dehydration, sepsis) is common. Occasionally, a patient will be diagnosed with MM by a kidney biopsy performed for unexplained AKI.

In addition to renal involvement, a paraprotein can result in non-renal AL amyloidosis (including cardiac involvement), cryoglobulinemia, hyper viscosity syndrome, and peripheral neuropathy.

49.3 Epidemiology

There are around 5500 new cases/year of MM in the UK [7]. It is the seventeenth most common cancer in the UK [8] and the second most common haematological malignancy. The reported international incidence for MM varies from 4 to almost 50 per million population/year, with the highest rates reported in high-income countries [9]. The median age at onset is 70 years, and it occurs more frequently in men and in African Americans [8]. The current overall survival from the first diagnosis is 4 years, and disease-free survival (from remission to relapse) is around 18 months. Outcomes are rapidly improving in this time period with the introduction of new therapies.

49.4 The Biology of Immunoglobulin Light Chains

The renal lesions associated with MM and MGRS are caused by clonal Ig, usually the light chain component; infiltration by clonal cells is rare. Igs are symmetrical molecules composed of two identical heavy chains (HCs) and identical two light chains (LCs), each containing variable and constant domains (▣ Fig. 49.1). Ig can be produced by all cells of B-cell lineage; however, the predominant source are plasma cells: each cell produces an Ig of unique specificity consisting of HCs and LCs of a single isotype. When a clone develops from sustained proliferation of a single aberrant plasma cell, there is usually excess production of clonal Ig; this molecule has no useful biological role.

There are two isotypes of LC, kappa (κ) and lambda (λ). There is a 2:1 ratio of κ:λ producing plasma cells in humans. Whilst the majority of produced LC is incorporated into the intact Ig molecule, around 40% is freely released κLC (a monomeric protein with a molecular weight (MW) of 22.5 Kd) or λLC (as a dimeric protein, MW 45 Kd), although oligomers and polymers of the clonal isotype are present in some patients (▣ Fig. 49.1). Renal involvement usually occurs because of interactions between LCs and resident renal cells. Different LCs exert differential pathogenicity due to their differing physico-chemical properties [10].

Serum free LCs (FLCs) are cleared by glomerular filtration at 40% for κFLC and 20% for λFLC, equating to half-lives of 2–3 hours and 4–6 hours, respectively, in patients with normal renal function. In contrast, IgG has a MW of 160 kDa and has minimal renal clearance, with a half-life of 21 days.

In complete renal failure, the half-life of serum FLC increases to 18 hours or more with slow clearance by the reticuloendothelial system. The relationship between the MW of LCs, renal clearance, and serum half-life is crucial in the development of AKI. Furthermore, because of the big differences in half-life between the serum FLC and

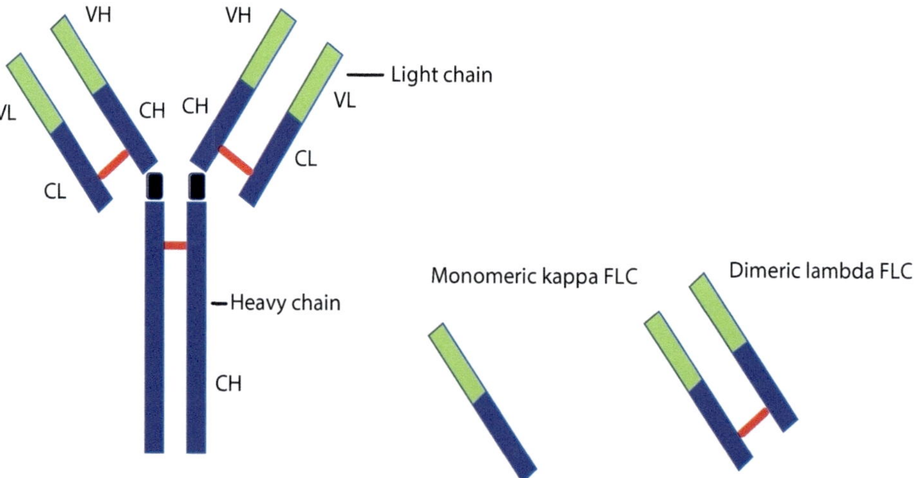

▣ **Fig. 49.1** Diagrammatic representation of intact immunoglobulin with monomeric kappa (k) and dimeric lambda (λ) FLC molecule. Each light chain consists of variable domain, VL, and one constant domain, CL. The heavy chain consists of a variable domain, VH, and three constant domains, CH

intact Ig, changes in involved serum FLC levels are a better marker of early disease response than intact (clonal) Ig.

Given the important role of kidneys in the clearance of FLCs, in patients with a low GFR, the normal serum free light chain (sFLC) ratio shifts up, because κFLC is differentially retained as it has a lower MW: this means that the upper limit of the normal range for the sFLC ratio in a patient receiving dialysis treatment is 3.17. The normal range ratio in normal kidney function is 0.26–1.65 [11].

49.5 Paraprotein-Related Renal Disease

The clonal proliferation of plasma cells or other cells of B-cell lineage can be malignant or non-malignant. The paraprotein produced in these cells can result in a diverse range of renal disorders. Whilst most paraprotein-related renal disease is due to the direct effects of the MIg LCs, it can also be due to intact Ig or HC Ig. Occasionally (e.g. C3 glomerulopathy), the renal disease is due to a distal effect of a MIg. The classification of paraprotein-related renal disease is shown in ◘ Fig. 49.2.

49.5.1 Monoclonal Gammopathy of Renal Significance-Associated Renal Disease

The term MGRS is used to describe a B-cell lineage clonal proliferation with: 1) one or more renal lesions caused by the produced MIg and 2) a clone that does not cause tumour complications or meet current haematological criteria for immediate specific therapy. Most of these patients have a low-grade clone consistent with that seen in MGUS; however, unlike in MGUS, the monoclonal protein causes end-organ damage. The renal lesion is a consequence of the physico-chemical properties of the clone rather than the nature of the underlying clonal lymphoproliferation. Renal disease secondary to MGRS is termed an MGRS-associated renal lesion.

The range of haematological disorders that can produce MGRS includes MGUS (although this is confusing as by definition it is not MGUS), smouldering multiple myeloma (SMM), smouldering Waldenström macroglobulinemia (WM), monoclonal B-cell lymphocytosis (MBL), low-grade chronic lymphocytic lymphoma (CLL), and other low-grade lymphomas.

The International Kidney and Monoclonal Gammopathy (IKMG) research group has proposed a classification system for MGRS-associated lesions based on immunofluorescence (IF) and the ultrastructural appearance of in situ deposits, categorised as organised and non-organised (◘ Fig. 49.3). This emphasises that MGRS can only be fully assessed by pathology departments that have available IF for a full panel of antibodies and electron microscopy (EM).

The deposition of the MIg can occur in the glomeruli, the tubulointerstitium, and/or the vasculature, with glomerular capillaries and mesangium, being a preferred site for deposition [12]. LC deposition in the kidney is most commonly seen, deposition of the whole Ig is less frequent, and monoclonal HC deposition is rare.

MGRS may be underappreciated in clinical practice since patients with renal dysfunction often have other plausible explanations for their deteriorating renal function, and the monoclonal protein is considered coincidental rather than causal [13]. Also, the disease spectrum is wide with manifestations ranging from laboratory results suggestive of a tubulopathy (e.g. Fanconi syndrome) to proteinuria and renal impairment, which is often progressive.

If a monoclonal protein is detected in patients with unexplained renal dysfunction or urinary abnormalities (proteinuria or haematuria), a complete haematologic workup must be carried out if a renal biopsy then shows a MGRS-associated renal lesion. A critical aspect of the renal biopsy is to correlate the specific Ig found in the kidney with the circulating paraprotein to ensure a direct link between the MG and renal lesion is established [14].

Treatment of MGRS-associated kidney disease is often indicated to preserve or restore kidney function and prevent recurrence after kidney transplantation.

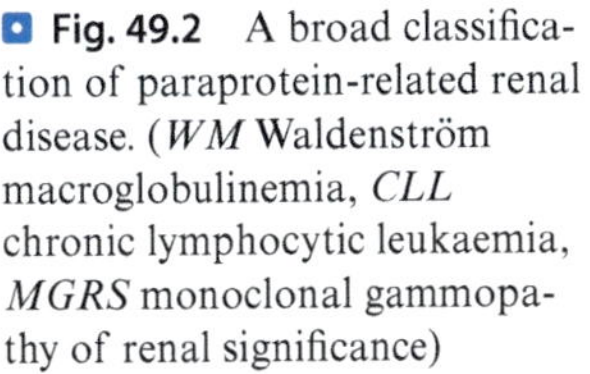

◘ **Fig. 49.2** A broad classification of paraprotein-related renal disease. (*WM* Waldenström macroglobulinemia, *CLL* chronic lymphocytic leukaemia, *MGRS* monoclonal gammopathy of renal significance)

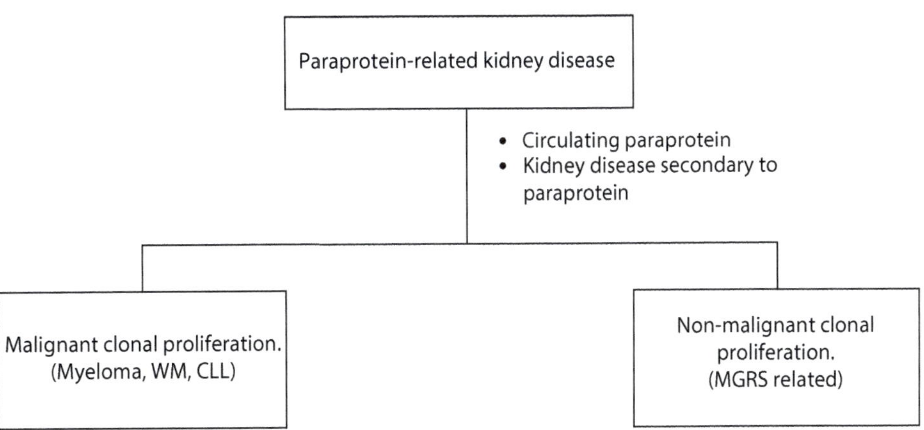

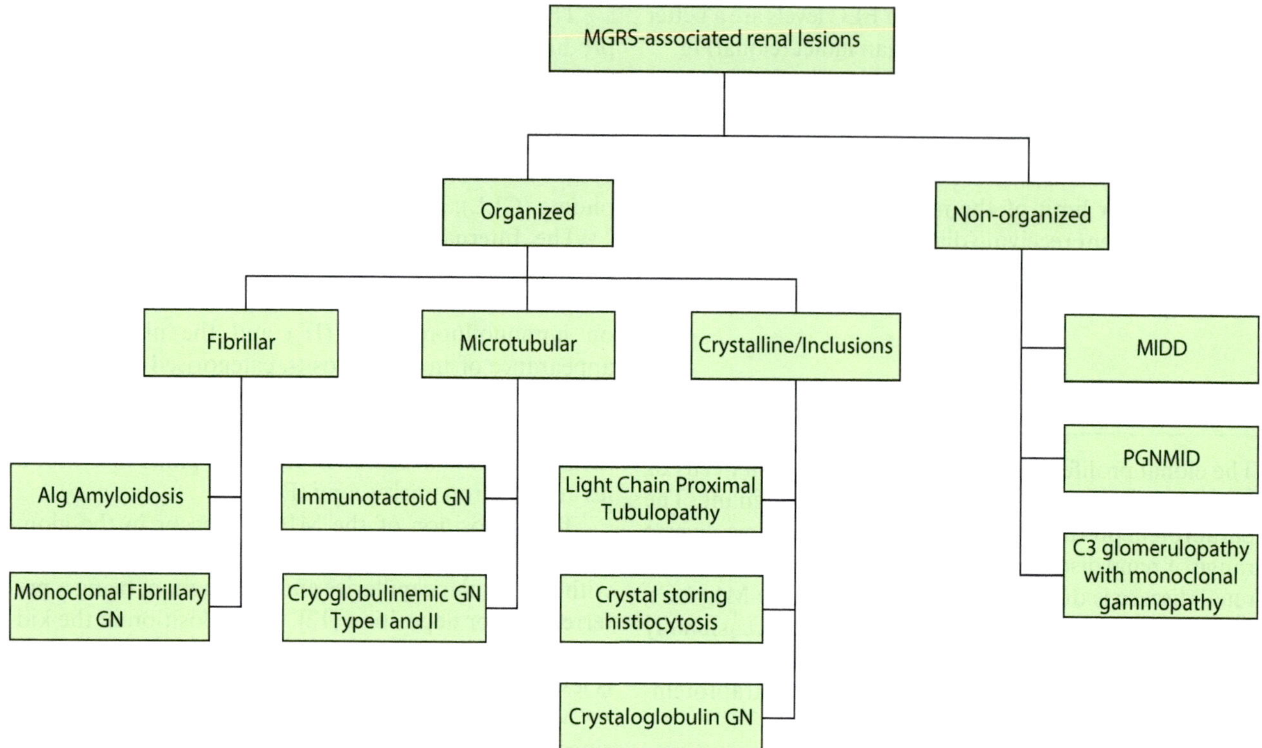

Fig. 49.3 Classification of MGRS-associated renal lesions based on the ultrastructural appearance of deposits. (Adapted with permission from Bridoux et al. (2015). *Ig* immunoglobulin, *AIg* immunoglobulin amyloidosis, *GN* glomerulonephriti, *MIDD* monoclonal immunoglobulin deposition disease, *PGNMID* proliferative glomerulonephritis with monoclonal immunoglobulin deposits)

The choice of chemotherapy regimen depends on the nature of underlying B-cell clone; i.e. lymphocytic or plasmacytic in origin [15]. The renal response strongly correlates with the nature of the haematologic response, and rapid suppression of Ig secretion with chemotherapy is required to improve outcomes [15]. For patients who have progressed to end-stage renal failure, kidney transplantation may be an option for those with a sustained haematologic response [16].

49.6 Pathogenesis of MM

Myeloma is a genetically complex disease and intra-clonal heterogeneity is a common feature [17]. A plasma cell becomes malignant through an accumulation of genetic hits across different cellular pathways, leading to dysregulation of the intrinsic biology of the cell over time [18].

There appears to be interplay between tumour cell genetics and the local microenvironment. The first oncogenic events may occur in the germinal centre during somatic hypermutation and isotype switching, and the plasma cell differentiates into a long-lived cell [19]. These initial mutations also occur in premalignant plasma cell dyscrasias (MGUS and SMM), suggesting they are necessary but not especially causative in the pathogenesis of MM.

Later oncogenic events include the following: mutations or expression-mediated activation of oncogenes, loss of function of onco-suppressor genes, overexpression of anti-apoptotic proteins, secretion of various cytokines, growth factors, and chemokines. Each of these processes may have a role in supporting cancer cell growth, survival, and resistance to therapies and occur in the bone marrow [18]. Genetic, epigenetic, and biological events occurring in the cancer clones and bone marrow microenvironment all play a role in pathogenesis [18].

49.7 Evolution and Development of Myeloma

MM almost always evolves from MGUS. Patients with MGUS have a 1% per year lifelong rate of malignant transformation; therefore, most individuals with MGUS do not develop MM. The risk of progression is related to the concentration of the monoclonal protein, sFLC ratio, BM plasmacytosis, proportion of phenotypically clonal plasma cells, and presence of immune paresis [20, 21]. The monitoring strategy for a patient with known MGUS will be determined by risk of progression.

The incidence of MGUS increases with age and is present in 3% of white individuals = > 50 years old [22]. About 80% of MM originates from non-IgM intact

Table 49.1 International Myeloma Working Group diagnostic criteria and classification for monoclonal gammopathy of undetermined significance and smouldering multiple myeloma

	Definition	Progression rate	Primary progressing events
Non-IgM MGUS	Serum monoclonal protein (non-IgM type) <30 g/L Clonal bone marrow plasma cells <10% Absence of end-organ damage, i.e. CRAB lesions or amyloidosis that can be attributed to the plasma cell proliferative disorder	1% per year	MM, solitary plasmacytoma, immunoglobulin-related amyloidosis
IgM MGUS	Serum IgM monoclonal protein <30 g/L Bone marrow lymphoplasmacytic infiltration <10% No evidence of anaemia, constitutional symptoms, hyperviscosity, lymphadenopathy, hepatosplenomegaly, or other end-organ damage that can be attributed to the underlying lymphoproliferative disorder	1·5% per year	Waldenström macroglobulinaemia, immunoglobulin-related amyloidosis
Light chain MGUS	Abnormal FLC ratio (<0·26 or >1·65) Increased level of the appropriate involved light chain (increased κ FLC in patients with ratio >1·65 and increased λ FLC in patients with ratio <0·26) No immunoglobulin heavy chain expression on immunofixation. Absence of end-organ damage such as CRAB lesions or amyloidosis that can be attributed to the plasma cell proliferative disorder Clonal bone marrow plasma cells <10% Urinary monoclonal protein <500 mg/24 h	0·3% per year	Light chain MM, immunoglobulin light chain amyloidosis
Smouldering MM	Both criteria must be met: Serum monoclonal protein (IgG or IgA) ≥30 g/L or urinary monoclonal protein ≥500 mg per 24 h and/or clonal bone marrow plasma cells 10–60% Absence of myeloma defining events or amyloidosis	10% per year in the first 5 years	MM

Adapted with permission from Rajkumar et al. (2014)

Ig MGUS and 20% from light chain only (LCO) Ig MGUS [23].

LCO MGUS has a lower rate of evolution to MM compared to intact Ig producing MGUS [24]. When IgM MGUS evolves into a disease, this is usually to WM; rarely IgM MGUS can progress to IgM myeloma [25, 26].

The diagnosis of MGUS requires the absence of end-organ damage attributed to the clone of B-cell lineage or the monoclonal gammopathy produced by the clone.

SMM is an intermediate asymptomatic clinical stage between MGUS and MM, and patients have a 10%/year risk of progression to MM within the first 5 years of diagnosis, which then progressively reduces but never disappears; therefore, SMM requires more frequent monitoring than MGUS [27].

It is important to note that not all patients with myeloma precursor diseases will develop overt MM. Refer to Table 49.1 for International Myeloma Working Group (IMWG) definition and diagnostic criteria for MGUS and SMM.

For MM, the diagnosis requires either a myeloma defining event (see ► Box 49.1) or a heavy tumour burden.

49.8 Diagnosis

The IMWG updated the diagnostic criteria for MM in 2015 (► Box 49.1). The revised criteria comprise the presence of clonal plasma cells and either a myeloma defining event of one or more of the classic 'CRAB' features of hyper**c**alcemia, **r**enal failure, **a**naemia, and/or destructive **b**one lesions or evidence of a heavy tumour burden defined by one or more of >60% plasma cells on BM biopsy, sFLC ratio of >100, or >1 focal bone lesion on MRI scan [28].

These criteria allow for the recognition and treatment of high-risk patients (i.e. patients with 80% risk of progression of SMM to MM within 2 years), in whom treatment would clearly be beneficial before serious end-organ damage has occurred.

The requirement for monoclonal protein as a part of diagnostic test criteria is not mandatory as 3% of MM patients have non-secretory MM (NSMM) characterised by no M-protein in the serum or urine on immunofixation at the time of diagnosis; 30% of these patients with NSMM have a normal FLC assay, despite clearly having MM as defined by other criteria.

49

Box 49.1 Revised International Myeloma Working Group Diagnostic Criteria for Multiple Myeloma. Reproduced with Permission from Rajkumar et al. (2014)

Definition of multiple myeloma:

Clonal bone marrow plasma cells ≥10% or biopsy-proven bony or extramedullary plasmacytoma▶ * and any one or more of the following myeloma defining events:

Evidence of end-organ damage that can be attributed to the underlying plasma cell proliferative disorder, specifically:

- Hypercalcaemia: serum calcium >0·25 mmol/L (>1 mg/dL) higher than the upper limit of normal or >2·75 mmol/L (>11 mg/dL).
- Renal insufficiency: creatinine clearance <40 mL per min† or serum creatinine >177 micromol/L (>2 mg/dl).
- Anaemia: haemoglobin value of >20 g/L below the lower limit of normal, or a haemoglobin value <100 g/L.
- Bone lesions: one or more osteolytic lesions on skeletal radiography, CT, or PET-CT▶ ‡.

Any one or more of the following biomarkers of malignancy:

- Clonal bone marrow plasma cell percentage* ≥60%.
- Involved: uninvolved serum free light chain ratio > =100§.
- >1 focal lesions on MRI studies. Each focal lesion must be 5 mm or more in size.
- *Clonality should be established by showing κ/λ-light chain restriction on flow cytometry, immunohistochemistry, or immunofluorescence
- †Measured or estimated by validated equations
- ‡If bone marrow has less than 10% clonal plasma cells, more than one bone lesion is required to distinguish from solitary plasmacytoma with minimal marrow involvement
- §These values are based on the serum Freelite assay (The Binding Site Group, Birmingham, UK). The involved free light chain must be ≥100 mg/L. The involved free light chain, either κ or λ, is the one that is above the normal reference range; the uninvolved free light chain is the one that is typically in or below the normal range.

49.9 Prognostic Factors

Prognosis in MM can be stratified by the International Staging System (ISS) and chromosomal abnormalities [29]. The ISS incorporates beta 2 microglobulin (B2M), serum albumin, and reflects tumour burden, renal function (as a function of B2M renal clearance), and patient fitness. BM karyotype, translocations, chromosome number, and gene expression profiling also have prognostic value [30].

Although detection of any cytogenetic abnormality is considered to suggest higher-risk disease, the specific abnormalities considered poor risk are cytogenetically detected chromosomal 13 or 13q deletion, t(4;14) and del17p, and detection by fluorescence in situ hybridization of t(4;14), t(14;16), and del17p [31].

Detection of 13q deletion by fluorescence in situ hybridization only, in the absence of other abnormalities, is not considered a high-risk feature.

49.10 Definition of Renal Failure in MM

The IMWG recommends using estimated glomerular filtration rates (eGFR) for the evaluation of renal function in patients with MM with a stable creatinine. An eGFR threshold of less than 40 ml/min/1.73m^2 has now been adopted to define renal impairment in MM consistent with evidence of renal end-organ damage that fulfils the diagnostic criteria.

The IMWG criteria has been recently updated to clarify that only renal failure caused by light chain cast nephropathy (based on typical histological changes or presumptive diagnosis based on the presence of high involved FLC levels, >1500 mg/l) is regarded as a myeloma defining event. The IMWG threshold for cast nephropathy is higher than that recommended by the International Kidney and Monoclonal Gammopathy (IKMG) Research group (>500 mg/L). The published literature indicates that the threshold sFLC at which there is a risk of MCN by the involved LC is 500 mg/L.

A renal biopsy should be reserved for diagnostic uncertainty, such as patients with an involved FLC level <500 mg/L and or heavy albuminuria, which may indicate the presence of a different renal pathology (e.g. AL amyloidosis) (◘ Fig. 49.4).

49.11 Impact of Kidney Disease on Prognosis

The survival of patients who present with impaired kidney function has been improved by the use of novel agents, in particular regimens that included the proteasome inhibitor bortezomib [32].

Dialysis has a major impact on the survival of patients with MM; however, survival is improving in patients with MM who require dialysis with a median overall survival of 14 months [4]. Over 50% of patients

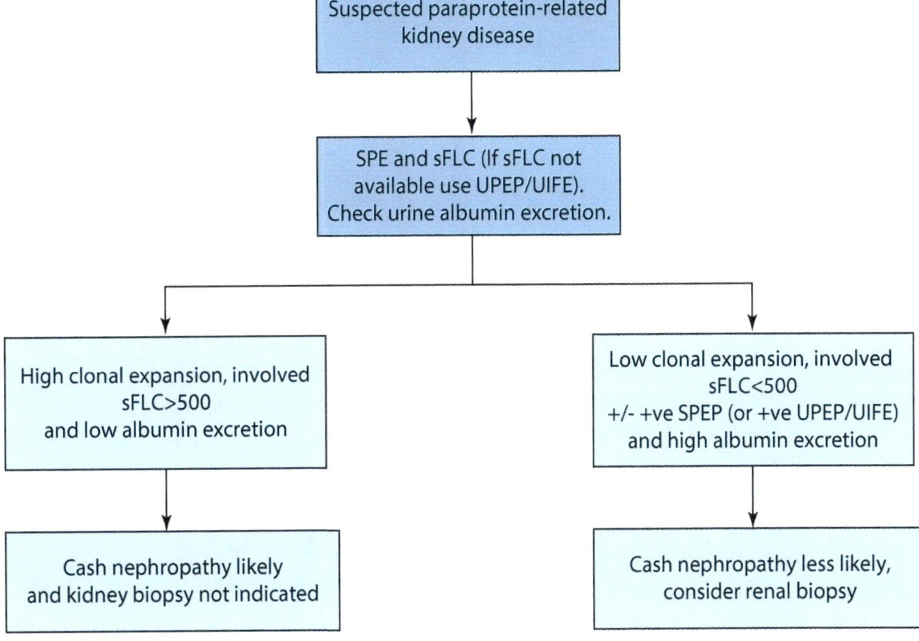

Fig. 49.4 Algorithm for evaluation of suspected paraprotein-related kidney disease. (*SPE* serum protein electrophoresis, *sFLC* serum free light chain, *UPEP* urine protein electrophoresis, *UIFE* urine immunofixation)

who present with AKI and require dialysis now recover independent renal function with an associated improvement in survival [33].

49.12 Pathogenesis of MM and Kidney Disease

Many patients with newly diagnosed MM have mild to moderate renal impairment, which is usually transient and reversible. This is generally a consequence of dehydration, infection, hypercalcemia, use of contrast agents, and /or prescription of non-steroidal anti-inflammatory drugs (NSAIDs). With more severe AKI, the dominant lesion is MCN; for patients who have dialysis-dependent AKI, MCN is present in 90%.

Serum FLCs are normally freely filtered by the glomerulus and reabsorbed in the proximal tubule via receptor-mediated endocytosis. MCN develops when an excessive load of the involved FLC overwhelms the capacity of the tubular cells to catabolise them, with subsequent significant level in the tubular fluid of distal nephron segments. Here, FLCs bind to Tamm-Horsfall protein (uromodulin), a glycoprotein synthesised by the cells in the medullary thick ascending limb of the loop of Henle to form tubular casts (Fig. 49.5). Light chains interact through their complementary determining region with a specific binding site on Tamm-Horsfall protein to form aggregates and casts that subsequently lead to the tubular obstruction of the distal tubule and the thick ascending loop of Henle.

Tubular obstruction increases intraluminal pressure, reduces GFR, and reduces interstitial blood flow, thus further compromising renal function [34]. The reduced tubular clearance of FLC further increases their concentration in the tubules and contributes to the vicious cycle that results in MCN (Fig. 49.6). This lesion can quickly progress to end-stage renal disease [34].

An involved free light chain level in excess of 500 mg/l can cause MCN [35]. However, most patients with levels >500 mg/L will not develop the lesion and require serum levels of several g/L of the involved LC before MCN develops. The threshold for cast formation is dependent on the structural features of the involved LC and cofactors that increase the likelihood of cast formation including low pH, dehydration, hypercalcemia, NSAIDs, diuretics, and radiological contrast media.

Light chain endocytosis may also cause acute tubular necrosis; aggregation of light chains after endocytosis may initiate a cascade resulting in tubular cell death [34]. Light chains may lead to functional impairment of tubular cells, in which case Fanconi syndrome may present. Focal loss of microvilli and inhibition of Na-K-ATPase may lead to reabsorption defects [36].

Some myeloma patients also have a urine concentration defect, probably due to tubulo-interstitial changes, and nephrogenic diabetes insipidus due to unresponsiveness to ADH, thus further promoting dehydration [37].

Hypercalcemia is an important common cause of renal impairment in MM. Hypercalcemia impairs renal concentrating ability. It causes vasoconstriction of renal vasculature and enhances diuresis, which may result in hypovolemia and prerenal azotemia [34]. Concentrated urine and reduced urine flow enhance cast formation, thus leading to further renal damage [34].

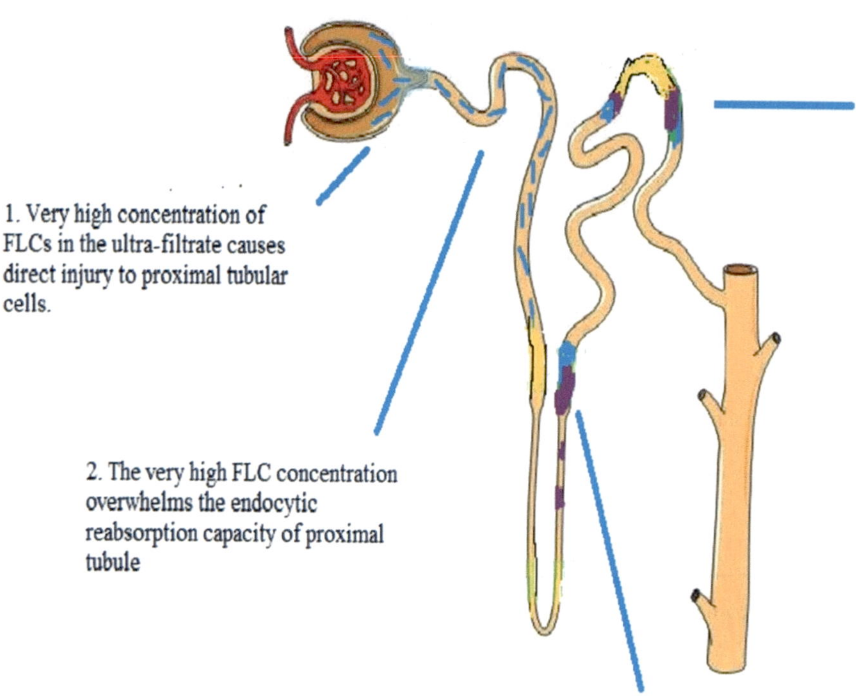

Fig. 49.5 Mechanism of FLC-induced AKI. *FLC* free light chain)

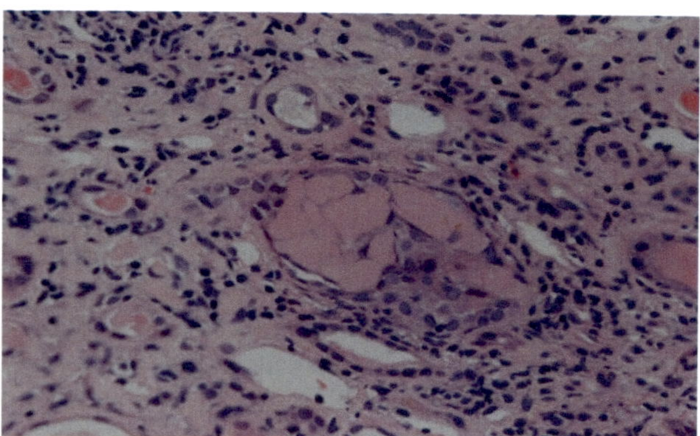

Fig. 49.6 The histological appearances of cast nephropathy. Typical appearance of myeloma cast nephropathy: tubules contain hard, often fractured, distal tubular protein precipitates (casts), consisting of uromodulin and free light chain and surrounding cellular reaction

49.13 Diagnostic Workup in Patients with Suspected MM

1. History and physical examination.
2. Routine testing.

   Full blood count with differential and peripheral blood film.

   Chemistry panel including calcium, creatinine, and eGFR.

   Serum protein electrophoresis (SPEP), immunofixation electrophoresis (IFE), and serum FLC.

   Nephelometric quantification of serum Igs.

   Routine urinalysis; 24-hour urine collection for proteinuria or quantification of proteinuria with albumin creatinine ratio (ACR) or protein creatinine ratio (PCR), urine electrophoresis, and immunofixation. Additional discrimination between glomerular and tubular proteinuria can be obtained through a PCR:ACR ratio
3. Bone marrow aspirate plus trephine biopsy with testing for cytogenetics, fluorescent in situ hybridisation and immunophenotyping.
4. Imaging: Bones; including spine, pelvis, skull, humeri, and femurs.

   The IMWG now recommend that either a PET-CT or low-dose whole-body CT or MRI of whole body or spine, be done in all patients with suspected myeloma. These approaches are far more sensitive than plain x-rays for the identification of lytic lesions.

SPEP tests for an intact Ig. If SPEP is positive, immunofixation will provide isotype characterization. SPEP is less sensitive than IFE for an intact Ig.

All patients should be tested for sFLC. If this test is not available, urinary protein electrophoresis (UPE) or urinary immunofixation electrophoresis (UIFE) for urinary LC (Bence Jones proteinuria) can be used.

The Freelite™ assay is the best validated and most widely used FLC assay [38]; the test measures sFLC to below the normal range on a single blood sample. Elevation of both isotypes of serum free LC occurs in patients with renal impairment. Hence, an abnormal ratio and elevation of the involved free LC are required for the diagnosis of a LC clone.

The haematological response to treatment is classified on the basis of serial monitoring of involved LC.

Occasionally, the sFLC assay can produce a false negative result as a consequence of antigen excess. If the test is negative and there is significant suspicion, then the laboratory should be informed and provided with a second sample that can be appropriately diluted.

Once a monoclonal protein is identified in a patient with AKI, an immediate referral should be made to a haematologist.

49.14 Management of Patients

49.14.1 MM and AKI

This is a medical emergency. The optimal management comprises early institution of novel antimyeloma therapy with good supportive care, to maximise restoration of kidney function. For patients who require dialysis, the primary goal should be independence from dialysis.

The initial evaluation of patients includes an assessment of eligibility for high-dose therapy and autologous stem cell transplantation (ASCT) based on age, frailty, performance status, and comorbidities to guide choice of chemotherapy.

Myeloma is usually regarded as a contraindication to kidney transplantation. However, there are reports of successful kidney transplantation, and this may be a treatment option for patients who sustain a complete remission and where the long-term haematological prognosis is good.

At some stage, most patients will require support for end-of-life care; some of these patients will be in end-stage kidney disease, and careful MDT involvement to include renal service staff will be required at these times.

49.14.2 Antimyeloma Therapy

Prompt commencement of disease-specific therapy is the single most important factor in the management of patients with MM. The introduction of novel agents, such as bortezomib, thalidomide, and lenalidomide, in the treatment of both transplant and non-transplant candidates has revolutionised the treatment.

Bortezomib does not require any dose reduction in renal impairment and is safe and effective in renal failure including dialysis. These drugs can maximise the likelihood of renal recovery with a major improvement in overall survival [32].

Steroids are cytotoxic for myeloma cells, and dexamethasone is the most effective steroid for rapid tumour kill, particularly when used in combination with other therapies. The most common dosing strategy is four-day pulses of 40mgs a day of dexamethasone, repeated weekly for three cycles, followed by less frequent pulses, depending on disease response and the combination regimen that is being followed. Smaller doses of dexamethasone are generally used in older patients.

A three-drug combination, including bortezomib and dexamethasone, is the standard of care for the induction treatment of adults with previously untreated MM and severe AKI, who are eligible for high-dose chemotherapy with haematopoietic stem cell transplantation. Three to six cycles of induction chemotherapy may be administered before proceeding to stem cell collection. High-dose stem cell therapy in transplant eligible patients is associated with improved disease-free survival.

Thalidomide in combination with an alkylating agent and a corticosteroid or bortezomib in combination with an alkylating agent and a corticosteroid are the standards of care for transplant ineligible patients.

49.14.3 Extracorporeal Removal of Serum Free Light Chains

Plasma exchange should not be performed for myeloma-induced renal disease as previous studies have failed to show a benefit of plasma exchange on patient and renal outcomes [39].

The pathological proteins in myeloma kidney are FLCs. These are distributed throughout the extracellular compartment in patients with MM. As a consequence, a short treatment such as plasma exchange will only remove a small amount of total FLC, with rapid re-equilibration of extravascular FLC from the extravascular to the intravascular compartment. This makes plasma exchange ineffective.

A high cut-off (HCO) dialyser can remove far more sFLC than plasma exchange. The membrane in this dialyser removes both FLC isotypes [40, 41]. A number of retrospective studies reported an increased proportion of patients with MM and dialysis-dependent AKI recovering independent kidney function compared to those historically reported. However, patients in these studies received novel chemotherapy (usually bortezomib based) and assessed the relationship between FLC level and renal function in dialysis-dependent patients treated with chemotherapy and HCO dialysis.

Two randomised controlled trials have been recently completed: the MYRE and EuLITE studies both reported no difference in renal recovery at 3 months in patients treated with HCO-HD compared to HF-HD. There was an increase in overall renal recovery in the MYRE study, but not in the EuLITE study, where there was an increased mortality reported by 2 years in patients who received HCO-HD.

There is not sufficient evidence of benefit to support the use of HCO-HD in routine clinical practice.

49.14.4 Supportive Care

Careful attention to fluid and electrolyte, infection, drug use, and bone management is mandatory. An individualised approach is required for provision of supportive care. For example, whilst a high oral fluid intake is important for the dilution of light chains to decrease the likelihood of ongoing cast formation and direct tubular toxicity, in patients with oligo-anuria or pre-existing cardiac disease this may require reassessment.

49.14.5 Fluid Balance and Acid-Base Status

As long as there are no contraindications, then the aim should be to maintain a urine output of 3 L a day. Salt loading should be avoided, as increased tubular NaCl concentrations can precipitate cast formation. Loop diuretics are contraindicated as they both increase intra-tubular sodium and lower intra-tubular pH. Animal and in vitro studies have indicated that casts are more likely to precipitate with a more acidic milieu.

Maintenance of adequate hydration, tissue oxygenation, avoidance of infection, and timely commencement of dialysis treatment should prevent the development of systemic acidosis.

49.14.6 Drugs

Drugs that can decrease renal perfusion are contraindicated, and all medications should be justified as clinically appropriate for the patient. Drugs should be adjusted for renal impairment; clinicians often overlook that most drug dose adjustments based on kidney function utilise the Cockroft-Gault calculation, not MDRD. In patients with rapidly progressive AKI, there should be an assumption that the GFR is <15 mls/min/1.73m^2 .

49.14.7 Preventing and Managing Bone Disease

Bone destruction and hypercalcaemia are very common in MM. Hypercalcemia is a consequence of osteoclast-mediated osteolysis and inhibition of osteoblast function. Intravenous bisphosphonates are a critical component of supportive care; in addition to treatment of hypercalcaemia, bisphosphonates reduce skeletal-related events and have anti myeloma properties [42]. Bisphosphonates are recommended for all MM patients requiring therapy, which should be continued with active disease and reassumed after disease relapse.

To prevent bone disease in patients with myeloma, zoledronic acid should be offered. If zoledronic acid is contraindicated or not tolerated, disodium pamidronate should be given. If zoledronic and disodium pamidronate are contraindicated, not tolerated or not suitable sodium clodronate should be offered [8].

The UK MRC IX trial showed that zoledronic acid was associated with better outcomes than clodronate; however, it should be avoided in patients with an eGFR <30 ml/min/1.73m^2.

At present, intravenous pamidronate at an adjusted dose should be used for the management of hypercalcaemia and to facilitate immediate bone stabilization in patients with an eGFR <30 ml/min/1.73m^2. If the kidney function does not subsequently improve to an eGFR of ≥30 ml/min/1.73m^2, a dialogue with haematology colleagues is recommended to produce an individualised risk assessment that can then be discussed with the patient.

49.14.8 Preventing Infection

Patients with MM are at increased risk of infections, as a consequence of disease-related immunodeficiency as well as anti-myeloma therapy. Humoral immunity can be overestimated by not accounting for the M-protein when interpreting the levels of intact Ig isotype. For example, patients with an intact IgG clone may have 'normal IgG' levels, but the major component of IgG may be clonal with no useful biologic activity, and there may be profound depression of humoral immunity.

Patients with MM develop suboptimal antibody responses; however, they should be offered seasonal influenza and pneumococcal vaccination. Patients with hypogammaglobulinemia and recurrent infections should be considered for intravenous Ig replacement therapy.

Antiviral prophylaxis is recommended after treatment with bortezomib or other proteasome inhibitors, in those on immunomodulatory drugs and high-dose steroids as these are associated with reactivation of varicella zoster. Antibacterial prophylaxis is commonly included in dexamethasone containing and multi agent regimens.

Consider testing for hepatitis B, hepatitis C, and HIV before starting treatment for MM.

49.14.9 Managing Peripheral Neuropathy

Peripheral neuropathy is an important toxicity of both thalidomide and bortezomib occurring in up to 50% of patients [43]. Peripheral neuropathy from thalidomide is cumulative, dose dependent, and usually permanent. Peripheral neuropathy from bortezomib is related to dose, schedule, and mode of administration and mostly reversible [29]. Patients receiving bortezomib who develop neuropathic pain should be considered for switching to subcutaneous injections and/or dose reduction. Those on a drug other than bortezomib should be considered for dose reduction. Prompt dose reductions are required with development of neuropathy of any grade with thalidomide.

49.14.10 Preventing Thrombosis

Immunomodulatory drugs (thalidomide, lenalidomide) when combined with steroids result in a marked increase in thromboembolic events. The rate of venous thromboembolism in these regimes ranges from 20 to 40% without prophylaxis [29].

For people with myeloma who are starting immunomodulatory drugs, thromboprophylaxis with either low-molecular-weight heparin at a prophylactic dose or vitamin K antagonists at a therapeutic dose to maintain an INR of 2–3 should be offered.

If low-molecular-weight heparin or vitamin K antagonists are contraindicated, low-dose aspirin should be considered [8].

Full anticoagulation should be considered in patients with nephrotic syndrome or heavy proteinuria, especially when commencing immunomodulatory drugs.

49.14.11 Managing Fatigue

If other treatable causes have been excluded, consider erythropoietin analogues adjusted to maintain steady state of haemoglobin at 110–120 g/litre, to improve fatigue in people with myeloma who have symptomatic anaemia [8].

49.15 Multidisciplinary Working in MM

Although MM is a haematological malignancy, it may present to a variety of specialties and when diagnosed will often require the input of a multidisciplinary team. Only when all members of this team are aware of MM as a potential diagnosis and recognise the urgency in prompt treatment will optimal care be delivered. It is important to emphasise that involvement of a speciality is dependent on a specific indication and involvement can occur anywhere from diagnosis through to end-of-life care.

There is evidence that the diagnosis of MM may be delayed when the initial presentation of the patient is to a nephrologist [44]. The multidisciplinary team who may be involved in the diagnosis and management of MM are shown in ▶ Box 49.2.

Box 49.2 Multidisciplinary and Medical Specialty Involvement in the Diagnosis and Management of MM

Multidisciplinary specialists

- Haematology clinical nurse specialists.
- Dialysis nurses.
- Research nurses.
- Pharmacists.
- Physiotherapists.
- Occupational therapists.
- Social workers.
- Psychologists.

Medical specialties

- General practitioners.
- Haematologists.
- Nephrologists.
- Neurosurgeons (to manage spinal cord compression).
- Clinical oncologists (radiotherapy to bone lesions).
- Palliative care specialists.
- Pain control specialist.

Tips and Tricks

1. If the sFLC results do not fit with the clinical picture, discuss with the laboratory about the possibility of antigen excess.
2. In new patients presenting with AKI who have an abnormal sFLC (>500 mg/L), commence dexamethasone treatment following discussion with haematology colleagues. Do not delay treatment whilst waiting for further diagnostic tests.
3. IF is required to rule out MGRS, many institutions don't routinely offer this test, and samples may need to be sent to an alternative laboratory. Always liaise with histology colleagues if you are performing a biopsy to look for MGRS to ensure the relevant test is requested. In addition, ensure that EM assessment is performed.

Case Study

Case 1

An 86-year-old African American man with a previous diagnosis of cardiomyopathy with congestive cardiac failure, chronic obstructive pulmonary disease, and prostate cancer presented to the hospital with pneumonia and AKI requiring dialysis.

On presentation, he had a haemoglobin of 109 g/L (normal range 130–180 g/L), and serum calcium level was normal. His urine dipstick was negative for blood and showed a trace of protein, and ACR was 8 mg/mmol. A renal tract USS was normal.

A myeloma screen showed an IgA Kappa paraprotein on immunofixation, and clonal Ig quantitation was 5.88 g/L. Serum Ig levels were normal; sFLC results showed evidence of FLC clonality with LC of 852.0 mg/l, λ LC of 18.59 mg/l, and a κ:λ ratio of 45.83.

Immunology profile revealed a negative ANCA and ANA, and complement levels were normal. A skeletal survey didn't show any lytic lesions; BM trephine biopsy showed a 20% clonal population of plasma cells consistent with a diagnosis of MM.

He was started on weekly bortezomib- (Velcade), cyclophosphamide-, and dexamethasone-based chemotherapy (VCD). At 1 month post presentation, he recovered independent renal function to an eGFR of 25 ml/min/1.73 m2.

The patient completed four cycles of VCD with a very good partial response (VGPR) (IgA paraprotein fell from 5.8 g/L to 0.4 g/L and κ LC fell from 852 mg/l to 80 mg/l); however, he developed a painful ulcer on the tip of the left hallux, which was slow to heal.

For cycle 5, he was switched to fortnightly bortezomib and dexamethasone; however, his chemotherapy had to be discontinued because of increasing foot pain, and as there was a concern this could be neuropathic. Despite stopping the chemotherapy, his symptoms did not improve.

He was then seen in the vascular clinic as an arterial duplex scan of left lower limb revealed >75% stenosis of left superficial femoral artery and occluded anterior tibial artery. A MRI foot ruled out osteomyelitis or any lytic lesion. Given his frailty and comorbidities, the vascular team decided to manage him conservatively.

His renal function slowly continued to improve (to an eGFR 40 ml/min/1.73 m2 at 8 months post presentation); however, he was becoming increasingly frail with time. From the haematological perspective, he continued to be in remission.

He developed gangrene in left hallux secondary to peripheral vascular disease and died 15 months later secondary to pneumonia.

This case illustrates that:

- MM commonly affects elderly people, acting as a chronic disease for the rest of the patients' life; patients may subsequently die of unrelated diseases.
- With prompt disease-specific management patients can recover independent renal function, although this may not be to their previous baseline.
- Myeloma has good disease outcomes for the very old and therefore full treatment may be indicated.

Case 2

A 67-year-old Caucasian man was admitted with a 2-month history of weight loss and left flank pain. On presentation, he had stage 3 AKI (MDRD eGFR 3 ml/min, creatinine 1500 micromol/l) and required dialysis. Haemoglobin was 81 g/L (haematinics normal), and calcium was normal. Urinalysis showed 2 + protein and 3+ blood and ACR 11.3 mg/mmol. The renal tract USS was normal.

An IgA lambda paraprotein was present on immunofixation, and clonal immunoglobulin quantitation was 26 g/L. Serum Ig showed immunoparesis (IgG 2.04 g/L, IgA 27 g/L, IgM 0.02 g/L), and sFLC results showed evidence of free LC clonality with κ LC of 15 mg/l, λ LC of 5835 mg/l, and a κ:λ ratio of 0.003. ANCA, ANA, and complement levels were normal.

A BM trephine biopsy showed neoplastic plasma cells accounting for 60–70% of the cellularity, and skeletal survey did not reveal any lytic lesion.

He received five cycles of VCD chemotherapy with a VGPR (IgA paraprotein fell from 26.6 g/L to 0.5 g/L, and serum free lambda light chain level fell from 5835 mg/l to 39 mg/l).

Within a month of starting chemotherapy, patient recovered independent renal function (to an eGFR 35 ml/min/1.73m^2) and reached a long-term steady state (of eGFR 75 ml/min/1.73m^2) at 8 months post presentation.

The patient underwent an ASCT after completing five cycles of VCD and is currently ten post-transplant and in remission.

This case illustrates that:

- Patients present with nonspecific symptoms and often there is a delay in presentation.
- ASCT is not a curative procedure but extends the length of time disease is controlled for, typically for 2 and a half years to 3 years.
- The renal response depends on the quality of the haematologic response, and rapid suppression of Ig secretion with chemotherapy improves outcomes.

Case 3

A 44-year-old lady known to the haematology team with MGUS (IgG lambda paraprotein on immunofixation, clonal Ig quantitation of 2 g/L, κ LC of 71 mg/L, λ LC of 16 mg/L, and κ:λ ratio of 4.32; bone marrow biopsy did not demonstrate neoplastic plasma cells, and skeletal survey showed no lytic lesions) was referred to the renal clinic with CKD stage 3 (eGFR 50 ml/min/1.73 m2) and ACR of 127 mg/mmol.

Her BP was suboptimal on four antihypertensive agents, and she had diet-controlled diabetes. A 24-hour blood pressure monitor showed persistently high blood pressure with an average reading of 184/109.

A renal tract USS was normal and causes of secondary hypertension were excluded. A renal biopsy after optimising her BP revealed chronic vascular change related to hypertension and diabetes with no paraprotein deposition.

This case illustrates:

- A patient with MGUS and chronic kidney disease unrelated to MGUS.
- Majority of patients with MGUS have an unrelated kidney disease.

Conclusion

The kidney is a major target organ in MM. Renal involvement with MM is the most common paraprotein-related renal disease. Patients with MM and severe AKI have poor outcomes; however, with the introduction of bortezomib and other novel chemotherapy agents, there are increased rates of renal recovery, and long-term survival is improving dramatically.

MGRS is rare but needs consideration as a diagnosis if there is a paraprotein and signs of kidney disease: a kidney biopsy is required to make the diagnosis.

Prompt and accurate care in MM with disease-specific management and supportive care is essential in achieving improved outcomes.

49.16 Resources and Patient Information in MM

A diagnosis of MM may be a shattering event for a patient, and there are a number of different areas where detailed and carefully targeted patient information will be required.

These include information about:

- The cause of the disease
- The consequences of the disease (e.g. renal failure, bone disease, anaemia).
- The supportive treatment options available (e.g. pain control).
- Chemotherapy, the various options available, and the side effects patient may experience.
- Renal impairment, including information about aspects of dialysis if required.
- Potential clinical trials.
- General supportive information that any patient with a potentially life-limiting condition might require (relating to social, psychological, or other palliative care issues).

There are a number of sources of such information and support for patients diagnosed with MM. Myeloma UK has a series of info guides, which are available online and are a useful resource for patients and health-care professionals (▶ www.myeloma.org.uk).

Questions

1. What are the indications for a kidney biopsy in patients with suspected paraprotein-related kidney disease?
2. Does a negative serum protein electrophoresis and sFLC exclude myeloma?
3. How do monoclonal proteins cause kidney disease in myeloma or other monoclonal gammopathies?
4. What factors are used to determine suitability for stem cell transplant in MM?
5. Which chemotherapy agent is first line in myeloma treatment and has improved renal outcomes for patients with AKI and MM?
6. What is the single most important determinant of renal recovery in MM patients with MCN?

Answers

1. A kidney biopsy is indicated in the setting of a progressive proteinuric CKD or AKI with non-light chain proteinuria. Also, if the involved sFLC<500 mg/L, as the likelihood of MCN is less and an alternative diagnosis like MGRS is high.
2. No, as 3% of MM patients have NSMM characterised ≥ 10% clonal plasma cells in the bone marrow and no M-protein in the serum or urine on immunofixation; 30% of these patients with NSMM have normal FLC assay.
3. The monoclonal proteins can cause kidney injury by intratubular cast formation, by direct tubular toxicity as in light chain proximal tubulopathy, or via deposition in different compartments of the kidney, i.e. in amyloidosis or monoclonal immunoglobulin deposition disease.

4. Frailty, performance status measures, and comorbidities are used to determine eligibility for stem cell transplant.
5. Novel chemotherapy agents especially bortezomib-based chemotherapy.
6. Prompt start of chemotherapy.

References

1. Lyratzopoulos G, Neal RD, Barbiere JM, Rubin GP, Abel GA. Variation in number of general practitioner consultations before hospital referral for cancer: findings from the 2010 National Cancer Patient Experience Survey in England. Lancet Oncol. 2012;13(4):353–65.
2. Yadav P, Cook M, Cockwell P. Current trends of renal impairment in multiple myeloma. Kidney Diseases. 2015;1(4):241–57.
3. Dimopoulos MA, Sonneveld P, Leung N, Merlini G, Ludwig H, Kastritis E, et al. International myeloma working group recommendations for the diagnosis and management of myeloma-related renal impairment. J Clin Oncol. 2016;34(13): 1544–57.
4. Evison F, Sangha J, Yadav P, Aung YS, Sharif A, Pinney JA, et al. A population-based study of the impact of dialysis on mortality in multiple myeloma. Br J Haematol. 2018;180(4): 588–91.
5. Bladé J, Fernández-Llama P, Bosch F, Montolíu J, Lens XM, Montoto S, et al. Renal failure in multiple myeloma: presenting features and predictors of outcome in 94 patients from a single institution. Arch Intern Med. 1998;158(17):1889–93.
6. Talamo G, Farooq U, Zangari M, Liao J, Dolloff NG, Loughran TP, et al. Beyond the CRAB symptoms: a study of presenting clinical manifestations of multiple myeloma. Clinical Lymphoma, Myeloma and Leukemia. 2010;10(6): 464–8.
7. MYELOMA INCIDENCE STATISTICS: CANCER RESEARCH UK [press release]. CANCER RESEARCH UK. 2015.
8. NICE. Myeloma: diagnosis and management (NG 35). NICE. 2016.
9. Ferlay J, Soerjomataram I, Dikshit R, Eser S, Mathers C, Rebelo M, et al. Cancer incidence and mortality worldwide: sources, methods and major patterns in GLOBOCAN 2012. International journal of cancer. 2015;136(5).
10. Basnayake K, Stringer SJ, Hutchison CA, Cockwell P. The biology of immunoglobulin free light chains and kidney injury. Kidney Int. 2011;79(12):1289–301.
11. Hutchison CA, Plant T, Drayson M, Cockwell P, Kountouri M, Basnayake K, et al. Serum free light chain measurement aids the diagnosis of myeloma in patients with severe renal failure. BMC Nephrol. 2008;9(1):11.
12. Kapoulas S, Raptis V, Papaioannou M. New aspects on the pathogenesis of renal disorders related to monoclonal gammopathies. Nephrologie & Therapeutique. 2015;11(3):135–43.
13. Glavey SV, Leung N. Monoclonal gammopathy: the good, the bad and the ugly. Blood Rev. 2016;30(3):223–31.
14. Rosner MH, Edeani A, Yanagita M, Glezerman IG, Leung N. Paraprotein–related kidney disease: diagnosing and treating monoclonal Gammopathy of renal significance. Clin J Am Soc Nephrol. 2016;11(12):2280–7.
15. Fermand JP, Bridoux F, Kyle RA, Kastritis E, Weiss BM, Cook MA, et al. How I treat monoclonal gammopathy of renal significance (MGRS). Blood. 2013;122(22):3583–90.
16. Herrmann SM, Gertz MA, Stegall MD, Dispenzieri A, Cosio FC, Kumar S, et al. Long-term outcomes of patients with light chain amyloidosis (AL) after renal transplantation with or without stem cell transplantation. Nephrology Dialysis Transplantation. 2011;26(6):2032–6.
17. Chapman MA, Lawrence MS, Keats JJ, Cibulskis K, Sougnez C, Schinzel AC, et al. Initial genome sequencing and analysis of multiple myeloma. Nature. 2011;471(7339):467.
18. Morgan GJ, Walker BA, Davies FE. The genetic architecture of multiple myeloma. Nat Rev Cancer. 2012;12(5):335.
19. Seifert M, Scholtysik R, Küppers R. Origin and pathogenesis of B cell lymphomas. Lymphoma: Springer; 2013. p. 1–25.
20. Cesana C, Klersy C, Barbarano L, Nosari AM, Crugnola M, Pungolino E, et al. Prognostic factors for malignant transformation in monoclonal gammopathy of undetermined significance and smoldering multiple myeloma. J Clin Oncol. 2002;20(6):1625–34.
21. Turesson I, Kovalchik SA, Pfeiffer RM, Kristinsson SY, Goldin LR, Drayson MT, et al. Monoclonal gammopathy of undetermined significance and risk of lymphoid and myeloid malignancies: 728 cases followed up to 30 years in Sweden. Blood. 2014;123(3):338–45.
22. Kyle RA, Therneau TM, Rajkumar SV, Larson DR, Plevak MF, Offord JR, et al. Prevalence of monoclonal gammopathy of undetermined significance. N Engl J Med. 2006;354(13): 1362–9.
23. Rajkumar SV, Dimopoulos MA, Palumbo A, Blade J, Merlini G, Mateos M-V, et al. International myeloma working group updated criteria for the diagnosis of multiple myeloma. Lancet Oncol. 2014;15(12):e538–e48.
24. Dispenzieri A, Katzmann JA, Kyle RA, Larson DR, Melton LJ III, Colby CL, et al. Prevalence and risk of progression of light-chain monoclonal gammopathy of undetermined significance: a retrospective population-based cohort study. Lancet. 2010;375(9727):1721–8.
25. Rajkumar SV, Dispenzieri A, Kyle RA, editors. Monoclonal gammopathy of undetermined significance, Waldenström macroglobulinemia, AL amyloidosis, and related plasma cell disorders: diagnosis and treatment. Mayo Clinic Proceedings; 2006:81(5):693–703. https://doi.org/10.4065/81.5.693.
26. Schuster SR, Rajkumar SV, Dispenzieri A, Morice W, Aspitia AM, Ansell S, et al. IgM multiple myeloma: disease definition, prognosis, and differentiation from Waldenstrom's macroglobulinemia. Am J Hematol. 2010;85(11):853–5.
27. Kyle RA, Remstein ED, Therneau TM, Dispenzieri A, Kurtin PJ, Hodnefield JM, et al. Clinical course and prognosis of smoldering (asymptomatic) multiple myeloma. N Engl J Med. 2007;356(25):2582–90.
28. Rajkumar SV, Dimopoulos MA, Palumbo A, Blade J, Merlini G, Mateos MV, et al. International Myeloma Working Group updated criteria for the diagnosis of multiple myeloma. Lancet Oncol. 2014;15(12)538–48.
29. Engelhardt M, Terpos E, Kleber M, Gay F, Wäsch R, Morgan G, et al. European Myeloma Network recommendations on the evaluation and treatment of newly diagnosed patients with multiple myeloma. Haematologica. 2014;99(2):232–42.
30. Fonseca R, Bergsagel P, Drach J, Shaughnessy J, Gutierrez N, Stewart AK, et al. International myeloma working group molecular classification of multiple myeloma: spotlight review. Leukemia. 2009;23(12):2210.
31. Munshi NC, Anderson KC, Bergsagel PL, Shaughnessy J, Palumbo A, Durie B, et al. Consensus recommendations for risk stratification in multiple myeloma: report of the international myeloma workshop consensus panel 2. Blood. 2011;117(18):4696–700.

32. Uttervall K, Duru AD, Lund J, Liwing J, Gahrton G, Holmberg E, et al. The use of novel drugs can effectively improve response, delay relapse and enhance overall survival in multiple myeloma patients with renal impairment. PLoS One. 2014;9(7):e101819.
33. Yadav P, Hutchison CA, Basnayake K, Stringer S, Jesky M, Fifer L, et al. Patients with multiple myeloma have excellent long-term outcomes after recovery from dialysis-dependent acute kidney injury. Eur J Haematol. 2016;96(6):610–7.
34. Dimopoulos M, Kastritis E, Rosinol L, Blade J, Ludwig H. Pathogenesis and treatment of renal failure in multiple myeloma. Leukemia. 2008;22(8):1485.
35. Hutchison CA, Batuman V, Behrens J, Bridoux F, Sirac C, Dispenzieri A, et al. The pathogenesis and diagnosis of acute kidney injury in multiple myeloma. Nat Rev Nephrol. 2012;8(1):43.
36. Guan S, El-Dahr S, Dipp S, Batuman V. Inhibition of Na-K-ATPase activity and gene expression by a myeloma light chain in proximal tubule cells. Journal of Investigative Medicine: the Official Publication of the American Federation for Clinical Research. 1999;47(9):496–501.
37. DeFRONZO RA, Cooke CR, Wright JR, Humphrey RL. Renal function in patients with multiple myeloma. Medicine. 1978;57(2):151–66.
38. Pratt G. The evolving use of serum free light chain assays in haematology. Br J Haematol. 2008;141(4):413–22.
39. Clark WF, Stewart AK, Rock GA, Sternbach M, Sutton DM, Barrett BJ, et al. Plasma exchange when myeloma presents as acute renal failure: a randomized, controlled trial. Ann Intern Med. 2005;143(11):777–84.
40. Hutchison CA, Cockwell P, Reid S, Chandler K, Mead GP, Harrison J, et al. Efficient removal of immunoglobulin free light chains by hemodialysis for multiple myeloma: in vitro and in vivo studies. Journal of the American Society of Nephrology: JASN. 2007;18(3):886–95.
41. Hutchison CA, Harding S, Mead G, Goehl H, Storr M, Bradwell A, et al. Serum free-light chain removal by high cutoff hemodialysis: optimizing removal and supportive care. Artif Organs. 2008;32(12):910–7.
42. Morgan GJ, Davies FE, Gregory WM, Szubert AJ, Bell SE, Drayson MT, et al. Effects of induction and maintenance plus long-term bisphosphonates on bone disease in patients with multiple myeloma: the Medical Research Council myeloma IX trial. Blood. 2012;119(23):5374–83.
43. Sonneveld P, Jongen JL. Dealing with neuropathy in plasma-cell dyscrasias. ASH Education Program Book. 2010;2010(1):423–30.
44. Kariyawasan CC, Hughes DA, Jayatillake MM, Mehta AB. Multiple myeloma: causes and consequences of delay in diagnosis. QJM. 2007;100(10):635–40.

Amyloidosis and the Kidney

Julian D. Gillmore and Helen J. Lachmann

Contents

M. Harber (ed.), *Primer on Nephrology*, https://doi.org/10.1007/978-3-030-76419-7_50

Learning Objectives

1. To understand the basis of amyloidosis, its clinical presentation, renal involvement, associations and management.

50.1 Introduction

Amyloidosis is the generic term for a group of diseases caused by misfolding and extracellular accumulation of proteins as fibrillar deposits that, when stained with Congo red, display pathognomonic green birefringence when viewed under crossed polarised light microscopy. Amyloidosis is remarkably diverse and can be hereditary or acquired, localised or systemic and lethal or merely incidental. So far, more than 30 different human proteins with in vivo amyloidogenic potential have been identified, of which 16 cause systemic amyloidosis. The classification of amyloid is based on the fibril protein, and different amyloidogenic proteins give rise to distinct but frequently overlapping clinical syndromes. The kidneys are frequently involved in systemic amyloidosis (Table 50.1), which, without treatment, is usually fatal. Current management of amyloidosis is dependent upon determining the fibril protein and reducing its abundance. This can result in regression of amyloid deposits, prevention or recovery of organ failure and improved survival.

Table 50.1 Systemic amyloidoses commonly associated with kidney involvement

Amyloid type	Fibril precursor	Note
AL	Light chain V region fragments	Sporadic, myeloma or plasma cell clone associated
AA	Serum amyloid A protein (SAA)	Sporadic, reactive to chronic inflammation
ALect2	Leukocyte chemotactic factor 2	Sporadic, more common in Mexican-Americans and south Asians
AApoAI	Apolipoprotein A-I	Familial
AApoAII	Apolipoprotein A-II	Familial
AApoAIV	Apolipoprotein A-IV	Familial
AApoCII	Apolipoprotein C-II	Familial
AApoCIII	Apolipoprotein C-III	Familial
ALys	Lysozyme	Familial
AFib	Fibrinogen Aα-chain	Familial
AGel	Gelsolin	Familial
ATTR	Transthyretin	Familial, kidney involvement/dysfunction unusual until late stage of disease
Aβ_2M	β2-microglobulin	Dialysis-related amyloidosis and familial

50.2 Aetiology and Pathogenesis

Amyloid formation occurs when a protein or peptide loses, or fails to acquire, its physiologic, functional folding and, in its misfolded state, undergoes fibril formation and extracellular deposition [1]. Amyloid deposits display distinctive ultrastructural (beta-sheet conformation) and tinctorial properties. The process of amyloid formation and deposition ultimately results in tissue damage and organ dysfunction (Fig. 50.1). The propensity of proteins to form amyloid fibrils in vivo is enhanced by the following:

- A pathologic and sustained increase in concentration of the protein. This is the case of the acute phase reactant serum amyloid A protein (SAA) in chronic inflammation and of β2-microglobulin in patients with end-stage renal disease (ESRD).
- Presence of an unstable mutant protein, favouring its misfolding and aggregation, as occurs in hereditary amyloidosis.
- Presence of an intrinsically unstable protein, favouring its misfolding and aggregation, as occurs with monoclonal immunoglobulin light chains in AL amyloidosis.
- Proteolytic remodelling of a protein, as in the case of the protease furin cleaving ABri and gelsolin and the β- and γ-secretases releasing amyloid-β (Aβ) peptides.
- Advancing age, as in the case of wild-type transthyretin and apolipoprotein A-I, both of which have intrinsic amyloidogenic properties and are associated with age-related amyloid deposition.

Frequently, a combination of these factors determines the amyloidogenicity of an individual protein. However, the inherent amyloidogenicity of a specific protein, per se, is not sufficient to account for amyloid deposition in vivo; undetermined environmental and genetic factors must be involved as only a minority of patients with long-lasting inflammation and persistent elevation of SAA levels develop AA amyloidosis [2], and, similarly, the disease-associated Val30Met mutation of transthyretin shows significant variation in penetrance and

50

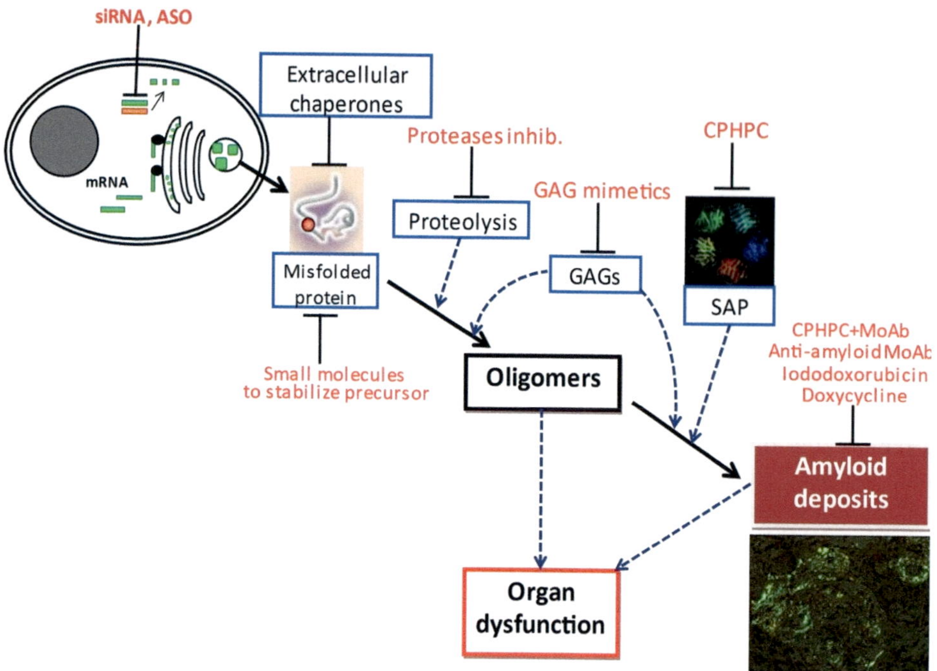

Fig. 50.1 Molecular events leading to amyloidosis. Interaction of the misfolded protein with the extracellular environment may result in proteolytic cleavage and binding to matrix components, such as glycosaminoglycans (GAGs) and collagen, that facilitate aggregation. Several lines of evidence support a role for extracellular chaperones in the in vivo clearance of aggregation-prone extracellular proteins. Serum amyloid P component (SAP) binds to amyloid fibrils and protects them from reabsorption. The organ dysfunction may result from the combined action of the cytotoxic pre-fibrillar aggregates and of the amyloid deposits. Several new therapeutic approaches have been recently developed. The synthesis of the amyloid protein can be silenced using RNA interference (siRNA) or antisense oligonucleotides (ASO). Small molecules capable of stabilising the amyloid precursor and preventing its misfolding and aggregation (diflunisal, tafamidis) are being tested in patients with ATTR amyloidosis. Inhibitors of proteases (secretase) and compounds interfering with the binding of GAGs to amyloid proteins (eprodisate) are being evaluated in trials. SAP can be cleared from amyloid deposits by using small palindromic drugs (CPHPC). The clearance of amyloid deposits can be promoted and accelerated by specific antibodies through passive and active immunotherapy. Small molecules, such as iododoxorubicin and doxycycline, have shown to be able to disrupt the amyloid fibrils and have been tested in clinical trials

clinical presentation among different ethnic groups and geographic areas [3].

50.2.1 Amyloid Structure

Electron microscopy and X-ray diffraction analysis reveal that amyloid deposits are composed of rigid, non-branching fibrils with an average diameter of 7–13 nm and a cross-β structure, in which the β-strands are perpendicular to the fibril axis and assemble into β-sheets [4]. Although, more recently, refined structural studies of amyloid fibrils by solid-state nuclear magnetic resonance spectroscopy and microcrystals of small amyloid-like peptides by X-ray diffraction analysis have revealed a degree of structural variation, the morphology and structure are remarkably consistent regardless of the constituent polypeptide.

50.2.2 Common Constituents of Amyloid Deposits

Serum amyloid P component, a glycoprotein of the pentraxin family, is synthesised by hepatocytes and binds reversibly to all amyloid, independent of the protein of origin, through a specific binding motif and protects amyloid fibrils from proteolytic degradation [5]. These properties make SAP a means of imaging amyloid deposits and a potential therapeutic target [6]. Other common elements found in amyloid deposits are proteoglycans, heparan sulphate (HS) and extracellular matrix components, such as laminin, entactin and collagen IV.

50.2.3 Organ Tropism

Amyloid deposition may occur in almost any organ. Nonetheless, specific amyloidogenic proteins tend favour deposition in defined organs, for example, the kidney for fibrinogen Aα chain and leukocyte chemotactic factor 2 and the joints and bones for wild-type β_2-microglobulin. In AL amyloidosis there is some evidence that the physicochemical characteristics (amino acid composition and conformation of the variable region) of the LC may be the most significant factor in determining the type and location of organ dysfunction.

50.3 Epidemiology

Systemic amyloidosis is a rare disease accounting for approximately 1 in 2000 deaths in the UK and presumably other developed countries [7]. Although cases of amyloidosis have been reported in children, it is predominantly a disease of mid to late life and accounts for 4% of adult renal biopsies and 1.6% of patients starting dialysis.

50.3.1 Systemic Amyloidosis Associated with Monoclonal LCs: AL Amyloidosis

The age-adjusted incidence of AL amyloidosis in the USA and UK has been estimated to be between 5.1 and 12.8 per million persons per year, and AL is the diagnosis in 40 to 60% of patients with amyloidosis seen at large referral centres. Approximately 60% of cases are men, and median age at presentation is 65 years; it can occur in young adults and is probably under-diagnosed in the elderly, among whom monoclonal gammopathies are most prevalent. AL amyloidosis develops in about 2% of individuals with monoclonal B-cell dyscrasias [7]. The B-cell dyscrasias underlying systemic AL amyloidosis can include almost any clonal proliferation of differentiated B-lymphocytes; 94% have an underlying clone of plasma cells [8, 9]. The clonal cell burden in AL amyloidosis is usually small and the plasma cell proliferation fraction similar to monoclonal gammopathy of unknown significance (MGUS). Only 10–20% of patients who are diagnosed with AL amyloidosis meet myeloma criteria. Progression of the underlying monoclonal gammopathy to overt myeloma is rare in systemic AL amyloidosis, which, in part, reflects patients' short survival.

50.3.2 Reactive Systemic AA Amyloidosis

The exact incidence of AA amyloidosis is unclear, but it accounts for 4% of the cases of amyloidosis seen at major referral centres. It is always a complication of inflammation, and the list of chronic disorders that can be complicated by AA amyloidosis is summarised in ► Box 50.1. In industrialised countries, inflammatory arthritides used to underlie 60%, but this is falling in the era of effective biologics [10]. For unexplained reasons the incidence of AA amyloid is much lower in the USA than in Europe. The median latency between the onset of inflammation and diagnosis of amyloid is approximately 17 years, but this varies from less than a year to decades. The median age at diagnosis is 50 years, but presentation in childhood, although becoming less common, is still recognised. As with all types of amyloidosis, AA appears slightly commoner in men who account for 56% of the largest characterised series [11].

50.3.3 Dialysis-Related Amyloidosis (DRA)

β_2-microglobulin amyloidosis occurs in patients who have been on dialysis for more than 6–10 years, or very occasionally in individuals with long-standing severe chronic kidney disease. β_2-microglobulin amyloid deposits have been reported in 20 to 30% of patients within 3 years of commencing dialysis for ESRD, but the incidence seems to have fallen by 80% between the 1980s and 1990s, reflecting improvements in technology with biocompatible and high-flux membranes [12].

50.3.4 Hereditary Systemic Amyloidosis

In the UK the prevalence of hereditary non-neuropathic systemic amyloidosis, which typically presents with renal dysfunction, appears to be in the order of 1.5 per million with most patients presenting in their sixth decade.

50.3.5 Leukocyte Chemotactic Factor 2 (LECT2) Amyloidosis

This is thought to be an acquired form of amyloid in specific populations and accounts for up to 2.5% of renal biopsies containing amyloid [13].

50

50.4 Clinical Features

50.4.1 Systemic Amyloidosis Associated with Monoclonal LCs: AL Amyloidosis

The clinical features of AL amyloidosis are protean as any organ other than the central nervous system can be directly involved (Table 50.2; Figs. 50.2 and 50.3).

50.4.2 Reactive Systemic AA Amyloidosis

The predominant clinical manifestations of AA amyloidosis are renal.

- More than 97% of patients present with proteinuric kidney dysfunction. Haematuria, tubular defects and diffuse renal calcification occur rarely. Just over 50% of patients have nephrotic syndrome at presentation. Approximately 10% of patients are in ESRF at diagnosis, and over 40% eventually progress to ESRF.
- The spleen is almost always infiltrated.
- Adrenal glands are involved in more than 33%, although hypoadrenalism is rare.
- Hepatosplenomegaly is seen at presentation in 9% of cases, but liver failure is exceptionally rare.
- Malabsorption occurs only in very advanced disease.
- Cardiac amyloidosis is seen in 2% and only in advanced disease.

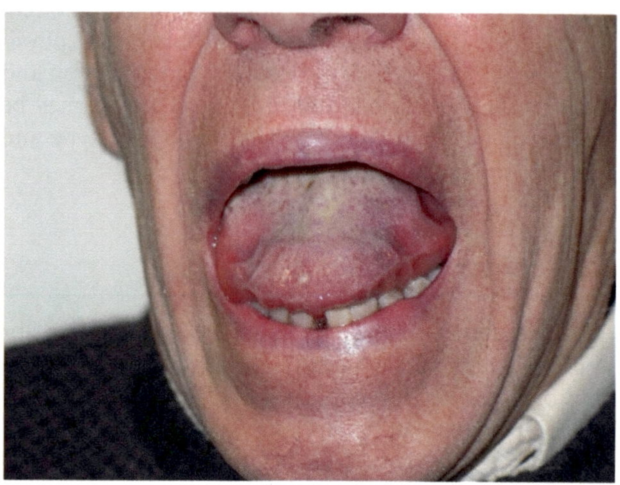

Fig. 50.2 Macroglossia present in approximately 10% of cases of AL amyloidosis

Table 50.2 Organ involvement in systemic AL amyloidosis

Organ system	Clinical manifestations
Non-specific	Fatigue and weight loss
Renal	Proteinuric renal disease in the context of a normal or low blood pressure is seen in >60%. In recent large studies, 44% of patients presented with chronic kidney disease (CKD) stage 1 or 2, and 16% with CKD stage 5; median proteinuria at presentation was 5–7 g/day and median serum albumin 21–28 g/L
Cardiac	Cardiac involvement is a major determinant of outcome and occurs in ~75% of patients at presentation, with approximately 30% presenting with congestive heart failure. Cardiac biomarkers provide a quantitative assessment of cardiac damage (troponin I or T) and wall strain (BNP, NT-proBNP) and are the most important predictors of outcome in amyloidosis. By using the cut-offs of 0.055 mcg/L for high-sensitivity troponin T and 332 ng/L for NT-proBNP, patients can be classified into three prognostic stages [33]
Hepatic	Hepatic amyloid is present in ~50% of patients. Despite substantial hepatomegaly liver function is often well preserved with modest elevation of ALP and GGT. Hyperbilirubinaemia is unusual but associated with a poor outcome (median survival of 4 months)
Gastrointestinal	Gut involvement may cause motility disturbances (often secondary to autonomic neuropathy), malabsorption, perforation, haemorrhage or obstruction
Peripheral neuropathic	Painful sensory polyneuropathy with early loss of temperature sensation, followed later by motor deficits, is seen in 10 to 20% of cases and carpal tunnel syndrome in 20%
Autonomic	Autonomic neuropathy leads to orthostatic hypotension, impotence and gastrointestinal disturbances
Soft tissue	Macroglossia occurs in 10% and is pathognomonic of AL-type amyloid (Fig. 50.2)
Skin	Skin involvement is common and usually takes the form of bruising spontaneously or after minor trauma (Fig. 50.3)
Haematological	An acquired bleeding diathesis may be associated with deficiency of factor X and factor IX or with increased fibrinolysis
Musculoskeletal	Articular amyloid is rare and may superficially resemble acute polyarticular arthritis, or it may present as asymmetrical arthritis affecting the hip or shoulder. Infiltration of the glenohumeral joint and surrounding soft tissues occasionally produces the characteristic 'shoulder pad' sign

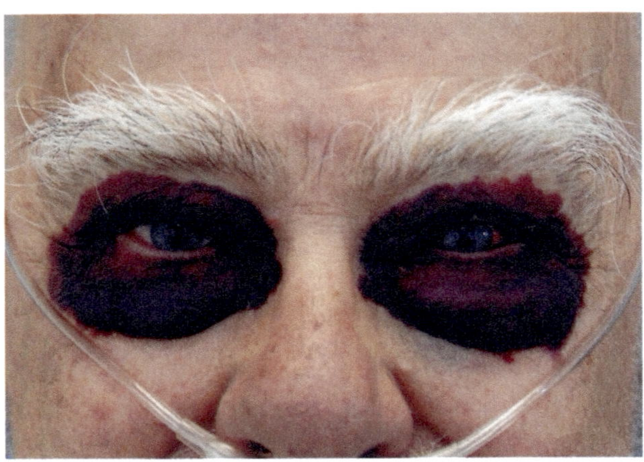

Fig. 50.3 Capillary fragility manifesting as periorbital bruising and conjunctival haemorrhage in AL amyloidosis

50.4.3 Dialysis-Related Amyloidosis (DRA)

β_2-microglobulin amyloidosis is preferentially deposited in articular and periarticular structures, and its manifestations are largely confined to the locomotor system [14].

- Carpal tunnel syndrome is usually the first clinical manifestation. Some individuals develop symptoms within 3 to 5 years of initiation of renal replacement therapy, and by 20 years the prevalence was almost 100%. Older patients appear to be more susceptible to the disease and tend to exhibit symptoms more rapidly.
- Amyloid arthropathy tends to occur a little later but eventually affects the most patients on dialysis. It affects the shoulders, knees, wrists and small joints of the hand and is associated with joint swelling, chronic tenosynovitis and, occasionally, haemarthrosis. Spondylarthropathies are also well recognised, as is cervical cord compression. Deposition within the periarticular bone produces typical appearances of subchondral erosions and cysts, which can contribute to pathological fractures particularly of the femoral neck, cervical vertebrae and scaphoid.

50.4.4 LECT2 Amyloidosis

Most patients are of Hispanic, Asian or Middle Eastern ancestry and present in the 6–seventh decades with slowly progressive renal impairment. Proteinuria tends to be low grade, and hypertension is well recognised [15]. Although splenic and adrenal amyloid deposits are visible on SAP imaging, clinically the disease appears to be renal isolated.

50.4.5 Hereditary Non-neuropathic Systemic Amyloidosis

50.4.5.1 Lysozyme Amyloidosis (ALys)

This typically presents in middle age with proteinuria, slowly progressive renal impairment and sometimes hepatosplenomegaly with or without purpuric rashes. In retrospect most recollect a long history of dry eyes and dry mouth. Substantial gastrointestinal amyloid deposits are common and important since gastrointestinal haemorrhage or perforation is a cause of death in these patients.

50.4.5.2 Apolipoprotein A-I Amyloidosis (AApoAI)

Depending on the mutation, patients can present with massive abdominal organomegaly, predominant cardiomyopathy or neuropathy. Most patients eventually develop renal failure, but despite extensive amyloid deposition, liver function is usually preserved. Additional features are hypertension, cholestasis and hypogonadism with infertility.

50.4.5.3 Fibrinogen a Alpha Chain Amyloidosis (AFib)

Patients with this form of hereditary amyloidosis frequently have no family history of similar disease and are readily misdiagnosed as having AL amyloidosis. Most patients present in their 6th–seventh decades with proteinuria or hypertension and progress to ESRD over 4–10 years [16]. Amyloid deposition is seen in the kidneys, characteristically localised to the glomeruli, spleen and rarely the liver, but is usually asymptomatic in the latter two sites.

50.4.5.4 Apolipoprotein A2 Amyloidosis (AApoA2)

The few kindreds described have slowly progressive proteinuric renal failure.

50.4.5.5 Gelsolin Amyloidosis (AGel)

This usually presents with corneal lattice dystrophy and progressive cranial neuropathy. Renal amyloid deposits are often subclinical but can occasionally cause ESRD.

50.4.5.6 Transthyretin Met30 (ATTR)

In addition to neuropathy and cardiac involvement, up to a third of cases have evidence of proteinuria and renal failure, and 10% eventually develop ESRD [17]. Gradually progressive autonomic neuropathy typically causes impaired bladder emptying, requiring indwelling urinary catheters.

50

50.5 Investigations

The diagnosis of amyloidosis relies on a high index of clinical suspicion. Amyloid can be asymptomatic until a relatively late stage and then present with highly variable or non-specific symptoms. Amyloidosis should be suspected in any patient with the following: non-diabetic nephrotic syndrome; non-ischemic cardiomyopathy, particularly if the echocardiogram suggests concentric hypertrophy; increased NT-proBNP in the absence of primary heart or renal disease; hepatomegaly or increased alkaline phosphatase without an imaging abnormality; peripheral and/or autonomic neuropathy; unexplained facial or neck purpura; and macroglossia. Any patient with suggestive features should undergo a biopsy to look for presence of amyloid deposits. Identification of amyloid should prompt a series of investigations to determine the amyloid fibril protein and organ involvement/dysfunction (■ Table 50.3).

50.5.1 Histology

The diagnosis of amyloidosis requires histological confirmation (■ Fig. 50.4). Subcutaneous fat biopsy (taken by aspiration of abdominal subcutaneous fat under local anaesthetic using a 14 gauge needle), screening rectal biopsy and labial salivary gland biopsy are between 60 and 80% sensitive. There have been concerns that organ biopsies in patients with amyloidosis carry an increased risk of haemorrhage, although firm evidence of this is lacking. Congo red staining of amyloid produces pathognomic apple green birefringence when viewed under cross-polarised light, and negatively stained electron microscopy reveals 8–15 nm diameter rigid, non-branching fibrils composed of twisted protofibrils of indeterminate length.

The main protein constituting the amyloid deposit can often be identified by immunohistochemistry, although this may be unreliable in AL and hereditary amyloidosis [18]. Laser microdissection (LMD)- and tandem mass spectrometry (MS)-based proteomic analysis can confirm the amyloid protein composition and has become the gold standard for identifying the amyloid fibril protein [19].

50.5.2 Imaging Amyloid Deposits

50.5.2.1 SAP Scintigraphy

SAP concentrates specifically in amyloid deposits of all types. Radiolabelled SAP scintigraphy has been used since 1988 in the UK for diagnosis and quantitative monitoring of amyloid deposits [20]. This safe, non-invasive method provides information on the presence, distribution and extent of visceral amyloid deposits, and serial scans monitor progress and response to therapy (■ Fig. 50.5). The method is not informative about amyloid deposition in the moving heart and is not commercially available.

50.5.2.2 Imaging the Heart

The classical two-dimensional Doppler echocardiographic appearance of cardiac amyloidosis is of concentric biventricular wall thickening with a restrictive filling pattern. Amyloid causes diastolic dysfunction with well-preserved contractility until a very late stage. The ECG in advanced disease may show small voltages and pathological 'Q' waves (pseudo-infarct pattern). The finding of abnormal gadolinium kinetics particularly global late gadolinium enhancement on cardiac magnetic resonance imaging has a high sensitivity and specificity for cardiac amyloidosis and has substantially contributed to diagnosis [21]. Scans following injection of technetium-99 m-labelled 3,3-diphosphono-1,2-propanodicarboxylic acid (^{99}Tc-DPD), an established bone tracer, are sensitive for detecting presence of cardiac ATTR amyloid deposits [22].

50.5.2.3 DNA Analysis

Hereditary amyloidoses are rare and often overlooked. Although all types are dominantly inherited, penetrance and expressivity are highly variable, and there is frequently no obvious family history. DNA analysis is mandatory in all patients with systemic amyloidosis whose fibril type cannot be confirmed by immunohis-

Table 50.3 Investigation and staging of patient discovered to have amyloid deposits

	Purpose and method	Note
Determining the amyloid type (i.e. amyloid fibril protein)		
	Clinical presentation/features	Soft tissue amyloid (macroglossia/periorbital bruising/jaw claudication) – Strongly suggestive of AL Amyloid cardiomyopathy – Likely AL/ATTR Amyloid neuropathy – Likely AL/ATTR Family history of amyloid – Likely hereditary amyloidosis
	Biochemical evaluation	Evidence of clonal dyscrasia (BJP, abnormal sFLC ratio, pp) – Suggestive (but not diagnostic) of AL Evidence of chronic acute phase response – Suggestive (but not diagnostic) of AA
	Immunohistochemistry	AA amyloidosis can be reliably excluded by negative immunohistochemical staining Sensitivity in AL and hereditary amyloidosis 70–90% (i.e. frequent false-negative staining)
	Mass spectrometry	Currently research technique. Likely gold standard in the future
	Genetic sequencing	Frequently required when immunohistochemistry +/– mass spectrometry non-diagnostic of amyloid type
Determining amyloidotic organ involvement		
	Clinical history and examination	Examine for macroglossia, carpal tunnel syndrome, postural hypotension, ecchymoses, ECOG performance status, 6-minute walk test
	SAP scintigraphy	To determine visceral organ involvement and whole body amyloid load; serial scanning for monitoring
	Cardiac evaluation	Echocardiography/cardiac MRI/Tc-DPD scintigraphy/NT-proBNP/troponin T
	Other organs	Quantification of proteinuria, renal function (GFR), liver function tests, tests of autonomic function
Characterising the underlying disease		
AL	Bone marrow biopsy	Include cytogenetic and flow cytometric analysis
	Serum immunoelectrophoresis	Monitor paraprotein throughout disease course
	Urine immunoelectrophoresis	Quantification of 24 hr. urine BJP, monitor BJP quantity throughout disease course
	Serum free light chain assay (sFLC)	sFLC should be monitored during therapy and throughout disease course
	Skeletal survey	Look for lytic lesions
	Lymph node biopsy CT scanning of the chest, abdomen and pelvis PET scanning	Where indicated (absence of plasma cell dyscrasia, suggestion of lymphoma, IgM paraprotein) Where indicated (absence of plasma cell dyscrasia, suggestion of lymphoma, IgM paraprotein) Where indicated (absence of plasma cell dyscrasia, suggestion of lymphoma, IgM paraprotein)
AA	Clinical syndrome	Rheumatoid arthritis, juvenile inflammatory arthritis, chronic infection, hereditary periodic fever
	Serological assays	Autoantibodies, CRP, SAA – SAA should be serially monitored throughout disease course
	Genetic sequencing	Sequencing of periodic fever genes (*MEFV, TNFRSF1A, MVK*)

BJP Bence Jones protein; *sFLC* serum free light chain; *pp.* paraprotein; *SAA* serum amyloid A protein; *CRP* C-reactive protein; *MRI* magnetic resonance imaging; *MEFV* familial Mediterranean fever gene; *TNFRSF1A* TRAPS gene; *MVK* mevalonate kinase gene

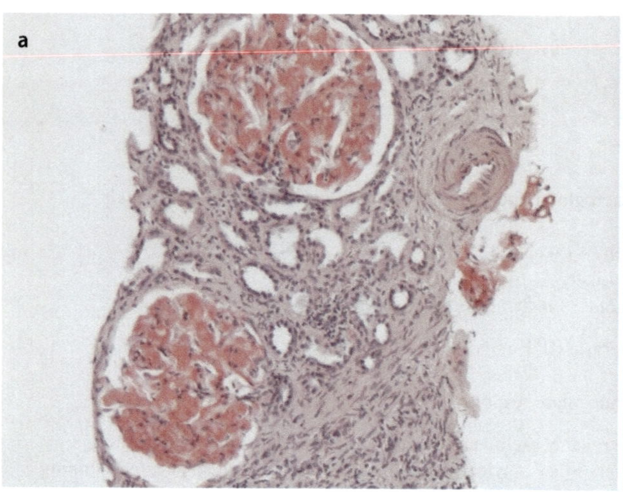

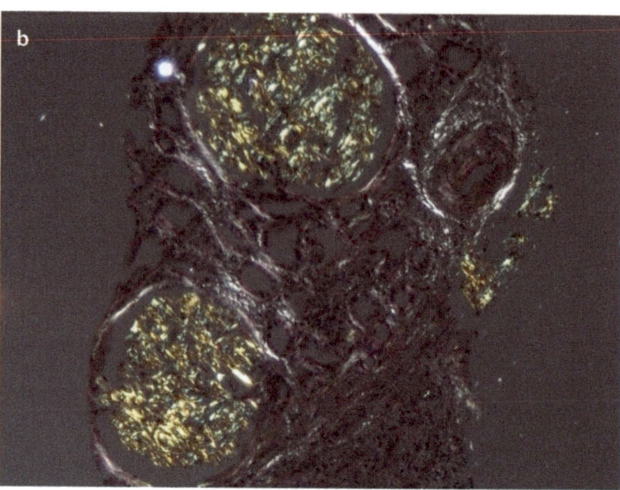

Fig. 50.4 Sections of renal biopsy stained with Congo red viewed under x10 magnification. **a** Amorphous deposits of eosinophilic material are seen within the glomeruli. **b** Pathognomonic apple green birefringence of amyloid deposits when viewed under cross-polarised light

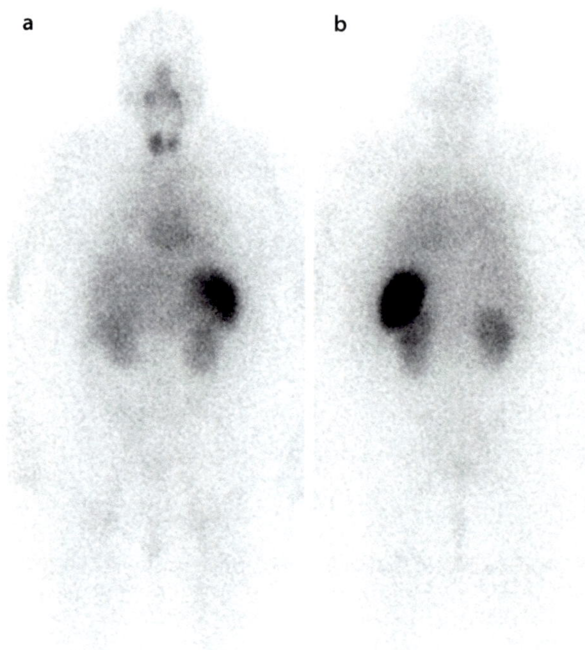

Fig. 50.5 SAP scintigraphy. **a** Anterior whole body SAP scan showing presence of AL amyloid deposits in the liver, spleen, kidneys and bones. **b** Serial SAP scans taken several years apart showing marked regression of liver amyloid

tochemistry or mass spectroscopy. Mutations encoding a number of amyloidogenic protein variants are known to cause hereditary amyloidosis, and both new variants and new amyloidogenic proteins are periodically identified [23].

50.5.3 Investigation of the Underlying Disease

50.5.3.1 AL Amyloidosis

All patients with AL amyloidosis should have the source of their amyloidogenic monoclonal light chain production investigated in detail. This should include a bone marrow examination, skeletal survey, serum and urine electrophoresis and immunofixation and serum FLC assay (Table 50.3).

AA Amyloidosis.

An attempt to characterise the underlying inflammatory disease should be made in all cases of AA amyloidosis, although it may be very difficult due to the diverse conditions involved (▶ Box 50.1 and Table 50.3). The precise cause of excessive SAA production remains undetermined in up to 25% of patients with AA amyloidosis.

Box 50.1 Inflammatory Conditions Which can be Complicated by AA Amyloidosis

Chronic inflammatory arthritides
Rheumatoid arthritis
Juvenile inflammatory arthritis
Ankylosing spondylitis
Psoriatic arthropathy
Reiter's syndrome

Vasculitides
Polyarteritis nodosa
Takayasu's arteritis
Behcet's disease
Systemic lupus erythematosus
Giant cell arteritis/polymyalgia rheumatica

Chronic infections
Bronchiectasis
Chronic cutaneous ulcers
Chronic pyelonephritis
Chronic osteomyelitis
Subacute bacterial endocarditis
Leprosy
Tuberculosis
Whipple's disease
HIV/AIDS

Inflammatory bowel disease
Crohn's disease
Ulcerative colitis

Systemic autoinflammatory diseases
Familial Mediterranean fever
Cryopyrin-associated periodic syndrome (CAPS)
TNF receptor-associated periodic syndrome (TRAPS)
Mevalonate kinase deficiency (MVK)
Schnitzler's syndrome
Adult-onset Still's disease

Neoplasia
Hodgkin's disease
Renal cell carcinoma
Adenocarcinoma of the lung, gut and urogenital tract
Basal cell carcinoma
Hairy cell leukaemia
Castleman's disease
Hepatic adenoma

Other
IV and subcutaneous drug abuse
Cystic fibrosis
Kartagener's syndrome
Epidermolysis bullosa
Hypogammaglobulinaemia
Cyclic neutropenia
Common variable immunodeficiency
Hyperimmunoglobulin M syndrome
SAPHO syndrome

50.6 Treatment and Outcome

50.6.1 Principles of Treatment

Therapies aimed at enhancing amyloid clearance are under development, but at present the treatment of all types of amyloid centres on slowing new amyloid formation by reducing the supply of the amyloid fibril precursor protein and supporting or replacing compromised organ function. Treatment therefore requires precise identification of the amyloid fibril type. Successful inhibition of amyloid formation can result in net amyloid regression [24]. Early diagnosis is the key to effective therapy. Clinicians should be aware that in the near future amyloid diseases are likely to be treated with combination approaches that reduce protein precursor production, prevent aggregation and induce fibril resorption.

50.6.2 Systemic AL Amyloidosis

The immediate goals of therapy are to rapidly eliminate production of misfolded amyloidogenic LCs with chemotherapy whilst minimising treatment toxicity and supporting target organ function [25]. Effective management of AL amyloidosis requires a multidisciplinary approach. Consensus criteria for hematologic and organ responses were updated at the 12th International Symposium on Amyloidosis. Achieving a hematologic response translates into improved overall survival. Although partial responses can be beneficial, complete clonal responses are associated with the best clinical outcomes. A new paradigm for the treatment of AL amyloidosis has been proposed, in which both the underlying hematologic disorder and the end organ damage can be monitored with FLC and cardiac biomarkers to optimise therapy and minimise toxicity.

Treatment regimens, generally administered by haematologists, have been adapted from those developed in multiple myeloma, although most patients with AL amyloidosis have a low-grade plasma cell dyscrasia and small clonal burden. Treatment for AL amyloidosis is highly individualised and is based on age, cardiac staging and regimen toxicities. Outcomes in AL amyloidosis have improved following introduction of effective chemotherapy regimens [26].

50.6.3 Response to Therapy in Patients with Renal Involvement

Close communication between the treating haematologist and nephrologist is crucial during chemotherapy for renal AL amyloidosis. Median survival in patients presenting with renal disease is between 2 and 3 years [27, 28]. Survival is strongly influenced by the degree of haematological response and the presence of cardiac amyloidosis but not by the degree of renal dysfunction at presentation [26]. More than 40% of patients eventually receive dialysis, and 13–26% of cases presenting with potentially salvageable renal function progress to ESRD within a median of 12 months. Renal function deteriorates in ~50% and improves in approximately a third of cases. Proteinuria of >5 g/day and an eGFR of <50 ml/min have been identified as the best predictors of progression to dialysis [29]. In a study of 298 patients who had received stem cell transplantation, a renal response was seen in 43% of patients at 24 months [30]. High-dose melphalan and stem cell rescue were associated with renal toxicity with 21% reaching ESRF over follow-up. The potential nephrotoxicity of lenalidomide has been recently reported and demands careful follow-up of renal function.

50.6.4 Reactive Systemic AA Amyloidosis

In AA amyloidosis the aim of treatment is complete biochemical control of the underlying inflammatory disease, often carried out by the treating rheumatologist. The choice of therapy depends on the underlying disease process, but therapeutic success must always be assessed by measurement of the acute phase response, ideally by serial SAA monitoring. Most patients with inflammatory arthritis have previously failed to respond to conventional disease-modifying anti-rheumatoid drugs, and many do well with anti-TNF therapies or other biologics, such as anti-CD20 antibodies or anti IL-1 or IL-6 therapies. In patients who fail to respond to these agents, there may still be a role for therapy with alkylating agents, such as chlorambucil or cyclophosphamide. A multidisciplinary approach involving the nephrologist and, most frequently, rheumatologist is beneficial.

Median SAA concentration has been shown to be a strong predictor of both survival and renal outcome; persistent complete suppression of inflammation with normal SAA levels is associated with an almost 18-fold lower risk of death than median SAA levels of >155 mg/L [11]. Median survival of 79–137 months has been recently reported in large series from Italy and the UK. Approximately 40% of patients will eventually require renal replacement therapy with a median time to dialysis from diagnosis of 78 months.

50.6.5 Dialysis-Related Amyloidosis (DRA)

The only effective treatment for DRA is successful renal transplantation, although drugs targeting the amyloid deposits are being tested. Serum levels of β_2-microglobulin fall rapidly following transplantation, and this is usually accompanied by an improvement in symptoms. This rapid response is probably due more to the anti-inflammatory properties of transplant immunosuppression and to discontinuation of dialysis than actual regression of deposits. In contrast to symptoms, radiological bone cysts heal slowly, and amyloid can be demonstrated histologically many years after renal transplantation. Attempts have been made to reduce DRA by altering the dialysis prescription. There is evidence that the risks of DRA are increased in patients dialysed using less 'biocompatible' membranes and that use of the more permeable membrane systems is relatively protective. Greater removal of β_2-microglobulin is attained in patients undergoing high-flux haemodiafiltration, and in the long term these patients may be less prone to DRA. The incidence of DRA appears to be falling, possibly reflecting the increasingly widespread use of such membranes. Surgery may be required to relieve carpal tunnel compression, stabilise the cervical spine or treat bone fractures.

50.6.6 Hereditary Non-neuropathic Systemic Amyloidosis

These diseases, particularly lysozyme and apolipoprotein A-I amyloidosis, tend to run very indolent courses, and, when renal failure is reached, transplantation can be successful with grafts surviving for decades. The rate of renal deterioration seems to be faster in fibrinogen amyloidosis, and the limited experience of renal transplantation suggests that amyloid deposition will cause graft loss after a median of ~7 years [16]. As fibrinogen is synthesised solely in the liver, combined hepatorenal transplantation offers the possibility of 'surgical gene therapy' and complete protection from recurrent amyloidosis. The limitation of this approach is the serious risks associated with combined transplantation.

50.6.7 Preservation and Replacement of Organ Function

Organs infiltrated by amyloid may fail acutely often without obvious provocation. Attention must to be paid to salt and water balance, maintenance of the circulating volume and prompt treatment of sepsis to reduce the risk of acute organ failure. Potentially nephrotoxic drugs, elective surgery and general anaesthesia are best avoided, unless there are compelling indications. There is a vogue for using doxycycline as antibiotic prophylaxis, given its postulated ability to destabilise amyloid structure [31].

Significant renal disease is present at diagnosis in at least 75% of patients with systemic amyloidosis. Nephrotic syndrome can be severe and difficult to manage in some patients who cannot maintain their intravascular volume. Infusions of salt poor albumin may be helpful in this regard.

Caution is required in the use of standard heart failure medications in patients with amyloidosis. Digoxin and calcium channel blockers have been associated with excess toxicity. Angiotensin-converting enzyme inhibitors can promote hypotension and should generally be avoided. Prophylactic amiodarone has been incorporated into therapy trials of amyloidosis to reduce the risk of sudden cardiac death if complex ventricular arrhythmias are detected on Holter ECG.

The use of beta blockers in patients with cardiac amyloid may be associated with increased mortality. Diuretics are the mainstay of therapy but should be used with caution as amyloidosis causes a restrictive cardiomyopathy and high filling pressures are required to maintain cardiac output. Alpha agonists such as midodrine can improve orthostatic hypotension. Implantable cardiac defibrillators have been used, but their efficacy in this disease remains controversial.

In highly selected younger patients with isolated irreversible cardiac failure, heart transplantation offers a possibility of long-term survival and has been performed in a small number of patients. The scarcity of donor hearts, the high transplant-related mortality and the risk of amyloid deposition in the graft make rigorous patient selection mandatory. In AL amyloidosis chemotherapy is required after cardiac transplantation to prevent graft amyloid or its progression in other organ systems.

50.6.8 Renal Dialysis

The outcome of AL amyloidosis patients on long-term dialysis is improving, but survival is reduced compared to age-matched non-diabetic patients with other diseases [32]. Patients who commenced dialysis after 2002 in the UK had a median survival of 43.6 months, whereas data from the USA and Italy report median survival of 10.4 to 11 months. The outcome in patients with other types of amyloid is more favourable. In AA amyloidosis the medians survival on dialysis has been reported as 17 months in earlier series and 69 months in more recent series with an incident mortality of 18% droping to 10% in subsequent years.

50.6.9 Renal Transplantation

Although early mortality is increased, due to sepsis and cardiac failure, long-term renal graft survival and rejection rates are comparable with other systemic diseases. Less than 10% of patients who reached ESRD due to AL amyloidosis receive a renal transplant; median patient and graft survival in these highly selected patients was 89 months [32]. In a few cases renal transplantation has been followed by autologous stem cell transplantation with stable renal function in 4/8 patients. Recent experience of renal transplantation in selected patients with AA amyloidosis has shown 5- and 10-year graft survival of 74% and 68%, respectively. These encouraging data have prompted use of living donor renal transplants. Most patients have a functioning graft until death, despite frequent histological presence of amyloid deposits in the renal allograft.

Further information about amyloidosis is available at ▶ www.myeloma.org.uk, ▶ www.ucl.ac.uk/medicine/amyloidosis/nac and ▶ www.mayoclinic.com/health/amyloidosis.

? Questions

1. How is amyloid type best determined?
2. What conditions underlie AL amyloidosis?
3. Do any types of amyloidosis show ethnic predisposition?
4. How important is the presence of cardiac amyloidosis?
5. What determines treatment choice in Al amyloidosis?

✓ Answers

1. The gold standard is by typing the deposits; probably the best technique is laser microdissection (LMD)- and tandem mass spectrometry (MS)-based proteomic analysis (available in a few centres) or immunohistochemistry.
2. In AL amyloidosis the fibril proteins are derived from monoclonal immunoglobulin light chains, and any haematological condition resulting in their production can be complicated by amyloid. The commonest underlying disorder is a monoclonal gammopathy, full-blown myeloma is seen less often and amyloidosis can complicate lymphomas and chronic lymphocytic leukaemia.
3. Generally not really. There are geographic hotspots where carriage of mutations underlying hereditary amyloidosis is relatively frequent.

   Acquired LECT2 amyloidosis predominantly affects individuals of Hispanic, Egyptian and South Asian descent.
4. Significant cardiac amyloidosis confers a poor prognosis without early effective treatment. The

best assessment is multimodality including biomarkers such as BNP, easily available tests including ECG and echocardiography and specialised cardiac MRI and DPD scintigraphy.

5. The aim of treatment is to obtain an early, complete and sustained clonal response with minimal treatment-related toxicity. Treatment is best handled by multidisciplinary teams, and choice of agents is highly individual depending on the specific underlying clonal disorder, organ function, presence of neuropathy and performance status.

References

1. Merlini G, Bellotti V. Molecular mechanisms of amyloidosis. N Engl J Med. 2003;349:583–96.
2. Obici L, Raimondi S, Lavatelli F, Bellotti V, Merlini G. Susceptibility to AA amyloidosis in rheumatic diseases: a critical overview. Arthritis Rheum. 2009;61:1435–40.
3. Saraiva MJ. Hereditary transthyretin amyloidosis: molecular basis and therapeutical strategies. Expert Rev Mol Med. 2002;2002:1–11.
4. Chiti F, Dobson CM. Protein Misfolding, Amyloid Formation, and Human Disease: A Summary of Progress Over the Last Decade. Annu Rev Biochem 2. 2017;86:27–68.
5. Pepys MB. Serum amyloid P component. In: Haeberli A, editor. Human Protein Data. Weinheim: Wiley-VCH Verlag GmbH; 1997.
6. Bodin K, Ellmerich S, Kahan MC, Tennent GA, Loesch A, Gilbertson JA, et al. Antibodies to human serum amyloid P component eliminate visceral amyloid deposits. Nature. 2010;468:93–7.
7. Pinney JH, Smith CJ, Taube JB, Lachmann HJ, Venner CP, Gibbs SD, et al. Systemic amyloidosis in England: an epidemiological study. Br J Haematol. 2013;161(4):525–32.
8. Kyle RA, Gertz MA. Primary systemic amyloidosis: clinical and laboratory features in 474 cases. Semin Hematol. 1995;32(1):45–59.
9. Wechalekar AD, Lachmann HJ, Goodman HJ, Bradwell A, Hawkins PN, Gillmore JD. AL amyloidosis associated with IgM paraproteinemia: clinical profile and treatment outcome. Blood. 2008;112:4009–16.
10. Lane T, Pinney JH, Gilbertson JA, Hutt DF, Rowczenio DM, Mahmood S, et al. Changing epidemiology of AA amyloidosis: clinical observations over 25 years at a single national referral Centre. Amyloid. 2017;24(3):162–6.
11. Lachmann HJ, Goodman HJB, Gilbertson JA, Gallimore JR, Sabin CA, Gillmore JD, et al. Natural history and outcome in systemic AA amyloidosis. N Engl J Med. 2007;356:2361–71.
12. Schwalbe S, Holzhauer M, Schaeffer J, Galanski M, Koch KM, Floege J. Beta 2-microglobulin associated amyloidosis: a vanishing complication of long-term hemodialysis? Kidney Int. 1997;52:1077–83.
13. Murphy CL, Wang S, Kestler D, Larsen C, Benson D, Weiss DT, et al. Leukocyte chemotactic factor 2 (LECT2)-associated renal amyloidosis: a case series. Am J Kidney Dis. 2010;56:1100–7.
14. Drueke TB. Beta2-microglobulin and amyloidosis. Nephrol Dial Transplant. 2000;15(Suppl 1):17–24.
15. Larsen CP, Ismail W, Kurtin PJ, Vrana JA, Dasari S, Nasr SH. Leukocyte chemotactic factor 2 amyloidosis (ALECT2) is a common form of renal amyloidosis among Egyptians. Mod Pathol. 2016;29(4):416–20.
16. Gillmore JD, Lachmann HJ, Rowczenio D, Gilbertson JA, Zeng CH, Liu ZH, et al. Diagnosis, pathogenesis, treatment, and prognosis of hereditary fibrinogen a alpha-chain amyloidosis. J Am Soc Nephrol. 2009;20:444–51.
17. Lobato L. Portuguese-type amyloidosis (transthyretin amyloidosis, ATTR V30M). J Nephrol. 2003;16:438–42.
18. Arbustini E, Morbini P, Verga L, Concardi M, Porcu E, Pilotto A, et al. Light and electron microscopy immunohistochemical characterization of amyloid deposits. Amyloid. 1997;4(3):157–70.
19. Vrana JA, Gamez JD, Madden BJ, Theis JD, Bergen HR 3rd, Dogan A. Classification of amyloidosis by laser microdissection and mass spectrometry-based proteomic analysis in clinical biopsy specimens. Blood. 2009;114:4957–9.
20. Hawkins PN, Myers MJ, Epenetos AA, Caspi D, Pepys MB. Specific localization and imaging of amyloid deposits *in vivo* using ^{123}I-labeled serum amyloid P component. J Exp Med. 1988;167:903–13.
21. Maceira AM, Joshi J, Prasad SK, Moon JC, Perugini E, Harding I, et al. Cardiovascular magnetic resonance in cardiac amyloidosis. Circulation. 2005;111:186–93.
22. Rapezzi C, Quarta CC, Guidalotti PL, Pettinato C, Fanti S, Leone O, et al. Role of (99m)Tc-DPD scintigraphy in diagnosis and prognosis of hereditary transthyretin-related cardiac amyloidosis. JACC Cardiovasc Imaging. 2011;4(6):659–70.
23. Rowczenio DM, Noor I, Gillmore JD, Lachmann HJ, Whelan C, Hawkins P, et al. Online registry for mutations in hereditary amyloidosis including nomenclature recommendations. Hum Mutat. 2014;35(9):E2403–E12.
24. Gillmore JD, Lovat LB, Persey MR, Pepys MB, Hawkins PN. Amyloid load and clinical outcome in AA amyloidosis in relation to circulating concentration of serum amyloid a protein. Lancet. 2001;358:24–9.
25. Vaxman I, Gertz M. Recent advances in the diagnosis, risk stratification, and Management of Systemic Light-Chain Amyloidosis. Acta Haematol. 2019;141(2):93–106.
26. Muchtar E, Dispenzieri A, Leung N, Lacy MQ, Buadi FK, Dingli D, et al. Depth of organ response in AL amyloidosis is associated with improved survival: grading the organ response criteria. Leukemia. 2018;32:2240–9.
27. Gertz MA, Leung N, Lacy MQ, Dispenzieri A, Zeldenrust SR, Hayman SR, et al. Clinical outcome of immunoglobulin light chain amyloidosis affecting the kidney. Nephrol Dial Transplant. 2009;24:3132–7.
28. Pinney JH, Lachmann HJ, Bansi L, Wechalekar AD, Gilbertson JA, Rowczenio D, et al. Outcome in renal AL amyloidosis following chemotherapy. J Clin Oncol. 2011;29(6):674–81.
29. Palladini G, Hegenbart U, Milani P, Kimmich C, Foli A, Ho AD, et al. A staging system for renal outcome and early markers of renal response to chemotherapy in AL amyloidosis. Blood. 2014;124(15):2325–32.
30. Havasi H, Doros G, Sanchorawala V. Predictive value of the new renal response criteria in AL amyloidosis treated with high dose melphalan and stem cell transplantation. Am J Hematol. 2018;93:E129–32.
31. Wechalekar AD, Whelan C. Encouraging impact of doxycycline on early mortality in cardiac light chain (AL) amyloidosis. Blood Cancer J. 2017;7(3):e546.
32. Pinney JH, Lachmann HJ, Bansi L, Wechalekar AD, Gilbertson JA, Rowczenio D, et al. Outcome in renal Al amyloidosis after chemotherapy. J Clin Oncol. 2011;29(6):674–81.
33. Dispenzieri A, Gertz M, Kyle R, Lacy M, Burritt MF, Therneau TM, et al. Serum cardiac troponins and N-terminal pro-brain natriuretic peptide: a staging system for primary systemic amyloidosis. J Clin Oncol. 2004;22:3751–7.

Thrombotic Microangiopathies

Neil S. Sheerin

Contents

M. Harber (ed.), *Primer on Nephrology*, https://doi.org/10.1007/978-3-030-76419-7_51

Learning Objectives

1. The combination of thrombocytopenia and microangiopathic haemolysis with a normal clotting screen is highly suggestive of a TMA.
2. TMAs can present with a wide range of clinical features including neurological involvement and acute kidney injury.
3. In patients with a suspected TMA, it is important to investigate thoroughly to identify the cause of the TMA.
4. TMAs should be treated as an emergency as they can be rapidly fatal.
5. The treatment required will depend on the clinical features at presentation, but urgent plasma exchange should be considered until TTP has been excluded.

In a patient with thrombotic microangiopathy endothelial dysfunction leads to the formation of thrombi in small vessels, platelet consumption, and mechanical damage to erythrocytes (microangiopathic haemolysis).

Haemolytic uraemic syndrome (HUS) is a form of TMA that is caused by Shiga toxin in 90% of cases with the remaining cases (atypical HUS) most commonly due to excessive complement activation. Kidney injury is the most common clinical feature.

Thrombotic thrombocytopenic purpura (TTP) is a form of TMA due to an inherited or acquired deficiency in ADAMTS13 which leads to the accumulation high molecular weight multimers of von Willebrand factor on the surface of endothelial cells and the formation of platelet-rich thrombi. Neurological disease is the most common clinical feature.

51.1 Introduction

Thrombotic microangiopathies (TMAs) are a group of rare diseases characterised by thrombocytopenia, microangiopathic haemolytic anaemia (MAHA), and occlusion of small vessels by thrombi, the site, and severity which determines the clinical presentation. A diagnosis of TMA should be considered in all patients presenting with a combination of thrombocytopenia and microangiopathic haemolytic anaemia as TMA can rapidly progress to organ failure and death. TMAs have been divided into two broad diseases, thrombotic thrombocytopenia purpura (TTP), and haemolytic uraemia syndrome (HUS), based on their clinical manifestations. TTP typically causes neurological disease whereas in HUS acute kidney, injury predominates. Although in many cases the diagnosis is clear, in other cases it is not possible to reliably distinguish between these diseases purely on clinical criteria as significant overlap can exist. As a better understanding of the molecular basis of TTP and HUS has developed, it is now possible to diagnose and differentiate between these diseases with greater accuracy, and classification of TMAs is now based on aetiology rather than clinical features. The early recognition of the clinical and laboratory features of a TMA by clinicians remains critically important to allow appropriate investigation and early initiation of treatment.

51.2 Clinical Features

The clinical features depend on the site of vascular occlusion with predominant involvement of the central nervous system in TTP and the renal vasculature in HUS. However, there is significant clinical overlap, and a classification based on aetiology rather than clinical features provides a better guide to prognosis and a rationale for therapy. TMA can also occur in a range of other clinical scenarios where features of the original disease may be evident. These are listed in ◘ Table 51.1.

51.2.1 Thrombotic Thrombocytopenic Purpura.

With the exception of the inherited form of TTP (Upshaw-Schulman syndrome) which usually occurs early in childhood TTP occurs predominantly in adults (90%), the features of TMA are present, and the thrombocytopenia is often profound, with platelet counts lower than in HUS. Neurological symptoms and signs are usually present and often severe and can include headache, focal neurological deficit, seizures, and reduced level of consciousness. Cardiac involvement can also occur in up to 40% of patients. Fever is frequently present, and renal impairment, including an abnormal

51

Table 51.1 Classification of HUS, TTP, and other TMA associated diseases

Reduced ADAMTS13 activity (TTP). Genetic (homozygotic or compound heterozygotic) Acquired (inhibitory autoantibody)
Shiga toxin-induced HUS Shiga toxin-producing *E. coli* and *Shigella dysenteriae* type 1
Atypical HUS due to disorders of complement regulation Genetic disorders of complement regulation Acquired disorders of complement regulation
Atypical HUS due to other genetic causes DGKε Defective cobalamin (B12) metabolism
TMA associated with pregnancy Preeclampsia/HELLP syndrome aHUS and TTP
TMA associated with other infections *Streptococcus pneumoniae* HIV Influenza Herpes viruses (CMV, EBV, HHV8) Hepatitis A and C
Drug-related TMA Chemotherapy (mitomycin, cisplatin, gemcitabine) VEGF inhibitors (bevacizumab, aflibercept) Anti-platelet drugs (ticlopidine, clopidogrel) Immunosuppressants (ciclosporin, tacrolimus, sirolimus) Interferons (α and β) Tyrosine kinase inhibitors (sunitinib, sorafenib) Antibiotics (penicillins, ciprofloxacin)
Malignancy-related TMA Epithelial malignancies (stomach, bowel, prostate, breast) Haematological malignancy
TMA related to malignant hypertension
TMA following bone marrow transplantation
TMA following solid organ transplantation Recurrent aHUS De novo TMA (drugs, ischaemia reperfusion injury) Antibody-mediated rejection

urinary sediment, can be present. The disease can progress rapidly with a high mortality associated with TTP without appropriate treatment and even with treatment a mortality of >10% is reported.

51.2.2 Haemolytic Uraemic Syndrome

Haemolytic uraemic syndrome is a group of diseases usually presenting with evidence of thrombocytopenia, microangiopathic haemolysis, and acute kidney injury. Although often thought of as a disease predominantly affecting children, it is clear that HUS can affect any age group, and this diagnosis should be considered in any patient presenting with a TMA and renal impairment.

51.2.3 Shiga Toxin-Associated HUS

This is the commonest form of HUS and is caused by gastrointestinal infection with bacteria that produce Shiga toxin, most frequently Shiga toxin-producing *Escherichia coli* (STEC). Farm animals are the natural reservoir for STEC, and infection occurs after direct contact or after consumption of undercooked meat or contaminated food products. Symptoms typically begin after a 4–7-day incubation period with the abrupt onset of diarrhoea, which is usually bloody (60%), and abdominal pain. The features of HUS develop in approximately 10% of people infected with STEC with development of thrombocytopenia, microangiopathic haemolysis, and acute kidney injury 2–10 days after the onset of diarrhoea, which may have resolved. Importantly 5–10% of patients with STEC HUS report no preceding gastrointestinal symptoms. In the acute phase, 50% of patients require dialysis, and there is a reported mortality of 1–2%. Neurological symptoms and signs are common and may be present in approximately 20–30% of patients. Although renal recovery is usual after the initial presentation, 40% of patients subsequently develop CKD or hypertension. In patients who progress to ESKD, kidney transplantation is an option as recurrence is very rare.

51.2.4 Atypical HUS

The clinical presentation of aHUS can be indistinguishable from other causes of TMA, with renal involvement predominating. Other organ involvement, including neurological and cardiac disease, can be present. Traditionally thought of as a disease primarily affecting children, all age groups can be affected. Preceding gastroenteritic symptoms are reported by 25% of patients with aHUS; therefore, the presence of diarrhoea is not a robust criteria to distinguish between atypical and STEC forms of HUS. A family history of aHUS may be present as may a history of previous episodes of TMA as aHUS can run a remitting, relapsing course.

Without treatment the prognosis is poor with 50% of patients progressing to renal failure or dying within 1 year of presentation. The severity of aHUS is influenced by the underlying genetic abnormality in complement regulation responsible for disease development (Table 51.2) [1]. Once a patient develops end-stage renal failure, the other features of the disease usually remit.

Table 51.2 Complement defects associated with TMA

Complement defect	Function of protein	Frequency	Rate of End-stage renal disease (ESRD)
Factor H mutations	Dissociation of convertases and cofactor for factor I-mediated cleavage and inactivation of C3b	15–30%	70–80%
CD46 mutations	Cofactor for factor I-mediated cleavage and inactivation of C3b	10–15%	20%
Factor I mutations	Serine protease degrading C3b to inactive smaller fragments	5–10%	50–80%
Factor B mutations[a]	Binds to C3b to form the alternative pathway C3 convertase	1–2%	70–80%
C3 mutations[a]	Pivotal complement protein at the convergence of the three activation pathways	5–10%	50–60%
Anti-factor H autoantibodies	Inhibit function of factor H	6–11%	40–60%

ESRD End-stage renal disease
[a]Denotes gain-of-function mutation

Recurrence after a kidney transplant is common and occurs in 80–90% of patients with certain mutations (Factor H, C3, Factor B), and a high rate of graft loss is reported if the disease recurs and is not treated appropriately [2]. Patients with no identifiable mutation have a lower but significant risk of relapse. The exception is patients with CD46 mutations who rarely develop recurrent disease. Previously, because of the risk of relapse, patients with aHUS were not considered for kidney transplant alone. The availability of therapeutic complement inhibition means that transplantation is now a viable option.

51.3 Epidemiology

TTP has an annual incidence of approximately 2–5 cases per million population, with over 90% of cases occurring in adults. The majority of cases (>95% in adults) are caused by an autoantibody that inhibits the function of ADAMTS13. The highest incidence is after the age of 40 years, and females are affected more commonly than males (2:1). Inherited deficiency in ADAMTS13 activity is rare (5% of cases) and usually presents in childhood.

STEC infection, typically serotype O157, is the commonest cause of HUS and accounts for 90% of cases of HUS. STEC HUS has an annual incidence of seven cases per million population. The incidence of STEC HUS is highest in the summer months. Other *E. coli* serotypes also cause HUS, including the serotypes O26, O111, O103, and O145, as can infection with other Shiga toxin-producing bacteria, particularly *Shigella dysenteriae* type 1, which is common in parts of Asia. The largest recorded outbreak of STEC HUS occurred in continental Europe, mainly Germany, in 2011 and was caused by *E. coli* O104 [3]. This outbreak was notable because of the high proportion of adults affected, the high mortality rate (4.3%), and the high proportion of patients with neurological sequelae.

Atypical HUS is less common and accounts for the remaining 10% of cases. Complement-mediated aHUS is the most common form and has an annual incidence of 0.4 per million population. It most commonly presents in childhood, but any age can be affected. Females are more frequently affected (approximately 60% of cases). Other inherited or secondary forms of aHUS are rare in the population as a whole.

51.4 Aetiopathology of the Thrombotic Microangiopathies

The vascular endothelium has a critical role in maintaining normal haemostasis. Activation or injury to the endothelium results in a reduction in endothelial anticoagulant activity and release of pro-thrombotic molecules. Activation of the coagulation cascade results in platelet aggregation and trapping of erythrocytes in a fibrin mesh, finally leading to thrombus formation. In the context of vascular injury, this will bridge any defect in the endothelium and vessel wall and, because coagulation is usually localised, will not result in detectable changes in coagulation tests or other haematological parameters.

In contrast in a TMA, there is widespread activation of the endothelium. There is no breach of the endothelium to bridge, but instead small vessels are occluded by thrombi causing ischaemic tissue injury. Because of the more extensive endothelial activation, haematological abnormalities are evident. Platelets are consumed within the thrombi, and a low platelet count ($<150 \times 10^9$/l) will usually be present. Platelets fall early in the disease, and although a normal platelet count can be present, significant TMA is unusual in the absence of thrombocytopenia. Erythrocytes are trapped within the thrombi and are also damaged as they pass over activated endothelium and through partially occluded vessels leading to microangiopathic haemolysis.

51.4.1 Thrombotic Thrombocytopenic Purpura

TTP is caused by a severe deficiency in the protease enzyme 'a disintegrin and metalloproteinase with a thrombospondin type 1 motif member 13' (ADAMTS13) which is responsible for cleaving von Willebrand factor (VWF). VWF is involved in haemostasis, and the surface expression of VWF on endothelial cells induces platelet aggregation and thrombus formation. VWF is initially produced as ultra-large multimers which are gradually broken down by ADAMTS13. If ADAMTS13 activity is reduced, multimers of VWF accumulate on the endothelial surface leading to platelet aggregation and thrombus formation [4]. Inherited TTP is rare accounting for 5% of all cases of TTP. It is due to a homozygous (or compound heterozygous) mutation in the *ADAMTS13* gene, and there is a high degree of penetrance. Inherited TTP accounts for a higher proportion of childhood TTP. More commonly (>90% of cases), TTP is due to an autoantibody that inhibits the function of ADAMTS13 [5].

TTP has also been linked to the platelet inhibitors ticlopidine and clopidogrel. This is a rare side effect which usually develops in the first few weeks after starting treatment. Autoantibodies to ADAMTS13 have been reported in some cases and plasma exchange may improve outcome.

51.4.2 Shiga Toxin-Associated HUS

Once ingested, STEC adheres to the intestinal epithelium and releases toxin. Shiga toxin is absorbed across the intestinal epithelium and transported to the target organ bound to erythrocytes and leukocytes. It exerts a cytotoxic effect by binding to globotriaosylceramide 3 (Gb3), which leads to endocytosis of toxin and retrograde transport to the endoplasmic reticulum where the toxin inhibits protein synthesis. This disrupts cell function, finally leading to cell death [6]. Gb3 receptors are highly expressed on glomerular endothelial cells, podocytes, and tubular cells; therefore, explaining why the kidney is the primary target of the disease. Shiga toxin-mediated injury and activation of endothelial cells produces a pro-thrombotic state with activation of the coagulation cascade, platelet and erythrocyte consumption, and the vaso-occlusive disease which typifies a TMA. HUS only develops in a minority of people infected with STEC suggesting that other genetic or environmental factors are important in determining whether HUS develops.

51.4.3 Atypical HUS

Atypical HUS was used to describe cases of HUS not caused by STEC infection. It is now clear that this represents a group of diseases with similar clinical features but different aetiologies. Most cases of aHUS are due to a genetic or acquired defect in the regulation of the complement cascade. Mutations in the complement control protein Factor H were first described in 1998 [7]. Since then loss-of-function mutations, polymorphisms, or antibodies that interfere with the function of complement inhibitors and gain-of-function mutations in complement activators have been identified in approximately 70% of patients with aHUS.

The complement cascade is a system of over 30 proteins and is a pivotal component of the innate immune system. It is activated by three distinct pathways, but it is the alternative pathway, with its continuous, low level of activation, that is critical in the development of aHUS. In the alternative pathway, activation of C3 occurs by spontaneous hydrolysis. Binding of Factor B to activated C3 results in further cleavage of C3 to produce C3a (an anaphylatoxin) and C3b which generates the C3 convertase of the alternative pathway (C3bBb). This cleaves more C3 with amplification by a system of positive feedback and generation of a C5 convertase. C5 is cleaved into C5a, a potent anaphylatoxin, and C5b which leads to the assembly of the membrane attack complex (MAC, C5b-9). The MAC forms a membrane-spanning lytic pore which when deposited in sub-lytic concentrations can alter cell phenotype. MAC deposited on endothelial cells induces a pro-thrombotic change resulting in a TMA.

In normal circumstances activation of complement is controlled by a series of cell membrane-bound and soluble inhibitors to prevent injury to autologous cells. If there is loss of function in one of these inhibitors, increased activation of complement occurs leading to endothelial cell damage and development of TMA. Loss of function is usually due to a mutation in one of the control proteins, most frequently Factor H, but also membrane cofactor protein (MCP, CD46) and Factor I. In addition gain-of-function mutations have been described in proteins involved in complement activation (Table 51.2) [8]. The disease usually follows an autosomal dominant pattern of inheritance with incomplete penetrance. Approximately 50–60% of people who carry a disease-associated mutation develop the disease. Other genetic and environmental factors influence disease development (a multi-hit hypothesis) including commonly occurring genetic variants in complement genes that predispose to disease in the presence of a pathogenic mutation [9]. Environmental triggers, including infection, pregnancy, transplantation, and drug exposure, are involved in triggering TMA in a patient with a genetic susceptibility. Another recognised cause of aHUS is autoantibodies that interfere with the function of complement regulators in particular anti-Factor H.

51.5 Diagnosis

The initial step is to diagnose the presence of a TMA. This is based on the clinical presentation and the presence of the characteristic biochemical and haematological changes which are summarised in ◘ Table 51.3. Once this has been established, the next step is to identify the cause of the TMA.

51.5.1 Thrombotic Thrombocytopenic Purpura

The diagnosis is made by testing ADAMTS13 activity, with severe deficiency (<5–10% activity), being associated with the disease. ADAMTS13 activity can also be low in TMA associated with autoimmune disease, pregnancy, and drugs and can be low in patients with malignancy or chronic infection without features of TMA. If low ADAMTS13 activity is found, the patient should be screened for inhibitory autoantibodies to ADAMTS13 or mutations in the *ADAMTS13* gene (in the absence of an inhibitor). It is critical to perform these tests before starting plasma-based therapies.

◘ Table 51.3 Laboratory investigation in suspected TMA

Test	Result in TMA
Full blood count	Anemia and thrombocytopenia
Blood film	Red cell fragmentation (schistocytes)
Reticulocyte count	Elevated
Lactate dehydrogenase	Raised due to release from damaged red cells
Liver function tests	Isolated raise in bilirubin due to haemoglobin degradation
Haptoglobin	Reduced due to trafficking of free haemoglobin
Creatinine	Elevated due to renal dysfunction
Coagulation screen	Normal (differentiating TMA from disseminated intravascular coagulation)
Direct antiglobulin test	Negative (differentiating TMA from immune hemolysis)
Urinalysis	Haemoglobinuria

51.5.2 Shiga Toxin-Associated HUS

STEC O157 can be identified after culture from the stool or from a rectal swab (which is a useful technique to obtain cultures in children or after diarrhoea has stopped). It is possible to test for the presence of Shiga toxin, and the gene encoding Shiga toxin can be detected by polymerase chain reaction. Infection can be confirmed by measuring the serological response to the O-serotype of Shiga toxin-producing *E. coli*; however, it is not possible to test for all serotypes. Renal biopsy is rarely necessary to confirm the diagnosis, but when performed arteriolar and glomerular capillary thrombosis is seen, with glomerular capillaries congested with fragmented erythrocytes. Acute tubular injury and mesangiolysis are commonly seen.

51.5.3 Atypical HUS

Initially aHUS is a diagnosis of exclusion in patients with a TMA, negative tests for STEC infection, and preserved ADAMTS13 protease activity. A low plasma C3 level is suggestive of aHUS, although C3 levels can be normal particularly in patients with CD46 mutations. Low concentrations of circulating Factor H or Factor I can be detected if the protein is not synthesised as a consequence of a mutation; however, mutations may result in normal quantities of non-functioning protein. Low cell surface expression of CD46 can be detected on peripheral blood mononuclear cells.

Genetic and immunological testing is usually required to identify the exact aetiology. Because of the time required to perform these tests, they are rarely useful in guiding initial diagnosis and treatment but should be performed in all patients with suspected aHUS. Screening for genetic or immune defects will identify a cause in approximately 70% of cases [1]. The remaining 30% of patients may have mutations in other genes, have a 'secondary TMA' (see below) or a disease without an identifiable cause. In some of these situations, patients may still respond to complement inhibition.

51

51.6 Treatment

51.6.1 Thrombotic Thrombocytopenic Purpura

Without treatment mortality in patients with TTP is high (over 90%). Plasma-based therapy, either exchange or infusion, is the mainstay of treatment, with plasma exchange generally being preferred in adults because of its ability to remove inhibitory autoantibodies [10]. Despite treatment mortality rate remains high (>10%). Early treatment (within hours) is important, and treatment should begin based on clinical and laboratory features before ADAMTS13 activity is known. It is less important to exclude aHUS as plasma therapy is an appropriate treatment for this condition. Plasma exchange should be with fresh frozen plasma (or equivalent product) and should be at least 1.5 plasma volume on a daily basis until a response is seen. Increasing the volume of exchange or twice-daily exchanges should be considered if no response is seen. Immunosuppression should be considered in patients with TTP. High-dose intravenous methylprednisolone followed by oral steroids should be started in patients with suspected TTP. Relapse after remission occurs in up to 30% of patients. A beneficial effect of rituximab (anti-CD20) has been reported, particularly in reducing the risk of relapse. Other drugs, including vincristine, cyclophosphamide, and cyclosporine A, have been used to treat TTP, but rituximab is now preferred. A monoclonal antibody that blocks the interaction between VWF and platelet glycoprotein 1b, caplacizumab, has shown promising results in recent trials [11].

51.6.2 Shiga Toxin-Associated HUS

In most cases this is a self-limiting disease, and treatment is supportive until resolution of the acute episode. In severe cases, this will include renal replacement therapy and when necessary other organ support. The use of antibiotics in STEC HUS is controversial. Some authors have reported a worse outcome with the use of antibiotics, possibly due to the increased release of Shiga toxin [12]. However, more recent reports from the German outbreak with STEC O104 suggest a better outcome after antibiotic treatment [13, 14]. Reports following the German outbreak and other studies have failed to show any beneficial effect of plasma exchange or other plasma-based therapy in the treatment of STEC HUS an observation supported by a Cochrane systematic review in 2009 [15].

A role for complement activation has been suggested in the pathogenesis of STEC HUS. This is supported by a report in 2011 of three patients with severe STEC HUS who responded to treatment with the complement inhibitor, eculizumab [16]. Future studies may define a role for complement inhibition in this disease, but at present the routine use of eculizumab in STEC HUS cannot be recommended.

51.6.3 Atypical HUS

Plasma therapy has until recently been the main therapy for aHUS. This is usually plasma exchange with fresh frozen plasma or equivalent. Plasma exchange, as opposed to plasma infusion, not only avoids problems of volume overload and hyperviscosity but will remove proteins with abnormal function and autoantibodies that may interfere with the function of normal proteins. As many as 40% of patients are resistant to plasma therapy and show signs of ongoing TMA and progressive organ damage despite treatment. Of the patients who respond in some cases, treatment can be withdrawn while others become dependent on plasma therapy to maintain remission.

Eculizumab is a monoclonal antibody that inhibits activation of C5 and is licenced for the treatment of aHUS. The first beneficial effects of eculizumab in aHUS were reported in 2009 [17, 18], and these reports have been confirmed in clinical trials [19]. Adolescent or adults patients with aHUS were enrolled in the initial trials with either plasma-resistant or plasma-sensitive aHUS, and eculizumab was very effective at inducing and maintaining remission. Kidney function also improved after eculizumab treatment. In these trials approximately 30% of patients did not have an identifiable defect in complement regulation but responded to treatment with eculizumab. Inhibition of C5 activity with eculizumab increases susceptibility to meningococcal infection. Vaccination with a tetravalent (ACWY) and anti-B serotype vaccine is mandatory prior to eculizumab use, and some centres recommend long-term antibiotic prophylaxis. Although life-long treatment with eculizumab was recommended in the initial licence, it is now clear that a significant proportion of patients can withdraw from treatment without relapse [20, 21].

51.7 Other Genetic Causes of HUS

51.7.1 HUS Due to Defective Cobalamin (B12) Metabolism

Methylmalonic aciduria and homocystinuria type C protein is involved in the metabolism of vitamin B12 (cobalamin). Homozygotic or compound heterozygotic mutations in the gene encoding this protein, *MMACHC*, causes an aHUS-like disease in addition to a wide range of other clinical features including neurological, cardiac, and pulmonary abnormalities. Biochemically patients have elevated plasma homocysteine, low methionine, and methylmalonic aciduria. Biochemical and genetic analysis is vital in patients presenting with a TMA, particularly if there are other clinical abnormalities. Patients usually present in childhood, and without treatment the prognosis is poor, with approaching a 100% mortality without treatment. Patients respond to treatment with hydroxocobalamin (B12) and betaine, and treatment can be initiated before the results of biochemical and genetic analyses are available.

51.7.2 HUS Due to Mutations in Diacylglycerol Kinase ε

Homozygous or compound heterozygous mutations in the lipid kinase diacylglycerol kinase ε can lead to atypical HUS. Patients usually present in childhood, significant proteinuria is common, there may be histological features of membranoproliferative glomerulonephritis, and the disease may follow a relapsing remitting course. There is no effective treatment, and patients commonly progress to CKD and ESRD at which stage transplant is an option as disease recurrence has not been reported.

51.7.3 HUS Due to Mutations in Other Genes

Genetic variants in thrombomodulin (*THBD*) have been reported in patients with atypical HUS [22]. Thrombomodulin is part of the coagulation pathway and enhances clot formation. It may also activate complement and possibly links these two pathways. New genes associated with atypical HUS are being identified, for example, *INF2* [23], which may provide insights into the pathophysiology of TMA as well as explaining the disease in some patients in whom no complement defect is identified.

51.8 HUS Occurring in the Context of Other Infections

51.8.1 HUS Following Streptococcal Infection

This is a rare form of HUS complicating infection with *Streptococcus pneumonia* (septicaemia, pneumonia with empyema and meningitis) accounting for 5% of childhood HUS [24]. Patients are usually young (<2 years), and the disease is associated with a high mortality (approximately 25%). The enzyme neuraminidase is produced by the bacteria and released into the plasma where it strips neuraminic acid residues from the glycocalyx of many cells including erythrocytes, platelets, and endothelial cells. This exposes the Thomsen-Friedenreich (T-) antigen which is recognised by naturally occurring antibodies that bind to the exposed antigen leading to endothelial and platelet activation and TMA. The presence of the antigen on erythrocytes explains why in this type of HUS, uniquely, the direct antiglobulin test (DAT, Coombes test) is positive. Treatment is supportive with the eradication of *Streptococcus pneumoniae* infection.

51.8.2 HUS Following HIV Infection

HUS was common in patients with HIV infection (2–7% of patients) before the introduction of highly active antiretroviral therapy (now <1%). Although other forms of HUS (e.g., STEC related) can occur in patients infected with HIV there appears to be a specific HIV-related form of HUS associated with high viral load, low CD4 counts, and opportunistic infection. The mechanism by which HIV induces a TMA is not known but is hypothesised that direct virus infection causes endothelial activation inducing a pro-thrombotic state.

51.9 TMAs Occurring in Association with Other Conditions

51.9.1 Pregnancy

There are a number of causes of a TMA either during pregnancy or in the post-partum period including pre-eclampsia, HELLP syndrome, TTP, and aHUS. Differentiating between these can be difficult because of significant clinical overlap.

Pregnancy can also unmask inherited ADAMTS13 deficiency, in which case disease occurs early in pregnancy. Approximately 20% of cases of aHUS occur in association with pregnancy, and these most commonly occur in the post-partum period. A significant proportion of women developing atypical HUS in association with pregnancy have a genetic defect in a complement regulator, suggesting pregnancy is the trigger for disease in women with a genetic predisposition.

51.9.2 Malignancy and its Treatment

HUS- and TTP-like syndromes are associated with disseminated adenocarcinoma (gastric, colonic, breast, and prostate) and haematological malignancies, and the

TMA can pre-date the diagnosis of malignancy. In addition drugs used in the treatment of these cancers can cause a TMA including mitomycin, gemcitabine, platinum-based drugs, tyrosine kinase inhibitors, and VEGF inhibitors (◘ Table 51.1). It can be difficult to determine whether the TMA is due to malignancy or its treatment. There is some evidence of a response to steroids and plasma exchange.

51.9.3 Drug-Induced TMA

The development of a TMA has been reported in association with the use of a range of drugs in addition to those used for the treatment of cancer (◘ Table 51.1). For some drugs this appears to be a direct effect on the endothelium as is the case for Interferon-β [25] and bevacizumab [26], while in the case of quinine, the TMA is due to the development of autoantibodies against platelet glycoproteins. The TMA induced by clopidogrel [27] and ticlopidine [28] leads to the production of antibodies against ADAMTS13 and a TTP-like disease which responds to plasma exchange. In some drugs the exact mechanism of TMA development is unknown, and management is supportive with the withdrawal of the causative drug.

51.9.4 Malignant Hypertension

Severe hypertension causing a TMA and atypical HUS due to an inherited defect in complement regulation can present with identical clinical features. Pre-existing hypertension and other features of hypertensive end-organ damage in this patient group make a secondary TMA more likely. However, if there is no improvement in laboratory parameters with control of blood pressure, treatment with eculizumab should be considered. This strategy avoids missing patients with a defect in complement regulation.

51.9.5 Solid Organ Transplantation

A TMA can occur after any solid organ transplant, most frequently after kidney transplantation. It can be due to a number of factors including calcineurin inhibitor toxicity, ischaemia reperfusion injury, antibody-mediated rejection, and infection. Complement mutations have been reported, in up to 30% from one series [29], possibly due to recurrence of previously undiagnosed atypical HUS. Complement inhibition should be considered particularly if there is uncertainty about the primary diagnosis or the TMA does not resolve with measures such as calcineurin inhibitor withdrawal.

51.9.6 Bone Marrow Transplantation

The development of a TMA has been reported in 10–40% of patients following allogeneic bone marrow transplantation. There are several factors that could contribute to this including graft versus host response, calcineurin inhibitor use, chemotherapy, and infection. Defects in complement regulation have also been reported and complement activation can be demonstrated in some cases. These observations have led to the use of eculizumab in this situation although evidence that this should be part of the management of this condition is still lacking.

51.9.7 Autoimmune Disease

TMA is seen in patients with systemic lupus erythematosus (SLE) and scleroderma renal crisis. In patients with anti-phospholipid antibody syndrome (APS), particularly catastrophic APS, antibodies bind to and activate platelets and endothelial cells leading to a pro-thrombotic state and a TMA. TMAs have also been described in patients with primary glomerular diseases including IgA nephropathy, FSGS, and ANCA-associated vasculitis.

Tips, Tricks, and Pitfalls

1. Consider a thrombotic microangiopathy in any patient presenting with unexplained thrombocytopenia.
2. In the presence of thrombocytopenia, check for haemolysis by requesting a blood film and measuring serum lactate dehydrogenase and haptoglobin. Also check the clotting profile and fibrinogen concentration as this will be abnormal if the patient has disseminated intravascular coagulation.
3. Make sure that you send off blood for ADAMTS13 activity and complement protein levels before you start plasma-based therapies. Once plasma infusion has been given, it is difficult to interpret the results, and diagnosis may be delayed.
4. Always send stool samples for STEC culture and for toxin PCR even if diarrhoea has stopped or the patient did not report diarrhoea at all. Diarrhoea will often stop before HUS develops, and 5–10% of cases STEC HUS have no diarrhoea. This may require discussion with your

microbiologist to arrange culture in the absence of diarrhoea.

5. Plasma exchange should be started as quickly as possible, ideally within 4 hours of presentation with suspected TTP. This may require transfer to a specialist centre where this treatment is available out of hours.
6. Patients with TMA are at relatively low risk of bleeding, and platelet transfusions should be avoided if possible as this may increase the risk of thrombosis and a worsening of disease severity.

Questions

1. Should plasma exchange be delayed until ADAMTS activity is known in patients with suspected TTP?
2. Why should stool be sent for testing in patients with suspected STEC HUS even if diarrhoea has resolved?
3. Does a negative stool culture exclude STEC HUS?
4. Can complement-mediated TMAs be identified by a low circulating C3 level?
5. What infections are more common in patients treated with eculizumab?

Answers

1. No. It is important to take blood for ADAMTS13 activity before starting plasma exchange, but treatment should be started as soon as possible as TTP can progress rapidly.
2. The diarrhoeal illness may have resolved by the time HUS develops, and some patients with STEC HUS report no diarrhoea at all. It is therefore important to send stool for culture and PCR in all cases of TMA. These cases should be discussed with a microbiologist.
3. No. As HUS can develop some time after the initial infection STEC culture can be negative by the time patients present. PCR can improve diagnosis rates, and serology can be informative in some cases.
4. No. C3 levels can be low in aHUS due to excessive activation of complement, but a normal C3 level does not exclude this. Also low C3 levels have been reported in some patients with STEC HUS.
5. The complement membrane attack complex is particularly important in defence against *Neisseria meningitidis* infection; therefore, patients on eculizumab are particularly susceptible to meningococcal infection. Patients on eculizumab should be vaccinated against meningococcus and long-term prophylactic antibiotics considered. Infection with other *Neisseria* species can also occur.

Case Study

Case 1

A 27-year-old man presented with severe abdominal pain. A diagnosis of pancreatitis was made was based on a raised amylase and pancreatic inflammation evident on imaging. No gall stones were identified and the patient did not drink alcohol. On admission he was thrombocytopenic with a platelet count of 62 x 10^9/l, his haemoglobin was low (109 g/l), and he had evidence of fragmentation on his blood film. His coagulation screen was normal. He was managed conservatively and the symptoms and laboratory abnormalities resolved. He presented again 9 months later again with pancreatitis and laboratory findings of thrombocytopenia and microangiopathic haemolytic anaemia.

Screening was performed for a genetic abnormality in complement regulation, and a pathogenic variant in *CD46* was identified making a diagnosis of complement-mediated aHUS most likely. This case demonstrates that TMAs can affect and organ and should be considered in patients presenting with thrombocytopenia and haemolysis. Although disseminated intravascular haemolysis can occur during the severe inflammatory response associated with pancreatitis, the normal clotting screen in this case makes it unlikely.

Case 2

A 58-year-woman presented to her local hospital with a 2-hour history of drowsiness and slurring of her speech. She was initially diagnosed as having had a CVA, but her admission blood demonstrated severe thrombocytopenia (platelets 9 x 10^9/ml) and evidence of haemolysis with anaemia (haemoglobin 97 g/l, LDH unmeasurable due to haemolysis, and fragmentation on the blood film). A diagnosis of TTP was made, and she was transferred to the closest hospital where plasma exchange was available. By the time she arrived, her level of consciousness had fallen, and she required ventilation to protect her airway. Blood for ADAMTS13 activity was taken and plasma exchange (1.5 x plasma volume initiated). She was given pulsed methylprednisolone. On day 3 she remained ventilator dependent. The frequency of plasma exchange was increased to twice daily, and she started a course of rituximab. After 7 days her platelet count started to improve; plasma exchange frequency was reduced to daily and finally stopped on day 18 after admission following normalisation of her platelet count and weaning from the ventilator. She was finally discharged from the hospital for further rehabilitation.

This case demonstrates how rapidly TTP can cause severe neurological disease, which can be fatal without treatment, and highlights the importance of rapid initiation of plasma exchange. It also demonstrates that after the acute phase, patients can be left with residual neurocognitive impairment.

Case 3

A 5-year-old boy developed abdominal pain and bloody diarrhoea 5 days after visiting a petting farm. The diarrhoea resolved, but 9 days after the onset of diarrhoea, he presented with pallor and reduced consciousness. He has a seizure in the emergency room and required ventilation. He was thrombocytopenic (platelets 43 x 10^9/l) and anaemic (haemoglobin 76 g/l) with evidence of haemolysis. He had acute kidney injury with a serum creatinine of 340 µmol/l and oligoanuria. He was started on peritoneal dialysis. STEC culture was negative but Shiga toxin PCR was positive. He remained dialysis dependent for 6 days and required blood transfusion on 2 occasions. Twelve days after admission, he was discharged from the hospital with no neurological deficit and improving renal function. This case is characteristic of STEC infection with a diarrhoeal illness preceding the onset of HUS. It emphasises the importance of STEC testing in all cases and potential for neurological involvement. The good outcome is normal after the acute phase, but these children require long-term monitoring because of the risk of CKD and hypertension.

Conclusion

A thrombotic microangiopathy can develop in a range of diseases and presents with a characteristic pattern of laboratory findings. The main diseases that cause a TMA, TTP and HUS, are rare diseases that can progress rapidly and without treatment are associated with a high morbidity and mortality. Therefore, early recognition that a TMA is present, and appropriate investigation to determine its cause is essential to make the diagnosis and to institute correct treatment, possibly with support from specialist centres.

References

1. Noris M, et al. Relative role of genetic complement abnormalities in sporadic and familial aHUS and their impact on clinical phenotype. Clin J Am Soc Nephrol. 2010;5(10):1844–59.
2. Noris M, Remuzzi G. Thrombotic microangiopathy after kidney transplantation. Am J Transplant. 2010;10(7):1517–23.
3. Frank C, et al. Epidemic profile of Shiga-toxin-producing Escherichia coli O104:H4 outbreak in Germany. N Engl J Med. 2011;365(19):1771–80.
4. Furlan M, et al. Deficient activity of von Willebrand factor-cleaving protease in chronic relapsing thrombotic thrombocytopenic purpura. Blood. 1997;89(9):3097–103.
5. Joly BS, Coppo P, Veyradier A. Thrombotic thrombocytopenic purpura. Blood. 2017;129(21):2836–46.
6. Obrig TG. Escherichia coli Shiga toxin mechanisms of action in renal disease. Toxins (Basel). 2010;2(12):2769–94.
7. Warwicker P, et al. Genetic studies into inherited and sporadic hemolytic uremic syndrome. Kidney Int. 1998;53(4):836–44.
8. Sanchez-Corral P, Melgosa M. Advances in understanding the aetiology of atypical Haemolytic Uraemic syndrome. Br J Haematol. 2010;150(5):529–42.
9. Esparza-Gordillo J, et al. Predisposition to atypical hemolytic uremic syndrome involves the concurrence of different susceptibility alleles in the regulators of complement activation gene cluster in 1q32. Hum Mol Genet. 2005;14(5):703–12.
10. Michael M, et al. Interventions for hemolytic uremic syndrome and thrombotic thrombocytopenic purpura: a systematic review of randomized controlled trials. Am J Kidney Dis. 2009;53(2):259–72.
11. Scully M, et al. Caplacizumab treatment for acquired thrombotic thrombocytopenic purpura. N Engl J Med. 2019;380(4):335–46.
12. Wong CS, et al. The risk of the hemolytic-uremic syndrome after antibiotic treatment of Escherichia coli O157:H7 infections. N Engl J Med. 2000;342(26):1930–6.
13. Menne J, et al. Validation of treatment strategies for enterohaemorrhagic Escherichia coli O104:H4 induced haemolytic uraemic syndrome: case-control study. BMJ. 2012;345:e4565.
14. Kakoullis L, et al. Shiga toxin-induced haemolytic uraemic syndrome and the role of antibiotics: a global overview. J Infect. 2019;
15. Michael M, et al. Interventions for haemolytic uraemic syndrome and thrombotic thrombocytopenic purpura. Cochrane Database Syst Rev. 2009;1:CD003595.
16. Lapeyraque AL, et al. Eculizumab in severe Shiga-toxin-associated HUS. N Engl J Med. 2011;364(26):2561–3.
17. Gruppo RA, Rother RP. Eculizumab for congenital atypical hemolytic-uremic syndrome. N Engl J Med. 2009;360(5):544–6.
18. Nurnberger J, et al. Eculizumab for atypical hemolytic-uremic syndrome. N Engl J Med. 2009;360(5):542–4.
19. Legendre CM, et al. Terminal complement inhibitor eculizumab in atypical hemolytic-uremic syndrome. N Engl J Med. 2013;368(23):2169–81.
20. Ardissino G, et al. Discontinuation of eculizumab maintenance treatment for atypical hemolytic uremic syndrome: a report of 10 cases. Am J Kidney Dis. 2014;64(4):633–7.
21. Fakhouri F, et al. Pathogenic variants in complement genes and risk of atypical hemolytic uremic syndrome relapse after Eculizumab discontinuation. Clin J Am Soc Nephrol. 2017;12(1): 50–9.
22. Delvaeye M, et al. Thrombomodulin mutations in atypical hemolytic-uremic syndrome. N Engl J Med. 2009;361(4):345–57.
23. Challis RC, et al. Thrombotic Microangiopathy in inverted Formin 2-mediated renal disease. J Am Soc Nephrol. 2017;28(4):1084–91.
24. Copelovitch L, Kaplan BS. Streptococcus pneumoniae-associated hemolytic uremic syndrome. Pediatr Nephrol. 2008;23(11):1951–6.
25. Kavanagh D, et al. Type I interferon causes thrombotic microangiopathy by a dose-dependent toxic effect on the microvasculature. Blood. 2016;128(24):2824–33.

26. Eremina V, et al. VEGF inhibition and renal thrombotic microangiopathy. N Engl J Med. 2008;358(11):1129–36.
27. Zakarija A, et al. Clopidogrel-associated TTP: an update of pharmacovigilance efforts conducted by independent researchers, pharmaceutical suppliers, and the Food and Drug Administration. Stroke. 2004;35(2):533–7.
28. Bennett CL, et al. Thrombotic thrombocytopenic purpura associated with ticlopidine. A review of 60 cases. Ann Intern Med. 1998;128(7):541–4.
29. Le Quintrec M, et al. Complement mutation-associated de novo thrombotic microangiopathy following kidney transplantation. Am J Transplant. 2008;8(8):1694–701.

Pregnancy and the Kidney

Hannah Blakey, Ellen Knox, Clara Day, and Graham Lipkin

Contents

M. Harber (ed.), *Primer on Nephrology*, https://doi.org/10.1007/978-3-030-76419-7_52

52

Learning Objectives

1. Chronic kidney disease, even CKD stage 1, is associated with substantially increased risk of adverse pregnancy outcome including pre-eclampsia, preterm delivery, and low birth weight. The risks are greater with an increasing severity of CKD and proteinuria.
2. Pregnancy frequently unmasks hitherto undiagnosed CKD. Persistent proteinuria (PCR >30 mg/mmol) and/or a serum creatinine >75 μmol/l identified before 20 weeks suggests CKD.
3. Contraception and pre-conception counselling are essential. Pregnancy planning should include substituting medications known to be teratogenic – including mycophenolate – for safer alternatives and optimizing underlying disease control.
4. During pregnancy, patients should be reviewed regularly by an obstetrician and nephrologist with experience in managing patients with renal disease in pregnancy ideally in a dedicated joint renal-obstetric clinic. It is important to establish close links with obstetricians and gynaecologists in your hospital but also with other obstetric units within the catchment of the renal unit. Clear referral guidelines and rapid access are important both for the management of patients with CKD or renal replacement therapy but also for the diagnosis and follow-up of patients presenting to obstetricians with renal disease.
5. All women with CKD should be offered low-dose aspirin from 12 weeks of pregnancy (unless otherwise contraindicated) to mitigate the risk of pre-eclampsia. Low molecular weight heparin prophylaxis is indicated for patients with nephrotic range proteinuria.

52.1 Introduction

Chronic kidney disease (CKD) is often clinically silent until renal function declines to less than 25% of normal. CKD stages 1 and 2 (normal or mildly impaired renal function with abnormal albuminuria or structural kidney damage) affect roughly 3% of women of childbearing age, whilst stages 3–5 (GFR <60 ml/min) affect just less than 1% of women in this age group [1]. Enhanced antenatal monitoring in pregnancy and increased complication rates offer an opportunity to identify women with hitherto unrecognised CKD in early pregnancy. Furthermore, around 20% of women who develop severe early-onset (<30 weeks) pre-eclampsia (PET) have underlying CKD as the predisposing cause. Whilst live birth outcomes have improved, pregnancies in women with CKD are at high risk for maternal and foetal morbidity and mortality. Their management is complex, and successful outcomes are optimised by thorough pre-conception counselling and collaborative antenatal care in dedicated renal-obstetric specialist clinics. This chapter explores maternal and foetal outcomes in women with CKD and offers guidance on optimal pregnancy management.

52.1.1 Physiological Changes in Pregnancy

Normal pregnancy results in profound changes in renal and cardiovascular physiology. These changes are mirrored in women with chronic kidney disease (CKD), albeit to a diminishing extent with the greater severity of CKD reflecting reduced renal reserve, and this may underlie frequent adverse pregnancy outcomes. It is important to recognise these changes in order to appropriately interpret the results of laboratory tests during pregnancy; the normal upper limit for serum creatinine falls to <75 μmol/l, normal serum sodium concentration falls by 5 mmol/l, and women develop a compensated respiratory alkalosis manifest by a fall in serum bicarbonate.

52.1.2 Cardiovascular Physiology in Normal Pregnancy [2]

Substantial vasodilatation leading to reduced systemic vascular resistance occurs within 4 weeks of conception reaching a nadir at 40–50% below baseline in the mid second trimester which is maintained until delivery. There is a contemporaneous increase in cardiac output of 40% (due to an increase in stroke volume in early pregnancy and increased heart rate later on). Consequently, in normal pregnancy blood pressure (BP) falls in the first and second trimesters (sometimes allowing withdrawal of antihypertensives), returning to pre-pregnancy levels in the third trimester. There is no physiological change in cardiac ejection fraction or normal range for central venous pressure or pulmonary capillary wedge pressure during the antenatal period. In later pregnancy, inferior vena cava compression by the gravid uterus may lead to 'supine hypotension'.

Plasma and extracellular fluid volume progressively rises from conception reaching 40 to 50% over baseline by 32 weeks. There is a lesser increase in red cell mass of 20 to 30%, driven by enhanced renal erythropoietin production resulting in mild dilutional anaemia. A mild degree of peripheral oedema is common in normal pregnancy.

52.1.3 Renal Haemodynamic and Structural Changes [2, 3]

Glomerular filtration rate (GFR) rises within 1 month of conception, peaks 40–50% above baseline levels by the early second trimester, and is sustained at this level until 1–2 weeks postpartum. The rise in GFR (hyperfiltration) is mediated by elevated renal plasma flow (RPF) in the first two trimesters resulting from both pre- and post-glomerular arteriolar dilatation and not by glomerular hypertension. This may explain why multiple pregnancy in women with normal kidney function or those with CKD 1 and 2 is not associated with renal damage. However, in the third trimester, RPF falls but GFR remains elevated: maintained by a modest increase in glomerular permeability and reduced intraglomerular oncotic pressure.

The mechanism of pregnancy-induced systemic and renal vasodilatation is incompletely understood, but the ovarian vasodilator hormone relaxin appears to mediate the upregulation of NO-dependent vasodilation via the NO-endothelin-B pathway [2].

Neither the MDRD nor the Cockcroft-Gault formulae are accurate in estimating GFR in pregnancy and should not be used. In an individual, GFR can be tracked across pregnancy by serial creatinine measurements.

52.1.4 Anatomical Changes in the Urinary Tract

The kidneys increase in size by 10% in pregnancy; the minimum normal bipolar length is 10 cm. Pregnancy-related hydronephrosis and hydroureter to the level of the pelvic brim are common, particularly on the right side (85%) secondary to reduced ureteric tone and peristalsis (progesterone-mediated) and compression against the pelvic brim by the gravid uterus. The dilated collecting system and ureter may hold 200–300 ml of urine resulting in urinary stasis; a potential reservoir for bacteria which may contribute to the increased risk of pyelonephritis in pregnancy. Differentiation of physiological hydronephrosis from true ureteric obstruction is difficult in pregnancy (see later). In early pregnancy, bladder wall relaxation induced by progesterone may lead to increased capacity although later in pregnancy the enlarging uterus may limit bladder volume. Urinary frequency, urgency, and nocturia are common in normal pregnancy and may be associated with urge incontinence.

52.2 Tubular Changes

52.2.1 Electrolyte Balance

Total body sodium increases by 3–4 mmol/day resulting in a net positive balance of 900–1000 mmol over the whole gestation (total body potassium increases by 320 mmol). Exquisite tubular control of sodium balance is achieved in pregnancy, despite the net increase of sodium filtration resulting from a 50% gestational rise in GFR. A fine balance of natriuretic factors (raised GFR, atrial natriuretic peptide, and progesterone) versus anti-natriuretic factors (aldosterone, deoxycorticosterone, and tubuloglomerular feedback) is felt to achieve this critical homeostatic task.

As a consequence of resetting of the hypothalamic osmostat, plasma osmolality falls by 10 (standard deviation 3) mOsmol/kg in normal pregnancy reflecting a fall in plasma sodium by 5 (2) mmol/l. This change occurs early in pregnancy and correlates closely with increased production of human chorionic gonadotrophin. Enhanced urate excretion in the first two trimesters of pregnancy leads to a fall in serum urate. In the third trimester, serum urate is restored to pre-pregnancy levels. This must be considered if urate levels are being considered as part of the assessment of pre-eclampsia (PET).

52.2.2 Acid-Base Balance

Progesterone stimulates the central respiratory centres leading to a chronic respiratory alkalosis in pregnancy. The kidney compensates leading to a fall in plasma bicarbonate level.

Pregnancy is associated with profound renal anatomical, haemodynamic, tubular, and cardiovascular changes. These have significant implications for the outcome of pregnancy in women with CKD.

52.3 Common Themes in the Care of Pregnant Women with Chronic Kidney Disease

52.3.1 Pre-Conception Counselling

Pregnancy decisions for women with CKD can be complicated by their pre-conceptions and those of other clinicians about risks to their health and that of their baby [4]. Major advances in obstetric monitoring and neonatal intensive care have dramatically improved maternal and foetal outcomes over the last 40 years, and the focus of advice for women with CKD is now shifting. Pre-pregnancy counselling should be offered to all women with CKD to allow shared and informed decision-making and an individualised management plan centred around their underlying disease aetiology, baseline renal function, obstetric history, and other comorbidities. It is optimally provided in a dedicated combined clinic led by an obstetrician and nephrologist who have experience of looking after women with renal disease in pregnancy. In this setting, the nephrologist and obstetrician learn to speak the same language and recognise each other's anxieties in the care of these patients. Moreover, the vast majority of women attending these clinics find them beneficial in their pregnancy decision-making process [4].

Counselling should cover:

1. Contraceptive advice
2. How pregnancy might affect maternal kidney function
3. How kidney disease might affect pregnancy outcomes
4. Optimal timing of pregnancy to improve maternal/foetal outcomes:

   In general, women with slowly progressive renal disease may be best advised to plan pregnancy earlier (rather than waiting a potentially long time before transplant is deemed necessary), and women with relapsing and remitting disease such as lupus have more favourable outcomes if pregnancy is delayed until a period of disease quiescence. Those with rapidly progressing renal disease or on dialysis may have better pregnancy outcomes if they wait to conceive until after a potential renal transplant (if likely to occur within the timeframe of being of childbearing age).
5. Modification of drug therapy to those known to be safe in pregnancy
6. Assessment of comorbidity, e.g. diabetes, cardiopulmonary disease, renal/bladder structure
7. General preparation for pregnancy:
   - Folic acid (400ug daily or 5 mg OD in those with diabetes mellitus, a previous child with a neural tube defect, or a BMI >30 g/m^2) at least 3 months prior to conception until 12 weeks of pregnancy.
   - Smoking cessation.
   - Weight loss (targeting an ideal BMI).

52.4 Hypertension in Pregnancy

The definitions of hypertension and classification of severity are listed in Table 52.1. BP measurement should be taken in a sitting position using a validated oscillometric device or manual reading to Korotkov 5. Hypertensive disorders in pregnancy affect 10% of women and are a major cause of maternal morbidity and a leading cause of maternal death worldwide. In a large meta-analysis of over 795,000 pregnancies, chronic hypertension was found to be strongly associated with adverse pregnancy outcomes including pre-eclampsia (incidence 25.9%; 95% C.I. 21.0–31.5%), Caesarean section (41.4%; 35.5–47.7%), preterm delivery (28.1%; 22.6–34.4%), and perinatal death (4.0%; 2.9–5.4%) [5]. Specific management of chronic essential or gestational hypertension is beyond the scope of this chapter, but guidelines are available from the UK National Institute for Health and Clinical Excellence [6].

Table 52.1 Definitions of hypertension and its severity in pregnancy [6]

Definition	Presentation	Significant Proteinuria[a]	Prevalence (%)
Chronic hypertension	<20 weeks	No	2
Gestational hypertension	>20 weeks	No	4–8
Pre-eclampsia (PET)	>20 weeks	Yes	4.1**/1.7***
PET superimposed on chronic hypertension	>20 weeks	Yes	<1
Hypertension severity		Systolic BP (mmHg)	Diastolic BP (mmHg)
Mild		140–149	90–99
Moderate		150–159	100–109
Severe		>160	>110

**First pregnancy, ***second pregnancy

[a]Significant proteinuria is >300 mg in a validated 24 h urine collection or urine PCR >30 mg/mmol

52.5 Blood Pressure Targets

There have been historic concerns that overzealous BP lowering during pregnancy for women with chronic essential or gestational hypertension may adversely affect foetal growth by reducing placental blood flow. However, a more recent meta-analysis of 49 RCTs showed that anti-hypertensive treatment for pregnant women with mild to moderate hypertension did not result in harm to the foetus [7]. These findings have been corroborated by the 2015 Chronic Hypertension in Pregnancy Study (CHIPS) [8], which assigned 987 pregnant women with chronic

Table 52.2 Impact of 'tight' vs 'less tight' BP control on pregnancy outcomes. Data from [8]

Outcome	'Less tight' control diastolic BP <100 $n = 493$	'Tight' control diastolic BP <85 $n = 488$	Odds ratio
Pregnancy loss or high-level neonatal care >48 hours	31.4%	30.7%	1.02 (0.77–1.35)
Birth weight < tenth percentile	16.1%	19.7%	0.78 (0.56–1.08)
Serious maternal outcomes (TIA, stroke, pulmonary oedema, renal failure, blood transfusion)	3.7%	2.0%	1.74 (0.79–3.84)
Severe hypertension (>160/110 mmHg)	40.6%	27.5%	**1.80 (1.34–2.38) *P* < 0.001**

or gestational hypertension to either 'tight BP control' (diastolic BP <85) or 'less tight control' (diastolic BP <100). Tight BP control was not associated with adverse maternal or foetal outcomes when compared with less tight control, although the mean BP difference between groups was small (<5 mmHg). Tight BP control did however reduce the risk of developing severe hypertension [8] (see Table 52.2). Post hoc analysis found that those women who went on to develop severe hypertension had significantly higher rates of foetal growth restriction, pre-eclampsia, and preterm delivery [9].

Prevention of severe hypertension in pregnancy therefore appears important in optimising maternal and foetal outcomes. In practice, initiating treatment in uncomplicated chronic mild hypertension to achieve a target BP of <140/90 is now recommended to reduce the risk of developing severe hypertension and its associated adverse pregnancy outcomes [10]. For those with target organ damage, including renal disease and/or proteinuria, a lower target of <130/80 is recommended.

52.6 Antihypertensive Drugs

All antihypertensive drugs cross the placenta and their half-life in pregnancy is reduced. Women with hypertension should receive pre-conception counselling and ideally be established pre-pregnancy on labetalol or nifedipine LA or converted as soon as pregnancy is confirmed.

Table 52.3 Antihypertensive agent use in pregnancy

Drug	Dose	Comments
Labetalol	100–400 mg orally twice to 4 times daily (max dose 1200 mg/day)	First line unless contraindications, e.g. asthma. Reduced half-life in pregnancy
Methyldopa	250–500 mg orally 2 to 4 times daily (max dose 2 g/day)	Slower onset of action. Tends to require higher doses to achieve target BP: Maternal side effects may limit dose
Nifedipine (LA)	Long-acting preparation preferred 30–120 mg/day	May aggravate pedal oedema
Angiotensin-converting enzyme inhibitors (ACEi) or angiotensin receptor blockers (ARB)		Teratogenic in second and third trimester No increased risk of teratogenicity if stopped in first trimester
Atenolol		Preferential use of labetalol May be associated with foetal growth restriction
Diuretics		Avoid in pregnancy May limit physiological increase in plasma volume

Comments on antihypertensive therapy in pregnancy are listed in Table 52.3. A large meta-analysis comparing different antihypertensive agents in pregnancy identified beta blockers, predominantly labetalol, to be better tolerated and more effective than methyldopa in controlling BP. Furthermore, a combination of beta blocker and calcium channel blocker was reported to be more effective in reducing the risk of severe hypertension and developing proteinuria and/or pre-eclampsia than methyldopa alone. There was insufficient evidence to detect any other significant differences in pregnancy outcomes between agents [7].

52.7 Angiotensin-Converting Enzyme Inhibitors

Outside of pregnancy, angiotensin-converting enzyme inhibitors (ACEi) or angiotensin receptor blockers (ARB) are used as first-line treatment for proteinuric

CKD. However, the continuation of ACEi or ARB in the second and third trimester is associated with a specific fetopathy comprising oligohydramnios, neonatal renal failure, neural tube defects, and cardiac abnormalities and should be avoided [11]. One American study involving almost half a million pregnancies revealed an increased risk of congenital malformations in hypertensive women exposed to ACEi in the first trimester. However, the magnitude was the same as those receiving other antihypertensives or no BP treatment at all. It therefore appears that hypertension per se in the first trimester is associated with an increased risk of birth defects with no additional adverse impact of ACEi *in the first trimester* [11].

As a rule, women with hypertension receiving ACEi who are considering pregnancy should be stabilised on antihypertensives known to be safe in pregnancy before conception. Some women may take some considerable time to conceive and those denied ACEi pre-pregnancy may consequently suffer an unnecessary renal decline, particularly those with proteinuric CKD. Women who have a strong indication for the use of ACEi, such as those with CKD and proteinuria, may be carefully counselled to continue on the ACEi until conception, at which point they should be converted to labetalol, long-acting nifedipine, or methyldopa.

52.8 Pre-Eclampsia

Pre-eclampsia (PET) is defined as de novo development of hypertension (BP >140/90) and either proteinuria (>300 mg/24 hrs) or evidence of thrombocytopenia, renal insufficiency, impaired liver function, pulmonary oedema, or cerebral symptoms (including visual disturbance) after 20 weeks' gestation [12].

In practice albeit rarely, PET can occur without proteinuria or with proteinuria preceding hypertension. PET is a common and potentially devastating multisystem capillary leak disorder, affecting around 5% of all pregnancies globally. Its features include the development of severe hypertension, cerebral oedema and fits (eclampsia), placental abruption and foetal growth restriction, the syndrome of abnormal liver function, low platelets and microangiopathy (HELLP), pulmonary oedema, and if neglected, maternal and foetal death. **It is important to remember that whilst BP may be controlled in severe PET, the only definitive treatment is delivery of the baby, without which the maternal condition will deteriorate.**

The pathophysiology of PET remains poorly understood, although abnormal maternal and foetal immune responses to pregnancy are likely to contribute. It is widely accepted that the placenta plays a central role in disease initiation, with placental mal-perfusion and ischaemia arising from abnormal placentation within the uterine wall. This may promote abnormal placental secretion of angiogenic factors leading to altered vascular endothelial growth factor (VEGF) signalling. In PET, there is increased expression of anti-angiogenic soluble fms-like tyrosine kinase-1 (sFlt-1) and reduced serum placental growth factor (PlGF) which act via functional VEGF deficiency to cause endothelial dysfunction (hypertension) and podocyte injury (proteinuria). A high ratio of sFlt-1 to PIGF has been associated with an increased risk of PET [13], and abnormal levels may precede the clinical onset of PET by several weeks. A recent study found a low sFlt-1/PIGF ratio was associated with a low risk of development of PET in the short term in cases where PET was clinically suspected [14]. NICE have since issued clinical guidance recommending the use of sFlt-1/PIGF assay in tandem with clinical review to help rule out PET in women suspected to have PET between 20 and 34 weeks +6 days gestation (NICE DG23): ▶ https://www.nice.org.uk/guidance/dg23/chapter/1-Recommendations. It should be noted that this assay is not currently widely available, and cannot be used for confirming or ruling in a diagnosis of PET. PlGF has also been reported as a promising biomarker for predicting the development of PET in those with CKD [15]. PlGF did not correlate with serum creatinine in study participants; however, the sample size and number of women with severe CKD were limited, so further study is required to assess the predictive value in women with CKD and whether the underlying renal impairment is a confounding factor and affects the interpretation of results.

52.9 Pre-Eclampsia in Patients with CKD

The incidence of PET in women with CKD is substantially increased, ranging from 20 to 60% depending on the severity of maternal renal dysfunction, baseline proteinuria, or pre-existing hypertension [4]. These patients often have a more severe clinical course with PET occurring earlier in pregnancy. Women with CKD are frequently hypertensive and have proteinuria; both of which commonly worsen in pregnancy as a consequence of pregnancy physiology. A key element of care of these women is to differentiate the onset of superimposed PET from the natural response of the damaged kidney to pregnancy physiology. Discriminatory factors are listed in Table 52.4. Sonographic assessment of uterine and umbilical artery blood flow at 20–24 weeks has predictive value for PET in women with CKD in pregnancy similar to that seen in the general population [16]. In practice the most important discriminatory test is time: PET often progresses over hours/days whereas pregnancy aggravated change in CKD occurs over weeks.

Table 52.4 Differentiation of pre-eclampsia from the effects of pregnancy in women with chronic kidney disease

	Pregnancy impact on CKD	Superimposed PET
Onset	<20 weeks	>20 weeks
Rate of change in BP/proteinuria	Weeks	Hours to days
Uterine artery Doppler velocimetry at 24 weeks	Normal	Abnormal 'notching' sometimes
Elevated transaminase and/or low platelets	No	Sometimes
Serum urate	High	High
sFlt/PlGF ratio[a]	Normal More evidence needed to assess impact of degree of renal impairment / CKD stage on sFlt-1 and PlGF levels	High
Treatment	Support/monitoring	Delivery (if severe)

[a]not currently used in routine clinical practice

52.10 Prevention of Pre-eclampsia in Women with CKD and/or Hypertension

52.10.1 Low-Dose Aspirin

An imbalance of vasodilator and vasoconstrictor prostaglandins contributes to abnormal placentation which led to trials of low-dose aspirin as prophylaxis for PET. Meta-analysis and systematic review of women at medium and high risk of PET treated with low-dose aspirin have shown significant maternal and foetal benefit with no evidence of increased risk of bleeding complications [17] see Fig. 52.1.

Current UK guidelines therefore recommend the use of low-dose aspirin (typically 75 mg daily) for all women considered to be at high risk of PET from 12 weeks gestation until delivery [18]. A recent large RCT however found that using a daily dose of 150 mg aspirin from 11–14 weeks until 36 weeks gestation for women considered to be at high risk of PET resulted in a significantly reduced incidence of early-onset pre-eclampsia when compared with a placebo [19]. This did not however specifically examine women with CKD, and current advice still recommends a 75 mg daily dose of aspirin.

No other interventions so far tested have shown a beneficial impact on the prevention of PET including anti-oxidants, folic acid, oral magnesium, fish oils, or calcium (in women with normal calcium intake).

52.10.2 Proteinuria

Significant proteinuria in pregnancy is >300 mg/24 hour or >30 mg protein/mmol creatinine in a 'spot urine' sample protein/creatinine ratio (PCR). Women should be screened for proteinuria at each antenatal visit using urine reagent tests assessed by an automated reagent reader

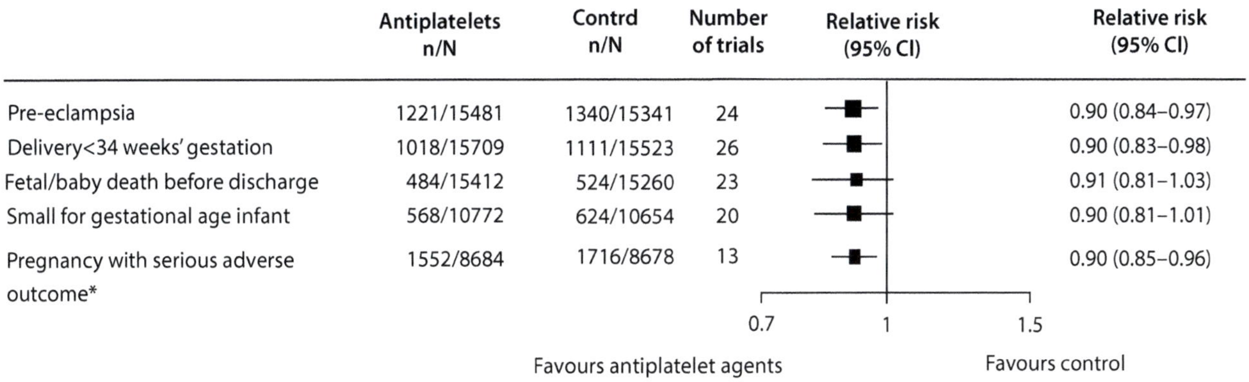

	Antiplatelets n/N	Contrd n/N	Number of trials	Relative risk (95% CI)
Pre-eclampsia	1221/15481	1340/15341	24	0.90 (0.84–0.97)
Delivery<34 weeks' gestation	1018/15709	1111/15523	26	0.90 (0.83–0.98)
Fetal/baby death before discharge	484/15412	524/15260	23	0.91 (0.81–1.03)
Small for gestational age infant	568/10772	624/10654	20	0.90 (0.81–1.01)
Pregnancy with serious adverse outcome*	1552/8684	1716/8678	13	0.90 (0.85–0.96)

Fig. 52.1 Relative risk of pregnancy outcomes for women treated with low-dose aspirin for primary prevention of pre-eclampsia. (Reproduced with permission from [17])

52

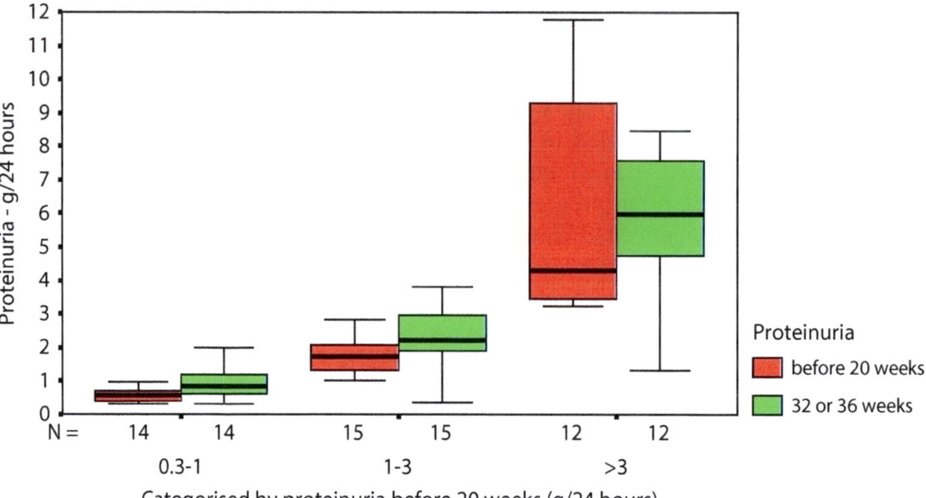

Fig. 52.2 Progression of proteinuria in women with CKD during pregnancy in absence of PET (From UK CORD Registry)

device which has far greater precision than manual readout. Moderate proteinuria detected early in pregnancy frequently progresses to heavy proteinuria, sometimes into the nephrotic range in the third trimester (see Fig. 52.2).

Pregnancy is a thrombophilic state, and heavy proteinuria substantially increases thromboembolic risk. In this setting, daily subcutaneous low molecular weight heparin (LMWH) (prophylactic dose) continued until 6 weeks postpartum is recommended. The threshold level of proteinuria to initiate treatment is unclear, though many authorities treat when proteinuria >2 g/24 h (PCR >200). Monitoring anti-factor Xa activity may improve safety in CKD (samples taken 3 hours after dose).

A high index of suspicion for a venous thromboembolic disease should be maintained in these women during pregnancy. The risks of foetal radiation exposure from V/Q or CTPA scanning are small when balanced against the risk of undiagnosed pulmonary embolism or blind treatment. Women treated with low-dose aspirin and LMWH are at high risk of symptomatic oesophageal reflux or peptic ulceration and should receive oral ranitidine which appears safe from the second trimester. Those women receiving long-term LMWH and/or steroids should receive calcium/vitamin D3 supplements as prophylaxis from bone mineral loss.

52.10.3 Urinary Tract Infection

Pregnant women are at increased risk of UTI. Mechanical compression from the gravid uterus can impede ureteric outflow, and progesterone-mediated smooth muscle relaxation leads to reduced ureteral peristalsis, ureteric dilatation, and urinary stasis. Asymptomatic bacteriuria is common (incidence 2–10% in normal pregnancy). If left untreated, up to one-third will go on to develop cystitis or pyelonephritis, which has been strongly associated with preterm delivery and poor perinatal outcomes [20]. Some women with CKD have urinary tract abnormalities (such as renal stone disease, reflux nephropathy, bladder dysfunction, and autosomal dominant polycystic kidney disease) which substantially increase their risk. Meta-analysis demonstrates that antibiotic treatment is highly effective in eradicating asymptomatic infection and preventing pyelonephritis, and treatment is associated with higher birth weight [21].

Urine should be sent for culture at each antenatal visit, and those with evidence of asymptomatic bacteriuria are treated empirically with antibiotics to reduce their risk of ascending infection and adverse pregnancy outcome. Strict prophylaxis from infection is vital in those with a history of recurrent UTI or abnormal urinary tract anatomy. The mainstay is the bladder toilet comprising at least 3 litre daily oral fluid intake, double micturition, and post-coital voiding. Those women with predisposing factors or who suffer more than one antenatal infection or persistent asymptomatic bacteriuria after two or more antibiotic courses should also receive nocturnal prophylactic antibiotics until 6 weeks postpartum. Cefalexin 250 mg nocte is effective and safe in all trimesters or, if allergic to beta lactam antibiotics, nitrofurantoin 50 mg nocte (the latter should be suspended around 36 weeks due to risk of haemolytic anaemia in some babies). Where possible, quinolones or gentamicin (risk of neonatal deafness) should be avoided if safer alternatives exist, based on antibiotic sensitivities. Co-amoxiclav use late in pregnancy may increase the risk of necrotising enterocolitis in preterm babies.

52.10.4 Renal Tract Obstruction Versus Physiological Hydronephrosis

Differentiating physiological hydronephrosis in pregnancy from ureteric obstruction can be challenging. In general, physiological hydronephrosis is asymptomatic, whereas acute obstruction is often associated with loin pain and tenderness. Pregnancy-related hydronephrosis tends to be right-sided and occurs from the second trimester onwards, whereas pathological hydronephrosis can affect either side and in any stage of pregnancy. Ureteric calculi are the commonest cause of urinary tract obstruction in pregnancy, associated with non-visible haematuria and renal colic, whilst urine in healthy women rarely contains red cells. A significant increase in plasma creatinine is suggestive of unilateral obstruction.

Imaging techniques may be helpful in differentiating. Ultrasonography is the first-line imaging modality for suspected obstructive uropathy in pregnancy, although up to 40% of nephrolithiasis cases may be missed if this is used alone. Measuring renal artery resistive index (RI) derived by Doppler ultrasound can be a useful adjunct; an RI >0.7 in the setting of unilateral hydronephrosis is suggestive of obstruction if contralateral RI is <0.7. Magnetic resonance urography (MRU) can be helpful (see ► Case 52.43.1 and ◘ Fig. 52.3a and b). Recent evidence shows this to be safe in pregnancy, even in the first trimester, although gadolinium contrast has been associated with birth defects and increased risk of stillbirth and should not be used at all [22]. Although MRU does not adequately image calculi, a ureteric filling defect or a level of ureteric 'cut-off' above the pelvic brim is suggestive of a stone. Faced with a critically ill pregnant woman with tender hydronephrosis, not settling with antibiotics, prompt relief of obstruction either by percutaneous nephrostomy (with antibiotic cover) or retrograde stent insertion (in the mid trimester of pregnancy) is required and can be lifesaving for the foetus and the mother.

52.11 Anaemia in Pregnancy

Women with CKD frequently fail to drive an adequate increase in red cell mass during pregnancy and may become increasingly anaemic. If required, IV iron replacement appears safe: the greatest experience is with IV iron sucrose ('Venofer'). Erythropoietin (EPO) alpha, beta, and gamma does not cross the placenta and is effective (usually requiring 50–100% dose increase) in women with CKD in pregnancy, targeting Hb 100–110 g/L. It remains unclear as to whether EPO increases the risk of or exacerbates hypertension in pregnancy, and BP requires close monitoring.

52.12 Chronic Kidney Disease in Pregnancy

Three percent of women of childbearing age have stage 1 or 2 CKD, whilst moderate to severe CKD (stages 3–5) affects around 1 in 150 women of childbearing age.

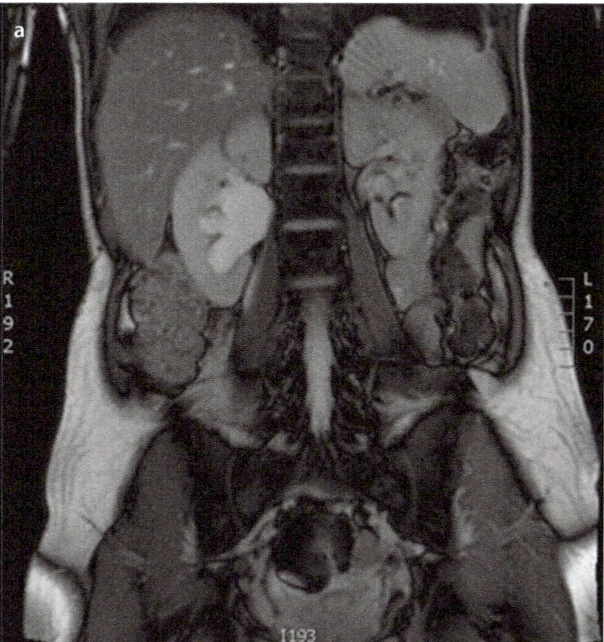

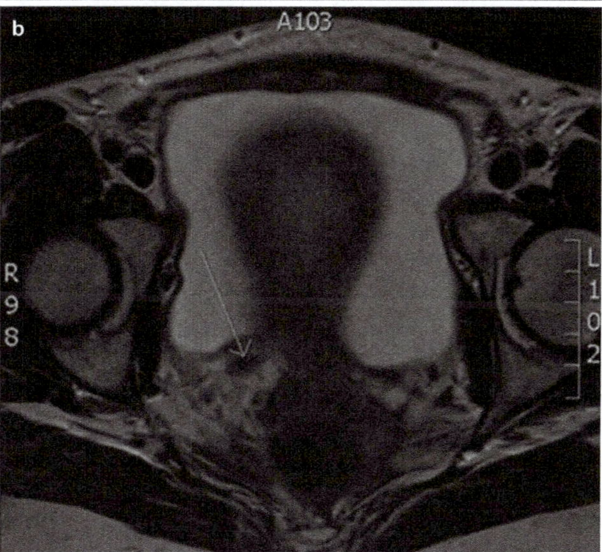

◘ **Fig. 52.3** **a** and **b**: A case of obstructive uropathy in pregnancy

Pregnancy places substantial physiological demands on the kidney which may explain why women at any stage of CKD experience a high risk of adverse maternal (sixfold) and foetal (twofold) outcomes [23]. The risk of maternal and foetal complications increases with poorer baseline renal function. The gestational rise in GFR is blunted in women with moderate CKD and often absent in those with creatinine >200 μmol/l [3]. Despite the high complication rate, most pregnancies that progress beyond the first trimester will result in a live birth. The key to optimising outcome is preparation with systematic pre-conception counselling and regular expert antenatal review ideally in combined renal-obstetric antenatal clinics.

52

52.12.1 Identification of Women with CKD in Pregnancy

Routine monitoring of urinalysis and BP in pregnancy frequently identifies previously unrecognised CKD (see ► Case 52.43.2). Persistent proteinuria (PCR >30 mg/mmol) and/or a serum creatinine >75 μmol/l identified before 20 weeks gestation is suggestive of CKD. Investigation by repeat serum creatinine, full blood count, tests of soluble immunology (antinuclear antibody, complements 3 and 4, antineutrophil cytoplasmic antibody), and baseline renal ultrasound is indicated. These findings put the pregnancy at high risk for complications and thus the need for enhanced antenatal monitoring and postpartum follow-up. Neither the MDRD nor Cockcroft-Gault equations accurately predict eGFR. Serial creatinine measurements should be used instead to avoid the risks of underestimating the degree of renal impairment.

52.13 Role of Renal Biopsy in Pregnancy

In pregnancy, proteinuria presenting for the first time after 20 weeks gestation is generally due to PET. Renal biopsy risks complications including foetal compromise. A meta-analysis of renal biopsies performed in pregnancy suggested an increased risk of complications compared with non-pregnant patients [24]. However, this analysis included historic series where biopsy was performed for the diagnosis of PET. Renal biopsy is technically difficult and uncomfortable for the patient after 20–24 weeks gestation. In highly selected cases of undiagnosed progressive kidney disease (before foetal viability, <26 weeks), early onset of nephrotic syndrome (<20 weeks), or unexplained AKI (<26 weeks), renal biopsy has a similar complication risk to the non-pregnant state. Histological diagnosis beneficially affects care in over one-third of cases, being safer than blind therapy [25]. Pregnant women with stable CKD and proteinuria or those presenting after 26 weeks should be observed carefully. In this situation renal biopsy should be deferred until stable postpartum [25].

52.14 Effect of Pregnancy on Maternal Kidney Function

Mild Renal Impairment (CKD Stages 1–2).

Pregnancy in women with stages 1 and 2 CKD pre-pregnancy or first trimester creatinine <110 μmol/l with low-level proteinuria (<1 g/24 hours) and absent/well-controlled hypertension appears to have little or no long-term adverse effect on renal function. A 2015 meta-analysis reported no significant difference in long-term adverse renal outcomes between pregnant women with mild CKD and non-pregnant controls with CKD (OR 0.96; 95 CI 0.69 to 1.35) [26]. Adverse renal outcomes were broadly defined however as doubling of creatinine, >50% decline in GFR, or reaching ESRD.

Moderate to Severe Renal Impairment (CKD Stages 3–5).

More advanced CKD pre-pregnancy and heavy proteinuria (>1 g/24 h) appear to be strong predictors of an irreversible decline in renal function associated with pregnancy.

In a landmark retrospective study, women who started pregnancy with moderate CKD (creatinine 124–168 μmol/L) had a 40% risk of deteriorating renal function during pregnancy, which persisted postpartum in half [27]. Two-thirds of those with severe CKD (antenatal creatinine >177 μmol/l) suffered a decline in renal function in the third trimester which persisted postpartum. A third deteriorated to the point of requiring dialysis. A subsequent prospective study confirmed adverse pregnancy outcomes of 49 women with moderate/severe pre-pregnancy CKD (mean creatinine 186 μmol/L and GFR 35+/−12 ml/min). Mean GFR fell from 35 before to 30 ml/min after pregnancy ($p < 0.001$). However, the rate of decline of GFR before and after pregnancy remained the same for this group. Those women with a pre-pregnancy GFR <40 ml/min and heavier proteinuria (>1 g/24 h) had an increased risk of accelerated deterioration in GFR post-pregnancy and progressed more rapidly to dialysis [28].

A more recent Italian cohort study reported similar outcomes [29], although the numbers of women studied with advanced renal impairment remain small and lack comparison with non-pregnant control groups. It is therefore unclear whether the decline seen in renal function is due to pregnancy alone or following the natural underlying disease course.

52.15 Effect of Maternal CKD on Pregnancy Outcomes

CKD has been widely reported as an independent risk factor for adverse maternal and foetal outcomes in pregnancy in recent meta-analyses [26] and cohort studies [29]. Zhang et al. reported significantly increased risks of pre-eclampsia (OR 10.36, 95% CI 6.28 to 17.09) and Caesarean section (OR 2.67, CI 2.01 to 3.54) in pregnancy with CKD, compared to pregnancies in women without CKD. Moreover, there were significantly increased odds of adverse foetal events for pregnancies in CKD, including preterm delivery (OR 5.72, 95% CI 3.26 to 10.03), small for gestational age/low birth

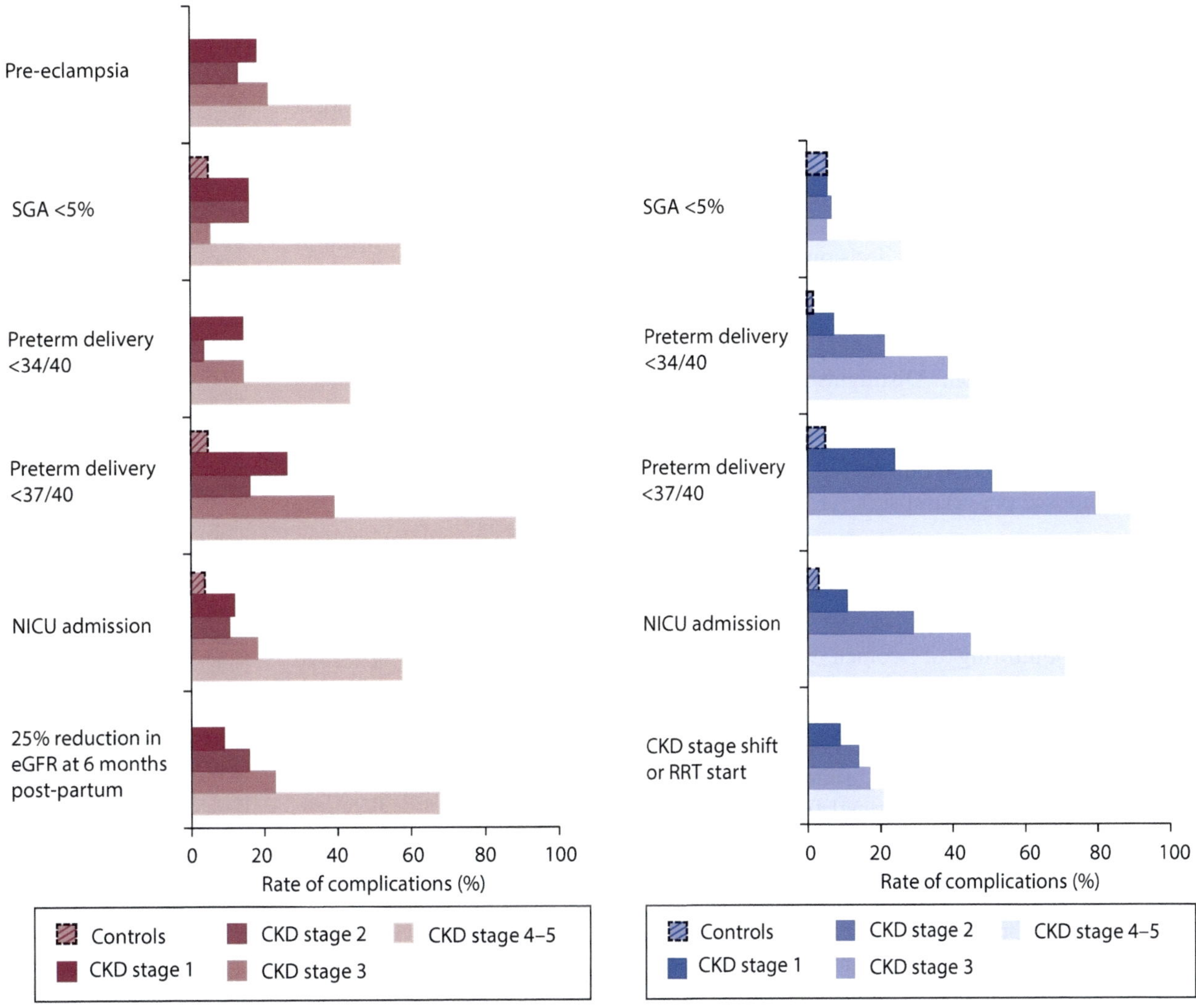

Fig. 52.4 Effect of maternal CKD on pregnancy outcome. Reproduced with permission from [4]. (Data taken from two cohort studies: [15, 29])

weight babies (OR 4.85, 95%CI 3.03 to 7.76), and failure of pregnancy (stillbirth, foetal death, and neonatal death) (OR 1.80, 95%CI 1.03 to 3.13) [26]. Absolute outcomes vary between studies, given differing cohort sizes, the heterogenous nature of renal disease, and local factors such as variance in thresholds for early delivery and referral to neonatal intensive care. Despite this, all adverse maternal and foetal outcomes become increasingly prevalent as renal function worsens – see Fig. 52.4.

In pregnant women with CKD, proteinuria (>1 g/24 hours) and hypertension are associated with adverse pregnancy outcomes, independently of renal disease severity. Proteinuria >1 g/24 h increases the need for neonatal intensive care (RR of 4.2), and hypertension is associated with an increased risk of preterm delivery (RR 7.2) and Caesarean section (RR 5.7) [30]. Interestingly, however, one study reported that CKD stage 1 is associated with adverse pregnancy outcome, even when hypertension, proteinuria, and systemic disease are absent (OR 1.88, 95%CI 1.27–2.79). This raises the suggestion that renal disease itself presents a "baseline risk" in pregnancy, regardless of CKD severity [29].

52.16 How Should CKD be Managed in Pregnancy?

All women with CKD or those identified with CKD in pregnancy should be referred promptly to an established renal-obstetric clinic to plan antenatal care. Assessment of renal function, degree of proteinuria (ACR or PCR), haemoglobin, urine dip and culture, BP measurement (24 h ambulatory BP can be helpful), and baseline renal ultrasound should be performed. All women with CKD should be offered daily low-dose aspirin, given their increased risk of pre-eclampsia and adverse foetal outcomes. NICE recommend aspirin is started at 12 weeks as pre-eclampsia prophylaxis although many experienced centres start earlier [6].

Monthly follow-up before 20 weeks gestation and fortnightly follow-up after 20 weeks (more frequent if deteriorating) is recommended. Weekly urinalysis and BP measurement in primary care after 20 weeks may identify early PET. Difficult decisions often need to be made about the timing of delivery, balancing the foetal risks of premature delivery against maternal health. This requires experienced obstetric, nephrological, and neonatal collaboration. Distinguishing the expected increase in urine protein excretion and BP in the late second/third trimester of pregnancy from pre-eclampsia is key (see ◘ Table 52.4: differential diagnosis of CKD vs superimposed pre-eclampsia).

52.17 Postpartum Care

Enhanced monitoring of women with CKD should continue postpartum, particularly in those with deteriorating renal function or nephrotic range proteinuria in pregnancy. All women with CKD should be seen in a combined renal-obstetric clinic around 4–8 weeks postpartum to assess changes in renal function, plan contraception, and arrange long-term renal follow–up. It can take 3 months for the physiological changes of pregnancy to disappear. Moreover, proteinuria, especially after severe PET, may take 6 months to return to baseline. The increased GFR of pregnancy returns to baseline 1–2 weeks postpartum leading to an expected rise in creatinine. It is vital that women with newly identified CKD in pregnancy are referred for postnatal nephrological investigation and follow-up. Breastfeeding in general should be encouraged if the baby is thriving and drugs changed to those known to have minimal breast milk excretion.

52.18 Management of Specific Kidney Diseases during Pregnancy

See ◘ Table 52.5

◘ **Table 52.5** Important points relating to specific kidney diseases during pregnancy

Condition	Possible complication needing monitoring	Key management points
Primary glomerulonephritis (including lupus nephritis)	Hypertension Proteinuria Disease flare/relapse	Treat BP (target <130/80 if evidence of renal impairment and/or proteinuria) and monitor If PCR >200, consider LMW heparin prophylaxis Significantly increased risk of PET if pre-existing hypertension and/or proteinuria Monitor renal function and proteinuria Differentiate from PET: See ◘ Table 52.4
Autosomal dominant polycystic kidney disease	Hypertension Recurrent UTI/cyst infection	Treat BP and monitor Bladder toilet advice and prophylactic antibiotics if evidence of >1 UTI in pregnancy Discuss 50% risk of inheritance
Reflux nephropathy	Recurrent UTI Hypertension	Bladder toilet, prophylactic antibiotics if evidence of >1 UTI in pregnancy Treat BP and monitor Screen baby for reflux
Renal calculi	Renal colic, UTI	High fluid intake, prophylactic antibiotics. MR urography may be helpful to exclude obstruction after the first trimester
Diabetic nephropathy	Risk of progressive CKD Hypertension Proteinuria	Assess comorbidity, maintain tight glycaemic control pre-pregnancy, antenatal, and postpartum Treat BP and monitor If PCR >200, consider LMW heparin prophylaxis Significantly increased risk of PET if pre-existing hypertension and/or proteinuria

52.18.1 Pregnancy in Women with Systemic Lupus Erythematosus

Lupus is predominantly a disease affecting women of childbearing age. Its management in pregnancy therefore requires special consideration. There remains a significant risk of foetal and maternal morbidity and mortality in patients with lupus; more so in those with lupus nephritis (even for those women with preserved renal function). Patients with active lupus (of any manifestation), active lupus nephritis, and/or hypertension have particularly high risk of adverse outcome. ◘ Table 52.6 presents results from a recent meta-analysis. Ideally, pregnancies should be planned in periods of quiescent

Table 52.6 Lupus and risk of adverse pregnancy outcome. (Data from [53])

Lupus factor	Pregnancy outcome	Odds ratio
Active or flaring lupus	Pre-eclampsia	12.7
	Emergency caesarean	19.0
	Early foetal loss	3.0
	Preterm delivery	5.5
Active lupus nephritis	Any adverse maternal outcome	5.3
Hypertension	Pre-eclampsia	4.8–7.3
Use of glucocorticoids ≥10–20 mg/day	Preterm birth	3.5

disease when maternal and foetal outcomes are significantly improved.

In the pregnant woman with lupus nephritis, there are various factors to consider:

1. Lupus itself does not appear to affect fertility (but prior the use of cyclophosphamide and/or advanced CKD may do). Appropriate contraception should be discussed with all women of childbearing potential. Combined oral contraceptives are probably best avoided in this group because of increased risks of hypertension and venous thromboembolic complications.
2. Lupus activity: maternal and foetal outcomes are significantly worse when lupus is active at conception. This applies to renal and non-renal manifestations and emphasises the need for early and frank discussion with all female patients of childbearing potential of the importance of planning pregnancy.
3. Background CKD: as with all pregnancies in women with CKD, the degree of chronic damage caused by previous active disease is an important factor and can influence maternal and foetal outcomes.
4. Flares: it remains unclear whether pregnancy itself increases the risk of lupus flare in the antenatal or early postnatal period. The risk is increased by any lupus activity within 6 months of conception, history of multiple flares, and discontinuation of hydroxychloroquine.
5. Medication: see the British Society of Rheumatology guideline on prescribing drugs in pregnancy and breastfeeding for detailed guidance [31]. Glucocorticoids, azathioprine, hydroxychloroquine, ciclosporin, and tacrolimus appear to be safe to use in pregnancy. Mycophenolate mofetil has been shown to be associated with various congenital abnormalities, particularly of the heart, palate, and face (which may be difficult to detect on a foetal ultrasound scan). It should ideally be stopped at least 3 months prior to conception and switched to an alternative agent such as azathioprine if necessary. Cyclophosphamide is associated with significant teratogenic and abortifacient effects and should not be used. Rituximab crosses the placenta especially in the third trimester and has been associated with neonatal B cell depletion and should probably be avoided in pregnancy. Antihypertensive medication may also need modification as discussed previously.
6. Antiphospholipid antibodies: these have been shown consistently to increase both the rate of pregnancy loss (typically after 10 weeks) and the risk of pre-eclampsia. There appears to be a hierarchy of effect with the presence of lupus anticoagulant being associated with more adverse events than anticardiolipin antibodies alone. In addition, higher titres of antiphospholipid antibodies increase the risk of adverse outcomes as does a history of previous thromboembolic events or pregnancy loss.
7. Lupus serology: women with high levels of anti-dsDNA antibodies or low complement are at greater risk of adverse pregnancy outcomes than patients with quiescent serology, but the presence of active disease with active serology gives by far the worst outcomes. It should be noted that complement levels are naturally raised in pregnancy so that trends in complement levels should be monitored in addition to absolute values.
8. Anti-Ro/SSA antibodies: these antibodies are associated with neonatal lupus and two main foetal complications:
   (a) Cutaneous neonatal lupus.
   (b) Cardiac complications such as heart block (around 1–2%) or endocardial fibroelastosis.

   Higher antibody titres and a history of cutaneous neonatal lupus in a previous pregnancy appear to be associated with an increased risk of cardiac complications. All lupus patients with the presence of anti-Ro/SSA antibodies should undergo foetal heart rate auscultation weekly from 16 weeks.

   The use of hydroxychloroquine in anti-Ro-positive mothers with a previous child affected by cardiac neonatal lupus has been shown to significantly reduce the risk of cardiac neonatal lupus in a subsequent pregnancy [32].
9. Other organ damage from lupus: pulmonary hypertension appears to be associated with antiphospholipid syndrome and can be fatal in pregnancy even with specialist management.

Bearing in mind the above factors, we recommend that all patients with lupus nephritis receive joint renal-obstetric pre-pregnancy counselling with experienced practitioners to enable tailored advice of individual risk of both maternal and foetal outcomes. In addition, this allows:

1. Discussion about lupus activity and planning therapy to achieve quiescence in preparation for pregnancy. Best outcomes result in those women with quiescent disease for >6 months on pregnancy safe drugs. Where there is uncertainty about activity of lupus nephritis (such as the presence of persistent proteinuria), a pre-pregnancy renal biopsy is helpful as a guide.
2. Medication changes:
   (a) Transfer from mycophenolate, cyclophosphamide, or rituximab when the disease is felt to be quiescent to azathioprine with a period of observation.
   (b) Cessation of ACE inhibitors or ARB and transfer to either labetalol or nifedipine for control of hypertension if necessary. This also allows re-establishment of a new baseline for proteinuria prior to pregnancy which makes interpretation of any subsequent rise in pregnancy easier (allowing for a further physiological rise). *In patients with significant proteinuria, one may recommend the continuation of ACEi or ARB until conception to allow anti-proteinuric benefit to continue.*
   (c) Discussion around the use of folic acid for prevention of neural tube defects and low-dose aspirin from conception to reduce the risk of pre-eclampsia in this high-risk group.
   (d) Hydroxychloroquine should be offered to (or continued in) all women with lupus in pregnancy. It reduces the risk of lupus flare and is also of benefit to anti-Ro-positive mothers in reducing the risk of cardiac neonatal lupus (as discussed above).

3. Consideration of the need for low molecular weight heparin. This should be used at a prophylactic dose (with factor Xa monitoring):
   (a) In all cases of significant proteinuria (PCR or ACR ≥200) whenever it develops in pregnancy.
   (b) When there is a previous history of venous thromboembolic disease.
   (c) When there is a history of significant pregnancy loss in the presence of antiphospholipid antibodies.
   (d) In patients currently anticoagulated with warfarin – patients should be switched to LMWH in pregnancy. The evidence for safety of direct orally acting anticoagulants is unclear, and patients should be converted pre-conception to alternative agents.

52.18.2 Diagnosis of Lupus Nephritis for the First Time in Pregnancy Presents Its Own Challenges

Occasionally a patient will present with an active urinary sediment and positive lupus serology for the first time in pregnancy. We would recommend a full immunology screen in any patient presenting with proteinuria prior to 20 weeks and at any stage when proteinuria is associated with haematuria or appears not to be typical for pre-eclampsia. The decision to perform a renal biopsy can then be a difficult one. Real-time, ultrasound-guided biopsy up to foetal viability can be very useful, both to confirm a renal diagnosis allowing appropriate intensity of treatment and to provide informed counselling to a woman. After viability, 'blind' treatment of assumed lupus nephritis may be required with induction of preterm delivery if a significant deterioration of renal (or extra-renal) parameters occur that require treatment contraindicated in pregnancy.

52.19 Pregnancy in Women Treated by Dialysis

Fertility in women treated by chronic dialysis is markedly reduced due to the complex interplay of biological and psychosocial factors, including decreased libido and disturbances of the hypothalamic-pituitary-gonadal hormonal axis (hyperprolactinaemia occurs in 70–90%), leading to irregular periods, anovulation, or amenorrhoea. Conception rates for women on dialysis have been reported as 1.4 pregnancies per 1000 patients per year, compared with the national rate of approximately 76 per 1000 patients per year [4]. Conception on peritoneal dialysis is 3 times less common than on haemodialysis.

A recent meta-analysis reported an increase in the number of successful pregnancies in dialysis patients over the last 15 years (574 pregnancies in 543 patients reported from 2000 to 2014) [33].

Pregnancy outcomes have also improved over the last 3 decades as a consequence of more intensive dialysis regimes, advances in obstetric/neonatal care, and a reduction in therapeutic termination. Conception rates and outcomes (including live birth rates) for women who progress to dialysis during pregnancy are superior to those already established on dialysis prior to pregnancy [34]. Nevertheless, pregnancy in women treated by dialysis is arduous, associated with high maternal and foetal morbidity, and pregnancy outcomes remain comparatively poor. See ◘ Table 52.7.

Table 52.7 Foetal and maternal outcomes in meta-analysis of pregnancies in women treated by dialysis. (Data from [33])

Pregnancy outcome	Incidence (%)
Preterm delivery (<37 weeks)	83 (median gestational age 33 weeks)
Low birth weight/IUGR	32
Requirement for NICU care	60
Stillbirth/neonatal death	18
Surviving infants	83
Maternal perinatal mortality	0.4

52.19.1 Diagnosis of Pregnancy

Diagnosis of early pregnancy in dialysis patients is difficult. Amenorrhoea or irregular periods are common, and urine pregnancy tests are often unreliable. Serum beta-HCG levels may be elevated in the absence of pregnancy. Trans-abdominal or the more sensitive transvaginal ultrasound is the most reliable pregnancy test in this population and allows assessment of gestation.

52.19.2 Pre-Pregnancy Counselling

Many women assume that it is impossible to conceive on dialysis. It is good practice to counsel women of fertile age treated by dialysis for the risks of pregnancy and routinely offer contraceptive advice. Any woman contemplating pregnancy should be offered combined renal-obstetric pre-conception counselling in a unit experienced in the care of such pregnancies and be managed under the supervision of a joint renal-obstetric antenatal service throughout pregnancy. For most women, delaying pregnancy until after a successful renal transplant with much improved prospects of a successful outcome is the optimum pre-conception advice. Pregnancy, even if unsuccessful, may lead to HLA sensitisation – reducing opportunities for subsequent transplantation, especially spousal donation.

52.20 Pregnancy Outcomes

52.20.1 Peritoneal Dialysis

There are some theoretical advantages of peritoneal dialysis over haemodialysis in pregnancy, including more gentle fluid, electrolyte and toxin removal, reduced hypotensive episodes, and no requirement for anticoagulation. However, reported outcomes between treatment modalities are similar. Peritonitis has been associated the with onset of spontaneous labour, and by the third trimester, peritoneal space for dialysis fluid is limited even on automated nocturnal treatment, often leading to reduced appetite. We do not recommend immediate switch of dialysis modality in early pregnancy but suggest the formation of AV fistula early in the second trimester to enable easy conversion to haemodialysis later in pregnancy if problems are encountered.

52.20.2 Haemodialysis

The literature is almost certainly influenced by publication bias in favour of successful outcomes and underreporting of spontaneous miscarriage. An attempt at rationalisation of contemporaneous data has been made recently in a systematic review of 126 heterogeneous studies of pregnancies (n = 574) in patients receiving haemodialysis or peritoneal dialysis (n = 543), reported between 2000 and 2014 [33].

Rates of adverse foetal outcomes, including low birth weight ($p = 0.017$) and preterm delivery ($p = 0.044$), were significantly reduced in those women undergoing more intensive dialysis schedules. Incidence of maternal perinatal mortality was low (0.4%). Maternal complications such as pre-eclampsia, hypertension, and anaemia are commonplace; however, exact incidence is difficult to define due to heterogeneity of studies and differences in definitions.

Polyhydramnios is widely reported and may underlie the high rate of spontaneous premature labour precipitating delivery. It is suggested that foetal osmotic diuresis secondary to high maternal urea may be the cause. An inverse correlation between pre-dialysis urea and successful outcome has been reported, leading to a recommendation to keep pre-dialysis urea <17 mmol/l [35].

The incidence of polyhydramnios and premature labour may be reduced by better solute control achieved by more prolonged dialysis. A recent cohort study compared outcomes of 22 pregnancies in women receiving intensive haemodialysis (mean 43 hours per week) with outcomes from 70 pregnancies of patients receiving 'standard' dialysis (mean 17 hours per week). The intensive dialysis group had a significantly higher live birth rate (86.4% vs 61.4%, $p = 0.03$) and a longer median duration of pregnancy (36 weeks vs 27 weeks, $p = 0.002$). Furthermore, a dose-response was found, with a longer duration of dialysis therapy associated with improved pregnancy outcomes [36].

It therefore appears that increasing hours of dialysis, whether by daily or nocturnal dialysis, is associated with better outcomes. The logistics of such therapy should be discussed with any woman undertaking pregnancy on dialysis and can be particularly difficult in those who already have caring responsibilities for other children or who remain in employment. We would recommend the commencement of intensive dialysis therapy from the second trimester and earlier if feasible.

52.21 Guidelines for Management of Pregnancy in Haemodialysis Patients

1. Offer contraceptive advice and pre-conception counselling for all women of childbearing age receiving dialysis.
2. Intravenous iron (after the first trimester) and ESA are widely used and are not associated with foetal abnormalities. Maintain haemoglobin 95–110 g/L. Monitor BP closely. ESA dose increase of 50–100% is usually required.
3. Folic acid and water-soluble vitamin supplementation are advised.
4. Dialysis dose: increase dialysis frequency to 6 times/week in early second trimester providing a minimum of 20 hours/week, keeping pre-dialysis urea below 17moml/l. There may be benefits in longer hours or daily nocturnal dialysis.
5. Maintain BP <140/90 to 130/80 mmHg.
6. Avoidance of intra-dialytic hypotension with careful and regular reassessment of dry weight.
7. Anticoagulation: low molecular weight heparin does not cross the placenta and is not associated with increased antepartum haemorrhage.
8. Treatment with daily low-dose aspirin from 12 weeks to reduce risk of pre-eclampsia.
9. Dialysate: try to mimic pregnancy physiology. Reduce dialysate sodium to 135 mmol/l, bicarbonate to 25 mmol/l, and calcium to 1.25 mmol/l. Serum phosphate levels frequently fall below normal on intensive treatment requiring dialysate phosphate supplementation and/or supplementary dietary advice.
10. Regular review by an experienced renal-obstetric multidisciplinary team to allow appropriate maternal and foetal monitoring and discussions with regard to optimal timing of delivery.
11. Meticulous management of other comorbidities such as diabetes, cardiovascular disease, and immune-related conditions by experienced teams.

The long-term outcome of children born to mothers on dialysis remains unknown. The immediate risks associated with prematurity are well characterised, and there is some evidence for increased long-term cardiovascular morbidity in babies born small for gestational age. Moreover, there may be a potential risk of renal impairment in children born to dialysing mothers [37].

In summary, pregnancy in the dialysis patient is increasingly common and appears to have better outcomes than previously noted – probably related to the provision of more frequent dialysis and better maternal and neonatal care. Nevertheless, pregnancy in this group of patients will require a considerable time commitment from the patient and medical staff, and pregnancy outcomes are less favourable than for those with a functioning transplant or with less severe CKD. Most women should be advised to defer pregnancy until after successful renal transplantation when a maternal and foetal outlook is improved. Pregnancy may however be a reasonable option in the highly motivated, counselled patient within an experienced environment.

52.22 Pregnancy Following Renal Transplantation

Renal transplantation rapidly restores fertility in women with ESRD, offering for many the first opportunity to conceive with a good chance of a successful pregnancy outcome. Nevertheless, these pregnancies are complex and at high risk for foetal and maternal complications. At least 50% of transplant pregnancies reported in the literature are unplanned. Best outcomes are most likely if early effective contraceptive advice is given on discharge post-transplantation, and women considering pregnancy are advised in a joint renal-obstetric pre-pregnancy counselling clinic. Appropriate antenatal care is best provided in a joint antenatal clinic managed by renal and obstetric doctors with significant experience in this area see ▸ Case 52.43.3.

52.23 The Evidence Base and Sources of Guidance

The evidence base to counsel women in guiding pregnancy management remains incomplete but has improved considerably recently. Many small single centre retrospective case series which may suffer from selection bias have been collated in a large meta-analysis [38]. The US National Transplant Pregnancy Registry employed voluntary submission, but three prospective registries collecting data on almost all transplants (two from the UK and one from Australia/New Zealand) have also been published [39–41] as well as a recent study reporting pregnancy outcomes from all kidney transplant patients in England using Hospital Episode Statistics data [42]. UK Kidney Association, American

Society of Transplantation Clinical Practice Guidelines and European Best Practice Guidelines advise clinicians [43, 44].

52.24 The Timing of Pregnancy in Relation to Transplantation

Guidelines recommend deferring pregnancy until at least 12 months post-transplantation. By this time, immunosuppressant doses should be at their nadir, and the risks of rejection and opportunistic infection (in particular cytomegalovirus which can affect the foetus) are remote. Meta-analysis however does not support a clear cut-off in the timing of conception post-pregnancy. The live birth rate for pregnancies <2y, 3–4y, and >4y post-transplant were reported to be 80%, 76%, and 75% respectively, whereas obstetric complications were significantly greater in earlier pregnancies [38]. In practice it is best to wait for stable well-preserved kidney function after conversion to treatment known to be safe in pregnancy.

52.25 Transplant Immunosuppression

Prednisolone crosses the placenta but with a maternal/cord blood concentration of 10:1 due to metabolism within the placenta. Daily doses of <15 mg per day have not been associated with teratogenicity or neonatal adrenal suppression. It is likely that steroids are associated with an increased risk of gestational diabetes. Glucose tolerance testing at 26 weeks is therefore advised.

Extensive human study both in and out of transplantation has shown no association between azathioprine and congenital abnormalities. Fetal myelosuppression is extremely unlikely if the total dose is <2 mg/kg and maternal white count is maintained within the normal range.

The calcineurin inhibitors (CNIs) ciclosporin and tacrolimus have not been associated with an increased risk of congenital abnormalities. Babies born to women taking ciclosporin may have a lower birth weight compared to those receiving prednisolone and azathioprine alone. This is likely to relate to a higher prevalence of hypertension and poorer renal function in this population. The dose of CNI required to maintain equivalent trough levels in pregnancy frequently requires dose adjustment, with a mean dose increase of 40% (increased volume of distribution in adipose tissue and red cells). Outcomes of pregnancies in women taking ciclosporin or tacrolimus are similar. Those treated with tacrolimus have a greater incidence of gestational diabetes (2–10%).

There is increasing evidence that mycophenolic acid (MPA) and mycophenolate mofetil (MMF) are teratogenic. Reports in renal transplant pregnancies identify a greater than expected first trimester spontaneous miscarriage rate of 40% (10–15% in the general population). In addition, an embryopathy comprising cleft lip and palate, ear, and cerebral abnormalities is reported in a quarter of exposed pregnancies [45], which may be difficult to detect on the foetal ultrasound scan. All women should be counselled for the risks of congenital abnormality at the time of transplantation and should practice secure contraception and undergo pre-pregnancy counselling if they wish to conceive. Women taking MMF or MPA should be advised to stop at least 3 months before planned conception (ideally 6 months) to enable transfer to alternative therapy (usually azathioprine) and assessment of stability, before attempting conception. There is a small but definite increased risk of rejection during this period, and this must be discussed.

52.26 Men and Mycophenolate

The European Medicines Agency (EMA) has recently updated their advice for men taking mycophenolate derivatives. Registry studies have not found significant evidence of increased risk of malformations or miscarriages in pregnancies affected by paternal exposure to mycophenolate. However, the risk of genotoxicity in spermatozoa cannot be ruled out, and men should therefore be informed of the theoretical risks of foetal exposure to mycophenolate. These risks should be weighed up against the risk of converting to alternative immunosuppressive treatment on an individualised basis, bearing in mind the stability of underlying immunological disease or renal transplant status. A summary of updated recommendations can be found at ▶ https://renal.org/wp-content/uploads/2018/02/Full-Update.pdf.

52.27 Early Pregnancy Outcomes

Pregnancy outcomes in renal transplant recipients have improved over the last three decades; in large part due to a reduction in 'therapeutic' terminations presumably as a consequence of greater medical confidence in pregnancy outcomes [41]. Despite this, UK data from 2001 to 2015 shows a significantly lower live birth rate of 68.5% for patients with a kidney transplant, compared to 79.6% in the general population ($p < 0.001$) [42]. The prevalence of spontaneous miscarriage (<20 weeks) was reported as 13.4% which is higher than background population rates (11.2%, $p = 0.043$). No cases of ectopic pregnancy were identified, reassuring given pelvic transplant and the likelihood that some women have had previous peritoneal dialysis-related peritonitis (although results rely on voluntary submissions and may be subject to reporting bias).

52.28 Maternal Outcomes of Pregnancies in Renal Transplant Recipients

Pregnancies progressing beyond the first trimester have a greater than 95% chance of a successful outcome with a live birth [39]. However, maternal complications such as pre-eclampsia and gestational diabetes are substantially increased for renal transplant recipients when compared to the general population (adjusted odds ratio for pre-eclampsia is 6.3 [40]). More than half of pregnancies are delivered by Caesarean section, with the risk increasing if delivery is prior to 37 weeks. Maternal outcomes are listed in ◘ Table 52.8 and provide important information for counselling transplant recipients contemplating pregnancy.

The UKOSS study importantly demonstrates a significant rise in serum creatinine in the third trimester which is exaggerated in women with a poor pregnancy outcome [40]. The cause of the rise is unexplained but is likely to result from a physiological decline in GFR rather than the adverse impact of superimposed PET. Proteinuria develops or increases in around a third of women sometimes to near nephrotic levels [40].

52.29 Foetal Outcomes

Foetal outcomes are listed in ◘ Table 52.9 . As compared with the general population, the adjusted odds ratio for preterm delivery is 12.7 [40]. The mean gestational age at birth is 36 weeks, being remarkably consistent between different registry series and meta-analyses. Over half of births are premature (<37 weeks), and consequently a significant proportion is born with low birth weight (<2.5 kg) and is small for their gestational age (birth weight < tenth centile). Many babies born to renal transplant recipients will therefore require neonatal intensive care.

Kidney transplant recipients with a GFR >90 appear to have less favourable pregnancy outcomes than non-transplanted patients with CKD stage 1. However, this effect levels out when only CKD stage 1 patients with progressive or immunologically mediated diseases (such as lupus and diabetes) are compared with kidney transplant patients. Outcomes are comparable between transplant and non-transplanted patients of all other CKD stages [46].

52.30 Long-Term Effect of Pregnancy on Graft and Patient Survival

Case-control studies show no evidence of an adverse impact of pregnancy on graft and patient survival in women with preserved kidney transplant function. However, those with more significant pre-pregnancy renal dysfunction are more likely to suffer pregnancy-related decline [47].

◘ **Table 52.8** Maternal outcomes of pregnancies in renal transplant recipients

	England Hospital Episode Statistics Study, 2016 [42]	UK Obstetric Surveillance Study, 2013 [40]	ANZDATA Registry Study, 2013 [41]	Meta-analysis, 2011 [38] %[C.I.]	UK Transplant Registry, 2007 [39]
Number of pregnancies reported (n)	569	105	692	4706	193
Acute rejection (%)		2		4.2	
Pre-eclampsia (%)		24	29	27 [25–29]	
Antenatal graft dysfunction (%)		38			30 (>20% rise in creatinine)
Gestational DM (%)	12.9	3	3	8 [6.7–9.4]	
New-onset proteinuria in absence of PET (%)		30			
Caesarean section delivery (%)	63.1	64		57 [55–59]	72 (87% if delivery <37 weeks)

Table 52.9 Foetal outcomes of pregnancies in renal transplant recipients

	England Hospital Episode Statistics Study, 2016 [42]	UK Obstetric Surveillance Study, 2013 [40]	ANZDATA Registry Study 2013 [41]	Meta-analysis, 2011 (CI) [38]	UK Transplant Registry, 2007 [39]
Live birth (%)	68.5	91	76	74 (72–75)	79
Gestational age (weeks)		36 (IQR 27–43)	35 + 5	36 (35–36)	36.8
Preterm birth (%)		52	54	46 (44–48)	50
Very preterm (<32 weeks) (%)		9	18		
Birth weight (g)		2483	2485	2420	2316 +/−80
Low birth rate (<2500 g) (%)		48	46		54
Very low birth rate (<1500 g) (%)		9	8		22
Small for gestational age (%)	9.3	24	25		
Need for neonatal ICU (%)		30			

52.31 Management of Declining Graft Function in Pregnancy

Despite immunological tolerance shown to the foetus, the reported incidence of rejection during pregnancy is similar to that in non-pregnant transplant recipients, 2–4% [38–40]. In early pregnancy, this is associated with volume depletion and failure to absorb immunosuppression due to hyperemesis. Physiological hydronephrosis of the transplant is common in pregnancy, but ureteric obstruction by the gravid uterus is thankfully rare. Unexplained transplant dysfunction before 28 weeks gestation should include consideration of renal biopsy as this may be safer than blind antirejection treatment. PET may explain transplant dysfunction later in pregnancy. Any decision must be carefully considered and the risk/benefit ratio discussed with the pregnant woman.

52.32 Factors Affecting Live Birth Rate

Risk factors for adverse pregnancy outcome (live birth or delivery <32 weeks) include:

1. Maternal age <20 or >35 years.
2. African-Caribbean ethnicity.
3. End-stage renal failure secondary to diabetes.
4. Poorer pre-pregnancy renal function.

The UK Transplant Registry identifies higher pre-pregnancy creatinine and systolic BP at conception with adverse transplant outcome. The odds ratio for preterm birth in those women with a creatinine of <150 mmol/l at conception is 0.2 as compared to those with a serum creatinine of >150. It appears that hypertension (even when controlled) has an even greater association with preterm birth (30-fold increased risk) as compared with normotensive transplant recipients [40].

52.33 Delivery

The pelvic transplant kidney does not impair vaginal delivery, nor is there evidence of damage to the transplant in the process. Nevertheless, two-thirds of deliveries are by Caesarean section. Delivery should be 'covered' with IV steroids and IV hydration.

It is advisable for obstetricians to plan Caesarean section delivery in advance by a discussion with the transplant surgeon, particularly where there may be anatomical challenges including simultaneous pancreas-kidney transplantation or those with abnormal urinary drainage.

52

52.34 Breastfeeding

Breast milk transfer from mothers taking low-dose prednisolone or azathioprine is safe. Azathioprine transfer in breast milk is very low and results in undetectable serum levels of the active metabolite 6-mercaptopurine in the baby. Recent data suggest a low-level transfer of both ciclosporin and tacrolimus into breast milk. Cord blood levels on the day of delivery approximate maternal levels. By 1 week, despite breastfeeding, tacrolimus drug levels are undetectable in the baby. *With careful neonatal blood level monitoring* and following discussion with the neonatologist, it is reasonable to allow breastfeeding [48].

52.35 Long-Term Outcome of Children Born to Renal Transplant Recipients

Both severe prematurity and intrauterine growth retardation are associated with neurocognitive impairment in babies born to women in the general population and may lead to increased long-term risk of cardiovascular disease. However, when compared to appropriate controls, there was no increased risk of neurodevelopmental delay or behavioural problems in babies born to renal transplant recipients taking ciclosporin [49]. Despite exposure to the potential nephrotoxic effects of CNIs throughout intrauterine growth, renal function and BP in children tested at mean of 2.5 years age are normal. Long-term follow-up studies of these children are required to detect any late complications of immunosuppressant drug exposure and explore a possible higher long-term risk of renal or cardiovascular disease.

52.36 Pregnancy after Kidney Donation

Counselling of women of childbearing age who wish to be live kidney donors should include any risks of donation upon subsequent pregnancy outcomes. A recent meta-analysis of medium and long-term health outcomes in living kidney donors found no significant evidence of an increased risk of gestational hypertension, low birthweight, or preterm birth in pregnancy. There is however evidence of an increased risk of pre-eclampsia (RR 2.12 [C.I. 1.06–4.27]) when compared to non-donor pregnancies [50]. Though the absolute risk remains relatively small, this increased risk should be discussed with any woman of childbearing age considering living kidney donation.

52.37 Management Guidelines for Renal Transplant Recipients in Pregnancy

1. Women should be offered contraception advice post-transplant and pre-conception counselling in a dedicated renal-obstetric antenatal clinic detailing known complication risks to mother and baby.
2. Women should have stable renal transplant function and ideally defer pregnancy until at least 1-year post-transplant.
3. Outcomes are best for those with pre-pregnancy serum creatinine <125 μmol/l and urine protein excretion <1 g/24 hours. In women with serum creatinine <125 μmol/l, there is no adverse effect of pregnancy on long-term graft or patient survival. Renal function may be adversely impacted on by pregnancy if serum creatinine exceeds 150–175 μmol/l.
4. BP should be maintained <140/90 mmHg pre-pregnancy on two or fewer drugs. Aim for a BP target of <140/90 during pregnancy.
5. Prednisolone, azathioprine, ciclosporin, and tacrolimus are safe in pregnancy.
6. Mycophenolate mofetil or mycophenolic acid appear to be teratogenic and should be stopped at least 3 months before pregnancy (ideally 6 months to ensure stable renal function). In most situations it is advisable to substitute with azathioprine. Women should be warned that there is a small risk of rejection.
7. Unless otherwise contraindicated, low-dose aspirin is recommended from the end of the first trimester until delivery in all women with a renal transplant in pregnancy as pre-eclampsia prophylaxis.
8. Those women with nephrotic range proteinuria (>2 g/24 hours or PCR >200) should in addition receive prophylactic daily low molecular weight heparin which may be monitored using Factor Xa activity (measured 3 hours after administration).
9. Breastfeeding is safe for babies of renal transplant recipients taking prednisolone and azathioprine and for those taking tacrolimus or ciclosporin, but drug levels in the baby should be monitored.

52.38 Contraception for Women with Chronic Kidney Disease

Whilst fertility is maintained to a variable degree in almost all women of childbearing age with CKD (including those with stage 4/5 CKD or those treated by dialysis), the risks of pregnancy are substantially increased. Unplanned pregnancy increases these risks still further;

around a third to a half of all pregnancies in patients with CKD are unplanned [4]. As such, informed contraceptive advice should be a standard of care for all women of fertile age with any degree of CKD and is an essential element of pre-conception counselling.

52.39 Contraception Counselling

For women with CKD, contraception should be safe and highly effective, and the choice of method must take into account comorbidities and existing drug treatments. Other considerations relevant to any woman include side effect profile, duration of action, reversibility, time to return of fertility, convenience, and protection from sexually transmitted infection (STI). Contraceptive counselling is of particular importance as part of a package of sexual health education for young women with CKD transitioning from paediatric to adult care.

52.40 Overview of Contraceptive Methods

There are few absolute contraindications to most forms of contraception in women with CKD, kidney transplant recipients, or those with lupus nephritis. See Table 52.10.

Barrier methods including male/female condoms provide protection from STIs but lack contraceptive efficacy, so it should be combined with other more effec-

Table 52.10 Comparison of forms of contraception with reference to women with CKD. (Reproduced with permission from [4])

Contraceptive method	Advantages	Disadvantages	Perfect use failure rate (%)	Typical use failure rate (%)
Barrier (male/female condoms)	Simple Protection from STI	Poorly effective Spermicide may increase risk of UTI in susceptible women –alters vulval bacterial flora	2 (male) 5 (female)	18 (male) 21 (female)
IUCD – Copper	Long-acting	Efficacy reduced by immunosuppression?		
IUS-levonorgestrel- releasing (Mirena®)	Long-acting Suitable for nulliparous	Effective Low risk of PID even in immunosuppressed	0.2	0.2
Combined (oestrogen/progesterone) Oral contraceptive (COC) COC patch or COC vaginal ring	Well tolerated	Contraindicated in thrombophilia (nephrotic/APS) Small adverse impact on hypertension? CNI interaction (monitor levels)	0.3	9
Standard progesterone only pill (POP) (Levonorgestrel)	Simple/reversible No impact on BP Safe in thrombophilia	CNI interaction (monitor levels) Efficacy reduced if taken 2 h late	0.3	9
Desogestrel	As for POP Efficacy maintained if taken up to 12 h late	CNI/mTORi interaction (monitor levels)		
Depot progesterone MPDA (depo-Provera®)	As for POP Effective for 3 months	3 monthly deep IM injection CNI/mTORi interaction (monitor levels) May add to risk of post-transplant/steroid-induced osteoporosis		
Progesterone-only subdermal implant Etonogestrel (Nexplanon®)	Compliance-effective for 3 years	Subdermal implantation	0.05	0.05
Female sterilisation/vasectomy	Highly effective/non-hormonal	Surgical procedure Tubal occlusion may now be performed using hysteroscopy without the need for incision or anaesthesia Should be considered irreversible	0.5	0.5

tive contraception. The spermicide, nonoxynol-9, alters periurethral microbial flora and may lead to recurrent urinary tract infections in those with predisposing factors such as reflux nephropathy or bladder dysfunction.

Long-acting reversible contraception includes depot progestogens, depot medroxyprogesterone acetate (DMPA) requiring 3-monthly deep IM administration, and etonogestrel (Nexplanon®) inserted subdermally by a trained operator, providing contraception for 3 years. The alternatives, intrauterine devices include copper coil or levonorgestrel releasing intrauterine system (LNG-releasing IUS, Mirena®). In our experience, these long-acting forms are forms are preferred by many women with CKD not contemplating pregnancy after counselling because of high efficacy and convenience. The Mirena IUS is associated with light menses or amenorrhoea and can be inserted in nulliparous women. Over 80% of women in the general population remain satisfied with these methods after 12 months.

52.41 Oral Contraceptives

The traditional progesterone-only 'mini pill' is effective if taken within a 2-hour window each day. Efficacy in practice is reduced and may not be adequate for women requiring a high level of security from pregnancy. Desogestrel 75 mcg (Cerelle, Cerazette®) has a different mechanism of action including inhibition of ovulation and has a 12-hour window of administration without loss of effectiveness. This is effective and well tolerated in women with CKD, including those immunosuppressed, although it can lead to irregular uterine bleeding.

In the general population, combined oral contraceptives (COCs) are the most commonly used form of reversible hormonal contraception and are well tolerated and highly effective and have a long history of safety. However, many women with CKD, especially those with treated hypertension, are advised against their use. Oestrogens should be avoided in those women at greater risk of venous thromboembolic disease (including those with antiphospholipid syndrome and nephrotic syndrome). The evidence of a hypertensive effect in women with CKD is limited, and experience suggests that any change in BP can be offset by a dose increase in antihypertensive treatment. As such the use of COC in women with CKD and controlled hypertension should not be considered an absolute contraindication.

52.42 Contraception for Patients with Lupus Nephritis and Renal Transplant Recipients

Women with lupus nephritis are often denied oestrogen-containing COC or intrauterine device/system contraception. Historic literature has led to the belief that oestrogens lead to a flare of lupus and may increase BP and that the IUD/S may not be effective or are associated with a high risk of pelvic infection in the setting of immunosuppression. These fears appear largely unfounded. A single blind study of 162 women with SLE and mild/quiescent disease randomised patients to COC, POP, or copper IUD. No pregnancies occurred over 12 months, and the incidence of lupus flare was the same across all groups. No episodes of PID occurred in those treated with the IUD [51]. A second randomised study of COCs vs placebo (exclusions included moderate/high anticardiolipin antibodies, lupus anticoagulant or history of thrombosis) in women with inactive or stable SLE [52] confirmed no increased risk of lupus flares with use of the COC. As such, women with mild or stable lupus can be safely treated with either the COC (in the absence of thrombotic risk factors, which includes nephrotic syndrome) or IUD/S.

In renal transplant recipients, the use of progestogens may alter CNI metabolism. Both increases and reductions in levels have been reported, which should therefore be monitored and doses adjusted accordingly. A small uncontrolled cohort study of COC use in renal transplant recipients using the COC pill or patch demonstrated contraceptive efficacy. However, 30% of women required alteration of antihypertensive therapy. No comparator group was included so causation is unproven. The COC should not be used as first-line in transplant recipients. However, in those who have controlled BP, with no other contraindication who have been intolerant or do not wish to use alternative methods, we cautiously allow their use in this population. The risk of pregnancy in this setting usually outweighs the risks of COC.

The IUD/S is widely used in another immunosuppressed population, those with HIV, and is not associated with an increased risk of pelvic infection or unplanned pregnancy. The LNG-releasing IUS is appropriate for use in selected women post-renal transplantation. We tend to avoid the use of DMPA because of the potential risk of exacerbating post-transplant osteoporosis although good evidence for this is lacking.

Contraception Tips and Advice

1. Contraceptive advice is an essential component of care of women with CKD.
2. There are few additional absolute contraindications to most forms of contraception in this population.
3. Desogestrel POP (Cerazette) is well tolerated by many patients with CKD and highly effective with less demanding compliance issues (12-hour window).
4. The LNG-IUS is effective and safe for women with kidney disease receiving immunosuppression including those with SLE or transplant recipients.
5. Where there is no increased risk of vascular thrombosis, the COC can be safely used in women with inactive or low activity SLE and is not associated with an increased risk of lupus flare.

Case Study

Case 1: Obstructive Uropathy and AKI in Pregnancy

A 35-year-old nulliparous female presented at 28 weeks pregnant with acute onset right flank pain. Blood tests revealed a stage 1 AKI (creatinine rise from a baseline of 50 to 90) and urine dipstick showed 4+ blood and 2+ leucocytes.

An abdominal ultrasound was performed which showed right-sided hydronephrosis. Given ongoing pain and AKI, an MRU was requested. This showed right-sided hydronephrosis (see ◘ Fig. 52.3a) and dilation of the right ureter to the level of the pelvic inlet where it narrowed. Beyond this there was an apparent filling defect at the VUJ, suggestive of a calculus (see ◘ Fig. 52.3b with an arrow showing filling defect).

The patient was treated with intravenous fluid and antibiotics and the stone spontaneously passed. The AKI resolved soon after and the pregnancy was able to continue to term.

Case 2: Newly Diagnosed Chronic Kidney Disease in Pregnancy

A 32-year-old female with no past medical history was referred to renal antenatal clinic at 19 weeks pregnant with heavy proteinuria (PCR 350) and invisible haematuria (3+ on dipstick). Blood pressure was mildly elevated (142/96 mmHg), so she was treated with labetalol. There were no other clinical features of pre-eclampsia, and the proteinuria was attributed to probable underlying renal disease.

Blood tests showed normal renal function (creatinine 55, GFR >90 ml/min), albumin 30, negative ANA, ANCA and paraproteins, and normal complements and dsDNA.

Careful discussion took place around the risks and benefits of doing a kidney biopsy. Given that immunology was all negative and there was no evidence of lupus or vasculitis, the decision was made to hold off biopsying in pregnancy. She was managed instead with prophylactic low molecular weight heparin (given the nephrotic range proteinuria) and low-dose aspirin for pre-eclampsia prophylaxis. Induced delivery took place at 38 weeks gestation due to rising proteinuria. A renal biopsy post-pregnancy showed focal and segmental glomerulosclerosis.

Case 3: Pregnancy in a Renal Transplant Recipient

A 28-year-old female with a background of ESRD secondary to membranous nephropathy treated with a living donor kidney transplant. Her baseline graft function was good (creatinine 85, eGFR 70), she had no proteinuria (ACR <1), and blood pressure was normal with no requirement for antihypertensive medication. She expressed a wish to conceive at 9 months post-transplant and was referred to the joint renal-obstetric pre-pregnancy counselling clinic. She was advised to wait until at least 1-year post-transplant prior to conceiving, but mycophenolate immunosuppression was switched to azathioprine in preparation. Tacrolimus and prednisolone were continued.

On confirmation of pregnancy at 12-month post-transplant, this patient was commenced on 75 mg aspirin as pre-eclampsia prophylaxis. Pregnancy initially progressed well with no change in graft function or blood pressure, and monthly monitoring took place in a joint renal-obstetric antenatal clinic. Gestational diabetes was diagnosed at 28 weeks after an abnormal glucose tolerance test, and treatment with metformin, and later insulin, was initiated.

Pregnancy continued uneventfully until around 32 weeks gestation, when creatinine began to rise to reach a peak of 120, and there was evidence of proteinuria (PCR 50–70). Blood pressure remained well controlled. She was admitted to the antenatal ward for closer monitoring and steroid treatment for foetal lung maturation in the event of premature delivery being required. Tacrolimus levels were slightly low, so the dose was increased. A transplant ultrasound scan was also carried out which showed normal graft perfusion and no evidence of obstruction. There was no further deterioration in proteinuria or renal function so she was discharged from the hospital but kept under thrice weekly outpatient monitoring for blood pressure, blood, and urine testing and underwent planned delivery at 37 weeks gestation. The deterioration in renal function and proteinuria were attributed to probable superimposed pre-eclampsia.

52

Questions

1. A 32-year-old female with a background of CKD secondary to lupus nephritis attends the nephrology clinic and expresses a wish to become pregnant. She has a baseline creatinine of 140 and an eGFR of 42. Urine ACR is 150. Her medication list includes mycophenolate mofetil, prednisolone, ramipril, and hydroxychloroquine.

   The patient wishes to know what the risks are to her health from pregnancy. What would you advise?
2. This patient also wishes to know what the potential risks could be to the baby. What would you tell her?
3. Which of her current medications can be continued and which would you stop?
4. Which additional medication(s) would you consider starting on confirmation of pregnancy?

Answers

1. CKD is an independent risk factor for adverse maternal outcomes in pregnancy, including significantly increased odds of developing pre-eclampsia and requirement for Caesarean delivery. The presence of proteinuria and hypertension increase the risks further. There is also an increased risk of a further decline in renal function post-pregnancy. Successful pregnancy is however possible and should ideally be planned in a period where lupus has been quiescent for a period of at least 6 months. Regular antenatal monitoring by a nephrologist and obstetrician will be required.
2. There are increased risks of adverse foetal outcomes in pregnancy in women with CKD. The risks increase incrementally with increasing severity of renal impairment and include preterm delivery, requirement for neonatal intensive care, and low birth weight.
3. Mycophenolate: stop at least 3 months prior to conceiving and switch to azathioprine. Prednisolone and hydroxychloroquine – continue. Ramipril – consider continuing until confirmation of pregnancy given underlying proteinuria. Alternatively could be switched to labetalol.
4. Folic acid should be commenced in the pregnancy planning period. Aspirin 75 mg daily from 12 weeks gestation as pre-eclampsia prophylaxis. Consider the need for low molecular weight heparin if urine ACR rises to a nephrotic range.

References

1. Coresh J, et al. Prevalence of chronic kidney disease in the United States. JAMA: J Am Med Associat. 2007;298(17):2038–47.
2. Odutayo A, Hladunewich M. Obstetric nephrology: renal hemodynamic and metabolic physiology in normal pregnancy. Clin J Am Soc Nephrol. 2012;7(12):2073–80.
3. Williams D, Davison J. Chronic kidney disease in pregnancy. Br Med J. 2008;336(7637):211–5.
4. Wiles KS, Nelson-Piercy C, Bramham K. Reproductive health and pregnancy in women with chronic kidney disease. Nat Rev Nephrol. 2018;14(3):165–84.
5. Bramham K, et al. Chronic hypertension and pregnancy outcomes: systematic review and meta-analysis. BMJ. 2014;348:g2301.
6. National Institute for Health and Care Excellence (NICE). Hypertension in pregnancy: diagnosis and management. 2011 [cited 2018 24/7/2018]; Clinical guideline (CG107)]. Available from: https://www.nice.org.uk/guidance/cg107/resources/hypertension-in-pregnancy-diagnosis-and-management-pdf-35109334011877.
7. Abalos E, Duley L, Steyn DW. Antihypertensive drug therapy for mild to moderate hypertension during pregnancy. Cochrane Database Syst Rev. 2014;2:CD002252.
8. Magee LA, et al. Less-tight versus tight control of hypertension in pregnancy. N Engl J Med. 2015;372(5):407–17.
9. Magee LA, et al. The CHIPS Randomized Controlled Trial (Control of Hypertension in Pregnancy Study): Is Severe Hypertension Just an Elevated Blood Pressure? Hypertension. 2016;68(5):1153–9.
10. Butalia S, et al. Hypertension Canada's 2018 guidelines for the management of hypertension in pregnancy. Can J Cardiol. 2018;34(5):526–31.
11. Li DK, et al. Maternal exposure to angiotensin converting enzyme inhibitors in the first trimester and risk of malformations in offspring: a retrospective cohort study. BMJ. 2011;343:d5931.
12. Roberts JM, et al. Hypertension in pregnancy report of the American college of obstetricians and gynecologists' task force on hypertension in pregnancy. Obstet Gynecol. 2013;122(5):1122–31.
13. Levine RJ, et al. Circulating angiogenic factors and the risk of preeclampsia. N Engl J Med. 2004;350(7):672–83.
14. Zeisler H, et al. Predictive value of the sFlt-1:PlGF ratio in women with suspected preeclampsia. N Engl J Med. 2016;374(1):13–22.
15. Bramham K, et al. Diagnostic and predictive biomarkers for pre-eclampsia in patients with established hypertension and chronic kidney disease. Kidney Int. 2016;89(4):874–85.
16. Piccoli GB, et al. Pre-eclampsia or chronic kidney disease? The flow hypothesis. Nephrol Dial Transplant. 2013;
17. Askie LM, et al. Antiplatelet agents for prevention of pre-eclampsia: a meta-analysis of individual patient data. Lancet. 2007;369(9575):1791–8.
18. Visintin C, et al. Management of hypertensive disorders during pregnancy: summary of NICE guidance. BMJ. 2010;341:c2207.
19. Rolnik DL, et al. Aspirin versus placebo in pregnancies at high risk for preterm preeclampsia. N Engl J Med. 2017;377(7):613–22.

20. Wing DA, Fassett MJ, Getahun D. Acute pyelonephritis in pregnancy: an 18-year retrospective analysis. Am J Obstet Gynecol. 2014;210(3):219 e1–6.
21. Smaill FM, Vazquez JC. Antibiotics for asymptomatic bacteriuria in pregnancy. Cochrane Database Syst Rev. 2015;8: CD000490.
22. Ray JG, et al. Association Between MRI Exposure During Pregnancy and Fetal and Childhood Outcomes. JAMA. 2016;316(9):952–61.
23. Nevis IF, et al. Pregnancy outcomes in women with chronic kidney disease: a systematic review. Clin J Am Soc Nephrol. 2011;6(11):2587–98.
24. Piccoli GB, et al. Kidney biopsy in pregnancy: evidence for counselling? A systematic narrative review. Bjog-an Inter J Obstet Gynaecol. 2013;120(4):412–27.
25. Day C, et al. The role of renal biopsy in women with kidney disease identified in pregnancy. Nephrol Dial Transplant. 2008;23(1):201–6.
26. Zhang JJ, et al. A systematic review and meta-analysis of outcomes of pregnancy in CKD and CKD outcomes in pregnancy. Clin J Am Soc Nephrol. 2015;10(11):1964–78.
27. Jones DC, Hayslett JP. Outcome of pregnancy in women with moderate or severe renal insufficiency. N Engl J Med. 1996;335(4):226–32.
28. Imbasciati E, et al. Pregnancy in CKD stages 3 to 5: fetal and maternal outcomes. Am J Kidney Dis. 2007;49(6):753–62.
29. Piccoli GB, et al. Risk of adverse pregnancy outcomes in women with CKD. J Am Soc Nephrol. 2015;26(8): 2011–22.
30. Piccoli GB, et al. Pregnancy and chronic kidney disease: a challenge in all CKD stages. Clin J Am Soc Nephrol. 2010;5(5):844–55.
31. Flint J, et al. BSR and BHPR guideline on prescribing drugs in pregnancy and breastfeeding-Part I: standard and biologic disease modifying anti-rheumatic drugs and corticosteroids. Rheumatology (Oxford). 2016;55(9):1693–7.
32. Izmirly PM, et al. Maternal use of hydroxychloroquine is associated with a reduced risk of recurrent anti-SSA/Ro-antibody-associated cardiac manifestations of neonatal lupus. Circulation. 2012;126(1):76–82.
33. Piccoli GB, et al. Pregnancy in dialysis patients in the new millennium: a systematic review and meta-regression analysis correlating dialysis schedules and pregnancy outcomes. Nephrol Dial Transplant. 2016;31(11):1915–34.
34. Jesudason S, Grace BS, McDonald SP. Pregnancy outcomes according to dialysis commencing before or after conception in women with ESRD. Clin J Am Soc Nephrol. 2014;9(1): 143–9.
35. Asamiya Y, et al. The importance of low blood urea nitrogen levels in pregnant patients undergoing hemodialysis to optimize birth weight and gestational age. Kidney Int. 2009;75(11): 1217–22.
36. Hladunewich MA, et al. Intensive Hemodialysis Associates with Improved Pregnancy Outcomes: A Canadian and United States Cohort Comparison. J Am Soc Nephrol. 2014;25(5): 1103–9.
37. Abou-Jaoude P, et al. What about the renal function during childhood of children born from dialysed mothers? Nephrol Dial Transplant. 2012;27(6):2365–9.
38. Deshpande NA, et al. Pregnancy outcomes in kidney transplant recipients: a systematic review and meta-analysis. Am J Transplant. 2011;11(11):2388–404.
39. Sibanda N, et al. Pregnancy after organ transplantation: a report from the UK Transplant pregnancy registry. Transplantation. 2007;83(10):1301–7.
40. Bramham K, et al. Pregnancy in renal transplant recipients: a UK national cohort study. Clin J Am Soc Nephrol. 2013;8(2):290–8.
41. Wyld ML, et al. Pregnancy outcomes for kidney transplant recipients. Am J Transplant. 2013;13(12):3173–82.
42. Sarween N, et al. pregnancy outcomes in renal transplant recipients in England over 15 years. Nephrol Dial Transplant. 2016;31:6–6.
43. McKay DB, et al. Reproduction and transplantation: report on the AST Consensus Conference on Reproductive Issues and Transplantation. Am J Transplant. 2005;5(7):1592–9.
44. Transplantation E.E.G.O.R. European best practice guidelines for renal transplantation. Section IV: Long-term management of the transplant recipient. IV.10. Pregnancy in renal transplant recipients. Nephrol Dial Transplant. 2002;17(Suppl 4):50–5.
45. Sifontis NM, et al. Pregnancy outcomes in solid organ transplant recipients with exposure to mycophenolate mofetil or sirolimus. Transplantation. 2006;82(12):1698–702.
46. Piccoli GB, et al. Outcomes of pregnancies after kidney transplantation: lessons learned from CKD. A comparison of transplanted, nontransplanted chronic kidney disease patients and low-risk pregnancies: a multicenter nationwide analysis. Transplantation. 2017;101(10):2536–44.
47. Levidiotis V, Chang S, McDonald S. Pregnancy and maternal outcomes among kidney transplant recipients. J Am Soc Nephrol. 2009;20(11):2433–40.
48. Bramham K. et al. Breastfeeding and tacrolimus: serial monitoring in breast-fed and bottle-fed infants. Clin J Am Soc Nephrol. 2013.
49. Nulman I, et al. Long-term neurodevelopment of children exposed in utero to ciclosporin after maternal renal transplant. Paediatr Drugs. 2010;12(2):113–22.
50. O'Keeffe LM, et al. Mid- and Long-Term Health Risks in Living Kidney Donors: A Systematic Review and Meta-analysis. Ann Intern Med. 2018;168(4):276–84.
51. Sanchez-Guerrero J, et al. A trial of contraceptive methods in women with systemic lupus erythematosus. N Engl J Med. 2005;353(24):2539–49.
52. Petri M, et al. Combined oral contraceptives in women with systemic lupus erythematosus. N Engl J Med. 2005;353(24): 2550–8.
53. Andreoli L, et al. EULAR recommendations for women's health and the management of family planning, assisted reproduction, pregnancy and menopause in patients with systemic lupus erythematosus and/or antiphospholipid syndrome. Ann Rheum Dis. 2017;76(3):476–85.

GPSR Compliance

The European Union's (EU) General Product Safety Regulation (GPSR) is a set of rules that requires consumer products to be safe and our obligations to ensure this.

If you have any concerns about our products, you can contact us on ProductSafety@springernature.com

In case Publisher is established outside the EU, the EU authorized representative is:

Springer Nature Customer Service Center GmbH
Europaplatz 3
69115 Heidelberg, Germany

Batch number: 10371111

Printed by Printforce, the Netherlands

Primer on Nephrology

Mark Harber
Editor

Primer on Nephrology

Second Edition

Volume II

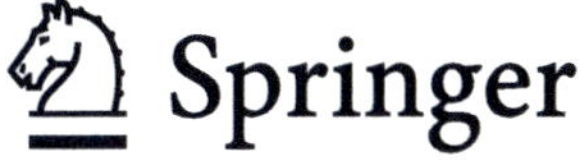

Editor
Mark Harber
Department of Renal Medicine
UCL
London, UK

ISBN 978-3-030-76421-0 ISBN 978-3-030-76419-7 (eBook)
https://doi.org/10.1007/978-3-030-76419-7

This Springer imprint is published by the registered company Springer Nature Switzerland AG
The registered company address is: Gewerbestrasse 11, 6330 Cham, Switzerland

Preface

The forerunner to *Primer in Nephrology*, *Practical Nephrology*, was published in 2014 and aimed to provide a clear, modern account of nephrology with a practical spin. The motivation for the book came from teaching and the acknowledgment that practical experience, examples of real-world nephrology (good and bad), and case discussions are an essential aspect of training. This edition of *Primer in Nephrology* is an update with the same ethos, but hopefully yet more experience imparted. In addition, much has happened both within and outside nephrology since 2014 that has transformed the practice, and this edition addresses major ongoing challenges for our patients and staff as well as key questions for us as nephrologists.

Our knowledge and understanding of acute kidney injury (AKI) have grown substantially, particularly the appreciation of the long-term impacts of moderate to severe AKI on renal function and frailty, with significant implications for patients who survive episodes of AKI. AKI is not only emerging as an important cause of chronic kidney disease (CKD) but CKD is also an important risk factor for AKI. In the context of a massive increase in the global prevalence of CKD, secondary to an aging population with multiple comorbidities, this represents a major test for nephrologists specifically and healthcare providers in general. By way of a medical counterattack, there have been many exciting new treatments in nephrology over the last few years. In particular, the development of GLA-1 receptor agonists and SGLT-2 inhibitors that significantly slow the progression of diabetic nephropathy and markedly mitigate the risk of cardiovascular comorbidities is particularly welcome. The observation that SGLT-2 inhibitors are equally effective in protecting non-diabetic patients with heavy proteinuria from renal progression and cardiovascular disease offers huge potential in combating progressive renal disease. The real challenge for us, however, is implementation of all the measures we know to prevent the development and severe consequences of CKD and cardiovascular co-morbidity. How do we as a specialty tackle major healthcare inequalities and ensure that patients from all backgrounds and in all communities are identified early, supported, and treated to deliver the best outcome?

The COVID-19 pandemic has shaken the world and pummeled health services. It has demonstrated the susceptibility of patients with end-stage renal disease, particularly those with no choice but to attend hospital dialysis as well as those who are immunosuppressed. It has highlighted the critical importance for our patients of prevention of infectious disease in the form of good infection control and vaccination. The early pandemic revealed nephropathies associations with this virus but most strikingly it has reminded us of the importance of appropriate fluid replacement in sepsis; when anxiety about wet lungs, and relative fluid restriction, contributed to a huge surge in hospital AKI. This unintended consequence, in turn, demonstrated the vulnerability of supply chains for acute renal replacement therapy and engendered an unprecedented cooperation between nephrologists and intensivists, working in a less rigid and more dynamic way across regions supporting colleagues outside usual arrangements. We have rapidly learned to assess patients in virtual clinics, been forced to become more fluent with setting ceilings of treatment and guiding patients and families through end-of-life care in profoundly stressful circumstances, as well as adapting to deliver background renal medicine including transplantation, and treatment of autoimmune diseases with the minimum possible risk. It has also reminded us of the selfless dedication, value, and, at times, vulnerability of frontline workers in the healthcare sector. We have learned a great deal over the last 2 years and adapted rapidly in our patient's interests. A key question is how many of the positive aspects of practice will we preserve post pandemic, and will we retain our capacity to innovate imaginatively when things normalize?

The above questions are germane to another, greater global crisis, that of the climate emergency. It is still very difficult to discuss the scientifically backed implications of global warming without seeming to resort to hyperbole. But the bottom line from the 6th International Panel on Climate Change was that "climate change is real, man made, rapid and unprecedented. That temperatures will continue to rise in all scenarios. Species extinction, widespread disease, unlivable heat, ecosystem collapse and cities menaced by rising seas will become painfully obvious before a child born today turns 30." Or put it another way, approximately 1 billion, nearly half the world's population of children, currently live in regions at extreme risk of environmental stresses from flooding to drought, extreme heat, ecosystem collapse, and famine. Low-income countries will bear the brunt initially, but high-income countries are already seeing extreme weather events and a dawning of the disorder this will cause. The multitude of ways climate change will affect patients with kidney conditions are not difficult to imagine, but supply-chain disruption including energy, food, and water will occur. In 2019, there were estimated to be approximately 80 million refugees or internally displace individuals. Extremes of heat, flooding, and famine will inevitably contribute to a huge increase in this number. Optimizing the care of patients with lifelong CKD or those receiving renal replacement therapy as the consequences of climate change or war, will become increasingly demanding, especially for those who are displaced or in high-risk regions. We face the most serious practical, ethical, and financial issues, many of which are not difficult to predict, and yet our collective response has thus far been grossly inadequate.

The healthcare sector is responsible for roughly 5% of CO_2 emissions, and nephrology has a disproportionately large carbon footprint, so we have a particular obligation to address this and start thinking sustainably. The good news is that, as recently demonstrated, we are at our best when free to innovate and invent. In this context, there are huge changes afoot in healthcare with rapidly developing alliances of like-minded people and green nephrology networks aimed at sustainable change and using the financial clout of the healthcare sector to catalyze change in providers. And then there is us, healthcare professionals who have had a crash course in supporting each other and remodeling, who like science, evidence, and facts, the wealth of which mean it is not difficult to predict the challenges ahead. As a profession, we are well regarded and have a responsibility to influence change and change the ethos of the institutions we work in with vigor and urgency.

I hope that this edition not only serves as a useful and engaging text on nephrology but also invites us all to ambitiously reassess practice with the aim of achieving the best possible experience and outcomes for our patients.

Mark Harber
Hampstead
London, UK

Acknowledgments

As with the previous edition, *Practical Nephrology*, I would like to thank again the generosity of the numerous authors who have contributed to this book. For most, clinical practice over the last 2 years has been particularly punishing and all consuming, so I remain especially indebted to all those authors have over the years taught me much of the nephrology I know and who contributed so generously and with such tolerance.

I am also particularly grateful to those who have very generously contributed to the additional material used in the book, especially Sue Car and Peter Topham, Steve Holt and Michael Ci, Mr. Peter Veitch, Arundi Mahendran, Justin Harris, Dominic Yu, Shella Sandoval, Ramesh Batra, Hannah Deltrey-King, Amanda Rea, and David Bishop who have produced videos that demonstrate procedures with much greater clarity than I could have achieved in prose and that I hope will assist doctors in carrying out these procedures with safety and confidence. I would particularly like to thank Paul Sweny for his mentorship and for the gift of his collection of clinical images accumulated over the years of frontline service. Histological images were generously provided by Lauren Heptinstall, Paul Bass, Alec Howie, Catherine Horsfield, and Mared Casey-Owen.

Once again, my heartfelt thanks to our patients who have contributed to this book in so many ways and who remain the key motivation behind this book.

Contents

Volume I

IV Hypertension and Renovascular Diseases

V Glomerular Diseases

Contributors

Ali Abdall-Razak, BSc Imperial College School of Medicine, London, UK
ali.abdall-razak14@imperial.ac.uk

Shahid Abdullah, MBBS, MRCP Salford Royal NHS Foundation Trust, Salford, UK
Manchester Royal Infirmary, Manchester, UK

Asmat Abro, MBBS, MRCP UCL Centre for Nephrology, Royal Free Hospital, London, UK
Department of Renal Medicine and Transplantation, Royal Free Hospital, London, UK
a.abro@nhs.net

Sarah Afuwape Department of Nephrology and Transplantation, Royal Free London NHS Foundation Trust, London, UK
sarah.afuwape@nhs.net

John Agar University Hospital Geelong and Deakin University School of Medicine, Barwon Health, Geelong, VIC, Australia
geerenal@ncable.net.au

Yogita Aggarwal University Hospitals of Coventry and Warwickshire NHS Trust, London, UK
Yogita.Aggarwal@uhb.nhs.uk

Nikita Agrawal North Middlesex University Hospital NHS Trust, London, UK
nikita.agrawal@nhs.net

Ammar Al Midani Department of Nephrology & Transplantation, Royal Free London NHS Foundation Trust, London, UK
ammar.almidani@nhs.net

Inji Alshaer North Middlesex University Hospital NHS Trust, London, UK
Inji.alshaer@nhs.net

Rakesh Anand, BSc, MSc, MBBS, MRCP Royal Free London NHS Foundation Trust, London, UK
rakesh.anand1@nhs.net

Marilina Antonelou Department of Renal Medicine, University College London and Royal Free London NHS Foundation Trust, London, UK
Department of Renal Medicine, University College London, London, UK
Marilina.antonelou@nhs.net

Ravi Armstron Johannesburg, South Africa

Caroline Ashley, BPharm (Hons), FFRPS, FRPharmS Department of Pharmacy, Royal Free London NHS Foundation Trust, London, UK
carolineashley@nhs.net

Domenico Bagordo, MD Nephrology Unit, Sapienza University of Rome, Rome, Italy
d.bagordo@ucl.ac.uk

Richard J. Baker, MBBChir, MA, FRCP, PhD Renal Medicine, St James's University Hospital, Leeds, UK
Richard-j.baker@nhs.net

Simon Ball Queen Elizabeth Hospital, Birmingham, UK
Simon.Ball@uhb.nhs.uk

Ravi Barod Royal Free London, London, UK
r.barod@nhs.net

Jonathan Barratt The John Walls Renal Unit, Leicester General Hospital, University Hospitals of Leicester, Leicester, UK
jb81@le.ac.uk

Chathurika Beligaswatta Department of Renal Medicine, UCL, London, UK
chathurika.beligswatta@nhs.net

Christopher O. C. Bellamy Department of Renal Medicine, Royal Infirmary of Edinburgh, Edinburgh, UK

Sanjay Bhagani Royal Free London Hospital, London, UK

Department of Infectious Diseases/HIV Medicine, Royal Free Hospital, London, UK
s.bhagani@nhs.net

Hannah Blakey Renal Department, Queen Elizabeth Hospital NHS Trust, Birmingham, UK
hannah.blakey2@uhb.nhs.uk

Sarah Blakey Hammersmith Hospital, Imperial College Healthcare NHS Trust, London, UK
sarahblakey@nhs.net

Detlef Bockenhauer University College London, Great Ormond Street Hospital, London, UK
d.bockenhauer@ucl.ac.uk

Ekaterini Boleti Kidney Cancer Centre, Royal Free Hospital, London, UK
ekaterini.boleti@nhs.net

John Booth Royal London Hospital, Department of Nephrology, London, UK
John.booth@bartshealth.nhs.uk

James Brown Department of Respiratory Medicine, Royal Free London NHS Foundation Trust, London, UK
james.brown13@nhs.net

Sinéad Burke Royal Free London NHS Foundation Trust, London, UK
sinead.burke@nhs.net

Áine Burns Royal Free Hospital, London, UK
Aine.burns@nhs.net

Michael X. Cai The Royal Melbourne Hospital, Melbourne, VIC, Australia
Michael.Cai@mh.org.au

Chris J. Callaghan, PhD, FRCS University Department of Surgery, Addenbrooke's Hospital, Cambridge, UK
chris.callaghan@gstt.nhs.uk

Stephanie Camilleri Mater Dei Hospital, Valletta, Malta
Stephanie.b.camillia@gov.mt

Ben Caplin, BSc (Hons), MBChB, PhD UCL Medical School, Royal Free Campus, London, UK
Department of Renal Medicine, UCL Medical School, Royal Free Campus, London, UK
Department of Renal Medicine, University College London, London, UK
b.caplin@ucl.ac.uk

Paul J. Champion de Crespigny The Royal Melbourne Hospital, Melbourne, VIC, Australia
Paul.ChampiondeCrespigny@mh.org.au

Melanie M. Y. Chan, MRCP UCL Department of Renal Medicine, Royal Free Hospital, London, UK
melanie.chan@nhs.net

Rawya Charif, MRCP, MD (Res) Imperial College Kidney and Transplant Centre, Imperial College Healthcare NHS Trust, Hammersmith Hospital, London, UK
Rawya.Charif@nhs.net

Lindsay Chesterton, FRCP, DM Department of Renal Medicine, Royal Derby Hospital, Derby, UK
lindsay.chesterton@nhs.net

Chee Kay Cheung University of Leicester, Leicester, UK
ckc15@le.ac.uk

Roohi Chhabra Royal Free Hospital, London, UK
roohi.chhabra@nhs.net

Stephanie M. Y. Chong Department of Nephrology, Royal Free Hospital, London, UK
Stephanie.chong1@nhs.net

Pratima Chowdary, MBBS, MRCP, FRCPath Katharine Dormandy Haemophilia and Thrombosis Centre, Royal Free London NHS Foundation Trust, London, UK
Department of Haematology, University College London, London, UK
P.chowdary@ucl.ac.uk

Paul Cockwell Department of Renal Medicine, Queen Elizabeth Hospital Birmingham, Birmingham, UK
Paul.Cockwell@uhb.nhs.uk

John O. Connolly, PhD, FRCP UCL Department of Renal Medicine, Royal Free Hospital, London, UK
johnconnolly@nhs.net

Thomas M. F. Connor Oxford Kidney Unit, Churchill Hospital, Oxford, UK
thomas.connor@ouh.nhs.uk

Bryan Conway Department of Renal Medicine, Royal Infirmary of Edinburgh, Edinburgh, UK
Bryan.Conway@nhslothian.scot.nhs.uk

Richard W. Corbett Hammersmith Hospital, Imperial College Healthcare NHS Trust, London, UK
rwcorbett@nhs.net

A. E. Courtney Regional Nephrology & Transplant Unit, Belfast City Hospital, Belfast, UK
aisling.courtney@belfasttrust.hscni.net

Jeff Cove Renal Psychology Service, Royal Free London NHS Foundation Trust, London, UK
j.cove@nhs.net

Alison Craik Freeman Hospital, Newcastle Upon Tyne, UK
alison.craik2@nhs.net

Jennifer Cross Royal Free London NHS Foundation Trust, London, UK

Royal Free Hospital, London, UK
jennifer.cross@nhs.net

John Cunningham UCL Centre for Nephrology, The Royal Free Hospital, London, UK

Sunil K. Daga, MBBS, MRCP (Nephrology), PhD Renal Medicine, St James's University Hospital, Leeds, UK
Sunildaga@nhs.net

Andrew Davenport UCL Centre for Nephrology, Royal Free Hospital, University College London Medical School, London, UK

University College London, London, UK
Andrewdavenport@nhs.net

Sara N. Davison University of Alberta, Edmonton, AB, Canada
Sara.davison@ualberta.ca

Clara Day Renal Department, Queen Elizabeth Hospital Birmingham, Birmingham, UK
clara.day@uhb.nhs.uk

Neeraj Dhaun, MD Centre for Cardiovascular Science, University of Edinburgh, The Queen's Medical Research Institute, Edinburgh, UK
bean.dhaun@ed.ac.uk

Geraint Dingley Wessex Kidney Centre, Portsmouth, UK

Philippa Dodd Whittington Hospital, London, UK
Phillipa.dodd@nhs.net

Gavin Dreyer Barts Health NHS Trust, London, UK

Peter J. Dupont, PhD, FRCPI Department of Renal Medicine, University College London, Royal Free Hospital, London, UK
pdupont@nhs.net

Cathy Egan Moorfields Eye Hospital, London, UK
cathy.egan@nhs.net

Nasirul Jabir Ekbal Royal Free London NHS Foundation Trust, London, UK
Nasirul.Ekbal@nhs.net

Timothy John Ellam Renal Services, The Newcastle upon Tyne Hospitals NHS Foundation Trust, Newcastle upon Tyne, UK
timothy.ellam@nuth.nhs.uk

Rhys Evans University College London, London, UK
rhys.evans@ucl.ac.uk

Stanley Fan Consultant Nephrologists, The Royal London Hospital, Barts Health NHS Trust, London, UK
fan.stanley@bartshealth.nhs.uk

John Feehally University of Leicester, Rutland, UK
jf27@leicester.ac.uk

Raymond Fernando, BSc, PhD Department of Renal Medicine, University College London & The Anthony Nolan Laboratory, Royal Free Hospital, London, UK
raymond.fernando@nhs.net

Richard S. Fish University Hospitals of North Midlands, Stoke-on-Trent, UK
rsfish@doctors.org.uk

Richard J. Fluck, FRCP, MA (Cantab), MBBS Department of Renal Medicine, Royal Derby Hospital, Derby, UK
richard.fluck@nhs.net

Suzanne H. Forbes, MBBS, MRCP, MD Department of Nephrology, The Royal London Hospital, Barts Health NHS Trust, London, UK
Suzanne.Forbes@bartshealth.nhs.uk

Antje Fürstenberg-Schaette Nephrology, Nierenzentrum Stendal-Gardelegen MVZ, Stendal, Germany

Alice Gage Royal Free London NHS Foundation Trust, London, UK
alice.gage1@nhs.net

Daniel Gale, MA, MB, BChir, PhD, FRCP Department of Renal Medicine, University College London, Royal Free Hospital, London, UK
d.gale@ucl.ac.uk

Jack Galliford, MBBS, FRCP Richard Bright Renal Unit, Southmead Hospital, Bristol, UK
Jack.Galliford@nbt.nhs.uk

David Game, MA, PhD, FRCP Department of Nephrology and Transplantation, Guy's Hospital, London, UK
David.Game@gstt.nhs.uk

Conall Mac Gearailt Galway University Hospital, Galway, Ireland
conall.macgearailt@hse.ie

Julian D. Gillmore UK National Amyloidosis Centre, University College London and Royal Free Hospital London NHS Foundation Trust, London, UK
j.gillmore@ucl.ac.uk

Jane Goddard Department of Renal Medicine, Royal Infirmary of Edinburgh, Edinburgh, UK
Unkn2134@meteor.com

Gabrielle Goldet Royal Free Hospital, London, UK
gabrielle.goldet@nhs.net

Antony Goode Department of Radiology, Royal Free Hospital, London, UK
Antony.goode1@nhs.net

Darren Green Vascular Research Group, Manchester Academic Health Sciences Center, University of Manchester, Salford Royal NHS Foundation Trust, Stott Lane, Salford, UK
Unkn524@meteor.com

George H. B. Greenhall, MRCP(Neph.), MBChB, MSc Department of Statistics and Clinical Research, NHS Blood and Transplant, Bristol, UK
georgegreenhall@nhs.net

Pooja Mehta Gudka Renal Services, Department of Pharmacy, Royal Free London NHS Foundation Trust, London, UK
Poojamehta.gudka@nhs.net

Angela D. Gupta, MD Texas Childrens Pediatric Urology Clinic, Houston, TX, USA
agupta45@jhmi.edu

Asheeta Gupta, BSc, BMedSci, BMBS, MRCPCH Department of Nephrology, Birmingham Women's and Children's NHS Foundation Trust, Steelhouse Lane, Birmingham, UK
asheeta.gupta@nhs.net

Sanjana Gupta, MBBS, MSc, MRCP, DPMSA Royal Free and Royal London Hospital, London, UK
University College London, London, UK
sanjana.gupta@ucl.ac.uk

Zoya Hameed, BSc, MBBS, MSc, FRCOphth Royal Free London NHS Foundation Trust, London, UK
Zoya.hameed@nhs.net

Sally Hamour Department of Renal Medicine, University College London and Royal Free London NHS Foundation Trust, London, UK
sallyhamour@nhs.net

Tanzina Haque Royal Free Hospital, London, UK
thaque@nhs.net

Mark Harber, MBBS, PhD, FRCP Department of Renal Medicine UCL, London, UK
mark.harber@nhs.net

Justin Harris Royal Free London NHS Foundation Trust, London, UK
justinharris@nhs.net

Gerlineke Hawkins-van der Cingel Royal Free London NHS Foundation Trust, London, UK
gerlineke.hawkins-vandercingel@nhs.net

Scott R. Henderson UCL Centre for Nephrology, Royal Free Hospital, London, UK
scotthenderson@nhs.net

Heidy Hendra Department of Nephrology & Transplantation, Royal Free London NHS Foundation Trust, London, UK
Royal Free London NHS Foundation Trust, London, UK
heidy.hendra1@nhs.net

Joanne Henry Department of Nephrology and Transplantation, Royal Free London NHS Foundation Trust, London, UK
joannehenry@nhs.net

Lauren Heptinstall Royal Free London NHS Foundation Trust, London, UK
lauren.heptinstall@nhs.net

Sarah Hildebrand Royal Free London NHS Foundation Trust, London, UK
sarah.hildebrand2@nhs.net

Peter Hill West London Renal and Transplant Centre, Hammersmith Hospital, Imperial College Health Trust, London, UK
peter.hill4@nhs.net

Aroon Hingorani UCL Division of Biosciences, London, UK
a.hingorani@ucl.ac.uk

Stephen G. Holt, BSc, MBBS, PhD, FRCP, FRACP The University of Melbourne, School of Medicine, Melbourne, VIC, Australia
steve.holt@mh.org.au

Sally-Anne Hulton, MBBCh, FCP(Paeds)SA, FRCPCH, MD Birmingham Women's Childrens and Children's NHS Foundation Trust, Birmingham, UK
sally.hulton@nhs.net

Rachel K. Y. Hung Department of Nephrology, Royal Free Hospital, London, UK
Royal Free Hospital, Department of Nephrology, London, UK
R.hung@nhs.net

Buddhika Illeperuma Royal Free London NHS Foundation Trust, London, UK
Buddhika.Illeperuma@nhs.net

Ferina Ismail, BSc, MBBS, MRCP, PhD Department of Dermatology, Royal Free London NHS Foundation Trust, London, UK
ferina.ismail@nhs.net

Alan Jaap Department of Diabetes, Royal Infirmary of Edinburgh, Edinburgh, UK
Unkn3134@meteor.com

Aneesa Jaffer Department of Nephrology & Transplantation, Royal Free London NHS Foundation Trust, London, UK
aneesa.jaffer@nhs.net

Paramjit Jeetley Department of Cardiology, Royal Free London NHS Foundation Trust, London, UK
paramjit.jeetley@nhs.net

Sarah Jenkins, FRCP Sheffield Kidney Institute, Sheffield, UK
sarah.jenkins@sth.nhs.uk

Jennie Jewitt-Harris Transplant Links, Camberley, UK
info@transplantlinks.org

Gareth Jones North Middlesex University Hospital NHS Trust, London, UK
gareth.jones14@nhs.net

Philip A. Kalra, MA, MB, BChir, FRCP, MD Vascular Research Group, Manchester Academic Health Sciences Center, University of Manchester, Salford Royal NHS Foundation Trust, Stott Lane, Salford, UK

Department of Renal Medicine, Salford Royal NHS Foundation Trust, Stott Lane, Salford, UK
philip.kalra@srft.nhs.uk

Nigel Suren Kanagasundaram The Newcastle upon Tyne Hospitals NHS Foundation Trust, Newcastle upon Tyne, UK
suren.kanagasundaram@newcastle.ac.uk

Zuze Kawale The Queen Elizabeth Central Hospital, Blantyre, Malawi

Maryam Khosravi Royal Free Hospital, London, UK
m.khosravi@ucl.ac.uk

Ed Kingdon Brighton and Sussex University Hospital Trust, Brighton, UK
Sussex Kidney Unit, Brighton and Sussex University Hospitals NHS Trust, Brighton, UK
ekingdon@nhs.net

David C. Kluth, MD Department of Renal Medicine, Royal Infirmary of Edinburgh, Edinburgh, UK
Centre for Cardiovascular Science, University of Edinburgh, The Queen's Medical Research Institute, Edinburgh, UK
David.Kluth@ed.ac.uk

Ellen Knox Obstetrics Department, Birmingham Women's Hospital, Birmingham, UK
ellen.knox1@nhs.net

Jeevan Kumaradevan Department of Radiology, Whittington Hospital, London, UK
jeevan.kumaradevan@nhs.net

Helen J. Lachmann UK National Amyloidosis Centre, University College London and Royal Free Hospital London NHS Foundation Trust, London, UK
h.lachmann@ucl.ac.uk

Chris Laing Department of Nephrology, University College London, London, UK
UCL Centre for Nephrology, Royal Free Hospital, London, UK
chris.laing@nhs.net

Katie Lane Guy's and St Thomas' NHS Foundation Trust, London, UK
Katie.Lane@nhs.net

Steven Law UCL Department of Renal Medicine, Royal Free Hospital, London, UK
stevenlaw@nhs.net

Ben Lindsey, FRCS Department of Vascular Surgery and Department of Renal Surgery, The Royal Free London NHS Foundation Trust, Hampstead, UK
ben.lindsey@nhs.net

Graham Lipkin Renal Department, Queen Elizabeth Hospital Birmingham, Birmingham, UK
graham.lipkin@uhb.nhs.uk

Mark A. Little Tallaght University Hospital, Dublin, Ireland
MLITTLE@tcd.ie

Rebecca Liu Royal Free Hospital, London, UK
rebecca.liu@nhs.net

Olivia Lucas Barts Cancer Centre, St Bartholomew's Hospital, London, UK
olivia.lucas@nhs.net

Valerie Luyckx University of Cape Town, Cape Town, South Africa
Harvard Medical School, Boston, MA, USA
valerie.luyckx@uzh.ch

Bernadette Lynch Galway University Hospital, Galway, Ireland
bernadette.lynch4@hse.ie

Douglas Macdonald Royal Free Hospital, Department of Gastroenterology, London, UK
douglasmacdonald@nhs.net

Iain C. Macdougall, BSc, MD, FRCP London, UK
iain.macdougall@nhs.net

Iain A. M. MacPhee St George's, University of London, London, UK
imacphee@sgul.ac.uk

Ciara N. Magee UCL Centre for Nephrology, Royal Free Hospital, London, UK
Ciara.magee@nhs.net

Hannah Maple, FRCS, PhD Department of Nephrology and Transplantation, Guy's Hospital, London, UK
Hannah.Maple@gstt.nhs.uk

Stephen D. Marks, MD, MSc, MRCP, DCH, FRCPCH Professor of Paediatric Nephrology and Transplantation, University College London Great Ormond Street Institute of Child Health and Great Ormond Street Hospital for Children NHS Foundation Trust, London, UK
stephen.marks@gosh.nhs.uk

Philip David Mason, BSc, PhD, MBBS, FRCP Oxford Kidney Unit, The Churchill Hospital, Headington, Oxford, UK
Phil.Mason@ouh.nhs.uk

Phil Masson Royal Free Hospital, London, UK
philip.masson@nhs.net

David Mathew Department of Nephrology & Transplantation, Royal Free London NHS Foundation Trust, London, UK
david.mathew2@nhs.net

Alexander P. Maxwell, MD, PhD, FRCP Regional Nephrology Unit, Belfast City Hospital, Belfast, Antrim, UK
Centre for Public Health, Queens University Belfast, Institute of Clinical Sciences, Block B, Royal Victoria Hospital, Belfast, Antrim, Ireland
a.p.maxwell@qub.ac.uk

Patrick H. Maxwell University of Cambridge, Cambridge, UK
Regius@medschl.cam.ac.uk

Stephen P. McAdoo Centre for Inflammatory Disease, Department of Medicine, Imperial College London, London, UK
s.mcadoo@imperial.ac.uk

Fiona McCaig Royal Free London NHS Foundation Trust, London, UK
fionamccaig@nhs.net

Adam McLean, MA, MBBS, FRCP, DPhil Imperial College Kidney and Transplant Centre, Hammersmith Hospital, Imperial College Healthcare NHS Trust, London, UK
AdamMclean@nhs.net

Breeda McManus Barts Health NHS Trust, London, UK
breeda.mcmanus@bartshealth.nhs.uk

Clare Melikian Department of Anaesthesia, Royal Free London NHS Foundation Trust, London, UK
c.melikian@nhs.net

Stephen Mepham Royal Free London NHS Foundation Trust, London, UK
stephen.mepham@nhs.net

Shona Methven, BSc, MBChB, MD, MRCP, FRCP(Edin) Aberdeen Royal Infirmary, Aberdeen, UK
shona.methven@nhs.net

Eve Miller-Hodges, MD Department of Renal Medicine, Royal Infirmary of Edinburgh, Edinburgh, UK

Centre for Cardiovascular Science, University of Edinburgh, The Queen's Medical Research Institute, Edinburgh, UK
Eve.miller-hodges@ed.ac.uk

Shabbir H. Moochhala UCL Department of Renal Medicine, Royal Free Hospital, Royal Free Hospital, London, UK

Royal Free Hospital, London, UK
smoochhala@nhs.net

Frances Mortimer Centre for Sustainable Healthcare, Oxford, UK
frances.mortimer@sustainablehealthcare.org.uk

Fliss E. M. Murtagh Hull York Medical School, University of Hull, Hull, UK
fliss.murtagh@hyms.ac.uk

Vasantha Muthu Muthuppalaniappan Royal Free Hospital, London, UK

Queen Elizabeth Hospital, Birmingham, UK
vasantha.muthuppalaniappan@nhs.net

Anna Nagy Royal Free Hospital, London, UK
anna.nagy@ucl.ac.uk

David Nicol Department of Urology, Royal Marsden Hospital & Institute of Cancer Research, London, UK
davidnicol@nhs.net

Dorothea Nitsch, MD, MSc Department of Non-Communicable Disease Epidemiology, Faculty of Epidemiology and Population Health, London School of Hygiene and Tropical Medicine, London, UK
dorothea.nitsch@lshtm.ac.uk

Aisling O'Riordan Department of Nephrology, St. Vincent's University Hospital, Dublin, Ireland
aisling.oriordan@svhg.ie

Thomas Oates Royal London Hospital, London, UK

Amin Oomatia, MRCP, MBBChir, MA (Cantab) Department of Nephrology, Royal Free London NHS Foundation Trust, London, UK
amin.oomatia@nhs.net

Mared Owen-Casey, MBBCh, FRCPath Histopathology Department, Betsi Cadwaladar University Health Board, Wrexham, UK
mared.owencasey@wales.nhs.uk

Padmasayee Papineni Northwick Park Hospital, London, UK
p.papineni1@nhs.net

Arum Parthipun Department of Radiology, Royal Free Hospital, London, UK
Arum.parthipun@nhs.net

Katharine Pates, MBBS, MBiochem Department of Renal Medicine, UCL Medical School, Royal Free Campus, London, UK
Unknown_54098@Meteor.com

Alan Patrick Department of Diabetes, Royal Infirmary of Edinburgh, Edinburgh, UK
Unkn5134@meteor.com

Ruth J. Pepper Royal Free Hospital, London, UK
UCL Centre for Nephrology, Royal Free Hospital, London, UK
r.pepper@ucl.ac.uk

Alfredo Petrosino Department of Nephrology, Royal Free Hospital, London, UK
alfredo.petrosino@nhs.net

Benedict L. Phillips, BSc (Hons), MSc, MRCS Renal and Transplant Surgery, Guy's Hospital, London, UK
benedict.phillips@nhs.uk

Jennifer Pinney Department of Renal Medicine, Queen Elizabeth Hospital Birmingham, Birmingham, UK
Jennifer.Pinney@uhb.nhs.uk

Liam Plant Department of Renal Medicine, Cork University Hospital & University College Cork, Cork, Ireland
william.plant@ucc.ie

Madhu Potluri, MBCHB, MRCP UK, MRCP Gloucestershire Hospitals NHS Foundation Trust, Cheltenham, UK
madhupotluri@nhs.net

Nithya Prasannan, MBBS, MRCP, FRCPath Katharine Dormandy Haemophilia and Thrombosis Centre, Royal Free London NHS Foundation Trust, London, UK
Department of Haematology, University College London, London, UK

Maria Prendecki Centre for Inflammatory Disease, Department of Immunology and Inflammation, Imperial College London, London, UK
m.prendecki@imperial.ac.uk

Zudin Puthucheary William Harvey Research Institute, Barts and The London School of Medicine and Dentistry, Queen Mary University of London, Royal London Hospital, Barts Health NHS Trust, London, UK
z.puthucheary@nhs.net

Ravindra Rajakariar Barts Health NHS Trust, London, UK
ravindra.rajakariar@bartshealth.nhs.uk

Gayathri Rajakaruna University College London, London, UK
g.rajakaruna@ucl.ac.uk

Ritika Rana Department of Renal Medicine, Queen Elizabeth Hospital Birmingham, Birmingham, UK
Ritika.Rana@uhb.nhs.uk

Andrew Ready University Hospital Birmingham, Birmingham, UK

Transplant Links, Camberley, UK
andrew.ready@uhb.nhs.com

James Ritchie Vascular Research Group, Manchester Academic Health Sciences Center, University of Manchester, Salford Royal NHS Foundation Trust, Stott Lane, Salford, UK
james.ritchie@nca.nhs.uk

Candice Roufosse Imperial College, London, UK
Candice.roufosse@nhs.net

Adam Rumjon, MBBS, PhD, MRCP North Middlesex University Hospital, Sterling Way, London, UK
adamrumjon@nhs.net

Gill Rumsby, PhD, FRCPath UCL Hospitals, London, UK
gill.rumsby@nhs.net

Omid Sadeghi-Alavijeh Royal Free Hospital, London, UK
omid.sadeghi-alavijeh@nhs.net

Alan D. Salama, MBBS, MA, PhD, FRCP University College London, London, UK

Royal Free Hospital, London, UK

UCL Department of Renal Medicine Royal Free Hospital, London, UK
a.salama@ucl.ac.uk

Nasreen Samad Consultant Nephrologists, The Royal London Hospital, Barts Health NHS Trust, London, UK
nareen.samad@bartshealth.nhs.uk

Jennifer Scott Trinity Health Kidney Centre, Dublin, Ireland

Haresh Selvaskandan The John Walls Renal Unit, Leicester General Hospital, University Hospitals of Leicester, Leicester, UK
haresh.selvaskandan@nhs.net

Claire C. Sharpe Department of Inflammation Biology, Faculty of Life Sciences and Medicine, King's College London, London, UK
Claire.sharpe@kcl.ac.uk

Neil S. Sheerin National Renal Complement Therapeutic Centre, Translational and Clinical Research Institute, Newcastle University, Newcastle upon Tyne, UK
neil.sheerin@ncl.ac.uk

Ali M. Shendi, MD Faculty of Medicine, Zagazig University, Zagazig, Egypt

Nephrology Unit, Internal Medicine Department, Faculty of Medicine, Zagazig University, Zagazig, Egypt
ali.shendi@zu.edu.eg

Kin Yee Shiu, MBBS, PhD, FRCP Department of Renal Medicine, University College London, Royal Free Hospital, London, UK
kinyee.shiu@nhs.net

Badri Shrestha, MD, FRCS Sheffield Kidney Institute, Sheffield, UK
badri.shrestha@sth.nhs.uk

Ruth Silverton University College London Medical School, Department of Postgraduate Medical Education, London, UK

Cambridge University Hospitals NHS Foundation Trust, Department of Renal Medicine, Cambridge, UK
ruth.silverton@doctors.org.uk

James Smith, BSc, MBChB, PhD, MRCP Abderdeen Royal Infirmary, Foresterhill, Aberdeen, UK
jsmith82@nhs.net

Reecha Sofat UCL Institute of Health Informatics, London, UK
r.sofat@ucl.ac.uk

Henry Stephens, BSc, PhD Department of Renal Medicine, University College London & The Anthony Nolan Laboratory, Royal Free Hospital, London, UK
h.stephens@ucl.ac.uk

Dinesha Himali Sudusinghe Faculty of Medical Sciences, University of Sri Jayewardenepura, Sri Lanka, Colombo, Sri Lanka

James Tomlinson Royal Free London NHS Foundation Trust, London, UK
James.tomlinson3@nhs.net

Charles R. V. Tomson, MA, BMBCh, FRCP, DM (Oxon) Newcastle upon Tyne Hospitals NHS Foundation Trust, Newcastle upon Tyne, UK

Freeman Hospital, Newcastle upon Tyne, UK
charles.tomson1@nhs.net

Caroline Tulley Royal Free London NHS Foundation Trust, London, UK
caroline.tulley@nhs.net

A. Neil Turner, PhD, FRCP Centre for Inflammation, University of Edinburgh, QMRI, Edinburgh, UK
neil.turner@ed.ac.uk

M. Umaid Rauf Royal Free Hospital, London, UK
m.rauf@nhs.net

Robert Unwin UCL Department of Renal Medicine, Royal Free Hospital, Royal Free Hospital, London, UK
robert.unwin@ucl.ac.uk

Diana Vassallo Vascular Research Group, Manchester Academic Health Sciences Center, University of Manchester, Salford Royal NHS Foundation Trust, Stott Lane, Salford, UK
Unk534@meteor.com

Stephen B. Walsh University College London, London, UK
stephen.walsh@ucl.ac.uk

Elizabeth R. Wan University College London, London, UK
e.mumford@nhs.net

Thuvaraka Ware Department of Nephrology, Royal Free Hospital, London, UK
Royal Free Hospital, London, UK
thuvaraka.ware@nhs.net

Christopher J. E. Watson, MA, MD, FRCS University Department of Surgery, Addenbrooke's Hospital, Cambridge, UK
cjew2@cam.ac.uk

Lakshman Weerasekara Royal Free London NHS Foundation Trust, London, UK
Lakshman.weerasjara@nhs.net

David C. Wheeler, MD, FRCP Department of Renal Medicine, UCL Medical School, Royal Free Campus, London, UK
d.wheeler@ucl.ac.uk

William White Departments of Acute Medicine & Nephrology, Royal London Hospital, London, UK
william.white9@nhs.net

Dilushi Wijayaratne Department of Renal Medicine, UCL, London, UK
Dilushi.Wijajaratne@nhs.net

Martin Wilkie, MD, FRCP Sheffield Kidney Institute, Sheffield, UK
Sheffield Teaching Hospitals NHS, Sheffield, UK
martin.wilkie@nhs.net

Eleri Williams, MB, BChir, MRCP Centre for Inflammation, University of Edinburgh, QMRI, Edinburgh, UK
eleri.williams@doctors.org.uk

Elizabeth Williams Homerton University Hospital, London, UK
eawilliams@doctors.org.uk

Jo Wilson Royal Free Hospitals London NHS Foundation Trust and University of Bath, London, UK
jo.wilson8@nhs.net

Dan Wood, PhD, FRCS (Urol) Adolescent Urology, University College London Hospitals NHS Foundation Trust, London, UK
dan.wood1@nhs.net

Nick Woodward, MBBS, MRCP, FRCR Department of Radiology, Royal Free London NHS Foundation Trust, London, UK
nick.woodward@nhs.net

Dominic Yu Royal Free London NHS Foundation Trust, London, UK
dominic.yu@nhs.net

Urology and Nephrology

Contents

Urology Renal Interface

Stephanie Camilleri, Jeevan Kumaradevan, Ravi Barod, and Mark Harber

Contents

M. Harber (ed.), *Primer on Nephrology*, https://doi.org/10.1007/978-3-030-76419-7_53

Learning Objectives

1. To appreciate the extent of renal urology interface and consider the opportunities to enhance multidisciplinary care.
2. To identify protocols and pathways that can be jointly agreed upon across the region for haematuria, renal stones, and renal masses.
3. To consider ways of providing bidirectional teaching between urologists and nephrologists.

53.1 Introduction

Many patients with significant urological disorders will, at some point, develop AKI or CKD. Patients with CKD 3 or above are likely to have need of nephrology input, and there is very substantial evidence that patients who 'crash-land' onto dialysis without prior engagement with a nephrologist have a significantly worse outcome. Some patients investigated by urologists for haematuria will have 'renal' causes such as glomerulonephritis, many patients with renal stones will have underlying metabolic causes, and some patients presenting to urologists will have underlying multisystem renal tumour syndromes. Congenital abnormalities of the kidney and urinary tract (CAKUT) are the commonest cause of the end-stage renal disease (ESRD) in children, and such patients often require intervention and long-term urological support. In this group and others, recurrent urinary tract infection can plague patients with repeated sepsis and progressive renal impairment, the solution to which may also involve urological intervention. Finally, the management of both lower and upper urinary tract obstruction is very dependent on the expertise of urologists. In short, there are many circumstances where the optimum care of patients depends on a slick interface between urology and nephrology, yet this is often somewhat less organised and efficient than it could be. Renal transplantation epitomizes the benefits of surgeons and physicians cohabiting the same world of work, sharing protocols and working in a close multidisciplinary fashion to provide best care. Given the mortality associated with AKI and CKD, there is a clear imperative to developing close links, joint protocols, and service-level agreements with urology services. The challenge is to establish and maintain these links.

Most of the conditions described above are covered in their specific chapters; what follows is a brief overview of potential links between our two specialities.

53.2 Haematuria

Haematuria is a common presenting feature of renal and urological diseases, and in the case of overt visible (macroscopic) haematuria, there is a widely accepted urological pathway for investigation (although a number of conditions that require nephrology input, shown in Table 53.1 can present with visible haematuria). There are many guidelines for the diagnosis and evaluation of non-visible (microscopic) haematuria [1] (an example of which is shown in Fig. 53.1).

Efficient urology departments have devised 'one-stop' urological assessments. The principle aim for urologists is to diagnose or exclude renal, upper tract, and bladder tumours as well as non-malignant causes of urinary tract bleeding. The aim for the nephrologist is to diagnose or exclude significant 'renal' disease without over investigating everyone. For patients who don't have an obvious urological cause the possibilities become (a) a glomerular cause, (b) myoglobinuria or haemoglobinuria, (c) missed urological cause or rarely, and (d) fictitious haematuria [2, 3]. Making a pathway that reliably identifies who needs which test is surprisingly problematic. The renal association has issued thoughtful guidelines on the investigation of visible and non-visible

Table 53.1 List of 'renal' causes for **visible (macroscopic)** haematuria

IgA nephropathy frequent cause, often associated with URT infection
Postinfectious GN globally common, urine typically cola coloured
Polyarteritis Nodosa
Goodpasture's disease usually associated with proteinuria
GPA/MPA (vasculitis)
Thin basement membrane disease may be associated with URT infection
Alport's syndrome may be associated with URT infection
Urinary tract infection
Renal vein thrombosis likely to be associated with proteinuria
Papillary necrosis single episode possibly with obstruction
Ruptured or bleeding cyst common in patients with ADPKD
Bleeding angiomyolipoma consider tuberosclerosis complex
Renal haemorrhage/infarction consider underlying thrombophilia or vasculopathy

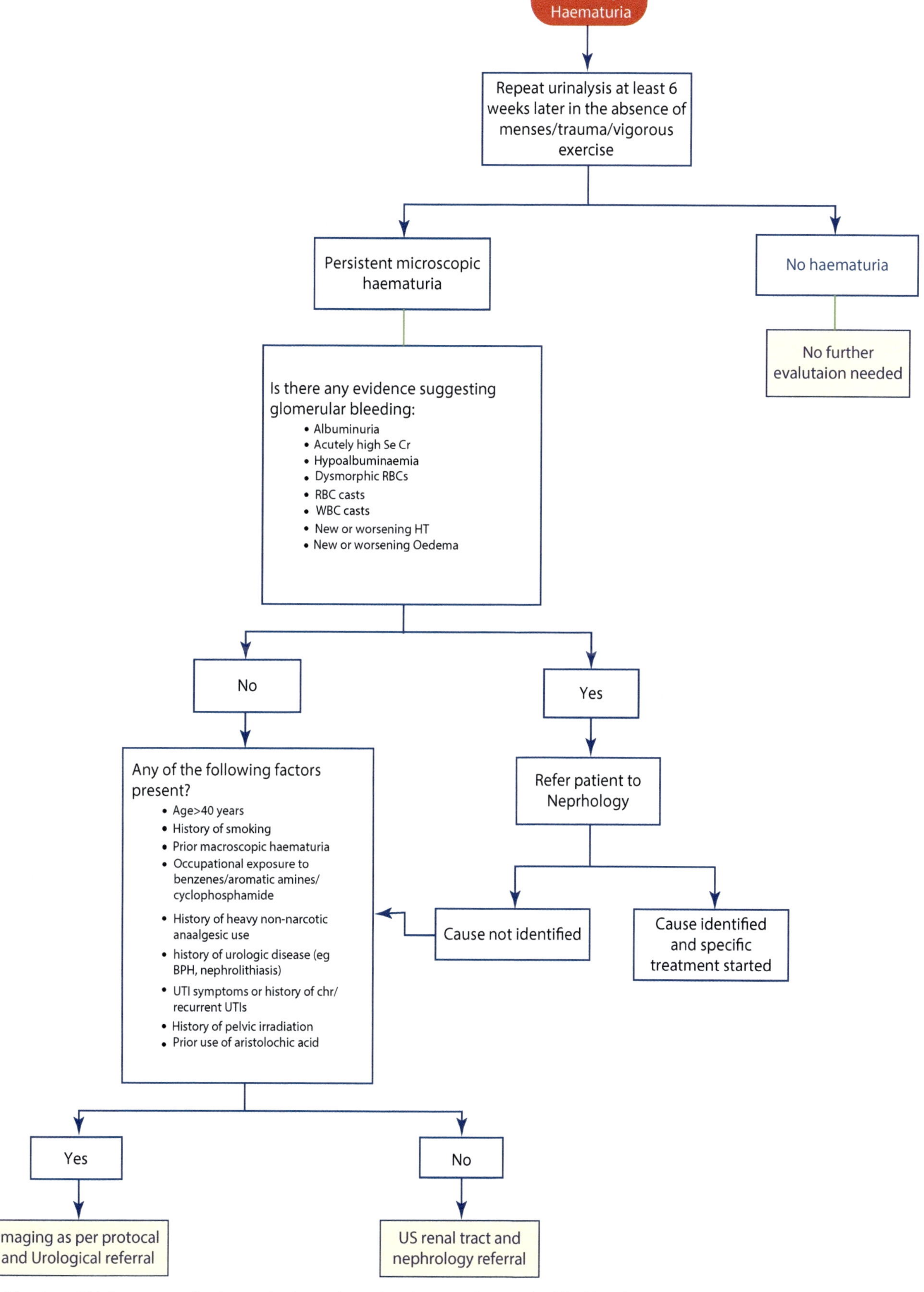

Fig. 53.1 This is one example of an evaluation pathway for adults with asymptomatic non-visible (microscopic) haematuria. There are many alternative versions of this; the principle is to embed a simple, robust method for identifying patients at risk of renal disease or conversely urological causes of haematuria so patients can be rapidly referred appropriately and also avoid unnecessary investigations

53

haematuria (see Chap. 2 on urine analysis), and it is commonly accepted that visible haematuria should be referred to a urologist for initial assessment (there are some caveats here, see below) [4]. Investigation of non-visible haematuria is complicated by the facts that (a) dipsticks are very sensitive (so guidelines usually recommend ignoring 'trace' and frequently 1^+) and (b) automated urine microscopy for RBC may be falsely negative if RBCs have time to haemolyse. Thus, for asymptomatic non-visible haematuria 2–3 positive dipsticks are recommended before referral having excluded urinary tract infection. Conventionally, patients over 40 are referred for upper tract imaging and cystoscopy to exclude a urological cause. What needs to be built into the urology and nephrology pathways is the identification of patients who are at increased *risk of renal disease* and malignancy, respectively. Therefore, for patients referred to urology, it would be very helpful to know that as part of the urological assessment:

1. eGFR is >60mls/min (or no significant drop in eGFR).
2. Urine albumin/creatinine ratio (ACR) or protein/creatinine ratio (PCR) is less than 30 or 50, respectively.
3. Blood pressure <140/90.
4. *Microscopy performed** [5, 6].

*Given that glomerular haematuria is distinct from non-glomerular haematuria and that dipstick positive haematuria without red blood cells might indicate a pigment nephropathy the addition of confirmatory microscopy or, ideally, phase-contrast microscopy to the end (or beginning) of a negative one-stop shop might genuinely improve the pathway. With or without this addition, convincing non-visible haematuria should be considered for nephrology review and in patients who trigger on the three screening tests above as being increased risk of renal disease, there needs to be a system for efficient nephrology referral.

Conversely, nephrologists need to be adept at spotting and confirming new haematuria in existing patients, requesting the appropriate imaging and referring. For a small subset of patients, such as those with aristolochic acid nephropathy, analgesic nephropathy, large exposure to cyclophosphamide, or those with renal tumour syndromes, there needs to be a clear plan for urological surveillance that follows the patient whether they have transitioned to dialysis or transplant or to another nephrologist. There will also be patients (particularly older patients and smokers) with chronic renal haematuria (such as IgA nephropathy) who may have increased haematuria. Thus, when possible it would be efficient to screen out patients with glomerular haematuria to avoid unnecessary cystoscopy. As alluded to above, perhaps the least invasive screening tool is phase-contrast microscopy; if the RBC are predominantly dysmorphic, then the cause is likely to be the underlying glomerular lesion, but if predominantly lower tract, it should provoke urological assessment.

The need for radiological evaluation of the upper urinary tract in patients with asymptomatic microscopic haematuria (AMH) is supported by all guidelines (see the end of chapter), but the recommended modality varies between them. The American Urology Association (AUA), American College of Radiology Appropriateness Criteria, and European Association of Urology (EAU) choose multiphase CT urogram as the preferred study (highest sensitivity and specificity). The CUA microscopic haematuria guidelines recommend renal ultrasonography as the first-line imaging method, with CT urography used in cases where additional tests are needed for abnormal or inconclusive findings [7].

In summary, confirmed asymptomatic non-visible haematuria is a non-specific sign with both urological and nephrological causes. Nephrologists need to refer patients at increased risk of malignancy, and urologists need to establish clear pathways to identify patients with increased risk of renal.

53.3 Renal Stones

The assessment and management of renal stones is covered in Chap. 55 However, in the context that there is a steadily growing incidence of stone formation (4.4% increase in 5 years in the UK) [8] resulting in roughly a 10% lifetime risk of stones in Western countries and with recurrence rates after an initial symptomatic stone event reported to be from 30 to 50% within 10 years of the first presentation, this is an increasingly common problem [6, 7]. Therefore, it is important to consider the ability of urologists and nephrologists to efficiently manage such patients. While some urologists have a specialist interest in metabolic stone disease, for most patients there is merit in referring to a specialized metabolic stone clinic with multidisciplinary review including radiology, dietetics, urology, and nephrology [9]. There are different models for this, but the most efficient ones probably don't involve nephrologists and urologists sharing the same consultation.

The key to investigation is deciding who is a **low-risk stone former** and who is a **high-risk stone former**. It is generally accepted that even low-risk first-time stone former should undergo a basic minimum metabolic evaluation, usually at the time of presentation in the emergency department. Fig. 53.2 shows how patients are assigned to either low- or high-risk groups and their

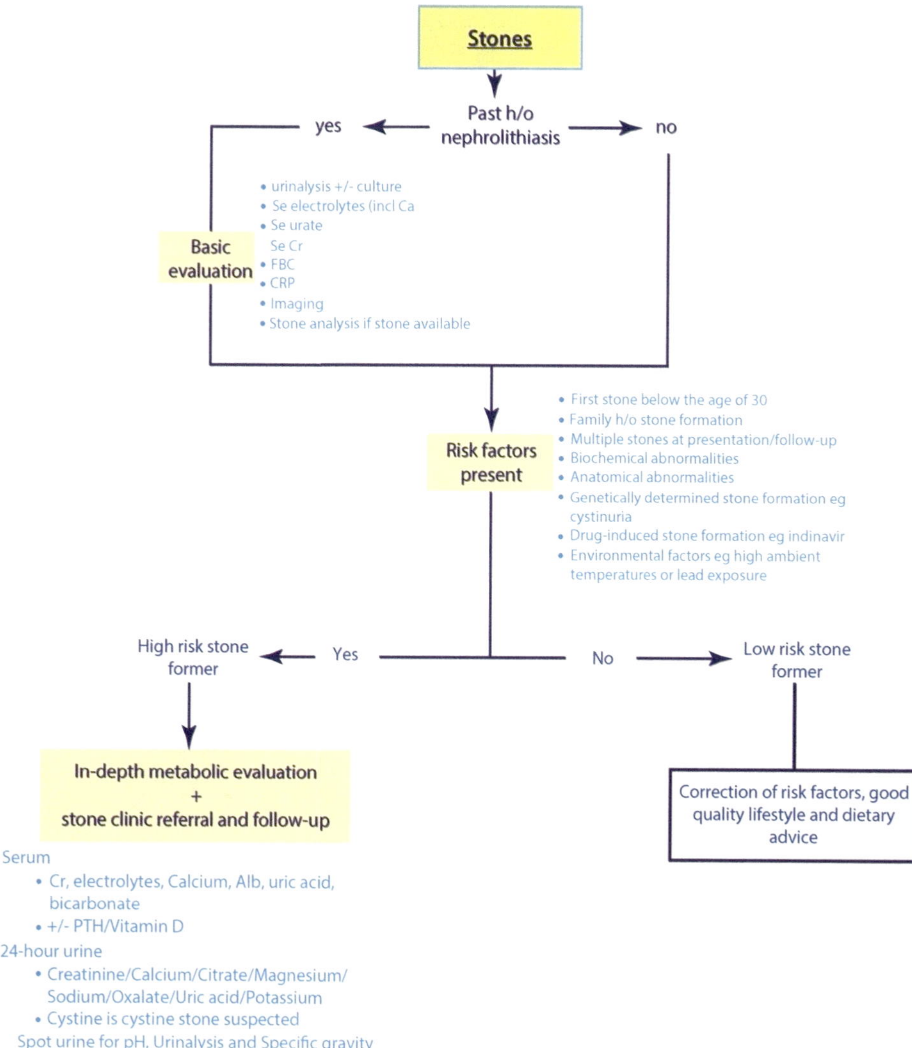

Fig. 53.2 Offers one structure for the investigation of stones based on risk. Patients who are low-risk stone formers will usually be managed in isolation by urologists but will need a robust system for reviewing results and offering good-quality advice on lifestyle changes or medical intervention. High-risk stone formers may need a referral to a metabolic clinic that can address risk factors for stone formation and management in more detail. This may be run by a urologist, nephrologist, or biochemist but needs clear referral guidelines and protocols that can be replicated

management thereof based on the EAU urolithiasis guidelines (▶ https://uroweb.org/guideline/urolithiasis/stone/#3).

The reason for mentioning these screening tests in this chapter is that anecdotally, basic and in-depth screening is frequently not achieved, and not all patients are referred appropriately.

There may also be other stone forming patients who warrant discussion or referral to nephrologists such as those with a single kidney, recurrent infections, nephrocalcinosis, sarcoidosis, and chronic gastrointestinal problems resulting in malabsorption, oxalate stones, and dehydration.

Typically, nephrologists offering long-term metabolic follow-up strive to encourage weight loss, appropriate dietary changes, and management of CKD. Urologists have a critical role in (see Fig. 53.3 resolving acute obstruction or recurrent stone-related UTIs very much in collaboration with nephrologists and microbiologists (Fig. 53.4). In short, nephrologists and urologists should make a point of formally liaising to agree to practice and audit adherence to guidance. We also have a responsibility to develop a system that reliably communicates between both specialities and offers a consistent, reliable, and patient-centred service.

53.4 Obstruction

The causes and management of urinary tract obstruction is covered in Chap. 57. Clearly it remains a common and important problem, and while the vast majority of urinary tract obstruction is managed by urologists and radiologists, nephrologists are frequently involved in managing patients who develop AKI/CKD or urosepsis in this context. Given that even relatively brief episodes of obstruction may cause nephron loss, obstruction and sepsis is a very bad combination compounding renal injury. Nephrologists have a key role in supporting and promoting rapid management of obstruction, particularly as such patients often present to non-renal specialists.

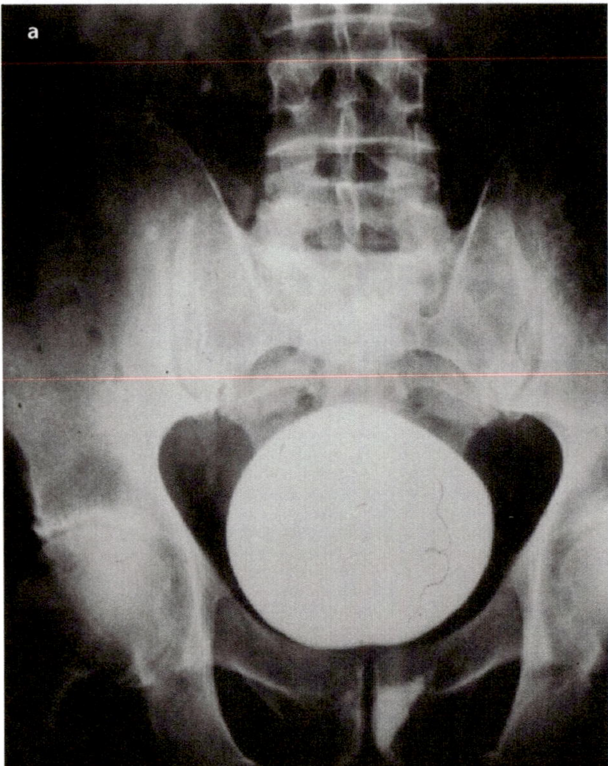

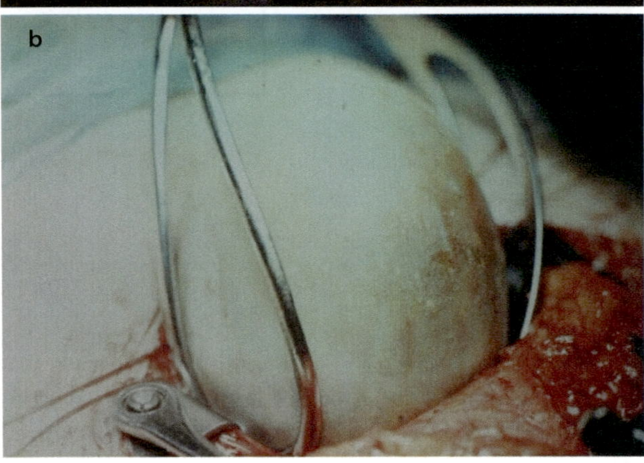

Fig. 53.3 **a**: A plain abdominal X-ray in a patient referred to nephrology with hypertension and non-visible haematuria. On direct questioning the patient also had bladder discomfort/strangury, frequency, and nocturia. The X-ray shows a large bladder stone that was (not surprisingly) causing obstruction. **b**: The stone was delivered by urologists using tools borrowed from obstetric colleagues

Renal and urology clinics that have ready access to non-invasive tests such as post-micturition residual volume measurements and flow studies are likely to speed the diagnosis of bladder outflow tract obstruction and expedite appropriate treatment.

Medical causes of obstruction such as retroperitoneal fibrosis (RPF) are best managed by a multidisciplinary team particularly if immunosuppression or biologicals are required. Patients with RPF (which can have a malignant aetiology) will often require stenting in the short term, but some without evidence of an inflammatory component won't benefit from immunomodulation and may benefit from ureterolysis rather than life-long stenting. Having a clear urological and renal

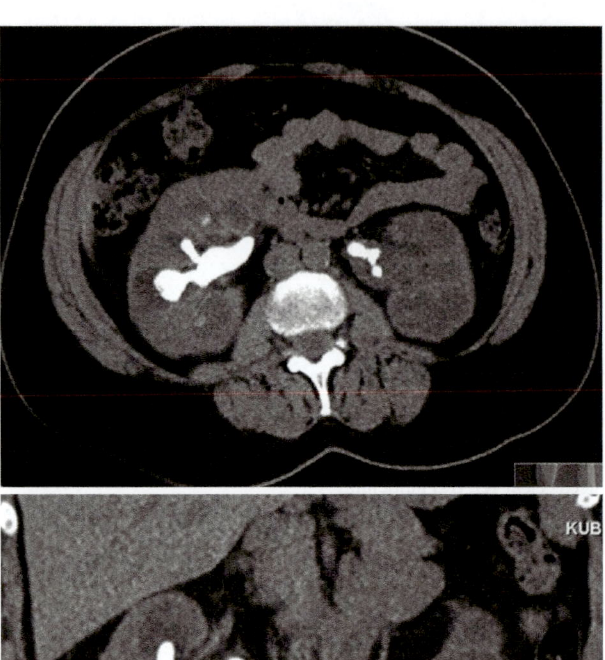

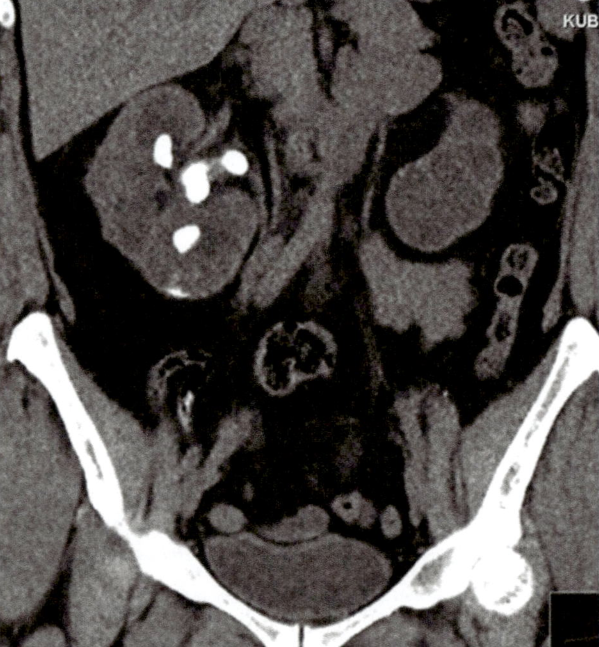

Fig. 53.4 A cross section and sagittal non-contrast CT of a patient with bilateral staghorn calculi and recurrent UTIs. The left kidney is shrunken and chronically dilated secondary to obstruction; the right kidney still has some functioning; the renal cortex is badly damaged. Urologists have a key role in treating obstructing and/or infected stones but in collaboration with microbiologists as multidrug resistance is not unusual in this setting. It is also important to collaborate early with nephrologists if the patient develops declining renal function. Metabolic screening may help reduce the risk of further stone development, but it may also have a role in reducing recurrence in a transplant

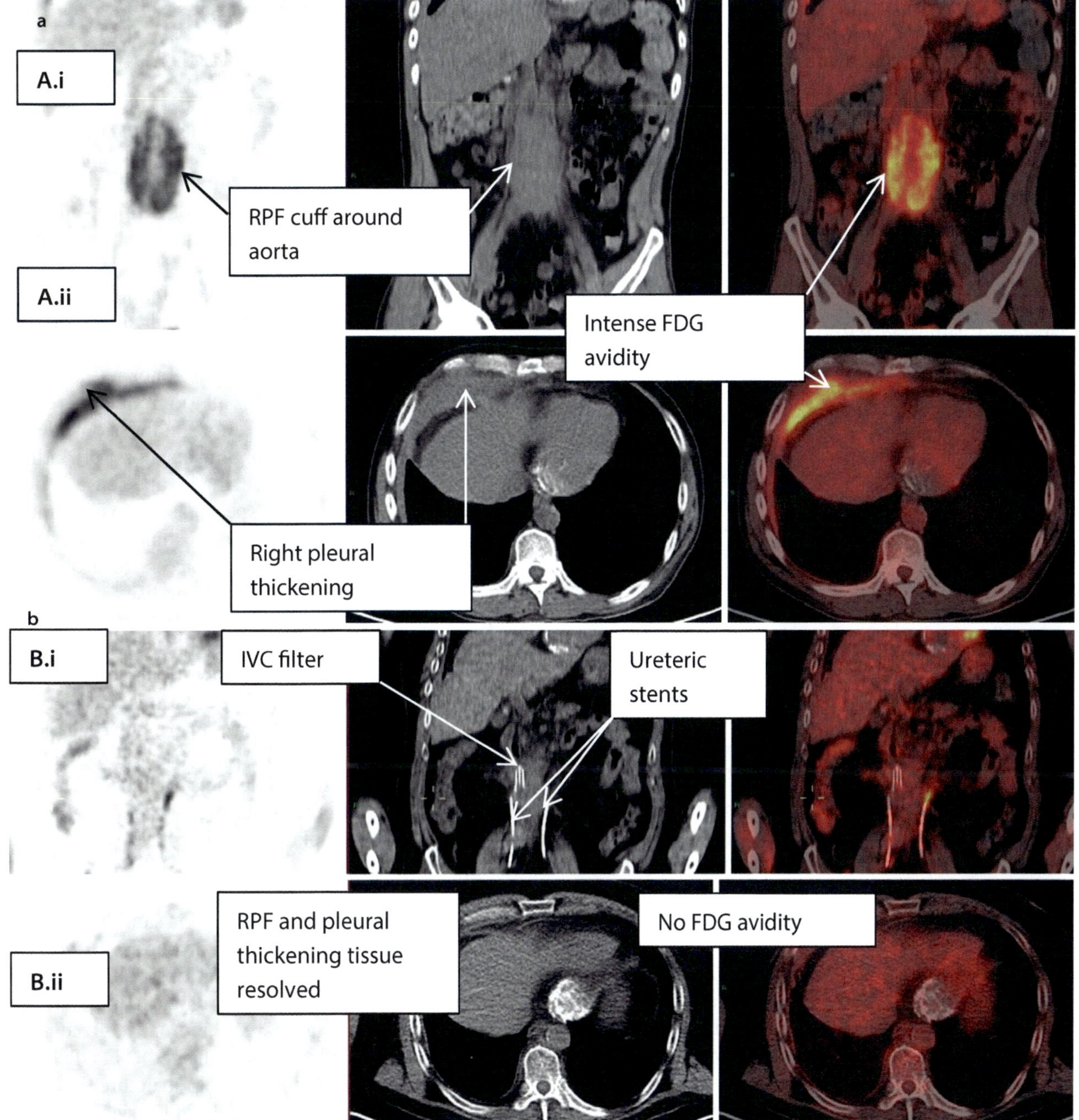

Fig. 53.5 FDG-PETCT imaging at **a** time of diagnosis and **b** following 1 year of treatment with weaning doses of prednisolone and maintenance methotrexate

pathway for MDT management of these patients is highly recommended (see Fig. 53.5)..

A Caucasian male in his 50s was under investigation for a cough and pleural thickening. On the day of an elective pleural biopsy, his serum creatinine was found to be 1100umol/L despite being 102umol/L only 4 weeks previously. He underwent emergency haemodialysis, and following CT imaging demonstrating evidence of RPF, bilateral ureteric stents were placed with good kidney function back to baseline after 4 weeks. An IVC filter was placed following confirmed PEs during the admission, likely caused by external IVC compression by the RPF mass. Histological analysis of a pleural biopsy revealed no malignant cells, fibrotic tissue with patchy small lymphoid aggregates, and only scanty IgG4-positive staining cells. A retroperitoneal soft tissue biopsy revealed a rich-plasma cell infiltrate but, again, only scanty IgG4-positive staining. He was treated with a weaning course of prednisolone and maintenance methotrexate.

This case emphasizes just how critical it is to have a multidisciplinary approach to complex conditions such as RPF to achieve an optimum outcome for the patient. With increasing knowledge some centres have also developed dedicated RPF multidisciplinary teams consisting of radiologists, urologists, nephrologists, gastrointestinal specialists, and vascular surgeons.

(images courtesy of Dr. Nemi Ganda and Dr. Tara Barwick).

One final area of overlap is the functional obstruction caused by high-pressure bladders. This is a critical and often delayed diagnosis in patients with CAKUT (see below); ensuring that a bladder is 'safe' at presentation and remains 'safe' is extremely important. Ready access to urodynamics service (usually run by urologists) with clear referral criteria needs to be established.

53.5 Congenital Abnormalities of the Kidney and Urinary Tract (CAKUT) (See ▶ Chapter 56)

Most patients with CAKUT are identified at birth or early childhood and invariably managed by paediatric urologists often requiring multiple complex surgical interventions. However, CAKUT is the cause of 40–50% of paediatric and 7% of adult end-stage renal disease worldwide, and whilst CAKUT is mostly sporadic, the increased recurrence risk of CAKUT among relatives has been confirmed in several studies and is estimated at 4–20%. Hence, not only do nephrologists need to offer follow-up/care due to risks of CKD/ESRF but often CAKUT is only the first manifestation of a complex systemic disease with a genetic predisposition. A precise genetic definition can help identify other subtle clinical features and give the patient and their family appropriate genetic counselling.

53.6 Recurrent, Persistent, and Complicated Urinary Tract Infection (UTI)

'Uncomplicated' UTIs describe infections in patients with no structural, functional, or predisposing abnormalities to developing further infections that are difficult to treat. This includes most UTIs in post-pubertal and premenopausal women, and their management is covered by well-established guidelines [10, 11]. However, recurrent UTIs amongst women along with UTIs in other patient groups can be very challenging in particular 'complicated UTI', i.e. patients not in the above group and in particular those with abnormal anatomy are often poorly managed. This all too frequently results in persistent or recurrent infections, admissions, development of multiresistant organisms, loss of kidney function, and occasionally death. In one sense it does not necessarily matter which specialist group champions this issue in a region, just as long as someone does, that they have clear referral pathways, access to urological, radiological, and microbiological expertise.

It should be possible to provide a 'one-stop shop' for women with recurrent but uncomplicated UTIs: offering a simple diagnostic screen, flow studies, and bladder emptying ultrasound. These investigations are relatively cheap and can be established by any urology or nephrology department with a will to do so. Clear and evidence-based patient information leaflets on strategies that reduce risk, when appropriate prophylactic antibiotics or topical hormone replacement may have a role in clinical management.

For a relatively small proportion of patients, cystoscopy, video urodynamics, and ureteric sampling may be required to establish a cause of urosepsis. Ultimately, treatment of bladder outflow tract obstruction, stones, and poor drainage may require urological intervention.

What is required is a clear and mutually agreed pathway for recurrent UTIs and complicated UTIs. Below is a suggested pathway that might help structure the development of a service. A recurrent UTI service needs to have the facility for rapid access and administrative support especially to obtain imaging and previous microbiology results. It also needs a mechanism for feedback of outcomes by a MDT (see blue lines) and robust audit of outcomes (UTI and microbiology resistance).

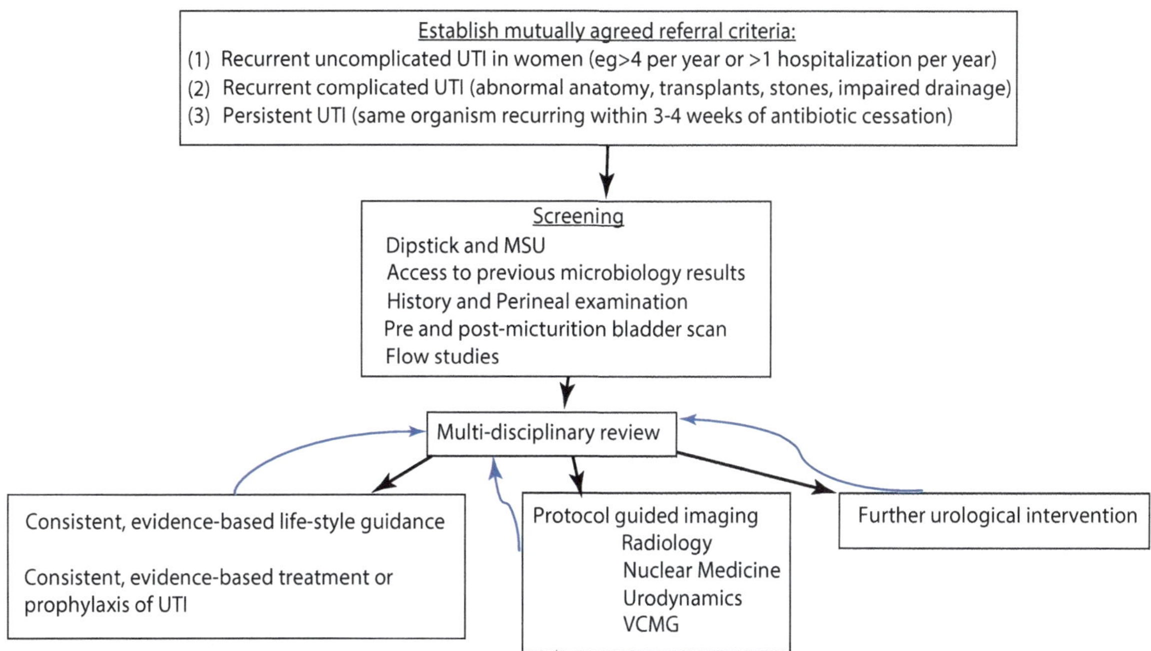

53.7 Renal Tumour Syndromes

Most urological cancers are diagnosed and managed solely by urologists [12]. However, there are several renal tumour syndromes (see below) that often first present to urologists. It is important to have a system that can identify such patients and have a referral pathway for syndromes with multi-organ involvement, usually to a renal geneticist.

Renal tumours with genetic predisposition:

- Von Hippel-Lindau disease.
- Birt-Hogg-Dubé syndrome.
- Hereditary papillary renal carcinoma,
- Hereditary leiomyomatosis and renal cell carcinoma.
- Succinate dehydrogenase-associated renal cancer.
- Tuberose sclerosis complex.
- BAP1 tumour predisposition syndrome.
- MiTF-associated cancer syndrome.

Due to the multifocality and often bilateral nature of such genetic disorders as well as the propensity for recurrent or de novo tumour formation, these patients often require recurrent interventions with nephron-sparing surgery (NSS)/ablation/single or even bilateral nephrectomy. Hence though urologists usually have the first-hand experience with such cases identification, early referral and long-term follow-up by nephrologists is of great importance as not only do some of these require specific treatments such as mTOR inhibition but also due to reduction in nephron mass and the risk of progressive CKD and end-stage renal failure [12].

The patient below presented at 34 with a renal cell cancer (RCC) of the left kidney and underwent a left nephrectomy. She was lost to follow-up but presented in a different country with hypertension and non-visible haematuria. The presence of a clear cell renal carcinoma at 34 is suspicious of a genetic renal tumour complex. Imaging of the remaining kidney demonstrated a significantly abnormal kidney with at least two masses with the characteristic of RCCs and multiple simple cysts (▫ Fig. 53.6). Von Hippel-Lindau syndrome was sus-

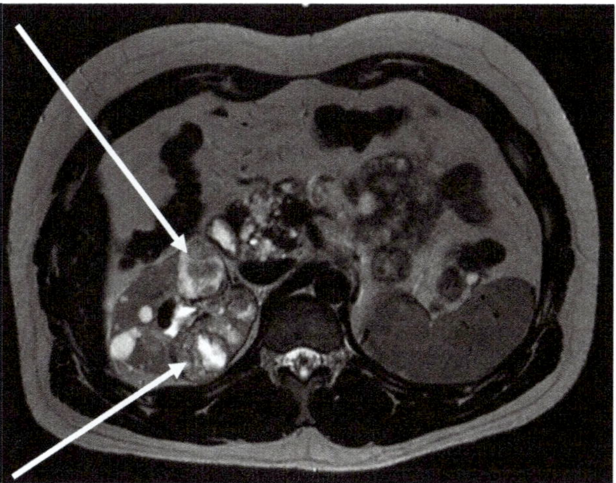

▫ **Fig. 53.6** MRI scan of patient with Von Hippel-Lindau syndrome

pected and while awaiting genetic testing a cerebellar haemangioblastoma was diagnosed on screening MRI.

As a part of a multidisciplinary review, the masses were monitored, and the patient was counselled and prepared for dialysis (including the formation of a fistula and vaccinations) with a clear plan for delayed transplantation. This case illustrates the critical importance of coordinating care, in this case among several specialities.

Similarly, some patients with large angiomyolipomas will be in greater need of radiologist and urologist follow-up (◘ Fig. 53.7(a–c)) or more need of a nephrologist (◘ Fig. 53.7(d)).

Beyond the relatively rare renal tumour syndromes, urologists are increasingly and more commonly, faced with elderly comorbid patients with CKD and renal tumours. The role of the nephrologist is no less critical in optimising renal function and assessing these patients for renal replacement therapy. Urologists, on the other hand, commonly run a low clearance pathway for such patients with eGFR <45 mL/min/1.73m^2 involving the use of DMSA scans to help decide on nephron-sparing surgery versus radical nephrectomy.

53.8 Renal Haemorrhage

Renal haemorrhage is relatively common in the setting of trauma (rarely requiring nephrology input) but thankfully uncommon in the spontaneous or postrenal

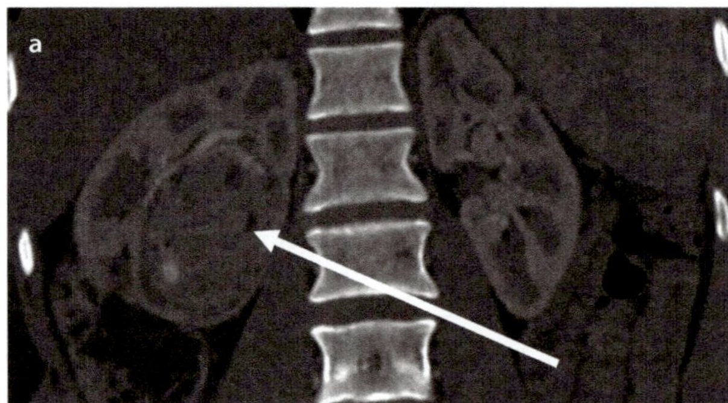

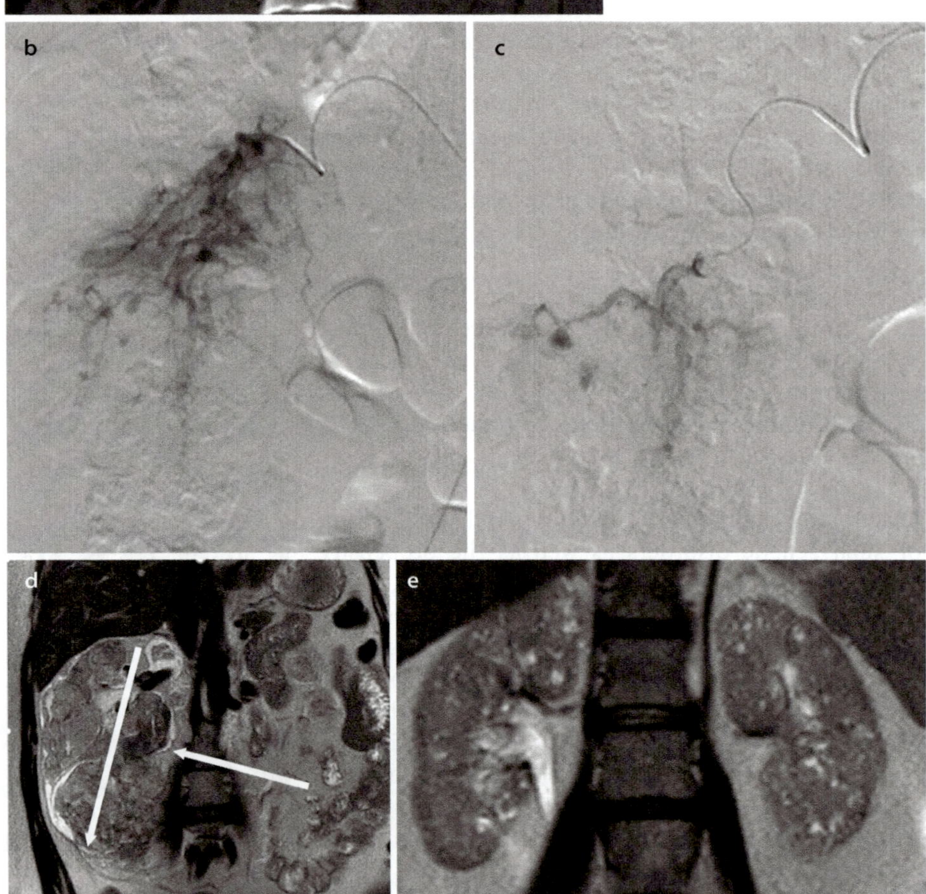

◘ **Fig. 53.7** **a** shows a large right-sided AML that was at moderate risk of bleeding. Following a MDT discussion, an angiogram was performed **b** and **c** shows post-embolization angiogram. **d** shows a massive right-side AML that had bled and could not be managed with mTOR inhibition. This kidney was surgically removed by a urologist following embolization. Conversely, **e** shows the incidental finding of multiple AMLs in a 39-year-old woman. The patient was transferred to a nephrologist with an interest in tuberous sclerosis complex (TSC) as there were no surgical concerns, screened for possible complications of TSC, and possible management with mTOR inhibition if the AMLs became sufficiently big

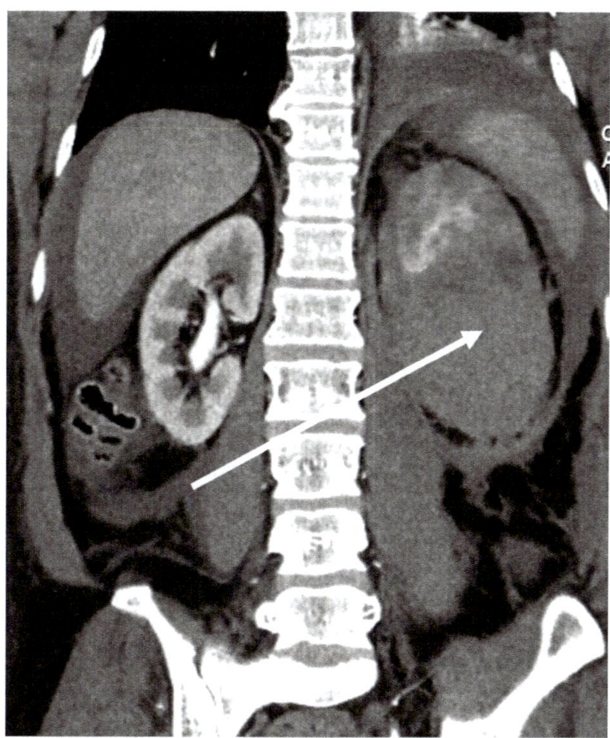

Fig. 53.8 Shows a large spontaneous renal bleed in a patient anticoagulated for a mechanical heart valve. The patient presented with all the features of Lenk's triad. In this case an urgent CT angiogram demonstrated a ruptured renal artery aneurysm which was embolised

biopsy setting. Spontaneous renal rupture is rare, and causes described include benign (often angiomyolipoma) and malignant (commonly RCC) lesions, vascular malformation, kidney infection, and blood dyscrasia, typically presenting with Lenk's triad: acute flank pain, tender flank mass, and clinical hemodynamic deterioration (Fig. 53.8).

Renal haemorrhage of any cause requires close liaison with urologists for optimal and timely interventions. The choice of therapeutic strategies for renal haemorrhage will vary according to the severity of haemorrhage, hemodynamic stability, and local resources. If there is no direct access to interventional radiology, then liaison with the urologist is even more critical, and a pre-agreed protocol and pathway for serious bleeds (e.g. post-biopsy) needs to be established.

Nephrologists may be involved in the management of ensuing AKI and exclusion or management of rare medical causes.

Tips and Tricks

- Make a point of liaising with the urologist in your catchment area and establish common protocols for (a) non-visible haematuria, (b) metabolic stone screening, (c) referral of patients with AKI or CKD, and (d) recurrent UTI clinic.
- Agree on audits of combined protocols with urologists and copying of discharge letters.
- Urology/radiology multidisciplinary meetings are a good place to learn some urology and identify patients who might benefit from a renal review.
- There is also a great opportunity for bidirectional teaching and learning from joint meetings with urologists and radiologists.

53.9 Summary

It is to the distinct advantage of our patients to forge close links, common protocols, and clear lines of communication between nephrologists and urologists (not just within the same hospital but in the renal catchment area of the hospital).

Questions

1. In a patient with non-visible haematuria, what features would suggest an increased risk of a renal cause?
2. What does a basic stone screen involve?
3. What characteristics define a high risk of metabolic stone disease?
4. What is Lenk's triad?
5. What % of ESRD is caused by CAKUT in (a) children and (b) adults?

Answers

1. Non-visible haematuria Is Suggestive of a Renal Cause in the Presence of
   - eGFR is <60mls/min (or with a significant drop in eGFR).
   - Urine ACR or PCR is more than 30 or 50, respectively.
   - Blood pressure >140/90.
   - Active urinary sediment on microscopy.
2. The Following Represents the Low-Risk Stone Formers Basic Screen
   - Urinalysis +/– culture.
   - Serum electrolytes + calcium.

- Serum urate.
- Serum Cr.
- FBC.
- CRP.
- Imaging.
- Stone analysis if a stone is available.

3. The Following
   - First stone <30 years of age.
   - Family history of stone formation.
   - Multiple stones at presentation or follow-up.
   - Biochemical or anatomical abnormalities predisposing to stone formation.
   - Drug-induced stone formation.
   - Genetically caused stones.

53

4. Features of renal haemorrhage (i) sudden onset flank pain, (ii) tender flank mass, and (iii) haemodynamic instability.
5. CAKUT is, by far, the commonest cause of ESRD in children at 40–50% and is probably the cause of ESRD in about 7% of adults. These patients have a high incidence and risk of UTIs, high pressure, or poor drainage urinary tracts. Those with augmented bladders and Mitrofanoffs or urinary diversions needed for catheterisation will need regular urology follow-up for the duration (Table 53.2).

Table 53.2 List of indications for specialist referral for investigation of women with risk factors for complicated UTI

Prior urinary tract surgery or trauma
Gross haematuria after resolution of infection
Previous bladder or renal calculi
Obstructive symptoms (straining, weak stream, intermittency, hesitancy), low uroflowmetry or high PVR
Urea-splitting bacteria on culture (e.g., *Proteus*, *Yersinia*)
Bacterial persistence after sensitivity-based therapy
Prior abdominopelvic malignancy
Diabetes or otherwise immunocompromised
Pneumaturia, faecaluria, anaerobic bacteria or a history of diverticulitis
Repeated pyelonephritis (fevers, chills, vomiting, CVA tenderness)
Asymptomatic microhaematuria after resolution of infection should be evaluated as per CUA guidelines

Guidelines on Investigation of Non-visible (Microscopic) Haematuria

- American Urological Association 2016. ▶ https://www.auanet.org/guidelines/asymptomatic-microhematuria-(amh)-guideline
- European Association of Urology 2019:
  - ▶ https://uroweb.org/guideline/non-muscle-invasive-bladder-cancer/#11
  - ▶ https://uroweb.org/guideline/upper-urinary-tract-urothelial-cell-carcinoma/
  - ▶ https://uroweb.org/guideline/primary-urethral-carcinoma/
  - ▶ https://uroweb.org/guideline/renal-cell-carcinoma/
- American College of Physicians 2016; (▶ http://annals.org/aim/fullarticle/2484287/hematuria-marker-occult-urinary-tract-cancer-advice-high-value-care)
- Joint Consensus Statement of the Renal Association.
- National Institute for Health and Care Excellence guidelines 2015 (▶ https://www.nice.org.uk/guidance/ng12/chapter/1-Recommendations-organised-by-site-of-cancer).
- Guidelines on surgical management of stones: AUA/Endourology Society Guideline: Published 2016 ▶ https://www.auanet.org/guidelines/stone-disease-surgical-(2016)#x3166.

References

1. https://www.uptodate.com/contents/etiology-and-evaluation-of-hematuria-in-adults?search=microscopic%20haematuria§ionRank=1&usage_type=default&anchor=H5&source=machineLearning&selectedTitle=1~150&display_rank=1#H5
2. Cohen RA, Brown RS. Clinical practice. Microscopic hematuria N Engl J Med. 2003;348:2330–8.
3. Yuste C, Gutierrez E, Sevillano AM, Rubio-Navarro A, Amaro-Villalobos JM, Ortiz A, et al. Pathogenesis of Glomerular Haematuria. World Journal of Nephrology. 2015;4.2:185–95. PMC. Web. 28 Aug. 2018.
4. Anderson JFD, Feehally J, Goldberg L, Kelly J, MacTier R. Joint consensus statement on the initial assessment of haematuria. Prepared on behalf of the Renal Association and British Association of Urological Surgeons. Available at: http://www.renal.org/docs/default-source/guidelines-resources/joint-guidelines/joint-guidelines-archieve/Haematuria_-_RA-BAUS_consensus_guideline_2008.pdf.
5. Grossfield GD, Wolf JS, Litwin MS, et al. Asymptomatic microscopic haematuria in adults: summary of the AUA best PracticePolicy recommendations. Am Fam Physician. 2001;63:1145–53.

6. Thaller TR, Wang LP. Evaluation of asymptomatic microscopic hematuria in adults. Am Fam Physician. 1999;60(4):1143–52, 1154.
7. Linder J, Bass EJ, Mosta H, Boorjiann SA. Guideline of guidelines: asymptomatic microscopic haematuria. BJU Int. 2018;121:176–83.
8. Heers H, Turney BW. Trends in urological stone disease. BJU Int. 2016;118(5):785–9.
9. Dion M, Ankawi G, Chew B, Paterson R, Sultan N, Hoddinott P, Razvi H. CUA guideline on the evaluation and medical management of the kidney stone patient – 2016 update. Can Urol Assoc J. 2016;10(11–12):E347–58. https://doi.org/10.5489/cuaj.4218. Published online November 10, 2016.
10. https://www.ncbi.nlm.nih.gov/pmc/articles/PMC3202002/
11. NICE guidance of treatment of UTI 2019.
12. Bratslavsky G, Linehan WM. Long-term Management of Bilateral, multifocal, recurrent renal carcinoma. Nat Rev Urol. 2010;7(5):267–75. https://doi.org/10.1038/nrurol.2010.44.

Urinary Tract Infection

Gayathri Rajakaruna, Ali M. Shendi, Stephen Mepham, and Mark Harber

Contents

M. Harber (ed.), *Primer on Nephrology*, https://doi.org/10.1007/978-3-030-76419-7_54

Learning Objectives

1. To identify the risk factors for and the impact of UTIs.
2. To illustrate the different sorts of UTI and different clinical presentations.
3. To appreciate the difference between uncomplicated and complicated UTI in terms of management.
4. To consider options for stream-lining referral and assessment of patients with recurrent, persistent, and complicated UTIs.
5. To inspire enthusiasm among nephrologists to teach, lead, and research in this area.

54.1 Introduction

Urinary tract infection *(UTI)* in vulnerable groups is responsible for considerable morbidity and mortality, but even in healthy individuals 'uncomplicated' UTIs (cystitis or pyelonephritis in a healthy woman) are responsible for a considerable health care burden [1]. In 2011 UTIs were responsible for 8.6 million visits a year in the USA, symptoms lasting an average of 6 days with 2–4 days of reduced activity and an estimated cost to the US economy of $2–4 billion per year. Patients with complicated UTIs and recurrent urosepsis in the setting of urological abnormality, transplantation, and antimicrobial resistance, are often seen by nephrologists and can represent a considerable challenge. Care pathways for these patients are often haphazard, without a clear structure, with patients commonly suffering care that is more disjointed than it should be.

54.2 Diagnosis and Definition

Bacterial UTIs are classically divided into 'uncomplicated', where patients are otherwise healthy individuals with no underlying structural or neurological lesions of the urinary tract with no other systemic diseases predisposing the host to bacterial infection and 'complicated' (essentially everyone else, i.e. UTIs in men, pregnancy, diabetics, transplantation, and anyone with an anatomically or functionally abnormal urinary tract).

Complicated UTI also occurs in patients in whom there may be residual inflammatory changes following recurrent infection or instrumentation, obstruction, stones, or anatomical or physiological abnormalities or pathological lesions. These interfere with the drainage of urine in part of the tract which encourages prolonged colonisation. Examples include acute and chronic pyelonephritis and perinephric, renal, and emphysematous abscesses.

There is a genuine clinical utility in dividing UTIs this way in terms of patient risk and overall management. Moreover, it is also useful to divide urinary tract infection into anatomical location: balanitis, urethritis, prostatitis, cystitis, and pyelonephritis, all of which can also be divided into acute or chronic.

The definition and diagnosis of UTIs are not always straightforward, for example, a poorly taken sample may be contaminated with perineal bacteria, whilst a delayed or un-refrigerated can yield a spurious result. Asymptomatic bacteriuria (ASB) is defined as the growth of bacteria from a well-taken sample in the absence of symptoms with or without associated pyuria. This commonly occurs in several patient groups including the elderly, pregnant women, transplant, and diabetic patients.

The laboratory definition of UTI derives from work in asymptomatic women with $\geq 10^5$ colony-forming units (cfu)/ml, and counts below this or 10^4 are rarely reported by laboratories. There is however good evidence that $\geq 10^2$ cfu is an appropriate diagnostic threshold in symptomatic patients. These groups include acutely symptomatic young women with counts of a single isolate ($>10^2$ cfu/mL), men ($\geq 10^3$ cfu/ml), renal transplant recipients ($\geq 10^2$ cfu/mL), and children (a carefully voided sample of $\geq 10^4$ or $\geq 10^3$ cfu/mL of a single species).

Recent antibiotics may inhibit culture; fastidious organisms may not grow or may be overwhelmed by other organisms with standard techniques. Urinary catheters, ileostomies, and urostomies will inevitably be colonised with bacteria and result in 'positive' cultures. Patients with neutropenia may have no pyuria, whilst pyuria may be caused by non-infectious disease. Urethritis and vaginitis can mimic the symptoms of cystitis, and symptoms of upper and lower UTI are often minimal in the elderly and immunocompromised. In short, urine cultures need to be interpreted thoughtfully to avoid over or underdiagnosis and treatment.

Distinguishing recurrent UTI (rUTI) from relapsed UTI is very important. rUTI is defined as the occurrence of two more UTIs within 6 months or three or more infections within a 12-month period. This can be a reinfection where recurrence occurs with a different organism or the same organism, however, with sterile urine on culture in between episodes. In contrast a relapse is defined as a recurrent UTI with the same organism from an intracellular uroepithelial organism usually occurring within 2 weeks. One in three women are known to have an acute UTI by the age of 24, and around 25% of these women are likely to have a recurrence within 6 months. Recurrences are common in sexually active or postmenopausal women. Recurrences are either due to exogenous organisms repeatedly introduced to the urinary tract system or due to recrudescence of endogenous organisms such as intracellular uropathogenic *E. coli* (UPEC) within transitional cells.

54.3 Balanitis

Acute balanitis is usually clinically obvious, but chronic balanitis, often associated with phimosis and diabetes, may not be. Recurrent short courses of antibiotics for presumed recurrent cystitis on the basis of positive cultures (usually without pyuria) is a good way of generating multi-resistant organisms. The diagnosis is usually obvious on inspection illustrating the importance of local examination and treatment usually involves circumcision.

54.4 Urethritis, Urethral Syndrome, and Vaginitis

These conditions may be misdiagnosed as cystitis on the basis of dysuria. Symptoms more suggestive of urethritis are the predominance of dysuria, with less frequency and urgency, often more gradual onset and more common in a sexually active patient, especially with new partner(s). If urethritis is secondary to *Chlamydia trachomatis* or *Neisseria gonorrhoeae*, then it is often associated with pyuria and should be detected by urinary antigen testing. Additional pathogens such as mycoplasma genitalium may be detected using a urethral specimen at a sexually transmitted disease clinic visit. Culture negative or low bacterial count bacteriuria associated urethritis/acute urethral syndrome is often not associated with pyuria is a poorly understood condition with a variety of aetiologies including autoimmune (e.g. Bechet's syndrome, Wegener's granulomatosis), mycobacterial, viral (e.g. *Adenovirus*) trauma, chemical, foreign body, strictures, and stones/crystalluria. Occasionally viral infections such as herpes simplex can present with culture-negative urethritis and can respond to prophylactic acyclovir. As a chronic condition, it is often difficult to diagnose and treat; referral to a urologist or genitourinary medicine colleague with a specialist interest is worth considering.

Vaginitis is another cause for dysuria misdiagnosed as UTI, and it is important to specifically ask about vaginal discharge (the absence of which has a good negative predictive value). Symptoms are often felt to be external and as with urethritis frequency and urgency may be absent. Candida, gonorrhoea, chlamydia, mycoplasma, and herpes simplex are all common causes.

54.5 Prostatitis

Acute prostatitis may present as a lower UTI, fever, and urethral obstruction. Urine dipstick and cultures will not distinguish from cystitis, and the suspicion may only be raised following a relapse of a UTI after a short course of antibiotics. The prostate is tender on palpation, and a raised prostatic specific antigen can be a useful clue.

Chronic prostatitis may also present with relapse of UTI after antibiotics, the prostate typically less tender with less dramatic inflammatory markers than with acute prostatitis. Midstream urine (MSU) taken after prostatic massage may reveal inflammatory cells on microscopy and occasionally the organism.

For both acute and chronic prostatitis, the empiric treatment is usually fluoroquinolones for 4 weeks, with cotrimoxazole and fosfomycin being useful alternatives.

54.6 Interstitial Cystitis (IC) and Overactive Bladder (OAB) Complex

Interstitial cystitis and OAB form a spectrum of chronic, poorly understood conditions that can cause profound and disabling lower urinary tract symptoms (LUTS). IC is associated with mast cell infiltrate and may be associated with sterile pyuria, forming an important part of the differential for recurrent UTI reviewed by Moutzouris [2]. From the nephrologist's point of view, it is important to exclude other pathologies such as low-grade chronic infection (especially in diabetics) which can present with IC/OAB symptoms, malignancy, stones, and other physiochemical causes such as radiation cystitis or ketamine-induced inflammation. An index of suspicion is required and early referral for cystoscopy and to a sympathetic specialist.

54.7 Epidemiology of Bacterial Cystitis and Pyelonephritis

In infancy bacteriura occurs in 1–2%, more commonly in boys for the first 3 months and more likely to be associated with bacteraemia and pyelonephritis. After this time girls are more commonly affected with a pre-school incidence of 4.5% compared to 0.5% in boys in whom UTI is very likely to be associated with a significant congenital abnormality.

In adults 84% of uncomplicated UTIs occur in women with 3% of American women seeking medical help for this per year. Fifty percent of women experience at least one symptomatic UTI in their lifetime and 20–25% of these having a recurrence within 6 months.

For a woman having a first-degree female relative with a history of UTI is a significant risk factor (OR ~ 2.5–4).

With increasing age, comorbidity, and institutionalization, the incidence of UTI increases dramatically with the female/male ratio reducing significantly. In postmenopausal women alone, the annual risk of UTI is around 10% with 5–15% of women over 60 having recurrent UTIs. UTIs are the commonest nosocomial infection (40%). Instrumentation is an important and potentially modifiable risk factor; a one off urinary catheterisation carries a 1% risk of UTI, but for hospital patients, an indwelling catheter has a 10% risk of UTI. Urinary tract infection is also very frequent in transplant recipients commonly exceeding 50% in the first year of transplantation with the highest risk in the first few weeks.

The risk factors for urinary tract infection are shown in ◘ Table 54.1 and explain much of the increase in old age and transplant recipients. In short, anything that reduces or circumvents the normal physiochemical barriers and innate immunity of the urinary tract becomes a significant risk factor.

◘ **Table 54.1** Risk factors for urinary tract infection and potential preventative interventions

Female sex	**Short urethral**
Old age	Potential impairment of any aspect of innate or physiochemical defences
Sexual intercourse especially with a new partner	This is a prominent risk factor
Use of diaphragm and spermicides	Possible impairment of protective microbiome (eg vaginal lactobaccili)
Previous UTIs	Consider antibiotic prophylaxis if frequent and conservative measures fail
First degree relative with UTI	
Urological instrumentation, intermittent self-catheterisation and ureteric stents	An important element of acute history. Exclude and or treat ASB prior to instrumentation, refresh ISC technique, minimize stent duration.
Catheterisation (especially indwelling but also convene catheters)	Avoid unnecessary catheterisation and minimise catheter duration where possible
Congenital abnormality of urinary tract	Impaired drainage, reflux, reduced barriers to bacterial entry.
Acquired abnormality of urinary tract	
Neurogenic bladder,	Consider indwelling self catheterisation (ISC)
Stones,	Where possible remove (rarely possible with nephrolithiasis or multiple stones)
Bladder diverticulum,	Consider surgical repair
Rectovesical fistula,	Consider surgical repair
Prolapse	Consider surgical repair
Obstruction	Restore free flow of urine, ideally avoiding foreign body
Ileal conduit	Diagnosis often difficult as urine universally infected/colonised in asymptomatic patients
Urethral strictures	Regular flow studies and post micturition bladder volumes with urological follow up
Prostatic enlargement	Flow studies and post micturition bladder volumes in elderly male with UTI
Oestrogen deficiency	Consider topical (but not systemic) HRT
Renal transplant	Very high incidence, progression to pyelonephritis common and may be asymptomatic
Pregnancy	Screening for and treating ASB, with subsequent follow up throughout pregnancy
Diabetes	Exclude autonomic bladder, consider attempts to improve glycaemic control
Lower socioeconomic status	
Mental impairment and institutionalization	
Insertive rectal intercourse	Insertive rectal intercourse and vaginal intercourse following rectal intercourse

Acute uncomplicated pyelonephritis in women is roughly 3 per 1000 person-years [3] with a peak age of 15–34. The host risk factors for acute and chronic pyelonephritis are almost identical to that of lower urinary tract infection, but diabetes, stones, pregnancy, and urinary tract abnormalities including transplantation are prominent. Emphysematous pyelonephritis (EPN) and xanthogranulomatous pyelonephritis (XPN) also have a very strong female predominance and a peak incidence in the sixth decade both being highly associated with diabetes (95% of EP) and stones [4].

Both lower and upper UTIs are almost exclusively the result of ascending infection of periurethral organisms, predominantly the patient's own bowel organisms with over 85% of infections being due to gram-negative bacilli. The vast majority (75–95%) of infections in uncomplicated upper and lower UTI are due to *Escherichia coli*. The remainder are due to other gram negatives (*Klebsiella pneumoniae*, *Proteus mirabilis*, *Citrobacter*, *Pseudomonas aeruginosa*, and other *Enterobacteriaceae*) or gram positives (*Staphylococcus saprophyticus*, *Enterococci*, Group B streptococci, *Staphylococcus aureus*). It is important to note that along with an increasing risk of resistance, this pattern of uropathogens significantly alters in complicated UTIs with a marked increase in other enterobacteria such as *Pseudomonas* (especially related to catheters), *Proteus* (especially related to stones), and enterococci. *Staphylococcus aureus* infection can result from ascending infection, but particularly in the setting of APN, it is critical to exclude a haematogenous source. Multiple infections from a variety of different gut organisms suggest repeated urinary tract introduction or, rarely, an anatomical connection between the gut and urinary tract. On the other hand, multiple infections with the same organism suggest a persistent nidus of infection or an organism particularly adept at causing UTIs, e.g. UPEC. A very small proportion of upper and lower UTIs are secondary to mycobacteria, fungal, and viruses (BKV, CMV, HSV and adenovirus) in the immunocompromised (▶ Chap. 94 Infections complications of transplantation).

54.8 Bacteria Virulence

Some UPEC have virulence factors that facilitate infection or avoid host defences. They include adhesins such as P, Type 1 and Dr. fimbriae, haemolysin, and factors that disrupt the integrity of the uroepithelium, impair ureteric peristalsis, complement resistance, and promote iron sequestration. Some pathogens have multiple virulence factors with some specifically facilitating cystitis but not APN with others promoting APN. Specifically three virulence factors are associated with APN; (a) mannose resistant P fimbriae (>90% of APN), (b) papGAP (class II) genotype, and (c) Dr. fimbriae which binds to decay-accelerating factor virulence in pregnancy and is associated with APN in pregnancy. While interesting, organisms are not routinely screened for these virulence factors; however, it does have clinical relevance in that sexual partners often have the same uropathogenic bacteria, and in the absence of good infection control, these organisms can be transmitted from patient to patient in the hospital setting.

54.9 Host Defences and the Urinary Microbiome

Most of our protection from UTIs comes from physiochemical barriers and, when infection occurs, the innate immune system. Acquired immunity (antibodies or cell-mediated) seems to count for very little in the way of defence or cure of UTIs. Our understanding of the host defences is continuously evolving with the evidence emerging regarding the urine microbioma. Contrary to our previous understanding that 'urine is sterile', it is now known that the normal urinary bladder has a microbiome and there are several commensal organisms in a healthy person's uroepithelium. Although it would be commonly assumed that these organisms are likely to be associated with bowel flora, in females these microbiota seem to be associated with vaginal flora. The implications for the existence of a commensal microbiota are not clear. However, it is thought that these commensals might outcompete pathogens and may play a role in regulation and maintenance of epithelial junctions, priming epithelial defences including immune defences, degradation of harmful compounds, and prevention of recurrent superficial bladder cancer, necessary for proper development of the urinary tract, including the uroepithelium, immune system, and peripheral nervous system within the bladder and surrounding tissues. ◘ Figure 54.1 shows the impact of impairing local barriers in the perineum on the propensity to UTI.

As shown in ◘ Table 54.2, there are a variety of antimicrobial peptides and anti-adhesion molecules as natural defences. In acute cystitis there may be a direct invasion of the uroepithelial cells, with the formation of intracellular bacterial colonies, which are semi-protected from antibiotics and the innate immune system and subsequently cause reinfection. In response, the superficial umbrella cells of the bladder wall exfoliate in part triggered by FimH bacterial adhesion. Macroscopically APN causes either focally or a diffuse enlargement of the kidney and localised bacterial infection, this may result in a lobar nephronia (see ◘ Fig. 54.2) intra-renal abscess, perinephric abscess, or papillary necrosis* (*in predisposed individuals (diabetes, sickle cell disease and anal-

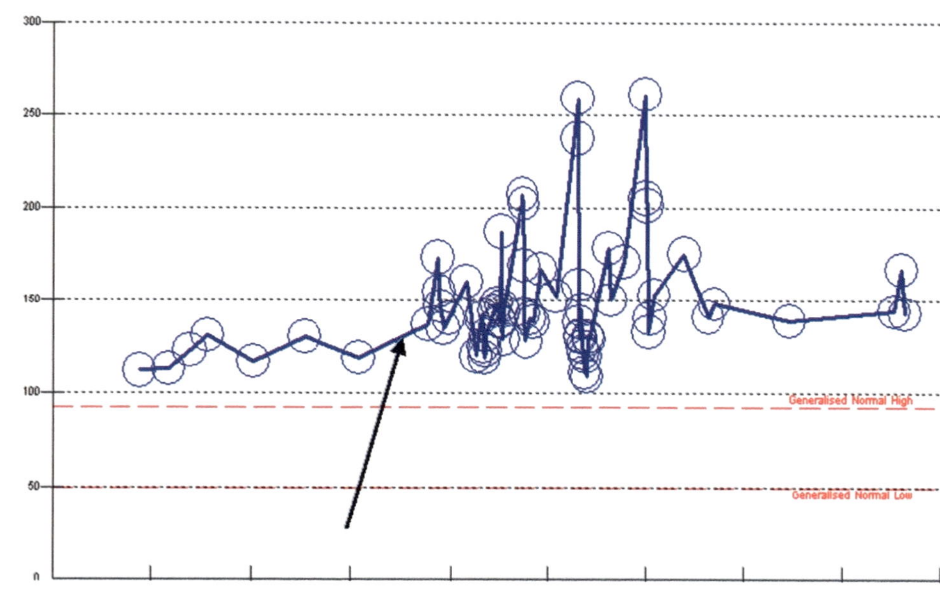

Fig. 54.1 The importance of normal mucosal barriers in preventing UTI. This renal transplant recipient had been free of UTIs since transplantation but was treated with topical imiquimod cream (arrow) for vaginal intra-epithelial neoplasia. This resulted in significant local inflammation and for 9 months she suffered recurrent severe UTIs reflected in recurrent deterioration in renal function (y-axis creatinine in μmol/L), despite prolonged courses of appropriate antibiotics. UTIs stopped with cessation of imiquimod and topical oestrogen cream

Table 54.2 Host defences against urinary tract infection

Urine:	
High osmolality	Ability to produce a concentrated high osmolality, acid urine with high flow rates is impaired in almost all forms of AKI and CKD. The presence of glycosuria, a nutrient for bacteria as well as impairing the function of neutrophils is an important risk factor in diabetic patients
Low pH	Potentially impaired in CKD and renal tubular acidosis
Urine flow	
Urine voiding	Complete bladder emptying is a crucial mechanism for controlling or eradicating bacteria hence the excess of UTI in male patients with BPH and incomplete voiding or those with bladder diverticulae, reflux to transplant or native kidneys. Bacteria can also commonly sequester in stones
Urinary tract mucosa (antibacterial peptides and cytokines)	The role of the mucosal barrier is illustrated by the increased incidence of UTIs in post-menopausal women and in those with local inflammation (see Fig. 54.1)
Anatomical barrier of male urethra	Both the male and female urethra offer an important defence against ascending infection, which is completely out flanked by instrumentation or catheterisation
FimH-mediated exfoliation of superficial epithelial cells	Shedding of infected 'umbrella cells' of transitional epithelium
Urinary inhibitors of bacterial adhesion:	
Tamm-Horsfall protein (uromodulin)	The impact of AKI or CKD is unknown but it seems likely that production of urinary inhibitors such as uromodulin may be impaired in this setting and urine concentrations of uromodulin are significantly reduced in older patients with a UTI
Mucopolysaccharides	
Lactoferrin	
Blood group P secretor status	
Antimicrobial peptides	α and β defensins, Catlicidin, Pentraxin related peptide-3 (PTX-3), Ribonuclease-7, Hepcidin
Innate immunity:	
Neutrophils (TLR4/CD14 pathway, IRF-3, CXCR1)	Neutropenia is a significant risk factor especially in the progression of lower UTI to systemic sepsis. Functional impairment of neutrophils and other aspects of innate immunity by steroids may also result in greater severity of UTI rather than increased risk

(continued)

Table 54.2 (continued)

Urine:	
Cytokines (IL-6, IL1β)	IL-6 produced by renal tubular epithelial cells is likely to be reduced in CKD and AKI
Macrophage/monocytes	The importance of macrophages is demonstrated by renal malacoplakia, a chronic granulomatous condition resulting from impairment of macrophage bactericidal activity
Acquired immunity:	
Humoral immunity	There is little evidence for a defensive role of either humoral or cell-mediated acquired immunity in UTI. Although antibodies can be generated following APN with septicaemia and globally immunosuppressed patients fare worse with septicaemia
Cell-mediated immunity	T and B cell immunity significantly impaired by a variety of immunosuppressive agents used in autoimmunity and transplantatio

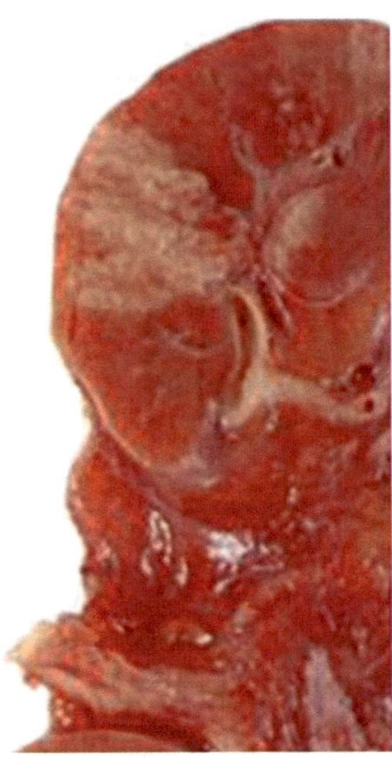

Fig. 54.2 Macroscopic section of kidney showing a wedge-shaped area of infection in acute pyelonephritis

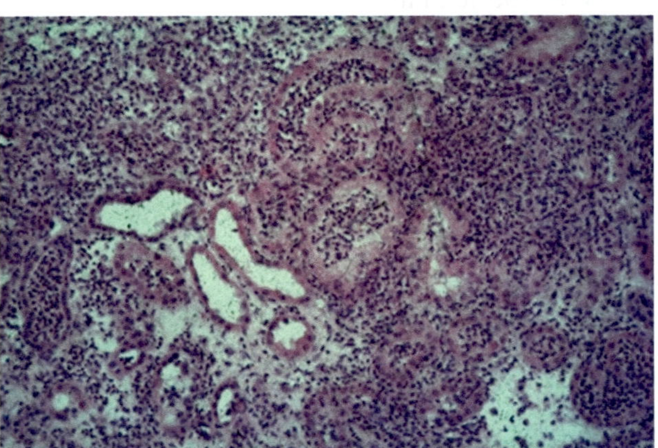

Fig. 54.3 Gross pyelonephritis at low power showing tubules full of neutrophils but also extensive inflammatory infiltrate of neutrophils, lymphocytes, macrophages, and eosinophils

gesic nephropathy). Microscopically there are sharply demarcated wedge-shaped areas of marked inflammation with polymorph infiltration of the tubules with relative sparing of the glomeruli (Fig. 54.3). Neutrophil and macrophage defences are increasingly important in managing established infection of the kidney and bladder.

54.10 Clinical Features of Acute Cystitis and Pyelonephritis

UTIs can present in a myriad of ways from asymptomatic bacteruria (ASB) on routine screening, acute cystitis, and acute pyelonephritis to life-threatening septicaemia but also and increasingly in the elderly and comorbid population with acute confusional state and AKI. Chronically, UTI can present with PUO, weight loss, anaemia, polyclonal gammopathy and raised inflammatory markers, mass in the kidney, or progressive chronic renal disease. A previous history of UTIs, diabetes, stones, ADPKD, abnormal urological anatomy, or instrumentation provides useful clues.

Acute cystitis in adults classically presents as sudden onset dysuria, frequency, and urgency with or without suprapubic tenderness, usually abrupt onset. The symptoms are usually accompanied by pyuria and bacteriuria. Patients often notice that their urine is cloudy and offensive and sometimes have macroscopic haematuria. However, as mentioned above, in the elderly or infirm, UTIs can manifest as non-specific decompensation. APN in adults is usually but not always preceded by the symptoms of lower UTI, associated with nausea, a fever, chills or rigors, flank pain, and/or costovertebral angle tenderness. Again, the elderly may present with acute confusion and significantly are much more likely to result in septicaemia and shock than in younger patients. There are no specific clinical features of EPN apart from the strong association with diabetes and the severity of the patient's condition, the diagnosis being made on imaging. Finally, APN can have no upper tract signs or symptoms, and it is not unusual to diagnose lower UTI but miss APN in the elderly, diabetic, transplants and even in healthy individuals resulting in an inappropriately short course of antibiotics.

Dipstick positivity for leucocytes (plus or minus nitrites) is often very helpful but can result in false-positives (especially from catheter and ileostomy samples) and negatives (especially in neutropenia). However, urinary dipsticks are a useful point of care test in patients with urinary symptoms. The four markers of blood, leucocytes, nitrite, and protein have an excellent negative predictive value of 98% for the absence of all four markers in one study, with a sensitivity and specificity of 98.3% and 19.2%, respectively. Although rare, white blood cell casts are highly suggestive of APN and can be very helpful if the diagnosis is uncertain. Modest proteinuria (<1 g) and haematuria is common.

The differential diagnosis of APN includes renal arterial or venous infarction, acute nephritis, perinephric abscess, and obstruction and or stones, pneumonia, or empyema and loin pain secondary to viral illness.

Only 25% of patients with APN have positive blood cultures, but 90–95% have positive MSU cultures. While there is an argument for treating a clear case of uncomplicated cystitis without sending MSU for culture [5], there is a strong argument for ensuring an MSU is sent before treatment of APN or any patient with a complicated/recurrent UTI as the risk of relapse, recurrence, or resistance is much higher.

When should imaging be considered? For uncomplicated cystitis and some who would argue a first episode of uncomplicated APN, imaging has a low diagnostic yield. However, for recurrent or complicated UTIs then imaging becomes increasingly critical. It is also indicated for patients presenting with sepsis or septic shock, a known or suspected urolithiasis, a urine pH of 7.0 or higher, or a new decrease in the glomerular filtration rate below 40 ml/min. AKI is often more dependent on the degree of sepsis than the extent of renal involvement. Renal function often appears normal in unilateral uncomplicated APN, and thus if AKI is present, it implies a severe infection and or obstruction.

A plain X-ray may show calcification or gross emphysematous pyelonephritis but is insensitive and should be combined with a renal ultrasound for the initial investigation of APN [6]. Renal ultrasound is critical to rule out bladder or renal obstruction (pyonephrosis or EP are both medical emergencies) and may also reveal nephronia, diffusely enlarged kidney, or renal/perirenal abscess. However, the most sensitive imaging for pyelonephritis is contrast CT KUB (Fig. 54.4) [7] especially for identifying perinephric stranding, focal infections, stones, and excluding emphysematous pyelonephritis (Fig. 54.5) or cystitis. Whilst MRI avoids the radiation dose of CT scanning and ionic contrast, it currently has no diagnostic advantage over CT scanning which remains more sensitive. Functional imaging such as gallium-CT, white blood cell, or PET scan can sometimes identify focal or diffuse renal infection in the kidney and is worth considering in patients with PUO or recurrent UTI to identify the source (Fig. 54.6). DMSA scanning is the most sensitive method for detecting scarring providing the patient has a reasonable GFR, and the scan is at least 3 months post APN [8]. In the context of a poor GFR, ultrasound scanning in skilled hands or CT may identify renal scarring. Establishing the presence of scarring can help make the diagnosis of APN as the cause of renal impairment in a new patient and is also helpful in monitoring progression in patients with recurrent upper UTI.

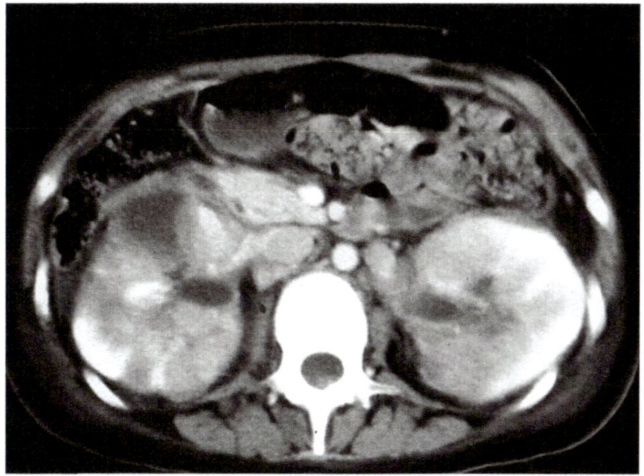

Fig. 54.4 CT KUB in a patient with acute pyelonephritis demonstrating gross swelling of the kidneys and very patchy nephrograms. (Courtesy of Dr. Ian Cropley)

Pyonephrosis (obstructed and infected upper tract) and EPN deserve special mention because of their extreme risk. EPN is a severe version of APN defined by the presence of gas with rapid deterioration, septicaemia, and high mortality. The vast majority of cases (90–95%) of cases occur in diabetics (who have a much higher rate of asymptomatic bacteruria), up to a third of cases may be associate with obstruction (pyonephrosis), and 5–8% can be bilateral [4]. The mortality of EPN has fallen from 78 to 13.5% in the last 4 decades, and this is probably attributable to earlier diagnosis with greater access to CT scanning and the combination of broad-spectrum antibiotics plus rapid medical drainage (large bore nephrostomy) (antibiotics alone (without

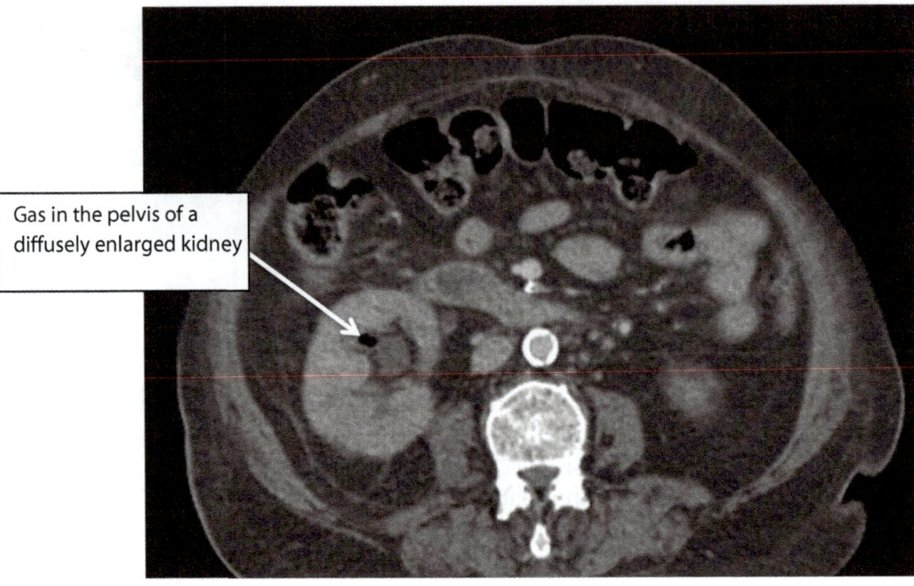

Fig. 54.5 CT KUB with enlarged kidney with fat stranding and free gas of emphysematous pyelonephritis

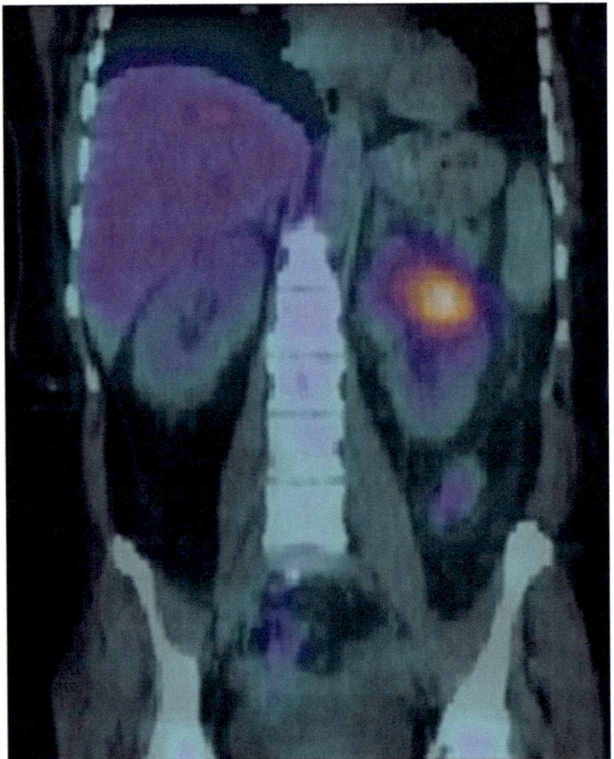

Fig. 54.6 CT gallium scan showing the focal area of inflammation due to pyelonephritis in a patient being investigated for pyrexia of unknown origin. (Courtesy of Dr. Ian Cropley)

drainage) is associated with a RR of death of 2.85) [9]. The choice between percutaneous drainage and surgical nephrectomy needs to be made on a case-by-case basis depending on the stability of the patient and the availability of experienced radiologists or surgeons; however, even if nephrectomy is appropriate, the patient can often be stabilized for this by a period of radiological drainage and antibiotics [4]. EPN and pyonephrosis constitute medical emergencies and require a rapid and multidisciplinary approach.

Subsequent imaging should be carried out in all cases of worsening condition or lack of improvement after 24 to 48 hours of initial therapy.

54.11 Treatment of Acute UTI

It is important to ensure the correct diagnosis and differentiate a patient likely to have uncomplicated UTI from those with complicated UTI, where the risks of treatment failure or more severe disease are much higher. Recommendations vary between countries and are influenced by local resistance patterns and tolerability. The principles treatment of uncomplicated UTI is summarised in a 2012 review [1]. Whilst 2011 US guidance is currently under review [10], recently published UK Guidance [11] are based on yearly Public Health England surveillance data [12].

54.12 Prevention and Treatment of Uncomplicated UTI

The approach to UTI prophylaxis includes taking a good history to look for predisposing risk factors and behaviours, adopting behavioural changes, and considering nonantibiotic and antibiotic prophylaxis. It is really important to limit advice to interventions known to reduce infections rather than give patients multiple suggestions of no proven benefit. Table 54.3 summarizes the different preventive measures for recurrent UTI according to their evidence of benefit.

Table 54.3 Prophylactic measures for recurrent UTI

Evidenced-based interventions	No evidence but seems sensible	No evidence
1. Increasing daily fluid intake by 1.5 L 2. Controlling blood glucose in diabetics 3. Antibiotic prophylaxis (regularly or post-coital) 4. Vaginal oestrogen 5. Avoidance of spermicides 6. Avoiding disruption of normal vaginal microbiota with harsh cleansers 7. Methenamine hippurate	1. Voiding after intercourse 2. Avoiding sequential anal and vaginal intercourse 3. Avoiding prolonged holding of urine 4. Habitual double micturition in patients with modest post-micturition residuals or those who have significant reflux	1. Cranberry juice 2. D-mannose 3. Intravesical hyaluronic acid

54.13 Conservative Measures

Good evidence exists for increasing daily fluid intake by 1.5 L, the avoidance of spermicides, controlling blood glucose in diabetics, and avoiding disruption of normal vaginal microbiota with harsh cleansers. In addition, despite the absence of supportive evidence, it is reasonable to advocate voiding after intercourse, avoiding sequential anal and vaginal intercourse and avoiding prolonged holding of urine. In patients with modest post-micturition residuals that do not require more definitive treatment or those who have significant reflux (and thus may have post-reflux residuals), there is a logical argument (although no evidence base) for recommending habitual double micturition, i.e. waiting for a brief period and attempting to pass more urine.

54.14 Nonantibiotic Measures

1. Vaginal Oestrogen. There is a significant rise in UTI in postmenopausal women due to the changes in vaginal microbiota away from lactobacillus-dominant environment to a more readily colonization by gram-negative pathogens due to the reduction in vaginal oestrogen and the increase in vaginal pH that occurs in menopause. Oestrogens are known to improve mucosal protection, reduce urethral pH, and promote protective lactobacilli. Atrophic urethritis and vaginitis can cause severe lower urinary tract symptoms in the absence of infection. Reviews of the literature show no evidence of benefit and the possible deterioration of symptoms with systemic hormone replacement therapy. Five RCTs on topical oestrogen therapy have been conducted so far showing that topical therapy is safe with no increased risk for recurrence of breast cancer, endometrial hyperplasia, or carcinoma. A meta-analysis concluded that vaginal oestrogen reduced rUTIs compared to placebo (RR 0.25, 0.13–0.50 [cream], RR 0.64, 0.47–0.86 (ring)) but is associated with vaginal irritation and poor adherence. Larger trials are needed, but we advocate a trial (3 months) of topical oestrogens in postmenopausal women with recurrent UTI especially if she has prominent symptoms of urethritis or vaginitis.
2. Methenamine Hippurate. This agent has been advocated to reduce urinary tract infections through urinary acidification through the production of formaldehyde. A 2012 Cochrane meta-analysis indicated a benefit in short term prophylaxis of less than 7 days in patients with normal urinary tracts.
3. D-Mannose. One trial reported efficacy comparable to nitrofurantoin prophylaxis [13]. Criticised for poor trial design and high selection bias [14], more studies are required.

Many other agents are under investigation, including lactobacillus vaginal pessaries, and *E. coli* vaccines (Uro-Vaxom® and vaginal vaccines) [15, 16].

Whilst non-steroidal anti-inflammatory agents are effective at relieving the symptoms of dysuria, they are currently not recommended as a stand-alone treatment due to an increased risk of progression to pyelonephritis. Currently, no evidence exists for intravesical hyaluronic acid, nor the previously much-celebrated cranberry juice which a Cochrane metanalysis has shown no significant reduction in symptomatic UTI overall or among specific at-risk groups in 24 studies with a total of 4473 patients [17].

54.15 Antibiotic Prophylaxis

There is good evidence from RCTs that antibiotic prophylaxis (either regularly or post-coital) is highly effective at reducing the frequency of recurrent UTIs (90–95% reduction) although on stopping the relapse rate is high (~50%). IDSA guidelines, and more recently NICE, recommend nitrofurantoin (50–100 mg. GFR >45 ml/min), trimethoprim (100 mg), or cephalexin (125 mg). In the USA, trimethoprim-sulfamethoxazole (240–480 mg) is given as an option, but not in the UK due to sulphonamide side-effect concerns. It is important to exclude an infection at the time of starting prophylaxis, and the choice of antibiotic will depend on several fac-

54

tors including local resistance profiles. Co-amoxiclav and fluoroquinolones both offer highly effective prophylaxis but are not recommended as first line due to the risks of resistance and altered bowel flora, whilst resistance develops quickly to fosfomycin (3 g every 10 days). There is no convincing evidence that rotating antibiotics (changing prophylactic antibiotics periodically) are beneficial; however, it may be helpful in preventing the long-term use of nitrofurantoin (which can rarely cause neuropathy and pulmonary fibrosis) especially in patients with renal impairment. Antibiotic prophylaxis always carries the risk of the development of antibiotic resistance and no lasting post-prophylaxis difference in rUTIs. Prophylaxis is also effective in patients carrying out intermittent self-catheterisation. In a randomised open-label study using daily prophylactic antibiotics vs control for 1 year, a 48% reduction in UTIs (1·3 cases per person-year (95% CI 1·1–1·6) versus 2·6 (2·3–2·9) (control) incidence rate ratio of 0·52 (0·44–0·61; $p < 0{\cdot}0001$) = 22 minor adverse events in prophylaxis group) was seen however with increased antimicrobial-resistant rates. NICE guidance in 2018 offers a very useful approach to individuals with recurrent UTI [11].

54.16 Antibiotic Treatment

There are a few guiding principles for the treatment of UTI: the quality of the diagnosis and sample is important before commencing treatment, not everyone needs treatment, and poor renal function significantly limits the penetration, usefulness, and safety of some antibiotics. An up-to-date appreciation of local levels of antibiotic resistance, previous resistance patterns in your patient, and a close liaison between nephrologist and microbiologist are extremely important. It is critical to distinguish between uncomplicated and complicated UTI in terms of treatment length, follow-up, and exclusion of reversible predisposing factors. Nice guidance for the treatment of uncomplicated lower urinary tract infection [11] is a very helpful guideline and is broadly similar to European and North American recommendations that aim to promote antibiotic stewardship and reduce collateral damage from antibiotics. Antibiotic recommendations for uncomplicated lower UTI in a woman from this guideline are 3 days of either nitrofurantoin (if eGFR >45 ml/min), trimethoprim, pivmecillinam, or a single dose of fosfomycin. The caveat being that choice should be informed by local resistance patterns [11].

Asymptomatic bacteruria (ASB) often should not be treated (especially if likely to be contaminated, catheter, urostomy or ileal loop-related samples), whereas in other groups such as pregnancy (where treatment of ASB reduces the rate of subsequent pyelonephritis from 20–35% to 1–4%) and pre-procedure prophylaxis before urological intervention likely to draw blood, treatment is mandatory. In other words treatment depends on the perceived risk; in healthy women while 50% of patients with ASB resolve spontaneously, the 50% that do develop cystitis rarely progresses to severe disease, so observation of ASB is reasonable unless the patient has a history of recurrent severe UTIs. Similarly, in the elderly ASB there is no strong evidence that treatment is beneficial. UTI is very common in renal transplantation, associated with detrimental effects, but there is no evidence that treatment of ASB is helpful in this setting. For other patients at risk of complicated UTI, such as those with abnormal anatomy, treatment greatly depends on the individual assessment. Tables 54.4a, b, c, d shows treatment options for UTIs.

54.17 Special Groups

54.17.1 Pregnancy

Progesterone-induced dilatation of the collecting system with decreased peristalsis partial obstruction from the gravid uterus contribute to a high (1–2%) rate of pyelonephritis [18]. 80–90% of pyelonephritis occurs in the last two trimesters and more commonly on the right (50% and 25% on the left and 25% bilateral) [18, 19]. ASB in early pregnancy is an important predictor with less than 1% of patients without ASB going on to develop pyelonephritis later in pregnancy compared to 20–40% of those with untreated bacteriuria early in pregnancy [19]. APN in pregnancy is associated with

Table 54.4a Treatment of asymptomatic bacteriuria (ASB)

Contaminated sample	Contaminated samples (mixed growth, multiple epithelial cells no pyuria) should not be treated
Healthy women	There is little convincing evidence for treating ASB in healthy women (despite a 50% chance of progressing to cystitis)
Elderly	Treatment of ASB in the elderly should be avoided as it makes no difference to morbidity or mortality
Indwelling catheters	Long-term indwelling catheters, urostomies, and ileal loops are universally contaminated with bacteria often associated with pyuria. Culture and treatment with antibiotics are unnecessary when the patient shows no sign of infection, and treatment is likely not only to fail to clear colonisation but almost guaranteed to generate increasing resistance
Urostomy/ileal loop	

Table 54.4b Asymptomatic bacteriuria special cases

Pregnancy	Treatment of ASB in pregnancy shown to reduce subsequent APN from 20–35% to 1–4% screening and treatment is mandatory with post-antibiotic follow up in pregnancy
Prior to urological intervention/surgery	Compelling evidence that treatment or prophylaxis directed at ASB in patients prior to urological surgery reduces the risk of urosepsis (not routine catheterisation)
Neutropenia	It is unclear if treatment of ASB in the neutropenic patient is beneficial
Transplantation	ASB is common with a high conversion to transplant pyelonephritis and high levels of antibiotic resistance. However there is currently no evidence showing the benefit of treating ASB. Stent removal should be considered urgently in the context of ASB. Anecdotally, ASB in patients with complex anatomy such as augmented bladders or reflux may behave differently and require more thought.
Complex uroanatomy	The role of treating ASB is unclear; there is a high risk of conversion to symptomatic complicated UTI in this group but little evidence that treatment of ASB has long-term benefits and these patients often have resistant organisms

Table 54.4c Common treatment options for uncomplicated cystitis

Treatment of uncomplicated cystitis. Typical first line treatment options for cystitis in women with normal anatomy.

Choice depends on knowledge of local resistance patterns.

Nitrofurantoin 100 mg twice daily for 3 days

Co-trimoxazole 960 mg twice daily for 3 days

Fosfomycin 3 g single dose

Pivmecillinam 400 mg twice a day for 3 days

increased risk of preterm delivery and small-for-dates infants (although it is not clear if this is causal) and sepsis syndrome with leaky lungs, stressing the importance of screening patients for ASB early in pregnancy. Consequently, aggressive treatment with good supportive care is important; however, antibiotic choices are limited somewhat. Fluoroquinolones and aminoglycosides are relatively contraindicated in pregnancy (although are probably safe), and sulfonamides should be avoided in the third trimester due to the risk of the grey baby syndrome. It is important to liaise with microbiology, but intravenous third generation cephalosporins or temocillin are reasonable first-line options assuming no previous resistance. Imaging by ultrasound is urgent, and it can be challenging to differentiate physiological dilatation from obstruction. If the patient's condition is not rapidly improving, then sequential ultrasound scanning sometimes helps to identify progressive dilatation.

Table 54.4d Treatment of acute pyelonephritis

Antimicrobial prescribing in acute pyelonephritis in non-pregnant women and men aged more than 16 years:

Most patients can be managed at home but need thoughtful assessment and early review. For those who are clinically sick should be admitted to a place of safety and if AKI associated with sepsis then should have urgent renal imaging (within 12 hours) to exclude obstruction. The choice of antibiotics will depend on local protocols, resistance patterns and in some cases availability. Typical oral treatment options in the UK are the following:

1. Cefalexin: 500 mg twice or three times a day (up to 1 to 1.5 g three or four times a day for severe infections) for 7 to 10 days
2. Co-amoxiclav (only if culture results available and susceptible) 500/125 mg three times a day for 7 to 10 days
3. Trimethoprim (only if culture results available and susceptible) 200 mg twice a day for 14 days
4. Ciprofloxacin (consider safety issues): 500 mg twice a day for 7 days

If the patient is nable to take oral antibiotics, or severely unwell treatment should initiated intravenously and rapidly. In the case of a sick patient it is critical to discuss local resistance patterns or previous recent cultures with microbiology department. Typical IV treatment options in the UK are the following:

Co-amoxiclav (only in combination or if culture results available and susceptible) 1.2 g three times a day

1. Cefuroxime 750 mg to 1.5 g three or four times a day
2. Ceftriaxone 1 to 2 g once a day
3. Ciprofloxacin (consider safety issues) 400 mg twice or three times a day
4. Gentamicin initially 5 mg/kg to 7 mg/kg once a day, subsequent doses adjusted according to serum gentamicin concentration
5. Amikacin initially 15 mg/kg once a day (maximum per dose 1.5 g once a day), subsequent doses adjusted according to serum amikacin concentration (maximum 15 g per course)

Remember also that readmission within 1–2 weeks of finishing antibiotics strongly suggests a persistent and deep-seated infection which requires imaging and careful consideration

Pyonephrosis and emphysematous pyelonephritis

These are medical emergencies

Radiological, microbiological and surgical liaison essential

High dose, broad-spectrum intravenous antibiotics and rapid drainage (usually radiological) of obstructed system has best outcome followed by antibiotics and nephrectomy compared to medical treatment alone. Minimum of 2 weeks treatment

54.17.2 Transplantation

UTI post-transplant is incredibly common and accounts for 40–50% of infectious complications commonly affecting >50% of transplant recipients, the majority of which occur within the first few months and with a high (30–40%) recurrence rate. ◘ Table 54.5 shows the risk factors for post-transplant UTI which have little to do with immunosuppression but mostly involve breaches of the normal physicochemical barriers. Not only the rate of ASB (50%) and cystitis high post-transplant but there is a high conversion rate to acute transplant pyelonephritis (ATPN)(18.7% in one study) [20]. There are several possible explanations for the high frequency of APN in transplants but near-universal reflux (85%) to the transplant kidney, the use of stents and catheters and the high prevalence of abnormal urinary tracts probably all contribute. The high incidence of ASB is a key element as in pregnancy the presence of ASB is a very strong risk factor for APN (RR 12–26). It is important to remember that hospitalized deceased donor kidneys may well have been exposed to bacteriuria and urosepsis with potential donor transmission. Patients receiving transplants abroad may come from areas with high levels of multi-resistant organisms, and there is an argument for prompt screening of urine or stool in patients from high-risk areas.

54

◘ **Table 54.5** Reported risk factors for urinary tract infection post -transplant

Risk Factor	Possible intervention
Donor infection	Culture perfusion fluid and donor urine
Female	
Old age	Impairment of normal physiochemical barriers and innate immunity
History of reflux	Thorough urological assessment pre-transplant
UTIs pre-transplant	Full urological assessment pre-transplant
ADPKD (native kidneys still in situ)	Consider native nephrectomy if recurrent serious UTIs
Diabetes	Exclude autonomic bladder and it seems sensible to attempt tight diabetic control
Long period on haemodialysis pre-transplant	Possibly related diseased underused bladder
Deceased donor	
Delayed graft function	Possibly related toduration of catheter, length of hospitalization or impairment of innate immunity
Acute rejection	Possibly related to the effect of high dose steroids on the innate immune system.
Chronic viral infection	
Reflux to transplant	Occasionally use of native ureter helpful
Ureteric stent	Consider early (2 weeks) removal, with rapid removal if ASB or symptomatic UTI
Indwelling catheter	Earliest possible removal
Dual kidney transplant	Sfbfn
Surgical manipulation of the Graf	Screening for ASB and appropriate prophylaxis

Clinically UTI in transplant recipients may present with classical LUTS and in the case of acute transplant pyelonephritis (ATPN), a tender kidney, fever, and sepsis (7% presenting with septicaemia). However, in immunosuppressed patients, the presentation can be subclinical presenting with unexplained graft dysfunction, and a high index of suspicion is required before giving a short course of antibiotics for a presumed lower urinary tract UTI. Having ruled out the obstruction with an USS, sometimes a CT scan (ideally with contrast) will pick up enlargement, perinephric stranding, or a nephronia, alternatively a CT gallium (not requiring ionic contrast) may identify ATPN in a patient with recurrent UTIs.

The impact of UTI post-transplant has not been absolutely clear partly because many studies have been based on positive cultures rather than clinical disease. It is increasingly clear however that ATPN undoubtedly results in frequent admission, temporary deterioration in function, late renal scarring, and poorer long-term patient survival [21]. ATPN is an independent risk factor for reduced function, rejection, and increasing evidence of graft dysfunction and graft loss [22, 23]. A Spanish study demonstrated 89% 1-year graft survival in those patients with ATPN compared to 96% in those without [24]. Another study demonstrated worse 5-year graft *and* patient survival following early ATPN [25]. It is also clear that rUTIs in RTRs have increased antimicrobial drug resistance, and inadequately treating UTI in RTRs is an effective way of generating multi-drug resistant organisms [26].

A meta-analysis of six studies demonstrated significantly less bacteriuria and 60% less bacteraemia in transplant patients receiving UTI prophylaxis in the early stages of a transplant [27]. This data is striking when one considers the universally high rates of antibiotic resistance in transplant recipients (frequently 100% for Septrin and >50% for beta-lactams and ciprofloxacin). In practical terms almost all patients will receive *Pneumocystis jirovecii* prophylaxis with Septrin, whether adding in a second agent for the early transplant period is beneficial is not clear. Nor is the optimum duration of prophylaxis clear or whether long-term prophylaxis for all transplant recipients is helpful but the pragmatic approach adopted by most units is to stop prophylaxis with Septrin when pneumocystis is felt to be lower risk and offer UTI prophylaxis only to those who declare themselves to have recurrent UTIs.

There is no clear guidance on screening but given the strong association of ASB with subsequent ATPN we routinely send MSUs each visit for the first 3 month and on any subsequent visit if the patient has symptoms or the dipstick is suggestive of a UTI. However, a study done by Origuen [28] have shown that there is no benefit in treatment of asymptomatic bacteruria in renal transplant patients. 112 patients with asymptomatic bacteruria two months post renal transplant randomised to receive treatment have shown no difference in occurrence of TPN at 2 years and current guidance is not to treat ASB in transplant recipients. Advice on the treatment of clinical UTIs in transplant recipients is not evidence based. Our policy is to accelerate ureteric stent removal in any new transplant with ASB or overt UTI and investigate for correctable risk factors such as poor bladder emptying in patients with recurrent, severe or later UTI. A study done looking early stent removal at 5 days without cystoscopy post-transplant vs late removal at 6 weeks post-transplant with cystoscopy in 227 patients showed that stent related complications were significantly higher in the late versus early stent removal groups (36 of 126 [28.6%] vs. 6 of 79 [7.6%]; $p < 0.001$) with a UTI incidence of 31 of 126 (24.6%) in the late group compared with 6 of 79 (7.6%) UTIs in the early group ($p = 0.004$) suggesting that early removal is a sensible manoeuvre [25, 29]

If clinically the patient has cystitis and is well, then a 5-day course of antibiotics is probably appropriate, but if there is a suggestion of ATPN, then 14 days of treatment is probably reasonable. Relapse and readmission following an inadequate course of antibiotics are not infrequent with transplant UTI. It is important to note that any patient returning within 2–3 weeks of their last day of antibiotics is likely to have a persistent, inadequately treated infection and requires rapid resolution of the anatomical cause and if the patient has a deep nidus, then a longer course of antibiotics may be required.

Due to the high rates of resistance to ciprofloxacin and amoxicillin-clavulanic acid, we do not use these as first line in transplant patients sick enough to require admission.

54.18 Infections and Complex Uroanatomy (See ▸ Chapter 56)

Urosepsis can be a significant problem in patients with complex uroanatomy. Recurrent infection, multiple drug resistance, and a high rate of progression to acute and chronic pyelonephritis are common. This is a complex and challenging area, and patients should be reviewed in with MDT meetings involving a specialist urologist, radiology, and urology nurse specialists. Patients should be offered streamlined pathways for acute deteriorations.

54.19 Infected Renal Cysts

Infection of renal cysts is relatively common in patients with polycystic kidney disease when the MSU may be negative and can be difficult to distinguish from a haemorrhage into a cyst. Macroscopic haematuria, flank pain, and lower urinary tract infection recurring after treatment or pyrexia of unknown origin are common presentations. Contrast CT scan may help the diagnosis but often fails to distinguish between infection, bleed, or chronic changes, and treatment is often empirical. Considering diagnostic aspiration of the offending cyst if the infection is not responding to treatment bearing in mind that whilst fluoroquinolones have good penetration, other antibiotics, e.g. aminoglycosides and beta-lactams, have poor penetration into renal cysts and may result in treatment failure. Some success has been claimed for the injection of antibiotics into a single infected cyst. More commonly, particularly in patients suffering recurrent post-transplant, UTI then native nephrectomy may be curative, but getting the correct kidney is crucial; it is not a small operation, and UTIs may continue post-operatively.

54.20 Renal and Perinephric Abscesses

Both renal and perinephric abscesses may occur secondary to haematogenous spread or as a complication of APN, but renal abscess is more likely to be due to the former (therefore search for distant source) and perinephric abscess the latter. In either case culture of *Staphylococcus aureus* or *Candida* species should provoke a fingertip search for the primary source. Both renal and perinephric abscesses may present as loin pain, fever, rigors, and tenderness in the costovertebral angle, or subacutely as a PUO, anaemia, and a raised acute phase response. A positive urine culture is highly likely with an untreated perinephric abscess although less so with a renal abscess and commonly negative if a patient has already received a course of antibiotics for presumed APN rapidly responding to treatment. CT scanning is the imaging of choice and should be considered early in a patient with presumed APN not responding to treatment. Perinephric abscess is usually contained within Gerota's fascia but can infiltrate locally into the diaphragm (hiccups), lung, psoas, and pelvis. Most renal abscesses respond to appropriate parenteral antibiotics without the need for percutaneous drainage, but the bigger the abscess, the less likely conservative management will be effective and percutaneous (especially if culture negative), or sometimes surgical drainage should be considered if the patient is failing to respond to treatment.

54

54.21 Chronic Pyelonephritis

Chronic pyelonephritis (CPN) can affect the kidneys in a variety of ways, most commonly focal scarring (see ◻ Fig. 54.7) following episodes of APN plus or minus papillary necrosis (particularly in diabetic patients) with the risk that sloughed necrotic papilla may then cause obstruction. It is also increasingly common to see patients (particularly diabetics) with progressive CKD secondary to subclinical, subacute pyelonephritis. Rarer but important presentations include Xanthogranulomatous pyelonephritis (XGN) or very rarely malakoplakia. The aetiological risk factors for CPN are similar to those for APN but are frequently associated with a failure of adequate resolution secondary to an abnormal urinary tract (particularly reflux in children), recurrent infection, impaired immunity, or inadequately treated infections. CPN where the infections have been resolved may be associated with salt wasting and relatively preserved urine volumes. The prevalence of ESRD secondary to CPN is not easy to determine; in the UK it is recorded as the cause of ESRD in ~10%, but this probably includes a whole mixture of pathologies including diabetic and reflux nephropathy.

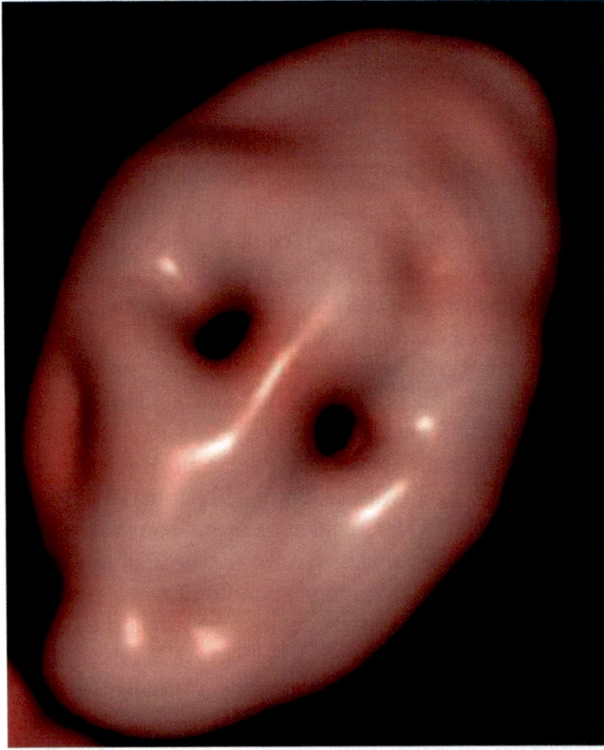

◻ **Fig. 54.7** CT Spect (DMSA) scan in a patient with recurrent ESBL UTIs. The patient incurred recurrent urosepsis with AKI in the setting of a urethral stricture recurrence and incomplete bladder emptying. The CT SPECT shows several holes (scars) secondary to previous episodes of pyelonephritis

54.22 Xanthogranulomatous Pyelonephritis (XPN)

XPN represents less than 1% of pyelonephritis; however, we are likely to see more of it in part because of the increased diagnosis with the ready availability of CT scanning but also because the risk factors of diabetes and nephrolithiasis are also increasing. XPN has been reported in all age groups but typically occurs in women with diabetes in their 60s and 70s, renal stones are extremely common (90%, staghorn in 73%), pyonephrosis in nearly 50%, and non-functioning kidney in a third [30, 31]. In 85% of cases, renal tissue is replaced diffusely by yellow tissue although, in 15% the lesions are focal. The yellow tissue is made up of chronic inflammatory tissue principally lipid-filled histiocytes and multinucleate giant cells as well as neutrophils and lymphocytes. The pathogenesis seems to require obstruction with failure to eradicate the chronic uropathogenic infection, whether diabetes merely predisposes to infection or handicaps the innate immune system in clearing the infection is not clear.

Patients classically present with fevers, weight loss, malaise, and sometimes loin pain. Recurrent UTI infection is common or pyuria in ~60%, and acute phase response is common as is raised polyclonal IgG. The non-specific nature of the symptoms means the diagnosis is often made while screening for, or confused with, malignancy and a preoperative diagnosis of XPN is made in less than 50% of cases. CT scanning is the imaging of choice, and the identification of stones is an important clue but MRI may be able to differentiate between XPN and renal cell cancer [31].

Treatment of diffuse XPN is supportive, antibiotics, and nephrectomy (there are no reported cases of renal recovery using a conservative approach, whereas some patients with focal XPN have achieved renal salvage with the removal of obstruction/stone and prolonged antibiotics. Either way treatment requires a coordinated approach with urologists, microbiologists, and radiologists, and a high index of suspicion of XPN is required in patients with diabetes, stones, and either general unwellness or something funny in the kidney.

54.23 Malakoplakia

Malakoplakia is a very rare condition involving the bladder, occasionally the ureters and kidneys (and very rarely other organs). It is a granulomatous condition resulting from defective lysozomal clearance of intracellular bacteria by macrophages [32]. Presentation is often non-specific and similar to XPN, i.e. fevers, recurrent UTIs, unexplained anaemia, and LUTS. Like XPN, malakoplakia is often mistaken as malignancy or tuberculosis, and the diagnosis is usually made by the histopathologist rather than the clinician. The condition may respond to a very long course of quinolones, but often surgery is also required.

54.24 Recurrent UTI Service

Recurrent urinary tract infection is common in healthy females and very common in patients with abnormal uroanatomy or renal transplants. A streamlined and thoughtful pathway for such patients is probably rarer than it should be, and it is not uncommon for patients to receive multiple courses of inappropriate or inadequate antibiotics and multiple hospital admissions before receiving optimum treatment. One approach to improving the patient experience is a dedicated service for recurrent UTIs, usually, but not exclusively, led by a urologist with specialist interest. ◘ Box 54.1 suggests a plan for initial investigations to consider in a one-stop visit, and ► chapter 53 provides a suggested scheme for setting up a recurrent UTI clinic including suggestions for referral criteria.

Box 54.1 Suggested Initial Investigations in One-Stop Shop

1. Full medical history (including LUT symptom scoring, stones, past history of UTIs, family, sexual and contraceptive history. Medication including anticholinergics and ketamine. Fluid intake and voiding diaries and history of previous microbiology results
2. Examination to include external genitalia and perineum to exclude phimosis, epididymitis, female genital mutilation, cystocele, rectocele, urethrocele, and exclusion of vaginitis
3. Urine dipstick for leucocytes and nitrites (including pH)
4. MSU (liaison with microbiology to culture and identify counts as low as $10^{2 \text{ or } 3}$)
5. STD screen (chlamydia, gonorrhoea, mycoplasma, HSV) if appropriate
6. Full blood count, ESR, urea, creatinine and electrolytes, random glucose, or HbA1c if diabetic
7. Urinary flow rate and post-micturition residue
8. Flexible cystoscopy if appropriate

These tests can be obtained in a single well-organised clinic, and it is especially helpful if previous culture results are available. Following this may be necessary to perform a cystogram to exclude reflux or diverticulae (see ◘ Fig. 54.8 and occasionally urodynamics. Further imaging with CT or CT gallium may be helpful to exclude upper tract abnormalities or locate a site of persisting infection.

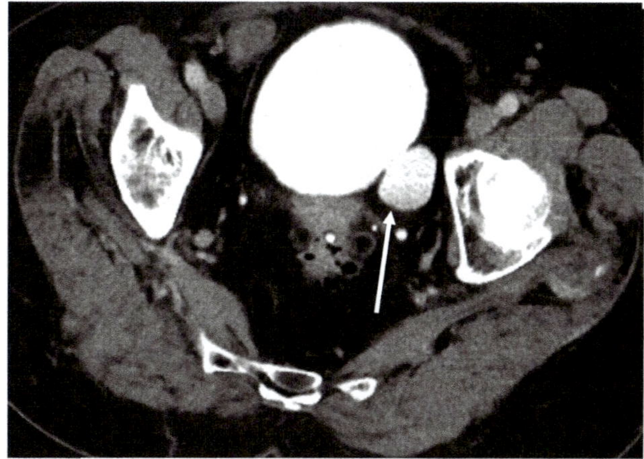

◘ **Fig. 54.8** Cystogram in a patient with recurrent UTIs demonstrating a large diverticulum (arrow) which was excised with the resolution of infections

A suggested pathway for setting up a recurrent UTI (rUTI) clinic with urologists/transplant surgeons, nephrologists, microbiologists/infectious disease specialists, and specialist nurses is shown in the chapter on the urology renal interface.

Patient information leaflets should be available and include basic self-help advice. ► http://www.nhs.uk/conditions/urinary-tract-infection-adults/Pages/Introduction.aspx, ► http://kidney.niddk.nih.gov/kudiseases/pubs/uti_ez/; ► http://www.nhs.uk/conditions/kidney-infection/Pages/Introduction.aspx; and ► https://www.guidelines.co.uk/urology/phe-uti-guideline/453379.article are useful sources for patient information and recommended as a first stop.

If avoidable or correctable causes have been treated, then well-documented trials of prophylactic antibiotics would be appropriate.

54.25 Catheter-Associated UTI (CAUTI)

CAUTI is a significant challenge for modern medicine and the commonest (40%) cause of nosocomial infection and contributes significantly to prolonged inpatient stay and morbidity. Diagnosing infection for patients with urethral and suprapubic catheters may be difficult as colonisation is extremely common and pyuria is not diagnostic (an absence of pyuria does however argue against infection). Clinically UTI may manifest with fever and rigors but in the absence of lower urinary tract symptoms may be non-specific such as acute confusion.

Despite the limited literature, a heroic attempt has been made to produce international guidelines on the diagnosis and treatment of CAUTIs and have resulted in a useful document addressing common issues [33].

54

Table 54.6 Diagnosis, treatment and management of CAUTI

Catheter avoidance	Develop indications for catheterisation with mechanisms promoting pause for thought. Catheterisation for incontinence should be a last resort. Ready access to bladder ultrasound scanning may significantly reduce the need for catheterization to exclude obstruction
Reduced duration	Systems (and culture) to ensure removal of catheters at the earliest opportunity. For in-patients the continued need for a catheter should be considered on a daily basis (as with intravenous access) ideally with an electronic alert
Drainage hygiene	Avoid disconnections of the catheter where possible and ensure catheter tubing and bag are below the level of the bladder; seems basic but stale urine flowing back into the bladder is not uncommon
Screening	There is no merit in screening asymptomatic patients with IDC an exception to this may be pregnant patients
Antibiotic prophylaxis	There is no evidence to support single dose antibiotics with insertion or removal of catheters unless part of a urological procedure likely to result in bleeding
Treatment	Cultures must be sent before commencing treatment. Best guess is to treat symptomatic CAUTIs for 7 days but longer (10–14 if slow response). Once on antibiotics then change of catheter makes sense and experience suggests this is helpful

Perhaps the most important issue related to catheters is whether the patient actually needs it and if so what is the minimum duration required. Institutional reform may be necessary to ensure catheters are only placed when essential, systems put in place, such as "catheter passports" [34] to ensure that the need for the catheter is constantly questioned and removed as soon as safe to do so are likely to have a significant impact on the numbers of CAUTIs (Table 54.6).

54.26 Tuberculosis of the Urinary Tract

The global incidence of TB peaked around 2003 and had plateaued or begun to decline by 2006 [35], but the incidence of TB in some localities such as the UK and particularly in London continues to rise. Approximately 20–25% of cases are extrapulmonary tuberculosis, and the genitourinary tract is the commonest site at 15–20% of these, although isolated genitourinary TB (GUTB) occurs in just 4% of patients.

54.27 Epidemiology

Up to 20% of patients with pulmonary TB are thought to have urogenital involvement [36] the vast majority of these cases are in or from developing countries. GUTB is twice as common in men for reasons that remain unclear. The incidence of extrapulmonary TB is significantly higher amongst dialysis patients and patients with ESRD presumably due to impaired cell immunity. Similarly, the incidence of all forms of TB is variously reported 20–70 times higher amongst transplant patients particularly in the first year of transplantation. However, recent registry data from the UK suggests much lower rates than this, although Asian origin remains a potent risk factor (approximately 10 x incidence compared to Caucasian recipients). Typically, GUTB accounts for 7–15% of TB cases amongst transplant recipients [36] although recent UK data suggests lower rates of GUTB.

54.28 Pathogenesis

Genitourinary disease is mainly secondary to haematogenous dissemination although the disease has been described after intravesical BCG especially in immunocompromised patients. In an immunocompetent person, tuberculous bacilli are trapped in periglomerular capillaries and are followed by granulomata formation. These are typically bilateral, cortical, and adjacent to the glomeruli and can remain dormant for decades. If the patient's immune competence is disturbed, these can progress with typical tuberculous granuloma with caseating necrosis, disseminating the viable organism into the proximal tubules and loop of Henley with the progression of the disease to the renal medulla.

54.29 Clinical Features of GUTB

The diagnosis of renal tuberculosis is often delayed because of insidious onset and non-specific symptoms. The classical symptoms of cystitis with sterile pyuria, weight loss, and fevers should rouse clinical suspicion, but other symptoms are pretty non-specific and include back, flank pain, suprapubic pain, haematuria, frequency, and nocturia. Calcification and fibrosis causing stricture formation (typically at the vesicoureteric junction) in the pelvicalyceal system may result in obstruction, atrophy, and auto-nephrectomy [37]. In the bladder the chronic inflammation causes fibrosis resulting in a thick-walled non-compliant small capacity storage unit causing secondary renal dysfunction (see Fig. 54.9).

Tubulointerstitial nephritis related to tuberculosis is a rare but more recognized manifestation of renal tuberculosis, which is part of the differential of granulomatous TIN although it is uncommon to identify acid-fast bacilli in biopsy specimens.

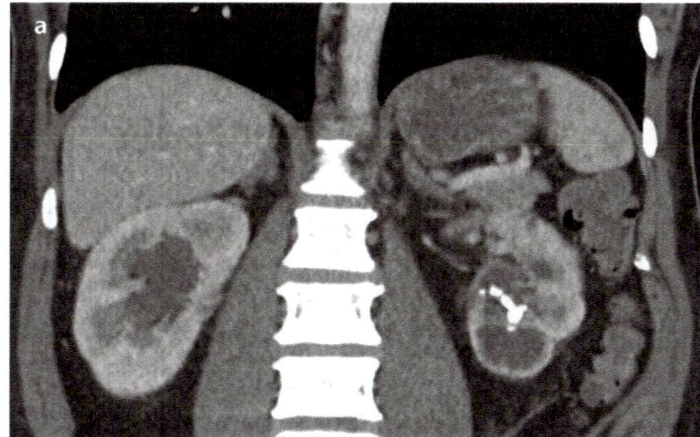

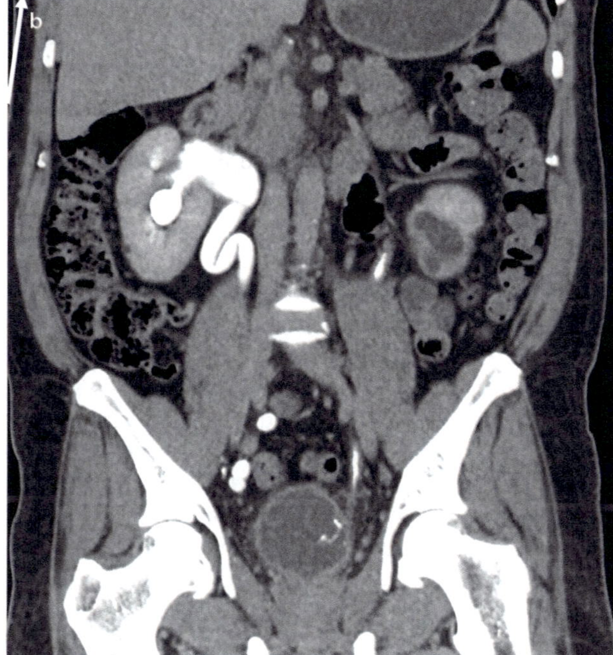

Fig. 54.9 a CT KUB demonstrating a small irregular left kidney with cortical thinning, calcification secondary to a TB abscess. The right kidney is obstructed on this view. b Demonstrates the cause of the obstruction as occurring somewhere in the distal ureter/vesicoureteric junction. The bladder is shrunken and irregular and calcified all classical features of mTB of the urinary tract

54.30 Investigations

Serial early morning urine samples (EMUs) for culture remain the standard for identifying patients with a sensitivity of 65% and a specificity of 100% (at least three samples should be obtained). Tuberculin skin tests and interferon release assays have a high false-negative rate in patients with ESRD due to impaired T cell immunity, and positive results indicated exposure not active disease. Cystoscopy and bladder biopsy may be worth considering in anyone with sterile pyuria; TB culture would need to be requested on biopsy samples. Calcification is common (>50%) with CT scanning having the highest sensitivity. Focal hypoperfusion creating a striated nephrogram and a moth-eaten calyx secondary to papillary necrosis is characteristic.

As the parenchymal granulomata coalesce CT can demonstrate a mass-like lesion with central low attenuation corresponding to tuberculoma with central caseous necrosis. Long-standing TB gives rise to renal parenchymal atrophy and stricture formation with thinning of cortices, multiple thin-walled cysts, progressive hydronephrosis, and dystrophic calcification involving the entire kidney which is the final product of end-stage renal tuberculosis.

Ureteral involvement initially is seen as mucosal irregularity creating a saw tooth ureter appearance. Stricturing and ureteral shortening which occurs as disease advances produces corkscrew ureter with calcifications along the ureter. Renal biopsy may show caseating granulomas, but it is very rare to see acid-fast bacilli.

54.31 Management

The aims of treatment are to render the patient non-infectious, preserve renal function, and address any complication from GUTB infection and should be done in the context of a multidisciplinary team including urology and TB specialists.

GUTB generally responds well to treatment because of the generally low mycobacterial load. Isoniazid and rifampicin penetrate well into cavitating lesions and a high concentration of isoniazid, rifampicin, and pyrazinamide is maintained in urine. With the increasing emergence of multi-resistant TB, sensitivity testing is essential. Surgery has an important part to play in current management. This includes nephrectomy and reconstructive surgery mainly related to strictures and augmentation of the bladder for small fibrotic bladders.

54.32 Fungal Urinary Tract Infections

Fungal urinary tract infections are rare in healthy community-based individuals but are more commonly found in hospitalized patients. The vast majority of these fungal UTIs are due to *Candida* species. The pathological nature of these infections is closely related to host factors and management is dependent upon the underlying condition of the patient in particular immune competence, glycaemic control, anatomy, and presence of foreign bodies (see Table 54.7). The incidence of fungal infections has increased in the context of extensive and prolonged use of broad-spectrum antibiotics, immunosuppressive medication, and cytotoxic drugs.

54.33 Epidemiology

Candida species usually exist as saprophytes of the skin, oropharynx, gastrointestinal tracts, and genital region and thus can contaminate as well as infect. Among

Table 54.7 Predisposing factors for candiduria and *Candida* urinary tract infections

Diabetes mellitus
Renal transplantation
Extremes of age
Instrumentation of the urinary tract
Female sex
Concomitant bacteriuria
Prolonged hospitalization
Congenital abnormalities of the urinary tract
Intensive care unit admission
Structural abnormalities of the urinary tract
Broad-spectrum antibiotics
Indwelling urinary tract devices
Bladder dysfunction
Urinary stasis
Nephrolithiasis

normal adults yeasts are encountered in <1% of clean voided urine specimens but account for up to 5–10% of positive urine culture results in tertiary care facilities, mostly in those with indwelling catheters. The incidence of infections in patients in burns units is threefold that in medical and surgical intensive care units [38]. One study in renal transplants recorded 3% of patients having candiduria within the first 2 years. Candiduria was three times more common in women, 60% associated with antibiotic use and 40% with catheters [39]. Community-acquired *Candida* infections are most common amongst patients with diabetes mellitus, those who are bedridden, and patients receiving antimicrobial therapy. The microbiology of candiduria is changing globally with <50% of urinary isolates now belonging to *Candida albicans.*

The environmental fungi such as *Blastomyces*, *Histoplasmosis*, and *Coccidioides* are found primarily in soil, environment, and guano. Although very serious infections, they rarely involve the renal tract, and if they do so, it is invariably via haematogenous spread, usually in the profoundly immunocompromised.

54.34 Pathophysiology

Candida species can cause antegrade and retrograde infections of the urinary tract. Antegrade infections are due to haematogenous spread of the organism and may involve multiple abscesses or fungal balls and should always prompt a vigorous search for a primary site and exclusion of endocarditis. Ascending infections start from a focus of colonization at or near the urethra. Candida species adhere poorly to bladder mucosa, so infection is usually dependent on the presence of urinary tract obstruction, concomitant bacterial urinary sepsis, or profound immune suppression.

54.35 Diagnosis of Fungal UTI

Distinguishing contamination from infection can be difficult and has significant implications although in the majority; candiduria does not represent infection. Infection is associated with typical and indistinguishable symptoms of cystitis, prostatitis, epididymo-orchitis, or APN. Oliguria, strangiuria, passage of particulate matter, and pneumaturia in the presence of a positive urine culture result can be a feature of more severe infection such as the presence of a fungal ball. Pyuria is suggestive (except in catheterised patients), but candida is frequently a co-infection with uropathogenic bacteria in which case ruling out the contamination is less straightforward and may be absent in neutropenia.

In the presence of a susceptible individual such as a critically ill patient or an immunocompromised patient, candiduria should be regarded as a marker of potential invasive candidiasis. A high index of clinical suspicion in such a scenario should follow with subsequent investigations with blood cultures, examination of the retina and skin, CXR, and ECHO cardiographs to identify disseminated infection. In selected patients a renal ultrasound should be carried out to rule out the presence of hydronephrosis/obstruction, a focal mass in the collective system. Further investigations with CT or MRI may be required to demonstrate the presence of a renal abscess, fungal balls, or non-functioning kidneys.

A pragmatic diagnostic approach to the finding of candiduria was expounded by Kauffman et al. [40]. In essence, suggesting repeating the sample (if absent then to ignore) and if persistent in a previously healthy individal, search for a predisposing condition such as diabetes, urological abnormality, or catheter (which should be changed). In the absence of any obvious abnormality in a well patient, it is reasonable to monitor but if candiduria is associated with a predisposing factor then this should be addressed.

54.36 Treatment

As stated above for asymptomatic candiduria in a previously healthy individual, the finding should be verified on a second carefully collected urine specimen. For persistent candiduria removal of a precipitating cause or treatment of underlying conditions is usually sufficient.

A review for the treatment of fungal infections is a useful reference (38). For patients with symptomatic candida cystitis, treatment is with fluconazole which is highly active against many *Candida* species including *Candida albicans*. It is well tolerated and inexpensive and is concentrated in the urine. For refractory bladder infection, flucytosine, or intravenous therapy with amphotericin B deoxycholate is used. Non-albicans species may need voriconazole, but caspofungin has no role to play due to limited urinary excretion. The presence of fungal balls, obstruction, and renal or prostatic abscesses may well need radiological or surgical intervention. Irrigation with amphotericin B deoxycholate, saline, or streptokinase have all been reported as therapy for fungal balls in combination with parenteral antifungals.

54.37 Summary

Urinary tract infection is a profoundly important problem with significant financial and medical implications. It is especially challenging in patients with abnormal anatomy and renal transplants, yet it remains a Cinderella subject, and the approach to patients with UTI is often less thoughtful than it could be. Nephrologists are in a good position to assist in the improvement of care of these patients.

Tips and Tricks

1. In CKD some antibiotics have very poor penetration into the urine so, for example, Septrin, trimethoprim and nitrofurantoin offer negligible prophylaxis or treatment in patients with significant renal impairment.
2. For cyst-based infection consider antibiotic penetration (fluoroquinolones).
3. Consider subclinical urosepsis/pyelonephritis in diabetic patients with unexpected deterioration in CKD and XPN in the same patients especially if constitutional symptoms, stones, interstitial cystitis, or mass in the kidney.
4. Treatment of uncomplicated UTIs follows well-documented guideline; treatment of complicated UTIs is more complex, and while long courses of antibiotics are not without risk, it is very common for patients to be undertreated and suffer relapses – identification and correction where possible of underlying predisposition is essential.
5. Consider establishing a recurrent UTI clinic if the current patient pathway is not robust or patient-centred.
6. It is very important to identify which patients with complicated urosepsis especially those with anatomical abnormalities and establish an early multidisciplinary review of management to avoid the revolving door of urosepsis following the recurrent inadequate course of antibiotics (see ◘ Fig. 54.10).
7. A patient who has returning symptoms within 2–3 weeks of stopping antibiotics, especially if with the same organism and increasing resistance, is likely to have a persistent infection and repeating the same experiment of a short course of antibiotics without resolving the cause or finding the nidus is likely to repeat the mistake. Patients returning with a second episode of urosepsis need a thoughtful sort out.

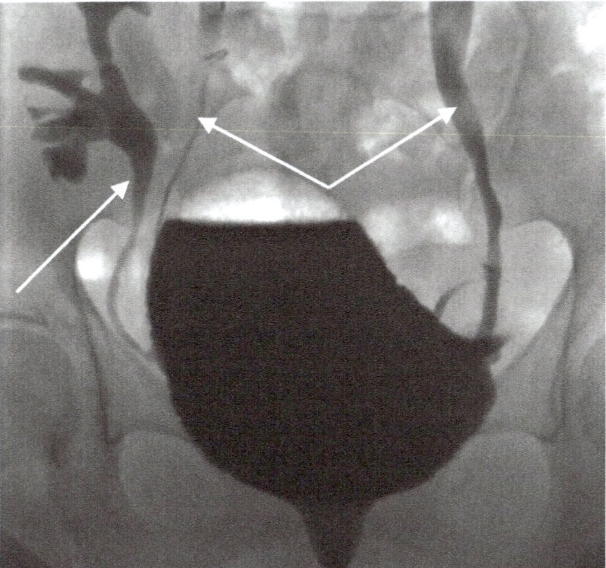

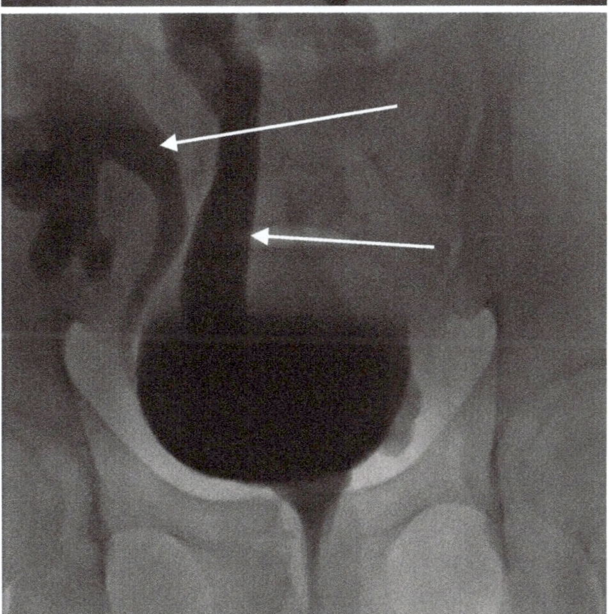

◘ **Fig. 54.10** Two examples of VCMGs in renal transplant recipients with recurrent UTIs. 10a VCMG Reflux to renal transplant and both native ureters. 10b Reflux to transplant kidney and gross reflux to right native ureter. Both cases had recurrent UTIs encouraged by abnormal reflux and storage of urine in ureters during micturition and free backflow to transplanted kidneys resulting in recurrent transplant pyelonephritis. In both cases the problem was only really appreciated following VCMG

54.37.1 Additional Resources

► http://cid.oxfordjournals.org.libproxy.ucl.ac.uk/content/50/5/625.full guidelines on catheters.

► www.nlm.nih.gov/medlineplus/ency/article/000483.htm catheter-related patient information leaflet.

54

Case Study

Case 1

An elderly gentleman was admitted to the hospital with chest pain. His referral letter mentioned that he was on a second course of antibiotics for a UTI. The patient had evidence of acute coronary syndrome but also a CRP of nearly 200 in the context of pyuria. His ACS was treated, and he was put on alternative antibiotics for a UTI. Looking back at his CRP for the preceding few months (◘ Fig. 54.11, the arrow indicates his admission CRP), it was apparent that he had recurrent or partially treated persistent UTI. His historical CRP, the fact that he is male and that he had been treated for several UTIs in the recent past is strongly suggestive of inadequate drainage and or a nidus of infection partially treated. He was found to have poor bladder emptying and a partially obstructed left kidney which was subsequently drained and infection treated with 2 weeks of intravenous antibiotics. In retrospect his recurrent infections were often associated with AKI and progressive renal impairment, identifying that this was not a straightforward UTI, by definition a complicated UTI would have prompted earlier exclusion of abnormal anatomy and avoidance of recurrent short 'uncomplicated' courses of antibiotics.

Case 2

A young woman 7-month postrenal transplant was admitted with urosepsis and rigors. She was treated with co-amoxiclav (initially intravenously) for 2 weeks and discharged with normal imaging and bladder emptying on ultrasound. She subsequently represented on multiple occasions within 1–3 weeks of discharge with the same clinical picture of a UTI with sepsis, settling

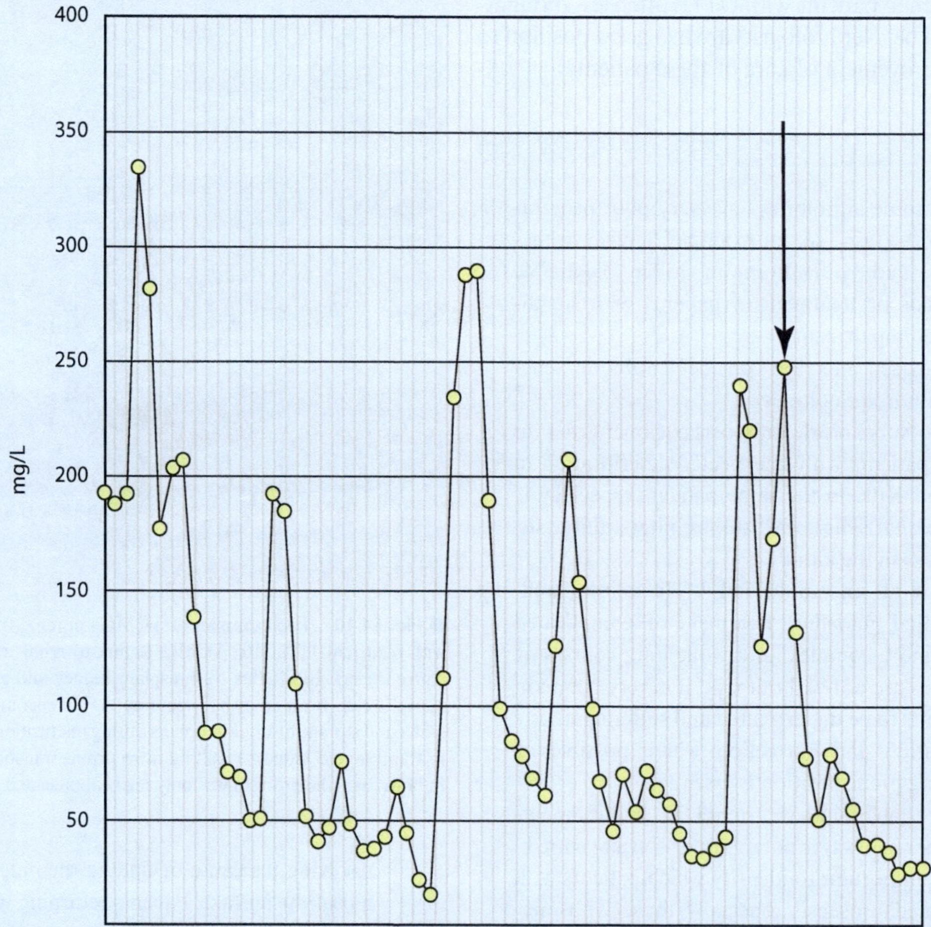

◘ **Fig. 54.11** CRP of a patient admitted with AKI on CKD secondary to UTI. The admission point is shown by the arrow with preceding CRPs

Klebsiella pneumoniae
ESBL confirmed.

	1)
Amikacin	(S)
Ampicillin	R
Augmentin	R
Aztreonam	(R)
Cefepime	(R)
Ceftriaxone	(R)
Ceftazidime	(R)
Cefuroxime	(R)
Cephalexin	R
Ciprofloxacin	(R)
Colistin	(S)
Cotrimoxazole	(R)
Ertapenem	(S)
Gentamicin	R
Levofloxacin	(R)
Meropenem	(S)
Nitrofurantoin	S
Piperacillin	(R)
Piperacillin/Tazoba	(I)
Temocillin	(S)
Tobramycin	(R)
Trimethoprim	R
Mecillinam	S
Polymixin	(S)
All penicllins	(R)
All cephalosporins	(R)
Fosfomycin	S
ESBL test.	(PO)

Fig. 54.12 *Klebsiella pneumoniae* resistance profile following 6 months of recurrent UTI with multiple courses of antibiotics

quickly on appropriate antibiotics. Some urine cultures were negative some demonstrated an increasingly resistant *Klebsiella pneumoniae* which eventually procured the resistance profile shown in Fig. 54.12. Despite normal ultrasound imaging, the fact that her symptoms recurred within 2 weeks of stopping antibiotics with the same but increasingly resistant organism is highly suggestive of an inadequately treated nidus of infection. A CT PET scan (Fig. 54.13) identified a focus of infection in the transplant kidney. She was treated with 6 weeks of IV temocillin in the community and had no further UTIs for 18 months.

This illustrates a couple of key points, firstly it is very easy to generate multi-resistant uropathogenic bacteria in 'complicated' UTI. Secondly the index of suspicion that there is a persistent infection should be very high if a patient represents within 2–3 weeks of completing their antibiotics.

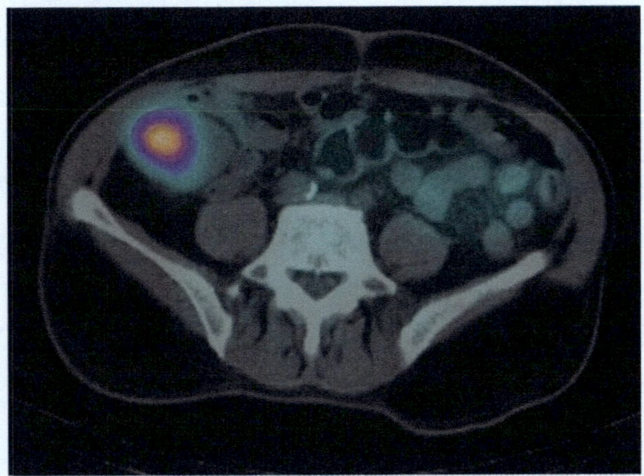

Fig. 54.13 PET CT scan demonstrating clear focus of infection in the upper pole of the transplanted kidney

Case 3

A renal transplant recipient with a past history of posterior urethra valves was seen in the clinic with a rising creatinine (Fig. 54.14) (dashed arrow). Biopsy and imaging at this stage revealed no obvious acute cause although it was in the context of high tacrolimus levels and persistent asymptomatic bacteruria (*E. coli*). Things appeared to settle, and then after missed appointments, the patient represented (solid arrow) with a marked deterioration in renal function and low tacrolimus levels. An urgent renal biopsy demonstrated a florid bacterial pyelonephritis. A MRI scan (Fig. 54.15) done at the time demonstrated multiple areas of inflammation and oedema consistent with pyelonephritis. At no stage did the patient have any symptoms, fever or graft tenderness and indeed remained very well with CRPs no greater than 30. Although current guidelines do not recommend treating ASB (except in pregnancy) it is important to be vigilant in patients with persistent pyuria and ASB, and ensure that there is not an ongoing nidus of infection in the kidney.

Case 4

A 65-year-old man presented with PCP as an AIDS-defining illness. He had a CD4 count of 20 and mildly abnormal renal function with a creatinine of 100mcmol/L. He was treated with co-trimoxazole and ARVs including tenofovir. At a follow-up clinic 5 weeks following ARV, he complained of bilateral loin pain and fevers. His creatinine has

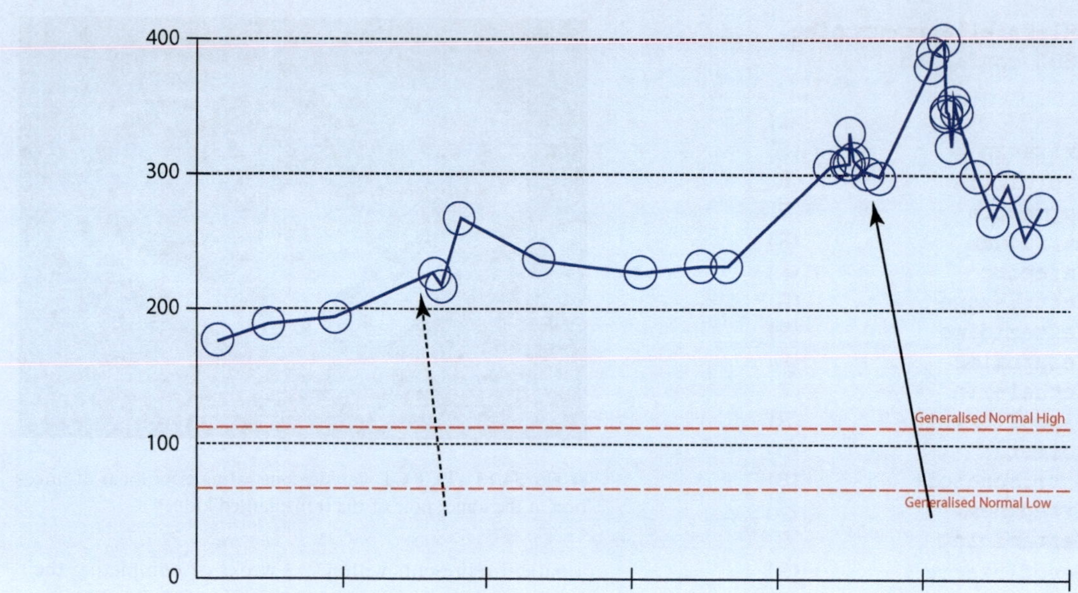

Fig. 54.14 Creatinine in a renal transplant recipient with persistent ASB

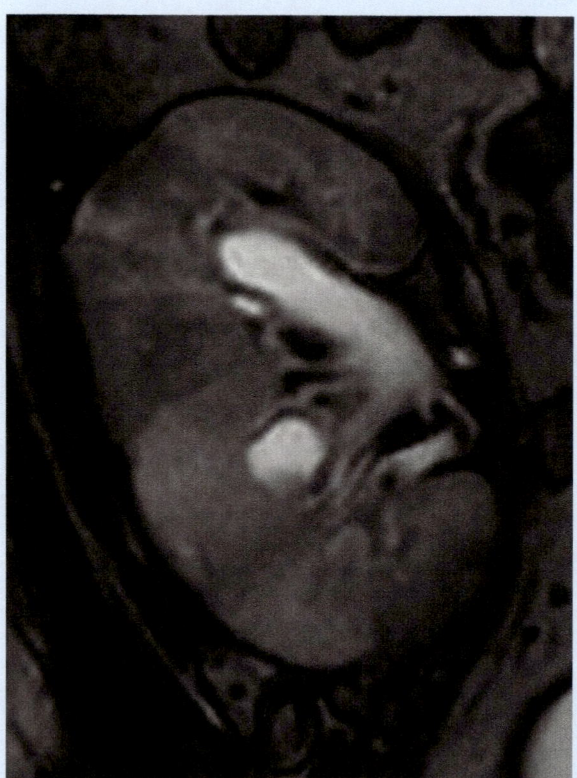

Fig. 54.15 MRI of the transplant kidney demonstrating heterogenous cortex with multiple wedge-shaped areas of oedema and inflammation consistent with ongoing infection

risen to 250mcmol/L; a CTKUB showed obstruction to the right ureter and bilateral renal enlargement. His right kidney was decompressed, and a renal biopsy demonstrated a florid interstitial nephritis with granulomata consistent with immune reconstitution syndrome and renal *Mycobacterium* infection. Although renal TB is typically clinically quiet, immune reactivation typically presents fairly acutely.

Case 5

A man in his 40s who had reached ESRD secondary to recurrent UTI, pyelonephritis, and scarring presented with a failing transplant secondary to recurrent episodes of urosepsis with different but increasingly resistant organisms. His native kidneys had previously been removed, but this failed to stop the infections. An ultrasound and cross-sectional imaging revealed no obvious nidus and his bladder appeared to empty well on USS. However, VCMG demonstrated gross reflux to his failing transplant and some pooling of urine in the bladder at the end of micturition as urine from the renal pelvis returned to the bladder. Given the loss of his native and transplant kidneys to recurrent urosepsis, his transplant kidney was surgically removed before relisting. Subsequent transplantation has been free from urosepsis demonstrating the importance of identifying and resolving problematic drainage problems.

Questions

1. What are the key virulence factors for UPEC causing acute pyelonephritis?
2. Is it recommended to start antibiotics whenever asymptomatic bacteruria detected?
3. When to recommend antibiotic prophylaxis for patients with recurrent UTI?
4. Is it sufficient to treat a case of emphysematous pyelonephritis with broad-spectrum antibiotics?
5. What is the diagnostic and therapeutic approach for a case with fungal UTI?

Answers

1. Pathogens can have virulence factors that facilitate infection or avoid host defences. Some specifically facilitate cystitis while others promote APN. Specifically three virulence factors are associated with APN: (a) mannose resistant P fimbriae (>90% of APN), (b) papGAP (class II) genotype, and (c) Dr. fimbriae which binds to decay-accelerating factor virulence in pregnancy and is associated with APN in pregnancy.
2. No, not all patients with asymptomatic bacteruria should be treated, and treatment depends on the perceived risk. Treatment is mandatory in pregnancy and pre-procedure prophylaxis before urological intervention, whereas ASB should not be treated if likely to be contaminated, catheter, urostomy, or ileal loop-related samples. In healthy women, observation of ASB is reasonable unless the patient has a history of recurrent severe UTIs. Similarly, in the elderly ASB, there is no strong evidence that treatment is beneficial. UTI is very common in renal transplantation, but there is no evidence that treatment of ASB is helpful in this setting.
3. Antibiotic prophylaxis is highly effective at reducing the frequency of recurrent UTIs, yet carries risk of inducing bacterial resistance. First, behavioural and personal hygiene measures should be implanted. If not effective or appropriate, vaginal oestrogen can be considered for postmenopausal women. If no improvement, consider single-dose antibiotic prophylaxis for exposure to an identifiable trigger or a trial of daily antibiotic prophylaxis if no improvement or no identifiable trigger.
4. No, antibiotics alone (without drainage) are not suitable to manage emphysematous pyelonephritis, as such approach is associated with a RR of death of 2.85, and the combination of broad-spectrum antibiotics plus rapid medical drainage (large bore nephrostomy) helps to improve the outcome. The choice between percutaneous drainage and surgical nephrectomy needs to be made on a case-by-case basis, and even if nephrectomy is appropriate, the patient can often be stabilized by a period of radiological drainage and antibiotics.
5. First, establishing a diagnosis of fungal UTI is paramount as in the majority of cases, candiduria does not represent infection but rather contamination. Generally, fungal UTIs are rare in healthy community-based individuals and more commonly found in hospitalized patients. Community-acquired *Candida* infections are most common amongst patients with diabetes mellitus, those who are bedridden, and patients receiving antimicrobial therapy. Infection is associated with typical and indistinguishable symptoms of cystitis, prostatitis, epididymo-orchitis, or APN. Asymptomatic candiduria in a previously healthy individual should be verified on a second carefully collected urine specimen. If absent then ignore. While for persistent candiduria in a previously healthy individual search for a predisposing condition such as diabetes, urological abnormality, or catheter (which should be changed). The removal of a precipitating cause or treatment of underlying conditions is usually sufficient, and in the absence of any obvious abnormality in a well patient, it is reasonable to monitor. In the presence of a susceptible individual such as a critically ill patient or an immunocompromised patient, candiduria should be regarded as a marker of potential invasive candidiasis. In selected patients, a renal ultrasound should be carried out to rule out the presence of hydronephrosis/obstruction, a focal mass in the collective system. Further investigations with CT or MRI may be required to demonstrate the presence of a renal abscess, fungal balls, or non-functioning kidneys.

References

1. Hooton TM. Clinical practice. Uncomplicated urinary tract infection. N Engl J Med. 2012;366(11):1028–37.
2. Moutzouris D-A, Falagas ME. Interstitial cystitis: an unsolved enigma. Clin J Am Soc Nephrol. 2009;4(11):1844–57.
3. Scholes D, Hooton TM, Roberts PL, Gupta K, Stapleton AE, Stamm WE. Risk factors associated with acute pyelonephritis in healthy women. Ann Intern Med. 2005;142(1):20–7.
4. Pontin AR, Barnes RD. Current management of emphysematous pyelonephritis. Nat Rev Urol. 2009;6(5):272–9.
5. Car J. Urinary tract infections in women: diagnosis and management in primary care. BMJ. 2006;332(7533):94–7.
6. McNicholas MM, Griffin JF, Cantwell DF. Ultrasound of the pelvis and renal tract combined with a plain film of abdomen in young women with urinary tract infection: can it replace intravenous urography? A prospective study. Br J Radiol. 1991;64(759):221–4.
7. Sandler CM, Amis ESJ, Bigongiari LR, Bluth EI, Bush WHJ, Choyke PL, et al. Imaging in acute pyelonephritis. American

54

College of Radiology. ACR Appropriateness Criteria. Radiology. 2000;215(Suppl):677–81.

8. Lavocat MP, Granjon D, Allard D, Gay C, Freycon MT, Dubois F. Imaging of pyelonephritis. Pediatr Radiol. 1997;27(2): 159–65.
9. Somani BK, Nabi G, Thorpe P, Hussey J, Cook J, N'Dow J. Is percutaneous drainage the new gold standard in the management of emphysematous pyelonephritis? Evidence from a systematic review. J Urol. 2008;179(5):1844–9.
10. Gupta K, Hooton TM, Naber KG, Wullt B, Colgan R, Miller LG, et al. International clinical practice guidelines for the treatment of acute uncomplicated cystitis and pyelonephritis in women: a 2010 update by the Infectious Diseases Society of America and the European Society for Microbiology and Infectious Diseases. Clin Infect Dis. 2011;52(5): e103–20.
11. No Title [Internet]. 2018 [cited 2019 May 4]. Available from: https://pathways.nice.org.uk/pathways/urinary-tract-infections.
12. English surveillance programme for antimicrobial utilisation and resistance (ESPAUR) report [Internet]. 2018 [cited 2019 May 4]. Available from: https://www.gov.uk/government/publications/english-surveillance-programme-antimicrobial-utilisation-and-resistance-espaur-report.
13. Kranjcec B, Papes D, Altarac S. D-mannose powder for prophylaxis of recurrent urinary tract infections in women: a randomized clinical trial. World J Urol. 2014;32(1):79–84.
14. Ahmed H, Davies F, Francis N, Farewell D, Butler C, Paranjothy S. Long-term antibiotics for prevention of recurrent urinary tract infection in older adults: systematic review and meta-analysis of randomised trials. BMJ Open. 2017;7(5):e015233.
15. Naber KG, Cho Y-H, Matsumoto T, Schaeffer AJ. Immunoactive prophylaxis of recurrent urinary tract infections: a meta-analysis. Int J Antimicrob Agents. 2009;33(2):111–9.
16. Wagenlehner FME, Naber KG. A new way to prevent urinary tract infections? Lancet Infect Dis. 2017;17(5):467–8.
17. Jepson RG, Williams G, Craig JC. Cranberries for preventing urinary tract infections. Cochrane Database Syst Rev. 2012;10:CD001321.
18. Hill JB, Sheffield JS, McIntire DD, Wendel GDJ. Acute pyelonephritis in pregnancy. Obstet Gynecol. 2005;105(1):18–23.
19. Archabald KL, Friedman A, Raker CA, Anderson BL. Impact of trimester on morbidity of acute pyelonephritis in pregnancy. Am J Obstet Gynecol. 2009;201(4):406.e1–4.
20. Pelle G, Vimont S, Levy PP, Hertig A, Ouali N, Chassin C, et al. Acute pyelonephritis represents a risk factor impairing long-term kidney graft function. Am J Transplant. 2007;7(4): 899–907.
21. Abbott KC, Swanson SJ, Richter ER, Bohen EM, Agodoa LY, Peters TG, et al. Late urinary tract infection after renal transplantation in the United States. Am J Kidney Dis. 2004;44(2):353–62.
22. El-Zoghby ZM, Stegall MD, Lager DJ, Kremers WK, Amer H, Gloor JM, et al. Identifying specific causes of kidney allograft loss. Am J Transplant. 2009;9(3):527–35.
23. Kamath NS, John GT, Neelakantan N, Kirubakaran MG, Jacob CK. Acute graft pyelonephritis following renal transplantation. Transpl Infect Dis. 2006;8(3):140–7.
24. Bodro M, Sanclemente G, Lipperheide I, Allali M, Marco F, Bosch J, et al. Impact of urinary tract infections on short-term kidney graft outcome. Clin Microbiol Infect. 2015;21(12):1104.e1–1104.e8.
25. Kroth LV, Barreiro FF, Saitovitch D, Traesel MA, d'Avila DOL, Poli-de-Figueiredo CE. Acute graft pyelonephritis occurring up to 30 days after kidney transplantation: epidemiology, risk factors, and survival. Transplant Proc. 2016;48(7):2298–300.
26. Britt NS, Hagopian JC, Brennan DC, Pottebaum AA, Santos CAQ, Gharabagi A, et al. Effects of recurrent urinary tract infections on graft and patient outcomes after kidney transplantation. Nephrol Dial Transplant. 2017;32(10):1758–66.
27. Green H, Rahamimov R, Gafter U, Leibovitci L, Paul M. Antibiotic prophylaxis for urinary tract infections in renal transplant recipients: a systematic review and meta-analysis. Transpl Infect Dis. 2011;13(5):441–7.
28. Origuen J, Lopez-Medrano F, Fernandez-Ruiz M, Polanco N, Gutierrez E, Gonzalez E, et al. Should asymptomatic bacteriuria be systematically treated in kidney transplant recipients? Results from a randomized controlled trial. Am J Transplant. 2016;16(10):2943–53.
29. Patel P, Rebollo-Mesa I, Ryan E, Sinha MD, Marks SD, Banga N, et al. Prophylactic ureteric stents in renal transplant recipients: a multicenter randomized controlled trial of early versus late removal. Am J Transplant. 2017;17(8):2129–38.
30. Li L, Parwani AV. Xanthogranulomatous pyelonephritis. Arch Pathol Lab Med. 2011;135(5):671–4.
31. Loffroy R, Guiu B, Watfa J, Michel F, Cercueil JP, Krause D. Xanthogranulomatous pyelonephritis in adults: clinical and radiological findings in diffuse and focal forms. Clin Radiol. 2007;62(9):884–90.
32. Sanchez LM, Sanchez SI, Bailey JL. Malacoplakia presenting with obstructive nephropathy with bilateral ureter involvement. Nat Rev Nephrol. 2009;5(7):418–22.
33. Hooton TM, Bradley SF, Cardenas DD, Colgan R, Geerlings SE, Rice JC, et al. Diagnosis, prevention, and treatment of catheter-associated urinary tract infection in adults: 2009 international clinical practice guidelines from the Infectious Diseases Society of America. Clin Infect Dis. 2010;50(5): 625–63.
34. Urinary Catheter Care Passport [Internet]. 2017 [cited 2019 May 4]. Available from: https://www.hps.scot.nhs.uk/web-resources-container/urinary-catheter-care-passport/.
35. Global tuberculosis report 2018 [Internet]. 2018 [cited 2019 May 4]. Available from: https://www.who.int/tb/publications/global_report/en/.
36. Abbara A, Davidson RN. Etiology and management of genitourinary tuberculosis. Nat Rev Urol. 2011;8(12):678–88.
37. Patterson IYL, Robertus LM, Gwynne RA, Gardiner RA. Genitourinary tuberculosis in Australia and New Zealand. BJU Int. 2012;109(Suppl 3):27–30.
38. Fisher JF, Sobel JD, Kauffman CA, Newman CA. Candida urinary tract infections--treatment. Clin Infect Dis. 2011;52(Suppl 6):S457–66.
39. Delgado J, Calvo N, Gomis A, Perez-Flores I, Rodriguez A, Ridao N, et al. Candiduria in renal transplant recipients: incidence, clinical repercussion, and treatment indication. Transplant Proc. 2010;42(8):2944–6.
40. Kauffman CA, Fisher JF, Sobel JD, Newman CA. Candida urinary tract infections--diagnosis. Clin Infect Dis. 2011;52(Suppl 6):S452–6.

Renal Stone Disease

Shabbir H. Moochhala and Robert Unwin

Contents

M. Harber (ed.), *Primer on Nephrology*, https://doi.org/10.1007/978-3-030-76419-7_55

Learning Objectives

1. To understand that renal stone disease is a symptom and therefore an underlying diagnosis should be sought.
2. To know the modifiable risk factors for stone disease and how to treat them.
3. To allow the reader to design an optimum clinical pathway in their clinical setting to identify and treat rarer types of stone disease.

55.1 Introduction

There has been a progressive increase in the global incidence of urinary tract stone disease, for reasons stated below, and as a consequence results in a considerable burden of disease. The combination of urinary tract stones, diabetes, anatomical abnormalites or urinary tract infection can be particularly damaging and difficult to manage. This chapter covers the causes and management of renal stones and emphasises the important role of nephrologists working together with urologists to provide and efficient and patient-centred service.

55.1.1 Changes in Epidemiology

Urinary tract stone disease is common, important, and increasing: the lifetime prevalence of stones is ~10% in developed countries, and it disproportionately affects people of working age. After passage of a first stone, the risk of recurrence is 40% at 5 years and 75% at 20 years [1]. The incidence of stone disease has always been higher in certain areas such as the Arabian Gulf countries but is increasing internationally [2, 3]. Some of this is due to improvements in stone detection using CT scanning, but changes in dietary and fluid intake habits [4–7] and increased rates of obesity and metabolic syndrome [7, 8] are more important contributors. The incidence of stones in children has increased by 19% in the last 15 years, the age at first presentation is reducing, and the traditional male/female ratio of 3:1 is changing to a greater proportion of women.

Stone disease is a major contributor to the total number of urological procedures performed in the UK, with an increase of 63% between 2000 and 2010 [3]. In 2009–2010 there were over 83,000 stone-related hospital attendances in England. This results in a major cost burden, with direct and indirect costs associated with kidney stones estimated at over $5 billion annually in the USA [9].

55.1.2 Associations with Other Disorders

There is increasing evidence that calcium renal stone disease is a generalised metabolic disorder in its own right, rather than simply an associated feature or merely a cause of urinary tract obstruction. Stone formers of all types:

1. Are at increased risk of developing CKD compared to non-stone formers (over 8-year follow-up) [10].
2. Have lower bone mineral density when compared with the general population [11].
3. Are associated with a higher incidence of metabolic syndrome and increased cardiovascular risk [12], with a 30% increased risk of myocardial infarction over a 9-year period [13].

55.2 Presentations

Stone disease is unusual in that the first presentation is rarely to a nephrologist. Patients with acute renal colic may present to A&E, "recurrent urinary tract infections" may be a presentation of ureteric stone disease in general practice, and stones found incidentally on imaging may be referred directly to a urologist. Patients who have suffered a previous stone are more likely to recognise the symptoms.

55.2.1 Common Presentations

- Visible haematuria (important differentials: tumour, infection, glomerular disease).
- Renal colic (implies *ureteric* stone). Important differentials: clots due to any other cause of haematuria; papillary necrosis; other causes of abdominal pain with incidental finding of stone.
- Dysuria, frequency, urgency (only for bladder stones, or suggestive of infection contributing to stone formation).
- Increasingly, as an incidental finding on CT or USS scanning for an unrelated indication.

55.2.2 Rarer Presentations

- AKI.
- Fever/septicaemia (pyonephrosis + obstruction).
- Recurrent UTI and xanthogranulomatous pyelonephritis.
- Other features of the underlying medical condition (e.g. hypercalcaemia/hyperuricaemia).

Differential diagnoses always include obstruction, infection, and tumour.

55.3 Pathophysiology

While traditional classification is by stone type, it is more useful to differentiate abnormal physicochemical properties of urine that may increase the risk of stone formation (**metabolic** causes) from **structural** causes. Within each category, causes can be genetic or acquired.

55

55.3.1 Metabolic Risk Factors

A recent survey of young stone formers found that 64% had a single metabolic risk factor, with 27% having more than one [14]. Below is a breakdown of the commonly found metabolic risk factors present in a typical cohort of stone formers:

Hypercalciuria	50%
Hypocitraturia	25%
Hypomagnesuria	10%
Hyperuricosuria	3%
Hyperoxaluria	1%

55.3.2 Structural Risk Factors

Any macro- or microanatomical defect causing stasis can also predispose to stones. These include the pelviureteric junction (**PUJ**) obstruction; vesicoureteric reflux; a malformed kidney, such as horseshoe or duplex; and medullary sponge kidney.

- **The medullary sponge kidney (MSK)** is characterised by congenital ectasia and cystic dilatation of the medullary collecting ducts, which is associated with hypercalciuria and hypocitraturia. There is often a family history and sometimes an association with hemi-hypertrophy. No genetic cause has yet been identified. Hence, both anatomical and biochemical features predispose to stone formation in MSK. MSK itself is not a cause of progressive CKD.

55.3.3 Genetic Causes and Rarer Stone Types

A family history is present in up to 50% of stone forming patients. Despite this, the genes contributing to renal stone risk are still largely unknown. In one series, 15% of stone disease was linked to 14 genes (Halbritter et al. 2015). However, some definite monogenic stone diseases are known; the most common in adult clinical practice[1] are:

- **Primary hyperoxaluria** (autosomal recessive; PH types 1, 2 and 3) *(CaOx)*.
- **Cystinuria** (autosomal recessive) *(Cystine)*.
- **Familial distal renal tubular acidosis** (autosomal recessive and dominant) *(CaPi)*.
- **Dent's disease** (X-linked recessive) *(CaPi and mixed CaPi/CaOx)*.

1 CaOx, calcium oxalate; CaPi, calcium phosphate

It is important to detect these conditions because:

- Primary hyperoxaluria and Dent's are associated with long-term progression to ESRD.
- There may be implications for other family members.
- They are potentially treatable, e.g. siRNA silencing technologies for primary hyperoxaluria.

More common genetic causes of calcium renal stone disease in adults are shown in ◘ Table 55.1.

55.3.3.1 Rarer Genetic Causes of Non-calcium Renal Stone Disease

Other even rarer causes of renal stones should always be considered in patients with radiolucent kidney stones, after excluding urate stones. These diagnoses are treatable but are often diagnosed late, leading to renal impairment in many cases. Further information on these conditions, registries and trials, can be obtained from the RareRenal website: ► rarerenal.org (◘ Fig 55.1 and ◘ Tables 55.2 and 55.3).

55.3.4 Causes and Pathophysiology of Metabolic Risk Factors

55.3.4.1 Hypercalciuria

Most hypercalciuria noted on screening is "idiopathic", i.e. not associated with hypercalcaemia. Idiopathic hypercalciuria is due to one or more of:

- **Increased calcium resorption from bone.** This account for the increased incidence of stones in postmenopausal women (especially where osteoporosis is treated with calcium and vitamin D supplements instead of hormone replacement therapy). Men with hypercalciuria are also often found to have **osteopaenia**, particularly of the lumbar spine, but the mechanism of this increase in bone loss is unknown.
- **Increased calcium resorption from the gut.**
- **Decreased calcium reabsorption in the nephron.** A common cause is excessive dietary sodium intake with low dietary potassium (i.e. diet lacking fresh fruit and vegetables), but rare genetic causes can cause a urinary "leak" of calcium, e.g. hereditary hypophosphataemic rickets with hypercalciuria (caused by defective proximal tubular sodium reabsorption via the transporter SLC34A3).

Before diagnosing idiopathic hypercalciuria, it is important to specifically exclude systemic hypercalciuric conditions such as **primary hyperparathyroidism** (~1% of hypercalciuria) and sarcoidosis. Primary hyperparathyroidism presents with often vague symptoms, not necessarily including stone disease, but with clear

■ **Table 55.1** More common genetic causes of calcium renal stone disease in adults

Disease	Stone composition	Inheritance	Defect	Diagnosis	Diagnostic clue	Treatment
Primary hyperoxaluria type 1 (80% of PH)	Calcium oxalate	Autosomal recessive	Alanine-glyoxylate aminotransferase 1 (AGT1 – Liver enzyme which converts glyoxylate to glycine)	Previously liver biopsy showing decreased AGT1 function. Nowadays mutation analysis of *AGXT* gene	Progressive chronic kidney disease; systemic deposition (oxalosis) when plasma oxalate >30 μM childhood presentation, urinary oxalate >0.7 mmol/24 h, 100% calcium oxalate stones	Combined kidney-liver transplantation. Trials of specific siRNA knockdown technologies are in progress. These target genes involved in oxalate production
Primary hyperoxaluria type 2 (10% of PH)	Calcium oxalate	Autosomal recessive	Hydroxypyruvate reductase (GRHPR – Converts glyoxylate to glycolate)	Mutation analysis of *GRHPR* gene	Milder phenotype than type 1 disease	Low oxalate diet
Primary hyperoxaluria type 3 (5–10% of PH)	Calcium oxalate	Autosomal recessive	4-Hydroxy-2-oxoglutarate aldolase	Mutation analysis of *HOGA1* gene	May present in adulthood; urinary oxalate 0.4–0.7 mmol/24 h	Low oxalate diet
Familial distal renal tubular acidosis	Calcium phosphate	Autosomal dominant/ autosomal recessive	Impaired activity of H-ATPase pump or AE1 chloride-bicarbonate exchanger	Mutation analysis	Normal anion gap metabolic acidosis	Potassium citrate

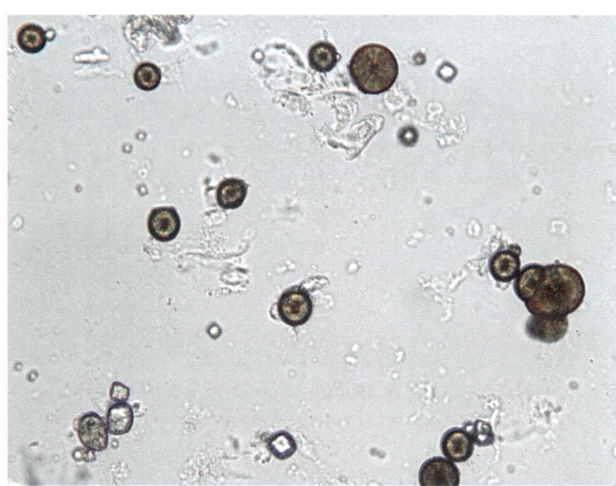

■ **Fig. 55.1** Light microscopy of 2,8-dihydroxyadenine crystals. Kindly provided by Vidar Edvardsson, MD and Runolfur Palsson, MD, Landspitali-The National University Hospital of Iceland, and the APRT Deficiency Programme of The Rare Kidney Stone Consortium

biochemical evidence: elevated PTH, inappropriately normal or raised plasma calcium, reduced plasma phosphate, and reduced TMPi/GFR (this is an index of PTH-induced reduced tubular phosphate reabsorption).

Treatments

Bisphosphonates reduce hypercalciuria due to bone loss and can be used if GFR >30 ml/min. They have the advantage of also inhibiting the crystallisation of calcium salts.

It is worth noting that vitamin D itself, given as **25-OH vitamin D** (e.g. cholecalciferol) without a calcium supplement, does not *usually* increase hypercalciuria. An important exception is *CYP24A1* loss of function (which is often undiagnosed) (see ■ Table 55.3). Restricting dietary calcium intake is *never* recommended.

Thiazide diuretics reduce hypercalciuria by inducing a mild volume depletion which encourages proximal tubular sodium and hence calcium reabsorption. They should be used only once a primary cause of hyper-

55

Table 55.2 Rarer genetic causes of non-calcium renal stone disease

Disease	Stone composition	Inheri-tance	Diagnosis	Diagnostic clue	Treatment
Cystinuria	Cystine	Autosomal recessive	Typical crystals, stone analysis	Often few; necessitates screening	Urinary alkalinisation, chelating agents
Xanthinuria (xanthine oxidase deficiency causes purine excretion as xanthine rather than uric acid)	Xanthine	Autosomal recessive	Hypouricaemia with hypouricosuria (i.e. under-production of uric acid)	Extreme hypouricaemia with radiolucent stones in person of middle eastern/ Mediterranean origin	Low purine diet and high fluid intake (allopurinol is not indicated)
Adenine phosphoribosyltransferase (APRT) deficiency	2,8-dihydroxyadenine	Autosomal recessive	Typical crystals, stone analysis, assay of enzyme activity in red cell lysates	Symptoms improve with allopurinol but not with alkalinisation (unlike uric acid stones)	Allopurinol 5–10 mg/kg/day (or febuxostat) completely prevents 2,8-DHA crystalluria

Table 55.3 Rarer genetic causes of calcium renal stone disease

Monogenic disease	Causative gene	Location of defect	Inheritance	Clues in addition to stone disease
Dent disease	CLCN5	Proximal tubule	X-linked recessive	Proximal tubulopathy, progressive CKD, predominantly calcium phosphate stone type
Hypophosphataemic nephrolithiasis/osteoporosis	SLC34A1 (sodium phosphate co-transporter)	Proximal tubule	Autosomal dominant	Phosphate wasting
Familial hypomagnesaemia, hypercalciuria, nephrocalcinosis ("FHHNC")	CLDN16, CLDN19 (claudins 16 and 19)	Thick ascending limb of Loope of Henle; distal tubule	Autosomal recessive	Renal magnesium wasting, nephrocalcinosis on imaging
Bartter syndrome	Various	Thick ascending limb of Loope of Henle	Autosomal recessive	Hypokalaemic alkalosis, presentation in infancy
Autosomal dominant hypocalcaemia	CASR (calcium-sensing receptor)	Parathyroid gland; thick ascending limb of Loope of Henle	Autosomal dominant	Stone formation usually only noted during inappropriate treatment with calcium/vitamin D
Vitamin D-induced hypercalcaemia	CYP24A1 (loss of function)	Mitochondria	Autosomal recessive	Unexpectedly high native vitamin D level, hypercalciuria, suppressed PTH with either hypercalcaemia or normocalcaemia, high 1,25-dihydroxy vitamin D. treat with fluconazole

calciuria has been excluded. Their tendency to cause increased urinary potassium loss results in mild potassium deficiency which can reduce the urinary excretion of citrate (a stone inhibitor). This effect can be lessened by combination with amiloride.

55.3.5 Hyperoxaluria

Hyperoxaluria is usually **secondary** to increased gut absorption:

- **Dietary**, due to excessive intake of oxalate-rich foods, e.g. chocolate, tea, bran, nuts, also spinach, and rhubarb.
- **Enteric hyperoxaluria** refers to increased intestinal absorption of oxalate due to:
- Inappropriately low calcium diet (sometimes, but incorrectly, advocated in hypercalciuria).
- Malabsorption due to small intestinal or pancreatic exocrine disease or surgery, e.g. inflammatory bowel disease, ileal resection, and Roux-en-Y gastric bypass for obesity. Malabsorption increases free fatty acid availability in the colon. The excess fatty acids preferentially complex with dietary calcium, reducing the calcium available for complexing with oxalate in the colon which is the main site of oxalate absorption.
- Megadose vitamin C (rare).
- Ethylene glycol toxicity (rare).

The **primary hyperoxalurias** (see table above) are caused by autosomal recessive defects in the enzymes that metabolise glyoxylate, causing metabolism to oxalate. **Type 1** is the more common form. Normal oxalate excretion is variably defined with an upper limit of ~0.4 mmol/24 h. Primary hyperoxaluria (PH) types 1 or 2 are only suspected when excretion exceeds 0.7 mmol/24 h and usually present in childhood. However, PH **type 3** may present in adulthood, suggesting that values >0.4 mmol/24 h should be also be followed up (and reviewed after dietary advice), even in the absence of a history of recurrent stones, and especially if any stone analysis reports a composition of 100% calcium oxalate. Note that only about 20% of excreted oxalate is dietary in origin, that a low calcium diet (never recommended in stone formers) can lead to an increase in absorption of dietary oxalate (see below), and that even small decreases in urinary oxalate can have a large impact on stone risk (due to the relatively small daily amount of oxalate excretion).

55.3.6 Mechanisms of Calcium Stone Formation

The three main mechanisms have some overlap between them:

1. **The free particle theory.** Crystals spontaneously precipitate in supersaturated urine.
2. **The fixed particle theory.** Crystals adhere to damaged tubular cell membranes.
3. **Randall's plaque theory.** Calcium phosphate is deposited in papillary interstitium, causing damage to overlying epithelium, to which calcium oxalate can then adhere.

These mechanisms are balanced by inhibitors of calcium stone formation:

1. **Citrate.** Hypocitraturia is the most easily measured and is currently the most clinically modifiable inhibitor. Citrate occurs naturally in fruit and fruit juices and is metabolised to bicarbonate. It is easily replaced orally as potassium citrate, e.g. in the management of distal renal tubular acidosis and sometimes in the medullary sponge kidney.
2. **Magnesium.** Although can sometimes participate in stone formation.
3. **Pyrophosphate.** A structural analogue of bisphosphonates.
4. **Tubular proteins** such as uromodulin (◘ Fig. 55.2).

55.3.7 Stone Types

Stones are made up of 90% mineral and the rest is water plus organic matrix (◘ Fig. 55.3).

- **Rare stone types: xanthine, 2,8-dihydroxyadenine (APRT), silica, ammonium urate, insoluble drugs** (indinavir, acyclovir, methyldopa, triamterene, sulphonamides). Stones due to protease inhibitors are actually large, often pure, crystals.

55.3.7.1 Urinary pH

This is an important factor that affects the solubility of many stones types and hence their formation, although calcium oxalate is pH-independent. Note that pH measured on the dipstick is unreliable; the most accurate assessment is by pH meter measured soon after voiding. As a guide, the normal pH range of early-morning urine sample is 5.3–6.8.

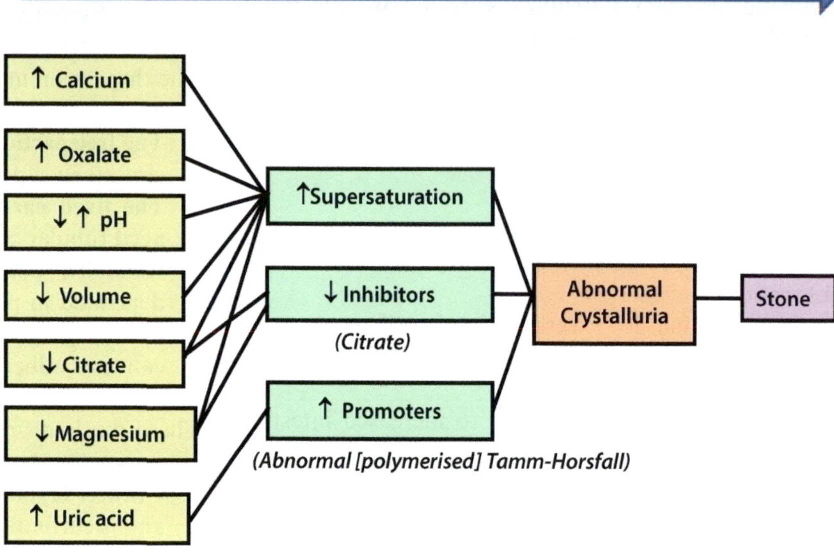

Fig. 55.2 Mechanisms of calcium stone formation

55

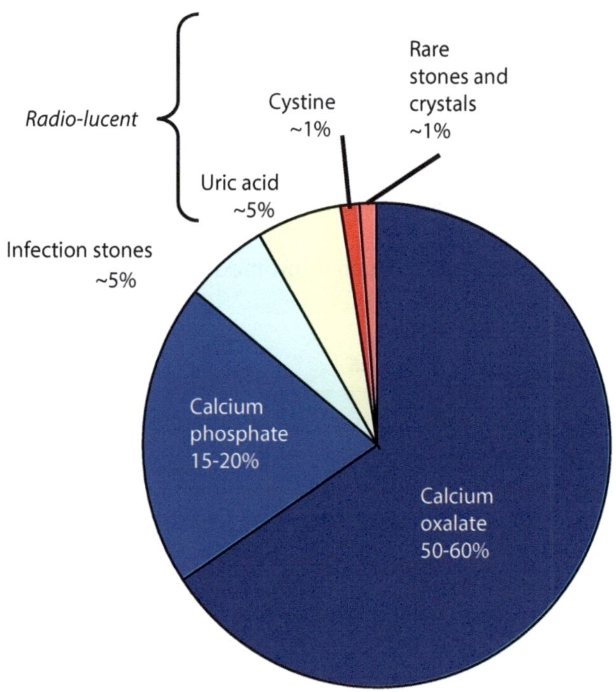

Fig. 55.3 Overall prevalence of stone types

55.3.7.2 Forming at Low pH (Uric Acid, Cystine)

- Acid urine (consistently less than pH 5.3) occurs in those with **metabolic syndrome** and/or obesity, who are also more likely to have hyperuricaemia, increasing their risk of uric acid stones. Patients with **ileostomies** are also at risk of forming uric acid stones from a combination of ileal losses of bicarbonate-rich fluid, leading to low urine volumes and acid urine.
- Cystine is increasingly soluble at higher pH, but this effect is overwhelmed if urinary cystine excretion is massive.
- Some drug-induced crystals: sulphonamides, e.g. co-trimoxazole.

55.3.7.3 Forming at High pH

- Calcium phosphate (pH >6.2) stones are suggestive of an acidification defect (deficient proton secretion in type 1 renal tubular acidosis).
- Magnesium ammonium phosphate ($MgNH_4Pi$; radio-opaque, pH >7.0) and ammonium urate (radiolucent) stones are caused by:
  - Infection with a urea-splitting organism – urease from *Proteus*, *Klebsiella*, or *Pseudomonas* species causes ammonia release.
  - Laxative abuse – this results in chronic potassium depletion and reduced urinary citrate excretion.
- Most drug-induced crystals typically form at higher pH:
  - Protease inhibitors.
  - Ciprofloxacin (pH >7.3).

55.4 Nephrocalcinosis

Nephrocalcinosis means a generalised increase in calcification of the renal parenchyma due to increased urinary excretion of calcium, phosphate, or oxalate. This is distinct from calcium renal stone disease which represents more discrete calcification, usually in the collecting system, although both conditions may coexist. It should be regarded as being a clue to an underlying cause of abnormal calcification.

Table 55.4 Causes of nephrocalcinosis

Cause	Disease	Location of nephrocalcinosis
Acute hyperphosphaturia	Acute phosphate nephropathy (due to sodium phosphate bowel prep), tumour lysis syndrome	Intracellular; cortical or medullary
Hypercalciuria + hypercalcaemia	Primary hyperparathyroidism (20% have nephrocalcinosis), sarcoidosis, vitamin D, or milk-alkali syndrome	Medullary
Hypercalciuria + normocalcaemia	Tubulopathies (dRTA, MSK)	Medullary
	Rarer tubulopathies (all causes listed in "genetic causes of calcium stones" table above)	Medullary
Hyperoxaluria	Primary or secondary hyperoxaluria (see above)	Medullary
Structural or other diseases	Severe disease of the renal cortex (chronic glomerulonephritis, renal allograft rejection, renal cortical necrosis), renal tuberculosis	Cortical
Drugs	Analgesic nephropathy (chronic papillary necrosis)	Medullary

Nephrocalcinosis *always* requires investigation because (a) there is a high likelihood of finding an underlying metabolic defect and (b) progression of the underlying disease process may cause renal failure. The calcium deposits are composed of calcium phosphate or calcium oxalate (the latter known as "oxalosis" especially if systemic) and once present are usually permanent, even if the cause is treated. The largest nephrocalcinosis registry [15] found that 97% of nephrocalcinosis affected the medulla and that these correlated with metabolic causes, most of which are also causes of calcium renal stone disease. The remaining 3% (cortical) comprised structural causes.

It is usually asymptomatic, but symptoms can occur due to the underlying cause or of hypercalcaemia itself (if present) or due to consequences including calcium renal stone disease and sometimes polyuria (medullary nephrocalcinosis affects concentrating ability) (Table 55.4).

55.5 Clinical Assessment

The aims of management are to treat the stone and to institute longer-term measures to reduce recurrence.

55.5.1 Rationale for Metabolic Screening

To a nephrologist, urinary tract stones are a symptom rather than a diagnosis, whose cause should be investigated. General advice to patients to reduce stone risk should of course be provided, but an individualised management plan is more likely to reduce recurrence. The high recurrence rate, rising incidence, number of procedures, and associated costs justify preventative strategies:

- 64% of young adult stone formers had a single metabolic risk factor, and 27% had more than one, the commonest being hypercalciuria and hypocitraturia [14].
- Screening reduces healthcare costs, by around £2000 per avoided surgical episode [16] as well as indirect costs (reduced sick pay, etc).
- The European Association of Urology (EAU) guidelines [17] recommend that first-time, solitary stone formers should have a basic metabolic screen and estimation of renal function. For recurrent stone formers/high-risk patients a more complete evaluation is recommended.

In many cases screening results will identify only subtle abnormalities. Validated algorithms (e.g. AP_{CaOx}, EQUIL, P_{sf}) have been developed which combine parameters to quantify the risk of recurrence in these patients. But even with this information, clinical evaluation of underlying conditions, diet, lifestyle, and medication is required in order to provide meaningful advice to the individual patient.

55.5.2 Practical Management

55.5.2.1 Acute Setting

In the acute situation, the priority is rapid imaging and diagnosis of urinary tract obstruction, as well as any accompanying AKI or infection. This will allow appropriate emergency treatment (see Urological Treatment ▶ Sect. 55.7.3).

55.5.2.2 Initial Investigations in the Urology Clinic

Initial investigations should occur in the urology clinic for all patients with confirmed stones but **not** in those who have had a procedure or acute renal colic within the last month. They should include:

One biochemistry blood sample for:

- Urea and electrolytes, venous bicarbonate, serum calcium, serum urate.

Two universal containers of urine for:

- Urine dipstick (pH estimation, blood, protein, nitrites/leucocytes) and then sent for culture.
- Qualitative cystine screen.

Stone analysis (of any collected stones; or give the patient a universal container and ask to sieve urine, especially if post procedure).

A mechanism should be in place for reviewing the results and making referrals for further screening where necessary. No studies have ascertained the sensitivity or specificity of this limited screen, and in our view, it forms the initial part of the advanced screen. It allows assessment of renal function and detection of obvious abnormalities including systemic acid-base abnormalities, hypercalcaemia, and urinary infections. Instituting this simple protocol will require a liaison with local urologists. Prioritisation for formal metabolic assessment can then occur from this initial screen, and the risk factors are listed in the table below (◘ Table 55.5).

◘ **Table 55.5** Suggested referral criteria for metabolic screening

Suggested referral criteria for metabolic screening
Any of the following:
1. First presentation at age <25
2. Bilateral or multiple stones (any age)
3. First stone episode with strong family history (any age)
4. Associated impaired renal function (eGFR <60 – Any age)
5. Any non-calcium stone (any age)
6. Single functioning kidney or renal transplant
7. Difficult surgical approach/high anaesthetic risk
8. Anatomical abnormality posing a high risk, e.g. renal malformation, ileostomy, some urinary diversion procedures
9. Coexisting severe bone disease
10. Potential live kidney donor with documented or incidental stone, risk factors, or strong family history
Table adapted from [18]

55.5.2.3 Full Metabolic Evaluation

An NIH Consensus Conference [19] had previously suggested fully investigating all stone formers, but this is not UK practice and is neither necessary nor cost-effective, as stones will not recur in a large proportion of cases. In theory, a full screen is only justified if the patient agrees that they will make long-term dietary and lifestyle changes and/or take drug treatment. On the other hand, research trials of new potential medications are available to particular subgroups of stone forming patients. A useful starting point is analysing stone composition where available, and this is advocated in the UK NICE guidelines (NICE guideline recommendation 1.7.1). Non-calcium stones and those with a single functioning kidney (see table above) should always be completely evaluated either due to an increased risk of recurrence or because the consequences of a recurrence are more severe.

Full metabolic evaluation should proceed as follows:

History and Examination

See the table below for history. The examination should include assessment of BMI, blood pressure, and exclusion of signs of underlying causes such as eating disorders (◘ Table 55.6).

Dietary Assessment

In the absence of a specialist dietician and week-long diet diary, focus on these important points:

- **Fluid intake and losses** – timing of intake throughout the day, type of fluid (water v tea, alcohol etc), activities causing sweating including frequent air travel, diarrhoea.
- **High animal protein** (meat, fish, and poultry) – diets high in animal protein ("high acid ash" diets) are associated with an increased risk of stone formation due to hypercalciuria, hyperuricosuria, hypocitraturia, and lower urinary pH.
- **High salt intake** – can lead to hypercalciuria, by decreasing proximal tubular calcium reabsorption. Salt intake must be reduced before considering thiazide therapy.
- **High-oxalate intake** – foods include bran, spinach, beetroot, okra, yams, soya beans and soya products, sesame seeds, nuts, peanut butter, chocolate, and tea/coffee (especially instant coffee) without milk.
- **Calcium intake** – dairy products, supplements. A common mistake is to decrease dietary calcium intake. This can lead to an increase in oxalate stone formation (due to decreased complexation in the colon) and if sustained, to osteoporosis.
- **Low fresh fruit and vegetable intake** – these are an important source of citrate, magnesium (inhibitors of calcium stone formation) and potassium (a promoter of urinary citrate excretion).

Table 55.6 How to take a history in patients with stone disease

	Item in history	Pathophysiological implications
Symptoms	Lower urinary tract symptoms	May indicate current stone as well as UTIs. UTI is a risk factor for struvite stones if urine is alkaline
	Chronic immobilisation/spinal injury	Hypercalciuria from bone loss; urinary stasis if neurogenic bladder
Stone history	Age of the first onset before age 30	Young age is suggestive of a genetic cause
	Unilateral or bilateral stone disease	Bilateral more likely to suggest an underlying metabolic or genetic cause
Past surgical and medical history	Number, type, and timing of previous stone episodes and procedures	Severity and consequences of recurrence; staghorn calculi suggest cystine or struvite stones
	Bowel surgery or inflammation (esp. ileostomy),malabsorption	May lead to secondary hyperoxaluria; also low urinary volume and acidic urine pH if high ileostomy losses
	Gastric banding/bariatric surgery causing small bowel malabsorption	May lead to secondary hyperoxaluria
	Anatomical renal tract abnormalities, e.g. medullary sponge kidney, horseshoe kidney, single functioning kidney, PUJ obstruction	MSK is associated with biochemical and anatomical risk factors. Horseshoe kidney may increase risk but also causes technical difficulties with urological treatment. Obstruction of a single functioning kidney will have more severe consequences
	Obesity/insulin resistance; gout	Associated with decreased urine pH, hence increased uric acid and mixed urate-calcium oxalate stone risk
	Hypertension	Associated with high salt diets causing hypercalciuria
Social history	Job	Deliberate restriction of fluid intake e.g. taxi drivers; working in hot conditions, e.g. cooks
	Betel nut chewing; chronic laxative or antacid abuse	Increased calcium and alkali absorption ("milk-alkali syndrome") leading to calcium phosphate stones (calcium hydroxide is often added to betel nuts or "paan")
	Regular strenuous exercise; frequent air travel	Increased free water loss
Family history	First degree relatives affected	Increased risk of monogenic stone disorder
Drugs and supplements	Excessive vitamin D supplements	Avoid in sarcoidosis. But the correction of hypovitaminosis D is not associated with increased stone risk
	Protease inhibitors	Risk of crystallisation
	Vitamin C in megadoses	Metabolised to oxalate
	Losartan	Commonly used drug which is uricosuric (not a class effect)

Further Biochemical Investigations

In addition to all the investigations mentioned above:

Spot urine in the universal container– for dipstick testing as above. Also retinol-binding protein if suspected proximal tubular disease (Fanconi/Dent's).

24 hr urine collections – Accurate collections are difficult but essential to avoid under–/over-collection, and over/covert influences on the result (by drinking more or altering diet). Optimum collections require:

- Clear instructions to perform collections while on the usual diet, fluid intake, and preferably during normal weekday activity.
- Avoiding collections if symptomatic urinary tract infection, known obstruction, oliguric (e.g. dialysis patient), or within 1 month of a stone episode or lithotripsy session.
- At least two (and preferably three [20] 24-hour collections).

Miscollection is identified by large discrepancies in creatinine excretion values between the two bottles and by obvious discrepancies between reported fluid intake and measured urine volume. Acidified (pH <4.0) samples prevent precipitation of calcium oxalate crystals which would cause underestimation of these metabolites. Most laboratories require separate acidic and plain collections.

■ **Serum Biochemistry**

Urea and electrolytes (baseline renal function), venous bicarbonate, and chloride (looking for hyperchloraemic metabolic acidosis); serum calcium, magnesium, phosphate, parathyroid hormone, and vitamin D; serum urate; serum glucose (features of metabolic syndrome).

Additional tests include coeliac serology and haematinics (if malabsorption suspected or diarrhoea present) and exclusion of autoimmune causes (if dRTA suspected).

■ **Analysis of Stone or Fragments**

55

The gold standard is infrared spectroscopy with supportive wet chemistry [21], but this is often not possible or available. Clues may be obtained from:

- **Urine microscopy** – looking for the presence of classic crystalluria. Some crystals are always abnormal (calcium phosphate crystals; hexagonal cystine crystals are pathognomonic of cystinuria). However, calcium oxalate and urate crystals can be a feature of normal urine.
- **Radiology evidence** – Hounsfield unit (HU) density on non-contrast CT KUB can differentiate between "soft" (e.g. urate) and "hard" (calcium) stones. Uric acid stones have a density of around 200–400 HU, while calcium oxalate monohydrate stones may have values of >1000 HU [22]. Plain KUB or the scout film from a CT KUB may show whether stones are radio-opaque or not and whether staghorn calculi are present.

Further Radiological Investigations

Anatomical and functional abnormalities of the urinary tract can also predispose to stone formation (see section above) or can increase the likelihood of stone complications (such as obstruction of a single functioning kidney). With the increasing use of non-contrast CT and ultrasound, anatomical abnormalities may be more readily noted.

Further Specific Investigations

After interpretation of the above results, further investigations may include:

- Urinary acidification testing.
- Screening for tubular proteinuria.
- Genotyping (RTA, PH, cystinuria).

55.5.3 Running a Medical Stone Clinic

Close clinical liaison between urologists, nephrologists, and radiologists is necessary. Initially, appropriate referral criteria (see ■ Table 55.4) must be agreed, with a mechanism for follow-up of basic screening tests previously requested in the urology clinic. There should preferably also be a system for longer-term follow-up of outcomes via the urology follow-up clinic, with re-referral to a nephrologist if indicated. For most patients only two clinic visits would normally be needed: an initial visit and a review with the results of screening tests. Further review visits may be indicated for certain patients, for example, if an underlying tubular disorder is diagnosed.

Benefits of the medical stone clinic:

- Identification of high-risk patients (e.g. those with an extensive family history of stone disease, bowel surgery, known underlying metabolic disorder).
- Increase in patient empowerment and understanding – in the case of recommended lifestyle/dietary changes, patients will need to understand and maintain these recommendations long-term.
- Allow a genetic diagnosis to be made (e.g. cystinuria, primary hyperoxaluria).
- Improve diagnosis of rarer stone types.
- Decide whether specific nephrological follow-up is indicated, e.g. for CKD or a tubular disorder.
- Assist urologists in determining risk (and hence follow-up arrangements) in specific cases, e.g. single functioning kidney.

55.5.4 Interpretation of Results and Assessment of Risk

Urinary pH

55.5.4.1 Consistently High Urinary pH

Look for:

- Renal tubular acidosis (perform urinary acidification testing).
- Recurrent urinary infection with a urea-splitting bacterium (perform MSU).
- Systemic alkalosis, e.g. chronic vomiting.
- Ongoing alkali treatment.

55.5.4.2 Consistently Low Urinary pH

This is an increasingly common finding, especially in obesity and metabolic syndrome. These conditions are themselves associated with an increased risk of all stone formation (see above), so it is common for acidic urine to be associated with calcium oxalate (but not calcium phosphate) stones, as well as uric acid stones, or a mixture of these types.

24-Hour Urine Collection Results

The "normal ranges" quoted for urinary metabolites are much more variable than for serum values, reflecting the normal response of the kidneys to daily variations in intake. Stone risk varies continuously with the concentration of each metabolite [23] and is affected by interactions between metabolites and by urine volume and supersaturation. Urine biochemistry must therefore be interpreted in relation to the history, clinical features, and serum biochemistry.

55.5.5 Should Urinary Metabolites be Measured as Concentrations or Total Daily Amounts?

There are four ways of measuring urinary metabolite excretion: average solute concentration over 24 hours (mmol/L) and the total amount excreted daily (mmol/day), as a molar ratio corrected for urinary creatinine excretion and as a fractional excretion relative to plasma concentration. The solute concentration may intuitively seem to be the most useful measure, but peak concentration (and hence supersaturation) varies greatly throughout the day. The nephron has a defined maximum excretion limit for some metabolites under normal circumstances, which is more easily expressed as a total daily amount and is subject to less variability than the concentration. Generally in UK practice, the total amount excreted daily is used for all metabolites except for monitoring of patients with cystinuria, where the aim is an average cystine concentration of less than ~1 mmol/L (243 mg/L). Molar ratios, e.g. oxalate/creatinine ratio (upper limit of normal = 38 μmol/mmol), can be useful as a first-line screening test, especially where 24-hour collections are not practical, e.g. young children (◘ Table 55.7).

55.6 Radiological Investigations

The traditional combination of the "kidneys, ureter, bladder" (KUB) radiograph and intravenous urography (IVU) has largely been replaced by the more modern imaging techniques of ultrasound (US), computed tomography (CT), and magnetic resonance imaging (MRI).

55.6.1 Plain Film Kidney/Ureter/Bladder (KUB) Radiograph

Even for radio-opaque stones, the sensitivity of KUB radiograph is as low as 19% [25], limiting its usefulness in patients with acute renal colic, obese patients, or those with pelvic vascular calcifications (phleboliths). A plain film KUB alone offers no information regarding urinary tract obstruction. However, in patients with known radio-opaque stone disease, KUB films can be reliably used for follow-up to determine stone size, growth, and clearance.

◘ **Table 55.7** 24-h urinary biochemical values and their interpretation

	"Normal" ranges (mmol/day)		Interpretation
	Male	Female	
Direct stone constituents			
Calcium	2.5–8.0 (2.5–6.0 in stone formers)	2.0–6.0	"Idiopathic" (i.e. non hypercalcaemic) hypercalciuria may be due to (a) renal calcium leak, sometimes caused by excessive dietary sodium intake, (b) increased calcium resorption from bones, and (c) increased intestinal absorption [24]. In dRTA, hypercalciuria only occurs when bicarbonate <20 mmol/l
Oxalate	0.15–0.45		Note that only 10–20% of oxalate is dietary in origin; the rest is the urinary end-product of glyoxylate metabolism. Excretion of 0.45–0.8 mmol/d suggests secondary (enteric) hyperoxaluria or type 3 primary hyperoxaluria. Excretion >0.8 mmol/d occurs in primary hyperoxaluria type 1 and 2
Urate (uric acid)	2.0–5.5	1.5–5.0	High values caused by: High purine diet (animal protein, beer), uricosuric drugs, increased protein catabolism, metabolic syndrome. Risk factor for uric acid and calcium oxalate stones. The risk of urate stones increases with higher urate excretion
Inhibitors of crystallisation			
Citrate	2.0–5.0	2.5–5.0	If very low investigate for dRTA. Low in chronic potassium depletion, e.g. high animal protein diet with little fruit/vegetables
Magnesium	2.5–8.5		Often reduced with chronic proton pump inhibitor usage, although not a directly proven stone forming mechanism. But if increased (e.g. excess magnesium trisilicate (antacid) intake) then can contribute to stone formation

(continued)

55

Table 55.7 (continued)

	"Normal" ranges (mmol/day)		Interpretation
	Male	Female	
Electrolytes			
Sodium	40–220 (highly variable depending on dietary sodium intake)		High sodium excretion can cause hypercalciuria due to decreased proximal tubular calcium reabsorption. Chronic diuretic therapy in steady state does not cause high urinary sodium
Potassium	25–125		Higher excretion with diets high in fresh fruit and vegetables. Usage together with urinary sodium in calculating urine anion gap to estimate ammonium secretion
Validation of collection			
Creatinine	9–21 (very variable depending on muscle mass)		The value should be very similar between 24 h collections in an individual patient
Volume	Dependent on fluid intake		Aim for a minimum of 2 L/day in divided amounts throughout the day for all patients, although cystinurics in particular require larger volumes in order to prevent supersaturation
Other risk factors and markers			
Phosphate	13–42		If high, suggests renal phosphate wasting usually due to proximal tubular cause
Urinary pH	*See above sections on urinary pH in "pathophysiology" and "interpretation"*		Average urinary pH over 24 h is more useful than spot urine pH which can be very variable (early-morning second void sample is better, but must be transported quickly to laboratory)
Urea			Sustained high excretion is suggestive of high protein intake

Note: variability in urine biochemistry occurs mainly due to physiological variations in day-to-day excretions but also due to under–/over-collection by the patient and differences in quality assurance between laboratories

55.6.2 Intravenous Urography (IVU)

Usually performed in conjunction with a "control" study (plain film KUB), the IVU was the initial investigation of choice prior to the advent of non-contrast CT. The control film is used to identify the presence of radio-opaque stones. The delayed post-intravenous contrast films demonstrate renal pelvicalyceal anatomy and the presence and level of obstruction and allow visualisation of contrast excretion into the collecting systems (e.g. allowing diagnosis of medullary sponge kidney).

55.6.3 Ultrasound (US)

Ultrasound is cheap and free of ionising radiation and importantly can also detect hydronephrosis but is very much operator-dependent. Stones are seen as hyperechoic (bright) foci with posterior acoustic shadowing (dark area behind the stone). Colour Doppler imaging sometimes shows a rapidly changing colour complex ("twinkling artefact") behind ureteric stones.

55.6.4 Computerised Tomography Kidney-Ureter-Bladder (CT KUB)

CT KUB has now replaced IVU as the gold standard investigation for detecting renal and ureteric stones. There is a slightly higher radiation dose (3.5 mSv; range 2.8–4.5) compared to that from an IVU (1.5 mSv), but nowadays low-dose scanning protocols can be used in many situations, giving a radiation dose equal to or even lower than that from an IVU. However, CT is used with caution in children, pregnancy, and routine frequent follow-up, in order to reduce the doses of ionising radiation in these groups (1 mSv exposure is associated with a 1 in 20,000 lifetime risk of cancer).

CT KUB has two other advantages over other modalities:

- Detection of the vast majority of "radiolucent" stones, which are not detectable on plain KUB films. An important exception is for stones (crystals) due to protease inhibitors (antiretrovirals) which are of similar density to soft tissue (e.g. the ureter) and are therefore not detectable on non-contrast CT, although obstruction secondary to such stones may be identified.

- Diagnosis of alternative pathologies that may have a similar presentation to renal colic, such as pancreatitis, leaking aortic aneurysm, cholecystitis, biliary colic, appendicitis, and diverticulitis.

Intravenous contrast may be administered in certain circumstances (the investigation is then called a CT urogram). Scanning in the urographic phase (10–15 minutes after injection) helps to outline the pelvicalyceal system and ureters. This may be useful to define whether a stone lies within or outside the ureter (the main cause of false positives on non-contrast CT KUB, particularly in thin subjects) and outline stones that are difficult to detect, such as protease inhibitor stones.

55.6.5 Magnetic Resonance Urography

After ultrasound, an MR urogram is a possible alternative investigation in children and pregnant women (but not in the first trimester) to identify the level of obstruction. T2-weighted static-fluid MR urogram does not require intravenous contrast and is useful in dilated systems. Stones are seen as areas of signal loss (black). Excretory MR urography can be performed after administering the gadolinium contrast agent, similarly to an IVU or CT urogram, with low GFR being a relative contraindication (◘ Table 55.8).

55.7 Treatment

Treatment strategies should combine treatment of the stone (medical or surgical) with preventative measures (dietary or medical) including treatment of any identified underlying cause. In general, stone forming patients will benefit from appropriate tailored lifestyle and diet advice, before pharmacotherapy. Follow-up should be approximately 6 months later, with repeat imaging/surgical follow-up if needed and with re-screening using 24-hour urinary collections to monitor metabolic abnormalities.

55.7.1 Dietary

Many of the recommended interventions are consistent with general healthy eating advice and can be combined by advocating Mediterranean-style diets such as the DASH (Dietary Approaches to Stop Hypertension) diet, modified to avoid high-oxalate vegetables and nuts. Formal dietetic intervention is recommended when the patient has other diagnoses that require conflicting diets. Most of these interventions are directed towards calcium stone disease:

▪ Fluid Intake

Drinking more fluid throughout the day is important (particularly in cystinuria where peak concentration is important), but this strategy is not adequate in isolation. Poor fluid intake is not by itself a cause of stones, since most people with low urine output do not suffer from stones. Trial evidence suggests that increasing urine volume to >2 L/day can reduce recurrence rates by 40–50% [5]. Fluid is best consumed as water, as other drinks tend to contain sugar. Tea or coffee should be taken with milk (which binds oxalate).

▪ Good Calcium Intake

A good intake of calcium, preferably as lower-fat dairy products such as bioactive yogurts, is beneficial in allowing enteric complexing of oxalate while maintaining bone health.

◘ Table 55.8 Comparison of imaging modalities and current usage in urinary tract stone disease

Imaging modality	Sensitivity for kidney stones (%)	Sensitivity for ureteric stones (%)	Specificity (%)	Modern-day usage
Plain abdominal ("KUB") radiograph	44–77	48	80–87	Follow-up of known radio-opaque stone disease
Intravenous urogram (IVU)	85	68	90	Visualisation of anatomy and exclusion of obstruction where CT is not available. Diagnosis of medullary sponge kidney. Diagnosis of protease inhibitor stones (or use CT urogram).
Ultrasound scan	55	73.3		Good for stones at the pelviureteric and vesicoureteric junctions; less good for other ureteric stones. Use in pregnancy
CT KUB	94	97	94–96	Gold standard investigation for almost all stones. Also identifies obstruction and non-renal tract pathology
MR urogram		94	100	Alternative to ultrasound in second and third trimesters of pregnancy

55

Low Oxalate Intake

Even small reductions in dietary oxalate can lead to a significant reduction in urinary oxalate excretion and hence stone risk. This is despite dietary oxalate accounting for only 10–20% of urinary oxalate excretion. Common oxalate-rich foods include bran, chocolate, nuts, and tea/coffee (without milk). Others include spinach, rhubarb, okra, beetroot, soya beans and tofu.

Reduce Dietary Fat

In the short term, this increases the efficacy of calcium and oxalate binding in the colon (by reducing free fatty acids) and in the long term reduces weight gain and risk of metabolic syndrome.

Reduce Animal Protein Intake

This will also help with uric acid stone formation. Aim for 150 g of animal flesh per day. There is no distinction between sources of protein for stone risk.

Other Measures

Increasing fruit and vegetable intake increases dietary potassium, magnesium, and citrate. Dietary sodium restriction will reduce calcium excretion and is essential prior to commencing thiazide diuretic therapy.

A patient information leaflet is available at ▶ https://www.baus.org.uk/_userfiles/pages/files/Patients/Leaflets/Stone%20diet.pdf (Table 55.9)

Table 55.9 Pharmacotherapy

Drug	Action	Stone type	Suggested dose	Cautions
Thiazide diuretics	Increase tubular reabsorption of calcium leading to reduced urinary excretion; increase magnesium excretion	Calcium stones	Indapamide 2.5 mg/day; chlorthalidone 25–50 mg/day; hydrochlorothiazide 50 mg/day [26]	Dose-dependent hypokalaemia, hyperglycaemia, hyperlipidaemia, and Hyperuricaemia, all of which can impact on stone risk
Magnesium supplements	Works as an oxalate binder in the gut	Calcium oxalate	500 mg/day	Diarrhoea can be a problem and if severe will negate the beneficial effect
Potassium citrate	(a) Alkalinises urine, (b) citrate is itself a calcium stone inhibitor, (c) alkalinising effect increases tubular reabsorption of urinary calcium	Uric acid, cystine	20 mmol tds (either as liquid or tablets where available, e.g. *Urocit-K*, *Effercitrate*)	Over-alkalinisation promotes the formation of calcium phosphate stones, even in calcium oxalate stone formers
Sodium bicarbonate	As above, but used where potassium salts not indicated or not available	Uric acid, cystine	Standard doses	Contributes to dietary sodium load
Pyridoxine	Reduces oxalate production in type 1 primary hyperoxaluria (certain mutations only)	Calcium oxalate	300 mg/day	
Allopurinol/febuxostat	Xanthine oxidase inhibitors	Uric acid	Standard doses	Allopurinol given during very high uric acid excretion can result in xanthinuria and xanthine stones
D-penicillamine Tiopronin (2-mercapto-propionylglycine) Captopril (but not other ACE inhibitors)	Cystine chelators which increase cystine solubility by forming a disulphide complex	Cystine	Standard doses	D-Penicillamine can cause bone marrow side effects, rash, nephrotic syndrome
Tamsulosin	α_1 (alpha −1) receptor blocker used as "medical expulsive therapy", relaxing urinary tract smooth muscle	Any	Standard doses	Postural hypotension

55.7.2 Combined Approaches for Particular Stone Types

- **Uric Acid Stone Formers**

Low purine-containing diet (commonest purine sources are meat, fish, seafood, pulses, and beer), alkali treatment (aim for urinary pH >6.2) with high fluid intake (aim for urine output >2.5 L/day). Add allopurinol if still forming stones.

- **Infection Stones (Calcium Phosphate or Magnesium Ammonium Phosphate)**

Cranberry juice is advisable since it is the only fruit juice that acidifies the urine, whereas all others alkalinise the urine. Prolonged antibiotic therapy may be needed since stones and fragments may contain organisms. Recurrent infections can sometimes be due to an obstructing stone of any type, so in this case, a full metabolic screen should be performed *after* the infection has been cleared.

- **Cystine Stones**

As urinary pH becomes more alkaline, insoluble cystine is more likely to dissociate to its more soluble ion. A urinary pH of >7.5 and urine output of >3 L/day (spread throughout the day) is optimal in reducing the urinary concentration of cystine to prevent precipitation. This can be augmented by:

- Titration of fluid and alkali therapy to maintain urine cystine concentration of <1 mmol/L (preferably <0.5 mmol/L).
- If necessary, the addition of a chelating agent which combines with cystine forming a soluble disulphide complex (see table above) while maintaining fluid and alkali therapy.

- **Xanthine Stones**

These require dilution with large amounts of fluid and consumption of a low purine diet. Xanthine oxidase catalyses the conversion of hypoxanthine to insoluble xanthine and of xanthine to uric acid. Stones occur due to a build-up of xanthine caused by allopurinol therapy in patients with high urate production of any cause (hence stop allopurinol) or rarely due to a deficiency of endogenous xanthine oxidase.

- **2,8-Dihydroxyadenine Stones**

Stones formed from this metabolite are effectively treated with allopurinol or febuxostat.

- **Ammonium Urate Stones**

In developed countries, this rare stone type is either an infection stone or a marker of laxative abuse or eating disorders. In the latter, the resulting metabolic acidosis results in an appropriate increase in urinary ammonium production to buffer the excess acid. In less developed countries, these stones may occur due to insufficient dietary phosphate resulting in increasing urinary ammonium production rather than phosphate to buffer acid.

55.7.3 Surgical Treatment of Ureteric and Renal Stones

55.7.3.1 Stones in the Ureter

All patients with a ureteric stone should be referred for urgent urological review even if they are asymptomatic, as there is a high chance of progressing to obstruction and/or infection and management is nicely covered in UK guidelines [27].

Treatment options are:

- **Direct treatment of the stone.** Lithotripsy (SWL) is the first choice for proximal ureteric stones less than 10 mm, and ureteroscopy for distal ureteric stones greater than 10 mm [17]. In all other cases, options will be determined by local expertise.
- If obstruction or infection is suspected, or if direct treatment is not possible, then **decompression of the kidney** should be performed as an interim measure, via either a percutaneous nephrostomy (under local anaesthetic) or JJ stent (a stent with two coiled ends placed in the ureter).
- **Medical expulsive therapy** with either a calcium channel blocker or alpha blocker (to relax the smooth muscle of the distal ureter and bladder trigone) is an option for lower ureteric stones. If the stone has not passed within 6 weeks, then definitive treatment is required.

55.7.3.2 Stones in the Kidney

Staghorn calculi, symptomatic stones, and those causing obstruction should always be treated. Increasingly, kidney stones are an incidental finding on imaging for other indications. Unlike ureteric stones, they are often asymptomatic or present subacutely with nagging back or flank pain. It is unclear whether small asymptomatic kidney stones should be observed or actively treated. A study looking at 300 men with a mean stone diameter of 10.8 mm over 3 years showed 77% progressed and 26% required surgical intervention [28]. All patients with kidney stones should be offered the urological review to consider the benefits of treatment or to allow urological follow-up (◘ Table 55.10).

Table 55.10 Treatment Algorithm for Surgical Management of Stones

Size of kidney stone	Position of stone	
	Kidney	Ureter
>2 cm	First choice: PCNL Second choice: URS or SWL	Not usually applicable
1–2 cm	First choice: SWL or URS Second choice: PCNL	First choice: URS Second choice: SWL
<1 cm	First choice: SWL Second choice: Flexi URS Third choice: PCNL	First choice: SWL Second choice: Flexi URS

PCNL percutaneous nephrolithotomy; *SWL* shock wave lithotripsy; *Flexi URS* flexible ureterorenoscopy

From: EAU Guidelines on Urolithiasis 2019, European Association of Urology (▸ https://uroweb.org/wp-content/uploads/EAU-Guidelines-on-Urolithiasis-2019.pdf) and NICE guideline [NG118] Renal and ureteric stones: assessment and management

55

55.7.4 Types of Surgical Intervention

55.7.4.1 Shock Wave Lithotripsy (SWL)

SWL uses acoustic energy to fragment calculi and is focused onto the stone by either ultrasound or fluoroscopy. It is performed as a day-case procedure and requires minimal analgesia. Each treatment lasts between 25 and 50 minutes and involves 3000 shocks delivered at a rate of between 60 and 120/minute.

The resulting numerous residual stone fragments can lead to sepsis/obstruction or act as foci for the development of new stones. An alternative therapy should be considered if the stone is large, hard, in a lower calyx (poor subsequent drainage) or in the lower ureter (difficult to localise) or if the patient is obese. SWL is contraindicated in urinary tract sepsis, obstruction, and pregnancy.

55.7.4.2 Rigid Ureteroscopy and Flexible Ureterorenoscopy

These endoscopic techniques now allow the whole urinary tract to be accessed. Rigid ureteroscopy is the treatment of choice for distal ureteric stones >10 mm [17] though can be considered for all ureteric calculi. It is more invasive with a higher risk of complications than SWL, although it is more likely to clear the stone in a single session and offers the advantage of allowing the collection of stone material for biochemical analysis.

Flexible ureterorenoscopy (often preceded by rigid ureteroscopy) can treat most stones in the kidney. Fragmentation of stones using a Holmium laser introduced via the scope is very effective even for hard stones, and the resulting fragments can then be removed via the scope, reducing the chance of distal obstruction. Postoperative stenting of the ureter is often performed, particularly where there is ureteric injury or a high risk of obstruction due to fragments or residual stones.

55.7.4.3 Percutaneous Nephrolithotomy (PCNL)

PCNL is indicated for large stones (>2 cm), stones that are difficult to access endoscopically (acutely angled lower pole or calyceal diverticulum), and where a single procedure to clear stones is preferable. A contrast imaging study allows planning of renal access, which in the UK is usually obtained by a radiologist. The tract is then dilated and a rigid nephroscope is inserted. The stone can either be grasped and removed whole or can be fragmented in situ prior to removal. A nephrostomy tube is usually then placed into the tract, which tamponades it and allows repeat access if needed. Complications include bleeding and occasionally sepsis. Despite the formation of the tract, PCNL results in minimal damage to the renal parenchyma with an average loss of <1% [29].

Open and Laparoscopic Stone Surgery

Only 47 open stone procedures were performed in England in 2010. Indications include failure of less invasive procedures, requirement for partial nephrectomy of a non-functioning moiety, or morbid obesity (Figs. 55.4, 55.5, and 55.6).

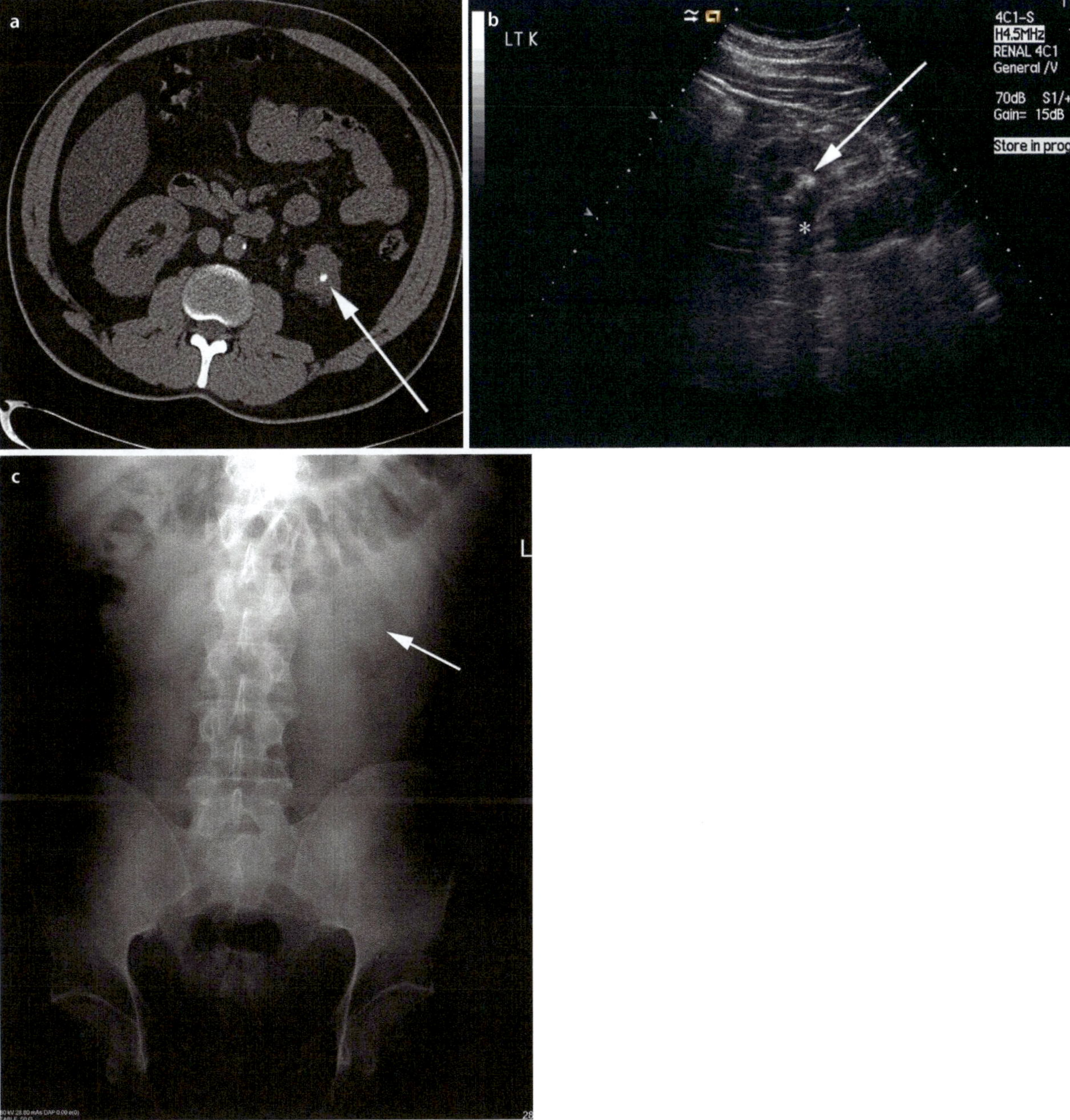

Fig. 55.4 Small left lower pole stone (arrow) visualised on different imaging modalities. **a** Axial non-contrast CT KUB is the most accurate at demonstrating the dense (i.e. white) stone. **b** The same stone is seen as a hyperechoic (i.e. bright) focus on ultrasound, with a posterior acoustic shadow (dark streak running vertically down underneath the stone, marked with an asterisk). **c** The stone is difficult to visualise on plain film. Overlying faeces/bowel gas and adjacent venous phleboliths can mask or mimic stones

55

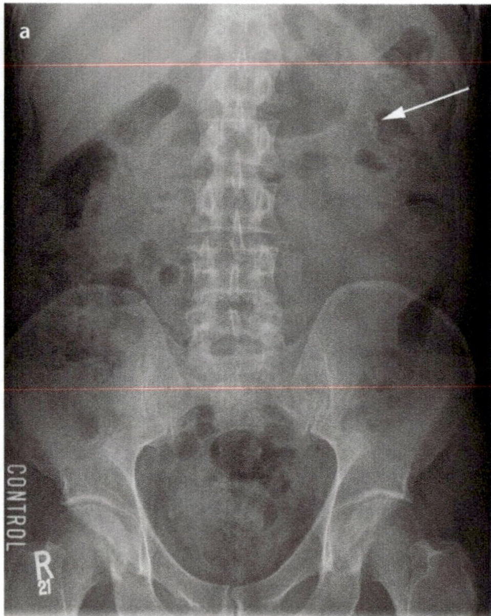

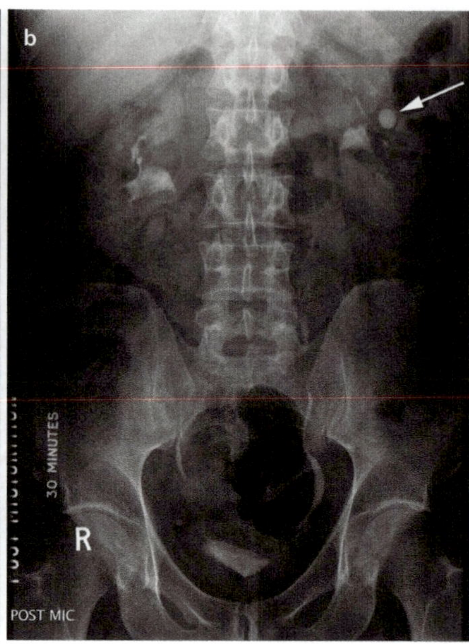

Fig. 55.5 Images from an intravenous urogram. **a** Pre-contrast control film shows a small cluster of stones in the left kidney (arrowed). **b** Film taken 30 minutes post-contrast, by which time the contrast has been excreted by the kidney into the pelvicalyceal systems and down into the bladder. The contrast outlines a rounded calyceal diverticulum in a similar position to the stones on the control film, i.e. the stones lie within a calyceal diverticulum

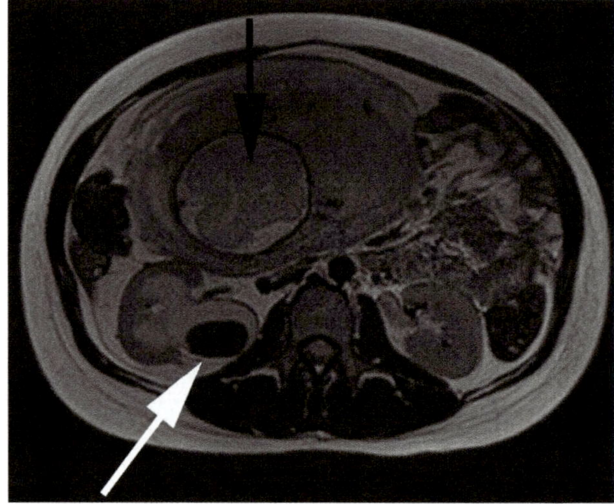

Fig. 55.6 Axial image from a non-contrast MR urogram in a pregnant patient. (Note that the foetal skull/brain is seen anteriorly; marked with a black arrow). This T2-weighted axial image shows a dilated right pelvicalyceal system with a large stone (dark in appearance and marked with a white arrow) in the renal pelvis

55.8 Conclusion

With the advent of new clinical guidelines and new medications for stone prevention, the clinical pathway for patients with kidney stone disease is changing to include a preventative aspect. Expertise in each centre will vary, and many urologists are skilled in the medical aspects of stone prevention and treatment, but links to multisystem conditions will need to be led by the nephrologist. Even simple screening of all new stone patients can pick up treatable conditions, e.g. cystinuria. Full investigation of every patient is neither possible nor desirable, and risk stratification can now be achieved, allowing prioritisation of patients. Even where no specific stone-modifying treatment is possible, benefits of screening can include detection of early cardiovascular and bone disease. Increasingly systems are available in each country, and internationally, to obtain advice and treatment for rarer stone diseases, and this together with potential diagnostic benefits for other family members makes identification of these conditions very worthwhile.

Tips and Tricks

Scenario	Top tips
"UTIs" diagnosed in a young man but never confirmed microbiologically	Symptoms may be due to spontaneously passed small stones. These can give dipstick abnormalities of haematuria, leucocytes and proteinuria, mimicking findings in infection
Bilateral stone disease	Suggests underlying metabolic/genetic rather than anatomical abnormality (although may co-exist)
Stones with proteinuria	Differential includes infection (albuminuria), Dent's disease (low molecular weight proteinuria)
Pure oxalate stones	Screen for primary hyperoxaluria, initially by measuring 24-hour urinary oxalate. 10% present in late adulthood, so look for a family history
Unusual combinations of stone types	Ammonium urate stones are suggestive of laxative abuse [21]. Silica/calcium/magnesium stones are suggestive of antacid abuse

Scenario	Top tips
Stone disease in potential kidney donor	Full metabolic evaluation is helpful in determining donation decision

Questions

True or False?
1. Which stone types are radiolucent?
2. Collecting a 24-hour urine specimen is mandatory in the assessment of all stone formers – true or false?
3. Which are the commonest genetic stone forming conditions?

Answers

1. All non-calcium stones are radiolucent, but cystine stones are very dense and can appear radio-opaque on a plain film. This classification is no longer clinically useful as it does not give a precise diagnosis, and all stones (except some pure drug crystals) are visible as densities on non-contrast CT scans.
2. False. The assessment process consists of history (especially gastrointestinal, dietary, and family history) and basic biochemical assessment (stone analysis, urine pH, acid-base status). Often a differential diagnosis can be made on this basis alone. It is important to note that 24-h urine collections are often inaccurately collected and are naturally diet-dependent and hence very variable and need to be interpreted in the overall clinical context.
3. Cystinuria is the commonest and is to an extent treatable. Like many monogenic stone forming conditions, it can present at any age, although usually in children and younger age groups. It is usually diagnosed biochemically and not by genetics. Other monogenic disorders are diagnosed by genetics especially if they give rise to calcium stones. Many of the rarer stone diagnoses are autosomal recessive and therefore do not always have a positive family history of stone formation.

Case Study

Case 1

Male, aged 48. First presentation aged 31 with a calcium phosphate stone.

PMH: Sjogren's syndrome.

Metabolic assessment: low serum bicarbonate level, low urinary citrate excretion.

Differential diagnosis: normal anion gap acidosis. The likeliest diagnosis in the case would be distal renal tubular acidosis, secondary to Sjogren's syndrome. This can be confirmed by demonstrating a failure to acidify the urine below pH 5.3 despite an oral acid load.

Treatment: immunosuppression, e.g. with mycophenolate. There can be coexisting osteomalacia which should be investigated and treated.

Case 2

Female, aged 34. First presentation aged 21 with bilateral stones and underwent several urological procedures.

PMH: Nil, very fit person. No medications. No family history. Normal diet.

Metabolic assessment: Serum calcium 2.43 mmol/l (normal) with parathyroid hormone 1.3 pmol/l (low) and elevated vitamin D (192 nmol/l). 24-hour urine collection showed high calcium excretion (14.5 mmol/24 h).

Differential: exogenous sources of vitamin D (e.g. sunbeds, high dose supplements) were excluded. Bone density was normal. Parathyroid disease is excluded due to the low PTH level, but exclusion of other hypercalcaemic disorders should be considered (despite normocalcaemia). In this case, there was no clinical evidence of sarcoidosis and no justification for the CT scan in this well person. The primary abnormality is the vitamin D excess, causing suppression of parathyroid hormone. This pattern fits with best with a vitamin D receptor abnormality. This can be confirmed by looking for an elevated 1,25-dihydroxy vitamin D or by finding a mutation in the CYP24A1 gene (the latter was found).

Treatment: fluconazole lowered the 1,25-dihydroxyvitamin D level.

Acknowledgements

- Benjamin Turney.
- Dariush Douraghi-Zadeh BSc, MB BS, FRCR.
- Navin Ramachandran BSc, MB BS, MRCP, FRCR.
- Darrell Allen FRCS (Urol), BSc.
- Giulia Magni.
- Omid Sadeghi-Alavijeh.
- Other acknowledgements for figures are in the text.

55

References

1. Worcester EM, Coe FL. Clinical practice. Calcium kidney stones. N Engl J Med. Sep 2;363(10):954–63. PubMed PMID: 20818905. Pubmed Central PMCID: 3192488. Epub 2010/09/08. eng.
2. Romero V, Akpinar H, Assimos DG. Kidney stones: a global picture of prevalence, incidence, and associated risk factors. Rev Urol. Spring;12(2–3):e86–96. PubMed PMID: 20811557. Pubmed Central PMCID: 2931286. Epub 2010/09/03. eng.
3. Turney BW, Reynard JM, Noble JG, Keoghane SR. Trends in urological stone disease. BJU Int. Apr;109(7):1082–7. PubMed PMID: 21883851. Epub 2011/09/03. eng.
4. Asplin JR. Obesity and urolithiasis. Adv Chronic Kidney Dis. 2009;16(1):11–20. PubMed PMID: 19095201. Epub 2008/12/20. eng.
5. Borghi L, Meschi T, Amato F, Briganti A, Novarini A, Giannini A. Urinary volume, water and recurrences in idiopathic calcium nephrolithiasis: a 5-year randomized prospective study. J Urol. 1996;155(3):839–43. PubMed PMID: 8583588. Epub 1996/03/01. eng.
6. Taylor EN, Fung TT, Curhan GC. DASH-style diet associates with reduced risk for kidney stones. J Am Soc Nephrol. 2009;20(10):2253–9. PubMed PMID: 19679672. Pubmed Central PMCID: 2754098. Epub 2009/08/15. eng.
7. Taylor EN, Stampfer MJ, Curhan GC. Obesity, weight gain, and the risk of kidney stones. JAMA. 2005;293(4):455–62. PubMed PMID: 15671430. Epub 2005/01/27. eng.
8. Jeong IG, Kang T, Bang JK, Park J, Kim W, Hwang SS, et al. Association between metabolic syndrome and the presence of kidney stones in a screened population. Am J Kidney Dis. Sep;58(3):383–8. PubMed PMID: 21620546. Epub 2011/05/31. eng.
9. Saigal CS, Joyce G, Timilsina AR. Direct and indirect costs of nephrolithiasis in an employed population: opportunity for disease management? Kidney Int. 2005;68(4):1808–1814. PubMed PMID: 16164658. Epub 2005/09/17. eng.
10. Rule AD, Bergstralh EJ, Melton LJ, 3rd, Li X, Weaver AL, Lieske JC. Kidney stones and the risk for chronic kidney disease. Clin J Am Soc Nephrol. 2009;4(4):804–811. PubMed PMID: 19339425. Pubmed Central PMCID: 2666438. Epub 2009/04/03. eng.
11. Lauderdale DS, Thisted RA, Wen M, Favus MJ. Bone mineral density and fracture among prevalent kidney stone cases in the third National Health and nutrition examination survey. J Bone Miner Res. 2001;16(10):1893–8. PubMed PMID: 11585355. Epub 2001/10/05. eng.
12. Domingos F, Serra A. Nephrolithiasis is associated with an increased prevalence of cardiovascular disease. Nephrol Dial Transplant. Mar;26(3):864–8. PubMed PMID: 20709737. Epub 2010/08/17. eng.
13. Rule AD, Roger VL, Melton LJ, 3rd, Bergstralh EJ, Li X, Peyser PA, et al. Kidney stones associate with increased risk for myocardial infarction. J Am Soc Nephrol. Oct;21(10):1641–4. PubMed PMID: 20616170. Pubmed Central PMCID: 3013539. Epub 2010/07/10. eng.
14. Spivacow FR, Negri AL, del Valle EE, Calvino I, Zanchetta JR. Clinical and metabolic risk factor evaluation in young adults with kidney stones. Int Urol Nephrol. Jun;42(2):471–5. PubMed PMID: 19653114. Epub 2009/08/05. eng.
15. Wrong O. Nephrocalcinosis. The Oxford Textbook of Clinical Nephrology. 3rd ed. Oxford1998. p. 1882–905.
16. Robertson WG. Is prevention of stone recurrence financially worthwhile? Urol Res. 2006;34(2):157–61. PubMed PMID: 16456694. Epub 2006/02/04. eng.
17. Türk C, Knoll T, Petrik A, Sarica K, Straub M, Seitz C. Guidelines on urolithiasis: European Association of Urology Guidelines. 2011;2012
18. Johri N, Cooper B, Robertson W, Choong S, Rickards D, Unwin R. An update and practical guide to renal stone management. Nephron Clin Pract. 116(3):c159–71. PubMed PMID: 20606476. Epub 2010/07/08. eng.
19. Consensus conference. Prevention and treatment of kidney stones. JAMA 1988;260(7):977–981. PubMed PMID: 3294456. Epub 1988/08/19. eng.
20. Hess B, Hasler-Strub U, Ackermann D, Jaeger P. Metabolic evaluation of patients with recurrent idiopathic calcium nephrolithiasis. Nephrol Dial Transplant. 1997;12(7):1362–8. PubMed PMID: 9249770. Epub 1997/07/01. eng.
21. Kasidas GP, Samuell CT, Weir TB. Renal stone analysis: why and how? Ann Clin Biochem. 2004;41(Pt 2):91–97. PubMed PMID: 15025798. Epub 2004/03/18. eng.
22. Bellin MF, Renard-Penna R, Conort P, Bissery A, Meric JB, Daudon M, et al. Helical CT evaluation of the chemical composition of urinary tract calculi with a discriminant analysis of CT-attenuation values and density. Eur Radiol. 2004;14(11):2134–2140. PubMed PMID: 15221262. Epub 2004/06/29. eng.
23. Curhan GC, Willett WC, Speizer FE, Stampfer MJ. Twenty-four-hour urine chemistries and the risk of kidney stones among women and men. Kidney Int. 2001;59(6):2290–2298. PubMed PMID: 11380833. Epub 2001/05/31. eng.
24. Sayer JA, Moochhala SH, Thomas DJ. The medical management of urolithiasis. Brit J Med Surg Urol. 2010;3(3):87–95.
25. Chan VO, Buckley O, Persaud T, Torreggiani WC. Urolithiasis: how accurate are plain radiographs? Can Assoc Radiol J. 2008;59(3):131–134. PubMed PMID: 18697719. Epub 2008/08/14. eng.
26. Reilly RF, Peixoto AJ, Desir GV. The evidence-based use of thiazide diuretics in hypertension and nephrolithiasis. Clin J Am Soc Nephrol. Oct;5(10):1893–903. PubMed PMID: 20798254. Epub 2010/08/28. eng.
27. Renal and ureteric stones: assessment and management. NICE guideline [NG118] Published date: 08 January 2019.
28. Burgher A, Beman M, Holtzman JL, Monga M. Progression of nephrolithiasis: long-term outcomes with observation of asymptomatic calculi. J Endourol. 2004;18(6):534–9.
29. Traxer O, Smith TG, Pearle MS, Corwin T, Saboorian H, CadedDU JA. Renal parenchymal injury after standard and mini percutaneous nephrostolithotomy. J Urol. 2001;165(5):1693–5.

Congenital Anomalies of the Kidneys and Urinary Tract

Melanie M. Y. Chan, Angela D. Gupta, Dan Wood, and John O. Connolly

Contents

M. Harber (ed.), *Primer on Nephrology*, https://doi.org/10.1007/978-3-030-76419-7_56

Learning Objectives

1. CAKUT is the leading cause of CKD and ESRD in children and adolescents with the median age patients require RRT of 31 years.
2. The pathogenesis of CAKUT is complex with a monogenic cause identified in approximately 20% of patients. Environmental factors including maternal diabetes, obesity, and exposure to teratogens such as ACE inhibitors are also thought to contribute.
3. Patients with CAKUT may have undergone multiple reconstructive and corrective surgeries as a child including bladder augmentation, ureteric reimplantation, and Mitrofanoff formation. It is essential that nephrologists are familiar with the long-term management and possible complications associated with such conditions.
4. Management of patients with CAKUT requires joint nephrology and urology multidisciplinary input with particular focus on the transition between paediatric and adult services.

56.1 Introduction

Congenital anomalies of the kidneys and urinary tract (CAKUT) encompass a diverse range of developmental malformations (▶ Box 56.1) and are an important cause of chronic kidney disease (CKD) and end-stage renal disease (ESRD) in children and young people. Although the majority of CAKUT occur as isolated malformations, a significant number of patients will have familial inheritance, and many cases occur as part of multisystem syndromes. With improvements in foetal screening and early urological management, the number of adults with CAKUT as a cause of CKD is likely to increase. Patients with CAKUT present a variety of clinical and management problems and are often cared for as part of a multidisciplinary team – involving a range of healthcare professionals. This is particularly important for young people making the transition from paediatric care to adult follow-up.

Box 56.1 Congenital anomalies of the kidneys and urinary tract

Renal parenchymal malformations	Renal agenesis, renal dysplasia, renal hypoplasia, multicystic dysplastic kidney
Abnormal renal embryonic migration	Ectopic kidney, pelvic kidney, horseshoe kidney, crossed fused renal ectopia
Anomalies of the collecting system and ureter	Duplex collecting system, ureteropelvic junction obstruction (UPJO), ectopic ureter, megaureter, ureterocele, vesicoureteral reflux (VUR)
Lower urinary tract malformations	Bladder exstrophy, bladder aplasia, posterior urethral valves

56.2 Epidemiology

CAKUT occur in approximately 3–6 per 1000 live births and collectively account for 20–30% of all congenital anomalies detected antenatally [1]. CAKUT usually occur in isolation although non-renal anomalies are seen in 30%, and it has been associated with over 200 different syndromes. Renal tract malformations account for up to 50% of all childhood CKD and are the leading cause of paediatric ESRD [2], placing a huge socioeconomic and educational burden on patients and their families. However, CAKUT is not just a paediatric disease; the median age for patients requiring renal replacement therapy (RRT) is 31 years, and as a group, they make up 4–5% of adults requiring RRT [3, 4].

56.3 Pathogenesis

The embryonic kidney is derived from the intermediate mesoderm and proceeds through three distinct developmental phases; the pronephros, mesonephros, and metanephros (▶ Box 56.2). The lower urinary tract forms from the endodermal cloaca which develops into the urogenital sinus (early bladder and urethra) and rectum. Urine is produced from 9 weeks, and nephrogenesis continues until approximately 36 weeks. Disruption of the tightly regulated process of renal and urinary tract development results in the many differing clinical manifestations of CAKUT, depending on the timing and location of the disruption. Environmental factors such as pre-gestational maternal diabetes mellitus [5] and obesity [6] have been shown to disrupt normal renal development.

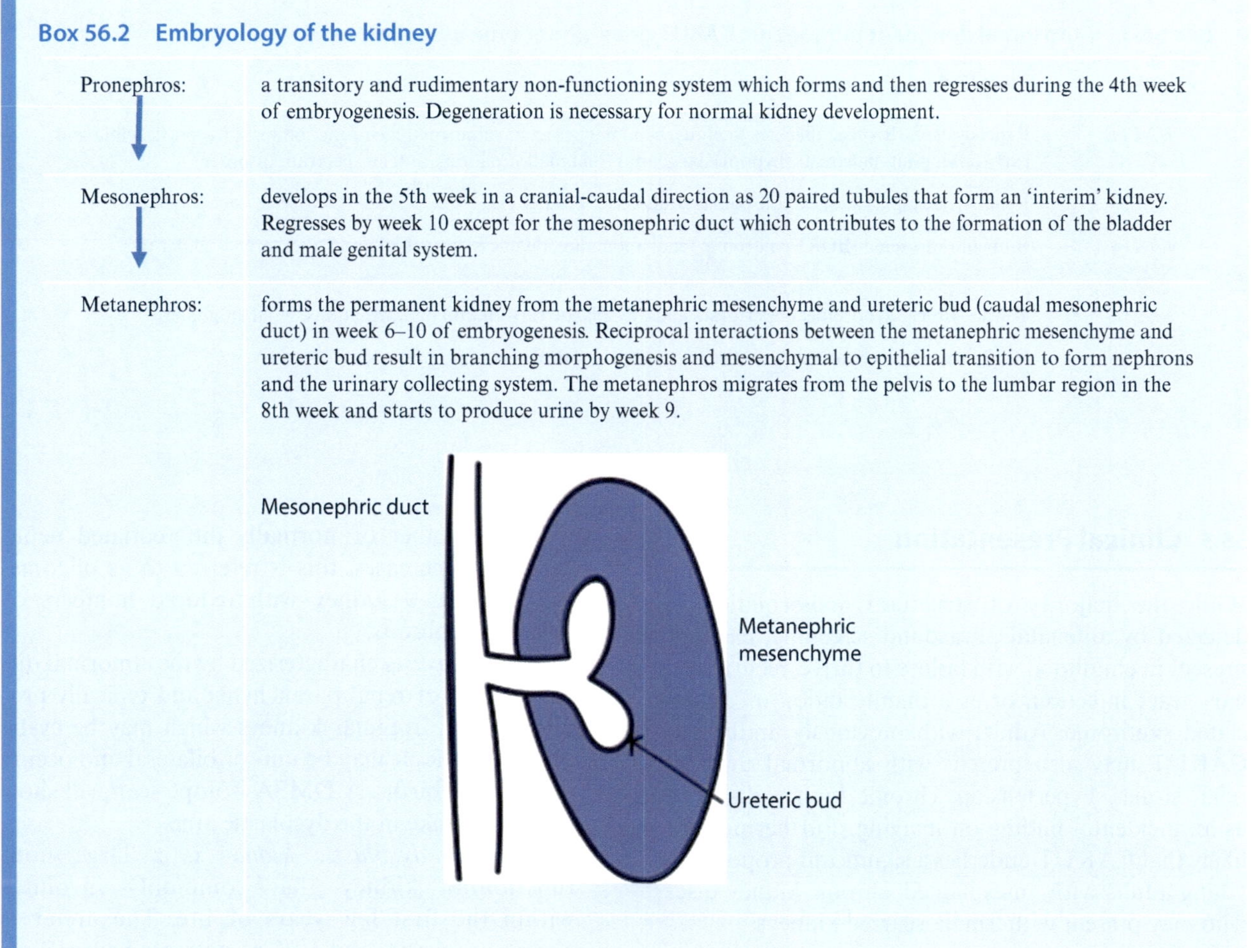

Box 56.2 Embryology of the kidney

Pronephros: ↓	a transitory and rudimentary non-functioning system which forms and then regresses during the 4th week of embryogenesis. Degeneration is necessary for normal kidney development.
Mesonephros: ↓	develops in the 5th week in a cranial-caudal direction as 20 paired tubules that form an 'interim' kidney. Regresses by week 10 except for the mesonephric duct which contributes to the formation of the bladder and male genital system.
Metanephros:	forms the permanent kidney from the metanephric mesenchyme and ureteric bud (caudal mesonephric duct) in week 6–10 of embryogenesis. Reciprocal interactions between the metanephric mesenchyme and ureteric bud result in branching morphogenesis and mesenchymal to epithelial transition to form nephrons and the urinary collecting system. The metanephros migrates from the pelvis to the lumbar region in the 8th week and starts to produce urine by week 9.

56.4 Genetics

Approximately 10–15% of patients with CAKUT report a family history, and up to 1 in 4 asymptomatic first-degree relatives have been shown to be affected with ultrasound screening [7]. Over 50 different CAKUT-causing genes affecting nephrogenesis have been reported, but the genotype-phenotype heterogeneity and incomplete penetrance seen means a monogenic cause can be identified in only approximately 20% of patients [1, 8–11]. Pathogenic variants identified in the transcription factors hepatocyte nuclear factor factor-1-beta (*HNF1B*) and paired box gene 2 (*PAX2*) are most frequently identified and are associated with renal cysts and renal hypodysplasia, respectively. ▶ Box 56.3 details the most frequent monogenic CAKUT syndromes associated with autosomal dominant inheritance that may be seen in the renal clinic.

Genetic testing is not currently routine clinical practice but should be considered if there is a family history of CAKUT or any associated eye, limb, ear, or genital anomalies. Similarly, hypomagnesaemia, deranged liver function tests, or early-onset diabetes in a patient with CAKUT might prompt testing for *HNF1B* variants which are the most frequent genetic diagnosis associated with CAKUT [12]. A molecular diagnosis can not only confirm a diagnosis for the patient, but also help inform prognosis and enable screening for extra-renal manifestations. In addition, it allows accurate counselling regarding recurrence risk in children as well as potentially permitting renal transplantation from a proven unaffected relative.

Box 56.3 Autosomal dominant monogenic CAKUT gene-phenotype associations

Gene	Phenotype
HNF1B	Renal cysts, early-onset diabetes mellitus, hypomagnesaemia, abnormal liver function tests, hyperuricaemia and early-onset gout, pancreatic hypoplasia, genital tract malformations, autism spectrum disorder.
PAX2	Renal hypodysplasia, optic coloboma, adult-onset FSGS.
EYA1 *SIX5*	Branchio-oto-renal (BOR) syndrome: renal anomalies, deafness, branchial anomalies, pre-auricular pits.
SALL1	Townes-Brocks syndrome: imperforate anus, dysplastic ears, thumb malformations, renal anomalies.
GATA3	HDR syndrome: hypoparathyroidism, sensorineural deafness, and renal anomalies.

56.5 Clinical Presentation

While the majority of structural malformations are detected by antenatal ultrasound screening, cases may present in childhood with failure to thrive, recurrent urinary tract infection, or as a manifestation of an associated syndrome. Adults with previously undiagnosed CAKUT may also present with abnormal urinalysis, renal stones, hypertension, chronic kidney disease, or as an incidental finding on imaging. Furthermore, it is likely that CAKUT underlies a significant proportion of young adults with 'unexplained' chronic kidney disease who may present with 'small, scarred kidneys'.

56.5.1 Renal Parenchymal Malformations

- *Bilateral renal agenesis* is incompatible with life and is characterized by absent kidneys on antenatal ultrasound, pulmonary hypoplasia, and Potter facies (flattened nose, recessed chin, low-set cartilage-deficient ears); a result of intrauterine compression from oligohydramnios. Siblings have an increased risk of occurrence (3–6%) which increases to 15% with a family history of renal agenesis.
- *Unilateral renal agenesis* occurs in 1 in 3000 live births. Typically, there is no ipsilateral ureter, and half of the bladder trigone is absent. In 10% of cases, the adrenal gland is also missing. Genital anomalies are commonly associated, and the remaining solitary kidney is usually hypertrophic and may be dysplastic. Ultrasound screening of first-degree relatives is advised.
- *Renal hypoplasia* describes a kidney that is two standard deviations below mean size for age with a reduced number of normally differentiated nephrons. In some cases, this is referred to as oligomeganephronia, a kidney with reduced numbers of enlarged nephrons.
- *Renal dysplasia* is characterized by the abnormal differentiation of renal parenchyma and typically produces small, irregular kidneys which may be cystic or multicystic. It may be uni- or bilateral and occurs in 2–4/1000 births. A DMSA isotope scan will show reduced uptake in the dysplastic area.
- *Multicystic dysplastic kidney* is a large nonfunctioning kidney that commonly involutes within the first few years of life. The ureter is absent or atretic, and 10% of patients have a family history.

Tips, Tricks, and Pitfalls: Dysplasia vs. Reflux

Renal dysplasia is often associated with the presence of vesicoureteric reflux (VUR) and controversy still exists as to whether renal scarring in the presence of VUR is congenital or acquired. Progressive scarring and renal failure were once considered chronic parenchymal infection (the so-called chronic pyelonephritis) as a consequence of VUR. However, in the 1980s emphasis was placed on scarring as a result of VUR itself and the progressive nature of the lesion associated with glomerular hyperfiltration, the so-called reflux nephropathy. The emphasis is changing again to the concept that scarring is often a consequence of renal dysplasia and that the reflux is a secondary feature. Thus, irregular kidneys with normal calibre ureters are more likely to be caused by primary dysplasia, and there may be no evidence of VUR.

56.5.2 Abnormal Embryonic Migration

- *Ectopic kidneys* fail to ascend correctly into the retroperitoneal renal fossa during development and can have a variable blood supply. They may remain in the pelvis, cross the midline, fuse (e.g. crossed fused ectopia), or fail to rotate medially. The incidence is approximately 1 in 1000 births and are usually asymptomatic. They may be associated with VUR or other genitourinary abnormalities.
- *Horseshoe kidney* is the most common fusion anomaly occurring in 1 in 10,000 live births, with fusion occurring at the lower pole in 90%. It is commonly associated with VUR and UPJO and may present with complications of reflux, obstruction, or stone formation.

56.5.3 Abnormalities of the Collecting System and Ureters

- *Ureteropelvic junction obstruction (UPJO)* is the most common cause of antenatally detected hydronephrosis and describes a partial or intermittent total blockage of urine where the ureter enters the kidney. It occurs in 1 in 500 live births. The abnormality is most commonly a congenital ureteric defect but occasionally may be due to extrinsic compression from an aberrant blood vessel or proximal ureteric kinking. Surgical intervention is indicated for pyelonephritis, renal stones, pain, or renal impairment. Occasionally a brisk diuresis (e.g. following consumption of alcohol or caffeine) may precipitate symptoms.
- *Duplex collecting systems* may be partial or complete and are the most common congenital anomaly of the urinary tract seen in up to 5% of the population in autopsy studies. They are more common in girls. Ectopic ureters are frequently associated with duplex systems and arise from the upper moiety. In males they are always supra-sphincteric but may insert into the posterior urethra, vas, or seminal vesicle. In females they may be either supra-sphincteric or sub-sphincteric in the urethra, uterus, or distal vagina. Ectopic ureters tend to be associated with a dysplastic upper pole and may be associated with a ureterocele (a cystic dilatation of the lower part of the affected ureter).
- *Megaureter* refers to a ureter that exceeds the upper limit of normal size (>7 mm), and management is guided by the presence or absence of reflux or obstruction. Primary dilatation usually results from abnormal ureteric musculature, and affected ureters may show an adynamic segment of ureteric wall. Outflow obstruction with secondary ureteric dilatation may be seen in conditions such as posterior urethral valves or neuropathic bladder. Initial reflux is likely, but subsequent bladder wall thickening may result in ureteric obstruction. Surgical correction is generally advised for symptomatic patients.

56.5.4 Lower Urinary Tract Malformations

- A variety of conditions give rise to bladder abnormalities or outflow obstruction which can have long-term consequences on both bladder and kidney function and thus quality of life. Kidney damage may be due to the effects of obstruction, but many cases are associated with abnormal kidney development. Bladder obstruction leads to bladder compensation with muscular hypertrophy. Further fibrosis leads to a non-compliant bladder with thickening and 'stiffening' of the bladder wall and may result in ureteric obstruction. In later stages the bladder may decompensate functioning as a floppy reservoir with little or no contractility. Regardless of bladder function, low-pressure storage and good drainage are essential. For some whose bladder has decompensated, intermittent self-catheterization may be necessary.
- *Posterior urethral valves (PUV)* are the most common cause of congenital bladder outflow obstruction in male infants occurring in 1 in 5000–8000 pregnancies. The obstruction is caused by a membrane that extends across the posterior urethra. It is most commonly suspected antenatally with bilateral hydroureteronephrosis, a thick-walled bladder, and dilated posterior urethra (known as the keyhole sign) but may present after birth with a poor stream, straining to void, palpable bladder, enuresis, or urinary sepsis. Rare adult cases with end-stage kidney disease are still reported. Management involves immediate catheterization and confirmation of the diagnosis with a micturating cystogram (MCUG) – followed by valve resection. Many patients continue to have bladder dysfunction after surgical correction which necessitates clean intermittent self-catherization. Those with associated renal dysplasia and ongoing severe bladder dysfunction are at increased risk of developing CKD.
- *Prune belly syndrome* predominantly occurs in males – diagnostic features include the partial aplasia or hypoplasia of the anterior abdominal wall muscles, gross dilatation of the bladder and ureters, and bilateral cryptorchidism. Men also characteristically have a dysplastic prostate and azoospermia. Although true outflow obstruction is sometimes present and should be corrected, the gross and irregular

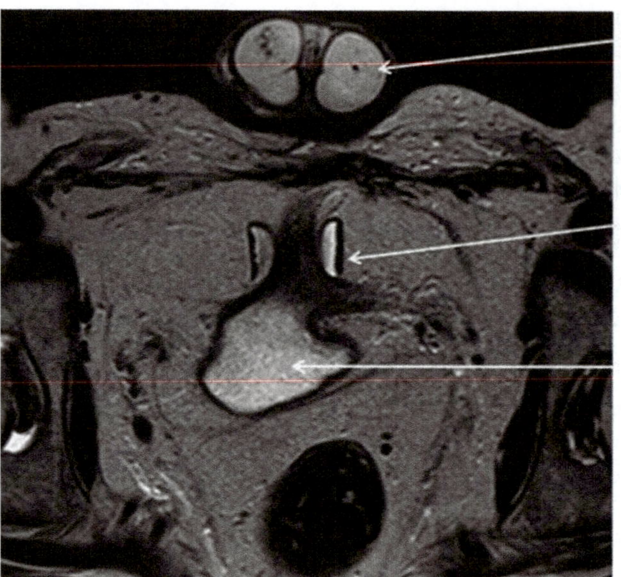

Fig. 56.1 MRI scan of the pelvis in a man with bladder exstrophy

dilation of the urinary tract that is characteristic of this syndrome is primarily caused by replacement of smooth muscle with fibrous tissue leading to aperistaltic ureters. Urodynamics are often difficult to interpret because of gross VUR, but typically there is a low-pressure bladder. With late presentation, some patients have detrusor instability. Surgical intervention may be indicated to optimize urinary drainage and prevent recurrent UTIs. Approximately 50% of patients who survive infancy will develop CKD with the severity and timing dependent on the degree of associated renal dysplasia present.

- *Bladder exstrophy* is a rare but significant congenital anomaly which occurs in 1 in 20,000–33,000 live births. The male to female ratio is 2:1 and offspring of affected individuals have an increased risk of 1 in 70 indicating some genetic predisposition. It is characterized by an open, 'inside-out' bladder which is fused with the lower abdominal wall and an open exposed dorsal urethra, requiring surgical reconstruction of the abdominal wall, bladder, bladder neck, and in a male infant, the penis. The reproductive, digestive, and urinary tracts as well as the abdominal wall and pelvic muscles are often affected. Occasionally, the more severe condition, cloacal exstrophy, is found; this is associated with other anomalies of the bowel or kidneys and may include neuropathic damage as a result of sacral agenesis or myelomeningocele. Only a third of patients empty their bladder via the urethra with the remainder requiring a urinary diversion (see Fig. 56.1). Long-term renal outcomes are generally good.
- *Neuropathic bladder dysfunction* can occur in patients with spina bifida, especially when associated with myelomeningocele. Approximately 30–40% of children will develop some degree of CKD, usually associated with a lack of coordination between the detrusor and external sphincter. Detrusor overactivity causes high functional bladder pressures with uncontrolled contractions against a closed sphincter, resulting in upper tract damage. Low bladder pressures with incomplete bladder emptying and urinary sphincter incompetence can also result in urinary stasis and recurrent infections. Early initiation of clean intermittent self-catheterization and the use of anticholinergics or botulinum toxin type A for high pressure or hyperreflexic bladders can help to preserve renal function and promote continence.
- *Urofacial or Ochoa syndrome* is an extremely rare autosomal recessive disease characterized by facial grimacing when attempting to smile and a neuropathic bladder. They are at risk of CKD.

56.6 Diagnosis and Monitoring

By the time an adolescent with CAKUT is seen in adult services, the diagnosis has usually been made, any corrective surgery is completed, and it is assumed that the urinary tract is not obstructed. It is important however that this be reviewed periodically and any increase in the frequency or severity of urinary tract infections or sudden decline in renal function should prompt further investigation for the presence of stones, obstruction, or dysfunctional bladder emptying (Box 56.4). Patients with dysfunctional bladder emptying will commonly carry out clean intermittent self-catheterization, and adherence to this should be confirmed. Routine monitoring of renal function, blood pressure, and proteinuria should also be carried out in line with CKD guidelines.

Box 56.4 Investigations used to monitor clinical status in CAKUT

Investigation	Indication
Ultrasound of kidneys, ureters and bladder	Diagnosis of CAKUT Exclude obstruction Assess residual volume (<100mls post-micturition)
CT KUB	Exclude stones
^{99}Tc-labeled MAG3 dynamic isotope scan +/− furosemide	Assess outflow obstruction
^{99}Tc-labeled DMSA static isotope scan	Assess renal scarring and divided function
Urodynamics with videocystometrogram (VCMG)	Bladder dysfunction Assess free urine flow rate (>15 ml/s), end filling pressures, bladder capacity and compliance
Loopogram	Exclude obstruction in patients with ileal conduits
^{51}Cr-EDTA isotopic GFR	Assess GFR in patients with reduced muscle mass, e.g. spina bifida

56.7 Treatment

Without careful bladder management progressive, kidney damage will be seen in the first 5 years of life in 30–40% of children. This can be dramatically reduced or delayed by ensuring the native or reconstructed bladder is compliant, has low pressure, and provides good drainage. Clean intermittent self-catheterization plays a central role and anticholinergic medication offers additional benefit by improving bladder capacity [13].

56.7.1 Ureterosigmoidostomy

Now rarely seen, this technique used until the 1970s, anastomosed the ureters directly onto the sigmoid colon, and was most commonly used in patients with bladder exstrophy. Progressive CKD, hyperchloraemic, hypokalaemic metabolic acidosis, kidney stones, infection, ureteral strictures, and increased risk for colonic carcinoma are important complications. Patients with ureterosigmoidostomy require annual flexible sigmoidoscopy.

56.7.2 Ileal Conduit (Urostomy)

The ureters are attached to an isolated segment of ileum and urine drains into a stoma bag. The ileal conduit is free flowing with rapid urinary transit and no reservoir (see ◘ Fig. 56.2). Metabolic complications are much less common, but hyperchloraemic metabolic acidosis can still occur as the bowel exchanges sodium and chloride for potassium and bicarbonate. Long-term complications of conduits include strictures, obstruction, calculi, vitamin B12 deficiency, and malignancy at the intestinal-ureteral anastomosis [14].

56.7.3 Neobladder (Bladder Reconstruction)

Bowel is used to augment or completely replace the native bladder. A Mitrofanoff channel using appendix or small bowel may also be necessary to allow bladder drainage. This provides a continent, cutaneous channel for catheterization. Complications include infection, mucus production, kidney stones, and CKD. Lifelong follow-up is needed to detect medical or surgical complications. Excess mucus production can be treated with regular bladder washouts.

56.8 Complications

56.8.1 Urinary Tract Infections

Recurrent UTIs may be associated with urinary stasis, vesicoureteral reflux, stones, obstruction, or inadequate self-catheterization. An increase in the frequency or severity of UTIs should prompt investigation for stones or obstruction including CT KUB, renal ultrasound, and post-micturition residual volume. Patients with reconstructed bladders often have abnormal urinalysis and positive urine cultures and should be advised to increase fluid intake and the frequency of self-catheterization if they have any signs of cloudy or offensive urine. Only symptomatic infections should be treated with antibiotics.

56.8.2 Stones

Kidney stones may form in the presence of infected urine and are typically magnesium ammonium phosphate (struvite) or calcium phosphate [15]. In 90% of patients, the infecting organism is *Proteus* species. Stones (usually calcium phosphate) are common in

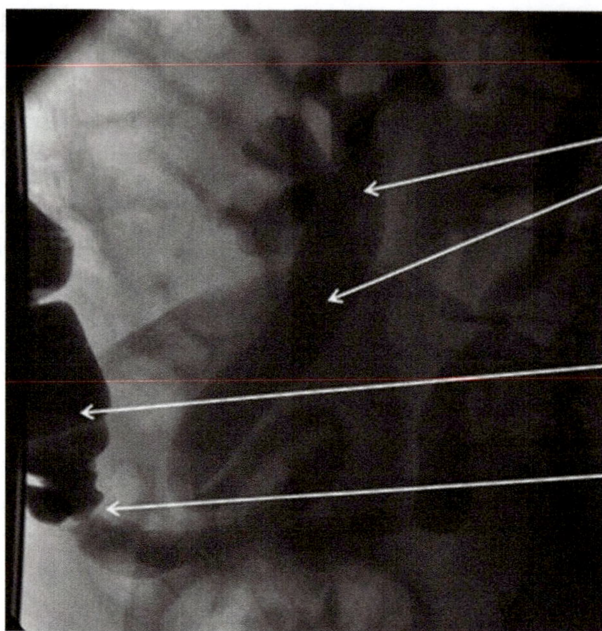

Fig. 56.2 Loopogram to examine an ileal conduit

56

cystoplasties and ileal conduits (5–30%) because of the alkaline environment. Upper tract stones must be suspected if UTIs recur or become more frequent; there is a sudden onset of severe pain and renal function suddenly deteriorates or there is an unexplained sterile pyuria.

56.8.3 Hypertension

Hypertension is common in the presence of scarred kidneys due to glomerular hyperfiltration and should be treated as per CKD guidelines. In patients with CKD secondary to obstruction, volume contraction may occur with subsequent normal or only mildly elevated blood pressure and diuretics should therefore be avoided.

56.8.4 Chronic Kidney Disease

The renal outcome of patients with CAKUT is similar whether there is primary renal dysplasia or abnormal bladder function. Predictive factors include GFR and degree of proteinuria. In young adults a GFR of less than 40mls/min/1.73m^2 and proteinuria greater than 100 mg/mmol are poor prognostic indicators [16]. ACE inhibitors or angiotensin receptor blockers (ARB) are preferred for patients with proteinuria and progressive renal failure. Interestingly, a 2018 study of 3198 adolescents with a diagnosis of CAKUT but normal renal function and blood pressure who were followed up for 30 years reported an increased risk for ESRD (HR 5.19) [17], highlighting the importance of long-term follow-up for patients even with normal renal function as an adolescent.

56.8.5 Acidosis and Bone Disease

There is often a metabolic acidosis disproportionate to the degree of renal impairment. Metabolic acidosis was particularly common with ureterosigmoidostomy. It is our practice to give sufficient sodium bicarbonate to correct the plasma bicarbonate into the normal range. In addition to the typical bone disease of progressive CKD, acidosis contributes significantly to osteomalacia.

56.8.6 Tubular Dysfunction

Renal failure secondary to obstruction can cause significant tubular injury which may cause problems with urinary concentration, acidification, and sodium reabsorption. In this situation nocturia and polyuria are frequently reported, and a 24-hr urine volume diary should be completed to assess this objectively. Patients who are salt depleted typically present volume contracted and should be advised to increase their salt intake with close monitoring on blood pressure.

56.9 Transplantation

Many young people with CAKUT will have received a renal transplant in childhood and subsequently transition into an adult transplant clinic for continued follow-up. Transition to adult services is known to be associated with increased graft loss among adolescents [18], and a specialist young person's service should be in place with support from a multidisciplinary team involving youth workers, clinical nurse specialists, and paediatric and adult nephrologists and urologists. Particular vigilance for recurrent urinary tract infections in patients with abnormal bladders is necessary. Any increase in frequency should prompt screening for stones in the graft or native kidneys and consideration of urodynamics. A significant post-micturition residual volume may require clean intermittent self-catheterization to ensure adequate bladder emptying.

Given the median age for reaching ESRD in patients with CAKUT is 31 years old [4], the majority of these patients will require assessment for transplantation within adult services and an algorithm to help guide pre-transplant assessment in patients with abnormal lower urinary tracts is given in ◘ Fig. 56.3. Thorough assessment of bladder function is key, and even patients with CAKUT and seemingly normal bladders should have a baseline postmicturition bladder ultrasound and urinary flow rate.

From our local experience, there was no difference in 10-year graft survival between patients with renal dysplasia and normal bladders (61%) compared to those with augmented bladders or urinary diversions (66%); however, longer-term follow-up did show an advantage in graft survival for patients with normal bladders [19].

Conclusion

CAKUT encompasses a diverse range of structural malformations which together account for up to 50% of CKD and ESRD in children and places a significant health, educational, and economic burden on young people and their families. Patients may have had significant urological intervention as a child or have associated extra-renal anomalies requiring joined up and holistic care, particularly through the transition to adult services. Long-term follow-up for both urological and CKD complications is necessary, as even patients with normal renal function in adolescence remain at increased risk of developing ESRD.

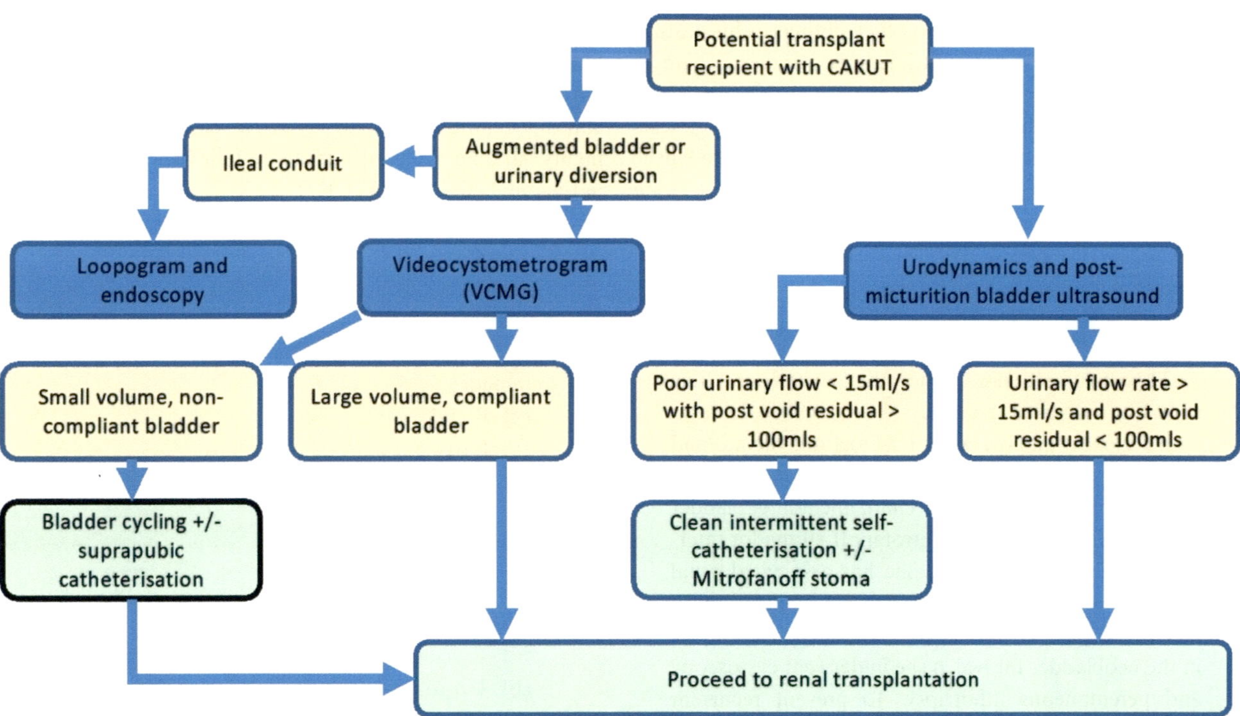

◘ **Fig. 56.3** A suggested algorithm for pre-transplant assessment of a patient with CAKUT and abnormal lower urinary tract

Tips, Tricks, and Pitfalls

1. CAKUT are the most common cause of CKD in childhood and are probably under-diagnosed in young adults. A careful history and investigation will improve diagnosis.
2. A detailed family history is always needed as there is a strong genetic predisposition to many CAKUT phenotypes.
3. Proteinuria is a key prognostic indicator and probably reflects hyperfiltration injury. Treatment goals should be as for other causes of proteinuric CKD.
4. When investigating possible renal tract obstruction, start distally, i.e. urethra, and work back towards kidneys.
5. Lifelong follow-up is usually needed. Pay particular care to metabolic complications in patients with bladder reconstructions, i.e. acidosis, stone disease and bone mineral metabolism.
6. Abnormal or reconstructed bladders may be of large capacity which can lead to functional obstruction at high volumes. In general bladder volumes should be kept low, i.e. less than 400 ml. This can easily be assessed with 24 or 48 h recording of urine volumes together with fluid intake. Many patients will have been instructed to drink large volumes, and this childhood habit can be hard to break!
7. Patients with reconstructed bladders or urinary diversions will often have abnormal urinalysis and culture-positive MSU. Only treat for UTI if symptomatic.

Case Study 1

A 25-year-old man is referred to general nephrology clinic with hypertension and proteinuria following a recent diagnosis of type 2 diabetes mellitus for which he takes metformin. He was previously fit and well and is asymptomatic. On specific questioning he mentions that his mother also has type 2 diabetes which was diagnosed at a similar age and he has no other siblings as his mother unfortunately suffered multiple miscarriages. There is nothing significant to find on clinical examination except for an elevated blood pressure of 146/95. Blood tests show normal renal function with mildly elevated liver function tests, hypomagnesaemia, and a raised urate level. HbA1c is mildly elevated at 50 mmol/mol. Urine PCR is 50 mg/mmol and a renal ultrasound shows bilateral cystic dysplastic kidneys. He is diagnosed with CAKUT. Given his diabetes, renal cysts, and blood test abnormalities, a blood sample is sent for sequencing and dosage analysis of *HNF1B*, and a heterozygous pathogenic variant is reported. The results are explained to him, and he is counselled that any future offspring will have a 50% chance of inheriting the variant but that the clinical manifestations of *HNF1B*-related disease are highly variable. He continues to be followed up annually in the renal clinic for his CKD.

Case Study 2

A 22-year-old woman attends the nephrology clinic reporting increased frequency of UTIs. She was born with a cloacal malformation (the rectum, vagina, and urethra drain into a single common channel) requiring reconstructive surgery as a child, including bladder augmentation, and uses a Mitrofanoff stoma for intermittent self-catheterization. She has associated renal dysplasia and CKD stage 3b. An ultrasound showed no hydronephrosis, but CT KUB demonstrated stones in the neobladder for which she underwent cystoscopy and percutaneous lithotripsy. To prevent recurrent stones, she was advised to increase fluid intake to 2–3 L/day, perform regular bladder irrigation to aid mucus clearance, and increase self-catheterization to every 3–4 hours.

Chapter Review Questions

1. Clinical manifestations of *HNF1B*-related disease include:
   (a) Renal cysts
   (b) Early-onset diabetes-mellitus
   (c) Neuropathic bladder
   (d) Hypomagnesaemia
   (e) All of the above

2. Which of the following statements is false with regards to prune belly syndrome?
   (a) It occurs exclusively in males.
   (b) Up to 50% will develop CKD depending on the degree of associated renal dysplasia and bladder dysfunction.
   (c) It is characterized by absent anterior abdominal wall muscles, gross dilatation of the bladder and ureters, and bilateral cryptorchidism.
   (d) It is usually associated with infertility.

3. UTIs in patients with augmented bladders may be associated with all of the following except:
   (a) Stones
   (b) A lack of symptoms
   (c) Poor bladder emptying
   (d) Mucus production

4. When assessing a patient with CAKUT for possible transplantation, the following are true except for:
   (a) It is essential to carry out a urinary flow rate and post-micturition bladder ultrasound in all patients.
   (b) Patients with small volume, non-compliant bladders should undergo bladder cycling +/– suprapubic catheterization.
   (c) Patients with post-void residual volumes of >100mls should be taught how to carry out clean intermittent self-catheterization.
   (d) Patients with ileal conduits require assessment with videocystometrogram (VCMG).

5. Complications seen in patients with urinary diversions include:
   (a) Hyperchloraemic metabolic acidosis
   (b) Stones
   (c) Malignancy
   (d) Vitamin B12 deficiency
   (e) All of the above

Answers

1. (**a**), (**b**), and (**d**). *HNF1B*-related disease is inherited in an autosomal dominant manner and has a variable phenotype which may include renal cysts, renal hypoplasia, single or duplex kidney, early-onset diabetes mellitus, pancreatic hypoplasia, abnormal liver function tests, hypomagnesaemia, early-onset gout, and genital tract malformations. It is not associated with a neuropathic bladder.
2. (**a**). Prune belly syndrome is seen predominantly in males; however, it can also rarely occur in females.
3. (**b**). Patients with urinary diversions and augmented bladders will often have an abnormal urinalysis and positive urine culture. Antibiotics should only be started in the presence of symptoms.
4. (**d**). Pre-transplant assessment of patients with ileal conduits requires a loopogram (contrast is injected into the conduit under fluoroscopy) to exclude obstruction or strictures and endoscopy to exclude malignancy at the intestinal-ureteral anastomosis.
5. (**e**). All the above can occur.

References

1. Nicolaou N, Renkema K, Bongers E, Giles R, Knoers N. Genetic, environmental, and epigenetic factors involved in CAKUT. Nat Rev Nephrol. 2015;11(12):720–31.
2. Chesnaye N, Bonthuis M, Schaefer F, Groothoff JW, Verrina E, Heaf JG, et al. Demographics of paediatric renal replacement therapy in Europe: a report of the ESPN/ERA-EDTA registry. Pediatr Nephrol. 2014;29(12):2403–10.
3. Wuhl E, van Stralen K, Wanner C, Ariceta G, Heaf J, Bjerre A, et al. Renal replacement therapy for rare diseases affecting the kidney: an analysis of the ERA-EDTA registry. Nephrol Dial Transplant. 2014;29:1–8.
4. Wuhl E, van Stralen K, Verrina E, Bjerre A, Wanner C, Heaf J, et al. Timing and outcome of renal replacement therapy in patients with congenital malformations of the kidney and urinary tract. Clin J Am Soc Nephrol. 2013;8(1):67–74.
5. Dart A, Ruth C, Sellers E, Au W, Dean H. Maternal diabetes mellitus and congenital anomalies of the kidney and urinary tract (CAKUT) in the child. Am J Kidney Dis. 2015;65(5):684–91.
6. In 't Woud S, Renkema K, Schreuder M, Wijers C, van der Zanden L, Knoers N, et al. Maternal risk factors involved in specific congenital anomalies of the kidney and urinary tract: a case-control study. Birth Defects Res Part A Clin Mol Teratol. 2016;106(7):596–603.
7. Bulum B, Ozcakar Z, Ustuner E, Dusunceli E, Kavaz A, Duman D, et al. High frequency of kidney and urinary tract anomalies in asymptomatic first-degree relatives of patients with CAKUT. Pediatr Nephrol. 2013;28(11):2143–7.
8. Hwang D, Dworschak G, Kohl S, Saisawat P, Vivante A, Hilger A, et al. Mutations in 12 known dominant disease-causing genes clarify many congenital anomalies of the kidney and urinary tract. Kidney Int. 2014;85(6):1429–33.
9. Vivante A, Kohl S, Hwang D, Dworschak G, Hildebrandt F. Single-gene causes of congenital anomalies of the kidney and urinary tract (CAKUT) in humans. Pediatr Nephrol. 2014;29(4):695–704.
10. Nicolaou N, Pulit S, Nijman I, Monroe G, Feitz W, Schreuder M, et al. Prioritization and burden analysis of rare variants in 208 candidate genes suggest they do not play a major role in CAKUT. Kidney Int. 2016;89(2):476–86.
11. Sanna-Cherchi S, Kiryluk K, Burgess K, Bodria M, Sampson M, Hadley D, et al. Copy-number disorders are a common cause of congenital kidney malformations. Am J Hum Genet. 2012;91(6):987–97.
12. Raaijmakers A, Corveleyn A, Devriendt K, van Tienoven TP, Allegaert K, Van Dyck M, et al. Criteria for HNF1B analysis in patients with congenital abnormalities of kidney and urinary tract. Nephrol Dial Transplant. 2015;30(5):835–42.
13. Woodhouse C, Neild G, Yu R, Bauer S. Adult care of children from pediatric urology. J Urol. 2012;187(4):1164–71.
14. Stein R, Schroder A, Thuroff JW. Bladder augmentation and urinary diversion in patients with neurogenic bladder: non-surgical considerations. J Pediatr Urol. 2012;8(2):145–52.
15. Seth JH, Promponas J, Hadjipavlou M, Anjum F, Sriprasad S. Urolithiasis following urinary diversion. Urolithiasis. 2016;44(5):383–8.
16. Neild GH, Thomson G, Nitsch D, Woolfson RG, Connolly JO, Woodhouse CR. Renal outcome in adults with renal insufficiency and irregular asymmetric kidneys. BMC Nephrol. 2004;5:12.

17. Calderon-Margalit R, Golan E, Twig G, Leiba A, Tzur D, Afek A, et al. History of childhood kidney disease and risk of adult end-stage renal disease. N Engl J Med. 2018;378(5):428–38.
18. Foster BJ, Dahhou M, Zhang X, Platt RW, Samuel SM, Hanley JA. Association between age and graft failure rates in young kidney transplant recipients. Transplantation. 2011;92(11): 1237–43.
19. Neild G, Dakmish A, Wood S, Nauth-Misir R, Woodhouse C. Renal transplantation in adults with abnormal bladders. Transplantation. 2004;77(7):1123–7.

Acquired Urinary Tract Obstruction/Obstructive Uropathy

Fiona McCaig, James Tomlinson, and Mark Harber

Contents

M. Harber (ed.), *Primer on Nephrology*, https://doi.org/10.1007/978-3-030-76419-7_57

57

Learning Objectives

1. To review the causes and impact of acute and chronic obstruction
2. To review the management of obstructed urinary tracts and appreciate some of the pitfalls
3. To establish the robust communication and protocols to ensure rapid diagnosis and management of aUTO

Definition

Acquired UTO is classified according to duration (acute or chronic) and by location (lower or upper tract). There is limited data on the incidence of acquired UTO, and part of the reason for this comes from the difficulty in accurately defining cases. Absolute acute lower urinary tract obstruction is clear-cut but, despite being frequent, tends to occur in the hospital setting merely as a transient phenomenon. Conversely many patients have some degree of chronic post-micturition residual, the clinical relevance of which is not clear in an asymptomatic patient with normal renal function. The diagnosis of upper tract obstruction normally relies on deterioration in renal function and the hallmark of hydronephrosis seen on imaging. But of course renal reserve means it is possible to lose up to ~50% of renal function before it becomes apparent biochemically, and imaging the upper tracts may also be problematic. ◘ Table 57.1 illustrates common examples of false positives and negatives, seen on imaging.

However, UTO often predisposes to renal impairment in the absence of obstructive uropathy via urosepsis or is superimposed on other renal diseases particularly in the elderly. In practical terms the definition of obstructive nephropathy is when UTO is the primary or contributing cause of renal damage.

◘ Table 57.1 Causes of dilated but non-obstructed and causes of obstructed but non-dilated upper tract

Common causes of dilated but non-obstructed kidneys	
Pregnancy obstruction	Physiological dilatation (effects of progesterone) and superimposed from the gravid uterus. R > L kidney
Extra-renal pelvis/ parapelvic cyst	Very common cause of apparent dilatation but the absence of dilated calyces key
Vesicoureteric reflux	Associated with (sometimes grossly) chronically dilated ureters
Renal transplant or ileal conduit loop	Typically mildly dilated in the setting of unrestricted reflux (may lessen post-voiding)
Megacalyces/ calyx	Congenital abnormalities mimicking obstruction
Postsurgical	Postoperative repair of PUJ obstruction
Following removal of obstruction	Temporary persistence of dilatation after natural passages of stone of clot
Causes of obstructed but non-dilated kidney	
Malignant encasement	Most commonly in the setting of transitional cell carcinoma but can occur with any local tumour
Obstruction with AKI	Overt dilatation may not be apparent in the setting of oliguric renal failure
Micro-obstruction	AKI in the setting of crystal nephropathy eg antivirals such as acyclovir (kidney may be "bright") and Orlistat (oxalate deposition)
Functional obstruction	High pressure bladder, detrusor instability

57.1 Epidemiology

Acquired UTO (aUTO) increases with age, in line with the prevalence of predominant causes: renal tract calculi, bladder outflow obstruction (BOO), and urological/gynaecological malignancies. Globally, conditions such as schistosomiasis and tuberculosis also contribute significantly (usually from middle age onwards). Benign prostatic hyperplasia (BPH) is a common cause of bladder outflow obstruction (BOO) in ageing men; autopsy studies have demonstrated almost universal benign prostatic hyperplasia (90%) beyond 80 years although only a proportion of these have symptoms, and it is not clear how many have clinically relevant obstruction. As mentioned above, accurate figures for acute or chronic UTO are difficult to come by, yet it is clear that with an ageing population UTO is responsible for a considerable and increasing healthcare burden. Moreover, from the nephrologist's point of view acquired UTO is an important treatable cause of AKI, CKD, and acute chronic CKD.

57.2 Causes

The causes of UTO can be divided into congenital (covered in the chapter on CAKUT) or aUTO. The causes of aUTO are multiple and can be divided up in a variety of ways, but in practical terms the most important element in terms of management is where the level of the obstruction is, i.e. upper or lower urinary tract. ◘ Table 57.2 illustrates the main causes of aUTO and divides upper and lower into intrinsic and extrinsic causes. Many of the likely causes may be suggested by the history but when this is not obvious, particularly in the setting of lower aUTO neurological and perineal examinations are very important (and too often neglected). It is important to note that apparent bilateral upper UTO can occur secondary to lower UTO pathology when there is (a) reflux to the native ureters or (b) when the bladder wall becomes

Table 57.2 Causes of Acquired Obstruction

Upper Tract Intrinsic	
Nephrolithiasis	Stones and occasionally crystals related to drugs (can be bilateral especially if chronic and sequential)
Blood clot	Any cause of upper tract bleeding (including biopsy)
Sloughed papilla	Any cause of papillary necrosis most commonly diabetes, sickle cell disease, analgesic nephropathy, pyelonephritis. See Figs. 57.1 and 57.2
Tumour	Benign or malignant (usually transitional cell carcinoma (TCC)) in ureter or bladder
Infection	Tuberculosis, BK virus infection in the immunosuppressed, fungal ball, schistosomiasis causing fibrotic contracted bladder (often bilateral upper tract obstruction)
Inflammatory	Vasculitis, chronic interstitial cystitis, malakoplakia
Ischaemic Ureter	Loss of lower pole artery (eg in transplantation or ischaemic insult to lower pole in native kidneys)
Obstructed stent	Blocked, especially retained or 'forgotten' stents
Upper tract extrinsic	
Pregnancy	Physiological dilation and obstruction from the gravid uterus
Retroperitoneal	Retroperitoneal fibrosis usually bilateral (see causes), retroperitoneal tumours (eg lymphoma, sarcoma) radiation fibrosis, extensive haematoma
Gynaecological	Cervical, ovarian or uterine malignancy, large benign gynaecological masses, endometriosis
Extensive prostatic carcinoma	Spread to and involvement of ureteric orifices
Extensive peritoneal malignancy or inflammation	Crohn's disease, abscess formation, pancreatic inflammation
Vessels	Retrocaval ureter (right side)
Ligation	Inadvertent ligation or occasionally use of native ureter in ESRD for transplanted kidney (whereby the native ureter is tied off)
Lower tract intrinsic	
Intraluminal urethral mass	Stone, clot, tumour (TCC), inflammatory, infections eg tuberculosis, acute non-specific urethritis, posterior urethral valves
Urethral stricture	Post-instrumentation, post-radiation, post-trauma, phimosis, chronic non-specific urethritis (gonococcal, chlamydial), female genital multilation
Bladder mass	Large stone(s) or bladder haematoma
Bladder wall involvement	Bladder cancer (TCC), schistosomiasis, tuberculosis, chronic interstitial cystitis
Bladder functional	Pain, prostatitis, immobility, confusional state, drugs (e.g. anticholinergics, analgesics, anti-dementia medication, anti-depressants, cessation or non-compliance with alpha blockers)
Neurological	Congenital neurological involvement eg spina bifida, dysfunctional bladder, acquired neurological conditions, autonomic neuropathy e.g. diabetes, peripheral neuropathy e.g. surgical (traumatic, tumour) or medical cord lesion eg multiple sclerosis, central nervous system pathology, e.g. cerebrovascular disease
Lower tract extrinsic	
Prostatic enlargement	Benign prostatic hypertrophy and prostatic malignancy
Perineal malignancy	Gynaecological and pelvic malignancy
Faecal impaction	Elderly and neurological pathology
Pelvic prolapse	Vaginal prolapse, cystocele, rectocele and enterocele

grossly hypertrophied and occludes the distal ureters. In these circumstances patients can present with upper UTO that does not improve on the catherisation of the bladder.

57.3 Pathophysiology of Urinary Tract Obstruction

Acute obstruction initially has a largely functional impact on tubular function and glomerular filtration, but if persistent, interstitial inflammation with tubular apoptosis and interstitial fibrosis with nephron loss and tubular dilatation follow. Following aUTO there is a drop in the hydraulic pressure differential across the glomerulus, resulting in reduced filtration fraction, a significant drop in renal blood flow within a few hours with further and an abrupt reduction in GFR. Urinary acidification deficits and urinary concentration deficits are common, usually only manifest when the obstruction is relieved but explain why it is possible to be polyuric in the face of partial obstruction.

57

These haemodynamic and tubular changes are initially fully reversible, but with ongoing obstruction, macrophage and other leucocytes infiltrate the kidney and progressive interstitial fibrosis ensues. Tubular dilatation may be seen incidentally on renal biopsy and hint at a degree of obstruction or reflux as an underlying cause. Ultimately the renal pelvis dilates further and the surrounding renal tissue diminishes resulting in a rind of end-stage kidneys around a grossly dilated pelvis. How rapidly irreversible damage occurs is not clear, but it seems sensible to relieve obstruction as soon as possible (see Case 4).

Relief of obstruction may result in hyperfiltration of remaining nephrons with glomerular enlargement and sclerosis (secondary FSGS).

57.4 Clinical Features of Urinary Tract Obstruction

The symptoms and signs of UTO depend to some extent on the underlying cause, duration, and completeness. The symptoms of acute lower tract obstruction are usually manifest by intense suprapubic discomfort with the patient being clear of the diagnosis; however, it may present merely as acute confusion or agitation (an important diagnosis to make and treat). Chronic lower tract obstruction is often much more insidious with lower urinary tract symptoms of nocturia, frequency, poor stream, and incontinence (particularly nocturnal enuresis); however, urinary tract symptoms of prostatic hypertrophy correlate poorly with obstruction [1].

Acute upper tract UTO may manifest as loin pain or renal colic if the cause is intraluminal such as stone or clot but is often clinically silent especially if the other kidney is healthy and unaffected. While complete bilaterally upper or lower UTO results in anuria, partial obstruction can result in polyuria (see above). So while urine output is rarely a critical symptom it does become one in a patient with a single functioning kidney, especially if the other kidney was lost due to obstruction, e.g. stones. Very rarely in pregnancy or following ligation of a ureter the renal pelvis may rupture causing a urinary leak. This is usually associated with intense pain that is constant rather than colicky.

Clinical features may also arise from the underlying pathology: back pain from retroperitoneal fibrosis; fevers with tuberculosis; malaise, anorexia, and weight loss with malignancy. Chronic UTO may also present with the symptoms of advanced CKD mimicking malignancy. Urosepsis is a common presentation of an obstructed or partially obstructed system, and partial obstruction must be ruled out in a patient with recurrent urosepsis.

The examination may reveal a distended palpable or visible, bladder, depending on the patient's habitus but equally may have a grossly hypertrophied wall without large capacity (25% of men with lower UTO do not have a raised post-micturiction volume). And occasionally an obstructed kidney can be palpated; however, the examination is not a sensitive tool for diagnosing obstruction. It is critical to ensure adequate examination of the perineum (excluding causes such as phimosis, urethral meatal stenosis, prostatic enlargement, pelvic malignancy, female genital mutilation) as well as a thorough neurological examination.

57.5 Diagnostic Tests

Imaging of the urinary tract with ultrasound or cross-sectional imaging is the definitive diagnostic test in the vast majority (but not all) cases, and rapid access to imaging in the form of ward or clinic-based bladder USS as well as upper tract scanning is therefore critical. Functional studies are also invaluable in a subset of patients with suspected obstruction, compliment imaging in the management of these patients, and also need to be readily accessible when appropriate.

57.5.1 Urodynamics

Urodynamics is a broad term used for the study of micturition. The term includes:

(a) Post-micturition residual volume and uroflowmetry (study of urinary flow)
(b) Cystometrography and voiding pressure/flow studies
(c) Video urodynamics
(d) Electromyography
(e) Urethral pressure profiling
(f) Ambulatory urodynamics

Rather confusingly 'urodynamics' is often used specifically to describe cystometrography, voiding pressure/

flow studies +/– urethral pressure profile which are used to establish the diagnosis of bladder outflow obstruction or lower urinary tract dysfunction (such as detrusor overactivity). Whatever the nomenclature, it is important to be clear what the diagnostic question is and therefore what test is most appropriate.

57.5.2 Bladder Ultrasound and Uroflow Studies

Portable ultrasound is cheap, non-invasive, and sensitive for detecting urine volumes pre- and post-micturiction. A persistent post-micturition residual (PMR) is really important to identify in recurrent urosepsis and may mean obstruction or detrusor failure. A residual <100mls is usually acceptable; however, it is dependent upon the expected bladder capacity. There is no consensus on what is an irrelevant PMR in the context of recurrent urosepsis, however, and a volume of 50–100mls may be relevant in this setting. Much of the data on the sensitivity and specificity of PMR and flow studies come from men with suspected bladder outflow obstruction (BOO). As mentioned above, in one study up to a quarter of men with BOO did not have a PMR and 50% of men with a PMR do not have an obstruction [2].

Flow studies/uroflowmetry provide a good screening test for bladder outflow obstruction. Patients are asked to drink until their bladders are comfortably full. Often drinking 500mls of water on arrival in the clinic will suffice, alternatively patients can be asked to attend the clinic with a full bladder. A minimum voided volume of 150mls is required to render any flow trace interpretable, therefore ensuring adequate pre-micturition bladder volume is important to build into the protocol. Both the voided volume and maximum flow rate (Q_{max}) are recorded as well as the shape/pattern of the graph and time taken to void. ◘ Figure 57.1a–e demonstrates different types of flow traces and their corresponding diagnosis. Most men with BOO have reduced flow rates, and very low flow rates are a sensitive test for BOO (90% of men with a Q_{max} of ≤10 ml/s have bladder outflow tract obstruction, but above this figure, a significant proportion of men with reduced flow rates do not have BOO [2]). Other causes of a low flow rate include detrusor failure and urethral stricture disease.

While they have their limitations, PMR and flow studies are simple non-invasive and cheap tests and easy to perform in the renal outpatient clinics (avoiding the need for a second hospital visit) and may have particular merit in following patients for dynamic changes.

57.5.3 Cystometry and Pressure/Flow Studies

Cystometrography and pressure/flow studies are invasive and should only be used when the diagnosis is in doubt or where the result of the test will influence the patient's management or provide useful prognostic information. Patients are advised to stop anticholinergic, B3 agonists, and alpha blocker medications approximately 1 week beforehand. Fine urethral/bladder and rectal catheters are placed with a small amount of discomfort. Warn fluid (either saline or contrast medium) is infused into the bladder, and pressure studies are recorded. The detrusor pressure is calculated from intra-vesical pressure minus intra-abdominal pressure (rectal catheter, vaginal vault, or intra-abdominal stoma) and should remain low during filling. The patient is asked to void with the catheters in situ to assess the detrusor pressure during micturition. The procedure usually takes approximately 30–60 minutes to perform. Cystometrography and pressure/flow studies are not routinely required to diagnose or institute treatment for bladder outflow obstruction in patients presenting with AKI secondary to high-pressure chronic urinary retention with upper tract dilatation. There may be a role in some patients presenting with very large residual volumes who are suspected of having atonic detrusor muscles or patients presenting for a re-do TURP. In these patients, urodynamic studies are sometimes useful in predicting whether outflow tract surgery (e.g. TURP) is likely to be successful in restoring voiding. The bladder outflow index nomogram demonstrates if the patient is obstructed; general indications for urodynamic cystometrography and pressure flow studies are listed in ◘ Table 57.3.

Bladder compliance is defined as the change in bladder pressure for a given change in volume, *V*/*P*. Under normal circumstances, the bladder is very compliant and may be filled with large volumes with very little increase in detrusor pressure. Poorly compliance occurs from fibrosis and reduced elasticity, e.g. radiation cystitis.

57.5.4 Videourodynamics or VCMGs (Video Cystometrography)

Cystometrography and pressure/flow studies can be combined with x-ray screening when radiological contrast medium is used to fill the bladder. This technique can be useful in demonstrating anatomical aspects of storage such as capacity, reflux, diverticula, incomplete emptying, hypermobility of the bladder neck during voiding, and intrinsic sphincter deficiency (see ◘ Fig. 57.2). The detrusor pressure during the voiding phase helps distinguish between bladder outflow obstruction (high detrusor pressure and low flow) and detrusor dysfunction (low detrusor pressure and low flow). Detrusor overactivity manifests as spikes of high detrusor pressure during filling. For men there are nomograms to help distinguish between BOO and detrusor dysfunction [1]. The diagnosis of a poorly compliant high-pressure bladder is critical as it is likely to result in loss of renal function and thus urodynamics can add vital information. Disadvantages include exposure to

57

a

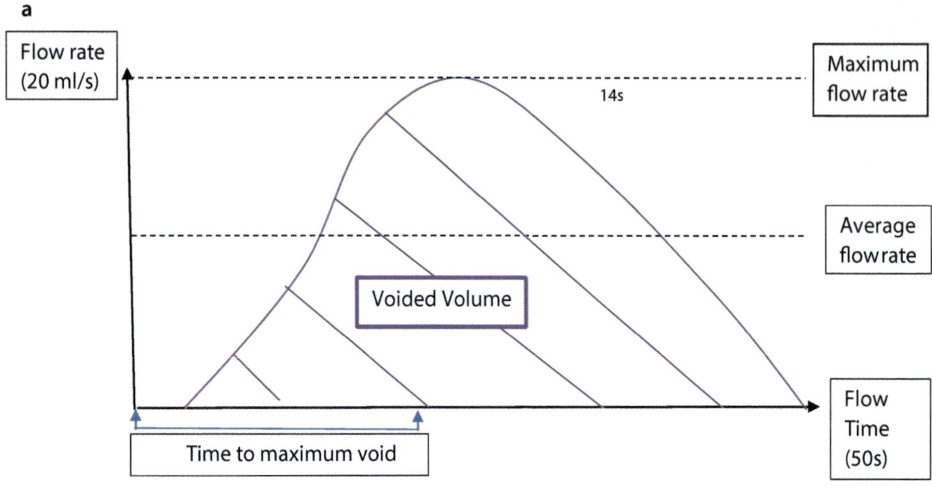

b

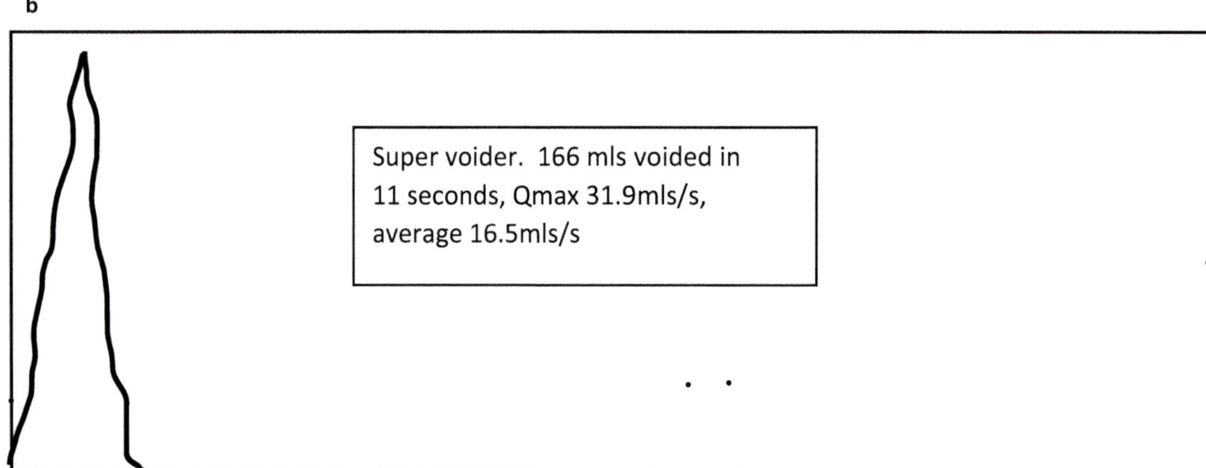

Fig. 57.1 Typical uroflowmetry traces. (**a**) Normal flow rate. (**b**) Flow rate of 'supervoider'. (**c**) Abdominal straining. (**d**) Bladder outflow obstruction (intermittent, prolonged trace). (**e**) Urethral stricture (flat box-like shape)

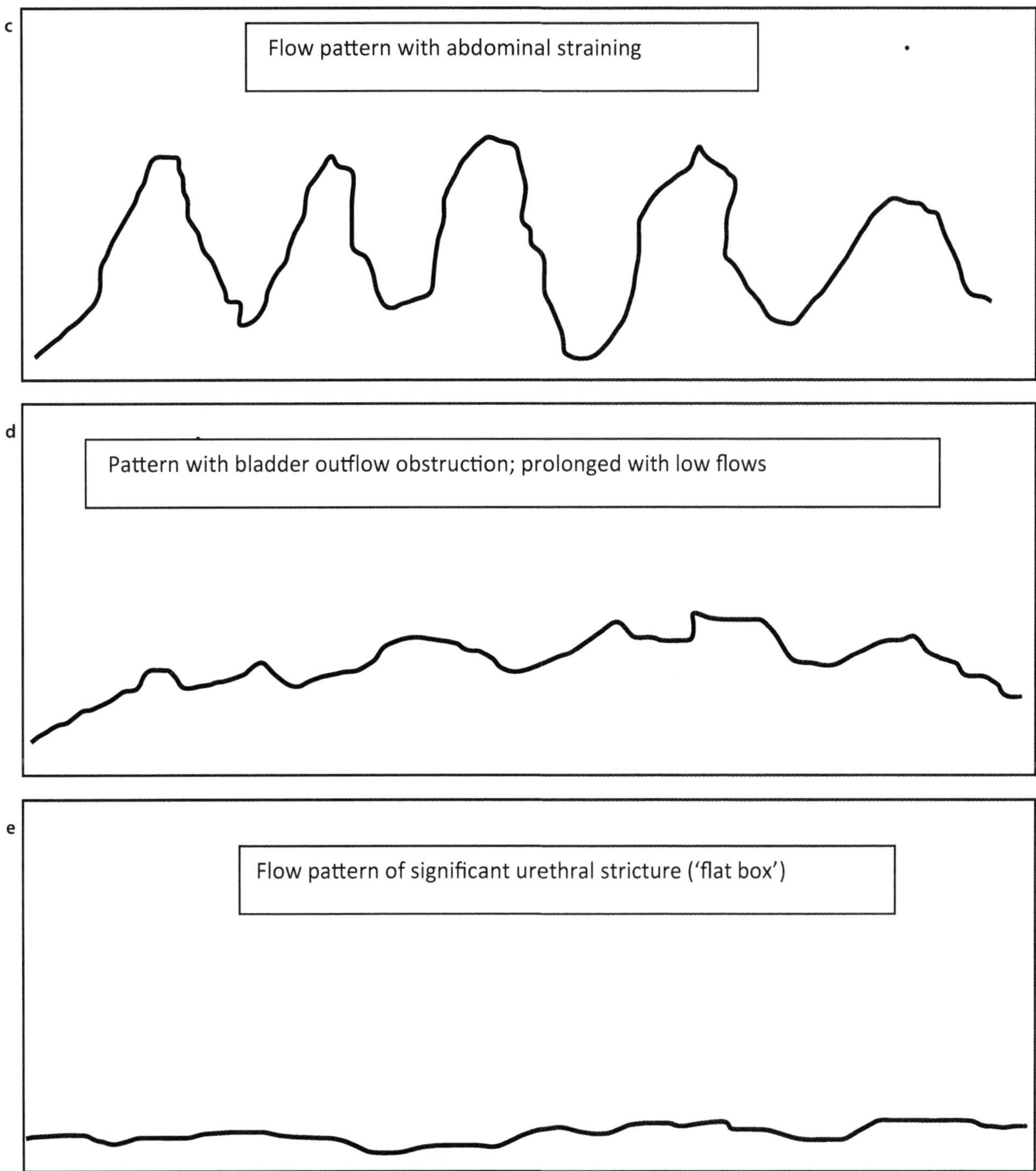

Fig. 57.1 (continued)

57

Table 57.3 Indications for cystometrography/voiding pressure flow studies in adults

Indication	Question to be answered
Clarification of diagnosis before invasive treatment	Is the patient obstructed and therefore is bladder outflow obstruction surgery likely to be successful. Urodynamic diagnosis of bladder outflow obstruction is associated with better outcomes from TURP and is the gold standard investigation
Lower urinary tract symptoms/ suspected bladder outflow obstruction	Failed medical therapy. Mixed symptoms, especially if marked storge symptoms. Particularly useful in young men
Urinary incontinence	Does the patient have detrusor overactivity/dysfunction or bladder outflow obstruction. Used when first-line therapy has failed, typically mixed storage and voiding symptoms
Neurological disorders (VCMGs)	Mismatch between symptoms and clinical assessment. Is there neurogenic bladder dysfunction, poor compliance and high storage pressures, with the attendant risk of renal damage. Detrusor sph
Vesicoureteric reflux (VCMGs)	Is reflux causing infection, scarring

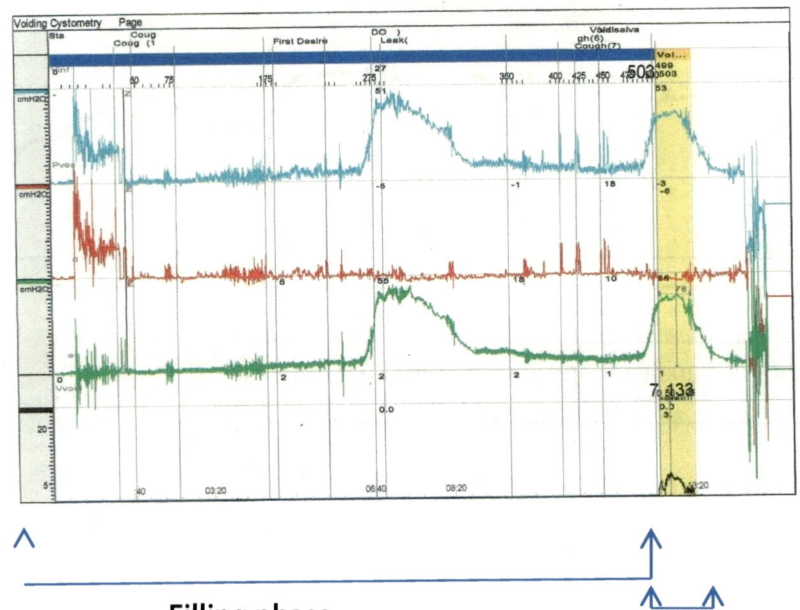

Blue line shows vesical pressure. Red line shows abdominal pressure. Detrusor pressure = pabdo- pves

Green line shows detrusor pressure. Detrusor overactivity and bladder outflow obstruction demonstrated.

Voiding phase

Filling & Storage Phase
Filling rate = 50mls/s
First desire to void 182mls (pdet 6cmH20)
Detrusor overactivity at 277mls/s
Significant associated incontinence
Normal desire to void = 349mls (pdet 17cmH20)
Strong desire to void = 499mls
Maximum cystometric capacity = 503mls

Voiding Phase
Voided volume = 133mls
Max flow rate = 6.3ml/s
pdet at max flow = 67cmH20
BOO index = 60 (obstructed)

Diagnosis: Detrusor overactivity, normal compliance with outflow obstruction

Fig. 57.2 Urodynamic trace divided into two parts – filling and storage phase (cystometrogram) and the voiding phase (voiding pressure flow study)

radiation, the use of contrast medium, greater expense, and more discomfort for the patient.

Bladder imaging may demonstrate a thickend bladder trabeculated bladder wall (≥5 mm) and diverticula. A thickened bladder wall is never normal and not to be dismissed.

57.6 Upper Tract Imaging

With the caveats shown in ◘ Table 57.1, radiological and/or nuclear medicine imaging are required to make or exclude a diagnosis of upper tract obstruction. The diagnosis may be obvious but becomes increasingly difficult in patients with poor renal function or abnormal anatomy consistent with long-standing pelvic dilatation or encasement.

57.6.1 Ultrasonography

Ultrasound is sensitive for upper tract dilatation in most patients, and imaging has significant advantages in terms of availability, cost, lack of contrast or ionising radiation, and ease of repeated measurements (for instance, in pregnancy). Gross obstruction can usually be relatively easily identified or excluded by nephrology trainees (see ◘ Fig. 57.3) and thus good practice when faced with a patient with AKI. AKI guidelines in the UK recommend upper tract ultrasound within 24 hours of unexplained AKI and within 6 hours in a septic patient if pyonephrosis is suspected (reflecting the seriousness of an infected obstructed system). A variety of enhanced US techniques may assist in the diagnosis or differentiation of obstruction [3]. Harmonic imaging (higher frequency ultrasound) is more sensitive for identifying stones and 3-dimensional ultrasound can generate multiplane cross-sectional imaging with enhanced definition and better characterisation and measurement of apparently dilated upper tract systems.

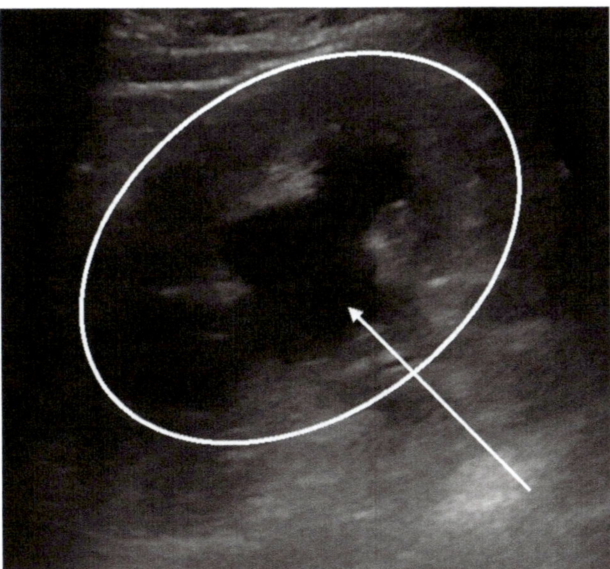

◘ **Fig. 57.3** Bedside ultrasound of a patient with AKI demonstrating marked pelvic and caliceal dilatation

57.6.2 Computer-Assisted Tomography

A plain CTKUB (kidney ureter bladder), i.e. without IV contrast, is also sensitive at picking up the pelvic obstruction, excluding extrarenal pelvis and is the modality of choice for renal stones. ◘ Figure 57.4 demonstrates a CT Urogram, i.e. with IV contrast, which has excellent spatial resolution including ureters and can demonstrate potential causes such as retroperitoneal fibrosis or malignancy. Late images (>2 minutes) may differentiate functional obstruction from dilatation. However, there is a significant radiation dose; ionic contrast is not welcome in patients with significant dysfunction and excretion urography becomes increasingly ineffective with falling GFR.

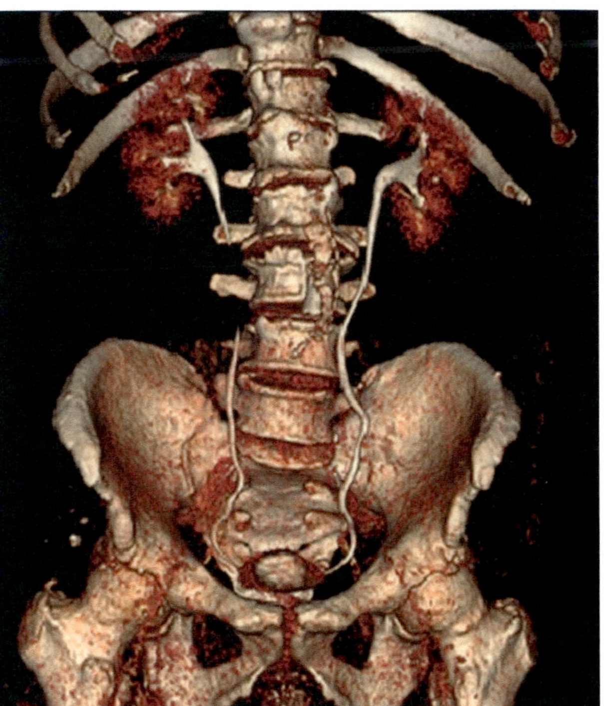

◘ **Fig. 57.4** CT Urogram of an unobstructed patient showing the delicacy of normal ureters in a non-dilated system with free flow of contrast to bladder

57.6.3 Magnetic Resonance Imaging

MR urography is increasingly finding a place in determining the cause and functional extent of obstruction. It has excellent contrast resolution with the pre-contrast T2-weighted images, but also post-contrast dynamic studies are possible in combination with loop diuretics and include the potential for divided GFR as well as the detection of functional obstruction similar (but probably superior) to MAG-3 diuretic renography [4, 5]. This is a useful imaging modality in pregnancy (see ◘ Fig. 57.5).

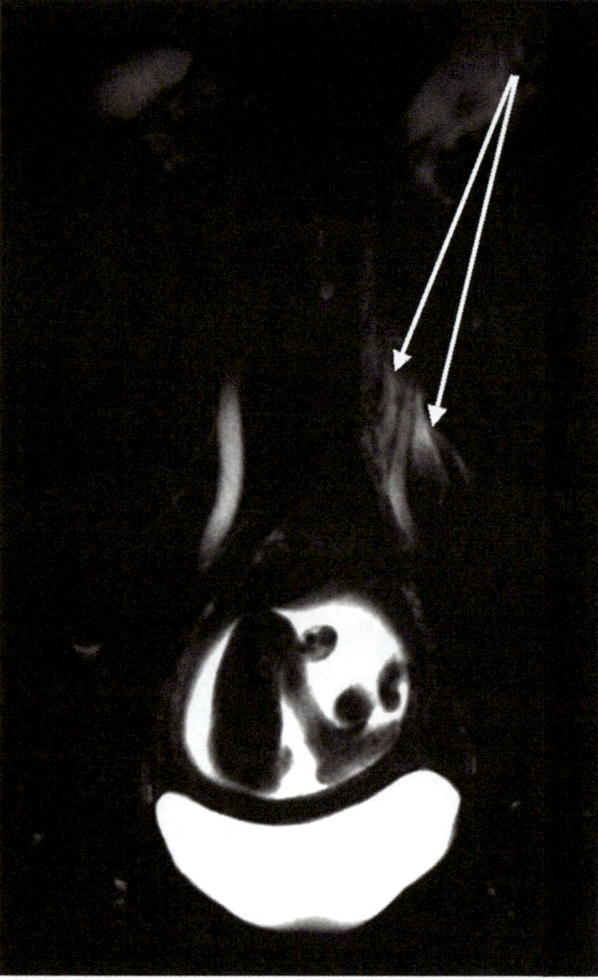

◘ **Fig. 57.5** Rupture of renal pelvis in preganancy. The patient presented at 24 weeks with left loin pain which progressed to very severe pain within the following 24 hours. A MRU demonstrated a normal ureter on the right but a spontaneous rupture of left renal pelvics and urinary leak (arrows). This is a very rare complication but worth considering in a patient with unexplained pain (urine is very inflammatory). In a non-pregnant patient, a MAG-3 with delayed films may also be diagnostic. (Image courtesy of Dr Stephanie Camillarie)

57.6.4 Nuclear Medicine Renography

Dynamic renography lacks the anatomical merits of cross-sectional imaging but brings divided function and a non-contrast functional assessment to the table. The sensitivity of the MAG3 renogram in obstruction is enhanced by IV loop diuretic 20 minutes before the injection of tracer (this is undermined by the patient routinely taking large doses of diuretics beforehand so best stopped on the day). The renogram may show progressive accumulation of tracer in the obstructed kidney. Diuretic renography can be invaluable to exclude or identify obstruction in patients with chronically "baggy" systems or those with encased and non-dilated upper tracts. It is also particularly useful in sequential monitoring of patients following stent removal; however, as with CT and MR urograms, sensitivity falls off sharply with poor renal function.

57.6.5 Whitaker Test

This test involves antegrade pressure measurements requiring a nephrostomy with pelvic and bladder pressure measurements as fluid is instilled at 10 ml/minute into the renal pelvis. A pressure differential between the pelvis and the bladder of >20 cm of water correlates with ureteropelvic or ureterovesical obstruction and can be combined with an antegrade study. The test was never intended as first line and is very rarely used now but may have merit in patients with suspected upper tract obstruction who have (a) severe renal impairment (when renogram unlikely to be helpful), (b) an equivocal diuretic renogram, and (c) intermittent obstruction particularly in the setting of the chronically dilated upper tract. The test may yet have a role when MRU is not available or tolerated [6, 7].

57.6.6 Trial of Nephrostomy or Stenting

A more pragmatic approach where there is significant doubt about drainage is to perform a nephrostomy (with antegrade study) or stent (antegrade or retrograde (with retrograde study) and monitor renal function for days (with the former) or weeks (with the later) (◘ Fig. 57.6). This is not an infrequent approach to rule out obstruction and is an effective treatment if there is obstruction, but is invasive, not without complications (see below) and can be falsely negative if there is acute tubular injury.

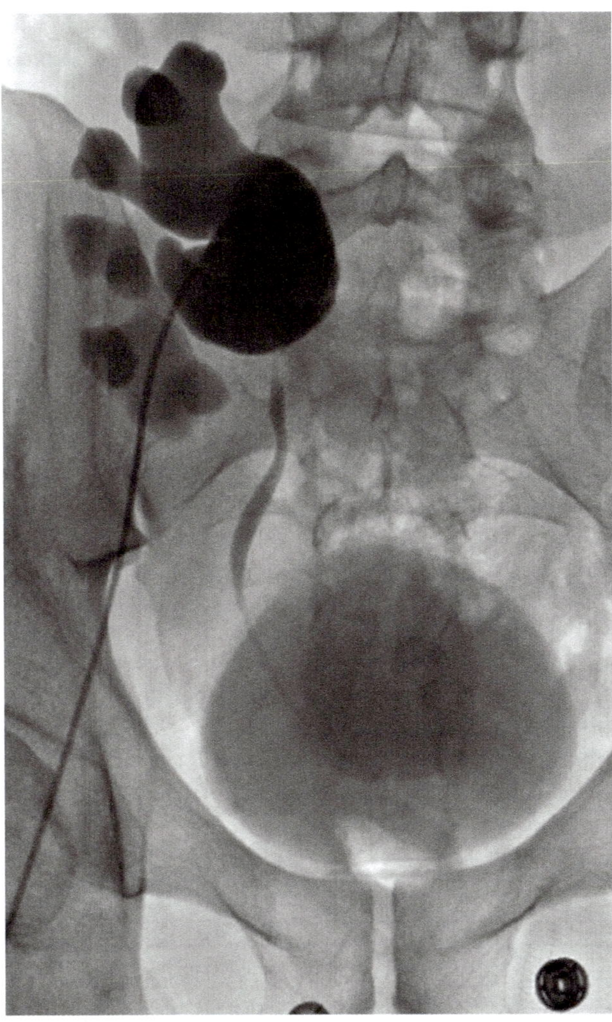

Fig. 57.6 A renal transplant with grossly dilated system but negative diuretic renogram showing apparent PUJ obstruction but good flow into the ureter and bladder. An antegrade stent was inserted to assess if the obstruction was contributing to graft dysfunction but failed to improve renal function over the following month

57.7 Treatment

57.7.1 Lower UTO

For lower urinary tract obstruction, decompression of an acutely obstructed bladder is urgent not only to relieve pain but also to prevent permanent damage to the bladder (equally important to identify and deal with treatable causes such as pain, anticholinergic medication, etc. (see Table 57.2) and to avoid recurrence on the removal of the catheter). If catheterisation is difficult, less experienced staff must be encouraged to escalate to more experienced staff as it is easy to generate life-long damage to the urethra, e.g. stricture disease. Suprapubic catheterisation, ideally under USS guidance, is the alternative if urethral catheterisation is not possible.

The treatment of long-term BOO needs careful thought and an accurate diagnosis is vital. For BPH there are a variety of options, but for severe disease then transurethral resection of the prostate, holmium laser enucleation, green light prostatectomy, Urolift, or occasionally open prostatectomy are definitive treatments but are not without complications including sepsis, bleeding, urethral stricture, incontinence, sexual dysfunction, and recurrence. A variety of minimally invasive surgical techniques are available but tend to have a lower success rate. Medical therapies can be very effective but require indefinite treatment. α-Blockers are usually first line (having a maximal effect in 2–3 days and significantly improving the success of trial without catheter (and possibly passage of ureteric stones)), but up to 33% of patients do not improve, and postural hypotension is a well recognised cause of discontinuation. Silodosin is more specific for the $\alpha 1_A$ receptor subtype predominating in the bladder neck/prostate and may be better tolerated in patients with hypotension. 5-α reductase inhibitors (5ARIs) reduce prostate size by 20–30% (but may be 3 months before clinical benefit evident) and can be used as monotherapy or in combination with alpha blockers but are associated with sexual dysfunction in around one in eight patients. There is significant data showing an additive benefit of combined therapy with an alpha blocker and 5ARIs. Large-scale trials have suggested an increased incidence of high-grade prostate cancer (Gleason 8-10) in patients taking 5ARIs but whether these findings translate into real effects on long-term cancer and survival outcomes continues to be debated. Patients and physicians need to understand that 5ARIs artificially reduce PSA readings by ~50% and therefore monitoring of PSA is important: the threshold for prostatic imaging and biopsy is therefore different when compared with the general population. A variety of other medical and surgical approaches are in the offing but not yet proven [8]. For those without BPH, the treatment depends on the diagnosis or exclusion of other causes such as urethral stricture, malignancy, detrusor dysfunction, or other neurological pathologies. Ultimately the bladder needs to be effectively drained and maintained at low pressure and options include a trial of α-blockers, intermittent self-catheterisation, indwelling urethral or suprapubic catheter, or urinary diversion such as an ileal loop or urostomy. Both anticholinergics and intra-detrusor botulinum toxin injections can be used to reduce bladder pressures.

57.7.2 Upper UTO

Pyonephrosis (emphysematous or otherwise) is a medical emergency and when suspected requires urgent imaging and decompression. Similarly, in patients with AKI and metabolic mayhem such as hyperkalaemia, acidosis, or pulmonary oedema, decompression is urgent (the alternative being dialysis followed by decompression) and the definitive treatment. In noninfected patients the time it takes humans with complete obstruction to go from reversible to irreversible kidney dysfunction is not clear. However, it seems likely given the reduction in blood flow and early infiltration of macrophages that subtle progression starts within days. Thus, prolonged delay in decompressing a healthy obstructed kidney does not seem prudent for someone likely to need their kidney in the future, and as the speciality involved in managing CKD, nephrologists should encourage timely decompression. The procedure of nephrostomy is very nicely described by Uppot [9]. ◘ Figure 57.7 shows a nephrostomy and nephrostogram demonstrating a tight stenosis of a transplant ureter. In essence, nephrostomy is not risk free with a mortality of 0.05–0.03% and transfusion requirement of 1–3%. Generally the sicker the patient (and the less experienced the operator), the greater the risk so optimising the patient, operator, and timing are important. Acute tubular injury, nephrostomy displacement, blockage, and misplacement are common reasons for failure to drain. Flushing the nephrostomy can usually rule out blockage, and a displaced catheter is often obvious, but repeat imaging is important to ensure that the nephrostomy catheter has not perforated the urinary tract.

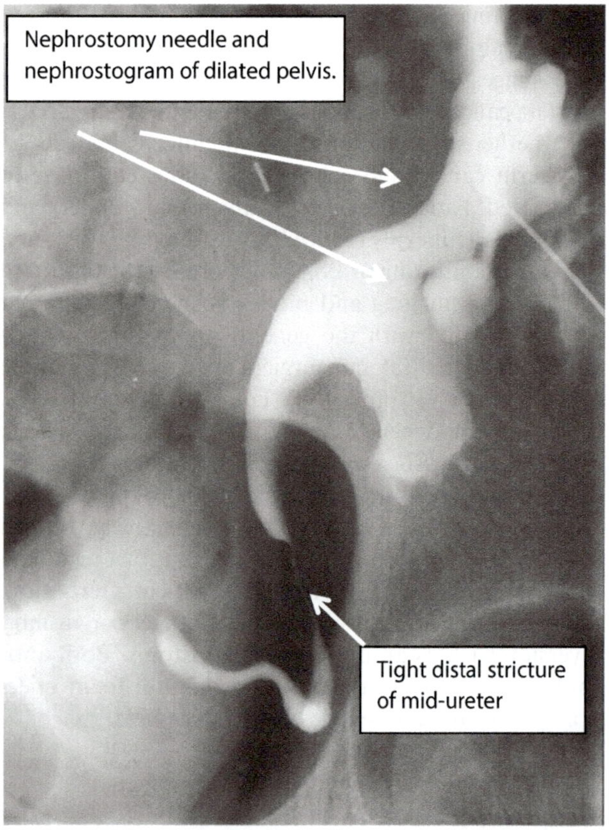

◘ **Fig. 57.7** Showing obstructed transplant kidney with nephrostomy and nephrostogram showing a tight stricture of the ureter in this case secondary to mycobacterium infection with BKV and ischaemic strictures important differentials

If possible an antegrade study is done at the time of the nephrostomy insertion, but often clot or ureteric oedema precludes a descent study, and often a better study is achieved a day or two later. Sepsis is a contraindication for antegrade studies or simultaneous insertion of ureteric stents. Balloon dilatation of a stricture is not universally successful [10]; strictures of less than 3-month duration have a higher patency rate (88%) than those >3 months (67%) with those over a year having poor rates (15%). Stricture length also appears to be important, greater than 2 cm having a poor long-term patency rate, and malignant strictures do predictably worse than benign ones. Ballooning is usually accompanied by stenting and stent removal several weeks later, at which time retrograde studies can be done to assess patency and the need for further stents or surgery. Given the significant recurrence rate, patients need a mechanism for monitoring either with bloods and repeat USS or renogram; if the patient has another normal kidney, then reliance on creatinine and eGFR is probably not sufficient.

57.8 Post-Obstructive Diuresis

Post-obstructive diuresis (POD) is a genuine phenomenon, in part related to acquired urinary concentrating defects (including early downregulation of aquaporin channels), high levels of urea acting as an osmotic diuretic as well as appropriate excretion of accumulated salt and water and can result in a massive diuresis. Without support this can result in a collapse in intravascular volume and further AKI. Conversely stage managed reduction in fluids is necessary to avoid perpetuating the polyuria for days. These patients are often managed by relatively junior non-renal medical staff; clear and constructive renal advice can help prevent avoidable complications and probably shorten length of stay. The first priority is to ensure adequate intravascular volume and regular reassessment followed by clear instructions for monitoring, including hourly urine output, pulse, blood pressure, accurate fluid balance, and daily weights. In practical terms if the patient is euvolaemic, then ml for ml fluid replacement of urine output on an hourly basis is probably the safest approach in the short-term, the choice of the replacement being governed by the electrolytes although the more physiological the solution the easier to manage. In the setting of a massive diuresis, the teams looking after the patient need to know that frequent testing of electrolytes (sodium, potassium, magnesium, calcium, and bicarbonate) is critical to avoid wild excursions of electrolytes or osmolality. In particular, the fractional excretion of potassium can be disproportionate because of high sodium delivery to the distal tubule. While this is often helpful in a patient with obstruction and life-threatening hyperkalaemia, patients with significant POD can become profoundly hypokalaemic quite quickly. Large volumes can ultimately perpetuate the diuresis in part by continued washout of the countercurrent multiplier, and if the diuresis is persisting and the patient is intravascularly replete, then a gentle and carefully monitored negative fluid balance (e.g. 50 or 100mls per hour negative) needs to be introduced.

57.9 Post-Obstructive Haemorrhage (Decompression Haematuria)

Post-obstructive haematuria can occur following sudden decompression of a chronically obstructed bladder. Although macroscopic this is usually self-limiting and managed either conservatively or with a 3 W catheter and irrigation. Very rarely haemorrhage can be extensive and can involve the upper tract in patients with secondary upper tract dilatation (◘ Fig. 57.8).

Serious post-decompression bleeding is very rare, and there is no evidence that clamping the catheter periodically during decompression has any protective effect.

57.10 Aortitis, Periaortitis, and Retroperitoneal Fibrosis (RPF)

Retroperitoneal inflammation of any cause has the potential to involve the ureters and result in upper tract obstruction. A collection of diseases are increasingly

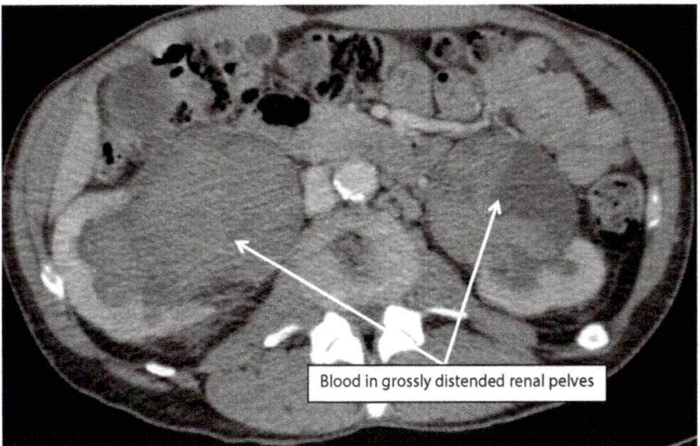

◘ **Fig. 57.8** Showing extensive upper tract blood clot and obstruction following urinary catheter decompression of a chronically obstructed bladder secondary to benign prostatic enlargement

◘ **Table 57.4** Causes of retroperitoneal fibrosis

Idiopathic retroperitoneal fibrosis	IgG-4 related disease associated with raised inflammatory markers, membranous glomerulonephritis, IgG-4 interstitial nephritis others, e.g. pancreatic, biliary, ENT, and orbital involvement
Secondary to aortitis	Atherosclerotic aneurysm (especially if leaking)
Periaortitis	May be IgG-4-related disease
Retroperitoneal infection	Tuberculosis
Medication	Methysergide, bromocriptine
Radiation to retroperitoneum	
Malignancy	8% including sarcoma and lymphoma
Trauma	With haematoma

recognised to cause this problem, and wider availability of ^{18}f-fluorodeoxyglucose (FDP) PET scanning and identification of IgG-4 related disease is advancing the diagnosis and management of this heterogenous group. The common causes/associations of retroperitoneal fibrosis are shown (◘ Table 57.4). It has become apparent that there is considerable overlap in some of the conditions and that a significant proportion of 'idiopathic' retroperitoneal fibrosis (70%) and a smaller but significant proportion of aortitis and periaortitis are associated with IgG-4 related disease.

Classically RPF secondary to atherosclerotic aortitis presents in the middle-aged smoker (strong male preponderance) with extensive macrovascular disease (asbestos exposure is also a risk factor as is HLA-DRB1*03 [11]) in the setting of an abdominal aortic aneurysm. However, RPF also occurs in the absence of aneurysmal dilatation but in the setting of the periaortitis involving vasculitis of the vasa vasorum with obliterative endarteritis or phlebitis. This is often associated with fibro-inflammatory reaction in the retroperitoneum with tissue encasing retroperitoneal structures including the ureters and left renal vein. Clinically this may present with back or abdominal pain, fatigue, anorexia, weight loss, ureteric colic, varicoele, or hydrocele with an inflammatory response (raised ESR and CRP), deep vein thrombosis, and renal impairment if ureteric drainage is compromised. Renal artery involvement may occur in up to a third of cases with fibro-inflammatory tissue reaching the hilum.

'Idiopathic RPF', i.e. those with no other obvious precipitant, has an incidence of approximately 1:100000, and 70% of these cases are associated with IgG-4 RD. In addition, 50% of IgG-4-related RPF cases have extraperitoneal involvement (pancreas, biliary tree, periorbital, thyroid, pericardium, skin, salivary glands, breast, and meninges). The pathology of IgG-4-related RPF differs from that of other causes in that there is dense inflammatory infiltrate with a high proportion of plasma cells (35–76% vs 0–10% in atheroma related RPF [12]), a significant proportion of which stain for IgG-4. Although serum levels of IgG-4 are usually hardly raised, a ratio of IgG-4/total IgG >0.3 is indicative.

Medial deviation of the middle third of the ureters is a classic finding but has poor sensitivity, and although US is excellent for diagnosing obstruction, it is not sensitive for examining the retroperitoneum and determining the underlying cause or extrarenal involvement. Therefore, cross-sectional scanning with contrast CT is the most helpful initial form of imaging. For those patients with evidence of periaortitis or idiopathic RPF in whom immunosuppression is planned, then ^{18}F-FDP-PET-CT is both sensitive and extremely useful for monitoring response to treatment whether it be renal or extrarenal (see ◘ Figs. 57.9 and 57.10).

57

The majority of patients with RPF seen by nephrologists have developed ureteric obstruction usually bilateral (70%), but renal artery and vein encasement as well as referral for management of large vessel vasculitis are also part of the case mix. The principles of management are similar and involve the decompression of the kidneys (almost exclusively via nephrectomies and antegrade stenting) and correction of any critical vascular pathology. Excluding any secondary cause, such as infection or malignancy, is critical, and biopsy of the RPF tissue mass is highly desirable where and when possible (including staining for plasma cells and IgG-4). FDP-PET scanning and acute phase markers suggestive of active inflammation, then a trial of immunosuppression is usually adopted. There is no consensus on this, but for 'idiopathic' or IgG-4-related RPF, medium-dose steroids with an antiproliferative such as azathioprine or mycophenolate mofetil are commonly adopted; symptoms, and ESR/CRP and PET scan response are all useful markers of disease activity. For RPF associated with a vasculitic aortitis steroids, methotrexate, azathioprine, mycophenolic acid, and cyclosphosphamide are all used. More recently anti-TNF monoclonal antibodies (infliximab and adalimumab) have been used with success in inflammatory aortitides such as Takaysu's aortitis [13].

The absence of an acute phase response or activity on FDP-PET scanning suggests a lack of inflammatory involvement, and immunosuppression is less likely to be helpful. Patients can be managed with retrograde stent changing, but this is not without complications, and blockade of one stent may be asymptomatic and go unnoticed resulting in permanent loss of renal function. Retrograde studies at the time of stent change may demonstrate free flow, but part of the pathogenesis lies in loss of ureteric peristalsis rather than occlusion or stenosis, so free flow may be falsely reassuring. If repeat imaging shows regression of the retroperitoneal mass and retrograde studies show free flow, stent removal may be justified, but a system of monitoring with US or diuretic renogram is critical. Where there is no evidence of FDG activity, acute phase response or a large burden of IS is required to maintain control; then ureterolysis with lateral or intraperitoneal transposition with an omental wrap is usually definitive but can result in devascularisation of the ureter.

The management of these patients requires cross-disciplinary care, and establishing smooth referral pathways, common guidelines, and an efficient multidisciplinary approach is the key to optimal care. Nephrology departments should ensure that such pathways and protocols are clearly established with local urologists, radiologists, and other specialists such as oncologists.

57.11 Malignancy

While obstruction secondary to malignancy is normally managed between urologists, oncologists, and palliative care teams, a significant proportion of these patients cross the paths of nephrologists, and it is worth special mention. Ureteric obstruction secondary to malignant invasion is associated with a very poor prognosis, and survival is typically between 3 and 7 months necessitating a thoughtful and holistic approach that is not always achieved in practice. If appropriate, and following a discussion of the options with the patient, their fitness and the stage of the malignancy, the first aim is to relieve the obstruction to the kidneys. Retrograde stenting is associated with a much higher (×3) rate of failure in the setting of external malignancy than with intrinsic obstruction such as stones, and this seems to be particularly bad with pelvic malignancies such prostate, bladder, and cervical malignancy (success rates of 15–21%) compared to colorectal or breast [14]. For this reason an antegrade approach is often adopted to drainage with percutaneous nephrostomy in the first instance. Antegrade stenting is either attempted simultaneously or subsequently when the patient is more stable. The decision to decompress both kidneys depends on the stability of the patient, their prognosis, whether the renal function needs to be maximised for chemotherapy, and whether there is felt to be associated sepsis. Both stenting and nephrostomy drains are associated with multiple complications and poor patient satisfaction.

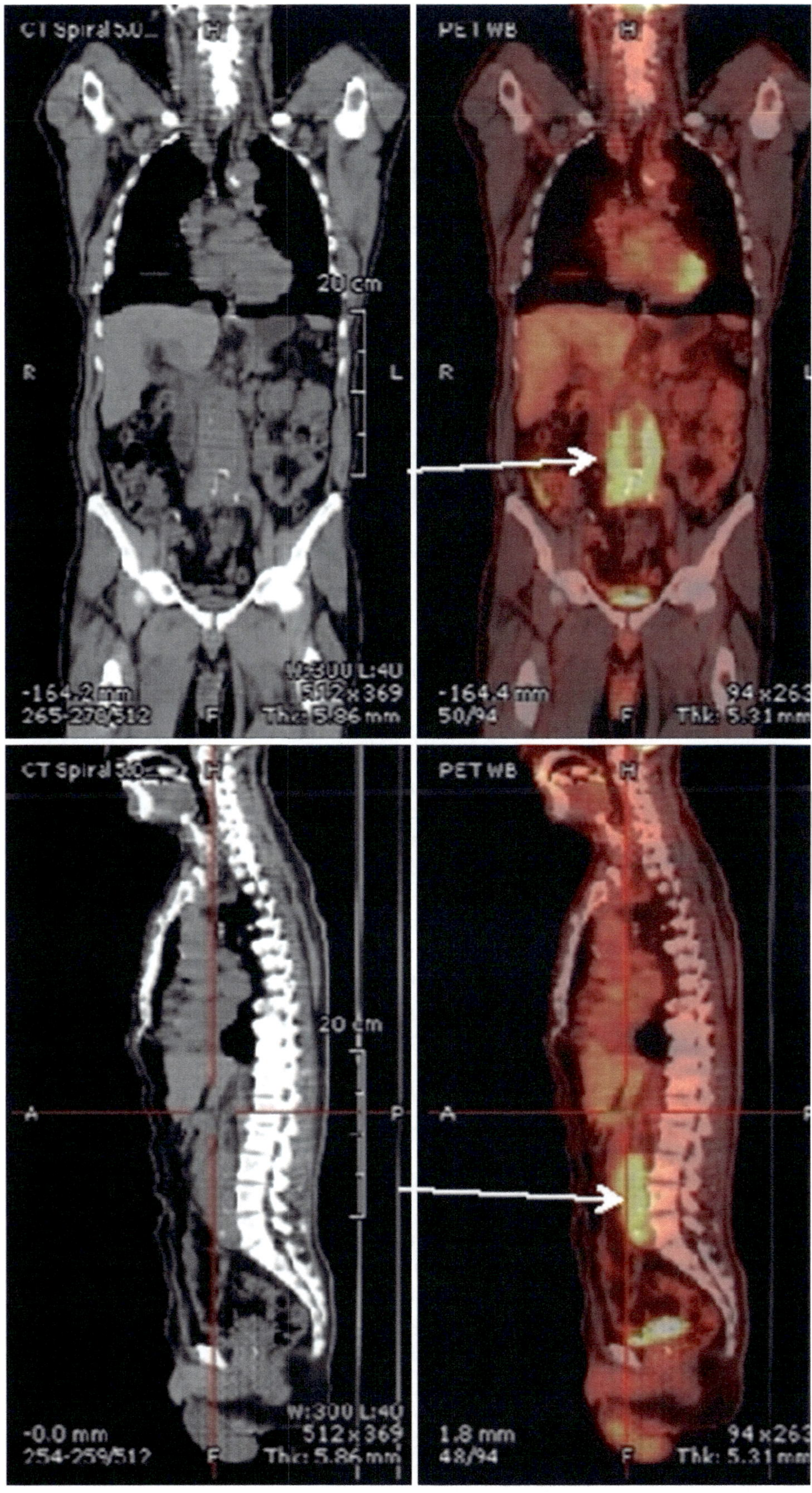

Fig. 57.9 PET-CT scan in a patient with idiopathic retroperitoneal fibrosis showing an intense inflammatory process (showing yellow) in the pre-lumbar region. This patient had high inflammatory markers which correlated well with subsequent PET-CT imaging following treatment

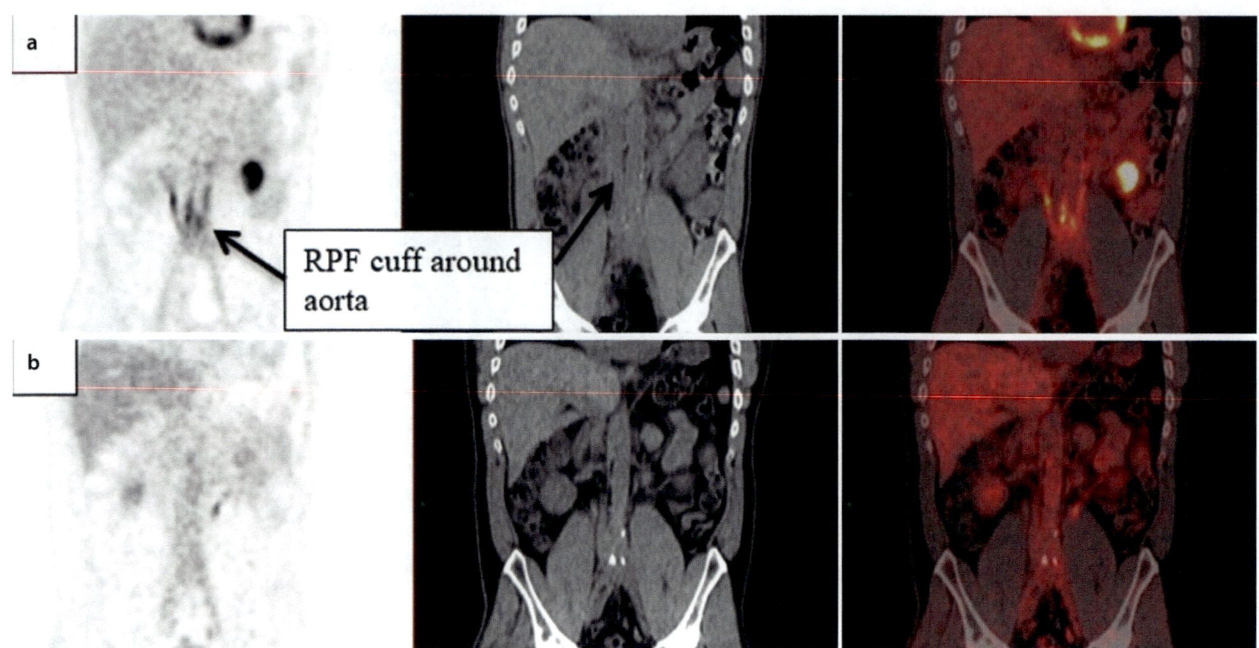

57

Fig. 57.10 PET-CT scan in a patient with idiopathic retroperitoneal fibrosis showing the intense inflammatory process (showing yellow) in the para-aortic and left renal region. (**a**) Before treatment. (**b**) After treatment

Long-term nephrostomy drains can become displaced, infected, and blocked or result in urinary leaks, all of which results in high readmission and reintervention rates. Similarly ureteric stents can become misplaced, blocked or encrusted, and cause irritation of the bladder (sometimes alleviated by antihcholinergics) [14]. There may occasionally be a benefit of metal stents in these patients, but they are not a panacea, and the evidence is not strong [15]. For a small group of patients with a prognosis of several months or more and with severe symptoms or urinary leak, surgical drainage may be appropriate such as ureterostomy, ureteric reimplantation, or conduit formation [16].

These are a complex group of patients facing a desperate time; an efficient, thoughtful, and multidisciplinary approach is required to avoid them spending much of their remaining time in hospital [17, 18].

Tips and Tricks

Urology MDT meetings are a good place to find patients with obstruction from stones, malignancy, retroperitoneal fibrosis, or recurrent UTIs due to poor drainage. Many of these patients have or are at risk of developing CKD. Renal involvement in or discussion of the urology MDT list is an easy way of facilitating nephrological input and joined up care, if needed.

Adding post-micturition residual measurements to a formal US request is non-invasive and helpful in those with recurrent UTIs or unexplained renal impairment. Better still, it is easy to train staff to accurately measure bladder residuals in the clinic and ward setting using simple handheld ultrasound devices. A post-void residual below 100mls is usually acceptable.

Urologists are well practiced at managing acute upper and lower tract obstruction, but a proportion of patients will have AKI that requires urgent nephrology input. Joint protocols including referral criteria for AKI in the context of obstruction, sepsis, and post-obstructive diuresis should be established.

Where there is diagnostic doubt about upper tract obstruction, then a combination of anatomical and functional scans are often complimentary, and serial scanning (e.g. USS with measurements, isotope renogram with divided function or MRU) may be necessary to decide on intervention. MRU is likely to become increasingly valuable at answering both anatomical and functional questions.

Upper tract obstruction may occur secondary to a hypertrophied bladder wall and may require stenting until the decompressed bladder allows remodelling of the bladder. However, functional upper tract obstruction can also occur without obvious BOO in the setting of detrusor dysfunction and a high-pressure bladder; renal function may not improve with stenting unless this is identified by urodynamics and treated accordingly.

Patients with upper tract obstruction secondary to malignancy face bleak times, and it is easy for the medical profession to make this worse either by under-treating obstruction or by intervening when not appropriate. Early thoughtful discussion of the patient's wishes and needs is key and should include 'what if AKI intervenes?', for example, if blocked nephrostomies or stents occur. Monitoring of renal function can often be done by the district nurse or family practitioner without the need to drag the patient repeatedly to multiple clinics.

57.12 Summary

Upper and lower UTO are a common cause of AKI, CKD, and urosepsis, all of which have significant risk and repercussions for patients. Achieving a rapid diagnosis and close liaison with urologists to achieve rapid acute and then definitive drainage is very important and not always accomplished but within the gift of nephrologists to deliver.

Case Study

Case 1

Obstetricians performed life-saving surgery on a 28-year-old woman following a torrential post-partum bleed, during which she became markedly hypotensive. She became oligo-anuric for a period after the surgery with an AKI (creatinine of 244 within 48 hours). An ultrasound scan demonstrated reduced perfusion to the right kidney and CT with contrast (◘ Fig. 57.11a) demonstrated an acutely enlarged right kidney with retained contrast and a dilated ureter. A diagnosis of ureteric ligation was made, and a right nephrostomy was performed with an antegrade study (◘ Fig. 57.11b) showing a grossly dilated right ureter with an abrupt obstruction. A renogram done at this time (◘ Fig. 57.11c) because of concerns regarding reduced perfusion demonstrates normal and rapid uptake of tracer in the left kidney but much reduced uptake in the right kidney. Over the next 15–20 minutes, the left kidney excretes the tracer whereas the right kidney continues to accumulate and retain tracer. Before definitive surgery, drainage from the nephrostomy stopped, and reimaging (◘ Fig. 57.11d) demonstrated a dilated renal pelvis and displacement of the nephrostomy tube (no longer draining) and an associated deterioration in renal function. A further nephrostomy was performed, and she subsequently underwent a ureteric reimplantation and removal of the stitch that inadvertently caught the lower ureter. A renogram done some months later (◘ Fig. 57.11e) showed 67% function on the left (arrow) and 33% on the right.

This case illustrates many points: ureteric obstruction must be rapidly excluded in AKI following abdominal or pelvic surgery. Acute obstruction cause swelling of the kidney and significantly reduced perfusion which suggests ongoing injury rather than a benign process secondary to obstruction. Nephrostomies are excellent treatments for acute upper tract obstruction but are best seen as a short-term bridge to definitive drainage; in this case the patient had to undergo another nephrostomy and period of obstruction following the displacement of the nephrostomy. Finally, periods of obstruction before definitive drainage may have a significant impact on the function of the kidney that is not always appreciated.

Case 2

A man aged 19 presented with end-stage renal disease with bilateral small kidneys and went on to have a cadaveric renal transplant within a year and was transferred to a new transplant unit as he started college. On transfer his creatinine was around 200 but progressively rose in the setting of variable tacrolimus levels, multiple investigations including, BKV and HLA antibody screening, and two renal biopsies over the space of a year were unremarkable, as were doppler ultrasounds and a MRA of the renal artery and vein. He had initially been unforthcoming about urinary symptoms, but on direct questioning it became apparent that he had enuresis most nights this, the fact that the cause of his original kidney disease was unknown and his age made a dysfunctional bladder a distinct possibililty. Video urodynamics demonstrated a high pressure, poorly compliant bladder with reflux into his transplant (◘ Fig. 57.12a–c).

He was treated with an anticholinergic and clean intermittent self-catheterisation (◘ Fig. 57.12d arrow) with almost immediate resolution of his enuresis and a progressive fall in creatinine (◘ Fig. 57.12d). In retrospect this diagnosis took too long to make and illustrates the point that it is important to always consider whether a patient may have a high-pressure bladder, especially if features suggestive of CAKUT such as previous posterior urethral valves or unexplained CKD early in life.

Case 3

A man in his late 40s presented with progressive left flank pain, significant weight loss, and retrograde ejaculation, in addition to pancreatitis 4 years previously. He was a smoker with a strong family history of cardiovascular disease (◘ Fig. 57.13).

This illustrates the importance of establishing not only the cause of the obstruction but the underlying aetiology to guide treatment of the cause as there are several causes of RPF including malignancy infection and autoimmune disease with very different management options.

Case 4

A 39-year-old man was admitted following a RTA with trauma to his left kidney. He had a major haemorrhage,

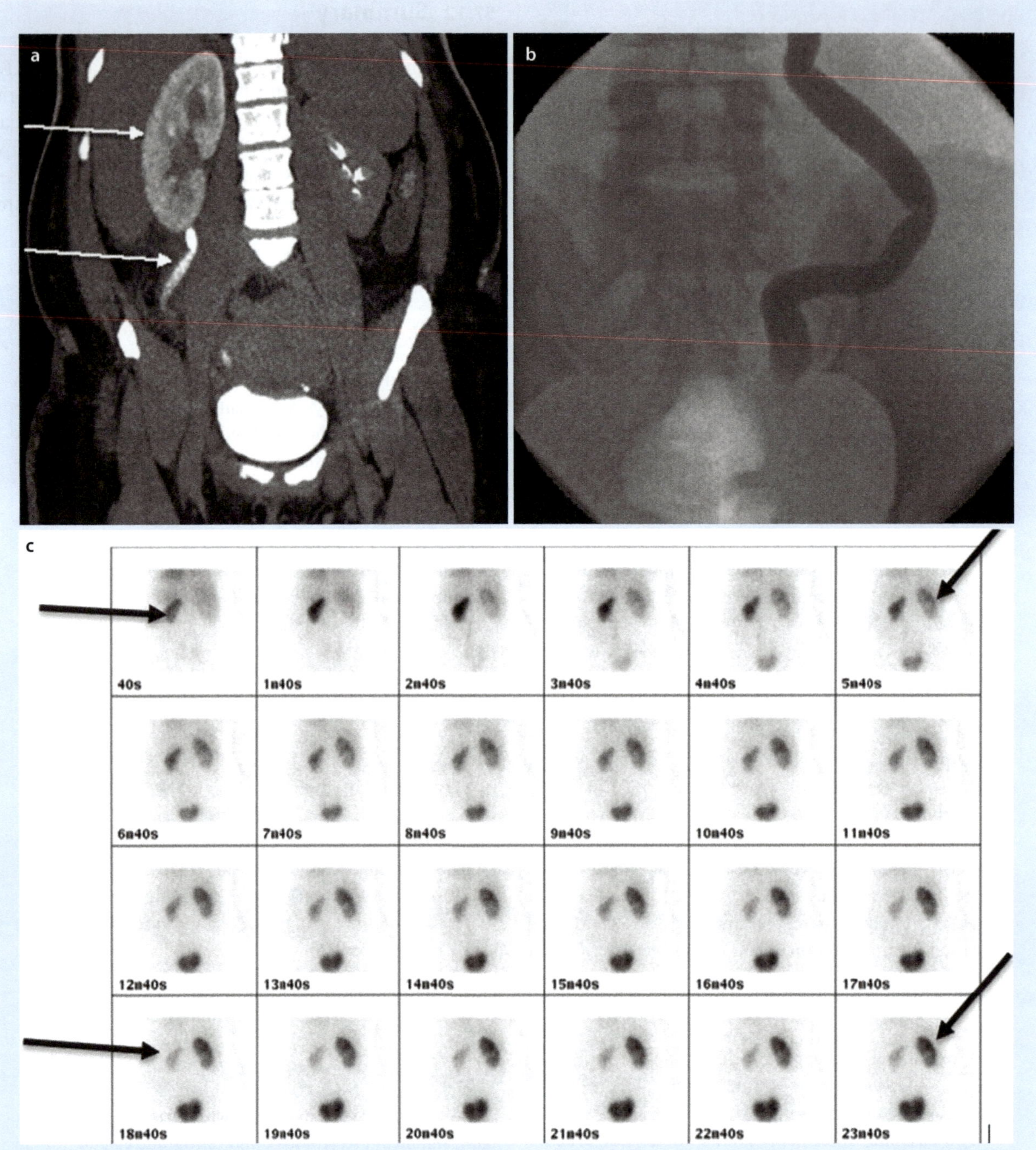

Fig. 57.11 (**a**) A CT with contrast demonstrated and enlarged right kidney with retention of contrast, dilated pelvis and a dilated right ureter. (**b**) A antegrade study following a nephrostomy showing a grossly dilated ureter with an abrupt stop at the point of the ligature. (**c**) Renogram showing delayed and then progressive uptake of istope in the right kidney. (**d**) CT scan showing right kidney reobstructed with clearly displaced nephrostomy. (**e**) A renogram performed several months after the original obstruction and subsequent surgical correction

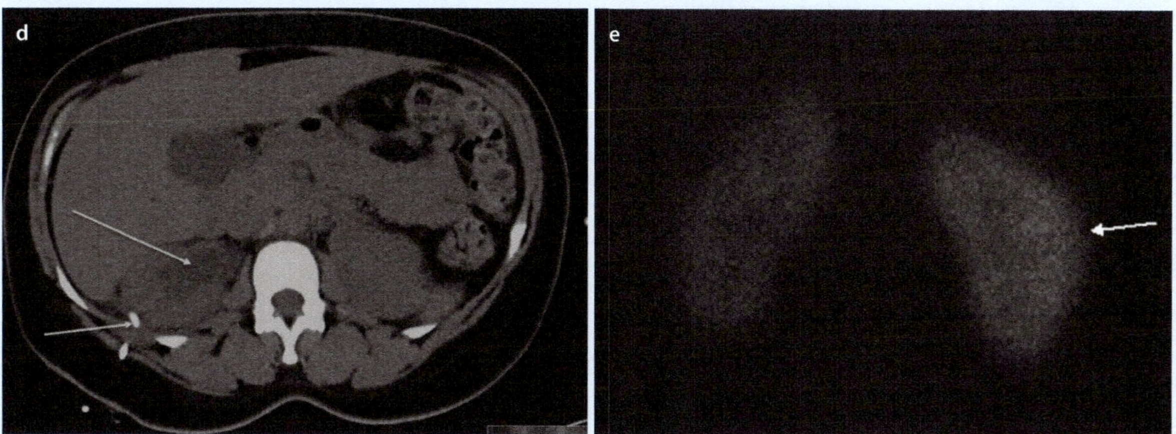

Fig. 57.11 (continued)

required embolization, and developed bilateral upper tract obstruction attributed to clots, requiring retrograde stenting. As he recovered, his urinary catheter was removed, but within a few hours he developed severe right loin pain. He was recatheterised, and two further attempted trials of voiding had identical outcomes; there was no evidence of neurological deficit. The clues here are that a 39-year-old failed trial without catheter (3 times) and that he developed severe loin pain on the side of the stent, implying transmitted bladder pressure and imaging focused on the upper tract at the time of obstruction (Fig. 57.14) demonstrated a thick-walled bladder (never normal!). He responded to alpha blockers which he required long term.

Case 5

Figure 57.15a shows the renogram of a man who presented with right loin pain (top). The estimated function of the kidneys at this time was 55% (left) and 45% (right) and demonstrates normal uptake and excretion of the left kidney (red), but an accumulation continued without excretion on the right (green) confirming obstruction. The non-contrast CT done at the time of presentation (Fig. 57.15a(i)) shows marked intra-renal dilatation secondary to pelvi-ureteric obstruction but with well-preserved renal cortex. Unfortunately the patient was lost to follow-up, but when seen 6 months later, the CT demonstrated almost complete loss of renal parenchymal tissue (Fig. 57.15b(ii)) and a renogram suggesting <5% function. This unfortunate case emphasizes that there may be a significant price in nephrons to pay for 'elective or routine' decompression of obstructed kidneys.

Figure 57.16 demonstrates the findings in a young man with sickle cell disease who presented with acute loin pain. An antegrade stent was placed to the relief the obstruction.

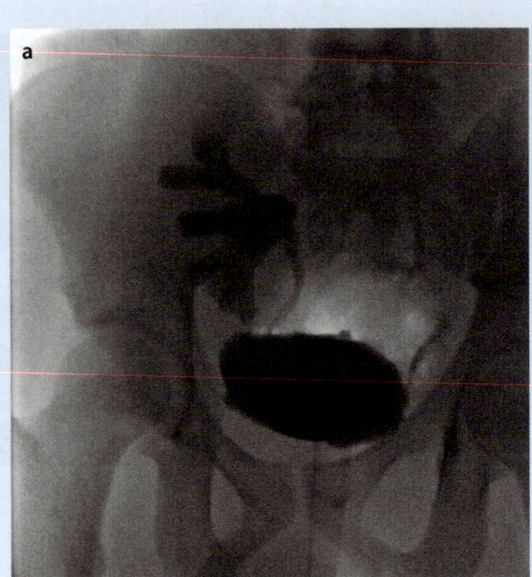

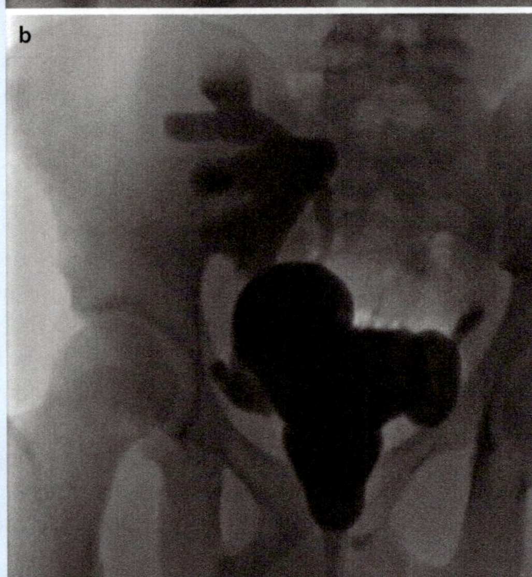

Fig. 57.12 (**a**) Shows a still from video urodynamics with reflux to the transplanted kidney and some to native ureter. (**b**) Shows more reflux with further filling and a distorted bladder. (**c**) Shows urodynamic traces with pressure measurements. Maximum and average flows for a young man were low at 14mls/s and 8.5mls/s respectively but pressures of 72 cm of water were generated in the bladder. (**d**) Sequential post-transplant creatinines in a patient with unknown cause of renal disease. Progressive rise in creatinine with no evidence of rejection or any abnormality on cross-sectional imaging. At the point indicated by the arrow, management for high pressure bladder was commenced

c

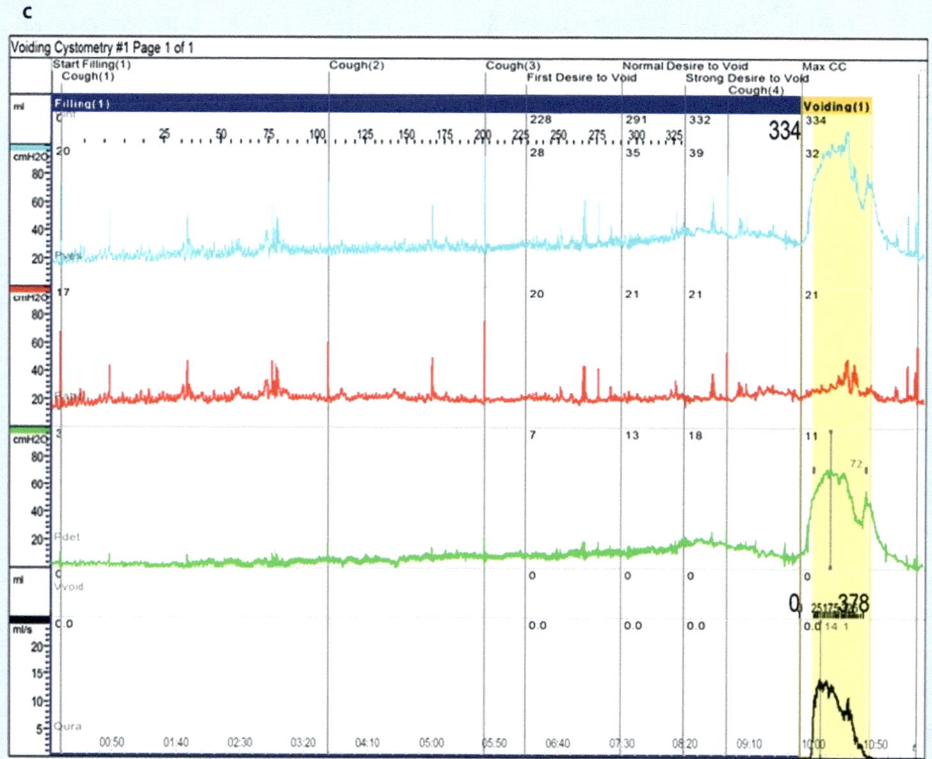

Voiding Cystometry #1

Voiding		
Patient Position		Sitting
Max Flow Rate	(ml/s)	14.1
Voided Voume	(ml)	377
Voided Time	(s)	45
Flow Time	(s)	44
Average Flow Rate	(ml/s)	8.5
Time to Max Flow	(s)	7
Max Pdet	(cmH2O)	72
Residual Urine	(ml)	-
Pdet at Opening	(cmH2O)	50
Pdet at Max Flow	(cmH2O)	60
Qura Delay	(s)	0.7
Pdet at Begin Flow	(cmH2O)	44
Pdet at Max Flow (p/Q)	(cmH2O)	61
Pdet at End Flow (p/Q)	(cmH2O)	52
Descending Slope	(cmH2O/ml/s)	0.7
A/G		Equivocal
A/G#	(cmH2O)	33.3

Fig. 57.12 (continued)

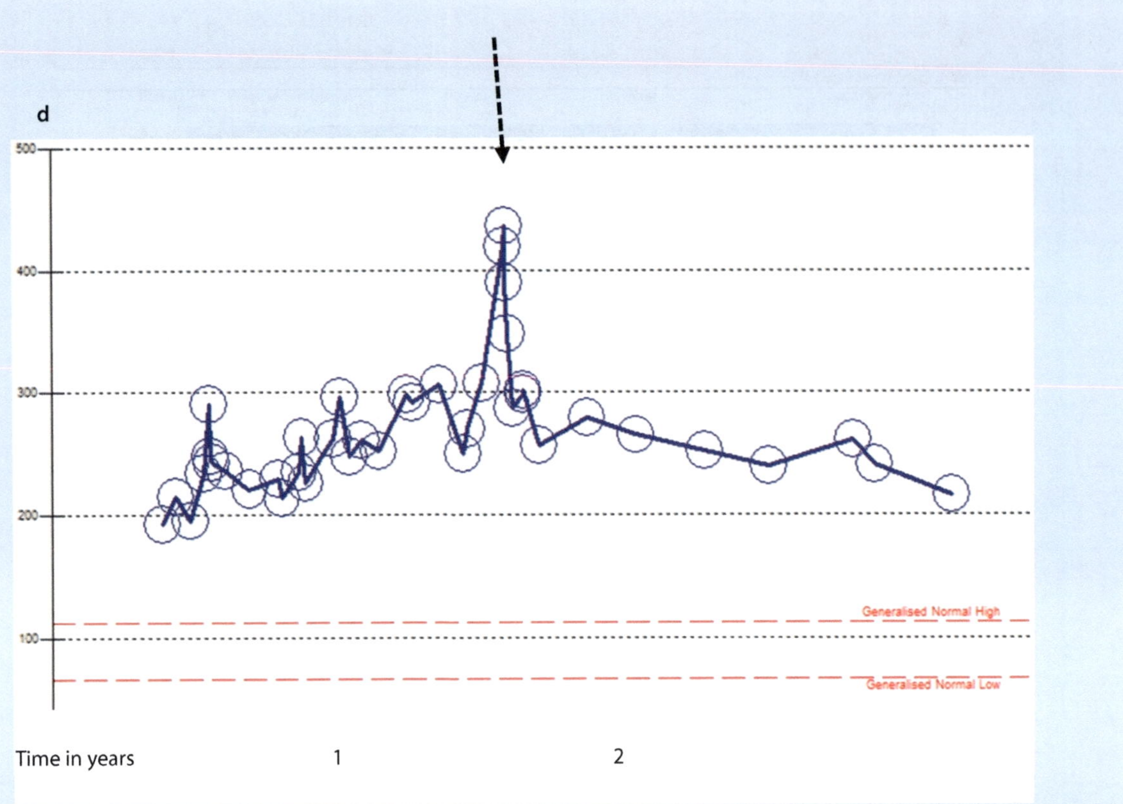

Fig. 57.12 (continued)

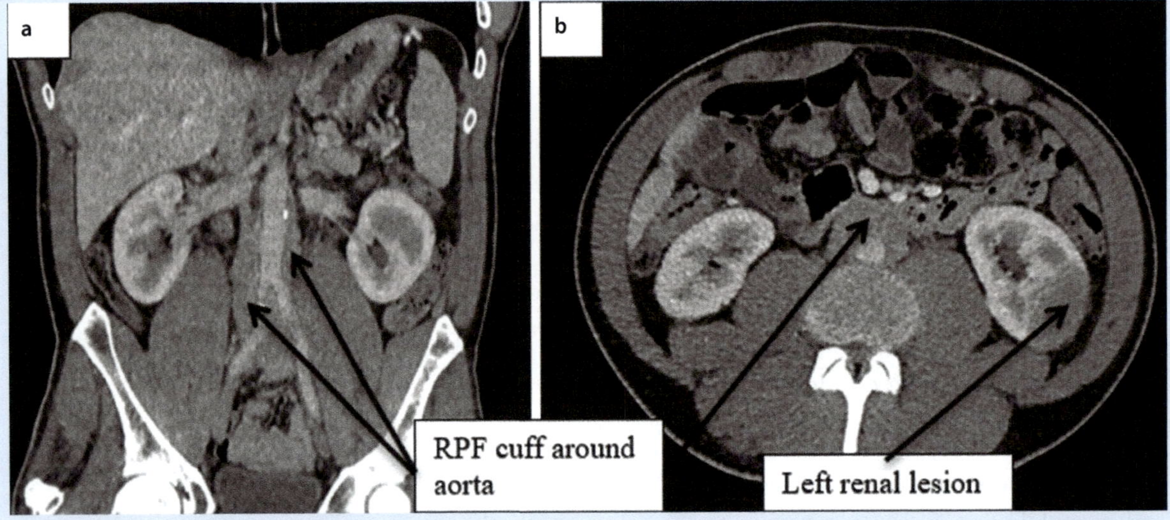

Fig. 57.13 (**a**) Contrast-enhanced CT abdomen and pelvis coronal (**a**) and axial (**b**) imaging revealed a circumferential cuff of RPF tissue around the abdominal aorta and involving the bifurcation into the iliac arteries. In addition a cortical left renal lesion was identified and was subsequently biopsied. Histological analysis revealed a fibrosing and necrotising granulomatous process with some plasma cells amounting to <30 / hpf. Screening for ANCA or TB-related disease was negative. (**b**) Coronal FDG PET-CT imaging. (**a**) Revealed avid tissue FDG uptake in the RPF peri-aortic cuff and left renal cortex lesion. (**b**) Follow-up imaging after 8 months of treatment with a weaning course of prednisolone and azathioprine revealed almost complete resolution. (Images courtesy of Nemi Ganda and Tara Barwick)

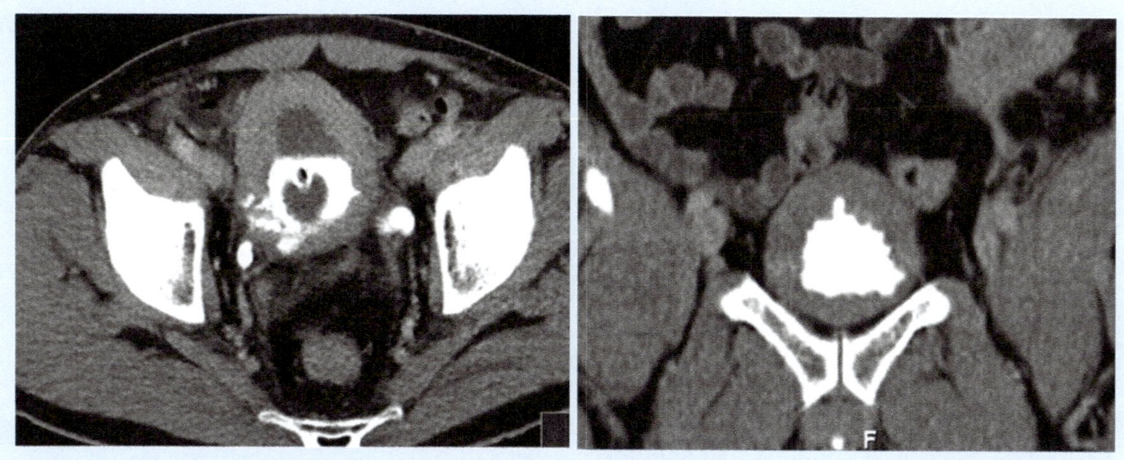

Fig. 57.14 CT Urogram demonstrating bladder thickening

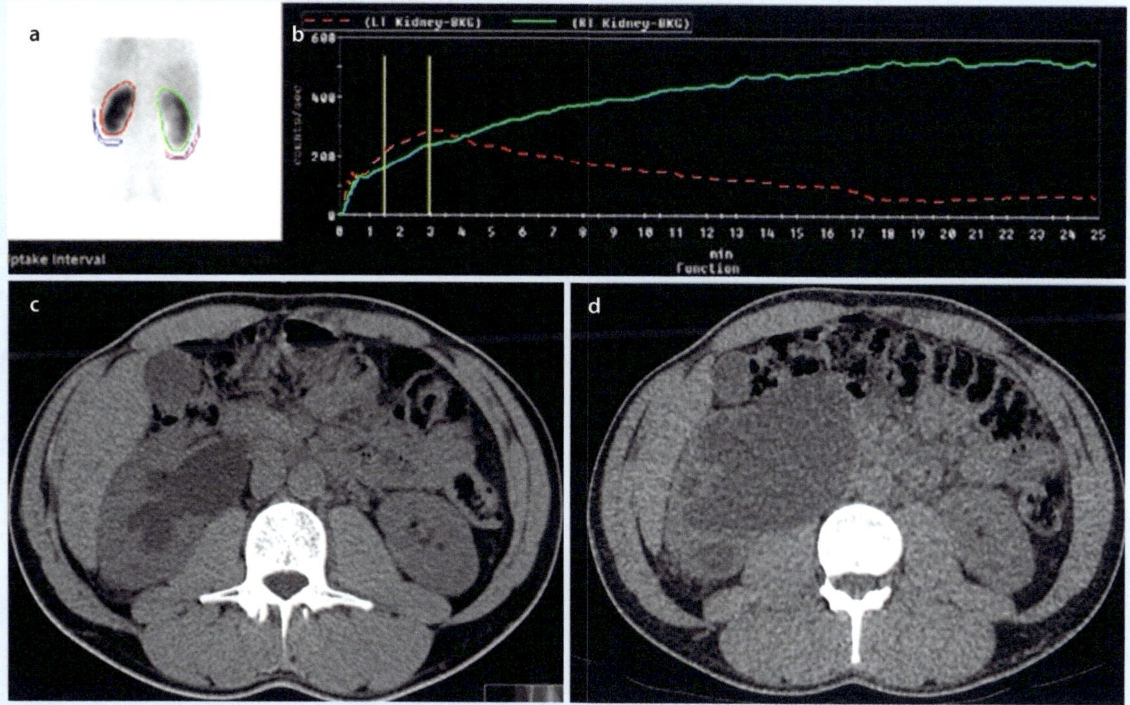

Fig. 57.15 (**a** and **b**) Renogram. (**b**) CTKUB (**c**) at presentation and (**d**) 6 months later

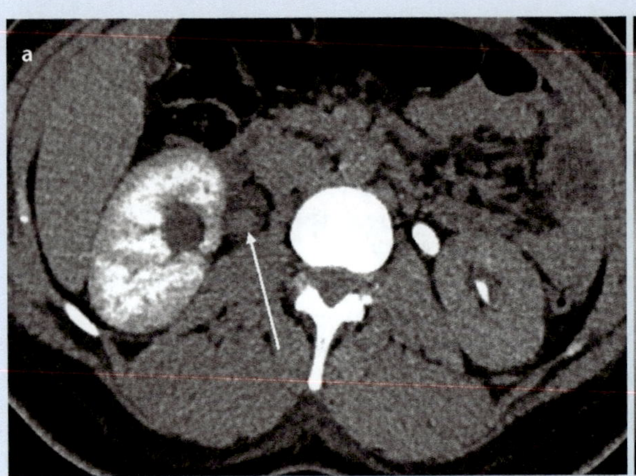

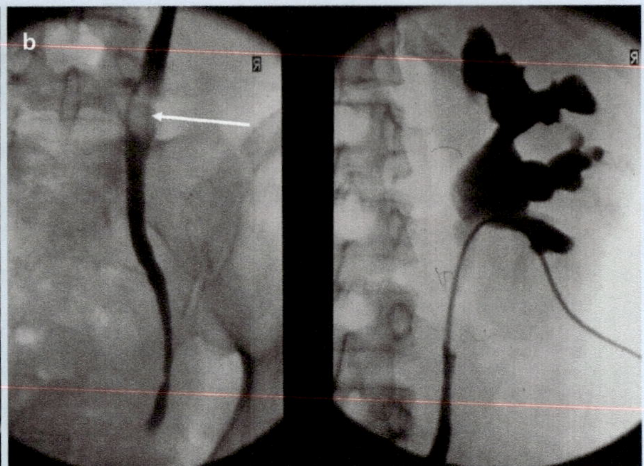

Fig. 57.16 (**a**) CT Urogram (with contrast) in a patient with HbSS who presented with loin pain and an AKI. It shows a sloughed papilla with dilatation of the ureter and pelvis. It also illustrates that in the acute setting an obstructed kidney retains contrast (i.e. is initially well perfused) but also enlarges possibly because of the tubular back leak and inflammatory cell infiltrate. (**b**) Nephrostomy and antegrade study in a patient with HbSS, demonstrating the hydronphrosis and a filling defect (sloughed papilla)

Chapter Review Questions

1. What % of men with a maximum urinary flow rate of <10 ml/s have bladder outflow tract obstruction?
2. What are the causes of upper tract urinary obstruction in the absence of a dilated system?
3. What radiological investigations are used to diagnose urinary tract obstruction in pregnancy?
4. Name the causes of retroperitoneal fibrosis?
5. What is an acceptable post-micturition volume?

Answers

1. Flow tests are simple outpatient tests to do, and 90% of men with a Qmax of 10mls/s or less have bladder outflow tract obstruction.
2. Obstruction concomitant with AKI (little urine produced), malignant encasement preventing dilatation, micro-obstruction (tubular obstruction typically secondary to crystals or cast).
3. Ultrasound is ubiquitous and safe but might have limited resolution in obese patients. MRI is thought to be safe and may better differentiate leaks. In an emergency then a CT may be necessary for urgent cross-sectional imaging, but it is clearly desirable to avoid this radiation exposure to the foetus if at all possible, similarly for nuclear medicine scans.
4. Idiopathic retroperitoneal fibrosis (secondary to aortitis, periaortitis including IgG-4-related disease). Retroperitoneal infection (e.g. tuberculosis), radiation to retroperitoneum, malignancy (including sarcoma, lymphoma), medications (methysergide and bromocriptine), trauma
5. There is not much consensus on this, but <100mls is usually acceptable; however, in the setting of recurrent UTI, <50mls might be more appropriate.

References

1. Nitti V. Pressure flow urodynamic studies: the gold standard for diagnosing bladder outlet obstruction. Rev Urol. 2005;7(Suppl 6):S14–21.
2. Abrams P. The diagnosis of bladder outlet obstruction: urodynamics. In: Cockett ATK, Khoury S, Aso Y, editors. Proceedings, the 3rd International Consultation on BPH. World Health Organization; 1995. p. 299–367.
3. Renjen P. Advances in uroradiologic imaging in children. Radiol Clin North Am. 2012;50:207–18.
4. Perez-Brayfield MR. A prospective study comparing ultrasound, nuclear scintigraphy and dynamic contrast enhanced magnetic resonance imaging in the evaluation of hydronephrosis. J Urol. 2003;170:1330–4.
5. Grattan-Smith JD. MR Urography anatomy and physiology. Pediatr Radiol. 2008;38(Suppl 2):S275–80.
6. Veenboer PW, de Jong TPVM. Antegrade pressure measurement as a diagnostic tool in modern pediatric urology. World J Urol. 2011;29:737–45.
7. Lupton EW, George NJ. The APR: 35 years on. BJU Int. 2010;105(1):94–100.
8. Parsons B. Emerging treatment options for benign prostatic obstruction. Curr Urol Rep. 2011;12:247–54.

9. Uppot R. Emergent nephrostomy tube placement for acute urinary obstruction. Tech Vasc Interv Radiol. 2009;12:154–61.
10. Robert A. Percutaneous ureteral interventions. Tech Vasc Interv Radiol. 2009;12:205–15.
11. Uibu T, Oksa P, Auvinen A, et al. Asbestos exposure as a risk factor for retroperitoneal fibrosis. Lancet. 2004;363:1422–142611.
12. Zen Y. Retroperitoneal fibrosis: a clinicopathologic study with respect to immunoglobulin G4. Am J Surg Pathol. 2009;33:1833–9.
13. Wren D. Takayasu arteritis: diagnosis, treatment and prognosis. Int Rev Immunol. 2012;31:462–73.
14. Wong LM, Cleeve LK, Milner AD, Pitman AG. Malignant ureteral obstruction: outcomes after Intervention. Have things changed? J Urol. 2007;178:178–83.
15. Sountoulides P. Current status for use of metal stents in the management of maligant ureteric obstruction. BJU Int. 2010;105:1066–72.
16. Woodhouse C. Supra-vesical urinary diversion and ureteric re-implantation for malignant disease. Clin Oncol. 2011;22: 727–32.
17. Kouba E. Management of urethral obstruction due to advanced malignancy: otimizing therapeutic and palliative outcomes. J Urol. 2008;180:444–50.
18. Liberman D. Renal and urologic problems: management of ureteric obstruction. Curr Opin Support Palliat Care. 2012;6:316–21.

Kidney Cancer

David Nicol, Peter Hill, and Ekaterini Boleti

Contents

M. Harber (ed.), *Primer on Nephrology*, https://doi.org/10.1007/978-3-030-76419-7_58

Learning Objectives

1. Kidney cancer is commonly diagnosed as an incidental finding with variable clinical significance.
2. Treatments include surveillance, surgery, percutaneous ablation, and systemic therapy based on the individual patient and tumour features.

58.1 Introduction

Primary malignancies involving the kidney fall into two discrete groups – arising either from the parenchyma or the urothelium lining the calyces or renal pelvis. Renal cell carcinoma (RCC) is the broad descriptor describing malignant parenchymal tumours.

58.2 Pathology

Parenchymal tumours generally arise from the tubular structures of the glomeruli and are described as adenocarcinomas. A number of discrete pathological subtypes have been described related to the cell of origin, histological appearance (architectural and cellular), and underlying genetic basis. These are outlined in the 2016 World Health Organization (WHO) classification [1]. In this most recent classification system, several new subtypes have been defined having been in the unclassified group in previous versions.

The commonest subtypes are clear cell RCC (CCRCC), papillary RCC (PRCC), and chromophobe RCC (ChRCC) with a range of other less common subtypes described (Table 58.1). The vast majority of patients with RCC have sporadic disease. CCRCC comprise the majority (65–70%) of tumours and are associated with tumour chromosomal mutations of 3p. Sporadic tumours are typically solitary although can be multifocal within the affected kidney in 4% and bilateral in up to 3% of cases. PRCC are the second largest group (15–20%) with two recognised subtypes. Type 1, associated with chromosome 7p, 17p, and 1q mutations, exhibits small basophilic cells with low nuclear grade and may be multifocal. Type 2 tumours, which are generally more aggressive and associated with 1p, 3p, and 5q changes have eosinophilic cells with higher nuclear grade. Small tumours less the 5 mm in maximum diameter with similar architecture and genetic alterations as type 1 and 2 papillary RCC tumours are regarded as benign adenomas and occur in over 20% of autopsies with a close examination of the kidneys. It is uncertain whether these constitute precursors of the larger malignant tumours with the same histological features. ChRCC (5–7%) typically stain with Hales colloidal iron. At times these tumours may be difficult to differentiate from oncocytomas – which are benign and have different underlying genetic changes. Collecting duct and renal medullary carcinomas are both uncommon with the latter almost exclusively found in patients with sickle cell trait or anaemia. The remaining tumour types are all relatively infrequent. Sarcomatoid changes can affect most forms of RCC and, rather than a discrete entity, is indicative of an aggressive often locally infiltrative phenotype with poor prognosis.

Table 58.1 Histological subtypes of RCC [1]

Existing renal cell tumour subtypes	Additional renal cell tumour subtypes in WHO 2016 [1]
Malignant Clear cell RCC	
Papillary RCC	MiT (microphthalmia transcription factor) translocation RCC
Chromophobe RCC	Tubulocystic RCC
Collecting duct carcinoma	Acquired cystic disease-associated RCC
Renal medullary carcinoma	Clear cell papillary RCC
Mucinous tubular and spindle cell carcinoma	Succinate dehydrogenase-deficient RCC
RCC, unclassified	Hereditary leiomyomatosis and RCC-associated RCC
Benign or low malignant potential	
Papillary adenoma	Multilocular cystic renal neoplasm of low malignant potential
Oncocytoma	

One specific tumour type (acquired cystic disease-associated RCC) is associated with end-stage renal disease [2]. These tumours arise in kidneys affected by an acquired cystic disease which is associated with dialysis. These tumours may exhibit combined features of clear and papillary tumours but without the typical chromosomal abnormalities affecting either clear (3p) or papillary (7p or 1q) RCC.

58.3 Staging

This is an important consideration that can dictate both treatment options and determine prognosis. The tumour node metastasis (TNM) staging classification is the most widely used system based on the size and local extent of the primary tumour as well as the involvement of regional lymph nodes and distant metastases [3]. The most recent classification is shown in ◘ Table 58.2a [3, 4].

Based on the TNM, four broad groups or stages are often considered in clinical practice ◘ Table 58.2b [4].

◘ **Table 58.2a** TNM staging of RCC [3]

Primary tumour (T):
TX: Primary tumour cannot be assessed
T0: No evidence of primary tumour
T1: Tumour <7 cm in greatest dimension, limited to kidney
T1a: tumour ≤4 cm, limited to the kidney.
T1b: tumour >4 cm but <7 cm, limited to the kidney.
T2: Tumour greater than 7 cm, limited to kidney
T2a: tumour 7–10 cm, limited to the kidney.
T2b: tumour >10 cm, limited to the kidney
T3: Tumour extends into major veins/adrenal/ perinephric tissue; not beyond Gerota's fascia
T3a: tumours with direct adrenal involvement/perinephric fat; not beyond Gerota's fascia
T3b: tumour extends into the renal vein(s) or IVC below the diaphragm
T3c: IVC involvement above the diaphragm
T4: Tumour invades beyond Gerota's fascia
N – Regional lymph nodes
NX: regional nodes cannot be assessed
N0: no regional lymph node metastasis
N1: metastasis in a single regional lymph node
N2: metastasis in more than one regional lymph node
M - distant metastasis
MX: Distant metastasis cannot be assessed
M0: No distant metastasis
M1: Distant metastasis

◘ **Table 58.2b** Clinical staging of RCC [4]

Stage	TNM
I	T1, N0, M0
II	T2, N0, M0
III	T1/2, N1+, M0 T3, N0+, M0
IV	T4, N0+, M0 T1+, N0+, M1

58.4 Epidemiology

Kidney cancer results in approximately 2% of all cancer deaths and is the 10 leading cause of cancer-related mortality. Reported worldwide incidence rates range from 0.6 per 100,000 to 14.7 per 100,000. In western nations the incidence is approximately 10 per 100,00, with a mortality rate of 3.5 per 100,000. Most tumours present in the fifth to seventh decades of life, with a median age at diagnosis of 66 years and a median age at death of 70 years. The incidence is two to three times higher in men and is slightly more common in blacks than in whites.

Over the past few decades, the incidence of renal tumours that are detected has increased although this now appears to be stabilising. It is likely that the increase purely reflects the increased availability and use of abdominal imaging for unrelated symptoms or conditions. Most RCC are detected as incidental findings, with a dramatic 'stage shift' in the modern era related to increased numbers of small T1 tumours now comprising the majority of cases. Interestingly the number of patients per head of population presenting with advanced or metastatic disease has remained essentially unchanged.

At autopsy, the incidence of renal tumours is approximately 2%. In general, the tumours are usually solitary but may be multifocal in 6–25% of patients. Associations have been described with cigarette smoking, obesity, diuretic use, exposure to petroleum products, chlorinated solvents, cadmium, lead, asbestos, ionizing radiation, high-protein diets, hypertension, and HIV infection.

Renal failure however has a much higher association which may be related to a number of factors. Firstly all stages of renal failure may occur with kidney cancer as a consequence of treatment. Patients requiring long-term dialysis who develop acquired renal cystic disease are at increased risk with rates 3–6-fold that of the general population. Acquired cystic disease-associated RCC is now a recognised discrete subgroup of RCC [2]. The duration of haemodialysis appears a specific risk possibly due to chronic repeated exposure to high HGF levels associated with renal failure and elevated with heparin used with haemodialysis. HGF is the ligand for cMET – a proto-oncogene associated with papillary RCC and is found in high concentrations in cysts associated with acquired cystic disease of the kidney also seen in dialysis.

58.5 Hereditary Disease

Hereditary syndromes account for up to 5% of RCC associated with specific germline mutations, pathological subtypes and systemic features [5, 6]. Patients typically present in their fourth decade and over 70% of

Table 58.3 Hereditary renal cancer syndromes. Other hereditary syndromes include Denys-Drash/Frasier and Li-Fraumeni and Lynch (MSH2) syndromes

Syndrome	Gene	Syndrome
VHL – von Hippel-Lindau syndrome	VHL	CCRCC, pheochromocytoma, retina angioma, haemangioblastoma
HLRCC – hereditary leiomyomatosis and renal cell cancer	Fumarate Hydratase (FH)	Papillary RCC Leiomyomatous skin lesions Uterine fibroids
BHD – Birt-Hogg-Dube syndrome	FLCN	RCC (chromophobe, CCRCC, papillary, oncocytomas) Lung cysts,
HPRCC – Hereditary papillary RCC	MET	Papillary RCC
Hereditary paraganglioma Phaeochromocytoma syndrome (succinate dehydrogenase (SDH) mutation)	SDHB	RCC – various Paraganglioma, phaeochromocytoma
TSC – tuberous sclerosis	TSC1 or TSC2	RCC Angiomyolipomas, lung lymphangiomyomatosis, facial angiofibromas
Chromosome 3p translocation Associated kidney cancer syndrome	3p loss (VHL + others, e.g. BAP1)	CCRCC
Cowden syndrome	PTEN	RCC – various Intestinal polyps, breast, uterine and prostate cancer
BAP1 cancer susceptibility tumour Predisposition syndrome	BAP1	Papillary and CCRCC

hereditary RCC tumours occur inpatients <45 years of age compared to <10% of sporadic tumours being in this age bracket. In addition to young age, family history, bilateral or multifocal RCC and presence of other manifestations of syndrome features should alert to the possibility of a hereditary basis. Genetic counselling and the availability of genetic analysis for testing a panel of genes should be offered to patients thought to be a risk of a hereditary cancer syndrome. Table 58.3 shows the more common hereditary renal cancer syndromes which all tend to be autosomal dominant.

Screening including genetic analysis should be offerred to patients with suspected hereditary RCC with referral to a multispeciality service for management of both renal and extrarenal manifestations where a specific syndrome is identified (eg VHL).

These patients may require multiple surgical interventions given the multifocal nature of the disease. Nephron-sparing approaches are generally recommended although these need to be appropriately timed to optimise long-term renal function [4].

58.6 Prognosis

Prognosis is linked to both TNM stage and histological criteria. For all stages comorbidities and performance status are also independent factors that influence survival. Survival in clinical trials is invariably better than usually seen in clinical practice due to their exclusion of patients with poor performance status.

Currently overall survival at 5 years for RCC is 49% representing an improvement over the past decade [4]. This change relates principally to the higher numbers of patients diagnosed with T1 tumours – many of which may not be clinically significant as well as the introduction of effective systemic agents to treat metastatic disease.

58.6.1 Histology

In patients with localised disease, histological features are used as a prognostic tool. Algorithms such as the Liebovich score are used with risk calculations based on tumour grade, histological subtype, lymphovascular invasion, tumour necrosis, as well as capsular and collecting system invasion. Using this system (and other scoring systems) patients can be grouped into low, intermediate, or high risk of recurrence with 5-year metastasis-free survival of 97%, 74%, and 31%, respectively [7].

58.6.2 Staging

The 5-year disease-specific survival rate in patients with T1 renal carcinoma is 95% and in those with stage T2 disease, 88%. Patients with T3 renal carcinoma have a 5-year survival rate of 59%, and those with T4 disease had a 5-year disease-specific survival rate of 20%.

Nodal and distant metastases have a marked effect on prognosis. Patients with regional lymph node involvement or extracapsular extension have a survival rate of 12–25%. Although renal vein involvement does not have a markedly negative effect on prognosis, the 5-year survival rate for patients with stage IIIB renal cell carcinoma is 18%. In patients with effective surgical removal of the renal vein or inferior vena caval thrombus, the 5-year survival rate is 25–50%.

With stage IV disease, 5-year survival rates for patients with stage IV disease are low (0–20%).

58.6.3 Metastatic Disease

Metastatic disease is present at diagnosis in over 30% of cases with a similar percentage of those having an undergoing surgery for localised disease subsequently develop metastases usually within 2 years [8].

In patients with metastatic disease, six prognostic factors have been identified for predicting survival in patients treated with current systemic agents [9]. The prognostic factors are as follows:

- Low Karnofsky performance status (< 80%)
- Anaemia
- Hypercalcemia
- Thrombocytosis
- Neutrophilia
- <1 year from diagnosis to treatment

These factors can be used to categorize patients into three risk groups. Patients in the favourable-risk group (zero risk factors) have a median survival of 43.2 months, and patients with an intermediate risk (1 or 2 risk factors) have a median survival of 22.5 months, whereas patients in the poor-risk group (3 or more risk factors) have a median survival of only 7.8 months.

Factors associated with increased survival in patients with a metastatic disease include a long disease-free interval between initial nephrectomy and the appearance of metastases, presence of only pulmonary metastases, and excellent performance status.

58.6.4 RCC with ESRF

An association has been demonstrated between end-stage renal failure (ESRF) and RCC. RCC arising in patients with ESRF seems to exhibit many favourable clinical, pathologic, and outcome features compared with those diagnosed in patients from the general population [10]. Consequently the RCC-specific survival for ESRF patients is substantially better than for other patients, independent of histological subtype. The data from this multi-institutional review whilst retrospective suggests that in most patients with ESRF, RCC, if treated, does not adversely affect their prognosis and consequently should not be viewed as a barrier to consideration of transplantation.

58.7 Diagnosis and Imaging

Diagnosis is generally based on one of several imaging modalities which may be used in combination for clarification of equivocal findings as well as staging. Typical findings are solid or complex lesions (containing solid and cystic components) demonstrating enhancement with intravascular injection of contrast agents. Other lesions which must be considered with such findings include complex benign cysts, arteriovenous malformations, angiomyolipomas, and inflammatory lesions including xanthogranulonatous pyelonephritis and malakoplakia. Cysts are the commonest parenchymal lesions detected in the kidney with benign simple cysts predominating. Tumours can also have cystic features related to central necrosis as well as malignancy within cyst walls. Bosniak described a classification of cyst features that is essentially a risk stratification tool for malignancy in evaluating renal cysts.

58.7.1 Ultrasound

Renal tumours typically appear as complex parenchymal lesions. These demonstrate solid features with variable amounts of fluid or anechoic components reflecting cystic carcinomas, necrosis, or haemorrhage. Angiomyolipomas may be differentiated from RCC on ultrasound based on their uniform hyperechoic appearance with the lack of the posterior shadowing seen

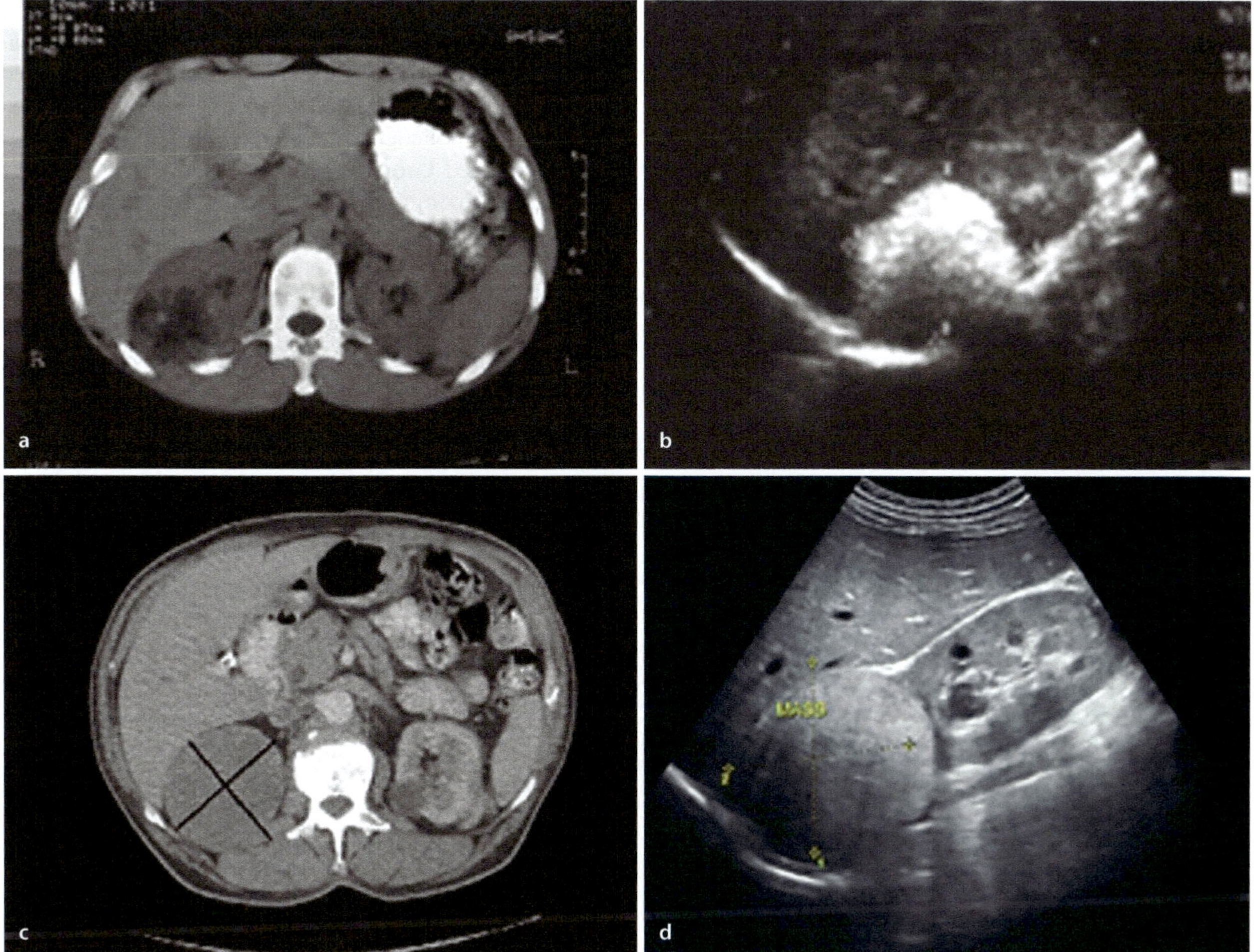

Fig. 58.1 Ultrasound and CT images of an angiomyolipoma showing typical fat density (**a**) and diffuse hyperechoic appearance (**b**) compared to RCC (**c** and **d**)

with calculi (Fig. 58.1). The use of Doppler is now a routine component of US imaging of renal lesions demonstrating internal blood flow. The addition of a microtubule contrast agent is a further recent addition that can be used to detect microvessels (with diameters as small as 40 μm) and quantitatively assess tumour perfusion of solid tumours. This relates to microbubbles remaining intravascular as they are resistant to extravascular diffusion.

58.7.2 Computerised Tomography(CT)

On CT (with pre- and post-contrast and delayed scans), renal tumours appear as solid or mixed lesions which demonstrate variable enhancement with an injection of iodine-based contrast media. Hyperdense cysts, which reflect haemorrhage into a benign cyst, may appear solid on a non-contrast CT but do not enhance with contrast. Angiomyolipomas may also appear as solid enhancing lesions but have a substantial or significant component reflecting the features of adipose tissue (Fig. 58.1). Other benign lesions including granulomatous pyelonephritis can be more difficult to distinguish on this and also other modalities.

58.7.3 Magnetic Resonance Imaging (MRI)

In the assessment of renal lesions, magnetic resonance imaging (MRI) is complementary to CT imaging. It has a role where intravenous contrast is problematic including contrast allergy and renal failure. It is also useful for staging purposes particularly in assessing tumour thrombus and the level of its proximal extension in the vena cava. MRI provides high inherent contrast between different forms of soft tissue. It has better contrast resolution but less spatial resolution than CT and hence is not as useful for sating of the primary lesion or procedural planning of nephron-sparing interventions.

Whole-body MRI also has greater sensitivity than other modalities such as PET and bone scan in the detection of bone metastases. It is also more sensitive than CT for cerebral secondary's but not as useful lung lesions.

58.7.4 Positron Emission Tomography(PET)

Imaging with 2-deoxy-2-[18F]-fluoro-D-glucose (FDG) and whole-body positron emission tomography scanning has been used in assessing renal tumours but lacks sensitivity compared to other imaging modalities. Newer radiotracers such as iodine-124-labelled antibody chimeric G250 (124I-cG250) which reacts with carbonic anhydrase-IX ('immuno-PET') may improve sensitivity. Whilst sensitivity may be low, its specificity is high, and a positive scan should be regarded as strongly suspicious for metastatic disease. It may be useful in the assessment of possible local recurrence which can be difficult with other modalities due to migration of other organs into the renal bed, scarring, and artefacts due to surgical clips. It also provides a mechanism to examine the whole body without risk of renal functional damage or contrast allergy.

58

58.7.5 Bone Scan

This may be used to diagnose or exclude bone metastasis. These typically produce lytic lesions on plain x-ray or CT. This reflects the osteolytic activity of RCC metastases with little co-existing osteoblastic response. In nuclear imaging studies, which reflect bone turnover and specifically osteoblastic activity, metastatic lesions may not be highlighted. Hence, a negative scan may not exclude the possibility of bone metastasis.

58.7.6 Biopsy

The use of biopsy varies in clinical practice although is increasingly utilised [11]. It has a clear role in metastatic disease in patients in whom treatment is planned without or prior to nephrectomy to establish a diagnosis and histological subtype. In this context biopsy of a metastatic lesion is preferred to the primary to exclude co-existing disease such as lung carcinoma. It has also been advocated in the assessment of equivocal or potentially benign lesions. HMB-45 (a melanocytic cell-specific monoclonal antibody) immunoreactivity is associated with angiomyelolipomas (AMLs) but not present in any malignant parenchymal tumours. Thus, it is a very specific marker to resolve radiologically indeterminate lesions where AML is suspected which occasionally occurs with tumours exhibiting diffuse hyperechoic features in US but without fat clearly being demonstrated on CT. It may also be considered with small solid renal masses if an oncocytoma is suspected. This requires an experienced Uropathologist as it may be difficult to distinguish an oncocytoma from a well-differentiated ChRCC.

Core biopsy (18 gauge needles) is preferred to provide an adequate sample for histological evaluation. Even with this non-diagnostic samples may occur in up to 20% of small masses. Due to low diagnostic yield, the biopsy is also not considered in the evaluation of cystic renal masses.

58.8 Treatment

58.8.1 Localised Disease

Surgical excision has been well established as the only potentially curative modality for RCC. The changing spectrum of disease presentation, particularly with respect to small incidentally detected tumours, has resulted in the increasing utilisation of nephron-sparing surgery including minimally invasive techniques as non-surgical ablative therapies (◘ Table 58.4).

58.9 Surgical Removal

Radical nephrectomy (RN) that encompassed removal of the tumour bearing kidney as well as the surrounding perinephric fat including the adrenal gland has been until recently the standard treatment option for most patients with localised tumours. A number of studies have now shown that removal of the adrenal gland does not confer any survival advantage – although is usually recommended with larger upper pole tumours [12]. Lymphadenectomy has also been variously advocated – although confounded by the diverse pattern of lymphatic drainage of the kidney. Published data suggests that for most renal tumours with clinically negative regional nodes, lymphadenectomy does not improve survival. In those with clinically enlarged nodes and no evidence of distant metastatic disease, however, resection of disease confirmed pathologically may confer a survival advantage. Whilst some centres advocate its use, its primary utility appears as a staging tool which may be of current significance with the evolution of systemic therapies and the definition of their role in the adjuvant setting.

Tumours with renal vein and vena caval extension can also be amenable to surgical excision. In the absence

Table 58.4 Treatment options for localised RCC

Modality	Advantages	Disadvantages	Clinical Setting
Radical nephrectomy	High probability of cure No risk of local recurrence Usually laparoscopic Minimal risk of peri-operative complications Minimal need for follow-up as local recurrence and metastatic risk low	Loss of renal function	T1–3
Partial nephrectomy	High probability of cure Preservation of renal function	Small risk of local recurrence requiring long-term follow-up Potential surgical risks of haemorrhage, urinary leakage Technically complex	T1a – elective (i.e. normal contralateral kidney) T1b, T2, T3 – imperative (i.e. impaired renal function where contralateral kidney compromised with a risk of end-stage renal failure with nephrectomy)
Radiofrequency ablation	Usually radiological procedure with sedation Preservation of renal function	Local failure 10–15% May prevent partial nephrectomy subsequently Requires ongoing follow-up	T1a + favourable features anatomically
Cryotherapy	Requires general anaesthesia Preservation of renal function	Local failure 10% May prevent partial nephrectomy subsequently Requires ongoing follow-up	T1a + favourable features anatomically
Surveillance	Avoids morbidity and mortality of interventional procedures Preservation of renal function	Small risk of metastatic disease Requires ongoing follow-up Anxiety related to untreated malignancy	T1a if comorbidities T1b+ – if elderly +/– major comorbidities

of metastatic disease, the removal of the tumour in conjunction with the tumour thrombus may be curative. This can be undertaken in a multidisciplinary setting combining standard urological techniques with those employed in liver transplantation for removal of tumours below the diaphragm or with minimal extension above this level. With the availability of veno-venous bypass, these tumours can be removed without the need for thoracic techniques. Tumours extending into the atrium, however, require a combined approach with cardiac surgery including the use of hypothermic arrest. Pre-operative embolization has been advocated as a preliminary to surgical intervention although recent publications fail to demonstrate any increase in survival or reduction in complications [4].

Laparoscopic techniques were introduced in 1991 for radical nephrectomy for RCC. Its role is now well established with oncological outcomes identical to standard open techniques. Laparoscopy may be limited by tumour size, volume of perinephric fat, previous surgery, and other contraindications to laparoscopy.

Partial nephrectomy (PN) entails excision of the tumour with preservation of the kidney. Wherever feasible this should be undertaken for patients with a solitary or functionally compromised contralateral kidney. Based on the favourable oncological outcomes reported in this setting for small T1 tumours, partial PN has been increasingly utilised over the past 2 decades in an elective setting with a normal contralateral kidney when this is anatomically favourable. A further factor has been the dramatic increase in the overall proportion as well as the size of T1 tumours related to earlier diagnosis of incidental masses with the widespread use of cross-sectional imaging for other medical conditions. PN has also been facilitated by the dissemination of robotically assisted laparoscopic techniques which has increased the feasibility of a minimally invasive approach – technically challenging with standard laparoscopy.

To date only a single randomised controlled trial has been reported comparing outcomes for RN and PN. The study recruited 541 patients with T1 tumours <5 cm in diameter with median follow-up over 9 years [13]. Recurrent disease was higher in the PN group although overall oncological outcomes were similar. Complications were more frequent with PN – with transfusions in 30% – twice that reported with RN. Most importantly overall survival including cardiovascular mortality was identical in both groups.

There are compelling arguments for PN over RN for many small renal tumours reflected in a progressive increase in its utilisation. Oncological outcomes with PN appears similar to that of RN based on retrospective series with cohorts often varying in terms of age, comorbidities, and tumour size [14]. Based on eGFR estimations, the risk of renal impairment is less with PN compared to RN. A number of studies have suggested that PN, with better eGFR outcomes, appear to be associated with a lower risk of adverse cardiovascular outcomes, although may be limited to younger patients. An analysis of US Medicare patients did not demonstrate an OS benefit for older patients (>75 years) with PN [15]. In a database comparison of patients undergoing PN for RCC with a non-cancer, healthy control group, overall survival was better in the cancer group, with survival in the RN cohort identical to non-cancer control [16] underscoring difficulties in comparing non-randomised cohorts. It has been suggested that the more pronounced deterioration of renal function after RN reduces survival. Patients with a normal pre-operative renal function and a decreased GFR due to surgical treatment, generally present with a stable renal function longer term [17]. These conflicting results indicate that unknown statistical confounders hamper the retrospective analysis of population-based tumour registries.

Thus, PN should be undertaken whenever possible for RCC with a solitary or compromised contralateral kidney to minimise the risk of dialysis and in cases of multifocal disease or RCC-related syndromes. PN can also be performed for many small T1 tumours based on tumour position within the kidney.

58.10 Ablative Therapies

Several forms of energy ablative therapies have been developed as alternative options for minimally invasive nephron-sparing treatment of small primary lesions. These are delivered via probes placed into renal masses either percutaneously with image-guided techniques or under direct vision via laparoscopy or open surgery.

58.10.1 Radiofrequency Ablation

Tumour ablation with RFA is achieved by heat generation from radiofrequency waves resulting in coagulative necrosis. It is best suited for smaller exophytic tumours (<3 cm) and has been generally delivered percutaneously.

58.10.2 Cryotherapy

This treatment involves the placement of several probes into the renal mass with tumour destruction by repeated freezing and thawing cycles. Most studies employing this have involved vision control either laparoscopically or with open surgery although percutaneous approaches under CT guidance have been reported. For selected tumours short to intermediate-term oncological outcomes are similar to partial nephrectomy with an upper treatment limit of 3–3.5 cm being recommended. Complications, which include bleeding, urinary leakage, and tumour persistence/recurrence, occur more commonly with a larger size as well as central tumours contacting the renal sinus.

Both RFA and cryotherapy are potentially suitable for small peripheral lesions. Studies have demonstrated successful eradication of tumours based on imaging studies although most studies have only short to intermediate-term follow-up [18]. Both modalities however do exhibit oncological failure in 10% or more of cases based on follow-up or investigational series where ablation was performed prior to surgical excision [19]. Complications which may require additional interventions include urine leakage, bleeding, abscess formation, and ureteric necrosis have been reported. In cases where tumour recurrence or persistence occurs following ablative therapy, retreatment has been described, where surgical intervention is undertaken for tumour persistence or recurrence PN may not be an option. Series reporting this scenario describe RN rather than PN as the outcome [20]. Whilst long-term efficacy with ablative therapies may be achieved, these modalities are at the present time best restricted to selected small lesions in older patients with comorbidities for whom treatment appears necessary where surgical intervention is associated with significant risk.

58.11 Active Surveillance

This is defined as initial monitoring of tumour size by serial imaging and delayed intervention for tumours exhibiting clinical progression based on size criteria. It is considered in which patients with small renal tumours

(<3–4 cm) who may have tumours unsuitable for ablative techniques, elderly, or with comorbidities. Studies reporting this experience suggest that in the short to intermediate term this is not associated with significant risks. In the largest series published similarly, the initial size and growth rates in benign lesions were similar to those in with histological features of RCC. Only three cases of metastatic disease were described after follow-up periods of 4, 9, and 11 years.

Thus, with short to intermediate periods of follow-up surveillance with selective use of surgical intervention, the risk of metastases and cancer-specific mortality appear extremely low. Consequently this is now viewed as a reasonable option for older patients or those with significant comorbidities.

58.12 Systemic Therapy

58.12.1 Chemotherapy

RCC exhibits little or no response to cytotoxic chemotherapy. This relates to the expression of the multidrug resistance (MDR) gene which encodes proteins which actively expel chemotherapeutic drugs from the cell. Efforts to bypass this mechanism have proven unsuccessful, and thus standard chemotherapy has no current role in the treatment of RCC with the possible exception of gemcitabine and doxorubicin for sarcomatoid tumours [4].

58.13 Targeted Therapies

The identification of genetic events associated with RCC and the effects on tumour cells and stromal elements, particularly angiogenesis, which are critical to progression has led to the development of a range of novel therapies specifically targeting tumour biology [21]. These drugs prolong survival in patients with metastatic disease. There is however no evidence to support their use in an adjuvant setting for localised disease [22].

58.13.1 Anti-VEGF Antibodies

Bevacizumab is a recombinant humanized monoclonal antibody which binds to VEGF-A isoforms preventing receptor activation. Neovascularisation, a prominent feature of RCC, is required tumour growth and progression. It relates to the dramatic upregulation of VEGF particularly in CCRCC associated with loss of pVHL, a protein which regulates VEGF production. Bevacizumab's effect is thus principally on the vascular stroma, as an inhibitor of angiogenesis, with a little direct effect on tumour cells. It is generally well tolerated with main toxicities being asymptomatic proteinuria (25%) and hypertension (14%) although thrombotic or haemorrhagic events are also noted. Bevacizumab has been used in combination with IFN-a based on a randomised phase III study that demonstrated statistically significant improvement in progression-free survival of patients with previously untreated metastatic RCC although no statistically superior overall survival. Similar results were observed in another study where it was combined with temsirolimus [23].

58.14 Multi-Targeted Receptor Kinase Inhibitors

58.14.1 Tyrosine Kinase Inhibitors (TKIs)

> Tyrosine kinase inhibitors(TKI's) are small molecules that target the adenosine triphosphate (ATP) binding site of transmembrane proteins and tyrosine kinases, which regulate the expression of angiogenic cytokines including VEGF.

Tyrosine kinases are enzymes that catalyze the transfer of the γ phosphate group from ATP to target proteins. They play an important role in diverse normal cellular regulatory processes. Tyrosine kinases can be classified as receptor protein kinases and nonreceptor protein kinases. The receptor tyrosine kinases are membrane-spanning cell surface proteins that play critical roles in the transduction of extracellular signals to the cytoplasm. There are 58 receptor tyrosine kinases that have been identified, and they are divided into some 20 subfamilies as defined by receptor and/or ligand. They are characterized by immunoglobulin-like sequences in their amino-terminal extracellular domains, a lipophilic transmembrane segment, and an intracellular carboxyl-terminal domain that includes the tyrosine kinase catalytic site. Nonreceptor tyrosine kinases, on the other hand, relay intracellular signals. Tyrosine kinases include members of the VEGF family and other angiogenic cytokines as well as their receptors.

TKIs are small molecules that target the ATP binding site of the kinase preventing phosphorylation. As TKIs are small and generally hydrophobic, they are able to pass through cell membranes with activity and thus target receptor and nonreceptor tyrosine kinases intracellular signalling pathways. There is now an increasing array of TKI's entering clinical practice – varying in the range and extent of the kinases they inhibit.

Numerous TKI's, which are oral medications, are now used in metastatic RCC with sunitinib, and pazopanib is the most widely used. As their target profiles differ, tumour sensitivity can vary between individuals. Side effects can also vary according to their specific targets but the commonest appear to be fatigue, oral and gut mucositis, dry, skin, palmar-plantar erythrodysaesthesia (hand-foot syndrome), leucopenia, thrombocytopenia, and altered taste [24]. Cardiotoxicity, although not common needs to be considered especially in patients with a previous history of cardiac problems. Thyroid dysfunction is also a well-recognised consequence and presents usually as hypothyroidism which may affect up to over 50% of patients. In cases of clinically overt disease, thyroxine supplements are used. Hypertension and proteinuria are also recognised side effects of TKIs. TKIs affect the glomerulus in the kidney which leads to proteinuria. Hypertension can develop as a result of renal injury and increased vascular resistance by reducing vasodilatation induced by nitric oxide and vascular rarefaction [reference]. It is suggested in patients who develop hypertension when being treated with TKIs have an improved prognosis [25].

58

Sunitinib malate inhibits c-KIT, FLT-3, PDGFR-b and VEGFR-2, FGFR-1, and IGFR-1 tyrosine kinases. It is currently commonly used for the first-line treatment of patients with advanced/metastatic RCC with good/intermediate prognosis criteria. This is based on a multicentre, randomised, study comparing sunitinib, and IFN-a in previously untreated patients with metastatic RCC. The objective response rates at the final analysis were 47% and 12% for the sunitinib and IFN-a arms, respectively. Progression-free survival was also significantly longer in the sunitinib group [11 months versus 5 months]. Overall survival was affected by crossover; however, in an exploratory analysis of patients who did not receive treatment post-study, the median overall survival with sunitinib was 28.1 months compared to 14.1 months in the IFN-a group.

Pazopanib, a newer oral TKI has a selective inhibitory effect on VEGFR-1, 2, 3, c-kit, as well as PDGFR--α/β. Based on a comparative study, it appears equivalent to sunitinib in terms of survival. It appears to be better tolerated and associated with a better quality of life than sunitinib.

Sorafenib, axitinib, and cabozantinib are other TKI's which have also been evaluated in CCRCC. Their effect on both overall and progression-free survival appear broadly equivalent to both sunitinib and pazopanib.

58.14.2 Mammalian Target of Rapamycin Inhibitors (MTORIs)

mTOR is a serine/threonine-protein kinase that together with Akt and MAPK regulates cell growth, growth proliferation, and angiogenesis. In RCC, through the synthesis of HIF-1, mTOR regulates the production of proteins involved in angiogenesis such as VEGF thus rendering mTOR an attractive target for the development of the relevant inhibitory agents [mTORIs]. The mTORIs have evolved from sirolimus, initially noted for its immunosuppressive activity and currently employed in renal and other solid organ transplantation. Two mTORIs have been used in RCC – orally administered everolimus and temsirolimus that is intravenously administered on a weekly basis. Pneumonitis is a rare but fatal complication of mTOR inhibitors and should be avoided in patients with existing lung disease such as pulmonary fibrosis or severe chronic obstructive pulmonary disease. Proteinuria may develop with mTOR inhibitors.

Temsirolimus is a water-soluble ester of sirolimus used in the first-line setting in patients with poor prognosis metastatic RCC. A large, randomised, phase III, international study which included 626 patients, mostly with poor prognosis criteria, was comprised of three arms. Temsirolimus, IFN-a, or their combination with a lower dose of temsirolimus. The primary endpoint of the study was overall survival, and temsirolimus demonstrated significantly longer overall compared to IFN-a alone [10.9 months versus 7.3 months], and combination therapy was significantly better than IFN-a alone [8.4 months versus 7.3 months]. Furthermore, temsirolimus demonstrated a better safety profile compared to the other two groups. However, side effects include fatigue, stomatitis, rash, hyperglycaemia, and hyperlipidaemia.

Everolimus, an oral second generation mTORI, is a sirolimus derivative, but unlike temsirolimus it does not convert into sirolimus in vivo. A randomised trial in patients who had failed TKI therapy with sunitinib, sorafenib, or both demonstrated a statistically improved progression-free survival of 4.1 months with everolimus compared to 1.9 months with placebo. As with other studies, survival analysis was affected by crossover from placebo to treatment with everolimus. Analysis of patients who did not cross over however estimated survival at 14.8 months with everolimus versus 10.0 months with placebo alone. Based on this evidence, everolimus is now used for the treatment of patients with advanced/metastatic RCC who fail TKI therapy.

58.15 Immunotherapy

The occasional dramatic regression reported with metastatic RCC stimulated the use of various immune therapy approaches to reproduce or accentuate this response on the basis that this was an immunological phenomenon.

> Immunotherapy treats cancer through stimulation of the patient's immune responses either via cytokine stimulation of the immune response or inhibition of regulatory control mechanisms of T lymphocytes.

58.15.1 Cytokines

Interferon-α (IFN-α) and interleukin-2 (IL-2), either alone or in combination, emerged in the 1980s as the first systemic treatments for metastatic RCC [26].

IL-2, a polypeptide lymphokine, is the principal stimulator of T-cell growth and may activate antitumour T cells and NK cells if present. IL-2 is produced by type 1 helper T lymphocytes causing activation and proliferation of the CD4 and CD8 lymphocyte population. A review of clinical results in 1714 patients with metastatic RCC treated with intravenous IL-2 monotherapy indicated an overall objective response rate of 15%. IL-2 can give response rates of up to 20% although only 5% of them will eventually be complete and long lasting [26].

IFN-α, a glycoprotein, is a potent immune effector agent with antiproliferative and immune-modulatory effects that increase the expression of cell surface antigens. Its effects include a combination of stimulation of cell-mediated cytotoxicity, a direct antiproliferative activity, and an effect on tumour circulation. Response rates are low at 10–15%, and unlike therapy with IL-2, incomplete and lasting remissions are not seen.

Neither IFN-α nor IL-2 are now regarded as a standard of care. Their role has largely been replaced by a number of drugs with a more specific activity.

58.15.2 Immune Checkpoint Inhibition

Recently therapies stimulating the immune system through drugs targeting T-cell checkpoint pathways have been introduced for metastatic RCC and include ipilimumab, nivolumab, pembrolizumab, and atezolizumab. Normally the immune response is tightly regulated to prevent autoimmune reactions. A broad class of extracellular 'checkpoint molecules' has been found to modulate T-cell responses to self-proteins. Many of these molecules also have a role in regulating T-cell responses to chronic infections and tumour antigens. Checkpoint molecules including programmed cell death 1 (PD-1) and cytotoxic T-lymphocyte-associated antigen 4 (CTLA4) are expressed on the surface of T cells. Blocking CTLA-4 (ipilimumab), PD-1 (nivolumab and pembrolizumab), PDL-1, as well as the PD-1 ligand(atezolizumab), restores tumour-specific T-cell immunity evoking an anticancer response.

These drugs are administered intravenously at weekly or greater intervals. These should be delivered at specialist centres given the significant toxicities which can occur. As a consequence of checkpoint inhibition, self-tolerance may be impaired, and consequently toxicities associated with these drugs are primarily autoimmune in origin. Almost any organ can be affected, although the skin, gastrointestinal including hepatotoxicity, pulmonary, and endocrine effects predominate [24]. Most of these side effects can be managed by treatment interruption or cessation immunosuppressive therapies when the severity warrants it. Endocrinopathies including hypophysitis, thyroid abnormalities, and adrenal crises can occur which may require hormonal treatments. Centres using immune checkpoint inhibitors have developed guidelines in collaboration with a number of specialists for the management of toxicities.

58.15.3 Nivolumab

Nivolumab is a human IgG4 antibody against PD1. A phase III trial randomized 821 patients with mRCC previously treated by one or two lines of antiangiogenic therapy [27]. Patients receiving nivolumab every 2 weeks experienced better clinical outcomes with a median OS of 25 months versus 19 months in patients given everolimus, with a response rate of 25% versus 5%.

58.15.4 Ipilimumab

Ipilimumab is a monoclonal anti-CTLA4antibody. The combination of ipilimumab and nivolumab has been compared to sunitinib as a first-line treatment of metastatic disease in intermediate and poor-risk patients [28]. After 25.2 months of follow-up, the objective response rate was 41.6% compared to 26.5% for sunitinib. Around 10% of patients receiving the combination therapy achieved complete response compared to only 1.2% of patients receiving sunitinib. Median PFS was 11.6 months for the nivolumab and ipilimumab combination versus 8.4 months with sunitinib. Significant toxicity was observed in 15% of cases including death in 1.5% of cases. As a result and thus patients who have treatment ceased because of toxicity should generally not be rechallenged with these drugs [28].

58.15.5 General Considerations on Systemic Therapy for Advanced/Metastatic RCC

Since the millennium considerable changes have occurred in the treatment of metastatic RCC beginning with the introduction of TKI's and mTOR inhibitors and the more recent and evolving entry of new immunotherapy agents. Clinical trials have been limited to two agents and largely to CCRCC with little evidence related to non-clear cell RCC. All groups of drugs have significant toxicities which can prevent or limit their use in specific patients. The fact that tumour resistance or intolerance to one agent in an individual may not be predictive of the effects of another within an individual patient is another consideration.

These treatments rarely yield complete responses and thus are not curative although, based on preliminary data, may show durable survival in a yet to be defined subset of patients. Healthcare economics are a further issue that will also influence their role in practice. All drugs are expensive and frequently exceed the recommended guidelines for funding agencies in terms of cost-benefit or cost/quality of life year (QALY). Thus, access is highly variable based on health care models [4].

Drug treatment of metastatic disease as well as drug treatment for high-risk localised and locally advanced disease is likely to remain highly topical and a constantly evolving process over the next decade. Issues to be resolved include the preferred systemic agents for specific tumour types and clinical scenarios, whether combinations of agents in series or parallel are preferred to single-agent therapy as well as the role of surgery together with its timing and combination with drugs in neoadjuvant or adjuvant settings.

58.16 Management of Patient Presenting with Metastatic Disease

The management of a patient presenting with metastatic RCC encompasses a number of issues including clinical staging, the primary tumour, localised treatments of specific metastases, and systemic therapy.

58.16.1 Clinical Staging and Diagnosis

Staging generally comprises CT scans of the chest abdomen and pelvis. If any cerebral or skeletal symptoms exist, then these need to be assessed with CT of the head and plain x-ray of the long bones to identify the need for urgent to avert a neurological event or pathological fracture. MRI may assist resolve equivocal CT findings of the axial skeleton. Biopsy should be undertaken and where feasible, a metastatic site is preferred to establish the histological subtype and exclude a co-existing malignancy.

58.16.2 Primary Tumour

In patients who are overtly symptomatic with significant haematuria or pain, nephrectomy should be considered as a palliative intervention, particularly in the patients with good performance status. In patients with poor performance or with extremely large metastatic burdens, this may not be feasible. Embolization of bleeding vessels is an alternative to surgery with bleeding although this may not control bleeding or require infarction of a large mass of tissue that may in itself result in substantial ongoing symptoms and morbidity.

Cytoreductive nephrectomy has been previously widely used based on two randomised controlled trials that demonstrated a survival benefit when nephrectomy is combined with IFN-α compared to IFN-α alone [29]. In these studies the survival advantage was only evident in patients with good performance status. This practice has continued as TKIs entered clinical practice with cytoreductive nephrectomy being a requirement for some trials evaluating these targeted therapies in view of their potential effects on wound healing. In intermediate or poor prognosis, patients' cytoreductive nephrectomy prior to sunitinib does not improve survival compared to treatment with sunitinib alone [30]. As performance status is a profound influence on prognosis, this study is consistent with the IFN studies in which nephrectomy only improved survival in patients who had good performance status.

The criteria for cytoreductive nephrectomy are shown in ◘ Table 58.7. In patients who do not have cytoreductive nephrectomy, this can be subsequently reconsidered. These are good performance status patients exhibiting a substantial response to systemic therapy particularly if the primary tumour is large.

58.16.3 Metastatic Sites

Specific intervention may need to be considered for metastatic deposits. These include intracerebral lesions, vertebral lesions if fracture or neurological compromise could occur, as well as femoral and humoral metastases. These can be treated with surgery or radiotherapy often in combination with initial surgical resection or stabilisation and subsequent radiotherapy.

58.16.4 Systemic Therapy

Metastatic RCC can follow an indolent course and in view of the toxicity, emergence of tumour resistance and non-curative nature of systemic therapy, patients can benefit from initial active surveillance with subsequent introduction of drug treatment when significant degree progression occurs. With this strategy selected patients with initial low volume metastatic disease can defer systemic treatment for over 12 months without compromising their long-term outcome [31]. Immediate treatment is advised however where there is an extensive multisite, progressive, or symptomatic disease. The initial choice of therapy will depend on the patient's prognostic category, comorbidities, as well as drug availability. Drug changes will subsequently be required due to either drug toxicity or the emergence of tumour resistance and progression.

Tips and Tricks

Small Renal Masses

The changing epidemiology of renal carcinoma has resulted in the commonest clinical scenario being a small incidentally detected lesion or small renal mass. This has resulted in a dramatic increase in the use of surgery and also ablative therapies to treat these lesions. Despite this the overall mortality related to RCC has not declined – suggesting that early intervention in these small lesions may represent overtreatment in many cases. Overall the options of radical nephrectomy, partial nephrectomy, tumour ablation, and surveillance (with selective use of intervention for rapidly enlarging lesions) all have to be associated with similar cancer-specific survival with incidentally detected tumours <3 cm in size. Each option is associated with specific implications which may drive the choice in individual patient circumstances.

Complex Lesions

Renal masses may be detected on imaging studies and need to be distinguished from renal cell carcinoma. Cysts are the commonest renal mass detected on imaging studies. The majority of these are benign and require no treatment or follow-up. Simple benign cysts are of fluid density, with thin walls and do not enhance with the injection of contrast media. However, many cystic structures have more complex features including solid elements which increase the possibility of an underlying or associated RCC. A risk stratification system, the Bosniak system(see ◘ Table 58.5), is used to direct management. This system is used in conjunction with clinical parameters in establishing the likely diagnosis and direct further treatment.

There are a number solid and complex lesions other than RCC that are detected on imaging studies. These may be differentiated on the basis of clinical history and specific imaging studies or investigations as outlined in ◘ Table 58.6. If there is clinical suspicion of these lesions, a tailored investigation may resolve the diagnosis and lead to more appropriate management. Nevertheless, at times this may not be possible and the diagnosis only established with surgical removal.

Renal Impairment

Renal impairment may be an important consideration in several aspects of the management of patients with renal cell carcinoma. This may limit the use of contrast agents although with the range of imaging modalities alternatives to CT may be employed, often in combination, to assess end-stage renal lesions. Renal failure may also be a consequence of treatment with loss of renal mass – although minimised the use of nephron-sparing techniques. At times significant renal impairment may delay consideration of surgical or ablative intervention. Where a patient presents with creatinine clearance of <30mls/min – a progressive deterioration in renal function is likely. In this scenario, particularly with smaller tumours, it may be more appropriate to undertake surveillance with a plan to intervene only if there is significant growth in size or if and when the patient becomes dialysis dependent. With the latter, patients may have the opportunity for planned dialysis access and avoiding temporary access with tunnelled dialysis lines and other external devices with their inherent complications. Similarly, patients, even with larger tumours, may be poor dialysis candidates with poor quality of life and potentially limited life expectancy related to cardiovascular and other comorbidities if end-stage renal failure were to occur. In these circumstances frank discussion with the patient may conclude with a nonoperative approach.

The end-stage renal failure population is also at higher risk of RCC – and if present may need to be considered in their suitability for transplantation. Historically arbitrary 'disease-free' intervals were mandated for patients with malignancy with the exception of epithelial-derived skin cancers. Better understanding of both the natural history and prognosis of kidney cancer, particularly T1 tumours, means that such an imposition is neither logical or appropriate. Given the high probability of 'cure' with surgical removal a history of T1 kidney cancer, this should not be a barrier to consideration. In situations where a patient with declining renal function has a potential donor with a potential T1 tumour, the possibility of pre-emptive transplantation with native nephrectomy 3–6 months later could be viewed as an option. This is highly unlikely to affect the oncological outcome even with immunosuppression and avoid the morbidity of a period on dialysis including that related to access as well as the accelerated cardiovascular complications associated with renal disease. With more advanced tumours, a judicious interval would seem appropriate with restaging after an interval of several years before considering transplantation.

58

Successful outcomes have been observed using kidneys from deceased and live donors following excision of small incidentally detected renal cell carcinoma. In patients electing radical nephrectomy for small renal masses the kidney, following excision of the tumour can be used as a novel form of altruistic organ donation [32]. With these donor sources, the risk of tumour recurrence is extremely low with patient survival significantly better than the alternative of long-term dialysis and graft outcomes similar to other sources of donor organs. Whilst controversial the presence of a small renal tumour should not prevent transplantation of a kidney from either deceased or potential live donors. In circumstances where patients elect for radical nephrectomy for small tumours, these kidneys should be considered for patients who may not otherwise have the opportunity of renal transplantation.

Systemic therapies of RCC may have implications for patients with impaired renal function. Some degree of renal insufficiency may be present in patients as a consequence of prior nephrectomy and other comorbidities with a small number also on haemodialysis. The degree of renal dysfunction may deteriorate in approximately 50% of patients with pre-existing renal insufficiency who receive a TKI – although usually resolves with dose modification. The effects of TKIs can be mitigated with the use of drugs such as ACE inhibitors, angiotensin receptor blockers, and calcium channel antagonists by their effects of vascular resistance.

Drugs with VEGF-related effects such as the TKIs and bevacizumab appear at higher risk of hypertensive side effects compared to other patients. Hypothyroidism, a recognised complication of sunitinib, also occurs more frequently with renal insufficiency.

The toxicities associated with mTOR inhibitors with metastatic RCC in the context of renal impairment reflect those seen in the transplant population with similar levels of renal dysfunction. In patients with RCC, these are associated with higher incidences of rash, infections, and dose interruptions than the patients with normal renal function, with no significant difference noted in the incidence of other toxicities.

There is relatively data related to drug toxicity for patients who are dialysis dependent. With sunitinib, and presumably other TKis, standard doses and pharmacokinetics appear similar to other patients. It does not appear dialyzable, and thus dosing can therefore be either before or after dialysis. Bevacizumab also does not appear affected by dialysis with similar pharmacokinetics in this group compared to patients with normal renal function.

Significant renal toxicity or complications have been reported with TKis and particularly sunitinib – probably reflecting the greater population exposed to this agent. Thrombotic-microangiopathic haemolytic anaemia is a recognised toxicity as well as acute interstitial nephritis and rhabdomyolysis. Toxicity may result in a need for dialysis in severe cases [33].

Table 58.5 Bosniak cyst classification; this was originally described on US criteria although features remain the criteria in radiological reporting with CT and MRI

Bosniak category	Description	Malignant risk
I	Thin-walled cyst without septae, calcifications, or solid components. It measures as water density and does not enhance	±0% Virtually nil
II	A cyst that may contain a few fine thin septae with possible perceived enhancement. Fine calcification or short segments of slightly thickened calcification may be present in the wall or septa. Uniformly high-attenuation lesions ≤3 cm that are well marginated and do not enhance (hyperdense cysts) are included in this category and do not require further evaluation	±1% Extremely unlikely
IIF	Cysts that may contain multiple hairline thin septa or minimal smooth thickening of their wall or septa. Perceived enhancement of their septa or wall may be present. Their wall or septa may contain calcification that may be thick and nodular, but no measurable contrast enhancement is present. These lesions are generally well marginated. Totally intrarenal nonenhancing high-attenuation renal lesions ≥3 cm are also included in this category. These lesions require follow-up surveillance studies to ensure they are benign. 'F' in this classification stands for 'follow-up'	5% Unlikely
III	'Indeterminate' cystic masses that have thickened irregular or smooth walls or septa in which measurable enhancement is present. Surgery is recommended for these lesions; whilst some will prove to be benign (haemorrhagic cysts, chronic infected cysts and multiloculated cystic nephroma), some will be malignant (cystic RCC and multiloculated cystic RCC)	35% Intermediate
IV	These are highly complex cystic lesions containing thickened irregular walls and solid components with a high risk of malignancy	90% High

Table 58.6 Solid and complex lesions detected on imaging studies which may be difficult to distinguish from RCC

Lesion	Clinical associations	Investigations
Angiomyolipomas	Tuberous sclerosis	US/CT/MRI – high fat content, diffuse echogenicity on US. Biopsy if uncertain and positive HMB-45 staining
Xanthogranulomatous pyelonephritis	Calculus Obstruction Diabetes Urinary infection	CT/Non-functioning kidney with calculi and dilatation of pelvicalyceal system
Abscesses	Sepsis possibly low grade and chronic Psoas irritation	CT - 'Rim' enhancement of complex (Bosniak IV)cyst Perinephric fat stranding and involvement or obscured anatomical planes with adjacent structures
Aneurysms and arteriovenous malformations	Previous biopsy or percutaneous nephrostomy	CT/MR angiography +/– formal angiography Doppler US
Transitional cell carcinoma of pelvicalyceal system	History of bladder cancer Analgesic nephropathy Lynch syndrome	CT Filling defects within the pelvicalyceal system Hydronephrosis Calyceal infundibula stenosis Urine cytology Ureteroscopy
Lymphoma	Clinical history	CT/MRI homogeneous infiltrative mass Biopsy
Secondary malignancy (rare)	Prior history of malignancy with risk of metastasis, e.g. melanoma, lung	Biopsy

Table 58.7 Criteria for consideration of cytoreductive nephrectomy for patients presenting with metastatic disease

Cytoreductive nephrectomy	Not for cytoreductive nephrectomy
Good performance status – ECOG 0 Symptomatic primary Asymptomatic primary with minimal, single site or modest pulmonary only metastatic disease Cases where a vast bulk of tumour burden relates to renal primary	ECOG performance status <1 Intermediate or poor prognosis Sarcomatoid tumour Large metastatic burden Regional nodal + distant metastases Nephrectomy would result in significant renal impairment

58

Case Study

Case 1

A 75-year-old man is referred with a creatinine of 190 mmol/l. Ultrasound reveals he has a 2 cm solid mass in his left kidney when he is investigated. Chest x-ray and liver ultrasound are normal. An MRI scan confirms the lesion is solid, and the radiologist suggests it may be a small renal cell carcinoma. The patient is observed and has a repeat ultrasound 3 months later which shows no change in the lesion. This is repeated 12 months later, and the lesion is 3 cm in size. In the intervening period, the patient's creatinine has deteriorated and is now 280 mmol/l. Further ultrasound is performed 6 months later with only marginal increase to 3.2 cm. At this stage he has developed symptoms of congestive cardiac failure related to coronary artery disease for which he is stented and placed on antiplatelet therapy. A further ultrasound 12 months later shows the renal lesion is 3.5 cm. This remains under observation with the patient dying 9 months later due to an acute coronary event. This case illustrates that surveillance is an appropriate option for an elderly patient with a small renal tumour. Biopsy is not undertaken as even if malignancy was confirmed this would not alter treatment. Small tumours even with slow growth have little potential for metastases or symptoms even if slow growth is observed.

Case 2

A 45-year-old man is referred after a chest x-ray reveals multiple pulmonary lesions consistent with metastases. Investigation of this with a CT reveals a 10 cm tumour in his left kidney. Biopsy of a lung lesion confirms metastatic clear cell RCC. He is commenced on sunitinib at a dose of 50 mg/day. His pulmonary metastases demonstrated very significant reduction in size on CT at 3 months. The primary tumour shows an only modest reduction in size. He continues with sunitinib with no further reduction in the size of the pulmonary metastases but develops recurrent episodes of macroscopic haematuria associated with intermittent left flank pain with these episodes. In view of these symptoms, he undergoes a left nephrectomy. The tumour is largely necrotic with only several sites of active disease. This case illustrates that in the absence of initial symptoms and large volume metastases, there was no indication for cytoreductive nephrectomy at presentation as systemic treatment was required. He responded to treatment in a typical fashion with a reduction in the size of metastases and subsequent stabilisation. Cytoreductive nephrectomy was required for symptom control but could also have been considered if he remained well in view of his response to drug treatment.

Conclusions

Whilst curative therapies have yet to be identified for RCC, the past decade has resulted in substantial changes in the understanding and management of this disease. These include a better understanding of the natural history of the disease with surveillance an appropriate option for selected patients with localised disease, emergence of nephron-sparing minimally invasive surgical techniques, and through translation of basic research identifying critical genetic events, signalling pathways, and tumour immunology, the emergence of targeted and immune therapies with demonstrable effects in many patients. Multidisciplinary care has become standard practice given the range of options now available for all disease stages with demonstrable effects on treatment decisions. Whilst diagnosis will largely occur in the community and general medical practice settings most patients, care should be based on review by specialist multidisciplinary teams comprising urologists, medical oncologists, radiologists, pathologists, and palliative care clinicians. Nephrologists must be regarded as important contributors to these teams and to the care of patients with renal tumours. Renal function is a key consideration in evaluating treatment options for individual patients. Expert advice required includes the accurate assessment of patient's renal function, potential for progressive decline, as well as an appraisal of the relative risks of the tumour and the consequences/risks associated with an intervention. Nephrological input should extend to the formal ongoing care of many patients with RCC many of whom will develop chronic renal failure in association with or as a consequence of their treatment. A further critical issue is the prognosis of patients with ESRF who develop RCC in the context of acquired cystic disease of the kidney. Nephrological involvement within multidisciplinary teams managing RCC is critical to ensure that ESRF patients who develop tumours are neither inappropriately considered for or, most importantly, not denied the opportunity of timely consideration of renal transplantation.

Chapter Review Questions

1. Will a biopsy reliably determine the diagnosis of kidney cancer?
2. Is MRI better than CT in evaluating a kidney mass detected on US?
3. Should patients with large renal tumours receive drug treatment after nephrectomy?
4. Are there curative treatments for metastatic kidney cancer?

Answers

1. A biopsy of a renal mass will be non-diagnostic in up to 20% of cases. This can relate to an inadequate sample or histological difficulties in distinguishing a low-grade malignancy from some benign tumours.
2. CT and MRI in general terms are equivalent in assessing a renal mass. There may be patient factors, such as contrast allergy or renal impairment which may limit the use of contrast which is necessary with CT.
3. Currently drug treatment is not used in an adjuvant setting (i.e. after surgery) in patients without metastatic disease.
4. Systemic drug treatments extend survival as tumour resistance almost inevitably occurs with time. When resistance emerges, patients may respond to another drug. Immunotherapy drugs may achieve a long-term response in a subset of patients.

References

1. Moch H, Cubilla AL, Humphrey PA, Reuter VE, Ulbright TM. The 2016 WHO classification of tumours of the urinary system and male genital organs-part a: renal, penile, and testicular tumours. Eur Urol. 2016;70(1):93–105.
2. Przybycin CG, Harper HL, Reynolds JP, Magi-Galluzzi C, Nguyen JK, Wu A, et al. Acquired cystic disease-associated renal cell carcinoma (ACD-RCC): a multiinstitutional study of 40 cases with clinical follow-up. Am J Surg Pathol. 2018;42(9):1156–65.
3. Paner GP, Stadler WM, Hansel DE, Montironi R, Lin DW, Amin MB. Updates in the eighth edition of the tumor-node-metastasis staging classification for urologic cancers. Eur Urol. 2018;73(4):560–9.
4. http://uroweb.org/wp-content/uploads/EAU-RCC-Guidelines-2018-large-text.pdf. 2018.
5. Hasumi H, Yao M. Hereditary kidney cancer syndromes: genetic disorders driven by alterations in metabolism and epigenome regulation. Cancer Sci. 2018;109(3):581–6.
6. Maher ER. Hereditary renal cell carcinoma syndromes: diagnosis, surveillance and management. World J Urol. 2018.
7. Tan MH, Kanesvaran R, Li H, Tan HL, Tan PH, Wong CF, et al. Comparison of the UCLA Integrated Staging System and the Leibovich score in survival prediction for patients with nonmetastatic clear cell renal cell carcinoma. Urology. 2010;75(6):1365–70; 70 e1–3.
8. Stewart SB, Thompson RH, Psutka SP, Cheville JC, Lohse CM, Boorjian SA, et al. Evaluation of the National Comprehensive Cancer Network and American Urological Association renal cell carcinoma surveillance guidelines. J Clin Oncol. 2014;32(36):4059–65.
9. Heng DY, Xie W, Regan MM, Harshman LC, Bjarnason GA, Vaishampayan UN, et al. External validation and comparison with other models of the International Metastatic Renal-Cell Carcinoma Database Consortium prognostic model: a population-based study. Lancet Oncol. 2013;14(2):141–8.
10. Neuzillet Y, Tillou X, Mathieu R, Long JA, Gigante M, Paparel P, et al. Renal cell carcinoma (RCC) in patients with end-stage renal disease exhibits many favourable clinical, pathologic, and outcome features compared with RCC in the general population. Eur Urol. 2011;60(2):366–73.
11. Marconi L, Dabestani S, Lam TB, Hofmann F, Stewart F, Norrie J, et al. Systematic review and meta-analysis of diagnostic accuracy of percutaneous renal tumour biopsy. Eur Urol. 2016;69(4):660–73.
12. Lam JS, Belldegrun AS, Pantuck AJ. Long-term outcomes of the surgical management of renal cell carcinoma. World J Urol. 2006;24(3):255–66.
13. Van Poppel H, Da Pozzo L, Albrecht W, Matveev V, Bono A, Borkowski A, et al. A prospective, randomised EORTC intergroup phase 3 study comparing the oncologic outcome of elective nephron-sparing surgery and radical nephrectomy for low-stage renal cell carcinoma. Eur Urol. 2011;59(4):543–52.
14. MacLennan S, Imamura M, Lapitan MC, Omar MI, Lam TB, Hilvano-Cabungcal AM, et al. Systematic review of oncological outcomes following surgical management of localised renal cancer. Eur Urol. 2012;61(5):972–93.
15. Sun M, Bianchi M, Trinh QD, Hansen J, Abdollah F, Hanna N, et al. Comparison of partial vs radical nephrectomy with regard to other-cause mortality in T1 renal cell carcinoma among patients aged >/=75 years with multiple comorbidities. BJU Int. 2013;111(1):67–73.
16. Shuch B, Hanley J, Lai J, Vourganti S, Kim SP, Setodji CM, et al. Overall survival advantage with partial nephrectomy: a bias of observational data? Cancer. 2013;119(16):2981–9.
17. Lane BR, Demirjian S, Derweesh IH, Takagi T, Zhang Z, Velet L, et al. Survival and functional stability in chronic kidney disease due to surgical removal of nephrons: importance of the new baseline glomerular filtration rate. Eur Urol. 2015;68(6):996–1003.
18. Atwell TD, Schmit GD, Boorjian SA, Mandrekar J, Kurup AN, Weisbrod AJ, et al. Percutaneous ablation of renal masses measuring 3.0 cm and smaller: comparative local control and complications after radiofrequency ablation and cryoablation. AJR Am J Roentgenol. 2013;200(2):461–6.
19. Leveridge MJ, Mattar K, Kachura J, Jewett MA. Assessing outcomes in probe ablative therapies for small renal masses. J Endourol. 2010;24(5):759–64.
20. Breda A, Anterasian C, Belldegrun A. Management and outcomes of tumor recurrence after focal ablation renal therapy. J Endourol. 2010;24(5):749–52.
21. Sanchez-Gastaldo A, Kempf E, Gonzalez Del Alba A, Duran I. Systemic treatment of renal cell cancer: a comprehensive review. Cancer Treat Rev. 2017;60:77–89.
22. Sun M, Marconi L, Eisen T, Escudier B, Giles RH, Haas NB, et al. Adjuvant vascular endothelial growth factor-targeted therapy in renal cell carcinoma: a systematic review and pooled analysis. Eur Urol. 2018.
23. Rini BI, Bellmunt J, Clancy J, Wang K, Niethammer AG, Hariharan S, et al. Randomized phase III trial of temsirolimus and bevacizumab versus interferon alfa and bevacizumab

in metastatic renal cell carcinoma: INTORACT trial. J Clin Oncol. 2014;32(8):752–9.
24. Pham A, Ye DW, Pal S. Overview and management of toxicities associated with systemic therapies for advanced renal cell carcinoma. Urol Oncol. 2015;33(12):517–27.
25. Miyake M, Kuwada M, Hori S, Morizawa Y, Tatsumi Y, Anai S, et al. The best objective response of target lesions and the incidence of treatment-related hypertension are associated with the survival of patients with metastatic renal cell carcinoma treated with sunitinib: a Japanese retrospective study. BMC Res Notes. 2016;9:79.
26. Coppin C, Porzsolt F, Awa A, Kumpf J, Coldman A, Wilt T. Immunotherapy for advanced renal cell cancer. Cochrane Database Syst Rev. 2005;(1):CD001425.
27. Ochoa CE, Joseph RW. Nivolumab in renal cell carcinoma: current trends and future perspectives. J Kidney Cancer VHL. 2018;5(1):15–8.
28. Motzer RJ, Tannir NM, McDermott DF, Aren Frontera O, Melichar B, Choueiri TK, et al. Nivolumab plus ipilimumab versus sunitinib in advanced renal-cell carcinoma. N Engl J Med. 2018;378(14):1277–90.
29. Galazi M, Rodriguez-Vida A, Josephides E, Chau NM, Chowdhury S. Cytoreductive nephrectomy: past, present and future. Expert Rev Anticancer Ther. 2014;14(3):271–7.
30. Mejean A, Ravaud A, Thezenas S, Colas S, Beauval JB, Bensalah K, et al. Sunitinib alone or after nephrectomy in metastatic renal-cell carcinoma. N Engl J Med. 2018;379(5): 417–27.
31. Rini BI, Dorff TB, Elson P, Rodriguez CS, Shepard D, Wood L, et al. Active surveillance in metastatic renal-cell carcinoma: a prospective, phase 2 trial. Lancet Oncol. 2016;17(9):1317–24.
32. Nicol D, Fujita S. Kidneys from patients with small renal tumours used for transplantation: outcomes and results. Curr Opin Urol. 2011;21(5):380–5.
33. Greef B, Eisen T. Medical treatment of renal cancer: new horizons. Br J Cancer. 2016;115(5):505–16.

Inherited Renal Tumour Syndromes

Thomas M. F. Connor

Contents

M. Harber (ed.), *Primer on Nephrology*, https://doi.org/10.1007/978-3-030-76419-7_59

Learning Objectives

1. Inherited cancer syndromes cause disease in a wide range of organ systems and are linked by mutations in related cellular pathways.
2. Von Hippel-Lindau (VHL) disease is caused by mutations in the *VHL* tumour-suppressor gene, which leads to activation of the intracellular hypoxia pathway and constitutive growth factor signalling.
3. Genetic testing and family screening can inform reproductive decisions and clarify the role of surveillance imaging.
4. Regular screening has significantly improved mortality and morbidity in affected patients.
5. mTOR inhibitors are now licensed for use in tuberous sclerosis where there have been shown to result in multisystem benefits, including shrinkage of large angiomyolipomas.

59.1 Introduction

Kidney cancer is among the most common adult malignancies [1]. The majority of cases will be detected and managed by urologists; however, in 3–5% of all cases of RCC, there is a major inherited predisposition. These complex cases may require additional input from nephrologists and clinical geneticists [2]. The presence of characteristic tumours or extra-renal signs may point to a diagnosis of a specific RCC susceptibility syndrome. It is important to recognise that renal cancer is only one aspect of these complex multisystem disorders and that optimal patient care requires long-term follow-up and the close liaison of a broad multispecialty team.

Kidney cancer is not a single disease, but comprises a number of histological subtypes. The Heidelberg classification system recognises five subtypes of malignant renal parenchymal neoplasm (Table 59.1).

Table 59.1 illustrates the seven genes that have been implicated in familial renal carcinoma. These genes are all implicated in two interrelated metabolic pathways. The most common cause of inherited RCC is von Hippel-Lindau (VHL) disease, which is caused by mutations in the *VHL* tumour-suppressor gene. VHL, FH, and SDHB all impact on the cellular response to changes in oxygen tension. TSC1 and TSC2, FLCN, and MET are all implicated in the activity of the nutrient-sensing pathway, which is centred on the mammalian target of rapamycin, mTOR.

59.2 Genetic Diagnosis

A comprehensive family history is an important step in the analysis of any disorder, whether or not it is known to be genetic. A family history is important because it can be critical in diagnosis, provide information about the natural history of a disease and variation in its expression, and clarify the pattern of inheritance.

The following key points are critical in taking a good family history:

- Detail all close family and their biological relation to the index case.
- Document consanguinity.
- Include miscarriages and stillbirths.
- Document the age of disease onset in each case.
- Find out the exact histological diagnosis.
- Detail all other potentially associated conditions in other systems, such as skin lesions, deafness, or pneumothorax.

A genetic disorder may be inherited from one or both parents' genes, or it may be caused by new mutations in the DNA during gametogenesis. Mutations can occur at meiosis and thus be passed on to every cell in the body or affect just the progeny of one mutant cell (somatic mutation). In kidney cancer, the same gene, commonly the

Table 59.1 Classification of renal cell tumours

Subtype	Percentage	Syndrome	Mutation
Clear cell	75–80%	Von Hippel-Lindau disease Familial Paraganglioma	*VHL* (loss of function) *SDHB* (loss of function)
Papillary type I	10–15% (Types 1 and 2)	Hereditary papillary renal carcinoma	*MET* (activating)
Papillary type II		Hereditary leiomyomatosis and renal cancer	*FH* (loss of function)
Chromophobe +/– oncocytic	5%	Birt-Hogg-Dubé	*FLCN* (loss of function)
Angiomyolipoma	<1%	Tuberous sclerosis complex	*TSC1* and *TSC2* (loss of function)

VHL tumour-suppressor gene, may be affected both by heritable mutations and by somatic mutations acquired during the lifetime of an individual.

Excepting translocations of chromosome 3, familial renal cancer is the result of single mutated genes. These conditions are all autosomal dominant; thus, each affected individual may have one affected parent, and there is a 50% chance that a child will inherit the mutated gene. However, autosomal dominant conditions may have reduced or variable penetrance, which means not all individuals who inherit that mutation go on to develop the disease or express the disease in the same way.

Most cases of familial kidney cancer are caused by the loss of function of a tumour-suppressor gene. In this situation an affected individual has one abnormal copy of the gene present in every cell in their body, but the remaining copy of the gene is sufficient for cells to behave normally. It is only when a cell develops a second, 'somatic', mutation in the normal copy that a tumour begins to develop.

Many of these disorders exhibit a correlation between the position of the mutation within the causative gene and the clinical signs observed; a genotype-phenotype correlation. This is best understood for VHL disease but is also true for less common conditions, such as BHD or HLRCC. Although genotype-phenotype correlations can aid clinical decision-making, it is not usual to alter screening guidelines.

59.3 Referral Criteria

These referral criteria are designed to pick up all individuals and families who may have a genetic predisposition to develop renal tumours or cysts. Ideally all patients with known polycystic syndromes and other genetic renal cystic diseases with cancer predisposition would be managed in a specialist renal genetics clinic. The following two key principles should guide referral:

1. The most important factor determining whether screening will be informative is the presence of renal disease in a first-degree relative.
2. Referral should be based on whether establishing a genetic diagnosis would lead either to the productive screening of the patient or other family members and/or affect reproductive decisions.

It is important to mention that the budget for genetic testing is usually held by the medical genetics service. This ensures that patients meeting criteria for a referral will receive appropriate counselling and that cascade testing of family members can be initiated. Consequently, patients should generally be referred to medical genetics or managed in a joint clinic. It is not advisable to collect blood samples for genetic testing in the absence of this support. Our own guidelines recommend referral in the following circumstances:

- Familial renal cell carcinoma
  - Positive family history, especially first-degree relative (e.g. parent or sibling)
- Young-onset renal tumour
  - < 45 years
- Multiple renal tumours
  - < 55 years
  - Clear cell carcinoma
  - Chromophobe
  - Oncocytoma
- Consider in patients with single tumours but a family history of
  - Renal tract anomaly
  - Renal cysts
  - Other renal disease/renal failure
- Recommendations for cancers in other organ systems (e.g. phaeochromocytoma, haemangioblastoma) are included in the relevant sections below.

59.4 Von Hippel-Lindau Syndrome: VHL Disease

59.4.1 Introduction and Epidemiology

VHL disease (Mendelian Inheritance in Man, MIM 193300) is a dominantly inherited familial cancer syndrome. It was named after Eugene von Hippel, who described angiomas in the eye in 1904, and Arvid Lindau, who described angiomas of the cerebellum and spine in 1927 [3]. The incidence of VHL disease is approximately 1 per 36,000 live births, with similar prevalence in both genders and across all ethnic backgrounds [4]. 80% of patients with VHL disease have a positive family history, but de novo *VHL* mutations and mosaicism are not uncommon.

59.4.2 Aetiology and Pathogenesis

VHL disease is caused by mutations in the *VHL* gene, which is located at 3p25 [5]. Mutation of the *VHL* gene is detected in nearly all VHL families and, importantly, the great majority (~90%) of nonfamilial clear cell renal cell cancer (CCRCC) [6]. VHL functions as a classical tumour-suppressor gene. Thus, tumour tissue in patients with VHL disease shows inactivation of the remaining normal *VHL* allele, either through mutation, deletion, or methylation.

The VHL protein binds to the hypoxia-inducible factor (HIF) and thereby mediates its degradation when intracellular oxygen levels are normal. HIF is a highly conserved transcription factor that mediates cellular adaptation to low levels of oxygen [7, 8]. Disruption of the VHL-HIF interaction results in the activation of HIF target genes, such as vascular endothelial growth factor (VEGF), that play a role in the growth and metastasis of primary tumours.

59.4.3 Clinical Features

The most frequent manifestations of VHL disease are retinal and central nervous system haemangioblastomas, CCRCC, and phaeochromocytomas (◘ Table 59.2 and ◘ Fig. 59.1). These are commonly multiple and develop at a younger age than similar sporadic tumours in the general population. Patients may also develop non-secreting neuroendocrine tumours of the pancreas, endolymphatic sac tumours (which can result in deafness), epididymal papillary cystadenoma (men), and cysts of the uterine broad ligament (women) [9]. In addition to tumours, patients develop multiple cysts of the kidney and other organs including the pancreas (◘ Fig. 59.1) [4]. Mortality is usually due to either metastasis of RCC or complications of CNS haemangioblastomas; however, following the introduction of systematic screening for tumour development, life expectancy of VHL patients has greatly improved.

There are now more than 350 distinct mutations in the VHL gene that have been linked to familial VHL disease, which demonstrates genotype and phenotype correlation [10]. The clinical phenotype is categorised on the basis of the incidence of haemangioblastoma, CCRCC, and phaeochromocytoma, as shown in ◘ Table 59.3. Different types of mutation variably affect VHL's many cellular functions, resulting in striking genotype-phenotype correlation.

59.4.4 Diagnostic Criteria

The diagnosis of von Hippel-Lindau disease is based on clinical criteria or genetic testing [2]. Patients with a family history, and a CNS (excluding retinal) haemangioblastoma, phaeochromocytoma, or CCRCC are diagnosed with the disease. Those with no relevant family history must have either two or more CNS haemangioblastomas or one haemangioblastoma of the CNS or retina and a visceral tumour. It is important to have a strong index of suspicion in patients who don't fulfil all the criteria and consider either genetic testing or continued surveillance.

59.4.5 Investigations

Mutation analysis is recommended to make a definitive diagnosis. There are a number of reasons why genetic testing for VHL disease is particularly successful:

- The *VHL* gene is small and so easier and cheaper to sequence.
- It is possible to identify a mutation in virtually all families.
- Almost all genetic variations in *VHL* are implicated in disease.
- Mutations have a high penetrance.
- Clinical screening of mutation carriers prevents serious consequences.
- Pre-implantation testing is entirely appropriate.

Screening for germline *VHL* mutations should also be considered in individuals with apparently sporadic cerebral and retinal haemangioblastoma since these are rare in the general population [11]. Direct sequencing is the gold standard for detecting germline *VHL* mutations and can identify the underlying abnormality in 86–100%.

◘ **Table 59.2** Manifestations of VHL disease

Manifestation	Percentage of patients with VHL disease exhibiting this feature	Mean age at diagnosis	Percentage of all cases due to mutations in *VHL*
CNS haemangioblastoma	Overall 60–80% Presenting feature in 40%	30	30%
Retinal angioma	45–60%	18	50%
Renal cell cancer	70% lifetime	45	1%
Phaeochromocytoma	0–20% depending on genotype Multifocal in 60% Malignant in 3%	30	10%

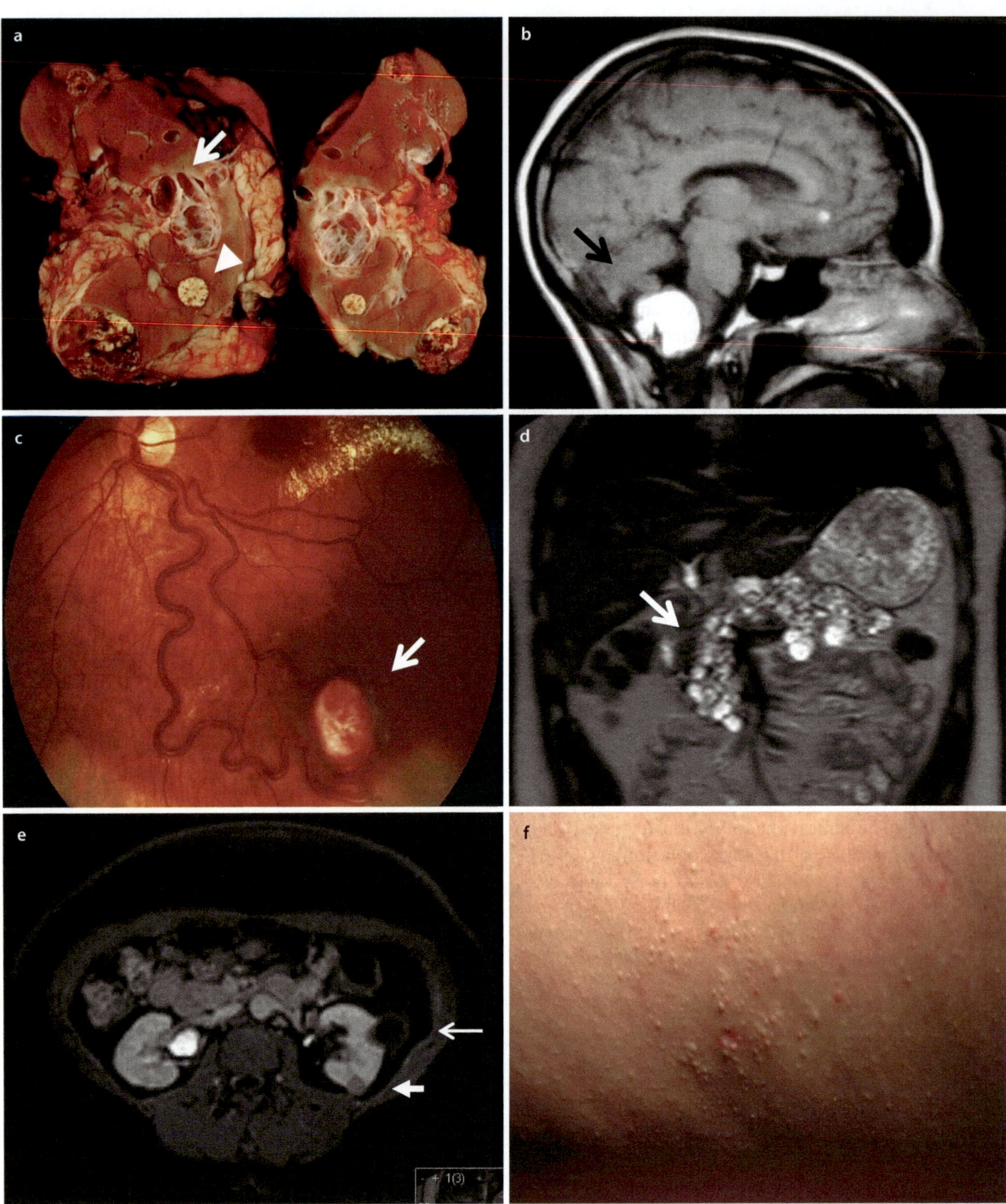

Fig. 59.1 Clinical manifestations of inherited renal tumour syndromes. (**a**) Nephrectomy specimen demonstrating multiple solid tumours (arrowhead) and cystic change (arrowed) in a patient with VHL disease. (**b**) Large cerebellar haemangioblastoma in a 35-year-old with VHL disease, arrowed (T1-weighted contrast-enhanced MRI). (**c**) Retinal photograph demonstrating a large retinal angioma in a patient with VHL disease. (Image courtesy of Professor Sue Lightman, UCL). (**d**) Multiple areas of cystic change in the pancreas of a 33-year-old with VHL disease, note possible soft tissue enhancement arrowed (T1-weighted contrast-enhanced MRI). (**e**) Multiple renal cysts in a 44-year-old patient with Birt-Hogg-Dubé syndrome. Note cyst with soft tissue component, blunt arrow, as well as a simple cyst, arrowed (T2-weighted contrast-enhanced MRI). (**f**) Characteristic skin lesions in a patient with Birt-Hogg-Dubé syndrome

Table 59.3 Classification of VHL families on the basis of tumour risk

Category	Risk of phaeochromocytoma	Risk of haemangioblastoma	Risk of renal cell carcinoma
1	Low	High	High
2A	High	High	Low
2B	High	High	High
C	Yes	No	No

High risk: tumour type observed in over 50% affected individuals
Low risk: tumour type observed in less than 5% of affected individuals
Yes: tumour type observed in all affected individuals
No: tumour type not observed in affected individuals

Table 59.4 Recommended screening programme in VHL disease

Associated tumours	Age range of onset (years)	Screening recommendations
Retinal hemangioblastoma	1–67 (mean 25)	From 5 years – lifelong Annual ophthalmic exam
CNS hemangioblastoma	9–78 (mean 33)	From 15 years – lifelong MRI brain and spine at baseline and MRI brain every 3 years
Pheochromocytoma	5–58 (mean 30)	From 11 years – lifelong Annual urine catecholamines or plasma metanephrines
Renal cell cancer	16–67 (mean 39)	From 15 years – lifelong Annual abdominal USS or MRI
Endolymphatic sac tumour	12–50 (mean 22)	See CNS hemangioblastoma
Pancreatic tumour	5–70 (mean 36)	See renal cell cancer
Cystadenoma	Unknown	None

'Mutation negative' patients should be screened with techniques capable of identifying deletions, such as multiplex ligation-dependent probe amplification (MLPA), quantitative southern blotting, and fluorescent in situ hybridization (FISH).

Screening for clinical manifestations in individuals who are known to carry a *VHL* mutation should begin in infancy. Current screening recommendations are detailed in Table 59.4. Early treatment reduces both morbidity and mortality [12]. Similarly, anyone at risk of inheriting a *VHL* mutation who has not had genetic testing performed should undergo regular clinical screening to identify tumours before they result in avoidable harm.

59.4.6 Management Issues in VHL Disease

59.4.6.1 Clear Cell Renal Cancer

VHL patients have a 70% risk of developing CCRCC by 60 years old [4] (Fig. 59.1a). The mean age of onset is 44 years, compared to 62 years for sporadic CCRCC in the general population, and asymptomatic tumours are frequently detected earlier (from adolescence onwards). Tumours are frequently multiple and bilateral in VHL disease, and histological examination often shows large numbers of microscopic tumour foci in apparently normal renal parenchyma. Renal cysts are also common in VHL patients and show a higher rate of malignant transformation than the simple cysts seen in the general population [9].

CCRCC probably originates from the distal renal tubule. These tumours are highly vascular, due to the overproduction of angiogenic growth factors [9]. *VHL* mutations linked to CCRCC (Type 1 and 2B, Table 59.3) show complete loss of the ability to regulate HIF consistent with HIF activation being critical in tumourigenesis. This may explain why targeted therapies that block the VEGF pathway have clinical activity as single agents in kidney cancer.

Nephron-sparing surgery is the optimum strategy for managing CCRCC in VHL disease. Many lesions are detected pre-symptomatically and do not require immediate intervention. Small tumours usually enlarge slowly (<2 cm/year) and can be monitored safely (typically at 6 monthly or annual intervals) until they reach 3 cm diameter [13]. Below 3 cm diameter, there is a low risk of metastasis, whereas tumours >3 cm have a 25% risk of metastasis [14]. Surgical treatment is with partial nephrectomy or alternative techniques, such as radiofrequency ablation, and should target as many smaller lesions as feasible in order to delay the need for re-operation.

Renal replacement therapy may be required if renal function has been reduced by repeated renal surgery. Renal transplantation has been undertaken successfully, and the subsequent immunosuppression does not appear to affect the course of VHL disease [15]. It has therefore been suggested that the usual tumour-free interval until an individual is accepted onto the transplantation waiting list can be shortened to 6 months for VHL patients with tumours <3 cm [2].

59.4.6.2 Renal Cysts

Renal cysts are found in 50–75% of patients with VHL disease (◘ Fig. 59.1a). The cysts are usually bilateral and multiple. Kidney shape usually remains normal, with normal renal function and preserved blood pressure. Renal cysts can be either simple or complex renal cysts, which combine cystic and solid components. Complex cysts are precursors to renal cell carcinoma and require close follow-up or surgery, depending on the degree of suspicion for cancer. In contrast to ADPKD, cyst infection does not occur in VHL disease whereas CCRCC is common (see above). Likewise, in contrast to ADPKD, pancreatic cysts can be numerous and scattered through the pancreas in VHL disease, whereas liver cysts show the opposite pattern in the two conditions.

59.4.6.3 Haemangioblastoma

Haemangioblastomas are the commonest manifestations of VHL disease, occurring in up to 80% of patients (◘ Fig. 59.1b). They are located most commonly in the cerebellum and retina [3, 4, 9]. They are cystic tumours of lipid-filled stromal cells embedded in a capillary network. Patients with cerebellar haemangioblastoma typically present with symptoms of increased intracranial pressure and limb or truncal ataxia. Hemangioblastomas are rarely malignant, but enlargement or bleeding within the CNS can result in neurological damage and death. The removal of asymptomatic tumours is not recommended. Complex lesions benefit from surgery in units with expertise in VHL disease.

Retinal angiomas are the most common presenting feature of VHL disease and lead to visual loss in 55% of patients with angiomas at 50 years (◘ Fig. 59.1c). Management is directed towards the identification of asymptomatic lesions and their treatment by laser photocoagulation or cryotherapy. Optic disc lesions are kept under surveillance because of the risk of optic nerve damage if they are treated.

VHL mutations are found in a third of all patients with CNS haemangioblastomas (◘ Table 59.2) [2]. This number is even greater in those with posterior fossa or spinal lesions and in those presenting at a young age (<40 years). Over half of all patients with retinal angiomas have *VHL* mutations. It is therefore recommended that all patients with these tumours are referred for genetic testing.

59.4.6.4 Phaeochromocytoma

Approximately 7–18% of VHL patients are afflicted with phaeochromocytomas, with a mean age of onset of 30 years [4]. Phaeochromocytomas are neoplastic intra- or extra-adrenal gland lesions that appear histologically as an expansion of large chromaffin positive cells, derived from neural crest cells [16]. Untreated phaeochromocytomas can result in severe, episodic hypertension and stroke, malignant hypertension, or death. Both intra- and extra-adrenal phaeochromocytomas can occur in VHL disease. The mechanism of phaeochromocytoma formation in VHL disease is likely to be different to that of other tumours in this syndrome and may be due to abnormal apoptosis during sympathetic neural development [16].

Up to 10% of patients with phaeochromocytomas have germline mutations in *VHL* (◘ Table 59.2) [2]. This proportion is higher in those with a positive family history, multifocal disease, and age of onset <45 years. Given that as many as 20% of apparently non-syndromic, phaeochromocytomas have an identifiable genetic cause it is advisable to refer these patients for consideration of genetic testing.

59.4.7 Novel Therapies

While surgery remains the mainstay of treatment for tumours in VHL disease, several new drug therapies have been developed. These therapies target the molecular consequences of VHL loss of function, in particular the stabilisation of HIF and consequent overproduction of secreted growth factors such as VEGF [8]. Current therapies have been designed to inhibit growth factor signalling using monoclonal antibodies and small molecule inhibitors [17]. These agents have all shown a consistent doubling of progression-free survival over prior standard of care treatments [8]. These drugs are generally well tolerated, as demonstrated by the quality of life improvement in clinical trials, and result in clinical benefit for in excess of 70% of patients treated.

Immunotherapy with programmed cell death 1 (PD-1) pathway inhibitors has also been developed in CCRCC [18]. These agents have been shown to be effective second-line agents for patients with poor prognosis metastatic CCRCC. Current trials are looking into combination therapy with agents that block the PD-1 pathway at multiple levels or in combination with inhibitors of growth factor signalling.

59.4.8 Follow-Up

VHL disease is a complex multisystem disorder that requires lifelong follow-up and the close liaison of a broad multispecialty team. Patients may have poor mobility and travel considerable distances therefore scans need to be closely coordinated with multidisciplinary appointments ideally on the same day with MDT discussion of management. The early diagnosis of most of the complications of VHL disease improves prognosis and reduces morbidity. All VHL patients and at-risk relatives should be entered into a comprehensive screening program in childhood, except where VHL disease has been excluded by molecular genetic testing.

59.5 Tuberous Sclerosis Complex

59.5.1 Introduction and Epidemiology

Tuberous sclerosis (MIM 605284) is an autosomal dominant genetic disorder with a birth incidence of 1:6000. It can affect virtually any organ system, and all racial and ethnic groups are affected equally. Males and females are affected equally. TSC has a highly variable phenotype, and two thirds of cases result from sporadic genetic mutations. TSC most often presents with neurologic symptoms in childhood [19, 20]. Renal lesions are the second most common finding and include multiple angiomyolipomas (80%) and cysts (50%), but early-onset RCCs have been reported. Renal failure is the most common cause of death for adult patients with TSC [20], and approximately 1% of the TSC population with normal intellect requires renal replacement therapy.

59.5.2 Aetiology and Pathogenesis

Tuberous sclerosis (MIM 605284) is a dominantly inherited familial cancer syndrome. Molecular genetic studies have identified at least two chromosomal loci for TSC, *TSC1* on 9q37 and *TSC2* on 16p13.3. Mutations in *TSC1*, which encodes the protein hamartin, are responsible for approximately 20% of cases. Mutations in *TSC2* account for the great majority of cases. *TSC2* encodes the protein tuberin and is adjacent to the polycystin-1 gene. Deletions of both *TSC2* and *PKD1* may account for the 2% of individuals with TSC who develop early-onset polycystic kidney disease [19].

Hamartin and tuberin form a heterodimer that interacts with Rheb, a Ras-family GTPase, preventing it from activating mTOR signalling (via mTORC1) [19]. Thus, mutations at the *TSC1* and *TSC2* loci result in a loss of inhibition of the mTOR nutrient and energy-sensing pathway that may explain their function as a tumour suppressor. The tuberous sclerosis proteins are also involved in the formation of the primary cilium that is disturbed in many forms of the renal cystic disease.

59.5.3 Clinical Features

TSC most often presents with neurological symptoms, and over 90% of affected individuals have subependymal nodules and/or cortical tubers on MRI. Approximately 90% of patients experience seizures, and virtually all subtypes of seizure have been reported [21]. About half of patients show cognitive impairment, autism, or other behavioural disorders. In approximately 10% of patients with TSC, the growth of subependymal tumours can cause hydrocephalus due to obstruction of CSF flow [19].

Renal cystic disease occurs in approximately half of patients with TSC. Renal cystic disease can be microcystic, and thus undetectable by standard imaging studies. Renal cysts arise from all parts of the nephron, including the glomerulus. TSC patients may have several risk factors for acute kidney injury, including the use of certain anticonvulsant and nonsteroidal anti-inflammatory drugs as well as rhabdomyolysis and hypoxia induced by prolonged seizures [20]. Both renal cystic disease and angiomyolipomas may contribute to chronic kidney disease (CKD) [22].

Skin lesions are present in 96% of individuals with TSC. The commonest finding is hypo-pigmented macules ('ash leaf spots'), which may require UV light (a Woods lamp) to visualise in fair-skinned individuals. Other skin lesions that comprise the diagnostic criteria include facial angiofibromas (adenoma sebaceum), periungual fibromas, and shagreen patches. Cardiac rhabdomyomas were the most frequent finding at routine antenatal ultrasound testing and are an indication for testing for TSC [21]. In all, 50–67% of children have evidence of one or more rhabdomyomas, and these may be associated with ECG abnormalities, including conduction defects and arrhythmias, and heart failure in infancy. Pulmonary involvement, specifically lymphangioleiomyomatosis (LAM) is the third most common cause of TSC-associated morbidity in approximately 35% of female TSC patients [20]. The female preponderance is not understood. Retinal hamartomas may occur in 40%. The commonest non-retinal findings on opthalmological examination include coloboma and papilloedema due to hydrocephalus.

59.5.4 Diagnostic Criteria

The diagnostic criteria for TSC are based on major and minor diagnostic features, shown in Table 59.5 [23]. Cases meeting these criteria fulfil a clinical diagnosis of TSC; the results of molecular genetic testing of the *TSC1* and *TSC2* loci are currently viewed as corroborative [19]. No single feature of TSC is diagnostic, and different manifestations of TSC appear at different developmental points from neonatal life to adulthood. Secure diagnosis usually requires assessment of all possible clinical features over a significant time period.

59.5.5 Investigations

Among patients meeting the clinical criteria for diagnosis of TSC, genetic testing is unable to locate the mutation in 15%. Patients with an inherited mutation tend to have less severe disease, as do those with mutations in *TSC1*. TSC may arise in individuals without identifiable mutations due to mosaicism or because of a mutation in an as yet unidentified locus.

59

Table 59.5 Diagnostic criteria for TSC [23]

Major criteria	Minor criteria
Facial angiofibroma or forehead plaque	Multiple, random dental pits
Nontraumatic ungula or periungual fibroma	Hamartomatous gastrointestinal or rectal polyps
Hypomelanotic macules (>3)	Bone cysts
Shagreen patch (connective tissue naevus)	White matter radial migration lines
Multiple retinal nodular hamartomas	Gingival fibromas
Cortical tuber(s)	Non-renal hamartomas
Subependymal nodule	Retinal achromic patch
Subependymal giant cell astrocytoma	'Confetti' skin lesions
Cardiac rhabdomyomas	Multiple renal cysts
Lymphangioleiomyomatosis	
Renal angiomyolipoma	

Two major features or one major with two minor features indicates *definite* clinical TSC
One major feature and one minor feature indicates *probable* TSC
One major or two minor features indicates *possible* TSC

All patients with TSC should be screened for renal involvement with MRI abdomen [24]. The combination of fat-suppressed and non-fat-suppfressed T2 signal on MRI is a very effective means of detecting both the macroscopic and microscopic adipose components of angiomyolipomas, and it is especially successful for the detection of those with minimal fat [20]. Renal ultrasound shows good sensitivity for cystic renal disease and most angiomyolipomas, except those which are 'fat poor'. CT is a reasonable alternative where MRI is contraindicated if concern remains after ultrasound. PET scans can be helpful because angiomyolipomas are generally not PET avid. Imaging should be repeated every 1–2 years when lesions have been identified, and every 3–5 years if no lesions are detected [24].

59.5.6 Management Issues in TSC

59.5.6.1 Renal Angiomyolipomas

Angiomyolipomas are the archetypal renal lesion in TSC, affecting up to 80% of patients [20]. They typically present in childhood, increasing during adolescence and stabilising in adulthood. These lesions are benign tumours composed of abnormal vessels, immature smooth-muscle cells, and fat cells. All cells in the lesion exhibit somatic mutations, which in addition to the germline mutation renders the cell deficient in tuberin or hamartin. Angiomyolipomas tend to grow slowly in adulthood (5% per year) and are usually asymptomatic. They may grow more rapidly and are more prone to rupture in pregnancy, so repeat imaging may be required. Given the likelihood of progressive CKD in patients with TSC, the management of these lesions should be conservative [20].

There are two main complications of angiomyolipomas: retroperitoneal haemorrhage and progressive CKD [19, 20]. Haemorrhage occurs due to the rupture of aneurysms within the disordered vasculature of these lesions. This risk is increased once they are >5 mm in diameter and is linked to greater tumour size (especially when >3 cm). Renal impairment is caused by the invasion of the normal renal parenchyma by both microscopic and macroscopic lesions [22].

Angiomyolipomas that are larger than 3 cm should now be treated medically with mTOR inhibitors [24]. Everolimus is licensed by the FDA and funded in the NHS, for the treatment of growing AMLs >3 cm. The greatest response to therapy occurs within the first year, followed by stabilisation [25]. Systemic therapy has been shown to benefit multiple TSC manifestations. It is advisable to prepare patients for the well-known adverse events linked to mTOR inhibitors, including mucositis, bone marrow suppression, and joint pain [25].

Embolization with beads is the current standard of care to control active bleeding. Corticosteroid therapy can reduce the subsequent post-embolisation syndrome. Nephron-sparing surgery is an alternative for acute haemorrhage, but nephrectomy should be avoided where possible.

59.5.6.2 Fat-Poor Angiomyolipomas

Solid lesions in the kidney of patients with TSC are a particular concern as they are difficult to image and may be malignant. Most are fat-poor angiomyolipomas (4.5% of all angiomyolipomas), but they can also rarely be oncocytomas or CCRCC [20]. Suspicious lesions should have repeat imaging to determine whether they are enlarging. These lesions should be referred to urology for consideration of diagnostic biopsy or nephron-sparing surgery.

Fat-poor TSC-associated angiomyolipomas can consist of a variety of cell types. Although very rare, the epithelioid type may exhibit an aggressive phenotype, with recurrence after surgery and metastasis [20, 22]. However, it is worth noting that the overall incidence of renal cell carcinoma in TSC is less than 2%.

59.5.6.3 Hypertension

Renal cystic disease is a significant risk factor for hypertension in this population and responds well to inhibition of the renin-angiotensin system [20]. Despite a significant burden of renal parenchymal abnormalities on imaging, renal function is often well preserved. An additional cause for hypertension is the use of adrenocorticotrophin hormone (ACTH) therapy to treat infantile spasms in some TSC patients [20]. This side effect can be ameliorated with diuretics with or without other agents.

59.5.6.4 Nephrolithiasis

Patients with TSC can be prone to nephrolithiasis both as a consequence of the disease and due to various medications used in this condition [20]. Reduced citrate excretion is the common mechanism, and nephrolithiasis can be treated with increased fluid intake and citrate supplementation where required. Direct uretoscopic stone removal is the preferred surgical therapy for nephrolithiasis in TSC [20]. Extracorporal shock wave lithotripsy (ESWL) may be associated with an increased risk of subcapsular haematoma formation, while percutaneous nephrolithotomy (PCNL) may be associated with an increased risk of haemorrhage due to distorted anatomy of the kidneys in TSC.

59.5.7 Follow-Up

TSC requires lifelong follow-up with regular imaging of the kidneys. Although renal angiomyolipomas are rare in the general population, only a minority of all cases are due to underlying TSC. Genetic testing is therefore not indicated in the absence of clinical criteria for TSC, in patients with angiomyolipomas. Now that mTOR inhibitors have emerged as a viable therapy in TSC, there is scope for involvement in nephrologists much earlier in the clinical course of these patients [25].

59.6 Birt-Hogg-Dubé Syndrome

59.6.1 Introduction and Aetiology

Birt-Hogg-Dubé (BHD) syndrome (OMIM #135150) is an autosomal dominant disease characterized by cutaneous fibrofolliculomas, pulmonary cysts, spontaneous pneumothorax, and renal cancer (◘ Fig. 59.1e) [26]. In 2001, a BHD-associated gene locus was localised to chromosome 17p11.2, and subsequently truncating germline mutations were identified in a novel gene, the FLCN (BHD) gene [27].

59.6.2 Clinical Features

BHD is probably under-diagnosed because of the wide variation in clinical presentation. Skin lesions (follicular hamartomas) are the most common manifestation, affecting 75% of patients and usually appearing in the third decade as whitish papules on the face and neck (◘ Fig. 59.1f). Similarly, 80% of adult BHD patients have multiple lung cysts on CT, but the lung parenchyma generally appears normal and lung function is usually unaffected [28]. The main problem associated with these cysts is a 50-fold increased risk of pneumothorax, with 24% prevalence of pneumothorax and a median age of 38 years. In some families, non-syndromic cystic lung disease or pneumothorax can be the only manifestation of BHD.

A quarter of patients with BHD develop RCC, which presents at an early age (mean age at diagnosis 50 years) [26, 28]. Chromophobe RCC and mixed chromophobe and oncocytic tumours are typical in BHD, although other histological subtypes can occur, including clear cell and papillary RCC. Somatic second mutations have been identified in BHD-associated renal tumours, consistent with a two-hit tumour-suppressor function; however, these were not seen in the skin tumours. BHD has also been reported in association with a range of tumours other than RCC; however, a causal relationship has not yet been proven [28].

59.6.3 Diagnostic Criteria

Criteria for the diagnosis of BHD have been proposed, to take into account the clinical variability seen with this condition (◘ Table 59.6; after [26]).

Table 59.6 Diagnostic criteria for BHD (adapted from [26])

Major criteria	Minor criteria
At least five fibrofolliculomas or trichodiscomas, at least one histologically confirmed, of adult onset	Multiple lung cysts: bilateral, basally located cysts with no other apparent cause, with or without spontaneous pneumothorax
Pathogenic *FLCN* germline mutation	Renal cancer: early-onset (<50 years) or multifocal or bilateral renal cancer of mixed chromophobe and oncocytic histology
	A first-degree relative with BHD

Patients should fulfil one major and two minor criteria for diagnosis

59.6.4 Management Issues in BHD

Surveillance for renal tumours is indicated in BHD, although the exact risk of occurrence is uncertain and may vary between different families. There are no established guidelines; current recommendations are for annual renal MRI starting at age 20, as ultrasound is insufficiently sensitive to detect small lesions [29]. As with other hereditary renal cancer syndromes, treatment consists of nephron-sparing surgery. It is important to determine the rate of tumour growth, although there is not yet enough evidence for the 3 cm threshold discussed earlier in relation to VHL disease.

Assessment of lung involvement by thoracic CT scan should be included at diagnosis; further investigation should be at the behest of a pulmonary physician. Treatment for pneumothorax in BHD does not differ from standard approaches. Current therapeutic options for skin involvement are limited, though the psychological burden should not be underestimated.

59.7 Hereditary Leiomyomatosis and Renal Cancer

59.7.1 Introduction and Aetiology

Hereditary leiomyomatosis and renal cell cancer (HLRCC) is an autosomal dominant disorder characterised by smooth-muscle tumours of the skin and uterus and/or renal cancer (OMIM 605839). In 2001, an HLRCC-associated gene locus was localised to chromosome 1q42-44, and subsequently heterozygous germline mutations were identified in the fumarate hydratase (*FH*) gene. Inactivating mutations have since been found in approximately 180 families worldwide [30].

59.7.2 Clinical Features

Skin lesions are the most prominent feature of HLRCC, with multiple benign leiomyomas occurring in all men and 55% of women by the age of 35 [31]. These tumours typically cause pain, usually in response to touch and changes in temperature. 79–100% of women with FH mutations have uterine leiomyomas, which are larger, more numerous, and of earlier onset than in the general population.

RCC develops in 20–25% of FH mutation-positive patients, with a median age of diagnosis around 42 years. Most importantly, HLRCC tumours may be very aggressive and metastasise early, unlike other types of hereditary renal cancer. Renal tumours seen in HLRCC have a distinct histology, described as the type II papillary or collecting duct subtype.

59.7.3 Diagnostic Criteria

Smit et al. have listed practical criteria for the diagnosis of HLRCC (Table 59.7) [32].

Table 59.7 diagnostic criteria for HLRCC. (Adapted from [32])

Major criteria	Minor criteria
Multiple cutaneous leiomyomas (histologically confirmed)	Surgical treatment of severely symptomatic uterine leiomyomas before the age of 40
	Type 2 papillary or collecting duct renal cell carcinoma before the age of 40
	A first degree relative who meets one of the above-mentioned criteria (leiomyomas in second-degree paternal relatives may be relevant).

Fulfilling major criteria indicates HLRCC with a high likelihood
HLRCC can be suspected when an individual meets ≥2 of the minor criteria

59

59.7.4 Management Issues in HLRCC

Screening with annual MRI should begin at age 18. Given their aggressive nature, all renal tumours will usually be treated surgically. Preclinical data demonstrating that *FH* loss of function activates pathways that include HIF and so overlap with those in VHL disease suggests that there may be value in using similar targeted therapies; however, clinical data in this area is still scarce.

59.8 Other Causes of Familial RCC

A number of other inherited disorders may be associated with renal tumours. In the absence of a genetic diagnosis, individuals with familial non-syndromic clear cell renal cancer should be referred to a renal genetics clinic for consideration of karyotype, *VHL*, and possibly *FLCN* sequence. If testing is normal, they and their first degree relatives should receive annual ultrasound from 25 to 60 years via their GP (no published evidence).

Individuals with early-onset, non-syndromic clear cell renal cancer should have Xp11.2 TFE3 translocation carcinoma is excluded. Affected family members should have karyotype assessed. There is no clear evidence to guide whether other family members should receive screening.

59.8.1 Hereditary Translocation of Chromosome 3

Another rare cause of familial RCC is the hereditary translocation of chromosome 3. The first to be described was a t(3;8)(p14;q24) translocation, and a further eleven cases have since been described [33]. When routine karyotype analysis identifies a chromosome 3 translocation in the context of familial RCC, this is likely to be the cause [2]. Such patients and their first degree relatives should be screened with annual renal MRI from age 20. By contrast, the risk of developing RCC for translocation carriers in the absence of a family history is probably low, and such individuals probably do not require screening.

59.8.2 Hereditary Papillary Renal Carcinoma

Hereditary papillary renal carcinoma (HPRC) is a dominantly inherited familial cancer syndrome characterised by a predisposition to develop multiple, bilateral papillary renal tumours (OMIM 605074). Linkage analysis in 1997 showed that this condition was caused by activating mutations in the c-*MET* proto-oncogene on 7q34 [34]. The renal tumours in HPRC have a distinct histological appearance, characterized as type 1 papillary, and have a better prognosis than type 2 papillary RCC [2]. 95% of sporadic tumours with this appearance show trisomy of chromosome 7, which includes both the MET and hepatocyte growth factor (HGF) genes.

HPRC is very rare (approximate incidence 1 per 10 million), but identification of germline MET mutations allows precise diagnosis and targeted surveillance of mutation carriers. Moreover, such molecular insights have facilitated the use of targeted oncological therapies [17].

59.8.3 Succinate Dehydrogenase

Germline mutations in three of the four subunits of succinate dehydrogenase (*SDHB*, *SDHC*, and *SDHD*) have been associated with familial head and neck paragangliomas and sporadic and familial phaeochromocytoma [35]. Subsequently, early-onset renal tumours were also found to develop in individuals with germline *SDHB* mutations. A variety of histological subtypes of RCC may be associated with *SDHB* mutations (and less frequently *SDHD*), and the lifetime risk of RCC in *SDHB* mutation carriers was estimated to be about 15% [36]. As with *FH* mutations, SDH inactivation results in HIF activation, which may contribute to tumour formation.

Case Study

A 42-year-old man moved into the region and was referred for follow-up in the renal transplant clinic. He had a history of renal transplantation after bilateral nephrectomy for CCRCC due to VHL disease. He was asking whether he still needed follow-up in the VHL clinic.

VHL is a multisystem familial cancer syndrome. Although his native kidneys have been removed, he remains at risk of retinal angiomas, CNS haemangioblastomas, and phaeochromocytomas. He needs ongoing screening for these conditions (◘ Table 59.4).

A 46-year-old woman with learning difficulties due to tuberous sclerosis is seen in the pre-dialysis clinic for education. What specific considerations need to be discussed?

Firstly, general considerations around capacity and consent to treatment relating to her learning difficulties may necessitate a formal best interest meeting. Secondly, progressive decline in eGFR and transition to dialysis will affect the clearance of any anticonvulsant medication she is on. Thirdly, the routine use of anticoagulation in haemodialysis may impact the specific risk of retroperitoneal haemorrhage due to renal angiomyolipomas.

Tips and Tricks

1. Effective management of inherited renal tumour syndromes involves liaison with a broad multidisciplinary team, including geneticists, neurologists, urologists, endocrinologists, respiratory physicians, dermatologists, and opthalmologists.
2. Patients can struggle with frequent hospital visits and appreciate the coordination of imaging and clinic appointments.
3. Imaging in these patients is complex and may take time to be reported formally for use by the MDT.
4. It is important to establish a good long-term relationship with affected individuals as they will need careful follow-up over many years.

59

Chapter Review Questions

1. What screening advice should you give to the brother of a patient with VHL disease who has refusing genetic testing?
2. Can nephron-sparing surgery be recommended for all patients with inherited renal tumour syndromes?
3. Should you perform genetic testing on a 66-year-old lady referred by their primary care physician with a single 17 mm angiomyolipomas?

Answers

1. First degree relatives are at 50% risk of developing VHL disease. The brother should therefore be offered the same screening as any affected individual (◘ Table 59.4). Refusal to engage with genetic testing highlights the role of skilled genetic counselling in cascade testing. It may become possible to make a diagnosis on clinical criteria, but genetic testing offers the only way to exclude the diagnosis.
2. Nephron-sparing surgery is recommended in inherited tumour syndromes predisposing to CCRCC, in order to delay the need for renal replacement therapy for as long as possible. It is not appropriate for some histological types of renal cancer, in particular type II papillary, which is associated with HLRCC.
3. Angiomyolipomas are common in the general population and rarely indicate a diagnosis of tuberous sclerosis. Hereditary renal tumours typically present at a young age (<45 years). It is very unlikely that a woman in her seventh decade would present with an inherited disease. The patient should be assessed for cutaneous features of TS, but she does not need genetic testing. Lesions of this intermediate size should be referred to the urology MDT to determine the timing of repeat imaging and plans for embolization.

References

1. UK, C.R., Kidney cancer - UK incidence statistics; 2011.
2. Maher ER. Genetics of familial renal cancers. Nephron Exp Nephrol. 2011;118(1):e21–6.
3. Melmon KL, Rosen SW. Lindau's disease. Review of the literature and study of a large kindred. Am J Med. 1964;36:595–617.
4. Maher ER. Von Hippel-Lindau disease. Curr Mol Med. 2004;4(8):833–42.
5. Latif F, et al. Identification of the von Hippel-Lindau disease tumor suppressor gene. Science. 1993;260(5112):1317–20.
6. Nickerson ML, et al. Improved identification of von Hippel-Lindau gene alterations in clear cell renal tumors. Clin Cancer Res. 2008;14(15):4726–34.
7. Kaelin WG Jr, Ratcliffe PJ. Oxygen sensing by metazoans: the central role of the HIF hydroxylase pathway. Mol Cell. 2008;30(4):393–402.
8. Linehan WM, et al. Molecular diagnosis and therapy of kidney cancer. Annu Rev Med. 2010;61:329–43.
9. Kaelin WG. Von Hippel-Lindau disease. Annu Rev Pathol. 2007;2:145–73.

10. Nordstrom-O'Brien M, et al. Genetic analysis of von Hippel-Lindau disease. Hum Mutat. 2010;31(5):521–37.
11. Neumann HPH, et al. Germ-line mutations in nonsyndromic pheochromocytoma. N Engl J Med. 2002;346(19):1459–66.
12. Lonser RR, et al. von Hippel-Lindau disease. Lancet. 2003;361(9374):2059–67.
13. Walther MM, et al. Renal cancer in families with hereditary renal cancer: prospective analysis of a tumor size threshold for renal parenchymal sparing surgery. J Urol. 1999;161(5):1475–9.
14. Herring JC, et al. Parenchymal sparing surgery in patients with hereditary renal cell carcinoma: 10-year experience. J Urol. 2001;165(3):777–81.
15. Goldfarb DA, et al. Results of renal transplantation in patients with renal cell carcinoma and von Hippel-Lindau disease. Transplantation. 1997;64(12):1726–9.
16. Lee S, et al. Neuronal apoptosis linked to EglN3 prolyl hydroxylase and familial pheochromocytoma genes: developmental culling and cancer. Cancer Cell. 2005;8(2):155–67.
17. Linehan WM, Srinivasan R, Schmidt LS. The genetic basis of kidney cancer: a metabolic disease. Nat Rev Urol. 2010;7(5):277–85.
18. Atkins MB, Tannir NM. Current and emerging therapies for first-line treatment of metastatic clear cell renal cell carcinoma. Cancer Treat Rev. 2018;70:127–37.
19. Crino PB, Nathanson KL, Henske EP. The tuberous sclerosis complex. N Engl J Med. 2006;355(13):1345–56.
20. Dixon BP, Hulbert JC, Bissler JJ. Tuberous sclerosis complex renal disease. Nephron Exp Nephrol. 2011;118(1):e15–20.
21. Yates JR, et al. The Tuberous Sclerosis 2000 Study: presentation, initial assessments and implications for diagnosis and management. Arch Dis Child. 2011;96(11):1020–5.
22. Siroky BJ, Czyzyk-Krzeska MF, Bissler JJ. Renal involvement in tuberous sclerosis complex and von Hippel-Lindau disease: shared disease mechanisms? Nat Clin Pract Nephrol. 2009;5(3):143–56.
23. Roach ES, Gomez MR, Northrup H. Tuberous sclerosis complex consensus conference: revised clinical diagnostic criteria. J Child Neurol. 1998;13(12):624–8.
24. Amin S, et al. The UK guidelines for management and surveillance of Tuberous Sclerosis Complex. QJM; 2018.
25. Samuels JA. Treatment of renal angiomyolipoma and other hamartomas in patients with tuberous sclerosis complex. Clin J Am Soc Nephrol. 2017;12(7):1196–202.
26. Menko FH, et al. Birt-Hogg-Dube syndrome: diagnosis and management. Lancet Oncol. 2009;10(12):1199–206.
27. Nickerson ML, et al. Mutations in a novel gene lead to kidney tumors, lung wall defects, and benign tumors of the hair follicle in patients with the Birt-Hogg-Dube syndrome. Cancer Cell. 2002;2(2):157–64.
28. Toro JR, et al. BHD mutations, clinical and molecular genetic investigations of Birt-Hogg-Dube syndrome: a new series of 50 families and a review of published reports. J Med Genet. 2008;45(6):321–31.
29. Freifeld Y, Ananthakrishnan L, Margulis V. Imaging for screening and surveillance of patients with hereditary forms of renal cell carcinoma. Curr Urol Rep. 2018;19(10):82.
30. Lehtonen HJ. Hereditary leiomyomatosis and renal cell cancer: update on clinical and molecular characteristics. Fam Cancer. 2011;10(2):397–411.
31. Alam NA, et al. Clinical features of multiple cutaneous and uterine leiomyomatosis: an underdiagnosed tumor syndrome. Arch Dermatol. 2005;141(2):199–206.
32. Smit DL, et al. Hereditary leiomyomatosis and renal cell cancer in families referred for fumarate hydratase germline mutation analysis. Clin Genet. 2011;79(1):49–59.
33. Woodward ER, et al. Population-based survey of cancer risks in chromosome 3 translocation carriers. Genes Chromosomes Cancer. 2010;49(1):52–8.
34. Schmidt L, et al. Germline and somatic mutations in the tyrosine kinase domain of the MET proto-oncogene in papillary renal carcinomas. Nat Genet. 1997;16(1):68–73.
35. Baysal BE, et al. Mutations in SDHD, a mitochondrial complex II gene, in hereditary paraganglioma. Science. 2000;287(5454):848–51.
36. Ricketts CJ, et al. Tumor risks and genotype-phenotype-proteotype analysis in 358 patients with germline mutations in SDHB and SDHD. Hum Mutat. 2010;31(1):41–51.

Internet Resources

Screening guidelines for VHL disease: https://www.vhl.org/handbook/vhlhb4.php#Suggested.

Patient information on VHL: https://www.vhl.org/healthcare/, https://www.vhlcg.com/80290/info.php?p=3.

Patient information on TSC: https://www.tuberous-sclerosis.org/?page_id=35, https://www.tsalliance.org/pages.aspx?content=133.

Patient information on BHD: https://www.bhdsyndrome.org/.

Patient information on HLRCC: https://hlrccinfo.org/.

Polycystic Kidney Disease

Alexander P. Maxwell

Contents

M. Harber (ed.), *Primer on Nephrology*, https://doi.org/10.1007/978-3-030-76419-7_60

Learning Objectives

1. Autosomal dominant polycystic kidney disease (ADPKD) is the most common genetic cause of the end-stage renal disease (ESRD).
2. ADPKD is a systemic disorder caused by either a *PKD1* or *PKD2* gene mutation that results in progressive cystic kidney enlargement.
3. The *PKD1* and *PKD2* genes encode the proteins polycystin 1 and polycystin 2 respectively. Polycystins are integral components of renal tubular cilia.
4. Knowledge of the pathophysiology of ADPKD has been translated into novel therapies being tested in clinical trials. Tolvaptan is now licensed for the treatment of patients with ADPKD.
5. The steady progression of ADPKD to ESRD over many years allows for optimal planning by multidisciplinary teams for eventual renal replacement therapy.

60.1 Introduction

Polycystic kidney disease is a Mendelian autosomal dominant disorder that is estimated to affect more than 12 million people worldwide and is responsible for up to 10% of patients with end-stage renal disease (ESRD) [1–4]. At-risk individuals with a family history of the disorder have a 50% chance of inheriting polycystic kidney disease [1]. It represents a major public health burden and is associated with reduced quality of life (QoL) [5, 6]. Autosomal dominant polycystic kidney disease (ADPKD) is characterized by the development and growth of multiple renal cysts resulting in a gradual increase in kidney size and associated hypertension [1, 7]. The enlarged kidneys may become symptomatic secondary to painful cyst expansion, haematuria, infection, and nephrolithiasis. ADPKD is a systemic disorder with other organ involvement including polycystic liver disease and a higher risk of cerebral haemorrhage from associated intracranial aneurysms [8].

Chronic kidney disease develops because the kidney cysts expand and destroy much of the renal parenchyma resulting in loss of nephrons [1, 7]. Glomerular hyperfiltration can maintain a relatively normal glomerular filtration rate into later adulthood when renal failure develops. ADPKD is not typically associated with elevated urinary protein excretion [9]. Unfortunately, no treatment has been proven to extend renal survival [1]. Improved understanding of the cell biology and pathophysiology of ADPKD is informing the design of clinical trials to establish if novel drugs can delay progression to ESRD [1, 7, 10].

Autosomal dominant polycystic kidney disease is a systemic disorder characterized by gradual cystic enlargement of both kidneys and is associated with slowly progressive chronic kidney disease in adults

60.2 Clinical Features

The spectrum of presentation of ADPKD is wide and includes both renal and extra-renal features.

60.2.1 Kidney Involvement

ADPKD can be discovered incidentally following imaging tests for other indications or following an ultrasound scan in persons with a positive family history who have requested screening (Figs. 60.1 and 60.2). Hypertension typically emerges in early adulthood and usually prior to the obvious increase in kidney size on clinical examination [11]. The hypertension is in part due to distortion of the renal microvasculature by cysts leading to activation of the renin-angiotensin-aldosterone system [11]. Other asymptomatic findings include urinary dipstick abnormalities (non-visible haematuria, proteinuria and/or leucocytes) and as a later feature the presence of abnormal renal function (elevated serum creatinine and reduced eGFR) [12].

Renal cysts may be symptomatic resulting in loin pain secondary to infection or haemorrhage resulting in rapid cyst expansion [1, 7]. Visible haematuria may be secondary to cyst rupture or kidney stone disease [12,

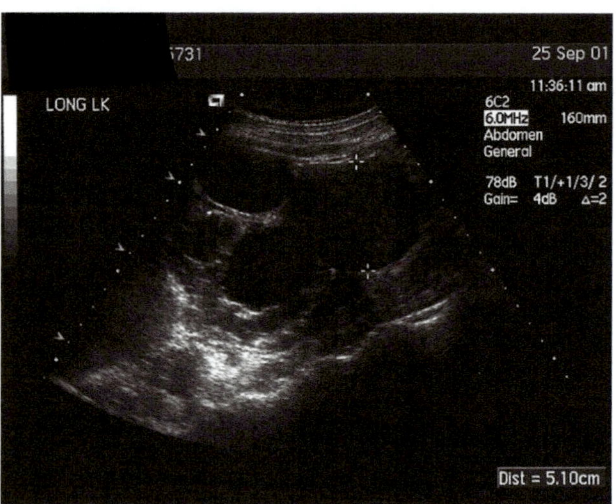

Fig. 60.1 Ultrasound scan of polycystic kidney. The scan demonstrates numerous fluid-filled renal cysts of varying diameter

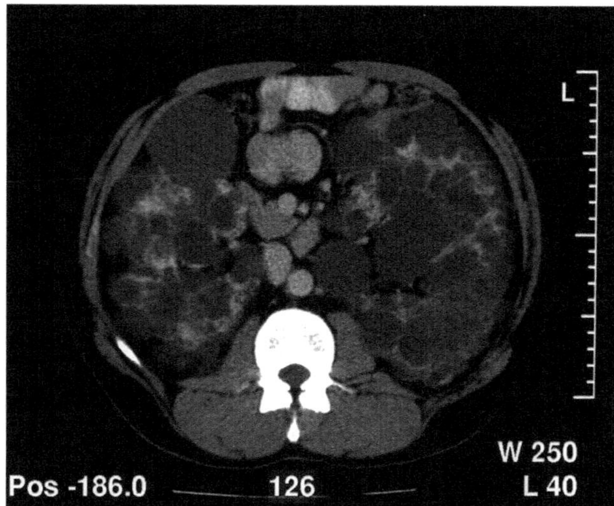

Fig. 60.2 CT scan of the abdomen. Massively enlarged polycystic kidneys occupy most of the abdominal cavity

13]. The cysts of PKD are not premalignant but can make the investigation and diagnosis of a coincidental renal cancer challenging, and malignancy should be considered if older patients present with new-onset haematuria.

The development of abnormal kidney function tends to be a later feature of ADPKD although several factors are reported to be associated with an earlier decline in GFR. These include inheritance of a *PKD1* mutation versus a *PKD2* mutation (as cysts develop earlier in persons with the *PKD1* genotype), a younger age at ADPKD diagnosis, hypertension from a younger age, male sex, hyperlipidaemia, sickle cell trait, large kidney volumes at diagnosis, and visible haematuria [14, 15]. Low birth weight may also be an independent risk factor [16]. When counselling individuals, it is often helpful to determine when any affected relatives were diagnosed or required renal replacement therapy. This can help when discussing the prognosis and possible requirement for renal replacement therapy. Unfortunately, this is not a completely reliable guide as there can be considerable variation in age at onset of ESRD, even between family members with the same documented *PKD* mutation [1, 8]. This heterogeneity in clinical course reflects modifying contributions from other genes as well as environmental factors that may be triggering the somatic mutational 'hits' on the normal copy of the *PKD* gene. At present, there are no useful urinary or plasma biomarkers, other than serum creatinine, that reliably predict the risk of progression in ADPKD [17]. Measurement of total kidney volume by MRI is a promising imaging biomarker to help predict progression to ESRD [8, 18].

60.2.2 Other Organ Involvement in ADPKD

Extra-renal features include cysts in other organs, most commonly the liver, but also in the pancreas, spleen, arachnoid membranes, and seminal vesicles. There is no relationship between ADPKD and polycystic ovarian syndrome [19].

Polycystic liver disease (PLD) is the most common extra-renal manifestation of ADPKD (present in up to 83% of affected individuals), and hepatic cysts can cause massive liver enlargement with abdominal pain, distension, early satiety, nausea, and vomiting [20]. It is uncommon for liver function tests (LFTs) to be abnormal due to the presence of cysts alone, and so alternative explanations such as liver cyst infection or biliary tract obstruction should be sought if elevated LFTs are detected [20, 21]. Symptoms of hepatic pain, compression of the inferior vena cava, or recurrent infection may require surgery [20]. Interestingly, women tend to have more severe liver cyst involvement than men, with multiparity and oestrogen exposure being recognised risk factors for PLD [1].

Intracranial aneurysms (ICAs) are perhaps the most feared extra-renal complication of ADPKD with the prevalence of ~5% in younger adults rising to over 20% in persons over 60 years of age [22, 23].

Patients with a family history of ICA or subarachnoid haemorrhage appear to be at greatest risk for ICA rupture [8, 24]. Screening for ICA remains controversial; definite indications for screening with MRI or CT include a personal or family history of rupture, presence of warning symptoms such as a headache or focal neurological deficit or for those in whom a loss of consciousness while working would place them or others at serious risk of harm [8]. At present screening is not recommended outside of these scenarios unless the patient requests an investigation. If an ICA is larger than 7–10 mm, there is an increased risk of rupture, but smaller ICAs are generally safely managed by interval scanning [25]. Intervention for smaller, asymptomatic ICAs is not without danger. The risk-benefit ratio of intervention mandates individual discussion with neurosurgical colleagues and careful explanation to patients. There are no randomised trials to determine the risk-benefit ratio of screening for ICA [26].

Other extra-renal manifestations of PKD include an increased risk of abdominal herniae (especially in those who elect to perform peritoneal dialysis), colonic diverticula, and various cardiac valvular lesions, the most common being mitral valve prolapse which occurs in up to 25% of persons with ADPKD [1, 8]. Occasional case reports of thoracic aortic aneurysms have been published, and it is worth bearing this in mind if a patient presents with back pain, hypotension, or chest pain for which no other obvious cause is apparent [27].

Fertility is not affected by the presence of ADPKD unless renal function is severely compromised. Women with normal blood pressure and renal function usually have uncomplicated pregnancies, but those with hypertension are at an increased risk of pre-eclampsia and progressive chronic kidney disease and so should receive counselling, ideally pre-conceptually, with an early discussion between nephrologists and obstetricians [28]. Hypertension should be managed using drugs that are not obviously teratogenic. Seminal or prostatic cysts can affect male fertility.

The ***psychological impact*** of living with ADPKD can easily be overlooked [5]. Some individuals may consider themselves as having an incurable illness or may fear rapid progression to ESRD, especially if other family members required renal replacement therapy at a young age [29]. The presence of chronic pain or discomfort from polycystic organs may contribute to depression [30]. Uncertainty concerning the prognosis of younger family members or children can also be a source of considerable psychosocial stress. Studies that incorporate the psychological impact of APDKD as part of the patient-reported outcome measures are important [31]. Patients should be counselled about the management of chronic pain and advised not to use NSAIDs and to limit dependence on opiates. The addition of a tricyclic antidepressant may be useful for both depression and pain.

60.3 Epidemiology

ADPKD affects all races equally with a frequently quoted prevalence of 1:400 to 1:1000 [32]. A more recent estimate, based on a meta-analysis of European studies, indicates that ADPKD prevalence is less than 5:10,000, i.e. it is a rare disease [33]. ADPKD is the fourth and fifth most common cause of ESRD in the USA [4] and UK [3], respectively. ADPKD may be clinically silent and it has been estimated that less than half of those affected are diagnosed during their lifetime [34]. Inheritance of *PKD1* mutations confers an earlier median age of onset of ESRD (54 years) than in those with *PKD2* mutations (74 years) [35]. Men tend to be more severely affected than women. Approximately 50% of individuals with ADPKD will require renal replacement therapy by 60 years of age [1, 36].

60.4 Genetics

Autosomal dominant polycystic kidney disease (ADPKD) is the most common inherited renal disorder and an important monogenic cause of hypertension [1, 37]. ADPKD is caused by germline mutations in either the *PKD1* gene (chromosome 16p13.3-p13.1) or *PKD2* gene (chromosome 4q21-q23). The *PKD1* and *PKD2* genes encode the proteins polycystin-1 and polycystin-2 [7, 8]. Mutations in *PKD1* and *PKD2* are responsible for ~80% and 15% of ADPKD cases, respectively [8, 38]. To date over 1500 unique mutations affecting the *PKD1* and *PKD2* genes have been characterised in various families (ADPKD Mutation Database ► http://pkdb.mayo.edu/). Mutations in the *PKD1* gene that are closer to the transcription start site (5′ end) potentially have a more severe effect on the translated polycystin-1 protein [39]. In general, mutations nearer the 5′ end of the gene are associated with a higher risk of intracranial haemorrhage compared to mutations closer to the 3′ end [40]. Since inheritance is autosomal dominant, there is a 50% chance of an affected child of either gender being born if a parent has ADPKD. This disorder has a very high penetrance (development of clinical disease in a genetically affected individual). A de novo mutation will be the cause in about 5% of those presenting with ADPKD, and up to 25% of affected individuals have no known family history of the condition [41]. Due to the large number of possible mutations within the genes and the difficulties inherent in assigning a causative role to some detected *PKD* gene sequence variants, confirmation by direct genetic sequencing of all individuals with the disorder remains challenging and furthermore, genetic testing may not be available in local clinical practice.

Of interest, even though all cells have a germline mutation, cysts only arise from a small percentage of tubular cells. It is believed that inheritance of a *PKD* mutation is a necessary but not sufficient factor for the PKD phenotype to manifest. One hypothesis is that a second somatic mutational 'hit' is needed on the 'normal' copy of the *PKD* gene before a cyst develops [42]. This could be another randomly occurring mutation in one of the *PKD* genes or a mutational 'hit' triggered by an environmental factor such as acute kidney injury [43]. Further somatic mutational events accumulate over time permitting the creation of multiple independent cellular clones that proliferate more rapidly and give rise to cysts (◘ Fig. 60.3a, b).

60.4.1 Genetic Testing

Careful attention to the ADPKD patient's family history can often provide a simple and reliable means of

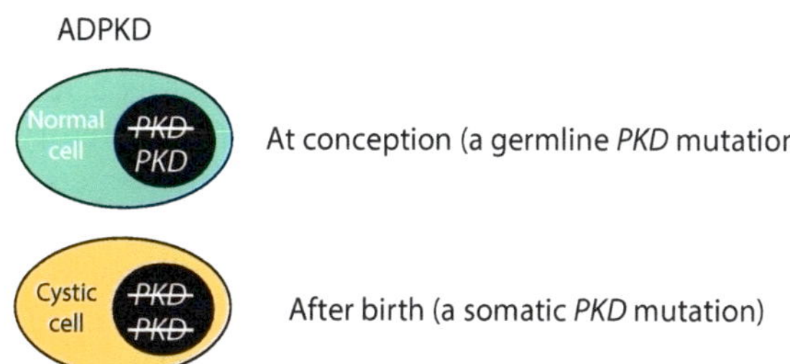

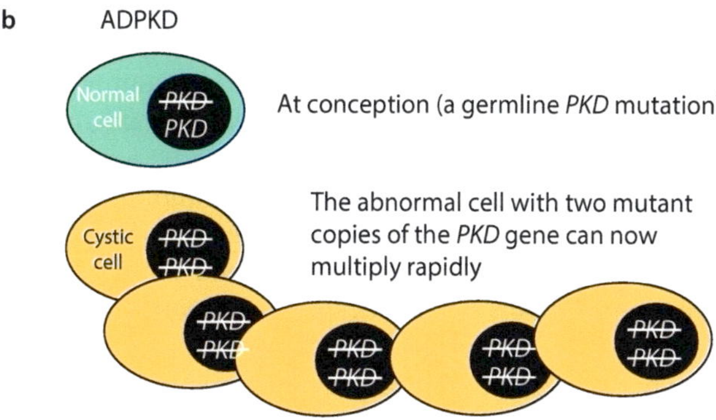

Fig. 60.3 Germline and somatic mutations of the *PKD* gene are required for kidney cyst formation. **a** Germline PKD mutation present at conception with subsequent somatic mutational event disrupting the 'normal' copy of the *PKD* gene. **b** The 'cystic' cell with mutations in both copies of the PKD gene has an altered phenotype. The 'cystic' cell has a growth advantage and proliferates resulting in the development of a kidney cyst

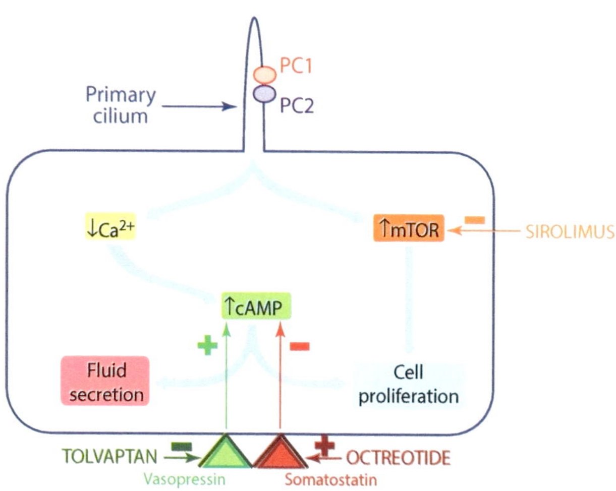

Fig. 60.4 Intracellular signalling disruption in ADPKD. Schematic of a renal tubular epithelial cell and its primary cilium. Mutations in the *PKD1* and *PKD2* genes lead to relative or absolute loss of function of the polycystin complex on the primary cilium. Reduced intracellular calcium influx occurs, and the compensatory increase in cAMP levels promotes fluid secretion and cell proliferation. Cell proliferation is also driven by upregulation of the mTOR pathway secondary to defective ciliary function. Vasopressin (antidiuretic hormone) acting through V2 receptors increases cAMP levels, while somatostatin inhibits cAMP generation. These main pathways are the targets of the therapeutic agents: sirolimus, tolvaptan, and octreotide. *cAMP* cyclic adenosine monophosphate, *mTOR* mammalian target of rapamycin, *PC1* polycystin-1, *PC2* polycystin-2

predicting the causative mutated gene (*PKD1* or *PKD2*). The family history of renal disease severity is predictive of the *PKD* mutation. A *PKD1* mutation is highly likely (positive predictive value 100%, sensitivity 72%) for patients with a family member with ADPKD who developed ESRD at <55 years of age. A *PKD2* mutation is predicted for a patient with at least one affected family member who continued to have sufficient renal function or developed ESRD when they were >70 years of age (positive predictive value 100%, sensitivity 74%) [44].

In practice there is clinical overlap between the phenotypes associated with *PKD1* and *PKD2* mutations, e.g. a patient with ESRD in their mid-60s may harbour either a *PKD1* or *PKD2* mutation. There can be extensive within-family variation in ADPKD with disease variability presumably reflecting the effects of other environmental, epigenetic, and genetic modifiers on disease progression. This variability in age-dependent clinical severity of ADPKD can make counselling individual family members very challenging.

Reliable genetic testing would provide a definite diagnosis in young adults or those individuals without a prior family history of ADPKD. Previously linkage-based diagnostic methods were used in large family pedigrees, but a direct mutation test is more practical. There are several unresolved technical challenges with the development of reliable and cost-effective mutation testing. These include the large size of the *PKD* genes and the multiple unique 'pathogenic' mutations identified already. Each allele (copy) of the *PKD* gene can have allelic heterogeneity that means both alleles must be screened. With the development of effective drug therapy for ADPKD, it has become more imperative to develop cost-effective molecular testing for this disease [38]. The next generation of DNA sequencing techniques will allow rapid analysis of individual patient's *PKD* genes and comparison of their sequence data with *PKD* mutation databases [45]. The UK Genetic Testing Network (▶ www.ukgtn.nhs.uk) does offer genetic testing for ADPKD. This genetics service may be particularly helpful when evaluating, as a potential living kidney donor, a young adult with a family history of ADPKD [46].

60.5 Pathophysiology

Abnormal function of the primary cilium of renal tubular cells appears to be an integral component of the pathophysiology of ADPKD that can be considered as one of the many ciliopathy disorders [47].

The primary cilium functions as a calcium-dependent mechanosensor, detecting urinary flow in the collecting tubules (■ Fig. 60.4). The integral membrane-spanning proteins, polycystin-1 (PC1) and polycystin-2 (PC2), are located within the primary cilia of renal tubular epithelial cells [48]. The polycystins, together with other cilia proteins, regulate cell-cell interactions, epithelial proliferation, and downstream signalling events. PC2 interacts with PC1 and operates as a non-selective calcium channel. This calcium influx from the extracellular to the intracellular compartment triggers cell signalling in response to the flow-dependent movement (mechanosensing) of the primary cilium. The protein products of *PKD* genes, PC1 and PC2, inhibit cystogenesis. Inactivating mutations in *PKD1* and *PKD2* encoding the polycystins lead to the ADPKD phenotype [1, 7, 49].

60

Several interrelated mechanisms have been proposed to explain why cysts form and grow. Firstly, the ability of the primary cilium to sense urinary flow is compromised because polycystin protein structure or function is disturbed. This leads to reduced intracellular calcium levels resulting in compensatory increases in second messengers such as cyclic AMP (cAMP) and upregulation of mammalian target of rapamycin (mTOR), STAT3, Wnt, β-catenin, and MAPK pathways that mediate cell growth and proliferation [1, 7].

Secondly, there is a change in the polarity of tubular cells such that the normal orientation of the mitotic spindle, which would permit tubular elongation without dilatation, is rearranged permitting tubular dilatation and the possibility of cyst formation [50, 51].

Thirdly, within cyst walls, the epithelial cells proliferate consequent to the activation of several mitogenic pathways, and the end-point of this is an outpouching from the parent tubule. This outpouching is the beginning of a cyst, and once its diameter exceeds 2 mm, it will eventually lose communication with the glomerular filtrate and become a separate fluid-filled cyst.

Fourthly, the accumulation of fluid within the cyst is promoted by the effect of antidiuretic hormone (ADH) on the transepithelial secretion of chloride with sodium and water following into the cyst. Abnormal fluid secretion into cysts is associated with translocation of the sodium-potassium-ATPase pumps to luminal membranes (rather than being limited to the basolateral membranes) [48]. Cyclic AMP-dependent chloride channels, such as the cystic fibrosis transmembrane conductance regulator (CFTR), also contribute to cyst growth. The epithelial cells lining the cyst develop a 'secretory phenotype', and further fluid accumulation expands the cyst. Thus, pathways leading to increased intracellular cAMP levels, upregulated and disorganised cell proliferation, and fluid accumulation in cysts as a result of both the action of ADH and change to a secretory phenotype have become potential therapeutic targets [52].

The net result of these processes over time is that while only a small number of tubules will generate cysts, those that do give rise to cysts that continually release cytokines and growth factors that stimulate inflammation and fibrosis. As the cyst continues to expand, adjacent structures such as blood vessels, lymphatics, and tubules are physically disrupted or obstructed, and the cycle of inflammation, hypoxia, and worsening tubular injury with atrophy continues [53]. The remaining glomeruli hyperfilter, but eventually enough parenchyma will have been damaged that there is a steady, irreversible decline in GFR of between 4.4 and 5.9 ml/min per year with the potential for progression to ESRD [54].

Unlike the liver, where a synthetic and secretory function is usually normal despite multiple hepatic cysts, the kidney is dependent on the maintenance of a delicate balance between blood supply, lymphatic flow, and tubular architecture in order to function. Combined with the limited regenerative capacity of the kidney compared to the liver, the importance of trying to slow the progression of renal damage is readily appreciated.

60.6 Diagnosis

Ultrasound is the safest and most cost-effective imaging technique to establish a diagnosis of ADPKD. Molecular genotyping has been uncommon in clinical practice outside of defined research projects. If there is no prior family history of PKD, the diagnosis can be challenging particularly in younger adults who have been referred for assessment with relatively few cysts in each kidney. In adults, the presence of ten or more cysts in each kidney is generally considered diagnostic of ADPKD in the absence of renal or extra-renal features of rarer cystic kidney disorders such as tuberous sclerosis complex or von Hippel-Lindau syndrome.

Age-dependent ultrasound criteria for the diagnosis of ADPKD in families with *PKD1* mutation have been in use since the 1990s [55]. These specified that a diagnosis of ADPKD is established in individuals with a *PKD1* mutation family history if the following age-dependent cyst numbers are present: 15–30 years of age with at least two unilateral or bilateral cysts, 30–59 years of age with at least two cysts in each kidney, and >60 years of age with at least four cysts in each kidney. In practice, it is often uncertain whether an individual presenting with

Table 60.1 Ultrasound criteria for diagnosis of ADPKD in persons with a positive family history

Age (years)	*PKD1* genotype	*PKD2* genotype	Unknown genotype
15–29	≥3 cysts[a] (94.3%)	≥3 cysts[a] (69.5%)	≥3 cysts[a] (81.7%)
30–39	≥3 cysts[a] (96.6%)	≥3 cysts[a] (94.9%)	≥3 cysts[a] (95.5%)
40–59	≥2 cysts in each kidney (92.6%)	≥2 cysts in each kidney (88.8%)	≥2 cysts in each kidney (90%)
≥60	≥4 cysts in each kidney (100%)	≥4 cysts in each kidney (100%)	≥4 cysts in each kidney (100%)

Adapted from Pei et al. [56]
All criteria have a 100% positive predictive value
[a]Unilateral or bilateral cysts

cystic kidneys has a family history of ADPKD secondary to a *PKD1* or *PKD2* mutation.

Revised age-dependent criteria for the diagnosis of ADPKD in families of unknown genotype were published in 2009 [56]. A diagnosis of ADPKD is established as follows: the presence of three or more cysts (unilateral or bilateral) in individuals 15–39 years of age, two or more cysts in each kidney in individuals 40–59 years of age, and four or more cysts in each kidney in persons >60 years of age (Table 60.1). If a family member is being considered as a potential living kidney donor, then the diagnosis of PKD is excluded if there are two or fewer cysts in individuals >40 years of age (despite the personal history of ADPKD). A diagnosis of ADPKD is almost certainly excluded when renal cysts are absent in individuals 30–39 years of age (false-negative rate 0.7%) [56]. One important caveat is that these criteria were developed using images from ultrasound scanners capable of detecting cysts >1 cm in diameter. Modern high-resolution ultrasound scanners can detect kidney cysts with diameters 2–3 mm [57].

60.6.1 ADPKD Diagnosis When Genotype Is Unknown

Up to 10–25% of individuals may be referred for assessment of ADPKD (e.g. multiple kidney cysts are present) but have no other family members known to be affected. Using ultrasound for the diagnosis of ADPKD is not sufficient because the age-dependent criteria were developed in individuals who had a 50% risk of ADPKD [55, 56]. In individuals with a negative family history, there is no definitive number of cysts that confirms a diagnosis of ADPKD. The presence of 10 or more cysts in each kidney makes the ADPKD more likely particularly if the kidneys are enlarged and liver cysts are present [57].

Genetic testing should be considered to confirm the diagnosis of ADPKD, especially if only a few cysts are present, with the proviso that genetic testing is not yet freely available and remains technically challenging partly because of the complex DNA sequence of the larger PKD1 gene and the growing number of pathogenic mutations within the PKD databases.

60.7 Differential Diagnosis

Multiple kidney cysts occurring at a young age, presence of developmental malformations, or the early onset of gout or type 2 diabetes should prompt consideration of alternative diagnoses to ADPKD and discussion with a clinical geneticist. Rarely individuals may have a deletion of both *PKD1* and the adjacent *TSC2* gene on chromosome 16p and express the tuberous sclerosis phenotype in addition to having a much earlier onset of ADPKD in infancy [58]. Others who possess mutations in both *PKD1* and *PKD2* also display more severe disease. The main differential diagnoses for ADPKD are listed in Table 60.2.

60.8 Treatment of Polycystic Kidney Disease

60.8.1 General Principles

Identification and treatment of hypertension, dietary salt restriction, avoiding excess dietary protein intake, early introduction of statin treatment, and efforts to correct disorders of bone mineral metabolism may all help to reduce the progression of ADPKD and decrease cardiovascular morbidity.

As the progression of ADPKD is driven in part by vasopressin (antidiuretic hormone), it is logical to advise affected individuals to stay well hydrated (to reduce antidiuretic hormone release). This strategy of maintaining a high oral fluid intake may be beneficial in the long-term management of ADPKD and is being studied in several clinical trials [1, 10].

Prompt treatment of cyst infections is most effective with lipid-soluble antibiotics that have better tissue penetration, e.g. ciprofloxacin or sulfamethoxazole-trimethoprim. Haematuria may be secondary to cyst rupture, but it is important to consider other diagnoses that may result in renal tract bleeding including nephrolithiasis and urological malignancy.

Table 60.2 Renal cystic disorders

Cystic kidney disorders			
Cystic kidney disease (*and mode of inheritance*)	**Incidence**	**Clinical features distinguishing from ADPKD**	**Comments**
Acquired cystic disease of the kidney (*not inherited*)	5–20% incident dialysis patients; up to 80–100% after 10 years on dialysis	Cysts develop as a consequence of ESRD due to other causes than ADPKD. Cysts within small or normal-sized kidneys	Cysts have premalignant potential (unlike those of PKD). New onset of haematuria in a dialysis patient should trigger the investigation for renal tract neoplasms
Tuberous sclerosis complex (AD)	1:6000	Characteristic skin lesions (facial angiofibromas, periungual fibroma, hypomelanotic macules, Shagreen patches); CND involvement (hamartomas astrocytoma): retinal hamartomas, developmental delay, epilepsy	Multiple renal cysts with benign angiomyolipomas that may harbour RCC. Mutations in *TSC1* and *TSC2* genes
Autosomal recessive polycystic kidney disease (AR)	1:20,000	Diagnosis in utero or infancy; Potter's phenotype; hepatic fibrosis, portal hypertension	Gene defect in *PKHD1* encoding polyductin May require liver and kidney transplantation
Von Hippel-Lindau disease (AD)	1:36,000	Retinal angiomas, cerebellar and spinal haemangioblastoma, renal tumours and phaeochomocytoma	Mutations in *VHL* gene associated with the development of RCC
Nephronophthisis (AR)	1:50,000–1:100,000	Retinal dystrophy, blindness, oculomotor apraxia, developmental delay (10% cases); kidneys often of normal size or small	Commonest genetic cause of renal failure in children. Multiple pathogenic mutations identified
Medullary cystic kidney disease (AD)	1:100,000	Hyperuricaemia, gout, medullary cysts	Serum creatinine often elevated prior to the later appearance of cysts. Associated with *UMOD* gene mutations
Polycystic liver disease (AD)	Unknown	Minor, if any, renal cystic involvement	Mutations in *PRKCSH* or *SEC63* genes
Renal cysts and diabetes syndrome MODY5 (AD)	Unknown	Renal cysts and diabetes syndrome. Pancreatic atrophy. May be associated with other structural genitourinary malformations	Mutations in *HNF1B* gene. Part of the maturity-onset diabetes of the young (MODY) spectrum
Birt-Hogg-Dubé syndrome (AD)	1:200,000	Presence of fibrofolliculomas on face and trunk	Mutation in gene encoding folliculin. May have recurrent pneumothoraces; associated with rare renal tumours

AD autosomal dominant, *AR* autosomal recessive, *CNS* central nervous system, *ESRD* end-stage renal disease, *RCC* renal cell carcinoma

60

60.8.2 Hypertension

The development of hypertension is almost universal in ADPKD and is typically present when the kidneys have increased in size but before renal failure is present. Loss of normal nocturnal dipping in blood pressure usually occurs before the emergence of more sustained hypertension. Antihypertensive treatment reduces the risk of hypertension-related complications in chronic kidney disease, but lowering blood pressure has not convincingly been demonstrated to retard the progression of ADPKD [59]. Hypertension will respond to renin-angiotensin axis blockade with ACE inhibitors or angiotensin receptor blockers (ARBs) [60]. The use of diuretics should be avoided because of the evidence that cyst growth is mediated by vasopressin (antidiuretic hormone). In theory, diuretic-induced intravascular volume depletion could accelerate cyst growth by increasing vasopressin levels.

60.8.3 Preparing for Renal Replacement Therapy

ADPKD is typically slowly progressive with a predictable individual rate of GFR decline. This allows for advanced planning for renal replacement therapy (RRT) [29]. The median age of ESRD onset for persons with the more prevalent *PKD1* gene defect is 54 years of age [61]. One of the advantages of prolonged follow-up of persons with ADPKD at nephrology clinics is the ability to plan the choice of RRT and optimal timing of RRT start.

Options for RRT include pre-emptive kidney transplant (living donor or listing for deceased donor transplant), haemodialysis, or peritoneal dialysis. Outcomes for persons with ADPKD who are successfully transplanted are generally more favourable than for any other common causes of ESRD such as diabetes or glomerulonephritis. There is obviously no risk of recurrent disease in the renal allograft.

60.8.4 Practical Implications for Renal Replacement Therapy in Persons with ADPKD

The *physical size of polycystic kidneys* may be a significant clinical issue when planning for pre-emptive transplantation. Accurate measurement of kidney size, employing MRI, or CT scanning, will allow the volume of each kidney to be assessed. Further discussion with the transplant surgery team is necessary to establish if there will be sufficient room in the pelvis for surgical placement of a transplanted kidney (■ Fig. 60.5). If not, then the patient will need counselling on the requirement for polycystic kidney nephrectomy and the attendant risks of this procedure. Surgeons may elect to perform a bilateral nephrectomy to ensure adequate space for transplant in either the left or the right iliac fossa. Either open or laparoscopic nephrectomy are surgical options.

Other *indications for nephrectomy* include recurrent kidney cyst infections, staghorn calculi, persistent severe cyst pain, or recurrent visible haematuria resulting in anaemia. The risk of kidney cancer is not increased in persons with polycystic kidney disease, but the diagnosis of cancer is challenging since symptoms of loin pain and visible haematuria are common and often reasonably attributed to ADPKD itself. Imaging of the kidneys to identify malignancy is also problematic since multiple simple and complex cysts already grossly distort the renal anatomy. Occasionally an incidental renal cell carcinoma is found on careful sectioning of a polycystic kidney following nephrectomy. The finding of an incidental cancer will mean delaying transplantation until further cancer workup is completed and a disease-free interval is recorded.

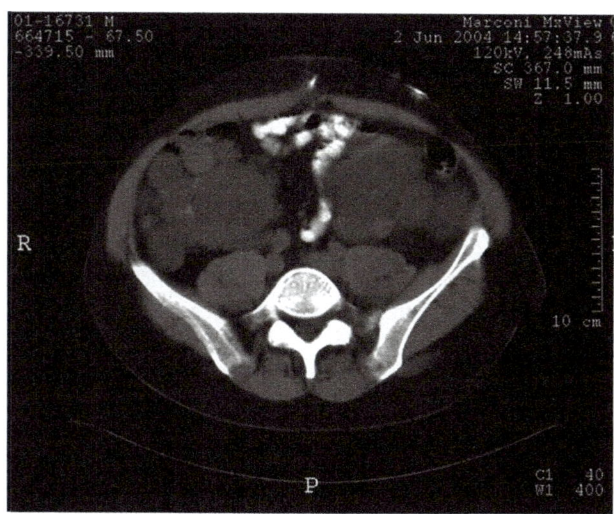

■ **Fig. 60.5** CT scan of the pelvis. Massively enlarged polycystic kidneys extend into the pelvis. Bilateral nephrectomy was subsequently undertaken to enable this patient to have a successful renal transplant procedure

Bilateral nephrectomy in ADPKD is a major procedure with considerable post-operative morbidity, and patients need to be advised concerning chest, wound, and retroperitoneal infections and the potential requirement for blood transfusion (with risk of HLA sensitisation) in the perioperative period. As the patient is anuric, they are rendered dialysis dependent, and only haemodialysis support is suitable in the post-op period. In view of these considerations, it is generally advisable to have established reliable vascular access, preferably by creating an arteriovenous fistula, prior to proceeding to nephrectomy. If a fistula has been fashioned, it may be several months before it is mature enough to be usable as vascular access. In the absence of a fistula (or arteriovenous graft), a tunnelled jugular vein catheter may be placed preoperatively. Haemodialysis support immediately post-bilateral nephrectomy can be complicated by difficulties establishing an accurate dry weight. It is important to account for the weight loss related to both the removal of the large kidneys (as much as 6–8 kg) and the loss of intravascular volume if there is continued oozing of tissue fluid from the retroperitoneal site of operation into a 'third space'. Post-operative ileus with intraluminal accumulation of fluid may also occur due to intraoperative bowel mobilisation.

Recovery from bilateral nephrectomy may take several months; therefore, in planning an elective living donor transplant procedure, it is generally prudent to wait for at least 3–6 months after nephrectomy before proceeding to transplantation.

The physical size of polycystic kidneys also has practical implications for the placement of a *peritoneal dialysis* catheter and subsequent effective peritoneal dialysis therapy. Enlarged kidneys may make it difficult to ensure appropriate placement of the catheter tip in the pelvis and increase the likelihood of migration of the catheter within the abdomen. Larger volumes of peritoneal dialysate in CAPD or APD regimens are also more likely to cause patient discomfort. The addition of peritoneal dialysate fluid can exacerbate the predisposition to abdominal herniae (which are more common in persons with ADPKD). Cyst pain and cyst infection in polycystic kidneys may mimic symptoms and signs of peritonitis and can lead to diagnostic dilemmas if peritoneal dialysate effluent cultures are negative. Rupture of a kidney cyst can occasionally lead to visible blood staining of peritoneal fluid. Although this is an alarming symptom for patients to experience, it is usually self-limiting and settles without need for intervention. Despite these potential complications, many patients will be able to tolerate peritoneal dialysis.

60.8.5 Assessment of a Potential Living-Related Kidney Donor When There Is a Family History of ADPKD

Adult offspring of an affected parent may be considered as potential living related kidney donors [62, 63]. All potential donors should be counselled about the possibility of an ADPKD diagnosis being established before embarking on assessment [62]. Typically, the affected parent will have a *PKD1* mutation, i.e. median age of onset of ESRD in their 50s. All potential living kidney donors will have detailed kidney imaging as part of their extended clinical assessment. A CT scan or MRI (undertaken to identify the number and calibre of kidney blood vessels) will also be able to exclude ADPKD in potential adult donors. There are published criteria for the diagnosis or exclusion of ADPKD using CT or MRI with >10 cysts confirming the diagnosis and <10 cysts excluding the disease [57]. For persons 40 years or older, with a first-degree relative with ADPKD, the finding of normal kidneys rules out ADPKD in the potential donor. Many transplant centres would still be reluctant to use a kidney from a younger relative under 30 years without first undertaking mutation screening of the first-degree relative with ADPKD and their potential living kidney donor. This may still not answer the question because up to 15% of persons with ADPKD will not have an identified pathogenic mutation following genetic screening [63].

60.9 Novel Therapies for ADPKD

Research to understand the cell biology of cyst growth coupled with studies using animal models of polycystic kidneys has been critical to the development of new drug treatments for ADPKD (◘ Fig. 60.4). Cyst growth can be slowed by blocking the cell membrane transporters that increase fluid secretion into cysts [1, 7, 48]. In vivo data demonstrated that blocking vasopressin V2 receptor would lower renal tubular epithelial cyclic AMP levels. V2 receptor blockade slowed the progression of renal disease in animal models of polycystic kidneys [1, 7]. Randomised controlled clinical trials of tolvaptan, a V2 receptor antagonist, demonstrated long-term efficacy measured by serial measurements of renal function and polycystic kidney volume by MRI scans [64–66]. In the UK, tolvaptan (a vasopressin antagonist) became the first NICE-approved treatment to slow the progression of cyst development and progression of renal failure in ADPKD. Tolvaptan can be prescribed for patients with ADPKD and CKD stages 2 or 3 with rapidly declining GFR. The main side effects of tolvaptan are thirst and polyuria. In the clinical trials of tolvaptan, liver function test (LFT) abnormalities were more common than placebo therefore monthly LFT monitoring is mandatory for the first 18 months of treatment.

Other clinical trials of drugs for ADPKD have been completed or are in progress. Therapeutic agents being studied include mTOR inhibitors, metformin, statins, tyrosine kinase inhibitors, and somatostatin analogues [1, 10, 67]. Continued research focused on the biology of ADPKD should ultimately translate into safe and cost-effective treatments that significantly extend renal survival.

60.10 Resources and Patient Information

- PKD charity ▸ https://www.pkdcharity.co.uk
- NHS Health A-Z: Polycystic Kidney Disease ▸ https://www.nhs.uk/conditions/autosomal-dominant-polycystic-kidney-disease-adpkd/
- Kidney Care UK: Polycystic Kidney Disease ▸ https://www.kidneycareuk.org/about-kidney-health/conditions/polycystic-kidney-disease-pkd/

Chapter Review Questions

1. For persons with ADPKD, why are diuretic drugs avoided (if possible) in treatment of hypertension?
2. What problems can be caused by very large polycystic kidneys?
3. Adult children of an affected parent with ESRD secondary to ADPKD are being considered as a potential living-related kidney donor. What kidney imaging is best to exclude ADPKD in the potential donors?
4. Tolvaptan (a vasopressin antagonist) is licensed for use in ADPKD to reduce the rate of cyst growth and slow the progression of renal failure. What issues are relevant in clinical practice?

Answers

1. Diuretics can trigger intravascular volume depletion and result in a rise in vasopressin (antidiuretic hormone) levels. Vasopressin stimulates the growth of cysts in ADPKD. Diuretics may accelerate cyst development resulting in more rapid progression of ADPKD.
2. Very large polycystic kidneys may extend into the pelvis limiting the space available for a kidney transplant. The surgical team may recommend a nephrectomy before the patient is listed for transplantation. Large polycystic kidneys may also interfere with the placement of a peritoneal dialysis catheter and limit the effectiveness of peritoneal dialysis exchanges.
3. An MRI or CT scan is helpful in determining is a first-degree relative is affected by ADPKD. A normal scan in a person >40 years of age rules out ADPKD in the potential donor. Many transplant centres are still reluctant to use a kidney from a younger donor <30 years of age without also undertaking gene mutation screening.
4. Tolvaptan blocks the action of vasopressin leading to troublesome symptoms of polyuria and thirst. Starting with the lowest recommended dose (45 mg morning and 15 mg evening) and allowing the person with ADPKD to get used to the symptoms is helpful before increasing to higher and more effective doses. In clinical trials, there was a higher incidence of liver function test abnormalities in patients treated with tolvaptan compared to placebo. Monitoring liver function tests every month for 18 months and then every 3 months is recommended best practice.

References

1. Cornec-Le Gall E, Alam A, Perrone RD. Autosomal dominant polycystic kidney disease. Lancet. 2019;393:919–35.
2. Spithoven EM, Kramer A, Meijer E, et al. Renal replacement therapy for autosomal dominant polycystic kidney disease (ADPKD) in Europe: prevalence and survival – an analysis of data from the ERA-EDTA registry. Nephrol Dial Transplant. 2014;29 Suppl 4:iv15–25.
3. UK Renal Registry Report. Available at: www.renalreg.com 2019.
4. United States Renal Data System. Available at: www.usrds.org 2019.
5. Simms RJ, Thong KM, Dworschak GC, Ong AC. Increased psychosocial risk, depression and reduced quality of life living with autosomal dominant polycystic kidney disease. Nephrol Dial Transplant. 2016;31:1130–40.
6. Eriksson D, Karlsson L, Eklund O, et al. Health-related quality of life across all stages of autosomal dominant polycystic kidney disease. Nephrol Dial Transplant. 2017;32:2106–11.
7. Bergmann C, Guay-Woodford LM, Harris PC, et al. Polycystic kidney disease. Nat Rev Dis Primers. 2018;4:50.
8. Chapman AB, Devuyst O, Eckardt KU, et al. Autosomal-dominant polycystic kidney disease (ADPKD): executive summary from a Kidney Disease: Improving Global Outcomes (KDIGO) Controversies Conference. Kidney Int. 2015;88:17–27.
9. Chapman AB, Johnson AM, Gabow PA, Schrier RW. Overt proteinuria and microalbuminuria in autosomal dominant polycystic kidney disease. J Am Soc Nephrol. 1994;5:1349–54.
10. Weimbs T, Shillingford JM, Torres J, et al. Emerging targeted strategies for the treatment of autosomal dominant polycystic kidney disease. Clin Kidney J. 2018;11(Suppl 1):i27–38.
11. Rahbari-Oskoui F, Williams O, Chapman A. Mechanisms and management of hypertension in autosomal dominant polycystic kidney disease. Nephrol Dial Transplant. 2014;29:2194–2.
12. Keenan D, Maxwell AP. Optimising the management of polycystic kidney disease. Practitioner. 2016;260:13–6.
13. Bhasin B, Alzubaidi M, Velez JCQ. Evaluation and management of gross hematuria in autosomal dominant polycystic kidney disease: a point of care guide for practicing internists. Am J Med Sci. 2018;356:177–80.
14. Schrier RW, Brosnahan G, Cadnapaphornchai MA, et al. Predictors of autosomal dominant polycystic kidney disease progression. J Am Soc Nephrol. 2014;25:2399–418.
15. Cornec-Le Gall E, Audrézet MP, Rousseau A, et al. The PROPKD score: a new algorithm to predict renal survival in autosomal dominant polycystic kidney disease. J Am Soc Nephrol. 2016;27:942–51.
16. Orskov B, Christensen KB, Feldt-Rasmussen B, Strandgaard S. Low birth weight is associated with earlier onset of end-stage renal disease in Danish patients with autosomal dominant polycystic kidney disease. Kidney Int. 2012;81(9):919–24.
17. Parikh CR, Dahl NK, Chapman AB, et al. Evaluation of urine biomarkers of kidney injury in polycystic kidney disease. Kidney Int. 2012;81(8):784–90.
18. Perrone RD, Mouksassi MS, Romero K, et al. Total kidney volume is a prognostic biomarker of renal function decline and progression to end-stage renal disease in patients with autosomal dominant polycystic kidney disease. Kidney Int Rep. 2017;2:442–50.

19. Abdul-Majeed S, Nauli SM. Polycystic diseases in visceral organs. Obstet Gynecol Int. 2011;2011:609370.
20. van Gulick JJM, Gevers TJG, van Keimpema L, Drenth JPH. Hepatic and renal manifestations in autosomal dominant polycystic kidney disease: a dichotomy of two ends of a spectrum. Neth J Med. 2011;69:367–71.
21. Judge PK, Harper CHS, Storey BC, et al. Biliary tract and liver complications in polycystic kidney disease. J Am Soc Nephrol. 2017;28:2738–48.
22. Xu HW, Yu SQ, Mei CL, Li MH. Screening for intracranial aneurysm in 355 patients with autosomal-dominant polycystic kidney disease. Stroke. 2011;42:204–6.
23. Cagnazzo F, Gambacciani C, Morganti R, Perrini P. Intracranial aneurysms in patients with autosomal dominant polycystic kidney disease: prevalence, risk of rupture, and management. A systematic review. Acta Neurochir. 2017;159:811–21.
24. Pirson Y, Chauveau D, Torres V. Management of cerebral aneurysms in autosomal dominant polycystic kidney disease. J Am Soc Nephrol. 2002;13:269–76.
25. Irazabal MV, Ill JH, Kubly V, et al. Extended follow-up of unruptured intracranial aneurysms detected by presymptomatic screening in patients with autosomal dominant polycystic kidney disease. Clin J Am Soc Nephrol. 2011;6:1274–85.
26. Chalouhi N, Chitale R, Jabbour P, et al. The case for family screening for intracranial aneurysms. Neurosurg Focus. 2011;31(6):E8.
27. Fukunaga N, Yuzaki M, Nasu M, Okada Y. Dissecting aneurysm in a patient with autosomal dominant polycystic kidney disease. Ann Thorac Cardiovasc Surg. 2012;18(4):375–8.
28. Vora N, Perrone R, Bianchi DW. Reproductive issues for adults with autosomal dominant polycystic kidney disease. Am J Kidney Dis. 2008;51:307–18.
29. EAF co-chairs, Harris T, Sandford R, et al. European ADPKD Forum multidisciplinary position statement on autosomal dominant polycystic kidney disease care: European ADPKD Forum and Multispecialist Roundtable participants. Nephrol Dial Transplant. 2018;33:563–73.
30. Youssouf S, Harris T, O'Donoghue D. More than a kidney disease: a patient-centred approach to improving care in autosomal dominant polycystic kidney disease. Nephrol Dial Transplant. 2015;30:693–5.
31. Cho Y, Sautenet B, Rangan G, et al. Standardised Outcomes in Nephrology-Polycystic Kidney Disease (SONG-PKD): study protocol for establishing a core outcome set in polycystic kidney disease. Trials. 2017;18(1):560.
32. Dalgaard OZ. Bilateral polycystic disease of the kidneys; a follow-up of two hundred and eighty-four patients and their families. Acta Med Scand Suppl. 1957;328:1–255.
33. Solazzo A, Testa F, Giovanella S, et al. The prevalence of autosomal dominant polycystic kidney disease (ADPKD): a meta-analysis of European literature and prevalence evaluation in the Italian province of Modena suggest that ADPKD is a rare and underdiagnosed condition. PLoS One. 2018;13(1):e0190430.
34. Lanktree MB, Haghighi A, Guiard E, et al. Prevalence estimates of polycystic kidney and liver disease by population sequencing. J Am Soc Nephrol. 2018;29:2593–600.
35. Hateboer N, v Dijk MA, Bogdanova N, et al. Comparison of phenotypes of polycystic kidney disease types 1 and 2. European PKD1-PKD2 Study Group. Lancet. 1999;353:103–7.
36. Torres VE, Harris PC. Autosomal dominant polycystic kidney disease: the last 3 years. Kidney Int. 2009;76:149–68.
37. Torres VE, Harris PC, Pirson Y. Autosomal dominant polycystic kidney disease. Lancet. 2007;369:1287–301.
38. Harris PC, Rossetti S. Molecular diagnostics for autosomal dominant polycystic kidney disease. Nat Rev Nephrol. 2010;6:197–206.
39. Hwang YH, Conklin J, Chan W, et al. Refining genotype-phenotype correlation in autosomal dominant polycystic kidney disease. J Am Soc Nephrol. 2016;27:1861–8.
40. Rossetti S, Burton S, Strmecki L, et al. The position of the polycystic kidney disease 1 (PKD1) gene mutation correlates with the severity of renal disease. J Am Soc Nephrol. 2002;13:1230–7.
41. Iliuta IA, Kalatharan V, Wang K, et al. Polycystic kidney disease without an apparent family history. J Am Soc Nephrol. 2017;28:2768–76.
42. Pei Y, Watnick T, He N, et al. Somatic PKD2 mutations in individual kidney and liver cysts support a "two-hit" model of cystogenesis in type 2 autosomal dominant polycystic kidney disease. J Am Soc Nephrol. 1999;10(7):1524–9.
43. Maxwell AP, Lewis G. Genetic renal abnormalities. Medicine. 2015;43:399–406.
44. Barua M, Cil O, Paterson AD, et al. Family history of renal disease severity predicts the mutated gene in ADPKD. J Am Soc Nephrol. 2009;20:1833–8.
45. Bergmann C. Recent advances in the molecular diagnosis of polycystic kidney disease. Expert Rev Mol Diagn. 2017;17: 1037–54.
46. Lentine KL, Kasiske BL, Levey AS, et al. KDIGO clinical practice guideline on the evaluation and care of living kidney donors, 2017. Transplantation. 2017;101:S1–109.
47. Hildebrandt F, Benzing T, Katsanis N. Ciliopathies. N Engl J Med. 2011;364:1533–43.
48. Ong AC, Harris PC. A polycystin-centric view of cyst formation and disease: the polycystins revisited. Kidney Int. 2015;88(4): 699–710.
49. Grantham JJ. Clinical practice. Autosomal dominant polycystic kidney disease. N Engl J Med. 2008;359:1477–85.
50. Fischer E, Legue E, Doyen A, et al. Defective planar cell polarity in polycystic kidney disease. Nat Genet. 2006;38:21–3.
51. Patel V, Li L, Cobo-Stark P, et al. Acute kidney injury and aberrant planar cell polarity induce cyst formation in mice lacking renal cilia. Hum Mol Genet. 2008;17:1578–90.
52. Chang MY, Ong ACM. Mechanism-based therapeutics for autosomal dominant polycystic kidney disease: recent progress and future prospects. Nephron Clin Pract. 2012;120:c25–35.
53. Grantham JJ, Mulamalla S, Swenson-Fields KI. Why kidneys fail in autosomal dominant polycystic kidney disease. Nat Rev Nephrol. 2011;7:556–66.
54. Klahr S, Breyer J, Beck G, et al. Dietary protein restriction, blood pressure control, and the progression of polycystic kidney disease modification of diet in renal disease study group. J Am Soc Nephrol. 1995;5:2037–47.
55. Ravine D, Gibson RN, Walker RG, et al. Evaluation of ultrasonographic diagnostic criteria for autosomal dominant polycystic kidney disease 1. Lancet. 1994;343:824–7.
56. Pei Y, Obaji J, Dupuis A, et al. Unified criteria for ultrasonographic diagnosis of ADPKD. J Am Soc Nephrol. 2009;20: 205–12.
57. Pei Y, Hwang YH, Conklin J, et al. Imaging-based diagnosis of autosomal dominant polycystic kidney disease. J Am Soc Nephrol. 2015;26:746–53.
58. Brook-Carter PT, Peral B, Ward CJ, et al. Deletion of the TSC2 and PKD1 genes associated with severe infantile polycystic kidney disease–a contiguous gene syndrome. Nat Genet. 1994;8:328–32.
59. Schrier RW, Abebe KZ, Perrone RD, et al. Blood pressure in early autosomal dominant polycystic kidney disease. N Engl J Med. 2014;371:2255–66.
60. Torres VE, Abebe KZ, Chapman AB, et al. Angiotensin blockade in late autosomal dominant polycystic kidney disease. N Engl J Med. 2014;371:2267–76.

61. Hateboer N, van Dijk MA, Bogdanova N, et al. Comparison of phenotypes of polycystic kidney disease types 1 and 2. Lancet. 1999;353:103–7.
62. British Transplant Society Guidelines. Guidelines for living donor kidney transplant. 2018. https://bts.org.uk/guidelines-standards/
63. KDIGO Living Donor Guideline. 2017. https://kdigo.org/guidelines/living-kidney-donor/
64. Torres VE, Meijer E, Bae KT, et al. Rationale and design of the TEMPO (tolvaptan efficacy and safety in management of autosomal dominant polycystic kidney disease and its outcomes) 3-4 study. Am J Kidney Dis. 2011;57:692–9.
65. Torres VE, Chapman AB, Devuyst O, et al. Tolvaptan in patients with autosomal dominant polycystic kidney disease. N Engl J Med. 2012;367:2407–18.
66. Torres VE, Chapman AB, Devuyst O, et al. Tolvaptan in later-stage autosomal dominant polycystic kidney disease. N Engl J Med. 2017;377:1930–42.
67. Brosnahan GM, Abebe KZ, Rahbari-Oskoui FF, et al. Effect of statin therapy on the progression of autosomal dominant polycystic kidney disease. A secondary analysis of the HALT PKD trials. Curr Hypertens Rev. 2017;13:109–20.

Other Cystic Kidney Diseases

Adam Rumjon

Contents

M. Harber (ed.), *Primer on Nephrology*, https://doi.org/10.1007/978-3-030-76419-7_61

Learning Objectives

1. Review the incidence and diagnostic criteria for simple renal cysts and acquired cystic kidney disease and their implications for renal transplantation, as both donor and recipient.
2. Outline the changes in classification in the autosomal dominant ciliopathies.
3. Highlight the increasing number of mutations implicated in the pathogenesis of the autosomal recessive ciliopathies and nephronophthisis.

61.1 Introduction

There are many causes of renal cysts that can present at varying phases through life including simple cysts, which remain the most common renal abnormality, through to multiple large cysts that may significantly impact on renal function. The main clinical difference in the cystic diseases affecting the kidney is the rate of cyst formation and growth, with simple cysts being by far the least aggressive and often not becoming radiologically evident on ultrasonography until the age of 40 years. The improved resolution afforded by CT and MRI scanning has resulted in the increasing detection in younger age groups throughout the general population [1].

> Many cystic diseases affect the kidney aside from autosomal dominant polycystic kidney disease, and as these are often diagnosed in the paediatric population, knowledge of these conditions is essential for the adult nephrologist.

61.2 Simple Cysts

Simple cysts are the most common renal masses, and in the vast majority of cases, they are unilateral and confined to the renal cortex. They are usually inadvertently discovered during the course of non-renal investigations and are most commonly found in the aging kidney. They are often associated with the male gender, smoking, hypertension, and an elevated body mass index [2]. The prevalence of simple cysts increases with advancing age, with fewer than 5% of under-40s affected compared to greater than 30% of the over-70s, suggesting that they are acquired over time, although the mechanism remains unidentified. These cysts tend to be unilateral and solitary with well-defined features [3]. They are typically considered to be of little relevance in healthy adults and tend to be small and slow-growing compared to the hereditary cystic diseases [4]. The ultrasound characteristics of simple cysts are well established (Bosniak category I) and are classically fluid-filled (without septations) with a smooth outline and posterior acoustic enhancement [5].

Using donor kidneys with small simple cysts (<5 mm) for transplantation is not considered to be a contraindication, and there is no evidence that these kidneys display an increased cystic growth rate post-transplantation [6].

61.3 Acquired Cystic Kidney Disease

Acquired cystic kidney disease (ACKD) is a non-heritable form of cystic kidney disease and is associated with chronic and end-stage kidney disease (▶ Box 61.1). In contrast to adult polycystic kidney disease, the kidneys are usually small or normal-sized, and typically greater than 25% of the renal parenchyma is replaced by cysts. The cysts are usually less than 5 mm in diameter and rarely exceed 30 mm [7]. The frequency of ACKD increases throughout the advancing stages of CKD and the duration of time spent on haemodialysis; up to one-third of patients are affected after 3 years of haemodialysis and >80% after 10 years [8]. Afro-Caribbean patients may be at higher risk of developing ACKD compared to Caucasians. Both men and women appear to be equally affected by ACKD, and there is no apparent correlation with the underlying renal condition [7]. Patients on peritoneal dialysis similarly develop ACKD, although it has been shown that the cysts can regress after successful transplantation. However, cysts can also appear in the failing graft and are subject to exactly the same consequences seen in native kidneys [9].

The pathology of ACKD is complex, but it is most likely that the cysts originate in the proximal tubules, and although the mechanism of cyst formation in CKD has not yet been fully elucidated, the process of their development may be driven by proto-oncogenes, which may subsequently be implicated in cystic transformation to renal cell carcinoma [10, 11].

In the early stages, acquired cysts are asymptomatic and are often inadvertently discovered from CT or ultrasound investigations for non-associated conditions. Patients less frequently present with symp-

Box 61.1 Diagnostic Criteria for Acquired Cystic Kidney Disease

Acquired cystic kidney disease [15]

- Minimum of 3 cysts
- Renal failure
- No cysts before onset of renal failure
- No family history or clinical features of other renal cystic disease
- Kidney usually small or normal size

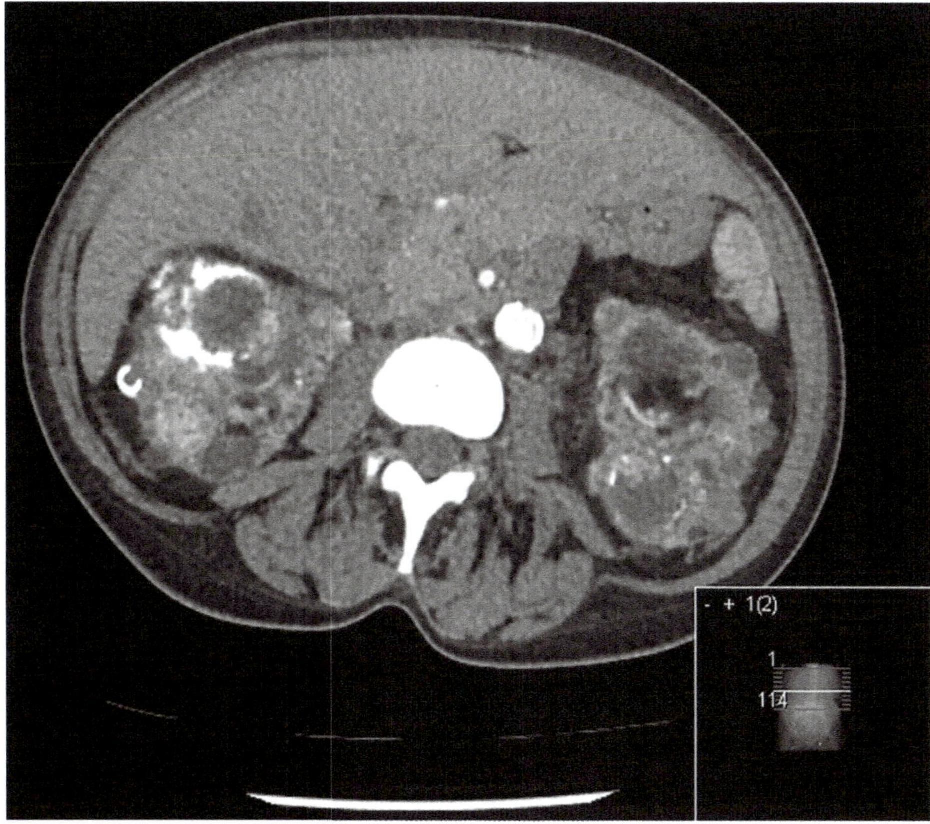

Fig. 61.1 Acquired cystic kidney disease in a patient who had been on dialysis for 11 years, who presented with erythropoietin resistance and haematuria. The scan shows the characteristic features of multiple complex cysts with extensive calcification

toms that are sometimes associated with more serious conditions, such as non-visible or visible haematuria, complicated urinary tract infections, loin pain, or inappropriate erythrocytosis, but the vast majority of ACKD runs a benign course [7]. However, the risk of malignant transformation is a concern, and the frequency of renal cell carcinoma (RCC) development is currently estimated to affect 1–3% of dialysis and renal transplant patients per year compared to the general population. In the transplant group, there is a preponderance towards males and Afro-Caribbean patients, with other risk factors including a longer dialysis vintage, increasing age (>65 years), and microscopic haematuria (Fig. 61.1) [12]. In the dialysis group, these tumours are often detected at a younger age, but the 5-year survival appears to be lower [13].

As of 2016, the World Health Organization included ACKD-associated RCCs as a distinct pathological subtype of RCC. These tumours typically have an eosinophilic and/or clear cytoplasm and prominent nucleoli, and calcium oxalate crystal deposition is very common [14]. They often affect both kidneys and are multi-focal, but frequently present at an early stage with low-grade disease [15]. Renal cell carcinoma remains a clinical concern with ACKD post-transplantation, so careful monitoring must be considered in these patients [16]. There is no established guidance on screening for ACKD in either dialysis or post-transplant patients despite the risk of malignant transformation. American investigators undertook a decision analysis to assess the benefit of CT/ultrasound screening in all dialysis patients three-yearly, which was increased to annually in those found to have ACKD, compared to a strategy of investigating only when clinically indicated. They found the greatest benefit in the youngest and healthiest patients with a life expectancy of at least 25 years and after factoring in the relatively low life expectancy of the average dialysis patient concluded that screening was not justified across the entire dialysis cohort [17].

A practical approach towards screening may include investigating those patients considered to have a life expectancy in excess of 10 years as well as high-risk individuals. If cysts are detected and are categorised IIF, III, or IV according to the Bosniak renal cyst classification system, then referral to the urological surgeons is indicated [18].

61.4 Hereditary Cystic Diseases/Ciliopathies

61.4.1 Autosomal Recessive Conditions

Ciliopathies are a collection of disorders characterised by nephronophthisis, cystic kidneys, or renal cystic dysplasia and include a range of conditions whose numbers continue to rise as mutations in the genes encoding components of the primary cilium are increasingly identified [19]. They tend to be monogenic autosomal recessive disorders and typically present in childhood. Hereditary renal cystic ciliopathies account for approximately 5% of CKD observed in the paediatric population. Although originally defined as distinct clinical entities such as nephronophthisis or nephronophthisis-associated multi-system disorders (e.g. Bardet-Biedl, Joubert, Meckel-Gruber, or Senior-Løken syndromes), the disease classification is now based on genetic characteristics [20]. In the renal tubules, the genetic alteration affects the function of the cilia and leads to dysregulated tissue growth and ultimately results in the formation of cysts. The ability of the tubules to concentrate urine is impaired leading to polyuria and in some instances results in a chronic tubulointerstitial nephropathy and end-stage kidney disease. The renal histopathological findings include the classic triad of tubular atrophy with thickening and disruption of the tubular basement membrane, interstitial fibrosis, and the presence of corticomedullary cysts [21].

The most common recessive renal ciliopathy resulting in childhood end-stage kidney disease is nephronophthisis, and to date, at least 20 identified gene loci and greater than 150 mutations have been identified. An *NPHP1* mutation is responsible for approximately 20—25% of cases, resulting in juvenile end-stage kidney disease by 13 years of age, whilst mutations in the other genes contribute fewer than 5% of cases each. The affected gene locus has an impact on the clinical phenotype, including the age of onset – *NPHP2* leads to infantile end-stage disease; *NPHP3* leads to adolescent end-stage disease. Though the renal features are reasonably characteristic, it is not unusual for mutations affecting the same gene to manifest phenotypes that are typical of several different clinical syndromes. The typical features associated with *NPHP1* include ocular disease (retinitis pigmentosa or coloboma) and possible neurological disease. Other forms of nephronophthisis have been associated with defects in the ophthalmic, musculoskeletal, and cerebellar systems, thus sharing similar features with some other related paediatric syndromes (◘ Table 61.1). Genetic screening may be diagnostic, but around 30% of affected individuals diagnosed with nephronophthisis do not have an identifiable genetic mutation, suggesting that a number of candidate genes have yet to be identified. If suspected, then renal imaging, retinal screening, and a renal biopsy are the recommended investigations in obtaining a clinical diagnosis. If renal failure has not developed by the age of 25 years, the diagnosis of nephronophthisis should be reassessed, and autosomal dominant tubulointerstitial kidney disease considered as an alternative.

◘ Table 61.1 Recessive ciliopathy syndromes associated with nephronophthisis

Bardet-Biedl syndromes (number of genes implicated: 21)	Retinitis pigmentosa, centripetal obesity, polydactyly, deafness, hypogonadism (males), and learning disability
Joubert syndromes	Cerebellar vermis hypoplasia, developmental delay, retinal dystrophy with dysregulated eye movements/nystagmus, coloboma, and renal dysplasia
Meckel-Gruber syndromes [13]	Renal dysplasia, polydactyly, encephalocoele, and hepatic ductal dysplasia and cysts
Senior-Løken syndromes [9]	Retinitis pigmentosa, retinal aplasia and phenotype of Leber's amaurosis, and renal dysplasia
Cogan syndrome	Liver fibrosis, hearing loss, and oculomotor apraxia

61.4.2 Autosomal Dominant Conditions

There are a number of rare autosomal dominant tubulointerstitial kidney diseases (ADTKD), which were previously labelled with inconsistent and confusing terms (◘ Table 61.2). They have now been simplified in line with current knowledge of the underlying genotypes associated with the disease subtypes [22]. These diseases are characterised by autosomal dominant inheritance, slowly progressive disease potentially resulting in adult-onset end-stage kidney disease, and the presence of medullary cysts in fewer than 50% of cases of imaged kidneys.

There are currently five known subtypes of ADTKD, the most studied of which is the *UMOD* gene encoding uromodulin (previously known as Tamm-Horsfall protein), which is the most abundant protein secreted in the urine and expressed exclusively in the epithelial cells of the TAL [23]. A *UMOD* mutation (ADTKD-UMOD) presents with hyperuricaemia and juvenile-onset gout and accounts for approximately 70% of all ADTKD. The resulting defects in tubular function may induce net urinary salt loss leading to volume contraction and compensatory reabsorption of urate in the proximal tubule; therefore, the hyperuricaemia seen in this condition is a result of urate underexcretion rather than excess production [24]. A clinical diagnosis is supported by a family history of autosomal dominant kidney disease and gout with minimal proteinuria and is confirmed by genetic testing. Xanthine oxidase inhibitors are useful in the treatment of gout, but there are

Table 61.2 Classification of autosomal dominant tubulointerstitial kidney disease

Gene/protein	Terminology	Previous terminology
MUC1/mucin 1	ADTKD-MUC1	MCKD1 (medullary cystic kidney disease type 1) MKD (mucin-1 kidney disease)
UMOD/uromodulin	ADTKD-UMOD	MCKD2 (medullary cystic kidney disease type 2) UKD (uromodulin kidney disease) UAKD (uromodulin-associated kidney disease) FJHN (familial juvenile hyperuricaemic nephropathy)
REN/preprorenin	ADTKD-REN	FJHN2 (familial juvenile hyperuricaemic nephropathy type 2)
HNF1β/hepatocyte nuclear factor 1ß	ADTKD-HNF1ß	MODY5 (maturity-onset diabetes of the young type 5) RCAD (renal cyst and diabetes syndrome)
SEC61A1/α1 subunit	ADTKD-SEC61A1	

far less data to suggest that they slow the progression of CKD in these patients, who may reach end-stage kidney disease in their early 30s [21].

Around 30% of ADTKD is accounted for by a *MUC1* mutation (encoding mucin 1), which phenotypically has a very strong resemblance to the clinical and histological features witnessed in nephronophthisis. However, the median age of onset of end-stage kidney disease in these patients is much later and typically occurs in their early 60s. There are no therapeutic targets although renal transplantation is curative for all variants of ADTKD.

The other forms of ADTKD are rare. A relative decrease in renin levels characterises the features seen in ADTKD-REN including childhood anaemia (via reduced erythropoietin), hypotension, polyuria, hyperuricaemia, and gout. HFN1β mutations (ADTKD-HFN1β) may result in disordered glucose metabolism and maturity-onset diabetes mellitus, renal magnesium wasting, and hyperuricaemia. If undiagnosed, those that receive a renal transplant may rapidly develop new-onset diabetes after transplantation (NODAT). Screening for HFN1β mutations should be considered in patients with end-stage kidney disease caused by dysplastic cystic kidneys [25].

61.5 Autosomal Recessive Polycystic Kidney Disease

Autosomal recessive polycystic kidney disease (ARPKD) arises as a result of a *PKHD1* mutation (which codes for fibrocystin). A second locus has been identified with mutations in the *DZIP1L* gene [26, 27]. The incidence is estimated at approximately 1 in 10,000 live births and is more frequently seen in Caucasians. The characteristic histological features are cystic dilatations of the renal collecting ducts and congenital hepatic fibrosis, and these manifest clinically as progressive renal dysfunction, haematuria, mild proteinuria, and chronic liver disease [28]. The renal cysts in ARPKD maintain their afferent and efferent channels and therefore remain open and are not discrete sacs separated from the renal tubular lumen, differentiating them from the cysts of ADPKD, von Hippel-Lindau disease, and tuberous sclerosis [29].

The vast majority of patients present before the age of 20. Around half of cases are diagnosed antenatally, and those who present in infancy typically have severe renal disease whereas those who are diagnosed in adulthood generally have symptoms related to congenital hepatic fibrosis [30]. The 1-year and 10-year survival of those who successfully negotiate infancy is 85% and 82%, respectively [31]. ARPKD frequently results in end-stage kidney disease (over half of patients require renal replacement therapy in childhood), and a proportion may have isolated hepatic fibrosis or Caroli's disease (congenital cystic dilatation of the intrahepatic biliary tree) with little or no renal involvement [32]. The diagnosis is predominantly achieved through clinical evaluation with dedicated imaging of the liver and kidneys. The features on standard second trimester ultrasonography include bilaterally large hyperechogenic kidneys with poor corticomedullary differentiation, and cystic kidneys (approximately 5 mm) are present in nearly a third of those cases. The liver may also be enlarged (increased echogenicity), but hepatic sequelae often develop later in life. Genetic testing can sometimes be used to confirm a clinical diagnosis of ARPKD or for genetic screening of siblings of a child with a known diagnosis. As no specific therapies have yet been identified, the management of ARPKD is largely supportive, and therapies that are broadly applicable to CKD remain the standard of care, such as the aggressive treatment of hypertension. As with the autosomal dominant form of polycystic kidney disease, the cysts can rupture and subsequently haemorrhage or become infected. ARPKD invariably involves the liver, and the development of portal hypertension can lead to splenomegaly, thrombocytopenia, and oesophageal varices. Ascending cholangitis carries a high mortality rate, especially after renal transplantation, and combined liver-renal transplantation should be considered in patients with significant portal hypertension [33].

61.6 Medullary Sponge Kidney

Medullary sponge kidney (MSK) is a rare and benign nephropathy that is characterised by congenital dilatation of the renal medullary collecting ducts and subsequent enlargement of the affected pyramids of the kidneys. It is usually an incidental finding affecting both kidneys although in a third of cases, it can present unilaterally. Up to 20% of patients with recurrent calcium nephrolithiasis have been observed to have MSK, and it can also manifest as a result of nephrocalcinosis or renal acidification (partial distal renal tubular acidosis) and concentration defects. Both adult males and females appear to be equally affected, and there is no racial preponderance. It is often asymptomatic, but when symptoms are present, then haematuria and urinary tract infections are most likely [34].

The cause of MSK is not fully understood but is likely to be related to an underlying developmental abnormality. Glial cell line-derived neurotrophic factor (GDNF) is essential for nephrogenesis, and mutations in *GDNF* have been associated with MSK [35]. The intravenous urogram remains the gold standard diagnostic tool and has much better sensitivity than a CTKUB for detecting cystic dilatation. Ten minutes after the administration of intravenous contrast medium, papillary precalyceal ectasia is seen when the contrast pools in the dilated papillary ducts, and a resultant 'brush-like' or 'bouquet' appearance is observed by radiography (Fig. 61.2). The utility of a CTKUB, however, lies in detecting medullary nephrocalcinosis, which often accompanies MSK but is not essential in making a diagnosis. The management revolves around treating and preventing complications of urinary tract infections or the formation of renal calculi. Hypercalciuria and hypocitraturia are very common findings, and thiazide diuretics and alkali citrate are sometimes used to correct these urinary electrolyte abnormalities [34].

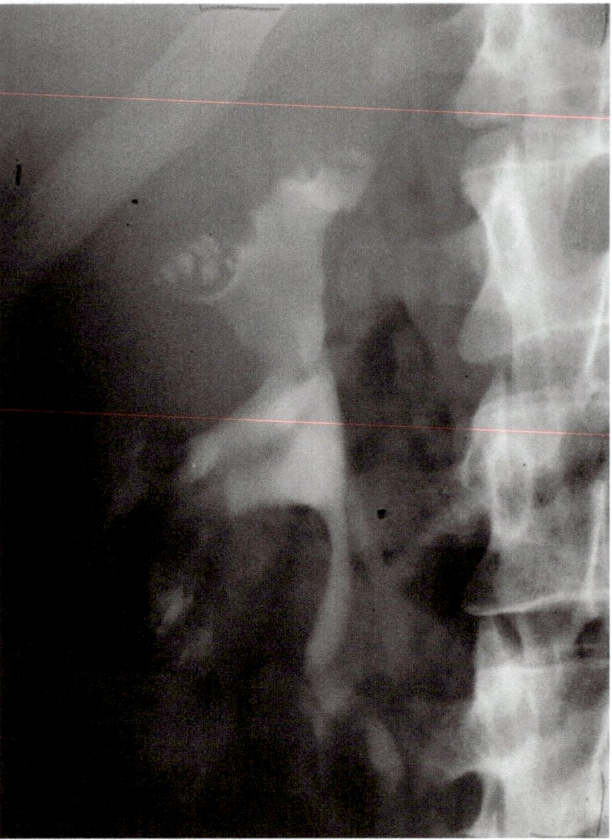

Fig. 61.2 Intravenous pyelogram in a patient with medullary sponge kidney showing the characteristic 'bunch of grapes' appearance

61

Conclusion

Ciliopathies are responsible for a significant burden of paediatric renal disease, and with increasing knowledge of the underlying pathophysiology of these diseases along with earlier detection and intervention, many patients will transition to adult renal services making knowledge of these conditions vital for the adult nephrologist. Some of these conditions may present in later life with little indication as to the cause, and a detailed family history alongside interpretation of the radiographic and histological findings may guide the diagnosis. Advances in next-generation sequencing and decrease in associated costs will inevitably enable genetic testing and identification of underlying germline predisposition and other associated genetic alterations. Given the potential for future studies to identify novel mutations, there is a need to consider prospective DNA sample collection for genetic testing when available. Ultimately, transplantation is curative of the underlying condition.

Tips and Tricks

- Kidneys with small simple renal cysts are not a contraindication to kidney donation.
- Clinicians should be mindful that acquired cystic kidney disease has the potential for malignant transformation especially in those patients who have undergone a prolonged period of haemodialysis.
- Inappropriate erythrocytosis is an important clue not to be overlooked.
- Nephronophthisis (autosomal recessive) is generally a disease of childhood, whereas ADTKD (autosomal dominant) often manifests in older age.
- A parent who is a carrier of the PKHD1 mutation (autosomal recessive PKD) may be able to donate their kidney to an affected child.
- Patients with undiagnosed ADTKD-HFN1β may rapidly develop NODAT.

Case Study

Case 1

A patient with a parapelvic cyst in the right kidney presented with fever and right loin pain. Cross-sectional imaging demonstrated a right hydronephrotic kidney that had developed after the cyst became infected and inflamed and caused obstruction of the kidney. The symptoms resolved following drainage of the cyst and antimicrobial therapy.

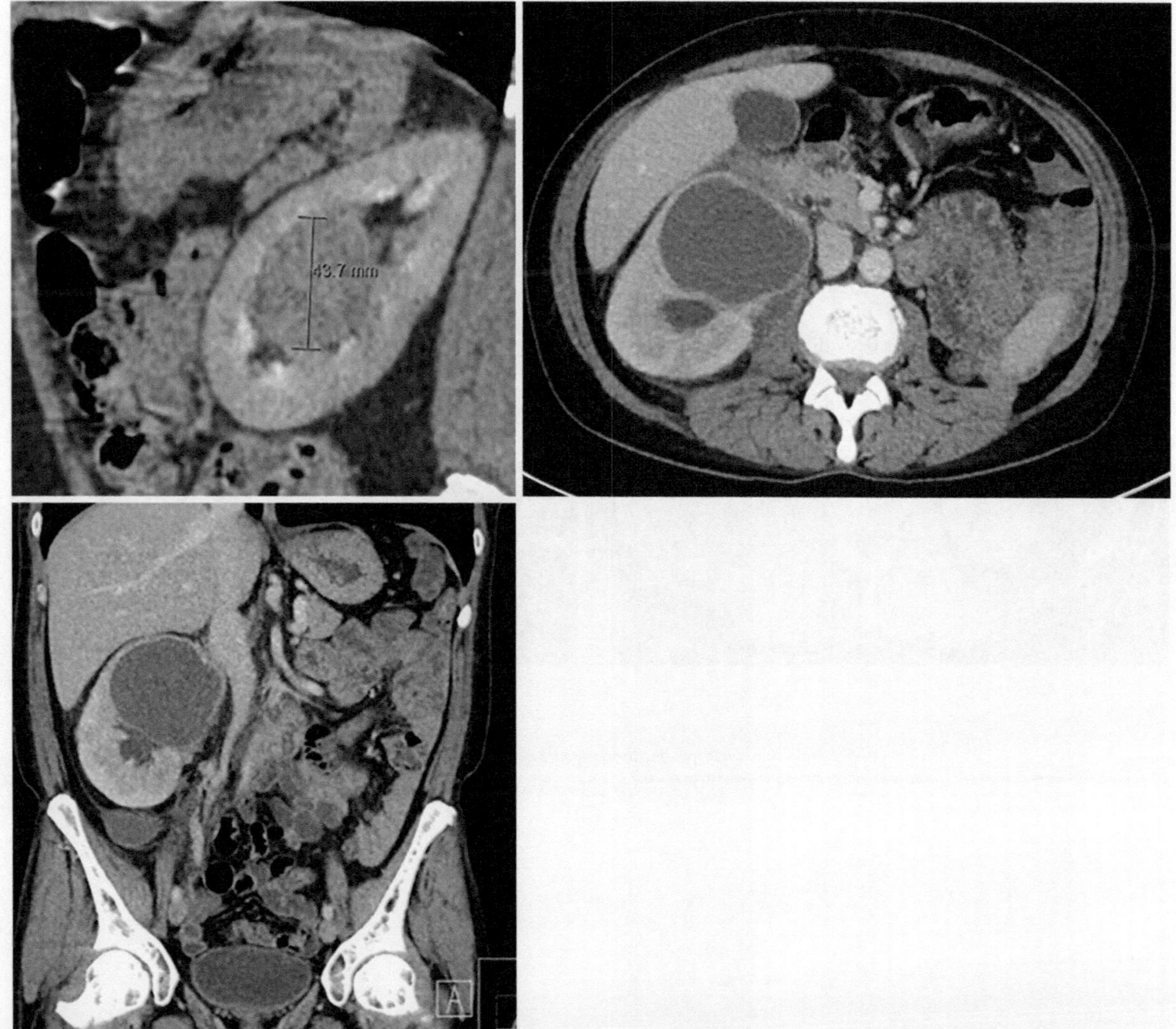

Case 2

A patient presented with loin pain as a result of a large simple renal cyst. There was resolution of the pain following aspiration of the cyst, but the symptom recurred with re-accumulation, and he was referred for surgical defenestration.

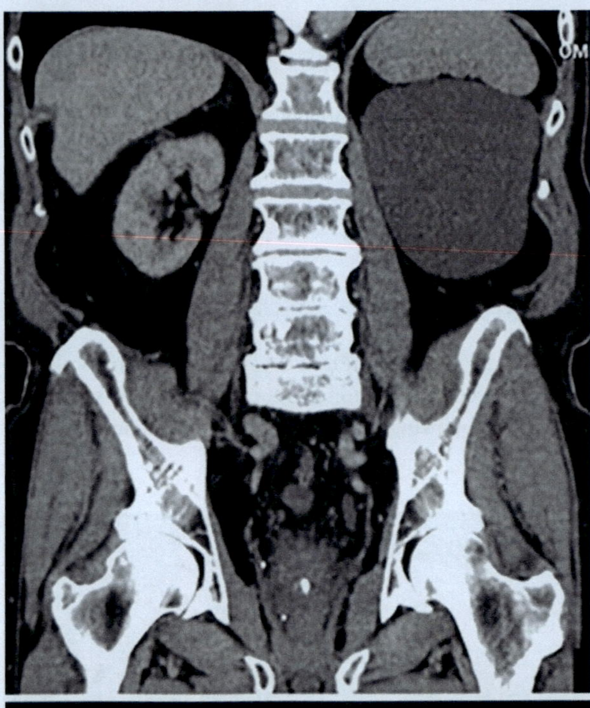

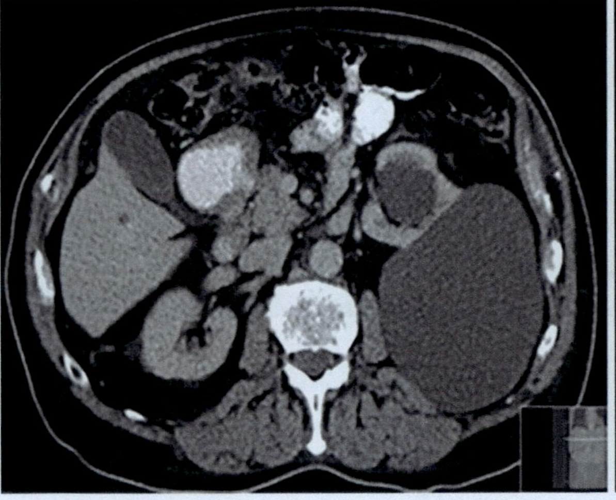

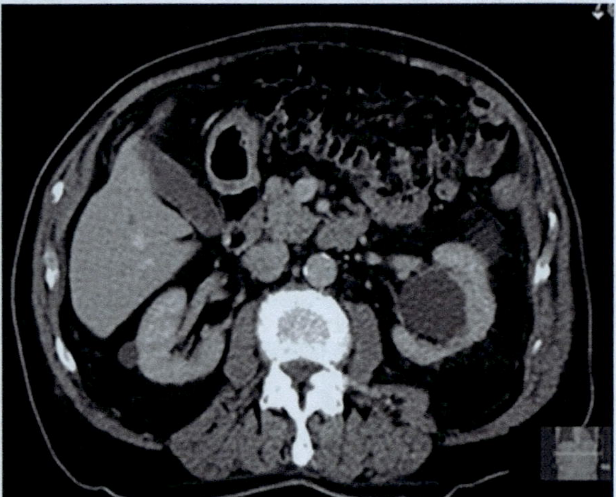

Chapter Review Questions

1. What is the risk of malignant transformation of acquired cystic kidney disease?
2. What are the main histological features of nephronophthisis seen on renal biopsy?
3. What genetic mutation is responsible for approximately 25% of nephronophthisis?
4. Which class of autosomal dominant tubulointerstitial kidney disease is most prevalent?
5. What urine electrolyte abnormalities are typically seen in medullary sponge kidney?

Answers

1. Malignant transformation of acquired cystic kidney disease is currently estimated to affect 1–3% of dialysis and renal transplant patients per year compared to the general population.
2. The classic triad of tubular atrophy with thickening and disruption of the tubular basement membrane, interstitial fibrosis, and the presence of corticomedullary cysts
3. *NPHP1* mutation
4. ADTKD-UMOD
5. Hypercalciuria and hypocitraturia

References

1. Rule AD, Sasiwimonphan K, Lieske JC, Keddis MT, Torres VE, Vrtiska TJ. Characteristics of renal cystic and solid lesions based on contrast-enhanced computed tomography of potential kidney donors. Am J Kidney Dis. 2012;59(5):611–8.
2. Lee YJ, Kim MS, Cho S, Kim SR. Association between simple renal cysts and development of hypertension in healthy middle-aged men. J Hypertens. 2012;30(4):700–4.
3. Eknoyan G. A clinical view of simple and complex renal cysts. J Am Soc Nephrol. 2009;20(9):1874–6.
4. Terada N, Arai Y, Kinukawa N, Terai A. The 10-year natural history of simple renal cysts. Urology. 2008;71(1):7–11; discussion -2.
5. Israel GM, Bosniak MA. An update of the Bosniak renal cyst classification system. Urology. 2005;66(3):484–8.
6. Srivastava A, Kumar A, Agarwal A. Donors with renal cysts: a dilemma in decision making. Transplant Proc. 2003;35(1):30–1.
7. Grantham JJ. Acquired cystic kidney disease. Kidney Int. 1991;40(1):143–52.
8. Matson MA, Cohen EP. Acquired cystic kidney disease: occurrence, prevalence, and renal cancers. Medicine (Baltimore). 1990;69(4):217–26.
9. Scandling JD. Acquired cystic kidney disease and renal cell cancer after transplantation: time to rethink screening? Clin J Am Soc Nephrol. 2007;2(4):621–2.
10. Herrera GA. C-erb B-2 amplification in cystic renal disease. Kidney Int. 1991;40(3):509–13.
11. Costa MZ, Bacchi CE, Franco M. Histogenesis of the acquired cystic kidney disease: an immunohistochemical study. Appl Immunohistochem Mol Morphol. 2006;14(3):348–52.
12. Klatte T, Marberger M. Renal cell carcinoma of native kidneys in renal transplant patients. Curr Opin Urol. 2011;21(5):376–9.
13. Truong LD, Krishnan B, Cao JT, Barrios R, Suki WN. Renal neoplasm in acquired cystic kidney disease. Am J Kidney Dis. 1995;26(1):1–12.
14. Moch H, Cubilla AL, Humphrey PA, Reuter VE, Ulbright TM. The 2016 WHO classification of tumours of the urinary system and male genital organs-part A: renal, penile, and testicular tumours. Eur Urol. 2016;70(1):93–105.
15. Fleming S. Renal cell carcinoma in acquired cystic kidney disease. Histopathology. 2010;56(3):395–400.
16. Schwarz A, Vatandaslar S, Merkel S, Haller H. Renal cell carcinoma in transplant recipients with acquired cystic kidney disease. Clin J Am Soc Nephrol. 2007;2(4):750–6.
17. Sarasin FP, Wong JB, Levey AS, Meyer KB. Screening for acquired cystic kidney disease: a decision analytic perspective. Kidney Int. 1995;48(1):207–19.
18. Rahbari-Oskoui F, Mittal A, Mittal P, Chapman A. Renal relevant radiology: radiologic imaging in autosomal dominant polycystic kidney disease. Clin J Am Soc Nephrol. 2014;9(2):406–15.
19. Online Mendelian Inheritance in Man, OMIM® Johns Hopkins University (Baltimore, MD): McKusick-Nathans Institute of Genetic Medicine; [cited 2020 June 14]. Available from: https://omim.org.
20. Devlin LA, Sayer JA. Renal ciliopathies. Curr Opin Genet Dev. 2019;56:49–60.
21. Hildebrandt F, Omram H. New insights: nephronophthisis-medullary cystic kidney disease. Pediatr Nephrol. 2001;16(2):168–76.
22. Eckardt KU, Alper SL, Antignac C, Bleyer AJ, Chauveau D, Dahan K, et al. Autosomal dominant tubulointerstitial kidney disease: diagnosis, classification, and management – A KDIGO consensus report. Kidney Int. 2015;88(4):676–83.
23. Gokhale JA, Glenton PA, Khan SR. Characterization of Tamm-Horsfall protein in a rat nephrolithiasis model. J Urol. 2001;166(4):1492–7.
24. Scolari F, Caridi G, Rampoldi L, Tardanico R, Izzi C, Pirulli D, et al. Uromodulin storage diseases: clinical aspects and mechanisms. Am J Kidney Dis. 2004;44(6):987–99.
25. Devuyst O, Olinger E, Weber S, Eckardt KU, Kmoch S, Rampoldi L, et al. Autosomal dominant tubulointerstitial kidney disease. Nat Rev Dis Primers. 2019;5(1):60.
26. Ward CJ, Hogan MC, Rossetti S, Walker D, Sneddon T, Wang X, et al. The gene mutated in autosomal recessive polycystic kidney disease encodes a large, receptor-like protein. Nat Genet. 2002;30(3):259–69.
27. Lu H, Galeano MCR, Ott E, Kaeslin G, Kausalya PJ, Kramer C, et al. Mutations in DZIP1L, which encodes a ciliary-transition-zone protein, cause autosomal recessive polycystic kidney disease. Nat Genet. 2017;49(7):1025–34.
28. Shaikewitz ST, Chapman A. Autosomal recessive polycystic kidney disease: issues regarding the variability of clinical presentation. J Am Soc Nephrol. 1993;3(12):1858–62.
29. Sweeney WE Jr, Avner ED. Diagnosis and management of childhood polycystic kidney disease. Pediatr Nephrol. 2011;26(5):675–92.
30. Guay-Woodford LM, Desmond RA. Autosomal recessive polycystic kidney disease: the clinical experience in North America. Pediatrics. 2003;111(5 Pt 1):1072–80.
31. Bergmann C, Guay-Woodford LM, Harris PC, Horie S, Peters DJM, Torres VE. Polycystic kidney disease. Nat Rev Dis Primers. 2018;4(1):50.
32. Gunay-Aygun M, Font-Montgomery E, Lukose L, Tuchman Gerstein M, Piwnica-Worms K, Choyke P, et al. Characteristics of congenital hepatic fibrosis in a large cohort

of patients with autosomal recessive polycystic kidney disease. Gastroenterology. 2013;144(1):112–21 e2.
33. Buscher R, Buscher AK, Weber S, Mohr J, Hegen B, Vester U, et al. Clinical manifestations of autosomal recessive polycystic kidney disease (ARPKD): kidney-related and non-kidney-related phenotypes. Pediatr Nephrol. 2014;29(10):1915–25.
34. Fabris A, Anglani F, Lupo A, Gambaro G. Medullary sponge kidney: state of the art. Nephrol Dial Transplant. 2013;28(5):1111–9.
35. Torregrossa R, Anglani F, Fabris A, Gozzini A, Tanini A, Del Prete D, et al. Identification of GDNF gene sequence variations in patients with medullary sponge kidney disease. Clin J Am Soc Nephrol. 2010;5(7):1205–10.

Patient Information and Guidelines

RaDaR National Renal Rare Disease Registry. https://rarerenal.org/patient-information/.

Genetic Disorders of the Glomerular Basement Membrane

A. Neil Turner and Eleri Williams

Contents

M. Harber (ed.), *Primer on Nephrology*, https://doi.org/10.1007/978-3-030-76419-7_62

Learning Objectives

1. A moderately detailed understanding of the second most common inherited cause of end-stage renal failure.
2. Understand when to implement treatments to slow its progression.
3. Recognise the possibility of COL4A3-5 mutations in CKD of unknown cause or unrecognised in other patients.
4. Understand uncertain risk to those carrying a normal copy of a COL4A3-5 gene alongside a copy with a significant mutation.

Basement membranes are specialised matrices found beneath epithelial and endothelial cell layers in all organs of the body. In the kidney, the glomerular basement membrane (GBM) forms part of the barrier between blood and filtrate.

Alport syndrome is the second most common genetic cause of renal failure. Blocking angiotensin effects seems to slow its progression. Thin basement membrane nephropathy is a common diagnosis in patients presenting with microscopic haematuria. This chapter reviews our current understanding of these conditions and mentions other less common inherited diseases of the GBM.

62.1 The Glomerular Basement Membrane: Components, Structure and Function

The GBM is part of the glomerular filtration barrier and lies between two layers of cells [1]. It is flanked on one side by endothelial cells that face the glomerular capillary lumen, whilst podocyte foot processes line the other side protruding into the urinary space. The GBM is thicker than other basement membranes, measuring 300–350 nm. In health, the function of the glomerular filtration barrier is to allow the passage of water and small solutes whilst preventing the passage of large proteins.

All basement membranes have four major protein components: (1) type IV collagen, (2) laminin, (3) nidogen and (4) heparan sulphate proteoglycans. Diseases occurring as a result of type IV collagen and laminin gene mutations have been described.

Type IV collagen is the major component of mammalian basement membranes [1], and abnormal type IV collagen is the culprit in most of the inherited GBM disease as we currently identify them.

There are six α chains, and each molecule of type IV collagen is composed of three of these chains. A triple helical structure is common to all collagens, but type IV collagens are characterised by non-collagenous interruptions in the helical structure and retention of non-collagenous domains at each end.

The six α chains (α1(IV) to α6(IV)) are encoded by *COL4A1* to *COL4A6* genes which are arranged in pairs as shown in ◘ Fig. 62.1. Each chain has a molecular weight of over 160,000, and the genes encoding them are large and complex.

The composition of the type IV molecule varies between different membranes. An α1-α2 (112) network is common to all basement membranes. The glomerular basement membrane in adults is mainly made from a network of α3α4α5 (345) molecules, which is also present in the eye, ear and lungs (◘ Fig. 62.2). A third network, found in Bowman's capsule, skin and other locations, contains α5-α6 molecules. The 112 network is the first formed during development, so that a later developmental switch is required to form the mature composition. In developing glomeruli, immature nephrons swap from the 112 network to the 345 network as the capillary loops form.

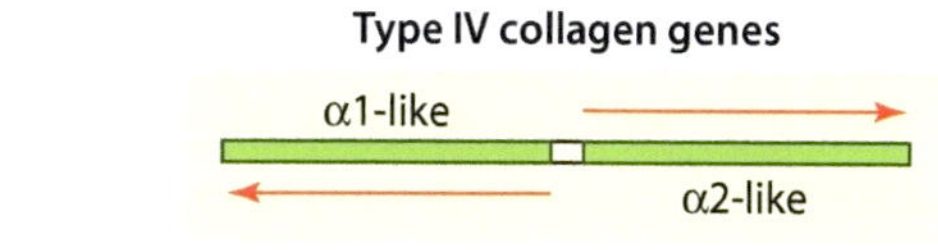

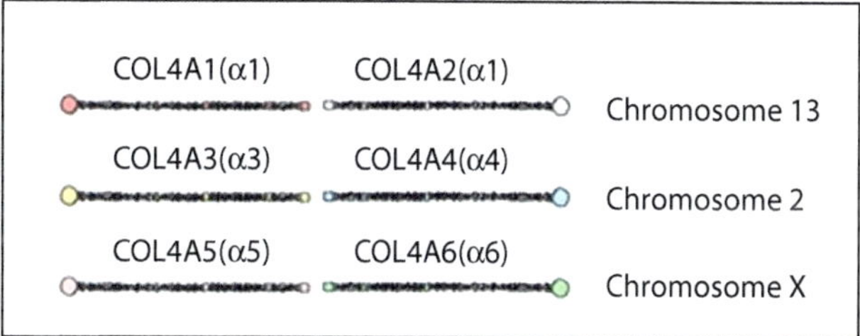

◘ **Fig. 62.1** The six type IV collagen genes and their chromosomal relationships. (Reproduced with permission from Neil Turner and ► www.edren.org)

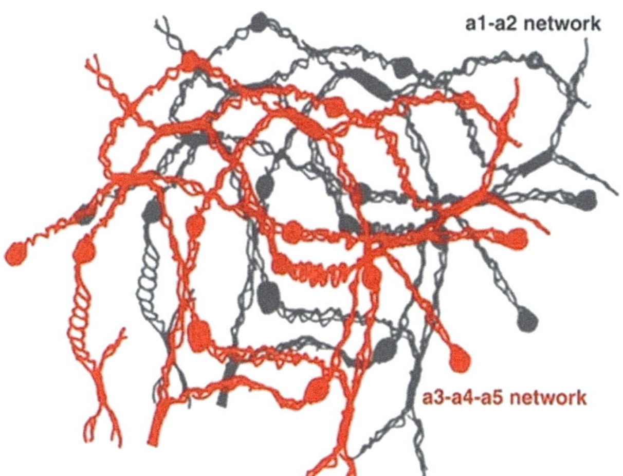

◘ **Fig. 62.2** Type IV collagen networks. The α3-α4-α5 is the major network in the GBM. (Reproduced with permission from Neil Turner and ► www.edren.org)

Laminins are large glycoproteins, made of one α, one β and one γ chain from the products of 5 *LAMA*, 4 *LAMB* and 3 *LAMC* genes. Laminin 521 (formed of the α5, β2 and γ1 chains) is the dominant component in adult GBM [1], but like collagen isoforms, this shifts developmentally, from 111 through 511 to the 521 network.

Laminins form a separate network in basement membranes that seems to assemble before the collagen network [1].

Nidogen (also known as entactin) is another universal component of basement membranes. It is a dumbbell-shaped molecule with two isoforms, nidogen 1 and 2, which can bind to both laminin and collagen. *NID* mutations have not yet been identified in human diseases, but deletion of both isoforms is lethal perinatally in mice and associated with abnormal basement membrane development [2].

The heparan sulphate proteoglycan (HSPG) *agrin* is the major HSPG in adult GBM. HSPGs are strongly anionic, giving an electronegative charge to GBM which has been thought to be functionally important. However, *AGRN* (agrin) mutations are associated with a congenital myasthenic syndrome but not renal disease.

Major conditions affecting the GBM are shown ◘ Table 62.1. This chapter considers only genetic causes.

Alport syndrome and thin basement membrane nephropathy are relatively common in renal practice. There is also a handful of rarer diseases.

62

62.2 Alport Syndrome

Is the prototypical basement membrane disease. In 1927, Cecil Alport described the condition that now bears his name, in a family with hereditary nephritis and deafness [3, 4].

◘ **Table 62.1** Diseases of the glomerular basement membrane

Inherited diseases of GBM	Acquired diseases of GBM
Alport syndrome	Anti-GBM (Goodpasture) disease
Thin basement membrane nephropathy	Fibrillary nephritis – deposition
Nail-patella syndrome	Inflammatory nephritis – holes in GBM
Pierson syndrome	
HANAC	

62.2.1 Epidemiology

Alport syndrome is the second only to ADPKD as most common inherited cause of renal failure. A prevalence of 1 in 5000 in Utah was reported in the late 1980s, but in most populations, the prevalence is much lower than this. Scandinavian studies found an incidence of 1 in 53,000 in Finland [5] and 1 in 17,000 in male births in southern Sweden. Europe-wide, the underlying primary renal disease is reported to be Alport syndrome in approximately 1% of patients reaching ESRF. In paediatric and adolescent populations, this proportion is closer to 2% [6].

Figures from the UK (◘ Fig. 62.3) are consistent with this and show that the proportion has remained stable over almost two decades, whilst the number of patients kept alive by dialysis and transplantation has only recently shown signs of plateauing.

62.2.2 Aetiology and Pathogenesis

The underlying defect in Alport syndrome is a mutation in one of the three genes encoding the α chains of the α345 type IV collagen molecule described above [3]. In the most common form of the disease, X-linked Alport syndrome, the mutation arises in the gene encoding the α5 chain, *COL4A5*, located on the long arm of the X chromosome.

62.2.2.1 X-Linked Alport Syndrome

Mutations in *COL4A5* were first described in the early 1990s [5] and paved the way for the discovery of hundreds of different mutations. A significant proportion of patients develop the disease as a result of de novo mutations. There are no documented hotspots, and most affected families carry unique mutations [7].

Jais (2000) [8] correlated the natural history of X-linked Alport syndrome with the type of underlying gene mutation in a large cohort of male patients. Large deletions, and nonsense mutations and frameshift mutations that led to early chain termination, were associated with a higher probability of reaching end-stage disease and hearing loss by the age of 30 than missense mutations. This has been confirmed by subsequent studies.

In X-linked Alport syndrome, affected men cannot give the disease to their sons, but all of their daughters will carry the affected gene. The offspring of these female carriers, male or female, have a one in two chance of inheriting the mutant gene.

Women who carry one copy of a defective *COL4A5* gene are at increased lifetime risk of developing significant renal disease. A few become severely affected, some

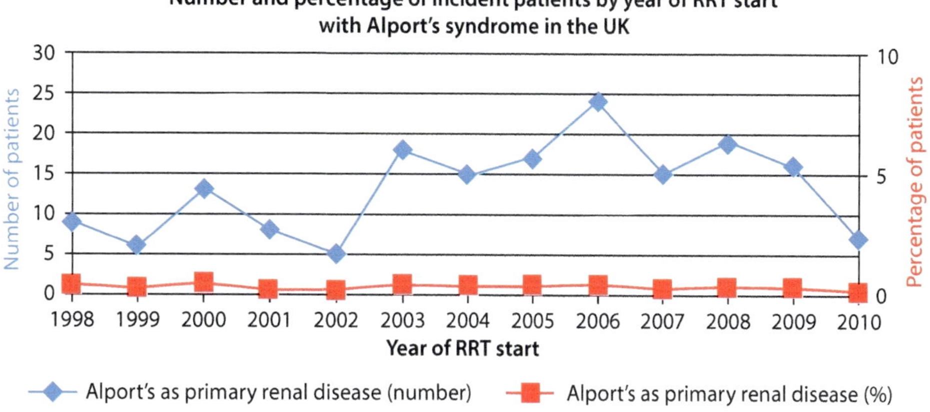

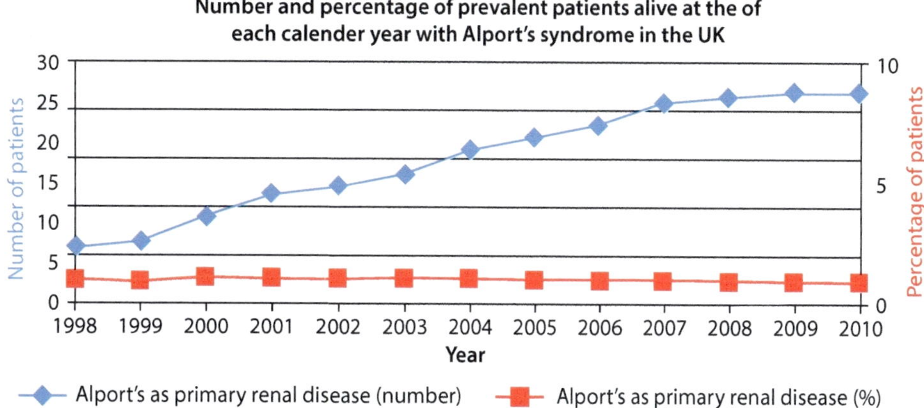

Fig. 62.3 Incidence and prevalence of Alport syndrome in UK RRT population. (Data from UK Renal Registry (▶ http://www.renalreg.com/))

developing significant manifestations in adolescence or early adulthood. This is discussed further below.

62.2.2.2 Autosomal Recessive Alport Syndrome

In the less common autosomal recessive form of the disease, the mutations occur in the genes encoding for the α3(IV) and α4(IV) chains, *COL4A3* or *COL4A4*, located on chromosome 2.

62.2.2.3 Having Both an Abnormal and a Normal Copy of an Autosomal Alport Gene

Carriers of abnormal autosomal Alport genes are at increased risk of renal disease. Although absolute risk is not characterised, the risk to autosomal carriers of *COL4A3/4* mutations seems probably less than that to female carriers of *COL4A5* mutations.

In some families, ESRF has occurred frequently enough that the label autosomal dominant has been applied. However, the disease in autosomal Alport single mutation carriers is generally much later in onset, usually weakly penetrant within families, and not consistently associated with deafness or other Alport features.

62.2.2.4 Unsuspected Alport Mutations

Through modern, less targeted genetic studies, unexpected Alport mutations are being reported repeatedly in two particular circumstances. The first is in those with familial renal disease without any characteristic features, where whole exome or whole genome sequencing has been carried out. Here, unexpected Alport mutations are a common or even the most frequent explanation (e.g [9].). The second is in nephrotic syndrome in childhood [10].

Reports are also appearing of various second mutations, often in a podocyte protein, that exacerbate the effect of a single *COL4* mutation.

62.2.3 Clinical Features

The genetic heterogeneity of Alport syndrome is reflected in the variable clinical course of the disease. The genetic basis and corresponding clinical features of Alport syndrome are summarised in Table 62.2. 'Classic' Alport syndrome refers to the X-linked disease in males and the autosomal recessive form in either sex.

Table 62.2 Incidence, affected gene and clinical features of Alport syndrome

Alport syndrome			
Inheritance	**Proportion of affected families**	**Affected gene**	**Clinical picture**
X-linked dominant	85%	*COL4A5*	Severe in male patients, progression to ESRF, high incidence of deafness
			No father-son transmission
			Variable course in females, with most never progressing to ESRF
Autosomal recessive	10–15%	*COL4A3/4*	Severe form of disease in homozygotes, male or female
			Haematuria in father of affected male
			Usually no overt disease in parents of patient
			Variable course in heterozygous carriers, rarely including progression to ESRF
Autosomal (other)	Uncertain	*COL4A3/4*	Male-to-male transmission
			Often no manifestations and when affected generally much milder than in X-linked or recessive disease
			Progression to ESRF (if at all) usually >50 years. No ocular involvement

62.2.4 Renal Disease

Persistent microscopic haematuria is the hallmark of classic Alport syndrome, when it is detectable in the first years of life. Episodes of macroscopic haematuria may occur in infancy or childhood. Dipstick haematuria is also found in 95% of female 'carriers' of X-linked disease [11].

Significant proteinuria typically appears in childhood or adolescence and becomes progressively more severe. It may become very severe. Nephrotic syndrome is increasingly recognised as a presenting feature, so that it is now appropriate to include *COL4* in gene panels for investigation of nephrotic syndrome in childhood [10].

In X-linked disease, affected males almost all eventually develop renal failure. The clinical course in autosomal recessive Alport syndrome for both males and females is essentially the same.

Other autosomal forms of Alport syndrome, including those labelled as autosomal dominant, generally have a more benign course. Progression to end-stage renal disease, if it occurs, is usually over the age of 50 years, and in most families, this is a very infrequent outcome [5, 12]. The co-inherited genes, or environmental factors that account for the increased incidence in some families, are the subject of current research.

62.2.5 Carriers and Heterozygotes

Female carriers of X-linked Alport syndrome had a significant rate of serious renal disease in Jais' 2003 study [7]: 12% progressed to end-stage renal failure by the age of 40 and 30% by the age of 60. These figures are likely to be higher than the true incidence because more severely affected individuals are more likely to be followed up, but most large centres have transplanted or dialysis patients with this background.

The phenotype for heterozygous carriers of autosomal recessive Alport syndrome is generally mild, but not consistently benign. Most are asymptomatic, and fewer seem to have microscopic haematuria. Comprehensive data is not yet available, but end-stage renal failure does occur with increased frequency in such carriers. Why should they have better outcomes than female carriers of X-linked disease? Perhaps the patchy absence of α5 expression (caused by lyonisation, the silencing of one X chromosome) is worse than consistent, evenly distributed under-expression.

Interestingly, there appears to be no correlation between the type of mutation and outcome in female carriers of X-linked disease. Perhaps a 'second hit' in these patients makes more difference than the underlying mutation.

The fact that autosomal mutations can occasionally cause dominantly expressed disease, albeit usually milder than classic Alport syndrome, suggests that there may be a gradation of mutation types and expression, or co-inheritance of other genes that influence outcome, or susceptibility to second hits to cause more severe renal damage. It is known that being a 'carrier' of an autosomal *COL4A3* or *COL4A4* mutation is associated with thin GBM nephropathy, which was historically characterised as a benign condition without long-term threat.

It is wise to be slightly guarded about long-term prognosis for carriers of mutations in autosomal *COL4* genes and definitely guarded about long-term prognosis for female carriers of *COL4A5* mutations.

62.2.6 Hearing Loss

The most common extra-renal manifestation is bilateral sensorineural deafness, the severity of which is variable. High-tone loss is the earliest change. Affected children are not born deaf; hearing loss is progressive during childhood or early adult years. In X-linked disease, 79% of males and 28% of females are said to be affected, although if females get hearing loss, it is usually much later. The degree of hearing impairment is varied too, but never complete, and with hearing aids, good communication is almost always preserved.

Males and females with autosomal Alport syndrome are affected in a similar manner to males with X-linked disease. The pathogenesis of hearing loss in Alport syndrome is not fully understood, but the 345 type IV collagen network is expressed in the cochlea.

62.2.7 Ocular

The most common eye finding is a dot-and-fleck retinopathy, which does not affect visual acuity [13]. Ocular involvement is seen in a third of males with X-linked disease; though as it is progressive, it depends on how severely affected or old the subject is when screened. Less common but much more specific is anterior lenticonus, in which the lens becomes misshapen as a consequence of thinning of the COL4A 345-containing lens capsule. This is typically a late change which occurs after years of renal failure. The retinopathy may be seen earlier, but it is often absent at the time the diagnosis is contemplated. It has been suggested that its appearance in a mutation-bearing parent may be helpful, though this has not been confirmed.

Ocular abnormalities have not been reported in non-recessive autosomal variants of Alport syndrome.

62.2.8 Contiguous Gene Syndromes

Leiomyomatosis is seen in a small proportion of patients with Alport syndrome, as a result of a large deletion involving the proximal (5′) end of the *COL4A5* gene which extends into the proximal part of the adjacent *COL4A6*. The oesophagus, tracheobronchial tree and female genital tract are affected [14]. As the leiomyomatosis component is dominantly expressed, female carriers are fully affected by it even when they have a mild renal phenotype.

AMEE (Alport syndrome, mental retardation, midface hypoplasia and elliptocytosis) is an even more rare contiguous gene deletion syndrome [11].

62.2.9 Differential Diagnosis

The principal differential diagnoses are other haematuric diseases, including TBMN, but also IgA nephropathy or other low-grade nephritis.

A common cause of mislabelling is the expectation of deafness at the time of presentation (it may only become apparent later) and the assumption that deafness with renal failure is always Alport syndrome. Other diseases in which deafness and renal failure occur are listed in ◘ Table 62.3.

◘ Table 62.3 Deafness and renal failure

Condition	Features
1. Alport syndrome	Progressive, high-tone deafness that is not present in early childhood *COL4A3-5* genes
2. Branchio-oto-renal syndrome	Renal hypoplasia or malformation. Other manifestations variable and may not be obvious: some or all of deafness, preauricular pits, abnormal pinnae, sinuses in the neck from branchial fistula (or scars from operation). *EYA*, *SIX1*, *SIX5* genes implicated
3. MYH9 mutations	Epstein-Fechtner syndrome; autosomal dominant renal disease – not necessarily glomerular?; with deafness, giant platelets. Epstein has no leucocyte inclusions, nor cataract formation
4. Mitochondrial DNA mutations	Look for other manifestations such as myopathy, diabetes and acidosis
5. Very small print	Other manifestations usually prominent; DIDMOAD syndrome with diabetes mellitus, diabetes insipidus, distal renal tubular acidosis with deafness, etc.
6. Coincidence	Deafness is the most common congenital abnormality

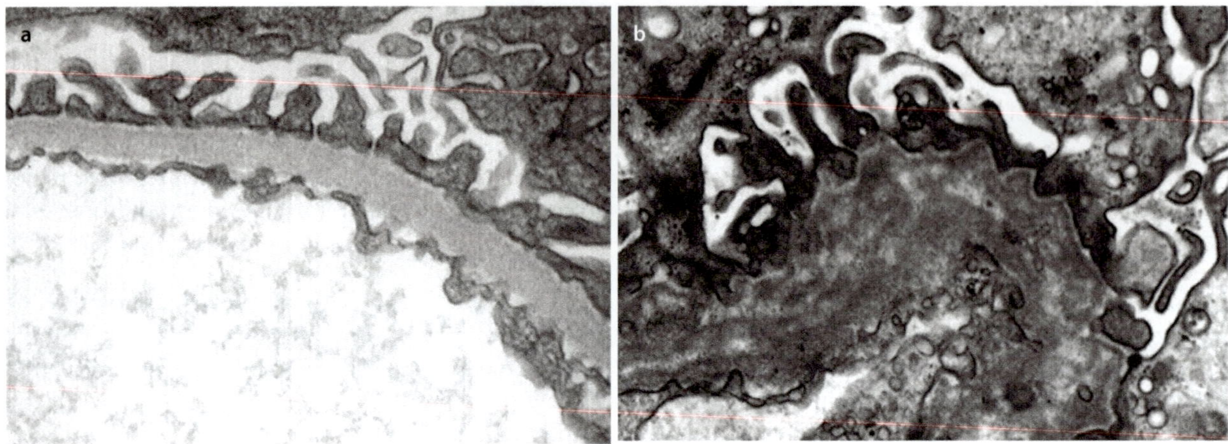

Fig. 62.4 Electron microscopy of the GBM in a normal kidney **a** and in Alport syndrome **b**

62.2.10 Investigations

Early diagnosis of Alport syndrome has become important now that there is evidence for benefit from treatment with ACE inhibitors [15].

Thirty years ago, criteria for diagnosing Alport syndrome for a research study were (1) positive family history, (2) sensorineural hearing loss, (3) ocular changes and (4) typical ultrastructural changes of the GBM [16]. Now however, modern genetic testing has reduced the primacy of both family history and biopsy. If you can demonstrate definitely pathogenic mutation(s) in COL4A3/4/5 in the presence of supportive features, family history and ultrastructure of glomeruli become optional.

Diagnoses in the clinical setting must now also be influenced by new appreciation of the wide range of effects associated with an Alport mutation beyond the classic Alport phenotype. Molecular testing is playing an increasing part.

Formal audiographic testing and ophthalmological referral have been historically recommended as part of diagnostic workup. But they are only reliable in most severe cases, which are often not the ones causing diagnostic difficulty. They are easy to justify if there are symptoms or signs.

62.2.11 Renal Biopsy

Light microscopy of glomerular tissue is mainly useful in ruling out other diagnoses. Changes seen are non-specific and in early disease may include podocyte hypertrophy and capillary wall stiffness. Focal segmental glomerulosclerosis (FSGS) is a common finding and is sometimes erroneously applied as a diagnostic label. Later in the disease process, diffuse glomerular sclerosis is seen.

In early disease, direct immunofluorescence studies are negative. Non-specific deposits of IgM and C3 may be seen in sclerosed glomeruli in more advanced disease [17].

Electron microscopy is required to demonstrate the sometimes dramatic changes in the GBM (Fig. 62.4). The normal architecture is destroyed, replaced by irregularly thickened GBM with multiple splits and lamellae. Not all patients exhibit such impressive ultrastructural changes, and those with earlier disease, or carriers, characteristically show thinning of the GBM. This can be the only abnormality in a significant proportion of adults with the disease, before irregular thickening, advancing to the characteristic and almost pathognomonic 'basket weave' pattern.

Indirect immunofluorescence for the presence of the (IV) collagen α3α4α5 network is possible and can be useful. In an affected patient, it may be negative for all three chains on architecturally preserved glomeruli, whilst positive on control sections. This means obtaining a biopsy early in the disease.

Presence of α3α4α5 chains cannot exclude the diagnosis however, as some mutations cause reduced level of α3α4α5 network rather than absence. Binding of antibodies to α3/4/5(IV) may be segmental in female carriers of X-linked disease, but is normal in carriers of autosomal disease and in patients with TBMN.

62.2.12 Genetic Testing

As newer techniques expand the possibilities and reduce the cost, genetic testing is rapidly becoming an integral part of diagnosing new families in developed countries. Sequencing of all three genes has become the current standard.

Genetic testing is not essential though. In many cases, the diagnosis and inheritance are obvious, and of course, the presence of a mutation does not preclude the presence of other conditions, so a renal biopsy may be necessary anyway. This perception is likely to shift further as the cost of genetic testing falls, and quality and experience rise, including discovery of genes associated with disease progression.

Genetic testing is most helpful in confirming a probable or likely diagnosis. It is less useful in 'possible' disease, as a negative result does not rule out the diagnosis. It is important to note that:

- Sequencing does not identify mutations in all cases, even when the diagnosis and inheritance pattern are certain. Success rate is however now high.
- As most mutations are unique to a family, the significance of a newly identified mutation may be uncertain. A large deletion or mutation affecting a key amino acid can be labelled as near-certain, but other types of mutation rely on computer prediction, analogy from other cases or in vitro studies. These may make a less certain prediction of relevance.

Once a mutation is identified in a family, it becomes much easier (and less costly) to identify other family members with the same mutation. This can also be done as an antenatal test or before implantation of embryos (preimplantation diagnosis).

Definite identification of carrier status is becoming valuable in screening potential living related donors. Both phenotype and long-term prognoses of carriers are variable (see above), so knowing the genetic status may be helpful in considering the risk of donation.

As more patients are sequenced, knowledge of the significance of gene variants is increasing rapidly. It is important that this knowledge is shared widely.

62.2.13 Skin Biopsy

As the 556 network of type IV collagen is expressed in epidermal basement membrane, it is an attractive idea that COL4A5 mutations (but not autosomal mutations, as α3 and α4 are not expressed in skin) could be detected by skin biopsy. Its use in diagnosis is however limited by technical difficulties and by the variability of α5(IV) expression in affected individuals [18].

Demonstration of α3(IV) or α5(IV) in glomeruli (see above) is more reliable if an early-stage biopsy is available, remembering that presence of antigen does not rule out the disease.

62.3 Treatment

62.3.1 Drug Therapy

Gross et al. published data in 2012 [15] implying substantial long-term benefits from the early use of ACE inhibitors in patients with AS. In this European longitudinal observational study of 283 patients with biopsy-proven or genetically identified AS, it seemed that males with X-linked AS, or homozygotes for autosomal AS, had end-stage renal failure substantially delayed by ACE inhibitors. Previous studies had demonstrated slowed progression in animal models.

Current recommendations [16] are to commence ACE inhibitors or angiotensin receptor blockers in any patient likely to have 'classic' Alport syndrome who has established proteinuria at any increased level, including children. Dose should be titrated to maximum tolerated, which may be less than full dose in young patients. Advice needs to be more nuanced in 'carriers' of abnormal Alport genes, in whom progression is likely to be slower, considering age, severity of proteinuria, whether any GFR has been lost and possibility of pregnancy.

The mechanism of action of ACE inhibitors in Alport syndrome is not fully understood, but may go beyond their well-recognised anti-hypertensive and anti-proteinuric effects. To date, no other therapies have been shown to improve outcome in man, but several add-on alternatives are under active consideration or study, including targeted genetic interventions.

62.3.2 Renal Transplantation

Patients with Alport syndrome benefit from renal transplantation with good long-term outcomes [19]. Recurrence of Alport syndrome in the transplanted kidney does not occur, providing the organ donor does not have the disease. However, two specific issues arise.

62.3.2.1 Living Donation

The use of Alport (usually female) carriers as live kidney donors to their affected relatives seems risky in the light of long-term data on risk to female carriers, but transplants have taken place [6]. Although it seems a less than perfect option, it could be considered in older donors with no proteinuria (in women, usually after child-bearing years) and if both donor and recipient fully understand and accept the increased risk of renal failure.

62.3.2.2 Post-transplant Anti-GBM Nephritis

This rare but devastating complication of renal transplantation in Alport syndrome was first described in 1982 [20], was always rare (probably well below 5%) but now seems to be even more rare. It is a consequence of the recipient generating an immune response to a molecule in the donor kidney that they have not encountered before. It is more likely if the underlying genetic defect is a gene deletion, so that the recipient has seen no protein, rather than a slightly changed one. In line with that, the target is usually the collagen chain that is affected by the mutation. As this is usually α5(IV), the resulting antibodies are likely to be different from the anti-α3 antibodies of spontaneous, autoimmune anti-GBM (Goodpasture) disease and may not be identified by specific anti-GBM antibody assays [21].

Immunofluorescence of the renal biopsy reveals that antibody fixation to the GBM is relatively common and in most cases is not associated with glomerular damage and does not progress to anti-GBM nephritis. Binding to Bowman's capsule is typically strong if antibodies are anti-α5 chain, whereas this membrane contains less α3(IV) than GBM as the Col(IV) 56 network is found here.

When the disease occurs, it is typically diagnosed months to years after a first transplant, weeks to months after a second and days to weeks after a third. There are haematuria and subsequently often proteinuria, with progressive graft dysfunction that is often initially attributed to rejection. Crescentic nephritis is seen, but lung haemorrhage is not a feature, in contrast to classic anti-GBM disease.

Once identified (usually late), the prognosis for graft survival is very poor, with failure ensuing in near to 90%. The risk of developing the disease again increases with subsequent transplants as described by Browne et al. [21]. In 16 cases of retransplantation, anti-GBM nephritis was seen in 15, with 12 of those grafts damaged irretrievably. Patients seeking retransplantation in this context, and their clinicians, need to be made fully aware of the slim chances of success.

No treatment has been proven to be effective, though sometimes recurrences have been unaccountably less severe and therapy apparently has been more effective. The use of anti-B-cell therapies apart from cyclophosphamide has not been extensively reported, but almost every other option has.

62.3.3 Thin Basement Membrane Nephropathy

Thin basement membrane nephropathy (TBMN) is a disorder in which the GBM is uniformly thinned. The earliest description is likely to date from 1926 [22]. In the past, it was commonly known as 'benign familial haematuria', though we now know that the condition does not always run a benign course.

62.3.4 Epidemiology

This condition is common. Though it is difficult to know the precise prevalence, it has been estimated to be 1%, though post-mortem and transplant data (definitely not synonymous with the general population) have suggested up to 9% [4, 23]. TBMN is the most common inherited renal condition and the most common cause of persistent glomerular haematuria. It is estimated that it is the underlying diagnosis in about a quarter of patients referred to nephrology services for investigation of asymptomatic haematuria [24].

62.3.5 Clinical Features

Microscopic haematuria is the sine qua non of TMN. Episodes of gross haematuria and flank pain also feature in some patients. Proteinuria is not a typical finding in children. Detectable proteinuria may occur in adults, hinting that this is not necessarily a benign condition. However, in the majority of cases, the disease does not lead to significant renal impairment. In a very small number of cases, progressive renal failure has been described without other obvious explanation. In contrast to Alport syndrome and the other rare inherited GBM diseases, extra-renal manifestations are not generally seen in TMN.

62.3.6 Differential Diagnosis

The differential diagnosis of TMN includes any condition that can cause isolated haematuria and therefore can be the early stage of any inflammatory glomerulonephritis. IgA nephropathy is the most likely alternative diagnosis in Europe. Alport syndrome should also be considered, and a family history sought. C3 hereditary nephritis, described in several Cypriot families, should also be considered in the differential of a familial haematuric syndrome [25].

62.3.7 Investigation

Histologically, there is thinning of the basement membrane in the absence of any other morphological changes. Normal GBM thickness is in the range of 350–450 nm. In TMN, this is reduced to less than 250 nm in greater than 50% of the GBM [26]. These findings are similar to those seen in early Alport syndrome, but distinct to the gross distortion of architecture seen later in some patients with Alport syndrome.

A genetic linkage to the *COL4A3* or *COL4A4* locus was identified in 40% of families with TBMN in one research study [27]. Matching mutations have been found in autosomal recessive Alport syndrome. Patients with TBMN who have such mutations can be regarded as carriers of the recessive form of Alport syndrome, with the less certain prognosis described above, and as studies of selected families who carry single copies of autosomal COL4 mutations sometimes show (above). However, the linkage studies, and unpublished observations, suggest that many cases of TBMN are not linked to Alport syndrome genes, and other explanations must pertain.

Perhaps we need to understand the condition better before genetic testing becomes a standard part of its investigation of TBMD. The balance of utility could change if there was proteinuria or loss of function, providing a stronger possibility of a diagnosis of Alport syndrome. That distinction may otherwise be difficult in the absence of a clear family history.

Immunohistochemical analysis of the distribution of type IV collagen chains has the disadvantages outlined under Alport syndrome.

62.3.8 Management

There is no specific treatment, though in the light of newer uncertainty about long-term prognosis, as outlined above for Alport carriers, long-term monitoring is indicated, e.g. annual blood pressure, urinalysis and occasional creatinine measurement, not necessarily by a nephrologist.

The uncertain long-term outcome of those who do have heterozygous *COL4* mutations, described above, suggests that if there is significant proteinuria, there are good reasons to favour ACE inhibitors [16]. More is likely to be learned in the future about underlying causes and outcomes in those without such mutations or where it is not yet studied. The same mostly upbeat, but slightly guarded, long-term prognosis, and recommendation for continuing occasional monitoring, applies to both.

62.3.9 Nail-Patella Syndrome (Hereditary Osteo-onychodysplasia)

Nail-patella syndrome (NPS) is a rare, autosomal dominant inherited condition in which renal involvement affects only a minority, but sometimes severely. Descriptions of patients with clinical findings similar to those seen in NPS date back to the early nineteenth century. The incidence is thought to be around 1 in 50,000 live births [28].

Nails and patellae exhibit some of the most striking changes, but other common abnormalities are outlined in ◘ Table 62.4.

Sweeney et al. looked at a group of 123 patients with NPS [29] and identified end-stage renal disease in only 2%. The prevalence is likely to have risen because of the availability of renal replacement therapy: proteinuria was much more common.

◘ Table 62.4 Clinical features of nail-patella syndrome

Nails	Dysplastic or hypoplastic nails, mainly affecting the thumbs and index fingers
Skeletal	Underdeveloped or absent patellae
	Elbow contracture
	Iliac horns (visible on X-rays)
Renal	Fibrillar collagen bundles within the GBM
Eyes	Open-angle glaucoma

The implicated gene is LMX1B, found on chromosome 9. LMX1B is a transcription factor that influences expression of multiple glomerular genes.

Light microscopy of renal tissue shows subtle and non-specific changes, the most common being focal thickening of the GBM. Electron microscopy is required to reveal the abnormal accumulation of fibrillar type III collagen in the GBM and mesangium. Type III collagen is an interstitial collagen not normally found in the kidneys. Renal disease in NPS is associated with abnormal accumulation of non-glomerular basement membrane components, unlike Alport syndrome where the defect is in a molecule native to the GBM.

62.3.9.1 LMX1B Mutations Without NPS

LMX1B is another gene that is being unexpectedly identified in the absence of recognised extra-renal features in blind sequencing approaches to the investigation of familial renal disease (e.g [30].).

62.3.10 *Laminin* Mutations, Pierson Syndrome and Proteinuria

In 1963, Pierson described siblings with eye abnormalities, congenital nephrotic syndrome and rapid development of end-stage renal failure. Forty years later, the genetic defect was localised to the *LAMB2* gene encoding the β2 chain of laminin [26], part of the dominant laminin 521 isoform that is the major laminin of adult GBM. β2 laminin is also found in other locations that mirror the clinical manifestations. Several ocular abnormalities have been described, with microcoria (fixed constriction of the pupil) being the most characteristic finding.

The original cohort described in the 1960s had severe disease, often fatal in infancy, but it is now appearing that milder mutations may have less florid systemic, predominantly renal phenotypes and indeed potential to exacerbate *COL4* mutations [31]. A role for LAMA5 mutations in proteinuric renal disease is also being suggested [32].

62.3.11 *COL4A1* Mutations and HANAC

Hereditary angiopathy with nephropathy, aneurysms and cramps (HANAC) has been associated with mutations in the COL4A1 gene, encoding the ubiquitous α1-chain of type IV collagen. Because this is such a universal and core basement membrane component, it understandable that only minor mutations are compatible with life.

Plaisier and colleagues [33] described a complex phenotype in which the renal manifestations were a relatively minor component and included haematuria, decreased GFR and renal cysts. Histological and ultrastructural analysis revealed normal appearances of the GBM, but the basement membranes of Bowman's capsule, renal tubules and interstitial capillaries showed irregular thickening and splitting. HANAC is therefore not a disease of the GBM itself, but of other basement membranes within the kidney.

HANAC should be considered in the differential diagnosis of unexplained haematuria in a 'syndromic' patient. Rare mutations associated with renal disease without obvious systemic phenotypes have been identified for this gene too [27].

62

Chapter Review Questions

1. What are the top 5 causes to explain deafness with renal failure?
2. What simple information do you want that could be very helpful?
3. What is the best diagnostic approach here?
4. What is the relevance of his mother remembering an episode of painless macroscopic haematuria as a baby?
5. What would you expect his urine to show now?
6. What do you think of her blood pressure?
7. What are the key differential diagnoses?
8. Why doesn't she have primary FSGS?
9. What management would you recommend and what advice would you give?
10. What is her long-term prognosis?
11. What could make the risk less (or more) acceptable?

Answers

1. Alport syndrome, branchio-oto-renal syndrome, Fechtner/Epstein syndrome (MYH9 mutation). Coincidence, especially if deafness congenital. Aminoglycosides – (Has anyone ever seen that with current aminoglycosides?)
2. Urine dipstick for clues to nature of renal disease
3. Repeat family history; urine dipstick parents and siblings. If positive for blood, consider renal biopsy (in relative) or genetic testing (in him).
4. This is a characteristic feature of Alport syndrome.
5. Probably still substantial blood and protein
6. It's normal for 17, a little below the 50th centile for a woman of that age.
7. Glomerulonephritis (IgA most likely); thin GBM nephropathy; Alport syndrome
8. Haematuria and not nephrotic
9. ACE inhibitor to max tolerated dose, long-term. Stop in pregnancy. Discuss contraception. Discuss risks of pregnancy whilst proteinuric another time.
10. Regardless of the underlying diagnosis and GFR, a PCR of 160 in your teens gives you a high chance of ESRF in later life. ACEi may reduce that.
11. Tubes tied or post-menopausal (no risk of stress from further pregnancies); no other renal risk factors; urgent need for renal transplant and no other donors

References

1. Miner JH. The glomerular basement membrane. Exp Cell Res. 2012;318(9):973–8.
2. Lennon R, Turner AN. Chapter 320 The molecular basis of GBM disorders. In: Turner AN, et al., editors. Oxford textbook of clinical nephrology. Oxford: OUP; 2015.
3. Alport AC. Hereditary familial congenital haemorrhagic nephritis. Br Med J. 1927;1:504–6.
4. Kashtan C. Alport syndrome and thin BM nephropathy. GeneReviews 2001, revised Nov 2015. www.ncbi.nlm.nih.gov/books/NBK1207.
5. Savige J, Ariani F, Mari F, et al. Expert consensus guidelines for the genetic diagnosis of Alport syndrome. Pediatr Nephrol. 2018. https://doi.org/10.1007/s00467-018-3985-4. [Epub ahead of print].
6. Gross O, Weber M, Fries JW, Müller GA. Living donor kidney transplantation from relatives with mild urinary abnormalities in Alport syndrome: long-term risk, benefit and outcome. Nephrol Dial Transplant. 2009;24(5):1626–30.
7. Jais JP, Knebelmann B, Giatras I, et al. X-linked Alport syndrome: natural history and genotype-phenotype correlations in girls and women belonging to 195 families: a "European Community Alport Syndrome Concerted Action" study. J Am Soc Nephrol. 2003;14(10):2603–10.
8. Jais JP, et al. X-linked Alport: natural history in 195 families and genotype-phenotype correlations in males. J Am Soc Nephrol. 2000;11:649–57.
9. Lin F, Bian F, Zou J, Wu X, et al. Whole exome sequencing reveals novel COL4A3 and COL4A4 mutations and resolves diagnosis in Chinese families with kidney disease. BMC Nephrol. 2014;15:175. https://doi.org/10.1186/1471-2369-15-175.
10. McCarthy HJ, RADAR the UK SRNS Study Group. Simultaneous sequencing of 24 genes associated with steroid-resistant nephrotic syndrome. Clin J Am Soc Nephrol. 2013;8(4):637–48. https://doi.org/10.2215/CJN.07200712. Epub 2013 Jan 24.
11. Vitelli F, Piccini M, Caroli F, Franco B, et al. Identification and characterization of a highly conserved protein absent in the

Alport syndrome (A), mental retardation (M), midface hypoplasia (M), and elliptocytosis (E) contiguous gene deletion syndrome (AMME). Genomics. 1999;55(3):335–40.

12. Pescucci C, Mari F, Longo I, Vogiatzi P, Caselli R, Scala E, Abaterusso C, Gusmano R, Seri M, Miglietti N, Bresin E, Renieri A. Autosomal-dominant Alport syndrome: natural history of a disease due to COL4A3 or COL4A4 gene. Kidney Int. 2004;65(5):1598–603.
13. Tan R, Colville D, Wang YY, Rigby L, Savige J. Alport retinopathy results from “severe” COL4A5 mutations and predicts early renal failure. Clin J Am Soc Nephrol. 2010;5(1):34–8.
14. Garcia-JTorres R, Cruz D, Orozco L, Heidet L, Gubler MC. Alport syndrome and diffuse leiomyomatosis. Clinical aspects, pathology, molecular biology and extracellular matrix studies. A synthesis. Nephrologie. 2000;21(1):9–12.
15. Gross O, Licht C, Anders HJ, et al. Early angiotensin-converting enzyme inhibition in Alport syndrome delays renal failure and improves life expectancy. Kidney Int. 2012;81(5):494–501.
16. Alport study group. Alport Syndrome – clinician recommendations. https://rarerenal.org/clinician-information/alport-syndrome. Accessed 30 July 2020.
17. Heidet L, Gubler MC. The renal lesions of Alport syndrome. J Am Soc Nephrol. 2009;20(6):1210–5.
18. van der Loop FT, Monnens LA, Schröder CH, Lemmink HH, Breuning MH, Timmer ED, Smeets HJ. Identification of COL4A5 defects in Alport’s syndrome by immunohistochemistry of skin. Kidney Int. 1999;55(4):1217–24.
19. Kashtan CE. Renal transplantation in patients with Alport syndrome. Pediatr Transplant. 2006;10(6):651–7.
20. McCoy RC, Johnson HK, Stone WJ, Wilson CB. Absence of nephritogenic GBM antigen(s) in some patients with hereditary nephritis. Kidney Int. 1982;21(4):642–52.
21. Browne G, Brown PA, Tomson CR, Fleming S, Allen A, Herriot R, Pusey CD, Rees AJ, Turner AN. Retransplantation in Alport post-transplant anti-GBM disease. Kidney Int. 2004;65(2):675–81.
22. Baehr G. Benign and curable form of hemorrhagic nephritis. JAMA. 1926;86:1001–4.
23. Tryggvason K, Patrakka J. Thin basement membrane nephropathy. J Am Soc Nephrol. 2006;17(3):813–22.
24. Topham P, Feehally J. Chapter 21.8.2 Thin membrane nephropathy. In: David AW, Timothy MC, John DF, editors. Oxford textbook of medicine. 5th ed. Oxford/New York: Oxford University Press; 2010.
25. Gale DP, et al. Identification of a mutation in complement factor H-related protein 5 in patients of Cypriot origin with glomerulonephritis. Lancet. 2010;376:794–801.
26. Zenker M, et al. Human laminin β2 deficiency causes congenital nephrosis with mesangial sclerosis and distinct eye abnormalities (Pierson syndrome). Hum Mol Genet. 2004;13:2625–32.
27. Gale DP, Oygar DD, Lin F, et al. A novel COL4A1 frameshift mutation in familial kidney disease: the importance of the C-terminal NC1 domain of type IV collagen. Nephrol Dial Transplant. 2016;31:1908–14.
28. Bongers EM, Gubler MC, Knoers NV. Nail-patella syndrome. Overview on clinical and molecular findings. Pediatr Nephrol. 2002;17(9):703–12.
29. Sweeney E, Fryer AE, Mountford RC, Green AJ, McIntosh I. Nail Patella Syndrome: a study of 123 patients from 43 British families and the detection of 16 novel mutations of LMX1B. Am J Hum Genet. 2001;69(Suppl):A72.
30. Edwards N, Rice SJ, Raman S, et al. A novel LMX1B mutation in a family with end-stage renal disease of ‘unknown cause’. Clin Kidney J. 2015;8:113–9.
31. Funk SD, Lin MH, Miner JH. Alport syndrome and Pierson syndrome: diseases of the glomerular basement membrane. Matrix Biol. 2018;71-2:250–61.
32. Braun DA, Warejko JK, Ashraf S, et al. Genetic variants in the LAMA5 gene in pediatric nephrotic syndrome. Nephrol Dial Transplant. 2019;34:485–93.
33. Plaisier E, Gribouval O, Alamowitch S, et al. COL4A1 mutations and hereditary angiopathy, nephropathy, aneurysms, and muscle cramps. N Engl J Med. 2007;357(26):2687–95.

Online Resources

www.rarerenal.org/clinician-information/alport-syndrome Part of the UK Strategy for Rare Kidney Diseases. Offers advice for clinicians and patients.

www.ncbi.nlm.nih.gov/books/NBK1207 GeneReviews on Alport and Thin BM Nephropathy. (Cliff Kashtan).

www.ncbi.nlm.nih.gov/books/NBK1132 GeneReviews on Nail Patella Syndrome. (Elizabeth Sweeney et al).

www.npsuk.org Patient-run site for Nail Patella Syndrome.

www.ncbi.nlm.nih.gov/books/NBK7046 GeneReviews on COL4A1-related disorders (Emmanuelle Plaisier and Pierre Ronco).

Anderson-Fabry Disease and Other Inherited Lipid Disorders of the Kidney

Thuvaraka Ware and Shabbir H. Moochhala

Contents

M. Harber (ed.), *Primer on Nephrology*, https://doi.org/10.1007/978-3-030-76419-7_63

Learning Objectives

1. To list the different ways AFD can affect the kidneys
2. To recognise the multisystemic features which might be diagnostic clues for AFD
3. To understand the challenges to a timely diagnosis and principles of multidisciplinary management

63.1 Introduction

Anderson-Fabry disease (AFD) is the second-most common of the lysosomal storage disorders (after Gaucher's disease) and the one most typically characterised by renal involvement.

It is a rare disease with a wide, multisystemic spectrum of clinical presentations. It is therefore important to consider it in the differential diagnosis of most patients with renal disease of unknown cause.

63.2 Pathophysiology

AFD is an X-linked, inherited disorder of the lysosomal enzyme *alpha-galactosidase A*. In the disease state, mutations in the *GLA* gene that codes for this enzyme result in a reduction in enzyme activity and intracellular accumulation of globotriaosylceramide (*Gb3*), a glycosphingolipid. This is responsible for the multisystem pathology seen in AFD.

Although the inheritance pattern was once considered to be X-linked recessive, and therefore the disease affecting males only, it is now recognised that reduced enzyme activity has significant pathological consequences even in females who carry one mutated and one wild-type copy of the GLA gene [1]. The phenotype in females is unpredictable but less severe as a rule (see Clinical Presentations, below). A case report [2] suggests the same genotype mutation in related family members can also present with variable renal pathology.

63.3 Epidemiology

AFD is underdiagnosed (see Diagnosis, below) and the true prevalence is not known. Estimates vary dramatically depending on the population and the method of analysis.

- An Italian screening study found (potentially disease-causing) GLA gene mutations in *1 in 3100* male neonates [3].
- An Australian study comparing the diagnosis rate of AFD with the birth rate for the same population group estimated a prevalence of *1 in 117,000* [4].
- A prospective, multicentre screening study in Argentina found the prevalence in their male dialysis cohort (9604 patients) to be *1 in 500* [5].

These numbers need to be taken with a pinch of salt: all of the large series are in Caucasian populations, and most of them only estimate male prevalence.

63.4 Clinical Features

AFD can be thought of as a glycolipid-associated multisystem vasculopathy. Glycosphingolipid deposits can be found in microscopic examination of most tissue types in AFD which explains the multisystemic manifestations seen in affected patients (Fig. 63.1). This includes cutaneous (Fig. 63.2), cardiovascular, neurological and cerebrovascular sequelae as well as renal. On pathological examination of the kidney, glycosphingolipid deposits are principally concentrated around the glomerulus and distal tubule [6]. As might be predicted therefore, the typical renal presentation is of isolated proteinuria and occasionally a urinary concentrating defect or Fanconi syndrome, in a young male, followed by progressive chronic kidney disease.

In the Fabry Outcome Survey (FOS) of 366 European patients with AFD, renal signs and symptoms were reported in 50% of patients. Proteinuria was observed in 44% of males and 33% of females [7]. Renal prognosis is variable between population studies and even within families. In a UK-only study of 98 hemizygous adult males (84% of whom had proteinuria), end-stage renal disease was present in 30%, whereas in FOS, it was seen in only 17% of adult males [8].

63.5 Diagnosis

This represents a challenge, as the vast majority of patients are not diagnosed at first presentation. In the Fabry Outcome Survey, the mean delay to diagnosis from initial symptom onset was 13 years for males and 17 years for females. For this reason, the most pressing clinical challenge is to consider the diagnosis in a wider cohort of patients [9]. Previously attention focused on diagnosis of AFD in dialysis patients, but these studies uniformly show diagnosis rates of <1% [10]. This compares to rates of 3–11% in patients with hypertrophic cardiomyopathy as their presentation.

In addition to those with a recognised family history, nephrologists should consider diagnostic testing for AFD in all patients with a typical renal presentation and

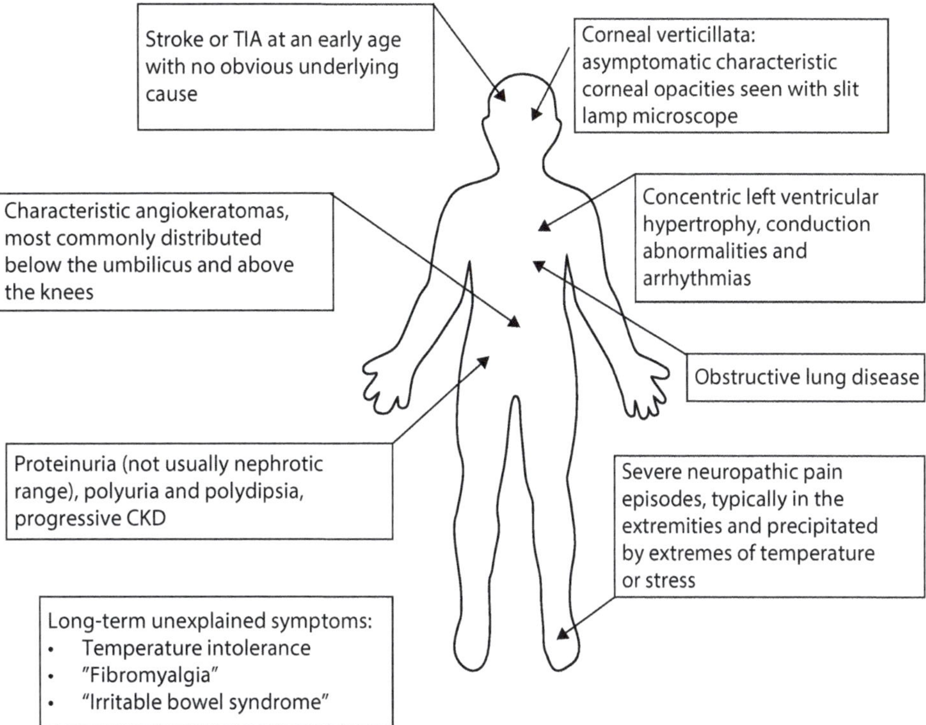

Fig. 63.1 Clinical manifestations of AFD

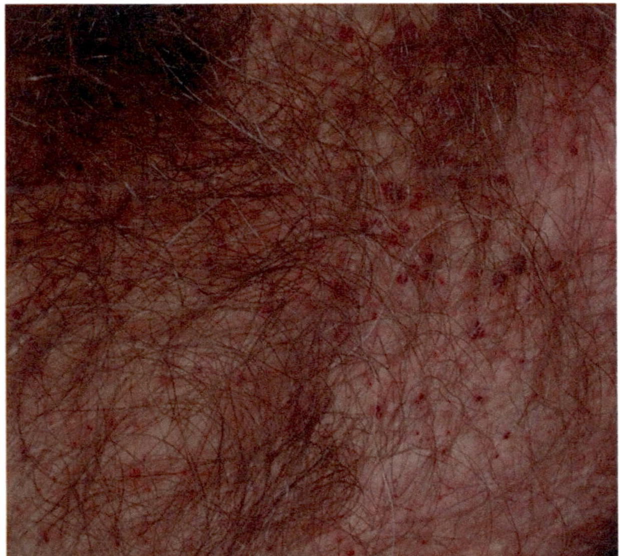

Fig. 63.2 Perineal angiokeratoma (see also ► Chap. 40)

one or more additional features as below. Often patients will have pre-existing diagnostic labels (e.g. chronic pain, fibromyalgia, irritable bowel syndrome) which might be a clue. This can also apply to renal diagnoses where there is no histopathology (e.g. ischaemic nephropathy, hypertensive renal disease). See Fig. 63.3 for a guide on when and how to test for AFD. A more comprehensive diagnostic algorithm for nephrologists is available at ► https://rarerenal.org/wp-content/uploads/2019/04/RA-RareRenal-Fabry-diagnosis-algorithm.pdf.

63.6 Investigations

63.6.1 Urine

Proteinuria is usually seen on dipstick. Nephrotic range proteinuria is rare. Oval fat bodies in the urine can often be seen as "Maltese crosses" under polarised light. This is a cheap, readily available and non-invasive test [11]. A cohort study of 39 AFD patients showed that podocyturia may be present prior to proteinuria [12].

63.6.2 Blood

Diagnosis is usually made by enzymatic activity testing in males. Variable phenotype means that these tests have much lower sensitivity in females and genetic analysis is normally required. In the UK, genetic testing for AFD is currently funded by industry partners when accessed via any of the 12 regional lysosomal storage disorders units or can be obtained via local clinical genetics services. The preferred enzymatic assay is leucocyte alpha-GAL-A activity (more sensitive than plasma activity). This is expressed as a percentage of normal. All affected men will have activity <35%, and the majority will have undetectable activity [13]. Suspected cases in women without a clear family history (or those with a family history and hoping to donate a kidney) should have molecular sequencing of the entire *GLA* gene, as most families have "private" mutations.

Fig. 63.3 When and how to test for AFD

Renal presentation
- Proteinuria
- Chronic kidney disease
- Urinary concentrating defect

Additional features
- Unexplained intermittent pain episodes (particularly abdominal or in the extremities)
- Intolerance to extreme temperatures or disorders of sweating
- Cutaneous vascular lesions
- Cardiac abnormalities under the age of 55 (particularly LVH or conduction defects)
- Stroke under the age of 55
- A family history of any kidney dysfunction of unknown aetiology or heart disease at young age
- Renal sinus cysts (yarapelvic cysts)

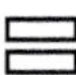

Tests
Males: Leucocyte alpha-GAL-A activity <35% normal
Females: GLA gene sequencing

63.6.3 Eyes

Referral for an ophthalmology opinion is appropriate in all cases where AFD is a possibility as verticillata (detectable on corneal slit lamp examination) is present in all affected males and most female carriers and they may also detect early cataracts.

63

63.6.4 Imaging

Renal sinus cysts (also known as parapelvic cysts) on ultrasound are seen in about 50% of patients with AFD.

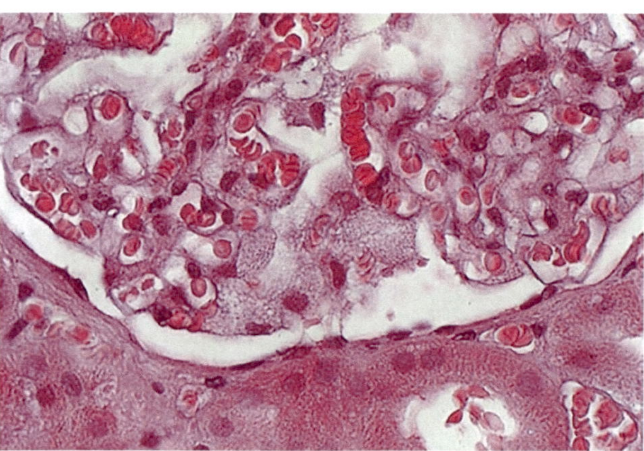

Fig. 63.4 Light microscopy showing characteristic showing enlargement of podocytes filled with clear vacuoles

63.6.5 Histopathology

As the diagnosis can be confirmed in both men and women on peripheral blood, there is no clear diagnostic role for renal biopsy. This should be reserved for cases where a second renal diagnosis is suspected in addition once the diagnosis of AFD is confirmed on blood (e.g. where there is severe nephrotic syndrome or rapidly progressive renal dysfunction).

However, as AFD disease is not often considered as the cause of proteinuric CKD, in some cases, it appears as an unexpected pathological diagnosis. Light microscopy shows foamy vacuoles in the podocytes and distal tubular epithelial cells (Fig. 63.4), and electron microscopy shows Gb3 deposits directly as membrane-bound lamellated structures known as "zebra bodies" [6] (Fig. 63.5). If electron microscopy is not available, then ask for toluidine blue staining, as this demonstrates glycolipid inclusion bodies.

63.7 Management

The two most important treatments in managing Fabry nephropathy are combined enzyme replacement and RAS inhibition. There are now some data from non-

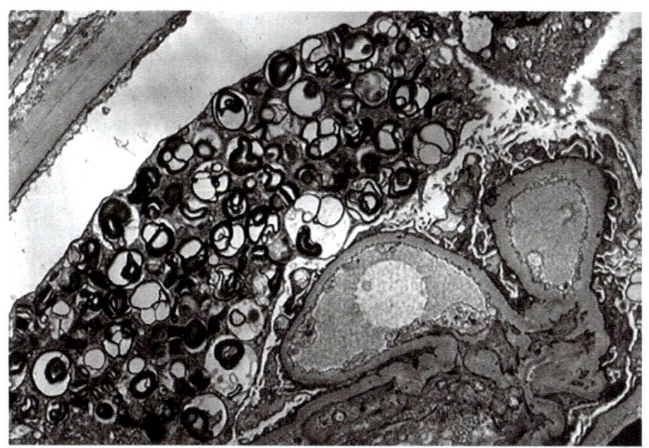

Fig. 63.5 Electron micrograph image showing the pathognomonic inclusions in lysosomes of multi-layered glycosphingolipids known as zebra bodies

controlled trials showing that RAS inhibitors reduce the rate of decline in GFR due to Fabry disease. Maximising RAS inhibition aiming for minimising proteinuria reduced GFR decline from 7.0 to 3.6 ml/min/yr [14]. There is growing evidence that disease-modifying enzyme replacement therapy may slow progression (see below), but in general, the strategies used in all CKD (e.g. control of hypertension and reduction of proteinuria with RAS blockade) are applicable. Clinical guidelines are available from KDIGO [15] and ERBP [16]. These advise patients to be managed in multidisciplinary expert centres, treat CKD and albuminuria according to standard guidelines and perform renal biopsy either for diagnostic purposes (e.g. if coexisting pathology is suspected) or as part of a clinical trial.

Care should be taken to monitor non-CKD renal outcomes. The incidence of urinary tract malignancy was nearly twice the rate expected in the general population, and the incidence of renal malignancy was three times this rate [17]. For this reason, we recommend monitoring for new-onset haematuria and a low threshold for renal imaging if there are suggestive symptoms.

63.8 Renal Replacement Therapy

63.8.1 Dialysis

Survival of AFD patients on haemo- or peritoneal dialysis is lower than in the dialysis population as a whole. European registry data up to 1994 estimated 3-year survival at 60% compared with 78% in the general dialysis population of comparable age [14]. The excess mortality appears to be attributable to cardiovascular risk associated with the disease.

63.8.2 Transplantation

Renal transplantation has been widely used in patients with ESRD due to AFD and is the preferred modality of renal replacement. The disease does not recur in the graft, but renal transplantation does not supply enough normal enzyme to ameliorate extra-renal manifestations. Graft survival in AFD patients is comparable to that in other non-diabetic ESRD cohorts. Patient survival is comparable to non-AFD patients (in a study with follow-up over 25 years; median follow-up 11.5 years) [18]. Excess mortality is due to increased cardiac and cerebrovascular risk. Given the variable clinical phenotype within families, genetic screening of potential live related donors is important, even where the donor is asymptomatic.

63.9 Enzyme Replacement Therapy (ERT)

There are two forms of recombinant alpha-galactosidase A commercially available for the treatment of AFD:

- Agalsidase alpha (from a genetically engineered human cell line)
- Agalsidase beta (from a hamster ovary cell line)

They are both given as an intravenous infusion every 2 weeks. In 2016, an oral pharmacological chaperone (migalastat) was licensed which can stabilise the activity of up to 30–50% of the mutant forms of alpha-galactosidase. Enzyme replacement therapy (ERT) is very expensive: £125,000/year per patient in the UK as of 2012. Furthermore, as with many rare diseases, the evidence base for its efficacy is limited. There have been at least 5 randomised, placebo-controlled trials in ERT for AFD including a total of approximately 200 patients. These trials have provided clear pathological evidence that ERT reduces disease activity but none of them have included renal outcomes in their primary analysis. Open-label extension of some of these trials has shown a trend towards reduced rate of renal progression (or a rate comparable to the normal population) if treated with ERT [19, 20]. It is important to note that some non-renal symptoms are more responsive to ERT than others, especially in children.

The Fabry Outcome Survey (FOS) of 560 male patients receiving ERT showed that lower baseline eGFR was associated with worse progression of renal disease compared to patients with a better baseline renal function [21]. Whilst this suggests patients who start ERT prior to significant renal impairment may derive the most benefit from it, the quality and rigour of this data is limited by the selection and reporting biases to which industry-sponsored surveys are subject. The benefits from ERT may also be difficult to distinguish from those of ACE inhibitors which a significant proportion of the FOS cohort were taking. Approximately 50% of younger Fabry patients have evidence of hyperfiltration (GFR > 130 ml/min) and may benefit from ACE inhibitors earlier in their disease course than previously recognised [22].

Expert consensus draws heavily on open-label studies that showed reduced pain, LV mass and reduced renal progression in patients on ERT. In the UK, AFD services including provision of ERT are commissioned nationally, and there are equivalent provisions in other EU member states. The therapy appears to be well tolerated, so the main restriction on its use outside of Europe will be related to cost. Advice on special cases, e.g. CKD stages 4 and 5 and dialysis patients, and when to stop ERT, can be obtained from the European Rare Kidney Disease Reference Network [23].

63.10 Multidisciplinary Care Team

A large part of the challenge of caring for patients with rare, multisystem disorders is building the appropriate network of colleagues to provide appropriate investigative and therapeutic expertise. Typically, a nephrologist will be one member of multidisciplinary team caring for patients with AFD. The team would ideally also include members from cardiology, neurology, gastroenterology, dermatology and ophthalmology operating in a joined-up way.

63

63.11 Other Inherited Lipid Disorders of the Kidney

63.11.1 Lecithin-Cholesterol Acyltransferase (LCAT) Deficiency

LCAT deficiency is a rare, autosomal recessive, inborn error of lipid metabolism. LCAT is a plasma enzyme involved in the esterification of cholesterol and the metabolism of HDL cholesterol. Multiple (>80) mutations of the LCAT gene have been identified leading to two main syndromes: fish eye disease (which does not have significant renal involvement) and familial LCAT deficiency. Affected patients typically have very low HDL cholesterol levels (although accelerated atherosclerotic disease is surprisingly uncommon), corneal opacities, anaemia and proteinuric renal disease, which can progress rapidly to end stage in early adulthood. Diagnosis is by enzymatic activity testing but may be suggested by renal biopsy findings which result from the deposition of Lp-X particles in the glomeruli resulting in mesangial expansion, thickening and double contouring of the GBM with foamy lipid deposition. Electron microscopy findings are more obvious; nascent HDL form rouloux and lipid deposition is seen in all compartments of the glomerulus [24].

There are no specific therapies available although there are reports of success with high-dose angiotensin receptor blockade and enzyme replacement is in development but not established therapy. Acquired LCAT deficiency has been reported secondary to autoantibodies, and treatment with B-cell-directed immunosuppression would be logical. The primary renal disease can recur after transplantation although it is not known how common this is.

63.11.2 Apoprotein E-Related Glomerular Disorders

Lipoprotein glomerulopathy (LPG) and Apo-E homozygote glomerulopathy are both inherited causes of lipid-related kidney disease [25].

63.11.2.1 Lipoprotein Glomerulopathy

This rare disease but probably underdiagnosed condition has predominantly been reported in Japan and East Asia but has been identified worldwide, sometimes as family clusters. The pathophysiology is not well understood, but the disease is seen in association with mutations in the apolipoprotein E gene impairing the LDL receptor.

It typically presents as proteinuric renal disease often as the nephrotic syndrome in association with disturbances of lipoprotein metabolism (raised triglycerides and type III hyperlipidaemia). Diagnosis is on renal biopsy, which shows dilated glomerular capillaries occluded by lamellated lipid deposits.. Most patients respond at least partially to standard lipid-lowering therapies and generic RAAS blockage, but there is no specific treatment, and approximately 50% reach end-stage kidney disease. Typically, the disease recurs very early after transplantation so making the diagnosis and counselling are important [26].

63.11.2.2 Apo-E Homozygote Glomerulopathy

Apo-E homozygote glomerulopathy is a very rare disease in patients with homozygote mutations of apo-E2 gene. Histological findings differ from LPG by having glomerulosclerosis that may be difficult to differentiate from diabetic nephropathy and more marked infiltration of foam-laden macrophages. A non-immune membranous pattern has also been described and is associated with renal disease that can progress to nephrotic syndrome and end-stage renal disease.

Conclusion

Anderson-Fabry disease and the other renal lipidoses are rare, but there is obvious benefit to improving awareness among a wide range of clinicians. Patients are often diagnosed late and may present to a variety of specialities. It is important to establish links between specialties so that ophthalmologists, cardiologists, neurologists and others are able to make the diagnosis and refer on to renal teams appropriately (and vice versa).

Case Study

A 30-year-old male teacher was incidentally found to have 2+ protein on urine dipstick on registration with a new GP practice. On review, he had a non-tender macular rash around his umbilicus and to his upper thighs. On questioning, he reported having very sharp, short-lived episodes of pain in his fingers, which he thought were related to periods of stress at work. His past medical history included irritable bowel syndrome. He also recalls an eye test a few years ago after which he was referred to ophthalmology – he missed this appointment. He was normotensive. Blood tests showed creatinine 130 umol/l with eGFR 40 ml/min, and there were no previous blood test results available. Urine protein/creatinine ratio was abnormal at 95 mg/mmol. ECG showed borderline changes consistent with LVH. He has been referred to the renal clinic.

This case seems like a non-specific presentation of proteinuric renal impairment in a young patient, but there are several clues that there might be an underlying chronic condition. The characteristic angiokeratomas of AFD often present in a swimsuit distribution. The asymptomatic corneal verticillata seen by the optician may have resulted in a diagnosis on consulting an ophthalmologist (provided drug causes of verticillata are excluded) especially if the IBS, rash and LVH had been present and noted at the time. Had he been seen by a neurologist, without consideration of his other symptoms, his neuropathic pain may also have been treated in isolation. A renal biopsy would have yielded non-specific changes at this point, and the diagnosis can be missed even on careful light microscopy (although zebra bodies would be seen on electron microscopy). A clinical suspicion of AFD is raised by careful consideration of all of the symptoms and signs over many years. By the third decade, many patients with classical Fabry disease will have chronic kidney disease, resulting in delayed commencement of ACE inhibitors and enzyme replacement.

Tips, Tricks and Pitfalls

- AFD should be in a differential list for any young person with CKD.
- Angiokeratomas in the swimsuit distribution are classical for AFD.
- Diagnostic clues for AFD include a history of LVH or stroke in a young person.

Chapter Review Questions

1. Anderson-Fabry disease is caused by a disorder of what enzyme?
2. What is the typical renal presentation of AFD?
3. What are the multisystemic features and non-specific diagnostic labels associated with AFD?
4. What are the typical histological findings on renal biopsy?
5. What are the mainstays of treatment of AFD and what optimises care for these patients?

Answers

1. Mutations in the GLA gene cause a reduction in the activity of the lysosomal enzyme alpha-galactosidase leading to AFD. This leads to intracellular accumulation of the glycosphingolipid globotriaosylceramide (Gb3).
2. Isolated proteinuria is the classical renal presentation, and infrequently this is associated with a urinary concentrating defect (or Fanconi syndrome).
3. The multisystemic features include neurological (stroke or TIA at a young age/neuropathic pain), opthalmological (corneal verticillata), cardiac (LVH, conduction abnormalities) and dermatological (angiokeratomas) presentations. Non-specific diagnostic labels are IBS, fibromyalgia and temperature intolerance.
4. Light microscopy can show foamy vacuoles in the podocytes and distal tubular epithelia cells. EM shows characteristic “zebra bodies” – Gb3 deposits that appear as membrane-bound lamellated

structures. Toluidine blue staining can show the glycolipid inclusion bodies.

5. RAS blockade (and other common strategies for preventing progression of CKD like managing hypertension) and enzyme replacement therapy (agalsidase alpha or agalsidase beta). Cross-disciplinary care is essential for ensuring appropriate and co-ordinated care.

Acknowledgements With thanks to Dr. Edward Stern for his contribution to the first edition of this chapter.

References

1. Wilcox WR, Oliveira JP, Hopkin RJ, et al. Females with Fabry disease frequently have major organ involvement: lessons from the Fabry Registry. Mol Genet Metab. 2008;93:112–28.
2. Mignani R, Moschella M, Cenacchi G, et al. Different renal phenotypes in related adult males with Fabry disease with the same classic genotype. Mol Genet Genomic Med. 2017;5(4):438–42.
3. Spada M, Pagliardini S, Yasuda M, et al. High incidence of later-onset Fabry disease revealed by newborn screening. Am J Hum Genet. 2006;79(1):31–40.
4. Meikle PJ, Hopwood JJ, Clague AE, et al. Prevalence of lysosomal storage disorders. JAMA. 1999;281(3):249–54.
5. Frabasil J, Durand C, Sokn S, et al. Prevalence of Fabry disease in male dialysis patients: Argentinean screening study. JIMD Rep. 2019;48(1):45–52.
6. Alroy J, Sabnis S, Kopp JB. Renal pathology in Fabry disease. J Am Soc Nephrol. 2002;13 Suppl 2:S134–8.
7. Mehta A, Ricci R, Widmer U, et al. Fabry disease defined: baseline clinical manifestations of 366 patients in the Fabry Outcome Survey. Eur J Clin Investig. 2004;34:236–42.
8. MacDermot KD, Holmes A, Miners AH. Anderson-Fabry disease in high-risk populations: a systematic review. J Med Genet. 2001;47(4):217–22.
9. Linthorst GE, Bouwman MG, Wijburg FA, et al. Screening for Fabry disease in high-risk populations: a systematic review. J Med Genet. 2010;47:217–22.
10. Sunder-Plassman G, et al., editors. Chapter 17, Fabry disease: perspectives from 5 years of FOS. Oxford: Oxford PharmaGenesis; 2006.
11. Selvarajah M, Nicholls K, Hewitson TD, et al. Targeted urine microscopy in Anderson-Fabry disease: a cheap, sensitive and specific diagnostic technique. Nephrol Dial Transplant. 2011;26(10):3195–202.
12. Fall B, Scott CR, Mauer M, et al. Urinary podocyte loss is increased in patients with Fabry disease and correlates with clinical severity of Fabry nephropathy. PLoS One. 2016;11(12):e0168346.
13. Germain DP. Fabry disease. Orphanet J Rare Dis. 2010;5(30). https://doi.org/10.1186/1750-1172-5-30.
14. Tsakiris D, Simpson HK, Jones EH, et al. Report on management of renal failure in Europe XXVI, 1995, Rare diseases in renal replacement therapy in the ERA-EDTA Registry. Nephrol Dial Transplant. 1996;11 Suppl 7:4–20.
15. KDIGO Kidney International, Meeting Report. Screening, diagnosis, and management of patients with Fabry disease: conclusions from a "Kidney Disease: Improving Global Outcomes" Controversies Conference. 2017;91(2):284–93.
16. https://academic.oup.com/ndt/article/28/3/505/1814362#85063236
17. Bird S, Hadjimichael E, Mehta A, et al. Fabry disease and incidence of cancer. Orphanet J Rare Dis. 2017;12:150.
18. Ersözlü S, Desnick RJ, Huynh-Do U, et al. Long-term outcomes of kidney transplantation in Fabry disease. Transplantation. 2018;102(11):1924–33.
19. West M, Nicholls K, Mehta A, et al. Agalsidase alfa and kidney dysfunction in Fabry disease. J Am Soc Nephrol. 2009;20:1132–9.
20. Germain DP, Waldek S, Banikazemi M, et al. Sustained, long-term renal stabilisation after 54 months of Agalsidase Beta therapy in patients with Fabry disease. J Am Soc Nephrol. 2007;18(5):1547–57.
21. Parini R, Pintos-Morell G, Hennermann JB, et al. Analysis of renal and cardiac outcomes in male participants in the Fabry outcome survey starting agalsidase alfa enzyme replacement therapy before and after 18 years of age. Drug Des Devel Ther. 2020;14:2149–58. https://doi.org/10.2147/DDDT.S249433.
22. Riccio E, Sabbatini M, Bruzzese D, et al.; on behalf of AFFIINITY Group. Glomerular hyperfiltration: an early marker of nephropathy in Fabry disease. Nephron. 2019;141(1):10–7.
23. Biegstraaten M, et al. Orphanet J Rare Dis. 2015;10:36. https://doi.org/10.1186/s13023-015-0253-6.
24. Hirashio S, Ueno T, Naito T, et al. Characteristic kidney pathology, gene abnormality and treatments in LCAT deficiency. Clin Exp Nephrol. 2014;18(2):189–93.
25. Saito T, Matsunaga A, Fukunaga M. Apolipoprotein E-related glomerular disorders. [Review]. Kidney Int. 2020;97(2):279–88.
26. Miyata T, Sugiyama S, Nangaku M, et al. Apolipoprotein E2/E5 variants in lipoprotein glomerulopathy recurred in transplanted kidney. J Am Soc Nephrol. 1999;10(7):1590–5. ev 2010;:CD006663.

Further Resources

The MPS Society (mpssociety.org.uk) and Metabolic Support (metabolicsupportuk.org) provide assistance for patients with Fabry in the UK. The Fabry Support and Information Group (www.fabry.org) is an international patient support group based in the USA. It includes links to a range of national organisations worldwide.

Inherited Metabolic Disease and the Kidney

Asheeta Gupta, Gill Rumsby, and Sally-Anne Hulton

Contents

M. Harber (ed.), *Primer on Nephrology*, https://doi.org/10.1007/978-3-030-76419-7_64

64.1 Introduction

A number of inherited metabolic diseases with renal manifestations were previously the remit of paediatric nephrologists, but as medical and scientific advances have improved the quality of life of these children, survival well into adult life is a reality. Therefore, adult nephrologists and their multiprofessional teams will be required to familiarise themselves with these conditions and provide continuing therapy. In some situations such as pregnancy, information is limited, and outcomes are less well known. Prospective data collection from rare disease registries will assist our understanding of the evolution of these conditions. This chapter focuses on two metabolic disorders that have varied presentations and will be seen in adult nephrology practice. The table of medications used more commonly in renal metabolic disorders in childhood may be of use in establishing dosage equivalence and palatability for the patient (Table 64.1).

Table 64.1 Electrolyte content of frequently used medications in paediatric nephrology practice

Phosphate supplementation		
Joulie's solution		
	1 ml contains:	Na = 0.76 mmol
		PO_4 = 0.98 mmol
Phosphate Sandoz (soluble)		
	1 tab contains:	PO_4 = 16 mmol
		K = 3 mmol
		Na = 20.4 mmol
Potassium supplementation		
Potassium chloride solution		
	1 ml contains:	K^{+1} = 1 mmol
		Cl^- = 1 mmol
Slow K tablets (MR-swallow whole)		
	1 tab contain:	K^{+1} = 8 mmol
		Cl^- = 8 mmol
Sando K tablets (soluble)		
	1 tab contains:	K^{+1} = 12 mmol
		Cl^- = 8 mmol
Calcium supplementation		
Calcium Sandoz liquid		
	1 ml contains:	Ca^{+2} = 0.5 mmol
Sandocal 400 tablets (soluble)		
	1 tab contains:	Ca^{+2} = 10 mmol
Sandocal 1000 tablets (soluble)		
	1 tab contains:	Ca^{+2} = 25 mmol
Magnesium supplementation		
Magnesiocard tablets		
	1 tab contains:	Mag = 2.5 mmol
		No phosphate
Magnesiocard tablets (soluble)		
	1 tab contains:	Mag = 7.5 mmol

Table 64.1 (continued)

		No phosphate
Magnesium glycerophosphate solution:		
	1 ml contains:	Mag = 1 mmol
		PO_4 = 1 mmol
Magnesium glycerophosphate		
	1 tablet contains:	Mag = 4 mmol
		PO_4 = 4 mmol
Bicarbonate supplementation		
Sodium bicarbonate solution		
	1 ml contains:	Na = 1 mmol
		Bicarb = I mmol
Sodium bicarbonate tablet 600 mg		
	1 tab contains:	Na = 7 mmol
		Bicarb = 7 mmol
Sodium bicarbonate capsule 500 mg		
	1 tab contains:	Na = 6 mmol
		Bicarb = 6 mmol
Citrate supplementation		
Sodium citrate mixture		
	1 mmol in 1 ml	
Potassium bitrate mixture BP		
(3 g in 10 ml)	1 mls contains:	K = 2.8 mmol
		Citrate = 1.15 mmol
		(equivalent to 3.45 mmol bicarb/ml)
Albright's solution		
	1 litre contains:	Na = 510 mmol
		K = 462 mmol
		Citrate = 636 mmol
		(equivalent to 1.9 mmol bicarb/ml)
	10 mls contains:	Na = 5 mmol
		K = 4 mmol
		Citrate = 6 mmol
		(equivalent to 1.9 mmol bicarb/ml)
Effercitrate (soluble tab)		
	1 tablet contains:	K = 14 mmol
		Citrate = 6 mmol
		(equivalent to 17 mmol bicarb/tab)
	i.e. 10 mls Albrights = 1 Effercitrate (except higher K^+)	

(continued)

Table 64.1 (continued)

Tricitrates oral solution (lemon flavour)		
	1 ml contains:	K = 1 mmol
		Na = 1 mmol
		Citrate = 0.7 mmol
		(equivalent to 2 mmol bicarb/ml)
This is an unlicensed medicine made by the pharmacy manufacturing unit of Guy's and St Thomas's Hospital and can be ordered from that department (telephone 0207 118 4992) or by contacting Order Processing Service, Pharmacy Production Unit, Pharmacy Department, St Thomas's Hospital, Westminster Bridge Road, London, SE1 7EH. Fax No: 0207 188 5013		

There are other, generally very rare, metabolic disorders that impact on the kidney shown in Table 2.

Table 64.2 An overview of the impact of rare metabolic disorders on the kidney

Fabry's disease	Lysosomal storage disorder	Commonest storage disorder in adulthood Proteinuria, IFTA, progressive CKD
Cystinosis	Lysosomal storage disorder	Fanconi syndrome, IFTA, glomerulosclerosis, interstitial crystals and giant multinucleate podocytes
Wilson disease	Disorder of copper metabolism	Fanconi syndrome
Tyrosinaemia	Disorder of tyrosine metabolism	Fanconi syndrome
Methylmalonic acidaemia	Organic acidaemias	AR, metabolic acidosis (high anion gap), hyperammonaemia, hypoglycaemia, IFTA, tubulointerstitial nephritis, progressive CKD early adulthood Liver or kidney transplant
Hereditary fructose intolerance	Disorder of fructose metabolism	Fanconi, hyperuricaemia, hypoglycaemia, metabolic acidosis, abnormal liver function, raised magnesium, raised lactate
Galactosaemia	Disorder of carbohydrate metabolism	Fanconi, hypoglycaemia, hypophosphataemia, metabolic acidosis, abnormal liver function
Glycogen storage disorders		IFTA, glomerulosclerosis, proteinuria or Fanconi Liver or combined liver kidney transplant
Cystinuria	Disorder of amino acid transport	Cystine stones (also elevated urinary lysine, ornithine, arginine)
Lysinuric protein intolerance	Disorder of amino acid transport	Generalised amino aciduria and phosphate wasting. Glomerulonephritis, chronic TIN
Xanthinuria	Disorder of purine (xanthine metabolism)	Xanthine stones
Lesch-Nyhan syndrome	Disorder of purine metabolism	Urate stones
Phosphomannomutase deficiency		Proteinuria and nephrotic syndrome

64

Learning Objectives

1. To understand the importance of compliance and monitoring therapy in cystinosis to manage the long-term complications
2. To describe the subtypes of primary hyperoxaluria, the investigation and targeted treatment
3. To recognise the importance of effective transition of patients affected by inherited metabolic conditions

64.2 Cystinosis

Cystinosis is an autosomal recessive lysosomal transport disorder characterised by the accumulation of cystine with subsequent crystal formation in tissues of the body. The cystinosis gene *CTNS*, located on chromosome 17p13, encodes the protein cystinosin which is primarily expressed at the lysosomal level [1].

64.2.1 Presentation and Investigation

A variety of clinical forms of the disease are noted [2]:

- The infantile form, common and with greater severity, presenting with early-onset Fanconi syndrome within the first year of life
- Juvenile cystinosis presenting with glomerular impairment in adolescence or early adult life without the development of severe tubulopathy
- Ocular cystinosis, less common, with no renal manifestations

The infant with cystinosis appears normal at birth and will develop appropriately up to 6 months of age before presenting with polyuria and polydipsia, unexplained fever, anorexia, constipation, vomiting with resultant dehydration and failure to thrive and signs of rickets (◘ Fig. 64.1). The key presenting features are hypokalaemia, hyponatraemia, hypophosphataemia, acidosis, generalised amino aciduria and glycosuria [3]. Caucasian infants typically have blond hair and blue eyes. At presentation, the glomerular filtration rate (GFR) in these children is normal. Cystine accumulation in the proximal tubular cells impairs oxidative phosphorylation and decreases the activity of Na-K-ATPase which reduces the gradient for sodium entry into the cells with decrease in sodium-coupled transport of other solutes, leading to the clinical presentation of Fanconi syndrome [4].

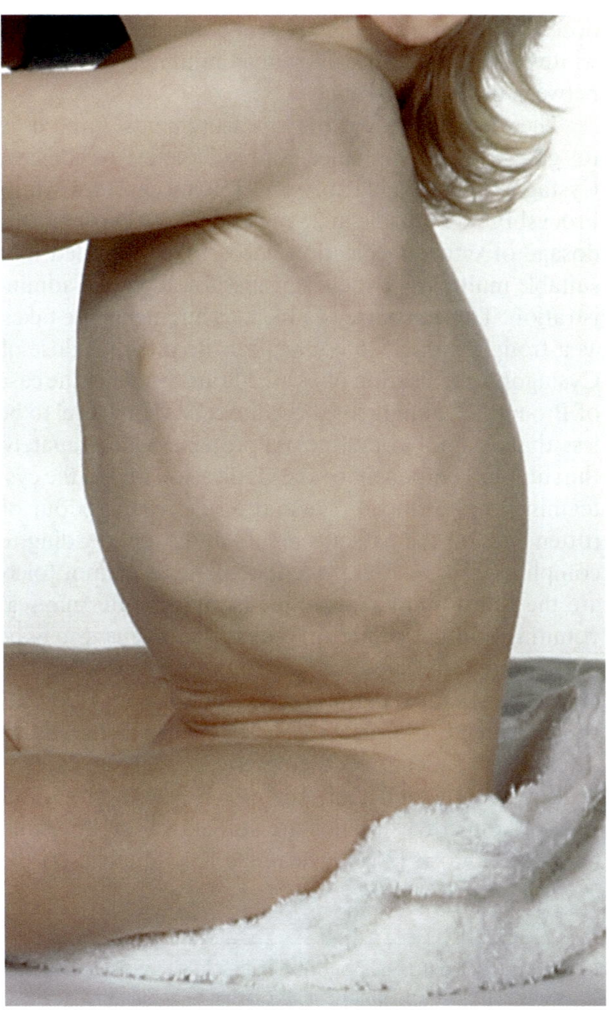

◘ **Fig. 64.1** Swollen costochondral junctions associated with rickets in cystinosis

64.2.1.1 Diagnosis

The diagnosis is made by the white blood cell cystine (WBC) assay which is typically 10–100 times above the normal range and with genetic confirmation. Antenatal testing of chorionic villi for specific mutations is available from 8 weeks gestation in suitable families or through measurement of cystine content in the amniotic fluid.

64.2.1.2 Genomics

Given the advances in genomics and the range of genetic tests now available, it is useful to recap what is now known about the underlying genetic causes of cystinosis. The *CTNS* gene contains 12 exons and is 26 kilobases in length [1, 5]. The condition is inherited in an autosomal recessive manner.

At present, 148 different pathogenic variants (including promotor variants) in *CTNS* have been reported in the Human Gene Mutation Database (HGMD) [6]. These variants are found in different combinations in individuals with cystinosis and vary across different geographical populations [1, 5–18]. There are no mutational hotspots within the gene, and types of pathogenic variant include missense, nonsense, insertions and deletions [13].

The most common pathogenic variant in Northern European and North American patients (50% of affected individuals) is the 57 kb deletion involving the first 10 exons of the *CTNS* gene. This variant represents a founder effect [7]. The same deletion has been described with a lower frequency in French, Italian, Canadian, Mexican and Turkish patients [19–21]. Another relatively common pathogenic variant is p.Trp138Ter.

There is much focus on developing a biochemical neonatal screening tool for cystinosis, to aid early identification and treatment. A promising candidate, sedoheptulose, has been found to be elevated in blood spots taken from patients homozygous for the 57 kb deletion in *CTNS* [22]. This method unfortunately fails to diagnose approximately 50% of cystinotic newborns in Northern Europe, America and the majority of those born in other parts of the world that do not carry that specific mutation [22].

64.2.2 Management

64.2.2.1 General

In early life, the importance of adequate correction of hydration and electrolyte imbalances are paramount to improve growth. Regular review of electrolytes and phosphate supplementation is required to prevent constipation from hypokalaemia and rickets from hypophosphataemia (◘ Fig. 64.1). To maintain adequate nutritional intake, gastrostomy or nasogastric feeding is required. Growth hormone therapy is beneficial once nutritional intake is optimised [23]. Carnitine supplementation has not been proven to have specific benefits except for restoring normal plasma concentrations. Indomethacin (1–3 mg/kg/day in two to three divided doses) is very useful in improving general wellbeing as well as reducing polyuria and may be given as a single dose at night to assist nocturia. It is not recommended when renal function is deteriorating and requires regular renal function monitoring.

Cysteamine, the main drug therapy for cystinosis, is effective in circumventing the defective lysosomal cystine carrier system, thereby reducing the cystine content of the lysosomes (◘ Figs. 64.2 and 64.3). The most commonly available form of administration is as cysteamine bitartrate (Cystagon®), administered orally at a dose of 60–90 mg/kg/day given every 6 hours [24]. A slow-release, enteric coated cysteamine formulation (Procysbi™) is now available. This is administered every 12 hours and has demonstrated non-inferiority when compared to Cystagon® with respect to its efficacy in lowering WBC cystine levels [24], whilst using 82% of the Cystagon® dose [25]. The 12-hourly administration is more likely to be favoured by patients from a compliance perspective but is more expensive. At commencement of therapy, the cysteamine dose must be prescribed at a quarter of the final intended maintenance dose and

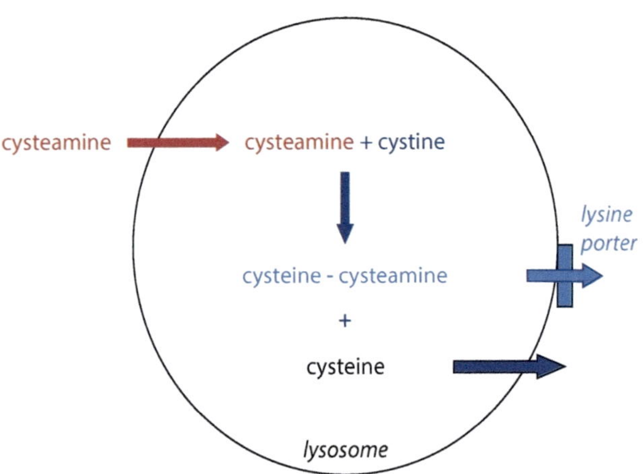

◘ Fig. 64.2 Schematic representation of action of cysteamine in cystine transport from the lysosome

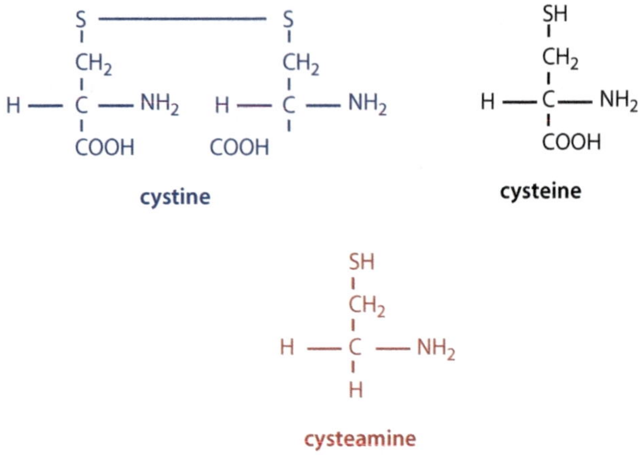

cystine

cysteine

cysteamine

◘ Fig. 64.3 Structural similarities between cystine and cysteamine

increased gradually over the first 2–4 weeks of therapy, to avoid nausea and neurological complications. The maintenance dose of Procysbi™ after initial escalation is 1.3 g/m^2 of body surface area per day divided into two doses. Dose adjustments are made according to blood white cell cystine levels, allowing a minimum of 2 weeks between dosing intervals.

The leukocyte cystine measurements are used to gauge the compliance and adequacy of dosing. Cystagon® is available in 50 and 150 mg capsules, whilst Procysbi™ is available in 25 mg and 75 mg capsules: the dosage of either medication needs to be rounded into suitable multiples of these capsules for adequate administration. The leukocyte cystine measurements are taken as a trough level 5.5–6 hours after the previous dose of Cystagon® medication or as a 12-hour trough in the case of Procysbi®, aiming for the white cell cystine level to be less than 2 nmol ½-cystine/mg protein.[1] Unfortunately, the sulphur component of the medication makes the cysteamine unpleasant to take and results in the odour of rotten eggs on the patient's breath and sweat, leading to compliance issues. Ten percent of patients cannot tolerate the full dose of cysteamine as many suffer nausea, vomiting and gastrointestinal upset, and thus it may be better to aim for suboptimal therapeutic levels that can at least be tolerated in the first instance. A pilot study has shown a trend towards lower levels of exhaled dimethyl sulphide in patients on the enteric coated versus conventional cysteamine formulation; however, the lower levels of dimethyl sulphide are still above the threshold to cause halitosis [26]. Cysteamine has no effect on the

1 *Note: Reference laboratories may report measurement for white cell cystine in units of half-cystine because initial methods of quantitation involved reduction of cystine and measurement of the reduced product, cysteine. The target white cell cystine level is less than 2 nmol ½-cystine/mg protein or less than 2 µmol/g cysteine protein.

Fanconi syndrome, but it does retard the rate of renal glomerular deterioration and improves linear growth in children [3, 27]. Gastrointestinal irritation is a common side effect of cysteamine treatment, and cases of peptic ulceration have been reported [28]. Concomitant use of proton pump inhibitors helps in preventing or alleviating some of these symptoms [29]. The optimal care of patients with cystinosis requires a multiprofessional team approach with referral to and advice from to centres specialising in the disorder.

64.2.2.2 Management of Progression of the Disease

The progressive effects of cystinosis on organ systems and the specific management are listed below:

- *Renal*

  The early renal features are those of Fanconi syndrome. Polyuria may result in the loss of up to 6 litres of dilute urine (<300 mosmol/litre) per day and poses a significant problem of enuresis in children and adolescents. There is a gradual decline in creatinine clearance over the years, and end-stage renal disease occurs at around 10 years of age in those not receiving cysteamine treatments [30]. The introduction of cysteamine has delayed the onset of end-stage renal failure (ESRF) by up to 10 years, in particular when administered as early as possible following the diagnosis and certainly before the age of 5 years [31]. Many well-managed patients will reach 25 years of age before requiring kidney transplantation [32]. Preemptive transplantation is the treatment of choice, and where this is not available, peritoneal dialysis or haemodialysis is appropriate prior to awaiting a renal transplant. Both cadaveric and living related donor kidneys perform well in patients with cystinosis [33] and may have lower rejection rates, perhaps suggesting less intense long-term immunosuppression. Heterozygous relatives are able to donate kidneys to their offspring. Native kidneys remaining in situ can persist with renal tubular Fanconi losses, and native nephrectomies may be required to control this. The donor kidney itself does not develop Fanconi syndrome. Cystine crystals do deposit in the donor kidney through invasion of host cells with crystals noted in the interstitium but not in the tubular epithelium. Renal transplantation does not correct the systemic metabolic defect of cystinosis.

- *Eyes*

  Cystine crystals deposit in most parts of the eye particularly the anterior chamber (◘ Fig. 64.4). The cornea is hazy by 20 years of age, and a band keratopathy can develop. Photophobia is particularly obvious in bright sunlight, and dark glasses are essential for all patients. Scarring can pre-dispose to glaucoma. Retinal damage with poor colour and night vision occurs in early adulthood [34]. Oral cysteamine does not improve the effects in the eye, but topically administered cysteamine 0.5% eye drops given 6–12 times per day are extremely useful. Intensive treatment with 2-hourly instillations of the drops can dramatically improve photophobia within weeks. The lower strength 0.1% cysteamine eye drops can be used but are less effective.

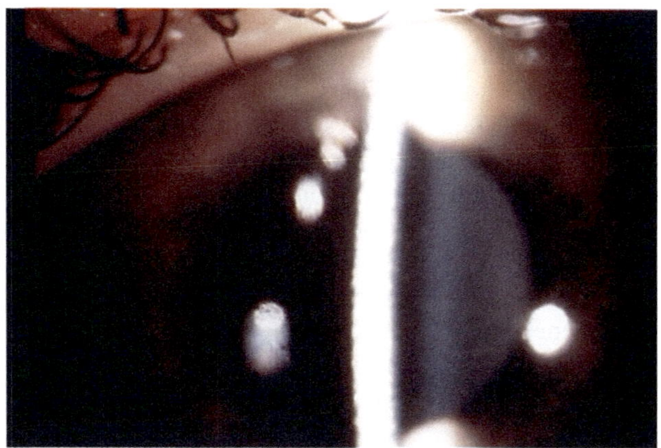

◘ **Fig. 64.4** Cystine crystals seen on slit-lamp examination of the eye

- *Endocrine Involvement*

  Hypothyroidism is documented pre- and post-renal transplant relating initially to the loss of thyroglobulin in the urine and subsequently to deposition of crystals in the thyroid gland. As a result, the majority of patients are on thyroid supplements from late childhood onwards [35]. Primary hypogonadism is recorded in males. Infertility is noted in all males, but ovulatory cycles are normal in female patients, and successful pregnancy outcomes are recorded. Specialist prenatal support is required. Diabetes post-transplant is common, with many patients requiring insulin treatment.

- *Gastrointestinal Complications*

  Seventy-five percent of patients develop feeding abnormalities due to reflux dysmotility and swallowing dysfunction [36]. Proton pump inhibitors can be helpful. Hepatosplenomegaly is common with gradual development of portal hypertension. Exocrine pancreatic insufficiency can develop which requires enzyme supplementation.

- *Haematological*

  Anaemia is commonly seen in patients with cystinosis as a result of cystine deposition in the bone marrow in addition to a reduction in erythropoietin protein production by the kidney. These patients also have hypocoagulability and platelet dysfunction [37].

- *Neuromuscular*

  Neurocognitive deficits have been recorded in children who show effects primarily with visuospatial functions [38]. A progressive myopathy with skeletal muscle wasting is particularly notable in adult life. This can contribute to oromotor dysfunction including dysphagia. Accessory muscles of the chest can be involved contributing to ventilatory restriction. In untreated patients, cerebral complications will result in encephalopathy with impaired cerebellar and pyramidal function [35, 36]. Idiopathic cranial hypertension is well recognised [39].
- *Cardiovascular*

  Arterial hypertension is noted secondary to a renin-dependent hypertension. This together with the hypercholesterolemia of cystinosis can result in early calcification of arteries, particularly coronary.
- *Bone Involvement*

  Bone mineral density is significantly reduced in adults and children after transplantation. The development of osteopaenia and bone fragility occurs irrespective of correction of metabolic mineral losses in earlier life. Dental issues may arise as a result.

Cysteamine treatment can provide salutary effects even when administered late to previously noncompliant patients with established complications such as severe encephalopathy. Cysteamine retards the development of serious late complications of cystinosis and ideally should be commenced immediately after birth and continued indefinitely [40]. The teratogenicity of oral cysteamine has not been determined in humans. The current advice is that women planning to conceive should stop cysteamine from the date of conception until after the pregnancy although there is a report of a woman receiving 300 mg of cysteamine three times daily throughout her pregnancy, who subsequently delivered a healthy infant [41]. Cysteamine should be recommenced soon after delivery, and breastfeeding is not advised.

64

64.2.3 Future Therapies

Current therapies for cystinosis do not offer a cure. Moreover, treatment with cysteamine imposes a significant burden on patients. Adherence to a strict 6-hourly or even 12-hourly dosing schedule, drug intolerability due to gastrointestinal side effects and halitosis are amongst the reasons for patients not adhering to treatment. Compliance is a major issue and is thought to be a problem in at least a third of patients [42] resulting in a progressive decline in growth and renal function [24]. Future therapeutic strategies are aimed at tackling these issues.

64.2.3.1 Cysteamine Prodrugs

Research approaches are investigating the use of prodrugs that have desirable properties in comparison to their parent drug. Several drugs have been developed to overcome side effects of cysteamine such as its bad taste, consequent halitosis and production of a longer half-life [43, 44]. An example of this is a prodrug targeting gamma-glutamyl transpeptidase (GGT), which has less toxicity and fewer gastrointestinal side effects in comparison to conventional oral cysteamine in mice models [45]. In vivo efficiency of these drugs has not been tested.

64.2.3.2 Stem Cell Transplant and Gene Therapy

Bone marrow transplantation to correct the genetic defect is under consideration [46]. Mouse models of cystinosis treated with wild-type allogeneic bone marrow and haematopoetic stem cells (HSC) have shown a multisystem reduction in cystine accumulation [47, 48]. However, tissue cystine levels still remained higher than in heterozygous carriers suggesting that cysteamine therapy may still be required to optimise cell cystine levels. Haematopoietic stem cell and progenitor cell lines have been isolated from mouse models of cystinosis. These cell lines have allowed transduction of human *CTNS* cDNA sequence using a self-inactivating lentiviral vector. Cell lines have then been transplanted into *ctns* -/- mice showing a significant multisystem decline in cystine content [49]. The use of autologous stem cells has the major advantage of dramatically reducing the immunosuppressive regimen and the risks of rejection and of developing graft-versus-host disease. No increased incidence of secondary tumours or unexpected toxicity was described [49].

64.3 Transition

Facilitating effective transition of paediatric patients to adult services has received much attention given the improvement in survival rates of patients diagnosed with cystinosis [50, 51]. Several documents now propose a framework for transition and allow physicians and multidisciplinary teams to incorporate crucial elements to aid this process [see additional reading].

Case Study

Case 1

A 17-year-old was screened for cystinosis antenatally as a result of a positive family history and an affected sibling. Genetic studies confirmed the 57 kb deletion in *CTNS*. She was commenced on cysteamine within 4 weeks of birth. Compliance with cysteamine therapy was reasonable for the first 4 years of life but then deteriorated, and despite significant multiprofessional and social services involvement, the adherence to the cysteamine therapy could not be improved. The renal function was noted to decline from the age of 8 years, and haemodialysis was commenced at age 10 years. She underwent a deceased donor renal transplant shortly thereafter. Despite on-going efforts at improving adherence, she refuses to take the cysteamine mediation regularly, and her white cell cystine levels have ranged from 0.4 in infancy to 15.2 with an average of 8 nmol/mg of protein, indicative of the poor level of adherence. More recently, she disclosed that she sometimes does not take her immunosuppressive therapy, but she has not presented with rejection. Her last recorded creatinine was 65 μmol/L (CKD stage 2 T, eGFR 77 ml/min/1.73 m2). She has significant visual impairment secondary to crystal deposition in the eyes and has short stature (height < 0.4th centile). She is developing hypophonia. At transition to adult services, despite intellectual ability to understand all the consequences, she refuses to take cysteamine medication, even the twice-daily preparation, because of the side effect of the sulphurous odour on her breath.

Learning Points

- This illustrates the impact of poor compliance and the requirement of a multidisciplinary approach in trying to tackle this.

Case 2

At transition, a 17-year-old girl with cystinosis demonstrated exemplary adherence to all her medications including cysteamine since her diagnosis at 13 months of age. Over the past 8 years, the white cell cystine level has ranged between <0.2 and 2.9, with an average of 1.55 nmol/mg of protein. She has chronic kidney disease (stage 2, current eGFR 52 ml/min/1.73 m^2) and requires thyroxine and electrolyte supplements for on-going Fanconi syndrome. Her weight falls on the 30th centile, with height on the 72nd centile. She is reviewed 3 monthly in clinic and remains asymptomatic, with no eye crystals demonstrated. She has achieved A grades in her school examinations and intends to embark on an intellectual career following university.

Learning Points

- This case demonstrates the positive effect of cysteamine compliance on growth and renal outcomes. Whilst the renal function will decline, the rate is slow, and renal replacement therapy would be expected only in the mid-20s.

Tips and Tricks

- The odour of the cysteamine medication influences compliance. The twice-daily preparation now available may facilitate improved adherence; however, patients still report their aversion to the smell and to the halitosis they experience.
- With poor oral and ophthalmic cysteamine compliance, the complications are devastating, leading to low self-esteem, depression, poor social integration and often unemployment.
- Cysteamine medication can be commenced soon after birth.
- Patients with cystinosis show good renal graft tolerance.

Advocacy support is available through ▶ www.cystinosisfoundation.org, the Cystinosis Foundation and the Cystinosis Research Network ▶ www.cystinosis.org which provide advice and support for affected families, as well as funding research.

64.4 The Primary Hyperoxalurias

The primary hyperoxalurias are inborn errors of metabolism of which three have been described at the molecular level (◘ Fig. 64.5). Primary hyperoxaluria type 1 (PH1) is caused by mutations in the *AGXT* gene which result in dysfunction of the vitamin B6 (pyridoxine)-dependent, liver-specific, peroxisomal enzyme alanine: glyoxylate

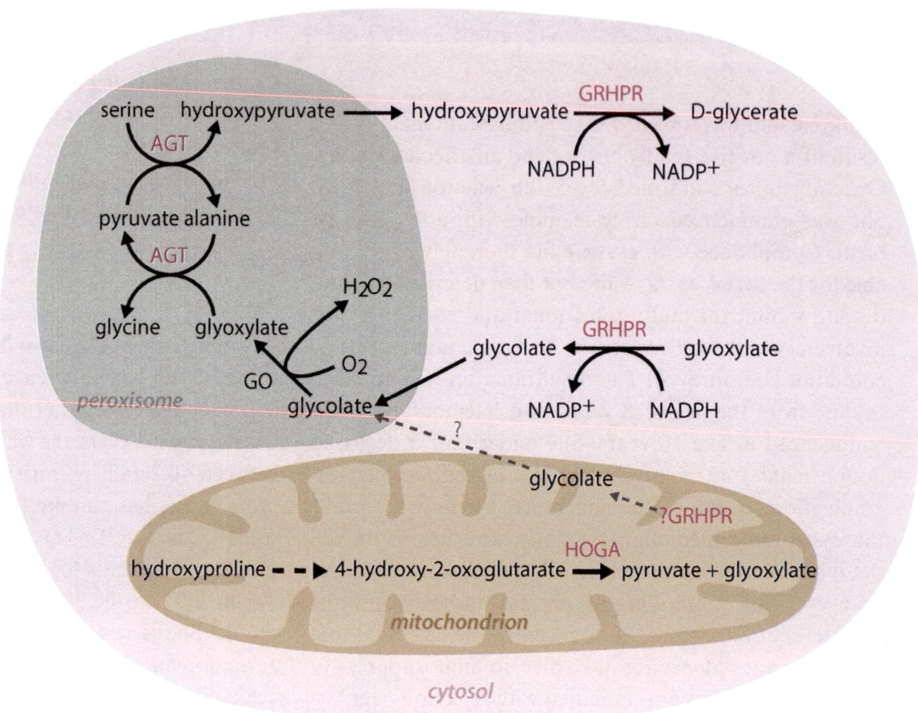

Fig. 64.5 The metabolic pathway of glyoxylate showing the relationship of the three enzymes AGT, GRHPR and HOGA. Lactate dehydrogenase (LDH) is a major contributor to oxalate production in types 1 and 2. The cause of elevated oxalate in PH3 is still unknown. GO, glycolate oxidase

aminotransferase (AGT) [51]. Primary hyperoxaluria type 2 (PH2) arises from mutations in the *GRHPR* gene with subsequent dysfunction of the enzyme glyoxylate/hydroxypyruvate reductase (GRHPR) [52]. Primary hyperoxaluria type 3 (PH3) arises from mutations in the *HOGA1* gene which encodes the mitochondrial enzyme 4-hydroxy-2-oxoglutarate aldolase (HOGA) [53].

Oxalate is derived principally from the diet and endogenous production following the metabolism of glyoxylate and ascorbic acid and is excreted primarily via the kidney. Hyperoxaluria can occur due to hyperabsorption of ingested oxalate, as seen in patients with bowel malabsorption, e.g. ulcerative colitis or Crohn's disease or following excess dietary intake. Less commonly, there is derangement of the normal metabolic pathways involving synthesis of oxalate by the action of lactate dehydrogenase (LDH) on accumulated glyoxylate (PH1 and PH2) and from the excessive production of 4-hydroxy-2-oxoglutarate (PH3), a metabolite of hydroxyproline, although the origin of oxalate in the latter disorder is as yet unclear.

64

As oxalate is poorly soluble, calcium oxalate calculi will form when the urine becomes supersaturated. Bidirectional transport of oxalate has been demonstrated in proximal renal tubular cells and in intestinal epithelia with evidence to suggest a role for the SLC26A6 apical membrane anion transporter in both enteric and renal oxalate transport. Calcium oxalate crystals form in the lumen of the renal tubules. These crystals then adhere to the tubular epithelium and are internalised into the cells with subsequent extrusion into the interstitial region where they cause an inflammatory reaction and subsequent nephrocalcinosis (Figs. 64.6, 64.7 and 64.8).

64.4.1 Presentation and Investigation

The primary hyperoxalurias show considerable genetic and phenotypic heterogeneity and can present in the following forms:

- Asymptomatic (picked up on family studies or stone picked up incidentally on imaging)
- Occasional passage of renal stones
- Recurrent urolithiasis
- Recurrent urolithiasis with the development of nephrocalcinosis and eventual progressive renal failure
- Infantile presentation with faltering growth, early nephrocalcinosis and rapid progression to end-stage renal failure

The investigation of any child or adult presenting with even the occasional passage of renal stones, but certainly for those presenting with nephrocalcinosis, must exclude PH as an underlying cause. Analysis of the renal stone, if available, providing it is done by a reliable centre, can be helpful, and stones are typically composed of 100% calcium oxalate, but in some cases may be mixed with calcium phosphate. In all such presentations, a **fresh** urine sample must be sent for urine oxalate/creatinine

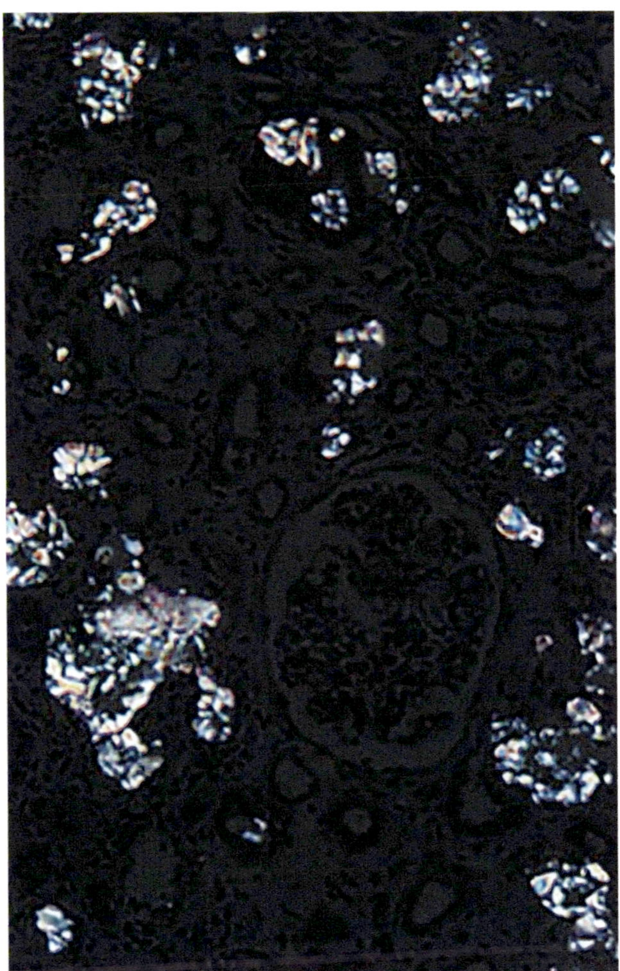

■ **Fig. 64.6** Oxalate crystals in PH demonstrated in a renal biopsy under polarised light

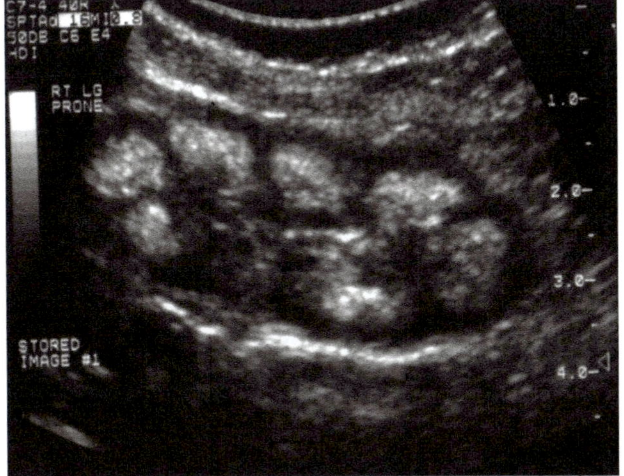

■ **Fig. 64.7** Renal ultrasound demonstrating marked nephrocalcinosis in a patient with primary hyperoxalosis

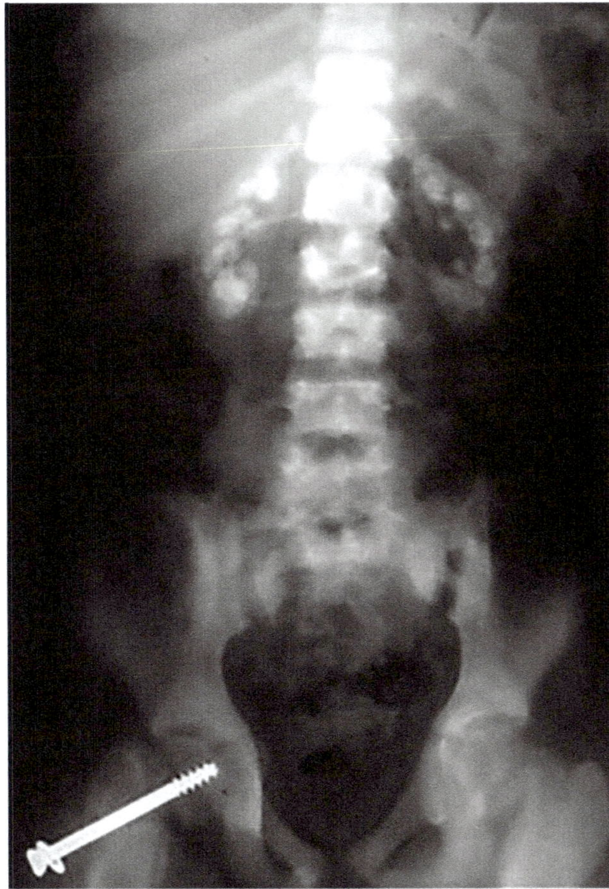

■ **Fig. 64.8** Abdominal X-ray demonstrating marked nephrocalcinosis and severe osteopaenia associated with PH1 in a 9-year-old

ratio in the first instance. If the sample is borderline or elevated, a 24-hour urine collection for oxalate excretion is required, and in some cases, three consecutive 24-hour urine collections, as there is marked variability in the excretion of oxalate on a day-to-day basis. During the 24-hour collection period, the urine collected must be placed into a container acidified with hydrochloric acid (obtained from the hospital Clinical Chemistry department). Acidification is required to improve oxalate solubility and also to prevent oxalogenesis from any ascorbate in the urine. For this reason, it is recommended that vitamin C supplements are discontinued prior to sample collection.

A urine oxalate (UOx) excretion of >0.7 mmol/1.73 m^2/day is likely to be due to a metabolic cause although some secondary cases due to Crohn's disease, short gut syndrome and pancreatic insufficiency have grossly elevated oxalate excretions >1 mmol/1.73 m^2/day. In children, the urinary oxalate/creatinine ratio is useful, but interpretation requires the use of age-related reference ranges, and

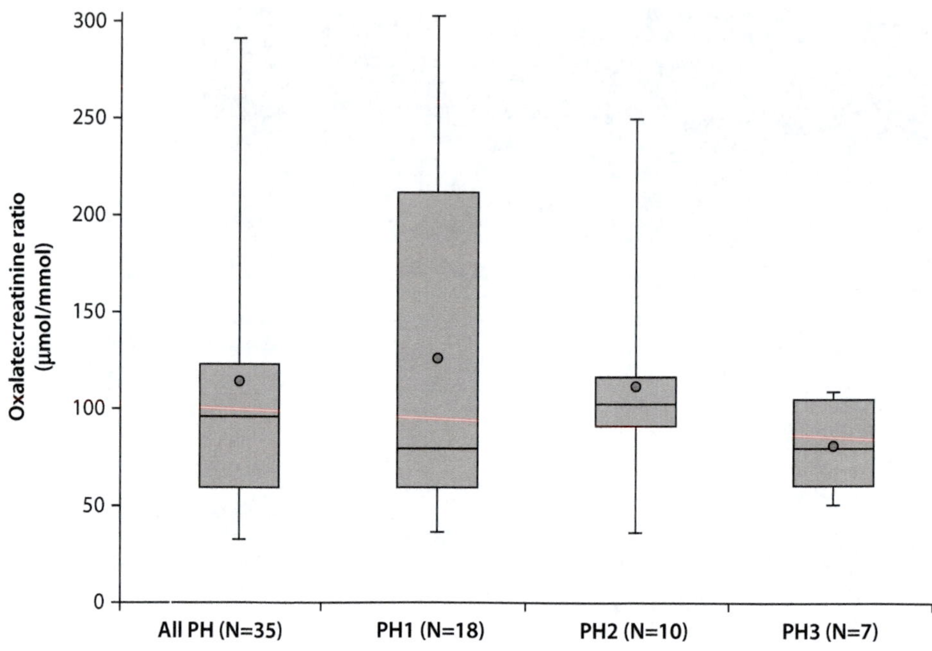

Fig. 64.9 Urine oxalate excretion in PH1, PH2 and PH3 illustrating overlap of urine oxalate/creatinine ratio. Box denotes interquartile range; whiskers denote the 2.5 and 97.5 centiles

ratios in early life are influenced by prematurity and nutrition, being higher in breastfed infants. Thus, urine oxalate itself cannot make a diagnosis of primary hyperoxaluria, and there is overlap between the three types of disorder (Fig. 64.9).

There are now additional urinary metabolites, known collectively as primary hyperoxaluria metabolites or PHM, that can be quantitated to give additional support to the diagnosis and type of PH. PHMs constitute glycolate, glycerate, dihydroxyglutarate and hydroxyoxoglutarate. Urinary glycolate excretion is raised in approximately two-thirds of cases of **PH1** but has a low diagnostic sensitivity and specificity as some of it is derived from dietary sources. A ratio of >193 umol/mmol creatinine had 100% specificity for PH1 but only 73% sensitivity (Woodward and Rumsby, submitted for publication). Excess urinary L-glycerate (>28 µmol/mmol) is a hallmark of **PH2**. This test can be performed as part of a routine organic acid screen, but false negatives can occur as a result of poor extraction and likely account for rare reports of normal glycerate excretion in genetically confirmed PH2 cases. More specific methodology shows elevation of L-glycerate in all patients tested. As the gene for **PH3** has been identified only relatively recently [53], the patient phenotypic characteristics are still being described. In addition to hyperoxaluria, the urine also shows the presence of 4-hydroxy-2-oxoglutarate and its metabolite dihydroxyglutarate. The former is unstable in unacidified urine and can sometimes be negative, whereas the latter appears to be consistently elevated.

The plasma oxalate level may not be raised unless there is marked nephrocalcinosis or a decline in the GFR has occurred. Note that all patients with end-stage renal failure from whatever cause demonstrate a raised plasma oxalate due to inadequate excretion but those with PH tend to be higher [54], with values in excess of 80 µmol/L almost certainly due to PH. The main value of plasma oxalate is assessing response to dialysis. Blood samples collected for oxalate analysis should be sent to the laboratory promptly for rapid separation and freezing to prevent oxalogenesis.

64

64.4.2 Genetic Testing

Any patient with a raised urinary oxalate in whom secondary causes have been excluded should be considered to have PH. If PHMs are available, the demonstration of raised glycolate, glycerate or dihydroxyglutarate can focus genetic testing to PH1, PH2 or PH3, respectively. In the absence of PHMs, initial testing should be for PH1 as this accounts for more than 80% of PH, followed by PH2 and PH3. Alternatively, with the new whole gene/exome sequencing, testing for all three at once may be cost-effective. Sibling and family screening is particularly beneficial and can identify asymptomatic cases which can allow the institution of appropriate therapy before symptoms arise [55].

64.4.3 Conservative Management

The key aims of therapy are to prevent systemic oxalate deposition with a high fluid intake accompanied by the administration of crystallisation inhibitors. A high urinary oxalate excretion has been linked with more progressive nephrocalcinosis and worse outcome [56, 57]. Recommendations for treatment are as follows:

- High fluid intake is mandatory, at least 3 litres/m^2/24 hours. This may require the placement of a nasogastric or gastrostomy feeding tube in infants in order to guarantee adequate hydration.
- Oral potassium citrate at a dose of 0.1–0.15 g/kg body weight per day (0.3–0.5 mmols/kg/day) to inhibit calcium oxalate crystallisation.
- The administration of pyridoxine to any patient with proven PH1 starting at a dose of 5 mg/kg/day up to 20 mg/kg/day with the intention of decreasing the urine oxalate excretion by at least 30%.

The alkalinisation of the urine with citrate reduces calcium oxalate saturation by forming complexes with calcium and by decreasing stone production. The potassium content needs review if the patient has a significantly reduced GFR. Pyrophosphate may also inhibit calcium oxalate crystallisation, and moderate doses of phosphate, 20–30 mg/kg/day, may be administered.

Vitamin B6 is a co-factor for AGT, and the administration of pyridoxine has been associated with a decrease in urine oxalate in about 30% of **PH1** patients. Some patients are extremely responsive to vitamin B6 at small doses such as 1 mg/kg/day or even a single 5 mg daily dose. In responsive patients, the pyridoxine dose can be reduced gradually to find the individual threshold of responsiveness using UOx:creat ratio as a guide. The absorption of vitamin B6 is variable, and some European centres assess plasma levels of vitamin B6 although there are no defined therapeutic levels. Sensory neurotoxicity is very rarely seen even at higher doses. A particular subset of patients with specific gene mutations, namely, p.Gly170Arg or p.Phe152Ile mutation, are more likely to respond to pharmacological doses of vitamin B6 and are predicted to have a better long-term outcome, an important reason to perform genetic mutation analysis [57–59].

Dietary restriction of oxalate is of limited use as the main source of oxalate is endogenous and the intestinal oxalate absorption in PH patients is lower than that of normal subjects [60]. Some experts recommend avoiding oxalate-rich foods in the diet such as dark chocolate, strawberries, spinach, rhubarb, beetroot, nuts and tea on a precautionary principle. Calcium intake should be normal, but excessive intake of vitamin C and vitamin D should be avoided. The gut bacterium *Oxalobacter formigenes* is able to metabolise oxalate in normal subjects, but there is limited evidence of its efficacy in reducing urine oxalate excretion in PH patients [61, 62].

64.4.4 Dialysis

Oxalate is generated at a rate of 4–7 mmols/1.73 m^2/day in contrast with clearance via conventional dialysis at a rate of 1–4 mmols/1.73 m^2/day, resulting in uncontrolled tissue accretion. Oxalate clearance on haemodialysis is greater than on peritoneal dialysis (120 mls/min on haemodialysis compared to 7 mls/min on peritoneal dialysis). Thus, standard haemodialysis programmes will result in a weekly clearance of oxalate of 6–9 mmol/1.73 m^2/week which is equivalent to 2–3 days of endogenous production of oxalate. Therefore, a combination of modalities, with intermittent daily haemodialysis and overnight peritoneal dialysis, enhances the overall clearance of oxalate and attempts to reduce the rebound which occurs after haemodialysis. These combination therapies with the use of high flux dialysers or long episodes of haemofiltration have all been advocated to improve oxalate removal [63–65]. The aim is to prevent the requirement for dialysis and to anticipate impairment in renal function with strategic planning for organ transplantation.

64.4.5 Transplantation

When the GFR falls below 60 ml/min/1.73 m^2, assessment for transplantation should take place initially with isolated liver transplantation being advised if the GFR continues to fall progressively below 60 ml/min/1.73 m^2 in patients with **PH1.** The liver is the only organ responsible for glyoxylate detoxification through the enzyme AGT. Thus, liver transplantation is a cure for PH1, but the native liver must be removed in order to avoid excessive oxalate production continuing [66–68].

Combined hepato-renal transplantation must be considered when the GFR falls below 40 ml/min/1.73 m^2 as there is a dramatic decrease in excretion of oxalate, with increase in plasma oxalate levels, resulting in systemic deposition of calcium oxalate in the heart (cardiomyopathy and conduction defects), vessel walls, skin (ulcerating lesions), nerves (peripheral neuropathy, mononeuritis multiplex), retina and joints (synovitis). The hepato-renal transplantation can be done simultaneously with excellent success even in small infants. A sequential procedure involving hepatic transplantation first, followed by a period of dialysis, with subsequent renal transplantation months later may be considered more appropriate in certain situations [69]. This type of approach can be useful if living related donors for split liver or kidney donation are being considered by relatives and when the patient has severe systemic oxalosis where a delay in the renal transplantation may be considered more conducive to successful final outcome after a period of some further dialysis to attempt to remove oxalate burden.

After combined hepato-renal transplantation, the urine oxalate can remain elevated for many years due to the slow resolubilisation of systemic calcium oxalate. These patients must still continue with a high fluid intake supported by the use of crystallisation inhibitors in order to protect the transplanted kidney from further calcium oxalate damage through stones or nephrocalcinosis [70]. Calcineurin inhibitors must be used with caution in order to minimise additional nephrotoxicity. The benefit of haemodialysis post-combined transplantation is still debated and currently should be limited to patients with acute tubulonecrosis or delayed graft function [71].

64.4.6 Management of Urolithiasis

Surgical intervention in the management of uncomplicated urolithiasis in PH patients should be limited. Extracorporeal shock wave lithotripsy (ESWL) was initially recommended in PH patients, but the calcium oxalate monohydrate stones typical of this disease are very hard and resistant to ESWL. Endoscopic stone removal allows direct visual control of removal of stone material, an advantage over ESWL where in situ fragmentation can leave gravel behind with subsequent formation of new stone matrix on these residues because of the on-going hyperoxaluria. Thus, endoscopic treatments such as semi-rigid ureterorenoscopy, flexible ureterorenoscopy and percutaneous nephrolithotomy are now procedures of choice [72, 73].

64.4.7 PH2

64

The overall long-term prognosis for patients with PH2 appears to be better than for PH1 and similar in outcome to the pyridoxine-sensitive PH1 genotypes, with the majority of patients presenting with urolithiasis. Nephrocalcinosis is less common but can occur in childhood and adult life [74]. End-stage renal failure tends to occur over 25 years of age and is now reported in around 25% of patients. The supportive management is the same as for PH1, but there is no rationale for the use of vitamin B6. Renal transplantation has been performed in some of these patients, but the majority will have a recurrence of their condition in the transplanted kidney. Success with combined hepato-renal transplantation has limited reporting [75].

64.4.8 PH3

The principles of management are the same, but in addition, a role of a vegetarian diet to reduce dietary hydroxyproline is being considered.

64.4.9 New Therapies and Future Strategies

The role of the innate immune system is being investigated in the pathogenesis of oxalate crystal-induced kidney injury, where the inflammasome describes a high molecular weight complex localised in the cytosol of cells, with signalling triggered via activation of toll-like receptors [76]. Approaches for therapy in PH1 include research into restoration of defective enzyme activity through chemical chaperones, hepatocyte cell transplantation and recombinant gene therapy for enzyme replacement. Substrate reduction therapy using RNA interference (RNAi) is a novel therapeutic approach currently being investigated in clinical trials. Glycolate is a substrate for glyoxylate production via the peroxisomal enzyme glycolate oxidase. Glycolate oxidase inhibition, initially studied using genetically modified mice, is now being evaluated using RNAi technology depleting the substrate for oxalate synthesis [77, 78] and directing a new approach to therapy in PH1 patients [79, 80]. Another chemically synthesised duplex RNA oligonucleotide conjugated to GalNac sugar residues inhibits the lactate dehydrogenase A (*LDHA*) gene and is being investigated as a therapeutic agent with potential use in PH1, PH2 and possibly PH3 [81].

Case Study

Case 1

A 14-year-old boy presented with a 3-month history of lethargy and pallor to his GP. A routine blood test demonstrated markedly deranged renal function, and an urgent referral was made to the tertiary renal service. The blood tests on admission revealed urea 57 mmol/l, creatinine 2070 μmol/l, Hb 6.8 g/dl, bicarbonate 9 mmol/l and PTH 896 ng/l. He was hypertensive but passing urine. The ultrasound scan of the kidneys showed marked nephrocalcinosis, and therefore urinary and plasma oxalate screening tests were sent, both of which were markedly raised: urine oxalate 440 mmol/mol creat (normal 2–83) and plasma oxalate 87 μmol/l (normal < 10). He was commenced on haemodialysis and pyridoxine.

After genetic studies confirmed PH1, workup for transplantation was undertaken, and he successfully received a cadaveric combined liver kidney transplant 8 months after presentation. His last plasma creatinine was recorded at 202 μmol/l at 12 years post-transplantation.

The presence of urine output resulted in a delayed presentation of renal impairment. The continued urine output provides some mechanism for oxalate removal, and, although systemic oxalosis was present, this was less severe. Post-transplant, the oxalate burden from the bones did not cause immediate tubular deposition and damage, hence a successful longer-term renal function.

Case 2

Following the presentation of case 1 above, his younger brother, then aged 8 years, underwent screening. The urinary oxalate was within the normal range, and the renal ultrasound scan was normal. However, as the phenotype of the disorder is so variable, genetic studies were undertaken. These tests confirmed that he had the same mutations as his brother (p.[Gly161Cys]; [Ser205Leu]) and thus has PH1. He continued with annual follow-up. On transfer to adult services at 18, and now at 26 years of age, he remains asymptomatic, with normal renal function and renal scan, and 24-hour urine oxalate measures consistently within the normal range, although at the upper limit at last collection U Ox 85 mmol/mol creat (normal 2–83).

Learning Points

- In this case, the marked nephrocalcinosis was the clue to the diagnosis differentiating it from other (more common) causes of renal failure.
- Although normal urinary oxalate is not typical in this disorder, it does occur, and genetic analysis should be used in suspicious cases or if a family history is suggestive.
- Despite identical gene mutations, there is marked phenotypic variability, with symptomatic presentation at variable ages. This young man requires annual follow-up for the rest of his life. He remains on pyridoxine and is advised to maintain a high fluid intake.

Tips and Tricks

1. Cases where stone analysis is inconclusive urine analysis should be undertaken. A fresh urine sample is required for a calcium/oxalate ratio. If further urine analysis is required due to an equivocal result, a 24-hour sample should be undertaken which will require acidification before testing. Vitamin C should also be discontinued prior to sampling.
2. Raised plasma oxalate is found in all patients with renal failure; thus, genetic testing must be carried out.
3. Surgical intervention in the management of uncomplicated urolithiasis in PH patients should be limited. When needed, endoscopic treatments such as semi-rigid or flexible ureterorenoscopy and percutaneous nephrolithotomy are now procedures of choice.
4. Pyridoxine is continued in mutations deemed to be sensitive. It is stopped post-liver transplant as the AGT activity is restored by the new graft.

64.5 Additional Information

Several national and international societies provide support for physicians and patients requiring more information on the primary hyperoxalurias. The European Hyperoxaluria Consortium, OxalEurope (▶ www.oxaleurope.org), provides contact details for clinicians and scientists, whilst the Oxalosis and Hyperoxaluria Foundation (▶ www.ohf.org) is an active organisation located in the United States providing regular updates for patients as well as physicians.

Chapter Review Questions

1. What are the key features of a patient presenting with infantile cystinosis?
2. What adjuvant therapy has been shown to reduce risk of gastric side effects from cysteamine therapy?
3. Is cysteamine therapy teratogenic?
4. In what setting is plasma oxalate measurement useful in primary hyperoxaluria?
5. Why is vitamin B6 a useful adjuvant treatment in primary hyperoxaluria type 1?

Answers

1. Infants develop appropriately up to 6 months of age before presenting with polyuria and polydipsia, unexplained fever, anorexia, constipation, vomiting with resultant dehydration and failure to thrive and signs of rickets. The key presenting features are hypokalaemia, hyponatraemia, hypophosphataemia, acidosis, generalised amino aciduria and glycosuria.
2. Proton pump inhibitors
3. The teratogenicity of oral cysteamine has not been determined in humans. The current advice is that women planning to conceive should forgo cysteamine from the date of conception until after the pregnancy although there is a report of a

woman receiving 300 mg of cysteamine three times daily throughout her pregnancy, who subsequently delivered a healthy infant. Cysteamine should be recommenced soon after delivery, and breastfeeding is not advised.
4. The plasma oxalate level may not be raised unless there is marked nephrocalcinosis or a decline in the GFR has occurred. Note that all patients with end-stage renal failure from whatever cause demonstrate a raised plasma oxalate due to inadequate excretion but those with PH tend to be higher, with values in excess of 80 μmol/L almost certainly due to PH. The main value of plasma oxalate is assessing response to dialysis. Blood samples collected for oxalate analysis should be sent to the laboratory promptly for rapid separation and freezing to prevent oxalogenesis.
5. Vitamin B6 is a co-factor for AGT, and the administration of pyridoxine has been associated with a decrease in urine oxalate in about 30% of primary hyperoxaluria type 1 patients. Pyridoxine is continued in mutations deemed to be sensitive. It is stopped post-liver transplant as the AGT activity is restored by the new graft.

64.6 Conclusion

This chapter highlights the improvements in identification and management of cystinosis and the primary hyperoxalurias enabling patients to reach adulthood. The multisystem manifestations have been summarised and key developments in treatment strategies highlighted. Continuing advances in genomics, together with information obtained from the rare disease registries, are adding to current knowledge of both conditions. Progress in this area forms the basis of developing new screening strategies and novel therapeutic interventions. Despite these advances, patients can experience significant psychosocial burden, and thus effective transition of these patients is crucial.

References

Cystinosis

1. Town M, Jean G, Cherqui S, Attard M, Forestier L, Whitmore SA, Callen DF, Gribouval O, Broyer M, Bates GP, van't Hoff W. A novel gene encoding an integral membrane protein is mutated in nephropathic cystinosis. Nat Genet. 1998;18(4):319.
2. Kalatzis V, Antignac C. Cystinosis: from gene to disease. Nephrol Dial Transplant. 2002;17(11):1883–6.
3. Gahl WA, Thoene JG, Schneider JA. Cystinosis. N Engl J Med. 2002;347(2):111–21.
4. Kalatzis V, Antignac C. New aspects of the pathogenesis of cystinosis. Pediatr Nephrol. 2003;18(3):207–15.
5. Anikster Y, Shotelersuk V, Gahl WA. CTNS mutations in patients with cystinosis. Hum Mutat. 1999;14(6):454.
6. The Institute of Medical Genetics in Cardiff. Human Gene Mutation Database [Internet]. 2018 [Date Accessed 28th June 2018]. Available from: http://www.hgmd.cf.ac.uk/ac/index.php.
7. Shotelersuk V, Larson D, Anikster Y, McDowell G, Lemons R, Bernardini I, Guo J, Thoene J, Gahl WA. CTNS mutations in an American-based population of cystinosis patients. Am J Hum Genet. 1998;63(5):1352–62.
8. Attard M, Jean G, Forestier L, Cherqui S, van't Hoff W, Broyer M, Antignac C, Town M. Severity of phenotype in cystinosis varies with mutations in the CTNS gene: predicted effect on the model of cystinosin. Hum Mol Genet. 1999;8(13):2507–14.
9. McGowan-Jordan J, Stoddard K, Podolsky L, Orrbine E, McLaine P, Town M, Goodyer P, MacKenzie A, Heick H. Molecular analysis of cystinosis: probable Irish origin of the most common French-Canadian mutation. Eur J Hum Genet. 1999;7(6):671.
10. Thoene J, Lemons R, Anikster Y, Mullet J, Paelicke K, Lucero C, Gahl W, Schneider J, Shu SG, Campbell HT. Mutations of CTNS causing intermediate cystinosis. Mol Genet Metab. 1999;67(4):283–93.
11. Anikster Y, Lucero C, Guo J, Huizing M, Shotelersuk V, Bernardini I, McDowell G, Iwata F, Kaiser-Kupfer MI, Jaffe R, Thoene J. Ocular nonnephropathic cystinosis: clinical, biochemical, and molecular correlations. Pediatr Res. 2000;47(1):17.
12. Phornphutkul C, Anikster Y, Huizing M, Braun P, Brodie C, Chou JY, Gahl WA. The promoter of a lysosomal membrane transporter gene, CTNS, binds Sp-1, shares sequences with the promoter of an adjacent gene, CARKL, and causes cystinosis if mutated in a critical region. Am J Hum Genet. 2001;69(4):712–21.
13. Kalatzis V, Cohen-Solal L, Cordier B, Frishberg Y, Kemper M, Nuutinen EM, Legrand E, Cochat P, Antignac C. Identification of 14 novel CTNS mutations and characterization of seven splice site mutations associated with cystinosis. Hum Mutat. 2002;20(6):439–46.
14. Kiehntopf M, Schickel J, Gönne BV, Koch HG, Superti-Furga A, Steinmann B, Deufel T, Harms E. Analysis of the CTNS gene in patients of German and Swiss origin with nephropathic cystinosis. Hum Mutat. 2002;20(3):237.
15. Mason S, Pepe G, Dall'Amico R, Tartaglia S, Casciani S, Greco M, Bencivenga P, Murer L, Rizzoni G, Tenconi R, Clementi M. Mutational spectrum of the CTNS gene in Italy. Eur J Hum Genet. 2003;11(7):503.
16. Heil SG, Levtchenko E, Monnens LA, Trijbels FJ, Van der Put NM, Blom HJ. The molecular basis of Dutch infantile nephropathic cystinosis. Nephron. 2001;89(1):50–5.
17. Kleta R, Anikster Y, Lucero C, Shotelersuk V, Huizing M, Bernardini I, Park M, Thoene J, Schneider J, Gahl WA. CTNS mutations in African American patients with cystinosis. Mol Genet Metab. 2001;74(3):332–7.
18. Kalatzis V, Cherqui S, JEAN G, Cordier B, Cochat P, Broyer M, Antignac C. Characterization of a putative founder mutation that accounts for the high incidence of cystinosis in Brittany. J Am Soc Nephrol. 2001;12(10):2170–4.
19. McGowan-Jordan J, Stoddard K, Podolsky L, Orrbine E, McLaine P, Town M, Goodyer P, MacKenzie A, Heick H. Molecular analysis of cystinosis: probable Irish origin of the most common French Canadian mutation. Eur J Hum Genet. 1999;7(6):671.
20. Anikster Y, Lucero C, Touchman JW, Huizing M, McDowell G, Shotelersuk V, Green ED, Gahl WA. Identification and detection of the common 65-kb deletion breakpoint in the

nephropathic cystinosis gene (CTNS). Mol Genet Metab. 1999;66(2):111–6.

21. Topaloglu R, Vilboux T, Coskun T, Ozaltin F, Tinloy B, Gunay-Aygun M, Bakkaloglu A, Besbas N, Van Den Heuvel L, Kleta R, Gahl WA. Genetic basis of cystinosis in Turkish patients: a single-center experience. Pediatr Nephrol. 2012;27(1): 115–21.
22. Wamelink MM, Struys EA, Jansen EE, Blom HJ, Vilboux T, Gahl WA, Kömhoff M, Jakobs CA, Levtchenko EN. Elevated concentrations of sedoheptulose in bloodspots of patients with cystinosis caused by the 57-kb deletion: implications for diagnostics and neonatal screening. Mol Genet Metab. 2011;102(3):339–42.
23. Wühl E, Haffner D, Offner G, Broyer M, van't Hoff W, Mehls O. Long-term treatment with growth hormone in short children with nephropathic cystinosis. J Pediatr. 2001;138(6):880–7.
24. Levtchenko EN, van Dael CM, de Graaf-Hess AC, Wilmer MJ, van den Heuvel LP, Monnens LA, Blom HJ. Strict cysteamine dose regimen is required to prevent nocturnal cystine accumulation in cystinosis. Pediatr Nephrol. 2006;21(1): 110–3.
25. Langman CB, Greenbaum LA, Sarwal M, Grimm P, Niaudet P, Deschenes G, Cornelissen E, Morin D, Cochat P, Matossian D, Gaillard S. A randomized controlled crossover trial with delayed-release cysteamine bitartrate in nephropathic cystinosis: effectiveness on white blood cell cystine levels and comparison of safety (vol 7, pg 1112, 2012). Clin J Am Soc Nephrol. 2013;8(3):468.
26. Besouw M, Tangerman A, Cornelissen E, Rioux P, Levtchenko E. Halitosis in cystinosis patients after administration of immediate-release cysteamine bitartrate compared to delayed-release cysteamine bitartrate. Mol Genet Metab. 2012;107(1):234–6.
27. Besouw M, Levtchenko E. Growth retardation in children with cystinosis. Minerva Pediatr. 2010;62(3):307–13.
28. Dohil R, Newbury RO, Sellers ZM, Deutsch R, Schneider JA. The evaluation and treatment of gastrointestinal disease in children with cystinosis receiving cysteamine. J Pediatr. 2003;143(2):224–30.
29. Dohil R, Fidler M, Barshop B, Newbury R, Sellers Z, Deutsch R, Schneider J. Esomeprazole therapy for gastric acid hypersecretion in children with cystinosis. Pediatr Nephrol. 2005;20(12):1786–93.
30. Manz F, Gretz N. Progression of chronic renal failure in a historical group of patients with nephropathic cystinosis. Pediatr Nephrol. 1994;8(4):466–71.
31. Brodin-Sartorius A, Tête MJ, Niaudet P, Antignac C, Guest G, Ottolenghi C, Charbit M, Moyse D, Legendre C, Lesavre P, Cochat P. Cysteamine therapy delays the progression of nephropathic cystinosis in late adolescents and adults. Kidney Int. 2012;81(2):179–89.
32. Markello TC, Bernardini IM, Gahl WA. Improved renal function in children with cystinosis treated with cysteamine. N Engl J Med. 1993;328(16):1157–62.
33. Cohen C, Charbit M, Chadefaux-Vekemans B, Giral M, Garrigue V, Kessler M, Antoine C, Snanoudj R, Niaudet P, Kreis H, Legendre C. Excellent long-term outcome of renal transplantation in cystinosis patients. Orphanet J Rare Dis. 2015;10(1):90.
34. Tsilou E, Zhou M, Gahl W, Sieving PC, Chan CC. Ophthalmic manifestations and histopathology of infantile nephropathic cystinosis: report of a case and review of the literature. Surv Ophthalmol. 2007;52(1):97–105.
35. Geelen JM, Monnens LA, Levtchenko EN. Follow-up and treatment of adults with cystinosis in the Netherlands. Nephrol Dial Transplant. 2002;17(10):1766–70.
36. Nesterova G, Gahl W. Nephropathic cystinosis: late complications of a multisystemic disease. Pediatr Nephrol. 2008;23(6):863–78.
37. Emadi A, Burns KH, Confer B, Borowitz MJ, Streiff MB. Hematological manifestations of nephropathic cystinosis. Acta Haematol. 2008;119(3):169–72.
38. Besouw MT, Hulstijn-Dirkmaat GM, van der Rijken RE, Cornelissen EA, van Dael CM, Walle JV, Lilien MR, Levtchenko EN. Neurocognitive functioning in school-aged cystinosis patients. J Inherit Metab Dis. 2010;33(6):787–93.
39. Dogulu CF, Tsilou E, Rubin B, FitzGibbon EJ, Kaiser-Kupper MI, Rennert OM, Gahl WA. Idiopathic intracranial hypertension in cystinosis. J Pediatr. 2004;145(5):673–8.
40. Gahl WA. Early oral cysteamine therapy for nephropathic cystinosis. Eur J Pediatr. 2003;162(1):S38–41.
41. Haase M, Morgera S, Bamberg C, Halle H, Martini S, Dragun D, Neumayer HH, Budde K. Successful pregnancies in dialysis patients including those suffering from cystinosis and familial Mediterranean fever. J Nephrol. 2006;19(5):677–81.
42. Kleta R, Bernardini I, Ueda M, Varade WS, Phornphutkul C, Krasnewich D, Gahl WA. Long-term follow-up of well-treated nephropathic cystinosis patients. J Pediatr. 2004;145(4):555–60.
43. McCaughan B, Kay G, Knott RM, Cairns D. A potential new prodrug for the treatment of cystinosis: design, synthesis and in-vitro evaluation. Bioorg Med Chem Lett. 2008;18(5):1716–9.
44. Omran Z, Kay G, Di Salvo A, Knott RM, Cairns D. PEGylated derivatives of cystamine as enhanced treatments for nephropathic cystinosis. Bioorg Med Chem Lett. 2011;21(1):45–7.
45. Frost L, Suryadevara P, Cannell SJ, Groundwater PW, Hambleton PA, Anderson RJ. Synthesis of diacylated γ-glutamyl-cysteamine prodrugs, and in vitro evaluation of their cytotoxicity and intracellular delivery of cysteamine. Eur J Med Chem. 2016;109:206–15.
46. Hippert C, Dubois G, Morin C, Disson O, Ibanes S, Jacquet C, Schwendener R, Antignac C, Kremer EJ, Kalatzis V. Gene transfer may be preventive but not curative for a lysosomal transport disorder. Mol Ther. 2008;16(8):1372–81.
47. Syres K, Harrison F, Tadlock M, Jester JV, Simpson J, Roy S, Salomon DR, Cherqui S. Successful treatment of the murine model of cystinosis using bone marrow cell transplantation. Blood. 2009;114(12):2542–52.
48. Yeagy BA, Harrison F, Gubler MC, Koziol JA, Salomon DR, Cherqui S. Kidney preservation by bone marrow cell transplantation in hereditary nephropathy. Kidney Int. 2011;79(11): 1198–206.
49. Harrison F, Yeagy BA, Rocca CJ, Kohn DB, Salomon DR, Cherqui S. Hematopoietic stem cell gene therapy for the multisystemic lysosomal storage disorder cystinosis. Mol Ther. 2013;21(2):433–44.
50. Doyle M, Werner-Lin A. That eagle covering me: transitioning and connected autonomy for emerging adults with cystinosis. Pediatr Nephrol. 2015;30(2):281–91.
51. Raina R, Wang J, Krishnappa V. Structured transition protocol for children with cystinosis. Frontiers in pediatrics. 2017;5:191.

The Primary Hyperoxalurias

51. Takada Y, Kaneko N, Esumi H, Purdue PE, Danpure CJ. Human peroxisomal L-alanine:glyoxylate aminotransferase: evolutionary loss of a mitochondrial targeting signal by point mutation of the initiation codon. Biochem J. 1990;268:517–20.
52. Cregeen D P, Williams E L, Hulton S A, Rumsby G. Molecular analysis of the glyoxylate reductase (GRHPR) gene and description of mutations underlying primary hyperoxaluria type 2. Human Mutation, Mutation in Brief [Online Journal)

2003 http://www.interscience.wiley.com/humanmutation/pdf/mutation/671.pdf.
53. Belostotsky R, Seboun E, Idelson GH, Milliner DS, Becker-Cohen R, Rinat C, Monico CG, Feinstein S, Ben-Shalom E, Magen D, Weissman I, Charon C, Frishberg Y. Mutations in DHDPSL are responsible for primary hyperoxaluria type III. Am J Hum Genet. 2010;87:392–9.
54. Barratt TM, Kasidas GP, Murdoch I, Rose GA. Urinary oxalate and glycolate excretion and plasma oxalate concentration. Arch Dis Child. 1991;66:501–3.
55. Rumsby G. An overview of the role of genotyping in the diagnosis of the primary hyperoxalurias. Urol Res. 2005;33:318–20.
56. Tang X, Bergstrath EJ, Mehta RA, Vrtiska TJ, Milliner DS, Lieske JC. Nephrocalcinosis is a risk factor for kidney failure in primary hyperoxaluria. Kidney Int. 2015;87:623–31.
57. Zhao F, Bergstralh EJ, Mehta RA, Vaughan LE, Olson JB, Seide BM, Meek AM, Cogal AG, Lieske JC, Milliner DS, Investigators of Rare Kidney Stone Consortium. Predictors of incident ESRD among patients with primary hyperoxaluria presenting prior to kidney failure. Clin J Am Soc Nephrol. 2016;11(1):119–26.
58. Williams EL, Acquaviva C, Amoroso A, Chevalier F, Coulter-Mackie M, Monico CM, Giachino D, Owen EP, Robbiano A, Salido E, Waterham H, Rumsby G. Primary hyperoxaluria type 1: update and additional mutation analysis of the AGXT gene. Hum Mutat. 2009;30:910–7.
59. Mandrile G, van Woerden CS, Berchialla P, Beck BB, Bourdain CA, Hulton SA, Rumsby G, on behalf of Oxal Europe Consortium. Data from a large European study indicate that the outcome of primary hyperoxaluria type 1 correlates with the AGXT mutation type. Kidney Int. 2014;86(6):1197–204.
60. Sikora P, von Unruh GE, Beck B, Feldkötter M, Zajaczkowska M, Hesse A, Hoppe B. [13C2]oxalate absorption in children with idiopathic calcium oxalate urolithiasis or primary hyperoxaluria. Kidney Int. 2008;73:1181–6.
61. Hoppe B, Groothoff JW, Hulton SA, Cochat P, Niaudet P, Kemper MJ, Deschênes G, Unwin R, Milliner D. Efficacy and safety of Oxalobacter formigenes to reduce urinary oxalate in primary hyperoxaluria. Nephrol Dial Transplant. 2011;26(11):3609–15.
62. Milliner D. Treatment of the primary hyperoxalurias: a new chapter. Kidney Int. 2006;70:1198–200.
63. Illies F, Bonzel KE, Wingen AM, Latta K, Hoyer PF. Clearance and removal of oxalate in children on intensified dialysis for primary hyperoxaluria type 1. Kidney Int. 2006;70:1642–8.
64. Hoppe B, Graf D, Offner G, Latta K, Byrd DJ, Michalk D, Brodehl J. Oxalate elimination via haemodialysis or peritoneal dialysis in children with chronic renal failure. Pediatr Nephrol. 1996;10:488–92.
65. Tang X, Voskoboev NV, Wannarka SL, Olson JB, Milliner DS, Lieske JC. Oxalate quantification in hemodialysate to assess dialysis adequacy for primary hyperoxaluria. Am J Nephrol. 2014;39(5):376–82.
66. Perera MT, Sharif K, Lloyd C, Foster K, Hulton SA, Mirza DF, McKiernan PJ. Pre-emptive liver transplantation for primary hyperoxaluria (PH1) arrests long-term renal function deterioration. Nephrol Dial Transplant. 2011;26:354–9.
67. Kemper MJ, Nolkemper D, Rogiers X, Timmermann K, Sturm E, Malago M, Broelsch CE, Burdelski M, Müller-Wiefel DE. Preemptive liver transplantation in primary hyperoxaluria type 1: timing and preliminary results. J Nephrol. 1998;11(S1):46–8.
68. Cochat P, Fargue S, Harambat J. Primary hyperoxaluria type 1: strategy for organ transplantation. Curr Opin Organ Transplant. 2010;15:590–3.
69. Ellis SR, Hulton SA, McKiernan PJ, de Ville de Goyet J, Kelly DA. Combined liver-kidney transplantation for primary hyperoxaluria type 1 in young children. Nephrol Dial Transplant. 2001;16:348–54.
70. Hoppe B, Latta K, von Schnakenburg C, Kemper MJ. Primary hyperoxaluria - the German experience. Am J Nephrol. 2005;25:276–81.
71. Harps E, Brinkert F, Ganschow R, Briem-Richter A, van Husen M, Schmidtke S, Nashan B, Fischer L, Kemper MJ. Immediate postoperative intensive care treatment for pediatric combined liver-kidney transplantation: outcome and prognostic factors. Transplantation. 2011;91:1127–31.
72. Türk C, Knoll T, Petrik A, Sarica K, Straub M, Seitz C. EAU guidelines on urolithiasis. European Association of Urology, The Netherlands; 2011.
73. Straub M, Gschwend J, Zorn C. Pediatric urolithiasis: the current surgical management. Pediatr Nephrol. 2010;25:1239–44.
74. Johnson SA, Rumsby G, Cregreen D, Hulton SA. Primary hyperoxaluria type 2 in children. Pediatr Nephrol. 2002;17(8):597–601.
75. Dhondup T, Lorenz EC, Milliner DS, Lieske JC. Combined liver–kidney transplantation for primary hyperoxaluria type 2: a case report. Am J Transplant. 2018;18(1):253–7.
76. Joshi S, Wang W, Peck AB, Khan SR. Activation of the NLRP3 inflammasome in association with calcium oxalate crystal-induced reactive oxygen species in kidneys. J Urol. 2015;193(5):1684–91.
77. Martin-Higueras C, Luis-Lima S, Salido E. Glycolate oxidase is a safe and efficient target for substrate reduction therapy in a mouse model of primary hyperoxaluria type 1. Mol Ther. 2016;24(4):719–75.
78. Dutta C, Avitahl-Curtis N, Pursell N, et al. Inhibition of glycolate oxidase with dicer-substrate siRNA reduces calcium oxalate deposition in a mouse model of primary hyperoxaluria type 1. Mol Ther. 2016;24(4):770–8.
79. Milliner DS. siRNA therapeutics for primary hyperoxaluria: a beginning. Mol Ther. 2016;24:666–7.
80. Hulton S, Frishberg Y, Milliner D, Hoppe B, Lorch U, Olgesbee D, Lieske J, Haslett P. A phase 1/2 trial of ALN-GO1, an investigational RNAi therapeutic for Primary Hyperoxaluria Type 1 (PH1). Pediatr Nephrol. 2016, 2016;(31):1763–3.
81. Chengjung L, Pursell N, Gierut J, Saxena U, Zhou W, Dills M. et al., Specific inhibition of hepatic lactate dehydrogenase reduces oxalate production in mouse models of primary hyperoxaluria. Mol Ther. 2018;26(8) https://doi.org/10.1016/j.ymthe.2018.05.016.

Supplementary Reading

Cystinosis

Ariceta G, Camacho JA, Fernández-Obispo M, Fernández-Polo A, Gamez J, García-Villoria J, Monteczuma EL, Leyes P, Martín-Begué N, Oppenheimer F, Perelló M. Cystinosis in adult and adolescent patients: recommendations for the comprehensive care of cystinosis. Nefrología (English Edition). 2015;35(3):304–21.

64

Emma F, Nesterova G, Langman C, Labbé A, Cherqui S, Goodyer P, Janssen MC, Greco M, Topaloglu R, Elenberg E, Dohil R. Nephropathic cystinosis: an international consensus document. Nephrol Dial Transplant. 2014;29(suppl_4):iv87–94.

Langman CB, Barshop BA, Deschênes G, Emma F, Goodyer P, Lipkin G, Midgley JP, Ottolenghi C, Servais A, Soliman NA, Thoene JG. Controversies and research agenda in nephropathic cystinosis: conclusions from a "Kidney Disease: Improving Global Outcomes" (KDIGO) Controversies Conference. Kidney Int. 2016;89(6):1192–203.

The Primary Hyperoxalurias

Cochat P, Hulton SA, Acquaviva C, Danpure CJ, Daudon M, De Marchi M, Fargue S, Groothoff JW, Harambat J, Hoppe B, Jamieson N, Kemper MJ, Mandrile G, Marangella M, Picca S, Rumsby G, Salido E, Straub M, van Woerden CS, on behalf of OxalEurope. Primary hyperoxaluria type 1: indications for screening and guidance for diagnosis and treatment. Nephrol Dial Transplant. 2012;27:1729–36.

Rumsby G, Hulton SA. Primary hyperoxaluria type 2. GeneReviews. 2017;

Chronic Kidney Disease

Contents

Chronic Kidney Disease: Epidemiology and Causes

Asmat Abro, George H. B. Greenhall, and Dorothea Nitsch

Contents

M. Harber (ed.), *Primer on Nephrology*, https://doi.org/10.1007/978-3-030-76419-7_65

Key Points of the Chapter

1. When considering risk factors of kidney disease, longitudinal data that investigate incidence of disease may be more useful than cross-sectional data assessing prevalence.
2. There is to date no firm evidence supporting blanket screening for kidney disease irrespective of underlying cause in the general population. However, for specific forms of kidney disease, there may be benefits of testing and early identification, for example, amongst people with diabetes.
3. Urinary testing for albuminuria is infrequently done in primary care, yet albuminuria is a key risk factor for poor health outcomes.

65.1 Introduction

Abnormalities of kidney function or structure lasting more than 3 months are considered as chronic kidney disease (CKD). CKD is then classified further into categories of risk and severity of function loss based on albuminuria and eGFR. The cause of kidney disease should be recorded as well, though only a subset of people in the general population are investigated as to the cause of their kidney function loss. Typically, people in the general population present with a decreased glomerular filtration rate (GFR less than 60 ml/min per 1.73 m^2). Urinary testing is infrequently done in general practice, and structural kidney problems are often only picked up during abdominal ultrasounds carried out for other reasons; hence, patients present less often with gross proteinuria or structural abnormalities.

CKD is increasingly recognised as worldwide health problem. This chapter reviews the epidemiology of CKD. As CKD is a silent disease and often asymptomatic until the presence of established renal failure, there are limited data on its natural history. This chapter aims to put the available data from routine health care and renal registries into context and discusses why screening for CKD has not been established in many health settings.

65.2 Incidence and Prevalence Explained Using Renal Replacement Therapy Data

Incidence of renal replacement therapy captures how many new people start chronic RRT per unit time (typically years) per million population. ◘ Figure 65.1 shows the change in the UK RRT incidence since 1990. The initial rise in incidence rate in the over 65 age group, which occurred due to acceptance of elderly for RRT, has plateaued, but there appears to be an upward trend in incidence rate in individuals between 45 and 65 years of age [1].

Prevalence refers to how many patients are on RRT at a given point in time. Prevalence data are affected by how many people start dialysis (incidence) and by how long people survive on RRT. Trends of prevalence are therefore much harder to interpret as there are a range of factors that impact on incidence of RRT and factors that impact on survival on RRT, both of which may

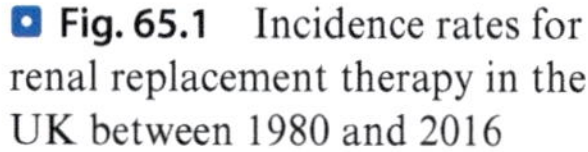

◘ **Fig. 65.1** Incidence rates for renal replacement therapy in the UK between 1980 and 2016

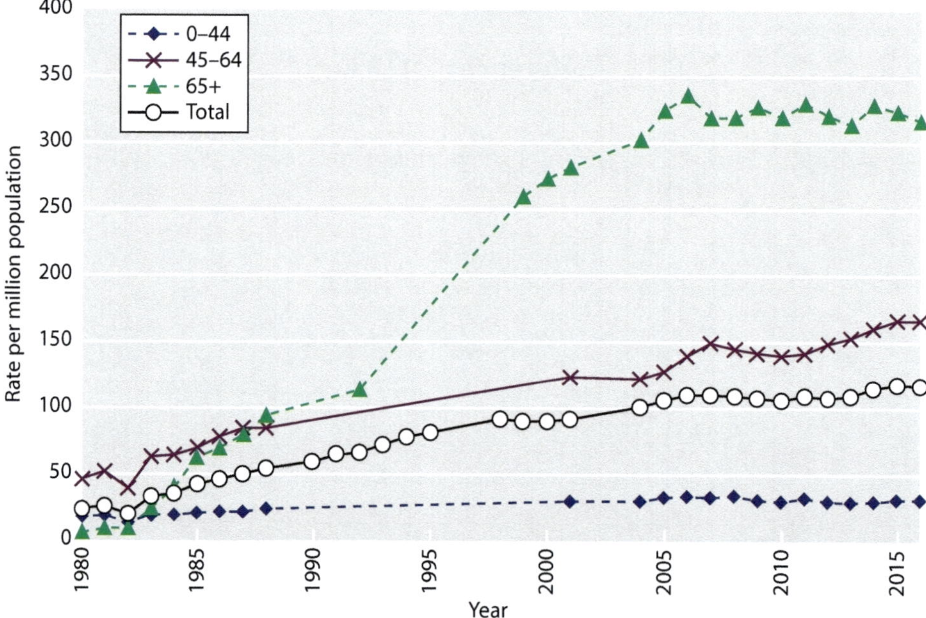

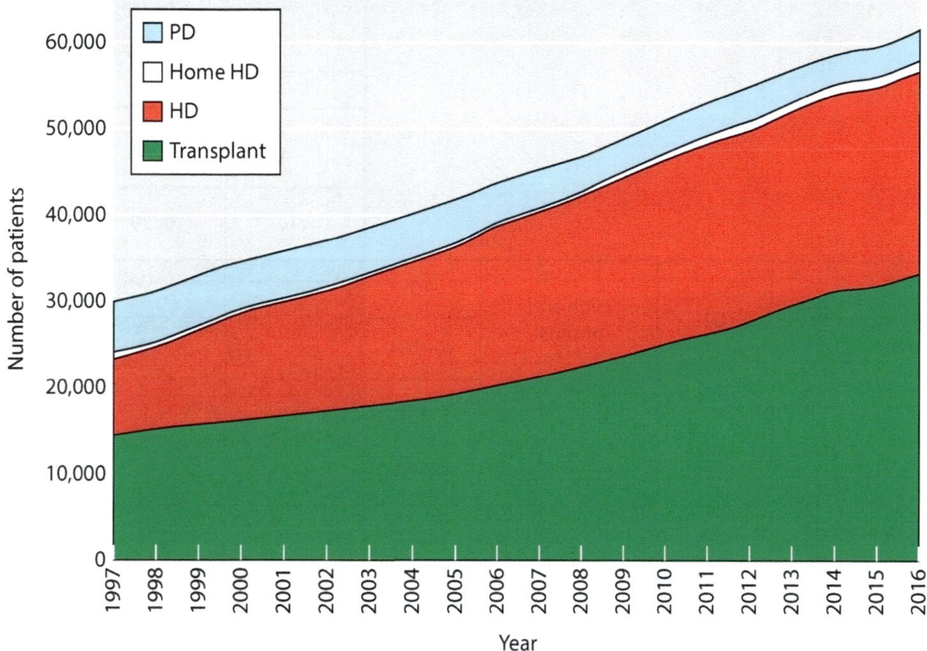

Fig. 65.2 Growth in prevalent patients by treatment modality at the end of each year 1997–2016

affect total prevalence figures. For example, in the UK, prevalence has increased each year by ~3–4%. When comparing RRT incidence with prevalence data over time, it becomes apparent that this yearly increase in prevalent patient numbers on dialysis has been mainly driven by improved survival and a larger surviving proportion of transplant patients because in the same time period, there has been an overall stable incidence of new RRT patients (Fig. 65.2) [2].

Prevalence data are useful to quantify costs to the health system; however, incidence data are more useful to understand underlying factors associated with increases in dialysis or transplant take-on over time.

65.2.1 Limitations of Using RRT Data

Most renal registries record and report the incidence of RRT for patients who have started and survived RRT for at least 90 days as these patients are assumed to have irreversible or established end-stage renal disease (ESRD). This 90-day rule originated in the USA where the government starts to pay for dialysis of patients when they are deemed to be chronic. Many other renal registries adopted the same rule to collect their national data to allow for international comparisons. However, collecting data only on people who survived more than 90 days on dialysis means that this measure does not capture the information of the incidence of dialysis, and it does not tell us how many patients in the population needed acute or chronic dialysis. Not every patient who needs dialysis may get started on dialysis, and not every patient started on dialysis will survive for 90 days. When making international comparisons of RRT incidence, investigators therefore have to make a series of assumptions with regard to the referral and availability of RRT, people with CKD stage 5 being started on dialysis, reversibility of the kidney problem, survival in the first 90 days of the dialysis (*numerator*) and the population (*denominator*).

Whether very elderly patients or those with other chronic conditions such as HIV, malignancy or severe cardiovascular disease are offered RRT depends to a large extent on available resources, national legislation with respect to life-prolonging therapy in the face of chronic disease and the degree of renal knowledge and ethical opinions of treating doctors.

65.3 Defining the Incidence and Prevalence of CKD in a Population

The term CKD covers a number of primary disease processes that result in structural and/or functional kidney abnormalities persisting for at least 3 months. There have been various staging systems over time. A widely used version was from NFK-KDOQI which subdivided CKD into five stages according to the eGFR. This staging was later superseded by the KDIGO CKD staging system (Fig. 65.3) which was based on solid epide-

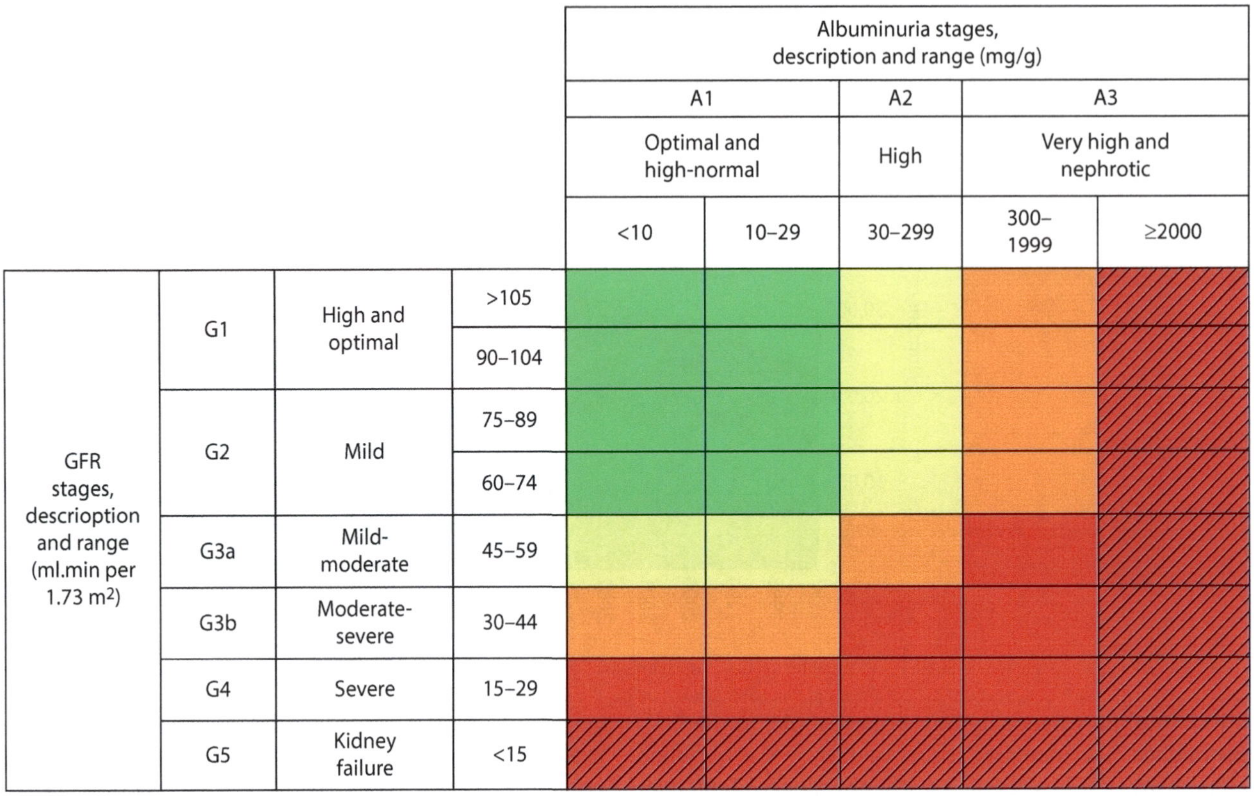

				Albuminuria stages, description and range (mg/g)				
				A1		A2	A3	
				Optimal and high-normal		High	Very high and nephrotic	
				<10	10–29	30–299	300–1999	≥2000
GFR stages, descrioption and range (ml.min per 1.73 m^2)	G1	High and optimal	>105					
			90–104					
	G2	Mild	75–89					
			60–74					
	G3a	Mild-moderate	45–59					
	G3b	Moderate-severe	30–44					
	G4	Severe	15–29					
	G5	Kidney failure	<15					

Fig. 65.3 Composite ranking for relative risks by GFR and albuminuria (KDIGO 2009). (Reproduced with permission from Kidney Disease: Improving Global Outcomes (KDIGO) CKD Work Group [3])

miological information on how single time point eGFR and albuminuria test results relate to later risk of cardiovascular disease and incidence of ESRD.

The incidence of CKD is much harder to ascertain than the incidence of RRT. In order to measure 'incidence of CKD', i.e. true new CKD cases in a perfect epidemiological cohort study, one would need to exclude those with CKD at baseline from our follow-up study. The follow-up requires re-measuring kidney function at regular time points on every participant using the exact same assay each time. This assumes a perfect measurement of CKD, but as we discuss below, this is not feasible. In order to have enough observations to understand the risk factors for incident ESRD, a very large study would be needed. For a million population in the UK, there would be about 150 incident RRT cases per year, so the cost of a proper research study just to define CKD incidence, and how this relates to RRT incidence, is prohibitive. To date, there is no universal screening for kidney disease in the general population at pre-specified time points in life. Due to the use of changing creatinine assays over time and testing of kidney function at irregular intervals according to patient need, the use of routine data is therefore challenging and relies on some untestable assumptions.

65.3.1 Limitations of Using CKD Definition and Staging

The biggest problem of the NKF-KDOQI system was that it did not reflect the true risk of who progresses to RRT and, of those identified, who has a treatable kidney problem. As mentioned before, pooled population-based studies looking at risks for ESRD and death in international studies provided evidence which led to the KDIGO staging of CKD to include albuminuria as an independent risk factor for RRT and low GFR; indeed, albuminuria is an equally strong or potentially stronger predictor of the risk of RRT than eGFR (Fig. 65.3). This is now firmly reflected in the risk system [3, 4] – a person with persistent albuminuria who has an eGFR >60 ml/min/1.73 m^2 has the same risk of ending up on dialysis as a person with already reduced eGFR but no albuminuria. However, in practice, the largest group of patients to come to clinical attention with CKD are those with reduced GFR (stages 3–5), for many of whom the causes are multifactorial, and for whom it is unclear whether detecting CKD has any implications on specialised kidney care. Most people with CKD stages 3–5 benefit from agressive cardiovascular risk management, as their risk of dying from cardiovascular disease is very high. The vast majority of these patients are frail elderly people who are traditionally managed by general practitioners and geriatricians. Unfortunately, the many patients with proteinuria/albuminuria and maintained renal function who may merit relatively more attention because there is a greater potential to prevent progression are often not detected as they are not tested for albuminuria.

The second issue is accuracy of measuring estimated GFR. The traditional indirect measure of GFR in clinical practice was the 24 h creatinine clearance. These 24 h urine collections are subject to substantial measurement error and not feasible in large studies. NHANES III was the first population-based survey that assessed renal impairment using a serum creatinine-based formula that had been validated for the US kidney patient population [5]. The typical eGFR formula requires simple input data such as the age, gender and ethnicity, in addition to serum creatinine. Because creatinine is a product of the endogenous muscle metabolism, these calculations assume the presence of a stable muscle mass. An investigation in standardisation of creatinine assays showed that the type of assay plays a role for an estimated GFR >60 ml/min per 1.73 m^2. Each of the available eGFR formulae has its own biases, e.g. the MDRD formula overestimates presence of CKD in older women and has not been validated in older age groups [6]. The CKD-EPI formula is thought to perform better in Western populations [7] but does not appear to work in less well-nourished populations in other parts of the world, and using the 'race' adjustment in the formula has been shown to lead to unintended health inequalities. The measurement error around an eGFR measurement ranges from ±20 ml/min relative to the gold-standard GFR measurement (with worse errors when eGFR is >60 ml/min), and so any survey using eGFR data will be imprecise by default [8]. Most epidemiologic studies only use a single time point eGFR, and the reported risk associations are to some degree affected by non-differential misclassification. Non-differential misclassification means that the observed associations for eGFR and spot urine or dipstick measurements will be imprecise and not capture true kidney function and true albuminuria perfectly. Hence, research studies underestimate the true degree of risk associations for the true underlying kidney function/damage. This is not a major problem for clinical practice as we use repeats of these imperfect test results to reduce measurement error for an individual patient. Of note is that the current KDIGO classification system is based on these imperfect test results.

Overall, despite above criticisms – in comparison with pure serum creatinine measurements and 24 h collections of urine, serum creatinine-based GFR estimates and urinary albumin/creatinine or protein/creatinine ratios seem to perform well to detect the presence of kidney disease.

65.4 What Influences Prevalence of CKD and Incidence of ESRD?

Many community-based surveys in the USA, the UK and elsewhere have highlighted that the prevalence of CKD is much higher than previously appreciated and appears to be increasing especially in countries with a rising prevalence of diabetes, hypertension, cardiovascular disease and obesity. An updated NHANES survey which used ACR ≥30mg/g and GFR <60 ml/min/1.73 m^2 showed that the prevalence of CKD in the USA has increased over the last 10 years by a factor of approximately 1.3; increases in prevalence of microalbuminuria were explained by increases in BMI, diagnosed diabetes and hypertension; however, only parts of the overall decrease in GFR were explained by the same factors. Cross-sectional data suggest that proteinuria has different prevalence in different ethnicities and that these differences already exist in childhood. Hispanic patients with CKD seem to have a faster decline of GFR when compared to non-Hispanic whites, when adjusting for diabetes. Whether these ethnic differences in albuminuria and proteinuria and disease progression are a function of a certain lifestyle or due to genetic differences remains unclear.

Most countries have similar CKD prevalence estimates but very different RRT incidences. For example, in the USA, the incidence of 90-day RRT is 340 pmp; in the UK, approximately 150 pmp; and in Germany, 180 pmp – again highlighting that CKD prevalence and RRT incidences are not measuring the same entity. Within the USA, the prevalence of CKD as measured by MDRD eGFR has remained stable over 10 years, whilst incidence of RRT increases in the same time period with a disproportionate number of patients with diabetic ERF [9]. In Caucasian populations, variation of RRT incidences is a function of the variation of differing age structures in the population. If this variation is removed via age/sex standardisation and restriction to those under 65 to account for a potential referral bias by age, then the residual variation is partially explained by varying RRT incidence of diabetic nephropathy [10].

65.5 Referral of Patients with CKD

CKD prognosis consortium data (◘ Fig. 65.4) shows that there are many more patients within primary care than seen by a nephrologist in secondary or tertiary care. It is very evident that for every 100 patients seen in primary care, there were 10 seen in clinics, and only 1 survives and reaches ESRD. To date, we do not know

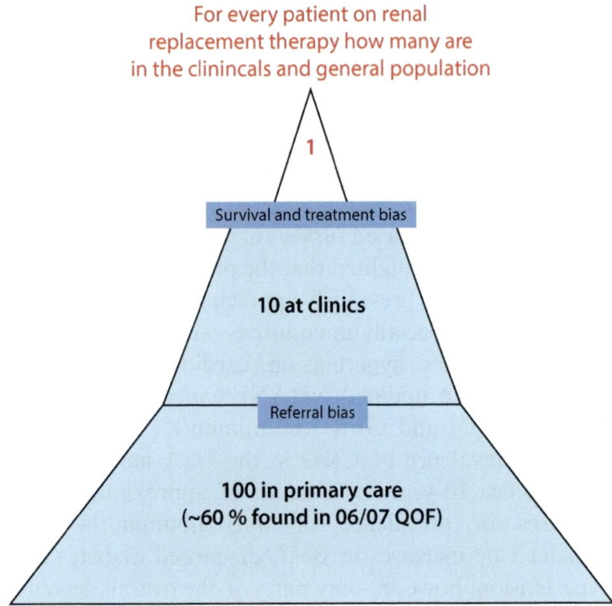

Fig. 65.4 CKD-ESRD spectrum: understanding biases in CKD and ESRD data due to referral and survival or treatment biases

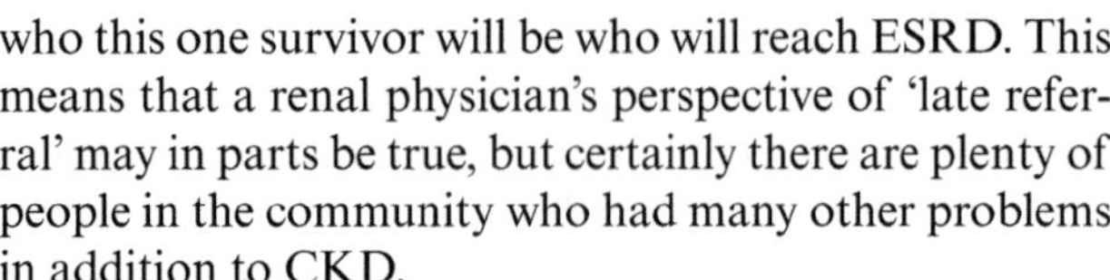

who this one survivor will be who will reach ESRD. This means that a renal physician's perspective of 'late referral' may in parts be true, but certainly there are plenty of people in the community who had many other problems in addition to CKD.

It is important to appreciate that as CKD gets worse, the risk profile of patients changes. Whilst most patients with CKD whom a general practitioner detects on screening will die before ever reaching RRT, patients with progressive renal disease who are seen by nephrologists may have been selected and therefore may show a better survival prognosis with consequently more people needing RRT.

Patients who were referred from primary care to renal services and who have CKD stage 4 show higher cumulative risks death or progression to ESRD than those with earlier CKD (Fig. 65.5) [11]. Almost 65% of patients with CKD stage 4 will have either a renal or a cardiovascular event over the ensuing 5 years. As the GFR falls below 20 ml/min per 1.73 m^2, the focus moves to treating the advanced CKD complications and planning for RRT.

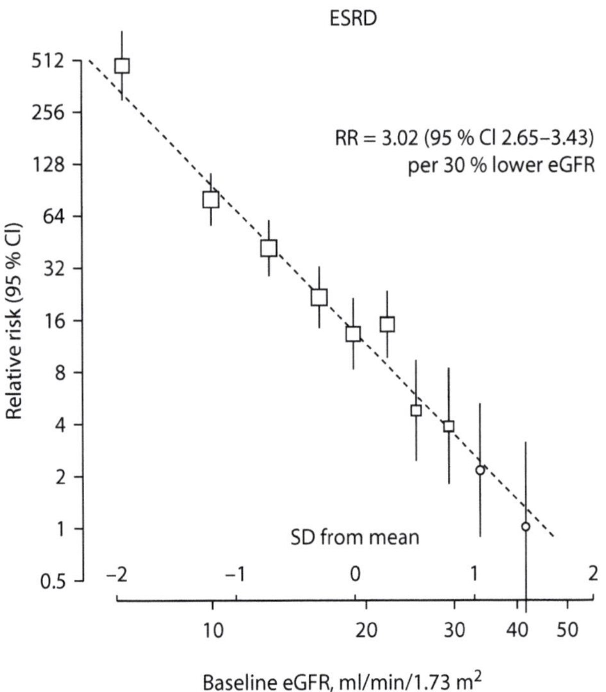

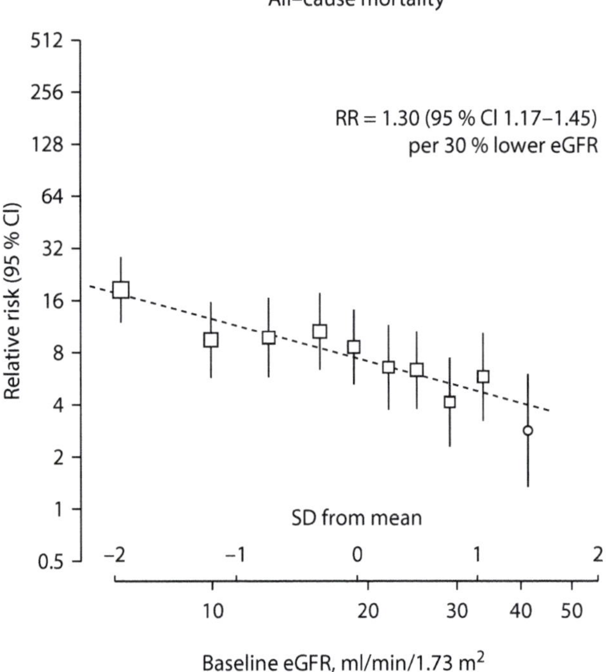

Fig. 65.5 Age- and sex-adjusted relative risk (*RR*) of end-stage renal disease (*ESRD*) and death in the Chronic Renal Impairment in Birmingham Study by baseline estimated glomerular filtration rate. Both the horizontal and vertical axes are shown on a logarithmic scale. The points in the right-hand panel have been adjusted so that the absolute mortality rates they represent are comparable with the absolute ESRD rates represented in the left-hand panel (thus, the point at which the two lines cross is the level of eGFR above which, in the CRIB cohort, the risk of death started to exceed the risk of ESRD). (Reprinted with permission from Landray et al. [11])

65.6 Understanding CKD Progression and the Issue of AKI

AKI is reported to complicate up to 5% of all hospital admissions. In a study of over five million hospital admissions in the USA, the AKI rate was 14.6 cases per 1000 discharges in 1992 and increased to 36.4 cases per 1000 discharges in 2001 [12] though case identification was incomplete. Applying laboratory definitions of AKI (an acute rise in serum creatinine), much higher incidences of AKI have been observed. In 2003, in a well-defined Scottish region, the incidences of AKI and acute-on-chronic kidney disease (ACKD) were 1811 and 336 per million population (pmp), respectively, each year. The median age for AKI was 76 years and for ACKD was 80.5 years. Sepsis was a precipitating factor in half of these patients [13]. The same authors repeated this study a few years later and found that the AKI incidence had risen to 2147 pmp per year. A higher proportion of patients with AKI were now referred to specialists, and treatment with RRT was almost four times more common. Whether this is due to true increases in AKI due to the changing population structure with more frail older patients being susceptible or whether this is due to increases in better testing for and coding of AKI due to physician awareness needs to be investigated further.

There is increasing evidence that AKI returning to a 'normal' baseline may not be benign but significantly predispose to CKD particularly in the context of multiple or severe episodes [14]. It is increasingly appreciated that AKI often occurs in patients with pre-existing CKD – so-called acute-on-chronic kidney disease. This is best thought of as an acute deterioration in renal function occurring in an individual with limited renal reserve, and not all of these acute-on-chronic declines in kidney function are reversible.

In summary, AKI is common, and its incidence appears to be rising in particular in the older population many of whom have CKD. Of course, AKI will impact on any epidemiological study of CKD progression. Emerging data suggest that the concept of 'slow CKD progression' through CKD stages 1–5 does not really hold up in the community setting. The idea of slow progression may very well be true for defined well-understood kidney disease entities. However, at the population level, it appears that CKD progression as a continuous phenomenon is not present in older people, whilst the risk of AKI in the context of acute illness is substantive due to a multitude of factors, which require further investigations as to their preventability.

65.7 Defining an Underlying Cause of CKD: Considerations and Causes Not to Miss

Figure 65.6 shows an approximate breakdown of CKD causes. Within the British white population, recorded primary causes of ESKD include in 20% diabetic nephropathy, in probably more than 15% severe CVD unrelated to diabetes, in 8% polycystic kidney disease and in autoimmune diseases, as, for example, glomerulonephritis or systemic lupus erythematosus (SLE), 30%. Ideally, the primary cause of CKD should be established in every patient, but a substantial percentage (20–30%) of registry returns worldwide have 'CKD unknown cause' as the reason for ESRD – partly because patients may present with small kidneys so it is not appropriate or possible for them to undergo a renal biopsy.

There are undoubtedly new renal diseases waiting to be discovered in the CKD population as illustrated by the recent discovery of C5 nephropathy in the Cypriot dialysis population, or the Mesoamerican nephropathy [15, 16]. Some authors refer to an epidemic of primarily tubulointerstitial chronic kidney disease (CKD) of unknown cause which has been acknowledged to cause an enormous number of early deaths in the last two decades in younger inhabitants in agricultural communities in low- and middle-income countries (LMICs) due to unavailability of diagnostic services and RRT. Whether this is one single disease entity of single causation or a mix of different diseases is unknown [17]. Due to the highly politicised nature of this problem as the hypothesised causes are often directly related to the livelihoods of affected populations, it has been difficult to carry out solid epidemiological research into causation. Most studies are cross-sectional and affected by reverse cau-

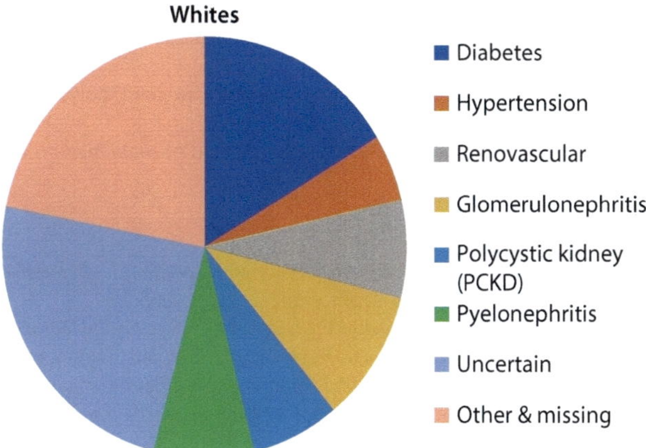

Fig. 65.6 Pie chart of recorded primary cause of kidney disease amongst people of white ethnicity using the UKRR 2016 data report

sality (i.e. presence of kidney damage affecting other biomarker assessments and risk factor reporting). There have been occupational cohort studies which often lose many participants over time and do not reflect the underlying populations as most agricultural workers are healthier than the average population (the so-called healthy worker effect). It has been difficult to perform screening tests as the natural history is not well understood, and this kidney disease has not shown association with traditional markers such as hypertension or proteinuria. The existing eGFR formulae have not been validated in affected populations.

In clinical practice, there are advantages to the patient in honing down the differential diagnosis in terms of (a) the possibility of an inheritable condition, (b) recurrent disease and (c) potential on-going treatment for systemic conditions. ▶ Box 65.1 shows some conditions worth considering in the patient first presenting with CKD in whom the diagnosis is not clear (obstruction and other obvious causes excluded) and a biopsy either non-diagnostic or inappropriate. This is not a comprehensive list, nor are most of these tests appropriate in most patients, but some in the right setting can be very suggestive of the underlying disease.

Box 65.1 Some Causes of ESRD to Consider (Beyond the Obvious) with Non-invasive Tests That May Make or Suggest the Diagnosis

Genetic causes

Nephronophthisis: AR, urinary concentrating defect, *medullary cysts, screening NPHP1* (and others) childhood and adolescent CKD
MCKD1: AD, urinary concentrating defect (polyuria), preserved renal size
MCKD2: AD, *gout in adolescence, high urate*
RCAD: AD, HNF1B *type 2 diabetes in youth* (MODY)
Thin basement membrane nephropathy: AD, haematuria and family history, *genotyping: COL4A3/4/5*
CFHR5 nephropathy: AD, *haematuria and macroscopic haematuria (in Cypriots)*
Branchio-oto-renal: AD, *pre-auricular pits, deafness, branchial clefts*
Alport's syndrome: X-linked (and AR), *deafness* (but not always), haematuria, retinal signs
Anderson-Fabry: X-linked, angiokeratomas, eye and heart signs, pain, *white blood cell alpha- galactosidase, urine for 'Maltese cross'*
Nail-patella syndrome: AD, *X-ray of pelvis (iliac horns), absent patellae and dystrophic nails (especially thumbs)*

Nephrocalcinosis and ESRD

Primary hyperoxalosis: Nephrocalcinosis, *oxalate levels, mutation analysis* AGAT
Adenine phosphoribosyltransferase deficiency: AR, nephrocalcinosis, *APRT enzyme level, stone analysis*
Dent's disease: X-linked, nephrocalcinosis, tubular proteinuria *proximal tubulopathy*
Cystinosis: AR, nephrocalcinosis, corneal crystals (photophobia), proximal tubulopathy

Infections

Tuberculosis: Sterile pyuria, early morning urines for TB culture, QuantiFERON assay, X-ray for calcinosis
Chronic pyelonephritis: Especially in diabetics, recurrent UTIs, *scarring* on DMSA (if function good enough) or USS/CT
Xanthogranulomatous pyelonephritis: Diabetes and stones (often staghorn), pyuria, recurrent UTIs, abnormal kidney on CT or MRI
HIV, hepatitis B and C: Serology and viral load, polyclonal gammopathy, hypocomplementaemia, large bright kidneys suggest HIVAN
Schistosomiasis: Obstructed system and or *small high-pressure bladder, serology, early morning urine for ova, cystoscopy and biopsy*

Tubulointerstitial nephritis

Heavy metal toxicity: Anaemia, rashes, *proximal tubular disorder/Fanconi syndrome, blood, urine or hair analysis (Ar, Cd, Pb)*
Lithium: Polyuria, nephrogenic diabetes insipidus
Analgesic nephropathy: *CT scan small, irregular kidneys with papillary calcification*
Balkan/aristolochic acid nephropathy: Endemic region, exposure to herbal remedies with aristolochic acid
IgG-4-related disease: 'Autoimmune' pancreatitis, sialadenitis, aortitis, retroperitoneal fibrosis, elevated IgG-4 ratio
Sjögren's syndrome: *Dry eyes and mouth, sterile pyuria, anti SS-A and SS-B (anti-Ro and anti-La) antibodies*, polyclonal gammopathy
Sarcoid: Raised serum ACEI, sterile pyuria, hypercalcaemia (especially with vitamin D supplements), positive gallium scan
Sickle cell nephropathy: HbSS or HbSC, *papillary necrosis*

Glomerular disease (significant protein or blood, dysmorphic RBC on microscopy)

IgA: Raised serum IgA may be a clue, ethnicity, history of chronic microscopic haematuria or episodes of synpharyngitic macroscopic haematuria
FSGS primary: Usually history of oedema, frothy urine, relatively rapid course (NPHS1, NPHS2, NPHS3, other genetic screening available)
FSGS secondary: Low birth weight, reduced nephron mass (e.g. subtotal nephrectomy), history of renal dysplasia, obesity, body building (anabolic steroids), sickle cell disease, HIV, CMV, parvovirus, congenital heart disease (cyanotic), heroin, interferons, lithium, pamidronate
Membranous primary: *Anti-phospholipase A2 receptor antibody*
Membranous secondary: Hepatitis B, C, HIV, schistosomiasis, *cryoglobulinaemia, hypocomplementaemia, positive rheumatoid factor*, rheumatological conditions (SLE, rheumatoid, Sjögren's syndrome)
MPGN primary and C3 glomerulopathies: Dense deposit disease: low C3, *partial lipodystrophy, Drusen* and retinal atrophy, *anti-C3Nef (80%)*, CFHR5 nephropathy: Cypriot ancestry, family history, synpharyngitic macroscopic haematuria
MPGN secondary: Hepatitis B, C, HIV, schistosomiasis, *cryoglobulinaemia, hypocomplementaemia, positive rheumatoid factor*, rheumatological conditions (SLE, rheumatoid, Sjögren's syndrome)
Light chain-related disease: *Igs, protein electrophoresis, Bence-Jones proteinuria, serum-free light chains* (abnormal ratio), skeletal survey, bone marrow biopsy
Amyloid: Usually *heavy proteinuria and normal-sized kidneys, macroglossia, abdominal fat or rectal biopsy*. Causes of AA amyloid, i.e. chronic infection or chronic inflammatory disease, history of IV or subcutaneous drug abuse, causes of AL amyloid (see above), serum *amyloid-P scan*
Systemic lupus erythematosus: Clinical features, *low complement, raised antinuclear antibody, double-stranded DNA antibody*, polyclonal gammopathy
Vasculitis: Extrarenal clinical features, raised inflammatory markers, *ANCA (MPO or PR3 positive)*
Goodpasture's syndrome: Always presents acutely but results in ESRD if diagnosis missed, *anti-GBM antibodies*

Episode(s) of AKI

Documented or presumed episodes of AKI: Severity of AKI (1–3, especially need for renal replacement), length and number of AKI, cancer therapy, major surgery (especially cardiac bypass or cross-clamping aorta/renal vessels), cardiac or liver disease, non-renal transplant, episodes of sepsis, haemolytic uraemic syndrome, episodes of nephrotoxic drugs including chemotherapy. Obtaining previous creatinines from previous hospital admissions invaluable

Miscellaneous

Diabetes: Proteinuria (evidence of progressive increase) and normal-sized kidneys, retinopathy, 20-year history for type 1 diabetes, other end-organ disease history
Radiation nephritis: Unequal-sized kidneys (if only one irradiated), low-grade TMA
Arterial/venous insufficiency: Unequal size, US/MRA-V of renal vessels, cholesterol emboli: episodes of low complement, eosinophilia, vascular intervention
Impaired drainage: Chronic obstruction usually obvious on imaging but dysfunctional high-pressure bladder may not be obvious, *history of enuresis*, UTIs or *posterior urethral valves*. Abnormal neurology, *thick bladder wall*, upper tract dilatation, high detrusor pressure on urodynamics
Cardiorenal syndrome: Evidence of right or left heart failure (systolic or diastolic dysfunction), often low blood pressure and 'saw-toothed' pattern to creatinine
Hepatorenal syndrome: Exclusion of other causes in patient with cirrhosis, ascites, low blood pressure

Aside from known individual causes in selected patients, there are also more population factors to consider. For example, individuals born in developing countries may be at increased risk of chronic kidney disease due to the high prevalence of poor maternal health and malnutrition leading to low birth weight, prematurity and smaller renal reserve. ▶ Box 65.2 shows the maternal factors affecting birth weight and prematurity [18].

Data from Pakistan suggest that South Asian children have higher blood pressure than white children in the USA, with also a relatively high prevalence of proteinuria. Data from the UK show convincingly that people who have low birth weight and gain weight in early adulthood will have a lower eGFR than people who are overweight in middle or older age [19]. In short, some patients may be preconditioned from birth to later reduced GFR, and superimposition of secondary causes such as hypertension, diabetes or even AKI such as post-streptococcal glomerulonephritis may result in a higher risk of CKD. This temporal delay in having kidney disease related to diabetes may in part be related to ethnicity. For example, South Asian patients seem to have a two to four times faster progression of diabetic nephropathy in comparison to their Dutch counterparts.

Box 65.2 Maternal Factors Associated with Low Birth Weight and Pre-term Birth

Maternal developmental and demographic characteristics

1. Maternal birth weight (<2.5 kg or >4.0 kg)
2. Age (<18 or >40 years)
3. Maternal height (145 cm)
4. Ethnicity
5. BMI (obesity, low BMI)

Pregnancy and medical conditions

1. Maternal medical conditions (diabetes, hypertension, kidney disease)
2. Pregnancy factors (pre-term birth, multiple pregnancies, pre-eclampsia and eclampsia, assisted conceptions, consanguinity)
3. Infections
4. Nutrient deficiency
5. Medications

Behavioural, socio-economic and environmental

1. Alcohol intake, tobacco use and substance abuse
2. Antenatal care
3. Childhood marriage
4. Socio-economic situation and education
5. Stress, war, environmental factors (famine)
6. Exposure to toxins

65.8 Prevention and Screening of CKD

According to the World Health Organization, coronary heart disease is now the leading cause of death worldwide with 60% of the global burden of heart disease in low- to middle-income countries. Some say that cardiovascular risk is very high in patients with CKD, which makes a strong argument for screening for CKD. However, from epidemiologic studies, it appears that a large proportion of people with CKD have to do with lifelong exposure to an adverse lifestyle, in particular, obesity. Hence, targeting common cardiovascular risk factors such as smoking, obesity, diabetes and hypertension is likely to prevent at least in parts CKD and development of renal failure.

Currently, there is no clear evidence showing that 'screening for CKD' should be done in all populations. There are several criteria that need to be fulfilled to qualify for screening. The condition should be an important health problem which kidney disease undoubtedly is. Its natural history should be understood – this is the case for people with type 1 diabetes, but less so for the general population where the importance of AKI has only been recognised in the past decade. There should be a recognisable early stage and an acceptable test – this is undoubtedly the case as we have eGFR and albuminuria tests. However, the key criteria to justify screening are that a condition must be treatable, and an outcome prevented, and treatment should be cost-effective. For many forms of common kidney disease, there is no strong evidence that treatment by nephrologists indeed prevents poor outcomes – evidence from a recent hypertension trial suggests that more intensive blood pressure treatment may in fact cause AKI [20]. There is good evidence that detecting and treating albuminuria and hypertension in the context of diabetes delays dialysis and that detecting people requiring referral for dialysis preparation on time may prevent an unplanned start to RRT [21]. However, considering the majority of patients identified in routine primary care, there is no strong evidence that detecting a mildly reduced eGFR in an older person who is already well managed in terms of cardiovascular risk either prevents poor outcomes or is cost-effective.

65

65.9 Summary

CKD is common and is associated with an increased risk of cardiovascular disease, mortality, progression to ESRD and AKI. There is very little understanding of the epidemiology of CKD progression in older people. Robust systems for identifying at-risk populations to prevent medication side effects, especially in the setting of acute illness, and higher awareness of albuminuria being a marker for progression to ESRD, may reduce the risk for these patients.

Chapter Review Questions

1. Why do trends on prevalence of RRT provide only limited information on causes of kidney disease?
2. Would you capture the entire population of patients with CKD by applying blood tests?
3. Who is at higher risk of death, a person with eGFR 50 ml/min without albuminuria or a person of the same age and sex with nephrotic syndrome but an eGFR of 88 ml/min?
4. In a given person, by how much can eGFR be wrong relative to the true (but unmeasured GFR) – and does that matter for clinical practice when looking at repeat measurements for that person?
5. Were the guidelines for CKD derived on two measurements of blood/urine more than 3 months apart?

Answers

1. RRT prevalence is not a good measure to use – that is, the number of people on dialysis or living with kidney transplants divided by the total population irrespective of the duration of RRT. The numerator of this figure is the number of patients

starting dialysis in that year, plus the number of people that were already on dialysis or living with a kidney transplant in that year, minus the people who died on dialysis or with a transplant. The numerator is affected by a range of factors, which include the causes that drive people to end up on dialysis or with a kidney transplant, but also importantly how long people survive on dialysis or with a transplant which may mask any important associations. It also does not capture people with kidney failure who are treated conservatively.

2. No, CKD is defined by both urine and blood tests.
3. The person with nephrotic syndrome has higher risk of death.
4. eGFR may be ±20 ml/min erroneous, with the error decreasing as GFR declines, i.e. the error is much less in people with advanced CKD, compared to those with normal renal function. However, repeated measurement of eGFR over time in the same patient is meaningful as this will map kidney function change over time, provided the muscle mass/nutrition and fluid status are in a steady state.
5. No, all the risk associations that underlie the guidelines derive from single time point measurements. Clinical populations who are seeking health care are quite different to cohort participants who are in steady state – often patients who seek help are unwell, which will mean that they are not in steady state, and therefore the 'chronicity' criterion was introduced based on clinical reasoning. The epidemiological data are clear that a random on-off measurement in steady state informs on risk – a second measurement is not needed.

References

1. Hole B, Gilg J, Casula A, Methven S, Castledine C. UK renal registry 20th annual report: UK renal replacement therapy adult incidence in 2016. Nephron. 2018;139(suppl1):13–46.
2. MacNeill S, Ford D, Evans K, Medcalf. UK renal registry 20th annual report: UK renal replacement therapy adult prevalence in 2016. Nephron. 2018;139(suppl1):47–74.
3. Kidney Disease: Improving Global Outcomes (KDIGO) CKD Work Group. KDIGO 2012 clinical practice guideline for evaluation and management of chronic kidney disease. Kidney Int. 2013;3(Suppl):1–150.
4. Levey AS, de Jong PE, Coresh J, El Nahas M, Astor BC, Matsushita K, et al. The definition, classification, and prognosis of chronic kidney disease: a KDIGO Controversies Conference report. Kidney Int. 2011;80(1):17–28.
5. Coresh J, Astor BC, Greene T, Eknoyan G, Levey AS. Prevalence of chronic kidney disease and decreased kidney function in the adult US population: Third National Health and Nutrition Examination Survey. Am J Kidney Dis. 2003;41(1):1–12.
6. Froissart M, Rossert J, Jacquot C, Paillard M, Houillier P. Predictive performance of the modification of diet in renal disease and Cockcroft-Gault equations for estimating renal function. J Am Soc Nephrol. 2005;16(3):763–73.
7. Matsushita K, Mahmoodi BK, Woodward M, Emberson JR, Jafar TH, Jee SH, et al. Comparison of risk prediction using the CKD-EPI equation and the MDRD study equation for estimated glomerular filtration rate. JAMA. 2012;307(18):1941–51.
8. Giles PD, Fitzmaurice DA. Formula estimation of glomerular filtration rate: have we gone wrong. BMJ. 2007;334(7605):1198–200.
9. Hallan SI, Coresh J, Astor BC, Asberg A, Powe NR, Romundstad S, et al. International comparison of the relationship of chronic kidney disease prevalence and ESRD risk. J Am Soc Nephrol. 2006;17(8):2275–84.
10. Group TEIS. Geographic, ethnic, age-related and temporal variation in the incidence of end-stage renal disease in Europe, Canada and the Asia-Pacific region, 1998–2002. Nephrol Dial Transplant. 2002;21(8):2178–83.
11. Landray MJ, Wheeler DC, Lip GY, Newman DJ, Blann AD, McGlynn FJ, Ball S, Townend JN, Baigent C. Prediction of ESRD and death among people with CKD: the chronic renal impairment in Birmingham (CRIB) prospective cohort study - American Journal of Kidney Diseases (ajkd.org). Am J Kidney Dis. 2004;43(2):244–53.
12. Xue JL, Daniels F, Star RA, Kimmel PL, Eggers PW, Molitoris BA, Himmelfarb J, Collins AJ. Incidence and mortality of acute renal failure in Medicare beneficiaries, 1992 to 2001. J Am Soc Nephrol. 2006;17(4):1135–42.
13. Prescott GJ, Metcalfe W, Baharani J, Khan IH, Simpson K, Smith WC, MacLeod AM. A prospective national study of acute renal failure treated with RRT: incidence, aetiology and outcomes. Nephrol Dial Transplant. 2007;22(9):2513–9.
14. Coca SG, Yusuf B, Shlipak MG, Garg AX, Parikh CR. Long-term risk of mortality and other adverse outcomes after acute kidney injury: a systematic review and meta-analysis. Am J Kidney Dis. 2009;53(6):961–73. https://doi.org/10.1053/j.ajkd.2008.11.034.
15. Gale DP, de Jorge EG, Cook HT, Martinez-Barricarte R, Hadjisavvas A, et al. Identification of a mutation in complement factor H-related protein 5 in patients of Cypriot origin with glomerulonephritis. Lancet. 2010;376(9743):794–801.
16. Gonzalez-Quiroz M, Pearce N, Caplin B, Nitsch D. What do epidemiological studies tell us about chronic kidney disease of undetermined cause in Meso-America? A systematic review and meta-analysis. Clin Kidney J. 2018;11(4):496–506.
17. Caplin B, Jakobsson K, Glaser J, Nitsch D, Jha V, Singh A, Correa-Rotter R, Pearce N. International collaboration for the epidemiology of eGFR in low and middle income populations – rationale and core protocol for the disadvantaged populations eGFR epidemiology study (DEGREE). BMC Nephrol. 2017;18(1):1.
18. Luyckx VA, Brenner BM, Luyckx VA, Brenner BM. Birth weight, malnutrition and kidney-associated outcomes—a global concern. Nat Rev Nephrol. 2015;11:135–49.
19. Silverwood RJ, Pierce M, Hardy R, Sattar N, Whincup P, Ferro C, Savage C, Kuh D, Nitsch D. Low birth weight, later renal function, and the roles of adulthood blood pressure, diabetes, and obesity in a British birth cohort. Kidney Int. 2013;84(6):1262–70. https://doi.org/10.1038/ki.2013.223.
20. The SPRINT Research Group. A randomized trial of intensive versus standard blood-pressure control. New Engl J Med. 2015;373:2103–16.
21. Black C, Sharma P, Scotland G, McCullough K, et al. Early referral strategies for management of people with markers of renal disease: a systematic review of evidence of clinical effectiveness, cost-effectiveness and economic analysis. Health Technol Assess. 2010;14(21):1–184.

Chronic Kidney Disease: Diagnosis and Assessment

James Smith, Shahid Abdullah, Charles R. V. Tomson, and Shona Methven

Contents

M. Harber (ed.), *Primer on Nephrology*, https://doi.org/10.1007/978-3-030-76419-7_66

Learning Objectives

1. Chronic kidney disease (CKD) is common and frequently managed by the non-nephrologist.
2. Accurate identification of those with CKD generally involves assessment of estimated glomerular filtration rate (eGFR), quantification of proteinuria, identification of non-visible haematuria and tailored assessment for structural and histological abnormalities.
3. eGFR can be calculated using formulae such as CKD-EPI, or rarely a formal GFR measurement may be required.
4. Proteinuria can be quantified using a spot urine sample analysed for protein/creatinine ratio or albumin/creatinine ratio; rarely, a 24-h urine collection is still required.
5. Risk stratification is essential to identify those at high risk of end-stage kidney disease. This can be calculated using routinely measured variables and online calculators.

66.1 Introduction

This chapter aims to provide a pragmatic approach to the assessment of patients with CKD.

We must correctly identify those with CKD and impart the information to the patient in an informative and appropriate way in order that we can then offer strategies to ameliorate the complications of CKD and prevent progression of the kidney disease.

66.2 Ascertainment of CKD

The diagnosis of CKD relies upon the accurate measurement of excretory kidney function and proteinuria, both of which have some pitfalls. Given that kidney disease is predominantly asymptomatic (in the early stages at least), healthcare providers must ensure that they correctly identify those with CKD in order to offer optimal care to those with CKD and reassure those who do not. To diagnose CKD, renal abnormalities must persist for more than 90 days. These abnormalities can be of renal function (e.g. reduction in eGFR, proteinuria or haematuria of renal origin) or renal structure, at a micro- or macroscopic level.

66

66.2.1 Estimating Glomerular Filtration Rate

While it is possible and sometimes useful to *measure* glomerular filtration rate (GFR) (see next section), in normal clinical practice, the techniques required to do this are time-consuming, expensive and unnecessary. A number of standardised equations have been derived which allow GFR to be *estimated* (eGFR).

eGFR equations rely on the measurement of an endogenous filtration marker, of which serum creatinine is the most common. The formulae generally include age, sex and race along with the filtration marker in order to take account of the effect of non-GFR determinants of serum creatinine level (e.g. muscle mass). The aim is to produce a more reliable estimate of GFR than would have been achieved by using the filtration marker alone. In the UK, national guidance recommends the use of the CKD EPI equation for creatinine-based eGFR, as this is less likely to misclassify individuals as having CKD, and is better at predicting risk of death or end-stage kidney disease than the widely used MDRD eGFR equation [1, 2].

Table 66.1 shows that the international CKD staging system is predominantly based on the level of a person's eGFR according to thresholds:

For certain individuals, the diagnosis of CKD based on eGFR using creatinine (even using the CKD-EPI equation) may be spurious. For example, young males with high muscle mass may have an elevated serum creatinine due to increased creatinine production, resulting in an *estimated* GFR less than 60 ml/min/1.73 m^2, often leading to referral to the nephrology clinic to identify the cause for their 'CKD'. In such situations, if the eGFR is persistently 45–59 ml/min/1.73 m^2 and there are no other markers of kidney disease, for example, proteinuria, non-visible haematuria, electrolyte disorders or structural renal abnormalities, a measurement of serum cystatin C can be used to re-calculate eGFR. This may be more reliable as it is not derived from muscle mass. If cystatin C eGFR is

Table 66.1 (Adapted from KDIGO 2012 clinical practice guideline for the evaluation and management of CKD) [3]

GFR stage	GFR (ml/min/1.73m^2)	Description
G1	≥90	Normal or high
G2	60–89	Mild decrease (relative to young adult level)
G3a	45–59	Mild to moderate decrease
G3b	30–44	Moderate to severe decrease
G4	15–29	Severe decrease
G5	<15	Kidney failure

>60 ml/min/1.73 m^2, a diagnosis of CKD should not be made [3]. If cystatin C testing is not available, a formal GFR measurement or 24-h creatinine clearance can be employed (see next section).

66.2.2 Measurement of Glomerular Filtration Rate in the Management of CKD

As indicated above, it is seldom necessary to measure glomerular filtration rate directly in routine clinical practice, but there are exceptions:

1. When eGFR is not felt to be precise enough to guide treatment decisions that carry significant risk of toxicity, for example, use of renally cleared drugs with a narrow therapeutic index such as cytotoxic chemotherapy
2. In assessing excretory kidney function prior to live kidney donation
3. To reassure patients with high muscle bulk, a high serum creatinine concentration and a low *estimated* GFR that excretory kidney function is normal when cystatin C testing is not adequate or feasible (e.g. for certain occupations where a diagnosis of CKD must be entirely excluded)

Measurement of GFR can be performed using isotopic methods (such as clearance of ^{125}I-iothalamate or Cr^{51}-EDTA) or using contrast media (such as iohexol). A systematic review with meta-analysis of cross-sectional diagnostic studies in 2014 compared these GFR measurement methods with renal inulin clearance (the historical gold standard) and supported their accuracy [4].

Alternatively creatinine clearance may be measured using 24-h urine collection and a serum creatinine measurement taken during the collection period. However, creatinine clearance overestimates GFR as a result of tubular creatinine secretion (approximately 15% in normal renal function, rising to 50% in advanced CKD). This can be corrected by the concurrent administration of a drug that blocks tubular creatinine secretion such as 48 h pretreatment with full-dose cimetidine.

66.2.3 Quantification of Proteinuria

Proteinuria is the cardinal feature of renal disease; therefore, the accurate identification and quantification of proteinuria is paramount in the management of patients with CKD.

A small amount of urinary protein is to be expected. Normal healthy adults excrete 40–80 mg of protein per day. This consists mostly of albumin (most of which is retained at the glomerulus, with a small amount passing through the glomerular basement membrane which is then mostly, but not fully, reabsorbed in the proximal tubule), plus low-molecular-weight proteins such as β2-microglobulin, α1-microglobulin, retinol-binding protein, etc. (filtered freely at glomerulus but not fully reabsorbed) and uromodulin (derived from tubular epithelial cells at loop of Henle).

Higher levels of proteinuria can also be physiological. Proteinuria may be a transient phenomenon after strenuous exercise in normal healthy adults, in which case it is usually very low grade and resolves spontaneously [5, 6]. Progression to permanent renal damage is rare in such cases. However, heavy exercise can also exacerbate proteinuria in patients with existing CKD [6]. Orthostatic proteinuria, more common in children and adolescents, is the presence of albuminuria in the context of an upright position, which disappears when supine. This is also considered benign.

Pathological proteinuria may be glomerular (predominantly albuminuria), tubular (as a result of the failure of tubular reabsorption of filtered low-molecular-weight proteins) or overflow (such as excess light chain excretion in myeloma which overwhelms the normal tubular reabsorptive capacity). Quantification of urinary protein using a total protein assay will take account of all of these varying proteins; however, measuring albuminuria will only give an indication of glomerular disease. The measurement of albumin is generally favoured in the biochemistry community as it is quantified using an immunoassay which has technical advantages over the less precise physicochemical assays used for total protein. It has also been said that albuminuria is the better test at low levels (<0.5 g/day total proteinuria equivalent) as the noise/signal ratio (with physiological proteins being the noise and the albuminuria being the signal) is superior. However, the early studies of diabetic nephropathy (from which this received wisdom emanated) did not measure total proteinuria, so no head-to-head comparison was made. This low-level albuminuria was previously known as 'microalbuminuria' which is a misleading term and should now be avoided.

Traditionally, proteinuria was measured using timed (usually 24-h) urine collections. However, these are cumbersome for the patient, doctor and laboratory and have generally been superseded by spot measurements of urine total protein/creatinine ratio (PCR) or urine albumin/creatinine ratio (ACR). The urine creatinine (the denominator) is used as a surrogate for urine flow rate to allow comparison between samples, with the assumption that creatinine excretion is constant over time. Generally, it is assumed that the *average* adult excretes around 10 mmol of urinary creatinine per day and so an ACR of 3 mg/mmol is said to equate to around 30 mg albuminuria per day. This gives reasonably reliable intra-individual comparisons; however, there is significant inter-individual variation in urinary creatinine excretion which is not taken into consideration with this approach. This may or may not be an important issue [7]. Ratios from spot urine samples become unreliable at very high protein excretion rates (such as >6 g/day), and a timed urine collection may still be indicated in these circumstances [8].

Dipsticks are no longer recommended for the quantification of proteinuria (unless laboratory quantification is not available in a resource-scarce healthcare environment); however, they still have utility to detect non-visible haematuria.

Quantitation of urine protein excretion is important in several clinical situations:

1. In patients with suspected glomerular disease, including the nephrotic syndrome. Quantification of albumin excretion is the most logical test to do in this situation, as this gives the best estimate of the severity of glomerular damage. However, there is much less convincing evidence to support changes in management at lower levels of albuminuria in glomerular disease, and so quantitation of total protein (which is cheaper and still takes account of albumin loss) is still widely used.
2. In patients with suspected tubular disease (either inherited, as in Dent's disease, or acquired, such as tubulointerstitial nephritis) – in this situation, specific assays for low-molecular-weight proteins that appear in the urine as a result of failure of tubular reabsorption (endocytic mechanism via megalin and cubilin receptors on proximal tubular cells) may be required, the commonest test being for retinol-binding protein. In addition, a large discrepancy between the results of a paired urine protein/creatinine ratio and albumin/creatinine ratio can provide indirect evidence of high levels of non-albumin proteinuria.
3. Amongst patients with diabetes mellitus, albuminuria of 30–300 mg/day equivalent (e.g. ACR of 3–30 mg/mmol or 30–300 mg/g), when present on repeated tests, is diagnostic of early diabetic nephropathy and should prompt treatment to prevent progressive nephropathy.

66

The 2012 KDIGO guidelines recommend that every description of kidney disease includes a quantification of albuminuria (A1–A3 depending on severity) [3] (◘ Table 66.2). The addition of albuminuria to the international CKD classification underlines the increasing appreciation of the importance of albuminuria in the diagnosis, management and prognostication in CKD.

The presence of low-level albuminuria (30–300 mg/day equivalent) is also associated with atherosclerosis and hypertensive vascular disease and has been shown to be a powerful predictor of cardiovascular disease (the risk extends into the 'normal' range) [9]. In this situation, low-level albuminuria probably reflects widespread endothelial dysfunction rather than indicating a specific kidney disease. It is unknown whether offering non-diabetic people with low-level albuminuria additional treatment to prevent vascular disease improves prognosis, when it would not otherwise be indicated by traditional risk factors. However, many such patients do have existing vascular disease and will benefit from interventions to reduce risk such as advice on exercise, smoking, correction of obesity, salt restriction, blood pressure-lowering drugs and lipid-lowering drugs.

Proteinuria that is caused by kidney disease, whether resulting from diabetes or from other disorders, is also strongly associated with an increased risk of cardiovascular disease. It is not known whether specific immunosuppressant treatment that reduces proteinuria caused by kidney disease results in a subsequent improvement in cardiovascular risk.

◘ **Table 66.2** Albuminuria categories in the 2012 KDIGO guidelines

	AER (mg/24 h)	ACR (mg/mmol)	ACR (mg/g)
A1	<30	<3	<30
A2	30–300	3–30	30–300
A3	>300	>30	>300

Adapted from KDIGO 2012 clinical practice guideline for the evaluation and management of chronic kidney disease (▶ http://www.kdigo.org/clinical_practice_guidelines/pdf/CKD/KDIGO_2012_CKD_GL.pdf)

AER albumin excretion rate, *ACR* albumin/creatinine ratio

66.3 Finding Patients with CKD

66.3.1 The Role of Automated eGFR Reporting

The widespread implementation of eGFR reporting (since 2006 in the UK) has revolutionised how CKD is perceived, diagnosed and managed by non-nephrologists (but has not been without its share of critics). It has allowed increased recognition in primary care and the subsequent improvement in the primary care management of CKD in the UK. There has also been an increase in the diagnosis of CKD, predominantly in the early stages (stage 3A, eGFR 45–59 ml/min/1.73 m^2). Conversely, late presentation of CKD (defined as starting renal replacement therapy (RRT) within 90 days of the first assessment by a nephrologist) has fallen significantly over recent years in the UK, and in 2015/2016, only 15.9% of incident patients starting RRT had presented within 90 days [10].

66.3.2 Screening Programmes

The principles of a screening programme were first outlined by the World Health Organization in 1968. An ideal screening programme should be based on a reasonably accurate screening test acceptable to the population. It should also be able to improve clinical outcomes without causing patient harm, in a cost-effective manner. It is important to consider potential harms associated with screening which include false-positive and false-negative results (leading to patient anxiety or false reassurance), unnecessary testing and treatment and disease labelling.

Kidney disease is amenable to screening as early CKD (the preclinical state) is usually asymptomatic and effective interventions exist (such as blood pressure control) to prevent progression of disease.

There are two main questions to consider regarding screening for CKD; firstly, what should we measure and in whom should we measure it? The obvious measurement is serum creatinine (and eGFR), but studies (such as PREVEND in the Netherlands) have also assessed albuminuria screening and found even low levels to be highly predictive of subsequent renal decline [11]. Secondly, should we screen the whole adult population or select high-risk patients? The Alberta Kidney Disease Network, in Canada, reported that screening with eGFR was not cost-effective [12]. However, this analysis is extremely dependent on the provision of primary healthcare in the host country, what proportion of patients already underwent testing and therefore what proportion would require additional screening to ensure population coverage. A Scottish study found that 42% of the adult population had had their serum creatinine checked in the preceding year – in the absence of a formal screening programme [13].

Several groups have now published on the potential benefits of systematic screening of existing laboratory databases to detect patients with progressive CKD and offer additional interventions. In the Kaiser Permanente system in Hawaii, for instance, the provision of unsolicited nephrology consultations based on the detection of high-risk patients, combined with triage of incoming nephrology consultations to prioritise patients at high risk of progressive CKD, reduced the rate of late referrals markedly, increased the proportion of patients starting haemodialysis with an arteriovenous fistula and increased the proportion of patients starting haemodialysis as an outpatient [14]. A similar programme in Birmingham, UK, in which a nephrologist screened all creatinine reports from patients with diabetes in a single laboratory database, identified those with low or deteriorating eGFR and wrote with unsolicited advice to the doctor who had requested the test, resulted in a fall in the number of patients with diabetes starting RRT [15]. Savings (both monetary and carbon) can be made by a system of electronic consultation, in which nephrologists are given full access to the primary care electronic record of patients with CKD [16].

In the UK at present, there is not a population screening programme for serum creatinine or urinary protein excretion, but regular estimation of kidney function is recommended in people at high risk of developing CKD [1], including those with:

- Diabetes mellitus
- Hypertension
- Previous acute kidney injury
- Heart failure
- Coronary, cerebral vascular or peripheral vascular disease
- Structural renal tract disease, recurrent renal calculi or prostatic hypertrophy
- Chronic multisystem diseases with potential renal involvement – e.g. systemic lupus erythematosus, rheumatoid arthritis and chronic diarrhoeal illnesses
- A family history of stage 5 CKD or hereditary kidney disease
- Regular use of drugs that can cause CKD, including nonsteroidal anti-inflammatory drugs, lithium and 5-aminosalicylate derivatives
- Proteinuria and/or otherwise unexplained haematuria

There is no evidence on which to base recommendations regarding the ideal interval between measurements. For most patients, an annual measurement is adequate; however, increasingly frequent monitoring will be required for those with advancing kidney disease (from eGFR<45 ml/min/1.73 m^2 onwards) and for those with heavy proteinuria (who are risk of more rapid progressive deterioration). The frequency should be tailored to the individual patient taking account of their treatment, prognosis and preference [1]. Screening for albuminuria is recommended in specific conditions (most notably diabetes mellitus), and we are likely to see increasing use of albuminuria as a screening test (and for prognostication) in conditions such as hypertension in the future.

66.4 Predicting Progression

66.4.1 Measuring Progression

Progression of CKD is often seen in the context of worsening of the primary renal disease, although there is some evidence to suggest that secondary changes (such as interstitial fibrosis, secondary FSGS), once established, can result in an inexorable decline in GFR even in the absence of on-going primary renal disease.

In routine clinical practice, changes in excretory kidney function are monitored by serial measurement of serum creatinine concentration. Assuming that the patient's creatinine generation rate has remained constant, a rise in serum creatinine concentration denotes a fall in GFR, and vice versa. However, this assumption does not always hold true. Creatinine generation rate falls in acute illness [17]. Even in chronic, stable disease, it is possible that some apparent alterations in GFR are in fact caused by alterations in tubular secretion of creatinine.

National guidance in the UK (NICE, 2014) recommends at least three eGFR readings over a period of not less than 90 days to identify rate of progression. Progression of CKD is said to be 'accelerated' if there are a sustained decrease in eGFR of 25% or more and a change in eGFR category within 12 months or a sustained decrease in GFR of 15 ml/min/1.73 m^2 per year [1]. KDIGO guidelines are congruent with NICE but define rapid progression as a sustained decrease in eGFR of 5 ml/min/1.73 m^2 [3].

66.4.2 Graphing eGFR over Time

Past performance is helpful in predicting progression of CKD. Graphical display of changes in eGFR over time provides a visual indication of rate of eGFR decline or conversely to show that an apparent recent deterioration in renal function is within the limits of previous fluctuations while also allowing response to treatment to be monitored. This may be useful for both clinicians and patients. Studies are underway to investigate the utility of providing primary care physicians with eGFR graphs when checking kidney function [18].

66.4.3 Prediction Equations

66

The Kidney Failure Risk Equations (KFRE), of which there are the 4-variable version (age, sex, eGFR and albuminuria) and the 8-variable version (as 4-variable, plus serum calcium, phosphate, bicarbonate and albumin), have been developed in recent years as tools to predict 2- and 5-year risk of end-stage kidney disease for patients with CKD 3–5 [19, 20]. Significant progress has been made in recent years in validating these equations in cohorts comprising hundreds of thousands of CKD patients across the world, demonstrating excellent discrimination in a diverse range of patient cohorts. These variables are routinely measured in clinical practice and could easily be incorporated in a laboratory reporting system. In addition, the Kidney Disease: Improving Global Outcomes (KDIGO) risk calculator (▶ http://www.kdigo.org/equation/) provides information on an individual's risk of ESKD and cardiovascular events while taking account of the competing risk of death, which the KFRE does not offer.

The importance of recognising and predicting progression of CKD lies both in stimulating clinician and patient to ensure that all possible measures are in place to retard CKD progression and in allowing sufficient time to prepare for renal replacement therapy in those patients in whom CKD progression is inexorable.

66.4.4 Risk Factors for Progression

Identifying, and correcting, modifiable risk factors for progressive loss of GFR in patients with CKD is the cornerstone of preventive management.

66.4.5 Proteinuria

The most well-established risk factor is proteinuria, and there is a strong dose-response relationship between the quantity of urinary protein and the rate of progression of renal decline. It is also very well established that low-level albuminuria is a risk marker for progressive kidney damage amongst patients with type 1 and type 2 diabetes and the same holds true for people without diabetes [21]. Evidence suggests that patients with heavy proteinuria but without overtly abnormal GFR had more rapid decline of kidney function than did those with moderately reduced GFR but mild proteinuria [22].

KDIGO have developed user-friendly 'heat maps' which stratify risk of developing progressive CKD and end-stage kidney disease according to eGFR and proteinuria. There is a powerful multiplicative relationship between reduced excretory function, proteinuria and risk (see ◻ Fig. 66.1). Interestingly, the 'heat maps' are also very similar for the outcomes of all-cause mortality, cardiovascular mortality and AKI [3].

66.4.6 Hypertension

Hypertension is common in CKD and is associated with poorer outcomes. Experimental studies have shown that, in CKD, systemic hypertension is transmitted to the glomeruli: the resulting glomerular hypertension is damaging to the kidney, resulting in glomerulosclerosis and accelerated decline in kidney function. There is a strong relationship between hypertension and proteinuria: interventions for the former will impact on the latter.

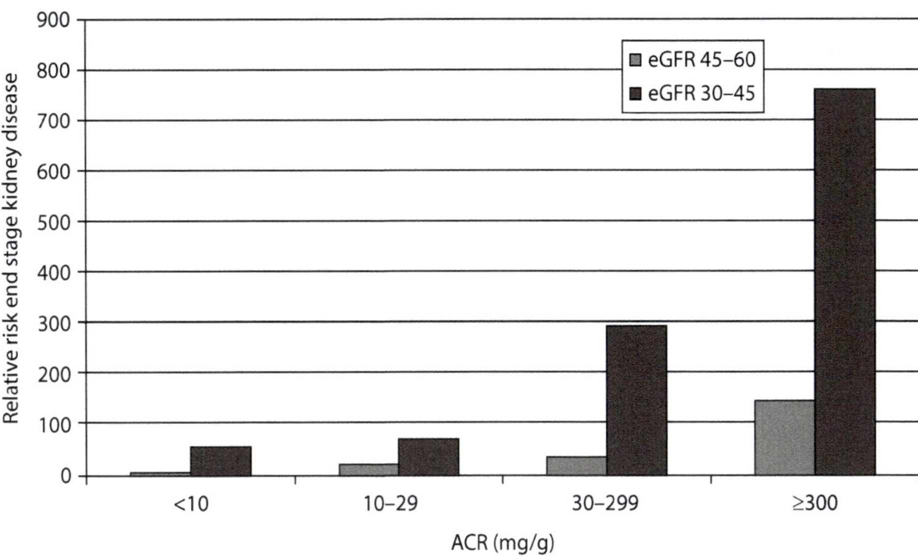

Fig. 66.1 Relationship between proteinuria and risk of end-stage kidney disease at moderately reduced eGFR. (Data adapted from KDIGO 2012 clinical practice guideline for the evaluation and management of chronic kidney disease with permission (▶ http://www.kdigo.org/clinical_practice_guidelines/pdf/CKD/KDIGO_2012_CKD_GL.pdf))

66.4.7 Others

Other potentially important modifiable risk factors include:

- Glycaemic control in diabetes
- High dietary protein intake
- Obesity
- High fructose intake
- Hyperuricaemia
- Low fluid intake
- Cigarette smoking
- Untreated urinary outflow tract obstruction
- Acute kidney injury (CKD increased risk of AKI and an episode of AKI may increase risk of subsequent CKD)

Non-modifiable risk factors include age, male gender and non-White ethnic origin.

There is good evidence that modification of risk factors can slow the progression of CKD which is a critical objective. In particular, there is now overwhelming evidence of benefit of therapeutic intervention in patients with hypertension, moderate to severe proteinuria, diabetes or heart disease. Part of the therapeutic endpoint is reduction in individual glomerular hyperfiltration and intraglomerular pressure. Inhibition of the renin-angiotensin system with ACEis and ARBs is well established in this area and has a marked benefit in terms of slowing progression of renal disease in patients with proteinuria and a significant survival advantage in those comorbid with cardiac disease. More recently, glucagon-like peptide 1 receptor agonists (GLP-1 RA) and sodium-glucose cotransporter 2 inhibitors (SGLT-2i) have both demonstrated marked renoprotective and cardioprotective effects. This has been reflected recently in both diabetic and renal (KDIGO 2020) guidelines for the management of diabetes in patients with CKD, both of which recommend metformin and SGLT-2 inhibition followed by GLP-1 RAs as primary therapies for type 2 diabetics and CKD [23, 24]. Moreover, it is clear that the benefit SGLT-2 inhibition in terms of cardiovascular and renal risk reduction is equally potent in non-diabetic patients with proteinuric CKD. In the DAPA-CKD study, the hazard ratio for a composite endpoint of a sustained decline in the estimated GFR of at least 50%, end-stage kidney disease or death from renal causes was 0.56 for those patients receiving SGLT-2i [25].

It is worth noting that both ACEi/ARBs and SGLT-2is are often appropriately stopped in the setting of AKI. However, they are not 'nephrotoxic agents' and in the majority of cases confer considerable morbidity and mortality benefit, especially in those with proteinuria or heart disease. Supporting colleagues in secondary care with the safe reintroduction of these disease-modifying agents is an important task.

66.5 How Do You Tell Your Patient That They Have CKD?

Although age-related reduction in GFR is common, it is not an inevitable consequence of ageing. Just as low bone density or high arterial blood pressure is common in older people, so is low GFR. Some commentators argue that 'labelling' older patients with a low GFR is an example of the medicalisation of normal old age. Given that older patients have higher absolute risks of cardiovascular disease and death, the finding that the *relative* risks of these events associated with a reduction in GFR are lower in older than in younger adults should not be seen as surprising nor as evidence that a low GFR is harmless. The association of anaemia, hypertension and hyperparathyroidism with reduced GFR is the same in older than in younger adults [26].

However, there is a legitimate concern that 'labelling' asymptomatic patients with the 'diagnosis' of CKD, based solely on the results of an estimate of GFR, could do harm. This partly depends on what is said to patients, how it is said and by whom.

Let us imagine a 76-year-old patient with a 15-year history of reasonably controlled hypertension, a 3-year history of type 2 diabetes, a urine albumin/creatinine ratio of 1.2 mg/mmol, no dipstick haematuria and an eGFR of 52 ml/min/1.73 m^2. She is seen by a general practitioner for medication review. She is told 'Your blood test shows that you have stage 3 chronic kidney disease. There are 5 stages, and if you reach stage 5 you will either die or need dialysis. I am going to refer you to a specialist, and they will probably send you an appointment'. One would expect that the patient will go home in a state of severe anxiety and spend the time while waiting for the appointment to come through worrying, writing her will, attributing every minor new symptom to kidney disease and asking for repeated checkups at the GP's surgery. If the same patient were seen by a GP or practice nurse and told 'As part of our routine checks for your high blood pressure and diabetes, the practice nurse did a blood test the last time you saw her. The blood test gives a rough estimate of how efficiently the kidneys are working to clear waste products from the bloodstream. This estimate is called the "eGFR". A healthy young person usually has an eGFR of around 100. Your eGFR was 52, so you have about 52% of the kidney function of a young healthy person. This is most likely due to "wear and tear" in the kidneys that has occurred over the years; we know that high blood pressure can make this type of wear and tear more likely. Luckily, there is a lot of reserve capacity in the kidneys, so you are unlikely to become unwell unless the kidney function gets a lot worse. I suggest that we repeat your blood test in 3 months' time. If the next eGFR is also below 60, that will mean that you will be said to have "stage 3 chronic kidney disease". When we use the word "chronic", we don't mean "bad", we just mean that the condition has persisted over the 3 months. So long as we keep your blood pressure and diabetes under control, it is unlikely that your kidney function will get significantly worse – but it's worth us keeping an eye on this every 6 months or so. Do you have any questions?' This patient may ask questions but is much less likely leave feeling anxious or 'labelled'. This may look like a long explanation but takes less than 90 seconds to say. If backed up by a patient information leaflet or, even better, an individualised care plan, this investment of time is likely to improve the patient's understanding of her condition and her adherence to recommended lifestyle and drug treatment and improve long-term outcomes.

66.6 Specialist Referral

Given the increasing ascertainment of CKD (and possibly a true increase in prevalence), the vast majority of patients with CKD are cared for in primary care. Most kidney units will have local guidelines for primary care providers regarding referral of patients with CKD. UK NICE guidance from 2014 provides some guidance with regard to indications for referral to renal services [1]:

1. GFR less than 30 ml/min/1.73 m^2 (GFR category G4 or G5), with or without diabetes
2. ACR 70 mg/mmol or more, unless known to be caused by diabetes and already appropriately treated
3. ACR 30 mg/mmol or more (ACR category A3), together with haematuria
4. Sustained decrease in GFR of 25% or more and a change in GFR category or sustained decrease in GFR of 15 ml/min/1.73 m^2 or more within 12 months
5. Hypertension that remains poorly controlled despite the use of at least four antihypertensive drugs at therapeutic doses
6. Known or suspected rare or genetic causes of CKD
7. Suspected renal artery stenosis

These groups will derive additional benefit from seeing the renal multidisciplinary team in a hospital setting. However, the person with stable CKD stage 3A without proteinuria and controlled blood pressure may find attendance at hospital clinics a stressful burden without any discernible improvement in outcome compared to the monitoring that can be provided in primary care.

66.7 Finding Patients with Treatable Causes

It is essential to pause (perhaps only briefly) to consider treatable causes before moving on to the next step in the assessment of a patient with CKD. The great majority of patients with CKD have nephrosclerosis in association with generalised vascular disease and hypertension. This is not associated with haematuria, and seldom with clinical proteinuria, although moderate increases in albumin excretion are common. Treatment requires control of cardiovascular risk factors and avoidance of further damage to the renal circulation, including avoidance of acute kidney injury and nephrotoxicity. However, it is dangerous to assume that CKD is due to nephrosclerosis without some effort to exclude causes that may require specific treatment – particularly because in some instances such treatment may be curative or at least prevent further deterioration. This aspect of management was not emphasised in the original 2002 classification of CKD, and it became commonplace to see patients being described as having 'CKD' as the sole diagnosis with no effort to exclude treatable causes. This was addressed to a certain extent in the 2012 KDIGO guidelines with the introduction of the CGA classification (*cause*, GFR, albuminuria) which re-emphasises the importance of seeking the cause of the kidney disease [3]. Often this will be apparent on detailed history and examination, and the clinical findings can be augmented by (a relatively small number of) investigations.

If your patient has blood and protein on dipstick urinalysis, this may be suggestive of a glomerular disorder, and a number of serological markers can be measured. Testing for myeloma may also be undertaken, but the yield is low in the absence of any suggestive features (such as hypercalcaemia and bone pain) [27]. The finding of a paraprotein band in the absence of any clinical features of myeloma may represent a monoclonal gammopathy of uncertain significance (MGUS) and lead to further investigations and anxiety, so the testing should not be undertaken routinely without careful consideration. However, there is increasing recognition of the entity of monoclonal gammopathy of renal significance (MGRS) which shares some features with MGUS but, in addition, results in progressive renal decline and histological evidence of monoclonal immunoglobulin deposition in the kidney. MGRS, in contrast to MGUS, requires haematological treatment [28].

It is equally important in a patient with established CKD to exclude any superimposed causes of an unexpected decline in function (see ◘ Table 66.3). Commonly, this may be an episode of hypotension or sepsis particularly in a patient receiving renin-angiotensin blockade, but sometimes important reversible causes

◘ Table 66.3 Common causes of acute on chronic deterioration in renal function

Pre-renal	
Reduced intravascular volume	Over-diuresis, non-renal losses (gastrointestinal), poor intake
Reduced cardiac output	Occult cardiac failure, dysrhythmia, cardiac event
Hypotension	Over-medication, sepsis, Addison's syndrome
Renovascular	Emboli, atherosclerotic renal artery stenosis, cholesterol emboli, renal vein thrombosis or inferior vena cava occlusion
Post-renal	Any cause of obstruction, most commonly prostatic hypertrophy in elderly men, anticholinergic medications, neurological causes, stones especially those with a history of nephrolithiasis. Relatively easily excluded by US of kidneys and post-micturition residual bladder volume
Renal	
Toxins endogenous	CKD patients more susceptible to all toxins: light chain (usually myeloma), rhabdomyolysis, tumour lysis syndrome, intravascular haemolysis, hypercalcaemia, enteric hyperoxaluria. Any form of acute sepsis
Toxins exogenous	NSAIDs, other medication that may have a direct toxic effect such as antivirals (e.g. acyclovir), antibacterials (e.g. aminoglycosides), chemotherapy, intravenous contrast
Interstitial nephritis	Usually drug induced in this setting, may also be progression of original disease (e.g. lupus, vasculitis, sarcoid)
Glomerulonephritis	Usually progression of original disease, e.g. flare of vasculitis, occasionally de novo glomerulonephritis such as IgA nephropathy, glomerulonephritis secondary to staphylococcal infection or amyloid may superimpose on background CKD (may be indicated by a bland urine developing haematuria or nephrotic range proteinuria, respectively)
Poorly controlled hypertension	May be associated with increase in proteinuria
Urosepsis	Apart from acute sepsis caused by UTIs decompensating CKD, pyelonephritis can be remarkably silent especially in patients who are immunocompromised or diabetic. This is a common and important cause of accelerated renal decline especially in patients with diabetes and may be suspected in the presence of sterile pyuria, mildly raised inflammatory markers (may be normal) and recurrent UTIs

intervene, and it is the nephrologist's job to identify these and postpone ESRD. Graphing reciprocal creatinine or log creatinine will highlight those that have deteriorated unexpectedly from their trajectory; this is not routine practice for most units but should be an absolute requirement of any new renal software.

66.8 Radiology

There is very little literature to guide a recommendation regarding who should undergo renal imaging in a cohort with CKD. NICE guidance from 2014 [1] suggests that imaging with an ultrasound should be considered for all patients with CKD who:

1. Have accelerated progression of CKD (defined as a sustained decrease in GFR of 25% or more and a change in GFR category within 12 months or a sustained decrease in GFR of 15 ml/min/1.73 m^2 per year)
2. Have visible or persistent non-visible haematuria
3. Have symptoms of urinary tract obstruction
4. Have a family history of polycystic kidney disease and are aged over 20 years
5. Have a GFR of less than 30 ml/min/1.73 m^2 (GFR category G4 or G5)
6. Are considered by a nephrologist to require a renal biopsy [2008, amended 2014]

This is not intended to be an exhaustive list, and clinical judgement will dictate other instances where a renal tract ultrasound is indicated. However, the salient point remains: the yield of structural abnormalities will be extremely poor in low-risk patients (e.g. those with stable CKD stage 3, negative urinalysis and no other history or symptoms suggestive of the causes listed above), and therefore they do not automatically require imaging of their renal tract. On the other hand, ultrasound scans are noninvasive, are relatively cheap, give some idea of prognosis depending on kidney size and can also assess bladder emptying which may impact on subsequent progression or transplantation.

66

Ultrasound scanning remains the initial radiological investigation of choice; it is cheap and noninvasive and in skilled hands can be very helpful in diagnosing CKD and excluding obstruction. The quality of the scanning is critical however, and 'normal kidneys' may well not be; there is considerable interobserver variation in sizes which might prejudice management. Any degree of hydronephrosis indicates obstructive nephropathy until proven otherwise: if there is a history of previous long-standing obstruction or reflux nephropathy, additional investigations (e.g. dynamic isotope renography or even a trial of nephrostomy drainage) may be required. The degree of dilatation is not a reliable predictor of the severity of obstructive nephropathy, and case series exist of obstructive nephropathy without any detectable dilatation, caused by encasement of the kidneys and ureters by tumour or fibrosis. Although hydronephrosis usually resolves after relief of obstruction (e.g. by catheter drainage in patients with bladder outflow obstruction), this can take several days, and patients may be left with CKD as a result of the chronic inflammation and fibrosis that results from prolonged renal tract obstruction.

Renal size and echogenicity are also helpful. Using ultrasound, renal size is usually estimated from the length from upper to lower pole; these measurements can be unreliable, however, particularly in the presence of obesity, and are operator-dependent. Renal length should ideally be reported relative to body height (as taller patients have longer kidneys [29]), but this is seldom done in routine practice. Increased echogenicity is a feature of chronic kidney disease and correlates with interstitial fibrosis [30].

Renal asymmetry (often defined as a discrepancy of renal length of >1 cm) can occur for several reasons, including:

- Renal artery stenosis
- Reflux nephropathy
- Renal parenchymal loss due to previous obstruction, e.g. due to stone disease
- Artefacts caused by observer error (e.g. failure to image the long axis of the kidney; inclusion of renal cysts)

Increased renal size can occur as a result of infiltration, for instance, by lymphoma or amyloidosis.

CT scanning gives more accurate information about renal volume, which in health is closely related to body surface area and is a better predictor of measured GFR than creatinine-based estimating equations [31]. Contrast-enhanced CT is occasionally valuable, for instance, in suspected renal embolism and in IgG4-related tubulointerstitial nephritis. MR is increasingly being used to calculate renal volume for various purposes including risk stratification in polycystic kidney disease to guide tolvaptan therapy [32] and also shows promise for the detection of fibrosis.

66.9 Renal Biopsy

The role of renal biopsy in the diagnosis of CKD remains poorly defined [33]. The decision to proceed to renal biopsy should be individualised based on benefits (usually to yield a diagnosis that would 'change' the management plan) and risks (mainly bleeding). There should be a clear understanding that the patient is willing and sufficiently fit to tolerate a potential change in management plan as well as the risks of the procedure itself. A good example would be a frail, elderly patient with suspected underlying glomerulonephritis in whom the risks of immunosuppression would be considerable even if renal biopsy yielded such a diagnosis.

Renal biopsy is usually performed percutaneously with ultrasound guidance. The major feared complication is that of significant bleeding; however, using modern equipment and real-time imaging, the risk is relatively low [34]. In some units, percutaneous biopsies are performed by interventional radiologists; however, a recent study showed that percutaneous renal biopsy performed by experienced nephrologists was not inferior to that performed by interventional radiologists with regard to specimen yield and post-biopsy complications [35]. Occasionally, transjugular, laparoscopic or open surgical approaches to renal biopsy are considered.

An important aspect in the planning of renal biopsies is the peri-procedure management of anti-platelet agents and systemic anticoagulation. Standard practice in many renal centres is to ask the patient to withhold anti-platelet agents for 7 days before an elective biopsy. However, a systematic review and meta-analysis showed that the rate of blood transfusion did not differ between patients in whom anti-platelet agents were held for ≥7 days pre-biopsy and those for whom the anti-platelet agents were discontinued for ≤7 days [36]. Observational data exists suggesting that continuing aspirin is safe in the context of renal biopsy, and this is standard practice in some centres [37].

For those where anticoagulation cannot be entirely discontinued (e.g. metallic valves), it is customary to stop warfarin and bridge with unfractionated or low-molecular-weight heparin. In the absence of supporting data in the context of renal biopsies, evidence-based guidelines on the perioperative management of antithrombotic therapy can be used as guidance [38]. Unfractionated heparin is usually stopped 4–6 h before procedure, while the last therapeutic dose of LMWH is given 24 h before procedure. Some renal centres advocate the administration of desmopressin 1-h pre-biopsy to reduce the risk of bleeding, but there is a lack of consensus regarding this [39].

66.10 Conclusion

The recognition of CKD has changed dramatically over the past 15 years with the introduction of eGFR reporting and increased awareness amongst non-nephrologists. It is no longer a collection of rare diseases looked after by specialists in hospital clinics; it is a common condition predominantly managed in primary care with appropriate support and input from nephrologists. Our current assessment strategies reflect these changes with greater emphasis on quantification of proteinuria, prognostication and risk stratification. The management of CKD is a rapidly evolving field, and there are now treatment strategies that substantially reduce the risk of renal progression and cardiovascular events with many exciting developments on the horizon for us and our patients.

Case Study

Case 1

A 38-year-old male, otherwise healthy, is referred to the kidney clinic due to an unexpected finding of a low estimated glomerular filtration rate (eGFR) of 55 ml/min/1.73 m^2. There are no historical measurements of renal function, but he has no personal or family history of kidney disease. He denies use of any recreational drugs including anabolic steroids or protein supplements. He is 95 kg and of athletic build. Blood pressure is 115/72 mmHg. Urinalysis is negative, and quantification of proteinuria using urine albumin/creatinine ratio (ACR) is normal. An ultrasound of his renal tract is normal. Therefore, there is no evidence of kidney disease other than an isolated low eGFR. The presumptive diagnosis is that the low eGFR is spurious and related to increased muscle mass (and hence increased production of creatinine) rather than reduced GFR. Further evaluation is required; 24-h creatinine clearance could be measured, which would demonstrate higher than normal creatinine generation in addition to normal creatinine clearance, or $eGFR_{cystatin}$ could be measured which does not rely on muscle mass and should confirm $eGFR_{cystatin}$ >60 ml/min/1.73 m^2. If required for employment purposes, isotopic testing can be used to measure the GFR.

Case 2

A 45-year-old man attends his primary care physician (PCP) for review of his recently diagnosed chronic kidney disease (CKD). He was found to have hypertension during opportunistic screening and therefore had urinalysis performed which showed protein 3+ and blood 1+, and urine ACR confirms significant albuminuria of 230 mg/mmol. eGFR is reduced at 35 ml/min/1.73 m^2. According to the international CKD staging system, he has CKD G3b, A3, cause unknown. His PCP calculates his risk of end-stage kidney disease (ESKD) using the online Kidney Failure Risk Equation calculator which estimates his 2-year risk of ESKD to be 10.8% and 5-year risk of ESKD to be 35.7% which is considered high risk. Therefore, his PCP explained this to the patient and arranged specialist referral to a nephrologist for investigation of the cause of his CKD and discussion regarding appropriate interventions to slow progression of his CKD.

Chapter Review Questions

1. What variables are included in the CKD-EPI eGFR formulae?
2. Approximately how much albumin will a person have excreted in 24 h if their ACR measures 3 mg/mmol (or 30 mg/g equivalent)?
3. What does the abbreviation CKD G3b, A2 represent when using the international CKD staging system?
4. What is the strongest risk factor for progression of chronic kidney disease?
5. How can predicted 5-year risk of end-stage kidney disease (ESKD) be calculated?

Answers

1. Age, sex, race (black or other) plus the filtration marker (either serum creatinine, cystatin C or both)
2. The crude assumption is that an average adult will excrete around 10 mmol/day or urinary creatinine and therefore ACR 3 mg/mmol is equivalent to 30 mg/24 h.
3. CKD G3b, A2 represents chronic kidney disease stage 3b (eGFR 30–44 ml/min/1.73 m^2) with albuminuria excretion of 30–300 mg/24 h.
4. The degree of urinary protein excretion is the single strongest risk factor for progressive CKD, with a clear dose-response relationship with heavier proteinuria leading to more rapid deterioration.
5. Online calculators are available such as ▸ http://kidneyfailurerisk.com which uses routinely measured variables (age, sex, geographical location, eGFR and ACR) to predict 2- and 5-year risk of ESKD or ▸ http://www.kdigo.org/equation/ which uses the same variables plus blood pressure, diagnosis of diabetes, smoking status and history of cardiovascular disease to predict 2- and 4-year risk of ESKD, death and cardiovascular events.

Tips and Tricks

- If a patient does not have expected muscle mass, e.g. as a result of an above-knee amputation, eGFR is not an accurate measure of excretory kidney function.
- If there is a large discrepancy between urine PCR and ACR, this suggests heavy non-albumin proteinuria, and myeloma (with overflow proteinuria caused by urinary light chains) should be excluded.
- If there is an unexpected finding of a low eGFR (in the context of a well patient), always repeat a few days later to ensure they do not have rapidly deteriorating renal function as rapidly progressive glomerulonephritis or tubulointerstitial nephritis can be clinically silent until advanced kidney disease occurs.
- The appearance of deteriorating renal function in the context of a UTI may be due to the effect of trimethoprim (blockade of tubular creatinine secretion leads to a rise in serum creatinine without fall in GFR).
- Unexplained CKD in an elderly man always warrants active exclusion of bladder outlet obstruction.

References

1. National Clinical Guideline Centre (UK). Chronic kidney disease (partial update): early identification and management of chronic kidney disease in adults in primary and secondary care. London: National Institute for Health and Care Excellence (UK); 2014.
2. Matsushita K, Mahmoodi BK, Woodward M, Emberson JR, Jafar TH, Jee SH, et al. Comparison of risk prediction using the CKD-EPI equation and the MDRD study equation for estimated glomerular filtration rate. JAMA. 2012;307(18):1941–51.
3. KDIGO. Chapter 1: Definition and classification of CKD. Kidney Int Suppl. 2013;3(1):19–62.
4. Soveri I, Berg UB, Björk J, Elinder C-G, Grubb A, Mejare I, et al. Measuring GFR: a systematic review. Am J Kidney Dis. 2014;64(3):411–24.
5. Heathcote KL, Wilson MP, Quest DW, Wilson TW. Prevalence and duration of exercise induced albuminuria in healthy people. Clin Invest Med. 2009;32(4):E261–5.
6. Shephard RJ. Exercise proteinuria and hematuria: current knowledge and future directions. J Sports Med Phys Fitness. 2016;56(9):1060–76.
7. Methven S, MacGregor MS, Traynor JP, O'Reilly DS, Deighan CJ. Reply to "Improving the interpretation of protein creatinine ratios. The impact of creatinine excretion.". Nephrol Dial Transplant. 2011;26(3):1109.
8. Methven S, MacGregor MS, Traynor JP, O'Reilly DSJ, Deighan CJ. Assessing proteinuria in chronic kidney disease: protein-creatinine ratio versus albumin-creatinine ratio. Nephrol Dial Transplant. 2010;25(9):2991–6.
9. Chronic Kidney Disease Prognosis Consortium, Matsushita K, van der Velde M, Astor BC, Woodward M, Levey AS, et al. Association of estimated glomerular filtration rate and albuminuria with all-cause and cardiovascular mortality in general population cohorts: a collaborative meta-analysis. Lancet. 2010;375(9731):2073–81.
10. Hole B, Gilg J, Casula A, Methven S, Castledine C. Chapter 1 UK renal replacement therapy adult incidence in 2016: national and centre-specific analyses. Nephron. 2018;139 Suppl 1:13–46.
11. Halbesma N, Kuiken D-S, Brantsma AH, Bakker SJL, Wetzels JFM, De Zeeuw D, et al. Macroalbuminuria is a better risk marker than low estimated GFR to identify individuals at risk for accelerated GFR loss in population screening. J Am Soc Nephrol. 2006;17(9):2582–90.
12. Manns B, Hemmelgarn B, Tonelli M, Au F, Chiasson TC, Dong J, et al. Population based screening for chronic kidney disease: cost effectiveness study. BMJ. 2010;341:c5869.
13. Gifford FJ, Methven S, Boag DE, Spalding EM, Macgregor MS. Chronic kidney disease prevalence and secular trends in a

UK population: the impact of MDRD and CKD-EPI formulae. QJM. 2011;104(12):1045–53.

14. Lee BJ, Forbes K. The role of specialists in managing the health of populations with chronic illness: the example of chronic kidney disease. BMJ. 2009;339:b2395.
15. Rayner HC, Hollingworth L, Higgins R, Dodds S. Systematic kidney disease management in a population with diabetes mellitus: turning the tide of kidney failure. BMJ Qual Saf. 2011;20(10):903–10.
16. Stoves J, Connolly J, Cheung CK, Grange A, Rhodes P, O'donoghue D, et al. Electronic consultation as an alternative to hospital referral for patients with chronic kidney disease: a novel application for networked electronic health records to improve the accessibility and efficiency of healthcare. Qual Saf Health Care. 2010;19(5):e54.
17. Wilson FP, Sheehan JM, Mariani LH, Berns JS. Creatinine generation is reduced in patients requiring continuous venovenous hemodialysis and independently predicts mortality. Nephrol Dial Transplant. 2012;27(11):4088–94.
18. Gallagher H, Methven S, Casula A, Thomas N, Tomson CRV, Caskey FJ, et al. A programme to spread eGFR graph surveillance for the early identification, support and treatment of people with progressive chronic kidney disease (ASSIST-CKD): protocol for the stepped wedge implementation and evaluation of an intervention to reduce late presentation for renal replacement therapy. BMC Nephrol. 2017;18(1):131.
19. The Kidney Failure Risk Equation [Internet]. Available from: http://kidneyfailurerisk.com/.
20. Tangri N, Stevens LA, Griffith J, Tighiouart H, Djurdjev O, Naimark D, et al. A predictive model for progression of chronic kidney disease to kidney failure. JAMA. 2011;305(15):1553–9.
21. Lambers Heerspink HJ, de Zeeuw D. Debate: PRO position. Should microalbuminuria ever be considered as a renal endpoint in any clinical trial? Am J Nephrol. 2010;31(5):458–61; discussion 468.
22. Turin TC, James M, Ravani P, Tonelli M, Manns BJ, Quinn R, et al. Proteinuria and rate of change in kidney function in a community-based population. J Am Soc Nephrol. 2013; 24(10):1661–7.
23. Buse JB, Weler D, Tsapai A, et al. 2019 Update to management of hyperglycaemia in type 2 diabetes 2018: a consensus report by the American Diabetes Association (ADA) and the European Association for the study of Diabetes (EASD). Diabetologia. 2020;63:221–8.
24. KDIGO 2020 clinical practice guideline for diabetes management in chronic kidney disease: improving global outcomes (KDIGO) diabetes work group practice guideline. 2020;98(4, Supplement):S1–S115. https://www.kidney-international.org/article/S0085-2538(20)30718-3/fulltext.
25. Heerspink HJL, Stefansson BV, Correa-Rotter R, Chertow GM, Greene T, Hou FF, Mann JFE, McMurray JJV, Lindberg M, Rossing P, Sjostrom CD, Toto RD, Langkilde AM, Wheeler DC, DAPA-CKD Trial Committees and Investigators. Dapagliflozin in patients with chronic kidney disease. N Engl J Med. 2020;383(15):1436–46.
26. Bowling CB, Inker LA, Gutiérrez OM, Allman RM, Warnock DG, McClellan W, et al. Age-specific associations of reduced estimated glomerular filtration rate with concurrent chronic kidney disease complications. Clin J Am Soc Nephrol. 2011;6(12):2822–8.
27. Doyle A, Soutar R, Geddes CC. Multiple myeloma in chronic kidney disease. Utility of discretionary screening using serum electrophoresis. Nephron Clin Pract. 2009;111(1):c7–11.
28. Leung N, Bridoux F, Hutchison CA, Nasr SH, Cockwell P, Fermand J-P, et al. Monoclonal gammopathy of renal significance: when MGUS is no longer undetermined or insignificant. Blood. 2012;120(22):4292–5.
29. Emamian SA, Nielsen MB, Pedersen JF, Ytte L. Kidney dimensions at sonography: correlation with age, sex, and habitus in 665 adult volunteers. AJR Am J Roentgenol. 1993;160(1):83–6.
30. Moghazi S, Jones E, Schroepple J, Arya K, McClellan W, Hennigar RA, et al. Correlation of renal histopathology with sonographic findings. Kidney Int. 2005;67(4):1515–20.
31. Johnson S, Rishi R, Andone A, Khawandi W, Al-Said J, Gletsu-Miller N, et al. Determinants and functional significance of renal parenchymal volume in adults. Clin J Am Soc Nephrol. 2011;6(1):70–6.
32. Irazabal MV, Rangel LJ, Bergstralh EJ, Osborn SL, Harmon AJ, Sundsbak JL, et al. Imaging classification of autosomal dominant polycystic kidney disease: a simple model for selecting patients for clinical trials. J Am Soc Nephrol. 2015;26(1):160–72.
33. Tomson CRV. Indications for renal biopsy in chronic kidney disease. Clin Med. 2003;3(6):513–7.
34. Scottish Renal Registry Report 2016: Section N.
35. Chung S, Koh ES, Kim SJ, Yoon HE, Park CW, Chang YS, et al. Safety and tissue yield for percutaneous native kidney biopsy according to practitioner and ultrasound technique. BMC Nephrol. 2014;15:96.
36. Corapi KM, Chen JLT, Balk EM, Gordon CE. Bleeding complications of native kidney biopsy: a systematic review and meta-analysis. Am J Kidney Dis. 2012;60(1):62–73.
37. Lees JS, McQuarrie EP, Mackinnon B. Renal biopsy: it is time for pragmatism and consensus. Clin Kidney J. 2018;11(5): 605–9.
38. Douketis JD, Spyropoulos AC, Spencer FA, Mayr M, Jaffer AK, Eckman MH, et al. Perioperative management of antithrombotic therapy: Antithrombotic Therapy and Prevention of Thrombosis, 9th ed: American College of Chest Physicians Evidence-Based Clinical Practice Guidelines. Chest. 2012;141(2 Suppl):e326S–50S.
39. Manno C, Bonifati C, Torres DD, Campobasso N, Schena FP. Desmopressin acetate in percutaneous ultrasound-guided kidney biopsy: a randomized controlled trial. Am J Kidney Dis Off J Natl Kidney Found. 2011;57(6):850–5.

Clinical Management of CKD: Prevention of Progression

Shahid Abdullah, Shona Methven, and Charles R. V. Tomson

Contents

M. Harber (ed.), *Primer on Nephrology*, https://doi.org/10.1007/978-3-030-76419-7_67

Learning Objectives

Reading this chapter will help practitioners to understand:

1. The importance of patient-centred care, taking into account co-morbidities other than chronic kidney disease and encouraging active participation by the patient in their own management
2. The importance of lifestyle advice to reduce the impact of obesity and hypertension on the progression of chronic kidney disease
3. The importance of blood pressure reduction for the prevention of progressive chronic kidney disease
4. The differentiation between acute haemodynamically mediated changes in glomerular filtration rate and progressive loss of glomerular filtration rate due to progressive structural kidney damage

67.1 Non-pharmacological Measures

67.1.1 Patient Activation

Patients with a chronic disease live with it 24 hours a day, 365 days a year, and interact with health professionals for a tiny fraction of that time – four 15-minute consultations per year for a patient with stable stage 4 CKD would probably be a generous estimate. There is a growing body of evidence that patients with chronic diseases who feel that they control their disease have better outcomes (e.g. adherence to drug treatment or dietary restrictions; lower consultation and hospitalisation rates) than those who feel that their disease controls them. Patient 'activation' and 'empowerment' are terms used to denote this sense of being in control. Sceptics might argue that both higher levels of patient activation and better outcomes might be caused by underlying factors such as educational attainment – and most would recognise the stereotype of the well-educated middle-class professional who attends an outpatient clinic armed with Internet printouts about their disease. However, there is also good evidence that specific interventions – such as provision of personalised care plans, education sessions or coaching – can increase patient activation, irrespective of baseline health literacy. One specific example of such an intervention in the UK is the PatientView (▶ www.patientview.org) which gives patients secure web-based access to their test results and clinic letters.

67.1.2 Co-operation with Primary Care and Other Secondary Care Disciplines

Many patients with CKD interact mainly with their primary care physician (PCP), with only intermittent input from a nephrologist. Increasing numbers of patients with CKD have one or more major active co-morbidities, including diabetes; peripheral, coronary and cerebral vascular disease; heart failure; and other age-related diseases including osteoarthritis and osteoporosis [1]. This system, even in a single-payer system like the UK NHS, generates the potential for waste, duplication and confusion. For instance, a nephrologist may repeat tests (creatinine, glycated haemoglobin, full blood count) that may have been performed recently by the PCP, subjecting the patient to unnecessary venepuncture and generating additional cost. Often this is done simply because the nephrologist and the PCP are using different information systems – so one-off investment in computerised linkage between these systems is likely to generate major savings and improvements in clinical care. The introduction of joint hospital clinics can reduce duplication within secondary care, the most common example being a joint kidney-diabetes clinic where patients can see physicians from both specialties and other members of the multidisciplinary team with cross-over, such as dieticians. Joint kidney/heart failure clinics are another good example, particularly because drugs used to treat heart failure (many of which can improve prognosis, reduce hospitalisation and improve quality of life) can appear to result in a reduction in kidney function, leading many non-specialists to discontinue such treatment unnecessarily. Such joint clinics can improve patient management, reduce waste and improve the patient pathway.

Clear communication between professionals is extremely important. It is commonplace, for instance, for recommendations to be made about changes in regular drug treatment when a patient attends a specialist clinic. Unless precise actions are specified, the GP may wait for the patient to request a new prescription, while the patient may be waiting to hear from the GP. The same is true of requests to monitor kidney function between visits; unless it is precisely specified who should arrange the blood test, and how the result should be brought to the attention of the right clinician, such arrangements can cause false reassurance. This is particularly true when test results need to be interpreted in the context of previous test results or recent changes in treatment – for instance, a GP may consider an Hb of 135 g/L normal, but in a patient on treatment with an erythropoiesis-stimulating agent, this result would usually trigger a dose reduction, depending on previous results and dose changes.

67.1.3 Salt Intake

There is overwhelming evidence in the general population that high dietary intake of salt (as sodium chloride) is associated with hypertension. Low dietary intake of

67

potassium also contributes to hypertension: the ratio of sodium to potassium intake is a better predictor of blood pressure.

The conventional wisdom, until recently, has been that high salt intake causes extracellular volume expansion and that hypertension results from this change in extracellular volume. Volume expansion, in turn, stimulates production of ouabain-like pressor hormones that restore sodium balance at the expense of higher blood pressure. However, it has been known for many years that positive sodium balance does not result in the expected change in body weight or extracellular volume. It is now clear that retained sodium is largely stored in non-osmotically active form by binding to polyanionic glycosaminoglycans, synthesised in response to positive sodium balance. The pathological consequences of non-osmotic salt storage are now being explored; they may include, for instance, changes in conduit artery function [2].

Many patients with CKD have 'salt-sensitive' hypertension. In patients with CKD, there is limited, observational evidence for the benefits of dietary salt restriction. Amongst patients with functioning kidney transplants, for instance, there was a positive association between 24 h urine sodium and blood pressure [3]. There is good evidence that dietary salt restriction amplifies the anti-proteinuric effect of renin-angiotensin system inhibition [4]. Most studies reporting an association between unusually low sodium intake and adverse outcomes can be explained by inadequately rigorous assessment of sodium intake or excretion or are confounded by the association between ill health and low dietary intake of all nutrients, including salt. However, there may well be a lower limit for safe intake [5]. In patients with diabetes mellitus, there is high-quality observational evidence that a **low** dietary salt intake may be associated with harm [6]. There are no prospective interventional studies on the effect of advice to reduce salt intake on 'hard' outcomes such as ESKD or death.

67.1.4 Water Intake

High water intake increases urine volume, but does not increase GFR. Recurrent severe dehydration may cause progressive CKD, in combination with heat and osmotic stress [7], although it remains uncertain whether 'Meso-American nephropathy' is fully explained by such exposure. In polycystic kidney disease, a fluid intake sufficient to suppress vasopressin secretion may reduce the rate of cyst growth [8]. In temperate climates, there is no evidence that drinking any more fluid than is required to prevent hypovolaemic dehydration protects against progression of non-polycystic CKD [9, 10].

67.1.5 Exercise

Physical inactivity is associated with increased mortality amongst patients with CKD, just as it is amongst patients without CKD. A systematic review found that regular exercise has significant benefits for physical fitness, walking capacity, blood pressure, health-related quality of life and some nutritional parameters for patients with CKD, but the effects on hard outcomes (e.g. hospitalisation, death) remain to be proved [11].

67.1.6 Weight Loss

Obesity increases the risk that a person will develop diabetes and hypertension – two major risk factors for CKD. Obesity may also directly cause glomerular hyperfiltration and increase the risk of albuminuria, 'sensitising' the kidney to hypertension. Amongst patients with CKD, there is good evidence that obesity is associated with an increased risk of progression [12]. However, there is no direct evidence from randomised controlled trials that weight loss improves kidney outcomes.

Estimation of GFR is complex in obese individuals. Use of the Cockcroft/Gault formula (which includes body weight) gives higher values of estimated creatinine clearance than the eGFR estimate derived from the MDRD or CKD-EPI formulae, but this is partly because the latter provide an estimate of GFR normalised to body size (in ml/min/1.73 m^2). An ideal filtration marker would be normalised not to body size, but to basal metabolic rate (as the best predictor of the rate of production of water-soluble waste products). Creatinine production cannot reliably be predicted from body weight in obese people – particularly not in those with advanced CKD, in whom sarcopaenic obesity is common.

67.1.7 Alcohol Intake

Contrary to common perception, there is no evidence that alcohol use or over-use is associated with an increased risk of kidney failure, other than in the setting of hepatorenal failure complicating alcoholic cirrhosis.

67.1.8 'Hard' Drug Use

Use of heroin, cocaine and other street drugs is associated with an increased risk of progressive CKD. Several causal pathways are involved [13].

67.1.9 Avoidance of Acute Kidney Injury Superimposed on CKD

'Primum non nocere' (first, do no harm)

Patients with CKD are at higher risk of developing AKI than the general population (although this may partly be due to the definition of AKI: the lower the initial GFR, the less of a change in GFR is required to cause a serum creatinine increment that qualifies as AKI); more likely to require RRT for AKI; and less likely to recover renal function. Having responsive systems in place to rapidly identify any deterioration and act upon it may substantially delay the need for dialysis or death. It is essential to identify or exclude reversible causes in patients who have unexplained deterioration in their CKD. Common examples of this are super-imposed obstructive uropathy (especially in elderly men), urinary tract infection, medication (TIN, direct toxic effect) and pre-renal causes including reduced intravascular volume and cardiac output. Avoiding or minimising any renal insult is paramount, especially those that are iatrogenic. Important examples are the avoidance of contrast nephropathy, the avoidance of over-diuresis and hypotension and dose adjustment of aminoglycosides.

Remember that not all changes in GFR truly reflect kidney 'injury'. For instance, initiation of ACEI, ARB or SGLT-2 inhibitors can cause a reduction in GFR due to changes in glomerular haemodynamics, but without causing any increase in markers of tubular injury [14]. If the reduction in GFR causes complications such as symptomatic uraemia, acidosis or hyperkalaemia, then dose reduction or cessation may be justified; in all other situations, the potential harm of a non-progressive reduction in GFR must be balanced against the possibility that the drug might be improving quality of life or prognosis.

67.2 Pharmacological Measures

67.2.1 Treatment of Anaemia

67

This is covered elsewhere (*cross-reference to anaemia chapter*).

67.2.2 Antiproteinuric Treatment

Albuminuria is a powerful marker of the severity of glomerular damage; non-albumin proteinuria helps to identify tubular damage. Proteinuria also causes tubular toxicity, contributing to progressive kidney injury. Reduction in proteinuria is a useful marker of the success of specific treatment for glomerulonephritis (e.g. steroid treatment in minimal change disease); but treatments that reduce proteinuria by reducing glomerular hyperfiltration also improve prognosis. As discussed elsewhere, glomerular hyperfiltration results from a combination of systemic hypertension, afferent arteriolar vasodilatation and efferent arteriolar vasoconstriction. Reducing any of these three components causes a reduction in proteinuria. This is combined with a non-progressive fall in GFR, but in the medium and long term, this is offset by a slowing or complete stabilisation of the progressive fall in GFR that would have occurred without treatment.

In this context, not all antihypertensive drug treatments are equal. Dihydropyridine calcium channel blockers, for instance, increase afferent arteriolar vasodilatation and can worsen proteinuria, particularly when systemic blood pressure remains above target [15].

67.2.3 Inhibitors of the Renin/Angiotensin/Aldosterone System

A clear understanding of the effects of angiotensin-converting enzyme inhibitors (ACEIs) and angiotensin receptor blockers (ARBs) on kidney function in CKD is important. They are the first line of drug treatment in patients with proteinuric CKD, particularly in the presence of hypertension. Although this is an oversimplification (and ignores, for instance, antifibrotic actions via TGF-beta), it is useful to assume that the protection that these drugs provide against progressive loss of renal function is associated with their capacity to reduce intraglomerular pressure by causing preferential vasodilatation of the efferent arteriole. (We explain this to patients by saying that the excess protein in the urine is a sign that there is high pressure in the kidney filters, caused by kidney disease, making the filters work harder than normal: reducing the pressure on the filters allows them to last for longer, 'giving the kidneys a rest'.) This haemodynamic action results in an acute fall in GFR. Post hoc analyses of trials amongst patients with diabetes show that the early fall in GFR and the early fall in albumin excretion are both predictive markers of long-term stability of kidney function [16]. However, it remains uncertain whether titrating antiproteinuric drug treatment against proteinuria results in better outcomes. Only one small trial has tested this strategy: titration of the dose of benazepril or losartan against proteinuria conferred greater benefit than standard doses, despite similar blood pressure control [17].

There are potential risks to maximising RAAS blockade: the RAAS plays an important part in autoregulation of renal blood flow and GFR, and acute hypotension and sepsis may be more likely to result in an acute fall in GFR in the presence of RAAS blockade. However, RAAS blockade may also protect against tubular injury, and further evidence is needed to guide decisions about whether to continue or discontinue these drugs during acute illness.

Dual blockade of the RAAS (by combining an ACEI and ARB or an ACEI and ARB with aliskiren) has been tested in several large trials (ONTARGET, VA NEPHRON-D, ALTITUDE) and, despite reduction in proteinuria, has not been shown to be of net benefit [18–20].

In the presence of renal artery stenosis, or other conditions causing generalised renal *under*-perfusion, GFR is maintained solely by intense vasoconstriction of the efferent arteriole. In this setting, ACEIs and ARBs can cause acute kidney injury, which may be irreversible despite withdrawal of the drug. Therefore, a serum creatinine and potassium measurement is generally recommended 7–10 days following the introduction or dose titration of RAAS blockade and drug withdrawal if serum creatinine has risen >20% or serum potassium >6.0 mmol/L.

Some clinicians have introduced 'sick day rules' for patients receiving RAAS blockade and counsel their patients to withhold these medicines if they have an acute intercurrent illness (the verbal warning may also be supported by written information). This intervention has some biological plausibility but has not been tested in a randomised controlled trial and may have unintended consequences, including reluctance to continue or resume treatment that is of undoubted prognostic benefit once the acute illness has resolved [21]. Amongst patients with heart failure with reduced ejection fraction, withdrawal of RAAS blockade may do more harm than good.

67.2.4 Sodium-Glucose Co-transport Inhibition

Glucose that is filtered at the glomerulus is normally reabsorbed with sodium (1:1) in the proximal tubule by the sodium-glucose co-transporter, SGLT-2. Hyperglycaemia stimulates increased activity of this co-transporter. This results in increased reabsorption of sodium in the proximal tubule and decreased delivery of sodium to the macula densa. The macula densa is responsible for tubulo-glomerular feedback – glomerular filtration rate increases in response to decreased sodium delivery and decreases in response to increased sodium delivery. This is the mechanism by which hyperglycaemia causes glomerular hyperfiltration. SGLT-2 inhibitors (canagliflozin, dapagliflozin, empagliflozin, sotagliflozin) improve glycaemic control and promote weight loss by increasing glucose loss in the urine, but also reduce blood pressure (partly by promoting sodium loss) and reduce glomerular hyperfiltration (by increasing tubulo-glomerular feedback). Recent randomised trial evidence suggests that these drugs reduce cardiovascular mortality and progression of CKD amongst patients with CKD and diabetes; their role in non-diabetic CKD is under investigation. SGLT2 inhibition is associated with an increased risk of urinary and genital infections, including Fournier's gangrene, and an increased risk of distal amputation [22]. Exactly when and in which patients these drugs are indicated remains uncertain. They are currently not licensed in advanced CKD.

67.2.5 Non-dihydropyridine Calcium Channel Blockers

Non-dihydropyridine calcium channel blockers (such as diltiazem) may also have a beneficial effect on proteinuria when used in conjunction with an ACEi. They are effective antihypertensive agents in renal disease and have a superior antiproteinuric effect when compared to dihydropyridine calcium channel blockers (such as amlodipine) and some advocate their greater use in renal disease [15].

67.2.6 Antihypertensive Treatment

Blood pressure targets (and the agents used to achieve them) should be individualised to the patient according to their age, comorbidity, risk of progression of CKD, presence of pre-existent cardiovascular disease and diabetes. The SPRINT study has reignited debate on how far blood pressure can safely be lowered, but also caused renewed attention on how BP is measured. All recent trials have used resting BP; SPRINT used the average of three measurements taken after 5 minutes of quiet rest. Treatment decisions based on 'casual' clinic measurements, taken as soon as the patient arrives in clinic, are indefensible. Excellent international guidelines written specifically for patients with CKD are available on this topic from the KDIGO website (▶ www.kdigo.org). Particular recommendations of note: a lower blood pressure target (≤130 mmHg systolic and ≤80 mmHg diastolic) is recommended if urine albumin excretion exceeds 30 mg/day (or equivalent) regardless of a co-existent diagnosis of diabetes. However, if urine albumin is <30 mg/day (or equivalent), then a less stringent blood pressure target of ≤140 mmHg systolic and ≤90 mmHg diastolic is recommended, regardless of a co-existent diagnosis of diabetes. These guidelines are currently under review.

67.2.7 Metabolic Acidosis

Metabolic acidosis is common in stage 4–5 CKD and is associated with multiple metabolic derangements including muscle wasting and loss of bone density and also with increased tubular ammoniagenesis, which may cause tubular damage and contribute to progressive loss of GFR. Several studies now support the hypothesis that correction of metabolic acidosis by sodium bicarbonate supplementation improves nutritional status and slows progression [23–25], and the KDIGO CKD guidelines suggest that patients with CKD and a serum bicarbonate concentration of <22 mmol/L should be treated to maintain serum bicarbonate within the normal range [26]. Larger studies, with hard endpoints, are awaited; the fact that sodium bicarbonate is so cheap means that such studies will require state funding.

There is some evidence that increased intake of sodium in the form of sodium bicarbonate does **not** result in volume expansion or worsening of hypertension amongst patients with CKD; these effects are only seen with increased sodium chloride intake. Although this has been known for more than 30 years [27, 28], the precise physiological explanation remains unclear but must relate in some way to renal chloride handling. Despite these observations, new drugs to correct acidosis without altering sodium balance are now being tested [29].

67.2.8 Hyperkalaemia

Hyperkalaemia is a common problem in CKD, particularly for people with diabetes who may have an element of type 4 renal tubular acidosis (hyporeninaemic hypoaldosteronism), but also in patients treated with RAAS blockade. Managed badly, this can result in multiple admissions with hyperkalaemia often with inappropriate doses of insulin and dextrose, stop-starting of important drugs and increased levels of anxiety. Pseudohyperkalaemia should be excluded. Careful, thorough culture-specific dietary advice is valuable in patients with persistent problems, and patient information leaflets should be readily available for those with minor hyperkalaemia. Correction of chronic acidosis (see above) and addition of diuretics are often very helpful medium-term solutions. In type 4 RTA, the renin production is suppressed by real or apparent volume expansion, and the addition of a thiazide diuretic (in full dose) can combat this and concurrently improve the hyperkalaemia. In those with recurrent hyperkalaemia who are taking RAAS blockade, a careful review of the balance of risk and benefit is required, once other reversible causes have been dealt with. Clear guidelines on acceptable and not-acceptable hyperkalaemia need to be available for those encountering patients with CKD.

Drugs that bind potassium in the gut (patiromer calcium [30]; sodium zirconium cyclosilicate [31]) have now been introduced into clinical practice and may allow continued use of RAAS inhibitors in the presence of CKD and allow better control of hyperkalaemia in advanced CKD; their role remains to be decided and will depend partly on cost.

67.2.9 Dyslipidaemia

Atherosclerosis and glomerulosclerosis share pathological characteristics, so many researchers have looked for a benefit of lipid-lowering therapy on the progression of kidney disease. Statins do appear to reduce albuminuria, although the effect is variable [32]. However, treating dyslipidaemia in CKD, using an HMG Co-A reductase inhibitor (statin), with or without a selective cholesterol absorption inhibitor (e.g. ezetimibe), has not been shown to retard the progression of CKD in the SHARP [33], PANDA [34] and PLANET [35] studies, respectively, and the lack of effect on progression has been confirmed in a recent meta-analysis, although the same study showed some reduction in all-cause mortality, attributable to a reduction in cardiovascular risk [32].

67.2.10 Hyperuricaemia

Gout is a common complication of CKD. Some researchers have hypothesised that hyperuricaemia also contributes to the pathogenesis of salt-sensitive hypertension and progressive loss of GFR, although it has not been shown that urate-lowering therapy improves blood pressure or slows progression.

Colchicine is preferable to NSAIDs or steroids for the treatment of acute attacks of gout amongst patients with CKD; 500micg twice daily is often enough while avoiding the diarrhoea that is common with higher doses. Colchicine can also be used for suppression of acute attacks during initiation of urate-lowering therapy. Long-term use of colchicine can cause peripheral neuropathy. Dose reductions or temporary cessation of interacting drugs may be required (including drugs cleared by cytochrome P450 3A4 and some statins).

Long-term urate-lowering therapy is often indicated solely for the prevention of recurrent attacks of gouty arthritis and to promote regression of tophaceous gout. Allopurinol can cause severe cutaneous adverse reactions (SCAR), which can be life-threatening; these occur when patients with CKD are started on the full starting dose of 300 mg daily and are vanishingly rare if the drug is started at 50–100 mg daily and then titrated monthly to achieve a target serum urate of <300 micmol/L, even if to a dose of 400 mg [36]. The HLA B*5801 allele, commoner amongst people of Han Chinese, Korean or Thai descent, confers greatly increased susceptibility to SCARs [37]. Febuxostat may be more effective than allopurinol but can also cause SCARs [38] and is associated with a higher risk of cardiovascular disease [39].

Uricosuric drugs are of limited utility amongst patients with CKD. However, losartan is uricosuric, and it makes sense to use this in preference to other ARBs in patients with gout.

67.2.11 Other Drug Therapy

It is important for prescribers to recognise impaired excretory renal function for two reasons: firstly, to avoid drug accumulation in renally cleared drugs (such as excess bleeding with low molecular weight heparins when eGFR<30ml/min/1.73m^2) and secondly, to avoid renal toxicity at inappropriate doses (such as gentamicin). In theory, calculated creatinine clearance is often preferred to eGFR for drug dosing purposes because it is not normalised to body surface area (and the Cockcroft/Gault formula is often specified in the Summary of Product Characteristics); in practice, neither formula is 100% reliable at the extremes of body size.

67.2.12 Fibrates

Most fibrates, with the possible exception of gemfibrozil, can cause a reversible increase in urea and creatinine concentration. In some patients, a progressive rise over time has also been demonstrated. Studies in people with normal kidney function have not demonstrated an effect of fibrates on isotopically measured GFR, but no such studies have been done in patients with CKD. Very few patients with CKD G3-5 were included in the FIELD and ACCORD studies. One study suggests that fibrates increase the rate of release of creatinine from muscle; this would explain a rise in creatinine, but not a progressive rise over time, nor a rise in serum urea concentration. In patients with CKD, it is probably safe to ignore a small, step-wise increase in serum creatinine concentration following the initiation of fibrate therapy, particularly if the serum urea concentration is unchanged; however, if there is a progressive rise in creatinine over time, particularly if accompanied by a rise in urea, the drug should be stopped.

67.2.13 Trimethoprim, Cimetidine and Antiretroviral Drugs

Trimethoprim, cimetidine and several antiretroviral drugs used in HIV treatment [40] inhibit the tubular secretion of creatinine. The use of trimethoprim in a patient with CKD can result in a marked rise (20–50%) in serum creatinine concentration and fall in *estimated* GFR, without any change in true GFR. A clinician who doesn't understand what is happening may think that the patient has acute kidney injury and arrange unnecessary admission, invasive investigations, etc. Although no systematic studies have been reported, in our experience, the serum creatinine can remain above baseline for at least 14 days after completion of a course of full-dose trimethoprim. Trimethoprim also reduces renal potassium excretion (through an amiloride-like action), and clinically apparent hyperkalaemia may be observed. This is of particular importance in patients with CKD and/or taking other drugs associated with hyperkalaemia (such as RAAS blockade, particularly if in combination with spironolactone) [41], and the balance of risk versus benefit should be considered before prescribing trimethoprim in this context. The effect is dose-dependent: high doses used for the treatment of *Pneumocystis* infection, for instance, are much more likely to cause hyperkalaemia.

67.2.14 Non-steroidal Anti-Inflammatory Drugs (NSAIDs)

NSAIDs inhibit the action of vasodilator prostaglandins that play a major role in maintaining GFR, particularly in the presence of pre-existing CKD. Therefore, all NSAIDs can cause salt and water retention, a fall in GFR and hyperkalaemia. These effects are amplified amongst patients with effective or true hypovolaemia, those on RAAS blockade and those in sepsis. These drugs must be used with great care in patients with CKD, who should be warned not to buy NSAIDs over the counter. However, an absolute 'ban' on prescription of these drugs in all patients with CKD is neither practicable nor justified. In some patients with severe osteoarthritis, for instance, in whom paracetamol is ineffective and opiate-based analgesics cause unacceptable adverse effects, it is reasonable to prescribe NSAIDs even in the presence of CKD4 *so long as* kidney function, blood pressure and fluid status are monitored carefully and regularly.

NSAIDs can also cause minimal change nephrotic syndrome and interstitial nephritis, but these are idiosyncratic reactions and may be drug-specific.

67.2.15 Aminoglycosides

As part of the drive to reduce hospital-acquired infections, such as *Clostridium difficile* infection, there has been a switch from broad-spectrum antibiotics to aminoglycoside antibiotics (especially gentamicin), with some hospitals seeing gentamicin prescribing doubling [42]. If monitored appropriately and dose alterations are made in light of changing renal function, gentamicin can be administered safely to patients with CKD. This requires multidisciplinary working between medical, nursing and pharmacy colleagues. The conventional wisdom is that nephrotoxicity is usually the result of cumulative exposure over several days and much more likely if high trough levels are allowed to occur. However, even single doses of gentamicin, when given as surgical prophylaxis, appear to be associated with an increased risk of acute kidney injury [43].

67.2.16 Antiviral Drugs

Several antiviral drugs are nephrotoxic; this is a particular concern during the treatment of human immunodeficiency virus infection. Tenofovir disoproxil causes cumulative tubular toxicity, with tubular proteinuria and phosphate wasting progressing to progressive CKD. Concurrent use of other antiretroviral drugs can increase the risk of toxicity. The choice of antiretroviral drugs should include individualised risk assessment but also depends on resources, as most of the less nephrotoxic drugs are more expensive [44]. Several antiretroviral drugs also inhibit tubular creatinine secretion without reducing GFR [40].

67.3 Clinical Management of CKD: Preparation for End-Stage Kidney Failure

67.3.1 Prediction of Outcome

67

Most people with CKD will never progress to end-stage kidney failure (ESKD), although many will die prematurely, predominantly from cardiovascular disease. It is therefore important to tailor management to the patient's individual risk of ESKD and death. These risks can be predicted with simple online tools using routinely available clinical information. The Kidney Failure Risk Equation (▶ http://kidneyfailurerisk.com) has been extensively validated and predicts the risk of kidney failure requiring dialysis or transplantation. The Kidney Disease: Improving Global Outcomes (KDIGO) risk calculator (▶ http://www.kdigo.org/equation/) provides information on an individual's risk both of ESKD and of death.

67.3.2 Multidisciplinary Education Programmes

Initiating renal replacement therapy (RRT) is a major life change, with practical, social, psychological and financial consequences as well as physical consequences. Physicians who focus solely on the physical consequences (e.g. treatment of anaemia, acidosis, hypertension and phosphate retention) are therefore missing the 'bigger picture' and, when patients don't always adhere to complex drug treatments, may blame the patient for 'poor compliance' when in reality, the patient is struggling to cope with other aspects of their life and accords low priority to drug treatments than might affect their health some time into the future (think of Maslow's hierarchy of needs – food is a basic need, but a low-potassium, low-phosphate, fluid-restricted diabetic diet accompanied by the correct timing of insulin therapy before the meal and a phosphate binder afterwards is a need of a different magnitude. It requires a complex interplay of financial resources, strict dietary modification, memory, eyesight, manual dexterity, time, organisation *and* patient motivation).

While there is no reason in principle why doctors should not be trained, and given time, to address the 'non-biological' aspects of coping with CKD and RRT, they are an expensive resource, and there is evidence that the most cost-effective way of preparing patients with CKD for major decisions about RRT is to provide a multidisciplinary clinic. Patients may meet other patients in small groups, including patients who have experienced various RRT modalities; nursing staff with expertise in patient education; psychologists; dietitians; and others. Several observational studies have found that patients who have attended a multidisciplinary clinic are better informed and better prepared for RRT than similar patients attending conventional medical clinics. A non-randomised comparison of a formal education programme ('RightStart') with standard care found improved morbidity and mortality over the first year after starting RRT [45]. A randomised trial in Canada amongst relatively low-risk patients with CKD not previously known to nephrologists found no clear evidence that multidisciplinary care slowed progression or improved management of complications compared to care by primary care physicians [46] but proved cost-effective largely due to a lower number of days in hospital; patients receiving multidisciplinary care reported a higher quality of life [47]. A recent randomised trial amongst Zuni Indians in New Mexico demonstrated that community-based coaching resulted in a significant increase in patient activation, with parallel improvements in body mass index, glycaemic control, inflammation and mental health [48].

67.3.2.1 Identification and Workup of Patients Suitable for Transplantation

This is an important area and often delivered in an inconsistent manner. For most young patients, pre-emptive transplantation (ideally with a live donor transplant) is the treatment of choice when approaching ESRD. For an older patient with asymptomatic CKD, at low risk of progression, the risks and benefits are more evenly balanced, even when eGFR is below 15. There are caveats and conditions around this, but early assessment and education of appropriately selected patients is important. Strategies to avoid blood transfusion and advice on contraception in women of child-bearing age are important to avoid sensitisation against HLA antigens.

67.3.2.2 Balancing the Burdens and Benefits of Renal Replacement Therapy: The Option of Active Supportive Care

Several observational studies have demonstrated that the initiation of dialysis treatment amongst older adults, particularly those with pre-existing co-morbidities including frailty, is associated with a reduction in functional status, a reduction in quality of life and a high burden of treatment. Elective initiation of dialysis even at an eGFR as low as 6 ml/min may not even prolong life in some elderly patients with co-morbidity [49]. For these reasons, the decision about whether or not to plan for dialysis treatment should ideally be made in advance (rather than waiting for a crisis, for instance, refractory hyperkalaemia or pulmonary oedema) and should take into account how the patient weighs up the burden of treatment with the possible extension of life [50]. Some patients may choose dialysis treatment; others may choose 'active supportive care' and should receive a package of care that includes on-going management of renal anaemia, acidosis and fluid balance, together with drug treatment for symptoms caused by uraemia.

Shared Decision-Making: Patient Decision Aids

Patients with CKD will be faced with numerous 'medical' decisions over the course of their life with CKD – some of which are listed in the ◘ Table 67.1. For some decisions, the choice is straightforward, because of strong evidence that the outcomes are better with one choice than with the other. In guidelines using the GRADE classification, these options will be given as level 1 Recommendations and will normally be supported by level A or B evidence. However, many other options are based on weaker evidence, will be given as level 2 Suggestions and will normally have level C or D evidence in support. The definition of a 'Suggestion' for patients is 'The majority of people in your situation would want the recommended course of action, but many would not'. For clinicians, the definition reads 'Different choices will be appropriate for different patients. Each patient needs help to arrive at a management decision consistent with her or his values and preferences'.

◘ Table 67.1 Examples of preference-sensitive decisions in CKD care

Clinical scenario	Options
Stable stage G3b CKD	Phosphate binder treatment Aspirin as primary prevention
Stable stage G4 CKD	Fistula construction (if HD would be preferred treatment option) vs wait and see if function declines
Young active patient with CKD: renal anaemia, Hb 9.5, adequate iron stores	Correction with ESA – target range 10–12 Correction with ESA – target range 12–13
Progressive CKD, currently stage 4	Conservative care or RRT Home-based or hospital-based RRT HD or PD (assuming not transplanted) Pre-emptive transplant listing
Plan for kidney transplantation	Perfectly matched ideal donor HLA-mismatched donor (specify acceptable degree of mismatch) 'Marginal' donor

Achieving high-quality shared decisions with patients about aspects of CKD care is morally the right thing to do, but there are also important pragmatic reasons. Patients who feel 'ownership' of the decision are more likely to implement it – improving adherence to treatment. Patients who are 'activated' to take control over their own treatment will require less support, in the medium term, than those who are the passive recipients of patriarchal, 'doctor knows best' care.

Achieving shared decision-making in practice is culturally disruptive both for care-givers and for patients. Doctors, for instance, have more knowledge about the risks and benefits of the various options than patients can possibly have; patients used to conventional medical care may well reply 'you're the doctor, you should know what's best for me'. Accepting these attitudes means that patients will probably spend more time researching their next holiday than they will researching their medical options.

67.3.2.3 Late Presentation

'Late presentation' is usually defined as the commencement of RRT within 3 months or less of the patient's first contact with a nephrologist. Late presentation is associated with higher costs, poorer outcomes and a greater chance of the patient being treated with hospital-based haemodialysis via a catheter – although with appropriate multidisciplinary input, other modalities can be successfully adopted. Although late presentation rates have fallen (partly as a result of better recognition and management of CKD), there is an irreducible minimum of late presenting patients. Some late presentation is attributable to poor medical management; some to patients not engaging with advice from healthcare professionals; and some, the irreducible minimum, to unavoidable acute and irreversible kidney failure, for instance, due to anti-GBM disease, vasculitis or myeloma.

Many such patients are elderly and frail with poor functional status. This group of patients, in whom the balance between burden and benefit of RRT is particularly finely balanced, are most in need of decisions that take their values and preferences into account; a decision about the benefits of providing acute renal replacement therapy must be made relatively promptly, frequently out-of-hours. These patients deserve careful and thoughtful assessment, and a decision to withhold or commence renal replacement therapy should be made at a senior level.

Conclusion

Management of CKD requires a holistic approach, considering the individual patient's risk of progression, their competing risks (particularly the risk of death from cardiovascular disease) and their values and preferences. Encouraging patients to become 'activated' in their own management is important, but can be difficult, particularly in the context of multimorbidity. Although new treatments to prevent progression of CKD are needed, effective deployment of the available treatments can slow progression and buy time for the planning of RRT amongst those in whom progression continues.

Case Study

Case Study 1

A 69-year-old female with type 2 diabetes mellitus (with retinopathy and peripheral neuropathy), ischaemic heart disease and systolic heart failure has been found to have worsening proteinuria. She has pitting oedema to the knees and sub-optimal blood pressure control (mean of two measurements after 5 minutes unattended quiet rest = 163/82 mm Hg). Currently, she is on aspirin, metformin, furosemide, lisinopril (10 mg/day) and bisoprolol. Dipstick urinalysis shows blood ++ and protein +++. Her serum creatinine is 150 μmol/L and eGFR 30 ml/min/1.73m^2. Serum potassium is 5.8 mmol/L and serum bicarbonate 19 mmol/L. Her early morning urine albumin/creatinine ratio (ACR) is 140 mg/mmol and was 70 mg/mmol 11 months previously, 33 mg/mmol 2 years previously, 7.8 mg/mmol 5 years previously and <3 mg/mmol 10 years previously. Serum albumin is normal. Renal immune screen is negative. Imaging of renal tract showed no hydronephrosis, with bipolar lengths of 105 and 103 mm. A recent echocardiogram showed impaired left ventricular function (ejection fraction 35%) with no valvular disease.

67

This clinical presentation is consistent with diabetic kidney disease although haematuria is unusual. Further urological testing may be required if haematuria persists or if other risk factors are present. A kidney biopsy would be unlikely to change management but should be kept under consideration, particularly if proteinuria does not improve with blood pressure control. Optimisation of blood pressure is important, but increasing the dose of lisinopril is likely to worsen hyperkalaemia. The patient should be offered loop diuretics, adjusted to control peripheral oedema; if necessary, a thiazide-type diuretic can be added to potentiate the loop diuretic. Diuretic treatment might result in a fall in serum potassium, in which case the lisinopril might safely then be increased if blood pressure is still above target. Sodium bicarbonate treatment should be considered to correct acidosis: this might help to correct hyperkalaemia. Diltiazem should be avoided because of the risk of bradycardia in combination with bisoprolol. Glycaemic control is also important, but metformin will have to be withdrawn if GFR continues to fall.

Case Study 3

A 75-year-old male with multiple co-morbidities including severe aortic stenosis, heart failure, chronic obstructive pulmonary disease and peripheral vascular disease has slowly progressive chronic kidney disease (CKD) G4, A2 with current eGFR of 16 (compared to 20 a year ago and 25 2 years ago). He lives alone, is independent and walks with a stick. His exercise tolerance is limited due to shortness of breath and pre-syncope; he uses a mobility scooter. Current blood pressure is around 85/50 mm Hg, on no blood pressure-lowering drugs.

The KDIGO risk calculator suggests a 4-year risk of renal replacement therapy of 20.2% and a 4-year risk of death of 54.2%, but does not take into account his severe aortic stenosis. He is judged too high risk for open valve surgery. Trans-catheter aortic valve replacement (TAVI) is an option, but carries a significant risk of precipitating kidney failure from contrast nephropathy. Decisions about whether to attempt TAVI therefore depend on his values and preferences with respect to surviving but remaining dialysis-dependent. The patient should be provided with adequate information in digestible portions to facilitate informed decision-making. A multidisciplinary approach is required. He may require several visits and considerable support to come to a decision.

Tips and Tricks

- Never give up on advising patients on lifestyle measures. Encourage obese patients to reflect on what has worked for them in the past: slimming clubs are often much more effective than dietetic advice from health professionals.
- Diuretics are a very useful add-on option in hypertension in patients with CKD; combinations of loop and thiazide-type diuretics can provide additional benefit even in advanced CKD. Diuretic treatment also often helps to offset a tendency to hyperkalaemia.
- Correction of acidosis with sodium bicarbonate is safe and well tolerated and does not exacerbate fluid overload or hypertension.
- It is seldom if ever a good idea to use the phrase 'If I was in your situation' or 'If you were my father/mother' when discussing options with a patient. It is unlikely that you will know enough about the patient's values and preferences to make a decision that will be right for them.

Chapter Review Questions

1. What is the best clinical approach if a patient with CKD stage G3b has persistent proteinuria (albumin/creatinine ratio persistently >70 mg/mmol) despite full dose of an ACEI? Usual clinic blood pressure, measured after 5 minutes of quiet rest, is persistently around 145/70 mm Hg.
2. Do statins slow the progression of chronic kidney disease in patients with hypertension and atherosclerosis?
3. Are non-steroidal anti-inflammatory drugs (NSAIDs) contraindicated in all patients with CKD?
4. What is the appropriate action if eGFR falls from 45 to 38 ml/min/1.73m^2 within 2 weeks of initiation of an ACEI in a patient with marked proteinuria (albumin/creatinine ratio 135 mg/mmol)? Serum potassium has remained well within the normal range.

Answers

1. The patient should be advised on dietary salt restriction: this can augment the antiproteinuric effect of an ACEI. A 24 h urine collection can be used to estimate daily sodium intake and guide therapy. If this is ineffective, then addition of a diuretic should be considered. A third option would be to add a non-dihydropyridine calcium channel blocker.
2. No: the balance of evidence suggests that statins do not affect progression of CKD; however, they do reduce the risk of cardiovascular events, which for many patients with CKD are more of a threat to future health than progressive kidney disease.
3. No; but they should be used with great caution because of their ability to reduce renal blood flow, reduce GFR and exacerbate hypertension, fluid overload and hyperkalaemia. A decision to prescribe these drugs (or to advise a patient to use NSAIDs bought 'over the counter') should be individualised and should always be accompanied by close monitoring for these complications.
4. The correct course of action would be to continue the drug but to repeat the eGFR measurement 2 weeks later. It is far more likely that this patient is demonstrating the expected, haemodynamically mediated reduction in GFR that the drug causes: in the long term, this reduction in GFR predicts long-term stability due to amelioration of pressure-related glomerular damage. A progressive fall in GFR should prompt consideration of alternative causes, including bilateral renal artery stenosis.

References

1. Barnett K, Mercer SW, Norbury M, Watt G, Wyke S, Guthrie B. Epidemiology of multimorbidity and implications for health care, research, and medical education: a cross-sectional study. Lancet. 2012;380(9836):37–43.
2. Lambers Heerspink HJ, Navis G, Ritz E. Salt intake in kidney disease--a missed therapeutic opportunity? Nephrol Dial Transplant. 2012;27(9):3435–42.
3. van den Berg E, Geleijnse JM, Brink EJ, van Baak MA, Homan van der Heide JJ, Gans RO, et al. Sodium intake and blood pressure in renal transplant recipients. Nephrol Dial Transplant. 2012;27(8):3352–9.
4. Lambers Heerspink HJ, Holtkamp FA, Parving HH, Navis GJ, Lewis JB, Ritz E, et al. Moderation of dietary sodium potentiates the renal and cardiovascular protective effects of angiotensin receptor blockers. Kidney Int. 2012;82(3):330–7.
5. Heerspink HL, Ritz E. Sodium chloride intake: is lower always better? J Am Soc Nephrol. 2012;23(7):1136–9.
6. Vallon V, Thomson SC. Anomalous role for dietary salt in diabetes mellitus? Nat Rev Endocrinol. 2011;7(7):377–8.
7. Gonzalez-Quiroz M, Smpokou ET, Silverwood RJ, Camacho A, Faber D, Garcia BR, et al. Decline in kidney function among apparently healthy young adults at risk of Mesoamerican nephropathy. J Am Soc Nephrol. 2018;29(8):2200–12.
8. El-Damanawi R, Lee M, Harris T, Mader LB, Bond S, Pavey H, et al. Randomised controlled trial of high versus ad libitum water intake in patients with autosomal dominant polycystic kidney disease: rationale and design of the DRINK feasibility trial. BMJ Open. 2018;8(5):e022859.
9. Wenzel UO, Hebert LA, Stahl RA, Krenz I. My doctor said I should drink a lot! Recommendations for fluid intake in patients with chronic kidney disease. Clin J Am Soc Nephrol. 2006;1(2):344–6.
10. Clark WF, Sontrop JM, Huang SH, Gallo K, Moist L, House AA, et al. Effect of coaching to increase water intake on kidney function decline in adults with chronic kidney disease: the CKD WIT randomized clinical trial. JAMA. 2018;319(18):1870–9.

11. Heiwe S, Jacobson SH. Exercise training in adults with CKD: a systematic review and meta-analysis. Am J Kidney Dis. 2014;64(3):383–93.
12. Herrington WG, Smith M, Bankhead C, Matsushita K, Stevens S, Holt T, et al. Body-mass index and risk of advanced chronic kidney disease: prospective analyses from a primary care cohort of 1.4 million adults in England. PLoS One. 2017;12(3):e0173515.
13. Bundy JD, Bazzano LA, Xie D, Cohan J, Dolata J, Fink JC, et al. Self-reported tobacco, alcohol, and illicit drug use and progression of chronic kidney disease. Clin J Am Soc Nephrol. 2018;13(7):993–1001.
14. Anders HJ, Davis JM, Thurau K. Nephron protection in diabetic kidney disease. N Engl J Med. 2016;375(21):2096–8.
15. Bakris GL, Weir MR, Secic M, Campbell B, Weis-McNulty A. Differential effects of calcium antagonist subclasses on markers of nephropathy progression. Kidney Int. 2004;65(6):1991–2002.
16. Holtkamp FA, de Zeeuw D, Thomas MC, Cooper ME, de Graeff PA, Hillege HJ, et al. An acute fall in estimated glomerular filtration rate during treatment with losartan predicts a slower decrease in long-term renal function. Kidney Int. 2011;80(3):282–7.
17. Hou FF, Xie D, Zhang X, Chen PY, Zhang WR, Liang M, et al. Renoprotection of Optimal antiproteinuric Doses (ROAD) Study: a randomized controlled study of benazepril and losartan in chronic renal insufficiency. J Am Soc Nephrol. 2007;18(6):1889–98.
18. Mann JF, Schmieder RE, McQueen M, Dyal L, Schumacher H, Pogue J, et al. Renal outcomes with telmisartan, ramipril, or both, in people at high vascular risk (the ONTARGET study): a multicentre, randomised, double-blind, controlled trial. Lancet. 2008;372(9638):547–53.
19. Fried LF, Emanuele N, Zhang JH, Brophy M, Conner TA, Duckworth W, et al. Combined angiotensin inhibition for the treatment of diabetic nephropathy. N Engl J Med. 2013;369(20):1892–903.
20. Parving HH, Brenner BM, McMurray JJ, de Zeeuw D, Haffner SM, Solomon SD, et al. Cardiorenal end points in a trial of aliskiren for type 2 diabetes. N Engl J Med. 2012;367(23):2204–13.
21. Martindale AM, Elvey R, Howard SJ, McCorkindale S, Sinha S, Blakeman T. Understanding the implementation of 'sick day guidance' to prevent acute kidney injury across a primary care setting in England: a qualitative evaluation. BMJ Open. 2017;7(11):e017241.
22. Chang HY, Singh S, Mansour O, Baksh S, Alexander GC. Association between sodium-glucose cotransporter 2 inhibitors and lower extremity amputation among patients with type 2 diabetes. JAMA Intern Med. 2018;178(9):1190–8.
23. de Brito-Ashurst I, Varagunam M, Raftery MJ, Yaqoob MM. Bicarbonate supplementation slows progression of CKD and improves nutritional status. J Am Soc Nephrol. 2009;20(9):2075–84.
24. Dubey AK, Sahoo J, Vairappan B, Haridasan S, Parameswaran S, Priyamvada PS. Correction of metabolic acidosis improves muscle mass and renal function in chronic kidney disease stages 3 and 4: a randomized controlled trial. Nephrol Dial Transplant. 2018.
25. Mahajan A, Simoni J, Sheather SJ, Broglio KR, Rajab MH, Wesson DE. Daily oral sodium bicarbonate preserves glomerular filtration rate by slowing its decline in early hypertensive nephropathy. Kidney Int. 2010;78(3):303–9.
26. Kidney Disease Improving Global Outcomes. KDIGO clinical practice guideline for the management of blood pressure in chronic kidney disease. Kidney Int Suppl. 2012;2(5).
27. Husted FC, Nolph KD, Maher JF. NaHCO3 and NaCl tolerance in chronic renal failure. J Clin Invest. 1975;56(2):414–9.
28. Weinberger MH. Sodium chloride and blood pressure. N Engl J Med. 1987;317(17):1084–6.
29. Bushinsky DA, Hostetter T, Klaerner G, Stasiv Y, Lockey C, McNulty S, et al. Randomized, controlled trial of TRC101 to increase serum bicarbonate in patients with CKD. Clin J Am Soc Nephrol. 2018;13(1):26–35.
30. Weir MR, Bakris GL, Bushinsky DA, Mayo MR, Garza D, Stasiv Y, et al. Patiromer in patients with kidney disease and hyperkalemia receiving RAAS inhibitors. N Engl J Med. 2015;372(3):211–21.
31. Packham DK, Rasmussen HS, Lavin PT, El-Shahawy MA, Roger SD, Block G, et al. Sodium zirconium cyclosilicate in hyperkalemia. N Engl J Med. 2015;372(3):222–31.
32. Zhang Z, Wu P, Zhang J, Wang S, Zhang G. The effect of statins on microalbuminuria, proteinuria, progression of kidney function, and all-cause mortality in patients with non-end stage chronic kidney disease: a meta-analysis. Pharmacol Res. 2016;105:74–83.
33. Haynes R, Lewis D, Emberson J, Reith C, Agodoa L, Cass A, et al. Effects of lowering LDL cholesterol on progression of kidney disease. J Am Soc Nephrol. 2014;25(8):1825–33.
34. Rutter MK, Prais HR, Charlton-Menys V, Gittins M, Roberts C, Davies RR, et al. Protection Against Nephropathy in Diabetes with Atorvastatin (PANDA): a randomized double-blind placebo-controlled trial of high- vs. low-dose atorvastatin(1). Diabet Med. 2011;28(1):100–8.
35. de Zeeuw D, Anzalone DA, Cain VA, Cressman MD, Heerspink HJ, Molitoris BA, et al. Renal effects of atorvastatin and rosuvastatin in patients with diabetes who have progressive renal disease (PLANET I): a randomised clinical trial. Lancet Diabetes Endocrinol. 2015;3(3):181–90.
36. Stamp LK, Chapman PT, Barclay ML, Horne A, Frampton C, Tan P, et al. A randomised controlled trial of the efficacy and safety of allopurinol dose escalation to achieve target serum urate in people with gout. Ann Rheum Dis. 2017;76(9):1522–8.
37. Jung JW, Song WJ, Kim YS, Joo KW, Lee KW, Kim SH, et al. HLA-B58 can help the clinical decision on starting allopurinol in patients with chronic renal insufficiency. Nephrol Dial Transplant. 2011;26(11):3567–72.
38. Drug, Therapeutics B. Latest guidance on the management of gout. BMJ. 2018;362:k2893.
39. White WB, Saag KG, Becker MA, Borer JS, Gorelick PB, Whelton A, et al. Cardiovascular safety of febuxostat or allopurinol in patients with gout. N Engl J Med. 2018;378(13):1200–10.
40. Yombi JC, Pozniak A, Boffito M, Jones R, Khoo S, Levy J, et al. Antiretrovirals and the kidney in current clinical practice: renal pharmacokinetics, alterations of renal function and renal toxicity. AIDS. 2014;28(5):621–32.
41. Crellin E, Mansfield KE, Leyrat C, Nitsch D, Douglas IJ, Root A, et al. Trimethoprim use for urinary tract infection and risk of adverse outcomes in older patients: cohort study. BMJ. 2018;360:k341.
42. Helps A, Deighan C, Gourlay Y, Seaton RA. Gentamicin and acute kidney injury requiring renal replacement therapy in the context of a restrictive antibiotic policy. J Antimicrob Chemother. 2011;66(8):1936–8.

43. Bell S, Davey P, Nathwani D, Marwick C, Vadiveloo T, Sneddon J, et al. Risk of AKI with gentamicin as surgical prophylaxis. J Am Soc Nephrol. 2014;25(11):2625–32.
44. Swanepoel CR, Atta MG, D'Agati VD, Estrella MM, Fogo AB, Naicker S, et al. Kidney disease in the setting of HIV infection: conclusions from a Kidney Disease: Improving Global Outcomes (KDIGO) controversies conference. Kidney Int. 2018;93(3):545–59.
45. Wingard RL, Pupim LB, Krishnan M, Shintani A, Ikizler TA, Hakim RM. Early intervention improves mortality and hospitalization rates in incident hemodialysis patients: RightStart program. Clin J Am Soc Nephrol. 2007;2(6):1170–5.
46. Barrett BJ, Garg AX, Goeree R, Levin A, Molzahn A, Rigatto C, et al. A nurse-coordinated model of care versus usual care for stage 3/4 chronic kidney disease in the community: a randomized controlled trial. Clin J Am Soc Nephrol. 2011;6(6):1241–7.
47. Hopkins RB, Garg AX, Levin A, Molzahn A, Rigatto C, Singer J, et al. Cost-effectiveness analysis of a randomized trial comparing care models for chronic kidney disease. Clin J Am Soc Nephrol. 2011;6(6):1248–57.
48. Nelson RG, Pankratz VS, Ghahate DM, Bobelu J, Faber T, Shah VO. Home-based kidney care, patient activation, and risk factors for CKD progression in Zuni Indians: a randomized, controlled clinical trial. Clin J Am Soc Nephrol. 2018;13(12):1801–9.
49. Verberne WR, Geers AB, Jellema WT, Vincent HH, van Delden JJ, Bos WJ. Comparative survival among older adults with advanced kidney disease managed conservatively versus with dialysis. Clin J Am Soc Nephrol. 2016;11(4):633–40.
50. Ladin K, Pandya R, Perrone RD, Meyer KB, Kannam A, Loke R, et al. Characterizing approaches to dialysis decision making with older adults: a qualitative study of nephrologists. Clin J Am Soc Nephrol. 2018;13(8):1188–96.

Thinking About the Future, Symptom Control and Other Aspects of Palliative Care in Advanced CKD

Fliss E. M. Murtagh, Jo Wilson, and Sara N. Davison

Contents

M. Harber (ed.), *Primer on Nephrology*, https://doi.org/10.1007/978-3-030-76419-7_68

Learning Objectives

1. To raise awareness of increasing need for a holistic approach to advanced care planning in patients with multiple comorbidity and frailty
2. To appreciate the need to identify patients who may need palliative and supportive care in a timely manner and have early open discussions about advanced care planning
3. To understand the common symptoms associated with advanced CKD and treatment options for these symptoms and the therapeutic options for management of pain in advanced CKD

68.1 Introduction

As we build healthcare services that are fit for future purpose, there are multiple challenges ahead. By 2040, we will have an increasingly aged population with a greatly increased number of deaths [1]. We are facing a rise in multimorbidity at all ages [2] but especially connected with deprivation [3]. We know that people with multimorbidity are more likely to die in hospital [4], but this is not where most people choose to be cared for towards the end of their life [4, 5].

68.2 Thinking About the Future

As CKD advances and life expectancy reduces, the priorities and preferences of people with CKD change. Many people with advanced CKD and their families place increasing priority on quality of life, symptom control and psychological/social concerns, over extension of life [6]. It is important, therefore, that renal professionals adjust the goals of care to match these changing priorities. This work involves understanding something of the priorities, preferences and psychosocial circumstances of the patient, relationships within the family and wider cultural and religious contexts, in order to support patients and families to plan ahead (advance care planning). Without planning ahead, the last months and weeks of life are likely to be much more difficult.

The fundamental purpose of an advance care plan is to represent the priorities of the patient in the face of future circumstances as health declines [7]. Without it, priorities are not met, preparation is denied and bereavement may be more traumatic. Patients with advanced CKD expect their doctors to talk about the future [8], yet advance care planning can be met with ambivalence by both patients and families [9]. Nevertheless, evidence shows that – with hindsight – it is valued for improving choice and enabling preparation [10]. There is evidence too that bereavement outcomes for families are improved with advance care planning [11].

Most patients with advanced CKD needing palliative care are older people with multimorbidity. They have variable and often complex needs with symptoms that are often unaddressed. Comorbidities such as stroke, Parkinson's disease and dementia can affect the individual's mental capacity to take part in decision-making. In such cases, assessing mental capacity and optimizing participation in decision-making where possible are important. Ascertaining whether any member of the family can legally and ethically represent the patient's best interests for medical decision-making is also a crucial part of patient care.

Although detailed evidence about palliative needs and interventions in advanced CKD remains limited, the symptom burden is high [12, 13], and the psychological and social impacts are considerable [14]. Extensive burdens are placed on people with CKD and their families, and complex transitions need to be negotiated. Dialysis is a demanding, time-intensive treatment, and as people approach the end of their life, the risks and benefits of dialysis need careful weighing. Communication is key, especially in relation to dialysis decision-making, treatments such as cardiopulmonary resuscitation and ward-based versus intensive management and advance care planning [15], yet it presents many challenges. This is especially true for those with multimorbidity, who may present with frequent hospital admissions and life-threatening complications. We know from a large US study among patients with end-stage renal disease who had been on dialysis for greater than 90 days that many are offered inhospital cardiopulmonary resuscitation (1.4 events per 1000 inhospital days). For the 22% who survived the hospital admission to discharge, post-discharge survival was just 5 months [16].

Providing high-quality palliative and supportive care to patients with advanced CKD has the potential to markedly improve patient outcomes but has not always received sufficient attention. It needs a systematic approach, relevant training and skills and dedicated resources.

68.3 Which Patients Need Palliative and Supportive Care?

Patients whose palliative and supportive care needs should be considered are those with CKD who:

- Have a high physical and/or psychological symptom burden that impacts significantly on quality of life
- Decline renal replacement therapy (dialysis or transplant) based on their own preferences

- Are advised against renal replacement therapy because the burden of frequent dialysis is felt to outweigh likely survival and quality of life benefits (a complex and difficult decision likely to apply more frequently to those with poor prognoses)
- Do not have the mental capacity to engage in dialysis
- Have been on dialysis but are now withdrawing or about to withdraw from dialysis
- Are on dialysis but with a poor prognosis, often because of comorbid conditions (especially cardiac disease)

It is vitally important for patients that their physical and psychological symptoms are assessed. In the face of serious illness, a holistic need assessment is advised in which the multidisciplinary care team, in partnership with the patient, considers the multifaceted nature of the patient's needs including physical, social, psychological and social aspects.

68.4 Palliative and Supportive Care Assessment

Palliative and supportive care assessment requires a holistic and patient-centred approach. It includes the detailed assessment of:

- Preferences for communication, involvement in decision-making and place of care
- Physical symptoms
- Physical functioning and rehabilitation needs
- Psychological symptoms and emotional well-being
- Social and occupational well-being
- Family communication and well-being and pre-bereavement care
- Planning ahead as the illness advances to maximize influence over quality of life and place of death in accordance with preferences.

Once these needs have been identified and assessed fully, appropriate interventions should then be implemented in a coordinated way. Coordination of care across providers is extremely important for high quality care.

68.5 Symptoms

Patients with advanced CKD are among the most symptomatic of any chronic disease group [17–19]. Excellent symptom management is therefore essential. For more robust individuals with limited comorbidity, dialysis may address some symptoms such as fatigue, anorexia, nausea and vomiting. However, it appears to do little to address symptoms in older, more frail patients or those with multimorbidity. For some patients, dialysis may add to overall symptom burden. Shared care involving multidisciplinary kidney teams (nephrologist, dietician, therapists and psychologists), general practice, and palliative care is essential to optimally manage the high symptom burden.

68.5.1 Symptom Prevalence

Recently, evidence on the epidemiology of symptoms has increased, and the prevalence and severity of individual symptoms are better understood [18–21]. Prevalence depends in part on the stage of CKD, whether a patient is receiving dialysis or not and the nature and extent of comorbid conditions. ◘ Figure 68.1 presents an overview of the prevalence of different symptoms, according to stage of CKD and management pathway.

This illustrates how prevalent the individual symptoms are, but multiple symptoms often interact [22] and persist over time [23]. Pain or nausea, for instance, are more burdensome for a patient who is not sleeping well with restless legs and a low mood.

68.5.2 Symptom Assessment

Symptoms are not assessed routinely or well by kidney professionals and are frequently under recognized [13, 24]. Patients do not always raise their symptoms for discussion spontaneously, partly because their symptoms are often from comorbid conditions and not the kidney disease itself and partly because professionals tend to focus more on biochemical markers and kidney management. Routine and proactive assessment of symptoms will help address this gap. An appropriate, clinically relevant and valid symptom score should be used systematically for all patients with CKD at regular intervals. There are three global symptom scores in regular use which have been adapted and validated specifically for use in those with renal disease:

- The renal version of the Palliative (or Patient) Outcome Scale – symptom module (POSs renal) [25] – developed in the UK
- The Edmonton Symptom Assessment Scale-revised: Renal (ESAS-r: Renal) [26] – developed in Canada
- The Dialysis Symptom Index (DSI) [27] – developed in the USA

All are patient-completed symptom scores which ask about the presence and severity of a range of symptoms common in CKD, and they can be downloaded for use from the relevant websites (see Internet Resources). There is also now a more 'global' assessment and

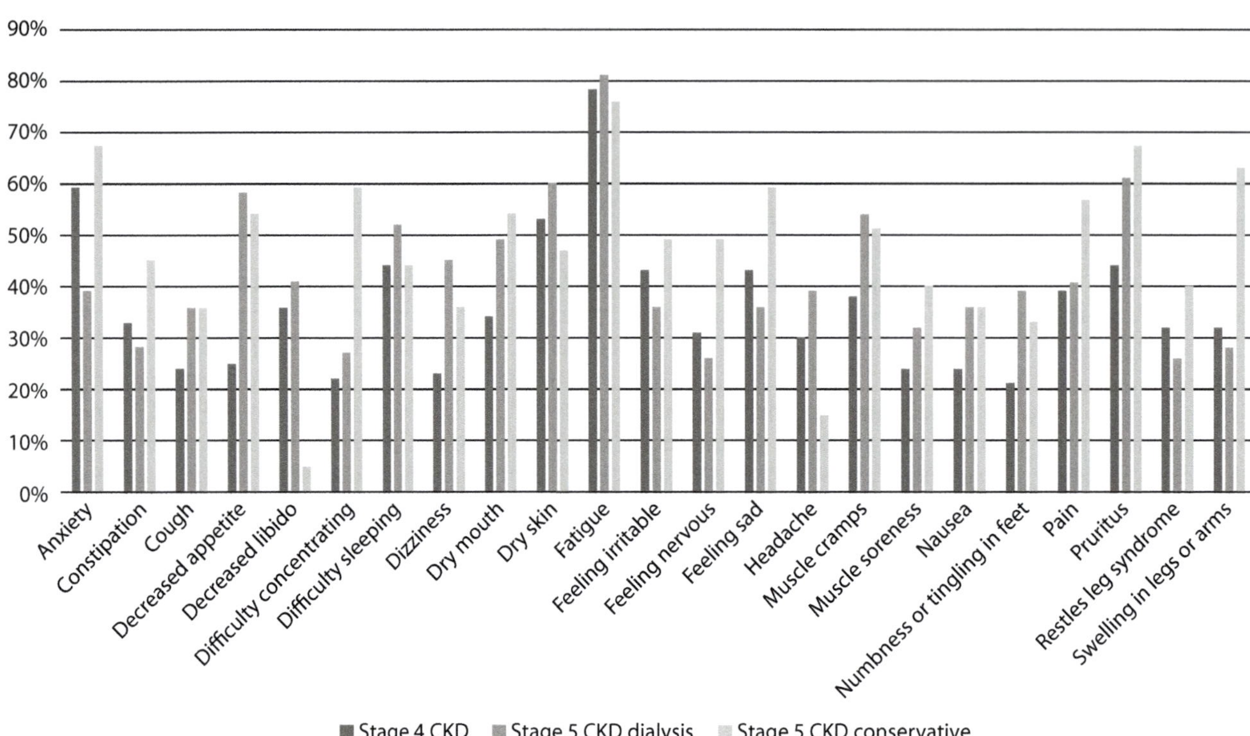

Fig. 68.1 Proportion (%) of patients with common symptoms in renal disease, by modality (weighted mean prevalence of symptoms, reported by Almutary et al. [18])

outcome measure specific for advanced CKD which includes symptoms *and* other issues, such as information needs, communication concerns and practical issues:

- The Integrated Palliative (or Patient) Outcome Scale (IPOS renal) [28] – developed in the UK (see Internet Resources)

68.5.3 Symptom Management

Once symptoms are identified, they need active management. It is important to consider non-pharmacological management, especially for symptoms such as itch which have high psychological and social impact. This chapter focuses predominantly on pharmacological management. The aim of symptom management is to control or ameliorate symptoms that adversely affect quality of life while avoiding drug toxicity. The use of medication in advanced CKD is challenging because of the pharmacokinetic impact of kidney failure. The evidence presented here applies to stages 4 or 5 CKD, when eGFR is $\leq$30 ml/min/1.73m^2. At these levels of kidney impairment, drug metabolism is significantly altered, and the risk of toxicity from accumulation of renally excreted drugs or their active metabolites is very high.

For those receiving dialysis, the effects of dialysis on the drug should be considered. Removal of a drug from the systemic circulation during dialysis is dependent on the following:

- The molecular size of the drug
- The water solubility of the drug
- The degree of protein binding of the drug
- Dialysis-related factors (such as frequency, duration, type of dialysis, type of dialyser membrane)

An up-to-date review of the effects of dialysis on drugs should be used for guidance on the effect of dialysis on medications, e.g. dialysis of drugs (updated annually and now available as an app).

68.5.4 Pain

Recent evidence shows that pain is common among dialysis patients [29], those managed without dialysis [30] and those withdrawing from dialysis [31]. The pharmacological management of pain in patients with advanced CKD has been extensively reviewed recently [32].

Acetaminophen (paracetamol) is the initial analgesic of choice for patients with advanced CKD. It is metabolized extensively in the liver with only 2–5% of the dose excreted unchanged in the urine, so no dose adjustments are required. The recommended maximum daily dose is 3000 mg given that liver injury can be seen with doses of <4000 mg. In emaciated patients, dosing should be reduced.

68.5.4.1 Which Opioids to Use?

Opioid metabolism takes place primarily in the liver to either active or inactive metabolites. The metabolites, and to varying degrees the parent drug, are usually excreted by the kidneys. These may accumulate in patients with advanced CKD. If a significant proportion of the unchanged opioid is excreted by the kidneys and/or the metabolites are active, then the opioid is highly likely to cause toxicity when the eGFR is <30 mL/min. Careful selection of opioids is therefore essential.

There are no opioids for mild to moderate pain considered suitable or safe for use in patients with advanced CKD, so it is recommended to add a very low dose of a stronger opioid to acetaminophen (paracetamol) if pain is inadequately treated. Opioids for mild to moderate pain have the same dose-dependent adverse effects as the strong opioids, and there is no evidence that these are less risky than strong opioids if the strong opioid is used at its lowest effective dose [32]. A recent study of 140,899 adult haemodialysis patients in the USA showed that the highest hazards for altered mental status, falls and fractures were associated with codeine rather than the strong opioids [33]. There is also no evidence that at equivalent analgesic efficacy, opioids for mild to moderate pain carry a lower risk of addiction than low-dose strong opioids.

All strong opioids should be used cautiously, with both dose reduction and increase in the dosing interval. Full details are available in a recent review [32]. Early review and regular monitoring should be undertaken, since accumulation and subsequent adverse effects can occur quickly (within hours). It is also strongly recommended to avoid the longer-acting preparations and use short-acting preparations whenever possible.

Alfentanil and fentanyl are cautiously recommended and are probably the best opioids to use in the last days of life when an injectable strong opioid is needed. Several clinical and practical considerations (other than safety) need to be taken into consideration; for instance, the short half-life of alfentanil makes it less practical for breakthrough pain, although it is appropriate for continuous infusion.

Transdermal fentanyl patches are useful earlier in the disease trajectory, but professionals unfamiliar with these should recognize that even the lowest strength patches represent a significant opioid dose, and careful titration of immediate acting oral opioids is usually needed before commencing them. Transdermal fentanyl can be used, provided there is careful titration of dose and early regular review to watch for accumulation. Transdermal buprenorphine is increasingly being used for patients with advanced CKD without reports of adverse effects, although the evidence to support this remains limited. For oral immediate-acting preparations, evidence is very limited; hydromorphone or oxycodone (at reduced doses) are likely to be better choices than morphine or diamorphine, although these may still accumulate.

68.5.4.2 Specific Types of Pain

Neuropathic pain Neuropathic (nerve) pain is unlikely to respond to opioids alone. Certain strong opioids may be more useful than others in neuropathic pain. For instance, methadone may be appropriate but should only be prescribed by someone experienced in its use (usually pain or palliative care specialists). Anticonvulsants (e.g. gabapentin and pregabalin) and antidepressants (e.g. tricyclic antidepressants) in low doses can be used effectively as adjuvant medications to improve neuropathic pain and should be started before considering opioids. A small study showed improvement in pain and quality of life scores for haemodialysis patients with diverse causes of neuropathic pain using gabapentin [34]. Gabapentin is almost exclusively cleared by the kidneys, and substantial dose reduction is required as kidney function declines to avoid toxicity. Adverse effects include somnolence, dizziness, peripheral oedema and gait disturbances. Although effective for neuropathic pain, tricyclic antidepressants appear to be less well tolerated than the gabapentinoids in patients with advanced CKD because of anticholinergic, histaminergic and adrenergic adverse effects causing symptoms such as dry mouth, orthostatic hypotension and somnolence. Patients with advanced CKD will often respond to lower doses of tricyclic antidepressant than those with normal kidney function.

Bone pain Bone pain is also unlikely to respond to opioids alone. Nonsteroidal anti-inflammatory drugs (NSAIDs) are likely to be beneficial for bone pain but carry a high risk of adverse effects in severe kidney failure, including risk of loss of any residual kidney function. This consideration may be critical and prevent the use of NSAIDs completely, but each case should be reviewed by an experienced clinician in order to make the best judgement. Sometimes, a short course of NSAIDs may be prescribed as a considered risk in the absence of any residual renal function or towards the very end of life.

68.5.5 Breathlessness

Breathlessness or dyspnoea in the patient with advanced CKD may be due to anaemia, pulmonary oedema (related to fluid overload or to coexisting cardiovascular disease) or comorbidity (cardiac or respiratory disease). It is important to identify the underlying cause, since treating this is almost always the most appropriate and effective first line of management. Diuretic use and fluid restriction may or may not be appropriate, depending on the clinical circumstances. Optimizing anaemia management may be helpful for some patients although the correlation between symptoms and the degree of anaemia is poor. If treatment of the underlying cause has been exhausted, then the situation may arise (particularly in far advanced disease or close to the end of life) where symptomatic measures to relieve breathlessness are required.

General measures, such as sitting upright rather than lying (which maximizes vital capacity), using a fan or stream of cool air which can provide effective symptom relief, inhaled oxygen if hypoxia is confirmed or suspected, and a calm, settled environment, are important. Physiotherapy and occupational therapy can help to maximize mobility and provide appropriate aids to improve function constrained by breathlessness. Breathlessness is very commonly associated with anxiety, often in an escalating cycle (anxiety causing worsening dyspnoea, which triggers worsening anxiety, and so on). Appropriate information, education and support of patient and family are therefore critical, and in advanced disease, an approach based on the Breathing, Thinking, Functioning clinical model may be helpful [35].

As prognosis worsens, general and non-pharmacological measures will have less to offer, and pharmacological measures become more appropriate. This applies only when treatment of the underlying cause of breathlessness has been exhausted. Untreated moderate or severe dyspnoea towards end of life is very distressing and should be treated as actively as pain or any other distressing symptom. Breathlessness is an increasingly important and dominant symptom in patients with advanced CKD towards the end of life, so it is important to discuss an individual's priorities pre-emptively so as to meet management preferences if they become symptomatic in the future.

Pharmacological treatments directed specifically at breathlessness include opioids and benzodiazepines (especially if there is associated moderate or severe anxiety). Low-dose opioids are helpful in relieving breathlessness near the end of life [36]. Strong opioids can be used to control breathlessness (following the pain guidelines), but note that doses should be much smaller (25–50% of those for pain), and if not initially effective, titration should be slower.

Benzodiazepines are useful when there is coexisting anxiety (as there often is) but again need to be used with considerable care and in much reduced doses. Shorter-acting benzodiazepines are recommended, such as lorazepam 0.5–1 mg orally or sublingually qds (if used sublingually, it has a quicker onset of action and may more readily restore a sense of control to the frightened and anxious patient). If the patient is in the last days of life, midazolam (at 25% of normal dose if eGFR is <10) can be given subcutaneously and titrated according to effect. Midazolam can be given every 2–4 hours, although CKD patients are sensitive to its effects and do not usually need frequent or large doses. A starting dose of 1 mg is recommended. If more than one or two doses are required, a subcutaneous infusion over 24 hours is most practical.

68.5.6 Constipation

Constipation is common among patients with CKD. The causes can be multifactorial, including fluid restriction, reduced mobility, medication (i.e. aluminium or calcium phosphate binders, iron supplements and opioids), poor dietary intake, reduced muscle tone through debility and dietary restriction of high potassium fruits and vegetables (reduced fibre content of food ingested).

Management requires detailed assessment, treatment of reversible causes where appropriate/possible and acute management to overcome current constipation (including rectal measures). Action to prevent further recurrence includes improving mobility and ensuring adequate dietary intake and including sufficient fibre and fluid (within the constraints of any reduced fluid intake). Osmotic laxatives such as polyethylene glycol or lactulose or peristaltic stimulants such as sennosides or bisacodyl may be used, sometimes in combination with a stool softener. Laxatives which contain magnesium, citrate or phosphate should be avoided in advanced CKD. Polyethylene glycol contains potassium so it is therefore better suited for short-term constipation which does not respond to other measures.

68.5.7 Nausea and Vomiting

Nausea and vomiting are extremely unpleasant symptoms. They may frequently be multifactorial. Assessment requires a thorough history including establishing the history and pattern of both nausea and vomiting separately. The relationship between the two should also be established, as well as the frequency and volume of vomits, whether there is associated constipation and a detailed medication history. Profound nausea and/or repeated vomiting will prevent absorption of any medications taken orally, and alternative routes (such as sublingual, rectal or subcutaneous routes) need to be considered, at least until nausea and vomiting are controlled.

The first step is to identify the specific cause where possible, since treatment specifically directed to the cause is most likely to succeed. If medication or toxins are causing nausea, then nausea is usually persistent and unremitting and sometimes unaccompanied by vomiting. Uraemia and a variety of drugs (including opioids, anticonvulsants, antibiotics and antidepressants) can cause this kind of persistent nausea. Gastroparesis or delayed gastric emptying (which may be caused by drugs such as opioids, as well as occurring secondary to diabetes mellitus) usually presents with a history of postprandial nausea or vomiting of undigested food which relieves nausea. Bloating, epigastric fullness, flatulence, hiccough or heartburn may accompany this. Nausea related to gastritis is often associated with heartburn, dyspepsia or epigastric pain. Constipation may exacerbate nausea and vomiting.

If gastroparesis or delayed gastric emptying is suspected, then metoclopramide to increase gastric motility is preferred. Metoclopramide needs 50% dose reduction in patients with CKD 4 and CKD 5 with an increased risk of adverse effects such as dystonia. If uraemia is a suspected cause, then haloperidol or possibly a 5HT3 (a serotonin receptor subtype) antagonist may be the best choice. The dose of haloperidol should be reduced, as there is increased cerebral sensitivity in renal failure. 5HT3 antagonists often cause moderate or severe constipation – this should be anticipated by co-prescribing of laxatives when appropriate. Drug-induced nausea can be relieved by stopping the causative drug. When this is not feasible, haloperidol is often effective. Gastritis (high risk in uraemia) may sometimes contribute to nausea and should be actively treated with a proton pump inhibitor, to help control related nausea. Towards the end of life, levomepromazine (a 'broad-spectrum' antiemetic which works on several of the relevant receptors) in low dose can be effective to control nausea and vomiting, but higher doses can be very sedative.

68.5.8 Pruritus

The cause of uremic pruritus has not yet been fully elucidated. Given the complexity in understanding the causes of pruritus in CKD, it is not surprising that it can be a difficult symptom to manage, with a variety of different treatments proposed, each of limited effectiveness.

The first step is to address possible contributing factors such as anaemia and iron deficiency or other causes of itch such as xerosis, allergies or drug hypersensitivities. Dry skin is particularly prevalent in older people and may cause or contribute to pruritus, so it should be treated actively. Appropriate skin care includes the liberal use of aqueous emollients and gentle soaps with no fragrances. Older people living alone may find it hard to apply emollients easily; spray applications are often helpful in this instance. Preventive measures, such as nail care (keeping nails short) and keeping cool (light clothing and tepid baths or showers), are useful concurrent measures.

It is hard to recommend specific pharmacological measures given the lack of strong evidence. Topical treatments such as capsaicin ointment 0.025% or 0.03%; pramoxine 1%, menthol/camphor/phenol 0.3% each, either separately or in combination with each other; and gamma-linolenic acid cream 2.2% can be tried. If systemic treatment is desired, gabapentin starting at 50–100 mg at night can be tried. A tricyclic antidepressant may be beneficial; mirtazapine has some evidence to suggest effectiveness at doses reduced for the degree of kidney impairment [37]. Although UVB light has good supporting evidence, its benefit is short-lived and may not be readily available. Antihistamines are widely used, but there is very little evidence to support their use.

68.5.9 Restless Legs

Restless legs syndrome (RLS) can be an extremely debilitating symptom for some patients with CKD. The formal International Restless Legs Syndrome Study Group (IRLSSG) criteria for diagnosis are:

- Urge to move the legs, usually with unpleasant sensations in the legs
- Worse during periods of rest or inactivity like resting or sitting
- Partial or total relief by physical activity
- Worse symptoms in the evening or night rather than the day

The exact cause for restless legs is not well understood, and multiple complex mechanisms likely play a role. It is widely accepted, however, that the dopaminergic system in the central nervous system is somehow disrupted. There is limited evidence in uraemic RLS that iron deficiency, low parathyroid hormone, hyperphosphatemia and psychological factors may all play a role. Treatment should involve correction of these factors and reduction of potential exacerbating agents, such as caffeine, alcohol, nicotine and certain drugs (topiramate, opioids, tricyclic antidepressants, selective serotonin uptake inhibitors, dopamine antagonists olanzapine and quetiapine).

There is very limited evidence about treatment of RLS in people with CKD, and much of the evidence is extrapolated from idiopathic RLS in the general population. Gabapentin or pregabalin, at the appropriately reduced dose, may be effective. Non-ergot dopamine agonists (pramipexole, ropinirole or transdermal rotigotine) may also be effective. There is uncertainty about the use of dopamine agonists long term due to augmentation (return of the symptom, often at a worse level after treatment has commenced). In treating restless legs, the choice of drug management should be tailored to the individual and will depend on the presence of other symptoms, age and tolerance of side effects. Gabapentin may be especially beneficial if the patients also have concomitant symptoms such as insomnia, pruritus and/or neuropathic pain.

68.6 Symptom Management at the End of Life

Traditionally, it was believed that a uraemic death was relatively symptom-free, but the evidence does not support this. Where studies have specifically reviewed end of life symptoms, it appears that a significant minority experience severe or distressing symptoms [38, 39]. Pain, breathlessness, nausea, retained respiratory tract secretions and terminal agitation can all be problematic.

These symptoms can be relatively well controlled in the majority of patients. Agitation usually responds to low disease of anxiolytics, such as midazolam. Retained respiratory tract secretions can be improved (although not always resolved) by glycopyrronium or hyoscine butylbromide, and treatment is optimal if commenced early. Pain or breathlessness can be effectively managed with opioids, and often only low doses are required. If a patient is on a regular strong opioid orally and can no longer take oral medication, then the total daily dose of strong opioid should be converted to the equivalent dose for subcutaneous fentanyl or alfentanil over 24 hrs and administered via subcutaneous infusion.

68.6.1 Care After Death

The care offered to the person and family at the time of death is hugely important and geographically informed as different countries have different laws and processes. Care after death can be informed by national guidance (see Internet Resources), but in summary, family needs to be supported to spend time with the person as they die and after death, according to cultural and family preferences. Families with limited socioeconomic resources, and those who stop work to care for the patient, have poorer bereavement outcomes [40]. Families need to be supported with information regarding the legal processes after death such as registration of the death, how to contact funeral directors and sources of support in bereavement.

68.7 Summary

Detailed and thorough holistic assessment of the palliative and supportive needs of those with advanced CKD and deteriorating health is essential This involves the assessment of mental capacity to be involved in decision-making, advance care planning, care at the time of death and support of the bereaved after death.

Symptom burden is high in this population, and there is evidence of under-prescribing and under-management. In those managed without dialysis, or in those withdrawing from dialysis, symptoms (whether caused by kidney disease or more commonly by comorbid conditions) need careful attention if optimal quality of care is to be achieved.

Symptom assessment should be an integral part of clinical assessment, alongside routine kidney care and review of biochemical markers. The use of a formal, validated symptom assessment tool will help this, and subsequent symptom management needs careful attention to detail and regular review. Towards the end of life, anticipatory prescribing (prescribing in advance of symptoms) is also recommended to ensure distressing symptoms are minimized.

Case Study

Case Study 1

Mr B is an 89-year-old gentleman with diabetic nephropathy. He has been on haemodialysis for 8 years (three times/week) and is admitted to hospital with 'all over' body pain and right stump pain (right above knee amputation 8 years earlier for peripheral vascular disease and critical ischaemia). The pain that has been present for several months in his amputated stump had worsened over the previous few days. There were no clinical signs of a deep vein thrombosis. There was no swelling, erythema or cellulitis of right stump. He received regular paracetamol, pregabalin was increased from 50 to 75 mg and oxycodone immediate release 2.5 mg 2–4 hourly as required was prescribed. The pain settled with three or four doses of oxycodone immediate release daily, and he was switched to oxycodone 5 mg slow release 12 hourly. He was also commenced on laxatives – sodium docusate 200 mg twice daily – to counter the constipating effect of the oxycodone.

Case Study 2

Mrs C is a 49-year-old lady, on haemodialysis three times a week, admitted to hospital with a lupus flare and chest infection, who then developed neutropenic sepsis (administered cyclophosphamide prior to this admission). She has active treatment for the sepsis, and this resolves, but she is experiencing ongoing severe and distressing pain around her jaw, neck and back secondary to her disease. It is 'all too much', and she expresses inability to go on with her treatment. Pain is the main cause of her distress, but she has reactions to a wide variety of drugs. Oxycodone is discontinued as it caused localized itching. Her pain is eventually improved with 1 mg alfentanil administered subcutaneously over 24 hours, and this is well tolerated.

A meeting is held with the patient, her son and family, the consultant and (at her request) the hospital chaplain. It is agreed that the treatment for the lupus is very arduous and almost as tough as the illness. Mrs C agrees to continue all active treatment, but that if her heart was to stop, she would not want resuscitation, and that her care should be managed on the ward (with no escalation to intensive care). The chaplain confirms that should Mrs C want this, that withdrawal of dialysis is not suicide but withdrawal of life-sustaining treatment and that Mrs C could rest assured that she will be supported should she choose to stop dialysis. The option of a hospice for symptom management was offered. The family agrees to respect any decision Mrs C makes in due course about not wanting any further treatment for her lupus or dialysis. Mrs C transferred to the hospice for continued symptom management and is content to continue regular dialysis now her pain is better controlled.

Case Study 3

Mr S is a 70-year-old gentleman. He has end-stage renal failure – his e-GFR is 11 mL/hour – and he has opted (after some discussion several months ago) to be managed with maximal conservative management (no dialysis and full supportive care). The main issues are interrupted sleeping pattern due to nocturia/frequent urination at night brought by furosemide (with known heart failure and a history of pulmonary oedema) and spinal/hip pain secondary to osteoarthritis. He then has a transient ischaemic episode and is admitted to hospital. On discharge he expresses a desire not to be admitted to hospital again and to receive end of life care at home. He is referred to the palliative care team for support, management of fatigue and pain control. The palliative care team meet him and ensured his wishes and preferences were recorded, alongside documentation of Do Not Attempt cardiopulmonary resuscitation, and liaise with the renal team and general practitioner to optimize his care and future plans. Over a subsequent weekend, the ambulance service is called as Mr S has upper abdominal pain and an upper gastrointestinal bleed. Mr S states again that he does not want 'tests and things', and home is where he wants to be, even if this means he has less time to live. The "as required" medicines for comfort at end of life are prescribed and made available in the house. Mr S is given 2.5 mg oxycodone subcutaneously stat for pain and 0.75 mg alfentanil over 24 hours via subcutaneous infusion to manage his ongoing pain. On review, he is pain free and settled. Regular mouth care and other nursing care are provided, and Mr S dies at home 4 days later with his family around him.

Chapter Review Questions

1. Why is it important to start thinking with patients and their families about their wishes and preferences as a patient's disease advances?
2. What medical, nursing and therapy decisions need to be considered as an advance plan of care is considered?
3. Think of a patient you have cared for who has experienced uraemic itch. How did you help the patient cope with this symptom? What might you do differently now?
4. Think of a patient for whom you have cared for until the point of death. What did you do after death to support the family? How did you ensure all those who were involved in their care were notified?

Answers

1. Without open discussion of prognosis and what to expect in the future, and consideration of an individual's preferences for care and treatment as they become less well, including what is realistically available, it will be very difficult to ensure that last months, weeks or days of life are lived as fully as possible, in the way that person prefers, despite the illness.
2. The main decisions to be considered are whether dialysis, active treatment of infections and other complications and resuscitation are likely to bring benefit and burden and how the individual regards each of these interventions. Place of care (and place of death) is also important to consider. Realistic understanding of what can and cannot be achieved or delivered in terms of healthcare is key, since unrealistic understanding will often lead to bitter disappointment or even anger. It is also important to involve family if possible, so that they too understand what is possible or not and why decisions may be made in one direction or another. A person with advanced CKD may become weak or confused as the illness advances;

clarifying how decisions will be made if this occurs is also important.

3. You may think more readily about contributing factors such as anaemia or iron deficiency. You will suggest that dry skin should be very actively treated; itch will not readily improve without active management of dryness. Advice on nail care and keeping cool are also helpful. There are a range of medications which you can consider, although evidence is limited, and it will be important to match the choice of one of these medicines to the individual.
4. Providing information, time and above all kindness is the most important considerations. Families may not have experienced the death of a family member before; they may be shocked, saddened, angry, upset or none of these. Different family members may have different emotions, and this can be hard for them to comprehend. Allowing time for questions and supporting through a follow-up visit or call can be helpful. The extent of support beyond the immediate post-death period may depend on bereavement risk factors; consider referral to bereavement support services if this is appropriate.

It is important to notify *all* the professionals involved in care so they are aware of the death.

References

1. Bone AE, Gomes B, Etkind SN, Verne J, Murtagh FE, Evans CJ, et al. What is the impact of population ageing on the future provision of end-of-life care? Population-based projections of place of death. Palliat Med. 2017:269216317734435.
2. Pefoyo AJ, Bronskill SE, Gruneir A, Calzavara A, Thavorn K, Petrosyan Y, et al. The increasing burden and complexity of multimorbidity. BMC Public Health. 2015;15:415.
3. Barnett K, Mercer SW, Norbury M, Watt G, Wyke S, Guthrie B. Epidemiology of multimorbidity and implications for health care, research, and medical education: a cross-sectional study. Lancet. 2012;380(9836):37–43.
4. Higginson IJ, Daveson BA, Morrison RS, Yi D, Meier D, Smith M, et al. Social and clinical determinants of preferences and their achievement at the end of life: prospective cohort study of older adults receiving palliative care in three countries. BMC Geriatr. 2017;17(1):271.
5. Davison SN. End-of-life care preferences and needs: perceptions of patients with chronic kidney disease. Clin J Am Soc Nephrol CJASN. 2010;5(2):195–204.
6. Steinhauser KE, Christakis NA, Clipp EC, McNeilly M, McIntyre L, Tulsky JA. Factors considered important at the end of life by patients, family, physicians, and other care providers. JAMA. 2000;284(19):2476–82.
7. Lund S, Richardson A, May C. Barriers to advance care planning at the end of life: An explanatory systematic review of implementation studies. PLoS One. 2015;10(2).
8. Davison SN. Facilitating advance care planning for patients with end-stage renal disease: the patient perspective. Clin J Am Soc Nephrol. 2006;1(5):1023–8.
9. Zwakman M, Jabbarian LJ, van Delden J, van der Heide A, Korfage IJ, Pollock K, et al. Advance care planning: a systematic review about experiences of patients with a life-threatening or life-limiting illness. Palliat Med. 2018;32(8):1305–21.
10. Schmidt RJ, Weaner BB, Long D. The power of advance care planning in promoting hospice and out-of-hospital death in a dialysis unit. J Palliat Med. 2015;18(1):62–6.
11. Song MK, Ward SE, Fine JP, Hanson LC, Lin FC, Hladik GA, et al. Advance care planning and end-of-life decision making in dialysis: a randomized controlled trial targeting patients and their surrogates. Am J Kidney Dis. 2015;66(5):813–22.
12. Murtagh FE, Addington-Hall J, Higginson IJ. The prevalence of symptoms in end-stage renal disease: a systematic review. Adv Chronic Kidney Dis. 2007;14(1):82–99.
13. Davison SN. Pain in hemodialysis patients: prevalence, cause, severity, and management. Am J Kidney Dis. 2003;42(6):1239–47.
14. Murtagh FE, Addington-Hall J, Edmonds P, Donohoe P, Carey I, Jenkins K, et al. Symptoms in the month before death for stage 5 chronic kidney disease patients managed without dialysis. J Pain Symptom Manage. 2010;40(3):342–52.
15. Davison SN, Torgunrud C. The creation of an advance care planning process for patients with ESRD. Am J Kidney Dis. 2007;49(1):27–36.
16. Wong SP, Kreuter W, Curtis JR, Hall YN, O'Hare AM. Trends in in-hospital cardiopulmonary resuscitation and survival in adults receiving maintenance dialysis. JAMA Intern Med. 2015;175(6):1028–35.
17. Murtagh FEM, Weisbord S. Symptoms in renal disease: their epidemiology, assessment and management. In: Chambers EJ, Germain M, Brown E, editors. Supportive care for the renal patient. 2nd ed. Oxford: Oxford University Press; 2010.
18. Almutary H, Bonner A, Douglas C. Symptom burden in chronic kidney disease: a review of recent literature. J Ren Care. 2013;39(3):140–50.
19. Senanayake S, Gunawardena N, Palihawadana P, Bandara P, Haniffa R, Karunarathna R, et al. Symptom burden in chronic kidney disease; a population based cross sectional study. BMC Nephrol. 2017;18(1):228.
20. Almutary H, Bonner A, Douglas C. Which patients with chronic kidney disease have the greatest symptom burden? A comparative study of advanced CKD stage and dialysis modality. J Ren Care. 2016;42(2):73–82.
21. Brennan F, Collett G, Josland E, Brown MA. The symptoms of patients with CKD stage 5 managed without dialysis. Prog Palliat Care. 2015;23(5):267–73.
22. Weisbord SD, Fried LF, Arnold RM, Fine MJ, Levenson DJ, Peterson RA, et al. Prevalence, severity, and importance of physical and emotional symptoms in chronic hemodialysis patients. J Am Soc Nephrol. 2005;16(8):2487–94.
23. Davison SN, Jhangri GS, Johnson JA. Longitudinal validation of a modified Edmonton symptom assessment system (ESAS) in haemodialysis patients. Nephrol Dial Transplant. 2006;21(11):3189–95.
24. Weisbord SD, Fried L, Mor MK, Resnick AL, Unruh ML, Palevsky PM, et al. Renal provider recognition of symptoms in patients on maintenance hemodialysis. Clinical Journal of the American Society of Nephrologists. 2007;2:960–7.
25. Murphy EL, Murtagh FE, Carey I, Sheerin NS. Understanding symptoms in patients with advanced chronic kidney disease managed without dialysis: use of a short patient-completed assessment tool. Nephron Clin Pract. 2009;111(1):c74–80.
26. Davison SN, Jhangri GS, Johnson JA. Cross-sectional validity of a modified Edmonton symptom assessment system in dialysis patients: a simple assessment of symptom burden. Kidney Int. 2006;69(9):1621–5.

27. Weisbord SD, Fried LF, Arnold RM, Rotondi AJ, Fine MJ, Levenson DJ, et al. Development of a symptom assessment instrument for chronic hemodialysis patients: the Dialysis Symptom Index. J Pain Symptom Manage. 2004;27(3):226–40.
28. Raj R, Ahuja K, Frandsen M, Murtagh FEM, Jose M. Validation of the IPOS-renal symptom survey in advanced kidney disease: a cross-sectional study. J Pain Symptom Manage. 2018;56(2):281–7.
29. Davison SN, Koncicki H, Brennan F. Pain in chronic kidney disease: a scoping review. Semin Dial. 2014;27(2):188–204.
30. Murtagh FE, Addington-Hall JM, Edmonds PM, Donohoe P, Carey I, Jenkins K, et al. Symptoms in advanced renal disease: a cross-sectional survey of symptom prevalence in stage 5 chronic kidney disease managed without dialysis. J Palliat Med. 2007;10(6):1266–76.
31. Germain MJ, Cohen LM, Davison SN. Withholding and withdrawal from dialysis: what we know about how our patients die. Semin Dial. 2007;20(3):195–9.
32. Davison SN. Clinical pharmacology: considerations in pain management in patients with advanced kidney failure. Clin J Am Soc Nephrol. 2018; in press.
33. Ishida JH, McCulloch CE, Steinman MA, Grimes BA, Johansen KL. Opioid analgesics and adverse outcomes among hemodialysis patients. Clin J Am Soc Nephrol CJASN. 2018;13(5):746–53.
34. Atalay H, Solak Y, Biyik Z, Gaipov A, Guney F, Turk S. Cross-over, open-label trial of the effects of gabapentin versus pregabalin on painful peripheral neuropathy and health-related quality of life in haemodialysis patients. Clin Drug Investig. 2013;33(6):401–8.
35. Spathis A, Booth S, Moffat C, Hurst R, Ryan R, Chin C, et al. The breathing, thinking, functioning clinical model: a proposal to facilitate evidence-based breathlessness management in chronic respiratory disease. NPJ Prim Care Respir Med. 2017;27(1):27.
36. Jennings AL, Davies AN, Higgins JP, Broadley K. Opioids for the palliation of breathlessness in terminal illness. Cochrane Database Syst Rev. 2001;(4):CD002066.
37. Davis MP, Frandsen JL, Walsh D, Andresen S, Taylor S. Mirtazapine for pruritus. J Pain Symptom Manage. 2003;25(3):288–91.
38. Cohen LM, Germain MJ. Measuring quality of dying in end-stage renal disease. Semin Dial. 2004;17(5):376–9.
39. Cohen LM, McCue JD, Germain M, Kjellstrand CM. Dialysis discontinuation. A 'good' death? Arch Intern Med. 1995;155(1):42–7.
40. Roulston A, Campbell A, Cairnduff V, Fitzpatrick D, Donnelly C, Gavin A. Bereavement outcomes: a quantitative survey identifying risk factors in informal carers bereaved through cancer. Palliat Med. 2017;31(2):162–70.

Internet Resources

Palliative Care Outcome Scale (POS-Renal and IPOS-Renal). London UK: Cicely Saunders Institute, King's College London [Last Accessed 30th October, 2018] Available from: http://pos-pal.org/index.php.

ESAS – Edmonton zone palliative care program and Northern Alberta renal program. Last Accessed 17th September, 2018. Available from: http://www.palliative.org/tools.html.

Care after death: guidance for staff responsible for care after death. 2nd edn. https://www.hospiceuk.org/what-we-offer/publications?cat=72e54312-4ccd-608d-ad24-ff0000fd3330. Last accessed 1st November 2018.

Transition of Adolescents with Nephrological Conditions

Stephen D. Marks

Contents

M. Harber (ed.), *Primer on Nephrology*, https://doi.org/10.1007/978-3-030-76419-7_69

Learning Objectives

- To facilitate transition of adolescents from paediatric to adult healthcare settings
- To investigate the different models of transition programmes
- To understand evidence-based guidelines for ensuring best practice for young adults going through the transition process

Definitions

- Adherence
  - Is the extent to which medication intake behaviour corresponds with the recommendations of the healthcare provider
- Adolescence
  - Is a transitional period of physical and psychological development following the onset of puberty during which a young person develops from a child into an adult
- Compliance
  - Is the extent to which patients follow recommendations of prescribers
- Concordance
  - Refers to an agreement between the prescriber and patient on the purpose and use of the medication
- Persistence
  - Is the length of time between the first and last dose, being applicable in the event that a patient discontinues treatment
- Transition
  - Has been described by the Department of Health as "a guided, educational, therapeutic process rather than an administrative event", and the National Services Framework emphasised that transition should be "a purposeful, planned process that addresses the medical, psychosocial and educational/vocational needs of adolescents and young adults with chronic physical and medical conditions as they move from child-centred to adult-oriented health care systems".

69.1 Introduction

There are differences in provision of healthcare depending on the modality of renal therapies and requirement for nephrological follow-up:

- End-stage kidney disease
  - Dialysis: home therapies with peritoneal dialysis and haemodialysis as well as in-centre haemodialysis (where there may be constraints on the availability of this provision in a satellite adult unit)
  - Renal transplantation
- Chronic kidney disease
- Other nephrological conditions from nephrotic syndrome, glomerular and tubular disorders, nephrolithiasis and nephrocalcinosis, systemic lupus erythematosus, vasculitis and hypertension

Whatever the chronic renal condition or replacement therapy, it is important to have smooth transition of care for adolescents between paediatric and adult nephrology services which involves a preparatory phase, the transfer event itself and post-transfer phase, and transition checklists can be useful for identifying the attainment of skills in young adult patients. The eventual transfer of care can be a stressful time for adolescents and their parents who may be known to the staff in the paediatric nephrology unit for many years, if not the whole of the young adult's life.

An ideal transition clinic should conform to the requirements or wishes of young adults with:

- Adequate consultation with professionals and patients
- Flexibility in the timing of transition
- A period of preparation for the young person and family
- Information transfer
- Monitoring of attendance until the young person is established in the appropriate adult-oriented service
- A cohort of young adults in the clinic at the same time
- Being seen by the same medical and nursing staff

The ideal immediate post-transfer scenario would consist of a specialist young adult clinic within the adult unit and run by the same core key personnel each time. The American Society of Adolescent Medicine recommended that services in any healthcare setting should be appropriate for both the chronological age of the patient and development attained. The ideal transition age is around 17–20 years from patient surveys of adolescent patients with chronic conditions but does change with availability of healthcare services throughout the world with many services aiming to transfer care prior to the age of 18 years.

Young adult patients may be expected to be independent and manage their own healthcare needs and take over the responsibility of their healthcare from their parent(s). There needs to be collaboration between patient, parent, children's and adults' services in order to obtain successful transition of adolescent patients. This is particularly important given that different adult specialists may work in different hospitals emphasising the importance of communication between various teams.

Young adults may also need to be educated about the causes of their renal condition and importance of medications (especially risks of non-adherence to immunosuppressive medications for renal transplant recipients) to improve adherence to therapy.

Renal transplant recipients need to know that non-adherence to immunosuppressive medications may result in renal allograft loss and the requirement for dialysis (although the young adult may never have had dialysis or may not remember their dialysis treatment if this was during their early childhood). It seems likely that poorly planned transition from paediatric to adult-oriented health services may be a contributing factor in medication non-adherence and missed clinics, whereas well-planned transition may improve clinical, educational and social outcomes for young people.

- Therefore the timing of transition should take into account chronological age/maturity, adolescent readiness, medical stability and psychosocial issues, and the duration of joint care can be individualised for each patient depending on need.

There are several different models of transition of young adults with renal disease, but each model should involve physicians, surgeons, nurse specialists, pharmacists and allied health professionals, including the psychosocial team and other multidisciplinary team members. All members of the multidisciplinary team should be trained in managing adolescents and involved in the transition process. Where possible a preparation period and education programme should be included in the transition process to enable the young patient to acquire the necessary knowledge and skills to function in an adult service, largely independent of parents and staff (where possible dependent on cognitive ability), before they are transferred.

The simplest model is a dedicated young adult clinic provided within the adult setting; the success of this model is dependent on a good co-ordinated transition process between the adult and paediatric services, such as meetings between the paediatric and adult clinic staff to plan coordinated care, and the involvement of nurse specialists and/or youth workers (who can escort young people to the adult clinics if required). Ongoing continuity can be provided where both paediatric and adult professionals provide ongoing care in a joint clinic from adolescence to adulthood allowing patients to benefit both from experts in paediatric diseases and the appropriate management of more pertinent adult issues, such as sexual health, fertility issues and cardiovascular disease. This model is used in the transitioning of adolescent renal transplant recipients where the joint clinic lasts for around 2 years (◘ Fig. 69.1). During the preparatory phase of transitioning, patients attend a special joint transition clinic at 3–4 monthly intervals in addition to both regular medical and adolescent clinic appointments. Educational sessions are available for both patients and their parents, and the transition clinic allows the development of a relationship and trust between the patient and adult team during the pre-transfer period and enables a joint decision on timing of transfer.

This model may involve access to a buddy scheme to foster peer support. Other transitioning models in North America include a generic transition team located within a children's hospital and consisting of dedicated nurse specialists who coordinate transitions for all patients in different specialities.

- There is a gap between provision of paediatric and adults' services, and it is important that young adults

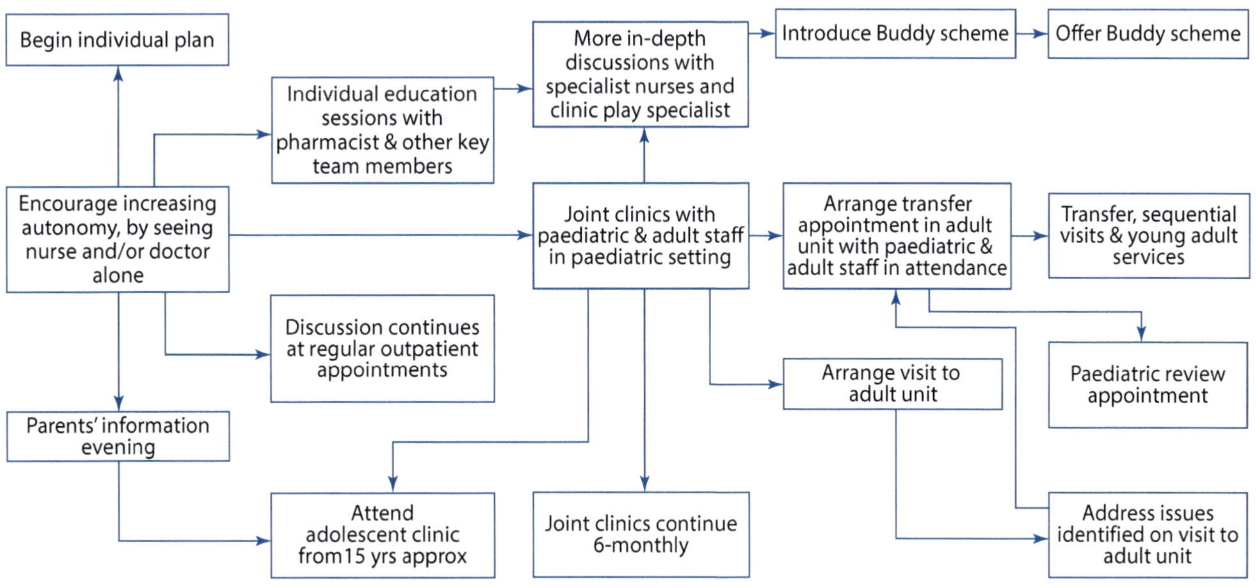

◘ **Fig. 69.1** Model of care for transitioning adolescents with renal disease

are prepared for the change from a parent-focused to patient-focused environment.
- One aspect of transition of adolescents with renal disease is that they may have complex healthcare needs, so they may be under different paediatric subspecialties, which should be transferred to adult specialists.
- There are various models of transitioning of patients which are as follows:
  - Paediatric service to adults' service
  - Paediatric service to transition clinic to adults' service
  - Paediatric service to adolescent service to young adults' service to general adults' service
- The children's clinic may take place in a small, playful yet noisy, child-friendly environment in a central children's teaching hospital.
- The adult clinic may take place in a different geographical location in a larger, more impersonal, quieter yet busier, individual-focused setting in a regional adult or local district general hospital.
- Clinic attendance may result in young adults being surrounded by much older patients whose disease experience may be very different from their own.

Adult clinic appointments may result in patients being less likely to see the same medical staff at each visit with possibly shorter consultations and less readily available support and advice from staff as there is usually an increased number of medical and nursing staff (who may not have come across their medical condition previously). There are various barriers to successful transition which can be overcome by careful preparation during the transitioning process, for example, joint transition clinics are useful in identifying issues and smoothing out these difficulties, visit to the adult unit and allocation of a key liaison member of staff during preparation for transfer.

69.2 Barriers to Successful Transition

There are several potential obstacles to successful transition be that relating to the young adult, parents or indeed paediatric and adult nephrologists, and it is important to identify any issues.
- Barriers from young adults:
  - Fear of the unknown
  - Reluctant to leave friends and healthcare personnel
  - Ongoing dependence on parents or guardians or other adults
  - Lack of maturity compared to peers
  - Adherence issues
- Barriers from parents
  - Overprotective and used to taking the lead in the paediatric setting
  - Reluctant to leave familiar staff and clinic surroundings
  - Resist attempts by the adult service to enhance the self-advocacy of their child if not adequately prepared
  - May have become aware of lack of confidence in adult staff by other health professionals
- Barriers from paediatric nephrologists
  - Attachment to patient
  - Lack of confidence in adult staff if aware of differences in the attitudes and priorities of adults' services
- Barriers from adult nephrologists
  - Lack of confidence in managing adolescents
  - Lack of training in child and adolescent development and the impact of chronic disease
  - Concern regarding different dynamics of consultation (such as not being used to the presence of parents)
  - Lack of confidence in paediatric staff if aware of differences in the attitudes and priorities of paediatric services (such as feeling that the paediatrician has not managed the patient correctly or transferred at the wrong time (too early or too late)
- Barriers from care delivery system
  - Time and financial constraints such as lack of funding and limited psychosocial resources in adult renal units
  - Shorter adult consultation times
  - Different location with difficult transition of medical files
  - Other location of adult unit

Tips, Tricks and Pitfalls

Establishing a working team and modus operandi is very helpful so that there are clear pathways and transition can start in a timely fashion but also be a clear and robust process.

Simple things like ensuring that data (such as anti-HLA antibody screening and radiology images) and information (key aspects of history, particularly adverse events (psychological or medical)) are transferred as important to build confidence in the process.

Patients who are struggling significantly with adherence or other aspects of engagement before transfer are unlikely to immediately transform behaviour on reaching another institution. Tackling adherence problems jointly in the transition work-up process *may* help the adult nephrologist and young adult continue to work on this rather than starting from scratch on transfer.

It is particularly important to ensure that care is coordinated and communication is good between other specialties before, during and after transition in patients who have several other comorbidities and specialist follow-up.

Case Study

- A 17-year-old young man with end-stage kidney disease on haemodialysis after failed renal transplant 2 years ago due to recurrent nephrotic syndrome post-transplant with underling focal and segmental glomerulosclerosis without identified genetic mutation is going through the transition process to an adult renal unit. He misses occasional haemodialysis sessions in the paediatric unit and voices concern about transition to an adult unit. However, when he attends his paediatric haemodialysis sessions, he is usually hypertensive with systolic blood pressures of 160–180 mmHg due to fluid overload from increased fluid intake; he is anuric with non-functioning renal transplant post-bilateral native nephrectomies. How do you manage this clinical situation?
  - It is important to work closely with this adolescent and his family to ensure that he understands his current clinical situation and the risks of hypertension as well as his underlying condition and future plans.
  - Utilising youth workers who can meet the young adult in the community and assist in introducing him to older haemodialysis patients in the adult renal unit who have gone through the transition process as part of a buddy system.
  - Involvement of transitional care staff in introducing him to the adult renal unit and staff.
  - Educational programme on risks of hypertension, alcohol, recreational drugs, sexually transmitted diseases and non-adherence to fluids, medications and haemodialysis sessions.
- A 16-year-old young lady who is 2 years post-pre-emptive living related renal transplantation for end-stage kidney disease due to congenital anomalies of the kidney and urinary tract with bilateral renal dysplasia has low trough tacrolimus levels and has missed her last two paediatric transplant outpatient clinic appointments. She now attends your clinic without an appointment to inform you that her last menstrual period was 3 months ago, but she normally menstruates regularly every 28 days. How do you manage this clinical situation?
  - The consultation should start positively with showing gratitude to the patient coming to clinic and being honest about her current status.
  - It is important to ascertain if she could be pregnant (and perform pregnancy test to confirm) and what her plans are if she was pregnant and check to see if she has stable renal allograft function together with acceptable trough tacrolimus level.
  - Liaise closely with adult renal unit staff about current and future management strategies, which would also involve obstetric and gynaecology staff if pregnancy is confirmed and change of immunosuppressive medications if proceeding with pregnancy.

69.3 Conclusion

Staff members of every adult nephrology unit should be trained in adolescent medicine and safeguarding with provision of their own transitional care pathways to ensure effective communication and collaboration with appropriate paediatric units and facilitate continuity of care with ongoing educational and social programmes. Successful transitioning involves input from both the paediatric and adult multidisciplinary teams with overlap between the two services. The duration of the preparatory phase and the timing of transition should be flexible and geared to the individual needs of the young adult looking specifically at chronological and developmental ages, maturity, medical stability and psychosocial issues.

Buddy systems and peer support can aid smooth transitioning with the promotion of patients attending a clinic with similar age groups, which can include the formation of a special young adult clinic.

Chapter Review Questions

1. Adolescence is a transitional period of physical and psychological development following the onset of puberty during which a young person develops from a child into an adult.
   A. True
   B. False
2. Are the terms patient compliance and medication adherence synonymous?
   A. Yes
   B. No
3. Which of the following can be barriers to successful transition?
   A. Young adults
   B. Parents
   C. Paediatric nephrologists
   D. Adult nephrologist
   E. All of the above

Answers

1. A. True
   - This is true as adolescence is a transitional period of physical and psychological development following the onset of puberty during which a young person develops from a child into an adult.
2. B. No
   - Compliance has been viewed as having the negative connotation that patients are submissive to medical professionals so the term adherence to medication is the preferred terminology which refers to how well patients implement the prescribed regimen.
3. E
   - There are various barriers to successful transition which can be overcome by careful preparation which includes barriers from young adults, parents, paediatric nephrologist, adult nephrologists and care delivery systems

References/Further Reading/Guidelines

1. Harden PN, Walsh G, Bandler N, Bradley S, Lonsdale D, Taylor J, Marks SD. Bridging the gap: an integrated paediatric to adult clinical service for young adults with kidney failure. BMJ. 2012;344:e3718. (published in print on 16 June 2012;344(7861): 51–5).
2. Marks SD. Chapter 292 The adolescent with renal disease: transition to adult services. In: Turner N, Lameire N, Goldsmith DJ, Winearls CG, Himmelfarb J, Remuzzi G, editors. Oxford textbook of clinical nephrology, vol. 3. 4th ed. Oxford University Press; 2016. p. 2527–9. isbn:978-0-19-959254-8.
3. Mistry RD, Bradley S, Harden P, Blunden M, Harber M, Chowdhury P, Fairchild V, Marks SD. Improving renal allograft survival by introducing a multicomponent transition programme for paediatric renal transplant recipients. Arch Dis Child. 2015;100(Suppl 3):A207–8.
4. Plumb L, Mistry R, Bradley S, Marks SD. Structure transition programme leads to improved renal allograft survival for adolescent renal transplant recipients transferring to adult nephrology. Pediatr Nephrol. 2016;31(10):1956–7.

Resources and Patient Information

Children and young people: transition to adult services. Royal College of Nursing. https://www.rcn.org.uk/library/subject-guides/children-and-young-people-transition-to-adult-services. Accessed 1 Mar 2019.

Children's transition to adult health services – from the pond into the sea. Care Quality Commission. https://www.cqc.org.uk/sites/default/files/CQC_Transition%20Report.pdf. Accessed 1 Mar 2019.

Helping adolescents transition to adult health care. American Academy of Pediatrics. https://www.aap.org/en-us/about-the-aap/aap-press-room/Pages/Helping-Adolescents-Transition-to-Adult-Health-Care.aspx. Accessed 1 Mar 2019.

Implementing transition care locally and nationally using the "Ready Steady Go" programme. NICE Guidance. https://www.nice.org.uk/sharedlearning/implementing-transition-care-locally-and-nationally-using-the-ready-steady-go-programme. Accessed 1 Mar 2019.

Transition and young adult – patient empowerment. British Association for Paediatric Nephrology and the Renal Association. https://renal.org/bapn/transition-young-adult. Accessed 1 Mar 2019.

Transition from children's to adults' services for young people using health of social care services. NICE guideline [NG43]. https://www.nice.org.uk/guidance/ng43 (accessed 1 March 2019).

Transition to adult services. Royal College of Paediatrics and Child Health. https://www.rcpch.ac.uk/resources/transition-adult-services. Accessed 1 Mar 2019.

Young adults and adolescents transition project. Royal College of Physicians. https://www.rcplondon.ac.uk/projects/young-adults-and-adolescents-transition-project. Accessed 1 Mar 2019.

Adherence and Kidney Disease

Sarah Afuwape, Joanne Henry, Pooja Mehta Gudka, and Mark Harber

Contents

M. Harber (ed.), *Primer on Nephrology*, https://doi.org/10.1007/978-3-030-76419-7_70

Learning Objectives

1. Understand the definition, prevalence and significance of treatment non-adherence among individuals with renal conditions and renal transplantations.
2. Understand the measurement of adherence and determine the multiple underlying factors for non-adherence including socioeconomic, individual and system-related factors.
3. Review specific educational and individual interventions aimed at improving non-adherence.

70.1 Introduction

70.1.1 Definition of Adherence

Adherence to medical therapy can be described as conformity to treatment with regard to timings, dosages, frequency and duration of treatment [1]. Formerly referred to as *compliance* and often used interchangeably, adherence is considered a more dynamic and complex behavioural and cognitive process which presumes agreement and collaboration between the patient and the prescriber about the prescriber's recommendations with the patient's informed choices. Contrastingly, compliance fails to acknowledge the collaborative component suggesting instead a passive and more submissive patient-prescriber relationship in which the patient merely follows the orders given by the prescriber [2]. Challenges with adherence have been observed in all situations where self-administration of treatment is required, regardless of the type of disease, its severity and accessibility to health resources [3]. It can include health behaviours and activities that extend beyond medication-taking including, for example, hospital appointment attendance and implementing a necessary lifestyle change, such as stopping smoking or improving a diet. Regardless of the required behaviour change, evidence suggests that a corroborative, supportive, patient-centred approach to treatment is most effective in producing sustained changes in adherence [4].

70.1.2 Prevalence of Poor Adherence

Rates of adherence vary widely between conditions and patient age with adolescence being a particularly high-risk period. The prevalence of poor adherence is sufficient to have a significant impact: one study estimated that 89,000 premature deaths per year could have been prevented in the USA by better adherence to anti-hypertensive medications alone [5]. In 2010, the National Health Service in England (NHSE) reported that the overall cost of pharmaceutical waste in the UK was approximately £300 million with an estimated 4 yearly increase of 11% [6]. Renal transplantation is considered the gold standard of treatment for end-stage renal failure but requires life-long adherence to immunosuppressant medication. Advancement in modern immunosuppressive therapy has delivered average live donor graft survival rates of 21 years and 10-year graft survivals of over 80% but only in the context of high levels of patient commitment and self-management [7–11]. Rates of immunosuppressant medication non-adherence (IMNA) range from 20% to 50% [12, 13] with studies showing a threefold increased risk of acute late rejection and sevenfold higher risk of graft failure [14–16] making it the commonest avoidable cause of graft loss. Among kidney transplant patients, IMNA is estimated at between 20% and 32% [6, 13] with one study documenting kidney transplant recipients (KTRs) having four times worse adherence compared with other solid organ transplants [17]. The reasons for this large discrepancy are not clear but validated in other studies suggest a great deal more needs to be done by renal units to address this.

70.2 Factors Associated with Non-adherence

Non-adherence is a complex and multifaceted behavioural concept [18]. The World Health Organisation has loosely categorised determinants of non-adherence into five broad dimensions: social and economic, health-system related, therapy related, condition related and individual related (Table 70.1) [19]. Furthermore, non-adherence can either be *unintentional* or *intentional*: the former is considered a passive process where patients fail to adhere to recommendations either due to forgetfulness, carelessness or any circumstances that may be beyond their control. It is predicted by medication beliefs, chronic disease and sociodemographic characteristics [1]. In contrast, intentional non-adherence indicates an active decision by the patient to forego treatment for a number of reasons, some of which are listed in Table 70.2. It is particularly problematic in older adults with one study showing intentional non-adherence to comprise approximately 50% of non-adherent behaviour among those over 65 years [20, 21]. Conversely, adolescence is also a very high-risk period; but include a sense of invulnerability, risk-taking behaviour and rebellion. Whatever the demographics, there are a number of situational risk factors for non-adherence including those listed in ► Box 70.1 [20, 22]; in particular it is

Table 70.1 Factors affecting non-adherence

Social and economic	Treatment-related	Health system/ prescriber-related	Individual-related	Condition-related
Socioeconomic variables (e.g. age, gender, ethnicity, social support, religious beliefs, employment status) Cost of treatment Peer pressure and social norms Access to alternative Treatments	Complex regimes Unwanted side effects Route of administration Polypharmacy Not seeing immediate benefits Frequent changes in treatment Duration of treatment	Collaborative approach Poor communication Lack of access to prescriber Lack of follow-up Service over- burdened Lack of training in appropriate interventions to improve adherence Irregular medication review	Poor understanding of requirements Health illiteracy Poor organisational skills Forgetting to take medication Inaccurate health beliefs about condition cause, chronicity and treatment efficacy Unhelpful illness-specific representations Cognitive deficits Poor motivation Low self-efficacy Negative previous experience of medication-taking	Characteristics of the disease, e.g. severity and chronicity Significant symptom distress High visibility of condition

Table 70.2 Unintentional and intentional non-adherence

Types of non-adherence and reason	
Unintentional non-adherence	**Intentional non-adherence**
Forgetting to take medications Running out of medications Difficulty with medication administration Misunderstanding about medication regimen	Skipping doses to make medication last longer Taking smaller doses to make medication last longer Altering dose of medications to suit own needs Stopping/reducing/increasing medication due to perceived improved symptoms without prescriber approval Stopped medication as thought to be ineffective

Adapted from "Unintentional non-adherence to chronic prescription medications: How unintentional is it really?" [1]

Box 70.1 Situational Risk Factors for Non-adherence

- Polypharmacy exists
- Complex treatment regimens
- Frequent and several changes to medication regimens, e.g. dose adjustments/frequency changes
- Fear exists of perceived risks with treatment, e.g. side effects/dependence
- Patient thinks the necessity of potential treatments outweighs benefits
- Illness beliefs vary from illness/treatment-related experiences
- Existence of inter-current physical and/or mental illness
- Financial constraints exist
- Inability to understand or interpret of health-related information (health literacy)
- Inadequate patient-practitioner relationship exists

important to remember that even the most conscientious patient can be destabilised by inter-current mental health issues or life events.

Health literacy has been an underappreciated aspect of adherence and is defined as "the personal characteristics and social resources needed for individuals and communities to access, understand, appraise and use information and services to make decisions about health" [23]. Influenced by general literacy and numeracy, health literacy has been found to be negatively associated with non-intentional non-adherence in renal transplant patients [24, 25]. Findings from an English observational study comparing health material demonstrated low levels of health literacy among the national adult working population, with 43% of adults reporting health information as too complex [26]. This proportion may well be much higher in patients from poor socioeconomic backgrounds and those whose first language differs from that of the healthcare providers. Half of the US population reads below seventh grade level (12 years);

none of the content from the top 10 reputable websites for live donor and deceased donor transplantation met the seventh grade reading level recommended by the National Institute of Health; the mean reading level corresponded to university level [27]. The Organisation for Economic Co-operation and Development (OECD) data offer guidance on individual countries.

Health Literacy Screening Tools ▶ healthliteracy.org.uk offers a comprehensive library of over 133 screening tools.

Taylor et al. (2016) conducted the only data of health literacy in the renal population using the Single-Item Literacy Screener (SILS) when investigating the prevalence and associations of limited health literacy using data from the UK-wide ATTOM program. They asked "How often do you need to have someone help you when you read instructions, pamphlets or other written material from your doctor or pharmacy?" Responses were given on a 5-point scale ranging from Never to Always, with responses "Sometimes", "Often" and "Always" suggestive of limited health literacy [28]. This question would fit discretely in a questionnaire.

▪▪ REALM-R

The rapid estimate of adult literacy in medicine (REALM-R) offers screening based on word recognition to identify patients at risk of poor health literacy skills. This version has eleven words the participants read out loud that are commonly experienced and expected to understand in the course of interacting with a healthcare professional in the clinical setting. A score of 6 or less indicates an at-risk patient. The response burden including explanation and delivery of the REALM-R takes less than 2 min to complete.

An appreciation of patients' health literacy can help tone our communication skills, regardless of media, to use appropriate language and recognise that our life-long patients have life-long learning needs and a shared understanding will help navigate and address some of the factors associated with non-adherence identified above.

70.3 Measuring Adherence

Several instruments exist to measure adherence, some with the aim of predicting future non-adherent behaviour. They can be loosely divided into *subjective*, *objective* and *biochemical* measures of adherence.

70.3.1 Subjective Ratings of Adherence

Self-report questionnaires provide an inexpensive method of adherence assessment; not surprisingly, their reliability is limited and tends to underestimate non-adherence [29]. Moreover, they are heavily reliant on respondents' memory for responses. Validated self-report questionnaires of non-adherence include the Medication Adherence Reporting Scale (MARS) [30] which contains items measuring both intentional and non-intentional forms of adherence.

In a cross-sectional survey of 24,000 patients with chronic illnesses and patients who self-identified as being persistent at taking their prescription medications, 70% reported at least one sign of unintentional non-adherence, whereas 37% reported at least one sign of intentional non-adherence [1]. Conversely, studies based on practitioners' assessments tend to overestimate poor adherence.

Continuous non-attendance to clinic visits can be used as a marker for adherence; however, it should be noted that non-adherence is also seen in 50% of patients who do attend clinics regularly. Personality traits such as those with "low openness" have also been used as tools for predicting adherence in patients, both of which have shown to be unreliable markers of adherence.

70.3.2 Objective Measures of Adherence

Non-attendance This is easy to identify and quantify with any booking system that records non-attendance or multiple clinic cancellations as in the obvious case of non-attendance for dialysis. A more subtle, less obvious form however is the patient who chooses to reduce their dialysis hours. Non-attendance is an alarm bell for non-adherence but does not necessarily equate to the same; there are transplant patients who stop attending for years but who continue to be extremely good at taking their medication. ◘ Figure 70.1 shows the creatinine graphs of four patients who lost transplant kidneys from late rejection in the context of non-adherence with immunosuppression. The two on the right attended very regularly with stable renal function and good tacrolimus levels but had life events that resulted in what was felt to have been unpredictable, non-adherence. The two on the left both had missed appointments (arrows) which were out of character, prior to presenting with late rejection. In these two patients, non-attendance was an important warning sign of non-adherence.

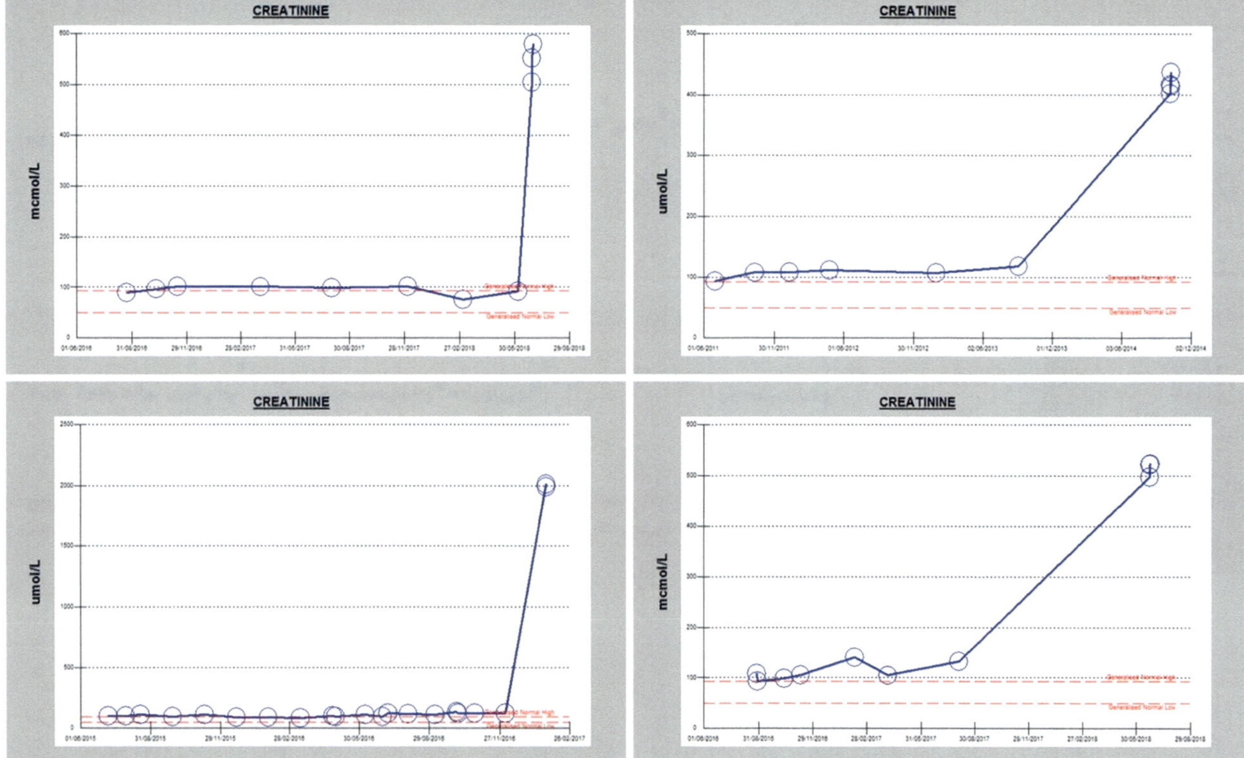

Fig. 70.1 Creatinine graphs on four KTRs with good function presenting with late rejection in the context of unrecordable tacrolimus levels. For the two patients on the right, there was very little warning of risk behaviour, and attendance had been excellent. However for the two patients on the left, non-adherence was evident in their non-attendance to clinic, a trigger for intervention potentially avoiding harm

70.3.2.1 Medication Monitoring

Pill counting is a traditional method favoured by healthcare professionals and used routinely in treatments regimes, for example, in TB and HIV treatment. Used on its own, it does not allow the practitioner to deduce adherence and can underestimate it. Pharmacy dispensing records have also been used as a method of auditing adherence. The frequency of repeat prescriptions collected has been audited [31]. This has not shown to be a reliable method as patients do not always visit the same pharmacy for all their medications. Moreover, lifestyle changes can lead to a change frequency of prescription refills, e.g. collecting medications earlier than needed due to an upcoming holiday, and could lead to an overestimation of adherence. As both look at the quantity of medications, neither method deduces the patient's patterns of medication administration nor shows any patterns of missed doses – both of which are essential in understanding poor adherence.

Electronic medication monitoring systems, e.g. Medications Event Monitoring Systems (MEMS) record the time and date of medication administration. Generally fitted within bottle caps or available as jackets for medication strips, they are better methods for understanding patients' medication administration patterns. They are more reliable compared to self-reporting and pill counting, but the risks of malfunction and high costs associated with their use make them an unpopular tool for assessing adherence. On its own, it is not reliable at assessing medications adherence as no record is made of whether the dose of medication is actually taken after the bottle has been opened [32, 33]. There are alternative MEMs on the market and example of which is shown below (Fig. 70.2).

With objective measures, there is a potential for the data to be "gamed" by a patient who may be aware of the assessments and wishes to keep non-adherence private; however a sudden improvement in tacrolimus levels in

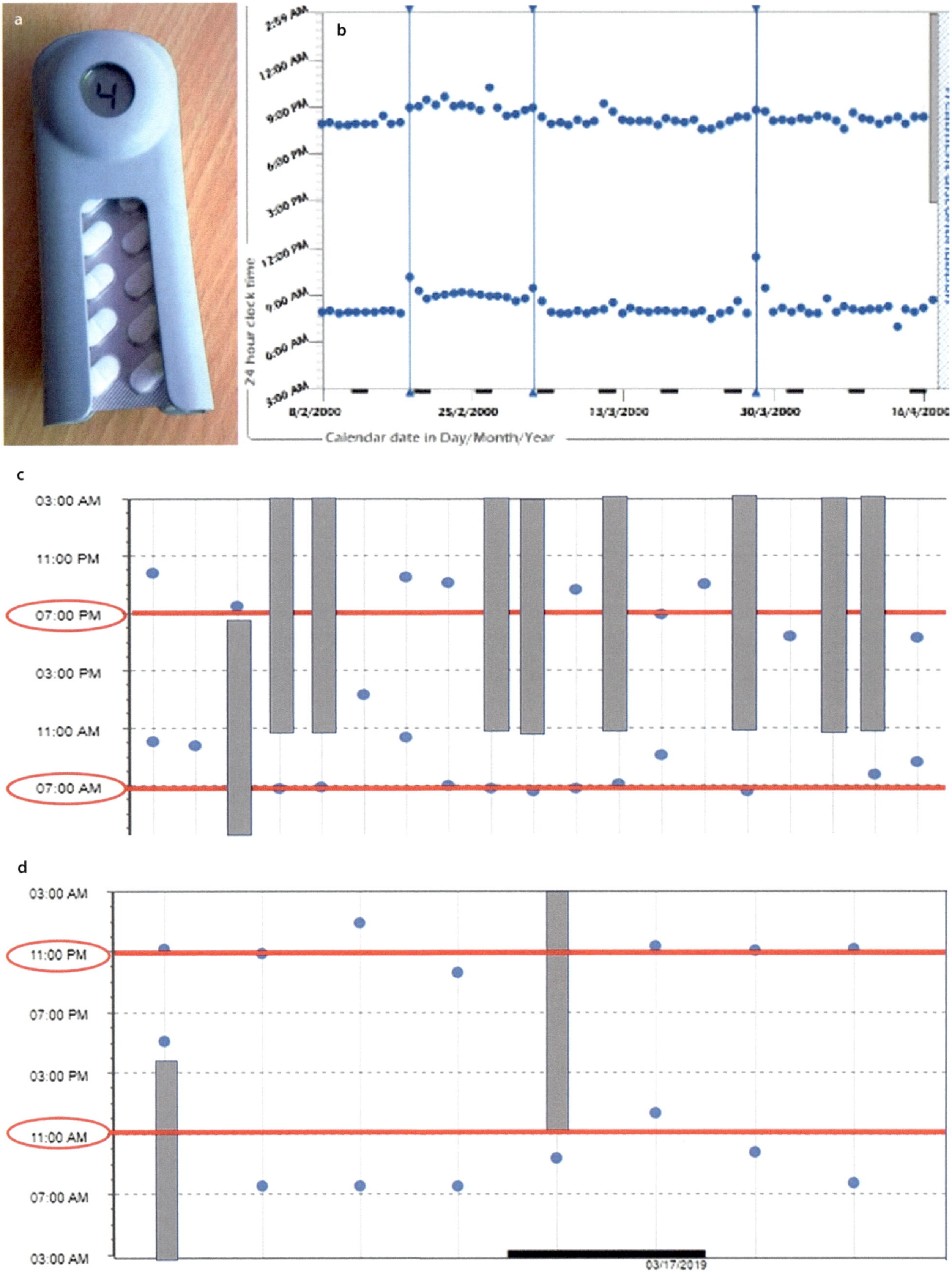

Fig. 70.2 Examples of MEMS. **a** Medication adherence monitor. **b** Monitoring record for an adherent patient. **c** MEMS output showing erratic timing of self-administration and multiple missed episodes. **d** Output from MEMS showing erratic timings of medications administration, which can be addressed at a more suitable time agreed with the patient to improve adherence

the setting of being monitored is in itself useful information and the start of a discussion. MEMS can give some insight into the pattern and severity of missed medication that may reveal potential solutions whether that be to do with lifestyle, rationalising medication burden or the need to discuss health beliefs and understanding of the need for medication. Crucially, just increasing the dose in patient (c) because of low levels seen in clinic is really not going to solve the problem and indeed may make things worse in periods when the patient is compliant.

MEMS are not widely adopted in clinical practice in part because of the expense, but it is likely that prices will reduce, and it is worth bearing in mind that not only the premature loss of a transplant due to non-adherence with medication is a tragedy and life shortening, but also a return to dialysis is extremely expensive.

70.3.3 Biochemical Markers of Adherence

There are a variety of established assays for therapeutic drug monitoring (TDM) discussed below in the context of transplantation, but one off assays (usually urine) can be invaluable when assessing adherence in patients with difficult to manage conditions such as multi-agent hypertension. Simply prescribing more when a patient is not taking medication is unlikely to help; identifying non-adherence and attempting to address the underlying cause are a more thoughtful strategy.

Monitoring tacrolimus trough levels in renal centres has long been used to indicate patients' level of adherence. Although tacrolimus trough level variation can be affected by other physiological or medical factors, tacrolimus 12-hour trough variability over a period of time (intra-patient variability, IPV) is significantly affected by adherence and a useful objective tool. It is calculated using the mean absolute deviation in trough tacrolimus levels. Studies have shown that high intra-patient variability in tacrolimus levels is associated with a higher risk of late rejection, development of donor-specific antibodies and poor graft and patient survival rates (◘ Fig. 70.3) [34, 35].

Calculation of tacrolimus IPV is a cheap, easy method of monitoring patients and identifying any high-risk patients during routine clinic visits, allowing practitioners to address reasons for non-adherence before graft function is compromised. Lastly, incidences of late antibody-mediated rejection, transplant glomerulonephritis, graft failure and death with/without function have also been routinely measured as indicators of adherence; unless there is a problem with absorption or increased metabolism, late rejection is likely to be related to poor adherence.

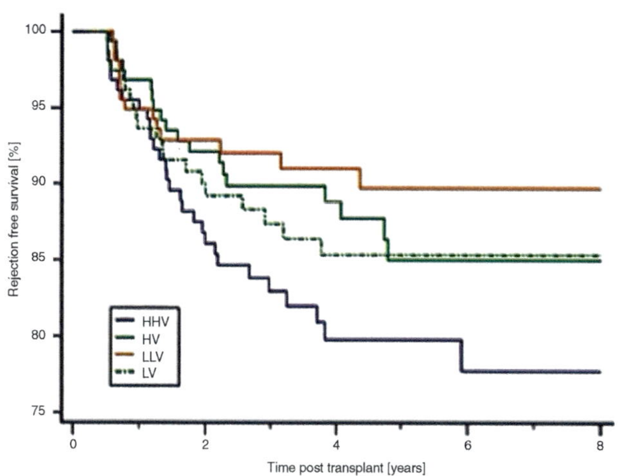

◘ **Fig. 70.3** Survival without rejection in patients with variable tacrolimus levels. Patients with very high variability (HHV) showed inferior survival rates compared to those with lower tacrolimus variability (LV, LLV) [34]. (Reproduced with permission from Wolters Kluwer Health, Inc.)

70.3.3.1 Interventions to Improve Non-adherence

An evaluation of all interventions is beyond the realm of this chapter, but a range of interventions have been described to improve medication adherence with varying rates of effectiveness [36]. Costa and Giardini et al. [18] in their comprehensive review of varying types of interventional tools and Low et al. who reviewed medication adherence interventions in kidney transplant recipients have examined and categorised interventions according to their primary components. Five categories of intervention have been identified, namely, *behavioural*, *educational*, *integrated care*, *self-management* and *risk communication* interventions. The characteristics and effectiveness of each are shown in ◘ Table 70.3. Irrespective of the disease, evidence suggests that the complex nature of non-adherence necessitates an intervention that targets multiple behavioural risk factors or combines behavioural, educational and emotional changes to be effective in improving short-term adherence [37]. Improvement in overall health literacy is an essential component to better patient understanding and sustained patient engagement.

70.4 Summary

Suboptimal adherence with medication and medical advice is very costly to the healthcare system and not infrequently tragic for patients with serious conditions.

Table 70.3 Characteristics of interventions aimed at improving medication adherence (in adult kidney transplant patients)*

	Type of intervention				
	Behavioural/ counselling	**Educational**	**Integrated care**	**Self-management**	**Risk communication**
Aim	To modify patients' behaviour towards a treatment/foster permanent optimal medication-taking behaviour [37]	To educate patients about their specific condition and how to take their medicines	Groups of techniques aimed at improving collaboration between healthcare providers to increase patients' overall satisfaction with healthcare and improve quality of care and of life	To promote sustainable patient involvement in their own disease and increase patient roles and responsibility	To communicate accurate information regarding risk to improve accurate appraisal and reduce intentional non-adherence
Intervention method	Cognitive behavioural strategies to alter dysfunctional thoughts, behaviours and emotions and promote positive changes to symptoms and treatment. Telephone follow-ups Home visits Electronic monitoring device	Patient-centred discussions to address ambivalence about medication-taking. Discusses and explores patients' health beliefs and knowledge [41]. Principles of shared decision-making are central	Multidisciplinary team (MDT) working with cohesive clinical pathways, integrated patient education and self-management support	Multi-component. Includes provision of information, practical and social support. targets problem-solving ability and coping skills	Techniques to improve risk communication with decision aids (e.g. pamphlets, videos, web-based tools) to indicate cost benefits of taking medication
Overall effectiveness	Variable results [42, 43] *[44, 45]. No significant difference between behavioural intervention and control group. *[46]. Significantly higher adherence in intervention group vs control	Interventions have improved knowledge in post-organ transplant patient but inconsistent findings of improved adherence among interventions using education or information only [47]. *[48] significant differences in adherence between intervention and control	Bodenheimer et al. [49]. Positive impact on patient care quality found in different chronic health conditions	Chodosh [50]. Improved HbA levels, systolic and diastolic blood pressure and pain in patients with chronic conditions Radhakrishnan (2012) [51]. No evidence for improved self-management activities in those with type II diabetes, heart disease and hypertension	Kuntz et al. [52]. Outcomes are variable. Improved understanding of risk demonstrated although inconsistently correlated with medication adherence

Adapted from *Interventional tools to improve medication adherence: review of the literature* [18]

It is also very common, and yet in general it is rare that we have robust systems to identify the issue and offer targeted support to mitigate the causes. Getting better at preventing non-adherence and the consequences is a challenge that we should take up.

Tips and Tricks

- A department that has a non-confrontational system for assessing barriers to compliance (in a non-confrontational way), for example, by routinely monitoring objective markers such as non-attendance, IPV tacrolimus levels and unrecordable levels, stands a better chance of avoiding unexpected tragedies.
- It is not sufficient to "diagnose" non-adherence alone; the key is to identify, among the very many reasons, why the patient is struggling with adherence and therefore can the route cause be tackled.
- Simplify medication regimens including the number of daily doses and number of concurrent medications where possible. Identify and discontinue all unnecessary medication.
- It is critically important to appreciate a patient's health literacy and provide education and support at an appropriate level.
- Effective communication is essential; discuss with patient the purpose of the medication and the expectations of the treatment (e.g. when/quantity to take, how to administer, time to onset of effect, expected treatment outcomes, method of monitoring effectiveness). Encourage patient to ask questions; adherence is much likely to be higher if patients fully appreciate the reasons and needs for medication. Relay this information to the patient's GP in a clear and timely manner so that shared decision-making can continue across all aspects of the patient's care.
- Provide leaflets and literature to aid understanding and memory about condition and treatment.
- Explore and address any possible barriers to obtaining and administering the medication (e.g. practical/financial issues, unhelpful health beliefs, concerns about side effects, perceived stigma of taking treatment, psychological distress or illness).
- Encourage use of individually tailored techniques (e.g. alarms on phones, dosette boxes, calendars, repeat prescriptions, pharmacy delivery service, free medicine reminder app).
- Where applicable, encourage family/social network involvement and peer support groups.

Case Study

Case 1

A 32-year-old female received a pre-emptive deceased donor kidney transplant f risk and achieved good renal function; however, after a 2-month period of clinic non-attendance, her creatinine rose from a baseline of 100 to 250 secondary to biopsy-proven rejection. She had low but none undetectable tacrolimus levels at the time but denied any non-adherence. Her transplant made a poor recovery following treatment but stabilised at a creatinine of 240. A further episode of non-attendance occurred, and she was eventually admitted with a rise in creatinine to 494. She attributed her non-attendance to unreliable hospital transport.

Her health literacy score was within the *normal* ranges on the REALM-R [38] (score = 7) and on the Single-Item Literacy Screener score (SILS) [39], meaning that her highest educational attainment was secondary education only. Her MARS score suggested that she often experienced some non-intentional non-adherence.

She reported having a needle phobia and often failed to administer her Aranesp injections to manage her anaemia. She used a dosette box to organise her immunosuppression and, as a reminder to take them, set twice daily alarms on her phone at 12 pm and 10 pm. However, she often missed her noon dose of tacrolimus as she usually slept through her alarm beyond midday. Believing it was then too late to take her medication, she took her 10:00 pm dose only. She also reported having difficulty coping with her condition and reported experiencing low mood from a recent bereavement.

Intervention

To help her needle phobia and promote self-administering, the specialist nurse prescribed and she was counselled on the use of the Aranesp SureClick which has a less visible needle. With discussion, her tacrolimus times were personalised to suit her schedule and altered to be taken at 12 am and 12 pm resulting in a significant improvement in her adherence and a stabilising of her tacrolimus levels. She was informed of and has been eligible for the hospital financial assistance scheme to support with travel costs. Lastly, she was referred to the renal clinical health psychology service for therapy to help manage her mood, increase coping skills and improve her needle phobia.

In this case, there were several factors leading to poor adherence, none of which were obvious or volunteered. Sadly, by the time that the non-adherence and causes were clearly identified, the graft was lost. Despite the very plausible explanations, her non-adherence should have triggered a more detailed assessment and intervention, possibly avoiding both rejection episodes.

Case 2

A 21-year-old man transferred from children services 3 years ago maintained good clinic attendance and gave the impression of being very diligent about taking his medication but had a medication lists that varied with what he appeared to be taking. REALM-R score of 3 indicates that he is at risk of low health literacy. He defied the SILS test as he indicated he never needs anyone to help reading instructions as he never reads them anyway. He trusts his transplant consultant and follows "whatever she tells him at their clinic consultation". This case illustrates an important point about assumed knowledge and understanding. Until this issue of health literacy was identified, multiple pointless unhelpful letters were sent, perhaps causing distress but certainly not achieving the changes in medication recommended. The intervention here was to simply consult the documentation detailing the barrier on his diagnosis and management list: "Any changes to his medications must be done face to face or by phone". This approach had the spin off effect of improving patient engagement generally.

Case 3

A 66-year-old diabetic woman received a dual kidney transplant. Initially her transplant did extremely well, but she had recurrent UTIs severe enough to require admission and a very high tacrolimus IPV, frequently ranging from relatively toxic levels to unrecordable. There were communication issues as English was not her first language, and this was felt to be contributing to the high IPV. Her bladder emptying was normal, and she was treated with prophylactic antibiotics. She had multiple episodes of AKI with high tacrolimus levels as an inpatient.

It became apparent that her very supportive daughter had moved out of the house once she had started her family, and the relationship had deteriorated significantly. While the daughter would attend and offer the tablets, it was clear that the patient would make a point of not taking them. Ultimately the transplant was lost to chronic rejection, and the patient deemed unfit for retransplantation. Only in retrospect was it apparent that her UTIs were not controlled because she was not taking prophylaxis; however the huge variation in tacrolimus levels especially the unrecordable levels as an outpatient and high levels when an impatient was a clear sign of poor adherence and an important warning signal. Earlier interventions with an interpreter and engagement with the family to identify the problem might have resulted in a different outcome.

Case 4

An 18-year-old boy was transferred from the paediatric hospital for transplant follow-up. His tacrolimus levels were highly variable with frequent low levels, and his attendance was erratic. He had a single parent who held down two jobs to make ends meet. The patient had some learning difficulties, and it became apparent that he had to take three buses to get to clinic. Although he could do this, it was a significant logistic and financial barrier for him. Variable or unrecordable tacrolimus levels when he attended provoked the need for frequent and early follow-up visits. When a youth support worker visited his home following a missed clinic appointment, she was struck by sea of tablets over his bedroom floor. His non-adherence was not wilful; had we measured his health literacy sooner, we would have identified his unintentional non-adherence. Indeed he was very keen to comply with medical instructions; it was consequent to the fact that he had never acquired the skills to organise his medication, when he was close to running out and therefore to initiate a request for more medication. He was offered support for travel, alerts/reminders for clinics and engagement with a youth support worker. His medication was delivered as a dosette box, and he was encouraged to use a direct line to contact the transplant team if he had issues. This illustrates the point that being frustrated and critical of a patients' compliance without understanding the reasons can be completely counterproductive and rarely helpful; the key is, where possible, to unpick the causes.

Case 5

A 59-year-old female received an aged-matched deceased donor dual cadaveric renal transplant. The kidney was a 2-0-1 mismatch with a baseline eGFR of >90 mls/min. The recipient did not speak English but had an engaged and supportive daughter who helped with her polypharmacy; however the support reduced over time with the responsibilities of a new mother. Over the years, the recipient experienced variable tacrolimus levels with multi-resistant urinary tract infections. High tacrolimus level coincided with inpatient episodes and infections.

Five years and 1 month post-transplant, the recipient experienced rejection with an eGFR of <15 mls/min as a consequence of donor-specific antibodies. She was treated with intravenous steroids, and medication was formally arranged in dosette boxes with reminder prompts from her daughter to adhere with treatment. With the failure to improve tacrolimus variability, dosage was converted to once daily to aid adherence. Five years and 7 months post-transplant, the recipient began and unplanned start onto dialysis treatment. Transplant failed.

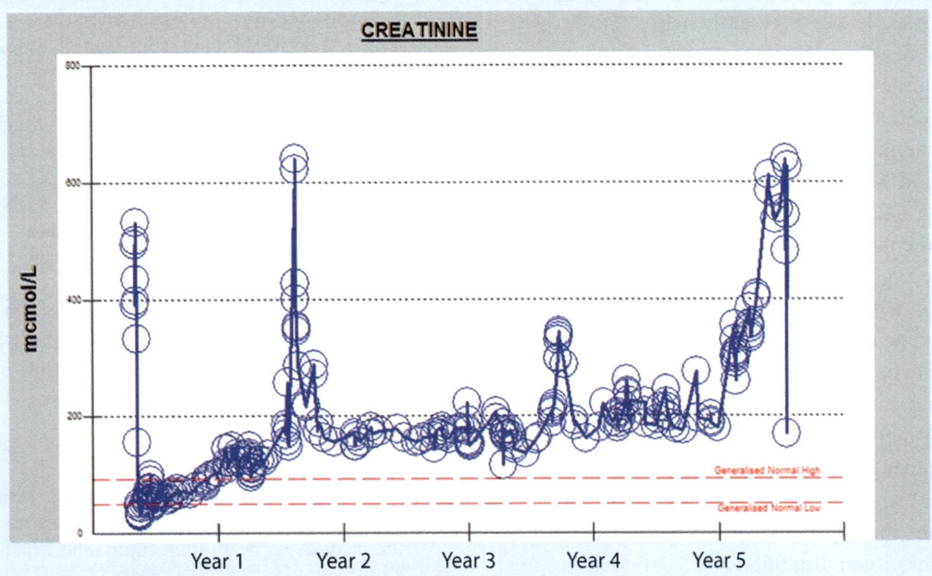

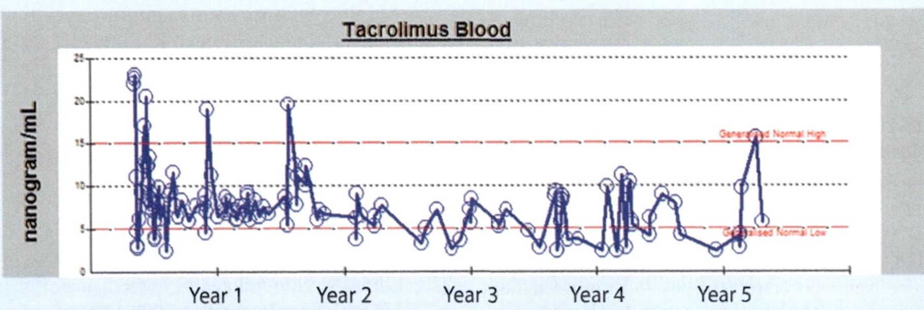

From the graphs, it is noticeable that the tacrolimus levels were very variably continued despite the dosette box with high levels during inpatient episodes. On reflection we should not have given once daily tacrolimus as it an expensive way of facilitating non-compliance particularly in a patient deliberately not taking prophylactic antibiotics and immunosuppression.

Chapter Review Questions

1. What are the main risk factors for poor adherence?
2. What markers can assist in identification of poor adherence?
3. What education level do I aim my health message?
4. What level of tacrolimus trough level variance is associated with a worse outcome?

Answers

1. The reasons why individuals take or forego their medication are varied. Non-intentional non-adherence implies a behaviour that is out of one's control and includes reasons such as forgetting or misunderstanding what is expected. Those patients who take many medicines, for example, can forget to take one medicine that they are not adverse to taking but actively chose not to take another medication that they believe gives them adverse side effects. Refer to Table 70.1 to help identify factors affecting poor adherence you may not have considered.
2. Adherence can improve or worsen over time. Sustained adherence requires excellent communication and patient education to ensure patients have a good understanding of their condition and the required treatment. Tailored treatment interventions are associated with ongoing adherence. Adopt system to calculate IPV and clinic non-attendance to identify those most vulnerable to graft loss. Include a question on adherence in your consultation. For example, "how many doses of your immunosuppressant have you missed in the last 2 weeks?"

   Reiteration from every member of the transplant team that a life event such as bereavement/

mental health can render us non-adherent with tragic consequences. Seek early help.

3. Aim all health education/opportunities at low health literacy level, as you reach all levels of education. Use short sentences avoiding big words; give a chunk of information and check if they understand what they are to do. For example, drink 2 l a day; never forget to take your medicines and come to clinic.
4. Evidence suggests that perceived social support is correlated with improved health outcomes when compared with no social support [40]. Friends and family members can potentially have a role in reminding patients to take their treatments, providing practical (e.g. collecting medications, accompanying patients to appointments) and emotional support. Social support is particularly helpful for those patients with physical, cognitive and/or emotional disabilities.

References

1. Gadkari AS, McHorney CA. Unintentional non-adherence to chronic prescription medications: how unintentional is it really? BMC Health Serv Res. 2012;12:98.
2. Vlasnik JJ, Aliotta SL, DeLor B. Medication adherence: factors influencing compliance with prescribed medication plans. Case Manager. 2005;16(2):47–51.
3. Roter DL, Hall JA, Merisca R, Nordstrom B, Cretin D, Svarstad B. Effectiveness of interventions to improve patient compliance: a meta-analysis. Med Care. 1998;36(8):1138–61.
4. Vlasnik JJ, Aliotta SL, DeLor B. Evidence-based assessment and intervention strategies to increase adherence to prescribed medication plans. Case Manager. 2005;16(2):55–9.
5. Cutler DM, Everett W. Thinking outside the pillbox--medication adherence as a priority for health care reform. N Engl J Med. 2010;362(17):1553–5.
6. Hazell BR, Ross Robson Pharmaceutical waste reduction in the NHS. Report. 2015.
7. Denhaerynck K, Manhaeve D, Dobbels F, Garzoni D, Nolte C, De Geest S. Prevalence and consequences of nonadherence to hemodialysis regimens. Am J Crit Care. 2007;16(3):222–35. quiz 36
8. Hardinger KL, Hutcherson T, Preston D, Murillo D. Influence of pill burden and drug cost on renal function after transplantation. Pharmacotherapy. 2012;32(5):427–32.
9. Couzi L, Moulin B, Morin MP, Albano L, Godin M, Barrou B, et al. Factors predictive of medication nonadherence after renal transplantation: a French observational study. Transplantation. 2013;95(2):326–32.
10. Russell C, Conn V, Ashbaugh C, Madsen R, Wakefield M, Webb A, et al. Taking immunosuppressive medications effectively (TIMELink): a pilot randomized controlled trial in adult kidney transplant recipients. Clin Transpl. 2011;25(6):864–70.
11. Goldfarb-Rumyantzev AS, Wright S, Ragasa R, Ostler D, Van Orden J, Smith L, et al. Factors associated with nonadherence to medication in kidney transplant recipients. Nephron Clin Pract. 2011;117(1):c33–9.
12. Helmy R, Duerinckx N, De Geest S, Denhaerynck K, Berben L, Russell CL, et al. The international prevalence and variability of nonadherence to the nonpharmacologic treatment regimen after heart transplantation: findings from the cross-sectional BRIGHT study. Clin Transpl. 2018;32(7):e13280.
13. Denhaerynck K, Dobbels F, Cleemput I, Desmyttere A, Schafer-Keller P, Schaub S, et al. Prevalence, consequences, and determinants of nonadherence in adult renal transplant patients: a literature review. Transpl Int. 2005;18(10):1121–33.
14. Belaiche S, Decaudin B, Dharancy S, Noel C, Odou P, Hazzan M. Factors relevant to medication non-adherence in kidney transplant: a systematic review. Int J Clin Pharm. 2017;39(3):582–93.
15. Dew MA, Dabbs AD, Myaskovsky L, Shyu S, Shellmer DA, DiMartini AF, et al. Meta-analysis of medical regimen adherence outcomes in pediatric solid organ transplantation. Transplantation. 2009;88(5):736–46.
16. Mathis AS. Managed care implications of improving long-term outcomes in organ transplantation. Am J Manag Care. 2015;21(1 Suppl):s24–30.
17. Dew MA, DiMartini AF, De Vito DA, Myaskovsky L, Steel J, Unruh M, et al. Rates and risk factors for nonadherence to the medical regimen after adult solid organ transplantation. Transplantation. 2007;83(7):858–73.
18. Costa E, Giardini A, Prados-Torres A, Cahir C, Marengoni A. Interventional tools to improve prescription and adherence to medical plans. Biomed Res Int. 2015;2015:602078.
19. Sabate E. Adherence to long-term therapies: evidence of action World Health Organization. 2003.
20. Mukhtar O, Weinman J, Jackson SH. Intentional non-adherence to medications by older adults. Drugs Aging. 2014;31(3):149–57.
21. Barber N, Parsons J, Clifford S, Darracott R, Horne R. Patients' problems with new medication for chronic conditions. Qual Saf Health Care. 2004;13(3):172–5.
22. Elliott R. Non-adherence to medicines: not solved but solvable. J Health Serv Res Policy. 2009;14(1):58–61.
23. World Health Organization. Health literacy and health behaviour 7th Global Conference on Health Promotion: track themes. 2015.
24. Demian MN, Shapiro RJ, Thornton WL. An observational study of health literacy and medication adherence in adult kidney transplant recipients. Clin Kidney J. 2016;9(6):858–65.
25. Patzer RE, Serper M, Reese PP, Przytula K, Koval R, Ladner DP, et al. Medication understanding, non-adherence, and clinical outcomes among adult kidney transplant recipients. Clin Transpl. 2016;30(10):1294–305.
26. Rowlands G, Protheroe J, Winkley J, Richardson M, Seed PT, Rudd R. A mismatch between population health literacy and the complexity of health information: an observational study. Br J Gen Pract. 2015;65(635):e379–86.
27. Zhou EP, Kiwanuka E, Morrissey PE. Online patient resources for deceased donor and live donor kidney recipients: a comparative analysis of readability. Clin Kidney J. 2018;11(4):559–63.
28. Taylor DM, Bradley JA, Bradley C, Draper H, Johnson R, Metcalfe W, et al. Limited health literacy in advanced kidney disease. Kidney Int. 2016;90(3):685–95.
29. Mahler C, Hermann K, Horne R, Ludt S, Haefeli WE, Szecsenyi J, et al. Assessing reported adherence to pharmacological treatment recommendations. Translation and evaluation of the Medication Adherence Report Scale (MARS) in Germany. J Eval Clin Pract. 2010;16(3):574–9.
30. Fialko L, Garety PA, Kuipers E, Dunn G, Bebbington PE, Fowler D, et al. A large-scale validation study of the Medication Adherence Rating Scale (MARS). Schizophr Res. 2008;100(1–3):53–9.

31. Grymonpre RE, Didur CD, Montgomery PR, Sitar DS. Pill count, self-report, and pharmacy claims data to measure medication adherence in the elderly. Ann Pharmacother. 1998;32(7–8):749–54.
32. Choo PW, Rand CS, Inui TS, Lee ML, Cain E, Cordeiro-Breault M, et al. Validation of patient reports, automated pharmacy records, and pill counts with electronic monitoring of adherence to antihypertensive therapy. Med Care. 1999;37(9):846–57.
33. Lee JY, Kusek JW, Greene PG, Bernhard S, Norris K, Smith D, et al. Assessing medication adherence by pill count and electronic monitoring in the African American Study of Kidney Disease and Hypertension (AASK) pilot study. Am J Hypertens. 1996;9(8):719–25.
34. Goodall DL, Willicombe M, McLean AG, Taube D. High intrapatient variability of tacrolimus levels and outpatient clinic nonattendance are associated with inferior outcomes in renal transplant patients. Transplant Direct. 2017;3(8):e192.
35. Shukeri WF, Zaini RH, Soon CE, Hassan MH. Overcoming airway challenges with the C-MAC((R)) video laryngoscope in a child with Goldenhar syndrome. Indian J Anaesth. 2016;60(11):868–9.
36. Neuberger JM, Bechstein WO, Kuypers DR, Burra P, Citterio F, De Geest S, et al. Practical recommendations for long-term management of modifiable risks in kidney and liver transplant recipients: a guidance report and clinical checklist by the Consensus on Managing Modifiable Risk in Transplantation (COMMIT) Group. Transplantation. 2017;101(4S Suppl 2):S1–S56.
37. Low JK, Williams A, Manias E, Crawford K. Interventions to improve medication adherence in adult kidney transplant recipients: a systematic review. Nephrol Dial Transplant. 2015;30(5):752–61.
38. Bass PF 3rd, Wilson JF, Griffith CH. A shortened instrument for literacy screening. J Gen Intern Med. 2003;18(12):1036–8.
39. Morris NS, MacLean CD, Chew LD, Littenberg B. The single item literacy screener: evaluation of a brief instrument to identify limited reading ability. BMC Fam Pract. 2006;7:21.
40. Wang HH, Wu SZ, Liu YY. Association between social support and health outcomes: a meta-analysis. Kaohsiung J Med Sci. 2003;19(7):345–51.
41. Ratanawongsa N, Karter AJ, Parker MM, Lyles CR, Heisler M, Moffet HH, et al. Communication and medication refill adherence: the diabetes study of Northern California. JAMA Intern Med. 2013;173(3):210–8.
42. George J, Elliott RA, Stewart DC. A systematic review of interventions to improve medication taking in elderly patients prescribed multiple medications. Drugs Aging. 2008;25(4):307–24.
43. Nieuwlaat R, Wilczynski N, Navarro T, Hobson N, Jeffery R, Keepanasseril A, et al. Interventions for enhancing medication adherence. Cochrane Database Syst Rev. 2014;11:CD000011.
44. Hardstaff R, Green K, Talbot D. Measurement of compliance posttransplantation--the results of a 12-month study using electronic monitoring. Transplant Proc. 2003;35(2):796–7.
45. Hardstaff R, Green K, Talbot D. Noncompliance postrenal transplantation: measuring the extent of the problem using electronic surveillance and nurse practitioner interviews. Transplant Proc. 2002;34(5):1608.
46. McGillicuddy JW, Gregoski MJ, Weiland AK, Rock RA, Brunner-Jackson BM, Patel SK, et al. Mobile health medication adherence and blood pressure control in renal transplant recipients: a proof-of-concept randomized controlled trial. JMIR Res Protoc. 2013;2(2):e32.
47. De Bleser L, Matteson M, Dobbels F, Russell C, De Geest S. Interventions to improve medication-adherence after transplantation: a systematic review. Transpl Int. 2009;22(8):780–97.
48. Chisholm MA, Mulloy LL, Jagadeesan M, DiPiro JT. Impact of clinical pharmacy services on renal transplant patients' compliance with immunosuppressive medications. Clin Transpl. 2001;15(5):330–6.
49. Bodenheimer T, Wagner EH, Grumbach K. Improving primary care for patients with chronic illness: the chronic care model, part 2. JAMA. 2002;288(15):1909–14.
50. Chodosh J, Morton SC, Mojica W, Maglione M, Suttorp MJ, Hilton L, et al. Meta-analysis: chronic disease self-management programs for older adults. Ann Intern Med. 2005;143(6):427–38.
51. Radhakrishnan K. The efficacy of tailored interventions for self-management outcomes of type 2 diabetes, hypertension or heart disease: a systematic review. J Adv Nurs. 2012;68(3):496–510.
52. Kuntz JL, Safford MM, Singh JA, Phansalkar S, Slight SP, Her QL, et al. Patient-centered interventions to improve medication management and adherence: a qualitative review of research findings. Patient Educ Couns. 2014;97(3):310–26.

Information and Guidelines: Useful Links

UK– Plain English guidelines offer free guides on how to write medical information – http://www.plainenglish.co.uk/files/medicalguide.pdf.

US – National Institute of Health. How to write easy-to-read health materials. https://medlineplus.gov/etr.html.

Adult Medication: Improving medication adherence in older adults. http://adultmeducation.com/index.html.

Healthliteracy.org.uk offers health literacy tool shed with 133 different tools, their domains and psychometrics. http://healthliteracy.bu.edu/all.

http://www.who.int/chp/knowledge/publications/adherence_report/en/.

A review of the published literature on the definitions, measurements, epidemiology, economics and interventions applied to several chronic conditions and risk factors.

Medicine reminders APP Free – Medisafe pill reminder and tracker available in English, Arabic, Danish, Dutch, Finnish, French, German, Hebrew, Italian, Japanese, Korean, Portuguese, Russian, simplified Chinese, Spanish and Turkish and is designed for users age 12 and above.

https://itunes.apple.com/gb/app/medicine-reminders-and-tracker/id573916946?mt=8.

Chronic Kidney Disease-Mineral and Bone Disorder (CKD-MBD)

Richard S. Fish, and John Cunningham

Contents

M. Harber (ed.), *Primer on Nephrology*, https://doi.org/10.1007/978-3-030-76419-7_71

Learning Objectives

1. To understand the dynamic between the kidney, skeleton and parathyroid glands in health and in the setting of CKD
2. To appreciate the risk factors and impact of an increasingly maladaptive response in advanced kidney failure
3. To discuss strategies to reduce the risk of severe bone disease or tertiary hyperparathyroidism

Definition

Chronic kidney disease-mineral bone disorder (CKD-MBD) is defined as:

A systemic disorder of mineral and bone metabolism due to CKD comprising either one or a combination of the following:

- Abnormalities of calcium, phosphorus, PTH or vitamin D metabolism
- Abnormalities in bone turnover, mineralization, volume, linear growth or strength
- Vascular or other soft tissue calcification

Clinical manifestations are very variable between subjects and are not reliably predictable from any given set of biochemical results. As such treatment strategies should be individualized.

71.1 Pathophysiology and Clinical Correlates

Normal mineral metabolism involves the integrated actions of the kidney, parathyroid glands, GI tract and bone. These organs act in linked fashion to maintain calcium and phosphate balance and the structural and metabolic integrity of the skeleton (see ◘ Fig. 71.1). CKD results in a number of disturbances to this system, ultimately resulting in CKD-MBD (see text and ◘ Fig. 71.2).

71.1.1 Biochemical Features

Failure of phosphate excretion and renal calcitriol production underlies many of the changes seen in early and late CKD. At early stages of CKD, changes in serum phosphate are minimized by adaptive increases of the phosphaturic hormones PTH and FGF-23 such that appropriate phosphate balance is initially maintained. Hyperphosphataemia is not usually present until the GFR drops to 30 ml/min or less (see ◘ Fig. 71.3), at which point the adaptive responses have been overwhelmed. These adaptive responses may then become increasingly maladaptive.

71.1.1.1 PTH

Decreased calcitriol and calcium, and increased phosphate, all increase synthesis and release of PTH. PTH promotes calcium and phosphate resorption from the bone, inhibits the sodium-phosphate cotransporter in the proximal tubule (promoting phosphate excretion) and by stimulating calcitriol production indirectly increases intestinal calcium and phosphate absorption. Sustained stimulation of the parathyroid glands results in hyperplasia and clonal proliferation of parathyroid cells which express fewer receptors for both vitamin D and calcium. PTH secretion may become uncontrolled (maladaptive) with resulting hypercalcaemia representing the transition from secondary (appropriate) to tertiary (inappropriate) hyperparathyroidism. Gross elevation of PTH is catabolic to the bone and has been implicated in cardiac fibrosis, left ventricular hypertrophy, hypertension, neuropathy and impotence. Bone marrow fibrosis as a result of hyperparathyroidism contributes to erythropoietin-stimulating agent (ESA) resistance.

71.1.1.2 Vitamin D

25-hydroxyvitamin D (calcidiol), generated in the liver from its precursor, vitamin D, is terminally activated by 25-hydroxyvitamin D-1α-hydroxylase (CYP27B1) to produce 1,25-dihydroxyvitamin D (calcitriol). The bulk of the hormonal form is synthesized in the kidney where production is stimulated by PTH and inhibited by FGF-23 and phosphate. Acting through the vitamin D receptor (VDR), circulating calcitriol acts to promote intestinal and renal absorption of calcium and phosphate and to inhibit PTH. Osteoblast activity is augmented and enhances bone remodelling and mineralization. A number of novel roles have been recently described for vitamin D and are discussed below.

71.1.1.3 FGF-23

FGF-23 is a hormone produced by osteocytes and induces phosphaturia by downregulation of proximal tubular sodium-phosphate cotransporters. In addition, FGF-23 decreases serum calcitriol by suppressing synthesis by renal 1α-hydroxylase (CYP27B1) and stimulating catabolism by 24-hydroxylase (CYP24A1). FGF-23 also negatively regulates PTH. Increasing levels of FGF-23 may become increasingly maladaptive and are associated with comorbidities including vascular calcification, left ventricular hypertrophy, endothelial dysfunction and progression of renal disease. Moreover, serum FGF-23 correlates strongly with mortality risk in both CKD and dialysis populations, and in this respect, FGF-23 is emerging as a powerful biomarker, and possible mediator, of adverse clinical outcomes in these

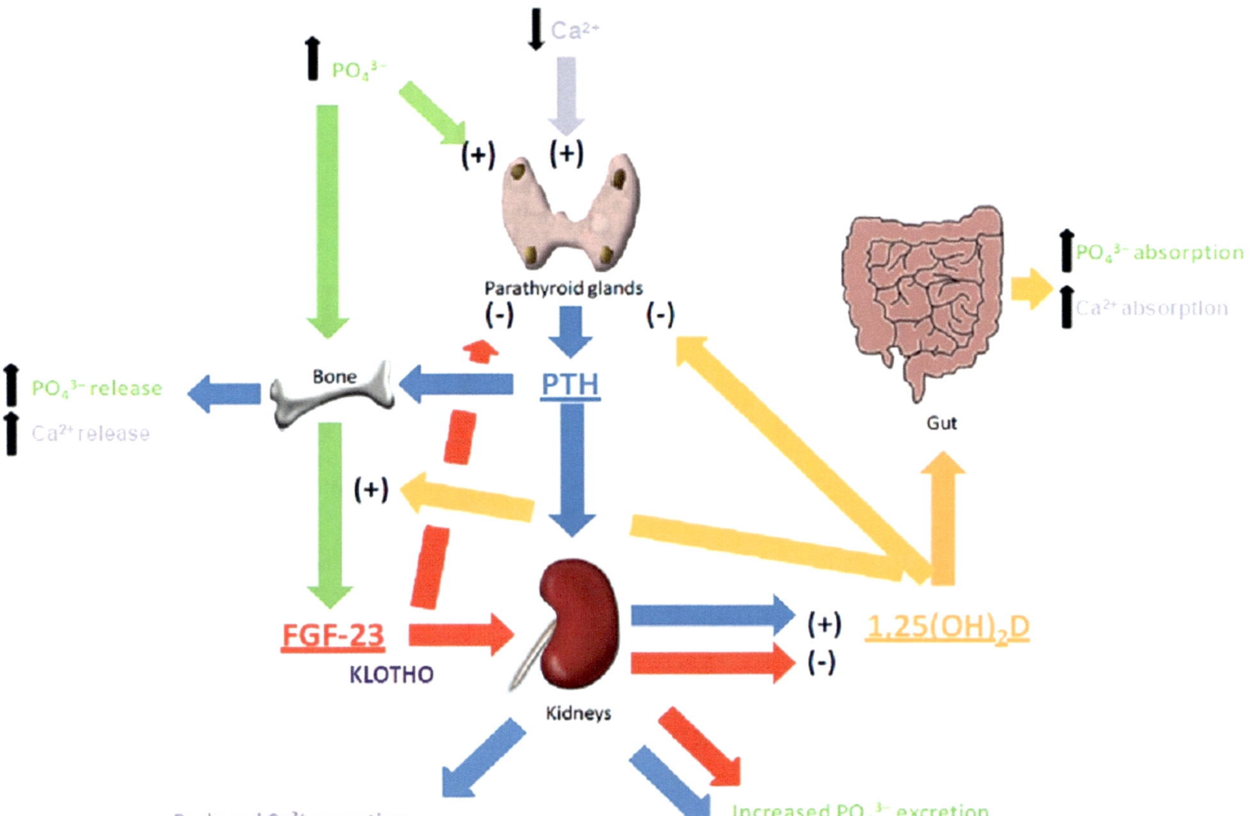

Fig. 71.1 Normal mineral metabolism
PTH release is stimulated by decreases in serum calcium or calcitriol or a rise in serum phosphate. The actions of PTH (blue arrows) are to (1) increase phosphate and calcium release from the bone; (2) enhance renal calcitriol production; (3) increase renal tubular calcium reabsorption; and (4) increase renal phosphate excretion
Calcitriol production is stimulated by PTH and inhibited by FGF-23. The actions of calcitriol (orange arrows) are to (1) increase intestinal calcium and phosphate absorption;(2) inhibit PTH release; and (3) enhance FGF-23 release
FGF-23 production and release are stimulated by increased phosphate and calcitriol. The actions of FGF-23 (red arrows) are to (1) enhance renal phosphate excretion; (2) inhibit renal calcitriol production; and (3) inhibit PTH release. FGF-23 requires its cofactor, klotho, to exert its biological effects in the kidney

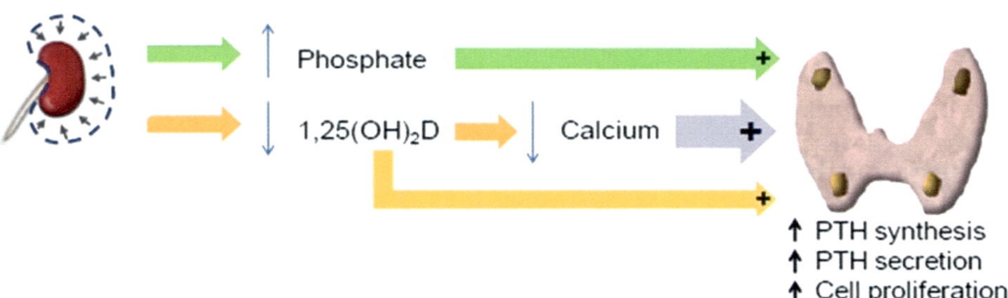

Fig. 71.2 Effects of advanced CKD on mineral metabolism
As glomerular filtration rate (GFR) declines, phosphate accumulates, and calcitriol production decreases with a consequent fall in calcium. These three effects all stimulate PTH synthesis and release. In addition prolonged stimulation results in clonal proliferation of parathyroid cells which express fewer receptors for both vitamin D and calcium. Ultimately the gland becomes unresponsive to these downregulators – tertiary hyperparathyroidism

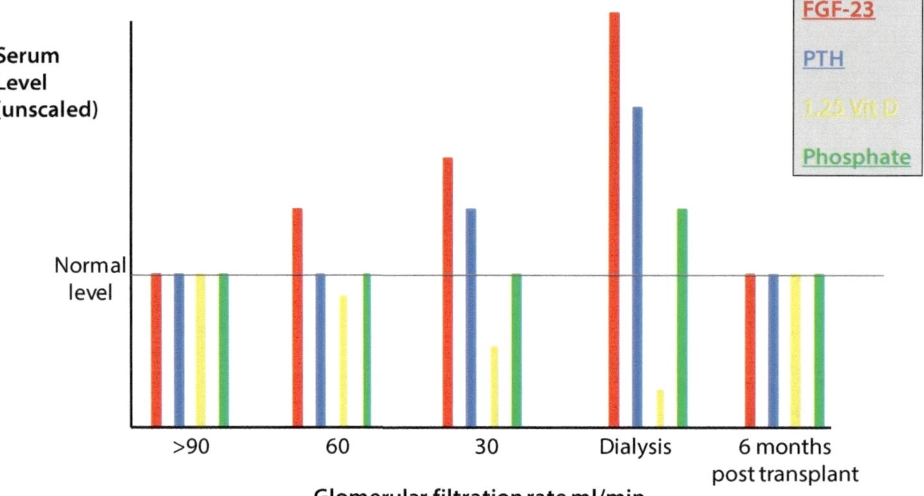

Fig. 71.3 Changes in CKD-MBD-associated biochemical parameters as CKD progresses and following transplantation FGF-23 begins to increase at very early stages of CKD with PTH beginning to climb somewhat later. These two adaptive responses keep serum phosphate levels within the normal range until GFR drops well below 30 ml/min. 1,25-dihydroxyvitamin D begins to fall at a GFR of around 60 ml/min. These changes are corrected with kidney transplantation (provided good function is obtained)

groups. The renal effects of FGF-23 require its cofactor klotho. Klotho itself decreases very early on in CKD.

71.1.2 Renal Bone Disease

The risk of fracture is elevated about fivefold in dialysis patients with the mortality rates following a fracture at least double those seen in the general population.

Renal osteodystrophy comprises alterations of bone morphology in patients with CKD and defines the skeletal component of the systemic disorder of CKD-MBD. It is only quantifiable reliably by bone histology, though bone biopsy is seldom done due to the invasive nature of the procedure and the expertise required for interpretation. Biochemical markers, especially PTH and bone-specific alkaline phosphatase (BALP), are used as surrogates for histology.

71.1.2.1 High Turnover (Hyperparathyroid) Bone Disease

This lesion is characterized by a PTH-driven increase in the activity of osteoblasts (direct) and osteoclasts (indirect) with disordered bone formation, accelerated resorption and evidence of fibrosis on bone biopsy. PTH and BALP are raised. Serum calcium concentrations are variable.

Overt symptoms are not usually apparent until disease is very advanced, at which point potential manifestations include bone pain and deformity, proximal muscle weakness and pruritus secondary to cutaneous mineral deposits. Hyperparathyroid bone disease leads to a marked increase in fracture rates, and children with hyperparathyroid bone disease also exhibit growth failure. Typical radiological features include subperiosteal reabsorption, often seen best in the middle and distal phalanges (see Fig. 71.4).

71.1.2.2 Adynamic Bone Disease (ABD)

This lesion is characterized by decreased bone cell activity, and typical biochemical findings include a raised calcium (adynamic bone buffers calcium poorly) and phosphate, with low normal PTH and BALP. Clinical symptoms are often absent, as are positive radiological findings. Fracture rates are increased, and fractures heal poorly. ABD associates with vascular calcification and high osteopenia risk post-transplantation.

71.1.3 Vascular Calcification (VC)

VC occurs frequently in patients at all stages of CKD, and its severity correlates with survival. Medial calcification of vessels predominates in CKD (compared to intimal disease which is the usual finding in the general population), which leads to arterial stiffening, an increase in afterload and subsequently left ventricular hypertrophy. In addition, calcification can make transplantation and vascular access for dialysis problematic and is probably involved in the development of calciphylaxis (see below). VC involves overlapping and integrated processes including loss of calcification inhibitors, a gain of calcification promoters, cellular apoptosis and a change in phenotype of vascular smooth muscle cells into bone-forming osteoblast-like cells.

Screening for VC is controversial, not least because there are no treatments proven to ameliorate the process.

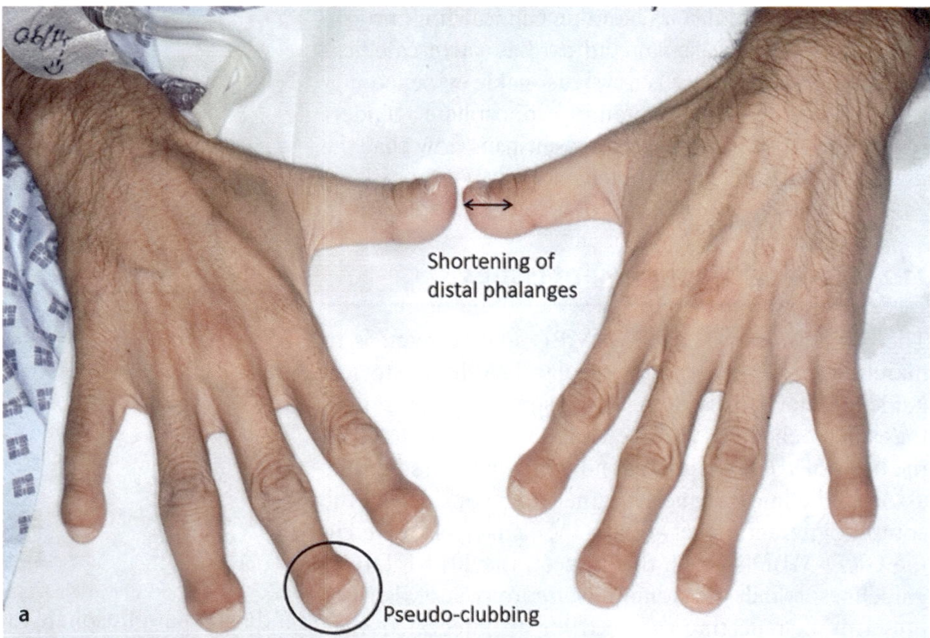

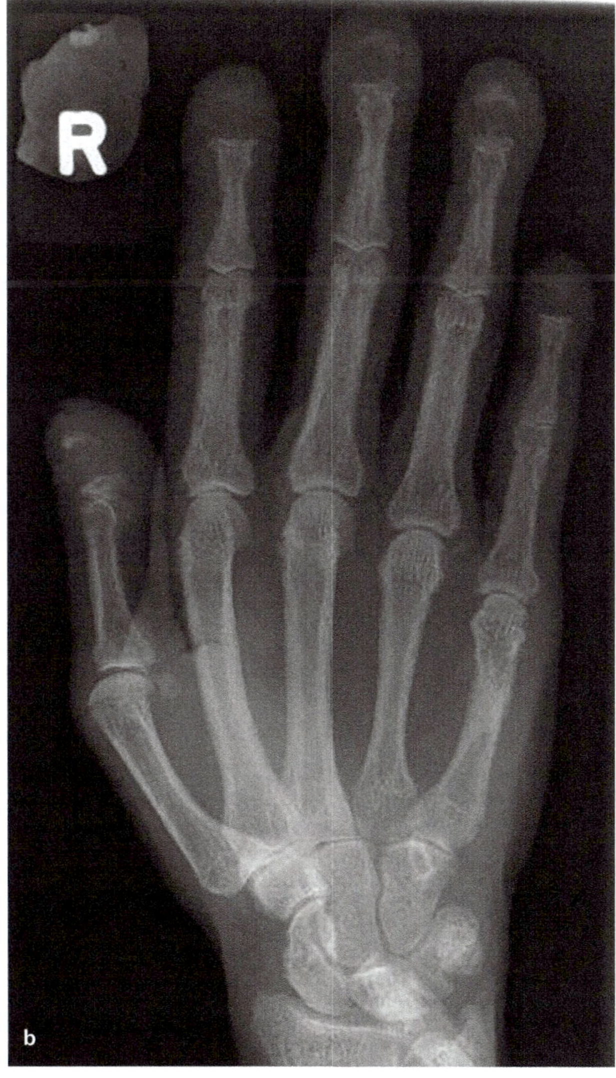

Fig. 71.4 **a** Pseudoclubbing in a patient with severe hyperparathyroid bone disease, **b** radiograph from the same patient showing severe subperiosteal resorption of all phalanges with almost complete loss of terminal phalanges. Image courtesy of Dr Saeed Al-Ghamdi

A lateral abdominal X-ray and an echocardiogram can be used to detect vascular and cardiac valve calcification, respectively. There is now reasonable evidence suggesting that calcium-containing phosphate binders contribute to VC, and expert consensus is now that the use of these agents be restricted.

71.2 General Management Issues

The prime objective of CKD-MBD management is to maintain bone and cardiovascular health. Historical guidelines have focused on setting suitable target ranges for each biochemical parameter and were often made on the basis of trials examining individual markers and the associated clinical sequelae, rather than considering the complex interaction between all the elements involved in the CKD-MBD axis. In this respect, the 2017 KDIGO guidelines, which are admirably rigorous, are also less prescriptive, reflecting the need for an integrated view taking account of trends rather than isolated results (◘ Table 71.1).

The guidelines highlight the fact that many therapeutic interventions influence more than one CKD-MBD parameter and suggest that this should be taken into account during management decisions. ◘ Table 71.2 summarizes the main treatment options available for CKD-MBD along with the expected outcomes of therapy.

71.2.1 Controlling Hyperphosphataemia

Although higher phosphate levels have been shown to associate with increased mortality in some epidemiological studies, there is currently no robust evidence to indicate that phosphate lowering measures improve outcomes. Nonetheless treatment of hyperphosphataemia is generally accepted as standard of care and universally practiced.

◘ **Table 71.1** KDIGO 2017 guidelines see ► www.kdigo.org

CKD stage	Serum phosphorus	Serum calcium	PTH
3–5	Lower towards normal range	Avoid hypercalcaemia	Optimal level is unknown but if level rising or above the upper limit of assay, assess for modifiable factors
5D	Lower towards normal range	Avoid hypercalcaemia	Maintain level at approximately 2–9 times the upper limit of the normal reference range and intervene if level rapidly changing to avoid progression to levels outside this range

◘ **Table 71.2** Effects of available treatments for CKD-MBD. The arrows refer to direction of travel in response to interventions

	Calcium	Phosphate	PTH
Calcium-based phosphate binder	↑↑	↓↓	↓↓
Calcium-free phosphate binder	↔	↓↓	↔
Active vitamin D (alfacalcidol/calcitriol)	↑	↑	↓↓↓
Calcimimetic	↓	↓	↓↓↓
Lower dialysate calcium	↓	↔	↑
Parathyroidectomy	↓	↓	↓↓↓

71.2.1.1 Diet

Phosphate is ubiquitous in the diet, and dietetic input to limit excessive phosphate intake should be a part of any management strategy. Many processed foods and drinks contain large amounts of added inorganic phosphate with the added hazard of extremely high bioavailability.

71.2.1.2 Phosphate Binders

Oral phosphate binders reduce intestinal absorption of phosphate by rendering dietary phosphate less absorbable. Broadly they can be divided into two classes – calcium based (generally cheap) and calcium free (generally expensive). These are suboptimal therapies, being bulky, unpalatable and of low potency, and all must be taken with meals to maximize efficacy. It is hardly surprising that compliance with phosphate binders is poor. To state the obvious, the best phosphate binder is one that the patient will take – and this may require a certain amount of trial and error at the outset.

Calcium-containing agents are relatively cheap and have the advantage that they will suppress PTH. However they augment the overall calcium burden, and numerous studies have linked their use to increased mortality. It is now suggested that the use of these compounds be limited. Some would avoid altogether.

Sevelamer is a calcium-free phosphate binder which when compared to its calcium-containing counterparts has been shown to slow progression of vascular calcification. In addition, it has the benefits of improving lipid profiles and having anti-inflammatory effects, thereby possibly conferring an advantage in terms of vascular health, although these benefits remain potential rather than actual.

Lanthanum carbonate is a calcium free binder with a high binding capacity offering a lower tablet burden. Like sevelamer, GI side effects are problematic, and both are considerably more expensive than the older calcium-based agents.

Aluminium-based binders, whilst available, cheap and effective, are rarely used because of concerns about aluminium toxicity to the CNS (aluminium encephalopathy-dialysis dementia) and to the skeleton (dialysis osteodystrophy, a form of low turnover adynamic bone disease). Both toxicities were seen in epidemic form in the 1970s until aluminium in tap water used to prepare dialysate and in aluminium-based phosphate binders was identified as the causative agent.

Iron-based binders are the newest class to emerge. These are relatively expensive at present but appear to be reasonably well tolerated and efficacious and have the added benefit of potentially improving iron levels and haemoglobin. Their use is likely to increase in the coming years.

In order to try and increase adherence to binder therapy, there is some evidence suggesting that an integrated, multidisciplinary team-led approach can be successful. Such strategies can in some cases involve phosphate binder prescribing by dieticians, who are well placed to tailor therapy to the dietary needs of the patient.

71.2.1.3 Dialysis

Standard markers of dialysis adequacy such as Kt/V calculations are not accurate markers of phosphate removal. The majority of phosphate resides in the intracellular compartment, and as such a significant rebound effect is seen upon completing a haemodialysis session. Longer hours or more frequent sessions (e.g. home dialysis) achieve greater overall phosphate removal although there are clearly practical considerations which limit these options.

71.2.2 Controlling Serum Calcium

The pathophysiology of CKD-MBD exerts downward pressure on serum calcium triggering an adaptive rise of PTH – secondary hyperparathyroidism. Patients with long-standing, previously unrecognized CKD can present with profound hypocalcaemia (<1.5 mmol/L in extreme cases). ECG abnormalities or physical signs of hypocalcaemia require intravenous treatment (see under parathyroidectomy), although if the patient is asymptomatic, oral supplementation with calcium and active vitamin D therapy is appropriate.

Hypercalcaemia is often iatrogenic during therapy with calcium-containing compounds (usually phosphate binders) or active vitamin D. Always check that the patient is only taking what you think they are! Other causes of hypercalcaemia should also be excluded. The treatment of autonomous hyperparathyroidism is discussed under PTH. For patients on dialysis, the calcium concentration of dialysate fluid is important. Typically dialysate calcium should be between 1.25 and 1.50 mmol/L (2.5 and 3.0 mEq/l), with the former being more suitable if calcium-based phosphate binders are used.

71.2.3 PTH

The optimal levels of PTH are unknown. Mild elevations in PTH seen in earlier stages of CKD may well be a beneficial, adaptive, physiological response to combat increasing phosphate levels. Furthermore some therapies designed to lower PTH may do so at the expense of elevating calcium and phosphate. The current consensus is therefore to intervene when PTH is consistently trending upward, rather than acting on isolated values, and to consider (and address) the potential impacts of treatment on the other CKD-MBD parameters (most importantly calcium and phosphate).

Management of an elevated and increasing PTH depends on the level of serum calcium. Most straightforward are those with low to low normal calcium. The appropriate intervention here is with active vitamin D therapy. Treatment options for replacing active vitamin D include the 1-alpha-hydroxylated analogues (calcitriol and alfacalcidol) and the newer vitamin D receptor agonists (paricalcitol, doxercalciferol (USA) and 22-oxacalcitriol (Japan)). Adequate phosphate controlling measures must first be in place whichever agent is used. The therapeutic window of these agents is small, and hence a low starting dose should be used (e.g. 0.25 μg/day alfacalcidol), with titration upwards according to target levels. Administration of iv therapy on dialysis days can aid compliance. Monthly monitoring of calcium and phosphate is essential.

Conversely, in those patients in whom PTH is elevated with an inappropriately raised serum calcium, autonomous hyperparathyroidism is present. Calcimimetics are the best option here. Cinacalcet and the newer intravenous agent, etelcalcetide, bind to and modulate the calcium-sensing receptor, increasing sensitivity to calcium. Consequently, reductions are seen in both serum PTH and calcium.

Calcimimetics can improve biochemical parameters and probably decrease the risk of fractures and parathyroidectomy in CKD patients. Cinacalcet is expensive, and in the UK, the National Institute for Clinical Excellence (NICE) currently only recommends its use for patients with refractory hyperparathyroidism with PTH exceeding 85 pmol/l who are not suitable for a parathyroidectomy. Etelcalcetide is an alternative agent for those not tolerating cinacalcet. Administration is thrice weekly on haemodialysis.

Low PTH usually results from oversuppression with either calcium-containing phosphate binders or active vitamin D agents, another cause of hypercalcaemia or a previous parathyroidectomy.

71.2.3.1 Parathyroidectomy

The main indication for a parathyroidectomy (in patients with CKD) is PTH-dependent hypercalcaemia refractory to other available measures. PTH concentrations will be grossly elevated (typically over 100 pmol/l) with raised calcium and usually increased phosphate and alkaline phosphatase. Conversely, if PTH is very high and if serum calcium is low or low normal, the patient requires further medical therapy with active vitamin D, not a parathyroidectomy.

Surgery requires localization of the parathyroid glands preoperatively and identification of any ectopic tissue. This can be achieved by nuclear medicine scans such as those using methoxyisobutyl isonitrile (MIBI). Subtotal parathyroidectomy is usually preferred over a total procedure. As with thyroid surgery, preoperative assessment by an ear, nose and throat clinician will depend on the local policy.

Unopposed bone uptake of calcium ('hungry bone syndrome') in the early postoperative phase is the most frequently seen complication and is highest in patients with severe disease. High doses of active vitamin D (e.g. 5 μg alfacalcidol/day) are administered for 5 days pre-procedure and decrease, but do not eliminate, the risk of post-operative hypocalcaemia. Intravenous calcium is needed in severe cases.

Following the procedure, careful monitoring of calcium is vital. A typical protocol would be to check blood calcium immediately after the operation, then 4 hourly for the first 24 h and 12 hourly for 2 days. A combination of oral calcium and active vitamin D (e.g. at least 2 g calcium and 2 μg alfacalcidol as starting doses) should be employed, with dose adjustments as appropriate. Calcium and vitamin D requirements decrease over time and can be titrated down in the outpatient clinic.

Severe hypocalcaemia (<1.8 mmol/L) post-operatively, or symptoms of hypocalcaemia, necessitates intravenous (iv) therapy. An initial 10 ml of 10% calcium gluconate (which contains 2.25 mmol calcium) over 2–3 min through a large vein (extravasation can lead to tissue necrosis), repeated if necessary, can be followed by an infusion of 50 ml of 10% calcium gluconate (10 mmol of calcium) in 500 ml of either 5% dextrose or 0.9% saline initially at 2 mmol/h. with adjustments as required. Two hourly clinical assessment and serum calcium measurement are appropriate during iv calcium infusion, and continuous cardiac monitoring is needed.

The other main post-operative complication is bleeding which can cause airway compression and compromise. This is a dangerous scenario necessitating immediate anaesthetic assistance.

71.3 Additional Considerations and Controversies

71.3.1 Native Vitamin D Therapy

Experimentally, vitamin D has been shown to protect against left ventricular hypertrophy, hypertension and renal fibrosis and to have regulatory functions in the immune system and tumourigenesis. It is now clear that the VDR is ubiquitous. Both autocrine and paracrine effects are demonstrable, in addition to classic endocrine effects of calcitriol, and it may therefore be appropriate to replace both 1,25-dihydroxyvitamin D and its precursor 25-hydroxyvitamin D in patients with CKD. Below 75 nmol/L is considered to represent insufficiency, but no definitive guidelines exist in relation to replacement of native vitamin D. A typical regime would be cholecalciferol 20,000 units taken orally once a week. Side effects are minimal, and no significant alterations in calcium or phosphate are seen.

71.3.2 Calciphylaxis

Calciphylaxis, or calcific uraemic arteriolopathy (CUA), is a relatively rare and often fatal complication of CKD-MBD. It is part of the spectrum of vascular calcification in advanced CKD, most often seen in the dialysis population. Initial presentation is with superficial, violaceous, painful, hyperaesthetic or pruritic skin lesions. Secondary infection and overwhelming sepsis can ensue. The most commonly affected areas are the thighs, buttocks and abdomen, although distal lesions are also seen.

The differential diagnosis is relatively wide and includes atheroembolic phenomena, severe ischaemic lesions and vasculitides. The definitive diagnostic investigation for calciphylaxis is a skin biopsy.

The most promising treatment is sodium thiosulphate. This leads to calcium exchange for sodium and results in the highly soluble compound calcium thiosulphate. Experience with its use is limited at present although increasing. A typical dosing regimen would be

25 g iv over 1 h immediately following haemodialysis for patients receiving thrice weekly haemodialysis. The experience in peritoneal dialysis patients and non-dialysis patients is extremely limited. Metabolic acidosis may complicate therapy and necessitate dose adjustment or termination of therapy. Anecdotal evidence also exists for emergency parathyroidectomy, cinacalcet, intensive dialysis and bisphosphonates. It is often exquisitely painful, and therefore regular review of analgesia is important. A referral to a pain specialist may be necessary.

There is an emerging link between warfarin and CUA which is thought to be due to the inhibition of the vitamin K-dependent calcification inhibitor matrix GLA protein. Many advocate withdrawing warfarin if CUA is a diagnostic possibility. In theory novel anticoagulant drugs (NOACs) should not be associated with this complication.

71.3.3 Bone Mineral Density and Fracture Prophylaxis

Dual-energy X-ray absorptiometry (DXA) is the conventional tool used to assess fracture risk and define bone mineral density (BMD) in the general population, though it has been considered less useful in those with CKD. However data have now emerged indicating that DXA can also predict fracture risk in patients with CKD 3–5. How to use this information remains somewhat controversial.

In patients with CKD stages 1–3, BMD assessment and treatment can proceed in the same way as those from the non-CKD population. Bisphosphonates and denosumab are safe and effective in these patients, with the proviso that denosumab is more likely to cause hypocalcaemia as the GFR falls.

Patients with CKD stages 3–5D represent a more difficult cohort. Their bone disease is more heterogeneous, and although treatment could be guided by bone biopsy, this is not always possible. Data concerning the efficacy of bisphosphonates and denosumab in this patient group are limited, and safety is questionable. A multidisciplinary approach is advised, if possible including bone specialists from any of rheumatology, endocrinology or nephrology.

71.3.4 The Transplant Patient

A well-functioning graft will often lead to normalization of calcium and phosphate, enhanced vitamin D production and often dramatic falls of PTH and FGF23. These advantages are somewhat countered by increased bone turnover and a decrease in BMD (particularly during the first 6 months post-transplant). Risk factors for this include an abnormal skeletal substrate from previous dialysis, steroid use and treatment with calcineurin inhibitors. Many transplant centres in the UK are now adopting 'steroid-sparing' protocols to address this and other complications of glucocorticoids.

The lifetime risk of sustaining at least one fracture is significant in transplant recipients. DXA scans may help predict this risk, but there is no robust evidence base to guide management. Early bone loss in these patients is preventable with bisphosphonates, but these agents are not proven to reduce fracture.

71.3.4.1 Avascular Necrosis

This debilitating condition has previously complicated up to 1% of transplant per year and is caused by ischaemic injury to bone parenchyma, particularly the femoral head. Steroid use is the biggest risk factor with others including a longer dialysis vintage, hyperparathyroidism, weight gain and trauma. Presentation is frequently with severe hip pain, especially on weight bearing. MRI is the investigation of choice to detect early disease. Plain X-rays are often normal initially. Steroids should be withdrawn if possible. The role for bisphosphonates is not certain. Orthopaedic surgery is usually required, with decompression procedures initially and ultimately joint replacement.

Tips and Tricks

1. When measuring PTH in the context of CKD, remember mild elevations (to within KDIGO guidelines) can be adaptive and may be beneficial.
2. A combination of diet, dialysis and binders is the most effective strategy for phosphate management, whereas active vitamin D and calcimimetics are most suitable for lowering PTH. Activated vitamin D therapy should not be introduced before phosphate controlling measures are in place.
3. Peri-parathyroidectomy management should be handled by a multidisciplinary team including physicians, endocrine and ENT surgeons, anaesthetists and radiologists. Preloading with calcium and active vitamin D (alfacalcidol) is essential (see text).
4. Total parathyroidectomy commits a patient to life-long risk of adynamic bone disease but also life-threatening hypocalcaemia if intake of alfalcidol and calcium supplements is interrupted. Ensuring that the importance of this medication is clear to the patient and medical contacts is an important responsibility of the renal team.

Case Study

A 56-year-old woman with type 2 diabetes, morbid obesity and CKD presented late to the renal unit in the context of poorly controlled diabetes, heavy proteinuria and other complications of diabetes. She was started on 1-alphacalcidol in the context of a low calcium and proceeded to dialysis via a tunnelled line (she refused a fistula or graft). She often had a raised phosphate which was felt to be dietary and started on calcium carbonate phosphate binders (2 three times a day). Within 24 months of starting, her PTH was significantly raised but in the context of calcium is still within the upper limit of normal. Her oral 1-alphacalcidol was switched to high dose intravenously three times a week on dialysis. Over the next 2 years, she had a variety of admissions for line sepsis and urinary tract infection and then was admitted with a non-ST elevation MI with high troponins and atrial fibrillation. At the time of her coronary angiogram, she was noted to have very calcified coronary vessels. At this point, she had a calcium of 2.71 mmol/L, a PTH six to eight times the upper limit of normal and a phosphate around 2.5 mmol/L. She was anti-coagulated but readmitted 4 weeks later following a fall and a fractured tibia; during her admission, she had severe pain in her thighs and lower abdomen with ischaemic patches consistent with calciphylaxis on biopsy. This was successfully treated with cinacalcet and sodium thiosulphate along with analgesia and meticulous wound care.

This case illustrates some of the issues predisposing to CKD-MBD and the need for long-term strategies to reduce the risk. Earlier referral might have slowed the rate of renal failure and permitted a little more patient education on low phosphate diet. She was almost certainly profoundly 25 OH vitamin D deficient at presentation and subsequently; correcting this before high-dose 1-alphacalcidol supplementation may have corrected the calcium without the same degree of phosphate retention. Poor dialysis via her line contributed to her high phosphate levels. Several features including her obesity, diabetes and subsequent tertiary hyperparathyroidism put her at risk of vascular calcification; in this setting, an alternative to a calcium-based phosphate binder might have been considered. In this context, the choice of warfarin for anticoagulation may well have precipitated calciphylaxis in a high-risk patient.

Chapter Review Questions

1. What are the physiological actions of PTH?
2. What are the physiological actions of FGF-23?
3. What is the increase in fracture risk for dialysis patients and fracture-associated mortality, compared to the general population?
4. What is calciphylaxis and what are the risk factors?

Answers

1. PTH acts to maintain calcium levels and is important in ensuring a dynamic skeleton. It releases both calcium and phosphate from the bone, increases production of renal calcitriol and increases renal tubular reabsorption of calcium and renal excretion of phosphate (via the proximal tubular sodium phosphate cotransporter). In the setting of tertiary hyperparathyroidism, maladaptive effects contribute to renal osteodystrophy, fractures, cardiac fibrosis, vascular calcification, hypertension, neuropathy and impotence.
2. FGF-23 acts to inhibit calcitriol production (decreasing 1α-hydroxylase and increasing metabolism), increase renal phosphate excretion (via the proximal tubular sodium phosphate transporter) and inhibit PTH release. Levels climb significantly with declining GFR and dialysis but fall after successful transplantation.
3. Fractures in the dialysis population are approximately five times more common than in the general population and are associated with roughly twice the mortality.
4. Calciphylaxis is a calcific uraemic arthropathy resulting small vessel ischaemia and infarction typically of the skin and subcutaneous tissue most commonly in the lower half of the body. It is extremely painful and associated with a high mortality. Risk factors for developing calciphylaxis include warfarin use, diabetes, obesity, Caucasian race, female gender and malnutrition.

Suggested Further Reading

British Renal Association guidelines for managing CKD-MBD available at www.renal.org.

Cunningham J, Zehnder D. New vitamin D analogs and changing therapeutic paradigms. Kidney Int. 2011;79:702–7.

Cunningham J, Locatelli F, Rodriguez M. Secondary hyperparathyroidism: pathogenesis, disease progression, and therapeutic options. Clin J Am Soc Nephrol. 2011;6:913–21.

Hruska K, Mathew S, Lund R, Fang Y, Sugatani T. Cardiovascular risk factors in chronic kidney disease: does phosphate qualify? Kidney Int Suppl. 2011;121:S9–13.

Hsu CY. FGF-23 and outcomes research – when physiology meets epidemiology. N Engl J Med. 2008;359:640–2.

KDIGO guidelines on CKD-MBD available at www.kdigo.org.

Miller PD. Diagnosis and treatment of osteoporosis in chronic renal disease. Semin Nephrol. 2009;29:144–55.

Moe SM, Chen NX. Mechanisms of vascular calcification in chronic kidney disease. J Am Soc Nephrol. 2008;19:213–6.

Ott SM. Bisphosphonate safety and efficacy in chronic kidney disease. Kidney Int. 2012;82:833–5.

Ross EA. Evolution of treatment strategies for Calciphylaxis. Am J Nephrol. 2011;34:460–7.

Resources for Patients

'Phosphorus and your CKD diet': available from the National Kidney Foundation at http://www.kidney.org.

Information from the UK National Kidney Federation concerning CKD-MBD available at: https://www.kidney.org.uk/help-and-info/medical-information-from-the-nkf-/medical-info-calcium-phosphate-index/.

Kidney Research UK factsheet on renal bone disease available at: http://www.kidneyresearchuk.org/health/factsheets/ckd-and-issues/bone-disease-in-chronic.php.

Anaemia Management in Chronic Kidney Disease

Iain C. Macdougall

Contents

M. Harber (ed.), *Primer on Nephrology*, https://doi.org/10.1007/978-3-030-76419-7_72

Learning Objectives

1. To understand the importance and implications of anaemia as a major complication of chronic kidney disease
2. To understand how best to diagnose and investigate this condition with regard to key laboratory tests
3. To understand how best to manage this condition, using erythropoiesis-stimulating agents, iron supplementation and blood transfusions
4. To learn about a potential new treatment for this condition (HIF prolyl hydroxylase inhibitors)

72.1 Introduction

Anaemia is a highly prevalent complication in patients with chronic kidney disease, occurring in around 5% of patients with CKD stage 3 and increasing to around 95% of patients on chronic haemodialysis. It is associated with a number of adverse outcomes, including death and nonfatal cardiovascular events, and it also has an adverse effect on patients' physical capacity and quality of life. Anaemic CKD patients also show a much increased requirement for red cell transfusions compared to those whose anaemia is corrected.

There is no absolute cut-off to define anaemia in the CKD population. The World Health Organisation just over half a century ago defined anaemia in males as indicating a haemoglobin concentration <13 g/dl and in females a haemoglobin concentration <12 g/dl. This was based on statistics from the general population. In the CKD population, an arbitrary definition of anaemia was a haemoglobin concentration <11 g/dl, based on previous guidelines for triggering the use of erythropoiesis-stimulating agent (ESA) therapy.

The remainder of this chapter will discuss the practical aspects of anaemia management, using a stepwise approach. The role of ESA therapy and iron supplementation will be discussed, as will the use of blood transfusions. Finally, some guidelines on anaemia management will be highlighted and referenced.

72.2 Practical Stepwise Approach to CKD Anaemia Management

Broadly speaking, a pragmatic approach to anaemia management in patients with chronic kidney disease should follow a stepwise approach using four steps:

- *Step 1: Exclude Other Causes of Anaemia*
  - Although the major cause of anaemia associated with chronic kidney disease is due to inappropriately low circulating erythropoietin levels [1], there are many other causes of anaemia, and these should be excluded before any consideration is given to using ESA therapy. These include chronic blood loss, nutritional deficiencies, haemolysis, sepsis and malignancy.
- *Step 2: Iron Management*
  - Iron deficiency is also an important contributory cause of anaemia in renal patients, and this too should be investigated and treated in any CKD patient found to be anaemic [2]. Intravenous iron therapy is widely used in the CKD population, particularly in haemodialysis patients where iron losses are unable to be matched by dietary or oral iron supplementation.
- *Step 3: ESA Therapy*
  - Since most patients with CKD anaemia have inappropriately low erythropoietin levels, it is logical to replace this with supplemental ESA therapy. The earlier agents were recombinant human erythropoietin (epoetin), although longer-acting EPO analogues have since become available. These agents have transformed the management of CKD anaemia, particularly in haemodialysis patients, many of whom were heavily transfusion-dependent prior to 1990 when ESA therapy first became available.
- *Step 4: Blood Transfusions*
  - Red cell transfusions are generally a last resort for patients actively bleeding or requiring an urgent top-up prior to a renal biopsy or a surgical procedure. Their role in chronic anaemia should be restricted to severe symptomatic anaemia unresponsive to ESA therapy or iron supplementation [3].

72.3 Excluding Other Causes of Anaemia

Data from the US National Health and Nutrition Examination Survey (NHANES 3) provide helpful information on the expected mean haemoglobin at various stages of CKD [4]. Anaemia is uncommon in CKD stages 1 and 2, starts to develop in early stage 3 and becomes highly prevalent in late stages 3, 4 and 5. The vast majority of patients on chronic dialysis are anaemic to a greater or lesser extent. Thus, CKD patients in stages 1, 2 and early stage 3 who are found to be anaemic require stringent investigations for other causes of anaemia, since renal anaemia alone is much less likely. 'Pure' renal anaemia is usually normochromic and normocytic, and either a low or high MCV or low MCH or MCHC strongly suggests other contributory causes.

Examination of the blood cell indices, white cell and platelet counts may be helpful (Table 72.1). In

Table 72.1 Abnormalities of MCV, MCH, MCHC and RDW

Low MCV	Iron deficiency
	Haemoglobinopathies
	Aluminium intoxication
	Sirolimus
High MCV	B_{12}/folate deficiency
	Hypothyroidism
	Alcohol
	Azathioprine
	Mycophenolate
	Myelodysplastic syndrome
Low MCH	Iron deficiency
	Haemoglobinopathies
High MCH, MCHC	Haemolytic uraemic syndrome
High RDW	Recent blood transfusion
	Iron therapy

previous times, a low MCV was suggestive of aluminium overload, either through poor quality dialysis or the use of aluminium-containing phosphate binders. Aluminium overload is no longer a problem in current times due to modern-day dialysis techniques. A low MCV can occur with sideroblastic anaemia (e.g. secondary to tuberculosis) and is also common in patients receiving sirolimus therapy; the exact cause of this is not known at the present time. There are quite a number of important causes of a high MCV that should be considered (Table 72.1). It is important to exclude B_{12} or folate deficiency, as well as hypothyroidism. Other causes of a raised MCV include drug therapy, notably azathioprine or mycophenolate, and in elderly patients, an elevated MCV (often very high) may be a feature of myelodysplastic syndrome.

In patients of certain ethnic backgrounds, e.g. Africans (sickle cell anaemia) and natives of some Mediterranean countries such as Greece (thalassaemia), haemoglobin electrophoresis should be performed to ascertain whether or not the patient has a haemoglobinopathy. In progressive iron deficiency, the red cells will become hypochromic and deficient in intracellular haemoglobin before the MCV becomes abnormal. A decreased MCH or MCHC therefore indicates long-standing iron deficiency; if a low MCV is also evident, then this suggests an even longer exposure to iron deficiency.

A sudden change in MCV or other red cell parameters (such as red cell width (RDW)) suggests that the patient may have been transfused. This is the most likely cause of a rapid increase or decrease in MCV as well as a sharp rise in RDW, both suggesting more than one population of circulating red cells.

Abnormalities of white cell count or platelet count suggest an underlying haematological disorder, which may justify a bone marrow examination if there is no other obvious cause.

72.4 Reticulocyte Count

In previous times, reticulocytes were counted under the microscope on a blood film. This was not only laborious for the haematology technician but was also very inaccurate. Modern-day automated blood count analysers now allow a very accurate reticulocyte count to be measured, and this is usually expressed in two ways: (1) absolute count and (2) percentage reticulocyte count of the total red cell population. The absolute count is generally more helpful, and a normal reticulocyte count in healthy individuals should be between 50 and 100×10^9/l. CKD patients may run reticulocyte counts of around 30–60 × 10^9/l, but clearly this may be higher if the patient is receiving high doses of all ESA therapy. Reticulocyte counts lower than 40–50 × 10^9/l on ESA therapy suggest a degree of bone marrow failure, and low reticulocyte counts may indicate a need for a bone marrow examination. Very low reticulocyte counts of <10 × 10^9/l suggest severe bone marrow failure, such as occurs with antibody-mediated pure red cell aplasia or aplastic anaemia. Antibody-mediated pure red cell aplasia is a complication of ESA therapy, caused by antibodies developing against the ESA that cross-react with endogenous erythropoietin, effectively shutting down red cell production in the bone marrow [5]. The condition is confirmed on bone marrow examination where absence or near absence of erythroid progenitor cells in the bone marrow is evident. Circulating anti-erythropoietin antibodies may be detectable by immunoassay, and the patient is often transfusion-dependent. The condition is managed by, firstly, stopping the ESA, transfusing as required to correct severe anaemia and then introducing immunosuppressive therapy such as prednisolone and ciclosporin (or cyclophosphamide) to suppress further antibody production [5]. A novel peptide-based ESA called peginesatide (see below), which does not cross-react with anti-erythropoietin antibodies, has been shown to 'rescue' patients with this condition [6].

Higher reticulocyte counts (e.g. >100 × 10^9/l) suggest an active bone marrow, but in the presence of anaemia, this indicates enhanced red cell loss, either due to haemolysis or bleeding.

CKD patients are also prone to a number of acute and chronic inflammatory conditions, and measurement of C-reactive protein may potentially suggest an underlying infective or inflammatory cause. Other clues may be a low serum albumin level or high ferritin level, since both of these laboratory parameters are part of the acute phase response. A well-recognised, but often ignored, cause of chronic inflammation is a failed kidney transplant, still in situ, which may potentially harbour a massive pool of pro-inflammatory cytokines.

A detailed history for possible causes of blood loss should be taken, and there may be a need for an upper gastrointestinal endoscopy, colonoscopy or even small bowel video capsule enteroscopy. A low ferritin level, particularly if this persists despite repeated top-up injections of intravenous iron, may provide additional impetus for subjecting the patient to more detailed gastrointestinal investigations.

If haemolysis is suspected, then a blood film may be useful to detect red cell fragments. A positive Coombs test may indicate an immune-mediated haemolysis, while a raised bilirubin or LDH level would also be consistent with a haemolytic process. A low serum haptoglobin level is highly suggestive of underlying haemolysis. Thus, any patient who does not appear to be bleeding but who has a high reticulocyte count and/or a normal or high ferritin level should be assessed for underlying haemolysis by measuring a bilirubin level, LDH, serum haptoglobins, blood film and Coombs test.

Other, more specialist, tests of causes of both renal impairment and anaemia may be indicated in certain circumstances, e.g. myeloma may induce both kidney and bone marrow disease, causing renal dysfunction and anaemia together. Thus, serum electrophoresis, looking for a paraprotein, and/or measurement of serum free light chains may be indicated.

72.5 Iron Management

72.5.1 Iron Deficiency: Absolute Versus Functional

For the last two decades, iron deficiency has been categorised as either *absolute* or *functional* [2]. *Absolute* iron deficiency implies that there is a deficiency in total body iron stores, such that there are inadequate levels of iron to supply the bone marrow. The two types of iron deficiency are often compared to a bank account. Absolute iron deficiency is when there is simply not enough money in the bank to be able to make a withdrawal.

Functional iron deficiency is a condition in which there are normal or even increased levels of total body iron stores, but there is a failure to be able to mobilise this iron for use by the bone marrow for erythropoiesis. To continue the bank account analogy, functional iron deficiency is illustrated by a condition in which there are ample amounts of money in a savings account, but this cannot be withdrawn on demand.

There are two types of *functional* iron deficiency. The first occurs when erythropoiesis is stimulated pharmacologically by ESA therapy. Such is the demand for iron that the iron supply becomes a rate-limiting step, and this is usually manifest by an increase in the percentage of hypochromic red cells.

The second type of *functional* iron deficiency occurs when there is an inflammatory blockade of iron release from its stores in the reticuloendothelial system. This is mediated by hepcidin, which is the master regulator of iron availability [7]. Hepcidin is upregulated in any acute or chronic inflammatory state, largely mediated via interleukin-6, although other pro-inflammatory cytokines may play a part. Hepcidin exerts its physiological effect by binding to the cellular iron export protein, ferroportin, thereby preventing any iron efflux from cells responsible for iron transport, such as duodenal enterocytes, macrophages, Kupffer cells and splenocytes. Since one of the major rate-limiting steps in this process is the absorption of iron from the gut, it is possible to circumvent this by the administration of intravenous iron.

72.5.2 Detection of Iron Deficiency

There is no ideal test to confirm or refute the diagnosis of iron deficiency. The exception to this is a very low serum ferritin level (e.g. <20 ug/l), which conclusively proves a diagnosis of absolute iron deficiency. There is no other cause of such a low serum ferritin level. However, the majority of patients have ferritin levels above this, and yet many of them are also iron-deficient. There are many other laboratory tests available for assessing iron status (◘ Table 72.2). Serum iron on its own is unhelpful, but its relationship to the total iron-binding capacity (TIBC) expressed as a percentage (transferrin saturation) may support a diagnosis of iron insufficiency.

Several studies have investigated the possible role of percentage hypochromic red cells as an indicator of functional iron deficiency, and in a ROC (receptor operator curve) analysis, this parameter was found to be the best in predicting a response to intravenous iron [8].

Serum transferrin receptor is used outside the renal setting, but unfortunately for patients receiving ESA therapy, it is less helpful. The two drivers of an increase in serum transferrin receptor are iron deficiency and increased erythropoiesis, and for patients receiving ESA therapy, this may be problematic. Erythrocyte zinc protoporphyrin levels remain a research investigation with

Table 72.2 Markers of iron status

Marker	Characteristics
Serum ferritin	Reasonable marker of iron stores, but artificially elevated in the presence of inflammation or liver disease
Transferrin saturation (TSAT)	Subject to considerable diurnal variation; widely used in the USA
Hypochromic red cells	Several studies suggest that this is the most sensitive/specific marker of iron deficiency but requires to be performed on a fresh blood sample and requires specific automated blood count analysers which are not widely available
Reticulocyte haemoglobin content (CHr)	Also a fairly sensitive/specific marker of iron deficiency but requires specific automated blood count analysers which are not widely available
MCV, MCH, MCHC	Abnormalities of these red cell indices will only occur in long-standing iron deficiency and therefore are not a sensitive marker of iron status
Serum transferrin receptor	Used outside the nephrology setting, but not helpful in patients receiving ESA therapy since this parameter will increase in either iron deficiency or enhanced erythropoiesis
Erythrocyte zinc protoporphyrin levels	Largely a research investigation with no practical applicability
Serum hepcidin levels	A novel biomarker of iron status which remains experimental
Bone marrow	Useful investigation, but invasive and not practical for repeat assessments

no clinical applicability. Bone marrow examination for stainable iron may be helpful but is clearly more invasive than the other laboratory tests. As previously mentioned, the red cell indices such as MCH and MCHC may indicate a long-standing iron deficiency. Measurement of serum hepcidin is a novel biomarker which has been investigated as a marker of iron insufficiency, but the results to date have been disappointing [9].

72.5.3 Iron Supplementation: Oral Versus Intravenous?

Oral iron supplementation is simple and cheap to administer, with a cost of only a few pence per week. Unfortunately, in many CKD patients, iron absorption is impaired due to hepcidin upregulation, and this renders oral iron supplementation ineffective. Although hepcidin levels progressively increase with worsening kidney function, it is largely in late stage 3 onwards that they reach a level when oral iron is most likely to be ineffective.

Iron requirements in haemodialysis patients are almost universally too great for oral iron supplementation to keep pace with the demand, and this patient population is usually treated with intravenous iron [2]. Non-dialysis CKD patients, those on peritoneal dialysis and kidney transplant recipients may receive oral iron first, although the other problem with this mode of administration is a high incidence of gastrointestinal side effects due to a local Fenton reaction at the site of the gastric or colonic mucosa. Compliance with oral iron supplementation is often poor due to these side effects. Finally, many drugs may interfere with iron absorption such as proton pump inhibitors (e.g. omeprazole), phosphate binders and certain antibiotics such as ciprofloxacin. Certain foodstuffs and tea may also impair dietary iron absorption.

If oral iron supplements are used, then the first choice is often ferrous sulphate. Attempts to reduce gastrointestinal side effects include taking iron supplements with meals, but this will also reduce their absorption. Other iron salts such as ferrous fumarate or ferrous succinate are sometimes reported as being better tolerated. The reason for this is that they contain lower amounts of elemental iron.

In recent times, ferric citrate has become available as an oral iron supplement in CKD patients. This was initially developed as a phosphate binder, but it subsequently became apparent that significant amounts of iron were absorbed, even in advanced or end-stage CKD.

Intravenous iron is, however, used widely in the CKD setting. Not only does this guarantee a readily available supply of iron, but it is extremely easy to administer to a haemodialysis population who already have vascular access in situ. Thus, intravenous iron is usually administered on dialysis.

There are several IV iron preparations available (Table 72.3). All of these have a core containing the iron salt, surrounded by a carbohydrate shell to allow the slow release of the iron (Fig. 72.1). The older iron preparations such as iron dextran carried a small but definite risk of anaphylaxis due to preformed dextran antibodies. This was more prevalent with high-molecular-weight iron dextran compared to low-molecular-weight iron dextran compounds, and the HMW dextran preparation (Dexferrum®) is no longer licensed.

Iron sucrose has been around for many years and is tried and tested in millions of doses worldwide. The dose usually administered is 100 or 200 mg, since tolerance at higher doses is reduced. Iron gluconate is not

Table 72.3 Requirements for a test dose and dosing schedule for various IV iron preparations licensed in the USA and Europe, as per the product label

IV iron preparation	Country/ region	Test dose required	Dosing schedule
Iron dextran – LMW (INFeD®)	USA	Yes	100 mg bolus injection or slow IV infusion of up to 20 mg/kg
Iron dextran – LMW (CosmoFer®)	Europe	No	100 mg bolus injection or slow IV infusion of up to 20 mg/kg
Iron sucrose (Venofer®)	USA	No	100–200 mg bolus over 5–10 min, respectively
Iron sucrose (Venofer®)	Europe	No	100–200 mg bolus over 5–10 min, respectively
Ferric gluconate (Ferrlecit®)	USA, Germany, Italy	No	62.5–12.5 mg bolus over 5–10 min
Ferumoxytol (Feraheme®)	USA	No	510 mg infusion over 30 min
Ferric carboxy-maltose (Ferinject®)	Europe	No	500 mg bolus over 6 min
Ferric carboxy-maltose (Ferinject®)	Europe	No	1 g infusion over 15 min (max 20 mg/kg)
Iron isomalto-side (Monofer®)	Europe	No	500 mg bolus over 30 min
Iron isomalto-side (Monofer®)	Europe	No	1 g infusion over 60 min (max 20 mg/kg)

LMW low molecular weight

licensed or marketed in the UK but is used widely in the USA, Italy and Germany.

There are three more recently approved IV iron preparations approved for use in either the USA or Europe. These include ferric carboxymaltose (Ferinject® in Europe or Injectafer® in the USA), iron isomaltoside (Monofer® in Europe only) and ferumoxytol (Feraheme® in the USA only). These newer IV preparations may be administered in a larger dose over a shorter period of time and do not require a test dose. There may be lower levels of free iron and oxidative stress with these newer preparations, although clinical and hard outcome data are lacking.

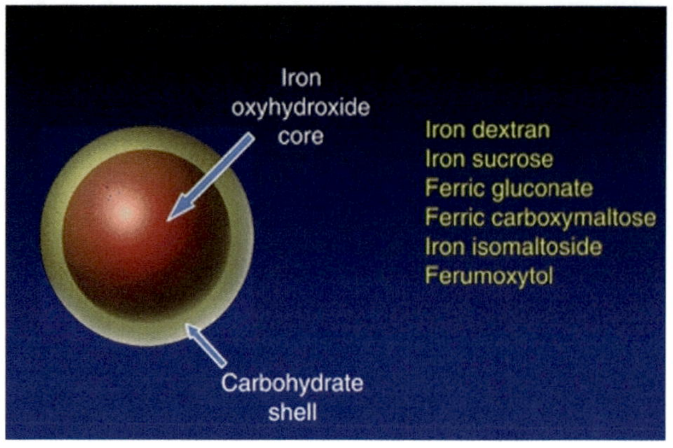

Fig. 72.1 IV iron preparations

In some countries, such as France and Spain, iron sucrose 'similars' are marketed. It is clear, however, that these products are very different from the iron sucrose originator (Venofer®), with different levels of oxidative stress and also different efficacy.

The choice of IV iron preparation depends on the patient population to be treated. Thus, iron sucrose (Venofer®) is often the IV iron of choice for haemodialysis patients (mainly due to cost), with boluses of 100 or 200 mg being administered once a month or once weekly depending on iron requirements. A recent randomised controlled trial (PIVOTAL, **P**roactive **IV** Ir**O**n **T**herapy in Haemodi**AL**ysis Patients) suggested that a proactive high-dose IV iron regimen (aiming to give 400 mg of iron sucrose a month with a safety cut-off of ferritin 700 ug/l and transferrin saturation 40%) reduced the risk of all-cause death, myocardial infarction and hospitalisation for heart failure, with no increase in infections or other safety concerns,

For non-dialysis patients, the choice of IV iron is a balance between patient convenience and cost. Traditionally, many such patients received repeated boluses of IV iron sucrose, 200 mg at a time, but often three separate visits were required to administer the required amount of IV iron. The newer IV iron preparations allow larger doses to be administered at a single visit, and thus doses of 500 or 1000 mg can be given as either a slow bolus injection or a fairly rapid IV infusion. Although the newer IV irons are slightly more costly, this is balanced by savings on repeated outpatient visits and transport costs.

72.6 Reactions to IV Iron

Over the years, IV iron administration has been notorious for causing immediate hypersensitivity-type anaphylactoid reactions. As previously mentioned, the iron dextran-containing preparation caused type I anaphylactic reactions, which resulted in several fatalities. The modern-day intravenous iron preparations do not usually induce anaphylactic reactions but may rarely cause hypersensitivity reactions. These include hypotensive episodes, characterised by sudden onset of dizziness and light-headedness and associated with a fall in blood pressure. This usually responds to lying the patient supine, and there is usually no need to give antiallergenic treatment such as adrenaline or steroids. The reaction is usually self-limiting after periods of a few minutes up to half an hour. Admission to hospital is not usually necessary.

These reactions to IV iron are rare but can be frightening for both the patient and the healthcare professional, and appropriate debriefing for the patient is important as they are likely to be dependent on further IV iron.

72.7 ESA Therapy

Erythropoiesis-stimulating agents remain the cornerstone of CKD anaemia management. They were introduced in 1990, and they transformed the management of anaemia in dialysis patients, many of whom were transfusion-dependent and iron overloaded.

72.8 Epoetins

The first generation of ESAs were the recombinant human erythropoietins, epoetin alfa (Eprex®) and epoetin beta (NeoRecormon®). Both products are fairly short-acting, with a plasma half-life of between 6 and 8 h, and this requires them to be administered by intravenous or subcutaneous injection two or three times weekly. Following the expiration of the patent for these products, several biosimilar epoetins have recently appeared on the market, including epoetin zeta (Retacrit®) and biosimilar epoetin alfa (Binocrit®). Another recombinant human erythropoietin (epoetin theta, Eporatio®) has also been licensed.

72.9 Darbepoetin Alfa

The main difference between darbepoetin alfa (*Aranesp*®) and the epoetins is the presence of an additional two N-linked carbohydrate chains to enhance the metabolic stability of the molecule in vivo. Thus, the intravenous half-life of darbepoetin alfa is approximately 25 h, while the subcutaneous half-life is between 48 and 70 h. This property allows less frequent dosing, and this product is effective once weekly or once every 2 weeks. Moreover, in some patients, once monthly dosing is possible.

72.10 Methoxy Polyethylene Glycol-Epoetin Beta

Methoxypolyethylene glycol-epoetin beta (CERA, Mircera®) was created by attaching a pegylation chain to the epoetin beta molecule. This considerably prolonged the circulating half-life of the molecule to around 130 h, which allows once monthly administration. This is particularly useful in non-dialysis patients.

72.11 Peginesatide

In March 2012, peginesatide was licensed as an ESA in the USA (Omontys®). Peginesatide is an EPO-mimetic peptide that has no structural homology with erythropoietin but shares the same biological and functional properties as the native or recombinant protein. Thus, it simulates erythropoiesis by binding to the erythropoietin receptor and evoking the same intracellular signalling cascade. Four large phase 3 clinical trials of this product were conducted (PEARL 1 and 2 EMERALD 1 and 2) [10, 11], allowing a cumulative exposure in approximately 2600 patients. As described above, in contrast to the other licensed ESAs, peginesatide does not cross-react with anti-erythropoietin antibodies, and thus this molecule may be used to 'rescue' patients who have developed an antibody-mediated pure red cell aplasia with the other ESAs [6]. In March 2013, following several severe reactions to peginesatide (including a few fatalities), however, the product was voluntarily recalled by the manufacturer and at the present time is no longer available.

The practical issues with the use of all ESAs are the trigger haemoglobin concentration for introducing therapy, the target haemoglobin range for treatment and the management of a poor response to ESA therapy.

Until recently, physicians had no reason to suppose that there was any clinically meaningful difference between short-acting and long-acting ESAs. However, a rigorous observational study from Japan examined nearly 200,000 haemodialysis patients comparing mortality outcomes and found results suggesting that there was a greater risk of all-cause death among patients treated with long-acting ESAs (such as darbepoetin and methoxy polyethylene glycol-epoetin beta) compared to the epoetins [12].

72.12 Trigger Haemoglobin Concentration

Four randomised controlled trials (US Normal Hematocrit Trial [12], CREATE study [13], CHOIR study [14] and the TREAT study [15]) all suggested potential safety concerns with the use of ESA therapy to normalise the haemoglobin concentration. The latter was the most scientifically robust and influential study, being a randomised double-blind, placebo-controlled trial in over 4000 non-dialysis diabetic CKD patients. The results of this trial compared various outcomes in two groups of patients, the first group being randomised to target a haemoglobin of 13 g/dl, while the second group received placebo, being rescued only if their haemoglobin fell below 9 g/dl. Targeting a higher haemoglobin concentration showed a significant reduction in the use of blood transfusions but only a modest improvement in quality of life. Against this was a significant increase in a number of adverse events, such as a doubling of stroke risk, doubling of venous thromboembolism, significant increase in arterial thromboembolism and a more than tenfold increase in cancer-related mortality in the subpopulation of patients previously diagnosed with a malignancy [15]. The results from this study suggest that for CKD patients, ESA therapy should be introduced somewhere around 9–10 g/dl, with the aim of preventing patients falling below 9 g/dl. This trigger haemoglobin concentration is somewhat lower than was previously recommended in both US and European clinical practice guidelines. Because of concerns about increasing tumour growth and worsening the risk of venous thromboembolism, ESA therapy should be used with caution in all patients with cancer, and the benefit to risk ratio should be carefully evaluated.

Table 72.4 Causes of hyporesponsiveness to erythropoiesis-stimulating agent therapy

Common	Iron deficiency
	Infection/inflammation
	Underdialysis
Less common	Blood loss
	Hyperparathyroidism
	Aluminium toxicity
	Vitamin B_{12}/folate deficiency
	Haemolysis
	Bone marrow disorders
	Haemoglobinopathies
	Angiotensin-converting enzyme inhibitors
	Carnitine deficiency
	Obesity (in subcutaneous administration)
	Anti-EPO antibodies (pure red cell aplasia)

72.13 Target Haemoglobin

The results of the TREAT study have also impacted on the target haemoglobin concentration. Whereas, previously, guidelines had suggested targeting a haemoglobin concentration of between 11 and 12 g/dl, this has now been reduced to around 10–12 g/dl. Indeed, the KDIGO Anemia Guideline published in 2012 suggests an upper limit of 11.5 g/dl [16] (see below).

72.14 Poor Response to ESA Therapy

There are two types of poor response to ESAs. The first is a failure to show an increase in haemoglobin concentration despite repeated increases in ESA dose. The second is characterised by a loss of response to treatment, again despite increased ESA doses. Both of these conditions require a careful systematic approach.

The causes of hyporesponsiveness to ESA therapy are several (Table 72.4). Investigating a patient who is showing hyporesponsiveness to ESA therapy demands a stepwise approach (Fig. 72.2). If the patient is self-injecting, adherence to therapy should be questioned and confirmed. The reticulocyte count may give a clue as to whether there is a primary problem with erythropoiesis or whether the bone marrow is already working overtime, but the red cell survival is reduced as a result of bleeding or haemolysis.

The possibility of either absolute or functional iron deficiency should be entertained, and a trial of IV iron may be indicated. A raised CRP may suggest active infection or inflammation, and this should be vigorously investigated. Occult conditions such as tuberculosis or malignancy may prove hard to elucidate. An increase in dialysis prescription and/or a change from conventional haemodialysis to haemodiafiltration may be of benefit. Screening for B_{12} or folate deficiency, blood loss or haemolysis may be indicated. A sharp fall in haemoglobin coupled with a very low reticulocyte count should alert the physician to the very rare condition of antibody-mediated pure red cell aplasia. Bone marrow examination may be required to exclude some haematological conditions such as myelodysplastic syndrome. A higher reticulocyte count makes it more likely that bleeding or haemolysis is the cause, and a full haemolytic screen and possible G-I investigations may be indicated.

Whereas, previously, physicians were happy to continue escalating the dose of ESA therapy, the randomised controlled trials mentioned above have suggested possible harm in using high doses in EPO-resistant patients. It is not clear whether the poor outcomes in this situation are due to the high doses of ESA therapy per se

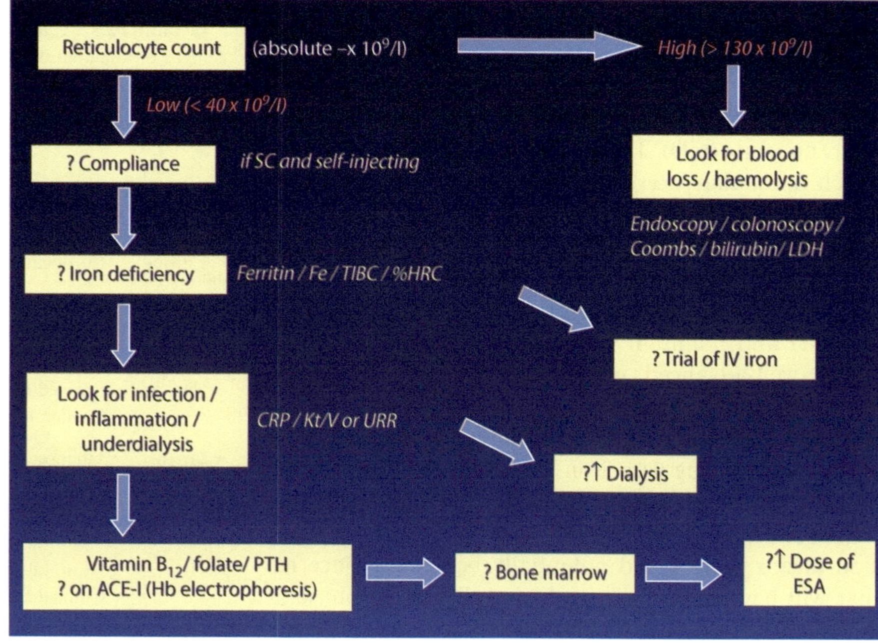

Fig. 72.2 Investigation of hyporesponsiveness to erythropoiesis-stimulating agent therapy. ACEI angiotensin-converting enzyme inhibitors, CRP C-reactive protein, ESA erythropoiesis-stimulating agent, Hb haemoglobin, PTH parathyroid hormone, URR urea reduction ratio

or whether this simply represents a 'sicker' group of patients. Nevertheless, repeated dose escalation is no longer advised, and a maximum dose of epoetin of around 15,000 units per week in divided doses seems reasonable. This translates into a weekly dose of approximately 75 ug of darbepoetin alfa or a monthly dose of approximately 300 ug of methoxy polyethylene glycol-epoetin beta.

72.15 Blood Transfusions

Prior to 1990, red cell transfusions were very frequently used in chronic haemodialysis patients. The advent of erythropoietin therapy led to a dramatic reduction in the incidence of transfusions, the annual report of the US Renal Data System (USRDS) in 2009 indicating a halving of blood transfusions from around 14% to around 7% over the first decade of ESA use, and during the same period, average haemoglobins increased by 2 g/dl [17].

Given the safety concerns associated with ESA therapy, red cell transfusions are once again being used more liberally in CKD patients. The major concerns associated with blood transfusion use are the fairly rare occurrence of transmission of infectious agents and some rare but life-threatening transfusion reactions, such as transfusion-related lung injury and transfusion-related acute circulatory overload, but the main concern with their use in CKD patients is the risk of HLA sensitisation [18].

Recent data from the USRDS confirm that this remains a problem, and HLA sensitisation is associated with a longer waiting time for kidney transplantation, reduced likelihood of receiving a kidney transplant and poor graft outcomes if transplanted. Thus, every attempt should be made to avoid blood transfusions where possible, particularly in younger patients.

The current 'catchphrase' in renal anaemia management is *individualisation of treatment*, and the balance between the use of ESA therapy and blood transfusions is a good example of this. For example, patients resistant to ESA therapy who are elderly and have no chance of receiving a kidney transplant should have a lower threshold for using red cell transfusions compared to a young patient who is keen to receive a transplant 1 day.

Blood transfusions may be used in either the acute or the chronic setting. Their use in an acute haemorrhagic state or immediately prior to any urgent surgical procedure is understandable and clearly appropriate.

Elective transfusion for chronic anaemia in the absence of active bleeding, however, is more controversial. A randomised controlled trial of two trigger haemoglobins for blood transfusion in the critical care setting (7 g/dl versus 10 g/dl) showed no benefit in transfusing patients when their haemoglobin fell below 10 g/dl [19], and this has resulted in a significant reduction in the trigger haemoglobin for transfusion to around 7–8 g/dl. Even in the cardiac setting, when patients may be suffering from acute coronary syndrome, the use of blood transfusion above a haemoglobin of 8 g/dl has been critically questioned.

Thus, in the absence of acute bleeding, there is little indication to transfuse a patient above 7–8 g/dl unless a surgical procedure is planned in which significant blood loss might be expected.

72.16 HIF Prolyl Hydroxylase Domain Inhibitors

A new class of drugs may shortly be available to treat CKD anaemia (refs). These are the HIF PHD inhibitors, which upregulate erythropoietin gene expression via a transcriptional mechanism and consequently enhance endogenous erythropoietin production instead of stimulating erythropoiesis via an exogenous ESA. Phase 2 trials confirmed the ability of these agents to correct anaemia and maintain haemoglobin, and phase 3 trials are well-advanced, with some reporting shortly. By impacting on other aspects of erythropoiesis, notably iron availability, they may potentially have the advantages of requiring less iron supplementation and of being effective in inflammatory states which normally induce EPO resistance, but the ubiquitous gene expression means there could potentially be safety concerns that will have to be examined carefully in the phase 3 trials.

72.17 Guidelines on Anaemia Management in CKD

Ever since ESA therapy was introduced, clinical practice guidelines on the management of anaemia in CKD patients have been devised in various parts of the world. Thus, US, European, UK (NICE), Australian, Canadian and Japanese anaemia guidelines have all been published (◘ Table 72.5). The guidelines have discussed most of the issues outlined in this chapter, focusing mainly on ESA and iron management, and there has been an evolution of recommendations over time. The current KDIGO Anemia Guideline was published in August 2012 [16], and it is likely that this will be revised and updated in the near future. Subsequent to the KDIGO Anemia Guideline publication, the European Renal Best Practice Group published a report of the latest recommendations [20]. Finally, the latest guideline update from NICE was published in 2015; a further limited update is pending as part of a more comprehensive guideline update on CKD in general.

◘ **Table 72.5** Clinical practice guidelines on the management of anaemia in chronic kidney disease

Region	Guideline	Year of publication
USA	National Kidney Foundation	1997
Europe	European Best Practice Guidelines	1999
Canada	Canadian Guidelines on Anemia	1999
USA	National Kidney Foundation	2001
Europe	Revised European Best Practice Guidelines	2004
Japan	Japanese Guidelines on Anemia	2004
Australasia	Caring for Australasians with Renal Impairment	2005
UK	National Institute for Health and Clinical Excellence	2006
USA	KDOQI Clinical Practice Guideline and Clinical Practice Recommendations for Anemia in Chronic Kidney Disease: 2007 Update of Hemoglobin Target	2007
Europe	European Best Practice Guidelines	2010
UK	National Institute for Health and Clinical Excellence (update)	2011
Global	KDIGO Clinical Practice Guideline for Anemia in Chronic Kidney Disease	2012
Europe UK	European Renal Best Practice position statement National Institute for Health and Clinical Excellence (update)	2013 2015

72.18 Conclusions

Anaemia management in chronic kidney disease has seen many changes over the last few decades. Prior to 1990, the mainstay of treatment was blood transfusions and/or iron supplementation. The introduction of ESA therapy in 1990 led to a dramatic reduction in the use of red cell transfusions, and at the same time iron supplementation was instituted more widely in order to maximise the response to ESAs (as well as to keep the doses and costs as low as possible). The results from the TREAT study strongly impacted on ESA use in CKD, encouraging more cautious use of ESA therapy. The PIVOTAL trial results in haemodialysis patients suggest that a more liberal approach to IV iron and a more conservative approach to ESA therapy may produce clinical benefits. Finally, other strategies for treating anaemia in CKD may soon be available, notably a new class of drugs called HIF PHD inhibitors, which are orally active and which enhance a patient's own endogenous production of erythropoietin.

Case Study

Case 1

A 35-year-old woman with advanced renal impairment (eGFR 28 ml/min) has a haemoglobin of 9.4 g/dl and a ferritin of 18 ug/L. There is no other obvious contributory cause for anaemia; vitamin B12 and folate levels are normal, as is her CRP.

She is clearly anaemic, and with this level of eGFR, her erythropoietin level is likely to be inadequate. However, she is also clearly iron-deficient, as indicated by her ferritin level, and she may well respond to iron supplementation alone without needing an ESA at this stage. Both oral and intravenous iron may be effective, although the latter is likely to be more effective and avoids problems of iron absorption and gastrointestinal side effects. It would be appropriate to give her 1 g of intravenous iron and assess the response 1–2 months later.

Case 2

A 56-year-old man was stable on epoetin therapy for quite some time with a haemoglobin maintained between 10 and 12 g/dl. Over the course of the next 3 months, however, his haemoglobin fell fairly rapidly to 7.3 g/dl despite two increases in his dose of epoetin. There was no obvious cause for this and no obvious source of bleeding.

This patient has lost his response to epoetin with no obvious cause, but he merits detailed investigations to find the cause. The most helpful test at this point would be his reticulocyte count. In this particular case, his reticulocyte came back at 280, with his ferritin level raised at 620 ug/L. The two most likely causes for the drop in haemoglobin in this particular case are bleeding and haemolysis since the reticulocyte count indicates increased bone marrow erythropoietic activity, and the ferritin excludes significant blood loss. Further investigations should include a haemolysis screen. In this particular case, his Coombs test came back positive, and a diagnosis of autoimmune haemolytic anaemia was made. Following steroid therapy, his haemoglobin response to epoetin was once again restored, and he was able to reduce his dose of epoetin back to baseline levels.

Case 3

A 67-year-old man on haemodialysis has been stable on epoetin therapy and supplemental IV iron for nearly 2 years, and unfortunately he develops a cough and a hoarse voice. He has been a heavy smoker for many years. A CT scan of his chest shows a lung malignancy, and you refer him to the oncologists. He is an educated man and knows that erythropoietin is a growth factor. He asks you whether or not there is any possibility that his lung cancer could be worsened by erythropoietin. What do you say to him?

This case illustrates the dilemma faced by doctors and patients regarding ESA management in the context of malignancy. In vitro data suggest strongly that erythropoietin will not cause an increase in his tumour growth, and randomised controlled trials in malignancy also suggest no increased in cancer growth provided his haemoglobin is kept within the appropriate target range of 10–12 g/dl. However, there is an enhanced risk (approximately double) of venous thromboembolism, which should be considered if he develops any symptoms suggestive of DVT or pulmonary embolus.

Key Author and Reference

Besarab et al.: US Normal Hematocrit Study

The first study to suggest possible harm in normalising haemoglobin. The primary endpoint was a composite of all-cause death and first non-fatal myocardial infarction.

Weaknesses include the patient population, which was restricted to haemodialysis patients with known cardiovascular risk. The study was stopped early at 29 months following safety concerns.

Drueke et al.: CREATE Study

Another study to examine the effects of normalising haemoglobin, this time in a non-dialysis CKD population. The primary endpoint was a composite of cardiovascular events. Significant benefits were seen in quality-of-life measures following full correction of anaemia, but there was a significantly faster need for dialysis treatment.

The main weakness of this study was that it ended up underpowered for the primary endpoint. Although the quality-of-life data were impressive, neither the patients not their treating physicians were blinded to the treatment allocation arm.

Singh et al.: CHOIR Study

Similar to CREATE, and published in the same issue of NEJM, the study also examined normalisation of haemoglobin in a non-dialysis CKD population. The primary endpoint was a composite of cardiovascular events, and there was a significant increase in event rate in patients randomised to the higher haemoglobin arm.

The main weaknesses of this study were that it was conducted exclusively in the USA and used much higher doses of epoetin than were used outside of the USA. The target haemoglobin was also changed after study initiation. However the signal of harm was undeniable, largely driven by death and heart failure hospitalisation.

Pfeffer et al.: TREAT Study

The final nail in the coffin for the use of higher haemoglobin targets and ESA doses. By far, the most scientifically robust of the four big trials, with a double-blind, placebo-controlled design in over 4000 patients.

The main findings were doubling of stroke risk, doubling of venous thromboembolism, increase in arterial thromboembolism and increase in cancer-related death in patients who had a previous malignancy. Both the primary endpoints in the trial were negative.

Very few weaknesses in the trial – the patient population was exclusively type II diabetics who were not on dialysis, but the concordance of results with the other trials suggests that the findings should not be restricted to this patient population.

Macdougall et al.: PIVOTAL Study

The only large randomised controlled trial of intravenous iron in haemodialysis patients with hard outcomes. Contrary to many opinions and observational data before the trial was conducted, a proactive high-dose IV iron regimen was superior to reactive low-dose IV iron in reducing all-cause mortality, myocardial infarction and hospitalisation for heart failure. There was no increase in the risks of hospitalisation or infections.

Weaknesses of this study were that only incident (up to 12 months) patients were included, and the study was conducted exclusively in the UK.

Chapter Review Questions

1. What is a reasonable reticulocyte count to expect from an average patient receiving ESA therapy?
   - A. 10–20
   - B. 20–40
   - C. 50–100
   - D. 100–150
   - E. 150–200

2. Which of the following statements are true in relation to the TREAT study?
   - A. There was a significant increase in the primary composite endpoint in patients randomised to darbepoetin versus placebo.
   - B. There was a significant increase in the risk of venous thromboembolism in patients randomised to darbepoetin versus placebo.
   - C. There was a significant increase in the risk of myocardial infarction in patients randomised to darbepoetin versus placebo.
   - D. There was a threefold increase in the risk of stroke in patients randomised to darbepoetin versus placebo.
   - E. There was a threefold increase in the risk of cancer in patients randomised to darbepoetin versus placebo.

3. Which of the following statements are true in relation to the PIVOTAL study?
   - A. There was a significant reduction in the risk of stroke in patients randomised to the high- versus the low-dose IV iron arm.
   - B. There was a significant reduction in the risk of myocardial infarction in patients randomised to the high- versus the low-dose IV iron arm.
   - C. There was a significant reduction in the risk of infections in patients randomised to the high- versus the low-dose IV iron arm.
   - D. There was a significant reduction in the risk of vascular access thrombosis in patients randomised to the high- versus the low-dose IV iron arm.
   - E. There was a significant reduction in the risk of overall hospitalisations in patients randomised to the high- versus the low-dose IV iron arm.

4. Which of the following statements is true about ferritin and transferrin saturation?
   - A. A very low ferritin (<20 ug/L) always indicates iron deficiency.
   - B. A ferritin of over 1000 ug/L excludes iron deficiency.
   - C. A ferritin of over 200 ug/L is optimal in haemodialysis patients.
   - D. A transferrin saturation of over 20% excludes iron deficiency.
   - E. The optimal transferrin saturation for haemodialysis patients is over 40%, if this can be achieved.

5. For an *average* CKD patient starting ESA therapy, which of the following statements is true?
   - A. A baseline erythropoietin level is sometimes helpful.
   - B. An increase in haemoglobin would be expected after 1 week.
   - C. It usually takes 4 weeks before there is a significant increase in haemoglobin.
   - D. The peak reticulocyte count is usually seen at 2 to 4 days.
   - E. The peak reticulocyte count is usually seen at 7 days.

Answers

1. (C) 50–100
2. (B) There was a significant increase in the risk of venous thromboembolism in patients randomised to darbepoetin versus placebo.
3. (B) There was a significant reduction in the risk of myocardial infarction in patients randomised to the high- versus the low-dose IV iron arm.
4. (A) A very low ferritin (<20 ug/L) always indicates iron deficiency.
5. (D) The peak reticulocyte count is usually seen at 2–4 days.

(a) For example, useful information and links to guidelines (the UK and global)
(b) Patient information leaflets, patient websites
(c) Useful resources
- ▸ https://www.nice.org.uk/guidance/ng8
- ▸ http://www.european-renal-best-practice.org/content/guidelines-topic-ckd-anaemia
- ▸ https://kdigo.org/guidelines/anemia-in-ckd/
- ▸ https://www.kidneycareuk.org/about-kidney-health/conditions/anaemia/
- ▸ https://www.niddk.nih.gov/health-information/kidney-disease/anemia

References

1. Caro J, Brown S, Miller O, et al. Erythropoietin levels in uremic nephric and anephric patients. J Lab Clin Med. 1979;93:449–58.
2. Macdougall IC. Monitoring of iron status and iron supplementation in patients treated with erythropoietin. Curr Opin Nephrol Hypertens. 1994;3:620–5.
3. Macdougall IC, Obrador GT, El Nahas M. How important is transfusion avoidance in 2013? Nephrol Dial Transplant. 2013;28:1092–9.
4. Astor BC, Muntner P, Levin A, et al. Association of kidney function with anemia: the Third National Health and Nutrition Examination Survey (1988–1994). Arch Intern Med. 2002;162:1401–8.
5. Rossert J, Casadevall N, Eckardt KU. Anti-erythropoietin antibodies and pure red cell aplasia. J Am Soc Nephrol. 2004;15:398–406.
6. Macdougall IC, Rossert J, Casadevall N, Stead RB, Duliege AM, Froissart M, Eckardt KU. A peptide-based erythropoietin-receptor agonist for pure red-cell aplasia. N Engl J Med. 2009;361:1848–55.
7. Ganz T. Hepcidin and iron regulation, 10 years later. Blood. 2011;117:4425–33.
8. Tessitore N, Solero GP, Lippi G, Bassi A, Faccini GB, Bedogna V, Gammaro L, Brocco G, Restivo G, Bernich P, Lupo A, Maschio G. The role of iron status markers in predicting response to intravenous iron in haemodialysis patients on maintenance erythropoietin. Nephrol Dial Transplant. 2001;16:1416–23.
9. Tessitore N, Girelli D, Campostrini N, Bedogna V, Pietro Solero G, Castagna A, Melilli E, Mantovani W, De Matteis G, Olivieri O, Poli A, Lupo A. Hepcidin is not useful as a biomarker for iron needs in haemodialysis patients on maintenance erythropoiesis-stimulating agents. Nephrol Dial Transplant. 2010;25:3996–4002.
10. Macdougall IC, Provenzano R, Sharma A, Spinowitz BS, Schmidt RJ, Pergola PE, Zabaneh RI, Tong-Starksen S, Mayo MR, Tang H, Polu KR, Duliege AM, Fishbane S, PEARL Study Groups. Peginesatide for anemia in patients with chronic kidney disease not receiving dialysis. N Engl J Med. 2013;368:320–32.
11. Fishbane S, Schiller B, Locatelli F, Covic AC, Provenzano R, Wiecek A, Levin NW, Kaplan M, Macdougall IC, Francisco C, Mayo MR, Polu KR, Duliege AM, Besarab A, EMERALD Study Groups. Peginesatide in patients with anemia undergoing hemodialysis. N Engl J Med. 2013;368:307–19.
12. Besarab A, Bolton WK, Browne JK, Egrie JC, Nissenson AR, Okamoto DM, Schwab SJ, Goodkin DA. The effects of normal as compared with low hematocrit values in patients with cardiac disease who are receiving hemodialysis and epoetin. N Engl J Med. 1998;339:584–90.
13. Drüeke TB, Locatelli F, Clyne N, Eckardt KU, Macdougall IC, Tsakiris D, Burger HU, Scherhag A, CREATE Investigators. Normalization of hemoglobin level in patients with chronic kidney disease and anemia. N Engl J Med. 2006;355:2071–84.
14. Singh AK, Szczech L, Tang KL, Barnhart H, Sapp S, Wolfson M, Reddan D, CHOIR Investigators. Correction of anemia with epoetin alfa in chronic kidney disease. N Engl J Med. 2006;355:2085–98.
15. Pfeffer MA, Burdmann EA, Chen CY, Cooper ME, de Zeeuw D, Eckardt KU, Feyzi JM, Ivanovich P, Kewalramani R, Levey AS, Lewis EF, McGill JB, McMurray JJ, Parfrey P, Parving HH, Remuzzi G, Singh AK, Solomon SD, Toto R, Investigators TREAT. A trial of darbepoetin alfa in type 2 diabetes and chronic kidney disease. N Engl J Med. 2009;361:2019–32.
16. National Kidney Foundation. KDIGO clinical practice guideline for anemia in chronic kidney disease. Kidney Int. 2012; 2:v–335.
17. US Renal Data System. USRDS 2009 Annual Data Report: Atlas of Chronic Kidney Disease and End-Stage Renal Disease in the United States. National Institutes of Health, National Institute of Diabetes and Digestive and Kidney Diseases; 2009.
18. Obrador GT, Macdougall IC. Effect of red cell transfusions on future kidney transplantation. Clin J Am Soc Nephrol. 2013;8:852–60.
19. Hébert PC, Wells G, Blajchman MA, Marshall J, Martin C, Pagliarello G, Tweeddale M, Schweitzer I, Yetisir E. A multicenter, randomized, controlled clinical trial of transfusion requirements in critical care. Transfusion Requirements in Critical Care Investigators, Canadian Critical Care Trials Group. N Engl J Med. 1999;340:409–17.
20. Locatelli F, Bárány P, Covic A, De Francisco A, Del Vecchio L, Goldsmith D, Hörl W, London G, Vanholder R, Van Biesen W, On behalf of the ERA-EDTA ERBP Advisory Board. Kidney disease: improving global outcomes guidelines on anaemia management in chronic kidney disease: a European Renal Best Practice position statement. Nephrol Dial Transplant. 2013;12: 1346–59. [Epub ahead of print].

Nutrition in Kidney Disease

Sinéad Burke

Contents

M. Harber (ed.), *Primer on Nephrology*, https://doi.org/10.1007/978-3-030-76419-7_73

Learning Objectives

1. Maintaining good nutritional status in CKD is complex and must balance sometimes competing priorities, including both patient-centred (e.g. QOL) and clinical end points.
2. Frailty is increasingly understood as an important predictor of mortality and morbidity in CKD, and inadequate nutritional intake is a modifiable risk factor for frailty.
3. Diabetes and CVD remain challenging long-term conditions which account for a high morbidity and mortality burden in CKD. Diet is an important component of management.
4. Related to this, the role of diet in the management of CKD mineral bone disorder (MBD) is not insignificant – the use of a dietary strategy in combination with optimal dialysis can assist with the high pill burden seen in managing this disorder (and CKD in general).
5. Long-term changes to diet are rarely simple and require skilled dietetic and sometimes psychology professionals to achieve using advanced motivational interviewing techniques.

73.1 Introduction

73.1.1 Nutrition in Kidney Disease: The Big Picture

Maintaining good nutritional status through the stages of chronic kidney disease is an important challenge to all clinicians working in this field. Malnutrition (both over- and undernutrition) accounts for a significant morbidity and mortality burden, notwithstanding the additional impact on quality of life in both physical and mental domains.

The public health burden of diabetes and cardiovascular disease is seen increasingly in people with kidney disease. This is of course in line with population trends and is disproportionately seen in minority ethnic groups, a global public health challenge.

The traditional approach to a 'kidney diet' focuses often on individual components: low potassium, low phosphate, low sodium, restricted volume and modified protein intake (depending on the stage of kidney disease), for example. There is a paucity of high-quality evidence supporting the role of such dietary restrictions in lowering mortality risk in CKD and ESKD [1]. Given the considerable burden of restricted diets on quality of life, there is a need for clinicians to understand their responsibility in ensuring that the benefit of a dietary approach is realised, without causing harm (outcome versus balancing measure). A good example of this is in the prescription of a low phosphate diet in a patient with malnutrition.

At the heart of the nutritional management of a patient with kidney disease or, indeed, any long-term condition is the need for a person-centred approach. This is the principle that people should be treated with dignity and treated as equals when delivering care. The clinician should consider the impact of health literacy, financial status, cultural practices and health beliefs (this is not an exhaustive list of all considerations required when supporting dietary change). Care should enable the person to be an active, not passive, participant [2]. This will facilitate more effective goal setting and achievement of treatment targets.

The value of objective measures of nutritional status is not to be overlooked. Where nutrition interventions are woven with other aspects of a treatment protocol, being precise about the magnitude of change in nutritional status is key. This helps to recognise the helpful interventions and make decisions on what is cost and clinically effective practice.

73.2 Undernutrition

Definition

WHO [3] describes the states of undernutrition: underweight, stunting and wasting, as well as deficiencies in vitamins and minerals. The term undernutrition is commonly replaced by malnutrition, although the latter refers to the disordered states of both under- and overnutrition.

Undernutrition not only carries a huge personal burden but also places an enormous financial strain on health care systems. Caring for malnourished people in a hospital setting can cost double what it costs in well-nourished people [3]. They are at higher risk of falls, fractures, functional deterioration and developing skin pressure areas. Malnourished individuals are more likely to require specialist dietetic input and interventions, such as artificial feeding. They exhibit higher levels of depression, and psychological support is important. Undernutrition increases the hospital length of stay for the reasons described above.

The International Society of Renal Nutrition and Metabolism (ISRNM) describe protein-energy wasting (PEW) as the 'state of decreased body stores of protein and energy fuels (body protein and fat masses)'. PEW is the recommended terminology for the state of undernutrition in people with CKD. It is observed in 20–54% of patients with CKD stages 4–5d and is one of the strongest predictors of morbidity and mortality [4]. The most severe PEW can be referred to as cachexia. PEW is both caused by and a cause of depression, cardiovascular disease, frailty and infection. The metabolic derangements which contribute to this state are complex and multiple, a very small number of which are outlined below.

Anorexia in CKD leads to a decreased intake of protein and calories and is a major cause of undernutrition. Anorexia is driven by key factors in CKD including but not limited to the following:

- Increased pro-inflammatory cytokines TNF and IL-6
- Changes in circulating appetite mediators such as ghrelin and leptin
- Nitrogen-derived uraemic toxins (the uraemic milieu)

Uraemia promotes poor nutritional intake via the suppression of appetite and taste changes. Factors promoting protein catabolism in preference to synthesis include insulin resistance, chronic inflammation and acidosis [5].

Dialysis itself causes the loss of small amounts of nutrients into the dialysate. Practically, people are sometimes too fatigued following dialysis to prepare a meal. Early satiety in people in PD is common due to the presence of a 'dwell' in the peritoneal cavity, as is the suppression of appetite via the absorption of glucose from PD solution. The number and magnitude of dietary restrictions cause an unintentional reduction in food intake as people feel overwhelmed by the question 'what can I eat'?

73.2.1 Screening and Diagnosis

At relative speed, all clinicians can look for symptoms of undernutrition when reviewing a patient in general practice, specialist clinic or on admission to hospital: low appetite, loss of (dry) weight, looser fitting clothes/rings/dentures, low mood, lethargy, loss of muscle strength [6].

Objective tools are needed, however, to triage the patients of greatest concern from within a larger cohort (such as a hospital ward or dialysis unit). The success of nutritional screening is driven by the speed, ease and sensitivity/specificity of the tool used.

There is often a two-stage approach:

1. Screening – designed to be carried out by any trained health care professional to highlight people who are at risk of undernutrition
2. Assessment – designed to more quantitatively measure the degree of nutritional deficit/functional deficit

It is considered best practice is screen the CKD population annually, approximately 3-monthly on maintenance haemodialysis or peritoneal dialysis, and on modality change. Nutritional screening in the acutely unwell should take place on admission to hospital wards (and weekly thereafter). Local practice varies, and this often depends on factors such as staffing and knowledge, as well as how much screening has been embedded in the practice of the multidisciplinary team. Screening usually comprises a temporal component such as percentage weight loss over a given period. It may aim to quantify the impact of acute illness such as infection. The main problem with tools based on weight or BMI is both the inability to quantify 'dry' weight and that it may mask undernutrition accompanied by volume overload (rampant in dialysis populations).

Nutrition assessment tools are not typically specific for use in CKD, but a number have been validated in the kidney disease population. As previously mentioned, these are best carried out by trained dietitians and often require those professionals to demonstrate their proficiency, including monitoring intra-rater and inter-rater variability. A sample of these tools is in ◘ Table 73.1.

73.2.2 Evidence-Based Interventions

Interventions to reduce undernutrition in the CKD population are typically inexpensive to implement and have significant benefits to the recipient.

Following are some examples [5]:

- Correction of metabolic acidosis
- Adequate small solute removal (if on dialysis)*
- Achievement of adequate protein intake
- Achievement of adequate calorie intake
- Supplementation with a water-soluble multivitamin for those on dialysis with poor oral intake or unusually high solute clearance
- Replacement of any other micronutrients such as zinc, selenium, and copper (if deficient)

Additionally, consider the following:

- Management of any focal inflammation that would increase nutritional requirements.
- Management of other comorbidities such as depression, congestive heart failure, and diabetes.
- Treatment of dental and periodontal disease. Tooth loss is correlated with a lower intake of protein and energy. Periodontal and dental disease has been demonstrated to be more prevalent with advancing CKD and is under-recognised and treated. During an admission to the hospital, ensuring a patient is wearing any dentures required can help to mitigate a reduction in oral intake. In the CKD setting, early management of periodontal disease to reduce the

Table 73.1 An overview of common nutrition assessment techniques in CKD

Technique	Advantages	Disadvantages
Dual-energy X-ray Absorptiometry (DEXA/DXA) and MRI	Gold standard for the assessment of lean/muscle mass	Costly and not always readily available in clinical practice
Upper arm anthropometry (UAA)	Good agreement with DEXA	Impacted by overhydration Needs good technique to minimise intra- and inter-rater variability
Subjective Global Assessment (SGA)	Semi-quantitative predictor of outcome Strongly associated with mortality in CKD	Need for training to reduce inter- and intra-rater variability If using the patient generated component, requires the patient to be able to self-report
Handgrip strength (HGS)	Simple, inexpensive, highly predictive of mortality	Intra-individual variability, significant difference if conducted pre- or post-HD
BIA-derived SMM	Objectively demonstrates changes over time Can distinguish between body compartments such as skeletal muscle mass (SMM) and fat mass (FM)	Best conduced >30 min following dialysis, therefore may be less practical
Malnutrition inflammation score	Predictive of QOL as well as mortality	Incorporates elements of the SGA so prone to the same limitations

impact of systemic inflammatory burden is supported by studies in this area [7].

*Malnutrition increases with failure to reach a Kt/V of 1.7 in PD patients, and the risk of death may increase threefold [8].

Practically, the use of high-protein/calorie, low-volume oral nutrition supplements is advisable when moderate to severe malnutrition is detected. In cases of mild malnutrition, providing recommendations of high-calorie and high-protein snacks and meals as well as fortifying food with extra protein or calories would be the first-line nutrition intervention. Other practical considerations would be determined by the initial nutritional assessment – for example, may indicate the need for financial support, the introduction of care in the home to help prepare meals.

In significant malnutrition, interventions that provide nutrition via an enteral feeding tube or parenteral nutrition may be indicated where the person is not able to meet estimated calorie and protein requirements with oral nutrition support and nutrition education; these are described in the section of this chapter: Nutrition in the Hospitalised CKD Patient.

Intradialytic amino acids and intradialytic parenteral nutrition are used with variable rates internationally. There have been inconclusive results as to their benefits, and there are known risks associated with their use. In selected cases, it may be helpful where oral nutrition support alone has not attenuated PEW development.

Interestingly, evidence supports that the route of administration of nutritional supplementation (that is, oral or parenteral) does not have any significant effect on the response to therapy if equal and adequate amounts of protein and calories are provided. This supports the value of an individualised approach to identify the most appropriate strategy for each patient.

Anabolic agents, growth hormones, as well as appetite stimulants need to be used with caution in the CKD population. Anti-inflammatory supplements (e.g. omega 3) are generally safe in this cohort. The efficacy of therapy is not well understood. Fish liver oils that are high in vitamin A should not be used in CKD due to the risk of hypervitaminosis A.

It is common practice to reduce dietary restrictions when someone is significantly undernourished, to encourage an increase in total calorie and protein intake. This is an example of prioritising the problem that presents the probable highest risk in that individual at the point of assessment.

73.2.3 Nutrition Is a Modifiable Risk Factor in Frailty

Frailty is a medical syndrome with multiple causes and contributors that is characterized by diminished strength, endurance and reduced physiologic function that increases an individual's vulnerability for developing increased dependency and/or death [9].

Frailty, both physical and cognitive, has become increasingly recognised for its role in the QOL of a person with CKD, as well as in clinical outcomes. It is also increasingly recognised. In the US Renal Data System Comprehensive Dialysis Study, frailty prevalence was 73% in over 1500 haemodialysis patients [10]. Crucially, frailty predicts higher mortality across all stages of CKD and in dialysis – in fact, this can cause a nine-fold increase in haemodialysis.

Identifying factors which increase the predisposition to frailty in the CKD population can inform interventions to attenuate its development. Known to be involved in frailty risk are inflammation and procoagulant factors – in this way, CKD itself, as a disease, increases frailty risk. Biochemical associations are observed, notably IL-6 (high levels seen alongside worsening frailty), where conversely increasing serum albumin presents with improving frailty [11].

Some of the broad sociodemographic/health behaviour determinants of frailty in the CKD population include age and worsening CKD, poor nutritional intake, smoking, psychiatric illness and comorbidities especially diabetes, cerebrovascular disease and chronic lung disease [12].

Nutrition is a modifiable risk factor for frailty; so, what are the interventions that make the difference? Morley and colleagues [9] suggested that vitamin D, physical activity, protein-calorie supplementation and reduction of polypharmacy may be beneficial in modifying the trajectory of frailty in the general population. The multidisciplinary team, including dietitians and physiotherapists, can be called upon to implement the above interventions.

Vitamin D, in the form of cholecalciferol, is routinely prescribed in advanced kidney disease and is relatively cheap. Most CKD patients under specialist care will be prescribed this; dose titration will be needed for those who remain deficient even after therapy has been commenced.

It should be noted that health care professionals, thought accepting of the benefit of physical activity in the CKD population, often lack the confidence to do so in clinical practice. This has been widely reported to be due to the concern about safety and the risk of adverse events, as well as not being certain of the 'dose' that is beneficial in this population [13]. Exercise is being increasingly promoted by nephrology teams, but is not embedded in care in the same way that it is done in populations such as those with cardiac or pulmonary diseases.

Studies have emerged in both CKD stage 3–5 and also in stage 5d that suggest that both aerobic and resistance training (individually or in combination) can be carried out safely so long as sensible precautions are taken – such as the patient ensuring they feel well enough to exercise, that they are not hypo- or hyperglycaemic (if relevant) and that their blood pressure is not uncharacteristically high or low. Some dialysis units promote the use of stationary cycles and resistance bands or offer group exercise training to patients, and this has been accepted as a good direction for holistic care.

Protein-calorie supplementation, as described elsewhere in this chapter, is a stalwart of dietetic practice in CKD. This often takes the form of liquid oral nutrition supplements. Their use is supported in both the general population and in dialysis settings where clinical outcomes impacted include increased nPNA, body weight, serum albumin and prealbumin and handgrip strength. Sometimes, this option is utilised for its practicality; many frail individuals will fatigue easily (such as when standing for long periods to prepare a meal or following dialysis), and the convenience of a ready-prepared product can overcome this. As always, this needs to be balanced with other nutritional challenges, such as the high phosphate additive load of processed meals. In the case of significant undernutrition, it would be prudent to favour the intervention allowing a higher protein and calorie intake, whilst monitoring serum phosphate levels.

Nutrition professionals can engage with the MDT including medical and pharmacy staff to rationalise medications. For example, poorly nourished individuals with a low oral intake are sometimes left on phosphate binders even after their phosphate has dropped to sub-normal levels. Similar can be seen in the overtreatment of diabetes – in ESKD and certainly, in frail individuals, controlling too tightly the glycaemic control increases falls risk and is detrimental to long-term outcomes. Both insulin and oral anti-hyperglycaemic agents can be down-titrated to allow glycated haemoglobin to sit around 58–68 mmol/mol [14].

Very importantly, a holistic management plan should include consideration of psychological and social support services [15]. It should seek out the input of a gerontology team or the person's family doctor where possible. When frailty is identified to be considerable, palliative care teams may be called upon.

73.3 Obesity

Obesity is prevalent in CKD, with a well-described 'paradox', or reverse epidemiology that appears to suggest that in certain cohorts, it can be protective. Certainly, there are some associations between elevated BMI and survival on haemodialysis specifically. Possible mechanisms are through bone strength, better stem cell mobilisation, haemodynamic tolerance and preserved energy stores [16]. There is data to suggest that this benefit is only seen where normal to high muscle mass coexists.

Some data supports that the U-shaped mortality curve exists for patients under 65 on HD but not over. Studies also suggest that obesity as a potential protective factor is less convincing the people on peritoneal dialysis. Furthermore, being morbidly obese has been shown to significantly reduce the chance of receiving a kidney donor [17].

In early CKD, obesity worsens cardiovascular health and can cause glomerular hyperfiltration, leading to raised interglomerular pressure. It is considered a risk factor for the progression of CKD to the end-stage, with increased inflammatory response and oxidative stress. In adults with CKD stage 1–4, the benefit for the reduction of proteinuria and hyperfiltration supports people losing excess body weight, but with careful attention to minimise the loss of lean muscle mass.

73.3.1 When Is Obesity a Problem?

The poorest outcomes are seen when inflammation is in conjunction with abdominal fat distribution and signs of wasting (sarcopenic obesity). For this reason, clinicians should seek to include assessments to determine the distribution/location of body fat, as well as identifying the presence of muscle wasting in the context of obesity [18]. This adds more to the clinical picture than BMI alone and allows the team to identify more readily the presence of abnormal peri-organ/intra-organ fat (API fat) as well as sarcopenia – both can exist independently of one another, but both pose a significant risk for poorer outcomes.

Figure 73.1 demonstrates two presentations of abdominal obesity, one with visceral/peri-organ fat and the other with a subcutaneous distribution of abdominal fat; the former being more dangerous due to the impact on circulating pro-inflammatory cytokine levels, among other factors.

It is theorised that people with obesity are protected from PEW by their excess weight and that this explains the obesity paradox. This is not universally true, and in situations where muscle wasting occurs despite high body weight, the term 'sarcopenic obesity' applies. This might be difficult to detect, however, tools for screening exist. For example, lower than expected handgrip strength (HGS) or bioimpedance measured lean mass can indicate sarcopenia in an individual.

In cases of significant central adiposity (particularly API fat), it is likely that losing weight will offer benefit, though no robust studies prove this theory at present.

73.3.2 Strategies for the Management of Obesity

This is a notoriously difficult area of clinical practice, and globally, strategies to reduce the accelerating numbers of both CKD and non-CKD individuals have not been successful at a population level. Further attention is required to how interventions in both CKD and then in dialysis specifically impact patient outcomes.

Experience and research in CKD and ESKD support the following non-surgical strategies:

- Calorie restricted diets (<1500 kcal and <900 kcal)
- Very low-calorie Diets (VLCD)
- Pharmacological agents
- Exercise participation
- Psychological support for managing other behaviour change – e.g. stress reduction, management of significant depression and addressing disordered eating

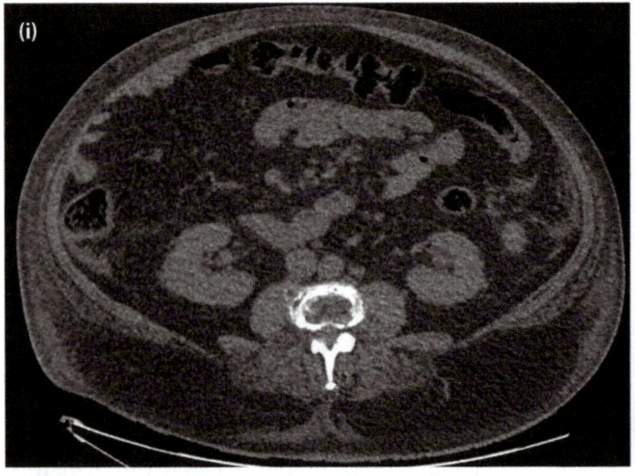

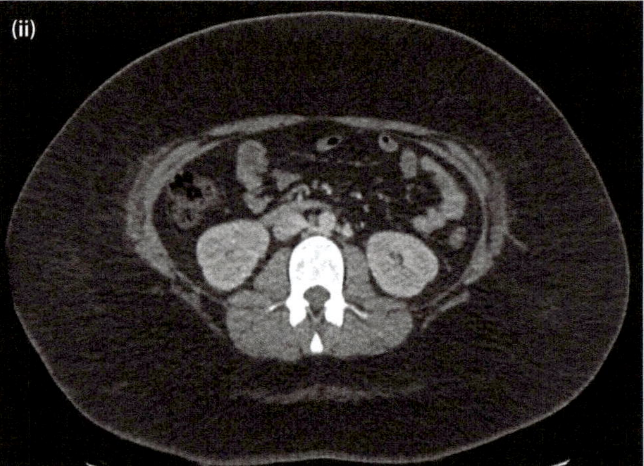

Fig. 73.1 Comparison of two types of abdominal obesity, showing (i) visceral/peri-organ fat distribution (ii) subcutaneous fat distribution

- MDT interventions, e.g. dietitian, doctor, physiotherapist, psychologist and the use of a motivational interviewing approach
- Optimisation of the management of other conditions which impact body weight such as thyroid function

There is evidence to support that those non-surgical interventions can work when well implemented; benefits include weight loss, improved reported QOL, lower BP and improved lipid profile. Generally, the challenge is with sustaining success or achieving the magnitude of weight loss to have the desired benefit, such a being listed for kidney transplantation. Adverse events are not significant, although in the case of VLCD's and pharmacological agents, there is an increased risk of electrolyte disturbances and renal oxalosis. The latter is of concern.

73.3.3 Bariatric Surgery Outcomes in CKD

Types of bariatric procedures include restrictive and malabsorptive, the former achieving weight loss of a smaller magnitude but with a better risk profile and the latter carrying greater risk but the potential for considerably more excess body weight loss.

Most used in CKD are the laparoscopic vertical sleeve gastrectomy, Roux-en-Y gastric bypass and the laparoscopic adjustable gastric band.

There is a suggestion that bariatric surgery significantly reduces eGFR decline in CKD patients [19].

People on dialysis who have bariatric surgery experience an acceptable cost/benefit ratio, although there is acknowledgement that the risk of perioperative complications is a little higher than those in the non-CKD population.

Nutritional challenges following bariatric surgery in the CKD patient include managing the recommendation of a high fluid intake with potential fluid restrictions (this has been evident in the development of renal stones in some patients). Assessing the post-operative diet contains adequate protein to avoid excess loss of lean mass, and monitoring for potential nutritional deficiencies is necessary. These may include vitamins, minerals and trace elements – commonly seen deficiencies in this group are iron, copper, zinc and selenium.

73.4 Diabetes

Tight glycaemic control in early CKD is part of the big picture of managing cardiovascular disease risk. Patients with diabetes will ideally be managed with a diabetes specialist team. Nutrition advice in diabetes (high fibre vegetables are promoted, for example) is often seen at odds with CKD advice (traditionally thought of as lower in vegetable intake), but in fact, the two can sit compatibly with the right support. As you will read in the section 'Managing Hyperkalaemia', fruit and vegetables with a higher fibre intake should not be over-restricted, and in fact, counselling should focus on lower fibre or less nutritive sources of potassium wherever possible.

Often diabetes in dialysis exhibits 'burnt out' status, and in approximately one-third of patients, medication needs to be reduced or stopped in order to manage frequently occurring hypoglycaemia [20]. This is thought to be contributed to by several factors including poor oral intake (anorexia or CKD +/– diabetic gastroparesis), reduced renal and hepatic clearance of insulin and decreased renal gluconeogenesis.

Diabetes in peritoneal dialysis presents a challenge; patients can be delivered between 80 and 330 g of glucose in a 24-hour period. Counselling patients about the impact of this on both glycaemic control and weight is advisable when they are preparing for/starting PD. The dietary contribution of low-fibre carbohydrate sources and refined sugars, particularly, should be limited in these patients. If not, fluid retention is observed, leading to volume overload. As above, high-fibre, low-GI sources are preferred and should still be eaten to avoid constipation.

Other practical considerations are the revision of meals and insulin timing. With overnight peritoneal dialysis regimes, patients can wake up with high blood sugars even if they have not eaten. This is due to the absorbed glucose from the peritoneal dialysate. Changing the timing of insulin is important here.

Diabetic gastroparesis is defined as delayed gastric emptying without mechanical obstruction [14]. Consequences are serious and include nausea, vomiting, postprandial discomfort or bloating. As it worsens, it can impact nutritional intake and lead to malnutrition. The ideal management plan should begin with consuming small meals more frequently. Textures that are more physically broken down such as minced food, or chewing very carefully can improve emptying times. Lower-fat and lower-fibre meals can assist gastric emptying, but this needs to be balanced with avoiding constipation. In the case of malnutrition, fat in liquid supplement form can help maintain calorie intake without exacerbating delayed gastric emptying. In very extreme cases of gastroparesis with malnutrition, diet in pureed or blended form or as an enteral tube feed is worth considering.

A person with gastroparesis usually has more difficulty achieving optimal glucose control as the timing of insulin with meals becomes more complicated – a postprandial dip in glucose is often observed.

73.5 Salt and Volume Overload

The regulation of salt and water is primarily the remit of the kidneys. Much has been said about the link between high salt intake in the pathogenesis of hypertension and fluid overload. Positive sodium balance raises the osmotic pressure. This then leads to an increased intake of water, which encourages hypervolaemia. Evidence also links high salt intake with the uraemic mediated pathways of proteinuria, oxidative stress, inflammation and endothelial cell damage.

In moderate CKD, sodium restriction can greatly enhance the benefits of RAAS blockade therapy. Conversely, high sodium intake limits the effects of this treatment which is well reported in the literature [21].

As CKD progresses, salt and volume overload are implicit in worsening hypertension and left ventricular hypertrophy (LVH). In haemodialysis patients, there has been data to suggest that across all levels of pre-dialysis blood pressure, chronic volume overload (measured by bioimpedance spectroscopy) is a risk factor for death [22]. Similarly, cardiovascular mortality in peritoneal dialysis patients is increased.

The most important drivers for thirst are salt intake and hyperglycaemia. Any attempts to moderate fluid intake in a patient without addressing these factors are futile.

Very strict sodium restriction is not recommended, due to the J-shaped mortality curve observed. WHO recommends a restriction of <6 g daily (ideally 4 g) for CVD risk reduction, and this is also the usual practice in the education of patients with CKD. This is referred to as a No-Added-Salt (NAS) diet.

Where possible, a 24-hour urine collection in the CKD population is the gold standard for assessing sodium intake. When so much salt is hidden in foods, self-reporting intake can be fraught with errors but can be used in conjunction with urine collection – for example, urine collection is able to confirm the effectiveness of a dietary intervention/confirm a change in reported sodium intake. There are a small number of tools validated in renal populations to assess sodium intake. These involve seeking out information about naturally occurring, added to food (often referred to as 'hidden') and that added to meals and food during cooking and serving.

Counselling around dietary reduction in sodium must be individualised, and this would begin with exploring the presence of barriers to reducing salt. Qualitative research conducted with UK dwelling Bangladeshi's, for example, revealed not only a culturally established taste for salt but also associations of status with salt intake [23]. Discussions of culturally acceptable ways to reduce salt that were led by the patient group led to this message being positively received.

Counselling on reducing fluid intake (in conjunction with sodium) is a common practice among all clinicians working in CKD. In most patients, this is not required until the patient reaches ESKD or if in AKI. It may also be indicated in a person suffering from nephrotic syndrome.

Strategies include the use of smaller cups, sucking ice chips slowly, swallowing tablets with food rather than liquid, monitoring liquid intake and avoiding high liquid content foods (e.g. soup, jelly, yoghurt, lettuce, melon, rice, pasta – N.B. practice on this varies widely, and wherever possible, this author recommends limiting drinks > food sources of fluid).

73.6 Chronic Kidney Disease Mineral Bone Disorder (CKD-MBD)

The management of CKD-MBD typically entails a multidisciplinary approach, but this chapter focuses on the role of diet/dietitians in this complex disorder. Good practice should include an integrated approach that considers diet, dialysis (when in stage 5d) and pharmacology. This is often called the 3D approach: diet, dialysis and drugs.

Dietary intake is the primary source of phosphate and should be carefully discussed to gather a full picture of potential areas to reduce phosphate load. Serum phosphate levels are maintained until quite late in CKD (unlike fibroblast-growth-factor 23, or FGF-23, which begins to rise earlier).

Phosphate is absorbed in the small intestine. Factors impacting net gastrointestinal absorption are:

- Phosphate amount
- Phosphate bioavailability (evidence supports < absorption with plant-based v animal-based phosphate sources and the most with inorganic phosphate additives)
- The presence of natural or pharmacological phosphate binders
- Vitamin D

There is variation in phosphate absorption between individuals. Phosphate absorption is not up- or down-regulated based on serum levels. Consideration of not only the phosphate content of the diet but also bioavailability is of value [24].

Good nutritional/dietetic management of hyperphosphataemia should include the following:

- Identification and reduction of phosphate additive containing processed foods – of which absorption is estimated at >90%. Examples are processed meats, cheeses, baked goods and beverages. It is common for these foods to be cheaper and therefore are frequently consumed – but particularly in Western diets.
- Limit the quantity of dairy-based food and drink (balance this with the need for adequate calories in undernutrition).
- Choosing animal foods with a lower phosphate-to-protein ratio.
- Choosing foods with the lowest phosphate bioavailability such as plant-based sources (phytates reduce phosphate absorption to about 40%) wherever possible.
- Review and education regarding the timing and dosing of phosphate binders to reflect phosphate intake. Identifying where a decreased dose of alfa-calcidol would enable target phosphate to be achieved without driving hyperparathyroidism.

When considering dietary phosphate restriction, it is important to note that the evidence behind its use is not high quality. Additionally, there are many factors in recommending dietary changes. Understanding what is financially and logistically possible when recommending a diet based on more fresh than prepared foods is vital. Working collaboratively with patients to facilitate change is supported. This may include negotiation around acceptable dietary changes as well as formulating a strategy to aid adherence with phosphate binders. As with all aspects of dietary counselling – aiming to choose no more than a few simple changes, driven by the patient based on the education provided is recommended.

73.7 Dietary Management of Hyper- and Hypokalaemia

73.7.1 Hyperkalaemia

Hyperkalaemia may present acutely (often as a result of haemolysis, acidosis or trauma) or be a chronic problem. The latter is more likely to require nutritional intervention.

Hyperkalaemia presents a significant challenge to renal clinicians as it tends to be common, and there is evidence that even small elevations over a long period of time carry an excess mortality risk [25].

The goals of nutrition therapy in the patient with hyperkalaemia may include:

- Enabling the ongoing use of nephro-protective RAAS inhibitors
- To delay the start of dialysis
- To reduce the mortality risk presented by chronic hyperkalaemia

An MDT approach to managing chronic hyperkalaemia is almost always needed. To illustrate this example, RAAS inhibitors increase circulating levels of potassium in the blood but have a potent antihypertensive and anti-inflammatory effect. Treatment with ACE inhibitors can also decrease frailty risk. In many cases, managing safe serum potassium levels by other strategies (such as diet) can allow a physician to maintain their patient on a nephro-protective anti-RAAS agent.

Intestinal absorption of dietary potassium is high, around 90%. Faecal excretion is thought to be no more than 15–20 mmol/day, but – importantly – appears to be at its highest when residual renal function is minimal. Some studies support that in HD patients, excretion of potassium by the bowel is up to 80% higher than in non-dialysis patients. It seems to be more a consequence of secretion of potassium into the rather than a reduced intestinal absorption. For this reason, constipation is possibly as important as high dietary potassium intake in net potassium balance.

Patients with CKD, particularly on dialysis, have been found to have a low intake of fruit and vegetable portions. The dietary fibre intake of individuals with CKD is some 10 g/day lower than the average intake, and observational studies in people with mild to moderate CKD demonstrated high fruit and vegetable consumption was associated with a 30% lower all-cause mortality [26].

Low consumption of fruit and vegetables in >8000 haemodialysis patients is associated with higher all-cause mortality [27]. This study did not measure serum potassium but pointed to the theory that traditional low potassium dietary modifications (lowering fruit and vegetable intake) could pose a detrimental effect. The purported wisdom is that asking people to avoid plant-based foods may lead to unfavourable metabolic changes such as the development of dyslipidaemia, hypertension and oxidative stress. This is in addition to constipation that is seen in as much as >50% of haemodialysis patients.

Well-designed, randomised controlled trials supporting the role of a diet low in potassium controlling hyperkalaemia have not been conducted in any significant number. In fact, early studies into the impact of low protein diets to delay kidney function decline demonstrated that even at very low levels of potassium ingestion, hyperkalaemia persisted. Despite this, reducing the potassium load in an individual's diet remains a widely adopted practice. It is certainly prudent to avoid a high potassium-to-fibre ratio, which would likely result in a net excess of body potassium.

Nutritional management of hyperkalaemia starts with a detailed dietary recall, targeted at known high-potassium food and drinks. It is more beneficial when the clinician involved has a good understanding of the potassium content of any food commonly consumed in various cultural diets.

Nutrition advice may include not only modification (reduction) of quantity/frequency of high-potassium foods and fibre content that promotes avoidance of constipation but also promotion of tight glycaemic control in diabetics (low-GI fire sources). This is particularly important in patients on peritoneal dialysis and following kidney transplantation.

Examples of dietary changes to reduce potassium intake:

- Avoiding salt substitutes, potassium-rich food additives
- Opting for fruit and vegetables rather than juices (also helps with limited fluid intake)
- Choosing low to moderate potassium fruit and vegetables as much as possible, and limiting the frequency of high-potassium fruits and vegetables
- Soaking pulses (e.g. chickpeas and lentils) and high-potassium vegetables prior to cooking them
- Boiling vegetables (once) and discarding the water – this should not be used for making gravies
- Limiting milk and milk products to some extent (will be dependent on the nutritional status of the individual
- Choose fewer high-potassium foods with lower nutritive value – potato crisps, chocolate, and Indian sweets from coconut milk

Wherever possible, take a pragmatic approach that enables a reasonable consumption of plant-based, fibre-rich, potassium-containing foods with regular monitoring of serum K levels and bowels. It is probably good practice to avoid very high-potassium foods, but understanding the lack of robust evidence for limiting fruit and vegetable intake, in fact, is understood to be detrimental to mortality risk.

73.7.2 Hypokalaemia

Hypokalaemia is just as dangerous as hyperkalaemia, and it can indicate a poor overall nutritional intake. This should be an immediate consideration of the MDT, particularly, if this is recurring in someone who has not changed modalities recently. Determining this requires a full nutritional assessment by a qualified nutritional professional.

Post kidney transplant rapid increases in daily urine output can drive a net loss of potassium resulting in a drop in serum levels. People who may have been following a low potassium diet whilst on dialysis or approaching ESKD may suddenly realise that their low potassium diet no longer serves a need, and in some cases, high-potassium foods may be encouraged for a brief period whilst potassium homeostasis re-equilibrates.

73.8 Nutrition in Hospitalised CKD Patients

Malnutrition on presentation to hospital is commonly described in the literature and, in most cases, worsens in hospital. Inflammatory, anorexia, uraemia, depression and unfamiliar foods are all examples of contributing factors to this problem.

The following section describes common nutrition-related challenges in the management of a hospitalised patient and is designed to prompt consideration of how optimising nutrition in such situations is important.

73.8.1 Nutritional Management of AKI

Although AKI can present in the community setting, in general, nutritional requirements are typically only impacted by AKI when the injury is catabolic in nature and significant. Sepsis, trauma, systemic diseases and acidosis are examples of clinical presentations which impact protein and calorie requirements with significance.

The need for nutritional input with AKI is seen in the hospital setting. A significant proportion (nearly half) of people admitted to hospital with AKI are severely malnourished [28]. Protein turnover is enhanced; this results in negative nitrogen balance. These patients are typically in stage 2 or 3 AKI.

Just as early identification of AKI is essential to an outcome, it is important to screen early for malnutrition that is either pre-existing when a person presents to the hospital or for malnutrition risk posed by the illness leading to the AKI.

The route of nutrition support is less important than that the patient achieves target protein, with sufficient calories to utilise the protein. People who are admitted to intensive care settings are almost always fed with an enteral feeding tube, particularly, if intubated or sedated. In order to avoid overfeeding, consideration would be required when patients are on propofol, as this delivers calories as fat. Where a patient is on CRRT, the net loss of amino acids is in the region of 10–15 g/day, which needs to be factored into nutrition delivery. CRRT also causes a loss of some vitamins and trace minerals; however, it is not known whether micronutrient supplementation meaningfully changes patient outcomes [29].

Typically, enteral nutrition needs to be low-volume, low-electrolyte, but nutrient-dense. In certain cases, parenteral nutrition may be indicated, but this would only be if the GI tract was not viable for use/required gut rest – this would typically be a result of the illness that preceded the AKI, rather than AKI itself.

As a patient recovers, the goal is to move back to oral diet. This should be supplemented to achieve target nutritional requirements. In hospital, this can be achieved practically by providing high protein and energy meal choices, snacks and drinks, as well as considering the environmental factors such as being sat out of bed to eat, being assisted with eating when this is difficult and food being presented attractively.

73.8.2 PD Peritonitis and Encapsulating Peritoneal Sclerosis (EPS)

During episodes of peritonitis, protein losses increase, although the magnitude is highly variable. There is evidence that malnutrition predicts the peritonitis rate [30].

Encapsulating peritoneal sclerosis may present as early fullness, loss of appetite, weight loss (can be masked by fluid overload or ascites), hypoalbuminaemia, raised CRP, nausea, vomiting, constipation or diarrhoea. Structural changes leading to ischaemia and loss of absorptive capacity are important here. The risk of bowel perforation and intra-abdominal sepsis is high. All of these have significant impact on the development of poor nutritional status.

The combination of GI symptoms, loss of appetite, inflammatory/catabolic state leads to the development of malnutrition.

Retrospective analyses of patients with EPS show a history of at least 10% dry weight loss over the previous 12 months [31]. We know that the risk of EPS increases over time on PD (in addition to the change of modality following time on PD). Any signs or symptoms of obstruction +/− significant changes in the nutritional status in a patient who has been on PD for >5 years should be a prompt to consider EPS as a possible diagnosis.

The nutritional management of EPS includes the use of oral, enteral tube feeding and parenteral nutrition. There is not clear preferred route in terms of patient outcome; rather, the percentage of nutritional requirements delivered is key. In essence, get the nutrition in, whatever the method that can safely achieve this. Factors such as QOL, prognosis of the patient, degree of cocooning (and likely malabsorption) and patient wishes need to be considered.

73.8.3 Refeeding Syndrome in CKD

NICE guidelines suggest that risk of refeeding syndrome can be identified by (a) little or no nutritional intake for >10 days, (b) BMI < 16 kg/m^2, (c) unintentional weight loss of >15% in 3–6 months or (d) low levels of phosphate, magnesium or potassium prior to feeding. Risk is also suggested by a combination of two or more of the following: (e) little or no nutritional intake for >5 days, (f) BMI <18.5 kg/ m^2, (g) unintentional weight loss of >10% in the past 3–6 months and (h) history of drug or alcohol abuse, with some medication such as insulin, chemotherapy, diuretics and antacids predisposing factors [32].

Refeeding syndrome is rarely reported in the CKD population. It is thought that this is because serum levels of potassium, phosphate and magnesium are higher in this group. It might also be purported that usually patients managed under specialist kidney services would be screened routinely, and as such, would hopefully not enter such a prolonged state of starvation before this is recognised.

Where refeeding syndrome risk is identified in an unwell individual, the management strategy should include the introduction of feeding at a rate of no more than 10 kcal/kg/day initially, monitoring of fluid balance closely to ensure circulatory volume is restored, supplementation of thiamine and vitamin B co-strong in oral or intravenous form and supplementation of multivitamin/trace element daily. Although rare in CKD, refeeding syndrome is a potentially fatal condition and requires attentive management.

73.8.4 Nutrition Post-transplantation

It continues to be recommended that during the immediate post-transplantation period, there should be attention to addressing metabolic abnormalities, electrolyte disturbances related to delayed graft function, issues with wound healing (requiring sufficient protein intake) and any gut disturbances (which may include constipation, diabetic gastroparesis and post-surgical ileus).

Grapefruit or grapefruit juice should be avoided for several hours following ciclosporin, tacrolimus or sirolimus. The pharmacokinetics is impacted; grapefruit juice increases the total area under the concentration-time curve (AUC) or peak concentration of these drugs [33]. The mechanism is the deactivation of intestinal cytochrome P450 34A. The impact of this overall is more important for regular grapefruit/grapefruit juice consumption.

When anti-rejection medication doses are at their highest, taking care to avoid infection by food-borne pathogens is important. Hygienic food storage and preparation is important here, as is avoiding unpasteurised products or probiotic food products. Cases of food poisoning following renal transplantation in the literature are limited. Most cases result in gastrointestinal effects which are self-limiting.

Risks to transplant graft function include those resulting from steroid-based immunosuppression and often influenced by nutrition, hypertension, diabetes (established and NODAT), dyslipidaemia, osteoporosis and obesity. In addition, at the time of transplantation, nutrition status at the extremes i.e. having PEW or morbid obesity leads to poorer clinical outcomes. As much as possible, this should be modified whilst a patient awaits a transplant, to prevent further weight gain in the obese, and weight loss in the undernourished.

73.8.5 Nutrition at the End of Life

Nutrition at the end of life is supportive and often for comfort. Invasive provision of nutrition such as via an enteral feeding tube or central venous catheter (for parenteral nutrition) is often not indicated if the patient is identified as likely being in their last hours or days. Any considerations to commence such an intervention during what is likely to be an individual's last 3 months of life should also be carefully weighed up to balance the benefits to the patient versus the potential to impact negatively on their quality of life [34].

Decisions on methods of nutrition support should be made with a multidisciplinary team and consider the patient's wishes. Where advanced care planning can be done with patients, it should include decisions about feeding – be it commencement, continuation or withdrawal of. If a valid advanced decision to refuse treatment (ADRT) exists around artificial feeding, this should be followed. This may include stopping any nutrition or hydration that had already begun before this information was known [35].

If there are no ADRT, making decisions in 'best interest' can be undertaken following proficient assessment of their mental capacity as well as consulting any persons with the authority to make decisions about their care. Independent advocates may be involved in certain circumstances. Clinicians have a responsibility to ensure that they are providing care in a patient's best interests but not care that is likely to be futile [35]. This means that decisions around feeding should be regularly reviewed in the context of any changes in clinical prognosis.

In circumstances where a person is reaching the end of their life, relaxing dietary restrictions, having their favourite foods and avoiding a dry mouth can be helpful and reassuring. In cases where modified texture diet/fluids had been recommended, it may be agreed with the expert evaluation by a speech and language therapist that the patient can accept any risk associated with having 'normal' diet and thin fluids. This is typically referred to as 'risk managed' feeding.

Case Study

Case 1

A 42-year-old man with a haemodialysis vintage of 6 years is presenting with consistently high potassium levels on monthly blood, in the region of 6.8–9.0 mmol/l pre-dialysis. He is a Black British man with a BMI of 32 kg/m^2. His family comprises a terminally ill wife for whom he cares, along with his two young children. He has a rising PTH with successive measures of 57, 69 and 72 mmol/l spanning the past 9 months. This is in the context of corrected calcium in range but a phosphate which is stable but consistently over 2.0 mmol/l. In your dialysis clinic, you wish to provide brief advice to ensure he is aware of the risks of these suboptimal results.

When prioritising nutritional issues here, the high BMI can be placed at the bottom of the list. BMI is distinctly unhelpful in people of African origin, who typically have high muscle mass. This may be overstating the magnitude of obesity. It is also not an urgent issue. The immediate concern is achieving safe potassium. With the family situation presented, it will be valuable to understand how much this man can realistically change in his current diet.

Is there a simple modification with a high likelihood of reducing potassium? Does he drink fruit juice frequently or pick up a chocolate bar or potato chips each time he comes to dialysis? Food and drink items that are lower in nutritional value (and importantly, fibre) should be limited before more nutritious food items.

Case 2

A 67-year-old female patient is admitted to a renal inpatient ward via ED having fallen twice since arriving home from her dialysis session that day, sustaining a cut to her head on the second fall. Her nutritional screening tool on admission indicates her weight has been unchanged in the past month; however, intradialytic weight gains are >4% of her body weight, and she reports poor oral intake of solid food. Your gut feeling is that she is clinically overhydrated but that she may have lost some 'flesh' weight.

You would seek to establish a clearer picture of nutritional status and the presence of overhydration. In addition to blood pressure and JVP, assessment methods could include measuring bioimpedance spectroscopy to look at the extracellular to total body water ratio (ECW:TBW), as well as looking at fat mass and lean body mass (low values would support the diagnosis of undernutrition). This method would be even more helpful if you had previous bioimpedance results to look at the trend for this individual.

Elevated N terminal pro-brain natriuretic peptide (NT pro-BNP) values can be interpreted as likely overhydration unless the person has had a recent cardiac event.

It would also be helpful to consolidate what you know about this lady's nutritional intake. A low intake of solids sometimes means a higher intake of fluid – for example, cups of tea and soup.

As you collate evidence of your diagnosis of undernutrition in the context of overhydration, your (nutritional) management plan could include commencement on low volume, high protein diet which may be food fortification through the hospital menu or the provision of sip feeds which are very concentrated – and can be delivered in 125 ml per portion or less. A dietetic referral will enable a more detailed exploration of the factors leading to poor oral intake in this case, which are likely to be multifactorial and may require assessment of the social environment, dentition, mental health status, uraemic factors (related to dialysis adequacy) and the persons functional status – to name a few.

Tips and Tricks

Nutrition is an important modifiable risk factor in frailty and sarcopenia. Markers of malnutrition such as reduced handgrip strength, SGA score indicating mild, moderate or severe malnutrition, low lean mass as measured by DEXA, bioimpedance or mid-arm muscle circumference strongly predict morbidity and mortality in CKD patients of all severity.

Early in CKD obesity, hypertension and diabetes are important targets for dietary intervention.

Low potassium is often a marker for malnutrition, and clinicians should consider referral to a dietitian rather than simply supplementing wherever this is possible.

Counselling people on fluid reduction is of little value without discussion of sodium restriction. Salt and volume overload can mask malnutrition and our ability to treat either requires us to clearly define where both are present. Care should be taken to establish this so that the appropriate intervention can be provided.

The burden of polypharmacy in the management of patients with CKD is well described. When managing CKD MBD, consider the use of a strategy involving a single binder type, timed with meals that are high in protein but low in readily absorbed phosphate additives.

Different priorities in diabetes management arise at different stages of the CKD disease pathway. Early in CKD tight control is recommended but as disease progression continues, there is a cohort of patients who will require a higher therapeutic target to minimise falls risk. These are typically frailer adults with poor nutritional status.

Although hyperkalaemia is undoubtedly not good for CKD patients, overtly restricting fruit and vegetables increases their risk of CVD. Refer to dietetic experts skilled in achieving a reduction in potassium intake whilst preserving valuable fibre, polyphenol, vitamin and mineral intake. Avoid making broad statements about cutting out fruit and vegetables to your patients, as the evidence does not support the role of a diet low in fruit and vegetables for reducing mortality risk in this group.

73.9 Conclusion

There is no single nutritional priority in the patient with CKD. At different stages, and guided by the aetiology of the condition, the focus may shift from an approach to attenuate disease progression (such as management of obesity, hypertension, diabetes) to the acute management of undernutrition in uraemic end-stage kidney disease. Making long-term dietary changes is not a simple undertaking and warrants consideration beyond the scope of this brief chapter.

Using the full MDT, but particularly experts in nutrition, to optimise conditions such as frailty, sarcopenia, obesity and undernutrition, in combination with pre-

73

venting disturbances of fluid and electrolyte balance is vital. Balancing achieving treatment targets with quality of life is an unending challenge in the management of the person with CKD.

Chapter Review Questions

1. In early CKD a restriction to how many grams of salt is recommended?
2. What is the risk of recommending a low potassium diet?
3. What is the most bioavailable/readily absorbed source of dietary phosphate?
   (a) Dairy products
   (b) Plant proteins (e.g. lentils)
   (c) Inorganic phosphate additives
   (d) Meat
4. What is sarcopenic obesity?

Answers

1. 4–6 g or 1 teaspoon daily (inclusive of all dietary salt, including what is in or added to foods in processing or at the table)
2. Compromising dietary fibre intake (as well as polyphenols, vitamins, minerals) → increased risk of all-cause mortality.
3. (c) inorganic phosphate additives
4. The loss of muscle strength in the presence of obesity.

References

1. Kalantar-Zadeh K, Tortorici AR, Chen JLT, Kamgar M, Lau W-L, Moradi H, et al. Dietary restrictions in dialysis patients: is there anything left to eat? Semin Dial. 2015;28(2):159–68. https://doi.org/10.1111/sdi.12348.
2. Morton RL, Sellars M. From patient-centred to person-centred care for kidney diseases. Clin J Am Soc Nephrol. 2019;14(4):623–5. https://doi.org/10.2215/CJN.10380818.
3. World Health Organisation. Malnutrition. April 2020. https://www.who.int/news-room/fact-sheets/detail/malnutrition.
4. Carrero JJ, Stenvinkel P, Cuppari L, Ikizler TA, Kalantar-Zadeh K, Kaysen G, et al. Etiology of the protein-energy wasting syndrome in chronic kidney disease: a consensus statement from the International Society of Renal Nutrition and Metabolism (ISRNM). J Ren Nutr. 2013;23(2):77–90. https://doi.org/10.1053/j.jrn.2013.01.001.
5. Wright M, Southcott E, MacLaughlin H, Wineburg S. Clinical practice guideline: undernutrition in chronic kidney disease. The Renal Association; 2019. https://renal.org/wp-content/uploads/2019/06/FINAL-Nutrition-guideline-June-2019.pdf
6. British Dietetic Association. 2019. https://www.bda.uk.com/resource/malnutrition.html.
7. Wahid A, Chaudhry S, Ehsan A, Butt S, Khan AA. Bidirectional relationship between chronic kidney disease and periodontal disease. Pak J Med Sci. 2013;29(1):211–5. https://doi.org/10.12669/pjms.291.2926.
8. Woodrow G, Fan SL, Reid C, Denning J, Pyrah AN. Clinical practice guideline on peritoneal dialysis in adults and children. 2017;18(333). https://doi.org/10.1186/s12882-017-0687-2.
9. Morley JE, Vellas B, Abellan van Kan A, Anker SD, Bauer JM, Bernabei R, et al. Frailty consenus: a call to action. J Am Med Dir Assoc. 2014;(6):392–7. https://doi.org/10.1016/j.jamda.2013.03.022.
10. Bao Y, Dalrymple L, Chertow GM, Kaysen GA, Johansen KL. Frailty, dialysis initiation and mortality in end-stage renal disease. Arch Intern Med. 2012;172(14):1071–7. https://doi.org/10.1001/archinternmed.2012.3020.
11. Johansen KL, Chertow GM, Jin C, Kutner NG. Significance of frailty among dialysis patients. J Am Soc Nephrol. 2017;18(11):2960–7. https://doi.org/10.1681/ASN.2007020221.
12. Wu PY, Chao C-T, Chan D-C, Huang J-W, Jung K-Y. Contributors, risk associates and complications of frailty in patients with chronic kidney disease: a scoping review. Ther Adv Chronic Dis. 2019;10. https://doi.org/10.1177/2040622319880382.
13. Jhamb M, McNulty ML, Ingalsbe G, Childers JW, Schell J, Conroy MB, et al. Knowledge, barriers and facilitators of exercise in dialysis patients: a qualitative study of patients, staff and nephrologists. BMC Nephrol. 2016;17:192. https://doi.org/10.1186/s12882-016-0399-z.
14. Joint British Diabetes Societies with the Renal Association. Management of adults with diabetes on the haemodialysis unit. 2016. http://www.diabetologists-abcd.org.uk/JBDS/JBDS_RenalGuide_2016.pdf.
15. Nixon AC, Bampouras TM, Pendleton N, Woywodt A, Mitra S, Dhaygude A. Frailty and chronic kidney disease: current evidence and continuing uncertainties. Clin Kidney J. 2018;11(2):236–45. https://doi.org/10.1093/ckj/sfx134.
16. Stenvinkel P, Lindholm B. JASN debates. Resolved: being fat is good for dialysis patients: the Godzilla effect. J Am Soc Nephrol. 2008;19(6):1059–64. https://doi.org/10.1681/ASN.2007090983.
17. Segev DL, Simpkins CE, Thompson RE, Locke JE, Warren ES, Montgomery RA. Obesity impacts access to transplantation. J Am Soc Nephrol. 2008;19(2):349–55. https://doi.org/10.1681/ASN.2007050610.
18. Stenvinkel P, Zoccali C, Ikizler TL. Obesity in CKD - what should nephrologists know? J Am Soc Nephrol. 2013;24(11):727–36. https://doi.org/10.1681/ASN.2013040330.
19. Chang AR, Grams ME, Navaneethan SD. Bariatric surgery and kidney related outcomes. Kidney Int Rep. 2017;2(2):261–70. https://doi.org/10.1016/j.ekir.2017.01.010.
20. Kalantar-Zadeh K, Derose SF, Nicholas S, Benner D, Sharma K, Kovesdy CP. Burnt-out diabetes: impact of chronic kidney disease progression on the natural course of diabetes mellitus. J Ren Nutr. 2009;19(1):33–7. https://doi.org/10.1053/j.jrn.2008.11.012.
21. McMahon EJ, Bauer JD, Hawley CM, Isbel NM, Stowasser M, Johnson DW, Campbell KL. A randomized trial of dietary sodium restriction in CKD. J Am Soc Nephrol. 2013;24(12):2096–103. https://doi.org/10.1681/ASN.2013030285.
22. Zoccali C, Moissl U, Chazot C, Mallamici F, Tripeppi G, Arkossy O, et al. Chronic fluid overload and mortality in ESRD. J Am Soc Nephrol. 2017;28(8):2491–7. https://doi.org/10.1681/ASN.2016121341.
23. De brito-Ashurst I, Perry L, Sanders TAB, Thomas JE, Yaqoob MM, Dobbie H. Barriers and facilitators of dietary sodium restriction amongst Bangladeshi chronic kidney disease patients. J Hum Nutr Diet. 2011;24(1):86–95.
24. Rastogi A, Bhatt N, Rossetti S, Beto J. Management of hyperphosphataemia in end-stage kidney disease: a new paradigm. J Ren Nutr. 2020:1–14. https://doi.org/10.1053/j.jrn.2020.02.003.

25. De Nicola L, Di Nullo L, Paoletti E, Cupisti A, Bianchi S. Chronic hyperkalaemia in non-dialysis CKD: controversial issues in nephrology practice. J Nephrol. 2018;31(5):653–64. https://doi.org/10.1007/s40620-018-0502-6.
26. Kelly JT, Palmer SC, Wai SN, Ruospo M, Carrero JJ, Campbell KL, Strippoli GFM. Clin J Am Soc Nephrol. 2017;12(2):272–9. https://doi.org/10.2215/CJN.06190616.
27. Saglimbene VM, Wong G, Ruospo M, Palmer SC, Garcia-Larsen V, Natale P, et al. Clin J Am Soc Nephrol. 2019;14(2):250–60. https://doi.org/10.2215/CJN.08580718.
28. Cano NJM, Aparicio M, Brunori G, Carrero JJ, Cianciaruso B, Fiaccadori E, et al. ESPEN guidelines on parenteral nutrition: adult renal failure. Available at: http://espen.info/documents/0909/Adult%20Renal%20Failure.pdf. Accessed 1 Feb 2020.
29. Oh WC, Rigby M, Mafrici B, Sharman A, Harvey D, Welham S, et al. Micronutrient loss in renal replacement therapy for acute kidney injury. Abstract – British Renal Society. Available at: https://britishrenal.org/ukkw2018-2/2015-abstracts/. Accessed 17 Jan 2020.
30. Prasad N, Gupta A, Sharma RK, Sinha A, Kumar R. Impact of nutritional status on peritonitis in CAPD patients. Perit Dial Int. 2007;27(1):42–7.
31. El-Sherbini N, Duncan N, Hickson M, Johansson L, Brown E. Nutrition changes in conservatively treated patients with encapsulating peritoneal sclerosis. Perit Dial Int. 2013;33(5):538–43. https://doi.org/10.3747/pdi.2012.00049.
32. National Institute for Clinical Excellence. Nutrition Support for adults: oral nutrition support, enteral tube feeding and parenteral nutrition. 2006. nice.org.uk/guidance/cg32.
33. Saito M, Hirata-Koizumi M, Matsumoto M, Urano T, Hasegawa R. Undesirable effects of citrus juice on the pharmacokinetics of drugs: focus of recent studies. Drug Saf. 2005;28(8):677–94. https://doi.org/10.2165/00002018-200528080-00003.
34. British Association for Parenteral and Enteral Nutrition. Ethics and clinically assisted nutrition or hydration approaching the end of life - decision tree. 2012. Available at: https://www.bapen.org.uk/resources-and-education/education-and-guidance/bapen-principles-of-good-nutritional-practice.
35. British Medical Association/Royal College of Physicians. Clinically Assisted Nutrition and Hydration in adults who lack the capacity to consent. 2020. Available at: https://www.bma.org.uk/media/1161/bma-clinically-assisted-nutrition-hydration-canh-full-guidance.pdf.

Patient Information and Guidelines

https://www.kidney.org/nutrition/Kidney-Disease-Stages-1-4.

Food with Thought (cookbook) available at: https://www.kidney.org.uk/diet-and-food.

http://edren.org/ren/edren-info/diet-in-renal-disease/.

https://www.niddk.nih.gov/health-information/kidney-disease/chronic-kidney-disease-ckd/eating-nutrition.

Pharmacology and the Kidney

Amin Oomatia and Caroline Ashley

Contents

M. Harber (ed.), *Primer on Nephrology*, https://doi.org/10.1007/978-3-030-76419-7_74

74

Learning Objectives

The kidney plays an important role in the handling of drugs in the body; therefore, patients with renal impairment will invariably require different dosage regimes to those with normal renal function [1]. Unfortunately, there are no absolute guidelines on how to adjust doses in renal impairment, and pharmaceutical company literature often excludes patients with renal impairment in the dosage guidelines. Where information can be found, the advice may not be specific and different texts may give different advice [2]. Therefore, it is important to have an understanding of the potential effects of renal impairment on the pharmacodynamic and pharmacokinetic properties of a drug so that appropriate dosing decisions can be made. Although a reduced GFR is the primary reason for reduced excretion of drugs in renal failure, absorption, distribution, protein binding, metabolism and pharmacodynamics are all relevant. Drugs can also often cause an acute kidney injury through varying mechanisms: glomerulonephritis, tubulointerstitial nephritis or even acute tubular necrosis, which can either be idiosyncratic or dose-dependent. Therefore, this chapter will cover the following:

1. Pharmacokinetics and how they alter in renal impairment
2. Drug metabolism and excretion and how they alter in renal impairment
3. The elimination of drugs by various modalities of renal replacement therapy
4. Prescribing in patients with acute kidney injury
5. Medication known to cause renal impairment

74.1 Absorption

Absorption of orally administered drugs may be reduced in patients with renal impairment as a result of:

1. Nausea, vomiting or diarrhoea associated with uraemia.
2. Hypoproteinaemic oedema of the gastrointestinal tract, e.g. in nephrotic syndrome.
3. Reduced intestinal motility and gastric emptying time, e.g. in uraemic neuropathy.
4. An increase in pH in the gut from increased gastric ammonia production in uraemia; this reduces the bioavailability of drugs requiring an acidic environment for absorption, such as ferrous sulphate [3, 4].
5. Co-administration of drugs which increase gastric pH, e.g. H_2 antagonists and proton pump inhibitors.
6. Co-administration of chelating agents such as those used as phosphate binders.

It is also speculated that the absorption of some drugs is increased as a result of both reduced activity of drug-metabolising enzymes in the intestine, although this increase may be offset by increased first-pass metabolism in the liver [4], and co-administration of drugs which increase gastric pH will increase the bioavailability of weakly acidic drugs [4].

Drug doses are not routinely altered to allow for these factors alone but if therapeutic levels of drugs are not being achieved or if a fast onset of action is required, a change of dose or a different route of administration may be required.

74.2 Distribution

Changes to the distribution of drugs in the body of patients with renal impairment may occur as a result of changes in the hydration state of the patient, alterations in protein binding and alterations in tissue binding.

The state of hydration of a patient is only important for drugs with a small volume of distribution (Vd) (<50 l), e.g. gentamicin [5]. In the presence of oedema, the Vd will be increased; conversely, in the presence of dehydration, the Vd will be reduced.

Protein binding is altered due to (1) hypoalbuminaemia, (2) uraemia and the accumulation of metabolites and endogenous substances which will compete with the drugs for binding to albumin and (3) altered structural arrangement of albumin possibly reducing the affinity or number of binding sites for drugs [3, 4]. Alterations in protein binding are clinically important for highly protein-bound drugs (>80%) [3]. A reduction in the bound drug in the plasma will result in a higher proportion of unbound, and therefore active, drugs in the plasma. However, as there is more unbound drug available for metabolism, this effect is usually transient.

For highly bound drugs, such as phenytoin, interpretation of drug level measurements can be problematic as total drug concentrations (bound and unbound) are usually reported, rather than only the free, unbound, drug. So a reported low phenytoin level may not necessarily be subtherapeutic, and free phenytoin levels should be measured where possible.

Where creatinine clearance is <10 ml/min or the patient is undergoing haemodialysis, phenytoin levels can be interpreted using an equation incorporating factors which take into account both altered serum albumin concentration and decreased binding affinity for this patient group:

$$\mathrm{Cp}_{\mathrm{normal}} = \mathrm{Cp}_{\mathrm{observed}} \frac{\left[(0.48)\times(1-0.1)\times \text{serum albumin}(\mathrm{g/dl})\right]}{4.4(\mathrm{g/dl})} + 0.1$$

where Cp_{normal} is the plasma drug concentration that would have been observed if the patient's serum albumin concentration had been normal and $Cp_{observed}$ is the observed plasma concentration reported by the laboratory.

Alterations in tissue binding may affect a drug's Vd. For the majority of drugs, this is not clinically relevant, although it is for digoxin [4]. The Vd of digoxin may be reduced by up to 50% in patients with CKD stages 4–5, and so both the loading and maintenance doses will need to be reduced to prevent toxicity.

74.3 Metabolism

Both phase I and phase II metabolism are generally slower in chronic kidney disease [4, 6]. The effect of this is to increase serum drug concentrations of the parent drug. Where drugs are usually metabolised to inactive metabolites, a slowing of biotransformation may lead to a higher prevalence of side effects and toxicity. The kidney itself is also the site of metabolism for some drugs, two important examples being the hydroxylation of 25-hydroxycholecalciferol to active vitamin D (1,25-dihydroxycholecalciferol) and the metabolism of insulin.

74.4 Elimination

The kidney eliminates drugs and metabolites by a combination of glomerular filtration, renal tubular secretion and resorption [4]. In renal impairment, all these functions are reduced, and while the reduction in glomerular filtration and tubular secretion results in higher plasma drug levels, reduced resorption will result in higher urinary concentrations of drug. The extent to which the profiles of drugs are affected depends on the percentage of active drug or active metabolite that would normally be excreted renally. For some drugs, the accumulation of active metabolites with different effects on the active parent may change the pharmacological response, a classic example being pethidine. In common with most opiates, pethidine produces CNS depression as a toxic effect, but the accumulation of the renally excreted, pharmacologically active metabolite norpethidine produces CNS stimulation and seizures [6].

74.5 Pharmacodynamics

Although there is a paucity of the literature on changes in the body's response to drugs in renal impairment, it is known that patients with uraemia have (1) increased sensitivity to drugs acting on the central nervous system, e.g. antipsychotics, opiates and benzodiazepines; (2) reduced sensitivity to some endogenous hormones such as growth hormone; (3) increased sensitivity to cholinesterase inhibitors; (4) increased risk of gastrointestinal bleeding with irritant drugs such as non-steroidal anti-inflammatory drugs; and (5) increased risk of hyperkalaemia with drugs such as potassium-sparing diuretics, ACE inhibitors and angiotensin receptor blockers [7].

74.6 Drug Metabolism in Normal and Impaired Kidney Function

In the normal kidney, molecular size, protein binding, lipid solubility and charge are all important factors in determining the elimination of drugs by the kidney.

Nonprotein-bound compounds up to a molecular size of 60 kD are filtered through the glomerulus. Smaller molecules are filtered more freely. Highly protein-bound substances may be filtered only if the protein binding is saturated, for example, in salicylate poisoning. Once filtered into the renal tubule, reabsorption may occur if the compound is nonpolar or lipid-soluble allowing it to diffuse readily across tubular cell membranes back into the plasma. Polar or water-soluble drugs remain in the glomerular filtrate and are excreted in the urine.

Urine pH can enhance or retard drug elimination from the normal kidney as acidic compounds become less ionic and more soluble in alkaline urine with the same applying to basic compounds in acidic urine.

Four other concepts are important in drug excretion by the kidney:

1. Volume of distribution (Vd)
2. Half-life ($t_{1/2}$)
3. Elimination rate constant (ke)
4. Steady-state concentration (Css) of a drug

The relationship between these variables is discussed below. Finally, drugs present in tubular fluid may affect the elimination of other compounds, for example, aspirin reduces methotrexate removal.

In considering the likelihood that excretion of an individual drug may be affected by kidney failure, the following factors need to be considered:

- *Size*: <60 kD filtered by the glomerulus.
- *Protein binding*: Only an unbound drug can be filtered, the more protein-bound a drug is, the less that drug is available for filtration; proteins can become saturated leaving the unbound drug to be filtered depending on its size.
- *Polarity or water/lipid solubility*: Polar/water-soluble drugs are usually not reabsorbed once filtered.
- *Charge*: Acidic drugs are excreted more efficiently in alkaline urine and basic compounds in acidic urine.

- *Volume of distribution* (Vd): A measure that relates the amount of drug in the body to the concentration in the blood. It is the theoretical volume required to distribute a drug at a defined concentration (measured in the blood) throughout the body.
- *Half-life* ($t_{1/2}$): Time taken for the plasma concentration to fall by half after absorption and distribution are complete.
- *Elimination rate* (*ke*): The proportion of the total amount of drug removed per unit time.
- *Proportion of the drug excreted by the kidney.*
- *Extent of liver metabolism and renal excretion of metabolites.*
- *Active secretion or reabsorption by the kidney.*

In considering drug metabolism in CKD, the most important point to remember is that both filtration and secretion of drugs fall in parallel and in proportion to the GFR. It is important to note that although serum creatinine is widely used as a surrogate measure of renal function, it is not sufficiently accurate and at the very least eGFR should be used to adjust dosing.

▪ Table 74.1 outlines the commonly used formulae for calculating eGFR. The Cockcroft and Gault formula, though crude, is based on age, sex and weight and current creatinine measurement and can be easily calculated at the bedside. It should not be used for patients with end-stage renal disease or receiving RRT. The ideal body weight is used for patients who are obese and is calculated as follows:

The MDRD (modified diet in renal disease) equation is more sophisticated and cannot be calculated so readily. However, there are websites that can perform the calculation within seconds, and as a result of the Renal NSF, most laboratories in the United Kingdom now routinely report MDRD eGFR both in primary and secondary care.

The CKD-EPI performed better than the MDRD Study equation, especially at higher GFR: lesser bias, improved precision and greater accuracy (percent of estimated GFR within 30% of measured GFR). However, no laboratory in the United Kingdom currently routinely reports CKD-EPI eGFRs.

74.7 Elimination of Drugs by Haemodialysis/Filtration and Peritoneal Dialysis

The same principles of drug elimination apply to dialysis and filtration membranes as to native kidneys. Drug removal follows first-order kinetics, and the amount of drug removed is determined by plasma concentration, the sieving coefficient or permeability of the membrane, the molecular weight of the drug and the extent to which it is bound to plasma proteins.

Newer "high-flux" dialysis membranes can remove larger molecules and are particularly useful when trying to remove middle molecules including β_2 microglobulin responsible for dialysis amyloid. Haemofilters remove molecules smaller than inulin (average molecular weight 5200 Da). This difference is especially important as most drugs which are not protein-bound are removed by haemodialysis including most antibiotics, but drugs such as vancomycin (1800 Da), amphotericin (960 Da) and erythromycin (734 Da) behave differently in haemodialysis, "high-flux" haemodialysis and haemofiltration. Just as in the native kidney, water-soluble drugs are more readily filtered than fat-soluble ones. When deciding on drug dosing regimens for patients on renal replacement therapy (RRT), it is essential to ascertain which mode of RRT the patient is receiving. This is because the different modalities all have differing solute clearance rates, which has major implications for drug dosing to ensure the patient is neither overdosed nor underdosed (see ▪ Table 74.2).

The plasma concentration of a drug is determined by its volume of distribution and tissue binding characteristics. Digoxin, phenytoin and antidepressants, for example, have large volumes of distribution with only very low plasma concentrations and are therefore hardly influenced by dialysis or filtration. Conversely, gentamicin has a very small Vd and negligible protein binding, so is removed extremely efficiently by dialysis.

Drugs are eliminated much less efficiently by the peritoneal membrane than by synthetic dialysis or filtration membranes. This poor permeability is used to advantage in treating peritonitis in peritoneal dialysis (PD) patients where antibiotics are injected into the peritoneal fluid.

There is one small advantage of ESRD in that reduced dosing of some antibiotics means that some patients can be easily managed with three times a week administration of antibiotics on haemodialysis, thus facilitating early discharge or avoiding daily outpatient administration of antibiotics. ▪ Figure 74.1 illustrates antibiotics that achieve therapeutic levels when given three times a week. Amikacin, gentamicin and vancomycin all require monitoring of drug levels to ensure therapeutic concentrations are reached and toxicity avoided, with trough levels usually being taken at the start of dialysis. Both dosage, which often depends upon body weight (or ideal body weight if obese), and target levels vary between units, and so prescribers should consult local guidelines or expertise for centre-specific protocols.

Table 74.1 Comparison of Cockcroft and Gault equation with MDRD equation for estimated GFR

Cockcroft and Gault equation	$Clcr = \frac{[140 - Age(years)] \times Weight(kg)}{Plasma\ creatinine(\mu mol/l)}$ NB. 1. For males, multiply above equation by 1.23 For females, multiply above equation by 1.04 2. Use ideal body weight in obesity (i.e. if patient's weight is >15% over IBW) 3. This equation can only be used if the plasma creatinine is stable (i.e. not varying by >40 μmol/l per day) 4. Do not use if: (i) Patient is <15 years or >90 years of age (ii) Patient has rapidly changing renal function (iii) Patient has a serum creatinine >350 μmol/l (iv) Patient is pregnant (v) Patient is an amputee (vi) Patient is severely wasted
MDRD equation	$GFR(ml/min/1.73\ 0.24\ m^2) = 175 \times \{[serum\ creatinine\ (mmol/l)/88.4] - 1.154\} \times \{age(years) - 0.203\} \times 0.742\ if\ female\ and \times 1.21\ if\ African\ American\ or\ African\ Caribbean$ Validated in Caucasians and African Americans Not yet validated in Asians and transplants Normalised GFR – reported as/1.73 m^2 Incorporated into Renal NSF and Renal Association guidelines Can be calculated from online websites, e.g. ► http://www.renal.org/eGFRcalc/GFR.pl
CKD-EPI equation	GFR = 141 × min(Scr/κ, 1)$^{\alpha}$ × max(Scr/κ, 1)$^{-1.209}$ × 0.993^{Age} × 1.018 [if female] _ 1.159 [if black], Where κ is 0.7 for females and 0.9 for males α is −0.329 for females and −0.411 for males min indicates the minimum of Scr/κor 1, max indicates the maximum of Scr/κ or 1
Ideal body weight (men) = 50 + 2.3 kg for every inch over 5 ft in height	
Ideal body weight (women) = 45.5 + 2.3 kg for every inch over 5 ft in height	

74.8 Electronic Prescribing

Both electronic records and prescribing are increasingly becoming common globally. Aside from the benefits of improving the efficiency of the clinical workforce, it has also resulted in far fewer prescribing errors. Birmingham University trust hospital, which has developed and implemented its own electronic prescribing system, has reported not only a reduction in the average length of stay for patients but also a significant decrease in its mortality rate compared to the ratios of standardized mortality rates across the country. Whilst there are no major studies looking specifically at the effect of electronic prescribing in renal patients, the benefits are likely to be twofold. By integrating patients' biochemical test records, prescribing systems can not only automatically calculate eGFR and thus alert prescribers to both contraindications for those with chronic kidney disease but also recommend dose adjustments. Furthermore, given the increasing occurrence of polypharmacy that is

Table 74.2 Approximate GFR for renal replacement modalities

Renal replacement therapy	Typical theoretical GFR achieved during therapy (ml/min)
Intermittent haemodialysis	150–200 during dialysis (0–10 between dialysis periods)
Continuous arteriovenous haemofiltration (CAVH)	10–15
Continuous venovenous haemodiafiltration (CVVH)	15–25
Continuous arteriovenous haemodiafiltration (CAVHD)	20–35
Continuous venovenous haemodiafiltration (CVVHD)	30–40
Continuous ambulatory peritoneal dialysis (CAPD) (4 exchanges daily)	5–10
Automated peritoneal dialysis (APD)	5–10

Data from Industry Submission, Renal National Service Framework (Acute Renal Failure) October 2003

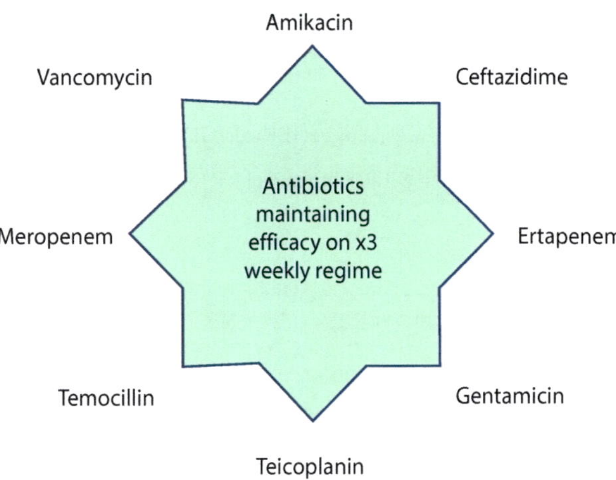

Fig. 74.1 Antibiotics that still achieve therapeutic levels when given three times a week post-haemodialysis

present in ageing and comorbid populations, electronic prescribing systems can also flag up potential drug interactions which may not necessarily be immediately apparent to the prescriber [8].

It is worth noting, however, that in many cases, it may still be clinically appropriate for many electronics alerts and warnings not to be heeded given that many drugs are used off-license or the benefits of the drug are deemed to outweigh the risks of side effects or adverse events. This is especially the case in patients with kidney disease.

Further still, there are often significant differences in published recommendations and resources for prescribing in renal failure [7]. Many units may thus differ on the dosing of various drugs depending on local guidelines, expertise and appraisal of published literature which may hinder "standardised" electronic prescribing programs, though these are likely to be circumvented by allowing local units some autonomy on specific alerts. As electronic prescribing systems are being increasingly implemented in primary and secondary care, it is likely that their use and utility will continue to evolve over the coming decade.

74.9 Prescribing in Acute Kidney Injury

From a drug's perspective, it is essential in AKI to review all the medications that a patient is taking, including those for comorbidities:

- Temporarily or permanently withdraw drugs that affect kidney haemodynamics especially NSAIDs and drugs blocking the renin-angiotensin system.
- Stop any nephrotoxic drugs and avoid prescribing nephrotoxic therapy.
- Review drugs that may have adverse effects in patients with AKI, for example, antihypertensives, metformin, statins and any drugs which may exacerbate hyperkalaemia.
- Ensure drug dosing is appropriate for the level of renal impairment or the type of renal replacement therapy used.

Caution should be taken with drug dosing in AKI. The use of eGFR and Cockcroft and Gault is unreliable in AKI as serum creatinine levels are regularly changing and their rate of change might not reflect current renal function. However, the daily assessment of renal function using eGFR or GFR may be an appropriate estimation for drug dosing, as long as the patient's prescription is reviewed each day.

In addition, review doses of medications as AKI resolves. This may happen quickly in patients with dehydration, where fluids can cause prompt reversal of the insult with renal function quickly improving. Underdosing of drugs such as antibiotics may have an adverse impact on the management of sepsis, and doses of low molecular weight heparins may need to be increased in VTE prophylaxis.

It is also worth bearing in mind that drugs are very commonly the primary or contributing cause of AKI. An obsessional medication history (prescribed and over the counter) with start dates, courses, dose increments and potential drug interactions is thus important and may involve contacting prescribers such as the patient's family practitioner or community pharmacy. Common drug causes of acute kidney injury by histological lesion are shown in Fig. 74.2. It is worth noting that some drugs cause an elevated serum creatinine without actually caus-

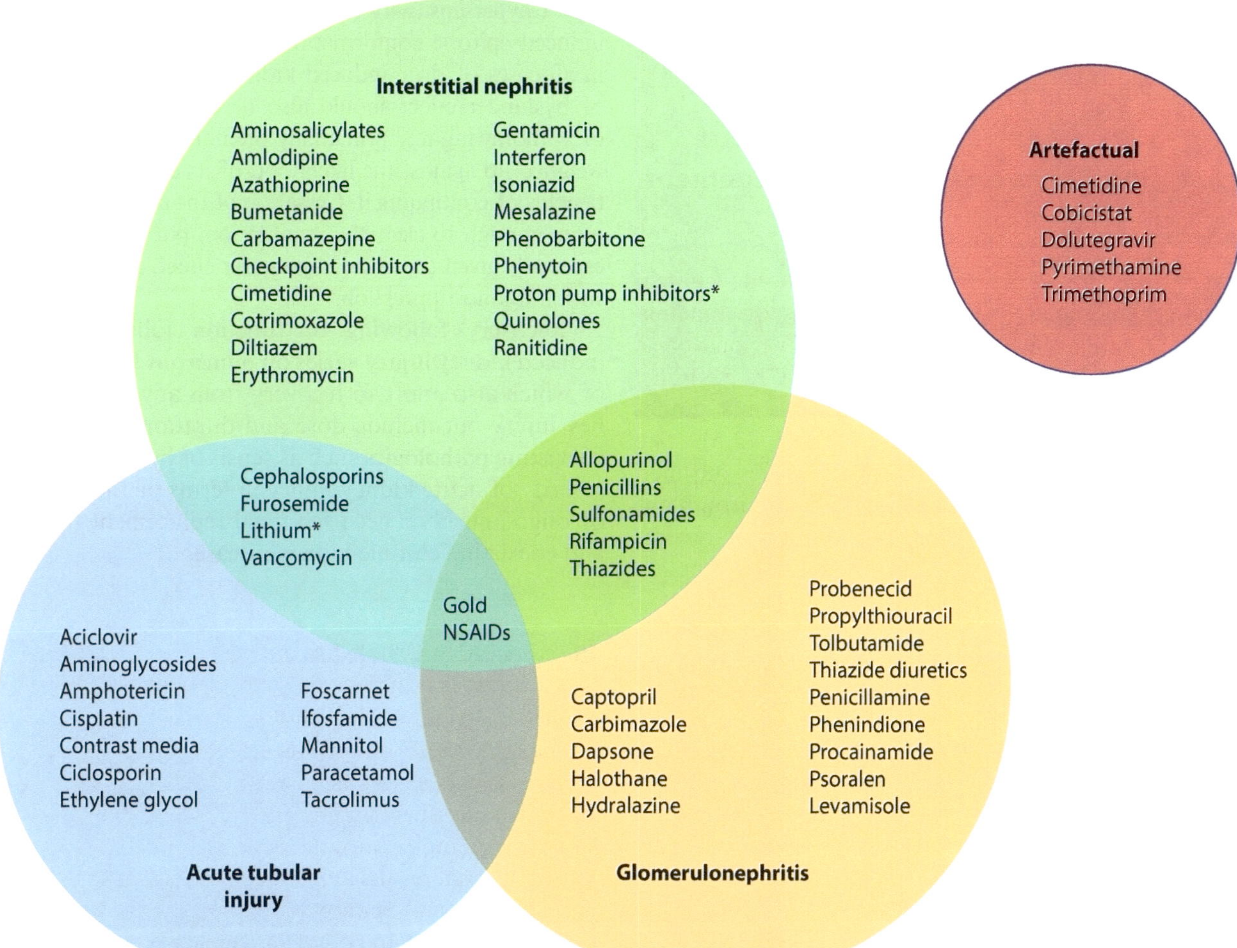

Fig. 74.2 Medication well documented to cause renal injury. In clinical practice, any drug could potentially cause an acute tubulointersitial nephritis – as this reaction is host-specific, but the drugs listed are commonly cited offenders.* Classically associated with chronic interstitial nephritis rather than acute

ing any renal injury. Creatinine excretion is mostly due to glomerular filtration but around 10% is also secreted by both anion and cation transporters in the proximal tubules. By competing for tubular secretion, drugs such as trimethoprim and cimetidine result in impaired urinary creatinine clearance, whereas other drugs such dolutegravir have the same effect but by direct inhibition of cation transporters such as OCT2 [9]. The consequent rise in serum creatinine resulting in an "artefactual" kidney injury. In these cases, serum urea will not be affected, nor will there be any abnormality on urinary dipstick testing. Both of these factors, in conjunction with a comprehensive drug history and clinical assessment, should prevent a misdiagnosis of an acute kidney injury.

The exact mechanism of renal injury can vary, and whilst it is usually dose-dependent, idiosyncratic reactions can occur. Drug-induced acute tubular necrosis (ATN) can occur as a result of various mechanisms which may be precipitated by coexisting conditions such as sepsis including renal ischaemia, interference of mitochondrial function increasing oxidative stress and tubular damage, direct tubular toxicity and even tubular precipitation of the drug resulting in crystal nephritis (see Fig. 74.3) [10]. Given that ischemia and necrosis often trigger the inflammatory cascade, it is not surprising to see the presence of immune cells in the interstitium surrounding the tubules on renal biopsy but this is often a mild tubulointerstitial nephritis (TIN) which is reactive and causative. Conversely, tubular damage and necrosis can occur as a result of TIN and may also be coexistent on a renal biopsy. Usually, the primary lesion predominates, but discerning the two entities may require clinic-histopathological correlation, especially if treatment other than drug withdrawal is being considered (see next paragraph).

The exact mechanisms for drug-induced immunological injury to the kidney, both glomerulonephritis and TIN, are not completely understood. There are multiple postulated mechanisms which are likely causative including direct

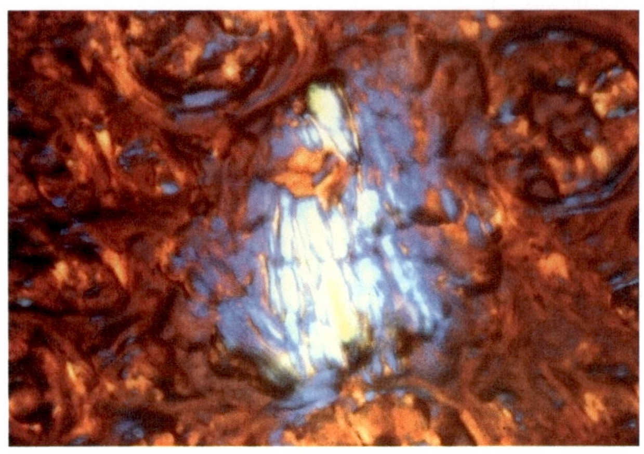

Fig. 74.3 Foscarnet crystals which have precipitated in renal tubules causing crystal nephritis. Acute tubular necrosis results from both obstruction and direct toxicity to the tubular epithelium

type I hypersensitivity reactions, antigenic mimicry, drug-induced epitope conformation change. In these cases, as in all cases of drug-induced kidney injury, the possibility of bystander effect should also be considered. The risks of withdrawing any potentially offending drug need to be weighed up against the likelihood of its causation and the benefits of continuing it. Cessation of the offending drug is often enough to clear the renal lesion, but clinicians may, especially given the risk of bystander effect, choose to treat with immunosuppression.

Recovery following of function following drug-induced kidney injury varies on numerous factors, many of which also apply to recovery from any form of kidney injury but include dose and duration of the drug, coexisting pathologies such as sepsis or hypotension, the severity of acute kidney injury in terms of the presence of oligo-anuria or need for renal replacement therapy, and coexisting chronic kidney disease.

Case Studies

Case 1: Drug Interaction

A 58-year-old 47 Kg female renal transplant recipient is seen in clinic where reports a tremor, headache and generally feeling unwell. She had an uneventful kidney transplant 22 years ago after reaching end-stage renal failure with chronic glomerulonephritis. Her baseline creatinine is usually 180. She had seen her GP 7 days ago with a fever, and he had given her a 7-day course of clarithromycin for a presumed chest infection.

Medication:

Adoport (Tacrolimus)	1.5 mg bd
Azathioprine	75 mg od
Prednisolone	5 mg od
Atorvastatin	10 mg nocte
Amlodipine	10 mg od
Aspirin	75 mg od
Omeprazole	20 mg od

Results:

Urea	24
Creatinine	370
Sodium	140
Potassium	5.8
Haemoglobin	15.5
WBC	10.0
Platelets	220

Tacrolimus trough level >30.

Questions

1. What has happened to cause the patient's kidney function to deteriorate and why?

   She was discharged after one week but one month later, she developed gout. Her GP treated her with colchicine and then started her on Allopurinol. Two weeks later, she developed shingles and was started on Aciclovir 800 mg five times a day for 10 days. A week later, she is admitted unwell, pyrexial and having seizures.

   Results

Urea	18
Creatinine	190
Sodium	140
Potassium	5
Haemoglobin	9.8
WBC	0.01
Plts	98

Tacrolimus trough 5.2

2. What has happened now?

Case 1: Answers and Learning Points

Answer to Question 1

- Tacrolimus nephrotoxicity caused by clarithromycin. Macrolides are inhibitors of Cytochrome P450 leading to vastly increased serum tacrolimus levels.
- Interestingly, although erythromycin and clarithromycin have this effect on tacrolimus, azithromycin appears not to, so it may be used safely in transplant patients.

Learning Points

- Transplant patients' renal function should always be compared to their baseline creatinine.
- Do not assume a transplant patient has normal renal function – they usually do not!
- Tacrolimus is metabolised by cytochrome P450, therefore subject to many drug-drug interactions. General physicians will not necessarily be aware of this fact, and so it is often the responsibility of the nephrologists to flag up potential interactions and to ensure enzyme inhibitors are not given. Important interactions and associated with tacrolimus are given below:
  - Tacrolimus levels are increased by cytochrome P450 inhibitors: grapefruit juice, erythromycin, clarithromycin (but NOT azithromycin), itraconazole, ketoconazole, miconazole, fluconazole, chloroquine, danazol, diltiazem, nicardipine, nifedipine, verapamil, high-dose methylprednisolone, progestogens (ethinyloestradiol, gestodene), cimetidine, ritonavir, protease inhibitors and grapefruit juice.
  - Tacrolimus levels are decreased by cytochrome P450 inducers: rifampicin, phenytoin, phenobarbitone, carbamazepine and isoniazid.
  - Increased risk of nephrotoxicity with amphotericin, aminoglycosides, vancomycin, cotrimoxazole, NSAIDs, ganciclovir and aciclovir.
  - Increased risk of hyperkalaemia with ACE inhibitors, angiotensin-II antagonists, potassium-sparing diuretics and potassium salts.
  - Increased risk of myopathy with HMG CoA reductase inhibitors.
  - Tacrolimus potentiates the effects of oral anticoagulants and antidiabetic drugs (though itself often causes or worsens diabetic control).

Answer to Question 2

- There is a major interaction between allopurinol and azathioprine leading to increased plasma levels of the azathioprine metabolite 6-mercaptopurine, which in turn leads to pancytopenia.
- The pancytopenia caused by this drug-drug interaction led to severe bone marrow and immune suppression and hence reactivation of the varicella zoster virus.
- Aciclovir toxicity due to a high dose being given to someone with renal impairment, leading to accumulation and seizures.

Learning Points

- Her estimated creatinine clearance is only 21 ml/min.
- For prescribing narrow therapeutic index drugs in patients with renal impairment, the Cockcroft and Gault equation is more accurate at estimating GFR than the MDRD equation.
- Aciclovir is excreted unchanged by the kidney. Renal clearance of aciclovir is substantially greater than creatinine clearance, indicating that tubular secretion, in addition to glomerular filtration, contributes to the renal elimination of the drug. The dose needs to be significantly reduced in patients with severe renal impairment to avoid accumulation and toxicity. In this patient a dose of 400 mg three times a day (rather than 800 mg 5 times a day) would have been sufficient.
- Aciclovir is also nephrotoxic per se in high dose, so the overdosage could have led to further deterioration of her graft function.

Case 2: Dose Change According to RRT

Mr. AA is a 61-year-old gentleman admitted with acute shortness of breath and abdominal pain.

He has a history of SLE diagnosed 10 years ago, with lupus nephritis (class IV) treated with Rituximab and Mycophenolate mofetil.

Reached ESRF last year and commenced on automated PD.

Had admission 4 weeks ago with PD peritonitis (*Strep sanguinis* sensitive to vancomycin).

Reported 8 kg weight loss over few months – CTCAP and BAL revealed chronic PCP.

Problems with this admission:

- *Pneumocystis jiroveci* pneumonia
- *Strep sanguinis* bacteraemia
- CMV colitis
- Candida sp. fungal peritonitis

He is prescribed the following medications:

- Cotrimoxazole
- Ceftazidime
- Daptomycin

74

- Ambisome, later switching to Caspofungin
- Ganciclovir

Over the course of his treatment, he is transferred to the ICU where he undergoes CVVHD.

On return to the ward, he is switched to intermittent haemodialysis, and then as his condition stabilises, he returns to receiving CAPD 4 × 2 L exchanges per day.

Question

- What doses would you prescribe for these drugs for each of the RRT modalities employed?

Effective GFRs on Renal Replacement Therapy

RRT	Effective GFR (ml/min)
Intermittent HD	250–300 whilst on machine (0–10 otherwise)
CAPD / APD	5–10
CAVHF / CVVHF	15–30
CAVHD / CVVHD	20–35

Case 2: Dose Change According to RRT: Answers and Learning Points

Ceftazidime	*2 g every 12 hour* Ceftazidime is < 10% protein bound, and so will be very readily removed by CHHVD	*Either 1 g every 24 hours or 2 g 3 ×/ week* In patients with ESRD, the half-life of ceftazidime increases from 2 hours to 25 hours. Hence it is possible to dose every 2–3 days at the end of each dialysis session	*1 g every 24 hours* Ceftazidime is recmoved by peritoneal dialysis Daily dosing rather than thrice weekly dosing is preferred in this modality	Ceftazidime is mainly excreted by the kidneys. About 80–90% of a dose appears unchanged in the urine within 24 hours
Daptomycin	*4–6 mg/kg every 24 hours, or 8 mg/kg every 48 hours* RRT should be initiated within 8 hours of administering a daptomycin dose to minimise the risk of accumulation	*4–6 mg/kg, 3 ×/ week post-HD* 50% of a dose is removed by a 4-hour haemodialysis session using a high-flux filter	*4 mg/kg IV every 48 hours* 11% of a dose is removed by peritoneal dialysis over 48 hours For treatment of PD peritonitis, penetration of daptomycin into the peritoneum following IV administration is poor. Hence administration via the IP route is preferred at a dose of *20 mg/L for 6 exchanges a day, or 25 mg/L for 4 exchanges a day*	Daptomycin is excreted mainly as unchanged drug via renal filtration with about 78% and 6% of a dose recovered in the urine and faeces, respectively

Ambisome	*1–3 mg/kg/day, maximum 5 mg/kg* Amphotericin is highly protein-bound and not removed by haemofiltration or haemodiafiltration	*1–3 mg/kg/day, maximum 5 mg/kg* Amphotericin is highly protein-bound and not removed by haemodialysis If given whilst the patient is undergoing dialysis, it should be administered into the venous return arm of the circuit. If given on the arterial side, as the Ambisome passes through the peristaltic pump, the micelles are smashed, releasing toxic doses of amphotericin	*1–3 mg/kg/day, maximum 5 mg/kg* Amphotericin is highly protein-bound and not removed by peritoneal dialysis	Liposomal amphotericin has a significantly different pharmacokinetic profile from the old water-soluble presentations of amphotericin B, with higher amphotericin plasma concentrations (Cmax) and increased exposure (AUC_{0-24}). Due to the size of the liposomes, there is no glomerular filtration and renal elimination of Ambisome, which avoids the interaction of amphotericin with the cells of the distal tubuli and thus reducing the nephrotoxicity seen with amphotericin
Caspofungin	*70 mg loading dose followed by 50 mg daily, thereafter* Caspofungin is 97% protein-bound, and is not removed by CVVHD or CVVH	*70 mg loading dose followed by 50 mg daily, thereafter* Caspofungin is 97% protein-bound, and is not removed by intermittent HD	*70 mg loading dose followed by 50 mg daily, thereafter* Caspofungin is 97% protein-bound, and is not removed by peritoneal dialysis	Plasma clearance of caspofungin is dependent on distribution rather than on biotransformation or excretion. Caspofungin undergoes spontaneous degradation; there is further slow metabolism of caspofungin by hydrolysis and *N*-acetylation and excretion in faeces and urine In established renal failure the AUC is increased by 30–49% but a change in dosage schedule is not required
Ganciclovir	*2.5 mg/kg twice daily* Ganciclovir is well-cleared by CVVHD / CVVH so may be safely given at a higher dose	*1.25 mg/kg once daily* For intermittent haemodialysis, the fraction of ganciclovir removed in a single dialysis session varies from 50% to 63% Daily doses of ganciclovir should be timed to be administered AFTER dialysis	*1.25 mg/kg once daily* There is evidence to suggest that ganciclovir (like aciclovir) is not as well cleared by peritoneal dialysis as it is by haemodialysis. Monitor for signs of toxicity, and if necessary, reduce dose to 1.25 mg/kg 3 ×/week	Renal excretion of unchanged drug by glomerular filtration and active tubular secretion is the major route (approximately 90%) of elimination of ganciclovir There have been reports of treatment failure when ganciclovir is prescribed at licensed doses. An alternative dosing strategy used by several units is:- GFR — Dose >50 — 5 mg/kg bd 25–50 — 2.5 mg/kg bd 10–25 — 2.5 mg/kg od <10 — 1.25 mg/kg od

Tips and Tricks for Prescribing for Patients with Renal Impairment

- A number of published tables that provide dosing guidelines exist to assist in dose modification (see below), but it is important to note that there often exist differing recommendations for dosage and dosing intervals. Individualisation of therapy should be based on pharmacokinetic principles whenever possible [7].
- Most texts use creatinine clearance (as calculated using Cockcroft and Gault) as an estimation of GRF for recommending doses [11].
- For most drugs, there is a broad creatinine clearance range for guidance on dosage, and so in practice, the variations of measurement will not change the recommendations [6], but it is important to consider the implications of under and overdosing for patients with GFR levels which are borderline.
- If non-renal clearance accounts for the elimination of more than 50% of a drug, then no adjustments need to be made to dose or frequency of administration.
- Dosages of toxic drugs which are mainly excreted in an active form by the kidney (i.e. as unchanged drug or active metabolites) may need to be modified to avoid accumulation.
- In renal failure, potentially toxic drugs should only be used if there is a specific indication for their use and if therapy can be monitored appropriately.
- If dose adjustment is required, then dose, dose interval or both can be adjusted to achieve the desired therapeutic effect. For example, with antibiotics, particular peak concentrations are required for optimal bacteriocidal or bacteriostatic effects, so typically the normal dose given less frequently is prescribed. Conversely, with digoxin, a steady plasma concentration is desirable, so the dosing interval remains at 24 hours, and the dose is reduced.
- Drugs that require therapeutic levels quickly may require a loading dose as the time taken to reach a steady state will be prolonged for drugs where the metabolism and excretion are slowed in renal impairment.
- Supplementary doses for RRT – some texts quote supplementary doses to be given after intermittent RRT. They will only be important for drugs with a low Vd and a narrow therapeutic range which are cleared efficiently by dialysis. In practice, it is better to adjust the timings of doses so that the next dose falls after the RRT session rather than add in extra doses.
- Always remember to use caution when using calculated eGFRs in patients for whom conventional formulae are likely to be inaccurate. Broadly speaking, this includes those patients with limb amputations, very low muscle mass (i.e. cachexia) or those with jaundice (as high bilirubin levels result in an underestimate of serum creatinine).

Chapter Review Questions

1. (a) *Calculate the renal function of the patients in the table below, using both MDRD (eGFR) and Cockcroft & Gault equations.*

Age	Gender	Race	Weight (kg)	Height (cm)	Serum Creatinine (μmol/L)	CrCl (ml/min) C&G equation	eGFR (ml/min/1.73m^2) MDRD equation
20	Male	Black	90	188	110		
75	Female	Caucasian	50	160	110		
86	Male	Caucasian	76	178	92		
54	Female	Black	106	165	82		

(b) Mr. NL is admitted with urinary sepsis and requires antibiotic therapy with gentamicin. He has previously undergone an above-knee amputation following a car accident. How would you assess his renal function in order to prescribe the gentamicin at the correct dose?

2. Mr. LB is admitted for a cadaveric renal transplant. He is HIV positive, and his antiretroviral treatment consists of:-
   Darunavir 800 mg od
   Lamivudine 100 mg od
   Ritonavir 100 mg nocte
   What immunosuppression regimen would you prescribe and at what doses?
3. (a) *Mr. AJ is admitted to the ICU with AKI stage 3 and sepsis. He is commenced on CVVHD. What dose of gentamicin would you prescribe for him?*
   (b) *Mr. AJ is later transferred to the renal ward where he still requires renal replacement therapy in the form of intermittent haemodialysis 3 days a week. What dose of gentamicin does he require now?*
4. Mrs. TH, a 61-year-old lady with type II diabetes and ESRD is admitted with a cold, ischaemic and very painful left leg. She is referred to the vascular surgeons but meanwhile requires urgent pain relief.
   (a) *What is your strong opiate of choice in patients with ESRD and why?*
   (b) *Which other analgesic preparations may be used in patients with renal impairment?*
5. Mrs. PC is a 49-year old lady with CKD stage 4 (eGFR 21ml/min) and a history of lupus nephritis, who is admitted with symptoms that included shortness of breath, chest pain particularly on inspiration, and haemoptysis. She was found to be D-dimer-positive, and CT pulmonary angiography (CTPA) confirmed the diagnosis of pulmonary embolus.
   (a) How would you initially treat her PE?

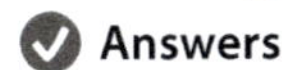

Answers

1. (a)

Age	Gender	Race	Weight (kg)	Height (cm)	Serum creatinine (μmol/L)	CrCl (ml/min) C&G equation	eGFR (ml/min/1.73 m^2) MDRD equation
20	Male	Black	90	188	110	*120*	*> 90*
75	Female	Caucasian	50	160	110	*29*	*40*
86	Male	Caucasian	76	178	92	*55*	*68*
54	Female	Black	106	165	82	*65 (IBW)* *115 (ABW)*	*76*

   (b) An above-knee amputation would remove a reasonable amount of the body's muscle mass and so would invalidate the usual equations used to estimate renal function. A 12- or 24-hour urine collection would enable a fairly accurate indication of creatinine clearance. Alternatively, the website ▶ https://clincalc.com/Kinetics/EBWL.aspx provides a means of estimating renal function in amputees and could be employed in this instance.
2. Mr. LB's ARV regimen includes a boosted protease inhibitor. This combination causes major inhibition of the cytochrome P450 system responsible for the metabolism of tacrolimus (and also ciclosporin and sirolimus), leading to toxic levels of tacrolimus. Hence, although each transplant unit has their own protocol for these cases, a typical tacrolimus regimen for a patient on a boosted PI is a loading dose of 1 mg, followed by a maintenance dose of 0.5 mg every 7–10 days, adjusted according to tacrolimus levels. Liaison with the HIV unit is essential, especially if they subsequently switch the patient to a different ARV regimen that does not include a boosted PI. If this occurs, the patient will revert to usual tacrolimus doses.
3. (a) Different hospitals have varying policies for aminoglycoside prescribing. However, most patients on CVVHD will be prescribed 5–7 mg/kg as an initial dose, since gentamicin is a small, highly hydrophilic drug which is very easily removed by dialysis. The next dose should not be given until a trough level has been measured, and the dose and dosing interval then adjusted accordingly.
   (b) Since a patient with ESRD effectively only has "renal function" when they are actually being dialysed, the pharmacokinetics of gentamicin change drastically in somebody undergoing intermittent haemodialysis. Here, it is standard practice to give a small dose of gentamicin, typically 2–2.5 mg/kg, at the end of each dialysis session. Larger doses are usually discouraged since the total exposure to the drug (i.e. the area under the curve) will be greatly increased leading to irreversible ototoxicity and vestibular damage. A trough level should be taken before the next dialysis session, but

the next dose should be given anyway to ensure continuity of therapy.

4. (a) Great care is required when prescribing opioids to patients with impaired renal function. There is increased permeability of the blood-brain barrier which leads to increased sensitivity to the CNS side effects of opioids e.g. drowsiness.

   Oxycodone: Oxycodone is metabolised in the liver to produce noroxycodone, oxymorphone and various conjugated glucuronides. These are then excreted along with any remaining unchanged drug in the urine. As the analgesic effects of the metabolites are clinically insignificant, the risks of toxicity are reduced with oxycodone. However, as the metabolites are not excreted and remain in circulation, the plasma concentration of the active drug may be increased and so dose initiation should follow a conservative approach in these patients. The recommended adult starting dose should be reduced by 50% (typically 1.25–2.5 mg) and with an increased dosing interval (2–3 times a day rather than 2–4 hourly), and each patient should be titrated to adequate pain control according to their clinical situation. It is partially removed by haemodialysis.

   PCA Devices: Oxycodone (60 mg in 60 ml) is the opiate of choice for use in PCA devices for patients with moderate to severe renal impairment.

   (b) *Transdermal Fentanyl*: mainly metabolised in the liver to inactive metabolites, is a useful strong opioid for patients with impaired renal function who have stable pain. It takes 3 days to reach a steady state. Patients require access to regular doses of immediate-release opioid during the first 12–24 hours and for breakthrough medication.

   Fentanyl can also be given transmucosally or sublingually for incident pain. It is rapidly absorbed and has a short half-life by these routes.

   PCA Devices: Fentanyl (25 mcg/ml) may also be used in PCA devices for patients with moderate to severe renal impairment.

   Transdermal buprenorphine is safe in renal impairment. Buprenorphine 35mcg/hr. is approximately half as strong as Fentanyl 25mcg/hr. Unlike Fentanyl, Transtec patches can be cut, so very small doses can be delivered to opioid naïve patients.

   Paracetamol is safe in moderate renal failure. Use up to 1 g QDS. In cases of severe renal impairment, the elimination of paracetamol is slightly delayed and metabolites may accumulate ⇒ max 1 g TDS, especially if given via the IV route.

   Methadone: Useful drug in renal impairment especially if pain is neuropathic as it is metabolised in the liver and predominantly excreted in faeces.

   Non-steroidal anti-inflammatory drugs (NSAIDs): NSAIDs are useful for nociceptive pain associated with tissue inflammation (e.g. arthritis). These drugs are usually contraindicated in patients with CKD who are not on dialysis due to the significant risk of causing deterioration in renal function. In patients with stable CKD stage 3 where there is a strong indication (e.g. severe arthritis), then a trial of NSAIDs with close monitoring of renal function may be appropriate. Ibuprofen 200–400 mg TDS is a reasonable first-line drug, with co-prescription of a proton-pump inhibitor where appropriate for gastric protection. NSAIDs may also be used in dialysis patients who are anuric (i.e. have no significant residual kidney function) although there is also an increased risk of gastrointestinal side effects.

   The following analgesics can also be used in renal impairment but less preferable than those listed above but their use may be necessary, for example, if the above drugs are not available or tolerated by patients.

   Morphine: Morphine and its active metabolites morphine-3-glucuronide and morphine-6-glucuronide have an extended elimination half-life and accumulate in patients with severe renal impairment. The half-life of morphine-6-glucuronide increases from 3–5 hours up to 50 hours in ESRD. The accumulation of morphine and its metabolites leads to toxic side effects including increased drowsiness, respiratory depression and coma. Long term use is contraindicated in moderate/severe renal impairment. Use only if no other opioid is available. Morphine and its metabolites are removed by dialysis.

   Tramadol: Approximately 30% of a dose is excreted in the urine as unchanged drug, and 60% is excreted as metabolites. One metabolite, O-desmethyl tramadol, is pharmacologically active.

   Codeine: The main metabolite of codeine is codeine-6-glucuronide, which has a similar potency to the parent drug and is renally excreted; 2–10% of a dose is metabolised to morphine, which accounts for most of the analgesic effect of codeine. Half-life is significantly prolonged in renal failure and there are case reports of extreme sensitivity. Main side-effects are confusion, respiration depression and constipation (increased K+ and problematic for PD patients).

Dihydrocodeine is a semi-synthetic derivative of codeine, with an analgesic effect independent of its metabolism to dihydromorphine.

5. (a) Use of treatment doses of LMWHs in patients with a creatinine clearance level <30 ml/minute is not officially recommended, as all LMWHs are cleared via the renal route so will accumulate in severe renal impairment. Available evidence demonstrates no accumulation in patients with creatinine clearance levels down to 20 ml/min. When required in these patients, LMWH treatment can be initiated with anti-Xa monitoring, if the benefit outweighs the risk, and the dose of LMWH should be adjusted, if necessary, based on anti-factor Xa activity.

   Treatment options for Mrs. PC are:

   1. Continuous infusion of unfractionated heparin (typically 30,000 units in 30 ml, i.e. 1000 units/ml) with the rate adjusted according to APTT levels. Target APTT ratio is 1.8–2.5
      - First APTT ratio should be measured 4–6 hours after bolus and start of UFH infusion
      - Repeat APTT ratio every 6 hours on the first day until 2 consecutive APTT ratios are in the therapeutic range or 6 hours after any dosage adjustment
      - Monitor once a day in stable patients, but more often in unstable patients

   This option does have the advantage that the effects wear off relatively quickly (the half-life ($t_{1/2}$) of UFH is dose-dependent; however, at therapeutic doses, the half-life is 4–90 min), and in cases of overdosage, heparin can be reversed with protamine. However, continuous heparin infusions have largely gone out of vogue since the advent of LMWH and given the need for frequent monitoring of levels and dose titration, which often leads to insufficient monitoring and the associated risks of over- or under-anticoagulation.

   2. Treatment with LMWHs. Since all LMWHs are cleared via the kidneys, they accumulate in severe renal impairment, and so all doses for treatment of PE/VTE must be adjusted accordingly. Tinzaparin is the LMWH closest in structure to unfractionated heparin, so it may be partially reversed with protamine. The other LMWHs require FFP in order to reverse their effects.
      - Tinzaparin should be prescribed at a dose of 125 units/kg once daily (dose based on actual body weight) in patients with a GFR <25 ml/min, including those who are dialysis-dependent.
      - Dalteparin – the dose for patients with GFR 15–30 ml/min is 200 units/kg once daily.
      - Enoxaparin – the dose for patients with GFR 15–30 mi/min is 100 units/kg once daily.

   In all cases, anti-factor Xa levels must be monitored and doses should be adjusted accordingly. It should be noted that even if initial anti-factor Xa levels are within the therapeutic range, with prolonged courses, accumulation can still occur over a period of weeks or months, leading to catastrophic bleeding. Hence, monitoring should continue throughout the course of treatment.

74.10 Useful Links

The following are useful websites and resources to consult when prescribing for patients with renal impairment:

- ▶ https://renaldrugdatabase.com/ – This is essentially an electronic version of the very comprehensive and widely used renal drug handbook [12] but is updated more regularly. The website requires subscription, but many renal units will have a departmental login,
- ▶ https://globalrph.com/drugs/renal-dosing-database/ – This is a free-to-use website which contains manufacturers' advice and recommendations for drug dosing in renal impairment for many drugs.
- ▶ https://www.hiv-druginteractions.org/checker – This is strictly speaking not a resource for drug interactions in renal impairment, but rather for HIV medication, but still very comprehensive and useful, especially when prescribing for patients with both renal impairment and HIV.

74.11 Summary

Drug dosing in patients with impaired renal function is a complex area. It is important to have an understanding of how drug handling may be altered in renal impairment and RRT and on the limitations of the calculations used to estimate renal impairment in order to help make informed decisions on drug doses. Where possible, textbooks on drug dosing in renal impairment should be consulted and, in addition, liaise with pharmacists with a special interest in the field who have clinical experience with these patients. In all cases, once a drug regimen has been prescribed, monitor the patient for efficacy, side effects and signs of toxicity.

74

References

1. Gabardi S, Abramson S. Drug dosing in chronic kidney disease. Med Clin North Am. 2005;89:649–87.
2. Cockwell P, Stringer S, M. J. Acute kidney injury. In: Walker R, editor. Clinical pharmacy and therapeutics. 5th ed. London: Churchill Livingstone; 2011. p. 255–71.
3. Ashford C. Clinical pharmacokinetics in renal impairment. In: Dhillon S, Kostrzewski AJ, editors. Clinical pharmacokinetics. London: Pharmaceutical Press; 2006. p. 53–78.
4. Matzke GR, Frye RF. Drug administration in patients with renal insufficiency minimising renal and extrarenal toxicity. Drug Saf. 1997;16:205–31.
5. Aronson JK. Drugs and renal insufficiency. Medicine (Baltimore). 2007;35:396–8.
6. Thompson CA. Better renal-function estimates not expected to alter drug dosing right away. Am J Heal Pharm. 2005;62: 2442–4.
7. Vidal L, Shavit M, Fraser A, Paul M, Leibovici L. Systematic comparison of four sources of drug information regarding adjustment of dose for renal function. BMJ. 2005;331:263.
8. Nuckols TK, et al. The effectiveness of computerized order entry at reducing preventable adverse drug events and medication errors in hospital settings: a systematic review and meta-analysis. Syst Rev. 2014;3:56.
9. Andreev E, Koopman M, Arisz L. A rise in plasma creatinine that is not a sign of renal failure: which drugs can be responsible? J Intern Med. 1999;246:247–52.
10. Ghane Shahrbaf F, Assadi F. Drug-induced renal disorders. J Ren Inj Prev. 2015;4:57–60.
11. Bauer L, Bailie GR, Uhlig K, Levey AS. Creatinine clearance versus glomerular filtration rate for the use of renal drug dosing in patients with kidney dysfunction. Pharmacotherapy. 2005;25:1286–7.
12. Ashley C, Dunleavey A. The renal drug handbook: the ultimate prescribing guide for renal practitioners. Boca Raton: CRC Press; 2018.

Coagulation in Kidney Disease

Nithya Prasannan, Suzanne H. Forbes, and Pratima Chowdary

Contents

M. Harber (ed.), *Primer on Nephrology*, https://doi.org/10.1007/978-3-030-76419-7_75

75

Learning Objectives

1. Basic understanding of current concepts around normal haemostasis and the pathophysiological abnormalities seen in CKD.
2. Description of bleeding complications and their prevalence in relation to renal dysfunction. An understanding of the practical steps that can be used in relation to the assessment and management of these complications.
3. An understanding of the epidemiology of thrombotic complications and the principles underlying their prevention and management. Information is provided about anticoagulation with both conventional indirect anticoagulants and the newer direct anticoagulants.

75.1 Introduction

Haemostasis is triggered by tissue injury, and the severity of the injury determines the magnitude of response (◘ Fig. 75.1). Primary haemostasis is characterised by platelet adhesion to subendothelial tissues following tissue trauma as a first step [1]. This is facilitated by circulating von Willebrand factor (vWF) anchoring collagen in subendothelial tissues with glycoprotein Ib (GPIb) receptors on the platelet surface. Subsequent platelet activation is brought about by the interaction of subendothelial collagen with platelet glycoprotein VI (GPVI) receptors, reinforced by activation by thrombin of platelet protease-activated receptors (PAR4). Platelet activation results in the release of platelet alpha and dense granule content including adenosine diphosphate (ADP) and thromboxane A2 generation, all of which are necessary for additional platelet recruitment and aggregate formation. Platelet aggregation is mediated by platelet glycoprotein IIb/IIIa (GPIIb/IIIa) receptors on adjacent platelets bridged by fibrinogen.

Secondary haemostasis is characterised by thrombin generation and fibrin clot formation and is brought about by exposure of tissue factor (TF) following tissue trauma [2]. TF is a transmembrane glycoprotein that acts as the cell surface receptor for factor VIIa. It is expressed constitutively in fibroblasts and smooth muscle cells around blood vessels, and expression can be induced on monocytes and endothelial cells. Thrombin generation is localised to phospholipid (PL) surface and in addition, requires calcium. The generation of thrombin is brought about by three enzyme complexes. In the initiation phase, the formation of extrinsic tenase complex (factor VIIa.TF.PL.Ca++) results in the production of small quantities of Xa, which activates small amounts of prothrombin to thrombin. These minute quantities of thrombin are necessary for priming the amplification pathway for an explosive thrombin generation, the thrombin burst crucial for fibrin clot formation. The small amounts of thrombin generated by the extrinsic tenase complex result in activation of cofactors V and VIII, activation of platelet membrane with exposure of phospholipids and activation of factors IX and XI. In the amplification phase, two complexes are responsible for the thrombin burst: intrinsic tenase (FIXa.FVIIIa.PL.Ca++) activating FX to FXa and prothrombinase complex (FXa.FVa.PL.Ca++) activating prothrombin to generate thrombin. This thrombin burst converts soluble fibrinogen molecules to insoluble fibrin meshwork that traps red cells and white cells, resulting in the formation of a blood clot.

Natural anticoagulants regulate thrombin generation spatially and temporally, thus limiting it to the site of tissue injury. These include tissue factor pathway inhibitor (TFPI), antithrombin (AT) and protein C and S and thrombomodulin. TFPI is a rapid and potent inhibitor of initiation through the formation of an inactive quaternary complex with FVIIa.TF.FXa. Activated serine proteases, including factors IXa, XIa, VIIa, Xa and thrombin, are inhibited irreversibly by AT, the principal physiological inhibitor of serine proteases in plasma. Its primary targets are FXa and thrombin, and interaction with heparin-like glycosaminoglycans (GAGs) increases its activity 2000- to 10,000-fold. Endogenous GAGs key to this interaction are heparan sulphate and dermatan sulphate expressed on the surface of the endothelial cells at the level of microcirculation. Cofactors FVa and FVIIIa are inactivated by the activated protein C with protein S as a cofactor, and activation of protein C by thrombin requires the former bound to endothelial protein C receptor and the latter to thrombomodulin on the endothelial surfaces.

In summary, blood coagulation is a complex biological system with numerous pathways and dysfunction in any pathway can potentially contribute to either bleeding or thrombosis.

75.2 Bleeding

Uraemia, in both acute and chronic renal failure, causes a bleeding tendency mediated primarily by platelet and endothelial dysfunction. Other contributing factors include reduced haematocrit, thrombocytopenia, comorbidities associated with bleeding, need for frequent procedures and use of antiplatelet agents and anticoagulants [3].

All aspects of primary haemostasis, including platelet adhesion, secretion and aggregation, are affected. A few essential mechanisms are elaborated in ◘ Table 75.1 [4, 5, 3]. It is believed that the uraemic substances present in the plasma mediate many of these abnormalities.

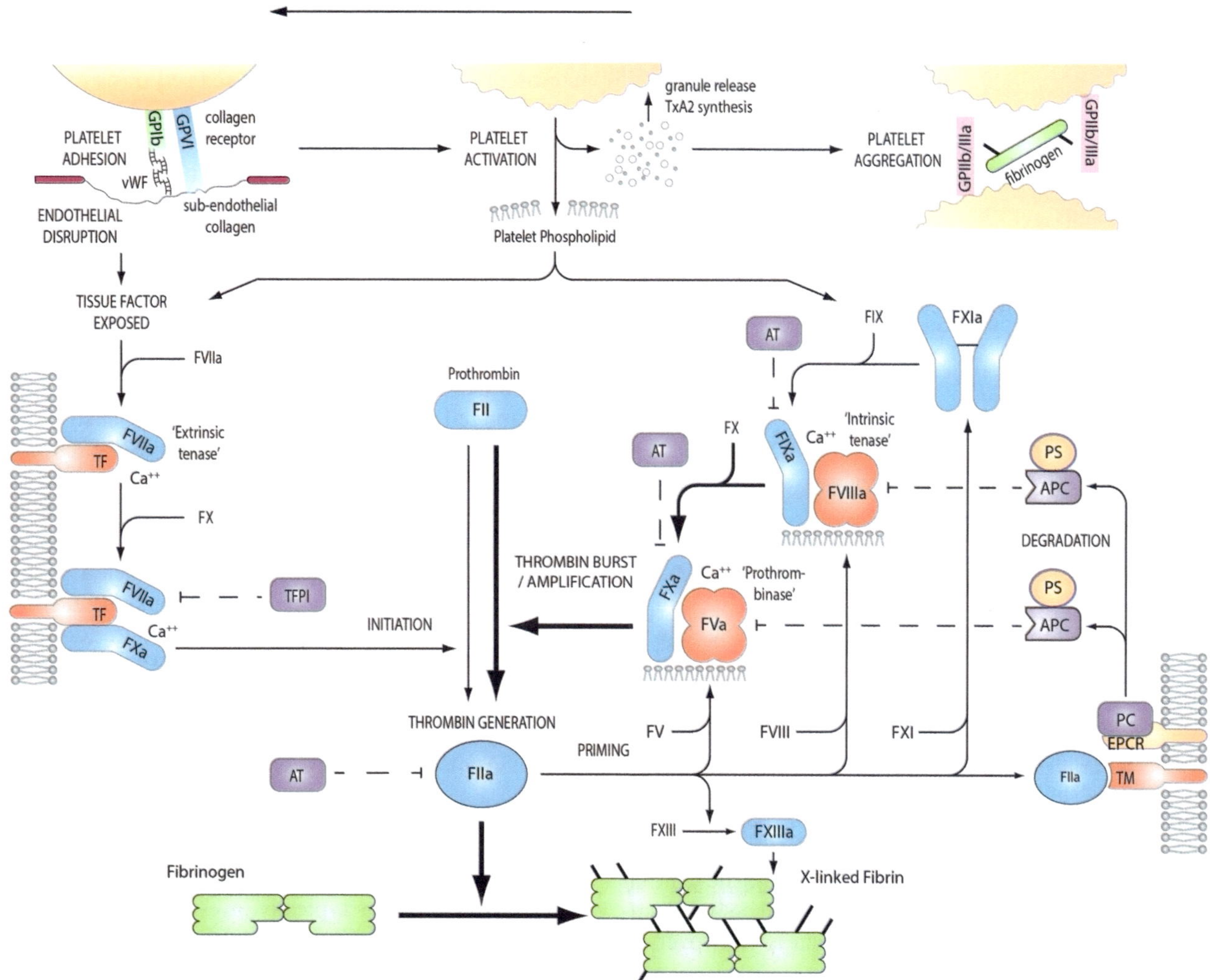

Fig. 75.1 Diagram of normal haemostasis. GPIb glycoprotein Ib, GPVI glycoprotein VI, vWF von Willebrand factor, TxA2 thromboxane A2, GPIIb/IIIa glycoprotein IIb/IIIa, TF tissue factor, AT antithrombin, TM thrombomodulin, EPCR endothelial protein C receptor, PC protein C, APC activated protein C, PS protein S. Primary haemostasis is characterised by vWF and collagen-mediated platelet adhesion at sites of trauma and subsequent platelet activation, which results in further platelet recruitment and provision of a phospholipid surface for thrombin generation. Secondary haemostasis begins with exposed tissue factor leading to the formation of the extrinsic tenase which activates factor X, initiating thrombin generation. Thrombin (FIIa) primes activation of the intrinsic factors V, VIII and IX resulting in the formation of prothrombinase which leads to a thrombin burst. Thrombin converts soluble fibrinogen into insoluble fibrin which is then cross-linked by activated factor XIII. Fibrinogen also facilitates platelet aggregation while thrombin also stimulates platelet activation via PAR4 receptors (not shown). Thrombin activates protein C via thrombomodulin. Activated protein C, with its cofactor protein S, negatively regulates thrombin generation. Only the principal anticoagulant proteins TFPI, antithrombin, protein C and S are shown (see text for further detail)

75.2.1 Clinical Presentation

Typically, the bleeding diathesis in patients with advanced chronic kidney disease (CKD) or end-stage renal disease (ESRD) presents as prolonged bleeding at sites of venipuncture, easy bruising, menorrhagia and gastrointestinal blood loss [3]. Other symptoms include procedure or trauma-related bleeding and, less commonly, spontaneous retroperitoneal or intracranial haemorrhages. Haemarthroses and spontaneous intramuscular haematomas are uncommon. Haemorrhagic pericardial and pleural effusions can still occur in underdialysed patients or those with advanced CKD stage 5 not on dialysis. Gastrointestinal (GI) and intracranial haemorrhage (ICH) in particular, remain significant causes of morbidity and excess mortality in patients with end-stage renal failure [6].

Mucosal bleeding commonly presents as increased physiological blood loss from the GI tract, which in healthy subjects is typically around 1 ml/day, but in uraemic patients can be as high as 4–6 ml/day [7]. In CKD patients, lower renal function was associated with

75

Table 75.1 Pathophysiology of bleeding diathesis

Site	Mechanism
Endothelium	↑ nitric oxide(NO) due to ↓ red cell scavenging and ↑ prostacyclin – result in abnormal platelet adhesion
	Anaemia – ↓ platelet interaction with vessel walls
Platelets	↓ Platelet activation due to ↓ TxA_2 production and abnormal intracellular Ca^{2+} mobilisation
	↓ Platelet aggregation due to ↓ ADP, epinephrine and serotonin pool in the platelets
	GPIIb/IIIa receptors show ↓ affinity for both vWF and fibrinogen
Clotting factors	↓ vWF activity with abnormal platelet adhesion at high shear

a higher risk of upper gastrointestinal bleeding with an incidence of 13.9 per 100 patient-years in patients with stage 5 CKD [8]. Data from the United States provides the breakdown of the aetiology for upper GI bleeding, with only a third being secondary to peptic ulcer disease with erosive gastritis, oesophagitis, vascular ectasia and angiodysplasia being relatively common [9, 10]. Indeed, capsule endoscopy in haemodialysis patients with obscure GI bleeding has shown erosions in the jejunum and vascular lesions in the ileum [11]. It is believed that platelet dysfunction contributes to this excessive bleeding, and the role of hypergastrinaemia is controversial [12, 13].

Patients with ESRD receiving maintenance dialysis have a higher incidence of both ischemic and hemorrhagic strokes compared with the general population. They have an eight-fold increase in acute ischemic stroke with higher in-hospital morbidity and mortality [14]. Also, a 20-fold increase in subdural haematomas was noted in patients on haemodialysis compared to the UK general population and was associated with poor outcomes [15].

Patients with renal disease often require invasive procedures, such as renal biopsies and vascular access procedures (temporary vascaths, tunnelled central catheters, fistula formation, PD catheter insertion) and so care should be taken to minimise any peri-procedural bleeding. Indeed, a retrospective cohort study of patients with stages 3 and 4 CKD undergoing coronary artery bypass grafting demonstrated significantly higher post-operative bleeding complications (8%) compared to normal renal function (3%) and higher 30-day mortality [16].

A systematic review published in 2012 attempted to identify risk factors for symptomatic bleeding in native kidney biopsy with an automated biopsy device under real-time ultrasonographic guidance [17]. The review spanned 31 years and included 9474 biopsies and showed macroscopic haematuria in 3.5%, red cell transfusion in 0.9%, and angiographic intervention in 0.6% of the cohort. The risk of bleeding was higher with a 14-gauge needle compared to smaller biopsy needles, in female patients, in patients with elevated serum creatinine or decreased haemoglobin and in patients with acute kidney injury. Mean systolic blood pressure above 130 mmHg and age over 40 were also associated with higher transfusion rates. In a single-centre retrospective review, where risk factors were controlled with bed rest for 24 h, desmopressin injections, red cell transfusions for prolonged bleeding time and antihypertensives for hypertension, the incidence of post-biopsy haematoma was 33.4%, and significant complications (blood transfusion, nephrectomy and angiography) were seen in 1.2% of patients [18].

Increasingly, renal biopsies are undertaken as a day case procedure with a smaller gauge biopsy needle followed by bed rest for 6 h post-procedure. In addition, control of blood pressure ensuring an SBP <140 mmHg and cessation of antiplatelets at least a week prior to the procedure seem to decrease the risk of bleeding.

75.2.2 Investigation of Platelet Dysfunction

Platelet dysfunction is typically investigated either with global tests, like bleeding time and PFA-100 (Platelet Function Analyser-100®, Dade Behring), or with more specific platelet function tests that include platelet aggregation studies, assays of granule content and release and flow cytometry [19].

The gold standard for the evaluation of platelet function is platelet aggregometry. In this test, platelets suspended in citrated plasma are activated with various agonists, and their ability to form aggregates is evaluated by the amount of light transmission. Investigations in uraemic patients in the pre-dialysis era revealed prolonged skin bleeding time and mildly impaired platelet aggregation to a range of platelet-activating agonists including ADP, epinephrine and collagen. In a small cohort, while a good correlation was noted between collagen-induced platelet aggregation, bleeding time, urea levels and clinical bleeding, the bleeding time unlike collagen-induced platelet aggregation appeared to better differentiate patients with clinically significant bleeding from non-bleeding patients [20].

The PFA-100® is a rapid test that assesses platelet-dependent primary haemostasis. It measures the time required for flowing whole blood to occlude a collagen and adenosine diphosphate (CADP) or collagen and epinephrine (CEPI) coated cartridge. Although this easy-to-perform test is popular, it requires specialised equipment. Prolonged closure times are seen in patients with platelet dysfunction and von Willebrand disease. In patients with mild inherited platelet dysfunction, the sensitivity and specificity of prolonged closure time were lower compared to platelet aggregation studies.

In a prospective cohort study of haemodialysis patients and control population, a comparison between PFA-100, platelet aggregation with ADP only and skin bleeding time demonstrated abnormalities in 60%, 40% and 20% of haemodialysis patients and 0%, 10% and 3% of the control population, respectively [21]. Subsequent studies in patients who have undergone renal biopsy post-transplant or for diagnostic purposes did not show any correlation between PFA-100 and post-procedural bleeding [22, 23].

Routine evaluation for the presence and severity of platelet dysfunction is neither feasible nor recommended. Skin bleeding time typically undertaken on the forearm is an invasive non-reliable test for assessing bleeding risk. Further, it has the potential for scarring, and patient acceptability is very low. In some centres, there has been increasing use of PFA-100 for assessing platelet dysfunction prerenal biopsy. It is important to note that the test is sensitive to mild abnormalities, and therefore, its use must be accompanied by an understanding of the limitations and ideally as part of agreed local protocols and algorithms. Where patients have significant bruising despite adequate dialysis, specialist opinion for a comprehensive evaluation of platelets function, including granule contents, is indicated.

There is increasing interest in whole blood viscoelastometric tests (ROTEM and TEG) that measure the rate of fibrin polymerisation [24]. These assays are helpful to avoid transfusion but are not validated for predicting bleeding risk, and are particularly poor at identifying platelet dysfunction. Similarly, there is increasing interest in global plasma assay, the thrombin generation assay, which assesses both hypocoagulability and hypercoagulability [25]. Similar to the viscoelastometric tests, it is sensitive to procoagulants and anticoagulants, but its ability to identify platelet abnormalities is limited.

75.3 Therapy for Uraemic Bleeding

Management of bleeding tendency in renal patients is dictated by the clinical presentation and the treatment of their underlying renal dysfunction. Broadly, treatments are aimed at long-term prevention of spontaneous bleeding, prevention of procedure-related bleeding or management of active bleeding [4].

75.3.1 Long-Term Prevention of Spontaneous Bleeding

Management of uraemia with either haemodialysis or peritoneal dialysis via the removal of toxins that impair platelet function results in partial correction of the platelet dysfunction. The correction lasts as long as the patients continue to be dialysed, and there is a suggestion that peritoneal dialysis may result in better improvement of platelet function. Anaemia increases the bleeding tendency through decreased platelet-vessel wall interaction, and a target haematocrit of >30% appears to be ideal. Erythropoietin and its analogues are used increasingly to maintain haemoglobin within the desired range. In rare cases, red cell transfusion may be appropriate, particularly in patients who are at high risk of bleeding and undergoing a closed procedure, where ongoing monitoring is not feasible.

75.3.2 Periprocedural Prophylaxis and Active Bleeding: Non-specific Interventions

In the setting of acute kidney injury or first presentation of end-stage renal failure, prevention and treatment of bleeding complications continue to be challenging particularly in the context of procedures such as renal biopsy or insertion of temporary vascular access. There is no consensus on the investigation and risk stratification of patients' bleeding tendency, nor are there any consensus guidelines on the role of desmopressin for prevention and management of procedural-related bleeding.

Desmopressin, cryoprecipitate and tranexamic acid have a non-specific prohaemostatic effect with some clinical benefit. Thrombocytopenia may also occur in uraemic patients. However, platelet transfusions are generally avoided as transfused platelets will acquire dysfunction similar to the patient's platelets and lead to the risk of alloimmunisation [26].

Desmopressin (DDAVP®) is an antidiuretic hormone analogue, specific to V2 receptors expressed on endothelial cells and the kidney collecting duct [27]. Activation of receptors on the endothelial cells stimulates the release of stored ultra-large vWF multimers and FVIII an hour after administration, and the antidiuretic effect, that can last up to 24 h is secondary to receptors on the collecting duct. In a randomised placebo-controlled study, desmopressin resulted in shortened skin bleeding times in all patients at 1 h with the effect lasting for at least 4 h in most cases [28]. It has been suggested that the released vWF multimers contribute to platelet aggregation. In patients with normal renal function, a randomised controlled trial of desmopressin administered pre-biopsy demonstrated decreased bleeding and haematoma size [29]. The standard dose is 0.3 mcg/kg administered either intravenously as slow bolus infusion or subcutaneously, 60 min pre-procedure. The effect decreases with repeat dosing, and fluid retention and hyponatraemia are potential risks. Patients are advised to restrict fluid intake to about 800 ml over 24 h. There is a small risk of hypotension, particularly when administered intravenously, and a slow rate of infusion is recommended. Indeed, because of this potential risk of hypotension, it is not recommended for use in patients with uncontrolled hypertension or at risk of cardiac events.

Cryoprecipitate contains vWF, fibrinogen, fibronectin and factor XIII. The administration of cryo has demonstrated a shortening of bleeding time and was used for both the prevention and management of bleeding [30]. This improvement has not been consistent across studies [31]. A typical dose is an adult will increase the fibrinogen by 1 g while concurrently increasing vWF and is ideally given pre-procedure.

Tranexamic acid (TXA) is a synthetic derivative of the amino acid lysine that inhibits fibrinolysis through reversible blockade of lysine binding sites on plasminogen molecules [32]. Randomised control trials in the context of trauma and post-partum haemorrhage demonstrated reduced death due to bleeding when administered within 3 h of bleeding onset. No increase in vascular occlusive events was seen, negating the previously held concern that TXA is associated with an increased risk of thrombosis [33, 34]. It is excreted mainly as an unchanged drug in the urine with a half-life of approximately 3 h. A typical dose is 1 g given IV every 6–8 h based on the indication, and often, this can be followed up with oral tranexamic acid for mucosal procedures. Higher TXA levels have been noted in patients with decreased renal function, and high doses have been associated with post-operative seizures, and therefore, dose reductions are indicated in renal dysfunction [35]. Typically, the interval is increased to 12–24 h in mild to moderate CKD, and both dose and frequency reduction is required in ESRD. The oral dose is 1 g, three to four times a day in the presence of normal renal function.

In rare instances, rFVIIa (NovoSeven®) has been used for the management of acute bleeding that is not responsive to standard measures. Increasingly, it is acknowledged that an excess risk of thrombosis might offset any potential benefit. The typical dose is 90 mcg/Kg as a single dose with doses repeated in two to three hours' time based on the clinical benefit.

Conjugated oestrogens (e.g., Premarin) have demonstrated a clinical effect in the management of recurrent bleeding and prevention of procedure-related bleeding. Their clinical use has declined over the years, but they may have a role in the management of obscure GI bleeding after extensive investigations have excluded a treatable bleeding lesion. The exact mechanism is poorly defined and suggested mechanisms include decreases in L-arginine (NO precursor) potentially increasing TxA2 and ADP. Also, oestrogens are associated with a reduction in AT and protein S levels and an increase in FVII concentrations. A dose of 0.6 mg/kg/day IV for 5 days starts shortening the BT as early as 6 h, but the peak effect is seen around 5–7 days after treatment initiation, and the effect lasts up to 2 weeks after cessation of treatment [31]. Transdermal patches and oral tablets also appear to be effective [36].

It is essential to appreciate that most of the suggested interventions correct bleeding diathesis partially, and procedures must only be performed after an appropriate risk assessment. In patients with a history suggesting a new onset of bleeding diathesis or procedures at high risk of bleeding, a comprehensive evaluation along with oestrogens started 5 days pre-procedure and desmopressin and tranexamic acid an hour pre-procedure may be considered.

In the management of patients with active bleeding, intervention with cryoprecipitate should be considered earlier rather than later, along with intravenous tranexamic acid in addition to standard resuscitation. Care should be taken to anticipate the volume required to administer some of these treatments, particularly in an anuric dialysis patient.

75.4 Thrombosis

Thrombotic complications are common in patients with CKD and ESKD and present as arterial thrombotic events (ATE), venous thromboembolism (VTE) or thrombosis related to vascular access for haemodialysis [3, 37]. Haemostatic changes described include elevated procoagulants, impaired natural anticoagulant pathways and a decrease in fibrinolytic activity and detailed in ◘ Table 75.2 [3, 37–39]. There are multiple reasons for the excess of arterial events, including accelerated atherosclerosis, hypertension, loss of normal vessel elasticity and vascular calcification that are covered in ▸ Chap. 37, Cardiology and the Kidney.

Table 75.2 Pathophysiology of the thrombotic tendency

Site	Mechanism
Endothelium	Endothelial cell and monocyte activation
	↓ Thrombomodulin leads to ↓ protein C activity
Platelets	↑ Platelet activation by uraemia/haemodialysis membranes
	↑ Thrombin generation, ↑ CRP/inflammatory cytokines
Coagulation and fibrinolysis	↑ Fibrinogen, FVII, FVIII, tissue factor pathway inhibitor (TFPI), vWF and tissue factor (TF)
	↑ Markers of coagulation activation, including D-dimers, thrombin-antithrombin complexes and plasmin-antiplasmin complexes
	↑ Lipoprotein(a) causes impaired fibrinolysis
	↓ Antithrombin (AT) in nephrotic syndrome
Other	Alteration of sphingolipids

75.4.1 Venous Thrombosis and VTE Prophylaxis

The risk of VTE is increased across the spectrum of renal disorders, including patients with mild renal impairment, nephrotic syndrome, renal transplant and dialysis [37]. In a cohort study with a mean follow up of 11.8 years, the incidence rates of VTE per 1000 person-years were 1.5, 1.9 and 4.5 for normal kidney function, mildly decreased kidney function and stage 3/4 CKD, respectively. Following adjustment for age, gender, race and centre, the relative risks were 1.28 for early CKD (stages I and II) and 2.09 for patients with stage III and IV CKD [40]. Further, mortality from pulmonary embolism was higher in patients with renal disease [41].

There are no consensus guidelines around VTE prophylaxis in patients with CKD. The accepted practice in many units is to use lower or half-dose LMWH for patients with CKD stages 4 and 5, which appears safe in terms of anti-Xa activity and accumulation. Accumulation is typically related to the type of LMWH, and pharmacokinetic studies have shown accumulation of enoxaparin in patients with CrCl <30 ml/min but not with prophylactic tinzaparin or dalteparin. Caution should be exercised in patients receiving antiplatelet agents, with anaemia, or those with any history of recent (within the last year) significant bleeding events, particularly GI bleeding. Routine monitoring for prophylactic doses is not indicated.

75.4.2 Nephrotic Syndrome

Thromboembolic disease is a significant complication in patients with nephrotic syndrome, presenting with both arterial and venous thromboembolic events, with the latter including deep venous thrombosis, pulmonary embolism, cerebral vein thrombosis and renal vein thrombosis. It is possible that these events, particularly renal vein thrombosis, are asymptomatic or overlooked, and a detailed history and focused investigations are beneficial. The prevalence of thrombosis is in part related to the underlying aetiology and is highest in patients with membranous glomerulonephritis and heavy proteinuria. A review of published case series suggests that this can potentially be seen in almost a third of patients [42]. A retrospective study of patients with nephrotic syndrome over a 10-year period revealed that the risk of thromboembolic events was highest in the first 6 months, with an event rate of 9.85% for VTE and 5.52% for ATE, and during follow-up, the annual incidence of objectively verified symptomatic thromboembolic events was 1.02% for VTE and 1.48% for ATE [43].

Several studies have been undertaken to understand the risk factors predictive of thrombosis and pathophysiologic mechanisms underpinning this increased risk. To date, an essential marker of thrombotic risk has been serum albumin with a level 28 g/L being identified in one study. Similarly, the ratio of proteinuria and serum albumin appears to be a good predictor of the VTE risk and a reduction of antithrombin by 75% or concurrent reduction of albumin to below 20 g/L appear to be predictive [44]. Pathophysiological mechanisms that potentially contribute include increased platelet reactivity due to increased thromboxane A2 synthesis secondary to hypoalbuminemia, increase in procoagulants (factor VIII, VWF and fibrinogen) and impaired anticoagulant activity secondary to a decrease in antithrombin due to glomerular loss and decreased fibrinolytic capacity due to elevated PAI-1 and loss of plasmin [44–46].

Despite the excess risk of VTE and ATE, there is no consensus on the role of prophylactic anticoagulation with practice varying from aspirin only through to warfarin and direct oral anticoagulants. Decisions typically tend to be individualised, and the following risk factors suggested as indicators for prophylactic anticoagulation: personal and family history, severity of hypoalbuminaemia (<20–25 g/l), magnitude of proteinuria (>10 g/24 h) and presence of membranous nephropathy [47]. Risk factors for bleeding preclude the use of prophylactic anticoagulation, and significant risk factors include the presence of hypertension, concomitant antiplatelet therapy, poorly controlled anticoagulation with warfarin, eGFR less than 30–60 ml/min, anaemia and previous bleeding. Although several bleeding risk scores have been developed based on the parameters described, the predictive value has not been high [48]. Indeed, this risk-benefit has been explored in a clinical decision model, and the model confirms that patients at high risk of bleeding in the presence of very low albumin do not benefit from prophylactic anticoagulation [49]. Symptomatic events are best treated initially with heparin followed by warfarin for a minimum of 3–6 months and potentially continued for the duration of the risk period. The low AT levels do not preclude treatment with low-molecular-weight heparin. There is increasing interest in using direct oral anticoagulants in this group of patients with their more stable dose-response relationship, with a few case reports of successful clinical use [50].

75.4.3 Vascular Access Thrombosis

Proper functioning of an arteriovenous fistula (AVF) is vital for hemodialysis, and the maturation of AVF following its creation is influenced by multiple factors. In addition to poor maturation, stenosis is not an uncommon complication. Other complications include fistulae thrombosis, AV graft thrombosis or thrombosis of a central venous catheter [51]. The thrombotic episodes are in part related to stenosis caused by fibromuscular and intimal hyperplasia facilitated by the shear created by fistulae, and the role of hypercoagulability is poorly defined. In a case-control study evaluating the importance of thrombophilia defects, an association between thrombophilia and access thrombosis was noted with an adjusted odds ratio of 2.4, and for each additional abnormality, the odds of access thrombosis increased significantly [52]. In patients with more than one episode of venous access thrombosis, screening for thrombophilia may be justified, but there is limited data on the management of identified abnormalities and outcomes. In addition, there are no prospective studies on the prophylactic use of anticoagulation to prevent access thrombosis, while there is a body of evidence around potential complications of anticoagulation in patients with ESKD. A Cochrane review on the use of antiplatelet and anticoagulants in vascular access thrombosis suggested a potential benefit with aspirin and dipyridamole and no benefit with warfarin [53]. Following the systematic review, another randomised controlled trial published in 2008 demonstrated a reduced frequency of early thrombosis with the use of clopidogrel, but there was no increase in the proportion of fistulae that became suitable for dialysis [54]. The long-term benefit on patency and suitability has not been demonstrated, and there continue to be ongoing concerns about the bleeding risk posed by these agents, preventing their routine use in clinical practice.

75.4.4 Atrial Fibrillation

Atrial fibrillation (AF) is the most common indication for anticoagulation in patients with and without renal impairment. In a Danish cohort study of atrial fibrillation, patients with non-end-stage CKD and kidney disease requiring renal replacement therapy (RRT), compared to patients with no renal disease reported an increased risk of stroke or systemic thromboembolism and bleeding. The event rate per 100 person-years for thrombosis for the three groups were 6.44, 5.61 and 3.61, respectively, and 8.77, 8.89 and 3.54, respectively, for bleeding [55]. In the same cohort, warfarin demonstrated a significantly decreased risk of stroke or systemic thromboembolism overall among CKD patients requiring RRT, with a nonsignificant reduction in patients with non-end-stage CKD. Aspirin demonstrated no additional benefit. Further, the risk of bleeding was higher with kidney disease and was highest in patients receiving both warfarin and aspirin [55]. In a Swedish cohort of established cardiovascular disease and AF, warfarin was associated with a lower 1-year risk for the composite outcome of death, MI and ischemic stroke without a higher risk of bleeding in consecutive acute MI patients with atrial fibrillation. This association was not related to the severity of concurrent CKD [56].

In a systematic review of ESKD and AF that included about 20 observational cohort studies, the association between warfarin and stroke, bleeding and mortality was reviewed. Warfarin was not associated with a statistically significant reduction in all-cause stroke, but a significant association with an increase in all-cause bleeding (HR 1.21) was noted, but surprisingly, there was no association with major bleeding or gastrointestinal bleeding [57]. In another systematic review of patients with AF and non-end-stage CKD, warfarin resulted in a lower risk of ischemic stroke/thromboembolism and mortality with no effect on major bleeding. In the same review, in patients with AF and end-stage CKD, warfarin had no effect on the risks of stroke and mortality but increased the risks of major bleeding [58].

The net clinical effect of warfarin treatment requires careful consideration in patients with chronic kidney disease. In CKD stage 5, the evidence of benefit for prevention of systemic thromboembolism in AF is not evident, but an increased risk of bleeding is well documented. It is common practice for anticoagulation in this group to be stopped. Part of the increased bleeding risk may be related to the labile control of anticoagulation. In addition, warfarin use also poses a risk in terms of vascular calcification, particularly calciphylaxis, a life-threatening complication with limited treatment options [59].

75.5 Anticoagulants in Renal Disease

The indications for anticoagulation in patients with renal disease while similar to the general population require an individualised risk-benefit assessment. The most common indications for consideration are AF and venous thrombosis for primary and secondary prevention of thromboembolic events, respectively. In addition, patients are also exposed to anticoagulants for haemodialysis and occasionally for management of recurrent vascular access thrombosis. Anticoagulants that are used in patients with renal disease include indirect anticoagulants and direct anticoagulants. Indirect anticoagulants include oral vitamin K antagonists like warfarin and parenteral heparins. Direct oral anticoagulants have been licensed in the last decade and include the thrombin inhibitor, dabigatran (Pradaxa®), and anti-Xa inhibitors, rivaroxaban (Xarelto®), apixaban (Eliquis®) and edoxaban (Lixiana®).

75.5.1 Warfarin

Warfarin is an indirect anticoagulant and mediates its action as a vitamin K antagonist. It decreases the synthesis of vitamin K-dependent coagulation factors (factors II, VII, IX and X and anticoagulant factors protein C and S) through interruption of the post-translational gamma-carboxylation of these factors which requires vitamin K-dependent carboxylase. It mediates its antithrombotic effect primarily through reduction of procoagulant FII, FX and concurrent reductions FVII, and FIX potentially contribute [60]. It is important to note that the antithrombotic effect of warfarin takes a minimum of 4–5 days to take effect, related to the long half-life of FX (27–48 h) and FII (42–72 h). Prolongation of prothrombin time can be seen earlier and is related to the short half-life of FVII (4–6 h) [61]. This delay in the onset of the antithrombotic effect prevents warfarin use for the immediate management of a thrombotic event.

Warfarin is rapidly absorbed with high bioavailability, and peak concentration is seen 90 min after oral ingestion with a mean circulating half-life of 40 h (15–60 h). The anticoagulant effect is mediated by a small fraction as most (97–99%) is protein-bound (mainly to albumin) and ineffective. Drugs that displace albumin-bound warfarin will increase the action of warfarin. Metabolism occurs mainly in the liver, involving the cytochrome P450, and drugs sharing the same pathway have an impact on the warfarin levels and INR.

Bleeding is the most significant complication of warfarin therapy [61, 60]. Bleeding can be from any site, and typical locations of bleeding include GI bleeding, urinary tract bleeding, menstrual bleeding and potentially fatal intracranial haemorrhage (ICH). Rare complications seen include skin necrosis usually observed between the third to the eighth day of therapy caused by extensive thrombosis of the venules and capillaries within the subcutaneous fat. The other complication is foetal warfarin syndrome, which follows warfarin administration to pregnant women between the sixth and twelfth week of gestation when warfarin that has crossed the placenta is teratogenic.

75.5.1.1 Monitoring and Dose Adjustments

The decrease in the procoagulants results in a prolongation of prothrombin time, and the degree of prolongation is related to reagent sensitivity. The international normalised ratio (INR) has been developed to address the impact of reagents on prothrombin time and allows comparability of the anticoagulant effect between labs and reagents. A target INR of 2–3 is typically indicated in patients anticoagulated with warfarin, and in rare instances, a higher target INR of 3–4 is recommended. The INR is a reflection of both the antithrombotic effect and risk of bleeding and represents the balance between vitamin K and warfarin on the production of active factors, and therefore, regular monitoring is required to ensure maximum efficacy and safety [61]. Indeed, the time in range is used as a marker of stability of anticoagulation control in patients, and poor control is predictive of adverse outcomes.

The delay in the onset of antithrombotic effect requires the use of rapidly acting anticoagulants like heparin for a minimum of 5 days and/or until the antithrombotic effect has been established as indicated by two consecutive INRs in the desired target range. In patients with AF, a gradual onset of an antithrombotic effect is reasonable, and warfarin doses are titrated into the target INR range slowly. Due to the indirect nature of the anticoagulant and antithrombotic effect, fast loading or frequent changes have no advantage and indeed contribute to overanticoagulation.

Warfarin dose changes must take into account the half-life of warfarin and half-life of coagulation factors, with the effect on INR seen up to 5 days and maximum effect seen 2–3 days after a dose change. Typically, in outpatient clinical practice, validated nomograms are used for adjusting warfarin dosing. Monitoring is generally undertaken every 2–3 days until INR is in the target range and, thereafter, frequency is decreased based on the stability of INR control. In the inpatient setting, daily monitoring is recommended to identify overanticoagulation. When dose changes are performed, they should be done in 5–20% increments based on the desired INR increase. There are several patient-related variables that affect the response to warfarin. Older patients tend to exhibit an exaggerated response to warfarin, in part because they tend to store less vitamin K than younger people. Patients with concurrent medical conditions affecting the liver or drugs that affect the metabolism of warfarin or vitamin K also have an impact on anticoagulation control.

75.5.1.2 Bleeding and Reversal of Warfarin Anticoagulation

Patients anticoagulated with warfarin can bleed due to an underlying pathology or secondary to overanticoagulation with high INR. Factors that increase bleeding may be related to the intensity of anticoagulation or patient-based risk factors [61]. The risk is higher when the target INR range is 3–4.5 when compared to INR range of 2–3. The risk of ICH appears to rise with patient's age, history of previous ischemic stroke and INR >4.0 and is highest in the first few months after initiation. The concurrent use of antiplatelet agents doubles the frequency of bleeding with no difference in the incidence of ICH. Polypharmacy, herbal and food supplements potentially can increase the effect of warfarin by either influencing the binding to albumin or warfarin metabolism. Therefore, it is crucial to monitor the INR a couple of weeks after the introduction of a new drug or a week after initiation of antibiotic therapy as the latter decrease the availability of vitamin K.

Other patient related factors that increase the risk of bleeding include age >75 years, cancer, occult pathologic lesions, hypertension and underlying CVD. Congestive heart failure, hepatic insufficiency, renal insufficiency and anaemia also appear to be associated with an increased risk. Thrombocytopenia and other inherited or acquired bleeding disorders are synergistic with warfarin and increase the risk of bleeding. Similarly, concurrent use of medications that impact platelet function can also increase the risk. Predisposition to falls with head trauma, alcoholism, poor compliance with medications increase the risk.

The degree of overanticoagulation and the presence and severity of bleeding dictate the reversal strategy to be implemented [60]. Non-bleeding patients are managed by the cessation of the drug and a small dose of vitamin K, given orally or IV if the INR >6.0. Interruption of dosing for a couple of days restores the coagulation factors over days. Oral vitamin K can achieve near-complete correction, dependent on the dose used and pre-treatment INR. Intravenous vitamin K has a rapid onset of action, and the effect is seen as early as 6 h with complete correction taking between 12 and 24 h and importantly lasts for days.

Minor bleeding can be managed by topical tranexamic acid or missing a couple of doses of warfarin if rebleeding is anticipated. In patients where bleeding is life or limb-threatening or has the potential to develop into significant bleeds, i.e. minor bleeding with high INR, or bleeding in enclosed spaces, rapid reversal of anticoagulation is indicated. This is typically achieved with prothrombin complex concentrates (e.g. Beriplex® /Octoplex®) [62]. PCCs are plasma-derived clotting factors that are rich in vitamin K-dependent coagulation factors (factors II, VII, IX and X and anticoagulant protein C and S). They are lyophilised preparations and can be administered intravenously after reconstitution over 5–10 min at a dose of 20–35 IU/Kg based on the INR. Repeat INR is recommended to confirm complete correction and assess the need for repeat doses. In addition, 5 mg of IV vitamin K needs to be administered simultaneously as the effect of PCCs is transient and related to the half-life of the coagulation factors infused. In the absence of PCCs, plasma at a dose of 15 ml/Kg may be used for correction, but the correction is slower and often incomplete.

75.5.2 Heparins

Parenteral indirect anticoagulants include unfractionated heparin (UFH), low-molecular-weight heparins (LMWH), fondaparinux and danaparoid [63]. Heparins and heparinoids mediate their anticoagulant activity by increasing the inhibitory activity of antithrombin (AT) by 2000–10,000-fold. AT is the principle serine protease inhibitor of blood coagulation, and the primary targets of the heparin/AT complex are FXa and thrombin, and it inhibits both equally.

75.5.2.1 Unfractionated Heparin

Pharmaceutical grade heparin is made from the porcine intestinal mucosa. UFH is a sulphated polysaccharide that is heterogeneous with respect to molecular size, anticoagulant activity and pharmacokinetic properties. UFH is administered as an intravenous (IV) infusion and occasionally into subcutaneous (SC) tissues.

Therapeutic anticoagulation for patients with renal impairment in the acute situation can be achieved either with IV UFH or SC LMWH. UFH has a short half-life of ~30–60 min at standard doses, but at high doses and in severe renal failure, the half-life may be prolonged. Rapid elimination via the reticuloendothelial system and through binding with other plasma proteins contributes to the majority of the clearance with a smaller component being renally excreted [64]. The administration of UFH is monitored by the APTT ratio, and the therapeutic ratios are determined locally. A prolonged baseline APTT makes monitoring challenging, and dose adjustments are best undertaken through the use of dosing nomograms [63].

A significant advantage of UFH is the short half-life that allows for rapid reversal of anticoagulation when needed in situations such as planned procedures or bleeding. The effect can also be reversed with protamine sulphate, which works by forming an inactive salt with heparin [62]. Major disadvantages include unpredictable response and the need for routine venipuncture for APTT monitoring and the higher incidence of heparin-induced thrombocytopenia described later. SC administration may avoid the wide fluctuations in APTT ratios but has the same disadvantages, and there are no nomograms for dose adjustment to achieve therapeutic range rapidly.

75.5.2.2 Low-Molecular-Weight Heparins and Fondaparinux

LMWHs are derived through the chemical or enzymatic depolymerisation of UFH. The mean molecular weight is third or less of UFH, and they inhibit FXa more than FIIa usually in a ratio of 2:1–4:1 in contrast to the 1:1 ratio of UFH. The various LMWHs differ, at least to some extent, in their pharmacokinetic properties and anticoagulant profiles, and therefore, these drugs are not clinically interchangeable. Anticoagulant response with LMWHs is more consistent due to good bioavailability after SC administration and the use of weight-adjusted doses results in more predictable blood levels. In addition to the predictable response, other advantages include convenient dosing regimes (once or twice daily), that do not require regular or routine monitoring.

Unlike UFH, LMWHs are predominantly cleared renally. The anti-IIa effect mediated by the higher molecular weight chains is cleared like UFH. The small molecules with predominant anti-Xa effect are cleared renally, almost around 90% and therefore accumulate in renal impairment primarily when used in therapeutic doses. In addition to the dose of LMWH, the type of LMWH determines the degree of accumulation with enoxaparin accumulating more than dalteparin and both more than tinzaparin. Therapeutic anticoagulation with LMWH, therefore, requires dose reduction as recommended by the manufacturer.

Fondaparinux is a synthetic AT-dependent selective FXa inhibitor. It has a half-life of 17 h in healthy adults, increasing to 29 h in moderate and 72 h in severe renal impairment and is generally not the first choice of anticoagulant.

Routine monitoring of anti-FXa levels is not required for prophylactic low-molecular-weight heparins (LMWH) but may be considered in patients with ESKD, especially in patients with CrCl <30 ml/min receiving therapeutic LMWH. This is particularly the case with enoxaparin to avoid overanticoagulation with high anti-FXa levels. When monitoring is undertaken, samples for peak anti-FXa levels 3–4 h post-administration are collected, and levels are usually between 0.4 and 1.0 U/ml for treatment doses. While the anti-FXa levels do not necessarily predict bleeding risk, supratherapeutic levels may contribute to an excess of bleeding from underlying lesions. For patients with severe renal impairment or who are unstable, the choice between UFH and LMWH is in part related to venous access for sampling, the type of LMWH and the lab facilities for anit-FXa monitoring and timely reporting. It is important to note that the effect of LMWHs is only partially reversed with protamine.

75.5.3 Haemodialysis Anticoagulation

Almost all haemodialysis patients require anticoagulation of the extracorporeal circuit to allow effective and efficient dialysis. For standard thrice weekly, four hourly haemodialyses, this equates to 26 full days of exposure to anticoagulation per annum. The choice is broadly split between unfractionated heparin (UFH) and low-molecular-weight heparin (LMWH). Single centre experience [65] and meta-analysis [66] suggested similar safety and efficacy, and many units use LMWHs as standard with no increase in adverse events. There is no requirement for regular monitoring of APTT or anti-FXa levels with this, and patients should start at the lowest dose, incrementing as required. The first dialysis session and ideally the first three dialysis sessions should be anticoagulant-free owing to excessive bleeding risk around this period of maximal uraemia. This has been discussed extensively in ▶ Chap. 12.

75.5.4 Direct Oral Anticoagulants (DOACs)

Currently, four DOACs that include one anti-thrombin inhibitor, dabigatran and three anti-Xa inhibitors, rivaroxaban, apixaban and edoxaban, are licensed for use in the prevention of stroke and systemic embolism in atrial fibrillation (AF), venous thromboembolism (VTE) prophylaxis in major orthopaedic surgery, treatment of acute VTE and prevention of recurrent VTE. Further, rivaroxaban is also registered for use in the prevention of cardiovascular deaths after acute coronary syndrome. Significant advantages of DOACs include their immediate action, fixed dosing, fewer drug and food interactions, and importantly, they do not require routine monitoring for therapeutic effect, unlike warfarin.

A meta-analysis demonstrated a favourable risk-benefit profile for all DOACs with significant reductions in stroke, intracranial haemorrhage and mortality, and with similar major bleeding as for warfarin, but with an excess of gastrointestinal bleeding seen in all DOACs except apixaban and edoxaban [67–72]. Although there is an overall decreased risk of major bleeding when compared to warfarin, because of renal excretion, decisions need to be individualised in patients with renal impairment.

Dabigatran etexilate is an oral prodrug of dabigatran, which binds and inhibits the active site of thrombin, including free and clot bound thrombin [73, 74]. This is a highly selective, competitive, rapid and reversible process. The absolute bioavailability of dabigatran following oral administration of dabigatran etexilate is ~6.5%, achieving peak levels within a couple of hours of ingestion with food delaying the peak effect. The volume of distribution exceeds the total body water volume suggesting moderate tissue distribution and a third is bound to plasma proteins. It is predominantly renally excreted, with 80% being excreted unchanged in the urine. The mean terminal half-life is about 12–14 h, and this increases after surgery and in patients with renal dysfunction. Interestingly, women have a 40–50% increased exposure after oral ingestion, but dosage adjustments are not required. Its clinical effect can be reversed by idarucizumab [75].

Rivaroxaban is an oral, direct Factor Xa inhibitor that inhibits selectively and reversibly free FXa activity and FXa associated with prothrombinase complex and clot [76]. It is rapidly absorbed with high bioavailability, and food slows its absorption, and the standard recommendation is for rivaroxaban to be administered with food. Peak levels are achieved around 2 h after ingestion, and half-life varies by age, ranging from 5 to 9 h in healthy young subjects and from 11 to 13 h in healthy elderly subjects. Two-thirds of the ingested dose undergoes metabolic degradation to inactive metabolites, and the final third is excreted unchanged by renal filtration and renal secretion. In patients with mild to moderate renal impairment, caution needs to be exercised, as a dose reduction is not recommended.

Apixaban, similar to rivaroxaban, is a selective FXa inhibitor [77]. It is also rapidly absorbed with a 50% bioavailability, and peak levels are achieved about 3 h post-dose. Food has no impact on its absorption, and it has a half-life of about 8–15 h and 87% is bound to plasma proteins. Drug elimination is by multiple routes with about half recovered unchanged in the faeces, a quarter excreted in the urine and the remainder metabolised and excreted through faeces. Dose reductions depend on the indication for anticoagulation, and it is not recommended for use in patients with CrCl <15 ml/min. Recent pharmacokinetic studies have suggested that low-dose apixaban does not accumulate in dialysis patients, and this may open the way for some centres using it in dialysis patients. Dose reductions with apixaban are indicated in patients with age ≥80 years, body weight ≤60 kg or serum creatinine ≥133 μmol/l.

Edoxaban is the newest available oral Xa inhibitor [78]. It is rapidly absorbed and reaches a peak concentration within 1–2 h and has an approximate half-life of 10–14 h. Its oral bioavailability is about 62%, and 55% is protein-bound. It is metabolised, but the majority (over 70%) is excreted unchanged into faeces and urine with about 35% eliminated via the kidneys. A dose reduction from 60 to 30 mg is recommended if patients have at least one of the following: CrCl 15–50 ml/min, bodyweight <60 kg or concomitant use of P-glycoprotein inhibitors. Its use is not recommended in patients with CrCL <15 ml/min.

Andexanet alfa, the universal antidote for anti-Xa inhibitors, has been licensed for reversing the effect of Xa inhibitors and requires IV administration [79].

Of note, DOACs are not licenced for patients >80 or at the extremes of weight (<60 kg or >130 kg). A summary of the dose adjustments in relation to renal function is presented in ◘ Table 75.3. A recent review addressed the issue of the choice of DOACs in patients with renal impairment [80]. In patients with a creatinine clearance of >50 ml/min, all DOACs can be prescribed as per license. In patients with mild renal impairment and creatinine clearance between 30 and 50 ml, all DOACs can be used with dose reductions as recommended by the manufacturer. None are indicated in patients with creatinine clearance <15 mL/min, and in patients with clearance between 15 and 29 mL/min Dabigatran is contraindicated, and anti-Xa agents can be used with dose reduction, and monitoring is preferred in these situations.

Table 75.3 Comparision of Direct Acting Oral Anticoagulants (DOACs) in renal disease

DOAC	CrCl	AF	VTE	Other considerations
Rivaroxaban	15–50 ml/min	15 mg OD	15 mg OD for 3 weeks then 20 mg OD	–
	<15 ml/min or on RRT	Contraindicated	Contraindicated	
Dabigatran	30–50 ml/min	150 mg BD	150 mg BD	Age ≥80 years: 110 mg BD Concomitant verapamil: 100 mg BD
	30–50 ml/min with high risk of bleeding	Consider 110 mg BD	Consider 110 mg BD	
	<30 ml/min or on RRT	Contraindicated	Contraindicated	
Apixaban	>30 ml/min	5 mg BD	5 mg BD	≥2 of age ≥80 years, weight ≤60 kg or creatinine >133: 2.5 mg BD
	15–29 ml/min	2.5 mg BD	5 mg BD (use with caution)	
	<15 ml/min or on RRT	Contraindicated	Contraindicated	
Edoxaban	15–50 ml/min	30 mg OD	30 mg OD	Weight <60 kg or concomitant use of P-glycoprotein inhibitors: 30 mg OD
	<15 ml/min	Contraindicated	Contraindicated	

75.6 Antiplatelet Therapy

The cardiovascular benefit of antiplatelets other than aspirin in renal disease, including clopidogrel and glycoprotein IIb/IIIa inhibitors including abciximab, eptifibatide and tirofiban, is the subject of considerable debate. Various definitions of bleeding outcomes and different trial durations limit the clinical relevance of currently available evidence.

A recent systematic review and meta-analysis suggested that the addition of glycoprotein IIb/IIIa inhibitors or clopidogrel in CKD patients with acute coronary syndromes or undergoing percutaneous coronary revascularisation procedures appears to increase major bleeding with little or no effect on myocardial infarction, death or coronary revascularisation; further, the authors were of the opinion that evidence was of poor quality with no risk stratification by the severity of renal dysfunction [81]. As platelet dysfunction is in part related to the severity of the renal disease, one would expect that the use of glycoprotein IIb/IIIa inhibitors to be associated with a higher risk of bleeding in patients on haemodialysis.

In haemodialysis patients, there is good evidence that the use of aspirin and/or clopidogrel is associated with a six-fold increase in major bleeding events [82]. International outcome data has also suggested that all-cause mortality, cardiovascular mortality and bleeding events are elevated in the context of oral antiplatelet/anticoagulant use in prevalent haemodialysis patients [83].

75.7 Heparin-Induced Thrombocytopenia (HIT)

HIT is an immune-mediated adverse drug reaction, caused by the development of IgG antibodies against the complex of heparin and platelet factor 4 (PF4) [84]. PF4 is a chemokine present in platelet alpha granules that promotes coagulation when released. The PF4/heparin/HIT-antibody complexes develop either on the surface of platelets or bind to platelets after formation via their Fc gamma receptors (FcγIIa). This binding results in cross-linking of receptors with secondary platelet activation, the release of platelet granule contents (including further PF4), membrane activation and microparticle formation, leading to platelet aggregation and thrombus formation [85]. Two types of heparin-induced thrombocytopenia are recognised: the first is HIT type I, mild thrombocytopenia that is nonimmune and self-limiting caused by heparin-associated platelet aggregation. The second is HIT type II, the classic immune-mediated adverse drug reaction described above.

75.7.1 Clinical Presentation

Thrombocytopenia, with or without thrombosis, is the classic manifestation of HIT. Atypical presentations have been described including an acute systemic reaction 5–30 min after UFH bolus, presenting with fever and chills and on occasions cardiorespiratory compromise or arrest [86]. Skin necrosis at heparin injection sites have also been reported that initially present as small erythematous painful nodules [87]. The thrombocytopenia of HIT typically develops between 5 and 14 days after starting treatment with heparin but may occur within 1 day if there has been exposure to heparin in the previous 100 days [88]. A 50% decrease in platelet count from baseline is a more sensitive clinical marker of HIT compared to a standard definition of thrombocytopenia. Severe thrombocytopenia is unusual with platelet counts below 20 × 10^9/L seen in fewer than 10% of cases. The median nadir is typically around 60 × 10^9/L, the platelet count in some cases may not fall below 100 × 10^9/L. Resolution of thrombocytopenia occurs over 1–2 weeks following heparin cessation.

Thrombosis that is potentially fatal occurs in over 50% of patients diagnosed with HIT, usually with the onset of thrombocytopenia, or on the day of platelet count reduction to >50% from baseline. Venous thrombotic events are more prevalent than arterial events and can present either in limbs or in the viscera. Historical series of untreated patients show a thrombosis risk of 5–10% per day in the first couple of days after discontinuation of heparin therapy, and the 30-day cumulative risk of new thromboembolism can be high at 50% [89]. Despite thrombocytopenia, bleeding is very uncommon due to platelet activation and platelet transfusions are not indicated, and if indicated for pre-procedure, extreme caution is advised.

Prospective and retrospective studies have demonstrated that symptomatic HIT is less common than the prevalence of heparin-induced antibodies (HIA) measured by Enzyme immunoassay (EIA), and the incidence is related to the underlying medical condition. In general medical patients, HIAs are seen in about 20% following heparin exposure with a range of 1.5–50% across various medical and surgical disorders [90]. In addition, LMWHs are associated with a five- to tenfold lower risk of developing HIAs compared to UFH. In a group of patients on haemodialysis, HIAs were seen in 8.1% of 1450 patients exposed to UFH and in 1.8% of 218 patients dialysed with LMWH [91]. In a retrospective cohort study with a mean follow up of 2.3 ± 1.4 years, peak titres were seen in the first 6 months with reduction in titres over time. There was no significant association between HIA and thrombocytopenia, with a non-significant association between thrombosis and high antibody titre [92]. In a prospective cohort study, EIA positivity at the end of 6 months was seen in 10.3% when UFH was used for haemodialysis with no association with arterial cardiovascular events, venous thromboembolism, vascular access occlusion or mortality [93].

75.7.2 Diagnosis

Thrombocytopenia is common in patients on dialysis or receiving heparin, and laboratory testing is required to confirm the diagnosis of HIT where clinical probability is moderate or high.

Investigations available include either functional assays or immunological assays [94]. Functional tests are performed on platelets and detect antibodies that induce heparin-dependent platelet activation and include 14C-serotonin release assay (SRA) and heparin-induced platelet activation assay (HIPA). They are specific and sensitive but require considerable expertise and are available only in selected labs. The immunological tests (enzyme immunoassays, EIAs) identify circulating anti-PF4/heparin antibodies, irrespective of their capacity to activate platelets [95]. EIAs are widely available, with high sensitivity and low specificity. Because of the low specificity of the EIA and the risk of bleeding with alternative anticoagulants if used empirically, clinical criteria remain important when electing to perform testing and interpreting results. Various scoring systems have been developed, including the '4Ts' (thrombocytopenia, timing, thrombosis and other causes of platelet fall) proposed by Warkentin for estimating the pretest probability of HIT [95].

The challenge for the nephrologists considering HIT in this population are multiple [87]. Mild to moderate thrombocytopaenia in the dialysis population is not uncommon with various mechanisms responsible, including increased platelet consumption, immunosuppression, drugs and uraemia [87]. Due to the intermittent nature of heparin exposure, there are reports of late diagnosis in the literature [96], further the decrease in platelet count may not be as precipitous.

75.7.3 Treatment of HIT

Treatment of HIT requires immediate withdrawal of all heparin, including heparin-containing flushes and catheters. Heparin cessation alone is not sufficient to prevent thrombosis and initiation of non-heparin parenteral anticoagulant is the standard of care [94]. The choice of anticoagulant is dictated by renal function, and in patients with normal renal function, argatroban or lepirudin or danaparoid are recommended, and fondaparinux has also been used [97]. In patients with impaired renal function, argatroban is the anticoagulant of choice as it cleared via the hepatobiliary system with a half-life of 40–50 min, with dialysis patients showing about a 20% increase in half-life. Oral vitamin K agonists are contraindicated in the acute phase due to the risk of necrosis/gangrene, as is platelet transfusion. Parenteral anticoagulants are continued until full recovery of platelet counts when conversion to warfarin may be initiated. The optimal duration of anticoagulation is unclear, with the risk of thrombosis believed to last between 4 and 8 weeks, although in general, 3–6 months is appropriate depending on other risk factors [98]. When HIT is suspected in a dialysis patient, dialysis needs to be performed heparin free. Other possibilities include regional citrate anticoagulation or prostaglandins. Other anticoagulation regimens utilised in dialysis typically include danaparoid or fondaparinux. The antibody positivity declines with time, and retesting should be done every few months until the test becomes negative. Once the antibodies disappear, recurrence is uncommon, and rechallenge with heparin is not unreasonable, although caution needs to be exercised and patients need to be monitored closely [91].

Case Study

Case 1

A patient with a history of recurrent DVTs is listed for a renal transplant. She is anticoagulated with warfarin with a target INR of 2–3. A perioperative bridging anticoagulation plan needs to be set up for the transplant.

Surgery in patients while therapeutically anticoagulated results in excessive bleeding and associated mortality and morbidity. It is imperative to know if the patient is scheduled for a cadaveric transplant in which case it is managed as an emergency or live-related donor transplant when an elective peri-operative bridging plan can be instituted. For an emergency transplant, anticoagulation with warfarin is reversed with prothrombin complex concentrate at a dose of 25–30 IU/kg along with vitamin K 5 mg IV. This will ensure the immediate complete reversal of anticoagulation for the surgery and in the post-operative period. For a planned procedure, warfarin typically is stopped five days pre-procedure, and therapeutic LMWH at a reduced dose as determined by the creatinine clearance is commenced three days before the procedure to bridge the loss of warfarin anticoagulant effect. This bridging decreases the duration that a patient is not therapeutically anticoagulated. The last dose of LMWH is administered 24 h pre-procedure. This briding ensures normal coagulation during the procedure and post-operative period with minimal risk of thrombosis. The highest risk of bleeding is on the first day post-surgery with the risk decreasing quite markedly 48 h post-procedure. Post-procedure, patients can receive a prophylactic dose of LWMH if there are no concerns about bleeding. Therapeutic anticoagulation can be started 24 h after a procedure with split-dose LWMH in patients at high risk of thrombosis, e.g. antiphospholipid syndrome patients with recurrent events or patients with a metallic mitral valve. Preferably therapeutic anticoagulation is initiated 48 h post-procedure when the risk of bleeding has decreased. In the first week post-procedure if there are any concerns about bleeding the initiation of anticoagulation should be postponed. Warfarin can be restarted once the patient is stable and off antibiotics. The patient should be continued on treatment dose LWMH until INR is in the target range.

Case 2

A patient with CrCl of 20 ml/min develops a suspected DVT and is started on reduced dose LMWH as per hospital policy. He has a history of severe epistaxis which has previously required red cell transfusions. A few days after starting anticoagulation, he develops epistaxis.

It is important to remember that epistaxis can be life-threatening. In addition to local causes, anticoagulation with LWMH and potentially renal impairment related platelet dysfunction are contributary. LMWHs are renally excreted and accumulation varies with different types of LMWHs, with enoxaparin demonstrating the maximum accumulation. As for any other epistaxis, local measures including compression and a nasal pack as needed are important. The need for reversal is dictated by the severity of the bleed. If the bleed is rapid, reversal with Protamine needs to be instituted. Protamine reverses up to 60% of LMWH, and is more effective in neutralising the anti-IIa effect in contrast to its limited efficacy against the anti-Xa effect. Tranexamic acid may also be given systemically to help stabilise the clot locally. If the bleed is less severe, missing a couple of doses of LWMH may be adequate. In this situation, measurement of anti-FXa levels to ensure there is no accumulation may be informative. Anticoagulation is typically restarted once bleeding has settled and pack removed. This can typically take between 1 and 3 days. When LMWH is reinitiated, consideration for the use of split doses needs to be given as this decreases the peak anti-Xa levels achieved. Consideration must also be given to monitoring the LWMH dosing with anti-Xa levels.

Case 3

A patient presents with upper gastrointestinal bleeding and is managed with fluid resuscitation, red blood cells, FFP and TXA. His admission blood results revealed elevated creatinine of 190 μmol/l, and examination and investigations demonstrated peripheral oedema, proteinuria and hypoalbuminemia with a diagnosis of Nephrotic syndrome. Shortly afterwards, a renal biopsy was performed, and post-procedure the patient developed haematuria which was monitored. The following day, the patient

75

complains of suprapubic pain and distension, and the nurses notice that his catheter is bypassing. His creatinine rises to 230 µmol/l.

In all probability, the acute deterioration is related to haematuria. Haematuria in this context can either cause ureteric obstruction or obstruction of a catheter. Further, the tranexamic acid might have contributed to the occlusion of the catheter. It is important to remember that tranexamic acid is generally contraindicated in the management of haematuria for its potential to stabilise a clot that is resistant to lysis with subsequent ureteric obstruction and clot colic or catheter obstruction. Tranexamic acid in this situation, if indicated, must be used with caution under close monitoring.

Tips and Tricks

1. Patients with renal disease are at increased risk of both bleeding and thrombosis.
2. Impaired primary haemostasis in particular impaired platelet function contributes to the bleeding tendency typically seen in patients with advanced kidney disease or ESRD. Clinically this presents as exaggerated bleeding post-procedure or excess physiological loss or excess loss from other pathological lesions.
3. The gold standard for the investigation of platelet dysfunction is platelet aggregometry with a panel of platelet-activating agonists. The PFA-100® is a rapid test that assesses platelet-dependent primary haemostasis and is sensitive to minor platelet dysfunction with the potential for overestimating the risk of bleeding when compared to the skin bleeding time.
4. Management of bleeding tendency is dictated by the clinical situation and includes long-term prevention of spontaneous bleeding via renal replacement therapy, prevention of procedure-related bleeding and management of active bleeding. Resuscitation of active bleeding is complicated by the patients' tolerance to the volume of transfused blood products.
5. Non-specific short term measures that improve platelet function and clot formation include desmopressin and cryoprecipitate. Tranexamic acid increases clot stability. Conjugated oestrogens also seem to be efficacious in the prevention and management of bleeding with the clinical effect seen as early as 6 h. They have a particular role in the management of obscure GI bleeding with no identifiable lesions.
6. Thrombotic complications in the form of arterial thrombotic events (ATE), venous thromboembolism (VTE) or thrombosis related to vascular access for haemodialysis are common in patients with CKD and ESKD.
7. Haemostatic changes described include elevated procoagulants, impaired natural anticoagulant pathways and a decrease in fibrinolytic activity. All of these changes contribute to the excess risk of venous thrombosis. Additional risk factors for arterial events include accelerated atherosclerosis, hypertension, loss of normal vessel elasticity and vascular calcification.
8. The risk of VTE is increased across the spectrum of renal disorders, including patients with mild renal impairment, nephrotic syndrome, renal transplant and dialysis. Prophylactic anticoagulation in nephrotic syndrome should be informed by an individualised risk-benefit assessment, and the evidence is against treatment in the presence of bleeding risk factors.
9. The haemostatic abnormalities that contribute to vascular access thrombosis are poorly defined, and while there is some suggestion that thrombophilic defects might increase the risk, anticoagulation with warfarin has not demonstrated clinical benefit. Similarly, antiplatelet therapy has demonstrated a physiological effect with no obvious clinical benefit. A role for routine prophylactic anticoagulation or antiplatelet therapy has not been established.
10. In patients with CKD and AF, the risk-benefit for anticoagulation is related to the severity of renal disease and requires careful consideration. In CKD stage 5, the evidence of benefit for prevention of systemic thromboembolism in AF is not evident, but an increased risk of bleeding is well documented.
11. Warfarin is the most commonly used anticoagulant in patients with renal disease, and the risk of bleeding with warfarin anticoagulation is related to the intensity of anticoagulation, the stability of INR control, presence of risk factors for overanticoagulation and patient-related variables.
12. Unfractionated heparin (UFH) has a short half-life of ~30–60 min at standard doses and is rapidly eliminated by the reticuloendothelial system. It is administered intravenously, and dose adjustments to achieve and maintain therapeutic APTT ratios are ideally made using a nomogram and regular monitoring.
13. Anticoagulant response with LMWHs is more consistent compared to UFH due to good bioavailability

after SC administration, and the use of weight-adjusted doses results in more predictable blood levels. The effects of LMWH can be measured with anti-FXa assays using product-specific calibrators.

14. Routine monitoring of anti-FXa levels is not required for prophylactic low-molecular-weight heparins (LMWH) but may be considered in patients with ESKD, especially in patients with CrCl <30 ml/min receiving therapeutic LMWH, particularly enoxaparin. Enoxaparin is the only LMWH with a licensed dose reduction for patients with CrCl <30 mL/min.
15. All DOACs can be prescribed as per license in patients with a creatinine clearance of >50 ml/min. In patients with mild renal impairment and creatinine clearance between 30 and 50 ml, all DOACs can be used with dose reductions as recommended by the manufacturer. All DOACs are contraindicated in patients with creatinine clearance <15 mL/min. When the creatinine clearance is between 15 and 29 mL/min, dabigatran is contraindicated as it is predominantly renally excreted, but anti-Xa agents can be used with dose reduction, and monitoring is preferred in these situations.
16. Heparin-induced thrombocytopenia is an immune-mediated adverse drug reaction associated with thrombocytopenia, with or without thrombosis. Atypical presentations include an acute systemic reaction 5–30 min after UFH bolus, presenting with fever and chills and rarely cardiopulmonary arrest. Other challenges to diagnosis include the wide prevalence of thrombocytopenia and the lack of precipitous drop in platelet count.

Chapter Review Questions

1. Can direct oral anticoagulants be prescribed in patients with renal disease?
2. A patient under investigation for renal impairment presents with pleuritic chest pain and shortness of breath and is diagnosed with a PE and is started on LMWH. The renal biopsy is planned for 2 weeks' time. What factors need to be considered?

Answers

1. All DOACs can be prescribed as per license in patients with a creatinine clearance of >50 ml/min. The renal excretion is variable across DOACs with Dabigatraon demonstrating 80% renal excretion; Rivaroxaban 30% renal excretion; Apixaban 25% renal excretion and Edoxaban demonstrating 50% renal excretion.
2. In patients with acute pulmonary embolism, the risk of embolisation is highest in the first month and decreases with increasing time. In this situation, the risk of interruption of anticoagulation versus the benefit of gathering additional information about the renal impairment needs to be considered. A repeat Doppler ultrasound of the initial venous thrombotic event might shed light on the potential for extension. An appropriate bridging plan also needs to be instituted.

Acknowledgements The authors wish to thank Duncan Brian, MBBS, MCRP, FRCPath, who wrote tirelessly for the chapter in the first edition of the textbook.

Disclosures No relevant disclosures.

References

1. Ruggeri ZM, Mendolicchio GL. Adhesion mechanisms in platelet function. Circ Res. 2007;100(12):1673–85. https://doi.org/10.1161/01.RES.0000267878.97021.ab.
2. Monroe DM, Hoffman M, Roberts HR. Platelets and thrombin generation. Arterioscler Thromb Vasc Biol. 2002;22(9):1381–9.
3. Pavord S, Myers B. Bleeding and thrombotic complications of kidney disease. Blood Rev. 2011;25(6):271–8. https://doi.org/10.1016/j.blre.2011.07.001.
4. Hedges SJ, Dehoney SB, Hooper JS, Amanzadeh J, Busti AJ. Evidence-based treatment recommendations for uremic bleeding. Nat Clin Pract Nephrol. 2007;3(3):138–53. https://doi.org/10.1038/ncpneph0421.
5. Noris M, Remuzzi G. Uremic bleeding: closing the circle after 30 years of controversies? Blood. 1999;94(8):2569–74.
6. Remuzzi G. Bleeding in renal failure. Lancet. 1988;1(8596):1205–8.
7. Sohal AS, Gangji AS, Crowther MA, Treleaven D. Uremic bleeding: pathophysiology and clinical risk factors. Thromb Res. 2006;118(3):417–22. https://doi.org/10.1016/j.thromres.2005.03.032.
8. Liang CC, Wang SM, Kuo HL, Chang CT, Liu JH, Lin HH, et al. Upper gastrointestinal bleeding in patients with CKD. Clin J Am Soc Nephrol. 2014;9(8):1354–9. https://doi.org/10.2215/cjn.09260913.
9. Yang JY, Lee TC, Montez-Rath ME, Paik J, Chertow GM, Desai M, et al. Trends in acute nonvariceal upper gastrointestinal bleeding in dialysis patients. J Am Soc Nephrol. 2012;23(3):495–506. https://doi.org/10.1681/asn.2011070658.
10. Sood P, Kumar G, Nanchal R, Sakhuja A, Ahmad S, Ali M, et al. Chronic kidney disease and end-stage renal disease predict higher risk of mortality in patients with primary upper gastrointestinal bleeding. Am J Nephrol. 2012;35(3):216–24. https://doi.org/10.1159/000336107.
11. Ohmori T, Konishi H, Nakamura S, Shiratori K. Abnormalities of the small intestine detected by capsule endoscopy in hemodialysis patients. Intern Med. 2012;51(12):1455–60.

12. Korman MG, Laver MC, Hansky J. Hypergastrinaemia in chronic renal failure. Br Med J. 1972;1(5794):209–10. https://doi.org/10.1136/bmj.1.5794.209.
13. Taylor IL, Sells RA, McConnell RB, Dockray GJ. Serum gastrin in patients with chronic renal failure. Gut. 1980;21(12):1062–7. https://doi.org/10.1136/gut.21.12.1062.
14. Alqahtani F, Berzingi CO, Aljohani S, Al Hajji M, Diab A, Alvi M et al. Temporal trends in the outcomes of dialysis patients admitted with acute ischemic stroke. J Am Heart Assoc. 2018;7(12). https://doi.org/10.1161/jaha.118.008686.
15. Power A, Hamady M, Singh S, Ashby D, Taube D, Duncan N. High but stable incidence of subdural haematoma in haemodialysis--a single-centre study. Nephrol Dial Transplant. 2010;25(7):2272–5. https://doi.org/10.1093/ndt/gfq013.
16. Anderson RJ, O'Brien M, MaWhinney S, VillaNueva CB, Moritz TE, Sethi GK, et al. Renal failure predisposes patients to adverse outcome after coronary artery bypass surgery. VA cooperative study #5. Kidney Int. 1999;55(3):1057–62. https://doi.org/10.1046/j.1523-1755.1999.0550031057.x.
17. Corapi KM, Chen JL, Balk EM, Gordon CE. Bleeding complications of native kidney biopsy: a systematic review and meta-analysis. Am J Kidney Dis. 2012;60(1):62–73. https://doi.org/10.1053/j.ajkd.2012.02.330.
18. Manno C, Strippoli GF, Arnesano L, Bonifati C, Campobasso N, Gesualdo L, et al. Predictors of bleeding complications in percutaneous ultrasound-guided renal biopsy. Kidney Int. 2004;66(4):1570–7. https://doi.org/10.1111/j.1523-1755.2004.00922.x.
19. Harrison P, Lordkipanidze M. Testing platelet function. Hematol Oncol Clin North Am. 2013;27(3):411–41. https://doi.org/10.1016/j.hoc.2013.03.003.
20. Steiner RW, Coggins C, Carvalho AC. Bleeding time in uremia: a useful test to assess clinical bleeding. Am J Hematol. 1979;7(2):107–17.
21. Zupan IP, Sabovic M, Salobir B, Ponikvar JB, Cernelc P. Utility of in vitro closure time test for evaluating platelet-related primary hemostasis in dialysis patients. Am J Kidney Dis. 2003;42(4):746–51.
22. Islam N, Fulop T, Zsom L, Miller E, Mire CD, Lebrun CJ, et al. Do platelet function analyzer-100 testing results correlate with bleeding events after percutaneous renal biopsy? Clin Nephrol. 2010;73(3):229–37.
23. Ranghino A, Mella A, Borchiellini A, Nappo A, Manzione AM, Gallo E, et al. Assessment of platelet function analyzer (PFA-100) in kidney transplant patients before renal allograft biopsy: a retrospective single-center analysis. Transplant Proc. 2014;46(7):2259–62. https://doi.org/10.1016/j.transproceed.2014.07.052.
24. Whiting D, DiNardo JA. TEG and ROTEM: technology and clinical applications. Am J Hematol. 2014;89(2):228–32. https://doi.org/10.1002/ajh.23599.
25. Hemker HC, Giesen P, Al Dieri R, Regnault V, de Smedt E, Wagenvoord R, et al. Calibrated automated thrombin generation measurement in clotting plasma. Pathophysiol Haemost Thromb. 2003;33(1):4–15. https://doi.org/10.1159/000071636.
26. Estcourt LJ, Birchall J, Allard S, Bassey SJ, Hersey P, Kerr JP, et al. Guidelines for the use of platelet transfusions. Br J Haematol. 2017;176(3):365–94. https://doi.org/10.1111/bjh.14423.
27. Kaufmann JE, Vischer UM. Cellular mechanisms of the hemostatic effects of desmopressin (DDAVP). J Thromb Haemost. 2003;1(4):682–9.
28. Mannucci PM, Remuzzi G, Pusineri F, Lombardi R, Valsecchi C, Mecca G, et al. Deamino-8-D-arginine vasopressin shortens the bleeding time in uremia. N Engl J Med. 1983;308(1):8–12. https://doi.org/10.1056/nejm198301063080102.
29. Manno C, Bonifati C, Torres DD, Campobasso N, Schena FP. Desmopressin acetate in percutaneous ultrasound-guided kidney biopsy: a randomized controlled trial. Am J Kidney Dis. 2011;57(6):850–5. https://doi.org/10.1053/j.ajkd.2010.12.019.
30. Janson PA, Jubelirer SJ, Weinstein MJ, Deykin D. Treatment of the bleeding tendency in uremia with cryoprecipitate. N Engl J Med. 1980;303(23):1318–22. https://doi.org/10.1056/nejm198012043032302.
31. Liu YK, Kosfeld RE, Marcum SG. Treatment of uraemic bleeding with conjugated oestrogen. Lancet. 1984;2(8408):887–90.
32. Dunn CJ, Goa KL. Tranexamic acid: a review of its use in surgery and other indications. Drugs. 1999;57(6):1005–32. https://doi.org/10.2165/00003495-199957060-00017.
33. Shakur H, Roberts I, Bautista R, Caballero J, Coats T, Dewan Y, et al. Effects of tranexamic acid on death, vascular occlusive events, and blood transfusion in trauma patients with significant haemorrhage (CRASH-2): a randomised, placebo-controlled trial. Lancet. 2010;376(9734):23–32. https://doi.org/10.1016/s0140-6736(10)60835-5.
34. Shakur H, Roberts I, Edwards P, Elbourne D, Alfirevic Z, Ronsmans C. The effect of tranexamic acid on the risk of death and hysterectomy in women with post-partum haemorrhage: statistical analysis plan for the WOMAN trial. Trials. 2016;17(1):249. https://doi.org/10.1186/s13063-016-1332-2.
35. Andersson L, Eriksson O, Hedlund PO, Kjellman H, Lindqvist B. Special considerations with regard to the dosage of tranexamic acid in patients with chronic renal diseases. Urol Res. 1978;6(2):83–8.
36. Stiles KP, Yuan CM, Chung EM, Lyon RD, Lane JD, Abbott KC. Renal biopsy in high-risk patients with medical diseases of the kidney. Am J Kidney Dis. 2000;36(2):419–33. https://doi.org/10.1053/ajkd.2000.8998.
37. Wattanakit K, Cushman M. Chronic kidney disease and venous thromboembolism: epidemiology and mechanisms. Curr Opin Pulm Med. 2009;15(5):408–12. https://doi.org/10.1097/MCP.0b013e32832ee371.
38. Contaifer D Jr, Carl DE, Warncke UO, Martin EJ, Mohammed BM, Van Tassell B, et al. Unsupervised analysis of combined lipid and coagulation data reveals coagulopathy subtypes among dialysis patients. J Lipid Res. 2017;58(3):586–99. https://doi.org/10.1194/jlr.P068833.
39. Dubin R, Cushman M, Folsom AR, Fried LF, Palmas W, Peralta CA, et al. Kidney function and multiple hemostatic markers: cross sectional associations in the multi-ethnic study of atherosclerosis. BMC Nephrol. 2011;12:3. https://doi.org/10.1186/1471-2369-12-3.
40. Wattanakit K, Cushman M, Stehman-Breen C, Heckbert SR, Folsom AR. Chronic kidney disease increases risk for venous thromboembolism. J Am Soc Nephrol. 2008;19(1):135–40. https://doi.org/10.1681/asn.2007030308.
41. Kumar G, Sakhuja A, Taneja A, Majumdar T, Patel J, Whittle J, et al. Pulmonary embolism in patients with CKD and ESRD. Clin J Am Soc Nephrol. 2012;7(10):1584–90. https://doi.org/10.2215/cjn.00250112.
42. Singhal R, Brimble KS. Thromboembolic complications in the nephrotic syndrome: pathophysiology and clinical management. Thromb Res. 2006;118(3):397–407. https://doi.org/10.1016/j.thromres.2005.03.030.
43. Mahmoodi BK, ten Kate MK, Waanders F, Veeger NJ, Brouwer JL, Vogt L, et al. High absolute risks and predictors of venous and arterial thromboembolic events in patients with nephrotic syndrome: results from a large retrospective cohort study. Circulation. 2008;117(2):224–30. https://doi.org/10.1161/circulationaha.107.716951.

44. Barbano B, Gigante A, Amoroso A, Cianci R. Thrombosis in nephrotic syndrome. Semin Thromb Hemost. 2013;39(5):469–76. https://doi.org/10.1055/s-0033-1343887.
45. Kerlin BA, Ayoob R, Smoyer WE. Epidemiology and pathophysiology of nephrotic syndrome-associated thromboembolic disease. Clin J Am Soc Nephrol. 2012;7(3):513–20. https://doi.org/10.2215/cjn.10131011.
46. Mirrakhimov AE, Ali AM, Barbaryan A, Prueksaritanond S, Hussain N. Primary nephrotic syndrome in adults as a risk factor for pulmonary embolism: an up-to-date review of the literature. Int J Nephrol. 2014;2014:916760. https://doi.org/10.1155/2014/916760.
47. Glassock RJ. Prophylactic anticoagulation in nephrotic syndrome: a clinical conundrum. J Am Soc Nephrol. 2007;18(8):2221–5. https://doi.org/10.1681/asn.2006111300.
48. Senoo K, Proietti M, Lane DA, Lip GY. Evaluation of the HAS-BLED, ATRIA, and ORBIT bleeding risk scores in patients with atrial fibrillation taking warfarin. Am J Med. 2016;129(6):600–7. https://doi.org/10.1016/j.amjmed.2015.10.001.
49. Lee T, Biddle AK, Lionaki S, Derebail VK, Barbour SJ, Tannous S, et al. Personalized prophylactic anticoagulation decision analysis in patients with membranous nephropathy. Kidney Int. 2014;85(6):1412–20. https://doi.org/10.1038/ki.2013.476.
50. Sexton DJ, de Freitas DG, Little MA, McHugh T, Magee C, Conlon PJ, et al. Direct-acting oral anticoagulants as prophylaxis against thromboembolism in the nephrotic syndrome. Kidney Int Rep. 2018;3(4):784–93. https://doi.org/10.1016/j.ekir.2018.02.010.
51. Siddiqui MA, Ashraff S, Carline T. Maturation of arteriovenous fistula: analysis of key factors. Kidney Res Clin Pract. 2017;36(4):318–28. https://doi.org/10.23876/j.krcp.2017.36.4.318.
52. Knoll GA, Wells PS, Young D, Perkins SL, Pilkey RM, Clinch JJ, et al. Thrombophilia and the risk for hemodialysis vascular access thrombosis. J Am Soc Nephrol. 2005;16(4):1108–14. https://doi.org/10.1681/asn.2004110999.
53. Osborn G, Escofet X, Da Silva A. Medical adjuvant treatment to increase patency of arteriovenous fistulae and grafts. Cochrane Database Syst Rev (Online). 2008;(4):Cd002786. https://doi.org/10.1002/14651858.CD002786.pub2.
54. Dember LM, Beck GJ, Allon M, Delmez JA, Dixon BS, Greenberg A, et al. Effect of clopidogrel on early failure of arteriovenous fistulas for hemodialysis: a randomized controlled trial. JAMA. 2008;299(18):2164–71. https://doi.org/10.1001/jama.299.18.2164.
55. Olesen JB, Lip GY, Kamper AL, Hommel K, Kober L, Lane DA, et al. Stroke and bleeding in atrial fibrillation with chronic kidney disease. N Engl J Med. 2012;367(7):625–35. https://doi.org/10.1056/NEJMoa1105594.
56. Carrero JJ, Evans M, Szummer K, Spaak J, Lindhagen L, Edfors R, et al. Warfarin, kidney dysfunction, and outcomes following acute myocardial infarction in patients with atrial fibrillation. JAMA. 2014;311(9):919–28. https://doi.org/10.1001/jama.2014.1334.
57. Tan J, Liu S, Segal JB, Alexander GC, McAdams-DeMarco M. Warfarin use and stroke, bleeding and mortality risk in patients with end stage renal disease and atrial fibrillation: a systematic review and meta-analysis. BMC Nephrol. 2016;17(1):157. https://doi.org/10.1186/s12882-016-0368-6.
58. Dahal K, Kunwar S, Rijal J, Schulman P, Lee J. Stroke, major bleeding, and mortality outcomes in warfarin users with atrial fibrillation and chronic kidney disease: a meta-analysis of observational studies. Chest. 2016;149(4):951–9. https://doi.org/10.1378/chest.15-1719.
59. Brandenburg VM, Kramann R, Specht P, Ketteler M. Calciphylaxis in CKD and beyond. Nephrol Dial Transplant. 2012;27(4):1314–8. https://doi.org/10.1093/ndt/gfs015.
60. Baglin TP, Keeling DM, Watson HG. Guidelines on oral anticoagulation (warfarin): third edition--2005 update. Br J Haematol. 2006;132(3):277–85. https://doi.org/10.1111/j.1365-2141.2005.05856.x.
61. Ansell J, Hirsh J, Hylek E, Jacobson A, Crowther M, Palareti G. Pharmacology and management of the vitamin K antagonists: American College of Chest Physicians Evidence-Based Clinical Practice Guidelines (8th edition). Chest. 2008;133(6 Suppl):160s–98s. https://doi.org/10.1378/chest.08-0670.
62. Makris M, Van Veen JJ, Tait CR, Mumford AD, Laffan M. Guideline on the management of bleeding in patients on antithrombotic agents. Br J Haematol. 2013;160(1):35–46. https://doi.org/10.1111/bjh.12107.
63. Garcia DA, Baglin TP, Weitz JI, Samama MM. Parenteral anticoagulants: antithrombotic therapy and prevention of thrombosis, 9th ed: American College of Chest Physicians Evidence-Based Clinical Practice Guidelines. Chest. 2012;141(2 Suppl):e24S–43S. https://doi.org/10.1378/chest.11-2291.
64. Hughes S, Szeki I, Nash MJ, Thachil J. Anticoagulation in chronic kidney disease patients-the practical aspects. Clin Kidney J. 2014;7(5):442–9. https://doi.org/10.1093/ckj/sfu080.
65. Nadarajah L, Fan S, Forbes S, Ashman N. Major bleeding in hemodialysis patients using unfractionated or low molecular weight heparin: a single-center study. Clin Nephrol. 2015;84(5):274–9. https://doi.org/10.5414/cn108624.
66. Lazrak HH, Rene E, Elftouh N, Leblanc M, Lafrance JP. Safety of low-molecular-weight heparin compared to unfractionated heparin in hemodialysis: a systematic review and meta-analysis. BMC Nephrol. 2017;18(1):187. https://doi.org/10.1186/s12882-017-0596-4.
67. Patel MR, Mahaffey KW, Garg J, Pan G, Singer DE, Hacke W, et al. Rivaroxaban versus warfarin in nonvalvular atrial fibrillation. N Engl J Med. 2011;365(10):883–91. https://doi.org/10.1056/NEJMoa1009638.
68. Giugliano RP, Ruff CT, Braunwald E, Murphy SA, Wiviott SD, Halperin JL, et al. Edoxaban versus warfarin in patients with atrial fibrillation. N Engl J Med. 2013;369(22):2093–104. https://doi.org/10.1056/NEJMoa1310907.
69. Granger CB, Alexander JH, McMurray JJ, Lopes RD, Hylek EM, Hanna M, et al. Apixaban versus warfarin in patients with atrial fibrillation. N Engl J Med. 2011;365(11):981–92. https://doi.org/10.1056/NEJMoa1107039.
70. Connolly SJ, Ezekowitz MD, Yusuf S, Eikelboom J, Oldgren J, Parekh A, et al. Dabigatran versus warfarin in patients with atrial fibrillation. N Engl J Med. 2009;361(12):1139–51. https://doi.org/10.1056/NEJMoa0905561.
71. Ageno W, Gallus AS, Wittkowsky A, Crowther M, Hylek EM, Palareti G. Oral anticoagulant therapy: antithrombotic therapy and prevention of thrombosis, 9th ed: American College of Chest Physicians Evidence-Based Clinical Practice Guidelines. Chest. 2012;141(2 Suppl):e44S–88S. https://doi.org/10.1378/chest.11-2292.
72. Ruff CT, Giugliano RP, Braunwald E, Hoffman EB, Deenadayalu N, Ezekowitz MD, et al. Comparison of the efficacy and safety of new oral anticoagulants with warfarin in patients with atrial fibrillation: a meta-analysis of randomised trials. Lancet. 2014;383(9921):955–62. https://doi.org/10.1016/s0140-6736(13)62343-0.
73. Burness CB, McKeage K. Dabigatran Etexilate. Drugs. 2012;72(7):963–86. https://doi.org/10.2165/11209080-000000000-00000.

74. Dabigatran eMCe. Dabigatran etexilate mesilate - Summary of Product Characteristics. 20 May 2019. https://www.medicines.org.uk/emc/product/6229/smpc. Accessed June 2019.
75. Pollack CV Jr, Reilly PA, van Ryn J, Eikelboom JW, Glund S, Bernstein RA, et al. Idarucizumab for dabigatran reversal - full cohort analysis. N Engl J Med. 2017;377(5):431–41. https://doi.org/10.1056/NEJMoa1707278.
76. Trujillo T, Dobesh PP. Clinical use of rivaroxaban: pharmacokinetic and pharmacodynamic rationale for dosing regimens in different indications. Drugs. 2014;74(14):1587–603. https://doi.org/10.1007/s40265-014-0278-5.
77. Watson J, Whiteside G, Perry C. Apixaban. Drugs. 2011;71(15):2079–89. https://doi.org/10.2165/11596820-000000000-00000.
78. Bounameaux H, Camm AJ. Edoxaban: an update on the new oral direct factor Xa inhibitor. Drugs. 2014;74(11):1209–31. https://doi.org/10.1007/s40265-014-0261-1.
79. Connolly SJ, Crowther M, Eikelboom JW, Gibson CM, Curnutte JT, Lawrence JH, et al. Full study report of andexanet alfa for bleeding associated with factor Xa inhibitors. N Engl J Med. 2019;380(14):1326–35. https://doi.org/10.1056/NEJMoa1814051.
80. Parker K, Thachil J. The use of direct oral anticoagulants in chronic kidney disease. Br J Haematol. 2018;183(2):170–84. https://doi.org/10.1111/bjh.15564.
81. Palmer SC, Di Micco L, Razavian M, Craig JC, Perkovic V, Pellegrini F, et al. Effects of antiplatelet therapy on mortality and cardiovascular and bleeding outcomes in persons with chronic kidney disease: a systematic review and meta-analysis. Ann Intern Med. 2012;156(6):445–59. https://doi.org/10.7326/0003-4819-156-6-201203200-00007.
82. Holden RM, Harman GJ, Wang M, Holland D, Day AG. Major bleeding in hemodialysis patients. Clin J Am Soc Nephrol. 2008;3(1):105–10. https://doi.org/10.2215/cjn.01810407.
83. Sood MM, Larkina M, Thumma JR, Tentori F, Gillespie BW, Fukuhara S, et al. Major bleeding events and risk stratification of antithrombotic agents in hemodialysis: results from the DOPPS. Kidney Int. 2013;84(3):600–8. https://doi.org/10.1038/ki.2013.170.
84. Horsewood P, Warkentin TE, Hayward CP, Kelton JG. The epitope specificity of heparin-induced thrombocytopenia. Br J Haematol. 1996;95(1):161–7.
85. Kelton JG, Warkentin TE. Heparin-induced thrombocytopenia: a historical perspective. Blood. 2008;112(7):2607–16. https://doi.org/10.1182/blood-2008-02-078014.
86. Davenport A. Sudden collapse during haemodialysis due to immune-mediated heparin-induced thrombocytopaenia. Nephrol Dial Transplant. 2006;21(6):1721–4. https://doi.org/10.1093/ndt/gfl124.
87. Dutt T, Schulz M. Heparin-induced thrombocytopaenia (HIT)-an overview: what does the nephrologist need to know and do? Clin Kidney J. 2013;6(6):563–7. https://doi.org/10.1093/ckj/sft139.
88. Warkentin TE, Kelton JG. Temporal aspects of heparin-induced thrombocytopenia. N Engl J Med. 2001;344(17):1286–92. https://doi.org/10.1056/nejm200104263441704.
89. Warkentin TE, Kelton JG. A 14-year study of heparin-induced thrombocytopenia. Am J Med. 1996;101(5):502–7.
90. Arepally GM, Ortel TL. Clinical practice. Heparin-induced thrombocytopenia. N Engl J Med. 2006;355(8):809–17. https://doi.org/10.1056/NEJMcp052967.
91. Syed S, Reilly RF. Heparin-induced thrombocytopenia: a renal perspective. Nat Rev Nephrol. 2009;5(9):501–11. https://doi.org/10.1038/nrneph.2009.125.
92. Maharaj S, Chang S, Seegobin K, Morales J, Aysola A, Rana F, et al. Temporality of heparin-induced antibodies: a retrospective study in outpatients undergoing hemodialysis on unfractionated heparin. Exp Hematol Oncol. 2018;7:23. https://doi.org/10.1186/s40164-018-0115-8.
93. Asmis LM, Segal JB, Plantinga LC, Fink NE, Kerman JS, Kickler TS, et al. Heparin-induced antibodies and cardiovascular risk in patients on dialysis. Thromb Haemost. 2008;100(3):498–504.
94. Cuker A, Arepally GM, Chong BH, Cines DB, Greinacher A, Gruel Y, et al. American Society of Hematology 2018 guidelines for management of venous thromboembolism: heparin-induced thrombocytopenia. Blood Adv. 2018;2(22):3360–92. https://doi.org/10.1182/bloodadvances.2018024489.
95. Warkentin TE, Greinacher A, Gruel Y, Aster RH, Chong BH. Laboratory testing for heparin-induced thrombocytopenia: a conceptual framework and implications for diagnosis. J Thromb Haemost. 2011;9(12):2498–500. https://doi.org/10.1111/j.1538-7836.2011.04536.x.
96. Hutchison CA, Dasgupta I. National survey of heparin-induced thrombocytopenia in the haemodialysis population of the UK population. Nephrol Dial Transplant. 2007;22(6):1680–4. https://doi.org/10.1093/ndt/gfm055.
97. Linkins LA, Dans AL, Moores LK, Bona R, Davidson BL, Schulman S, et al. Treatment and prevention of heparin-induced thrombocytopenia: antithrombotic therapy and prevention of thrombosis, 9th ed: American College of Chest Physicians Evidence-Based Clinical Practice Guidelines. Chest. 2012;141(2 Suppl):e495S–530S. https://doi.org/10.1378/chest.11-2303.
98. Watson H, Davidson S, Keeling D. Guidelines on the diagnosis and management of heparin-induced thrombocytopenia: second edition. Br J Haematol. 2012;159(5):528–40. https://doi.org/10.1111/bjh.12059.

Dialysis

Contents

Prevention of Infection in Kidney Patients

Caroline Tulley, Gerlineke Hawkins- van der Cingel, and Mark Harber

Contents

M. Harber (ed.), *Primer on Nephrology*, https://doi.org/10.1007/978-3-030-76419-7_76

76

Learning Objectives

This chapter will discuss the following elements in the prevention of infections in renal patients:

1. Core principles of infection prevention and control
2. Specific important organisms including multidrug-resistant organisms (MDRO)
3. Access-related infections
4. Prevention of other important healthcare-associated infections
5. Preventing the spread of blood-borne viruses
6. Vaccine-preventable diseases (including travel health)
7. An approach to prevention of Covid-19 infection

76.1 Introduction

In 2009, infection was the second most frequent prevalent cause of death in those undergoing dialysis and the most frequent cause of death in those with a renal transplant. To put in perspective, in renal patients, sepsis accounts for 30% of hospital admissions [1]. It is salutary to remember that approximately 7–10% of *all* hospital admissions develop at least one hospital-acquired infection and in ICU this rises 1 in 3 patients. Furthermore, it is particularly chastening to note that in the first wave of Covid-19, up to 11% of patients acquired their Covid infection whilst in UK hospitals for other reasons. Renal patients are particularly vulnerable in part because of their frequent and chronic interaction with the healthcare system.

Antimicrobial resistance is currently responsible for 700,000 deaths per year, but this is estimated to rise to ten million every year by 2050 exceeding global deaths from cancer and at the time of writing 4–5 times the number that have succumbed to Covid-19 in the first 10 months of 2020. It is particularly telling and alarming that the first reports of both vancomycin-resistant enterococci (VRE) and vancomycin-resistant *Staphylococcus aureus* (VRSA) came from renal patients, and renal patients are also likely to be particularly impacted by the rise in AMR.

As our antibiotic armamentarium diminishes, one of our most important weapons against infection is now prevention.

76.2 Core Principles of Infection Prevention and Control

The prevention of infection is core to the provision of any healthcare. The following are essential to prevent infections in the healthcare environment:

1. Hand hygiene
2. Personal protective equipment (PPE)
3. Sharps disposal
4. Cleaning and decontamination
5. Surveillance and feedback
6. Education of healthcare workers and patients
7. Early and prompt recognition and treatment of infection
8. Isolation of patients with potential or confirmed significant cross-transmissible pathogens

In the United Kingdom, healthcare workers (HCW) are required by law to have appropriate supplies of hand decontamination, PPE and sharps disposal.

76.2.1 Hand Hygiene

Despite advances in healthcare delivery and technology, *the single most effective method to prevent onward transmission of infection in healthcare settings is hand hygiene.* Yet audits continue to show poor performance with hand hygiene among otherwise highly educated medical staff. The World Health Organization is promoting the five moments (Figs. 76.1 and 76.2) – (i) before patient contact, (ii) before an aseptic task, (iii) after body fluid exposure, (iv) after patient contact and (v) after contact with patient surroundings – of hand hygiene worldwide and have reviewed the evidence extensively [2]. Resources to help develop hospital and unit campaigns are located at ▸ http://www.npsa.nhs.uk/cleanyourhands/ and ▸ http://www.who.int/gpsc/5may/en/.

Normal human skin is colonized with multiple bacteria, and the bacterial counts on the hands of HCW have been estimated at 4×10^4 CFU/cm^3: Transient organisms – for example, *S. aureus*, gram-negative bacilli or yeasts – are most frequently acquired by direct contact with patients or healthcare environment and are very amenable to removal by cleaning (Fig. 76.3). Only occasionally do HCW's hands become persistently colonised with these organisms.

In outbreaks, contaminated hands are responsible for transmitting infections. Hand decontamination can reduce significantly gastrointestinal infections, respiratory infections [3, 4] and transmission of multidrug-resistant organisms in high-risk areas (e.g. ICU or renal dialysis units) [5]. In one study, the introduction of readily available alcohol-based hand rubs reduced new nosocomial acquired MRSA by 21% and VRE by 41% [6]. The English government policy 'bare below the elbows', as it is popularly known, endorses rolled-up sleeves, no wristwatches, no false nails or nail varnish and only a simple wedding band to assist in hand hygiene.

Your 5 Moments for Hand Hygiene

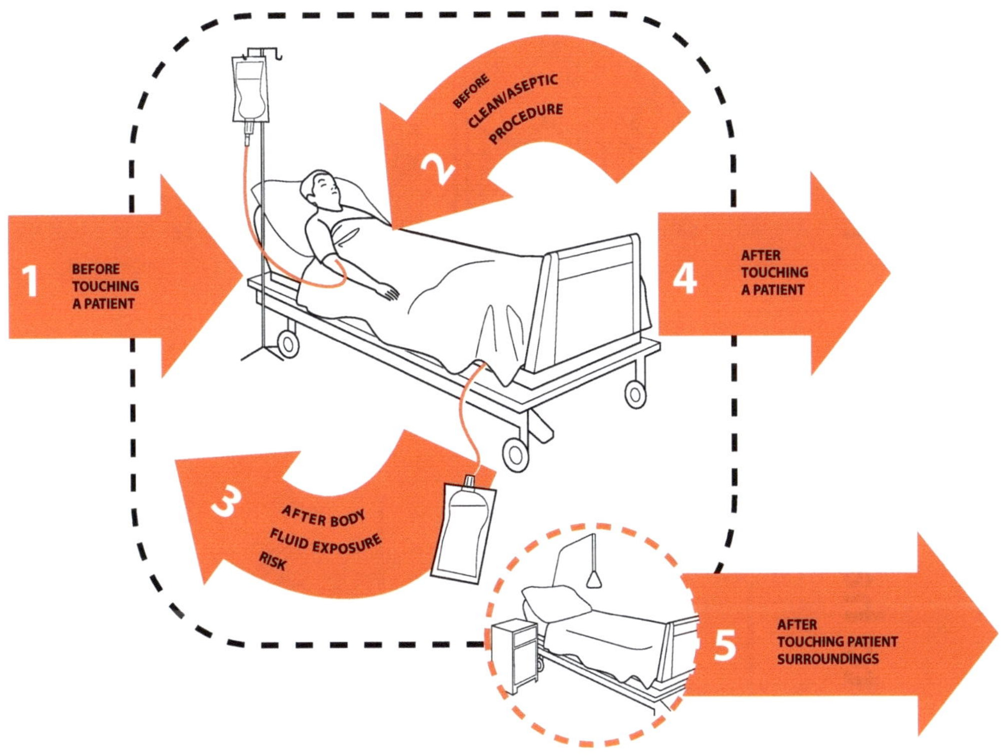

1 BEFORE TOUCHING A PATIENT	WHEN?	Clean your hands before touching a patient when approaching him/her.
	WHY?	To protect the patient against harmful germs carried on your hands.
2 BEFORE CLEAN/ ASEPTIC PROCEDURE	WHEN?	Clean your hands immediately before performing a clean/aseptic procedure.
	WHY?	To protect the patient against harmful germs, including the patient's own, from entering his/her body.
3 AFTER BODY FLUID EXPOSURE RISK	WHEN?	Clean your hands immediately after an exposure risk to body fluids (and after glove removal).
	WHY?	To protect yourself and the health-care environment from harmful patient germs.
4 AFTER TOUCHING A PATIENT	WHEN?	Clean your hands after touching a patient and her/his immediate surroundings, when leaving the patient's side.
	WHY?	To protect yourself and the health-care environment from harmful patient germs.
5 AFTER TOUCHING PATIENT SURROUNDINGS	WHEN?	Clean your hands after touching any object or furniture in the patient's immediate surroundings, when leaving – even if the patient has not been touched.
	WHY?	To protect yourself and the health-care environment from harmful patient germs.

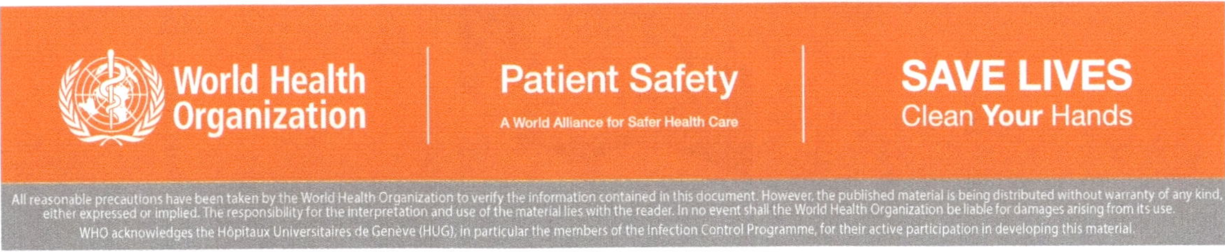

May 2009

Fig. 76.1 World health organisation 'your 5 moments for hand hygiene' points at which hands should be cleaned

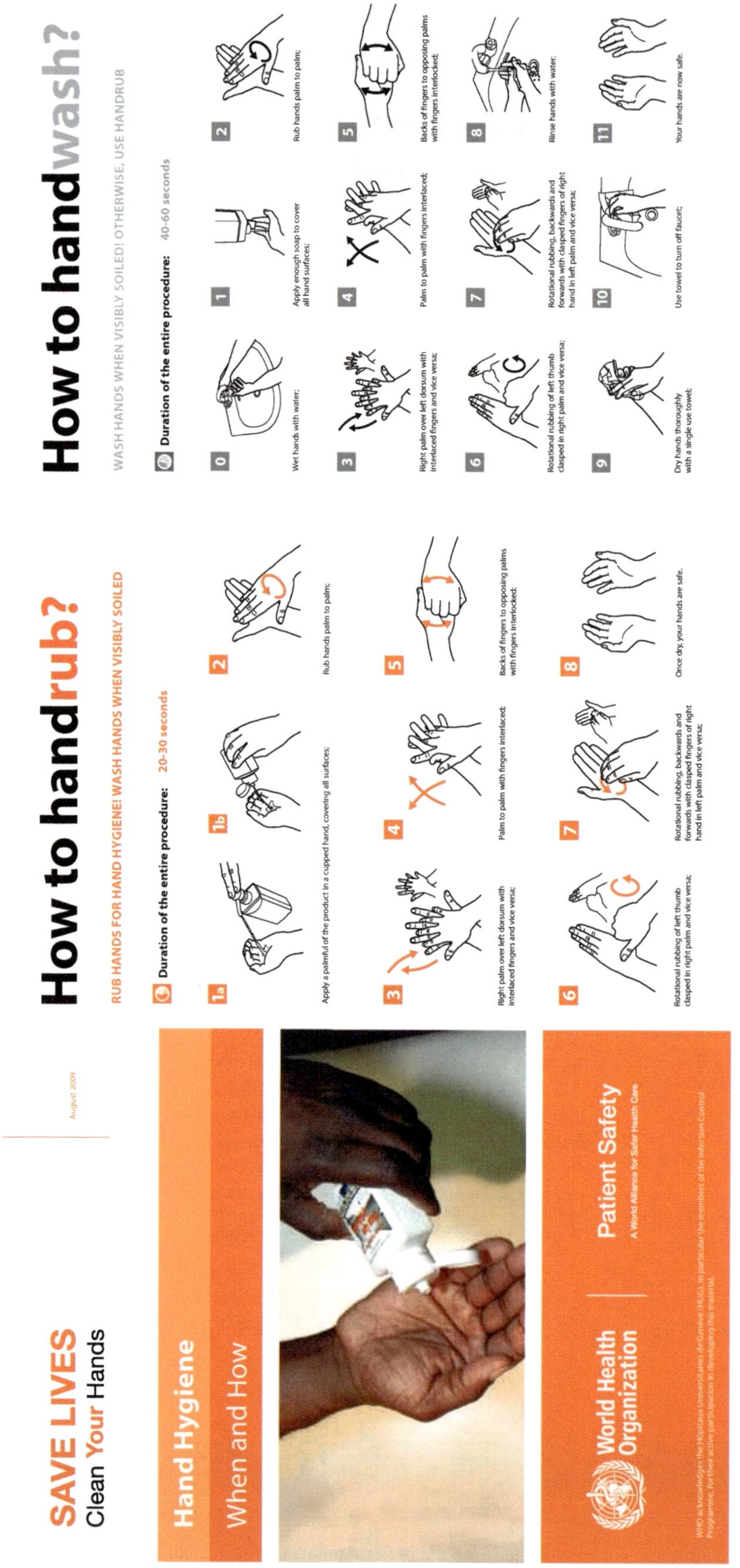

Fig. 76.2 World health organisation guidance on hand washing technique

Clean hands
are safer hands.
Are yours clean?

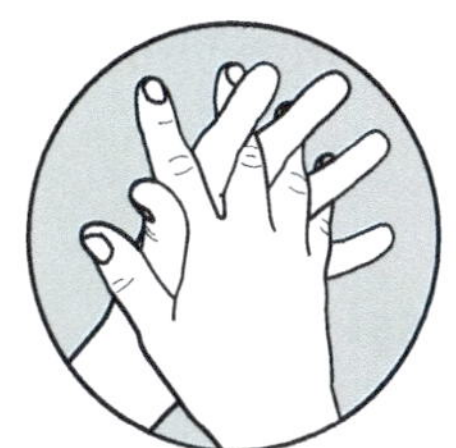

All reasonable precautions have been taken by the World Health Organization to verify the information contained in this document. However, the published material is being distributed without warranty of any kind, either expressed or implied. The responsibility for the interpretation and use of the material lies with the reader. In no event shall the World Health Organization be liable for damages arising from its use.

Fig. 76.2 (continued)

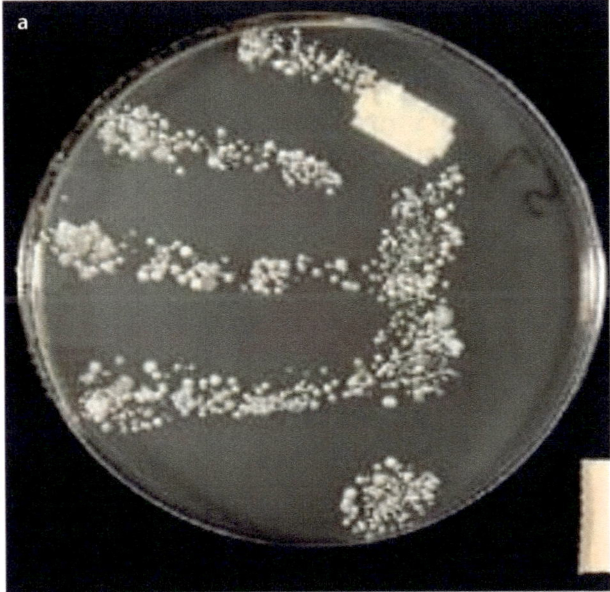

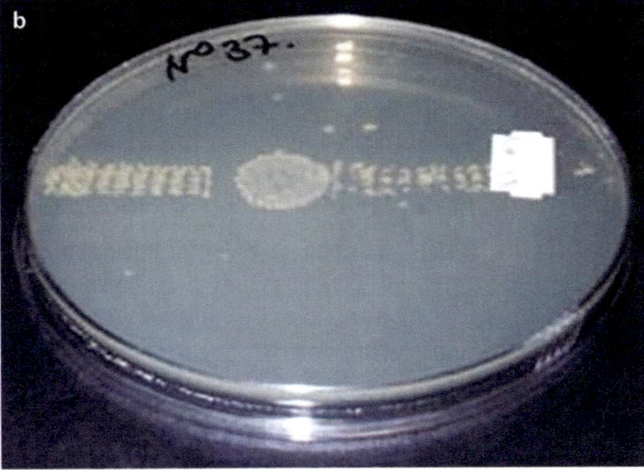

Fig. 76.3 **a** Hand print and **b** watch print from medical staff on a renal ward round. The watch imprint illustrates the very real importance of 'bare below the elbow'

76.2.2 Personal Protective Equipment (PPE)

Whilst there are no definitive studies proving the benefit for individual PPE, expert opinion (and common sense) consistently suggests that it protects patients and HCW, both in hospitals and community settings from the transmission of microorganisms. The Covid-19 pandemic has brought PPE to the forefront of current infection control policy, with new WHO [7] and UK Department of Health guidance [8] advocating the use of PPE as an important measure in both maintaining healthcare practitioner safety and minimising Covid-19 transmission in healthcare settings.

The specific PPE required needs to be matched to both the clinical environment and what procedures are being undertaken. At present, current UK guidance recommends fluid resistant surgical masks are worn at all times whilst delivering face to face healthcare. A particulate filter respiratory mask should be used if performing aerosol-generating procedures (AGPs) or where there is a risk of other respiratory infections related to certain respiratory diseases, for example, multidrug-resistant tuberculosis.

Where exposure to bodily fluids or non-intact skin is likely, gloves and aprons are recommended. Gloves reduce the risks of transmission of microorganisms to patients and staff but should be single-use and discarded after each care activity to prevent colonisation from one site to another. Nitrile gloves are now considered standard within the United Kingdom to prevent latex allergies. It is uncertain whether aprons provide any significant protection to prevent cross-transmission of HCAI and microorganisms.

If AGPs or extensive splashing of blood or body fluids are anticipated, fluid repellent gowns should be used.

Gowns are also useful to prevent transmission of multidrug-resistant organisms in high-risk areas – and have been shown to prevent the acquisition of VRE. Eye and face protection (with goggles or visors) are indicated for surgical teams, during AGPs, or for those at risk of occupational exposure to blood-borne infections.

Lastly, ensuring adequate training of healthcare professionals in donning and doffing of PPE is important to minimise the risk of self-contamination. Resources demonstrating the correct use of PPE can be found at ▶ https://www.cdc.gov/coronavirus/2019-ncov/hcp/using-ppe.html.

76.3 Sharps Disposal

The incidence of sharps injuries varies across clinical settings, and data suggests that 16% of occupational injuries in hospitals are attributable to sharps, 43% related to nurses and 24% medical staff. Sharps injuries are predominantly related to the administration of medication into intravascular lines. The average risk of transmission of blood-borne pathogens following a single exposure of a positive source patient are as follows [9]:

- Hepatitis B virus 33.3% (1 in 3)
- Hepatitis C virus 3.3% (1 in 30)
- Human immunodeficiency virus 0.31% (1 in 319)

Sharps should be (a) minimally handled, (b) not recapped and (c) immediately disposed of in an appropriate sharps container. The sharps container should be located in a safe location that avoids spillage and is out of reach of children. It should not be filled above the fill line and be closed and appropriately disposed of when the fill line is reached.

76.3.1 Surveillance

Surveillance of HCAI is the systematic, active ongoing observation of the occurrence and distribution of HCAI. The purpose of surveillance is to detect unusual levels or changes in incidence or prevalence of infection, to identify multidrug-resistant organisms and outbreaks and to apply and then assess control measures. Within renal settings, it is the routine collection of data on HCAI – particularly, catheter-related bloodstream infections (CRBSI), peritoneal dialysis infections and multidrug-resistant organisms. After analysis of this data, it must be fed back to renal clinicians and nursing staff. Surveillance, feedback and control programmes have been repeatedly demonstrated to reduce the incidence of infections [10].

Bloodstream infections can be captured using laboratory data with simple databases set up to determine the number of infections per week in each area. Particular resistant organisms should be highlighted and surveyed. Antibiotic surveillance should be considered – either using consumption or prescription data to determine the antibiotics being used and whether they are according to local policies.

The CDC and KDOQI recommend that CVC infection rates in each unit are fed back on a 6 monthly basis at a trust-wide and local level. Root cause analysis is a very useful tool for the investigation of bacteraemias and will often show where system failures have occurred. It is recommended that units monitor their PD infection rates and perform a root cause analysis on all episodes of peritonitis to determine if there was a preventable factor involved [11].

Screening of patients for BBV and CRE when they return from high-risk countries or institutions is an intrinsic part of avoiding local outbreaks; it is a lot easier to isolate a single inpatient until CREs excluded than to prevent spread when a patient is only isolated after a positive screen.

76.3.2 Important Microorganisms Including Multidrug-Resistant Organisms (MDRO)

For both HD and PD patients, *S. aureus* is a common and life-threatening pathogen. In HD patients, this organism can cause exit-site infections, CRBSI and fistula infections. *Staphylococcus aureus* bacteraemias (SAB) are associated with significant mortality (19% at 12 weeks in a retrospective review of 210 HD patients) and morbidity with approximately 30% of SAB leading to a deep-seated complication such as osteomyelitis, endocarditis and septic arthritis [12]. Each SAB was estimated to cost $24,034 in this study. Recommendations for SAB treatment state that these infections should be given at least 14 days of an intravenous (IV) beta-lactam antibiotic or a glycopeptide if the bacteria are methicillin-resistant. The combination of two or more antimicrobial agents is generally not recommended, except in severe methicillin-resistant *S. aureus* (MRSA) infections (e.g. endocarditis, prosthetic joint infections). Where there is a focus of infection identified, this should be drained or removed, including the prompt removal of vascular access devices. Prolonged treatment (4–6 weeks) may need to be administered if the focus of infection is unable to be removed, or evidence of endocarditis or osteomyelitis is present.

Staphylococcus aureus nasal carriage is much higher in the dialysis population than in the general public. Infection rates in carriers are 2–12 times higher than in non-carriers [13], and a substantial proportion are endogenous infections. Studies have shown both in PD and HD patients that in the short-term, intranasal mupirocin can eradicate carriage. A meta-analysis suggested an 80% risk reduction in *S. aureus* infections in dialysis patients associated with mupirocin use but only included two randomised trials, and the benefits were predominantly related to exit-site infections [14]. A comprehensive review states that for decolonisation to be effective in dialysis patients, repeated courses are needed to prevent recolonisation and reinfection [15]. This strategy would be likely to increase mupirocin resistance but few studies have looked at this in the long term. Previous guidelines recommended an approach of regular screening and decolonisation. Updated 2017 UK PD renal association guidelines support consideration of decolonisation protocols in conjunction with local microbiology protocol [16]; however, such an approach does not form part of the 2019 UK HD guidelines [17].

Population-based surveillance data collected in the United States showed that dialysis patients are 100 times more likely to acquire an invasive infection caused by methicillin-resistant *S. aureus* (MRSA) than individuals in the general population. In 2005, dialysis patients accounted for 15% of all invasive infections caused by MRSA reported to CDC. MRSA infections have fewer antibiotic treatment options and those available are less effective than the beta lactams. There is also evidence of reduced susceptibility to vancomycin amongst MRSA strains leading to poorer clinical outcomes. *Dialysis patients who are colonised with MRSA should be dialysed in isolation.*

Other organisms which commonly cause access-related infections include skin commensals such as *S. epidermidis*, which stick to intravascular devices, also enterococci, gram-negative organisms such as *Pseudomonas aeruginosa* and *Enterobacter* sp. Occasionally, *Candida* spp. can cause CRBSIs. Many of these infections will necessitate line removal as the most important element of source control.

The majority of peritoneal dialysis infections are caused by gram-positive organisms, particularly *S. aureus*, coagulase-negative staphylococci and *Corynebacterium* sp. Gram-negative organisms, particularly *P. aeruginosa*, make up about 30% of infections, with fungi causing about 3%. When a polymicrobial infection is diagnosed, clinicians must rule out intra-abdominal pathology, such as intestinal perforation.

Gram-negative infections are important infections in renal patients contributing to vascular access devices, peritoneal infections and urinary tract infections, particularly in the transplant population. Increasing antibiotic resistance is seen in these organisms both in the community and healthcare settings. Over 20% are routinely resistant to fluoroquinolones (e.g. ciprofloxacin), and 10% are resistant to third-generation cephalosporins usually signifying the carriage of resistance genes such as extended-spectrum beta-lactamases (ESBLs) or AmpC. Whilst carbapenems have been the empirical choice for treating resistant gram negatives, their increased use in response to the rising prevalence of ESBLs over the past decade has led to the emergence of carbapenem-resistant *Enterobacteriaceae* (CRE). Subsequent antimicrobial treatment options in CRE are sparse, limited to either polymyxins or tigecycline, to which further resistance is reported.

Diarrhoea in healthcare settings is predominantly a result of norovirus or *Clostridium difficile*. To prevent these infections, patients with diarrhoea should be isolated promptly within healthcare settings, and appropriate PPE worn. Prompt diagnosis requires stool samples to be processed for both pathogens. In addition, *hands should be washed with soap, and water as alcohol hand gel does not kill the spores of C. difficile or norovirus effectively; therefore, staff and relatives need access to appropriate handwashing.* The healthcare environment should be cleaned with an appropriate chlorine-based product.

The spores of *C. difficile* are transmissible and contaminate the environment, where they survive for long periods and once ingested the spores germinate in the gut; therefore, thorough cleaning of the environment is essential to prevent cross-transmission within hospitals [18]. Antibiotics disturb the normal gut flora, third-generation cephalosporins, clindamycin and ciprofloxacin are particularly implicated – allowing the proliferation of the *C. difficile* bacteria which produce two toxins – A and B. These toxins cause diarrhoea and colitis with clinical presentations ranging from mild diarrhoea to severe colitis with dehydration, pseudomembranous colitis, megacolon and perforation. There is substantial registry evidence that patients with CKD and ESRD are at greater risk of acquiring *C. difficile* and have mortality that is significantly worse at approximately twice that of the general population. Antimicrobial stewardship is therefore particularly essential in the prevention of *C. difficile* – for our patients; the narrowest spectrum agent should be used for the shortest duration possible. Local antibiotic policies should be followed and high-risk antibiotics usually restricted to certain conditions or with the approval of the local infection expert. Another risk factor for *C. difficile* infection has consistently been the prior use of proton pump inhibitors; however, there is no evidence that stopping these drugs once started reduces infections. Lactobacilli and other related probiotics have long been hypothesised to have a role in the prevention of *C. difficile* infection, but the evidence is still preclinical and no randomised controlled trial has demonstrated a statistically significant preventative effect to date. Initial treatment of *C. difficile* diarrhoea should be with metronidazole; severe or relapsing disease should be treated with oral vancomycin. Fidoxamicin is the first in its class of macrocylic antibiotics that has recently been licensed based on two randomised control trials. These demonstrated that fidoxamicin was non-inferior to vancomycin in the treatment of *C. difficile* infection but more importantly reduced the risk of recurrence (10% versus 30%) [19, 20]. However, before hospital staff are able to prescribe it, local decision-makers will need to review the evidence, the benefits and the cost increase, in comparison to the other available drugs.

76.4 Access-Related Infections

Infection constitutes the most challenging and life-threatening complication of vascular access and accounts for the excess mortality seen in patients using catheters when compared to fistulas.

There is a hierarchy of infection risk in decreasing order [21, 22] from

- Temporary catheters (27.1 events/100 patient months)
- Tunnelled cuffed catheters (4.2 events/100 patient months)
- Arteriovenous grafts (AVG) (0.9 events/100 patient months)
- Arteriovenous fistula (AVF) (0.5 months/100 patient months)

Among non-tunnelled lines, femoral catheters have the highest infection rates (7.6 episodes/1000 catheter days) compared with internal jugular (5.6 episodes/1000 catheter days) and subclavian catheters (2.7 episodes/1000 catheter days). For long-term catheters, particularly those that are cuffed and/or surgically planted, the hub is a major source of colonisation.

As the infection rates in CVCs are 4–5 times higher than AVF, there is a global drive to increase the percentage of patients using AVF. The UK Renal Association guidelines recommend that 65% of all incident haemodialysis patients should commence dialysis on an AVF and 85% of all prevalent patients should receive dialysis via a functioning AVF.

76.4.1 Prevention of CVC Infections

It is imperative that all measures are taken to drive down the infection risk from vascular access. Evidence-based policies must be firmly embedded throughout the renal unit and describe the actions from when the catheter is first inserted to its ongoing day-to-day care, by both HCW and patients. Evidence-based reviews have established that CVC infections are reduced when the insertion and continuous care of CVC are performed by competent experienced HCW [23]. These points are summarized in Table 76.1.

Table 76.1 Prevention of line infections

Insertion	Use a tunnelled catheter
	Avoid the femoral site when possible
	Clean the skin with >0.5% chlorhexidine preparation with alcohol
	Use maximum barrier sterile precautions (sterile gloves, gowns, and full body drape)
Continuing care	Patient education – advise patient not to touch line or get it wet
	Consider using a chlorhexidine impregnated dressing at the exit site during the first 3–6 months
	When accessing the line, clean the hubs with >0.5% chlorhexidine solution
	Use an antimicrobial locking solution and monitor for side effects
	Consider using an antimicrobial preparation at the exit site, particularly in high risk patients (check the preparation will not affect the integrity of the catheter)
	Monitor the exit site for infection and ensure policies are in place for prompt antibiotic treatment

The use of antibiotic prophylaxis is not currently recommended in the CDC or KDOQI guidelines, and a recent retrospective study confirmed that the infection rate directly following the procedure is so low as to render antibiotic prophylaxis unnecessarily.

No recommendation on coated long-term dialysis catheters can be made at present. Short-term lines coated with chlorhexidine and silver can reduce catheter colonisation and infections in intensive care and haemotology patients, but there is limited evidence in renal patients. A trial of minocycline and rifampicin coated catheters in patients with acute renal failure showed a decrease in infections (0/66 versus 7/64 in those without an impregnated line) with lines in situ for a mean duration of 8 days in each group [24].

Evidence-based guidelines state that CVC should be inserted using maximum sterile barrier precautions (sterile gloves, gowns, and full-body drapes). The skin should be cleaned with >0.5% chlorhexidine preparation with alcohol (if allergic to chlorhexidine then less effective agents such as poviodine/alcohol or 70% alcohol may be used) and allowed to dry [23]. The environment should be suitable from a ventilation and cleanliness perspective for sterile procedures. A sterile, transparent semi-permeable dressing should be used to cover the catheter site as this allows clear visibility of the site [23]. However, if there is bleeding or oozing, a gauze dressing should be used until this resolves.

All the different elements of care required for the scrupulous management of CVC's after insertion are brought together in the UK Saving Lives High Impact Intervention audits. Anybody who is going to have contact with the CVC or vascular access site must perform adequate hand hygiene and then put on clean (for aseptic non-touch technique) or sterile gloves. The CDC, KDOQI and UK guidelines recommend the use of chlorhexidine-based preparations for skin antisepsis and hub cleaning prior to access with reduced rates of catheter colonisation and CRBSIs compared to other agents [25]. Catheter dressings are generally changed once a week but should be changed immediately if they are wet, soiled or loose.

Currently, chlorhexidine-impregnated dressings are not recommended for routine use by KDOQI or the Renal Association guidelines [14, 26]. Updated CDC guidelines only recommend the use of chlorhexidine impregnated sponge in adult patients with temporary short-term catheters [27].

The current CDC guidelines recommend the use of povidone-iodine antiseptic ointment or bacitracin/gramicidin/polymyxin B ointment at the exit site at end of each dialysis session if the ointment does not interact with the catheter material as per manufacturers recommendations [23]. Topical povidone-iodine ointment applied to non-tunnelled catheter exit sites has been shown to decrease exit-site infections and BSIs. Topical mupirocin ointment was effective in preventing SA exit-site infections and BSIs [28]. A double-blind randomized clinical trial involving 169 patients with cuffed catheters assessed an antibiotic ointment containing polymyxin B, bacitracin and gramicidin and showed a decrease in infections from 34% to 12% ($p = 0.0007$), reduction in bacteraemias from 2.48 per 1000 catheter days to 0.63 ($p = 0.0004$), as well as a significant survival advantage for patients in the intervention group (3 deaths compared to 13 in 6 months) [29].

Inspection of the exit site should be documented at each dialysis session. A scoring system (for example, the MR VICTOR tool) can be extremely useful. This stands for Multiracial Visual Inspection Catheter Tool Observation Record and was developed by Waterhouse et al. at the Central Manchester University Hospitals NHS Foundation Trust. It gives an objective score, which can then be used to guide further management and prompt antibiotic treatment if necessary.

Multiple studies have evaluated the use of antimicrobial catheter lock solutions to prevent BSIs in haemodialysis patients. Agents used in these locks include antibiotics, such as gentamicin (with and without citrate), cefotaxime, cefazolin (with gentamicin) and vancomycin (with gentamicin), and non-antibiotic antimicrobial agents, such as citrate with and without taurolidine. A marked reduction in CRBSI's is associated with the use of antimicrobial lock solutions (range: 51–99%) [30]. However, many of the studies performed have been small and heterogeneous not only in the chosen lock intervention but also by what other infection prevention measures were in place during the study. Currently, CDC recommends against the routine use of antimicrobial lock solutions for the prevention of CRBSIs but recommends them for patients with multiple episodes of line sepsis despite optimal adherence to full aseptic technique [23]. Some centres have described resistance developing to gentamicin after long-term use [28], and one centre discontinued their use of gentamicin locks after a number of patients presented with serious complications of infections with gentamicin resistant organisms. One solution would be to use a non-antibiotic antimicrobial lock (e.g. citrate), and a meta-analysis found about a 50% decrease in CRBSIs with such locks [30]. The Renal Association guidelines recommend the use of a preventative catheter lock but comment that is it still unclear which is the optimal solution [14].

76.4.1.1 Peritoneal Dialysis (PD)

Technical failure remains a significant problem with PD, and PD-related infection commonly contributes to this. The most common routes of infection involve the catheter as a portal of entry and comprise of intraluminal and periluminal entry. Intraluminal spread of organisms can occur after touch contamination at the time of catheter connection. Periluminal infection occurs when there is exit-site infection, which can then spread along the tunnel. Occasionally, infections are caused by the transmigration of organisms across the intestinal wall.

76.4.1.2 Insertion of PD Catheter

The use of prophylactic antibiotics has been shown to be beneficial in randomised controlled trials, and although the optimal regime is still not completely clear, the ISPD guidelines recommend a single dose of vancomycin before skin incision [31–32], and the European Best Practice guidelines recommend a dose of either vancomycin or a first-generation cephalosporin [33].

The 2019 ISPD guidelines state that no particular catheter type has been proven to be the best [34]. A Cochrane review did not find any advantage for straight versus coiled catheters, double-cuffed versus single cuffed and medical versus lateral incision [35]. Since this review, a large retrospective study found there was a trend towards a lower rate of exit-site infections when a double-cuffed catheter was used, as compared to the single-cuffed catheter. However, most of the reduction was from *S. aureus* infections and was greater before the introduction of changes to exit-site care and the use of topical antibiotics [36].

76.4.1.3 Connection Methods

The initial connection method involved conventional spike connection systems; however, these have been shown in several studies to increase peritonitis rates [31]. A double-bag system with the flush before fill technique should be used to reduce the risk of contamination.

76.4.1.4 Exit-Site Preparations

It is a more accepted practice amongst PD patients to routinely use antimicrobial ointment at the exit site. A number of studies have proven a benefit in reducing catheter site infections and peritonitis caused by gram-positive organisms by placing mupirocin on the exit site [31]. Bernadini et al. compared mupirocin and gentamicin and found that both agents decreased *Staphylococcus* infections, but as expected, gentamicin decreased gram-negative catheter infections and peritonitis [37]. Increasing mupirocin resistance has been of concern in some units and associated with treatment failure [31]. However, it is not reported to be a significant problem despite routine use in others.

76.4.1.5 Invasive Procedures

PD patients undergoing colonoscopy are at risk of developing enteric peritonitis, and so appropriate IV antibiotics (for example, ampicillin, gentamicin and metronidazole) should be given prior to the procedure [31]. The abdomen should be emptied of fluid prior to procedures.

76.4.1.6 Prevention of Fungal Peritonitis

The majority of cases of fungal peritonitis are preceded by a course of antibiotics. The mortality of fungal peritonitis is high and requires prompt catheter removal. Randomised trials have shown a benefit when antifungals are used as prophylactic agents for PD patients on antibiotics, both with oral nystatin and fluconazole [31]. Further observational studies have found that in units where there is a high background rate of fungal peritonitis, prophylaxis was useful but in units with low background rates, it was not. Current ISPD guidelines support the use of antifungal prophylaxis during antibiotic therapy for peritonitis [38].

76.4.1.7 Preventing Fistula and Graft Infections

As discussed above, the best option for permanent access for a dialysis patient is a native AVF. From an infection point of view, native fistulae have lower infection rates than grafts. A large Canadian prospective cohort study found a 19.7% probability of polytetrafluroethylene (PTFE) graft infections compared with 4.5% for autogenous AV fistula [39]. Higher rates of infection in graft versus fistulae have been also seen in a number of observational studies, and many guidelines (K/DOQI, Canadian Society for Nephrology and European Best practice guidelines for Haemodialysis) recommend native AV fistulas as the best option, then a graft and a tunnelled line as a last resort.

There is evidence that as with lines, the lower extremities should be avoided as infection rates are higher. An American centre reported a high rate of graft loss and infection (27%) in 30 patients over a 7-year study period [40]. Another smaller study reported a higher infection rate in polyurethane grafts versus PTFE grafts, particularly, when they are placed in the thigh. There is now some controversy as to whether a femoral graft or a long-term tunnelled line is the best option for patients who have exhausted all other possibilities.

There is some evidence that preoperative antibiotics for graft access procedures decrease early infection rates. A randomized trial, using 750 mg vancomycin or no antibiotics, in just over 500 patients showed a sixfold decrease in those who received antibiotics [41]. In our centre, antibiotics are given pre graft insertion but not for a native AVF formation.

For native AVF, there is a growing body of evidence that the needling technique can influence infection rates. Standard recognised techniques include area puncture, rope ladder cannulation and the buttonhole (BH) technique. In the last of these, a sharp needle is used to create a tract along the same path each time, until the tract can be cannulated with a blunt needle. However, some studies have reported an increase in infections with this technique. In 2010, a report by van Loon et al. found more infections in patients using the BH technique, compared to those using rope ladder [42]. It is important for a single person to create the tract, thus causing less trauma and haematoma formation. The need for an excellent aseptic technique when removing the scab of the tract should not be underestimated. Another study reported an increase in septic events in those on extended hours home HD using the BH technique. Applying topical mupirocin to the BH site at the end of each dialysis session has been to lower the increased risk of SAB [43].

76.5 Prevention of Other Important Healthcare-Associated Infection

Renal patients are at risk of other HCAI. Between 20% and 30% of catheterized patients develop bacteriuria, 2–6% develop symptoms of a UTI. The risk of infection will be affected by the method and duration of catheterisation, the quality of catheter care and host susceptibility. The need for insertion of and care of the catheter must be documented and regularly reviewed. The catheter must be removed when no longer needed. ◘ Table 76.2 outlines tips to prevent infections. ◘ Table 76.3 outlines the management of common infections in renal patients.

Table 76.2 Tips and tricks in preventing infection in renal patients (excluding infections that predominantly occur in the immediate post-transplant period)

Infection associated risk	Method of prevention	Approach
All infections	Hand hygiene, cleaning and decontamination, safe sharps disposal	Policies, guidelines, education, training competency assessment Regular audit and feedback
Clostridium difficile	Antimicrobial stewardship Isolation of symptomatic patients Hand hygiene using soap and water Environmental cleaning with chlorine-based product	Policies, guidelines, education Ward based antimicrobial rounds Regular audit and feedback
Dialysis vascular access device	Device insertion and care protocols Patient education	Staff education, competency assessment and audits of practice
Urinary catheters	Device insertion and care protocols, including regular review of the need for catheter	Staff education, competency assessment and audits of practice
Influenza	Vaccination Post exposure prophylaxis	Annual vaccine recommended
Pneumococcal disease	Vaccination	23 serotype PPV Vaccine every 5 years recommended
VZV	Screening and active vaccination Passive vaccination	Consider pre-immunosuppression active vaccine Post exposure VZIg
Hepatitis B	Screening and vaccination	If negative, vaccinate prior to starting haemodialysis If positive, pretreatment or early antiviral treatment, refer to a specialist Maintain adequate infection control
TB	Screening and treatment	Interferon gamma releasing assay (IGRA) prior to immunosuppressants Treatment if IGRA positive
Tropical diseases	Appropriate vaccination, prophylaxis and education	Refer to travel clinic prior to travel abroad

Table 76.3 Common infection syndromes in renal patients and their empiric management

Infection type	Management
Vascular access device	Send blood cultures, line site swab Remove VAD if sepsis not responding to fluid and antibiotics Send catheter tip for culture Start empiric antimicrobials, covering MRSA if known MRSA positive or unit MRSA prevalence >10%
Staphylococcus aureus bacteraemia	Needs IV antibiotics (2 weeks minimum) Use beta-lactam antibiotics for MSSA wherever possible Remove infected source, e.g. line, graft Monitor for evidence of spread to other organs, e.g. heart, bone, joint Length of treatment decided by time for fever to defervesce, repeat blood cultures being negative and absence of focus of spread
Lower respiratory tract	Obtain sputum for culture, blood cultures if febrile Nasopharyngeal swab for respiratory viruses – isolate in flu season until result available Consider acute and convalescent serology – *Mycoplasma* *Consider legionella urinary antigen testing* Start empiric therapy according to local guidelines – for example, amoxicillin and clarithromycin Empiric oseltamivir in flu season if not vaccinated Further investigations if not improving at day 3–4 (e.g. bronchoscopy, induced sputum for tuberculosis, and other agents if post-transplant)

(continued)

Table 76.3 (continued)

Infection type	Management
Skin and Soft Tissue	MRSA screen Isolate suspected streptococcal infection for initial 24 hours of treatment (rapidly progressive, ascending lymphangitis) Obtain tissue samples for culture if exposed ulcer/bone Aspirate joint prior to antibiotics Empiric treatment according to local guidelines Tailor treatment with culture results Consider X-ray of affected limb +/– MRI scan for deep collections/osteomyelitis – especially if diabetic
Urinary T	Send urine culture prior to therapy Review previous cultures if available to tailor treatment (especially where multidrug- resistant organisms may be present) Initial treatment according to local empiric guidelines
Diarrhoea	Isolate patient Send stool samples prompt for GI pathogens (*Salmonella, Shigella, E. coli* 0157*, Campylobacter*), *C. difficile* and Norovirus testing Rehydrate the patient and monitor renal function X-ray abdomen and consider CT abdomen if toxic megacolon suspected Consider empirical treatment of *C. difficile* infection if severe disease
Infective Eocarditis	3 × Blood cultures, consider HACEK[a] organisms where necessary CVC removal if infected MRSA screen Empiric therapy for *S. aureus(*including MRSA if known positive or high MRSA prevalence >10% on unit) and streptococci Await blood culture results for final therapy Echocardiogram – determine effect and suitability for emergency valve replacement Specialist infection and cardiology input
Disseminated infections, e.g. TB, viruses, fungi, tropical	Discussion with specialist infection unit

[a]Haemophilus (Haemophilus parainfluenzae, Haemophilus aphrophilus, Haemophilus paraphrophilus), Actinobacillus (Actinobacillus actinomycetemcomitans, Aggregatibacter aphrophilus), Cardiobacterium hominis, Eikenella corrodens, Kingella kingae

76.6 Preventing the Spread of Blood-Borne Viruses (BBV)

In response to a viral hepatitis outbreak in renal units in the United Kingdom in the 1960s, the Rosenheim report set out guidelines for the prevention and control of infection in dialysis units, which are just as relevant today [44]. The recently updated 2019 UK renal association guidelines outline optimal management for control of hepatitis B and C and HIV within dialysis units [45] and should be consulted alongside the 2018 KDIGO guidelines for Hepatitis C [46].

Incidence of HBV and HCV diagnosed in patients attending dialysis units over the last three decades has dramatically reduced. The introduction of universal infection control precautions, with the basic premise that all patients could be infectious, has played a major role in this. Such infection control procedures mandate precautions that effectively prevent the transfer of blood or bloodstained fluid between patients. Care with parenteral medicines is also critical, meaning medicine vials should be discarded after single use and multi-use vials avoided.

Dialysis machines must always be decontaminated between patients according to the manufacturer's instructions and local protocol. Patients with acute infections are more infectious than those with chronic disease as the viral loads tend to be higher, so precautions must be taken to monitor those at the highest risk of acquiring BBV infections.

Current guidelines recommend that patients infected with hepatitis B (or those at high risk of new HBV infection) should be dialysed on a separate machine. This machine must be thoroughly decontaminated before it can be used in the 'general pool' again. Patients who are positive for HBV should be dialysed in a segregated area away from the main dialysis unit, with dedicated separate staff where possible. In contrast, the use of dedicated dialysis machines for HIV- and HCV-positive patients is not required, provided excellent universal infection control precautions between patients are maintained. Segregation of HIV-positive patients should be based on a local risk assessment.

External transducer protectors on the blood circuit pressure monitoring lines should be inspected at the end of each dialysis session to ensure no breach. Machines must be correctly disinfected in between patients. This will including cleaning of the external surfaces with low-level disinfectant, unless there has been obvious blood spillage when a stronger disinfecting agent such as hypochlorite solution (at least 500 p.p.m) should be used, as long as this is not detrimental to the machine [46]. If there is a concern that there has been leakage into the internal fluid pathways, the machine must be taken out of service until it can be dismantled and disinfected.

Some patients may undergo treatment with antiviral drugs and may clear their BBV infection in the case of both HCV and HBV, but not HIV. The local virology specialist should be consulted about such patients to see what testing is required and when they can be managed as 'non-infectious'.

Prior to a patient starting dialysis, it is also recommended that their BBV status is known for HBC, HCV, HIV and human T Cell lymphotrophic virus (HTLV). Patients requiring dialysis prior to the results of their HBsAg test should be dialysed in a segregated area until their result is known to be negative. Those who are HBV surface antigen negative and non-immune should be given a course of vaccination and the surface antibody level checked. Responders are those who have a level of >100 mIU/ml. Non-responders to the vaccine should be monitored thrice monthly for HBsAg, and booster doses are given accordingly, and responders 6 monthly. Occult HBV infection can occur. This is the presence of HBV DNA by PCR in the absence of detectable HBSag, and so, PCR testing can be used to enhance surveillance and as a measure of 'infectivity'.

Patients should be monitored thrice monthly for HCV. In high-risk patients (e.g. immunosuppressed patients, those who have returned from a high-risk country, have had a renal transplant, those with high-risk behaviour, e.g. intravenous drug abuse), the HCV RNA should be checked, as well as antibodies to HCV, to detect early infection. Only those with risk factors for HIV (such as intravenous drug abuse) should be monitored for HIV. Patients with abnormal serum aminotransferase levels should have HBsAg and HCV RNA testing [46].

When patients return from dialysing abroad, they need to have a risk assessment for potential exposure to BBV whilst on holiday. If they have returned from a high-risk country, they need to be dialysed in a separate area for a period of enhanced surveillance (this is also a good time to screen for CRE). A suitable surveillance scheme of testing and a list of high-risk countries can be found in the UK Department of Health good practice document [47]. Patients should be screened for HBV and HCV on return, and the test for HCV should be a sensitive combined HCV Ab/Ag or HCV RNA test. Patients only need to be tested for HIV if the risk assessment merits testing. During this time, patients' status on the transplant list may need to be reviewed.

If a new patient is identified as being infected with HBV or HCV, there needs to be a period of enhanced surveillance of all non-immune patients who had shared a dialysis session with the infected patients since their last negative test. Such programmes should be discussed with the local infection control and virology specialist.

All staff members in contact with patients' blood and bloodstained fluid on the dialysis units should be vaccinated against HBV. Immunisation is also recommended for carers of patients on haemodialysis.

76.6.1 Vaccine Preventable Diseases (Including Travel Health)

Reduced response rates to vaccinations have been reported in individuals with CKD and postrenal transplant. Therefore, where possible, individuals should be vaccinated as early as possible in their treatment of CKD, before renal replacement therapy and transplantation. However, even though the response rates can be lower than healthy adults, some vaccines (particularly Influenza) should still be administered every year at all stages as the protection provided by vaccination is essential for the immunocompromised. Guidelines will undoubtedly emerge once a vaccine is available for SARS-CoV-2 (Covid-19), and it seems likely that patients with ESRD would be offered vaccination.

Live vaccines are contraindicated in those who are pregnant or immunosuppressed. The UK Department of Health Green book defines 'high-dose' steroids as ≥40 mg prednisolone daily use for more than 1 week compared to CDC guidelines of prednisolone 20 mg or more daily for >14 days. It is generally accepted that this state of immunosuppression remains for at least 1 month in corticosteroids use.

The recommended vaccinations for patients with chronic disease and immunosuppression are outlined in ◘ Table 76.2. The important characteristics of some vaccines are considered here.

The 23 serotype polysaccharide pneumococcal vaccine (PPV) is an inactivated polysaccharide vaccine which covers 23 serotypes of *Pneumococcus*, accounting for 88% of all pneumococcal infections [48]. It is recommended for patients with chronic disease every 5 years.

Influenza vaccines are inactivated vaccines that are required annually as the composition of these vaccines changes yearly based on expert group consensus of circulating strains. Household contacts and carers should also be vaccinated to ensure adequate protection especially in those who show poor seroconversion [49]. The nasal spray flu vaccine is an attenuated vaccine and not suitable for immunocompromised renal patients.

Varicella zoster vaccine is a live attenuated vaccine that has been contraindicated for use in patients who are immunosuppressed but may be given to those with autoimmune diseases prior to immunosupressants [49]. Varicella zoster vaccine in those with auto-immune disease has been shown to reduce infection risk by 51% and postherpetic neuralgia by 66% three years post-vaccination. Varicella zoster immunoglobulin (VZIG) should be considered in immunosuppressed patients who are exposed to cases of zoster infection, both chickenpox and shingles, from 48 h prior to rash developing until crusting of vesicles. VZIG use does not preclude infection, and therefore, if these patients develop early signs of infection, they should be given empirical antivirals. Immunoglobulin use alters the normal immune response to vaccines, and therefore, use of vaccines should be delayed until 3 months after Ig administration [45]. Our practise is not to suspend patients on the waiting list post-VZV vaccination, but to give acyclovir if transplanted within 2 weeks of vaccination.

76.6.1.1 Tuberculosis

Up to 10% of patients with latent TB infection (LTBI) develop reactivation of the disease. The use of immunomodulatory drugs in rheumatological or autoimmune diseases allow reactivation of LTBI to occur, through dysregulation of the granulomatous process.

Prior to starting immunosuppressive therapy, individuals should be assessed for active and latent TB. An accurate history of previous TB exposure, diagnosis or treatment should be taken and a clinical examination performed to look for signs of active TB, particularly, lymphadenopathy. A chest X-ray should be performed to determine whether there are radiological appearances of active or old TB. If there are signs of active TB, referral to a TB specialist physician is recommended.

For those with no TB history and no active TB on chest radiograph, further tests should be performed. The current UK guidelines recommend the use of blood interferon gamma release assays (IGRA) to diagnose LTBI in immunocompromised patients, as they are appear to be more sensitive in this population [50]. IGRAs are in vitro blood tests using antigens that detect a T cell response to TB antigens by releasing measured interferon-gamma.

Positive IGRA tests require prompt treatment for LTBI in those due to undergo immunosuppressive treatment if the risk of treatment (mainly hepatotoxicity) is less than the risk of reactivation. Those deemed at high risk of hepatotoxicity should be monitored 3–4 monthly and warned of TB symptoms. Standard LTBI therapy is 3 months of combination rifampicin and isoniazid or alternatively 6 months of isoniazid monotherapy [50].

Vaccination against TB uses a live attenuated vaccine derived from *Mycobacterium bovis* that confers up to 70–80% protection depending on individual response [50]. It is generally not recommended over the age of 16 years, and as it is, a live vaccine is also contraindicated in individuals on immunosuppressive therapy.

76.7 Persistent Bacterial Infections

A not infrequent, but under-recognised, clinical scenario in modern medicine is that of persistent bacterial infection. This is covered here in a chapter on infection control because inadequately treated, and hence, persistent infections predispose to MDR organisms and *c.difficile.*

Classically, this presents in patients who present with evidence of sepsis the source of which may or may not be obvious but responds, initially, to antibiotics. Typically, patients then represent 1–3 weeks following cessation of the antibiotics. The time to recurrence may depend on several factors but a virulent organism is likely to represent sooner than a more indolent organism. The underlying problem is a deep-seated infection, which has received an inadequate course of antibiotics and/or the cause of the infection (foreign body, inadequate drainage) has not been resolved. Renal patients are particularly prone to this in part because of the high prevalence of intravenous lines, comorbidity and urinary tract abnormalities predisposing to 'complicated UTIs'.

Risk factors for persistent infection include:

1. Presence of a foreign body (cardiac valve, pacing equipment, prosthesis, any metal work (embolization coils, orthopaedic rods, dialysis access, stents, implants, stones)
2. Poor vascular perfusion (peripheral vascular disease with osteomyelitis, infected calcified or abnormal heart valves, infected atrial or pulmonary thrombi)
3. Poor drainage (inadequate urinary tract drainage, inadequate biliary tract drainage)
4. *Inadequate penetration of antibiotics (to cysts or abscess)*
5. *Poor compliance*

Clues to persistent infection:

1. Recurrent symptoms or admission within days to four weeks following completion of antibiotics
2. Recurrent culture of the same organism
3. The presence of a multiresistant organism in the setting of recent antibiotics
4. Persistent pyuria
5. Chronically raised CRP, normocytic anaemia or polyclonal gammopathy

Identification of persistent infection is not only important to make the correct diagnosis and avoid a recurrence and readmission but also because it is very easy to generate multiresistant organisms without sorting the underlying problem. This is particularly common in the setting of 'complicated UTIs' and requires an astute assessment of the problem as well as good antimicrobial stewardship by nephrologists.

76.8 Patient Education

Patients and their carers should receive education about hand hygiene and when to use different types of hand decontamination and their role.

Patients should be educated on the ability to challenge their HCW – in a recent study, only 16% of patients (independent of MRSA status) tried to ask medical personnel to wash hands during their last stay in the hospital. However, when doctors and nurses invite patients to challenge, it increases those challenging 2.5-fold.

Patients should be given written and verbal information about care of all devices (CVC, PD etc) when it is being inserted. When patients regularly attend for dialysis with wet or soiled dressings, further education is a key part of preventing exit-site infections and CRBSIs.

PD patients need to fully understand how to use an aseptic technique for when they connect up their dialysis fluid. Published studies have demonstrated how the training programme can influence rates of exit-site infections and peritonitis [31].

76.8.1 Embedding Infection Control Excellence in the Renal Department

Ignaz Semmelweis (1818–1865) was a Hungarian physician who discovered that the rate of puerperal sepsis (and death) could be dramatically reduced by ensuring effective handwashing. Sadly, his colleagues and peers were offended by the implication that they might be responsible for the high rate of death, mocked him and rejected his theory of contamination and the cure, handwashing. Semmelweis, ultimately had a nervous breakdown and died in a lunatic asylum. The reason for mentioning this is that the greatest obstacle to achieving really good infection control is always senior staff. To achieve anything approaching zero avoidable nosocomial infections, the heads of departments have to invest seriously in the ethos of infection control. Senior doctors who flout sensible protocols are the biggest and most consistent threat to an infection avoidance culture. ◘ Figure 76.4 illustrates a banner made by renal staff to remind both patients and medical staff of the need for infection control.

Regular audits of hospital-acquired infections, handwashing, timely removal of unnecessary lines and catheters all help guide performance. Getting patient representation on the audit committee and comparing local with regional and national infection rates is a good way to focus the mind. Root-cause-analysis (RCA) of any hospital-acquired MRSA septicaemia, *C. difficile*, and generation or spread of ESBL/CREs are helpful and educational reviews to accumulate and act on.

Microbiology/nephrology MDTMs can be an effective way of overseeing antibiotic stewardship as well as support for the management of complex infections.

76.9 An Approach to Prevention of Covid-19 Infection

Both kidney transplant recipients and patients who are on immunosuppressive medication for their underlying renal disease are at increased risk of a severe clinical course of Covid-19 infection.

In the United Kingdom, around 10% of haemodialysis patients have had confirmed Covid-19 infection, with a mortality of 25% [51]. It is clear that dialysis units are prone to outbreaks both among patients and staff working in dialysis units [52].

Communication and education for both patients and staff are paramount; Covid-19 is likely to be even more stressful for patients than staff, and the clearer the communication and support for patients, the better. Different formats and languages should be provided to educate patients about the symptoms of Covid-19 infection, hand hygiene, social distancing, PPE and new renal unit protocols.

76.9.1 The Haemodialysis Unit

Considerations to prevent the spread of infection in the haemodialysis unit are as follows:

76.9.1.1 Social Distancing

All efforts should be made to avoid contact where possible; i.e. eradicate time spent in communal waiting areas, increase the space between dialysis stations, use 'one way' systems and separate entrances/exits for Covid-19-positive patients.

76.9.1.2 Transport

Many patients require transport to and from the dialysis unit; this is a potential source of exposure. Working together with patients and transport providers should reduce transmission of infection by using private transport where possible, isolating those with suspected infection and cohorting confirmed Covid-19 cases. If hospital or public transport is used, this must be with social distancing; wearing a facemask is also recommended.

NHS
Royal Free London
NHS Foundation Trust
Infection control is a priority, gel hands on entering and leaving the ward
world class expertise local care

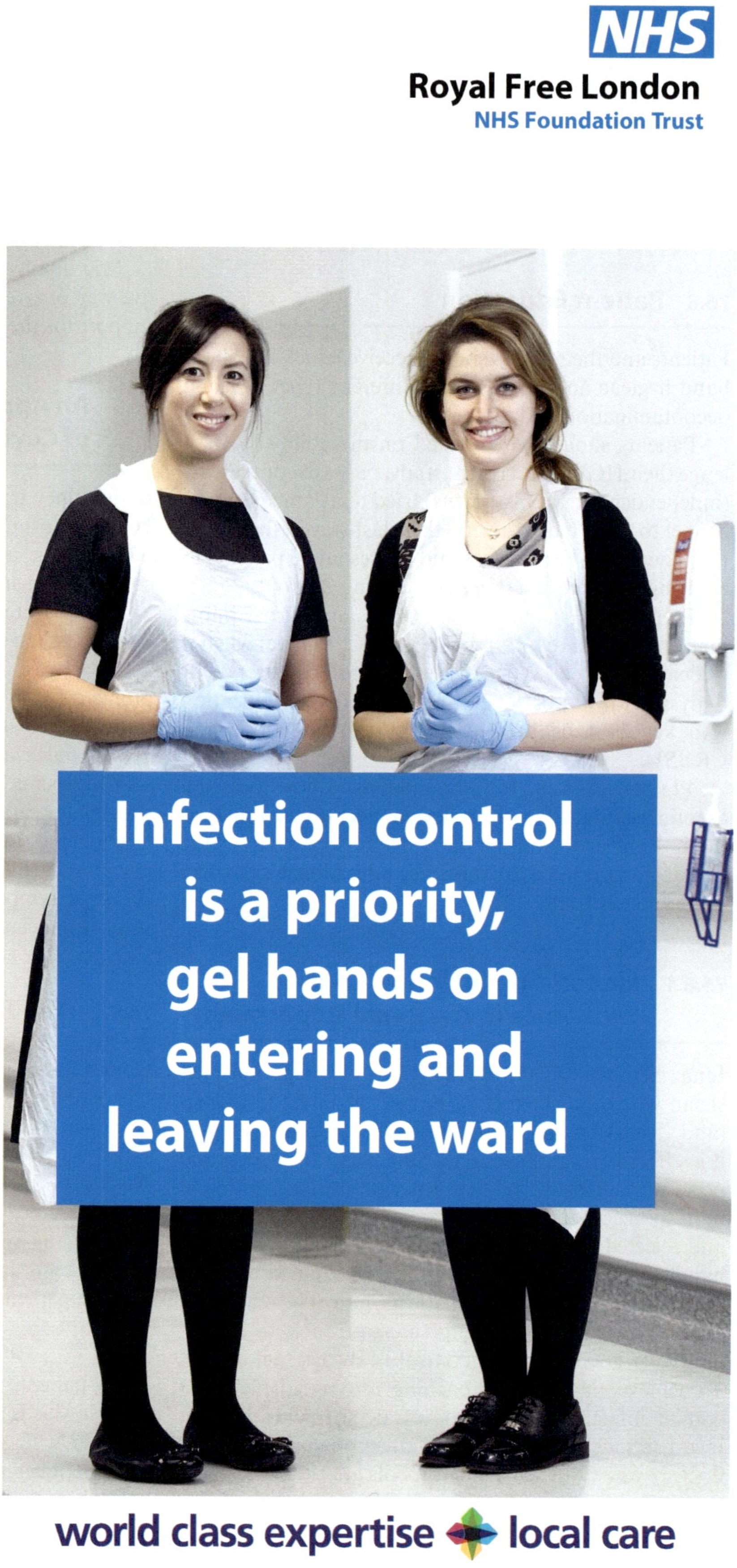

Fig. 76.4 Example of a banner at ward entrance

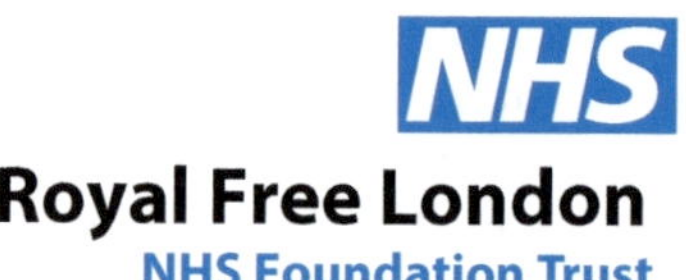

■ **Fig. 76.4** (continued)

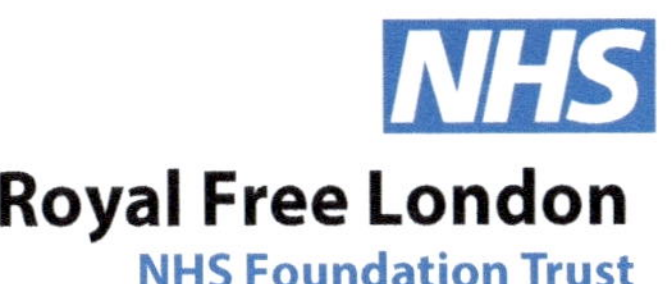

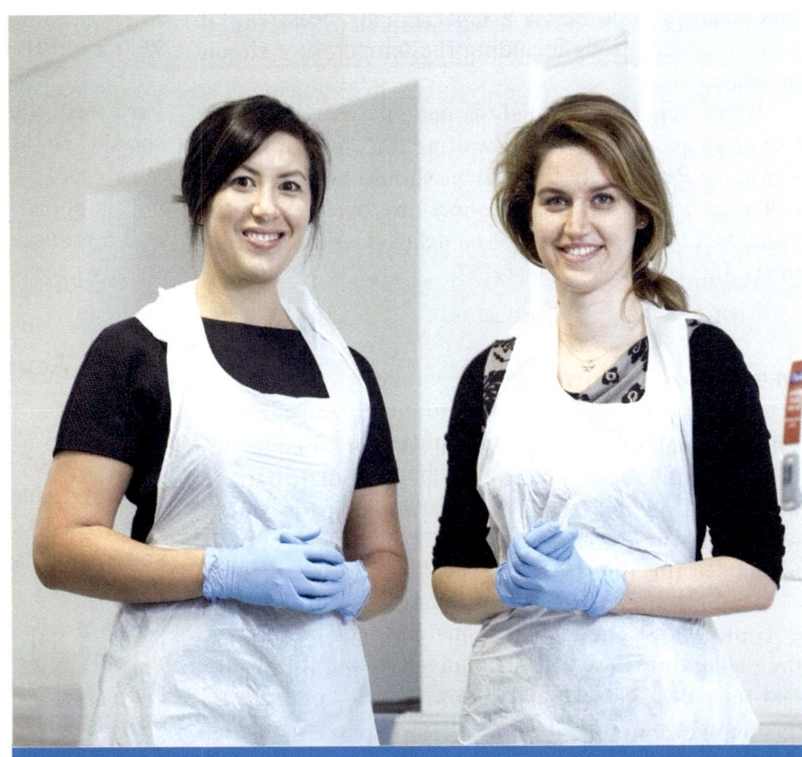

Infection control is a priority, gel hands on entering and leaving the ward

world class expertise local care

76.9.1.3 Triage

Patients should be asked to contact the unit in advance of their dialysis session if they have symptoms or have had contact with a confirmed or suspected case of Covid-19. An initial telephone assessment should be completed to identify if the patient is so unwell as to require emergency medical review. If well enough to attend dialysis, this ideally should be via a separate entrance/area. On arrival, observations including the temperature should be recorded.

Rapid screening of dialysis patients with suspected Covid-19 is vital. Whilst awaiting the results of the Covid-19 PCR swab, the patient should be dialysed in isolation or in a suspected cohort or Covid-19-positive patients. Dialysis should not be delayed whilst awaiting the results of screening tests [52].

76.9.2 Cohorting

The following should be provided: an area for cohorting proven positive cases, an area in which to isolate patients whilst awaiting test results or quarantining post-contact with a known positive case and facilities to protect other patients at this time [53].

Methods for cohorting include the following: using a separate dialysis unit for patients with Covid-19 infection, dialysing COVID-19-positive patients on a separate shift – ideally the final shift of the day to allow for thorough decontamination. Isolation rooms can be used if sufficiently available or temporary screens to separate the cohorts [53, 54].

76.9.2.1 Testing and Surveillance

Regular surveillance swab testing of dialysis patients is advised; with increased frequency depending on local infection levels.

Contact tracing on the dialysis unit should include patients dialysed on the same shift, those who shared transport or a waiting room for >15 min. These patients should be isolated for 14 days and tested on days 0, 7 and 14 [53].

76.9.2.2 Staffing and PPE

It is now recommended that all patients and staff wear surgical masks throughout dialysis. Having observed the high rates of staff infection, enhanced PPE (eye/face protection, FFP2/FFP3 mask, a long-sleeved fluid-repellent surgical gown and gloves) should be worn by staff caring for patients with confirmed or suspected Covid-19 infection. An FFP3 mask should always be worn during an aerosol-generating procedure, e.g. cardiopulmonary resuscitation [53].

Standard PPE (eye/face protection, fluid-resistant surgical mask, plastic apron and gloves) should be used for all other patient care [53].

Careful cleaning of the dialysis station and surrounding area with appropriate cleaning products should be completed after the patient has left the station.

76.9.3 Peritoneal Dialysis

Peritoneal dialysis patients can remain at home so should be at less risk than haemodialysis patients. Where possible, home therapies should be encouraged and supported with a focus on increased telemedicine and a reduction in home visits to only those which are strictly necessary [54].

76.9.4 Acute Transplantation

Although most transplant programs were suspended at the height of the pandemic, protocols have been developed to enable the resumption of kidney transplantation:

Covid-19 secure areas must be provided for recipient and donor assessment, transplantation and follow-up. Live donors and recipients must be tested in advance and asked to self-isolate between testing and admission to hospital. Deceased donors should be tested and recipients receive rapid (<1 h) COVID-19 testing prior to transplantation.

Additionally, patients should be counselled on an individual basis regarding the risks and benefits of proceeding with transplantation accounting for the local current Covid-19 prevalence. The induction and maintenance immunosuppression should also be reviewed on an individual basis.

Waiting list patients should be suspended if they have tested positive for Covid-19 until they are swab negative and fully recovered.

76.9.5 Outpatient Services Including Transplant Follow-Up

Aiming to reduce face-to-face consultations should reduce the risk of transmission to patients using measures including phone and video consultation, local phlebotomy services and electronic prescriptions/delivery services will contribute to decreased exposure for vulnerable patients.

When in-person appointments are required, the social distancing and transport procedures as above should be arranged.

76.10 Summary

Infections are frequent and life-threatening in renal patients and excellent infection control measures are paramount in looking after these patients. Simple, proven measures can reduce the risk of infections in these patients and can save money, hospitalization and lives. These measures should be performed on all patients at all times. Nephrologists have a particularly important responsibility in protecting our patients who are at high risk and minimising the risk of developing AMR.

Case Study

A patient who was 8 years post-renal transplant previously stable presented repeatedly with fevers and severe joint pains; each spike of CRP correlates with an admission. Multiple cultures were performed on many occasions; joint aspirations were negative and imaging unhelpful. She would improve within a few days and then be discharged. The clue here was the rapid recovery at each admission. This might possibly have happened if the patient had given immunosuppression such as steroids each admission in the context of a non-infective inflammatory condition or following removal of a drug that was restarted in the community but this remote possibility was not the case but the patient had received antibiotics on each occasion. In short, this pattern could not be due to anything other than a persistent, antibiotic bacterial infection. Ultimately, following culture of a fastidious commensal bacteria, her asymptomatic vascular graft was removed with a resolution of joint symptoms and fevers.

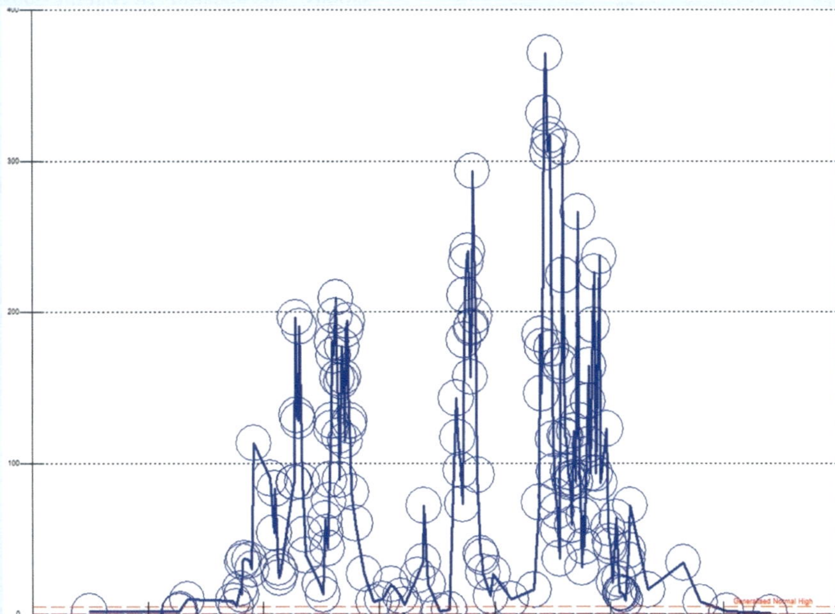

Whilst it was surprisingly difficult to prove infection and identify the source, this is not a rare scenario, and a patient who responds to antibiotics with a recurrence of symptoms within 2 weeks of ceasing antibiotics is likely to have a persistent unresolved infection.

76

Chapter Review Questions

1. What is the risk of transmission of hepatitis B/C or HIV following a needle-stick injury?
2. What percentage of renal admissions are due to sepsis and what % of patients acquire a nosocomial infection?
3. What are the relative rates of infection related to AV fistulas, AV grafts, tunnelled dialysis lines and temporary lines?
4. What is the risk of deep-seated infection (endocarditis or osteomyelitis) following a *S. aureus* bacteraemia?
5. What is the greatest obstacle to good infection control?

Answers

1. The risk of transmission of hepatitis B is approximately 1:3, hepatitis C 1:30 and HIV approximately 1:300.
2. Approximately 30% of renal admissions are due to infection; between 7% and 10% of patients acquire infection in hospital.
3. Approximately figures for infection are AVF 0.5 per 100 patient months, AVG 0.9 per 100 patient months, tunnelled lines 4.2 per 100 patient months and 27 per 100 patient months with temporary femoral lines having the highest rate.
4. Approximately one-third of patients will develop a deep-seated infection such as endocarditis, and this has a mortality of 30–50% in dialysis patients.
5. Probably, buy in and uptake by senior members of the team. It is critical that senior members of the department promote and contribute actively to an infection control ethos; units where this happens are likely to have a better outcome for their patients, units where senior staff don't get it, will not.

Acknowledgements Thanks and acknowledgement to Sophie Collier and Susan Hopkins for their contribution to the first edition.

References

1. Sarnak MJ, Jaber BL. Mortality caused by sepsis in patients with end-stage renal disease compared with the general population. Kidney Int. 2000;58(4):1758–64.
2. World Health Organization & WHO Patient Safety. WHO guidelines on hand hygiene in health care. World Health Organization; 2009.
3. Shahid NS, et al. Hand washing with soap reduces diarrhoea and spread of bacterial pathogens in a Bangladesh village. J Diarrhoeal Dis Res. 1996;14(2):85–9.
4. Luby SP, et al. Effect of intensive handwashing promotion on childhood diarrhea in high-risk communities in Pakistan: a randomized controlled trial. JAMA. 2004;291(21):2547–54.
5. Cardoso CL, et al. Effectiveness of hand-cleansing agents for removing Acinetobacter baumannii strain from contaminated hands. Am J Infect Control. 1999;27(4):327–31.
6. Gordin FM, et al. Reduction in nosocomial transmission of drug-resistant bacteria after introduction of an alcohol-based handrub. Infect Control Hosp Epidemiol. 2005;26(7):650–3.
7. World Health Organization Guidelines. Rational use of personal protective equipment (PPE) for coronavirus disease (COVID-19): interim guidance 2020.
8. Department of Health. COVID-19 guidance for the remobilisation of services within health and care settings: infection prevention and control (IPC) recommendations' August 2020.
9. Pratt RJ, et al. The epic project: developing national evidence-based guidelines for preventing healthcare associated infections. Phase I: guidelines for preventing hospital-acquired infections. Department of Health (England). J Hosp Infect. 2001;47 Suppl:S3–82.
10. Public Health Laboratory Service AIDS and STD Centre. Occupational transmission of HIV. London; 1999.
11. Haley RW, et al. Update from the SENIC project. Hospital infection control: recent progress and opportunities under prospective payment. Am J Infect Control. 1985;13(3):97–108.
12. Piraino B, et al. Peritoneal dialysis-related infections recommendations: 2005 update. Perit Dial Int. 2005;25(2):107–31.
13. Engemann JJ, et al. Clinical outcomes and costs due to Staphylococcus aureus bacteremia among patients receiving long-term hemodialysis. Infect Control Hosp Epidemiol. 2005;26(6):534–9.
14. Simor AE. Staphylococcal decolonisation: an effective strategy for prevention of infection? Lancet Infect Dis. 2011;11(12):952–62; Fluck R, Kumwenda M. Renal association guidelines - vascular access for haemodialysis. 2011.
15. Tacconelli E, et al. Mupirocin prophylaxis to prevent Staphylococcus aureus infection in patients undergoing dialysis: a meta-analysis. Clin Infect Dis. 2003;37(12):1629–38.; Woodrow GADS. Clinical practice guidelines: peritoneal dialysis. UK Renal Association. 2010.
16. Woodrow G, et al. Renal Association Clinical Practice Guideline on peritoneal dialysis in adults and children. BMC Nephrol. 2017;18:333.
17. Ashby D, Borman N, Burton J, et al. Renal association clinical practice guideline on haemodialysis. BMC Nephrol. 2019;20:379.
18. Public Health England and Department of Health and Social Care Clostridium difficile infection: how to deal with the problem. 2008. Guidance overview: - GOV.UK (www.gov.uk).
19. Cornely OA, et al. Fidaxomicin versus vancomycin for infection with Clostridium difficile in Europe, Canada, and the USA: a double-blind, non-inferiority, randomised controlled trial. Lancet Infect Dis. 2012;12(4):281–9.
20. Louie TJ, et al. Fidaxomicin versus vancomycin for Clostridium difficile infection. N Engl J Med. 2011;364(5):422–31.
21. Klevens RM, et al. Dialysis surveillance report: National Healthcare Safety Network (NHSN)-data summary for 2006. Semin Dial. 2008;21(1):24–8.
22. Hannah EL, et al. Outbreak of hemodialysis vascular access site infections related to malfunctioning permanent tunneled catheters: making the case for active infection surveillance. Infect Control Hosp Epidemiol. 2002;23(9):538–41.
23. O'Grady N, Mary Alexander, Burns L, Dellinger E, Garland J, O'Heard S, Lipsett P, Masur H, Mermel L, Pearson M, Raad I, Randolph A, Rupp M, Saint S and the Healthcare Infection Control Practices Advisory Committee (HICPAC) Guidelines for the preventions of intravascular catheter-related infections.

2011. Clin Infect Dis. 2011 May 1; 52(9): e162–e193. https://doi.org/10.1093/cid/cir257.
24. Chatzinikolaou I, et al. Antibiotic-coated hemodialysis catheters for the prevention of vascular catheter-related infections: a prospective, randomized study. Am J Med. 2003;115(5):352–7.
25. Chaiyakunapruk N, et al. Chlorhexidine compared with povidone-iodine solution for vascular catheter-site care: a meta-analysis. Ann Intern Med. 2002;136(11):792–801.
26. KDOQI clinical practice guideline for vascular access: 2019 update Am J Kidney Dis. 2020 Apr;75(4 Suppl 2):S1–S164. https://doi.org/10.1053/j.ajkd.2019.12.001. Epub 2020 Mar 12.
27. O'Grady N, Mary Alexander, Burns L, Dellinger E, Garland J, O'Heard S, Lipsett P, Masur H, Mermel L, Pearson M, Raad I, Randolph A, Rupp M, Saint S and The Healthcare Infection Control Practices Advisory Committee (HICPAC). Updated recommendations on the use of Chlorhexidine-impregnated dressings for prevention of intravascular catheter-related infections. Clin Infect Dis. 2017;52(9):e162–e193.
28. Lok CE, Mokrzycki MH. Prevention and management of catheter-related infection in hemodialysis patients. Kidney Int. 2011;79(6):587–98.
29. Lok CE, et al. Hemodialysis infection prevention with polysporin ointment. J Am Soc Nephrol. 2003;14(1):169–79.
30. Yahav D, et al. Antimicrobial lock solutions for the prevention of infections associated with intravascular catheters in patients undergoing hemodialysis: systematic review and meta-analysis of randomized, controlled trials. Clin Infect Dis. 2008;47(1):83–93.
31. Piraino B, et al. ISPD position statement on reducing the risks of peritoneal dialysis-related infections. Perit Dial Int. 2011;31(6):614–30.
32. Figueiredo A, et al. Clinical practice guidelines for peritoneal access. Perit Dial Int. 2010;30(4):424–9.
33. Dombros N, et al. European best practice guidelines for peritoneal dialysis. 3 peritoneal access. Nephrol Dial Transplant. 2005;20(Suppl 9):ix8–ix12.
34. Crabtree J, et al. ISPD guidelines/recommendations: creating and maintaining optimal peritoneal dialysis access in the adult patient: 2019 update. Perit Dial Int. 2019;39(5):414–36.
35. Strippoli GF, et al. Catheter-related interventions to prevent peritonitis in peritoneal dialysis: a systematic review of randomized, controlled trials. J Am Soc Nephrol. 2004;15(10):2735–46.
36. Nessim SJ, Bargman JM, Jassal SV. Relationship between double-cuff versus single-cuff peritoneal dialysis catheters and risk of peritonitis. Nephrol Dial Transplant. 2010;25(7):2310–4.
37. Bernardini J, et al. Randomized, double-blind trial of antibiotic exit site cream for prevention of exit site infection in peritoneal dialysis patients. J Am Soc Nephrol. 2005;16(2):539–45.
38. Szeto C-C, et al. ISPD guidelines / recommendations. ISPD catheter- related infection recommendations: 2017 update. Perit Dial Int. 2017;37:141–54.
39. Churchill DN, et al. Canadian hemodialysis morbidity study. Am J Kidney Dis. 1992;19(3):214–34.
40. Englesbe MJ, et al. Single center review of femoral arteriovenous grafts for hemodialysis. World J Surg. 2006;30(2):171–5.
41. Zibari GB, et al. Preoperative vancomycin prophylaxis decreases incidence of postoperative hemodialysis vascular access infections. Am J Kidney Dis. 1997;30(3):343–8.
42. van Loon MM, et al. Buttonhole needling of haemodialysis arteriovenous fistulae results in less complications and interventions compared to the rope-ladder technique. Nephrol Dial Transplant. 2010;25(1):225–30.
43. Nesrallah GE, et al. Staphylococcus aureus bacteremia and buttonhole cannulation: long-term safety and efficacy of mupirocin prophylaxis. Clin J Am Soc Nephrol. 2010;5(6):1047–53.
44. Report of the Rosenheim Advisory Group. Hepatitis and the treatment of chronic renal failure. London: Department of Health and Social Security; 1972.
45. Renal Association. Clinical practice guideline management of blood borne viruses within the haemodialysis unit. Renal Association; 2019.
46. KDIGO. 2018 clinical practice guideline for the prevention, diagnosis, evaluation, and treatment of hepatitis C in chronic kidney disease. Kidney Int Suppl. 2018;8(3):91–165.
47. Department of Health (UK). Good practice guidelines for renal dialysis/transplantation units, Prevention & control of Blood-borne virus infection, Addendum Guidelines for dialysis away from base 2010.
48. Jadoul M, Cornu C, van Ypersele de Strihou C. Universal precautions prevent hepatitis C virus transmission: a 54 month follow-up of the Belgian Multicenter study. The Universitaires Cliniques St-Luc (UCL) collaborative group. Kidney Int. 1998;53(4):1022–5.
49. Health, D.o. Immunisation against infectious disease – 'The Green Book' - 2006 updated edition. 2nd ed; 2007.
50. NICE guideline: Clinical diagnosis and management of tuberculosis, and measures for its prevention and control. 2011.
51. UK Renal Registry. COVID-19 surveillance report for renal centres in the UK: all regions and centres. Bristol: The Renal Association; 2020. https://renal.org/covid-19/data/
52. The Renal Association. Recommendations for minimising the risk of transmission of COVID-19 in UK adult haemodialysis units. KQuIP COVID-19 HD Ensuring Patient Safety Work Stream. Version 2. September 2020.
53. NICE. COVID 19 rapid guideline: dialysis service delivery. NICE guideline [NG160]. Published 20 March 2020. Last updated 11 September 2020.
54. Ikizler TA, Kliger AS. Minimizing the risk of COVID-19 among patients on dialysis. Nat Rev Nephrol. 2020;16:311–3. https://doi.org/10.1038/s41581-020-0280-y.

Setting Up and Running a Haemodialysis Service

Gavin Dreyer, Ravindra Rajakariar, Breeda McManus, Zuze Kawale, Ravi Armstron, and Valerie Luyckx

Contents

M. Harber (ed.), *Primer on Nephrology*, https://doi.org/10.1007/978-3-030-76419-7_77

Learning Objectives

1. To understand the different options for funding sustainable haemodialysis services
2. To understand the core resources required to initiate and operationalise a haemodialysis service
3. To understand the requirements for a safe haemodialysis water plant
4. To understand the core aspects of multidisciplinary staffing and delivery of clinical care on a haemodialysis unit
5. To understand the challenges of setting up a haemodialysis unit in LLMIC settings

77.1 Introduction

As the global requirement for renal replacement therapy (RRT) increases and with haemodialysis still the most prevalent global modality of RRT [1], understanding the unique challenges of establishing haemodialysis services is an increasingly important part of global nephrology care. The challenges and methods of setting up haemodialysis services in high-income countries (HIC) and low- and low-middle-income countries (LLMIC) have important similarities but significant differences.

Establishing a high-quality haemodialysis service requires multi-professional expertise, sustainable funding and an understanding of the clinical and economic context of where the service is to be located. Sustainability of any RRT service is key; therefore, consideration and planning of a haemodialysis service well in advance is imperative. Transparent priority setting is required based on reliable local data to determine not only the need but also the opportunity costs of an RRT service.

When setting up a haemodialysis service, it must be recognised that haemodialysis treatment is only part of the journey for patients with kidney disease which will include, but not be limited to, regular laboratory testing, reliable access to medication, affordable transportation, dialysis access surgery, acute hospital resources for intercurrent medical problems, provision of renal transplantation and palliative care.

It can not be overstated that prevention of kidney disease and its progression is the most cost-effective and life-sustaining approach, but inevitably, a proportion of patients will reach end-stage kidney disease (ESKD). Others may need temporary dialysis support if they develop acute kidney injury (AKI), and these patients should have timely access to haemodialysis including catheter placement.

Financial considerations will determine the model of care that can most sustainably be provided in any given health setting, but this must always be balanced with the provision of a safe and high-quality clinical service which provides both an excellent patient experience and excellent clinical outcomes. Large inequities and catastrophic health expenditures (CHE), defined as a health expense greater than 10% or 25% of household income [2] or 40% of non-food expenses [3], arise where dialysis is only affordable to those few who can meet the out of pocket costs; therefore, government oversight is important in planning any RRT service. In addition to ensuring sustainable infrastructure and consumable supplies for haemodialysis, establishing clinical guidelines and clinical governance structures are an important part of establishing haemodialysis services in any setting to ensure that safety and quality are prioritised alongside capacity and funding. Haemodialysis services consume water and electricity at high rates and many of the consumable supplies used cannot be recycled. Ensuring that the environmental impact of a haemodialysis service is considered during its commission is a novel but important consideration given the rapidity of climate change and the growth of haemodialysis services [4, 5].

This chapter will describe the major components required to set up a haemodialysis service and will also provide an overview of the unique challenges of establishing a haemodialysis service in LLMIC.

77.2 Should Haemodialysis Be Provided?

Availability of an intervention does not mean equity of access, and many patients with kidney failure die without ever having had or been referred for RRT [6]. The ethical dilemmas presented by RRT and faced by governments, healthcare workers, patients and families in both HIC and LLMIC should not be underestimated. A preliminary policy framework highlighting considerations in the planning provision of RRT is discussed elsewhere and summarised in Table 77.1 [7].

The out-of-pocket costs for one cardiovascular medication for 1 month, across 18 LMICs, was on average 1.8 days' wages [8]. It is therefore obvious that given that the costs of dialysis are exponentially higher, the risk of catastrophic health expenditure (CHE) is almost inevitable. For example, the average out of pocket (OOP) cost of haemodialysis across Africa ranges from USD 100 to 350 per treatment where no government subsidy exists. In India, where costs are significantly lower, 11.1% of patients experience CHE per dialysis session [3]. In Cameroon, dialysis is subsidized by the state, requiring an OOP cost of USD 40 per treatment (required a minimum of 8 times per month) [9]. With the minimum wage of USD 50 per month, even this reduced cost is unsustainable for most patients. In South Africa, dialysis is provided at no cost for those meeting eligibility criteria, but among children attending haemodialy-

Table 77.1 Policy options for dialysis coverage

Dialysis policy strategy	Expected health benefits for patients	Potential harm and burdens	Impact on autonomy	Impact on equity	Expected efficiency
Universal coverage for AKI and ESKD	Potential for all to benefit	Diversion of funds to kidney disease away from other diseases (opportunity costs)	Patient autonomy respected	Good for kidney failure patients however kidney disease prevention programs often not in place	Expensive
Government subsidy for AKI and ESKD	Potential for all to benefit	Diversion of funds to kidney disease away from other disease	Patient autonomy respected if they can afford co-payment	Tends to favour those with resources to pay	Expensive
Universal coverage for AKI only	Saves lives of patients with AKI	Diversion of funds to kidney disease away from other disease	Respected for patients with AKI	ESKD patients not dialyzed	More cost effective than dialysis for ESKD, short term treatment, may not require much infrastructure
State coverage under limited conditions	Benefit for those eligible to receive treatment	Ineligible patients die	Needs rationing and clear guidance for this	May exacerbate inequities especially for poor, vulnerable, sick	Prioritise peritoneal dialysis (cheaper) Prioritise Transplant (most cost-effective)
No state coverage	Access limited to rich few	Inadequate informed consent will lead to CHE and death	Restricted to rich	Exacerbates inequity	Left to market forces

Adapted from Luyckx et al. [7] with permission, presented in part at ICCEC Oxford, 2018

77

sis, the average family spent 27.1% of their income on transport to and from dialysis [10]. Other barriers to care include gender, extremes of age and geographical location [11, 12].

Ideally, a formal Health Technology Assessment (HTA) should be conducted when RRT provision is being considered, as has been exemplified by Thailand, to objectively determine options, projected costs and affordability [13]. Governments may feel pressured by industry, powerful people and patient advocates to provide RRT even where opportunity costs are very high and at times choose to do so. Governments in some countries may also not be able to restrict the provision of dialysis in the private sector. Under these circumstances, dropout rates tend to be high and outcomes are poor [6, 14]. Under all circumstances, however, where dialysis is provided, it is essential that the service provided is safe and of acceptable quality.

77.3 Haemodialysis Service Capacity

Planning services to allow for increased growth in the number of patients requiring haemodialysis is essential to avoid imbalances between supply and demand and thus having to make hard choices as to which patients to accept and which to decline for haemodialysis. It is common that once dialysis starts, there is an increase in patients which then slows over time [15]. Using local or national epidemiological and renal registry data can help model likely growth in the requirement for services over time and will be an important part of any business case at the outset of a new dialysis program [16].

Initial capital costs (haemodialysis machines, water plant and premises) may be high and should be considered alongside human resources, consumable costs, maintenance costs and all ancillary services that support patients receiving haemodialysis. Alternative funding

Table 77.2 Options for locating a haemodialysis service

	Advantages	Disadvantages
Hospital-based haemodialysis	Lower overheads and cost-efficiency Better for complex and unstable patients Close to emergency medical services and clinical staff	Providing individualised care is more challenging Can be far from patients houses (long transport time)
Satellite haemodialysis	Closer to patients homes Provides capacity in a stretched hospital Haemodialysis service More individualised care	Limited access to emergency medical staff Capital costs can be high Less flexibility with staffing
Home haemodialysis	Provides the ultimate in patient independence and flexibility Allows for more frequent dialysis which leads to improved health outcomes. This can be delivered daily/alternate days/short hours dialysis	Not suitable for most patients and challenging to achieve in LLMIC Only suitable for most stable patients
Community-based/ shared haemodialysis	Promotes out of hospital environment for haemodialysis Individualised design of unit	Capital cost of premises and high running costs No access to emergency medical staff
Remote, portable haemodialysis	Provides haemodialysis close to the patients home where it might not otherwise be possible Promotes patient independence	Risk of adverse dialysis events without direct clinical supervision High initial set-up costs Higher cost of delivering supplies and maintenance

models such as private-public partnerships initiatives are increasingly popular options to avoid high capital costs in LLMIC [17]. Limited healthcare resources may require a different model of care to be considered, for example, twice weekly compared to thrice weekly haemodialysis or shorter dialysis sessions to accommodate more patients [6]. Thus far, evidence supports twice-weekly haemodialysis in selected patients [18], although patient safety must be monitored when making these decisions.

If resources cannot keep up with demand, a clear and transparent process will need to be developed, with meaningful community and stakeholder engagement to develop criteria for eligibility for dialysis. Where possible, peritoneal dialysis services should be initiated in parallel with haemodialysis services to allow decisions about the treatment of ESKD to be made as equitably as possible. In South Africa, for example, all patients with AKI have access to haemodialysis, but patients with ESKD must go through a rationing process as described by Moosa et al. [11]. This process is challenging, but transparent guidelines are important to optimize equity, to communicate with patients and to reduce the moral distress of individual physicians who otherwise would have to take the full responsibility of declining patients for dialysis [7]. When developed in a transparent way with inclusion and opportunities for feedback from all stakeholders, appeals by patients can be objectively evaluated and decisions have been upheld in court [11].

77.4 Physical Location and Security of Haemodialysis Services

There are several options for locating a haemodialysis service. The main objective is to ensure 'the delivery of high-quality clinically appropriate forms of dialysis which are designed around individual needs and preferences and are available to patients of all ages throughout their lives.' Geographic location is dependent on current demand as well as anticipated growth based on available epidemiological data.

The location of the unit should be a site that will best serve the needs of access for the majority of the renal patient population in its catchment area (Table 77.2). Patient-centred considerations should focus on reducing travel time and promoting easy physical access to haemodialysis units, in terms of public and private transport, for patients with mobility challenges and ease of access to emergency and elective health services. Haemodialysis facilities should ideally be located on the ground floor allowing easy access to less mobile patients. Haemodialysis modalities will generate a range of CO_2, and this should be considered in the wider context of climate change and global health [4].

Haemodialysis patients can be remarkably well and entirely self-caring or heavily dependent on clinical staff for their care and treatment. Patients with ESKD treated with haemodialysis can have rapidly changing health needs; therefore, services must include flexibility to adapt to changing patient needs.

77.5 Functional and Safety Considerations

77.5.1 Utilities

Provision of reliable power, water, telephone and internet services will have different challenges across geographical areas. Haemodialysis units and patients must have emergency contingency plans in place in the event of failure of technical equipment, extreme weather conditions and other unexpected events (including non-payment of utilities) that may temporarily prevent haemodialysis delivery to an established cohort of patients. Where possible, this should include plans to move patients to another nearby haemodialysis centre [19]. An on-site generator and high volume water storage area may be required if power and water are so unreliable as to regularly compromise the delivery of haemodialysis. Providing access by lifts to a dialysis unit will require stairs to be built as well in case of power failure. Both lifts and stairs should be designed to transport bed or stretcher bound patients.

Theft of dialysis consumables, machines or other hardware can compromise the continuity of care. Dialysis units should have robust locks, and a plan should be made at each unit to ensure that it is secure for any period when it is not staffed.

77.6 Treatment Area and Patient Stations

The nurse's station should be centrally located with a clear line of sight to all patients. Staff must be able to see patients in the dialysis area; balancing adequate observation with patient privacy. Utility areas, equipment storage and maintenance areas should be located to enable ease of access from patient treatment stations. The layout should enable patients to talk to each other and for nurses to be able to call for assistance from one station to another. This is particularly important if patients are dialysing under special circumstances, for example, inside rooms because of infection or on a unit where haemodialysis patients are treated separately if they have blood-borne viruses such as hepatitis B. When patients return from a period abroad, they will need to be treated on an isolated machine due to the risk of acquired viral infection. Regular testing for hepatitis B, C and HIV should be undertaken, and agreement with local infection control colleagues will determine when a patient can be returned to a standard haemodialysis treatment machine [20].

Unit layout needs to be balanced with patient privacy, the capacity of the unit and its physical space. Each patient should have a personal space around their dialysis station and the entire space around a single treatment station should ideally be in the region of 10 m^2 which should allow for access in an emergency [21]. There should be sufficient space allowed for chairs to be fully reclined and for nurses to carry out procedures, with a slightly larger space allowed if beds are used instead of chairs. In an open ward, patients should be provided with curtains to draw around them should additional privacy be required or if this is not practical, mobile screens should be provided. Providing patients with a dialysis chair or bed will depend on the physical condition of the patient. Independent and physically well patients should be offered a chair, whereas those who are frail or acutely unwell may need a bed. Avoiding beds for all patients will encourage a feeling of independence rather than dependence.

77.7 Occupational Health and Safety

Adequate staffing is of paramount importance to ensure the health and well-being of staff and an enthusiastic and motivated workforce. Legal requirements for occupational health in a dialysis unit will need to be considered in local contexts. All staff should receive vaccination against hepatitis B [22] and be trained in manual handling including the use of hoists, particularly, as patients receiving haemodialysis are increasingly frail and obese.

There should be one hand basin between two stations, as well as an alcohol hand rub dispenser, a wall-mounted soap dispenser, a towel dispenser, a clinical and non-clinical waste bin and a sharps bin. The floor should be slip-resistant and easily cleanable as the risk of spillage of body fluids and contaminants is high.

77.8 Functional Areas

A typical HD centre will need the functional areas shown in ◘ Table 77.3.

Table 77.3 The main functional areas of a haemodialysis unit

Patient facilities	Entrance and waiting room Toilets (male and female) Main clinical treatment room(s) Kitchen area for refreshments
Staff facilities	Consulting rooms for clinical staff Changing, shower, kitchen and toilet facilities (appropriately separated) Nursing offices Staff common/restroom Receptionist and admin staff area Cleaner's room and equipment Nurses station in the main clinical treatment area
General areas	Clean and dirty utility areas for specimen preparation and discarding of waste Staff training room Secure storage for medical notes and medications
Technical areas	Main water treatment plant Technician's rooms Dialysis machine storage room Dialysis consumable storage area Electrical and IT distribution rooms

77.9 Patient Safety

Haemodialysis units should make provision for the treatment of unwell patients and medical emergencies. A resuscitation trolley including a defibrillator and basic airway support should be available on a dialysis unit and staff should receive regular at least basic life-support (BLS) training as well as having access to telephones to call emergency services. Clinical protocols and policies for the acutely unwell haemodialysis patient as well as for the management of common problems during haemodialysis such as hypotension and cramps should be available and medications made available on the unit to treat them. In addition, a range of commonly used therapeutic agents including antibiotics, oxygen and intravenous fluids should be available within the haemodialysis unit. Sufficient space around each haemodialysis patient should be available to ensure that resuscitation equipment can easily be brought to the patient's bedside should this be needed.

Contingency for evacuation in the event of a fire should be clearly documented and staff and patients equally aware of any plan, particularly, for any patients who will be more challenging to evacuate due to frailty, language barriers or limited mobility. All doors, corridors and access areas must be correctly sized to accommodate bed-bound patients and to avoid injury as well as obstruction to patient, staff and visitor flow. A plan for how to manage violent and aggressive patients should also be adopted in each unit [23]. A reporting mechanism for medical incidents on the dialysis unit can help plan for staff training and provisions of relevant clinical services.

Table 77.4 Potential contaminants in haemodialysis water

Type of contaminant	Examples
Organic contaminants	Chorine, chloramines, pesticides and herbicides
Inorganic contaminants	Sodium, potassium, calcium, magnesium, aluminium, lead, zinc, copper, iron, tin, fluoride, arsenic, sulphate and other trace elements
Microbial contaminants	Fungus, yeast, algae, bacteria and endotoxins

77.10 Minimum Requirements for Safe and Adequate Delivery of Haemodialysis

77.10.1 Water Treatment Unit

Water plants are a vital and complex part of any haemodialysis unit [24, 25]. Haemodialysis patients are exposed to large volumes of water around 600 L/week and nocturnal haemodialysis patients around 850 L/week. Organic, inorganic and microbial products can cause significant damage to dialysis patients' health (see Table 77.4).

Table 77.5 lists the major components of a haemodialysis water plant. The size of a haemodialysis unit will dictate the scale and complexity of the associated water plant.

The distribution loop can either be a direct feed or indirect feed into the haemodialysis treatment area. Direct feed delivers straight from RO to the loop, and excess unused water goes back to the RO. Indirect feed has a storage tank after the RO from which the water goes to the loop; excess and unused water goes back to the storage tank. Direct feed is preferred since bacterial contamination is reduced. However, in units with irregular water supply, indirect feed is preferred to prevent dialysis cessation due to water shortage (see the example from Malawi later in this chapter). The storage tank should have the capacity to supply adequate water for all the machines until the completion of dialysis (Fig. 77.1).

77

Table 77.5 The major components of a haemodialysis water system

Component	Function	Monitoring	Action
Sediment filter	Removes macroscopic particles, suspended and colloidal matter	Daily – pressures should be monitored at the inlet and outlet of the filter; as particulate matter accumulates, the pressure difference increases	Increase in pressure difference above the manufacture's set value indicates filter replacement required
Softener	Removes calcium and magnesium from incoming water in exchange for sodium	Daily/before starting the shift – check hardness of water and brine tank salt level. Regeneration cycle at pre-set intervals, when dialysis not performed.	Higher values indicate inadequate regeneration – increase contact time, higher water quantity than the softener capacity, fouling of resin due to iron – resin change
Carbon filtration	Removes organic contaminants chlorine and chloramines, by passing the water through activated carbon by adsorption	Daily/before starting the shift – check for chlorine levels immediately after sampling as chlorine levels drop if delayed. Carbon beds to be monitored to prevent breakthrough (a process where chlorine molecules reach the outlet of the bed without finding an active site). Monitoring of inlet and outlet pressures of carbon bed at constant flow rate	Increase in pressure drop indicates fouling (suspended particles in water), decrease in pressure drop indicates channelling (carbon particles not packed uniformly). For either condition back flushing should be done, back flushing prolongs bed life. Two carbon beds in series recommended
Reverse osmosis (RO)	Removes inorganic and microbial contaminants	Daily – Conductivity, temperature and pressure	Increase in pressure should prompt membrane cleaning according to manufacturer's guidelines. If cleaning fails to restore performance, membranes should be replaced
Deionizer	Removes cations and anions, deionizer is used to polish the water when RO alone cannot reduce the contaminants to desired levels	Monthly - bacteria and endotoxin levels post deionizer and endotoxin filter. Low flow rates can lead to bacterial growth	Deionizer tanks should be replaced periodically even if resin not exhausted to prevent bacterial growth
Ultraviolet irradiator	Ultraviolet mercury vapour lamp emitting 254 nm wavelength which kills bacteria by penetrating the cell wall	Ultraviolet intensity meter should be calibrated to ensure required dose is delivered, if low visual alarm should indicate low intensity	Quartz sleeve should be cleaned periodically to avoid biofilm growth which makes the UV less effective. UV device to be replaced annually or every 8000 h clocked. UV size to be appropriate according to the quantity of water flow
Endotoxin filters	Endotoxin filters remove endotoxins and bacteria, and must be followed after UV	Ensure medical grade endotoxin filters are used, which are free from preservatives, which requires 500–1000 gallons to rinse out if not rinsed adequately can cause severe adverse reactions (FDA, 1989). Inlet and outlet pressures should be monitored every day before shift start	If inlet and outlet pressures are the same, it indicates water flowing around the membrane, not through the membrane. If there is great difference between inlet and outlet pressure from the manufactures recommendation, this indicates clogging of the membranes. Membrane change is required

Monthly water samples from the loop for endotoxin test should be done. Weekly loop disinfection with heat prevents biofilm growth. Multiple sampling ports are required in the distribution loop for water testing. For new systems, weekly bacterial testing should be performed, until a pattern of compliance is established [26]. Alcohol can be used outside the sampling port if allowed to dry completely before sampling.

The target microbial counts in haemodialysis water should be <100 CFU/ml but may vary by region. The endotoxin content in haemodialysis water should be less than 0.25 EU/ml and again may vary by region. An intervention to the haemodialysis water purification system may be required when the performance of these indicators is 50% of acceptable limits [25]. Sites for testing water at different points in the haemodialysis water

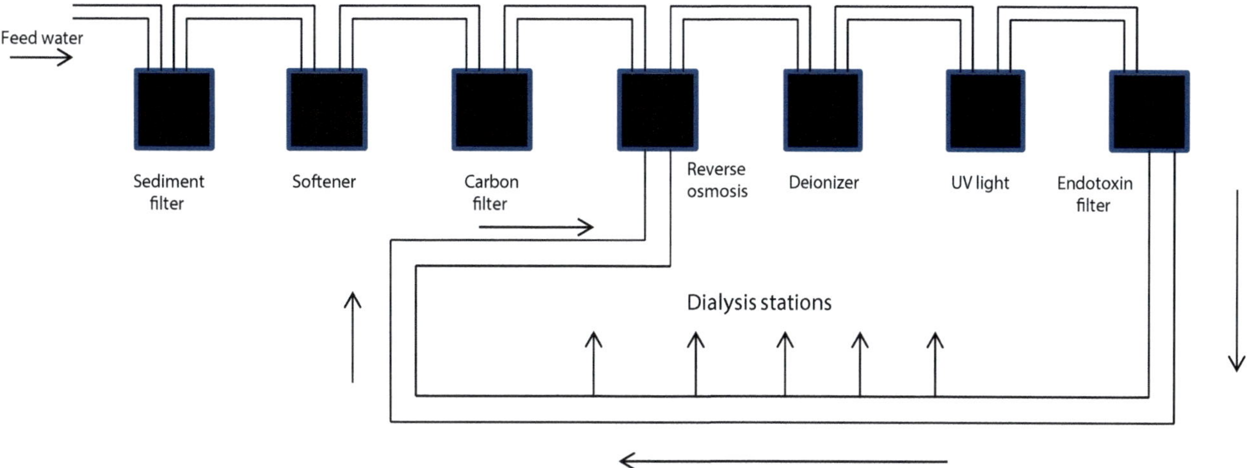

Fig. 77.1 An example of a direct feed haemodialysis system

purification system can be found in online reference documents [25].

If decontamination is not correctly completed, a biofilm can develop, which, once established is difficult to eradicate. If so, the entire distribution loop should be replaced. If loop material is compatible, 2–3% citric acid before disinfection may help to remove biofilm.

77.11 Maintenance, Documentation and Servicing

Annual service, repairs and maintenance should be done by professionally trained personnel as per the manufacturer's guidelines. Logbook should be maintained to assess water treatment performance. Dialysis units should have written policies that describe actions to be taken when an abnormality is detected in the water treatment system. Where water quality is not ideal, consideration should be given to preferential use of low flux dialyzers because of the lower risk of endotoxin contamination of the patients [27].

The tables below outline maximum allowable levels of water contaminants in a haemodialysis water system (see Tables 77.6 and 77.7).

Table 77.6 Maximum allowable levels of toxic chemicals and dialysis fluid electrolytes in dialysis water

Contaminant	Maximum concentration mg/L (unless otherwise stated)
Contaminants with documented toxicity in haemodialysis	
Aluminium	0.01
Total Chlorine	0.1
Copper	0.1
Fluoride	0.2
Lead	0.005
Nitrate (as N)	2
Sulphate	100
Zinc	0.1
Electrolytes normally included in dialysis fluid	
Calcium	2 (0.05 mmol/L)
Magnesium	4 (0.15 mmol/L)
Potassium	8 (0.2 mmol/L)
Sodium	70 (3.0 mmol/L)

Adapted from Water for Haemodialysis and Related Therapies [25]

77.12 Haemodialysis Machines

There are a wide variety of haemodialysis machines available through multiple providers. Their functionality will vary depending on the make, model and unit cost of the machine. Consideration will need to be given to whether a unit wants to provide haemodialysis, haemodiafiltration or both and whether more unstable patients will be treated which may require additional functionality from the machines and thus potentially higher cost. Financial contracts to purchase machines require sustainable financial models as well as maintenance costs built into the contract. Different types of machines and different brands of haemodialysis machine manufacturers will have discrete advantages, and some may be more appropriate for high- versus low-income settings. For

77

Table 77.7 Maximum allowable levels of other trace elements in dialysis water

Contaminant	Maximum concentrations (mg/l)
Antimony	0.006
Arsenic	0.005
Barium	0.1
Beryllium	0.0004
Cadmium	0.001
Chromium	0.014
Mercury	0.0002
Selenium	0.09
Silver	0.005
Thallium	0.002

Adapted from Water for haemodialysis and related therapies [25]

healthcare providers in LLMIC, identifying a contract which may not require an upfront cost in full for the machines and/or water plant could be beneficial.

77.13 Consumable Equipment

The consumables required to complete a successful haemodialysis session may differ depending on the type of dialysis machine used. Other items such as basic needles and syringes will be generic. To achieve a complete dialysis circuit, the following dialysis specific consumables will be required:

- Needles – specific for arterio-venous fistulae (different gauges are available)
- Haemodialysis filters – different surface areas and properties are available (e.g. low flux vs high flux)
- Bloodlines to connect the patient to the haemodialysis machine
- Plastic clamps (often part of the haemodialysis tubing)
- Saline solution and administration sets

Generic equipment including blood pressure machines, body weight scales, sharp disposal bins, general waste points and linen will be required on a daily basis. Heparin or other locking solutions are necessary for patients with a haemodialysis catheter. Dialysate solutions contain different biochemical compositions, predominantly varying around K^+ and Ca^{2+} – if resources restrict the variety of dialysate solutions available, a pragmatic choice may be to choose a bicarbonate dialysate with 2 mmol/L potassium and 1.25 mmol/L calcium concentration, although caution must be exercised in patients at risk of hypokalaemia. Bicarbonate cartridges or solutions will be required and may differ by machine manufacturer.

77.14 Dialysis Staff

To deliver good quality dialysis, dialysis staff must be well trained, fully competent and familiar with dialysis, dialysis access and acute complications which may occur on dialysis. In some settings, a nephrologist may not always be on-site (and this may not always be needed), but should be available by telephone or by internet, and there should be an identified doctor on-site who can step in for emergencies or be contacted if dialysis is occurring in a remote unit.

77.15 Vascular Access

Quality haemodialysis is not possible without a reliable vascular access. Trained personnel capable of placing these catheters, arterio-venous fistulas or grafts, including senior nurses, radiologists and surgeons should be part of a haemodialysis team. Other hospital personnel must be aware of the importance of protecting venous access in all patients with kidney disease. The non-dominant arm should be saved, and patients must be clearly instructed to refuse intravenous access or blood draws in that arm except in life-threatening emergencies.

77.16 Basic Medications for Haemodialysis Patients

Basic medications are required to maintain haemodialysis patients feeling as well as possible. These medications should be included in costing calculations of a haemodialysis service as the out-of-pocket costs for patients, if additional to those of dialysis and transportation, are often prohibitive.

Erythropoietin is necessary to avoid the need for blood transfusions which are costly, a scarce resource, and may lead to infection or development of antibodies which might preclude transplantation. In addition to erythropoietin, intravenous iron should be available to optimize haemoglobin levels and reduce erythropoietin dose.

Phosphate binders are necessary to control serum phosphate, which is likely to be less well controlled in patients dialyzing twice compared with three times weekly. Most patients will have an elevated blood pressure or other common comorbidities; therefore, access to basic medication for blood pressure, diabetes, HIV and cardiovascular care should be ensured.

77.17 Laboratory Tests

For adequate monitoring of dialysis quality and patient well-being, access to basic laboratory testing must be included on cost estimates for dialysis and must be provided within the dialysis package.

77.18 Dialysis Prescription

Dialysis prescriptions should be adapted to each patient, ideally, using a standard dialysis order sheet. This should include dialysis time, dialysis filter, anticoagulant prescription, dialysis access, blood flow rate, potassium, calcium and bicarbonate dialysate bath and most importantly the patient's target dry weight.

77.19 Infection Control

Developing a culture of hygiene and infection prevention will help reduce the transmission of infection through dialysis units. Ensuring staff and patients have access to running water soap and alcohol gel for hand hygiene is vital. Handwashing units must be highly visible and regularly maintained. Each unit will also need to have treatment protocols for episodes where infection prevention procedures have not been successful. Further details of this are covered. Any allergies should be clearly documented on the dialysis order sheets.

77.20 Clinical Protocols

Ideally, protocols should be in place in all haemodialysis units, for as many of the following protocols listed in Table 77.8.

77.21 Additional Considerations for a Haemodialysis Unit

77.21.1 Haemodialysis Schedule

Haemodialysis should be prescribed ideally 3 times a week for 4 h or at a minimum, 2 × 4–5 h per week per patient. Twice weekly schedules should occur on Mon/Thurs, Tues/Fri or Weds/Sat or Sun/Weds depending on

Table 77.8 Suggested clinical and non-clinical protocols for a haemodialysis unit

Clinical protocols	
Dialysis prescription	Determination of dry weight, Blood flow, Ultrafiltration rate
Management of vascular access including	Hygiene Clinical Assessment of AVF/access for puncture Needle sizes and placement Management of catheter infections Management of catheter flow problems Emergencies and non-functioning access
Managing the complications of ESKD	Management of anaemia Management of calcium-phosphate balance Nutrition, volume intake
Managing common scenarios on haemodialysis	Hypotension and hypertension (both acute and long-term) Shortness of breath Chest pain, arrhythmias Avoiding disequilibrium in uremic patients Bleeding Hyperkalaemia Volume overload Fever
Frequency and type of lab tests	Haemoglobin, electrolytes, calcium, phosphate, parathyroid hormone, iron status, albumin, viral infection surveillance
Infection prevention and control	Hygiene, hand hygiene Management of patients with chronic infections: hepatitis B, hepatitis C and HIV
Guidelines for emergencies	Patient preparedness self-if dialysis sessions may be missed dialysis Staff preparedness – emergency procedures, telephone numbers of local police, rescue, transport services
Non-clinical protocols	
Ordering and purchasing of consumable supplies	Lead time for delivering Raising purchasing requests
Patient eligibility for haemodialysis treatment	Including those with hepatitis B, hepatitis C and HIV
Managing medical records	Dialysis session record sheets Patient files (electronic or paper, ideally both)
Water system maintenance	Protocols for acceptable levels of chemicals and bacteria in water, frequency of filter changes, daily monitoring RO system
Machine maintenance	Service logs Maintenance schedule Ordering spare parts

dialysis unit opening times/days, such that patients have the shortest possible intervals between treatments. These schedules are difficult to achieve if most other patients dialyse 3 times a week. Operational pragmatics and capacity issues may require most patients to be treated with haemodialysis twice rather than thrice a week. The former model can allow more patients to be treated but at the cost of a lower delivered dialysis dose and risk of complications. Volume status, potassium, acid-base status and phosphorus must be regularly monitored to assess dialysis quality in patients dialyzing twice per week. If dialysis quality is inadequate, dialysis time should be increased or the third dialysis added per week where possible.

Dedicated training for patient self-care in a centre-based dialysis unit should be a vital part of any dialysis unit. Empowerment of patients to be independent not only helps with their experience but also reduces the need for trained staff, a significant component of the cost of a dialysis session. It is important to determine whether offering evening shifts for dialysis will be practically achievable. This will depend on transport to the unit, willingness of staff and patients to attend as well as safety and security. Evening haemodialysis treatment offers patients a more independent lifestyle with the opportunity to work during the day.

77.21.2 Staffing

The staffing of a haemodialysis unit should revolve around the core principle of patient-centred, quality care delivered by an expert multidisciplinary team [28]. Depending on the setting, this will include a range of staff giving direct haemodialysis care and indirect care. Staffing ratios recommendations may be available through local guidance and will be context-specific based on locally available expertise. Within each group of staff, leadership roles should be established as well as line management principles to ensure the quality of service delivery.

Direct clinical staff usually comprise of registered nurses, health care assistants dialysis support workers who are responsible for the direct connection and disconnection of patients to the haemodialysis machine and the nursing care through a dialysis session.

Indirect haemodialysis staff includes equipment technicians who would be responsible for maintaining the water plant and the haemodialysis machines and should be on call to cover for emergencies. Dietitians will advise about dietary modification including salt, water and bone mineral metabolism. A social worker, counsellor and psychologist can provide holistic care around some of the non-medical aspects of a haemodialysis patient's life. A vascular access nurse coordinator is a highly specialised post and should work in conjunction with haemodialysis nurses, nephrologists and vascular access surgeons to plan the creation and monitoring of permanent haemodialysis access. An administrator role is beneficial to assist with the administration of the day to day running of the service, transport booking and dealing with other administration tasks.

In some settings, more specialised staff such as vascular access nurses and dietitians may not be available, and the roles of these individuals may need to be taken on by more senior nurses or doctors on a haemodialysis unit.

The entire multidisciplinary team should be trained in all aspects of their work, appraised regularly and supported to further develop their careers and skills.

77.21.3 Clinical Governance

Collection of relevant clinical and non-clinical data and reporting of safety and outcome measures is the responsibility of all the clinical staff who work in any dialysis unit. Locally agreed parameters for data collection can then be compared over time, against other units, nationally and internationally.

A lead clinician for audit and governance should be identified and become responsible for collating and reporting the data. Mechanisms for delivering a change in the service based on audit performance needs to be established. Audit is an important part of governance and should be regular and could include infection rates in a dialysis unit, episodes of falls, vascular access and transplant listing as examples.

77.22 Clinical Guidelines

There are many available online guidelines from local and international organisations for many of the clinical and non-clinical aspects of establishing and maintaining a haemodialysis service (see ▶ Box 77.1). Each dialysis unit should agree on which guidelines they will use and will need to identify how or if these guidelines should be adapted for the local clinical context. Where guidelines do not exist for a given setting, they should be developed by the local clinical team using experience and information from the global nephrology community. A standardized set of guidelines for setting up a haemodialysis unit in LLMIC are under development by the International Society of Nephrology [29].

Box 77.1 Global Organisations for Nephrology and Haemodialysis

Kidney Organisations with Additional Resources

- International Society of Nephrology - ▶ https://www.theisn.org/
- International Society for Haemodialysis - ▶ http://www.ishd.org/
- European Association of Nephrology, European Dialysis and Transplant Association - ▶ http://web.era-edta.org/
- American Society of Nephrology - ▶ https://www.asn-online.org/
- United Kingdom Renal Association - ▶ https://renal.org/

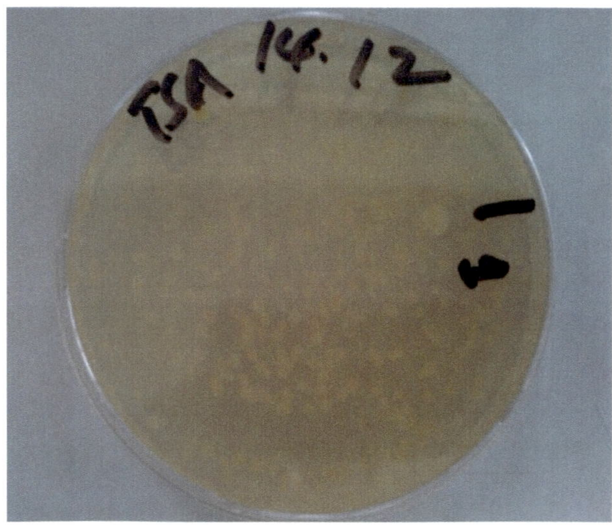

Fig. 77.2 *Pseudomonas aeruginosa* cultures from dialysis water at the QECH dialysis unit. Cultured on Tri Soy Agar plates

77.22.1 Setting Up a Dialysis Unit in an LLMIC: Developing a New Haemodialysis Unit in Malawi

Several of the authors of this chapter have been directly involved in setting up a new haemodialysis unit in Blantyre, Malawi. In this section, we describe the challenges and successes of establishing a haemodialysis unit in an LLMIC setting.

In 2011, Malawi (population 16.8 million) commissioned its second haemodialysis unit in the commercial city of Blantyre [30]. Prior to this, haemodialysis and peritoneal dialysis had been available uninterrupted since 1998 and free at the point of access in the country's capital Lilongwe. Funding for haemodialysis since the inception of the programme is met by the government of Malawi through the Ministry of Health. The Blantyre unit was opened with donated machines and a water plant that was 12 years old and part of the original donation in 1998. The entire haemodialysis system was upgraded in 2014 through a public-private initiative with Fresenius Medical Care in South Africa and included a water plant, five machines and five dialysis chairs [31]. This upgraded haemodialysis unit provides sustainable haemodialysis services for both end-stage kidney disease and acute kidney injury. Treatment is still free at the point of access unlike many other countries in sub-Saharan Africa. The majority of patients receive twice weekly haemodialysis which has allowed for more patients to be treated.

Twenty patients with end-stage kidney disease are treated, and since 2014, all cases of acute kidney injury have been treated with haemodialysis where it was indicated. The cost of haemodialysis provision reduced dramatically with the new machines from approximately $18,000 to $8000 per patient per year with ESKD. The unit is supported by a Sister Renal Centre link with the Barts Health NHS Trust as part of the programmes of the International Society of Nephrology [32]. The quality of life of haemodialysis patients in Malawi is in line with other global settings [33].

The development of this unit was been extremely challenging. When the unit was first set up in 2011, there had been no water sterilization, and the entire unit was contaminated with a biofilm of *Pseudomonas aeruginosa* (Fig. 77.2). This delayed the start of dialysis by 1 year and required chemical decontamination of the water plant and pipes (Figs. 77.3 and 77.4). Currently, in Malawi, there is still very limited access to laboratory tests for renal function or more specialist tests such as bone mineral disorders. Ancillary medications such as vitamin D analogues, intravenous iron and erythropoietin are not routinely available.

The leading cause of death in haemodialysis patients treated on the Blantyre unit is infection related, particularly, those using temporary vascular access catheters. Even though haemodialysis was provided free at the point of access, the second most common cause of death was lack of funds for transport to dialysis. This is a very real consideration even when the direct cost of haemodialysis to the government or the patient is relatively low. There is no reliable access to vascular access surgery; rather, this occurs on an ad hoc basis usually through visiting specialists, and therefore, haemodialysis catheter infections are common. Data collection is challenging due to lack of internet services and computers; however, the unit eventually plans to submit data to the pan African renal registry.

Transplantation is not yet viable in Malawi, and a live donor transplant overseas costs approximately $25,000 directly to the patient with no option currently for government support.

77

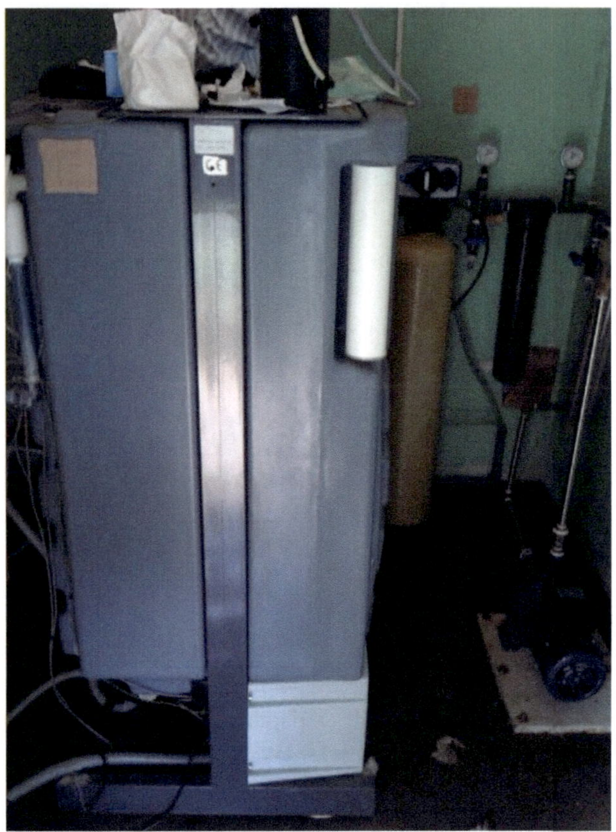

■ **Fig. 77.3** 350 L storage tank, pump and 10 micron filter in the first iteration of the Blantyre haemodialysis unit

The ethical challenges around patient selection for dialysis have caused significant psychological distress among staff and patients. Building psychological resilience within a dialysis unit in resource-limited settings is extremely important as these choices are very difficult and occur on a frequent basis. Establishing transparent and clear guidelines regarding access to dialysis is necessary. Policy makers often do not want to appear to be restricting access to treatment to anyone and therefore are reluctant to develop such documents. Such guidelines, however, would reduce the moral distress of individual healthcare workers and family members at the bedside and improve transparency and the perception of fairness in decision-making for scarce resource allocation [7].

77.23 Concluding Remarks

How a haemodialysis unit is developed, staffed and run will be very context-specific and depend on finances, clinical expertise, available space and equipment. Determining the rationale for building a haemodialysis unit, its sustainable use within the wider context of the local health system and economy are essential considerations. Haemodialysis services should ideally provide treatment for both acute and end-stage kidney disease. There are country-specific guidelines available for fur-

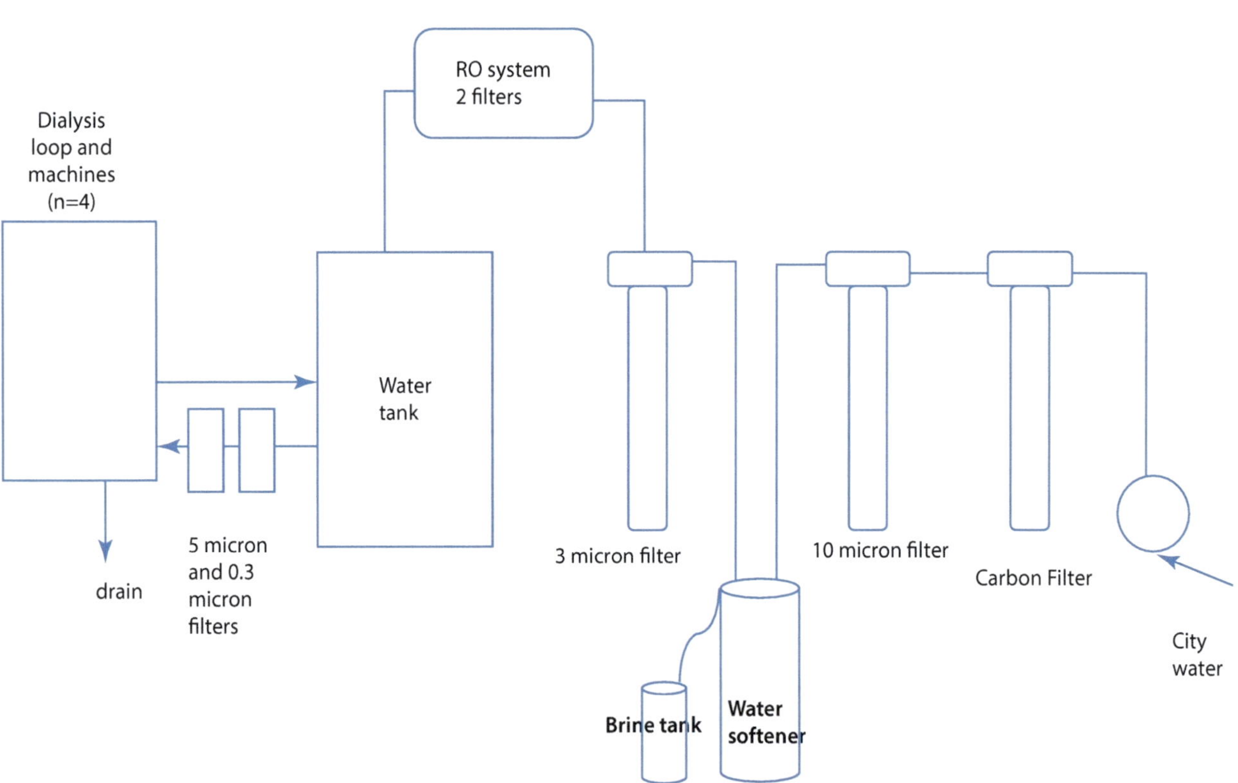

■ **Fig. 77.4** Schematic diagram of the water plant in the first iteration of the Blantyre haemodialysis unit. ■ Figures 77.3 and 77.4 demonstrate an indirect feed system

ther reference which could form the basis of an operational plan for a new haemodialysis unit. Sharing experiences around the challenges and successes of developing haemodialysis units through platforms such as the International Society of Nephrology will be a powerful addition to the existing information about this process.

Chapter Review Questions

1. List the core components of a haemodialysis water purification system?
2. What is the difference between a direct and indirect water feed system?
3. List the main members of a haemodialysis multidisciplinary team and briefly outline their role
4. What are the major benefits of an in hospital compared to satellite haemodialysis unit?
5. What are the major functional elements of a haemodialysis unit?

Answers

1. Sediment filter – removes macroscopic particles from water
   Water softener – removes calcium and magnesium from water in exchange for sodium
   Carbon filtration – removes organic contaminants, e.g. chlorine
   Reverse osmosis – removes inorganic and microbial contaminants
   De-ionizer – removes cations and anions
   UV irradiator – UV lamp to kill bacteria
   Endotoxin filters – removes endotoxin and bacteria
2. Direct feed delivers straight from RO to the loop and excess unused water goes back to the RO. Indirect feed has a storage tank after the RO from which the water goes to the loop, excess and unused water goes back to the storage tank. Direct feed is preferred since bacterial contamination is reduced. However, in units with irregular water supply, indirect feed is preferred to prevent dialysis cessation due to water shortage (see the example from Malawi later in this chapter).
3. Nephrologist/physician – directs clinical care of patients, coordinates MDT members, prescribes and modifies haemodialysis regimen
   Dialysis nurse – delivers haemodialysis sessions, holistic care of patient while on haemodialysis
   Dialysis technician – responsible for maintenance and upkeep of dialysis machines and water plant
   Dietitian – responsible for supporting haemodialysis patients with dietary changes related to ESKD
   Social worker – responsible for supporting haemodialysis patients with changing personal circumstances such as housing, finance caused by ESKD
   Psychologist – supports the psychological well-being of haemodialysis patients
   Vascular access surgeon – responsible for creating sustainable vascular access for haemodialysis including but not limited to arterio-venous fistulae
   Vascular access nurse – responsible for monitoring and maintaining vascular access
4. Lower overheads and cost-efficiency
   Better for complex and unstable patients
   Close to emergency medical services and clinical staff
   Can be used to provide haemodialysis in acute kidney injury as well as ESKD
5. Basic utilities – power and water
   Haemodialysis water plant and piping
   Haemodialysis machines and chairs/bedsNursing station
   Storage areas for consumable equipment/medicines
   Emergency medical/cardiac arrest trolley
   Curtains for privacy
   Rubbish bins
   Sinks for handwashing
   Staff rest room
   Toilets for staff and patients
   Isolated area for patients with blood-borne viruses

References

1. Liyanage T, Ninomiya T, Jha V, et al. Worldwide access to treatment for end-stage kidney disease: a systematic review. Lancet. 2015;385:1975–82.
2. Wagstaff A, Flores G, Hsu J, et al. Progress on catastrophic health spending in 133 countries: a retrospective observational study. Lancet Glob Health. 2018;6(2):e169–79.
3. Kaur G, Prinja S, Ramachandran R, et al. Cost of hemodialysis in a public sector tertiary hospital of India. Clin Kidney J. 2018;11:726–33.
4. Connor A, Lillywhite R, Cooke MW. The carbon footprints of home and in-center maintenance hemodialysis in the United Kingdom. Hemodial Int. 2011;15:39–51.
5. Connor A, Mortimer F, Tomson C. Clinical transformation: the key to green nephrology. Nephron Clin Pract. 2010;116:c200–5.
6. Ashuntantang G, Osafo C, Olowu WA, et al. Outcomes in adults and children with end-stage kidney disease requiring dialysis in sub-Saharan Africa: a systematic review. Lancet Glob Health. 2017;5:e408–17.
7. Luyckx VA, Miljeteig I, Ejigu AM, et al. Ethical challenges in the provision of dialysis in resource-constrained environments. Semin Nephrol. 2017;37(3):273–86.
8. van Mourik MSM, Cameron A, Ewen M, et al. Availability, price and affordability of cardiovascular medicines: a comparison across 36 countries using WHO/HAI data. BMC Cardiovasc Disord. 2010;10:25.

77

9. Tchape ODM, Tchapoga YB, Atuhaire C, et al. Physiological and psychosocial stressors among hemodialysis patients in the Buea Regional Hospital, Cameroon. Pan Afr Med J. 2018;30:49.
10. Bello A, Sangweni B, Mudi A, et al. The financial cost incurred by families of children on long-term dialysis. Perit Dial Int. 2018;38(1):14–7.
11. Moosa MR, Maree JD, Chirehwa MT, et al. Use of the 'accountability for reasonableness' approach to improve fairness in accessing dialysis in a middle-income country. Joles JA, ed. PLoS One. 2016;11:e0164201.
12. Ulasi I. Gender bias in access to healthcare in Nigeria: a study of end-stage renal disease. Trop Dr. 2008;38:50–2.
13. Teerawattananon Y, Luz A, Pilasant S, et al. How to meet the demand for good quality renal dialysis as part of universal health coverage in resource-limited settings? Health Res Policy Syst. 2016;14:21.
14. Olowu WA, Niang A, Osafo C, et al. Outcomes of acute kidney injury in children and adults in sub-Saharan Africa: a systematic review. Lancet Glob Health. 2016;4:e242–50.
15. Chuengsaman P, Kasemsup V. PD first policy: Thailand's response to the challenge of meeting the needs of patients with end-stage renal disease. Semin Nephrol. 2017;37(3):287–95.
16. Davids MR, Caskey FJ, Young T, et al. Strengthening renal registries and ESRD research in Africa. Semin Nephrol. 2017;37(3):211–23.
17. Morad Z, Choong HL, Tungsanga K, Suhardjono. Funding renal replacement therapy in Southeast Asia: building public-private partnerships in Singapore, Malaysia, Thailand, and Indonesia. Am J Kidney Dis. 2015;65(5):799–805.
18. Yan Y, Wang M, Zee J, et al. Twice-weekly hemodialysis and clinical outcomes in the China dialysis outcomes and practice patterns study. Kidney Int Rep. 2018;3:889–96.
19. Dries D, Reed MJ, Kissoon N, et al. Special populations. Chest. 2014;146:e75S–86S.
20. Good Practice Guidelines for Renal Dialysis/Transplantation Units. Prevention and Control of Blood-borne Virus Infection. Addendum Guidelines for dialysis away from base (DAFB). 2010.
21. Indian Society of Nephrology Standard of care for maintainance hemodialysis in India.
22. Clinical Practice Guideline Management of Blood Borne Viruses within the Haemodialysis Unit. 2018. https://ukkidney.org/sites/renal.org/files/FINAL-BBV-Guideline-June-2019.pdf.
23. Feely MA, Albright RC, Thorsteinsdottir B, et al. Ethical challenges with hemodialysis patients who lack decision-making capacity: Behavioral issues, surrogate decision-makers, and end-of-life situations. Kidney Int. 2014;86(3):475–80.
24. Hoenich N, Mactier R, Morgan I, et al. 2016 Guideline on water treatment systems, dialysis water and dialysis fluid quality for haemodialysis and related therapies. Clinical Practice Guideline.
25. ISO13959. Water for haemodialysis and related therapies. 2014; 2014.
26. http://www.aami.org/index.aspx.
27. Glorieux G, Neirynck N, Veys N, et al. Dialysis water and fluid purity: more than endotoxin. Nephrol Dial Transplant. 2012;27(11):4010–21.
28. The Renal Team A Multi-Professional Renal Workforce Plan BRS Mission Statement Recommendations for Renal Workforce Planning.
29. The International Society of Nephrology. https://www.theisn.org/focus/eskd-focus.
30. Dreyer G, Dobbie H, Banks R, Allain T, Gonani A, Turner NLV. Supporting Malawi's dialysis services in the international community. Br J Ren Med. 2012;17:24–6.
31. Craik A, Hemmila U, Mtekateka M, Kawale Z, Kalata O, Lusungu M, Kamwenda V, Dreyer G, Evans R. Partnerships to improve the detection and management of kidney disease globally. Br J Ren Med. 2016;21:107–11.
32. The ISN Sister Renal Centre Programme. http://src.theisn.org/.
33. Masina T, Chimera B, Kamponda M, et al. Health related quality of life in patients with end stage kidney disease treated with haemodialysis in Malawi: a cross sectional study. BMC Nephrol. 2016;17:61.

Vascular Access: Improving Outcomes for Haemodialysis Patients

Lindsay Chesterton, Ben Lindsey, and Richard J. Fluck

Contents

M. Harber (ed.), *Primer on Nephrology*, https://doi.org/10.1007/978-3-030-76419-7_78

Learning Objectives

1. To emphasise the importance of a multidisciplinary approach to the challenges of vascular access.
2. To identify key areas of the organisational pathway that need to be present in order to pursue definitive vascular access wherever possible for HD patients.
3. To understand the terms used in vascular access such as patency, assisted patency and the anatomical location of various access options thereby assisting communication amongst the MDT.
4. To understand the endovascular techniques employed to maintain vascular access patency and rescue thrombosed access when required.
5. To understand the surgical techniques used in access creation, maintaining patency, managing pseudoaneurysms and steal syndrome.

Although it is widely accepted that vascular access is of paramount importance in the delivery of high-quality haemodialysis (HD) care, obtaining and maintaining access can be time-consuming and resource-intensive. The data supporting definitive vascular access (arteriovenous fistula (AVF) or arteriovenous graft (AVG)) are considerable. Central venous catheters (CVCs) are associated with the highest risk of mortality and changing from a CVC to definitive access results in increased survival [1].

The Renal Association guidelines recommend that 65% of incident patients and 85% of prevalent HD patients should have definitive vascular access [2]. AVFs are advocated above AVG in view of their greater patency rates and reduced requirements for intervention [3]. Reducing vascular access morbidity and mortality is a considerable challenge that requires a multifaceted approach. This chapter aims to address the principles of access planning, monitoring and surveillance; reduce access-related harm and provide tips on vascular access organisation.

78.1 Establishing New Access for HD

78.1.1 Planning Access

It is generally recommended that AVFs are created well in advance of anticipated use, often 3–12 months prior to HD initiation [2]. However, renal function does not always decline in a linear, predictable pattern, and primary failure following AVF creation can occur in up to 50% of cases [4]. It has been demonstrated that older age, coronary/peripheral vascular disease and ethnicity are all factors likely to predict primary failure in the USA [5]. Furthermore, there may be a higher incidence of primary failure in those with small diameter forearm veins, previous central venous line placement and collateral vein development. Variation in theatre slot availability as well as in-centre organisation will inevitably influence the timing of the decision to embark upon access surgery. It is important to identify more challenging cases in advance rather than presume that the search for definitive vascular access will be futile. For example, a study of older patients (aged 65–94 years) demonstrated excellent patency rates in AVF at 12 months [6]. If HD is their modality of choice, older patients should not be precluded from receiving the gold standard therapy of definitive access.

Israeli data suggested that even in older patients >80 years, most had vasculature suitable for AVF creation [7], and even in older patients starting with a CVC, there is an advantage to switching to a AVF at a later stage as demonstrated by a Korean study [8]. The principal aim is to maximise the number of patients successfully starting HD and maintained with a durable, working AVF whilst minimising either unused access or access-related morbidity. Essential components of the vascular access planning process include patient education, modality selection, vein preservation and ideally an adequately resourced and flexible surgical referral pathway.

78.1.2 Decision-Making and Planning Ahead in Both Modalities

Patient empowerment and involvement in decision-making is a mandatory ingredient in the management of chronic illnesses, and HD is no exception. Education is an essential, early component in the battle against CVCs. It has been suggested that CVCs should be presented as temporary measures that are undesirable for long-term use [9]. The reason patients choose to decline definitive access is multifaceted but it appears to include poor previous experiences, incomplete understanding and, understandably, the desire to 'maintain the status quo and live on a day-to-day basis' [10]. It is important to ensure that patient choice is based upon a clear understanding of the risks and benefits of a CVC versus definitive access. These cultural considerations and societal expectations are global. Patient preference for a catheter varies across countries, ranging from 1% of HD patients in Japan and 18% in the USA, 42% in Belgium and 44% in Canada [11] yet the DOPPS data would suggest that the benefits of AVF are global in distribution including China, Singapore and Japan [12]. The dialysis unit 'culture' regarding access may also be important in understanding reasons for reduced rates of AVF prevalence. The acquisition and maintenance of cannulation skills are essential in a busy HD unit. Obtaining and preserving definitive vascular access for all patients (wherever possible) should be of the utmost importance in the nursing and medical care of HD patients and the message is reinforced at every opportunity by every member of the team.

Even in those patients that initially opt for PD, vascular access planning may also be applicable. Both forms of renal replacement therapy are complementary in an integrated care model of chronic kidney disease (CKD) management, yet PD to HD switch rates of over 35% have been reported in the USA [13]. Patients on PD with either a steady, predictable decline inadequacy/ultrafiltration or a wish to switch to HD can be identified in advance. Planning ahead to ensure HD initiation with definitive access is an important component of optimal care.

AVFs are not without their disadvantages. Primary failure rates, post-operative infections, 'steal' syndrome and requirements for sometimes repeated interventions in order to maintain access patency are all associated with morbidity. Furthermore, there is concern that AVF may have a deleterious effect upon cardiac status resulting in high-output cardiac failure. However, a study of almost 5000 US incident HD patients demonstrated that AVFs (as compared to CVCs) were strongly associated with reduced cardiovascular mortality [14]. In addition, if there is concern about heart failure, either as pre-existing or new comorbidity, due consideration should be given to either PD or adapted HD schedules such as more frequent dialysis.

78.1.3 Surgical Considerations

78.1.3.1 Sites

There are a few basic principles that surgeons follow in order to deliver usable vascular access. The concept of maintaining venous capital is paramount; the dialysis population is getting older with more challenging vascular anatomy, and dialysis units may have increasing numbers of patients whose vascular access options are becoming increasingly limited. It is, therefore, the responsibility of the surgical and nephrology team to consider the short- and long-term consequences of each access attempt.

A methodical approach to access is recommended, with the principle of starting peripherally in the non-dominant arm. The ideal AVF for dialysis will be no more than 6 mm below the skin, have a blood flow of at least 600 ml/min and be 6 mm in diameter (Rule of 6s) [15]. Clinical history and examination should identify patients with previous CVCs and thus risk of central vein stenosis. Ipsilateral access surgery with coexisting central stenosis will often result in limb swelling and primary AVF failure. Therefore, if access surgery is contemplated, every effort should be made to avoid the side of an occlusion or consider preoperative venoplasty. Assuming that both arm native options would be utilised prior to using a prosthetic graft, a sequence hierarchy for upper limb access would be as follows:

1. The upper limb vascular access hierarchy (◘ Fig. 78.1)
   - 1.1 Anatomical snuffbox (radiocephalic)
   - 1.2 Wrist (radiocephalic or ulna-basilic)
   - 1.3 Forearm (radiocephalic)
   - 1.4 Antecubital fossa (brachiocephalic or brachio-brachial)
   - 1.5 Brachiobasilic (single or stage two)
   - 1.6a Forearm loop AVG (onto brachial vein (vena comitans) cephalic vein or basilic vein)
   - 1.6b Brachio-axillary AVG (onto basilic, brachial or axillary vein)

In addition to the general principles described above, the vascular access surgeon needs to be able to think creatively in order to avoid prosthetic materials, avoid CVC insertion and deliver robust access. A fistula has the greatest chance of maturing if there is good inflow, low-pressure run-off and has a technically faultless tension-free anastomosis.

78.1.3.2 Mapping and Terminology

Clinical examination is satisfactory in those patients that have easily palpable arteries and obvious veins. However, duplex ultrasound permits a thorough evaluation of vascular anatomy and allows future access procedures to be planned at the same time. Measurements of vein calibre following application of an arm tourniquet have been proposed, but there is no standardisation of this method. Generally, a vessel diameter of >0.2 cm is deemed suitable for AVF creation. Duplex scanning provides information on axillary (or femoral) vein filling, and the reassuring finding of phasic flow changing with respiration reduces the suspicion of there being a downstream central venous (or pelvic vein) stenosis.

A multidisciplinary approach is key. The experienced and integrated vascular technologist will anticipate questions from surgeons. For example, they will not only confirm the presence of a recurrent cephalic arch stenosis but also contemplate surgical solutions. If planning a cephalic vein turndown procedure, they may check if the axillary or brachial veins are patent and anatomically suitable. The surgeon can then successfully redirect the fistula flow via a low resistance route to the right atrium via a tension-free anastomosis (see ◘ Fig. 78.6b for more information). The vascular technologist will also gain an understanding of favourable and unfavourable anatomy such as detecting the 12% of the population with a high bifurcation of the brachial artery. This may

78

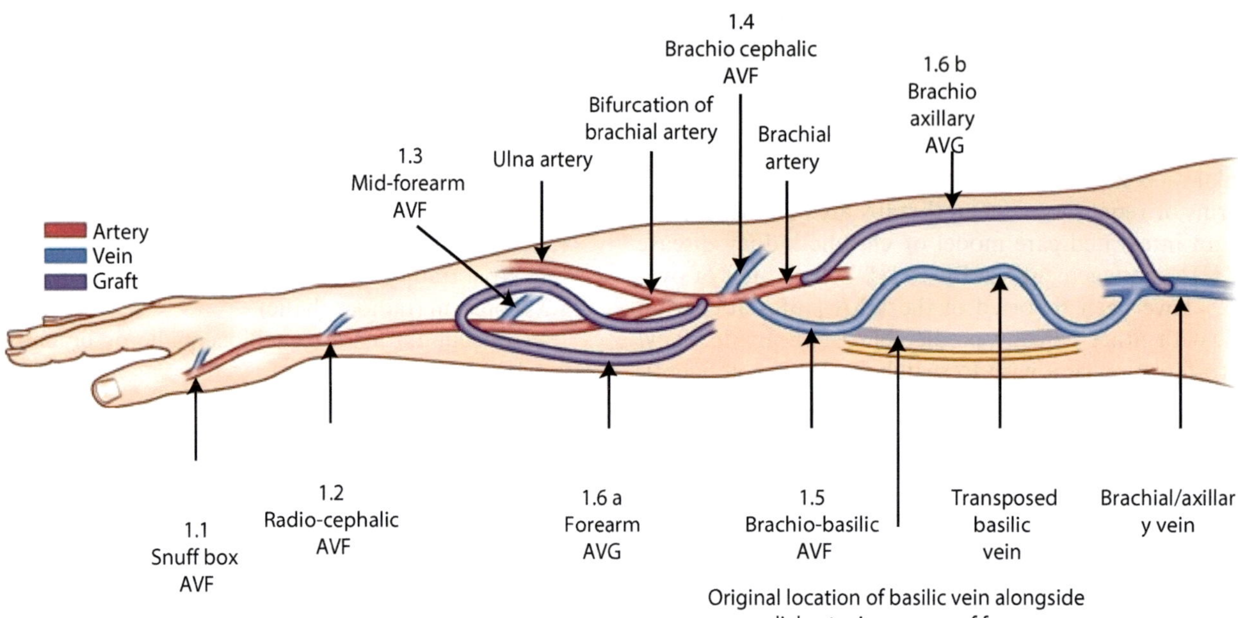

Fig. 78.1 The upper limb vascular access hierarchy

occur at shoulder level, requiring the surgeon to ensure that the dominant artery is identified at the antecubital fossa maximising inflow and therefore likelihood of fistula maturation. Venous anatomy may be very variable; sometimes, the basilic vein enters the brachial vein very low in the upper arm rendering it useless for the purpose of creating a usable length of brachiobasilic AVF.

It is important that there is a standardised terminology, particularly, when vascular access is being discussed between radiologists, nephrologists, surgeons, vascular technologists and dialysis nurses. The surgical author would like to recommend the following terms when referring to the fistula itself – upstream and downstream which are easy to remember if the direction of flow in a functioning fistula is used as the reference point. This is in preference to the anatomical terms proximal and distal, which may be misleading and confusing when describing the components of a fistula that impact upon function. However, the terms proximal and distal should be retained when describing anatomy and pathology relating to the artery.

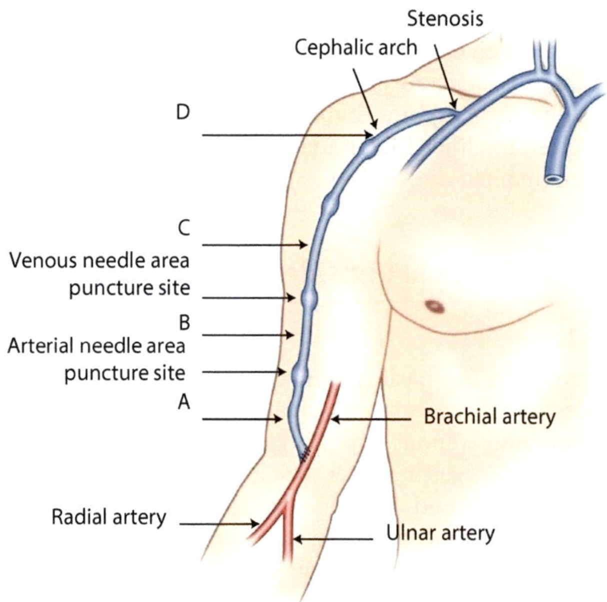

Fig. 78.2 Anatomy of an AVF including needling sites and a cephalic arch stenosis

Fistula Terminology (Fig. 78.2)

For example, point A in Fig. 78.2 is downstream to the anastomosis but upstream from the arterial needling point. Point B is downstream from the arterial needling point but upstream from the venous needling point, and C is downstream from the venous needling site. In order to demonstrate how confusing anatomical rather than functional terms can be, point C is anatomically proximal to the venous needling site but functionally upstream from the stenosis downstream in the cephalic arch at D and yet distal to it anatomically!

It is worth stating that duplex scanning of AVF can be complex, particularly, when trying to investigate problematic fistulas and close communication with the surgical team using this clearly agreed that terminology can maximise the information gleaned from a scan.

78.1.3.3 Surgical Techniques, Anaesthesia and Special Considerations

◘ Figure 78.3a shows the starting point of a generic native AV fistula with the pre-op direction of flow shown with arrows. 'End to side' anastomoses are created between the venous and arterial circulations, and the unused end of the vein is tied off as shown in ◘ Fig. 78.3b. The joint is sutured using fine prolene sutures which are akin to the fishing line (◘ Fig. 78.3c) and requires natural thrombosis along the joint and in the stitch holes to make the anastomosis leak proof. At the wrist, the length of the arteriotomy and thus the length of the anastomosis may be between 10 and 15 mm, whereas at the antecubital fossa, a maximum of 5 mm is recommended in order to limit the likelihood of 'steal syndrome' (see ◘ Fig. 78.9a for more information). It is helpful from the start to proactively manage patient expectations and concerns. Generally, only half of native AV fistula procedures will result in a usable fistula, and those that fail will do so as a result of non-maturation or thrombosis. The occlusive clot formed is not the type that results in life-threatening emboli but remains in situ. When a newly formed fistula fails, it will usually do so covertly. A rare exception is fistula thrombosis as a result of arterial thrombosis, in which case the hand may become acutely ischaemic and the patient may require a surgical thrombectomy. Patients with small and diseased arteries are more challenging, with the more distal AVFs (snuffbox, forearm) being less likely to mature and the more proximal ones (brachiocephalic) more likely to steal.

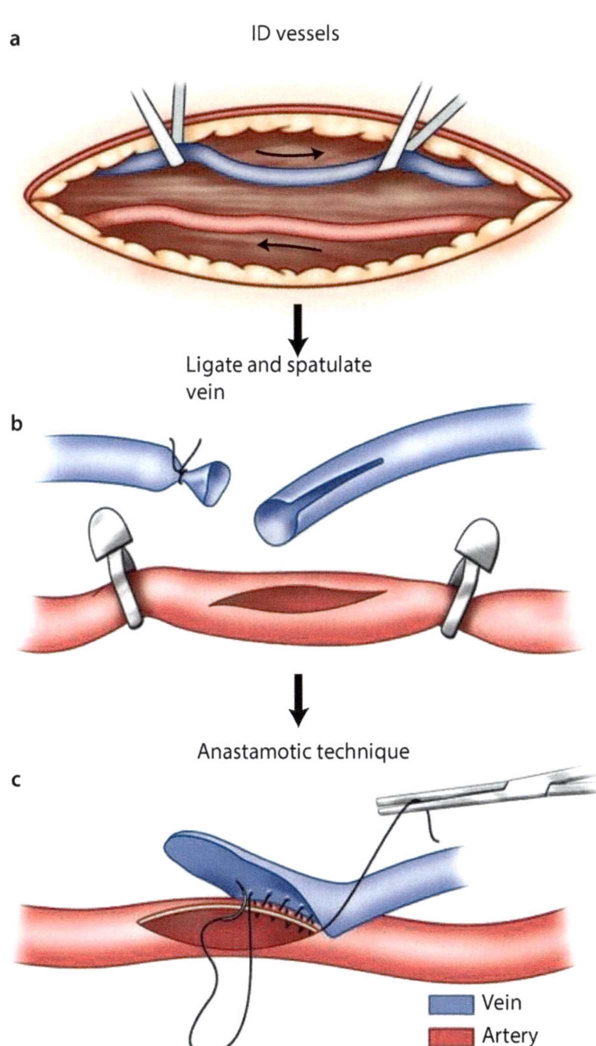

◘ **Fig. 78.3** Surgical techniques during AVF creation

Other Surgical Considerations: Patients Presenting at a Late-Stage Requiring RRT

Why do nephrologists place tunnelled CVCs in patients that require non-emergency RRT but do not have definitive access? There are several potential explanations. First, the recent Australian (IDEAL) study highlighted that early initiation of RRT is not associated with survival benefits and patient safety factors notwithstanding, it may be prudent to delay RRT until definitive access can be obtained [16]. PD can be a very useful tool in the battle to avoid CVCs, even in those patients that present at a late stage of their CKD, and should be a consideration at all stages of the RRT patient journey. Last, AVG may be a useful method of obtaining definitive vascular access, even in those requiring urgent HD initiation. Furthermore, a randomized controlled trial (RCT) has demonstrated that early needling of an AVG resulted in reduced incidences of bacteraemia when compared to a CVC [17].

It would be ideal if acute PD could be offered to patients who present with advanced CKD requiring urgent RRT. This is probably most frequently achieved following HD via a temporary line, after which, PD catheter insertion is carried out as a local anaesthetic (LA) or general anaesthetic (GA) procedure. Immediacy of use is essential, and the preferred approach is either percutaneous medical or laparoscopic insertion. The pneumoperitoneum required for laparoscopic insertion will predictably place a higher demand on the anaesthesia team. The technique requires the PD catheter to be placed through an 8 mm trocar that has been passed obliquely through the abdominal wall as well as following along the pre-peritoneal course. This affords a seal which will allow low-volume exchanges to commence immediately.

Patients that cannot have a GA, if not too obese, can have the procedure done under LA, and this requires some practical surgical attention to detail to maximise the likelihood of this being immediately usable.

Late-presenting patients not suitable for acute PD will have either a CVC or an AVG for immediate dialysis, which very much depends upon unit policy, and appropriately trained personnel.

The common upper limb sites for AVG are the forearm loop and the straight brachio-axillary graft (BAG) – options 1.6a and 1.6b respectively, in ◘ Fig. 78.1. The majority of cases need either a GA or a regional anaesthetic (RA) in the form of either an axillary or supraclavicular arm block. Even after RA block, placement of a brachioaxillary graft often requires local top-up LA infiltration to anaesthetise the proximal incision which is unavoidably made through the territory of the intercostobrachial nerve. A forearm loop has the advantage that it may be undertaken under RA.

Graft technology is moving on rapidly. It is a general belief that an AVG cannot be utilised for 2 weeks, following which the haemostatic rind will have formed appropriately and the post-operative subcutaneous oedema will have resolved, thereby permitting palpation of the graft. However, it is the surgical author's practice to use AVG immediately, encouraging very oblique cannulation with ultrasound guidance to ensure that there are no failed puncture attempts, i.e. only two punctures per dialysis session. Great care is required post decannulation to press exactly over the point at which the needle enters the graft. This practice will reduce the number of patients requiring a temporary CVC when presenting with an unsalvageable access.

Surgeons anastomosing a forearm loop graft onto a vein at the antecubital fossa do so in the hope that the vein will then arterialise. This could be a cephalic vein, basilic vein or as a last resort one of the brachial artery vena comitans as listed in ◘ Fig. 78.1 (option 1.6a). Future thrombosis/failure and unsuccessful salvage of the forearm graft may then permit the immediate anastomosis of the previously arterialised downstream vein onto the brachial artery and the fistula may be needled immediately. Similarly, if the graft has been anastomosed to the deeper veins, these can be superficialised, joined to the brachial artery and in some cases needled immediately. In cases with only a short distance of arterialisation, possibly as a result of multiple tributaries, alternative access will be needed whilst further maturation takes place.

Leg loops are associated with a much higher risk of infection because they are being needled below the level of both the waste as well as the waist. The keyword of caution for any surgeon putting these in is to assume that a proportion of leg loops will need to be taken out. For this reason, it is always important to anastomose them to the superficial femoral artery (SFA) rather than the common femoral artery (CFA). This means that if entire graft removal is mandated for early sepsis, ligation of a mycotic superficial femoral artery can be affected, with a lower likelihood of limb loss than would be associated with ligation of the more proximal common femoral artery above the origin of the profunda femoris.

Patients who require new vascular access mandating anaesthetic input will, by definition, be well advanced in their access career. The factors that contribute to traditional native AV access failure will also be those that make anaesthesia challenging. Nephrologists should always plan ahead and wherever possible ensure that the HD patient is as biochemically stable and as euvolaemic as possible in a timely fashion. New access attempts are probably best performed electively wherever possible. Communicating with your anaesthetists and surgeons is vital.

78.1.4 Assisted Patency

Primary failure of an autogenous AVF, defined as an access that never provided reliable HD postsurgical creation, occurs in up to 50% of cases [4]. Access which is patent but unusable for successful HD (non-functional) is frustrating for patients, surgeons and nephrologists alike, but measures can be undertaken to maximise success rates, thereby ensuring durable AVFs are ready for cannulation at an appropriate time for HD initiation.

Primary patency is often defined as the time interval between access placement and intervention to maintain or re-establish patency following failure or thrombosis. Assisted patency is the use of endovascular/surgical measures to maintain patency prior to thrombosis, and secondary patency can be defined as the interval from the access creation until access abandonment [18]. The increase in blood flow that characterises a developing AVF is often apparent in the first 2 weeks, and inadequate AVF maturation often relates to insufficient arterial inflow or non-ligated side branches [19]. The American Vascular Surgery guidelines recommend monitoring of new access at 4 weeks to ensure patency and appropriate maturation, and if not, then intervention should be considered [20]. This requires an individualised approach but usually includes (1) duplex scanning, (2) radiological angioplasty or (3) surgical intervention such as revision using one of the techniques in this chapter or a very simple tributary ligation. Following this algorithm, 92% of non-functional access became usable [21]. Post-operative exercises have long been promoted to aid maturation but the data remains controversial. Nonetheless, gentle exercises do not appear to cause harm.

In addition, if the access is too deep (>1 cm), it is also rendered non-functional. In our experience, access needs to be clinically assessed within 48 h postoperatively and is then assessed at weekly intervals, often with the adjunct of portable ultrasound to assess vessel diameter and depth. If the access is not maturing successfully, fistulography is performed with a view to correcting inflow/outflow stenoses if present and technically feasible. Other potential corrective measures are discussed first at a multidisciplinary team meeting.

78.1.5 First Use

The optimal timing of the initial AVF cannulation is not known. Traditionally, an experienced dialysis nurse/nephrologist assessed a fistula and deemed it to be suitable for first use if it was sufficiently palpable and had a relatively straight venous segment of sufficient length (10 cm) for two needles, an adequate diameter for needle insertion (>4 mm) and a uniform thrill to palpation [22]. It became common practice to delay cannulation to allow AVF to mature further. However, as discussed, AVFs that are going to mature usually do so within the first 2–4 weeks, failure is often due to anatomical reasons, and watchful, hopeful waiting is often not going to alter maturation by itself.

There is often a major concern that inappropriate cannulation may predispose to access failure due to thrombosis or extrinsic compression from haematoma/infection. However, the DOPPS study demonstrated that early cannulation (<4 weeks) in Japanese units was not associated with access failure [23].

If early cannulation is deemed desirable, factors such as clinical examination, vessel diameter and depth are all considered. Only experienced dialysis nurses, often with the use of ultrasound, will cannulate at an early stage in our unit and the ensuing HD session will take place with reduced blood pump speeds and measures to prevent intradialytic hypotension in order to reduce the thrombosis risk.

Although there is no 'right answer', there is a clear mandate that cannulation before 6 weeks may be both successful and advantageous, particularly, if the patient is receiving HD via a CVC. Reducing exposure to CVC complications will always be beneficial.

78.2 Maintaining the Current Vascular Access

So, your patient has opted for HD, agreed to a fistula, has had mapping; the AV anastomosis has been created; the AVF has been assessed and has had radiological intervention to assist development; the AVF is of sufficient calibre to withstand HD, and the AVF has been successfully needled. Which measures can we employ to maintain patency and increase AVF longevity?

78.2.1 Needling Technique

▫ Figure 78.4 shows the three main cannulation techniques for vascular access. These are rope ladder (▫ Fig. 78.4a), area puncture (▫ Fig. 78.4b) and buttonholing (▫ Fig. 78.4c).

Area puncture describes cannulation in a restricted area and is the least favoured technique due to the possibility of aneurysm development at the puncture site and stenoses in adjacent areas. The rope-ladder technique (needling is progressively moved up and down the length of the fistula) is widespread across the United Kingdom and has been utilised since the 1980s with the intention of reducing aneurysm development.

Buttonholing, a technique only applied to AVF, in which blunt needles are inserted into a preformed tract, has become increasingly popular due to reports of patient comfort and technical ease. Patient cannulation anxiety, bleeding times, haematoma formation, aneurysm development and radiological interventions were all reduced in buttonholed AVF [24]. It is important to note that the incidence of infection in buttonholed AVF may be higher and meticulous aseptic procedures are required. It is also important to note that AVG should only be cannulated by the rope ladder technique in order to avoid weakening the AVG integrity. For further information, we suggest accessing the British Renal Society and Vascular Access Society of Britain and Ireland best practice guidelines for cannulating/needling AVF and AVG.

78.2.2 Monitoring the Physical Examination

Vascular access monitoring and surveillance are common components of any strategy to minimise thrombosis and thereby maintain AVF/G patency and are often used interchangeably. However, monitoring is the evaluation of the vascular access by physical examination to detect signs that suggest the presence of dysfunction, and surveillance is the periodic evaluation of the vascular access by using tests that may involve special instrumentation for which an abnormal test result suggests the presence of dysfunction [15].

Physical examination is an extremely important component of vascular access care [25]. As previously discussed, the development of successful access can often be predicted from the physical examination by

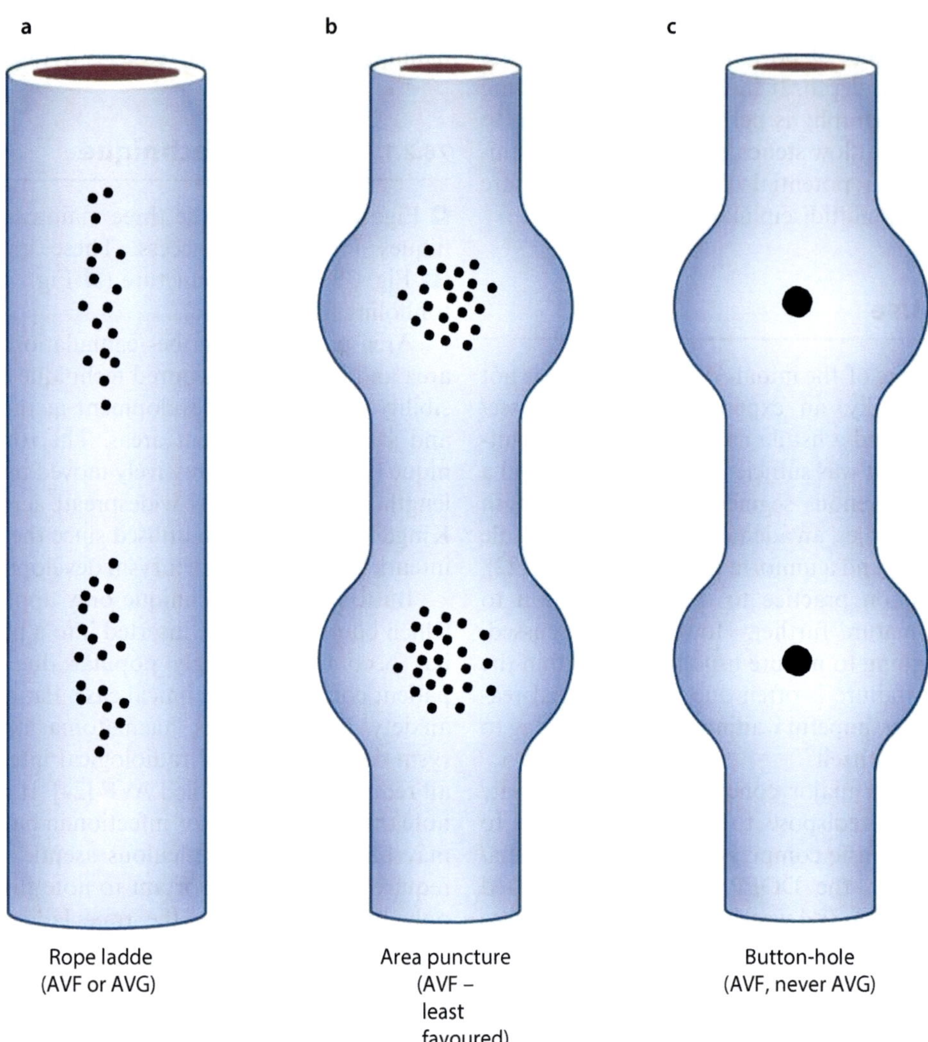

Fig. 78.4 Access cannulation techniques: **a** rope ladder **b** area puncture **c** button-hole

experienced dialysis nurses [22]. So, how should a fistula be examined?

A normal mature AVF has a soft pulse and is easily compressible. There is a palpable thrill and/or audible bruit throughout the length of the fistula as well as throughout the cardiac cycle. When the extremity is elevated, the AVF will usually partially collapse.

With inflow stenosis, the access may be flat and collapse excessively upon elevation. There may also be palpable stenoses in the juxta-anastomotic area. The thrill may be weak, the bruit may be high pitched, or the pulse may be weak or difficult to compress in the juxta-anastomotic or cannulation areas.

In contrast, an outflow stenosis is recognised with the following features: (1) arm swelling, (2) no partial vein collapse upon arm elevation, (3) palpation of stenotic segments in the venous region beyond the cannulation area and (4) abnormal thrill/bruit/pulse (weak and/or discontinuous bruit with only a systolic component or a weak or resistant pulse that is difficult to compress) in the venous region beyond the cannulation area [25].

With experience, it is therefore possible to use physical examination as the first step in the identification of inflow/outflow dysfunction, which when combined with a full fistula history will inform the clinician as to whether a radiological or a surgical solution is required.

78.2.3 Surveillance

There is considerable controversy regarding access surveillance. The basic tenet is that the longevity of thrombosed but rescued access is shorter than the long-term patency of a patent, yet stenosed access that undergoes angioplasty [15]. It is therefore proposed that surveillance would allow the detection of subclinical stenoses with haemodynamic significance, thereby leading to judicious endovascular intervention, resulting in fewer incidences of thrombosis and therefore greater access longevity.

Interventions to remedy subclinical stenoses, either through surgical or endovascular means, are associated with patient morbidity, require experienced vascular surgeons or interventional radiologists and can be expensive. Therefore, we will now discuss some of the techniques, advantages and disadvantages of access surveillance.

78.2.3.1 Intra-Access Flow (QA)

There are several methods of measuring intra-access blood flow (QA, ml/min) including Doppler ultrasound, ultrasound dilution, haematocrit dilution, thermal dilution and effective ionic dialysance. Only the widely available techniques of Doppler ultrasound, ultrasound dilution and effective ionic dialysance will be discussed here.

Vessel diameter can be measured with duplex scanning, and when combined with Doppler-derived velocity, intra- access flow can be calculated. However, it should be emphasised that Doppler ultrasound measurements are subject to operator error, turbulent blood flow and variability in the cross-sectional area of the vascular access.

The Transonic™ device utilises ultrasound dilution techniques to measure QA. Measurements are taken within the first hour of dialysis to minimise the effects of reduced cardiac output. The blood pump is stopped, and the arterial and venous lines are reversed from their normal position. Photometric flow sensors attached to an electronic flow metre are then clipped onto the reversed lines. The blood pump is restarted, a saline bolus is injected into the reversed venous line, and the intra-access blood flow is calculated. The error of duplicate measurements in the same patient is small, but the technique requires dedicated, expensive equipment and interrupts the delivered HD therapy [26, 27].

Ionic dialysance techniques can be used to measure QA. Access recirculation results in a dilution of the urea content of the dialyser arterial line and is inversely proportional to QA. It has since been validated that needle reversal, without injection of diluents, can measure QA by observing the effect on dialysate urea concentrations, a technique known as effective ionic dialysance (EID) [27]. This has been successfully validated against the Transonic™ device and has the advantage of being cheap, reproducible, non-operator dependent and easily performed in a busy dialysis unit.

Is Access Surveillance Useful?

Access guidelines recommend monthly measurement of access flow in AVF and AVG. Angiography is recommended if intra-access flow in AVF decreased to <500 ml/min or >20% from baseline or if AVG flow <650 ml/min or >20% from baseline [28].

The question remains, does access surveillance ultimately result in reduced access thrombosis and increased access longevity or just predict angiographically identified stenoses with attendant morbidity and overzealous intervention? The data is conflicting, often based on non-randomised studies using different access surveillance techniques in a mixture of fistulas and grafts.

Early and late access failure is often due to different anatomical reasons. Early fistula maturation failure is usually due to inflow stenosis at the juxta-anastomotic site. Late failure of autogenous AVF/G is usually, but not always, due to the appearance of outflow stenoses that reduce flow and increase the risk of thrombosis. The underlying mechanism is thought to be the marked increase in shear stress in the thin-walled outflow vein, triggering focal fibromuscular hyperplasia resulting in a fibrotic venous lesion [29].

Patent Yet Stenosed AVG: Is Intervention Useful?

Small studies initially demonstrated successful outcomes following angioplasty in terms of thrombosis reduction in AVG [30], but randomised controlled trials utilising either ultrasound dilution or duplex Doppler US did not show a benefit of access surveillance in AVG survival [31].

In our practice, although AVGs are subject to surveillance, the QA does not always predict subclinical stenosis, and other functional measurements are just as important in deciding upon the merits of endovascular intervention.

Patent Yet Stenosed AVF: Is Intervention Recommended?

In contrast, a prospective controlled study by Tessitore and colleagues utilising UDT and clinical examination in AVF did show increased access survival [32], and other studies have demonstrated that corrective treatment to haemodynamically significant stenoses improved patency and reduced thrombosis [33]. Although not a RCT, a clinically relevant 5-year controlled cohort study in 197 mature AVF analysed the efficacy of clinical monitoring, QA surveillance and elective stenosis repair. AVF loss and access-related costs were significantly reduced, but these effects were only observed in the first 3 years after fistula maturation [34]. More recently, an RCT of QA-based surveillance combining Doppler ultrasound and ultrasound dilution has demonstrated a reduction in thrombosis frequency, cost-effectiveness and improved secondary patency in autologous AVF [35].

Intervention in all access without good cause to suggest access dysfunction does not appear to be recommended. Analysis of >40,000 patients with an AVG or AVF did not demonstrate an overall benefit at 12 months of routine access surveillance/angioplasty repair. However, in those patients with low QA or new access, angioplasty (as opposed to non-intervention) did improve access survival [36, 38].

78.2.4 If a Subclinical Stenosis Is Suspected: What Next?

Once access dysfunction is suspected, the next step is often but not always an endovascular intervention. Informed consent is essential, and the risks of discomfort, bruising, contrast reactions (including the effect on residual renal function), infection and vessel rupture should all be explained.

Complication rates are low; studies report vessel rupture and free perforation in <1%. The surgical author suspects the incidence is higher having surgically explored a number of AVF following failed intervention and discovered defects in the fistula wall.

78.2.4.1 Percutaneous Fistuloplasty

A pathogenic stenosis is often defined as one which reduces the vessel diameter by >50%, thereby reducing the cross-sectional area by 75%, the critical point at which blood flow is dramatically reduced [26]. Fistuloplasty is undertaken in a stepwise manner under aseptic conditions (◘ Fig. 78.5a). The vascular access is entered percutaneously, the stenosis is identified with angiography, and conventional angioplasty balloons are inflated to dilate the stenosis. High inflation pressures are often required to overcome the fibrotic nature of the stenosis. After fistuloplasty, the remainder of the outflow and the central veins are imaged with venography. Surveillance tests should return to baseline following radiological intervention.

78.2.4.2 Other Endovascular Techniques to Maintain Access Patency

Newer technologies including cutting, high pressure and drug-eluting balloons are providing vascular radiologists with alternative tools to treat stenoses, but there is a lack of evidence to define their exact role in the treatment algorithm. They are often reserved for resistant lesions because of the increased likelihood of vessel rupture [37].

Bare-metal stents (BMS) should probably only be used in the treatment of resistant venous stenoses. A covered stent may be required to control an angioplasty-induced rupture. Stent placement for early recurrent stenosis (<6 months) in AVF and AVG doubled the interval between interventions. Stent grafts (a metal stent with PTFE covering the internal and/or external surface) may be very useful for failing or thrombosed access with resistant stenoses [38] or recurrent cephalic arch stenoses. The RESCUE investigators suggest that stent-graft use provided better patency than angioplasty when

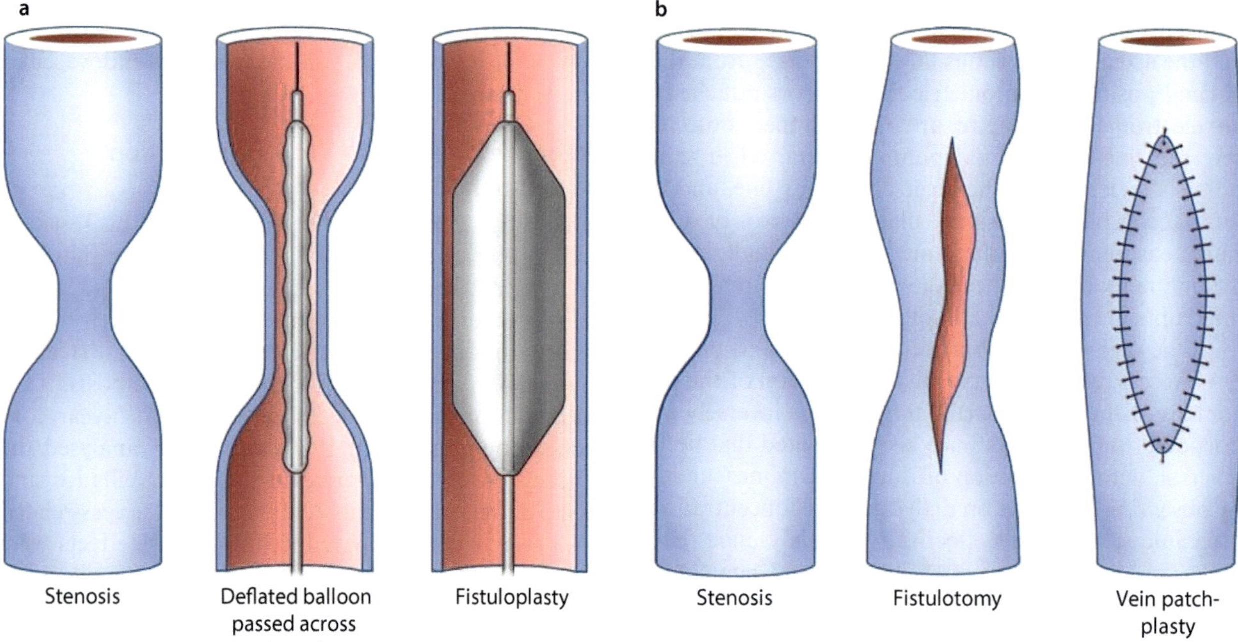

◘ **Fig. 78.5** **a** Fistuloplasty **b** surgical techniques to manage AVF stenoses

treating in-stent stenosis [39]. However, there are risks to consider including stent migration/shortening/fracturing and the induction of intimal hyperplasia leading to recurrent stenosis.

Surgical Techniques to Maintain Patency

Peripheral stenoses that recur despite sequential fistuloplasties need a different approach. This can be with either a surgical patch fistuloplasty – also termed a patch venoplasty (◘ Fig. 78.5b) – or a more complex surgical solution in the form of either a bypass (jump graft ◘ Fig. 78.6a) or re-routing (◘ Fig. 78.6b). A good example of the latter is the cephalic vein 'turn-down' for cephalic arch stenosis in which the fistula is divided upstream from the cephalic arch and anastomosed onto the axillary, brachial or basilic vein providing a low-resistance path back to the right atrium (◘ Fig. 78.6b).

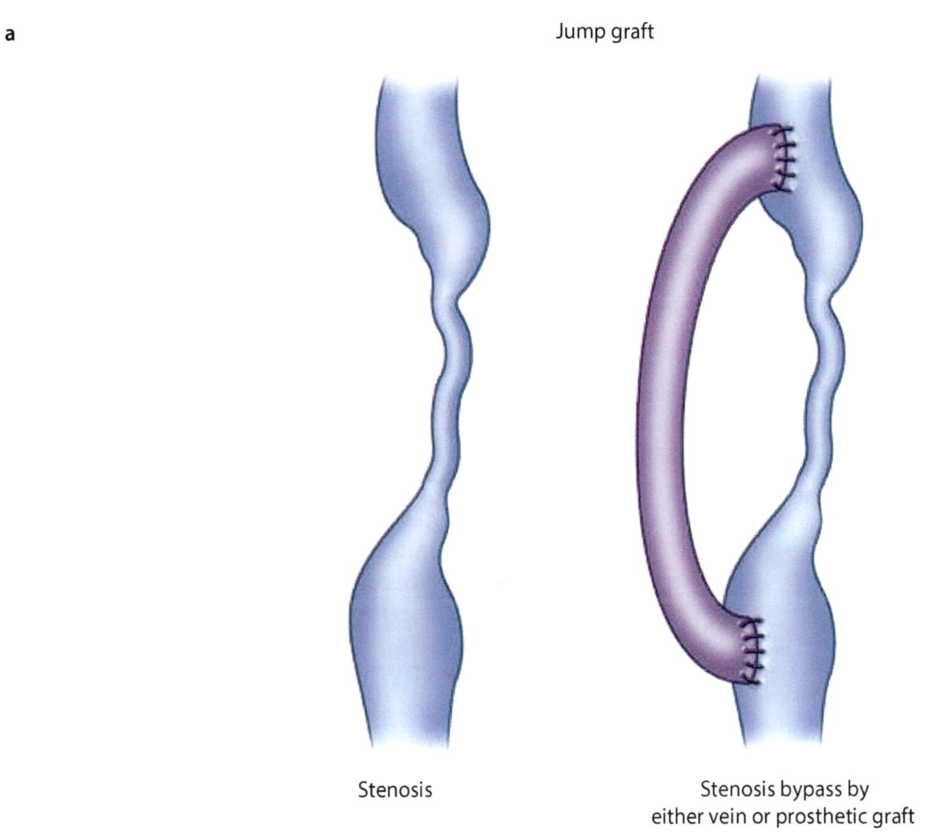

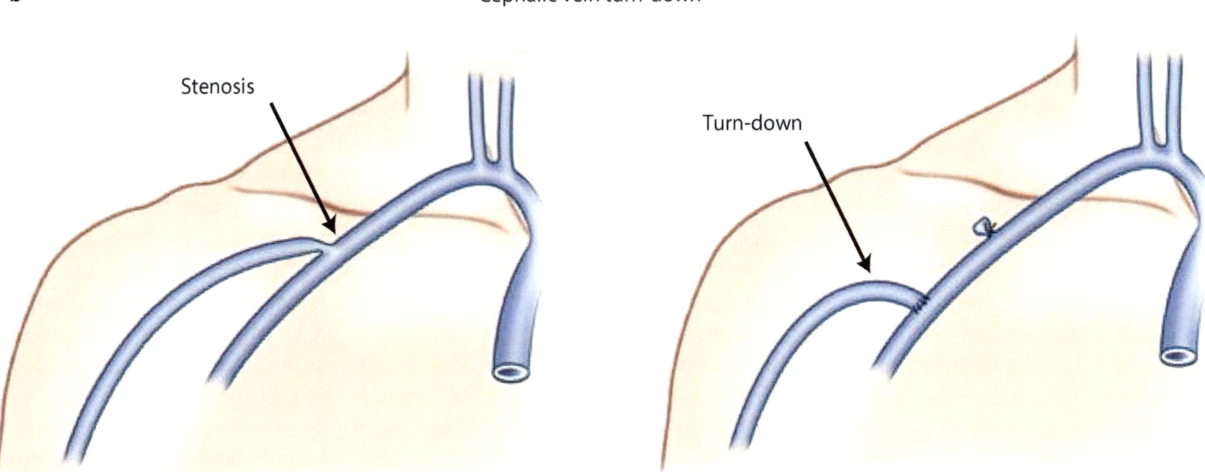

◘ **Fig. 78.6** Further surgical techniques to manage AVF complications: **a** jump graft **b** cephalic vein turndown

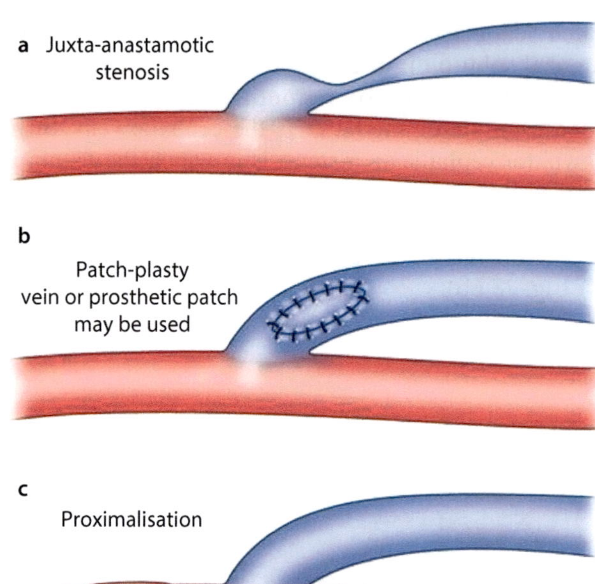

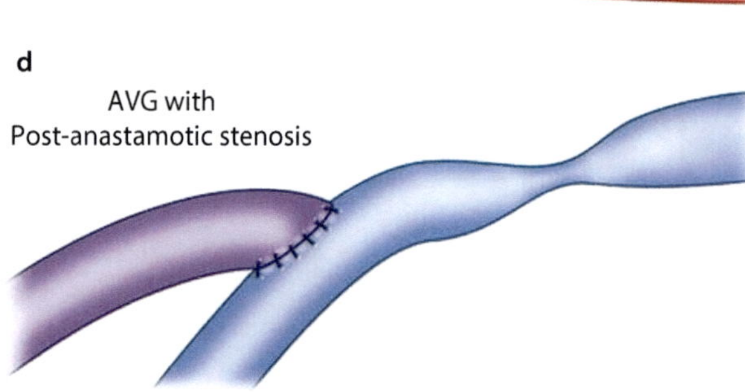

Fig. 78.7 Surgical techniques to manage juxta-anastomotic stenosis, **a** stenosed AVF, **b** utilising native venous or prosthetic patch tech-niques, **c** proximalising the venous circulation, **d** an AVG with a post-anastomotic stenosis

Juxta-Anastomotic Stenosis

In radiocephalic AVF, 55–75% of stenoses occur in the area just beyond the anastomosis (juxta-anastomotic) as shown in Fig. 78.7a. In native elbow AVFs, (brachiocephalic and brachiobasilic), 45% of stenoses are juxta-anastomotic, and the remainder tend to be at the junction between the superficial and deep veins. In AVG, 85% of the stenoses are found in the venous outflow region 2 cm downstream from the venous landing site of the prosthetic graft (Fig. 78.7d). Changes in the flow pattern as well as wall compliance mismatch are attributed to the cause of stenoses in these regions. Many of these can be treated in the first instance with fistuloplasty (Fig. 78.5a); however, a proportion of these will recur or be resistant to endovascular treatment and so should be treated with open surgery in the form of vein patch plasty (Figs. 78.5b and 78.7b) or proximalisation of the anastomosis (Fig. 78.7c).

No comparative studies exist between the endovascular and open treatments. If the puncture stretch is short, an endovascular approach is a justifiable first choice.

Access Monitoring and Surveillance: A Summary

To conclude, there is emerging data to support a tailored radiological/surgical intervention programme in individualised patients in order to maintain access patency and longevity. Our key recommendation is that all the available information is utilised in the decision to perform angioplasty in patent, yet failing access. This includes the physical examination; information on needling difficulties, i.e. difficult needle insertion, elevated venous/arterial pressures, and flow rates as well as information from surveillance tests. Recurrent lesions, particularly, if recurring at a rapid rate, should be discussed in a multidisciplinary meeting, ideally with vascular interventional radiologists, nephrologists and vascular surgeons in order to ascertain a treatment plan that is individualised for the patient, their dialysis vintage, previous access attempts and anticipated access longevity.

78.2.5 Thrombosed Access

Unfortunately, despite physical examination and surveillance, thrombosis, either predictable or unpredictable, will still occur. The steps to attempt to rescue thrombosed access are as follows.

78.2.5.1 Recognition and Patient Safety

Thrombosed access is usually recognised by either the patient (no longer aware of a ‘buzz’ in their access) or by the dialysis unit staff (no thrill or bruit; clinical detection of thrombus or inability to cannulate the access). If patients are encouraged to check their access is buzzing on a daily basis, then it is wise to suggest that it is done in the morning rather than the evening! This will increase the likelihood that the access can be salvaged on the same day. Prompt action is required to prevent access and patient-related harm.

The first consideration is patient safety; the degree of fluid overload and the presence of hyperkalaemia should be identified, and if necessary, placement of a temporary CVC may be required for HD prior to attempted salvage. In addition, it is prudent to ascertain the presence of any thrombocytopenia and coagulopathy. Informed consent should be obtained for endovascular thrombectomy as well as angioplasty. The additional complications include the risk of distal arterial thrombus if the anastomosis is involved and of pulmonary embolus (PE) (0–7% reported). Most vascular radiologists and surgeons would accept that many patients undergoing radiological de-clotting of a fistula will have multiple subclinical, asymptomatic PEs. Particularly in those patients with poor cardiopulmonary reserve, it may be prudent to consider the potential impact of thromboembolism, but the literature and our experience appear to support the benefits of access salvage in the majority of cases.

78.2.5.2 Contraindications

Contraindications to thrombectomy are few. Immature AVFs that have never been cannulated are relatively poor candidates for de-clotting due to technical and anatomical factors and should be assessed on a case-by-case basis. Local infection may preclude thrombectomy due to the risks of sepsis from infected thrombi entering the circulation, but it is important to note that thrombosis frequently presents with localised erythema, pain and tenderness, and a senior opinion should be obtained in these circumstances. These signs and symptoms are almost always the results of chemical phlebitis due to thrombosis rather than a bacterial, infective process.

Large aneurysms (in which thrombus extraction is technically more difficult and less likely to be complete) and huge clot burden (>100 ml) are relative contraindications due to the high risk of PE [40]. Other centres quote contraindications that include the presence of a right-to-left intracardiac shunt, pulmonary hypertension or surgical revision <30 days before intervention. Chronic, organised thrombus is often hard on palpation, and less amenable to successful rescue thrombectomy. Ideally, access salvage should be attempted within 48 h of thrombosis.

AVG thrombectomy has a higher success rate due to the absence of aneurysmal segments, and the synthetic graft material allows a more aggressive technical approach. The decision to attempt percutaneous thrombectomy rests between the patient, nephrologist, interventional radiologist and the surgeon.

78.2.5.3 Thrombectomy-Treatment Techniques

Techniques are highly dependent upon individual operators and centres, patient circumstances and equipment availability. The procedure is usually performed with patients fully monitored (pulse oximetry, blood pressure and continuous electrocardiography). Prophylactic antibiotics may or may not be required. Percutaneous thrombectomy involves three stages. Firstly, the thrombus is removed, sometimes with a mechanical device; secondly, the cause of the thrombus, usually an outflow stenosis, is dealt with; and lastly, a fistulogram is performed from the arteriovenous anastomosis to the superior vena cava. Success rates vary according to the mechanical device that is utilised and the case mix that is attempted, but access patency is reported to be >80%, >60% and >40% at 30 days, 3 and 6 months, respectively. Other complications include puncture site haematomas, vessel dissection or rupture, infection and contrast reactions. Some centres do not use mechanical devices but hope that once flow is re-established, autolysis occurs. If not, surgical thrombectomy should be considered. Intravenous heparin is a useful tool to clear residual thrombosis, and some centres recommend HD post-radiological thrombectomy. These decisions should be individualised and undertaken by a senior clinician as the data is limited. Some centres routinely warfarinise patients for 6–12 months post-salvage of a thrombosed fistula.

78.2.5.4 Thrombolysis

Thrombolytic drugs alone have reduced in popularity as single agents for thrombosed access since the introduction of mechanical thrombectomy but remain a useful tool when combined with mechanical devices in maximising thrombus clearance and reducing procedural times. Urokinase and tissue plasminogen activator (tPA) can be used for infusion thrombolysis. Antegrade vascular access is obtained as close to the arteriovenous anastomosis as possible, and the thrombolytic drug is infused directly into the vascular access via a multiple side-hole catheter. Doses and infusion times vary (3–20 h). Usual contraindications to thrombolytic agents apply.

It is still not clear if a radiological or a surgical approach is best to deal with the thrombosed AVF or AVG. Clinical practice varies within each renal unit, and access to either experienced vascular radiologists or vascular surgeons probably dictates the preferred approach. It is likely that a combined approach is probably best with each patient undergoing fistulography in a combined theatre and angiography suite.

Maintaining vascular access is time-consuming but rewarding. However, it is important to accept that long-term patency is not guaranteed despite radiological/surgical intervention. In these circumstances, planning for new access whilst utilising the existing, failing access may be beneficial in some individualised patients in order to avoid CVCs. There is insufficient evidence to suggest any further generalisations.

78.3 Reducing Risk

There is no denying that all vascular access for HD has risks. It is important that all members of the MDT including patients receiving HD are vigilant and educated in recognizing potential challenges. More frequent HD schedules may indeed result in increased access interventions but the other benefits certainly appear to outweigh these challenges. Education, meticulous needling, early recognition of complications and prompt action are paramount. The BRS/VASBI guidelines are a useful resource for further information and advice on quality improvement projects in this area of fundamental importance.

78.3.1 Pharmaceutical Therapies to Reduce Access Thrombosis

It is well recognised that access thrombosis is associated with morbidity and hospitalisations. Anticoagulants and anti-platelet agents are often prescribed to prevent thrombosis, but the data supporting this therapeutic approach are limited. A large study of HD patients prescribed aspirin, clopidogrel or warfarin concluded that these medications were associated with higher mortality [41]. A recent meta-analysis evaluated ten trials in patients with AVF or AVG thrombosis and concluded that anti-platelet agents reduced the risk of thrombosis in AVF (but not AVG) without an increase in bleeding events [42]. Further trials are required in order to fully understand the risk/benefit ratio of anticoagulants/anti-platelet agents in HD patients in order to prevent access thrombosis.

Ad-hoc analysis from the SHARP and AURORA trials would suggest that only modest benefits in terms of access longevity would be conferred by statins [43]. Fish oils were not found to be beneficial in the recently published FAVOURED trial [44].

78.3.2 Infection

Clinical risk associated with infected definitive access still exists, albeit at a lower rate than in those with CVCs. The usual approach is to identify infection at an early stage (erythema, tenderness, presence of pyrexia, etc. in the presence of negative blood cultures), swab and commence empirical antibiotic therapy as per local unit guidelines, which are then tailored to positive microbiology specimens. Prompt treatment is recommended as metastatic spread from AVF can still occur. The presence of aneurysms, infected thrombi or localised abscess formation may all increase the risk of AVF rupture, and early vascular surgical assessment is suggested as AVF ligation may be required [2].

As discussed previously, buttonholing may be advantageous but does appear to confer an elevated risk of infection. Meticulous care is required during cannulation, and infectious complications can be reduced following dialysis staff education [45]. Some centres use topical mupirocin ointment over buttonholes, although data supporting this approach are limited.

Superficial AVG infection should be swabbed and treated promptly with broad-spectrum antibiotic therapy and then treatment should be tailored to the causative organism. More extensive AVG infection can lead to bacteraemia, sepsis and death, and a combined antibiotic and surgical approach is often required for complete resolution. Subclinical infection is a difficult problem, occurring in abandoned and non-functioning grafts. It may present with erythropoietin resistance or elevated C-reactive protein and may require specialist radiological imaging in order to identify the source of the infection. AVG removal may be needed but can be difficult for technical reasons.

78.3.3 Mechanical Issues

The development of complications in an established AVF or AVG is predictable, and their management reflects an understanding of the basic rules of physics.

78.3.3.1 True Aneurysms, Pseudoaneurysms, Bleeding and Ruptures

A true aneurysm represents the dilatation of all the layers of the arterial wall. This may occur in a patient with poorly controlled blood pressure with other vascular risk factors. Generalised thinning and stretching of the AVF wall will, according to Laplace's law, continue to result in further expansion (◘ Fig. 78.8a). Usually, a pseudoaneurysm or false aneurysm will only form as a result of a downstream stenosis causing resistance to flow and elevation of AVF pressure. This will be evident on examination by detecting the replacement of a thrill with a pulse.

A false aneurysm is a contained persistent leak from a needle site (◘ Fig. 78.8b) or a fistuloplasty injury (◘ Fig. 78.8c), resulting in haematoma outside the arterial wall. Unlike the true aneurysm described above, it does not have a true wall. Common causes include failure to compress accurately and/or for long enough following decannulation combined with the presence of a downstream stenosis. It follows that inadvertently putting the dialysis needle through the back wall of the fistula will result in either a large haematoma ('blown' fistula ◘ Fig. 78.8d) or if more contained a pseudoaneurysm (◘ Fig. 78.8b). The likelihood of any of these bleeding complications following puncturing/decannulating of an AVF will be significantly greater in the presence of a downstream stenosis. Prolonged bleeding times post dialysis and elevated venous pressures during HD are often late warning signs of downstream stenosis.

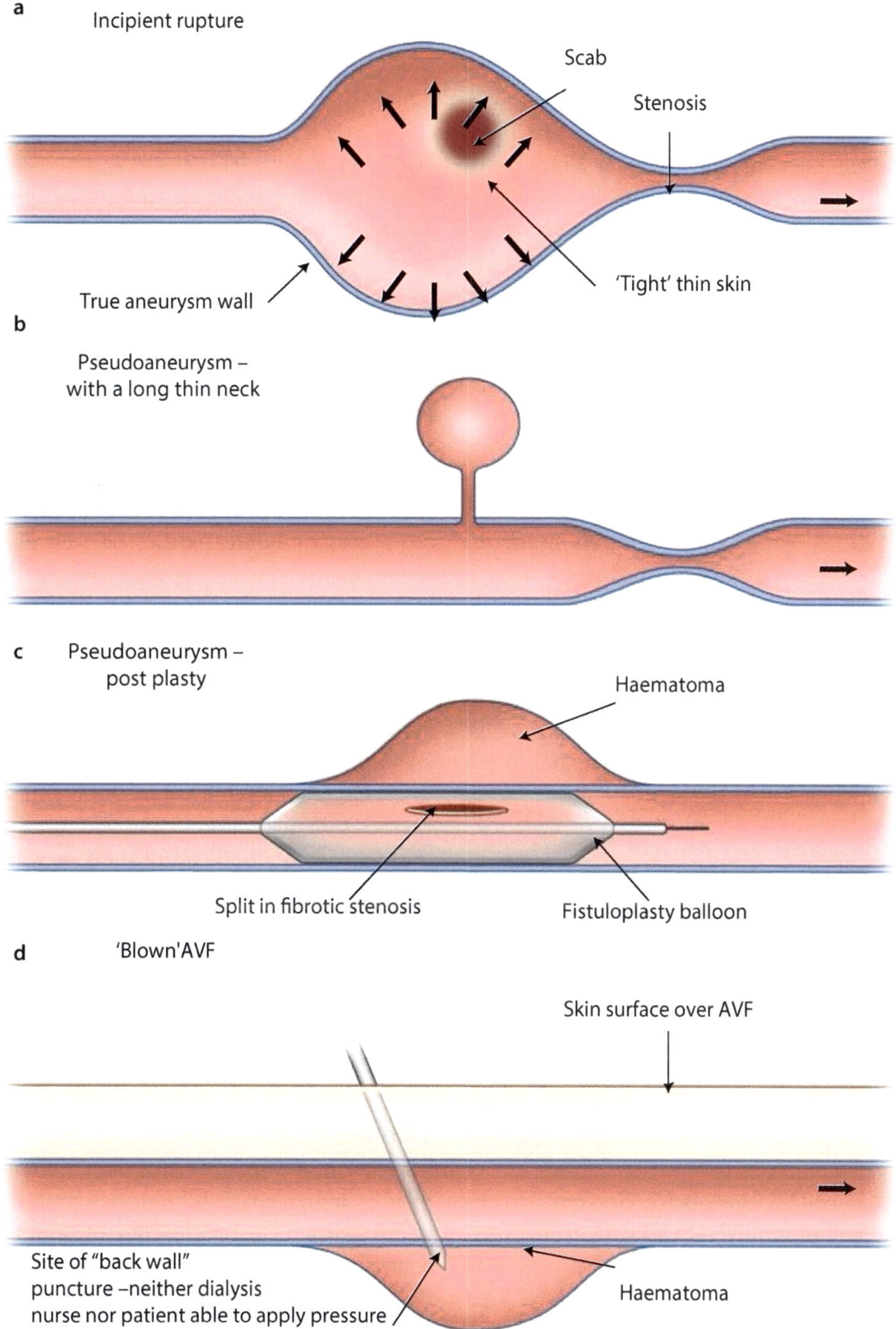

Fig. 78.8 Other AVF complications: **a** Incipient rupture in a true aneurysm, **b** pseudoaneurysm post HD cannulation, **c** pseudoaneurysm following fistuloplasty, **d** haematoma formation following inadvertent puncture of the posterior aspect of the AVF wall

78.3.3.2 Signs of Incipient AVF Bleed/Rupture

A serious clinical finding is a large black scab over an AVF aneurysm or needling site. These patients should be referred immediately to the vascular access team – night or day. It is important to make a surgeon take responsibility for this potentially life-threatening scenario. Options include AVF ligation, or if time allows, fistuloplasty to the downstream stenosis and then either rest or surgically fix the AVF. Surgical repair includes excising the scab as well as the surrounding unhealthy tissue. In practice, this means excision of a wedge or ellipse of skin and weak fistula wall before affecting a primary repair.

Extravasation of contrast during a fistuloplasty will be managed with reinflation of the balloon for a few minutes. If the leak fails to seal and there is increasing pain and swelling, a covered stent may be placed across the split.

Pseudoaneurysms often spontaneously thrombose once the downstream lesion is dealt with. In the presence of a long thin neck as shown in ◘ Fig. 78.8b, ultrasound-directed compression may work, and injection of thrombin may be tried. AVG pseudoaneurysms may be treated with stent grafts or surgical excision/ligation and interposition of a new AVG section.

Multiple aneurysms or large serpiginous fistulas may need surgical revision which may simply be replacement with a PTFE graft if the arterial inflow and venous outflow are satisfactory. Alternatively, the aneurysms themselves may be resected, the technical details of which are beyond the scope of this handbook. Other considerations for surgical referral include true aneurysms with thin, shiny, atrophic skin +/− ulceration, spontaneous bleeding, rapid increase in the size of the AV access, infection, limited section for cannulation and cosmetic appearances [46]. The emergency response to bleeds is very important. Patients should be aware of the potential for complications and resources are available to help patients, carers and staff to recognise warning signs. Further information can be found at the NHS Improvement site.

78.3.3.3 Central Venous Stenosis

Symptomatic central venous stenosis (CVS) should be suspected in patients with a history of CVC placement and the development of ipsilateral arm, breast, face or neck swelling and the development of collateral veins. Many patients with ipsilateral access will have dysfunctional AVF with reduced access flows potentially resulting in recirculation or aneurysmal development [47].

Treatment of CVS is based on limited data, and the options include conventional angioplasty, bare-metal stents (BMS) and covered stents.

Symptomatic central venous obstruction can also be managed surgically, commonly by vascular access ligation. However, managing the obstruction and retaining vascular access is also an option with the selective, judicious use of PTFE bridge grafts, although data is limited.

78.3.4 Surgical Solutions to Ischaemic Complications

78.3.4.1 Ischaemic Monomelic Neuropathy

This is a rare cause of immediate post-op pain following vascular access formation that involves surgery at the elbow. It is probably caused by damage or change to the blood flow to the median or ulna nerves. Despite the patient having a warm hand and radial pulse, the symptoms are similar to ischaemia. It is generally agreed that the best chance of reversing the proposed local neural ischaemia is to maximise flow into the forearm by immediately ligating the fistula with minimal dissection.

78.3.4.2 Steal Syndrome

Steal syndrome is an uncommon but important complication of access surgery, occurring in approximately 3–5% of all HD patients in the USA. Symptoms and signs of ischaemia develop if the AVF prevents sufficient arterial circulation from reaching the distal limb (hand/lower leg). Proximal AVF/G are more likely to steal because they comprise large calibre low- resistance veins. It is the artery/vein calibre mismatch that causes steal. This explains why it is more common in elbow rather than wrist fistulas, and in female patients with diabetes who have small arteries. Choice of anatomical site, awareness of comorbidities as well as minimising the brachial arteriotomy (4–5 mm) may reduce the likelihood of steal.

Four clinical stages of steal are recognised:

- Stage 1 tends to be mild with symptoms of coldness and possibly numbness being experienced from midway or towards the end of a dialysis session as circulating volume along with blood pressure start to fall.
- Stage 2 is the same as one but is experienced from the onset of the dialysis session.
- Stage 3 may render full dialysis sessions intolerable resulting predictably in greater intravascular volumes.
- Stage 4 is severe with ischaemic pain at rest off dialysis and may be complicated by digital necrosis. A diagnosis of stages 3 and 4 is confirmed not only with clinical examination but also with a digital pressure <50 mmHg or a digit/brachial index <0.6.

Management of Steal

Stages 1 and 2 may resolve over weeks or months and may be managed with analgesia and gloves. As well as vessel calibre mismatch, 20% of significant cases have been shown to be as a result of poor arterial inflow. Reduced arterial circulation (less than triphasic flow on duplex scanning) should lead to consideration of proximal arterial imaging to detect a treatable arterial stenosis. This reinforces the value of careful preoperative evaluation and the benefit of confirming triphasic flow on duplex scanning prior to theatre.

Surgical Treatments

◘ Figure 78.9a shows a BCF stealing blood from both the radial and ulnar arteries. The vein appears to be large compared to the artery. The simplest treatment is to ligate the AVF and start again at another site or revise it to make the diameter/length of the anastomosis smaller.

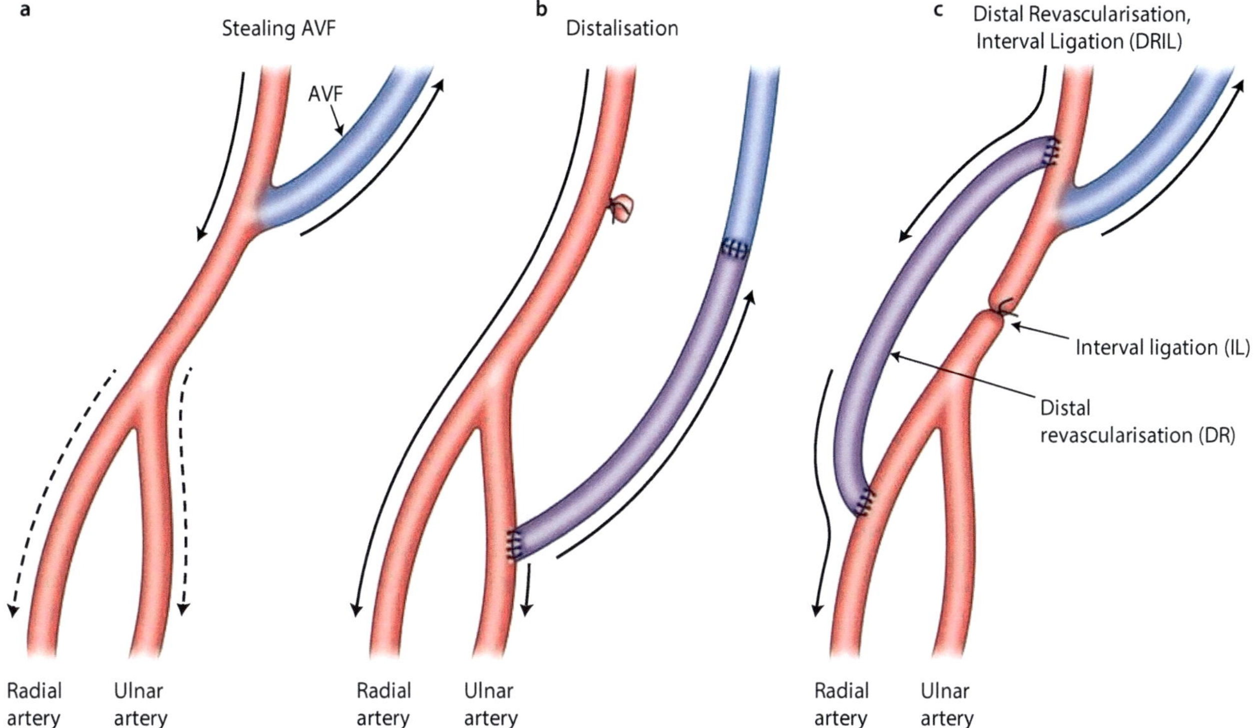

Fig. 78.9 Surgical techniques to manage steal syndrome: **a** AVF resulting in steal syndrome, **b** distalisation of the venous circulation, **c** distal revascularisation and interval ligation (DRIL)

Figure 78.9b demonstrates distalisation which can be done with either vein or a short externally supported graft. The origin of the fistula has been moved onto one of the forearm arteries 2–5 cm below the level of the elbow crease, in this case, the ulna artery.

Figure 78.9c illustrates the DRIL procedure. Distal revascularisation and interval ligation are often discussed but seldom undertaken.

The principle is the same as distalising the origin of the fistula in Fig. 78.9b by physically proximalising the arterial flow to the hand with the bypass graft (distal revascularisation). For this to work, there must be a reasonable distance between the new origin of the forearm blood flow and the origin of the fistula – probably 5 cm. Some surgeons believe that by ensuring this, the second part of the procedure, the interval ligation (IL) of the brachial artery, does not need to be done. If IL is not performed and symptoms persist, scanning will confirm retrograde flow stealing blood from the forearm arteries through the non-ligated brachial artery.

78.4 Conclusion

Definitive access is the cornerstone of optimal HD delivery. Obtaining AVF/AVG for the majority of our HD patients is a worthy, not necessarily elusive goal that is of paramount importance. Clinical examination and surveillance in combination with co-ordination and teamwork from vascular radiologists and surgeons are essential components in the maintenance of vascular access.

Important Learning Points

- 'Fistulas first, lines last' culture should resonate throughout the dialysis unit.
- Patient education regarding vascular access including the risk/benefits of AVF versus CVCs should begin at an early stage.
- Patients should be referred for vascular access in a timely fashion.
- It is recommended that AVFs are placed in the forearm if anatomically and technically possible.
- Once definitive access is created, monitoring is essential, and failing to mature AVF should be considered for endovascular intervention or surgical revision.
- AVF should be monitored and subject to surveillance. The suspicion of failing access should prompt consideration of endovascular intervention with angioplasty.
- Insufficient data exists to recommend agents for preventing access-related thrombosis.
- Reducing vascular access morbidity is time-consuming but rewarding and is associated with a

reduction in hospitalisations and mortality. Definitive vascular access provision requires communication and co-ordination amongst patients, dialysis unit staff, nephrologists, vascular radiologists, vascular surgeons and anaesthetists.

78

Chapter Review Questions

1. State the 'Rule of 6s' when applied to arteriovenous fistula (AVF) development
2. Given the greater diameter of vessels in the upper arm, it is advantageous to use more proximal veins first when creating vascular access.
3. Assisted patency does not have any benefit in AVF that fail to mature.
4. The needling technique of choice for arteriovenous grafts is button-hole.
5. Name the 4 grades of steal syndrome.

Answers

1. The ideal AVF for dialysis should be no more than 6 mm below the skin, have a blood flow of at least 600 ml/min and be 6 mm in diameter.
2. We believe this is false. Given the access that will be needed for a patient throughout their lifetime, it is very important that the forearm veins are utilised first wherever possible. In addition, steal tends to occur less frequently with the forearm vessels.
3. Assisted patency is beneficial in AVF that fail to mature but it is important to evaluate each occasion on individual merits. Endovascular and surgical options are available but local expertise and the risks vs benefits should be carefully considered.
4. This is false. It is vital that AVG are NEVER button-holed. This is because the button-hole would weaken the wall integrity and lead to rupture.
5. Stage 1 – symptoms of cool circulation towards the end of diaysis; stage 2- same as stage 1 but experienced at the onset of dialysis; stage 3- symptoms that preclude full dialysis resulting in reduced ultrafiltration and risk of fluid overload; stage 4- severe ischaemic pain even when not on dialysis and may manifest as digital necrosis.

Case Study

1. A young patient who presented late opted for PD but developed complications. A planned transition to HD was pursued and a RCF created. He became uraemic due to non-concordance and a decision had to be made whether to needle his 4 week old AVF or place a tunnelled line. What would you do?
   He underwent successful needling of his AVF and shortly after received a renal transplant.
2. An elderly patient aged 88, fit, active and independent opted for HD. He underwent successful AVF (BCF) surgery and is receiving good quality HD 3 years later.
3. A gentleman commenced HD via his R BCF. Due to needling difficulties, fistulography was performed and demonstrated a significant brachiocephalic stenosis which was successfully angioplastied. A week later, he presented with a very oedematous (non-pitting), erythematous, non-tender right arm. Repeat fistulography identified recurrent stenosis and a stent graft was deployed. 3 years on, the AVF is performing well. It is important to note that venous obstruction may cause erythema.

Acknowledgements With grateful thanks to Dr. Pete Bungay and Cathryn James for their help with preparing the manuscript, to our dedicated vascular access team for their ongoing hard work and attention to detail, and to our dialysis patients and staff for their participation in the pursuit of definitive vascular access.

References

1. Lacson E Jr, Wang W, Lazarus JM, Hakim RM. Change in vascular access and mortality in maintenance hemodialysis patients. Am J Kidney Dis. 2009;54(5):912–21.
2. Fluck R, Kumwenda M. Renal association clinical practice guide- line on vascular access for haemodialysis. Nephron Clin Pract. 2011;118(Suppl 1):c225–40.

3. Pisoni RL, Young EW, Dykstra DM, Greenwood RN, Hecking E, Gillespie B, Wolfe RA, Goodkin DA, Held PJ. Vascular access use in Europe and the United States: results from the DOPPS. Kidney Int. 2002;61(1):305–16.
4. Allon M, Robbin ML. Increasing arteriovenous fistulas in hemodi- alysis patients: problems and solutions. Kidney Int. 2002;62(4):1109–24.
5. Lok CE, Allon M, Moist L, Oliver MJ, Shah H, Zimmerman D. Risk equation determining unsuccessful cannulation events and failure to maturation in arteriovenous fistulas (REDUCE FTM I). J Am Soc Nephrol. 2006;17(11):3204–12.
6. Jennings WC, Landis L, Taubman KE, Parker DE. Creating func- tional autogenous vascular access in older patients. J Vasc Surg. 2011;53(3):713–9.
7. Olsha O, Hijazi J, Goldin I, Shemesh D. Vascular access in hemodialysis patients older than 80 years. J Vasc Surg. 2015;61(1):177–83.
8. Ko GJ, Rhee CM, Obi Y, Chang TI, Soohoo M, Kim TW, Kovesdy CP, Streja E, Kalantar-Zadeh K. Vascular access placement and mortality in elderly incident hemodialysis patients. Nephrol Dial Transplant. 2020;35(3):503–11.
9. Rehman R, Schmidt RJ, Moss AH. Ethical and legal obligation to avoid long-term tunneled catheter access. Clin J Am Soc Nephrol. 2009;4(2):456–60.
10. Xi W, Harwood L, Diamant MJ, Brown JB, Gallo K, Sontrop JM, MacNab JJ, Moist LM. Patient attitudes towards the arteriovenous fistula: a qualitative study on vascular access decision making. Nephrol Dial Transplant. 2011;26(10):3302–8.
11. Fissell RB, Fuller DS, Morgenstern H, Gillespie BW, Mendelssohn DC, Rayner HC, Robinson BM, Schatell D, Kawanishi H, Pisoni RL. Hemodialysis patient preference for type of vascular access: variation and predictors across countries in the DOPPS. J Vasc Access. 2013;14(3):264–72.
12. Yap HY, Pang SC, Tan CS, Tan YL, Goh N, Achudan S, Lee KG, Tan RY, Choong LH, Chong TT. Catheter-related complications and survival among incident hemodialysis patients in Singapore. J Vasc Access. 2018;19(6):602–8.
13. Guo A, Mujais S. Patient and technique survival on peritoneal dial- ysis in the United States: evaluation in large incident cohorts. Kidney Int Suppl. 2003;88:S3–12.
14. Wasse H, Speckman RA, McClellan WM. Arteriovenous fistula use is associated with lower cardiovascular mortality compared with catheter use among ESRD patients. Semin Dial. 2008;21(5):483–9.
15. III. NKF-K/DOQI clinical practice guidelines for vascular access: update 2000. Am J Kidney Dis. 2001;37(Suppl 1): S137–81.
16. Cooper BA, Branley P, Bulfone L, Collins JF, Craig JC, Fraenkel MB, Harris A, Johnson DW, Kesselhut J, Li JJ, Luxton G, Pilmore A, Tiller DJ, Harris DC, Pollock CA. IDEAL study. A random- ized, controlled trial of early versus late initiation of dialysis. N Engl J Med. 2010;363(7):609–19.
17. Aitken E, Thomson P, Bainbridge L, Kasthuri R, Mohr B, Kingsmore D. A randomized controlled trial and cost-effectiveness analysis of early cannulation arteriovenous grafts versus tunneled central venous catheters in patients requiring urgent vascular access for hemodialysis. J Vasc Surg. 2017;65(3):766–74.
18. Huijbregts HJ, Bots ML, Wittens CH, Schrama YC, Moll FL, Blankestijn PJ, ; CIMINO study group. Hemodialysis arteriove- nous fistula patency revisited: results of a prospective, multicenter initiative. Clin J Am Soc Nephrol 2008;3(3): 714–719.
19. Beathard GA, Settle SM, Shields MW. Salvage of the nonfunction- ing arteriovenous fistula. Am J Kidney Dis. 1999;33(5):910–6.
20. Sidawy AN, Spergel LM, Besarab A, Allon M, Jennings WC, Padberg Jr FT, Murad MH, Montori VM, O'Hare AM, Calligaro KD, Macsata RA, Lumsden AB, Ascher E, ; Society for Vascular Surgery. The Society for Vascular Surgery: clinical practice guide- lines for the surgical placement and maintenance of arteriovenous hemodialysis access. J Vasc Surg 2008;48(5 Suppl):2S–25.
21. Beathard GA, Arnold P, Jackson J, Litchfield T, ; Physician Operators Forum of RMS Lifeline. Aggressive treatment of early fistula failure. Kidney Int 2003;64(4):1487–1494.
22. Robbin ML, Chamberlain NE, Lockhart ME, Gallichio MH, Young CJ, Deierhoi MH, Allon M. Hemodialysis arteriovenous fistula maturity: US evaluation. Radiology. 2002;225(1):59–64.
23. Saran R, Dykstra DM, Pisoni RL, Akiba T, Akizawa T, Canaud B, Chen K, Piera L, Saito A, Young EW. Timing of first cannulation and vascular access failure in haemodialysis: an analysis of practice patterns at dialysis facilities in the DOPPS. Nephrol Dial Transplant. 2004;19(9):2334–40.
24. van Loon MM, Goovaerts T, Kessels AG, van der Sande FM, Tordoir JH. Buttonhole needling of haemodialysis arteriovenous fistulae results in less complications and interventions compared to the rope-ladder technique. Nephrol Dial Transplant. 2010;25(1):225–30.
25. Tessitore N, Bedogna V, Melilli E, Millardi D, Mansueto G, Lipari G, Mantovani W, Baggio E, Poli A, Lupo A. In search of an optimal bedside screening program for arteriovenous fistula stenosis. Clin J Am Soc Nephrol. 2011;6(4):819–26.
26. Vesely TM. Optimizing function and treatment of hemodialysis grafts and fistulae. Semin Intervent Radiol. 2004;21(2):95–103.
27. Mercadal L, Hamani A, Béné B, Petitclerc T. Determination of access blood flow from ionic dialysance: theory and validation. Kidney Int. 1999;56(4):1560–5.
28. Vascular Access 2006 Work Group. Clinical practice guidelines for vascular access. Am J Kidney Dis. 2006;48(Suppl 1): S176–247.
29. Swedberg SH, Brown BG, Sigley R, Wight TN, Gordon D, Nicholls SC. Intimal fibromuscular hyperplasia at the venous anastomosis of PTFE grafts in hemodialysis patients. Clinical, immunocytochemi- cal, light and electron microscopic assessment. Circulation. 1989;80(6):1726–36.
30. Martin LG, MacDonald MJ, Kikeri D, Cotsonis GA, Harker LA, Lumsden AB. Prophylactic angioplasty reduces thrombosis in vir- gin ePTFE arteriovenous dialysis grafts with greater than 50% ste- nosis: subset analysis of a prospectively randomized study. J Vasc Interv Radiol. 1999;10(4):389–96.
31. Moist LM, Churchill DN, House AA, Millward SF, Elliott JE, Kribs SW, DeYoung WJ, Blythe L, Stitt LW, Lindsay RM. Regular monitoring of access flow compared with monitoring of venous pressure fails to improve graft survival. J Am Soc Nephrol. 2003;14(10):2645–53.
32. Tessitore N, Mansueto G, Bedogna V, Lipari G, Poli A, Gammaro L, Baggio E, Morana G, Loschiavo C, Laudon A, Oldrizzi L, Maschio G. A prospective controlled trial on effect of percutaneous transluminal angioplasty on functioning arteriovenous fistulae sur- vival. J Am Soc Nephrol. 2003;14(6): 1623–7.
33. Tonelli M, Jindal K, Hirsch D, Taylor S, Kane C, Henbrey S. Screening for subclinical stenosis in native vessel arteriovenous fis- tulae. J Am Soc Nephrol. 2001;12(8):1729–33.

34. Tessitore N, Bedogna V, Poli A, Mantovani W, Lipari G, Baggio E, Mansueto G, Lupo A. Adding access blood flow surveillance to clinical monitoring reduces thrombosis rates and costs, and improves fistula patency in the short term: a controlled cohort study. Nephrol Dial Transplant. 2008;23(11):3578–84.
35. Aragoncillo I, Abad S, Caldés S, Amézquita Y, Vega A, Cirugeda A, Moratilla C, Ibeas J, Roca-Tey R, Fernández C, Macías N, Quiroga B, Blanco A, Villaverde M, Ruiz C, Martín B, Ruiz AM, Ampuero J, de Alvaro F, López-Gómez JMJ. Adding access blood flow surveillance reduces thrombosis and improves arteriovenous fistula patency: a randomized controlled trial. Vasc Access. 2017;18(4):352–8.
36. Chan KE, Pflederer TA, Steele DJ, Lilly MP, Ikizler TA, Maddux FW, Hakim RM. Access survival amongst hemodialysis patients referred for preventive angiography and percutaneous transluminal angioplasty. Clin J Am Soc Nephrol. 2011;6(11):2669–80.
37. Bittl JA. Venous rupture during percutaneous treatment of hemodi- alysis fistulas and grafts. Catheter Cardiovasc Interv. 2009;74(7):1097–101.
38. Bent CL, Rajan DK, Tan K, Simons ME, Jaskolka J, Kachura J, Beecroft R, Sniderman KW. Effectiveness of stent-graft placement for salvage of dysfunctional arteriovenous hemodialysis fistulas. J Vasc Interv Radiol. 2010;21(4):496–502.
39. Falk A, Maya ID, Yevzlin AS, RESCUE Investigators. A prospective, randomized study of an expanded polytetrafluoroethylene stent graft versus balloon angioplasty for in-stent restenosis in arteriovenous grafts and fistulae: two-year results of the RESCUE study. J Vasc Interv Radiol. 2016;27(10):1465–76.
40. Bent CL, Sahni VA, Matson MB. The radiological management of the thrombosed arteriovenous dialysis fistula. Clin Radiol. 2011;66(1):1–12.
41. Chan KE, Lazarus JM, Thadhani R, Hakim RM. Anticoagulant and antiplatelet usage associates with mortality among hemodialysis patients. J Am Soc Nephrol. 2009;20(4):872–81.
42. Coleman CI, Tuttle LA, Teevan C, Baker WL, White CM, Reinhart KM. Antiplatelet agents for the prevention of arteriovenous fistula and graft thrombosis: a meta analysis. Int J Clin Pract. 2010;64(9):1239–44.
43. Herrington W, Emberson J, Staplin N, Blackwell L, Fellström B, Walker R, Levin A, Hooi LS, Massy ZA, Tesar V, Reith C, Haynes R, Baigent C, Landray MJ, SHARP Investigators. The effect of lowering LDL cholesterol on vascular access patency: post hoc analysis of the Study of Heart and Renal Protection. Clin J Am Soc Nephrol. 2014;9(5):914–9.
44. Irish AB, Viecelli AK, Hawley CM, Hooi LS, Pascoe EM, Paul-Brent PA, Badve SV, Mori TA, Cass A, Kerr PG, Voss D, Ong LM, Polkinghorne KR, Omega-3 Fatty Acids (Fish Oils) and Aspirin in Vascular Access Outcomes in Renal Disease (FAVOURED) Study Collaborative Group. Effect of fish oil supplementation and aspirin use on arteriovenous fistula failure in patients requiring hemodialysis: a randomized clinical trial. JAMA Intern Med. 2017;177(2):184–93.
45. Labriola L, Crott R, Desmet C, André G, Jadoul M. Infectious com- plications following conversion to buttonhole cannulation of native arteriovenous fistulas: a quality improvement report. Am J Kidney Dis. 2011;57(3):442–8.
46. Shah R, Vachharajani TJ, Agarwal AK. Aneurysmal dilatation of dialysis arteriovenous access. Open Urol Nephrol J. 2013;6:1–5.
47. Kundu S. Central venous obstruction management. Semin Interv Radiol. 2009;26(2):115–21.

Additional Resources

MAGIC – Managing Access by Generating Improvements in Cannulation. Joint quality improvement project using the BRS and VASBI Clinical \Practice Recommendations for needling AVF and AVG for HD (thinkkidneys.nhs.uk).

Resources to support management of life threatening bleeds from arteriovenous fistulae and grafts (improvement.nhs.uk).

Vascular Access: Haemodialysis Catheters

Madhu Potluri, Dominic Yu, Justin Harris, and Jennifer Cross

Contents

M. Harber (ed.), *Primer on Nephrology*, https://doi.org/10.1007/978-3-030-76419-7_79

Learning Objectives
1. Indications for CVC catheters
2. Anatomical site selection and how to perform insertion of haemodialysis catheter
3. Complications of haemodialysis catheter
4. Haemodialysis catheter repair and removal
5. Indications for HeRO® Graft

79.1 Introduction

79

UK Renal Registry data suggests that approximately 20% of patients present to renal services with dialysis dependant renal failure without the opportunity to create timely native AV access. Many studies have drawn attention to the potentially serious complications associated with central venous dialysis catheters (CVC) [1]. These include the risk of thrombosis and infection septicaemia, deep-seated metastasis infection and central venous stenosis [2, 3].

Dialysis using a catheter is also associated with a lower survival than that with definitive AV access which was shown in the published 2009 DOPPS (Dialysis Outcomes and Practice Patterns Study) study by Pisoni et al. (20% mortality in facilities that had more than 20% catheter usage adjusted for case mix).

In addition, CVC access is associated with lower blood flow rates compared with fistulae or grafts [4, 5] and shorter access survival [6–9].

Haemodialysis catheters come in two basic forms, tunnelled and non-tunnelled or temporary. They are made of silicone and polyurethane with a polyester cuff designed to promote tissue growth to both fix and seal the catheter in the tunnel. A variety of coatings are now available on the surface of catheters designed to reduce infective complications and reduce clotting of lines including heparin, rifampicin, minocycline and silver or copper nanoparticles. All catheters have at least two ports, traditionally marked with a red and blue hub. The red or arterial port terminates at least 2 cm proximal and pulls blood from the patient, and the blue or venous port terminates distally and is used for the return of blood to the patient. The distance between the ends reduces direct return of blood between these two ports (recirculation). How long a catheter continues to function adequately with an effective blood pump of at least 300 mls/min is highly variable. The vast majority of dialysis catheters require some sort of intervention to maintain flow over a 12-month period and the majority of line failures relate to infection.

79.2 Preparation for Line Insertion

Patients should be prepared for line insertion with education describing the procedure they are about to undergo specifically discussing possible complications both short and long term including pain, haematoma, rarely pneumothorax or haemothorax. The National Kidney Federation (UK) provides a patient information leaflet (PIL) for central venous catheters and is a useful resource:

▶ http://www.kidney.org.uk/Medical-Info/haemodialysis/dialysis-line-insertion.html

In the United Kingdom, DOH guidance suggests that this information should be delivered by an individual who is trained in line insertion. All line insertion should be performed using strict aseptic technique (see infection chapter) with an assistant under direct vision using screening or ultrasound guidance to avoid insertion complications [1]. Additionally, all patients who have tunnelled haemodialysis catheter insertion must undergo *Staphylococcus aureus* screening, prior to insertion and eradication if found positive (see infection chapter). Alternatively, patients can be decolonised blindly, without screening, prior to catheter insertion; this may be particularly relevant for the acute presentations of end-stage renal failure. Approximately a third of patients with *S. aureus* septicaemia develop endocarditis, and approximately a third of these patients die, so having a robust process for screening or treating blindly is essential. Prophylaxis with antibiotics is not recommended for line insertion by the UK Renal Association as no benefit has been demonstrated on a review of current literature. A record of all line insertion and any complications or concerns should be made in the patient's medical record.

79.3 Catheter Selection

Tunnelled dialysis catheters have demanding requirements that exceed all other CVC including delivering volume flow of 300–400 mls/min at moderate pressure gradients without obstructing, minimizing trauma to the vein, resisting occlusion by biofilm/clot/ lumen collapse or kinking, prevention of infection, resistance to antiseptic agent deformation and radio-opacity for site confirmation.

- *Split-Cath_ III™ (Medcomp):* dual-lumen catheter with end and side ports
- *HemoSplit™ (bard access systems):* pre-curved dual lumen catheter with end and side ports
- *Tesio twin catheter (Medcomp):* two separate catheters, with end and side ports
- *Permcath™ (Quinton instruments):* dual-lumen catheter with end ports

There are many commercially available tunnelled dialysis catheters and a similar number of publications extolling the virtues of one catheter over another, but these data are conflicting. There is little compelling evidence that one dialysis catheter has significant advantage over others as evidenced by the variety that are currently in use in units around the world. In your choice of a dialysis catheter, you should consider whether its length is appropriate for the anatomical position (18 cm right internal jugular, 22 cm left internal jugular, to achieve a tip position at the confluence of the internal jugular and the right atrium, 28 cm for femoral approach, to achieve a tip position in the distal inferior vena cava). The longer, the narrower and the greater the bends in the path of a catheter, the lower the volume flow achieved. Invariably, right-sided internal jugular lines have better volume flows than left for those reasons. The true blood flow rate displayed on the dialysis blood pump is generally lower than the actual blood flow rate achieved partly because of negative pressure exerted as blood is sucked through using the rolling pump system that partially deforms the flexible catheter. This effect may reduce actual volume flow by as much as 25%, thus reducing dialysis efficiency. An elevated haematocrit will also have the effect of reducing effective volume flow by increasing viscosity and thus resistance to flow. Commercial line packs vary in the technical ease of insertion and the equipment that is included in the line pack. Many lines include features that may reduce infection rates (coating/nano-impregnation of silver or copper, heparin or even bismuth) features that reduce biofilm formation, antimicrobial hubs and the presence of subcutaneous cuffs [10]. Most catheters for chronic dialysis, both single and dual lumen, have side holes in addition to end holes. The position of the catheter holes is relevant to line flow rate and catheter dysfunction related to the formation of clots in addition to the migration of line locks and the development of biofilm for a review of the factors affecting line performance (for a review on the subject Ref Seminars in Dialysis Volume 21 issue 6 pg 503–590) [11].

79.4 Choosing a Tunnelled CVC Position (KDOQI vascular access guidelines 2006) [1]

Insertion positions are described in descending order of preference:

1. *The right internal jugular vein* is the optimal position for insertion of a tunnelled CVC catheter as there is a straight anatomical run from this position to the SVC/atrial confluence where the catheter tip should sit (figure of CXR with optimal position). This position minimises the risk of central vein stenosis (10%) [12].
2. *The left internal jugular vein* has a serpiginous course, and catheters tips commonly lie against the wall of the innominate vein/SVC which can intermittently occlude side and end ports resulting in poor dialysis flow rates; in addition, this position is also associated with higher rates of central vein stenosis and thrombosis [13].
3. *The femoral vein catheter insertion* is easily accessible, and a 28 cm line ought to be used to try and place the tip in the distal IVC as the calibre of the vessel increases as you ascend. Flow problems encountered in the first week of insertion in this position are commonly related to inadequate line length. Femoral tunnelled CVC are more likely to become infected (19.8% risk of bacteraemia [14]), and the risk of gram-negative/gut-related organisms is increased because of the proximity to the groin. During hip flexion/walking, femoral catheters kink/dislodge, and they have a higher failure rate in this position with an overall patency rate of approximately 2 months. Unwitnessed bleeding from end ports is a greater risk in femoral catheters as a result of the relatively hidden position, and DVT is common on the side of the catheter [15].
4. *Translumbar vein catheter insertion* should only be performed by specialist interventionalists. It is not a routine site of insertion as it is technically demanding, has a high early failure rate, is associated with a

poor flow and the risk of thrombosis extending to the IVC and has an increased risk of infection compared with upper body access [16].

5. *Transhepatic vein catheter insertion* should only be considered in a specialist centre where there is experience of this technique in this patient group. The technique utilises the hepatic venous sinus to gain entry to the venous drainage vessels to the IVC but requires a needle and Seldinger wire to be inserted through the liver tissue which is not uncommonly associated with significant bleeding. In a small series of transhepatic line insertion, 29% experienced a complication including intraperitoneal haemorrhage, catheter migration and catheter thrombosis [17].
6. *Intratrial catheter insertion* involves the direct insertion of a CVC under general anaesthesia into the right atrium) [18]. This technique is rarely used and should not be considered in centres that have not used this access in the past.
7. *Subclaviancatheter insertion* access is associated with the highest rate of stenotic complication at 50% and should be avoided where possible [19].

79

In the setting of Acute Kidney Injury intensive care units and multi-organ failure related to sepsis syndrome, you may require short-term vascular access. This should be placed with a full aseptic technique and does not require antibiotic prophylaxis.

The femoral vein is most commonly used for temporary access, and bleeding complications are less likely in this site; however, large unnoticed bleeds occur with insertion sites above the inguinal ligament where blood tracks back and upwards into the retroperitoneum and are not outwardly visible and may only become evident when the patient is hypotensive/shocked or develops an unexplained ileus. For an average adult, the minimum length of a femoral catheter should be 25 cm to ensure that the tip lies in the distal inferior vena cava [20].

This risk of infection which is more likely to be with a gram-negative organism rises exponentially after a period of 5 days of temporary access at the femoral site. In prescribing dialysis therapy, you should consider dialysing daily and replacing it with a permanent catheter if practicable. Alternatively, femoral temporary catheters should be removed electively at day 5, and careful consideration should be given to prophylactic heparin to avoid deep vein thrombosis which is increased in hospital patients and still further in those with femoral access. Thereafter, the right internal jugular and left internal jugular are used, and the external jugular and subclavian routes should be avoided.

79.5 Catheter Insertion Procedure (See Video on Line Insertion)

Catheters are inserted using the Seldinger technique of needle followed by a curve ended guidewire. Insert link for Justins DVD of catheter insertion. The straight end of the guidewire should not be used to guide the catheter as it is associated with an increased risk of mediastinal trauma and atrial puncture than the curved wire tip which is designed for the purpose and is much softer. The catheter tip should be at least at the caval/atrial junction to ensure adequate blood flow. Positioning the line tip deep within the atria may be associated with irritation of the mitral valve and result in atrial and ventricular tachyarrhythmias. Temporary dialysis catheters tend to be more rigid than tunnelled catheters and are associated with an increased risk of vein and atrial trauma, so atrial placement of temporary catheters should therefore be avoided.

The position of all lines inserted into the thorax should be checked by screening or chest X-ray prior to use to ensure that the line has been correctly inserted into the vein and advanced adequately, to confirm there are no kinks and exclude haemo- or pneumothorax or pneumomediastinum all of which are rare but accepted complications of line insertion. Though tunnelled lines are fixed in position by the subcutaneous cuff and two hub stitches initially, line tip retraction is common when patients move from the horizontal to the vertical position immediately after insertion, and a perfect tip position while supine may require advancement when vertical making a CXR or fluoroscopic imaging while standing invaluable, so this can be corrected before line use. If a line has inadvertently been placed in an arterial position, do not use the line, and do not remove the line without consulting a surgeon who may be required to control bleeding after line removal. The cause of a newly placed catheter failing to deliver adequate flow in the first week is usually related to a malposition, too short, too long, the proximity of side holes against a vein wall with 'sucking' or a clot in the lumen because of inadequate locking at the time of placement or after use. Dialysis catheters tend to 'prove' or harden after insertion in the first 48 h, and not uncommonly, the line may have a poor volume flow during the first dialysis session only to settle subsequently with no specific intervention. Distinguishing these catheter problems is not possible without a chest X-ray.

79.6 Complications of Catheter Insertion

The large bore of dialysis catheters and the coagulopathy associated with renal failure increase the probability and potential consequences of trauma to the vein; inadvertent arterial puncture, massive extravasation of blood or mediastinal or right atrial perforation is greater. These risks are associated with the introducer, wire, tissue expander and line itself. If an introducer needle is placed in an artery, this should be obvious in all but the most shocked and hypoxic patients but processing a sample for blood gas analysis if there is doubt can be helpful. The needle should be removed and direct finger pressure placed on the access site for 10 min. Insertion of access into the external jugular vein rather than the internal increases the probability of lacerating the subclavian vein particularly with the more rigid temporary catheters because of the 90-degree angle of incidence at the confluence and should thus generally be avoided. Unwitting insertion of a line into an artery can result in massive neck, thoracic, or retroperitoneal bleeding. In such an event, the catheter should not be used or locked and a vascular surgeon should be consulted before removal as bleeding is often a greater issue after removal than at the time of insertion. Any CVC insertion can result in a haemothorax and the development of a new ipsilateral pleural effusion soon after line placement with SOB ought to alert you to the possibility of a haemothorax from a catheter malplacement and communication into the mediastinum. Finally, air embolus, though rare, is more common during the insertion of dialysis catheters because of their greater calibre. This can be avoided by placing the line with a patient in a head-down position, ensuring that during the line insertion that the clamps on the ports are sealed, asking the patient to slowly breathe out during line insertion and passage of the introducer sheath. Finally, during difficult CVC insertion, where multiple attempts have been made to site the line, it is possible to cannulate both artery and vein creating an artificial communication between the two resulting in a fistulous communication. This can result in a bruit over the area and aneurysmal dilatation of the vessel. This can usually be rectified using occlusion devices such as Amplatz wires, onyx or thrombin instillation. Occasionally, a formal surgical procedure may be required.

79.7 Catheter Locks

At the end of each dialysis session, both arterial and venous ports are locked with an anticoagulant/antimicrobial which is designed to prevent thrombus or fibrin formation [1].

The ideal lock solution should prevent line occlusion, not migrate from the line lumen to the systemic circulation and resist planktonic organisms and sessile organisms existing in a biofilm.

It is important, given its frequent use that it is safe, relatively low in cost and simple to use. Currently, there are a variety of catheter locks (citrate, taurolidine, low-dose gentamicin, heparin), but there is insufficient data to compare different strategies for optimal approach, and therefore, larger randomised controlled trials in haemodialysis population are required.

In the inter-dialytic period, inevitably, some of the anticoagulant is lost in equilibrium with blood; this is greatest with dense locking agents such as 46% citrate. This equilibration occurs soon after the line lock is placed [21]. The anticoagulant lost is replaced by blood and its clotting factors potentially resulting in thrombosis of the catheter tip and catheter dysfunction eventually culminating in occlusion [1].

If the catheter is in the superior vena cava, this increases the risk of fibrin deposition and tip thrombosis. Line manipulation may be possible to place the line tip caval/atrial junction or beyond into the right atrium [22]. There is little evidence to suggest that using thrombolytics as a lock contributes to medium-term resolution of a dysfunctional catheter as the thrombolytic effect is limited to the interior of the lumen and will not disrupt either biofilm or external ball valve clot, and therefore, its expense in regular use cannot be justified.

The current practice in our centre is to use a 46% concentrated citrate solution as a lock and to salvage occluded catheters using alteplase (t-PA) 8 mg as an online infusion via the heparin infusion device into the venous trap before the kidney which has the advantage of low relative cost, a longer duration of action and greater efficacy compared with other agents [23, 24].

Exclusion Criteria for t-PA Infusion

- Bleeding diathesis
- History of active peptic ulceration (<3 months)
- CVA/TIA
- Recent haemorrhage or surgery (<7 days)
- Untreated proliferative diabetic nephropathy

Techniques for fibrin or thrombus removal that have gone out of favour recently are the endoluminal catheter brush [25]. This device can be inserted, gently up to the tip of the catheter and slightly beyond. On gentle withdrawal, any fibrin may be dislodged enough to improve blood flow through the catheter [25].

Failure of the measures, described so far, to restore adequate blood flow should prompt review of the need for line exchange. Exchange in the same position over a wire can result in the new line following the path of the previously established fibrin sheath and may result in a rapid return of line dysfunction. The general experience of other salvage techniques such as line stripping or thrombectomy have been largely unsuccessful and are associated with an increased risk of infection and are not commonly practised in our institution. There is little evidence that anticoagulation with coumarin-based agents is the mechanism of obstruction in infrequently simple thrombin mediated clot production, and there is substantial evidence of an augmented bleeding risk in dialysis dependant patients, and the practice is not recommended.

79.8 Catheter Complications

Catheters are associated with various complications due to long-term use (>3 weeks), such as catheter-related bacteraemia, occlusion secondary to fibrin or thrombus, central vein stenosis or catheter extrusion.

The frequency and severity of complications are dependent on the frequency of catheter insertions and duration of dwell time.

79.9 Catheter Occlusion

Catheters may be occluded in various ways [1]:

1. Intraluminal occlusion by thrombus which may cause partial or complete occlusion and usually results from failure to completely exclude blood from the lumen at the time of locking (wrong lock volume, failure to flush with online fluid or saline prior to lock, failure to fully clamp lines prior to lock, ingress of blood as a result of inter-dialytic lock migration).
2. Catheter tip thrombus of fibrin at the tip may cause complete occlusion or act like a ball valve.
3. Fibrin sheath (sleeve): fibrin adheres to the external surface of the catheter, thrombus trapped between sheath and catheter tip.
4. Fibrin tail (fibrin flap): fibrin adheres to CVC end causing 'ball valve' effect.
5. Mechanical bend or kink can be identified on a chest X-ray and is often an early cause of catheter malfunction.
6. Catheter migration is common in obese individuals or those with large abdomens or chests.

Catheter dysfunction as a result of partial or complete occlusion is common. In general, this is manifest as poor blood flow, increased line arterial or venous pressure, deteriorating clearance and increased recirculation see table below. Luminal clots can often be managed if identified early by a high pressure flush using a very small syringe (small surface area plunger means that the small fluid volume is ejected with greater force and can be more effective in dislodging a small luminal clot than a 20 mls syringe. First, check that the line has not moved or been kinked since insertion, by inspecting the line, looking for an externalised cuff. Perform a chest X-ray to confirm there are no kinks and identify the position of the line tip. If these are in place, then it is likely that the line has developed a clot or a biofilm. Thrombosis of a dialysis catheter can either be within the lumen of the line, encircling the external surface of the line, mural and adherent to the wall of the vessel or a ball of clot adherent to the tip acting as a ball valve occluding the line during aspiration. Clots on lines are probably much more common than we realize and often give rise to no clinically evident problems. The incidence of pulmonary embolus as a result of line thrombosis appears low, and the greater risk is associated with an infected clot which may result in mycotic pulmonary emboli. Clots can be delineated using Doppler ultrasound in many cases or echocardiography in the case of the right atrial clots or using digital subtraction angiography. Management of an incidentally identified large ball clot (>2 cm) in the right atrium attached to the line tip while investigating line dysfunction is unclear from the literature. A reasonable approach is to remove the line and consider the risk-benefit ratio of systemic anticoagulation for 6 months and repeat echocardiography to monitor the size and stability of the thrombus at an interval of 1 week. The safety and efficacy of thrombolytics in this setting are unclear. In the setting of significant bleeding risk, some patients have been managed with thrombectomy rather than anticoagulation.

A biofilm often forms in and around the catheter starting at the hub and progressing down the length of the line. Biofilm is produced by the interaction of microbial glycocalyx with fibrin, fibronectin and extracellular polysaccharides [1]. This does not usually happen overnight and nursing staff have often identified these problems for days or weeks before the line fails completely so it typically affects the more proximal venous/blue lumen before the arterial/red giving rise to the observation that the lines had to be 'reversed' on dialysis sessions for a period prior to failure of line volume flow. If you suspect a biofilm or clot/thrombus, then this can be disrupted using a thrombolytic. You can either infuse the thrombolytic systemically in 20 ml of saline throughout the dialysis session using the heparin syringe driver. Alternatively, arrange for a day case admission to administer the drug down each lumen over 4 h. Both appear to be efficacious and safe [26].

Thrombolytics are contraindicated in patients with a bleeding diathesis, recent haemorrhagic stroke, recent surgery, proliferative retinopathy or malignant hypertension.

Signs of Catheter Dysfunction

- *Blood flow rate <300 ml/min*
- *Arterial pressure <−250 mmHg*
- *Venous pressure >250 mmHg*
- *Conductance <1.2 (ratio of blood pump flow to the value of prepump pressure)*
- *URR <65% or KT/V <1.2*
- *Unable to aspirate blood freely (late sign)*
- *Frequent pressure alarms (not responsive to patient repositioning or catheter flushing)*

79.10 Catheter Infection

Line infection is the most common and potentially most important complication of a long-term dialysis catheter. Catheter-related infection is one of the commonest reasons for access loss. (See access related infection Chap. 77.)

Catheters may be colonized by bacteria soon after insertion [27], and bacteria commonly colonise the catheter hub, and colonisation of the catheter or the relatively immunologically shielded catheter biofilm results in apparent bacterial resistance to systemic antimicrobial therapy [28].

At the first sign of a local exit-site infection characterised by redness, tenderness and discharge, the wound should be swabbed, and empiric flucloxicillin 500 mg PO QDS should be given for 10 days. If MRSA +ve, then IV vancomycin as per local policy should be given for three sessions according to levels (15–20). Antibiotics should be modified in light of culture results.

Exit-site infection if treated late or inadequately can progress to involve the tunnel. This is associated with neovascularisation of the tunnel wall which may be detected with ultrasound scan and is a reliable sign of tunnel infection and precedes abscess formation. The presence of a tunnel infection requires parenteral antibiotics (such as vancomycin or gentamicin with levels). Line removal should be considered if this has not settled after 14 days of antibiotics or if it recurs after cessation of antibiotics or if the organism at the exit site is a pseudomonas or yeast or other slime former with a predilection for plastic [1].

Although bacteraemia may result from the progression of an exit-site infection, to involve the tunnel and progress to systemic bacteraemia with circulating organisms, specific line related bacteraemia can occur in the absence of symptoms. The commonest organisms identified are skin commensals such as coagulase-negative staphylococci (CNS) and *Streptococcus viridans*. In a dialysis patient with a line in situ who has no obvious chest or abdominal complaint, then it is reasonable to assume that fever even in the absence of an exit site or tunnel infection represents systemic bacteremia related to the line. The exit site should be swabbed, blood cultures and CRP should be taken, and empiric antibiotics should be administered according to the likely culprit. We use flucloxicillin 1 g QDS and gentamicin (MRSA negative) and vancomycin and gentamicin (MRSA +ve). Line removal is essential in the event of *S. aureus*, *Candida albicans* and *Pseudomonas* species as the line is unlikely to be cleared and will act as a reservoir of organisms. The longer the line is left in situ, the greater the risk of metastatic deep-seated infective complications. In an uncomplicated infection with an indolent organism, parenteral treatment should continue for a minimum of 14 days. If the CRP fails to fall or there is persistent bacteraemia in the face of sensitive antibiotics it suggests, there is either a deep-seated infection (discitis, endocarditis, osteomyelitis, paraspinal, psoas or other abscess are the most common) or that the catheter is colonised and should be replaced. Investigations should be tailored to the clinical situation. Deep-seated infection often declares itself. Ask patients if they have back pain, are breathless or have other sites of pain to focus the hunt for deep-seated infection and remember to identify any old PTFE access still in situ. Investigations to consider are CXR, TTE, complement, rheumatoid factor, MRI back which is much more sensitive than plain X-ray or CT in detecting discitis.

79.11 Central Vein Stenosis

Endothelial injury occurs with recurrent short-term central venous catheter placements [29, 30], over time, the vein wall thickens and is invaded by smooth muscle cells, and collagen accumulates with overlying thrombus [31].

Central vein stenosis is defined as 50% narrowing of the diameter of the vessel and is more common in patients of African or Caribbean origin. [31]

Most frequently, it can cause massive head and neck swelling and upper limb or breast oedema rendering the subsequent creation of definitive access in the upper body difficult.

Additional symptoms or signs may include [31]:

- Pleural effusion [32]
- Venous collateral formation (upper chest, neck, shoulder and upper arm) [31]
- Increased risk of infection [31]
- Thrombosis of AVF [15]
- Increasing length of time to establish haemostasis post dialysis (possible central or peripheral venous stenosis
- Headaches
- Nose bleeds

Central vein stenosis is most prevalent at these sites in descending order:

- Subclavian vein (up to 50% [19] due to direct injury to vein due to anatomical curvature of the junction between subclavian, inominate and superior vena cava [6]).
- Left internal jugular vein (due to complex anatomy with several angulations in its course and due to overlying structures such as brachiocephalic artery and aorta which can cause extrinsic compression, this route is not preferred [31]).
- Right internal jugular vein (approximately 10% [12, 13]).

Stenosis can be functional due to the catheter itself contributing to the reduction of lumen diameter and removal can resolve symptoms this is often temporary, however.

79.12 Investigations

If symptoms of superior vena cava obstruction and/or swelling of the unilateral arm become apparent, then the patient should undergo a magnetic resonance venogram to confirm the diagnosis if this is available. Ultrasound scan is usually unhelpful as the views of the deep thoracic great veins are impaired by the overlying anterior thoracic cage. However, a normal polyphasic atrial waveform on the duplex excludes the possibility of central venous stenosis of greater than 80% [33].

Fluroscopic venography is useful if an interventional procedure with venoplasty is planned. In general, the use of venous stents is discouraged as they frequently obstruct with clot and if a line is required through them, the incidence of SVC stent colonisation is high.

79.13 Management of Central Vein Stenosis

Not all >50% stenotic lesions [31] require intervention. Only consider intervention if the patient is symptomatic or dialysis adequacy is impaired [31, 34] (see ◘ Fig. 79.1).

Lesions commonly progress and the management is percutaneous central venoplasty without a stent [1, 31] (see ◘ Fig. 79.1). These lesions tend to be recurrent, and repeat percutaneous venoplasty is required between 3 and 6 months [35, 36].

In 2006, the K/DOQI guidelines recommended that stent placement should be considered if there is acute elastic recoil of the vein (which had greater than 50 per cent stenosis) after angioplasty [31], or if there is recurrent stenosis within a 3-month period post-angioplasty [31].

Surgery is reserved as the last resort for recurrent stenosis or severe head and neck oedema with respiratory embarrassment. This approach requires bypassing the occluded segment to the atrium [37] or ipsilateral femoral vein via tunnelled subcutaneous graft [38]. Additionally, as a final measure, if the patient has an ipsilateral ateriovenous fistula, it can be occluded to rapidly relieve symptoms [31].

79.13.1 HeRO® Graft (Merit Medical)

The HeRO® (Haemodialysis Reliable Outflow) graft has been developed over the last 10 years for patients with severe central vein stenosis who have exhausted all other access.

It is viable long-term access for haemodialysis that benefits patients with unsuitable venous anastomosis points, by crossing a stenosed central vein. It is composed of polytetrafluoroethylene graft anastomosed to a peripheral artery, e.g. brachial at one end and a titanium hub which joins a silicone tube which sits in the right atrium. It can be then used after a suitable healing period just like any AV Graft by inserting dialysis needles.

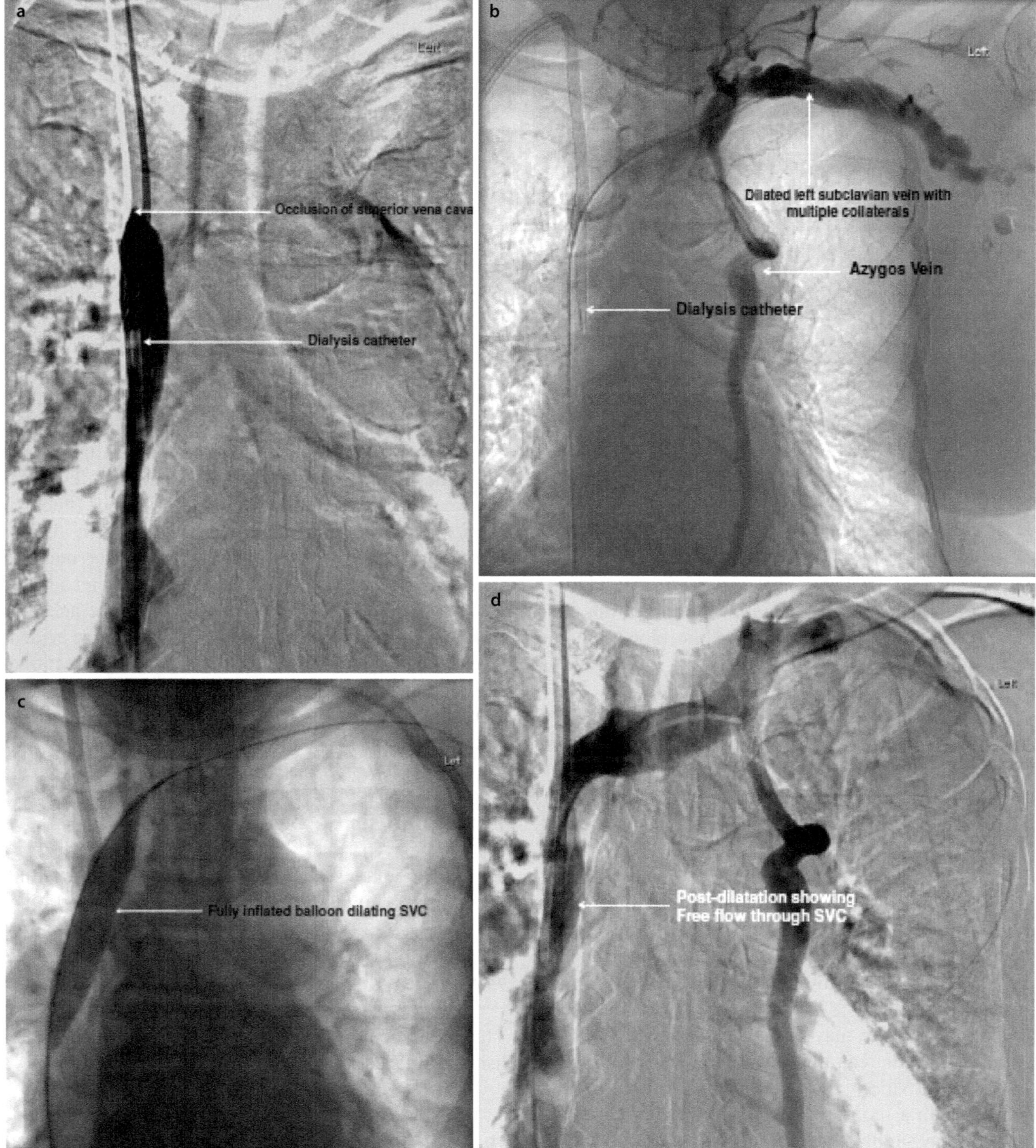

◻ **Fig. 79.1** **a** Central venogram from the femoral route showing complete occlusion of the superior vena cava (SVC) in a patient with a right internal jugular dialysis line complaining of marked facial swelling and headaches worse on wakening **b** guidewire and a catheter having crossed the obstruction radiocontrast dye fails to pass into the SVC but outlines the grossly enlarged azygous vein, **c** dilatation by 10 mm balloon across SVC stenosis, **d** post-dilatation flow through SVC with symptomatic relief, **e** MRV in a patient with SVC stenosis and failed attempts at internal jugular line insertion

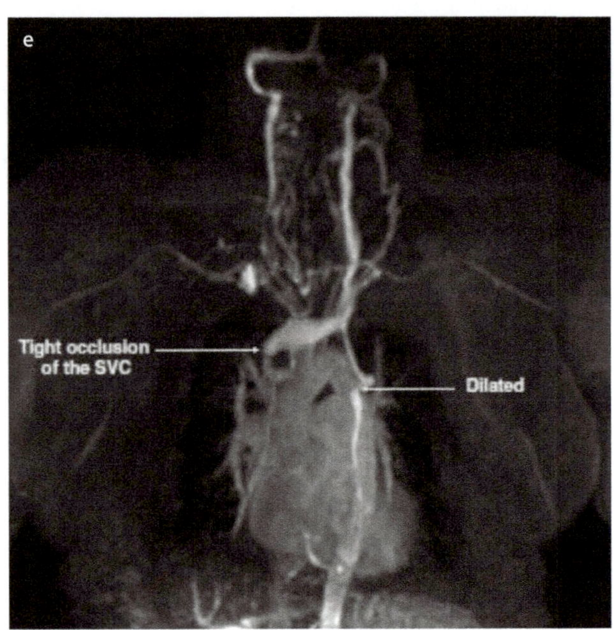

79

▣ **Fig. 79.1** (continued)

Patient factors that enable success for the HeRO® graft are brachial artery diameter >3 mm, cardiac ejection fraction of >20% and a systolic blood pressure >100 mmHg.

79.14 Removal of Haemodialysis Catheters

Removal of a venous dialysis catheter may be necessary because definitive access has been created and reliably used for 14 days, of line-associated sepsis, a tunnel infection or an exit-site infection that has failed to resolve despite 10–14 days of an appropriate antibiotic or finally a proximal line leak. In the setting of *S. aureus* bacteraemia, the removal of the catheter is an emergency and should be achieved without delay to reduce the risk of metastatic seeding.

This procedure may be undertaken in a treatment room in a ward area rather than in a theatre setting (see line removal video). New CVC that has been in place for less than a month or in which a tunnel infection is present may simply be removed by gentle pulling as the cuff may not be adherent to surrounding tissues. If any resistance is met, then a formal skin incision with cuff exposure and dissection as demonstrated in the attached video clip will be required. The critical point is to be aware at all times identifying, occluding and keeping hold of the proximal line portion preferably with a pair or arterial clamps during removal to avoid retraction of the open line inside the patient risking air embolus, haemorrhage and line loss into circulation all of which are recorded.

79.15 Dialysis Catheter Repair

The catheter may become extruded and is defined as cuff being visible outside of the tunnel and commonly occurs because the cuff or tunnel has been colonised with bacteria or there is a low-grade tunnel infection. Unfortunately, this cannot be repaired and attempts to replace the catheter in the tunnel are likely to be associated with a tunnel infection and potentially an episode of septicaemia. Patients with an extruded cuff should receive a single dose of parenteral antibiotics (flucloxicillin/vancomycin and gentamicin), they can dialyse through the line, and arrangements should be made to remove the line and replace it with a new catheter, ideally, in a new tunnel. Catheters may be damaged, cracked or split or dilated and leak which may only become evident when the catheter is in use, which poses a bidirectional contamination risk. This may be repaired if the split is 4.5 cm distal to the hub in the extension pieces (see Catheter Repair Procedure Video).

79.16 Dialysis Catheter Insertion

This video demonstrates the preparation and procedure of an internal jugular tunnelled dialysis line insertion.

79.17 Dialysis Catheter Removal

This video demonstrates the safe removal of an established tunnelled dialysis line.

79.18 Dialysis Catheter Repair

This video demonstrates the technique for repairing a split dialysis catheter.

Case Study

Case 1

An 80-year-old male needed left-sided access due to stenosis in the right internal jugular vein. Tunnelled line inserted in radiology (fluoroscopy), using the Seldinger method and screening. Guidewire was inserted via left internal jugular into the brachiocephalic trunk and then what was thought to be the upper SVC/RA. At this point, the patient developed some mild chest discomfort but was maintaining oxygenation at 98% at room air.

A left-sided haemodialysis catheter was inserted. The patient then complained of severe chest pain with radiation to the interscapular region and became haemodynamically unstable.

It became apparent that the patient had developed a haemo-pneumothorax and had to undergo an urgent chest drain. It became evident, with further screening, that the guidewire initially perforated the SVC creating a small deficit which was further enlarged by the large bore dilator which was fully inserted into the left internal jugular vein.

He was then transferred to a cardiothoracic unit where the dialysis catheter was removed in the operating room.

This case illustrates just how easy it can be to do harm to the patient if simple rules of the technique of haemodialysis catheter insertion are not followed. The guidewire should never be forced through a vein and instead should glide through with minimal effort; additionally, the large bore dilator and peel-away sheath should never be inserted beyond a few cm (<3 cm) into a central vein.

Case 2

A woman who presented with acute renal failure had a 20 cm femoral haemodialysis catheter insertion for acute haemodialysis. On day 5, the catheter was exchanged over the guidewire and continued to be used for 48 h till experiencing line-flow problems which necessitated a new femoral catheter. Once again, the catheter was exchanged over the guidewire.

Over the next few days, the patient experienced right-sided posterior headaches, and on CT imaging, a radio-opaque object was identified in the right sigmoid sinus. A plain CXR showed guidewire in the right internal jugular vein entering the cranium. The patient then required interventional radiology to retrieve the displaced/migrated guidewire and the headaches resolved.

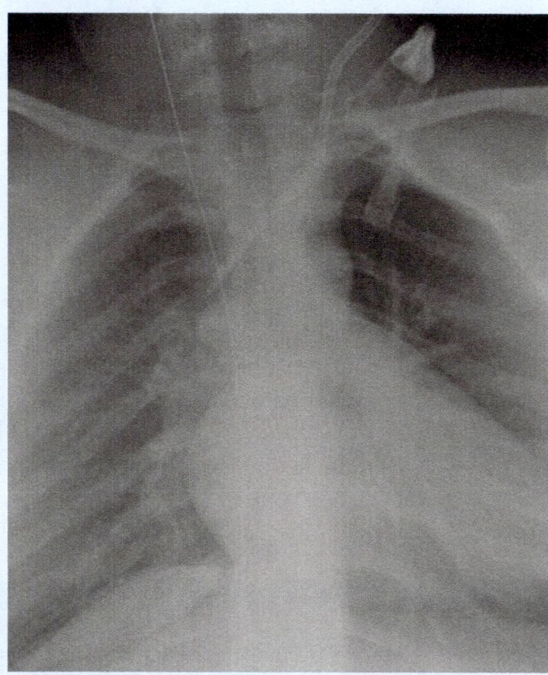

This 'Never Event' illustrates it is critical to ensure that (a) there is plenty of wire beyond the dilator or line when the dilator or line is being introduced to ensure the wire is not pushed in, which can easily happen particularly if there is rapid venous bleeding when the dilator is removed and the line is being introduced rapidly. (b) Needles and guidewire should be accounted for at the end of each procedure; if the guidewire is retained, then this needs to be identified and a management plan agreed with interventional radiology and vascular surgery.

Case 3

A 45-year-old dialysis patient on anticoagulation who declined fistula formation presented with recurrent chest infections characterised by minor haemoptysis, sputum and raised inflammatory markers. Each episode settled with 7–10 day courses of antibiotics but recurred within a short period thereafter. His chest X-rays were consistent with right upper lobe infection but otherwise not remarkable.

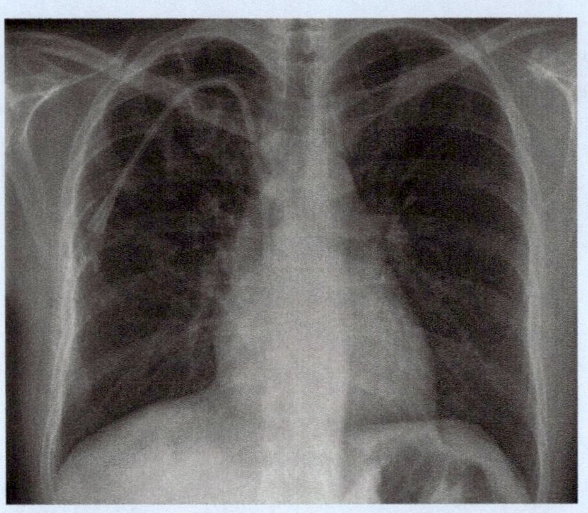

A CT chest demonstrated multiple cavitating lesions (arrowed) consistent (and a large pleural effusion) with infected pulmonary emboli with the line as the source.

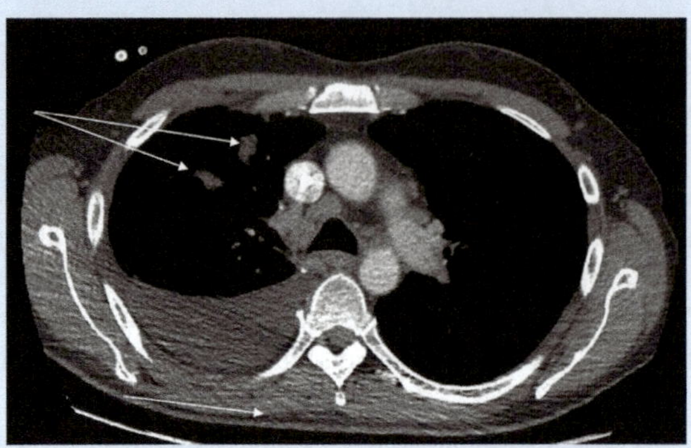

A fistula was created and used within 3 weeks, and the lines were removed under prolonged antibiotic cover.

There are several reasons for recurrent/persistent chest infections, but in a dialysis patient with lines, a high index of suspicion of infected pulmonary emboli is warranted if a chest infection is slow to resolve or recurs despite an 'adequate' course of antibiotics.

Tips

- Ensure guidewire is free moving whilst dilating the internal jugular/femoral vein to reduce complication.
- Do not insert more than 13 cm of the guidewire into the internal jugular to avoid complications such as perforation of the atrium and SVC.
- Do not insert a large-bore dilator and peel away the sheath fully to the hilt into the vein as this runs a high risk of vein rupture. Instead, only a few centimetres of dilator should be inserted into the vein to allow passage of peel-away sheath into vein uninterrupted.
- Use Tesio twin catheters for femoral tunnelled line insertion and tunnel onto the anterior abdominal wall to avoid infection complications, although the patient must be counselled for DVT as a complication.

79.19 Conclusion

Haemodialysis catheters offer a temporary but safe method of providing access for haemodialysis, provided a few simple rules are followed in the technique of insertion and removal by a skilled operator. They are temporary by their nature and are a bridge towards definitive access.

Chapter Review Questions

1. What are the signs of dialysis catheter dysfunction?
2. What is the commonest cause of catheter loss?
3. What reasons are there for a failure of resolution of infection on treating line-related sepsis?
4. What concerns are there in placing a temporary dialysis line for a renal transplant recipient with AKI?

Answers

1. Poor outflow and inflow (i) blood flow rate <300 ml/min, (ii) arterial pressure <−250 mmHg.
   (iii) Venous pressure >250 mmHg, (iv) unable to aspirate blood freely, (v) low ratio of blood pump flow to prepump pressure (conductance ratio <1.2).
   (vi) URR <65% or KT/V <1.2.
   (vii) Frequent pressure alarms (not responsive to patient repositioning or catheter flushing).
2. Infection is the Achilles heel of dialysis lines.
3. Apart from the certainty of knowing that the correct antibiotic is being administered, the commonest cause for relapse is a deep-seated infection. This can be almost anywhere but endocarditis and pacing wire infection, discitis or prosthesis infection, infected embolus such as displaced fibrin sheath or line embolus. The latter may present initially as a chest infection with an under impressive CXR.

4. Avoid and alert ICU teams to avoid placing the catheter on the same side as the transplant because of the risk of causing a DVT involving the transplanted vein.

References

1. KDOQI Vascular Access Guidelines 2006.
2. Caruana RJ, Raja RM, Zeit RM, Goldstein SJ, Kramer MS. Thrombotic complications of indwelling central catheters used for chronic hemodialysis. Am J Kidney Dis. 1987;9: 497–501.
3. Bander SJ, Schwab SJ. Central venous angioaccess for hemodialysis and its complications. Semin Dial. 1992;5:121–8.
4. Depner TA. Catheter performance. Semin Dial. 2001;14(6): 425–31.
5. Atherikul K, Schwab SJ, Twardowski ZJ, et al. What is the role of permanent central vein access in hemodialysis patients? Semin Dial. 1996;9:392–403.
6. Fan PY, Schwab SJ. Vascular access: concepts for the 1990s. J Am Soc Nephrol. 1992;3:1–11.
7. Windus DW. Permanent vascular access: a nephrologist's view. Am J Kidney Dis. 1993;21:457–71.
8. Suhocki PV, Conlon PJ Jr, Knelson MH, Harland R, Schwab SJ. Silastic cuffed catheters for hemodialysis vascular access: thrombolytic and mechanical correction of malfunction. Am J Kidney Dis. 1996;28:379–86.
9. Schwab SJ. Assessing the adequacy of vascular access and its relationship to patient outcome. AmJ Kidney Dis. 1994;24: 316–20.
10. Lok CE, Mokrzycki MH. Prevention and management of catheter-related infection in hemodialysis patients. Kidney Int. 2011;79:587–98.
11. Sem Dial. 2008;21(6):503–90.
12. Schillinger F, Schillinger D, Montagnac R, Milcent T. Post catheterisation vein stenosis in haemodialysis: comparative angiographic study of 50 subclavian and 50 internal jugular accesses. Nephrol Dial Transplant. 1991;6(10):722.
13. Vanholder R, Ringoir S. Vascular access for hemodialysis. Artif Organs. 1994;18:263–5.
14. Merrer J, De Jonghe B, Golliot F, Lefrant JY, Raffy B, Barre E, Rigaud JP, Casciani D, Misset B, Bosquet C, Outin H, Brun-Buisson C, Nitenberg G, French Catheter Study Group in Intensive Care. Complications of femoral and subclavian venous catheterization in critically ill patients: a randomized controlled trial. JAMA. 2001;286(6):700.
15. Maya ID, Allon M. Outcomes of tunneled femoral hemodialysis catheters: comparison with internal jugular vein catheters. Kidney Int. 2005;68(6):2886.
16. Lund GB, Trerotola SO, Scheel PJ Jr. Percutaneous translumbar inferior vena cava cannulation for hemodialysis. Am J Kidney Dis. 1995;25:732–7.
17. Smith TP, Ryan JM, Reddan DN. Transhepatic catheter access for hemodialysis. Radiology. 2004;232(1):246–51. Epub 2004 May 20.
18. Villagrán Medinilla E, Carnero M, Silva JA, Rodríguez JE. Right intra-atrial catheter insertion at the end stage of peripheral vascular access for dialysis. Interact CardiovascThorac Surg. 2011;12(4):648–9. Epub 2011 Jan 10.
19. K/DOQI clinical practice guidelines and clinical practice recommendations 2006 updates hemodialysis adequacy peritoneal dialysis adequacy vascular access. Am J Kidney Dis. 2006;48(Suppl 1):S1.
20. Kelber J, Delmez JA, Windus DW. Factors affecting delivery of high-efficiency dialysis using temporary vascular access. Am J Kidney Dis. 1993;22:24–9.
21. Agharazii M, Plamondon I, Lebel M, Douville P, Desmeules S. Estimation of heparin leak into the systemic circulation after central venous catheter heparin lock. Nephrol Dial Transplant. 2005;20:1238–40.
22. Vesely TM. Central venous catheter tip position: a continuing controversy. J Vasc Interv Radiol. 2003;14:527–34.
23. Dowling K, Sansivero G, Stainken B, et al. The use of tissue plasminogen activator infusion to re-establish function of tunneledhemodialysis catheters. Nephrol Nurs J. 2004;31:199–200.
24. Savader SJ, Ehrman KO, Porter DJ, Haikal LC, Oteham AC. Treatment of hemodialysis catheter associated fibrin sheaths by rt-PA infusion: critical analysis of 124 procedures. J Vasc Interv Radiol. 2001;12:711–5.
25. Tranter SA, Donoghue J. Brushing has made a sweeping change: use of the endoluminal FAS brush in haemodialysis central venous catheter management. Aust Crit Care. 2000;13:10–3.
26. Hilleman D, Campbell J. Efficacy, safety, and cost of thrombolytic agents for the management of dysfunctional hemodialysis catheters: a systematic review. Pharmacotherapy. 2011;31(10):1031–40.
27. Raad I, Costerton W, Sabharwal U, Sacilowski M, Anaissie E, Bodey GP. Ultrastructural analysis of indwelling vascular catheters: a quantitative relationship between luminal colonization and duration of placement. J Infect Dis. 1993;168:400–7.
28. Lewis K. Riddle of biofilm resistance. Antimicrob Agents Chemother. 2001;45:999–1007.
29. Forauer AR, Theoharis C. Histologic changes in the human vein wall adjacent to indwelling central venous catheters. J Vasc Interv Radiol. 2003;14(9 Pt 1):1163.
30. Hernández D, Díaz F, Rufino M, Lorenzo V, Pérez T, Rodríguez A, De Bonis E, Losada M, González-Posada JM, Torres A. Subclavian vascular access stenosis in dialysis patients: natural history and risk factors. J Am SocNephrol. 1998;9(8):1507.
31. Central vein stenosis associated with dialysis access. Gerald A Beathard, MD, PhD. www.UptoDate.com
32. Wright RS, Quinones-Baldrich WJ, Anders AJ, Danovitch GM. Pleural effusion associated with ipsilateral breast and arm edema as a complication of subclavian vein catheterization and arteriovenous fistula formation for hemodialysis. Chest. 1994;106(3):950.
33. Rose SC, Kinney TB, Bundens WP, Valji K, Roberts AC. Importance of Doppler analysis of transmitted atrial waveforms prior to placement of central venous access catheters. J Vasc Interv Radiol. 1998;9(6):927.
34. Levit RD, Cohen RM, Kwak A, Shlansky-Goldberg RD, Clark TW, Patel AA, Stavropoulos SW, Mondschein JI, Solomon JA, Tuite CM. Asymptomatic central venous stenosis in hemodialysis patients. Trerotola Radiol. 2006;238(3):1051.
35. Surowiec SM, Fegley AJ, Tanski WJ, Sivamurthy N, Illig KA, Lee DE, Waldman DL, Green RM, Davies MG. Endovascular management of central venous stenoses in the hemodialysis patient: results of percutaneous therapy. Vasc Endovasc Surg. 2004;38(4):349.
36. Beathard GA. Percutaneoustransvenous angioplasty in the treatment of vascular access stenosis. Kidney Int. 1992;42(6):1390.
37. El-Sabrout RA, Duncan JM. Right atrial bypass grafting for central venous obstruction associated with dialysis access: another treatment option. J Vasc Surg. 1999;29(3):472.
38. Ayarragaray JE. Surgical treatment of hemodialysis-related central venous stenosis or occlusion: another option to maintain vascular access. J Vasc Surg. 2003;37(5):1043.

Complications of Maintenance Haemodialysis and How to Avoid Them

Nigel Suren Kanagasundaram and Timothy John Ellam

Contents

M. Harber (ed.), *Primer on Nephrology*, https://doi.org/10.1007/978-3-030-76419-7_80

Learning Objectives

To understand, recognize, treat and prevent some of the main complications encountered in chronic haemodialysis practice.

80.1 Introduction

Maintenance haemodialysis (HD) poses some of the greatest technical, logistical and clinical challenges in renal practice. The HD population is highly vulnerable and places a disproportionate strain on hospital resources in comparison to their overall numbers. For instance, end-stage renal disease (ESRD) patients suffer more frequent and prolonged admissions than the general hospital population and although much of the burden may be due to non-renal morbidity, such as cardiovascular disease and infections, complications of vascular access are a dominant contributor. This chapter will cover some of the most significant complications that can arise in the HD population and how they might be prevented or mitigated. Organisational structure can play a key role and is discussed, in detail, elsewhere in this textbook. The range of topics covered is by no means comprehensive but have been chosen to reflect those complications that have the greatest impact on the HD population or which require specific considerations to mitigate or manage.

80.2 Blood Pressure and Fluid Management

Cardiovascular disease is one of the leading causes of death in HD patients and will be discussed later in this chapter; blood pressure (BP) and fluid management will be covered separately as they extend beyond pure cardiovascular risk to other aspects of HD pathophysiology. An added complexity is the cyclical nature of both BP and fluid status over the course of a week; the asymmetric weekly HD schedule not only causes difficulties in interpreting findings but also has a real clinical impact with, for instance, highest mortality around the time of the first session of the week, following the longest inter-dialytic gap.

80.2.1 Aetiology

At least 75% of incident HD patients are reported to be hypertensive. As well as pre-existing essential hypertension, other factors such as salt and water retention, increased activity of the sympathetic and renin-angiotensin-aldosterone systems, and arterial stiffness (due to vascular calcification) may play a role. Increased intracellular calcium, due to hyperparathyroidism, and erythropoiesis-stimulating agents, may contribute. Of these, salt and water retention is probably most important.

Evidence in support of this includes the association between high inter-dialytic weight gains and hypertension in some (but not all) studies, a higher prevalence of hypertension at dialysis initiation (volume control presumably improving as therapy progresses) and the finding that drug-free hypertensive control can be achieved by optimising extracellular fluid volumes with long session HD. Even in the absence of clinical signs, volume overload can be detected in hypertensive HD patients using sensitive experimental techniques.

80.2.2 Measurement of BP

Pre- and post-HD BP measurements may not be representative of overall control. The former tend to be higher than mean BP [1] due to increased salt and water accumulation between sessions, pretreatment patient anxiety and the omission of antihypertensive drugs before HD to minimise the risk of intra-dialytic hypotension (IDH). BP tends to fall during HD due to volume removal; post-HD readings, although more representative of inter-dialytic control [2], may underestimate mean BP, though [1].

Ambulatory BP recording may be most representative of overall control and may be useful in defining 'systolic load' and in picking up blunted nocturnal dipping [3], but there is still some evidence of intra-individual variability [4].

Home BP monitoring is a cheap, practical alternative to ambulatory recording and can be useful in clarifying overall control [5].

80.2.3 Assessing Volume Status

This is one of the commonest clinical challenges in HD and is compounded by different interpretations of what actually defines 'dry weight' – for instance, 'normotension' without symptomatic hypovolaemia, 'normotension' without antihypertensive drugs or the absence of clinically detectable oedema. However, there is enough nuance to make a comprehensive definition, problematic. For instance, an oedema-free state does not necessarily mean that dry weight has been reached. Clinically, evident peripheral oedema may have other causes – right heart failure, drugs, venous insufficiency, liver failure, etc. – meaning that attempts to achieve an oedema-free state may be poorly tolerated. An ultrafiltration (UF) rate that is excessive for an individual patient may cause hypotension even though they remain fluid overloaded. A highly individualized interpretation of dry weight may be needed and will depend on overall BP control, patient tolerability and clinical signs and symptoms. Perhaps the most important element of volume management – and akin to intravenous fluid resuscitation in other clinical circumstances – is an assessment of the therapeutic response; repeated assessment and reassessment may be needed to ensure that treatment goals are being achieved.

Re-evaluation of dry weight should routinely be undertaken every quarter, in stable patients, and when other clinical circumstances require it (for instance, after hospitalization when there may have been considerable loss of lean body mass).

In terms of complementary technologies, bioimpedance plethysmography, inferior vena cava diameter measurement, measurement of atrial and brain natriuretic peptides and blood volume monitoring have all been employed to improve the assessment of volume status. Their role in routine clinical practice remains unclear at this stage although bioimpedance seems to have the better supportive evidence base at this stage [6]. Clearly, sufficient experience and expertise in using these tools are needed for results to be meaningful and interpretable within the clinical context.

80.2.4 Target BP

Correlation between BP and cardiovascular mortality remains unclear in the HD population although studies of better design and longer duration have tended to show a stronger relationship. For instance, a prospective cohort study of 432 ESRD patients (261 HD) with mean follow-up of 41 months found that each 10 mmHg rise in the averaged mean arterial pressure (MAP) was independently associated with the presence of concentric left ventricular hypertrophy and a deterioration in other echocardiographic indices [7]. An averaged MAP >106 mmHg was also associated with the development of clinical cardiac failure or ischaemic heart disease. In other work, an increased mortality was seen with post-dialysis hypertension (>180 mmHg systolic or >110 mmHg diastolic) [8]. J-shaped mortality curves complicate the interpretation of these findings.

In one study, the lowest mortality was found in those with a pre-dialysis systolic BP of 160–189 mmHg [9]. Those with a pre-dialysis systolic BP <110 mmHg and diastolic BP <50 mmHg had the highest risk of death. The relationship between low pre-HD systolic BP and mortality seemed strongest in the presence of congestive cardiac failure [8]. A pre-dialysis SBP <120 mmHg for both incident and prevalent patients [10] and achievement of a goal pre-BP <140/90 mmHg [11] were also associated with increased mortality.

Some have suggested a changing relationship between BP and mortality with dialysis vintage with a low BP associated with increased risk of death in the first 2 years but with hypertension associated with an increased mortality in those surviving ≥3 years [12].

Loss of nocturnal dipping and increased pulse pressure may be associated with worse outcomes but their use as clinical management targets remains unclear.

80.2.5 Management

It is possible to achieve good BP control solely by correction of extracellular volume overload with long hours of HD. Thrice weekly sessions of 8 h each lower the risk of IDH and allow 90% of patients to be antihypertensive-free [13]. Constrained capacity prevents similar programmes in most units although home therapy conducted on nocturnal or short, frequent schedules may circumvent these resource issues. In practice, though, most patients will be receiving 'standard' HD schedules, in-centre or in satellite facilities, delivered for about 4 h, thrice weekly. Attempts to regain control of the extracellular fluid space can be complex and prolonged.

The first step is to identify patients who might be volume loaded. The only evidence for this might be persisting hypertension without any clinical evidence of pulmonary or peripheral oedema. Patients with pre- and post-dialysis BPs consistently >160/90 and / or >140/90, respectively, may benefit from BP control. Others who may breach these thresholds more intermittently might benefit from inter-dialytic BP assessment, through primary care-, self- or ambulatory-BP monitoring, although the former does not lend itself to the assessment of diurnal variation. The latter may be most beneficial if there is a suspicion of hypotension. If discrete readings are consistently >140/85 or the mean ambulatory reading is >130/80 without evidence of hypotension, patients may benefit from augmented BP management.

80.2.6 Salt and Fluid Restriction

The initial steps should be to review the dialysate sodium prescription and dietary salt and fluid intake – see Table 80.1.

A net intra-dialytic sodium gain should be avoided by re-setting the dialysate sodium towards the individual's pre-dialysis serum sodium. Sodium profiles should generally be avoided as most result in sodium loading. Where dialysate sodium needs to be reduced, this should be undertaken cautiously to reduce the risks of cramps

Table 80.1 BP and volume control – salt and water management (see text for further details)

Review dialysate sodium prescription	Reduce dialysate sodium towards usual pre-dialysis sodium by 1 mmol/L every 2 weeks Avoid sodium profiling
Review dietary salt intake	Reduce daily sodium intake to 80–100 mmol (a 'no added salt' diet) Beware hidden salt – encourage food label checking Avoid potassium-containing salt substitutes If cardiac failure, aim for tighter restriction
Review fluid restriction	Aim for inter-dialytic weight gain ≤3% 'active' body weight If non-obese, active and actual body weight are pragmatically equivalent If obese, active body weight = 25*height^2 (weight in kg, height in meters; 'fat-free' BMI assumed as 25)

Box 80.1 BP and Volume Control – Salt and Water Restriction and Patient Education (See Text for Further Details)

Emphasise the key role of sodium in hypertension, volume overload, thirst

Differentiate between sensations of thirst and dry mouth

Review drugs that may be contributing to dry mouth

Patient tips and tricks to manage restrictions:

- Check the sodium content of processed food
- Take tablets with food where possible
- Use small volume cups
- Sip and savour; don't gulp
- Use ice cubes, ice lollies, sweets or gum (n.b. sugar content), mouthwashes, artificial saliva
- Use a pre-filled measuring jug or similar receptacle to help guide daily fluid intake

and hypotension. A unit-wide reduction in dialysate sodium (from 141 mmol/L to 138) has been associated with improved BP [14] and should be considered where standard prescriptions risk sodium imbalance.

Dietary sodium intake should be restricted to 80–100 mmol/day. Even tighter restrictions are needed for those with cardiac failure.

Accounting for urine output, fluid restriction should limit inter-dialytic weight gains to ~3% of 'active' body weight. This will usually work out at an allowable weight gain of 2.5 kg. Diuretics may help limit the degree of fluid restriction by increasing urine output. When daily urine output is >1 litre, strict restriction is unnecessary but vigilance for falling volumes over the course of time should be maintained.

Patient education (see ▶ Box 80.1) is usually delivered by renal dietitians and dialysis nursing staff. The central role of sodium in hypertension, volume overload and – immediately relevant to the patient –thirst should be emphasised. It is useful to ask patients to try to differentiate between the sensations of a dry mouth, per se, and thirst as the former may have another cause (see below).

Medical staff play a role in re-enforcing the above but also in reviewing drugs that might be contributing to a dry mouth (review anti-cholinergic agents but others (e.g. proton pump inhibitors), also carry this side effect – check the formulary) and in considering ACE inhibitors which may ameliorate thirst.

80.2.7 Identification of Goals

Identify a BP/fluid management goal for each stage of management and continue to re-evaluate progress on these goals, ensuring that these are communicated to the patient and amongst all relevant staff. Echocardiography may reveal left ventricular hypertrophy which may require more aggressive BP management using ACE inhibitors or angiotensin 2 receptor blockers.

A number of clinical scenarios are given in Table 80.2.

The development of hypotensive symptoms, especially during dialysis, should not be assumed to be a result of excessive, overall BP control or overaggressive target weight reduction. Consider the contribution from mistimed or inappropriate antihypertensive therapy, excessive ultrafiltration rates and over-rapid reductions in the target weight.

80.2.8 Target Weight Reduction

Cautious reductions in target weight should be the initial step in achieving BP/fluid control (see Table 80.2) unless hypertension or fluid overload is severe. These rates are usually well tolerated but might need to be sustained over a period of weeks to months to take effect. If even these are poorly tolerated, more cautious decrements (e.g. 0.1 kg/week) can be tried. Changes at the

Table 80.2 BP and fluid management – example treatment goals (see text for further details)

Goal	Actions	Trigger for re-evaluation	The next steps
1. Pre- and post-BP consistently <160/90 and <140/90, respectively	Nurse-led: Reduction of target weight by 0.1 kg/session in 2 week cycles Review of salt and fluid intake – seeking dietetic help if necessary Re-evaluation of control after each 2 week cycle Repeat cycles whilst goals still not met	Nurse-led feedback if: Failure to achieve goals after pre-defined number of treatment cycles (e.g. 3 or 4) Haemodynamic instability during HD Pre-HD BP <120/50	Medical review of: Rate of target weight reduction – consider more cautious/aggressive approach Antihypertensive drugs Are timing or dose contributing to haemodynamic instability? Can target weight reduction, alone, achieve goals or is drug treatment necessary? Supplementary measures to reduce haemodynamic instability, e.g. Cooled dialysate (e.g. 35 °C) Intra-HD blood volume monitoring to guide UF profiling Increased session duration/frequency (if patient willing) Isolated UF with isovolaemic/low UF HD Need for inter-dialytic BP measurement to help re-evaluate BP goals
2. Correction of non-life-threatening clinical volume overload	Medic-led: Reduction of target weight by 0.1 kg/session in 2 week cycles Review of salt and fluid intake – seeking dietetic help if necessary Re-evaluation of volume status after pre-defined period	Nurse-led feedback if: Haemodynamic instability during HD Pre-HD BP <120/50	Medical review of: Rate of target weight reduction – consider a more cautious approach Antihypertensive drugs Supplementary measures to reduce haemodynamic instability
3. Achievement of mean ambulatory BP <130/80	Medic-led: Reduction of target weight by 0.1 kg/session in 2 week cycles Review of salt and fluid intake – seeking dietetic help if necessary Re-evaluation of ambulatory BP profile after pre-defined period	Nurse-led feedback as '2'	Medical review as '1' (including repeat inter-dialysis BP profiling)
4. Weaning of antihypertensive –medications	Medic-led: Weaning of antihypertensive drugs Reduction of target weight by 0.1 kg/session in 2 week cycles if required to maintain BP goals Review of salt and fluid intake – seeking dietetic help if necessary Re-evaluation of BP control and need for further drug reduction	Nurse-led feedback if: Failure to maintain BP control Haemodynamic instability during HD Pre-HD BP <120/50	Medical review of: Rate of target weight reduction – consider more cautious / aggressive approach Antihypertensive drugs Need for inter-dialytic BP measurement to help re-evaluate treatment goals
5. Control of severe hypertension	Medic-led: Initiation of antihypertensive medication Review of salt and fluid intake – seeking dietetic help if necessary Re-evaluation of BP control (e.g. at every session) Reduction in target weight if clinically volume overloaded	Nurse-led feedback if: Over-correction of BP below pre-defined limits	Medical review of: Rate of BP correction The potential to wean antihypertensive drugs once BP control is well established

end of the weekly dialysis cycle may be better tolerated when patients will have less fluid to lose after the short inter-dialytic gap.

Intra-dialytic hypotension, regardless of cause, is a distressing symptom that may jaundice a patient's view on future attempts at target weight reduction. A careful, incremental wean of antihypertensives may be needed as target weight is reduced to reduce its risk. Similarly, antihypertensives may need to be taken after HD, again to improve haemodynamic tolerability.

An important complicating factor in knowing when the true target weight has been reached is the lag phenomenon between the achievement of acceptable extracellular fluid volume and improvements in BP [15]. A failure to appreciate this risks 'overshoot' and IDH.

The logistics of achieving therapeutic goals can be difficult to sustain on a busy dialysis unit, especially if the time course over which it is to be delivered is prolonged. This is particularly so given the need for timely and regular re-evaluation, prompt troubleshooting and weaning of antihypertensives. Some driver to propel an individual patient down their defined treatment pathway is highly desirable and may come in the form of a quality assurance programme or by one or a small group of allied healthcare professionals (e.g. nurse practitioners). Successful management of hypertension is entirely possible on a 'standard' HD schedule provided a sustained and consistent effort can be made [16].

80.2.9 Use of Antihypertensives

Despite attempts at target weight reduction, BP goals may not be achieved. In these circumstances, once daily preparations are desirable to aid concordance. Administration after HD can minimise the risk of IDH – doses should be kept as low as possible for similar reasons. If BP rises, reduce the target weight in the first instance rather than increasing antihypertensives.

The choice of antihypertensive depends both on coexistent diseases and specific issues relevant to HD (see Table 80.3).

Table 80.3 Use of antihypertensives

Class	Advantages	Disadvantages	Dialysability[c]
Beta-blockers	Block sympathetic over-activity which may be more pronounced in ESRD Beneficial post-MI Beneficial in left ventricular systolic dysfunction (although should be started cautiously)	Can cause hyperkalaemia May promote IDH[a] by blocking baroreceptor response to reduced plasma volume Short-acting agents, administered in the morning, may promote IDH.	Most removed Carvedilol, Bisoprolol: not significantly dialysable
Calcium channel blockers		May promote IDH by blocking reflex arteriolar vasoconstriction	Not significantly dialysable
Alpha blockers		May promote IDH through vasodilation	Not dialysed
ACE inhibitors and angiotensin-2 receptor blockers	Beneficial in ventricular impairment May reduce left ventricular mass in HD patients [57, 58] May help preserve residual renal function	Can cause hyperkalaemia Can cause severe hypotension in the setting of volume depletion May blunt the response to erythropoiesis stimulating agents ACE inhibitors[b] can cause anaphylaxis when AN69 membranes are used	ACE inhibitors: Ramipril removed by HDF / high flux HD but not by HD; lisinopril, captopril, perindopril, enalapril also removed by low flux HD Angiotensin 2 receptor blockers: not significantly dialysable
Clonidine	Can aid BP control when drug concordance otherwise poor (see text)		Not significantly dialysable

[a] *IDH* intra-dialytic hypotension
[b] Although thought to be a bradykinin-mediated phenomenon, there are occasional reports of similar reactions occurring with the concurrent use of angiotensin-2 receptor blockers
[c] See also ▶ www.renaldrugdatabase.com

80.2.10 Refractory Hypertension

Hypertension refractory to volume removal and antihypertensives requires a review of drug concordance (feedback from primary care or the dispensing pharmacist can give useful insights), of sodium gains (dietary, intradialytic) and of over-the-counter medication which may be contributing to hypertension (e.g. non-steroidal anti-inflammatory agents). Longer-acting agents, administered once daily, can aid drug concordance as can the regular provision of drugs via pill organisers. For those who remain non-concordant with drugs, the administration of long-acting agents (e.g. ACE inhibitors, calcium channel blockers) on the renal unit after dialysis can provide some level of BP control. Regimes comprising a combination of lisinopril, amlodipine and/or transdermal clonidine (patches of the latter, changed every week) [17] have proved successful. However, if patients become haemodynamically unstable for any reason, it should be remembered that drug levels will persist at therapeutic levels for ~8 h after patch removal and, thereafter, will decline only slowly over several days. Such patients who have also lost capacity are at additional risk if patch removal is neglected.

Consider renin-mediated hypertension and the need for high dose renin-angiotensin system modifying agents – doses may be limited by hyperkalaemia, though. Consider, also, a switch to peritoneal dialysis in those who have difficulty with volume control – problems with the concordance with sodium and fluid restrictions – may also foretell future problems with the new modality, whose suitability will therefore require careful evaluation.

It is important to bear in mind the dialysis 'lag phenomenon' in which hypertension may respond to fluid removal only after days to a fortnight or more, arguing for a slow and gradual reduction in target weight over the course of weeks rather than days.

Total nephrectomy is only very rarely needed to control BP but can be effective where hypertension has been severe, complicated and resistant to fluid and drug management.

80.2.11 Intra-dialytic Hypertension

Intra-dialytic hypertension complicates between 8% and 30% of dialysis sessions [18] and is a marker for worse outcomes [19]. It is more common in patients who are young, have pre-existing hypertension or have high inter-dialytic weight gains. Possible mechanisms include sympathetic hyper-reactivity [20], an increased cardiac output [21] or hyper-reactivity of the renin-angiotensin system in response to fluid removal [22]. Iatrogenic contributors include over-rapid correction of the haemoglobin by erythropoietin and related agents, high dialysate sodium concentrations and the prescription of antihypertensive agents that are removed during dialysis (see ◘ Table 80.3). A short-acting ACE inhibitor, such as captopril, or clonidine, a centrally acting vasodilator, can be used if severe (e.g. SBP >180 mm Hg). Drug therapy could be administered pre-dialysis if hypertension predictably develops during treatment sessions.

80.3 Intra-dialytic Hypotension

Intra-dialytic hypotension (IDH) is a frequent complication of HD and may be more common in those with lower body mass, cardiac disease, older age and higher volume removal. As well as symptoms of hypotension, patients may experience yawning, cramps, and nausea and vomiting although many remain asymptomatic. Patients with IDH have higher morbidity and mortality [23, 24], and many end up in a vicious cycle of repeated episodes, leading to saline infusion, saline-induced hypertension, drug therapy, drug-induced inhibition of protective reflexes (such as tachycardia, vasoconstriction) and further IDH. IDH also increases the risk of AV access thrombosis.

IDH is multifactorial. An inability to adequately increase arteriolar tone and a reduction in left ventricular function during treatment may contribute [25]. Impaired myocardial reserve, rather than myocardial ischaemia seems to be important [26]. Patients at risk of IDH are often diabetic, have autonomic neuropathy or have cardiac disease (especially left ventricular dysfunction and diastolic dysfunction). Antihypertensive drugs inhibiting protective reflexes, the ingestion of food (causing splanchnic vasodilatation) [27] and high inter-dialytic weight gains may also contribute. Organ ischaemia leads to the release of adenosine which inhibits noradrenaline release [28]. Uraemia, itself, may increase the production of nitric oxide [29] which may also be increased following a hypotensive episode [30]. Attenuated vasopressin secretion in response to fluid removal has also been implicated [31].

Attributes of the HD prescription, itself, contributing to IDH include warm dialysate, low dialysate sodium and a high UF rate. Rapid reductions in plasma osmolality at the start of HD can lead to a fall in plasma volume and hypotension; although conventionally regarded as being caused by the diffusion of uraemic toxins, this could also, theoretically, result from glucose shifts in those with significant hyperglycaemia. Finally, bioincompatible membranes and the use of acetate buffer (a vasodilator) may have contributed to the risk of IDH, at least historically.

The differential diagnosis of IDH includes cardiac ischaemia/myocardial infarction (consider these if episode associated with chest pain or shortness of breath), pericardial effusion or haemorrhage (consider these especially if uraemic pericarditis is possible – anticoagulation-free HD is mandated until resolution), cardiac dysrhythmias, dialyser membrane reactions (which may also be associated with wheezing and dyspnoea), GI bleeding or other haemorrhages, bloodline disconnection or needle dislodgement, massive haemolysis, air embolism or sepsis. Patients who have recently undergone dialysis catheter insertion may have developed a tension pneumothorax or cardiac tamponade from myocardial or mediastinal injury. Hypotension from excessive or over-rapid ultrafiltration remains the most common cause of IDH, though.

80.3.1 Immediate Management

The patient should be placed in Trendelenburg position, blood-flow (Qb) should be reduced, UF should be discontinued or reduced and, if these measures fail to resolve the episode, a saline bonus should be administered (e.g. 100 mL 0.9% saline). Boluses should be repeated, as necessary, bearing in mind that salt loading will promote hypertension and volume overload. There is, currently, no evidence for the use of intravenous albumin in IDH. IDH should correct quickly, with the above physical measures and with the administration of two or three boluses of saline if it has been caused by excessive ultrafiltration – if not, the differential diagnosis should be urgently re-evaluated.

Following an episode of IDH, the patient's target weight and antihypertensive therapy should be reviewed.

80.3.2 Prevention

Low peri-HD BPs (<120/60) should prompt an evaluation of overall control even in the absence of overt symptoms.

The slow, cautious approach to target weight reduction, described above, will help minimise the impact of over-enthusiastic UF. Longer times mean lower UF rates and with evidence that UF rates >10 ml/h/kg are associated with an increased risk of both IDH and mortality [6], slower volume removal should remain a key treatment goal. Patient education is key to both inter-dialytic fluid gains and acceptance of prescribed session times.

Attempts at initiating HD infrequently or for short durations can lead to resistance when more intensive treatment is needed so patients on such incremental schedules should be counselled on the likely need for more intensive prescriptions as residual renal function declines.

Unit-wide adoption of dialysate temperatures no greater than 36 °C may be of benefit in reducing the population incidence of IDH [6]. An individualized approach may be needed with further cooling for those with refractory IDH or a raised dialysate temperature for those, conversely, who are intolerant of it.

There remains, however, considerable uncertainty around the use of unit-wide dialysate sodium settings and at what level these should be applied; although evidence points to improved fluid gains and hypertensive control with lower settings (see also above), there is also at least some association with worse outcomes, possibly as a result of an increased incidence of IDH [6].

80.3.3 Assessment of Recurrent IDH

Table 80.4 details initial steps to be taken if IDH is frequent and recurring.

If IDH persists despite these measures, drug treatment can be considered (see also Table 80.4) and if required:

- *Sequential Ultrafiltration and No UF/Low UF HD*

Start with isolated UF before HD as plasma solute concentrations will be at their highest levels and will hence promote vascular refilling when fluid removal is at its greatest. The technique tends to prolong HD times to maintain dialysis adequacy which may not be possible due to constrained capacity or patient choice.

- *Dialysate Sodium Management*

Controlled trials have shown a reduction in hypotensive episodes but increased thirst and fluid gains. Sodium profiles should, therefore, be used only cautiously in selected patients, as a last resort to maintain HD and in a pattern that minimises net sodium gain (the time-averaged dialysate sodium equating to the pre-HD serum sodium).

Conversely, there may well be an advantage in setting individual dialysate sodium prescriptions according to the patient's pre-dialysis serum sodium. Although this may not be achievable for every patient, a clear and consistent discrepancy – either contributing to fluid gains and thirst or, conversely, dialysis intolerance through IDH, cramping, etc. – may well require specific management.

- *Peritoneal Dialysis*

This may need to be considered if the patient is suitable.

Table 80.4 Assessment of recurrent intra-dialytic hypotension (IDH) – see text for further details

Assessment	Comment	Action
Initial assessment		
Review target weight	Clinical evaluation of volume status Review pre-, post-HD BPs Consider inter-dialytic BP profiling to confirm overall BP control, variability of BP over a 24 h cycle	If clearly volume deplete, increase target weight by, for example, 0.5–1.0 kg If clinically euvolaemic and BP control acceptable, consider cautious increments in target weight (e.g. 0.1 kg / session for 2 weeks) with evaluation of response – repeat as required
Review antihypertensive therapy		Reschedule short-acting drugs after HD Review BP control over the inter-dialysis cycle (from inter-dialytic BP profile) for targeted rescheduling of drugs according to need (e.g. skewed towards greater nocturnal / non-HD day control)
Review UF rate	Should not exceed 10 ml/kg body weight/hour Consider blood volume monitoring	Review sodium load, fluid restriction Consider increased session duration and/or frequency (e.g. if on home HD) Ultrafiltration profiling may help mitigate periods of greatest fall in blood volume A threshold fall in blood volume may be defined below which the patient develops IDH[a]
Replace acetate with bicarbonate dialysate	Largely an historical issue, now	
Avoid food intake during and in the hour before dialysis	There is no clear evidence of benefit from caffeine ingestion before or during HD	
Consider position	Dialyse in a leg up position in the dialysis chair / in a bed	
Correct anaemia if present		
Lower dialysate temperature	May be uncomfortable if too cool Vasoconstriction may increase the regional blood flow differential and hamper solute clearances from under-perfused tissues – watch the *equilibrated* Kt/V	
If IDH continues to recur despite these measures:		
Review cardiac function[b]	Consider occult cardiac ischaemia Left ventricular systolic or diastolic function may be managed with non-HD RAS[c] modifying drugs if BP profile allows Cooled dialysate can augment myocardial function Anaemia should have been corrected by this stage Consider cardiac monitoring or 24 ECG for occult dysrhythmias	

Table 80.4 (continued)

Assessment	Comment	Action
Check adrenal function/ adequacy of steroid replacement		
Consider drug therapy		Oral midodrine (a selective alpha 1 adrenergic agonist) 2.5 mg pre-HD with doses increased, as required, to increase peripheral vascular resistance and BP during treatment May be particularly effective in autonomic neuropathy [59] A mid-session supplemental dose may be needed (it is dialysable) Use with caution in the presence of CV & vascular disease; contraindications include aortic aneurysm, cardiac conduction abnormalities, CCF, MI, urinary retention, serious prostate disorders, blood vessel spasm, cerebrovascular occlusion, proliferative diabetic retinopathy Carnitine (20 mg/kg/session, iv) or sertraline (50 to 100 mg/day, PO) have little evidence to support their routine use

[a]Unless 'fuzzy logic' feedback systems are in place that can automatically intervene (e.g. discontinuation of UF, or saline bolus), a so-called 'crash crit' is rarely practical on a busy HD unit; in addition, there is wide intra- as well as inter-individual variability in this threshold, which requires ongoing reassessment
[b]Increasing dialysate calcium (ref) (e.g. to 1.50 mmol per litre) can improve cardiac performance but needs to be undertaken with caution because of the risks of worsening mineral metabolic control
[c]*RAS* renin-angiotensin system

80.4 Post-dialysis Fatigue

The post-treatment hangover is one of the most troublesome symptoms for patients and adds, considerably, to the attrition of dialysis. Two potential contributors include high dialysis intensity and post-treatment hypotension. Other potential causes of post-dialysis fatigue to consider include hypoglycaemia and hypokalaemia [19].

Strategies to address dialysis intensity include stepwise decrements in the intensity of the thrice-weekly dialysis prescription and, particularly, if in-centre capacity allows it or the patient is a home HD candidate, more frequent, low intensity and/or long hours schedules.

Hypotension may be managed by supporting haemodynamics during treatment by cooling dialysate, adding an ultrafiltration profile, upwards adjustment of the dialysate sodium to reflect physiologically higher pre-dialysis serum sodiums, if relevant, and/or adding or substituting periods of isolated ultrafiltration to allow more tolerable fluid removal. A better appreciation of post-dialysis blood pressure drops can be achieved through non-dialysis records – either ambulatory or manual – although the latter also has the advantage of being able to delineate postural changes, too.

Other measures to address post-dialysis fatigue include L-carnitine supplementation although its precise role in routine practice is unclear [19].

80.5 Pruritus

Again, this symptom can be intrusive and unpleasant and can lead to significant sleep disturbance, mood disorders and complications such as nodular prurigo and super-added skin infections.

If symptoms clearly associate with dialysis (with symptoms developing during or immediately after treatment), consider reactions to the dialyser or other components (e.g. the dialyser sterilant, heparin, dressings and adhesive tapes, latex from rubber gloves, antiseptic solutions, dialysis needles, etc.). Otherwise, ensure good control of phosphate, calcium, PTH and magnesium and explain the association between hyperphosphataemia and itching. In the absence of disordered bone chemistry, consider other, non-renal causes (e.g. hypothyroidism, hyperglycaemia, liver disease, skin disorders or allergic reactions to other products, etc.), although uraemic pruritus is the most likely aetiology. The latter can be addressed through the liberal use of topical emollient creams in affected areas and after bathing/showering, to prevent drying of the skin. Ensure good dialysis adequacy and consider a switch to haemodiafiltration. Low strength (e.g. 0.025%) capsaicin ointment may be tried over affected areas with the usual caveats around avoiding contact with broken skin, wounds, catheter exit sites, fistula needling sites and mucous membranes.

Drug therapy may prove necessary (e.g. gabapentin, anti-histamines). A baseline ECG, repeated after drug initiation and after each dose increase is advisable to ensure that the QT interval is not increasing with therapy. For refractory cases, consider dermatology input, particularly if there is doubt about the diagnosis or for consideration of phototherapy.

Studies of the κ-opioid receptor agonist, nalfurafine (given iv, post-dialysis), have yielded positive results [32]. Ondansetron (a selective 5-hydroxytryptamine 3-antagonist), topical tacrolimus, thalidomide, long-chain essential fatty acids and oral activated carbon have been used in experimental settings and are discussed in more detail in Ref. [32].

80.6 Restless Leg Syndrome

Another complication that can dominate the patient experience, restless legs, should be distinguished from cramps, both of which have a tendency to manifest at night. Although functional iron deficiency can contribute, it may be worthwhile pushing iron stores to the upper limits of the target range (e.g. serum ferritins of 700 ug/L rather than 200 ug/L) whilst also aiming to control hyperparathyroidism – another potential contributory factor. Thereafter, a dopamine receptor agonist such as pramipexole or gabapentin or a low-dose benzodiazepine could be tried with the usual caveats around checking QT intervals for the former two and on the risk of over-sedation for the latter two.

80.7 Cardiovascular Disease in the Haemodialysis Patient (see Wheeler and Caplin)

Cardiovascular disease (CVD) accounts for around 50% of all deaths on dialysis [33]. Although deaths from myocardial infarction (MI) are more common than in the non-dialysis population, there is a particular preponderance of sudden cardiac arrest and arrhythmia. The incident dialysis population has a higher burden of traditional cardiovascular (CV) risk factors with the individual patient often carrying more than one. Around 40% of patients enrolled on the HEMO study had a diagnosis of ischaemic heart disease (IHD) [34] whilst the USRDS reported a 10% annual incidence of MI or angina [33]].

Beyond the traditional risk profile, there are a number of factors, unique to the ESRD patient, that may be contributory.

For instance, the presence of chronic kidney disease, per se, has been found to be an independent risk factor for coronary artery disease. This seems to be true for even modest dysfunction but as disease advances to end-stage, oxidant stress and a pro-inflammatory state may contribute to accelerated atherosclerosis. As a reflection of this, a raised C-reactive protein is associated with an increased risk of CVD in HD patients [35]. Finally, as well as an increased burden of intimal atherosclerotic disease, the disordered mineral metabolism of advanced CKD also increases the risk of vascular calcification, which also affects the arterial media.

▶ See Chap. 37 Wheeler and Caplin

▶ Box 80.2 details a number of scenarios where coronary artery disease should be suspected even in the absence of symptoms typical of MI or angina. It should be remembered that the process of HD is a haemodynamic stressor that may reveal manifestations of coronary artery disease when none may be present between sessions. Any HD patient developing new manifestations that might represent CAD should be considered for further evaluation – electrocardiography, echocardiog-

Box 80.2 Possible Presentations of Coronary Artery Disease in the HD Patient (See Text for Further Details)

- Recurrent intra-dialytic hypotension
- Persisting inter-dialytic hypotension
- Dysrhythmias
- Exertional dyspnoea
- Persisting symptoms of heart failure despite the achievement of assumed target weight
- Difficulty achieving dry weight due to hypotension
- The incidental finding of ventricular dysfunction (for instance, during renal transplant recipient workup), especially, if progressive or known to be recent
- The finding of regional wall motion abnormalities on echocardiography

raphy and, potentially, stress imaging, myocardial perfusion studies or coronary angiography. Local expertise and opinion will determine the appropriate approach.

Even accounting for these non-typical presentations, a high prevalence of occult coronary artery disease and silent ischaemia [36] have been found. This is a particular concern in the dialysis population but there is no evidence, currently, to support routine screening of the asymptomatic patient. With ESRD regarded as a coronary artery disease equivalent in much the same way as diabetes mellitus, all HD patients should be considered for preventative management (see below). An exception to this is the HD patient who is active on the renal transplant waiting list who should undergo re-screening on a regular basis. Our own practice is for the annual review of cardiac risk using a simple risk stratification scoring tool that incorporates both clinical and symptom indices. An abnormal score or changing echo- and electro-cardiography requires further cardiac evaluation, initially with stress imaging.

80.7.1 Prevention

All HD patients should be considered for risk factor modification. As well as a healthy lifestyle and diet, the following, specific measures should be considered:

80.7.1.1 Weight Loss

Optimising weight in clinically obese patients may help BP control and facilitate renal transplant wait listing. Nutritional programmes combined with the use of orlistat have proved effective in CKD patients [37].

80.7.1.2 Smoking Cessation

This should be strongly encouraged, recruiting patients onto formal smoking cessation programmes, where necessary. The smoking status of patients should be recorded as a matter of course.

80.7.1.3 Exercise

Physical exercise capacity and muscle strength are reduced in dialysis patients who may well benefit from structured, intra-dialytic exercise programmes. The evidence base is discussed in further detail in current UK Renal Association guidance along with practical tips on the institution of in-house programmes and on patient selection [6].

80.7.1.4 Diabetic Management

Attendance for HD, thrice weekly, detracts from the logistics and (patient) acceptability of non-renal clinic review. This may be especially relevant for routine diabetes management. UK-based guidance [38] recommends that local diabetic services should retain responsibility for diabetic management and relevant screening programmes and, whilst they should remain cognizant of dialysis schedules, a dialysis link worker should provide an additional safety net to ensure treatment and screening plans are executed. The guidance also recommends that all patients have access to a diabetes specialist nurse (ideally, via renal services) and that those with labile control should be under specialist diabetic services (rather than primary care).

There are two other practical considerations.

Firstly, the insulin prescription should be reviewed in relation to the weekly dialysis cycle as low dialysate glucose may lower requirements on dialysis days.

Secondly, questions have been raised about the accuracy of the glycosylated haemoglobin (HbA1c) in monitoring diabetics with ESRD. A variety of factors can affect interpretation – interference with assays from carbamylation of haemoglobin in urea-rich environments (HPLC – high-performance liquid chromatography-based assays prevent this), reduced red cell life spans, rapid erythropoiesis after augmentation of anaemia management, haemoglobinopathies and the effect of blood transfusions. HbA1c levels between 6% and 7% do, however, appear to reflect the degree of diabetic control although values >7% may underestimate it [39]. Glycosylated albumin has been mooted as a more accurate method of monitoring, but lack of widespread use and of familiarity amongst healthcare teams limit its utility at this time. Despite these cautions, the HbA1c is still a useful tool for monitoring overall diabetic control with the following recommendations [38]:

- The target HbA1c in patients should be individualised, but if the patient is on hypoglycaemia inducing treatment, this should be aimed at between 7.5% and 8.5% (58–68 mmol/mol).
- Reduction in treatment should be considered for patients with an HbA1c <7.5% (<58 mmol/mol) on treatments associated with increased risk of hypoglycaemia.

The impact of this degree of control does come with caveats, though:

- As yet, it is unclear if good control affects the rate of progression of other microvascular complications of diabetes in HD patients
- It is also unclear whether this will have any impact on the development of overt cardiovascular disease, particularly given the importance of vascular calcification in its aetiology
- The risk of hypoglycaemia in the more vulnerable patient requires a degree of compromise on overall diabetic control

80

Despite the reasonable utility of the HbA1c, it should not, however, take primacy over the mainstay of control – self-assisted monitoring of blood glucose.

Further recommendations on anti-diabetic therapies, diet and nutrition, and management of diabetic complications are also included in the joint guidance [38].

80.7.1.5 Lipid Lowering Therapy

There is currently no consistent evidence supporting the initiation of statins as primary prophylaxis in dialysis patients [40]. The decision to start treatment should be discussed on a case-by-case basis and be guided by patient choice, tablet burden and the likelihood that any marginal benefit might actually be realized in the context of severe comorbidity. A marked elevation in LDL cholesterol (e.g. >> 2.6 mmol/L) or secondary prevention in the face of established vascular disease may sway the treatment choice in favour of statin treatment. Current UK guidance is that further monitoring (of total and LDL cholesterol) is not warranted as higher doses of statins are inadvisable due to the increased risk of adverse effects [40]. It would seem reasonable to leave pre-existing statin prescriptions unchanged provided these are being tolerated.

80.7.1.6 Vitamin Supplements

Hyperhomocysteinaemia is a potential risk factor for CVD in ESRD but there is no current evidence supporting homocysteine-lowering interventions (vitamins B6, B12 and folic acid) to improve outcomes [41]. Nevertheless, modern, high flux dialysis treatments do lead to the loss of water-soluble vitamins – previous recommendations were that these should be replaced as a matter of routine although more recent guidance suggests a more nuanced approach, targeting those with particularly high clearances (e.g. on overnight or frequent treatment schedules) or low dietary intake [42]. Unit practice, however, should also reflect their confidence that insidious undernutrition and higher clearances will be recognized in a timely fashion – any doubts about the robustness of surveillance may argue for blanket prescriptions to all maintenance HD patients.

80.7.1.7 Anaemia Management (► See Chap. 72)

This is discussed in more detail elsewhere in this textbook, but the importance of a robust anaemia management system that avoids wide fluctuations in haemoglobin levels cannot be overemphasised.

80.7.1.8 Aspirin (► See Chaps. 37 and 75)

Although ESRD may be considered to be a coronary heart disease equivalent, the theoretical risks of antiplatelet therapy in those with no prior history are not insignificant given that the pre-existing combination of uraemic platelet dysfunction and intra-dialytic anticoagulation already increase the risk of bleeding. In addition, the balance of risk and benefit may not favour the routine use of aspirin in primary prophylaxis except for those in the general population at highest risk. Given these considerations, aspirin should generally be confined to secondary prevention for those HD patients with established vascular disease.

80.7.1.9 Secondary Prevention in Patients with Established Coronary, Cerebral or Peripheral Arterial Disease

As well as statin therapy, patients should be prescribed aspirin (at low dose – 75 to 150 mg/day), beta-blockers and ACE inhibitors unless contraindicated in line with usual practice in the non-CKD population. Clopidogrel seems to be a safe alternative in those intolerant of aspirin. In HD patients receiving dual antiplatelet therapy following, for instance, percutaneous coronary intervention, intra-dialytic anticoagulation should be reviewed to ensure that the balance between extra-corporeal circuit patency and the risk of bleeding complications remains appropriate.

80.7.2 Acute Management of Acute Coronary Syndromes

HD patients with acute coronary syndrome have a worse prognosis than non-dialysis patients – this is most likely due to the higher rates of atypical presentation and consequently delayed diagnosis, under-use of diagnostic tools and failure to implement the full gamut of available treatments [43]. HD patients are less likely to present with chest pain or typical ST-segment changes on ECG [44]. HD patients with acute pulmonary oedema are often assumed to have volume overload, per se, rather than an acute coronary event – a high index of suspicion should be maintained with pointers towards the alternative aetiology including the acuteness of the presentation in an HD patient with no clear history of fluid indiscretion and otherwise well-controlled inter-dialytic weight gains. Further diagnostic difficulties can include prior electrocardiographic changes (particularly ST-segment changes resulting from left ventricular hypertrophy) that may confuse interpretation of the acute ECG (this may be mitigated by digitalizing all ECG records – these are routinely scanned into the patient record in our practice) and baseline elevations of both serum creatine kinase and troponin T in ESRD. The use of serial measurements of cTnI may be most specific in the ESRD population. To help mitigate the risk of delayed diagnosis,

HD patients should be routinely advised to inform any non-renal admitting medical teams to make early contact with the on-call renal service so the most appropriate management can be discussed.

The presence of ESRD should not limit available treatment options for HD patients. One caveat, though, is the use of high-dose low-molecular-weight heparin (LMWH) which should be used with caution due to unpredictability of action in advanced renal failure and the attendant increased bleeding risk. Although dose reduction and anti-factor Xa activity monitoring may help mitigate this, the combination of LMWH with dual antiplatelet therapy is potent and may cause serious bleeding complications. Our approach is to recommend substitution of unfractionated for low-molecular-weight heparin as the former is much more readily monitored and its shorter duration of action makes it much more readily reversed simply by stopping the infusion.

80.7.3 Management of Cardiac Failure

Treating volume overload may improve ventricular performance by altering cardiac haemodynamics along the starling curve. Clearly, this should be the focus of initial attempts at treating heart failure. Once a clinically euvolaemic state has been achieved, further assessment and treatment will be required if ventricular performance has failed to improve. Maximal doses of ACE inhibitors and beta-blockers should be considered in those with ventricular dysfunction, ideally with input from cardiology and particularly for those with severe cardiac dysfunction. Potassium control and the effects on blood pressure may limit the drug doses and scheduling. An aldosterone receptor antagonist such as eplerenone might be considered for those who are haemodynamically unstable on first-line therapies. A low threshold for investigation for occult coronary artery disease should be maintained especially if the cardiac changes and/or symptoms are known to be recent.

80.7.4 Sudden Cardiac Death

Sudden cardiac arrest is the most common cause of cardiac death in HD patients. It is more likely to occur around the time of the first HD session of the week [45]. Most episodes are thought to be triggered by myocardial ischaemia in the context of a structurally abnormal heart and produce ventricular dysrhythmias. Risk factors may include coronary artery disease and myocardial structural and functional changes. Features of the dialysis prescription that seem to add to risk include rapid solute shifts and high UF rates. Specifically, low dialysate potassium (<2 mEq/L [46]), especially when used, inappropriately, when the pre-dialysis serum potassium is well controlled, may be important as may a low calcium dialysate. In addition, a dialysis session duration <3.5 h and ultrafiltration requirements >5.7% of the post-HD weight were specific associations in DOPPS [47].

For patients with recurrent IDH, there should be a high index of suspicion that episodes might be due to dysrhythmias. Intra-dialytic cardiac monitoring and 24 h ECG recordings should be considered. The finding of a significant dysrhythmia or (survival of) sudden cardiac arrest, should prompt a comprehensive evaluation including an assessment for underlying coronary artery disease or cardiac structural abnormality, review of potentially arrhythmogenic drugs, modification of dialysate potassium and calcium settings and alteration of the dialysis prescription to mitigate high UF rates. Appropriate patient education should be undertaken if inter-dialytic fluid gains are excessive and should incorporate a review of the dialysate sodium prescription and dietary salt intake. Other measures to ameliorate haemodynamic intolerance of HD are described above, under 'Intra-dialytic hypotension', and should include consideration of a transfer to peritoneal dialysis.

Preventative measures should include prescriptions of adequate HD session duration (≥4 h), careful justification of low dialysate potassium and calcium prescriptions (avoiding them where possible by review of drugs, dietary intake, etc.) and attention to inter-dialytic weight gains.

Finally, it should be noted that the incidence of cardiovascular events is far higher in the weeks after first dialysis initiation [48] – as well as careful attention to volume management, strong consideration should be given to an incremental approach to prescribing dialysis intensity.

80.8 Infection Control (▶ Chap. 76)

Infection control covers a number of different aspects of HD care.

80.8.1 Blood-Borne Virus Protection

Measures to prevent the spread of blood-borne viruses (BBVs) – specifically, hepatitis B and C, as well as HIV – are covered in detail, elsewhere [49] ▶ Chap. 76, but include:

- Hygienic precautions to prevent viral transfer directly or form contaminated equipment
- The avoidance of multi-dose drug vials

- Serological surveillance
- Vaccination programmes
- The safe use of equipment in those with positive BBV serology or whose status is unknown
- Enhanced surveillance after identification of a new case of BBV positivity or of possible exposure
- Approach to surveillance after dialysis abroad

Our own approach acknowledges that even ideal systems can fail as a result of human error in a busy, high turnover service. A positive test or possible exposure requires contact tracing that may extend outside the immediate service to other dialysis units whose own patients may have visited during the period of exposure or who have accommodated local patients for holiday HD. Renal IT systems may help in linking machine use with individual patient sessions but failed hardware that is exchanged in the middle of a session may not be captured. Ultimately, because enhanced surveillance relies on the reassurance that these human processes are failsafe, our own practice is to undertake regular audits of staff understanding of protocol as well as spot checks of both staff knowledge and hygienic precautions. Because the scope of contact tracing is that much greater for serology that is checked less frequently, our own practice is for 3 monthly surveillance for both hepatitis B and C.

80.8.2 Vascular Access

Optimising vascular access is covered in detail, elsewhere in this textbook. Where dialysis catheters cannot be avoided, robust infection control methods should include surveillance of connection technique and infection rates (methicillin-sensitive and methicillin-resistant *Staphylococcus aureus*, *Clostridium difficile*). Our own armamentarium includes antimicrobial catheter locks and tunnelled dialysis catheter exit site patches (the latter as secondary prevention after exit site infection or catheter-related bacteraemia, even if this occurred with a previous line).

80.8.3 Prevention and Treatment of Infective Episodes

Infection is a major cause of morbidity and mortality in HD patients.

Although primary care is often the main drive to recruit at-risk groups (such as the HD population) to national vaccination programmes, it is recommended that an impetus be applied from renal services, too, to ensure that patients who may rarely engage with general practice are appropriately covered. Maintaining adequate dialysis and nutritional intake are key factors in minimizing the risk of infective complications and in ensuring that HD patients are physiologically equipped to survive an episode when it arises. Although resources are available to aid antimicrobial drug dosing in HD (see Ref. [51] and ▶ www.renaldrugdatabase.com), our own experience of a collaborative approach between renal services, microbiologists and renal pharmacists can help ensure well-targeted and appropriate treatment.

80.9 Intra-dialytic Symptoms

80.9.1 Muscle Cramps

Cramps are a common complication of HD treatment and seem to arise, predominantly, as a result of plasma volume changes and hyponatraemia. The preponderance of symptoms towards the end of dialysis increased frequency when dialysate sodium is low or ultrafiltration requirements are high and improvements with sodium profiling seem to support this assertion. Lower limb involvement is most common but cramps can also affect the upper limbs and abdomen.

The risk of cramping can be reduced through measures that reduce the risk of intra-dialytic hypotension (see above) and by cautiously increasing the dialysate sodium. The latter manouevre does, however, risk a net sodium gain which can promote the vicious cycle of thirst, high fluid intake and high ultrafiltration requirements. Prophylactic quinine should be avoided because of the risk of serious side effects, in particular, cardiac arrhythmia associated with QT interval prolongation. Other potential pharmacological treatments have been explored (carnitine or vitamin E supplementation, short-acting benzodiazepines, carbamazepine, amitryptiline, gabapentin, etc.), but none are underpinned by a sufficiently robust enough evidence base to support their routine use.

80.9.2 Nausea, Vomiting and Headaches

These common intra-dialytic complications can be manifestations of intra-dialytic hypotension. If there is no evidence of haemodynamic instability, the most likely cause seems to relate to over-vigorous solute removal leading to compartmental fluid shifts – effectively, a *forme fruste* dialysis disequilibrium syndrome. As with intra-dialytic hypotension, though, there is a broad differential diagnosis that should be considered; these include significant pathologies (particularly neurological), metabolic disturbances (hyponatraemia, hypernatraemia, hypoglycaemia) or drug removal (e.g. beta-blockers).

Where symptoms are an obvious manifestation of intra-dialytic hypotension, these should be managed and prevented as described, above.

Where symptoms may be a result of over-vigorous solute removal, it would be appropriate to reduce the intensity of HD by reducing blood flow, dialysate flow and/or membrane surface area in the first instance. Attempts should be made to preserve treatment duration both to maintain dialysis adequacy (which should be kept under close surveillance during this process) and to minimise ultrafiltration rates.

If symptoms prove refractory to these measures, consider a switch to haemodiafiltration, to increased dialysis frequency (if there is spare capacity, in-centre, or a possibility of home treatment) or to peritoneal dialysis.

These measures may also help ease the post-dialysis fatigue (or 'hangover') that features prominently amongst patients' own concerns (see also above).

80.10 Dialysis Disequilibrium Syndrome

The syndrome consists of a variety of neurological manifestations developing during or straight after HD and ranging from the *forme fruste*, described above (under 'Intra-dialytic symptoms' – 'Nausea, vomiting and headaches') to agitation, confusion, visual disturbances, seizures, coma and death. It is most likely to occur as a result of rapid changes in plasma osmolality, leading to compartmental water shifts and cerebral oedema.

Patients at risk include those with a pre-dialysis urea >50 mmol/L especially in the presence of severe metabolic acidosis, in the elderly and in those with a pre-existing neurological disorder. Typical patients at risk include those initiating renal replacement therapy for the first time by HD, existing HD patients who dialyse after prolonged non-attendance and peritoneal dialysis patients who are switching to HD due to poor clearances.

80.10.1 Differential Diagnosis

The differential diagnosis includes pathologies and metabolic disturbances that might develop or be exacerbated during or immediately after dialysis, e.g.:

- Hypo–/ hyper-natraemia
  - Incorrect setting of dialysate Na^+
  - Machine calibration errors
- Hypoglycaemia
  - Low dialysate glucose exacerbating:
    - Reduced insulin metabolism/anti-diabetic drug accumulation in ESRD
    - Coexistent sepsis
- Intra-cerebral haemorrhage/expanding subdural haematoma
  - Due to intra-dialytic anticoagulation
- Cerebral infarction
  - Due to intra-dialytic hypotension
- Hypertensive encephalopathy
  - Due to intra-dialytic exacerbation of pre-existing severe hypertension
- Uraemic encephalopathy
- Hypocalcaemia
  - Increased binding of Ca^{2+} to albumin after correction of severe metabolic acidosis (intravenous pre-dialysis pretreatment with calcium (e.g. 10 mL 10% calcium chloride) should be considered in those at risk; ionized Ca^{2+} should be checked, urgently, post-HD to guide further replacement)

The differential diagnosis should be swiftly limited by immediate assessments (e.g. absence of hypertensive retinopathy, hypoglycaemia, electrolyte disturbance) but may require further evaluation (e.g. CT brain) or simply, time (uraemic encephalopathy and dialysis disequilibrium may be difficult to differentiate although the former would improve with dialysis and the latter with time elapsed after it).

80.10.2 Prevention

Preventative strategies centre around delivering a minimal, safe dialysis dose. This can be achieved, for instance, by limiting the initial session duration to 2 h at a low blood flow (e.g. ≤200 ml/min), low dialysate flow (e.g. 300 ml/min) and with a low membrane surface area. Blood and dialysate flow can also be administered in a concurrent rather than countercurrent direction to minimise concentration gradients. Haemofiltration or sequential isolated ultrafiltration with low dose IHD may help sustain plasma osmolality.

There is an obvious need to balance the risks of rapid solute removal against inadequate clearances. For those deemed to be at high risk for dialysis disequilibrium, urgent post-dialysis blood should be sent to ensure that metabolic control is adequate enough to tide the patient over to the next planned session. Contingency should at least be considered to repeat treatment within a few hours in case clearance has been inadequate. These highest-risk patients may be best managed as in-patients but all who are thought to be at risk should be managed in a hospital setting (i.e. with access to medical staff), preferably within an acute care environment where nurse-patient ratios may be more optimal.

Subsequent sessions should be delivered on a daily basis with increasing intensity of the prescription until metabolic control is established – generally in the order of 3– 4 days.

80.10.3 Treatment

If high-risk patients develop symptoms suggestive of severe dialysis disequilibrium (e.g. agitation, confusion, seizures, reduced conscious level), HD should be stopped. The role of measures to increase plasma osmolality is unclear (e.g. iv mannitol or 50% dextrose) and may compound potential differential diagnoses (see above).

80.11 Needle Dislodgement

Blood losses may be undetected and potentially fatal. Bleeding from the patient's AV access will occur regardless of whether arterial, venous or both needles are dislodged, and it may be significant if it is not quickly stemmed. Perhaps, the biggest danger, though, is of losses through a displaced venous return as venous pressure alarms do not reliably differentiate between atmospheric and downstream venous pressures. With extracorporeal blood flows of 350–400 mL/min, exsanguination may swiftly occur. Arterial needle dislodgement, in isolation, should not lead to significant losses through the extracorporeal circuit; downstream air leak detector alarms should protect the patient from air embolism.

Patients at risk include those who are obtunded or agitated. Others at risk include those with excessive sweating, which may affect the adhesive properties of dressings and tape, and those on long-duration, nocturnal treatment (although the risks during the latter may be obviated by using single needle treatment – alarms will trigger during the arterial phase). The needle sites of at-risk patients should be kept under regular surveillance during treatment by dialysis staff. Where dialysis staff are not present (e.g. in the home setting) or where patients are at particular risk, blood leak alarms (similar to nocturnal enuresis pads) may be a valuable adjunct.

All patients should, however, be considered to be at some level of risk, and where privacy allows, the needled portion of their access should be kept visible (an 'airline seatbelt' policy).

80.12 Air Embolism

This rare complication is potentially fatal and requires swift action to save life. On the HD unit, the venous system is the initial route of air entry and is almost universally in the setting of a veno-venous dialysis catheter. Air embolism via AV access is highly unlikely (as vascular pressures significantly exceed atmospheric pressures) unless there is an accidental 'push' of air through it. This is likely to be a result of human error rather than a machine problem if air leak detectors in the extracorporeal blood circuit are functioning.

Excluding the risks associated with dialysis catheter insertion or removal, maintenance HD patients are vulnerable to air embolism:

- When sat up (as most are when dialyzing) as central venous pressures are lower
- Through catheter fracture or deliberate/accidental incision
- Through catheter extrusion – the subcutaneous tunnel may provide a ready portal to the venous system
- Through loose connections, either of the blood lines at the start of dialysis or of the caps at the end

Entry of air bubbles into the pulmonary arterial tree can occlude vessels, increase right heart pressures and ultimately reduce cardiac output due to reduced venous return to the left heart. Smaller gas bubbles in the pulmonary micro-circulation can lead to endothelial damage which can, in turn, produce bronchoconstriction, ventilation-perfusion mismatching and non-cardiac pulmonary oedema.

A significant venous air embolism that reaches the systemic arterial circulation can cause organ ischaemia, including myocardial and cerebral. A potentially fatal dose has been estimated to be 300–500 mL introduced at >100 mL/sec [51] when the filtering capacity of the pulmonary circulation is exceeded. This dose may be much lower if paradoxical embolism, with direct right-to-left communication with the arterial circulation, occurs. Air bubbles may also rise to enter the cerebral venous circulation retrogradely in an upright patient, potentially compromising cerebral perfusion and causing neurological injury.

The clinical features of air embolism may be:

Organ specific depends on the pattern of organ ischaemia when gas enters the vasculature but can include:

- Acute neurology
- Livedo reticularis
- Coronary insufficiency

Cardio-respiratory

- Dyspnoea, wheeze, lung crepitations, tachypnea, tachycardia, central chest pain, hypotension, signs of acute right heart failure
- There may be a 'gasp' reflex, thought to be caused by air entering the pulmonary circulation
- There may be a churning, systolic-diastolic 'millwheel' murmur caused by gas trapped within the right ventricle

The diagnosis of air embolism is largely one of exclusion but maintaining a high index of suspicion in the correct clinical context is vital as it is a differential diagnosis that is often not considered. As well as the clinical features, described above, aspiration through the most downstream limb of an in situ dialysis catheter (the venous lumen should be closest to the pulmonary circulation) might draw back air if performed swiftly or if the gas bolus is large. A range of investigations (ECG, chest X-ray and urgent echocardiography, if available) should be undertaken to help rule out alternative diagnoses but may also reveal corroborative findings (right heart strain, localized radiographic oligaemia, or air in the pulmonary vasculature or ventricle, for instance). Subsequent investigations, such as CT scanning may also reveal evidence of vascular gas.

In terms of treatment, the potential source of air entry should be isolated, immediately (e.g. clamp lines or catheter, shut down blood pump, place a secure airtight dressing over catheter exit sites). The patient should be placed in the left lateral decubitus head down position to allow gas to accumulate in the right ventricular apex rather than large pulmonary arteries or cerebral venous circulation. Aspiration of gas through an in situ dialysis catheter should be attempted immediately after the diagnosis has been entertained and again once the left lateral decubitus head down position has been obtained (using the most downstream lumen). Closed chest massage, in the event of cardio-respiratory arrest, may allow larger gas bubbles to be broken down. Supportive management should be initiated (high flow oxygen, haemodynamic support, ventilatory support, etc.). Where the diagnosis of air embolism is established and has caused cardio-respiratory or specific organ compromise, particularly neurological, early initiation of hyperbaric oxygen therapy should be considered [52].

Air embolism can be prevented through secure connection technique of blood lines and caps to dialysis catheter lumens, at the start and after HD treatment, respectively. Patients with dialysis catheters should be advised on the correct care of their access including how to troubleshoot a fractured, open or extruded line - airtight dressings, spare catheter caps and clamps should be readily accessible to the patient when at home or on holiday.

80.13 Dialyser Reactions

These may be divided into type A and type B reactions.

Type A (anaphylactoid) reactions occur usually occur within the first few minutes of dialysis with venous return of blood to the systemic circulation and may be caused by:

- Chemical products used in dialyser manufacture, sterilization (e.g. ethylene oxide) or re-processing (e.g. bleach, hydrogen peroxide, formaldehyde) that have been inadequately rinsed out
- Acetate-containing dialysate (now rarely used)
- The combined use of acrylonitrile AN-69 membranes and ACE inhibitors, which enhances bradykinin generation
- AN-69 ST membranes, whose electronegative charge is markedly reduced by surface treatment with a biocompatible polymer, carries a significantly lower incidence of anaphylactoid reactions
- Bacterial fragments, from contaminated water, inadequate sterilization of reused dialysers can produce the same clinical picture.

Symptoms range from the relatively modest (wheeze, urticarial rash, burning at the access needle site, chest or back pains, headaches, gastrointestinal symptoms, flushing, fevers and other allergic manifestations) to cardiovascular collapse and death.

If a type A reaction is suspected, dialysis must be stopped and the return of blood prevented by clamping the venous blood line. Blood in the dead space of the dialysis catheter or needles should be aspirated before administering saline flushes or drugs. The reaction should be treated with intravenous hydrocortisone, intravenous antihistamines, nebulized bronchodilators and supportive measures initiated as required (which may include circulatory or ventilatory support).

Eosinophilia, elevated serum tryptase and total IgE may support the diagnosis, but are not always present. Dialyser rinsing and (if relevant) re-processing technique should be reviewed. The combined use of ACE inhibitors and AN-69 membrane material should be identified. Dialysate should be sent for sensitive culture and endotoxin counts. If no clear cause can be found, at the next session, switch to another membrane material, sterilized using an alternative technique (e.g. gamma irradiation, steam). Ensure the dialyser is well rinsed with at least 2 litres of priming fluid before the patient is connected. Keep intravenous steroids and anti-histamines to hand. Pretreatment with these agents should be considered if the previous reaction was severe. When starting treatment, keep blood flow low (Qb 50–100 ml/min) until venous return to the systemic circulation has been established for several minutes without incident.

Type B reactions are generally less severe and usually occur later in treatment – between 15 and 30 min after starting. They are thought to be caused by complement activation after exposure of blood to cellulose membrane surfaces with free hydroxyl groups. Typical clinical features include chest pain, back pain, nausea and vomiting. Severe, anaphylactoid reactions are rare.

Dialyser reuse, ethylene oxide sterilization and use of unmodified cellulose membranes are rare in contemporary practice, so dialysis reactions are an uncommon occurrence. Nevertheless, allergic reactions can occur even with polysulphone dialysers or on exposure to other components of the dialysis process such as heparin [6]. This possibility should be considered in any patient becoming acutely or recurrently unwell on dialysis.

80.14 Acute Haemolysis

This should be part of the differential diagnosis of chest pain, back pain or dyspnoea, developing during HD. The potential that acute haemolysis could cause rapid and fatal hyperkalaemia requires a high index of suspicion and swift diagnosis.

80

Most episodes are due to some aspect of the HD process, itself:

- Mechanical trauma from ill-fitting roller pumps, kinked blood lines, narrowed blood line lumens caused by poor manufacture*
- Chemical contamination* of dialysate with formaldehyde, bleach, copper (leached from pipework) chloramine, nitrates
- Heat-mediated due to incorrectly set dialysate temperature
- Osmotic injury from hypotonic dialysate caused by incorrect proportioning of concentrates and water

HD may decompensate pre-existing conditions:

- e.g. cooling of blood in the extracorporeal circuit may exacerbate cold agglutinin disease if temperatures fall low enough

The diagnosis can be suggested by a port wine appearance of blood in the venous return and can be confirmed, rapidly, by the finding of a pink supernatant in a centrifuged specimen (most HD units should have a centrifuge on-site). Point-of-care testing may allow rapid detection of a reduced haematocrit. Corroborative evidence can be found in the FBC and blood film, but these should not be regarded as the initial investigative tools due to the critical delays in obtaining results.

The simultaneous development of symptoms in more than one patient dialyzing at the same time should immediately raise the possibility of acute haemolysis of a system-wide aetiology. Examples are asterisked (*) above, but human error or misunderstanding may be propagated across more than one HD machine.

The approach to early discontinuation of HD for the patient developing chest pain or dyspnoea during treatment (see below) should afford some protection whilst assessment is underway. However, if the diagnosis is even suspected, HD must be stopped, immediately, with the venous return clamped to prevent extracorporeal blood from reaching the patient. Treatment should be discontinued, immediately, across the dialysis shift, if a system-wide problem is suspected.

Immediately after clamping, the dead space within the dialysis catheter and AV fistula needles should be aspirated then locked. Unless or until alternative vascular access can be established, AV fistula needles should be kept in situ in case of the urgent need to treat hyperkalaemia or transfuse blood. As well as the FBC, biochemistry should also be sent, urgently, along with a group and save sample in case of the need for blood transfusion.

Acute intra-dialytic haemolysis requires the immediate attention of senior medical, nursing and technical staff to investigate aetiology and manage logistics. Contact with other, local dialysis units and intensive care units should be made as a contingency in case of a system-wide problem that requires alternative venues for renal replacement therapy.

80.15 Differential Diagnosis of Chest Pain Developing During Dialysis

Coronary artery disease remains the primary differential due to its prevalence amongst the ESRD population. This may be precipitated by the haemodynamic stress of treatment and may not necessarily be associated with overt intra-dialytic hypotension. Dysrhythmias, to which HD patients are also prone, may manifest as chest pain.

Other alternative diagnoses, with particular relevance to the HD population, include air embolism, pulmonary embolism (for instance, from a clot adherent to a dialysis catheter or from AV access, particular after an endovascular intervention), acute haemolysis, pneumothorax (after dialysis catheter insertion) and dialyser reactions.

Unless transient and self-limiting, it is probably safer to wash-back and discontinue HD whilst the episode is under assessment although this needs to be judged on a case-by-case basis and may depend on the urgency of the need for dialysis (for instance, the dangerously hyperkalaemic patient may need to persist with HD whilst augmenting haemodynamic tolerability by temporarily discontinuing ultrafiltration). If HD is terminated, urgent blood should be sent to confirm the biochemical safety of early discontinuation of the session.

80.16 Differential Diagnosis of Dyspnoea Developing During Dialysis

Patients who are fluid overloaded will be dyspnoeic before dialysis is commenced, and this should improve as ultrafiltration progresses. The differential diagnosis of dyspnoea developing or worsening during dialysis includes coronary artery disease, dysrhythmia, air or pulmonary embolism, pneumothorax, dialyser reactions, anaphylaxis due to an administered drug (e.g. intravenous iron), cardiac tamponade, acute haemolysis or bacteraemia. The decision on whether to continue HD depends on the urgency of the need for dialysis and the likely aetiology. If HD is terminated, urgent blood should be sent to confirm the biochemical safety of early discontinuation of the session.

80.17 Systemic HD Care

The chapter, to this point, has focused on some of the most significant complications that can arise in the HD population and specific measures by which they might be prevented or mitigated. This second and final section will examine some of the more important systems that may be put in place that can help augment the quality of HD care as a whole. Rather than addressing individual complications, these measures help ensure a safe environment within which the HD patient can be treated.

Beyond these preventative strategies, all those dealing with HD patients should also be aware of the widespread impact that an isolated breach of process might produce; unusual patterns of clinical presentation or results might just point towards a system-wide problem that requires urgent attention. Although some such problems can be detected and minimised by routine reporting (e.g. staphylococcal bacteraemia rates, water quality feedback), others may require intuition and individual vigilance (e.g. haemolytic complications, iatrogenic hypernatraemia caused by incorrect machine calibration). The importance of a senior, multidisciplinary approach to tackle these problems cannot be overstated.

80.18 Convective Therapies

Many of the retained solutes implicated in the pathology of the uraemic state are middle molecular weight molecules (0.5–5 kDa, such as B2M), which are not readily cleared by conventional diffusion dialysis. Since increasing small solute clearance above currently established targets does not improve patient outcomes, attention has focused on the potential benefits of convective therapies (haemofiltration and haemodiafiltration), which are better able to remove middle molecular weight molecules.

Convection depends on the transmembrane pressure (TMP) and the sieving coefficient (a property of the individual membrane for that solute) = [solute] ultrafiltrate / [solute] plasma. The closer this ratio is to 1, the more complete the removal of that particular solute. Two other factors influence convection. The first of these is protein adsorption to the membrane, which increases resistance to the transfer of both water and solutes of all sizes. The second factor is concentration polarisation, caused by the slower movement of larger molecules across the dialysis membrane. This leads to the accumulation of these large solutes at the surface of the membrane, impeding the movement of smaller molecules into the dialysate compartment. The large molecule concentration gradient, developing across the hollow fibre, encourages movement back into the centre of the fibre as well as across the membrane. This phenomenon can be minimised with the use of pre-dilutional fluid replacement, high blood flows and lower UF rates.

Pure convective treatment (i.e. haemofiltration) is less efficient at removing small molecules as it does not have the power of the concentration gradient behind it. This disadvantage is circumvented by the addition of diffusive removal (i.e. with haemodiafiltration, HDF). Based on replacement volumes delivered in clinical trials of HDF, a minimum volume of 22 L/session has been recommended by some, though the benefits of this are still uncertain (see below). Higher replacement volumes may be accompanied by greater albumin losses; selection of an appropriate membrane is important, with sufficient permeability to facilitate convective solute removal whilst minimizing albumin loss. This is an area of ongoing technological development [53].

Pre-and post-dilutional approaches to replacement of substitution fluid (i.e. upstream and downstream of the membrane respectively) can be applied. The main disadvantage of post-dilutional replacement is haemoconcentration. High transmembrane pressures can also lead to membrane fibre rupture and increased albumin leakage. Transmembrane pressures should, therefore, be kept at less than 400 mmHg. Haemoconcentration should also be limited by keeping the filtration fraction at 50% or less. The filtration fraction (FF) can be calculated as follows:

$$\text{FF} = \text{ultrafiltration flow rate} / \text{plasma flow rate, where plasma flow rate} = \text{Qb} * (1 - \text{haematocrit}), \text{ and Qb is the delivered extracorporeal blood flow.}$$

The minimum Qb to keep the FF at 50% or less can therefore be calculated as:

$$\text{Minimum Qb} = \text{UFR} / 0.5 * (1 - \text{haematocrit})$$

Some worked examples follow:

$$\text{Haematocrit} = 0.3, \text{UFR} = 60\,\text{mL} / \text{minute}, \quad \text{Target FF} = 50\%$$

$$\text{Minimum Qb} = 60 / 0.5 * 0.7 = 171\,\text{mL} / \text{min}$$

$$\text{Haematocrit} = 0.4, \text{UFR} = 120\,\text{mL} / \text{min}, \quad \text{Target FF} = 50\%$$

$$\text{Minimum Qb} = 400\,\text{mL} / \text{min}$$

The main disadvantage of pre-dilutional replacement is the expense of extra substitution fluid requirements. Mid-dilution HDF is said to minimise the disadvantages and maximise the advantages of the other replacement techniques. Unfortunately, it requires a special filter allowing the infusion of replacement fluid at the mid-point in the dialyser. Mixed pre- and post-dilution can also be delivered, with some machines having the capability to adjust the ratio automatically according to transmembrane pressures. The substitution fluid required for HDF is now, almost invariably, produced online to ultrapure standards through sterilizing ultrafilters.

In terms of the evidence base, three randomized controlled trials of HDF versus HD failed to show a significant benefit in terms of mortality. However, a fourth trial and a pooled analysis of all studies did report a survival advantage, with 14% and 23% reductions in risk of total and cardiovascular mortality, respectively [54]. There is also some evidence that HDF is accompanied by improved haemodynamic stability during treatment sessions, though this may simply reflect cooling or sodium loading via replacement fluid. A criticism of the evidence supporting HDF is that most of the studies reported outcomes on a per-treatment basis, with censoring of those patients not able to continue HDF treatment. Since frailer patients may not have sustained adequate blood flows to support larger convection volumes, adverse outcomes in the HDF arm may have been missed.

The reduced costs of HDF with the online production of substitution fluid makes the technique a much more attractive option despite the current lack of definitive evidence of superiority. Although absolute indications for initiating HDF have yet to be defined, the presence or prevention of beta 2 microglobulin amyloidosis, haemodynamic instability or patients with no clear prospect of renal transplantation who are likely to survive 2 years or more would seem reasonable circumstances to consider the technique [6].

80.19 Water Quality

On a standard treatment schedule, HD patients are exposed to at least 350 L of water per week, separated from their bloodstream only by the semipermeable membrane. For those receiving convective therapies or whose dialysers are reprocessed, water exposure will be direct.

Potential sources of harm include:

- Aluminium intoxication syndrome - aluminium is added to remove colloidal substances from the mains water supply. The syndrome may manifest as encephalopathy, bone disease or erythropoietin resistance but is now much less common since the introduction of reverse osmosis; HD patients are still at risk from marked variability in water supplier practices, though.
- Chloramine-induced haemolysis and methaemoglobinaemia – added to mains water for microbial control, the removal of both chloramine and chlorine by HD water treatment processes also renders the product water vulnerable to microbial growth.
- Fluoride-induced bone disease – added to mains water, fluoride can also be fatal in high concentrations.
- Microbial contamination – can produce pyrogenic reactions when contamination is heavy but even low levels of bacterial growth may contribute to long-term morbidity. Chronic inflammation (as evidenced by a raised plasma CRP or interleukin-6 level) is common in the chronic HD population and may be associated with an increased risk of long-term morbidity. This may be a consequence of low-level microbial contamination of the dialysate. Bacterial products such as endotoxin fragments, peptidoglycans and bacterial DNA can all induce cytokines and are able to cross even low flux dialysers.

80.19.1 Quality Assurance

A comprehensive and detailed overview of requirements is given in the joint UK Renal Association – Association of Renal Technologists guideline [55], but a few points need to be drawn out.

80.19.1.1 Communication

Clear lines of communication should be established with the local water provider to ensure early warning of variations in water content due to both changes in water treatment practice by the supplier as well as seasonal fluctuations. The biggest threats to the dialysis patient are the deliberate additives to mains water rather than existing contaminants.

Clear lines of communication should also be established with the HD unit institution's own Estates Department to ensure changes in the process do not have an impact upon the provision of dialysis water. As an example, *Legionella* preventative practice may involve the use of hydrogen peroxide which can cause both methaemoglobinaemia and haemolysis. Hydrogen peroxide is not well removed by reverse osmosis.

Clear responsibilities should be defined. The monitoring programme should include technical variables (e.g. water plant pressures and conductivity), chemical monitoring and microbiological surveillance. The output from these monitoring programmes should be reported on a regular basis to the clinical lead for HD. For all monitored variables, action plans should be available in the event of deviations from expected results. These outputs should, therefore, include documentation of action plans – a good disinfection schedule, for instance, should be reactive to microbial counts with an action level of 50% of the maximum allowable limit.

80.19.1.2 Technique

The recommended techniques for monitoring should be used to ensure that they are of sufficient enough sensitivity to detect problems, early. For example, water culture should use techniques most suited for growing fastidious, waterborne organisms (e.g. membrane filtration) using a low nutrient medium (e.g. Reasoner's 2A agar) at a lower incubation temperature (e.g. 25 °C) for longer periods (e.g. 7 days). Endotoxin assays should use the limulus amoebocyte lysate assay.

80.19.1.3 Hardware

The primary water treatment processes are discussed in detail in the joint UK Renal Association – Association of Renal Technologists guideline [55]. A few relevant highlights, follow:

- Deionisers provide an excellent environment for microbiological growth so downstream control measures are needed.
- A robust programme of deioniser replacement is required as exhausted resins can release toxic ions (e.g. fluoride) when other ions with higher affinity are present in the supply of water.
- Carbon beds (which remove organic compounds, chlorine and chloramines) should be replaced, regularly, to prevent their exhaustion.
  - They should be placed upstream of the reverse osmosis unit as chlorine can cause degradation of the RO membrane.
  - Because of the serious implications of chloramine escape past an exhausted carbon bed, two carbon filtration units are usually placed in series as a safety measure.
- Carbon beds provide a good environment for microbiological growth so downstream control measures will be needed.
- Water softeners are needed in hard water areas to remove both calcium and magnesium – these are best placed upstream of the reverse osmosis unit to prevent degradation of its membrane by these salts.
- An extra filtration step may be needed to help augment microbial control – for instance, point of use endotoxin filters at the dialysis machine.

80.19.1.4 Ultrapure Versus Standard Quality Water

UK guidelines, in keeping with others, suggest the following:

- Standard delivery of water for dialysis:
  - Bacterial colony counts <100 colony forming units/mL
  - Endotoxin count <0.25 IU/mL
- Ultrapure delivery:
  - Bacterial colony counts <0.1 colony forming units/mL
  - Endotoxin count <0.03 IU/mL

Some, but by no means all, studies have shown that a switch from standard to ultrapure dialysis may reduce levels of inflammation in chronic HD patients. Its use may improve anaemia management, help prevent dialysis-related amyloidosis and improve nutritional status. There is no clear evidence of benefits in terms of other clinical outcomes, though.

Although ultrapure water is a prerequisite for convective therapies and dialyser reprocessing, it is desirable for all given the relative ease of its provision when water plant hardware and maintenance are already providing good quality water. There are some practical highlights to consider:

- Maintenance and disinfection programmes should be robust.
- The water pipe connecting the main water delivery circuit to the HD machine is a weak link and vulnerable to contamination – these should be replaced/disinfected on a regular basis.

- Point-of-use, pre-dialyser endotoxin filters should be replaced, regularly, according to manufacturers' instructions but more frequently if downstream water quality deteriorates.
- Care should be taken in the preparation of concentrates, especially bicarbonate concentrates, which are especially prone to microbial growth – when using bicarbonate concentrate, as a matter of course, containers should be disposed of at the end of the dialysis unit working day.
- Samples should be tested by the most sensitive, recommended techniques but also when they are likely to yield the worst results (just prior to routine system disinfections and at the far end of the water loop).

It should be remembered, though, that culture and endotoxin assays only detect a proportion of cytokine-inducing substances that may be present – yeasts, peptidoglycans and other bacterial fragments will not be picked up.

80.20 Care of Haemodialysis Inpatients

The chronic HD patient suffers more frequent and prolonged hospital admissions than the general hospital population. This in-patient stays place the HD patient at risk for a number of reasons:

- Inappropriate care of vascular access.
- Undernutrition.
- Inappropriate drug dosing.
- The burden of transfer to and from the HD unit for regular sessions, especially if from an outside hospital – opportunities for comprehensive clinical evaluation when an HD in-patient attends, briefly, for their routine session, are limited.

In-patient care of the HD patient with a non-renal problem should be at least overseen (remotely or in-person) by renal services and where necessary through joint care. Patients should be advised that if they are admitted, either as an emergency or electively, to another department or hospital, local healthcare teams should be making prompt contact with the on-call renal team. They, in turn, should be discussing the need for transfer for renal unit care with the senior nephrologist on duty. It may be better for a patient to transfer their home team (e.g. their general surgical team) than risk the vagaries of remote renal care.

One caveat to transfer of in-patients to the renal unit from outside hospitals is the potential for their arrival with an unheralded critical illness. It is our practice for physiological severity scoring of all potential in-patient transfers from other hospitals to allow triage towards either critical care or the renal unit. Even if patients are not diverted for critical care, an understanding of physiological instability can highlight the need for added vigilance and ensure the early involvement of critical care outreach teams.

Finally, an under-recognised problem for the in-patient HD patient is the potential for under-prescription and under-delivery of the dose of dialysis [56]. The sicker chronic HD patient may, in urea kinetic terms, be closer to the patient with AKI than their stable, out-patient counterpart. Loss of lean body mass and changes in volume status can affect V (the volume of distribution of urea), and patients can become markedly hypercatabolic. In addition, HD patients admitted with vascular access problems are also, clearly, at risk of inadequate dialysis. For this reason, it is recommended that in-patients on chronic HD, unless entirely clinically stable with documented dialysis adequacy, should have the adequacy of their dialysis prescription and its delivery reviewed at each session until clinically stable.

80.21 Organization of the HD Service Will Be Covered by Roger Greenword

The 'conveyor belt' nature of in-centre HD provision serves the core function of delivering the HD prescription in an efficient and timely fashion. However, care requirements that are divergent from the routine can be vulnerable to these immediate priorities. The challenge for a busy HD service, therefore, is how the complexity of individualised care can be accommodated amongst the logistics of HD delivery and the over-arching strategic and organizational goals of the service as a whole. One particular issue is the need to break down those domains of HD care that are traditionally deemed to be exclusively 'nursing' in nature and those deemed to be predominantly 'medical' to ensure that holistic, multidisciplinary care can be delivered.

80.21.1 The HD Clinic

Traditionally viewed as the domain where medical therapy is defined and delivered, this can be vulnerable to a number of factors:

- Inadequate capacity may limit frequent enough follow-up to meet medical care needs. Assuming that most stable HD patients will need a review on a 3-month basis, but that some will need much more frequent follow-up, our own practice is to organize HD clinic capacity to allow an average of five clinic appointments per annum.

- Discordant record-keeping – multiple different sources of the clinical record are a risk to patient care. A clear understanding is needed, across the multidisciplinary team as to what are acceptable points of documentation and what are not. Progress towards fully integrated electronic health records will mitigate this problem but renal-specific functionality is currently delivered by specific software that is not immediately visible within the entirety of the hospital record.
- Non-attendance – coordinating clinic visits with dialysis sessions (before, during or after) can help. Again, enough HD clinic capacity is needed to ensure that there is enough flexibility to allow this degree of coordination – it should be remembered that dialysis shifts may not coordinate with physicians' routine clinic working patterns.
- Adherence to a strategic 'tick list' – there is much anecdotal and some more robust evidence to suggest that senior allied healthcare practitioners are more likely to achieve patient care targets than training grade medical staff. The available resource will clearly dictate how the HD clinic service is staffed (with nurse practitioners, senior medical staff, trainee medical staff under supervision, etc.) but our experience is, that a 'tick box' clinic proforma is rarely a satisfactory solution for a deficient strategic drive or inadequate experience. The removal of certain patient care pathways from the domain of the HD clinic (e.g. vascular access surveillance), with the drive provided by healthcare professionals dedicated to the task, may be beneficial.
- Communicating the individualized care plan – certain aspects of the care plan will need to be delivered by HD unit nursing staff. Examples include:
  - Once off extra blood tests
  - Regular monitoring with non-standard bloods (e.g. ANCA monitoring in vasculitis patients)
  - Blood pressure and fluid management programmes

  Our own practice uses a dialysis communications section in the HD nursing record that contains all current requirements and can include the need for feedback on the success or failure of a particular course of action. Each HD session requires a sign off that these requirements have been checked. Automated (electronic) alerts would represent a more elegant augmentation to cohesive, multidisciplinary team communications.

80.21.2 The Multidisciplinary Team (MDT) Meeting

The opportunity for MDT discussion of individual patients should be welcomed with some evidence that these produce greater success in achieving treatment goals.

As well as problems specific to that individual patient, topics covered include BP and fluid management, access to transplantation, urea kinetic modelling (and vascular access) and blood review. It can also be a useful opportunity to review modality and, for instance, ensure that suitable candidates for HDF, home HD and in-patient, self-care programmes, are identified. Encouraging participation in in-centre, self-care programmes can yield benefits for both the patient and the service as a whole (for instance, by providing a stepping stone towards home HD).

Renal IT systems play a critical role in, for instance, identifying outliers who may need more individualized attention.

80.21.3 The 'HD Committee'

As well as individual patient care, provided through the HD clinic and MDT meeting, there is a need to assure safe delivery and development of the service as a whole. The 'HD committee' – whether virtual or real – can be a useful forum for reporting of, for instance, regular infection control audits and water quality results and discussion of unit developments and new protocols.

80.21.4 Management of Intercurrent Problems

Attendance for thrice-weekly sessions places a heavy burden on patients when transport to and from the dialysis unit and recovery times are factored in. It is, therefore, unsurprising that main centre HD patients tend to seek the advice of renal unit doctors for unrelated medical problems. It is difficult to offer advice on how this should be managed as this will depend on available staffing resources. However, the use of HD nurses for triaging activities can place them in a difficult position if the wrong call is made. The use of a senior nurse to filter requests for assessment can mitigate the extra burden on a perhaps limited medical resource, but to some extent, there has to be an acceptance that certain facets of primary care will have to be undertaken on the dialysis unit. Nevertheless, there are key primary care functions (e.g. vaccinations and certain screening programmes) that require the relationship between the HD patient and the general practitioner to be maintained. This contact should be strongly encouraged.

80

Chapter Review Questions

1. A patient develops chest pain and dyspnoea 1 h into a dialysis session. You attend to assess but on arrival find the patient dialysing at the next station has developed similar symptoms. How should you proceed?
   - Simultaneous symptoms in two patients raise the possibility of haemolysis.
   - Immediately stop HD on both patients; clamp/aspirate don't wash back.
   - Look for evidence of haemolysis in venous line; centrifuge.
   - Simultaneously need to assess for other causes (examination, ECG, urgent bloods, chest radiograph..); two dialysis patients with chest pain are not that remote a possibility.
   - Send blood for group and save blood film, haemoglobin, urgent potassium (point of care if available).
   - If serious suspicion, cease dialysis immediately on other asymptomatic patients in the same facility. The situation will potentially need rapid escalation planning for safe dialysis provision in alternate facilities.
2. Shortly after the commencement of dialysis, a patient becomes acutely unwell and short of breath. The nurses found his tunnelled dialysis catheter disconnected from one of the blood lines and promptly clamped this before washing back through the other line. On your arrival, he is sat up gasping, distressed. What will you do? What physical findings may be present?
   - Supine left lateral decubitus position.
   - High flow oxygen.
   - Attempt to aspirate air from distal catheter lumen.
   - Critical care circulatory/respiratory support as necessary.
   - ECG, chest radiograph.
   - Consider hyperbaric oxygen if ongoing compromise (may attempt to confirm extent with CT).
   - Possible physical signs: churning 'millwheel' murmur, wheeze, crepitations, focal neurology, livedo.
3. A holiday patient is admitted from your dialysis unit with a fever and dyspnoea occurring on their first dialysis visit. They are treated with antibiotics and seem to be settling. No source of infection is evident clinically and it is considered possible they may have a dialysis catheter-related infection. 48 h later on the next dialysis session the patient again feels less well and is febrile. How may you investigate?
   - Differential diagnosis is infection versus dialyser reaction; may be hard to distinguish.
   - Line infection can cause pyrexia in the context of line use; send further cultures, consider echocardiogram for endocarditis, and monitor further for any pyrexias occurring between HD sessions.
   - Look for eosinophilia; consider sending tryptase.
   - Try a different dialyser type at the next session.
   - Confirm not AN69 ACEi combination.
   - Establish the patient's normal dialyser type.

Bibliography

1. Coomer RW, Schulman G, Breyer JA, et al. Ambulatory blood pressure monitoring in dialysis patients and estimation of mean interdialytic blood pressure. Am J Kidney Dis. 1997;29(5):678–84.
2. Kooman JP, Gladziwa U, Bocker G, et al. Blood pressure during the interdialytic period in haemodialysis patients: estimation of representative blood pressure values. Nephrol Dial Transplant. 1992;7(9):917–23.
3. Baumgart P, Walger P, Gemen S, et al. Blood pressure elevation during the night in chronic renal failure, hemodialysis and after renal transplantation. Nephron. 1991;57(3):293–8.
4. Peixoto AJ, Santos SF, Mendes RB, et al. Reproducibility of ambulatory blood pressure monitoring in hemodialysis patients. Am J Kidney Dis. 2000;36(5):983–90.
5. Agarwal R, Andersen MJ, Bishu K, et al. Home blood pressure monitoring improves the diagnosis of hypertension in hemodialysis patients. Kidney Int. 2006;69(5):900–6.
6. Ashby D, Borman N, Burton J, et al. Renal Association clinical practice guideline - haemodialysis. 2019 [cited 2019 21st October]. Available from: https://renal.org/wp-content/uploads/2019/07/FINAL-HD-Guideline.pdf.
7. Foley RN, Parfrey PS, Harnett JD, et al. Impact of hypertension on cardiomyopathy, morbidity and mortality in end-stage renal disease. Kidney Int. 1996;49(5):1379–85.
8. Port FK, Hulbert-Shearon TE, Wolfe RA, et al. Predialysis blood pressure and mortality risk in a national sample of maintenance hemodialysis patients. Am J Kidney Dis. 1999;33(3):507–17.
9. Kalantar-Zadeh K, Kilpatrick RD, McAllister CJ, et al. Reverse epidemiology of hypertension and cardiovascular death in the hemodialysis population: the 58th annual fall conference and scientific sessions. Hypertension. 2005;45(4):811–7.

10. Li Z, Lacson E Jr, Lowrie EG, et al. The epidemiology of systolic blood pressure and death risk in hemodialysis patients. Am J Kidney Dis. 2006;48(4):606–15.
11. Tentori F, Hunt WC, Rohrscheib M, et al. Which targets in clinical practice guidelines are associated with improved survival in a large dialysis organization? J Am Soc Nephrol. 2007;18(8):2377–84.
12. Stidley CA, Hunt WC, Tentori F, et al. Changing relationship of blood pressure with mortality over time among hemodialysis patients. J Am Soc Nephrol. 2006;17(2):513–20.
13. Charra B, Calemard E, Ruffet M, et al. Survival as an index of adequacy of dialysis. Kidney International. 1992;41(5):1286–91.
14. Thein H, Haloob I, Marshall MR. Associations of a facility level decrease in dialysate sodium concentration with blood pressure and interdialytic weight gain. Nephrol Dial Transplant. 2007;22(9):2630–9.
15. Charra B, Bergstrom J, Scribner BH. Blood pressure control in dialysis patients: importance of the lag phenomenon. American Journal of Kidney Diseases. 1998;32(5):720–4.
16. Ozkahya M, Toz H, Unsal A, et al. Treatment of hypertension in dialysis patients by ultrafiltration: role of cardiac dilatation and time factor. Am J Kidney Dis. 1999;34(2):218–21.
17. Ross EA, Pittman TB, Koo LC. Strategy for the treatment of noncompliant hypertensive hemodialysis patients. Int J Artif Organs. 2002;25(11):1061–5.
18. Chen J, Gul A, Sarnak MJ. Management of intradialytic hypertension: the ongoing challenge. Semin Dial. 2006;19(2):141–5.
19. Polkinghorne KR, Kerr PG. Acute complications during hemodialysis. In: Johnson R, Feehally J, Floege J, Tonelli M, editors. Comprehensive clinical nephrology. 6th ed. Elsevier; 2018. p. 1090–102.
20. Ligtenberg G, Blankestijn PJ, Oey PL, et al. Reduction of sympathetic hyperactivity by enalapril in patients with chronic renal failure. N Engl J Med. 1999;340(17):1321–8.
21. Gunal AI, Karaca I, Celiker H, et al. Paradoxical rise in blood pressure during ultrafiltration is caused by increased cardiac output. Journal of Nephrology. 2002;15(1):42–7.
22. Rahman M, Dixit A, Donley V, et al. Factors associated with inadequate blood pressure control in hypertensive hemodialysis patients. Am J Kidney Dis. 1999;33(3):498–506.
23. Shoji T, Tsubakihara Y, Fujii M, et al. Hemodialysis-associated hypotension as an independent risk factor for two-year mortality in hemodialysis patients. Kidney Int. 2004;66(3):1212–20.
24. McIntyre CW. Recurrent circulatory stress: the dark side of dialysis. Semin Dial. 2010;23(5):449–51.
25. Nette RW, van den Dorpel MA, Krepel HP, et al. Hypotension during hemodialysis results from an impairment of arteriolar tone and left ventricular function. Clin Nephrol. 2005;63(4):276–83.
26. Poldermans D, Man in't Veld AJ, Rambaldi R, et al. Cardiac evaluation in hypotension-prone and hypotension-resistant hemodialysis patients. Kidney Int. 1999;56(5):1905–11.
27. Barakat MM, Nawab ZM, Yu AW, et al. Hemodynamic effects of intradialytic food ingestion and the effects of caffeine. J Am Soc Nephrol. 1993;3(11):1813–8.
28. Shinzato T, Miwa M, Nakai S, et al. Role of adenosine in dialysis-induced hypotension. J Am Soc Nephrol. 1994;4(12):1987–94.
29. Noris M, Benigni A, Boccardo P, et al. Enhanced nitric oxide synthesis in uremia: implications for platelet dysfunction and dialysis hypotension. Kidney Int. 1993;44(2):445–50.
30. Yokokawa K, Mankus R, Saklayen MG, et al. Increased nitric oxide production in patients with hypotension during hemodialysis. Ann Intern Med. 1995;123(1):35–7.
31. van der Zee S, Thompson A, Zimmerman R, et al. Vasopressin administration facilitates fluid removal during hemodialysis. Kidney Int. 2007;71(4):318–24.
32. Evenepoel P, Kuypers DR. Dermatologic manifestations of chronic kidney disease. In: Johnson R, Feehally J, Floege J, Tonelli M, editors. Comprehensive clinical nephrology. 6th ed. Elsevier; 2018. p. 1013–21.
33. Collins AJ, Foley RN, Herzog C, et al. Excerpts from the US renal data system 2009 annual data report. Am J Kidney Dis. 2010;55(1 Suppl 1):S1–420. A426–427.
34. Cheung AK, Sarnak MJ, Yan G, et al. Cardiac diseases in maintenance hemodialysis patients: results of the HEMO Study. Kidney Int. 2004;65(6):2380–9.
35. Busch M, Franke S, Muller A, et al. Potential cardiovascular risk factors in chronic kidney disease: AGEs, total homocysteine and metabolites, and the C-reactive protein. Kidney Int. 2004;66(1):338–47.
36. Kremastinos D, Paraskevaidis I, Voudiklari S, et al. Painless myocardial ischemia in chronic hemodialysed patients: a real event? Nephron. 1992;60(2):164–70.
37. MacLaughlin HL, Cook SA, Kariyawasam D, et al. Nonrandomized trial of weight loss with orlistat, nutrition education, diet, and exercise in obese patients with CKD: 2-year follow-up. Am J Kidney Dis. 2010;55(1):69–76.
38. Frankel A, Kazempour-Ardebili S, Bedi R, et al. Management of adults with diabetes on the haemodialysis unit. 2016 [cited 2019 21st October]. Available from: https://renal.org/wp-content/uploads/2017/07/jbds-ip-management-of-adults-with-diabetes-on-the-haemodialysis-unit-1.pdf.
39. Joy MS, Cefalu WT, Hogan SL, et al. Long-term glycemic control measurements in diabetic patients receiving hemodialysis. Am J Kidney Dis. 2002;39(2):297–307.
40. Wanner C, Tonelli M, Kidney Disease: Improving Global Outcomes Lipid Guideline Development Work Group M. KDIGO Clinical Practice Guideline for Lipid Management in CKD: summary of recommendation statements and clinical approach to the patient. Kidney Int. 2014;85(6):1303–9.
41. Nigwekar SU, Kang A, Zoungas S, et al. Interventions for lowering plasma homocysteine levels in dialysis patients. Cochrane Database Syst Rev. 2016;5:CD004683.
42. Wright M, Southcott E, MacLaughlin H, et al. Renal Association clinical practice guideline - undernutrition in chronic kidney disease. 2019 [cited 2019 21st October]. Available from: https://renal.org/wp-content/uploads/2019/06/FINAL-Nutrition-guideline-June-2019.pdf.
43. Stenvinkel P, Herzog CA. Cardiovascular disease in chronic kidney disease. In: Johnson R, Feehally J, Floege J, Tonelli M, editors. Comprehensive clinical nephrology. 6th ed. Elsevier; 2018. p. 942–57.
44. Herzog CA, Littrell K, Arko C, et al. Clinical characteristics of dialysis patients with acute myocardial infarction in the United States: a collaborative project of the United States Renal Data System and the National Registry of Myocardial Infarction. Circulation. 2007;116(13):1465–72.
45. Bleyer AJ, Hartman J, Brannon PC, et al. Characteristics of sudden death in hemodialysis patients. Kidney Int. 2006;69(12):2268–73.
46. Pun PH, Lehrich RW, Honeycutt EF, et al. Modifiable risk factors associated with sudden cardiac arrest within hemodialysis clinics. Kidney Int. 2011;79(2):218–27.
47. Jadoul M, Thumma J, Fuller DS, et al. Modifiable practices associated with sudden death among hemodialysis patients in the Dialysis Outcomes and Practice Patterns Study. Clin J Am Soc Nephrol. 2012;7(5):765–74.

48. Eckardt KU, Gillespie IA, Kronenberg F, et al. High cardiovascular event rates occur within the first weeks of starting hemodialysis. Kidney Int. 2015;88(5):1117–25.
49. Garthwaite E, Reddy V, Douthwaite S, et al. Renal Association clinical practice guideline - management of blood borne viruses within the haemodialysis unit. 2019 [cited 2019 21st October]. Available from: https://renal.org/wp-content/uploads/2019/06/FINAL-BBV-Guideline-June-2019.pdf.
50. Ashley C, Dunleavy A. Renal drug handbook. Radcliffe Medical Press; 2014.
51. Orebaugh SL. Venous air embolism: clinical and experimental considerations. Crit Care Med. 1992;20(8):1169–77.
52. Blanc P, Boussuges A, Henriette K, et al. Iatrogenic cerebral air embolism: importance of an early hyperbaric oxygenation. Intensive Care Med. 2002;28(5):559–63.
53. Maduell F, Ojeda R, Arias-Guillen M, et al. A new generation of cellulose triacetate suitable for online haemodiafiltration. Nefrologia (Engl Ed). 2018;38(2):161–8.
54. Peters SA, Bots ML, Canaud B, et al. Haemodiafiltration and mortality in end-stage kidney disease patients: a pooled individual participant data analysis from four randomized controlled trials. Nephrol Dial Transplant. 2016;31(6):978–84.
55. Hoenich N, Mactier R, Morgan I, et al. Guideline on water treatment systems, dialysis water and dialysis fluid quality for haemodialysis and related therapies. 2016 [cited 2019 21st October]. Available from: https://renal.org/wp-content/uploads/2017/06/raandartguidelineversion-12647da131181561659443ff000014d4d8–2.pdf.
56. Kanagasundaram NS. Hemodialysis adequacy and the hospitalized end-stage renal disease patient--raising awareness. Semin Dial. 2012;25(5):516–9.
57. Cannella G, Paoletti E, Delfino R, et al. Prolonged therapy with ACE inhibitors induces a regression of left ventricular hypertrophy of dialyzed uremic patients independently from hypotensive effects. Am J Kidney Dis. 1997;30(5):659–64.
58. Tai DJ, Lim TW, James MT, et al. Cardiovascular effects of angiotensin converting enzyme inhibition or angiotensin receptor blockade in hemodialysis: a meta-analysis. Clin J Am Soc Nephrol. 2010;5(4):623–30.
59. Prakash S, Garg AX, Heidenheim AP, et al. Midodrine appears to be safe and effective for dialysis-induced hypotension: a systematic review. Nephrol Dial Transplant. 2004;19(10):2553–8.

Hemodialysis Prescription

Andrew Davenport

Contents

M. Harber (ed.), *Primer on Nephrology*, https://doi.org/10.1007/978-3-030-76419-7_81

Learning Objectives

- To understand the principles of and factors affecting hemodialysis clearance.
- To cover the ways of measuring hemodialysis clearance and potential limitations.
- To appreciate the need for tailored and responsive dialysis prescription.

81.1 Introduction

81

Chronic hemodialysis has evolved over half a century from a fairly crude life-saving treatment for the privileged few to a way-of-life treatment for approximately 4.35 million patients globally. Historically, the dialysis prescription was largely generic (typically 4 hours three times a week), but since the measurement of dialysis clearance/dose in the 1980s [1], it has become increasingly apparent that one size does not fit all and that chronic underdialysis has a poor outcome (Figs. 81.1 and 81.2 which illustrate the acute and chronic ends of the underdialysis spectrum). It has also become clear that residual renal function has huge benefits [2] and hemodialysis prescription can be tailored on the basis of residual renal function to the patient's potential advantage.

Assessment of dialysis clearance is based on measuring the removal of waste products of cell metabolism which accumulate in patients with chronic kidney disease. Urea is produced from the breakdown of proteins and recycling of amino acids. Although there is debate as to the toxicity of urea, urea is used as a surrogate measure of retained azotemic molecules [3]. Even though most laboratory assays report a composite of urea and some other small nitrogenous compounds, including ammonia, measurement of urea is still more reliable than that of creatinine. Increasingly, sophisticated and routine assessment of dialysis clearance, alongside measurement of residual

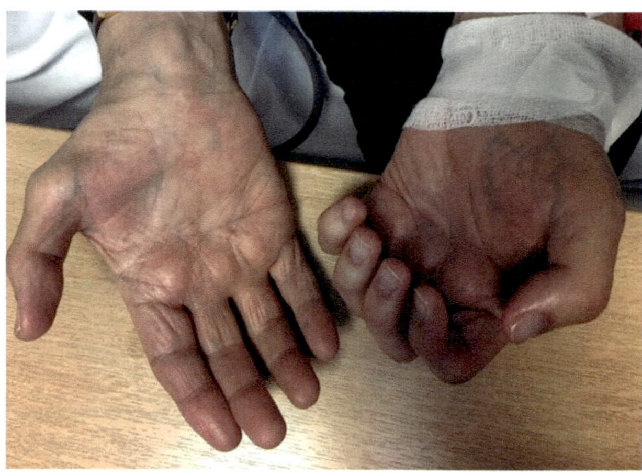

Fig. 81.2 Signs of dialysis amyloid (flexion contractures and carpal tunnel deposition) in an anuric patient who had been on dialysis for 17 years. The patient had no residual renal function, chronically high β_2M, and evidence of neuropathy. Dialysis amyloid illustrates the other, much more chronic end of the spectrum of 'underdialysis'. Although, this patient received regular dialysis with reasonable urea clearance on standard dialysis, it was not sufficient to clear middle molecules

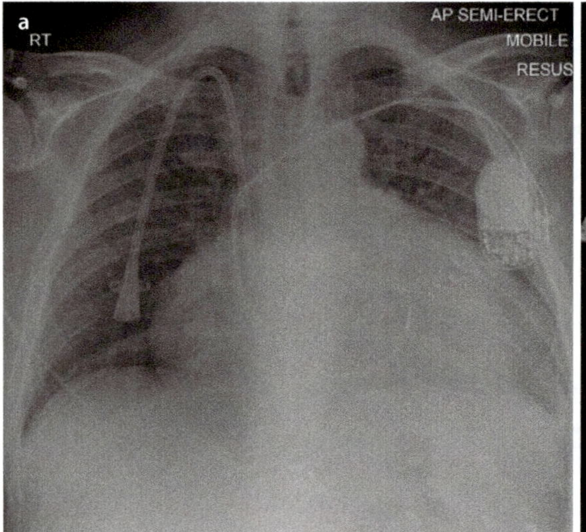

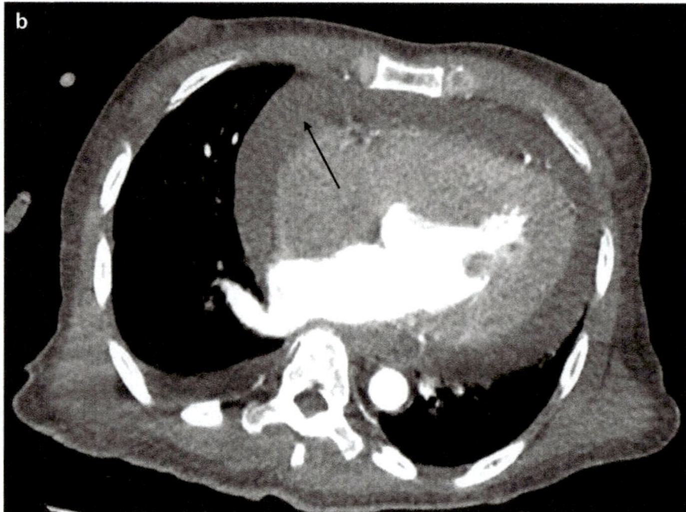

Fig. 81.1 **a**, **b** Show a CXR and CT chest, respectively of a patient who found dialysis difficult and repeatedly curtailed dialysis sessions or missed them altogether. The CXR is highly suggestive of a gross pericardial effusion, in this case due to uremia pericarditis secondary to chronic underdialysis. Uremic pericarditis is, perhaps, the most overt clinical presentation of chronic underdialysis and is associated with a high mortality. **b** CT chest of a patient with uremic pericarditis. The black arrow shows a large, circumferential pericardial effusion secondary to chronic underdialysis. This condition can resolve with intensive, careful dialysis, but prevention is considerably better than cure. Therefore, monitoring and appreciation of underdialysis should provoke an early assessment of the causes and potential solutions

renal function permit a more nuanced and bespoke prescription for patients requiring chronic dialysis.

81.2 Diffusive Dialyzer Clearance

Urea is a small uncharged molecule that readily diffuses. Diffusion is dependent on the concentration gradient which is increased by faster counter current blood and dialysate flow, dialyzer surface area, narrow-diameter capillary fibers reducing the distance molecules have to move, and resistance to passage through the wall of the capillary fiber. Each dialyzer comes with a manufacturer's measurement of ex vivo urea clearance at different blood pump and dialysate speeds for different sized dialyzers (KoA), but this clearance is greater than that in clinical practice, as it is not derived from experiments using human plasma.

81.3 Convective Dialyzer Clearance

Convective clearance is generated by applying an external hydrostatic pressure that drives water across the dialyzer membrane, and membrane permeability to water is termed hydraulic permeability, and differs with dialyzer membrane's composition and structure. Whereas molecular size is important for diffusion, with urea (MWt 64 d) moving 18 times faster than β2-microglobulin (MWt 11, 800 d), provided that the molecule can pass through the membrane, then convective clearance will be the same, so convective clearance will be similar for both urea and β2-microglobulin using a high-flux dialyzer. Dialyzer flux, which depends on membrane pore size, is now defined according to the clearance of β2-microglobulin.

During a standard hemodialysis treatment, there will be some convective exchange if there has been ultrafiltration. In addition, depending upon dialyzer hydraulic permeability, there may be internal diafiltration, which can be as much as 6–9 L during a four-hour dialysis session. Convective movement will potentially reduce the concentration gradient and may have a small effect in reducing diffusive clearance.

81.4 Sessional Dialyzer Clearance

The National Cooperative Dialysis Study (NCDS) was the first prospective dialysis study to examine the effect of urea clearance by randomizing patients to a lower and higher time averaged blood urea nitrogen target. During a 12-month follow-up, more patients dropped out of the study or had hospital admissions in the higher time averaged urea group. Gotch and Sargent subsequently reviewed the data, and developed the concept of dialyzer urea clearance, which only required pre- and post-dialysis blood sample, compared to three samples need to calculate time-average urea [1]. To be able to compare urea removal during dialysis (Kt) between patients, they argued that urea body distribution was equivalent to the volume of body water (V). This was estimated using equations derived from anthropometric measurements in healthy subjects.

81.5 Kt/Vurea Model

The simplest model of dialyzer urea removal is to calculate the urea reduction ratio (URR); however, this does not take into account any additional clearance from ultrafiltration losses. This led to the development of a first-generation equation to estimate Kt/V taking into account ultrafiltration losses. Single pool Kt/V (spKt/V) assumes that urea is distributed equally throughout body water and during the dialysis session urea is removed equally from body water. As this is not the case some advocate the use of a dual pool Kt/V model (dpKt/V) (◘ Fig. 81.3) [4, 5].

However, during dialysis blood supply to the skin and internal organs (muscle, heart, liver, kidney, and gastrointestinal tract) falls, and blood pools in the larger capacitance veins, such that shortly after the end of the dialysis session, plasma urea concentrations rebound upward (see ◘ Fig. 81.4).

To compensate for this effect, firstly, it is important to minimize this effect by taking precautions when taking the "post-dialysis" blood sample by using the slow-flow method, whereby blood flow is slowed down to allow for plasma urea concentration to re-equilibrate before blood sampling. Thus, a further revised equation was developed to take into account urea equilibration (eKt/V) to compensate for the differential removal of urea from body tissue compartments [7].

All these equations are based on the premise that patients dialyze three times a week, and that blood samples are taken pre- and post- midweek dialysis session. To allow comparison between patients dialyzing more or less frequently the concept of standardized Kt/V (stdKt/V) was introduced. To calculate stdKt/V, the derived stdK is multiplied by time (10,080 minutes per week) and adjusted by V.

As many patients now start dialysis with residual renal function, this has led to the practice of incremental dialysis, with patients bringing in 24-hour urine collections which are used to calculate urinary urea clearance (Kr). This is then adjusted according to the volume of urea distribution (body water) to estimate the equivalent urinary renal clearance (EKRc) [8].

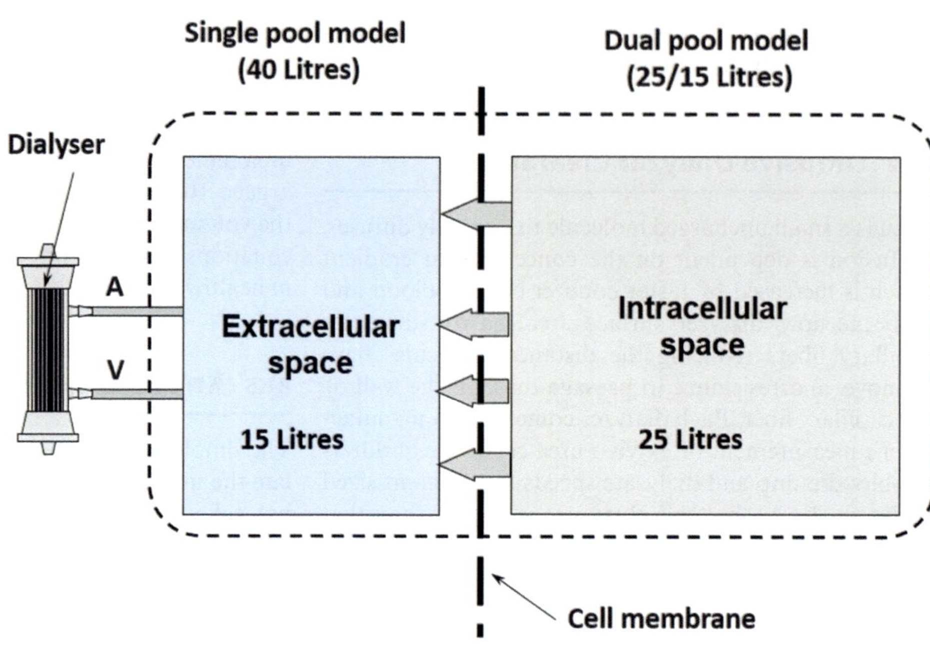

Fig. 81.3 A schematic of the difference between the single and dual pool model of urea clearance, illustrating the potential for rapid removal of urea (and other small molecules) from the extracellular space, but more limited, and slower access to the larger intracellular space. Single-pool modeling assuming a singular fluid pool, dual-pool modeling endeavors to account for the difference between these two pools

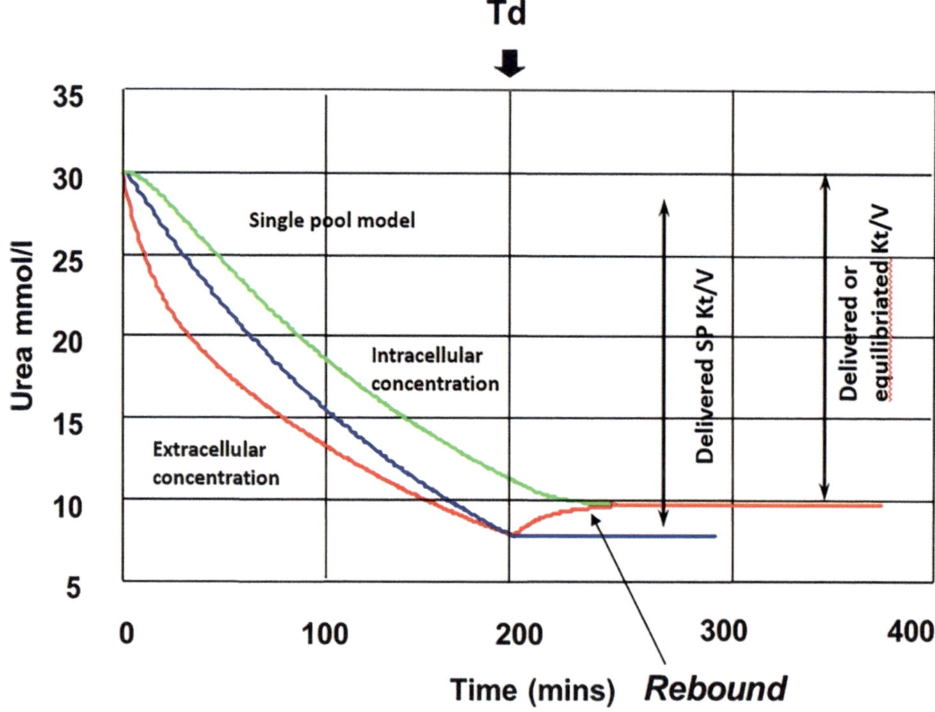

Fig. 81.4 Urea clearance curves demonstrating extracellular and intracellular clearance of urea (using a single pool model) with rebound of urea on cessation of dialysis. Sampling a later urea yields the equilibrated Kt/V which will be less of an underestimate that the spKt/V derived from an immediate post-dialysis urea [6]

81.6 Alternate Methods of Estimating Urea Clearance

Advances in dialysis machine technology can be used to estimate urea clearance, termed online clearance. One method is to use changes in dialysate conductivity. Although different in molecular weight, sodium and urea have almost identical diffusion coefficients at 37 °C (Na^+: 1.94 × 10^{-5} cm^2/s, Urea: 2.20 × 10^{-5} cm^2/s). By comparing the changes in dialysate conductivity of fresh and spent dialysate to short-term pulses of a change in dialysate sodium, designed to achieve a detectable diffusion of sodium ions across the dialyzer membrane, it is then possible to estimate urea clearance.

To prevent a positive sodium balance, pulses alternate between increased and decreased sodium concentrations. The frequency of pulses can be altered from every 12 to 30 minutes. Another method is based on ultraviolet light (UV) optical sensors, using C band: 280 nm −100 nm light-emitting diodes, measuring urea by absorbance in the spent dialysate.

81.7 Errors in Calculating Kt/V

One of the major technical errors in calculating dialyzer Kt/V is failure to allow sufficient time for urea to re-equilibrate when taking the post-dialysis blood sample, so obtaining a lower post-dialysis urea concentration, and thus, an inflated dialyzer Kt/V.

V is traditionally estimated using anthropometric equations which are based on healthy subjectsmainly Europeans from the 1950s. Body composition changes with age, gender, and ethnicity, and as adipose tissue contains less water than muscle this leads to an overestimation of V in large obese patients, and unsderestimation of V in small male patients, and also women. Thus, if all patients were to achieve the same Kt/V, then men would receive relatively more dialyzer clearance than women for any given weight, and heavier men more dialyzer clearance than lighter men. This inequality of V can be overcome using either bioimpedance to actually measure total body water, or scale Kt to total energy expenditure, or body surface area.

Online clearance methods tend to overestimate dialyzer urea clearance, as the intermittent method based on changes in sodium diffusion will potentially miss falls in blood pump speed or dialysate flow in between measurements, and the UV absorbance method will also measure other nitrogen containing molecules in addition to urea.

Urine output and urinary urea excretion fall in 24 hours post a hemodialysis session, and then start to increase. As such urine collections made after a dialysis session will underestimate residual renal function.

81.8 Incremental Dialysis for Solute Clearances

The majority of patients starting hemodialysis have some residual renal function. Currently, no dialysis treatment effectively removes protein-bound solutes. However, as the rate of production of these solutes is relatively slow, even a small amount of residual renal function is sufficient to clear these protein-bound toxins by renal tubule organic acid transporters. As such, there is an advantage to preserving residual renal function for as long as possible [9–14]. It is now recognized that during a standard hemodialysis session, the blood supply to the kidney falls and as there is no renal autoregulation, episodes of intra-dialytic hypotension risk acute ischemic damage to the kidney and premature loss of residual renal function [15].

This has led to a return to initiating hemodialysis in an incremental fashion, so starting dialysis once or twice weekly and for less than the standard 4 hours according to residual renal function [11–13]. The key is to sum residual renal function (KRU) to dialyzer urea clearance [8].

The 2006 KDOQI adequacy guideline advises against hemodialysis dose reduction for patients with a KRU of <2 ml/min/1.73 m^2,and recommends a sessional spKt/Vurea target 1.93 for a 3.5-hour dialysis session and 1.68 for a twice-weekly schedule for those with a KRU >2 ml/min/1.73 m^2), and a KRU > 3 ml/min/1.73 m^2 for twice-weekly 3.5-hour HD sessions to achieve an equivalent stdKt/Vurea of 1.2 [6]. In addition to advising against an incremental approach for patients with a residual renal function of a KRU of <2 ml/min, equally one has to consider patient volume status, and as such less frequent dialysis is not advised for patients with compromised cardiac function or have a residual urine output of <600 ml/day, or inter-dialytic weight gains of ≥3.5% [11].

As dialyzer urea clearance is not biologically equivalent to the residual renal clearance, one cannot simply add the time-averaged residual urea clearance (KRU) to the time-averaged dialysis urea clearance (Kdurea) as this would underestimate the contribution of KRU to overall clearance. There are proposed methods to add Kdurea to KRU by converting intermittent Kdurea to an equivalent continuous KRU or vice versa, so that they then may be added together [8].

81.8.1 Equivalent Renal Urea Clearance (EKRurea, ml/min)

EKRurea is the ratio of the net urea generation rate (G, mg/min) to time-averaged urea concentration (TACurea, mg/ml). To compare averaged renal urea clearance and dialysis urea clearance between patients, EKRurea should be normalized to a standardized urea volume (V, L) of 40 L to become corrected EKR (EKRc, ml/min/40 L). The same correction can be used to normalize KRU to a standardized urea volume of 40 L deriving corrected Kr (Krc, ml/min/40 L).

To prescribe Kt/Vurea corresponding to Krc and adjusting for dialysis sessions per week, European clinical guidelines advise using the Casino and Lopez nomogram (Figure) or an estimate using the following equations [8]:

$$\text{Weekly thrice EKRc} = 1 + \left(10 \times \text{eKt}/\left(\text{Vurea}\right)\right) + \text{Krc}$$

$$\text{Weekly twice EKRc} = 1 + \left(6 \times \text{eKt}/\left(\text{Vurea}\right) + \text{Krc}\right)$$

This target EKRc was derived from achieving a weekly thrice eKt/Vurea of 1.2 (regarding eKt/V urea 1.16 as the standard dose from the HEMO study), which is approximately 13 ml/min/40 L. This target is slightly higher than the target EKRc of 11 ml/min/40 L derived from earlier studies. Notably, these values remain similar for different dialysis schedules.

81.9 Augmented Dialysis

Although incremental dialysis is often interpreted as less dialysis than the traditional thrice weekly 4-hour sessions, incremental dialysis also includes increasing the amount of dialysis to more frequent or longer dialysis sessions to account for loss of residual renal function [16]. This increase in dialysis is also termed augmented dialysis, to include introducing hemodiafiltration, higher permeability dialyzers, adsorption or displacement techniques designed to increase clearance of middle-sized solutes and protein-bound solutes to compensate for the loss of residual renal function.

81.10 Interpreting Adequacy in Hemodialysis Patients

It must be remembered that Kt/V is a measure of urea clearance, and as such is only an aspect of the dialysis prescription. In the original National Cooperative Dialysis Study, patients became unwell with a sessional target of 0.9 or less. Over time the target has increased by consensus from 1.2 to 1.4. Achieving a sessional target of 1.4 does not necessarily mean that dialysis clearance of the waste products of metabolism is adequate. Urea is a small molecule with a rapid diffusion coefficient, other molecules diffuse more slowly, and may be predominantly intracellular or protein bound, and as such will have a much lower clearances than urea. So, although a Kt/V below target is likely to provide inadequate clearance, achieving a target Kt/V does not imply adequate clearance. In addition, one has to consider the patient as a whole, as patients with a low protein intake, low muscle mass who are physically inactive will generate fewer waste products of metabolism compared to a patient with a high-protein diet who is physically active with preserved muscle mass, and as such will need greater dialytic clearances.

81.11 Alternative Methods of Assessing Adequacy of Dialyzer Clearance

Traditionally, dialyzer clearance (Kt) has been adjusted for body water (V). However, this adjustment leads to a lower effective dose of dialysis delivered to women compared to men, and lighter men compared to heavier men. The generation of waste products of metabolism depend upon both basal metabolic rate (BMR) and active energy expenditure (AEE). The majority of dialysis patients are elderly and with additional comorbidities, and as such although total energy expenditure (TEE) is greater than BMR, BMR has accounted for 80% or more of TEE. As such, it has been suggested that as BMR is related to body surface area (BSA), scaling Kt for BSA would provide some groups, for example, women with an equivalent amount of dialysis. AEE is associated with appendicular muscle mass, and as such for men, who typically have more muscle mass, scaling Kt for BSA still leads to a lower effective dialysis dose for smallmen compared to larger men.

81.12 Adjusting Kt/V Targets for Individual Patients

Although the concept of a target Kt/V was to provide an equivalent dose of dialysis for all patients, there are several major confounders, and as such some patient groups receive a greater dialysis dose than others. As such it is important to recognize that some patient groups require a greater dose of dialysis above the standard target sessional Kt/V to guard against delivering a lower effective dialysis dose. The groups most at risk of receiving less dialysis, and as such require a delivered Kt/V above target include women, small men, patients who have less comorbidity, and those who are physically active and at work.

A key element of this whole process is patient engagement; if the only way to achieve adequate dialysis is to increase the dialysis time, then we have a moral obligation to explain to the patient (and possibly their family), why this is important and what, if any, the alternatives are. Dialysis patients are in a vulnerable position and most of the time have pretty limited control over their situation. Engaging with patients over the options for best treatment is much more likely to succeed than a purely prescriptive approach. Similarly, while it is relatively clear how much dialysis is required to keep a patient well for a significant proportion of elderly dialysis patients' life expectancy is very poor and there is an important balance to be made between what might appear to be optimum treatment to increase quantity of life and quality of life. There is no formula for this, just patient–doctor dialogue.

81.12.1 Equations

$$\text{URR} = (\text{pre urea concentration} - \text{post urea concentration}) * 100 / \text{pre urea concentration}$$

$$\text{Single pool Kt/V (spKt/V)}$$

$$\text{spKt/V} = -\text{natural logarithm}(1 - \text{URR})$$

First-generation equation

$$\text{spKt/V} = -\text{In}\left(\left(\begin{matrix}\text{Urea concentration post /}\\ \text{Urea concentration pre}\end{matrix}\right) - 0.008 * t - 1 * \text{UF/W}\right),$$

t – dialysis session time hours.

UF – ultrafiltration volume L.

W – post-dialysis weight kg.

Second-generation Kt/V equation

$$\text{spKt/V} = -\text{In}\left(\left(\begin{matrix}\text{Urea concentration post /}\\ \text{Urea concentration pre}\end{matrix}\right) - 0.008 * t\right) + (4 - 3.5 * \text{R}) * \text{UF/W}.$$

R = URR.

Equilibrated Kt/V.

Rate adjustment method

$$\text{eKt/V} = \text{spKt/V} - 0.6(\text{spKt/V})/\text{time hours} + 0.03$$

Standardized Kt/V

$$\text{stdKt}/V = \frac{10{,}080 \times \frac{1 - e^{-\text{eKt}/V}}{t}}{\frac{1 - e^{-\text{eKt}/V}}{eKt/V} + \frac{10{,}080}{Ft} - 1}$$

t = treatment time, min; V = modeled two-pool post-dialysis volume, mL; F = frequency of treatment per week; Uf = weekly fluid gain between dialyses, mL.

Urinary urea clearance (Kr)

$$\text{Urinary urea clearance}(\text{Kr}) = \frac{U \times V}{P}$$

U = Urinary urea nitrogen concentration of interdialytic urine sample (mg/dL).

V = Urine volume excretion rate during interdialytic collection (ml/min).

P = Time-averaged serum urea nitrogen concentration during interdialytic collection (mg/dL).

Variable volume model, with Kr

$$\text{stdKt}/V = \frac{Eq.6}{1 - \frac{0.74}{F}\left[\frac{Uf}{V}\right]} + Kr\frac{10{,}080}{V}$$

81.13 Summary

There is clearly a need to tailor dialysis on the basis of residual renal function, habitus, volume status, and many other aspects including patient preference [17]. Modern dialysis machines are able to document the delivery of dialysis in terms of urea clearance (and fluid removal). The challenge for a nephrologist looking after a heterogeneous group of patients is how to identify, recommend, and deliver the best bespoke dialysis for them.

81

Case Study

A 67-year-old male patient was reviewed in dialysis clinic with a Kt/V of 1.0 despite 4 hours of dialysis three times a week. He was dialyzing via a line having been very reluctant to have an AV fistula, with a medium kidney (dialyzer), dialysate flows (Qd) of 800 ml/min and an arterial flow (Qb) of 250 ml/min. He was extremely reluctant to increase his dialysis time and the question was whether he would benefit from using a bigger dialyzer. Unfortunately, dialyzer urea clearance is limited by the lowest factor Qb/KoA/Qd and as ◘ Fig. 81.5 illustrates, increasing the kidney size when the Qb is 250mls is a very inefficient way of increasing clearance.

It was possible to explain to the patient and his partner that the factors that influence, providing enough dialysis to keep him well are his weight (which was relatively fixed), the time on dialysis, and a combination of the dialyzer characteristics and blood flow. In practical terms the only two modifiable factors were increasing time or improving his access, which would likely have other benefits. After a discussion between him and his wife he elected for a fistular formation which eventually delivered a Qb of 380 ml/min, permitted the use of a larger dialyzer, and delivered much better clearance.

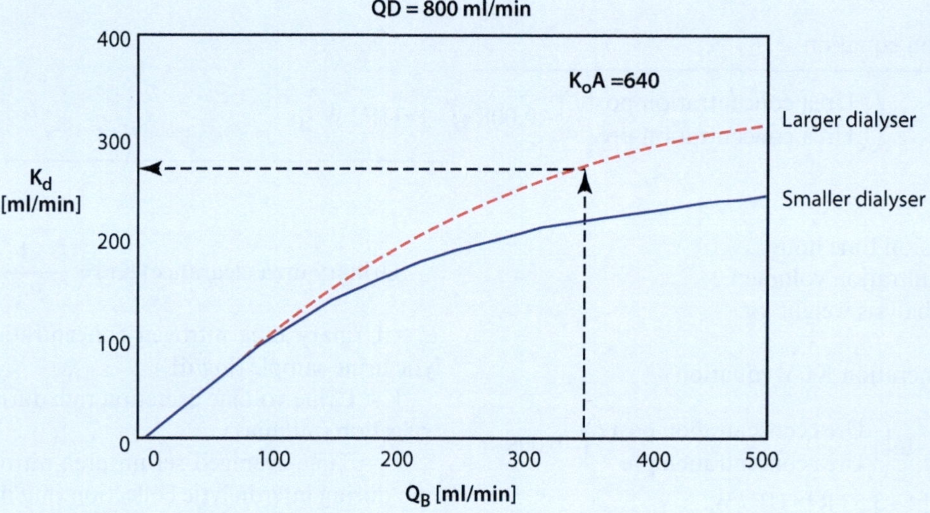

◘ **Fig. 81.5** The relationship between blood flow (Qb) and clearance at a fixed dialysate flow (Qd) for different sized kidneys (dialyzers). Larger dialyzers add very little at low blood flows, but offer a significant benefit when blood flows are higher (e.g., 350/ml/min)

Tips and Tricks

Supporting and training dialysis staff in measurement and recording of dialysis clearance is a critical first step and includes, ensuring appropriately delayed post-dialysis urea sampling, identification of aspects of dialysis that interfere with delivery (such as intermittent attendance), identification of recirculation, skilled needling etc. In short, having accurate data on which to make management decisions is essential.

Monitoring residual urine output and factoring this into dialysis clearance are both important and a reminder that despite being on dialysis, attempts should be made to avoid nephrotoxins and to preserve residual renal function [18].

Engaging staff in the goals and opportunities for achieving good clearance is also important and assists greatly in delivering patient education and engagement in their own treatment. Multi-disciplinary team meetings offer a good opportunity for discussing the options and teaching.

Questions

1. What happens to urine output after dialysis and why does it matter?
2. What is the relevance of residual renal function?
3. What is the KoA of a dialyzer?
4. What are the sizes of urea and β_2-microglobulin (β_2M) molecules?

Answers

1. Urine output drops postdialysis, a combination of reduced renal perfusion during dialysis and reduction in intravascular volume. This matters because urine collections post dialysis we underestimate

residual renal function, and perhaps, because it reminds us that dialysis itself can be damaging to renal function.

2. Residual renal function has huge value and loss of residual renal function is associated with worse mortality. Both blood pressure and volume control are important, permitting greater oral intake and potentially fewer dialysis sessions for longer. Residual renal function is associated with improved anemia control, better nutrition, and critically, the removal of middle molecules.
3. It is the manufacturer's estimate of urea clearance characteristics for a dialyzer at specified pump speeds and dialysate flow rates. It is derived from performance ex-vivo.
4. Urea is 64 daltons and β_2M 11,800 daltons. β_2M is derived from the MHC class 1 present on all nucleated cells. Because of its size it is not well cleared by conventional dialysis and therefore, accumulates, potentially forming amyloid fibrils which can cause dialysis amyloid. There are of course, many middle molecules that are well cleared by the kidney, but less well so by conventional dialysis. The fact that β_2M is ubiquitous and relatively easy to measure makes it a useful marker.

References

1. Lowrie EG, Laird NM, Parker TF, Sargent JA. Effect of the hemodialysis prescription of patient morbidity: report from the National Cooperative Dialysis Study. N Engl J Med. 1981;305(20):1176–81. PubMed PMID: 7027040.
2. Termorshuizen F, Dekker FW, van Manen JG, Korevaar JC, Boeschoten EW, Krediet RT, et al. Relative contribution of residual renal function and different measures of adequacy to survival in hemodialysis patients: an analysis of the Netherlands Cooperative Study on the Adequacy of Dialysis (NECOSAD)-2. J Am Soc Nephrol. 2004;15(4):1061–70. PubMed PMID: 15034110.
3. Meyer TW, Sirich TL, Fong KD, Plummer NS, Shafi T, Hwang S, et al. Kt/Vurea and nonurea small solute levels in the hemodialysis study. J Am Soc Nephrol. 2016;27(11):3469–78. PubMed PMID: 27026365.
4. European Best Practice Guidelines Expert Group on Hemodialysis ERA. Section I. Measurement of renal function, when to refer and when to start dialysis. Nephrol Dial Transplant. 2002;17(Suppl 7):7–15. PubMed PMID: 12386205.
5. Hemodialysis Adequacy Work G. Clinical practice guidelines for hemodialysis adequacy, update 2006. Am J Kidney Dis. 2006;48(Suppl 1):S2–90. PubMed PMID: 16813990.
6. National Kidney F. KDOQI clinical practice guideline for hemodialysis adequacy: 2015 update. Am J Kidney Dis. 2015;66(5):884–930. PubMed PMID: 26498416.
7. Tattersall JE, DeTakats D, Chamney P, Greenwood RN, Farrington K. The post-hemodialysis rebound: predicting and quantifying its effect on Kt/V. Kidney Int. 1996;50(6):2094–102. PubMed PMID: 8943495.
8. Casino FG, Lopez T. The equivalent renal urea clearance: a new parameter to assess dialysis dose. Nephrol Dial Transplant. 1996;11(8):1574–81. PubMed PMID: 8856214.
9. Wang AY, Lai KN. The importance of residual renal function in dialysis patients. Kidney Int. 2006;69(10):1726–32. PubMed PMID: 16612329.
10. Shafi T, Jaar BG, Plantinga LC, Fink NE, Sadler JH, Parekh RS, et al. Association of residual urine output with mortality, quality of life, and inflammation in incident hemodialysis patients: the Choices for Healthy Outcomes in Caring for End-Stage Renal Disease (CHOICE) Study. Am J Kidney Dis. 2010;56(2):348–58. PubMed PMID: 20605303. Pubmed Central PMCID: 2910835.
11. Obi Y, Rhee CM, Mathew AT, Shah G, Streja E, Brunelli SM, et al. Residual kidney function decline and mortality in incident hemodialysis patients. J Am Soc Nephrol. 2016;27(12):3758–68. PubMed PMID: 27169576.
12. Lin X, Yan Y, Ni Z, Gu L, Zhu M, Dai H, et al. Clinical outcome of twice-weekly hemodialysis patients in shanghai. Blood Purif. 2012;33(1-3):66–72. PubMed PMID: 22212562.
13. Hanson JA, Hulbert-Shearon TE, Ojo AO, Port FK, Wolfe RA, Agodoa LY, et al. Prescription of twice-weekly hemodialysis in the USA. Am J Nephrol. 1999;19(6):625–33. PubMed PMID: 10592355.
14. Obi Y, Streja E, Rhee CM, Ravel V, Amin AN, Cupisti A, et al. Incremental hemodialysis, residual kidney function, and mortality risk in incident dialysis patients: a cohort study. Am J Kidney Dis. 2016;68(2):256–65. PubMed PMID: 26867814.
15. Daugirdas JT, Greene T, Rocco MV, Kaysen GA, Depner TA, Levin NW, et al. Effect of frequent hemodialysis on residual kidney function. Kidney Int. 2013;83(5):949–58. PubMed PMID: 23344474. Pubmed Central PMCID: 3855839.
16. Rocco MV, Lockridge RS Jr, Beck GJ, Eggers PW, Gassman JJ, Greene T, et al. The effects of frequent nocturnal home hemodialysis: the frequent hemodialysis network nocturnal trial. Kidney Int. 2011;80(10):1080–91. PubMed PMID: 21775973. Pubmed Central PMCID: 3569086.
17. Tangvoraphonkchai K, Davenport A. Incremental Haemodialysis – a European perspective. Semin Dial. 2017;30(3):270–6.
18. Tangvoraphonkchai K, Davenport A. Increasing Haemodialytic clearances as residual renal function declines: an incremental approach. Blood Purif. 2017;44(3):217–26.

Providing a PD Service

Paul J. Champion de Crespigny, Michael X. Cai, and Stephen G. Holt

Contents

M. Harber (ed.), *Primer on Nephrology*, https://doi.org/10.1007/978-3-030-76419-7_82

Learning Objectives

This chapter hopes to help its readers create or improve their PD programs by collecting together helpful hints and tips acquired by the authors in a number of centers worldwide.

82.1 Introduction

Home-based dialysis therapies support superior quality of life and allows for flexibility not afforded by center-based dialysis hemodialysis (HD) treatment. Peritoneal dialysis (PD) is an essential part of a thriving home-based dialysis program and, in some places, may be the only practical dialysis modality. A key driver for this is that in many parts of the world, but not all, PD is considerably cheaper than assisted HD [1]. It is noteworthy that countries that have implemented a "PD first"' policy, there has been considerable success in both limiting the expansion in healthcare budgets compared with predictions, and brought equitable and affordable dialysis to many of the population [2]. Although there are some issues around providing enough trained personnel for catheter insertion and complications, especially in remote regions, PD is generally working well in many regions. When considering the value for more economically developed regions there is some evidence that transplant outcomes may be superior when transitioning from PD compared with coming from HD [3, 4]. A prerequisite for a successful PD program is support from colleagues within the renal department for a PD program. Perhaps, surprisingly, some nephrologists still believe that PD is a second-tier or inadequate treatment option, and in some way inferior to HD. This may be because of past experience in units with limited expertise or interest in PD as a valid form of renal replacement therapy (RRT). In such cases, belief in the value of PD may only emerge with evidence of good clinical outcomes and patient satisfaction. Education of all medical and nursing staff that PD is a valid, effective, and suitable dialysis choice is critical if a program is to be viable. The overemphasis on infection risks which some detractors point to is largely mitigated by the excellent results of CQI processes which have reduced peritonitis rates in many areas [5]and perhaps, more worrying infection risk among those who develop blood stream infection in HD [6]. Equally, some patients may be better suited to HD, and it is important to deliver a balanced and objective view of all modalities when advising patients of their options, considering all modalities in the continuum of RRT experienced by patients over a dialysis career. In addition, it is rare that the benefits of dialysis in any form outweigh those obtained by transplantation when successful, so increasing transplant rates need to be factored into the equation. It is also increasingly recognized that small solute transport as measured by Kt/V or creatinine clearance, may not be the best objective measure to judge a RRT modality and there may be some groups that could preferentially benefit in terms of quality of life, independent of comorbidities, for example, in independent elderly patients [7], those with severe congestive cardiac failure [8], or cirrhosis with ascites [9]there is evidence emerging of the advantages of PD in these groups.

Nevertheless, a 'try PD first' policy where there is genuine clinical equipoise is sensible because residual renal function (RRF) is important for the success of PD, and loss of native function may render PD more difficult at a later date in the patient's journey through end-stage kidney disease [10]. Some of the barriers preventing consideration of PD, especially for the elderly, can be overcome using different systems. For example, non-disconnect continuous ambulatory peritoneal dialysis (CAPD) systems, in-center intermittent automated peritoneal dialysis (IPD), or assisted automated peritoneal dialysis (APD) (aka continuous cycling peritoneal dialysis (CCPD)) can be performed, where a peripatetic healthcare professional will assist the patient at home [11]. If it is clear that PD is not possible, then home-based (particularly nocturnal) HD may be another good option. Interest is also increasing in more "portable" hemodialysis machines that combine the ease and simplicity of an "APD-like" setup with a hemodialysis machine that is smaller and easier to move around than traditional machines, although uptake probably depends upon reimbursement and economics. There is also renewed interest in adsorption systems capable of online fluid regeneration and we may see developments in this area in the relatively near future [12].

Increasingly, home therapy units do (and our view should) combine expertise in both modalities (PD and HD), as well as promoting transplantation wherever possible, but it is helpful to have a combined HD/PD home dialysis team. This approach has a number of advantages, and the continuity of care, familiarity, and trust that exists between patients and the home therapy team is conducive to excellent results. Additionally, once patients become institutionalized in a satellite or an in-center HD unit, the advantage and incentive to try home dialysis frequently wanes.

There are numerous informative and helpful resources and guidelines freely available to help set up a PD service. Some of these are listed in ▶ Box 82.1.

Box 82.1 Useful Resources with Guidelines and Training Information

Guidelines

- ▶ http://www.cari.org.au/guidelines.php
- ▶ http://www.csnscn.ca/site/c.lnKKKOOvHqE/b.8079309/k.799F/Guideline_Document_Library.htm

- ▶ http://www.european-renal-best-practice.org/content/ebpg-european-best-practice-guidelines-documents
- ▶ http://www.ispd.org/lang-en/treatmentguidelines/guidelines
- ▶ http://www.kidney.org/professionals/kdoqi/guidelines_updates/doqi_uptoc.htmL#pd
- ▶ http://www.renal.org/Clinical/GuidelinesSection/Guidelines.aspx
- ▶ http://www.kdigo.org/guidelines/topicsummarized/CPG%20Summary%20by%20Topic_Peritoneal%20Dialysis.html

Selected patient & training information

- ▶ http://kidney.niddk.nih.gov/kudiseases/pubs/peritoneal/
- ▶ http://www.ispd.org/lang-en/educational-material/materials
- ▶ http://www.kidneyatlas.org/book5/adk5-04.ccc.QXD.pdf
- ▶ http://www.renalweb.com
- ▶ http://www.bjrm.co.uk/patient-information.aspx

82.2 Survival on PD vs HD

A number of studies have attempted to compare differences in survival between dialysis modalities, but these are all confounded by indication bias. No studies have successfully randomized individuals between modalities, 95% of NECOSAD participants refused dialysis modality randomization [13]. Nevertheless, results of such comparisons have been debated at length, but neither modality appears to be able to claim a clear advantage across all age groups. However, some studies claim evidence for an early survival advantage for some groups of patients who start PD compared with those starting HD. This may disappear and reverse with time on dialysis, but results from many, but not all, studies suggest that for at least 2 years PD may have some advantages [14]. The groups that appear to have the best survival on PD (compared to HD) are young patients (aged below 45 years), and those who subsequently receive a kidney transplant. Elderly diabetic individuals may appear to do worst in large registry studies, but this effect may be historical and the use of icodextrin in this population may have removed this disadvantage [15].However, weighing up the advantages and disadvantages of different modalities in elderly patients of requires considerable thought and discussion [16]. Elderly patients with CKD and on dialysis have more severe comorbidities than aged matched controls and this includes cognitive impairment and frailty that may preclude good outcomes no matter what the modality of renal replacement therapy. Furthermore, it is debatable whether urea kinetic modeling as targets is as relevant to an the elderly population [17], a population largely excluded from controlled studies, and the studies validating small solute targets which were mainly performed on younger cohorts. Thus, in many cases, PD is a highly appropriate modality for elderly patients, improving quantity of life with acceptable quality. Indeed the latest ISPD guidelines no longer suggest measuring routine small solute targets.

There appears to be a slower decline in RRF for patients starting PD compared to HD [18] and CAPD may be better than APD in this regard [19], although this may relate to membrane transport characteristics and baseline residual renal function [20]. Those patients who are struggling with little or no residual renal function and who face long years on dialysis without transplantation may benefit from extended hours or overnight HD, as the metabolic correction achieved with these techniques is unparalleled. The long-term outcome benefits are confined to younger patients with little hope of transplantation due to immunological issues and selection bias remains a clear confounder [21].

There are also differences in patient preference and belief systems that may inform dialysis modality choice [22, 23]. Perceptions and real and misinterpreted advantages and disadvantages are commonplace when delivering pre-dialysis education [24].

Any long-term quality of life or survival benefits of hemodiafiltration (HDF) over PD or standard HD remain unclear, but might only occur in a subset of patients using high volumes of convective fluid exchange [25].

While home HD may be feasible for many patients, it is also technically more complex and generally takes longer to learn. The simplicity, safety, and ease of use of PD therapies is an attraction for many patients. In addition, improvements in quality of life for patients on PD has been repeatedly shown across many age groups [7].

82.3 Patient Selection

There are some data suggesting that young, fit patients with meaningful RRF have a survival advantage on PD, providing solute clearances are achieved. Some registry studies have reported that there are some patients who appear to have worse outlook on PD (e.g., elderly diabetic females). However, the reasons for these differences are not clear, and there are many patients who appear to do very well on PD, confounding the generalizations of aggregate data analysis. More recently, these differences have been shown to have been mitigated with the use of

Icodextrin [15, 26]. Thus, decisions regarding modality should simply be carefully considered by clinicians and patients, weighing such aspects as quality of life, daytime activities, dexterity an eyesight, body habitus, past abdominal surgery, and aims of therapy. Clinician preference is a large factor in this decision-making process [27], so staff education around knowledge of the key advantages and benefits of PD is highly likely to influence patient acceptance of this modality. Patient reported outcomes are generally favourable for PD [28].

Past HD is not a contraindication to PD, but such patients are often anuric and frequently need higher-dose APD to obtain sufficient clearance and UF targets above 750 mL [29]. The use of PD as a modality of last resort for patients who have exhausted vascular access options can create additional issues, often compounded by the pressure to succeed. Again, this argues in favor of PD as the initial renal replacement modality so that vascular access options can be preserved until required. Nevertheless, PD may be tried in these circumstances and especially if transplantation remains an option, or if the alternative is a heroic vascular access procedure that has multiple complications and a limited.

It is important to ascertain whether PD is likely to be successful. There are a few absolute contraindications to peritoneal dialysis and these are usually related to abdominal suitability (see KDOQI guidelines ▶ Box 82.1 for an extensive review of contraindications and relative contraindications). For example, PD is not usually attempted in patients who have a stoma, previous significant abdominal surgery, or known intra-abdominal adhesions. Similarly, tuberculous or fungal peritonitis and encapsulating peritoneal sclerosis (EPS) are relative contraindications to recommencing PD (although it may be preferable to continue PD, while the EPS is being treated [30]).

There are currently no good diagnostic/prognostic tools to determine if patients are suitable or trainable for PD, and assessment is largely subjective. However, visual acuity, dexterity, muscle strength (to lift the bags), a clean home environment, family support, a history of poor compliance with treatment, dementia, and clinically active psychiatric illness will likely influence the final decision [31]. There is increasing interest in frailty indices to facilitate decision-making at all stages of renal replacement therapy selection. There are tools currently being evaluated that formalize some of these assessments, but they are time-consuming and neither fully validated nor widely used [32]. The most practical and useful approach often is to obtain the views of experienced PD nursing staff combined with a careful clinical appraisal. The opinion of an experienced physiotherapist or psychologist can also be useful in particular circumstances.

Even if potential barriers to home-based therapies are identified, many perceived or potential problems can be addressed. Examples include the assisted home therapies, the training of staff in care homes, or the development of overnight in-center dialysis facility.

Case Study 82.1

Ken is a 65-year-old male with end-stage kidney disease secondary to Type II diabetes and hypertension. His diabetes was complicated by proliferative retinopathy, treated with laser photocoagulation. He had an appendectomy in his twenties for a ruptured appendix. He lives at home alone in a rural property. He drives and enjoys the company of friends. On examination, he weighs 95 kg with increased abdominal girth. After dialysis education, he realized that his nearest hemodialysis center is a 1-hour drive away and 4 hours' drive away from a tertiary hospital. He would like to have peritoneal dialysis, but have been told that he is not a good candidate for PD.

Questions:

1. Does Ken have any contraindications to PD?
2. Is his physical remoteness a barrier to success in PD?

Answers:

Poor vision, possible abdominal adhesions from previous abdominal surgery, and obesity are NOT absolute contraindications to peritoneal dialysis.

1. Poor vision has been previously viewed as a contraindication to PD because of the loss of stereoscopic vision to perform safe connection/disconnections. Assist devices such as PeriSafe® could help visually impaired patients to perform a safe connection.
2. Adhesiolysis can be performed at the same time as insertion of PD catheter. The rate of catheter malfunction in patients with previous abdominal surgery, having undergone adhesiolysis, has been shown to be the same to those without previous abdominal surgery.
3. Central obesity can be problematic for exit site placement. Presternal exit site can be fashioned via a long subcutaneous tunnel to help patient visualize exit site.

In addition to the issues discussed above, providing clinical support could be problematic because of Ken's physical remoteness. Upskilling of local healthcare professionals may reduce patient's need to travel for clinical assessment or troubleshooting. Specialist consultation via telemedicine can supplement local healthcare as required. Newer generations of automated peritoneal dialysis machines bundled with remote monitoring capabilities can further reduce the need for patients to travel.

82

82.4 Sodium Removal

Sodium removal can also be a challenge in PD patients, especially those without residual renal function [33]. Control of plasma volume related to sodium removal can be difficult in PD. It is often more of an issue in APD compared to CAPD due to the peritoneal transport characteristics associated with each modality. However, while the fluctuations in plasma volume are usually less in PD than with HD, the relationships between fluid overload, malnutrition, and inflammation appear complex. Data on biomarkers of fluid overload (e.g., NT and BNP) in HD compared to PD are conflicting and difficult to interpret with confidence [34].

Cases Study 82.2

A 34-year-old female with diabetes is having a problem with blood pressure. She is on APD using 12 L of 2.5% loaded on the machine and using 7.2 L over 9 hours, no tidal. The fill volumes are 1.8 L and she ultrafilters 300 ml from this. She has a daytime fill of icodextrin, 1 L fill during the day with an initial drain of 1200 ml. She passes 410 ml of urine during the last 24-hour collection. The 24-hour dialysate sodium concentration is 132 mmol/L and urine sodium 70 mmol/L. How much sodium can she consume without being in a positive sodium balance?

Answer

	OUT			IN			Difference
	Vol out (L)	[Na]	Total Na out	Vol in (L)	[Na]	Total Na in	mmol
APD	12.3	132	1623.6	12	132	1584	39.6
Day dwell	1.2	132	158.4	1	132	132	26.4
Urine	0.41	70	28.7				28.7
Sodium balance							94.7

The average sodium intake in many Westernized countries is ~170 mmol/day (Australia). Obligate intake is ~25 mmol/day and a really strict diet might provide 70–80 mmol/day. In this case, sodium intake exceeded what could be removed (~95 mmol). Dietary review improved her blood pressure by limiting salt intake.

82.5 Dialysate Calcium

Dialysate calcium varies across a number of company's products. Generally, PD dialysate calcium is ~1.25 mmol/L, but there are dialysate calcium concentrations of 1.0 and 1.75 mmol/L. The choice of calcium in the dialysate bags is predicated upon trying to obtain a neutral body calcium content. A number of calcium mass balance experiments have been performed over the years, especially in hemodialysis [35]. However, while this is useful, it generally measures changes in the miscible pool of circulating calcium across the dialysis session and it is hard to extrapolate the effects to PD, additionally the absorption of calcium is much more dependent upon calcitriol dose [36].In PD, the UF rate is the major determinant of calcium flux, such that calcium balance requires a higher dialysate calcium. If UF is likely to be higher [37, 38], especially in shorter dwell cycles as most calcium will be removed by small pores and some from large pores bound to albumin, more calcium ions are removed by CAPD compared with APD [39]. Dialysate calcium will modify PTH as expected and low dialysate calcium can be another driver to hyperparathyroidism [40]. There is some evidence for bone changes and higher mortality with higher dialysate calcium [41]. Recent data has implicated some calcium pathways in EPS and this may be an issue that needs to be explored further [42–44].

82.5.1 Obesity

Obesity is sometimes, but often inaccurately, cited as a contraindication to PD as many obese patients perform peritoneal dialysis very effectively. The reverse epidemiology of patients with an elevated body mass index is well known in dialysis patients generally [45], but not all studies suggest that the same is true for PD [46]. Conversely, there is no data to indicate that weight loss in obese patients improves outcomes. Nevertheless, data is sparse, and it is not possible to determine whether this is due to lack of effect, or simply lack of evidence. Whereas, most studies agree that being malnourished is an adverse prognostic sign for all modalities of RRT [47].

Potential problems in those with higher BMIs include reduced catheter survival, a more rapid decline in RRF, increased risks of peritonitis, and higher intra-abdominal pressures [48], not to mention more difficulty getting transplanted.

Weightgain after starting PD is common, but importantly appears to be similar in HD patients, and perhaps more likely related to loss of uremia-associated anorexia. PD is often blamed for such weightgain, but the use between 1000 and 7000 liters of PD fluid per year equates to around 15–150 kg of glucose passing through the abdomen, some of which is absorbed and adds to calorie intake. Glucose absorption depends on dialysate volumes, dialysate concentrations, peritoneal transport characteristics, surface area, and dwell time. Nevertheless, on an average glucose absorbed adds an extra ~500 kcal/day, equivalent to a daily intake of ~2 chocolate bars. More use of icodextrin may prevent some, but not all of this glucose exposure [49]. DEXA scanning looking at fat gain in patients starting renal replacement therapy, suggests that the gain in HD and PD is equivalent [48], although intra-abdominal fat accumulation is probably higher in PD patients [50]. Interestingly, this may be subject to genetic influences mediated by mitochondrial efficiency [51].

82.5.2 Diabetics

Diabetic status has been linked with higher transport status in some studies, but this has not been subsequently substantiated [52].Changes in the peritoneum caused by years of exposure to excess glucose in diabetes does change the peritoneum even before PD fluid is used. These changes are similar to those observed by glucose-based PD fluids and generally, result in higher transport characteristics. Thus, the reasons that some studies have not reported higher transport characteristics may reflect differences in the duration of diabetes and diabetic control. However, there are advantages to using non-glucose solutions (e.g., icodextrin) in diabetic patients with improved fluid status [53], better glucose control [54], and lower incidence of technique failure and all-cause mortality [26].

Glucose monitoring in PD is important, and it is vital that diabetic patients receive instruction on how to measure blood sugar and change their diabetic medication at the start of PD. In addition, patient–son nocturnal APD will need to adjust their insulin regimens to account for the overnight glucose absorption. This makes insulin requiring diabetes, slightly more complex and a risk if there is a problem with the APD machine overnight, as often a long-acting insulin dose needs increasing overnight in anticipation of the PD glucose load. If the APD is subsequently not delivered, then the risks of hypoglycemia are enhanced.

Icodextrin may be absorbed by the peritoneal lymphatic system and metabolized by circulating maltase enzymes, leading to accumulation of maltose in the circulation. This will interfere with blood glucose measurement in monitors detecting glucose dehydrogenase pyrrolate, leading to false high readings in the face of hypoglycemia [55, 56]. Such potentially dangerous situations can be avoided by using glucose oxidase-based assay monitors instead.

It should also be noted that icodextrin may lead to low amylase levels, potentially interfering with a possible diagnosis of pancreatitis, and plasma lipase should be used instead [57].

82.5.3 Heart Failure

The community prevalence of congestive cardiac failure (CCF) in Western society is increasing due to aging, associated comorbidities, and improved survival after cardiac events. Interestingly, there appears to be an epidemic of heart failure occurring in South East Asia [58]. Many acute hospital admissions involve decompensated heart failure, sometimes resistant to diuretics. This poses a symptom and economic burden on health services which is increasing. In relatively large studies in patients with heart failure, PD was effective therapy in preventing readmission, and improving symptomatic NYHA classification, cardiac function and survival [59–61] . The particular use of Icodextrin has been used successfully to treat resistant CCF [62], presumably due to its ability to effectively remove salt and water over a long dwell through small pores. In many cases, PD also allows reinstatement of other heart failure therapies like ACEI/ARB, spironolactone, or beta blockers because of potassium removal. Additionally, there is some economic data suggesting that this strategy is also cost saving [63].

82.5.4 Cardiac Surgery

Cardiac surgery is common in dialysis patients who have worse outcomes than patients without renal impairment. Many cardiac surgeons suggest that patients will require hemodialysis or hemodiafiltration postoperatively. However, there is no evidence to suggest that continuation of peritoneal dialysis (usually APD) is not equally as successful postoperatively. In fact, there may be advantages to continuing with PD with shorter high-dependency stays [64]. However, the main issues usually relate to leakage through intercostal drains that inadvertently breach the peritoneum.

82

82.5.5 Cirrhotic Patients

Peritoneal dialysis in cirrhotic patients can be successful, although complications do sometimes occur. Specific issues include bleeding from abdominal wall collaterals after peritoneal dialysis catheter insertion, early leakage due to high intra-abdominal pressure, and large protein losses [9, 65]. However, if such problems can be managed for the first few weeks, patients often tolerate the process well, and the protein leak, while initially high, often reduces with continued treatment [66], and renal vein and IVC pressure may be reduced by draining tense ascites. There appears to be no difference in peritonitis free survival [9]. If synthetic function is poor then prognosis is often limited and dialysis may not be appropriate, so as with cardiac failure case selection is the key to successful therapy.

82.5.6 Lung Disease

Conflicting data from small studies suggest either no or small (usually insignificant) changes in lung function testing (FEV_1, FVC, TLC, and DLCO) in patients with PD fluid present in the abdomen [67, 68]. Even if changes are identified, it appears lung function can then improve with time [69]. It would seem reasonable to expect patients with mild to moderate airways disease to successfully perform peritoneal dialysis and lung disease per se should not discourage a trial of PD where appropriate, and avoiding overfilling the abdomen. Intraperitoneal pressure can be simply measured and keeping maximum filing pressure below ~15–18 mmH_2O may be sensible.

82.5.7 Vascular Access

We advocate a PD first policy and there is rarely a need to form a 'backup' arteriovenous fistula (AVF) at the time of PD catheter insertion [70]. However, there is a recent vogue to use PD as a short term 'bridging" therapy, often with assisted or intermittent IPD to allow definitive vascular access with a mature fistula to be established. This is an excellent technique, since PD catheters can be used more or less immediately and minimize the very real risk of damage to large veins and blood stream infection associated with temporary or tunneled hemodialysis lines [71]. It also means that patients may try peritoneal dialysis, and some may find that they get on well with this technique, and have an AVF to fall back on should PD not be successful. There is also increasing interest in combined PD with a weekly HD session to augment clearances and fluid removal [72].

Occasional patients 'run out" of traditional HD access slots and then heroic efforts are made to make grafts and place tunneled lines via circuitous routes into part of the venous system. These patients sometimes tolerate PD well as access of last resort [73].

82.5.8 Dementia

Patients with dementia can do well on PD provided someone else performs the exchanges. This responsibility usually falls to a spouse, and consideration must be given to respite and support as the demands are on top of what is often a demanding and progressively deteriorating process. Nursing homes sometimes offer a PD service. Alternatively, intermittent thrice-weekly overnight APD may be possible with good residual renal function (5–6 mL/min/1.73m^2 residual GFR) [74]. Assisted PD programs may also be able to adapt to these circumstances [75].

82.5.9 Diverticular Disease

An incidental finding of diverticular disease (DD) is common and the incidence increases with age, which can be problematic. In one Swedish study, more than one diverticulum was found in 42% of patients and 18% had more than ten diverticula [76].The incidence of enteric peritonitis in this study was 26% at 2 years, and patients who had more than ten diverticula had the highest risk of peritonitis. In a more recent study in Chinese patients, the finding that diverticular disease was associated with a higher risk of enteric peritonitis was replicated [77]. Both studies showed that the more extensive the diverticular disease, the higher the risk. Patients with diverticula in the ascending colon appear to be at highest risk and a history of recurrent problems with diverticulitis should alert the clinician that PD might not be a suitable option. On the other hand, many elderly patients have subclinical diverticular disease and prospective investigation is likely not to be cost-effective. Our strategy is to disregard a diagnosis of diverticular disease unless a patient has had multiple admissions, but to warn the patient of the potential of a problem and to encourage dietary fibre.

82.5.10 Appetite and Constipation

Poor appetite is common in PD and can lead to protein energy malnutrition and combined with protein loss in dialysis effluent may mean that protein requirements are not being met in some PD patients [78]. There may also be more GI symptoms including nausea, vomiting, bloating early satiety, and reflux. The reasons for this are not entirely clear although, such patients do have reduced gastric emptying, low ghrelin levels, and more pro-inflammatory cytokines.

Constipation is the most common of all complications experienced in PD patients. It is also the most troublesome in terms of catheter problems (poor drainage, catheter malposition, and technique failure). Patients should have one or two soft bowel motions daily and predisposing factors like hypothyroidism, hypercalcemia, and drugs should be corrected before using laxatives. The use of opiates, 5HT-3 antagonists, calcium antagonists, and iron preparations are common drugs that cause constipation and are to be avoided, if possible, in PD patients. Some studies suggest exercise helps promote a regular bowel action. The idea is good, except that many patients find regular exercise difficult.

The regular use of fiber or bulk-forming laxatives (e.g., methylcellulose, ispaghula) or osmotic laxatives (e.g., macrogols, lactulose, or polyethylene glycol) are useful, especially in patients with diverticular disease and may reduce peritonitis, although this may not be by avoiding constipation [79]. Common additions are stool softeners (e.g., docusate) which have a detergent effect (thereby incorporating more water and fats in stool increasing softness), but there is poor evidence for its efficacy. Stimulant laxatives (e.g., senna or bisacodyl) may be used in patients with slowed bowel transit, but this can precipitate peritonitis in some cases due to increasing intraluminal pressure and bacterial translocation. So, care is needed. There has been intense debate over whether regular use of senna leads to increased incidence of melanosis coli, but this has not been substantiated in humans [80].

82.5.11 Hernias

Hernias are more common in some patients (e.g., age, polycystic kidney disease, and raised body mass index), but there is no correlation between dwell volume and hernias. Umbilical hernias are more common than inguinal or incisional and most are present before starting dialysis [81]. Hernias usually worsen with PD fills. It is therefore suggested that, when possible, hernias are repaired extraperitoneally if possible before starting dialysis, and PD is delayed postoperatively for ~4 weeks. Repairing hernias in patients on dialysis can be difficult and sometimes ineffective. Occasionally patients will need transfer to hemodialysis temporarily, but continuing PD with low volumes, long hours on APD is also often possible. But it is wise to discuss this issue with the surgical team prior to planning this [82].

82.5.12 Starting PD

There are no data to support starting any dialysis modality early (according to eGFR) [83, 84]. Rather, the decision to start dialysis should rest on discussions between physician and patient regarding symptoms, volume control, and biochemistry. Knowledge of local issues and available catheter insertion techniques will facilitate decision-making. For example, where there is an active catheter insertion service under local anesthetic, there are often shorter delays in insertion. The Moncrief–Popovitch implantation method allows a catheter to be inserted with the distal component buried in a subcutaneous pocket. Prompt externalization of this portion of the catheter under local anesthetic is then performed when needed. Using the residual renal function and starting on a low dialysis prescription is likely to be advantageous and incremental dialysis [85] has become popular.

82.5.13 Acute PD

A number of studies now indicate that insertion and commencement of PD may be performed rapidly for acute kidney injury (AKI) as well as the initial mode of RRT for patients who are likely to need long-term dialysis (Acute Start PD, ASPD) [86]. While there can be an increased incidence of mechanical complications with the latter option, no long-term outcome differences have been demonstrated.

For AKI, high-dose dialysis involves APD with fluid volumes up to 44 L over 24 hours, with short dwell times (<50 min) and 18 to 22 exchanges a day. For ASPD, a 7- to 10-day catheter rest is desirable if possible but, where necessary, low volume APD can be used while the patient is supine in bed. An ASPD program includes overnight exchange of ≥12 L of PD fluid for at least 12 hours, with fill volumes of 1.2–1.5 L and a high-tidal APD (e.g., 50% to 75%).

82.6 PD Team

The 'PD team' is vital and in many units the PD nurses shoulder the responsibility for day-to-day patient care. Numerous studies validate the advantages of chronic disease management by the nursing team [87]. The late, lamented Dimitrios Oreopoulos suggested that nurses need to have the following qualities: "compassion, empathy, patience, and love", but the benefits of an enthusiastic and experienced nurse who is able to relate to patients and make independent decisions are vital. Peritoneal dialysis is relatively straightforward to teach and to learn, so a lack of previous experience should NOT preclude working on a PD unit. There are published training pathways for PD nurses, teaching the rudiments takes little time and experience is quickly gained (45). The best PD programs promote a holistic service rather than simply focusing upon dialysis-related problems. An ability to empathize and give advice on other issues (especially diabetes and vascular problems) empowers patients to seek initial advice from the PD team, often about problems that require a multi-professional approach.

Nurses on the ward are frequently required to care for PD patients and to troubleshoot problems out-of-hours. Thus, adequate training of the ward team is an essential feature of a successful program. It is vital that the ward-based team feels included as part of the home therapies team for patients.

One advantage of PD is that dietary restrictions are often less rigorous. This is particularly with respect to removal of potassium and fluid, although sodium and phosphate removal is often more difficult. However, protein energy malnutrition is widely prevalent in all dialysis patients, regardless of dialysis modality [88]. Thus, dietary advice and direction are important. Since dietetics resources are usually limited, an efficient alternative is for PD nurses and many doctors to provide generic advice (backed up with appropriate written literature), reserving a longer, more focused appointment with the dietician for specific problems (e.g., fluid and/or electrolytes). In addition, there are useful roles for the pharmacist, social worker, counselor, and psychologist within the PD team.

82.7 Patient Training

The training period will often influence a patient's acceptance of home therapies. A poor experience may well act as a long-term deterrent. Having a well-structured curriculum and consistency of implementation is paramount. The value of retraining or a technique check at intervals, especially after a peritonitis episode, is also helpful. There is a limit to what patients can absorb and teaching of ~3 key messages a day (certainly <7) can actually facilitate training. The ISPD guidelines set out recommendations for patient [89] and trainee training [90], and there are a variety of web-based resources available to help (◘ Table 82.1). There is also some evidence that training patients in their own environment is advantageous and that longer training may reduce complications [89].

Whether to start patients on CAPD or APD may be guided by economics, APD being a more expensive modality. If APD is chosen, confidence can often be enhanced by modest initial aims for clearance and fluid removal.

It is important to recognize that patients (and caregivers) develop technique fatigue and, if possible, offer some form of respite if this occurs, such as assisting patients (equally their caregivers) to take a holiday. A CAPD exchange can be performed anywhere that is clean, free from draughts, and where there is a place to wash hands. In contrast, hemodialysis needs to be planned and usually booked well ahead, especially in periods of high demand such as school holidays and long weekends. Peritoneal dialysis supplies can easily be transported by car and heating the PD fluid can be done via a device that plugs into a car 'cigarette lighter" socket if required. CAPD is possible without electricity, even while camping. For longer trips, supplies can be ordered in advance and delivered to a holiday address for the cost of delivery. For the few countries that are not serviced by a fluid supplier, neighboring countries might deliver the bags or the patient can arrange for shipment of their supplies.

In a well-adjusted PD patient, dialysis is an accepted part of day-to-day life and patients can travel, spend nights with their family and friends, work, and play sports. Often, patients are apprehensive on their first visit to a home therapy unit even if they have been aware for years that dialysis is a possibility. Starting is a daunt-

Table 82.1 Common key performance indicators. Targets are gleaned from published guidelines or suggested from experience

KPI	Common targets
Antibiotic prophylaxis before catheter insertion	100%
Exit site prophylaxis prescribed (either exit site or nasal prophylaxis)	100%
Exit site infection	90% exit site score <2
Peritonitis rate: Number of episodes of peritonitis / ((sum of months on peritoneal dialysis for all patients)/12)	<0.3 episodes/pt year
Culture negative peritonitis	<20%
Primary peritonitis cure rate	>80%
Adequacy: Kt/V_{urea} > 1.7 or total creatinine clearance >50 L/week/1.73m^2	No longer considered useful KPI
Hemoglobin: 100-120 g/L (or according to national guidelines)	80%
Time on therapy: Number of months for 50% of patients to come off PD, excluding transplantation, renal recovery or lost to follow up.	48 months
Peritoneal function (e.g., PET) and adequacy is measured at baseline and then at least yearly or as appropriate.	>90% initial testing (unless palliative PD/heart failure PD)
Technique survival (death and transplant censored):	1 year >80% (90%) 3 years >60% (75%) 5 years >40% (65%)
Patient survival at 1 year (may depend on age and comorbidity):	>70–90%

ing prospect and many fear their life will change dramatically. Discussing how to fit dialysis around their individual routine helps them understand that PD can be flexible and that they can still enjoy life.

Patients will also be concerned that having a catheter and being on an APD machine will prevent a healthy sex life. Patients rarely feel comfortable initiating this topic, so having an open discussion about sexuality is important. We advise at least a week of abstinence while the exit site heals, but thereafter, there is no contraindication to having sex either with or without fluid in, on or off an APD machine. It is important to appreciate that sexual dysfunction is common in ~70% of dialysis patients [91], but that dialysis modality does not appear to be important in this problem [92]. Medication may sometimes be blamed, with betablockers commonly implicated. Psychological issues are also important, so referral for psychological, endocrinological, pharmacological, or physical treatments are often appropriate [93]. Many female patients on hemodialysis do not menstruate, but it is more frequent than with PD. Ovulatory cycles may restart with initiation of dialysis and this can sometimes be associated with blood in the PD fluid and while pregnancy is rare, it can occur. It is usually associated with fetal growth retardation, premature delivery, or stillbirth. There is also a high incidence of maternal preeclampsia. Patients that get pregnant on PD are probably best managed by conversion to daily HD. Therefore, it is important to discuss contraceptive options, when appropriate.

Swimming with a catheter is encouraged in well-maintained swimming pools (with precautions) once the exit site has healed. Colostomy bags can be supplied which encase the whole catheter to keep the exit site and catheter dry. After swimming, the patient is advised to ensure the exit site has not been moistened and to perform normal exit site care. Swimming in the sea and fresh water is permitted with the above caveats, but increased gram-negative infection has been reported after this practice, so it is important to be aware of local conditions and obvious pollution risks. Spas or saunas are not recommended.

Patients are encouraged to shower daily, gently washing their exit site and over their PD catheter with soap and water. Drying is performed with a fresh clean cloth every time. Hot baths are discouraged, but colostomy bags can be supplied for occasional use.

Other common misperceptions are that alcohol is prohibited, pets must be given away or destroyed, and that young children are not allowed in bed with parents/grandparents who are dialyzing. Companion animals are popular, and 40% to 65% of households in the US and Europe have a much-loved domestic animal, and while extra care is needed, keeping animals should not be discouraged. There are some distinctly unhygienic homes where animals are allowed to roam freely and where few surfaces are kept clean. In such environments, any home therapy would be challenging, but only small modifications are usually needed for home therapies to successfully coexist with pets. (to put this in context, zoonotic microorganisms make up only a tiny fraction (<1%) of all infectious complications [94]. Pets should be kept out of the room when connecting or disconnecting and the APD machine should always be protected specifically from cats which like lying on the warm fluid and playing with the lines.

Home therapy is eminently suited to patients in regional and rural areas. While the trainer is ideally at the home, a residential training facility can also suffice, where patients can be taught about complications, and when and how to seek help. Twenty-four-hour assistance and guidance should be available via a home therapy unit, an after-hours backup (e.g., hospital ward or on-call service), or a dialysis company for machine issues. During training, patients are taught how to recognize contamination, exit site issues, and peritonitis. For remote patients, the local or regional medical services can be educated in emergency care of a PD patient with access to a renal center for after-hours support.

Patients should be supplied with antibiotics, peritonitis policies, and contact phone numbers to take to their local medical service. There are a number of new technology-based innovations currently being assessed to improve contact with remote patients, such as internet-based two-way cameras, but their practicality is unproven. In the meantime, telephones and e-mail are the usual routes of communication. We have found that e-mail has been a useful aid of communication between patients (especially deaf patients), home therapy nurses, and various medical staff. Written responses reduce "translational errors" and can usually be provided within 48 hours. Some patients take an avid interest in their own biochemistry, we encourage this and results can be quickly transmitted via e-mail, an approach beginning to be recognized by funding agencies.

Case Study 82.3

Sue is 59-year-old, started peritoneal dialysis 1 month ago. She has IgA nephropathy and hypertension. Her appetite and energy level have improved significantly since starting dialysis. She was seen in PD clinic for the first time. BP was 180/105 mmHg, she had mild ankle edema. Her serum tests showed: sodium 135 mmol/L, potassium 4 mmol/L, creatinine 750 μmol/L, urea 22 mmol/L, albumin 30 g/L, and phosphate 2.2 mmol/L.

Which of the following statements are true or false?

1. She is volume overloaded, higher glucose strength dialysates should be used to remove excess fluid.
2. She should be counseled on dietary potassium restriction.
3. A low-protein diet is appropriate to prolong residual renal function.
4. Increased daily volume is indicated because of her high serum creatinine.

Answers:

1. False. The patient has evidence of volume overload, or more specifically sodium and water overload. It is likely that she has good residual renal function. Education regarding high salt content in processed foods is of paramount importance and often a neglected part of education. In the first instance, diuretic should be used to increase urinary salt loss. Better dialysate drainage by addressing bowel habits could also improve net volume loss through PD. Increased glucose strength dialysate should NOT be used as the first line of treatment as it increases patient's glucose load and is deleterious to the peritoneal membrane.
2. False. Compared to hemodialysis where dietary potassium restriction is almost universal, PD is more efficient in potassium removal. Hyperkalemia is seen much less frequently in PD. Foods with high fiber and low sodium content (e.g., fruits and vegetables) are often potassium rich. In the absence of significant hyperkalemia, patients should be encouraged to have fruits and vegetables.
3. Controversial. There have been several observational studies and small randomized controlled trials to address this issue. While there is limited evidence to suggest that low-protein diet protects the loss of residual renal function in PD, other studies suggest that protein restriction (<0.8 g/kg/day) results in moderate malnutrition and reduction in serum albumin. It is our opinion that protein restriction is not indicated in PD as protein malnutrition could lead to malnutrition–inflammation complex, which can accelerate the development of cardiovascular disease.
4. False. A high serum creatinine is a function of muscle production and clearance. On its own, it does not indicate dialysis adequacy. Furthermore, the patient's uremic symptoms have improved. The assessment of adequate dialysis should be based the combination of uremic symptom control, adequacy studies, goals of care, and biochemical parameters.

82.8 Pregnancy and PD

There are more than 40 reported published cases of successful pregnancy in women receiving renal replacement therapy with PD [95, 96]. There has been a progressive improvement in the outcomes of pregnancies in women on dialysis over the last three decades. The conception rate in women with ESRF is reported to be in the range 0.3–2.1% [97]. There is likely to be significant under reporting of pregnancies because of unrecognized pregnancy losses and unreported terminations of pregnancies. Although it has been considered preferable for patients with end-stage renal failure to undergo pregnancies post-renal transplant, women over the age of

30 years run the risk of completing families in their late 30s or 40s, which carries increased risk of fetal and maternal adverse outcomes. Counseling patients and their families by a nephrologist or physician with obstetric medicine experience is essential. Such discussions should address risks, taking into account patient's plans for a family, medical status, age, wishes with respect to numbers of children, and potential adverse genetic outcomes. Such discussions can then consider all options including preemptive renal transplantation, dialysis, and other forms of assisted reproduction including surrogacy. Deferring pregnancy until women have a successful transplant usually defers pregnancy by at least 2 years in patients aged in their late third and fourth decades and therefore, increases maternal age with an associated increased maternal risk.

Low-dose aspirin is recommended to reduce the risk of preeclampsia in pregnant patients with increased risk of preeclampsia such as those suffering from most forms of renal disease, however, there is no evidence for routinely prescribing aspirin for pregnant dialysis patients including those on PD [98]. A large number of prescribed and non-prescribed medications can be harmful to the fetus. Examples are angiotensin-converting enzyme (ACE) inhibitors and angiotensin receptor (ARB) blockers which should be discontinued before or shortly following conception. Beta blockers are relatively contraindicated late in pregnancy [99].

Target weight in dialysis patients needs to be reviewed regularly during pregnancy. Dry weight can fall in the first trimester due to hyperemesis gravidarum and nearly, always, needs to be increased in the second and third trimesters.

The EDTA registry [100] has reported a successful pregnancy rate of 23% and higher rates are reported. The Australian and New Zealand Registry data suggests conception on HD is higher in HD compared to PD patients [101]. A US survey of pregnancy and ESRD suggested 1.1% of reproductive-aged women receiving PD conceived vs 2.4% on HD. Hypotheses for differential fertility rates include fluid in the abdominal cavity and hypertonic dextrose solutions interfering with ovum transit, and inadequate dialysis. Once conception is successful infant survival is similar in PD and HD.

Modes of contraception need to be considered given the low, but not negligible spontaneous pregnancy rates in dialysis patients. The advantages of depot contraception and intrauterine contraceptive devices should be considered. Real life data for the failure rate of the oral combined contraceptive pill suggest poor adherence. ESRD patients have chronically increased levels of beta-human chorionic gonadotrophin and thus, the diagnosis of pregnancy can be complicated [102].

Women on dialysis have at least a two-fold increased risk of developing adverse maternal outcomes including gestational HT, preeclampsia, eclampsia, and maternal mortality [103]. As terminations of pregnancy are likely to be under reported, the published data is likely to underestimate adverse outcomes. Furthermore, there may be a significant incidence of undiagnosed and unrecognized spontaneous abortions.

There are reports of PD patients suffering from peritonitis and exit site infections in pregnancy, although, whether such infections have an increased incidence is difficult to ascertain.

A majority of published successful pregnancies in dialysis patients were preterm births. A higher rate of small for gestational aged babies were born to mothers on PD compared with HD [103] with no evidence of a difference in the incidence of congenital abnormalities.

Improved outcomes in pregnancies in patients on dialysis have been associated with achieving greater clearances with the delivery of more dialysis. A disadvantage of peritoneal dialysis is the difficulty increasing clearances. It has been suggested that the dose of PD can be increased by increasing dialysate volume to as high as 22 liters/day. Alternatively, a combination of HD and PD has been used. HD is associated with more variability of blood pressure than in PD patients which might result in poorer placental blood flow.

At 37 weeks gestation or just beyond, most clinicians recommend patients with no maternal or fetal complications should be delivered. Such decisions should be made by a multidisciplinary team. Planned induction allows the patient to drain the peritoneal cavity, and to ensure the patient is well dialyzed prior to delivery. The mode of delivery (vaginal or cesarean section), should be decided on obstetric grounds. Vaginal delivery is preferred in a complicated term pregnancy. Post-partum, a complicated pregnancy, which occurs in many dialysis patients, can take months for stabilization and resolution of complications.

Breast feeding is an appropriate option for mothers receiving dialysis and should be encouraged [104].

Post-partum adjustment of the dry weight, residual urine monitoring, blood pressure, and a complete review of drug treatment, with special attention to the antihypertensive agents and ESAs, are necessary. Postnatal depression is relatively common in women with medical comorbidities and should be considered. Pregnancy may result in a loss of residual renal function which can adversely affect PD outcomes in the long term.

Successful outcomes in pregnancy in dialysis patients require a multidisciplinary team of maternal-fetal medicine, renal, and obstetric medical physicians working with many other members of the healthcare team including dialysis nurses, social workers, dieticians, and other healthcare professionals. Frequent monitoring and review of blood pressure, target weight, clinical sigs, fetal growth, biochemical features as well as other investigations enable optimization of pregnancy outcomes, resulting in longer durations of pregnancy to achieve optimal pregnancy outcomes in women with end-stage renal failure. Combination therapy with PD and HD has not been studied and may be an appropriate option in selected patients.

Case Study 82.4

Charlotte is a sales assistant in a department store, aged 28 years, has end-stage renal failure due to IgA glomerulonephritis and is on peritoneal dialysis. She has a longstanding hyperlipidemia for which she takes rosuvastatin. She would like to have a pregnancy and asks you if it is possible while she is on PD.

Questions:

1. Is it possible for Charlotte to conceive while on PD?
2. Can Charlotte continue on PD during pregnancy?
3. What medications would you consider initiating if she chooses to embark on a pregnancy?
4. What medications would you consider stopping?

82

Answers:

1. Fertility is reduced in all dialysis patients. PD patients are less fertile than HD patients. Spontaneous pregnancies do occur and effective contraception needs to be considered in all premenopausal women who are not trying to become pregnant.
2. For dialysis adequacy reasons, most patients are converted to HD in pregnancy. A combination of HD and PD can be considered, but is relatively uncommon.
3. It is essential that all women who may become pregnant take prepregnancy folic acid for neural tube indications. Aspirin prepregnancy can be considered, but given the incidence of gastritis in dialysis patients, aspirin may be best avoided. Conversely, while not proven, aspirin would be recommended for dialysis patients by most obstetric physicians in pregnancy, commencing before 14 weeks gestation and preferably in the first weeks of pregnancy, to reduce the risk of preeclampsia.
4. On the basis of current knowledge, statins should be ceased prepregnancy with the current recommendation being 3 months prepregnancy. Concerns have been raised about a potentially adverse effect of statins on neural development. Trials of statins in pregnancy have been discussed. Statins are currently considered contraindicated in pregnancy.

   ACEI/ARBs are controversial. ACEs and ARBs have been reported to cause acute renal failure in neonates when taken in the third trimester and should not be continued once a patient is pregnant. There is no good evidence of teratogenesis, although there have been concerns that they may cause a decrease in fertility/early pregnancy loss, for which there is not good data. Dialysis patients have decreased fertility, so leaving patients off ACEs and ARBs for a prolonged time may have a negative impact on the mother's health status with a potential negative impact on subsequent pregnancy outcomes. Our recommendation is that patients continue ACEs and ARBs until they know they are pregnant and stop these agents as soon as they know they are pregnant, which is usually well before 10 weeks gestation.

Case Study 82.5

Henrietta is aged 28, on PD for end-stage renal failure related to multisystem lupus who is determined to have her first pregnancy. She has moderate ongoing arthritis and a history of pericarditis, requiring ongoing immunosuppression. She is negative for anticardiolipin antibodies, has no lupus anticoagulant, and is ENA negative. She is active on the cadaveric donor transplant list. A 40-year-old fellow worker is considering donating a kidney. Charlotte seeks your assistance as to whether she should embark on a pregnancy now or wait until she has a transplant. Her current medications are phosphate binders, perindopril, mycophenolate mofetil, low dose prednisone, and hydroxychloroquine.

Questions:

1. Should PD patients have children?
2. Should Henrietta have a pregnancy now or wait until she has a functioning renal transplant?
3. Should Henrietta be on the combined contraceptive pill?

Answers:

1. As medical practitioners, our role is to educate patients as to the potential risks of pregnancy. Once the patient has been educated, our role is to support their decision as best we can. Patients will often make different decisions to what we consider we might make in the same position.
2. Timing of pregnancy is difficult for dialysis patients. A consideration is whether patients are advantaged having children younger or later, given the increased incidence of pregnancy complications with age including preeclampsia and genetic abnormalities. There are, however, advantages of having a pregnancy with near normal function. It is, therefore, a decision that must be made considering the patient's medical and social situation.

   Most nephrologists recommend patients do not become pregnant for 12–24 months posttransplant.
3. Given Henrietta is taking mycophenolate, which is teratogenic, (approximately 25% incidence), highly reliable contraception is strongly recommended. Hydroxychloroquine is recommended for patients with lupus embarking on and during pregnancy. ACE inhibitors should be ceased, at the latest, as soon as the patients know they are pregnant.

   Real-life data with fertile women shows that over 3 years, more than 10% of women will become pregnant when taking the combined contraceptive pill. The combined contraceptive pill should be considered unreliable. Long-acting progestogens and IUDs are the most reliable contraceptives.

82.9 Catheter Insertion

Recent guidelines on PD access have been produced which set out good practice and have a number of excellent tips on advanced techniques that can be applied to get well functioning catheters which function well for the long term [105]. Not all of these guidelines will be practical or applicable, in all parts of the world and it should be noted that regional solutions will often depend upon local expertise and enthusiasm. In our view there is no one "correct way" of enabling PD access and while best practice guidelines may be helpful for low volume, high cost centers, there should be a recognition that this may not be possible in renal replacement programs.

82.10 Techniques

An essential element to a successful PD program is a catheter insertion service that is readily available and can place a PD catheter when needed and within a reasonable timescale. There are a variety of techniques used to insert catheters; which include a "blind" Seldinger techniques and variations (including using radiological guidance), peritoneoscopic or laparoscopic techniques, or open surgical techniques such as mini-laparotomy with or without omentectomy.

The physician-inserted local anesthetic (LAPD) Seldingerinsertion [89]is a valuable technique particularly when setting up a PD service. The procedure is relatively simple to learn and quickto perform, improves PD program capacity, and allows rapid decisions on when and how to start patients. Acute start PD can replace or at least offer an alternative to the common default option of HD, and additional advantages include the fact that LAPD can generally be done in a procedure room or as a daycase, which makes it cheaper and faster than many other techniques. Many of these advantages are shared by similar techniques such as radiologically placed catheters, which have the advantage of real-time imaging. However, like surgically placed catheters, involvement of individuals, and units outside the renal unit often increase the complexity of achieving the same result.

Peritoneoscopic techniques have become popular in some units and are similar in many ways to the LAPD procedure, except that visual confirmation of positioning is available, although there is a distinctly steep learning curve for those unfamiliar with looking down the scope. Disadvantages are pain from gaseous distension of the abdomen, longer operating times, higher start-up costs (peritoneoscope, light source, and other equipment), higher on-going costs (sterilization of equipment and more expensive kits), and greater technological demands. There are other hidden costs, including sterilization and the loss of fibers after recurrent sterilization, necessitating replacement at some point. The fact that the scopes and other equipment requires sterilization between cases limits operating numbers, due to the turnaround.

82.10.1 Antisepsis

Prior to insertion, patients should be decolonized by application of nasal mupirocin and an antiseptic wash. The bowel should be emptied by use of a laxative and antibiotics should be given preoperatively [106].

Chlorhexidine in alcohol is extremely irritant to the peritoneum and has been shown to cause chemical peritonitis in animals similar to that seen in encapsulating peritoneal sclerosis, a feared, but rare, complication of PD (see complications) [107]. However, in a drive towards eradication of hospital-acquired infection chlorhexidine has achieved widespread use. In PD patients, this antiseptic agent should be used carefully if at all, and no alcoholic chlorhexidine should go near the PD catheter or contaminate the peritoneum. It is recommended that only aqueous iodine is used on or near the ends of catheters and chlorhexidine is only used for hand hygiene and/or skin preparation, but not as a spray around surfaces and equipment.

82.10.1.1 LAPD (◘ Figs. 82.1, 82.2, 82.3, 82.4, and 82.5) (and See Video)

There are a number of governance and liaison issues before this service can commence. As with all procedures, consent should be obtained, see example, and a surgical "time out" must be performed before commencing the procedure [108].

- Surgical backup is potentially required should unforeseen complications arise. With proper identification of suitable patients, this is not usually a significant problem. However, a named surgeon should be consulted when the procedure is given governance approval for the procedure, and a surgical team should potentially be available to advise and help, on the rare occasion a bowel perforation occurs. Most surgeons do not regard the technique as particularly difficult, so do not usually object to physicians performing the procedure themselves, and it frees up their time for more challenging surgery.
- Anaesthetic approval is usually sought during governance approval for such a procedure, and is important as patients may require significant opiates and/or benzodiazepines and are generally left with an unsupervised airway after the procedure. However, the process involved is very much conscious sedation: patients are rousable, with typical doses of intravenous sedation being 25–50 mg of pethidine or equivalent opiate and 1–2 mg of midazolam. The procedure can be done without sedation, but both patients and operators may be less comfortable in such a situation. During the procedure it is important to have an assistant monitoring the patient and the level of sedation and oxygen saturations and blood pressure. We would also always have flumazenil and naloxone to hand should this become necessary.
- Infection control units are frequently keen for this procedure to be performed in the sterile environment of an operating theatre. This is not absolutely required, but is welcomed if available, a clean procedure room is enough. Much more important are adequate anti-infective precautions. Evidence-based recommendations include nasal decolonization with mupirocin ointment to the nose for some days prior to the procedure, washing with antibacterial soap and bowel cleansing with aperients. Preoperative antibiotics are also important [105].

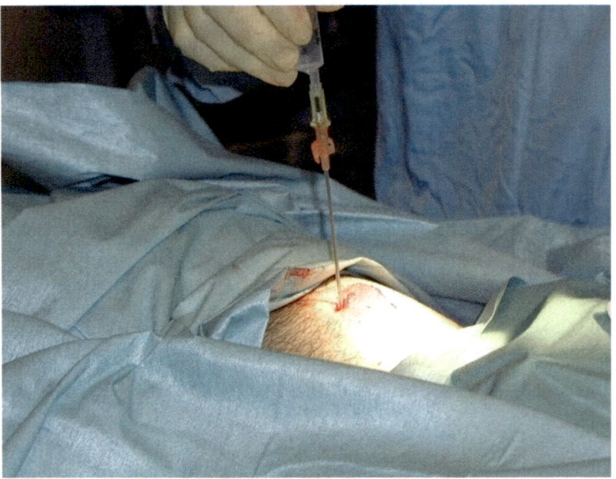

◘ **Fig. 82.1** Using local anesthetic in this needle, anesthetize the area around the rectus sheath. Advance the needle gently through the linea alba into the peritoneum. Two distinct "pops" may be felt as each of these layers is passed. After the second "pop", **stop**. Do not advance the needle further. Instead, advance the blunt sheath, beyond the needle tip and into the peritoneal space, angling the needle slightly downward toward the pubic symphysis. Withdraw the needle and leave the sheath in situ

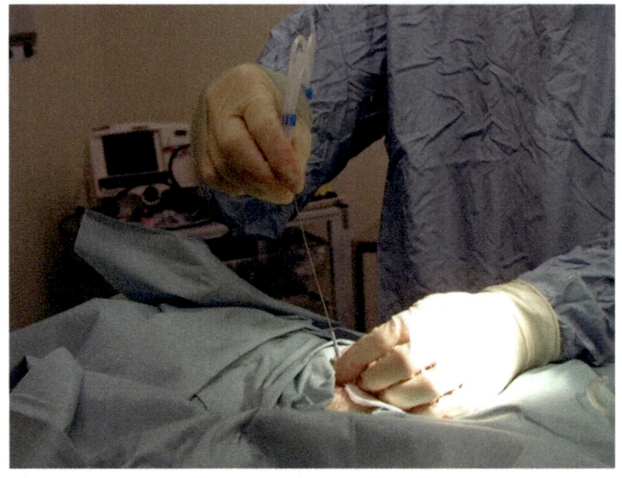

◘ **Fig. 82.2** Confirmation that the correct space has been entered can be achieved by flushing fluid under gravity into the abdominal cavity or passing a wire down the needle. It should pass imperceptibly beyond the sheath and deep into the pelvis. If it does not do so, remove and repeat the insertion process or abandon the attempt at this stage

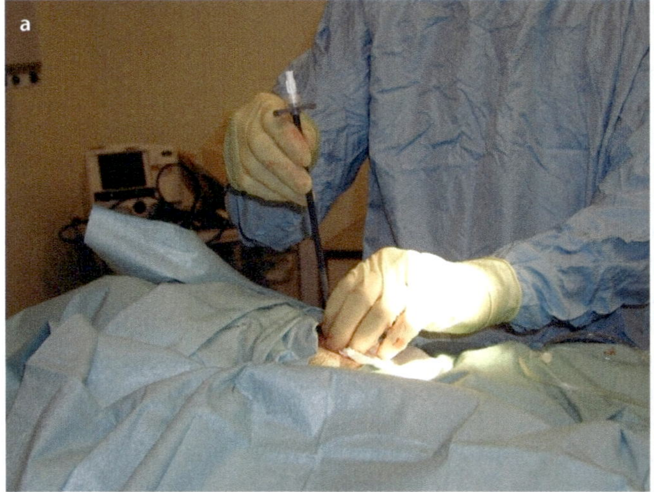

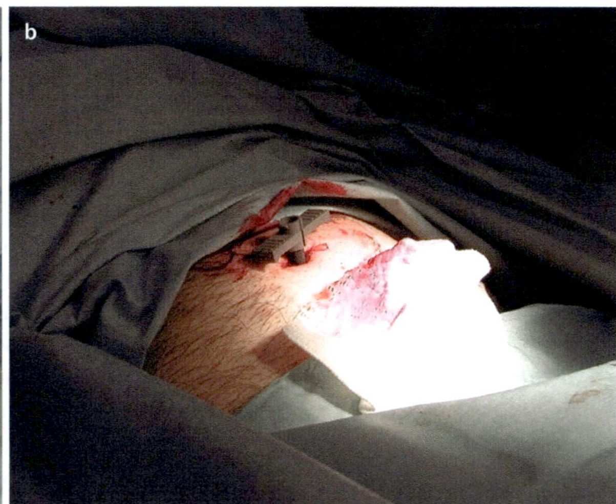

Fig. 82.3 **a**, **b** Once the abdomen is filled with ~700–800 mL of fluid, insert a J-tipped floppy guide wire into the abdominal cavity. Overcoming the resistance and inserting more of the wire makes it curve into the pelvis. The tract is then dilated and a peel-away sheath and dilator are advanced along the wire into the peritoneum, angled slightly down into the pelvis. The dilator is removed, leaving the sheath in situ

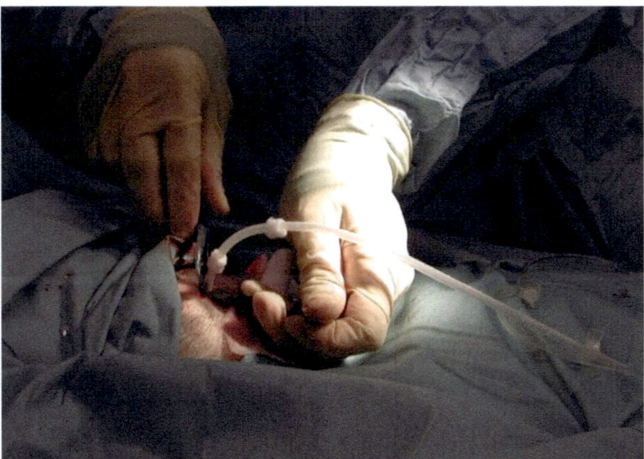

Fig. 82.4 The PD catheter can be simply fed down the sheath. The inner cuff is pushed with forceps down to the rectus sheath. The tunnel can then be fashioned by locating the exit site below the incision (so that the exit site is down-facing) and at least 3 cm from the distal cuff

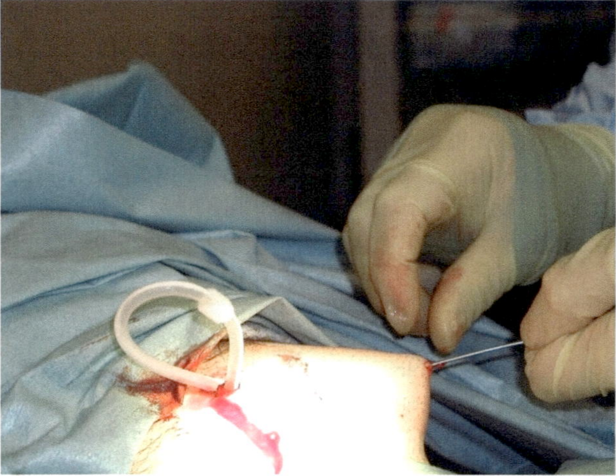

Fig. 82.5 Once the exit site has been anaesthetized the subcutaneous tract between the exit site and the incision site can also be infiltrated with lignocaine. The exit site is either made by scalpel incision or with a sharp tunneling tool, and the distal end of the catheter can be pulled through the subcutaneous tunnel and out of the exit site. The catheter is then fit with a plastic or titanium connector for the transfer set, which is then firmly attached

- Mark the position of the patient's belt line and the planned exit site with the patient standing. It is important to avoid placing the exit site over the belt line and to ensure it is visible to the patient. The patient is asked to empty their bladder prior to the procedure. An empty bladder should be confirmed by ultrasound. If necessary, a urinary catheter (*per urethra*)can be passed.
- The patient should be positioned on a trolley or table. They do not have to be completely flat (some patients with severe heart failure may be unable to lie completely flat). It is important to be able to feel the midline. If there is a large abdominal apron this can be taped in place centrally to ensure the midline is found.
- Intravenous drugs are then administered, including an antiemetic, antibiotics, and sedation, with reversal agents to hand (e.g., flumazenil and naloxone) if needed.
- The abdomen is shaved if necessary (ideally with a surgical shaver and not a razor) and cleaned with chlorhexidine or iodine solution. Locate the insertion site around 2–3 cm below the umbilicus in the midline and allow this to dry before draping the area.

Inject the skin at the insertion site with local anesthetic and make a 1–2 cm horizontal incision in the skin of the abdominal wall. Achieve hemostasis with gauze. Inject local anesthetic deeper, anesthetizing a tract all the way down to the rectus aponeurosis and, if possible, to the peritoneal surface. Blunt dissect with forceps though the fat layer down to the linea albato create a tract. Use the same technique to explore the fat space above and lateral to the insertion site where the catheter will turn in the subcutaneous tunnel. Insert the long needle with plastic sheath through the entry wound and down onto the linea alba, which can be appreciated by a smooth, slippery, and slightly hard feel at the end of forceps or needle. Using local anesthetic in this needle, anesthetize the area around the rectus sheath. Advance the needle gently through the linea alba into the peritoneum. Two distinct "pops" may be felt as each of these layers is passed. After the second "pop", **stop**. Do not advance the needle further. Instead, advance the blunt sheath, beyond the needle tip and into the peritoneal space, angling the needle slightly downwards towards the pubic symphysis (◘ Fig. 82.1). Withdraw the needle and leave the sheath *in situ*. Confirmation that the correct space has been entered can be achieved by flushing fluid under gravity into the abdominal cavity or passing a wire down the needle. It should pass imperceptibly beyond the sheath and deep into the pelvis (◘ Fig. 82.2). If it does not do so, remove and repeat the insertion process or abandon the attempt at this stage.

- Fill the abdomen through the advanced needle with 0.9% Saline (NS) or PD fluid. (The acidity of NS is said to be potentially harmful to the peritoneal surface, but stickiness of PD fluid may be problematic in itself. It is suggested that a single small volume of NS is unlikely to do damage.)The NS should flow freely into the abdomen under gravity, and not need any significant pressure. Further, 5–10 mL of lignocaine into this space at this point sometimes assists to ensure that the procedure continues without discomfort. If the patient experiences pain on filling or after<200 mL has been infused, it is likely the preperitoneal space has been entered. In that case, stop the infusion, aspirate as much fluid as possible, and try to re-enter the peritoneal space by reintroducing the needle slightly caudally, or abandoning the procedure in favor of a radiologically-assisted or surgical approach. This method is most challenging in very obese subjects, or where there is a large abdominal apron that flops to one side. Care should be taken to try to keep the abdominal apron central during insertion. An appreciation that the abdominal fat will move the catheter when the patient stands will enhance catheter placement.
- Once the abdomen is filled with ~700-800 mL of fluid, insert a J-tipped floppy guide wire into the abdominal cavity. Slight discomfort around the rectum or base of the penis sometimes occurs when the wire is in the pouch of Douglas, and some resistance to insertion is often felt here. Overcoming the resistance and inserting more of the wire makes it curve into the pelvis. The tract is then dilated and a peel-away sheath and dilator are advanced along the wire into the peritoneum, angled slightly down into the pelvis. The dilator is removed, leaving the sheath in situ (◘ Fig. 82.3a, b). Before placing the catheter into the abdomen, the cuffs should be soaked in saline (dry cuffs inhibit fibroblast growth, delaying healing). The PD catheter can then be simply fed down the sheath (◘ Fig. 82.4). Push the inner cuff with forceps down to the rectus sheath. The tunnel can then be fashioned by locating the exit site below the incision (so that the exit site is down-facing) and at least 3 cm from the distal cuff. The belt line has been pre-marked and this should be avoided for the exit site. Once the exit site has been anesthetized the subcutaneous tract between the exit site and the incision site can also be infiltrated with lignocaine. The exit site is either made by scalpel incision (◘ Fig. 82.5) or with a sharp tunneling tool, and the distal end of the catheter can be pulled through the subcutaneous tunnel and out of the exit site. The catheter is then fitted with a plastic or titanium connector for the transfer set, which is then firmly attached. All joints must be carefully tightened, and a cap placed on the transfer set. An absorbent/antibiotic cuff (e.g., Biopatch®)can be placed over the exit site which can usefully absorb any exudate. The catheter should then be immobilized for 2 weeks if possible. Do not put sutures at the exit site, if possible, but suture the entry site.
- A Moncrief–Popovitch modification for catheter implantation is a useful technique when a patient wishes to do PD, but the time frame for use is unknown, as a catheter can be placed for future use [109]. The process is similar to that described above except that the catheter is brought out through an incision more proximal to the entry site and a pouch is created to keep the (eventually external) portion of the catheter subcutaneous until needed (◘ Fig. 82.6). A further minor procedure is required to externalize the catheter. This involves anesthetizing the skin at the exit site down to the catheter in the subcutaneous layer (avoid puncturing the catheter with the anesthetic needle). Forceps are used to grab the catheter

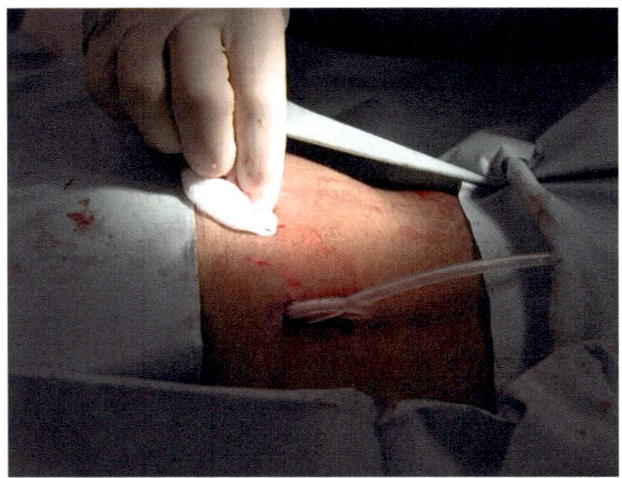

Fig. 82.6 A Moncrief–Popovitch modification for catheter implantation is a useful technique when a patient wishes to do PD, but the time frame for use is unknown, as a catheter can be placed for future use. The catheter is brought out through an incision more proximal to the entry site and a pouch is created to keep the (eventually external) portion of the catheter subcutaneous until needed

and pull it out through the anterior abdominal wall. The catheter is immobilized as far as possible to ensure that it moves as little as possible at the exit site, but the catheter may be used immediately.

82.10.2 Catheters

There are a number of catheters on the market, most have two cuffs and commonly come in the straight and "swan-neck" varieties, with a curled or straight intraperitoneal segment (Fig. 82.7). Even well-placed catheters can migrate and, in most PD programs where peritonitis rates are low, this, along with omental wrapping is perhaps the main practical catheter problem, when constipation has been eliminated. Whether to use a coiled or straight tipped catheter is also a difficult issue, as there are no randomized trials of sufficient power to draw a definitive conclusion. A meta-analysis of what data are available suggests that coiled catheters may have a greater technique failure rate than straight-tipped catheters, mainly because of catheter migration. However, coiled catheters probably have a lower incidence of infusion- and drainage-related pain, thus, at this stage the choice remains one of preference [110].

82.11 Governance

In any unit a process of continuous quality improvement and governance needs to be in place. Standard, generic policies should be adapted to local needs as experience develops. However, it is vital that protocols are agreed upon and uniformly followed in order to obtain consistent results. It is also important to define key competencies for nursing staff. Such performance standards need to be examined and compared regularly at all levels in order to ensure patients continue to receive optimal care and to identify potential and actual issues requiring intervention.

At a minimum the following standard operating procedures should be addressed:

1. PD catheter insertion and postoperative care.
2. CAPD exchange—prescription and recording, and management.
3. APD exchange—prescription and recording management.
4. PD access insertion pathway.
5. PD fluids ampling.
6. Review and monitoring policy.
   (a) Peritoneal equilibration and adequacy testing.
   (b) Transfer line change.
   (c) Exit site scoring and care.
7. Peritonitis protocol.
8. Antibiotic loading procedure.

82.11.1 Key Performance Indicators and Continuous Quality Improvement

As alluded to above, it is important to audit results and be prepared to make changes when necessary. Most governance structures collect and audit data on exit site and peritonitis rates, time on therapy, drop-out rate, and technique survival. Once the home therapies unit is well established, aspirational targets are important, and every effort should be made to try to achieve these. However, limiting PD only to those patients whom you are confident will succeed ("cherry picking") will limit program growth. Equally, not everyone is suited to PD: a balance needs to be struck. Continuous quality improvement (CQI) is the cycle of plan, check, and act that is widely used to improve quality and is well suited to a PD program. Key performance indicators (KPIs) are often used to judge the success of a program and common KPIs are listed in Table 2together with possible targets. Patient complaints and feedback are often helpful (if at times painful).

82.11.2 Finance

Costs of dialysis and remuneration vary worldwide, but a number of studies suggest that PD is a cheaper dialysis modality than HD. There is also a distinction between

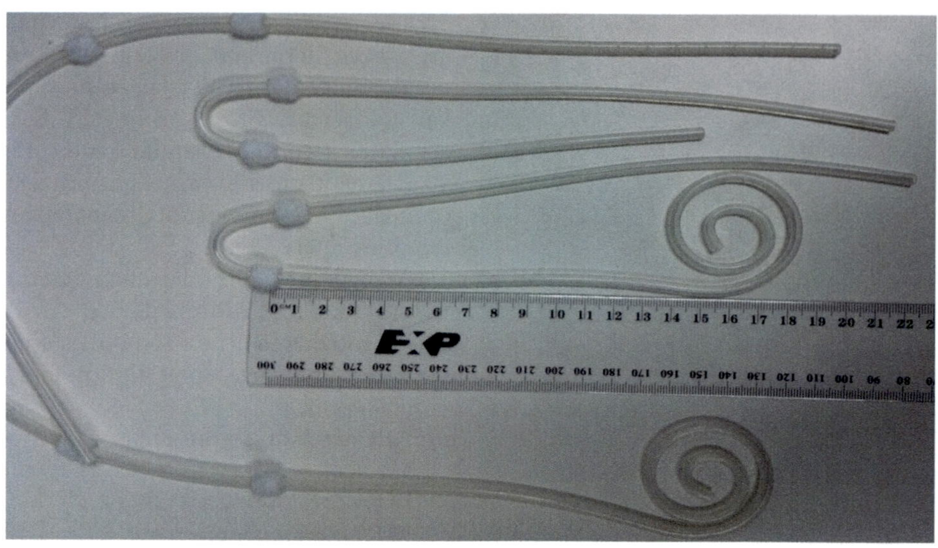

Fig. 82.7 There are a number of catheters in the market, most have two cuffs and commonly come in the straight and "swan-neck" varieties

APD and CAPD, costing approximately 38% and 56% less than hospital-based HD, respectively [111, 112]. In some countries, prices are set by the government, but in others, local contracts may be drawn up. In such cases, negotiations should deliver the essentials of the program to required specifications. Effective negotiations involve a mix of administration, medical, and nursing staff who meet to define critical needs and desired objectives before meeting with the PD company responsible for supplying services. Legal opinion on contracts is often very helpful, as is ensuring that a business-oriented person familiar (and ideally experienced) with dialysis contracts is engaged.

82.11.3 Knowing When to Give Up

Knowing when to give up PD is important. There are currently no data to suggest that fear of EPS should initiate stopping PD after a certain time [113]. It may be possible to predict a slow decline in patients with loss of the ability to ultrafilter or a change in transport characteristics (e.g., a rising D_{creat}/P_{creat} on repeated transport testing). Anticipating change to another modality facilitates retraining and readjustment, and this is facilitated by early identification of failing PD. However, patients themselves often resist change because of a personal bond with medical and/or nursing staff and fear of a new dialysis modality. The physician must recognize when the technique is failing and not persist until the patient needs urgent transfer. Some units advocate the addition of a single HD session with continued PD as a way of making the transition. However, this can be expensive and impractical, taking another dialysis slot which can be ill-afforded. An advantage to having an integrated home therapies team is that the same familiar and trusted team can seamlessly transfer patients to home-based HD when transfer is needed. This might not be possible, of course, if the patient's comorbidities, mental or physical or social, are driving the change.

82.12 Summary

Setting up a new PD service is a rewarding and interesting venture. It relies heavily on multi-disciplinary care and the key assets are an integrated and motivated team. A successful program is greatly facilitated by the ability to insert functioning PD catheters in a timely fashion. Continuous quality improvement is important to refine the program and ensure optimal results are maintained.

Acknowledgments We are indebted to Anabelle Ryan and Prof Lawrie McMahon who contributed to this chapter in the first edition of this book.

References

1. Karopadi AN, Mason G, Rettore E, Ronco C. Cost of peritoneal dialysis and haemodialysis across the world. Nephrol Dial Transplant. 2013;28:2553–69.
2. Chuengsaman P, Kasemsup V. PD first policy: Thailand's response to the challenge of meeting the needs of patients with end-stage renal disease. Semin Nephrol. 2017;37:287–95.
3. Goldfarb-Rumyantzev AS, Hurdle JF, Scandling JD, Baird BC, Cheung AK. The role of pretransplantation renal replacement therapy modality in kidney allograft and recipient survival. Am J Kidney Dis. 2005;46:537–49.

4. Thomson BK, MAJ M, Marek C, Bloch M, Weernink C, Shoker A, et al. Peritoneal dialysis versus hemodialysis in patients with delayed graft function. Clin Transpl. 2013;27:E709–14.
5. Mudge DW, Boudville N, Brown F, Clayton P, Duddington M, Holt S, et al. Peritoneal dialysis practice in Australia and New Zealand: a call to sustain the action. Nephrology (Carlton). 2016; https://doi.org/10.1111/nep.12731.
6. Lata C, Girard L, Parkins M, James MT. Catheter-related bloodstream infection in end-stage kidney disease: a Canadian narrative review. Can J Kidney Heal Dis. 2016; https://doi.org/10.1186/s40697-016-0115-8.
7. Brown EA, Johansson L, Farrington K, Gallagher H, Sensky T, Gordon F, et al. Broadening Options for Long-term Dialysis in the Elderly (BOLDE): differences in quality of life on peritoneal dialysis compared to haemodialysis for older patients. Nephrol Dial Transplant. 2010;25:3755–63.
8. Puttagunta H, Holt SG. Peritoneal dialysis for heart failure. Perit Dial Int. 2015;35 https://doi.org/10.3747/pdi.2014.00340.
9. Nader M, Aguilar R, Sharma P, Krishnamoorthy P, Serban D, Gordon-Cappitelli J, et al. In-hospital mortality in cirrhotic patients with end-stage renal disease treated with hemodialysis versus peritoneal dialysis: a nationwide study. Perit Dial Int. 2017;37:464–71.
10. Diaz-Buxo JA, Crawford-Bonadio T. The continuum home program concept. Clin Nephrol. 2008;69:326–30.
11. Povlsen JV, Ivarsen P. Assisted automated peritoneal dialysis (AAPD) for the functionally dependent and elderly patient. Perit Dial Int. 2005;25:S60–3.
12. Salani M, Roy S, Fissell WH. Innovations in wearable and implantable artificial kidneys. Am J Kidney Dis. 2018;72: 745–51.
13. Korevaar JC, Feith GW, Dekker FW, Van Manen JG, Boeschoten EW, Bossuyt PMM, et al. Effect of starting with hemodialysis compared with peritoneal dialysis in patients new on dialysis treatment: a randomized controlled trial. Kidney Int. 2003;64:2222–8.
14. Li PKT, Chow KM. Peritoneal dialysis-first policy made successful: perspectives and actions. Am J Kidney Dis. 2013;62:993–1005.
15. Wang IK, Lin CL, Yen TH, Lin SY, Sung FC. Comparison of survival between hemodialysis and peritoneal dialysis patients with end-stage renal disease in the era of icodextrin treatment. Eur J Intern Med. 2018;50:69–74.
16. Brown EA, Finkelstein FO, Iyasere OU, Kliger AS. Peritoneal or hemodialysis for the frail elderly patient, the choice of 2 evils? Kidney Int. 2017; https://doi.org/10.1016/j.kint.2016.08.026.
17. Corbett RW, Brown EA. Conventional dialysis in the elderly: how lenient should our guidelines be? Semin Dial. 2018; https://doi.org/10.1111/sdi.12744.
18. Jansen MAM, Hart AAM, Korevaar JC, Dekker FW, Boeschoten EW, Krediet RT. Predictors of the rate of decline of residual renal function in incident dialysis patients. Kidney Int. 2002;62:1046–53.
19. Michels WM, Verduijn M, Grootendorst DC, le Cessie S, Boeschoten EW, Dekker FW, et al. Decline in residual renal function in automated compared with continuous ambulatory peritoneal dialysis. Clin J Am Soc Nephrol. 2011;6:537–42.
20. Johnson DW, Mudge DW, Sturtevant JM, Hawley CM, Campbell SB, Isbel NM, et al. Predictors of decline of residual renal function in new peritoneal dialysis patients. Perit Dial Int J Int Soc Perit Dial. 2003;23:276–83.
21. Culleton BF, Walsh M, Klarenbach SW, Mortis G, Scott-Douglas N, Quinn RR, et al. Effect of frequent nocturnal hemodialysis vs conventional hemodialysis on left ventricular mass and quality of life: a randomized controlled trial. J Am Med Assoc. 2007;298:1291–9.
22. Walker RC, Howard K, Morton RL, Palmer SC, Marshall MR, Tong A. Patient and caregiver values, beliefs and experiences when considering home dialysis as a treatment option: a semi-structured interview study. Nephrol Dial Transplant. 2016;31:133–41.
23. Walker RC, Morton RL, Palmer SC, Marshall MR, Tong A, Howard K. A discrete choice study of patient preferences for dialysis modalities. Clin J Am Soc Nephrol. 2018;13:100–8.
24. Lee MB, Bargman JM. Myths in peritoneal dialysis. Curr Opin Nephrol Hypertens. 2016; https://doi.org/10.1097/MNH.0000000000000274.
25. Gatti E, Ronco C. Seeking an optimal renal replacement therapy for the chronic kidney disease epidemic: the case for online hemodiafiltration. Contrib Nephrol. 2011;175:170–85.
26. Han SH, Ahn SV, Yun JY, Tranaeus A, Han D-S. Effects of icodextrin on patient survival and technique success in patients undergoing peritoneal dialysis. Nephrol Dial Transplant. 2012;27:2044–50.
27. Clark MD, Szczepura A, Gumber A, Howard K, Moro D, Morton RL. Measuring trade-offs in nephrology: a systematic review of discrete choice experiments and conjoint analysis studies. Nephrol Dial Transplant. 2018;33:348–55.
28. Sukul N, Zhao J, Fuller DS, Karaboyas A, Bieber B, Sloand JA, et al. Patient-reported advantages and disadvantages of peritoneal dialysis: results from the PDOPPS. BMC Nephrol. 2019;20:1–10.
29. Brown EA, Davies SJ, Heimbürger O, Meeus F, Mellotte G, Rosman J, et al. Adequacy targets can be met in anuric patients by automated peritoneal dialysis: baseline data from EAPOS. Perit Dial Int J Int Soc Perit Dial. 2001;21(Suppl 3):S133–7.
30. Brown EA, Bargman J, van Biesen W, Chang M-Y, Finkelstein FO, Hurst H, et al. Length of time on peritoneal dialysis and encapsulating peritoneal sclerosis — position paper for ISPD: 2017 update. Perit Dial Int. 2017;37:362–74.
31. Oliver MJ, Garg AX, Blake PG, Johnson JF, Verrelli M, Zacharias JM, et al. Impact of contraindications, barriers to self-care and support on incident peritoneal dialysis utilization. Nephrol Dial Transplant. 2010;25:2737–44.
32. Van Munster BC, Drost D, Kalf A, Vogtlander NP. Discriminative value of frailty screening instruments in end-stage renal disease. Clin Kidney J. 2016; https://doi.org/10.1093/ckj/sfw061.
33. La Milia V, Di Filippo S, Crepaldi M, Andrulli S, Del Vecchio L, Scaravilli P, et al. Sodium removal and sodium concentration during peritoneal dialysis: effects of three methods of sodium measurement. Nephrol Dial Transplant. 2004;19:1849–55.
34. Paniagua R, Ventura M-J, Avila-Díaz M, Hinojosa-Heredia H, Méndez-Durán A, Cueto-Manzano A, et al. NT-proBNP, fluid volume overload and dialysis modality are independent predictors of mortality in ESRD patients. Nephrol Dial Transplant. 2010;25:551–7.
35. Basile C. Calcium mass balances in bicarbonate hemodialysis. Int J Nephrol. 2011;2011:10–3.
36. Gotch FA, Kotanko P, Thijssen S, Levin NW. The KDIGO guideline for dialysate calcium will result in an increased incidence of calcium accumulation in hemodialysis patients. Kidney Int. 2010;78:343–50.
37. Simonsen O, Venturoli D, Wieslander A, Carlsson O, Rippe B. Mass transfer of calcium across the peritoneum at three different peritoneal dialysis fluid Ca2+ and glucose concentrations. Kidney Int. 2003;64:208–15.

38. Eddington H, Hurst H, Ramli MT, Speake M, Hutchison AJ. Calcium and magnesium flux in automated peritoneal dialysis. Perit Dial Int. 2009;29:536–41.
39. Hamada C, Tomino Y. Transperitoneal calcium balance in anuric continuous ambulatory peritoneal dialysis and automated peritoneal dialysis patients. Int J Nephrol. 2013;2013:863791.
40. Sánchez C, López-Barea F, Sánchez-Cabezudo J, Bajo A, Mate A, Martínez E, et al. Low vs standard calcium dialysate in peritoneal dialysis: differences in treatment, biochemistry and bone histomorphometry. A randomized multicentre study. Nephrol Dial Transplant. 2004;19:1587–93.
41. Young EW, Albert JM, Satayathum S, Goodkin DA, Pisoni RL, Akiba T, et al. Predictors and consequences of altered mineral metabolism: the dialysis outcomes and practice patterns study. Kidney Int. 2005;67:1179–87.
42. Zavvos V, Buxton AT, Evans C, Lambie M, Davies SJ, Topley N, et al. A prospective, proteomics study identified potential biomarkers of encapsulating peritoneal sclerosis in peritoneal effluent. Kidney Int. 2017;92:988–1002.
43. Cai MMX, Wigg B, Smith ER, Hewitson TD, McMahon LP, Holt SG. Relative abundance of fetuin-A in peritoneal dialysis effluent and its association with in situ formation of calciprotein particles: an observational pilot study. Nephrology. 2015; https://doi.org/10.1111/nep.12350.
44. Smith ER, Hewitson TD, Cai MMX, Holt SG. Fetuin-A in the peritoneal effluent of patients with encapsulating peritoneal sclerosis—more than a protein? Kidney Int. 2017;92:1289–90.
45. Kalantar-Zadeh K, Block G, Humphreys MH, Kopple JD. Reverse epidemiology of cardiovascular risk factors in maintenance dialysis patients. Kidney Int. 2003;63:793–808.
46. de Mutsert R, Grootendorst DC, Boeschoten EW, Dekker FW, Krediet RT. Is obesity associated with a survival advantage in patients starting peritoneal dialysis? Contrib Nephrol. 2009;163:124–31.
47. Chan M, Kelly J, Batterham M, Tapsell L. Malnutrition (subjective global assessment) scores and serum albumin levels, but not body mass index values, at initiation of dialysis are independent predictors of mortality: a 10-year clinical cohort study. J Ren Nutr. 2012; https://doi.org/10.1053/j.jrn.2011.11.002.
48. Johnson DW. What is the optimal fat mass in peritoneal dialysis patients? Perit Dial Int J Int Soc Perit Dial. 2007;27(Suppl 2):S250–4.
49. Cho K-H, Do J-Y, Park J-W, Yoon K-W. Effect of icodextrin dialysis solution on body weight and fat accumulation over time in CAPD patients. Nephrol Dial Transplant. 2010;25:593–9.
50. Woodrow G, Oldroyd B, Turney JH, Tompkins L, Brownjohn AM, Smith MA. Whole body and regional body composition in patients with chronic renal failure. Nephrol Dial Transplant. 1996;11:1613–8.
51. Fernström A, Hylander B, Moritz A, Jacobsson H, Rössner S. Increase of intra-abdominal fat in patients treated with continuous ambulatory peritoneal dialysis. Perit Dial Int J Int Soc Perit Dial. 1998;18:166–71.
52. Rumpsfeld M, McDonald SP, Purdie DM, Collins J, Johnson DW. Predictors of baseline peritoneal transport status in Australian and New Zealand peritoneal dialysis patients. Am J Kidney Dis. 2004;43:492–501.
53. Davies SJ, Woodrow G, Donovan K, Plum J, Williams P, Johansson AC, et al. Icodextrin improves the fluid status of peritoneal dialysis patients: results of a double-blind randomized controlled trial. J Am Soc Nephrol. 2003;14:2338–44.
54. Paniagua R, Ventura M-J, Avila-Díaz M, Cisneros A, Vicenté-Martínez M, Furlong M-D-C, et al. Icodextrin improves metabolic and fluid management in high and high-average transport diabetic patients. Perit Dial Int J Int Soc Perit Dial. 2009;29:422–32.
55. Wens R, Taminne M, Devriendt J, Collart F, Broeders N, Mestrez F, et al. A previously undescribed side effect of icodextrin: overestimation of glycemia by glucose analyzer. Perit Dial Int. 1998;18:603–9.
56. Zhou H, Cui L, Zhu G, Jiang Y, Gao X, Zou Y, et al. Survival advantage of normal weight in peritoneal dialysis patients. Ren Fail. 2011;33:964–8.
57. Wang R, Leesch V, Turner P, Moberly JB, Martis L. Kinetic analysis of icodextrin interference with serum amylase assays. Adv Perit Dial. 2002;18:96–9.
58. Lam CSP. Heart failure in Southeast Asia: facts and numbers. ESC Hear Fail. 2015;2:46–9.
59. Courivaud C, Kazory A, Crépin T, Azar R, Bresson-Vautrin C, Chalopin JM, et al. Peritoneal dialysis reduces the number of hospitalization days in heart failure patients refractory to diuretics. Perit Dial Int. 2014; https://doi.org/10.3747/pdi.2012.00149.
60. Grossekettler L, Schmack B, Meyer K, Brockmann C, Wanninger R, Kreusser MM, et al. Peritoneal dialysis as therapeutic option in heart failure patients. ESC Hear Fail. 2019;6:271–9.
61. Mehrotra R, Kathuria P. Place of peritoneal dialysis in the management of treatment-resistant congestive heart failure. Kidney Int Suppl. 2006;103:S67–71.
62. Sánchez JE, Ortega T, Rodríguez C, Díaz-Molina B, Martín M, Garcia-Cueto C, et al. Efficacy of peritoneal ultrafiltration in the treatment of refractory congestive heart failure. Nephrol Dial Transplant. 2010;25:605–10.
63. Jose ES, Ortega T, Rodr C, Beatriz D, Mart M, Garcia-Cueto C, et al. Efficacy of peritoneal ultrafiltration in the treatment of refractory congestive heart failure. Nephrol Dial Transplant. 2010;25:605–10.
64. Kumar VA, Ananthakrishnan S, Rasgon SA, Yan E, Burchette R, Dewar K. Comparing cardiac surgery in peritoneal dialysis and hemodialysis patients: perioperative outcomes and two-year survival. Perit Dial Int J Int Soc Perit Dial. 2012;32:137–41.
65. Ruiz SR, Vilchez EG, Frías TPG, Velázquez TMM, Martos LB, Salcedo TJ, et al. Short reviews. The role of peritoneal dialysis in the treatment of ascites. Nefrologia. 2011;31(6):648–55. https://doi.org/10.3265/Nefrologia.pre2011.Jun.10901.
66. Ros Ruiz S, Gutiérrez Vilchez E, García Frías TP, Martín Velázquez TM, Blanca Martos L, Jiménez Salcedo T, et al. The role of peritoneal dialysis in the treatment of ascites. Nefrol Publicación Of La Soc Española Nefrol. 2011;31:648–55.
67. O'Brien AA, Power J, O'Brien L, Clancy L, Keogh JA. The effect of peritoneal dialysate on pulmonary function and blood gasses in C.A.P.D. patients. Ir J Med Sci. 1990;159:215–6.
68. Ulubay G, Sezer S, Ulasli S, Ozdemir N, Eyuboglu OF, Haberal M. Respiratory evaluation of patients on continuous ambulatory peritoneal dialysis prior to renal transplantation. Clin Nephrol. 2006;66:269–74.
69. Singh S, Dale A, Morgan B, Sahebjami H. Serial studies of pulmonary function in continuous ambulatory peritoneal dialysis. A prospective study. Chest. 1984;86:874–7.
70. K/DOQI: KDOQI Clinical Practice Guidelines and Clinical Practice Recommendations for Diabetes and Chronic Kidney Disease. Am J Kidney Dis. 2007;49:S12–154.
71. Fernández-Cean J, Alvarez A, Burguez S, Baldovinos G, Larre-Borges P, Cha M. Infective endocarditis in chronic hae-

82

modialysis: two treatment strategies. Nephrol Dial Transplant. 2002;17:2226–30.
72. Suzuki H, Hoshi H, Inoue T, Kikuta T, Tsuda M, Takenaka T. Combination therapy with hemodialysis and peritoneal dialysis. Contrib Nephrol. 2012;177:71–83.
73. Solá L, Noboa O, Fleitas G, Laborda R, Quintero V. Transfer to peritoneal dialysis due to vascular access complications. Perit Dial Int. 2007;27:S18.
74. Guest S, Akonur A, Ghaffari A, Sloand J, Leypoldt JK. Intermittent peritoneal dialysis: urea kinetic modeling and implications of residual kidney function. Perit Dial Int J Int Soc Perit Dial. 2012;32:142–8.
75. Dimkovic N, Aggarwal V, Khan S, Chu M, Bargman J, Oreopoulos DG. Assisted peritoneal dialysis: what is it and who does it involve? Adv Perit Dial. 2009;25:165–70.
76. Tranaeus A, Heimbürger O, Granqvist S. Diverticular disease of the colon: a risk factor for peritonitis in continuous peritoneal dialysis. Nephrol Dial Transplant. 1990;5:141–7.
77. Yip T, Tse KC, Lam MF, Cheng SW, Lui SL, Tang S, et al. Colonic diverticulosis as a risk factor for peritonitis in Chinese peritoneal dialysis patients. Perit Dial Int J Int Soc Perit Dial. 2010;30:187–91.
78. Setyapranata S, Holt SG. The gut in older patients on peritoneal dialysis. Perit Dial Int. 2015;35 https://doi.org/10.3747/pdi.2014.00341.
79. Afsar B, Elsurer R, Bilgic A, Sezer S, Ozdemir F. Regular lactulose use is associated with lower peritonitis rates: an observational study. Perit Dial Int. 2010;30:243–5.
80. Leung L, Riutta T, Kotecha J, Rosser W. Chronic constipation: an evidence-based review. J Am Board Fam Med. 2011;24:436–51.
81. García-Ureña MÁ, Rodríguez CR, Ruiz VV, Hernández FJC, Fernández-Ruiz E, Gallego JMV, et al. Prevalence and management of hernias in peritoneal dialysis patients. Perit Dial Int. 2006;26:198–202.
82. Shah H, Chu M, Bargman JM. Perioperative management of peritoneal dialysis patients undergoing hernia surgery without the use of interim hemodialysis. Perit Dial Int J Int Soc Perit Dial. 2006;26:684–7.
83. Oh K-H, Hwang Y-H, Cho J-H, Kim M, Ju KD, Joo KW, et al. Outcome of early initiation of peritoneal dialysis in patients with end-stage renal failure. J Korean Med Sci. 2012;27:170–6.
84. Cooper BA, Branley P, Bulfone L, Collins JF, Craig JC, Fraenkel MB, et al. A randomized, controlled trial of early versus late initiation of dialysis. N Engl J Med. 2010;363:609–19.
85. Sandrini M, Vizzardi V, Valerio F, Ravera S, Manili L, Zubani R, et al. Incremental peritoneal dialysis: a 10 year single-centre experience. J Nephrol. 2016; https://doi.org/10.1007/s40620-016-0344-z.
86. Gabriel DP, Caramori JT, Martim LC, Barretti P, Balbi AL. High volume peritoneal dialysis vs daily hemodialysis: a randomized, controlled trial in patients with acute kidney injury. Kidney Int Suppl. 2008;73:S87–93.
87. Wong FKY, Chow SKY, Chan TMF. Evaluation of a nurse-led disease management programme for chronic kidney disease: a randomized controlled trial. Int J Nurs Stud. 2010;47:268–78.
88. Kopple JD. McCollum award lecture, 1996: protein-energy malnutrition in maintenance dialysis patients. Am J Clin Nutr. 1997;65:1544–57.
89. Bernardini J, Price V, Figueiredo A. Peritoneal dialysis patient training, 2006. Perit Dial Int J Int Soc Perit Dial. 2006;26: 625–32.
90. Blake PG, Breborowicz A, Han DS, Joffe P, Korbet SM, Warady BA. Recommended Peritoneal Dialysis Curriculum for Nephrology Trainees. The International Society for Peritoneal Dialysis (ISPD) standards and education subcommittee. Perit Dial Int. 2000;20:497–502.
91. Katz A. What have my kidneys got to do with my sex life?: the impact of late-stage chronic kidney disease on sexual function. Am J Nurs. 2006;106:81–3.
92. Fryckstedt J, Hylander B. Sexual function in patients with end-stage renal disease. Scand J Urol Nephrol. 2008; https://doi.org/10.1080/00365590802085877.
93. Ayub W, Fletcher S. End-stage renal disease and erectile dysfunction. Is there any hope? Nephrol Dial Transplant. 2000;15:1525–8.
94. Broughton A, Verger C, Goffin E. Pets-related peritonitis in peritoneal dialysis: companion animals or trojan horses? Semin Dial. 2008;23:306–16.
95. Wiles K, de Oliveira L. Dialysis in pregnancy. Best Pract Res Clin Obstet Gynaecol. 2019;57:33–46.
96. Thiam C, Lim S, Wah FK. Pregnancy and peritoneal dialysis: an updated review. Emj Eur Med J. 2018;74:74–84.
97. Jesudason S, Grace BS, McDonald SP. Pregnancy outcomes according to dialysis commencing before or after conception in women with ESRD. Clin J Am Soc Nephrol. 2014; https://doi.org/10.2215/CJN.03560413.
98. Mone F, O'Mahony JF, Tyrrell E, Mulcahy C, McParland P, Breathnach F, et al. Preeclampsia prevention using routine versus screening test-indicated aspirin in low-risk women a cost-effectiveness analysis. Hypertension. 2018; https://doi.org/10.1161/HYPERTENSIONAHA.118.11718.
99. Pucci M, Sarween N, Knox E, Lipkin G, Martin U. Angiotensin-converting enzyme inhibitors and angiotensin receptor blockers in women of childbearing age: risks versus benefits. Expert Rev Clin Pharmacol. 2015; https://doi.org/10.1586/17512433.2015.1005074.
100. Successful pregnancies in women treated by dialysis and kidney transplantation. Report from the Registration Committee of the European Dialysis and Transplant Association. Br J Obstet Gynaecol. 1980; https://doi.org/10.1111/j.1471-0528.1980.tb04434.x.
101. Shahir AK, Briggs N, Katsoulis J, Levidiotis V. An observational outcomes study from 1966-2008, examining pregnancy and neonatal outcomes from dialysed women using data from the ANZDATA registry. Nephrology. 2013; https://doi.org/10.1111/nep.12044.
102. Potluri K, Moldenhauer J, Karlman R, Hou S. Beta HCG levels in a pregnant dialysis patient: a cautionary tale. NDT Plus. 2011; https://doi.org/10.1093/ndtplus/sfq195.
103. Piccoli GB, Minelli F, Versino E, Cabiddu G, Attini R, Vigotti FN, et al. Pregnancy in dialysis patients in the new millennium: a systematic review and meta-regression analysis correlating dialysis schedules and pregnancy outcomes. Nephrol Dial Transplant. 2016;31:1915–34.
104. Balzer MS, Gross MM, Lichtinghagen R, Haller H, Schmitt R. Got milk? Breastfeeding and milk analysis of a mother on chronic hemodialysis. PLoS One. 2015; https://doi.org/10.1371/journal.pone.0143340.
105. Crabtree JH, Shrestha BM, Chow KM, Figueiredo AE, Povlsen JV, Wilkie M, et al. Creating and maintaining optimal peritoneal dialysis access in the adult patient: 2019 update. Perit Dial Int. 2019;pdi.2018.00232.
106. Jose MD, Johnson DW, Mudge DW, Tranaeus A, Voss D, Walker R, et al. Peritoneal dialysis practice in Australia and New Zealand: a call to action. Nephrology. 2011;16:19–29.

107. Povlsen JV, Ivarsen P. How to start the late referred ESRD patient urgently on chronic APD. Nephrol Dial Transplant. 2006;21(Suppl 2_:ii56–9.
108. Braaf S, Manias E, Riley R. The 'time-out' procedure: an institutional ethnography of how it is conducted in actual clinical practice. BMJ Qual Saf. 2013; https://doi.org/10.1136/bmjqs-2012-001702.
109. Brum S, Rodrigues A, Rocha S, Carvalho MJ, Nogueira C, Magalhães C, et al. Moncrief-Popovich technique is an advantageous method of peritoneal dialysis catheter implantation. Nephrol Dial Transplant. 2010;25:3070–5.
110. Hoff CM. Experimental animal models of encapsulating peritoneal sclerosis. Perit Dial Int. 2005;25(Suppl 4):S57–66.
111. Xie J, Kiryluk K, Ren H, Zhu P, Huang X, Shen P, et al. Coiled versus straight peritoneal dialysis catheters: a randomized controlled trial and meta-analysis. Am J Kidney Dis. 2011;58:946–55.
112. Baboolal K, McEwan P, Sondhi S, Spiewanowski P, Wechowski J, Wilson K. The cost of renal dialysis in a UK setting–a multicentre study. Nephrol Dial Transplant. 2008;23:1982–9.
113. Brown EA, Van Biesen W, Finkelstein FO, Hurst H, Johnson DW, Kawanishi H, et al. Length of time on peritoneal dialysis and encapsulating peritoneal sclerosis: position paper for ISPD. Perit Dial Int J Int Soc Perit Dial. 2009;29:595–600.

Peritoneal Dialysis Prescription

Stanley Fan and Nasreen Samad

Contents

M. Harber (ed.), *Primer on Nephrology*, https://doi.org/10.1007/978-3-030-76419-7_83

Aims

1. To be able to describe the different types of PD modality.
2. To understand the parameters required to write an APD prescription.
3. To understand how and when to escalate a PD prescription as part of Incremental PD.
4. To be confident using Urgent Start PD for patients that present acutely with ESRD requiring dialysis.

83.1 Introduction

83

Peritoneal dialysis (PD) is performed by filling the peritoneal cavity with dialysis fluid, allowing this to dwell before draining the fluid out, and repeating the process with fresh dialysate. Solute transfer is by diffusion and convection transport, while water moves across the osmotic or oncotic gradient.

Traditionally, there has been great emphasis on measuring and optimizing solute and water clearance to ensure patients are "adequately" dialyzed. There is increasing understanding that quality of life (QoL) issues may be more paramount for many patients. For some patients, increasing clearance through more onerous dialysis prescriptions may not be appropriate.

The rates of solute transport (membrane function) across the peritoneum evolve. Membrane function is defined by the rate of equilibration of either creatinine or glucose over 4 hours (D/Pcr or D_0/D_4glc) and is measured during a peritoneal equilibration test (PET). Osmotic conductance (i.e., the rate of water transfer across an osmotic gradient) can also be defined using modified PETs.

This chapter aims to describe the methods of assessing patients and how dialysis prescription can be adjusted during the patients' PD life span to optimize peritoneal solute and fluid clearance while balancing quality of life issues.

83.2 PD Modalities

83.2.1 Continuous Ambulatory Peritoneal Dialysis (CAPD)

CAPD was introduced in 1976 by Popovich and Moncrief [1]. Patients using this modality usually perform 4 (although this can be 1–5) exchanges throughout the day. Each exchange procedure takes approximately 20–40 minutes depending on how well the PD catheter functions (typically a 20-minute drain-out time followed by 10 minutes drain-in time). The dwell times can be flexible and altered according to patient lifestyle (Fig. 83.1). We usually advise dwell times to be at least 3 hours. Day dwells of 6–8 hours are acceptable.

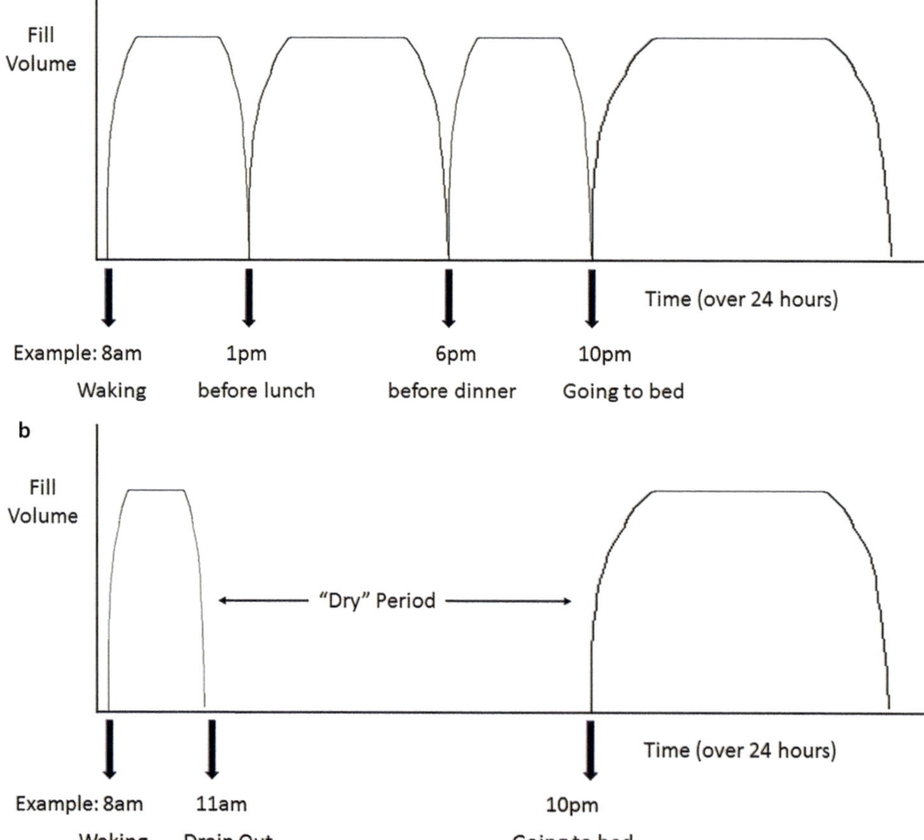

Fig. 83.1 Examples of continuous ambulatory peritoneal dialysis (CAPD). **a** Classic program with exchanges throughout the day with a longer night dwell. **b** Flexible exchanges with incremental CAPD (1–3 daytime dwells can be as short as 3 hours)

Patients who have fewer than 4 exchanges per day often have a period of "Dry Day" (they drain out and remain "dry" until they are due their next exchange). CAPD offers flexibility for patients although, as peritoneal membrane transport increases, long day dwells are likely to result in poor ultrafiltration.

83.2.2 Types of Automated Peritoneal Dialysis (APD)

Continuous cyclic peritoneal dialysis (CCPD) is the most common form of automated peritoneal dialysis. This modality was introduced in 1981 by Diaz–Buxo [2]. The use of a machine automates the PD exchanges while the patient sleeps and leaves a "last fill" at the end of the program so patients continue to dialyze during the day (◘ Fig. 83.2). The system gained immediate popularity to treat infants and children. Its use has also grown with adult patients [3], as it allows patients to be free from PD exchanges during the day and larger volumes are also better tolerated in the supine position. CCPD can often achieve greater solute clearance than CAPD. To increase dialysis further, day exchanges can be introduced (either manually or using the APD machine to deliver an exchange in the evening).

Nocturnal intermittent peritoneal dialysis (NIPD) patients have treatment periods at night, but are "dry" during the day. This modality is particularly common for patients who have significant residual renal function. It is, therefore, popular for incident patients who otherwise feel bloated and nauseous with day time dwells. Over time, patients tolerate day dwells and "progress" onto CCPD if solute clearances are inadequate.

Tidal peritoneal dialysis consists of exchanges in which the peritoneal cavity always contains some dialysate, a feature that minimizes drainage pain or alarms for patients that have PD catheter problems (e.g.,malpositioned catheter which results in large residual peritoneal volumes at the end of a drain cycle) [4].

A modified form of APD described as "Adapted APD" has been described recently [5]. During a 9–10 hours APD session, the machine is programmed to perform a mixture of short dwells with small-fill vol-

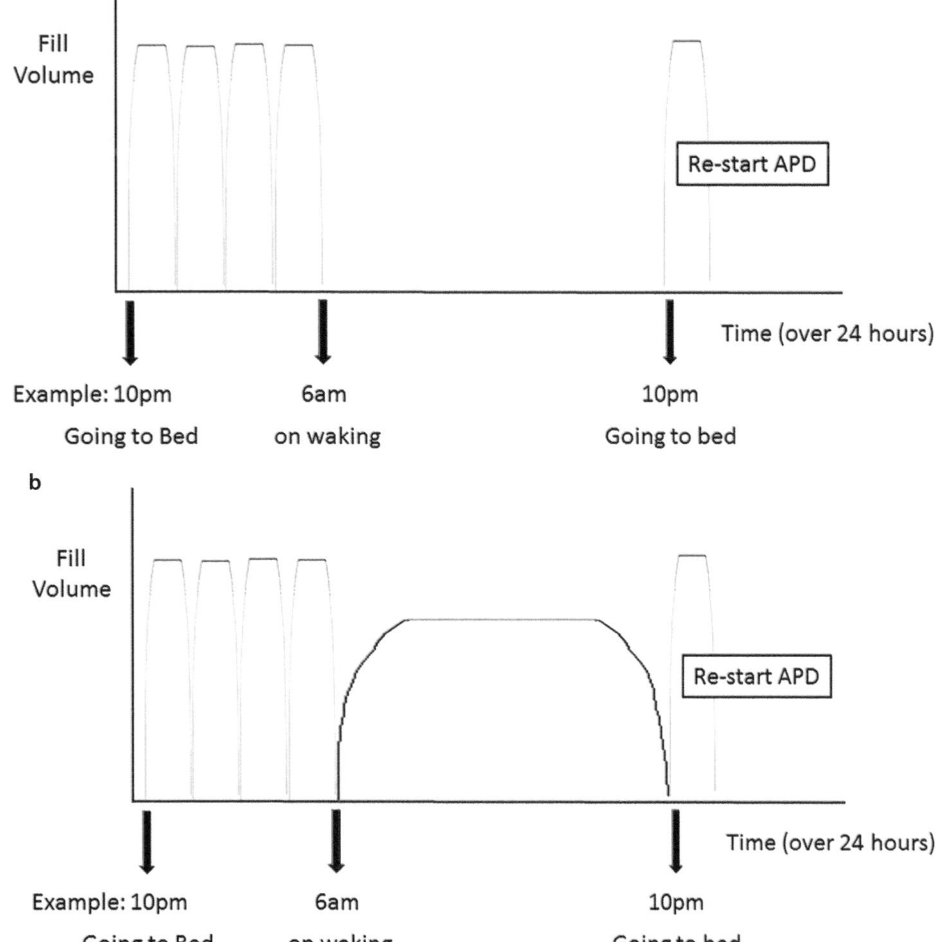

◘ **Fig. 83.2** Examples of different forms of Automated Peritoneal Dialysis (APD) **a** Example of typical nocturnal intermittent peritoneal dialysis (NIPD). Dialysis occurs only at night (is "dry" during the day) **b** Example of typical continuous cyclic peritoneal dialysis (CCPD). Dialysis occurs at night and during day (programmed to have last fill at the end of night cycles) **c** Example of typical tidal automated peritoneal dialysis (APD). Dialysis occurs at night, but machine is programmed to cycle without completely emptying peritoneum between cycles **d** Example of adaptive automated peritoneal dialysis (aAPD). Cycles at night are a mixture of short small and large long cycles. (can be with day dwell, if required)

Fig. 83.2 (continued)

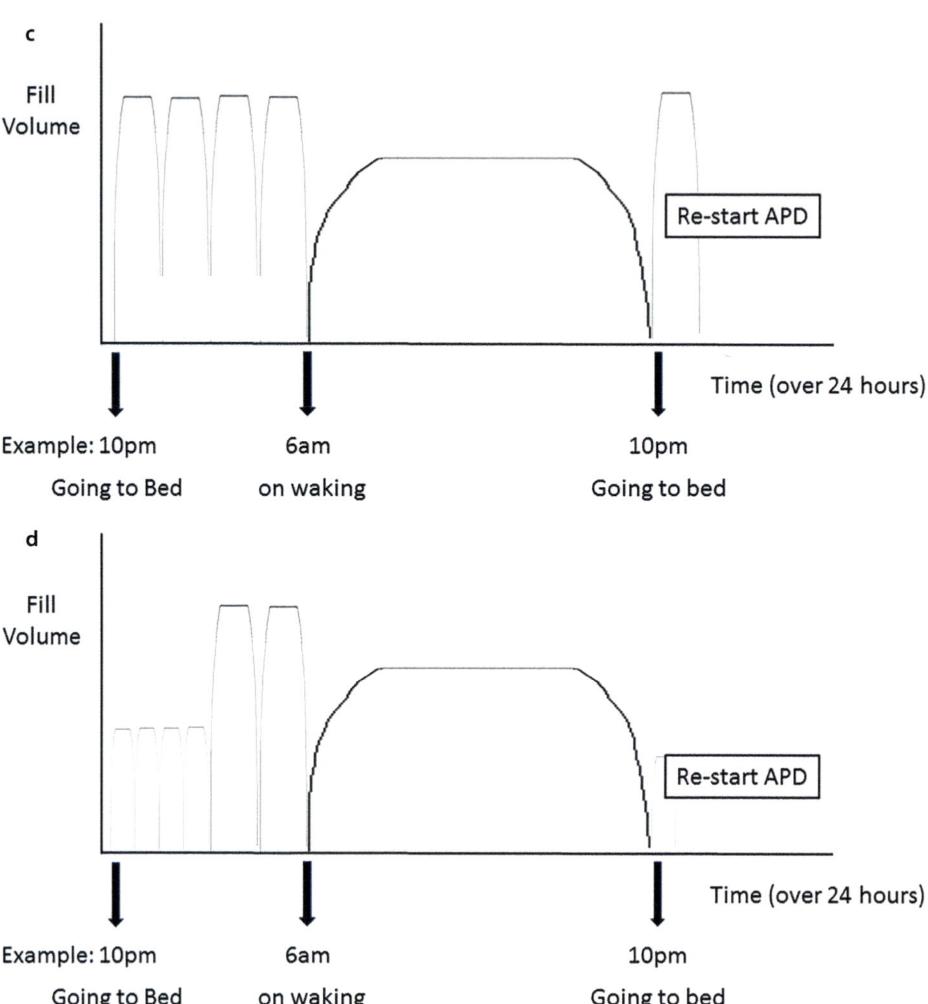

umes to promote ultrafiltration and longer dwells and larger fill volume to promote removal of uremic toxins. This has been shown to result in improved dialysis efficiency in terms of UF, KT/V, and phosphate and sodium dialytic removal without incurring any extra financial cost.

83.2.3 Assisted Peritoneal Dialysis (aAPD)

This form of PD is suitable for, but not limited to, elderly patients who are unable to perform peritoneal dialysis by themselves [6]. External Health Care Assistants (HCA) or nurses are employed to connect and disconnect patients to and from a cycler, set up the machine, or perform CAPD exchanges. Often the HCAs also help perform routine monitoring (weight and blood pressure) and inject erythropoiesis stimulating agents (ESAs). Assisted PD can be provided by family members, paid homecare nurses, visiting health care professionals and staff in rehabilitation centers, retirement homes, nursing homes, and chronic-care dialysis units [7].

There remains a debate about the cost-effectiveness of this modality treatment if health care assistants or nurses are employed to deliver the assistance [8]. A European Survey [9] suggested that the incremental cost associated with providing home care visits eliminates the savings traditionally associated with PD compared within hospital HD, but, of course, the level and cost of providing the assistance can vary widely. Moreover, the cost of transport for elderly dependent patients can be expensive, but not always included in the Service Line Reporting Cost for HD [10].

83.2.4 Hybrid (Combination) Peritoneal and Hemodialysis

Combination (hybrid) therapy with peritoneal and hemodialysis has been reported in Japan [11, 12], United States [13], and United Kingdom [14]. This treatment is uncommonly practiced, although the additional HD sessions (once or twice a week) can be used to increase weekly small solute or water clearance on top of that achieved by PD alone. However, exposing patients to the risks of both HD and PD has deterred the adoption of this therapy.

The reported use of hybrid dialysis is probably the highest in Japan. Interestingly, its use has been promoted as a method to reduce the incidence of symptomatic encapsulating peritoneal sclerosis (EPS). It is well known that discontinuation of PD can be a trigger that precipitates EPS. Thus, proponents of hybrid dialysis claim that continuing PD even at infrequent exchanges during the transition period prevents this disease.

83.2.5 Urgent Start Peritoneal Dialysis

Dialysis is initiated in different settings. Most commonly for PD is an elective start of dialysis in a patient that has end stage renal failure (ESRF). However, PD can be used "acutely" for:

1. Patients that have acute (reversible) renal failure requiring dialysis.
2. Patients that present acutely with chronic ESRF (Urgent Start PD).

It is beyond the scope of this chapter to discuss PD for Acute Kidney Injury, although it is frequently used in health care services with limited access to HD. Readers are referred to excellent review articles [15–17].

Urgent Start PD is increasingly adopted in many centers and is dependent on a flexible PD team to deliver expedited pre-dialysis education. Barriers and obstacles can usually be overcome if patients undergoing Urgent Start PD have good home support and a motivated patient.

Minimally invasive methods of PD catheter insertion are preferred, as these permit use of small-volume PD almost immediately (preferably after 24 hrs). To reduce the incidence of sub-cutaneous fluid leaks at catheter insertion site, incremental dialysis with strict adherence to "bed rest" during dialysis are important. We start with fill volumes <1.5 L. For convenience, we often use a cycler machine at night and limit the duration of APD to ≤8 hrs (shorter hours will improve adherence to bed rest).

Psychological and emotional support for these patients is critical as these patients are often "in denial" or "in shock" over their sudden diagnosis of ESRF. A personalized, incremental extended training program should be tailored to suit the patient. Small amounts of information may need to be delivered multiple times over a prolonged period for the patient to acquire all the skills and confidence to perform their dialysis at home. We particularly find that aAPD can be very useful, as it permits us to teach different aspects of a PD syllabus [18] incrementally:

1. Connection and disconnection techniques (with sterile technique and appropriate handwashing.
2. Setting up APD cyclers (if patient opts for APD vs CAPD).
3. PD catheter exit site care.
4. Managing PD-related infections (peritonitis and exit site infections).
5. Dietary restrictions for dialysis patients.
6. Lifestyle changes to adapt to limitations (physical and practical) imposed by medical conditions. This might include holidays, sex, and exercise limitations.

For patients starting electively on PD, these topics are often taught over a 3–5 day "training program". The reader is referred to the excellent ISPD guidelines suggesting a suitable syllabus for patients and caregivers. For Urgent Start PD patients, this training is best delivered incrementally over a prolonged period of time.

83.3 Choice of PD Modality

Studies suggest no difference in outcomes for death or technique failure resulting from the selection of CAPD or APD as initial PD modality. No difference was found from the United States Renal Data System on 66,381 incident patients on chronic peritoneal dialysis when adjusted for demographic, clinical, laboratory, and dialysis facility characteristics [3]. We have also observed that while there is impairment in quality of life (QoL) both for patients and caregivers at the start of dialysis therapy, with careful selection of patients, education, and support the Δ QoL for patients on CAPD vs APD were not different [19]. In fact, it was striking that despite having to help perform PD, there was some improvement in the QoL of caregivers (reflected by an improvement in the social functioning of caregivers after dialysis was initiated).

Hence, the choice of PD modality depends on several factors (◘ Table 83.1) which include:

(a) Social reasons and patient-related factors like employment, need for caregiver to do PD, housing situation, and the ability to cope with exchanges and cyclers. As APD provides freedom from doing any exchanges during day time, this tends to be selected by patients with employment and for patients who require assistance with their PD exchanges (e.g., assisted APD). However, some patients may find APD more technically challenging and find their sleep disturbed because of multiple cycler alarms.
(b) Peritoneal membrane characteristics. Patients with high peritoneal membrane transport characteristics particularly benefit from the use of APD. There is historical evidence that, in an era when APD was not readily available, CAPD patients that are high

Table 83.1 Comparison of advantages and disadvantages between CAPD and APD

CAPD	APD
Easy technique	More difficult technique
Daytime exchange can be difficult if working	No or only 1 daytime exchange
Poor UF if patient has high membrane transport characteristic; resulting in fluid overload and inadequate solute clearance. High transport status has been associated with higher technique failure in CAPD	Easier to achieve high UF, particularly for patient with high transport status (although the effects of sodium sieving needs to be considered). Association between high transport status and PD technique failure does not appear to exist
Increasing exchange volume increases intraperitoneal pressure when patient is ambulant	Intraperitoneal pressure lower when patient supine, thereby, permitting larger dwell volumes
Increased risk of hernia and leaks	If NIPD or small volume dwells are used during the day, there is less risk of hernia and leaks
Ease of travel	Can travel with machine but patients often revert to CAPD
6–10 liters of fluid used/day	10–15 liters of fluid used/day
Less storage space required	More storage space required
Cheaper	More expensive

transporters have higher mortality/ technical failure [20]. But this association is no longer true for more recent PD patients where APD utilization is much higher [21].

83

(c) Dialysis adequacy including the effect of residual renal function. Residual renal function has an important role in contributing to the overall adequacy of dialysis [22]. It may be difficult to provide adequate dialysis to anuric patients on CAPD [23]. But it has been shown that a high proportion of anuric patients can achieve adequate dialysis and ultrafiltration on APD [24].

83.4 Empiric Starting PD Prescription

At our institution, dialysis modality is chosen by patients.

For adult patients, empiric prescription for CAPD is generally based on patient size (weight). A typical protocol being:

- If weight >60 Kg start 4 × 2 liter exchanges.
- If weight <60 Kg start 4 × 1.5 liter exchanges.

For children, fill volume can be chosen by measuring primary pressure [25].

For incident PD patients selecting APD, our PD prescription is determined by patient size (weight) and residual renal function (RRF):

- If weight >60 Kg start with four 2 liter fill volume for 8 hours.
- If weight <60 Kg start with four 1.5 liter fill volume for 8 hours.
- If patient is anuric (e.g., patients transferring from hemodialysis) a last fill (1.5–2 liters depending on patient size) is included in PD prescription.

It is important to remember that these are set as guidelines, but prescription should be individualized for patients' unique circumstances. The choice of glucose concentration or use of Icodextrinis determined by how much ultrafiltration is required to achieve. This is discussed in the following section.

83.5 How to Adjust PD Prescription

PD prescription can be adjusted to

1. Suit changes in patient lifestyle. It is important to remember that switching to CAPD is possible to facilitate patient holidays.
2. Increase solute clearance.
3. Increase ultrafiltration.

Although solute clearance and ultrafiltration are listed separately, they are intricately linked. Increasing ultrafiltration/drain volume will, of course, also increase solute clearance through convection. An important exception is if very short dwells are performed in APD. In this scenario, water clearance via aquaporins can result in water, but not solute clearance and this phenomenon is measured as sodium sieving.

As a rule of thumb, dialysis volume and cycles are adjusted to optimize solute clearance whereas, fluid composition (tonicity) is changed to adjust ultrafiltration. The exception is for patients who have a high transport status. These patients lose the osmotic gradient and so dialysis cycles must be adjusted to shorter dwell times like switching the patient from CAPD to APD.

83.5.1 Dialysis Adequacy in Anuric Patients

There continues to be a debate about the effectiveness of PD in anuric patients. CANUSSA showed that residual renal function (RRF) is one of the most important determinants of patient survival [22]. However, this does not automatically mean that survival will be prolonged by switching patients to HD (the same relationship between RRF and survival also exists in HD [26]). In the absence of RCT on the subject, we can only interpret the non-randomized observational outcomes. EAPOS showed that anuric >70% anuric patients can achieve the small clearance target of >60 L/wk./1.72m^{2}BSA [27]. In addition, 2-year patient survival was 78% (although switching to HD according to clinical need was permitted) [24] and this compares favorably with the NECOSAD study of incident PD patients where 2 year survival was 77% [28].

We conclude that automatic switching of anuric patients to HD is not warranted, but anuria should alert the clinician to carefully consider a transition on an individual basis. Not only will QoL issues be paramount, but particular emphasis should be placed on fluid balance; EAPOS showed a strong association between poor UF (<750 ml/d) and reduced survival. This is also supported by the NECOSAD study, where total fluid removal was the only significant predictor of technique survival (RR = 0.79 at 500 ml/d).

83.5.2 Treatment for Hyperkalemia and Hypercalcemia

The rate of potassium removal with PD is much slower than with HD, and the latter, is therefore, recommended for patients with severe (life-threatening) hyperkalemia. However, rapid cycles of hypertonic glucose can induce convective loss of potassium and hyperglycemia that helps drive potassium into cells, thereby lowering serum potassium. While the high ultrafiltration risks cardiovascular instability, this strategy can be useful if there are delays initiating HD.

Commercially available PD solutions contain 1–1.75 mmol/l of calcium. Exchanges with calcium dialysate of 1–1.25 mmol/l will cause net efflux of calcium into dialysis fluid [29]. Successful treatment of acute hypercalcemia using in hospital prepared calcium-free dialysate has also been reported in adult and pediatric populations [30].

83.6 Sodium Sieving

Sieving of sodium is defined as the drop in the dialysate–plasma ratio of sodium (D/P Na) that occurs during the initial phase of a dialysis exchange with a hyperosmolar dialysis solution.

Water moves across the peritoneal membrane via different "pores". Sodium cannot follow water through aquaporins although over a long dwell, sodium concentrations will equilibrate through the other pores. At the beginning of a dwell with hypertonic glucose, there is rapid water entry into the peritoneal cavity via aquaporin. If dwell times are kept very short, high ultrafiltration is possible, but with relative low sodium removal. This may lead to an increased incidence of hypertension [31] and the patient may remain overhydrated despite the high ultrafiltration.

Long daytime dwells with Icodextrin PD solutions will have minimal sodium sieving and is particularly useful for APD patients [32].

83.7 Peritoneal Dialysis Fluid

83.7.1 Glucose

Glucose is the most commonly used osmotic agent and is available in different concentrations. Glucose-based dialysis solutions are at risk of caramelization (thereby generating glucose degradation products) during heat sterilization. Sole use of lactate as the buffer in PD solutions also means the infused solutions are acidic. This has led to the development of "biocompatible" solutions. Sodium bicarbonate is kept separate from other constituents of dialysate to avoid precipitation and the section of the bag containing glucose can now be sterilized at very low pH, minimizing the generation of GDPs. Prior to infusing into the patients, the different sections of the bag (containing sodium bicarbonate vs glucose and other constituents are mixed).

GDPs are potentially toxic to peritoneal membrane and leukocytes in vitro, although clinically significant benefits of using "biocompatible solutions" on membrane function and peritonitis rates are not yet conclusively proven [33]. Studies suggest that Bicarbonate–/lactate-buffered solutions are safe, well tolerated and physiologically balanced alternates to conventional lactate-based solutions [34]. They can be particularly useful for patients who develop infusion pain or discomfort when using "standard" glucose bags. The balANZstudy [35] has been recently published. While it did not show a difference in the rate of decline of residual renal function between conventional solution and a "biocompatible" solution, there was a significant difference though to the time to anuria and time to first peritonitis episode in favor of the biocompatible solution. Use of biocompatible solutions is likely to depend on assessment of cost effectiveness.

83.7.2 Glucose Polymer Icodextrin (Extraneal)

Icodextrin has a mean molecular weight of 13000–19000 daltons and has same osmolality as plasma at 290 mosmols. Icodextrin has a high reflection coefficient (σ). Reflection coefficient is described as permeability of solute, where reflection coefficient is greater and the permeability of solute is less. This allows the solute to stay longer in the dialysate. Icodextrin has been found to be safe and provides patients with greater fluid removal and small solute clearance [36].

83.7.3 Amino Acids (Nutrineal)

A 1.1% amino acid mixture is available and has similar osmolality as 1.36% glucose. Studies indicate that treatment with a daily exchange of this amino acid-based PD solution is safe and may provide nutritional benefits for malnourished PD patients [37]. However, no appreciable improvements were seen in well-nourished patients [38]. Nevertheless, advocates have suggested routine use of this (and Icodextrin) permits dialysis regimens that are low in glucose [39] (with potential, although not conclusively proven clinical benefits).

83.8 PD Clearance Targets

Different organizations have a general agreement about PD clearance targets. These are listed in ▫ Table 83.2. We direct the reader to the websites that provide justification for these recommendations. However, it is important to understand that peritoneal clearance of solute is not equivalent to residual renal function. Preservation of residual renal function is therefore of utmost importance in the clinical care of patients on peritoneal dialysis.

Equally, achieving the clearance targets is not the sole aim of clinicians looking after PD patients and the new ISPD guidelines emphasis that holistic approach incorporating Patient Reported Outcome Measures (PROMS) should be used to judge quality of life. The burden of the dialysis and negative impact on quality of life should be considered when prescribing PD [40]. Increased use of APD with Icodextrin and glucose permits anuric patients to achieve these targets, but if peritoneal membrane is changing, continuing peritoneal dialysis may not be appropriate [41].

83.9 Ultrafiltration Targets

The European guidelines setting of ultrafiltration target has been controversial. Perhaps, the term "target" is inappropriate, but measuring 24-hour UF can be useful especially if patients are anuric.

1. Overhydrated patients: If UF is <1 L, dialysis prescription is "inappropriate". But if UF is >1 L, overhydration may be secondary to non-compliance to salt and therefore, it is difficult for the patient to maintain a strict fluid restriction.
2. Euvolemic patients with poor ultrafiltration are at risk of malnutrition resulting from extreme restrictions in diet and fluid intake.

▫ Table 83.2 PD clearance targets set by different Guideline Groups

	CrCl	KT/V	UF	Ref:
KDIGO	None	>1.7/wk		▸ http://www.kidney.org/professionals/kdoqi/guidelines
EBPG	None except >45 L/wk for APD	>1.7/wk	1.0 L/24 hours in anuric patients	▸ http://www.european-renal-best-practice.org/content/ebpg-european-best-practice-guidelines
UK-RA	>50 L/wk	>1.7/wk		▸ http://www.renal.org/Clinical/GuidelinesSection/PeritonealDialysis

KDIGO Kidney Disease Improving Global Outcomes, *EBPG* European Best Practice Guidelines, *UK-RA* UK Renal Association

It is important to maintain fluid balance as increased fluid leads to rise in blood pressure, left ventricular hypertrophy, and increased mortality [42].

83.10 Summary

Peritoneal Dialysis is an effective method to achieve solute and water clearance. Its utilization is particularly appropriate for incident dialysis patients with significant residual renal function. Patients can be maintained on PD by adjusting PD modality and prescriptions as described above, thereby, permitting many anuric patients to achieve "adequate" ultrafiltration and solute clearances. An elective and planned switch to hemodialysis should be considered for those that appear "under dialyzed". However, a holistic approach is important; other aspects of patient's well-being, long-term prognosis from other comorbidities, and patient's perspective should be considered in deciding whether switching from PD to hemodialysis is appropriate.

Case Study 83.1

Male, 45-year-old Caucasian with biopsy proven IgA disease has declining kidney function. He expressed a wish to remain independent and have a home dialysis treatment. Home hemodialysis was considered, but he opted to have peritoneal dialysis.

When his eGFR fell to 7 ml/min, he become mildly symptomatic. A double-cuff coiled PD catheter was inserted by Seldinger technique under local anesthesia as a day case. The PD catheter dressing was undisturbed for 1 week. During this time, he was advised to avoid showering (to have sponge baths). On Day 7, he was taught how to perform his PD catheter exit site care and apply Mupirocin (2%) ointment to the exit site. He was permitted to shower. On day 14, he was recalled to start APD training. This lasted 3 days and was uneventful.

At the end of his training, he was reassessed. His blood test results included: K = 3.5 mmol/L, bicarbonate 19 mmol/L, urea = 23 mmol/L, and creatinine 720 μmol/L. Clinically, he was euvolemic.

His APD prescription was: 8 hours at night: 2 L fill volume, and 4 cycles with 75% tidal. No last fill. He was prescribed a biocompatible PD fluid. He was set a target weight range of 72–75 kg. He was instructed to use 1.36% glucose bags if he was "at target". If his weight increased above target, he was instructed to use 5 L of 2.27% glucose and 2.5 L 1.36% glucose bags. If he remained above or below target for 3 consecutive days, he was instructed to come to the PD unit for urgent assessment.

When he was reviewed after 6 weeks, he was asymptomatic. He had minimal alarms at night and his urine output was maintained.

Over the next 12 months, he continued to work full time. He had spent the summer holiday in Europe on APD with PD fluids delivered to his rented holiday home. He was also taught to perform CAPD so that he was able to spend long weekends away from home (he would carry the necessary bags in his car). Unfortunately, his urine output had reduced; his total kt/v was consistently <1.7 and his dietary protein intake was also falling. He was using 2.27% glucose bags regularly to maintain euvolemia despite strict salt restriction and increasing his frusemide dose to 250 mg/d.

His dialysis prescription was initially increased by removing the "tidal" option. Work schedule meant that he did not want to extend his APD duration. His PET revealed him to be an LA transporter with D/Pcr = 0.6 & good UF capacity (4 hour UF with 2.27%glc was 150mLs). He agreed to start a daytime last fill (icodextrin). He struggled with the 2 L-fill volume of his PET test, so we initiated at a volume of 1.4 L increasing by 200mLs every four weeks until he reached 2 L-daytime fill volume.

His target weight range was increased to 76–80 kg (this included the 2 kg increment from his day dwell).

Shortly after he reached his daytime fill volume of 2 L, he was reviewed at the clinic. He was generally tolerant of this, but he complained it was particularly difficult for him to exercise in the gym. It was agreed that he could "drain empty" prior to going to the gym (in the evenings after work).

He was maintained on this flexible APD/CAPD prescription for another four months when he underwent a successful cadaveric renal transplant.

Learning points:

1. Incremental PD prescription. Starting with "tidal" can minimize APD alarms that might otherwise disrupt sleep.
2. Empower patients to adjust "tonicity" of APD fluids according to target weight range.
3. Anticipate and monitor for loss of residual renal function, which will require escalation of PD prescription.
4. Be flexible with PD prescription. Patients can have a combination of APD / manual exchanges and CAPD to suit patient needs (including travel).

83

Case Study 83.2

A 47-year-old Asian lady is referred to the Renal Unit by her General Practitioner. She presented with uremic symptoms and blood tests revealed eGFR was 9 ml/min. She had a normochromic, normocytic anemia (Hb was 82 g/L). She was admitted as an emergency (Day 0) and found to be moderately fluid overloaded (raised JVP of 4 cm and edema extending to mid-shin). Her BP was 190/110 mmHg. Her serum K was 5.9 mmol/L and bicarbonate 14 mmol/L. An ultrasound of her kidneys confirmed small (8 cm) kidneys without scars. Her only significant past medical history was that she developed hypertension during the third trimester of her only pregnancy. She had normal vaginal delivery and has had no previous abdominal surgery.

On admission, she had expedited pre-dialysis counseling and she expressed a desire to have home dialysis (APD). Based on directed questioning, although she was living in a small two-bed apartment, her home situation was deemed to be suitable for APD. A home visit was not felt to be necessary; importantly, she had good support from her husband and 22-year-old son who was living at home.

Despite initiating oral sodium bicarbonate and a low K diet on admission, on Day 2, her serum K increased to 6.2 mmol/L. She also remained fluid overloaded and BP was 160/95, despite high dose loop diuretics and antihypertensive medications. A decision to initiate dialysis was made. She was not in respiratory distress, not hypoxic, and able to lie relatively flat in bed. Her options were:

1. Optimize her fluid and biochemistry prior to PD catheter insertion by "temporary" HD either via a femoral dialysis catheter or tunneled HD catheter.
2. Proceed with PD catheter insertion and initiate PD within 36 hours.

We elected to proceed with "Urgent Start" PD. She received potent laxatives for "pre-procedure bowel prep" followed by daily oral potassium binder (patiromer). The next morning (Day 3), a PD catheter was inserted by Seldinger technique. Pre- and post-procedure K remained between 6.0 and 6.2 mmol/L. We initiated low dose acute PD that night (8–12 hours after insertion). For convenience, we used an APD machine to deliver 5 cycles of 1.2 L PD fluid over 8 hours. During her dialysis, she was on "strict bedrest", using a bedpan when necessary. In the morning, she was "dry" (no last fill) and was permitted to mobilize normally.

Over the next 48hours, she continued on this dialysis regimen and was taught how to safely connect and disconnect herself from the APD machine. She was discharged on Day 6 (3 days after PD catheter insertion) with arrangements for home aAPD to start within 48 hours of discharge. Her APD prescription was: 8 hours, 4 cycles, 1.5 L fill volume, no tidal, no last fill. She was under instruction to remain in bed during her dialysis. The aAPD healthcare assistant (HCA) helped "clean" and set up the APD machine. Importantly she also provided psychological and emotional support. One week after PD catheter insertion, the patient was taught to look after her own PD catheter exit site. She was booked for "full" APD training and the HCA visits were withdrawn after 2 weeks. Her APD prescription was revised to: 8 hours, 4 cycles, 2 L fill volume, 75% tidal (she was developing drainage pains and alarms), and no last fill.

Learning points:

1. Expedited pre-dialysis education and assessment can permit "late-presenters" starting on PD electively.
2. Home visits prior to initiating "Urgent Start PD" are not always required if home support from family is strong.
3. PD can be initiated within 24 hours of minimally invasive methods of PD catheter insertion. These include PD catheters inserted by Seldinger technique and laparoscopic methods of "surgical" insertions.
4. "Urgent Start" PD prescription entails incremental dialysis prescription *and* training. Patients should adhere to strict bedrest during dialysis for the initial 72 hours. aAPD can be very useful to provide emotional and psychological support permitting expedited discharge from hospital.

Case Study 83.3

A 72-year-old African-Caribbean man with long standing diabetes mellitus type 2 presented with CKD stage 5. He was known to have diabetic retinopathy and peripheral vascular disease (intermittent claudication worse on the left and amputation of left second toe from previous infection/gangrene). He lived alone (divorced with one daughter who had her own family, but tries to support him at home). He initially declined dialysis, but when he became uremic (nausea) and developed significant edema extending to above knees with increasing breathlessness (including orthopnea), his daughter convinced him to reconsider. He still refused hemodialysis, but agreed to a trial of PD. After 3 days of intravenous high dose diuretics, he was able to lie flat for PD catheter insertion.

We initially planned for CAPD (2 exchanges: overnight icodextrin with another 3-hour CAPD dwell in the morning). However, it soon became apparent that his exchange technique was poor despite several attempts at training. We arranged for him to have aAPD. The HCA visited him in the evening (7–9 pm) to setup the APD machine and connect the patient. The patient was felt to be safe to disconnect in the morning and leave the machine to be cleaned by the HCA. To minimize the restriction after being "connected" to the APD machine, we relocated his bed to the living room and provided him with an "extension line" (1.8 m) so he could move around his living room while connected to his APD machine.

His initial aAPD dialysis prescription was: 10 hours 2 L fill volume 5 cycles with 75% tidal with 1.5 L last fill using extraneal. He was given a target weight range of 92–95 kg. As he was living alone, it became clear that diet included substantial processed foods. He was therefore, expected to use 10 L of 2.27% glucose dialysate.

During first clinic review, he complained about feeling very uncomfortable at night. It transpired that his weight had increased to 98 kg and he was using a combination of 3.86% & 2.27% glucose on the APD machine. When details of his dialysis were downloaded and examined, it became apparent that his final drain in the morning was >3300mLs. The use of high glucose concentration bags on a tidal prescription had resulted in "overfill". Removing tidal option improved his symptoms.

At subsequent clinic reviews, he was finding the aAPD onerous. He still got tired easily, but his edema was much improved allowing him to regain mobility. He felt the dialysis was restricting his life too much. He wanted to spend more time with his grandchildren and his church. We agreed to reduce his aAPD to 6 days/week (allowing him 1 day off dialysis).

His daughter requested to be trained to do CAPD. We arranged holiday CAPD fluid to be delivered to the Caribbean where he enjoyed a 2-week holiday. Over the next 18 months, he had only one episode of PD peritonitis that resolved quickly with antibiotics. He did not require hospital admission and remained self-caring at home. He was eventually admitted with worsening ischemia of his left leg. He declined amputation and opted instead for conservative care. He became overtly septic and confused. Peritoneal dialysis was discontinued.

Learning points:

1. Assisted APD program can deliver good quality of life to many patients with modest increase in peritonitis risk.
2. "Overfill" can be an issue with tidal APD, if high glucose dialysate is used.
3. End-of-life care is particularly important when managing frail elderly patients. Note: There was no emphasis on dialysis adequacy (kt/v) for this man. Instead, the aim was to achieve sufficient salt and fluid removal for him to maintain mobility and allow him to travel.

Question 1

A 63-year-old woman with diabetic nephropathy chooses to have automated peritoneal dialysis (APD) when she reaches end-stage kidney disease. A peritoneal dialysis catheter was inserted under local anesthetic, and after a 2-week break-in period she successfully completes her APD training. Her starting prescription: 8 hours APD with 4 cycles each 2 L fill volume (using dianeal 1.36% glucose bags) and 1.5 L last fill with extraneal. Unfortunately, she represents 1 week later complaining of multiple alarms at night and pain during drain out. The PD nurses have already asked her to take more laxatives, but this has not resolved her problem. What do you recommend:

1. Switch to continuous ambulatory peritoneal dialysis (CAPD)
2. Switch the dianeal to physioneal
3. Reprogram APD machine to include tidal (starting at 75%)
4. Switch her 1.36% glucose bags to 2.27% glucose bags

Answer

Options 1, 3, and 4 may alleviate the problem. The most likely cause of her problem is drainage issue from her PD catheter. Selecting option 1 and 3 depends on patient choice. Tidal option will mean the APD machine does not try to continue draining after a certain percent of dwell is drained. At 75% with 2 L fill volume, the APD machine will drain 1.5 L then switch to "fill mode." This should minimize the number of alarms. Figure 83.3 gives a depiction of a PD drain cycle (A) with tidal set at 75% that drains well. A subsequent cycle (B) is without tidal. The consequence of the intermittent drain is that the patient awoke with discomfort, and the third dwell (C) had to be shortened (reducing dialysis efficiency).

Switching to 2.27% glucose may alleviate the issue by allowing greater ultrafiltration (UF). If UF with a 2.27% glucose dwell is 200 mLs (10%), the intra-abdominal volume at the end of the cycle will be 2.2 L. If the drainage alarms and pain occur when 400 mL is retained, with 2.2 L at the start of the drain, 1.8 L will be drained before alarms or pain starts. Many APD machines are set to allow switch from "drain out" to "drain-in" if resistance to drainage is encountered after drainage of 85% of fill volume (which for a 2 L fill = 1.7 L). Hence the use of 2.27% glucose will alleviate her alarms and pain. However, this is not a recommended reason for using greater tonicity glucose bags.

Switching from a high glucose degradation product (GDP), low pH solutions (e.g., dianeal) to a more biocompatible solutions (Physioneal 40) can alleviate drain-in discomfort and pain. But would not help pain during drain-out caused by PD catheter problems.

Question 2

The above case continues. The patient opts to continue on APD so she has 75% tidal added to her APD program. She finds the alarms and end-of-drain pains are now tolerable. She returns to work as a lawyer. Her initial target weight was set at 72 kg but over the next 2 months, she finds that her weight has increased to 75 kg. She has mild pitting edema extending to mid shins. She has increased her APD to use Physioneal 40 2.27% glucose bags at night. Her overnight UF is 200 mLs, initial drain 1.3 L, and her urine output is 700 mLs on frusemide 250 mg/d. Suggest appropriate investigations to guide treatment options.

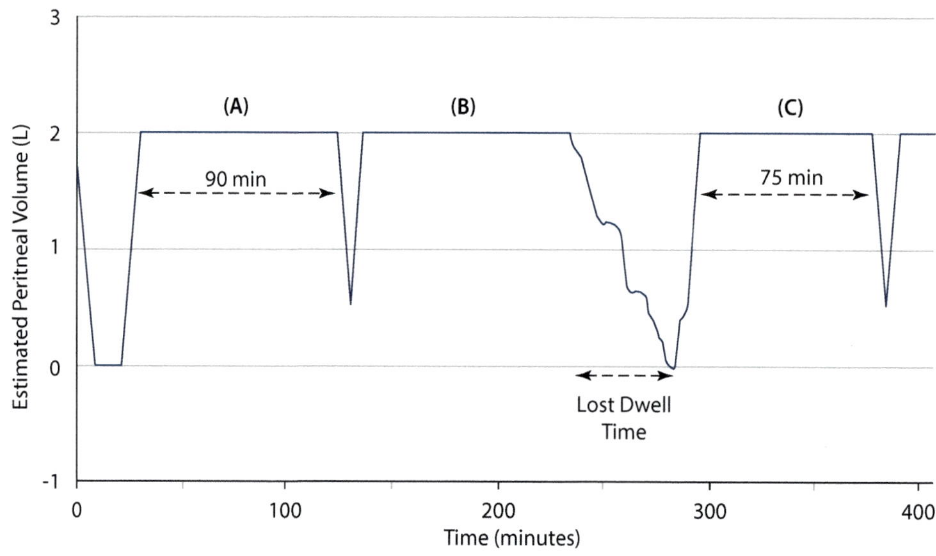

Fig. 83.3 APD machine report of patient's overnight dialysis session

Time	Urea (mmol/L)	Creatinine (µmol/L)	Glucose (mmol/L)	Sodium (mmol/L)
Serum	15.8	478	5.8	138
Overnight (6hrs)	16.1	415	27	133
0hr	3.8	90	96.2	134
4hr	14.2	372	32	133

4hr UF with 3.86% glucose was 500mL. Dialysate/Plasma creatinine = 0.78 (High Average Transporter)

- **UF > 400mL therefore not UF Failure**

Retained abdominal volume (R) can be calculated:

Amount of creatinine in abdomen after overnight dwell is drained: 415xR

=

Amount of creatinine in abdomen immediately after 2L of fresh dialysate is infused: 90 x (2000 + R)

- **Retained abdominal Volume = 553mL.** Retained abdominal volume > 300mL (15% of 2L fill volume) is likely to trigger APD alarms.

Fig. 83.4 Modified PET result

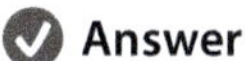

Answer

Peritoneal equilibration test (PET) with abdominal X-ray (AXR) would be my choice.

A UF of 200 mLs after 4 cycles of 2.27% glucose dwells is low. It would be unusual to have developed UF failure this early suggesting PD catheter drain issue. The retained abdominal dialysate volume at the end of a drain can be calculated using the "overnight" and "0-hour" samples from a PET. A modified PET (using 3.86% instead of 2.27% glucose for the 4-hour dwell) was performed (Fig. 83.4); if there is no significant retained dialysate volume, then a modified PET is better at identifying cases of UF failure (4-hour UF <400 mL with 3.86% glucose dwell or <100 mL with 1.36% glucose).

AXR is a simple noninvasive investigation to determine is the PD catheter is "malpositioned." Increasing laxatives is indicated as the patient had high retained dialysate volume even if her AXR was "normal" (PD catheter appeared to be in good position and not significant constipation).

Unfortunately, despite several days of good bowel movement, drainage remained poor. The patient was referred to surgeons for laparoscopic PD catheter surgery on the assumption that she had omental wrapping of her PD catheter.

Question 3

The case continues. While waiting for surgery, she started to use 3.86% glucose bags on her APD. But she was admitted via A&E with discomfort and breathlessness in the night. Chest X-ray did not show evidence of significant pulmonary oedema or pleural effusion, but she had significant vulval edema. Why was she breathless and how could this have been avoided?

Answer

It is likely she has abdominal overfill caused by use of 3.86% glucose dwells with tidal settings (Fig. 83.5). In the example given, the increased intra-abdominal pressure has caused splinting of diaphragm and inguinal hernia leading to subcutaneous leaking into vulva. A 3.86% glucose dwell induced UF of 300 mLs over 2-hour dwell time. If tidal option is selected, this will lead to increasing accumulation of intra-abdominal fluid that is drained only in the morning (last drain).

Tidal option should have been disabled when 3.86% glucose dwells are used on APD.

Question 4

The case continues.

The patient was admitted and switched temporarily to hemodialysis (HD) via a tunneled HD catheter. She

APD cycle	Drain In volume	2hr UF	Drain Out with 75% tidal	End-of cycle abdominal volume
Initial Drain	--	--	1.3L	0.2Ls
Cycle 1	2L	0.3L	1.5L	1L
Cycle 2	1.5L	0.3L	1.5L	1.3L
Cycle 3	1.5L	0.2L	1.5L	1.5L
Cycle 4	1.5L	0.1L	--	3.1L

Hypothetical abdominal volumes if 3.86% glucose dwells are used with tidal setting. Note 2hr UF reduces with each cycle as intra-abdominal pressure increases reducing UF.

Fig. 83.5 Example of OverFill with 3.86% glucose APD and Tidal

underwent laparotomy. Her PD catheter was found to be “wrapped by omentum.” The tip of her PD catheter was released and an omentectomy was performed. Her right inguinal hernia was also repaired. She was keen to return to PD as soon as possible as she finds it difficult work while on HD. Please advise a plan to restart PD.

Answer

There is no absolute rule about when to return to PD after hernia repair. But general rule is to minimize abdominal pressures in the first few weeks to reduce risk of leaks and recurrence of hernia. This has to be balanced by need to maintain adequate dialysis (her 24-hour urine output was only 700 mL). Her PD catheter was not replaced, so concern about exit site leak was reduced although there is still potential of leaks at laparoscopic port sites.

It was important to consult the patient about how to resume APD. We opted to restart APD 5 days post-operative:

8-hour 4 cycles, 1.5 L fill volume with 75% tidal (using 1.36% glucose). No last fill (Dry Day).

This dialysis program only uses 4.9 L fluid so a single 5 L APD was required. But this gives only modest dialysis clearance. The patient therefore agreed to have hybrid dialysis with once a week (Sat) HD until the APD program gradually increased over the next 3 weeks. Important consideration was the fact that she wanted to delay removing her THL until she was confident that her repositioned PD catheter was working. This permitted HD access for once-a-week HD (on Saturday) allowing her to return to work immediately.

Her drainage was good and she tolerated APD without tidal. She returned to her original APD program over the next 3 weeks.

References

1. Popovich RP, Moncrief JW, Nolph KD, Ghods AJ, Twardowski ZJ, Pyle WK. Continuous ambulatory peritoneal dialysis. Ann Intern Med. 1978;88(4):449–56.
2. Diaz-Buxo JA, Farmer CD, Walker PJ, Chandler JT, Holt KL. Continuous cyclic peritoneal dialysis: a preliminary report. Artif Organs. 1981;5(2):157–61.
3. Mehrotra R, Chiu YW, Kalantar-Zadeh K, Vonesh E. The outcomes of continuous ambulatory and automated peritoneal dialysis are similar. Kidney Int. 2009;76(1):97–107.
4. Juergensen PH, Murphy AL, Pherson KA, Chorney WS, Kliger AS, Finkelstein FO. Tidal peritoneal dialysis to achieve comfort in chronic peritoneal dialysis patients. Adv Perit Dial. 1999;15:125–6.
5. Fischbach M, Issad B, Dubois V, Taamma R. The beneficial influence on the effectiveness of automated peritoneal dialysis of varying the dwell time (short/long) and fill volume (small/large): a randomized controlled trial. Perit Dial Int. 2011;31(4):450–8.
6. Brown EA, Dratwa M, Povlsen JV. Assisted peritoneal dialysis: an evolving dialysis modality. Nephrol Dial Transplant. 2007;22(10):3091–2.
7. Povlsen JV, Ivarsen P. Assisted automated peritoneal dialysis (AAPD) for the functionally dependent and elderly patient. Perit Dial Int. 2005;25(Suppl 3):S60–3.
8. Mendelssohn DC. A skeptical view of assisted home peritoneal dialysis. Kidney Int. 2007;71(7):602–4.
9. Dratwa M. Costs of home assistance for peritoneal dialysis: results of a European survey. Kidney Int Suppl. 2008;108: S72–5.
10. Oliver MJ, Quinn RR, Richardson EP, Kiss AJ, Lamping DL, Manns BJ. Home care assistance and the utilization of peritoneal dialysis. Kidney Int. 2007;71(7):673–8.
11. Fukui H, Hara S, Hashimoto Y, et al. Review of combination of peritoneal dialysis and hemodialysis as a modality of treatment for end-stage renal disease. Ther Apher Dial. 2004;8(1): 56–61.
12. Kawanishi H, Moriishi M. Clinical effects of combined therapy with peritoneal dialysis and hemodialysis. Perit Dial Int. 2007;27 Suppl 2:S126–9.

13. Agarwal M, Clinard P, Burkart JM. Combined peritoneal dialysis and hemodialysis: our experience compared to others. Perit Dial Int. 2003;23(2):157–61.
14. McIntyre CW. Bimodal dialysis: an integrated approach to renal replacement therapy. Perit Dial Int. 2004;24(6):547–53.
15. Cullis B, Abdelraheem M, Abrahams G, et al. Peritoneal dialysis for acute kidney injury. Perit Dial Int. 2014;34(5):494–517.
16. Cullis B, Ponce D, Finkelstein F. What is the adequate dose for peritoneal dialysis in acute kidney injury: lower the bar or shift the goalposts? Perit Dial Int. 2017;37(5):491–3.
17. Gabriel DP, Nascimento GV, Caramori JT, Martim LC, Barretti P, Balbi AL. High volume peritoneal dialysis for acute renal failure. Perit Dial Int. 2007;27(3):277–82.
18. Figueiredo AE, Bernardini J, Bowes E, et al. A syllabus for teaching peritoneal dialysis to patients and caregivers. Perit Dial Int. 2016;36(6):592–605.
19. Fan SL, Sathick I, McKitty K, Punzalan S. Quality of life of caregivers and patients on peritoneal dialysis. Nephrol Dial Transplant. 2008;23(5):1713–9.
20. Brimble KS, Walker M, Margetts PJ, Kundhal KK, Rabbat CG. Meta-analysis: peritoneal membrane transport, mortality, and technique failure in peritoneal dialysis. J Am Soc Nephrol. 2006;17(9):2591–8.
21. Johnson DW, Hawley CM, McDonald SP, et al. Superior survival of high transporters treated with automated versus continuous ambulatory peritoneal dialysis. Nephrol Dial Transplant. 2010;25(6):1973–9.
22. Bargman JM, Thorpe KE, Churchill DN. Relative contribution of residual renal function and peritoneal clearance to adequacy of dialysis: a reanalysis of the CANUSA study. J Am Soc Nephrol. 2001;12(10):2158–62.
23. Van Biesen W, Vanholder R, Veys N, Lameire N. Peritoneal dialysis in anuric patients: concerns and cautions. Semin Dial. 2002;15(5):305–10.
24. Brown EA, Davies SJ, Rutherford P, et al. Survival of functionally anuric patients on automated peritoneal dialysis: the European APD Outcome Study. J Am Soc Nephrol. 2003;14(11):2948–57.
25. Fischbach M, Terzic J, Laugel V, Escande B, Dangelser C, Helmstetter A. Measurement of hydrostatic intraperitoneal pressure: a useful tool for the improvement of dialysis dose prescription. Pediatr Nephrol. 2003;18(10):976–80.
26. Shafi T, Jaar BG, Plantinga LC, et al. Association of residual urine output with mortality, quality of life, and inflammation in incident hemodialysis patients: the Choices for Healthy Outcomes in Caring for End-Stage Renal Disease (CHOICE) Study. Am J Kidney Dis. 2010;56(2):348–58.
27. Brown EA, Davies SJ, Heimburger O, et al. Adequacy targets can be met in anuric patients by automated peritoneal dialysis: baseline data from EAPOS. Perit Dial Int. 2001;21(Suppl 3):S133–7.
28. Jager KJ, Merkus MP, Dekker FW, et al. Mortality and technique failure in patients starting chronic peritoneal dialysis: results of the Netherlands cooperative study on the adequacy of dialysis. NECOSAD Study Group. Kidney Int. 1999;55(4):1476–85.
29. Armstrong A, Beer J, Noonan K, Cunningham J. Reduced calcium dialysate in CAPD patients: efficacy and limitations. Nephrol Dial Transplant. 1997;12(6):1223–8.
30. Querfeld U, Salusky IB, Fine RN. Treatment of severe hypercalcemia with peritoneal dialysis in an infant with end-stage renal disease. Pediatr Nephrol. 1988;2(3):323–5.
31. Rodriguez-Carmona A, Fontan MP. Sodium removal in patients undergoing CAPD and automated peritoneal dialysis. Perit Dial Int. 2002;22(6):705–13.
32. Boudville NC, Cordy P, Millman K, et al. Blood pressure, volume, and sodium control in an automated peritoneal dialysis population. Perit Dial Int. 2007;27(5):537–43.
33. Fan SL. Should we use biocompatible PD solutions for all patients? Perit Dial Int. 2009;29(6):630–3.
34. Pecoits-Filho R, Tranaeus A, Lindholm B. Clinical trial experiences with Physioneal. Kidney Int Suppl. 2003;88:S100–4.
35. Johnson DW, Brown FG, Clarke M, et al. Effects of biocompatible versus standard fluid on peritoneal dialysis outcomes. J Am Soc Nephrol. 2012;23(6):1097–107.
36. Wolfson M, Piraino B, Hamburger RJ, Morton AR. A randomized controlled trial to evaluate the efficacy and safety of icodextrin in peritoneal dialysis. Am J Kidney Dis. 2002;40(5):1055–65.
37. Jones M, Hagen T, Boyle CA, et al. Treatment of malnutrition with 1.1% amino acid peritoneal dialysis solution: results of a multicenter outpatient study. Am J Kidney Dis. 1998;32(5):761–9.
38. Kopple JD, Bernard D, Messana J, et al. Treatment of malnourished CAPD patients with an amino acid based dialysate. Kidney Int. 1995;47(4):1148–57.
39. le Poole CY, van Ittersum FJ, Weijmer MC, Valentijn RM, ter Wee PM. Clinical effects of a peritoneal dialysis regimen low in glucose in new peritoneal dialysis patients: a randomized crossover study. Adv Perit Dial. 2004;20:170–6.
40. Brown EA, Blake PG, Boudville N, et al. International Society for Peritoneal Dialysis practice recommendations: Prescribing high-quality goal-directed peritoneal dialysis. Peritoneal Dialysis International. 2020;40(3):244–53. https://doi.org/10.1177/0896860819895364.
41. Davies SJ, Brown EA, Frandsen NE, et al. Longitudinal membrane function in functionally anuric patients treated with APD: data from EAPOS on the effects of glucose and icodextrin prescription. Kidney Int. 2005;67(4):1609–15.
42. Ates K, Nergizoglu G, Keven K, et al. Effect of fluid and sodium removal on mortality in peritoneal dialysis patients. Kidney Int. 2001;60(2):767–76.

Complications of Peritoneal Dialysis

Sarah Jenkins, Badri Shrestha, and Martin Wilkie

Contents

M. Harber (ed.), *Primer on Nephrology*, https://doi.org/10.1007/978-3-030-76419-7_84

Learning Objectives

1. Peritoneal dialysis is limited by technique failure (TF).
2. The most important causes of TF include infection (peritonitis, exit site and tunnel infection), problems with the catheter, and limitations in solute and fluid removal.
3. Each centre should audit peritoneal infection rates as well as the success and complications of catheter insertion on a regular basis and undertake root cause analysis to better understand causes and remediable actions.
4. Regular multidisciplinary meetings should consider patient progress including the adequacy of solute clearance and volume management. These meetings should also consider patient requirements for support and how that changes over time.
5. Guidelines to support patient management are available at ▶ ISPD.org.

Case Study

Peritoneal Access

A 54-year-old male with progressive kidney disease is admitted to hospital feeling unwell. It is clear that he will need to start dialysis within the next few weeks. He works full time and is keen to remain as independent as possible. What considerations will you have as you plan his dialysis? How will you involve him in those discussions? What approach will you use for access placement and what will determine when dialysis can start?

Infection

A 74-year-old lady who has been on PD for 20 months presents with a 3-hour history of cloudy dialysate and abdominal pain. What initial assessment will you make and samples will you arrange? What will be your initial therapy and how will you assess response? At your unit, how frequent is PD peritonitis and what are the key steps that can be taken to reduce the rate?

Ultrafiltration

A 20-year-old student has recently transferred from HD to PD in order to have more time to attend college. At the first clinic attendance you note evidence of volume overload and poor blood pressure control. How will you go about assessing the patient and their therapy to inform decisions that can be made to resolve the problem?

84.1 Introduction

For many patients, peritoneal dialysis (PD) is an excellent therapy in which they can take control of their own care and remain independent from hospital. Outcomes are at least equal, if not better, for patients on peritoneal dialysis compared with hemodialysis (HD) [1] – however, most of the data is from registries. Only one randomized controlled trial has been published that compared dialysis modalities - however it was unable to recruit a sufficient number of patients [2]. A whole range of factors influence the comparison including comorbidity, age, residual renal function, late presentation, and the access used for HD. In general, effective management requires a multidisciplinary team-based approach that adheres to guidance produced by the International Society of Peritoneal Dialysis (▶ Box 84.1) underpinned by regular audit. Optimal care requires regular review of patient progress that includes problem-solving and prescription management, ultimately planning transfer to HD in those for whom PD is becoming no longer viable [3].

The likelihood of a particular PD-related complication is influenced to some extent by the time that the patient has been on PD, and a schema is presented in ◘ Fig. 84.1. Patients may discontinue PD for a range of reasons including access-related and mechanical complications, infection, problems with ultrafiltration and solute clearance as well as psychosocial problems [4]. This is described broadly as technique failure (TF) and is the primary outcome measure of the international Peritoneal Dialysis Outcomes and Practice Patterns Study [5]. Commonly emphasis is placed on the risk that patients on PD face without due recognition of the complications that are associated with HD. Although peritonitis is the most common complication of PD, bacteremia is rare and hospitalization for infection is similar between the modalities [6]. Low infection rates are possible based on regular education of patients and staff. When it comes to the important issue of access there is an appreciation of the difficulties that can occur when PD catheters don't work properly, but the burden is similar to that experienced by HD patients requiring revision of their vascular access [7]. Encapsulating peritoneal sclerosis (EPS) is a dreaded potential complication of PD, but is exceptionally rare in the early years of PD, and is declining in incidence [8]. It is by no means as frequent a risk factor as the major causes of adverse outcome that affect our patients [9].

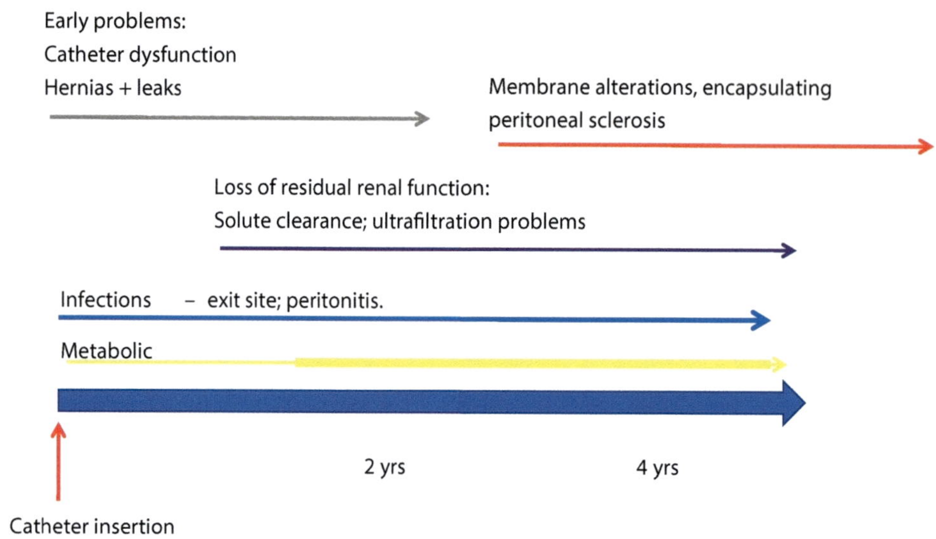

Fig. 84.1 A graphic demonstration of the time line of PD-related complications

84

> **Box 84.1 Guidelines Published by the International Society of Peritoneal Dialysis (available at ▶ www.ISPD.org)**
>
> - Peritoneal Dialysis for Acute Kidney Injury2020 update
> - ISPD Cardiovascular and Metabolic Guidelines in Adult Peritoneal Dialysis Patients 2015
>   - Part I – Assessment and Management of Various Cardiovascular Risk Factors
>   - Part II – Management of Various Cardiovascular Complications
> - Length of Time on Peritoneal Dialysis and Encapsulating Peritoneal Sclerosis: Position Paper for ISPD: Update 2017
> - ISPD Catheter-Related Infection Recommendations: 2017 Update
> - ISPD Peritonitis Recommendations: 2016 Update on Prevention and Treatment 2016
> - Creating and Maintaining Optimal Peritoneal Dialysis Access in the Adult Patient: 2019 Update.
> - A Syllabus for Teaching Peritoneal Dialysis to Patients and Caregivers 2016
> - ISPD recommendations for the evaluation of peritoneal membrane dysfunction in adults: Classification, measurement, interpretation and rationale for intervention 2021
> - ISPD practice recommendations: Prescribing high-quality goal-directed peritoneal dialysis 2020

84.2 Peritoneal Dialysis-Associated Infection

84.2.1 Prevention of PD-Associated Infection

In the early days of PD, infection was a common and difficult problem with peritonitis occurring every few months. Considerable attention has been given to this complication resulting in a marked improvement. Over the last 3 decades technical developments have included the change from glass bottles to plastic bags, improved systems (with the disconnect system and flush-before-fill), and more recently, the use of prophylactic antibacterial creams at the exit site. Emphasis has been placed on the importance of training for staff, patients, and carers and the role of audit to understand infection rates and causative organisms (Fig. 84.2). There is evidence that the degree of nursing experience and patient training methods influence the risk of PD infections which should be based on the principles of adult education. Refresher courses are recommended for patients 3 months after initial training and routinely thereafter at a minimum of once a year as well as following hospitalization, episodes of peritonitis and catheter infection or if there is a change in dexterity, vision, or mental acuity. International society for peritoneal dialysis (ISPD) has published an open access curriculum for patient training [10].

▶ Box 84.2 summarizes multidisciplinary team-based initiatives that have an impact on preventing peritoneal dialysis-associated infection. Peritonitis rates are reported as episodes per patient-year of therapy with the best centers having rates that are less than 0.3 (equivalent to 1

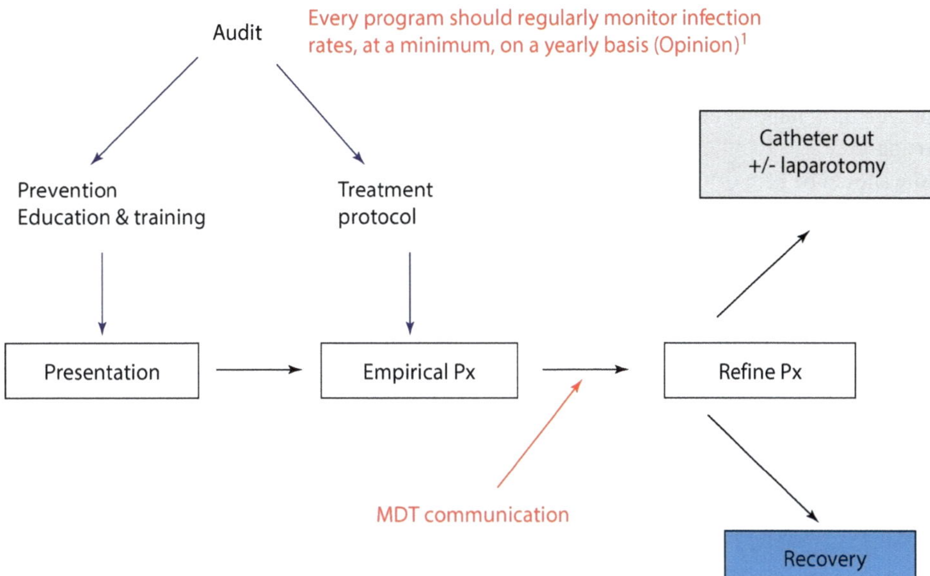

Fig. 84.2 A schema describing optimal prevention and management of PD peritonitis

infection per 36 months of treatment). For example, data from the French registry showed that half of the patients did not experience this complication in 31 months [11]. There are many publications on PD-associated infection, but few randomized controlled trials. The best resources are the guidelines from the ISPD [12] which are free to download from ▶ www.ispd.org (▶ Box 84.1).

An important part of infection prevention relates to the procedures for catheter placement and techniques focused on the prevention of exit site infection. Catheter placement should be governed by clear protocols [13] with the exit site location being selected preoperatively in discussion with the patient so that it is placed in a suitable position that is not at risk of abrasion from the belt and is easy for the patient to attend to. Recommendations regarding post-operative management of the PD catheter in order to minimize the risk of exit site infection are summarized in ▶ Box 84.3. There is good evidence for the preventative use of antibiotic creams at the exit site with meta-analysis showing benefit for mupirocin use on both exit site infection and peritonitis due to *Staphylococcus aureus* [14].

Box 84.2 Methods for Reducing the Risk of PD Peritonitis

- Catheter-related interventions
  - Double-cuffed catheter
  - Careful catheter insertion protocols as outlined in the ISPD guidance
- Systems
  - Flush-before-fill technology
  - Avoiding spike systems
- Antibiotic prophylaxis
  - Before catheter insertion
  - As part of exit site care
  - Before interventional procedures – e.g., colonoscopy
- Training
  - Careful training and directed retraining for patients and staff
  - Clear points of contact for patients, careers, and staff
  - Clear protocols for the management of PD-related infection and contamination events that are accessible and easily understood
- Review
  - Regular audit or continuous quality improvement (at least annually) to be presented at unit meetings
  - Regular multidisciplinary team meetings to review patient care, developing problems, and practice development requirements
  - Regular update of unit protocols in the light of new developments or data presented from the audit meetings

Box 84.3 Strategies to Prevent Exit Site Infection

- Dressings should be done by a trained dialysis nurse using sterile technique until the exit site is healed
- If possible, do not remove dressing for 5 days post-insertion
- The exit site should be kept dry until well healed – avoid baths and showers for this period
- Once the exit site is well healed, the patient should be taught how to perform exit site care
- The catheter should be kept immobile to avoid pulling and trauma to the exit site
- If possible, avoid using the catheter until healed – if earlier use is required low dialysate volumes are necessary, with the patient supine to reduce the risk of leaks.

Adapted from reference [13]

84.2.2 PD Peritonitis

PD peritonitis is the leading cause of TF and confers an increased mortality risk; if severe and prolonged, it can be associated with peritoneal membrane damage. It is diagnosed by the presence of abdominal pain and cloudy dialysate effluent that has a leucocyte count greater than 100/mm^3. In APD with rapid cycling there may be a lower cell count; therefore, a differential count of >50% neutrophils is considered diagnostic. It is possible to overlook the diagnosis of peritonitis in automated peritoneal dialysis (APD) patients if the effluent line runs straight to a drain without collecting in a bag and leucocyte esterase sticks are sometimes used by patients to test the effluent dialysate. Patients presenting with peritonitis range from the mildly unwell, who can be managed easily as an outpatient, to those with marked features of systemic sepsis requiring admission to hospital. The principal sources of contamination include a break in the sterile technique and infection at the exit site – others are organisms within the catheter biofilm, transmural migration of organisms across the bowel wall and rarely hematogenous spread or vaginal leak.

Root cause analysis should be performed after every episode of peritonitis to understand modifiable risk factors as much as possible and plan an intervention strategy. There are a number of potentially modifiable risk factors associated with PD peritonitis including depression, hypoalbuminemia, hypokalemia, constipation, exit site colonization, infection, connection methodology, technique errors, prolonged antibiotics, and medical procedures.

It is important that peritonitis is diagnosed promptly so that appropriate treatment can be started immediately and therefore the patient and their carers require clear contact details of the unit. The health care team should be experienced in the diagnosis and management of peritonitis, supported by evidence-based protocols. Presentation to the incorrect hospital department can potentially lead to misdiagnosis and inappropriate management. A suitable technique for dialysate sampling is required in order to maximize the opportunity for identifying the causative organism. The recommended approach to dialysate sampling is either the inoculation of blood culture bottles or centrifugation of 50 mL of peritoneal effluent at 3000 g for 15 minutes, followed by resuspension of the sediment in 3–5 mL of sterile saline and inoculation of this material both on solid culture media and into a standard blood culture medium [12].

The differential diagnosis of cloudy dialysate fluid includes noninfectious causes such as chemical and allergic peritonitis, hemoperitoneum, malignancy, and chylous effluent. A dialysate sample should ideally be taken after a 2-hour dwell and samples taken from a "dry" abdomen can give a spuriously elevated WCC.

Inability to identify the causative organism has implications for primary cure with most studies showing poorer outcomes where the organism has not been identified. Causes of sterile peritonitis include poor dialysate sampling and culture techniques, as well as recent courses of antibiotics – for example, the treatment of an exit site infection (▶ Box 84.4). It is important to have a low threshold for the possibility of surgical peritonitis in a PD patient since this can pose diagnostic and therapeutic challenges and may occur in 10% of the cases, resulting from inflammation, perforation, or ischemia of intra-abdominal organs. There are several possible pitfalls in the diagnosis of that complication including the innocent finding of air under the diaphragm of patients on PD, the possibility that serum amylase may be spuriously low in patients on icodextrin, and poor diagnostic sensitivity of CT scanning. Delays in institution of appropriate treatment, particularly surgical intervention, lead to increased morbidity and mortality [15].

The nature of organisms causing PD peritonitis has changed over the last 3 decades. Whereas gram-positive organisms were the commonest, their relative frequency has been reduced by improvements in technology and technique as demonstrated by a 25-year single-center experience from Brazil [16]. As a result, patients presenting with PD peritonitis are more likely than previously to have gram-negative infections, which needs to be considered when designing treatment protocols. It is important that individual centers examine their own patterns of infection, causative organisms, and sensitivities and adapt protocols as necessary for local conditions.

Box 84.4 Causes of Culture Negative Peritonitis

- In appropriate sampling or culture technique
- Presence of antibiotics – e.g., treatment for an exit site infection
- Fastidious organisms, e.g., fungi or *Mycobacterium tuberculosis*
- Chemical or allergic peritonitis, e.g., due to antibiotic allergy
- Intra-abdominal disease – e.g., carcinoma or lymphoma

84.2.3 Treatment of PD Peritonitis

The ideal antibiotic should give broad coverage of organisms, avoid disturbing normal bacterial flora, have a low side-effect profile, should not provoke the emergence of resistant organisms, and be convenient to administer and cheap. This will be influenced by the pharmacokinetic and pharmacodynamic profile as well as the potential side effects of particular antibiotics [17]. A number of factors impact on the choice of antibiotics that are used to treat peritonitis including the emergence of vancomycin-resistant enterococci, reports of vancomycin-intermediately sensitive *S. aureus*, methicillin resistance and gram-negative enteric bacteria such as *E. coli* and *Klebsiella pneumoniae* that produce Extended Spectrum β-Lactamases (ESBL) and carbapenemases [12, 18] as well as concern regarding the impact of aminoglycosides on residual renal function.

Initial empirical treatment for PD peritonitis should cover both gram-positive and gram-negative organisms and be governed by an understanding of local organisms and their sensitivities. The ISPD infection guidelines recommend possible antibiotic schedules including either the combination of a third-generation cephalosporin (ceftazidime) or an aminoglycoside for gram-negative cover with a first-generation cephalosporin (cephazolin) or vancomycin for gram-positive cover [12]. A Cochrane systematic review favored a vancomycin-based regimen; however, the evidence was graded as low quality [19]. It is important to liaise with the local microbiological team regarding the most appropriate protocol. Treatment should be adjusted once the organism has been identified and for detailed discussion the reader should access the guideline. Emphasis should be on preservation of the peritoneal membrane and the overall health of the patient rather than persisting with PD where the infection is not responding to treatment. It is recommended that the PD catheter should be removed if the patient does not respond within 5 days of treatment (▶ Box 84.5), however there should be a low threshold to remove it earlier if the patient is significantly unwell. It is often appropriate to consider returning to PD with a new catheter once the infection has cleared. Vancomycin and aminoglycoside doses require adjustment based on antibiotic levels due to complex pharmacodynamics which are influenced by a range of factors including patient size, dialysate flow rates, peritoneal membrane characteristics, the molecular weight of the antibiotic, degree of residual renal function, whether the patient is on continuous ambulatory peritoneal dialysis (CAPD) or APD, and whether it is administered continuously or intermittently [20].

Box 84.5 Indications for PD Catheter Removal for Peritoneal Dialysis-Associated Infections

- Refractory peritonitis (failure to clear up after 5 days of appropriate antibiotics).
- Relapsing, recurrent, or repeat peritonitis
  - In appropriate circumstances consider simultaneous removal and reinsertion.
- Refractory exit site and tunnel infection with evidence of dacron cuff infection on ultrasound scan
- Fungal peritonitis
- Catheter removal may also be considered for
  - Peritonitis associated with an exit site or tunnel infection due to *S. aureus* or *Pseudomonas species*
  - Mycobacterial peritonitis
  - Multiple enteric organisms

Adapted from Ref. [12]

84.3 Exit Site Infection (ESI)

The importance of ESI is that it is a risk factor for PD peritonitis. Once the exit site has become colonized with infecting organisms, eradication may be problematic and require prolonged courses of antibiotics. Strategies to reduce the risk of this complication are essential and are summarized in the appropriate guideline from the ISPD [21]. These start before the catheter is placed with a careful discussion with the patient regarding the location of the exit site, catheter placement protocols to minimize the risk of infection, and a rigorous approach to postoperative exit site care. Exit site prophylaxis with antibacterial creams have been demonstrated to have an impact on both exit site and peritonitis rates, in particular with gram-positive organisms [14]. A positive nose swab for *Staphylococcus aureus* is associated with an increased likelihood of developing an exit site infection.

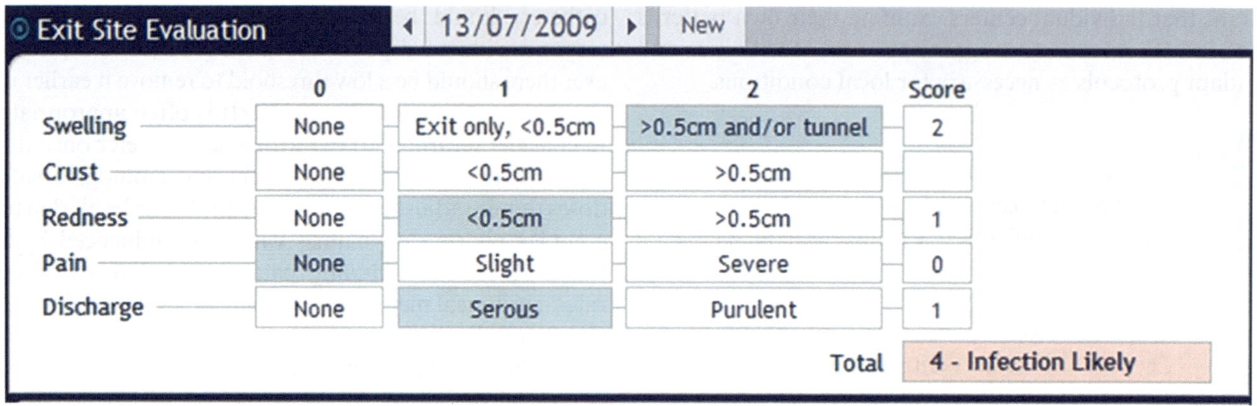

Fig. 84.3 Exit site scoring using the ISPD recommended system [22]

Although purulent drainage from the exit site indicates the presence of infection, erythema is not specific. The identification of an organism in the absence of inflammation indicates colonization, and does not require treatment. An exit site scoring system recommended by the ISPD is based on the presence of swelling, redness, pain, and discharge [22] (Fig. 84.3).

Treatment of an infected exit site requires appropriate antibiotics based on swab results and a prolonged course of antibiotics may be necessary. Infecting organisms are most commonly *Staphylococcus aureus*, *Staphylococcus epidermidis*, *Pseudomonas aeruginosa,* and *Escherichia coli*. For chronic exit site infections, a combination of synergistic antibiotics is preferred to avoid the development of resistance. Response may be slow, appearances may change only gradually and deroofing of the tunnel with exteriorization or shaving of the cuff may be required. A variety of topical agents are used to clean the exit site according to custom and practice and these include sodium hypochlorite, povidone iodine, chlorhexidine, non-antibacterial, and antibacterial soap; however, care should be taken not to use agents that are potentially damaging to the skin. International variation in the use of such agents is reported from the international peritoneal dialysis outcomes and practice patterns study (PDOPPS) [23]. A tunnel infection may present as exit site discharge, erythema, edema, or tenderness over the subcutaneous pathway but is often clinically occult. *Staphylococcus aureus* and *Pseudomonas aeruginosa* exit site infections are very often associated with concomitant tunnel infections and are the organisms that most often result in catheter infection-related peritonitis; aggressive management is always indicated for these organisms. Ultrasound examination of the dacron cuffs and tunnel can assist in diagnosis and aid in making decision on removal of catheter. Catheter removal is required in non-responsive tunnel infections. Presence of fluid around the dacron cuffs is associated with a tunnel infection and consideration should be given to removal of the catheter.

Exit site infection, unresponsive to antibiotics, can be treated with exteriorization of the catheter, shaving of the superficial cuff, splicing of the catheter, or relocation of the exit to a distant site using extended catheter (presternal or upper abdominal).

84.4 Audit Standards for PD-Related Infection

These are presented as continuous quality improvement in the 2016 ISPD infection guideline and are summarized in ▸ Box 84.6 [12].

Box 84.6 Selected Continuous Quality Improvement Measures to Prevent Peritonitis [12]

- Each PD center should have a continuous quality improvement (CQI) program in place to reduce peritonitis rates.
- Multidisciplinary teams running CQI programs in PD centers should meet and review their units' performance metrics regularly.
- Every program should monitor, at least on a yearly basis, the incidence of peritonitis.
- The parameters monitored should include the overall peritonitis rate, peritonitis rates of specific organisms, the percentage of patients per year who are peritonitis-free, and the antimicrobial susceptibilities of the infecting organisms.
- Peritonitis rate should be standardly reported as number of episodes per patient-year.
- Organism-specific peritonitis rates should be reported as absolute rates, i.e., as number of episodes per year.

84.5 Peritoneal Access-Related Problems

An adequately functioning PD catheter (PDC) is essential for successful PD and when the catheter does not work sufficiently this can prevent patients from receiving their chosen therapy and increase costs for health care systems. The UK Renal Registry reported considerable variation in 1 year catheter failure for 2015 with rates varying between 0 and 40% with the median being 13% [7]. Although it might appear that PDC are frequently causing problems and requiring replacement or repositioning it is relevant to note that vascular access causes at least as much of a problem for patients on HD [24]. PDC problems contribute significantly to early peritoneal TF [25] and therefore regular audit of primary catheter function and associated mechanical complications is essential to ensure that high standards are maintained. Systematic review has not demonstrated differences in outcome for PD catheters placed using the percutaneous, surgical method or laparoscopic methods [26–28] but does report advantage for the advanced laparoscopic technique that includes rectus sheath tunnelling and adjunctive procedures compared with basic laparoscopy with the caveat that only cohort studies were available for the analysis [29]. The medical Seldinger technique performed under local anesthetic has the advantage of being able to be performed by a nephrologist or specialist nurse, giving the control of catheter placement to the medical team, but it is not suitable for patients who have had previous lower abdominal surgery or in the obese. On the other hand, advanced laparoscopic techniques ensure that the catheter is placed in the pelvis and that necessary adjunctive interventions are performed. Whichever method is used, it is important that there is a team-based approach, that the service is responsive and that there is good availability of surgical support when required.

84.6 Common Catheter-Related Complications

The main complication of PDC is dysfunction. Since a PD catheter requires a flow of up to 300 ml/min it is necessary that the side holes are not obstructed and that the tip is well placed in the sump of the pelvis where the residual dialysate will be retained. If it is not appropriately placed this will result in a large residual volume reducing effective clearance and ultrafiltration, while increasing intra-abdominal pressure and associated complications. APD is more demanding on catheter function than CAPD and poor flows result in drainage alarms on the machine. This can be managed to some extent by the use of a tidal prescription (where a small amount of fluid is left in situ at the end of a dwell), however, if there are problems with clearance or ultrafiltration the catheter may need to be repositioned or replaced. Good early catheter function is essential if PD is to be used as treatment for patients presenting late with advanced uremia requiring dialysis.

Catheter dysfunction has several common causes including migration, which can be diagnosed by a plain abdominal film (Fig. 84.4), as well as fecal loading which is commonly cited and often treated with beneficial results. Adequate bowel preparation is an essential part of the catheter insertion protocol. An uncommon cause of catheter dysfunction is the omental wrap which can be diagnosed and treated by laparoscopy. Catheter obstruction may result from fibrin or blood clots which can be resolved by the use of a urokinase lock into the catheter. Of course, catheter dysfunction is not easy to define, being described in practice more by the impact on the patient or nursing staff rather than objective measurements of flow.

Patients may complain of pain on inflow or drainage of PD fluid, which may be due to a local irritant effect of the dialysis fluid, a consequence of negative pressure

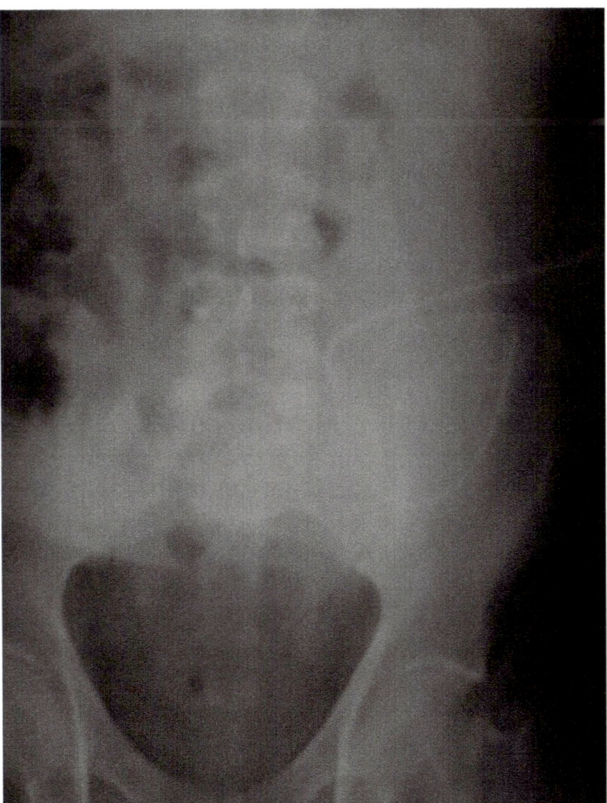

Fig. 84.4 Plain abdominal X-rays demonstrating the PD catheter located in the pelvis **a** and the tip having migrated out of the pelvis **b**

(suction) particularly in APD or a mechanical consequence of tube position. Tidal APD is commonly used to reduce drainage pain, combined with avoiding a "dry day" by leaving a residual volume of approximately 200 ml in the peritoneal cavity. The use of more biocompatible neutral pH dialysates may ameliorate inflow pain possibly due to less chemical irritation of the membrane resulting in reduced stimulation of nociceptors. The position of the tube in the pelvis can lead to mechanical irritation which may be resolved by tube repositioning. Unfortunately, it is challenging to prove this etiology and some patients may be discouraged from persisting with PD.

84.7 Audit Standards for Catheter Placement

The minimization of catheter-related complications requires care and attention from the operator in the context of a consistent team-based approach supported by clear guidelines and protocols [30]. These describe the conditions necessary for optimal catheter function with minimization of complications. The only registry that reports primary catheter function is the French Speaking Registry, and this gives really excellent catheter function data [11]. However, in reality, many centers describe results that are considerably lower. The ISPD audit standards for catheter placement include a 1-year catheter survival of at least 80% and peritonitis within 30 days of catheter insertion of less than 5% [30] and this is audited by the UK Renal Registry [7]. There is an advantage in using an earlier time-point such as 3 months post catheter insertion as an audit measure since it provides more proximate data for clinical teams to use in their quality assurance.

84.8 Surgical Complications of PD

The surgical complications related to the insertion of the PD catheter can lead to morbidity, seriously compromise outcomes and result in loss of confidence for patients. Early complications include hemorrhage, perforated viscus, wound infection, catheter obstruction and displacement, and dialysate leak. Later complications include external cuff extrusion, dialysate leaks, hernias, erosion of abdominal organs, hemoperitoneum, and chylous effluent. Independent of the insertion technique, the operator must be able to recognize and manage the complications promptly and effectively. Preoperative evaluation and identification of potential risk factors are essential to prevent them [31].

84.9 Hemorrhage

Intraperitoneal hemorrhage may arise from trauma to the omental or mesenteric vessels, particularly during closed or blind insertion. This usually presents with blood staining of the effluent, which may be heavy. Slight bleeding may be treated expectantly; however, heavy bleeding, particularly in association with hypotension, will require return to theater for localization of the source of the bleeding and hemostasis. Extraperitoneal bleeding may be obvious from the wound edge (main wound or exit site) or an enlarging wound hematoma. Skin edge bleeding can be dealt with using either additional sutures or local injection with a local anesthetic solution containing adrenaline. Failure to evacuate a hematoma predisposes to delayed wound healing, dehiscence and infection with potential risk of tunnel infection and peritonitis.

84.10 Hematoperitoneum

Hemoperitoneum can appear dramatic, but generally settles spontaneously without the patient suffering harm. There is a long list of possible causes, summarized in an excellent review article [32]. There are rare occasions when it can signify a significant intraperitoneal hemorrhage, for example, following the rupture of a splenic artery aneurysm, although most commonly the cause is a bleed from a peritoneal capillary or due to either ovulation or retroperitoneal menstruation in women. In one series, the incidence of hemoperitoneum was 6%. Seventy percent of these did not require any active intervention apart from addition of heparin to the dialysate, with 20% requiring active intervention for significant hemorrhage and the remaining 10% having significant intra-abdominal pathology but minor hematoperitoneum [33]. Blood transfusion may be required with severe bleeding due to follicular or ovarian cyst rupture or coagulopathies.

84.11 Perforation or Laceration

Perforation of bowel and urinary bladder is a well-recognized but rare complication of closed PDC insertion, and it can also occur with open insertion. Injuries to liver, a polycystic kidney, aorta, mesenteric artery, and hernial sac have all been reported. Predisposing factors include abdominal adhesions and distensions due to paralytic ileus or bowel obstruction, and unconscious, cachectic, or heavily sedated patients. The bladder is at risk of injury if it is of high volume, for example in patients with chronic bladder outflow obstruction, and this can be avoided by preoperative voiding confirmed by ultrasound examination. Evidence of peritonitis associated with contaminated effluent is an indication for laparotomy and repair of the perforation. Delayed perforation of intestine, bladder, and vagina caused by pressure necrosis and erosion from an unused catheter has been described.

84.12 Wound Infection

Although unusual, this is a serious complication, which may lead to catheter loss. Usual organisms are *Staphylococcus aureus* and *Pseudomonas* species. Contamination of the wound should be prevented by strict adherence to aseptic technique, prophylactic antibiotics, and meticulous hemostasis. Treatment of established infection requires antibiotics, surgical drainage, and possibly catheter removal for intractable infection involving the catheter. ESI or peritonitis directly as a consequence of catheter placement should be a rare event. Treatment of catheter associated infections is summarized in the relevant ISPD guideline [21].

84.13 Hernias

It is estimated that between 10 and 20% of the CAPD population develop hernias due to raised intra-abdominal pressure associated with PD, which can be inguinal, umbilical and pericatheter in location. Part of the preoperative assessment of the prospective PD patient is to assess for the presence of hernias since these can be repaired at the time of catheter placement. However, often these are not present at the time of catheter insertion and develop later, more commonly in patients who use larger intraperitoneal volumes and in those with adult polycystic kidney disease.

Elective hernia repair should be undertaken if possible and if the peritoneum remains intact and the hernia repair is not extensive, disruption of PD is not required. A small volume and short cycle dwell regimen can be continued postoperatively. However, where the peritoneum is breeched during hernia repair, change to hemodialysis for at least 3 weeks to allow healing of the peritoneum is required since leakage of dialysis fluid through the hernia wound encourages infection of mesh used to reinforce the repair. Pericatheter hernias, which usually occur in the midline, are difficult to manage without removing the catheter. Any attempt to repair a pericatheter hernia leaving the catheter intact will either compromise the hernia repair or the catheter function. Meticulous attention to the technique in placement of the catheter will usually prevent such hernias from developing. Paramedian placement of the PDC reduces the incidence of pericatheter hernias.

84.14 Leaks

A dialysate leak can occur months or even years after starting PD in up to 25% of catheters placed through the mid-line, but is less common with a paramedian incision and has been reported in 7.4% of cases following a laparoscopic PD catheter insertion [34]. Clinically, leakage presents as clear dialysis fluid around the catheter at its exit site or as a localized swelling and edema of the abdominal wall due to infiltration with fluid (peaud'orange). The passage of dialysis fluid through a patent processus vaginalis may lead to gross scrotal and penile oedema in the male and labial oedema in the female. Occasionally, the oedema may be so marked that it is not possible to decide the side of origin of the leak. Hydrothorax, in a patient on PD, can result from leak of fluid through a congenital pleura-peritoneal communication or an acquired diaphragmatic hernia, which presents with chest pain and dyspnea. It is important to note that this complication may be silent; therefore, to exclude this, careful chest examination including percussion should be performed routinely in patients who are new to PD. If an effusion is found, the diagnosis is suggested by biochemical characteristics of aspirated fluid including a relatively high glucose (dialysate /serum ratio), low protein or LDH concentration in the pleural fluid and confirmed by an ultrasound, CT (Fig. 84.5), or an MR scan. An isotope scan (peritoneo-scrotogram or pleural scintigraphy) will delineate the side of the leak (Fig. 84.6a and b) which if negative allows the therapy to be continued while other causes are pursued.

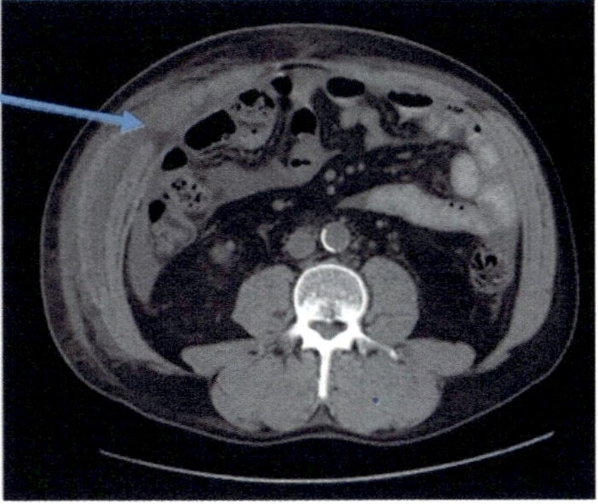

Fig. 84.5 A peritoneal leak demonstrated on CT scan in a patient on peritoneal dialysis following a failed renal transplant

a

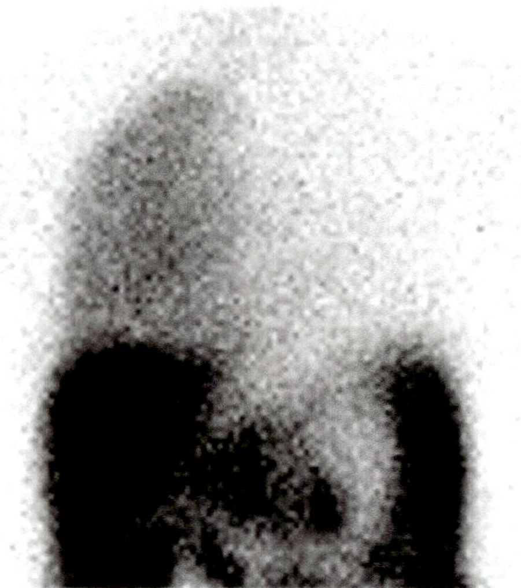

b

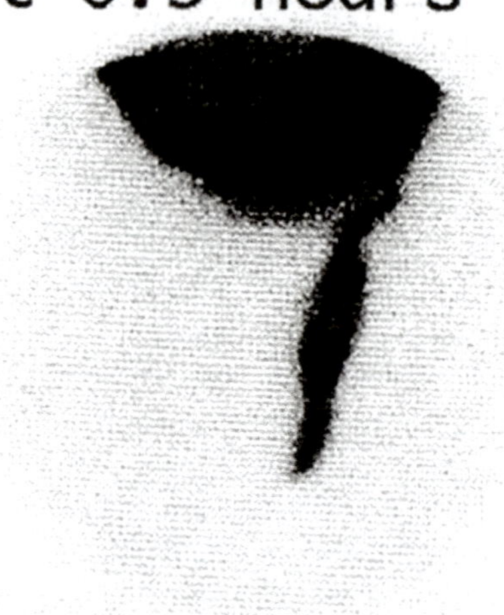

Fig. 84.6 **a** Scintigraphy – a positive study from a peritoneal dialysis patient with a pleural effusion, **b** Scintigraphy demonstrating peritoneal fluid leaking into the scrotum

Securing the PD catheter tightly at the deep cuff level or rectus sheath tunnelling reduces the risk of early leak and is recommended if there are plans to use the catheter early [35]. Early leaks can be managed by temporary discontinuation of PD, however, catheter replacement may be required. In a leak through patent processus vaginalis, PD should be discontinued until the oedema has subsided and then repair should be undertaken as for an inguinal hernia. If possible, the patient should be temporarily converted to hemodialysis for about 2 weeks following repair. Several approaches have been used to treat pleural leaks, although often the patient will require transfer to hemodialysis.

84.15 External Cuff Extrusion

Location of the subcutaneous cuff close to the exit site may lead to its protrusion, which can result either if the catheter becomes inadvertently pulled or may occur spontaneously due to its shape memory that tends to straighten the catheter. This complication can be avoided by placing the external cuff approximately 2–3 cm deep to the skin. If the subcutaneous cuff of the catheter begins to extrude, it may result in a persistent exit site infection. In the absence of signs of tunnel or deep cuff infection, removal of the subcutaneous cuff (shaving) allows the exit site infection to resolve in 50% of the cases unresponsive to antibiotic treatment. Failure of the infection to resolve mandates removal of the catheter.

84.16 Chylous Effluent

Chylous ascites, as defined by the presence of chylomicrons causing cloudiness of the effluent, is a rare entity which can occur with either no identifiable cause or in association with intra-abdominal malignancies (lymphoma and ovarian carcinoma), cirrhosis of liver, chronic pancreatitis, amyloidosis, cardiac failure, and patients on calcium channel blockers. In cases with no obvious cause, microtrauma to the peritoneal lymphatics is presumed to be the etiology, where improvement has been reported with cessation of PD, administration of medium chain triglycerides and octreotide. Continued loss of lymph (lymphocytes and fat) leads to malnutrition and immunosuppression, which may necessitate discontinuation of PD.

84.17 Indications for Catheter Removal

Catheter removal maybe required for malfunction which can result from intraluminal obstruction with blood or fibrin clots, omental tissue incarceration, catheter tip migration out of the pelvis with poor drainage, a catheter kink, catheter tip caught in an adhesion following severe peritonitis, or an accidental break. Indications for removal of a functioning catheter include severe, unresponsive or recurrent peritonitis, peritonitis due to exit site and/ or tunnel infection, persistent exit site infection, tunnel infection with abscess, late recurrent dialysate leak, atypical peritonitis, bowel perforation, severe abdominal pain due to the catheter impinging on internal organs, and catheter cuff extrusion with infection.

84.18 Metabolic Complications of Peritoneal Dialysis

The majority of PD exchanges rely on hypertonic glucose solutions to provide osmotic clearance of water in combination with a buffer for acid base correction. Perhaps, unsurprisingly, this process can lead to metabolic complications that can have either systemic or local effects on the peritoneal membrane. Components of PD fluid other than glucose can also have metabolic consequences and these will be considered. The potential for PD to cause adverse effects resulting in morbidity and mortality underlines the need to prescribe and manage PD responsibly. Research is a priority to identify mechanisms to ameliorate these complications.

84.19 Systemic Metabolic Complications of Peritoneal Dialysis

The use of glucose as the osmotic agent in PD leads to the absorption of approximately 800 g of glucose per week. In healthy people an excess of glucose will be utilized and stored as glycogen or later as lipids. It is therefore reasonable to propose that PD patients may manage excess glucose in this manner resulting in an increase in fat mass or body weight. However, the relationship between glucose exposure, fat mass, and body weight is not consistent suggesting that many factors influence metabolism in this group of patients.

Dialysis has the potential to impact on appetite in several ways. Leptin, the product of the Ob gene, is secreted by fat cells and regulates food intake and energy expenditure in animal models. Whether the hyperleptinemia observed in uremic patients is involved in the anorexia that is often identified in this group is unclear. Studies have observed that in PD patients, particularly those with diabetes, leptin levels and body fat content increase. In those who lost lean body mass, higher leptin and initial CRP levels were recorded [36]. It is of interest that insulin has been identified as a regulator of leptin gene expression. With chronic hyperinsulinemia, leptin levels can increase significantly.

The impact of glucose-based PD on the glucose-insulin system has been investigated [37]. Galach et al. studied 3.86% glucose dwells lasting 6 hours in 13 non-diabetic patients who were clinically stable and fasting. Significant increases in plasma glucose and insulin were identified. Insulin resistance was noted in the majority of patients although they were, in general, able to control the glucose peaks related to PD. Disruption of the glucose insulin axis is one factor defining the metabolic syndrome. Other elements include hypertension, raised BMI, depressed high density lipoprotein levels, and raised triglycerides. Metabolic syndrome had been identified in approximately 50% of PD patients and is recognized as a risk factor for cardiovascular death [38]. The management of metabolic syndrome in PD patients is challenging as it can at least in part be attributed to the effects of exposure to hypertonic glucose dialysis solutions. Advice includes increased exercise to limit the effect of absorbed glucose and consequent fat deposition, often difficult to follow for patients with comorbid conditions. Pharmaceutical management of dyslipidemia is advisable as is BP control through appropriate salt water balance and use of hypotensive agents. Techniques to limit glucose exposure in peritoneal dialysis include the appropriate scheduling of exchanges, the use of non-glucose based fluids and optimization of residual renal function. As yet there are no controlled trials to guide the management of this complex metabolic problem; however, recommendations are made in the relevant ISPD guideline [39].

84.20 Long-Term Changes to the Peritoneal Membrane: Impact on Ultrafiltration Capacity and Patient Outcome

The Cardiff peritoneal biopsy registry explored the relationship between peritoneal structural changes and membrane functional in patients on PD [40]. Most prominently was the development of submesothelial fibrosis which increased significantly with the duration of PD, for example, 180 μm (micron) in those 0 to 24 months and up to 700 μm in those on PD for 97 months. Vascular abnormalities were also a prominent finding with degrees of vessel wall thickening and capillary dilation which was graded from 1 to 4 according to the degree of subendothelial hyaline material, luminal distortion or obliteration. The findings suggested a causal relationship between the vasculopathy and the membrane thickening implying that vasculopathy may result in relative ischemia exacerbating the fibrosis.

From the clinical perspective, long-term changes to the peritoneal membrane are demonstrated by a time-dependent increase in solute transfer associated with a decline in ultrafiltration capacity (the amount of water moving across the membrane in response to a particular glucose concentration over a defined time) occurring after about 4 years of treatment. In a study of 210 consecutive patients commencing PD, peritoneal kinetics stabilized in the first 6 months of treatment but thereafter there was a time dependent increase in solute transport which became significant at 42 months. In that study, high solute transport (measured using the peritoneal equilibration test[1]) and earlier loss of residual renal function were associated with poor outcome in patients on CAPD [41]. The patients with increasing solute transport had earlier loss in residual renal function and had been exposed to significantly more hypertonic glucose during the first 2 years of treatment that preceded the increase in solute transport. This was associated with greater achieved UF compensating for reduced residual renal function. This finding was confirmed in a 2003 report in which early and higher dialysate glucose exposure, which was in the context of higher comorbidity and lower residual renal function, was associated with a more rapid deterioration in membrane function [42]. Thus, the changes in the structural-functional relationship of the membrane could be predicted to some extent by clinical factors present within the first year. Patients with PD technique survival beyond 5 years were more likely to have preserved residual renal function, maintained nutrition, and medium small solute transport characteristics [43]. The coupling between the increase in D/P creatinine and the reduction in UF is due to the earlier loss of the osmotic gradient leading to reduced aquaporin mediated water transport and increased water reabsorption. Importantly, a group of patients develop a disproportionate fall in UF with time on PD due to a marked loss of UF capacity which may be an important marker of significant membrane damage. This has been confirmed in studies that examined changes in the sodium "dip" which is the dialysate to plasma sodium ratio after a 1-hour dwell using a hypertonic solution. Loss of this sodium dip is a marker of a reduction in water movement through water only pores and is likely to be a marker of peritoneal fibrosis, correlating with the subsequent development of EPS [44]. Icodextrin and automated peritoneal dialysis can be used to improve volume status in patients with higher transport status who have insufficient urine volume and there is evidence from various reports of the benefits of this approach, in particular a meta-analysis suggesting that the adverse effect of the high transport status on outcome has been mitigated in recent years [45].

With time on, PD patients are often prescribed increasing glucose loads. The chicken and egg question has been whether increased glucose load results in changes to the membrane leading to impaired ultrafiltration or whether impaired ultrafiltration related to membrane changes comes first causing physicians to increase the glucose concentrations in the patients' prescription. A retrospective analysis of prospectively gathered data from PD patients by Davies et al. [46] provided supporting evidence that the primary event is the exposure of the peritoneal membrane to hypertonic glucose which in turn contributes to changes in membrane function. A cohort of patients who had performed continuous PD for 5 years were identified and divided into those who had stable membrane function and those with increasing membrane transport characteristics. When these two groups were compared the patients with increasing membrane transport were noted to have experienced earlier loss of residual renal function and were exposed to higher glucose loads to compensate for this in advance of the recorded changes in membrane characteristics.

Concern has persisted regarding cytotoxic components of the dialysis fluid. Using in vitro techniques including cell growth inhibition and assessment of advanced glycosylation end-products (AGEs) formation, Wieslander and colleagues demonstrated that the low pH of glucose dialysates causes significant cytotoxicity, with glucose degradation products (GDP) and to a lesser extent osmolality and the presence of lactate also causing damage [47]. GDP are formed by the exposure of the dialysate glucose to heat during sterilization. The condensation of a carbonyl group on these sugars with a reactive amino group of a protein produces AGEs. In vivo studies have confirmed that the interaction of the AGE with the receptor (RAGE) leads to damage of the peritoneum in humans. Uremic patients' peritoneum already shows changes of fibrosis, angiogenesis, and RAGE activation. Those patients exposed to peritoneal dialysis with glucose-based fluids demonstrated further increase in these parameters. The AGE molecules have a physical effect on the structure of the membrane causing disruption to the matrix of the membrane as well as a functional effect. The AGE / RAGE interaction triggers cellular signal pathways involved in inflammation and fibrosis.

The observed long-term changes in the integrity of the peritoneal membrane have led to the development of dialysis solutions that are intended to be more "biocompatible" utilizing a neutral pH, and lower concentrations of glucose degradation products and in some cases bicarbonate as a buffer. This development requires more

1 The peritoneal equilibration test measures the dialysate to plasma ratio of creatinine (D/P creatinine) at the end of a 4-hour dwell using a dialysate with a 2.27% glucose concentration.

complex (and consequently expensive) technology, including the use of twin chamber bags to separate the buffer from the electrolyte components until mixing just prior to use, and to allow the glucose to be heat sterilized at a lower pH than conventionally which reduces the formation of GDPs. Several studies have tested these more biocompatible solutions by examining their impact on biomarkers of peritoneal membrane integrity or inflammation, and on clinical aspects including UF, residual renal function, and solute transport [48]. The BalANZ study is the largest randomized controlled trial of biocompatible peritoneal dialysate vs. standard dialysate to date [49] recruiting 185 incident peritoneal dialysis patients to this 2-year study. Patients were randomized 1:1 to receive either a neutral pH, lactate buffered, low GDP Balance solution (Fresenius Medical Care, Bad Homburg, Germany) or a conventional, standard, lactate-buffered PD solution. The primary outcome measure was the difference in the slope of the decline in residual renal function and this was not met. However, there was a significant difference between the groups, both in time to anuria ($p = 0.009$) and time to first peritonitis episode ($p = 0.01$) in favor of the more biocompatible solution. Indeed, the peritonitis rate in the biocompatible group was 0.30 vs. 0.49 ($p = 0.01$) episodes per year. In addition, there was a significant reduction in overall infection in the biocompatible group (4 non-PD infections out of 91 patients vs. 20 out of 91 in the control group). Thus, the biocompatible group demonstrated meaningful benefits in terms of infection and time to anuria compared with the control solution. Systematic review has confirmed that the use of biocompatible solutions is associated with better preservation of residual renal function [50].

84.21 Encapsulating Peritoneal Sclerosis

Encapsulating peritoneal sclerosis (EPS) is a rare but potentially devastating complication of peritoneal dialysis (PD). Diagnostic criteria have been published by the ISPD and are based on a combination of clinical features (such as the presence of inflammation, disturbance of gastrointestinal function) supported by confirmatory imaging (◘ Fig. 84.7) or laparotomy [51]. Onset is often insidious, presenting with nonspecific features of inflammation, weight loss and abdominal discomfort. Patient experience attests to often delayed diagnosis and a sense of "not being heard" by the medical team [52]. In full-blown form it causes failure of the gastrointestinal tract and death. Its sporadic nature, the difficulty in early diagnosis, as well as the lack of suitable animal models, means that at present the understanding of risk factors is incomplete and evidence-based therapies are lacking.

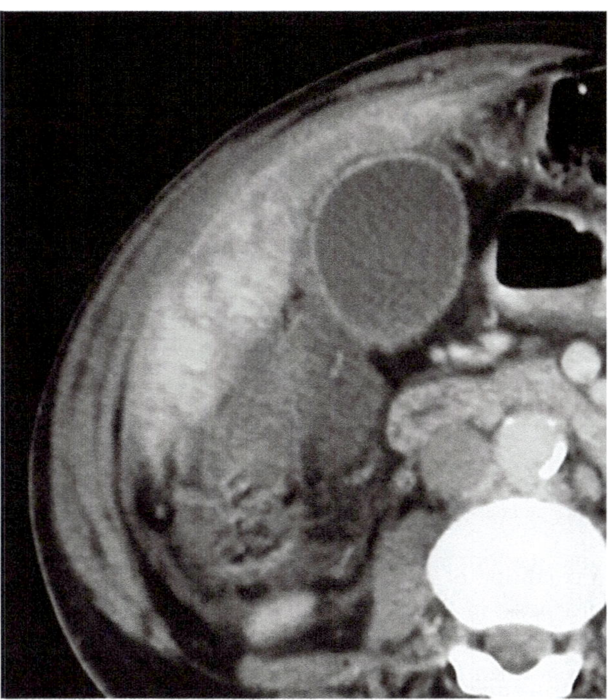

◘ **Fig. 84.7** CT scan from a patient with encapsulating peritoneal sclerosis demonstrating peritoneal thickening and cocoon formation

In some patients EPS seems to be a self-limiting condition that can be managed with appropriate nutritional support; whereas in others, the progression is rapid with the development of obstructive features and in these cases there is growing evidence that timely surgical intervention can be successful.

The Scottish Renal Registry reviewed all cases of encapsulating peritoneal sclerosis (EPS) [53] identified in Scotland from January 1, 2000, until December 31, 2007, and found an overall rate of 1.5%, however, the incidence increased with time on PD, reaching 8.1% (95% confidence interval: 3.6–17.6%) for those with 4 to 5 years exposure to the therapy. The Scottish data gave a similar prevalence of EPS to other key papers published since the Millennium of approximately 2–3% [54, 55], generally higher than that reported in earlier papers.

In the Scottish study, at diagnosis, 26% were on PD, whereas 63% were diagnosed within 1 year and 72% within 2 years of stopping PD; in 50% of the cases, patients had received a renal transplant before the diagnosis of EPS. Patients were likely to have discontinued PD because of ultrafiltration failure or inadequate dialysis and 65% of the cohort had used high-strength dextrose (3.86%) and 98% had used icodextrin, whereas no patients had used "bio-compatible" dialysis fluids exclusively. The cumulative risk is modest at 2.6% by 5 years, reflecting the reality that few patients continue PD beyond 4 years (◘ Fig. 84.8), and thus in a sense EPS is

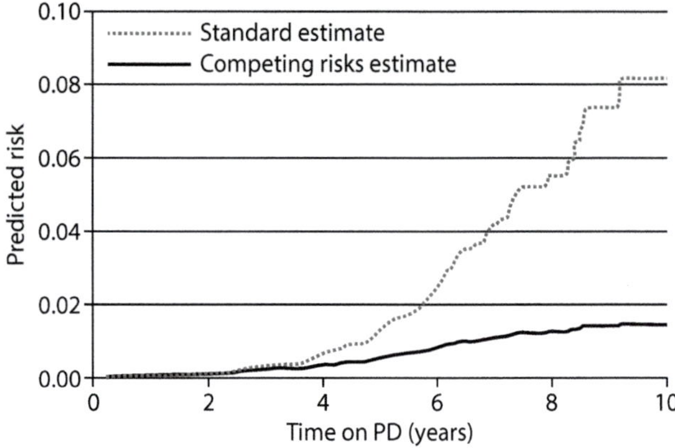

Fig. 84.8 Risk of encapsulating peritoneal sclerosis calculated using 'standard' and competing risks approaches (from Ref. [56])

a condition of survivors damaging the otherwise good prognosis in this younger group of patients. A recent analysis has demonstrated that EPS risk estimates are lower when calculated using competing risk of death analyses [56]. The mortality rate was 42% within 1 year of diagnosis, with the median survival from diagnosis being 180 days (range 1 to 1075).

84

Several cohort studies since the millennium [57–61] suggested either an increased disease frequency or at least an improved rate of diagnosis of PD-associated EPS, however more recently the Dutch EPS Registry reports a decline in incidence from 0.85% in 2009 to 0.14% in 2014 [8]. The reason for these changes is likely to be multifactorial and represents the influence of altered clinical management on a range of risk factors that are considered to be clinically relevant. These are reviewed in the latest ISPD guideline on this topic [9], and include PD exposure (time on PD), dialysate glucose concentrations and the possibility that icodextrin has a role as well as an association with discontinuing PD, and possibly renal transplantation. Good quality information on treatment for EPS is lacking and is based on case series reports; including nutritional optimization, the use of immunosuppressant agents, tamoxifen, and specialist surgery if clinical features fail to resolve with focused nutritional and medical treatment. The surgical method combines enterolysis with excision of the diseased peritoneum and cocooning membrane and should be performed at dedicated national centers [62]. Major outstanding questions remain around risk factors, diagnosis and treatment and large prospective studies are required.

Chapter Review Questions

1. What factors influence the decision around the most appropriate catheter insertion technique?
2. A patient on peritoneal dialysis is being treated with intraperitoneal antibiotics for an episode of peritonitis – what other treatment should be considered?
3. A patient who has previously been well on peritoneal dialysis starts to develop oedema and weight gain – what is the most likely explanation?
4. A patient on automated peritoneal dialysis who has lost residual renal function has become under dialysed. What is the first step?
5. You are tasked to develop quality improvement systems for your PD unit. What should you focus on?

Answers

1. Randomised controlled trials do not show advantage for one technique over another, although cohort studies suggest advantages for the laparoscopic insertion combined with advanced techniques. It is important that the catheter insertion pathway is responsive to need and is individualised. In other words for individuals within the normal body mass ranges who have not had previous lower abdominal surgery a percutaneous insertion under local anaesthetic by an expert operator is a good option – whereas in more complex cases surgical approaches will be necessary.
2. It is important to prescribe antifungal therapy for the duration of the antibiotics to reduce the risk of subsequent fungal peritonitis. This can either take the form of oral nystatin or fluconazole.
3. It is likely that the residual renal function has fallen. This can be measured using a 24 hour urine collection. If the patient is still passing urine one step that can be taken is to increase oral diuretic doses up to 240 mg of furosemide in divided doses (morning and lunch). A second step is to ensure that fluid is not being absorbed from any of the dialysis exchanges. The third step is to adjust the PD prescription to improve ultrafiltration.
4. The easiest course of action is to add a day time exchange if they do not have one already. Subsequent to that, it may be necessary to increase the volume of the overnight exchanges. This is guided by the patient's small solute transport status.
5. The two key areas to focus on are access and infection. You should ensure that regular audit of peritonitis and exit site infection rates are being conducted and shared with the team with a focus on root cause analysis to under stand the causes of individual cases. It is also important to audit the outcome of peritoneal dialysis catheter insertion. Important audit targets are 0.5 episodes of peritonitis per year for patient at risk (see ► ispd.org for guideline documents); for catheter patency the following guidance has been given – "Catheter patency at 12 months of > 95% for advanced laparoscopic placement and > 80% for all other catheter insertion methods". There is a value in auditing at 3 months post insertion since 1 year is rather too long to wait.

References

1. Yeates K, Zhu N, Vonesh E, Trpeski L, Blake P, Fenton S. Hemodialysis and peritoneal dialysis are associated with similar outcomes for end-stage renal disease treatment in Canada. Nephrol Dial Transplant. 2012;27(9):3568–75.
2. Korevaar JC, Feith GW, Dekker FW, van Manen JG, Boeschoten EW, Bossuyt PM, et al. Effect of starting with hemodialysis compared with peritoneal dialysis in patients new on dialysis treatment: a randomized controlled trial. Kidney Int. 2003;64(6):2222–8.
3. Nataatmadja M, Cho Y, Johnson DW. Continuous quality improvement initiatives to sustainably reduce peritoneal dialysis-related infections in Australia and New Zealand. Perit Dial Int. 2016;36(5):472–7.
4. Kolesnyk I, Dekker FW, Boeschoten EW, Krediet RT. Time-dependent reasons for peritoneal dialysis technique failure and mortality. Perit Dial Int. 2010;30(2):170–7.
5. Perl J, Davies SJ, Lambie M, Pisoni RL, McCullough K, Johnson DW, et al. The peritoneal dialysis outcomes and practice patterns study (PDOPPS): unifying efforts to inform practice and improve global outcomes in peritoneal dialysis. Perit Dial Int. 2016;36(3):297–307.
6. Williams VR, Quinn R, Callery S, Kiss A, Oliver MJ. The impact of treatment modality on infection-related hospitalization rates in peritoneal dialysis and hemodialysis patients. Perit Dial Int. 2011;31(4):440–9.
7. Hole B, Caskey F, Evans K, Fluck R, Kumwenda M, Steenkamp R, et al. UK renal registry 19th annual report: chapter 12 multisite dialysis access audit in England, Northern Ireland and Wales in 2015 and 2014 PD one year follow-up: national and Centre-specific analyses. Nephron. 2017;137(Suppl 1): 269–96.
8. Betjes MG, Habib SM, Boeschoten EW, Hemke AC, Struijk DG, Westerhuis R, et al. Significant decreasing incidence of encapsulating peritoneal sclerosis in the dutch population of peritoneal dialysis patients. Perit Dial Int. 2017;37(2):230–4.
9. Brown EA, Bargman J, van Biesen W, Chang MY, Finkelstein FO, Hurst H, et al. Length of time on peritoneal dialysis and encapsulating peritoneal sclerosis - position paper for ISPD: 2017 update. Perit Dial Int. 2017;37(4):362–74.
10. Figueiredo AE, Bernardini J, Bowes E, Hiramatsu M, Price V, Su C, et al. A syllabus for teaching peritoneal dialysis to patients and caregivers. Perit Dial Int. 2016;36(6):592–605.
11. Verger C, Ryckelynck JP, Duman M, Veniez G, Lobbedez T, Boulanger E, et al. French peritoneal dialysis registry (RDPLF): outline and main results. Kidney Int Suppl. 2006;103:S12–20.
12. Li PK, Szeto CC, Piraino B, de Arteaga J, Fan S, Figueiredo AE, et al. ISPD peritonitis recommendations: 2016 update on prevention and treatment. Perit Dial Int. 2016;36(5):481–508.
13. Crabtree JH, Shrestha BM, Chow KM, Figueiredo AE, Povlsen JV, Wilkie M, et al. Creating and maintaining optimal peritoneal dialysis access in the adult patient: 2019 update. Perit Dial Int. 2019;39(5):414–36.
14. Xu G, Tu W, Xu C. Mupirocin for preventing exit-site infection and peritonitis in patients undergoing peritoneal dialysis. Nephrol Dial Transplant. 2010;25(2):587–92.
15. Shrestha BM, Brown P, Wilkie M. Surgical peritonitis in patients on peritoneal dialysis. Perit Dial Int. 2008;28(4):331–4.
16. Moraes TP, Pecoits-Filho R, Ribeiro SC, Rigo M, Silva MM, Teixeira PS, et al. Peritoneal dialysis in Brazil: twenty-five years of experience in a single center. Perit Dial Int. 2009;29(5): 492–8.
17. Van Biesen W, Veys N, Vanholder R, Lameire N. Peritoneal-dialysis-related peritonitis: the art of rope-dancing. Nephrol Dial Transplant. 2002;17(11):1878–82.
18. Toleman MA. The future of peritoneal dialysis in a moving landscape of bacterial resistance. Perit Dial Int. 2017;37(2): 134–40.
19. Ballinger AE, Palmer SC, Wiggins KJ, Craig JC, Johnson DW, Cross NB, et al. Treatment for peritoneal dialysis-associated peritonitis. Cochrane Database Syst Rev. 2014;4:CD005284.
20. Bailie GR, Eisele G. Pharmacokinetic issues in the treatment of continuous ambulatory peritoneal dialysis-associated peritonitis. J Antimicrob Chemother. 1995;35(5):563–7.
21. Szeto CC, Li PK, Johnson DW, Bernardini J, Dong J, Figueiredo AE, et al. ISPD catheter-related infection recommendations: 2017 update. Perit Dial Int. 2017;37(2):141–54.
22. Schaefer F, Klaus G, Muller-Wiefel DE, Mehls O. Intermittent versus continuous intraperitoneal glycopeptide/ceftazidime treatment in children with peritoneal dialysis-associated peritonitis. The Mid-European Pediatric Peritoneal Dialysis Study Group (MEPPS). J Am Soc Nephrol. 1999;10(1):136–45.
23. Boudville N, Johnson DW, Zhao J, Bieber BA, Pisoni RL, Piraino B, et al. Regional variation in the treatment and prevention of peritoneal dialysis-related infections in the Peritoneal Dialysis Outcomes and Practice Patterns Study. Nephrol Dial Transplant. 2019;34(12):2118–26.
24. Oliver MJ, Verrelli M, Zacharias JM, Blake PG, Garg AX, Johnson JF, et al. Choosing peritoneal dialysis reduces the risk of invasive access interventions. Nephrol Dial Transplant. 2012;27(2):810–6.
25. See EJ, Johnson DW, Hawley CM, Pascoe EM, Badve SV, Boudville N, et al. Risk predictors and causes of technique failure within the first year of peritoneal dialysis: an Australia and New Zealand dialysis and transplant registry (ANZDATA) study. Am J Kidney Dis. 2018;72(2):188–97.
26. Boujelbane L, Fu N, Chapla K, Melnick D, Redfield RR, Waheed S, et al. Percutaneous versus surgical insertion of PD catheters in dialysis patients: a meta-analysis. J Vasc Access. 2015;16(6):498–505.
27. Tullavardhana T, Akranurakkul P, Ungkitphaiboon W, Songtish D. Surgical versus percutaneous techniques for peritoneal dialysis catheter placement: a meta-analysis of the outcomes. Ann Med Surg (Lond). 2016;10:11–8.
28. Xie H, Zhang W, Cheng J, He Q. Laparoscopic versus open catheter placement in peritoneal dialysis patients: a systematic review and meta-analysis. BMC Nephrol. 2012;13:69.
29. Shrestha BM, Shrestha D, Kumar A, Shrestha A, Boyes SA, Wilkie ME. Advanced laparoscopic peritoneal dialysis catheter insertion: systematic review and meta-analysis. Perit Dial Int. 2018;38(3):163–71.
30. Crabtree J, Shrestha B, Chow KM, Figueiredo A, Povlsen J, Wilkie M, Abdel-Aal A, Cullis B, Goh BL, Briggs V, Brown E, Dor F. Creating and maintaining optimal peritoneal dialysis access in the adult patient: 2019 update. Perit Dial Int. 2019 - *in press* Peritoneal Dialysis International.
31. Campos RP, Chula DC, Riella MC. Complications of the peritoneal access and their management. Contrib Nephrol. 2009;163:183–97.
32. Lew SQ. Hemoperitoneum: bloody peritoneal dialysate in ESRD patients receiving peritoneal dialysis. Perit Dial Int. 2007;27(3):226–33.
33. Greenberg A, Bernardini J, Piraino BM, Johnston JR, Perlmutter JA. Hemoperitoneum complicating chronic peritoneal dialysis: single-center experience and literature review. Am J Kidney Dis. 1992;19(3):252–6.

34. Keshvari A, Najafi I, Jafari-Javid M, Yunesian M, Chaman R, Taromlou MN. Laparoscopic peritoneal dialysis catheter implantation using a Tenckhoff trocar under local anesthesia with nitrous oxide gas insufflation. Am J Surg. 2009;197(1):8–13.
35. Sharma AP, Mandhani A, Daniel SP, Filler G. Shorter break-in period is a viable option with tighter PD catheter securing during the insertion. Nephrology (Carlton). 2008;13(8):672–6.
36. Stenvinkel P, Lindholm B, Lonnqvist F, Katzarski K, Heimburger O. Increases in serum leptin levels during peritoneal dialysis are associated with inflammation and a decrease in lean body mass. J Am Soc Nephrol. 2000;11(7):1303–9.
37. Galach M, Waniewski J, Axelsson J, Heimburger O, Werynski A, Lindholm B. Mathematical modeling of the glucose-insulin system during peritoneal dialysis with glucose-based fluids. ASAIO J. 2011;57(1):41–7.
38. Park JT, Chang TI, Kim DK, Lee JE, Choi HY, Kim HW, et al. Metabolic syndrome predicts mortality in non-diabetic patients on continuous ambulatory peritoneal dialysis. Nephrol Dial Transplant. 2010;25(2):599–604.
39. Wang AY, Brimble KS, Brunier G, Holt SG, Jha V, Johnson DW, et al. ISPD cardiovascular and metabolic guidelines in adult peritoneal dialysis patients Part II – management of various cardiovascular complications. Perit Dial Int. 2015;35(4):388–96.
40. Williams JD, Craig KJ, Topley N, Von Ruhland C, Fallon M, Newman GR, et al. Morphologic changes in the peritoneal membrane of patients with renal disease. J Am Soc Nephrol. 2002;13(2):470–9.
41. Davies SJ, Phillips L, Russell GI. Peritoneal solute transport predicts survival on CAPD independently of residual renal function. Nephrol Dial Transplant. 1998;13(4):962–8.
42. Davies SJ. Longitudinal relationship between solute transport and ultrafiltration capacity in peritoneal dialysis patients. Kidney Int. 2004;66(6):2437–45.
43. Davies SJ, Phillips L, Griffiths AM, Russell LH, Naish PF, Russell GI. What really happens to people on long-term peritoneal dialysis? Kidney Int. 1998;54(6):2207–17.
44. Morelle J, Sow A, Hautem N, Bouzin C, Crott R, Devuyst O, et al. Interstitial fibrosis restricts osmotic water transport in encapsulating peritoneal sclerosis. J Am Soc Nephrol. 2015;26(10):2521–33.
45. Brimble KS, Walker M, Margetts PJ, Kundhal KK, Rabbat CG. Meta-analysis: peritoneal membrane transport, mortality, and technique failure in peritoneal dialysis. J Am Soc Nephrol. 2006;17(9):2591–8.
46. Davies SJ, Phillips L, Naish PF, Russell GI. Peritoneal glucose exposure and changes in membrane solute transport with time on peritoneal dialysis. J Am Soc Nephrol. 2001;12(5):1046–51.
47. Wieslander A, Linden T, Kjellstrand P. Glucose degradation products in peritoneal dialysis fluids: how they can be avoided. Perit Dial Int. 2001;21(Suppl 3):S119–24.
48. Pajek J, Kveder R, Bren A, Gucek A, Ihan A, Osredkar J, et al. Short-term effects of a new bicarbonate/lactate-buffered and conventional peritoneal dialysis fluid on peritoneal and systemic inflammation in CAPD patients: a randomized controlled study. Perit Dial Int. 2008;28(1):44–52.
49. Johnson DW, Brown FG, Clarke M, Boudville N, Elias TJ, Foo MWY, et al. Effects of biocompatible versus standard fluid on peritoneal dialysis outcomes. J Am Soc Nephrol. 2012;23(6):1097–107.
50. Seo EY, An SH, Cho JH, Suh HS, Park SH, Gwak H, et al. Effect of biocompatible peritoneal dialysis solution on residual renal function: a systematic review of randomized controlled trials. Perit Dial Int. 2014;34(7):724–31.
51. Kawaguchi Y, Kawanishi H, Mujais S, Topley N, Oreopoulos DG. Encapsulating peritoneal sclerosis: definition, etiology, diagnosis, and treatment. International Society for Peritoneal Dialysis Ad Hoc Committee on Ultrafiltration Management in Peritoneal Dialysis. Perit Dial Int. 2000;20(Suppl 4):S43–55.
52. Hurst H, Summers A, Beaver K, Caress AL. Living with encapsulating peritoneal sclerosis (EPS): the patient's perspective. Perit Dial Int. 2014;34(7):758–65.
53. Brown MC, Simpson K, Kerssens JJ, Mactier RA. Encapsulating peritoneal sclerosis in the new millennium: a national cohort study. Clin J Am Soc Nephrol. 2009;4(7):1222–9.
54. Kawanishi H, Kawaguchi Y, Fukui H, Hara S, Imada A, Kubo H, et al. Encapsulating peritoneal sclerosis in Japan: a prospective, controlled, multicenter study. Am J Kidney Dis. 2004;44(4):729–37.
55. Summers AM, Clancy MJ, Syed F, Harwood N, Brenchley PE, Augustine T, et al. Single-center experience of encapsulating peritoneal sclerosis in patients on peritoneal dialysis for end-stage renal failure. Kidney Int. 2005;68(5):2381–8.
56. Lambie M, Teece L, Johnson DW, Petrie M, Mactier R, Solis-Trapala I, et al. Estimating risk of encapsulating peritoneal sclerosis accounting for the competing risk of death. Nephrol Dial Transplant. 2019;34(9):1585–91.
57. Korte MR, Sampimon DE, Lingsma HF, Fieren MW, Looman CW, Zietse R, et al. Risk factors associated with encapsulating peritoneal sclerosis in Dutch EPS study. Perit Dial Int. 2011;31(3):269–78.
58. Johnson DW, Cho Y, Livingston BE, Hawley CM, McDonald SP, Brown FG, et al. Encapsulating peritoneal sclerosis: incidence, predictors, and outcomes. Kidney Int. 2010;77(10):904–12.
59. Lambie ML, John B, Mushahar L, Huckvale C, Davies SJ. The peritoneal osmotic conductance is low well before the diagnosis of encapsulating peritoneal sclerosis is made. Kidney Int. 2010;78(6):611–8.
60. Gayomali C, Hussein U, Cameron SF, Protopapas Z, Finkelstein FO. Incidence of encapsulating peritoneal sclerosis: a single-center experience with long-term peritoneal dialysis in the United States. Perit Dial Int. 2011;31(3):279–86.
61. Balasubramaniam G, Brown EA, Davenport A, Cairns H, Cooper B, Fan SL, et al. The pan-Thames EPS study: treatment and outcomes of encapsulating peritoneal sclerosis. Nephrol Dial Transplant. 2009;24(10):3209–15.
62. Kawanishi H, Banshodani M, Yamashita M, Shintaku S. Surgical treatment for encapsulating peritoneal sclerosis: 24 years' experience. Perit Dial Int. 2018;39(2):169–74.

Transplantation

Contents

Setting-Up and Running a Renal Transplant Unit

Andrew Ready and Jennie Jewitt-Harris

Contents

M. Harber (ed.), *Primer on Nephrology*, https://doi.org/10.1007/978-3-030-76419-7_85

Case Study

MK is a 46-year-old farm manager in a LMIC. He is married to CK, and they have two children. His job provides a reasonable wage, and he considers himself secure and fortunate. However, at the age of 35, he was diagnosed with CKD of unknown cause. He progressed quickly to end stage and, being close to a dialysis unit, was commenced on hemodialysis. Although this kept him alive, he suffered chronic ill health, forcing him to miss work and put his income in jeopardy.

Moreover, MK had to pay for his dialysis and soon developed financial difficulties. He had seen dialysis patients reach the stage where they were unable to afford treatment, withdrew from dialysis and died. MK and his wife worried that he would suffer the same fate, and the stress affected the whole family. When they heard that a renal transplant was possible locally, CK immediately put herself forward as a living donor. CK was suitable, and KP underwent a successful living donor renal transplant from his wife. Within weeks he was able to return to work. Eight years later, he remains well, and despite having to pay for his medication, his financial state has improved as he has returned to regular work and been promoted. CK says that the transplant allowed them to become a normal family again. She remains well with no regrets about giving a kidney. She says that the best sound she knows is when her husband gets up in the night to pass urine. When she hears that she knows all is well in her world.

Learning Objectives

1. To recognize the need for development of renal transplantation in LMIC.
2. To identify safe stepwise plan toward performing units' first renal transplant.
3. To highlight the importance and value of developing a strong mentoring relationship with individuals from establishing a transplant unit.
4. To define continued unit development onward from the time of first transplantation to routine transplant practice and doing so in a way that incorporates comprehensive clinical governance.
5. To emphasize the critical importance of team working in renal transplantation.

85.1 Introduction

Successful renal transplantation (RTx) has been possible for more than 50 years, and in high-income countries (HIC), it is no longer an experimental procedure but a standard therapy. Advances in RTx have paralleled those in dialysis, so in HIC, virtually everyone reaching end-stage renal failure (ESRF) receives dialysis or RTx. Few die as a direct result of lack of treatment.

Unfortunately, in low- and middle-income countries (LMIC), this situation is frequently reversed. Only a minority of patients progressing to ESRF receive adequate Renal Replacement Therapy (RRT) [1], while the number transplanted in LMIC is small and unevenly distributed. This situation should not be viewed over-critically since LMICs have faced many challenges, including the overwhelming effect of infectious disease, which has required prioritization of limited resources. Since RRT is expensive and open-ended it was perhaps inevitable that its provision would lag behind other considerations.

Nevertheless, such prioritization now risks failing the growing burden of chronic kidney disease (CKD) in LMIC and the opportunity presented by RTx for patients to return to a near-normal and productive life. While accurate registry data from LMIC is sparse [2, 3] it is generally accepted that the incidence of CKD in LMIC is considerable. While the mean global prevalence of CKD is estimated to be 8–16% [4], it is undoubtedly higher in LMIC. This excess may relate to an increased predisposition to CKD in certain ethnic groups and the impact of higher incidences of diabetes and hypertension. In some regions, causes such as herbal and environmental toxins are more common, while elsewhere local causes drive CKD [5]. These factors are amplified by poverty, with the poorest populations carrying the highest risk [4]. The effect of CKD is compounded by disease presenting in younger patients [6] and at a more advanced stage. Hence young individuals are lost from the workforce and their families.

There is now an increasing awareness of these issues, particularly in middle-income countries. This development is prompted by increasing wealth, often from natural resources, along with epidemiological changes in which the growth of an educated middle class, combined with the availability of web-based information, has led to a growing awareness of CKD, its causes, and treatment options. Consequently, efforts are increasingly directed to making RRT more widely available.

While these factors have led to the development of dialysis in LMIC [5], its provision is far from adequate. Dialysis availability is at best patchy [7], and is associated with an unequal distribution of nephrologists [8], and variable access to medications and services [9]. The quality of dialysis is often suboptimal [10, 11] and pediatric dialysis units almost nonexistent. As such, the perceived quality of health infrastructure supporting

CKD care has been rated poor to extremely poor in over 40% of low-income countries [12]. Nevertheless, a start has been made and progress must be encouraged with an emphasis on increasing nephrology support and the availability of high-quality dialysis.

Even so, dialysis should not be the definitive treatment for ESRF in LMIC any more than it is in HIC. Dialysis is life-saving but compared to RTx provides an inferior quality of life, reduced survival, increased co-morbidity, and is more expensive [5]. Where the healthcare providers cover costs, the funding of complex infrastructure and running costs soon strain economies. Where out-of-pocket payment is required from patients, financial hardship is likely, and accounts of patients dying for lack of funds to maintain dialysis costs, as per the included case history, are not unusual [13]. When the relatively small number of transplants performed in LMIC are compared with the number of patients receiving dialysis [5], it is clear that the benefits of RTx are disproportionately under-delivered in LMIC, even though it represents the most cost-effective treatment [14].

Once the need to provide treatment for ESRF has been recognized, the pressure should mount to make RTx more available, and the reasons why it is not available should be examined.

Reasons often include the lack of trained personnel, inadequate infrastructure, poor financing, cultural factors, and the legal environment, amplified by poverty and inadequate health policies [15]. When compounded by commercial incentives favoring dialysis and geographical remoteness, inadequate access to transplantation has been almost inevitable for much of the world's population [14]. Hence, change is needed before transplantation becomes readily available, and change takes time.

Initially, the provision of transplantation can be met by CKD patients going abroad for transplantation. Indeed, formal arrangements in which governments send donor-recipient pairs abroad to undergo transplantation have been relatively frequent. If done in an ethically appropriate fashion, this may be successful for some individual patients, but overall, this option has serious drawbacks [16] related to outcomes, ethical accountability, and cost. It is not the answer to the rapidly growing number of patients diagnosed with CKD.

85.2 Developing New Transplant Units

Due to growing clinical need and lack of suitable alternatives, it seems that the third decade of the twenty-first century will witness growing demands to establish new RTx units in LMIC. For those developing such units, the task may appear daunting. The barriers mentioned must be overcome and complex skills, developed over many decades, acquired quickly. However, decades of transplant evolution have created well-structured management plans, and there is no need for the process to be reinvented, although adaptations may be needed to address local requirements. A checklist of the key stages that should be worked through toward a first transplant is shown in ▶ Box 85.1.

Even so, the process of developing genuinely sustainable transplant programs is complex and requires years of concerted effort. When faced with such a task, it is advisable to start making long-term plans before any transplants are performed, even though the temptation to rush to transplant may feel irresistible. Performing transplants is an intensive process and risks diverting energies from long-term planning toward short-term gains with the objective to treat many patients into the future, not merely a few now.

At an early stage of this planning process, it is appropriate to confront the negatives that most new units face. Often, on top of the list, is a lack of confidence that the task can be achieved. Perhaps, other developments have not been achievable. Why should this be any different? As a counter, it must be emphasized that the clinical

Box 85.1 Key Stages Toward First Transplant

- Establish the local clinical need and develop an outline plan
- Investigate other transplant centers in your region and establish how they got started
- Define the main challenges
- Discuss with local and national policy makers
- Establish the core members of the clinical transplant team
- Develop links to wider transplant services
  - Nursing, histocompatibility, pathology, radiology. operating theaters
- Recruit wider support to help development – patients, legal opinion, management
- Approach a mentor/support transplant team to establish a long-term partnership
- Agree the skillsets and services that are needed
- Establish legal and ethical framework
- Identify and workup patients and living donors first with mentor support
- Develop a realistic timescale for first transplants and steps needed toward this goal

need presented by CKD is so substantial that development is desperately needed. With proper planning, team working, confronting the economic difficulties, and by harnessing patients' voices, initial steps may be taken with heightened confidence that success is possible—as it has been elsewhere. A concern previously encountered at developing centers is that transplantation may be too complicated for their LMIC environment. However, neither the surgical techniques nor medical management required are beyond the capabilities of clinicians and healthcare professionals in National Centers in LMICs. Indeed, it is these healthcare teams who are best placed to adapt and deliver services for their populations.

From the outset, planning must recognize that transplantation is a multidisciplinary process, demanding an initial team of clinicians drawn from the principal areas of nephrology and surgery (vascular or urology). This team forms a core group of enthusiastic clinicians who can drive the development process and recruit members of the broader transplant team. From this core group, it is useful for a lead clinician, or 'local champion' to emerge and take organizational responsibility. This person will likely be a nephrologist. Such clinicians are likely to have developed local renal services and are the natural advocates of their CKD patients. They also have a duty of care to their dialysis patients that includes moving treatment toward RTx. However, the champion could equally be a surgeon, perhaps with transplant experience from working in a preexisting transplant unit. Less important than the specialty is that the champion takes the transplant process forward, orchestrating systematic development, ensuring appropriate communication with stakeholders, putting in place the mentoring, training, and support needed and assembling the required resources.

The core group will also likely be charged with distilling the clinical and economic arguments into a business case to share with Ministers of Health or equivalent policymakers. In this process, clinicians are the principal advocates for their patients' needs and must lobby governments for the provision of transplantation services and the legal infrastructure needed. In countries where governments cover the cost of dialysis, the decision to extend cover to include transplantation is not difficult since overall care costs are reduced. However, where patients fund dialysis through out-of-pocket payments, governments may be less eager to support transplantation if this requires additional central expenditure. Government/ministerial support is therefore critical to addressing the financial barriers, and clear and persuasive arguments must be included in business cases [5]. Government support may also be required for the development of legislative changes required for transplantation [16].

In constructing such proposals, it is also important to define the clinical need and to provide appropriate timescales, recognizing that program development invariably takes longer than expected. Realistic estimates help avoid later misunderstandings about the pace of progress.

It is also essential to recognize that initial transplants will most likely be from living rather than deceased donors [16]. Deceased donor transplantation is, on balance, a too complex starting point for most developing units [5]. Deceased donation requires additional infrastructure and intensive care units, which are often sparse in LMIC. Facilities to make the diagnosis of brain death may be limited while histocompatibility services are generally lacking. A deceased donor program may also face conflicting cultural attitudes toward death and national legislation requirements. With these significant challenges, it is more appropriate to start with living donation. Furthermore, as living donation can be planned, this facilitates the organization of surgical, nephrology, and nursing skill transfer with mentoring support. Also, the legal and cultural challenges to living donation are usually less than for a deceased donor program.

Once a living donor-based business plan has been successfully developed, and support approved, a reasonable next step is to begin identifying suitable recipients from the local dialysis population and begin discussions with potential donors. As part of this process, it is realistic to initially identify potential donors and recipients who have the lowest levels of complexity and so the highest chance of success. These are likely to be recipients who are well on dialysis, or possibly pre-dialysis. Donors should be healthy individuals, probably first-degree relatives who are eager to donate to their loved one. In both donors and recipients, there should be a minimum of anatomical complexity, with standard BMIs, healthy iliac vessels in recipients and standard renal, ureteric, and vascular anatomy in donors.

As such clinical issues are addressed, it is vital that the ethical issues inherent in transplantation, and particularly living donation, are recognized and openly confronted. The ethical challenges of transplantation are well known [14, 16], and all activity must comply with the internationally recognized Declaration of Istanbul [17]. To ensure that the ethical issues of living donor transplantation are upheld, early in unit development, an ethics committee should be assembled [18] for the discussion of general program policies and to implement a process for the review of all living donor cases. The committee must be responsive to issues that are ubiquitous to transplantation, including the avoidance of coercion and payment for donation, ensuring competency to consent to donation and that consent is fully informed. The committee should be composed of healthcare professionals and lay members who can assess the issues from a neutral standpoint with decision-making removed from the transplant team to avoid conflict of interest. It is also valuable to include a psychologist who can review patients, and particularly potential living donors, and report concerns back to the committee.

It is then necessary to start educating staff in the proposed unit regarding matters of RTx since it is unlikely that they will have any direct experience of the specialty. This includes nurses (operating theatre, HDU and post-op ward), pharmacists, intensive care unit staff, and also administrative staff who are likely to come into contact with transplant patients.

Fledgling units in LMIC will likely be geographically isolated from other transplant units. However, there is no need to undertake development in isolation as many existing units in HIC are willing to share their experience. Initial observational visits to such units can provide a rapid update in techniques and protocols. Also, most HIC, including the UK, have National Transplant Guidelines, including for living donation. These documents are invaluable in directing unit and protocol development and are usually available online [19].

However, visiting units and reviewing guidelines are rarely adequate when the time comes to start transplanting. Therefore, once the time is approaching for a program to 'go live', it is essential to identify experts early in the process with whom to collaborate and obtain mentorship. Only with the combination of support and teaching that comes with well-delivered mentorship will the first series of transplants occur with the required combination of safety and learning. It is important to avoid the mistake of assuming that the mentorship or support needed is only surgical. The support needed for nephrology work-up and post-tx management is also vital for the long-term success of the program, as is mentorship in nursing and other related services such as radiology, anesthetics and pathology. In preparation for this event, it is necessary to work with a mentoring team to finalize program structure, share the clinical assessment of the potential donor-recipient pairs and to assemble sufficient personnel 'on the ground' to perform the first transplants. The first cases are best done by the mentoring team as 'demonstration cases' (◘ Fig. 85.1), with access open to all members of the local team, allowing previously theoretical concepts to become a reality.

To ask professionals from elsewhere to invest time and energy in developing a program in a distant location may seem a difficult request. However, the transplantation community is global and increasingly looks toward assisting colleagues who wish to develop programs, and several options are available. These include global initiatives by the international transplantation and nephrology societies [14, 20], which encourage training fellowships and long-term twinning between developed and developing centers. Individual established units may be able to provide mentoring support, and personal links made by LMIC clinicians during training in HIC

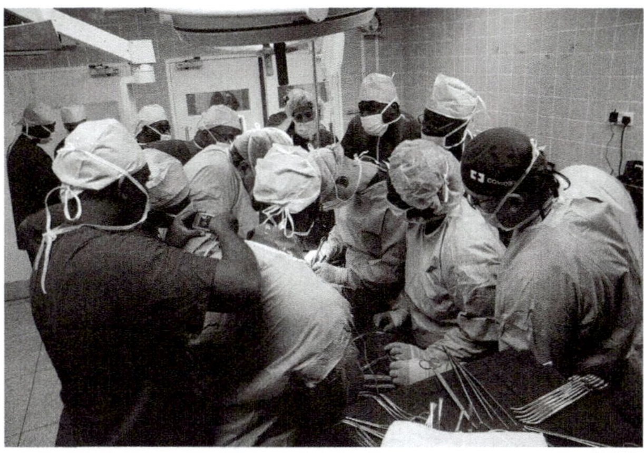

◘ **Fig. 85.1** Ghana's first transplant, performed at the Korle Bu Hospital, Accra by the Transplant Links mentoring team

can provide the catalyst for mentoring relationships to develop. Support is also available through independent groups such as our own Transplant Links Community which, funded by charitable donations and supported by experienced NHS transplant clinicians, has been mentoring developing units through skill transfer for more than a decade [21]. With all of these options, an initial approach is all that is required. From there, a lasting mentoring relationship can develop from which a new transplant program can emerge.

85.3 The Extended Transplant Team

Once these factors have been addressed, it is again important to recognize that transplantation is a multidisciplinary process, and it is necessary to develop the extended team (◘ Fig. 85.2). While many hospital departments will have a place in transplant management, the more specific members of the extended team include:

▪ Histocompatibility

Histocompatibility testing is required for tissue typing patients before transplantation to assess matches between recipients and donors. It is also used to assess the presence of preformed donor-specific antibodies before transplantation, as reflected in the pretransplant, antibody crossmatch, and to monitor donor-specific antibodies after transplantation.

Histocompatibility services are costly and require specialist infrastructure and expertise. It is unlikely that a preexisting local histocompatibility laboratory will be available or that stakeholders will want to invest resources into developing such a facility before transplantation is established. It Is likely, therefore, that histocompatibility testing will initially be outsourced to an existing laboratory, even in another country. This option

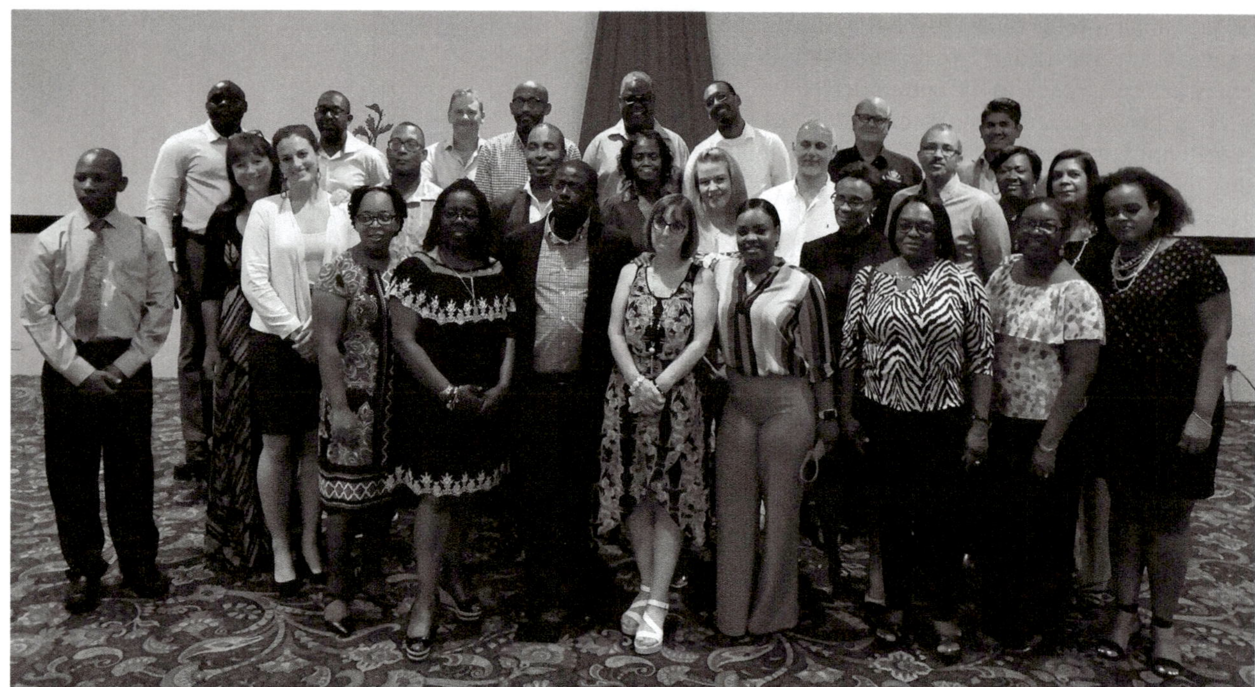

Fig. 85.2 The transplant team of the University Hospital of the West Indies, Kingston, Jamaica, together with the visiting Transplant Links mentoring team

can work well using courier services for sample transfer. Nevertheless, arrangement for distant assays should be made in advance of any transplants to ensure that the services are reliable and timely and included in the overall budget.

▪ Pharmacy

The hospital pharmacy must be involved at an early stage of transplant unit development to source immunosuppression and other essential drugs. Sources should be reliable and sustainable since patients will require a consistent source of immunosuppression for the duration of their transplant.

The cost of immunosuppression can be a challenge for units in LMIC, although, the cessation of dialysis may offset these costs. Nevertheless, this is only a minor concession if patients are required to cover immunosuppression cost themselves. Pharmacists may be able to identify the cheapest options available, and many immunosuppressive agents have now fallen from patent restrictions, with good quality cheaper and bioequivalent generic versions being produced. However, these agents are not always readily available in LMIC [16] and may need to be actively sourced.

▪ Pathology Services

A full range of easily accessible pathology services is essential to support the activity of a renal transplant unit, including:

▪▪ Histology

The rapid reporting of renal biopsies is required both before and after transplantation. Before transplantation, native biopsies define the cause of CKD and are particularly important in identifying conditions such as focal segmental glomerulosclerosis (FSGS) that may recur in a transplant. Posttransplant, percutaneous graft biopsies are essential to identify acute rejection, both cellular and antibody-mediated. Also, to identify the cause of chronic graft dysfunction.

Therefore, a pathologist with expertise in renal histopathology must be included in the transplant team. If not, the services of such an individual should be secured, even at a distance, before transplants are performed.

▪▪ Biochemistry

Most units will have access to clinical biochemistry, but it is essential to ensure that renal function tests, and other biochemical tests, are available 24 hours per day, 7 days a week. It is also vital that arrangements are made for assays of drug levels, particularly of the critical dose immunosuppressants. Initially, such drug levels may be devolved to laboratories with preexisting assays. However, for long-term sustainability, such assays should be available in-house.

▪▪ Microbiology

Infectious diseases constitute the most common complications after renal transplantation. As such, close liaison with the microbiology laboratory is essential, and program requirements should be discussed with the resident microbiologist.

A review of the extensive range of infectious complications in transplantation is beyond the scope of this chapter but are well-described elsewhere [22, 23]. However, microbiology support is essential for the pretransplant screening of recipients, for pathogens that may become reactivated following immunosuppression, as well as for donors, for pathogens that may be transmitted to the recipient.

Posttransplantation, microbiology is crucial for the identification and management of infections. These may be precipitated by immunosuppression and may be due to bacterial, viral, fungal, and parasitic causes [24, 25] rarely encountered in immunocompetent individuals. At the time of writing, the COVID-19 viral pandemic has reinforced the continuing threat from infectious diseases. Consideration of this virus will, no doubt, need to be included into transplant practice, although how, remains to be determined.

Recognition of the clinical manifestations of infection, which may be atypical, as well as a high index of suspicion linked with close cooperation between transplant clinician and microbiologists, are essential if early diagnosis of infection is to be achieved.

▪ Radiology and Interventional Radiology

Radiology services are critical in support of renal transplantation, and sophisticated imaging is an essential part of the preoperative assessment of both recipients and living donors. Following transplantation, ultrasound scanning is the fundamental means of reviewing transplants to define the cause of graft dysfunction. After that, interventional radiology techniques may be required to remedy both vascular and ureteric complications. Descriptions of these techniques are beyond the scope of this text, but are widely available elsewhere [26, 27].

▪ Patient Facilities

In the current era, isolation wards are not required for posttransplant patients. However, the highest standard of surgical ward is necessary with nursing support sufficient for regular monitoring of vital signs, fluid balance and daily weights. Since it is also likely that transplant recipients, and possibly living donors, will need a short postoperative period of high dependency/intensive care, discussions should occur with ICU staff before any transplants are performed. Clinical space will also be required in a clinic setting for the assessment of patients, with areas suitable for discussions with donors and recipients and their families. Indeed, having a physical space designated as the transplant unit helps to establish and normalize the place of transplantation in the hospital.

▪ Operating Theaters

A standard operating theatre with a full range of vascular surgical instruments is required to perform a renal transplant. However, provision must also be made for sterile ice and refrigerated sterile preservation fluids used for graft perfusion. Additional surgical instruments may be needed for ex vivo revision of the kidney (bench-work) before implantation occurs.

It is recognized that surgeons develop preferences for instruments and techniques, and beyond these basic facilities, it would be appropriate to liaise with mentors to determine specific requirements. In the same way, although the general anesthetic for renal transplants is mostly routine, as per major abdominal surgery, liaison between the mentoring teams and local anesthetists helps determine any additional mentoring requirements. Certainly, some modifications to normal intraoperative management is required, particularly in maintaining careful fluid balance, and most units have welcomed the input of an experienced RTx anesthetist during early mentoring.

Specific operating theatre considerations are required for living donor nephrectomy. This procedure can be performed as an open operation or laparoscopically. The International standard is now the laparoscopic approach, either fully laparoscopic or via a hand-assisted technique, and so, on balance, this technique should be adopted by developing units. Specialist laparoscopic equipment will be required including both hardware (monitor, insufflators, etc.) and disposable instruments. While this may have cost implications, the laparoscopic approach gives the best outcome for donors with reduced inpatient stays and less postoperative morbidity. It is, therefore, likely to be a more acceptable option for potential donors, so encouraging increased donation. Nevertheless, laparoscopic donor surgery is a complex discipline in which many choices are available regarding the approach, technique and instrumentation. Again, these matters should be clarified with mentors well in advance of any proposed donor surgery.

▪ Transplant Coordinators

As a unit develops, the number of patients under review grows, and managing the assessment and follow up process becomes more complicated. Invariably, these tasks outgrow the capability of clinicians to provide an appropriate overview. Consequently, these matters are usually addressed by transplant coordinators who ensure that investigations are performed, results are reviewed, and patients progress through the transplant pathway in an efficient and timely fashion. Coordinators inevitably become the primary interface between the patients and the program and the appropriate personnel to provide education and information to patients and the wider public.

Coordinators are usually recruited from nursing staff and information is widely available regarding such posts [28], which can be adapted toward local requirements. Ideally, the first transplant coordinator should be recruited at the commencement of a new transplant program, or at least early in the process.

85.4 Working Toward the First Transplant

As elements of the transplant team are assembled and potential donors and recipients are assessed and discussed with mentoring teams, it becomes appropriate to define a date for initial transplants to occur. It is worth considering that this process often takes longer than expected, so it is essential to allocate a suitable and mutually agreed lead time during which it is important to engage with mentors, discuss patients and identify any outstanding investigations. The availability of internet video conferencing facilitates this process.

Once all these tasks have been completed, arrangements can be made to bring the mentoring and local teams together to focus on performing the transplants. The ideal workload is perhaps three or four living donor cases over 1 week, including an initial day for patient review and several days after surgery to ensure that any early postoperative issues are addressed. During this period, all other matters should be excluded allowing focus on transplantation and learning from the procedures that are occurring. This event is an opportunity for broader teaching, ranging from in-theatre discussions with operating room staff, to patient bedside conversations with junior staff and formal lectures. Time can also be allocated for discussions with program stakeholders, including hospital management, patient groups, and government representatives.

After the focus of the 'transplant week' has subsided, it is necessary to ensure that adequate patient follow-up occurs. The details of both recipient and donor follow-up can be based on guidance provided by mentoring clinicians and published guidelines adapted to local requirements. In short, living donors will be usually reviewed at 4–6 weeks. A review of postoperative recovery is made, and renal function tests performed to ensure the satisfactory function of the remaining kidney. Other investigations include urinalysis and baseline blood pressure measurements. Most units then review living donors indefinitely to ensure that any potential risk to the remaining kidney is identified and managed as early as possible.

For recipients, follow-up will require regular visits to a transplant clinic, often starting twice weekly and then after longer intervals as progress occurs. Surveillance is maintained for evidence of infection and impaired graft function. Immunosuppressive drug levels must be assessed, and if graft dysfunction is suspected ultrasound scanning and graft biopsy will be required.

Mentors should continue to be involved in follow up, and again this can be facilitated by video conferencing. Further visits by mentors may be required if reversional surgery becomes necessary, as well as for further transplants until skill transfer is safely completed. This partnership process is normally expected to continue over a few years.

In this context, it is essential to recognize that complications can and do occur in all transplant programs, and such events should not deter progress. Nevertheless, such events should occur at an expected rather than an excessive rate, and from the outset, a registry of results should be maintained. Where possible, outcomes should be published as a record of progress and as encouragement for other developing units [29].

Following an initial series of successful transplants, it is also important to reinforce the benefits of transplantation back into the local community, as part of improving general and transplant-related health literacy [30]. It is appropriate to work with media to develop positive narratives encouraging further growth of transplantation and support of donation. It is also important to work with patients whose voices can eloquently demonstrate not only the clinical benefits of RTx but also the broader quality of life and family benefits (as in the case history). These voices are vital in reinforcing the benefits of transplantation, not only to the public but also politicians who may still have reservations reconciling the cost of transplantation against other healthcare pressures.

Then, having done the first transplants, a period of reflection is appropriate during which changes can be made in response to any perceived weakness in the program, before the team takes a collective deep breath and starts the mentoring cycle over again. After that, the cycle can repeat as necessary, with gradually reducing external support, ultimately leaving the unit self-reliant and sustainable [21].

If this development plan is adopted, the demand for RTx will likely increase, and an upscaling of resources will be required. Also, as experience grows, cases of increased complexity will be considered, together with the need to extend the service to children and adolescents at the earliest opportunity. Pediatric transplantation has additional complexity, but this should not deter units from providing appropriate care to children and adolescents with CKD. Ultimately, consideration will move toward the development of deceased donor transplantation. As discussed, this is a complex process but is possible in the setting of LMIC, albeit requiring substantial input and planning.

85.5 Developing Clinical Governance

Once the work of establishing a transplant program has been accomplished, attention must be increasingly given to ensuring that the program is well-managed. In essence, that appropriate clinical governance is incorporated into routine working to ensure that outcomes are optimized at both unit and individual patient levels.

Developing such clinical governance is an additional task, but this is a critical component of mature units. The effort given over to developing the elements of clinical governance will be more than repaid in the outcomes obtained. The sharing of clinical governance task by members of the team, through joint outcome meetings and other governance matters, helps create the structure and bonds needed for good teamwork. The shared responsibility of such tasks quickly becomes second nature and embedded within the unit's organizational framework.

The principal elements of clinical governance can reasonably be considered in three main areas.

1. The development of a service framework for the entire unit.

   This covers the development of appropriate patient pathways toward transplantation and including optimal waiting time to transplantation, identifying means of reducing preoperative complications and optimizing long-term transplant function. Proper levels of communication between the clinical teams and patients must be assured, while setting the appropriate interdependencies with other services and providers. In essence, this provides the bridge from the initial transplants to a fully functioning renal transplant unit with a full appreciation of the many facets of care required to provide the best outcomes for the patients it serves.

   Such frameworks do not need to be reinvented. Comprehensive guidance for such matters is widely available online with prominent examples being NHS England Adult Kidney Transplant Service Specifications [31] and the KDIGO guidelines for the Living Kidney donor, transplant candidate, and transplant recipient [32].

2. The identification of outcome metrics.

   Once a unit service framework has been developed, it is vital to continually monitor transplant outcomes to ensure that the best results are both obtained and then maintained. To do this, the most critical outcome metrics should be identified and applied to the unit's patients. The most widely used outcome measures are readily available online. They will also be used by mentoring teams in their units and guidance on implementing such surveillance will be available from transplant mentors.

   Metrics include those that focus on early transplant outcomes and therefore relate to events in the preoperative, perioperative and early postoperative phases of the transplant process. These include such measures as delayed graft function, renal vein thrombosis, and other causes of early graft loss, acute rejection, and early readmission rates. The collection of accurate 30-day graft and recipient outcomes is, therefore, a good starting point in developing a unit's clinical governance portfolio.

   In many countries, including the UK, there is significant variation in these outcomes between individual units even though longer-term results, for example, at 1 and 5 years show significantly less variation. In response to this early variation between units, in the UK and other HIC's more complex statistical means have become increasingly used to identify when such variation reaches unacceptable levels. In particular, this has involved the widespread adoption of CUSUM analyses. CUSUM (or cumulative sum control chart) is a sequential analysis technique that uses the cumulative sum of deviations from a target point and is typically used for monitoring change detection. The method is now used extensively to monitor the progress of many processes, both biological and nonbiological. In transplantation, CUSUM offers the ability to monitor the outcomes of several units and will create a signial when any outcome is unacceptable compared to comparitor units. The generation of a signal by a unit's outcomes will then indicate the needs to review working and make the changes necessary to return to the targeted outcome levels. A further, in-depth consideration of CUSUM theory and methodology is beyond the scope of this chapter. However, CUSUM monitoring of 30-day graft and patient outcomes has become a mandatory requirement for renal transplant units in the UK [33] and is also widely used in North America [34]. Furthermore, for ease of illustration, this type of data can also be presented as funnel plots as shown in ▫ Fig. 85.3.

   It is also essential that surveillance of longer-term outcomes is undertaken, which will reflect sustained optimal transplant management, both of the graft and recipient. Again, examples of long-term metrics are widely available and include: patient and graft survival at 1 and 5 years, graft function at similar time points, hospital readmission rates (for example at 30/180/365 days) and other markers of recipient wellbeing, such as blood pressure and diabetic status.

3. Assessing individual outcomes.

   Once the service framework and unit performance surveillance are underway, it is vital to assess outcomes on a case-by-case basis. Regular unit transplant clinical governance meetings should be held at which individual case histories should be reviewed. Any adverse issues identified should be included in an appropriate audit cycle with lessons learned reflected by necessary changes to unit protocol and then sub-

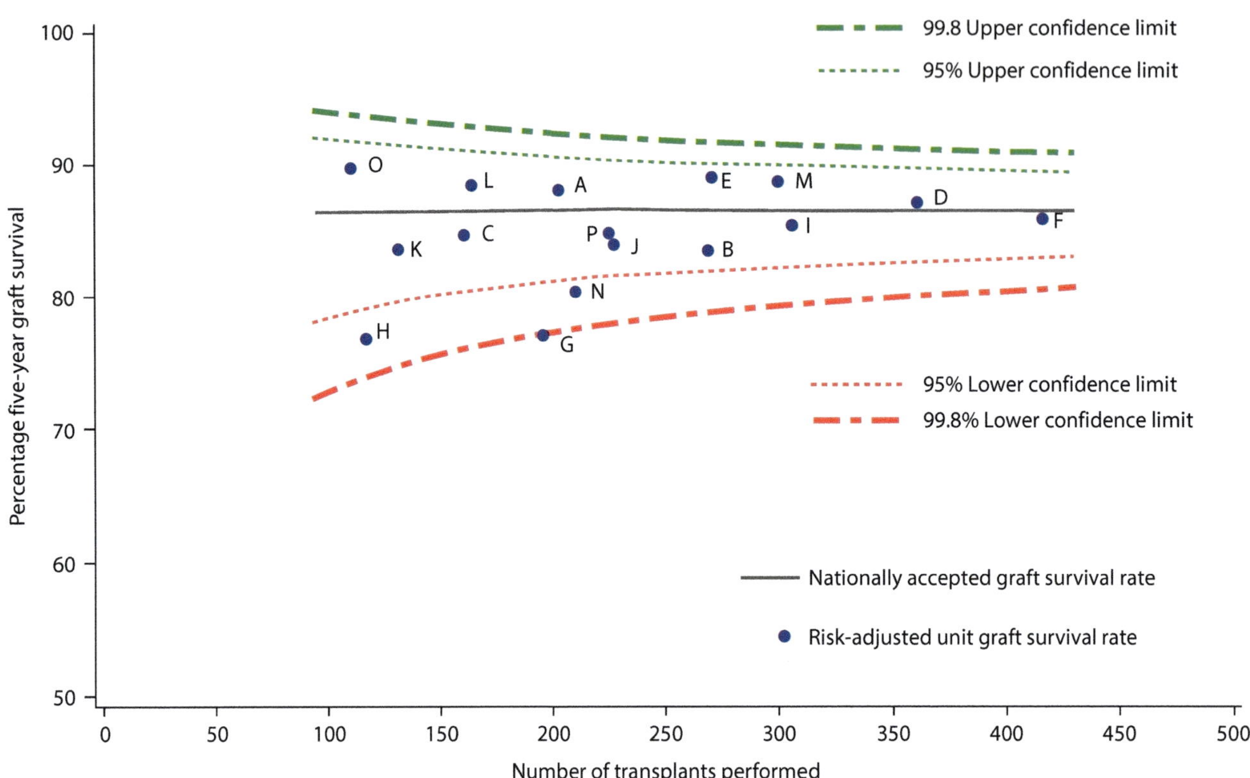

Fig. 85.3 Funnel plot of five-year graft survival rates of first adult renal transplants for a series of anonymized units. The majority of units' results fall comfortably within the accepted confidence levels and approximate to the nationally-defined target outcome. However, Unit G's performance is falling below the lower 98.5% confidence limit. This outcome will trigger a 'signal' indicating that this unit needs to review its practice and implement changes to restore outcomes to more acceptable levels

ject to ongoing review. In instances where significant issues arise in an individual case, e.g., unexpected early graft loss, careful analysis of the potential cause by way of a root cause analysis [35] should be undertaken, with any lessons learned again being reflected in appropriate changes in unit working.

Finally, once data become increasingly available, it is appropriate to construct a national transplant registry running in parallel to registries of CKD and dialysis outcomes.

It is recognized that establishing comprehensive clinical governance may be viewed as a complicated process. However, as previously stated, the information and tools required to set up and develop good clinical governance are widely available, often online and easily accessible. Also, mentoring groups will be fully aware of such matters and can guide how this matter may be taken forward.

Conclusion

In conclusion, the pivotal factor for a successful transplant program is multidisciplinary team working. Furthermore, it is not sufficient for the individual team components to be merely present and there must be a high level of connectivity between them underpinned by well-defined leadership. Against this background, program development requires the input of enthusiasm and energy, supported by the output of accurate outcome data, preferably in national registries [16]. Long-term patient care must be assured if optimum transplant outcomes are to be obtained and securing the provision of immunosuppression is an absolute requirement. Finally, RTx should strive to become an integral, rather than a competing part of a comprehensive healthcare system that includes broader CKD management and robust preventive measures for acute kidney injury and CKD.

Definitions

Low- and middle-income countries – Low-income countries are defined as those with a GNI per capita, calculated using the World Bank Atlas method of $1025 or less in 2018; lower middle-income economies are those with a GNI per capita between $1026 and $3995; upper middle-income economies are those with a GNI per capita between $3996 and $12,375.

End-Stage Renal Failure – The last stage of chronic kidney disease where suvival becomes dependent on dialysis or a kidney transplant (renal replacement therapy).

Deceased donation – Donation of an organ or tissue from someone who has already died.

Living donation – Donation of an organ from a living person.

BMI – Body Mass Index

HDU – High Dependency Unit

Immunosuppression – Medication to suppress the immune system that is essential to prevent rejection of the transplanted organ.

FSGS – Focal segmental glomerulosclerosis

KDIGO – Kidney Disease Improving Global Outcomes

Tricks and Tips

1. From the outset, keep as much outcome data as possible. It is easier to collect data prospectively than to go back and identify data retrospectively.
2. Multidisciplinary team working is the key to successful transplantation. Transplant programs are not the property of any individual. They are the shared outcome of well-organized teamwork.
3. Communication is paramount, with patients, team members, government representatives, mentors. Transplantation is a complex multiple-stage process and errors are likely to occur unless clear communication has happened between the interlinking stakeholders.
4. The use of modern technology, and in particular video-conferencing, enhances the ability of fledgling units to utilize the experience of established units throughout the world.
5. The development of transplantation invariably requires the support of both public and government. Eloquent patients' voices are far more persuasive, and emotive, giving the transplant message than the voices of clinicians.
6. Both donors and recipients need to receive a large amount of complex information as they prepare for transplantation. This must be presented in terms understandable by the layperson while simultaneously providing accurate clinical information on both the benefits and risks of transplantation. Only in this way can they go forward with confidence and in the context of fully informed consent.
7. The transplant ethics committee is an invaluable resource which provides reassuring support when difficult decisions need to be addressed.

Questions

1. What are the key challenges in starting a new kidney transplant program?
2. What are the key elements of a successful start to a new kidney transplant program?
3. Are all hospitals in LMIC suitable for the development of renal transplant services?
4. Must live donor nephrectomy only be performed laparoscopically?
5. Transplant Links is mentioned as an organization that can offer support to new and developing kidney transplant centers. Can I get in touch with clinicians who may be willing to assist with skill transfer in a developing center through Transplant Links?

Answers

1. The key challenges are gaining the governmental and managerial long-term support for the program, and ensuring all the crucial multidisciplinary team members are fully committed to the success of the project.
2. The key elements are good advice and support from multidisciplinary mentors; meticulous planning for the first series of transplants, and a high level of posttransplant support and advice; good data collection and review and sharing of case studies; careful selection of early cases to maximize success and learning before approaching more complex cases; and accepting that development of the program takes place over a number of years and that a slow and safe start is preferable to high early numbers and failures.
3. Probably not. Successful renal transplantation requires several specialist services, not the least of which is a preexisting nephrology service with patients receiving dialysis. Also, there is a requirement for specialist imaging and pathology services and operating departments equipped for the

development of laparoscopic donor surgery. It is most likely that these facilities will be found in national centers of excellence. So, it is in such institutions that renal transplant programs are most likely to be established and able to flourish. Even so, the development of the process of renal transplantation is complex and such centers as these will still benefit from mentor support at early stages to devise a plan for the development of renal and associated services. Once developed, such units can then be at the center of a hub-and-spoke network for referral of patients from other areas. With time, and as national pressures for renal transplantation increase, additional units may be established based on the initial development experience.

4. For many years live donor nephrectomy was performed as an open operation via a loin incision. However, this procedure was associated with considerable postoperative pain and a high incidence of wound complications. Also, and a delayed return to normal activities and employment. Laparoscopic donor nephrectomy reduces postoperative hospital stays, minimizes wound pain and complications and promotes early return to activities and employment. As such, the laparoscopic approach has become the internationally accepted method for donor nephrectomy. In live donor transplantation the welfare of the donor, who is undergoing surgery for the benefit of another, is paramount. The laparoscopic approach to donor surgery supports this ideal. Accordingly, this should be the method chosen by centers developing renal transplant programs. This approach does require additional surgical skills. However, through mentoring, these may be readily acquired by surgeons performing laparoscopic procedures in general surgical or urological practice. Time spent in learning these skills will be well rewarded in improved donor outcomes. It also results in an increased willingness of individuals to present as potential donors knowing that the procedure they will undergo will have a lesser impact upon their lives and wellbeing.
5. Transplant Links is a multidisciplinary group of nephrologists, surgeons, nurses, operating theatre technicians, pathologists, and other associated specialties, willing to share their skills and experience with developing transplant centers. New approaches are welcomed and contact can be made via the website at ▶ www.transplantlinks.org

References

1. Aviles-Gomez R, Luquin-Arellano VH, Garcia-Garcia G, Ibarra-Hernandez M, Briseño-Renteria G. Is renal replacement therapy for all possible in developing countries? Ethn Dis. 2006;16(2 Suppl 2):S2–70-2.
2. Davids MR, Eastwood JB, Selwood NH, Arogundade FA, Ashuntantang G, Benghanem Gharbi M, Jarraya F, MacPhee IA, McCulloch M, Plange-Rhule J, Swanepoel CR, Adu D. A renal registry for Africa: first steps. Clin Kidney J. 2016;9(1):162–7.
3. Bello AK, Levin A, Lunney M, Osman MA, et al. Status of care for end stage kidney disease in countries and regions worldwide: international cross sectional survey. BMJ. 2019;367:l5873.
4. Jha V, Garcia-Garcia G, Iseki K, Li Z, Naicker S, Plattner B, Saran R, Wang AY, Yang CW. Chronic kidney disease: global dimension and perspectives. Lancet. 2013;382(9888):260–72.
5. Muralidharan A, White S. The need for kidney transplantation in low- and middle-income countries in 2012: an epidemiological perspective. Transplantation. 2015;99(3):476–81.
6. Bamgboye EL. The challenges of ESRD care in developing economies: sub-Saharan African opportunities for significant improvement. Clin Nephrol. 2016;86(Supplement 1):18–22.
7. Barsoum RS, Khalil SS, Arogundade FA. Fifty years of dialysis in Africa: challenges and progress. Am J Kidney Dis. 2015;65(3):502–12.
8. Osman MA, Alrukhaimi M, Ashuntantang GE, Bellorin-Font E, Benghanem Gharbi M, Braam B, et al. Global nephrology workforce: gaps and opportunities toward a sustainable kidney care system. Kidney Int Suppl (2011). 2018;8(2):52–63.
9. Htay H, Alrukhaimi M, Ashuntantang GE, Bello AK, Bellorin-Font E, Jha V, et al. Global access of patients with kidney disease to health technologies and medications: findings from the Global Kidney Health Atlas project. Kidney Int Suppl (2011). 2018;8(2):64–73.
10. Jha V, Chugh KS. The practice of dialysis in the developing countries. Hemodial Int. 2003;7(3):239–49.
11. Bamgboye EL. Hemodialysis: management problems in developing countries, with Nigeria as a surrogate. Kidney Int Suppl. 2003;83:S93–5.
12. Bello AK, Alrukhaimi M, Ashuntantang GE, Bellorin-Font E, Benghanem Gharbi M, Braam B, Feehally J, Harris DC, et al. Global overview of health systems oversight and financing for kidney care. Kidney Int Suppl (2011). 2018;8(2):41–51.
13. Alasia DD, Emem-Chioma P, Wokoma FS. A single-center 7-year experience with end-stage renal disease care in Nigeria-a surrogate for the poor state of ESRD care in Nigeria and other sub-Saharan African countries: advocacy for a global fund for ESRD care program in sub-Saharan African countries. Int J Nephrol. 2012;2012:639653.
14. Garcia GC, Harden P, Chapman J. The global role of kidney transplantation. Transplantation. 2012;93:337–41.
15. Bamgboye EL. Barriers to a functional renal transplant program in developing countries. Ethn Dis. 2009;19(1 Suppl 1):S1. -56-9
16. Muller E, White S, Delmonico F. Regional perspective: developing organ transplantation in sub-Saharan Africa. Transplantation. 2014;97:975–6.
17. Participants in the International Summit on Transplant Tourism and Organ Trafficking Convened by the Transplantation Society and Inter- national Society of Nephrology, Istanbul,

Turkey, 2008. The Declaration of Istanbul on organ trafficking and transplant tourism. Transplantation. 2008;86:1013.
18. Casares M. Ethical aspects of living-donor kidney transplantation. Nefrologia. 2010;30(Suppl 2):14–22.
19. Andrews PA, Burnapp L, eds. British Transplantation Society / Renal Association UK Guidelines for Living Donor Kidney Transplantation 2018. Available at BTS https://bts.org.uk/wpcontent/uploads/2018/03/BTS_RA_LDKT_Guidelines_FINAL_12.03.18.pdf.
20. Feehally J, The International Society of Nephrology (ISN). Roles & challenges in Africa and other resource-limited communities. Clin Nephrol. 2016;86(Supplement 1):3–7.
21. Ready AR, Nath J, Milford D, Adu J, Jewitt-Harris J. Establishing sustainable kidney transplant programmes in developing world countries: a ten-year experience. Kidney Int. 2016;90(5):916–20.
22. Anastasopoulos NA, Duni A, Peschos D, Agnantis N, Dounousi E. The spectrum of infectious diseases in kidney transplantation: a review of the classification, pathogens and clinical manifestations. In Vivo. 2015;29(4):415–22.
23. Pérez JL, Ayats J, de Oña M, Pumarola T. The role of the clinical microbiology laboratory in solid organ transplantation programs. Enferm Infecc Microbiol Clin. 2012;30(Suppl 2): 2–9.
24. Wołyniec W, Sulima M, Renke M, Dębska-Ślizień A. Parasitic infections associated with unfavourable outcomes in transplant recipients. Medicina (Kaunas). 2018;54(2):27.
25. Fabiani S, Fortunato S, Bruschi F. Solid organ transplant and parasitic diseases: a review of the clinical cases in the last two decades. Pathogens. 2018;7(3):65.
26. Knipe H, Bickle I. Renal transplant available at Radiopaedia. https://radiopaedia.org/articles/renal-transplant?lang=gb
27. Nadalo LA, Lin EC, et al. Imaging in kidney transplantation complications available at Medscape: https://emedicine.medscape.com/article/378801-overview.
28. UK ODT Clinical. Role of transplant recipient co-ordinator. Available at ODT Clinical: https://www.odt.nhs.uk/odt-structures-and-standards/organ-donation-retrieval-and-transplantation-teams/role-of-transplant-recipient-co-ordinator/.
29. Osafo C, Morton B, Ready A, Jewitt-Harris J, Adu D. Organ transplantation in Ghana. Transplantation. 2018;102(4): 539–41.
30. Jewitt-Harris J, Ready A. Optimising Health Literacy for improved clinical practicies. Health Literacy in kidney transplantation in developing countries Editors Vassilios Papalois and Maria Theosopoulou IGI GLobal 2018.
31. NHS England adult kidney transplant service. https://www.england.nhs.uk/wp-content/uploads/2017/05/service-spec-adult-kidney-transplant-service.pdf.
32. KDIGO Guide lines. https://kdigo.org/guidelines/.
33. Collett D, Sibanda N, Pioli S, Bradley A, Rudge C. The UK scheme for mandatory continuous monitoring of early transplant outcome in all kidney transplant centres. Transplantation. 2009;88(8):970–5.
34. Axelroda DA, Guidingerb MK, Metzgerc RA, Wiesnerd RH, Webbe RL, Merione RM. Transplant center quality assessment using a continuously updatable, risk-adjusted technique (CUSUM). Am J Transplant. 2006;6:313–23.
35. NHS Improvement. https://improvement.nhs.uk/resources/root-cause-analysis-using-five-whys/.

Further Information

www.transplantlinks.org
https://renal.org/

Assessment of the Potential Transplant Recipient

Heidy Hendra, David Mathew, Jeff Cove, Paramjit Jeetley, Clare Melikian, Aneesa Jaffer, and Ammar Al Midani

Contents

We would like to dedicate a special thank you to Dr Albert Power and Dr Peter Dupont for their significant contribution to the first edition of this chapter.

M. Harber (ed.), *Primer on Nephrology*, https://doi.org/10.1007/978-3-030-76419-7_86

Learning Objectives

1. To understand the importance of surgical, psychological, anesthetic, and medical assessment of renal patients for potential kidney transplantation
2. To cover the assessment of cardiovascular, neoplastic, and infectious risk in the recipient and as a consequence of transplant surgery and immunosuppression
3. To appreciate the balance between risk and benefit for a renal transplant recipient and to be able to communicate this risk as well as re-evaluate
4. To recommend structures that can deliver robust and thoughtful assessments of potential recipients

86.1 Introduction

Renal transplantation can have multiple benefits in terms of life expectancy (see Fig. 86.1), quality of life, and very substantial health care saving but it is not without risks. In the UK, the patient's survival rate at 1 year for deceased donors is 97% which of course means a 3% mortality. Conversely, roughly 7% of patients die while on the waiting list and 7% are removed as no longer suitable, illustrating that all patients considered for renal transplantation require a thoughtful preoperative or continuing assessment. This assessment needs to ascertain their fitness to undergo surgery under general anesthesia and to optimize the therapeutic impact of a scarce and precious resource. This chapter will review the practical aspects of delivering such an assessment with reference to available evidence and guidelines [2–5].

86

For further information please see the following website:

- BTS: ► https://bts.org.uk/guidelines-standards/
- ERA-EDTA: ► https://www.era-edta.org/en/erbp/guidance/
- CARI: ► https://www.cariguidelines.org
- KDIGO: ► https://kdigo.org/guidelines/

Definitions

Assessment of potential transplant recipients encompasses evaluation and assessment to determine the suitability of a patient with end-stage renal failure to receive kidney transplantation. During the process, it will also investigate and optimize any potentially reversible risk factors that can affect peri- and post-operative outcomes.

86.2 Service Structure

There are many different models for transplant assessment, but it is important to remember that it is a continuous process from progressive CKD to transplant assessment, activation, and re-evaluation until transplanted. However, the nitty-gritty of formal transplant assessment is best delivered as a streamlined and ideally "one-stop" outpatient service (see Fig. 86.2). This will require a multi-disciplinary approach with input from a nephrologist, transplant surgeon, and clinical nurse specialist as a minimum. Clinical psychology review can be invaluable for patients with issues with adherence to treatment or adjustment to their diagnosis of end-stage kidney failure; an anesthetic review should be requested

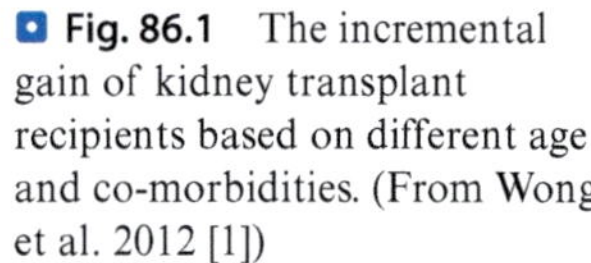

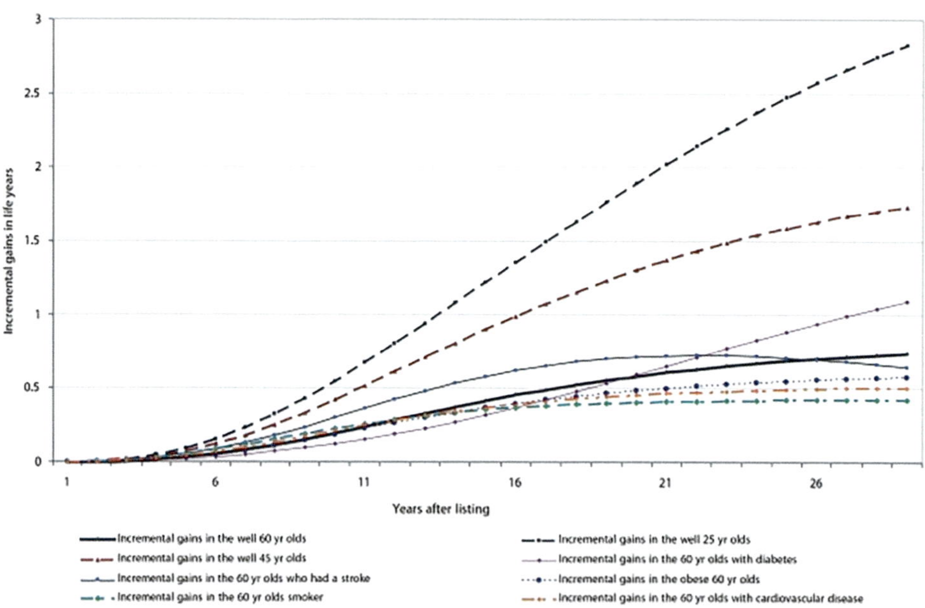

Fig. 86.1 The incremental gain of kidney transplant recipients based on different age and co-morbidities. (From Wong et al. 2012 [1])

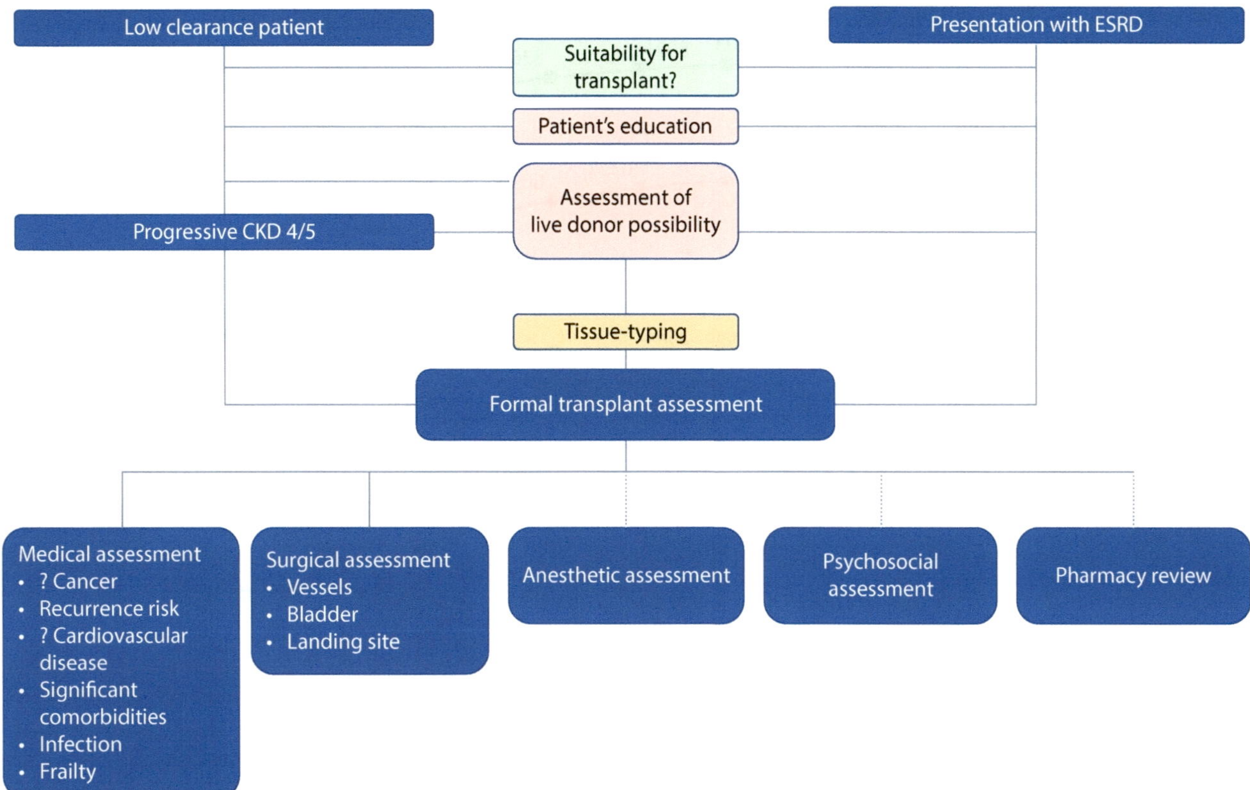

Fig. 86.2 A schematic of one model of transplant assessment. Patients present either through the CKD clinic under nephrologists in a more or less predictable manner or have first presentation at end-stage renal disease. Either way, assuming irreversible disease, a critical question is whether the patient might benefit from transplantation and whether they have potential live donors. Basic transplant workup screening can be done at this stage and then patients seen in a formal transplant assessment clinic. Medical and surgical assessments can be combined with a consent clinic

for patients with significant co-morbidity and a pharmacy review of potential medication issues is sometimes required.

For patients with potential live donors, the participation of a specialized live donor coordinator team and an efficient tissue-typing laboratory are vital in reducing the time between patient referral and transplantation.

For those patients who are suitable for transplantation either now or pending further tests, the one-stop shop is an ideal opportunity for a consent clinic. This is usually performed after the surgical assessment and gives the opportunity to discuss risks and potential complications in the cold light of the day, perhaps with family present rather than first addressing these issues for the first time in the middle of the night prior to an acute transplant.

Patients with complex cardiac histories or positive cardiac screening tests often need input from a cardiologist in determining optimal management. This may be best handled through a regular joint cardiology/nephrology meeting. Complex recipients or those with significant co-morbidity should be reviewed in dedicated multi-disciplinary team meetings with input from senior anesthetic staff and from the patient's primary nephrologist. These MDTMs need to meet frequently enough not to significantly delay a decision and the outcome needs to be carefully recorded. If the consensus is that a patient is not suitable for transplantation, this needs to be communicated sympathetically and the focus should then be on maximizing quality of life and health on dialysis.

For those patients suspended pending investigations, recovery from illness or to achieve an appropriate level of fitness or weight, there needs to be a very clear timeline for reassessment. In the UK, there are almost two-thirds as many patients on the suspended list as on the active list (see Fig. 86.3) and this raises concerns. If this represents a proportion of patients waiting excessive periods for tests and reassessment then this is unlikely to be good for the majority of those patients. In the UK, the ATTOM study identified a significant impact of limited health literacy as a risk factor for reduced likelihood to be on the transplant waiting list for a deceased donor transplant (HR 0.68), for receiving a living donor transplant (HR 0.41), or for receiving a transplant from any donor type (HR 0.65). Intervention is needed to improve this area [7].

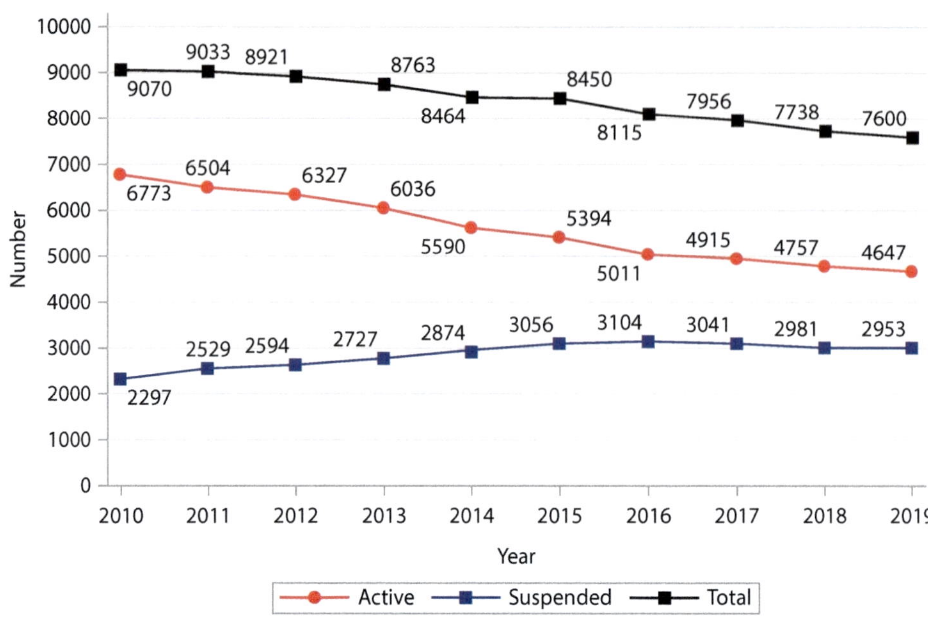

Fig. 86.3 ODT NHS BT annual report on kidney transplantation 2018–19 demonstrating an encouraging fall in the active waiting list but a very large number (roughly 3000) of patients suspended [6]

Once on the transplant list, it is essential that recipient contact details are up to date since the transplant offer often occurs outside of normal working hours. In addition, there is a need for an awareness of the changing clinical course of each recipient on the transplant waiting list to ensure that those who become medically unfit or who are traveling abroad are suspended from the national deceased donor list in a timely way. It is to no one's advantage to call in a patient for a transplant offer or indeed transplant a patient who has clearly unfit for transplantation. A dedicated transplant list coordinator at the transplanting center can ensure that waitlist maintenance is carried out to a high standard and that the local list aligns with that of the national organ allocation service.

86

86.2.1 When to Assess and Activate the Patient on the Transplant List?

The first part of this question is pretty straightforward; for patients who are likely to need chronic renal replacement therapy the question is "might they benefit from transplantation?" If the answer is yes or possibly, they should be assessed with alacrity and worked up in a timely fashion.

Choosing the time of activation is a bit more nuanced. The European Best Practice Guidelines (2000) recommend transplant wait-listing in patients with an eGFR consistently <20 ml/min and predicted to be within 6 months of needing RRT. Judging this latter criterion necessarily involves a degree of subjectivity particularly given that transplant organs are a scarce resource with a limited half-life and there is variation in practice; in the UK pre-emptive activation rates range from 33% to 57% (average of 44%). While this variation probably represents institutional ethos or efficiency there are clearly patients with an eGFR < 20 ml/min but a slow trajectory and may not need to be listed straight away, particularly elderly and co-morbid patients with relatively stable kidney function, for whom the risk-benefit is more marginal. Conversely, for a young person with progressive disease (for example with heavy proteinuria) who has most to gain from a transplant, it makes sense to activate relatively early.

86.3 Surgical Assessment

In some units, patients are primarily assessed for transplantation by surgeons rather than clinicians but either way, the key questions remain the same, that is:

1. Is the patient fit enough for a transplant and
2. Are they likely to gain from a transplant in terms of improved quality or quantity of life

There are however several specific surgical aspects to this equation that may not be at the forefront of a medical assessment:

1. Is a transplant technically possible in terms of (a) vessels, (b) space, (c) urinary drainage (e.g., functioning bladder), or (d) non-hostile abdomen
2. Is the patient fit enough to (a) tolerate a standard surgical transplant, (b) a transplant that incurs significant surgical complications (for example the need for reoperation(s))

Table 86.1 Surgical assessment and investigations in pre-transplant assessment

Surgical assessment	Investigations
Space for the kidney: previous transplants or APKD	CT scan without contrast
Technical difficulty: previous pelvic radiotherapy, multiple abdominal surgeries (stoma – EVAR)	Mitigate the technical problems by going to opposite iliac fossa or intra-abdominal
Iliac arteries: history of PVD, long-term DM, smoking, stroke, IHD or non-palpable pulses, and presence of a bruit	Doppler scan, MRA, or CT angiogram
Iliac veins: Previous femoral lines, history of DVT/PE, and previous transplant	Doppler scan
Bladder: History of reflux, PUV, bladder dysfunction, bladder or ureter surgery, or long history of HDx and anuria	Ultrasound scan, urodynamic study

Some of these questions, such as whether there is enough space in a patient with large ADPKDs or enough uncalcified vessel to plump in the kidney are relatively easy to determine if the question has been asked. However, others are less clear cut, for example, it may be impossible to know how "hostile" an abdomen and pelvis are post-radiotherapy until surgery is attempted and while a frail patient might manage an uncomplicated kidney transplant, the risks escalate rapidly for prolonged stays and re-exploration. What is clear is that to attempt a transplant and have to abandon it as it is not technically possible is a tragedy and everything should be done to try and mitigate the risk of this in advance.

Combining surgical assessment with pre-consent is a good model for ensuring important surgical issues are not missed (see Table 86.1), are appropriately planned for, and discussed openly with the patient.

86.3.1 Vessels

A recent meta-analysis seems to confirm the clinical impression that aortoiliac calcification in renal recipients is associated with an increased risk of mortality and graft loss [8]. Severe PAD at the time of transplant can lead to acute graft failure due to poor anastomoses, cholesterol emboli, or hypoperfusion [9] and other complications such as dissection of iliac and prolonged warm ischemic time, critical lower limb ischemia. Postoperatively PAD may lead to transplant renal artery stenosis and subsequent hypertension and progressive renal failure [10].

A focused history of risk factors for developing peripheral vascular disease (PVD), a history of macrovascular disease (cerebrovascular, PVD, or cardiac vascular disease), or a long history of CKD and dialysis with hyperparathyroidism or a high calcium burden suggesting the possibility of heavily calcified vessels.

Therefore, all potential transplant recipients should have an assessment of all peripheral pulses especially those in the lower limbs, and auscultation for carotid bruits. The presence of normal pedal pulses in the absence of symptoms of claudication makes the presence of moderate-to-severe disease less likely and maybe enough to confirm that renal transplantation is technically feasible.

Most centers would not offer transplantation to the patient with bilateral, diffuse circumferential calcification of the iliac arteries. In contrast, short-segment arterial stenosis that can be treated with endovascular techniques would not be an absolute contraindication for transplantation. Some European centers have started to perform aorto-bifemoral bypass graft for symptomatic patients with severe iliac disease to bridge end-stage renal disease patients with severe iliac calcification to kidney transplantation [11].

Many transplant centers advocate adjunctive vascular imaging particularly in higher risk groups, although there is no consensus on modality. Doppler ultrasonography (USS) is highly operator-dependent with variable sensitivity and specificity reaching 91% and 93% respectively in one study [12] while another suggested a positive predictive value of just 60% [13].

Conventional angiography remains the gold standard test that allows for intervention on any identified flow-limiting lesions. However, it is invasive and carries the risk of contrast-induced nephropathy. As there tends to be a low incidence of aortoiliac disease in younger patients (1.9% in those <40 years old), angiography is best reserved for symptomatic patients [14].

Non-invasive angiography using magnetic resonance angiography (MRA) or CT angiography (CTA) has increased in popularity with the ability to deliver high-quality, three-dimensional imaging of pelvic and lower limb vasculature. In pre-dialysis high-risk patients (10 years of diabetes and smoking), a plain CT is the modality of choice to determine the extent of vascular calcification of the pelvic vessels to assess the best landing zone and inform the surgical decisions about allograft placement (see Fig. 86.4). Contrast-enhanced angiographic sequences (CTA) can deliver 96% sensitivity and 97% specificity but can miss short stenoses. Unlike CT scanning, MRA avoids the use of ionizing radiation and

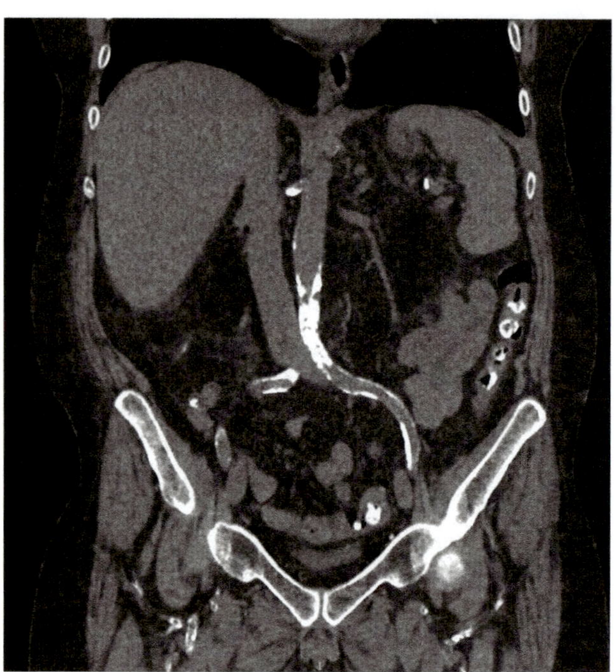

■ Fig. 86.4 A non-contrast CT scan of abdomen and pelvis in an ex-smoker with diabetes and PVD showing severe circumferential calcification of iliacs and aorta. This scan had to be reviewed with the radiologist to identify potential landing spots

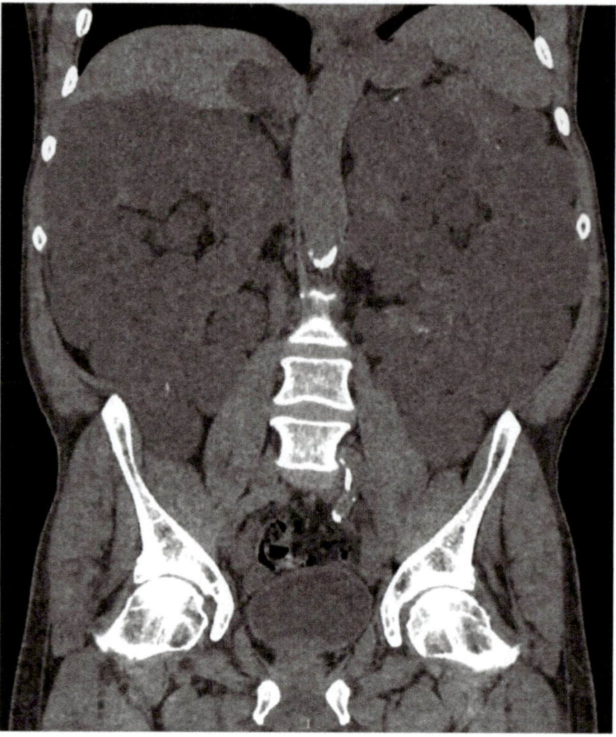

■ Fig. 86.5 CT scan of abdomen and pelvis showing: APKD extending into both right and left iliac fossae, it also shows a calcified left internal iliac artery. The latter making the right nephrectomy more appealing in terms of creating a good landing site for a transplanted kidney

has a sensitivity of 97% and specificity of 99% but has a higher false-positive rate.

It is also important to at least consider evaluation of venous drainage particularly in patients who have had dialysis access issues with multiple femoral lines, retroperitoneal fibrosis, pelvic radiation, or surgery. This is not just the adequacy of venous drainage but whether a patient has extensive collaterals, which may make surgery more hazardous. MR Venography can be very helpful if there is concern on this front.

86.3.2 Space

The second key issue for surgeons after blood supply is space and position. The main contenders for abdominal real estate are as follows:

1. Polycystic kidneys
2. Previous renal transplants
3. Stomas
4. Hernias

These should all be readily apparent at the time of surgical assessment and need to be incorporated into a plan. For example, with very large polycystic kidneys that overwhelm any potential landing sites, a non-contrast CT (see ■ Fig. 86.5) will usually make it clear but often the "rule of fist" can one fit a surgeon's fist below the native kidney, is sufficient. If there is not enough room to implant a transplant with the existing native kidneys then the timing of nephrectomy becomes complex in pre-emptive patients without a live donor, who is likely to be precipitated onto dialysis following a nephrectomy. A planned nephrectomy at the time of transplant has been done but is not widely popular given the prolonged combined operation and anesthetic time as well as risks of complications. A plan for nephrectomy clearly needs to be a discussion between the patient, surgeon, and nephrologist.

Previous transplants if in situ clearly need to be considered and if necessary imaged prior to transplant or elective nephrectomy.

Equally, stomas and hernias may provide immense technical challenges and pre-planning and discussion is key.

86.3.3 Bladder Drainage and Pressures

The third major concern for surgeons (and physicians) is the suitability of the bladder – whether it is too small, does not drain effectively, has high pressure, or is damaged in a way that is conducive to urosepsis. Therefore, it is important to consider formal urological assessment for patients with structural urinary tract abnormalities, those with a history of recurrent urinary tract infection, vesico-ureteric reflux, significant lower urinary tract symptoms, or abnormal bladder imaging. These candidates should be referred to a urologist with experience in transplant issues and may require urodynamics. For anuric patients, it may be appropriate to defer urological surgery until after the transplant is performed but where possible it is important to identify patients at risk of recurrent urosepsis or a high-pressure, poorly-functioning bladder early in their workup.

In those candidates where bladder cancer is suspected (heavy smoker, cyclophosphamide exposure, aristolochic acid nephropathy) then screening with cystoscopy is advised.

86.3.4 The Hostile Abdomen

In patients who have had extensive abdominal surgery, sclerosing peritonitis or abdominopelvic irradiation transplant surgery may be extremely challenging or impossible. Surgical assessment in workup should identify such patients and provoke thoughtful planning. This may result in specifications such as whether the transplant should be intra or extraperitoneal, that a deceased donor transplant would only be done in daylight hours, and perhaps only if senior surgeons were available. A decision may be made to only accept a standard criterion, DBD donor to minimize the risk of delayed graft function or other technical problems. The surgical assessment permits these decisions to be made with forethought and carefully documented.

86.3.5 Obesity

Obesity deserves a special mention in part because of the growing prevalence and in part because of the challenges it generates for the surgeon and more importantly the patient.

Obese transplant recipients have a slightly increased risk of graft loss, but it is important to note that they experience similar survival to recipients with normal BMI [15]. Postoperatively obesity, unsurprisingly, is associated with a higher incidence of new-onset post-transplant diabetes mellitus, lymphoceles, increased length of stay, and wound infections [16].

In the UK, fully adjusted hazard ratios for graft survival and patient survival did not differ across BMI bands in transplanted patients, up to BMI >40 kg/m^2. Yet, despite this, in the UK surgical cut-off for BMI varies from 30 to 40 between units, resulting in a somewhat arbitrary post-code lottery for access to the waiting list. In our view, obesity needs to be viewed as another co-morbidity and in an otherwise fit patient a rigid BMI cut-off value may not be appropriate particularly given that BMI is a crude indicator of adiposity failing to distinguish where the excess weight is distributed. In short, centers that limit transplants to those meeting arbitrary levels of body mass, rather than adopting an individualized assessment approach, maybe unfairly depriving many patients of the survival and quality of life benefits derived from kidney transplantation.

A robotic kidney transplantation programme may represent an opportunity to remove the arbitrary selection criteria of BMI and holds promise for reducing perioperative surgical risks and units should consider offering patients referral to centers that are able to transplant very high BMI patients, particularly if the alternative is to never be listed.

In selected candidates, active weight loss programmes with dietetic and physiotherapy input may be required as well as bariatric surgery prior to transplantation although criteria vary across transplant centers. However, if an obese patient has the potential to have and benefit from a transplant, then the approach to their obesity needs to be decisive; it is all too common for years to pass while waiting in vain for a dialysis patient to achieve sufficient weight loss, this is neither fair nor good practice.

86.4 Medical Assessment

Beyond the technical elements of placing a kidney, medical key aspects of a potential recipient need to be assessed. Broadly these can be divided into cardiovascular, malignancy, recurrent disease, and other factors including frailty, significant medical conditions, and psychological issues.

86.4.1 Cardiovascular Risk Assessment

This is perhaps one of the biggest issues for transplant workup; the evidence base is limited and despite careful preselection, cardiovascular disease remains the most common cause of death with a functioning graft at all times following transplantation (38% of cases) and particularly within the first 12 months [17].

There are some key elements that are considered when making an assessment of cardiac risk for patients undergoing pre-transplant assessment:

1. The patient is fit enough to be subjected to the rigors of general anesthesia, transplant surgery, and the perioperative period
2. The patient will survive long enough post-transplantation to justify allocation of a precious resource

The latter point is relevant as despite careful preselection cardiovascular disease still remains a common cause of death with a functioning graft in the transplant population [18].

Screening tends to focus on the assessment of coronary artery disease whereas the prevalence of all forms of cardiac disease is higher in patients with advanced renal disease (see Fig. 86.6). This includes coronary disease, arrhythmia, heart failure, and valvular heart disease and the prognosis is not only worse in the general population but also with the severity of CKD [19, 20]. While screening is a valuable risk stratification tool for surgery, interventions to modify risk while common in clinical practice are not well supported by randomized trial evidence (Table 86.2).

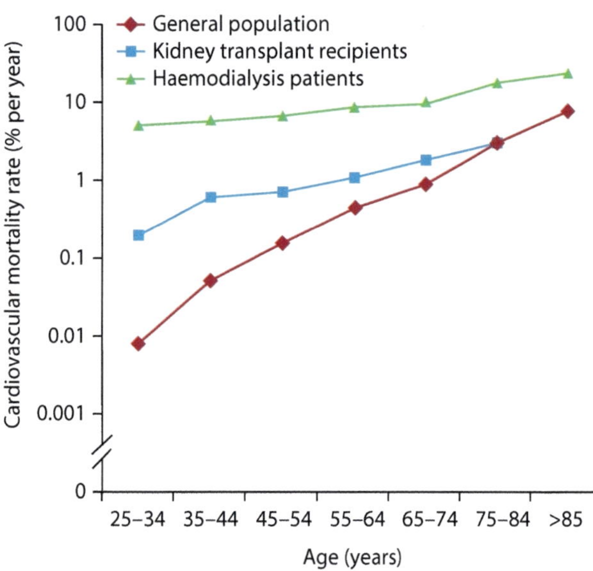

Fig. 86.6 Comparative cardiovascular mortality for patients with renal replacement therapy and the normal population

Table 86.2 Randomized control trials on screening and intervention in patients with stable coronary artery disease

Study	*n*	Population	*P* value
COURAGE	2287	Known CAD	0.62
DIAD	1123	Type 2 Diabetes	0.73
CARP	510	Treatable lesions prior to vascular surgery	0.92
Manske et al. [21]	26	Treatable lesions prior to transplantation	<0.01
ISCHEMIA-CKD	777	Known CKD with moderate-severe ischemia on functional imaging	0.95

COURAGE - Boden WE et al. NEJM 2007; DIAD – Young LH, et al. JAMA 2009; CARP - McFalls EO et al. NEJM 2004; ISCHEMIA-CKD - Bangalore et al. NEJM 2020

Non-invasive Cardiac Assessment

Standard screening tests such as 12-lead ECG, chest X-Ray, and trans-thoracic echocardiography (TTE) are sufficient in patients who are younger (<50 years old) with good effort tolerance with no cardiac symptoms and no history of diabetes. TTE can be particularly useful for the assessment of left and right ventricular dysfunction and valve disease.

Coronary Assessment

In addition to conventional risk factors such as hypertension and diabetes, the pathophysiology and pattern of coronary artery disease (CAD) in advanced CKD are made more complex by renal-specific risk factors. These include abnormalities in calcium and phosphate metabolism, homocysteine, and uremic factors. As a result, there is an increase in prevalence and complexity of CAD in the recipient population which would be in keeping with patterns of disease seen in much older patients without CKD (see Fig. 86.7).

86.4.1.1 Screening for CAD

Patients with significant risk factors for CAD such as diabetes should be considered for further testing either with anatomical or functional/physiological imaging.

Functional imaging involves inducing ischemia within the myocardium by subjecting it to either exercise or pharmacological stress. Exercise stress testing is more helpful as objective data on effort tolerance, symptoms and the induction of arrhythmia on exertion provide additional information. This combined with cardiac imaging can provide a comprehensive pre-anesthetic assessment. Exercise treadmill testing (ETT) without adjunctive imaging is much less accurate for CAD so is not recommended.

Functional imaging modalities include stress echocardiography which relies on the assessment of regional wall motion pre- and post-stress; myocardial perfusion imaging (MPI) which uses comparative radio-nucleotide tracer uptake pre-and post-stress and cardiac MRI (CMR) which uses perfusion mapping techniques to assess ischemia. The relative advantages and disadvantages are outlined in Table 86.3.

Stress echocardiography (SE) and myocardial perfusion imaging (MPI) have comparable accuracy in observational studies but comparative reviews suggest SE is more accurate (sensitivity 0.8 vs 0.69, specificity 0.89 vs 0.77 for SE and MPI, respectively) [22]. To its advantage, SE also provides additional information such as baseline and dynamic ventricular function, valve and pulmonary pressure assessments.

Anatomical imaging with cardiac CT or invasive coronary angiography allows visualization of the ves-

86

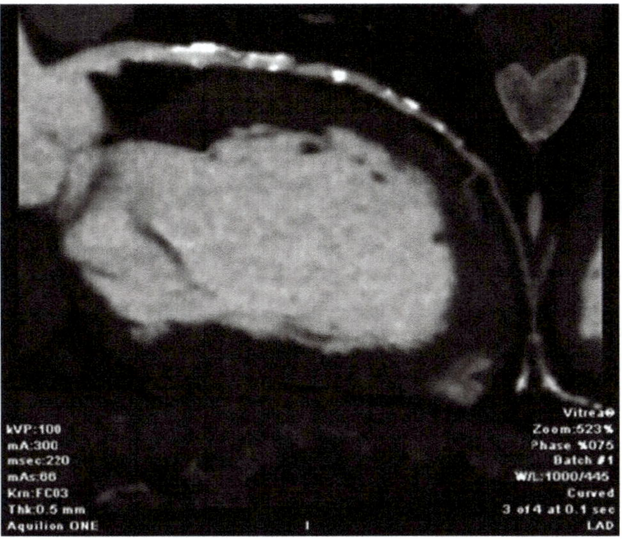

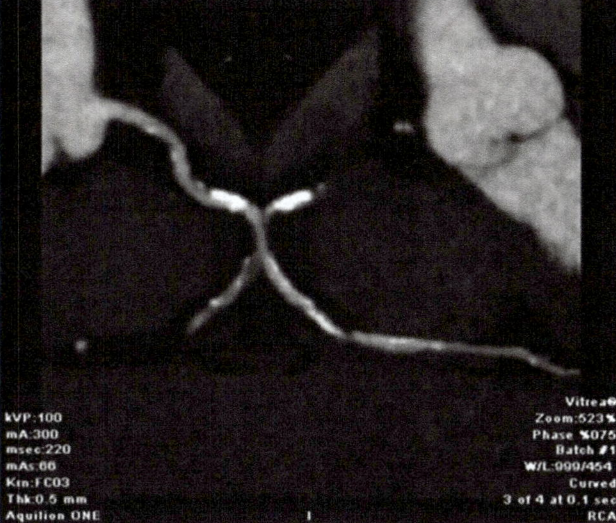

Fig. 86.7 Diffuse, severe, calcified multi-vessel CAD seen in an asymptomatic young patient with advanced CKD undergoing cardiac CT as part of pre-transplant assessment. The pattern of disease is commonly seen in much older patients in the non-CKD population

Table 86.3 Relative merits of non-invasive functional imaging techniques to assess for coronary artery disease in patients with advanced CKD

Modality	Advantages	Disadvantages
Myocardial perfusion imaging	Non-invasive Assess ischemic burden Prognostic value Pharmacological stress Assess functional status with exercise	Ionizing radiation Attenuation artefact Reduced sensitivity and specificity in CKD population "Balanced ischemia" phenomenon ?Reduced effects of vasodilator stress
Stress echocardiography	Non-invasive Higher specificity than MPS Non-ionizing radiation Prognostic value Assessment of myocardial viability and contractile reserve Assess functional status with exercise	Image quality Target heart rate not achieved can be challenging Dobutamine intolerance
Cardiac MRI	Non-invasive Assess structure, tissue characterization, and perfusion Non-ionizing radiation	Risk of nephrogenic systemic fibrosis Smaller evidence base

sels. Coronary CT is challenging due to the increased prevalence of coronary calcium in the CKD population and the risk of contrast nephropathy. Invasive coronary angiography, however, can be performed with lower doses of contrast and can be comprehensive with intracoronary imaging but has associated procedural risks (Table 86.4).

While the assessment of coronary disease is helpful in preoperative risk, coronary intervention to modify risk is controversial. Recent data has shown no benefit in patients with CKD undergoing percutaneous revascularization compared to medical therapy even when moderate-to-severe ischemia is demonstrated on functional imaging [23].

Current guidelines for non-cardiac surgery suggest that prognostic disease, i.e., left main stem involvement or severe three-vessel coronary disease should be revascularized [24]. There is no clear evidence base for other significant diseases and decisions are generally made on a case-by-case basis taking into account ischemic burden, symptoms, risk profile, and duration of dual antiplatelet therapy post-procedure.

86.4.1.2 Valvular Heart Disease

As with the assessment of valve disease in the native population, careful assessment of the valve as well as the impact on cardiac chambers is key. The best modality for this is echocardiography.

In valvular regurgitation, an important factor is also the volume status of the patient. It is well recognized that the severity of valvular regurgitation will be more if the patient is volume overloaded with dilatation of the ventricle causing annular dilatation. Meticulous fluid balance and modification of the dialysis regime can significantly reduce the degree of regurgitation optimizing the cardiac function (◘ Fig. 86.8a, b). Surgical or percutaneous intervention should therefore be discussed with a full multi-disciplinary team, and the patient fully optimized before prior to its undertaking.

◘ **Table 86.4** Relative merits of anatomical imaging to assess coronary artery disease in patients with advanced CKD

Modality	Advantages	Disadvantages
Cardiac CT	Cross Sectional Imaging Good negative predictive value Low radiation with new protocols and machines	Ionizing radiation Requires iodinated contrast Calcium burden high in renal population Requires low heart rates and beta-blockade No functional assessment of ischaemia
Invasive Angiography	"Gold standard" for identifying CAD Can proceed to PCI Invasive pressures assessed Intra-coronary physiology can be assessed – FFR	Risk of complication from invasive procedure Radiation exposure Use of iodinated contrast Expensive

86

Valvular stenosis, particularly left-sided can be accelerated with heavy calcification and full assessment with more frequent surveillance should be carried out in moderate and severe diseases.

The ideal preoperative tool is dynamic assessment with SE with the patient rendered euvolemic. Symptoms, effort tolerance, and pre- and post-valve, ventricular, and pulmonary artery pressure assessments can all be carried out using this technique. This can then inform anesthetic, surgical, and cardiology teams as to the risk of surgery and indications for intervention if needed.

86.4.1.3 Left Ventricular Disease

Given the prevalence of coronary disease in the renal population, ischemic cardiomyopathy is a significant cause of left ventricular systolic dysfunction. However, there also exists a complex interaction between the myocardium and volume status of patients with renal disease leading to non-ischemic cardiomyopathy.

The aetiology of such LV dysfunction may be related to conventional causes, e.g., alcohol, drug-induced, genetic but can be all related to chronic volume overload. Rendering the patient euvolemic can have an impressive effect on LV function. Moreover, renal transplantation has been shown to improve LV function from baseline with no other optimization being used [25].

Hence it is crucial to fully assess patients with baseline LV function and to understand the etiology including detailed history and screening blood tests. Cardiac MRI can be useful for LV tissue characterization but is limited by the risks of gadolinium contrast.

SE is invaluable for assessing baseline function and looking for regional wall motion abnormality. Exercise or pharmacological stress can then be performed to

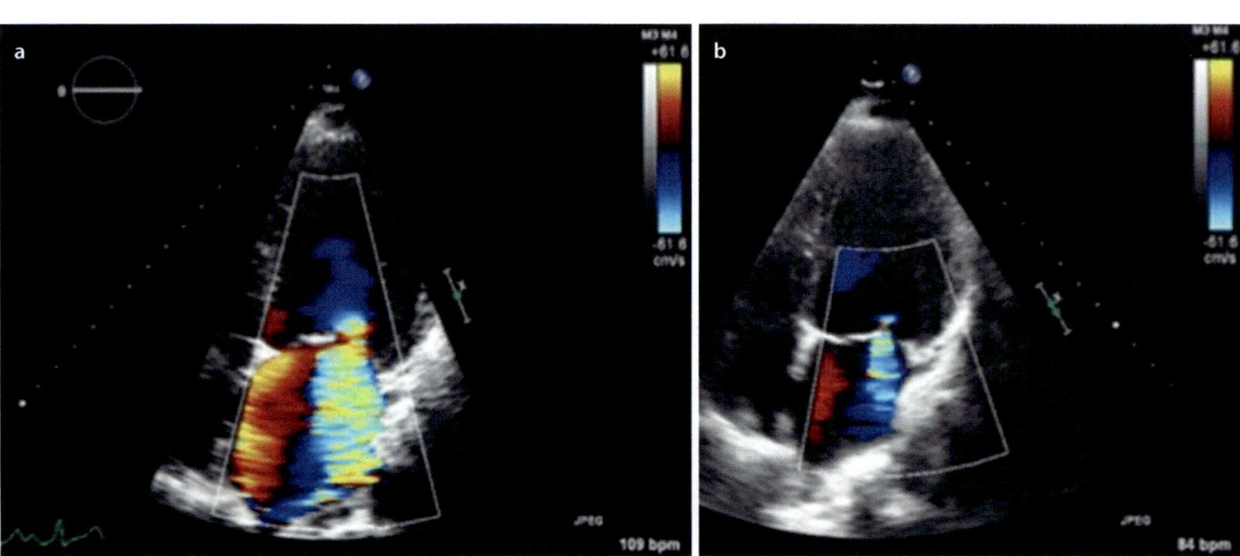

◘ **Fig. 86.8** **a** Severe mitral regurgitation seen in a patient with severe CKD. **b** Marked reduction in degree of mitral regurgitation in the same patient once rendered euvolemic

look for ischemia and also to detect regional and global LV systolic function from an abnormal baseline. The demonstration of the contractile reserve may support the decision to proceed to transplantation and may be a tool to predict recovery of LV function post-surgery.

The recipient population for renal transplantation has a significant cardiovascular risk profile. Assessment of risk should be as comprehensive as possible and primarily involve non-invasive techniques with both rest and stress imaging. Caution should be used in the echo assessment of these patients ensuring euvolemic status as far as possible.

Decisions regarding interventional procedures remain controversial and should be made using a multidisciplinary team.

86.4.2 Cerebrovascular Disease

It is reasonable to anticipate that patients with prior cerebrovascular events (transient ischemic attacks and/or strokes) are at heightened risk of further events postoperatively and that secondary prevention (e.g., use of antiplatelet agents, control of hypertension and dyslipidemia) would be of benefit. In patients with a prior history of TIA or stroke, carotid Doppler ultrasonography can stratify the risk of perioperative stroke but has no role in asymptomatic patients [26]. Moreover, there is no association demonstrated between carotid Doppler and post-transplant risk of stroke [12]. Current recommendations suggest delaying transplant for patients diagnosed with TIA and stroke 3 and 6 months after the acute event respectively [14]. This is based on expert opinion only and on available data from the general population demonstrating poorer outcomes in non-cardiac surgery within 12 months of acute stroke or TIA. These concerns must be balanced with long-term benefits and mortality reduction associated with transplantation, particularly in highly sensitized patients [13].

86.4.3 Recurrent disease

The leading cause of long-term allograft failure after chronic rejection is recurrent disease, which is responsible for around 15% of all graft loss. Recurrence of original disease in a transplant roughly doubles the risk of graft loss but this hides a huge variation in risk. In some conditions, recurrent disease can be catastrophic in terms of rapid graft loss and the majority of others result in reduced graft survival. So, while the primary renal disease is frequently unclear (undiagnosed in 25% of ESRD patients), striving to make a diagnosis where possible or at least exclude a few critical conditions that might preclude transplantation is a key part of the assessment process. This is particularly the case in young patients who have incurred a rapid presentation of CKD. Most conditions with potential for shortening graft survival don't preclude transplantation and can be managed and mitigated post-transplant but need to be part of the consent process and compared with the standard outcome; in the UK 10-year graft survival for patients with ADPKD (which does not recur) is c.85%. Key conditions are listed in ◘ Table 86.5.

86.4.4 Malignancy

Dialysis patients have an increased incidence of cancer compared to the general population with particularly high rates of renal cell carcinoma. This phenomenon has been linked to the relative immunoparesis associated with ESRD and its effect on anti-tumor surveillance. However, at present, there is no evidence that transplant wait-listed patients should have increased surveillance compared to their age-matched general population counterparts. The persistent pharmacological immunosuppression required for successful transplantation further disrupts innate anti-tumor and antiviral surveillance and has been linked to the increase in cancer risk following transplantation. Awareness of the potential for occult malignancy is therefore crucial prior to transplant listing (▶ Box 86.1) and appropriate investigations instituted early.

Box 86.1 Symptoms Suggestive of Underlying Malignancy that Warrants Directed Investigation

- Symptoms suggestive of malignancy
  - Unexplained weight loss (i.e., unrelated to dialysis adequacy, caloric intake)
  - Erythropoietin resistance
  - Treatment-resistant iron deficiency
  - Unexplained fevers (i.e., not related to underlying renal disease, infection, dialyzer)
  - Organ-specific symptoms (e.g., abdominal pain, bleeding per rectum, hemoptysis)

Current UK and European guidelines recommend waiting at least 2 years between successful tumor treatment/remission and transplantation, with a 5-year period being recommended for specific malignancies (e.g., colorectal cancer, breast cancer, and melanoma). These are based on data showing that 53% of recurrences occur in transplanted patients within 2 years of their cancer treatment, 34% within 2–5 years, and 13% if >5 years following treatment [40]. Renal cell carcinomas occur six times more frequently in ESRD patients compared to the general population but appropriately

Table 86.5 Primary renal diseases associated with significant rates of disease recurrence and which may lead to graft loss

Primary renal disease	Notes
Atypical Haemolytic Uremic Syndrome (aHUS)	Genotypic assessment is essential in stratifying recurrence risk post-transplantation (highest with factor H & I mutations which may have recurrence rates of 80% and devastating outcomes). Strenuous efforts should be made to identify the cause if suspected as a primary disease with genotype testing, anti-factor H antibodies, and exclusion of other less troublesome causes of microangiopathic hemolytic anemia in the native kidneys. The introduction of post-transplant eculizumab (humanized anti-C5 monoclonal antibody) has transformed the outcomes of patients with pathogenic factor H and I mutations and needs to be pre-planned (with appropriate vaccinations during workup) or instituted rapidly if the diagnosis declares itself post-transplant. *(see Chap. 51 on HUSSheerin)*
Focal segmental glomerulosclerosis (FSGS)	Overall 10-year graft survival for patients with FSGS in the UK is 66% but the diagnosis of FSGS is a mixed bag. 35–55% recurrence reported in adults although accurate diagnosis is vital especially in distinguishing primary from secondary forms [27, 28] Predictors include childhood presentation (<15 years old) and aggressive disease (heavy proteinuria, <3 years to reach ESRD). A history of prior recurrence post-transplant conveys an 80% risk of recurrence in subsequent allografts; early graft loss from recurrent FSGS is considered by some an absolute contraindication to further transplantation. In general, idiopathic forms of FSGS (30% recurrence risk overall) are much more likely to recur than familial forms; risk factors include age at diagnosis of native disease, white race, BMI, and native nephrectomy [29]. An important exception is those with heterozygous NPHS2 mutations – these are associated with a high risk of recurrence (65%); homozygous or complex heterozygous have much lesser risk (8%) so genetic screening is important. Idiopathic FSGS that results in recurrence in renal transplant is associated with a fivefold higher risk of graft loss [29]. It is important to consider family history when assessing the risks for live-related donors. Although routine use of plasma exchange or rituximab to reduce the risk of recurrence is not advised [4], plasma exchange and steroids are probably the treatment of choice *(see chapter on FSGS Mason)*
Membranoproliferative glomerulonephritis (MPGN) (immune complex-mediated)	Overall a primary diagnosis of MPGN impacts graft survival with a 10-year graft survival of around 70%. But the MPGN diagnosis is a very mixed bag and it is therefore worth considering genetic screening. Recommend investigation for infective, autoimmune, or paraprotein mediated causes prior to transplant as this can affect the risk of recurrence. Predictors of recurrence include pediatric presentation and the presence of crescentic GN on original biopsy
MPGN (C3 Glomerulonephritis including dense deposits disease/ DDD)	Dense deposit disease has a high recurrence rate and can occur very early (within days) with an average 10-year graft survival of around 56% (but worse figures: 30% 5-year survival, have been reported elsewhere). Consider genetic screening for complement disorder and C3NF antibodies to guide treatment and inform risk of recurrence. There is no proven treatment for recurrence, although removal of C3NeF with plasma exchange and anti-B cell strategies have been tried. There are case reports with the successful use of anti-C5 monoclonal antibodies. Recurrence in patients with CFHR5 nephropathy appears to be very common Loss of prior graft due to C3 Glomerulopathy indicates a high risk of recurrence in subsequent transplants. *(see chapter on MPGN Gale)*
Primary and Secondary hyperoxaluria	Primary hyperoxaluria type 1 is an absolute contraindication to renal transplantation unless combined with a liver transplant (100% recurrence rate leading to graft loss in the absence of a liver transplant). Screening for this disorder should be considered for all young patients with ESRD secondary to stones. Isolated kidney transplant should not be excluded in candidates with secondary hyperoxaluria or primary hyperoxaluria which is correctable (pyridoxine-responsive). The risk of recurrence should be considered, and high oxalate levels should be corrected prior to transplantation to reduce oxalate burden (dialysis, diet control, and pyridoxine treatment) [4]. *(see chapter on stones Moochhala)*
Alport's disease	De novo post-transplant anti-GBM disease can occur in up to 3% of mostly males with underlying Alport's disease. Given the low incidence, renal transplantation is not contraindicated. Screening for autoantibody levels postoperatively is advised, with early biopsy and treatment. Graft loss due to anti-GBM disease in this setting is a contraindication to further transplantation
Systemic sclerosis/ Scleroderma Renal Crisis	Risk of recurrence seems very low (approximately 3%) assuming the disease is quiescent; typically, in first year with a prodrome of anemia, pericardial effusion, and skin disease [30]. Typically, after dialysis is initiated, the transplant is not initiated for a minimum of 6 months due to the possibility of renal recovery. In our experience, the use of calcineurin inhibitors has not provoked recurrence The key is to avoid uncontrolled hypertension and ACE inhibitors should be continued peri-operatively or reintroduced early. High-dose steroids should be used with caution. The 5-year graft survival is 57% and patient survival is 73% at 5 years [30]

Table 86.5 (continued)

Primary renal disease	Notes
Lupus Nephritis	Although recurrence is uncommon (<5%) 10-year graft survival for lupus patients in the UK is reduced by72%, although this may not all be due to recurrent disease. Most clinicians would not list a patient until the disease is in clinical remission for at least 6 months It is important to consider that lupus can be associated with an increased risk of thrombotic events in patients with anti-cardiolipin antibodies, lupus anti-coagulant, or beta- 2 glycopeptide antibodies. Recurrent anti-phospholipid syndrome can be catastrophic and therefore all patients should be screened prior to transplantation to guide perioperative management *(see Lupus chapter Daun)*
Anti-GBM disease	Recurrence post-transplantation is exceptionally rare when given at least a 6-month interval prior to transplantation to allow anti-GBM antibodies to become persistently negative
Anti-Neutrophil Cytoplasmic Antibody (ANCA) Vasculitis	The recurrence rate is between 1% and 22% with time to relapse ranging between few days up to 13 years (mean time 22–31 months) [31]. ANCA positivity at the time of transplantation is not predictive and relapses have occurred with negative ANCA titers at the time of transplantation. Relapse of ANCA vasculitis may mimic infections and other complications of immunosuppressive therapy and therefore continuous monitoring is recommended Perhaps surprisingly, in the UK, 10-year graft survival for patients with granulomatous polyangiitis is no different to ADPKD (84%)
Membranous Nephropathy (MN)	MN is the second most common cause of nephrotic-range proteinuria in allograft recipients. Recurrent disease is common with a wide variability (10–45%) occurring in early and late phases [32] with a reduced overall graft survival of 76% at 10 years which probably reflects a wide range depending on primary etiology M-type phospholipase A2 receptor (PLA2R) antibodies, implicated in the pathogenesis of primary MN, have been identified as a risk factor for recurrence when circulating at the time of transplantation. Persistent detection of PLA2R antibodies is a marker for worsening the clinical course of recurrent MN [33]. It is therefore important to measure PLA2R levels at the time of transplantation and periodically thereafter It has been suggested that recurrence rates are higher in live donor transplants, but no significant difference has been proven Causes of secondary MN should be investigated prior to consideration for transplantation A high rate of de novo disease MN has been identified at 2–9% at 2 years post-transplantation [34].*(see membranous chapter Salama)*
Recurrent UTI/ urinary tract dysfunction	UTIs are the most common infection post-transplantation and may contribute to graft injury or loss. Reflux to the native or transplant ureter is shown to be contributory to recurrent UTIs in the immunocompromised transplant recipient and consideration of native nephroureterectomy may be required, particularly in the presence of voiding dysfunction A high-pressure dysfunctional bladder will be equally effective at damaging a transplant as a native kidney. Patients with CAKUT (the commonest cause of CKD in children and young adults) are, particularly at risk. Voiding dysfunction should be ruled out by means of pre- and post-micturition US, flow rate studies, micturating cystourethrography, or video-urodynamics as needed
Stones	As noted above, primary hyperoxaluria is an absolute contraindication for kidney only transplantation and needs to be excluded in a patient with multiple stones. Enteric oxalosis is not a contraindication but the cause needs to be diagnosed and pancreatic insufficiency or other causes managed 2,8-Dihydroxyadenine stones although rare, will recur and are easily prevented with xanthine oxidase inhibitors providing the diagnosis is made Other stones recur less frequently but urosepsis related to stones is highly likely to recur if native stones have a chronic subclinical infection
Diabetic nephropathy	In the tacrolimus era, histological evidence of diabetic nephropathy is seen in the allografts of about 52% of transplant recipients with diabetes at baseline [35]. This is a major contributor to graft failure by 10 years Simultaneous Pancreas-Kidney (SPK) is another option for patients with type 1 diabetes or those with type 2 diabetes who meet certain criteria (mainly insulin-dependent for over 1 year). Other options include pancreas after kidney transplant (PAK) or pancreas transplant alone (PTA) for those patients who have already received living or deceased donor kidney transplants Ten-year allograft survival rates are 69% for SPK, 44% for PAK following living donor kidney transplant, and 42% for PAK following deceased donor transplant [36]. Both patient and kidney allograft longevity are maximized by achieving insulin-free state New diagnosis of diabetes post-transplantation needs to be considered post-transplantation for all patients due to high corticosteroid burden and the diabetogenic properties of immunosuppressants. Twelve-year graft survival has been shown to be 48% for those who developed post-transplant diabetes compared to 70% for non-diabetics [37]. Traditional risk factors for non-transplant patients (increased age, obesity, family history, African American, Hispanic, and southeast Asian Race) also predispose transplanted patients to post-transplant diabetes

(continued)

Table 86.5 (continued)

Primary renal disease	Notes
IgA nephropathy (IgAN)	Histological recurrence with IgAN is common (>50%) but occurs late (>5 years). It was previously thought that recurrence was not clinically significant and rarely led to graft loss. Recent retrospective studies with a longer duration of follow-up have however demonstrated that this is not the case and 10-year graft survival in the UK is significantly reduced by 75% The following risk factors have been identified [38]: 1. Time post-transplantation (rate of recurrence increases with time) 2. Presence of specific Human leukocyte antigen (HLA) genotypes 3. Zero mismatch kidneys 4. High serum IgA levels pre and at 6 months post-transplant 5. Steroid-free maintenance immunosuppression (there is increasing circumstantial evidence that maintenance steroids reduce the risk of graft loss (HR 0.66)) Furthermore, features of native IgAN can also help predict the risk of recurrent disease in renal allograft. A patient reaching ESRD by 30 from IgA or with crescentic IgA would be of much greater concern than a patient reaching ESRD in their 60s with a non-proliferative pattern on biopsy
Amyloid	Risk of recurrence of AA amyloidosis is related to the degree of activity of the underlying disease. Rates of infection and cardiovascular complications are higher in these patients AL amyloidosis also recurs and can cause graft failure. A recent series suggests improving outcomes with no graft failures among 22 renal allografts after 48 months follow-up
Multiple myeloma	Previously considered an absolute contraindication to transplantation. Recent advances in therapeutic regimens mean durable remissions are more likely and transplantation may be appropriate in selected individuals with a good prognosis (e.g., good response to chemotherapy with further therapeutic options available or durable complete remission following autologous stem cell transplant). Long-term outcome data is limited but monitoring trends in serum-free light chains is critical
Sickle cell disease	Transplant outcomes for patients with SCD have been grim and underappreciated; retrospective data from London demonstrated death censored 10-year graft survival of only 19% and very high mortality. Of note those patients who received regular exchange blood transfusion (EBT) the 10-year outcome was 38% compared to 0% for those who did not. A pre-transplant plan with hematologists is essential and preoperative transfusion or exchange transfusion to maintain HbS <20% advised together with 40% FiO_2 to reduce the risk of sickle crisis seems sensible. The use of hydroxyurea and or EBT should be actively considered in all patients with a high sickle percentage
Lipoprotein glomerulopathy	Very limited data, with only six cases of patients who have received a renal transplant. Recurrent disease is reported in all but one case. There is no proven therapeutic intervention
Fibrillary glomerulonephritis	Limited data is available. Recurrence rate around 50% but relatively benign course when compared to native kidney, except when monoclonal gammopathy is present [39]
Eating disorders	Anecdotally ESRD secondary to eating disorders (recurrent pre-renal AKI) has a significant risk of recurrence, particularly if the transplant course is complicated and stressful. High serum bicarbonate (≥30 mmol/L) in the 6 months prior to transplantation might be a warning signal

Abbreviations: *HUS* hemolytic uraemic syndrome, *FSGS* focal segmental glomerular sclerosis, *MPGN* membranoproliferative glomerulonephritis, *PH1* primary hyperoxaluria type 1, *GBM* glomerular basement membrane, *ESRD* end-stage renal disease

treated, small (<3 cm), non-metastasized lesions do not preclude transplant listing after 2 years of surveillance as the risk of subsequent recurrence is very low.

Previous post-transplant lymphoproliferative disease (PTLD) is not a contraindication to transplant listing and good outcomes are reported following re-transplantation using conventional immunosuppression [41]. Current UK guidelines advocate a period of at least 1 year from the control of PTLD to re-transplantation to minimize recurrence risk and a 10% recurrence rate is a ball-park figure. It would seem prudent to reimage and check EBV PCR before relisting.

Specific guidelines vary by region for the minimum interval recommended between the treatment of a specific malignancy and transplantation. Both European and American guidance is based on observed rates of recurrence from registry data; a summary of both is included in Table 86.6 [40, 44].

86.4.5 Infection

Infection is the second leading cause of death with a functioning graft and, therefore, treating underlying

Table 86.6 Summary of American and European Guidelines for the minimum time period between the diagnosis and treatment of malignancy and renal transplantation [42, 43]

	American Society of Transplantation	European Best Practice Guidelines for Renal Transplantation
Less Than 2 Years	Incidentally Discovered Renal Cancers <5 cm In-situ Bladder Cancer Basal Cell Carcinomas	Incidentally Discovered Renal Cancer In-situ carcinomas Small Single Focal Neoplasms Low-Grade Basal Skin Cancers
At Least 2 Years	Wilms Tumor Bladder Cancer Symptomatic Renal Cancers Carcinoma of the Uterine Body Testicular Cancer Thyroid Cancer Kaposi or Other Sarcomas Some Early Stage Breast Cancers Prostate Cancer Hodgkin's or non-Hodgkin's Lymphoma Leukemia In situ or very thin melanoma Lung cancer	Most Other Common Cancers
More Than 2 Years	Cervical Cancer (2–5 years, depending on the case) Duke A or B1 Colon cancer	Malignant melanoma Breast Carcinoma Colorectal Carcinoma Non-in situ Carcinoma of the Uterus
At Least 5 Years	Invasive or >5 cm Renal Cancers Invasive Breast Cancer Colon Cancer Malignant Melanoma	Diffuse Bladder Cancer Non-in situ Cervical Cancer Colorectal Cancer
Contraindicated	Liver Cancer (unless also undergoing liver transplantation)	Diffuse Cancers of the Prostate

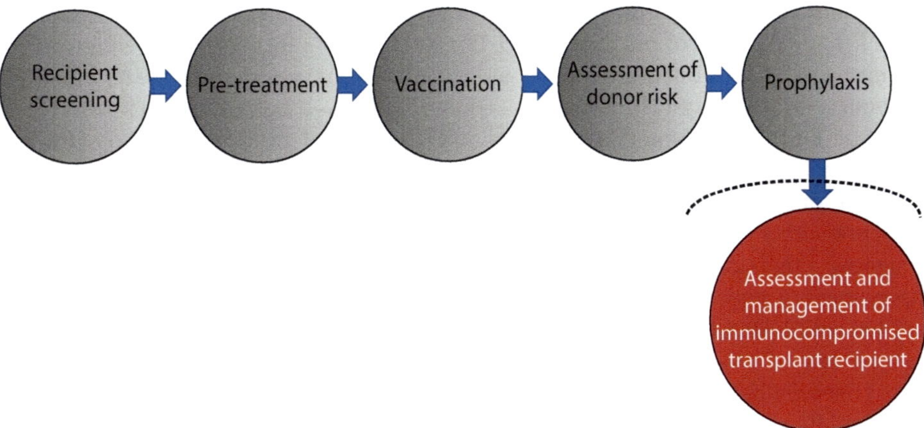

Fig. 86.9 Elements of infection control in a transplant service

infections, vaccination, and prophylaxis are key components of transplant workup (see Fig. 86.9). Patients undergoing workup for transplantation should be screened for any occult or latent infection which might be exacerbated by immunosuppression and which may require treatment before transplantation or prophylactic therapy post-transplantation and therefore it is important to include this workup in the transplant assessment clinic (▶ Box 86.2). Periodontal disease should be screened and treated prior to transplantation [4].

For the same infectious agent, there tends to be a hierarchy of virulence post-transplant with primary infections being worse than re-infections, which are more virulent than reactivations.

Box 86.2 Principal Infections Screened for in the Pre-transplant Assessment

- Infection
  - Tuberculosis (TB) (including past exposure) and *Mycobacterium avium-intracellulare* infection (MAI)
  - Hepatitis B
  - Hepatitis C
  - Human immunodeficiency virus (HIV)
  - Herpes simplex virus (HSV)
  - Human T-cell lymphotropic virus (HTLV)
  - Cytomegalovirus (CMV)
  - Epstein-Barr virus (EBV)

86.4.5.1 Tuberculosis

The frequency of active TB is 20–74 fold higher in solid organ transplant recipients compared to the general population, with an incidence rate of 0.5–15% among kidney transplant population, and the commonest form of acquisition is a reactivation of latent TB [45]. The majority of post-transplant TB manifestations are extra pulmonary and it can cause graft loss in up to a third of the case.

All transplant candidates should be assessed for a history of prior TB exposure including country of origin, a full contact (household, institution), and travel history. Heightened awareness is needed for patients deriving from areas of high endemicity (e.g., Africa, South Asia, Eastern Europe) (see ◘ Table 86.7). This should be accompanied by an up-to-date chest radiograph to look for any evidence of old, healed TB. Equivocal cases require specialist evaluation with the aid of interferon-gamma release assays/ IGRA (e.g., QuantiFERON-Gold or T-SPOT.TB) and consideration of CT imaging to demonstrate focal disease and/or lymphadenopathy. Conventional tuberculin skin testing performs poorly in patients with ESRD and cannot be relied on to direct diagnosis, therefore 2010 UK guidelines recommend assessment of patients who are on renal transplant waiting list with IGRA [47]. A meta-analysis in 2015 showed similar rate of sensitivity (50–53%) and specificity (67–69%) between both IGRA methods [48].

The UK guidelines recommend a 6-month course of treatment for active TB and consideration for similar treatment in cases of latent TB as directed by specialist review. Following completion of a 6-month course of treatment, surveillance is recommended but there is no evidence to support further treatment in the absence of disease reactivation [47].

◘ Table 86.7 Countries with a high burden of TB (>40 cases per 100,000 population) for the period 2016–2020

Africa	Angola Democratic Republic of the Congo Ethiopia Kenya Mozambique Nigeria South Africa Tanzania	Central African Republic Congo Lesotho Liberia Namibia Sierra Leone Zambia Zimbabwe
Asia	Southeast Asia, e.g., Indonesia, Myanmar, Philippines, Thailand, Vietnam, South Korea, Cambodia	China
	Bangladesh	Papua New Guinea
	India	Pakistan
Europe	Russian Federation	
Central & South America	Brazil	

Adapted from the WHO Tuberculosis report 2020 This list is not exhaustive and readers are encouraged to visit the relevant website: ► https://www.who.int/tb/publications/global_report/en/ [46]

Post-transplant chemoprophylaxis (6 months of isoniazid& pyridoxine) is advocated for all recipients from areas of high TB endemicity but is not needed for patients from low-risk countries or for those who have been previously fully treated for TB. List of high-burden countries defined by WHO for the period 2016–2020 can be found in ◘ Table 86.7 [46]. However, since exposure in childhood/young age is the source of latent TB, cautious interpretation of this list is needed, and careful consideration of the past history of TB in each country should be exercised.

86.4.5.2 Atypical Mycobacterial Infection

Non-tuberculous mycobacteria infection, such as *Mycobacterium avium and M. intracellulare* (both known as *Mycobacterium avium-intracellulare* infection (MAI)), is a rare complication post-transplantation with incidence ranging between 0.16% and 0.55% [49]. Treatment is empirical with antituberculosis therapy and reduction of immunosuppression. There is no data on the risk of recurrence or reactivation in patients who have suffered MAI previously, e.g., in the context of HIV disease and who subsequently progress to renal transplantation.

86.4.5.3 Hepatitis B

All potential transplant recipients should have full HBV serology performed – hepatitis B surface antigen (HBsAg), hepatitis B core antibody (HBcAb), and hepatitis B surface antibody level (HBsAb). This allows for the identification of occult infection as well as stratifying the risk of viral reactivation and donor-derived HBV infection.

All HBsAg +ve patients should have further investigations including HBeAg, HBeAb, HDV Ab serology, HBV DNA levels as well as liver disease staging. Treatment with tenofovir or entecavir should be initiated as indicated prior to transplantation [50].

Patients with evidence of chronic HBV infection (HBsAg +ve and HBcAb +ve) require a formal hepatological assessment to determine the need for nucleoside/nucleotide analog treatment prior to transplantation. Monitoring of liver enzymes, HBV DNA, and alfa-fetoprotein levels is recommended every 3–6 months coupled with 6–12 monthly liver USS. Chronic active HBV infection does not preclude transplantation, but patients are at risk of post-transplant reactivation and require indefinite antiviral therapy. Lamivudine is associated with a high risk of resistance (70% at 5 years) and the choice of agent (e.g., lamivudine, entecavir, tenofovir) is determined by viral resistance patterns.

All potential transplant recipients with evidence of past infection/ exposure (HBsAg –ve, HBV DNA –ve, and HBcAb +ve) must have HBV DNA and HDV serology testing. Among transplant recipients who are HBcAb +ve and have HBsAb titer <100 IU/mL, vaccination should be considered to boost the HBsAb titer and minimize the risk of reactivation. The risk of reactivation is low (1–2%) in patients with past cleared HBV infection and limited duration of post-transplant antiviral prophylaxis course, e.g., lamivudine (for duration 6–12 months) or surveillance (e.g. monthly testing for HBsAg for the first 6 months) are both reasonable approaches [50].

Regardless of treatment or prophylaxis regime, regular serology monitoring including HBV DNA and HBsAg should be performed every 3 months in the first year and then every 6 months for individuals receiving a graft from an HBc Ab +ve donor [50].

86.4.5.4 Hepatitis C

All potential transplant recipients should be screened for HCV antibody at the time of assessment and those with positive antibody tests should have an HCV RNA and genotypic assay performed. HCV infection per se is *not* a contraindication to renal transplantation; however, accelerated HCV-related hepatic fibrosis was seen in immunosuppressed individuals and overall 10-year survival is approximately 15% lower in HCV+ renal transplant recipients compared to those who are HCV-ve in the pre-DAA-era. Nevertheless, the survival advantage conferred by transplantation compared to remaining on dialysis still prevails in HCV+ recipients.

All HCV+ patients are required to have formal hepatological assessment and they also should be evaluated for the presence of cirrhosis using either non-invasive staging methods or on occasional, liver biopsy. Those without cirrhosis can undergo isolated kidney transplantation while those with decompensated cirrhosis should be referred for combined liver-kidney transplantation [51].

Treatment of HCV using interferon-based regimens post-transplantation is contraindicated due to the significant risk of precipitating acute rejection. Interferon-free agents such as the direct-acting antiviral agents (DAAs)-based regime have transformed this as they enable HCV clearance before or after transplantation.

In the last few years, there has been a significant revolution in the practice of transplanting kidney from hepatitis C positive donor following the availability of DAA treatment, which is safe and highly effective as it provides a high cure rate. DAA has been shown to cause 57% lower risk of death in HCV seropositive recipients who received kidney from seropositive donors compared to mortality rate in the pre-DAA era [52].

86.4.5.5 HIV

In the current era of highly active antiretroviral therapy (HAART) and modern transplant immunosuppression protocols, the outcomes of renal transplantation in HIV+ individuals are similar to those in HIV-ve patients. However, outcomes are poorer for recipients with HIV and HCV co-infection [53]. Although HIV infection is not a contraindication to transplantation, disease remission is essential prior to transplant listing (▶ Box 86.3).

HIV+ patients have a higher cumulative incidence of acute rejection (approximately double non-HIV patients) reaching 31% in one study [55].

The interaction between calcineurin inhibitors (CNIs) and protease inhibitors is extremely potent with significant prolongation of CNI half-life (e.g., some patients only require 0.5 mg tacrolimus weekly). This combination is best avoided where possible and our practice is to move patients to a raltegravir-based regimen when resistance patterns permit and in the absence of a protease inhibitor standard doses of CNI can be used. Either way early, close consultation with

Box 86.3 HIV-Specific Assessment for Transplant Candidates (See Guidelines for Details) [54]

In selected cases, solid organ transplantation may be appropriate for patients with fully suppressed HIV RNA (<50 copies/mL)and a CD4 cell count between 100 and 200 cells/μL

Patients with HIV RNA levels <200 copies/mL may be considered suitable for solid organ transplantation if otherwise well and fully adherent with their medications

Patients with advanced cervical/anal intraepithelial neoplasia (CIN/AIN III) or carcinoma in-situ should receive treatment prior to transplantation

History of extra-cutaneous Kaposi sarcoma, Castleman's disease, human herpes virus 8 (HHV8)-related primary effusion lymphoma or Epstein-Barr virus (EBV)-related lymphoma are contraindications for transplantation

the treating HIV Medicine team is essential. Some patients may require a dose-finding trial of immunosuppression on some regimens with monitoring of HIV viral load.

At present, UK guidelines recommend informing live donors factors that can affect recipient mortality/morbidity, for example, positive viral serology such as recipient HIV+ status [56]. This remains very controversial but to withhold information from a donor has legal (and trust) implications. Some units take the view that it is sufficient to inform the prospective donor that the recipient is at increased risk of complications without disclosing the HIV status.

86

86.4.5.6 HTLV Infection

HTLV-1 is endemic in some areas of the world (e.g., Caribbean, Japan, South America). In the general population, the virus is associated with an increased risk of adult T-cell leukemia–lymphoma (ATL) and the development of HTLV-1 associated myelopathy - tropical spastic paraparesis (HAM – TSP) (lifetime risk approximately 5% and 2%).

The median duration of HAM-TSP development post-renal transplantation in HTLV+ recipients is 3.8 years [57]. It remains unclear whether the risk of disease is increased by immunosuppression and increasingly recipient HTLV antibody positivity is felt not to be a contraindication to transplantation. Where available, it is worth considering screening for viral RNA although the impact of transplantation in viremic patients is not known.

86.4.5.7 Herpes Simplex (HSV)

Commonest route of symptomatic HSV disease in transplant recipients is via reactivation of latent viruses, especially in early phase post-transplantation and following antirejection therapy. Primary HSV infection post-transplantation is rare and, however, carries a risk of lethal fulminant hepatitis; therefore, it is important to ascertain the immunity of all transplant recipients prior to transplantation. This is particularly important in centers employing a policy of surveillance and pre-emptive treatment rather than prophylaxis for CMV (valganciclovir offers some protection). HSV is the commonest form of encephalitis in transplant recipients.

86.4.5.8 Cytomegalovirus (CMV)

Recipient status is important to know prior to transplantation but does not affect the decision to list. There is the real prospect of CMV vaccination and if trials are successful then vaccination of both CMV –ve and CMV +ve recipients may become routine.

86.4.5.9 Varicella Zoster (VZV)

Around 3% of patients are not immune and risk significant mortality if they contract VZV post-transplantation. Disease presentation can range from dermatomal to disseminated zoster with or without visceral involvement. Patients must be screened pre-transplant and vaccination with two doses of live vaccine seems to offer good protection. This should be given at least 4 weeks prior to transplantation [4]. Non-immune patients receiving a transplant should be given aciclovir prophylaxis.

86.4.5.10 Epstein-Barr Virus (EBV)

EBV seronegative transplant recipients (10% of adults, 50% of children) are at risk of primary EBV infection, which conveys a significant risk (10- to 76-fold) of subsequent development of PTLD [58]. The role of monitoring of viral load post-transplantation remains unclear (high viral load $>10^5$ copies/ml is associated with PTLD, but the positive predictive value is poor).

Intravenous immunoglobin and/or antiviral therapy have been suggested as prophylactic strategies but are of unproven value.

86.4.5.11 Strongyloides

Strongyloides stercoralis is an intestinal nematode that can persist in the human host for decades after the initial infection and can progress to fulminant hyper-infection syndrome in immunocompromised hosts. Hyper-infestation syndrome is rare but carries a high mortality and is avoidable. Patients who have traveled to or resided in endemic regions (South America, Africa, Southeast Asia) should be screened for strongyloides pre-transplant (serology +/− stool) and treated if positive. Ivermectin 200 mcg/kg OD orally for 2 days is the current recommended first-line treatment. Some units in endemic areas simply treat all patients. Either way, units need to have a robust policy to avoid hyper-infestation post- transplant.

86.4.5.12 Schistosomiasis

Schistosomiasis is a chronic parasitic infection with worms of the trematode family common in Africa, South America, and Southeast Asia. Infection can be associated with higher incidence of urinary tract infection, obstructive uropathy, and an increased risk of bladder malignancy. Serological screening is indicated for individuals from endemic areas. The main concern is a dysfunctional bladder and the risk of cancer post-transplant. Treatment is with praziquantel.

86.4.5.13 Toxoplasma

T. gondii is an intracellular protozoan parasite, with members of the cat family being the definitive hosts. The value of screening recipients for toxoplasma status is controversial but is potentially useful in identifying patients at risk, especially seronegative recipients with seropositive donors, and can help in establishing the diagnosis by showing seroconversion. It is also important to caution patients who are negative about handling cats and cat litter.

86.4.5.14 Syphilis

Syphilis infection is often asymptomatic, however can cause cardiac and neurological disease after transplantation. Screening for latent syphilis is initially with a rapid plasma reagin (RPR) assay. If the results are positive, the patient should undergo a specific treponemal test (fluorescent treponemal antibody absorption test or microhemagglutination assay for *Treponema pallidum*) to determine whether the RPR result is biologically false-positive. If the RPR result is low-titer and the patient has received appropriate treatment for syphilis in the past, the patient is unlikely to have latent infection. However, any other positive RPR assay result with positive treponemal test results should be considered an indication of active (presumably latent) syphilis and should be treated. Standard treatment is with benzathine penicillin G 2.4 million units IM given weekly for three doses. Ceftriaxone or doxycycline is alternative treatment for those who are allergic to penicillin.

86.4.5.15 Trypanosoma cruzi (Chaga's disease)

Trypanosomiasis is endemic in Central and South America. The infection can be present as latent disease for decades. Reactivation usually occurs in the first year post-transplantation and it can be asymptomatic or presented with fever, skin, cardiac, and neurology involvement [4]. Patients who have resided in endemic areas should be screened (serology) and monitored for reactivation post-transplantation.

86.4.5.16 Coccidioides

Coccidioidomycosis is a fungus endemic in the southwestern United States. Symptoms including severe pulmonary infection or extrapulmonary dissemination. Serological screening and secondary prophylaxis for coccidioidomycosis in transplant recipients are recommended for transplant candidates and recipients as approximately 50% of coccidioidal infections in transplant recipients are due to reactivation of pre-existing disease.

86.4.5.17 Histoplasmosis

Histoplasmosis is a fungal infection caused by the dimorphic saprophytic fungus *Histoplasma capsulatum*, which is endemic in the Central United States, South America, the Caribbean, Africa, and Asia. Median time from transplantation to diagnosis is 27 months [59] and in the face of immunosuppression, progressive disseminated disease may develop and is associated with a high mortality rate (20% or more). Serological screening should be considered to identify patients at risk of reactivation post-transplantation (although the risk is low even in seropositive individuals).

86.4.5.18 Human Herpes Virus-8

HHV-8 is associated with the development of Kaposi's sarcoma (KS). Transplantation-associated KS occurs in around 0.2–5% of transplant recipients [58]. Testing for

HHV-8 is not widely available but a history of previous KS should be noted as a significant factor for recurrence.

Vaccinations

Patients who are asplenic or will receive Eculizumab should receive pneumococcal, Haemophilus influenza and meningococcal vaccinations (see Table 86.8 for details).

Live vaccinations should be administered at least 4 weeks prior to transplantation.

86.4.6 Frailty

Frailty, defined as decline in physiological reserve and therefore reduced ability to respond to stressor events, has emerged as a better predictor for outcome post-transplantation compared to the sole use of ageism. It has higher prevalence in CKD population requiring dialysis with > 60% and this is influenced by multiple factors such as sarcopenia, malnutrition, infection and inflammation, cognitive impairment, physical inactivity, vitamin D deficiency, metabolic acidosis, and cellular

Table 86.8 List of infections that should be treated or controlled pre-transplant and vaccinations either recommended or to be considered on the grounds of common sense

Hepatitis C RNA positive	Attempt to eradicate infection and achieve sustained virological response using directly acting agents (DAAs) before listing
Hepatitis B	Universal vaccination of non-immune CKD patients (and ESRF), prelisting assessment and stable virological control of hepatitis B with antivirals
HIV Ab positive	Undetectable viral load and $CD4^{+}$>100 (ideally 200) and no opportunistic infections for 6 months prior to listing
VZV Antibody negative	Vaccination (live vaccine) of the 3% of ESRF population negative for VZV with live vaccine. Prophylaxis with acyclovir if transplanted within 2 weeks of vaccination
Influenza	Annual vaccination with quadrivalent vaccine
MMR (live vaccine)	If not previously vaccinated, vaccinate 1 month pre-transplant. Testing and vaccination of all women of childbearing age pre-listing if Rubella IgG negative
Diphtheria, tetanus and pertussis	If not previously vaccinated, vaccinate pre-transplant and routine boosters 5–10 yearly
Polio (inactivated)	Routine vaccination if not previously vaccinated; can be given post-transplant but *not live vaccine*
Human Papilloma virus	Girls and boys eligible for local vaccination programme should be strongly encouraged to take this up. No evidence yet for a benefit in older females to prevent CIN, or to prevent anogenital warts in women or men, but worth considering especially in those likely to receive high levels of immunosuppression
CMV	Early vaccine studies looking encouraging, large scale studies pending
Pneumococcal	Vaccination according to national guidelines ideally pre-transplant
Haemophilus influenzae B	Consider pre-transplant in those with pulmonary pathology (can also be given post-transplant)
Meningococcal meningitis	Vaccination according to national guidelines
Recurrent UTI	Patients with recurrent UTI before transplantation are highly likely to have significant urosepsis after transplantation - where possible the cause should be identified and treated pre-listing (NB. Persistent pyuria also needs explaining even if not associated with overt sepsis)
Tuberculosis	Screening in patients with ESRF by Mantoux or interferon-ϒ release assays (IGRA) often negative due to diminished T cell response.
StrongyloidesAb positive	If treatment history not clear, especially if eosinophilia, treat with Ivermectin 200 mg/kg/day for 2 days (blind treatment is routine practice in many endemic countries)
SchistosomiasisAb positive	Treat with two doses of 20 mg/kgpraziquantel

senescence [60]. The Clinical Frailty Score (CFS), which is used widely in the UK, describes a 9- point frailty score with higher score indicating higher frailty status.

Frailty is associated with 94% increased risk of delayed graft function [61], 61% higher risk of early hospital readmission [62], as well as 2.17-fold higher risk of death following kidney transplantation [63]. However, certain patients with frailty have also been shown to experience improvement in physical and health-related quality of life (HRQOL) [64], frailty status [65] as well as survival [66] post-transplantation.

Establishing a robust system, with integrating frailty screening in transplant assessment clinics as a start, is essential to recognize a cohort of patients that would benefit from transplantation from those that would have greater risk of morbidity and mortality should they proceed with transplantation. It is also important that regular monitoring of CFS assessment is in place to identify any changes during the waiting list period, as more than half experienced changes between evaluation and transplantation, and this transition is associated with mortality and longer length of stay [67]. Further research is needed to investigate whether the current frailty screening measures are sufficient to determine transplant outcomes in waiting list patients whether there are any reversible factors influencing frailty that can be identified and reversed prior to entering transplantation, and whether there are biomarkers that can help in making this decision [60].

86.4.7 Pulmonary Issues

Patients with poor respiratory function, as well as those with multiple co-morbidities, represent higher risk candidates for surgery and formal anesthetic review may be required. Poor candidates for renal transplant include those on home oxygen therapy, uncontrolled asthma, severe corpulmonale, severe COPD, pulmonary fibrosis, and restrictive disease [4, 68].

Pulmonary hypertension in patients with ESRD and advanced CKD is associated with time on dialysis, systolic and diastolic heart dysfunction, obstructive sleep apnoea, pulmonary embolism, and smoking. This results in decreased post-transplant survival as well as early allograft dysfunction in deceased donor transplants [69]. These patients should be treated prior to transplantation when possible.

Cigarette smoking is associated with an increased risk of death post-transplant [70]. The effects of smoking appear to dissipate after 5 years, so patients should be counseled to quit prior to transplantation and encouraged to abstain thereafter.

Pulmonary function tests should be carried out on all candidates with impaired functional capacity, respiratory symptoms, or known underlying respiratory disease. Chest radiograph is recommended on all candidates, with CT chest recommended for those with a current or previous heavy use of tobacco.

86.4.8 Gastrointestinal (GI) Issues

All candidates should be evaluated for the presence of GI and liver disease. Routine liver screens should be performed on all candidates and any abnormal findings must be addressed prior to transplantation.

Symptomatic peptic ulcer disease which has not been previously diagnosed should be investigated with an OGD and H. Pylori testing. They should be fully treated prior to transplant. Repeat OGD is not required for those who have been previously diagnosed.

Candidates with inflammatory bowel disease (IBD) should ideally be assessed in conjunction with their gastroenterologist, particularly with regards to the timing of transplant. Transplant should be delayed during an active flare-up. All candidates with IBD should be screened for bowel cancer prior to transplant.

Candidates with active diverticulitis should be delayed until their flare-up is treated. Routine screening is not advised.

Candidates with pancreatitis should not be transplanted for a minimum of 3 months after symptoms have resolved. This should not preclude them from future transplantation.

Symptomatic gall stone and gall bladder disease should delay transplantation until symptoms have been resolved. In those candidates with recurrent cholecystitis, cholecystectomy is recommended prior to transplantation. Routine screening in absence of symptoms is not required.

86.4.9 Miscellaneous

Finally, an awareness of the recipient's cultural and religious beliefs may influence the practicalities of transplantation. As an example, patients who are Jehovah's Witnesses may consent to transplantation but religious objections to the use of blood products may render such surgery high-risk, and careful preoperative counseling is recommended.

86.5 Anesthetic Assessment

86.5.1 Preoperative Assessment

While cardiovascular assessment of the transplant recipient has been covered elsewhere in this chapter there are several specific considerations given to the anesthetic assessment including:

1. Cardiopulmonary risk
2. SVC obstruction and access issues
3. Intubation hazard

86.5.1.1 Cardiovascular Risk

Kidney transplant surgery is classed by the European Society of Anaesthesiology as an "intermediate risk" procedure (in a standard patient), associated with a 1–5% 30-day risk of cardiovascular death and myocardial infarction [24]. Key cardiovascular hazards for the anesthetist to consider (prior to transplant call) in a renal patient are as follows:

1. Ischemic heart disease
2. Impaired left ventricular function (systolic and diastolic)
3. Pulmonary hypertension
4. Aortic stenosis
5. Idiopathic hypotension

86

The incidence of aortic valve calcification in dialysis patients is double that of the general population and the severity of which is proportional to time spent on dialysis [71]. Specific considerations for the patient with aortic stenosis related to anesthesia include avoidance of systemic hypotension as this will result in myocardial ischemia and therefore decreased contractility [72]. These patients are also at increased risk of new-onset tachyarrhythmia which may reduce coronary artery filling time in diastole and should therefore be promptly treated [72]. Preoperative intervention, e.g., valve surgery or TAVI, may be warranted.

Another consideration is the renal patient with pulmonary hypertension. As the right heart output (and therefore left heart output) is affected by increased pulmonary vascular resistance it is important to minimize factors predisposing to this related to surgery and anesthesia; such factors increasing pulmonary vascular resistance include hypoxia, hypercarbia, acidemia, and pain [73]. Increases in minute volume made by the anesthetist may prevent hypercarbia and dialysis pre-surgery may assist with acidosis. Systemic vasopressors, e.g., noradrenaline, are required in the event of right heart decompensation [73].

Guidelines on preoperative assessment of patients for non-cardiac surgery exist and incorporate functional assessments such as the "Duke Activity Status Index", a self-assessment questionnaire that provides some quantitative information assessing functional and therefore cardiac status [74]. However, there appears to be a lack of confidence in the application of these guidelines to an end-stage renal population. This uncertainty was highlighted by a 2019 survey of practice in the UK which demonstrated considerable variation between centers in the investigations used to assess cardiopulmonary function in potential kidney transplant recipients [75].

In an effort to better predict reserve in frailer, comorbid patients cardiopulmonary exercise testing has been used to assess outcomes in transplant-listed patients in the UK. It has demonstrated that those with a reduced cardiac reserve defined by a low "anaerobic threshold" have increased mortality [76].

In addition, patients with low cardiac reserve see an improvement in 5-year mortality after transplant [76]. A systematic review in 2016 however suggests that further work is needed in the context of renal transplant to assess (a) reduction in postoperative mortality, (b) length of stay, or (c) mobility post-transplant before this assessment can be routinely applied to a preoperative assessment [77].

86.5.1.2 Superior Vena Cava Obstruction and Central Vein Access

Haemodialysis patients have an increased incidence of Superior Vena Cava Obstruction (SVCO) requiring preoperative venoplasty. If the condition cannot be optimized by this approach, then elective tracheostomy postoperatively (the surgeon may encounter multiple collaterals) with respiratory wean in the intensive care unit may be necessary. Plans for limiting fluid loading, in favor of inotropes, and operating in a head-up position with table tilt at 15° are important considerations to prevent laryngeal edema and inability to extubate.

It is not unusual for central veins (and peripheral veins) to be exhausted following a career of kidney disease. This may make anesthetic monitoring and fluid resuscitation difficult and again something to factor in.

86.5.1.3 Difficult Airways

Some renal conditions are associated with high-grade airways risk and difficult intubation. For example, PR3 Vasculitis is associated with tracheal malacia and stenosis and scleroderma with reduced mouth opening.

86.5.1.4 Chronic Hypotension

A small but significant proportion of dialysis patients have chronic, non-volume-related, hypotension; the etiology of which is poorly understood and even more poorly corrected. It is a real challenge to anesthetize a patient with a systolic of 70 mmHg and avoid hypoperfusion injury to the transplant. A clear plan needs to be concocted in advance, usually involving perioperative inotropes, very careful intravascular monitoring, elective ICU admission, and how long inotropic support will be continued.

86.5.2 Perioperative Management

Perioperative planning of dialysis and fluid balance is a vital consideration for the renal transplant recipient. As with preoperative cardiovascular assessment, there is significant variation in practice within the UK.

Dialysis for solute removal and optimization of acid-base is often performed on the day of surgery, particularly when delayed graft function is expected, how high the potassium and how fluid overloaded the patient is. Avoidable dialysis, usually because of a mildly elevated potassium, may increase the cold ischemia time and leave the patient intravascularly deplete, risking hypoperfusion of the transplant and if there is doubt then an early discussion is wise. If a patient does require dialysis, we will typically leave the patient at least a kilo over their dry weight.

Intraoperative management is focused on maintaining fluid balance such that perfusion is maintained to the denervated graft in order to reduce delayed graft function while minimizing the risk of pulmonary edema. Assessment of fluid status intraoperatively is challenging, particularly in the presence of hypotension as a pharmacological consequence of anesthesia. Tools available include blood pressure/mean arterial pressure and central venous pressure monitoring. Assessment of stroke volume variation (SVV) allows dynamic assessment of response to intravenous fluid administration allowing clinicians to optimize cardiac output using the principle of the Starling curve (see Fig.86.10).

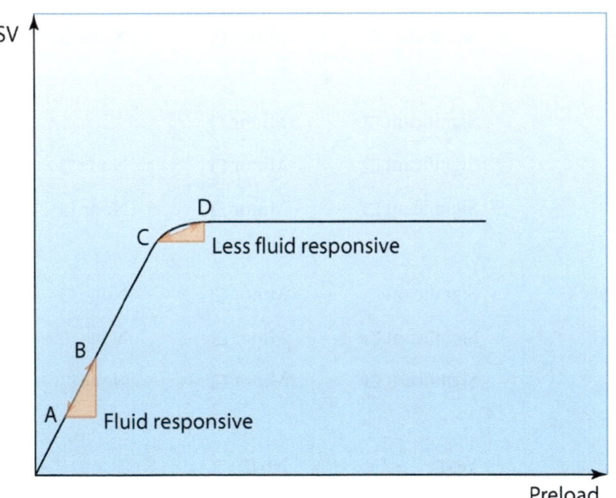

Fig. 86.10 Frank–Starling curve

Clinical work has demonstrated the use of SVV monitoring to be associated with reduced intraoperative fluid administration, reduced exposure to vasoactive drugs, and reduced incidence of postoperative pulmonary edema [78].

86.6 Pharmacy Review

This is a useful check to add to the recipient workup. It enables a specific assessment of the patient's

1. Previous and current adherence with medication, their ability to organize, and manage medication as well as their understanding of the importance of post-transplant medication.
2. Pre-identification of any allergies and necessary alternatives
3. Identification of key drug interactions such as protease inhibitors and tacrolimus
4. Identification of drugs that will need rapid dose increase with improving eGFR for example levetiracetam or lamivudine

86.7 Psychological Assessment

Successful transplantation is utterly dependent on adherence with immunosuppressive medication and regular clinic follow-up. Recipients will need to withstand the psychological "stress" this entails and have at least an informal assessment of their readiness for transplantation prior to listing. Formal psychological review allows for the time and expertise to explore any issues regarding treatment adherence (medication, dialysis session attendance, etc.) and diagnosis of covert psychiatric disease or substance misuse problems. Cultural barriers to adherence or unusual health beliefs may also be identified and challenged where appropriate. Early recognition of these problems may allow for appropriate treatment and prevent premature graft loss. A suggested screening tool is appended below.

Adherence Issues *Problems identified with*:	Extent of problems		
Attending previous medical appointments or dialysis sessions	Significant □	Minor □	None □
Taking current or previous medications	Significant □	Minor □	None □
Future adherence (e.g., being able to attend frequently)	Significant □	Minor □	None □
Other	Significant □	Minor □	None □
Health Beliefs *Problems Identified With*:			
Unhelpful or harmful health beliefs re medications	Significant □	Minor □.	None □
Unhelpful or harmful health beliefs re medical care/surgery	Significant □	Minor □	None □
Unrealistic beliefs regard medical outcomes	Significant □	Minor □	None □
Other	Significant □	Minor□	None □
Motivation for Transplant			
Were clear motivations identified for transplant?	Yes □	No □	
Were any de-motivators for transplant identified?	Significant □	Minor □	None□
Other motivational issues	Significant □	Minor □	None□
Motivation category Independence & Freedom □ subcategories: work □ finances □ travel □ other □ state			
Maintain own medical health □			
Commitments □ subcategories: dependents □ Significant other □ other □ state			
Other:			
If live-related problems identified with accepting/receiving kidney from live donor□state			
Understanding of Transplant & After-care problems:			
Knowledge of the kidney and its role in maintaining health	Significant □	Minor □	None □
The concept of the immune system	Significant □	Minor □	None □
The purpose & role of antirejection medications	Significant □	Minor □	
The need for high level of medical concordance (taking meds)	Significant □	Minor □	None □
The need for high level of clinic attendance post-transplant	Significant □	Minor □	None □
Other	Significant □	Minor □	None □
Psychological & Mental Health *Problems with*:			
Current Psychological or mental health *tick if depression*□	Significant □	Minor □	
Previous psychological or mental health *tick if depression*□	Significant □	Minor □	None □
Other	Significant □	Minor □	None □
Social Support & Coping Resources problems with:			
Lack of coping skills (e.g., cannot identify ways of coping with a setback)	Significant □	Minor □	None □
Lack of supportive others (e.g., cannot name one supportive other)	Significant □	Minor □	None □
Social problems (income/housing/immigration status/, etc.)	Significant □	Minor □	None □
Overall Outcome			
Psychologically suitable for transplant with no psychology input	Yes □	No □	
Psychologically suitable for transplant with psychology input in session	Yes □	No □	
Psychologically suitable for transplant with further post-session input	Yes □	No □	
Psychologically unsuitable for transplant at present time	Yes □	No □	
Courtesy of Dr Jeff Cove, Consultant Clinical Psychologist, Renal Unit, Royal Free Hospital			

86.8 Patient Education

Group education sessions prior to transplantation may be helpful in addressing patient fears, correcting misconceptions, and building confidence. Involvement of peers who have been through donor nephrectomy or renal transplantation is especially useful in this regard. It is important to discuss what happens on the day of the transplant, the implications for the patient (and their family) in terms of length of stay, possible complications, and likely graft survival rates. It is also important to discuss the different types of deceased donor transplants.

It is equally important to remember that health literacy levels are often much lower than perceived by medics; serious thought needs to be given to the nature of the information given to patients and their families. The critical importance of having up-to-date contact details, a plan for getting to the hospital, and care of any dependents are all important issues for patients to take on.

Needless to say, it is critical to explore the options for live donor transplantation, and where there is a live donor available and worked up, it is important to discuss the option of suspending the recipient from the deceased donor list with both donor and recipient. For many donor-recipient pairs, this is acceptable as a way of freeing up a deceased donor kidney for others without a live donor. Patient education sessions or newsletters are also a very good place to discuss any clinical trials that are in progress and give patients the opportunity to consider these in a calmer setting than the night of the transplant.

86.9 Pre-activation Checklist

See ▶ Box 86.4.

Box 86.4 Pre-activation Checklist

- Contact details up to date?
- Psychological assessment
- Patient education
- Consent given for data retention by NHS Blood & Transplant?
- HLA typing complete?
- HLA antibody screening up to date?
- Has the cause of ESRD been identified? Is genetic testing or biopsy required?
- Counseling of disease recurrence post-transplant
- Virology screen (HIV/Hep B/Hep C/HTLV/CMV/VZV/EBV/HSV/Rubella)
- Other infectious diseases (VDRL, toxoplasma, strongyloides, schistosomiasis, etc.)
- Vaccinations
- CXR
- 12 lead ECG
- Echocardiogram (where applicable)
- Cardiac stress testing (where applicable)
- Pulmonary function testing and CT scan (where applicable)
- Assessment of peripheral vascular disease and surgical assessment of vessels
- Counseling to quit smoking (where applicable)
- Assessment of GI and liver disease
- Assessment of urological disease
- Considerations for obesity (where applicable)
- Age and gender-appropriate malignancy screening (PSA, Cervical smear, Mammography)
- Frailty Screening

Tips, Tricks, and Pitfalls

- Cardiovascular disease is highly prevalent in the renal population with age being a poor discriminator for risk
- Imaging with echocardiography should be interpreted in the context of the patient's fluid status
- Surgical or percutaneous interventions to modify risk should be considered on a case-by-case basis with discussion in a multi-disciplinary setting
- To identify risk, endeavor to avoid hemodynamic instability and factor the pros and cons of anticoagulation

Case Study

Case 1

A 67-year-old retired female German teacher with ESRD secondary to ADPKD was assessed for transplantation. She had been on dialysis for 6 months where dialysis staff felt she was managing well. A thallium stress test was normal and her exercise tolerance was good (she walked every day with her husband). All routine screening tests were satisfactory as was the surgical review. She had a very supportive husband who accompanied her to dialysis and clinic visits, who also kept accurate records of her medication. She was activated on the transplant list and received a good deceased donor offer. The following morning, she was agitated and confused on the ward. Screening for an acute cause of delirium was negative but a CT head revealed marked cerebral atrophy. As acute events from the transplant settled, it became apparent that her short-term memory was very poor and she had a poor cognitive function which did not improve. In clinic and at admission for the transplant her husband had answered the majority of questions for her, unintentionally concealing significant cognitive impairment. This illustrates the complexity of ensuring that all aspects of frailty are considered and monitored as frailty is often progressive.

A mental test score at the time of listing (repeated either annually or at the time of transplant) would have detected this.

Case 2

A 41-year-old mother of three with type 2 diabetes and a BMI of 46 kg/m^2 who was established on dialysis was assessed for transplantation. All screening tests were satisfactory, but her obesity was felt to be a contraindication for transplantation. The patient was informed of this and told that she could not be activated until she had lost 25 kg and advised to diet and exercise more. She died on dialysis 7 years later secondary to calciphylaxis.

In a different scenario, she was assessed and felt to be too obese for transplantation however, it was acknowledged that losing weight on dialysis is difficult and that she had tried many times before to lose weight without success. The plan was for her to receive direct input from renal dietitians, advice on a realistic incremental exercise she could do locally, and her family was engaged in trying to support her. A timeline of 6 months was fixed for review with the plan to refer for bariatric referral if poor progress had been made. The MDTM discussion also obtained a second opinion from a center with capacity to robotic surgery and an upper BMI threshold of 40 kg/m^2. Her progress was reviewed, and she achieved the target for robotic transplant surgery within 9 months and had a successful transplant at another center, has a BMI that continues to improve with a change in diabetic medication and is now working full time.

This case reminds us that it is pretty rare to find an obese patient who has not tried many times before to lose weight and asking them to repeat the same strategy without a significant change is unlikely to be successful. It also illustrates the importance of having a thoughtful timetable for targets, tests, and early review to avoid patients being trapped in permanent transplant assessment workup.

Case 3

A 36-year-old patient with a background of lupus and anti-cardiolipin antibodies was reviewed in the complex patient meeting. She had lost her first transplant with primary non-function secondary to renal vein thrombosis at the age of 32. She was very highly sensitized with a CRF of 98% and because of SVC obstruction, she was dialyzing via a leg graft which was felt to be her last viable access. Her mean systolic blood pressure was 82 mmHg and she was fully anticoagulated.

The key issues addressed were the following:

1. Risk of laryngeal edema and failure to extubate with fluid loading
2. Risk of hypoperfusion secondary to low arterial pressure and restrictions on fluid loading
3. Risk of recurrent disease (lupus) and clotting secondary to anti-cardiolipin
4. Difficult access for anesthetic monitoring
5. Increased risk of rejection and ability to biopsy in a patient returning to anticoagulation post-transplant

A senior anesthetist reviewed the patient and arranged a Doppler vascular survey, her recent MRV was also reviewed for access options. The operation and after-care would be 15° head-up tilt with careful monitoring of fluid status and oesophageal Doppler. By prior agreement, the patient would be transferred to ITU for inotropic support and close monitoring.

Her lupus was assessed to be in remission but her anti-cardiolipin antibodies remained high and her risk of thrombosis was deemed to be very significant. An anticoagulation plan was made with a senior hemophilia consultant for correction of warfarin on the day and graded reintroduction of anticoagulation postoperatively involving low molecular weight heparin and factor Xa monitoring (but not IV unfractionated heparin).

It was agreed that only standard-criteria donor (SCD) kidneys would be accepted to reduce the chance of DGF and the need for surveillance biopsies. Surgery was to be performed in daylight hours with two experienced surgeons and a senior anesthetist. A timeline was set for a return of these opinions and the plan discussed with the patient and her family with realistic risks of complications including the need for an intraoperative tracheostomy if laryngeal edema compromised extubation.

A complex patient MDTM is extremely helpful in assessing patients like this, ensuring several minds can anticipate problems and consider solutions including second opinions.

Conclusion

Workup of an otherwise healthy potential recipient for transplantation is fairly straightforward and should be considered early in a patient approaching end-stage renal disease. The pros and cons of transplantation become more balanced in patients with significant co-morbidity and it is important to build a robust service that permits swift surgical, medical and if necessary, anesthetic review. Definitive tests or opinions need to be sort in a timely fashion and the patient kept abreast of the process. Similarly, frail patients on the transplant list need regular review by their nephrologist to ensure that patients who are no longer suitable on the list are suspended appropriately.

Good coordination of this process is key and the difference between swift thoughtful patient-centered and considered assessment versus potentially delayed access to transplantation or inappropriate listing with the possibility of avoidable harm should be recognized.

Chapter Review Questions

1. Which stress test is suitable for asymptomatic patients?
2. What is the outcome of renal transplantation in HIV+ individuals compared to HIV −ve patients and does this outcome change if the patient is co-infected with HCV at the same time?
3. How does frailty negatively affecting transplantation outcomes?
4. When assessing a patient with a past history of malignancy for transplantation which cancers require a minimum of 5 years between successful treatment and listing according to the European Best Practice Guidelines?
5. Pulmonary hypertension and aortic stenosis are common co-morbidities in renal patients undergoing transplant. What specific intraoperative complications may occur with each and how might patients be optimized/managed?

Answers

1. Stress echocardiography (SE) and myocardial perfusion imaging (MPI) are suitable for asymptotic patients. They have comparable accuracy in observational studies; however, reviews suggest stress echocardiography is more accurate (sensitivity 0.8 vs 0.69, specificity 0.89 vs 0.77 for SE and MPI, respectively) and it can provide additional information such as baseline and dynamic ventricular function, valve, and pulmonary pressure assessments
2. The outcomes of renal transplantation in HIV+ individuals are similar to those in HIV-ve patients in the current HAART era, while the outcomes are poorer for recipients with HIV and HCV co-infection. However, it is important to note that the rate of rejection of HIV+ recipients is double to non-HIV patients
3. Frailty is associated with 94% increased risk of delayed graft function, 61% higher risk of early hospital readmission, as well as 2.17-fold higher risk of death following kidney transplantation
4. Invasive Cervical Cancer, Breast Cancer Stage 0–4
5. *Aortic Stenosis*

   Complications—New-onset arrhythmia and systemic hypotension leading to ischemia and perpetuating hypotension

   Management—Preoperative valve intervention, avoidance of systemic hypotension, and prompt treatment of tachyarrhythmia

   Pulmonary hypertension

   Complications—Acidaemia, hypercarbia, and pain leading to increased pulmonary vascular resistance and decompensation

   Management—Preoperative dialysis and increased ventilation to optimize acid-base and minimize hypercarbia. Adequate analgesia. Systemic vasopressors to manage decompensation

References

1. Wong G, Howard K, Chapman JR, Chadban S, Cross N, Tong A, Webster AC, Craig JC. Comparative survival and economic benefits of deceased donor kidney transplantation and dialysis in people with varying ages and co-morbidities. PLoS One. 2012. https://doi.org/10.1371/journal.pone.0029591.
2. Chris Dudley PH. Assessment of the potential kidney transplant recipient. Ren. Assoc. 2011.
3. European Renal Best Practice Transplantation Guideline Development Group. ERBP guideline on the management and evaluation of the kidney donor and recipient. Nephrol Dial Transplant. 2013.
4. Chadban SJ, Ahn C, Axelrod DA, et al. KDIGO clinical practice guideline on the evaluation and management of candidates for kidney transplantation. Transplantation. 2020. https://doi.org/10.1097/TP.0000000000003136.
5. Campbell S, Pilmore H, Gracey D, Mulley W, Russell C, McTaggart S. KHA-cari guideline: recipient assessment for transplantation. Nephrology. 2013. https://doi.org/10.1111/nep.12068.
6. NHS Blood and Transplant. Annual Report On Kidney Transplantation - Report For 2018/2019. 2019.
7. Taylor DM, Bradley JA, Bradley C, et al. Limited health literacy is associated with reduced access to kidney transplantation. Kidney Int. 2019. https://doi.org/10.1016/j.kint.2018.12.021.
8. Rijkse E, van Dam JL, Roodnat JI, Kimenai HJAN, IJzermans JNM, Minnee RC. The prognosis of kidney transplant recipients with aorto-iliac calcification: a systematic review and meta-analysis. Transpl Int. 2020. https://doi.org/10.1111/tri.13592.
9. Shishehbor MH, Aksut B, Poggio E, Flechner SM. Presence of peripheral artery disease in renal transplant outcomes - Don't throw the baby out with the bath water. Vasc Med. 2017. https://doi.org/10.1177/1358863X17703195.

10. Erwin PA, Goel SS, Gebreselassie S, Shishehbor MH. Restoration of renal allograft function: Via reduced-contrast percutaneous revascularization of transplant renal artery stenosis. Tex Heart Inst J. 2015. https://doi.org/10.14503/THIJ-13-4059.
11. Davins M, Llagostera S, Jimenez R, Rosales A, Romero JM, Diaz M. Aortofemoral bypass to bridge end-stage renal disease patients with severe iliac calcification to kidney transplantation. Vascular. 2009. https://doi.org/10.2310/6670.2009.00044.
12. Currie IC, Wilson YG, Baird RN, Lamont PM. Detection of sub-critical arterial stenoses by hyperaemic Doppler. Eur J Vasc Endovasc Surg. 1996. https://doi.org/10.1016/S1078-5884(96)80131-6.
13. AbuRahma AF, Jarrett K, Hayes JD. Clinical implications of power Doppler three-dimensional ultrasonography. Vascular. 2004. https://doi.org/10.1258/rsmvasc.12.5.293.
14. Brekke IB, Lien B, Sødal G, Jakobsen A, Bentdal, PP, Flatmark A, Fauchald P. Aortoiliac reconstruction in preparation for renal transplantation. Transpl Int. 1993. https://doi.org/10.1007/BF00336361.
15. Hill CJ, Courtney AE, Cardwell CR, et al. Recipient obesity and outcomes after kidney transplantation: a systematic review and meta-analysis. Nephrol Dial Transplant. 2015. https://doi.org/10.1093/ndt/gfv214.
16. Bardonnaud N, Pillot P, Lillaz J, Delorme G, Chabannes E, Bernardini S, Guichard G, Bittard H, Kleinclauss F. Outcomes of renal transplantation in obese recipients. Transplant Proc. 2012. https://doi.org/10.1016/j.transproceed.2012.09.031.
17. Awan AA, Niu J, Pan JS, Erickson KF, Mandayam S, Winkelmayer WC, Navaneethan SD, Ramanathan V Trends in the causes of death among kidney transplant recipients in the United States (1996-2014). Am J Nephrol. 2018. https://doi.org/10.1159/000495081.
18. Steenkamp R, Pyart R, Fraser S. UK renal registry 20th annual report: Chapter 5 survival and cause of death in UK adult patients on renal replacement therapy in 2016: National and centre-specific analyses. Nephron. 2018. https://doi.org/10.1159/000490963.
19. Foley RN, Parfrey PS, Sarnak MJ. Epidemiology of cardiovascular disease in chronic renal disease. J Am Soc Nephrol. 1998. https://doi.org/10.1016/s0021-9150(00)81051-5.
20. USRDS (United States Renal Data System). 2018 annual data report – Chapter 4: Cardiovascular disease in patients with CKD. 2018.
21. Manske CL, Wang Y, Rector T, Wilson RF, White CW. Coronary revascularisation in insulin-dependent diabetic patients with chronic renal failure. Lancet. 1992. https://doi.org/10.1016/0140-6736(92)93010-K.
22. Wang LW, Fahim MA, Hayen A, Mitchell RL, Lord SW, Baines LA, Craig JC, Webster AC. Cardiac testing for coronary artery disease in potential kidney transplant recipients: a systematic review of test accuracy studies. Am J Kidney Dis. 2011. https://doi.org/10.1053/j.ajkd.2010.11.018.
23. Bangalore S, Maron DJ, O'Brien SM, et al. Management of coronary disease in patients with advanced kidney disease. N Engl J Med. 2020. https://doi.org/10.1056/NEJMoa1915925.
24. Kristensen SD, Knuuti J, Saraste A, Anker S, Bøtker HE, et al. 2014 ESC/ESA guidelines on non-cardiac surgery: cardiovascular assessment and management: The Joint Task Force on non-cardiac surgery: cardiovascular assessment and management of the European Society of Cardiology (ESC) and the European Society of Anaesth. Eur Heart J. 2014;35: 2383–431.
25. Wali RK, Wang GS, Gottlieb SS, et al. Effect of kidney transplantation on left ventricular systolic dysfunction and congestive heart failure in patients with end-stage renal disease. J Am Coll Cardiol. 2005. https://doi.org/10.1016/j.jacc.2004.11.061.
26. Ricotta JJ, Aburahma A, Ascher E, Eskandari M, Faries P, Lal BK. Updated society for vascular surgery guidelines for management of extracranial carotid disease. J Vasc Surg. 2011. https://doi.org/10.1016/j.jvs.2011.07.031.
27. Canaud G, Zuber J, Sberro R, et al. Intensive and prolonged treatment of focal and segmental glomerulosclerosis recurrence in adult kidney transplant recipients: a pilot study. Am J Transplant. 2009. https://doi.org/10.1111/j.1600--6143.2009.02580.x.
28. Hickson LJ, Gera M, Amer H, et al. Kidney transplantation for primary focal segmental glomerulosclerosis: outcomes and response to therapy for recurrence. Transplantation. 2009. https://doi.org/10.1097/TP.0b013e31819f12be.
29. Uffing A, Pérez-Sáez MJ, Mazzali M, et al. Recurrence of FSGS after kidney transplantation in adults. Clin J Am Soc Nephrol. 2020. https://doi.org/10.2215/CJN.08970719.
30. Pham PTT, Pham PCT, Danovitch GM, Gritsch HA, Singer J, Wallace WD, Hayashi R, Wilkinson AH. Predictors and risk factors for recurrent scleroderma renal crisis in the kidney allograft: case report and review of the literature. Am J Transplant. 2005. https://doi.org/10.1111/j.1600-6143.2005.01035.x.
31. Sagmeister MS, Grigorescu M, Schönermarck U. Kidney transplantation in ANCA-associated vasculitis. J Nephrol. 2019. https://doi.org/10.1007/s40620-019-00642-x.
32. Sprangers B, Lefkowitz GI, Cohen SD, Stokes MB, Valeri A, Appel GB, Kunis CL. Beneficial effect of rituximab in the treatment of recurrent idiopathic membranous nephropathy after kidney transplantation. Clin J Am Soc Nephrol. 2010. https://doi.org/10.2215/CJN.04120609.
33. Gupta G, Fattah H, Ayalon R, et al. Pre-transplant phospholipase A2 receptor autoantibody concentration is associated with clinically significant recurrence of membranous nephropathy post-kidney transplantation. Clin Transpl. 2016. https://doi.org/10.1111/ctr.12711.
34. Berger BE, Vincenti F, Biava C, Amend WJ, Feduska N, Salvatierra O. De novo and recurrent membranous glomerulopathy following kidney transplantation. Transplantation. 1983. https://doi.org/10.1097/00007890-198304000-00010.
35. Stegall MD, Cornell LD, Park WD, Smith BH, Cosio FG. Renal allograft histology at 10 years after transplantation in the tacrolimus era: evidence of pervasive chronic injury. Am J Transplant. 2018. https://doi.org/10.1111/ajt.14431.
36. Fridell JA, Niederhaus S, Curry M, Urban R, Fox A, Odorico J. The survival advantage of pancreas after kidney transplant. Am J Transplant. 2019. https://doi.org/10.1111/ajt.15106.
37. Kumar EP. Posttransplantation diabetes mellitus after renal transplantation – a brief overview. Int J Transplant Plastic Surg/ 2019. https://doi.org/10.23880/IJTPS-16000S1-004.
38. Avasare RS, Rosenstiel PE, Zaky ZS, Tsapepas DS, Appel GB, Markowitz GS, Bomback AS, Canetta PA. Predicting post-transplant recurrence of iga nephropathy: the importance of crescents. Am J Nephrol. 2017. https://doi.org/10.1159/000453081.
39. Czarnecki PG, Lager DJ, Leung N, Dispenzieri A, Cosio FG, Fervenza FC. Long-term outcome of kidney transplantation in patients with fibrillary glomerulonephritis or monoclonal gammopathy with fibrillary deposits. Kidney Int. 2009. https://doi.org/10.1038/ki.2008.577.
40. Penn I. The effect of immunosuppression on pre-existing cancers. Transplantation. 1993. https://doi.org/10.1097/00007890-199304000-00011.

41. Johnson SR, Cherikh WS, Kauffman HM, Pavlakis M, Hanto DW. Retransplantation after post-transplant lymphoproliferative disorders: an OPTN/UNOS database analysis. Am J Transplant. 2006. https://doi.org/10.1111/j.1600--6143.2006.01543.x.
42. Kasiske BL, Cangro CB, Hariharan S, et al. The evaluation of renal transplantation candidates: clinical practice guidelines. Am J Transplant. 2001;1:3–95.
43. European best practice guidelines for renal transplantation (Part 1). Nephrol Dial Transplant. 2000. https://doi.org/10.1093/ndt/15.suppl_7.3.
44. Maisonneuve P, Agodoa L, Gellert R, et al. Cancer in patients on dialysis for end-stage renal disease: an international collaborative study. Lancet. 1999. https://doi.org/10.1016/S0140-6736(99)06154-1.
45. Muñoz P, Rodríguez C, Bouza E. Mycobacterium tuberculosis infection in recipients of solid organ transplants. Clin Infect Dis. 2005. https://doi.org/10.1086/427692.
46. WHO. WHO | Global tuberculosis report 2019. World Heal Organ. 2020. ISBN: 9789241565714.
47. Milburn H, Ashman N, Davies P, Doffman S, Drobniewski F, Khoo S, Ormerod P, Ostermann M, Snelson C. Guidelines for the prevention and management of Mycobacterium tuberculosis infection and disease in adult patients with chronic kidney disease. Thorax. 2010. https://doi.org/10.1136/thx.2009.133173.
48. Ferguson TW, Tangri N, MacDonald K, et al. The diagnostic accuracy of tests for latent tuberculosis infection in hemodialysis patients: a systematic review and meta-analysis. Transplantation. 2015. https://doi.org/10.1097/TP.0000000000000451.
49. Abad CL, Razonable RR. Non-tuberculous mycobacterial infections in solid organ transplant recipients: an update. J Clin Tuberc Other Mycobact Dis. 2016. https://doi.org/10.1016/j.jctube.2016.04.001.
50. British Transplantation Society. Guidelines for hepatitis B & solid organ transplantation. 1st ed; 2018.
51. Kidney Disease: Improving Global Outcomes (KDIGO) Hepatitis C Work Group. KDIGO 2018 clinical practice guideline for the prevention, diagnosis, evaluation, and treatment of hepatitis C in chronic kidney disease. Kidney Int Suppl. 2018. https://doi.org/10.1016/j.kisu.2018.06.001.
52. Axelrod DA, Schnitzler MA, Alhamad T, et al. The impact of direct-acting antiviral agents on liver and kidney transplant costs and outcomes. Am J Transplant. 2018. https://doi.org/10.1111/ajt.14895.
53. Xia Y, Friedmann P, Yaffe H, Phair J, Gupta A, Kayler LK. Effect of HCV, HIV and coinfection in kidney transplant recipients: Mate kidney analyses. Am J Transplant. 2014. https://doi.org/10.1111/ajt.12847.
54. The British Transplantation Society. Kidney & pancreas transplantation in patients with HIV. 2nd ed; 2015.
55. Stock PG, Barin B, Murphy B, et al. Outcomes of kidney transplantation in HIV-infected recipients. N Engl J Med. 2010. https://doi.org/10.1056/NEJMoa1001197.
56. British Transplantation Society (BTS)/ The Renal Association (RA). Guidelines for living donor kidney transplantation. 4th ed; 2018.
57. Yamauchi J, Yamano Y, Yuzawa K. Risk of human T-cell leukemia virus type 1 infection in kidney transplantation. N Engl J Med.. 2019. https://doi.org/10.1056/NEJMc1809779.
58. Kotton CN, Fishman JA. Viral infection in the renal transplant recipient. J Am Soc Nephrol. 2005. https://doi.org/10.1681/ASN.2004121113.
59. Assi M, Martin S, Wheat LJ, et al. Histoplasmosis after solid organ transplant. Clin Infect Dis. 2013. https://doi.org/10.1093/cid/cit593.
60. Wu HHL, Woywodt A, Nixon AC. Frailty and the potential kidney transplant recipient: time for a more holistic assessment? Kidney360. 2020. https://doi.org/10.34067/kid.0001822020.
61. Garonzik-Wang JM, Govindan P, Grinnan JW, et al. Frailty and delayed graft function in kidney transplant recipients. Arch Surg. 2012. https://doi.org/10.1001/archsurg.2011.1229.
62. McAdams-Demarco MA, Law A, Salter ML, Chow E, Grams M, Walston J, Segev DL. Frailty and early hospital readmission after kidney transplantation. Am J Transplant. 2013. https://doi.org/10.1111/ajt.12300.
63. McAdams-Demarco MA, Law A, King E, et al. Frailty and mortality in kidney transplant recipients. Am J Transplant. 2015. https://doi.org/10.1111/ajt.12992.
64. McAdams-DeMarco MA, Olorundare IO, Ying H, et al. Frailty and postkidney transplant health-related quality of life. Transplantation. 2018. https://doi.org/10.1097/TP.0000000000001943.
65. McAdams-DeMarco MA, Ying H, Thomas AG, et al. Frailty, inflammatory markers, and waitlist mortality among patients with end-stage renal disease in a prospective cohort study. Transplantation.. 2018. https://doi.org/10.1097/TP.0000000000002213.
66. Reese PP, Shults J, Bloom RD, Mussell A, Harhay MN, Abt P, Levine M, Johansen KL, Karlawish JT, Feldman HI. Functional status, time to transplantation, and survival benefit of kidney transplantation among wait-listed candidates. Am J Kidney Dis. 2015. https://doi.org/10.1053/j.ajkd.2015.05.015.
67. Chu NM, Deng A, Ying H, Haugen CE, Garonzik Wang JM, Segev DL, McAdams-Demarco MA. Dynamic frailty before kidney transplantation: time of measurement matters. Transplantation. 2019. https://doi.org/10.1097/TP.0000000000002563.
68. Knoll G, Cockfield S, Blydt-Hansen T, Baran D, Kiberd B, Landsberg D, Rush D, Cole E. Canadian Society of Transplantation consensus guidelines on eligibility for kidney transplantation. CMAJ. 2005. https://doi.org/10.1503/cmaj.051291.
69. Zlotnick DM, Axelrod DA, Chobanian MC, Friedman S, Brown J, Catherwood E, Costa SP. Non-invasive detection of pulmonary hypertension prior to renal transplantation is a predictor of increased risk for early graft dysfunction. Nephrol Dial Transplant. 2010. https://doi.org/10.1093/ndt/gfq141.
70. Kasiske BL, Klinger D. Cigarette smoking in renal transplant recipients. J Am Soc Nephrol. 2000;11(4):753–759. https://doi.org/10.1681/ASN.V114753.
71. Lentine KL, Costa SP, Weir MR, et al. Cardiac disease evaluation and management among kidney and liver transplantation candidates: A scientific statement from the American Heart Association and the American College of Cardiology Foundation. J Am Coll Cardiol. 2012. https://doi.org/10.1016/j.jacc.2012.05.008.
72. Brown J, Morgan-Hughes NJ Aortic stenosis and non-cardiac surgery. Contin Educ Anaesth Crit Care Pain. 2005 https://doi.org/10.1093/bjaceaccp/mki001.
73. Pritts CD, Pearl RG. Anesthesia for patients with pulmonary hypertension. Curr Opin Anaesthesiol. 2010. https://doi.org/10.1097/ACO.0b013e32833953fb.
74. Fleisher LA, Fleischmann KE, Auerbach AD, et al. 2014 ACC/AHA guideline on perioperative cardiovascular evaluation and management of patients undergoing noncardiac surgery:

a report of the American college of cardiology/American heart association task force on practice guidelines. J Am Coll Cardiol. 2014. https://doi.org/10.1016/j.jacc.2014.07.944.
75. Morkane CM, Fabes J, Banga NR, Berry PD, Kirwan CJ. Perioperative management of adult cadaveric and live donor renal transplantation in the UK: a survey of national practice. Clin Kidney J. 2019. https://doi.org/10.1093/ckj/sfz017.
76. Ting SMS, Iqbal H, Kanji H, et al. Functional cardiovascular reserve predicts survival pre-kidney and post-kidney transplantation. J Am Soc Nephrol. 2014. https://doi.org/10.1681/ASN.2013040348.
77. Moran J, Wilson F, Guinan E, McCormick P, Hussey J, Moriarty J. Role of cardiopulmonary exercise testing as a risk-assessment method in patients undergoing intra-abdominal surgery: a systematic review. Br J Anaesth. 2016. https://doi.org/10.1093/bja/aev454.
78. Fabes J, Al Midani A, Sarna A, Hadi D, Banga N, Jones G, Berry P, Wittenberg M. Implementation of a novel algorithm to optimise fluid and vasopressor therapy in renal transplantation.

Transplant Donor Selection

Nikita Agrawal, Alison Craik, Gareth Jones, and Inji Alshaer

Contents

M. Harber (ed.), *Primer on Nephrology*, https://doi.org/10.1007/978-3-030-76419-7_87

Learning Objectives

1. This chapter aims to cover the selection of kidneys for transplantation based on function but also on the risk associated with deceased donors.
2. The outcomes of recipients getting extended criteria donor (ECD) kidneys are consistently lower than those receiving SCD kidneys; nevertheless they are still superior to outcomes if the patients were to remain on dialysis while on the transplant waiting list.
3. There is potential to do real harm by the transmission of infection, malignancy, or a badly damaged renal transplant, and having a system that consistently evaluates and reduces that risk is essential. The varying appetite for patients (and doctors) for risk needs to be appreciated and managed on an individual basis.
4. The assessment of a potential live kidney donor is a complex process that should evaluate the physical health of the donor, their suitability to undergo major abdominal surgery, the suitability of the donor to be left with a single kidney long term, the quality of the donor organ and any risk to the recipient of receiving the organ.

Tips and Tricks

1. Never transplant an organ from a donor with unexplained encephalomyelitic disease
2. Utilize the CKD EPI eGFR and KDPI calculators to assess the quality of deceased donor kidney offers
3. Discuss complex cases with colleagues and consider liaising directly with donor ICU teams to clarify the source of any systemic infections or uncertain donor diagnoses.
4. Consult guidelines such as those released by SaBTO regarding risks of malignancy/infection transmission from transplanted organs (▶ https://www.odt.nhs.uk/transplantation/tools-policies-and-guidance/sabto/)
5. See Top tips for selecting donor organs (Table 87.1) for an overview of some pertinent points discussed in this chapter.

Accepting kidneys for transplantation is not only based on function but also on the risk associated with donors. It is important to consult guidelines, for example, 'Safety of blood, tissues and organs' (SaBTO), when receiving deceased donor offers.

Table 87.1 Top tips for selecting donor organs

Most consistent donor indicator of long-term graft outcome	**Age**
Primary CNS brain tumors	Risk of transmission is low (~1.5%) with low-grade malignancy and lack of craniotomy/shunting
DCD vs. DBD donors	Long-term outcomes are similar in donors aged under 60 years old and cold ischemic time under 12 hours
Creatinine in potential donors	Terminal creatinine is a poor indicator of outcome and admission values may give a better insight eGFR gives a more accurate assessment of kidney function in elderly donors
Hepatitis B sAg +ve donors	Can be safely utilized in sAg recipients or patients with prior infection (cAb +ve) with sAb levels over 1000 IU/L
Hepatitis B cAb+ve/sAg −ve donors	Can be safely utilized in sAg +ve recipients or recipients with sAb over 1000 IU/L through prior exposure or vaccination
Hepatitis C ab +ve donors	Should only be considered for patients who are hepatitis C PCR positive. In this subgroup, the outcome is similar to receipt of hepatitis C negative kidney
Pediatric donors	Under 2 or less than 10 kg – Avoid 2–5 year. or 10–15 kg – En-bloc transplant 5–10 or 15–35 kg – Single transplant mainly Over 10 or over 35 kg – Single transplant
Elderly donors	Donors over 60 should be used with caution unless age-matched Beware additional comorbidities Consider dual transplant if eGFR<60 ml/min
Donors not suitable for a named recipient	Ask whether the kidney could be offered to an alternative recipient within your unit

87.1 Introduction

No doubt that every good transplant starts with a good operation and every good transplant operation, starts with a good donor. Donor selection is one of the most important factors for long-term graft survival and short-term outcomes in renal transplantation. The offer of a "perfect" donor is rare and evaluation should be undertaken on the balance of risk and benefit to the recipient. When assessing the donor offer, the clinician should always consider whether the donor is safe to transplant a kidney from and whether the kidney is suitable for the intended recipient. In the case of living donation, the safety and long-term impact of donation on the donor also needs to be considered.

Recipient safety should always be the front and foremost consideration when considering a donor for a recipient. The risk appraisal always considers transmissible factors, such as infection and malignancy, but will also consider the organ anatomy and retrieval, where multiple vessels or damage to the organ may confer considerable risk to the recipient. The suitability of the organ for the recipient should take into accounts both donor and recipient factors. While a young pre-emptive recipient should be matched with a suitably young donor that will provide a high level of graft function for optimal long-term graft survival, an older recipient or patients with high levels of sensitization or limited dialysis access may consider higher risk donors where the focus may not necessarily be on optimal long-term graft survival.

When matching the donor to recipient, the potential benefits of transplantation can be overstated and transplantation at any cost should be avoided. This is particularly relevant in the case of the high-risk recipient where the combination of sub-optimal donors with sub-optimal recipients often provides a sub-optimal result. Contrary to perceived wisdom, the marginal recipient often requires more optimal donor organs to limit the risk of evolving complications, prolonged hospital stay, and subsequent poor long-term outcomes.

87.2 Selection of the Deceased Donor

The offer of a deceased donor kidney frequently comes at the most inopportune time and acceptance is usually combined with the pressure of minimizing cold ischemic times. These factors can often lead to the refusal of a donor where careful consideration may uncover a kidney with good long-term outcomes. It is also important to avoid a "herd mentality" where the refusal to accept a donor by one unit is followed by refusal in other units on the ground that the previous unit did not want it. Although the reason for refusal may be valid, it is important to take a fresh look at each offer and evaluate the risk of the donor in combination with the circumstances of the recipient. In the case of donors who have been declined by a number of centers and are not suitable for your named recipient, it is always prudent to ask whether the offer would still stand for other recipients within your unit. In this case, the balance of risk may be different for an alternative recipient and most donor coordination teams would prefer seeing an organ allocated in a timely fashion rather than discarded.

Achieving a consensus on the suitability of organs for transplantation has always proven difficult. The first attempt at consensus on the contraindications to organ donation in the UK was by Gore et al. in 1992 [1]. More recent guidance from the UK on the absolute contraindications to donation is listed in ▶ Box 87.1 [2].

Box 87.1 Contraindications to Solid Organ Donation. Modified from Organ Donation and Transplantation Clinical Guidance 2020 [3]

General complete contraindications

- Age > 85 years
- Any cancer with evidence of spread outside affected organ (including lymph nodes) within 3 years of donation (however, localized prostate, thyroid, in situ cervical cancer, and non-melanotic skin cancer are acceptable)
- Melanoma (except completely excised Stage 1 cancers)
- Choriocarcinoma
- Active hematological malignancy (myeloma, lymphoma, leukemia)
- Definite, probable, or possible case of human TSE, including CJD and vCJD, individuals whose blood relatives have had familial CJD, other neurodegenerative diseases associated with infectious agents
- TB: active and untreated
- HIV disease (but not HIV infection)
- A history of infection with Ebola virus
- Bacillus anthracis (Anthrax)
- Dengue virus
- Middle East Respiratory Syndrome
- Severe Acute Respiratory Syndrome (SARS)
- Rabies
- Yellow fever
- Viral hemorrhagic fevers including Lassa, Ebola, Marburg, and CCHF viruses
- Chikungunya virus (donation can be considered 6 months post-recovery)
- Progressive multifocal leukoencephalopathy (PML)
- Zika virus (donation may be considered 6 months after recovery)

General relative contraindications

- Lyme disease
- Listeria
- MMR- acute
- Aspergillosis and ongoing systemic fungemias

Renal specific contraindications

- Chronic kidney disease (CKD stage 3B and below, eGFR<45)

- Long-term dialysis (that is, not acute relating to acute illness)
- Renal malignancy (prior kidney tumors of low-grade and previously excised would not exclude donation)
- Previous kidney transplant (> 6 months previously)

87.2.1 Donors with Infection

One area where clinical judgment should be exercised is the issue of infection in the donor and on the whole, undiagnosed or uncontrolled sepsis should be considered as a contraindication to donation. Although some centers will consider organs from donors with bacteremia of known antibiotic sensitivity, it is inadvisable to utilize donors with infection localized to the organ or sepsis from multi-resistant organisms. Fungal sepsis also presents the potential for metastatic infection and donors with known fungal sepsis, most particularly aspergillus, should not be utilized.

In 2017, the advisory committee on the safety of blood, tissues, and organs (SaBTO) published guidance to keep the infection risk passed through transplanted organs to an acceptable minimum to warrant the safety of transplantation. Donors with chronic viral infections or past exposure to viruses may be considered donors in specific situations. All donors in the UK are currently screened for hepatitis B, hepatitis C, HIV, and HTLV. The utilization of organs from virally infected donors varies according to local policy. In the setting where there are potential risks from donor infection, the recipient must be appropriately counseled to allow them to make an informed decision regarding transplantation.

87.3 Hepatitis B Positive Donors

Hepatitis B virus (HBV) has a prevalence of 0.1–0.5% in the UK [4] with significant variation across different communities and higher rates in populations from sub-Saharan Africa and Asia. Although the rate of chronic hepatitis is higher when exposure occurs at a young age, most adults will not develop chronic hepatitis after initial exposure but will have serological evidence of prior exposure (HBcAb +ve, HBsAg −ve). Chronic HBV and evidence of past infection are not contraindications to transplant but careful consideration of the serological status of both donor and recipient must be made. Vaccination or revaccination should be considered for all transplant recipients prior to transplantation.

87.3.1 HBsAg +Ve Donors

The use of HBsAg +ve kidneys in naïve recipients leads to universal infection with a high risk of subsequent morbidity and should be avoided. In recipients who are already HBsAg +ve and on antiviral treatment for Hepatitis B, the receipt of an HBsAg +ve kidney can reduce waiting time with a low risk of subsequent complications. The theoretical risk of transmission of resistant Hepatitis B strains appears to be low but recipients should receive antiviral therapy with a lower rate of viral resistance, rather than Lamivudine.

The utilization of HBsAg +ve kidneys donated to patients with previous exposure to hepatitis (HBcAb +ve) or vaccination (HBcAb -ve, HBsAb +ve) is now accepted practice, with a low risk of acquiring de novo HBV. Studies investigating the potential risks of HBV transmissions in this setting have varied in their use of antiviral prophylaxis and HBV immunoglobulin (HBIG) and there is no definitive consensus on the use of these treatments. Our local policy is to utilize HBsAg +ve kidneys for recipients who are HBsAg +ve. If no recipients are found, the kidneys may be offered to patients who have prior exposure to hepatitis B (HBcAb +ve), with the administration of HBIG at the time of transplantation and a further dose at day 5 if HBsAb levels are below 500 IU/L. Entecavir is our preferred choice of antiviral, which is usually continued for at least 1 year post-transplant. If the HBV resistance status of the donor is known, antivirals should be tailored as necessary.

87.3.2 HBsAg -Ve, HBcAb +Ve Donors

Prior infection with Hepatitis B is uncommon in the UK and only accounts for around 2% of cadaveric donors. The rates of HBc Ab sero-positivity are much higher in Asia and Africa. HBV can reactivate in recipients transplanted from HBcAb +ve donors, irrespective of donor HBsAb status. A review of nine studies, including a total of 1385 kidney transplant recipients who received a transplant from an HBsAg -ve, HBcAb +ve donor, calculated rates of recipient HBV seroconversion post-transplantation [5]. The overall rate of HBV seroconversion of any HBV serological marker was 3.2%. The authors reported that no patient with evidence of seroconversion developed hepatitis, graft failure, or had higher mortality compared to those without evidence of seroconversion. These studies suggest that HBcAb +ve, HBsAg -ve donors can be safely used in renal transplant recipients who are HBsAb +ve from either vaccination or prior infection with HBV. Our local practice is to administer HBIG at the time of transplantation and a further dose at day 7 post-transplant if repeat HBsAb levels are <500 IU/L. We commence Lamivudine prophylaxis just prior to transplantation and continue for 1 year; however, the optimal duration is unknown.

Recipients of hepatitis B kidneys, either HBcAb +ve/sAg -ve or HBsAg +ve, should have long-term surveillance of hepatitis serology and liver function tests. Our local protocol is to perform monthly hepatitis serology for 3 months followed by further serology every 3 months.

87.4 Hepatitis C Positive Donors

The estimated prevalence of chronic hepatitis C infection is 0.2% of the UK population, with intravenous drug abuse a leading cause for infection [6]. It is estimated that around two-thirds of chronic hepatitis C infections remain undiagnosed.

The long-term graft and patient survival are similar for HCV-positive patients in receipt of a kidney from an HCV-positive donor when compared to an HCV-negative donor [7].

With the development of highly effective direct-acting antivirals (DAAs) donors with hepatitis C can provide an additional source of transplantable kidneys but careful selection of potential recipients is required prior to utilization of these organs. The use of hepatitis C positive donor kidneys into recipients who are hepatitis C negative was not recommended due to a high risk of virus transmission and associated worse outcomes [8]. However, in the USA and the UK programmes are now in place to offer kidneys from hepatitis C positive

donors to naïve recipients in the context of post-exposure prophylaxis or post-infection treatment. Three small pilot trials, of a total of 38 patients combined, have demonstrated that while the majority of recipients had a transient viremia, sustained virological suppression was demonstrated in 100% of patients with no serious adverse treatment effects [9–11].

Unlike hepatitis B, antibodies against hepatitis C are not protective, and experience from prison populations and patients with HIV has shown that RNA-negative patients may become re-infected after repeat exposure. One study showed that four out of five patients who were RNA negative at the time of transplantation from a hepatitis C positive donor subsequently became RNA positive with associated abnormalities in liver function [12]. There is a theoretical risk of altering outcomes with different genotypes of hepatitis C, but the type and number of genotypes of hepatitis C do not appear to affect long-term outcomes post-transplantation [13].

87.5 HIV-Positive Donors

The UK population prevalence of HIV is around 0.16%, with an estimated 7% of HIV-infected individuals undiagnosed [14].

Transplantation of kidneys from HIV-positive donors into HIV naïve recipients is associated with a high risk of infection and subsequent complications. Therefore, HIV-positive kidneys should not be transplanted to HIV naïve recipients. Over the last decade, a number of authors have reported good medium-term outcomes of HIV-positive patients receiving kidney transplants. The transplantation of patients with HIV generated interest in transplanting kidneys from HIV-positive donors to HIV-positive recipients. Although transplantation between HIV-positive donors and recipients would have the benefit of increasing the donor pool, there is a risk of co-infecting patients with different genotypes or resistant viruses that might adversely affect the recipient or accelerate their HIV-associated disease. Kidney transplantation from HIV + ve donor to HIV + ve recipient remains experimental and experience is limited to a small number of studies. A case series of 51 patients in South Africa demonstrated 5-year graft survival of 79% and patient survival of 84% [15]. John Hopkins is in the process of a randomized controlled trial to assessing outcomes in kidney recipients from HIV + ve compared to HIV -ve donors.

Consideration of HIV-infected donors would require careful assessment of the donor risk with attention to the viral genotype of both donor and recipient, assessment of the risk of viral resistance, and exclusion of donors with unusual infections, malignancy, or any AIDS-defining illness. In the 6 months prior to death, viral load should have been demonstrated to be below 50 copies/ml and CD4 count above 200/μL [16]. Transplantation of HIV-positive live donor to HIV-positive recipient is rare because of the concerns of HIV-associated CKD in the donor (which is probably a higher risk in patients of African origin) but has been done in carefully selected highly motivated pairs with careful counseling.

87.6 HTLV Positive Donors

Prevalence rates of HTLV-1 vary markedly across the globe; high in Japan (10%) the Caribbean (3–6%) and sub-Saharan Africa but with extremely low prevalence rates in the USA and Europe. Transmission of HTLV-1 from donor to recipient is associated with a very poor outcome with progressive neurological decline or lymphoma. The difficulty lies in knowing what the risk of transmission is. In the case of a positive HTLV antibody screening (potentially false positive), confirmatory testing of HTLV specific antibodies or RNA is required. The lack of access to these tests in the time frame required has precluded the use of such donors. However, in the USA of 1408 donors screened 22 positive but only 5 HTLV-2 and 1 HTLV-1 were confirmed on specific antibody testing. The UNOS database showed no transmission to 162 recipients from 134 positive donors and in 2009 screening for HTLV-1 in cadaveric donors was abandoned in the states. It remains in place in the UK, but in one study of 1844 donors screened, four were positive and eight recipients had no transmission, so the lack of rapid RNA testing probably results in wasted organs.

87.7 Donors with Malignancy

The overall risk of developing cancer from a transplanted organ from a donor not known to have active or past malignancy is low and has been estimated at 0.06% based on UK registry data from 2001–2010, which looked at 30,765 transplants from almost 14,986 donors [17]. Nonetheless, this is an increasing consideration given the ongoing shortage of organs and increasing reliance on older donors, with potentially higher rates of undetected malignancy. Hence thorough donor evaluation with blood work and radiological screening is important. The transmission of donor-derived cancer is considered a serious adverse event by the EU donor directive and must be reported [18].

Donor origin cancers (DOCs) in transplant recipients can be transmitted with the graft at transplantation (potentially unknown), termed donor transmitted cancers (DTCs), or if they develop subsequently from the graft de novo, are called donor-derived cancers (DDCs). In a recent systematic review looking at all DOCs in kidney transplant recipients, in the published literature up to August 2019 (including 234 recipients in all), the most commonly transmitted cancers were lymphomas (20.5%), renal cell cancer (17.9%), melanomas (17.1%) and nonsquamous cell lung cancer (5.6%). The median time to cancer diagnosis in these recipients was 7 months (IQR 3–17), with the diagnosis being made by 2 years post-transplant in 84% of recipients. Of these melanoma and lung cancer had the worst prognosis with a 5-year overall survival of 43% and 19%, respectively [19]!

The issue of purposefully utilizing donors with known malignancy though has been the subject of significant debate, with clinicians having to balance the benefits of transplantation and coming off dialysis versus the risk of cancer transmission and remaining on the waiting list. The UK SaBTO (Advisory Committee on the Safety of Blood, Tissues, and Organs) 2014 guidelines are amongst several worldwide that have subdivided different cancers by their varying transmission risk rate into those that are as such absolutely contraindicated, and those carrying a high, intermediate, low or minimal risk of transmission (see ◘ Tables 87.2 and 87.3) to help guide clinicians.

Overall, any active cancer with metastatic spread outside the organ or an active hematological malignancy is an absolute contraindication to transplantation. Further, donors with a past medical history of cancers with a high risk of late recurrence or high transmission rates such as malignant melanoma, sarcoma, choriocarcinoma, and most higher-grade breast cancers, are also best avoided.

On the other hand, donors who have very localized low-grade disease, especially with a long interval (more than 5 years) of supervised recurrence-free survival and considered cure rate of over 99% could well be considered for patients who require urgent lifesaving transplantation. Also donors with cancers with minimal/low transmission rates (see ◘ Table 87.2) including non-melanoma non-metastatic skin cancers in situ and resected solitary low-grade renal cell carcinoma <2.5 cm could be considered. Similarly, donors with low-grade hematological malignancies such as monoclonal gammopathy of unknown significance, whose median survival is in the range of 13 years, could also be considered.

Moreover, if kidney donors with malignancy are used, it is wise to discuss the donor with an oncologist or expert in the malignancy involved and, if possible, discuss the risk of recurrence with the clinician who has cared for the donor.

Donors with primary CNS cancers can also be a potential source of transplantable organs. A series by Kauffman et al. looked at 397 donors with CNS tumors and found no evidence of transmission, although the histological grade of the tumor was unknown, a proportion of the tumors were benign, and follow-up was only 36 months [20]. A subsequent study of donors with malignant CNS tumors found a transmission rate of 7% in patients who did not have risk factors while patients with risk factors, defined as (1) extensive craniotomy, (2) ventriculoperitoneal shunting, (3) cerebellar lesions or (4) high-grade tumors, had a transmission rate of 53% with a high rate of mortality [21]. Subsequent guidance stratified the risk of transmission based on the malignant grade of tumor with WHO grade I and II having low risk of transmission and higher-grade tumors or patients with prior surgery/shunting having high risk (>10%). A more recent publication of the UK experience found no evidence of transmission of primary CNS malignancy from 179 donors where 24 donors had grade IV gliomas and 9 had medulloblastomas, although no details of surgical intervention were recorded [22]. A

Table 87.2 Recommendations for the use of organs from donors with non-CNS cancers

Risk of organ transplantation from donor	Risk of cancer transmission quantified	Non-CNS malignancy within donor
Absolute contraindications		Active cancer which spreads outside the organ Active hematological malignancy
High risk	(>10% risk of transmission)	Melanoma: Without spread (except as below) Breast: Cancer other than those identified below Colon: Cancer other than those identified below Kidney: Renal cell cancer >7 cm or stages 2–6 Sarcoma: >5 years previously and resected Small cell cancer: Lung/neuroendocrine Lung cancer: Stage I to IV
Low risk	(0.1–2% risk of transmission)	Melanoma: Superficial spreading type with tumor thickness <1.5 mm with curative surgery and cancer-free period of >5 years Breast: Stage 1, hormone receptor negative with curative surgery and cancer-free period of >5 years Ovary: Curative surgery and cancer-free >10 years Colon: Adenocarcinoma with curative surgery and cancer-free period of >5 years Thyroid: Solitary papillary carcinoma 0.5–2.0 cm Thyroid: Minimally invasive follicular carcinoma 1.0–2.0 cm Kidney: Resected solitary renal cell carcinoma >1.0 cm and < 2.5 cm and Fuhrman grade 1/2 Prostate: Gleason >6 Treated gastrointestinal stromal cancers
Minimal risk	(<0.1% risk of transmission)	Skin: Basal cell carcinoma Skin: Squamous cell carcinoma with no metastases Skin: Non-melanoma skin cancer in situ Uterine cervix: In situ cancer Thyroid: Solitary papillary carcinoma (<0.5 cm) Thyroid: Minimally invasive follicular carcinoma (<1.0 cm) Bladder: Superficial non-invasive papillary carcinoma Kidney: Resected solitary renal cell carcinoma <1.0 cm and Fuhrman grade 1/2 Prostate: Gleason <6 or > 6 with curative treatment and cancer-free >3 years

Modified from SaBTO guidance 2014 [18]

Table 87.3 Recommendations on the use of organs from donors with CNS tumors

Risk of organ transplantation from donor	Risk of cancer transmission quantified	CNS malignancy within donor
Absolute contraindications		Primary cerebral lymphoma All secondary intracranial tumors
Intracranial tumors with an intermediate risk of cancer transmission	(2.2% with an upper 95% CI of 6.4%)	WHO grade 4 tumors and equivalents including: Glioblastoma Medulloblastoma Choriocarcinoma
Intracranial tumors with a low risk of transmission include	(<2%)	WHO grade 3 and equivalents including: Anaplastic astrocytoma Anaplastic oligodendroglioma Anaplastic oligoastrocytoma Ependymoma

Modified from SaBTO guidance 2014 [18]

subsequent risk analysis of this data with application of the 95% confidence limits suggested that the risk of transmission of a primary brain malignancy is up to 1.5% with up to 6.4% transmission risk for high-grade tumors and an additional 8 years life for the recipient when utilizing a kidney with a primary CNS malignancy over waiting for a donor without [23].

Overall, donors with CNS tumors should be considered if the tumor is of primary CNS origin and not a secondary deposit or lymphoma. The risk of transmission is generally small, with the increasing risk associated with higher WHO-grade tumors, as reflected in the SaBTO guidance (◘ Table 87.3). Moreover as emphasized in subsequent European guidance, the presence of additional risk factors including previous surgery, chemo-radiotherapy, or shunting would shift the risk grading for each of the WHO-grade tumors up further. Such that WHO grade III tumors categorized as low transmission risk in SaBTO guidance, would convert to being high risk of transmission in the presence of any of these risk factors [24].

The risk of utilizing such kidneys from donors with a known history of malignancy has to be balanced against the risk to the recipient of continuing to wait on the transplant waiting list for another better offer, where there is considerable morbidity and mortality associated with ongoing dialysis.

In summary, when considering a potential organ donor with active malignancy, donor-related issues to consider include the type and extent of the tumor, its risk of transmission based on available evidence, and in cases of historical malignancies the timing of the tumor, any treatment received, tumor-free interval and whether the tumor is associated with late recurrence. All recipients must be thoroughly counseled of the risks of accepting that individual transplant kidney (especially if from a high-risk donor) and this discussion documented.

Recipient factors to weigh include the desires of the recipient, their comprehension of the risks, and the alternatives for them if transplantation is deferred, as well as post-transplant malignancy screening and potential treatment options if the tumor is transferred [24]. When donors with malignancy are considered, a number of clinicians will choose higher risk or older patients as recipients of these kidneys.

87.7.1 Marginal and Expanded Criteria Donors

There are multiple variables to consider when a deceased donor offer comes up and each one may have an impact on the outcome of the transplant.

Not only are we concerned about the risk the kidney may pose to the recipient (e.g., risk of transferring malignancy or infection as discussed above), but also whether the kidney is likely to have good graft function and consequent long-term graft survival. Certain risk factors have been associated with both primary nonfunction (non-function of graft post-transplantation despite adequate perfusion on ultrasound) and delayed graft function (need for dialysis within the first 14 days post-transplantation, with consequent RRT independence).

Though it is widely accepted that donor age is still the most important predictor of long-term graft survival, a number of authors have looked at donor variables when compared to long-term outcome post-transplantation with a view to predicting graft and patient survival by donor characteristics.

An early study of 5129 French cadaveric kidney recipients found that graft survival was greater in donors who were male, between the ages of 6 and 50, died from cranial injury rather than cerebral hemorrhage, and were CMV seronegative [25].

A further review of 29,068 first cadaveric kidney recipients in the USA looked at the donor factors associated with increased risk of graft loss or death post-transplant and found that donor age less than 10 and over 40, a history of hypertension, death from cerebrovascular disease, or terminal creatinine over 1.5 mg/dl were associated with greater risk [26].

These factors were then used to define expanded criteria donors (ECDs) where the recipients of these kidneys had a 70% higher risk of graft loss (RR 1.7) than low-risk donors (i.e., SCDs).

The criteria for ECD were as follows:

- Either donor age over 60
- Or donor age between 50 and 59 with more than two of the other three risk factors (hypertension, creatinine over 130 umol/l, or cerebrovascular cause of death).

Though outcomes of recipients getting ECD kidneys are consistently lower than those receiving SCD kidneys, nevertheless they are still superior to outcomes if the patients were to remain on dialysis while on the transplant waiting list [27].

This distinction between standard and ECDs is clearly important in terms of outcomes, however, it is still a rather crude tool for assessing the overall quality of any given kidney donor offer, as it is really only accounting for four donor variables. Moreover, not all SCDs are equal and some actually have a lower quality compared to ECDs when more factors are considered.

87.7.1.1 Kidney Donor Profile Index

Of greater practical use in terms of predicting the longevity of deceased donor kidneys is the Kidney Donor Profile Index (KDPI), which numerically quantifies (on a continuous scale) the quality of deceased donor kidneys relative to all other recovered kidneys in the USA in the previous year [28]. With higher KDPI values denoting lower donor quality and reduced predicted graft survival. For instance, if the donor has a KDPI of 80%, this means their kidney would have a higher risk of graft failure than 80% of all kidney donors recovered the previous year in the USA.

The KDPI is derived from the Kidney Donor Risk Index (KDRI) and is basically a remapping of the KDRI from a relative risk scale to a cumulative percentage scale.

The KDRI was originally devised by Rao et al. in 2009 [29] using US registry data from 1995 to 2005 for first-time-deceased donor transplants and takes into account ten different, variably weighted, donor characteristics which were all found to associate independently with graft failure/death- including donor age, race, history of hypertension or diabetes, last serum creatinine, a cerebrovascular cause of death, height, weight, donation after cardiac death and hepatitis C virus status. The original also included four transplants factors that adversely affected graft survival including the degree of HLA mismatch, CIT > 20 hours, single kidney, and non-en-bloc kidney transplants. These factors tend not to be used in the current KDPI, as all this information may not be available pre-transplantation when this score is generally used to assess donor quality. These factors are all listed in ◘ Table 87.4.

87

Though the KDRI was devised based on US data from 1995 to 2005, it has stood the test of time and not been shown to be meaningfully improved by additional data from 2000–2016 [30]. It has also been validated in European and Asian populations now [31, 32]. As such it provides a valuable tool for deceased donor assessment, and as discussed, more donors with higher KDPIs are being considered for transplantation given the ongoing shortage of organs.

◘ **Table 87.4** Factors associated with increased risk of graft loss post cadaveric renal transplant

Donor factors	Transplant factors
Increasing donor age – over 50 African American donor Serum creatinine over 1.5 mg/dL Donor hypertension Donor diabetic Cerebrovascular cause of death Decreasing donor height below 170 cm Decreasing donor weight below 80 kg Donation after cardiac death Donor HCV-positive	Increasing HLA mismatch Cold ischemic time over 20 hours Single kidney transplant Non-en-bloc transplant

Modified from Rao et al. [29]

87.7.1.2 Donor Serum Creatinine

Caution should be used when utilizing creatinine as a predictor of graft outcome with consideration of the donor's circumstances and body habitus. Terminal creatinine does not consistently predict outcome after transplantation but is dependent on the circumstances of the donor and whether they have suffered acute kidney injury (AKI) during their care prior to donation.

In addition, normal serum creatinine in elderly patients may be associated with a low level of renal function due to reduced muscle mass and clinicians should not be lulled into a false sense of security by values within the accepted normal range. In this situation, consideration of a calculated GFR may help evaluate the function of the donor's kidneys, although these methods are still imperfect. Our local practice is to consider donors over 60, with an eGFR over 60 ml/min (by the CKD EPI equation and based on the best creatinine), suitable for single donation, while an eGFR between 40 and 60 ml/min should be considered for dual transplant, and kidneys with a value under 40 ml/min are not utilized.

Many deceased donors have suffered an AKI in the context of their last illness. Deceased donor AKI is associated with organ discard and DGF [33]. In a large UK multicentre study [34], looking at deceased donor transplants from 2003–2013, graft failure at 1 year was greater for donors with AKI than for those without (graft survival 89% vs. 91%, $p = 0.02$; odds ratio (OR) 1.20 [95% confidence interval (CI): 1.03–1.41]). DGF rates increased with donor AKI stage ($p < 0.005$), and primary non-function (PNF) rates were significantly higher for AKIN stage 3 kidneys (9% vs. 4%, $p = 0.04$). Analysis of the association between AKI and recipient eGFR suggested a risk of inferior eGFR with AKI kidneys versus no AKI ($p < 0.005$; OR 1.25 [95% CI: 1.08–1.31]). They also reported a small reduction in 1-year graft survival of kidneys from donors with AKI. Their recommendation was AKI stage 1 or 2 kidneys should be used; however, caution is advised for AKI stage 3 donors.

Experience from the native AKI literature shows that younger patients are more likely to recover kidney function after AKI than older patients [35]. In this situation, a younger donor with a rising creatinine or filter dependency due to a known insult may be a suitable donor but an elderly donor in the same situation may not.

This data may support use of donors with an elevated terminal creatinine; however, caution must still be exercised when considering donors with an elevated admission creatinine which may indicate pre-existing irreversible renal dysfunction.

87.7.1.3 DCD Donors

The majority of deceased donations occur after brain death and are classified as DBD, previously known as heart-beating donors. With the increasing focus on maximizing the number of potential donors and pressure on resources for managing potential donors, there has been a significant increase in the utilization of Donors after Cardiac Death (DCD) in the past decade; previously known as non-heart-beating donors. Though there was initial skepticism about their use, the patient and graft survival as well as function in DCD kidney recipients are found to be comparable from 3 months onwards with DBD recipients [36–39] and this holds up to 10 years later [40].In the short term though, DCD kidneys are slower to start functioning with a higher rate of delayed graft function (OR 2.4) over recipients of DBD kidneys [38], which patients need to be consented for. They are also more sensitive to increasing cold ischemic time compared to DBD kidneys [39]. Moreover, we have mounting data to suggest that graft outcomes are more closely associated with the quality of donor as opposed to the mode of donation [41]. With transplantation from deceased donors after circulatory death with extended criteria, DCD recipients having similar graft survival and function to extended criteria DBD recipients [40]. It is important to remember though that not all DCD kidneys are the same and Maastricht categories I, II, and V (uncontrolled DCD) have a higher rate of primary nonfunction and delayed graft function when compared to Maastricht categories III and IV (controlled DCD). This is particularly important when the warm ischemic time is prolonged, with times over 40 minutes associated with a high rate of primary non-function [37]. Overall, DCD kidneys provide comparable results to DBD transplants but the utilization of donors with long cold ischemic time and prolonged warm ischemic time should be considered higher risk.

87.7.2 Pediatric Donors

A number of authors have reported excellent outcomes of kidneys from pediatric donors but there is considerable variation over the criteria for utilization and when kidneys should be transplanted as single kidneys or en-bloc. With transplantation as single pediatric kidneys maximizing resource utilization, and as en-bloc pediatric kidneys maximizing graft function. The use of KDPI is also not validated for pediatric donors making comparisons to SCDs more challenging [42]. Different groups have looked at the weight of the donor [43, 44], age of the donor [45, 46], and size of the kidney as methods for differentiating how to utilize the kidneys.

From data between 1995–2007, Kayler et al. [43] found that single pediatric kidney transplant recipients from >35 kg pediatric donors had similar 1 year graft survival as standard criteria adult kidneys. However, below 35 kg, one-year graft survival from single pediatric kidneys was inversely proportional to weight, with the relative risk of graft loss compared to ideal donors increasing by 20% for donors 25–35 kg, 30% for donors 20–24 kg, 50% for donors 10–19 kg and 110% for donors under 10 kg. Specifically, they reported that recipients of a single kidney from donors less than 10 kg had function equivalent to extended criteria transplants.

Bhayana et al. looked exclusively at outcomes of kidneys from pediatric donors less than 5 years of age when transplanted as either single or en-bloc kidneys (with mean donor weights of 15.8 vs. 12.5 kg). During the first 6 months post-transplant, the risk of graft loss was higher in kidneys from donors under 5-year-olds with the greatest graft loss occurring in the single transplanted kidneys. However, graft function in pediatric kidneys improved with time, up to 36 months post-transplant. Function was best in the en-bloc kidney group throughout the study but single pediatric kidney had an equivalent function to a standard adult donor at 1 year [36].

Though registry studies have shown worse outcomes with smaller donors than bigger pediatric donors [43], a study by Maluf et al. showed that when this was stratified based on center volume, the outcomes of the pediatric donors at high volume centers actually varied little by donor size [47].

A recent Chinese study by Zhu et al. found comparable results from single kidney transplantation into selected adult recipients of very small pediatric donor kidneys (Small Kidney Group- aged 8–36 months) versus older pediatric donors (Big Kidney Group-aged 3–12 years) with a median follow-up time of just over 2 years [48]. One-year graft survival and death-censored graft survival in the SKG were 89.1% and 100%, respectively, comparable to the results in the BKG (92.9% and 98.2%). One year later, the graft and patient survival rates in both groups remained unchanged. This is especially striking given that 28% of the SKG group and 59% of the BKG were DCDs.

Overall, increasingly successful outcomes are being seen for intermediate- to long-term graft survival with pediatric donors (though notably, early graft loss due to vascular/urological complications is higher than with SCD kidneys). On the whole, pediatric kidneys from bigger donors have better outcomes. Similarly, though pediatric en-bloc transplants provide better outcomes than single transplants especially when looking at very young/<5 kg pediatric donors, if the recipient selection is appropriate, and if these transplants are carried out at specialist high volume centers with expertise in this practice, the outcomes of even single kidney transplants from such donors can be successful.

In the UK transplants from pediatric donors <2 years old are reserved for transplanting at specialist centers only to optimize outcomes. Generally, we transplant en-bloc, kidneys from donors who are 2–5 years old or 10–15 kg in weight. Meanwhile kidneys from donors who are 5–10 years old or weigh 15–35 kg can usually be transplanted as single kidneys, and still achieve good long-term graft survival. Our local practice is to choose recipients of lower body weight and body mass index to limit the mismatch of vessel size and reduce the risk of complications associated with increasing body habitus.

87.7.3 Older Donors

Donor age is the strongest predictor of long-term kidney transplant outcomes with increasing age associated with lower long-term graft survival [29, 49]. However, older donors present one solution to the limited number of potential organ donors and are increasingly offered as potential kidney donors, with a proportion of kidney donors aged ≥70 years in one European study more than doubling in the time period of 2007–2016 compared to 1997–2006 (15.4% compared with 6.7%) [50].

Kidneys from donors over 70 years of age have a lower graft survival and function when compared to donors between 50 and 69 years of age [51], although the impact on death-censored graft survival was minimal in older recipients. In addition, recipients of kidneys from donors over 70 years of age have lower overall survival. Therefore, it has been suggested that donors over 70 should be allocated to older recipients where the donor-recipient age gap is lower.

Another method would be to increase the transplanted nephron mass and utilize two kidneys for one recipient (dual transplants). Some transplant centers have reported encouraging results for kidneys from >80-year-old donors with graft survival rates comparable to kidneys from younger donors by using pre-implantation biopsies and proceeding with either single or dual-kidney transplantation or discarding the organs, depending on the biopsy results [52]. Although this method can increase the transplanted kidney function, it is important to remember that the operative time, recovery time, and risk of complications are also increased and careful recipient selection is required to make sure the recipient is suitably robust. Dual transplants should be avoided in younger recipients where vascular access should be preserved for future transplants.

Overall, older donors present a useful resource for expanding the donor pool but careful selection of recipient and donor should be employed. Age matching of donor and recipient provides one method for allocating these extended criteria organs but care should be exercised when transplanting extended criteria organs into extended criteria recipients particularly in donors with additional comorbidities such as diabetes, hypertension, or vascular disease.

Renal function may provide a guide to allocation but the association of age with lower muscle mass and muscle metabolism makes utilization of creatinine alone inaccurate. Our policy is to consider dual transplants from donors with an eGFR under 60 ml/min. Donors with eGFR under 40 ml/min or eGFR over 40 ml/min with additional comorbidities are not utilized. Although both creatinine and calculated GFR may be affected by AKI in the donor, delayed graft function in donors over 60 years of age has a significantly negative impact on long-term graft survival, and such kidneys maybe best avoided [53].

87.7.4 Summary

Whenever considering a donor with a high-risk history or of extended criteria, the recipient should receive sufficient and accurate information for them to make an informed decision over whether to proceed with transplantation from that donor. The information should be received at the earliest time point prior to transplantation with a discussion of whether patients would wish to accept a high-risk or extended criteria donor prior to transplant listing. It has been suggested that this discussion should probably not only occur at the time of donor offer, when there may be a bias toward transplantation but preferably at the time of listing when a more rational and informed decision can be made.

87.8 Selection of the Live Donor

Live donor kidney transplantation provides the optimal treatment for patients with end-stage kidney failure. Live donor transplantation not only provides the best long-term graft and patient survival but also allows for a timely and elective procedure that can enable the recipient to avoid dialysis and lengthy waiting lists. In addition, the offer of a live donor kidney can facilitate desensitization protocols for overcoming immunological barriers and enable paired and pooled schemes for achieving compatible matches in patients who may not otherwise achieve a suitable transplant.

The evaluation of the donor has to consider the suitability of the kidney for the recipient but must also consider the safety aspects of the donor who is undergoing investigation and operation for the well-being of another person. In addition to the short-term issues of peri- and post-operative safety, the assessor must consider the long-term impact on the health of the donor and their ability to live with only a single kidney. Long-term follow-up of live donor patients has shown the operative risk of death to be 3.1 per 10,000 [54] and long-term mortality similar to age-matched controls within the general population [54, 55]. When renal function is considered, the incidence of end-stage renal failure was similar to that of the general population and eGFR was 64 ml/min or 76% of pre-donation GFR, after a median of 12 years post-donation [55]. At the time of assessment, 7.5% of patients had new-onset hypertension, 11.5% had microalbuminuria and 1.2% had macroalbuminuria. Other studies have estimated the excess risk of hypertension to be around 5% when compared to the general population and 14% of live donors develop microalbuminuria. Although these studies are reassuring and give some guidance to potential kidney donors, the issue of the correct control group still needs to be addressed and future studies will need to focus on the risk of long-term complications in live donors when compared to healthy donors who were unable to donate for reasons other than renal or physical wellbeing. Only then will we know the true increased risk to donors post-donation.

The assessment of a potential live donor should always include adequate counseling of the risks of living donation and potential outcomes for the recipient. Information should be imparted in multiple formats with written and audiovisual information used to supplement any office visits. The risk of donation should highlight potential outcomes for the kidney with special reference to long-term graft survival, the risk of graft loss from rejection, primary non-function of the kidney, and the risk of recurrent disease. Specific risks to the donor should always be highlighted, with particular reference to patients with pre-existing medical issues such as hypertension and obesity which may impact the well-being of the donor in the long term. The aim of the assessment process is to enable the donor to make a judgment on the risks of donation and be able to provide informed consent. Although very few issues are clear-cut contraindications to donation, the clinician must be aware of the emotion and context of the donation. While a parental donor may wish to consider a moderate level of risk in order to donate to a sick child, this level of risk would probably be inappropriate for an altruistic donor. In these situations, the live donor team should help guide the donor to make the correct decision for their individual situation.

It is very important to prepare both donor and recipient for the rare possibility of adverse outcomes, such as the loss of the transplanted kidney, loss of donor or recipient peri-operatively, or an inability to transplant the retrieved kidney. In the latter situation, the donor should be asked how they wish the kidney to be handled and whether they want the kidney to go to another donor or auto-transplanted back to themselves. Ideally, both donor and recipient should have separate clinical advocates to act on their behalves and make appropriate judgments to suit their respective wards. The discussion regarding donation should be undertaken with the donor in the absence of the recipient, and often the donor's family, to avoid any coercion. The final stage in the assessment process should involve an independent review of the donor's and recipient's understanding of the process, with particular relevance to adverse outcomes and evidence of potential coercion. Although coercion is classically thought of as financial, the emotional pressure of family or sick dependents should not be underestimated.

87.8.1 Choosing the Potential Live Donor

All potential transplants recipients should be asked whether they have any possible live donors. The response to this question will vary from no donors to a multitude of family and friends who wish to be considered as potential donors. Any prospective donors should then undergo a process of medical screening and blood group analysis to start the process of choosing a live donor. The medical screening should focus on potential contraindications to donation, such as diabetes, resistant hypertension, renal disease, or significant cardio/respiratory disease. Tissue typing can also be undertaken at this point to evaluate the immunological suitability of the donor. It is important to remember that any comparison of blood group and tissue typing between donor and recipient may uncover a disparity in the perceived genetic relationship between donor and recipient. This is most particularly relevant when tissue typing father and child where non-paternity can be found in roughly 10–20% of the population. Therefore, it is important to counsel the donor and recipient about the possible outcomes of the test and ask both if they would wish to be aware of the result in a situation where no genetic link is found.

The selection of the donor is usually made on immunological grounds where the best matched individual proceeds as a donor. This selection also has to be tempered by the physical circumstances of the donor and a poorer matched but physically fit donor may be selected over a better-matched donor with other significant comorbidities that may impact their ability to donate or the long-term survival of the graft. The advent of blood group incompatible transplantation and the long-term risk to the recipient from sensitization have also tempered the selection of donors. In this situation, a better-matched blood group incompatible transplant may be a more optimal donor to a poorly matched blood group compatible donor. Even in the situation where only a single blood group compatible donor is available, the risk of a poorly matched kidney in a young recipient who may need subsequent re-transplantation is considerable. In these circumstances, compatible but poorly matched donor and recipient pairs should be considered for **paired and pooled donations** to see whether the recipient can achieve a better-matched kidney transplant from a donor of similar physical characteristics. In most paired and pooled schemes, the physical characteristics of the donor match can be controlled for with age the most common variable.

87.8.2 Altruistic Donors

Altruistic or Good Samaritan donors are increasingly common referrals to transplant units. Altruistic donors provide the potential to transplant urgent or high-risk patients who may have been waiting for some time while also allowing domino transplants within paired and pooled donations that can set off chains of live donor transplants. Such transplants have similar outcomes to other forms of living donation.

Altruistic donation has previously been limited to non-directed altruistic donation (NDAD) where the donor and recipient are unknown to each other. As living donation and altruistic donation have increased with time, the concept of directed altruistic donation (DAD) has started to emerge. In this situation, potential altruistic donors can come forward to donate to recipients that they are aware of but have no formal relationship with. Although DAD does have the potential to increase kidney donation, this form of donation has a number of ethical and regulatory concerns. As with all living donations, the gift has to be altruistic with no gain, financial or otherwise, to the potential donor. In this case, the donor should not donate to seek any form of long-term gain or relationship with the recipient. The selection of recipients for this form of donation also raises significant ethical issues. While a donation to a casual acquaintance or work colleague who has kidney failure may be acceptable, the advertising of a kidney through a paid agency or internet site is probably not. In addition, the selection of potential recipients through a "beauty parade of most deserving candidates" raises significant ethical and moral issues.

The assessment of potential altruistic donors should follow the rigorous physical process required for all live donors. The evaluation should also include some exploration of the motivation for donation. Although the UK regulatory authorities have removed the mandatory status for psychological evaluation of potential altruistic donors, it is probably best practice for these donors to be evaluated by a person experienced in personal assessment that has sufficient time and skill to explore the motivation for and understanding of altruistic donation. Most donors are motivated to help their fellow humans and some donors may have a previous history of medical altruism, such as blood or bone marrow donation. Caution should be exercised with donors who have recently had major life events, such as significant loss or separation, where donors may be looking for absolution of previous events. In addition, young altruistic donors provide significant vexation for the clinician where a kidney of excellent function is offered but the donor may not be of sufficient emotional maturity or far enough into their "life experience" to fully understand the consequences of donation. It is always important to reaffirm that kidney donation can only be undertaken once and any future partner, child, or family member who develops kidney failure would be unable to receive a kidney if they have already donated to another person.

87.8.3 Assessment of the Potential Live Donor

The assessment of a kidney donor is a complex process that should evaluate the physical health of the donor, their suitability to undergo major abdominal surgery, the suitability of the donor to be left with a single kidney long term, the quality of the donor organ, and any risk to the recipient of receiving the organ. It is important to remember that a donor is always giving altruistically and may often be the financial breadwinner of a household. Any workup process should aim to minimize disruption to the work schedules and compact the investigations into as few days as possible. This is particularly relevant when donors have traveled from overseas to donate and may have left families or businesses back in their own country. Overseas donors may be on short visas and any workup should be planned in advance of their arrival.

Current best practice consists of a single day of donor assessment with subsequent medical and surgical review. Donors and recipients should then have time to digest the information before proceeding to independent assessment under the Human Tissue Act. Minimal suggested donor evaluation investigations are listed in ▶ Box 87.2.

Box 87.2 Suggested Minimal Investigations for Donor Assessment

Physical
- Office Blood pressure measurements × 2
- Urinalysis × 2
- Full medical history
- Physical examination

Hematology
- Full blood count
- Clotting
- Blood group and antibody screen

Biochemistry
- Urea, electrolytes, creatinine, and eGFR
- Calcium and phosphate
- Liver function
- Fasting glucose and lipids
- Urine protein estimation (ACR/PCR or 24-hour urine)

Endocrine
- Thyroid function

Infection Risk–Virology
- Hepatitis B sAg and cAb
- Hepatitis C
- HIV
- HTLV
- CMV
- EBV

Infection Risk—Microbiology
- Syphilis
- Toxoplasma
- Malaria—if from at-risk country

Imaging
- Chest X-ray
- EDTA GFR
- CT or MR angiography
- (DMSA)

Malignancy Risk
- PSA – if male
- Recent mammography in females over 50
- Recent cervical smear

Cardiovascular Assessment
- ECG
- Stress testing in high risk or elderly donors

87.8.4 Specific Points in the Workup Process

The live donor assessment is rigorous with around 30–40% of potential donors ruled out during the assessment process. The most common reasons for declining donors after the assessment stage are(1) insufficient renal function, (2) poorly controlled hypertension, and (3) anatomic abnormalities with the kidney that are picked up during scanning. The assessment process is multifaceted and each individual donor often presents their own idiosyncratic issues. Most national transplant bodies will provide guidance on the assessment process for living donation and recommendations for acceptability. In the UK, the British Transplant Society provides guidance for the assessment of donors which are freely available on their website. This guidance is detailed and covers a number of different situations. For the sake of brevity, this chapter will only cover some of the more common problems encountered.

87.8.5 Kidney Function and the Acceptable Level to Donate

The assessment of renal function prior to donation should be undertaken by a referenced measurement of glomerular filtration rate, i.e., chromium EDTA. Estimated methods such as CKD EPI, MDRD, or Cockroft and Gault are not sufficiently accurate to predict GFR and should not be relied upon. Although creatinine clearance may give an estimation of renal function and 24-hour collections are useful for measuring urinary protein excretion, the variable logistics and room for errors in performing these tests make them unsuitable for the accurate representation of true GFR.

The renal function of a prospective donor must be sufficient for a person to be able to donate a kidney and not be at risk from clinically significant renal failure over their lifetime. The level of GFR at which an individual person can donate their kidney has been achieved by extrapolation of a number of estimates. In the UK, the

Table 87.5 Acceptable GFR by donor age prior to donation

Age (years)	Threshold GFR (ml/min/1.73 m^2)	
	Male	Female
20–29	90	90
30–34	80	80
35	80	80
40	80	80
45	80	80
50	80	80
55	80	75
60	76	70
65	71	64
70	67	59
75	63	54
80	58	49

Reproduced from the UK Guidelines for living donor kidney transplantation [2]

guidance suggests that any person who donates a kidney should be left with sufficient renal function to achieve a GFR of 37.5 ml/min/1.73 m^2 by the age of 80 years. The most recent UK guidance is based on the data from Ibrahim et al. [54] where all donors had to achieve a baseline GFR of at least 80 ml/min/1.73 m^2 and rate of decline post-donation was 0.6 ml/min/1.73 m^2 per year. The acceptable rate of decline was then increased to 0.9 ml/min/1.73 m^2 per year to allow for safe variation and further data showing that the rate of decline of renal function in renal donors may be between 0.4–0.8 ml/min/1.73 m^2 per year. The last two factors are that renal function is grossly stable until the age of 40 before declining in a predictable fashion and after donation, there is a compensatory increase in function after donation to achieve a level of 75% of the original function (although this does not necessarily apply to patients over 60). Therefore, until the age of 40, a donor has to achieve a measured GFR of greater than 80 ml/min/1.73 m^2, but after that, there is a reduction in this limit by 0.9 ml/min/1.73 m^2 per year (Table 87.5).

Any estimate of a donor's kidney function should also take into account the divided split in function between kidneys. Most centers perform a nuclear medicine scan to assess the divided function of the two kidneys, the presence of scars, and drainage of the kidney (if a dynamic scan is performed). Some units prefer to rely on the length or volume of the kidneys on cross-sectional imaging to guide whether nuclear medicine assessment of divided function is necessary. Either way, the total GFR should be interpreted with the split function to decide the level of function that will be left with the donor and the function to be transplanted to the recipient.

87

87.8.6 Obesity

Obesity is an increasing problem with donor body mass index is slowly increasing with time. Increasing size of the donor is associated with an increase in the rate of surgical complications and the long-term risk of post-donation from hypertension and proteinuria. In addition, obesity is a significant risk factor for diabetes and its associated long-term complications.

Obese donors should be carefully assessed and counseled about their individual risk with strict weight loss targets given to donors who wish to progress. The risk of regaining weight after donation should also be highlighted and long-term lifestyle measures should be implemented prior to donation. Some donors have opted for bariatric surgery prior to donation but the risk of this technique in donors has not been established and certain procedures may increase long-term renal risk.

Each donor should be assessed individually with the limits of the body mass index and sex fat distribution (i.e., males tend to have a greater proportion of intra-abdominal fat than females) borne in mind. Although there is no specific cutoff for donation and surgical practice varies between centers, it is wise to counsel and try weight loss techniques in any donor with BMI kg/m^2 over 30, given the long-term increased risk of kidney disease in the context of obesity as well as the short term increased risk of perioperative complications (based on extrapolation of data on very obese donors) [2]. Moreover, such donors must also undergo a careful perioperative evaluation to exclude cardiovascular, respiratory, or kidney disease.

At a BMI over 35 kg/m^2 most centers would not proceed to donation unless there are extenuating circumstances, as data on the safety of kidney donation in the very obese are limited.

87.8.7 Hypertension

Hypertension is common with around a quarter of the general population lying within the hypertensive range and only one-third of patients adequately treated. Hypertension is a known risk factor for proteinuria and the progression of chronic kidney disease. In addition, hypertension can be an indicator of renal disease. The presence of hypertension is a risk for cardiovascular events and patients with hypertension may be at greater risk of cardiovascular events during the peri-operative period. Hypertension in the donor may be worsened by a donor nephrectomy and is a recognized risk factor for reduced long-term survival of the transplanted kidney. Donors should be screened for hypertension with office blood pressure readings and treated in accordance with local guidance.

Donors with readings over 140/90 should be assessed with repeated readings and a 24-hour ambulatory blood pressure measurement. If found to achieve the diagnostic criteria for hypertension, donors should initiate lifestyle changes and consider pharmacological therapy if indicated.

Donors with known hypertension should have office and ambulatory blood pressure measurements to assess their level of control. If donors have controlled blood pressure on one or two antihypertensive agents, they may be suitable for donation if they do not have evidence of target end-organ damage but should be counseled for the small risk of worsening hypertension and proteinuria after donation. Lifestyle measures, such as smoking cessation, exercise, and weight loss, should be initiated before and after donation to minimize risk. Our local practice is to perform ECG and echo assessments for left ventricular hypertrophy, retinal examination for evidence of hypertensive retinopathy, and screen for microalbuminuria. If patients are found to have evidence of target end-organ damage or uncontrolled hypertension, they are advised against donation.

87.8.8 Hematuria

Asymptomatic nonvisible hematuria affects 2.5% of the UK adult male population but the prevalence increases with age and has been estimated to be present in 22% of males over the age of 60. Although there are national guidelines for the significance and management of hematuria in the general population, the guidance is based on risk assessment and probability of finding significant disease which does not necessarily apply to a potential donor. In living donation, the purpose of the investigation is to rule out any significant transmissible disease while also prognosticating for the future of the donor post unilateral nephrectomy.

All donors should have at least two urine dipstick analyses performed on two separate occasions. A positive result should be considered at any level of positivity, including trace hematuria (corresponding to 1–5 red cells/microliter), as glomerular pathology has been identified in potential live kidney donors at even this low threshold. Initial investigations should aim to rule out reversible causes, such as infection, exercise, or menstrual contamination. In the event of persistent positive dipstick analysis, donors should undergo further evaluation with urine cytology and renal tract imaging to rule out common urological causes including nephrolithiasis and urothelial malignancy. Cystoscopy should be performed in all patients over 40 with persistent hematuria and considered in those less than 40 in the presence of further risk factors for urothelial malignancy including smoking, exposure to aniline dyes, analgesics, or cyclophosphamide.

All patients with persisting nonvisible hematuria will require a renal biopsy to rule out significant glomerular pathology if they wish to progress as a donor. This investigation is particularly pertinent to donors who are giving to a relative where the underlying cause of kidney failure is undiagnosed or possibly inherited. Given that a native renal biopsy carries significant risk and non-donor patients in the same situation with normal renal function in the absence of hypertension and proteinuria would not undergo a biopsy, the potential kidney donor is putting themselves at risk purely for the wish to donate. This balance of risk should be explained to the potential donor with a full explanation of the potential complications of kidney biopsy, including the small risk of damage to or loss of the kidney. If the donor decides to proceed to a renal biopsy, the kidney that is to be donated should be biopsied in order to reduce any long-term structural risk to the donor in their remaining kidney.

Glomerular pathology has been reported in eight out of ten donors who undergo a biopsy for isolated hematuria prior to donation [56] and 46% of nephrology patients presenting with asymptomatic nonvisible hematuria alone. Post-donation, persistent hematuria with dysmorphic red cells on cytology is associated with a higher incidence of proteinuria and declining renal function [57]. Patients who are found to have abnormal renal biopsies, other than thin basement membrane disease, should be ruled out as potential donors due to the risk of progressive renal pathology.

It is estimated that 10–50% of renal biopsies for persistent asymptomatic microscopic hematuria are reported as thin basement membrane disease [2], but the question of whether these patients should be considered as donors remains a contentious issue. First, the course of thin basement membrane disease may not be entirely benign with 10–20% of patients developing proteinuria and 5% having subsequent renal impairment- biopsy findings of FSGS like lesions are associated with progression to ESRF. Secondly, the diagnosis of thin basement membrane disease can be indistinguishable from the early or carrier status of Alport syndrome. In the case of the latter, potential donors with carrier status for X-linked Alport syndrome have a 15% chance of end-stage renal failure by the age of 60 and should not proceed to donation [58]. For this reason, any mother or sister who intends to donate to a patient with Alport syndrome should be offered genetic counseling, screening for known Alport mutations, and a renal biopsy prior to donation. This advice also applies to female extended family members where there is a family history of Alport syndrome. In the case of autosomal recessive Alport syndrome, family members can proceed to donation post-biopsy if they have only a single mutation (i.e., heterozygous) of COL4A3 or COL4A4 without proteinuria, hypertension, low GFR, or significant chronic damage on their biopsy [58].

Donors who are found to have thin basement membrane disease on biopsy should undergo genetic screening to rule out mutations associated with X-linked Alport syndrome [58]. If the screening is negative, donors may progress to donation in the absence of hypertension, proteinuria, family history of deafness, family history of renal disease, and significant scaring on a renal biopsy. A referral to a clinical geneticist should be considered, especially if the underlying cause of renal failure in the recipient is not fully defined or the donor is of Cypriot origin, where higher incidence of renal impairment with thin basement membrane disorder has been reported.

87.8.9 Diabetes

87

Due to the increased propensity to renal failure, patients with diabetes or those with impaired glucose tolerance have historically been ruled out from donation. A single study from Japan [59] has looked at donors who had impaired glucose tolerance or diabetes when undergoing an oral glucose tolerance test prior to kidney donation. Donors with no evidence of secondary complications, an HbA1c under 6.5%, and no albuminuria were allowed to donate after careful counseling. When compared to donors with normal glucose tolerance, there was no significant difference between the groups in survival to 20 years and renal disease at a median follow-up of 88 months. Although this data is encouraging and may suggest that donation in groups with impaired glucose tolerance or well-controlled diabetes is safe, the follow-up period is relatively short and the cohort of donors with diabetes was newly diagnosed at donation and may not have had sufficient time to develop significant complications. A further study [60] looked at the development of diabetes post-donation in donors who had a normal oral glucose tolerance test at the time of donation. After a follow-up of almost 18 years, 5% of the donors had developed diabetes. The main risk factors were body mass index over 30 kg/m^{2}and donating to a relative with type 1 diabetes. At the time of follow-up, there were a greater proportion of donors with hypertension (71% vs. 36%) and proteinuria (19% vs. 4%) in the group with diabetes compared to those without diabetes. The rate of decline in renal function post-donation was the same in both groups. Another similar study [61] looked at the incidence of diabetes post kidney donation and its association with decline in kidney function.

After a similar follow-up period of 18 years,7% of donors developed DM while the incidence of DM was 14.5% at 30 years of follow-up. During the follow-up period, higher percentage of diabetic donors developed hypertension (60.2% vs. 25.7%), proteinuria (16.8% vs. 5.4%), and hypertension or proteinuria (64.7% vs. 28.1) in comparison with nondiabetic donors. The rate of decline in renal function post-donation was significantly higher in the diabetic group with both hypertension and proteinuria in contrast to nondiabetic (1.10 ml/min/year vs. 0.09 ml/min/year) and only 0.08 for nondiabetic donors.

Although these studies may suggest that the risk of donation in patients with diabetes is low, it is important to remember that the follow-up time was short and the donors studied donated on average only 9 years after the diagnosis of diabetes (or impaired fasting glucose tolerance) [61]. From epidemiological studies of patients with diabetes, the incidence of end-stage renal disease in type 1 diabetics is between 4% and 17% at 20 years and 0.8% at 10 years in the UKPDS type 2 diabetes cohort. In light of the propensity for higher blood pressure and risk of proteinuria post-donation, there is likely to be a higher risk of chronic kidney disease or end-stage renal failure in donors with diabetes. Therefore, potential donors with diabetes should generally be ruled out from donation.

The diagnosis of diabetes or impaired glucose tolerance is fairly clear-cut, but the issue remains whether the clinician can predict which donors are likely to develop diabetes post-donation with a higher long-term risk from chronic kidney failure. The risk of diabetes is increased when a family member has diabetes, which may be pertinent to a donor who is giving a kidney to a family member with end-stage renal failure secondary to diabetic nephropathy. The overall risk of developing diabetes is increased two- to threefold if any first-degree relative has diabetes. If both parents have diabetes, the risk is increased five to six fold with some South Asian patients having up to 80% lifetime risk of developing diabetes in this situation. In addition, certain ethnic groups with higher rates of end-stage renal failure also have higher rates of diabetes, such as South Asian and Caribbean groups. The prospective Nurses' Health Study showed that females from an African American, Asian or Hispanic background have a relative risk of 2.2 for developing diabetes when compared to white

Americans. Therefore, these at-risk groups should be carefully screened for the presence of diabetes and their lifetime risk considered in conjunction with their lifestyle and anthropometrics.

Women with a history of gestational diabetes are at higher risk of developing type 2 diabetes with the incidence varying between 2.6% and 70% and the greatest risk occurring within the first 5 years post-pregnancy. A further study estimated the risk to be 19% by 9 years post-partum. Due to this much higher risk of diabetes, donors with gestational diabetes should normally be ruled out from donation. Individual donors with high body mass index or adverse anthropometrics (i.e., waist-hip ratios or waist measurements) may also be at greater risk of diabetes.

All donors should be screened for their risk of diabetes with fasting blood sugar. Donors with normal fasting blood glucose of 5.5 mmol/l or less have a low chance of developing diabetes of around 4% over 9 years. Fasting glucose of 5.6–6.9 mmol/l indicates impaired glucose tolerance while a value over 7 mmlo/l is indicative of diabetes mellitus. Donors with impaired glucose tolerance and a family history of diabetes have a 30% five-year risk of developing diabetes and should probably be ruled out of donation. All patients with fasting values in the impaired glucose tolerance range, a family history of diabetes or obesity should undergo a formal oral glucose tolerance test. Two-hour values over 11.1 mmol/l are indicative of diabetes and the donor should be ruled out. Two-hour values between 7.8 and 11.0 mmol/l are indicative of impaired glucose tolerance. A meta-analysis of six trials estimated the annual risk of developing diabetes in this group ranges from 3.6% to 8.7%. Overall, most clinicians would rule out donors with impaired glucose tolerance due to their much greater lifetime risk of developing diabetes, especially if they have other risk factors. If donors still wish to proceed in the face of impaired glucose tolerance, they should be fully cognizant of the risks with full documentation of the discussion. KDIGO approves donation from prediabetes or type 2 diabetes candidates based on individualized demographic and health profile in relation to the transplant program's acceptable risk threshold. Thorough counseling among these candidates is recommended about the potential progression over time which may lead to end-organ complications [62].

Although metabolic parameters allow for clear guidance on the risk of donation, young family members of diabetic recipients, such as children, present a greater challenge when considering donation. If a young adult in their twenties presents for donation to a diabetic father, the young donor may well have a normal oral glucose tolerance test and relatively normal anthropometrics. In this situation, the lifetime risk of diabetes in a donor with a strong family history of diabetes may be up to 80%. Donation should be cautioned and the long-term risk to the donor made clear with strict adherence to exercise, healthy lifestyle, and maintenance of normal body habitus.

87.8.10 Nephrolithiasis in Potential Donors

The prevalence of symptomatic renal stones in a UK population is around 3–5% with 5% of donors found to have asymptomatic renal stones at assessment. The utilization of cross-sectional imaging techniques for donor evaluation has led to a greater discovery of asymptomatic renal stones.

Any donor with a previous history of renal stones or asymptomatic stones on imaging should undergo a full metabolic and urological evaluation to assess the risk of recurrent stone formation. The metabolic screen would include 24-hour urine collections for calcium, oxalate, citrate, and urate, an early morning urinary pH, and qualitative screen for cystinuria initially; alongside serum calcium and urate levels. In the event of a significant or uncorrectable abnormality, donation is contraindicated. Donors with bilateral renal stones, a significant stone burden, or frequent recurrent stones should also be ruled out from donation. If the chemical composition of the stone is known, donors with struvite, cystine, or uric acid stones should be ruled out unless there are obvious reversible causes for the uric acid stones and the urinary urate load is low with a pH over 6.5 [62].

Donation may be considered in potential donors with minor or correctable metabolic abnormalities, e.g., isolated hypocitraturia, isolated hypercalciuria, isolated hyperuricosuria, particularly if the history of calculus disease is very limited. Donation may be considered where factors that have previously put the patient at risk of stone formation, e.g., diet or medication, have been successfully modified, urine pH has been corrected to normal (preferably using a pH meter rather than dipstick testing), and 24-hour urine levels have demonstrated to a return to the normal range. In such cases, careful counseling of the donor is mandatory before surgery.

Donors with a previous history of stones or low volume unilateral stones without an identifiable metabolic cause can be considered kidney donors. The risk of further stones should be fully discussed with the donor and lifestyle changes or therapy initiated to reduce the risk of future stone formation. The kidney with stones is usually removed for donation, allowing sufficient renal function in the remaining kidney. Our local practice is to remove the stones ex-vivo with a small ureteroscope prior to implantation.

87.8.11 Genetic Causes of Kidney Failure

All steps should be undertaken to identify the cause of end-stage renal failure in any potential kidney transplant recipient. In the presence of an inherited cause of renal failure, either monogenic or polygenic, a detailed family history should be elucidated and referral to a clinical geneticist considered. If a genetic abnormality in the recipient has been identified, screening the potential donor for the same defect can be considered to mitigate the risk of donation.

87.9 Adult Polycystic Kidney Disease

The most common cause of inherited renal failure is adult polycystic kidney disease APKD affects 1:1000–1:2000 individuals and leading cause of ESRD in ~10% of UK patients receiving renal replacement therapy [2]. Any related donors should undergo detailed imaging for cysts in the kidney and other organs. The international diagnostic criteria for polycystic kidney disease should be applied to screen donors whose relatives have adult polycystic kidneys and caution exercised with the offspring and young relatives of polycystic kidney sufferers. A negative renal ultrasound beyond the age of 40 years excludes disease. However, CT or MRI scans should be performed for candidates with negative ultrasound, aging 20–40 years old.

Other inherited conditions where renal failure may occur are summarized in ▣ Table 87.6. In most such cases, the donation should be precluded if a predisposition to the disease is identified within the prospective donor.

Particular care should also be exercised in donors related to recipients who have primary FSGS, HUS, or Alport syndrome, where the risk of similar disease in the donor is high.

▣ Table 87.6 Inherited conditions associated with risk of renal failure

Mode of genetic transmission	Examples of inherited conditions associated with renal failure
Autosomal dominant	ADPKD Renal cysts and diabetes Von Hippel Lindau disease Familial hemolytic uremic syndrome Familial FSGS Tuberose sclerosis complex ADTKDs Nail patella syndrome
Autosomal recessive	ARPKD Alport syndrome Familial nephrotic syndrome
X-linked	Alport syndrome Fabry disease Dent disease
Polygenic	VUR FSGS IgA nephropathy

Modified from the UK Guidelines for living donor kidney transplantation [2]

87.9.1 Cardiovascular Suitability for Donation

Live donor nephrectomy is a major intra-abdominal operation that is associated with significant cardiac stress. It is important to preclude any form of cardiac disease that may put the potential donor at significant risk. For this reason, any patient with overt cardiac disease should probably be ruled out from donation to avoid any unnecessary and avoidable cardiac events. All donors should be screened for occult cardiac disease through evaluation of clinical symptoms and scoring of known cardiovascular risk factors. Donors should routinely have an electrocardiogram and cholesterol estimations performed as part of their workup. The donor's exercise tolerance, symptoms of cardiac disease, smoking history, and family history of cardiac disease should be recorded to assess risk.

On the whole, most donors who can achieve four METS (gentle swimming, gentle cycling, or singles tennis) without other risk factors and a normal ECG are usually suitable as donors. The bar for further cardiac evaluation with stress testing should be set low and our local practice is to perform either exercise testing or stress echocardiography on any potential donor over 50 with other risk factors or an abnormal ECG.

87.9.2 Pregnancy Post-Donation

Women of childbearing age are often considered potential kidney donors. Pregnancy is known to have significant effects on the kidney which may be exacerbated post unilateral nephrectomy. A number of small series have looked at the effect of donation on pregnancy and have not found any significant effects of kidney donation on pregnancy outcome, hypertension or proteinuria. A further Norwegian registry study found a higher incidence of pre-eclampsia in pregnancies post-donation compared to pregnancy prior to donation (5.7% vs. 2.6%) but no other differences in maternal or fetal outcome were found. Another retrospective postal survey from the USA found a significantly higher rate of fetal loss (19% vs. 11%), gestational hypertension (5.7% vs. 0.6%), pre-eclampsia (5.5% vs. 0.8%) and proteinuria (4.3% vs. 1.1%) in mothers post-donation. Although the data from the last study does suggest an increased risk to the mother and fetus from pregnancy, it should be highlighted that a number of donors did not respond and some who did respond were asked to describe pregnancies that had occurred some decades prior.

When considering all these studies, there is insufficient data to be definitive about the risk of pregnancy post-donation but there does not seem to be a reduction in fetal outcomes. There may be a marginally higher incidence of hypertension, proteinuria, and pre-eclampsia but further detailed studies are required.

87.9.3 Consent and How Much Should the Donor Know?

All donors should be given enough detail to provide full and informed consent to donation. The donor should be aware that they may withdraw their consent and progression to donation at any time, including the day of transplantation. The provision of information should be in verbal, written, and other multimedia formats. This information should focus on the risk of donation and its long-term consequences but should also include detail on the outcomes for the transplanted kidney. This aspect is particularly important when the donor is giving to a recipient with a high risk of recurrent diseases, such as HUS, FSGS, and dense deposit disease. In addition, donors should be made aware of any issues that might materially affect the lifespan of the transplanted kidney. This situation can lead to significant ethical debate over informed consent and whether the donor should be made aware of significant medical conditions in the recipient, such as HIV and hepatitis C. At present, it is considered the best medical practice that the donor is made aware of these issues and the recipient should disclose their status to the donor prior to donation.

87.9.4 Which Kidney to Remove

The choice of the kidney to be removed should be discussed with the donor and agreed well ahead of the day of surgery. The balance of which kidney is donated is often based on anatomical considerations for donor and recipient, as well as the function of the remaining kidney. The left kidney is most often removed at donor nephrectomy due to the additional length of the vessels, ease of access to the kidney, and the overall lower divided function of the left kidney. The presence of renal stones, multiple vessels, multiple ureters, and cortical lesions may necessitate the removal of an alternative or functionally larger kidney. In this situation, the function of the remaining kidney should be considered where the single kidney function is sufficient to maintain long-term kidney function without the risk of significant or symptomatic kidney disease.

87.10 Summary

Thus living kidney donation provides the best long-term outcomes for patients with end-stage kidney failure. The selection of the donor is crucial to both the long-term outcome of the transplanted kidney and the safety of the procedure. The process of donor evaluation contains a number of clinical and ethical facets but the final outcome of live donor transplantation is often rewarding for all.

87.11 Conclusion

A pre-emptive live donor kidney transplant (LDKT) provides superior patient and graft survival when compared with deceased donor kidney transplants- hence the importance of early identification of possible live donors and a streamlined donor assessment process. The pooled sharing scheme has successfully increased the proportion of LDKTs occurring in the UK. Nonetheless, there are still significant numbers on the deceased donor waiting list, whose morbidity and mortality rise with increasing time on dialysis. System-wide it is thus imperative we safely maximize the utilization of deceased organs. Tools such as the KDPI can aid in the assessment of the quality of the deceased donor kidney offered, while the SaBTO guidance can help ensure that malignancy/infection transmission risk via donated kidney is kept at an acceptable minimum.

87

Case Study

Case 1

A 34-year-old male patient is on the transplant list for the last 5 years. He received three doses of HBV vaccination and the last HBsAb titer was 1000 IU/L. A deceased kidney was offered to him. The donor has HBsAg +ve. He was reluctant to accept this offer. It is important to explain that he has a low risk of acquiring de novo HBV.

The utilization of HBsAg +ve kidneys donated to patients with previous exposure to hepatitis (HBcAb +ve) or vaccination (HBcAb -ve, HBsAb +ve) is now accepted practice.

Case 2

A 19-year-old woman on peritoneal dialysis was seen in the transplant assessment clinic. Her sister who joined her in the clinic showed interest in live kidney donation. She would like more information about the long-term risks of kidney donation on her kidney function. It is important to illustrate that the incidence of end-stage renal failure in kidney donors is similar to that of the general population.

Case 3

A 39-year-old male patient on hemodialysis was seen in the assessment clinic. His 59-year-old mother was keen to donate to him. She has had Type II DM for the last 5 years, which is well controlled on one oral agent. This highlights that diabetic donors with no evidence of secondary complications, an HbA1c under 6.5%, and no albuminuria were allowed to donate after careful counseling.

Chapter Review Questions

1. Is transplanting a kidney from an HBsAg positive donor to an HBsAg negative recipient permitted?
2. What is the risk of transplanting HCV-positive donor kidneys into HCV-negative recipients?
3. Can organs from donors with brain tumors be used?
4. Can patients with diabetes mellitus safely donate a kidney?
5. What is the risk of pregnancy post kidney donation?

Answers

1. The use of HBsAg +ve kidneys in naïve recipients leads to universal infection with a high risk of subsequent morbidity and should be avoided. The utilization of HBsAg +ve kidneys donated to patients with previous exposure to hepatitis (HBcAb +ve) or vaccination (HBcAb -ve, HBsAb +ve) is now accepted practice, with a low risk of acquiring de novo HBV.
2. The recent widespread availability of interferon-free DAA therapy has revolutionized the landscape in respect to the treatment of hepatitis C viremia, offering the prospect of a cure in the vast majority including kidney transplant recipients. KDIGO guidelines recommend consideration of DAA treatment in all HCV-positive transplant candidates either pre- or post-transplantation, with treatment decisions made on an individual patient basis. Three small pilot trials, of a total of 38 patients combined, have demonstrated that while the majority of recipients had a transient viremia, sustained virological suppression was demonstrated in 100% of patients with no serious adverse treatment effects. Larger trials are awaited.
3. Overall, donors with CNS tumors should be considered if the tumor is of primary CNS origin and not a secondary deposit or lymphoma. The risk of transmission is generally small, with increasing risk associated with higher WHO-grade tumors.
4. In light of the propensity for higher blood pressure and risk of proteinuria post-donation, there is likely to be a higher risk of chronic kidney disease or end-stage renal failure in donors with diabetes. Therefore, potential donors with diabetes should generally be ruled out from donation.
5. There is insufficient data to be definitive about the risk of pregnancy post-donation but there does not seem to be a reduction in fetal outcomes. There may be a marginally higher incidence of hypertension, proteinuria, and pre-eclampsia but further detailed studies are required.

References

1. Gore SM, et al. BMJ. 1992;305:406.
2. BTS/RA Living donor kidney transplantation guidelines. British transplantation society. 2018. https://bts.org.uk/wp-content/uploads/2018/07/FINAL_LDKT-guidelines_June-2018.pdf.
3. ODT clinical guidelines- POL188/13- Clinical contraindications to Approaching Families for Possible Organ Donation 2020. https://nhsbtdbe.blob.core.windows.net/umbraco-assets-corp/19976/pol188.pdf.
4. https://www.hse.gov.uk/biosafety/blood-borne-viruses/hepatitis-b.htm
5. Mahboobi N, et al. Transpl Infect Dis. 2012;14(5):445–51.

6. https://assets.publishing.service.gov.uk/government/uploads/system/uploads/attachment_data/file/798270/HCV_in-England_2019.pd
7. Morales JM, et al. Kidney Int. 1995;47:236.
8. Morales JM, et al. Am J Transplant. 2010;10:2453.
9. Sise ME, et al. Kidney Int Rep. 2020;5(4):459–67.
10. Reese PP, et al. Ann Intern Med. 2018;169(5):273–81.
11. Durand CM, et al. Ann Intern Med. 2018;168(8):533–40.
12. Natov SN, et al. Kidney Int. 1999;56:700.
13. Muller E, et al. New Eng J Med. 2010;362:2336.
14. https://assets.publishing.service.gov.uk/government/uploads/system/uploads/attachment_data/file/858559/HIV_in_the_UK_2019_towards_zero_HIV_transmissions_by_2030.pdf
15. Selhorst P, et al. N Engl J Med. 2019;381(14):1387–9.
16. https://bts.org.uk/wp-content/uploads/2016/09/05_BTS_Kidney_HIV-1.pdf
17. Desai R, Collett D, Watson CJ, Johnson P, Evans T, Neuberger J. Cancer transmission from organ donors-unavoidable but low risk. Transplantation. 2012;94(12):1200–7. https://doi.org/10.1097/TP.0b013e318272df41. PMID: 23269448.
18. SaBTO guidelines 2014. Transplantation of organs from patients with cancer or a history of cancer.
19. Eccher A, et al. J Nephrol. 2020; https://doi.org/10.1007/s40620-020-00775-4.
20. Buell JF, et al. Transplantation. 2003;76:340.
21. Watson CJ, et al. Am J Transplant. 2010;10:1437.
22. Warrens AN, et al. Transplantation. 2012;93:348.
23. Busson M, et al. J Urol. 1995;154:356.
24. European Committee (Partial Agreement) on Organ Transplantation. Guide to the quality and safety of organs for transplantation. 2018. https://www.edqm.eu/en/reports-and-publications.
25. Port FR, et al. Transplantation. 2002;74:1281.
26. Schold JD, et al. Am J Transplant. 2005;5:757.
27. Hamed MO, et al. Am J Transplant. 2015;15(6):1632–43.
28. U.S. Department of Health and Human Services. Organ procurement and transplantation network: KDPI calculator. 2020. https://optn.transplant.hrsa.gov/resources/allocation-calculators/kdpi-calculator//https://optn.transplant.hrsa.gov/resources/guidance/kidney-donor-profile-index-kdpi-guide-for-clinicians.
29. Rao PS, et al. Transplantation. 2009;88(2):231–6.
30. Zhong Y, et al. Transplantation. 2019;103(8):1714–21.
31. Lehner LJ, et al. Nephrol Dial Transplant. 2018;33(8):1465–72.
32. Han M, et al. Clin Transpl. 2014;28:337–44.
33. Hall IE, et al. Am J Transplant. 2015;15(6):1623–31.
34. Boffa C, et al. Am J Transplant. 2017;17(2):411–9.
35. Cho YW, et al. New Eng. J Med. 2009;338:221.
36. Nicholson ML, et al. Kidney Int. 2000;58:2585.
37. Kokkinos C, et al. Transplantation. 2007;83:1193.
38. Summers DM, et al. Lancet. 2010;376:1303.
39. Summers DM, et al. Lancet. 2013;381:727.
40. Bell R, et al. Nephrol. Dial Transplant. British transplantation society. 2019;34(10):1788–98. https://bts.org.uk/wp-content/uploads/2016/09/15_BTS_Donors_DCD-1.pdf.
41. Transplantation from deceased donors after circulatory death BTS guidelines 2013.
42. Rogers J, et al. J Am Coll Surg. 2019;228(4):690–705.
43. Kayler LK, et al. Am J Transplant. 2009;9:2745.
44. Zhang R, et al. Clin J Am Soc Nephrol. 2009;4:1500.
45. Bhayana S, et al. Transplantation. 2010;90:248.
46. Chavalitdhamrong D, et al. Transplantation. 2008;85:1573.
47. Maluf DG, et al. Am J Transplant. 2013;13:2703–12.
48. Zhu L, et al. Transplantation. 2019;103(11):2388–96.
49. Dayoub JC, et al. Exp Gerontol. 2018;110:230–40.
50. Echterdiek F, et al. Front Immunol. 2019;10:2701. Published 2019 Nov 27
51. Lapointe I, et al. Transpl Int. 2013;26:162.
52. Ruggenenti P, et al. Am J Transplant. 2017;17:3159–71.
53. Segev D, et al. JAMA. 2010;303:959.
54. Ibrahim H, et al. New Eng J Med. 2009;360:459.
55. Koushik R, et al. Transplantation. 2005;80:1425.
56. Kido R, et al. Am J Transplant. 2010;10:1596.
57. Savige J, et al. J Am Soc Nephrol. 2013;24:364.
58. Okamoto M, et al. Transplanation. 2010;89:1391.
59. Ibrahim H, et al. Am J Transplant. 2010;10:331.
60. Jiang H, et al. Am J Transplant. 2009;9:1853.
61. Ibrahim HN, Berglund DM, Jackson S, Vock DM, Foley RN, Matas AJ. Renal Consequences of Diabetes After Kidney Donation. American journal of transplantation : official journal of the American Society of Transplantation and the American Society of Transplant Surgeons. 2017;17(12):3141–8. https://doi.org/10.1111/ajt.14416.
62. KDIGO. Clinical practice guideline on the evaluation and care of living kidney donors 2017.

Running a Living Donor Programme

A. E. Courtney

Contents

M. Harber (ed.), *Primer on Nephrology*, https://doi.org/10.1007/978-3-030-76419-7_88

Learning Objectives

1. Living donor transplantation is associated with significantly better graft and patient survival than deceased donor transplantation
2. Outcomes for living donors are good, the absolute risk of serious morbidity and mortality is small
3. Physician belief and attitude to risk is an important factor in equity of access to living donor transplantation

88.1 Introduction

Kidney transplantation is the optimum form of renal replacement therapy (RRT) for patients with end-stage renal disease (ESRD) [1, 2]. The benefits compared to maintenance dialysis therapy, in terms of patient survival, quality of life, and more broadly healthcare economy, are universally accepted. Despite advances in haemodialysis over the past decades, with better molecular clearance, shorter hours, less stringent dietary restriction, and the use of recombinant erythropoietin, it remains non-physiological and suboptimal compared to normal renal function. The deficits are felt by patients, in terms of quality of life, and measured by professionals, in terms of "quantity" of life. To term dialysis therapy as *"renal replacement"* therapy belies its limitations.

A successful kidney transplant offers substantial benefits compared to dialysis, and represents a much closer approximation to true renal replacement with excretion of waste products, regulation of electrolytes and other substances, and synthesis of important hormones. Although it cannot be considered curative, (with the possible exception of transplantation between identical twins), it offers hope of a normal, or near normal, life expectancy.

Transplantation from a living donor is associated with better graft and patient survival than that from a deceased donor [3, 4]. This persists despite adjustment in analysis for the other factors known to influence outcomes, and is consistently reported in different countries and healthcare settings. For example, in multi-variant analyses of all recipients of a first renal transplant between 1998 and 2000 in the UK, the actual 10-year patient survival was 75% in those who received a deceased donor organ compared to 90% in those who had a living donor [5]. It is noteworthy that at this time the vast majority of deceased organs came from standard criteria, donation after brainstem death donors, i.e., the kidneys transplanted in this cohort would be anticipated to provide better renal function and survival than those currently being implanted, given the change in donor demographics. In the latest reported outcomes from the UK, those who received a deceased donor transplant were twice as likely to be dead within 5 years than those who received a kidney from a living donor; 5-year patient survival 87% and 94%, respectively [6].

> Living donor transplantation is the optimal form of treatment for end-stage renal disease, with significantly better patient survival than after deceased donation.

88.2 What Makes Living Donor Transplantation Better?

The reasons for the better outcomes associated with living donor transplantation can be categorized into donor and recipient factors. In essence, both are more likely to be of better "quality" than in deceased donation.

88.2.1 Donor

"Injury" to a deceased donor kidney can occur in the premortal period, at time of death, and in the post-donation stage.

The demography of donors has changed substantially from the early years of transplantation. As a representative example, in Northern Ireland, in the first two decades of transplantation, the average age of deceased donors was 32 years and 75% were male. The efficacy of road safety and drink-driving campaigns is one of the reasons that has contributed to the great reduction in this cohort of donors, (in the UK in 2017–2018 only 3% of deceased donors died because of trauma), and the average age of donors has risen substantially [7]. Additionally, often those that die have preexisting comorbidities such as hypertension or diabetes mellitus. Overall the kidneys now available for transplantation from deceased donors are much more likely to have established chronic damage.

A physiological calamity has occurred in all deceased donors, so inevitably there is a degree of insult to renal function at the time of death. The extent of this is impossible to definitively establish, a substantial proportion of kidneys that are offered for donation are declined as the clinical impression is that they may have irreversible damage; despite this careful consideration, some kidneys that are transplanted never work (primary non-function) as the peri-mortal insult is too great.

In comparison to living donor transplants, deceased donor organs have prolonged cold ischaemia given the obvious inability to organize the transplant in advance. This adds further to the "injury" to a deceased donor kidney.

Mistakenly, some assume that closer HLA matching between donor and recipient contributes to better outcomes after living donation. On the contrary, on average deceased donor transplants are more closely matched to the recipient, (as it remains a cornerstone of allocation policies, and the persistent gap between the number of people waiting for a transplant and the annual donation rate ensures there is almost always someone for whom a particular organ will be close immunological match). Furthermore, a substantial minority of living donors are genetically unrelated to their recipient, though of course even a sibling may be completely mismatched if they have inherited the different HLA haplotype from each parent.

88.2.2 Recipient

The greatest difference in the "quality" of the recipient in living donation relates to the timing of transplantation. Given the limitations of dialysis alluded to above, it is unsurprising that the longer a recipient has been dialysis-dependent before transplantation, the poorer the outcome afterwards. This length of time is the strongest independent *modifiable* risk factor for renal transplant outcome. Having an available living donor offers the opportunity for a preemptive transplant (i.e., avoidance of dialysis altogether). Until such a time as there may be enough deceased donors to avoid a prolonged wait for a suitable organ, living donor transplantation offers a distinct advantage. This is especially true for patients with diabetic nephropathy (who typically have limited survival on dialysis), multiple comorbid potential recipients, and older individuals all of whom will particularly benefit from minimization of time on dialysis. In the UK, 40% of living donor transplants in 2017–2018 were preemptive compared to 16% from deceased donation [5].

A small but important exemption to the premise of a "healthier" recipient cohort in living donor transplantation is the group with such complexity that they are considered unsuitable for an emergency surgical procedure. With a carefully planned elective transplant from a living donor, they can potentially benefit from transplantation, without this option the risks are prohibitive. A critical aspect of embarking on such transplantation is careful and explicit counselling of both the potential donor and recipient, and consensus among the whole transplant team that this is a reasonable option. One of the challenges facing the transplant community is that the outcome measures of transplantation are classically graft and patient survival at various predefined time points. A true measure of the "success" of a transplant programme would take into account the whole ESRD population; excellent outcome results can be achieved by considering only fitter candidates as eligible, but such an approach risks inequity of access for those whose survival after transplantation will be less good, but still better for that individual than remaining on maintenance dialysis.

88.3 What Are the Associated Risks of Living Donation?

The risks of donating and living with one kidney are never zero. They can be categorized according to the temporal association with donation.

88.3.1 Short-Term Risks

This relates to complications that are inherent to (i) administration of any general anaesthesia, (ii) any surgical procedure, i.e., pain, nausea, infection, thrombosis, nerve injury, and (iii) a nephrectomy, i.e., vascular, bowel, splenic, or thoracic injury.

Initial concerns that laparoscopic, rather than open nephrectomy, would be associated with poorer outcomes for both donor and recipient have not been substantiated, and almost all centres now offer minimally invasive surgery for donors. Laparoscopic donor nephrectomy is considered as intermediate surgery. The risk of a major complication, including conversion to an open operation, is generally 1–2% [8]. The risk of death is typically quoted as 1 in 3000, based on the data reported on over 6000 living donors in the USA [9].

88.3.2 Medium-Term

Following the initial recovery period after nephrectomy, few living donors have any persistent issues. For the minority that do, one of the commonest for men who have had a left kidney removed is testicular discomfort. The venous drainage of the left testes is conventionally into the left renal vein, the disruption to this can result in venous engorgement of the testes, manifest as swelling and tenderness. This typically settles over a few weeks or months as collateral drainage develops, with supportive treatment only required.

Development of an incisional hernia may complicate recovery. The incidence of this varies depending on the type of nephrectomy, i.e., hand-assisted rather than total laparoscopic, and the approach for the hand-port, e.g., subcostal versus midline. More unusually, there may be a hernia at a port site. Surgical repair is usually mandated for hernia repair, unless symptoms are minimal.

Persistent pain and symptoms of irritable bowel can also be issues for a small minority of donors.

While not sinister, the added morbidity of these medium-term complications is unwelcome for previously healthy donors.

88.3.3 Long-Term Risks

Concerns relate to the risk of (i) hypertension, (ii) renal failure, and (iii) premature death.

The challenge in drawing conclusions about the risk of hypertension after donation is that many reports are observational, and lack a control group [10]. There may be an additional risk, over and above that related to aging, but the magnitude remains unclear, particularly in non-White donors. Long-term prospective and controlled studies are awaited.

There are similar challenges in terms of adequate comparative control cohorts when considering the likelihood of renal failure after living kidney donation. Two studies published in 2014 attempted to answer this question and both reported an increased relative risk of ESRD in living donors [11, 12]. In the Norwegian group, with a follow-up of 15 years, the cause of renal failure in donors was immunologically mediated disease; notably over 80% of donors were a first-degree relative of the recipient [11]. The follow-up period in the United States cohort was shorter at 7.5 years, and two-thirds of donors were genetically related to their recipient [12]. The relative risk of ESRD was eight times greater than controls. There were anxieties expressed about the validity of the control groups in both of these studies, however it is generally accepted that there is an increased long-term risk of ESRD to an individual who donates compared to the risk if he/she does not donate.

Crucially however the absolute risk in all studies remains very low, 0.47% in the Norwegian cohort and 0.1% in the American report. The distinction between relative and absolute risk is important; for example, if an individual's lifetime risk of renal failure is 0.05%, then even a tenfold increase in *relative* risk, means that the absolute risk of end-stage disease is 0.5%, or there is a 99.5% probability that he/she will have self-supporting renal function for the remainder of his/her life.

There is a plethora of online calculators available to estimate the lifetime risk of ESRD. The limitations of these must be appreciated if applying them in clinical practice, and it is important that there is understanding of the population on which the estimates are based, including age and ethnicity. Johns Hopkins School of Medicine has produced a number of "risk" calculators [13], which are freely available; applicability to a specific individual must be considered on a case-by-case basis. Notably the "post-donation risk of ESRD in living kidney donors" tool is based on those already "passed" as suitable to donate.

Just as there is well-established consensus on the short-term risks that are quoted to living donors, similarly there was an agreed mantra for the long-term survival, namely that compared to an age- and gender-matched general population, living donors had at least equivalent, if not better survival. A number of publications reported this outcome, one study confirming this involved more than 3500 living donors and was published in 2009 [14]. As with the risks of hypertension and renal failure, the validity of comparison with the general population is limited by the inclusion in the latter group of people who by virtue of comorbidities or lifestyle would not have been considered suitable to donate. Several large studies have made admirable efforts to recruit *healthy* non-donors as a control group, and have reported no increase in premature mortality in donors [9, 15]. There has not been replication of the increase in cardiovascular or all-cause mortality reported in the Norwegian study [11].

There are good maternal and foetal outcomes reported in pregnancies after living donation. The relative risk of pre-eclampsia is considered approximately twofold higher than in a healthy non-donor, and there may be an increased risk also of gestational hypertension [16]. Interestingly, the evidence does not indicate an increased risk of low-birth weight or prematurity and it is postulated that the mechanism of pre-eclampsia in this setting is different (i.e., not related to placental insufficiency) and subsequently not deleterious to foetal outcome.

The applicability of historic studies to today's potential living donors is uncertain, as the living donor demographic has evolved over time, most particularly in the twenty-first century. As the recipient age has increased, so too has the age of the peer group of siblings, partners, and friends that volunteer. Long-term outcomes in older donors cannot be known as such people did not donate previously. Similarly donors now are more likely to be obese (approximately a quarter of all donors in the USA), have impaired glucose metabolism, and hypertension than those historically considered. There is less stringent exclusion of those with other conditions, such as renal calculi, and again comparable donors were not included in the published outcome reports. Risks of renal failure vary between racial groups, another factor now to be considered and for which long-term data are scarce.

Overall, there must be appreciation of the limitations of available data on long-term outcomes for living donors, but also of the excellent outcomes for those who have donated after assessment according to national and internationally agreed guidelines. A systematic review and meta-analysis, which included approximately 118,000 donors and a similar number of non-donors, has concluded that, despite higher diastolic blood pressure readings, lower estimated glomerular filtration rates, increased relative risk for ESRD and, in females, pre-eclampsia, the absolute risks for such adverse outcomes in living donor is low [16]. When assessed with due diligence the long-term outcomes for the donor population are very good, and although the risks are not zero, they are low or very low.

88.4 How Should a Potential Living Donor be Assessed?

Since it is not possible to eliminate risk, the purpose of assessment is to ensure, as far as possible, that the risks for a particular individual in being a living donor are acceptably low [17]. It is equally true that it is not essential for someone to have "perfect" health in order to be a donor. The three critical areas to be addressed are:

1. Suitability for general anaesthesia/surgery
2. Suitability to be left with one kidney
3. Suitability of kidney for transplant into recipient

The commonest increased peri-operative risks relate to obesity and continued cigarette smoking. Previous venous thromboses do not preclude donation but may alter anti-coagulant management at the time of surgery. There is no particular reason to deviate from established protocols of cardiovascular or anaesthetic risk assessment in living donors. Such guidelines have been well considered by a number of experts, agreed by relevant professional bodies, and are designed to maximize patient safety [18]. Additional investigation, because the procedure involves a living donor, is unlikely to be beneficial in assessment and may actually be detrimental, acting as an unmerited barrier to donation.

Consideration of long-term risks to renal function is an important aspect of assessment. Firstly, it must be established that there are two kidneys and no current concern in relation to renal function. Secondly, there needs to be determination of any particular risks for this individual in terms of the development of renal disease in the long term, which means that he/she should not be left with a single kidney. One increasingly frequent concern is obesity in the potential donor. Persistent hyperfiltration in a single kidney, together with the concomitant higher risk of hypertension and diabetes, will compromise long-term function. While some individuals are sufficiently motivated to lose a substantial quantity of weight to permit donation, sustaining such weight loss lifelong is crucial.

The final part of the assessment process mandates consideration of three areas (i) technical feasibility of donation and implantation; (ii) the risk of transmissible disease (either malignancy or infection); and (iii) the compatibility at blood group and HLA loci between donor and recipient.

Highly skilled surgical teams rarely decline a donor on solely on a technical basis as there are a number of reconstructive techniques and options to overcome vascular complexity (for example, the use of bifid and trifid "trousering" if multiple arteries, or the interposition of internal iliac artery or cadaveric donor vessels). With the possibility of living donor exchange programmes in many countries, the finding of incompatibility does not preclude donation as it did historically, provided that the donor is willing for entry into such a sharing scheme.

There are broadly comparable national guidelines for assessment of potential living donors. The typical minimal assessment process is depicted in ◘ Fig. 88.1. How this is organized varies between centres. It is possible to have a streamlined donor journey, which is popular with potential donors [19]. Additional investigations are required if initial screening reveals another potentially relevant pathology. One example would be the finding of a renal calculus on imaging, (the sensitivity of current CT imaging results in a high detection rate of tiny calculi), which requires a metabolic stone profile to be completed to assess the risk of future stone formation.

88.5 Why Is There Variation in Rates of Living Kidney Donation?

The accepted unit of measurement of living donation is number of living donors per million population per annum. There is substantial variation within and between countries in living donor rates, illustrated in ◘ Fig. 88.2 [20]. Social and cultural attitudes, together with the deceased donation rate may explain some of the international variation, but the deviation within a country requires consideration of additional factors [21].

In the UK, there is notable regional difference in living donor rates depicted in ◘ Fig. 88.3 [6]. The comprehensive Access to Transplantation and Transplant outcome Measures (ATTOM) study from the same country, reported that the significant factors associated with a reduced likelihood of receiving a living compared to deceased donor transplant were older age, Asian and black ethnicity, being divorced/separated, lower educational attainment, not owning a car or home (as a recognized measure of socioeconomic deprivation), and geographical location [22]. While some of these are intuitive, other are not; in a healthcare system that is free at

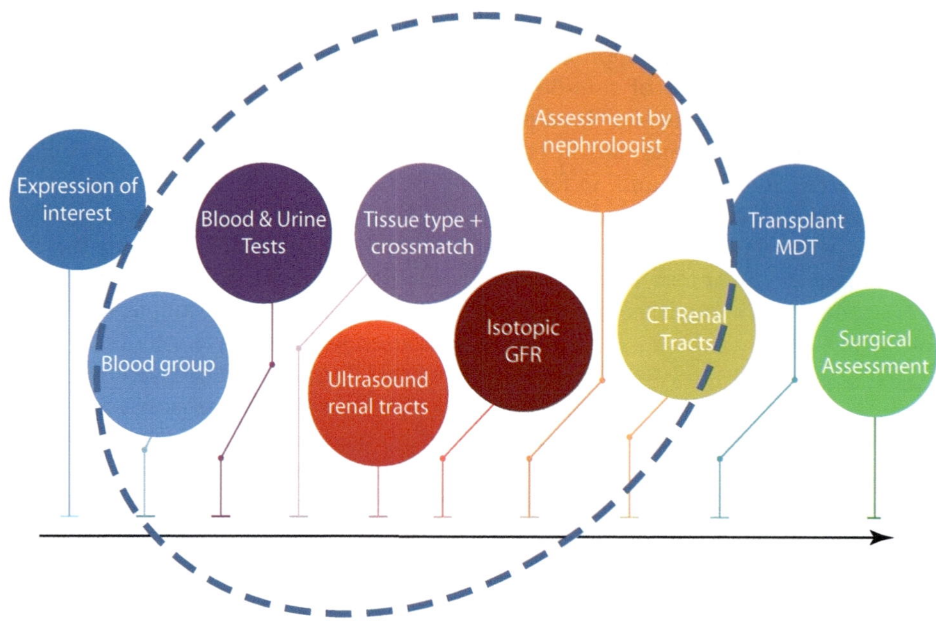

Fig. 88.1 Process involved in living donor assessment (*It is possible to have all those included in the circle carried out in a single day)

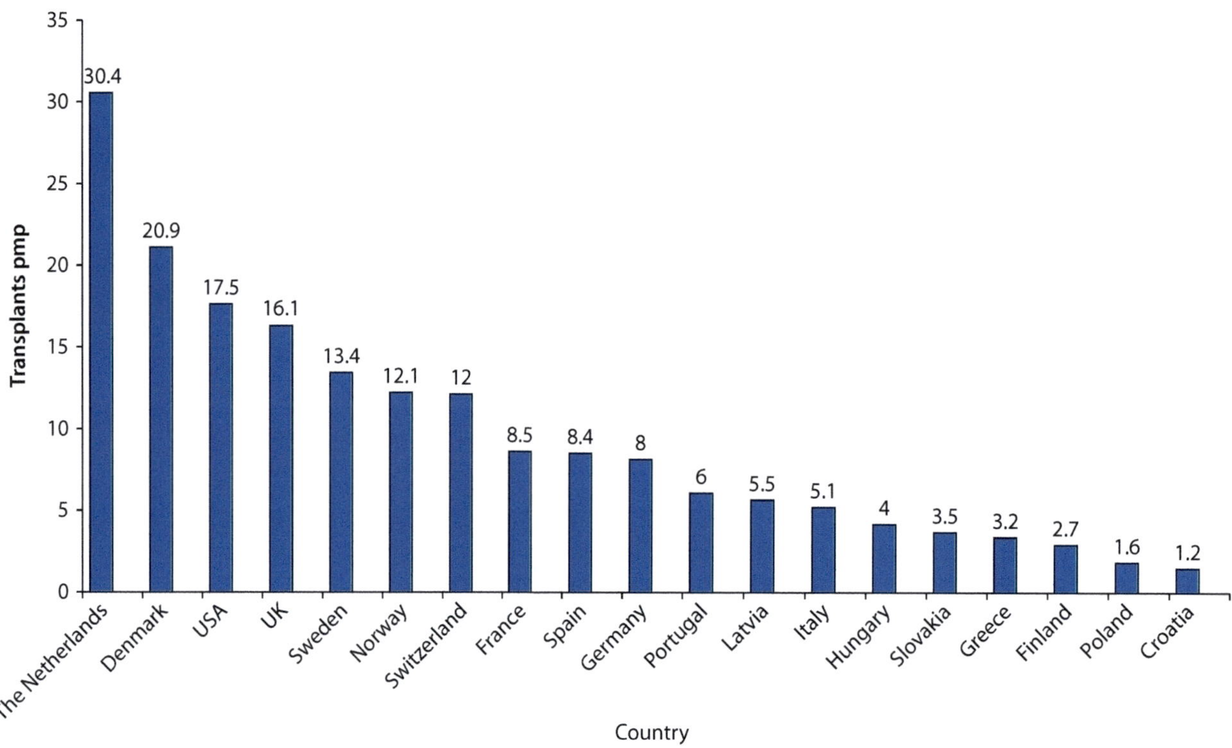

Fig. 88.2 Living donor transplant rates in Europe and the USA 2015

the point of delivery, why does socioeconomic status impact on accessing living donation? And why are people living in Northern Ireland significantly more likely to receive the optimal treatment for ESRD, compared to the equivalent person living in England, Scotland, or Wales?

There is well-developed literature, particularly in oncology, describing the factors that influence treatment

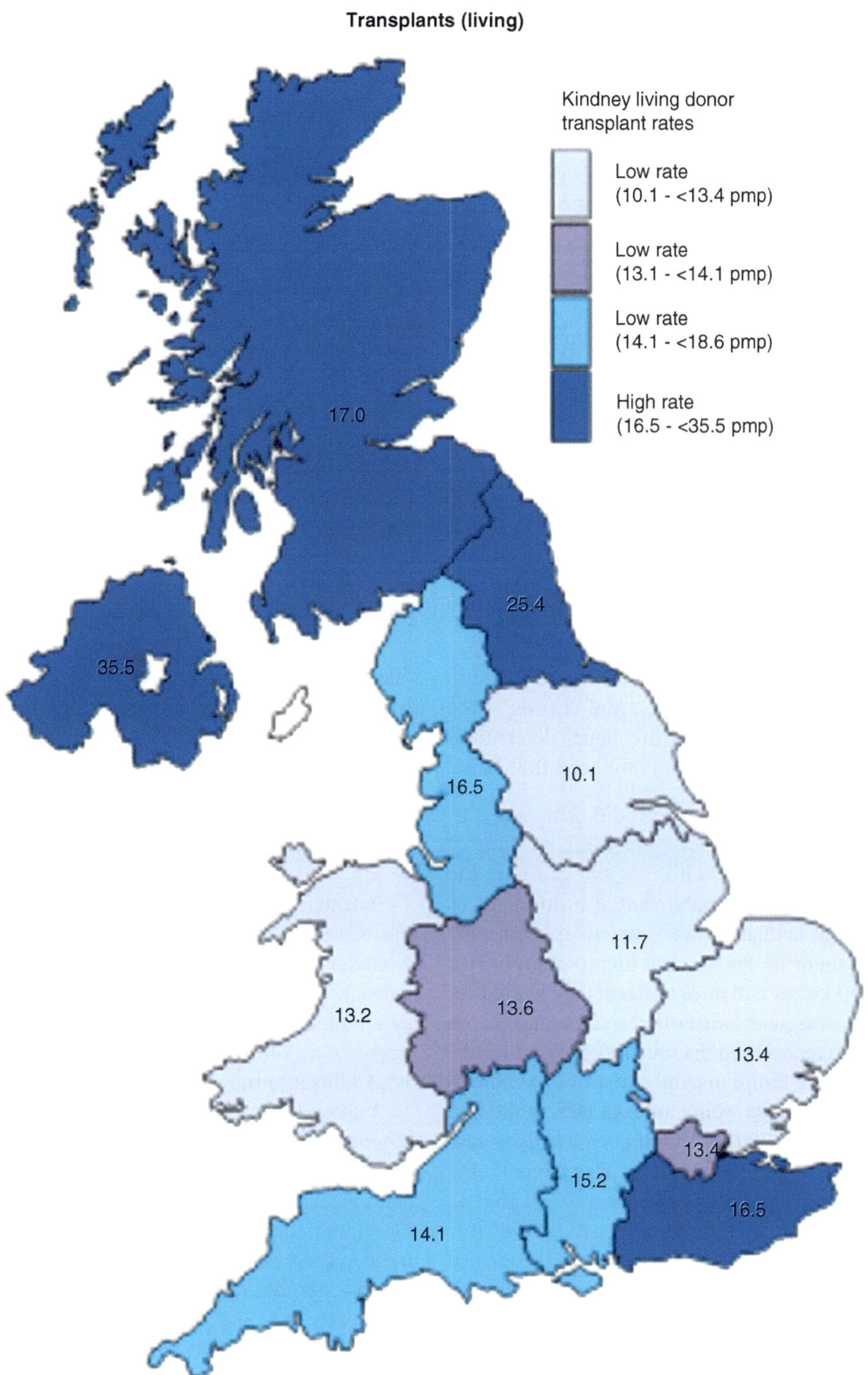

Fig. 88.3 Geographical variation in the living donor rate per million Population in the UK in 2017–2018

decision-making. These can be categorized into physician, patient, and contextual elements [23].

In terms of circumstantial factors, the availability of care, the payment system for such care and geographical proximity all influence what treatment option is chosen. In living donation it is critical to make it as easy as possible for people to donate. One aspect is making the assessment process straightforward, with compression of tests and evaluation into a minimum number of hospital visits. Making it as simple as possible reduces the days a potential donor has to take off work, avoids long delays with the associated uncertainty, and reduces donor fatigue and drop out [19]. Other important elements are clear communication with potential donors, ensuring timely reimbursement, ready support throughout the process, and making the donor feel special. Assessment and donation is inevitably anxiety inducing, minimization of this by a strong supportive team throughout an efficient donor journey will result in an increased living donor rate.

Patient factors are important in treatment decision-making, and a critical element is personal beliefs. These are influenced by ethnicity and cultural background, and previous health-related experiences. Ultimately a key determinant in what a patient believes depends on the information he/she has been given, and how this has been communicated. If the superiority of living versus deceased donation is explained this influences both the potential donor and recipient (almost uniquely in this treatment decision there are two "patients" involved). Both are likely to think differently about living donor transplantation if they know that the outcomes with living and deceased organs are not equivalent.

One of the critical inputs therefore into what a potential donor or recipient believes, and choses, is the physician belief. In every aspect of life, belief determines behaviour. If a nephrologist is not convinced that living donor transplantation is significantly better for his/her patient, then the patient is less likely to receive a living donor transplant. If he/she is not convinced that being a living donor is safe, then the patient is less likely to receive a living donor transplant. Undoubtedly living donor transplantation is risky, and for people who are by nature risk-averse, then it is a professionally uncomfortable area to be involved in [24]. The ability to balance risk objectively is an essential skill to enable the best treatment decision to be made for patients.

Even greater disparity than that between healthcare professionals is the difference in attitude to risk by potential living donors compared to the transplant team. The motivation of being able to make a transformational difference to the life of someone whom they care for dearly, clearly impacts on what is considered acceptable risk [25]. Similarly, what is counted as "success" by a donor and recipient is typically different from the medical staff. For the vast majority, being a living donor is a very positive, life-affirming, experience. Even nondirected altruistic donors, where the recipient is unknown, usually always "gains" in terms of self-esteem and well-being.

Transplant teams that understand and are comfortable in balancing relative risks of donation versus not donating for each particular individual, will have an associated higher rate of living donation than those that do not.

Case Studies

A 65-year-old man, whose only medical history was of paroxysmal atrial fibrillation, was assessed as a potential living kidney donor for his son. Imaging revealed a small stone in the left kidney and three stones in the right kidney. Although no metabolic propensity for stone formation was found, it was considered that the risks of symptomatic stone disease in the future were too great to allow him to donate. His 30-year-old son had returned to dialysis 4 years earlier, having ESRD since childhood and two previous transplants, one from his mother. There were no siblings, and because of chronic mental illness he had no close friendships. After the initial denial of donation, his father came back to the transplant team contenting that he had never had any symptomatic renal stone disease, that his son (who was highly sensitized) had no other possible living donors and very limited deceased donor options, and that he considered the personal risks were very acceptable given the potential to help his son. After careful counselling he was accepted as a donor, but they were HLA incompatible. A suitably matched pair was identified in the national Kidney Sharing Scheme; his son received a kidney from a 26-year-old donor, had an uncomplicated course, and 5 years later has a creatinine of 89 μmol/l. His father still has never had a symptomatic renal stone.

Potential donors concept of what is acceptable risk may be very different to that of the transplant team. The psychological benefits of donation can be easily underestimated. Kidney sharing schemes (paired/pooled exchanges) are an important contribution to living donor transplant programmes, offering possibilities for transplantation in those difficult to transplant.

A 38-year-old woman volunteered to donate to her 42-year-old sister who had widespread complications associated with a 35-year history of diabetes mellitus. These included 3 years of dialysis dependency and a below knee amputation because of osteomyelitis. The potential donor was advised of the higher risk of a poor outcome for her sister, but remained keen to help her only sibling particularly since she had a young family. The transplant procedure went well. The later post-transplant course was complicated by acute cellular rejection following steroid withdrawal, with a good response to enhanced immunosuppression but development of life-threatening *Pneumocystis jiroveci* pneumonia. Transplant function recovered, and after discharge following a prolonged hospitalization, she was reasonably well for some time, but 2 years later required an amputation of her remaining lower limb to manage distal necrosis. Three years after transplantation she died suddenly when out shopping. The medical team considered this to be a very disappointing transplant course following living donation, with almost 20% of her relatively short posttransplant survival being spent in hospital. Her family considered it a huge success. Her husband stated that her "final three years were so much better than the previous three years on dialysis", and compared to those days "she was hardly at the hospital at all". He was immensely grateful to the transplant team.

Outcomes for patients, particularly with diabetes, on dialysis are poor. Preemptive transplantation is common in living donor transplantation, but uncommon when there is reliance on deceased donation. What patients consider as success in transplantation may differ from that of medical professionals.

88.6 Conclusion

There is a significant survival advantage in graft and recipient survival with living compared to deceased donor transplantation. Outcomes for donors are good when the assessment is conducted in accordance with established guidelines. Appreciation of the benefits of living donor transplantation by the transplant team, and facilitation of the process to make it easy for potential donors, will result in an increased number of living donor transplants.

Tips and Tricks

1. Patients and their families need to be aware of the difference in transplant outcomes between living and deceased donor transplantation. The chances of being alive 5 years later are significantly higher after receipt of a living donor kidney.
2. The best outcomes after transplantation are facilitated by preemptive transplantation. Early preparation is required to achieve this. It is most important that those patients who inevitably will progress to end-stage renal disease, are aware at an early stage that living donation is the preferred option.
3. If the concept of living donor transplantation is introduced only when renal failure is at an advanced stage, it is less likely that there will be a suitable donor available to permit a timely transplant.
4. The risks of donating and living with a single kidney are never zero, but when assessment is in accordance with national guidelines, it remains very safe.
5. The difference between relative and absolute risks of a poor outcome needs to be appreciated—the relative risk of ESRD is increased for living donors, but the absolute risk is low.
6. It is not necessary to be "perfectly" healthy to donate a kidney; there are medical conditions that will not impact on suitability to donate or live with one kidney.
7. The attitude of healthcare professionals to risk should not contribute to inequity of access to living donor transplantation.

Chapter Review Questions

1. What are the options when an otherwise suitable potential living donor is incompatible either in blood group or HLA type with the intended recipient?
2. Is it possible for a living donor to give a kidney to a stranger?
3. If someone who donates a kidney later develops kidney failure, are the treatment options the same as anyone else with kidney failure?
4. Is there a particular role for living donation in complex patients?

Answers

1. In most countries there are two possible options to enable living donor transplantation when straightforward direct donation is prohibited by the presence of antibodies. The first is a sharing scheme whereby kidneys are shared /swapped/ exchanged between pairs when the donor is suitable to donate but the kidney is not a good option for his/her intended recipient. The organization of these schemes differs across countries but the concept and outcomes are comparable. If a compatible match cannot be identified then in some cases it is possible to lower antibodies levels sufficiently in the recipient prior to surgery to allow an antibody-incompatible transplant to proceed. There are increased risks associated with this type of transplant.
2. Yes, if someone is suitable to donate a kidney, but does not personally know anyone with kidney failure, it is possible for him/her to donate to a stranger. This has been termed nondirected altruistic donation, Good Samaritan, or stranger dona-

tion. Typically such individuals have a pattern of altruistic behaviour.

3. Yes, a donor who develops renal disease or whose remaining kidney has to be removed for any reason has the same options as anyone else with ESRD. In many jurisdictions, however previous donors receive priority listing for a suitable transplant.
4. Yes, in patients with particular anaesthetic, surgical/technical, or immunological challenges, the chances of a successful transplant are enhanced by an elective procedure with appropriate expertise available. In some cases the risks of an emergency operation are considered prohibitive, and a living donor transplant is the only alternative to maintenance dialysis.

References

1. Tonelli M, Wiebe N, Knoll G, et al. Systematic review: kidney transplantation compared with dialysis in clinically relevant outcomes. Am J Transplant. 2011;11(10):2093–109.
2. Laupacis A, Keown P, Pus N, et al. A study of the quality of life and cost-utility of renal transplantation. Kidney Int. 1996;50:235–42.
3. Legendre C, Canaud G, Martinez F. Factors influencing long-term outcome after kidney transplantation. Transpl Int. 2014;27(1):19–27.
4. Terasaki PI, Cecka JM, Gjertson DW, Takemoto S. High survival rates of kidney transplants from spousal and living unrelated donors. N Engl J Med. 1995;333(6):333–6.
5. Annual report on kidney transplantation 2011/2012, NHS Blood and Transplant. https://nhsbtdbe.blob.core.windows.net/umbraco-assets-corp/1284/activity_report_2011_12.pdf Accessed 15 October 2018.
6. Annual report on kidney transplantation 2017/2018, NHS Blood and Transplant https://nhsbtdbe.blob.core.windows.net/umbraco-assets-corp/12256/nhsbt-kidney-transplantation-annual-report-2017-2018.pdf. Accessed 15 October 2018.
7. Annual activity report organ donation and transplantation, NHS Blood and Transplant https://nhsbtdbe.blob.core.windows.net/umbraco-assets-corp/12300/transplant-activity-report-2017-2018.pdf. Accessed 15 October 2018.
8. Kortram K, Ijzermans JN, Dor FJ. Perioperative events and complications in minimally invasive live donor nephrectomy: a systematic review and meta-analysis. Transplantation. 2016;100(11):2264–75.
9. Segev DL, Muzaale AD, Caffo BS, et al. Perioperative mortality and long-term survival following live kidney donation. JAMA. 2010;303(10):959–66.
10. Boudville N, Prasad GV, Knoll G, et al. Meta-analysis: risk for hypertension in living kidney donors. Ann Intern Med. 2006;145(3):185–96.
11. Mjøen G, Hallan S, Hartmann A, et al. Long-term risks for kidney donors. Kidney Int. 2014;86(1):162–7.
12. Muzaale AD, Massie AB, Wang MC, et al. Risk of end-stage renal disease following live kidney donation. JAMA. 2014;311(6):579–86.
13. The Epidemiology Research Group for organ transplantation, Johns Hopkins School of Medicine. http://www.transplantmodels.com/. Accessed 15 October 2018.
14. Ibrahim HN, Foley R, Tan L, et al. Long-term consequences of kidney donation. N Engl J Med. 2009;360(5):459–69.
15. Garg AX, Meirambayeva A, Huang A, et al. Cardiovascular disease in kidney donors: matched cohort study. BMJ. 2012;344:e1203.
16. O'Keeffe LM, Ramond A, Oliver-Williams C, et al. Mid- and long-term health risks in living kidney donors: a systematic review and meta-analysis. Ann Intern Med. 2018;168(4):276–84.
17. British Transplant Society. United Kingdom guidelines for living kidney transplantation 4th ed. March 2018. https://bts.org.uk/wp-content/uploads/2018/07/FINAL_LDKT-guidelines_June-2018.pdf. Accessed 15 October 2018.
18. De Hert S, Staender S, Fritsch G, et al. Pre-operative evaluation of adults undergoing elective noncardiac surgery. Updated guideline from the European Society of Anaesthesiology. Eur J Anaesthesiol. 2018;35:407–65.
19. Graham JM, Courtney AE. The adoption of a '1-day assessment' model in a living kidney donor transplant program: a quality improvement project. Am J Kidney Dis. 2018;71(2):209–15.
20. European Directorate for the Quality of Medicines & HealthCare of the Council of Europe. Newsletter transplant international figures on donation and transplantation 2015. https://www.edqm.eu/sites/default/files/newsletter_transplant_volume_21_september_2016.pdf. Accessed 15 October 2018.
21. Arunachalam C, Garrues M, Biggins F, et al. Assessment of living kidney donors and adherence to national live donor guidelines in the UK. Nephrol Dial Transplant. 2013;28(7):1952–60.
22. Wu DA, Robb ML, Watson CJ, et al. Barriers to living donor kidney transplantation in the United Kingdom: a national observational study. Nephrol Dial Transplant. 2017;32(5):890–900.
23. Tariman JD, Berry DL, Cochrane B, et al. Physician, patient, and contextual factors affecting treatment decisions in older adults with cancer and models of decision making: a literature review. Oncol Nurs Forum. 2012;39(1):E70–83.
24. Young A, Karpinkski M, Treveaven D, et al. Differences in tolerance for health risk to the living donor among potential donors, recipients and transplant professionals. Kidney Int. 2008;73(10):1159–66.
25. Maple NH, Hadjianastassiou V, Jones R, et al. Understanding risk in living kidney donor nephrectomy. J Med Ethics. 2010;36(3):142–7.

Tissue Typing: Crossmatch, Antibodies, and Risk Analyses of Transplant Rejection

Henry Stephens, Raymond Fernando, Peter J. Dupont, and Kin Yee Shiu

Contents

M. Harber (ed.), *Primer on Nephrology*, https://doi.org/10.1007/978-3-030-76419-7_89

Learning Objectives

1. To understand the importance of ABO and HLA compatibility in renal transplantation.
2. To learn to interpret HLA typing and crossmatch data provided by the tissue-typing laboratory.
3. To review approaches to surmounting immunological barriers to renal transplantation including augmented immunosuppression, desensitization, paired donor exchange schemes, and acceptable mismatch schemes.
4. To review strategies for prevention of sensitization in patients with chronic kidney disease, ESRD, and following failure of the transplanted kidney.

89.1 Introduction

For the majority of suitable patients with end-stage renal disease (ESRD), transplantation offers a significant survival advantage, improved quality of life, and a substantial saving in terms of annual medical care. In countries with limited or no chronic dialysis provision, transplantation may offer the only hope of survival for patients with ESRD. However, in every country with a transplant program, the demand for kidney transplants continues to outstrip supply with the consequence that many patients fail to be transplanted in a timely fashion or at all. The two principal immunological barriers to solid organ transplantation (SOT), namely blood group incompatibility and HLA incompatibility have restricted access to transplantation. In the last two decades, strategies to expand the pool of donors have become increasingly commonplace and include the use of blood group-incompatible (ABOi) transplants, HLA-incompatible transplants (HLAi), acceptable mismatch schemes, and paired exchange programs.

89.2 ABO Blood Groups and ABO Incompatibility

The ABO blood group locus consists of three alleles A, B, and O, of which A and B code for oligosaccharide glycosyltransferase. The O allele does not encode for this glycosyltransferase, and thus blood group O patients do not express the antigen. The blood group antigens are expressed almost universally on human tissue, most notably on erythrocytes and endothelial cells. There are a variety of blood group subtypes associated with varying levels of blood group expression, most notably blood group A is divided into A_1 and A_2, the latter having much lower tissue expression and therefore potentially less immunogenicity.

Blood groups might not matter much but for the fact that, from infancy, humans naturally develop anti-blood group (isohaemagglutinins) antibodies (IgG and IgM), probably as a cross-reactivity response to bacteria.

Table 89.1 shows standard blood group compatibilities for renal transplantation.

In the early days of kidney transplantation, some ABOi transplants were done knowingly and there have been unfortunate examples of inadvertent ABOi transplantation since then; in both cases, the outcomes were usually disastrous. There are two main consequences of anti-donor blood group antibodies for renal transplantation. The first is that crossing the ABO barrier may result in hyperacute or accelerated rejection and graft loss. In hyperacute rejection anti-blood group, antibodies bind to the vascular endothelium, activate complement and platelets resulting in hypoperfusion of the kidney (which may go blue and flaccid on release of clamps). Engorgement of the capillaries occurs (glomerular and peri-tubular), with aggregation of erythrocytes and thrombosis which then spreads down the vascular tree to include afferent arterioles resulting in interstitial hemorrhage and infarction (Fig. 89.1).

Not all forbidden ABOi transplants meet this fate. A proportion experiences initial function but goes on

Table 89.1 ABO blood groups and compatibility in renal transplantation

Blood group	Antibody	Compatibility as donor	Compatibility as recipient
A_1	Anti-B	Recipient A	A or O donors
A_2	Anti-B	Recipient A (potentially (O or B))	A or O donors
B	Anti-A	Recipient B	B or O donors (potentially A_2)
AB	Nil	Recipient AB	A, B or O (universal recipient)
O	Anti-A and anti-B	AB, A, B, O (universal donor)	O (potentially A_2)

There is a window in infancy before anti-AB antibodies are generated and ABOi transplantation has been done in this setting. Although expression of A-Ag is much lower in A_2, their suitability as a donor depends on recipient anti-A titers; high levels still represent a barrier

NB potentially any blood group combination is compatible for SOT if the recipient anti-blood group antibody titer is sufficiently low

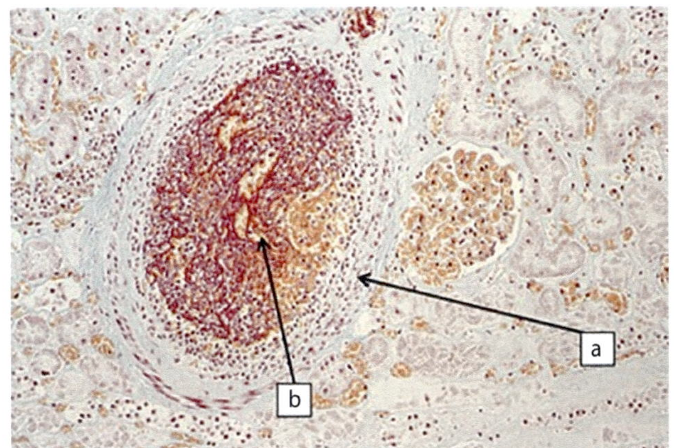

Fig. 89.1 Hyperacute rejection in the setting of ABOi transplantation. Section of an arteriole (*a*) with acute thrombus occluding entire vessel (*b*)

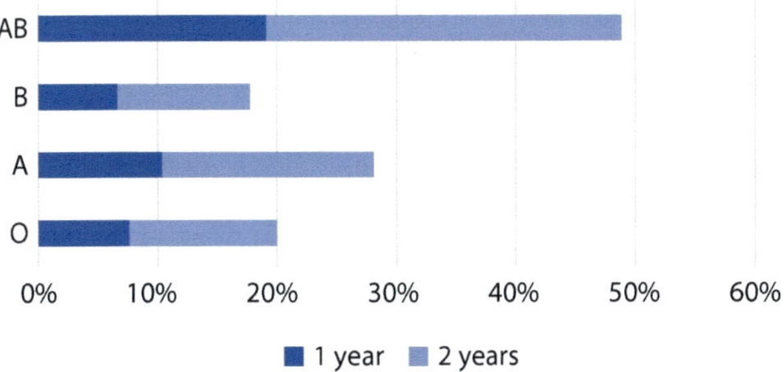

Fig. 89.2 Organ procurement and transplantation network data showing percentage of deceased donor kidney transplant recipients transplanted within 1 and 2 years of being listed (2011–2014 cohort) based on recipient blood group (based on OPTN data as of September 4, 2020)

to develop accelerated rejection with oliguria within the first few days (rarely beyond 2 weeks post-transplant) as a result of antibody-mediated rejection. Thus, for truly ABOi kidney transplantation, the outcome is graft loss or a significant risk of poor function. However, a proportion of apparently ABOi transplants can occur without adverse outcomes if the titer of anti-blood group antibodies is naturally low or can be rendered low prior to transplant.

The second consequence of the ABO barrier is the impact on waiting times for recipients of different blood groups. The waiting times for patients in the USA are shown in Fig. 89.2 [1] and show a similar pattern to those in Europe, namely, that patients with blood group B and O are likely to wait substantially longer than those with blood group AB or A. Strategies to overcome this disparity and that of having an ABOi live donor are discussed later.

89.3 Human Leukocyte Antigens (HLA) and Tissue Typing

The primary roles of tissue-typing laboratories providing a service to solid organ transplant units are as given below:

1. Facilitate the allocation of transplants by HLA typing and matching recipients and donors.
2. Identify unacceptable donor HLA antigens which could contribute to acute rejection by screening and defining HLA antibodies.
3. Provide a 24 h on-call service.
4. Prevent hyperacute rejection by performing a pre-transplant crossmatch.
5. Post-transplant surveillance of donor-specific HLA antibodies (DSAs).
6. Facilitate live donor transplantation.
7. Provide risk assessments of immunological rejection of renal transplants.

89.3.1 HLA Polymorphism

The genes encoding classical antigen-presenting HLA class I (-A, -B, -C) and class II (-DR, -DQ,-DP) molecules are the most polymorphic in the human genome, and thousands of molecular variants have now been described (see ► www.ebi.ac.uk/imgt/hla). There are numerous methods available to define HLA alleles, ranging from serotyping protein phenotypes to genotyping DNA with PCR and sequence-specific primers (SSP) or oligonucleotide probes (SSOPs), as well as direct sequencing of HLA genes [2]. The quickest methods are serotyping and PCR-SSP, which can be performed within 4 h and are suitable for relatively small numbers of test samples and on-call typing of deceased donors. PCR-SSP typing can also cover all classical class I (HLA-A, HLA-B, and HLA-C) and class II (HLA-DR, HLA-DQ, and HLA-DP) gene loci. Real-time PCR platforms and kits are now available for even more rapid (2 h) full molecular typing of all relevant HLA class I and II gene loci. Other techniques using HLA SSOPs ligated to polymer microspheres in solid-phase immunoassays (SPI) or direct sequencing of PCR-amplified HLA genes are more laborious to perform but generate better allele resolution and have the capacity for high-throughput typing.

89.3.2 HLA Nomenclature

The ever-increasing number of molecularly-defined HLA alleles has required establishing a rational system of nomenclature. The current international WHO-recognized scheme uses a basic four-figure system to define alleles that have been typed using DNA-based techniques, with the name of the HLA locus followed by an asterisk and at least four digits. The first two digits designate the broad HLA type (e.g., HLA-A*02), roughly equivalent to the serologically defined allotype (HLA-A2); the third, fourth, and sometimes fifth digits separated by a colon (e.g., HLA-A*02:01) are used to designate individual amino-acid differences [3]. With some HLA alleles, further digits have been introduced to define non-coding, silent, or synonymous nucleotide base changes, as well as intronic, 5′- and 3′-prime polymorphism, if available. Relatively rarely, alleles are unexpressed or "null", while others are low producers or are secreted; these are given the prefixes N (e.g., HLA-A*02:15 N), L or S, respectively [3]. When the molecular HLA typing method does not provide allele-level resolution, a "string" of HLA alleles are sometimes reported (e.g., HLA-A*02:01/02/03), but these all relate to primary molecular group (HLA-A*02) or allotype (HLA-A2) for the purposes of HLA matching and organ sharing.

Table 89.2 HLA-A, HLA-B and HLA-DR matching for cadaver renal transplants used in the UK organ sharing Scheme (2019)

HLA match level	HLA-A, HLA-B, HLA-DR mismatch (mm)	Possible HLA-A, HLA-B, HLA-DR (mm) combinations
1	000	000
2	[0 DR and 0/1 B] or [1 DR and 0 B]	100, 010, 110, 200, 210, 001, 101, 201
3	[0 DR and 2 B] or [1 DR and 1 B]	020, 120, 220, 011, 111, 211
4	[1 DR and 2 B] or [2 DR]	021, 121, 221, 002, 102, 202, 012, 112, 212, 022, 122, 222

The UK matching algorithm (2019) is weighted to prioritize difficult to match, highly sensitized, and patients with long waiting times. Points are allocated by both a donor and recipient clinical risk index combination, waiting time from earliest of dialysis or activation on the list, age difference, difficulty to HLA match, default HLA matchability for rare HLA antigens, level of HLA sensitization as well as organ donor versus recipient location [4]

89.3.3 HLA Matching

In the UK, the national deceased donor kidney sharing scheme matches all potential recipients for broad groups of related HLA-A, HLA-B, and HLA-DR alleles, largely based on the original serologically defined allotypes which share common structural and genetic features. Patient selection and organ offers are based on four levels of HLA-A, HLA-B, and HLA-DR matching (Table 89.2), but due consideration is also paid to the patient's reported antibody profiles to all HLA class I and II proteins, namely HLA-A, -B, -C, -DR, -DQ and -DP.

These HLA match levels were established from computational modeling of death-censored renal transplant survival data collected in the period of modern molecular HLA typing (in the UK since 1998), and are weighted for better matching of HLA-DR and HLA-B which have a greater effect on transplant survival. After donor and recipient match levels are established, ranked offers are made on the basis of points allocated for other relevant variables as given in Table 89.2 [4]. HLA-C, HLA-DQ and HLA-DP donor and recipient types are also compared in the matching algorithm, in order to exclude offers being made to recipients with pre-formed antibodies to any mismatched antigens encoded by these HLA loci.

There is considerable variation in HLA allele frequencies between different ethnic groups. The UK organ donor pool is highly representative of northern European populations, while the transplant waiting lists of patients in end-stage renal failure can have a mixed ethnic composition of Caucasoids, Africans, and Asians, particularly in large contemporary urban centers such as London. To compensate for any lack of accessibility of well-matched organs, the UK sharing scheme has introduced a rational HLA matching default system, whereby alleles common in Africans such as HLA-B53 are considered a match for B51 because of structural similarities; DR9 which is common in Oriental populations is now considered a match for DR4 which is similar and much more common in Caucasoids [4].

89.3.4 HLA Antibody Screening

Antibodies directed against mismatched donor HLA (anti-HLA antibodies) are associated with both acute and chronic transplant rejection. Serum can be tested for the presence of these antibodies using one of several assays. Cellular-based assays utilizing complement-dependent lymphocytotoxicity (CDC) to determine whether recipient serum lyses donor lymphocytes are historically the standard test for HLA antibodies and continue to be used in crossmatching. As T cells express HLA class I and B cells express HLA class I and II it is possible to determine if there are class I or II antibodies (or both).

Two refinements of the above cellular-based assay have come into common practice. Firstly, by using a panel of accurately HLA typed cells representative of the usual donor population, it is possible to define a patient's panel reactive antibody (PRA) percentage, and this indicates the probability of the patient will have a positive crossmatch with an unrelated donor. Secondly, using fluorescent labeling of antibodies and flow cytometry, but still using donor cells, it is possible to detect lower levels of antibodies that bind to the cells, and also to determine if these can bind complement. T- and B-cell flow crossmatching (FCXM) is now recognized to be the most accurate, reliable, and informative crossmatch test or risk analysis of graft rejection to perform just prior to a transplant proceeding.

In the last 20 years, SPI using Luminex beads coated with HLA antigens have transformed the ability to routinely screen and test for HLA antibodies in potential recipients: HLA proteins are bound to fluorescently labeled polystyrene microspheres or beads. Beads are coated with all major classical class I (HLA-A, HLA-B, and HLA-C) and class II (HLA-DR, HLA-DQ, and HLA-DP) antigens. The serum is added, followed by a further fluorescent label, and the resulting array can be computationally analyzed for the presence of specific anti-HLA antibodies by determining which beads have antibodies bound to them. The bead arrays are usually performed initially as an HLA screen (sensitive but less specific) in those being considered for renal transplant and then if positive, using single antigen beads, to determine more precisely the HLA antibody profile [5]. It should be noted that the mean fluorescent intensity (MFI) levels detected on beads represent the amount of antibody bound relative to the total HLA antigen present on a given bead, but as this varies between beads it should not necessarily be considered a measure of antibody titer. Nevertheless, the ability of Luminex single antigen beads to identify epitope-specific antibodies [5] that react with groups of HLA antigens or cross-reactive groups (CREG), as well as antibodies to HLA-C, HLA-DQ, and HLA-DP which are known to contribute to transplantation rejection [5], has helped in evaluating the risk of rejection of renal transplants allocated on the basis of HLA-A, HLA-B, and HLA-DR matching. There are also SPI assays for complement (C1q and C4d) binding HLA antibodies, although the relevance of these antibodies alone in predicting graft outcome is debatable [5].

The clinical relevance of antibodies detected using Luminex is still under scrutiny. Various correlations between MFI, antibody level, crossmatch results and clinical outcomes have been described [5, 6]. However, cut-off/threshold MFI values for HLA antibodies and antigens can vary between transplant centers. Nevertheless, consensus guidelines developed by an international group of experts in the field [5] are summarized below. See also the detailed national guidance for the UK last updated in 2016, including a table defining the immunological risk assessment based on the antibody screening result and crossmatch [7].

1. At least one SPI should be used to detect and characterize HLA class I and II antibodies. Laboratories must be able to define HLA-A, B, C, DR, DQ, and DP antibody specificities. Regular testing (typically every 3 months or after a sensitizing event) should take place pre-transplant.
2. The use of SPI can be supplemented with cell-based CDC and flow cytometry to fully define complex profiles and to examine correlations between all three methods, and the likelihood of a positive crossmatch and risk categories should be established - this is currently center-specific so local data should be examined.
3. Donor-specific HLA antibodies (DSAs) detectable by CDC and a positive flow crossmatch should be avoided due to their strong correlation with antibody-mediated rejection and graft loss unless some form of HLA antibody removal is achieved before transplantation.
4. "Virtual crossmatching": a renal transplant can be performed before a prospective crossmatch result is available (or completely in the absence of one being performed) if single antigen bead screening for antibodies to all class I and II HLA loci is negative if agreed with clinical users and regulatory bodies.
5. In high-risk transplant recipients (with pre-formed DSA and/or positive crossmatch before desensitization) there should be an agreed timetable of post-transplant monitoring for the development of antibodies. Consideration should be given to protocol/surveillance biopsies especially in the first 3 months post-transplantation.
6. Intermediate risk transplant recipients (with historic DSA but currently negative) should be monitored for antibody development in the first month post-transplant. If DSAs emerge, patients should be monitored closely for the development of proteinuria or declining transplant function with a low threshold for transplant biopsy.
7. Low-risk patients (unsensitized, first transplant) should be screened for DSA at least 3–12 months after transplant. If DSAs emerge, the intensity of monitoring should be stepped up and one should have a low threshold for performing a biopsy of the transplanted kidney.
8. Auditing crossmatch results conducted in the presence of Luminex-defined DSAs can assist in determining which MFI levels are likely to correlate with positive crossmatches, with most laboratories reporting HLA antibodies >2000 MFI as being unacceptable, although this is case variable and dependent on the overall antibody profiles and CREGS detected.

89.4 Crossmatching

This is the definitive pre-transplantation cell-based test which together with information derived from HLA antibody screening provides a comprehensive assessment of the immunological risk of graft rejection. The target cells in a crossmatch are donor lymphocytes derived from peripheral blood, spleen, or lymph node. T cells are used for the detection of donor HLA class I-specific antibodies and B cells for both class I and II antibodies. The CDC crossmatching detects both HLA-specific and non-HLA-specific complement-fixing antibodies of IgG and IgM classes. By contrast, crossmatching with flow cytometry is more sensitive and specific and is generally used to identify both complement-fixing and non-complement-fixing IgG. Both tests can be performed concurrently with fresh and selected historical recipient sera to provide a more comprehensive risk assessment of rejection. Autoreactive antibodies bind to both autologous and allogeneic lymphocytes but are largely irrelevant to transplant outcome and can be identified and excluded by performing an autologous crossmatch of recipient cells with relevant historic recipient sera, in addition to the allogeneic crossmatch of recipient sera with donor cells (Table 89.3). The interpretation of crossmatch is complex and relies on careful selection and inclusion of positive and negative control sera, comparing test results with pre-established cut-offs of serum reactivity, consideration of sensitizing events (previous transplants, recent blood transfusions, and infections), and the selected recipient's known HLA antibody profiles as determined with SPI, together with the HLA class I and II mismatch between potential donor and recipient [7].

89.4.1 Virtual Crossmatch

A standard pre-transplant crossmatch takes 4–6 h and this tends to contribute to prolonging cold-ischemia time (CIT). This is particularly important in kidneys that are not local and are already at risk of long CIT and those from donors that have died a cardiac death (DCD). If the crossmatch turns out to be positive, the process has to start again for the next recipient who, through no fault of their own, will receive a kidney with an even longer CIT and statistically less good outcome. There are several ways the tissue-typing service can help to reduce the CIT including declaring unacceptable antigens (so avoiding inappropriate allocation) and performing a "virtual crossmatch" [8], where the recipient antibody profile as defined by Luminex SPI is used to predict the outcome of formal crossmatching. It is more difficult to predict the crossmatch result in sensitized patients and therefore full crossmatching using CDC and preferably flow cytometry should take place prior to proceeding with transplantation. Typical inclusion criteria for virtual crossmatch are shown in ▶ Box 89.1.

89

Table 89.3 Interpretation of allogeneic and autologous crossmatch (CDC or flow cytometry)

Allogeneic T Recipient sera ± Donor T cells	Allogeneic B Recipient sera ± Donor B cells	Autologous T Recipient sera ± Recipient T cells	Autologous B Recipient sera ± Recipient B cells	Crossmatch interpretation
–	–	–	–	–ve
–	–	±	±	–ve
–	–	±	–	–ve
–	–	–	±	–ve
±	±	±	±	–ve or +ve[a]
–	±	–	±	–ve or +ve[a]
±	±	–	–	+ve
–	±	–	–	+ve
±	–	–	–	–ve or +ve[b]

[a]Recipient sera reactive with autologous cells may mask genuine alloreactive HLA DSAs; immediate review of historic HLA antibody screening and recent sensitization events are advised before overall interpretation of crossmatch is given

[b]Recipient sera reactivity with donor T cells alone indicates non-HLA antibodies which may be irrelevant, but a review of historic HLA antibody screening and any recent sensitization events is essential

Box 89.1 Suggested Criteria for Virtual Crossmatch

1. Well-documented anti-HLA antibody profile including historical sensitization
2. No recent sensitizing events (e.g., transplantation or withdrawal of IS in a failed transplant, pregnancy, transfusion, or recent infection)
3. Up-to-date antibody screening of patient samples every 3 months (for at least 6–9 months)
4. If anti-HLA antibodies are present, then stable and declining levels with the exclusion of current MFI >1500 (conservative) or >2000 (less so)
5. Close liaison between tissue typing and clinicians

Some schemes exclude women of child-bearing age but it is only those who are at risk of becoming pregnant, i.e., sexually active and not using reliable contraception, that is at risk of sensitization, so a fairer approach uses an individualized assessment

89.5 Non-HLA Antibodies

A variety of non-HLA antibodies have been implicated in the development of acute rejection and chronic graft deterioration (see Table 89.4) where there are pathological features of antibody-mediated rejection (AMR) in the absence of anti-HLA antibodies [9, 10]. Genome-wide analysis of deceased donor kidney transplant recipient pairs demonstrated that the genetic mismatch of non-HLA haplotypes is associated with increased graft loss, and this occurs independent of HLA incompatibility [11]. Antibodies against mismatched non-HLA epitopes were found in the serum of 25 patients who had histological evidence of chronic AMR.

An important target for non-HLA antibodies appears to be the endothelium or antigens expressed there [10]. Pre-transplant donor-reactive anti-endothelial cell antibodies (AECA) are associated with increased early rejection and are found more commonly in patients with early graft failure. Anti-angiotensin receptor antibodies have been shown to associate with both severe vascular rejection and malignant hypertension in the absence of HLA DSA [12]. Successful treatment reducing the risk of graft loss in patients with AT1R-Ab and rejection has included plasmapheresis, IVIG, and the angiotensin receptor blocker losartan.

Major histocompatibility complex class I-related chain A (MICA) is a highly polymorphic antigen, against which alloantibodies are present in around 10–15% of patients pre-transplantation and have been

Table 89.4 Non-HLA antigens associated with rejection in renal transplant

Anti-angiotensin type 1 receptor antibodies	Activating IgG engages AT1 receptor and causes vasoconstriction and endothelial activation with a phenotype of earlier, AR, hypertensive encephalopathy, and worse graft survival
Anti-endothelial cell antibodies (AECA)	Associated with higher rejection and poorer outcome if de novo
MHC class I chain-related (MICA) antibodies	Associated with AR and worse outcome in some studies
Anti-perlecan (anti-LG3) antibodies	Associated with vascular rejection
Anti-vimentin antibodies	No difference in early rejection or graft survival post-renal transplant but increased IgG against vimentin associated with interstitial fibrosis and tubular atrophy
Anti-collagen antibodies	Predominantly associated with lung transplant (collagen V Ab). Increased risk of transplant glomerulopathy in renal transplants with collagen IV Ab and collagen IV specific CD4+ T cells
Anti-alpha-galactose	Hyperacute rejection in xenotransplants

associated with rejection and worse graft outcome if specific to the donor's mismatched MICA antigens even in the absence of any DSAs [9].

Screening for non-HLA antibodies should be considered in patients with early or aggressive AMR despite adequate immunosuppression and with no identifiable DSA. These patients are relatively rare but will potentially need a second transplant if the cause is not identified. Similarly, patients with recurrent FSGS as the cause for graft failure may be worth screening for AT1R antibodies, as the presence of these appears to be associated with the risk of FSGS recurrence.

89.6 Sensitization

Individuals become sensitized to foreign donor HLA primarily by transplantation, pregnancy, and transfusion. Less frequently, sensitization may occur following exposure to microorganisms and allergens, presumably due to cross-reactivity. These antibodies are more commonly IgM. In the UK, approximately a quarter of the patients on the waiting list are sensitized.

Sensitized patients have a higher acute rejection rate and greater risk of graft loss. A high PRA is a useful biomarker for rejection and graft loss, as is DSA. In one study, 50% of those with a PRA >50% had acute rejection. In another study of over 5300 patients, 2-year graft survival was significantly lower at 76.5% in those with anti-HLA Ab to class I and II pre-transplant (but negative CDC crossmatch) compared to 87.5% without [13]. De novo donor-specific antibodies also augur poor outcomes with a six- to nine-fold greater risk of graft loss. A quarter of such grafts are lost within 3 years of the appearance of DSA, with chronic rejection the mechanism in 76% [14].

89.6.1 Risk Factors for Sensitization

Transplantation and graft failure are probably the greatest risk factors for sensitization; these and other factors are shown in supplementary ◘ Table 89.7. DSA appears in 11% of previously unsensitized patients in the first year post-transplant and 20% by 5 years [14]. In the UK, 52% of re-transplants are sensitized compared with 15% on the waiting list who have never received a transplant. In a review of nearly 16,000 patients from the Scientific Renal Transplant Database comparing PRA prior to the first transplant with PRA on relisting for a second transplant, 50% of patients became sensitized (PRA > 30%) and 34% highly sensitized. Risk factors include younger age of recipient, episodes of acute rejection, number of HLA mismatches, and weaning of immunosuppression on return to dialysis. Those matched for HLA-A and HLA-B were at relatively low risk (10%) [15]. Several studies have reported a significant increase in DSA following transplant nephrectomy. This may be because the transplanted kidney adsorbs DSA or because nephrectomy is often performed due to a late flare of rejection following immunosuppression withdrawal [15]. This late effect was highlighted in another study showing a 70% sensitization rate following graft loss, but for 80% of these patients, sensitization was not apparent until later [16].

Blood, platelet, or buffy coat transfusions are an important risk factor for allosensitization. Studies show approximately 20–30% of the patients became sensitized [17]. The introduction of erythropoietin has reduced the need for transfusions and roughly halved the rate of sensitization secondary to transfusion. Universal leukodepletion, implemented in many countries to reduce the risk of infections such as CMV, prion transmission, and transfusion reaction, has also reduced rates of allosensitization in potential transplant recipients. Although it does not prove causality, a review of over 2000 transplants in Ireland demonstrated a significantly worse 1-year graft survival (83% vs. 94%) in those who received a blood transfusion at the time of transplant compared with those who did not [18].

Pregnancy is a sensitizing event. On the UK waiting list, the male and female sensitization rates are 17 and 33%, respectively. It is often difficult to define these events as subclinical pregnancies/early miscarriages can result in sensitization but are often not recognized or recorded. This is a clinically relevant issue for units adopting a virtual crossmatch policy as significant AMR has occurred in this setting.

89.6.2 Prevention of Sensitization

Sensitization to common antigens may substantially impact a patient's survival and quality of life. For this reason, prevention of sensitization is paramount, and policies to reduce sensitization need to be embedded in unit policy and culture. Prevention is better than cure and a patient's prospects are likely to be enhanced in a unit with a thoughtful approach to avoiding sensitization. Strategies that should be considered for prevention are shown in supplemental ◘ Table 89.11.

89.6.2.1 Transfusion Avoidance

As discussed above, even with universal leukodepletion, transfusion risks sensitization. In many circumstances, this is unavoidable but systematic and careful erythropoiesis-stimulating agent (ESA) use and iron management have been demonstrated repeatedly to reduce transfusion requirements. Audit and, if necessary, upgrading of practice are important. Transfusion policies must be mindful of need and responsive enough to differentiate between patients who may receive a transplant in the future and those for whom this is not an issue.

Where transfusion is predictable, one option is autologous transfusion using intraoperative salvage. Alternatively selecting blood matched for HLA class I has been shown to prevent sensitization [19]. Both of these strategies require protocols and significant organization but are achievable. Where transfusion is unpredictable, there is some evidence that CNI can reduce sensitization. In one study, ciclosporin given for 2 weeks reduced sensitization rates from 30% to 10% although the ciclosporin was started 4 days before the transfusion [17], and clearly this strategy would not be appropriate for patients who may be unstable or septic. Again, this approach requires a protocol that ensures safe CNI dosing and monitoring but is worth considering particularly in young patients with a career of renal replacement ahead of them. Although not a controlled study, the impact of this is demonstrated by a pediatric series in France where pre-transplant blood transfusion was standard practice: the introduction of ciclosporin cover for transfusions was associated with substantially improved 1- and 5-year deceased donor graft survival (78% to 96% and 64% to 90% respectively) [20].

89.6.2.2 Avoidance of Allosensitization Following Transplantation

Rejection is an important risk factor for sensitization and for this reason alone worth avoiding. There is of course a price to pay for very low rejection rates; immunosuppressive (IS) protocols with very low AR rates increase the risk of over-immunosuppressing patients, putting them at risk of malignancy and opportunistic infection. Interestingly, despite higher rejection rates, Belatacept, a newer immunosuppressant agent which blocks co-stimulation of the T cell, seems to result in lower-level sensitization and seems effective at preventing de novo antibody production (which may explain higher rates of post-transplant lymphoproliferative disease in EBV-naïve patients). On the other hand, units employing minimal IS regimens may have some significant advantages in terms of side effects but will inevitably risk sensitization and can expect higher levels of AMR.

The best of both worlds may be a system that emphasizes patient education and adherence while modulating CNI levels to ensure patients are not inadvertently exposed to low IS levels. Risk stratification is also extremely important; an elderly unsensitized well-matched patient who has had previous IS is less likely to need the same level of immunosuppression as a young, poorly-matched recipient. Intelligent dosing of IS with clearly targeted drug levels is very helpful in avoiding under- or over-immunosuppression.

In this context, choosing the appropriateness of transplanting a poorly-matched live or deceased donor kidney is a complex issue. In an elderly patient, less likely to be sensitized and less likely to have a second transplant, a poor match may be entirely appropriate. For a young recipient who is likely to need a second or third transplant in the future, matching becomes more important. There are no hard-and-fast rules and each individual case needs to be considered on its merits. Projected life expectancy and a working knowledge of common HLA antigens all need to be considered. For a young recipient with several potential live donors, avoidance of common antigens (e.g., A2, A1, B7, and B44 in Caucasians) with a view to minimize the impact of future sensitization may be an important consideration.

89.6.2.3 Removal of Kidney or Reduction in IS Following Failed Graft

When a graft fails and the patient returns to dialysis, there is often a dilemma as to whether to leave in place a graft that is still producing significant quantities of urine (normally associated with improved survival and quality of life) or to put the patient through a graft nephrectomy. As discussed above, there is good evidence that patients not sensitized when recommencing dialysis become sensitized with reduction in IS, whereas those where IS is maintained do not [15, 21]. Enthusiasm for maintaining full-dose IS needs to be tempered with the fact that the commonest cause of death in transplant patients returning to dialysis is sepsis.

A pragmatic approach may be to maintain IS in a young patient who is likely to receive a transplant in the near future especially if there are potential live donors. For those who are oliguric and expecting to wait for a second transplant, then maintaining IS until (and for 2 weeks after) graft nephrectomy may be rational especially if the graft contains common antigens.

For those not suitable for re-transplantation, sensitization is not an issue but rejection can be associated with EPO-resistance, malaise, macroscopic haematuria, and increased investigations.

89.7 Improving Graft Numbers and Outcomes in the Context of ABOi or HLAi

Patients of certain blood groups or those with difficult to match HLA types, or who have been previously sensitized can be disadvantaged in access to transplantation, with longer waiting times and thereby negative impact on quality of life as well as patient survival. For patients waiting for a kidney transplant, there are a range of options to reduce waiting time on the list, reduce the risk of rejection as well as improve graft outcome post-transplant. These strategies are predominantly used to get around ABO incompatibility (summarized in ◘ Table 89.5) and also to help sensitized patients with HLA incompatibility. The frequency at which HLA types occur in the national population has the potential to skew the matching of donor organs towards certain population groups, and away from those with less common HLA types, for example, due to their ethnic background (for the relative frequencies of HLA type in the UK see ◘ Table 89.6). Achieving a fair allocation policy for the limited resource of organs is challenging, but there has been a trend to changing national allocation schemes in many countries in order to lessen the importance of blood group and HLA matching and thereby improve access for disadvantaged patient groups [22].

Table 89.5 Approaches to ABOi transplantation

1. National allocation schemes diverting O donors to B recipients	Effective at assisting long wait patients difficult to match
2. National or local allocation of A_2 or A_2B deceased donors to B recipients	Relies on recipient having consistently and naturally low anti-A antibody titers (most advocate ≤1:4)
3. National paired exchange/pooled donation scheme	Requires considerable administration but has the potential for greatest benefit especially if altruistic donors are directed to the scheme
4. ABOi transplantation	Maximum pre-treatment titers of ≤1:128–1:256 are commonly accepted

This has led to a reduction in the disparity previously seen, although not in all countries. National ethical, medical, and population engagement is needed in order to improve equity of access.

89.7.1 National Allocation Schemes for ABOi Transplantation

The disparity in waiting times for different blood groups has led some allocation schemes to divert a proportion of blood group O donors to blood group B recipients. This strategy can significantly improve group B waiting times with minimal impact on blood group O recipients.

National allocation of A_2 or A_2B deceased donors to blood group B recipients with consistently low anti-A titers has also been tried and permits some redistribution from blood group A recipients to blood group B. There is a need to define the blood group A subtype of the deceased donor rapidly and pre-screen blood group B recipients for anti-A titer initially and maintain ongoing surveillance of titers (see below). These requirements, together with the need for central administration of both these aspects, have meant that this practice is not widespread. However, it is worth considering for young blood group B patients on the waiting list who are running out of access or with high matchability scores, i.e., anticipating a very long wait. In the UK, registered patients with anti-A titers of ≤1:4 were allocated blood group A without recommendation for augmented immunosuppression or additional antibody removal.

89

89.7.2 Paired Exchange/Pooled Donation

Approximately a third of medically fit live donors are ABOi or HLAi for their potential recipients. Paired exchange programs permit the recipient to benefit by receiving a third-party kidney from a similarly incompatible donor-recipient pair. Where more than two pairs are involved, this is known as pooled donation. South Korea and Holland take the credit for first trialing early paired exchange kidney programs for patients with blood group- or HLA-incompatible live donors. Since then programs have also become established in the UK, Australia, and the USA. There are clear advantages of this system for individual recipients and the renal population as a whole, the main one being that donors previously not eligible to donate can contribute to the donor pool (see Fig. 89.3a). Competition for deceased donor transplants is also reduced. Moreover, it is likely that a standard live donor transplant is likely to have significantly lower risk, expense as well as a better outcome than a transplant requiring desensitization.

In a further refinement of paired exchange, national schemes may use a non-directed altruistic donor to start a chain of transplants. A single altruistic donor can donate to one individual, or if they donate into the paired/pooled scheme, this can facilitate multiple further transplants (see Fig. 89.3b). In one estimate, if fully implemented in the USA, paired donation could result in 1500 extra renal transplants a year.

The logistics of paired exchange/pooled donation are significant. Donors and recipients need to be in robust health, thoroughly worked up, and committed. Withdrawal of a single individual breaks the whole chain and is very disruptive. For this reason, it is unusual to have more than three pairs involved. In simultaneous exchanges, the live donor team is in close communication with the coordinating body, and surgeons phone the other surgical teams to commence donor nephrectomy once all donors are safely anesthetized, but sometimes it is necessary to stagger the operations on different days for practical reasons.

Although rare, it is very important to elicit in advance of donor nephrectomy the donor's wishes were something to go wrong with the chain. For example, if the other donor incurs a problem and cannot donate or the donor's recipient incurs a problem and cannot receive the other donor's kidney, donors should stipulate whether they would still be happy to donate as planned, to donate to the deceased donor pool or to have the kidney re-implanted.

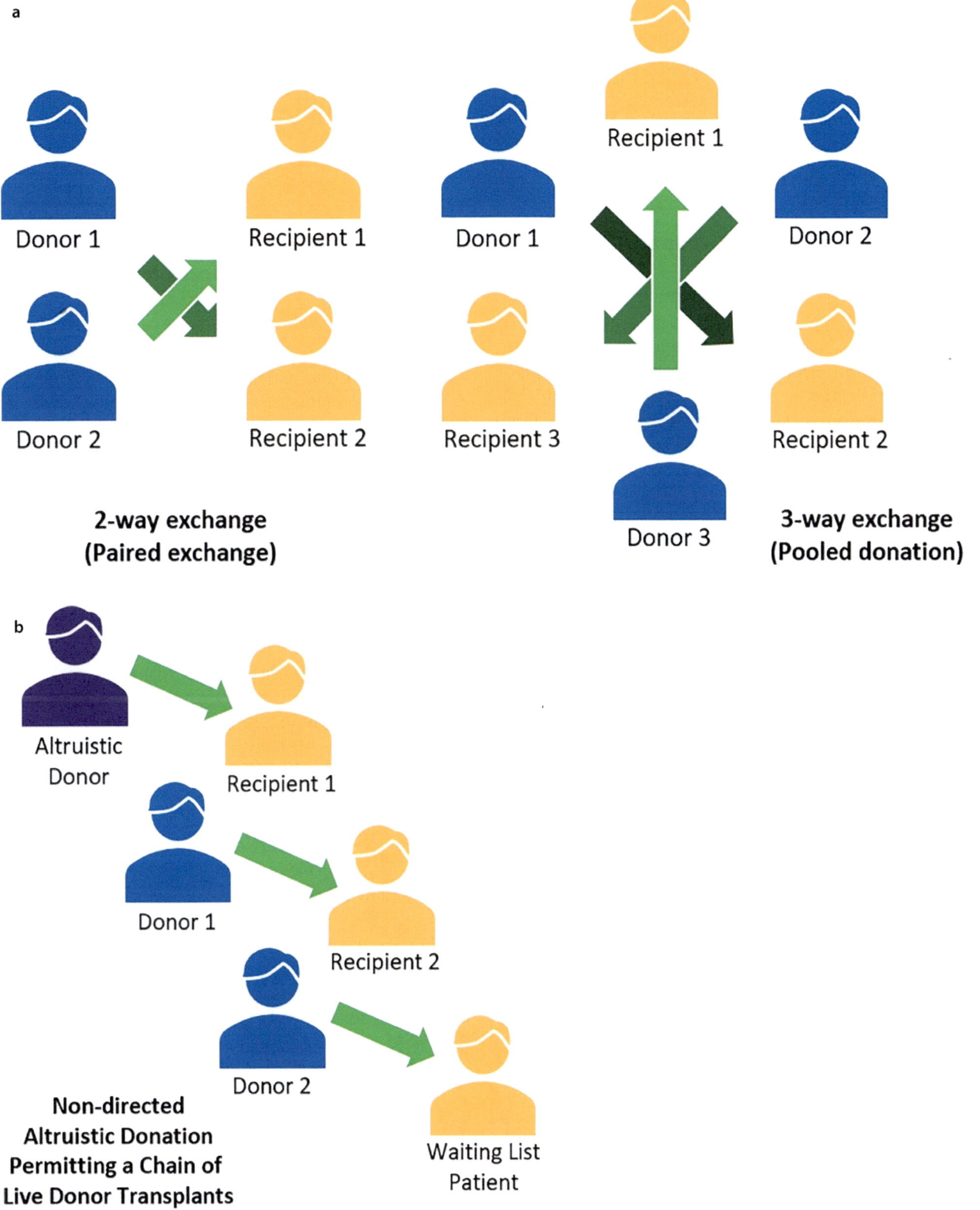

Fig. 89.3 **a** Two-way (paired) or three-way (pooled) exchange between recipients with incompatible donors. **b** Domino paired exchange with a single altruistic donor permitting three live donor transplants

Two groups of recipients fare notably less well in paired exchange—those with blood group O and those who are highly sensitized. Such patients with a donor in the pool are less likely to be selected and may be frustrated by missing out on repeated but increasing numbers of altruistic donors. This problem may be addressed by increasingly sophisticated allocation combining ABOi transplantation and paired exchange.

89.7.3 Blood Group-Incompatible Transplantation

In 1981, an inadvertent ABOi transplant was rescued with plasma exchange. This was followed in 1985 by the first successful elective ABO-incompatible transplant. Subsequently, the first successful ABOi transplant program was set up in Japan. Since then, ABOi live donor transplants have become routine in several countries. UK-based guidelines for ABOi transplantation are available on ► www.hta.gov.uk.

The most fundamental aspect of ABOi renal transplantation is the baseline maximum anti-A or anti-B titer: early data from Japan showed a 10-year graft survival of 20% for those with titers of ≥1:128 versus 60% for those with titers less than this and humoral rejection rates of 71% versus 24%, respectively [23]. Subsequent experience has confirmed this and most ABOi programs do not stray beyond a maximum titer of 1:128–256. Acceptable levels on the day of transplant vary between programs ranging from ≤1:4 to ≤1:32. In this setting, it appears that long-term ABOi graft survival is improving.

However, it is worth noting that the literature and individual experience is complicated by well-documented variation in isohaemagglutinin assays between different institutions and techniques. The commonest technique is erythrocyte isohaemagglutination using donor serum in serial dilutions but even this has considerable inter-observer variation. More recently some groups are using flow cytometry using formalin-fixed A or B erythrocytes, incubated with recipient serum and then with anti-human IgM or IgG FITC-conjugated antibodies.

As high-titer ABOi have such an adverse outcome, it is critical to have a close relationship with the lab providing ABO Ab titers. Stringent governance processes must be established for the audit and delivery of reliable titers. In addition, an ABOi program requires access to same-day anti-A/B titers to plan further Ab removal peritransplant or postpone the transplant if titer has not reached the minimum pre-agreed threshold. In practical terms regimens using antibody removal usually, but not always, employ augmented immunosuppression commencing before, or at the time of, initial plasma exchange (see supplemental ◘ Table 89.8). It is helpful to monitor anti-blood group titers pre- and post-removal sessions of each antibody to predict achievement of target titer and quantify rebound in antibody levels. The decision to proceed with transplant is usually made on the antibody titer post-removal either the day before the transplant or on the morning of the transplant if the assay turnaround time is swift.

89.7.4 Strategies for the Management of the HLA and Non-HLA Sensitized Patient

There are several approaches to facilitate transplanting of highly sensitized patients which broadly fall into two groups (supplemental ◘ Table 89.9). The first is organizational approach usually through national allocation bodies to find a donor without forbidden antigens through either paired or pooled donation or utilizing an altruistic donor (directly or through a chain) as described above. The second approach is to desensitize the patient by a combination of antibody removal and reduction in production. The former has the advantage of lower immunosuppression burden but may necessitate a longer wait on dialysis. For either approach, it is critical to have an accurate picture of the patient's sensitization including a database of historical peak antibody levels, sensitizing events, and a robust system for DSAb screening (minimum monthly) and post sensitizing event (usually at 14 days). It is worth bearing in mind that historically positive T or B cell CDC crossmatches associated with anti-HLA, even if negative at the time of transplant, are associated with a very poor outcome [24]. In the USA, cohort data suggest that live donor transplantation following desensitization is a better strategy than continuing on dialysis with 5-year patient survival with transplantation 85.7% compared to 30.5% for dialysis only patients, or 49.1% for patients who had dialysis followed by HLA compatible transplant [25].

In contrast, analysis of a cohort in the UK found there was no survival advantage between undergoing HLAi transplantation compared to waiting longer on dialysis for an HLA compatible transplant [26]. It is also worth pointing out that transplantation across the HLAi barrier is associated with worse graft survival than transplantation across the ABOi barrier: in a large UK registry analysis of 879 transplants, 5-year graft survival was 71% for HLAi compared to 88% ABOi transplant recipients [27]. Therefore, the decision of whether to proceed remains a clinical one, depending on local expertise and experience with dialysis outcomes, desensitization programs, and the anticipated wait for a suitable donor.

For those on the deceased donor list, allocation is often skewed in favor of highly sensitized patients via a points scheme, but such patients still face a very considerable wait. A more proactive approach adopted by Eurotransplant characterizes HLA antigens to which a highly sensitized patient is not sensitized and records these as acceptable mismatches. This successful program resulted in 60% of recruited patients being transplanted within 2 years and is a cheaper solution with a better outcome than desensitization programs [28].

89.7.4.1 Desensitization Strategies

A variety of desensitization studies have been published over the last 15 years. Almost all suffer from being single center, numerically small, non-randomized, retrospective, and with only short-term follow-up but illustrate that positive crossmatches can often be overcome with reasonable short-term outcomes but at the expense of acute rejection [AR] rates of 36% and acute AMR rates of 25% [29, 30]. In longer-term follow-up, higher rates of chronic AMR are seen, with transplant glomerulopathy (TG) occurring in 40–55% of patients [29, 30]. Better outcomes were seen in a series of live donors undergoing desensitization for positive crossmatch when class II donor-specific antibodies were avoided (85.3% graft survival compared to 62.6% in those who had class I DSA only) and was similar to those with negative crossmatch [31]. Given the increasing association between acute AMR, subsequent chronic AMR, TG, and overall poor outcome, such strategies need to be approached with caution. A careful assessment of the risks is required, with protocols based on local experience and individualized patient care.

The approaches used are generally: (1) augmented immunosuppression targeting the cells which are responsible for antibody production and also effector T cells, in the recognition that these patients are at increased risk of both AMR and ACR; (2) therapies that interfere with or target the mechanisms by which antibodies cause damage, including complement; and (3) removal of antibody using extracorporeal techniques. Finally, combined transplantation with either liver or stem cell transplantation is not at the stage where it would be recommended except for those patients in whom these are separately indicated.

89.7.4.2 Augmented Immunosuppression

Patients at intermediate risk, e.g., patients with class I or II DSA who have a current negative flow and CDC crossmatch but who may have a historical B-cell-positive crossmatch, or who are only flow crossmatch-positive (CDC negative) may not require full desensitization. Merely augmenting immunosuppression, by increasing the treatment at induction for example with lymphocyte depleting therapy and continuing with a combination of tacrolimus, mycophenoate mofetil, and steroids may be enough for many patients. These patients are undoubtedly at increased risk of AMR and early graft loss, but the data guiding how much immunosuppression to give to whom is very weak, and a significant increase in IS is not without its risks. In short, if the transplant is felt to be a good kidney and an acceptable immunological risk, then proceeding with transplantation with appropriate clinical caution is reasonable. This should be accompanied by appropriate post-transplant antibody monitoring, possibly protocol or low threshold for biopsy, as well as a discussion of the risks and benefits with the patient.

89.7.4.3 Reduction in Anti-HLA Antibody Production

Depleting antibodies such as ATG and Campath-H1 (alemtuzumab) will markedly reduce the number of helper T cells and B cells and hopefully DSA as a consequence. In addition, rituximab, a humanized anti-CD20 mAb, is highly effective at depleting B cells and is often used as preconditioning in live donor ABOi and HLAi transplants. Used as an alternative to splenectomy, ABOi outcomes with rituximab seem to be as good while being less invasive. Efficacy of depletion can be easily monitored by staining for co-expressed CD19. However, mature plasma cells (the source of DSAb) do not express CD20, and memory B cells appear to be less effectively depleted, so the precise role of rituximab (apart from removing potentially allogeneic naïve B cells) remains unclear. Almost all studies have been non-randomized, but one randomized controlled trial in 50 HLAi patients, patients treated with rituximab had lower rates and magnitude of HLA rebound post-transplant, but no difference in DSA persistence (although MFIs were lower) and no difference in AMR or 5-year graft survival [32].

An alternative approach has been to use the proteasome inhibitor bortezomib which induces apoptosis of active plasma cells and is licensed for the treatment of multiple myeloma. While bortezomib has been used as rescue therapy for AMR, in the context of desensitization uncontrolled studies have shown it can modestly lower anti-HLA Abs in patients waiting for renal transplant and permit transplantation if used in combination with rituximab with plasmapheresis without the use of IVIg or with rituximab and high-dose IVIg. However long-term data is still lacking and it is not clear what the proteasome inhibitor is adding to an already significant immunosuppression protocol [33]. Furthermore, bortezomib is expensive and has significant side effects including neuropathy. As yet, there are no RCTs to support its use in desensitization protocols.

89.7.4.4 Intravenous Immunoglobulin (IVIg)

IVIg has a variety of immunomodulatory effects including induction of apoptosis in B cells, inhibition of complement activation (C3b and C4b) and neutralization (C3a and C5a), up-regulation of FcϒIIB inhibitory receptors on B cells, neutralization of anti-HLA Ab via anti-idiotype effect and binding of Fc receptors on other immune cells. The fact that IVIg is not grossly immunosuppressive and contains protective antibodies against common microbes is obviously appealing. IVIg has been used in two ways – high-dose or repeated low doses. The high-dose approach uses 2 g/kg of IVIg combined with plasma exchange or plasmapheresis (PE) with transplant proceeding under a variety of other induction agents if the crossmatch becomes negative. This approach has also permitted relative desensitization of sensitized patients on the deceased donor list. In a rare randomized controlled trial (RCT), monthly IVIg × 4 doses resulted in a doubling of the transplant rate for such patients (from 17% to 39%) [34]. Various groups have adopted this approach with some success but typically encountered very high AR rates with AMR in excess of 20%. Short-term outcomes look promising but long-term data are lacking.

The low-dose approach involves giving lower doses of IVIg (100 mg/kg) repeatedly after PE as part of pre-transplant desensitization protocol. While it seems counter-intuitive to give IVIg and then PE this expensive agent out again, there is evidence that IVIg alone is much less effective. Similarly, antibody removal with PE alone tends to up-regulate antibody production, whereas IVIg administration has a suppressive feedback effect on antibody production. This approach is usually combined with augmented IS, particularly depleting antibodies for induction. Short-term graft survival rates are acceptable, but AR and AMR rates remain very high, and there is concern about long-term outcomes.

89 Although IVIg is not significantly immunosuppressive, it is not completely without risk. In particular, high-dose IVIg can cause AKI and arterial and venous thrombosis. Allergic reactions are also fairly frequent and can be severe if the patient is IgA deficient.

89.7.4.5 Removal of Anti-HLA Antibodies

The half-life of antibodies is approximately a month, thus any desensitization strategies that merely target production risk early AMR from pre-existing antibodies. Therefore antibody removal is now almost universally part of any desensitization and ABOi programs where the peak titer is above the threshold and is probably essential in this setting. The majority of programs use PE as it is readily available and cheap. Immunoabsorption (IA) used to a degree in Japan and Europe is much more expensive but cleaner and more efficient. A comparison between the techniques is shown in supplemental ◻ Table 89.10.

Both techniques have been used acutely in highly sensitized patients offered deceased donor kidneys to render the crossmatch negative (usually followed by ATG induction and further antibody removal post-transplant). In one study using IA, 5-year graft survival and death-censored graft survival were 63 and 76%, respectively; however, 25% of patients still incurred AMR.

89.7.4.6 Complement Inhibition

An alternative approach to antibody removal is to disrupt the terminal cascade of complement and thus hope to prevent the pathological effect of DSAb. Eculizumab, an anti-C5a monoclonal antibody licensed for the treatment of paroxysmal nocturnal haemoglobinuria, has been shown in just one non-randomized retrospective study to dramatically reduce the rate of AMR and TG in live donor crossmatch-positive transplants from 41% and 36% to 8% and 7% at 1 year in historical versus eculizumab treated, respectively [35]. The same group has subsequently reported high rates of chronic AMR despite C5a-inhibition. The inhibition of the complement approach remains appealing, but currently, eculizumab remains excessively expensive with the duration of treatment unknown; it impairs immunity to encapsulated bacteria and its use cannot be currently recommended. Other less expensive and safer strategies are likely to be more effective.

89.7.4.7 Combined Liver-Kidney Transplant (CLK)

This strategy has been employed with some success in very limited numbers [36] following the observation that anti-HLA antibodies reduce following a liver transplant possibly because the liver acts as a "sink". However, a review of nearly 2500 CLK transplants done for other reasons demonstrated significantly reduced patient and graft survival for sensitized patients [37]. Furthermore, there are significant risks associated with CLK and ethical issues related to using liver transplants for this purpose, limiting this approach to sensitized patients who require a liver transplant for other reasons.

89.7.4.8 Stem Cell Transplant

Chimerism has been documented to occur post-transplant and to correlate with significantly reduced rejection. Hemopoietic stem cell transplantation (HSCT) has recently been combined with HLAi kidney transplantation [38]. Sensitized patients with HLAi-incompatible donors were given non-myeloablative treatment, including total body irradiation, then donor stem cell transplant contemporaneous with a live donor kidney transplant. The outcome was apparently durable chimerism, minimal AMR in the face of minimal maintenance immunosuppression. Although tolerance in this setting is a highly desirable outcome, the long-term outcomes remain unknown and the place of combined HSCT and kidney transplant is yet to be determined. Nevertheless, this approach is worth considering in patients with a suitable donor and another indication for HSCT such as myeloma or sickle cell disease.

89.8 Summary

One argument for desensitization is the better survival with a transplant than on hemodialysis, and this may be true depending on the degree of immunological risk; however returning to dialysis following a failed transplant results in a significant survival disadvantage compared with wait-listed patients [39]; in addition, treatment of AMR is difficult, hazardous and sorely lacking in an evidence base.

The immunological rules of engagement in SOT have been learned by trial and quite a lot of error; breaching these rules enters "tiger territory" and should not be done lightly or without due governance.

Case Study

The following cases illustrate the importance of discussions between clinicians and the tissue-typing team—each case should be decided on its merits, and an over-cautious approach can delay transplantation for an individual.

Case 1

You are offered a kidney from the national allocation scheme to a 55-year-old female patient who has a PRA of 83% and has been waiting for 7 years for a transplant. She is currently on hemodialysis. The donor is 45 years old, and the HLA mismatch is 100.

Both full flow and CDC crossmatches are carried out, and these are the results:

- T cell flow crossmatch—Positive (on current and historical serum samples)
- B cell flow crossmatch—Negative
- T and B cell CDC crossmatch—Negative
- Autologous crossmatch—Negative
- HLA antibody testing -Positive screen, but no evidence of donor-specific antibody (i.e., no DSA) on single antigen bead testing

Question: Should transplantation proceed, and if so, should immunosuppression be augmented?

Answer: The interpretation of the above results would be "standard risk", and the transplant should proceed. The positive T cell flow crossmatch and HLA antibody screen may be due to non-complement activating HLA antibodies or non-HLA antibodies, which show in vitro activity but have less significance in vivo. The decision as to whether to augment immunosuppression is less clear—as the patient was highly sensitized, with a long waiting time and with multiple T cell flow crossmatches being positive, in this case, the clinical and tissue-typing team considered the patient to be at higher risk, and the transplant proceeded with ATG induction to augment standard immunosuppression.

Outcome: Excellent graft function, serum creatinine 90mcmol/L, but with CMV viraemia and PCP pneumonitis as complications.

Case 2

Jacqui is 50 years old and Afro-Caribbean, with a PRA of 69%. She has been waiting for four and a half years on the transplant waiting list after her previous transplant failed. She is offered a 210 mismatch kidney from a 52-year-old DBD donor.

A full crossmatch (flow and CDC) is performed:

- T and B cell flow crossmatches—Negative on the current sample (positive on historical serum sample)
- T and B cell CDC crossmatch—Negative, autologous crossmatch negative
- HLA Ab screen—Positive, and there was a Class I DSA
- Jacqui also had a B52 class II Ab and the donor was B52, but as she had a rare B53 tissue type, this was not thought to be a mismatch in the donor allocation scheme or a DSA

On the basis of the tissue-typing assessment, this patient is at *intermediate risk* of rejection, due to the historical positive flow crossmatch and presence of a class I DSA.

The team discusses whether to avoid transplantation, taking into account the following factors: her long waiting time, her tissue type, and whether it would be easy to avoid these mismatches in the future; together with consideration for enhanced immunosuppression, proactive monitoring both clinically and with antibody testing post-transplant. At this stage, is it useful to calculate her relative chance of transplantation— this can be done through a calculator available from NHSBT, and showed that her chance of being transplanted 1 year after waitlisting was 1%, at 3 years only 6%, and at 5 years only 20%.

This information helps the team to counsel the patient and decide whether to go ahead with the transplant, taking into account the increased risk.

Case 3

John is 35 and has had three previous transplants which all failed. He is highly sensitized with PRA of 99% and has been on the waiting list for 8 years. He is offered a 210 mismatch kidney from a 51-year-old DBD donor.

Both full flow and CDC crossmatches are carried out, and these are the results:

- T and B cell flow crossmatch— Negative (on current and historical serum samples)
- T and B cell CDC crossmatch— Negative
- Autologous crossmatch— Negative
- HLA Ab testing showed the presence of two weak class I DSAs and one weak class II DSA, all below the standard cut-off.

This is a standard risk transplant, and it proceeded with standard immunosuppression. There was delayed graft function, and a biopsy at one week showed no rejection. Repeat biopsy on day 14 showed C4d positive AMR, in association with a steep rise in two class I DSA and a class II DSA.

The learning points from this case were that one of the class I DSA was against a mismatch from the first transplant John had had, as well as present on the current transplant. Secondly, more proactive monitoring of the DSAs post-transplant may have precipitated earlier repeat biopsy so that treatment could have started earlier.

Chapter Review Questions

1. What are the risk factors for sensitization to HLA antigens and how can this risk be mitigated or avoided?
2. What strategies are available to circumvent the barriers of HLA or ABO incompatibility?
3. Which patients are suitable for "virtual crossmatch" and what are the advantages of this approach?
4. How does the pre-transplant crossmatch assist with risk assessment prior to proceeding to transplantation?
5. What is the clinical relevance of antibodies to non-HLA antigens in renal transplantation?

Answers

1. Sensitization to HLA antigens most commonly occurs following previous transplantation, pregnancy, and blood transfusion. Risk factors for transplant-related sensitization include younger recipients, multiple mismatches, acute rejection episodes, non-adherence to medication, and following graft failure when immunosuppression is reduced as patients return to dialysis. The risks can be mitigated by ensuring adequate immunosuppression, and considering continuing low-dose immunosuppression and/or graft nephrectomy post-graft failure. Sensitization due to transfusion can be reduced by reviewing transfusion policies to reduce/avoid transfusion or for those who require transfusion and awaiting a transplant, by using a short course of CNI. Risk stratification of patients is important to determine how best to mitigate or avoid the risks.

89

2. To reduce immunosuppressive burden, patients who have an HLAi or ABOi live donor will benefit from a national allocation approach which finds a suitable donor who does not have forbidden antigens. This is done through paired or pooled donation, or an altruistic donor. Alternatively, desensitization strategies to remove preformed antibody and reduce their production can mean that transplantation across HLAi or ABOi barrier is possible. However, patients who undergo transplant following a positive crossmatch and desensitization are still at increased risk of acute rejection (both cellular and antibody-mediated) and chronic antibody-mediated rejection, and require closer monitoring and typically ongoing increased immunosuppression. For patients awaiting a deceased donor, national allocation schemes do prioritize highly sensitized patients, but long waits are still likely. In some cases, proceeding with careful selection and avoidance of forbidden antigens may be better for an individual.
3. Virtual crossmatching is suitable for both non-sensitized and sensitized patients who have well-characterized anti-HLA antibody profile, with up-to-date antibody testing and no recent sensitizing events. If donor-specific anti-HLA antibodies are present in the most recent serum screened, then these need to be of a low relative titer as measured on the Luminex platform (<1,000 MFI for example), as well as being stable or declining, to accurately predict a negative retrospective bench crossmatch. The tissue-typing unit must liaise

closely with clinicians, to establish an evidence-based threshold for current or most recently detected donor-specific HLA antibodies. Virtual crossmatching is completed much more quickly than formal crossmatching, which reduces the cold-ischemia time and thereby potentially improves graft outcome.

4. Where pre-transplant crossmatching results in a positive cell-based CDC crossmatch, transplantation should not proceed (unless HLA antibody removal is first undertaken and achieved, e.g., desensitization for a live donor transplant). In patients with known donor specific antibodies with a positive T and B cell flow crossmatches, but negative CDC crossmatch, the risk of rejection is intermediate. This can aid discussion with the patient as to whether to proceed, as well as post-transplant surveillance planning.
5. Several non-HLA antibodies have been identified with acute rejection and chronic graft deterioration in patients without evidence of anti-HLA antibodies.

Tips and Tricks

Prevention of sensitization is extremely important therefore identify and flag any patient (particularly young) likely suitable for a transplant and ensure measures are put in place to avoid sensitization.

Establish a thoughtful transfusion policy including responsive ESA and iron dosing and transfusion avoidance, and consider HLA-compatible elective transfusion, autologous transfusion, and intraoperative erythrocyte salvage.

Consider transplant nephrectomy under IS in recipients with failed transplants who are suitable for further transplantation and a policy of encouraging contraception in women of child-bearing age with CKD.

Paired exchange/pooled donation and acceptable mismatch programs are much cheaper and likely to have better patient and graft survival than desensitization programs. Therefore, patients with incompatible live donors should be encouraged to enter paired exchange programs for blood group- and HLA-incompatible donors, especially where the recipient is young. Some donors feel uncomfortable with the paired exchange concept, and it is often helpful to have donors who have had a good experience with paired exchange talking at patient education sessions.

Close ties with the tissue-typing department are essential for virtual crossmatch programs as well as discussing safety and interpretation of crossmatch.

For any ABOi or desensitization programs, it is essential to have a good service-level agreement for screening and rapid turnaround times.

89.9 Seminal Papers

No. 5 (Tait et al., 2013): A concise yet in depth review written by a well-recognised international group of experienced H&I scientists, with up to date recommendations on all aspects and applications of measuring antibodies to HLA and their relevance in managing organ transplants.

No. 6 (Sullivan et al., 2017): An excellent insight into the technical complexities of the modern methods used to detect HLA antibodies, written by the Emory University group in Atlanta (USA) who are recognised as leading experts in this field.

Conclusion

Renal transplantation remains the gold standard renal replacement therapy option. Transplant clinicians have to work closely with tissue-typing specialists to ensure that donors and recipients are as well-matched as possible and that prognostic factors such as HLA incompatibility and either pre-existing or de novo HLA and non-HLA antibodies are recognized. They also need to regularly review and potentially individualize immunosuppression protocols to reduce the risk of rejection and avoid sensitization to potential future kidneys. This needs to be balanced against the risk of over-immunosuppression. The risk of sensitization (and therefore the increased risk of rejection and reduced graft survival) needs to be considered before, during, and after kidney transplantation in all patients with chronic kidney disease. Various approaches are used, including national organ allocation schemes, donor exchange schemes, desensitization protocols, and deciding acceptable mismatches in order to both optimize the ABO and HLA compatibility. However, the importance of matching has to be weighed against inequities in access to transplantation for certain patient groups. New allocation strategies have evolved that reduce the number of patients who face extended waits for transplantation, recognizing that even a less well-matched kidney may improve patient survival and quality of life compared to remaining on dialysis.

Supplementary Material

Table 89.6 Major HLA-A, HLA-B, and HLA-DR antigens or allotypes used for renal transplant matching and their relative frequencies (%) in the UK population

HLA-A		HLA-B		HLA-DR	
Antigen	%	Antigen	%	Antigen	%
A1	34	**B5** (B51, B52)	19	**DR1**	19
A2	50	**B7**	27	**DR2** (DR15, DR16)	29
A3	26	**B8**	25	**DR3**	27
A9 (A23, A24)	17	**B12** (B44, B45)	33	**DR4**	35
A10 (A25, A26, A34, A66)	9	**B13**	4	**DR5** (DR11, DR12)	16
A11	12	**B14** (B64, B65)	7	**DR6** (DR13, DR14)	23
A19 (A30, A31, A32, A33, A74)	19	**B15** (B62, B63, B75, B76, B77)	12	**DR7**	26
A29	8	**B16** (B38, B39)	5	**DR8**	4
A28 (A68, A69)	7	**B17** (B57, B58)	9	**DR9**	2
		B18	8	**DR10**	1
		B21 (B49, B50)	4	**DR51**	29
		B22 (B54, B55, B56)	4	**DR52**	58
		B27	9	**DR53**	57
		B35	13		
		B37	3		
		B40 (B60, B61)	13		
		B41	1		
		B47	1		
		B53	1		
		B70 (B71, B72)	1		
		Bw4	62		
		Bw6	86		

HLA allotypes used in matching renal transplants are given in bold with relevant related subtypes in parentheses. HLA allotype frequencies are derived from 10,000 UK deceased solid organ donors collected between 1994 and 2009 [40]. Other HLA-A and HLA-B allotypes that are included in the UK matching algorithms but occur at <1% frequency are A36, A43, A80, B42, B46, B48, B59, B67, B73, B78, B81, B82, and B83

89

Table 89.7 Risk factors for sensitization following transplantation

1. Blood transfusion	This is probably still significant despite the protective effect of IS
2. Young recipient	Vigorous immune system
3. Multiple mismatches	Consistent finding
4. Sensitized patient	High PRA to most HLA antigens
5. Deceased donor transplant	Possible also delayed graft function
6. HLA class II mismatch	DQ mismatch may be a particular risk
7. Acute rejection episodes	Significant risk factor
8. Withdrawal of immunosuppression	Following failure of transplant or in context of infection/malignancy
9. Non-compliance	A perennial problem causing AR and chronic low-level sensitization

Table 89.8 Common protocols for ABOi

Splenectomy/PE/augmented IS	Splenectomy now superseded by less invasive medical treatments
Rituximab*/PE/augmented IS	Rituximab is usually given a month before transplant (14 days before antibody removal), *final crossmatch needs to be done *before* rituximab
Rituximab*/immunoabsorption	Immunoabsorption is more expensive than plasma exchange but avoids perturbing coagulation
Standard treatment plus PE	ABOi transplants are being done for medium to low titers with only PE as additional treatment or with IVIg plus plasma exchange but without rituximab
Protocols using plasma exchange (PE) must monitor clotting and fibrinogen, correcting with fresh frozen plasma before surgery or invasive procedures	
Most protocols aim to keep anti-blood group titers down to acceptable levels for the first two weeks using post-transplant antibody removal if necessary. Beyond this, "accommodation" seems to occur whereby ABOi antibodies appear not to cause graft damage possibly through isotype switching	

Table 89.9 Options for the sensitized patient

Institutional strategies	
Paired donation	Combined with ABOi transplant programs
Acceptable mismatch programs	For example, Eurotransplant program defining non-sensitized antigens
Desensitization	
Increased immunosuppression	Potent induction agents (e.g., ATG) with higher maintenance IS
Reduction in B cells	Rituximab (role unclear) (crossmatch needs to be done *before* rituximab)
IV immunoglobulin	Low-dose IVIg 100 mg/kg, high-dose 2 g/kg plus or minus plasma exchange
Antibody removal	Plasma exchange, protein A or Ig-Therasorb®
Proteosome inhibition	Bortezomib
Complement inhibition	Eculizumab
Combined liver-kidney transplant	
Combined stem cell transplant	Mixed chimerism to prevent rejection of live donor kidney in highly sensitized

Table 89.10 Comparison of plasma exchange (PE) and immunoabsorption (IA) techniques

Plasma exchange	
Advantages	Cheap, readily available, and local know-how
Disadvantages	Removal of clotting and complement factors, thrombocytopenia, anemia, monitoring of clotting and fibrinogen with a need to reverse anticoagulation prior to surgery, reactions to fresh frozen plasma if required (especially if IgA deficient), moderate efficacy
Immunoabsorption	
Advantages	Highly efficient, no interference with clotting, complement, platelets, or erythrocytes
Disadvantages	Expensive, specialized columns and expertise, limited availability

Table 89.11 Strategies for avoiding allosensitization

Transfusion policy avoiding transfusion	Compelling evidence that overall transfusions can be reduced
Recipient-specific elective transfusion	Transfusions matched for HLA class I (A and B)
Post-transfusion immunosuppression	2 weeks of immunosuppression with CNI where appropriate
Autologous blood transfusion	Intraoperative blood harvesting, pre-emptive autologous storage
Avoidance of pregnancy in patients with a significant risk of ESRD	Where possible and appropriate, the importance of contraception should be emphasized in all women of child-bearing age likely to receive a transplant
Avoidance of rejection	An important cause of sensitization and risk of protocols focusing on minimal immunosuppression as well as patients at risk of poor compliance
Continued immunosuppression in failed grafts	Weaning immunosuppression has a significant risk of sensitization, maintenance seems to be preventative therefore worth considering in a patient likely to be re-transplanted soon
Graft nephrectomy	To be considered if risk to benefit ratio in favor of immunosuppression wean and further transplant considered

References

1. http://optn.transplant.hrsa.gov data accessed September 8, 2020.
2. Bunce M, Young NT, Welsh KI. Molecular HLA typing – the brave new world. Transplantation. 1997;64(11):1505–13.
3. Marsh SGE, Albert ED, Bodmer WF, Bontrop RE, Dupont B, Erlich HA, et al. Nomenclature for factors of the HLA system, 2010. Tissue Antigens. 2010;75(4):291–455.
4. Watson CJE, Johnson RJ, Mumford L. Overview of the evolution of the UK kidney allocation schemes. Curr Transplant Rep. 2020;17:140–4.
5. Tait BD, Susal C, Gebel HM, Nickerson PW, Zachary AA, Claas FHJ, et al. Consensus guidelines on the testing and clinical management issues associated with HLA and non-HLA antibodies in transplantation. Transplantation. 2013;95(1):19–47.
6. Sullivan HC, Gebel HM, Bray RA. Understanding solid-phase HLA antibody assays and the value of MFI. Hum Immunol. 2017;78:471–80.
7. The detection & characterisation of clinically relevant antibodies in allotransplantation. Guidelines & Standards - British Transplantation Society (bts.org.uk). Retrieved from https://bts.org.uk/wpcontent/uploads/2016/09/06_BTS_BSHI_Antibodies-1.pdf
8. Taylor CJ, Kosmoliaptsis V, Sharples LD, Prezzi D, Morgan CH, Key T, et al. Ten-year experience of selective omission of the pretransplant crossmatch test in deceased donor kidney transplantation. Transplantation. 2010;89(2):185–93.
9. Cox ST, Stephens HA, Fernando R, Karasu A, Harber M, Howie AJ, Powis S, Zou Y, Stastny P, Madrigal JA, Little AM. Major histocompatibility complex class I-related chain A allele mismatching, antibodies, and rejection in renal transplantation. Hum Immunol. 2011;72:827–34.
10. Zhang Q, Reed EF. The importance of non-HLA antibodies in transplantation. Nat Rev Nephrol. 2016;12(8):484–95. https://doi.org/10.1038/nrneph.2016.88.
11. Reindl-Schwaighofer R, Heinzel A, Kainz A, et al. Contribution of non-HLA incompatibility between donor and recipient to kidney allograft survival: genome-wide analysis in a prospective cohort. Lancet. 2019;393(10174):910–7. https://doi.org/10.1016/S0140-6736(18)32473-5.
12. Dragun D, Muller DN, Brasen JH, Fritsche L, Nieminen-Kelha M, Dechend R, et al. Angiotensin II type 1-receptor activating antibodies in renal-allograft rejection. N Engl J Med. 2005;352:558–69.
13. Susal C, Dohler B, Opelz G. Presensitized kidney graft recipients with HLA class I and II antibodies are at increased risk for graft failure: a collaborative transplant study report. Hum Immunol. 2009;70(8):569–73.
14. Everly MJ, Rebellato LM, Haisch CE, Ozawa M, Parker K, Briley KP, et al. Incidence and impact of de novo donor-specific alloantibody in primary renal allografts. Transplantation. 2013;95(3):410–7.
15. Augustine JJ, Woodside KJ, Padiyar A, Sanchez EQ, Hricik DE, Schulak JA. Independent of nephrectomy, weaning immunosuppression leads to late sensitization after kidney transplant failure. Transplantation. 2012;94(7):738–43.
16. Scornik JC, Kriesche H-UM. Human leukocyte antigen sensitization after transplant loss: timing of antibody detection and implications for prevention. Hum Immunol. 2011;72(5):398–401.
17. Raftery MJ, Lang CJ, O'Shea JM, Varghese Z, Sweny P, Fernando ON, et al. Controlled trial of azathioprine and cyclosporin to prevent anti-HLA antibodies due to third-party transfusion. Nephrol Dial Transplant. 1988;3(5):671–6.
18. O'Brien FJ, Lineen J, Kennedy CM, Phelan PJ, Kelly PO, Denton MD, et al. Effect of perioperative blood transfusions on long term graft outcomes in renal transplant patients. Clin Nephrol. 2012;77(6):432–7.
19. Magee BA, Martin J, Cole MP, Morris KG, Courtney AE. Effects of HLA-matched blood transfusion for patients awaiting renal transplantation. Transplantation. 2012;94(11):1111–6.
20. Niaudet P, Dudley J, Charbit M, Gagnadoux MF, Macleay K, Broyer M. Pretransplant blood transfusions with cyclosporine in pediatric renal transplantation. Pediatr Nephrol. 2000;14(6):451–6.
21. Knight MG, Tiong HY, Li J, Pidwell D, Goldfarb D. Transplant nephrectomy after allograft failure is associated with allosensitization. Urology. 2011;78(2):314–8.
22. Wu DA, Watson CJ, Bradley JA, Johnson RJ, Forsythe JL, Oniscu GC. Global trends and challenges in deceased donor kidney allocation. Kidney Int. 2017;91(6):1287–99.
23. Shimmura H, Tanabe K, Ishikawa N, Tokumoto T, Takahashi K, Toma H. Role of anti-A/B antibody titers in results of ABO-incompatible kidney transplantation. Transplantation. 2000;70(9):1331–5.
24. Ten Hoor GM, Coopmans M, Allebes WA. Specificity and Ig class of preformed alloantibodies causing a positive crossmatch in renal transplantation. The implications for graft survival. Transplantation. 1993;56(2):298–304.
25. Montgomery RA, Lonze BE, King KE, Kraus ES, Kucirka LM, Locke JE, et al. Desensitization in HLA-incompatible kidney recipients and survival. NEJM. 2011;365(4):318–26.
26. Manook M, Koeser L, Ahmed Z, Robb M, Johnson R, Shaw O, et al. Post-listing survival for highly sensitised patients on the UK kidney transplant waiting list: a matched cohort analysis. Lancet. 2017;389(10070):727–34.
27. Pankhurst L, Hudson A, Mumford L, Willicombe M, Galliford J, Shaw O, et al. The UK National Registry of ABO and HLA antibody incompatible renal transplantation: Pretransplant factors associated with outcome in 879 transplants. Transplant Direct. 2017;3(7):e181-e.
28. Claas FHJ, Rahmel A, Doxiadis IIN. Enhanced kidney allocation to highly sensitized patients by the acceptable mismatch program. Transplantation. 2009;88:447–52.
29. Marfo K, Lu A, Ling M, Akalin E. Desensitization protocols and their outcome. Clin J Am Soc Nephrol. 2011;6(4):922–36.
30. Gloor JM, Winters JL, Cornell LD, Fix LA, DeGoey SR, Knauer RM, et al. Baseline donor-specific antibody levels and outcomes in positive crossmatch kidney transplantation. Am J Transplant. 2010;10(3):582–9.
31. Bentall A, Cornell LD, Gloor JM, Park WD, Gandhi MJ, Winters JL, et al. Five-year outcomes in living donor kidney transplants with a positive crossmatch. Am J Transplant Off J Am Soc Transplant Am Soc Transplant Surg. 2013;13(1):76–85.
32. Jackson AM, Kraus ES, Orandi BJ, Segev DL, Montgomery RA, Zachary AA. A closer look at rituximab induction on HLA antibody rebound following HLA-incompatible kidney transplantation. Kidney Int. 2015;87(2):409–16.
33. Aubert O, Suberbielle C, Gauthe R, Francois H, Obada EN, Durrbach A. Effect of a proteasome inhibitor plus steroids on HLA antibodies in sensitized patients awaiting a renal transplant. Transplantation. 2014;97(9):946–52.
34. Jordan SC, Tyan D, Stablein D, McIntosh M, Rose S, Vo A, et al. Evaluation of intravenous immunoglobulin as an agent to lower allosensitization and improve transplanta-

tion in highly sensitized adult patients with end-stage renal disease: report of the NIH IG02 trial. J Am Soc Nephrol. 2004;15(12):3256–62.
35. Stegall MD, Diwan T, Raghavaiah S, Cornell LD, Burns J, Dean PG, et al. Terminal complement inhibition decreases antibody-mediated rejection in sensitized renal transplant recipients. Am J Transplant Off J Am Soc Transplant Am Soc Transplant Surg. 2011;11(11):2405–13.
36. Gutierrez A, Crespo M, Mila J, Torregrosa JV, Martorell J, Oppenheimer F. Outcome of simultaneous liver-kidney transplantation in highly sensitized, crossmatch-positive patients. Transplant Proc. 2003;35(5):1861–2.
37. Askar M, Schold JD, Eghtesad B, Flechner SM, Kaplan B, Klingman L, et al. Combined liver-kidney transplants: allosensitization and recipient outcomes. Transplantation. 2011;91(11):1286–92.
38. Leventhal J, Abecassis M, Miller J, Gallon L, Tollerud D, Elliott MJ, et al. Tolerance induction in HLA disparate living donor kidney transplantation by donor stem cell infusion: durable chimerism predicts outcome. Transplantation. 2013;95(1):169–76.
39. Kaplan B, Meier-Kriesche H-U. Death after graft loss: an important late study endpoint in kidney transplantation. Am J Transplant. 2002;2(10):970–4.
40. NHS Blood and Transplant [PDF File]. HLA Antigen Frequencies in UK Solid Organ Donor Population. https://www.odt.nhs.uk/transplantation/pathology-services/histocompatibility-and-immunogenetics/. Retrieved from https://nhsbtdbe.blob.core.windows.net/umbraco-assets-corp/2925/antigen.pdf.

Useful Websites

British Transplantation Society: Detection & characterisation of clinically relevant antibodies in allotransplantation. https://bts.org.uk/wp-content/uploads/2016/09/06_BTS_BSHI_Antibodies-1.pdf

British Transplantation Society: Guidelines for Living Donor Kidney Transplantation https://bts.org.uk/wp-content/uploads/2018/07/FINAL_LDKT-guidelines_June-2018.pdf

NHS Blood and Transplant: Chance of a transplant calculator https://www.odt.nhs.uk/transplantation/tools-policies-and-guidance/calculators/

Surgical Aspects of Kidney and Pancreas Transplantation

Benedict L. Phillips, Chris J. Callaghan, and Christopher J. E. Watson

Contents

M. Harber (ed.), *Primer on Nephrology*, https://doi.org/10.1007/978-3-030-76419-7_90

Learning Objectives

1. Understand how abdominal organs are retrieved from living and deceased donors, including the relevant anatomy and donor types
2. Understand the various organ preservation techniques, including preservation fluids and novel technologies
3. Understand the absolute and relative contraindications to donation
4. Understand the complex nature of donor and recipient selection
5. Understand the basic surgical technique of kidney and pancreas implantation, and the complications of surgery

Kidney transplantation is the preferred treatment of end-stage renal failure for the majority of patients suffering from this disease, with prolonged life expectancy and improved quality of life when compared to other forms of renal replacement therapy [1, 2]. Selected patients with renal failure due to diabetes also benefit from simultaneous pancreas and kidney (SPK) transplantation or pancreas after live donor kidney transplantation. Transplantation of pancreatic islets combined with a kidney from the same donor is another option for diabetic patients, but with less likelihood of insulin independence. However, transplantation of these organs has a higher incidence of death and morbidity in the short term, and it is, therefore, crucial that potential recipients are adequately assessed preoperatively in order to minimize risks and determine those most likely to benefit from transplantation. As part of this process, careful assessment of surgical considerations is essential.

Organ transplantation is a complex process, and good recipient outcomes are reliant on a carefully orchestrated and interrelated chain of events. This begins with the assessment of a potential donor, followed by meticulous surgery to recover the donor organs, optimal organ preservation and storage, and timely organ implantation. From a surgical perspective, this process continues with recipient postoperative care and the detection and management of surgical complications, the majority of which present within 3 months of transplantation.

90

90.1 Deceased Donor Kidney and Pancreas Recovery

In most Western countries, deceased donors provide the majority of transplanted kidneys. Even with increasing live donation rates, deceased donors will remain an essential source of organs with the ability to transplant two kidneys from one donor. The technical difficulties and morbidity associated with removing part of the pancreas from a live donor mean that the majority of pancreas transplantation is from deceased organ donors.

90.2 Organ Recovery Techniques

The evidence base for different organ recovery techniques is lacking, and therefore, there is significant variability between surgeons. The description given below is of a technique favored by the authors, though many other acceptable approaches have been described. Iatrogenic damage to kidneys occurs in approximately 7% of organs recovered [3] and is a common cause of organ decline [4]. Kidney damage is less likely to take place when the donor is young, slim, and female, and when organ recovery is performed by experienced multi-organ retrieval teams. Damage is more common during recovery from donation after circulatory death (DCD) donors [3].

Recovery of kidneys from donation after brain death (DBD) donors is performed via a midline laparotomy and median sternotomy. Methodical inspection of the abdominal and thoracic viscera is necessary to identify any pathology which contraindicates donation. The right colon and duodenum are mobilized medially. An arterial cannulation site is dissected out (e.g., the right common iliac artery or distal abdominal aorta), taking care to identify and preserve any right-sided lower polar renal arteries that may occasionally originate from the right common iliac artery. Further dissection of the liver hilum or peri-pancreatic tissues is then performed, as necessary (see below).

Once these preparations have been completed, systemic heparinization of the donor is achieved with a bolus of 300 IU/kg of heparin intravenously. When the heparin has circulated adequately, a large cannula (e.g., 20 Fr diameter) is introduced into the arterial cannulation site and secured. The donor's descending thoracic aorta is cross-clamped, preservation fluid is started via the arterial cannula, and blood and preservation fluid exit the circulation via a venting site (either an incision in the right atrium of the heart or a separate cannula in the inferior vena cava). The abdomen and peri-renal areas are packed with saline ice slush to ensure rapid cooling of the kidneys, pancreas, and liver.

After 3–4 L of preservation fluid has run through, the kidneys can be explanted. The left renal vein is divided at its confluence with the inferior vena cava (IVC) and reflected laterally. The abdominal aorta is then split in the midline from the bifurcation to just above the origin of the superior mesenteric artery. On the left, the entire lateral patch of the abdominal aorta is dissected posteriorly and laterally, leaving the patch intact to preserve any unrecognized polar arteries. A plane is then developed posterior and lateral to the kidney, and a 2–3 cm cuff of peri-ureteric tissue is included with the ureter to prevent damage to the ureteric blood supply. Both ureters are identified at the pelvic brim and divided. On the right, the IVC is divided inferiorly at the level of the confluence of the common iliac veins and superiorly between the infra-hepatic IVC and the confluence of the right renal vein. The right abdominal aortic patch and entire IVC are then removed with the right kidney, as above. Once removed, kidneys are placed in bowls of saline ice slush to prevent rewarming and enable back-table inspection.

Safe recovery of the pancreas is a more challenging procedure due to the fragile nature of the organ, its complex vascular anatomy, and its proximity to the liver and major vascular and gastrointestinal anatomical structures. Damage to the pancreas during organ recovery occurs in approximately 50% of cases and is most common in concomitant liver donation, aberrant arterial anatomy, and raised donor body mass index [5]. Prior to heparinization, and in addition to the above dissection, the DBD pancreas donor requires dissection of the hepatic hilum to identify the gastroduodenal and splenic arteries, as well as the portal vein. The common bile duct should be ligated and divided in this phase of the procedure. Aortic cannulation, heparinization, cross-clamping, perfusion, and venous venting should proceed as above, and the lesser sac and peri-pancreatic tissues should be packed with iced saline. If a cannula is placed in the portal circulation to perfuse the liver, it should be placed directly in the portal vein 1 cm superior to the donor duodenum, with the inferior part of the portal vein left unobstructed to drain freely into the peritoneum.

The pancreas should be explanted before the kidneys. The gastroduodenal artery should be ligated after the pancreas is perfused, and the splenic artery transected near its origin. The portal vein is divided at the level of the gastroduodenal artery, leaving a 1 cm length with the pancreas. The duodenum should be stapled just distal to the pylorus. Using the spleen as a handle, the pancreas is mobilized medially. The proximal jejunum is stapled, the origin of the transverse mesocolon divided, and the root of the mesentery is stapled and divided. Finally, the superior mesenteric artery is transected at its origin on the aorta and the pancreas removed. The right common, external, and internal iliac arteries and veins should be removed to enable vascular reconstruction of the pancreas.

Recovery of the pancreas and kidneys from controlled (Maastricht category III [6]) (Table 90.1) DCD donors uses a 'super-rapid' retrieval technique to minimize warm ischemic damage. The abdomen is entered rapidly, and cannulation of the right common iliac artery is performed before median sternotomy, cross-clamping of the descending thoracic aorta, venous venting, and packing the abdomen with ice. Although some centers insert a double-balloon triple-lumen catheter via the femoral artery to perfuse the kidneys in a kidney-only DCD donor, results appear to be inferior to the open cannulation technique [6]. The abdominal organs are covered with ice slush during perfusion, and organ recovery began immediately after the preservation fluid has run through. Although the basic principles of retrieval of organs from DCD and DBD donors are similar, the lack of arterial pulsation in the DCD donor makes identification of vascular structures difficult, and surgical injuries are more likely to occur [3].

Table 90.1 Modified Maastricht categories of DCD donation

Category	Circumstance	Description
I (uncontrolled)	Found dead IA. Out-of-hospital IB. in-hospital	Sudden unexpected cardiac arrest without any attempt of resuscitation
II (uncontrolled)	Witnessed cardiac arrest IIA. Out-of-hospital IIB. in-hospital	Sudden unexpected irreversible cardiac arrest with unsuccessful resuscitation
III (controlled)	Withdrawal of life-sustaining therapy	Planned withdrawal of life-sustaining therapy
IV (uncontrolled controlled)*	Cardiac arrest while brain-dead	Sudden cardiac arrest after brain death diagnosis during donor management but prior to organ recovery

Adapted from Thuong et al. [6]

[a]IV can also include the brain-dead donor who, for relative preference or other reasons, undergoes a DCD III-type withdrawal process. Because they are certified dead already, they can be heparinized before the withdrawal of treatment, and can therefore be considered more 'controlled' than III

Organs from DCD donors inevitably undergo a period of warm ischemia, and prolonged warm ischemia is expected to lead to poor subsequent graft outcomes. Warm ischemic limits vary between organs and are likely to vary between donors. Although guidelines for acceptable warm ischemic thresholds exist [7], the evidence-base supporting these is limited. The authors' opinions on these issues are detailed below.

90.3 Organ Assessment

Once explanted, the organs should be placed in a bowl of ice saline slush to facilitate further cooling and inspection. The kidneys and pancreas are assessed for quality of perfusion, anatomy, the presence of damage, and pathology (e.g., tumors). Kidneys from DCD donors are often patchily perfused and require additional perfusion on the back table. The pancreas should be inspected to determine the degree of fat infiltration, and the jejunum should be opened to enable flushing with preservation fluid and then re-stapled shut. Organs should then be packed in bags containing preservation fluid and stored in iceboxes. The role of machine perfusion techniques for the kidneys is expanding and is discussed below. Machine perfusion of the pancreas has not, to date, proved successful.

Any damage, perfusion defects, anatomical abnormalities, or pathology must be clearly documented and communicated to the implanting team. Decisions regarding the usability or the need for complex reconstruction are best made by an experienced implanting surgeon.

90.4 Organ Preservation and Storage

90.4.1 Scientific Basis of Organ Preservation Techniques

Organ preservation techniques are used to maintain organ function before transplantation and thus enable organ transport, cross-matching, and recipient preoperative preparations. In the absence of warm oxygenated blood, cells convert to anaerobic metabolism, leading to progressive cellular acidosis, cellular damage as loss of energy substrates leads to failure of membrane pumps (e.g., the Na^+/K^+-ATPase), cell swelling, membrane disruption, and activation of cellular autolysis.

Organ preservation aims to inhibit this process and can be broadly categorized into either static cold storage (SCS) or machine perfusion techniques.

SCS is currently the predominant technique due to its simplicity, efficacy, and relatively low cost. Preservation by machine perfusion involves attaching the organ to a perfusion machine through which preservation fluid or blood is circulated.

Preservation fluids used for SCS are perfused at 4 °C as soon as possible after cessation of circulation. There are numerous types of preservation fluids, but in the UK the most commonly used are the University of Wisconsin (UW) solution (ViaSpan, SPS-1, Belzer-UW), Marshall's hyperosmolar citrate solution (Soltran), histidine-tryptophan-ketoglutarate solution (Custodiol-HTK), and Celsior solution. Their principles of action are similar, namely, (1) cooling, to reduce cellular metabolism (10% of normal at 4 °C); (2) use of an osmotic agent (e.g., lactobionate, mannitol) to reduce cellular edema; (3) presence of a buffer to reduce intracellular acidosis (e.g., phosphate, bicarbonate); and (4) use of electrolytes to maintain the intracellular ionic composition (Table 90.2).

90.4.2 Use of Preservation Fluids for Cold Storage

The choice of preservation fluid is dictated by many factors including efficacy, the organs concerned, expected cold ischemic time, type of donor, cost, availability, and ease of use. All fluids are perfused via intravascular cannula at 4 °C as soon as possible after the loss of organ circulation in the donor.

Table 90.2 Common preservation fluids and their composition

Preservation fluid	Ionic composition	Buffer	Osmotic agents	Additional constituents
UW	Low Na^+, high K^+	Phosphate	Hydroxyethyl starch, lactobionate, raffinose	Glutathione[a], allopurinol[a], adenosine[b], insulin, dexamethasone
Marshall's HOC	Medium Na^+ and K^+	Sulfate, citrate	Mannitol	
HTK	Low Na^+ and K^+	Histidine	Mannitol	Tryptophan[c], ketoglutarate[b]
Celsior	High Na^+, low K^+	Histidine	Lactobionate, mannitol	Glutathione[a], glutamate[c]

Adapted from Saeb-Parsy et al. [8]
[a]Antioxidant
[b]Metabolic substrate
[c]Amino acid

A meta-analysis of 15 prospective comparative studies has demonstrated that for SCS of deceased donor kidneys, the rates of delayed graft function (DGF) posttransplantation are similar with UW, HTK, and Celsior [9]. A UK registry analysis has shown no difference in outcomes between Marshall's hyperosmolar citrate solution and UW with regard to primary nonfunction, DGF, acute rejection, 1-year graft function, and graft survival [10]. Marshall's solution is considerably cheaper than the UW solution. When cold ischemic times exceed 20 hours, renal graft survival from DBD donors decreases, with a 4% increase in the risk of graft failure at 1-year posttransplant with every additional hour of SCS [8]. Some studies have suggested that perfusion with UW may be advantageous if cold ischemic time is expected to exceed 24 hours [11].

The evidence for pancreas preservation fluids is limited. UW is currently the most common preservation fluid in both the USA and the UK, but HTK is becoming increasingly popular. Only one randomized trial has been conducted comparing HTK and UW preservation of pancreases, and although this showed equivalent graft outcomes, the study was underpowered [12]. However, a large risk-adjusted US registry analysis showed that use of HTK as a preservation fluid instead of UW was associated with poorer pancreas graft survival [13]. Small randomized trials have demonstrated that pancreas graft outcomes after perfusion with Celsior are equivalent to those with UW, especially when cold ischemic times are short.

90.4.3 Machine Perfusion Techniques

The ability to perfuse organs via a machine prior to transplantation has been present for many decades, but interest in these techniques has undergone a resurgence due to the increasing age and comorbidities of deceased donors along with higher rates of DGF due to rising DCD donor numbers. Anticipated physiological advantages of machine perfusion include thorough blood washout, removal of metabolic waste, provision of nutrients, vascular access for the administration of immunomodulatory or cytoprotective drugs, and assessment of organ viability.

Machine perfusion can be broadly divided into hypothermic (4 °C) and normothermic (35–37 °C) techniques. Oxygen can be delivered to the organ during both hypothermic and normothermic machine perfusion. Normothermic perfusion may have advantages over hypothermic machine perfusion (HMP), due to the restoration of aerobic metabolism and cellular energy stores [14]. However, it is more complex and costly due to the need for a warming circuit. With both techniques, the main expected benefit would be reduced DGF rates. The latest generation of hypothermic perfusion machines are portable, relatively simple to use, and require minimal maintenance. All machine perfusion devices remain costly and complex when compared to SCS.

Two recent trials have compared HMP to SCS in deceased donor kidney transplantation [15, 16]. Moers et al. conducted a randomized controlled trial in continental Europe, including kidneys from both DBD and DCD donors. Overall, DGF was significantly reduced in machine-perfused kidneys, with similarly beneficial effects in kidneys from both types of deceased donors. Follow-up has shown superior 3-year graft survival in machine-perfused kidneys from DBD donors, but not those from DCD donors [17]. HMP had an especially beneficial effect on 3-year graft survival in kidneys from extended criteria donors (donor age > 60 years or age 50–60 years with at least two of the following characteristics: history of hypertension, death due to cerebrovascular cause, terminal serum creatinine >132 μmol/L).

In contrast, a randomized controlled trial from the UK of HMP in kidneys from controlled (Maastricht category III) DCD donors only, showed no improvement in DGF rates when compared to SCS [16]. The discrepant results between the two trials may be explained by the following: (1) the European study did not have a standardized protocol for either the cold storage preservation solution or recipient immunosuppression; (2) the rate of DGF was surprisingly high in the European DCD cold storage group (70%), in which most kidneys were preserved with HTK; (3) in the UK trial the kidneys were placed on machine perfusion after arriving at the implanting center, while in the European trial they were placed on the machine at the retrieving centre.

Normothermic perfusion of organs can be performed in situ (in DCD donors) or ex vivo. The in situ technique, termed normothermic regional perfusion, involves rapid placement of large cannula in a major artery and vein of a DCD donor and perfusing the donor's abdominal organs via an extracorporeal membrane oxygenator (ECMO) circuit. Restoration of warm, oxygenated blood flow to abdominal organs is expected to allow the restoration of intracellular energy stores and reversal of intracellular acidosis. Although technically challenging and costly, this technique is increasingly used in Spain and France and is currently undergoing clinical evaluation in the UK.

In contrast to the in situ technique, ex vivo normothermic machine perfusion (EVNP) involves placing arterial and venous cannulae into an isolated organ after removal from the donor and attaching it to an ECMO circuit. This is less technically challenging than the in situ approach and has the advantage of enabling the organ to be assessed while warm, oxygenated blood circulates [18–20]. EVNP has been used to increase the number of DCD kidney transplants by assessing their viability prior to transplantation [21]. The ability of EVNP to reduce the rate of DGF in DCD kidney transplantation, compared to SCS, is being investigated in a randomized controlled trial in the UK [22].

In contrast to renal transplantation, ex vivo pancreatic machine perfusion (both hypothermic and normothermic) remains experimental [23]. The pancreas is not readily amenable to back-table perfusion due to the complexity and delicacy of its arterial supply. However, transplantation of pancreases from DCD donors treated with normothermic regional perfusion has been performed [24].

90.5 Deceased Donor Kidney Transplantation

90.5.1 Donor Selection

The assessment of potential deceased donors is often challenging due to time constraints, lack of access to preoperative imaging, difficulties obtaining medical records out-of-hours, alterations in donor physiology due to brain death or post-resuscitation, and comorbidities associated with an aging deceased donor population. Deceased donor selection criteria are dependent on local waiting list pressures, perception of risk by the assessing clinicians, recipient characteristics, and unit experience. Donor selection issues are complex, with a spectrum of risks that are difficult to accurately assess. The authors' views are presented, but it remains the responsibility of the implanting team (and the informed recipient) to decide whether the risks associated with transplantation outweigh the benefits of using that particular organ. General and organ-specific contraindications to donation in the UK are listed in ► Box 90.1. Well-controlled HIV-positive donors may donate to HIV-positive recipients [25]. There is controversy regarding the use of donors with high-grade primary intracranial malignancies (e.g., glioblastoma), though the UK guidance has recommended cautious use of these donors after careful recipient assessment and counseling [26].

Box 90.1 Contraindications to Donation in the UK

Contraindications to all organ donation

Age equal or greater than 85 years

Primary intra-cerebral lymphoma

All secondary intracranial tumors

Any active cancer with spread outside affected organ within the last 3 years

Poorly-controlled HIV disease

Definite, probable, or possible transmissible spongiform encephalopathy, including CJD and vCJD, family history of familial CJD, and other neurodegenerative diseases associated with infectious agents

Malignant melanoma (other than local and completely excised cancers, e.g., superficial spreading type with tumor thickness < 1.5 mm with curative surgery and cancer-free period of >5 years)

West Nile Virus infection

Active hematological malignancy (myeloma, lymphoma, leukemia)

Active and untreated TB

Ebola virus infection

Contraindications to kidney donation

The need for long-term dialysis (not acute renal failure requiring dialysis/filtration)

Chronic renal impairment (eGFR <45 mL/min/1.73 m^2)

Renal malignancy (excluding history of low-grade and completely excised tumors)

Contraindications to pancreas donation

Insulin-dependent diabetes (excluding ICU-associated insulin requirements)

Type 2 diabetes

Donor BMI >40 kg/m^2

DBD donors of age equal or greater to 66 years

DCD donors of age equal of greater than 56 years

Adapted from the NHSBT ODT Directorate document 'Contraindications to Organ Donation' 2018

Donor history, examination findings, and relevant investigations are collected by the donor coordinator. Factors particularly relevant to kidney transplantation include donor age, cause of death, baseline and pre-retrieval renal function, virology, and donor past medical history (e.g., hypertension, diabetes, malignancy, significant systemic disease). The UK Kidney Donor Risk Index (UKKDRI) was developed to quantify donor risk based on variables demonstrated to influence transplant outcomes [27]. This has recently been revised to incorporate other donor risk factors [28].

The authors have the same selection criteria for DBD and controlled (Maastricht III [6]) DCD kidney donors. UK data demonstrates that adults receiving a first kidney transplant from DCD donors have equivalent graft survival to those receiving a kidney from a DBD donor [29]. Many units will decline potential controlled DCD kidney donors that do not progress to circulatory arrest within 1 or 7 hours of treatment withdrawal. The authors believe that it is reasonable to wait much longer, though logistical issues (e.g., organ recovery team availability) become increasingly important. Significant hypotension (<80 mmHg systolic blood pressure) following the withdrawal of life-sustaining treatment may be associated with poor early transplant outcomes [30].

Kidneys from deceased donors with moderate age-related disease may be suitable for implantation into one recipient, i.e., double adult kidney transplantation. As the age of deceased donors increases, this has the advantage of potentially increasing the donor pool, though prospective randomized data supporting double kidney transplantation are lacking. Some units advocate routine histological assessment of kidneys from older deceased donors (e.g., those over 60 years old) with the aim of identifying kidneys with underlying age-related impairment prior to transplantation. However, the evidence for widespread use of preimplantation kidney biopsies to direct organ utilization is equivocal [31]. Performing preimplantation kidney biopsies also requires access to histopathology expertize out of hours.

90.5.2 Surgical Aspects of Recipient Selection

The main surgical issues to consider when determining if a potential recipient is suitable for kidney transplantation are the presence of iliac vessel vasculopathy, sufficient space in an iliac fossa for a graft, coagulopathy, peritoneal diseases, and the state of the bladder.

Unexpected inability to implant a kidney is a deeply upsetting event for both the potential recipient and the surgeon and usually occurs because of unrecognized severe iliac arterial disease. It is therefore essential that risk factors for arterial disease are identified and that patients with possible arterial disease are thoroughly evaluated to prevent inappropriate listing. These risk factors include age, smoking history, diabetes, renal failure due to renovascular disease or hypertension, known peripheral vascular disease (intermittent claudication), long duration of hemodialysis, and poor calcium and phosphate control. All patients should have a careful clinical assessment of their femoral artery pulses, and those with risk factors or abnormal examination findings should undergo duplex scanning of the iliac arteries and/or a non-contrast CT scan, depending on the index of suspicion. If a sufficient segment of disease-free common or external iliac artery cannot be identified, transplantation is usually precluded, though innovative techniques to solve this problem have been described [32]. Intraperitoneal placement onto the abdominal aorta and IVC may be another option in those with severe iliac arterial disease.

A history of previous DVT or PE or a previous long-term femoral venous dialysis catheter requires an iliac vein duplex to ensure that the veins are patent and thrombus-free. The presence of thrombus in the common or external iliac veins is a contraindication to placement of a kidney on that side, and a previous femoral vein thrombosis is a relative contraindication to ipsilateral transplantation.

Patients with polycystic kidney disease should be assessed carefully to ensure that there is sufficient space in at least one iliac fossa for a proposed kidney transplant. The presence of a palpable kidney well below the level of the anterior superior iliac spine (ASIS) on both sides suggests that pre-listing native nephrectomy may be required. Patients with kidneys just below the ASIS may be managed by puncturing the lower pole cysts at the time of transplant, though in general this should be avoided due to the small risk of introducing infected cyst fluid into the transplant operative field. CT imaging of the abdomen and pelvis can be used to assess native kidney size in patients with polycystic kidney disease where the examination findings are unclear. Other indications for native nephrectomy prior to listing for kidney transplantation include recurrent hematuria or pyelonephritis and severe uncontrollable proteinuria or hypertension.

Those with a previous kidney transplant in situ can have a subsequent graft placed on the opposite side, assuming that there are no other surgical contraindications. Patients with grafts in both sides require transplant nephrectomy in one iliac fossa before listing; occasionally, there may be sufficient space below a proximally placed shrunken graft to enable transplantation without nephrectomy, but radiological confirmation with a CT scan is required first.

Long-term anticoagulation requires reversal at the time of transplant, and a protocol for managing this should be in place at listing. Patients who have lost a graft due to venous or arterial thrombosis should be investigated for the presence of procoagulant states before relisting, although a negative result may be falsely reassuring. The need for postoperative anticoagulation needs careful consideration. Advice from hematology colleagues is required. In general, a previous thrombosis without a clear cause identifies the recipient at high risk for future thrombotic events, and management should be adjusted accordingly. On admission for transplantation, reversal of warfarin may be achieved with small doses of vitamin K, fresh frozen plasma, or clotting factor concentrates (e.g., Octaplex, Beriplex). The reversal of newer direct oral anticoagulants (e.g., dabigatran, rivaroxaban, apixaban) is complex and should be considered prior to listing. Hematology advice should be followed.

The INR should be below 1.6 before starting surgery, and further clotting factors and additional units of cross-matched blood should be available intraoperatively. Anticoagulation with an intravenous heparin infusion can be started during surgery, although it may be deferred until a couple of hours after completion of surgery, depending on the indication for anticoagulation and the degree of bleeding encountered during surgery. Patients receiving heparin infusions are at high risk of postoperative bleeding and often require a return to theatre in the early postoperative period; close monitoring on the ward or high dependency unit is essential.

Patients with severe peritoneal diseases such as encapsulating peritoneal sclerosis require careful assessment pre-listing. Extraperitoneal placement of kidney grafts is essential due to the difficulties in entering the intraperitoneal space, but separating the thickened, diseased peritoneum from the extraperitoneal tissues can be challenging. The extra time required to achieve this should be factored into the expected cold ischemic time of the graft, and kidneys with prolonged ischemic times prior to implantation should be avoided in this patient group. The presence of nonabsorbable mesh in the abdominal wall can make extraperitoneal graft placement difficult, and patients with a previous mesh inguinal hernia repair should have the kidney placed on the opposite side. Beware of the patient who has had a laparoscopic inguinal hernia repair; meshes placed via this approach are often large, may cover both inguinal regions, and the scar gives no indication of the side of the operation. The original operation note must be reviewed.

Most transplant units do not require formal assessment of bladder capacity and urodynamics prior to listing for kidney transplantation, as this is difficult in patients with oligo/anuria and bladder adaptation usually occurs posttransplant. In patients with urological abnormalities contributing to their renal failure, close liaison with urological surgeons may be necessary to plan the best method of achieving urinary outflow from a proposed graft. There is usually a relatively straightforward technique to achieve this, e.g., anastomosis of the transplant ureter to an ileal conduit, intraoperative placement of a suprapubic catheter in those with known bladder outflow obstruction, or cutaneous transplant ureterostomy in patients with the previous cystectomy without reconstruction.

90.5.3 Implantation Techniques

90.5.3.1 Single Kidney Transplantation

Kidneys retrieved from deceased donors often require extensive surgical preparation (benchwork) before they are suitable for implantation. Fat is removed from the surface of the kidney to check the adequacy of parenchymal perfusion and identify any possible tumors. The arterial patch should be inspected for vascular disease and the presence of accessory renal arteries. Dissection of the renal vein and artery is then performed to identify aberrant vascular anatomy and repair any damage that might have occurred during retrieval. A cuff of tissue should be left around the ureter to prevent damage to the ureteric blood supply. After benchwork, the kidney is returned to SCS or machine perfusion, awaiting the recipient.

Open surgical techniques to implant the donated kidney are most widely practiced, although there is increasing interest in laparoscopic and robotic-assisted techniques. The open approach is described in detail below.

The recipient is placed supine on the operating table, and a urethral catheter is inserted into the bladder. Prophylactic antibiotics should be given prior to knife-to-skin. In adult recipients, the standard implantation technique is an extraperitoneal approach via a groin incision. Not only is this the simplest approach to the iliac vessels and bladder, but it also facilitates postoperative percutaneous biopsy as intraperitoneal structures such as the bowel are pushed medially. After the extraperitoneal plane is developed, the external iliac artery and vein are dissected free, with ligation of neighboring lymphatic vessels. After the vein is clamped, and the kidney is wrapped in a cold swab in the correct orientation (ureter caudally), an end-to-side anastomosis between the renal vein and the external iliac vein is performed with a continuous nonabsorbable monofilament suture. The external iliac artery is then clamped, and the aortic patch containing the renal artery (or arteries) is anastomosed end-to-side, again with a continuous nonabsorbable monofilament suture. Alternative arterial inflow sites include the common iliac artery (end-to-side) or the internal iliac artery (end-to-end) (◘ Fig. 90.1). The venous and arterial anastomoses take approximately 30–40 min; once completed the vascular clamps can be released, and the kidney is perfused with recipient blood. The sight of copious volumes of urine emanating from the transplant ureter is especially gratifying but unfortunately is uncommon in deceased donor kidney transplantation. As long as renal perfusion is good, with excellent blood flow palpable in the renal artery, the presence or absence of urine at this stage is immaterial.

Once hemostasis has been achieved, the ureteric anastomosis to the bladder can be performed. Identification of the bladder can be facilitated by inflating the bladder with colored saline, e.g., methylene blue. There are many different ureteric anastomotic techniques, but most transplant surgeons favor an extravesical anastomosis, e.g., the Lich-Gregoir technique. This involves dissect-

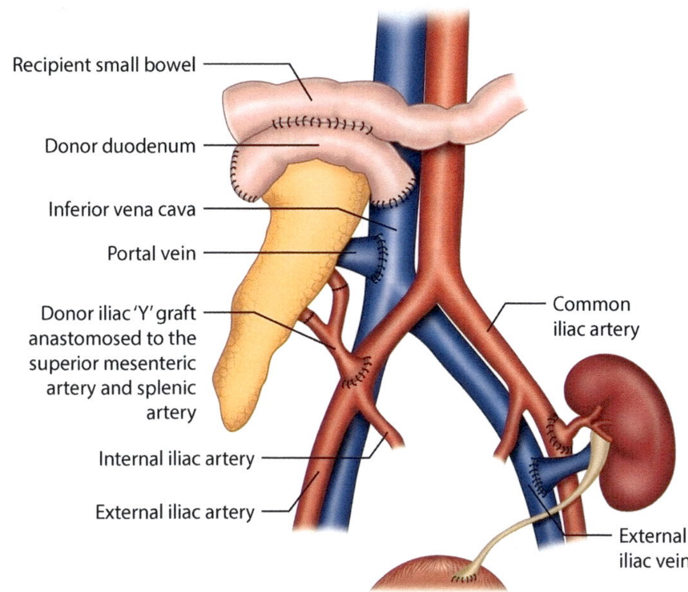

Fig. 90.1 Surgical anatomy of pancreas and kidney transplantation. Diagram of the authors' preferred technique for deceased donor pancreas and kidney transplantation. *1* common iliac artery, *2* internal iliac artery, *3* external iliac artery, *4* external iliac vein, *5* donor iliac 'Y' graft anastomosed to the superior mesenteric artery and splenic artery, *6* portal vein, *7* inferior vena cava, *8* donor duodenum, and *9* recipient small bowel (Image courtesy of Mr. Simon Harper, Cambridge Transplant Unit, with permission)

ing through the muscular layer of the bladder, making a small (7–10 mm diameter) hole in the mucosa, and performing an anastomosis between the spatulated ureter and the bladder mucosa. Routine placement of a ureteric stent reduces the rate of urine leaks and ureteric stenosis by approximately 75%. Early removal (<15 days) of ureteric stents following kidney transplantation may reduce the incidence of UTI [33].

Once the ureteric anastomosis is complete, perfusion and hemostasis of the kidney should be reassessed. If both are satisfactory, optional further steps include biopsy of the kidney and placement of a drain.

90.5.3.2 Double Adult Kidney Transplantation

When both kidneys are available from a deceased donor, and the expected function of a single kidney transplant is thought to be unacceptably low, double kidney transplantation can be performed. The technique favored by the authors is described. Both kidneys can be implanted into one iliac fossa in order to reduce operative (and cold ischemic) time and to preserve the contralateral iliac fossa for any future transplant. The right iliac fossa is favored due to the ease of access to the common iliac vein if required.

The incision is slightly larger for double kidney transplantation, but otherwise, the initial dissection is identical to single kidney transplantation. Both kidneys can usually be implanted onto the external iliac artery and vein, but in small recipients, or when both kidneys are large, dissection, and control of the common iliac artery and vein (and occasionally the inferior vena cava) are required. The first kidney to be implanted should be placed as cranially (proximally) as possible. The choice of which kidney to implant first is dictated predominantly by the length of the available ureter (the kidney with the longest ureter should be implanted first), though when both kidneys have long ureters then vascular anatomy should be considered. The venous and arterial anastomoses are performed in the usual manner and the kidney is re-perfused. The distal vein and artery can then be clamped and the second kidney implanted while the proximal kidney remains perfused. The authors favor two separate vesicoureteric anastomoses. Alternatively, one ureter may be implanted onto the native ureter. Patients with oligo/anuria pretransplant may have the native ureter ligated proximally, followed by an end-to-end ureteric anastomosis. A side-to-end ureteric anastomosis can be considered in patients with high native urine output to avoid native hydronephrosis.

90.5.3.3 Robotic-Assisted Kidney Transplantation (RAKT)

Robotic-assisted surgery has been successfully implemented in various surgical fields, most notably in prostatectomy [34]. RAKT provides a means of minimally invasive recipient surgery and is said to be particularly advantageous in obese patients [35]. There are multiple approaches to RAKT, and the authors, therefore, describe the generic concepts. Ports are placed through the anterior abdominal wall (8–12 mm diameter) for direct visualization of the surgical field. Access to the iliac vessels is gained via the transabdominal approach. An incision of approximately 7–8 cm is required to insert the graft into the surgical field prior to the vascular anastomosis. This incision can be placed in the upper or lower midline, or via a Pfannenstiel incision. A transvaginal approach has also been described. The arteries and veins are anastomosed to the recipient iliac vessels robotically. Regional hypothermia (e.g., ice slush jacket) of the kidney can be used during the vascular anastomoses, in order to reduce the effect of prolonged anastomosis times. After reperfusion, a ureteric anastomosis is performed over a stent. Early graft outcomes appear equivalent to open surgery thus far, though the number of centeres performing RAKT is small at present. Most centeres that perform RAKT use the technique for live donor kidney transplantation at present, as access to the robot and the appropriately trained theatre staff can be challenging out-of-hours. It remains to be seen whether RAKT becomes widely used in deceased donor kidney transplantation.

90.5.4 Postoperative Surgical Complications

Complications that require surgical interventions after kidney transplantation include bleeding (5–10%), renal artery/vein thrombosis (2–3%), infected deep and superficial wound collections (5–10%), lymphocele (5–10%), transplant renal artery stenosis (1–2%), major urinary complications (leak/stenosis) (2–3%), and incisional hernia (1–7%). Their frequency is highly variable and is dependent upon many factors such as the quality of the donor organs, the presence of recipient comorbidities, surgical technique, and the intensity of perioperative immunosuppression.

Blood loss during kidney transplantation is inevitable, with an average hemoglobin drop of about 20–30 g/L (in part due to volume expansion and hemodilution). Ongoing significant postoperative bleeding presents as a spectrum of disorders ranging from a gradual fall in hemoglobin concentrations in the days after the operation to progressive hemodynamic instability, to catastrophic exsanguination leading to cardiac arrest. Any suspicion of bleeding mandates prompt resuscitation and surgical review. Bleeding is a clinical diagnosis, and suspicion should lead to a return to theatre. CT scanning to detect perinephric hematomas may be of use in patients with subtle hemoglobin drops, but ultrasonography is generally misleading for the investigation of bleeding and can miss large bleeds. Drains can become blocked with clots, and the lack of a bloody drain output does not exclude bleeding.

Renal artery/vein thromboses usually present within 5–10 days of the operation with a sudden drop in urine output. Venous thromboses may also lead to pain, graft tenderness, and hematuria. Ultrasound or contrast-enhanced CT scanning may detect the thrombus, and emergency return to theatre is warranted, though the condition is almost always irreversible and graft nephrectomy is the most likely outcome. Technical failings are thought to be the underlying cause, though hypercoagulable states should be considered.

Infected superficial wound infections (outside the muscle layer) can present with wound cellulitis, discharge, and occasionally graft dysfunction. Diagnosis is clinical, though a contrast-enhanced CT scan is useful to exclude a deep component. Treatment requires laying open of the wound (either on the ward or in theater), evacuation of the abscess cavity, and appropriate intravenous antibiotics. When a deep (perinephric) collection is present, graft dysfunction and malaise are more common, though immunosuppressed patients can have often surprisingly large collections with minimal symptoms or signs. The authors generally favor operative washout of deep collections rather than radiologically guided drains, as open surgery enables thorough lavage, closure of fascial defects, and open graft biopsy if needed. Intravenous antibiotics are also needed.

Collections of lymphatic fluid around the kidney (lymphoceles) are common posttransplant and may come from a disrupted donor or recipient lymphatics. These are often detected on postoperative ultrasound scans and do not require treatment unless they are associated with graft dysfunction or significant compression of vital structures (e.g., iliac or renal veins). Radiologically guided aspiration and fluid biochemistry and culture are essential to differentiate between a lymphocele, urinoma (urine leak), and an infected deep collection. Simple aspiration may be successful, though recurrent lymphoceles require placement of a radiological drain. Instillation of sclerosants (e.g., povidone-iodine) has been described, but the authors avoid this approach due to the risk of introducing infection around the kidney. Laparoscopic or open surgical drainage may be required for lymphoceles failing to respond to percutaneous drainage.

Transplant renal artery stenosis presents weeks to months postoperatively with deteriorating renal function and refractory hypertension. The diagnosis may be suggested by ultrasound scanning, but the definitive diagnosis relies on digital subtraction angiography. Treatment options include radiological angioplasty or stenting, or surgical vascular reconstruction. Angioplasty has a risk of recurrence, while surgery is technically challenging. Treatment preferences vary between surgeons, and cases should be discussed between disciplines before intervention.

Major ureteric complications (ureteric stenoses or urinary leaks) are rare postoperatively, but can be a significant source of morbidity and even graft loss. Contributing factors include poor surgical technique, damage to lower polar renal arteries (which supply the transplant ureter), BK virus infection, and failure to use a ureteric stent. Urine leaks commonly manifest within days of transplantation with leakage of straw-colored fluid through the wound with high creatinine content on biochemical analysis. Occasionally, fluid aspirated from deep collections turns out to be urine on analysis. The patient should have a urethral catheter inserted to decompress the bladder, and imaging should be performed to identify the site of the leak (e.g., cystogram or nephrostogram). Leaks from the ureteric anastomosis are best treated with a return to theatre and ureteric reimplantation. Ureteric stenoses present with graft dysfunction with a dilated pelvicalyceal system on ultrasonography. A nephrostomy should be inserted and a nephrostogram performed to locate the stenotic area (usually at or near the site of the ureteric anastomosis). Blood and urine should be sent for BK viral loads and decoy cells, respectively. Distal ureteric stenoses can be treated with a variety of techniques including ureteric reimplantation, Boari flap, bladder mobilization, and bladder hitch, and anastomosis of the ipsilateral native ureter to the transplant renal pelvis.

An incisional hernia is a protrusion of body cavity contents thorough its containing fascial layers at the site of surgery. The rate of incisional hernia is significantly lower using the traditional extraperitoneal approach, relative to the intraperitoneal approach [36]. Risk factors for incisional hernia following kidney transplantation include recipient obesity, age, and reoperation.

Iatrogenic injury to the lateral femoral cutaneous nerve can occur during kidney transplant and is commonlyneurapraxia related to stretching of the nerve from retractors placed near the inferior wound margin. This results in meralgia paraesthetica, a condition characterized by pain, paresthesia, and loss of sensation in the outer thigh [37]. Femoral nerve injury has also been described after kidney transplantation, though this is rare.

90.6 Pancreas Transplantation

90.6.1 Donor Selection

Selection criteria for pancreas donors are more restrictive than kidney donors, with an upper age limit of approximately 60 years of age. General and specific contraindications to pancreas donation are listed in ▶ Box 90.2. High body mass index (BMI) is strongly associated with reduced pancreas graft survival, and the majority of pancreas donors have a BMI less than 30 kg/m^2.

A large US registry analysis identified the following donor risk factors for 1-year pancreas graft loss: (a) increasing age, (b) male sex, (c) non-white race, (d) high BMI, (e) low height, (f) cerebrovascular accident as the cause of death, (g) prolonged cold ischemic time, (h) DCD donor, and (i) elevated serum creatinine [38]. Surprisingly, donor serum amylase/lipase, smoking or alcohol history, and cocaine use were not associated with poorer pancreas graft outcomes, though this may be because current clinical practice restricts the use of grafts from donors with some of these characteristics.

Most transplant surgeons avoid using pancreases from donors with a heavy alcohol history, though accurate estimation of alcohol intake in deceased donors is difficult. A recent registry analysis indicates that high alcohol intake (>21 units per week) in deceased donors has no effect on pancreas graft survival indicating that these donors can be considered acceptable [39].

Simultaneous pancreas and kidney transplants from DCD donors have similar graft survivals to those from DBD donors, with roughly equivalent donor selection criteria [40]. Acceptable warm ischemic limits for controlled DCD donors have not yet been fully defined, but most centers would decline pancreases after more than 30 min of severe hypotension or hypoxia after withdrawal of life-supporting treatment.

Perhaps the most important factor in donor pancreas selection, and the most difficult to quantify at present, is the appearance and 'feel' of the gland. Pancreases with significant intrapancreatic fat infiltration or fibrosis are believed to have poor outcomes if transplanted, though objective evidence quantifying this risk is lacking. Assessment by an experienced surgeon is a key component in successful pancreas transplantation.

90.6.2 Surgical Aspects of Recipient Assessment

The assessment of potential candidates for pancreas transplantation is highly complex. Major issues in the assessment include determining the patient's cardiorespiratory fitness and selecting the appropriate type of transplant from the myriad of options available. The surgical aspects of recipient assessment prior to pancreas transplantation include assessment of vasculopathy, investigating procoagulable states, and consideration of the ability to close the abdomen post-transplant (i.e., BMI and abdominal girth). Broad acceptance criteria for candidates for SPK transplantation, pancreas-after-kidney (PAK) transplantation, and pancreas transplantation alone (PTA) are outlined in ▶ Box 90.2.

Box 90.2 Recipient Selection for Pancreas Transplantation

Patients are considered for pancreas transplantation on the following basis:

PTA: patients with recurrent life-threatening hypoglycemia (requiring third-party assistance) but normal or near-normal renal function

SPK transplant: patients with renal failure (GFR < 20 mL/min/1.73 m^2 or on dialysis) and insulin-dependent diabetes

PAK transplant: patients with stable, functioning kidney transplants, and insulin-dependent diabetes

The majority of patients have type I diabetes, but some insulin-dependent type II diabetes patients of low BMI (<30 kg/m^2) may also be suitable; patients with type II diabetes and a BMI >30 kg/m^2 are not eligible for pancreas in the UK

Relative contraindications to pancreas transplantation

BMI > 30 kg/m^2

Insulin requirements >1.5 units/kg/day

Extensive aorto-iliac disease

Pancreas transplantation is a major undertaking, with operations lasting from 4 to 12 hours and blood losses of 1–2 L or more. Adequate cardiorespiratory reserve is, therefore, necessary to cope with these intraoperative demands and the physiological stresses that postoperative complications may place on the recipient. Thorough cardiac assessment is especially important given the high rate of asymptomatic coronary artery disease in the diabetic population; investigations should therefore include an echocardiogram and cardiac stress test (e.g., myocardial perfusion scan or dobutamine stress echo), with lung function tests in those with respiratory symptoms. Cardiology advice is often necessary and coronary angiography is frequently required pre-listing.

Patients with insulin-dependent diabetes and renal failure have a variety of choices and careful assessment and counseling are required. These choices include SPK transplantation, kidney transplantation alone (deceased or live donor, if available), and PAK transplantation. In this patient group, long-term survival after SPK or live donor kidney transplantation is superior to that following deceased donor kidney transplantation [41]. Patient survival after SPK transplantation compared to that of the pancreas after live donor kidney (PALK) transplantation is reasonably similar, with superior pancreas graft survival in the SPK group [42, 43]. The availability of a suitable live donor, the requirement for glycemic control, local waiting times for pancreas transplantation, difficulties with vascular access, and the characteristics of the potential live donor are factors to be considered when deciding between these options.

Other issues must also be considered before listing a potential recipient for pancreas transplantation. Meticulous examination of the lower limbs is necessary to detect peripheral vascular disease and foot ulcers. The presence of peripheral vascular disease should prompt radiological investigation of the aortoiliac system to exclude significant diseases that might prevent organ implantation. Foot ulcers must be healed before listing to prevent sepsis posttransplantation. Implantation of a pancreas and a kidney into recipients with a BMI of more than 30 kg/m^2 may make abdominal closure difficult and is associated with an increased incidence of abdominal sepsis. Potential recipients with BMI >30 kg/m^2 and significant central obesity should not be listed until they lose weight.

Pancreas allograft thrombosis occurs in 5–10% of patients posttransplant and is one of the most common causes of early graft loss. Careful evaluation of the potential recipient is necessary to detect procoagulant states. Detection of clotting abnormalities, or a history of thromboembolic disease, may not preclude listing for transplantation but should prompt the use of a more aggressive anticoagulation regimen posttransplant.

90

90.6.3 Implantation Techniques

It is essential that the pancreas is assessed by the implanting surgeon as soon as it arrives at the implanting center; cold ischemic time has a strong influence on graft survival, and preparation of the pancreas for implantation often takes more than an hour. The pancreas is a delicate organ with a complex blood supply, and damage during organ recovery is common; repair is often needed. Implantation requires vascular reconstruction with donor vessels (usually the bifurcation of the common iliac artery), and these are commonly diseased or may also be damaged during recovery. Assessment of the degree of fatty infiltration of the pancreatic parenchyma is important, as fatty pancreases have a high rate of reperfusion pancreatitis and poor graft survival. These complexities at least partly explain the high rate of discard of recovered pancreases (up to 50%).

Preparation of the pancreas prior to implantation begins with removal of the spleen and ligation of the splenic hilar vessels, removal of extrapancreatic fat, and shortening of the attached duodenum/jejunum. The common bile duct and inferior mesenteric vein are ligated. The portal vein must be dissected free of tissue, and an extension graft of the donor iliac vein may be needed if it is too short, though many surgeons prefer to avoid these as they may be associated with an increased risk of vein thrombosis. The standard arterial reconstruction technique is to anastomose the donor external iliac artery to the pancreatic superior mesenteric artery stump, and the donor internal iliac artery to the splenic artery. This 'Y-graft' reconstruction enables a single, larger arterial anastomosis between the donor's right common iliac artery and the recipient's vessel on implantation. Although the gastroduodenal artery can be used as an additional arterial inflow to the pancreas, it is usually ligated.

Pancreatic implantation techniques are highly variable and depend primarily on the means by which the pancreatic venous and exocrine secretions are drained. The pancreatic venous outflow can go directly into the systemic circulation (e.g., via a pancreatic portal vein anastomosis with the IVC, right common or external iliac veins), or via the portal circulation by anastomosis of the pancreatic portal vein with the recipient's superior mesenteric vein. Portal drainage is technically challenging, though it has the advantage of enabling physiological insulin delivery to the liver. This was thought to improve posttransplant lipid profiles and graft survival, though this has not been borne out in practice. The overwhelming majority of the UK surgeons, therefore, prefer systemic venous drainage (◘ Fig. 90.1).

The exocrine secretions of the pancreas can be drained into either the gut or the bladder; both are technically straightforward. Bladder drainage enables the monitoring of graft function by measuring urinary amylase (early rejection leads to a drop in urinary amylase by more than 25% from baseline), but the secretion of bicarbonate-rich fluid and activated enzymes into the bladder can lead to acidosis, dysuria, and reflux pancreatitis. Disabling symptoms lead to a significant proportion of patients with bladder-drained pancreatic grafts requiring conversion to enteric drainage. The disadvantages of enteric drainage include the inability to monitor exocrine function and leakage of small bowel contents if the anastomosis between the donor duodenum and the recipient small bowel breaks down. Most UK surgeons currently prefer enteric drainage for SPK transplants in order to avoid the morbidities associated with bladder drainage and because early pancreatic rejection is usually associated with renal allograft dysfunction and is marked by rising serum lipase and amylase levels. Bladder drainage of PAK and PTA transplants is attractive due to the difficulties of detecting early rejection in pancreas-only enteric-drained grafts. Bladder-drained pancreases are placed 'head down' as opposed to the 'head up' position as seen in ◘ Fig. 90.1.

A common approach for implantation of a systemic-enterically drained pancreas as part of an SPK is as follows. A long midline laparotomy is performed, and the right colon mobilized medially. The IVC and right common iliac artery are dissected free. An end-to-side anastomosis between the pancreatic portal vein and lower IVC is performed. The arterial Y-graft is then anastomosed end-to-side with the right common iliac artery. Reperfusion characteristically results in significant graft bleeding, and the surgeon, anesthetist, and theatre team must be appropriately prepared. The recipient's insulin infusion should be stopped at reperfusion as graft insulin is produced almost immediately, and maybe excessive causing hypoglycemia. Once hemostasis is achieved, the recipient's small bowel can be anastomosed side to side with donor duodenum, either directly or as a Roux-en-Y loop. After further hemostasis, the kidney can be implanted; this can be placed intraperitoneally or extraperitoneally in the left iliac fossa.

90.6.4 Postoperative Surgical Complications

Early complications (within 1 month) after pancreas transplantation are common, with up to one-third of recipients requiring a return to the theater during their index admission. Common causes of re-laparotomy include bleeding, pancreatic leaks, peri-pancreatic collections, and leakages of gastrointestinal contents. Late complications that require surgery include those associated with bladder drainage. Graft thrombosis is common after pancreas transplantation (5–10%) and can present at any point after implantation, although it most frequently occurs within the first month. Spinal cord ischemia is an under-recognized but significant early complication in pancreas transplantation, with an estimated risk of 1:500.

Intra-abdominal bleeding is common due to the friable nature of the pancreas, the multiple anastomoses required for perfusion, and the need for anticoagulation to reduce the risk of graft thrombosis. As with kidney transplantation, bleeding can present with a gradual, progressive drop in hemoglobin concentration over a number of days, sudden catastrophic hypovolemic shock, or variations between the two. Again, bleeding is a clinical diagnosis, but CT scanning may be useful in subtle cases. Resuscitation and return to theatre for re-laparotomy, washout, and hemostasis are essential. Do not rely on drain output; drains can block. Enteric-drained pancreases can present with gastrointestinal bleeding; these most commonly come from the anastomosis to the donor duodenum or the entero-enterostomy of a Roux-en-Y loop and require the anastomosis to be taken down and the bleeding controlled.

A number of complications after pancreas transplantation present in similar ways, with abdominal pain over the graft, fever, vomiting, and raised serum amylase/lipase and inflammatory markers. Differential diagnoses include graft pancreatitis, leakage of enzyme-rich pancreatic fluid, and the presence of an infected peri-pancreatic collection. Raised blood glucose is uncommon with these disorders. A contrast-enhanced CT scan may identify an infected collection amenable to radiological drainage, but often the radiological findings are indistinct. Severe abdominal pain that does not settle rapidly with nonoperative management (i.e., gut rest, intravenous fluids, analgesia, and antibiotics), is an indication for re-laparotomy, washout, sampling of intra-abdominal fluid, and placement of drains. If the pancreas has been drained via the enteric route, all GI anastomoses must be checked carefully for the presence of an enteric leak. A significant enteric leak in a septic patient may also be an indication for graft pancreatectomy, especially if the leak is not amenable to repair.

Graft thrombosis (either venous or arterial) presents with abdominal pain, raised blood glucose, and characteristically normal serum amylase. Other causes for a raised blood glucose such as steroids, total parenteral nutrition, and elevated tacrolimus levels should be considered, but with a low threshold for urgent contrast-enhanced CT scanning to check the perfusion of the graft [44]. In a patient with significant abdominal pain, any perfusion defects on CT should prompt a return to theatre to inspect the graft. The presence of significant graft ischemia requires graft pancreatectomy. Patients with small perfusion defects and minimal pain can be fully anticoagulated, and occasionally graft function settles.

As discussed in the above section, bladder drainage of pancreatic exocrine secretions leads to the loss of enzyme- and bicarbonate-rich fluid in the urine, leading to significant dysuria and acidosis in 20–30% of patients. Also, urinary tract infections can lead to severe reflux pancreatitis. Inability to control these symptoms with simple measures such as antibiotics, oral bicarbonate, or urinary catheterization is an indication for re-laparotomy to convert to enteric drainage.

The rate of incisional hernia formation following laparotomy is 2–20%, though there is concern that immunosuppressed patients are at higher risk [45]. Elective repair is considered in those with intractable symptoms or significant risk of hernia incarceration or strangulation.

90.7 Live Donor Kidney Transplantation

90.7.1 Donor Selection

Deceased donor and living donor assessments are very different. As there is no physical benefit to the live donor in donating an organ, the priority with live donor assessment is to minimize donor risk. This includes the short-term risks associated with major surgery (with an estimated mortality of 1 in 3000 [46]) and the long-term implications of living with one functioning kidney [47]. Female living donors have a slightly higher risk of gestational hypertension and pre-eclampsia [48]. Also, the additional time and resources available make the investigation and quantification of expected live donor graft function more complete. From a potential recipient's perspective, the advantages of transplantation with a live donor kidney include superior graft survival, the opportunity for preemptive transplantation, antibody-incompatible or paired-exchange techniques, and planned preoperative optimization. Selected specific surgical issues of live donor assessment are discussed below; comprehensive guidelines for live donor assessment are available elsewhere (▶ www.bts.org.uk).

Deciding which kidney to remove can be challenging, but the basic principle of minimizing harm to the donor (rather than maximizing graft outcome in the recipient) should be adhered to. Investigation of anatomy requires cross-sectional imaging with either CT or MRI. Multiple renal arteries and veins are common. Single vessels are preferable, but not essential. When single vessels are present, the left kidney is preferred due to its longer vein and increased ease of implantation in the recipient. Kidneys with two or three renal arteries can be used with good outcomes, though specialized arterial reconstruction techniques may be necessary (see below). Small lower polar arteries that are unlikely to be able to be reconstructed are a relative contraindication to donation, as lower polar vessels supply the ureter and an increased rate of ureteric complications in the recipient is expected. The presence of a large lumbar vein, retroaortic vein, or double cava are not contraindications to donation. Quantifying split function is not necessary in all cases, but DMSA scanning should be requested if there is a significant size differential, if stones are present, or if anatomical parenchymal abnormalities are noted. If there is a significant difference in split function (e.g., >10%) the kidney with superior function should remain with the donor.

The presence of renal calculi is not a contraindication to donation, though careful assessment and review by a urologist are essential. As mentioned, DMSA scanning is recommended to detect renal scarring and to quantify split function, and a metabolic screen should be performed to identify underlying metabolic abnormalities. Kidneys with small stones (less than 1 cm diameter) in donors with no metabolic abnormalities can be donated. The stone can usually be removed using endoscopic techniques after donation and should be sent for analysis. If the stone is unable to be removed, then a careful radiological follow-up of the recipient is required. Metabolic abnormalities of the donor require a specialist opinion; donation is not necessarily precluded.

Renal cysts are common, with 10% of those over 50 years of age having one or more simple cysts. Potential donors with a family history of polycystic kidney diseases require careful consideration, and potential donors under 40-years-old with one or more cysts should undergo genetic testing. Polycystic disease is unlikely in those aged 40–59 years if they have less than two cysts in each kidney. Over 59 years, up to four cysts in each kidney are acceptable [49].

90.7.2 Surgical Aspects of Recipient Assessment

The principles of assessing potential recipients of live donor kidneys are the same as those of deceased donor kidneys. Recipients with significant surgical risks or major cardiorespiratory morbidities are better candidates for implantation with live donor kidneys rather than deceased donor kidneys, as transplantation can be performed on an elective basis. This enables preoperative medical and anesthetic optimization and risk reduction.

90.7.3 Live Donor Nephrectomy Techniques

Until the late 1990s, live donor nephrectomy was an open procedure, most commonly performed via a flank incision through the retroperitoneum. Since then, the introduction of laparoscopic technology has seen a marked expansion in the number of available donor nephrectomy techniques. Laparoscopic options now include totally laparoscopic, hand-assisted transperitoneal (when one of the operator's hands is present throughout the procedure), and hand-assisted nephrectomy via a retroperitoneal approach. Right nephrectomy, donor obesity, and kidneys with multiple vessels are no longer a contraindication to laparoscopic surgery.

Meta-analyses of studies comparing open and laparoscopic techniques have shown that operative and warm ischemic times are lower with open nephrectomy, but that blood loss is less with the laparoscopic approach [50, 51]. There were early concerns that the raised intra-abdominal pressure necessary for laparoscopic surgery would result in poorer graft outcomes due to reduced renal blood flow, but these have proven to be unfounded. The most significant advantages of laparoscopic nephrectomy are a shorter hospital stay, a faster return to work (by 2.5 weeks), and less pain postoperatively (including chronic wound pain). Conversion to open surgery is needed in approximately 1% of laparoscopic procedures. Mini-incision open nephrectomy does not appear to be superior to laparoscopic surgery.

New techniques continue to be developed. Abdominal scarring can be minimized by utilization of a totally laparoscopic approach with the extraction of the kidney via the vagina or by using a single port in the umbilicus through which the laparoscope and working instruments are placed. Robotic-assisted laparoscopy has also been described, though lengths of stay were similar to a traditional laparoscopic method [52]. The cost of robotic equipment remains high, though the cost is likely to fall as alternative models become available.

Ultimately, the central tenet of live donor surgery is to protect the safety of the donor. Reassuringly, laparoscopic nephrectomy is not associated with an increased rate of postoperative complications [50, 51]. Because patient mortality after live donor nephrectomy is extremely rare, lack of statistical power has meant that mortality differences have not been able to be detected between the two techniques. The decision on which donor nephrectomy technique is used should therefore be determined by the experience and preference of the surgeon.

90.7.4 Implantation Techniques

The technique of live donor kidney implantation is very similar to that of deceased donor kidney transplantation, with a few notable exceptions; the renal vein is shorter, and the renal artery has no aortic patch (and hence is also shorter). As a result, vascular anastomoses are more challenging technically.

To overcome these obstacles, many surgeons favor mobilizing the common and external iliac arteries and veins. This requires dissection, ligation, and division of the internal iliac vein, enabling the common and external iliac veins to be elevated considerably. When one large renal artery is present, either an end-to-side anastomosis with the external iliac artery or an end-to-end anastomosis with the divided proximal end of the internal iliac artery can be performed. When multiple renal arteries are present, the authors favor using the excised distal internal iliac artery and its major branches as a graft for back-table reconstruction, with subsequent implantation on to the remaining proximal end of the internal iliac artery [53].

Postoperative surgical complications are very similar to those of deceased donor kidney transplantation, except in limited regards. Rates of bleeding are higher in live donor kidney recipients undergoing antibody-removal protocols for ABO- or HLA-incompatible grafts, and lymphocele rates may also be higher.

90.7.5 Patient Safety Systems in Organ Transplantation

Systems to improve patient safety in organ transplantation can be categorized into organizational, data monitoring, and perioperative systems.

Organizational systems include the reconfiguration of local organ retrieval teams into consultant-led National Organ Retrieval Service teams in April 2010. This occurred in response to the publication of the Organ Donation Taskforce Report in 2008. As part of this process, data on injuries to organs at recovery are collected at a national level, and teams involved in organ recovery are contracted to the Service on the basis of maintaining low rates of damage. It is still too early to determine if this reconfiguration has resulted in lower rates of damage.

Data monitoring on graft and patient survival is carried out by NHS Blood and Transplant for every UK transplant unit. Those units with high rates of graft or patient loss are required to explain the clinical reason behind such results, and consistently poor results may lead to an inspection. Unit closure may be recommended if remedial measures are not undertaken. In the USA, outcome monitoring is undertaken by the Scientific Registry of Transplant Recipients (► www.srtr.org).

Perioperative systems designed to improve patient safety include the use of the World Health Organisation (WHO) checklist [54]. Checklists vary between NHS Trusts, but all have three basic components. The first occurs prior to anesthesia and aims to determine if the correct patient is present and that they have been consented and marked appropriately for the correct operation. After the induction of anesthesia (but before surgery starts), the surgical and anesthetic teams again check that the correct patient is present and that the necessary instruments and other equipment are in place. Plans for antibiotic and venous thromboembolic prophylaxis are also checked. Before the patient leaves theater, the team should check that swab and instrument counts are correct and that any special instructions for staff in theatre recovery areas have been clearly documented. Prior to organ transplantation, the operating surgeon should also ensure that the correct organ is in theatre and that virology, ABO compatibility, and tissue-typing cross-match results are appropriate.

Despite having these systems in place, errors can occur. This is of particular concern in transplantation, where patient safety errors can have life-threatening consequences for multiple patients. It is expected that systems to reduce the likelihood of these mistakes occurring will continue to evolve.

Case Study

A 45-year-old male suffered a hypoxic brain injury following hanging and was identified as a potential donation after circulatory death (DCD) donor by the intensive care unit. CT of the brain showed loss of grey/white matter differentiation in keeping with generalized hypoxia. The donor was a smoker, but with no history of malignancy, hypertension, or diabetes, and with a terminal serum creatinine of 367 μmol/L on admission, and 120 μmol/L at the time of referral for donation 2 days later.

The right kidney was accepted for transplantation into a 65-year-old female on hemodialysis. The recipient's 63-year-old husband had been successfully worked up for live donation in the next few weeks. During a clinic appointment, the patient and surgeon had decided to consider potential deceased donor kidney offers on an individual basis if this possibility arose before the live donor kidney transplant had taken place. A detailed discussion between the surgeon, nephrologist, and potential recipient was undertaken, in order to decide whether to proceed with deceased donor transplantation or to continue with live donor transplantation. The recipient chose to proceed with the deceased donor transplant, based on her own preferences.

Flow cytometric crossmatch was negative and induction immunosuppression was with basiliximab, tacrolimus, mycophenolate mofetil, and corticosteroid, according to local policy. The kidney was implanted into the right iliac fossa after 16 hours of cold ischemia time. Time-zero kidney biopsy showed acute tubular necrosis.

Postoperatively, the recipient was oliguric, and an urgent ultrasound of the graft was requested to rule out renal artery/vein thrombosis. The graft was globally perfused, with patent vessels. After returning to the ward, the patient required dialysis during the first postoperative week for hyperkalemia. A transplant biopsy was arranged on the seventh postoperative day for delayed graft function. The biopsy showed acute tubular necrosis once again, and no evidence of acute rejection. Graft function improved in the next few days, and the patient became dialysis-independent. She was discharged after 10 days in the hospital. The patient was able to return to voluntary work in a charity shop after 3 months.

Chapter Review Questions

1. The difference between Donation after Brain Death (DBD) and donation after circulatory death (DCD) is that the latter donor undergoes a significant period of renal warm ischemia during organ retrieval.
   (a) True
   (b) False

2. Donation after circulatory death (DCD) is considered 'controlled' if there is planned withdrawal of life-sustaining therapy.
   (a) True
   (b) False

3. Which of the following statements about adult kidney transplantation is false?
   (a) A first kidney transplant from a DCD donor has equivalent graft survival to a transplant from a DBD donor in the UK
   (b) The standard open implantation technique is an extraperitoneal approach via a groin incision
   (c) Transplant ureteric stents are routinely inserted intraoperatively to reduce urological complications
   (d) In double kidney transplantation, both grafts can be implanted in one iliac fossa to reduce operative time
   (e) Renal vein thrombosis is often detected on postoperative ultrasound scans and does not require treatment unless associated with graft dysfunction

4. Which of the following statements about pancreas transplantation is false?
   (a) Pancreas transplantation is only considered in patients with diabetes mellitus type I
   (b) Organ assessment by an experienced surgeon is a key component in pancreas transplantation
   (c) Graft thrombosis is a major cause of early graft loss
   (d) The donor duodenum is anastomosed to the bladder or the bowel of the recipient
   (e) Early complications necessitating return to theatre occur in one-third of pancreas transplant recipients

5. Which of the following statements about live kidney donation is false?
   (a) Living donation has an estimated early postoperative mortality of 1 in 3000
   (b) Potential living donors require a CT or MRI to assess renal anatomy
   (c) In live donor assessment, the kidney with the better function should ideally be chosen for a donation
   (d) Female living donors have a higher risk of gestational hypertension and pre-eclampsia
   (e) Laparoscopic donor nephrectomy is associated with shorter hospital stay and reduced pain when compared to open donor nephrectomy

Answers

1. True
2. True
3. E is false – renal vein thrombosis is not a common finding on postoperative ultrasound and emergency return to theatre is warranted
4. A is false – pancreas transplantation is considered in patients with insulin-dependent type II diabetes of low BMI (<30 kg/m^2)
5. C is false – the kidney with the better function should ideally remain with the donor

References

1. Valderrabano F, Jofre R, Lopez-Gomez JM. Quality of life in end-stage renal disease patients. Am J Kidney Dis. 2001;38(3):443–64.
2. Wolfe RA, Ashby VB, Milford EL, Ojo AO, Ettenger RE, Agodoa LY, Held PJ, Port FK. Comparison of mortality in all patients on dialysis, patients on dialysis awaiting transplantation, and recipients of a first cadaveric transplant. N Engl J Med. 1999;341(23):1725–30.
3. Ausania F, White SA, Pocock P, Manas DM. Kidney damage during organ recovery in donation after circulatory death donors: data from UK National Transplant Database. Am J Transplant. 2012;12(4):932–6.
4. Callaghan CJ, Harper SJ, Saeb-Parsy K, Hudson A, Gibbs P, Watson CJ, Praseedom RK, Butler AJ, Pettigrew GJ, Bradley JA. The discard of deceased donor kidneys in the UK. Clin Transpl. 2014;28(3):345–53.
5. Ausania F, Drage M, Manas D, Callaghan CJ. A registry analysis of damage to the deceased donor pancreas during procurement. Am J Transplant. 2015;15(11):2955–62.
6. Thuong M, Ruiz A, Evrard P, Kuiper M, Boffa C, Akhtar MZ, Neuberger J, Ploeg R. New classification of donation after circulatory death donors definitions and terminology. Transpl Int. 2016;29(7):749–59.
7. Reich DJ, Mulligan DC, Abt PL, Pruett TL, Abecassis MM, D'Alessandro A, Pomfret EA, Freeman RB, Markmann JF, Hanto DW, Matas AJ, Roberts JP, Merion RM, Klintmalm GB. ASTS recommended practice guidelines for controlled donation after cardiac death organ procurement and transplantation. Am J Transplant. 2009;9(9):2004–11.
8. Saeb-Parsy K, Watson C, Bradley JA. Organ preservation in renal transplantation. Br J Renal Med. 2007;12(4):1–6.
9. O'Callaghan JM, Knight SR, Morgan RD, Morris PJ. Preservation solutions for static cold storage of kidney allografts: a systematic review and meta-analysis. Am J Transplant. 2012; 12(4):896–906.

10. O'Callaghan JM, Knight SR, Morgan RD, Morris PJ. A national registry analysis of kidney allografts preserved with Marshall's solution in the United Kingdom. Transplantation. 2016;100(11):2447–52.
11. Opelz G, Dohler B. Multicenter analysis of kidney preservation. Transplantation. 2007;83(3):247–53.
12. Schneeberger S, Biebl M, Steurer W, Hesse UJ, Troisi R, Langrehr JM, Schareck W, Mark W, Margreiter R, Konigsrainer A. A prospective randomized multicenter trial comparing histidine-tryptophane-ketoglutarate versus University of Wisconsin perfusion solution in clinical pancreas transplantation. Transpl Int. 2009;22(2):217–24.
13. Stewart ZA, Cameron AM, Singer AL, Dagher NN, Montgomery RA, Segev DL. Histidine-tryptophan-ketoglutarate (HTK) is associated with reduced graft survival in pancreas transplantation. Am J Transplant. 2009;9(1):217–21.
14. Bagul A, Hosgood SA, Kaushik M, Kay MD, Waller HL, Nicholson ML. Experimental renal preservation by normothermic resuscitation perfusion with autologous blood. Br J Surg. 2008;95(1):111–8.
15. Moers C, Smits JM, Maathuis MH, Treckmann J, van Gelder F, Napieralski BP, van Kasterop-Kutz M, van der Heide JJ, Squifflet JP, van Heurn E, Kirste GR, Rahmel A, Leuvenink HG, Paul A, Pirenne J, Ploeg RJ. Machine perfusion or cold storage in deceased-donor kidney transplantation. N Engl J Med. 2009;360(1):7–19.
16. Watson CJ, Wells AC, Roberts RJ, Akoh JA, Friend PJ, Akyol M, Calder FR, Allen JE, Jones MN, Collett D, Bradley JA. Cold machine perfusion versus static cold storage of kidneys donated after cardiac death: a UK multicenter randomized controlled trial. Am J Transplant. 2010;10(9):1991–9.
17. Moers C, Pirenne J, Paul A, Ploeg RJ. Machine perfusion or cold storage in deceased-donor kidney transplantation. N Engl J Med. 2012;366(8):770–1.
18. Hosgood SA, Barlow AD, Hunter JP, Nicholson ML. Ex vivo normothermic perfusion for quality assessment of marginal donor kidney transplants. Br J Surg. 2015;102(11):1433–40.
19. Hosgood SA, Nicholson ML. The first clinical case of intermediate ex vivo normothermic perfusion in renal transplantation. Am J Transplant. 2014;14(7):1690–2.
20. Hosgood SA, Nicholson ML. First in man renal transplantation after ex vivo normothermic perfusion. Transplantation. 2011;92(7):735–8.
21. Hosgood SA, Thompson E, Moore T, Wilson CH, Nicholson ML. Normothermic machine perfusion for the assessment and transplantation of declined human kidneys from donation after circulatory death donors. Br J Surg. 2018;105(4): 388–94.
22. Hosgood SA, Saeb-Parsy K, Wilson C, Callaghan C, Collett D, Nicholson ML. Protocol of a randomised controlled, open-label trial of ex vivo normothermic perfusion versus static cold storage in donation after circulatory death renal transplantation. BMJ Open. 2017;7(1):e012237.
23. Barlow AD, Hamed MO, Mallon DH, Brais RJ, Gribble FM, Scott MA, Howat WJ, Bradley JA, Bolton EM, Pettigrew GJ, Hosgood SA, Nicholson ML, Saeb-Parsy K. Use of ex vivo normothermic perfusion for quality assessment of discarded human donor pancreases. Am J Transplant. 2015;15(9): 2475–82.
24. Minambres E, Suberviola B, Dominguez-Gil B, Rodrigo E, Ruiz-San Millan JC, Rodriguez-San Juan JC, Ballesteros MA. Improving the outcomes of organs obtained from controlled donation after circulatory death donors using abdominal normothermic regional perfusion. Am J Transplant. 2017;17(8):2165–72.
25. Canaud G, Avettand-Fenoel V, Legendre C. HIV-positive-to-HIV-positive kidney transplantation. N Engl J Med. 2015;372(21):2069.
26. Warrens AN, Birch R, Collett D, Daraktchiev M, Dark JH, Galea G, Gronow K, Neuberger J, Hilton D, Whittle IR, Watson CJ. Advising potential recipients on the use of organs from donors with primary central nervous system tumors. Transplantation. 2012;93(4):348–53.
27. Watson CJ, Johnson RJ, Birch R, Collett D, Bradley JA. A simplified donor risk index for predicting outcome after deceased donor kidney transplantation. Transplantation. 2012;93(3):314–8.
28. National Health Service Blood and Transplant. Online https://www.odt.nhs.uk/statistics-and-reports/slides-and-presentations/. Accessed on 24 June 2018.
29. Summers DM, Johnson RJ, Allen J, Fuggle SV, Collett D, Watson CJ, Bradley JA. Analysis of factors that affect outcome after transplantation of kidneys donated after cardiac death in the UK: a cohort study. Lancet. 2010;376(9749):1303–11.
30. Peters-Sengers H, Houtzager JHE, Heemskerk MBA, Idu MM, Minnee RC, Klaasen RW, Joor SE, Hagenaars JAM, Rebers PM, van der Heide JJH, Roodnat JI, Bemelman FJ. DCD donor hemodynamics as predictor of outcome after kidney transplantation. Am J Transplant. 2018;18(8):1966–76.
31. Wang CJ, Wetmore JB, Crary GS, Kasiske BL. The donor kidney biopsy and its implications in predicting graft outcomes: a systematic review. Am J Transplant. 2015;15(7):1903–14.
32. Frost J, Thiyagarajan UM, Bagul A, Nicholson ML. Renal transplantation with arterial inflow from an axillofemoral graft. Transplantation. 2011;92(4):e20–2.
33. Thompson ER, Hosgood SA, Nicholson ML, Wilson CH. Early versus late ureteric stent removal after kidney transplantation. Cochrane Database Syst Rev. 2018;1: Cd011455.
34. Hameed AM, Yao J, Allen RDM, Hawthorne WJ, Pleass HC, Lau H. The evolution of kidney transplantation surgery into the robotic era and it prospects for obese recipients. Transplantation. 2018;10:1650–65.
35. Oberholzer J, Giulianotti P, Danielson KK, Spaggiari M, Bejarano-Pineda L, Bianco F, Tzvetanov I, Ayloo S, Jeon H, Garcia-Roca R, Thielke J, Tang I, Akkina S, Becker B, Kinzer K, Patel A, Benedetti E. Minimally invasive robotic kidney transplantation for obese patients previously denied access to transplantation. Am J Transplant. 2013;13(3):721–8.
36. Simson N, Parker S, Stonier T, Halligan S, Windsor A. Incisional hernia in renal transplant recipients: a systematic review. Am Surg. 2018;84(6):930–7.
37. Tomaszewski KA, Popieluszko P, Henry BM, Roy J, Sanna B, Kijek MR, Walocha JA. The surgical anatomy of the lateral femoral cutaneous nerve in the inguinal region: a meta-analysis. Hernia. 2016;20(5):649–57.
38. Axelrod DA, Sung RS, Meyer KH, Wolfe RA, Kaufman DB. Systematic evaluation of pancreas allograft quality, outcomes and geographic variation in utilization. Am J Transplant. 2010;10(4):837–45.
39. Motallebzadeh R, Aly M, El-Khairi M, Drage M, Olsburgh J, Callaghan CJ. High alcohol intake in deceased donors has no effect on pancreas graft survival: a registry analysis. Transpl Int. 2017;30(2):170–7.
40. Qureshi MS, Callaghan CJ, Bradley JA, Watson CJ, Pettigrew GJ. Outcomes of simultaneous pancreas-kidney transplantation from brain-dead and controlled circulatory death donors. Br J Surg. 2012;99(6):831–8.
41. Salvalaggio PR, Dzebisashvili N, Pinsky B, Schnitzler MA, Burroughs TE, Graff R, Axelrod DA, Brennan DC, Lentine

90

KL. Incremental value of the pancreas allograft to the survival of simultaneous pancreas-kidney transplant recipients. Diabetes Care. 2009;32(4):600–2.
42. Poommipanit N, Sampaio MS, Cho Y, Young B, Shah T, Pham PT, Wilkinson A, Danovitch G, Bunnapradist S. Pancreas after living donor kidney versus simultaneous pancreas-kidney transplant: an analysis of the organ procurement transplant network/united network of organ sharing database. Transplantation. 2010;89(12):1496–503.
43. Wiseman AC. Pancreas transplant options for patients with type 1 diabetes mellitus and chronic kidney disease: simultaneous pancreas kidney or pancreas after kidney? Curr Opin Organ Transplant. 2012;17(1):80–6.
44. Powell FE, Harper SJ, Callaghan CJ, Shaw A, Godfrey EM, Bradley JA, Watson CJ, Pettigrew GJ. Postoperative CT in pancreas transplantation. Clin Radiol. 2015;70(11):1220–8.
45. Smith CT, Katz MG, Foley D, Welch B, Leverson GE, Funk LM, Greenberg JA. Incidence and risk factors of incisional hernia formation following abdominal organ transplantation. Surg Endosc. 2015;29(2):398–404.
46. Segev DL, Muzaale AD, Caffo BS, Mehta SH, Singer AL, Taranto SE, McBride MA, Montgomery RA. Perioperative mortality and long-term survival following live kidney donation. JAMA. 2010;303(10):959–66.
47. Ibrahim HN, Foley R, Tan L, Rogers T, Bailey RF, Guo H, Gross CR, Matas AJ. Long-term consequences of kidney donation. N Engl J Med. 2009;360(5):459–69.
48. Reese PP, Boudville N, Garg AX. Living kidney donation: outcomes, ethics, and uncertainty. Lancet. 2015;385(9981):2003–13.
49. Pei Y, Obaji J, Dupuis A, Paterson AD, Magistroni R, Dicks E, Parfrey P, Cramer B, Coto E, Torra R, San Millan JL, Gibson R, Breuning M, Peters D, Ravine D. Unified criteria for ultrasonographic diagnosis of ADPKD. J Am Soc Nephrol. 2009;20(1):205–12.
50. Nanidis TG, Antcliffe D, Kokkinos C, Borysiewicz CA, Darzi AW, Tekkis PP, Papalois VE. Laparoscopic versus open live donor nephrectomy in renal transplantation: a meta-analysis. Ann Surg. 2008;247(1):58–70.
51. Wilson CH, Sanni A, Rix DA, Soomro NA. Laparoscopic versus open nephrectomy for live kidney donors. Cochrane Database Syst Rev. 2011;Nov 9(11):Cd006124.
52. Gorodner V, Horgan S, Galvani C, Manzelli A, Oberholzer J, Sankary H, Testa G, Benedetti E. Routine left robotic-assisted laparoscopic donor nephrectomy is safe and effective regardless of the presence of vascular anomalies. Transpl Int. 2006;19(8):636–40.
53. Firmin LC, Nicholson ML. The use of explanted internal iliac artery grafts in renal transplants with multiple arteries. Transplantation. 2010;89(6):766–7.
54. Haynes AB, Weiser TG, Berry WR, Lipsitz SR, Breizat AH, Dellinger EP, Herbosa T, Joseph S, Kibatala PL, Lapitan MC, Merry AF, Moorthy K, Reznick RK, Taylor B, Gawande AA. A surgical safety checklist to reduce morbidity and mortality in a global population. N Engl J Med. 2009;360(5):491–9.

Management of the Acute Transplant

Hannah Maple, Rawya Charif, Jack Galliford, Adam McLean, and David Game

Contents

M. Harber (ed.), *Primer on Nephrology*, https://doi.org/10.1007/978-3-030-76419-7_91

Learning Aims

- To understand the relevant aspects of the preoperative management of patients who are called in for a kidney transplant, including aspects of the organ offer
- To understand the basic principles of crossmatching and immunosuppression as relevant to the perioperative period
- How to manage a newly transplanted patient from the time they leave theatre until discharge
- To understand the basic principles of rejection and what to look out for in the perioperative period
- To be able to troubleshoot common issues post-transplant, including fluid management, delayed graft function, and poor urine output

91.1 Introduction

Over the last 70 years kidney transplantation has moved from being a novel, exciting, and dangerous new therapy for end-stage renal disease (ESRD) to becoming a routine and common operation performed across many parts of the world. Transplantation confers many benefits over dialysis, including longevity and quality of life, and cost savings to the National Health Service (NHS). Transplantation has evolved considerably since its infancy and in addition to spanning a breadth of medical topics it routinely involves ethical, legal, and psychological issues related to both donors and recipients.

Kidney transplantation has been a successful venture that has almost come full circle, such that it now operates in an environment not to dissimilar to the formative years; one which again looks to push the boundaries of what is deemed possible and acceptable. We are able to transplant immunologically challenging patients with multiple grafts, overcome blood group and immunological barriers, and give opportunities to both adults and children with anatomical complexities. We remove kidneys from living donors laparoscopically or robotically for the benefit of their loved ones, strangers, and people they meet on the Internet, either directly or as part of a kidney exchange programme. Transplantation continues to be an extremely exciting area to practice nephrology and this is likely to be the case for many years to come.

While each transplant centre performs different aspects of kidney transplantation in its own way, there are a number of legal requirements, protocols, and guidelines that provide a framework upon which localized practices are based. In addition to maintaining standards across the field, maximising equity of access and optimising outcomes, these relatively strict rules and recommendations are intended to protect the field of transplantation in its entirety. This is because it relies upon the generosity of donors, living or deceased. Any activity that is deemed reckless, unfair, or unjust risks jeopardising the delicate relationship between donors and the transplant community. It is therefore paramount that clinicians remain diligent about maintaining standards of practice and are not seen to abuse the trust placed in them by the general public.

It is not possible to outline or justify the many different approaches to the acute transplant patient within this chapter. It is therefore intended to provide a broad overview of current principles and practices within the UK, which collectively has excellent outcomes for both living and deceased donor kidney transplantation. Living donor transplant outcomes remain superior to those from deceased donors in terms of both graft and patient survival (98% vs. 94% 1 year and 92% vs. 87% 5-year graft survival; 99% vs. 97% 1 year and 94% vs 87% 5-year patient survival, respectively) [1]. This chapter will outline the perioperative management of the transplant recipient and will discuss pertinent issues for the acutely transplanted patient.

Definitions

Acute Transplant: the chapter refers to the time from organ offer to pre-, peri- and postoperative transplant management until discharge from hospital.

Delayed Graft Function (DGF): for the purposes of clinical trials and data collection is often defined as the need for dialysis in the first week after transplantation. However, in reality, a patient may need dialysis early postop for hyperkalaemia despite a reasonable transplant urine output or if they have a good native urine output, may manage without dialysis despite the graft not making urine for several days or longer. Therefore when managing an individual patient, DGF is usually considered a composite of a failure of urine production reasonably attributed to the transplant together with a failure of the serum creatinine to fall.

91.2 Preoperative Management

91.2.1 Identification of Potential Recipients

Potential recipients of deceased donor organs are identified in one of two ways. The most common is through NHS Blood and Transplant (NHSBT) who telephone the transplant centre with a named offer for a particular individual. The second is through local identification of a recipient from a "matching run", a document sent by NHSBT with a list of potential recipients who have been matched against a particular donor. The local clinicians then choose a recipient, a decision which is most commonly based on donor and recipient characteristics and the circumstances in which that organ has been offered. In 2019, the allocation policy in the UK was changed to reflect the changing donor pool and to address some of the inequities observed in the previous Scheme [2]. Organs are allocated on the basis of a number of different factors, with long waiters (over 7 years), highly sensitized patients and those who are difficult to match being prioritized.

At the time of organ offering NHSBT will refer the clinician to the Core Donor Data Form (CDDF) and the Medical and Social History (MaSH) forms. These are populated by the Specialist Nurses for Organ Donation (SNODs) who approach the family and obtain consent for donation. It must be emphasized that while the clinical information and blood results relevant to the donor's admission may be accurate, the past medical history relies upon hospital records, the patient's GP and their family. Consequently this can be very variable in terms of accuracy. Key pieces of information to consider on the CDDF include the circumstances surrounding the admission and death, past medical history (with a specific focus on history or symptoms of malignancy or infection), blood results, the urine dip and urine output. Where available, a historic creatinine is useful in contextualizing any acute kidney injury and may help determine whether or not the kidneys will be implanted as singles or as a dual transplant (where both kidneys are transplanted into a single recipient). The donor's virological status for CMV, hepatitis, and HIV is usually confirmed by the time of donation; however, the EBV is often awaited. It is important to note the absence of this information, and have a plan to find out the result, especially if the intended recipient is EBV naïve.

91.2.2 Calling in Potential Recipients

91

The importance of time in kidney transplantation cannot be emphasized enough. It is well documented that outcomes are closely related to the cold ischaemic time (CIT), which is the time between the organ being flushed with cold preservation fluid at retrieval to when it is reperfused with the recipient's blood. Prolonged CIT is associated with increased ischaemia-reperfusion injury to the graft, and increased risk of delayed graft function, which is most damaging to kidneys retrieved from donors donating after circulatory death (DCD donors) and expanded criteria donors [3, 4]. This results in poorer long-term outcomes, such as graft survival. There is therefore an onus on the transplant team to prepare the recipient such that they can proceed to theatre as soon as possible.

Common reasons for a prolonged CIT include organs being rerouted from another centre, for reasons such as the organ being rejected for damage or other abnormalities, unexpected issues with the intended recipient and an unexpected positive crossmatch. Occasionally, where the allocation policy allows, the issues listed above may lead to the kidney remaining with the original transplant centre who must then try to find another recipient as soon as possible. There are also some circumstances that justify calling in two recipients for one kidney and this is typically with the intention of reducing the CIT, in the event that the first recipient is unable to have the transplant. The commonest reason for this is when there is a moderate to high probability that the crossmatch will be positive. Thankfully this is becoming increasingly unnecessary as advances in tissue typing allow greater accuracy in determining exactly which HLA specificities a patient has allo-antibodies against. These specificities are then registered as "unacceptable" (unacceptable donor antigens or UDAs within the UK system) with NHSBT so that the patient will not be offered organs carrying those HLA antigens. Issues with an unexpected positive crossmatch therefore most commonly occur with patients who are highly sensitized with low-level donor-specific antibodies which are thought to be of low clinical significance. It may be unclear from the available data whether the cross-match (especially the more sensitive flow cross-match) will be positive or not and this situation may therefore justify calling in a backup recipient.

More commonly there is usually plenty of time between being offered a kidney and the operation going ahead. Despite this, most recipients are called into the hospital as soon as the offer has been made available in order to prepare them adequately prior to transplantation. The transplant surgical team commonly juggle a number of different factors when planning the timing of the transplant. These include the likely arrival time of the kidney, the CIT at the point of arrival, theatre availability, surgeon availability, and other organs that may have been accepted. Recipient-related factors include travelling time, whether the patient has been adequately fasted and whether dialysis is required prior to surgery. Typically patients are asked to come to the hospital as soon as possible and to fast from that point onwards. If it is likely that the transplant is some hours away (i.e., the retrieval is yet to start) then the rules regarding fasting may be relaxed.

There are a number of different views towards dialysing patients immediately before they undergo a kidney transplant. The most obvious indication (and the one that leads to the least amount of debate) is hyperkalaemia, and different anaesthetists will have different cut-offs in terms of what they would like the potassium to be. Some surgeons become uncomfortable with very uraemic patients, as there is a concern regarding bleeding due to platelet dysfunction. This is less of an issue in those dialysing regularly, but may prove a problem in preemptive patients who have not been seen or had blood tests recently. Where patients will be in receipt of a good (commonly DBD) kidney, which is expected to have immediate graft function, there is more leeway to forego dialysis. If not, the situation then arises as to whether a patient should undergo their first session of haemodialysis immediately prior to surgery, and the general consensus is that this should only happen if absolutely necessary. Patients should not have any fluid removed during preoperative dialysis as this may cause issues with haemodynamic instability intraoperatively.

91.2.3 Preoperative Checks

The main purposes of the preoperative checks are to ensure, as much as is feasibly possible, that the patient is physically fit enough to undergo a transplant and that there are no contraindications or issues that may impact their early posttransplant clinical course. Most of these issues will or should have been carefully thought through by the physician activating the patient on the transplant list long before the day of transplantation. However, given that the average waiting time is in the region of 2 years [1] and that transplant centres vary on how regularly waitlisted patients are reviewed, it is important to confirm that nothing significant has changed and that previously controlled medical conditions remain so.

It is important to perform a final brief review of a number of issues including:

(i) *Primary renal diagnosis*

1. *Focal and Segmental Glomerulosclerosis (FSGS)*
   FSGS is the most important primary glomerular disease with known risk of significant recurrence posttransplant. It may recur aggressively and very early in paediatric recipients, but also in adults, presenting with proteinuria and progressive graft dysfunction [5]. Care should be exercised in accepting a primary underlying renal diagnosis of "hypertension", especially in patients of African, Afro-Caribbean, or African American ethnic origin as this may conceal an underlying diagnosis of FSGS. A positive family history of renal disease or known significant proteinuria as part of the original presentation is an important pointer. Treatment is usually with higher doses of calcineurin inhibitors, steroids, and plasma exchange.
2. *Atypical haemolytic uraemic syndrome (aHUS)*
   aHUS caused by genetic abnormalities in complement control proteins can recur early posttransplant, requiring treatment with eculizumab. In the UK, this is authorized in liaison with the National Renal Complement Therapeutics Centre (▶ www.atypicalhus.co.uk). If the diagnosis was not known pretransplant and not obvious posttransplant, sometimes plasma exchange is used pending confirmatory tests.
3. *Membranoproliferative glomerulonephritis (MPGN)*
   Recurrence of the complement-related MPGN spectrum is common posttransplant, especially the type II dense deposit type associated with acquired activating auto-antibodies against the complement system (C3 nephritic factors). Recurrent C3 glomerulopathy may be eligible for treatment with eculizumab (▶ www.atypicalhus.co.uk). Recurrent idiopathic or immune complex related MPGN is more common and there is no proven treatment. Sometimes increased background immunosuppression is tried (anti-metabolite and/or steroids), or addition of cyclophosphamide or plasma exchange.
4. *Other glomerular diseases*
   Almost all glomerular diseases may recur posttransplant. This is most commonly seen at ultrastructural level in IgA nephropathy and membranous nephropathy, but this very rarely results in a significant clinical impact in the early posttransplant period. Systemic diseases (diabetes, amyloid, Anderson-Fabry, sarcoidosis) may also affect the late course of transplant function.
5. *Primary hyperoxalurias*
   These inherited defects of glyoxalate metabolism can recur with rapid oxalate deposition early posttransplant, often triggered by reduced graft function from other causes leading to reduced oxalate clearance. When the diagnosis is known, liver transplantation is usually performed in advance of kidney transplant to correct the underlying condition. If undiagnosed, posttransplant management of high oxalate levels is important to prevent significant renal damage, and a plan for intermittent haemodialysis may be appropriate to reduce the total body and plasma oxalate burden. The role of novel RNA interference treatment (e.g., Lumasiran) in this setting is not yet known.

6. *Lower urinary tract abnormalities*
Congenital or surgical abnormalities of the bladder and urethra present a significant technical challenge to transplant surgeons and place patients at increased risk of complications after their transplant. Such patients should have had careful planning during the transplant workup phase to ensure that any necessary investigations (in terms of assessing bladder, urethral, or alternative channels of urine outflow such as ileal conduits for their anatomical and functional status) have been undertaken prior to activation on the transplant list. These complex and often difficult to interpret assessments cannot be easily undertaken in the time-limited context of deceased donor organ transplantation but at least need to be flagged and planned for before urethral catheter removal. It is worth noting that lower urinary tract issues may not be immediately obvious before the transplant, especially in patients who are anuric.

(ii) *Coronary artery disease*
All patients with renal impairment are at significantly increased risk of coronary artery disease with a 10- to 100-fold higher risk of death due to cardiovascular disease compared to age-matched controls [6]. This is contributed to by age, dialysis, and other risk factors, such as hypertension, diabetes, and obesity. Although the renal transplant surgical procedure is not usually a very prolonged or difficult operation from an anaesthetic point of view, peri- or posttransplant coronary ischaemia or myocardial infarction remains an important and difficult-to-manage complication in transplant recipients. Units will usually have a local protocol for attempting to identify clinically silent coronary artery disease in high-risk populations (such as diabetics) prior to listing for transplant. It is important that these investigations remain up to date (in accordance with local and/or national guidelines) and that the results are available out of hours.

Patients with known severe left ventricular dysfunction are at particular risk in the immediate posttransplant period as they may not be able to sustain the traditional aggressive fluid loading used to encourage prompt graft function, and poor graft perfusion due to pump failure can leave them at increased risk of delayed graft function.

(iii) *Peripheral vascular disease (PVD)*
Atheromatous disease, which is very common in renal patients, can cause problems with the arterial anastomosis at the time of surgery, especially when there is circumferential calcification of the iliac vessels. The main issue is in identifying a landing site for the transplant artery and an area to place the arterial clamps. Transplant units vary in their preoperative assessment of PVD prior to surgery with some undertaking no formal imaging of the vessels if the clinical examination is normal and the patient is asymptomatic. Imaging options include duplex ultrasound and non-contrast CT. The latter is commonly reserved for individuals with known PVD, diabetics and those who may have had multiple transplants into both groins. Haemodialysis access procedures involving the proximal leg vessels (such as thigh Gore-Tex grafts) are usually distal to the normal sites of arterial vascular anastomosis, but need to be known about prior to surgery.

(iv) *Venous anatomy*
Although much rarer than arterial atheromatous disease, venous occlusive disease of the proximal leg veins secondary to DVT or the use of femoral dialysis catheters may determine the site of transplant implantation. It is preferable to avoid the use of femoral lines on the side of the transplant.

(v) *Previous transplant history*
A careful history in relation to previous transplantation is necessary, as any previous graft will (by definition) have failed or be failing. The cause of previous graft failure will often have an impact on the initial immunosuppressive regimen used, and the location of these kidneys will need to be considered by the transplant surgeons.

Other pertinent questions to ask upon the patient's arrival to hospital are whether they produce urine and if so, how much, and whether they have had any urological issues. If patients have been anuric for many years they may have a very small bladder that is difficult to find at the time of surgery. It is also helpful to know whether they have developed any new symptoms of peripheral vascular disease (such as intermittent claudication) and whether they have recently had any issues with infections, including dental and skin infections, such as ulcers.

Patients should undergo a full examination including their cardiorespiratory and vascular systems, abdominal examination including the groins for pulses, examination of the mouth for dental abscesses and the feet for ulcers. Preoperative investigations should include blood tests, urinalysis, and a chest X-ray if not performed recently. The main blood tests of interest are the full blood count to assess for anaemia, thrombocytopenia, and signs of infection and the renal function to assess the need for dialysis pre-transplant. A coagulation screen is also important, especially in patients who are anticoagulated who may need their INR reversing preoperatively.

91.2.4 The Cross-Match (See ► Chap. 67)

▪ Blood Group Compatibility

It is the responsibility of the transplant team to double-check donor–recipient blood group compatibility. This is usually done by the consultant surgeon who confirms this with the anaesthetist and theatre team ahead of the transplant going ahead by correlating the paperwork that comes with the kidney with the group and save sample collected from the recipient.

▪ Standard Cross-Matching

Prior to understanding the importance of antibodies, hyperacute, antibody-mediated rejection was the leading cause of immediate graft failure in kidney transplantation. It is now well known that the presence of preformed, complement fixing, donor-specific antibodies (almost always directed against HLA antigens) was driving this process [7]. Since this discovery, it has been a standard practice to undertake some form of assessment of the presence of preformed donor-specific antibodies (dsAb) prior to proceeding with the kidney transplant operation. The modalities for doing this have grown progressively in their complexity and sensitivity, with the division of the target cells into T- and B-cell cross-matches (assumed to present class I and class I and II molecular targets for dsAb binding, respectively), the use of techniques to remove the effects of IgM dsAb (generally although not universally believed to be of little clinical significance), the development of flow-cytometric cross-matches (which will detect the binding of dsAb which cannot mediate in vitro cytotoxicity), and most recently the use of recombinant HLA molecules bound to tagged flow-cytometry beads [8]. The significance of low-level dsAb is currently debated. It is clear that outcomes are better in non-sensitized recipients and that while some antibodies that are detectable by the highly sensitive recombinant/solid-phase assays (without resulting in a positive cross-match) may not be acutely harmful to the graft, they are important markers of medium-term risk [9].

▪ Non-HLA Antibodies

Donor-specific antibodies directed against non-HLA antigens do exist and are not detected by assays based on recombinant HLA targets. Early antibody-mediated rejection due to such antibodies is rare [10], but as outcomes in renal transplantation improve, the relative significance of this pathway is increasing [11], as is interest in the detection of non-HLA antibodies.

▪ Virtual Cross-Matching (See ► Chap. 67)

The term "virtual crossmatch" is applied to the use of antibody data, detected by the highly sensitive solid-phase/recombinant target platforms, to predict crossmatch outcome based on a comprehensive knowledge of the specificity of any detected antibody, and the potential reactivity with a donor of a given HLA type [12]. This has allowed the confident recognition of the complete absence of HLA-specific antibodies in unsensitized individuals, allowing the transplant procedure to go ahead without the need for a laboratory crossmatch taking place, which potentially reduces the CIT for deceased donor transplants. It relies on a recent recipient serum sample being held in the tissue typing lab for analysis.

▪ Surgical Preparation of the Organ

Assuming that the patient is medically fit and the crossmatch is negative, the final hurdle is the confirmation that the retrieved organ is suitable for transplantation. Ahead of the kidney departing the retrieval hospital the SNOD will commonly notify NHSBT of the donor anatomy, which is then communicated to the transplant surgeon at the implanting centre. In the event that issues have been identified intraoperatively (i.e., a lesion on the kidney, obvious retrieval damage, or evidence of poor perfusion) it is not uncommon for the retrieval surgeon to call the accepting kidney surgeon while still in theatre with the donor. Photos can be confidentially sent to the implanting surgeon if requested.

Once the organ has arrived at the implanting centre it must be prepared for implantation; a process commonly known as "benching". Benching the kidney involves a global assessment of the organ, looking specifically at the parenchyma of the kidney (and to confirm the absence of suspicious lesions), the perfusion, and the vascular and ureteric anatomy. In the event that a lesion is identified it is imperative that the implanting surgeon notifies the other implanting centres receiving the other organs immediately. Assuming there are no issues with the kidney the vessels are dissected free from neighbouring fat and soft tissues, including part of the adrenal gland which often comes with the kidney. The fat surrounding the kidney is also removed, however the area between the infero-medial aspect of the kidney and the ureter (known as the "golden triangle") is left. This is because the vessels providing blood to the ureter area are commonly located in this fat and need to be preserved.

91.3 Immunosuppression (See ► Chap. 70)

The choice of immunosuppressive drugs used for the initial posttransplant period will be determined by local protocols, often with different regimens aiming to address different levels of immunological risk. Improvements in immunosuppressive strategies and the associated reduction in allograft rejection and minimization of side effects have been central to the improved survival seen in renal transplantation. Due to the range of drugs available and possibly the different stakeholders in each transplant unit, there is considerable variation of immunosuppression protocols between units, despite the UK National Institute for Health and Clinical Excellence (NICE) guidelines [13]. The commonly used drugs are described here briefly.

91.3.1 Calcineurin Inhibitors (CNIs)

Within the modern era of renal transplantation CNIs have become the mainstay of immunosuppression and their use can be credited with decreased rates of rejection and better short- and long-term survival in the last decade. The pharmacokinetics of CNIs can be monitored with 12-hour trough values. Elevation or depression of immunosuppressive drug concentrations can be toxic and predispose to graft dysfunction, infection, and neurotoxicity, whereas subtherapeutic values can predispose to rejection. It is therefore important to remember that a number of other drugs can interfere with the metabolism of CNIs via the cytochrome P450 pathway.

The last 20 years of clinical research in transplant immunosuppression have been dominated by a still-unresolved debate about the extent to which the undoubted short-term benefits of CNI use (in terms of acute rejection and graft survival) are undermined by the long-term consequences of chronic CNI toxicity. High-dose cyclosporin-based regimens are undoubtedly associated with essentially universal medium- and long-term graft dysfunction associated with histological changes attributable to CNI toxicity [14]. It is not clear whether tacrolimus, which is moderately more effective and less nephrotoxic, suffers from the same long-term disadvantages. Attempts to develop CNI-free regimens (at least those based on sirolimus plus MMF) have been broadly unsuccessful in terms of high rejection rates and poor graft survival [15].

91.3.1.1 Tacrolimus (FK506)

91

Tacrolimus is a macrolide antibiotic which has immunosuppressive properties. It exerts its effects by bonding to an immunophilin (FK506-binding protein (FKBP)). This complex then inhibits calcineurin phosphatase, which in turn inhibits calcium-dependent events, such as interleukin-2 gene transcription, nitric oxide synthase activation, cell degranulation, and apoptosis [16]. Tacrolimus is more effective in preventing acute rejection than its predecessor cyclosporin (CyA) [17, 18] and has been found to result in superior graft survival [19]. As a consequence it is the de facto CNI agent of choice.

In addition to the benefits on rates of acute rejection and graft survival, tacrolimus also has a preferable cardiovascular profile than CyA in terms of blood pressure and lipids. However, it is associated with a higher rate of new onset diabetes after transplantation (NODAT) due to peripheral insulin resistance. This problem can be diminished by the avoidance of long-term steroid exposure. A non-generic, modified release version of tacrolimus (Advagraf) and an expanding range of generic slow-release versions offer once-daily dosing regimens.

91.3.1.2 Ciclosporin or Cyclosporin (CsA or CyA)

Ciclosporin has a similar mode of action to tacrolimus. The modern formulation Neoral is a microemulsion and provides more reliable absorption from the gastrointestinal tract. Long-term side effects specific to ciclosporin are hirsutism, hypertension, dyslipidaemia, and gum hypertrophy (especially in conjunction with calcium antagonists).

91.3.2 Antiproliferative Agents

91.3.2.1 Mycophenolic Acid (MPA/MMF/Myfortic)

Mycophenolic acid (MPA) is a noncompetitive and selective antagonist to inosine monophosphate dehydrogenase, which is an enzyme important in the de novo synthesis of purines. The concentrations of MPA, although not commonly measured, can be monitored with 12-hour tough levels or with longer area under the curve sampling and calculation to avoid side effects (leucopenia, infection, and gastrointestinal upset) while maintaining effective immunosuppression. MMF is recommended by NICE as an initial option to prevent organ rejection in adults having a kidney transplant when it is used as part of an immunosuppressive regimen [13]. The inclusion of MMF in the optimum arm of the SYMPHONY study [19] has cemented its widespread in regimens including an antiproliferative agent.

91.3.2.2 Azathioprine

Azathioprine is derived from 6-mercaptopurine, which interferes with DNA synthesis. Together with corticosteroids, it provided the mainstay immunosuppressive agent until the introduction of CyA in the 1980s and subsequently became part of standard triple therapy immunosuppression with both steroids and CyA thereafter. Despite NICE recommendations for azathioprine use in low-risk transplantation, it has been abandoned by many units in favour of mycophenolate mofetil. In female transplant recipients planning a pregnancy, MMF is normally switched to azathioprine in advance.

91.3.3 mTOR Inhibitors (Rapamycin: Sirolimus and Everolimus)

Rapamycin also binds to FK-binding protein and inhibits cytokine-induced signal transduction pathways by impairment of progression through the G1 phase of the cell cycle. Consequently it inhibits the proliferation of T cells. Rapamycin does not produce the long-term nephrotoxicity associated with CNIs and therefore has been used as a replacement for CNIs in both the acute and chronic settings. It has also been used in association with CNIs in place of antiproliferative drugs. Although the predominant benefit is the reduction of calcineurin toxicity, it has been shown to be superior to CyA and steroids (both with and without azathioprine) in the prevention of acute rejection [20, 21], but this may be associated with an increased risk of infection (especially infections associated with delayed wound healing) [22].

Blocking mTOR has been shown to reduce tumorigenesis in vitro, and anecdotal reports do exist in vivo such as in Kaposi's sarcoma. Side effects include hyperlipidaemia; proteinuria with associated focal glomerular sclerosis; marrow suppression (mostly erythropoietin-requiring anaemia), especially when used in combination with MPA; lymphocoele formation; poor wound healing; testicular atrophy in men; and cystic ovaries. In some patients with a low glomerular filtration rate (GFR), rapamycin has been associated with proteinaceous bronchiolitis. In addition, poor wound healing has made this drug difficult to use in the immediate postoperative period.

91.3.4 Corticosteroids (Prednisolone, Methylprednisolone)

Corticosteroids act as agonists of glucocorticoid receptors at low doses, but at higher doses their effects become non-specific and receptor independent. It is a great pity that corticosteroids, which have been the mainstay of immunosuppression throughout the evolution of transplantation, are associated with deleterious side effects such as susceptibility to infection, weight gain, NODAT, hypertension, hyperlipidaemia, and osteopenia. The increased cardiovascular risk and death associated with steroid side effects have led many transplant centres to reduce or avoid steroid exposure in the immediate postoperative period or alternatively to withdraw steroids at a later date after successful transplantation.

Attempts to run long-term steroid-free maintenance regimens from CyA-based immunosuppressive platforms were associated with inferior graft survival [23], but the availability of tacrolimus and MMF has allowed the development of steroid-free long-term regimens with excellent outcomes [24] despite the slightly increased rejection risk associated with early steroid withdrawal, even under "modern" immunosuppression [25].

91.3.5 Induction Agents: Monoclonal and Polyclonal Antibodies

NICE recommends the use of Basiliximab (a monoclonal antibody) at induction when used as part of an immunosuppressive regimen that includes a CNI [13]. While commonly used as an alternative, T cell depleting antibody therapy is not risk-free, and while units will have well-developed protocols, it is important to consider the pros and cons of these agents for the individual due to be transplanted, ideally as part of their workup. These are covered in ▶ Chap. 70 on transplant immunosuppression.

91.3.6 Data Collection

Once the renal transplant recipient is discharged to outpatient follow-up in the transplant clinic, it is important that baseline information is easily available. An overview of relevant information is provided in ◘ Table 91.1.

91.3.7 In Recovery

In the immediate postoperative period, the recipient should undergo a careful volume status assessment, including a review of anaesthetic charts, for an estimation of fluid balance. The significance of pre-transplant urine volume/anuria is important to acknowledge when interpreting the immediate postoperative urine output. Recipients of living donor kidneys can pass significant volumes of urine in the hours immediately after a transplant. Physical examination of the patient should include their chest (to assess for evidence of fluid overload) and the legs to confirm distal perfusion. A discussion with the surgical team or review of the operative note should highlight any intraoperative difficulties and specific areas of consideration/concern postoperatively.

If consistent with local institutional practice, an ultrasound of the graft in recovery is extremely useful for establishing a baseline and allowing prompt return to theatres for reexploration in the (extremely rare) event of impaired perfusion following wound closure. This is typically caused by direct compression of the graft or vessels in recipients who have had a large kidney

Table 91.1 Data collection

Recipient details	Primary renal diagnosis
	Renal replacement therapy timeline (include positive confirmation if pre-emptive transplant)
	CMV, EBV, HIV, VZV status
	Hypertension history (including drugs)
	Vascular history (coronary/cerebral, peripheral)
	Dry weight pre-transplant
Donor details	Live vs deceased donor (Deceased after cardiac death (DCD) vs deceased after brain death (DBD))
	Donor age
	Cause of death
	Donor comorbidity (hypertension, diabetes, renal impairment)
	Cold ischaemic time
	Surgical warm ischaemic time (and pre-agonal WIT for deceased donors with prior out-of-hospital arrest and agonal WIT for DCDs)
	Number of arteries, veins and ureters
	Surgical comments on: on-table perfusion, any vessels sacrificed and the bladder
	Presence of (and plan for) ureteric stent
	Infections bacterial or viral
Transplant details	HLA matching (A:B:DR)
	Presence of any repeat mismatches
	Any known antibody incompatibility (ABO, HLA) and what/whether desensitization was undertaken
	Induction immunosuppressive therapy (if used)
	Maintenance immunosuppression used (and planned)
	Prompt vs delayed graft function
	Problems or issues with wound
	Rejection episodes
Discharge details	Creatinine at discharge
	Weight at discharge
	Drug levels (including trend) at discharge
	Prophylaxis for opportunistic infection given
	Dialysis access (venous lines/PD catheter) action and plan

implanted into a narrow pelvis, where positioning has been difficult or where torsion of the vessels has occurred.

Clinical investigations should include an urgent potassium, which is essential to determine dialysis requirement, especially if no urine is forthcoming. A chest x-ray for fluid balance assessment and confirmation of the correct positioning of the central line is also necessary.

When there is primary graft function the initial urine output is often high. It is not uncommon for loop diuretics and / or mannitol to be administered at the time of the anastomosis or reperfusion in theatre despite the complete lack of evidence suggesting any benefit. Attention should also be paid to blood loss from surgical drains (if placed), and the patient should be haemodynamically stable prior to return to the transplant ward.

91.3.8 The First 24 Hours

Recipients with primary graft function are usually straightforward to manage during the initial post-transplant period with the focus being on maintaining satisfactory fluid balance, administration of immunosuppression, and vigilance for early surgical complications. Common practice is to provide intravenous fluid (usually crystalloid) to match the urine output, but care must be taken to factor in the volume of other fluids being administered intravenously (blood, other colloids, and intravenous drugs) or by mouth, since overenthusiastic fluid administration leading to overload is a common problem. As soon as the patient is able to mobilize, daily weights are a helpful check on the tendency to overfill the recently transplanted (and can be compared to the pre-transplant weight or dialysis target dry weight). Patients are swiftly moved onto oral fluids as soon as they are able to match their urine output orally. A close eye needs to be kept on fluid balance around the time that intravenous fluids are removed to ensure the patient remains adequately hydrated.

Autoregulation of renal blood flow is impaired after even short periods of cold ischaemia, so the graft needs to be protected from hypoperfusion by ensuring an adequate blood pressure (aiming for mean arterial pressure of at least 65 mmHg). If this cannot be achieved with the establishment of adequate intravascular fluid volume, then pressor agents may be used; some units still use dopamine (at or slightly above the traditional "renal" dose of 2–5 μg/kg/h), although the formal evidence that this agent has any renal protective effect other than the promotion of diuresis in this context is limited [26, 27].

Recipients who remain oliguric posttransplant or whose urine output declines steadily after an initial period (of typically 2–6 hours) of reasonable urine output require careful management. A "pre-renal, renal, post-renal" approach to assessing oliguria or anuria after a transplant provides a system for excluding common causes. An ultrasound of the graft and chest X-ray should be arranged, and after a careful clinical assessment of fluid balance and assessment for evidence of bleeding, a fluid challenge (usually 250–500 ml) should be given. If the recipient is adequately filled and not bleeding, a furosemide infusion may help manage hyperkalaemia and avoid acute dialysis but does not shorten the AKI, and it is important to ensure intravascular volume is adequately maintained. The use of potassium binders, such as sodium zirconium cyclosilicate, is an increasingly popular way to manage hyperkalaemia in patients whose transplant is anticipated to start functioning adequately in the next few days. Assuming the patient is adequately filled and the ultrasound and doppler demonstrate adequate perfusion of the graft the patient can be assumed to be in DGF. Serial ultrasounds over subsequent days will provide further reassurance that the graft is perfused.

91.3.9 The First Week

Obsessive attention should be paid to urine output, haemoglobin, serum creatinine, and clinical examination directed towards the wound and fluid balance in the first week after transplantation. Monitoring of these parameters is likely to occur several times a day and night. Ideally the creatinine should fall by 50% on a daily basis and failing that, a fall by >10% is also acceptable, as this is acknowledged to be greater than the variability of the laboratory analyser. Should creatinine not fall, or worse rise, then addressing the volume status is paramount. It is an unfortunate paradox that CNIs have a narrow therapeutic window and are nephrotoxic at high doses so drug levels should be performed regularly (12-hour trough) and dose adjustments made if necessary. A transplant USS will ensure that perfusion is adequate and exclude obstruction. If all of these are addressed systematically and the creatinine remains suboptimal, then renal allograft biopsy remains the gold standard for diagnosis and is performed as either an open or percutaneous procedure according to local protocols. A post-perfusion biopsy in theatre (called a "time zero biopsy") is often very helpful in determining the severity of AKI and degree of chronic damage. Should the paired kidney be transplanted in the same unit, it is often helpful to compare patients as the kidneys are likely to behave similarly and this may guide the timing of a biopsy.

Baseline samples should be taken during the early posttransplant period for analysis of proteinuria and samples stored for the presence of anti-HLA antibodies, as these may be invaluable in establishing a time frame if subsequent problems with recurrent proteinuric disease or antibody-mediated rejection occur.

In the case of delayed graft function (DGF), it can be several weeks before independent kidney function is achieved, and regular dialysis may be required during this period. This can be a frustrating time for patients and physician alike. It is important to always contemplate the possibility of early rejection, which can be confirmed or excluded by a biopsy. Should the patient still require regular dialysis, biopsies should be performed approximately weekly to further confirm that there is no rejection. Continued vigilance towards urine output, fluid balance, weight, tacrolimus levels and allograft perfusion is essential.

Over the course of the first week the various items of surgical paraphernalia may be removed, including surgical drains, the central line, peripheral cannulae and finally the catheter, which is typically removed on day 5, although sometimes earlier in living donor transplantation. Patients with a stent usually have this removed around 6 weeks after their transplant. This is either done in theatre or in outpatients under local anaesthetic via a flexible cystoscopy with antibiotic cover. Some stents are magnetic and can be removed in clinic using a specially designed magnet which is inserted per urethra. If a patient requires a general anaesthetic for removal of their line or peritoneal dialysis catheter then it is not unreasonable to take the stent out while they are asleep.

91.3.10 Early Graft Dysfunction

Early complications are predominantly based around poor or reducing urine volumes (◘ Table 91.2), the failure of the creatinine to fall at a desirable rate, wound infections, catheter problems, and fluid balance difficulties. The catheter is usually removed in the first few days after transplantation, although this is often prolonged if intra-operatively there are surgical concerns about the bladder anastomosis- or patient-related issues that may put pressure on the bladder anastomosis.

The commonest infections encountered within the immediate posttransplant period are wound, urine, and chest. While antibiotics are usually given at induction, local protocols will vary with regard to further postoperative antibiotics. A high index of suspicion should be maintained throughout the postoperative course. Basal atelectasis is common following a general anaesthetic and is exacerbated by being in bed for prolonged periods of time, immobility and pain. Patients

Table 91.2 Early oliguria post-renal transplant

Clinical symptoms suggestive of bleeding or graft thrombosis such as pain over graft/abdomen and presence of blood in the surgical drain	
Risk factors—difficult anastomosis, multiple vessels, procoagulant state, patient with small pelvis	
Clinical signs suggestive of hypovolaemia, bleeding, or graft thrombosis such as hypotension, tachycardia, graft tenderness, and frank haematuria	
Exclude blocked catheter and clot retention	
Urgent ECG, CXR, bloods. Consider cross-matching four units of type-specific blood if bleeding is suspected.	
Venous gas for potassium and haemoglobin	
With hypotension	*Without hypotension*
Resuscitate IV	Fluid challenge if clinical evidence of hypovolaemia
If evidence of bleeding with falling Hb, transfuse and call a surgeon for urgent review. Keep the patient nil by mouth and ask the nursing staff to prepare the patient for theatre	Treat hyperkalaemia if present Bladder washout +/– change of catheter if in clot retention by surgical team Urgent USS for graft perfusion and patency of vessels and exclude obstruction
If deranged clotting or thrombocytopenia, consider FFP and platelets	Evidence of graft thrombosis (i.e., presence of reversed diastolic flow on USS) – contact the surgical team urgently and prepare the patient for theatre
Urgent USS/CT for perfusion and evidence of haematoma and exclude obstruction (e.g., compression from haematoma) may be indicated but should not delay surgery if the patient is unstable	If reduced cortical perfusion/no flow in diastole with patent large vessels, consider intraparenchymal pathology such as AMR Check for DSA and pro-thrombotic screen
If hypovolaemia and bleeding excluded, consider other causes for hypotension such as cardiac causes	

should be encouraged to ensure they can take regular deep breaths and cough reasonably comfortably, and if not they should be encouraged to ask for more analgesia. Early mobilization with the aid of physiotherapists also reduces the risks of developing chest sepsis. Early mobilization also helps to counteract the gastrointestinal effects of opiate medications, such as constipation and ileus. All of these infections will usually respond to broad-spectrum antibiotics but those with a more significant wound infection may need further surgical intervention.

91.3.11 Delayed Graft Function (DGF)

Failure of the transplanted kidney to function promptly as a consequence of acute tubular injury is common within the deceased donor kidney transplant population, and occurs most commonly in grafts exposed to extended cold and / or warm ischaemia and in kidneys from expanded criteria donors. DGF also occurs in living donor kidney transplantation, however this is extremely rare. It is imperative that living donor kidney recipients are rigorously assessed and investigated if there is any evidence of oliguria or anuria in the hours posttransplant. A surgeon should be actively involved with a low threshold for taking the patient back to theatre in order to confirm perfusion of the graft. Ultrasound findings consistent with DGF demonstrate perfusion and raised resistive indices, which are non-specific. It is not uncommon for oliguria to develop progressively after a few hours of urine production postoperatively and is thought to be a consequence of the reperfusion phase of ischaemia-reperfusion injury. A common reaction to DGF is to reduce the exposure to CNIs, although evidence that this is effective is marginal [28, 29].

Care must be taken to avoid overfilling the oliguric recipient and regular fluid balance assessments are necessary to monitor this. Dialysis should be instituted in a timely fashion if required and careful, repeated assessments of the patient and the graft should be undertaken to exclude other causes of graft dysfunction which may supervene before the onset of function. Investigations are likely to include repeated ultrasound scans and regular biopsies, with the first biopsy taking place on postoperative day 7 and then at weekly intervals until function is established.

91.3.12 Thrombosis and Anticoagulation

Transplant arterial or venous thrombosis remains a rare but difficult to manage complication. Patients at risk include those with a known pro-thrombotic tendency, although the predictive value of standard tests for thrombophilia is low [30] and the causative role of thrombophilia in hypercoagulability in kidney transplant recipients is unclear [31]. Other factors include the anatomical position of the kidney and the possibility of a haematoma causing compression of the vessels. Prolonged CIT also predisposes patients to thrombosis. Prophylaxis with low-dose aspirin is known to be effective [32], although this carries an increased risk of bleeding should an early biopsy be required. Heparin (usually subcutaneous unfractionated or low-molecular weight (LMW)) is also used, with due appreciation needed of the effects of low-GFR on clearance of LMW heparins. The initiation of anticoagulation is a matter for careful discussion with the surgeons involved in the procedure and should be based on the amount of intraoperative blood loss and the perceived chances of postoperative bleeding, an assessment of the patient's risk of thrombosis or bleeding based on their past medical history, the anatomy of the graft and the early postoperative platelet count.

The commonest signs of arterial or venous thrombosis are changes to the urine output. Abrupt anuria with little pain is typically characteristic of an arterial thrombosis which may also be accompanied by platelet consumption with peripheral thrombocytopenia and absence of parenchymal perfusion on ultrasound scan. By this stage there is a real risk of losing the graft and while surgical strategies are deployable, most commonly an operation results in a graft nephrectomy. Sudden onset pain and swelling over the graft and oliguria prior to anuria is more characteristic of venous thrombosis. The patient may also get macroscopic haematuria. The pain is typically caused by an increase in pressure within the kidney which is at risk of rupture. The ultrasound will demonstrate reversal of flow in diastole.

In both situations, the availability of a prior baseline ultrasound is extremely helpful to allow assessment of the extent to which factors such as body habitus, juxtaposition of vessels, and existing variation in regional perfusion and pulse pressure may influence the reliability of ultrasound-derived information. The assessment of graft perfusion by CT scan with contrast provides more objective information that can be derived from ultrasound, but risks precipitating or prolonging AKI and, more importantly, delaying a return to theatre. Contrast-enhanced ultrasound may offer a rapid, bedside test with greater sensitivity than doppler ultrasound, but the availability of this is variable.

91.3.13 Acute Cellular Rejection (ACR)

The increasing use of biological induction therapy combined with the use of high-efficacy agents such as tacrolimus and mycophenolate has been associated with a sharp reduction in the incidence of early acute cellular rejection (◘ Fig. 91.1) [19]. This does, however, still occur, even in recipients not obviously at high risk as a result of prior sensitization, history of previous immunological graft loss, low CNI levels, or young recipient age. In grafts with immediate function, the onset of graft dysfunction due to cellular rejection can vary from the indolent (over several days) to the very rapid, with rising creatinine and falling urine volume. Despite several decades of endeavour, no non-invasive test has proved to have sufficient predictive value to replace the creatinine as screening modality, and transplant biopsy as the definitive investigation, for cellular rejection [33].

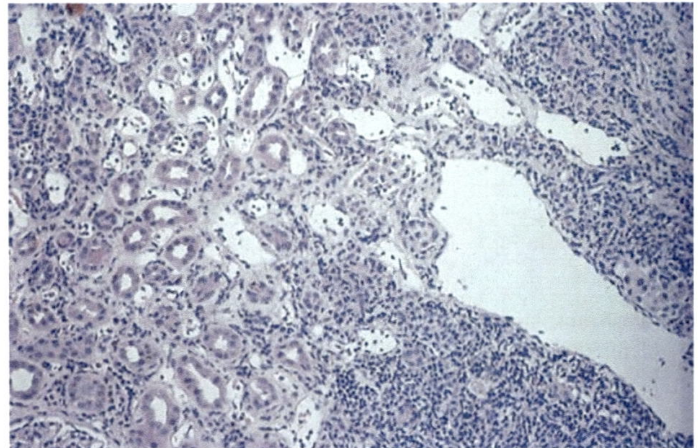

◘ **Fig. 91.1** Low-powered view of acute cellular rejection showing cellular infiltrate with lymphocytes invading tubules (tubulitis). Differential diagnosis is shown in ◘ Table 91.3

The timing of a transplant biopsy in the early postoperative period is largely determined by the desirability of maintaining anticoagulation in the initial posttransplant period and the potential difficulty of managing post-biopsy haemorrhage in a potentially unstable early postoperative window. Seven days posttransplant is generally considered a safe time point for percutaneous biopsy. Prior to this, and especially in the first 3–4 days, consideration should be given to open biopsy as the safest method of obtaining a definitive tissue diagnosis for graft dysfunction, with the added benefit of allowing direct examination of the graft and vessels which will encompass important parts of the differential diagnosis of early graft dysfunction (◘ Table 91.3 and ◘ Figs. 91.1 and 91.2).

91.3.14 Acute Antibody-Mediated Rejection

Acute antibody-mediated rejection remains a rare complication except in the context of planned (or unwitting) transplantation against a preexisting donor-specific antibody barrier, be that a HLA or non-HLA protein, or ABO-blood group antigens. The reducing incidence of cellular rejection makes this an increasingly important cause of early graft dysfunction [35]. The

Table 91.3 Differential diagnosis of cellular infiltrates in transplant biopsies, see [34]

T cell rejection (ACR)	Tubulitis (Fig. 91.1) with or without vascular (Fig. 91.2) and glomerular involvement. Typically interstitial infiltrate is lymphocytic but may also contain eosinophils, neutrophils, and macrophages. More likely in under patients who are immunosuppressed, commonest cause of interstitial infiltrate
Polyoma virus nephropathy	BKV (95%) or JC (≤5%), interstitial infiltrate typically rich in plasma cells, enlarged atypical tubular nuclei but may be indistinguishable from ACR thus SV40 large T antigen stain critical in all presumed ACR. BKV is more likely in over immunosuppressed
Posttransplant lymphoproliferative disorder (PTLD)	More common in the graft early on EBV D+/R-, monotonous diffuse infiltrate suggestive, immunohistochemistry (EBNA) staining critical
Cytomegalovirus nephropathy	A rare cause of interstitial nephritis, other end-organ damage usually apparent before renal involvement. Viral inclusion bodies may be seen in glomerular and tubular cells with enlarged "owl's eye" effect. Extensive infiltrate uncommon
Bacterial Pyelonephritis	Neutrophil casts in tubules highly suggestive but may coexist with ACR. Positive urine culture helpful but can frequently occur in the absence of positive MSU, especially after short course of antibiotics. Cellular infiltrate pleomorphic including neutrophils and the second commonest cause and more likely in those with recent UTIs especially if recurrent, diabetes, abnormal bladder, and stent in situ
Mycobacterial infection	Ethnicity and country of origin may indicate high risk, often associated with granulomas (acid-fast bacilli rarely seen)
Recurrent disease	Important to consider in patients with an original disease associated with acute interstitial nephritis such as sarcoid, vasculitis, SLE but all unusual in the early stages of a transplant due to augmented immunosuppression
Allergic interstitial nephritis	Common transplant drugs such as septrin, proton pump inhibitors, azathioprine, and penicillins may all cause an interstitial nephritis confused with ACR
ACR: Acute Cellular Rejection	

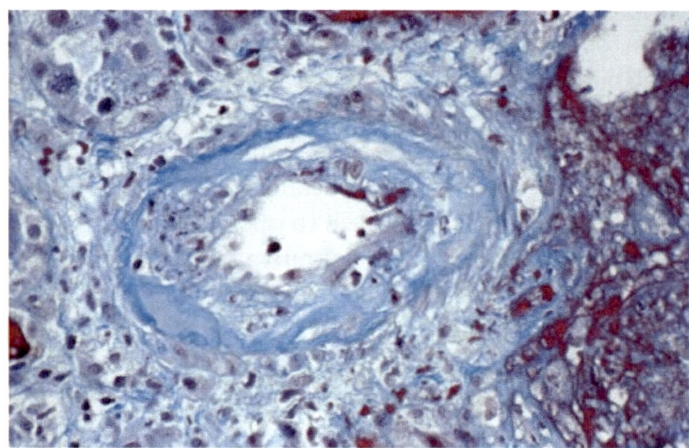

Fig. 91.2 Vascular rejection: arteriole showing lymphocytic infiltrate under the endothelium of the vessel

91

presentation may often be dramatic, with sudden onset anuria, often presaged by macroscopic haematuria. Classically, graft dysfunction will be preceded by the development of rapidly rising levels of donor-specific antibodies, as assessed by fluorescence intensity on solid-phase bead-based Luminex assay.

With improvements in tissue typing, much of which has occurred alongside the development of solid-phase antibody assays, there has been improved detection of both preformed and de novo anti-HLA antibody which is associated with AMR. Controversy remains regarding the practical importance of these tests in the absence of a positive flow or cytotoxic cross-match, but undoubtedly their presence should raise suspicion of AMR. A renal allograft biopsy remains the gold standard for diagnosis (Fig. 91.2), either open or percutaneous in accordance with local protocols. If a biopsy is contraindicated (i.e., due to proximity in time to surgery, overlying bowel, patient fitness, anticoagulation, risk of graft rupture), then presumptive therapy may be advised. Most protocols use a combination of intravenous corticosteroids and plasma exchange with or without the addition of intravenous immunoglobulin and mono- or polyclonal antibody therapy.

In the presence of early AMR refractory to standard therapy, the complement inhibitor eculizumab and proteasome inhibitor bortezomib are potential therapies still undergoing evaluation.

91.3.15 Urine Outflow Obstruction

If the patient is catheterized, then always ensure the catheter is not blocked, either by external pressure (lying on catheter or it being clamped accidentally) or clot retention. The latter will require either a catheter change or flushing which should be performed by a transplant surgeon, with care not to impact on the vesicoureteric anastomosis. Irrigation of the bladder can not only jeopardise the bladder anastomosis but make fluid balance incredibly difficult to record and can be complicated by hyponatraemia. It is sensible to record the urine output and empty the chamber of the catheter bag prior to performing a bladder washout in order to minimize confusion. Instrumentation of a renal patient's urethra, which often has not had urine passage, may not be straightforward and can lead to false passages which should also be considered in terms of catheter placement. In elderly anuric men on dialysis, prostatic obstruction may only declare itself after renal transplantation and should be anticipated.

91.4 Other Postoperative Considerations

91.4.1 Hypotension

The crucial differential diagnosis for the hypotensive patient in the early posttransplant period lies between haemorrhage and sepsis. In the former case, the patient will usually be peripherally shutdown and cold, while in the latter they will be vasodilated and hot. Beyond basic clinical examination, including close attention to the contents of surgical drains, an ultrasound will demonstrate peri-transplant haematoma, but cannot easily detect retroperitoneal haemorrhage. A CT scan will demonstrate this clearly but has the disadvantage of exposing the recently transplanted kidney to a contrast load and may also delay a return to theatre. Should the patient be unstable then a CT should not delay urgent surgical reexploration.

When a CVP line is present, the response of the central venous pressure to fluid bolus administration can be used to gauge adequacy of filling, although the common complications in dialysis patients of thoracic vein stenosis or thrombosis and cardiac ventricular dysfunction / poor ventricular compliance may need to be borne in mind. It is often helpful to discuss the patient's prior behaviour on dialysis (in terms of the BP response to fluid loading) with the physician who looked after them on dialysis.

Patients with diabetes (or other primary renal diseases associated with autonomic dysfunction) will often have marked postural falls in BP in the early transplant period, and care must be taken on their initial postoperative mobilization to avoid significant hypotensive episodes which may be sufficient to cause falls or compromise graft perfusion.

Cyto-depleting induction therapies, whether monoclonal (alemtuzumab) or polyclonal (anti-thymocyte globulins), may be associated with a cytokine release syndrome presenting with hypotension, rigors, thrombocytopenia, and occasionally a brisk spike in temperature. If not already given as part of the induction regimen, IV steroids (100 mg hydrocortisone) and IV antihistamines will usually control the reaction which is relatively short-lived (1–3 h).

91.4.2 Hypertension

The almost universal tendency to strive for a high urine output during the initial posttransplant period makes fluid overload with associated hypertension an extremely common phenomenon in the first few days posttransplant. Beyond attempting to avoid the all-too-common scenario of a patient with high blood pressure after intravenous administration of excess fluid, patients will often require staged reintroduction (or commencement) of antihypertensive medication. ACE inhibitors and angiotensin receptor blockers are often viewed with anxiety in the early postoperative period because of the theoretical risk of interfering with intrinsic homeostatic responses to volume stress in a kidney which is recovering from ischaemia-reperfusion injury, but the definite long-term benefits of these agents, which interrupt the renin/angiotensin system [36], do make them attractive agents even in the early postoperative period. The suggestion that non-dihydropyridine calcium channel antagonists, such as verapamil and diltiazem, have a protective effect against CNI toxicity has made these popular agents for use in early posttransplant hypertension. In any event, agents which are very long-acting and renally excreted (such as atenolol) or liable to produce sharp drops in BP on first administration (such as standard-release nifedipine) should be avoided.

A proportion of recipients (especially the young and often in patients of Afro-Caribbean ethnic origin) will respond to volume depletion with a marked vasoconstrictor response accompanied by significant arterial hypertension. In this context, carefully controlled vasodilatation (with low-dose nitrates or other vasodilators) accompanied by cautious fluid replacement ("dilate-and-fill") will result in resolution of the hypertension, the vasoconstriction, and hopefully the associated hypoperfusion of the graft.

Careful attention to fluid balance with gradual reversion to a euvolaemic state (which may require careful use of loop diuretics) after any overenthusiastic initial fluid loading will usually bring the blood pressure under control, although the vasoconstrictor effects of calcineurin inhibitors mean that most transplant recipients require long-term antihypertensive medication.

91.4.3 Accelerated-Phase Hypertension/ Thrombotic Microangiopathy (TMA)

Hypertension associated with failure of microvascular endothelial homeostatic protection mechanisms is a rare but always challenging and complex event early posttransplantation. The differential diagnosis includes the extreme manifestation of CNI toxicity, recurrence of underlying atypical HUS / complement regulatory disease, and antibody-mediated rejection. Although moderate degrees of thrombocytopenia are common after cyto-depleting induction therapies, any fall in platelet count should trigger a request for examination of a peripheral blood film, LDH, and whatever serves as the local haemolysis screen. This is because the presence of RBC fragments or evidence of haemolysis gives early warning of microangiopathy. Consideration should also be given to the primary renal diagnosis since atypical HUS is difficult to diagnose and will frequently be labelled as "hypertensive nephropathy". Onset at a young age and a positive family history are important clues.

In the presence of established TMA, careful attention to CNI levels, an urgent search for donor-specific and anti-phospholipid antibodies, evidence of lupus or lupus-associated autoimmune disease, and the consideration of the possibility of recurrent atypical HUS or active hepatitis C should all be undertaken. If correction of fluid overload and control of hypertension using renin/angiotensin blockade do not result in resolution of the TMA, then plasma exchange with FFP infusion should be considered and, in the UK, discussion with the National Renal Complement Therapeutics Centre (▶ www.atypicalhus.co.uk) regarding the use of eculizumab.

Heparin-induced thrombocytopenia (HIT) may mimic the clinical presentation of posttransplant TMA but is an even rarer entity. Most of transplant recipients (with the exception of those preemptively transplanted) will have had ample heparin exposure prior to transplantation, and the absence of catastrophic reaction to heparin when stable on dialysis means that the many alternative causes of thrombocytopenia in the early posttransplant period are overwhelmingly more likely than HIT to be the explanation of a low platelet count in this situation.

91.4.4 Sepsis

In addition to the posttransplant infections mentioned above relating to surgery, transplant recipients are at risk of a spectrum of other infections related to immunosuppression.

Significant CMV disease prior to 3 months posttransplant remains rare, although it is more commonly seen in patients given T-cell depletion induction without CMV prophylaxis. It is easily diagnosed and treated using modern PCR-based diagnostics and the highly orally active agent valgancyclovir. Local protocols may involve the administration of prophylactic antiviral therapy after determination of risk by donor and recipient CMV status or may avoid prophylaxis in favour or serial monitoring of posttransplant recipient CMV PCR levels. It is important to familiarize yourself with the local protocol as there are variations, and should a serial monitoring approach be relied upon it is crucial to know who is responsible for ordering and checking results.

It is usual for prophylaxis to *Pneumocystis jirovecii* (previously known as *Pneumocystis carinii* or PCP) to be used universally with septrin or inhaled pentamide. TB prophylaxis should be considered and usually instituted in patients with previous history of TB and in patients deemed at high risk of developing TB posttransplant, such as those of Indoasian ethnic origin. Together with these approaches, the progressive reduction in the amount of corticosteroid administered during the early posttransplant period over the last three decades (even in those regimens not focussed on steroid avoidance) has altered the landscape of early posttransplant sepsis, with herpes virus reactivation and fungal sepsis becoming much less common.

Current immunosuppressive regimens are highly potent and effective, but leave patients a relatively low risk of significant early sepsis, except in the context of recipients at risk of chronic or recurrent urosepsis (such as those with polycystic kidney disease or abnormal lower urinary tract anatomy), respiratory tract sepsis (bronchiectasis, pulmonary scarring secondary to pulmonary-renal inflammatory disease, or, most dangerously, lung transplant recipients with their risk of fungal or multi-resistant bacterial colonization) or those exposed to de novo infection from contaminated organs. Positive perfusion fluid culture results should be treated with great seriousness, as representing a very high-risk situation.

91.4.5 Proteinuria

Moderate (presumably predominantly tubular) proteinuria is very common in the immediate posttransplant period as a consequence of the tubular injury during the cold ischaemic phase, but persistent, significant early proteinuria (protein/creatinine ratio >100 mg/mmol) indicates major glomerular pathology, with recurrent focal and segmental glomerulosclerosis (FSGS) the most important underlying cause. Membranous nephropathy and complement-abnormality-associated MPGN can recur posttransplant, but usually with a timescale presenting beyond the initial transplant admission. When associated with delayed graft function, this can be a difficult diagnosis to establish. Early biopsy may not detect focal glomerular scarring at an early stage, and electron microscopy may be required to identify the associated podocytopathy.

In the presence of established, or probable, recurrent FSGS, the main current therapeutic option is high doses of calcineurin inhibitors, steroids and aggressive plasma exchange.

91.4.6 Discharge Planning

Patients facing discharge after successful kidney transplantation have to cope with a range of important challenges and tasks.

The first of these will be a new and often complex drug regimen which will often include agents with a narrow therapeutic index and important toxicities. The discharge drug combination must be reviewed carefully with the patient to ensure they understand what the different drugs are for, how they should be taken and which may be subject to changes. Particular attention should be paid to immunosuppressive agents with regard to the importance of taking these in a regular manner, not missing doses, and when to delay morning doses of twice-daily drugs to allow measurement of trough drug levels. Patients need to know not to take additional drugs without prior discussion with the transplant unit because of the risk of drug interactions.

The second of these will be the amount of fluid the patient needs to drink to ensure the kidney remains well perfused. Patients are commonly fluid restricted prior to their transplant and the need to drink significantly higher volumes of fluid can often be challenging. Exacerbating this is that the recently transplanted kidney often takes several weeks to acquire the ability to regulate urine concentration adequately, and patients will often be discharged during a polyuric phase with high volume, low concentration urine. Patients therefore need to understand the importance of identifying and reacting to developing fluid depletion (or overload) which can be most accurately anticipated after discharge by asking patients to check a daily weight and adjust their salt and water intake accordingly. Recipients who were oliguric or anuric prior to transplantation may also suffer with increased urinary frequency as their bladder adjusts and adapts to the presence of urine, so they ought to be warned about this and strategies provided for retraining their bladder.

Patients transplanted preemptively need to understand that the early post-discharge period will involve much more frequent hospital attendance with disruption to their day-to-day activities than they were experiencing in the pretransplant period. Those who were on dialysis will be able to set this intensity of supervision off against the time they gain from being dialysis-independent, but they need to understand that early surveillance in the transplant clinic may be much less predictable and regular than dialysis treatments.

A clear and brief summary of the postoperative course, including whether graft function was immediate or delayed, details of any surgical complications, rejection episodes, or infections; and the patient's weight, graft function, and CNI trough levels at discharge, is necessary to ensure effective transfer of care to the transplant clinic. This is especially the case if the patient will be followed up away from the transplant centre. A clear pathway for managing surgical complications should be in place to ensure that any issues can be managed appropriately and in a timely fashion.

91.5 Cases

Case History 1: Early Rise in Creatinine

A 50-year-old Caucasian male, primary disease, IgA nephropathy 90 kg, native urine output 1 litre per day received a preemptive living unrelated transplant from a 50-yr-old female friend. The HLA mismatch was 1–2-1, CMV D-R+, EBV D + R+. The recipient had historical low level anti-HLA antibodies which were not donor-specific. He was given basiliximab induction. The cold time was 4 hours and there were no intraoperative complications (no significant hypotension or bleeding, etc). His maintenance immunosuppression was tacrolimus (aim level 10–12), mycophenolate 1 g bd, and prednisolone 20 mg od.

He passed good urine volumes (as is common in preemptive transplantation), with minimum drain output. In patients who are oligo-anuric pretransplant, the postoperative urine output is a very good guide to transplant function. In patients with "normal" pre-transplant urine output, one relies more on the blood test results. Patients with complex anatomy (e.g., multiple or small vessels and difficult anastomoses) need to be monitored closely with

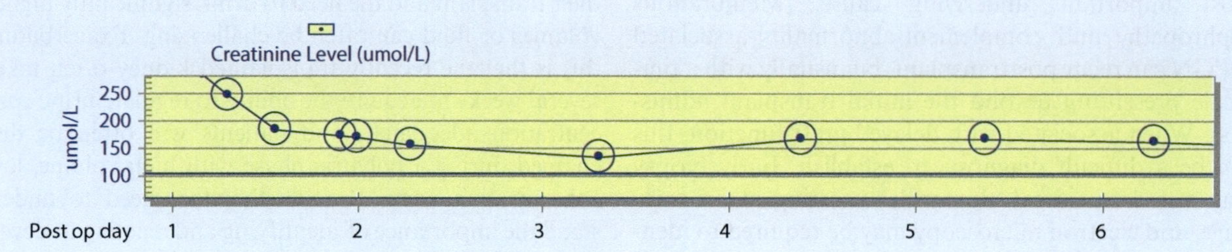

Fig. 91.3 Case 1, serum creatinine plot (μmol/l) against time (days)

more frequent scans. This case was straightforward with one artery and one vein.

He appeared to be making good progress until at day 4 his creatinine had risen from 133 to 166 (Fig. 91.3).

The causes of a raised creatinine at this stage were considered:

(1)	Volume depletion	Fluid balance charts reviewed (approximately 5 litres in and out), clinical assessment = euvolaemic; 3 kg above preop weight
(2)	Surgical complication (a) Vascular (b) Urine outflow blockage	No clinical suggestion, ultrasound good perfusion No hydronephrosis or collection on ultrasound
(3)	Tacrolimus toxicity	Level 14.1 on day 2 = above target range but not toxic
(4)	Other medication	No new changes (e.g. no new ACE inhibitor)
(5)	Urine leak	No clinical suggestion; minimal fluid in drain
(6)	Intrinsic kidney problem	Too early for recurrent IgA; consider rejection

The raised creatinine was confirmed on a repeat sample and a transplant biopsy was performed on day 5.

The verbal report of the biopsy was severe tubulitis, haemorrhage, oedema, eosinophilic infiltrations, mild peritubular capillaritis, no glomerulitis, vascular inflammation (V2 and V1 lesions), good background kidney, and moderate to severe acute tubular injury. Banff Category 2B.

The patient was treated with ATG and made a good recovery. The treatment of rejection is considered in another chapter but this case illustrates the stepwise nature of assessment in the early transplant period. Early aggressive rejection was not predicted in this case, but with a thorough systematic approach the diagnosis was quickly established.

Case 2: Urine Leak

91

A 49-year-old Caucasian female with primary disease reflux nephropathy and native urine output 1 litre received a preemptive 52-year-old deceased female's (DCD) kidney. Cause of death was intracranial haemorrhage, and cold ischaemic time 11 hours. There was a single artery on a patch and single renal vein. There were no intraoperative complications. The HLA mismatch was 1–1-1, CMV D + R+, EBV D + R+.

The operation appeared to have gone well. An ultrasound in recovery (normal practice) showed good perfusion with mild hydroureter. This was not thought to have been significant. She was passing 150–200 ml urine per hour which was replaced intravenously. That evening her urine output fell to 50 ml/hr. A fluid balance assessment was performed which was satisfactory (6 litres input, 3 litres urine output, 200 ml in drain). An urgent ultrasound scan was reported as normal (no mention of hydroureter). She was given further fluid boluses without any response and these were then stopped.

Careful fluid balance was maintained, drain output was 50–100 ml in 24 hrs, and drain was removed on day 3. A further scan at day 4 was unremarkable. Her urine output gradually increased. Serous fluid leaked through her wound on day 7 and an ultrasound reported "a small subcentimetre seroma inferior to the abdominal wall and a further small subcentimetre seroma seen inferior to the kidney. The bladder is noted to be a thin walled with the distal end of the stent visualized. The proximal end of the stent could not be visualized on this study".

Her creatinine did not fall and so a biopsy was performed on day 8 and a CT arranged for on day 9. The verbal report for the biopsy was florid glomerulitis and also

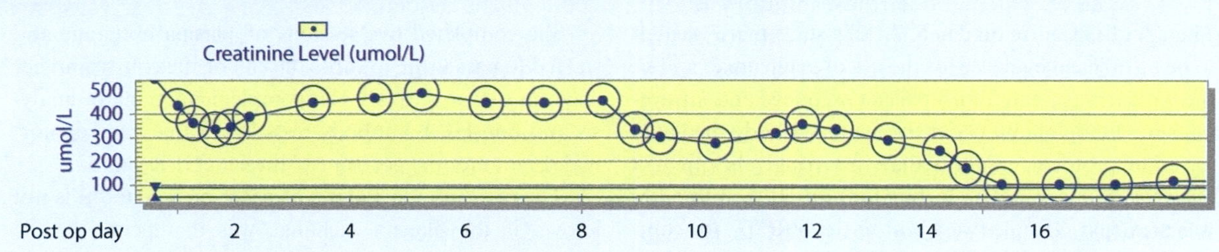

Fig. 91.4 Case 2, serum creatinine plot (μmol/l) against time (days)

peritubular capillaritis, and in one slide a focus highly suspicious for a v1 lesion. This was treated with pulsed methylprednisolone and a check for donor specific antibodies (negative, C4d subsequently negative). The CT showed a 2.7 cm (depth) × 7.1 cm (trans) collection between the bladder and rectus sheath, as well as a rectus sheath haematoma. Her creatinine started to improve (Fig. 91.4).

On day 10 she complained of severe flank pain adjacent to the graft and her stent was removed. On day 11 she then complained of clots in her urine and lower abdominal swelling and increased fluid from the wound (which now had a stoma bag on it). Ultrasound showed a collection between the bladder and rectus which was increasing in size. Fluid from the bag on the abdominal wall was sent for creatinine level: this was found to be 4800 μmol/l (serum 356 μmol/l) confirming a urine leak/ urinoma.

A urinary catheter was inserted, she was treated with broad spectrum antibiotics and she returned to theatre for exploration and reimplantation of the transplant ureter. Urine leak is infrequent post transplant but must be considered when drain or wound output is more than expected, and with collections not typically a lymphocele.

Case 3: Early Thrombotic Microangiopathy:? Cause

A 33-year-old African female, 120 kg (BMI 39), end-stage kidney disease of uncertain cause (presumed hypertension), oligoanuria on haemodialysis for five years received a deceased donor (DBD) kidney from a 80 kg 55-yr-old male, cause of death intracranial haemorrhage. The HLA mismatch was 0–1-0, CMV D + R+, EBV D + R+. She had no anti-HLA antibodies on multiple screening tests. The cold ischaemic time was 7 hrs. There were no surgical complications but there was a short period of hypotension intraoperatively treated with fluid boluses and metaraminol. She was given basiliximab induction and conventional triple therapy with tacrolimus, mycophenolate and steroids. Surgery was concluded at around 9 pm.

A postoperative ultrasound was planned the following day but the patient remained olioganuric while the paired kidney, which had already been transplanted in another patient on the ward was producing 400 ml/hr. of urine. Therefore an urgent scan was requested overnight which was unremarkable. The patient had a good blood pressure and was considered to be well filled with fluid, her haemoglobin was stable and lactate normal.

She was dialysed for hyperkalaemia on day 1 and another ultrasound later that day was unremarkable. She remained oligoanuric while the paired kidney continued to make good urine volumes and so she returned to theatre for exploration on day 2. The kidney appeared well perfused and an open biopsy was performed. This showed a diffuse glomerulitis, with thrombi in occasional capillary loops and glomerular hila. There was no crescents. There was very focal peritubular capillaritis. There was acute tubular injury but no tubulitis and no arteritis. There was around 5% interstitial fibrosis. Conclusion: acute thrombotic microangiopathy (TMA). Her platelet count fell from around 250 pre-transplant to 126 on day 3. Her LDH was mildly raised at 220. Her haemoglobin was stable and there were no red cell fragments on blood film.

Causes for a TMA were considered. Her blood pressure was 100/60 so hypertension was discounted. Her tacrolimus level on day was 15.9, which is higher than target [10–12] but not very high. Nonetheless there was a small dose reduction in tacrolimus. In case this was an early antibody mediated rejection, an urgent donor-specific antibody test was performed which was negative. The C4d staining on the biopsy came back as negative on day 4. Because the patient had not had a biopsy of her native kidneys, consideration was given that she might have an underlying complement pathology or coagulopathy. Testing was arranged for antiphospholipid and anticardiolipin antibodies, ADAMTS-13 and these were normal. Her case was discussed with the National Renal Complement

Therapeutics Centre on day 5. At this stage there was felt to be insufficient evidence for the use of eculizumab and so the patient was treated with plasma exchange and intravenous immunoglobulin under the acute antibody-mediated rejection protocol, mindful that this could also treat a recurrent primary TMA. Testing for non-HLA antibodies was arranged. Samples were sent to the NRCTC for complement regulator mutation analysis. She was vaccinated for meningococcus in case eculizumab would be given in the future.

She completed five sessions of plasma exchange and started to pass urine towards the end of the course and her creatinine started to fall. Her complement regulator analysis and non-HLA antibody tests later came back as normal. Eight months posttransplant her eGFR was 50.

The cause of the TMA was never proven and it is not known if the plasma exchange was therapeutic or the recovery was coincidental. This case shows the methodical approach to attempt to reach a diagnosis, and empirical treatment decisions when faced with an early TMA.

Tips and Tricks: Five Common Mistakes and How to Avoid Them

1. *Missing retroperitoneal haemorrhage*
   This commonly occurs because the retroperitoneum is a relatively hidden space and patients may not complain of pain in the presence of a significant haematoma. While ultrasound is the main traditional form of imaging for the recent renal transplant, it is not however a sensitive modality for the identification of retroperitoneal haemorrhage whi+ch, if progressive, can lead to pressure on the renal vessels.

   In cases where the patient's Hb is dropping without an obvious reason, a CT scan with contrast is required to exclude significant haemorrhage around or behind the graft. This is not an easy request to submit because of the risk of nephrotoxicity from x-ray contrast, especially in the context of delayed or suboptimal graft function. However remember that contrast nephrotoxicity is a transient phenomenon; kidney transplant vein thrombosis is usually forever. If at CT with contrast is indicated for the purposes of bleeding the risks of contrast are justified.
2. *Failing to anticipate changes in Tacrolimus absorption*
   Tacrolimus is absorbed throughout the GI tract (even from the oral mucosa, although this is not a reliable route). As well as first-pass metabolism in the liver, there is significant degradation of tacrolimus within small bowel mucosa, so that intercurrent events which prevent the drug from reaching the small intestine, or reduce the time it spends there, will lead to increased tacrolimus levels. Two common scenarios are:
   (i) A postoperative ileus following transplantation is associated with high tacrolimus levels due to reduced transit of the drug through to its sites of metabolism in the small bowel combined with efficient absorption from the gastric mucosa. This leads to reduction in the dose around postoperative day 4–5, just as the ileus is resolving. The patient then goes home about day 7 with tacrolimus levels which are falling sharply and is underdosed during the second posttransplant week, a period of high risk of acute cellular rejection in grafts undertaken without the cover of induction therapy.
   (ii) Diarrhoeal episodes are frequently associated with decreased tacrolimus breakdown (due to reduced exposure to the small intestinal mucosa combined with efficient absorption within the large intestine). When combined with the metabolic consequences of intravascular volume depletion, this may commonly present with significant hyperkalaemia (overriding the effects of gastrointestinal K^+ loss) and significant graft dysfunction.

   Cyclosporin is predominantly absorbed from the small intestine and is less prone to these effects than tacrolimus.
3. *Not knowing important interactions with Calcineurin inhibitors*
   Calcineurin inhibitors (cyclosporin and tacrolimus) have a narrow therapeutic index and are principally metabolized by the cytochrome P450 3A4 enzymes. Drugs which affect this system can significantly alter blood levels.

   The commonest interactions leading to high levels and toxicity are from CYP 3A inhibition by macrolide antibiotics (especially erythromycin, with clarithromycin exerting a smaller but still significant effect), azole antifungal agents (most commonly fluconazole), and the now rarely prescribed Cimetidine. There is a clinically significant effect of co-administration of CNI's with grapefruit juice (presumably via inhibition of enteric CYP3A4), which patients are encouraged to avoid. Less commonly, reduction in CNI levels can follow induction of cytochrome P450 by phenytoin, carbamazepine, or rifampicin.

4. *Overfilling the recipient with delayed graft function*
   Delayed graft function is not a life-threatening complication of transplantation, however significant fluid overload is. Fluid overload in a renal patient, who may well have impaired cardiac performance commonly due to coronary vascular disease or chronic uraemic myocardial dysfunction (often diastolic ventricular relaxation impairment), can rapidly result in life-threatening pulmonary oedema. In this context they will require dialysis / ultrafiltration as an emergency, which is always best avoided postoperatively. Less medically concerning, although uncomfortable for the recipient, is severe peripheral tissue salt and water accumulation as a result of overenthusiastic fluid administration in pursuit of a reassuringly high initial urine volume.
5. *Failure to react fast enough to sudden oligoanuria*
   The most helpful investigation in this scenario is an ultrasound as it rarely proves unhelpful and often is reassuring if not diagnostic. Common causes include:
   (i) Renal artery or vein thrombosis: While this is relatively rare, it is a highly important cause of allograft loss and requires a swift response. It should therefore remain top of the list of differential diagnoses to exclude. A high index of suspicion for thrombosis and early involvement of a transplant surgeon may negate the need for a scan and instead result in an expedited return trip to the operating theatre. Thrombosis is more commonly seen in those with a prothrombotic tendency and while early anticoagulation is likely to be protective this needs careful consideration and negotiation with the surgical team postoperatively.
   (ii) Obstruction: This is usually due to issue with the catheter, such as external compression or an intraluminal obstruction, most commonly from a blood clot. As mentioned above, a careful bladder washout by a transplant surgeon usually rectifies the problem, however if persistent haematuria with clots is ongoing then urological input and irrigation may be necessary, via a three-way catheter.
   (iii) Antibody-mediated rejection. Can be detected clinically with pain over the allograft and/or macroscopic haematuria. More prevalent in sensitized recipients (commonest causes of sensitization being pregnancy and previous transplantation, particularly when re-transplantation occurs across a repeat mismatch) and associated with graft loss as well as suboptimal outcomes both acute and chronically.

91.6 Quiz

Question 1: What information is not commonly available on the Core Donor Data Form (CDDF) issued by NHS Blood and Transplant when offering an organ?

(a) Donor blood group
(b) Detailed past medical history
(c) Donor virology, including hepatitis, HIV and CMV status
(d) The blood results taken from the patient on admission
(e) The cause of death

Answer: B

The details pertaining to the donor's detailed medical history is found on the Medical and Social History (MaSH) form. While a summary is available on the CDDF, more detailed information can commonly be found on the MaSH form. It is important to review both forms to make sure that there is nothing that is a contraindication to donation.

Question 2: Which of the following primary causes of renal disease do not recur in a kidney transplant?

(a) Focal and Segmental Glomerulosclerosis (FSGS)
(b) Atypical haemolytic uraemic syndrome (aHUS)
(c) Membranoproliferative glomerulonephritis (MPGN)
(d) All of the above
(e) None of the above

Answer: E

FSGS, aHUS, and MPGN can all recur in kidney transplants and patients with these conditions should be counselled and consented appropriately prior to undergoing transplantation.

Question 3: True or false

If a patient is passing urine after a transplant, then that confirms adequate perfusion of the newly transplanted kidney.

Answer: False

Some ESRD patients continue to pass urine while on dialysis. The presence of urine in the catheter bag after the transplant needs to be interpreted within the context of each individual patient. The absence of urine after a living donor kidney transplant is alarming and should be considered an emergency.

Question 4: True or false

Tacrolimus exerts its effects by binding to the IL-2 receptor of T cells.

Answer: False

Tacrolimus is a macrolide antibiotic which exerts its effects by bonding to an immunophilin (FK506 binding protein (FKBP)) inside the T cell. This complex then inhibits calcineurin phosphatase, which in turn inhibits calcium-dependent events, including interleukin-2 gene transcription.

Question 5: When is a biopsy for delayed graft function (DGF) most commonly indicated?

(a) Day 0
(b) Day 2
(c) Day 5
(d) Day 7
(e) Day 10

Answer: D

Delayed graft function is defined as the need for dialysis within the first seven days following a kidney transplant. Most units undertake biopsies to confirm the presence of DGF on day 7, unless the patient demonstrates clear evidence that the kidney is starting to work. The main alternative diagnosis to exclude is rejection.

Conclusion

The perioperative period following kidney transplantation can vary considerably between patients and is related to both donor and recipient factors. A structured and systematic approach to the acutely transplanted patient is useful for working through the list of most likely postoperative issues, including fluid balance, rejection, recurrence of primary disease and surgical complications. The current era of transplantation involving the use of kidneys from marginal donors makes the diagnosis of DGF much more common than vascular thrombosis, however any abrupt reduction in urine output must be acted upon immediately in conjunction with the transplant surgeons in order to exclude vascular compromise and potential graft loss.

References

1. NHS Blood and Transplant. Organ Donation and Transplantation Activity Report 2018/19. 2019.
2. NHS Blood and Transplant. Kidney Transplantation: Deceased Donor Organ Allocation. POLICY POL 186/10 ed2019.
3. Summers DM, Johnson RJ, Hudson A, Collett D, Watson CJ, Bradley JA. Effect of donor age and cold storage time on outcome in recipients of kidneys donated after circulatory death in the UK: a cohort study. Lancet. 2013;381(9868):727–34.
4. Siedlecki A, Irish W, Brennan DC. Delayed graft function in the kidney transplant. Am J Transplant. 2011;11(11):2279–96.
5. Cravedi P, Kopp JB, Remuzzi G. Recent progress in the pathophysiology and treatment of FSGS recurrence. Am J Transplant. 2013;13(2):266–74.
6. Glicklich D, Vohra P. Cardiovascular risk assessment before and after kidney transplantation. Cardiol Rev. 2014;22(4):153–62.
7. Patel R, Terasaki PI. Significance of the positive crossmatch test in kidney transplantation. N Engl J Med. 1969;280(14):735–9.
8. Gebel HM, Bray RA, Nickerson P. Pre-transplant assessment of donor-reactive, HLA-specific antibodies in renal transplantation: contraindication vs. risk. Am J Transplant. 2003;3(12):1488–500.
9. Tait BD, Süsal C, Gebel HM, Nickerson PW, Zachary AA, Claas FH, et al. Consensus guidelines on the testing and clinical management issues associated with HLA and non-HLA antibodies in transplantation. Transplantation. 2013;95(1):19–47.
10. Amico P, Hönger G, Bielmann D, Lutz D, Garzoni D, Steiger J, et al. Incidence and prediction of early antibody-mediated rejection due to non-human leukocyte antigen-antibodies. Transplantation. 2008;85(11):1557–63.
11. Cardinal H, Dieudé M, Hébert MJ. The emerging importance of non-HLA autoantibodies in kidney transplant complications. J Am Soc Nephrol. 2017;28(2):400–6.
12. British Transplantation Society. The detection & characterisation of clinically relevant antibodies in allotransplantation. 2015.
13. National Institute for Health and Care Excellence. Immunosuppressive therapy for kidney transplant in adults. 2017.
14. Nankivell BJ, Borrows RJ, Fung CL, O'Connell PJ, Allen RD, Chapman JR. The natural history of chronic allograft nephropathy. N Engl J Med. 2003;349(24):2326–33.
15. Srinivas TR, Schold JD, Guerra G, Eagan A, Bucci CM, Meier-Kriesche HU. Mycophenolate mofetil/sirolimus compared to other common immunosuppressive regimens in kidney transplantation. Am J Transplant. 2007;7(3):586–94.
16. Thomson AW, Bonham CA, Zeevi A. Mode of action of tacrolimus (FK506): molecular and cellular mechanisms. Ther Drug Monit. 1995;17(6):584–91.
17. Pirsch JD, Miller J, Deierhoi MH, Vincenti F, Filo RS. A comparison of tacrolimus (FK506) and cyclosporine for immunosuppression after cadaveric renal transplantation. FK506 Kidney Transplant Study Group. Transplantation. 1997;63(7):977–83.
18. Vincenti F, Jensik SC, Filo RS, Miller J, Pirsch J. A long-term comparison of tacrolimus (FK506) and cyclosporine in kidney transplantation: evidence for improved allograft survival at five years. Transplantation. 2002;73(5):775–82.

19. Ekberg H, Tedesco-Silva H, Demirbas A, Vítko S, Nashan B, Gürkan A, et al. Reduced exposure to calcineurin inhibitors in renal transplantation. N Engl J Med. 2007;357(25):2562–75.
20. Kahan BD. Efficacy of sirolimus compared with azathioprine for reduction of acute renal allograft rejection: a randomised multicentre study. The Rapamune US Study Group. Lancet. 2000;356(9225):194–202.
21. MacDonald AS. A worldwide, phase III, randomized, controlled, safety and efficacy study of a sirolimus/cyclosporine regimen for prevention of acute rejection in recipients of primary mismatched renal allografts. Transplantation. 2001;71(2):271–80.
22. Alangaden GJ, Thyagarajan R, Gruber SA, Morawski K, Garnick J, El-Amm JM, et al. Infectious complications after kidney transplantation: current epidemiology and associated risk factors. Clin Transpl. 2006;20(4):401–9.
23. Kasiske BL, Chakkera HA, Louis TA, Ma JZ. A meta-analysis of immunosuppression withdrawal trials in renal transplantation. J Am Soc Nephrol. 2000;11(10):1910–7.
24. Borrows R, Chan K, Loucaidou M, Lawrence C, Van Tromp J, Cairns T, et al. Five years of steroid sparing in renal transplantation with tacrolimus and mycophenolate mofetil. Transplantation. 2006;81(1):125–8.
25. Woodle ES, Peddi VR, Tomlanovich S, Mulgaonkar S, Kuo PC. A prospective, randomized, multicenter study evaluating early corticosteroid withdrawal with Thymoglobulin in living-donor kidney transplantation. Clin Transpl. 2010;24(1):73–83.
26. Dalton RS, Webber JN, Cameron C, Kessaris N, Gibbs PG, Tan LC, et al. Physiologic impact of low-dose dopamine on renal function in the early post renal transplant period. Transplantation. 2005;79(11):1561–7.
27. Grundmann R, Kindler J, Meider G, Stöwe H, Sieberth HG, Pichlmaier H. Dopamine treatment of human cadaver kidney graft recipients: a prospectively randomized trial. Klin Wochenschr. 1982;60(4):193–7.
28. Andrés A, Budde K, Clavien PA, Becker T, Kessler M, Pisarski P, et al. A randomized trial comparing renal function in older kidney transplant patients following delayed versus immediate tacrolimus administration. Transplantation. 2009;88(9):1101–8.
29. Wilson CH, Brook NR, Gok MA, Asher JF, Nicholson ML, Talbot D. Randomized clinical trial of daclizumab induction and delayed introduction of tacrolimus for recipients of non-heart-beating kidney transplants. Br J Surg. 2005;92(6):681–7.
30. Ghisdal L, Broeders N, Wissing KM, Saidi A, Bensalem T, Mbaba Mena J, et al. Thrombophilic factors do not predict outcomes in renal transplant recipients under prophylactic acetylsalicylic acid. Am J Transplant. 2010;10(1):99–105.
31. Sáez-Giménez B, Berastegui C, Loor K, López-Meseguer M, Monforte V, Bravo C, et al. Deep vein thrombosis and pulmonary embolism after solid organ transplantation: an unresolved problem. Transplant Rev. 2015;29(2):85–92.
32. Robertson AJ, Nargund V, Gray DW, Morris PJ. Low dose aspirin as prophylaxis against renal-vein thrombosis in renal-transplant recipients. Nephrol Dial Transplant. 2000;15(11):1865–8.
33. Williams WW, Taheri D, Tolkoff-Rubin N, Colvin RB. Clinical role of the renal transplant biopsy. Nat Rev Nephrol. 2012;8(2):110–21.
34. Haas M, Loupy A, Lefaucheur C, Roufosse C, Glotz D, Seron D, et al. The Banff 2017 Kidney Meeting Report: revised diagnostic criteria for chronic active T cell-mediated rejection, antibody-mediated rejection, and prospects for integrative endpoints for next-generation clinical trials. Am J Transplant. 2018;18(2):293–307.
35. Willicombe M, Roufosse C, Brookes P, Galliford JW, McLean AG, Dorling A, et al. Antibody-mediated rejection after alemtuzumab induction: incidence, risk factors, and predictors of poor outcome. Transplantation. 2011;92(2):176–82.
36. Paoletti E, Bellino D, Marsano L, Cassottana P, Rolla D, Ratto E. Effects of ACE inhibitors on long-term outcome of renal transplant recipients: a randomized controlled trial. Transplantation. 2013;95(6):889–95.

Resources and Patient Information

https://www.odt.nhs.uk/statistics-and-reports/annual-activity-report/ – The annual activity report from NHS Blood and Transplant provides a comprehensive update on organ donation rates, transplant waiting list figures and transplant activity for the previous financial year.

https://www.odt.nhs.uk/transplantation/tools-policies-and-guidance/policies-and-guidance/ – The ODT clinical website pages on policies and guidelines provide more detailed information regarding patient selection, organ allocation, and various other topics relevant to transplantation.

https://www.kidneycareuk.org – the home page of a leading kidney patient support charity providing useful information and advice about transplantation and kidney disease in general.

https://bts.org.uk/ – the home page of the British Transplantation Society with links to information and resources for patients and professionals, clinical guidelines and standards.

Renal Transplant Rejection

Philippa Dodd, Candice Roufosse, and Mark Harber

Contents

M. Harber (ed.), *Primer on Nephrology*, https://doi.org/10.1007/978-3-030-76419-7_92

Learning Objectives

1. To appreciate the risk factors associated with acute and chronic rejection
2. To explore the pathophysiology and diagnosis of acute and chronic rejection
3. Evaluation of treatment options and outcomes for rejection

Definitions

Renal allograft rejection manifests clinically as graft dysfunction evidenced by a rise in serum creatinine and an increase in urinary protein loss. From a clinical point of view, the time frame between transplantation and the onset of rejection defines either its acute or its chronic nature. For the pathologist however, activity and chronicity are graded in the renal allograft biopsy according to the scores for inflammation and scarring respectively, using the Banff Classification of renal allograft rejection [1], without reference to time posttransplantation. Subclinical rejection is defined as histological evidence of rejection in the absence of graft dysfunction, a pathologic entity identified by so-called protocol biopsy which is not performed in all transplant centres. In the absence of clinical graft dysfunction as well as robust data proving that treatment of subclinical lesions improves outcomes, how to manage this problem in the clinical practice of transplantation remains controversial.

Hyperacute rejection – occurs almost immediately upon reperfusion of the transplanted donor kidney on the operating table following cross-clamp release. This phenomenon is reflective of the interaction of recipient derived, usually high titre, preformed donor-specific anti-HLA antibody (DSA) with donor allo-antigens and associated complement activation. Or in the context of blood group incompatible (ABOi) transplantation.

Acute rejection—occurs within days (early or accelerated) or weeks (late) posttransplantation and may be antibody mediated or T-cell mediated.

- **Acute *antibody*-mediated rejection (AMR)** – occurs most often as a consequence of immunologic memory sustained through previously sensitizing events such blood transfusions, pregnancy, or previous transplant episodes. It may also occur in the face of high numbers of HLA donor and recipient mismatches and subsequent generation of de novo DSA.
- **Acute *T-cell* mediated rejection (TCMR)**—also known as cellular rejection, is the most common form of acute rejection and results either from direct interaction between recipient T cells and donor antigen expressed on donor cells or recipient T-cell interaction with donor alloantigen presented by recipient antigen-presenting cells (APCs).

Sub-acute rejection—usually occurs between three and six months posttransplantation, although it can occur at any point in the posttransplant period. It too may be antibody- or T-cell mediated. Where antibody-mediated rejection is concerned, graft dysfunction is most often reflective of the production of de novo DSA against donor antigen.

Chronic *T-cell* mediated rejection (cTCMR) – has relatively recently been recognized as a pathologic entity by the Banff working group and is characterized by marked tubulointerstitial inflammation in a scarred renal cortex with tubulitis and arterial intimal thickening and inflammation.

Chronic *antibody* mediated rejection (CAMR)—occurs months or years posttransplantation. Repeated or persistent immunologic injury has been strongly implicated in its development but the precise relationship between acute and chronic antibody-mediated rejection remains unclear. Its definition as a clinical-pathological entity has changed over time but the majority agree that the presence of glomerular double contouring, peri-tubular capillary basement membrane multi-lamination, interstitial fibrosis, tubular atrophy and vascular intimal hyperplasia are diagnostic histological features [2].

92.1 Introduction

Once the technical aspects of vascular surgery required for kidney transplantation were overcome, the immune response to the transplanted organ became the principal barrier to transplantation. And once Medawar, Billingham, and Brent demonstrated the immunological nature of rejection the next barrier was finding immunosuppression powerful enough to prevent graft destruction without killing the patient. In the early 1960s patients were subjected to enormous doses of steroids with predictable side effects and very poor graft and patient survival. Further understanding of the impact of sensitization and anti-HLA antibodies, led by Terasaki [3] in this era provided an explanation for and subsequent avoidance of hyperacute rejection and immediate allograft loss. Graft survival rates improved with the addition of 6-mercaptopurine and azathioprine [4] but it was only with the introduction of calcineurin inhibitors that acute rejection rates fell significantly [5]. Today, induction agents are in common-place use (anti-CD25mAb or depleting antibodies) combined with a maintenance regimen consisting of tacrolimus and mycophenolate mofetil often in combination with corticosteroids.

92.2 Pathogenesis of Rejection

The normal response of the host to foreign antigens is the presentation of foreign peptides by host antigen-presenting cells (APCs) via major histocompatibility complex (MHC) molecules to host T cells via the T-cell receptor. In transplantation this normal immunological response is known as *indirect* presentation. However, unique to transplantation is the addition of donor APCs which can also present peptides to recipient T cells (known as *direct* presentation). Donor APCs can present (a) donor peptides (b) recipient peptides but via foreign MHC, therefore overcoming acquired tolerance and (c) the MHC of donor APCs can activate recipient T cells without peptide. This may all seem rather abstract but the MHC is extraordinarily polymorphic and MHC is highly expressed; the combination of high density, polymorphic allo-antigens and *direct* plus *indirect* presentation is thought to explain the extremely high frequency of recipient T cells that can recognize and react to donor antigens compared to conventional antigens. The corollary of this is that the alloimmune response, left unchecked is exceptionally vigorous.

The second, real-world element to rejection is sensitization to donor antigens following prior exposure to foreign tissue types. This most frequently results following previous transplantation, pregnancy, blood transfusion, or more rarely following infection. This can result in a very powerful amnestic response from T cells, natural killer cells, macrophages and B cells with the generation of donor-specific antibodies which may be complement fixing. An amnestic response is particularly problematic as donor-specific IgG antibodies are likely to be high avidity and previous T- and B-cell clonal expansion engenders a rapid and vigorous immunological response. With this in mind, the nature and timing of rejection fits into clinical paradigms.

92.2.1 Hyperacute Rejection

Hyperacute rejection is the catastrophic fixation of preformed, high titre and complement fixing antibodies to the renal vascular endothelium. Fibrin thrombi form in small vessels resulting in occlusion of the blood supply. This either results from a blood group incompatible transplant or secondary to blood group incompatible or very high levels of donor-specific antibodies. It declares itself to the unhappy surgeon in theatre on release of vascular clamps with a blue, floppy, and unsalvageable kidney.

92.2.2 Acute T-Cell-Mediated Rejection (Cellular Rejection)

Acute cellular rejection represents the infiltration of T cells (CD3+) which include both cytotoxic ($CD8^+$) and T helper cells ($CD4^+$) that recruit the whole panoply of the immune system including macrophages, B cells, eosinophils and NK cells. It is associated with inflammation in three compartments, to a greater or lesser degree, namely tubules (Banff lesions score t1-3), interstitium (Banff lesions score i1-3), and arteries (Banff lesions score v1-3) (Fig. 92.1).

Immune invasion of the tubulointerstitium is the most common finding in early rejection, vascular involvement suggests more severe rejection and ranges from intimal arteritis (T cells invading the vascular intima, underneath the endothelium) (Fig. 92.2) to severe transmural inflammation and fibrinoid necrosis (Fig. 92.3).

92.2.3 Acute Antibody-Mediated Rejection

Acute antibody-mediated rejection (AMR) can occur in the context of a memory response if the patient is sensitized, so risk factors include a high CRF, previous positive cross-matches (CDC or flow) or simply as part of an unchecked primary alloimmune response. Rapid ("accel-

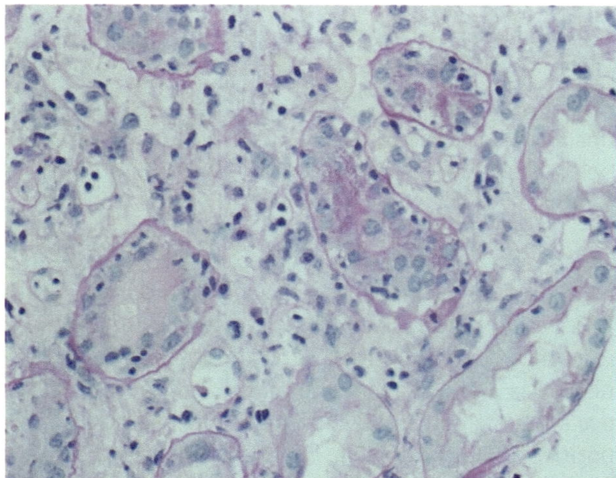

Fig. 92.1 T-cell mediated rejection, tubulointerstitial type (Banff 1): Lymphocytes and monocytes are present in the interstitium (Banff lesion score i) and within the confines of the tubular basement membranes (Banff lesion score t). PAS stain; tubular basement membranes stain bright pink

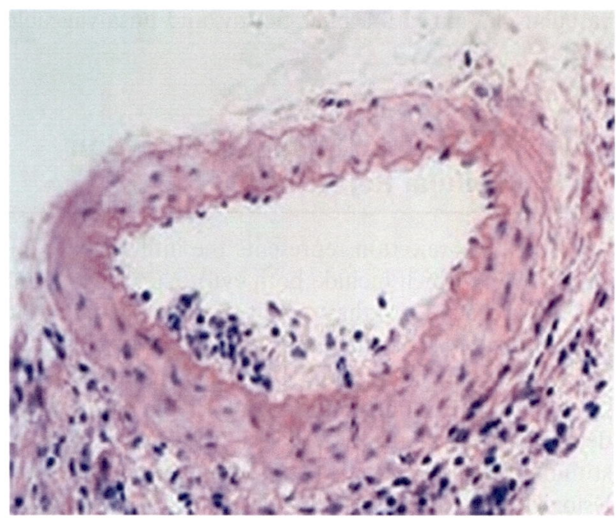

Fig. 92.2 T-cell mediated rejection, vascular type (Banff 2A): Lymphocytes and monocytes are present in the arterial intima, underneath the endothelium, occupying a limited circumference of the artery (Banff lesion score v1). H&E stain

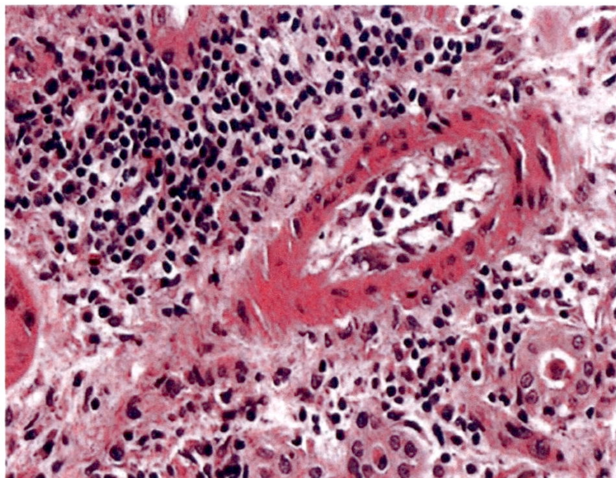

Fig. 92.3 T-cell mediated rejection, vascular type (Banff 2B): Lymphocytes and monocytes are present in the arterial intima, underneath the endothelium, occupying the full circumference of the artery (Banff lesion score v2). H&E stain

erated rejection") tends to occur in the context of a memory response to donor specific antibodies or non-HLA antibodies. The effector response to memory responses is faster than that of primary immune responses and as such acute rejection is more likely to occur in the setting of donor-specific sensitization, a positive CDC crossmatch, current or historical positive flow crossmatch and non-donor sensitization. The underlying disease process results from the fixation of donor-specific antibodies to the endothelium of renal arteries and microcirculation (glomerular and peritubular capillaries). This recruits leucocytes and NK cells with release of IFN-γ, and leads to activation of the endothelium and platelets with or without the fixation of complement which can be detected by the deposition of C4d in the peritubular capillaries. This can develop into a thrombotic microangiopathy initially indistinguishable from recurrent aHUS. Neutrophils in the peritubular capillaries are a useful early histological finding. The interstitial capillaritis may lead to interstitial haemorrhage (Fig. 92.4a–c).

92.2.4 Chronic Antibody-Mediated Rejection

Chronic antibody-mediated rejection (CAMR) has perhaps belatedly been recognized as the commonest cause of renal allograft loss. While the mechanisms of acute rejection are reasonably well defined those underlying CAMR remain less so and histological definitions have changed over time to reflect an improved understanding in this field. It is broadly accepted, largely from published data correlating the development of chronic rejection with acute rejection episodes, that CAMR results from recurrent "waves" of acute/sub-acute/chronic donor-specific (usually anti-HLA) antibody deposition and injury. Although, the lack of observed response to treatment with immunotherapies (as discussed later in this chapter) is strongly suggestive that additional cellular and molecular mechanisms are at play.

Endothelial cell activation resulting from deposition of immunoglobulin and complement is thought to lead to lying down of new basement membrane layers around peritubular capillaries and glomerular capillary loops. In glomeruli, this leads to double contouring on light microscopy and the pathognomonic multilayering of basement membranes seen on electron microscopy (Fig. 92.5a, b)—referred to as transplant glomerulopathy, which results in progressive occlusion of the vascular lumen and ischemia of the remaining nephrons. This is associated with progressive fibrosis and chronic inflammation of the interstitium as well as tubular atrophy causing a relentless fall in GFR usually accompanied by significant proteinuria.

92.3 Epidemiology and Risk Factors for Rejection

While rejection has always been an issue the clinical presentation and timeline has changed significantly since the dawn of transplantation (Fig. 92.6). The avoidance of unintentional blood group incompatible transplantation and CDC crossmatch incompatible transplantation has largely eliminated hyper-acute rejection and diminished acute antibody-mediated rejection.

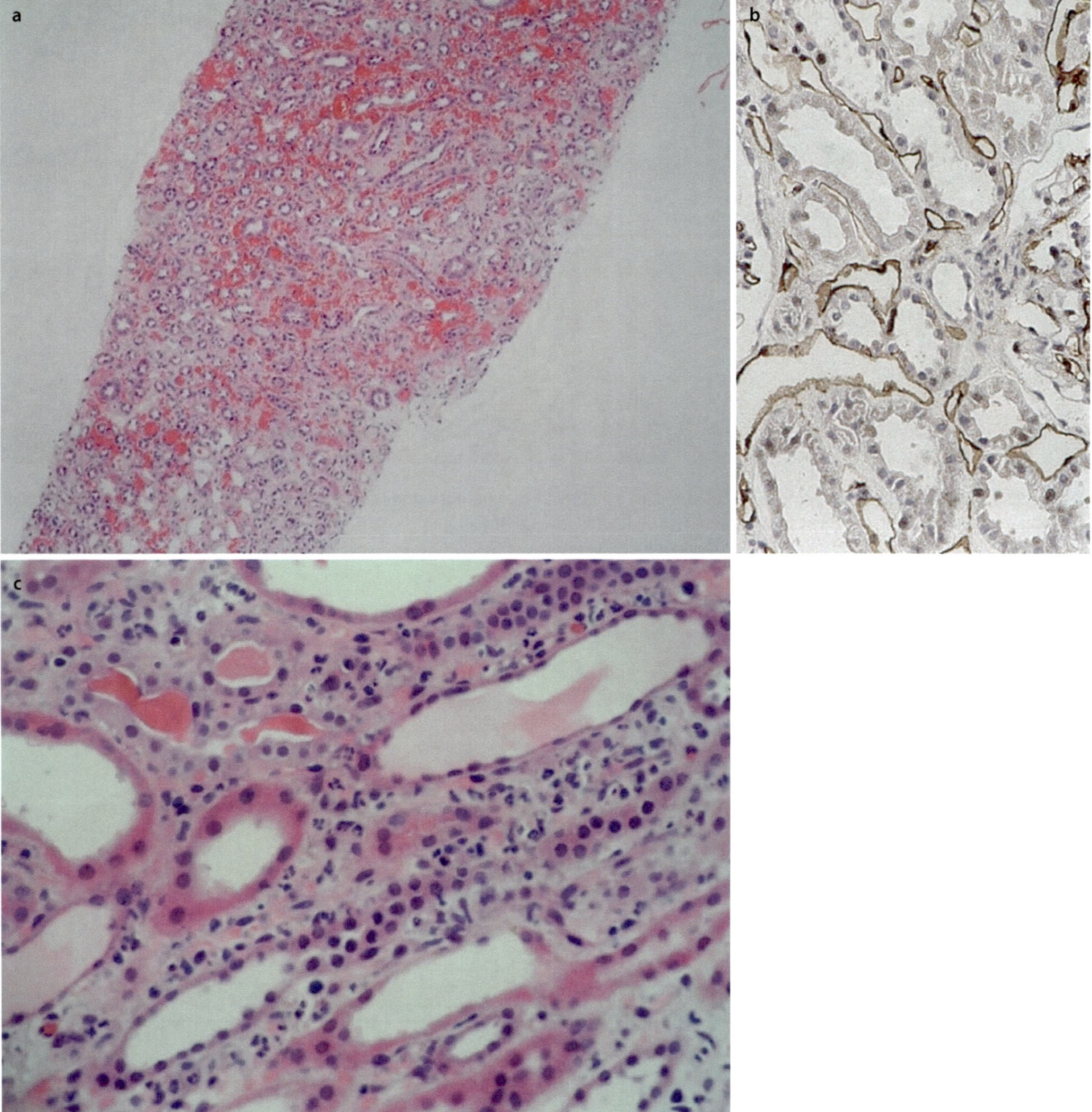

Fig. 92.4 (**a**, **b**) Acute antibody-mediated rejection with interstitial haemorrhage (H&E, on the left) and positive staining for complement factor 4d along the peritubular capillary endothelium on the right (C4d immunoperoxidase). (**c**) H&E section showing neutrophils in the capillaries between the tubules (peritubular capillaritis)

Since the symphony Elite study, acute rejection rates with tacrolimus, mycophenolate mofetil, and anti-CD25 mAb regimens, are in the mid-teens, units using depleting antibodies routinely achieve acute rejection rates in single figures. However, early success has left us with a larger proportion of chronic antibody-mediated rejection (CAMR).

With modern tissue-typing, regular antibody screening and good governance around blood group cross-matching hyperacute rejection should now be a "never event" and fortunately this irredeemable complication is extremely rare now. The role of antibody pre-screening and risk is nicely reviewed by Gebel et al. [6].

Prior to the "modern immunosuppressive era" acute rejection (AR) remained very common with rates of up to 50% biopsy proven rejection in the USA in the 1980s and early 1990s. Three large RCTs published in the

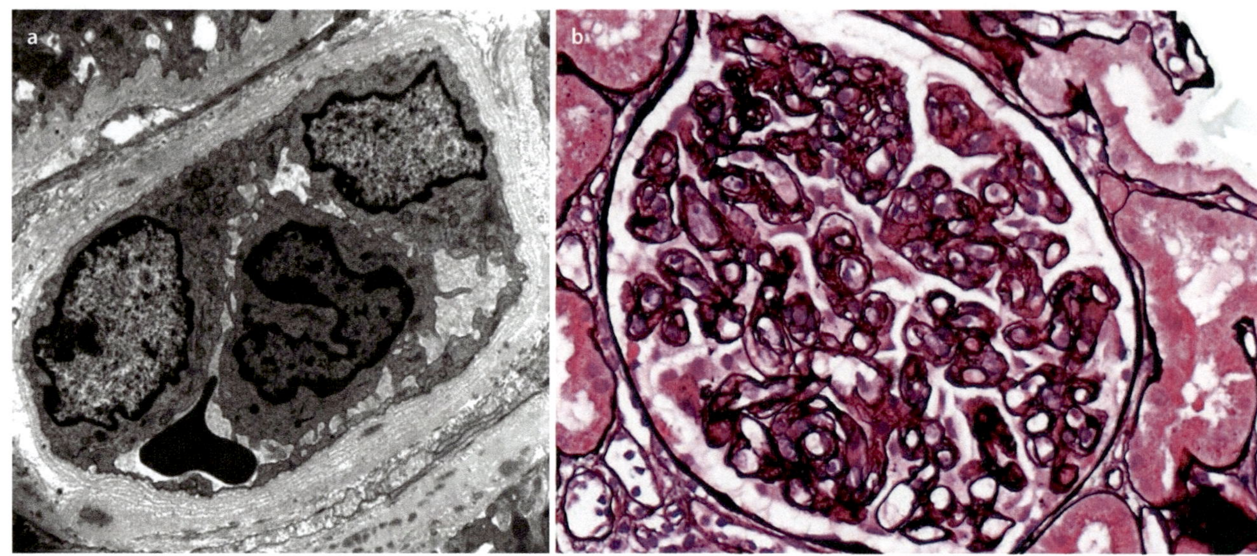

Fig. 92.5 (**a**) Electron micrograph of a peritubular capillary showing multiple layers of basement membrane, a typical finding in chronic antibody-mediated rejection (top). (**b**) Glomerulus with double contours along capillary walls, typical appearances of transplant glomerulopathy (right, silver stain)

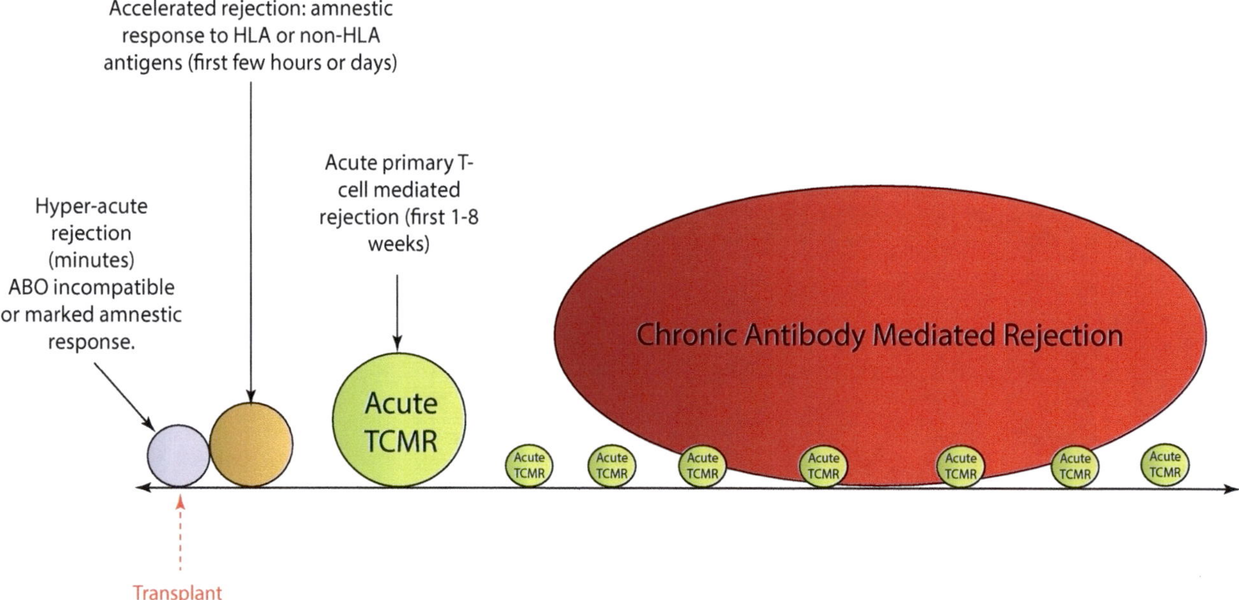

Fig. 92.6 Timeline of rejection. Hyperacute rejection when the transplant goes black on the operating table should now be a "never event". Accelerated rejection is still a useful term in that early aggressive rejection within the first few days is likely to represent a memory or amnestic response to HLA or non-HLA antigens. The majority of T-cell mediated rejection (TCMR) occurs within the first two months of an uncomplicated transplant. However, late acute TCMR and occur at any stage of a stable transplant, this may be obvious or subclinical but almost invariably results from underdosing of immunosuppression from non-adherence or medical error. Chronic antibody-mediated rejection is now thought to be the commonest cause of graft loss and can occur and progress at any stage of the transplant

1990s demonstrated reduction in AR with MMF versus AZA (for review, see reference [7]. Registry data from over 66,000 transplant in the USA seemed to confirm the benefit of mycophenolate mofetil over azathioprine in terms of acute rejection (15.5% versus 24.7%, respectively) and a further study in the elderly demonstrated reduced early AR with MMF (24%) versus AZA (28%) but also a significant reduction in late rejection after 12 months (2.3% versus 12.6%) [8].

Tacrolimus also resulted in better AR rates than cyclosporin (4–17% versus 14–20%, respectively). The requirement of ATG to treat rejection the first year was lower with tacrolimus and mycophenolate mofetil (6%) compared to Tacrolimus and azathioprine (13%) or cyclosporine and mycophenolate (12.6%). A meta-analysis of 30 studies and over 4000 patients in 2005 showed a RR of AR of 0.69 and steroid resistant AR 0.49 with tacrolimus compared with cyclosporine [9].

The use of tacrolimus and mycophenolate mofetil was embedded in practice following the Elite Symphony Study [10] which demonstrated an acute rejection rate of 17% in patients receiving anti-CD25mAb induction and triple therapy with steroids, mycophenolate, and "low dose" tacrolimus versus other regimens with rates of 29–43%. Nonetheless, even in this "modern era," early acute rejection has clear risk factors which relate broadly to:

1. Immunological barriers (mismatch and sensitization)
2. Host factors
3. Immunosuppression

92.3.1 Immunological Barriers

European registry data from 1995 to 2004 showed five-year outcomes of 80% for 000 mismatched grafts compared with 70% for 222 mismatched transplants although the difference was less significant for live donor transplants [11]. The implication here is that the worst outcomes are related to alloimmune damage.

It is not just the degree of mismatch but also the specific HLA antigens involved that determines outcome; the immunological hierarchy is broadly accepted to run DR > B > A in terms of outcome. In a retrospective review of over 1300 patients treated with anti-CD25mab, tacrolimus and mycophenolate mofetil and early steroid withdrawal showed that there was a significant difference in acute biopsy-proven rejection between those with no DR mismatches and no or only one B mismatch and those with a DR and/or two B mismatches (Henry Stephens, Personal communication) (Table 92.1).

Table 92.1 Acute renal transplant rejection rates based on mismatch

Mismatch	ACR
000 mm	7%
0DR ± 0/1Bmm (100, 010, 110, 200, 210)	11.7%
0DR ± 2B or 1DR ± 0/1Bmm (020, 120, 220, 001, 101, 201, 011, 111, 211)	15.3%
1DR ± 2B or 2DRmm (021, 121, 221, 002, 102, 202, 012, 112, 212, 022, 122, 222)	17.7%

NHSBT organ matching scheme 2006–2019. (*ACR* acute rejection rates)

92.3.2 Sensitization

The rules that have evolved on what is a negative or safe crossmatch, what is intermediate and what is high risk or unsafe derive entirely from the predicted allo-immune response to the donor antigens. Thus, by definition, patients with positive crossmatches and high levels of DSA are at very high risk of rejection and patients who are highly sensitized may find themselves effectively precluded from transplantation because the risk of rapid and severe rejection is unacceptably high.

Patients with lower levels of DSA that do not result in a positive crossmatch may be transplanted but significantly higher rates of acute antibody rejection (AMR) have been reported in retrospective analyses of patient cohorts, with detrimental effects on overall rates of allograft survival [12–14]. One such study reported more than double the incidence, 63% versus 26%, of AMR in those with low level DSA as compared to those without. At five years posttransplantation, allograft survival in those with DSA who experienced AMR was significantly inferior to those with DSA who experienced no AMR (68% versus 87%, $p = 0.002$). Interestingly, allograft survival in those without DSA was comparable to those with DSA but no AMR (89% versus 87%) [12].

Those who do not have DSA but who are highly sensitized to many other HLA antigens also tend to do less well in terms of both rejection episodes and long-term allograft survival when compared to unsensitized counterparts but outcomes are reported to be better when compared to those sensitized by DSA [13]. The accepted theory underlying this pertains to the notion that HLA antigens share epitopes which allows binding, albeit with variable avidity, of nonspecific HLA antibodies to multiple antigenic epitopes expressed on the renal allograft with resultant immune activation and allograft injury.

92.3.3 Host Factors

Outside the setting of sensitization, older patients have a lower rate of acute rejection, and increased rate of CMV reactivation and reduction in vaccine response, consistent with the idea that the reduction in rejection rates in older patients is secondary to immune senescence. Conversely, a young patient with a low immunosuppressive burden has a much higher relative risk of rejection. High intra-patient tacrolimus trough level variation in young adults seems to be particularly hazardous (see below).

Despite initial concerns that patients with controlled HIV would be over-immunosuppressed with transplant immunosuppression, HIV consistently confers a near doubling of acute rejection rates, somewhere in the region of around 30–40%. The reason for this is intriguing but not clear; it may be a combination of chronic immune dysregulation and low exposure to tacrolimus in patients on protease inhibitors.

While there is an increased incidence of acute rejection associated with CMV viremia and attributed to an antiviral pro-inflammatory milieu (interferon-γ treatment is contra-indicated in renal transplantation for this reason), the majority of CMV viremia follows, not proceeds treatment for rejection and is likely a consequence of an escalation in immunosuppression. However, it is clear that rejection is sometimes precipitated by immunosuppression reduction (ISR) in the face of troublesome primary CMV infection, as is the case with ISR to treat BK virus nephropathy.

92.3.4 Immunosuppression

Induction immunotherapy serves largely to ameliorate T-cell alloresponses involved in direct allorecognition encountered early in the post-transplant period. Randomized control trials and meta-analyses indicate that induction therapy plus conventional oral therapies offer superior outcomes to conventional therapies alone [14–16]. Published data regarding the optimal prophylactic induction therapy to prevent rejection remains controversial.

Induction agents can be broadly divided into cell depleting and non-depleting agents. Lymphocyte depleting agents including rabbit anti-thymocyte globulin—rATG, a polyclonal antibody targeted against numerous human T-cell antigens including MHC, alemtuzumab—Campath-1H, a monoclonal anti-CD52 antibody which is pan-lymphocyte depleting, belatacept, a CTLA-4-Ig which inhibits CD80/CD86 co-stimulation required for T-cell activation and rituximab a monoclonal anti-CD20 antibody which targets B-cells. Non-depleting agents include basiliximab and daclizumab both monoclonal antibodies which act as antagonists to CD25, the IL-2 receptor, activation of which is critical to T-cell expansion.

B-cell depletion using rituximab has not been shown to offer effective induction of immunosuppression over standard therapies and head-to-head comparison of T-cell depleting versus non-depleting agents have revealed conflicting results. In high immunologic risk renal transplants and ABOi, rATG proved superior when compared to anti-IL2 agents in preventing rejection at 1 year [17]. Early outcomes comparing alemtuzumab and rATG show no difference in rejection rates between these two agents. However, late acute rejection is more common with alemtuzumab (although not significantly different) and it appears that the beneficial effects may be lost over time with an increased risk of death and allograft failure at five years post-transplant in alemtuzumab treated patients (25.9% versus 22.9%) [18]. The evidence for low immunologic risk transplants is less clear. Some studies demonstrate a lower incidence of acute rejection, death and graft loss with rATG but at the expense of increased infection rates, others show no superiority of rATG over IL-2 antagonists and a similarity in adverse events.

In steroid-free protocols, at 12 months alemtuzumab was demonstrated to be superior to IL-2 antagonists (5% versus 17%, $P = <0.001$) in preventing rejection episodes. At 3 years, in the low risk groups treated with alemtuzumab, significant reduction in the incidence of acute rejection, graft loss and death was observed (10% versus 22%, $P = 0.003$) when compared to basiliximab but in high-risk patients there was no differences observed between rATG and alemtuzumab (18% versus 15%,) [19].

CNIs are difficult to beat in their ability to suppress rejection. CNI-free initial regimens are associated with high acute rejection rates that have, in the case of mTOR inhibitors precluded their de novo use. Belatacept (CTLA4-Ig competitive agonist for CD28, blocking co-stimulation via CD80 and CD86) in combination with MMF and prednisolone incurred rejection rates of 22–17% compared to those on a CNI with 7%. The CTOT-16 trial with belatacept and MMF but no steroids or CNI was stopped early due to rejection rates of >30% in the non-CNI arm [20].

One other compelling piece of data relates to transplant outcomes based on immunosuppression levels at one year. In a retrospective study of registry data, those patients with tacrolimus levels of ≤ 5 at one year had significantly worse outcome at five years and this was exacerbated by low MPA doses and improved by higher MPA doses implying that failure to control the alloimmune response is highly dependent on background immunosuppression levels (◘ Fig. 92.7).

An important caveat is that while acute rejection rates are undoubtedly lower with induction agents Tacrolimus and MPA there is little evidence of long-term benefit from these regimens in low or standard risk recipients [21].

92.3.5 Non-adherence

The commonest cause of late rejection is undoubtedly non-adherence which may either manifest as an abrupt, often irreversible deterioration in renal function in the context of acute rejection, unrecordable CNI levels, secondary to complete discontinuation of immunosuppres-

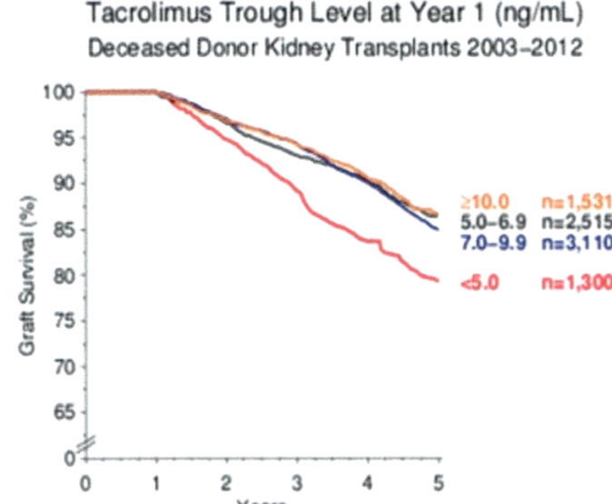

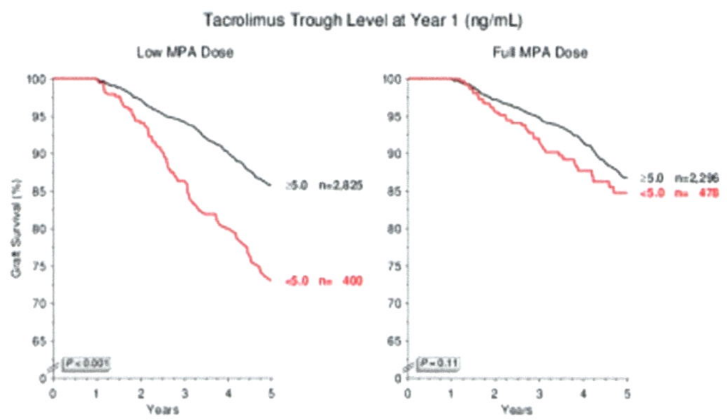

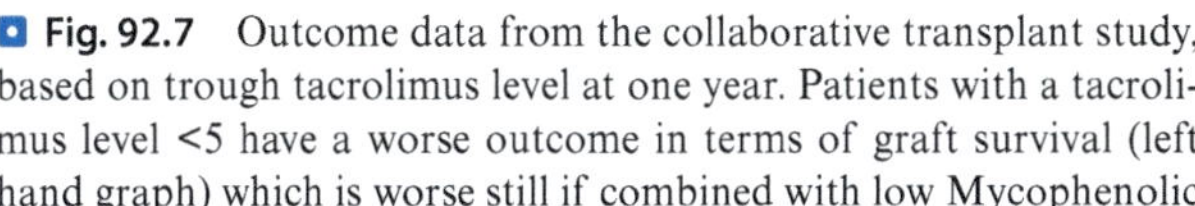

Fig. 92.7 Outcome data from the collaborative transplant study, based on trough tacrolimus level at one year. Patients with a tacrolimus level <5 have a worse outcome in terms of graft survival (left hand graph) which is worse still if combined with low Mycophenolic acid (MPA) doses (middle graph). High doses of MPA had a protective effect for those patients with a low tacrolimus trough levels. (Thanks to G Opelz for permission to reproduce this data)

sion. Possibly much more frequent than catastrophic abrupt cessation is the chronic intermittent subtherapeutic exposure due to multiple and frequent missed doses. Patients with high trough tacrolimus variability fit this pattern and have been shown to have worse rejection-free survival (78% vs 90% at 8 years) [20] or a combination of adverse outcomes [22].

92.4 Diagnosis

Historically in the early days of transplantation patients may notice a tender swollen kidney, oliguria or a temperature but these days this is pretty unusual unless there has been a complete withdrawal of immunosuppression. A version of this occurs in patients with a failed transplant who return to dialysis and have a wean of immunosuppression. This may result in disproportionate anaemia, an unexplained CRP and tender ("hot") kidney. More frequently the diagnosis is suggested simply by a rising creatinine or delayed graft function and failure of creatinine to fall, unexplained hypertension, proteinuria or perhaps the appearance of a new donor-specific antibody. A Doppler ultrasound may show a deterioration in perfusion index and reverse diastolic flow but this is not specific for rejection. A variety of biomarkers have been mooted to avoid the need for biopsy but as yet, none have made it to clinical practice. Ultimately, the definitive diagnosis rests on a renal biopsy although it is not infrequent to for patients to be treated blindly for rejection on best-guess speculation if a biopsy is not feasible. The disadvantage of this approach is that it is not clear that rejection was the correct diagnosis and the patient has been committed to a substantial increase in immunosuppression, moreover, a biopsy after high dose steroids is often much more difficult to interpret. Additionally, renal biopsy allows for the identification of immunosuppression-related toxicity such as that caused by CNIs as well as pathologies other than rejection such as recurrent disease and infection including BK nephropathy. It is also beneficial from a prognostic point of view allowing assessment of the degree of established scarring which often informs treatment decisions.

A single core has a sensitivity of around 91% whereas 2 cores, closer to 99% sensitivity. Clearly the size of the core and while the diagnosis may be made on a fragment >10 glomeruli and >2 vessels (as endarteritis is a focal process) is thought to be an adequate sample [23]. Given the importance of peritubular capillary basement membrane multilayering for a diagnosis of CAMR, a sample for electron microscopy should be standard or considered for biopsies beyond the acute first few months of a transplant.

However, in the context of an adequate biopsy prior to treatment the diagnosis is usually fairly clear. The Banff Classification for Allograft Pathology has evolved with the science and offers a standardization that facilitates an assessment of all compartments and comparative research. The Banff Classification comprises six categories shown in Table 92.2:

Table 92.2 Banff classification of renal allograft rejection

1.	Normal
2.	Antibody mediated rejection
3.	Borderline
4.	T cell-mediated rejection
5.	Interstitial Fibrosis and Tubular Atrophy
Other	E.g. BK virus

The rejection categories are established by specific thresholded combinations of individual Banff lesion scores, which are graded zero (if normal) to 3. Activity scores grade degrees on inflammation present: Tubulitis (t), arteritis (v), glomerulitis (g),peritubular capillaritis (ptc), interstitial inflammation (i, ti, ifta). Chronicity scores establish degree of scarring/new basement membrane present: tubular atrophy (ct), interstitial fibrosis (ci), intimal fibrosis (cv), glomerular basement membrane double contouring (cg),, peritubular capillary basement membrane lamellation (PTCML). There are also Banff lesion scores for extent of C4d staining (C4d), mesangial matrix expansion (mm) and degree of arteriolar hyalinosis (ah).

It is important to consider the differential diagnosis of a cellular infiltrate which includes:

1. BK virus nephropathy,
2. Other viral nephropathies (rarely CMV or adenovirus),
3. Lymphoma (monotonous infiltrate, may stain for EBV antigens)
4. Allergic tubulointerstitial nephritis (perhaps eosinophil rich but not specific)
5. Recurrent disease (recurrent TIN rare)
6. Pyelonephritis (common)
7. Tuberculosis (granulomas)

Rejection-mediated glomerulopathy has the important differential diagnosis of recurrent disease or de novo primary or secondary glomerulonephritis.

92.5 Treatment

92.5.1 Acute Rejection

The treatment of rejection episodes focusses largely on augmentation of immunotherapies in one form or another. High dose, often intravenous steroids are the backbone of treatment with variable use of T-cell depleting agents and implementation of antibody removal techniques such as plasma exchange and ivIg in the case of AMR but the evidence base for the best treatment is very poor.

Our policy is to obtain a transplant biopsy if at all possible prior to initiating treatment in order to avoid unnecessary IS acutely and a long-term escalation in the absence of rejection, to exclude BKV nephropathy and other potential causes of graft dysfunction such as pyelonephritis that are unlikely to benefit from a huge increase in IS.

92

Treating sub-clinical rejection remains controversial, the largest RCT involving contemporary IS (tacrolimus and MMF) in over 200 patients showed no benefit from treating sub-clinical rejection found on protocol biopsy [24].

For biopsy-proven acute TCMR and AMR high-dose steroids are most commonly used and work by blocking the synthesis and release of pro-inflammatory cytokines (IL-1, TNF-α) and inhibit IL-2 production by T cells. Steroids are usually given as IV bolus doses (typically 3–5 mg/kg or more typically as 500 mg daily for 3–5 days of methylprednisolone, or as high-dose oral 100–200 mg tapering over days). The evidence base for dose, route, and duration is very weak. Steroids are typically accompanied by an increase in antiproliferative (usually MMF) and CNI dose (usually tacrolimus) and long-term low-dose oral steroids. High dose steroids successfully treat acute rejection in roughly 60–70% of cases.

Thymoglobulin (ATG) is the most commonly used alternative treatment for rejection. Doses range from 1.5–3 mg/kg from 5–10 days (intention to treat). It has to be given via a central line and can be associated with significant allergy (particularly those who have had exposure/allergic to rabbits).

A meta-analysis of 11 studies comparing polyclonal and monoclonal antibodies for the treatment of AR concluded that polyclonal antibodies (ATG, ALG and OKT3) are probably better than steroids at treating acute TCMR (RR 0.5) and preventing subsequent rejection (RR 0.7) but the studies were of poor quality [25]. Neither anti-CD-25mAb nor Rituximab have any benefit in the setting of TCMR but Alemtuzumab (humanized anti-CD52 mAb) has been used as rescue therapy, is simpler to give than ATG; it does not require a central line (indeed can be given subcutaneously) and is a shorter course. To date there is not convincing prospective RCT demonstrating a benefit of depleting antibodies over high-dose steroids for the treatment of AMR. Even with access to high-dose steroids and ATG in the 1990s acute rejection had a significant impact on outcome with US registry date of over 63,000 transplants showing that AR conferred a relative risk for graft loss of 5.2.

In the setting of acute antibody mediated rejection plasma exchange and IVIg are both commonly used. It may seem counterintuitive (and expensive) to administer both IVIg and plasma exchange which removes Ig but it is important to note that lowering plasma IgG (either via plasma exchange or IgG endopeptidase (Imlifidase)) results in increased production of antibody so any benefit of plasma exchange alone is short-lived. IvIg suppressed the upregulated production, alternatively depleting remove B lymphocytes and further production, while plasma exchange removed preexisting donor-specific antibodies that would persist despite depleting antibodies or increased IS. It is important to note that plasma exchange can be associated with post-biopsy bleeding if clotting not supported and IVIg can result in arterial thrombosis if given in high concentrations. An important and noble attempt was made to address the potential for CD20 depletion in the setting of acute antibody-mediated rejection in the RITUX ERAH study. This French multicenter double-blind placebo-controlled phase III study compared steroids, plasma exchange and IVIg against this treatment plus rituximab for acute AMR. There were 19 patients in each group and there was no benefit at one year with the addition of rituximab [26].

Other agents such as Bortezomib Eculizumab, anti-IL-6 and IgG endopeptidase have all been promoted as treatments for acute rejection but to date none have been proven in prospective RCTs.

Our practice is to treat all but the most severe grades of acute rejection with three pulses of methylprednisolone initially, along with an increase in MPA and Tacrolimus dose. If there is a high level of DSA or evidence of AMR then the steroids are often combined with plasma exchange. In the setting of AMR or failure of TCMR to respond on repeat biopsy we have a low threshold for a treatment course of ATG. ATG is withheld if total lymphocyte count is ≤0.1 or given at half-dose if 0.2 but with an intention to treat for 7–10 days. Response to treatment is followed closely with renal biopsy unless rapid improvement. All patients return to PCP prophylaxis following treatment of acute rejection for a minimum of six months (or until CD4 count ≥200), enhanced BKV monitoring (PCR fortnightly) and CMV PCR monitoring (minimum of weekly if not receiving prophylaxis).

92.5.2 Chronic Antibody-Mediated Rejection

While steroids, depleting antibodies and ivIg/plasma exchange are commonly used and perceived to have some efficacy in the setting of acute rejection the therapeutic options for chronic antibody-mediated rejection are largely nonexistent. A thoughtful and comprehensive consensus document on the treatment of chronic (and acute) AMR, in 2019 summed the current situation thus:

> Currently, there are no approved therapies and treatment guidelines are based on low-level evidence. The number of prospective randomized trials for the treatment of AMR is small, and the lack of an accepted common standard for care has been an impediment to the development of new therapies". Furthermore, "there was no conclusive evidence to support any specific therapy. As a result, the treatment recommendations are largely based on expert opinion [27].

This reflects rather badly on the transplant community in terms of decent RCTs although there have been several noble attempts to address treatment options in a scientific manner. It is clear that this is a critically important issue. The RituxiCAN-C4 Trial (see ClinicalTrials.gov for study design) aimed to evaluate the effectiveness of anti-CD20 therapy in those with biopsy proven C4d+ CAMR. An interim analysis of the data revealed it to be underpowered for measurement of the primary outcome and as such recruitment to the trial was halted. Exploratory analyses revealed that optimization of immunosuppression with tacrolimus, MMF, and prednisolone resulted in favourable outcomes, although ***not*** with use of rituximab [28]. The OuTSMART Trial (▶ trialsjournal.biomedcentral.com) has been designed to test whether a routine screening programme for HLA antibody in all kidney transplant recipients is useful by comparing blinding versus unblinding of HLA antibody status. Additionally, it is designed to test whether those found to be HLA antibody positive experience a reduction in graft failure rates with the introduction of a standard optimization treatment protocol. The trial data is yet to be reported.

Graft survival of patients with and without DSA has been reported at 63% and 83% ($P = 0.0001$), respectively, and the hazard ratio for graft loss after developing de novo DSA =7.7 resulting in a 10-year graft survival of 27% versus 80%. Transplant glomerulopathy (TG) has a particularly poor prognosis; a recent meta-analysis of studies comprising 6783 patients gave a medium graft survival of 3.11 years following the diagnosis of TG, 15 years less than those patients without (18.82 years) [29]. In short, trying to combat a memory response to highly expressed HLA is very difficult and currently there is no effective treatment. The trick is prevention, that is, avoiding pre-sensitization and posttransplant sensitization. A unit that achieves low sensitization rates will have significantly better outcomes for their patients.

92.6 Summary

Despite advances in immunosuppression and immunehistocompatibility graft rejection remains a significant clinical issue, both for those who are highly sensitized and for the significant number of patients who lose transplants prematurely from CAMR. There remain a few absolutes: the quest for a clinically relevant alternative test to a diagnostic renal biopsy remains a quest; good biopsies with experienced interpretation remain essential for patient management. Prevention is better than cure for all forms of rejection but most particularly those forms with little effective treatment. Finally, it is likely that inadequate immunosuppression is the principle cause of late acute rejection and CAMR so identifying and tackling causes of non-adherence or inadequate immunosuppression should be a major focus of clinical care.

Tips and Tricks

Take a sample for electron microscopy when performing a biopsy on an established renal transplant; it will help to establish a diagnosis of recurrent GN or a definitive diagnosis of CAMR.

Establishing sampling for DSA at the time a renal transplant biopsy performed is very helpful to ensure the diagnosis of AMR or CAMR can be advanced if suggested by the biopsy.

High tacrolimus trough level variance (and unrecordable levels), as well as missed clinics offer important and stark warnings of impending CAMR or late T-cell mediated rejection and it is important to try and work with the patient to alter behaviour to prevent this outcome. While changing behaviour is often difficult it is likely to be more impactful and less dangerous than trying to treat transplant glomerulopathy or severe late TCMR.

Case Study

A 43-year-old man with ESRD secondary to IgA nephropathy and a stable renal transplant nine years earlier presented having not attended clinic for a year. His creatinine had gone from a baseline of 105 to 400 (see ◘ Fig. 92.8) with an undetectable tacrolimus level and urine PCR of 420. He admitted that he had missed his IS for the preceding two weeks. He received pulsed methylprednisolone on the basis of a biopsy that demonstrated an intense cellular infiltrate with tubulitis, interstitial oedema, acute tubular injury, and moderate chronic damage (IFTA 55%), but no obvious signs of AMR and C4d were negative. Tacrolimus and MPA doses were increased. However there was a new DSA to a class II antigen with an MFI of 18 000. There was some initial improvement in function followed by a drift upwards. Plasma exchange was initiated and a discussion was had about repeating three pulses of methylprednisolone or the use of ATG. Given the DSA and in the context of another biopsy demonstrating on-going cellular rejection (but 65% IFTA) he was treated with a 10-day course of ATG.

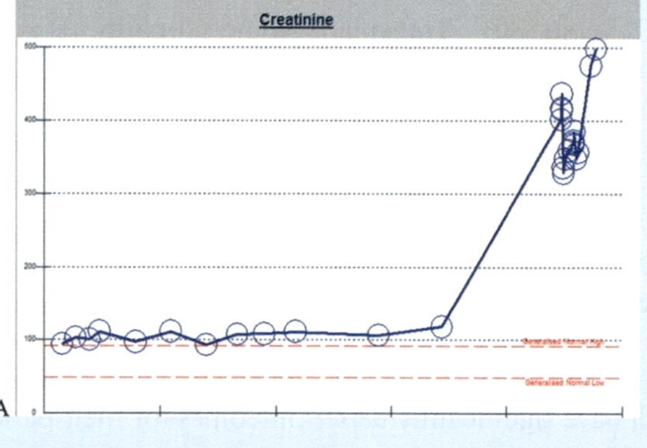

◘ **Fig. 92.8** Creatinine time plot

There was no further improvement in transplant function and he required dialysis within three weeks. On dialysis he developed high-level CMV viremia and was admitted with colitis and pneumonitis followed by two episodes of shingles.

Late rejection invariably results from inappropriately reduced immunosuppression and probably due to delayed diagnosis has a poor outcome. Making an assessment of whether treatment will be successful or not and whether to escalate further or stop is very tricky but it was clear that this patient had missed two previous clinic appointments and it is likely that he had missed IS for longer than two weeks. He had high level DSA, significant proteinuria and IFTA, all giving a poor medium-term prognosis for the transplant. What is clear is that a marked escalation of IS caries a significant risk of infectious complications and is the commonest cause of death on returning to dialysis, furthermore, ATG is not a treatment for non-compliance.

A 67-year-old woman with ESKD secondary to diabetic nephropathy received a DBD kidney transplant. She had been previously sensitized due to pregnancy with a historic DQ class II DSA which was not detectable at the time of transplantation. Flow and CDC crossmatch were both negative prior to transplantation. She received IL-2 induction therapy followed by standard triple immunotherapy with Tacrolimus, MMF, and corticosteroids on a tapering regimen. She achieved immediate graft function and was discharged on day 6 with a serum creatinine of close to 100umol/L. She suffered superficial wound infection and received a prolonged course of antibiotics. Her renal function remained stable on serial monitoring for a number of weeks with consistently therapeutic Tacrolimus levels.

At four weeks post-transplant, she was noted to have a slightly elevated creatinine from her baseline measuring 120umol/L and a rise in her CRP from <5 to 25. Urine dip was positive for leucocytes and protein. Pending urine culture and quantification of urinary protein excretion she underwent ureteric stent removal following concerns regarding early urinary tract infection. Her serum creatinine continued to increase 30–50 points on each serial measurement thereafter. Urine PCR was recorded at 220 and culture was negative for organisms. She was referred for an USS of her transplant kidney following concerns regarding ureteric outflow obstruction following the stent removal. Her USS showed no evidence of hydronephrosis and no extension of her wound infection.

However, concurrent measurement of class I and class II DSA revealed a recurrence of her class II DQ antibody with an MFI >16000 and well as de novo class I (B) and class II (DP) DSA. Urgent renal transplant biopsy revealed C4d+ and peritubular capillaritis consistent with AMR. She received three pulses of high-dose methylprednisolone, followed by up-titration in the dose of her oral corticosteroids as well as plasma exchange and iv Ig. She recovered her function to baseline with largely undetectable DSA thereafter.

In her case, acute rejection resulted from a memory response to class II HLA antigen the detection of de novo DSA likely resulting from recognition of shared antigenic epitopes. The question here is whether she would have benefitted from induction with a lymphocyte depleting agent such as ATG to prevent the aforementioned. This can often be a difficult decision to make. In her case, older age and underlying diabetes already predispose her to increased risk of infection related to immunosuppression. Furthermore, she suffered complications related to wound infection and as such lymphocyte depleting agents were also avoided as part of her treatment of AMR. Augmentation of immunosuppression in any case was necessary to treat rejection. Some may argue that the long-term burden of high-dose steroids, plasma exchange and IVIg is less than that imposed by lymphocyte depleting agents. Others would disagree and as we have discussed the evidence base for existing approaches is weak. The debate goes on but clearly highlights the need for individualized approaches to immunotherapy in transplantation.

Chapter Review Questions

1. What are the features of chronic antibody-mediated rejection?
2. What are the features of acute antibody rejection?
3. What are the risk factors for late rejection and chronic antibody-mediated rejection?
4. What are the risk factors for acute antibody-mediated rejection?
5. What treatment strategies are employed to treat chronic antibody-mediated rejection?

Answers

1. Thickening of the peritubular capillary and glomerular basement membranes—manifesting as double contouring on light microscopy and the pathognomonic multilayering and double contouring seen on electron microscopy. As such, examination of renal tissue by electron microscopy is critical to diagnosis. Endovascular neo-intimal thickening of renal vasculature and subsequent interstitial fibrosis and tubular atrophy.
2. Intimal or transmural arteritis. Inflammatory cell infiltration into peritubular capillaries—so-called peritubular capillaritis. Mononuclear cell infiltration within glomerular capillaries and endothelial cell enlargement—so-called glomerulitis. Positive C4d staining identified either by immunoperoxidase or immunofluorescence within peritubular and glomerular capillaries. It should be noted that the Banff Classification of transplant rejection also recognizes C4d negative AMR as a pathologic entity. In severe cases thrombotic microangiopathy (TMA) and interstitial haemorrhage may be evident.
3. The number and severity of acute rejection episodes. Sub-therapeutic immunosuppression as a result of non-adherence to immunotherapies is the leading cause. High variability in Tacrolimus trough levels suggestive of long-standing inter-

mittent non-adherence as opposed to total cessation of immunotherapy is most common in clinical practice. Immunosuppression reduction in the face of viral infection such as BK viral nephropathy or CMV infection is also contributory in this context.

4. Number of donor/recipient HLA mismatches as well as the specific antigens that are mismatched (DR > B > A). Sensitization and subsequent immunologic memory to previously encountered HLA are widely accepted to increase risk. Both donor-specific- and non-donor-specific HLA antibody confer a higher risk of rejection. The use of non-depleting anti-lymphocyte induction agents have been associated with a higher incidence of rejection at one year in high immunological risk groups.
5. Optimization of oral immunosuppression is often trialled but with little or no effect on graft survival. Most, if not all, would balance the risk of augmented immunotherapy against the risk of infection and/or malignancy while considering the degree of currently irreversible vasculopathy and parenchymal fibrosis. Control of secondary risk factors such as BP and urinary protein excretion is aimed at prolonging the time taken to reach end-stage disease. Some exciting preclinical data is emerging that focuses on inhibition of the pro-fibrotic pathways that contribute to the development of this pathology but are a long way from implementation into clinical practice. Importantly no treatment has been shown to be effective and as such prevention rather than cure remains the focus for specialists in this field.

Acknowledgement Acknowledgement and thanks to Dr. Adam McLean for contribution of material to this chapter.

References

1. Roufosse, et al. A 2018 reference guide to the Banff classification of Renal Allograft pathology. Transplantation. 2018;102:1795–814.
2. Nankivell BJ, Alexander SI. Rejection of the kidney Allograft. N Engl J Med. 2010;363:1451–62.
3. Patel R, Terasaki PI. Significance of the positive crossmatch test in kidney transplantation. N Engl J Med. 1969;280(14):735–9.
4. Murray, et al. Prolonged survival of human-kidney homografts by immunosuppressive drug therapy. N Engl J Med. 1963;268:1315–23.
5. Calne RY, et al. Cyclosporin A in patients receiving renal allografts from cadavers. Lancet. 1978;2:1323–7.
6. Gebel HM, et al. Pre-transplant assessment of donor-reactive, HLA-specific antibodies in renal transplantation: contraindication vs. risk. Am J Transplant. 2003;3(12):1488–500.
7. Knight SR, Russell NK, Barcena L, Morris PJ. Mycophenolate mofetil decreases acute rejection and may improve graft survival in renal transplant recipients when compared with azathioprine: a systematic review. Transplantation. 2009;87:785–9.
8. Meier-Kriesche HU, Morris JA, Chu AH, Steffen BJ, Gotz VP, Gordon RD, Kaplan B. Mycophenolate mofetil vs azathioprine in a large population of elderly renal transplant patients. Nephrol Dial Transplant. 2004;19(11):2864–9.
9. Webster AC, RRS T, Chapman JR, Craig JC. Tacrolimus versus cyclosporin as primary immunosuppression for kidney transplant recipients. Cochrane Database Syst Rev. 2005:CD003961.
10. Ekberg, et al. Calcineurin inhibitor minimization in the Symphony study: observational results 3 years after transplantation. Am J Transplant. 2009;9(8):1876–85.
11. Oplez, et al. Effect of human leukocyte antigen compatibility on kidney graft survival: comparative analysis of two decades. Transplantation. 2007;84(2):137–43.
12. Patel, et al. Renal transplantation in patients with pre-transplant donor-specific antibodies and negative flow cytometry cross matches. Am J Transplant. 2007;7:2371–7.
13. Amico, et al. Clinical relevance of pretransplant donor-specific HLA antibodies detected by single-antigen flow-beads. Transplantation. 2009;87:1681–8.
14. Gibney, et al. Detection of donor-specific antibodies using HLA-cated microspheres: another tool for kidney transplant risk stratification. Nephrol Dial Transplant. 2006;21:2625–9.
15. Webster, et al. Interleukin 2 receptor antagonists for renal transplant recipients: a meta-analysis of randomized trials. Transplantation. 2004;77(2):166–76.
16. Szczech, et al. Effect of anti-lymphocyte induction therapy on renal allograft survival: a meta-analysis. J Am Soc Nephrol. 1997;8(11):1771.
17. Brennan, et al. Rabbit antithymocyte globulin versus basiliximab in renal transplantation. N Engl J Med. 2006;355(19):1967–77.
18. Koyawala, et al. Comparing outcomes between antibody induction therapies in kidney transplantation. J Am Soc Nephrol. 2017;28(7):2188–200.
19. Hanaway, et al. Alemtuzumab induction in renal transplantation. N Engl J Med. 2011;364(20):1909–19.
20. Mannon RB. Avoidance of CNI and steroids using belatacept-results of the clinical trials in organ transplantation 16 trial. Am J Transplant. 2020;[record in progress]:18
21. Opelz G, Dohler B, Collaborative Transplant Study. Influence of immunosuppressive regimens on graft survival and secondary outcomes after kidney transplantation. Transplantation, 87(6). 2009:795–802.
22. Goodall, et al. High intrapatient variability of tacrolimus levels and outpatient clinic nonattendance are associated with inferior outcomes in renal transplant patients. Transplant Direct. 2017;3(8):e192.
23. Shuker N, et al. A high intrapatient variability in tacrolimus exposure is associated with poor long-term outcome of kidney transplantation. Transpl Int. 2016;29:1158–67.
24. Nankivell, et al. Does tubulitis without interstitial inflammation represent borderline acute T cell mediated rejection? Am J Transplant. 2019;19(1):132–44.
25. Rush D, Arlen D, Boucher A, et al. Lack of benefit of early protocol biopsies in renal transplant patients receiving TAC and MMF: a randomized study. Am J Transplant. 2007;7:2538–45.
26. Webster AC, Wu S, Tallapragada K, Park MY, Chapman JR, Carr SJ. Polyclonal and monoclonal antibodies for treating

acute rejection episodes in kidney transplant recipients. Cochrane Database Syst Rev. 2017;7(7):CD004756. https://doi.org/10.1002/14651858.CD004756.pub4.
27. Sautenet B, Blancho G, Büchler M, et al. One-year results of the effects of Rituximab on acute antibody-mediated rejection in renal transplantation: RITUX ERAH, a multicenter double-blind randomized placebo-controlled trial. Transplantation. 2016;100(2):391–9.
28. Schinstock, et al. Recommended treatment for antibody-mediated rejection after kidney transplantation: the 2019 expert consensus from the Transplantation Society Working Group C. A. Transplantation. 2020;104:911–22.
29. Shiu KY, Stringer D, McLaughlin L, et al. Effect of optimized immunosuppression (including Rituximab) on anti-donor Alloresponses in patients with chronically rejecting renal allografts. Front Immunol. 2020;11:79.
30. Kovács G, Devercelli G, Zelei T, Hirji I, Vokó Z, Keown PA. Association between transplant glomerulopathy and graft outcomes following kidney transplantation: a meta-analysis. PLoS One. 2020;15(4):e0231646.

Immunosuppression for Renal Transplantation

Iain A. M. MacPhee

Contents

M. Harber (ed.), *Primer on Nephrology*, https://doi.org/10.1007/978-3-030-76419-7_93

Learning Objectives

To appreciate that the choice of immunosuppressive drug regimen should balance the risk of rejection with the risk of immunosuppression-related and drug-specific toxicities within an individual patient.

To emphasize that the risk of acute rejection is greatest in the early period after transplantation; immunosuppression should be tailored across time.

1. To emphasize that immunosuppressive drugs have a narrow therapeutic index and it is therefore important to take care with factors that influence their pharmacokinetics and have systems in place to protect patients
2. To emphasize that in using therapeutic drug monitoring, ensure that you understand what you are measuring and the evidence base to guide selection of optimal drug blood or plasma concentration

93.1 Introduction

Acute rejection tends to occur during the first three months after renal transplantation and is uncommon later than this; unless compliance is poor or immunosuppressive therapy is reduced excessively. This drives the general principle of more intensive immunosuppression during the early period after transplantation with minimization in the longer term to reduce toxicity but aiming to effectively suppress chronic rejection. The allograft response is mediated by immune mechanisms designed to clear intracellular pathogens. Inhibition of this response was never going to come at no expense. The main complications of the immunosuppressed state are caused by infection with intracellular pathogens, most commonly viruses, and virally induced malignancy.

93.1.1 Therapeutic Drug Monitoring (TDM)

The immunosuppressive drugs all have a narrow therapeutic index with wide variation between individuals in the blood concentration achieved by a given dose. This has led to routine use of TDM for the calcineurin inhibitors and mTOR inhibitors, while use for mycophenolate is controversial. Area under the concentration-time curve (AUC) predicts efficacy. The correct term for quantity of drugs in blood is "concentration" rather than "level". The usual sample required is EDTA-anticoagulated blood to allow assay in whole blood or plasma. Clinicians should know which assay their laboratory uses to measure drug concentrations and understand the performance characteristics. Assays based on high performance liquid chromatography (HPLC) tend to give less variable results than immunoassays and only measure the parent drug while some immunoassays also measure cross-reacting metabolites. In general, it is easier to set up a system for same-day reporting of results using an immunoassay where samples are processed in parallel rather than in sequence. Initial set-up costs are higher for HPLC and running costs are higher for immunoassay, but which ever assay is adopted it is essential to have a robust service that can deliver accurate, reliable results in a timely fashion.

93.2 Generic Immunosuppression

Recently, the patents for a number of the widely used immunosuppressive drugs have expired leading to the availability of less costly generic preparations. Regulatory approval for generic drugs requires single-dose bioequivalence studies in normal human volunteers with no requirement for testing in renal transplant recipients. The generic preparations are not tested for bioequivalence to each other and therefore, patients should not be sequentially changed from one preparation to another as this may lead to fluctuations in drug exposure. The calcineurin inhibitors should be prescribed by brand. This is less of an issue for the other generic drugs with the exception of ensuring that mycophenolate mofetil and enteric-coated mycophenolate sodium are not interchanged [1].

93.3 Specific Drugs

An excellent review on the immunosuppressive drugs is provided in Ref. [2] The age of the reference is an indication of how little the pallet of available immunosuppressive drugs has changed recently.

93.3.1 Induction Agents

The term induction agent is used for therapeutic antibodies given to most patients around the time of the transplant when the risk of rejection is greatest. These agents either block cell receptors (non-lytic induction) or deplete cells (lytic induction).

93.3.2 Anti-CD25 Antibody

The reduction in incidence of acute rejection without an increase in the infectious complication rate when the CD25 antibodies were introduced is almost unique in the development of immunosuppression, although it is less clear whether this translates into improved long-term outcome [3]. Basiliximab, the only currently available drug in this class, is a chimeric antibody that binds to the alpha chain of the interleukin-2 (IL-2) receptor which is only expressed on activated T-lymphocytes. Two doses of 20 mg are given intravenously, prior to revascularization of the transplant and then four days later. There is concern that generation of human anti-chimeric antibody (HACA) precludes the reuse of basiliximab in subsequent transplants but there are no strong supporting data for this view. Basiliximab is not an effective treatment for acute rejection.

93.3.3 Lytic Induction

93.3.3.1 Polyclonal Anti-T-lymphocyte Antibodies

Antithymocyte globulin (ATG) is produced by immunization of rabbits with human thymocytes and anti-lymphocyte globulin (ALG) in horses immunized with human lymphocytes. The resulting immunoglobulin preparations have a broad range of specificities and deplete most haematopoietic cells. They also contain antibody to intercellular adhesion molecules that may explain the observed inhibition of ischemia-reperfusion injury, although this has not been shown to translate into improved transplant outcome. ATG/ALG are effective agents for both induction and the treatment of severe or steroid-resistant acute rejection. They are potently immunosuppressive with increased incidence of infectious and malignant complications. Exposure to these foreign proteins can generate anaphylactic reactions and neutralizing antibodies that preclude redosing with the same agent, as well as serum-sickness 1–2 weeks following re-exposure. Cross-linking of cellular receptors on first dosing can activate cells prior to lysis causing cytokine release syndrome which can be minimized by giving intravenous steroid and antihistamine prior to the first dose and infusing the ATG slowly over at least six hours.

For induction therapy with ATG, 1–1.5 mg/kg/day is infused intravenously for 3–9 days after transplantation and 1.5 mg/kg/day for 7–14 days to treat acute rejection, based on ideal rather than actual weight. Infusion through a central venous cannula is recommended but a large peripheral vein is an acceptable alternative. A 0.22 μm inline filter should be used to remove particulate material. Therapy is best monitored by the extent of depletion of CD3 positive peripheral blood lymphocytes (T-lymphocytes). The normal range is 1–30 cells/μL with a suggested algorithm for pre-dose count <10 cells/μL: omit dose, 10–20 cells/μL: 50% usual dose and >20 cells/μL: full dose. In the event of severe haematological toxicity: platelet count $<50 \times 10^9$/L or white blood cell count $<2 \times 10^9$/L omit dose, platelet count 50–75 $\times 10^9$/L or white blood cell count 2–3 $\times 10^9$/L give 50% usual dose [4]. Mycophenolate or azathioprine may need to be discontinued during ATG treatment to avoid severe haematological toxicity.

93.3.3.2 Alemtuzumab

Alemtuzumab (previously known as Campath-1H) is a humanized monoclonal antibody specific for CD52 that causes sustained depletion of a broad spectrum of peripheral blood mononuclear cells including T- and B-lymphocytes and natural killer (NK) cells. Low rates of acute rejection and low financial cost have driven widespread use. Peripheral blood lymphocyte counts take between three months and one year to return to normal. A single intravenous dose of 30 mg delivered lower rates of acute rejection than basiliximab in low immunological risk patients treated with tacrolimus and mycophenolate and early steroid withdrawal (5% versus 17% $p < 0.001$ at one year) balanced by increased incidence of infection. Efficacy and safety in high risk patients were equivalent to ATG [5]. Subcutaneous administration reduces the risk of cytokine release syndrome. Late episodes of acute rejection beyond the initial three-month period are more frequent in alemtuzumab-based regimens than with other induction agents. Planned follow-up schedules need to take account of this to avoid late diagnosis of episodes of acute rejection. Antibody-mediated autoimmunity, including haemolytic anaemia, thrombocytopaenia, and hyperthyroidism, is a rare complication of alemtuzumab therapy. There are some data to suggest an increased propensity to antibody-mediated rejection in alemtuzumab-treated patients, perhaps suggesting loss of regulation of B-lymphocytes.

93.3.3.3 Rituximab

Rituximab, a chimeric monoclonal antibody specific for CD20 that depletes B-lymphocytes but not plasma cells, has been used primarily as an induction agent in antibody-incompatible transplantation. Typically, a single dose of 375 mg/m^2 given 2–4 weeks before transplantation results in depletion of circulating B-lymphocytes for 6–9 months without significant hypogammaglobulinaemia [6]. Rituximab given at the time of transplantation has no impact on acute rejection. Use in heavily immunosuppressed patients leads to increased incidence of infectious complications including the rare but serious progressive multifocal leucoencephalopathy. Binding of rituximab to B-lymphocytes can cause a false positive B-cell lymphocyotoxic or flow-cytometry cross-match which can be overcome by removing the CD20 antibody with pronase.

93

93.3.3.4 MuromonabCD3 (OKT-3)

This murine monoclonal antibody to the CD3 component of the T-lymphocyte receptor complex activates and then depletes T-lymphocytes often causing severe cytokine release syndrome with pulmonary oedema. It is an extremely effective immunosuppressant with a consequent high incidence of infectious and malignant complications that has led to a decline in use. A typical regimen would be 5 mg daily given intravenously for 7–14 days, monitored as described above for ATG [7].

93.4 Small Molecule Drugs (Maintenance Immunosuppression)

93.4.1 Calcineurin Inhibitors

The calcineurin inhibitors (CNI), tacrolimus and ciclosporin, are the mainstay of most current immunosuppressive regimens. Toxicity, in particular nephrotoxicity, has led to a widespread aspiration to avoid CNIs but their effective control of both early acute rejection and chronic antibody-mediated rejection has maintained their place in the absence of equally effective alternatives. They bind to intracellular proteins, cyclophilin for ciclosporin and FK-binding protein 12 for tacrolimus and the resultant complex inhibits the phosphatase calcineurin that is required to activate the transcription factor nuclear factor of activated T-lymphocytes (NF-AT). Inhibition of NF-AT blocks the production of IL-2. Tacrolimus has generally been found to be more effective than ciclosporin in preventing rejection but there are published studies showing equal efficacy to microemulsion ciclosporin. Nephrotoxicity is manifest both as a reversible renal vasospastic response without histological change that may be ameliorated by the coprescription of calcium channel blockers and a more chronic arteriopathy (◘ Fig. 93.1a) with renal fibrosis. Acute tubular toxicity may be manifest as tubular vacuolation and haemolytic uraemic syndrome can develop secondary to CNIs (and mTOR inhibitors) (◘ Fig. 93.1b). The CNIs are probably equally nephrotoxic. While it might be considered logical, delayed introduction of CNI in patients with delayed graft function does not improve outcomes [8]. The CNIs are diabetogenic, tacrolimus more so than ciclosporin with approximately two-fold higher incidence of Post-transplant diabetes mellitus (PTDM) [9]. CNIs are also neurotoxic, tremor being a common problem and epilepsy or encaphalopathy with reversible white matter changes associated with high levels (◘ Fig. 93.2).

The CNIs are metabolized in the enterocyte and liver by the oxidative enzymes cytochrome P450 (CYP) 3A4 and 3A5 with metabolites excreted in bile and are transported by P-glycoprotein (P-gp) encoded by the *ABCB1* gene (previously known as *MDR1*). Oral bioavailability is only 25–30%, in part due to the active barrier to drug absorption formed by drug metabolism and transport out of the enterocyte. As a consequence, equivalent exposure when given intravenously requires 30% of the oral dose for ciclosporin and 20% for tacrolimus. Inhibitors of these proteins,e.g., macrolide antibiotics (erythromycin, clarithromycin) and imidazole antifungals (fluconazole, ketoconazole) increase the oral bioavailability by approximately twofold. Inducers of CYP and P-gp; e.g., rifampicin, carbamazepine, phenytoin; reduce CNI exposure. If possible, interacting drugs should be avoided. If their use is essential, a 50% change in CNI dose with careful monitoring and return to the original dose on stopping therapy usually maintains blood concentrations in the therapeutic range. Patients taking CNIs should avoid grapefruit which significantly inhibits CYP3A leading to increased CNI exposure. This advice on interacting agents also applies to the mTOR inhibitors (see below).

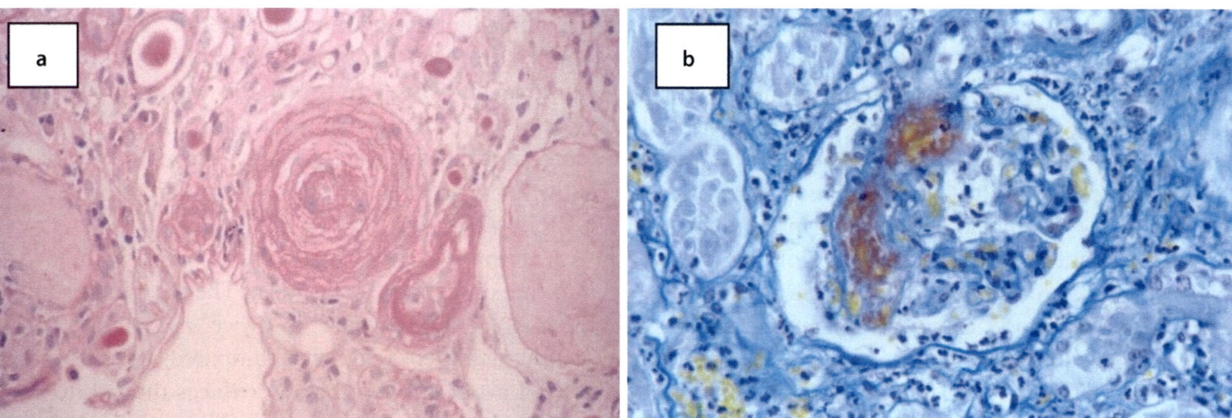

◘ **Fig. 93.1** Severe arteriopathy in a patient with sustained high ciclosporin blood concentrations (**a**). (**b**) showing a glomerulus with thrombosis in the capillary loops in the setting of ciclosporin-induced thrombotic microangiopathy

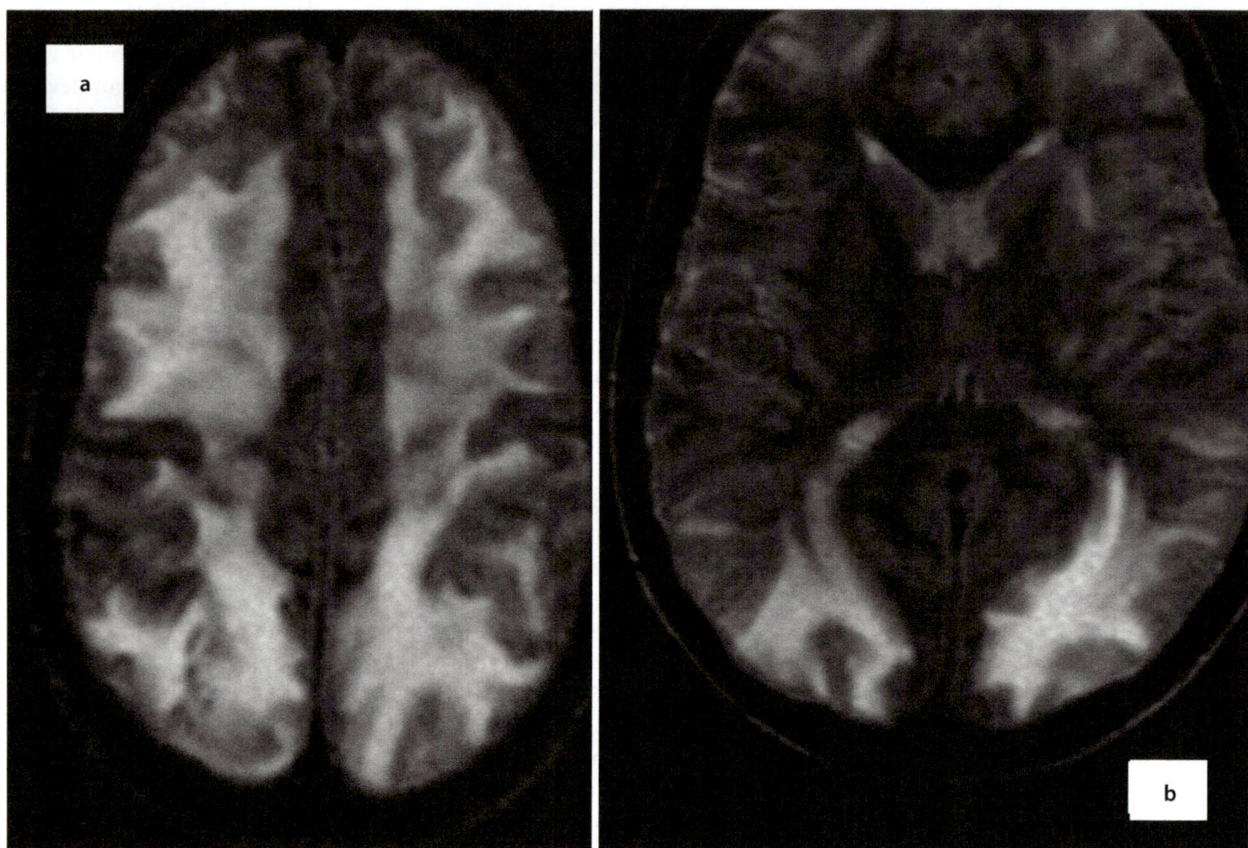

Fig. 93.2 (a) Extensive white mater changes throughout the brain in a patient on ciclosporin and marked drop in conscious level requiring ventilation. (b) Showing a more representative degree of CNI neurotoxicity which can mimic posterior reversible leucoencephalopathy syndrome (PRES) and is part of the differential in hypertensive patients

93.5 Tacrolimus

Tacrolimus is now the most widely used of the CNIs. It is available as a twice-daily immediate release formulation (Prograf™ and a number of generic preparations) and the once-daily sustained release preparations (Advagraf™ and Envarsus™). Maximum blood concentration for the immediate release formulations occurs at 1–2 hours after dosing and elimination half-life is 3.5–40 hours (usually towards the upper end of this range). Advagraf™ delivers a similar pharmacokinetic profile to the immediate release formulations with slightly later and lower Cmax. Envarsus™ delivers a profile with significantly delayed and reduced Cmax and while this has theoretical benefit in terms of toxicity, it remains to be demonstrated. Most tacrolimus in blood (95%) is in erythrocytes and of the 5% in plasma 99% is protein-bound. Blood concentration measurements in anaemic patients should be interpreted with caution in view of the large proportion of the drug in the erythrocyte compartment. It is important that patients take tacrolimus either one hour before or two hours after eating for all preparations. Food markedly reduces tacrolimus absorption, reducing peak concentration and AUC, but with relatively little change in the trough concentration. It is possible to be falsely reassured by trough concentrations in the therapeutic range in patients who take tacrolimus along with food. There is generally less absorption of tacrolimus following the evening dose, possibly due to food intake during the day. Exposure is increased by fasting which is of particular relevance in the immediate post-transplant period when the first sample after transplantation should be interpreted with caution as it is likely to overestimate exposure when the patient starts eating again. Diarrhoea usually increases tacrolimus absorption, possibly through loss of the active barrier to drug absorption formed by CYP3A4/3A5 and P-gp.

93

There are several drug-specific toxicities with tacrolimus that differ from ciclosporin. The most important of these is PTDM which is twice as common with tacrolimus-based regimens compared to ciclosporin. Steroid avoidance (see below) reduces the risk to some extent but does not eliminate it. Neurotoxicity is common, usually manifest by paraesthesia or tremor which resolves on dose reduction. Delirium is an occasional problem with CNIs which can induce acute neurotoxicity manifesting as confusion, epilepsy and white matter changes on MRI (◘ Fig. 93.1). The acute CNI neurotoxicity seems to be relatively idiosyncratic and may necessitate not only dose reduction but occasionally conversion to a non-CNI regimen. Hypertension is common but not universal. There is more functional effect on the renal tubule than with ciclosporin with greater incidence of hyperkalaemia and hypophosphataemia. Hyperkalaemia, acidosis (both common in the setting of high blood concentration, hypertension and hypercalciuria are in part, secondary to activation of the renal sodium chloride co-transporter and can be managed with dose reduction or thiazide diurectics. Serum phosphate concentrations below 0.32 mmol/L constitute a medical emergency and may cause skeletal muscle weakness and cardiac dysfunction. Patients will often still be adhering to the low phosphate diet that they took while on dialysis and this advice should be reversed to a high phosphate diet with the addition of oral phosphate supplements (40–100 mmol phosphate daily in divided doses). Hypophosphataemia may also be a consequence of uncontrolled hyperparathyroidism causing phosphaturia on return of renal function after transplantation. Cosmetic effects are uncommon with the exception of occasional hair loss. This is often noticed 2–3 months after transplantation and tends to resolve. Initial reassurance is appropriate with change to an alternative agent if hair loss continues. Tacrolimus is a macrolide with potential cross-reaction for allergy to the macrolide antibiotics (e.g., erythromycin, clarithromycin).

An initial oral dose of 0.1–0.2 mg/kg daily is followed by dose adjustments based on whole blood concentrations. Some immunoassays perform poorly at the lower end of the therapeutic range which is an important issue if aiming at a target of 3–7 ng/mL as attempted in the Symphony study [10]. Given the time to reach steady state after a dose change, blood concentration should not be measured more frequently than on alternate days. AUC over 24 hours correlates with efficacy. Trough concentrations measured either 12 hours (±2 hours) after dosing with twice-daily preparations or 24 hours (±2 hours) for once daily provide a reasonable surrogate measure for AUC, although the reported strength of the relationship is variable [11]. However, unlike ciclosporin, there is no practically applicable alternative sampling strategy that is more predictive. There are no published studies that have compared different ranges for target tacrolimus blood concentration. Excellent results were achieved in *de novo* patients in the Symphony study where the stated target was 3–7 ng/mL but the range actually achieved was closer to 5–10 ng/mL [10]. At concentrations above 15 ng/mL there is increased risk of toxicity, in particular PTDM. Based on these data, the therapeutic range lies between 5 and 15 ng/mL for *de novo* patients over the first three months after transplantation and 3–10 ng/mL subsequently, probably closer to 5 than 10 ng/mL.

Patients with genetic origin in sub-Saharan Africa (Black) require, on average, two-fold higher doses of tacrolimus to achieve target blood concentration than individuals from other ethnic groups. The difference lies in the absorption phase with no difference in exposure after intravenous administration and the same elimination half-life when compared to Caucasians [12]. Some transplant centres use a higher than standard initial dose of tacrolimus in Black patients (e.g., 0.3 mg/kg) to avoid delay in achieving target blood concentrations in a group with a higher than average risk of acute rejection. Individuals from other ethnic groups who are predicted to express functional CYP3A5 through possession of at least one wild-type *CYP3A5*1* allele have a twofold higher dose requirement for tacrolimus (◘ Figs. 93.2 and 93.3) An initial daily dose of 0.3 mg/kg in CYP3A5 expressers and 0.15 mg/kg in non-expressers (homozygous for the *CYP3A5*3* mutation) allowed earlier attainment of target blood concentrations when compared to a standard initial dose of 0.2 mg/kg. Unfortunately, the study did not have sufficient statistical power to determine reduction in acute rejection or toxicity and demonstration of improved outcome is required before application of this pharmacogenetic strategy in routine practice [13].

93.6 Ciclosporin

Ciclosporin was initially formulated in corn oil as Sandimmun™ with subsequent development of microemulsion preparations such as Neoral™ (confusingly branded as Sandimmun Neoral™ in some countries) to reduce variability in absorption. Ciclosporin microemulsion is administered twice daily at an initial total daily dose of 5–10 mg/kg. Peak blood concentration is at around two hours with elimination half-life of 6–20 hours. Most ciclosporin in blood is present in erythrocytes (60–70%) with only 4% in the plasma of which 60–70% is protein bound.

Ciclosporin is measured in whole blood. TDM was traditionally based on 12-hour post dose (trough or C0) blood concentrations. However, C0 is a relatively poor predictor of AUC. Differences in drug absorption rather than rate of elimination explain most of the interpatient variability in ciclosporin exposure. Blood concentrations measured two hours after drug dosing (C2), during the absorption phase, provide a significantly better estimate of AUC. C2 monitoring is challenging logistically with a requirement to collect samples in the time interval of 15 min before or after the two hours post-dose

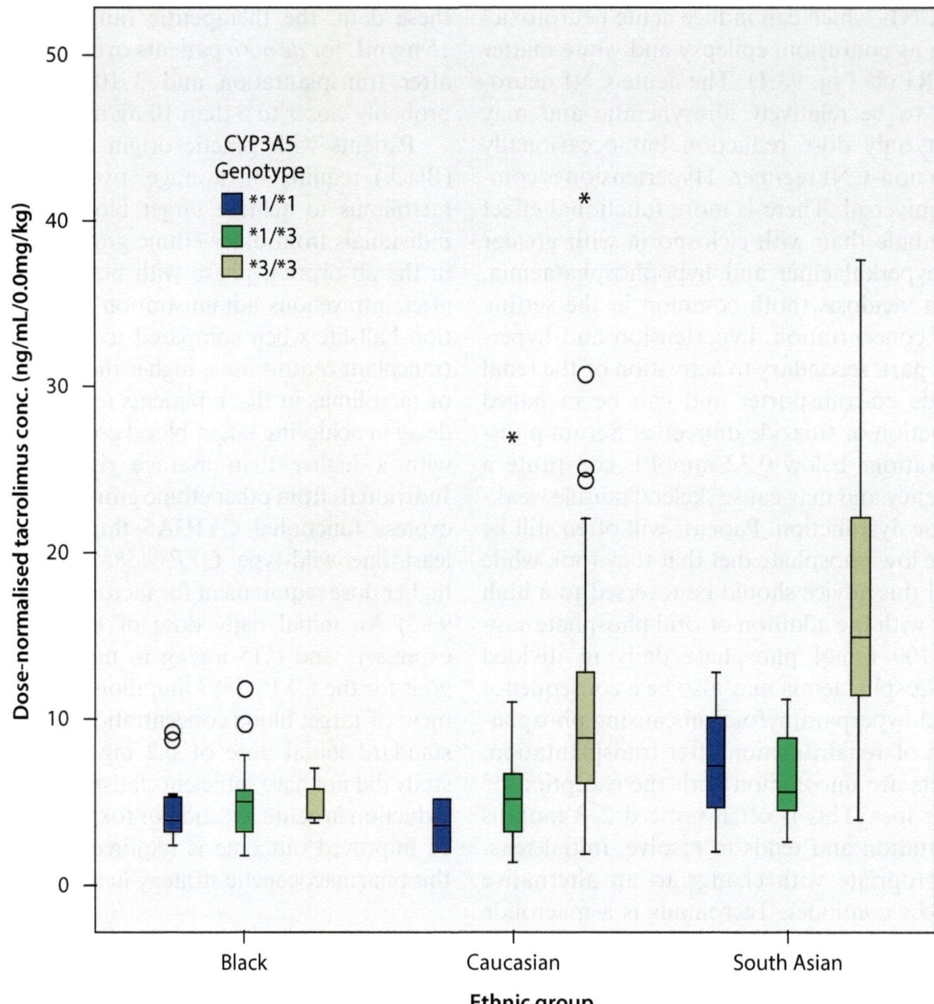

Fig. 93.3 Influence of ethnic group and *CYP3A5* genotype on tacrolimus exposure. Dose-normalized blood concentration for patients genotyped at the CYP3A5*1/*3 locus. Individuals with at least one wild-type **1* allele (**1/*1 or *1/*3*) are functional CYP3A5 expressers and individuals homozygous for the mutant *3 allele (**3/*3*) are functional non-expressers. (MacPhee, unpublished data)

time to maintain a 10% margin for error [14]. Ciclosporin concentration in samples collected two hours post-dose is usually above the range of detection of standard assays. The laboratory needs to be informed that a C2 sample has been sent and requires a validated dilution method.

The conventional therapeutic range for ciclosporin C0 concentrations is 150–300 μg/L during the first three months after transplantation and 100–200 μg/L thereafter. A regimen based on mycophenolate and anti-CD25 induction therapy delivered similar results with the lower target of 50–150 μg/L [10]. A target range of 75–125 μg/L from month 12 after renal transplantation delivered a lower rate of malignancy than 150–250 μg/L without increased risk of rejection [15]. A randomized controlled trial of two different ranges for C2 concentrations delivered good results with: 1600–2000 μg/L during month 1, 1400–1600 μg/L during month 2, 1200–1400 μg/L during month 3, 800–1000 μg/L in months 4–6 and 600–800 μg/L thereafter [16].

There are several drug-specific toxicities with ciclosporin that differ from tacrolimus. Hypertension is almost ubiquitous in ciclosporin-treated patients and seems to be commoner than with tacrolimus. Hyperuricaemia is common with increased incidence of gout. In treating gout, beware of using allopurinol in patients on azathioprine (see below). Cosmetic impact tends to be greater with hypertrichosis, gingival hyperplasia (see Fig. 93.5) and apparent coarsening of facial features. Co-prescription of dihydropyridine calcium channel blockers (e.g., nifedipine, amlodipine) increases the incidence of gingival hyperplasia. The most appropriate management of gingival hyperplasia is replacement of ciclosporin with an alternative agent, usually tacrolimus or sirolimus rather than use of antibiotics or dental hygiene measures as is sometimes advocated.

93.7 Choice of Calcineurin Inhibitor

Tacrolimus is now the most widely used CNI for *de novo* renal transplant recipients. Tacrolimus provides lower rates of acute rejection and better cosmetic tolerability than ciclosporin. The principal disadvantages of tacrolimus are a twofold higher rate of PTDM when compared to ciclosporin and more neurotoxicity. While it was hoped that sirolimus would be a less diabetogenic alternative to the CNIs, it is probably as diabetogenic as tacrolimus. Ciclosporin may be the correct CNI to use in patients at high risk of PTDM and there is evidence for reversal of diabetes on switching therapy from tacrolimus to ciclosporin [17]. The dose of ciclosporin required to achieve the therapeutic range is approximately 30-fold higher than that for tacrolimus [18].

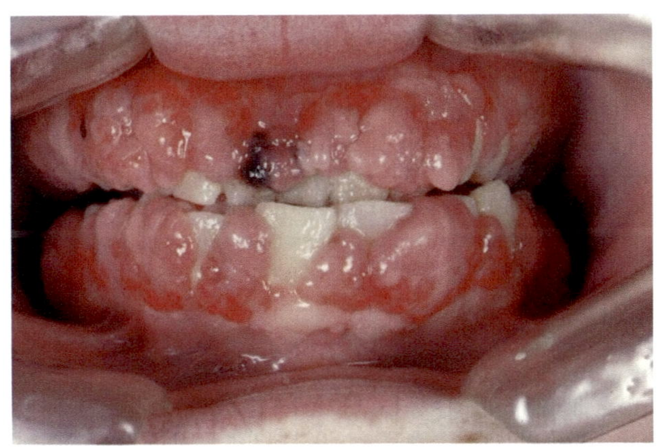

◘ **Fig. 93.4** Gingival hyperplasia in a transplant recipient on ciclosporin which resolved completely on conversion to tacrolimus

93.8 Intrapatient Variability in CNI Exposure

Patients who have greater variability in exposure to ciclosporin or tacrolimus across time (intrapatient variability) have poorer outcomes than those with less variability [19]. Intrapatient variability can be calculated as average percentage deviation from mean exposure: (((Xmean – X1) + (Xmean – X2)……… + (Xmean – Xn))/*n*)/Xmean * 100 or as the coefficient of variation (CV %). Examples of patients with high or low intrapatient variability are shown in ◘ Fig. 93.4 and 93.5) Patients with a high level of variability are likely to be exposed to periods of low drug exposure predisposing to rejection, or high exposure with the risk of nephrotoxicity. A high level of intrapatient variability may be a marker of poor compliance with drug doses, timing, or separation from food. Variable intake of enzyme inducers and inhibitors may also be a factor in variable first-pass metabolism. Drug formulation can impact on intrapatient variability and formulations conferring less variability are preferable.

93.9 Antiproliferative Agents

93.9.1 Mycophenolate

Mycophenolate inhibits inosine monophosphate dehydrogenase, an enzyme involved in purine synthesis. This reduces proliferation of both T- and B-lymphocytes and suppresses expression of some intercellular adhesion molecules. Mycophenolate is more potent than azathioprine in preventing acute rejection in CNI-treated patients [20]. The commonest dose-limiting toxicities are gastrointestinal upset (typically diarrhoea) and myelosuppression. Mycophenolate is the most

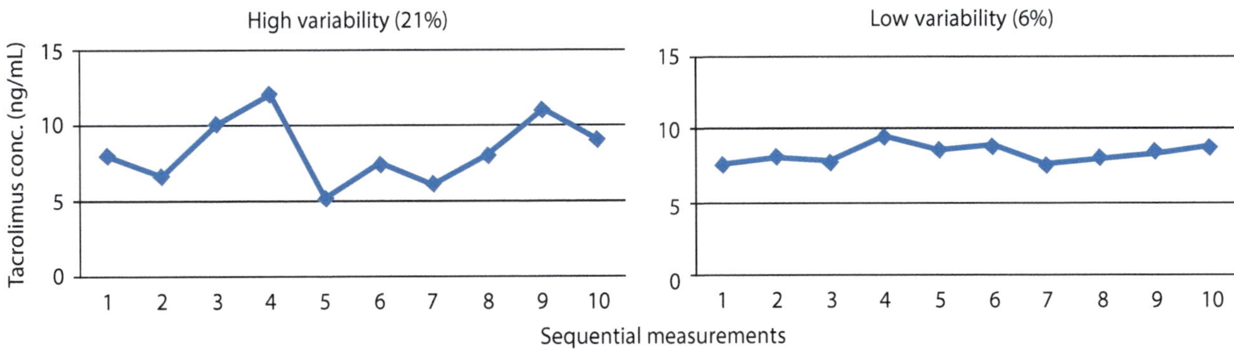

◘ **Fig. 93.5** Intrapatient variability. Intrapatient variability was calculated using the formula: (((Xmean – X1) + (Xmean – X2)……… + (Xmean – Xn))/*n*)/Xmean * 100. Examples are shown of patients with high and low degrees of variability

pharmacologicaly complex of the immunosuppressive drugs and poor understanding of the basic pharmacology often leads to irrational prescribing practice [21]. The active agent mycophenolic acid (MPA) is available as the morpholinoethyl ester pro-drug, mycophenolate mofetil, or as enteric-coated mycophenolate sodium (MPS). The ester group of MMF is removed in the gut and only MPA and not MMF is measurable in blood after oral administration. Equivalent MPA exposure is achieved with 1 g of MMF or 720 mg of MPS. It is important to ensure that the correct preparation and dose are prescribed. Mycophenolate is well absorbed (oral bioavailability close to 100%) with initial peak concentration in the blood at around two hours for MMF, occurring later and with more variability for MPS. MPA is highly protein-bound (97–98%) and a number of factors that are common in renal transplant recipients reduce the level of protein binding with an increase in the "free" fraction. MPA is glucuronidated in the liver with most metabolized to the inactive phenolic glucuronide (MPAG) and a small proportion metabolized to the acyl glucuronide which has some pro-inflammatory effects. MPAG is excreted either in urine or by active transport into bile by the drug transporter ABCC2(formerly known as MRP2). Elimination half-life is around 17 hours. Renal impairment or inhibition of ABCC2 by ciclosporin (but not tacrolimus or sirolimus) results in accumulation of MPAG. Intestinal bacteria remove a proportion of the glucuronide moieties resulting in a second peak of MPA absorption at around eight hours after administration due to enterohepatic recirculation that comprises 30–50% of AUC. High plasma concentrations of MPAG displace MPA from protein binding sites leading to an increase in the "free" fraction. Other factors increasing the "free" fraction include low plasma albumin concentration, uraemia and acidaemia. Somewhat counterintuitively, total MPA rather than the "free" fraction predicts efficacy. Increase in the "free" fraction results in increased rate of glucuronidation with reduced total plasma MPA concentration. High plasma concentrations of MPAG result in increased secretion into bile, explaining the increased gastrointestinal toxicity experienced by patients with factors leading to reduced binding of MPA to albumin. Key practical consequences of this complex pharmacology are:

1. MPA exposure for a given dose is 1.5- to 2-fold higher in patients treated with tacrolimus or sirolimus than in patients treated with ciclosporin due to inhibition of enterohepatic recirculation by ciclosporin. The standard maintenance dose of 1 g MMF daily was established in ciclosporin treated patients and is not appropriate for patients not coadministered ciclosporin.
2. Patients not treated with ciclosporin experience more gastrointestinal toxicity than those treated with ciclosporin.

Conditions that increase the "free" fraction of MPA result in reduced efficacy with increased gastrointestinal toxicity. Total plasma MPA increases with time after transplantation as renal function improves [22]. The empirical dosing regimen that delivers MPA concentrations consistently in the target range of 30–60 mg.L/hr for ciclosporin-treated patients is 1.5 g MMF twice daily for 30 days then reduced to 1 g twice daily and for tacrolimus or sirolimus-treated patients: 1 g twice daily for 30 days dropping to 500 or 750 mg twice daily (or equivalent MPS doses). In patients treated with mycophenolate and steroid without CNI or mTOR inhibitor, blood MPA exposure should be in the upper end of the therapeutic range (45–60 mg.L/hr). There is no evidence to support increased mycophenolate dosing in black patients that is sometimes advocated.

The role of therapeutic drug monitoring for mycophenolate is controversial. There is no single time point for blood sampling that is sufficiently predictive of AUC to be useful on an individual patient basis. Mycophenolate is measured in plasma, usually from EDTA-anticoagulated blood. The most practically applicable limited sampling strategies for estimating AUC are based on three blood samples collected over two hours. A Bayesian estimator for use with samples collected at various time points after drug dosing is available online at: ▶ https://pharmaco.chu-limoges.fr. The equations used to estimate AUC, based on samples collected predose and 0.5 and 2 hours after dosing in the FDCC study are shown in Table 93.1 [23]. This is impractical for routine measurement at all clinic visits but can be useful in the event of rejection or toxicity. There is no established limited sampling strategy to estimate AUC for MPS rendering TDM impractical. There is no evidence that dose-splitting to three or four times daily dosing reduces toxicity or preserves efficacy. The limited sampling strategies for estimation of AUC only apply to twice-daily dosing. Full blood count should be monitored weekly during the first month of treatment, twice-monthly during the second and third months, and then monthly throughout the first year. Dose reduction should be considered when the white blood cell count falls below 4×10^9/L or platelets below 100×10^9/L.

It is extremely important to remember that mycophenolate mofetil is associated with a high risk of

Table 93.1 Algorithms for calculating AUC for MPA from blood samples collected 0, 0.5, and 2 hours after drug administration

1. For fasted adults on MMF+ Tacrolimus:	
AUC = 7.75 + 6.49 × C0 + 0.76 × C0.5 + 2.43 × C2	$r^2 = 0.862$
2. For fasted adults on MMF+ CsA:	
AUC = 11.34 + 3.1 × C0 + 1.102 × C0.5 + 1.909 × C2	$r^2 = 0.752$
3. For not fasted pediatric patients on MMF and Tacrolimus:	
AUC = 10.01391 + 3.94791 × C0 + 3.24253 × C0.5 + 1.0108 × C2	$r^2 = 0.800$
4. For fasted pediatric patients on MMF and CsA:	
AUC = 18.609 + 4.309 × C0 + 0.536 × C0.5 + 2.148 × C2	$r^2 = 0.72$

Algorithms used in the FDCC study [23]

teratogenicity 23–27% compared to 2–3% for other immunosuppression, and spontaneous abortion rates of 45–49% versus 12–33%. Congenital abnormalities most commonly relate to ear defects but include cardiac, other ear nose and throat and renal abnormalities. Women of child bearing age need to be clearly advised of these risks and the need for robust contraception while on and for 90 days after stopping Mycophenolate.

93.9.2 Azathioprine

While azathioprine has been largely superseded by mycophenolate for *de novo* transplants, it remains a well-tested and useful agent. Azathioprine is a pro-drug that is metabolized to the purine analogue 6-mercaptopurine that inhibits DNA synthesis inhibiting the proliferation of rapidly dividing cells. There is also inhibition of intracellular signalling via the CD28 costimulatory pathway. In the early posttransplant period mycophenolate is more effective than azathioprine in preventing acute rejection but longer term benefit is less clear. Azathioprine offers a well-tolerated, once-daily treatment option after the immediate posttransplant period. The primary toxicities are dose-dependent myelosuppression and idiosyncratic hepatotoxicity. Full blood count and liver blood tests should be monitored, weekly for at least the first four weeks after initiation followed by a reduced frequency but not less than every three months. Dose reduction should be considered with white blood cell counts below 4 × 10^9/L or platelets below 100 × 10^9/L or evidence of hepatic injury.

Azathioprine is well absorbed orally with no need to adjust the dose for intravenous administration. Azathioprine is metabolized by 6 thiopurine-S-methyltransferase. (TPMT). 6-mercaptopurine has a short half-life of 38–114 min but the 6-thioguanine nucleotides persist in the tissues allowing once-daily dosing. A typical initial daily dose is 1–3 mg/kg body weight with dose adjusted according to toxicity. One in 300 individuals carry homozygous mutant alleles for the TPMT gene resulting in loss of enzyme activity and accumulation of azathioprine leading to toxicity [24]. In some specialties, testing for erythrocyte TPMT content (avoiding assay within 30–60 days of blood transfusion) or genotyping for mutant alleles has become standard practice prior to initiating azathioprine treatment. This practice has not been adopted widely for transplantation, possibly due to very close monitoring around the time of starting treatment that allows timely dose reductions in response to haematological toxicity. Measurement of azathioprine in blood is not useful but measurement of 6 thioguanine nucleotides has been used for TDM.

One of the most important drug interactions in immunosuppressed patients is the inhibition of metabolism of azathioprine by allopurinol or febuxostat used to treat gout, a common complication in renal transplant recipients. While some would advocate the use of low-dose azathioprine in this situation, avoidance of the combination is the safest option with use of mycophenolate in patients with gout.

93.9.3 Leflunomide

Leflunomide is an orally active pyrimidine synthesis inhibitor with a long elimination half-life that is licensed for treatment of rheumatoid arthritis. A derivative FK-778 was tested in renal transplant recipients and found to have equivalent efficacy to mycophenolate but development was discontinued. Leflunomide has activity against BK polyomavirus, offering an option in refractory cases.

93.10 Mammalian Target of Rapamycin (mTOR) Inhibitors

The mTOR inhibitors (sirolimus and everolimus) inhibit a transcription factor that is at a pivotal point in a number of intracellular signalling pathways including the response of T-lymphocytes to cytokines and pro-fibrotic processes such as wound healing. They come with the advantages of not being nephrotoxic or causing hypertension but do seem to be as diabetogenic as tacrolimus. Medium term (3–5 years) graft function and histological changes on protocol biopsy were better in sirolimus than in ciclosporin treated patients [25]. They are less potent than CNIs in *de novo* patients and less effective at preventing the generation of *de novo* donor-specific antibodies in the longer term. They bind to the same immunophilin, FKBP-12, as tacrolimus but do not compete functionally with tacrolimus, as was initially feared would be the case. This is a difficult class of agent to use due to tolerability with 30% of patients in most trials of sirolimus discontinuing the drug due to toxicity. They are metabolized by CYP3A4 and CYP3A5 so the advice on interacting drugs provided for the CNIs also applies to the mTOR inhibitors.

93.10.1 Sirolimus

Sirolimus, previously known as rapamycin, has a long elimination half-life of around 60 hours that may be perceived as a benefit in allowing once-daily dosing with simplicity potentially improving compliance. A counter argument is that achieving steady state after a dose change takes several days and leads to slow response to TDM. The half-life in children is much shorter (closer to 10 hours) and twice-daily dosing may be appropriate. While sirolimus is not nephrotoxic itself, inhibition of P-gp enhances entry of the CNIs to renal tubular epithelial cells, potentiating CNI nephrotoxicity. Although not directly nephrotoxic the antiproliferative activity of the mTOR inhibitors delays recovery from acute tubular necrosis so they are not an ideal agent in patients with delayed graft function.

93 Most patients become hyperlipidaemic due to changes in lipid distribution. While it is uncertain whether this confers increased atherosclerotic risk, it is likely to trigger prescription of lipid lowering treatment. Haematological toxicity including thrombocytopaenia and anaemia is common, particularly in patients taking another antiproliferative agent. Proteinuria is often exacerbated, probably through inhibition of vascular endothelial growth factor (VEGF) and mTOR inhibitors should be avoided when 24-hour urinary protein exceeds 800g [26]. Mouth ulcers, rashes and ankle oedema are common. Mouth ulcers probably occur more frequently in patients not on steroid treatment. Dose reduction and topical dental steroid paste can help with healing. Severely disabling lymphoedema is a rare complication that does not always resolve on drug discontinuation. Pneumonitis is a rare but serious complication presenting with dyspnoea, dry cough, fever, or generalized fatigue that can mimic a number of other opportunistic infections or malignancy leading to delayed diagnosis. mTOR inhibitors should be avoided in individuals with preexisting lung disease where the incidence is increased. Late switch and significantly impaired renal function have also been identified as risk factors for pneumonitis. Typical investigation findings are: bronchiolitis obliterans, organizing pneumonia and lymphocytic alveolitis. Diagnosis is based on a high index of suspicion with thoracic CT scanning and possibly bronchoscopy to confirm the diagnosis. Pneumonitis usually resolves on drug discontinuation and it is best to discontinue mTOR inhibitors in patients with respiratory pathology of uncertain aetiology. Reduced fertility in both sexes has been reported.

The therapeutic range for sirolimus, 24 hours post-dose (trough), measured in whole blood is probably 10–15 ng/mL during the first three months after transplantation and then 5–10 ng/mL [27]. The high rate of acute rejection for sirolimus-treated patients in the Symphony study suggests that a target of 4–8 ng/mL is insufficient for *de novo* patients [10]. *CYP3A5* expressers have reduced exposure to sirolimus but not everolimus which may explain the higher sirolimus dose requirement in Black patients.

93.10.2 Everolimus

Everolimus was derived from sirolimus by conjugation of a 2-hydroxyethyl group resulting in a molecule with a shorter elimination half-life of 18–35 hours requiring twice-daily dosing. While there are suggestions from clinical trials that tolerability may be better than for sirolimus, this may just reflect lower target drug exposure (whole blood 12 hours after dosing (trough concentration 3–8 ng/mL) and it would be anticipated that it will share the benefits and problems of sirolimus. While the European license for sirolimus indicates use instead of a CNI, clinical trials with everolimus have generally used it with low-dose CNI.

93.10.3 The Place of mTOR Inhibitors in the Immunosuppressive Regimen

Use in *de novo* renal transplant recipients without a CNI has fallen from favour due to increased rate of acute rejection when compared to CNI-based regimens and impaired wound healing, particularly in obese patients, and increased incidence of lymphoceles.

Alternative strategies involve *de novo* use of low-dose mTOR inhibitor along with a CNI or initial use of a CNI with later switch to a mTOR inhibitor. The optimal time to switch from CNI to mTOR inhibitor is probably between six weeks and six months after transplantation as late conversion, beyond one year after transplantation, does not result in improved renal function. An abrupt switch from CNI to mTOR inhibitor reduces the risk of infection due to over-immunosuppression noted in early studies where the therapies were overlapped. Consideration should be given to discontinuing mTOR inhibitors prior to elective surgery and substituting a CNI, followed by reinstatement after six weeks to allow wound healing.

Incidence of malignancy is reduced by treatment with sirolimus. Treatment with sirolimus often causes regression of Kaposi sarcoma and reduces the rate of recurrence of non-melanoma skin cancer [28]. This is probably the immunosuppressive class of choice in patients with previous malignancy. The mTOR inhibitors inhibit cyst growth in patients with autosomal dominant polycystic kidney disease, in particular the growth of hepatic cysts which may be helpful in patients suffering significant symptoms due to mass effect.

93.11 Corticosteroids

Corticosteroids are part of the physiological mechanism to control inflammation and reduce the risk of autoimmunity in times of stress or trauma. As such, corticosteroids have a broad spectrum of anti-inflammatory and immunosuppressive activity that inhibits the innate immune response to ischaemia-reperfusion injury in the peri-transplant period. Data from steroid withdrawal studies suggest that steroids may help to control chronic rejection, perhaps by regulating the response to episodic inflammatory stimuli such as infection. The wide ranging toxicity of steroids has led to progressive reduction in their use over time. They have an adverse influence on cardiovascular risk factors, including: glucose intolerance, hypertension, an adverse impact on lipid profile and increased appetite predisposing to obesity. Osteoporosis, cosmetic effects due to redistribution of body fat, and acne are feared by patients and striae for which there is limited treatment and camouflage, commonly causes long-term cosmetic distress (◘ Fig. 93.6).

Avascular necrosis (AVN) is an important long-term complication (◘ Fig. 93.7), often resulting in hip replacement at an early age and seems to be dose dependent being less common with daily doses of prednisolone below 20 mg.

Administration of steroid in the morning rather than in the evening can reduce the tendency to sleep disturbance when high doses are given. Most immunosuppressive regimens include a bolus of high dose intravenous steroid at the time of transplantation followed by oral prednisolone. In a study of steroid

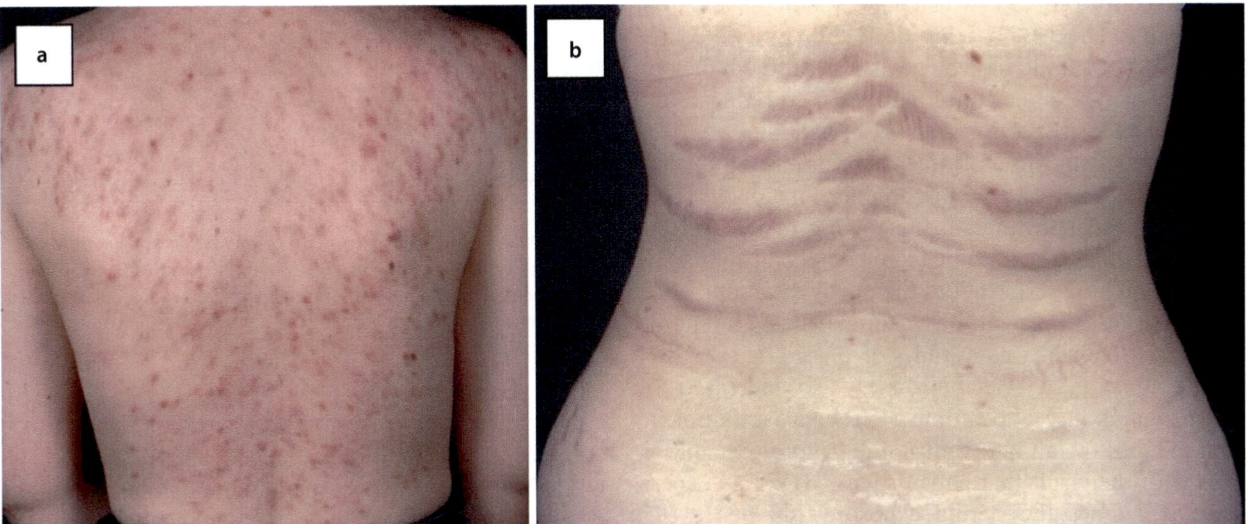

◘ **Fig. 93.6** (**a**) Extensive acne eruption in a patient on steroids. (**b**) Striae following high-dose oral steroids

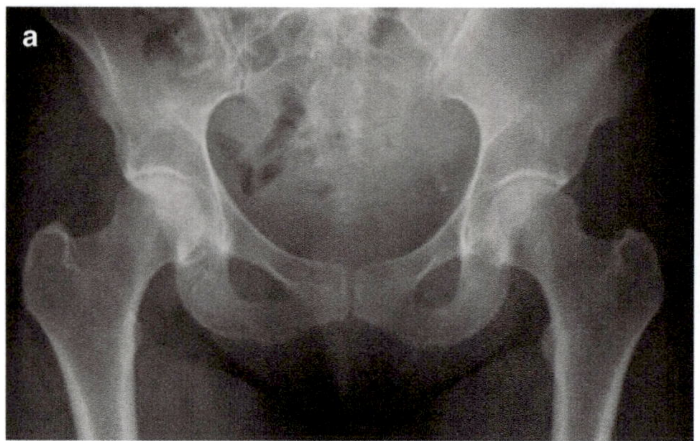

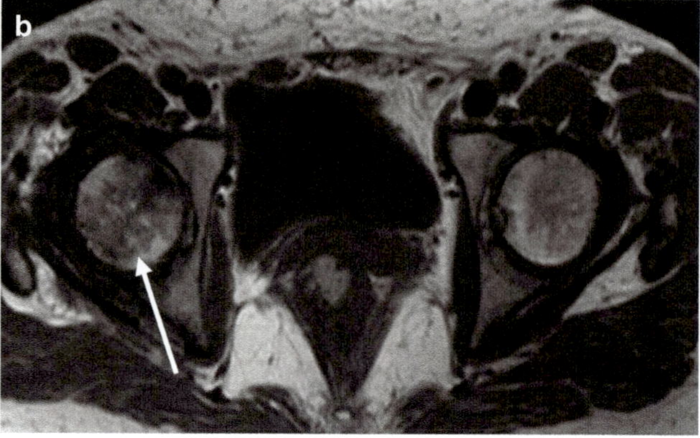

Fig. 93.7 (**a**) Pelvic X ray of a patient with patient with a long history of vasculitis and a renal transplant who presented with right hip pain. The X ray demonstrates relatively mild osteoarthritis of the right hip. However, given an extensive exposure to steroids there was a strong clinical suspicion of avascular necrosis and a MRI (**b**) demonstrated AVN of the right hip. (**b**) Avascular necrosis of right femoral head (arrow)

minimization with the aim of reducing the risk of PTDM, there was only a statistically significant reduction in the group given no steroid, including omission of the intravenous bolus at the time of surgery and not in the group where steroid was discontinued after day 7; and this came at the expense of an increased rate of acute rejection [29].

Prednisolone is well absorbed with maximum blood concentration at 1–2 hours after dosing and an elimination half-life of 2.5–4.5 hours. The current standard maintenance dose of prednisolone is 5 mg once daily, which is only marginally higher than what would be considered replacement for physiological glucocorticoid requirement. This does raise the question as to whether a meaningful therapeutic effect is being delivered. However, prednisolone exposure in renal transplant recipients is up to 50% greater for a given dose than in normal control subjects which may explain the apparent therapeutic effect of a 5 mg dose [30]. Enteric-coated prednisolone should be avoided as it has little impact on the risk of peptic ulceration and leads to reduced and unpredictable drug absorption (Fig. 93.8).

The following doses of other steroids have equivalent glucocorticoid effect to 5 mg prednisolone: hydrocortisone 20 mg, methylprednisolone 4 mg or dexamethasone 0.75 mg. A key point to remember in managing patients on long-term steroid therapy is the suppression of the hypothalamic–pituitary–adrenal axis. The steroid dose must be increased at times of physiological stress, including surgery. Metabolism is also increased by agents that induce cytochrome p450 (such as rifampicin) and reduced by inhibitors most notably protease inhibitors with the result that patients with HIV may experience 2–3 times the steroid exposure and hence side effects.

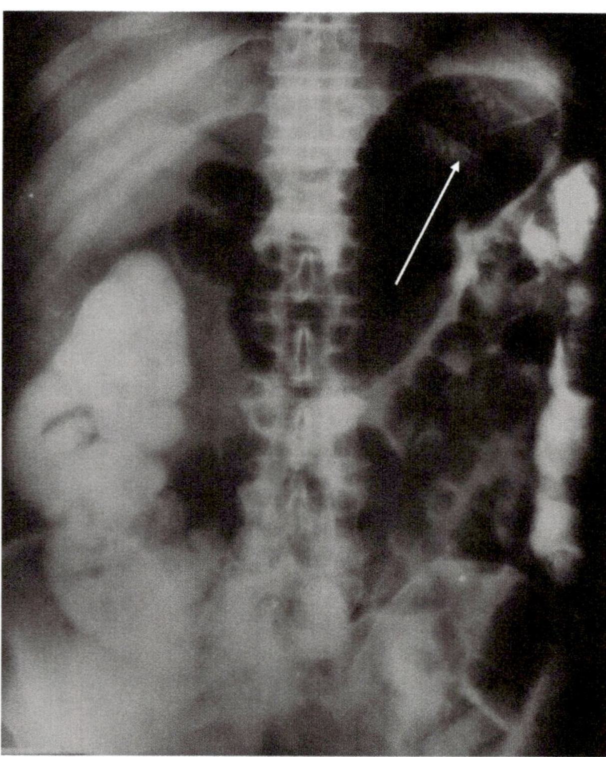

Fig. 93.8 Enteric-coated prednisolone has been shown in small studies to result in erratic absorption and exposure. The abdominal X-ray demonstrates multiple retained enteric-coated prednisolone tablets in the stomach of a patient with a recent renal transplant

93.12 Belatacept

Belatacept, a fusion protein between a modified CTLA4/CD152 molecule and a human immunoglobulin domain, blocks the co-stimulatory signal delivered to T-lymphocytes via CD28. Clinical trials testing it as an

93

alternative agent to CNI in de novo renal transplant recipients found better renal function and less interstitial fibrosis with tubular atrophy in protocol biopsies than in ciclosporin-treated patients but at the expense of more acute rejection and Post-Transplant Lymphoproliferative Disorder (PTLD). Emerging data suggest less generation of de novo donor-specific antibodies. Most of the patients with PTLD were Epstein–Barr virus naive leading to the recommendation to avoid belatacept in this patient group [31]. Provision of facilities for monthly intravenous infusions is an important consideration.

93.13 Choosing the Optimal Drug Combination

With the array of immunosuppressive drugs available, there will never be a clinical trial comparing all possible permutations, and a number of different approaches that may be equally effective are employed by different transplant centres. The most influential recent trial is the Symphony study which concluded that a regimen based on CD25 antibody induction, low-dose tacrolimus, mycophenolate, and steroid was the most effective regimen on the basis of a low rate of acute rejection and the best preserved renal function when compared to similar regimens based on ciclosporin or sirolimus rather than tacrolimus. An important caveat that tends to be "glossed over" in discussions of the study is that the low-dose tacrolimus group had significantly more PTDM than the other groups [10].

There are several important drug interactions between the immunosuppressive drugs. High-dose steroid therapy reduces the oral bioavailability of tacrolimus (and possibly ciclosporin but not sirolimus), most likely through induction of CYP3A. Tacrolimus dose may need to be increased during treatment for rejection to maintain therapeutic blood concentrations. It is sometimes necessary to reduce tacrolimus dose following steroid withdrawal. Ciclosporin but not tacrolimus increases sirolimus exposure. Sirolimus reduces tacrolimus exposure.

93.14 Treatment of Rejection

93.14.1 Acute T-Lymphocyte-Mediated Rejection

Most cases of T-lymphocyte mediated acute cellular rejection (Banff grade I) respond to high-dose steroid. The route of administration does not impact on efficacy but dyspeptic problems with oral regimens based on starting doses of 200 mg prednisolone daily have led to limited current use. The conventional dose of intravenous methylprednisolone is 500 mg–1000 mg daily for three days. There is no evidence that daily doses greater than 500 mg add any benefit but do carry the theoretical risk of increased toxicity, including avascular necrosis which is exposure-related. It is conceivable that lower doses, e.g., 60 mg of oral prednisolone daily would be effective but evidence for this is lacking. More severe rejection with vascular involvement (Banff grade II or III), is often treated with a more potent agent such as ATG. However, there is no evidence for this approach and severe rejection is often steroid-responsive. An alternative approach is to treat with steroid and reserve the more potent agents for biopsy-confirmed ongoing rejection after five days.

93.14.2 Acute Antibody-Mediated Rejection (AMR)

AMR is more challenging to treat than T-lymphocyte mediated rejection. Treatment is aimed at removal of circulating donor-specific antibody and prevention of re-synthesis. Most antibody removal regimens comprise plasma exchange and intravenous immunoglobulin (IVIG) [32]. Rituximab or ATG are used to deplete B-lymphocytes aiming to prevent ongoing antibody secretion. Agents that specifically target antibody-secreting plasma cells has been a deficiency in the immunosuppressive armamentarium that has recently been addressed by the introduction of bortezomib with promising preliminary data on treatment of AMR. Eculizumab, an antibody to the C5 component of complement inhibits formation of the membrane attack complex and has been effective in reversal of AMR but is extremely financially expensive.

93.14.3 Chronic Antibody-Mediated Rejection (CAMR)

There is no well-established treatment for CAMR. Deterioration in renal function may be slowed or prevented by optimizing immunosuppression with tacrolimus, mycophenolate, and steroids. Studies investigating B-lymphocyte targeted therapies including rituximab, IVIG, and plasma exchange are underway.

93.14.4 Increase in Maintenance Immunosuppression

Recurrent episodes of acute rejection carry poorer prognosis for long-term graft survival than single episodes. An episode of acute rejection indicates under-immunosuppression requiring an increase in intensity of the maintenance regimen after reversal of the acute episode. Changing from ciclosporin to tacrolimus or replacing azathioprine with mycophenolate have been shown to reduce the incidence of recurrent rejection. If rejection occurs following steroid or CNI withdrawal, the drug should probably be reintroduced.

93.15 Compliance

Poor compliance with immunosuppression often starts at the level of prescribing, with different lists of drugs held at the transplant centre and General Practitioner that may then differ from what the patient is actually taking. Even the best-organized patients find rigid adherence to complex immunosuppressive regimens challenging and in some healthcare systems the cost of purchasing drugs is a major barrier. Poor compliance becomes more common with time after transplantation and should be considered in any patient with a late episode of acute rejection or high levels of tacrolimus variability; that is highly variable 12/24-hour trough blood concentrations. Electronic monitoring can, sometimes help provide a focus of discussion regarding missed or erratic medication as well as an opportunity to discuss solutions (◘ Fig. 93.9).

There is no single measure that has been shown to have a major impact on compliance but a battery of complementary approaches probably helps. Polypharmacy is inevitable and drug regimens should be simplified where possible, avoiding nonessential treatments. Once-daily dosing has been shown to improve compliance in other therapy areas but robust data for renal transplant recipients are awaited. Education on the reason for taking drugs and possible side effects on starting treatment with a check that the patient knows what drugs they are taking and the doses at routine clinic visits helps to reinforce the importance of compliance. Written medication cards, dosette boxes, or daily alarms on mobile phones set for times when medication is due are useful aids to compliance.

93.16 Avoidance of Inadvertent Drug Interactions

93

Immunosuppressed patients should be advised to discuss any over-the-counter medications or prescriptions by other clinical teams before starting treatment. Communication with other healthcare professionals needs to emphasize the need for careful checking before starting or stopping a drug that impacts on the metabolism of immunosuppression to reduce the risk of serious toxicity or avoidable rejection. Common errors include the CYP3A inducer St. John's wart and the CYP3A inhibiting macrolide antibiotics that are widely used in the community.

93.17 Immunosuppression in the Elderly

As with all body systems, the immune system ages. Elderly transplant recipients have a lower incidence of acute rejection with significantly higher rates of infection and death with a functioning graft (unsurprisingly). There is a tendency to more severe immunosuppressive drug complications. In the absence of specific clinical trial data to guide practice, it would be logical to err on the side of using less potent immunosuppressive drug regimens in the elderly [33].

93.18 Immunosuppression and Pregnancy

Prior to conception, treatment should be established with a regimen based on ciclosporin, tacrolimus, azathioprine, or corticosteroids for which there has been no reported increased incidence of foetal malformations or teratogenicity. These drugs are present in breast milk and breast feeding is best avoided. While the infant is exposed to very low blood concentrations, immaturity of the cytochrome P450 system risks drug accumulation. Mycophenolate and sirolimus are contraindicated due to teratogenicity. Reduced haematocrit and serum albumin concentrations in pregnancy result in reduced whole blood concentrations with preserved unbound "free" drug. This makes interpretation of TDM difficult and blood concentrations at the lower end of the therapeutic range should be tolerated to avoid toxicity [34].

93.19 Immunosuppressive Drug Interaction with Anti-retrovirals

Treatment with ritonavir, a potent inhibitor of cytochrome P4503A, vastly prolongs elimination half-life of the CNIs. Patients may need as little as 1 mg tacrolimus once weekly to maintain blood concentrations within the target range. The long-term effects of this pharmacokinetic pattern are uncertain and alternative regimens that do not include ritonavir, e.g., by using raltegravir or dolutegravir, should be used if possible. In patients who cannot be switched from a protease

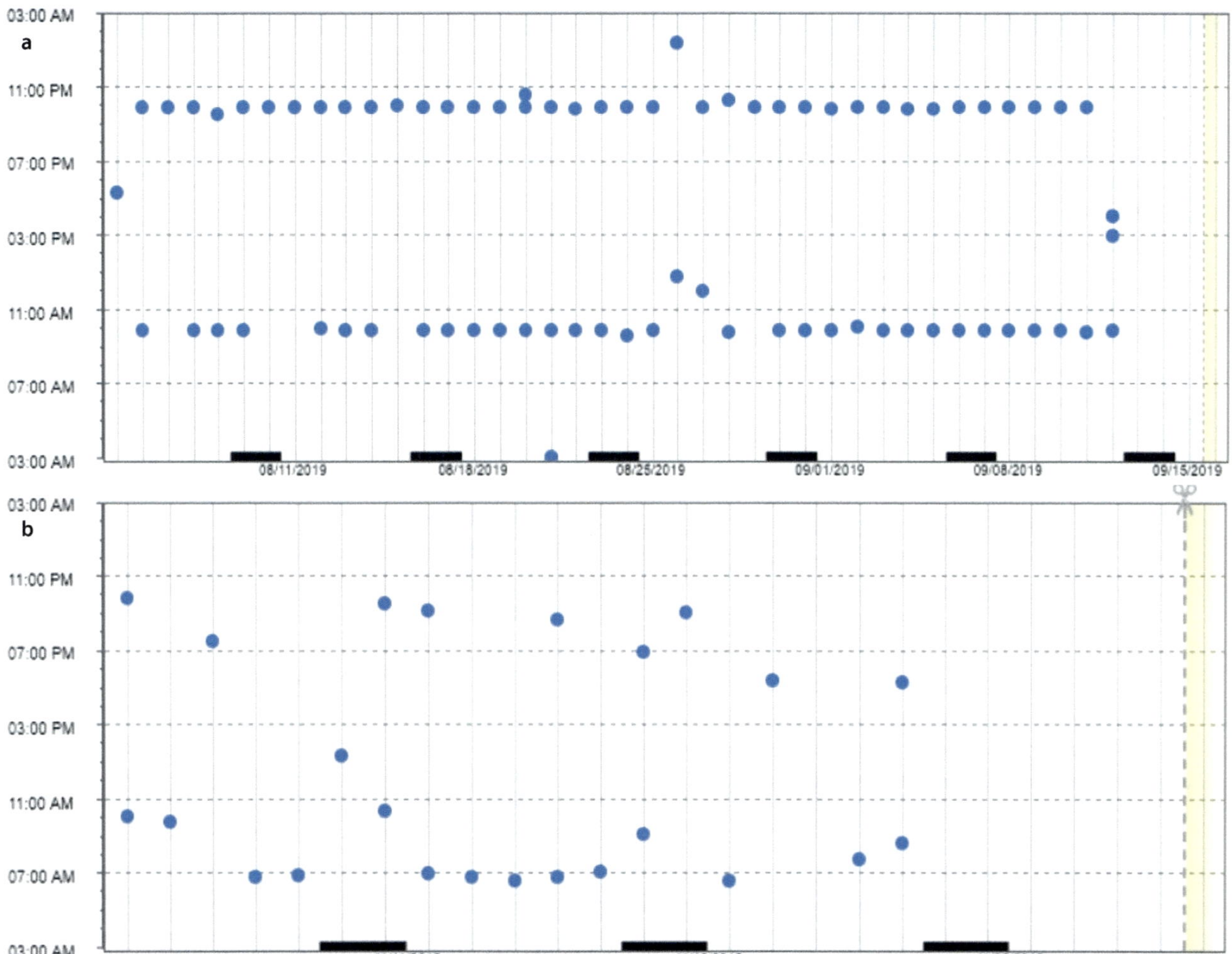

Fig. 93.9 (**a**) Electronic monitoring of tacrolimus in a patient who had low 12-hour trough variability (15%) showing occasional missed or delayed doses but otherwise very regular adherence to tacrolimus prompted by a mobile phone alarm. (**b**) Electronic monitoring on another patient who had tacrolimus variation of 42%, demonstrating multiple missed doses a greater proportion of which were in the afternoon

inhibitor then clear instructions for transplant IS doses are essential. One approach is to prescribe 2 mg of tacrolimus as a single dose at the time of transplant with 1 mg per week thereafter and a booster dose of 0.5 mg in the first week or two of the transplant if required. Ultimately the maintenance dose may reduce from 1 mg to 0.5 mg and the number of days between dosing vary based on blood concentrations.

93.20 Withdrawal of Immunosuppression After Transplant Failure

In the absence of published data on management of immunosuppression around the time of transplant failure, an empirical approach is required. If retransplantation is feasible either preemptively or with an identified suitable live donor, immunosuppression should be continued to avoid immunological sensitization. Preservation of a low-level of residual renal function in the transplant kidney may usefully contribute to dialysis adequacy, in particular for patients on peritoneal dialysis. Staged withdrawal of immunosuppression seems logical. Azathioprine or mycophenolate can be stopped abruptly followed by gradual reduction in CNI or mTOR inhibitor dose till withdrawn. Steroid withdrawal is more difficult due to potential hypoadrenalism and prednisolone should probably not be withdrawn more rapidly than 1 mg per month. If hypotension or hypoglycaemia occur, the steroid dose should be increased to the last tolerated dose with attempt at dose reduction over a longer time period.

Case Study

Case 1

A 64-year old nondiabetic Caucasian male with end-stage kidney failure due to IgA nephropathy was transplanted six months previously with a live donor kidney from his wife that was mismatched at both HLA DR alleles. Initial immunosuppressive drug regimen was Basiliximab induction with tacrolimus, mycophenolate and prednisolone triple therapy. He had gained 10 kg in weight following transplantation and prednisolone was weaned by 1 mg every two weeks from three months after transplantation with a maintenance regimen of tacrolimus immediate release 4 mg twice daily and mycophenolate mofetil 500 mg twice daily. When he attended the clinic one month ago serum creatinine had risen from 84 μmol/L to 147 μmol/L. Transplant ultrasound scan was normal and biopsy confirmed the presence of Banff 1a acute cellular rejection. He was treated with high-dose intravenous methylprednisolone and prednisolone was reintroduced at 20 mg once daily with a plan to reduce the dose by 5 mg every two weeks to a maintenance dose of 5 mg once daily. He now has a fasting blood glucose of 15 mmol/L.

How would you optimize his immunosuppressive drug regimen to manage his Post-Transplant Diabetes Mellitus (PTDM)?

Considerations:

1. Is steroid withdrawal feasible? In view of previous acute rejection on steroid withdrawal this would carry significant risk of acute rejection.
2. Consider switch from tacrolimus to ciclosporin with awareness that this is a slightly less potent immunosuppressant with some increase in risk of further acute rejection.
3. An alternative would be to minimize tacrolimus exposure, aiming for trough blood concentrations close to 5 μg/L. Need to ensure that local assay has appropriate performance in this range.
4. Mitigate risk of acute rejection on changing steroid or calcineurin inhibitor by optimizing mycophenolate exposure using therapeutic drug monitoring.
5. Reinforce importance of weight loss.

Case 2

A 54-year-old female who was transplanted 10 years previously on treatment with Ciclosporin microemulsion 100 mg twice daily and Azathioprine 75 mg once daily with stable serum creatinine of around 80 μmol/L reported three episodes of acute gout over the last year. She has been consistently hyperuricaemic. What do you need to take into account in planning preventive treatment for gout?

Considerations:

1. Allopurinol inhibits the metabolism of azathioprine and the combination is potentially hazardous. Changing to mycophenolate would allow the use of allopurinol.
2. Ciclosporin blocks the renal elimination of urate more than the other immunosuppressive agents. Consider a change from ciclosporin to tacrolimus or sirolimus.
3. If antihypertensive therapy is needed consider use of losartan which has some uricosuric effect.
4. Provide appropriate dietary advice

Seminal Papers

Ekberg H, Tedesco-Silva H, Demirbas A et al. Reduced exposure to calcineurin inhibitors in renal transplantation. N Engl J Med 2007;357: 2562–2575.

This is the key publication that supports the current most widely used immunosuppressive drug regimen for renal transplantation based on tacrolimus, mycophenolate, and steroids. It demonstrated superior outcomes in terms of rate of acute rejection and renal function in patients treated with "low-dose" tacrolimus compared to those treated with ciclosporin or sirolimus-based regimens. There are some weaknesses in the study including a sirolimus target range that was probably sub-therapeutic and use of an inappropriately high mycophenolate dose in patients not treated with ciclosporin which probably underlies the high rate of diarrhoea in these groups. The greater incidence of PTDM in the tacrolimus treated patients compared to those on ciclosporin is underplayed. The blood concentrations achieved for both "low-dose" tacrolimus and ciclosporin were significantly greater than the planned therapeutic range.

Hanaway MJ, Woodle ES, Mulgaonkar S et al. Alemtuzumab induction in renal transplantation. N Engl J Med 2011;364: 1909–1919.

Randomized controlled trial of lytic induction therapy.

A blinded, randomized clinical trial of mycophenolate mofetil for the prevention of acute rejection in cadaveric renal transplantation. The Tricontinental Mycophenolate Mofetil Renal Transplantation Study Group. Transplantation 1996;61: 1029–1037.

This study indicated increased efficacy of mycophenolate in preventing acute rejection when compared to azathioprine and highlighted the risk of invasive CMV disease with overexposure to mycophenolate.

93.21 Governance and Education with Transplant Immunosuppression

Drug errors posttransplant are common and can have serious consequences. Patients whose first language is not the language of the transplant unit are particularly at risk and need targeted support. Pictures of commonly used drugs, replacement of terms like "b.i.d" with "twice a day" and an insistence on patients bringing and showing their medication are all helpful.

Metabolism of CNIs and mTORi via the Cytochrome p450 system presents a huge risk of drug interactions; Inhibitors such as imidazole anti-fungals (e.g., fluconazole), protease inhibitors, macrolides (e.g., erythromycin), and grapefruit juice producing toxic concentrations, inducers such as rifampicin or phenytoin and carbamazepine will result grossly sub-therapeutic concentrations unless adjustment is made. As a general rule, if use of a potent inducer or inhibitor of cytochrome P450 is unavoidable, CNI or mTOR dose should be immediately adjusted up or down by twofold followed by further adjustments based on TDM. It is important to remember to revert to the original dose on stopping the interacting drug. The best solution to this and other interactions is an effective electronic prescribing system with alerts for key interactions. Coaching patients to question whether any new prescription will interact with their transplant drugs is helpful and flagging potential hazard drugs on their drug list (e.g.,"azathioprine 50 mg once a day (allopurinol contra-indicated")) is worth considering. Azithromycin is a useful macrolide that does not appear to significantly inhibit CNI/mTORi metabolism.

Anticipation of drug interactions is important; a patient on a protease inhibitor is likely to need approximately 1% of the usual dose of tacrolimus. Therefore, on listing a patient with HIV on a protease inhibitor stipulating an appropriate starting dose (e.g., 2 mg as a single dose on day of transplant and 1 mg weekly thereafter depending on blood concentration) can prevent gross overdosing. Similarly if HIV medication is changed, anti-TB or other interacting medication is started or stopped, there must be systems in place for clear and rapid communication with the transplant team and thence close monitoring of drug concentrations.

Tacrolimus undergoes redistribution a few days post-transplant often resulting in a drop in blood concentration. Fasting early after the transplant with gradual increase in food intake probably also contributes. Broadly speaking, if a concentration is in the therapeutic range or below it, on day 3 it will be subtherapeutic by day 5 if no increases are made. A high concentration at day 3 is likely to spontaneously move down towards the therapeutic range by day 5. A high concentration at day 5 is likely to be genuinely too high and may need adjustment down.

Further tips and tricks are offered in ◘ Table 93.2.

◘ **Table 93.2** "Tips of the trade" for transplant immunosuppression

Scenario	Salutary tips
Therapeutic Drug Monitoring (TDM)	Know the assay that your lab uses. If sending a C2 sample for ciclosporin, let the lab know as they will need to run the assay on a diluted sample.
Generic immunosuppression	Prescribe calcineurin inhibitors by brand to avoid inadvertent switching between non-bioequivalent preparations.
Calcineurin inhibitors	Tacrolimus gives less rejection Ciclosporin gives less diabetes
Tacrolimus and food	Reinforce importance of taking tacrolimus 1 hour before or 2 hours after eating. Food reduces the peak concentration more than the trough which may lead to falsely reassuring trough concentrations in the therapeutic range.
Mycophenolate dose	Lower doses are required in patients not treated with ciclosporin. The dose required to maintain therapeutic total MPA concentration in blood falls as transplant function improves. Dose requirement is higher during the first month after transplantation than subsequently.
Therapeutic drug monitoring for mycophenolate	Trough blood concentrations are of little value. Assay based on multiple samples is logistically demanding but is useful on a targeted basis for patients with rejection or toxicity.
Azathioprine	Avoid co-prescription of allopurinol or febuxostat. Changing to mycophenolate allows safe use of allopurinol.
Sirolimus	In the event of respiratory presentations, have a high index of suspicion for pneumonitis. If any doubt, discontinue sirolimus.
Prednisolone	Avoid enteric-coated prednisolone as it inhibits absorption and increases variability in drug exposure.
Acute rejection	Severe rejection is often steroid-responsive. May be prudent to reserve highly potent drugs such as ATG for steroid-resistant rejection.
Immunosuppression in HIV infected patients	Try to get the patient onto a regimen that does not require protease inhibitors

Chapter Review Questions

1. What happens to plasma total mycophenolic acid (MPA) concentration in patients with a deterioration in renal function?
2. Which immunosuppressive drugs are contraindicated in pregnancy?
3. What happens to tacrolimus exposure in patients with diarrhoea?
4. What are they key differences between ciclosporin and tacrolimus?
5. What are the key contraindications to sirolimus?

Answers

1. Total MPA concentration is decreased due to an increase in the unbound "free" fraction with more rapid glucuronidation with biliary excretion of the metabolite which causes diarrhoea.
2. Mycophenolate, sirolimus, everolimus
3. Tacrolimus absorption is usually increased with diarrhoea.
4. Tacrolimus is a more potent immunosuppressive agent, has fewer cosmetic side-effects and contributes to hypertension less than ciclosporin. Tacrolimus is more diabetogenic and causes neurotoxicity and hyperkalaemia more commonly. Ciclosporin has more impact on urate elimination than tacrolimus.
5. Preexisting lung disease, significant proteinuria, possibly renal impairment.

References

1. van GT. European Society for Organ Transplantation Advisory Committee recommendations on generic substitution of immunosuppressive drugs. Transpl Int. 2011;24:1135–41. https://doi.org/10.1111/j.1432-2277.2011.01378.x.
2. Halloran PF. Immunosuppressive drugs for kidney transplantation. N Engl J Med. 2004;351:2715–29.
3. Adu D, Cockwell P, Ives NJ, Shaw J, Wheatley K. Interleukin-2 receptor monoclonal antibodies in renal transplantation: meta-analysis of randomised trials. BMJ. 2003;326:789.
4. Peddi VR, Bryant M, Roy-Chaudhury P, Woodle ES, First MR. Safety, efficacy, and cost analysis of thymoglobulin induction therapy with intermittent dosing based on CD3+ lymphocyte counts in kidney and kidney-pancreas transplant recipients. Transplantation. 2002;73:1514–8.
5. Hanaway MJ, et al. Alemtuzumab induction in renal transplantation. N Engl J Med. 2011;364:1909–19. https://doi.org/10.1056/NEJMoa1009546.
6. Clatworthy MR. Targeting B cells and antibody in transplantation. Am J Transplant. 2011;11:1359–67. https://doi.org/10.1111/j.1600-6143.2011.03554.x.
7. Norman DJ, et al. A randomized clinical trial of induction therapy with OKT3 in kidney transplantation. Transplantation. 1993;55:44–50.
8. Kamar N, et al. Impact of early or delayed cyclosporine on delayed graft function in renal transplant recipients: a randomized, multicenter study. Am J Transplant. 2006;6:1042–8.
9. Kasiske BL, Snyder JJ, Gilbertson D, Matas AJ. Diabetes mellitus after kidney transplantation in the United States. Am J Transplant. 2003;3:178–85.
10. Ekberg H, et al. Reduced exposure to calcineurin inhibitors in renal transplantation. N Engl J Med. 2007;357:2562–75.
11. Brunet M, et al. Therapeutic drug monitoring of tacrolimus-personalized therapy: second consensus report. Ther Drug Monit. 2019;41:261–307. https://doi.org/10.1097/FTD.0000000000000640.
12. Mancinelli LM, et al. The pharmacokinetics and metabolic disposition of tacrolimus: a comparison across ethnic groups. Clin Pharmacol Ther. 2001;69:24–31.
13. Birdwell KA, et al. Clinical pharmacogenetics implementation consortium (CPIC) guidelines for CYP3A5 genotype and tacrolimus dosing. Clin Pharmacol Ther. 2015;98:19–24. https://doi.org/10.1002/cpt.113.
14. Levy G, Thervet E, Lake J, Uchida K. Patient management by Neoral C(2) monitoring: an international consensus statement. Transplantation. 2002;73:S12–8.
15. Dantal J, et al. Effect of long-term immunosuppression in kidney-graft recipients on cancer incidence: randomised comparison of two cyclosporin regimens. Lancet. 1998;351:623–628, S0140-6736(97)08496-1 [pii]. https://doi.org/10.1016/S0140-6736(97)08496-1.
16. Stefoni S, et al. Efficacy and safety outcomes among de novo renal transplant recipients managed by C2 monitoring of cyclosporine a microemulsion: results of a 12-month, randomized, multicenter study. Transplantation. 2005;79:577–83., 00007890-200503150-00010 [pii].
17. Wissing KM, et al. Prospective randomized study of conversion from tacrolimus to cyclosporine A to improve glucose metabolism in patients with posttransplant diabetes mellitus after renal transplantation. Am J Transplant. 2018;18:1726–34. https://doi.org/10.1111/ajt.14665.
18. Higgins RM, et al. Conversion between cyclosporin and tacrolimus--30-fold dose prediction. Nephrol Dial Transplant. 1999;14:1609.
19. Borra LC, et al. High within-patient variability in the clearance of tacrolimus is a risk factor for poor long-term outcome after kidney transplantation. Nephrol Dial Transplant. 2010;25:2757–63. gfq096 [pii]. https://doi.org/10.1093/ndt/gfq096.
20. A blinded, randomized clinical trial of mycophenolate mofetil for the prevention of acute rejection in cadaveric renal transplantation. The Tricontinental Mycophenolate Mofetil Renal Transplantation Study Group. Transplantation. 1996;61:1029–37.
21. Tett SE, et al. Mycophenolate, clinical pharmacokinetics, formulations, and methods for assessing drug exposure. Transplant Rev (Orlando). 2011;25:47–57. S0955-470X(10)00075-3 [pii]. https://doi.org/10.1016/j.trre.2010.06.001.
22. Kuypers DR, et al. Twelve-month evaluation of the clinical pharmacokinetics of total and free mycophenolic acid and its glucuronide metabolites in renal allograft recipients on low dose tacrolimus in combination with mycophenolate mofetil. Ther Drug Monit. 2003;25:609–22.
23. van GT, et al. Comparing mycophenolate mofetil regimens for de novo renal transplant recipients: the fixed-dose concentration-controlled trial. Transplantation. 2008;86:1043–51. https://doi.org/10.1097/TP.0b013e318186f98a. 00007890-200810270-00006 [pii].

24. Evans WE. Pharmacogenetics of thiopurine S-methyltransferase and thiopurine therapy. Ther Drug Monit. 2004;26:186–91.
25. Mota A, et al. Sirolimus-based therapy following early cyclosporine withdrawal provides significantly improved renal histology and function at 3 years. Am J Transplant. 2004;4:953–61.
26. Diekmann F, et al. Predictors of success in conversion from calcineurin inhibitor to sirolimus in chronic allograft dysfunction. Am J Transplant. 2004;4:1869–75.
27. Campistol JM, et al. Practical recommendations for the early use of m-TOR inhibitors (sirolimus) in renal transplantation. Transpl Int. 2009;22:681–87. TRI858 [pii]. https://doi.org/10.1111/j.1432-2277.2009.00858.x.
28. Hoogendijk-van den Akker JM, et al. Two-year randomized controlled prospective trial converting treatment of stable renal transplant recipients with cutaneous invasive squamous cell carcinomas to sirolimus. J Clin Oncol. 2013;31:1317–23. https://doi.org/10.1200/JCO.2012.45.6376.
29. Vincenti F, et al. A randomized, multicenter study of steroid avoidance, early steroid withdrawal or standard steroid therapy in kidney transplant recipients. Am J Transplant. 2008;8:307–16.
30. Potter JM, McWhinney BC, Sampson L, Hickman PE. Area-under-the-curve monitoring of prednisolone for dose optimization in a stable renal transplant population. Ther Drug Monit. 2004;26:408–14.
31. Vincenti F, et al. Ten-year outcomes in a randomized phase II study of kidney transplant recipients administered belatacept 4-weekly or 8-weekly. Am J Transplant. 2017;17:3219–27. https://doi.org/10.1111/ajt.14452.
32. Archdeacon P, et al. Summary of FDA antibody-mediated rejection workshop. Am J Transplant. 2011;11:896–906. https://doi.org/10.1111/j.1600-6143.2011.03525.x.
33. Shi YY, Hesselink DA, van Gelder T. Pharmacokinetics and pharmacodynamics of immunosuppressive drugs in elderly kidney transplant recipients. Transplant Rev (Orlando). 2015;29:224–30. https://doi.org/10.1016/j.trre.2015.04.007.
34. Hebert MF, et al. Interpreting tacrolimus concentrations during pregnancy and postpartum. Transplantation. 2013;95:908–15. https://doi.org/10.1097/TP.0b013e318278d367.

Links

British Transplantation Society Guidelines and Standards. https://bts.org.uk/guidelines-standards/

KDIGO guidelines for the management of the transplant recipient. kdigo.org/guidelines/transplant-recipient/

Infectious Complications of Transplantation

Rhys Evans, Sanjay Bhagani, Tanzina Haque, and Mark Harber

Contents

M. Harber (ed.), *Primer on Nephrology*, https://doi.org/10.1007/978-3-030-76419-7_94

94.1 Introduction

Posttransplant infection is a common cause of graft deterioration, morbidity, and mortality. It is also responsible for delayed discharge, multiple, and often prolonged admissions and thus a significant clinical challenge. Infections may be preexisting in the recipient, nosocomial, or opportunistic or uniquely in transplantation infections can be donor-derived. For each of these categories it is often possible to significantly reduce the jeopardy and thus the adverse consequences by identifying patients at risk. As always, clinical vigilance is vital, but equally important is the establishment of robust clinical systems for prevention, screening, and rapid treatment. ◘ Figure 94.1 shows the elements of a transplant service required to minimize or prevent infectious complications posttransplant.

94.2 Donor Infections

A variety of infections can be transmitted from the donor to the recipient of a kidney transplant with outcomes that range from mildly troublesome to fatal. To avoid this, transplant programs institute a variety of screening procedures (see ◘ Table 94.1) based on national guidelines but it is important to note that screening for donor infection is not absolute; infections can be missed. Following the death of two recipients from disseminated donor derived nematode infection (*Halicephalobus gingivalis*) UK national guidelines stated that "Transplant surgeons must consult with microbiologist/virologist or infectious disease team about any donor offer that has evidence of infection". In the majority of cases, the cause and management of sepsis in a donor is straightforward and low risk but legal responsibility emphasizes the need for careful clinical assessment of infectious risk. Donor serum usually accompanies the organ and thus can be tested by the receiving unit for any serology felt to be relevant. It is worth considering whether other samples may be helpful from the donor for additional screening.

94.2.1 Recipient Infections Pretransplant: Treatment, Vaccination and Prophylaxis

For the same infectious agent there tends to be a hierarchy of virulence posttransplant with primary infections being worse than re-infections, which are more virulent than reactivations. Risk stratification is therefore highly important; identification and eradication or control of infection as well as vaccination pre-listing and appropriate prophylaxis posttransplant is not always done as well as it might be yet is not complex.

◘ Table 94.2 Shows infections that should be treated or controlled pretransplant and vaccinations either recommended or to be considered on the grounds of common sense. It is also worth considering vaccination for patients who are likely to travel. For example, if a patient on the waiting list has family in a yellow fever region

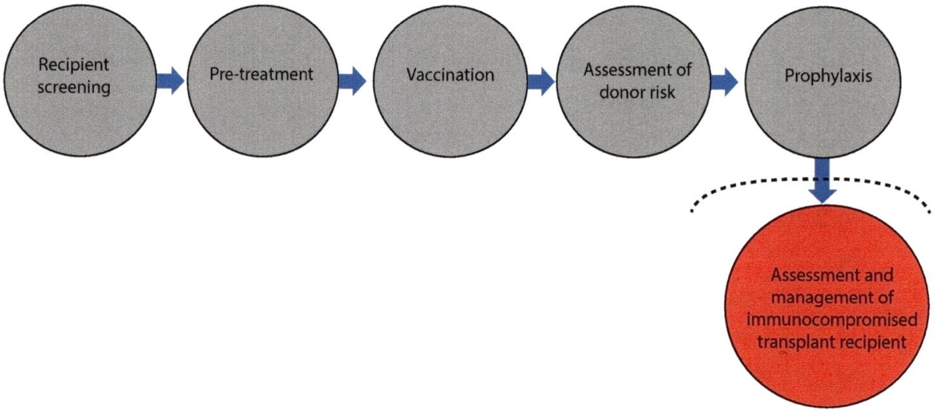

◘ **Fig. 94.1** Elements of infection control in a transplant service. Assessing patients for transplantation affords time to ensure appropriate screening for current infections or potential reactivation for example screening and irradiation of strongyloides is very straightforward and eradicates the risk of strongyloides hyperinfestation syndrome. Obtaining a record, and where appropriate boosters, of childhood and routine adult vaccinations in particular live vaccines (such as rubella in women of child-bearing age, zoster vaccination in those eligible) and human papilloma virus vaccination are all worth striving for. The importance of appropriate donor screening and assessment cannot be over-stated both in terms of avoiding transmission of serious infection but also avoiding discard of potentially valuable organs with manageable infections. National guidelines offer clear protocols for infection prophylaxis which can be individualized but need to be reliably implemented and units need protocols to minimize nosocomial infections following surgery. Finally, the transplant service needs to be able to offer rapid and thoughtful assessment of RTRs with infections, and offer early advice and/or transfer when patients present to other departments or institutions

Table 94.1 Donor screening

History of donor	At-risk behavior, country of origin, occupation, and travel
History from donor hospital	Presenting illness (NB. Beware undiagnosed meningo-encephalitis or flaccid paralysis[a]), evidence of undiagnosed nosocomial infection (CRP, WBC), treated nosocomial infection (UTI, pneumonia, bacteraemia - virulent vs non-virulent, antibiotic history and duration – discuss with microbiology in donor hospital if not clear). Blood cultures, MSU/CSU, respiratory viral PCR screen, line and wound swabs, post-mortem findings.
CXR	Active consolidation (or previous TB). Review other recent imaging.
Mini-laparotomy	A rummage mostly to exclude malignancy but also gross infection/lymph nodes
Perfusion fluid	Cheap and important test especially if virulent organism (e.g., if candida or staphylococcus aureus is cultured, may lead to mycotic aneurysm)
Viruses:	
1. *HIV 1&2 Ab*	Seroconversion window - HIV RNA not routinely available but testing should be considered for high-risk donors although fourth generation tests include HIV 1&2 antibody and p24 Antigen have high sensitivity. Some HIV donors may be suitable for HIV recipients IF infection is controlled and resistance history readily available
2. *Hepatitis B Surface and Core Ab*	Seroconversion window - Hepatitis B DNA not routinely available but testing should be considered for high-risk donors
3. *Hepatitis C Ab*	Seroconversion window - Hepatitis C RNA not routinely available but testing should be considered for high-risk donors, potential donors for Hepatitis C recipients
4. *HTLV 1&2 Ab*	Pro-viral DNA or RNA not routinely available; NB. Caution if Ab positive and signs of disease
5. *CMV Ab*	Routinely checked on all donors
6. EBV Ab	Not routinely done prior to donation but assume >95% adult donors positive (can be done at recipient centre)
7. HSV Ab	Not routinely done but essential if encephalitis (check for HSV DNA in CSF)
8. VZV Ab	Assume >95% adult donors positive
9. HHV-8 Ab	Not routinely done, possible merit in donors from endemic regions (e.g., North African countries)
10. HHV-6 Ab	Not routinely done
11. BKV serology	Not routinely done, assume 70% seropositive
12. West Nile virus (WNV)	Consider screening (Nucleic acid testing) in endemic areas, especially if undiagnosed encephalitis
Bacteria:	
1. *Syphilis serology*	Old versus current infection versus Yaws, if in doubt assume real and treat recipient with penicillin
2. Tuberculosis	Interferon release assays rarely done on donors but worth considering in live donors if from endemic regions
Fungi:	
1. Histoplasmosis Ab	Consider in donors from endemic regions: Africa, Australia, Eastern Europe, North/South America
2. Coccidioides Ab	Consider in donors from endemic regions: Central, South America and Southern USA
Parasitic:	
1. Toxoplasma Ab	Routine screening
2. Strongyloides Ab	Consider in endemic regions Sub-Saharan Africa, South-East Asia, Central and S. America, Eastern Europe
3. Trypanosoma cruzi Ab	Consider in donors from endemic regions Central and South America
4. Leishmania serology	Consider screening donors from endemic regions
5. Malaria antigen and film	Consider screening donors in or recently from endemic regions
Communication between recipient Hospitals: A unit identifying an infection acquired from a donor have a duty to relay this rapidly to other recipient units	

[a]Donor transmission of Rabies, WNV, LCMV has an extremely poor outcome
Communication between receiving units

Table 94.2 Pre-treatment and vaccination

Hepatitis C RNA positive	Attempt to eradicate infection and achieve sustained virological response using directly acting agents (DAAs) before listing.
Hepatitis B	Universal vaccination of non-immune CKD patients (and ESRF), prelisting assessment and stable virological control of hepatitis B with antivirals.
HIV Ab positive	Undetectable viral load and $CD4^{+}$ > 100 (ideally 200) and no opportunistic infections for 6 months prior to listing.
VZV Antibody negative	Vaccination (live vaccine) of the 3% of ESRF population negative for VZV with live vaccine. Prophylaxis with acyclovir if transplanted within 2 weeks of vaccination.
Influenza	Annual vaccination with quadrivalent vaccine
MMR (live vaccine)	If not previously vaccinated, vaccinate 1 month pre-transplant. Testing and vaccination of all women of child bearing age pre-listing if Rubella IgG negative
Diphtheria, tetanus and pertussis	If not previously vaccinated, vaccinate pretransplant and routine boosters 5–10 yearly
Polio (inactivated)	Routine vaccination if not previously vaccinated; can be given post-transplant but *not live vaccine*.
Human Papilloma virus	Girls and boys eligible for local vaccination programme should be strongly encouraged to take this up. No evidence yet for a benefit in older females to prevent CIN, or to prevent anogenital warts in women or men, but worth considering especially in those likely to receive high levels of immunosuppression.
CMV	Early vaccine studies looking encouraging, large scale studies pending.
Pneumococcal	Vaccination according to national guidelines ideally pre-transplant
Haemophilus Influenzae B	Consider pre-transplant in those with pulmonary pathology (can also be given post-transplant)
Meningococcal meningitis	Vaccination according to national guidelines.
Recurrent UTI	Patients with recurrent UTI before transplantation are highly likely to have significant urosepsis after transplantation - where possible the cause should be identified and treated pre-listing (NB. Persistent pyuria also needs explaining even if not associated with overt sepsis)
Tuberculosis	Screening in patients with ESRF by Mantoux or interferon-ϒ release assays (IGRA) often negative due to diminished T cell response.
Strongyloides Ab positive	If treatment history not clear, especially if eosinophilia, treat with Ivermectin 200 mg/kg/day for 2 days (blind treatment is routine practice in many endemic countries)
Schistosomiasis Ab positive	Treat with two doses of 20 mg/kg praziquantel

then it makes sense to offer (this live) vaccine before transplantation. It is important that, non-specific clinical features such as unexplained splenomegaly, lymphadenopathy, persistently raised CRP, eosinophilia, polyclonal gammopathy (in the absence of autoimmunity) all need explaining before listing. In patients who have previously been clobbered with immunosuppression or chemotherapy, or in those with recurrent viral (e.g., herpes) or bacterial infections, it is important to check Immunoglobulin levels and lymphocyte subsets. It is worth noting that immunosuppression posttransplant reduces seroconversion rates to around 50% of that achieved by control patients but the evidence suggests that a second dose of vaccine such as influenza offers no extra benefit [1]. Nonetheless, it is clear that vaccination has benefit, saves lives and should be built into any transplant program [2].

There are several sets of guidelines* recommending posttransplant prophylaxis and Table 94.3 illustrates the main recommendations. As with pretransplant vaccinations, units are frequently inconsistent about some areas of posttransplant prophylaxis such as TB prevention, culture of perfusate and hepatitis B follow up. A hardy system to ensure that patients are appropriately considered for posttransplant prophylaxis in line with local policy is critical to ensure patient safety.

Table 94.3 Infection prophylaxis post Renal Transplant

CMV	Pre-emptive monitoring or prophylaxis (see text). Valgancyclovir 900 mg daily if normal renal function (450 mg possibly as effective and less side-effects), dose adjusted if GFR <60.
HSV Ab negative	*Essential* if NOT receiving Valgancyclovir prophylaxis for CMV. Valacylovir 500 mg twice a day or Acyclovir 200 mg three times a day for 1 month regardless of donor HSV status.
HSV Ab positive	If history of recurrent cold sores pre-transplant, likely to be worse post-transplant. Acyclovir 200 mg od prophylaxis.
VZV Ab negative	Administer varicella zoster immunoglobulin if significant exposure to chicken pox or shingles (within 7 days of exposure)
Hepatitis B core Ab positive donor	HBV immunoglobulin (HBIG) at transplant (HBIG 4000 IU iv stat & measure HBsAb levels at day 7 and repeat dose if levels are <500 IU/L); Start lamivudine 2–3 days before or at least on the day of transplant; Monitor HBsAg regularly
Hepatitis B core Ab positive recipient	Lamivudine prophylaxis 2 to 3 days before or immediately after transplantation. Monitor HBsAg regularly.
Hepatitis B surface Ag positive donor	HBV vaccination for recipients pre-transplant. HBIG (HBIG 4000 IU iv stat) at transplant, measure HBsAb levels at day 5 and repeat dose if levels are <500 IU/L. Monitor HBsAb levels weekly and repeat HBIG to maintain levels >500 IU/L during the first month post-RT. Start antiviral prophylaxis 2 to 3 days before or immediately after transplantation. Preferred drug is entecavir. Obtain donor HBV treatment status if available and modify antiviral prophylaxis accordingly if there is a risk of drug resistance. Monitor HBsAg regularly.
Hepatitis B surface Ag positive recipient	Start antiviral therapy preferably 2–3 weeks prior to or at least immediately after transplantation. Entecavir is the preferred option.
Wound prophylaxis	Local policy
UTI prophylaxis	Co-trimoxazole (Trimethoprim/sulphamethoxazole/Septrin) (as part of universal pneumocystis jirovecii prophylaxis), some units give additional UTI prophylaxis (see chapter on UTI)
Bacterial growth in perfusate	Treatment on basis of culture but consider long course if virulent organism e.g., Staphylococcus aureus, pseudomonas
Mycobacterium	Six months of isoniazid 300 mg od and pyridoxine 10-25 mg od in high risk, no need to treat those who have fully completed treatment course. Prophylaxis against Non-tuberculous mycobacterium not currently recommended
Pneumocystis jirovecii	First choice: Co-trimoxazole 480 mg od or 960 mg 3 x per week for 3–6 months OR until CD4$^+$ count >200 if depleting antibodies or late immunosuppression (*also gives co-prophylaxis against toxoplasmosis, nocardia, listeria and UTI*). Allergy to co-trimoxazole/second line: monthly nebulised pentamidine 300 mg, dapsone 50-100 mg daily (if not G6PD deficient), Atovaquone 1500 mg daily. Prophylaxis is recommended for recipients exposed to cases of PCP
Candida sp.	Fluconazole 200-400 mg daily, itraconazole 200 mg twice a day, voriconazole 200 mg twice a day
Coccidioides immitis	Fluconazole 200-400 mg if past history or positive serology

NB Perfect aseptic technique for line/catheter insertion, prompt line drain and catheter removal, chest physiotherapy and early mobilisation as well as appropriate isolation and infection control measures for in-patients.

A robust system is needed for identifying patients with communicable infections such as any rash, shingles, viral respiratory tract infections and seeing them in isolation in out-patients.

94.2.2 Time-Line for Posttransplant Infections

Although not absolute, there is a clinically helpful time-line for infections posttransplant expounded by Rubin [3].

0–2 weeks: infections are mostly a direct result of surgery, i.e., chest and wound infection, line associated sepsis and occasionally bacterial infection derived from the donor (positive perfusate culture, donor UTI, donor bacteremia or unexplained meningo-encephalitic illness).

1–4 weeks: predominantly nosocomial infections related to stay and hospitalization, i.e., UTI, line and PD catheter associated infection, clostridium difficile.

Oral and oesophageal candidiasis is also common at this stage especially in patients on steroids. Of the herpes viruses, primary HSV is unusual in presenting at this early stage. Other viruses such as transmitted WNV can also present at this time.

4–26 weeks: is the period dominated by opportunistic infections related to the heaviest period of immunosuppression. Most Herpes viruses (reactivation and infection), e.g., CMV (in the absence of prophylaxis typically at 40 days), EBV, HSV, VZV (shingles), HHV-8/7/6. Respiratory viruses may present with chest involvement. Invasive fungal infections such as Candida or Aspergillus tend to present in this period, as may mycobacterium TB. Parasitic infections such as reactivation of strongyloides or toxoplasmosis tend to occur early. UTIs remain very common and, in the absence of prophylaxis, PCP presents in this period.

>26 weeks: periodic viral reactivation of HSV or VZV (shingles) can occur at any stage and a small proportion of patients develop very high levels of EBV viremia often many years posttransplant. Viral warts are also common in the first year. Late onset CMV presents usually within the 8 weeks following cessation of prophylaxis (oro-genital HSV may also recur). Incidental infections such as listeria, legionella, and respiratory viral infection can occur at any time. CMV, EBV, VZV, and HSV negative patients can acquire primary infection many years posttransplant particularly if they have a young family or become exposed to young children. MTB tends to present relatively early in the course of a transplant, NMTB tends to present later. Cryptococcus tends to present late and PJP can occur at any stage although risk diminishes with time. NB Hepatitis B and C reactivation can occur at any time especially after cessation of prophylaxis in hepatitis B and promoted by the use of steroids.

94.2.3 Urinary Tract Infection

UTI posttransplant is very common and associated with a significant morbidity, hospitalization, and graft loss and by definition constitutes "complicated UTI". UTI posttransplant is covered in more detail in ▸ Chap. 54 but it is worth emphasizing that: (a) patients with abnormal anatomy and recurrent UTI pretransplant are likely to have significant problems with urosepsis posttransplant unless the underlying cause is resolved; (b) as transplant UTIs are by definition "complicated" short courses of antibiotics may result in partially treated and recurrent infections (with high risk of generating multiple admissions and highly resistant organisms); and (c) patients with recurrent or severe urosepsis need prompt assessment in a urology-radiology-nephrology MDT.

94.2.4 Specific Infectious Agents

There are several good guidelines for the management of post-transplant infection, Improving Global Outcomes (KDIGO) Transplant Work Group, Improving Global Outcomes (KDIGO) Transplant Work Group [4] is clear and helpful.

94.2.4.1 Cytomegalovirus (CMV)

CMV is a beta herpes virus and the commonest opportunistic infection posttransplant: about 40–50% of renal transplants develop viremia and it represents a significant challenge in some organ transplant recipients.

CMV has a seroprevalence of 45–100% with higher rates in Africa, lower rates in Northern Europe and USA, and increasing prevalence with age. Transmission can be via saliva, urine, sexual contact, breast feeding, placental transmission, blood transfusion, or transplantation. In the immunocompetent host primary infection is usually asymptomatic although it can present as a mononucleosis-like illness, following which the virus undergoes a prolonged period of latency but can become reactivated by a variety of mechanisms including "stress", sepsis, and immunosuppression. For example, TNF-alpha released by rejection or infection can activate the Major immediate early promoter (MieP) of CMV and induce intracellular replication. Transplant recipients (and occasionally, it is worth remembering, patients immunosuppressed for autoimmune conditions) can have a primary infection (D+/R−), reinfection (with a different strain)(D+/R+), or reactivation (D−/R+).

The risk of viremia is very strongly associated with D+/R− status, but in addition the use of depleting antibody induction, acute rejection, poor graft function, and older donor age are known risk factors. In renal transplants predominantly induced with anti-IL2-R mAb and no prophylaxis, viremia occurred in 70% of D+/R−, 53% D+/R+, 44% of D−/R+ and none of the D−/R−. The peak viral load is also significantly higher in the D + R− patients [5].

Clinical characteristics: Many patients who have viremia are asymptomatic but there is a strong correlation between viral load and symptoms. The clinical characteristics of CMV infection in the immunocompromised are shown in ◘ Table 94.4. Viremia and clinical features usually occur between 4 and 12 weeks (typically 6) posttransplant but it is easy to be caught out by disease occurring outside this period (a) following treatment of late rejection (b) after cessation of prophylaxis (c) and in D−/R− transplants following primary exposure sometimes years later.

The kinetics of viral replication has clinical relevance; primary infection is associated with a doubling time of 1.5 days versus 2.7 days for reactivation. This means that a CMV naïve patient can go from asymp-

Table 94.4 Clinical characteristics of CMV infection post-transplant

CMV viraemia	Often asymptomatic. Commonly associated with leucopenia or myelosuppression before developing CMV syndrome.
CMV Syndrome	Temperature > 38 °C for at least 2 days in the absence of another cause, plus CMV DNA viraemia and either neutropenia, thrombocytopenia, lymphocytosis, myalgia, headache or arthralgia.
Pneumonitis	Interstitial pneumonitis with early desaturation. Can be rapidly progressive and may have co-infections such as PJP.
Upper GI	Gastritis/Duodenitis common symptoms in early primary infection, mouth ulcers and oesphagitis.
Lower GI*	Colitis - often bloody and may be fulminant.
Hepatitis	Raised transaminases and flu-like illness
Pancreatitis	Asymptomatic with raised amylase to fulminant pancreatitis
Encephalitis/ Meningitis	Usually late feature in the context of high viral load
Retinitis	Usually a late, perhaps chronic manifestation in profoundly immunocompromised patients
Myocarditis	Usually late
Nephritis	Relatively rare but can result in graft failure or native kidney loss. May have characteristic 'owl's eye' appearance in biopsy
Cystitis	Relatively rare following SOT but can occur post-BMT

NB peripheral blood is usually, but not always, positive for CMV DNA in the presence of end-organ disease

tomatic with a low detectable viral load to significant end organ disease within a week. A patient with primary infection often presents with CMV syndrome and flu-like illness that can progress rapidly to gastritis, colitis (often bloody), pneumonitis, and other end-organ involvement. This is usually associated with very high viral loads. Patients with reactivation or reinfection *may* have a less fulminant course with isolated colitis or pneumonitis without an obvious full-blown viral syndrome. Either way, end-organ damage can progress rapidly and can occur with only low-level viremia or very rarely in the absence of viremia; therefore, a high index of suspicion is required. CMV often co-associates with other infections and HHV-6 and EBV viremia may also be present.

The diagnosis of CMV infection is based on the detection of virus either by antigenemia or detection and quantification of CMV nucleic acid testing by real-time quantitative PCR. In practice most laboratories now use real-time PCR and should adhere to universal diagnostic standards. This technique is highly reproducible and concerns that PCR would result in false positives has not been our experience.

Although viremia is common, with modern management clinical disease affects only about 8% of renal transplant recipients and the vast majority of this is CMV syndrome, however, when end-organ disease occurs it can be devastating and rapidly progressive. Pneumonitis may present with shortness of breath and oxygen desaturation post-exercise and may progress swiftly from mild dyspnoea to marked desaturation. Chest X ray (see Fig. 94.2) or CT scan may show signs of an interstitial lung disease but there is a wide differential, so it is essential to get samples, rapidly, (ideally a broncho-alveolar lavage) where possible or treat blindly (covering CMV) or both. It is important to note that CMV infection predisposes to other infections and viral pneumonitis can coexist with Pneumocystis pneumonitis. Meningitis and encephalitis may present with classic symptoms and signs, or epilepsy and impaired cognition. It can be diagnosed from PCR on CSF so ensuring the appropriate sample is taken at the time of lumbar puncture is important. Where possible, with tissue invasive disease such as gastritis, colitis (Fig. 94.3), and nephritis (Fig. 94.4), biopsy, culture, and PCR are critical given the wide differential. The presence of viral inclusions and detection of CMV antigen and DNA in biopsy tissue are considered diagnostic of CMV end-organ disease. However, the pancreas and retina are less appealing biopsy targets: ophthalmologists can normally make a firm clinical diagnosis (although vitreous fluid can be tested for CMV DNA) and CMV pancreatitis is usually, therefore, a presumptive diagnosis based on viremia and clinical findings.

In short, it is important to have a high index of suspicion in any transplant with end-organ disease, with rapid requesting and processing of blood or any other tissue for CMV PCR and if possible/appropriate, sending a biopsy to virology as well as histopathology departments.

Beyond the direct effects of the virus, CMV infection has been implicated in several indirect consequences including: (a) increased cellular rejection; (b) increased infection by other microbes; (c) increased mortality; and (d) worse graft survival [6, 7]. This is not without controversy. For instance, studies showing an association with acute cellular rejection have not always differentiated cause and effect, and a significant proportion (80% in our experience) of acute rejection precedes CMV viremia so much of this association may simply be a response to increased immunosuppression. CMV viremia is immunomodulatory and may predispose to EBV and

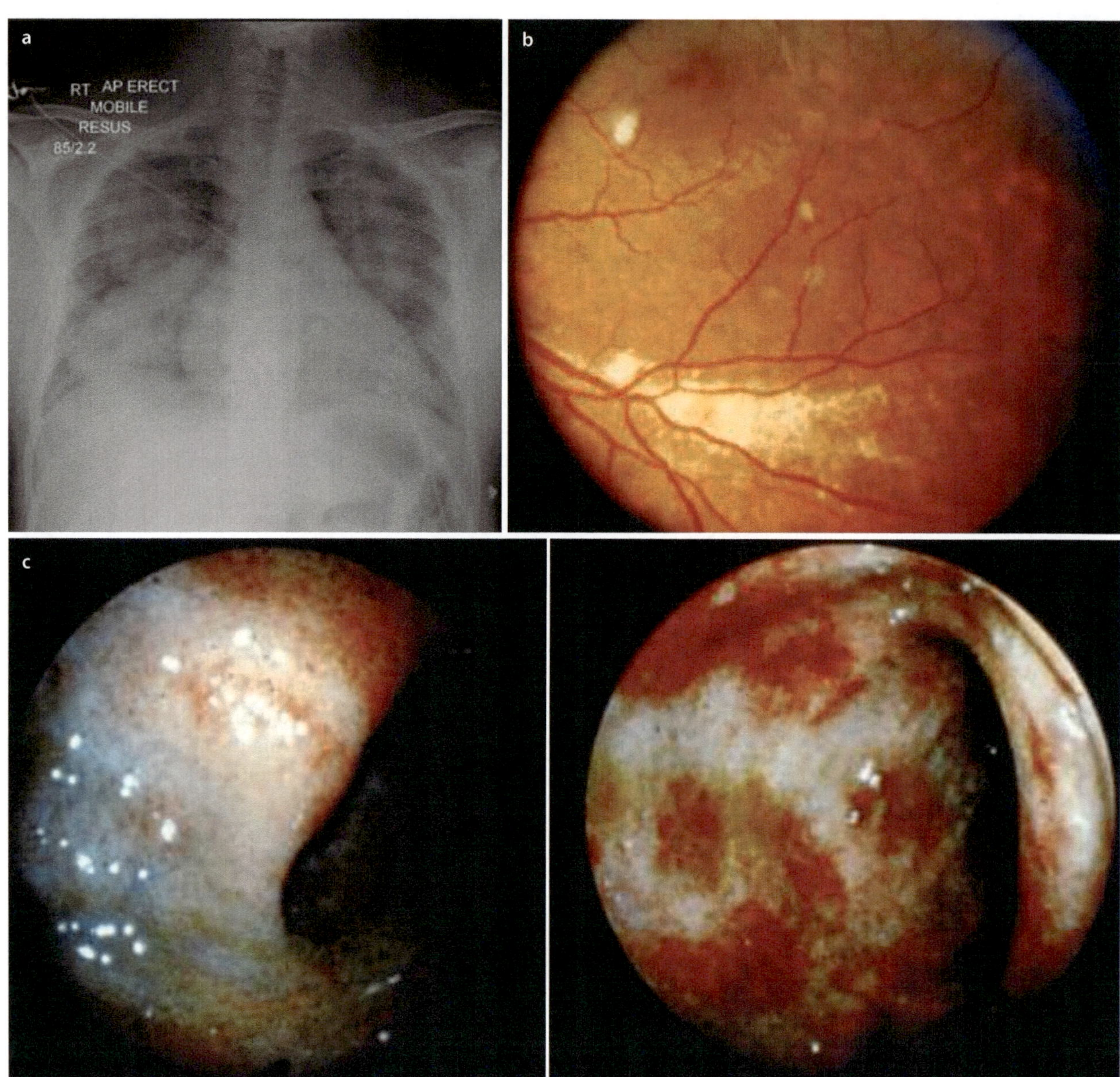

Fig. 94.2 **a** CMV pneumonitis in a renal transplant recipient. The patient had minimal constitutional illness, a dry cough and presented severely hypoxic. The differential is large (see table x) including pulmonary oedema but the peripheral sparing goes against this despite the cardiomegaly. There were very low levels of CMV viremia but BAL was positive and there was a very rapid improvement in clinical condition with IV gancyclovir. **b** Early CMV retinitis. **c** CMV colitis in a renal transplant recipient presenting with abdominal pain and bloody diarrhea. This patient also had only low levels of viremia and the diagnosis was made on biopsy

HHV-6 viremia, as well as an increase in fungal infections although again, CMV may be a biomarker of over immunosuppression. Some studies have shown increased mortality and worse four-year graft survival has also been shown [8], however a UK study based on serology in 10,000 transplants showed no effect on patient or allograft survival [9]. A detailed analysis is beyond the scope of this chapter but what is clear is that overt CMV disease is nasty and best avoided.

There are a variety of recommendations on the prevention and treatment of CMV posttransplant [4, 10, 11] and the 2011 BTS guidelines nicely summarize the current evidence [12]. For kidney transplantation most guidelines favor universal prophylaxis (for D+/R− or any positive recipients), especially following depleting antibodies. This is, in part, based on meta-analyses of prophylaxis and preemptive studies demonstrating benefit of both but a reduction in all-cause mortality with prophylaxis [13]. Most of the studies in the meta-analyses have short follow up and very few patients in the preemptive arm. Guidelines mostly acknowledge that preemptive therapy is probably equally appropriate

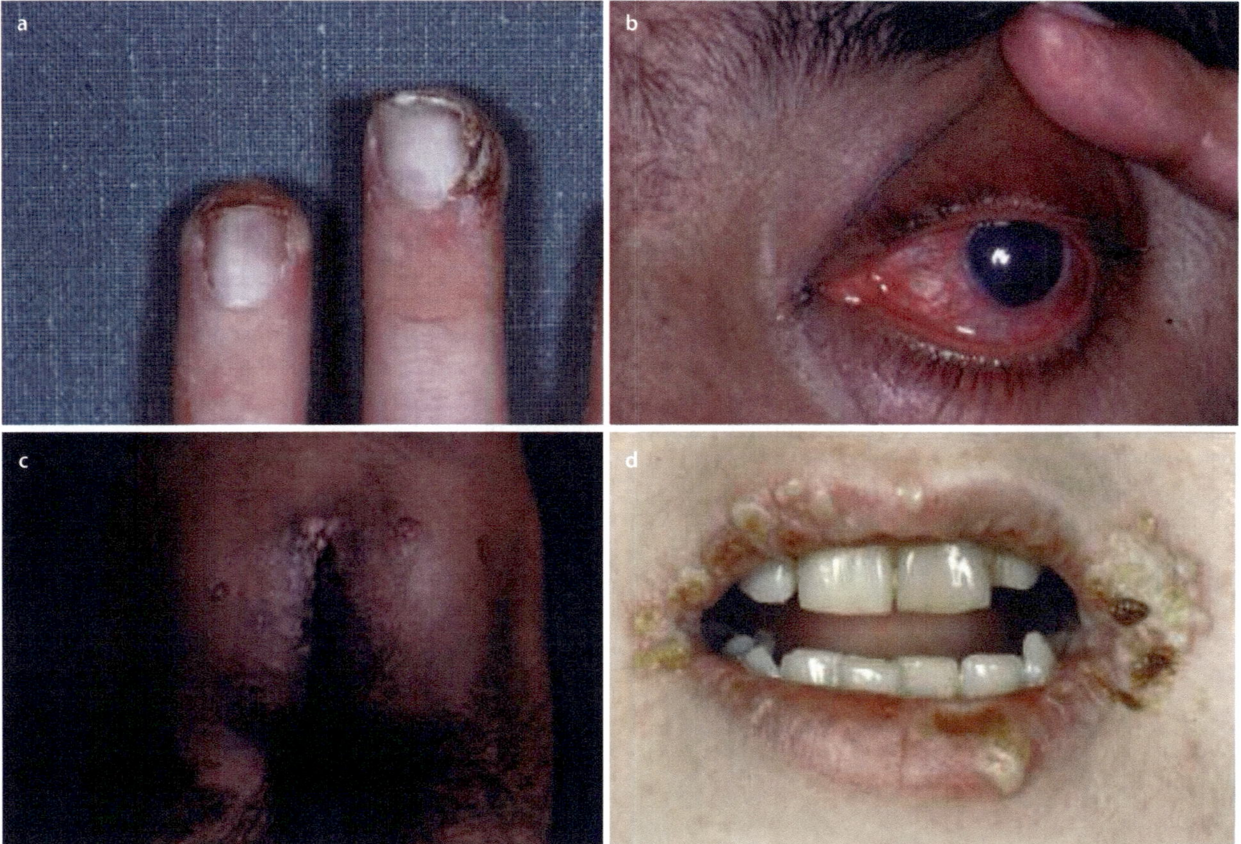

Fig. 94.3 Herpes simplex virus **a**, herpetic whitlow **b**, Herpes ophthalmitis **c**, perineal HSV **d**, extensive labial HSV

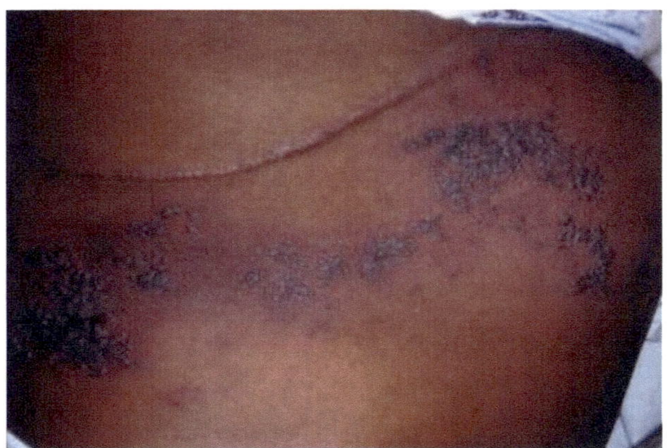

Fig. 94.4 Herpes Zoster reactivation (Shingles)

if the logistics can be robustly managed [the case for preemptive over prophylaxis is eloquently argued by Thomas Reischig [14]] and the prevailing opinion is moving towards equal recommendation for preemptive and prophylaxis.

The main advantages of universal prophylaxis include ease of administration and co-prophylaxis against over viruses (such as primary HSV), with disadvantages including drug side-effects (especially leucopenia) and the concern of late onset disease. The advantages of preemptive approach include limiting drug exposure to those that need it, encouraging immunity due to antigen exposure, and the near complete absence of late disease. The disadvantages of preemptive therapy include the extra vigilance required and the lack of co-prophylaxis.

To summarize the current guidelines [4, 10–12] on prevention, most recommend prophylaxis with valganciclovir (superior to acyclovir, valacyclovir, or oral ganciclovir) starting within 10 days of transplant for D+/R− and R+ patients. Based on the findings of the IMPACT study [15], which showed a reduced rate of late onset CMV disease with 200 compared to 100 days treatment (16% versus 37%), the guidelines tend to favor treatment for 200 days in D+/R− and in those who have received depleting antibodies such as ATG. The dose recommended for those with normal renal function is 900 mg per day but 450 mg appears to be as effective, and causes much less leucopenia, but potentially increases the risk of resistance [16]. Further dose reduction for renal impairment is required. The risk of CMV disease in D−/R− is so low as to not require CMV prophylaxis but does therefore mandate anti-HSV prophylaxis. Clinicians need to be vigilant to CMV on cessation of prophylaxis and have a system of monitoring patients at this time as well as being alert to the possibility of viral resistance, or non-compliance during prophylaxis.

Our experience of the preemptive approach has been very positive with CMV syndrome developing in only 4.9%, end-organ disease in approximately 1%, and only 2.3% with late onset viremia (first episode after 90 days) [5]. There are some important cautions included in ◘ Table 94.5. Preemptive therapy relies on robust monitoring and reporting as well as a good relationship with your virology department. Because of the rapid doubling time of primary infection we ensure twice weekly CMV monitoring for the first 8 weeks (longer if has had an episode of viremia) and weekly for a further 4 weeks. An email reporting service to the transplant team, with clear lines of responsibility works well and we give D+/R− patients 3 days of valgancyclovir on discharge to start if viremia is detected as an outpatient. Patients admitted to other hospitals or under other teams may be at risk as monitoring and reporting can breakdown and it is important to have a strategy for these patients.

Finally, it is clear that some patients such as those D+/R− who have viremia after depleting antibodies or who are high immunological risk (i.e., have had early rejection) and therefore cannot risk ISR are highly likely to have recurrent viremia after completion of treatment and it may be worth considering converting to prophylaxis after treatment with the advantage that the recipient will have developed some immunity with the first episodes of viremia.

Treatment: In asymptomatic serologically positive R+ patients with viral counts below 3000 genomes/ml

◘ **Table 94.5** A. Universal Prophylaxis (especially if received depleting antibodies). B. Pre-emptive therapy

A	
Valgancyclovir 900 mg/450 mg daily (dose adjusted for GFR)	
D+/R−, D+/R+ and D−/R+: 200 days for D+/R−, 100 days for R+	Late onset disease biggest hazard. Ensure robust monitoring on cessation of prophylaxis. Resistant CMV and non-compliance may rarely result in disease in prophylactic period if no routine monitoring. Leucopenia common side effect.
Partial prophylaxis (if not received depleting antibodies)	
D+/R− 200 days, no prophylaxis for R+	Numerically, D+/R+ and D−/R+ account for more viraemia than D+/ R− . Requires good monitoring of CMV PCR for R+ group and the ability to safely run two different approaches.
D−/R−	No prophylaxis for CMV but HSV negative recipients must have at least 1 month of anti-HSV prophylaxis and irradiated blood products
B	
D+/R−, D+/R+ and D−/R+: No prophylaxis	1. HSV prophylaxis in HSV negative recipients for at least 1 month (e.g., valacyclovir)
	2. Robust monitoring (guidelines at least weekly) ideally twice weekly especially in D+/R− and those receiving depleting antibodies for first 3 months from transplant or treated rejection episode. Rapid turnaround time and reporting (e.g., email alerts to transplant team).
	3. Twice weekly monitoring for those with viraemia and in those successfully treated
	4. System to ensure patients admitted to other hospitals or units are identified, and monitored appropriately.
	5. Issue patients with 3 day starter pack of valgancyclovir to take if develops viraemia
	6. Start treatment at any positive for D+/R− and at local threshold for R+ (e.g., 3000 copies per ml).
Hybrid prophylaxis (if received depleting antibodies or high immunological risk)	
D+/R−: No prophylaxis initially, prophylaxis following treatment of viraemia	D+/R− patients with primary infection following depleting antibody are highly likely to relapse following treatment as are those who have had rejection and cannot safely tolerate ISR. For these patients it may be worth considering prophylaxis after successful treatment.

Table 94.6 Risk Factors for the Development of Kaposi's Sarcoma post-transplant

Serostatus of Donor/ Recipient	Data suggesting both that reactivation and primary infection at transplant are significant risk factors.
Geographical location	Mediterranean, Middle East, Eastern Europe, and Sub-Sahara Africa
Burden of Immunosuppression	Overall burden of immunosuppression important especially depleting mAb
Age of recipient	>50 years
Homosexual Males	Multiple partners
Transfusion	In high prevalence areas

our practice is to reduce the overall burden of immunosuppression (CNI if level high, anti-proliferative if not). We treat reactivation if viremia of >3000 genomes/ml or evidence of end-organ disease. As a unit that practices preemptive therapy, CMV naïve patients with a positive donor are discharged with 3 days of valgancyclovir (starter pack) to take if there is a single positive PCR of any level to avoid delay in treatment (also worth considering post-prophylaxis).

First-line treatment of significant viremia or CMV disease should be with valgancyclovir or IV gancyclovir (especially the latter if any doubt about absorption) dose adjusted for eGFR (see Table 94.6). In patients who have not recently undergone rejection it is advisable to reduce any anti-proliferative agent or consider stopping altogether if serious disease. Treatment of CMV disease should be continued for at least 3 weeks even if early elimination of viremia and our practice is to continue treatment until two negative PCRs in everyone. Relapse is common, especially the D+/R− and in those who have received depleting antibodies. There is insufficient evidence to support the use of IVIg (CMV-Ab enriched or otherwise), which is expensive and a scarce resource, but it is likely to be relatively harmless and might be worth considering in a tight corner. It is important to ensure PCP prophylaxis continues and G-CSF can be helpful in the face of neutropenia.

Viral resistance is much more common in the D+/R− subgroup (up to 10%) with prolonged treatment and the use of depleting antibodies. Apart from this high-risk group, a strong indication of resistance is failure to clear the virus by 3 weeks and mutation analysis should be requested in this setting. Mutations in UL97 kinase and UL54 DNA polymerase genes are recognized markers of resistance and it is important to note that as gancyclovir, cidofovir, and foscarnet all target UL54 DNA polymerase, resistance to gancyclovir can lead to cross resistance to cidofovir and foscarnet. The latter two drugs are reserved as second-line drugs and generally reviled by nephrologists because of their high rate of nephrotoxicity; nonetheless they can be life-saving in extreme disease (doses for both need to be carefully adjusted for GFR and pre-hydration essential). Letermovir, recently used in a clinical trial of CMV prophylaxis in bone marrow transplant patients acts on CMV-terminase complex [17]. Maribavir, an oral anti-CMV drug, inhibits UL97 kinase enzyme activity and affects CMV DNA synthesis, viral gene expression, encapsidation, and viral capsid egress. Maribavir is active in vitro against CMV resistant to gancyclovir, foscarnet, or cidofovir and has been used for treating resistant and refractory CMV infection [18].

Leflunomide and mTOR inhibitors theoretically both have anti-CMV properties and there are case reports of some success using leflunomide to treat-resistant CMV in SOT. However, there is likely to be reporting bias, and as yet no RCTs to support the use of leflunomide as treatment.

The circumstantial evidence in favor of a clinically relevant anti-CMV effect of mTOR inhibitors is more convincing and there are many studies that show significantly reduced rates of CMV infection in *de novo* kidney transplants receiving mTOR inhibitors [19]. The evidence that mTOR inhibitors are helpful in treatment of CMV infection again degenerates to anecdote with small cases series. Our experience, and a niche that may prove important, is in those patients with persistent or resistant CMV who cannot tolerate further reduction in immunosuppression. Swapping tacrolimus for sirolimus or adding sirolimus to tacrolimus in high immunological risk patients with dose reduction of the CNI can be effective at clearing CMV and simultaneously avoiding rejection.

With modern management, CMV disease (the majority being CMV syndrome) affects only about 8% of renal transplants. In our experience of a preemptive approach, treatment was required in 63% of D+/R−, 22% of D+/R+ and 18% of D−/R+ for viremia, and end organ disease occurred in only 1%.

94.2.5 Herpes Simplex Virus: HSV 1 and 2

Reactivation of HSV in the form of nasolabial cold sores or genital ulcers is relatively common but can be very aggressive in significant immunocompromise (see Fig. 94.3). Patients may give a history of previous cold sores and, if frequent pretransplant, are highly likely to recur posttransplant. This can be prevented with ready access to topical acyclovir or low dose oral acyclovir prophylaxis (e.g., 200 mg daily). Treatment with oral acyclovir, valacyclovir, or famciclovir is highly effective but should start early and dose adjustment for GFR is important. It can also affect the cornea and conjunctiva presenting as a red eye/keratitis and progressing to a dendritic ulcer with potential sight loss (◘ Fig. 94.3) and any painful red eye should have viral swabs and rapid ophthalmology review.

Very rarely, seronegative patients can develop a fulminant primary HSV infection. This has been reported with both HSV1 and HSV2 and has a very high mortality. A high fever is universal, but skin lesions are present in only half the patients, which may explain delay in diagnosis. The patient may seem better than their fever would imply initially but without treatment pancytopenia, gastric ulceration, and acute hepatitis (CT imaging may appear as abscesses), rapidly progress to encephalopathy, coagulopathy, and death. The diagnosis can be made by detecting HSV DNA in blood, CSF, swabs, and biopsies. However, onset to death is rapid, so a high index of suspicion is important and early empirical treatment critical. CMV prophylaxis with valgancyclovir is essentially protective against primary HSV but in those HSV negative patients not having CMV, prophylaxis should be given either as acyclovir or valacyclovir (regardless of donor status). There is no consensus on duration of prophylaxis but our practice is to give valacyclovir 500 mg bid for the first month of transplant. HSV is very sensitive to acyclovir and, as mentioned above, any suspicion of fulminant HSV should prompt rapid IV treatment (10 mg/kg tid), reduction in antiproliferatives, and placement on a high dependency unit.

94.2.6 Varicella Zoster Virus (VZV)

Reactivation with herpes zoster (shingles) is markedly more common in transplant recipients (10×) than the general population, occurring in roughly 10% of patients in the first 5 years (◘ Fig. 94.4) [20] but more commonly still in those receiving anti-lymphocyte depleting antibodies. As neuralgia precedes the rash the diagnosis can be initially missed and should be considered in anyone with new onset severe, otherwise unexplained pain. Treatment is with early acyclovir or valacyclovir for 7 days, analgesia, surveillance for secondary infection, and usually reduction in anti-proliferatives.

Primary infection is potentially life-threatening in solid organ transplant recipients and about 3–5% of the adult population are VZV naïve; others bear a similar risk if hypogammaglobulinemic. Identification of naïve patients on the waiting list is mandatory and vaccination should be robustly embedded in any pretransplant program, although the evidence is that as a community, we are very poor at doing this. The vaccine is usually given as two doses, 4–8 weeks apart, and as it is a live vaccine, we offer acyclovir to any patient receiving a transplant within 2 weeks of the vaccination.

Conversely, elderly patients may be offered Zoster vaccination as part of a national program, this is ideal while on the waiting list but contra-indicated in RTRs who are immunocompromised. Patients unlucky enough to get primary varicella infection while under the influence of significant immunosuppression can present with pneumonitis, hepatitis, ulcerative gastritis, and colitis. Pancreatitis, encephalitis, meningitis, and DIC can follow swiftly and have a mortality of 5–30% (particularly if developing pneumonitis or encephalitis. Treatment of primary chickenpox should be with rapid initiation of IV acyclovir (10 mg/kg tid adjusted for GFR) for 7–10 days, usually until all the lesions have crusted over. Treatment may need to be continued longer (2–3 weeks) for CNS involvement or disseminated infection. Of course, it is more desirable to avoid anxious visits to the ICU, and seronegative patients should be identified, advised to avoid exposure, and given clear (written) advice on what to do if exposed either to chickenpox or shingles (often unwittingly in the transplant clinic waiting room). If pretransplant serostatus is not known, an urgent VZV IgG test is required to establish VZV immune status.

1. Attend hospital within 24 hours (up to 7 days of exposure) for varicella zoster immune globulin (VZIG; 1000 mg IM adult dose). If a second exposure occurs after 3 weeks, a further dose may be required.
2. If VZIG unavailable or exposed patient cannot be given an IM injection (bleeding disorder), IVIg can be used (0.2 g per kg body weight).
3. Despite having VZIG, patients can still develop clinical chickenpox, particularly if household contact. These patients should receive IV acyclovir promptly.

94.2.7 Epstein-Barr Virus (EBV)

A gamma-herpes virus with 95% seroprevalence worldwide, mostly acquired asymptomatically in childhood, or as infectious mononucleosis (IM) in 25% during puberty. It immortalizes B-cell lines and remains mostly latent with occasional lytic cycles and shedding mostly in saliva in healthy individuals. Given the prevalence of EBV infection, primary infection following transplantation is common in a seronegative recipient. Viremia is common posttransplant occurring in roughly 50% of all patients but this is usually asymptomatic. Occasionally patients may present with IM or non-specific viral illness, but the greatest concern is the propensity for EBV to induce posttransplant lymphoproliferative disorder

(PTLD). Ninety percent of early PTLDs are EBV positive and a primary infection posttransplant confers a 10- to 75-fold risk of PTLD (greater still if concomitant CMV infection and/or the use of depleting antibodies). There is also data to support EBV viremia preceding development of PTLD, however recent guidelines make the reasonable point that there is no evidence to support the routine monitoring of EBV levels post-renal transplant [21, 22].

The Renal Association Guidelines [22] however do recommend EBV PCR monitoring in D+/R− patients for the first year and following treatment for rejection. Despite the lack of evidence, risk stratification is key and it is worth considering monitoring: (1) D+/R− patients (especially if received depleting antibodies); (2) patients who are viremic pretransplant (usually previous transplants); (3) those with previous EBV + ve Lymphoma; (4) following treatment of rejection; and (5) possibly at annual review as a surrogate marker of over immunosuppression—a small percentage of patients develop very high levels asymptomatically with increasing time posttransplant. In the absence of convincing evidence, it is our practice to monitor the above groups. Stable patients with viremia are monitored as follows but with the acknowledgment that many patients may have stable high levels of EBV viremia for years, seemingly without any adverse effects and screening is not cost neutral:

- Levels of <10,000 monitor 3-monthly *initially*
- Levels of 10,000–50,000 monitor 6–8-weekly *initially* and consider ISR
- Levels of >50,000 gentle ISR monitor 4-weekly *initially*

While it is common sense, and our practice, to reduce immunosuppression in the presence of persistent high level EBV viremia, there is negligible evidence to support ISR in the absence of lymphoma and there is a risk of late rejection so should be undertaken cautiously. There is no convincing evidence on favor of prophylaxis.

94.2.8 Human Herpes Virus 6 (HHV-6)

The prevalence of HHV-6 infection is very high with >90% of the population infected in early childhood. Reactivation of HHV-6 is very common in the early posttransplant period often as a co-infection with CMV and HHV-7 [23] with clinical manifestations from asymptomatic viremia or a self-limiting viral illness, to more disseminated disease with pneumonitis, encephalitis, lymphadenopathy, and bone marrow suppression. As most units do not screen for HHV-6 and the vast majority of patients are either asymptomatic or settle spontaneously, treatment is not usually required but there are case reports of death secondary to HHV-6 and it worth considering as a diagnosis in a patient with unexplained viral illness. Treatment if required is ganciclovir or valgancyclovir, exclusion of coexistent CMV, and reduction in immunosuppression.

94.2.9 Human Herpes Virus 7 (HHV-7)

Reactivation of childhood-acquired virus may occur early posttransplant either asymptomatically or with a nonspecific viral illness, but severe disease is extremely rare. Management involves exclusion of more likely infections, then immunosuppression reduction and, if necessary, treatment with foscarnet or cidofovir.

94.2.10 Human Herpes Virus 8 (HHV-8)

The main clinical manifestation of HHV-8 primary infection, reactivation or reinfection in solid organ transplants is the development of Kaposi's sarcoma. Although HHV-8 infection does occur sporadically, there is a significant geographical bias in the seroprevalence of HHV-8 with the Mediterranean, Eastern Europe, the Middle East, and Sub-Sahara Africa having high rates. The role of immunosuppression is profound in that the prevalence of KS in SOT is 500 times that of the general population; occurring in 0.5% of transplant recipients from Northwestern Europe and up to 5% of transplant recipients in Saudi Arabia. Known risk factors for posttransplant KS are shown in ◘ Table 94.6 [24].

Clinical presentation is predominantly cutaneous involvement with red/purple/black nodules (see ◘ Fig. 94.5) typically on the lower body, initially often associated with lower limb oedema, which may precede the development of skin lesions. Visceral involvement may also occur including lymphadenopathy, pulmonary nodules, chylous pleural effusions, and gastrointestinal involvement. Clinical presentation is usually within the first year but it is not unusual for the diagnosis of visceral KS to be delayed particularly in the setting of GI involvement. The mortality associated with KS particularly with visceral involvement is around 10% and graft loss is common as a consequence of ISR.

Serology is rarely helpful in the diagnosis and donors are not currently screened, however it might be worth considering donor and recipient screening in high prevalence areas to identify risk. Histology is the gold standard for diagnosis; any suspicious lesion should be biopsied and a high index of suspicion is important par-

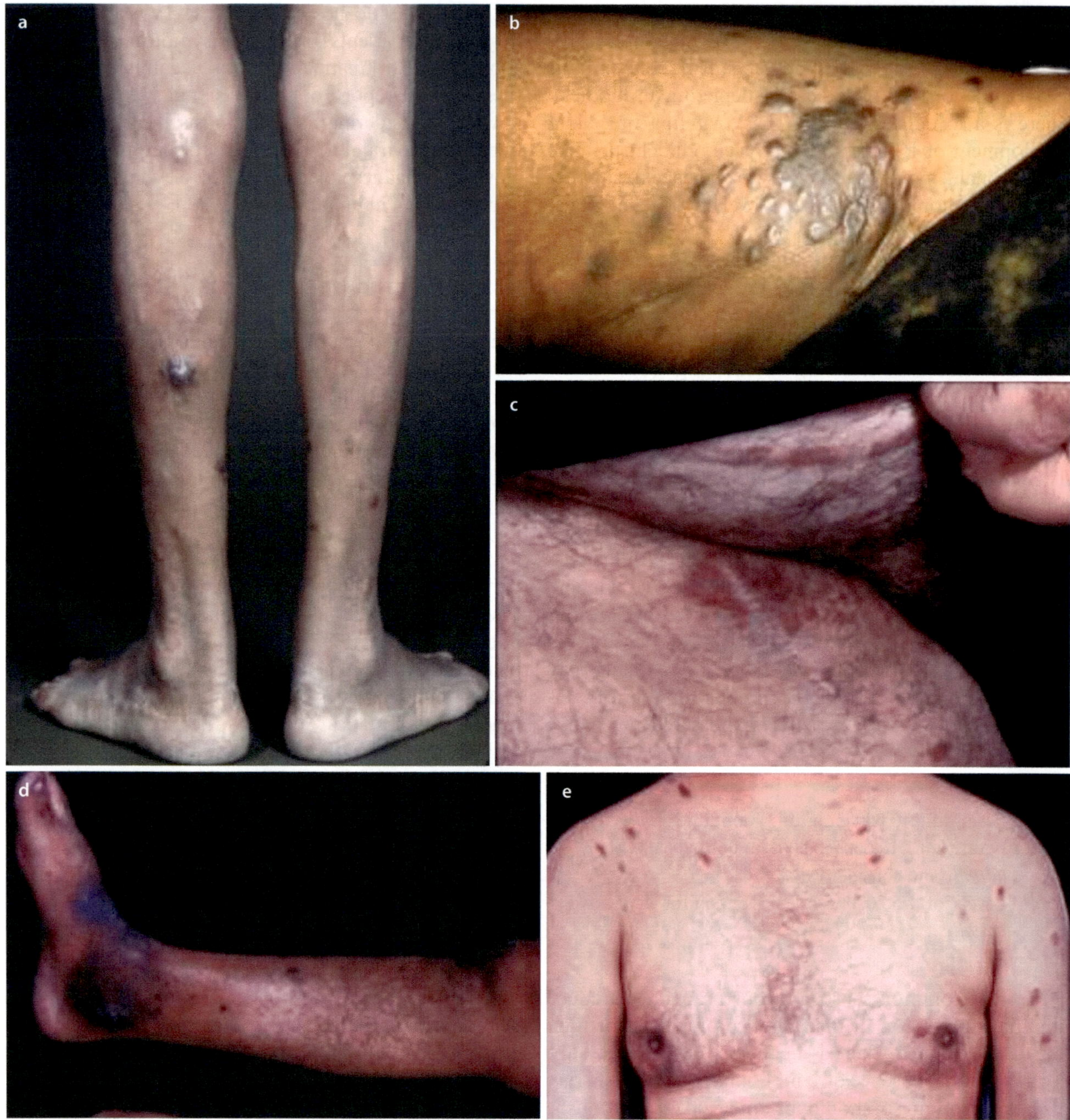

Fig. 94.5 a–e Multiple cutaneous manifestations of Kaposi's sarcoma

ticularly for gastrointestinal involvement. PCR for HHV-8 may be considered as a tool to monitor response to treatment for visceral KS, although will not be helpful in the absence of viremia.

Treatment is with reduction in immunosuppression, or complete cessation if life threatening visceral involvement or progressive disease. The reduction of immunosuppression required to induce remission often results in graft loss and conversion from CNI to mTOR inhibitor (with anti-VEGF activity) has had some significant success [25] although this is not universal. With aggressive, unresponsive disease, antivirals (foscarnet, cidofovir) and chemotherapy such as bleomycin, adriamycin, and taxols have been tried with variable success.

Our practice is to stop the anti-proliferative agents initially and if no response within 2–4 weeks, or significant visceral involvement convert non-proteinuric patients from their CNI to a mTOR-inhibitor. If intolerant of mTOR-inhibitor then proceed with a step-wise reduction in CNI, ideally with slow small cuts rather than large cuts, if the disease permits [26].

KS can recur in a second transplant; we aim to avoid heavy induction and plan for an early switch to an mTOR-inhibitor if possible.

94.2.11 Polyoma Viruses: Polyomavirus Hominis 1 (BK) and 2 (JC)

BK and JC are usually picked up in childhood remaining latent in the presence of a normal immune system but can cause significant nephropathy (polyoma virus associated nephropathy, PVAN) in renal transplants (although very rarely in other transplants), and JC virus is the causative agent in progressive multifocal leucoencephalopathy.

94.2.11.1 BKV

Is a double stranded DNA virus, acquired mostly in childhood with seroprevalence in excess of 85%. It remains latent in the renal tubular and uroepithelial cells, and 7–20% of immune competent individuals intermittently shed virus but there is no evidence of pathological consequences of BK infection in the general population. In RTR, infection results in nephropathy in 1–10% of recipients with high risk of graft loss, as well as causing ureteric strictures and hemorrhagic cystitis (most common in BMT).

The incidence of PVAN seems to have genuinely increased in the last 30 years and registry data from the US organ procurement and transplant network suggests current rates of 6% PVAN by 5 years (the vast majority occurring in the first 2 years) [27]. The main risk factor appears to relate to the total burden of immunosuppression (use of depleting antibodies, treatment of acute rejection and combination of tacrolimus and mycophenolic acid). However, it is extremely rare to get PVAN in other SOT (e.g., cardiac/lung) with much higher levels of IS, in part because the renal tract is the site of latency for BKV. Trauma to the uroepithelium during renal transplantation or ureteric stent placement, in addition to other known risk factors such as D+ R−, episodes of acute rejections, deceased donor, and viral co-infection, may contribute to infection and epithelial cell injury/division necessary for BKV growth. It is also possible that some serotypes are more virulent and may cause a reinfection. There is a clinically important natural history to PVAN; 20–40% of RTR have viruria, which precedes the 5–15% of those that get viremia by 4–6 weeks, and PVAN by 12 weeks [28], thus offering a window for detection and prevention.

There are usually no clinical features associated with BKV infection in RTR except a deterioration in renal function or ureteric obstruction, so screening and biopsy are critical.

Due to its poor specificity and the increasing availability of PCR to detect BK DNA, undertaking urine cytology (papanicolaou stain) to identify the viral cytopathic effect in "decoy cells" (detached tubular epithelial cells with viral nuclear inclusions) is rarely done in the modern era. Measuring serum BKV DNA is now the mainstay of BKV detection, and >10 [4]copies/ml of BKV DNA is a sensitive and specific marker of PVAN with a high negative predictive value. Consequently the KDIGO guidelines recommend screening plasma for BKV DNA, monthly for 3 months, followed by 3-monthly for 12–24 months [4]. Plasma BKV DNA screening should also be done in the context of an unexplained rise in creatinine or ureteric obstruction. Not everyone with viremia develops PVAN so the gold standard for diagnosis is histological evidence of polyoma virus with viral cytopathic changes, nuclear inclusion, interstitial infiltrate and tubulitis, granulomas may also be present (◘ Fig. 94.6). It is confirmed by positive simian virus large-T antigen (SV40) staining. However, the infection is patchy, and tends to initially involve the col-

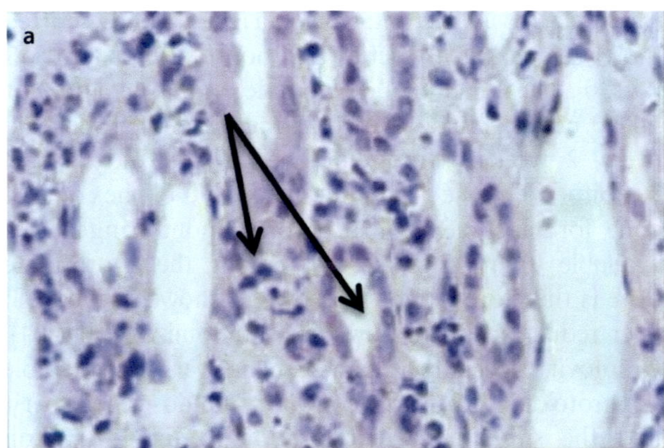

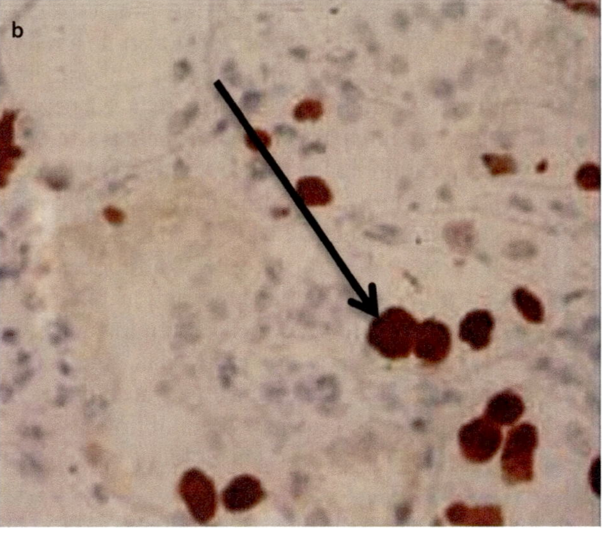

◘ **Fig. 94.6** BKV Nephropathy **a** cellular infiltrate and nuclear inclusions; **b** diagnosis of BKV confirmed by positive SV40 staining

lecting tubules, which lie deeper in the kidney, and the disease may be missed early on (in up to one-third), especially if the biopsy sample is small or superficial. In addition, initial views of the biopsy may appear identical to the tubulitis of acute cellular rejection, so all biopsies with a cellular infiltrate should be stained for SV40 with urgency to avoid increasing IS when reduction is necessary.

Treatment. It is important to note that there are no substantial data in support of any treatment of PVAN apart from ISR. Although not the subject of a RCT, pre-emptive ISR has been associated with viral clearance in 80–95% and a reduction in death-censored graft survival. A variety of protocols have been suggested for ISR in the face of viremia [28, 29] but essentially start with halving either mycophenolic acid or azathioprine and if no reduction in viremia either reduction in CNI or stopping the anti-proliferative altogether. Rapid and abrupt cuts in IS are more likely to be associated with rejection and differentiating the main pathological process even with SV40 staining can be very difficult.

A variety of drugs have been tried on the basis of theoretical or *in vitro* anti-polyoma activity and reported mostly as small case series and non-randomized trials [28, 30]. These include Leflunomide (usually at a dose of 20–60 mg/day), cidofovir (0.25 mg/kg with probenecid every 2 weeks), fluroquinolones, IVIg, and mTOR inhibitors. The use of Leflunomide is out of the comfort zone for most nephrologists, drug monitoring is not available to most units, and judging the appropriate dose is therefore tricky. Moreover, it showed no benefit over reduction in IS alone in a randomized trial [31]. Cidofovir, especially at high dose, has very considerable nephrotoxicity, pre-hydration with IV fluids is necessary, and the subsequent deterioration in renal function causes further diagnostic difficulty. A small trial of lower dose cidofovir did, however, demonstrate a reduction in graft loss [32] and brincidofovir, an oral lipid ester prodrug of cidofovir, which has reduced nephrotoxicity, is undergoing phase II trials. There is some evidence that fluroquinolones reduce viremia but there is no evidence currently of improved clinical outcomes. Given the seroprevalence of BKV infection, IVIg contains high titres of neutralizing BKV antibodies, and would seem a harmless therapeutic option but it is a scarce resource without an evidence base for improved graft outcomes, and it is not clear what significance humoral immunity has in clearing an intracellular virus. The data for conversion to mTOR inhibitors as treatment is also poor but there is quite a lot of circumstantial evidence that mTORi may reduce the risk of PVAN by roughly a half that of other IS regimens [27] possibly by inhibiting cell cycle progression and not disabling BKV-specific T cell responses to the same degree. In short, there is a shocking lack of decent evidence to support treatment of PVAN when appropriate ISR has failed. Our practice, and that of some others [29], if PVAN persists following ISR or there has been a rejection episode, is to introduce a mTORi (if proteinuria <0.5 g/l), ultimately aiming for mTORi monotherapy.

Original reports recounted grim outcomes in terms of graft survival and roughly 50% of grafts with PVAN were lost, however greater awareness and better screening seem to be improving the outcome. A histological grading system (A-C) for PVAN has been devised based on the amount of cellular involvement and the extent of interstitial fibrosis and atrophy (reviewed in [29]). This system has since been modified [33], but the original take home message remains that grade A is associated with 13% graft loss and grade C 100% graft loss, i.e., early detection and ISR is likely to be dramatically more helpful than applying toxic medication for advanced disease. Limited data suggests a recurrence rate of about 20% but loss of a second graft seems rare. There seems no evidence to remove the failed graft but persistent viremia is a likely risk factor and removal of IS until an immune response suppresses viremia would seem very prudent.

94.2.11.2 JCV

Is a viral infection commonly acquired asymptomatically early in life reaching 50% seroprevalence by middle age, viruria can be detected in normal individuals, and viremia has been detected in 5% of transplant patients. Despite this, clinically apparent reactivation in the form of progressive multifocal leucoencephalopathy (PML) is very rare in transplantation. A caveat here is that the risk of PML is clearly related to the burden of immunosuppression, cases have been reported in patients with SLE following rituximab and in transplants following belatacept, as well as less specific depleting antibodies. PML has a wide differential and may be confused with CNI toxicity. The treatment is with staged immunosuppression reduction mindful of IRIS with rapid withdrawal. Cidofovir has been used with limited success. The issue of re-transplantation is a moot point, often PML from whatever cause is an absolute contraindication but it might be considered once there is good evidence of immune recovery in the absence of further depleting antibodies and following counselling.

94.2.12 Respiratory Viruses

A number of respiratory viruses infect RTR (see ◘ Table 94.7), can cause asymptomatic or minor infection sometimes with prolonged shedding, but can also result in devastating respiratory illness and death. Apart

Table 94.7 Respiratory viruses in renal transplant recipients

Respiratory Syncytial Virus (paramyxovirus)	Common respiratory infection post SOT, can progress to pneumonitis/bronchiolitis. Ribavirin (IV or inhaled) can be used (no RCTs) alone or with IVIg and reduction in immunosuppression. Consider palivizumab.
Coronavirus (SARS-Coronavirus)	Coronavirus can cause URTi and LRTi, relevant in heavily immunosuppressed patients. SARS Coronovirus carries a significant risk of ARDS and mortality. Currently no treatment for coronovirdae infections so emphasis on avoidance, ISR and supportive care.
Adenovirus	May be shed for long periods from upper airway. Serotypes 1 and 2 associated with pneumonia. Supportive and reduction in IS (cidofovir can be used for disseminated infection).
Rhinovirus	Predominantly URTi but can cause LRTi, currently no effective treatment.
Parainfluenzae virus	URT and LRT infection as well as asymptomatic shedding, no effective treatment.
Influenza A and B (orthomyxovirus)	Influenza can cause considerable morbidity among SOT. Vaccination effective in SOT (less so in first 6 months post -transplant) and should be offered annually. Widespread resistance to M2 inhibitors (amantadine and rimantadine) - not recommended. Primary treatment with Oseltamivir 75 mg bid for 5 days. Prophylaxis should be considered for significant RTR contacts (Oseltamivir 75 mg od for 10 days)
Metapneumovirus	URTi and LRTi currently no effective treatment.
Bocovirus	URTi, clinical relevance unclear
Enteroviruses	URTi and LRTi as well as meningitis and encephalitis

from influenza, for most of these viruses there is either no effective antiviral or antivirals that have only modest efficacy. Management therefore relies on good housekeeping in terms of annual influenza vaccination (measles vaccination if not previously done), ensuring staff and patient hand hygiene is taught (and practiced), and the ability to isolate potentially infectious patients. Rapid nucleic testing of nasopharyngeal swabs is important to avoid inappropriate antibiotics and admitting an infectious patient into an open transplant ward.

Beyond specific antivirals, therapy is supportive care, treating secondary bacterial infections, and immunosuppression reduction. IVIg has been used in patients with severe infections and worth considering in patients with severe disease.

Parvovirus B-19 is a single-stranded DNA virus acquired by respiratory transmission although can be transmitted via transfusion or with the donor organ. Acute infection is with fever, arthritis, rash, and sometimes with an acute aplastic crisis with marked anemia (thrombocytopenia and leucopenia also common). Nephrotic syndrome secondary to a collapsing focal segmental glomerulopathy is also reported. Diagnosis can be made serologically with IgM but PCR for viral DNA is more sensitive and permits monitoring of response. Viremia can persist in RTR for a prolonged period of time posing infection risk to others. Treatment of aplastic anemia or glomerulonephritis is with IVIg 0.4 g/Kg over 5 days.

94.2.13 Human Papillomavirus (HPV)

HPV is an important cause of morbidity posttransplant both in terms of viral cutaneous and anogenital warts, as well as skin, vulval, and perianal malignancy (Fig. 94.7). The skin manifestations and management of viral warts are discussed in Chap. xxxx (renal skin disease), and it is worth remembering that HPV has been detected in the majority of posttransplant squamous cell and basal cell carcinomas [34]. Posttransplant patients have much higher incidence of HPV infection with pro-oncogenic serotypes 16 and 18. Registry data shows a substantial excess of cervical and anal precancer (approximately ×10) and a 50–100-fold increase in vulval pre-malignancies, most alarmingly at an average age of 37, approximately 25 years younger than the general population. HPV vaccination of schoolgirls may help reduce the incidence in women, but as yet there is no data to support the routine vaccination of patients on the waiting list. Many countries have guidelines recommending cervical screening posttransplant but in the UK the evidence is that the uptake is extremely poor at around 10% and something we could be much better at [35]. There is a strong argument for screening within a year of becoming sexually active or after acquiring a new partner.

94.2.14 Hepatitis E (HEV)

Hepatitis E is an RNA virus transmitted by the fecooral route due to poor hygiene in resource poor countries (genotype 1, 2), but in Western countries mainly from eating undercooked meat (predominantly genotype 3) and from blood donors. In the UK, it is recommended that HEV-screened blood components should be used for RTR. HEV is usually a self-limiting infection in healthy people but is associated with high mor-

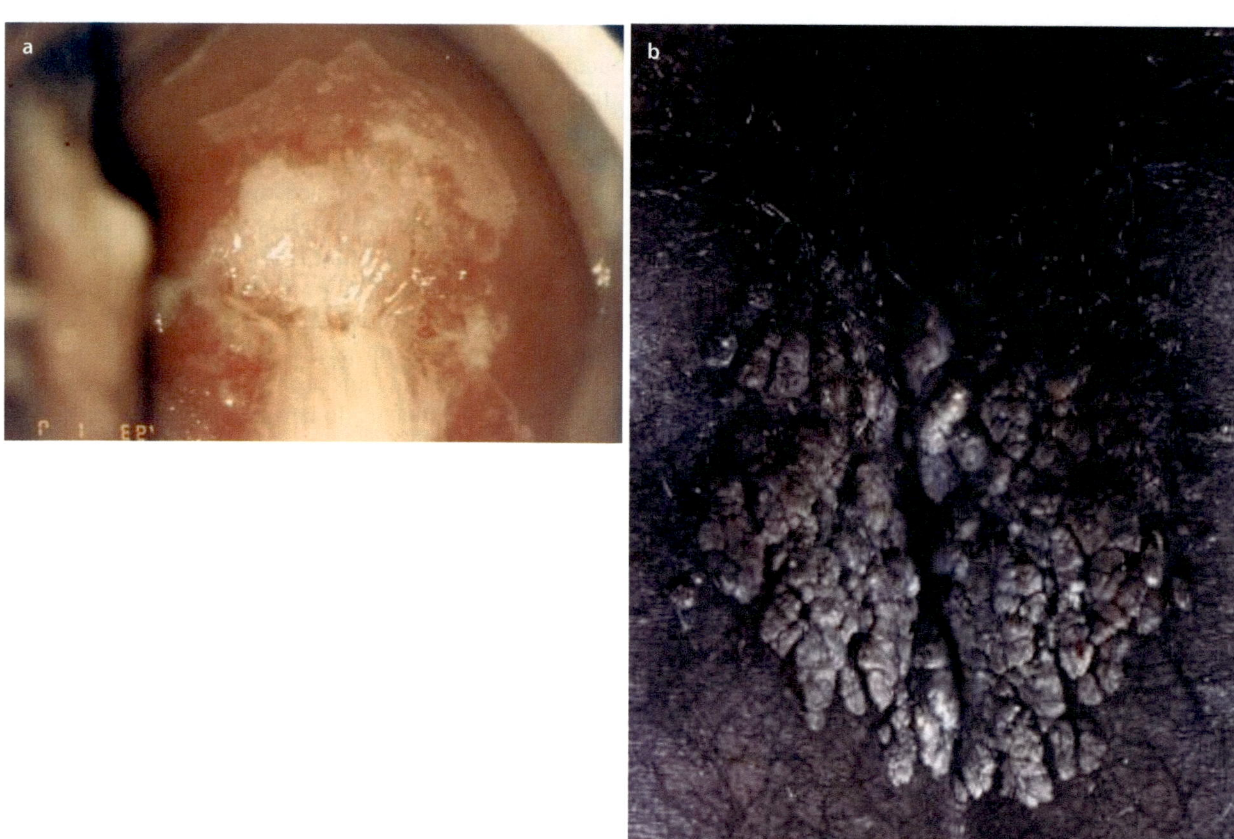

Fig. 94.7 **a** Colposcopy showing CIN3 in a 30-year-old renal transplant patient with human papilloma virus infection. **b** Perianal warts secondary to human papilloma virus infection in a renal transplant recipient

tality with acute hepatic failure in patients with preexisting chronic liver disease or pregnancy. Recent data suggests, however, that it may be associated with chronic sub-clinical hepatitis in solid organ transplants. In France the seroprevalence pretransplant is 14% but reactivation has not been demonstrated. A recent UK study screening nearly 900 liver, kidney, and bone marrow transplant patients detected hepatitis E RNA in only 0.46% (none of them RTRs) suggesting a pretty low incidence and prevalence in the first 90 days of transplantation in the UK. For those who do contract hepatitis E, >50% of *de novo* cases posttransplant are asymptomatic with the rest having hepatitis. Approximately 40% of these patients clear the virus spontaneously but 60% do not, and go on to have chronic infection with abnormal LFTs and occasionally rapid progression to cirrhosis. However, the overall prevalence of chronic infection is not known and making the diagnosis is important as clearance of the virus may prevent cirrhosis and, if suspected, the diagnosis can be made on RNA from blood or stool. Treatment is with immunosuppression reduction or, failing that, success has been reported with pegalated interferon or ribavirin [36]. Treatment is continued until RNA is undetected in stool.

94

94.2.15 Bacteria

94.2.15.1 Legionella

Cell-mediated immunity appears particularly important in the defence against legionella pneumophila and consequently SOT recipients are at substantial risk if exposed (usually from contaminated air-conditioning systems or water tanks and in outbreaks). High fever and cough with flu-like symptoms are the norm. The CXR may show focal, nodular, lobar, or diffuse consolidation sometimes with cavitation. Urine legionella antigen testing is quick (but only detects Legionella pnuemophilia serotype 1 infections)) unlike paired legionella serology which is rarely helpful in real time. As with mycoplasma and chlamydia, PCR for legionella can be done on BAL or sputum samples. The sensitivity of PCR testing is lower in sputum specimens.

Treatment is with macrolides (ideally azithromycin as does not inhibit cytochrome p450), fluroquinolones, rifampicin or dual therapy in sick patients.

Since tests may not be diagnostic, "atypical" pathogen cover should be considered (ideally with a macrolide) for SOT recipients with a lower respiratory tract infection.

94.2.15.2 Listeria

Listeria monocytogenes is an environmental gram-positive bacillus, contracted orally from pets, domestic animals, or unpasteurized or poorly kept foods and consequently can occur in outbreaks as well as sporadically. Listeria infection is associated with a high mortality especially in the immunocompromised as intracellular and normally eradicated by cell-mediated immunity, which is disabled in SOT. It is the commonest cause of bacterial meningitis in SOT and in addition has tropism for brain parenchyma. Incubation is within 24 hours of ingestion, symptoms developing within a week. Clinically presentation is nonspecific: fever possibly following a diarrheal illness, malaise, meningitis (50%), or encephalitis with abscess (10%) (◘ Fig. 94.8) [37]. Diagnosis is typically made on blood culture or examination and culture of CSF.

Treatment is with intravenous ampicillin (2 g every 4 hours). Gentamycin (3 mg/kg in three divided doses) is usually added in for immunocompromised patients.

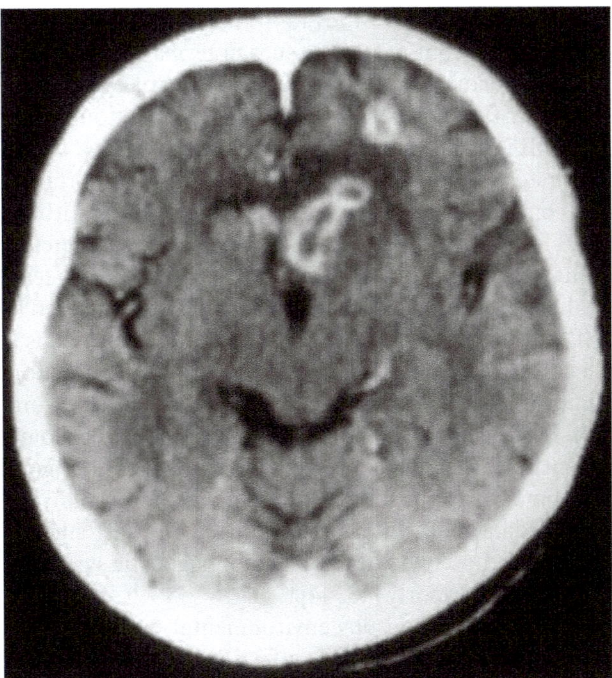

◘ **Fig. 94.8** Listeria causing a ring-enhancing space occupying lesion (SOL) in a recipient 6 years posttransplant

Trimethoprim-sulphamethaxozole (septrin) is an alternative for penicillin allergic patients.

94.2.15.3 Nocardia

Nocardia is a rare but serious opportunistic infection posttransplant caused by actinomycetes nocardia species mostly acquired by inhalation, occasionally via skin inoculation. The incidence in the reported literature is around 1% but this probably represents reporting bias and the evidence is that it is less common, in part because of universal prophylaxis with septrin. A review of the English literature case reports following renal transplantation shows a huge variation in onset from 4 weeks to 22 years, which most likely reflects the importance of environmental exposure [38].

The vast majority of cases present with or have primary pulmonary involvement and a significant proportion of these go on to have disseminated disease with a predilection for brain and cutaneous involvement (◘ Fig. 94.9). Pulmonary involvement does not typically present as classical pneumonia but fever is common and lung nodules and cavities are common. Cerebral involvement may be insidious and nonspecific with headaches, confusion, focal neurological signs, and is also associated with a fever [38].

Norcardia, especially disseminated disease, is associated with a significant mortality (17%) and early diagnosis with biopsy of unexplained skin nodules or other accessible lesions essential. Treatment for early pulmonary disease is with Sulphonamides, usually Trimethoprim/sulphamethoxazole 15 mg/kg/day. For severe pulmonary or any cerebral involvement, imipenem and amikacin are added in, with the caveat that some nocardia species have resistance and biopsy with culture and sensitivities is very important. Treatment must be prolonged to 6–12 months for pulmonary and 9–12 for cerebral involvement [39].

94.2.16 Mycobacteria: TM and Non-tuberculous Mycobacterium (NTM)

The incidence of active TB in RTRs in Western countries has been reported to be between 0.3% and 1%, which is 20–70× higher than the general population, and in Asia rates have been consistently higher at 5–15%. A recent registry study from the UK of over 30,000 RTRs suggests a much lower rate (0.03%) in the first year for Caucasian patients although the risk bias Asian patients persists with a rate about 10 times this (0.3%). Apart from country of origin, diabetes, chronic liver disease, and the burden of immunosuppression (e.g., the use of depleting antibodies) are significant risk factors [40, 41].

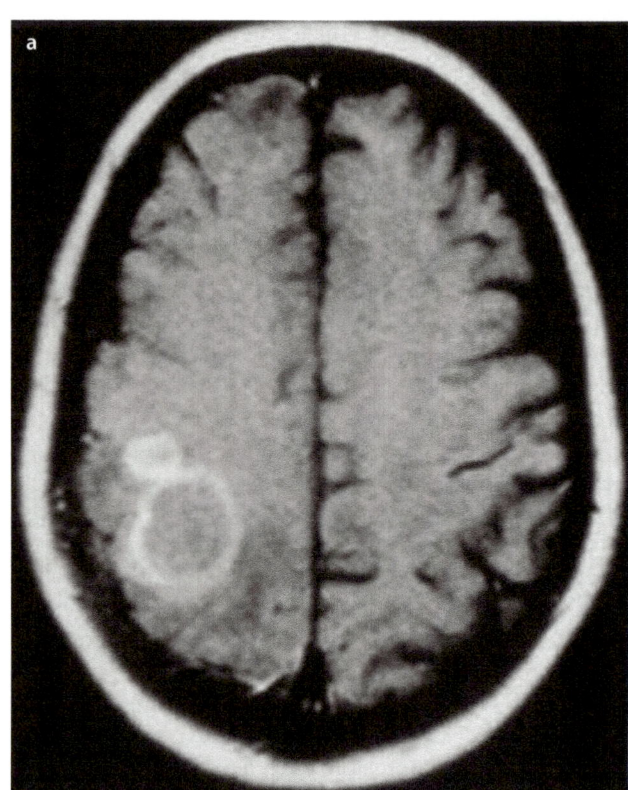

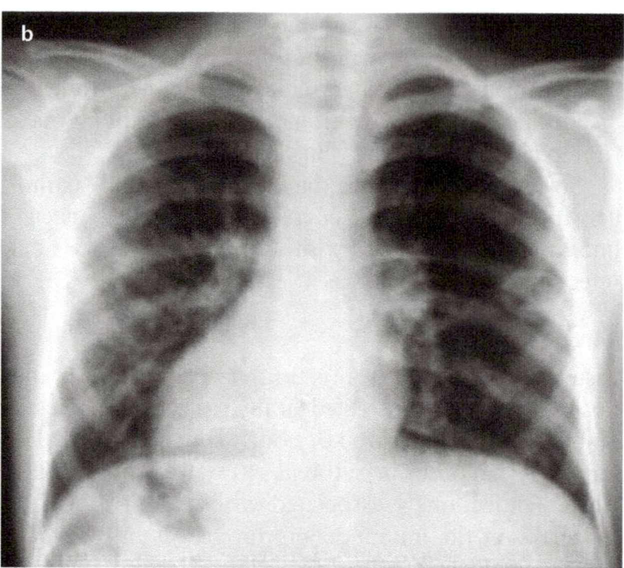

Fig. 94.9 Nocardia causing **a** a ring-enhancing SOL on CT **b** multiple cavities on CXR

Screening pretransplant is difficult as tuberculin skin tests, e.g., Mantoux test, while helpful if positive, often result in false negatives in patients with ESRD and patients with previous BCG may have false positives. CXR with signs of previous TB are clearly helpful and Interferon gamma release assays may be helpful but do not distinguish between previous exposure and active disease, but again can be negative in patients with ESRD or posttransplant [42].

UK guidelines are to offer prophylaxis for 6 months with 300 mg isoniazid (and pyridoxine prophylaxis) for patients from high risk countries (we avoid this if the patient has hepatitis or underlying chronic liver disease).

The peak incidence of clinical TB is in the first 12 months at an average of about 10–12 months posttransplant with the majority of infections thought to be reactivation with roughly 10% due to primary infection (a very small percentage of which are donor derived). Fever appears to be a prominent feature occurring in 70% with weight loss and asthenia. Strikingly, up to two-thirds of patients present with extrapulmonary disease (compared to 15% in the general population) (Fig. 94.10) [43] and consequently tissue biopsy and ensuring procedurists send a sample for mycobacterial staining, PCR and culture is important in making the diagnosis. In immunocompromised patients, mycobacterial burden is often high and mycobacterial blood cultures may be helpful, especially in the setting of disseminated atypical mycobacterial infections (e.g., *Mycobacterium avium–intracellulare* complex infections; see below).

Management for MTB in SOT is the standard anti-TB treatment but presents issues in terms of drug interactions, the main one being the induction of cytochrome p450 by rifampicin resulting in marked reduction in CNI levels. It is usual to have to triple the dose of CNI within the first 2 weeks of rifampicin-based therapy. Importantly, the converse is true when rifampicin is stopped with the need for significant dose reduction. It is critical therefore to have close liaison between the infectious disease team and the nephrologist. Treatment is often accompanied by ISR but this needs to be done with caution if the TB is in a neurological site as Immune Restitution Inflammatory Syndrome (IRIS) may result in paradoxical deterioration despite adequate anti-TB therapy. Outcome from a recent retrospective analysis in France suggests a good outcome with a mortality of 6%, much improved on historical data, with little or no impact on graft survival except for those who develop hemophagocytic syndrome which augurs poorly [43, 44].

NTM are ubiquitous environmental pathogens that can become opportunistic infections in SOT. Donor-derived NTM has been documented but is rare. The overall incidence of NTM is not clear but there are case

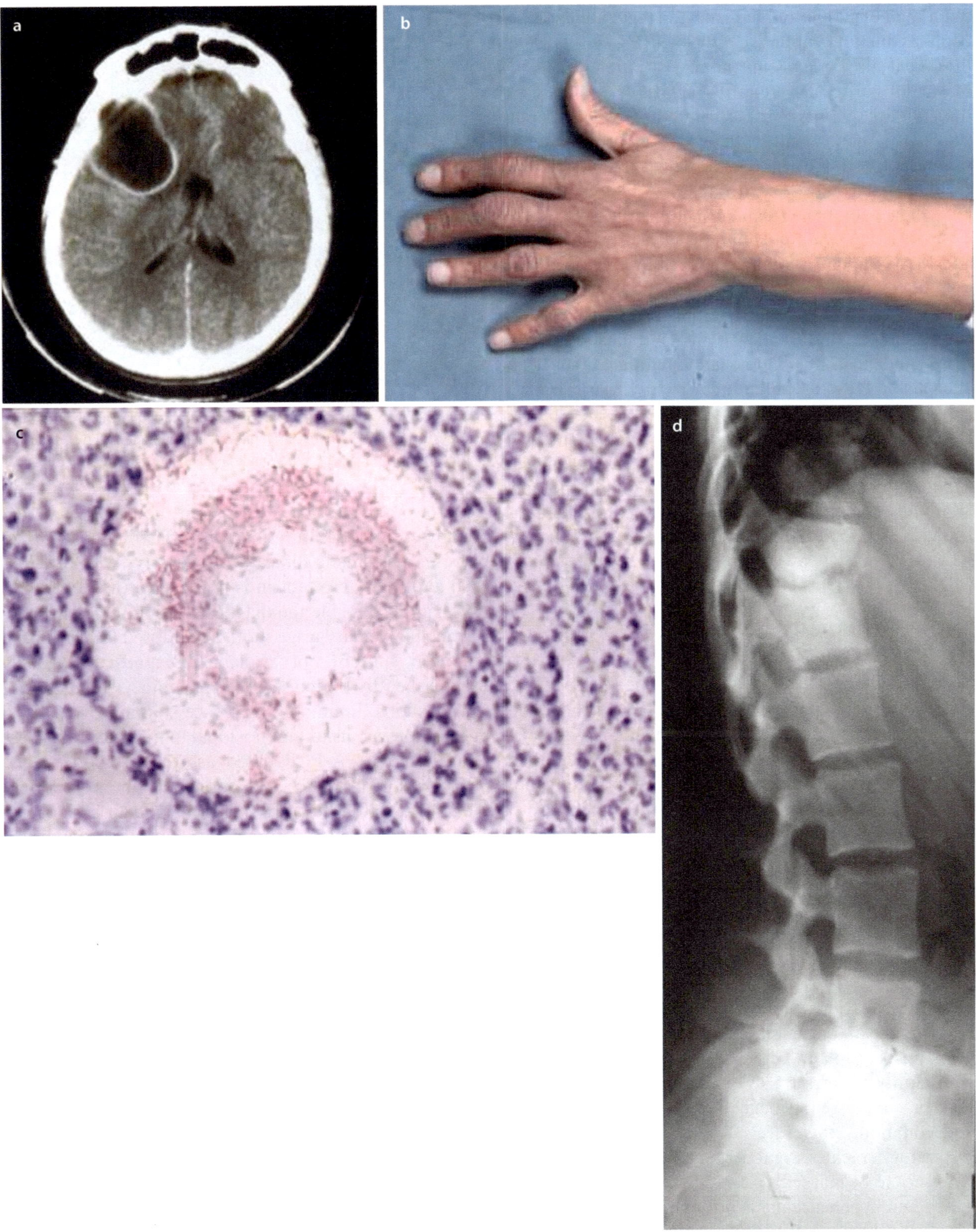

Fig. 94.10 **a** Frontotemporal Tuberculoma in a transplant recipient presenting with erratic behavior **b** Metacaropophalangeal and wrist swelling secondary to atypical mycobacterium **c** skin biopsy showing copious acid fast-bacilli **d** lumbar spine X-ray showing destruction of disc and lumbar vertebral secondary to mycobacterium infection

reports of infection in renal transplants by many NTM species, but the commonest appear to be *M. chelonae*, *Mycobacterium avium* complex (MAC), M. kansasii and M.xenopi with an average presentation 2 years post-transplant [45]. In SOT transplants (excluding lung transplants), the majority of disease is extra-pulmonary (CXR normal). Presentation may be cutaneous with erythematous nodules, and tenosynovitis and arthritis are also common, often at more than one site. Constitutional symptoms may be absent. M. abscessus and MAC are more common in recipients with chronic lung disease where colonization is facilitated. Therefore making the diagnosis of NTB infection in this setting can be difficult and the American Thoracic Society has issued guidelines involving a combination of consistent clinical and radiological findings, exclusion of other diseases, and culture of BAL or biopsy specimen [46]. Debridement may be necessary for cutaneous involvement and first-line agents often involve Azithromycin, Ethambutol, and Rifabutin, but treatment is a specialist area and requires liaison with the Infectious Diseases team.

94.2.17 Fungi

94.2.17.1 Pneumocystis Jirovecii (PJ)

PJ is an important opportunistic fungal infection, acquired asymptomatically (mostly in childhood), causing disease, mostly in the form of a severe pneumonia (PCP) in the immunocompromised through reactivation as well as primary or reinfection. In the absence of prophylaxis, rates of 5–15% occur in SOT and known risk factors include (1) use of steroids; (2) burden of immunosuppression and/or $CD4^{+}$ count <200; (3) rejection episodes (especially repeated); and (4) CMV viremia. There are now several reports of outbreaks, and respiratory transmission among transplant patients is clearly possible.

The incubation is thought to be about 7–8 weeks and cases are rare in the first month, but can also occur many years posttransplant. Clinically, onset is often insidious with slowly progressive dyspnoea and fever (although may be suppressed), cough if present is unproductive and commonly there are no chest signs or fine basal inspiratory crackles. A moderate fever is common, CRP tends not to be markedly elevated whereas LDH is often raised and hypercalcemia is not unusual. Beta-d-glucan appears to be very sensitive for PCP and relatively specific whereas glactomannan is less helpful. An invaluable early sign is desaturation on exertion and should be assessed in anyone with apparently mild dyspnoea. CXRs are often normal in early disease; CT scan has a much higher sensitivity showing classical ground-glass shadowing (see Fig. 94.11), and should be requested if any exercise desaturation is demonstrated. The diagnosis is often made clinically but there is a wide differential and high-dose septrin is not without its side effects so if at all possible the diagnosis should be confirmed. Bronchoalveolar lavage should be pressed for early if an induced sputum not available. Diagnosis is usually established by the presence of pneumocystis cysts with silver stains. Immunofluorescence staining of cell wall glycoproteins using monoclonal antibodies increases sensitivity. DNA-PCR-based assays of blood, saliva, and sputum are under evaluation. Cysts may be present for 7 days after starting treatment and in some cases even after 3 weeks of treatment. Therefore, empirical treatment should not be withheld while awaiting diagnostic tests. Rarely, a biopsy (transbronchial or open lung biopsy) may be required if progressive disease with no diagnosis or improvement with empirical treatment.

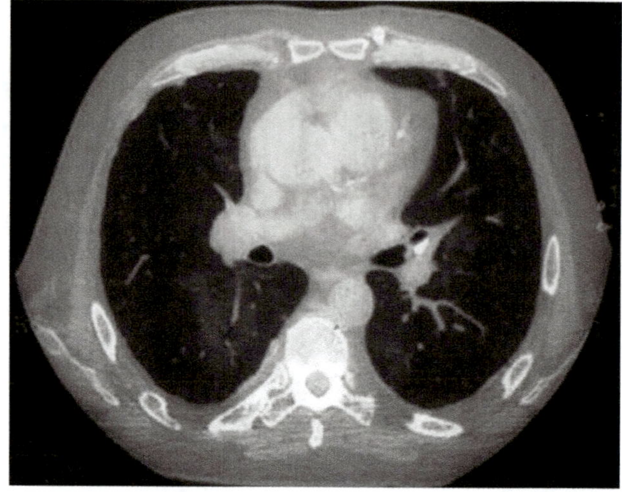

Fig. 94.11 CT scan showing ground-glass shadowing of pneumocystis jirovecii infection in a patient who had steroid treatment for late rejection but no PCP prophylaxis. The chest X-ray was normal

Prophylaxis against PCP is covered in Table 94.3 and is highly effective at reducing incidence of PCP. Various guidelines recommend prophylaxis from 4 months up to 12 months. It is common practice to give at least 6 months prophylaxis following T-cell depleting antibody and most units using Campath-H1 continue until $CD4^{+}$ count is >200; similarly, we check the $CD4^{+}$ count at the time of stopping prophylaxis on all our patients. In addition, it is important to have a system that considers every patient treated for rejection as restarting prophylaxis at time zero. Septrin is usually prescribed at 480 mg daily or 960 mg three times a week, which has the considerable advantage of offering co-prophylaxis against toxoplasma, nocardia, listeria and some protection against UTI (alternatives, that do not offer the same co-prophylaxis are shown in Table 94.3). Recent evidence of outbreaks has resulted in the sensible recommendation that patients exposed to the sentinel case should be offered prophylaxis, and patients with PCP should be isolated until completed 7 days of treatment [47].

First-line treatment for PCP is Septrin at 15 mg/kg/day in divided doses [48], this requires a large volume of intravenous fluid and can be problematic in patients with poor renal function. Septrin has good oral bioavailability and mild to moderate disease can be treated orally. Alternatives include iv pentamidine (associated with numerous complications including infusion-induced hypoglycemia, renal impairment, acute pancreatitis, etc), primaquine, and clindamycin, or (for milder disease) dapsone and atovaquone. Extrapolating from HIV literature, high-dose oral steroids are also recommended and should be started early (intravenous or oral prednisolone 40 mg bid, tapered over 10 days). It is common practice to reduce overall immunosuppression simultaneously and to restart prophylaxis following successful treatment.

Treatment is for a minimum of 2 weeks, three if severe disease.

94.2.17.2 Invasive Fungi

A variety of other fungal infections occur in RTR, with the burden of immunosuppression (especially the use of depleting antibodies), multiple rejection episodes, high-dose steroids (compromising the innate immune system), CMV viremia, and diabetes being significant risk factors. Consequently the majority of serious fungal infections occur within the first 12 months, cryptococcal infection being an important exception. Compared to other SOTs, RTRs are relatively spared from fungal infections but rates of 2–14% have been reported, with rates in pancreas recipients much higher [49]. In a review of nearly 100 RTR with invasive fungal infection, *Candida, Cryptococcus, and Aspergillus* are the three commonest [50]. Fungal infections may be trivial colonizations, but all of the fungi discussed below can cause invasive disease with high mortality and early diagnosis is critical. Azoles used to treat several fungal infections have a profound inhibitory effect on cytochrome p450, consequently in the absence of close monitoring, starting an azole is highly likely to render a fungemic patient CNI toxic.

94.2.17.3 Candida

Infection by candida is the commonest fungal infection in RTR usually presenting with oro-genital involvement (see ◘ Fig. 94.12), especially in the setting of steroid exposure (and/or diabetes) but also accounting for 60% of invasive fungal infections. Beyond mucocutaneous infection, candida can involve the gut, severe oesophagitis being particularly common (see ◘ Fig. 94.12b), urinary tract, lungs (focal cavity or pneumonitis), central nervous system and heart valves.

Prophylaxis with Nystatin 1 ml qds is pretty effective at preventing oral candidiasis as long as patients take it (we discontinue prophylaxis when steroids stopped or down to 5 mg), as is oral fluconazole 50 mg od. Distinguishing colonization from UTI or respiratory tract infection can be tricky and a judgement call must be made, but biopsy proven tissue involvement or positive blood cultures need rapid treatment. *Candida albicans* is sensitive to azoles but *C. glabrata* and *C. krusei* are often resistant. Treatment for oesophageal or systemic involvement is with fluconazole or caspofungin, voriconazole, posaconazole, amphotericin.

94.2.17.4 Aspergillosis

Aspergillus niger is common as a harmless tongue infection (see ◘ Fig. 94.13b), whereas *A. fumigatus* and *A. flavus* are responsible for 12% of invasive fungal infections (0.7% of RTR). As with other fungal infections, risk factors are total burden of immunosuppression, diabetes, chronic liver disease and CMV viremia, but exposure to building works and smoking marijuana have also been implicated. The commonest presentation is with pneumonia but rhinocerebral (see ◘ Fig. 94.13), sinus, gut, and skin involvement can also occur. Dyspnoea, unproductive cough and fever are usual, hemoptysis, which may be torrential, can occur. While the classical appearance on CT scan of pulmonary nodules with a "halo" sign is suggestive of angio-invasive aspergilliosis, patients may often present with infiltrates or consolidation. Where there is a high index of suspicion for invasive aspergillosis (e.g., non-response to broad spectrum antibiotics), a broncho-alveolar lavage or transbronchial biopsy may be required. Serum galacotomannans, though useful, may have low sensitivity and specificity in SOT recipients. BAL galactomannans may have better specificity in this setting. Culture and cytology/histopathological findings are more specific.

Treatment for invasive disease is with iv voriconazole, which is more effective than liposomal amphotericin—an alternative is caspofungin or a combination with immunosuppression reduction. In the context of an aspergilloma with invasion into preexisting cavitatory lung disease, pulmonary artery embolization or surgical resection may be required. Surgical debridement may also be required in patients with invasive aspergillosis where there is impending massive hemorrhage or in the case of rhinosinusitis. Mortality is high and the emphasis should be on early diagnosis and aggressive treatment. Duration of therapy will depend on clinical response.

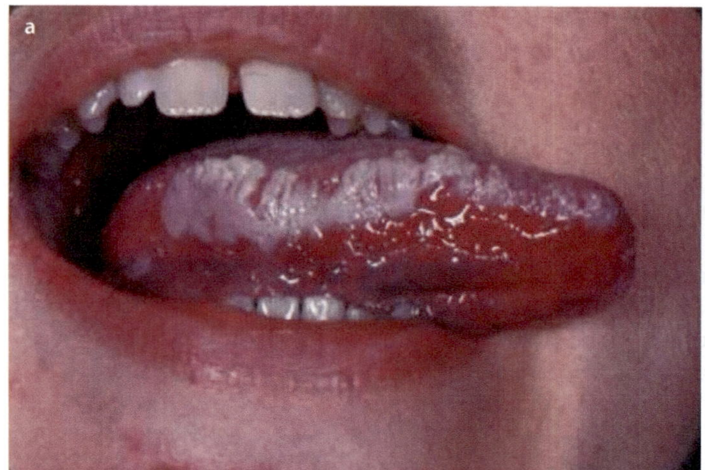

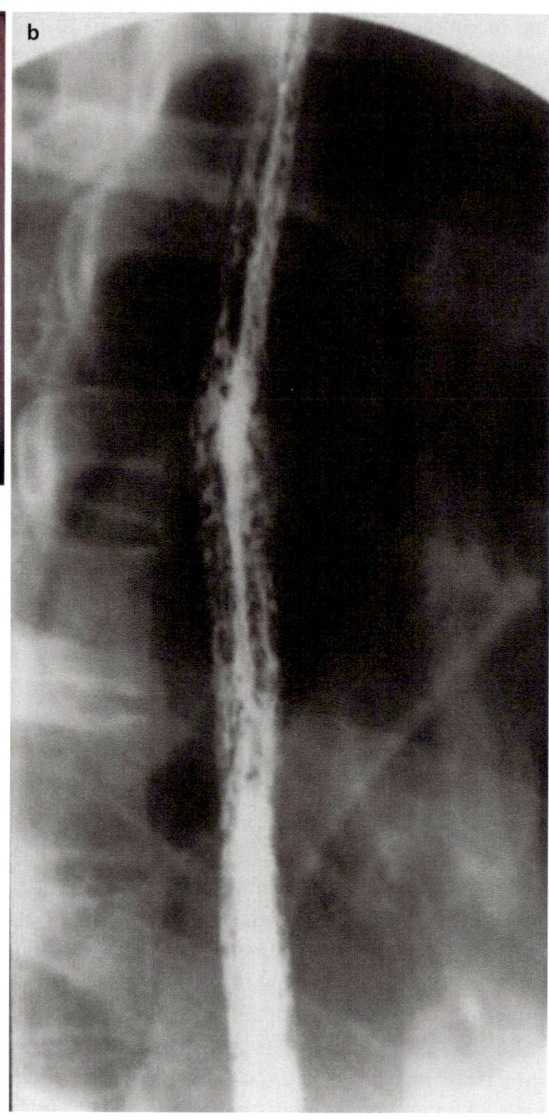

Fig. 94.12 **a** Oral candid adherent to the tongue **b** Barium swallow showing extensive oral candidiasis. The patient who was on large doses of steroids presented with severe retrosternal chest pain with oral candidiasis

94.2.18 *Cryptococcus Neoformans* (CN)

CN is an opportunistic environmental pathogen with highest risk of exposure related to birds and bird guano. Historical data suggests infection rates of 2–3.5% in RTR and this appears to be higher than in other SOT, and accounts for 19% of invasive fungal infections, although this may reflect previous use of higher doses of steroids and clinical experience suggests much lower rates in RTR than this currently. Patients may show signs of neurological, pulmonary and cutaneous involvement. Pneumonia has no characteristic features but dyspnoea and cough are common, x-rays may show either nodule(s) or lobar consolidation. Cutaneous involvement occurs in 10–20% and is a very useful diagnostic focus [51]. Meningoencephalitis often has an indolent and nonspecific presentation resulting in delayed diagnosis with headaches (over weeks), irritability, and confusion in the absence of classical signs of meningism, but ultimately progressing to a reduction in consciousness and or focal cranial nerve palsies. It is an important diagnosis not to miss and a high index of suspicion is required; at lumber puncture, high opening pressure, moderate elevation of CSF protein, and low white cell counts (predominantly lymphocytes) with low CSF:serum glucose ratio are characteristic but not specific findings. An Indian-Ink stain and cryptococcal antigen (CrAg) test must always be requested in this setting. A serum CrAg test is a useful to perform, and is almost always positive in meningeal and disseminated disease.

94

Treatment of *Cryptococcus* infection in RTR is associated with a high rate of IRIS (5–11%) presenting

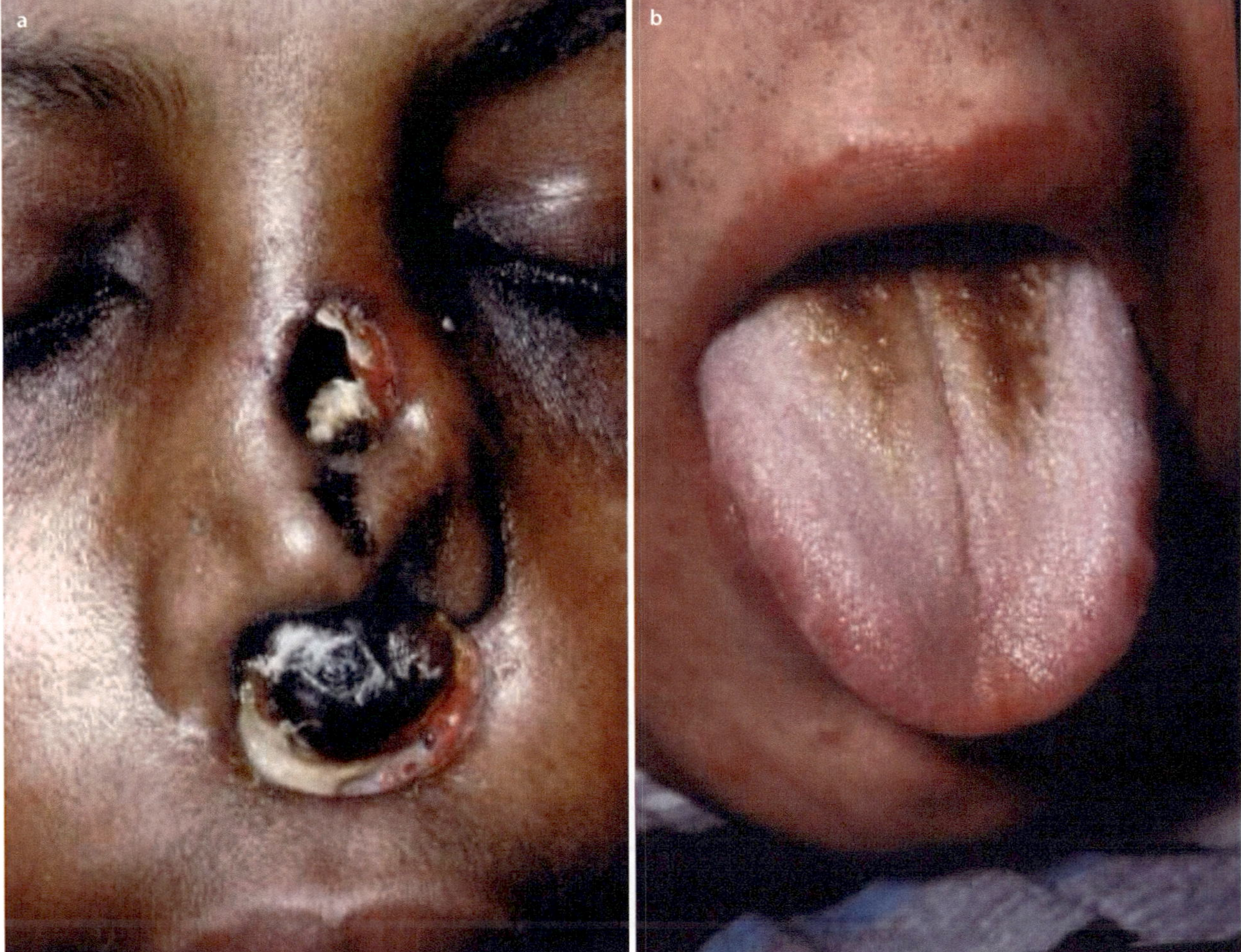

Fig. 94.13 *Aspergillus* infection: **a** invasive nasopalatal *Aspergillus* infection and **b** *Aspergillus niger* infection of the tongue

roughly 5 weeks after reduction in immunosuppression and clinicians must be aware of the risk of associated hydrocephalus with a low threshold for reimaging.

Initial treatment is with liposomal amphotericin and flucytosine for the first 2 weeks, followed by high-dose fluconazole (400 mg day) for 8 weeks. This should be followed by secondary prophylaxis with fluconazole 200 mg/day for at least 12 months (or lifelong if peripheral blood CD4 cells remain <200).

Morbidity and mortality in crypotococcal meningitis is mainly associated with raised intracranial pressure (as a result of CSF absorption blockade) and repeated lumber punctures to remove CSF may be required in the first 2 weeks of therapy.

94.2.19 Mucormycosis

Mucormycosis is a rare opportunistic fungal infection most commonly documented in debilitated and poorly controlled diabetics but also in renal transplants (1% of invasive fungal infections). Risk factors include prolonged neutropenia, diabetes and iron-chelation therapy as well as immunosuppression. Mucocutaneous, particularly orofacial, rhinocerebral, and pulmonary involvement are commonest and because of the propensity to invade vessels, a fatal outcome from pulmonary hemorrhage and dissemination is common (Fig. 94.14). Treatment is with IV Liposomal amphotericin (with posaconazole as an alternative or dual therapy) and surgical resection of pulmonary and extrapulmonary tissue is important. The mortality from mucormycosis in RTR remains the highest of any fungal infection at over 50%.

94.2.20 *Histoplasma Capsulatum* and *Coccidioides Immitis*

These are endemic fungi that are responsible for <4% of invasive fungal infections in SOT but with a very high mortality. Both fungi occur in SW USA, Central and

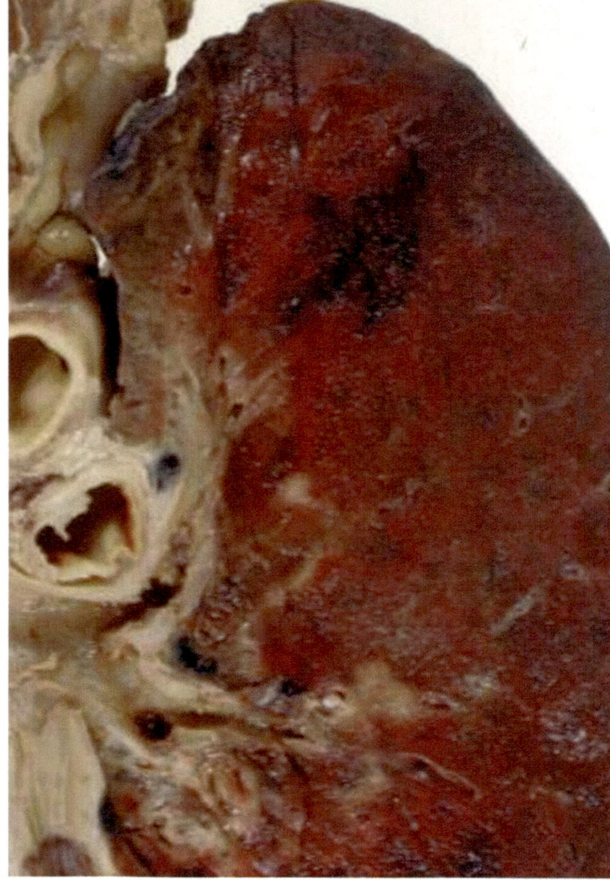

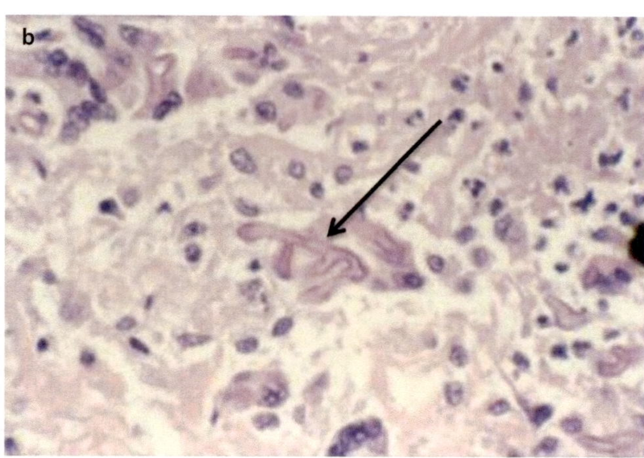

Fig. 94.14 **a** Postmortem specimen showing the lung with hemorrhage secondary to vessel involvement of a transplant patient with mucormycosis. **b** Biopsy showing invasive mycelium

South America but Histoplasma is also reported in Europe, Asia, and Africa. Outbreaks of both conditions have been described in RTRs and rare cases of donor-derived infection have also been reported, however the majority of infections appear to be reactivation (occurring within 6 months) or primary infections (occurring at any stage).

The main exposure risk for Histoplasma is bird or bat guano. Histoplasmosis in RTR may present with fever, cellulitis, mouth ulcers, oronasopharyngeal, pulmonary, or meningeal involvement [52]. Fungal cultures may take weeks and as with other fungal infections biopsies can be very helpful. Urine antigen screening has a high (>90%) sensitivity but is not widely available. Histopathological examination may show characteristic intracellular organisms.

In immunocompetent individuals, coccidioidomycosis almost exclusively causes pulmonary disease but in SOT 75% is extra-pulmonary, commonly involving liver, bone marrow, and meninges [53]. Guidelines do not recommend serological screening but some authors advocate this for donor and recipient in endemic regions.

First-line treatment for both fungi is with liposomal amphotericin, with itraconazole as second line for Histoplasmosis, fluconazole, or caspofungin for coccidioidomycosis, and accompanied by ISR. As fatal relapses can occur it is usual to treat with an azole for at least a year, and after meningeal involvement, usually for life.

94.2.21 Cryptosporidiosis

Cryptosporidium parvum (associated with drinking water, swimming pools, and livestock) can cause chronic disabling diarrhea in RTRs, which is watery/mucoid and associated with abdominal pain. In most individuals it is a self-limiting illness; patients are not normally screened but in one study of SOTs with diarrhea 20% of cases were attributed to cryptosporidium, so is probably underdiagnosed in most practice [54]. Cryptosporidium

Ag testing by ELISA is highly sensitive with a good specificity and worth considering in any RTR with culture negative diarrhea not responsive to replacement of the usual suspect medications. There is no specific treatment but spiramycin, nitrzoxamide, and paromomycin have been tried with some success but relapses can occur.

94.2.22 Parasites

94.2.22.1 Toxoplasmosis

Toxoplama gondii is an opportunistic parasite, which can cause disease in RTR through reactivation, primary infection, and occasionally through donor transmission. Risk factors include seronegative status of recipient, seropositive donor, burden of immunosuppression (CD4 counts below 200), lack of septrin prophylaxis and exposure to cats. Reactivation and donor-derived infection tend to present within the first 3 months of a transplant with pneumonitis (two-thirds) or neurological involvement (two-thirds) (90% at post mortem); cardiac involvement also occurs. Fever is common but neurological symptoms are nonspecific with headache, confusion, and ultimately coma [55]. Serology is only really helpful in diagnosing risk, as seroconversion is often slow and rarely helpful in making the diagnosis. The diagnosis may be made by contrast CT or MRI scanning showing multiple ring-enhancing lesions and an appropriate radiological response after 2–3 weeks of treatment. CNS ring-enhancing lesions in SOT recipients may be due to a number of causes, and if an appropriate response to treatment is not seen, a stereo-tactic brain biopsy may be required. When safe to do so, lumbar puncture and CSF toxoplasma DNA detection by PCR is highly sensitive and specific for CNS toxoplasmosis.

Septrin prophylaxis for PCP is very effective at preventing toxoplasmosis but reactivation can occur on stopping. Treatment is with pyrimethamine 200 mg loading dose followed by 50–75 mg daily and folinic acid plus sulfadiazine 4–6 weeks OR Septrin 5 mg/kg for 30 days. The mortality remains high at 50–65%, those with primary infection being particularly at risk [56].

In RTRs cerebral toxoplasmosis is rarely a problem but as always those who are naïve are particularly at risk. Checking toxoplasma serology prior to transplant is good, better still is to advise those who are naïve to avoid adopting cats or pet litter in general.

94.2.23 Strongyloides Stercoralis

Strongyloidiasis infection in the setting of SOT is a very rare but serious condition with mortality of around 50%. Strongyloides is endemic in large areas of the tropics and sub-tropics. Initial infection is via larval penetration of the skin and usually asymptomatic. Larvae migrate to the pulmonary vessels and then via swallowed sputum to the duodenum and jejunum where mature female larvae shed eggs. Importantly infection can remain quiescent for over 30 years so a history of living in an endemic area is as important as being transplanted in an endemic area.

Reactivation and hyper-infestation can occur in those with previous exposure once significantly immunocompromised, usually within 6 months, sometimes within the first month, but occasionally years after a transplant. Presentation tends to be predominantly respiratory and gastrointestinal with abdominal pain, diarrhea, nausea, vomiting, and abdominal distension, which may be due to ileus. Respiratory involvement is with tachypnoea, dyspnoea, fever, and cough and ARDS occurs in about two-thirds. The CXR is usually abnormal with diffuse or patchy infiltrates. Eosinophilia, although a very helpful clue, is often not present [57].

The diagnosis may be made by visualizing larvae in sputum or stool, but there is a high false-negative rate and multiple stool samples may be necessary. Duodenal aspiration, bronchoalveolar lavage and the Enterotest (a piece of string taped to the nose passing into the duodenum then withdrawn for microscopy) all have their supporters and are all worth considering if there is clinical suspicion.

Treatment is with Ivermectin (200 mcg/kg often for 5–7 days in hyperinfestation or 2 days in others) along with broad-spectrum antibiotics if there is evidence of gut translocation. Patients can deteriorate very rapidly with hyper-infestation either via ARDS or recurrent gram-negative septicemia as the larvae burrows into the gut. Early identification is therefore critical and a sensible approach is to check strongyloides serology in all patients from endemic areas pre-listing. If positive, or with unexplained eosinophilia, stool should be screened for ova, cysts, and parasites, and an ID opinion should be sought with regards to blind eradication.

94.2.24 Chagas Disease (*Trypanosoma Cruzi*)

Trypanosoma cruzi is endemic in central and south America and can cause disease in RTR by reactivation (20% of seropositive patients) or through donor-derived infection (20% of seropositive donors) [58]. Infection results in fever, myocarditis, meningo-encephalitis or cutaneous involvement such as panniculitis, typically within a year of transplant [59]. Pretransplant serology

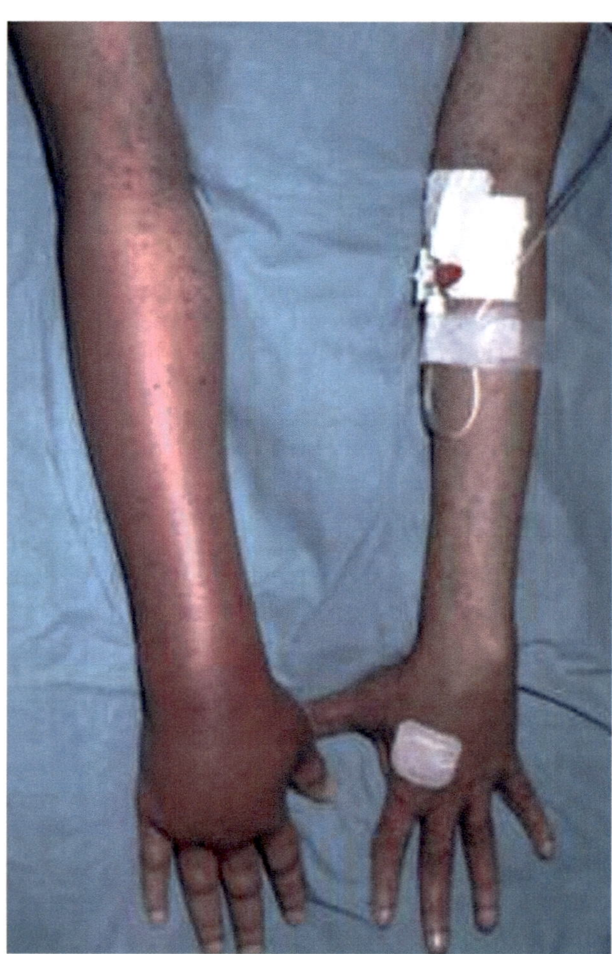

Fig. 94.15 Hyperinfestation with Norwegian Scabies

or treatment is not currently recommended, in part because of the toxicity of treatment, but undertake close surveillance posttransplant for D+ or R+. Treatment is with Benznidazole 5–7 mg/kg /day or Nifurtimox 8–10 mg/kg/day for 8 weeks in the context of parasitemia.

94.2.24.1 Scabies

This can result in hyper-infestation and severe secondary bacterial infection (Fig. 94.15) but the pruritus may be subdued and the source of the cellulitis not immediately apparent.

94.3 Syndromes

There are a variety of clinical scenarios in the immunocompromised with a wide differential diagnosis. Tables 94.8, 94.9, 94.10, 94.11, and 94.12 show the differential diagnosis for diarrhea, chest infiltration, nodules, CNS space occupying lesions and meningoencephalitis. A useful diagnostic sieve for such presentations is (a) could this be non-communicable for example drug-related or malignancy? (b) if infection related then could this be (i) viral? (ii) bacterial? (iii) fungal? (the main candidates tend to be candida, aspergillus, cryptococcus neoformans and less commonly histoplasmosis) (iv) protozoal/helminths?

Table 94.8 Differential diagnosis of diarrhea in SOT recipients

Medication:	
Immunosuppression	Mycophenolic acid (may develop overtime), tacrolimus (NB diarrhea increases tacrolimus levels), mTORi, functional hypoadrenalism following long-term steroids.
Antibiotics	
Miscellaneous	Laxatives, colchicine, metformin
Infectious opportunistic:	
Viral:	
CMV[a]	Usually but not always, associated with CMV viraemia, diarrhea often bloody
Norovirus	Seasonal, nausea, and vomiting prominent
Rotavirus	
Coxsackie[a]	
HSV[a]	
Adenovirus[a]	
Bacterial:	
Clostridium difficile	Early isolation and screening of *C.difficile* toxin especially if extensive antibiotic exposure
Listeria[a]	
MAI[a]	
Salmonella[a]	
Yersina[a]	
E.Coli[a]	
Campylobacter	
Bacterial overgrowth	Particularly in patients with diabetes or bowel surgery
Parasitic:	Cryptosporidium
Microsporidium[a]	
Isospora belli	
Giardia lamblia	
Strongyloides[a]	
Entamoebae histolytica[a]	

[a]Can result in disseminated disease

Table 94.9 Differential diagnosis of pulmonary infiltrates in SOT recipient

Infection:	
Bacteria	Conventional bacteria, Mycobacteria, Nocardia
Viruses	CMV, Community respiratory viruses (influenza, parainfluenza, RSV)
Fungi	Aspergillus, Pneumocystis, Cryptococcus
Protozoal/ Helminth	ARDS secondary to hyper-infestation syndrome
Fluid:	
ARDS	Sepsis, allergic reaction to anti-CD25mAb, ATG, OKT-3, Campath-H1
Fluid retention/ cardiac failure	Left ventricular failure, diastolic dysfunction, transplant renal artery stenosis (flash pulmonary oedema
Pulmonary hemorrhage	
Medication:	
mTOR-inhibitor	mTORi induced pneumonitis; opportunistic infection less likely if CD4+ count >200, (if in doubt stop mTOR and treat with steroids)
Other	Azathioprine, cyclophosphamide, nitrofurantoin

Table 94.10 Differential diagnosis of pulmonary nodule in SOT recipient

Infective:	
Bacterial abscess	Nocardia, legionella, gram positive (staph aureus, rhodocuccus equi), gram negative (enterobacteriaceae, pseudomonas aeruginosa, kebsiella pnumoniae), anaerobes and septic emboli.
Myco-bacteria	Mycobacterium tuberculosis and non-TB myycobacteria
Fungal	Aspergillus, Cryptococcus, histoplasmosis, coccidiodomycosis and paracoccidiodomycosis, PJP
Malig-nancy:	
PTLD	May or may not be associated with EBV viraemia
KS	Usually multiple, may be associated with chylous effusion, HHV-8 PCR positive
	Donor derived malignancy

Table 94.11 Differential diagnosis of focal CNS Lesion in SOT

Viral:	
PML	JC Polyoma virus solitary or multiple white matter changes (no mass effect)
EBV	Usually part of PTLD
Bacterial:	
Typical bacterial abscess	e.g., *Staph. aureus*, *Strep. viridans*, *Strep. milleri*
Listeria	Usually brainstem meningoencephalitis but can form focal lesions
Nocardia	Focal lesions (often associated with abnormal CXR)
Mycobacteria	
TB	>6 months, usually reactivation of latent TB. Single or multiple SOL may or may not enhance
Fungal:	
Aspergillus	Multiple lesions common.
Candida	Usually meningitis but can cause microabscesses
Coccidiodo-mycosis	
Mucor mycoses	Usually very aggressive with vascular invasion
Histoplasmo-sis	Can present in anyway mTB can
Parasitic:	
Toxoplasmo-sis	Primary infection or reactivation, single or multiple ring enhancing lesions
Malignancy:	
PTLD	
Donor derived tumor	Fortunately rare but important to consider in recipients of deceased donor kidneys
CNI Toxicity	
	White matter changes can mimic SOL

Table 94.12 Differential diagnosis of meningo-encephalitis in SOT: Infective

Viral:	
HSV	Important comments, in particular clinical characteristics and diagnostic tests
VZV	Systemic infection usually apparent with cutaneous or pulmonary involvement
CMV	Usually accompanied by viraemia and other systemic evidence of infection.
EBV	Can present as meningo-encephalitis or SOL as part of PTLD.
HHV-6	
Bacterial:	
Listeria monocytogenes	May have chest involvement
Others	Typical bacterial infections including *Strep. Ppneumonniae*, *Neisseria meningitides*, group B *Strep*, *Haemophilus influenzae*, and gram negatives
Mycobacteria:	
Fungal:	Cryptococcus
	Coccidiodes
Parasitic:	Toxoplasmosis
	Trypanosoma cruzi
Differential diagnosis of meningo-encephalitis in SOT: non-infective	
Medication:	
CNI neurotoxicity	Best seen on MRI with white matter changes consistent with PRES
Anti-virals	Acyclovir induced neurotoxicity more likely in renal impairment due to renal excretion

94.4 Summary

The unique nature of solid organ transplantation means that many of our patients go from relatively normal host defences to being profoundly immunocompromised overnight. There are clear guidelines and usually ample opportunity to prepare patients in terms of vaccination and pretreatment before this moment and plan post-transplant prophylaxis the implementation of which is key for a transplant service. The introduction of potentially infected donor tissues also adds another unique element to patient management and careful scrutiny of donor history is essential. Finally, the impaired response of RTRs to infection and the often, atypical presentation of opportunistic infections make it critical that patients are encouraged to present early if unwell and that teams not used to transplantation or managing the immunocompromised, rapidly liaise with the transplant team.

Case 1

A 71-year-old woman with ESRD secondary to MPO positive vasculitis presented 18 months after a deceased donor renal transplant with weight loss, anorexia, and multiple nonspecific symptoms stretching back 5 months. She was born in Malaysia but spent all of her adult life in the UK and not had any significant recent travel. On examination she was afebrile, without lymphadenopathy, chest signs, organomegaly, or any other significant findings. She had excellent renal function, was mildly anemic and had a modest CRP of 30. It was clear that something was very amiss but with no clear focus and the differential, given the duration of symptoms was between adverse drug reaction, malignancy (especially PTLD), recurrence of vasculitis and infection of which tuberculosis, given the chronicity, seemed most likely. Her chest X-ray demonstrated a cavitating upper lobe lesion which was smear positive for acid fast bacilli on induced-sputum without the need for bronchoscopy. She had not been given TB prophylaxis with her transplant in part as she had not developed TB despite heavy immunosuppression for her vasculitis. However, she gave a clear history of exposure to TB in childhood, the burden of immunosuppression with her transplant was greater than that for her vasculitis and there is a significant impairment of immune response with age.

Case 2

A 30-year-old woman underwent a deceased donor transplant. Initially things went well but she developed a fever and a progressive rise in CRP 6 days posttransplant. There was no obvious focus, multiple cultures were negative and the patient appeared well, but her liver function tests became increasingly abnormal with a marked coagulopathy. A CT scan demonstrated multiple microabscesses. She rapidly deteriorated and a laparoscopic liver biopsy demonstrated an acute hepatitis which was positive for HSV on immunoperoxidase. The recipient, and donor, were HSV negative and despite the absence of an obvious source she was started on acyclovir prior to the liver biopsy and the patient made a fully and rapid recovery. However, this case illustrates that while fulminant hepatic failure from primary HSV is very rare, herpes virus infections can be very dangerous when acquired posttransplant. HSV negative patients should receive anti-viral prophylaxis at the time of transplant (Fig. 94.16).

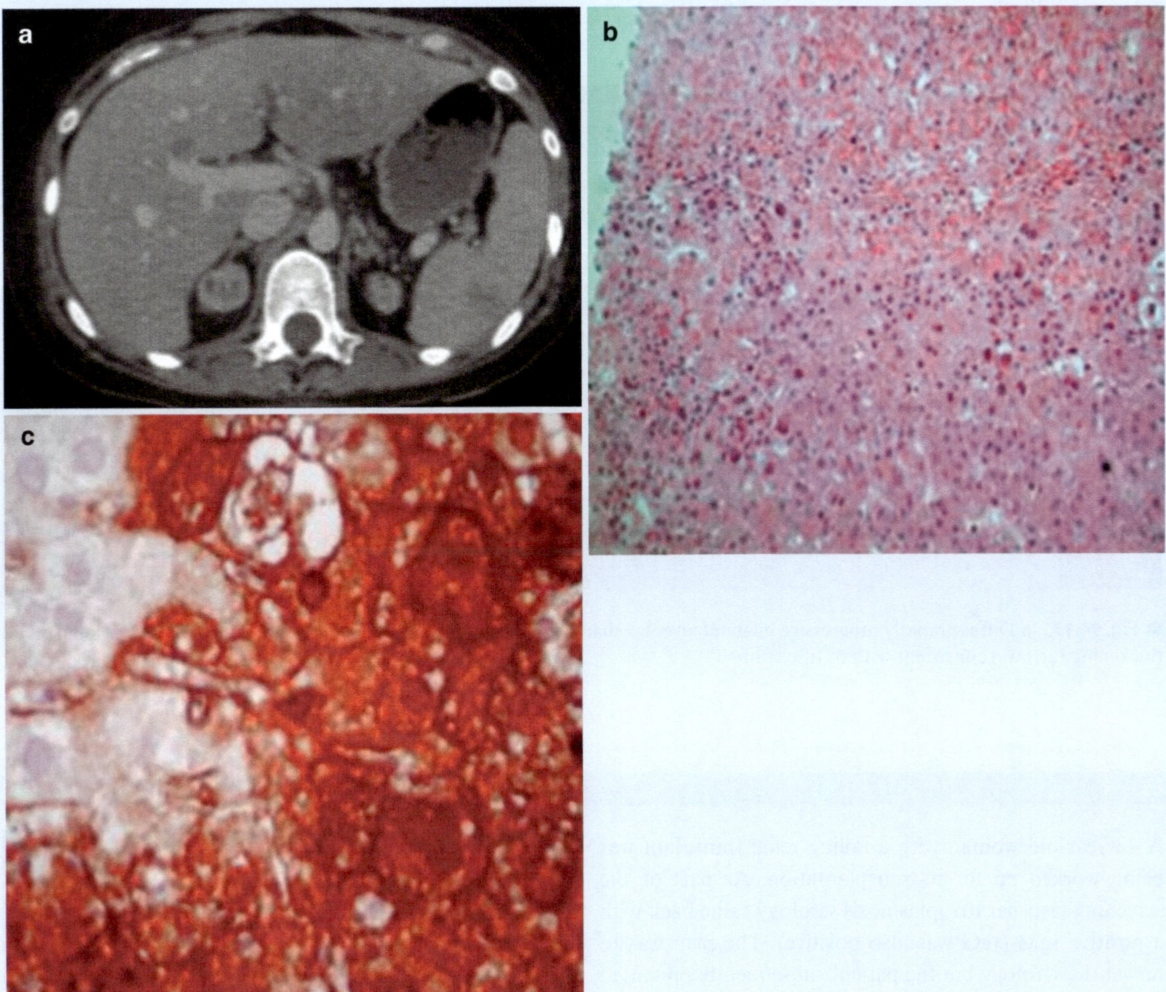

Fig. 94.16 **a** CT demonstrating multiple "microabscesses" secondary to HSV necrosis. **b** Liver biopsy demonstrating multinucleate giant cells, apoptotic cells and necrotic areas. **c** Liver biopsy Immunoperoxidase with livid staining for HSV

Case 3

HIV-positive patient 6 weeks posttransplant three-day history of SOB and abdominal pain with diarrhea . Originally from Tunisia with end-stage renal disease secondary to HIVAN. The patient had well-controlled disease on ART (abacavir/lamivudine/raltegravir) with a CD4 count of 340 (17%) and undetectable viral load. The patient was on Co-trimoxazole PCP prophylaxis and was CMV IgG positive with a CMV negative donor. The patient became progressively more breathless over a few hours with a CXR that showed marked diffuse alveolar shadowing (3a). The patient stabilized on oxygen and broad-spectrum antibiotics but had an abrupt, hypotensive episode overnight which responded to fluids. Cross-sectional imaging demonstrated pan-colitis with no obvious perforation (3b). The differential diagnosis remained fairly broad but pretransplant eosinophilia raised the prospect of helminth hyperinfestation and sigmoid biopsies confirmed the diagnosis. Strongyoides hyperinfestation, will often present, as in this case, with episode gram-negative bacteremia and often a very rapid deterioration which is completely preventable if patients are treated prior to transplantation (◘ Fig. 94.17).

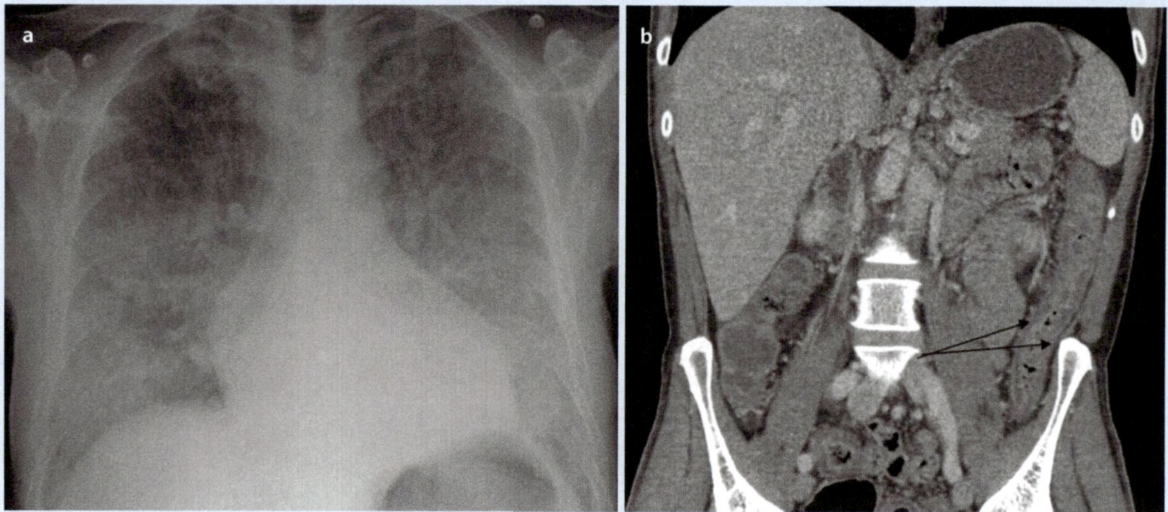

◘ **Fig. 94.17** **a** Diffuse rapidly progressive bilateral alveolar shadowing with a normal JVP consistent with ARDS. **b** Colonic mural thickening (arrows) consistent with diffuse colitis

Case 4

A 43-year-old woman with a failing renal transplant was being worked up for re-transplantation. As part of the screening tests her toxoplasmosis serology came back with a positive IgM (IgG was also positive). The plan was to repeat the serology but the patient subsequently presented with confusion, multiple brain lesions and extensive oedema.

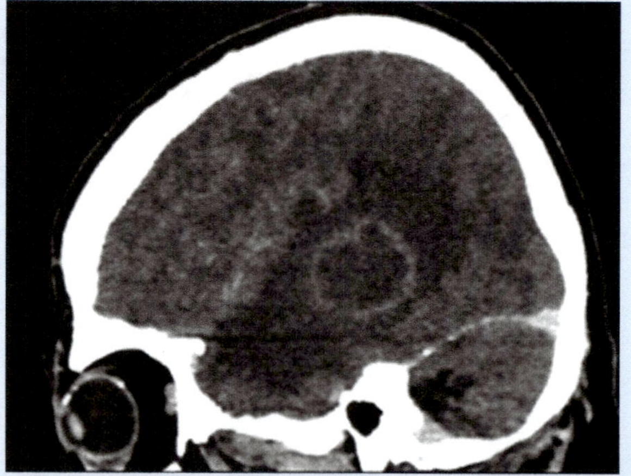

94

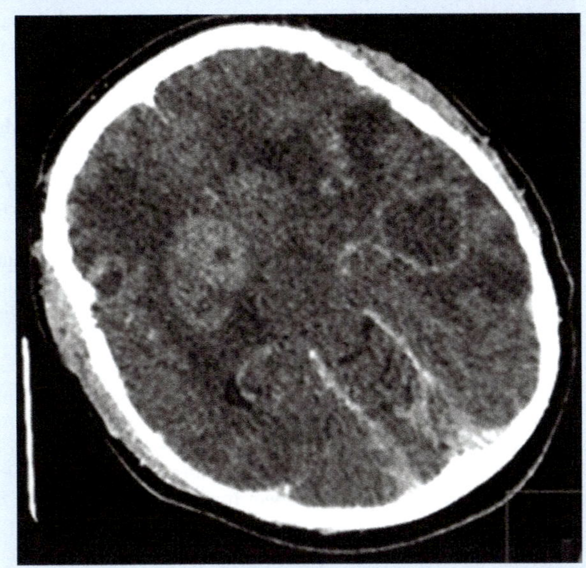

The working diagnosis was cerebral toxoplasmosis and the patient treated with dexamethasone for cerebral oedema and pyrimethamine and sulfadiazine with rapid initial improvement. However, improvement stalled, and subsequent scans demonstrated improvement in oedema but no reduction in lesion size. Eventually in the face of failure to respond a brain biopsy demonstrated lymphoma. This rather sad case illustrates a very important point viz.; in an immunocompromised patient it is absolutely essential to get tissue as soon as possible (sent to the histopathology AND virology AND microbiology) and always keep an open mind as to the potential disease process.

Tips and tricks for the management of posttransplant infec tion

1. There is considerable merit in a robust system for properly screening patients on the waiting list (and live donors) with appropriate vaccination, treatment, and plans for prophylaxis.
2. Travel and country of origin history of recipient and, if possible, the donor, should be obtained especially if investigating a fever posttransplant.
3. Culture of perfusion fluid and retention of donor serum, for serology screening if necessary, are cheap strategies that may help identify donor infections. Donor-derived infections must be reliably communicated to the transplant hub and onto the teams of other recipients.
4. Robust strategies need to be in place to ensure appropriate prophylaxis, dose and duration, with extension for those receiving depleting antibodies, those with low Igs or CD4+ counts, and those receiving treatment for late rejection.
5. A close relationship with virology and microbiology departments is vital and rapid alert systems (such as email alerts for viremia or positive MSUs) are invaluable.
6. Many opportunistic infections have atypical presentations and in the absence of diagnosis or improvement with empirical therapy biopsy (for histology and culture) may be critical.

Questions

1. Which is more sensitive for PCP infection? Galactomannan or Beta-d-glucan?
2. What else does co-trimoxazole offer prophylaxis against apart from PCP?
3. Which vaccinations are NOT suitable for post-transplant administration?
4. What alternative treatment options are there for CMV infection?
5. Whose responsibility is it to ensure no significant transmission of infection to donors?

Answers

1. Beta-d Glucan appears to be much more sensitive (and probably more specific) for PCP than galactomannan. Exertional desaturation, CRP higher than anticipated by overall condition and fever, raised LDH and calcium are also indicative.
2. Co-trimoxazole also covers toxoplasmosis, nocardia, listeria and has reduces the incidence of UTI.
3. Live vaccines attenuated vaccines viz. measles mumps rubella, yellow fever, chicken-pox and zoster vaccinations, small po, rotavirusx vaccine, oral polio vaccine, intranasal influenza, oral typhoid and BCG vaccination.
4. All treatments suppress CMV rather than cure. Valgancyclovir (oral) and ganciclovir (IV) are the mainstay of treatment options along-side immunosuppression reduction (ISR). IVIg may have a place in controlling viremia and helpful when ISR

is not possible. Foscarnet and cidofovir are both licenced but have considerable toxicity. Letermovir has recently been licenced and maribavir is in phase three trials. Conversion of antiproliferative or CNI to an mTOR inhibitor may be helpful.

5. Well, everyone's really. In the UK the legal responsibility lies with the surgeon but we are a team.

References

1. Manuel O, et al. Immunogenicity and safety of an intradermal boosting strategy for vaccination against influenza in lung transplant recipients. Am J Transplant. 2007;7:2567–72.
2. Hurst FP, Lee JJ, Jindal RM, Agodoa LY, Abbott KC. Outcomes associated with influenza vaccination in the first year after kidney transplantation. Clin J Am Soc Nephrol CJASN. 2011;6:1192–7.
3. Rubin RH. Infectious disease complications of renal transplantation. Kidney Int. 1993;44:221–36.
4. Kidney Disease: Improving Global Outcomes (KDIGO) Transplant Work Group. KDIGO clinical practice guideline for the care of kidney transplant recipients. Am J Transplant. 2009;9 Suppl 3:S1–155.
5. Atabani SF, et al. Cytomegalovirus replication kinetics in solid organ transplant recipients managed by preemptive therapy. Am J Transplant. 2012;12:2457–64.
6. Sagedal S, et al. Impact of early cytomegalovirus infection and disease on long-term recipient and kidney graft survival. Kidney Int. 2004;66:329–37.
7. Opelz G, Döhler B, Ruhenstroth A. Cytomegalovirus prophylaxis and graft outcome in solid organ transplantation: a collaborative transplant study report. Am J Transplant. 2004;4:928–36.
8. Kliem V, et al. Improvement in long-term renal graft survival due to CMV prophylaxis with oral ganciclovir: results of a randomized clinical trial. Am J Transplant. 2008;8:975–83.
9. Johnson RJ, Clatworthy MR, Birch R, Hammad A, Bradley JA. CMV mismatch does not affect patient and graft survival in UK renal transplant recipients. Transplantation. 2009;88:77–82.
10. Fischer SA, Lu K, AST Infectious Diseases Community of Practice. Screening of donor and recipient in solid organ transplantation. Am J Transplant. 2013;13 Suppl 4:9–21.
11. Kotton CN, et al. International consensus guidelines on the management of cytomegalovirus in solid organ transplantation. Transplantation. 2010;89:779–95.
12. Andrews PA, Emery VC, Newstead C. Summary of the British transplantation society guidelines for the prevention and management of CMV Disease after solid organ transplantation. Transplantation. 2011;92:1181–7.
13. Hodson EM, Ladhani M, Webster AC, Strippoli GFM, Craig JC. Antiviral medications for preventing cytomegalovirus disease in solid organ transplant recipients. Cochrane Database Syst Rev. 2013:CD003774. https://doi.org/10.1002/14651858.CD003774.pub4.
14. Reischig T, et al. Long-term outcomes of pre-emptive valganciclovir compared with valacyclovir prophylaxis for prevention of cytomegalovirus in renal transplantation. J Am Soc Nephrol JASN. 2012;23:1588–97.
15. Humar A, et al. Extended valganciclovir prophylaxis in D+/R− kidney transplant recipients is associated with long-term reduction in cytomegalovirus disease: two-year results of the IMPACT study. Transplantation. 2010;90:1427–31.
16. Kalil AC, Mindru C, Florescu DF. Effectiveness of valganciclovir 900 mg versus 450 mg for cytomegalovirus prophylaxis in transplantation: direct and indirect treatment comparison meta-analysis. Clin Infect Dis. 2011;52:313–21.
17. Marty FM, et al. Letermovir prophylaxis for cytomegalovirus in hematopoietic-cell transplantation. N Engl J Med. 2017;377:2433–44.
18. Avery RK, et al. Oral maribavir for treatment of refractory or resistant cytomegalovirus infections in transplant recipients. Transplant Infect Dis. 2010;12:489–96.
19. Nashan B, et al. Review of cytomegalovirus infection findings with mammalian target of rapamycin inhibitor-based immunosuppressive therapy in de novo renal transplant recipients. Transplantation. 2012;93:1075–85.
20. Gourishankar S, McDermid JC, Jhangri GS, Preiksaitis JK. Herpes zoster infection following solid organ transplantation: incidence, risk factors and outcomes in the current immunosuppressive era. Am J Transplant. 2004;4:108–15.
21. Parker A, et al. Management of post-transplant lymphoproliferative disorder in adult solid organ transplant recipients – BCSH and BTS Guidelines. Br J Haematol. 2010;149:693–705.
22. Baker RJ, Mark PB, Patel RK, Stevens KK, Palmer N. Renal association clinical practice guideline in post-operative care in the kidney transplant recipient. BMC Nephrol. 2017;18:174.
23. Tong CY, Bakran A, Williams H, Cheung CY, Peiris JS. Association of human herpesvirus 7 with cytomegalovirus disease in renal transplant recipients. Transplantation. 2000;70:213–6.
24. Hosseini-Moghaddam SM, Soleimanirahbar A, Mazzulli T, Rotstein C, Husain S. Post renal transplantation Kaposi's sarcoma: a review of its epidemiology, pathogenesis, diagnosis, clinical aspects, and therapy. Transplant Infect Dis. 2012;14:338–45.
25. Stallone G, et al. Sirolimus for Kaposi's sarcoma in renal-transplant recipients. N Engl J Med. 2005;352:1317–23.
26. Zmonarski SC, Boratyńska M, Puziewicz-Zmonarska A, Kazimierczak K, Klinger M. Kaposi's sarcoma in renal transplant recipients. Ann Transplant. 2005;10:59–65.
27. Dharnidharka VR, Cherikh WS, Abbott KC. An OPTN analysis of national registry data on treatment of BK virus allograft nephropathy in the United States. Transplantation. 2009;87:1019–26.
28. Kuypers DRJ. Management of polyomavirus-associated nephropathy in renal transplant recipients. Nat Rev Nephrol. 2012;8:390–402.
29. Suwelack B, Malyar V, Koch M, Sester M, Sommerer C. The influence of immunosuppressive agents on BK virus risk following kidney transplantation, and implications for choice of regimen. Transplant Rev (Orlando, FL). 2012;26:201–11.
30. Hilton R, Tong CYW. Antiviral therapy for polyomavirus-associated nephropathy after renal transplantation. J Antimicrob Chemother. 2008;62:855–9.
31. Guasch A, et al. Assessment of efficacy and safety of FK778 in comparison with standard care in renal transplant recipients with untreated BK nephropathy. Transplantation. 2010;90:891–7.
32. Kuypers DRJ, et al. Adjuvant low-dose cidofovir therapy for BK polyomavirus interstitial nephritis in renal transplant recipients. Am J Transplant. 2005;5:1997–2004.
33. Nickeleit V, et al. The Banff working group classification of definitive polyomavirus nephropathy: morphologic definitions and clinical correlations. J Am Soc Nephrol JASN. 2018;29:680–93.
34. Harwood CA, et al. Human papillomavirus infection and non-melanoma skin cancer in immunosuppressed and immunocompetent individuals. J Med Virol. 2000;61:289–97.

35. Courtney AE, Leonard N, O'Neill CJ, McNamee PT, Maxwell AP. The uptake of cervical cancer screening by renal transplant recipients. Nephrol Dial Transplant. 2009;24:647–52.
36. Kamar N, et al. Hepatitis E virus and the kidney in solid-organ transplant patients. Transplantation. 2012;93:617–23.
37. Eckburg PB, Montoya JG, Vosti KL. Brain abscess due to listeria monocytogenes: five cases and a review of the literature. Medicine (Baltimore). 2001;80:223–35.
38. Yu X, et al. Nocardia infection in kidney transplant recipients: case report and analysis of 66 published cases. Transplant Infect Dis. 2011;13:385–91.
39. Clark NM, Reid GE, AST Infectious Diseases Community of Practice. Nocardia infections in solid organ transplantation. Am J Transplant. 2013;13(Suppl 4):83–92.
40. Singh N, Paterson DL. Mycobacterium tuberculosis infection in solid-organ transplant recipients: impact and implications for management. Clin Infect Dis. 1998;27:1266–77.
41. Atasever A, et al. Tuberculosis in renal transplant recipients on various immunosuppressive regimens. Nephrol Dial Transplant. 2005;20:797–802.
42. Currie AC, Knight SR, Morris PJ. Tuberculosis in renal transplant recipients: the evidence for prophylaxis. Transplantation. 2010;90:695–704.
43. Canet E, Dantal J, Blancho G, Hourmant M, Coupel S. Tuberculosis following kidney transplantation: clinical features and outcome. A French multicentre experience in the last 20 years. Nephrol Dial Transplant. 2011;26:3773–8.
44. British Thoracic Society Standards of Care Committee and Joint Tuberculosis Committee, et al. Guidelines for the prevention and management of Mycobacterium tuberculosis infection and disease in adult patients with chronic kidney disease. Thorax. 2010;65:557–70.
45. Piersimoni C. Nontuberculous mycobacteria infection in solid organ transplant recipients. Eur J Clin Microbiol Infect Dis. 2012;31:397–403.
46. Griffith DE, et al. An official ATS/IDSA statement: diagnosis, treatment, and prevention of nontuberculous mycobacterial diseases. Am J Respir Crit Care Med. 2007;175:367–416.
47. Yazaki H, et al. Outbreak of Pneumocystis jiroveci pneumonia in renal transplant recipients: P. jiroveci is contagious to the susceptible host. Transplantation. 2009;88:380–5.
48. Martin SI, Fishman JA, AST Infectious Diseases Community of Practice. Pneumocystis pneumonia in solid organ transplant recipients. Am J Transplant. 2009;9 Suppl 4:S227–33.
49. Hagerty JA, Ortiz J, Reich D, Manzarbeitia C. Fungal infections in solid organ transplant patients. Surg Infect. 2003;4:263–71.
50. Neofytos D, et al. Epidemiology and outcome of invasive fungal infections in solid organ transplant recipients. Transplant Infect Dis. 2010;12:220–9.
51. Medical Complications of Kidney Transplantation. CRC Press. Available at: https://www.crcpress.com/Medical-Complications-of-Kidney-Transplantation/Ponticelli/p/book/9780415417150. Accessed 1st Feb 2019.
52. Rappo U, et al. Expanding the horizons of histoplasmosis: disseminated histoplasmosis in a renal transplant patient after a trip to Bangladesh. Transplant Infect Dis. 2010;12:155–60.
53. Blodget E, et al. Donor-derived Coccidioides immitis fungemia in solid organ transplant recipients. Transplant Infect Dis. 2012;14:305–10.
54. Arslan H, et al. Etiologic agents of diarrhea in solid organ recipients. Transplant Infect Dis. 2007;9:270–5.
55. Renoult E, et al. Toxoplasmosis in kidney transplant recipients: report of six cases and review. Clin Infect Dis. 1997;24:625–34.
56. Martina M-N, et al. Toxoplasma gondii primary infection in renal transplant recipients. Two case reports and literature review. Transpl Int. 2011;24:e6–12.
57. DeVault GA, et al. Opportunistic infections with Strongyloides stercoralis in renal transplantation. Rev Infect Dis. 1990;12:653–71.
58. Riarte A, et al. Chagas' disease in patients with kidney transplants: 7 years of experience 1989–1996. Clin Infect Dis. 1999;29:561–7.
59. Kocher C, et al. Skin lesions, malaise, and heart failure in a renal transplant recipient. Transplant Infect Dis. 2012;14:391–7.

Long-Term Management of Kidney Transplant Recipients

Richard J. Baker and Sunil K. Daga

Contents

M. Harber (ed.), *Primer on Nephrology*, https://doi.org/10.1007/978-3-030-76419-7_95

Learning Objectives

To describe key aspects of long-term management of kidney transplant recipients

1. Optimizing graft function
2. Prevent and improve morbidity and mortality of transplant recipients
3. Managing failing grafts and preparing for the next steps

95.1 Introduction

The advent of ciclosporin in the 1980s markedly improved renal transplantation outcomes, and by 1990 the 1-year graft survival rate approached 90%. Over the last three decades, the long-term graft survival rates have slowly improved but more importantly, the number of transplants being performed has risen markedly [1, 2]. This had led to a burgeoning number of prevalent KTRs who are increasingly elderly and co-morbid. Caring effectively for this population not only presents a significant medical challenge but also mandates well-organized delivery mechanisms to ensure that effective interventions are widely achieved.

Anecdotal evidence suggested that renal transplantation provided a better outcome for a given patient, and this was confirmed in longitudinal studies looking at the functional performance and quality of life in KTRs. More recently, robust evidence has emerged that patients who undergo renal transplantation not only enjoy a better quality of life, which is dialysis-free but also live longer as shown in Fig. 95.1 for patients in the USA [3–5]. One of the principal benefits of successful renal transplantation seems to be a reduction in the rate of cardiac events when compared to the wait-listed population [6, 7].

Although the transplant will fail in about 50% of all KTRs, the other half will die with a functioning transplant (Fig. 95.2). The principal causes of death are vascular disease, neoplasia, and infection. For this reason, it is essential to provide lifelong follow-up in clinics that specialize in both preventing and treating these diseases. There are detailed guidelines available from KDIGO and the Renal Association [8, 9].

The marked improvement in short-term graft survival has, in turn, generated a welcome new challenge– the problem of maximizing long-term transplant outcomes. This involves three principal concerns in addition to standard general medical care:

- Optimizing the survival of the graft by preventing and treating the pathological processes that cause graft damage.
- Preventing premature patient morbidity and mortality due to cardiovascular disease, neoplasia, and infection, all of which are exacerbated by immunosuppressive drugs.
- Managing the failing transplant with appropriate introduction of medications and timely discussion of options for renal replacement therapy including re-transplantation if applicable.

95.2 Optimizing Graft Function

95.2.1 Definition

These are measures taken before and after kidney transplantation that increases half-life of a kidney graft; by

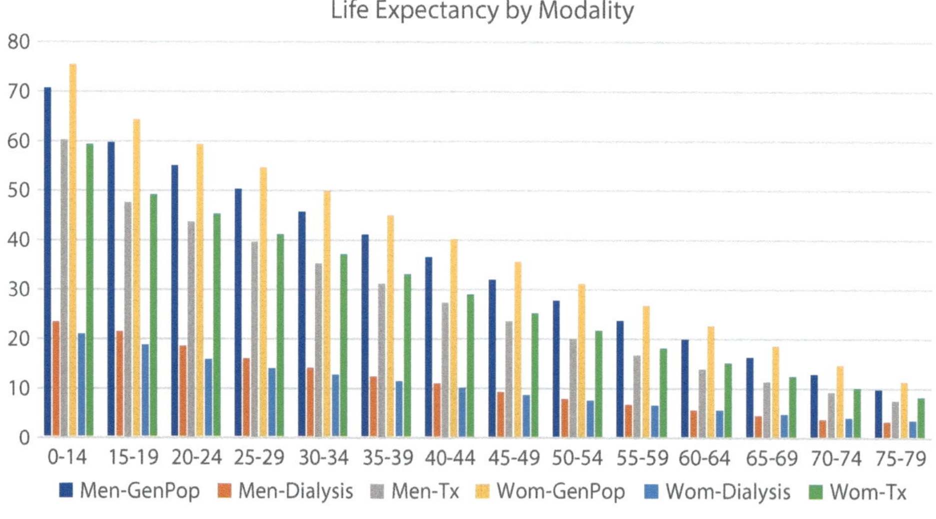

Fig. 95.1 Expected survival in years (y-axis) by modality, patient age, and sex (x-axis) –from USRDS 2018 Annual Data Report

95

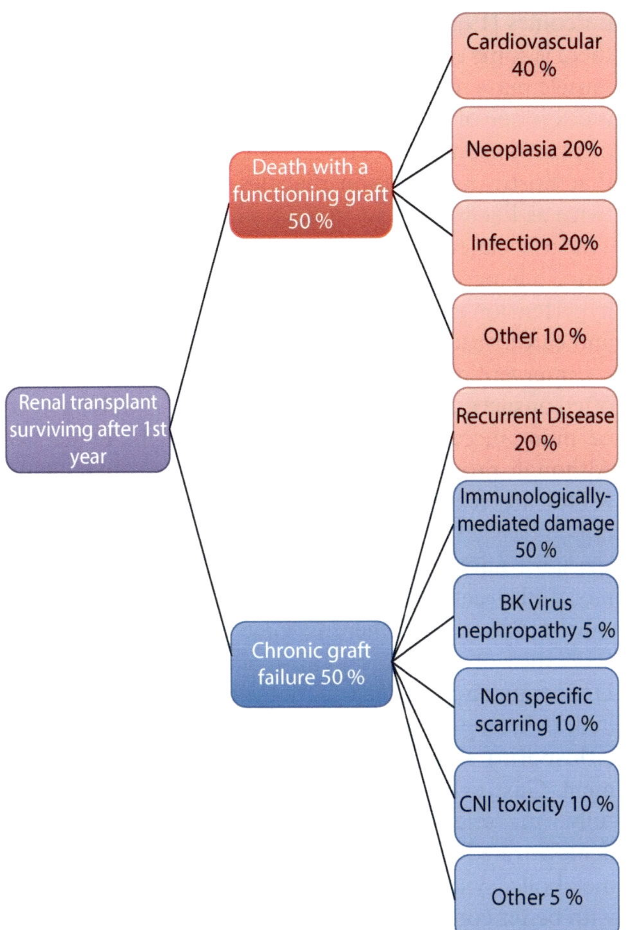

Fig. 95.2 Outcomes of Renal Transplantation

preventing and managing pathological process that cause premature graft failure.

Optimizing the survival of the graft starts prior to transplantation and forms one of the cornerstones of low clearance care. In particular, early discussion of potential living donors is required. Patients will generally obtain better outcomes in the following circumstances:

1. Living donor kidneys
2. Preemptive transplantation
3. Accurate and frequent determination of sensitization status

95.2.2 Epidemiology and Differential Diagnosis of Chronic Graft Failure

Factors associated with chronic graft failure are shown in Table 95.1. These factors can be broadly divided into immunological factors, related to the alloimmune response, and nonimmunological causes. Inevitably there is some overlap in the following section and later discussion of risk factors for vascular disease, but an attempt has been made to discuss the relationship to graft outcomes in the next section in contrast to cardiovascular morbidity and mortality in the later section.

Table 95.1 Factors associated with graft failure

Nonimmunological	Immunological
Donor-derived damage	Episodes of rejection
"Extended criteria" donors	HLA matching
Ischemia reperfusion injury	Allosensitization
Poor graft function	
High pulse pressure	
Hypertension	
Proteinuria	
Viral infection	
Hyperfiltration	
CNI toxicity	
Hyperlipidemia	
Recurrent disease	
De novo glomerular disease	
Poor adherence	

95.2.2.1 Nonimmunological Causes of Graft Failure

Donor-Derived Damage and Hyperfiltration

One of the most powerful predictors of poor outcomes is increasing donor age (See Fig. 95.3) [10]. In normal subjects, aging kidneys show increasing amounts of glomerulosclerosis and arteriosclerosis, which is manifested clinically by a fall in GFR of approximately 10% every decade after the age of 40. Consequently, it is perhaps not surprising that older kidneys perform worse since the delivered "nephron dose" is lower. The remaining functioning nephrons are then subjected to "hyperfiltration" with glomerular hypertension leading to glomerulosclerosis and the development of chronic graft damage. Perhaps, the best circumstantial evidence to support this assertion is the demonstration that low-weight kidneys transplanted into heavy KTRs are associated with worse graft outcomes and increasing proteinuria [11].

Poor Graft Function

In most renal diseases impaired renal function is a predictor of poor long-term outcome, and transplantation is no exception. The creatinine level at 1 year is a good predictor of long-term outcome although the predict-

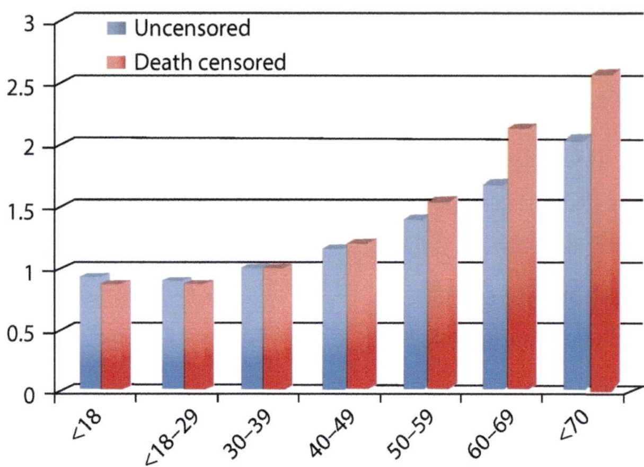

Fig. 95.3 Relative risk of graft loss by donor age from 108,118 DBD donors transplanted between 1995 and 2008 (UNOS)

ability of this marker is limited since it is not very specific and a significant number of grafts which fail have a good early function [12].

Hypertension

The link between hypertension and poor graft outcome was first established by analyzing registry data, but initially, no account was taken of graft function, which affects blood pressure control. However independent analysis established a definite link between blood pressure control and graft outcomes and furthermore that improving blood pressure control (Systolic Blood pressure below 140 mm Hg) is associated with better graft outcomes [13–15]. There is also an association between wider pulse pressures and both patient and graft survival [16]. Unfortunately, there are no prospective randomized controlled studies demonstrating that improved blood pressure control is associated with better graft function and the choice of agent should be determined by side effects with the emphasis on achieving the blood pressure goal [17]. The UK Registry data suggests that most renal units are very poor at ensuring good blood pressure control in KTRs and once again is essential to put an infrastructure in place to ensure firstly accurate ascertainment of blood pressure and secondly a robust monitoring system to effect changes, predominantly with medications (see below).

Body Mass Index

Registry data from the USA has demonstrated a clear association between elevated recipient BMI and adverse outcomes including graft function. However, there is no clear cut-off at which mortality and morbidity rates suddenly increase and the metanalysis of the available studies suggests a limited effect on graft outcome [18]. Recent data from the UK also suggests a limited effect on graft outcomes [19]. BMI is a poor indicator of obesity, and there is some evidence that waist circumference and lean muscle mass may be more informative. High body mass index is one of the main risk factors for the development of posttransplant diabetes mellitus, and there is evidence that posttransplantation diabetes mellitus (PTDM) is twice as likely to occur in KTRs with a BMI > 30 [20]. The associated metabolic syndrome of insulin resistance, hyperuricemia, hyperglycemia, obesity, and hypertension is also associated with premature graft loss and cardiovascular disease [21, 22].

Interventions in these patients are possible, though often unsuccessful, and preventing weight gain is likely to be more successful than subsequent weight reduction. Although more physically active than dialysis patients, KTRs are relatively inactive compared to the general population [23]. Preemptive interventions by dietitians or specialist nurses in the clinic should be encouraged and mood disorders should be treated. Immunosuppression can be altered, and there is some evidence that steroid avoidance or withdrawal can reduce early weight gain. Unfortunately, evidence for longer-term benefit is limited. Orlistat may be used although CNI levels (especially ciclosporin) should be closely monitored during treatment. Gastric bypass surgery has also been used successfully in selected patients. A single-center study demonstrated that the implementation of guidelines for metabolic syndrome control in KTRs was associated with better control of metabolic syndrome and improved graft stability [24].

Proteinuria

Increasing levels of proteinuria, even appearing as early as 3 months after transplantation, have been shown to have adverse effects on transplant function as well as other vascular outcomes [25, 26]. These observations have been made independent of the cause of proteinuria, and it is likely that the etiology is multifactorial, e.g., transplant glomerulopathy, recurrent and de novo glomerular disease. Since ACEi's and ARB's reduce proteinuria and have been shown to slow the deterioration of function in other renal diseases, it seems logical to use them as the agents of choice in hypertensive KTRs accepting that there will be a small reduction in hemoglobin and an elevation in potassium levels. However, a prospective randomized controlled trial failed to show any beneficial effect of ramipril on outcomes in KTRs with proteinuria [27] and a metanalysis failed to demonstrate any benefit of the ACE blockade on transplant outcomes [28]. Immunological activation should be assessed in proteinuric patients by testing for donor-specific anti-HLA antibodies, as positive DSA in presence of proteinuria is an adverse phenotype [29].

Viral Infection

Infection with cytomegalovirus (CMV), BK virus, or adenovirus may have an adverse effect on transplant outcomes including graft survival. These infections are discussed further in the chapter on "INFECTIOUS COMPLICATIONS OF TRANSPLANTATION" by Evans et al. Measures to prevent, rapidly diagnose, and treat opportunistic infections are central to successful management.

CNI Toxicity

The nephrotoxicity of calcineurin inhibitors became apparent soon after their introduction in the mid-1980s. Perhaps the best illustration is the incidence of chronic kidney disease in recipients of non-renal solid organ transplants who also have histological evidence of CNI toxicity [30]. Typical changes on renal biopsy include eccentric nodular arteriolar hyalinosis and interstitial fibrosis, typically in a striped pattern. While it is established that high levels of CNIs are associated with nephrotoxicity, there remains some controversy over the role of chronic low-level exposure. Proponents of chronic CNI toxicity cite the almost universal incidence of histological CNI nephrotoxicity amongst recipients of KTRs with type 1 diabetes who underwent annual protocol renal biopsies following simultaneous pancreas and kidney transplantation [31]. A meta-analysis of trials involving early CNI withdrawal seems to support the idea that early CNI withdrawal leads to better function [32]. In contrast, a large study, which meticulously studied both clinical and biopsy data from failed renal allografts, found very little evidence of CNI toxicity as a cause of graft loss [33]. There have been several trials looking at CNI avoidance by different means and while some have demonstrated early small benefits in terms of renal function, none has yet demonstrated improved graft survival [34, 35]. Despite this uncertainty, there is agreement that exposure to CNIs should be minimized with tapering of target levels in the chronic phase after transplantation. Our routine practice is to maintain CNIs aiming for low serum levels after 1 year (ciclosporin 50–100 ng/ml, tacrolimus 5–9 ng/ml) and consider withdrawal when biopsies (as indicated for graft dysfunction) show changes of IFTA or arteriolar hyalinosis without immune-mediated damage (see below) [36].

Hyperlipidemia

Hyperlipidemia is a well-established risk factor for both coronary and other vascular diseases. Epidemiologic data suggest that by 1 year after transplantation, 90% of KTRs have a total cholesterol >5.0 mmol/l and an LDL fraction >2.6 mmol/l. The prevalence of hypertriglyceridemia is also high following renal transplantation. These lipid abnormalities are largely due to the effects of immunosuppressive drugs. Both steroids and CNIs (ciclosporin more than tacrolimus) increase cholesterol levels, while sirolimus causes elevations in triglyceride levels. Given the incidence of cardiovascular disease in the ESRD population, KTRs should be treated as high-risk patients with low intervention thresholds for lipid treatment.

A randomized controlled trial of treatment of hypercholesterolemia with fluvastatin in KTRs did show some significant benefits in secondary cardiac outcomes although the primary composite vascular outcome measure fell short of significance [37]. Interestingly there was no effect on graft survival in this study. Metanalysis suggests an effect of cardiovascular outcomes but not on graft survival [38]. As a result, there have been widespread recommendations to treat hypercholesterolemia and recent guidelines suggested treating all KTRs over 30 years old with statins irrespective of serum cholesterol [39]. In the absence of hard evidence, our practice is pragmatic, aiming for total cholesterol below 4.0 mmol/l in secondary prevention and below 5.0 mmol/l in primary prevention. Successful treatment is generally accomplished with statins and ezetimibe. These drugs must be used judiciously since there are significant interactions with both immunosuppressive drugs, especially ciclosporin, and with amlodipine. For patients taking ciclosporin, it is advisable to avoid simvastatin and prescribe either atorvastatin or pravastatin.

Recurrent Disease

A distinction must be made between histological recurrence on biopsy and graft failure due to recurrent disease. In most glomerular diseases histological recurrence is quite common, but graft loss has a significantly lower incidence. The best data, from Australia and New Zealand, recorded the rate of graft loss after 10 years due to recurrent disease as follows [40] (◘ Table 95.2):

Other important recurrent diseases include diabetic nephropathy, primary oxalosis, hemolytic uremic syndrome, and Fabry's disease. Recurrent diseases are discussed further elsewhere in relevant chapters about the primary disease.

◘ Table 95.2 Recurrent disease post-kidney transplantation

Mesangiocapillary glomerulonephritis type I	14.40%
Focal segmental glomerulosclerosis	12.70%
Membranous nephropathy	12.50%
IgA nephropathy	9.70%
Pauci-immune crescentic glomerulonephritis	7.70%
Other types together	3.10%

Poor Adherence

Poor adherence is widely acknowledged to be associated with poor graft outcomes. It has been speculated that this may contribute to insidious chronic antibody-mediated graft loss. Factors associated with poor adherence include:

1. Older children and young adults
2. The time of transition between pediatrics and adult clinics
3. High variability in immunosuppression levels between visits
4. High non-attendance rates at outpatient clinic appointments
5. Admission of poor adherence

Innovative practices to improve outcomes include the appointment of youth key workers, the use of smartphone technology, and the establishment of transition clinics for adolescents and young adults.

95.2.2.2 Immunological Graft Loss

Episodes of Rejection

Since episodes of rejection lead to tissue damage and loss of functioning nephrons, it is perhaps not surprising that they are linked to poorer long-term outcomes [41, 42]. It is possible that some very pure forms of mild acute cellular rejection (BANFF 1) are not so harmful, but generally, rejection is best avoided [43]. Whatever immunosuppression protocol is being used, centers should generally aim for 12-month rejection rates of less than 15% in standard-risk patients. Diagnosis and management of rejection are discussed in detail in chapter "Rejection in Renal Transplantation" by Dr. McLean.

HLA Matching

The first successful renal transplants were carried out between identical twins, and with the discovery of HLA antigens, it became clear that better matching led to less rejection and better outcomes. Better HLA matching was shown to be more influential than increasing cold ischemia times, and this underpinned the rationale for national and regional sharing schemes. However, as immunosuppression has become more effective and acute rejection rates have decreased, the influence of HLA matching has waned. This is well illustrated by the excellent survival of living unrelated donor grafts which is similar to that of haploidentical siblings despite more HLA mismatches.

Allosensitization

Some KTRs have preexisting sensitization to donor antigens, and this is usually the result of previous transplantation, blood transfusion, or pregnancy. In such cases, there is an increased risk of rejection and outcomes are generally poorer [44]. It is increasingly recognized that KTRs develop de novo donor-specific antibodies after receiving a renal transplant [45].

95.2.3 Monitoring in the Clinic

Meticulous monitoring of graft function is an essential component of transplant care particularly in the first few months after the operation. Despite extensive efforts to develop other techniques (see ▶ Box 95.1), serum creatinine remains the gold standard for measuring transplant function. Many centers use one of the MDRD or CKD-EPI equations to estimate glomerular filtration rate (eGFR) for their transplant patients which helps to communicate function to KTRs, but these equations have not been fully validated in the transplant population.

Serum creatinine level is influenced by a number of factors and clinical reaction should be proportional to the degree of rise from baseline. Fluctuations of 10–20% from baseline are not uncommon, and evaluation should be conditioned by clinical risk (i.e., high immunological risk, difficult surgical procedure, multiple vessels, etc.). After such a rise in creatinine, it is usually advisable to repeat the blood test in 2–3 days to see that it is not part of an upwards trend. In the meantime, the patient should be advised to increase their fluid intake. Greater concern should be addressed to larger rises (i.e., >20%) and consistent increases by smaller percentages. Even in a steady-state, the creatinine level will vary and variation by up to 10% of the baseline is to be expected.

There are certain drugs that if taken concurrently will elevate the serum creatinine level and some of these may be taken after transplantation (e.g., trimethoprim, cotrimoxazole, cimetidine, and pyrimethamine). Generally, these drugs will only cause minor perturbations in serum creatinine.

Box 95.1 Methods for Monitoring Transplant Function

Blood

Serum creatinine – still the most widely used

Avntibody monitoring – good evidence that anti-donor HLA antibodies are associated with poor outcomes

Lymphocyte subset analysis – some evidence that certain phenotypic markers are associated with good function

Genomic, transcriptomic and proteomic approaches – currently a highly active research field

Urine

Urine albumin/creatinine ratio (ACR) or urine protein/creatinine ratio (PCR) – even low levels of proteinuria (PCR > 30) are associated with poor graft and vascular outcomes

Genomic, transcriptomic, and proteomic approaches – currently a highly active research field

Graft tissue

Protocol biopsy

- Light microscopy – championed by some enthusiasts but probably not effective with more potent modern immunosuppression and lower rejection rates
- Genomic, transcriptomic, and proteomic analysis

"For cause" biopsy

- Light microscopy – the gold standard for unexplained graft dysfunction. Immunohistochemistry (including C4d, SV40) and electron microscopy
- Genomic approaches

The serum creatinine level should be closely monitored in clinic since it is relatively sensitive to acute changes in renal function. It is also useful for monitoring long-term graft function. When reviewing long-term trends in creatinine (or calculated eGFR), it is worth bearing in mind some potential pitfalls detailed above.

If after consideration of these factors the elevation in creatinine level is deemed genuine, then further investigation is required. An algorithm for investigating transplant dysfunction is shown in ◘ Fig. 95.4. Renal biopsy remains the gold standard in the investigation of transplant dysfunction; however, it entails a low rate of morbidity and should not be undertaken lightly. Transplant biopsy may also be considered for isolated proteinuria with stable creatinine levels. This is warranted by the strong association between proteinuria and adverse graft and patient outcomes [13, 26]. Occasionally, a biopsy may be merited by the detection of high-level BK viremia or the presence of DSAs for similar reasons.

The interpretation of the renal biopsy requires a multidisciplinary meeting with input from clinicians, histopathologists, and clinical scientists. Various lesions on renal biopsy have been classified by the consensus of a group of experts in the BANFF classification [46]. This classification is continually evolving and now includes limited molecular analysis. ◘ Table 95.3 shows the current BANFF scoring system with clinicopathological correlations of different parameters that are scored by light microscopy. It is important to remember that other important findings may be present that are not part of the BANFF criteria:

1. Pyelonephritis
2. BK virus nephropathy
3. Thrombotic microangiopathy
4. De novo or recurrent glomerular disease
5. Calcification
6. Posttransplant lymphoproliferative disorder
7. Interstitial nephritis (antibiotics, PPI, azathioprine)

In certain circumstances, the interpretation of immunofluorescence, immunoperoxidase, or electron microscopy may be useful (e.g., SV-40 staining for BK nephropathy and C4d staining). There is increasing enthusiasm for electron microscopy in interpreting transplant biopsies, particularly multilayering of basement membranes due to CAMR (transplant glomerulopathy). This will require a separate core to be sent off in saline to the laboratory for rapid processing.

The rationale for a transplant renal biopsy for a declining renal function is twofold. First, an assessment can be made of the amount of chronic damage, predominantly judged by the degree of interstitial fibrosis and tubular atrophy (IFTA), which informs the long-term prognosis [47]. This information can be used by both patient and clinician to inform future strategies for renal replacement therapy. The second potential benefit is to plan an intervention to slow the decline of renal function. Unfortunately, the evidence base for such interventions is poor with few prospective trials of KTRs stratified by diagnosis.

95.2.4 Management of Late Graft Dysfunction

Another essential component of posttransplant care is the development of an infrastructure that can respond to changes in function and investigate them promptly. The solution may be provided by doctors, specialist nurses, or even a computer-based algorithm, but crucially it must react in a timely fashion. Missing a single

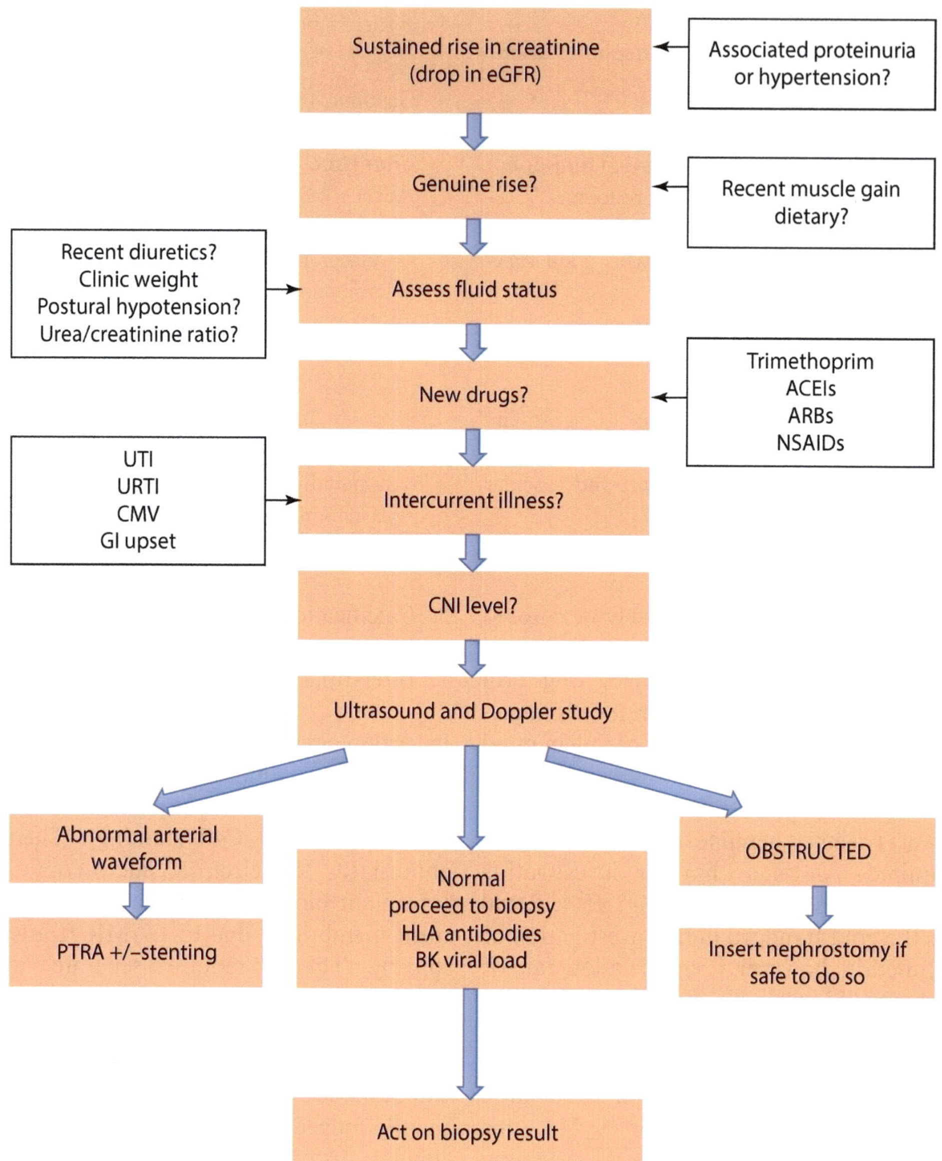

Fig. 95.4 Algorithm for investigation of transplant dysfunction

elevated creatinine level in a patient on a three-monthly follow-up can potentially result in graft loss. Results that come back later than the usual 24 h cycle such as CMV titers and microbiological culture results are particularly challenging. It is essential that robust mechanisms are put in place to ensure the widespread dissemination of such information (e.g., group emails to transplant teams or computer-generated alerts). Once identified, graft dysfunction requires rapid investigation with appropriate treatment. The causes of chronic transplant dysfunction are shown in Table 95.3.

A brief guide to treatment options is shown in Table 95.4.

The terms chronic rejection and chronic allograft nephropathy (CAN) were widely used to describe all grafts failing slowly without evidence of recurrent disease or other distinct pathologies. However, these terms have been widely criticized since it was felt that they had become too readily used as a "one size fits all" diagnosis without any consideration of the underlying pathophysiology, which in turn led to therapeutic nihilism. Analysis from the tissue of failed graft reveals significant heterogeneity [33], and it seems sensible not to label grafts as having "CAN". The term chronic allograft dysfunction is a better term since it describes a functional deterioration without any allusion to the underlying pathology. In some biopsies, there is evidence of coincident fibrointimal hyperplasia ("cv" lesions) (see Fig. 95.5) or arteriolar hyalinosis ("ah" lesions). Arteriolar hyalinosis is usually caused by either diabetes, hypertension or CNI toxicity.

Table 95.3 Causes of late graft dysfunction

Cause	Investigation	Treatment
Transplant renal artery stenosis	Doppler U/S	Angioplasty +/– stenting
	MR/CT angiogram	
	Angiography	
Chronic antibody-mediated rejection (CAMR)	Renal biopsy and anti-HLA antibody screening	Intensification of immunosuppression
Chronic cellular rejection	Renal biopsy	Intensification of immunosuppression
CNI toxicity	Renal biopsy and levels	Dose reduction
Viral nephropathy (BK, CMV, adenovirus, EBV)	Renal biopsy and blood PCR	Supportive
De novo glomerulonephritis	Renal biopsy	Disease specific
Recurrent disease	Renal biopsy	Disease specific
Thrombotic microangiopathy	Renal biopsy and blood film findings	Alteration of drug therapy and possibly plasma exchange or eculizumab
Diabetic nephropathy	Renal biopsy	Vascular risk factors and tight diabetic control
Nonspecific scarring (IFTA)	Renal biopsy	Vascular risk factors and CNI reduction or withdrawal
Infiltration (e.g., PTLD)	Renal biopsy, bone marrow, and cross-sectional scanning	Reduced immunosuppression and specific anti-tumor therapy
Transplant glomerulopathy	Renal biopsy and anti-HLA antibody screening	Intensification of immunosuppression and anti-proteinuric therapy
Ureteric stenosis or obstruction	Ultrasound, MR urogram	Nephrostomy, ureteric stenting, and possibly reconstruction
	Nephrostogram	
Extrinsic ureteric compression	Ultrasound, CT scan, MR Urogram	Nephrostomy, ureteric stenting, and relief of obstruction
	Nephrostogram	

Since these KTRs have a fairly pure form of fibrosis without any evidence of immune-mediated damage, most clinicians will opt to reduce or even withdraw CNIs. This is based on evidence that KTRs exposed to CNIs have almost universal changes of CNI toxicity, including interstitial fibrosis and arteriolar hyalinosis on protocol biopsy by 1-year after transplantation [31]. There is limited evidence that avoiding CNIs is helpful but also conflicting evidence from both large randomized controlled studies and meta-analysis that the best results are obtained by KTRs who continue to take CNIs [48, 49]. However, it should be noted that no trials of intervention have been limited to those KTRs with biopsy-proven IFTA lesions only, and forthcoming trials will need to stratify patients according to their diagnoses. Possible approaches to treating IFTA are shown in Table 95.4. An exciting recent development has been the potential to predict the development of IFTA at 1 year using gene expression analysis at 3 months in unscarred grafts, thus raising the possibility of preemptive therapy in such patients (i.e., substitution of CNI) [50].

95.3 Optimizing Kidney Transplant Recipient

95.3.1 Definition

These are measures taken to improve patient survival defines optimal care of kidney transplant recipient.

Kidney transplantation offers best survival advantage to patients with renal failure (Fig. 95.1), about half of the kidney transplant recipients die with a functioning graft. The causes of death in transplant recipients are shown in Fig. 95.2.

Table 95.4 Treatment strategies posttransplant biopsy for chronic allograft dysfunction/new-onset proteinuria

Diagnosis and treatment	
Current immunosuppression	**Possible new strategy**
Recurrent glomerulonephritis	
Any	Similar to native disease
Principally IFTA (high "ct" and "ci" scores) +/– CNI toxicity (high "ah" score)	
Prednisolone and azathioprine	No change
	Conservative measures only (e.g., BP control, ACEi/ARB, lipid treatment)
Prednisolone, azathioprine, and ciclosporin	Withdraw CNI
	Substitute MMF for Aza, and then if tolerated reduce CNI by 25% every 2 weeks
CNI monotherapy	Start MMF and prednisolone, and withdraw CNI as above
	OR substitute mTORi for CNI if eGFR >30 and PCR < 50, and add prednisolone 5 mg
Prednisolone and CNI	Start MMF, and withdraw CNI as above
	OR substitute mTORi for CNI if eGFR >30 and PCR < 50, and add prednisolone 5 mg
CNI and MMF	Start prednisolone and withdraw CNI as above
	OR substitute mTORi for CNI if eGFR >30 and PCI < 50 and add prednisolone 5 mg
Prednisolone, CNI, and MMF	Increase MMF to max dose, and withdraw reduced CNI by 25% every 2 weeks – Alternatively consider mTORi for CNI if eGFR >30 and PCR < 50
Acute immune-mediated (high "i", "t", and "v" scores)	
Any	Admit for MethylPred X3, and increase baseline immunosuppression
Chronic antibody-mediated rejection – Microvascular inflammation (high "g", "ptc", "C4d", and "cg" scores)	
Prednisolone and azathioprine	Add CNI (tacrolimus if DM risk low)
Prednisolone, azathioprine, and ciclosporin	Substitute tacrolimus for ciclosporin and MMF for Aza
CNI monotherapy	Add MMF and prednisolone 0.1 mg/kg od
Prednisolone and CNI	Add MMF
CNI and MMF	Add prednisolone, and maximize MMF
Prednisolone, CNI, and MMF	Increase MMF to max dose

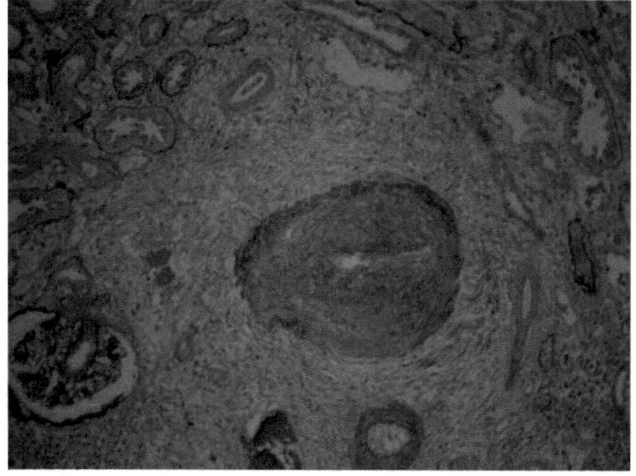

Fig. 95.5 Vascular fibrointimal hyperplasia ("cv" lesion)

95.3.2 Cardiovascular Risk

Half of all KTRs will die with a functioning transplant, and approximately half of these deaths (i.e., 25% overall) will be due to vascular disease. It is important that the renal transplant clinic actively promotes good vascular health. Healthy living should be encouraged with exercise, weight loss, smoking cessation, and patient-specific dietary advice. There are comprehensive guidelines available for this purpose [8, 9]. Epidemiological studies in KTRs suggest that risk factors for vascular disease are similar to the general population including diabetes, cigarette smoking, and hyperlipidemia. In a similar fashion to CKD renal function is a strong determinant of cardiovascular risk [51]. In this study, once the eGFR dropped below 45 ml/min/1.73 m^2, there was a 15% increase in both the death rate and the incidence of cardiovascular disease with each 5 ml/min drop in eGFR.

95.3.2.1 Hypertension

Hypertension occurs in approximately 70% of KTRs due to a number of reasons:

- Suboptimal graft function
- The presence of native kidneys with activation of the RAS and overactive sympathetic activity
- Immunosuppressive medications, especially CNIs and steroids
- High BMI
- Transplant renal arterial disease
- Allografts from hypertensive donors

Higher blood pressures are not only linked to graft loss but also vascular events. Furthermore, registry data suggest that when blood pressure control improves, then this will result in decreased rates of vascular events as well as improved long-term graft outcomes [15]. Clinic readings are often high, and it is essential to develop methods for regular and accurate BP measurement. For this purpose, home blood pressure monitoring and 24-hour continuous ambulatory monitoring may be useful, especially in cases of white coat hypertension.

Treatment consists of lifestyle modification and drug treatment. Unfortunately, there is a dearth of high-quality trial data in this area. A meta-analysis of the existing trial evidence suggested that there was little to choose between agents with perhaps a slight advantage to calcium channel blockade [17]. Existing studies have rarely targeted specific subgroups of KTRs although a study looking at the use of ramipril in proteinuric KTRS showed no benefit [27]. The clinical priority should be achieving the target by whatever means is best tolerated (Clinic blood pressure < 130/80 mmHg or 125/75 if proteinuric [PCR > 50]). The UK Renal Registry data suggest that compliance with this standard in the UK is currently poor.

Immunosuppressive drugs such as corticosteroids, ciclosporin, and tacrolimus contribute to hypertension, and modification of IS may benefit blood pressure control. However, such considerations will usually be secondary, and the effective use of antihypertensive agents remains the cornerstone of treatment.

Transplant renal artery stenosis is an important cause of hypertension in KTRs and usually occurs between 3 months and 2 years after transplantation. It should be suspected in patients with refractory hypertension, and there may be clinical evidence of salt and water retention. Ultrasound Doppler studies are more useful than in native kidneys and may show the typical "parvus tardus" waveform. MRA scans are also useful, and although they tend to be too sensitive, they do have a high negative predictive value. Definitive treatment requires angiography with angioplasty +/− stenting.

95.3.2.2 Posttransplant Diabetes Mellitus (PTDM) or New-Onset Diabetes after Transplantation (NODAT)

The development of new-onset diabetes after transplantation (PTDM) is an increasing problem and is associated with significantly increased morbidity and mortality [52, 53]. In the USA, up to 40% of adult KTRs develop PTDM within 3 years of transplantation. Risk factors for PTDM include:

1. Increasing donor age – older donors increase risk
2. Obesity – higher BMIs increase risk possibly related to increased secretion of adiponectin
3. Previous gestational diabetes
4. Ethnicity – more common in Asian and black recipients
5. Certain HLA types (HLA-B13, B15, B27, and B42) and other genetic polymorphisms
6. Family history of diabetes
7. HLA matching and donor characteristics
8. Viral infection – up to four times more common in HCV + ve KTRs, probably since HCV decreases hepatic insulin sensitivity
9. Type of underlying native renal disease – commoner in ADPKD
10. Medications – associated with steroid usage, sirolimus, and CNIs especially tacrolimus

Five-year patient survival drops from 93% to 87% for those KTRs who develop PTDM, and median graft survival also falls from 11 to 8 years. Prevention involves identifying susceptible individuals using the risk factors above and counseling regarding lifestyle modification, especially postoperative weight gain. Predictive risk scores have been proposed based on the preoperative characteristics, but they lack precision. Random glucose measurements should be checked before listing for transplantation, and if necessary fasting readings or a glucose tolerance test should be performed. Both high glucose levels prior to transplantation and high levels during the first seven postoperative days are associated with the subsequent development of PTDM after transplantation. Whether screening waiting list patients with a glucose tolerance test is cost-effective remains to be evaluated.

In certain cases, it may be justified to modify the immunosuppressive regime to minimize the future risk of PTDM, e.g., steroid avoidance or switching the CNI from tacrolimus to ciclosporin since tacrolimus has been shown to be more diabetogenic than ciclosporin [54]. Recently, an RCT demonstrated that switching from tacrolimus to ciclosporin could significantly reduce the incidence of PTDM in the first year after transplantation [55].

An interesting strategy under investigation is the early introduction of hypoglycemic agents such as vildagliptin, empagliflozin, and pioglitazone in KTRs with early hyperglycemia and the results of trials are eagerly awaited to see if this will reduce the incidence of PTDM. Another trial has suggested that the early provision of long-acting insulin infusions to KTRs with postoperative hyperglycemia reduces the incidence of PTDM at 1 year, possibly by "resting" pancreatic beta cells, and this strategy is being tested in a prospective multicenter RCT [56].

After transplantation, random glucose readings should be regularly checked although these may not identify some patients. Most cases of PTDM occur in the 12 months following transplantation, so testing should be most frequent during this time. Fasting glucose measurement or HbA_1C can be checked, but an oral glucose tolerance test is the most sensitive method. While hyperglycemia should be treated, PTDM should not be diagnosed until 3 months after transplantation when immunosuppressive medications are stable as some cases will remit.

If KTRs are maintained on steroids, then doses should be tapered as rapidly as possible. Unfortunately, PTDM often occurs in KTRs with poor function that has been repeatedly exposed to pulsed high-dose steroids for episodes of rejection. Once identified, prompt referral to the diabetic services is required. Severe hyperglycemia will require insulin, but lesser degrees can be treated safely with short-acting sulfonylureas [52]. If renal function permits (eGFR > 45 ml/min/1.73 m^2), then diabetes may be treated with metformin and newer agents such as glinides, thiazolidinediones, and DPP4 inhibitors can be used at lower eGFR. There is limited evidence for the use of GLP-1 receptor antagonists and SGLT-2 inhibitors and they are contraindicated in moderate to severe renal failure. There is some evidence that intense lifestyle modification may be helpful.

95.3.2.3 Lipids

There is epidemiological evidence that hyperlipidemia is linked to cardiovascular events after renal transplantation. As stated above a prospective RCT has shown that treatment with fluvastatin resulted in a reduction in cardiovascular events, although the primary outcome measure fell short of significance [37]. Approximately, half of all KTRs have hypercholesterolemia, and guidelines advise that they should be treated as high-risk patients for cardiovascular disease [8, 9].

95.3.2.4 Lifestyle

Cigarette smoking is strongly linked to adverse outcomes after renal transplantation, and thorough efforts should be made to facilitate smoking cessation. Both bupropion and varenicline may be prescribed although dose adjustments may be necessary if renal function is significantly reduced (eGFR < 30 ml/min/1.73 m^2).

95.3.3 Cancer

Immunosuppressive drugs work by interfering with lymphocyte activation and subsequent clonal proliferation. This is necessary to prevent the immune response against the alloantigens on foreign tissue. However, this effect is nonspecific and thus affects the protective function of lymphocytes against pathogens and neoplasia. Lymphocytes are particularly important in the defence against intracellular pathogens such as viruses and fungi. Immunosurveillance of epithelial surfaces forms one of the principal mechanisms of defence against neoplasia, particularly, cancers that occur in virally transformed cells (e.g., HPV in the skin, anal, cervical, and vulval cancer). As a result, KTRs are inevitably exposed to increased risks of cancer [57]. Other mechanisms also contribute to the increased risks of neoplasia observed in KTRs:

1. Reduced Immunosurveillance (as above)
2. Reduced immune response against viral cofactors, e.g., HPV, EBV, and HHV-8
3. Direct oncogenic effects of immunosuppressant, e.g., impaired DNA repair
4. Increased solar exposure including ozone effects
5. Increasing age
6. Increased survival posttransplantation
7. Evolution of more potent immunosuppressive drugs

Overall KTRs are exposed to approximately double the cancer risk of controls in the normal population. Standard incidence rates compared to the general population for specific cancers are shown in ◘ Table 95.5 [58, 59]:

The incidence of de novo malignancies increases with time after the transplantation. However, different tumors characteristically develop at different intervals after transplantation, e.g., PTLD at a mean of 32 months, epithelial tumors 69 months, and anogenital cancers 96 months. It is important to distinguish the difference between relative risks and absolute risks, since although KTRs often have very significant increases in relative risk, the absolute risk may still be very small (e.g., Kaposi's sarcoma). Unfortunately, KTRs also tend to develop more aggressive forms of cancer and conse-

Table 95.5 Relative risk of cancer posttransplant

Cancer	Relative risk	Associated virus
Kaposi's sarcoma	61	HHV8
Skin	13.9	HPV
Non-Hodgkin lymphoma	7.5	EBV
Anus	5.8	HPV
Vulva	7.6	HPV
Lip	16.8	HPV
Lung	2.0	
Kidney	4.7	
Colorectal	1.2	
Pancreas	1.5	
Hodgkin's lymphoma	3.6	EBV
Melanoma	2.4	
Other gastrointestinal, laryngeal, bladder, testis, sarcomas, penis, thyroid, and other hematological cancers	Mild increase	
Breast and prostate	Mild decrease	

quently have worse outcomes compared to controls in the normal population [60]. However, with the rapid advances being made in oncology and new staging systems (including genotyping) it must be acknowledged that there is a great deal of uncertainty regarding outcomes in KTRs.

The risks associated with different immunosuppressive agents are difficult to study, but both CNIs are certainly linked epidemiologically to higher cancer rates and have also been shown to be oncogenic in animal models. A randomized controlled trial of KTRs treated with ciclosporin administered in either a high- or low-dose regime showed a significant reduction in neoplasia in the latter group [61].

Cancer screening remains a controversial subject with wide variations in global practice. The UK guidelines advise screening in line with the routine national guidelines for the prostate, bowel; breast, and cervical cancer (see ▶ http://www.cancerscreening.nhs.uk).

95.3.3.1 Skin Cancer

Skin cancer is by far the most common form of malignancy after transplantation. In Australia and New Zealand, approximately, 40% of KTRs suffer from skin cancer 10 years after successful transplantation and 82% by 20 years (c.f. 25% and 61%, respectively, in the European and North American populations). Squamous cell (SCC) and basal cell (BCC) carcinomas make up the majority of these tumors, and they are similar to those in the general population in terms of appearance and location. However, they often exhibit aggressive biological features under immunosuppression, so early diagnosis and treatments are essential. Metastatic SCC has a particularly bad prognosis with a 3 years survival of only 29%.

Important cofactors in the development of cutaneous malignancies include the following:

- Ethnicity and coloring – unusual in non-Caucasians
- Fairer skin coloring
- Concomitant infection with human papilloma virus (HPV)
- Older average age of KTRs
- Childhood sun burning
- Intensity and duration of immunosuppression
- Geographical location
- Solar exposure
- Previous BCC, SCC, or actinic keratoses
- Exposure to voriconazole

Treatment involves early recognition and specialist referral. Given that more than half of all KTRs will eventually develop some form of cancer, most of which will be skin cancer; early detection of malignancy should form one of the keystones of the annual review clinic. As a bare minimum, this should include an examination of all sun-exposed areas, and some centers have established joint clinics with dermatologists. Certainly, a rapid referral system should be available for suspicious lesions. Most lesions require excision and biopsy followed by treatment along with the following principles:

1. *Reduction in Immunosuppression.* Most centers will stop any antiproliferative agent if used and otherwise reduce CNI levels. Patients with widespread or metastatic disease will often be on steroids alone or rarely on no immunosuppression at all.
2. Evidence from the original trials involving sirolimus in renal transplantation suggested that there was a reduction in the incidence of non-melanoma-type skin cancers (NMSCs). More importantly, recent evidence suggests that KTRs who develop a first SCC will reduce the risk of developing further SCCs by approximately half if their CNI is switched to sirolimus [62]. It is our practice to offer sirolimus to all KTRs who develop NMSCs as an alternative to CNIs. Whether it is beneficial to convert older cohorts of patients who are on azathioprine and steroids to sirolimus is uncertain. This issue has been clouded by the increased overall mortality associated with sirolimus in registry data [63].

3. Oral retinoids such as acitretin have been shown in some studies to reduce the incidence of further SCCs. However, these drugs have significant side effects, and it is important to monitor liver function tests and lipids.

95.3.3.2 Posttransplant Lymphoproliferative Disease (PTLD)

The lymphomas which occur after transplantation having different characteristics from those occurring in the general population [64]. Ninety-three percent are non-Hodgkin lymphomas (c.f 65%), and they are predominantly large cell types, composed of B cells. T-cell PTLD is very rare and carries a poor prognosis. The pathogenesis is usually thought to involve EBV-driven proliferation of B cells although a minority of tumors are EBV negative. Virally transformed lymphocytes escape the immune system due to the effects of immunosuppressive drugs on Immunosurveillance (e.g., cytotoxic $CD8^+$ T cells). Molecular studies have revealed that most tumors are derived from host tissue although donor-derived disease can occur in the renal allograft, and these are more likely to occur early (◘ Fig. 95.6).

The spectrum of the disease runs the gamut of a benign infectious mononucleosis-like pattern to highly malignant monoclonal lymphomas. Fifty percent of cases present with extranodal disease, most often in the GI tract, lungs, skin, or CNS. Tumors not associated with EBV tend to present later and have a worse prognosis. The incidence in KTRs is approximately 1–2% overall, but this represents a significant increase in risk compared to an age-matched population.

Risk factors for the development of PTLD include the following:

- Overall immunosuppressive burden – T-cell-depleting agents (e.g., OKT3, Thymoglobulin) are strongly linked to an increased relative risk of PTLD (78% increase in risk compared to no induction agent) [65]. Registry data suggest that alemtuzumab is associated with only a minimally increased risk (15% increases). The co-stimulatory blocker, belatacept, is also associated with PTLD, especially when an EBV + ve graft is implanted into an EBV – ve recipient. There is limited registry data suggesting that tacrolimus is associated with more PTLD than ciclosporin.
- EBV serostatus – EBV – ve KTRs are more than 20 times more likely to develop PTLD when receiving an EBV + ve graft. This is a particular problem when adults donate to children (belatacept is now contraindicated in EBV D+/R- transplants for this reason).
- Younger age – the relative risk of lymphoma is 260 in children <10-years-old compared with peers (RR for transplant recipients >60 is 8); this may relate to lower rates of EBV seropositivity.
- Time after transplantation – most common in the first year but can occur at any time.
- HLA mismatch – particularly at the HLA-B locus.
- Ethnicity – more common in Caucasians.

Early diagnosis requires a high index of suspicion with an aggressive investigation of unexplained weight loss, fevers, abdominal pain, etc. usually with cross-sectional imaging (see ◘ Fig. 95.7). EBV viral load measured by PCR is useful although the positive predictive value is low. Early PTLD is much more likely to originate in the transplanted organ than late PTLD. Roughly 25% of PTLDs are gut related and 10–20% is CNS related. Tissue biopsy excision is essential (c.f. fine needle aspira-

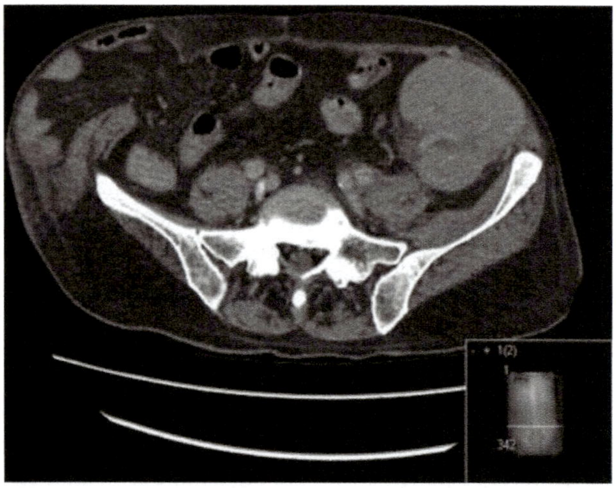

◘ **Fig. 95.6** CT scan showing marked enlargement of transplant kidney secondary to lymphomatous infiltration

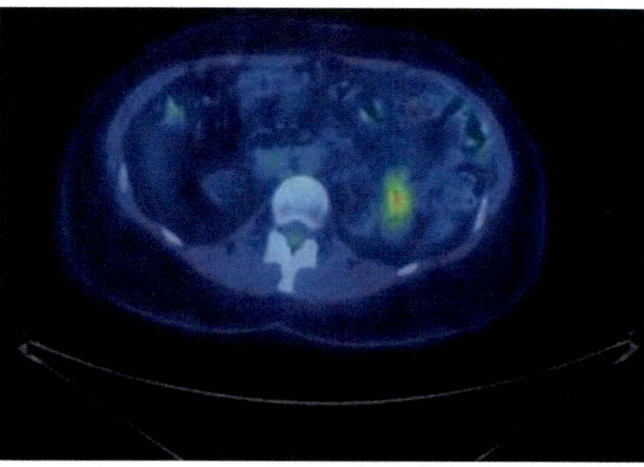

◘ **Fig. 95.7** CT gallium scan showing small bowel PTLD in a patient with weight loss, fevers but negative cross-sectional and luminal imaging

tion), and requires extensive expert evaluation to determine morphology, immunoglobulin gene rearrangements, clonality, and evidence of EBV infection. Treatment should be planned in association with the hematology/oncology MDT in accordance with current guidelines [66]. Specific imaging of different organ systems may be necessary (e.g., MRI in CNS disease). The determination of EBV viral loads, LDH, and paraproteins in blood may also be useful in monitoring disease activity and response. There is little evidence that preemptive therapy of EBV with antiviral agents (e.g., valganciclovir) is beneficial in EBV D^+/R^- cases. Research is ongoing with preemptive rituximab in such patients with increasing EBV viremia.

Surgical excision of the tumor may be possible, but the principal form of treatment is a reduction in immunosuppressive therapy. This intervention may be effective on its own especially in limited low-grade EBV-positive polyclonal disease where baseline immunosuppression at diagnosis is high.

Most clinicians will immediately stop any antiproliferative agent and reduce the dose of any CNI (e.g., by 50%). In extensive or nonresponsive disease, patients are often maintained on steroids alone (0.1 mg/kg PO daily). A study of 135 patients with PTLD treated with ISR demonstrated very good survival rates, especially in EBV-positive, polyclonal tumors, even in those with CNS involvement. The conclusion of the experience was that ISR should be gradual and not only precipitous in order to avoid rejection but also to achieve better response rates.

Adverse prognostic indicators include the following:
- Age < 60
- Poor performance status
- Elevated LDH
- Hypoalbuminemia
- EBV negative recipient
- Monoclonality
- Monomorphic histology
- B symptoms (fevers, night sweats, and weight loss)
- Greater than one site involved
- Involvement of the allograft or bone marrow
- CNS involvement
- Advanced stage
- Poor response to immunosuppression reduction

Disease with adverse prognostic characteristics will require further treatment which usually involves treatment with rituximab. A good initial response to rituximab is a good prognostic sign and complete responses can be consolidated with further rituximab while poorer responders are usually given additional chemotherapy (e.g., CHOP) [67]. There is good evidence that the use of rituximab is associated with improved outcomes in the modern era. There is no evidence to support antiviral therapy to treat established PTLD.

A further option now available in some countries including the UK is the transfer of allogeneic EBV-specific T cells. A phase two study of 33 patients with PTLD who had failed conventional treatment reported 50% response, most of which translated into complete remission and further studies are ongoing [68].

95.3.3.3 Other Solid Tumors

The management of other solid tumors in KTRs should begin with prevention. There is some contention over the best screening policy for KTRs, but the minimum is screening according to the NHS cancer screening guidelines for the general population. This usually includes:
- Breast cancer screening with mammography for those over 50
- Cervical screening at 3-yearly intervals for those over 25, then at 5 yearly intervals between 50 and 64
- Bowel cancer screening by fecal occult blood or colonoscopy testing every 2 years from 55 to 69

There is no evidence to support widespread PSA screening for prostate cancer, ultrasound of kidneys or indeed any other procedure in the general KTR population. Individualized approaches may be appropriate in specific cases, e.g., KTRs with previous tumors or von Hippel–Lindau disease.

When diagnosed, cancers should be managed along conventional lines with referral to cancer MDTs. However, as a general principle, the burden of immunosuppression should be reduced. Reducing immunosuppression is an important principle when cancer (or a precancerous lesion) is diagnosed and the necessity is often deemed to be proportionate to the relative risks of cancer under these drugs, i.e., more important for skin cancer and non-Hodgkin's lymphoma than for breast or prostate. This approach seems sensible although it assumes that biological effects of immunosuppression are similar in the genesis of cancer and the maintenance phase.

The risks of malignancy approximate to the cumulative burden of immunosuppression both before (e.g., for autoimmune disease) and after transplantation. The following observations relate to specific immunosuppressive agents:

1. CNIs – these agents have been shown to accelerate the metastatic spread of tumors in animal models. A prospective RCT comparing two different target levels of ciclosporin resulted in a significantly higher incidence of cancers in the high-dose group, especially skin cancer [66]. KTRs that develop cancers should either have CNIs reduced or withdrawn.

2. Antiproliferative agents – these drugs are linked to the development of neoplasia and are generally the first drugs to be stopped when cancer develops. There is limited circumstantial evidence that mycophenolic acid compounds are less carcinogenic than azathioprine, especially in skin cancer.
3. Prednisolone – generally thought to be the safest agent in KTRs with cancer and consequently is often used as immunosuppression and sometimes as monotherapy in severe diseases.
4. Sirolimus – has been shown to inhibit tumor growth in animal models. In prospective studies of sirolimus as a substitute for ciclosporin, the rates of both de novo skin and non-cutaneous tumors were 4% versus 9.6%. This finding has been consolidated in further trials, especially with respect to skin cancer. Similar findings have been observed with everolimus. Recently, a randomized controlled study has demonstrated that patients who develop squamous cell cancer have approximately half the risk of developing a second lesion if they are converted from CNIs to sirolimus [67]. Anecdotal evidence suggests sirolimus may also have specific benefits in patients with Kaposi's sarcoma and renal cell carcinoma, but these remain to be proven. Extrapolation to other solid tumors is a matter of speculation and there are concerns over registry data suggesting higher mortality in KTRs treated with sirolimus [68].

95.3.4 Infection

Infections, both opportunistic and otherwise, are a cause of significant morbidity and mortality posttransplant. This subject is covered in the chapter on "INFECTIOUS COMPLICATIONS OF TRANSPLANTATION' by Evans et al.

95.3.5 Other Morbidities

95.3.5.1 Mineral and Bone Disorders after Transplantation

Renal bone disease is a complex entity in KTRs and represents the sum of pretransplant disease superimposed with posttransplant factors such as corticosteroid usage. Most KTRs suffer loss of bone volume, abnormalities of mineralization, and low burn turnover. Bone biopsy studies reveal a decrease in bone formation and mineralization in the face of persistent bone resorption. KTRs have nearly four times the rate of fractures after transplantation compared to healthy individuals, a rate 30% higher than comparable dialysis patients in the first 3 years after transplantation [69]. While bone mineral density can be measured by DEXA scan, there is limited evidence that measurements can predict future fractures, particularly in those with eGFRs below 30 ml/min/1.73 m^2. Newer methods of bone evaluation such as high-resolution peripheral quantitative computed tomography (HRpQCT) may prove more promising [70]. See chapter on Chronic Kidney Disease Mineral and Bone Disorder (CKD-MBD) by Torres and Cunningham for details.

Osteoporosis

KTRs that either have or have significant risk factors for developing osteoporosis should be considered for steroid avoiding immunosuppression. For patients with established osteoporosis, the first-line agents are oral weekly bisphosphonates for those with eGFR > 30 ml/min/1.73 m^2. Calcium and vitamin D supplements may also be used although definitive proof of benefit in terms of fracture prevention is absent for any agent. Denosumab also decreases bone resorption, significantly increases BMD, and decreases the risk of fractures in women with osteoporosis. It is also effective at reducing fracture risk in patients with impaired kidney function. Denosumab is not renally cleared, which makes it more attractive than bisphosphonates in patients with significant graft dysfunction, although there are little data of its use in KTRs [70].

Avascular Necrosis

Avascular necrosis or osteonecrosis was previously more common in the era of prolonged high-dose oral steroids and may also be linked to high serum PTH levels. Symptoms usually appear within 12 months of transplantation with stiffness and reduced mobility of the joint. Commonly affected joints are the femoral heads, femoral condyle, tibial plateau, body of the talus, and the humoral head in order of descending frequency. The diagnosis is made with X-rays and MRI scanning the latter being much more sensitive (see ◘ Figs. 95.8a, b). Active treatment of femoral AVN consists of core decompression and if that fails total hip replacement.

Vitamin D Deficiency

Vitamin D levels are commonly reduced in KTRs. One study revealed almost universal vitamin D deficiency or insufficiency among 244 KTRs. These observations are more intriguing given the multiple nonskeletal effects of the vitamin [71]. In severe deficiency or insufficiency with musculoskeletal symptoms, it is our practice to prescribe over-the-counter preparations of vitamin D3 25 µg (1000 IU) daily for a few months and then reassess.

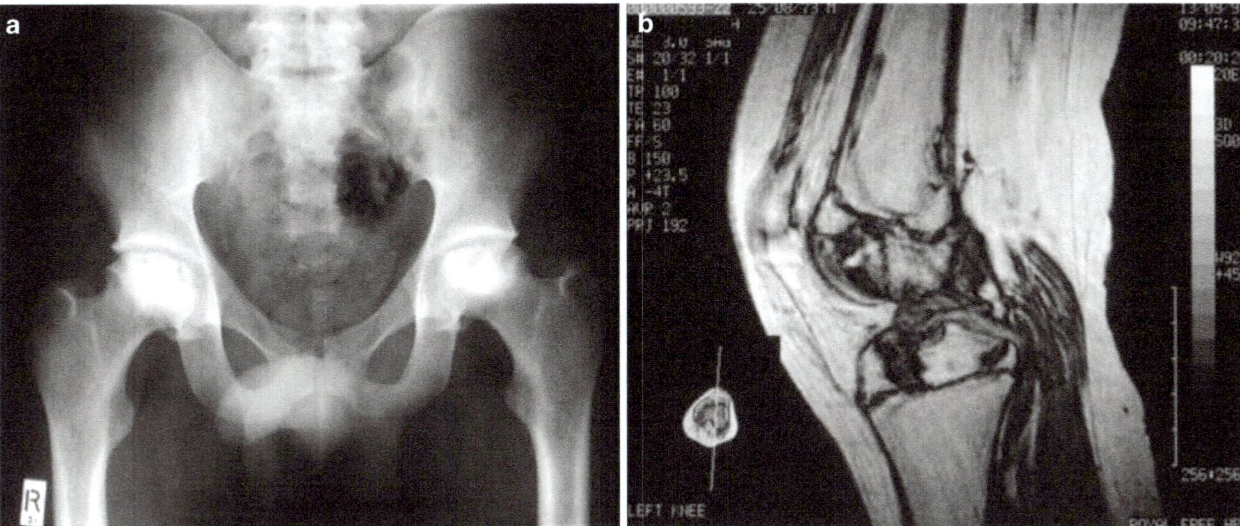

Fig. 95.8 a Late radiological appearance of bilateral avascular necrosis of the hips showing collapse of the acetabular heads and secondary osteoarthritis. b Extensive avascular necrosis of the knee in a young patient with knee pain but normal plain knee X-ray

Persistent Hyperparathyroidism

It is advisable to treat severe hyperparathyroidism prior to transplantation since there is some evidence that parathyroidectomy may be harmful to graft function. However, cinacalcet is safe to use in KTRs if tolerated but caution should be exercised with high doses. PTH levels usually decrease in the months following renal transplantation, but in up to 25% of KTRs, tertiary hyperparathyroidism persists often associated with hypercalcemia. Intriguingly, this clinical occurrence has been linked with calcifications on protocol biopsies and poor graft outcomes [72]. Data from bone biopsies in such patients is conflicting with a high bone turnover state in some patients but a low bone turnover state in others. In patients with a low bone turnover state, treatment with either cinacalcet or parathyroidectomy might theoretically provoke adynamic bone disease. However, most centers consider partial parathyroidectomy or cinacalcet therapy to avoid significant hypercalcemia and its attendant complications.

Gout and Urate

Gout is common after transplantation (see Figs. 95.9a, b), in part due to CNIs, and may cause significant morbidity. Hyperuricemia increases the risk of gout and may also be linked with increased rates of cardiovascular disease. Important drug interactions alter the strategy for managing gout in KTRs, and in particular, it is important to avoid the combination of allopurinol and azathioprine. CNIs are associated with higher uric acid levels and may contribute to the development of gout.

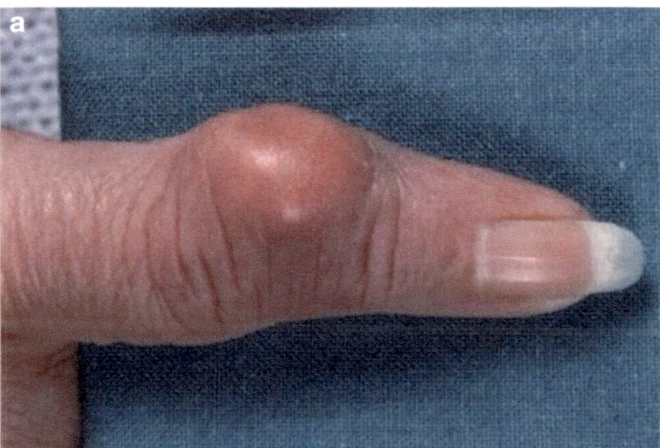

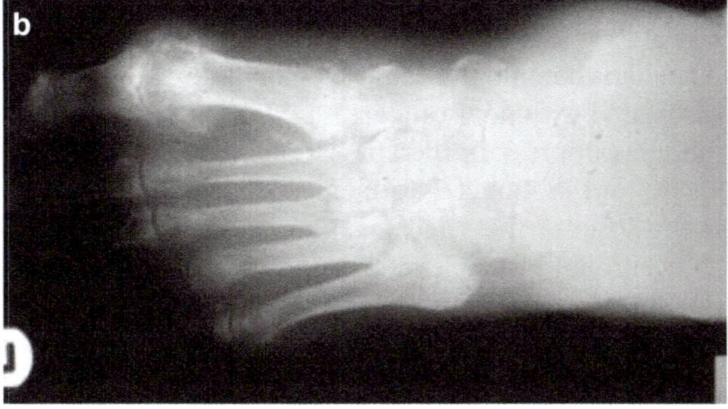

Fig. 95.9 a Showing gouty tophus in a transplant recipient on CNIs and diuretics. b Showing destructive changes of gout in the first metatarsal

Nonsteroidal anti-inflammatory drugs are generally avoided for acute flares. Acute attacks should be treated with short 5-day courses of steroids or colchicine. Both allopurinol and febuxostat may be used as prophylaxis

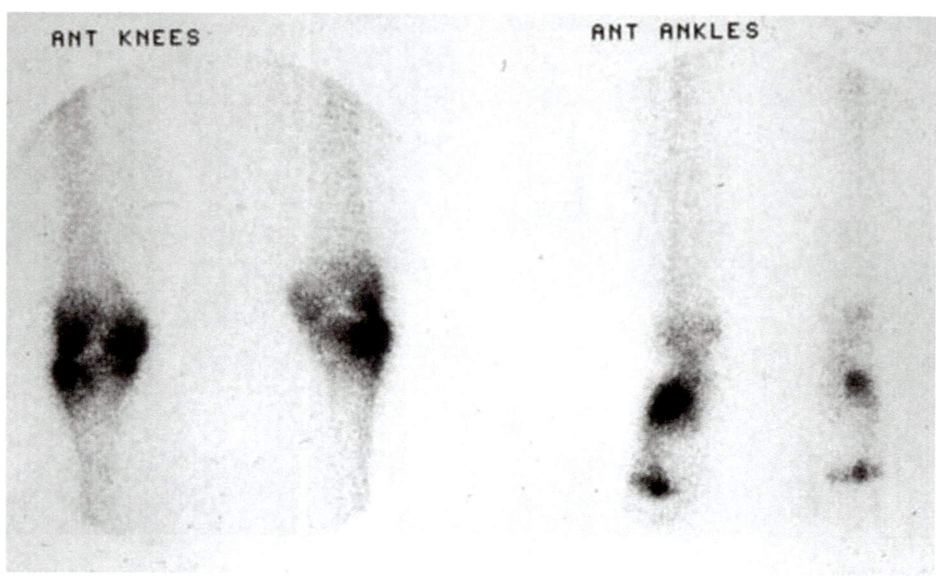

Figs. 95.10 Bone scan showing CNI-induced knee and ankle injury

for recurrent gout. Both agents should be used with azathioprine, and caution should be exercised when using febuxostat in those with eGFRs below 30 ml/min/1.73 m^2. Losartan (c.f. other ARBs) may be useful as an antihypertensive agent since it reduces serum uric acid levels.

Calcineurin Inhibitor-Induced Bone Pain

CNIs may cause bone pain which preferentially affects bones in the lower legs. Bone marrow edema can be demonstrated on the MRI scanning or bone scan (Fig. 95.10), and treatment involves reducing CNI levels and the use of dihydropyridine calcium antagonists.

95.3.5.2 Hematological

Anemia is common in the KTR population and may be associated with poor outcomes [73]. It is exacerbated by immunosuppressant therapy, especially antiproliferative agents and sirolimus. Treatment may involve a reduction in the doses of these agents but more commonly follows conventional principles consisting of iron and erythropoietin administration.

Polycythemia is common after renal transplantation and may be associated with significant morbidity and mortality [74]. Studies have shown that ACEIs and ARBs are associated with a drop-in hematocrit of around 10% in KTRs, and these should be used as first-line agents for those with hematocrits above 52% for men and 49% for women. Venesection and aminophylline may be used in refractory or intolerant patients [75].

95.3.5.3 Reproductive Function

Female fertility returns rapidly after successful renal transplantation. Given the risks to the mother, transplant and fetus of early pregnancy, women of childbearing age, and their partners need to be counseled about a potential pregnancy, immediately posttransplant, and the importance of having reliable mechanisms of contraception if not abstinent. It is recommended to wait at least 12 months after successful transplantation before conception to allow for stabilization of immunosuppression levels and allograft function. Pregnancies in KTRs should be deemed above-average risk since they are associated with increased rates of maternal hypertension (80%), pre-eclampsia (30%), prematurity (40%), low birth weight (50%), and cesarean section (60%) [76, 77]. The rate of live births is approximately 80%, the remainder resulting in miscarriages and occasionally stillbirths. The risk of pregnancy to allograft function is probably small as long as there is good baseline function (eGFR > 40 ml/min, PCR < 50 and well-controlled blood pressure). However, in some cases, particularly, KTRs with suboptimal baseline function, the effects of hyperfiltration, and potential alterations in the metabolism of immunosuppressive drugs (especially CNIs) can cause graft dysfunction. Preconception counseling should be carried out, and care of pregnancy should be in conjunction with the obstetric team. CNI levels should be monitored regularly.

The effects of immunosuppression, the choice of contraception, and breastfeeding are covered elsewhere. Mycophenolate compounds have been shown to be teratogenic in females and should be stopped prior to attempts at conception. Recommendations have also been made that male KTRs on these drugs should use barrier methods of contraception despite no documented evidence of harm [78].

Outcomes of pregnancies fathered by male KTRs are similar to the general population. Sirolimus and presumably other m-TORis are associated with oligospermia, which appears to be reversible on cessation of treatment.

95.3.6 Annual Review Clinics

A number of the issues discussed in this chapter are conveniently addressed in an annual review clinic. Any appropriately skilled healthcare worker, but usually a specialist nurse, can lead such a clinic. Appointments can be for longer time periods than those routinely allocated for doctor-led appointments to permit more comprehensive enquiry. Issues that can be addressed include:

1. Skeletal health including PTH with the use of DEXA scanning when appropriate
2. Psychosexual and social issues, which are surprisingly common if sought with an empathetic approach
3. Affective and anxiety disorders
4. Cancer screening review and skin surface examination
5. Comprehensive cardiovascular review including the arrangement of glucose tolerance tests, fasting lipid profiles, smoking cessation, and blood pressure monitoring by either home or ambulatory monitoring
6. Exercise activity and potential
7. Medication review with the pharmacist
8. Vaccination
9. Overall balance of immunosuppression (years' post-transplant, total burden of immunosuppression, immunoglobulins, $CD4^+$ and $CD8^+$ counts vs. mismatch, rejection episodes, sensitization, donor-specific HLA antibodies, and nonspecific HLA antibodies).

95.4 Management of the Failing Allograft

95.4.1 Definition

A failing allograft is a situation where a kidney transplant recipient will require further renal replacement therapy (RRT) within the next 6 months.

95.4.2 Epidemiology

Approximately, half of all renal allografts functioning at 1 year will eventually fail. Management of the failing allograft should be along similar lines to the management of native disease with the timely provision of education about different forms of renal replacement therapy. Preemptive re-transplantation should always be the treatment of choice if the patient is fit enough and the operation is technically feasible. Consideration for re-transplantation should be carried out by the specialist MDT when the transplant function falls below 20 ml/min/1.73 m^2. This is usually best accomplished by transferring the patient to a specialist low clearance clinic; however, there appears to be reluctance on behalf of both KTRs and their doctors to make this change. There is a perception on both sides that this represents a therapeutic failure, but it is important to emphasize the positive factors, specifically the alleviation of symptoms and the possibility of re-transplantation.

Evidence suggests that care of the failing transplant is not always carried out well [79]. In the USA, 13.1% of the adult waiting list was for re-transplantation in 2015, compared to 16.1% in 2005 and the actual re-transplantation rate was 13.2% ($n = 2354$) in adults [80]. The consideration for children and young people is more pertinent since they may require multiple renal transplantation operations during their lifetime. This was emphasized by a Dutch study of 249 RTR, all transplanted under the age of 15 years, which showed that after a mean follow up of 25 years of follow up, 36%, 34%, 17%, and 5% had been transplanted two, three, four, and five or more times, respectively [81]. Consequently, it is important to ensure that the pathway is as smooth as possible and to minimize the time spent on dialysis where possible.

KTRs with an estimated glomerular filtration rate (eGFR) less than 30 mls/min/1.73 m^2 contributed 13.3% of the UK transplant population in 2015 according to the 19th UKRR report [82]. This represents nearly 4500 patients with Stage IV-T and Stage V-T chronic kidney disease. Evidence from the UK Renal Registry demonstrates that the care of these patients is suboptimal. For example, across the UK, 16% of these patients have a hemoglobin of less than 100 g/L and less than a quarter achieved satisfactory blood pressure control (<130/80 mmHg).

Data from the USAdescribed nearly two-thirds of failing adult transplant patients commencing hemodialysis with intravenous catheters which are disappointing since they are nearly all under regular renal review [83]. These issues with patient care will be exacerbated by the continuing expansion of this population group which will make management increasingly difficult unless resources are allocated accordingly. As a result of the successful increase in deceased donor renal transplantation rates in the UK, the prevalent adult transplant population has increased from 19,074 in 2005 to 32,624 in 2015. To meet this challenge some units have established transplant low clearance clinics to facilitate better management of this patient population.

Outcomes after the failure of a transplant are generally poor. A meta-analysis of 40 studies in adults revealed that the mortality rate in the first 12 months following renal allograft failure was approximately 12% for the first 12 months dropping to around 6% for the next 3 years [84]. Even among the cohort who are fit enough relisted outcomes are inferior compared with transplant naïve patients, a recent study from Spain demonstrating a 50% increase in mortality [85]. The psychological effects of renal allograft failure cannot be overstated and detailed psychological studies have described the devastating effects of renal allograft failure, likening the process to a disenfranchized grief reaction (i.e., where the griever is not recognized as an individual who can and should grieve). Despite these observations, there is still data to suggest the benefit of a second preemptive transplant with improved patient and graft outcomes [86, 87].

95.4.3 Management Aspects

95.4.3.1 Starting Renal Replacement Therapy (RRT)

There is a published guidance for the management of the failing KTR which contains many sensible recommendations although it is conspicuous that the evidence levels are low [88]. There is little evidence to guide the timing of dialysis initiation after renal transplantation. Limited data in KTRs with failing grafts have revealed an association between higher eGFR at initiation and worse outcomes [89]. It seems sensible that renal replacement therapy should be commenced for symptoms or fluid control.

95.4.3.2 Graft Nephrectomy

Indications for graft nephrectomy are well established but it should be appreciated that there is a mortality rate of up to 1.5% at 30 days [90]. There is evidence that graft nephrectomy is associated with a risk of sensitization to human leukocyte antigens (HLA) [91]. However, interpretation of this data is confounded by other factors:

- The indication for nephrectomy is often the result of a clinical syndrome caused by antibody-mediated rejection
- Perioperative transfusion may occur
- Intracapsular nephrectomy leaves increased allogeneic material compared to extracapsular extraction
- Variation in immunosuppression withdrawal protocols around the time of nephrectomy
- Loss of the "sponge" effect as the graft no longer "mops up" antibodies

95.4.3.3 Managing Immunosuppression Medications

The correct strategy for weaning immunosuppression (IS) is not clear and there are conflicting priorities. Interpreting the outcome of IS withdrawal is complicated by concurrent nephrectomy which often occurs. There are no prospective randomized trials of IS withdrawal but several retrospective studies suggesting that nephrectomy is associated with a rise in donor-specific anti-HLA antibodies [92]. Another important study from the Cambridge group demonstrated the association of increasing HLA mismatches with donor-specific sensitization, with each mismatch increasing the chance of developing donor-specific antibodies by 41% 1 year after relisting [93]. This finding underpins the importance of avoiding mismatches in any patient who is likely to require more than one transplant. They also observed that graft nephrectomy was associated with an odds ratio of 3.42 for the development of DSAs. Interestingly remaining on immunosuppression was associated with significantly less risk of developing subsequent DSAs. Taken together these results suggest that if a second transplant is likely to occur within 12 months (e.g., live donor or high priority deceased donor renal transplant after early failure) then immunosuppressive therapy should be maintained. This is a complex clinical decision due to the infection risks on dialysis therapy and should be made according to individual circumstances by the transplant team in a timely fashion and documented before the initiation of renal replacement therapy.

95.4.3.4 Managing Immunological Aspects of Listing

When patients are relisted for a second transplant then they will often have a number of unacceptable antigens listed in the recipient registry and these are based on the following categories:

- Antigens that correlate with anti-HLA antibodies detected in serum screening samples that are above a locally agreed threshold (Mean Fluorescence Intensity – MFI)

- Antibodies that have previously been detected but are no longer present (Historic antibodies)
- Antigens to be avoided since they are present in future potential live donors
- Antigens that were present on a previous graft that has never been detected in serum

Local practice varies and it is essential to establish good communication with your local Histocompatibility and Immunogenetics (H&I) Laboratory in order to understand these processes. Most units in the UK are looking at less conservative strategies to increase the chances of transplantation in highly sensitized patients in the first two categories. Scrutiny of the literature suggests that the last category may be unnecessarily conservative since experimental data does not support a strong effect [94]. It is practically important since removing undetected HLA mismatches may considerably increase the chances of a patient receiving a second or subsequent transplant. More importantly, it emphasizes the need of maintaining an ongoing dialog with your H&I Laboratory.

Living donor transplantation has evolved considerably over the last decade with the establishment of living donor sharing schemes and the burgeoning of both blood group incompatible and HLA-incompatible transplantation. This is important since some patients who are being evaluated for re-transplantation may well have been informed that potential donors were unsuitable at the previous time of consideration and it may worthwhile revisiting the subject of living donation. It is sensible to check blood group antibody titers (i.e., Anti-A1 titres and anti-B titers in a blood group O recipient) since they can often below. In addition, pairs who were previously deemed incompatible may be reconsidered for the living donor sharing scheme and it is notable that this route now contributes more 10% of the overall live donor activity in the UK.

Tips, Tricks, and Pitfalls to Optimize Outcomes after Renal Transplantation

1. Maximize living donation rates – 1-year and 5-year first graft survival rates for living donation are 98% and 93% in the UK (c.f. 94% and 86% for cadaveric grafts (NHSBT 2018)).
2. Maximize preemptive donation rates – Preemptive transplantation results in approximately a 25% reduction in the rates of both graft and patient loss for both cadaveric and living donor transplants.
3. Avoid sensitization – Sensitization to HLA molecules reduces the chances of transplantation and impair graft outcomes, irrespective of whether sensitization is donor-specific or not.
4. Avoid rejection – Episodes of rejection are associated with increased long-term rates of graft loss.
5. Minimize ischemia reperfusion injury – Longer cold ischemic times decrease graft survival; critical times appear to be greater than 18 h in DBD grafts and greater than 12 h for DCD grafts.
6. Ensure rigorous monitoring and an efficiently organized clinic infrastructure – It is essential that the monitoring process is sensitive to changes in essential parameters and that a prompt response occurs.
7. Maximize adherence – While firm data is lacking, many experts agree that non-adherence contributes to many cases of graft loss.
8. Ensure robust systems for vaccination, prophylaxis, early diagnosis, and treatment of post-transplant infections.
9. Timely investigation of suboptimal function – Rising creatinine, the development of proteinuria, or de novo donor-specific anti-HLA antibodies.
10. Regularly evaluate the need for immunosuppression – Graft immunogenicity reduces over time, and reassessment should be carried out to minimize side effects.
11. Aggressively treat cardiovascular risk factors – KTRs should be treated as high-risk patients for vascular disease.
12. Ensure compliance with local cancer screening guidelines.
13. Establish a specialist long-term transplant clinic.

Case Study

Summary of figures used to illustrate in this chapter are cases with

1. Gradual transplant graft dysfunction and proteinuria – ◘ Fig. 95.5 illustrates IFTA and arterial hyalinosis. Such findings are frequently encountered in biopsies in patients with long-standing transplant kidneys. Management is usually BP control and wean off CNI. Based on current immunosuppression, other options are summarized in ◘ Table 95.4.
2. A transplant recipient presenting with weight loss needs urgent investigations that includes EBV PCR and 3-cavity CT scan to look for PTLD which could be early on donor-derived (◘ Fig. 95.6) or later in time that typically involves small bowel which is difficult to pick on conventional CT scan and one needs high index of suspicion with PET scan (◘ Fig. 95.7).

95.5 Conclusions

Long-term management of kidney transplant recipients requires a multidisciplinary approach with three key clinic organization – *Long -erm follow-up clinic* focusing on measures to optimize graft and patient survival focusing on medical aspects of monitoring and management; *annual review clinic* focusing on holistic needs, preventative and lifestyle measures; and finally a *transplant low clearance clinic* to manage failing transplant kidney, complications of advance CKD, prepare and timely RRT including preemptive transplantation, and manage immunosuppressive medications appropriately.

Chapter Review Questions

1. What determines better long-term kidney transplant graft survival and how would you improve this at your center?
2. What determines better long-term patient survival and how would you improve this at your center?
3. What are your preemptive rate for second-time transplant and how well are your patients' parameter when they start RRT?

Answers

1. A range of factors determines graft longevity and are broadly divided into recipient and donor factors. Tools to select donor's kidneys are slowly improving and with pre-implantation biopsy score may address some of these aspects. Key modifiable factors in recipients are summarized in ◘ Table 95.1. Careful management of BMI, BP, and adherence/toxicity of immunosuppressive medications during clinic visits is critical. Regular visits and vigilance of other factors such as viral activation particularly BKV and early immunological injury such as albuminuria are important lead and should follow with early histological diagnosis, and management could save loss of graft function.
2. The main etiologies for mortalities of kidney transplant recipients are CV disease, infection, and malignancies. Aggressive management of modifiable cardiovascular risk factors such as hypertension, obesity, smoking, and diabetes should be part of clinic review. A multidisciplinary team with dietetic review and specialist nurse review for preventative measures such as vaccine, skin check, and bone health in addition to mental health are vital part of long-term management. A collaborative work with other medical specialties is another key to success in improving patient survival. Lastly, empowering patients in self-management and involving in their care through home BP, weight monitoring, and access to patient's results improve patient activation and outcomes.
3. Managing a failing transplant in the conventional clinic lacks appropriate focus and is associated with poor preemptive transplant rate and worse biochemical and hematology parameters compared to other renal patients starting RRT. Other key components are measuring sensitization, managing immunosuppressive medications, and working closely with colleagues at the transplant immunology lab to complete the transplant work-up.

References

1. Byrne C, Caskey F, Castledine C, Davenport A, Dawnay A, Fraser S, Maxwell H, Medcalf JF, Wilkie M, Williams AJ. 20th Annual Report of the Renal Association. Bristol, UK. NEPHRON. 2018;139(suppl1).
2. Hart A, Smith JM, Skeans MA, Gustafson SK, Wilk AR, Robinson A, et al. OPTN/SRTR 2016 annual data report: kidney. Am J Transplant. 2018;18(Suppl 1):18–113.
3. McDonald SP, Russ GR. Survival of recipients of cadaveric kidney transplants compared with those receiving dialysis treatment in Australia and New Zealand, 1991–2001. Nephrol Dial Transplant. 2002;17(12):2212–9.
4. Oniscu GC, Brown H, Forsythe JL. Impact of cadaveric renal transplantation on survival in patients listed for transplantation. J Am Soc Nephrol. 2005;16(6):1859–65.
5. Wolfe RA, Ashby VB, Milford EL, Ojo AO, Ettenger RE, Agodoa LY, et al. Comparison of mortality in all patients on dialysis, patients on dialysis awaiting transplantation, and recipients of a first cadaveric transplant. N Engl J Med. 1999;341(23):1725–30.
6. Meier-Kriesche HU, Schold JD, Srinivas TR, Reed A, Kaplan B. Kidney transplantation halts cardiovascular disease progression in patients with end-stage renal disease. Am J Transplant. 2004;4(10):1662–8.
7. Tonelli M, Wiebe N, Knoll G, Bello A, Browne S, Jadhav D, et al. Systematic review: kidney transplantation compared with dialysis in clinically relevant outcomes. Am J Transplant. 2011;11(10):2093–109.
8. Improving Global Outcomes (KDIGO) Transplant Work Group. KDIGO clinical practice guideline for the care of kidney transplant recipients. Am J Transplant. 2009;9(Suppl 3):S1–155.
9. Baker RJ, Mark PB, Patel RK, Stevens KK, Palmer N. Renal association clinical practice guideline in post-operative care in the kidney transplant recipient. BMC Nephrol. 2017;18(1):174.
10. Tullius SG, Tran H, Guleria I, Malek SK, Tilney NL, Milford E. The combination of donor and recipient age is critical in determining host immunoresponsiveness and renal transplant outcome. Ann Surg. 2010;252(4):662–74.
11. Giral M, Foucher Y, Karam G, Labrune Y, Kessler M, de Ligny BH, et al. Kidney and recipient weight incompatibility reduces long-term graft survival. J Am Soc Nephrol. 2010;21(6):1022–9.
12. Hariharan S, McBride MA, Cherikh WS, Tolleris CB, Bresnahan BA, Johnson CP. Post-transplant renal function in the first year predicts long-term kidney transplant survival. Kidney Int. 2002;62(1):311–8.
13. Cherukuri A, Tattersall JE, Lewington AJ, Newstead CG, Baker RJ. Resolution of low-grade proteinuria is associated with

improved outcomes after renal transplantation-a retrospective longitudinal study. Am J Transplant. 2015;15(3):741–53.
14. Mange KC, Cizman B, Joffe M, Feldman HI. Arterial hypertension and renal allograft survival. JAMA. 2000;283(5):633–8.
15. Opelz G, Dohler B. Improved long-term outcomes after renal transplantation associated with blood pressure control. Am J Transplant. 2005;5(11):2725–31.
16. Kruger B, Dohler B, Opelz G, Kramer BK, Susal C. Pulse pressure and outcome in kidney transplantation: results from the collaborative transplant study. Transplantation. 2019;103(4):772–80.
17. Cross NB, Webster AC, Masson P, O'Connell PJ, Craig JC. Antihypertensives for kidney transplant recipients: systematic review and meta-analysis of randomized controlled trials. Transplantation. 2009;88(1):7–18.
18. Hill CJ, Courtney AE, Cardwell CR, Maxwell AP, Lucarelli G, Veroux M, et al. Recipient obesity and outcomes after kidney transplantation: a systematic review and meta-analysis. Nephrol Dial Transplant. 2015;30(8):1403–11.
19. Arshad A, Hodson J, Chappelow I, Inston NG, Ready AR, Nath J, et al. The impact of donor body mass index on outcomes after deceased kidney transplantation – a national population-cohort study. Transpl Int. 2018;31(10):1099–109.
20. Shah T, Kasravi A, Huang E, Hayashi R, Young B, Cho YW, et al. Risk factors for development of new-onset diabetes mellitus after kidney transplantation. Transplantation. 2006;82(12):1673–6.
21. Hricik DE. Metabolic syndrome in kidney transplantation: management of risk factors. Clin J Am Soc Nephrol. 2011;6(7):1781–5.
22. Pedrollo EF, Correa C, Nicoletto BB, Manfro RC, Leitao CB, Souza GC, et al. Effects of metabolic syndrome on kidney transplantation outcomes: a systematic review and meta-analysis. Transpl Int. 2016;29(10):1059–66.
23. Takahashi A, Hu SL, Bostom A. Physical activity in kidney transplant recipients: a review. Am J Kidney Dis. 2018;72(3):433–43.
24. Houri I, Tzukert K, Levi IM, Aharon M, Bloch A, Gotsman O, et al. Implementation of guidelines for metabolic syndrome control in kidney transplant recipients: results at a single center. Diabetol Metab Syndr. 2015;7:90.
25. Cherukuri A, Welberry-Smith MP, Tattersall JE, Ahmad N, Newstead CG, Lewington AJ, et al. The clinical significance of early proteinuria after renal transplantation. Transplantation. 2010;89(2):200–7.
26. Halimi JM, Laouad I, Buchler M, Al-Najjar A, Chatelet V, Houssaini TS, et al. Early low-grade proteinuria: causes, short-term evolution and long-term consequences in renal transplantation. Am J Transplant. 2005;5(9):2281–8.
27. Knoll GA, Fergusson D, Chasse M, Hebert P, Wells G, Tibbles LA, et al. Ramipril versus placebo in kidney transplant patients with proteinuria: a multicentre, double-blind, randomised controlled trial. Lancet Diabetes Endocrinol. 2016;4(4):318–26.
28. Hiremath S, Fergusson DA, Fergusson N, Bennett A, Knoll GA. Renin-angiotensin system blockade and long-term clinical outcomes in kidney transplant recipients: a meta-analysis of randomized controlled trials. Am J Kidney Dis. 2017;69(1):78–86.
29. Fotheringham J, Angel C, Goodwin J, Harmer AW, McKane WS. Natural history of proteinuria in renal transplant recipients developing de novo human leukocyte antigen antibodies. Transplantation. 2011;91(9):991–6.
30. Ojo AO, Held PJ, Port FK, Wolfe RA, Leichtman AB, Young EW, et al. Chronic renal failure after transplantation of a nonrenal organ. N Engl J Med. 2003;349(10):931–40.
31. Nankivell BJ, Borrows RJ, Fung CL, O'Connell PJ, Allen RD, Chapman JR. The natural history of chronic allograft nephropathy. N Engl J Med. 2003;349(24):2326–33.
32. Webster AC, Lee VW, Chapman JR, Craig JC. Target of rapamycin inhibitors (sirolimus and everolimus) for primary immunosuppression of kidney transplant recipients: a systematic review and meta-analysis of randomized trials. Transplantation. 2006;81(9):1234–48.
33. El-Zoghby ZM, Stegall MD, Lager DJ, Kremers WK, Amer H, Gloor JM, et al. Identifying specific causes of kidney allograft loss. Am J Transplant. 2009;9(3):527–35.
34. Durrbach A, Pestana JM, Florman S, Del Carmen RM, Rostaing L, Kuypers D, et al. Long-term outcomes in belatacept- versus cyclosporine-treated recipients of extended criteria donor kidneys: final results from BENEFIT-EXT, a phase III randomized study. Am J Transplant. 2016;16(11):3192–201.
35. Sawinski D, Trofe-Clark J, Leas B, Uhl S, Tuteja S, Kaczmarek JL, et al. Calcineurin inhibitor minimization, conversion, withdrawal, and avoidance strategies in renal transplantation: a systematic review and meta-analysis. Am J Transplant. 2016;16(7):2117–38.
36. Dudley C, Pohanka E, Riad H, Dedochova J, Wijngaard P, Sutter C, et al. Mycophenolate mofetil substitution for cyclosporine a in renal transplant recipients with chronic progressive allograft dysfunction: the "creeping creatinine" study. Transplantation. 2005;79(4):466–75.
37. Holdaas H, Fellstrom B, Jardine AG, Holme I, Nyberg G, Fauchald P, et al. Effect of fluvastatin on cardiac outcomes in renal transplant recipients: a multicentre, randomised, placebo-controlled trial. Lancet. 2003;361(9374):2024–31.
38. Palmer SC, Navaneethan SD, Craig JC, Perkovic V, Johnson DW, Nigwekar SU, et al. HMG CoA reductase inhibitors (statins) for kidney transplant recipients. Cochrane Database Syst Rev. 2014;Jan 28(1):Cd005019.
39. Wanner C, Tonelli M. KDIGO clinical practice guideline for lipid management in CKD: summary of recommendation statements and clinical approach to the patient. Kidney Int. 2014;85(6):1303–9.
40. Briganti EM, Russ GR, McNeil JJ, Atkins RC, Chadban SJ. Risk of renal allograft loss from recurrent glomerulonephritis. N Engl J Med. 2002;347(2):103–9.
41. Cole EH, Johnston O, Rose CL, Gill JS. Impact of acute rejection and new-onset diabetes on long-term transplant graft and patient survival. Clin J Am Soc Nephrol. 2008;3(3):814–21.
42. Hariharan S, Johnson CP, Bresnahan BA, Taranto SE, McIntosh MJ, Stablein D. Improved graft survival after renal transplantation in the United States, 1988 to 1996. N Engl J Med. 2000;342(9):605–12.
43. Famulski KS, Einecke G, Sis B, Mengel M, Hidalgo LG, Kaplan B, et al. Defining the canonical form of T-cell-mediated rejection in human kidney transplants. Am J Transplant. 2010;10(4):810–20.
44. Pankhurst L, Hudson A, Mumford L, Wilcombe M, Galiford J, Shaw O, et al. The UK National Registry of ABO and HLA antibody incompatible renal transplantation: Pretransplant factors associated with outcome in 879 transplants. Transplant Direct. 2017;3(7):e181.
45. Wiebe C, Gibson IW, Blydt-Hansen TD, Karpinski M, Ho J, Storsley LJ, et al. Evolution and clinical pathologic correlations of De Novo Donor-specific HLA antibody post kidney transplant. Am J Transplant. 2012;12(5):1157–67.
46. Roufosse C, Simmonds N, Clahsen-van Groningen M, Haas M, Henriksen KJ, Horsfield C, et al. A 2018 reference guide to the Banff classification of renal allograft pathology. Transplantation. 2018;102(11):1795–814.

47. Farris AB, Colvin RB. Renal interstitial fibrosis: mechanisms and evaluation. Curr Opin Nephrol Hypertens. 2012;21(3): 289–300.
48. Ekberg H, Tedesco-Silva H, Demirbas A, Vitko S, Nashan B, Gurkan A, et al. Reduced exposure to calcineurin inhibitors in renal transplantation. N Engl J Med. 2007;357(25):2562–75.
49. Sharif A, Shabir S, Chand S, Cockwell P, Ball S, Borrows R. Meta-analysis of calcineurin-inhibitor-sparing regimens in kidney transplantation. J Am Soc Nephrol. 2011;22(11): 2107–18.
50. O'Connell PJ, Zhang W, Menon MC, Yi Z, Schroppel B, Gallon L, et al. Biopsy transcriptome expression profiling to identify kidney transplants at risk of chronic injury: a multicentre, prospective study. Lancet. 2016;388(10048):983–93.
51. Weiner DE, Carpenter MA, Levey AS, Ivanova A, Cole EH, Hunsicker L, et al. Kidney function and risk of cardiovascular disease and mortality in kidney transplant recipients: the FAVORIT trial. Am J Transplant. 2012;17(10):1600–6143.
52. Conte C, Secchi A. Post-transplantation diabetes in kidney transplant recipients: an update on management and prevention. Acta Diabetol. 2018;55(8):763–79.
53. Jenssen T, Hartmann A. Post-transplant diabetes mellitus in patients with solid organ transplants. Nat Rev Endocrinol. 2019;15(3):172–88.
54. Webster AC, Woodroffe RC, Taylor RS, Chapman JR, Craig JC. Tacrolimus versus ciclosporin as primary immunosuppression for kidney transplant recipients: meta-analysis and meta-regression of randomised trial data. BMJ. 2005;331(7520):810.
55. Wissing KM, Abramowicz D, Weekers L, Budde K, Rath T, Witzke O, et al. Prospective randomized study of conversion from tacrolimus to cyclosporine a to improve glucose metabolism in patients with posttransplant diabetes mellitus after renal transplantation. Am J Transplant. 2018;18(7):1726–34.
56. Hecking M, Haidinger M, Doller D, Werzowa J, Tura A, Zhang J, et al. Early basal insulin therapy decreases new-onset diabetes after renal transplantation. J Am Soc Nephrol. 2012;23(4): 739–49.
57. Au E, Wong G, Chapman JR. Cancer in kidney transplant recipients. Nat Rev Nephrol. 2018;14(8):508–20.
58. Collett D, Mumford L, Banner NR, Neuberger J, Watson C. Comparison of the incidence of malignancy in recipients of different types of organ: a UK registry audit. Am J Transplant. 2010;10(8):1889–96.
59. Engels EA, Pfeiffer RM, Fraumeni JF Jr, Kasiske BL, Israni AK, Snyder JJ, et al. Spectrum of cancer risk among US solid organ transplant recipients. JAMA. 2011;306(17):1891–901.
60. D'Arcy ME, Coghill AE, Lynch CF, Koch LA, Li J, Pawlish KS, et al. Survival after a cancer diagnosis among solid organ transplant recipients in the United States. Cancer. 2019;125(6):933–42.
61. Dantal J, Hourmant M, Cantarovich D, Giral M, Blancho G, Dreno B, et al. Effect of long-term immunosuppression in kidney-graft recipients on cancer incidence: randomised comparison of two cyclosporin regimens. Lancet. 1998;351(9103):623–8.
62. Euvrard S, Morelon E, Rostaing L, Goffin E, Brocard A, Tromme I, et al. Sirolimus and secondary skin-cancer prevention in kidney transplantation. N Engl J Med. 2012;367(4):329–39.
63. Knoll GA, Kokolo MB, Mallick R, Beck A, Buenaventura CD, Ducharme R, et al. Effect of sirolimus on malignancy and survival after kidney transplantation: systematic review and meta-analysis of individual patient data. BMJ. 2014;349:g6679.
64. DeStefano CB, Desai SH, Shenoy AG, Catlett JP. Management of post-transplant lymphoproliferative disorders. Br J Haematol. 2018;182(3):330–43.
65. Bustami RT, Ojo AO, Wolfe RA, Merion RM, Bennett WM, McDiarmid SV, et al. Immunosuppression and the risk of post-transplant malignancy among cadaveric first kidney transplant recipients. Am J Transplant. 2004;4(1):87–93.
66. Parker A, Bowles K, Bradley JA, Emery V, Featherstone C, Gupte G, et al. Management of post-transplant lymphoproliferative disorder in adult solid organ transplant recipients – BCSH and BTS guidelines. Br J Haematol. 2010;149(5):693–705.
67. Trappe RU, Dierickx D, Zimmermann H, Morschhauser F, Mollee P, Zaucha JM, et al. Response to rituximab induction is a predictive marker in B-cell post-transplant lymphoproliferative disorder and allows successful stratification into rituximab or R-CHOP consolidation in an international, prospective, Multicenter phase II trial. J Clin Oncol Off J Am Soc Clin Oncol. 2017;35(5):536–43.
68. Barrett AJ, Prockop S, Bollard CM. Virus-specific T cells: broadening applicability. Biol Blood Marrow Transplant. 2018;24(1):13–8.
69. Stavroulopoulos A, Cassidy MJ, Porter CJ, Hosking DJ, Roe SD. Vitamin D status in renal transplant recipients. Am J Transplant. 2007;7(11):2546–52.
70. Bouquegneau A, Salam S, Delanaye P, Eastell R, Khwaja A. Bone disease after kidney transplantation. Clin J Am Soc Nephrol. 2016;11(7):1282–96.
71. Cianciolo G, Galassi A, Capelli I, Angelini ML, La Manna G, Cozzolino M. Vitamin D in kidney transplant recipients: mechanisms and therapy. Am J Nephrol. 2016;43(6):397–407.
72. Gwinner W, Suppa S, Mengel M, Hoy L, Kreipe HH, Haller H, et al. Early calcification of renal allografts detected by protocol biopsies: causes and clinical implications. Am J Transplant. 2005;5(8):1934–41.
73. Yabu JM, Winkelmayer WC. Posttransplantation anemia: mechanisms and management. Clin J Am Soc Nephrol. 2011;6(7):1794–801.
74. Vlahakos DV, Marathias KP, Agroyannis B, Madias NE. Posttransplant erythrocytosis. Kidney Int. 2003;63(4):1187–94.
75. Malyszko J, Oberbauer R, Watschinger B. Anemia and erythrocytosis in patients after kidney transplantation. Transpl Int. 2012;25(10):1013–23.
76. Deshpande NA, James NT, Kucirka LM, Boyarsky BJ, Garonzik-Wang JM, Montgomery RA, et al. Pregnancy outcomes in kidney transplant recipients: a systematic review and meta-analysis. Am J Transplant. 2011;11(11):2388–404.
77. Sibanda N, Briggs JD, Davison JM, Johnson RJ, Rudge CJ. Pregnancy after organ transplantation: a report from the UK transplant pregnancy registry. Transplantation. 2007;83(10):1301–7.
78. Midtvedt K, Bergan S, Reisaeter AV, Vikse BE, Asberg A. Exposure to mycophenolate and fatherhood. Transplantation. 2017;101(7):e214–e7.
79. Baker RJ, Marks SD. Management of chronic renal allograft dysfunction and when to re-transplant. Pediatr Nephrol. 2019;34(4):599–603.
80. Hart A, Smith JM, Skeans MA, Gustafson SK, Stewart DE, Cherikh WS, et al. OPTN/SRTR 2015 annual data report: kidney. Am J Transplant. 2017;17(Suppl 1):21–116.
81. Ploos van Amstel S, Vogelzang JL, Starink MV, Jager KJ, Groothoff JW. Long-term risk of cancer in survivors of Pediatric ESRD. Clini J Am Soc Nephrol. 2015;10(12):2198–204.
82. Sharples E, Casula A, Byrne C. UK renal registry 19th annual report: chapter 3 demographic and biochemistry profile of kidney transplant recipients in the UK in 2015: national and centre-specific analyses. Nephron. 2017;137(Suppl 1):73–102.
83. Chan MR, Oza-Gajera B, Chapla K, Djamali AX, Muth BL, Turk J, et al. Initial vascular access type in patients with a failed renal transplant. Clin J Am Soc Nephrol. 2014;9(7):1225–31.
84. Kabani R, Quinn RR, Palmer S, Lewin AM, Yilmaz S, Tibbles LA, et al. Risk of death following kidney allograft failure: a sys-

tematic review and meta-analysis of cohort studies. Nephrol Dial Transplant. 2014;29(9):1778–86.
85. Hernandez D, Muriel A, Castro de la Nuez P, Alonso-Titos J, Ruiz-Esteban P, Duarte A, et al. Survival in Southern European patients waitlisted for kidney transplant after graft failure: a competing risk analysis. PLoS One. 2018;13(3):e0193091.
86. Johnston O, Rose CL, Gill JS, Gill JS. Risks and benefits of preemptive second kidney transplantation. Transplantation. 2013;95(5):705–10.
87. Girerd S, Girerd N, Duarte K, Giral M, Legendre C, Mourad G, et al. Preemptive second kidney transplantation is associated with better graft survival compared with non-preemptive second transplantation: a multicenter French 2000-2014 cohort study. Transpl Int. 2018;31(4):408–23.
88. Andrews PA. Summary of the British Transplantation Society guidelines for management of the failing kidney transplant. Transplantation. 2014;98(11):1130–3.
89. Molnar MZ, Streja E, Kovesdy CP, Hoshino J, Hatamizadeh P, Glassock RJ, et al. Estimated glomerular filtration rate at reinitiation of dialysis and mortality in failed kidney transplant recipients. Nephrol Dial Transplant. 2012;27(7):2913–21.
90. Ayus JC, Achinger SG, Lee S, Sayegh MH, Go AS. Transplant nephrectomy improves survival following a failed renal allograft. J Am Soc Nephrol. 2010;21(2):374–80.
91. Del Bello A, Congy-Jolivet N, Sallusto F, Guilbeau-Frugier C, Cardeau-Desangles I, Fort M, et al. Donor-specific antibodies after ceasing immunosuppressive therapy, with or without an allograft nephrectomy. Clin J Am Soc Nephrol. 2012;7(8):1310–9.
92. Lachmann N, Schonemann C, El-Awar N, Everly M, Budde K, Terasaki PI, et al. Dynamics and epitope specificity of anti-human leukocyte antibodies following renal allograft nephrectomy. Nephrol Dial Transplant. 2016;31(8):1351–9.
93. Kosmoliaptsis V, Gjorgjimajkoska O, Sharples LD, Chaudhry AN, Chatzizacharias N, Peacock S, et al. Impact of donor mismatches at individual HLA-A, -B, -C, -DR, and -DQ loci on the development of HLA-specific antibodies in patients listed for repeat renal transplantation. Kidney Int. 2014;86(5):1039–48.
94. Tinckam KJ, Rose C, Hariharan S, Gill J. Re-examining risk of repeated HLA mismatch in kidney transplantation. J Am Soc Nephrol. 2016;27(9):2833–41.

Teaching, Training and Collaboration

Contents

International Health Partnerships: Developing Nephrology in Low- and Middle-Income Countries

John Feehally

Contents

M. Harber (ed.), *Primer on Nephrology*, https://doi.org/10.1007/978-3-030-76419-7_96

Learning Objectives

1. The practice of nephrology is markedly different in low and middle income countries (LMIC) compared to high income countries (HIC)
2. In LMIC where renal replacement therapy for end-stage renal disease is unaffordable, major gains in kidney health can be made through prevention, early detection and low cost management of both CKD and AKI
3. The International Society of Nephrology, and other professional organisations, have long established capacity building programs, including fellowships and sister centers, making a significant impact on the growth of nephrology in LMIC
4. Nephrologists from HIC can contribute much, and also learn much, from being involved in these capacity building programs

96.1 Introduction – Health Care Challenges in Low-and Middle-Income Countries

Most who read this book will be honing their skills as physicians in High-Income Countries (HIC) such as the UK. They will plan their continuing education and professional development to equip them for practicing nephrology in an arena of high resource, high opportunity, and high expectations among patients, professional colleagues, and policymakers. Debates about the quality of health care quality in HIC settings typically revolve around speed and equity of access to health care and all necessary health technologies, including high-cost drugs.

But most of the world's population live in low-and middle-income countries (LMIC), where health care budgets are mere fractions of those in HIC. Primary concerns for health care in such settings typically include fundamentals such as delivering adequate immunization strategies and other approaches to containing communicable disease, underpinned by the provision of clean water, and sufficient food. The growing challenge of non-communicable disease (NCD) in LMIC is beginning to be appreciated.

96.2 Kidney Disease a Low Priority in LMIC

In HIC, discussion about the quality of kidney care emphasizes issues such as equitable access to dialysis and transplantation for end-stage kidney disease (ESKD), affirming patient choice, and making very high-cost therapies such as eculizumab available to all who need them. In LMIC, many of these issues patterns of nephrology are typically viewed as an inappropriate, unaffordable, complex, demanding form of health care delivering low health gain to small numbers of people at high cost.

As a consequence ensuring that appropriate attention is given to kidney disease in LMIC requires strong advocacy. Governments associate kidney care with the high costs of long-term dialysis for ESKD; it should be emphasized to them that even when chronic dialysis is unaffordable, living donor transplantation may still be a justifiable therapy for ESKD. The point should also be made that prevention and early detection are cost-effective approaches to chronic kidney disease (CKD) especially when part of a coherent approach to all NCDs. And emphasizing the health gain achieved by effective prevention, early detection, and management of AKI, including, e.g., the availability of antivenom to treat snakebite (a major cause of AKI in several parts of the world), and the justifiable cost of short-term dialysis for reversible AKI.

96.3 Global Health

The concept of global health now has wide worldwide acceptance as a practical and academic discipline that is a force for good. At its best, it should be leading to evidence-based health care development which optimizes the resources and opportunities in LMIC under the leadership and delivery of those born and living there. To retain the focus on this goal, it is useful to recall the origins of the global health movement, and the stages through which it has evolved. One realistic (some might say cynical) insight reminds us that global health started with the need to understand and treat tropical diseases to protect the health of expatriate colonials, and later, the health of the workers on whom colonial profiteering depended. The next phase of global health was often characterized by HIC 'experts' telling LMIC health leaders what should be done, followed by a stage where health improvement in LMIC was being led by HIC 'experts.' But of course, the aim of 'mature' global health is that LMIC leaders and experts lead projects in their own countries and regions.

96.4 Varying Resources and Opportunities in LMIC

There is a wide range of socioeconomic circumstances between and within countries under the LMIC 'umbrella.' On the one hand, there are 31 low-income countries (defined by the World Bank by gross national income (GNI) per capita of ≥\$1045) that have very low health care budgets. On the other hand, there are a number of upper middle-income countries, including notably China and India, which have rapidly expanding economies and can offer in their major sites world-class facilities delivering health care delivery and biomedical research as good as those in most HIC, yet other parts of those countries have a limited economy, marked poverty, and access only to the most basic of health care. There are marked differences in the processes for driving up the quality of kidney care between these two extremes within LMIC.

Overall among LMIC, there is a predictable association between GNI and health expenditure. Distressing reports may emerge from many LMICs of major illness requiring out-of-pocket payment which may have catastrophic effects on families who sell all they have to support the treatment of a family member.

From their limited resources, LMIC seek to enhance health care for all their citizens and now do so in the context of the United Nations 2030 Sustainable Development Goals, and the call for Universal Health Coverage as a human right.

96.5 Opportunities for Health Care Improvement in LMIC: The Role of International Health Partnerships

Faced with such a gulf in wealth, resources, and opportunity, how can HIC nephrologists make any meaningful contribution to health care growth in LMIC? There are in fact a number of available opportunities through partnerships both for individual nephrologists and for the renal centers where they work.

96.5.1 Partnerships with HIC Governments

A detailed discussion of the nature of the government-level HIC and LMIC partnerships for health care improvement is beyond the scope of this chapter. They may include the offer of expert advice, e.g., to support health policy planning, as well as direct aid to support health infrastructure education and training. While some such provision by HIC has a purely philanthropic basis, geopolitical requirements may often add a *quid pro quo* in which investment in health care is given in exchange for advantageous access for a HIC to valuable assets within an LMIC (mineral rights or strategic military access might be examples).

The use and misuse of direct donations for LMIC projects from HIC governments continue to be politically charged. Skeptics point to poor return on investment; critics note that donations without sustainable increases in skills capacity or empowerment of those receiving the support are at high risk of providing a disappointing return.

96.5.2 Partnerships with Higher Education Institutions

Increasing numbers of universities in HIC have well-established global health programs which have given growing academic respectability to the understanding of global health issues and offer practical as well as theoretical opportunities for global health improvement. Some universities (particularly in North America) invest substantially in a sustained presence 'on the ground' with the goal of helping to drive sustainable change in the quality of health care. Nephrology is on occasion part of such programs, which are typically broad in scope.

96.5.3 Partnership Through Professional Organizations and Through Individuals

Opportunities to enhance kidney care in LMIC through international partnerships often begin with individual contacts, which trigger a cycle of development. A young LMIC physician who gains an opportunity to go abroad for fellowship training in nephrology returns home with new skills and energy to develop nephrology services. The relationship with the HIC center where that physician was trained, and especially with the individual's mentor, can then form the basis for continuing support: further individuals may go from the LMIC to the same HIC center to train, encouraged by the enthusiasm and expertize of the returning fellow. The emerging LMIC renal center may then develop a partnership with that or another HIC center, or a well-developed LMIC center, growing in due course into a recognized center of excellence, able in turn to be a beacon of high-quality clinical care, education, and training.

While some young LMIC physicians are successful on their own in developing an opportunity for fixed-term training experience in a center of excellence, most need some external support. Organizations arranging such international training fellowships are the key catalyst. The International Society of Nephrology has had a fellowship program for 30 years, and smaller fellowship programs are now also offered by the International Society for Peritoneal Dialysis and the International Pediatric Nephrology Association among others. The Royal College of Physicians of London runs a Medical Training Initiative providing a variety of assistance, particularly with visa and work permit arrangements for fellow coming to the UK.

Successful fellowship applications require a training program agreed by the fellow and the host center which reflects the needs of the fellow, the needs of the home institution when the fellow returns, and the training capacity of the hosting center.

In the early years of such fellowship programs, almost all fellows went for training in HIC, and some training offered was unfortunately not relevant to the home country (e.g., training in laboratory research when there was no immediate prospect of such work being possible on return)) and as a consequence, a significant number of fellows stayed to pursue their career in the HIC and never returned home. In the current model of ISN Fellowship training, an applicant must give a commitment to returning home immediately after the fellowship, and provide evidence that a position in the home institution has been reserved for them. Such measures are critical to assuring that a fellowship taken up in a HIC is not being used as an opportunity to leave home permanently. The steady growth in nephrology worldwide over recent years now means that an increasing number of fellowships can be offered in training centers in the same region as the applicant's home. This increases the relevance of training, by ensuring more experience in types of kidney disease seen in their home country, as well as minimizing language and cultural barriers to training. In these circumstances, the proportion of fellows returning home becomes close to 100%.

A crucial element for most clinical training fellows is the opportunity for hands-on clinical care, including relevant practical skills; by contrast, observer status has more limited educational value. Unfortunately, regulatory arrangements make it increasingly difficult to obtain approval for hands-on training in some HIC (e.g., USA) and require a long lead time in others to obtain necessary documentary approvals (e.g., UK).

Application for fellowship training is competitive, inevitably so because funds are limited. A consequence is that successful candidates are typically high-quality individuals with leadership potential as well as clinical commitment. This is strategically correct, ensuring that the future leaders of the speciality are being given the best training opportunities. The success of such an approach is shown in the disproportionately large proportion of former ISN Fellows who go on to become professors of medicine, deans of medical schools, and take up senior government positions in health planning and policy.

96.5.4 International Society of Nephology (ISN) Capacity Building Programs for LMIC

As well as a fellowship program similar to those of a number of other professional organizations in nephrology, ISN has a unique portfolio of LMIC capacity-building programs ► www.theisn.org/programs, broader in range and scale than those offered by any other specialist medical society.

ISN has developed the Sister Center concept to a point where up to 50 center pairs are being supported by ISN at any one time: the emerging center in LMIC, the supporting center usually in an HIC, but increasingly now in an upper middle-income country where there are centers of excellence able to give such support. ISN provides funds for interchange of personnel and expertize between a pair of centers over a six-year period.

The ISN also supports educational events by covering the costs of overseas speakers to support local teaching faculty, and can arrange on request for a senior nephrologist with relevant expertize (an 'educational ambassador') to spend a period of several weeks at an emerging LMIC center to help support the introduction of a new aspect of clinical service. ISN also offers start-up funding for small clinical research projects, and mentors those receiving such grants, to help build research capacity.

This portfolio of ISN programs has made a measurable impact [1], and while never the only factor in the growth of nephrology in any LMIC, testimonial continues to point the high respect for these programs in LMIC.

It is also important that the focus on capacity building is not narrowed to emphasize only training for physicians. In LMIC, there will never be enough physicians, strengthening even more the important roles for all members of a multidisciplinary care team – among others including nurses, technicians, dietitians, physiotherapists, and social workers. To ensure proper support and training for those professional groups may be more challenging, e.g., from the point of view of language, but the challenges must be overcome.

96.6 Opportunities for Young HIC Physicians to Be Involved in LMIC Nephrology

A young nephrologist in an HIC may be fortunate enough to train in a center involved in the ISN programs or other similar efforts. Meeting peers from LMIC when they come to train, and hearing from them of the challenges, and of the impact of the work being done, may be the first trigger to young HIC nephrologist to seek an opportunity to visit an LMIC center.

Opportunities to arrange this within postgraduate training are belatedly beginning to improve. Some nephrology training program directors in the UK are now approving periods up to 12 months spent in LMIC as an appropriate addition to training experience. There are also now some sources of funding to which application can be made to fund such a period abroad, e.g.,the ISN 'reverse fellowship' scheme. In the North America, for the first time, some training programs are likely to approve periods of a few months visiting an LMIC.

96.6.1 NOT a One-Way Experience

Whether based on an individual or organizational relationships between colleagues in HIC and LMIC, it is important not to misunderstand the development of these international partnerships as 'one way' – the expertize of the HIC being shared with the LMIC partner. There is also a wealth of wisdom, experience, and insight to be gained for those in HIC who welcome fellows from LMIC for training and for those based in the HIC supporting center who visit the emerging center. The insights this provides into the challenges and demands of clinical care and development in LMIC can be transformative.

96.6.2 Personal Commitment – Not 'Physician Tourism'

When HIC nephrologists first have opportunities to become involved in nephrology in LMIC, they do well to reflect on their role and limitations. Initial visits to LMIC will expose them to an environment which is utterly unfamiliar from many socioeconomic and cultural perspectives. Many aspects of 'good care' which they have been trained to take for granted may be absent; e.g., the prompt availability of laboratory testing or imaging, freedom from explicit discussion with patients about availability of complex therapies, the affordability of even simple treatments. As a consequence, LMIC physicians develop highly tuned clinical skills, not least because of the very large numbers of patients they see. Short visits, e.g., of a few weeks' duration, should be regarded as opportunities to listen, learn, and acclimatize; humility is a valuable asset. If such a visit is to be the beginning of a fruitful partnership, this will be steadily built by mutual trust and respect. Such involvement can be a uniquely rewarding part of an HIC nephrologist's professional life.

96.7 Other Health Care Resources

This discussion has emphasized the importance of sustainable capacity building through education and training as the key building block for the successful growth of nephrology (and other medical specialties) in LMIC. It is here that individual physicians, especially through channels such as the ISN can most contribute. But investing in workforce capacity is only one aspect of supporting sustainable nephrology development, others include the strengthening of infrastructures such as hospital and clinic buildings, as well as provision, maintenance, and replacement of medical equipment, and uninterrupted availability of drugs and other medical supplies. While governments and other HIC investors may be able to support infrastructure growth, the sustainable provision of equipment and supplies must be the responsibility of each LMIC government and develops in the context of a modest health care budget on which there are many demands.

HIC nephrologists are understandably attracted by the possibility of contributing to infrastructure, e.g., by offering used hemodialysis machines to support a burgeoning dialysis facility in an LMIC. But, as well as the high cost of transport to get such equipment to the receiving LMIC, it is not a meaningful gift without the technical expertize to maintain machines in working order, or a sustainable program for machine replacement and consumable supplies if those who start chronic treatment are to continue. Transported hemodialysis machines still packaged are not an unfamiliar sight in LMIC hospitals.

96.8 Nephrology on the Move Worldwide

The steady growth in nephrology expertize worldwide over the last two decades has been impressive and encouraging. Centers offering kidney care are increasing in number in most countries in the world. A cadre of young committed nephrologists and other renal health professionals is emerging, not least due to the efforts of the ISN and other organizations committed to sustainable capacity building.

There are growing and exciting opportunities for nephrologists and other health professionals in HIC to build partnerships with colleagues in LMIC, to learn from them, to encourage, and to support them. And thus to accelerate the growing access to care for people with kidney disease all over the world.

Chapter Review Questions

1. When RRT is unaffordable in LMIC, what is the role of nephrology?
2. How can nephrology fellowship training be made appropriate for LMIC?
3. What are the roles of HIC nephrologists in capacity building in LMIC?

Answers

1. Prevention, early detection and simple treatments, are cost-effective approaches which can improve outcomes in both CKD and AKI in LMIC.
2. Fellowship training should be 'hands on' and clinically relevant. This is often better provided, not in a remote HIC, but in another center in the region, so that a fellow is trained in a relevant clinical challenges in the same culture and language contexts.
3. HIC nephrologists can support directly by training fellows, giving sister center support, or travelling to educate. HIC nephrologists will also learn much from the experience and insight of working with LMIC colleagues.

References

1. Feehally J, Brusselmans A, Finkelstein FO, et al. Improving global health: measuring the success of capacity building programs: a view from the International Society of Nephrology. Kidney Int Suppl. 2016;6:42–51.

Further Reading

Global challenges in kidney health.

Harris D, Davies SJ, Finkelsein FO, et al. Increasing access to integrated ESKD care as part of universal health coverage. Kidney Int. 2019;95(4S):S1–S33.

Levin A, Tonelli M, Bonventre J, et al. Global kidney health 2017 and beyond: a roadmap for closing gaps in care, research, and policy. Lancet. 2017;390:1888–917.

Mehta RL, Cerdá J, Burdmann EA, et al. International Society of Nephrology's 0by25 initiative for acute kidney injury (zero preventable deaths by 2025). Lancet. 2015;385(9987):2616–43.

Education and Training in Nephrology

Ruth Silverton

Contents

M. Harber (ed.), *Primer on Nephrology*, https://doi.org/10.1007/978-3-030-76419-7_97

97

Learning Objectives

1. To illustrate the current state of nephrology training globally.
2. To understand the relevant educational theories underpinning postgraduate medical training.
3. To recognize some of the modes of learning that can be utilized through nephrology training.
4. To be aware of educational program design and specific case studies and resources for education relevant to nephrology training.

Definitions

- Andragogy: 'The art and science of helping adults learn' [2]
- Constructive alignment: The process of aligning the teaching and assessment with the intended outcomes for the learner.
- Formative assessment: Assessment for the purpose of learning
- Summative assessment: Assessment of learning
- Reflective practice: The study of a situation, your role within it, and other relevant forces, either at the time or after it has occurred, to increase self-awareness and learning

97.1 Introduction

The healthcare workforce is the foundation for any healthcare system. To ensure the sustainability of this workforce there must be an environment of continual training and education; allowing for regular progression from junior to senior clinician and up-to-date, evidence-based practice from all doctors. With the increasing global burden of CKD, advances in dialysis therapies, and awareness of the impact of AKI, the continuing education and training of nephrologists worldwide is paramount.

Medical education as an independent specialty has been growing in recent years.

The global online environment allows exchange of best practices and ongoing dialogue around education and training modalities. This has expanded both the reach and content of the field of medical education, with an increasing understanding and dissemination of educational theories and training methods.

There are training and educational challenges across all International Society of Nephrology (ISN) regions in the world [1]. This chapter will outline the current state of training globally. We will explore up-to-date educational theory and practice and make recommendations as to how different techniques may be implemented into training program development within resource variable settings.

Using case studies and resources from colleagues and centers around the globe, this chapter will analyze some exemplars of education in practice. With worldwide technological advances, a more global training ground for medical professionals is emerging. Toward the end of the chapter, you will find a list of currently available online resources and platforms; a growing pool of training and educational opportunities available for the training nephrologist.

97.2 Specialty Training: The International Picture

There are 1.87 nephrology trainees per million population (PMP) worldwide [1]. However, there is enormous variation in the concentration between low-and high-income areas, ranging from 0.18 to 6.03 trainees PMP, respectively. Nephrology training programs exist in 79% of countries worldwide, from 97% of high-income countries to only 41% of low-income countries [1].

In the USA in 2018, only 60.1% of nephrology fellowship matches were filled [3]. In the UK, fill rates for training posts in 2017 were 74%, down from 100% in 2013 [4]. The reasons behind the low numbers of nephrology trainees within these two health care settings are likely multifactorial; perceived workload and work–life balance and lack of role models have all been mentioned [4]. In lower-income countries, the availability of time and resources for educational provision in addition to enormous service needs is likely an important determinant.

Although it is hoped that formal training schemes offer the benefits of quality assurance and evaluation, curriculum mapping, and ring-fenced educational time, it is important to acknowledge that learning occurs in all settings. Those doctors, junior or senior, managing renal patients outside a traditional training program continue to learn.

Here is the challenge; in order to produce a sustainable kidney care system, we must *'Scale up the current nephrology workforce through training qualified providers by implementing evidence-based, competence-based, and community-oriented curriculums'* [1]

97.3 Educational Theory

The exploration of a social science such as education, within a book containing such advanced and complex medical sciences, may seem counterintuitive. However, there is a necessary symbiosis between the two in order to reach the desired outcome: the qualified nephrologist able to provide independent patient care.

There is a multiplicity of theoretical approaches to adult learning. I hope that the three briefly described below will provide food for thought and a gateway into our consideration of nephrology training specifically.

- **Social Constructivism**: The idea that learning is affected by people, and mediated by the culture and community in which the social interaction takes place. Acknowledging that learners bring their own experiences and existing knowledge and that they construct their learning through problem-solving and social interaction.

  The multidisciplinary dimension of nephrology, and the consistent attendance of patients with renal dysfunction but as yet undiagnosed pathologies, lend themselves to regular learning in this way.
- **Experiential Learning:** Learners have an experience; they reflect on the experience and form abstract concepts – the potential learning. They then test these concepts in their next experience and cement the learning.

  There is a necessity for nephrology trainees to undertake practical procedures. This may vary by setting, but the insertion of dialysis lines and performances of renal biopsy are two examples. Each time the trainee performs a procedure – be that in a simulated fashion, under guidance, or independently, they should be encouraged to reflect on the experience to embed their learning.

  > Dr Dan Cooper – UK Nephrology Trainee *"Consultant supervision of practical procedures is hugely valuable to highlight different techniquse and help guide reflection on means of improvement"*

  The use of portfolios can be effective in this setting. Either online or paper; the assimilation of the regional nephrology curriculum, records of assessments, procedures, and experiences, along with a space to collate reflections is a useful tool.

> **A note on reflection:**
> Although the evidence for direct improvement in patient outcome as a result of reflective practice is lacking, there is acceptance amongst clinicians and educationalists alike that the process offers enormous benefit. Not only as part of the experiential learning cycle mentioned above, but to enable learning as a result of challenging incidents. See resource 2.

- **Communities of Practice**: A network of people sharing a mutual purpose. A trainee moves from the periphery to the core of the community through time and interaction, as they learn the languages, behaviors, and knowledge of the specialty.

Many of the references within the chapter will provide further reading around the theoretical underpinning of medical education; Tim Swanwick's 'Understanding Medical Education' [5] is a particularly comprehensive yet digestible resource.

97.4 Workplace-Based Learning

> William Osler *"He who studies medicine without books sails unchartered sea, but he who studies medicine without patients does not go to sea at all"*

Apprenticeship is an almost ancient entity in many practical vocations. The wide variety of specialties within the medical sphere has resulted in varying amounts of this model persisting; surgery remaining closer to the traditional model and medical specialties, including nephrology, veering away.

> Dr Sarah Gleeson, Advanced nephrology and general medicine trainee, New Zealand: *"The most effective learning I have had is through on the job teaching. If someone can teach you more about something you've read about and are trying to understand, within the clinical context, it sticks forever. It's also the most challenging – both the trainee and supervisor need to have the time and mental space for it."*

In postgraduate nephrology training, there exists a delicate balance between service and education provision in the workplace. Below is a schematic based on the Royal College of Physicians 'Never too busy to learn' document [6], highlighting some examples of opportunities for on the job teaching/learning:

Utilizing brief moments	**Huddles:** The congregating of the full nephrology clinical team or MDT (face-to-face or virtually) to discuss a topic before the day begins: This could be the inpatient list, a specific patient safety issue, new practical technique, or hospital guideline. Different team members can facilitate these short huddles to provide additional learning in communication and team management. **Debrief:** The moments between patients, or immediately following a procedure, offer the opportunity for effective learning through debrief. Initiated by trainee or senior clinician, informally discussing the case can initiate the reflective cycle and embed learning more deeply than observation alone.
Learning with patients	**The flipped ward round:** Consider a busy ward round, usually run by the most senior clinician and passively attended by other members of the team: There is huge opportunity here for workplace-based learning. With planning and prewarning to allow for any preparation, the ward round can be flipped, with the nephrology trainee and their team (medical, nursing, and allied healthcare) running it and the consultant observing. This flipped and active bedside learning promotes the members of the team to share their underlying knowledge to problem solve and create management plans in an active manner. Combining service provision and ensuring patient safety through the presence of a senior clinician, the trainee can enter the *zone of proximal development* [7]); the space in which, through the guidance, and support of others, their learning occurs.
Learning through caring	**The Schwartz Round:** These structured forums were established by Ken Schwartz in Boston. Available to all staff, clinical, and nonclinical, they are based on the emotional and relational aspects of healthcare. A trained facilitator leads panel members to share an experience on a theme and encourages the audience to then share their thoughts and feelings. When considering the holistic care needed for both our patients and for trainees, these forums aim to cultivate compassionate staff through allowing them to feel supported in their work.
Learning through assessment	Learning in the workplace can also occur as a result of formative assessment. With many formal training programs utilizing these assessments to monitor competence and make decisions about trainee progression. Ring-fencing time for feedback after the observed assessment is paramount for learning and can be challenging in a busy clinical environment. However, if the training culture allows an open dialog; either trainee or supervisor can acknowledge a potential opportunity for formative assessment and this can be coordinated around patient and service pressures.

A Word About Competence and Entrustable Professional Activities:

In many countries, nephrology training has moved from time based to competency based, a reversion to the apprenticeship style model discussed previously. In the UK, this is seen through the entry of doctors not into the start of a training program, but the appropriate level of training, taking into account experience, or 'competence,' gained elsewhere.

However, the assessment of individual, measurable performance entities does not necessarily equal a capable, independent practitioner. This is where supervision becomes an essential adjunct to workplace-based learning and assessment.

Entrustable professional activities are the units of professional activity necessary within a specialty or department [8]. For example; performing a renal biopsy, taking a history, and writing an acute hemodialysis plan may all be individual competencies assessed as 'pass' for a trainee within the workplace. However, the assessment and management of an acute admission of dialysis requiring acute kidney injury of unknown etiology would be the entrustable professional activity (EPA). Necessitating those individual competencies to be combined and performed under pressure, with appropriate communication skills and teamwork.

These are important ideas to consider for both supervisor and trainee; the possession of the individual competence bricks does not equate to a stable building.

97.5 Supervision

Over recent years, many parts of the world have seen a shift from traditional pedagogical approaches in medical education to an emphasis on andragogy; takeswith experience providing the basis for learning experiences. Irrespective of resource setting, technological access, and training structure, the cornerstone of a successful training pathway is the presence of consistent and supportive supervision and mentorship to guide trainees through their learning. When provided effectively, postgraduate supervision has been shown to improve both the performance of the trainees and the patient outcome measures [9, 10].

Don't forget the students….

It is important to mention, although we are considering postgraduate training of nephrologists, supervision within the specialty includes undergraduate students. A recent study exploring the reasons behind the reduction in numbers of application to nephrology, highlighted that lack of early clinical exposure and role models within medical school had an impact [4]. Both junior and senior nephrologists have an important part to play in providing this exposure for students in order to maintain the workforce required in the future. As discussed in 'Training the teacher' below, for the continuation of qualified nephrologists, learning to supervise and teach is as essential as the nuts and bolts of glomerular pathophysiology.

Many types of supervision should take place throughout training, focusing on the development, performance, or both.

With well-being and morale an increasing concern with respect to trainee quality of life, and continuation in post [11], supervision has an essential role to play in encouraging and providing learning, preventing stress, and facilitating reflective practice. Whether informal, clinical, educational, or remedial supervision, there are multiple conceptual frameworks that can be drawn on [12]. One example is 'the seven C's' framework, outlined below. This is a narrative-based approach to supervision that is transferrable to all settings.

Conversation	Supervision should use open conversation to resolve problems, rather than through the one-way dissemination of advice.
Curiosity	A supervisor should remain curious, exploring what the supervisee already knows, what they have considered, and what could be explored further.
Contexts	The context of a problem is often more important than the content. Such as the beliefs of the patient or supervisee, the pressures, and needs of the organization, or the impact of conflicting values.
Complexity	Problems brought to supervision are often complicated; with multiple levels involving any combination of knowledge, practical, communication, ethical, or personal aspects. Supervision should be an opportunity for a trainee to increase their understanding of the situation and plan the next steps in learning and action, rather than having a 'quick fix' found.
Challenge	There is a necessity for honesty, frankness, and risk-taking by both supervisor and supervisee
Caution	In addition to the above, supervision also needs cautiousness and respect in order to take place within the limits of the supervisee's individual capacities and producing an optimum and not detrimental amount of challenge.
Care	Most essentially, supervision demands attentiveness, care, and positive regard.

Launer [12]

97.6 Simulation and Technology in Training

Simulation is an increasingly advocated educational tool for clinical learning. The replication of a clinical environment, or scenarios in situ, can be used for learning around management, treatment, and communication skills. The association of medical education in Europe has produced a two-part guide on simulation in healthcare education which is available online [15].

Simulation can be utilized to train competence in procedural skills prior to patient interaction and to progress team-based management and communication skills in multiple settings. Case study 2 describes a minimal resource procedural simulation and resource 1 introduces a freely accessible online simulation program:

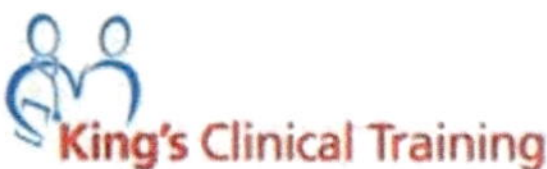

IN SITU SIMULATION TEAM TRAINING FOR THE MANAGEMENT OF MEDICAL EMERGENCIES OCCURRING ON HAEMODIALYSIS

A practical guide

Kathryn Watson[1]
Simon Calvert[2]
Tunjil Lasoye[3]
Alexandra Rankin[4]

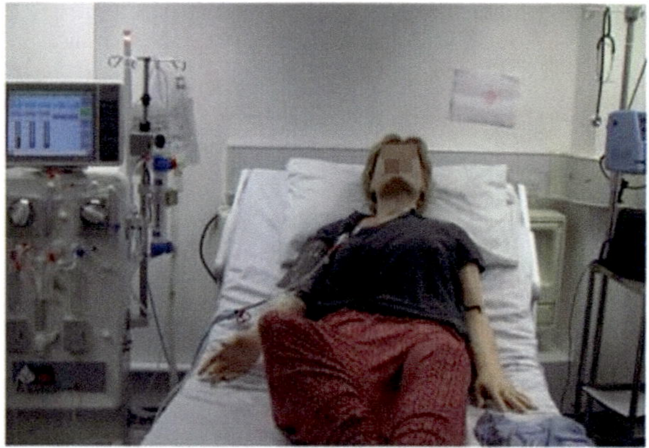

[1] SpR Renal and Educational Fellow; [2] Consultant in Emergency and Critical Care, Associate director of Medical Education; [3] Director of Medical Education; [4] Consultant Nephrologist;
King's College Hospital London NHS Foundation Trust

The use of technology to facilitate teaching is happening as early as primary school level in many countries. Although caution and criticality are necessary to ensure confidentiality and evidence-driven learning, there is vast potential through the rapid connections the internet offers. #NephTwitter is a hashtag on the Twitter platform which opens an online gateway into a world of FOAMed (Free Open-Access Medical Education). There is a global community of nephrologists who share cases, discussions, and insights over the world wide web. This community of practice has huge potential for learning. NephJC, the international online journal club, is discussed in more detail in case study 3.

97.7 Training the Teacher

The need to communicate well and provide patients with the information they need, in an understandable and digestible way, is an accepted and substantial part of nephrology. Between the complexities of glomerular diseases, the modes of renal replacement therapies, and the precision of transplantation, all trainees should be developing the skills of communication and education. In addition, the need to equip trainees with the skills to be teachers, or facilitators of learning, within clinical education is becoming more apparent. From medical student presence on the ward round to colleague preparation for professional exams and multidisciplinary discussions over coffee, there is huge scope for formal and informal teaching and supervision experience for nephrology trainees.

As this chapter outlines, medical education is a distinct subject, and incorporating it into training, rather than assuming clinical competence equates to teaching skill, is important.

> Abraham Flexner *"Medical education is not just a program for building knowledge and skills in its recipients… it is also an experience which creates attitudes and expectations"*

There are multiple options for developing the educator; from well-supervised delivery in the local context to local/national or international courses and qualifications (many of which can be completed via online distance learning cross-continent, see resource 3). Within the UK, taking time out of official training programs to pursue postgraduate qualifications in healthcare professions education is becoming increasingly common, allowing a break from the pressures of service provision and the development of a new skill. For those remaining within full-time clinical training, the development and delivery of local short courses by experienced clinical educators can begin an impactful cycle perpetuating a culture of education within a training program and department.

97.8 Instructional Design and Program Development

Irrespective of the setting, as demonstrated above, nephrology training necessitates knowledge of acute and chronic renal pathologies, procedural skills, multidisciplinary team working and adaptable communications and teaching skills. Aligning these necessary outcomes with the provision of learning is the starting point for training program design. With knowledge of the underpinning educational theories and the different modalities of facilitating learning, a setting-specific training program can be curated.

Instructional design is the consideration of how all the necessary material will be taught [13]. As with several aspects of education discussed in this chapter, there are multiple models of instructional design that can be used as guides. The cyclical ADDIE model demonstrates the process well:

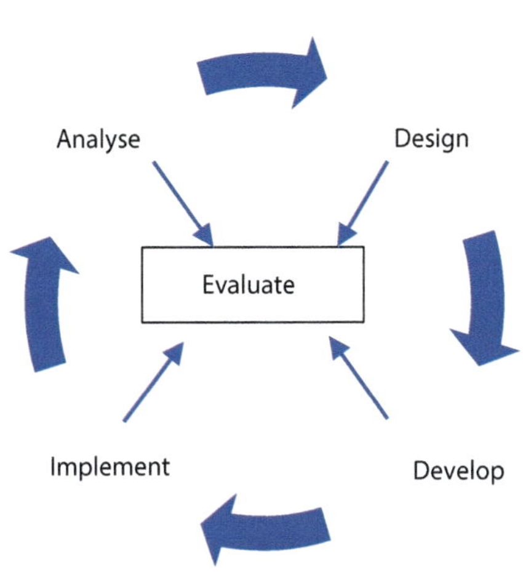

Once the 'what' of the regional nephrology curriculum is known, it's time to consider the 'how':

Analyse:

- What do the trainees feel they need? A focus group can be useful.
- What is the programme aiming to achieve?

Design:

- What opportunities do you have to deliver the programme?
- Get creative considering the methods of teaching, assessment and evaluation you can include.

Develop:

- Move the programme from the theoretical design to a delivered entity.
- Can you use a small group of trainees to pilot new elements or give feedbackto the overall design?

Implement:

- Roll out the programme.

Evaluation

- Remember to evaluate at all stages; keeping the process iterative and responsive to feedback.

Conclusion

Although the difficulties facing trainees and training program leaders across the ISN nations are many and varied; there are transferrable concepts that can lead to successful education while maintaining patient-centered care. Through a broad understanding of education theory and concepts, context-specific training can be designed from the most formal to most informal of training programs.

Tips

- Cultivating a culture of education within the provision of service and developing an enriched training program is likely to result in improved trainee experience, better staff recruitment, and retention, and ultimately improve patient care.
- Forming a robust supervisory relationship and agreeing a personal development plan, within the context of the national training curriculum, local hospital resources, and individual trainee's needs,

Chapter Review Questions

1. What percentage of countries currently have an official nephrology training program?
2. What is an entrustable professional activity?
3. What are the 7 C's of supervision?
4. What is FOAMed?
5. What does ADDIE stand for?

Answers

1. 79%
2. A key task of a specific specialty (e.g., nephrology) that a trainee can be trusted to perform, once the component competencies have been demonstrated.
3. Conversation, curiosity, contexts, complexity, challenge, caution, care
4. Free open access medical education
5. Analysis, design, develop, implement, evaluate

Case Studies and Resources

Case Study 1 – Communities of Practice: The Renal SpR Club

> Dr Toby Humphrey, Renal Clinical Research Fellow UK *"Attendance at conferences, combining socialising with learning, enthuses me around all aspects of nephrology"*

This registrar club is an offshoot of the wider UK Renal Association. It has been established for over 20 years and is trainee led. Primarily an online network disseminating educational training and job opportunities among the SpR workforce, there is also a biannual face-to-face meeting which combines current evidence-based practice information with the development of social connections.

From a financial perspective, this is a relatively resource low requirement and has the potential to foster learning in a social context and create a community of practice within the national trainee cohort.

Case Study 2 – Simulation

Micheal Mrug and colleagues [14] developed an inexpensive tool for the simulation of real-time percutaneous renal biopsy. Porcine or bovine kidneys were placed in a turkey breast (all purchased from a local butcher's shop). Ultrasonography revealed very similar images to those in humans, the resistance of the tissue to the biopsy needle and the needle images on USS were also representative of the human procedure. The model remained in good condition to allow multiple attempts. This is just one example of the innovative and novel approaches possible to train in nephrology procedural skills.

Learning from simulation does not necessitate high-tech models, intense resources, or complex teaching programs. The replication of a practical procedure through the use of everyday items facilitates an experiential learning cycle for a trainee and provides an opportunity for formative assessment of competence in an environment safe for both trainee and patient cohorts.

Case Study 3 – The Online Environment

NephJC is an online journal club which has been running on Twitter since 2014. The self-proclaimed mission is to 'increase free open access medical education (FOAMed) pertaining to nephrology, hypertension, and transplantation.' A fortnightly journal club takes place on the Twitter platform at three different times, to allow for truly international participation. Via the hashtag #NephJC, the social media environment is utilized to facilitate the age-old flipped classroom model of journal clubs of old. The article to be discussed is disseminated via the @NephJC Twitter handle, and all are welcome to use the designated 'classroom' time online to critically debate the methods, results, and interpretations of the article.

Resource 1 – Simulation and Interprofessional Education

Nowhere is the multidisciplinary element of nephrology more evident than in hemodialysis units. A freely accessible in situ hemodialysis team simulation training guide by Kathryn Watson et al is available on the Renal Association UK website. Containing seven simulation scenarios for main hemodialysis units and three specifically for satellite units, with two associated workshops, it is an invaluable resource.

From setting up weekly or monthly sessions for junior trainees to familiarize themselves with a unit to amending the satellite scenarios to represent the elements most pertinent to local trainees, this offers a simulation outline to constructively align with your nephrology curriculum and trainee learning needs.

► https://renal.org/wp-content/uploads/2019/01/In-situ-haemodialysis-team-simulation-training-_A--practical-guide.pdf

Resource 2 – Reflection on Action

► https://www.aomrc.org.uk/wp-content/uploads/2018/09/Reflective_Practice_Toolkit_AoMRC_CoPMED_0818.pdf

The Academy of Royal Colleges and Conference of Postgraduate Medical Deans of the UK have produced a reflective practice toolkit. Beneficial to both trainees and trainers. It offers templates based on the multiple styles of reflection to suit the specific doctor and is an accessible document to facilitate deeper learning for nephrology trainees.

Resource 3 – Training the Teacher

Faimer (Foundation for the advancement of international medical education and research) is a nonprofit organization that aims to improve the health of all, by improving health professions education. Their website: ► www.faimer.org contains a wealth of information, providing a list of master's programs in health professions education across 31 different countries, along with the information on the foundation's international fellowship in medical education.

References

1. Osman MA, Alrukhaimi M, Ashuntantang GE, Bellorin-Font E, Benghanem Gharbi M, Braam B, et al. Global nephrology workforce: gaps and opportunities toward a sustainable kidney care system. Kidney Int Suppl. 2018;8(2):52–63.
2. Knowles MS. The modern practice of adult education: from pedagogy to andragogy, 2e. New York: Cambridge Books; 1980.
3. Nair D, Pivert KA, Baudy A, et al. Perceptions of nephrology among medical students and internal medicine residents: a national survey among institutions with nephrology exposure. BMC Nephrol. 2019;20:146. https://doi.org/10.1186/s12882-019-1289-y.
4. Karangizi AHK, Chanouzas D, Mahdi A, Foggensteiner L. How can we make renal medicine careers more appealing to UK trainees? Clin Kidney J. 2019;12(5):756–759. https://doi.org/10.1093/ckj/sfz002.
5. Swanwick T, Forrest KAT, O'Brien BC. Understanding medical education: evidence, theory, and practice. 3rd ed. Hoboken: Wiley-Blackwell; 2018. https://doi.org/10.1002/9781119373780.
6. Basheer H, Allwood B, Lindsell C-M, Freeth D, Vaux E, Royal College of Physicians. Never too busy to learn. London: RCP; 2018.
7. Kuusisaari H. Teachers at the zone of proximal development. Teach Teach Educ. 2014;43:46–57.
8. Cate OT. A primer on entrustable professional activities. Korean J Med Educ. 2018;30(1):1–10. https://doi.org/10.3946/kjme.2018.76.
9. Farnan JM, Petty LA, Georgitis E, et al. A systematic review: the effect of clinical supervision on patient and residency education outcomes. Acad Med. 2012;87(4):428–42. https://doi.org/10.1097/ACM.0b013e31824822cc.
10. Proctor B. Training for the supervision attitude, skills and intention. In: Cutcliffe J, Butterworth T, Proctor B, editors. Fundamental themes in clinical supervision. London: Routledge; 2001. p. 25–46.
11. Rich A. Viney R. Needleman S, et al. 'You can't be a person and a doctor': the work–life balance of doctors in training—a qualitative study. BMJ Open. 2016;6e013897.
12. Launer J. In: Swanwick T, editor. 'Supervision, mentoring and coaching' in understanding medical education. Hoboken: Wiley – Blackwell; 2018. p. 182–9.
13. Merrill MD, Drake L, Lacy MJ, Pratt J. Reclaiming instructional design. Educ Technol. 1996;36(5):5–7.
14. Mrug M, Bissler JJ. Simulation of real-time ultrasound-guided renal biopsy. Kidney Int. 2010;78:705–7.
15. Motola I, Devine LA, Chung HS, Sullivan JE, Barry Issenberg S. Simulation in healthcare education: a best evidence practical guide. AMEE Guide No. 82. Med Teach. 2013;35(10):e1511–30. https://doi.org/10.3109/0142159X.2013.818632.

Climate Change, Sustainability, and Nephrology

Frances Mortimer and John Agar

Contents

M. Harber (ed.), *Primer on Nephrology*, https://doi.org/10.1007/978-3-030-76419-7_98

Learning Objectives

1. Describe the global environmental crisis and its implications for human health and survival.
2. Discuss the contributions of the health sector and kidney services to environmental degradation.
3. Articulate the need to embed environmental measures in governance, innovation, and procurement of kidney services.
4. Identify examples of good practice in improving the environmental impact of dialysis.
5. Outline how the principles of sustainable healthcare can guide innovation toward high-value, sustainable kidney care.

98.1 Introduction: The Scale and Gravity of the Global Environmental Crisis

The stable climate of the Holocene epoch, spanning the 11,700 years since the last ice age, has provided a "safe space" in which human civilizations have evolved. Widespread, biodiverse habitats have supported food production, allowing the development of agricultural, and urban societies all around the world [1].

In the last few decades, human activities have expanded to such an extent that three-quarters of all land and two-thirds of marine environments are "severely altered" as a result. Over one-third of all the land surface and 75% of all freshwater resources are now used for agriculture [2].

Land clearance and fossil fuel combustion have altered the global carbon cycle, increasing the carbon dioxide in Earth's atmosphere from approximately 280 ppm in pre-industrial times to over 400 ppm today [3], trapping heat and raising the average surface temperature of the planet by about 1.0 °C above preindustrial levels [2]. Despite international agreements, greenhouse gas emissions have doubled since 1980 [2] and continue to rise, rapidly closing the window for action to stabilize global temperatures below 1.5 °C above preindustrial levels [4].

Meanwhile, each year, 4.8–12.7 million metric tonnes of plastic [5] and 300–400 million tons of heavy metals, solvents, toxic sludge, and other wastes from industrial facilities are allowed to enter the oceans, creating ocean "dead zones." [2]

The impacts of these human-made changes to land use, climate, and oceans are combining to drive a rate of global species extinction (known as the sixth-mass extinction) that is tens to hundreds of times faster than the average over the last 10 million years and continues to accelerate. At least 680 vertebrate species have been lost since 1500 as a result of human activities and a further one million animal and plant species are threatened with extinction [2].

The 2005 Millennium Ecosystem Assessment report warned that "human activity is putting such strain on the natural functions of Earth that the ability of the planet's ecosystems to sustain future generations can no longer be taken for granted" [6]. Urgent action to eliminate greenhouse gas emissions and restore ecosystems is now a matter of survival. Within this decade, every part of society - including healthcare - must find ways to operate sustainably.

98.2 First Do No Harm? Kidney Care Is Part of the Problem

Global healthcare creates an annual carbon footprint of 2 billion tonnes of carbon dioxide equivalents (CO_2e). This equates to ~4.4% of global net greenhouse gas (GHG) emissions and is equivalent to the annual GHG emissions of 514 coal-fired power plants [7]. If the global healthcare sector was a country, it would be the fifth-largest GHG emitter on the planet, ranking just behind Japan.

As well as climate change, healthcare contributes to plastic waste [8], air, and water pollution (including with biologically active pharmaceutical products), deforestation (e.g., for rubber plantations to supply glove manufacture), and depletion of scarce minerals for use in surgical instruments.

Global dialysis is a multi-billion-dollar healthcare treatment. While the number of patients currently on dialysis is difficult to confirm, most estimates suggest upward of three million currently access some form of dialysis. A further estimated 4–5 million lack access to supportive care and die in renal failure [9]. The global financial spend and carbon footprint of kidney care/dialysis is, however, impossible to estimate due to stark differences in access, availability, treatment modality, practice models, site of delivery, equipment, funding, and monetary value.

A study of the carbon footprint of a renal service in the UK in 2010 found that 66% of the carbon footprint was attributable to the provision of hemodialysis and peritoneal dialysis (about 7 tonnes CO_2e per patient per year), 27% to inpatient care, and 6% to outpatient care [10]. The carbon footprints of kidney transplantation and management of kidney disease in primary care (particularly, the manufacture of pharmaceuticals) are also likely to be significant but were not included in this study. Analysis of the data suggests that kidney care is a carbon-intensive specialty in relation to the number of patients treated.

In addition to its carbon footprint, dialysis impacts on the environment through the consumption of large amounts of water, energy, and single-use equipment and through the generation of plastic waste. The use of PVC plastic results in additional harms via the release of environmental pollutants in its manufacture and disposal, as well as leaching of endocrine-disrupting phthalates into patients' bloodstreams during use.

98.3 Embedding Environmental Impact in Management and Procurement of Kidney Services

Service management and innovation within kidney care do not currently prioritize improvements to the environmental impact. Given the scale of the environmental crisis and its implications for human survival and wellbeing, this needs to change. A culture of continual improvement in the value that services provide should be required, thereby maximizing health outcomes while reducing environmental, social, and financial costs (the "triple bottom line" of sustainability).

Work is needed to refine consistent methods for measuring and comparing the environmental costs of kidney services and the products they rely upon (as well as for assessing their social impacts on staff, patients, and communities). However, starting from today, the tendering process for kidney services should require suppliers to provide data on water consumption, energy demand, and waste management along with estimates of the carbon impact of their wares.

Box 98.1 Sustainable Value in Healthcare [11]

$$\text{Sustainable value} = \frac{\text{Outcomes for patients and populations}}{\text{Environmental + social + financial impacts (the 'triple bottom line')}}$$

98.4 Improving Resource Efficiency in Dialysis

Hemodialysis and peritoneal dialysis together account for the majority of kidney care's environmental impact. In hemodialysis, innovative practices have been shown to yield clear efficiency gains – whether in consumption of single-use items, energy and water use, food, transport, or waste management. To date, these practices have yet to be widely adopted.

98.4.1 Reduction in Dialysis Consumables

The supply of pharmaceuticals and medical equipment together contribute over half of the carbon footprint of kidney services [10]. The GHG emissions associated with dialysis consumables arise during their manufacture and transport as well as their disposal (which is counted separately, contributing a further 10% to the carbon footprint of care). Therefore, reducing consumption avoids more GHG emissions than recycling waste at the end of the process. The design of dialysis systems to minimize the volume of consumables could be incentivized through partnership with industry and by including metrics on consumables in the tendering process.

The following case studies illustrate two different approaches to reducing the carbon footprint associated with the supply of acid concentrate for dialysis.

Case Study 1 – Infrastructure: Central Acid Delivery – St Luke's Hospital, Bradford, UK [12, 13]

- Installation of two storage tanks for acid concentrate with pressurized loops to convey the acid to the dialysis machines (cost = £44,000 in 2009) enabled fortnightly bulk deliveries.
- Central delivery eliminated the use and disposal of 30,000 individual plastic 6 L canisters per year while reducing acid wastage (from leftover acid in the canisters after treatments).
- Savings were 16 tonnes of CO_2e, 4.2 tonnes of plastic, and £23,072 per year (return on investment 163% at five years).

Case Study 2 – Procurement: Concentrated Acid Solution – East Kent Hospitals University NHS Foundation Trust, UK [13, 14]

- Procurement of acid in a more concentrated form (44:1 rather than the previous 34:1 solution) reduced the size of canisters from 6 liters to 4.7 liters, with no change in cost.
- The smaller canisters avoided the transport of 81 tonnes of liquid per year over a distance of 1334 km, saving 16 tonnes CO_2e.

(NB. Even greater efficiencies are possible by procuring acid concentrate in dry powder form and mixing on site.)

98.4.1.1 Process Innovations

Because of the number of almost identical dialysis treatments taking place in a unit each year, small changes to staff or patient routines which eliminate the unnecessary opening of equipment (such as saline bags or dressing packs) can multiply up into significant resource savings [15].

98.4.2 Saving Water

Hemodialysis requires large volumes of water. Producing the 120 liters of dialysate required for a typical four-hour session can require approximately 400 liters of mains water – for a unit providing 200 patients with three sessions per week, that amounts to 12.5 million liters of water annually. An important step in the water purification process is reverse osmosis (RO), which removes dissolved ions and salts. Currently, many RO systems reject up to two-thirds of the water processed, and this (still drinking quality) water is typically sent down the drain.

Options for Water-Saving:

- Review of dialysis prescriptions to optimize dialysis flow rates [16]
- Upgrade of RO to a more efficient system
- Re-presentation to/recirculation of RO reject water through the RO [17, 18]
- Collection of RO reject water for multipurpose reuse: instrument sterilizing services, laundry, janitor use, gardens, nondrinking domestic use, or water troughs (farm animals) [17, 18]

98.4.3 Minimizing Energy Use

Sustainable building design can significantly reduce the energy needed for heating, cooling, lighting, and ventilation. Even in existing buildings, installing window shades, insulation, or more efficient lighting can reduce energy demand. Efficient appliances such as fridges and computers can also make an impact, as can making sure that lights and equipment are switched off when not needed.

There are further opportunities to minimize energy use for dialysis itself, through procurement of energy-efficient machines (including RO systems), optimizing dialysis flow rates [16], and heat disinfection cycles [19].

98.4.4 Renewable Energy Generation [20]

Some energy demand is inevitable and kidney services can contribute to clean energy generation both at dialysis centere and for home-dialysing patients.

Case Study 3: Photovoltaic Energy Generation

- The installation of a 24 m^2, 3 kWh solar array, and inverter (cost = AU$16,219 in 2012) augmented power to a four -chair home HD training unit, reduced power costs by 76.5%
- The expected return on investment is one-third of the lifespan of the array.

98.4.5 Travel

Staff and patient travel contributes significantly to both GHG emissions and air pollution from healthcare, particularly, where distances are further. Travel for dialysis can be minimized by supporting patients to dialyse at home (although GHG savings on travel may be outweighed by increases in other resource use), by siting dialysis units close to where people live, and by coordinating treatment times and patient transport routes [15]. Active travel and other low-carbon transport choices can be encouraged and facilitated, particularly for staff.

98.4.6 Responsible Waste Disposal

In a circular economy, products and materials are retained within the system through reuse, repair, remanufacturing, or (in the last resort) recycling into materials

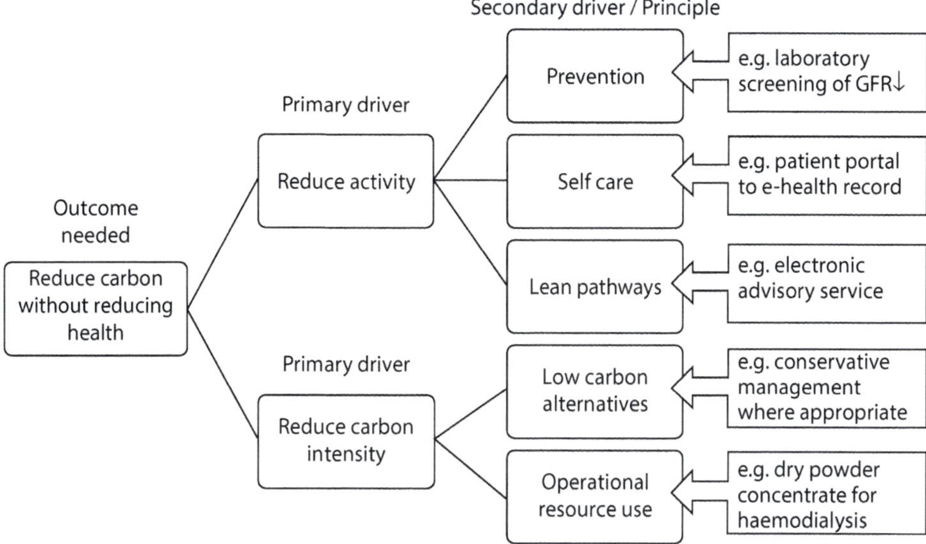

Fig. 98.1 Principles of sustainable clinical practice [23]

of the same or highest possible value. Moving from our current linear economy (resource extraction > manufacture > use > disposal) requires rethinking product design to ensure that equipment is durable, able to be disinfected, and reused and eventually disassembled into separate materials for recycling. This is an endeavor which the kidney care community could undertake in partnership with its suppliers.

In the meantime, the priority remains to reduce consumption where possible and to separate/sterilize waste to enable the least environmentally harmful disposal method. Where it is not possible to convert used dialysis products into plastics of the same grade (recycling) or lower (downcycling [21, 22]), efforts can be made to recover the embedded energy, for example through waste-to-energy incineration.

A significant barrier to the growth of recycling worldwide is the lack of demand for recycled products. Healthcare organizations can help to create this demand by purchasing products that are made from, or packaged in, recycled materials.

98.5 Clinical Transformation to Sustainable Models of Care

While sustainability efforts to date have focused on the operational efficiencies in the provision of hemodialysis, given the global scale of kidney disease and the need for urgent decarbonization, more fundamental changes are needed to the design and delivery of care.

Principles of sustainable healthcare have been developed to guide this transformation: minimizing demand and low-value activity through *prevention, patient self-care,* and *"lean" service design*, while prioritizing the use of *resource-efficient interventions* and maximizing *operational efficiencies* (Fig. 98.1).

98.5.1 Low-Carbon Alternatives: Prioritizing High-Value, Resource-Efficient Interventions

Kidney replacement therapies (KRT) account for the majority of the carbon footprint of renal services. There is currently no definitive data allowing comparison of the carbon footprints of different modes of KRT, particularly, when considering variations in resource use between different countries. The carbon footprint of hemodialysis per patient per year has been estimated at 4000–7000 kg CO_2e [3] in the UK and 10,000 kg CO_2e in Australia [4] – equivalent to driving 55,000 km in an average-sized petrol car [24]. The larger carbon footprint in Australia is likely to be influenced by distance and geography, e.g., the distances over which water is sourced and the transport distances for consumables.

The carbon footprint of peritoneal dialysis has been estimated at 1700 kg CO_2e in China [25] but the true figure is likely to be higher as the study did not include the carbon footprint of the manufacture of the dialysis fluids.

The carbon footprint of transplantation and immunosuppression has not been estimated. Extrapolating from financial modeling, it is likely that transplantation is more carbon-efficient over 10 years than either haemodialysis or peritoneal dialysis.

Home hemodialysis had a higher carbon footprint than in-center HD in a 2011 study [26] because of the increased frequency of dialysis sessions, but this may have changed with the introduction of more efficient home dialysis systems.

The integration of carbon footprint analysis into health technology appraisal would be a welcome development, and would help to inform environmentally sound decisions – not just about KRT, but on investigations and interventions throughout the renal pathway [27]. While environmental efficiency would not be the only factor, it should be considered alongside other factors in decision-making. Even if environmentally more costly, home therapies can score well on other aspects of sustainable value, offering both health and social benefits to many patients and their families.

Finally, in many countries, there is scope to improve patients' quality of life and to minimize environmental, social, and financial costs by improving shared decision-making between patients and professionals. This should include allowing and supporting people to choose conservative management where this offers comparable health outcomes and/or aligns with their values.

98.5.2 Lean Service Design

The Covid-19 response has highlighted opportunities to create leaner services through moving information rather than people, built on prior examples of good practice. Particular opportunities to streamline care sit at the interface of different parts of the system: coordination between primary and secondary care and between nephrology and related specialties (e.g., combined clinics). Cost and environmental savings occur across the patient pathway as a whole but may fall asymmetrically in different parts of the service: if so, we should not allow this to be a barrier to adoption.

Case Study 4: Electronic Consultation as an Alternative to Hospital Referral for Patients with Chronic Kidney Disease – Bradford, UK [28]

- Electronic sharing of primary care electronic health records with the nephrology service was introduced to 17 general practices. Participating general practitioners (GPs) attended education workshops.
- Outpatient referrals were reduced by almost half. GPs reported that the service was convenient, provided timely and helpful advice, and avoided outpatient referrals. Specialist recommendations were well followed, and GPs felt more confident about managing chronic kidney disease in the community.

98.5.3 Supporting Patient Empowerment and Self-Care

Attending to patient preference/ shared decision-making is discussed above. Another important opportunity is empowering patients to take an active role in comanaging their disease, thereby improving patient experiences and outcomes and potentially reducing future healthcare demand. Services can support this through patient education, peer support, care planning, and shared care records (such as PatientView, which gives patients direct access to live test results, clinic letters, and other information and is used in almost all adult kidney units in the UK [29]). These should be flexible systems that are responsive to patient-initiated contact.

98.5.4 Reducing Demand

Stemming the tide of kidney disease requires intervening upstream of the clinic door (or electronic advice portal). Already much work has been done to enable the identification of chronic kidney disease at an earlier stage and provide guidance and support for appropriate management in primary care. Programs to improve management and outcomes from acute kidney injury have also been initiated.

There is a need for ongoing improvements in these areas, fostering collaboration, and bidirectional learning between kidney services and primary care. Further investment is required in both healthcare and societal measures to tackle risk factors such as diabetes, hypertension, and environmental factors and to increase understanding of kidney health.

98.6 Summary

Early work in sustainable kidney care has already identified many practical innovations which preserve finite resources while maintaining or improving health outcomes, which services are encouraged to adopt. In addition, there is a need for collective agreement on parameters for assessing and driving improvement in the sustainability of kidney services.

Definitions

Carbon Footprint - the sum of GHG emissions attributable to a given process. Six different types of gases are commonly included; as each has a different global warming potential, the quantities are expressed in "carbon dioxide equivalents" (CO_2e).

Circular Economy – an economic system that eliminates waste and pollution, keeping products and materials in use

Downcycling – the recycling of waste where the recycled material is of lower quality and functionality than the original material

Greenhouse gas – any gas that is capable of absorbing infrared radiation, thereby trapping heat in the atmosphere. The increase in greenhouse gases, especially carbon dioxide, in Earth's atmosphere are responsible for global heating or climate change.

Ecosystem – a community of plants and animals interacting with each other in a given area and with their nonliving environments

Lean – an approach to management which focuses on optimizing flow of value across the whole system and eliminating waste

Linear Economy – an economic system in which raw materials are collected, then transformed into products that are used until they are finally discarded as waste

Patient Empowerment – a process through which people gain greater control over decisions and actions affecting their health (WHO 1998)

Photovoltaics – the conversion of light into electricity

Recycling – the process of converting waste materials into new materials and objects

Renewable Energy – energy from natural sources which would not run out, such as the sun, wind, rivers, or ocean waves and tides.

Social impact – an impact (positive or negative) on the social circumstances of people affected by a process or service (such as patients, carers, staff, communities)

Sustainable healthcare – healthcare that meets the needs of populations now without compromising the health or healthcare of current and future generations

Sustainable value – the value provided by health services, expressed in terms of health outcomes achieved for patients and populations against the environmental, social, and financial costs

Triple bottom line – the environmental, social, and financial costs or impacts of an organization or service

Waste-to-energy – the process of generating electricity +/– heat energy from the primary processing (often incineration) of waste.

Tips

Measure and reduce energy, water, and waste in your unit. Make sure these measures are included when procuring dialysis services.

Look for opportunities to avoid unnecessary opening or use of items in routine dialysis setup – the impact will quickly multiply up with thousands of treatments taking place in each unit every year.

Tricks and Pitfalls

Try not to focus too heavily on waste disposal – you can have a greater impact on reducing environmental impact through preventing unnecessary waste in the first place.

Chapter Review Questions

1. Why is environmental sustainability relevant to kidney care?
2. How do I balance the needs of my patients against the needs of wider society and the environment?

Answers

1. Natural systems provide the fundamental conditions for life, including oxygen, water, food, and a stable climate. These systems are currently being disrupted on a global scale, threatening the health, and well-being of whole populations. All sectors have a responsibility to urgently address their environmental impact, including healthcare.
2. You may not have to. There is huge potential to improve patient care through the adoption of sustainable approaches, including primary and secondary prevention, supporting patients to comanage their conditions, attending to patient preference, improving efficiency, and minimizing unnecessary travel.

Acknowledgments Thank you to Sarah Peters for help in collating material.

References

1. Rockström J, Steffen W, Noone K, Persson A, Chapin FS 3rd, Lambin E, Lenton TM, Scheffer M, Folke C, Joachim Schellnhuber H, et al. Planetary boundaries: exploring the safe operating space for humanity. Ecol Soc. 2019;14(2):32.
2. IPBES. Summary for policymakers of the global assessment report on biodiversity and ecosystem services of the Intergovernmental Science-Policy Platform on Biodiversity and Ecosystem Services; 2019.

3. Dlugokencky EJ, Hall BD, Montzka SA, Dutton G, Mühle J, Elkins JW. Atmospheric composition [in *State of the Climate in 2018,* Chapter 2: Global Climate]. Bull Am Meteorol Soc. 2019;100(9):S48–50.
4. Intergovernmental Panel on Climate Change. Special report: global warming of 1.5C; 2018.
5. Jambeck JR, et al. Marine plastic. Plastic waste inputs from land into the ocean. Science. 2015;347:768–71.
6. The Board of the Millennium Ecosystem Assessment. Living beyond our means: natural assets and human well-being. Summary for policy makers; 2005.
7. Arup & HCWH. Health care's climate footprint. Climate-smart health care series. Green Paper Number One; 2019.
8. Rizan C, Mortimer F, Stancliffe R, Bhutta MF. Plastics in healthcare: time for a re-evaluation. J R Soc Med. 2020;113(2):49–53.
9. Barraclough KA, Agar JWM. Green nephrology. Nat Rev Nephrol. 2020;16(5):257–68.
10. Connor A, Lillywhite R, Cooke MW. The carbon footprint of a renal service in the United Kingdom. QJM. 2010;103(12): 965–75.
11. Mortimer F, Isherwood J, Wilkinson A, Vaux E. Sustainability in quality improvement: redefining value. Future Healthcare J. 2018;5(2):88–93.
12. Central Delivery of Acid for Haemodialysis. Bradford Teaching Hospitals NHS Foundation Trust & Centre for Sustainable Healthcare. https://map.sustainablehealthcare.org.uk/bradford-teaching-hospitals-nhs-foundation-trust/systematic-review-dialysis-prescriptions-use-dialys. Last accessed 12.7.2020.
13. Mortimer F, Dixon J, Gilmour F, Stoves J, Owen A, Connor A, Campbell F. Cutting the carbon cost of dialysis: efficient delivery of acid concentrate. Br J Renal Med. 2014;19(2):21–3.
14. 44:1 Haemodialysis Concentrate Solution. East Kent Hospitals University NHS Foundation Trust & Centre for Sustainable Healthcare. https://map.sustainablehealthcare.org.uk/east-kent-hospitals-university-nhs-foundation-trust/441-haemodialysis-concentrate-solution. Last accessed 12.7.2020.
15. Carbon reduction at a renal unit through sustainable action planning. Royal Cornwall Hospitals NHS Trust & Centre for Sustainable Healthcare. 2012. https://map.sustainablehealthcare.org.uk/royal-cornwall-hospitals-nhs-trust/carbon-reduction-renal-unit-through-sustainable-action-planning. Last accessed 12.7.2020.
16. Systematic review of dialysis prescriptions (use of dialysate autoflow facility). Bradford Teaching Hospitals NHS Foundation Trust & Centre for Sustainable Healthcare. https://map.sustainablehealthcare.org.uk/bradford-teaching-hospitals-nhs-foundation-trust/systematic-review-dialysis-prescriptions-use-dialys. Last accessed 12.7.2020.
17. Agar JWM. Reusing and recycling dialysis reverse osmosis system reject water. Kidney Int. 2015;88:653–7.
18. Connor A, Milne S, Owen A, Boyle G, Mortimer F, Stevens P. Toward greener dialysis: a case study to illustrate and encourage the salvage of reject water. J Ren Care. 2010;36(2):68–72.
19. Nystrand R. Heat disinfection in dialysis. Spektrum der Dialyse & Apherese. 2015;5(1):1–5.
20. Agar JWM, Perkins A, Tjipto A. Solar-assisted hemodialysis. CJASN. 2012;7(2):310–4.
21. Deakin University Media Release [25.10.2017]. Deakin University, Waurn Ponds, Victoria, Australia. Found at: https://www.deakin.edu.au/about-deakin/media-releases/articles/deakin-project-uses-plastic-dialysis-waste-to-produce-durable-concrete. Last accessed 01.07.2020.
22. Conference Program and Abstract Book: Victorian Renal Clinical Health Network. Page 16. Published by Safer Care, Victoria. 2017. Found at: https://www2.health.vic.gov.au/hospitals-and-health-services/safer-care-victoria/safer-care-publications/vrcn-conference-abstract-book-29-aug-2017. Last accessed 01.07.2020.
23. Mortimer F. The sustainable physician. Clin Med. 2010;10(2):110–1.
24. Based on an emissions factor of 0.18084 kg CO2e/km for an average car. Source: UK Government emission conversion factors for greenhouse gas company reporting; 2019.
25. Chen M, Zhou R, Du C, Mend F, Wang Y, Wu L, Wang F, Xu Y, Yand X. The carbon footprints of home and in-center peritoneal dialysis in China. Int Urol Nephrol. 2017;49(2):337–43.
26. Connor A, Lillywhite R, Cooke MW. The carbon footprint of home and in-center maintenance hemodialysis in the United Kingdom. Hemodial Int. 2011;15(1):39–51.
27. Tomson C. Reduciong the carbon footprint of hospital-based care. Future Hosp J. 2015;2(1):57–62.
28. Stoves J, Connolly J, Cheung CK, et al. Electronic consultation as an alternative to hospital referral for patients with chronic kidney disease: a novel application for networked electronic health records to improve the accessibility and efficiency of healthcare. Qual Saf Health Care. 2010;19:e54.
29. https://ukkidney.org/patients/patientview.

Supplementary Information

M. Harber (ed.), *Primer on Nephrology*, https://doi.org/10.1007/978-3-030-76419-7

Index

A

B

C

D

E

H

I

J

K

L

M

N

O

P

Q

R

S

T

U

V

W

X

Z

GPSR Compliance

The European Union's (EU) General Product Safety Regulation (GPSR) is a set of rules that requires consumer products to be safe and our obligations to ensure this.

If you have any concerns about our products, you can contact us on ProductSafety@springernature.com

In case Publisher is established outside the EU, the EU authorized representative is:

Springer Nature Customer Service Center GmbH
Europaplatz 3
69115 Heidelberg, Germany

Batch number: 10371111

Printed by Printforce, the Netherlands